OPTUM360°®

EXPERT

ICD-10-CM Expert for Hospitals

The complete official code set

Codes valid from October 1, 2020 through September 30, 2021

Value-Added Content — Just For Our Customers

Scan the QR code below with your phone or tablet to access value-added content.

Check back often for new content that supports and expands on the details in this ICD-10 code set.

Can't scan?

Then go to

optum360coding.com/icd-10-extra/

Publisher's Notice

Acknowledgments

Marianne Randall, CPC, *Product Manager*
Anita Schmidt, BS, RHIA, AHIMA-approved ICD-10-CM/PCS Trainer, *Subject Matter Expert*
Karen Krawzik, RHIT, CCS, AHIMA-approved ICD-10-CM/PCS Trainer, *Subject Matter Expert*
Leanne Patterson, CPC, *Subject Matter Expert*
LaJuana Green, RHIA, CCS, *Subject Matter Expert*
Jacqueline R. Petersen, RHIA, CHDA, CPC, *Subject Matter Expert*
Stacy Perry, *Manager, Desktop Publishing*
Tracy Betzler, *Senior Desktop Publishing Specialist*
Hope M. Dunn, *Senior Desktop Publishing Specialist*
Katie Russell, *Desktop Publishing Specialist*
Kate Holden, *Editor*

Our Commitment to Accuracy

Optum360 is committed to producing accurate and reliable materials.

To report corrections, please email accuracy@optum.com. You can also reach customer service by calling 1.800.464.3649, option 1.

Copyright

Made in the USA
ISBN 978-1-62254-523-0

Anita Schmidt, BS, RHIA, AHIMA-approved ICD-10-CM/PCS Trainer

Ms. Schmidt has expertise in ICD-10-CM/PCS, DRG, and CPT with more than 15 years' experience in coding in multiple settings, including inpatient, observation, and same-day surgery. Her experience includes analysis of medical record documentation, assignment of ICD-10-CM and PCS codes, and DRG validation. She has conducted training for ICD-10-CM/PCS and electronic health record. She has also collaborated with clinical documentation specialists to identify documentation needs and potential areas for physician education. Most recently she has been developing content for resource and educational products related to ICD-10-CM, ICD-10-PCS, DRG, and CPT. Ms. Schmidt is an AHIMA-approved ICD-10-CM/PCS trainer and is an active member of the American Health Information Management Association (AHIMA) and the Minnesota Health Information Management Association.

Karen Krawzik, RHIT, CCS, AHIMA-approved ICD-10-CM/PCS Trainer

Ms. Krawzik has expertise in ICD-10-CM, ICD-9-CM, CPT/HCPCS, DRG, and data quality and analytics, with more than 30 years' experience coding in multiple settings, including inpatient, observation, ambulatory surgery, ancillary, and emergency room. She has served as a DRG analyst and auditor of commercial and government payer claims, as a contract administrator, and worked on a team providing enterprise-wide conversion of the ICD-9-CM code set to ICD-10. More recently, she has been developing print and electronic content related to ICD-10-CM and ICD-10-PCS coding systems, MS-DRGs, and HCCs. Ms. Krawzik is credentialed by the American Health Information Management Association (AHIMA) as a Registered Health Information Technician (RHIT) and a Certified Coding Specialist (CCS) and is an AHIMA-approved ICD-10-CM/PCS trainer. She is an active member of AHIMA and the Missouri Health Information Management Association.

2021 ICD-10-CM Official Guidelines for Coding and Reporting

Optum360 is pleased to provide you with this 2021 ICD-10-CM code book that INCLUDES the 2021 Official Guidelines for Coding and Reporting.

Contents

Preface

ICD-10-CM Official Preface

This FY 2021 update of the International Statistical Classification of Diseases and Related Health Problems, 10th revision, Clinical Modification (ICD-10-CM) is being published by the United States government in recognition of its responsibility to promulgate this classification throughout the United States for morbidity coding. The International Statistical Classification of Diseases and Related Health Problems, 10th Revision (ICD-10), published by the World Health Organization (WHO), is the foundation of ICD-10-CM. ICD-10 continues to be the classification used in cause-of-death coding in the United States. The ICD-10-CM is comparable with the ICD-10. The WHO Collaborating Center for the Family of International Classifications in North America, housed at the Centers for Disease Control and Prevention's National Center for Health Statistics (NCHS), has responsibility for the implementation of ICD and other WHO-FIC classifications and serves as a liaison with the WHO, fulfilling international obligations for comparable classifications and the national health data needs of the United States. The historical background of ICD and ICD-10 can be found in the Introduction to the International Classification of Diseases and Related Health Problems (ICD-10), 2010, World Health Organization, Geneva, Switzerland.

ICD-10-CM is the United States' clinical modification of the World Health Organization's ICD-10. The term "clinical" is used to emphasize the modification's intent: to serve as a useful tool in the area of classification of morbidity data for indexing of health records, medical care review, and ambulatory and other health care programs, as well as for basic health statistics. To describe the clinical picture of the patient the codes must be more precise than those needed only for statistical groupings and trend analysis.

Characteristics of ICD-10-CM

ICD-10-CM far exceeds its predecessors in the number of concepts and codes provided. The disease classification has been expanded to include health-related conditions and to provide greater specificity at the sixth and seventh character level. The sixth and seventh characters are not optional and are intended for use in recording the information documented in the clinical record.

ICD-10-CM extensions, interpretations, modifications, addenda, or errata other than those approved by the Centers for Disease Control and Prevention are not to be considered official and should not be utilized. Continuous maintenance of the ICD-10-CM is the responsibility of the aforementioned agencies. However, because the ICD-10-CM represents the best in contemporary thinking of clinicians, nosologists, epidemiologists, and statisticians from both public and private sectors, when future modifications are considered, advice will be sought from all stakeholders.

All official authorized addenda since the last complete update (October 1, 2020) have been included in this revision. For more detailed information please see the complete official authorized addenda to ICD-10-CM, including the "ICD-10-CM Official Guidelines for Coding and Reporting," and a description of the ICD-10-CM updating and maintenance process.

How to Use ICD-10-CM Expert for Hospitals 2021

Introduction

ICD-10-CM Expert for Hospitals: The Complete Official Code Set is your definitive coding resource, combining the work of the National Center for Health Statistics (NCHS), Centers for Medicare and Medicaid Services (CMS), American Hospital Association (AHA), and Optum360 experts to provide the information you need for coding accuracy.

The International Classification of Diseases, 10th Revision, Clinical Modification (ICD-10-CM), is an adaptation of ICD-10, copyrighted by the World Health Organization (WHO). The development and maintenance of this clinical modification (CM) is the responsibility of the NCHS as authorized by WHO. Any new concepts added to ICD-10-CM are based on an established update process through the collaboration of WHO's Update and Revision Committee and the ICD-10-CM Coordination and Maintenance Committee.

In addition to the ICD-10-CM classification, other official government source information has been included in this manual. Depending on the source, updates to information may be annual or quarterly. This manual provides the most current information that was available at the time of publication. For updates to the source documents that may have occurred after this manual was published, please refer to the following:

- **NCHS, International Classification of Diseases, Tenth Revision, Clinical Modification (ICD-10-CM)**

  https://www.cdc.gov/nchs/icd/icd10cm.htm

  https://www.cms.gov/medicare/icd-10/2021-icd-10-cm

- **CMS Inpatient Prospective Payment System Proposed Rule, FY2021**

  https://www.cms.gov/medicare/acute-inpatient-pps/fy-2021-ipps-proposed-rule-home-page

- **CMS Inpatient Prospective Payment System Proposed Rule, FY 2021 — Proposed, version 38, MS-DRG grouper software, Definitions Manual files and Medicare Code Editor (MCE) Files**

  https://www.cms.gov/Medicare/Medicare-Fee-for-Service-Payment/AcuteInpatientPPS/MS-DRG-Classifications-and-Software

- **CMS Risk Adjustment Model, version 24**

  https://www.cms.gov/Medicare/Health-Plans/MedicareAdvtgSpecRateStats/Risk-Adjustors.html

- **CMS Long-term Care Hospital Prospective Payment System Proposed Rule and Data Files, FY 2021**

  https://www.cms.gov/medicaremedicare-fee-service-paymentlongtermcarehospitalppsltchpps-regulations-and-notices/cms-1735-p

- **AHA Coding Clinics**

  https://www.codingclinicadvisor.com/

- **Additional specialty-specific resources will also be provided on our product updates page at Optum360coding.com, which can be accessed at the following:**

  https://www.optum360coding.com/ProductUpdates/

  Password: Hospital21

The official NCHS ICD-10-CM classification includes three main sections: the guidelines, the indexes, and the tabular list, all of which make up the bulk of this coding manual. To complement the classification, Optum360's coding experts have incorporated Medicare-related coding edits and proprietary features, such as supplementary notations, coding tools, and appendixes, into a comprehensive and easy-to-use reference. This publication is organized as follows:

What's New for 2021

This section provides a high-level overview of the changes made to the ICD-10-CM official code set for fiscal 2021, identifying codes that have been added and deleted from the classification, codes that had validity changes as a result of these additions and deletions, as well as codes that had revisions to their descriptions. All changes are based on the 2021 official addendum, posted June 30, 2020, by the National Center for Health Statistics (NCHS), the agency charged with maintaining and updating ICD-10-CM. NCHS is part of the Centers for Disease Control and Prevention (CDC).

Conversion Table

The conversion table was developed by National Center for Healthcare Statistics (NCHS) to help facilitate data retrieval as new codes are added to the ICD-10-CM classification. This table provides a crosswalk from each FY 2021 new code to the equivalent code(s) assigned prior to October 1, 2020, for that particular diagnosis or condition. For the full conversion table, including code crosswalks before October 1, 2020, refer to the 2021 Conversion Table zip file at https://www.cms.gov/medicare/icd-10/2021-icd-10-cm.

10 Steps to Correct Coding

This step-by-step tutorial walks the coder through the process of finding the correct code — from locating the code in the official indexes to verifying the code in the tabular section — while following applicable conventions, guidelines, and instructional notes. Specific examples are provided with detailed explanations of each coding step along with advice for proper sequencing.

Official ICD-10-CM Guidelines for Coding and Reporting

This section provides the full official conventions and guidelines regulating the appropriate assignment and reporting of ICD-10-CM codes. These conventions and guidelines are published by the U.S. Department of Health and Human Services (DHHS) and approved by the cooperating parties (American Health Information Management Association [AHIMA], National Center for Health Statistics [NCHS], Centers for Disease Control and Prevention [CDC], and the American Hospital Association [AHA]).

Indexes

Index to Diseases and Injuries

The Index to Diseases and Injuries is arranged in alphabetic order by terms specific to a disease, condition, illness, injury, eponym, or abbreviation as well as terms that describe circumstances other than a disease or injury that may require attention from a health care professional.

Neoplasm Table

The Neoplasm Table is arranged in alphabetic order by anatomical site. Codes are then listed in individual columns based upon the histological behavior (malignant, in situ, benign, uncertain, or unspecified) of the neoplasm.

Table of Drugs and Chemicals

The Table of Drugs and Chemicals is arranged in alphabetic order by the specific drug or chemical name. Codes are listed in individual columns based upon the associated intent (poisoning, adverse effect, or underdosing).

External Causes Index

The External Causes Index is arranged in alphabetic order by main terms that describe the cause, the intent, the place of occurrence, the activity, and the status of the patient at the time the injury occurred or health condition arose.

Index Notations

With

The word "with" or "in" should be interpreted to mean "associated with" or "due to." The classification presumes a causal relationship between the two conditions linked by these terms in the index. These conditions should be coded as related even in the absence of provider documentation explicitly linking them unless the documentation clearly states the conditions are unrelated or when another guideline specifically requires a documented linkage between two conditions (e.g., the sepsis guideline for "acute organ dysfunction that is not clearly associated with the sepsis"). For conditions not specifically linked by these relational terms in the classification or when a guideline requires explicit documentation of a linkage between two conditions, provider documentation must link the conditions to code them as related.

The word "with" in the index is sequenced immediately following the main term, not in alphabetical order.

Dermatopolymyositis M33.9Ø
with
myopathy M33.92
respiratory involvement M33.91
specified organ involvement NEC M33.99
in neoplastic disease — *see also* Neoplasm D49.9 *[M36.Ø]*

See

When the instruction "see" follows a term in the index, it indicates that another term must be referenced to locate the correct code.

Hematoperitoneum — *see* Hemoperitoneum

See Also

The instructional note "see also" simply provides alternative terms the coder may reference that may be useful in determining the correct code but are not necessary to follow if the main term supplies the appropriate code.

Hematinuria — *see also* Hemaglobinuria
malarial B5Ø.8

Default Codes

In the index, the default code is the code listed next to the main term and represents the condition most commonly associated with that main term. This code may be assigned when documentation does not support reporting a more specific code. Alternatively, it may provide an unspecified code for the condition.

Hemiatrophy R68.89
cerebellar G31.9
face, facial, progressive (Romberg) G51.8
tongue K14.8

Parentheses

Parentheses in the indexes enclose nonessential modifiers, supplementary words that may be present or absent in the statement of a disease without affecting the code.

Pseudomeningocele (cerebral) (infective) (post-traumatic) G96.198
postprocedural (spinal) G97.82

Brackets

ICD-10-CM has a coding convention addressing code assignment for manifestations that occur as a result of an underlying condition. This convention requires the underlying condition to be sequenced first, followed by the code or codes for the associated manifestation. In the index, italicized codes in brackets identify manifestation codes.

Polyneuropathy (peripheral) G62.9
alcoholic G62.1
amyloid (Portuguese) E85.1 *[G63]*
transthyretin-related (ATTR) familial E85.1 *[G63]*

Shaded Guides

Exclusive vertical shaded guides in the Index to Diseases and Injuries and External Causes Index help the user easily follow the indent levels for the subentries under a main term. Sequencing rules may apply depending on the level of indent for separate subentries.

Hemicrania
congenital malformation QØØ.Ø
continua G44.51
meaning migraine — *see also* Migraine G43.9Ø9
paroxysmal G44.Ø39
chronic G44.Ø49
intractable G44.Ø41
not intractable G44.Ø49
episodic G44.Ø39
intractable G44.Ø31
not intractable G44.Ø39
intractable G44.Ø31
not intractable G44.Ø39

Following References

The Index to Diseases and Injuries includes following references to assist in locating out-of-sequence codes in the tabular list. Out-of-sequence codes contain an alphabetic character (letter) in the third- or fourth-character position. These codes are placed according to the classification rules — according to condition — not according to alphabetic or numeric sequencing rules.

Carcinoma (malignant) — *see also* Neoplasm, by site, malignant
neuroendocrine — *see also* Tumor, neuroendocrine
high grade, any site C7A.1 (*following* C75)
poorly differentiated, any site C7A.1 (*following* C75)

Additional Character Required

The Index to Diseases and Injuries, Neoplasm Table, and External Causes Index provide an icon after certain codes to signify to the user that additional characters are required to make the code valid. The tabular list should be consulted for appropriate character selection.

Fall, falling (accidental) W19 ☑
building W2Ø.1 ☑

Tabular List of Diseases

ICD-10-CM codes and descriptions are arranged numerically within the tabular list of diseases with 19 separate chapters providing codes associated with a particular body system or nature of injury or disease. There is also a chapter providing codes for external causes of an injury or health conditions, a chapter for codes that address encounters with healthcare facilities for circumstances other than a disease or injury, and finally a chapter for codes that capture special circumstances such as new diseases of uncertain etiology or emergency use codes.

Code and Code Descriptions

ICD-10-CM is an alphanumeric classification system that contains categories, subcategories, and valid codes. The first character is always a letter with any additional characters represented by either a letter or number. A three-character category without further subclassification is equivalent to a valid three-character code. Valid codes may be three, four, five, six, or seven characters in length, with each level of subdivision after a three-character category representing a subcategory. The final level of subdivision is a valid code.

Boldface

Boldface type is used for all codes and descriptions in the tabular list.

Italics

Italicized type is used to identify manifestation codes, those codes that should not be reported as first-listed diagnoses.

Deleted Text

~~Strikethrough~~ on a code and code description indicates a deletion from the classification for the current year.

Key Word

Green font is used throughout the Tabular List of Diseases to differentiate the key words that appear in similar code descriptions in a given category or subcategory. The key word convention is used only in those categories in which there are multiple codes with very similar descriptions with only a few words that differentiate them.

For example, refer to the list of codes below from category H55:

√4th H55 Nystagmus and other irregular eye movements
√5th H55.Ø Nystagmus
H55.ØØ Unspecified nystagmus
H55.Ø1 Congenital nystagmus
H55.Ø2 Latent nystagmus
H55.Ø3 Visual deprivation nystagmus
H55.Ø4 Dissociated nystagmus
H55.Ø9 Other forms of nystagmus

The portion of the code description that appears in **green font** in the tabular list helps the coder quickly identify the key terms and the correct code. This convention is especially useful when the codes describe laterality, such as the following codes from subcategory H4Ø.22:

√6th H4Ø.22 Chronic angle-closure glaucoma
Chronic primary angle-closure glaucoma
√7th H4Ø.221 Chronic angle-closure glaucoma, right eye
√7th H4Ø.222 Chronic angle-closure glaucoma, left eye
√7th H4Ø.223 Chronic angle-closure glaucoma, bilateral
√7th H4Ø.229 Chronic angle-closure glaucoma, unspecified eye

Tabular Notations

Official parenthetical notes as well as Optum360's supplementary notations are provided at the chapter, code block, category, subcategory, and individual code level to help the user assign proper codes. The information in the notation can apply to one or more codes depending on where the citation is placed.

Official Notations

Includes Notes

The word INCLUDES appears immediately under certain categories to further define, clarify, or give examples of the content of a code category.

Inclusion Terms

Lists of inclusion terms are included under certain codes. These terms indicate some of the conditions for which that code number may be used. Inclusion terms may be synonyms with the code title, or, in the case of "other specified" codes, the terms may also provide a list of various conditions included within a classification code. The inclusion terms are not exhaustive. The index may provide additional terms that may also be assigned to a given code.

Excludes Notes

ICD-10-CM has two types of excludes notes. Each note has a different definition for use. However, they are similar in that they both indicate that codes excluded from each other are independent of each other.

Excludes 1

An EXCLUDES 1 note is a "pure" excludes. It means "NOT CODED HERE!" An Excludes 1 note indicates mutually exclusive codes: two conditions that cannot be reported together. An Excludes1 note indicates that the code excluded should never be used at the same time as the code above the Excludes1 note. An Excludes1 is used when two conditions cannot occur together, such as a congenital form versus an acquired form of the same condition.

An exception to the Excludes 1 definition is when the two conditions are unrelated to each other. If it is not clear whether the two conditions involving an Excludes 1 note are related or not, query the provider. For example, code F45.8 Other somatoform disorders, has an Excludes 1 note for "sleep related teeth grinding (G47.63)" because "teeth grinding" is an inclusion term under F45.8. Only one of these two codes should be assigned for teeth grinding. However, psychogenic dysmenorrhea is also an inclusion term under F45.8, and a patient could have both this condition and sleep-related teeth grinding. In this case, the two conditions are clearly unrelated to each other, so it would be appropriate to report F45.8 and G47.63 together.

Excludes 2

An EXCLUDES 2 note means "NOT INCLUDED HERE." An Excludes 2 note indicates that although the excluded condition is not part of the condition it is excluded from, a patient may have both conditions at the same time. Therefore, when an Excludes 2 note appears under a code, it may be acceptable to use both the code and the excluded code together if supported by the medical documentation.

Note

The term "NOTE" appears as an icon and precedes the instructional information. These notes function as alerts to highlight coding instructions within the text.

Code First/Use additional code

These instructional notes provide sequencing instruction. They may appear independently of each other or to designate certain etiology/manifestation paired codes. These instructions signal the coder that an additional code should be reported to provide a more complete picture of that diagnosis.

In etiology/manifestation coding, ICD-10-CM requires the underlying condition to be sequenced first, followed by the manifestation. In these situations, codes with "In diseases classified elsewhere" in the code description are never permitted as a first-listed or principal diagnosis code and must be sequenced following the underlying condition code.

Code Also

A "code also" note alerts the coder that more than one code may be required to fully describe the condition. The sequencing depends on the circumstances of the encounter. Factors that may determine sequencing include severity and reason for the encounter.

Revised Text

The revised text ▶◀ "bow ties" alert the user to changes in official notations for the current year. Revised text may include the following:

- A change in a current parenthetical description
- A change in the code(s) associated with a current parenthetical note
- A change in how a current parenthetical note is classified (e.g., an Excludes 1 note that changed to an Excludes 2 note)
- Addition of a new parenthetical note(s) to a code

Deleted Text

~~Strikethrough~~ on official notations indicate a deletion from the classification for the current year.

Optum360 Notations

AHA Coding Clinic Citations

Coding Clinics are official American Hospital Association (AHA) publications that provide coding advice specific to ICD-10-CM and ICD-10-PCS.

Coding Clinic citations included in this manual are current up to the second quarter of 2020.

These citations identify the year, quarter, and page number of one or more *Coding Clinic* publications that may have coding advice relevant to a particular code or group of codes. With the most current citation listed first, these notations are preceded by the symbol **AHA:** and appear in purple type.

> **I15.1 Hypertension secondary to other renal disorders**
> **AHA:** 2016, 3Q, 22

Definitions

Definitions explain a specific term, condition, or disease process in layman's terms. These notations are preceded by the symbol **DEF:** and appear in purple type.

> ✓5th **M51.4 Schmorl's nodes**
> **DEF:** Irregular bone defect in the margin of the vertebral body that causes herniation into the end plate of the vertebral body.

Coding Tips

The tips in the tabular list offer coding advice that is not readily available within the ICD-10-CM classification. It may relate official coding guidelines, indexing nuances, or advice from *AHA's Coding Clinic for ICD-10-CM/PCS*. These notations are preceded by the symbol **TIP:** and appear in brown type.

> ✓5th **B97.2 Coronavirus as the cause of diseases classified elsewhere**
> **TIP:** Do not report a code from this subcategory for COVID-19; refer to U07.1.

Icons

Note: The following icons are placed to the left of the code.

● **New Code**
Codes that have been added to the classification system for the current year.

▲ **Revised Code Title**
Codes that have had a change to their description or validity change for the current year. For additional information on codes with validity changes, see the "What's New" section.

☑ **Additional Characters Required**

✓4th This symbol indicates that the code requires a 4th character.

✓5th This symbol indicates that the code requires a 5th character.

✓6th This symbol indicates that the code requires a 6th character.

✓7th This symbol indicates that the code requires a 7th character.

> ✓5th **H60.3 Other infective otitis externa**
> ✓6th **H60.31 Diffuse otitis externa**
> **H60.311 Diffuse otitis externa, right ear**
> **H60.312 Diffuse otitis externa, left ear**
> **H60.313 Diffuse otitis externa, bilateral**
> **H60.319 Diffuse otitis externa, unspecified ear**

✓x7th **Placeholder Alert**
This symbol indicates that the code requires a 7th character following the placeholder "X". Codes with fewer than six characters that require a 7th character must contain placeholder "X" to fill in the empty character(s).

> ✓x7th **T16.1 Foreign body in right ear**

This manual provides the most current information that was available at the time of publication. Except where otherwise noted, the icons and/or color bars reflect edits associated with the inpatient prospective payment system (IPPS). Because the fiscal 2021 IPPS final rule was not available at the time this book was printed, the edits in this manual are based on the proposed, version 38, MS-DRG grouper software, Definitions Manual files, and Medicare Code Editor (MCE) files, published with the fiscal 2021 IPPS proposed rule.

In an effort to provide the most current edit information, Optum360 has provided a searchable data file that includes the final edit designations for all ICD-10-CM codes based on the fiscal 2021 IPPS final rule official files, effective October 1, 2020. The edits included in the data file are as follows:

- Age
- Sex
- Hospital-acquired condition (HAC)
- CC
- MCC
- HIV
- Manifestation code
- Unacceptable diagnosis
- Questionable diagnosis

This data file can be accessed at the following:

https://www.optum360coding.com/ProductUpdates/
Title: "2021 ICD-10-CM for Hospital IPPS Data File"
Password: Hospital21

Note: The following icons are placed at the end of the code description.

Age Edits

N **Newborn Age: 0**
These diagnoses are intended for newborns and neonates and the patient's age must be 0 years.

> **N47.0 Adherent prepuce, newborn** N ♂

P **Pediatric Age: 0-17**
These diagnoses are intended for children and the patient's age must be between 0 and 17 years.

> **L21.1 Seborrheic infantile dermatitis** P

M **Maternity Age: 9-64**
These diagnoses are intended for childbearing patients between the age of 9 and 64 years.

O02.9	**Abnormal product of conception, unspecified**	M♀

A **Adult Age: 15-124**
These diagnoses are intended for patients between the age of 15 and 124 years.

R54 Age-related physical debility A
Frailty
Old age
Senescence
Senile asthenia
Senile debility
EXCLUDES 1 *age-related cognitive decline (R41.81)*
sarcopenia (M62.84)
senile psychosis (F03)
senility NOS (R41.81)

Sex Edits

♂ **Male diagnosis only**

Q98.0	**Klinefelter syndrome karyotype 47, XXY**	♂

♀ **Female diagnosis only**

N35.12	**Postinfective urethral stricture, not elsewhere classified,** female	♀

H1-H14 **Hospital Acquired Condition (HAC)**
These codes identify conditions that are high cost or high volume or both, are either a complication or comorbidity (CC) or major complication or comorbidity (MCC) that as a secondary diagnosis results in assignment of a case to a higher-paying MS-DRG. These conditions are reasonably preventable through the application of evidence-based guidelines. If the condition is not present on admission (meaning it developed during the hospital admission), the case will not group to the higher-paying MS-DRG based solely upon the reporting of the HAC code. Many of these HACs are conditional, and are based on reporting the specific diagnosis code(s) in combination with certain procedure codes.

Note: Hospital-acquired conditions do not impact MS-LTC-DRG assignment.

The comprehensive list of HAC tables that coincide with these icon numbers appears in appendix G of this book.

N15.1	**Renal and perinephric abscess**	MCC H6

CC **CC Condition**
This symbol designates a complication or comorbidity diagnosis that may affect DRG assignment. A complication or comorbidity diagnosis, CC condition, is defined as a significant acute disease, a significant acute manifestation of a chronic disease, an advanced or end-stage chronic disease, or a chronic disease associated with systemic physiological decompensation and debility that have consistently greater impact on hospital resources.

A comprehensive list of ICD-10-CM codes considered a CC appears in appendix E of this book.

G90.59	**Complex regional pain syndrome I of other specified site**	CC

MCC **MCC Condition**
This symbol designates a major complication or comorbidity diagnosis that may affect DRG assignment. An MCC condition meets the same criteria as a CC condition but is associated with a higher acuity level and hospital resource consumption is expected to be higher than that for a CC condition. There are fewer conditions that meet the criteria as an MCC than those for a CC condition.

A comprehensive list of ICD-10-CM codes considered an MCC appears in appendix D of this book.

√7th **S35.238**	**Other injury of inferior mesenteric artery**	MCC

Note: The assignment of an MS-DRG or MS-LTC-DRG often depends on the presence or absence of a secondary diagnosis code that is designated as an MCC or CC. However, in some instances the MCC or CC designation for that secondary diagnosis code is negated due to its relationship with the principal diagnosis; this is referred to as CC exclusion. The ICD-10 MS-DRG Definitions Manual included with the IPPS final rule provides a list of all principal diagnosis codes that would render ineffective the MCC/CC designation for a particular ICD-10-CM code when used as a secondary diagnosis. Optum360 has provided this CC exclusion list in an easily searchable data file, which can be accessed at the following:

https://www.optum360coding.com/ProductUpdates/
Title: "2021 ICD-10-CM for Hospitals CC Excludes Data File"
Password: Hospital21

HIV **HIV-related Condition**
This symbol indicates that the condition is considered a major HIV-related diagnosis. When the condition is coded in combination with a diagnosis of human immunodeficiency virus (HIV), code B20, the case will move from MS-DRG/MS-LTC-DRG 977 to MS-DRGs/MS-LTC-DRGs 974-976.

G96.9	**Disorder of central nervous system, unspecified**	HIV

HCC **CMS-HCC Condition**
Identify conditions that are considered a CMS-HCC (hierarchical condition category) diagnosis.

The HCC codes represented in this manual have been updated to reflect the 2021 Initial ICD-10-CM Mappings for CMS-HCC Model v24. Midyear final mappings were not available at the time this publication went to print; refer to the following CMS website for final mappings: https://www.cms.gov/Medicare/Health-Plans/MedicareAdvtgSpecRateStats/Risk-Adjustors.html.

Y62.2	**Failure of sterile precautions during** kidney dialysis and other perfusion	HCC

SW **Severe Wound Diagnosis**
This symbol indicates that the condition is considered a severe wound diagnosis. Depending on the facility from which the patient is discharged, these conditions may not require that the payment rate for that admission be adjusted.

A comprehensive list of ICD-10-CM codes considered a severe wound diagnosis appears in appendix K of this book.

L89.014	**Pressure ulcer of right elbow,** stage 4	MCC H4 HCC SW

Color Bars

Manifestation Code

Codes defined as manifestation codes appear in italic type, with a blue color bar over the code description. A manifestation cannot be reported as a first-listed code; it is sequenced as a secondary diagnosis with the underlying disease code listed first.

G32.89 ***Other specified degenerative disorders of nervous system in diseases classified elsewhere***
Degenerative encephalopathy in diseases classified elsewhere

Unacceptable Principal Diagnoses

Unacceptable principal diagnoses will appear with a purple color bar over the code description. These codes do not describe a current illness or injury, but a circumstance which influences a patient's health status. They are considered an unacceptable principal diagnosis for *inpatient* admission.

√7th **T48.5X5** Adverse effect **of other anti-common-cold drugs**

Questionable Admission Diagnoses

Questionable admission diagnoses will appear with a yellow color bar over the code description. These codes, although not unacceptable as a PDx, may be considered a "questionable admission" when used as PDx in an acute care hospital.

E66.Ø9 **Other obesity due to excess calories**

Wrong Procedure Performed Edit

An orange color bar over the code title indicates the Wrong Procedure Performed edit. This edit was created to identify cases in which wrong surgeries occurred. Any claim with a code from Y65.51-Y65.53 will be denied and returned to the provider. A surgical or other invasive procedure is considered to be a wrong procedure if one of the following is true:

- The procedure was performed on the wrong site.
- The procedure was performed on the wrong patient.
- The incorrect procedure was performed on a patient.

Y65.51 **Performance of wrong procedure (operation) on** correct patient
Wrong device implanted into correct surgical site
EXCLUDES 1 *performance of correct procedure (operation) on wrong side or body part (Y65.53)*

Unspecified Diagnosis

Codes that appear with a gray color bar over the alphanumeric code identify unspecified diagnoses. These codes should be used in limited circumstances, when neither the diagnostic statement nor the documentation provides enough information to assign a more specific diagnosis code. The abbreviation NOS, "not otherwise specified," in the tabular list may be interpreted as "unspecified."

GØ3.9 **Meningitis, unspecified** MCC
Arachnoiditis (spinal) NOS

Footnotes

Certain codes in the tabular section have a numerical superscript located to the upper left of the code. This numerical superscript corresponds to a specific footnote description.

For example:

[1] **R57.1** Hypovolemic **shock** MCC HCC

For convenience, the footnote descriptions are provided on the front cover.

The following list also provides the footnote descriptions of all numerical superscripts found in the Tabular List of Diseases:

1 These codes are considered major complication/comorbidity (MCC) conditions only if the patient is discharged alive.

2 This condition is considered an MCC only when reported as an initial encounter for an open fracture (7th character B or C specific to category).

3 This condition is considered a CC only when reported as an initial encounter for a fracture (7th character A, B, or C specific to category) or a subsequent encounter for nonunion or malunion fracture (7th character K, M, N, P, Q, or R specific to category).

4 This condition is considered a CC only when reported as a subsequent encounter for a nonunion or malunion fracture (7th character K, M, N, P, Q, or R specific to category).

5 This condition is considered a CC only when reported as an initial encounter or subsequent encounter (7th character A or D).

6 This condition is considered an HCC when reported as initial encounter (7th character A, B, or C specific to category).

7 This condition is considered an HCC when reported as initial encounter (7th character A or B specific to category) or as a sequela.

8 This condition is considered an HCC when reported as a sequela.

Chapter-Level Notations

Chapter-Specific Guidelines with Coding Examples

Each chapter begins with the Official Guidelines for Coding and Reporting specific to that chapter, where provided. Coding examples specific to inpatient care settings have been provided to illustrate the coding and/or sequencing guidance in these guidelines.

Muscle and Tendon Table

ICD-10-CM categorizes certain muscles and tendons in the upper and lower extremities by their action (e.g., extension or flexion) as well as their anatomical location. The Muscle/Tendon table is provided at the beginning of chapter 13 and chapter 19 to help users when code selection depends on the action of the muscle and/or tendon.

Note: This table is not all-inclusive, and proper code assignment should be based on the provider's documentation.

Appendixes

The additional resources described below have been included as appendixes for the *ICD-10-CM Expert for Hospitals*. These resources further instruct the professional coder on the appropriate application of the ICD-10-CM code set.

Appendix A: Valid 3-character ICD-10-CM Codes

The user may consult this table to confirm that no further specificity, such as the use of 4th, 5th, 6th, or 7th characters or placeholders (X), is necessary. All ICD-10-CM codes that are valid at the three-character level are listed.

Appendix B: Pharmacology List 2021

This reference is a comprehensive but not all-inclusive list of pharmacological agents used to treat acute and/or chronic conditions. Drugs are listed in alphabetical order by their brand and/or generic names along with their drug action and indications for which they may commonly be prescribed. Some drugs have also been mapped to their appropriate long-term drug use Z code.

Appendix C: Z Codes for Long-Term Drug Use with Associated Drugs

This resource correlates Z codes that are used to identify current long-term drug use with a list of drugs that are typically categorized to that class of drug.

Note: These tables are not all-inclusive but list some of the more commonly used drugs.

Appendix D: Major Complication and Comorbidity (MCC) Code List
This is a full listing of conditions considered to be major complications and/or comorbidities that when present as a secondary diagnosis may affect DRG assignment under the Medicare Severity DRG (MS-DRG) system.

Note: This resource provides the most current MCC information that was available at the time of publication using the proposed, version 38, MS-DRG grouper software and Definitions Manual files published with the fiscal 2021 IPPS proposed rule.

Appendix E: Complication and Comorbidity (CC) Code List
This is a full listing of conditions considered to be complications and/or comorbidities that when present as a secondary diagnosis may affect DRG assignment under the MS-DRG system.

Note: This resource provides the most current CC information that was available at the time of publication using the proposed, version 38, MS-DRG Grouper software and Definitions Manual files published with the fiscal 2021 IPPS proposed rule.

Appendix F: Present on Admission (POA) Tutorial
This tutorial walks the coder through the process of assigning the appropriate present-on-admission (POA) indicator for inpatient codes based on the POA reporting guidelines. Detailed scenarios for a variety of situations are provided and discussed.

Appendix G: Hospital Acquired Conditions
This comprehensive table displays codes that identify conditions that are considered reasonably preventable when occurring during the hospital admission and may prevent the case from grouping to a higher-paying MS-DRG. Many of these HACs are conditional and are based on reporting the specific diagnosis code(s) in combination with certain procedure codes, which are also noted in this table.

Note: This resource provides the most current HAC information that was available at the time of publication using the proposed, version 38, MS-DRG Grouper software and Definitions Manual files published with the fiscal 2021 IPPS proposed rule.

Appendix H: Centers for Medicare & Medicaid Services (CMS) Hierarchical Condition Categories (HCC) (CMS-HCC)
This resource provides the framework behind CMS's Medicare Advantage (MA) program, a risk-adjustment model developed as a means of compensating health care plans with large numbers of Medicare Part C beneficiaries. It includes a brief synopsis of the evolution of the program from its inception; insight into the various elements needed to predict risk, including the principles used to develop the hierarchical condition categories (HCCs), one of the fundamental components of the risk adjustment model; and a description of the audit process used to ensure the accuracy of payments made to MA plans.

Appendix I: Long-term Care Hospital Prospective Payment System Overview
The long-term care hospital prospective payment system (LTCH PPS) provides payment rates for LTCH facilities certified by Medicare as LTCH with an average length of stay (LOS) of 25 days or longer. This resource summarizes the certification qualifications for LTCH facilities, payment methodology, and current fiscal year PPS updates.

Appendix J: Long-Term Care Hospital Quality Reporting Program
The LTCH QRP is a mandatory reporting component for LTCH facilities certified by Medicare as LTCH with an average LOS of 25 days or longer. Much of the current QRP for LTCH, like other post-acute care providers, is based upon the requirements of the 2014 IMPACT Act. This resource summarizes the current QRP requirements for facilities certified as LTCH under Medicare, including required data set items and market-basket payment impact.

Appendix K: Severe Wound Diagnosis Codes by Category
This resource includes a full listing of codes identified as severe wound diagnoses that may allow certain discharges from LTCHs a temporary exception from the site-neutral payment rate.

Illustrations

This section includes illustrations of normal anatomy with ICD-10-CM-specific terminology.

What's New for 2021

Official Updates

The official ICD-10-CM addendum identifies changes to the ICD-10-CM code set for fiscal 2021, effective October 1, 2020, to September 30, 2021. These changes were made by the agency charged with maintaining and updating the ICD-10-CM code set, the National Center for Health Statistics (NCHS), a section of the Centers for Disease Control and Prevention (CDC). A summary of the changes is provided below:

39 Codes with a Change in Validity

Note: Validity changes are the result of codes being added to or deleted from the classification. Codes that change from valid to invalid allow the creation of a new subcategory to which new codes can be assigned that provide greater detail about the condition. Codes that change from invalid to valid are the result of codes being deleted from a subcategory in the classification, when the detail provided in those codes is no longer required.

Valid to Invalid

A84.8	B60.0	D59.1	D72.1	D84.8	E70.8	E74.8
G11.1	G71.2	G96.0	G96.19	G96.8	H18.50	H18.51
H18.52	H18.53	H18.54	H18.55	H18.59	J82	J84.17
K20.8	K20.9	K21.0	K59.8	K74.0	M92.50	M92.51
M92.52	N18.3	O99.89	R51	R74.0	T86.840	T86.841
T86.842	T86.848	T86.849	Y77.1			

Invalid to Valid

No applicable codes

19 Codes Deleted from the Classification

Q51.2Ø Other doubling of uterus, unspecified

T4Ø.4X1A Poisoning by other synthetic narcotics, accidental (unintentional), initial encounter

T4Ø.4X1D Poisoning by other synthetic narcotics, accidental (unintentional), subsequent encounter

T4Ø.4X1S Poisoning by other synthetic narcotics, accidental (unintentional), sequela

T4Ø.4X2A Poisoning by other synthetic narcotics, intentional self-harm, initial encounter

T4Ø.4X2D Poisoning by other synthetic narcotics, intentional self-harm, subsequent encounter

T4Ø.4X2S Poisoning by other synthetic narcotics, intentional self-harm, sequela

T4Ø.4X3A Poisoning by other synthetic narcotics, assault, initial encounter

T4Ø.4X3D Poisoning by other synthetic narcotics, assault, subsequent encounter

T4Ø.4X3S Poisoning by other synthetic narcotics, assault, sequela

T4Ø.4X4A Poisoning by other synthetic narcotics, undetermined, initial encounter

T4Ø.4X4D Poisoning by other synthetic narcotics, undetermined, subsequent encounter

T4Ø.4X4S Poisoning by other synthetic narcotics, undetermined, sequela

T4Ø.4X5A Adverse effect of other synthetic narcotics, initial encounter

T4Ø.4X5D Adverse effect of other synthetic narcotics, subsequent encounter

T4Ø.4X5S Adverse effect of other synthetic narcotics, sequela

T4Ø.4X6A Underdosing of other synthetic narcotics, initial encounter

T4Ø.4X6D Underdosing of other synthetic narcotics, subsequent encounter

T4Ø.4X6S Underdosing of other synthetic narcotics, sequela

490 New Codes Added to the Classification

A84.81 Powassan virus disease

A84.89 Other tick-borne viral encephalitis

B6Ø.ØØ Babesiosis, unspecified

B6Ø.Ø1 Babesiosis due to Babesia microti

B6Ø.Ø2 Babesiosis due to Babesia duncani

B6Ø.Ø3 Babesiosis due to Babesia divergens

B6Ø.Ø9 Other babesiosis

D57.Ø3 Hb-SS disease with cerebral vascular involvement

D57.Ø9 Hb-SS disease with crisis with other specified complication

D57.213 Sickle-cell/Hb-C disease with cerebral vascular involvement

D57.218 Sickle-cell/Hb-C disease with crisis with other specified complication

D57.413 Sickle-cell thalassemia, unspecified, with cerebral vascular involvement

D57.418 Sickle-cell thalassemia, unspecified, with crisis with other specified complication

D57.42 Sickle-cell-thalassemia beta zero without crisis

D57.431 Sickle-cell thalassemia beta zero with acute chest syndrome

D57.432 Sickle-cell thalassemia beta zero with splenic sequestration

D57.433 Sickle-cell thalassemia beta zero with cerebral vascular involvement

D57.438 Sickle-cell thalassemia beta zero with crisis with other specified complication

D57.439 Sickle-cell thalassemia beta zero with crisis, unspecified

D57.44 Sickle-cell thalassemia beta plus without crisis

D57.451 Sickle-cell thalassemia beta plus with acute chest syndrome

D57.452 Sickle-cell thalassemia beta plus with splenic sequestration

D57.453 Sickle-cell thalassemia beta plus with cerebral vascular involvement

D57.458 Sickle-cell thalassemia beta plus with crisis with other specified complication

D57.459 Sickle-cell thalassemia beta plus with crisis, unspecified

D57.813 Other sickle-cell disorders with cerebral vascular involvement

D57.818 Other sickle-cell disorders with crisis with other specified complication

D59.1Ø Autoimmune hemolytic anemia, unspecified

D59.11 Warm autoimmune hemolytic anemia

D59.12 Cold autoimmune hemolytic anemia

D59.13 Mixed type autoimmune hemolytic anemia

D59.19 Other autoimmune hemolytic anemia

D72.1Ø Eosinophilia, unspecified

D72.11Ø Idiopathic hypereosinophilic syndrome [IHES]

D72.111 Lymphocytic Variant Hypereosinophilic Syndrome [LHES]

D72.118	Other hypereosinophilic syndrome
D72.119	Hypereosinophilic syndrome [HES], unspecified
D72.12	Drug rash with eosinophilia and systemic symptoms syndrome
D72.18	Eosinophilia in diseases classified elsewhere
D72.19	Other eosinophilia
D84.81	Immunodeficiency due to conditions classified elsewhere
D84.821	Immunodeficiency due to drugs
D84.822	Immunodeficiency due to external causes
D84.89	Other immunodeficiencies
D89.831	Cytokine release syndrome, grade 1
D89.832	Cytokine release syndrome, grade 2
D89.833	Cytokine release syndrome, grade 3
D89.834	Cytokine release syndrome, grade 4
D89.835	Cytokine release syndrome, grade 5
D89.839	Cytokine release syndrome, grade unspecified
E70.81	Aromatic L-amino acid decarboxylase deficiency
E70.89	Other disorders of aromatic amino-acid metabolism
E74.810	Glucose transporter protein type 1 deficiency
E74.818	Other disorders of glucose transport
E74.819	Disorders of glucose transport, unspecified
E74.89	Other specified disorders of carbohydrate metabolism
F10.130	Alcohol abuse with withdrawal, uncomplicated
F10.131	Alcohol abuse with withdrawal delirium
F10.132	Alcohol abuse with withdrawal with perceptual disturbance
F10.139	Alcohol abuse with withdrawal, unspecified
F10.930	Alcohol use, unspecified with withdrawal, uncomplicated
F10.931	Alcohol use, unspecified with withdrawal delirium
F10.932	Alcohol use, unspecified with withdrawal with perceptual disturbance
F10.939	Alcohol use, unspecified with withdrawal, unspecified
F11.13	Opioid abuse with withdrawal
F12.13	Cannabis abuse with withdrawal
F13.130	Sedative, hypnotic or anxiolytic abuse with withdrawal, uncomplicated
F13.131	Sedative, hypnotic or anxiolytic abuse with withdrawal delirium
F13.132	Sedative, hypnotic or anxiolytic abuse with withdrawal with perceptual disturbance
F13.139	Sedative, hypnotic or anxiolytic abuse with withdrawal, unspecified
F14.13	Cocaine abuse, unspecified with withdrawal
F14.93	Cocaine use, unspecified with withdrawal
F15.13	Other stimulant abuse with withdrawal
F19.130	Other psychoactive substance abuse with withdrawal, uncomplicated
F19.131	Other psychoactive substance abuse with withdrawal delirium
F19.132	Other psychoactive substance abuse with withdrawal with perceptual disturbance
F19.139	Other psychoactive substance abuse with withdrawal, unspecified
G11.10	Early-onset cerebellar ataxia, unspecified
G11.11	Friedreich ataxia
G11.19	Other early-onset cerebellar ataxia
G40.42	Cyclin-Dependent Kinase-Like 5 Deficiency Disorder
G40.833	Dravet syndrome, intractable, with status epilepticus
G40.834	Dravet syndrome, intractable, without status epilepticus
G71.20	Congenital myopathy, unspecified
G71.21	Nemaline myopathy
G71.220	X-linked myotubular myopathy
G71.228	Other centronuclear myopathy
G71.29	Other congenital myopathy
G96.00	Cerebrospinal fluid leak, unspecified
G96.01	Cranial cerebrospinal fluid leak, spontaneous
G96.02	Spinal cerebrospinal fluid leak, spontaneous
G96.08	Other cranial cerebrospinal fluid leak
G96.09	Other spinal cerebrospinal fluid leak
G96.191	Perineural cyst
G96.198	Other disorders of meninges, not elsewhere classified
G96.810	Intracranial hypotension, unspecified
G96.811	Intracranial hypotension, spontaneous
G96.819	Other intracranial hypotension
G96.89	Other specified disorders of central nervous system
G97.83	Intracranial hypotension following lumbar cerebrospinal fluid shunting
G97.84	Intracranial hypotension following other procedure
H18.501	Unspecified hereditary corneal dystrophies, right eye
H18.502	Unspecified hereditary corneal dystrophies, left eye
H18.503	Unspecified hereditary corneal dystrophies, bilateral
H18.509	Unspecified hereditary corneal dystrophies, unspecified eye
H18.511	Endothelial corneal dystrophy, right eye
H18.512	Endothelial corneal dystrophy, left eye
H18.513	Endothelial corneal dystrophy, bilateral
H18.519	Endothelial corneal dystrophy, unspecified eye
H18.521	Epithelial (juvenile) corneal dystrophy, right eye
H18.522	Epithelial (juvenile) corneal dystrophy, left eye
H18.523	Epithelial (juvenile) corneal dystrophy, bilateral
H18.529	Epithelial (juvenile) corneal dystrophy, unspecified eye
H18.531	Granular corneal dystrophy, right eye
H18.532	Granular corneal dystrophy, left eye
H18.533	Granular corneal dystrophy, bilateral
H18.539	Granular corneal dystrophy, unspecified eye
H18.541	Lattice corneal dystrophy, right eye
H18.542	Lattice corneal dystrophy, left eye
H18.543	Lattice corneal dystrophy, bilateral
H18.549	Lattice corneal dystrophy, unspecified eye
H18.551	Macular corneal dystrophy, right eye
H18.552	Macular corneal dystrophy, left eye
H18.553	Macular corneal dystrophy, bilateral
H18.559	Macular corneal dystrophy, unspecified eye
H18.591	Other hereditary corneal dystrophies, right eye
H18.592	Other hereditary corneal dystrophies, left eye
H18.593	Other hereditary corneal dystrophies, bilateral
H18.599	Other hereditary corneal dystrophies, unspecified eye
H55.82	Deficient smooth pursuit eye movements

J82.81	Chronic eosinophilic pneumonia
J82.82	Acute eosinophilic pneumonia
J82.83	Eosinophilic asthma
J82.89	Other pulmonary eosinophilia, not elsewhere classified
J84.17Ø	Interstitial lung disease with progressive fibrotic phenotype in diseases classified elsewhere
J84.178	Other interstitial pulmonary diseases with fibrosis in diseases classified elsewhere
K2Ø.8Ø	Other esophagitis without bleeding
K2Ø.81	Other esophagitis with bleeding
K2Ø.9Ø	Esophagitis, unspecified without bleeding
K2Ø.91	Esophagitis, unspecified with bleeding
K21.ØØ	Gastro-esophageal reflux disease with esophagitis, without bleeding
K21.Ø1	Gastro-esophageal reflux disease with esophagitis, with bleeding
K59.81	Ogilvie syndrome
K59.89	Other specified functional intestinal disorders
K74.ØØ	Hepatic fibrosis, unspecified
K74.Ø1	Hepatic fibrosis, early fibrosis
K74.Ø2	Hepatic fibrosis, advanced fibrosis
MØ5.7A	Rheumatoid arthritis with rheumatoid factor of other specified site without organ or systems involvement
MØ5.8A	Other rheumatoid arthritis with rheumatoid factor of other specified site
MØ6.ØA	Rheumatoid arthritis without rheumatoid factor, other specified site
MØ6.8A	Other specified rheumatoid arthritis, other specified site
MØ8.ØA	Unspecified juvenile rheumatoid arthritis, other specified site
MØ8.2A	Juvenile rheumatoid arthritis with systemic onset, other specified site
MØ8.4A	Pauciarticular juvenile rheumatoid arthritis, other specified site
MØ8.9A	Juvenile arthritis, unspecified, other specified site
M19.Ø9	Primary osteoarthritis, other specified site
M19.19	Post-traumatic osteoarthritis, other specified site
M19.29	Secondary osteoarthritis, other specified site
M24.19	Other articular cartilage disorders, other specified site
M24.29	Disorder of ligament, other specified site
M24.39	Pathological dislocation of other specified joint, not elsewhere classified
M24.49	Recurrent dislocation, other specified joint
M24.59	Contracture, other specified joint
M24.69	Ankylosis, other specified joint
M24.89	Other specific joint derangement of other specified joint, not elsewhere classified
M25.39	Other instability, other specified joint
M25.59	Pain in other specified joint
M25.69	Stiffness of other specified joint, not elsewhere classified
M26.641	Arthritis of right temporomandibular joint
M26.642	Arthritis of left temporomandibular joint
M26.643	Arthritis of bilateral temporomandibular joint
M26.649	Arthritis of unspecified temporomandibular joint
M26.651	Arthropathy of right temporomandibular joint
M26.652	Arthropathy of left temporomandibular joint
M26.653	Arthropathy of bilateral temporomandibular joint
M26.659	Arthropathy of unspecified temporomandibular joint
M8Ø.ØAXA	Age-related osteoporosis with current pathological fracture, other site, initial encounter for fracture
M8Ø.ØAXD	Age-related osteoporosis with current pathological fracture, other site, subsequent encounter for fracture with routine healing
M8Ø.ØAXG	Age-related osteoporosis with current pathological fracture, other site, subsequent encounter for fracture with delayed healing
M8Ø.ØAXK	Age-related osteoporosis with current pathological fracture, other site, subsequent encounter for fracture with nonunion
M8Ø.ØAXP	Age-related osteoporosis with current pathological fracture, other site, subsequent encounter for fracture with malunion
M8Ø.ØAXS	Age-related osteoporosis with current pathological fracture, other site, sequela
M8Ø.8AXA	Other osteoporosis with current pathological fracture, other site, initial encounter for fracture
M8Ø.8AXD	Other osteoporosis with current pathological fracture, other site, subsequent encounter for fracture with routine healing
M8Ø.8AXG	Other osteoporosis with current pathological fracture, other site, subsequent encounter for fracture with delayed healing
M8Ø.8AXK	Other osteoporosis with current pathological fracture, other site, subsequent encounter for fracture with nonunion
M8Ø.8AXP	Other osteoporosis with current pathological fracture, other site, subsequent encounter for fracture with malunion
M8Ø.8AXS	Other osteoporosis with current pathological fracture, other site, sequela
M92.5Ø1	Unspecified juvenile osteochondrosis, right leg
M92.5Ø2	Unspecified juvenile osteochondrosis, left leg
M92.5Ø3	Unspecified juvenile osteochondrosis, bilateral leg
M92.5Ø9	Unspecified juvenile osteochondrosis, unspecified leg
M92.511	Juvenile osteochondrosis of proximal tibia, right leg
M92.512	Juvenile osteochondrosis of proximal tibia, left leg
M92.513	Juvenile osteochondrosis of proximal tibia, bilateral
M92.519	Juvenile osteochondrosis of proximal tibia, unspecified leg
M92.521	Juvenile osteochondrosis of tibia tubercle, right leg
M92.522	Juvenile osteochondrosis of tibia tubercle, left leg
M92.523	Juvenile osteochondrosis of tibia tubercle, bilateral
M92.529	Juvenile osteochondrosis of tibia tubercle, unspecified leg
M92.591	Other juvenile osteochondrosis of tibia and fibula, right leg
M92.592	Other juvenile osteochondrosis of tibia and fibula, left leg
M92.593	Other juvenile osteochondrosis of tibia and fibula, bilateral
M92.599	Other juvenile osteochondrosis of tibia and fibula, unspecified leg
NØØ.A	Acute nephritic syndrome with C3 glomerulonephritis
NØ1.A	Rapidly progressive nephritic syndrome with C3 glomerulonephritis
NØ2.A	Recurrent and persistent hematuria with C3 glomerulonephritis

NØ3.A	Chronic nephritic syndrome with C3 glomerulonephritis
NØ4.A	Nephrotic syndrome with C3 glomerulonephritis
NØ5.A	Unspecified nephritic syndrome with C3 glomerulonephritis
NØ6.A	Isolated proteinuria with C3 glomerulonephritis
NØ7.A	Hereditary nephropathy, not elsewhere classified with C3 glomerulonephritis
N18.3Ø	Chronic kidney disease, stage 3 unspecified
N18.31	Chronic kidney disease, stage 3a
N18.32	Chronic kidney disease, stage 3b
N61.2Ø	Granulomatous mastitis, unspecified breast
N61.21	Granulomatous mastitis, right breast
N61.22	Granulomatous mastitis, left breast
N61.23	Granulomatous mastitis, bilateral breast
O34.218	Maternal care for other type scar from previous cesarean delivery
O34.22	Maternal care for cesarean scar defect (isthmocele)
O99.891	Other specified diseases and conditions complicating pregnancy
O99.892	Other specified diseases and conditions complicating childbirth
O99.893	Other specified diseases and conditions complicating puerperium
P91.821	Neonatal cerebral infarction, right side of brain
P91.822	Neonatal cerebral infarction, left side of brain
P91.823	Neonatal cerebral infarction, bilateral
P91.829	Neonatal cerebral infarction, unspecified side
R51.Ø	Headache with orthostatic component, not elsewhere classified
R51.9	Headache, unspecified
R74.Ø1	Elevation of levels of liver transaminase levels
R74.Ø2	Elevation of levels of lactic acid dehydrogenase [LDH]
S2Ø.213A	Contusion of bilateral front wall of thorax, initial encounter
S2Ø.213D	Contusion of bilateral front wall of thorax, subsequent encounter
S2Ø.213S	Contusion of bilateral front wall of thorax, sequela
S2Ø.214A	Contusion of middle front wall of thorax, initial encounter
S2Ø.214D	Contusion of middle front wall of thorax, subsequent encounter
S2Ø.214S	Contusion of middle front wall of thorax, sequela
S2Ø.223A	Contusion of bilateral back wall of thorax, initial encounter
S2Ø.223D	Contusion of bilateral back wall of thorax, subsequent encounter
S2Ø.223S	Contusion of bilateral back wall of thorax, sequela
S2Ø.224A	Contusion of middle back wall of thorax, initial encounter
S2Ø.224D	Contusion of middle back wall of thorax, subsequent encounter
S2Ø.224S	Contusion of middle back wall of thorax, sequela
S2Ø.3Ø3A	Unspecified superficial injuries of bilateral front wall of thorax, initial encounter
S2Ø.3Ø3D	Unspecified superficial injuries of bilateral front wall of thorax, subsequent encounter
S2Ø.3Ø3S	Unspecified superficial injuries of bilateral front wall of thorax, sequela
S2Ø.3Ø4A	Unspecified superficial injuries of middle front wall of thorax, initial encounter
S2Ø.3Ø4D	Unspecified superficial injuries of middle front wall of thorax, subsequent encounter
S2Ø.3Ø4S	Unspecified superficial injuries of middle front wall of thorax, sequela
S2Ø.313A	Abrasion of bilateral front wall of thorax, initial encounter
S2Ø.313D	Abrasion of bilateral front wall of thorax, subsequent encounter
S2Ø.313S	Abrasion of bilateral front wall of thorax, sequela
S2Ø.314A	Abrasion of middle front wall of thorax, initial encounter
S2Ø.314D	Abrasion of middle front wall of thorax, subsequent encounter
S2Ø.314S	Abrasion of middle front wall of thorax, sequela
S2Ø.323A	Blister (nonthermal) of bilateral front wall of thorax, initial encounter
S2Ø.323D	Blister (nonthermal) of bilateral front wall of thorax, subsequent encounter
S2Ø.323S	Blister (nonthermal) of bilateral front wall of thorax, sequela
S2Ø.324A	Blister (nonthermal) of middle front wall of thorax, initial encounter
S2Ø.324D	Blister (nonthermal) of middle front wall of thorax, subsequent encounter
S2Ø.324S	Blister (nonthermal) of middle front wall of thorax, sequela
S2Ø.343A	External constriction of bilateral front wall of thorax, initial encounter
S2Ø.343D	External constriction of bilateral front wall of thorax, subsequent encounter
S2Ø.343S	External constriction of bilateral front wall of thorax, sequela
S2Ø.344A	External constriction of middle front wall of thorax, initial encounter
S2Ø.344D	External constriction of middle front wall of thorax, subsequent encounter
S2Ø.344S	External constriction of middle front wall of thorax, sequela
S2Ø.353A	Superficial foreign body of bilateral front wall of thorax, initial encounter
S2Ø.353D	Superficial foreign body of bilateral front wall of thorax, subsequent encounter
S2Ø.353S	Superficial foreign body of bilateral front wall of thorax, sequela
S2Ø.354A	Superficial foreign body of middle front wall of thorax, initial encounter
S2Ø.354D	Superficial foreign body of middle front wall of thorax, subsequent encounter
S2Ø.354S	Superficial foreign body of middle front wall of thorax, sequela
S2Ø.363A	Insect bite (nonvenomous) of bilateral front wall of thorax, initial encounter
S2Ø.363D	Insect bite (nonvenomous) of bilateral front wall of thorax, subsequent encounter
S2Ø.363S	Insect bite (nonvenomous) of bilateral front wall of thorax, sequela
S2Ø.364A	Insect bite (nonvenomous) of middle front wall of thorax, initial encounter
S2Ø.364D	Insect bite (nonvenomous) of middle front wall of thorax, subsequent encounter
S2Ø.364S	Insect bite (nonvenomous) of middle front wall of thorax, sequela

S20.373A Other superficial bite of bilateral front wall of thorax, initial encounter
S20.373D Other superficial bite of bilateral front wall of thorax, subsequent encounter
S20.373S Other superficial bite of bilateral front wall of thorax, sequela
S20.374A Other superficial bite of middle front wall of thorax, initial encounter
S20.374D Other superficial bite of middle front wall of thorax, subsequent encounter
S20.374S Other superficial bite of middle front wall of thorax, sequela
T40.411A Poisoning by fentanyl or fentanyl analogs, accidental (unintentional), initial encounter
T40.411D Poisoning by fentanyl or fentanyl analogs, accidental (unintentional), subsequent encounter
T40.411S Poisoning by fentanyl or fentanyl analogs, accidental (unintentional), sequela
T40.412A Poisoning by fentanyl or fentanyl analogs, intentional self-harm, initial encounter
T40.412D Poisoning by fentanyl or fentanyl analogs, intentional self-harm, subsequent encounter
T40.412S Poisoning by fentanyl or fentanyl analogs, intentional self-harm, sequela
T40.413A Poisoning by fentanyl or fentanyl analogs, assault, initial encounter
T40.413D Poisoning by fentanyl or fentanyl analogs, assault, subsequent encounter
T40.413S Poisoning by fentanyl or fentanyl analogs, assault, sequela
T40.414A Poisoning by fentanyl or fentanyl analogs, undetermined, initial encounter
T40.414D Poisoning by fentanyl or fentanyl analogs, undetermined, subsequent encounter
T40.414S Poisoning by fentanyl or fentanyl analogs, undetermined, sequela
T40.415A Adverse effect of fentanyl or fentanyl analogs, initial encounter
T40.415D Adverse effect of fentanyl or fentanyl analogs, subsequent encounter
T40.415S Adverse effect of fentanyl or fentanyl analogs, sequela
T40.416A Underdosing of fentanyl or fentanyl analogs, initial encounter
T40.416D Underdosing of fentanyl or fentanyl analogs, subsequent encounter
T40.416S Underdosing of fentanyl or fentanyl analogs, sequela
T40.421A Poisoning by tramadol, accidental (unintentional), initial encounter
T40.421D Poisoning by tramadol, accidental (unintentional), subsequent encounter
T40.421S Poisoning by tramadol, accidental (unintentional), sequela
T40.422A Poisoning by tramadol, intentional self-harm, initial encounter
T40.422D Poisoning by tramadol, intentional self-harm, subsequent encounter
T40.422S Poisoning by tramadol, intentional self-harm, sequela
T40.423A Poisoning by tramadol, assault, initial encounter
T40.423D Poisoning by tramadol, assault, subsequent encounter
T40.423S Poisoning by tramadol, assault, sequela
T40.424A Poisoning by tramadol, undetermined, initial encounter
T40.424D Poisoning by tramadol, undetermined, subsequent encounter
T40.424S Poisoning by tramadol, undetermined, sequela
T40.425A Adverse effect of tramadol, initial encounter
T40.425D Adverse effect of tramadol, subsequent encounter
T40.425S Adverse effect of tramadol, sequela
T40.426A Underdosing of tramadol, initial encounter
T40.426D Underdosing of tramadol, subsequent encounter
T40.426S Underdosing of tramadol, sequela
T40.491A Poisoning by other synthetic narcotics, accidental (unintentional), initial encounter
T40.491D Poisoning by other synthetic narcotics, accidental (unintentional), subsequent encounter
T40.491S Poisoning by other synthetic narcotics, accidental (unintentional), sequela
T40.492A Poisoning by other synthetic narcotics, intentional self-harm, initial encounter
T40.492D Poisoning by other synthetic narcotics, intentional self-harm, subsequent encounter
T40.492S Poisoning by other synthetic narcotics, intentional self-harm, sequela
T40.493A Poisoning by other synthetic narcotics, assault, initial encounter
T40.493D Poisoning by other synthetic narcotics, assault, subsequent encounter
T40.493S Poisoning by other synthetic narcotics, assault, sequela
T40.494A Poisoning by other synthetic narcotics, undetermined, initial encounter
T40.494D Poisoning by other synthetic narcotics, undetermined, subsequent encounter
T40.494S Poisoning by other synthetic narcotics, undetermined, sequela
T40.495A Adverse effect of other synthetic narcotics, initial encounter
T40.495D Adverse effect of other synthetic narcotics, subsequent encounter
T40.495S Adverse effect of other synthetic narcotics, sequela
T40.496A Underdosing of other synthetic narcotics, initial encounter
T40.496D Underdosing of other synthetic narcotics, subsequent encounter
T40.496S Underdosing of other synthetic narcotics, sequela
T86.8401 Corneal transplant rejection, right eye
T86.8402 Corneal transplant rejection, left eye
T86.8403 Corneal transplant rejection, bilateral
T86.8409 Corneal transplant rejection, unspecified eye
T86.8411 Corneal transplant failure, right eye
T86.8412 Corneal transplant failure, left eye
T86.8413 Corneal transplant failure, bilateral
T86.8419 Corneal transplant failure, unspecified eye
T86.8421 Corneal transplant infection, right eye
T86.8422 Corneal transplant infection, left eye
T86.8423 Corneal transplant infection, bilateral
T86.8429 Corneal transplant infection, unspecified eye
T86.8481 Other complications of corneal transplant, right eye
T86.8482 Other complications of corneal transplant, left eye

T86.8483 Other complications of corneal transplant, bilateral

T86.8489 Other complications of corneal transplant, unspecified eye

T86.8491 Unspecified complication of corneal transplant, right eye

T86.8492 Unspecified complication of corneal transplant, left eye

T86.8493 Unspecified complication of corneal transplant, bilateral

T86.8499 Unspecified complication of corneal transplant, unspecified eye

U07.Ø Vaping-related disorder

U07.1 COVID-19

VØØ.Ø31A Pedestrian on foot injured in collision with rider of standing electric scooter, initial encounter

VØØ.Ø31D Pedestrian on foot injured in collision with rider of standing electric scooter, subsequent encounter

VØØ.Ø31S Pedestrian on foot injured in collision with rider of standing electric scooter, sequela

VØØ.Ø38A Pedestrian on foot injured in collision with rider of other standing micro-mobility pedestrian conveyance, initial encounter

VØØ.Ø38D Pedestrian on foot injured in collision with rider of other standing micro-mobility pedestrian conveyance, subsequent encounter

VØØ.Ø38S Pedestrian on foot injured in collision with rider of other standing micro-mobility pedestrian conveyance, sequela

VØØ.841A Fall from standing electric scooter, initial encounter

VØØ.841D Fall from standing electric scooter, subsequent encounter

VØØ.841S Fall from standing electric scooter, sequela

VØØ.842A Pedestrian on standing electric scooter colliding with stationary object, initial encounter

VØØ.842D Pedestrian on standing electric scooter colliding with stationary object, subsequent encounter

VØØ.842S Pedestrian on standing electric scooter colliding with stationary object, sequela

VØØ.848A Other accident with standing micro-mobility pedestrian conveyance, initial encounter

VØØ.848D Other accident with standing micro-mobility pedestrian conveyance, subsequent encounter

VØØ.848S Other accident with standing micro-mobility pedestrian conveyance, sequela

VØ1.Ø31A Pedestrian on standing electric scooter injured in collision with pedal cycle in nontraffic accident, initial encounter

VØ1.Ø31D Pedestrian on standing electric scooter injured in collision with pedal cycle in nontraffic accident, subsequent encounter

VØ1.Ø31S Pedestrian on standing electric scooter injured in collision with pedal cycle in nontraffic accident, sequela

VØ1.Ø38A Pedestrian on other standing micro-mobility pedestrian conveyance injured in collision with pedal cycle in nontraffic accident, initial encounter

VØ1.Ø38D Pedestrian on other standing micro-mobility pedestrian conveyance injured in collision with pedal cycle in nontraffic accident, subsequent encounter

VØ1.Ø38S Pedestrian on other standing micro-mobility pedestrian conveyance injured in collision with pedal cycle in nontraffic accident, sequela

VØ1.131A Pedestrian on standing electric scooter injured in collision with pedal cycle in traffic accident, initial encounter

VØ1.131D Pedestrian on standing electric scooter injured in collision with pedal cycle in traffic accident, subsequent encounter

VØ1.131S Pedestrian on standing electric scooter injured in collision with pedal cycle in traffic accident, sequela

VØ1.138A Pedestrian on other standing micro-mobility pedestrian conveyance injured in collision with pedal cycle in traffic accident, initial encounter

VØ1.138D Pedestrian on other standing micro-mobility pedestrian conveyance injured in collision with pedal cycle in traffic accident, subsequent encounter

VØ1.138S Pedestrian on other standing micro-mobility pedestrian conveyance injured in collision with pedal cycle in traffic accident, sequela

VØ1.931A Pedestrian on standing electric scooter injured in collision with pedal cycle, unspecified whether traffic or nontraffic accident, initial encounter

VØ1.931D Pedestrian on standing electric scooter injured in collision with pedal cycle, unspecified whether traffic or nontraffic accident, subsequent encounter

VØ1.931S Pedestrian on standing electric scooter injured in collision with pedal cycle, unspecified whether traffic or nontraffic accident, sequela

VØ1.938A Pedestrian on other standing micro-mobility pedestrian conveyance injured in collision with pedal cycle, unspecified whether traffic or nontraffic accident, initial encounter

VØ1.938D Pedestrian on other standing micro-mobility pedestrian conveyance injured in collision with pedal cycle, unspecified whether traffic or nontraffic accident, subsequent encounter

VØ1.938S Pedestrian on other standing micro-mobility pedestrian conveyance injured in collision with pedal cycle, unspecified whether traffic or nontraffic accident, sequela

VØ2.Ø31A Pedestrian on standing electric scooter injured in collision with two- or three-wheeled motor vehicle in nontraffic accident, initial encounter

VØ2.Ø31D Pedestrian on standing electric scooter injured in collision with two- or three-wheeled motor vehicle in nontraffic accident, subsequent encounter

VØ2.Ø31S Pedestrian on standing electric scooter injured in collision with two- or three-wheeled motor vehicle in nontraffic accident, sequela

VØ2.Ø38A Pedestrian on other standing micro-mobility pedestrian conveyance injured in collision with two- or three-wheeled motor vehicle in nontraffic accident, initial encounter

VØ2.Ø38D Pedestrian on other standing micro-mobility pedestrian conveyance injured in collision with two- or three-wheeled motor vehicle in nontraffic accident, subsequent encounter

VØ2.Ø38S Pedestrian on other standing micro-mobility pedestrian conveyance injured in collision with two- or three-wheeled motor vehicle in nontraffic accident, sequela

VØ2.131A Pedestrian on standing electric scooter injured in collision with two- or three-wheeled motor vehicle in traffic accident, initial encounter

VØ2.131D Pedestrian on standing electric scooter injured in collision with two- or three-wheeled motor vehicle in traffic accident, subsequent encounter

VØ2.131S Pedestrian on standing electric scooter injured in collision with two- or three-wheeled motor vehicle in traffic accident, sequela

VØ2.138A Pedestrian on other standing micro-mobility pedestrian conveyance injured in collision with two- or three-wheeled motor vehicle in traffic accident, initial encounter

V02.138D Pedestrian on other standing micro-mobility pedestrian conveyance injured in collision with two- or three-wheeled motor vehicle in traffic accident, subsequent encounter

V02.138S Pedestrian on other standing micro-mobility pedestrian conveyance injured in collision with two- or three-wheeled motor vehicle in traffic accident, sequela

V02.931A Pedestrian on standing electric scooter injured in collision with two- or three wheeled motor vehicle, unspecified whether traffic or nontraffic accident, initial encounter

V02.931D Pedestrian on standing electric scooter injured in collision with two- or three wheeled motor vehicle, unspecified whether traffic or nontraffic accident, subsequent encounter

V02.931S Pedestrian on standing electric scooter injured in collision with two- or three wheeled motor vehicle, unspecified whether traffic or nontraffic accident, sequela

V02.938A Pedestrian on other standing micro-mobility pedestrian conveyance injured in collision with two- or three wheeled motor vehicle, unspecified whether traffic or nontraffic accident, initial encounter

V02.938D Pedestrian on other standing micro-mobility pedestrian conveyance injured in collision with two- or three wheeled motor vehicle, unspecified whether traffic or nontraffic accident, subsequent encounter

V02.938S Pedestrian on other standing micro-mobility pedestrian conveyance injured in collision with two- or three wheeled motor vehicle, unspecified whether traffic or nontraffic accident, sequela

V03.031A Pedestrian on standing electric scooter injured in collision with car, pick-up or van in nontraffic accident, initial encounter

V03.031D Pedestrian on standing electric scooter injured in collision with car, pick-up or van in nontraffic accident, subsequent encounter

V03.031S Pedestrian on standing electric scooter injured in collision with car, pick-up or van in nontraffic accident, sequela

V03.038A Pedestrian on other standing micro-mobility pedestrian conveyance injured in collision with car, pick-up or van in nontraffic accident, initial encounter

V03.038D Pedestrian on other standing micro-mobility pedestrian conveyance injured in collision with car, pick-up or van in nontraffic accident, subsequent encounter

V03.038S Pedestrian on other standing micro-mobility pedestrian conveyance injured in collision with car, pick-up or van in nontraffic accident, sequela

V03.131A Pedestrian on standing electric scooter injured in collision with car, pick-up or van in traffic accident, initial encounter

V03.131D Pedestrian on standing electric scooter injured in collision with car, pick-up or van in traffic accident, subsequent encounter

V03.131S Pedestrian on standing electric scooter injured in collision with car, pick-up or van in traffic accident, sequela

V03.138A Pedestrian on other standing micro-mobility pedestrian conveyance injured in collision with car, pick-up or van in traffic accident, initial encounter

V03.138D Pedestrian on other standing micro-mobility pedestrian conveyance injured in collision with car, pick-up or van in traffic accident, subsequent encounter

V03.138S Pedestrian on other standing micro-mobility pedestrian conveyance injured in collision with car, pick-up or van in traffic accident, sequela

V03.931A Pedestrian on standing electric scooter injured in collision with car, pick-up or van, unspecified whether traffic or nontraffic accident, initial encounter

V03.931D Pedestrian on standing electric scooter injured in collision with car, pick-up or van, unspecified whether traffic or nontraffic accident, subsequent encounter

V03.931S Pedestrian on standing electric scooter injured in collision with car, pick-up or van, unspecified whether traffic or nontraffic accident, sequela

V03.938A Pedestrian on other standing micro-mobility pedestrian conveyance injured in collision with car, pick-up or van, unspecified whether traffic or nontraffic accident, initial encounter

V03.938D Pedestrian on other standing micro-mobility pedestrian conveyance injured in collision with car, pick-up or van, unspecified whether traffic or nontraffic accident, subsequent encounter

V03.938S Pedestrian on other standing micro-mobility pedestrian conveyance injured in collision with car, pick-up or van, unspecified whether traffic or nontraffic accident, sequela

V04.031A Pedestrian on standing electric scooter injured in collision with heavy transport vehicle or bus in nontraffic accident, initial encounter

V04.031D Pedestrian on standing electric scooter injured in collision with heavy transport vehicle or bus in nontraffic accident, subsequent encounter

V04.031S Pedestrian on standing electric scooter injured in collision with heavy transport vehicle or bus in nontraffic accident, sequela

V04.038A Pedestrian on other standing micro-mobility pedestrian conveyance injured in collision with heavy transport vehicle or bus in nontraffic accident, initial encounter

V04.038D Pedestrian on other standing micro-mobility pedestrian conveyance injured in collision with heavy transport vehicle or bus in nontraffic accident, subsequent encounter

V04.038S Pedestrian on other standing micro-mobility pedestrian conveyance injured in collision with heavy transport vehicle or bus in nontraffic accident, sequela

V04.131A Pedestrian on standing electric scooter injured in collision with heavy transport vehicle or bus in traffic accident, initial encounter

V04.131D Pedestrian on standing electric scooter injured in collision with heavy transport vehicle or bus in traffic accident, subsequent encounter

V04.131S Pedestrian on standing electric scooter injured in collision with heavy transport vehicle or bus in traffic accident, sequela

V04.138A Pedestrian on other standing micro-mobility pedestrian conveyance injured in collision with heavy transport vehicle or bus in traffic accident, initial encounter

V04.138D Pedestrian on other standing micro-mobility pedestrian conveyance injured in collision with heavy transport vehicle or bus in traffic accident, subsequent encounter

V04.138S Pedestrian on other standing micro-mobility pedestrian conveyance injured in collision with heavy transport vehicle or bus in traffic accident, sequela

V04.931A Pedestrian on standing electric scooter injured in collision with heavy transport vehicle or bus, unspecified whether traffic or nontraffic accident, initial encounter

V04.931D Pedestrian on standing electric scooter injured in collision with heavy transport vehicle or bus, unspecified whether traffic or nontraffic accident, subsequent encounter

V04.931S Pedestrian on standing electric scooter injured in collision with heavy transport vehicle or bus, unspecified whether traffic or nontraffic accident, sequela

V04.938A Pedestrian on other standing micro-mobility pedestrian conveyance injured in collision with heavy transport vehicle or bus, unspecified whether traffic or nontraffic accident, initial encounter

V04.938D Pedestrian on other standing micro-mobility pedestrian conveyance injured in collision with heavy transport vehicle or bus, unspecified whether traffic or nontraffic accident, subsequent encounter

V04.938S Pedestrian on other standing micro-mobility pedestrian conveyance injured in collision with heavy transport vehicle or bus, unspecified whether traffic or nontraffic accident, sequela

V05.031A Pedestrian on standing electric scooter injured in collision with railway train or railway vehicle in nontraffic accident, initial encounter

V05.031D Pedestrian on standing electric scooter injured in collision with railway train or railway vehicle in nontraffic accident, subsequent encounter

V05.031S Pedestrian on standing electric scooter injured in collision with railway train or railway vehicle in nontraffic accident, sequela

V05.038A Pedestrian on other standing micro-mobility pedestrian conveyance injured in collision with railway train or railway vehicle in nontraffic accident, initial encounter

V05.038D Pedestrian on other standing micro-mobility pedestrian conveyance injured in collision with railway train or railway vehicle in nontraffic accident, subsequent encounter

V05.038S Pedestrian on other standing micro-mobility pedestrian conveyance injured in collision with railway train or railway vehicle in nontraffic accident, sequela

V05.131A Pedestrian on standing electric scooter injured in collision with railway train or railway vehicle in traffic accident, initial encounter

V05.131D Pedestrian on standing electric scooter injured in collision with railway train or railway vehicle in traffic accident, subsequent encounter

V05.131S Pedestrian on standing electric scooter injured in collision with railway train or railway vehicle in traffic accident, sequela

V05.138A Pedestrian on other standing micro-mobility pedestrian conveyance injured in collision with railway train or railway vehicle in traffic accident, initial encounter

V05.138D Pedestrian on other standing micro-mobility pedestrian conveyance injured in collision with railway train or railway vehicle in traffic accident, subsequent encounter

V05.138S Pedestrian on other standing micro-mobility pedestrian conveyance injured in collision with railway train or railway vehicle in traffic accident, sequela

V05.931A Pedestrian on standing electric scooter injured in collision with railway train or railway vehicle, unspecified whether traffic or nontraffic accident, initial encounter

V05.931D Pedestrian on standing electric scooter injured in collision with railway train or railway vehicle, unspecified whether traffic or nontraffic accident, subsequent encounter

V05.931S Pedestrian on standing electric scooter injured in collision with railway train or railway vehicle, unspecified whether traffic or nontraffic accident, sequela

V05.938A Pedestrian on other standing micro-mobility pedestrian conveyance injured in collision with railway train or railway vehicle, unspecified whether traffic or nontraffic accident, initial encounter

V05.938D Pedestrian on other standing micro-mobility pedestrian conveyance injured in collision with railway train or railway vehicle, unspecified whether traffic or nontraffic accident, subsequent encounter

V05.938S Pedestrian on other standing micro-mobility pedestrian conveyance injured in collision with railway train or railway vehicle, unspecified whether traffic or nontraffic accident, sequela

V06.031A Pedestrian on standing electric scooter injured in collision with other nonmotor vehicle in nontraffic accident, initial encounter

V06.031D Pedestrian on standing electric scooter injured in collision with other nonmotor vehicle in nontraffic accident, subsequent encounter

V06.031S Pedestrian on standing electric scooter injured in collision with other nonmotor vehicle in nontraffic accident, sequela

V06.038A Pedestrian on other standing micro-mobility pedestrian conveyance injured in collision with other nonmotor vehicle in nontraffic accident, initial encounter

V06.038D Pedestrian on other standing micro-mobility pedestrian conveyance injured in collision with other nonmotor vehicle in nontraffic accident, subsequent encounter

V06.038S Pedestrian on other standing micro-mobility pedestrian conveyance injured in collision with other nonmotor vehicle in nontraffic accident, sequela

V06.131A Pedestrian on standing electric scooter injured in collision with other nonmotor vehicle in traffic accident, initial encounter

V06.131D Pedestrian on standing electric scooter injured in collision with other nonmotor vehicle in traffic accident, subsequent encounter

V06.131S Pedestrian on standing electric scooter injured in collision with other nonmotor vehicle in traffic accident, sequela

V06.138A Pedestrian on other standing micro-mobility pedestrian conveyance injured in collision with other nonmotor vehicle in traffic accident, initial encounter

V06.138D Pedestrian on other standing micro-mobility pedestrian conveyance injured in collision with other nonmotor vehicle in traffic accident, subsequent encounter

V06.138S Pedestrian on other standing micro-mobility pedestrian conveyance injured in collision with other nonmotor vehicle in traffic accident, sequela

V06.931A Pedestrian on standing electric scooter injured in collision with other nonmotor vehicle, unspecified whether traffic or nontraffic accident, initial encounter

V06.931D Pedestrian on standing electric scooter injured in collision with other nonmotor vehicle, unspecified whether traffic or nontraffic accident, subsequent encounter

V06.931S Pedestrian on standing electric scooter injured in collision with other nonmotor vehicle, unspecified whether traffic or nontraffic accident, sequela

V06.938A Pedestrian on other standing micro-mobility pedestrian conveyance injured in collision with other nonmotor

	vehicle, unspecified whether traffic or nontraffic accident, initial encounter
V06.938D	Pedestrian on other standing micro-mobility pedestrian conveyance injured in collision with other nonmotor vehicle, unspecified whether traffic or nontraffic accident, subsequent encounter
V06.938S	Pedestrian on other standing micro-mobility pedestrian conveyance injured in collision with other nonmotor vehicle, unspecified whether traffic or nontraffic accident, sequela
Y77.11	Contact lens associated with adverse incidents
Y77.19	Other therapeutic (nonsurgical) and rehabilitative ophthalmic devices associated with adverse incidents
Z03.821	Encounter for observation for suspected ingested foreign body ruled out
Z03.822	Encounter for observation for suspected aspirated (inhaled) foreign body ruled out
Z03.823	Encounter for observation for suspected inserted (injected) foreign body ruled out

47 Code Descriptions Revised

Note: Each code is listed with its revised description only. Please refer to the full FY 2021 official addenda code files at Conversion Table zip file at https://www.cms.gov/medicare/icd-10/2021-icd-10-cm for the specific changes made to the codes listed.

D57.411	Sickle-cell thalassemia, unspecified, with acute chest syndrome
D57.412	Sickle-cell thalassemia, unspecified, with splenic sequestration
D57.419	Sickle-cell thalassemia, unspecified, with crisis
H55.81	Deficient saccadic eye movements
Q51.21	Complete doubling of uterus
Q51.22	Partial doubling of uterus
Q51.28	Other and unspecified doubling of uterus
Y92.002	Bathroom of unspecified non-institutional (private) residence as the place of occurrence of the external cause
Z68.1	Body mass index [BMI] 19.9 or less, adult
Z68.20	Body mass index [BMI] 20.0-20.9, adult
Z68.21	Body mass index [BMI] 21.0-21.9, adult
Z68.22	Body mass index [BMI] 22.0-22.9, adult
Z68.23	Body mass index [BMI] 23.0-23.9, adult
Z68.24	Body mass index [BMI] 24.0-24.9, adult
Z68.25	Body mass index [BMI] 25.0-25.9, adult
Z68.26	Body mass index [BMI] 26.0-26.9, adult
Z68.27	Body mass index [BMI] 27.0-27.9, adult
Z68.28	Body mass index [BMI] 28.0-28.9, adult
Z68.29	Body mass index [BMI] 29.0-29.9, adult
Z68.30	Body mass index [BMI] 30.0-30.9, adult
Z68.31	Body mass index [BMI] 31.0-31.9, adult
Z68.32	Body mass index [BMI] 32.0-32.9, adult
Z68.33	Body mass index [BMI] 33.0-33.9, adult
Z68.34	Body mass index [BMI] 34.0-34.9, adult
Z68.35	Body mass index [BMI] 35.0-35.9, adult
Z68.36	Body mass index [BMI] 36.0-36.9, adult
Z68.37	Body mass index [BMI] 37.0-37.9, adult
Z68.38	Body mass index [BMI] 38.0-38.9, adult
Z68.39	Body mass index [BMI] 39.0-39.9, adult
Z68.41	Body mass index [BMI] 40.0-44.9, adult
Z68.42	Body mass index [BMI] 45.0-49.9, adult
Z68.43	Body mass index [BMI] 50.0-59.9, adult
Z68.44	Body mass index [BMI] 60.0-69.9, adult
Z68.45	Body mass index [BMI] 70 or greater, adult
Z68.51	Body mass index [BMI] pediatric, less than 5th percentile for age
Z68.52	Body mass index [BMI] pediatric, 5th percentile to less than 85th percentile for age
Z68.53	Body mass index [BMI] pediatric, 85th percentile to less than 95th+percentile for age
Z68.54	Body mass index [BMI] pediatric, greater than or equal to 95th percentile for age
Z88.1	Allergy status to other antibiotic agents
Z88.2	Allergy status to sulfonamides
Z88.3	Allergy status to other anti-infective agents
Z88.4	Allergy status to anesthetic agent
Z88.5	Allergy status to narcotic agent
Z88.6	Allergy status to analgesic agent
Z88.7	Allergy status to serum and vaccine
Z88.8	Allergy status to other drugs, medicaments and biological substances
Z88.9	Allergy status to unspecified drugs, medicaments and biological substances

Proprietary Updates

The following proprietary features have also been added:

- New definitions that describe, in lay terms, a specific condition or disease process
- New coding tips that provide coding advice beyond the code classification
- Updated *AHA Coding Clinic* references through second quarter 2020

Conversion Table of ICD-10-CM Codes

At the time of printing, the Centers for Medicare and Medicaid Services (CMS) had not released the 2021 conversion table. Please see the product update page on optum360coding.com for a PDF of the 2021 conversion table. The password for obtaining your update is: **Hospital21**

10 Steps to Correct Coding

Follow the 10 steps below to correctly code encounters for health care services.

Step 1: Identify the reason for the visit or encounter (i.e., a sign, symptom, diagnosis and/or condition).

The medical record documentation should accurately reflect the patient's condition, using terminology that includes specific diagnoses and symptoms or clearly states the reasons for the encounter.

Choosing the main term that best describes the reason chiefly responsible for the service provided is the most important step in coding. If symptoms are present and documented but a definitive diagnosis has not yet been determined, code the symptoms. *For outpatient cases, do not code conditions that are referred to as "rule out," "suspected," "probable," or "questionable."* Diagnoses often are not established at the time of the initial encounter/visit and may require two or more visits to be established. Code only what is documented in the available outpatient records and only to the highest degree of certainty known at the time of the patient's visit. For inpatient medical records, uncertain diagnoses may be reported if documented at the time of discharge.

Step 2: After selecting the reason for the encounter, consult the alphabetic index.

The most critical rule is to begin code selection in the alphabetic index. Never turn first to the tabular list. The index provides cross-references, essential and nonessential modifiers, and other instructional notations that may not be found in the tabular list.

Step 3: Locate the main term entry.

The alphabetic index lists conditions, which may be expressed as nouns or eponyms, with critical use of adjectives. Some conditions known by several names have multiple main entries. Reasons for encounters may be located under general terms such as admission, encounter, and examination. Other general terms such as history, status (post), or presence (of) can be used to locate other factors influencing health.

Step 4: Scan subterm entries.

Scan the subterm entries, as appropriate, being sure to review continued lines and additional subterms that may appear in the next column or on the next page. Shaded vertical guidelines in the index indicate the indentation level for each subterm in relation to the main terms.

Step 5: Pay close attention to index instructions.

- Parentheses ( ) enclose nonessential modifiers, terms that are supplementary words or explanatory information that may or may not appear in the diagnostic statement and do not affect code selection.
- Brackets [ ] enclose manifestation codes that can be used only as secondary codes to the underlying condition code immediately preceding it. If used, manifestation codes must be reported with the appropriate etiology codes.
- Default codes are listed next to the main term and represent the condition most commonly associated with the main term or the unspecified code for the main term.
- *"See"* cross-references, identified by italicized type and "code by" cross-references indicate that another term *must be referenced* to locate the correct code.
- *"See also"* cross-references, identified by italicized type, provide alternative terms that may be useful to look up but *are not mandatory*.
- "Omit code" cross-references identify instances when a code is not applicable depending on the condition being coded.
- "With" subterms are listed out of alphabetic order and identify a presumed causal relationship between the two conditions they link.
- "Due to" subterms identify a relationship between the two conditions they link.
- "NEC," abbreviation for "not elsewhere classified," follows some main terms or subterms and indicates that there is no specific code for the condition even though the medical documentation may be very specific.
- "NOS," abbreviation for "not otherwise specified," follows some main terms or subterms and is the equivalent of unspecified; NOS signifies that the information in the medical record is insufficient for assigning a more specific code.
- *Following* references help coders locate alphanumeric codes that are out of sequence in the tabular section.
- Check-additional-character symbols flag codes that require additional characters to make the code valid; the characters available to complete the code should be verified in the tabular section.

Step 6: Choose a potential code and locate it in the tabular list.

To prevent coding errors, always use both the alphabetic index (to identify a code) and the tabular list (to verify a code), as the index does not include the important instructional notes found in the tabular list. An added benefit of using the tabular list, which groups like things together, is that while looking at one code in the list, a coder might see a more specific one that would have been missed had the coder relied solely on the alphabetic index. Additionally, many of the codes require a fourth, fifth, sixth, or seventh character to be valid, and many of these characters can be found only in the tabular list.

Step 7: Read all instructional material in the tabular section.

The coder must follow any Includes, Excludes 1 and Excludes 2 notes, and other instructional notes, such as "Code first" and "Use additional code," listed in the tabular list for the chapter, category, subcategory, and subclassification levels of code selection that direct the coder to use a different or additional code. Any codes in the tabular range AØØ.Ø- through T88.9- may be used to identify the diagnostic reason for the encounter. The tabular list encompasses many codes describing disease and injury classifications (e.g., infectious and parasitic diseases, neoplasms, symptoms, nervous and circulatory system etc.).

Codes that describe symptoms and signs, as opposed to definitive diagnoses, should be reported when an established diagnosis has not been made (confirmed) by the physician. Chapter 18 of the ICD-10-CM code book, "Symptoms, Signs, and Abnormal Clinical and Laboratory Findings, Not Elsewhere Classified" (codes RØØ.-–R99), contains many, but not all, codes for symptoms.

ICD-10-CM classifies encounters with health care providers for circumstances other than a disease or injury in chapter 21, "Factors Influencing Health Status and Contact with Health Services" (codes ZØØ–Z99). Circumstances other than a disease or injury often are recorded as chiefly responsible for the encounter.

A code is invalid if it does not include the full number of characters (greatest level of specificity) required. Codes in ICD-10-CM can contain from three to seven alphanumeric characters. A three-character code is to be used only if the category is not further subdivided into four-, five-, six-, or seven-character codes. Placeholder character X is used as part of an alphanumeric code to allow for future expansion and as a placeholder for empty characters in a code that requires a seventh character but has no fourth, fifth, or sixth character. Note that certain categories require seventh characters that apply to all codes in that category. Always check the category level for applicable seventh characters for that category.

Step 8: Consult the official ICD-10-CM conventions and guidelines.

The *ICD-10-CM Official Guidelines for Coding and Reporting* govern the use of certain codes. These guidelines provide both general and chapter-specific coding guidance.

Step 9: Confirm and assign the code.

Having reviewed all relevant information concerning the possible code choices, assign the code that most completely describes the condition.

Repeat steps 1 through 9 for all additional documented conditions that meet the following criteria:

- They exist at the time of the visit *AND*
- They require or affect patient care, treatment, or management

Step 10: Sequence codes correctly.

Sequencing is the order in which the codes are listed on the claim. List first the ICD-10-CM code for the diagnosis, condition, problem, or other reason for the encounter/visit that is shown in the medical record to be chiefly responsible for the services provided. List additional codes that describe any coexisting conditions. Follow the official coding guidelines (see the guidelines, section II, "Selection of Principal Diagnosis"; section III, "Reporting Additional Diagnoses"; and section IV, "Diagnostic Coding and Reporting Guidelines for Outpatient Services") on proper sequencing of codes.

Coding Examples

Diagnosis: Anorexia

Step 1: The reason for the encounter was the condition, anorexia.

Step 2: Consult the alphabetic index.

Step 3: Locate the main term "Anorexia."

Step 4: Two possible subterms are available, "hysterical" and "nervosa." Neither is documented in this instance, however, so they cannot be used in code selection.

Step 5: The code listed next to the main term is called the default code selection. Because the two subentries (essential modifiers) do not apply in this instance, the default code (R63.Ø) should be used.

Step 6: Turn to code R63.Ø in the tabular list and read all instructional notes.

Step 7: The Excludes 1 note at code R63.Ø indicates that anorexia nervosa and loss of appetite determined to be of nonorganic origin should be reported with a code from chapter 5. The diagnostic statement does not describe the condition as anorexia nervosa, however, and does not indicate that the anorexia is of a nonorganic origin. There is no further division of the category past the fourth-character subcategory. Therefore, code R63.Ø is at the highest level of specificity.

Step 8: Review of official guideline I.C.18 indicates that a symptom code is appropriate when a more definitive diagnosis is not documented.

Step 9: The default code, R63.Ø Anorexia, is the correct code selection.

Repeat steps 1 through 9 for any concomitant diagnoses.

Step 10: Since anorexia is listed as the chief reason for the health care encounter, the first-listed, or principal, diagnosis is R63.Ø. Note that this is a chapter 18 symptom code but can be assigned for both inpatient and outpatient records since the provider did not establish a more definitive diagnosis, according to sections II.A and IV.D.

Diagnosis: Acute bronchitis

Step 1: The reason for the encounter was the condition, acute bronchitis.

Step 2: Consult the alphabetic index.

Step 3: Locate the main term "Bronchitis."

Step 4: There is a subterm for "acute or subacute." Additional subterms are not included in the diagnostic statement.

Step 5: Review the instructional notes. Nonessential modifiers (with bronchospasm or obstruction) are terms that do not affect code assignment. Since no other subterms indented under "acute" apply here, the code listed next to this subentry—in this case J2Ø.9—should be chosen.

Step 6: Turn to code J2Ø.9 in the tabular list and read all instructional notes.

Step 7: The Includes note under category J2Ø lists alternative terms for acute bronchitis. Note that the list is not exhaustive but is only a representative selection of diagnoses that are included in the subcategory. The Excludes 1 note refers to category J4Ø for bronchitis and tracheobronchitis NOS. There are several conditions in the Excludes 2 notes that, if applicable, can be coded in addition to this code.

Note that the codes included in J2Ø represent acute bronchitis due to various infectious organisms that could be selected if identified in the documentation. In this case, the organism was not identified and there is no further division of the category past the fourth character subcategory. Therefore, code J2Ø.9 is at the highest level of specificity.

Step 8: Review of official guideline I.C.10 provides no additional information affecting the code selected.

Step 9: Assign code J2Ø.9 Acute bronchitis, unspecified.

Repeat steps 1 through 9 for any concomitant diagnoses.

Step 10: In the absence of additional diagnoses that may affect sequencing, code J2Ø.9 should be sequenced as the first-listed, or principal, diagnosis.

Diagnosis: Cerebellar ataxia in myxedema

Step 1: The reason for the encounter was the condition, cerebellar ataxia.

Step 2: Consult the alphabetic index.

Step 3: Locate the main term "Ataxia."

Step 4: Available subterms include "cerebellar (hereditary)," with additional indented subterms for "in" and "myxedema," all essential modifiers that are included in the diagnostic statement. Two codes are provided, EØ3.9 and G13.2, the latter of which is in brackets.

Step 5: Note the nonessential modifier (in parentheses) after the subterm cerebellar includes the term "hereditary." Because it is in parentheses, this term is not required in the diagnostic statement for this subentry to apply. The brackets around G13.2 identify this code as a manifestation of the condition described by code EØ3.9 and indicate that the two must be reported together and sequencing rules apply.

Step 6: Locate codes EØ3.9 and G13.2 in the tabular list, and read all instructional notes.

Step 7: For code EØ3.9, there are no instructional notes in the tabular list at the category EØ3 or code level that indicate that this condition should be coded elsewhere in the classification or that additional codes are required. Without further information from the diagnostic statement, myxedema, not otherwise specified (NOS), is appropriately reported with code EØ3.9 Hypothyroidism, unspecified, according to the inclusion term at this code.

Code G13.2 in the tabular list has an instructional note to "Code first underlying disease," which includes conditions found in category EØ3.-. Based on this note, codes EØ3.9 and G13.2 are to be coded together, with G13.2 listed only as a secondary diagnosis. This correlates with what the alphabetic index indicated. As there is no further division of codes in category G13 beyond the fourth character, G13.2 is at the highest level of specificity.

Step 8: Although there are some general conventions, such as how to interpret brackets in the alphabetic index, no chapter-specific guidelines apply to this coding scenario.

Step 9: Assign codes EØ3.9 Hypothyroidism, unspecified, and G13.2 Systemic atrophy primarily affecting the central nervous system in myxedema.

Repeat steps 1 through 9 for any concomitant diagnoses.

Step 10: Based on the alphabetic index and tabular instructional notations, code EØ3.9 should be sequenced as the first-listed, or principal, diagnosis followed by G13.2 as a secondary diagnosis.

Diagnosis: Decubitus ulcer of right elbow with skin loss and necrosis of subcutaneous tissue

Step 1: The reason for the encounter was the condition, decubitus ulcer.

Step 2: Consult the alphabetic index.

Step 3: Locate the main term "Ulcer."

Step 4: For the subterm "decubitus," there is no code provided or additional subterms indented, but a cross-reference is listed.

Step 5: The italicized cross-reference instructs the coder to "*see* Ulcer, pressure, by site."

Repeat steps 3 through 5 for the cross-reference.

Step 3: Locate the main term "Ulcer."

Step 4: Review the subentries for the subterm "pressure." The next level of indent lists either the site of the ulcer or the specific stage of the ulcer (stage 1–4, unstageable, and unspecified stages). The diagnostic statement provides the site, right elbow, and the extent of tissue damage (skin loss and necrosis of subcutaneous tissue) but does not specifically state that the ulcer is stage 1, stage 2, etc. Nonessential modifiers (in parentheses) at each stage include a description of the typical extent of damage at each stage. For example, stage 1 describes "pre-ulcer skin changes limited to persistent focal edema." Based on the documentation in the record, the coder can correlate the documentation to the nonessential modifiers and choose the specific stage from the index. The coder can also go directly to the body site, choosing the stage of the ulcer after reviewing the code options and instructional notations in the tabular list.

The diagnostic statement indicates that the extent of the damage to the elbow includes skin loss and necrosis of subcutaneous tissue, coinciding with the nonessential modifier next to the subentry "stage 3." The body site of elbow (L89.Ø-) is listed as another level of indent with other body sites.

Step 5: Note that code L89.Ø is followed by a dash and an additional-character-required icon, which indicate that more characters are needed to complete the code. From here, the tabular listing for L89.Ø- can be consulted.

Step 6: Locate code L89.Ø- in the tabular list and read all instructional notes.

Step 7: The tabular listing at category L89 has an Includes note for "decubitus ulcer," which confirms that category L89 is the appropriate category to represent what is documented in the diagnostic statement.

Several Excludes 2 notes are also listed at the category level. Excludes 2 notes represent conditions that can occur concomitantly with the decubitus ulcer and can be coded in addition to code L89, if supported by the documentation.

The subcategory codes under L89.Ø indicate that the fifth character describes laterality. Locate the right elbow at subcategory L89.Ø1. See that an additional sixth character to specify the stage of the ulcer is now needed to complete the code. The stage can be determined either by the specific documentation of the stage (e.g., stage 1, stage 2) or, in this case, a description that matches one of the inclusion terms that follow each stage code. For example, the diagnostic description in this case of "skin loss and necrosis of the subcutaneous tissue" matches the inclusion term under L89.Ø13 Pressure ulcer of right elbow, stage 3. No additional characters are required because code L89.Ø13 is at its highest level of specificity.

Step 8: The official guidelines contain quite a bit of information relating to pressure ulcers in chapter-specific guideline I.C.12 as well as information in general guideline I.B.14. These and any other pertinent guidelines should be reviewed to ensure appropriate code assignment.

Step 9: Assign code L89.Ø13 Pressure ulcer of right elbow, stage 3.

Repeat steps 1 through 9 for any concomitant diagnoses.

Step 10: Since the decubitus ulcer is listed as the chief reason for the health care encounter, the first-listed, or principal, diagnosis is L89.Ø13. However, according to the code first instructional note at the L89 category level, gangrene (I96) would be sequenced before the pressure ulcer if it were documented.

Diagnosis: Emergency department visit for bimalleolar fracture of the right ankle due to trauma

Step 1: The reason for the encounter was the condition, bimalleolar fracture.

Step 2: Consult the alphabetic index.

Step 3: Locate the main term "Fracture." Note that many main terms represent fractures: "Fracture, burst,""Fracture, chronic,""Fracture, insufficiency,""Fracture, nontraumatic NEC,""Fracture, pathological," and "Fracture, traumatic." Since the diagnostic statement specifically states that this fracture was the result of trauma, the main term "Fracture, traumatic" should be used.

Step 4: Subterms that should be referenced are "ankle" and "bimalleolar (displaced)," which lists code S82.84-.

Step 5: A nonessential modifier (in parentheses) next to the term bimalleolar for "displaced" indicates that S82.84- is the default category unless the fracture is specifically identified as "nondisplaced."

Note that code S82.84- is followed by a dash and an additional-character icon, both of which indicate that more characters are required. From here, the tabular list can be consulted.

Step 6: Locate code S82.84- in the tabular list and read all instructional notes.

Step: 7 The instructional notes at category S82 indicate that fractures not specified as displaced or nondisplaced default to displaced and that fractures not designated as open or closed default to closed. Additional instructional notes can be found at the category level but none pertain to the current scenario.

Read through the subcategory codes under S82.84, and note that the sixth character specifies displaced or nondisplaced and laterality. Based on the index nonessential modifier (displaced) and the code note at category S82, code selection should identify a displaced fracture of the right side. A displaced bimalleolar fracture of the right lower leg is coded to S82.841.

To complete the code, a seventh character must be assigned to identify the type of encounter (initial, subsequent, or sequela) and whether the fracture is open or closed. Most of the codes in category S82 require a seventh character represented in the list at the category level. However, it is important to note that some subcategories have their own specific set of seventh characters. In this instance, subcategory S82.84- does not have a unique set of seventh characters and the list provided at the category level should be used. Without documentation of the fracture being open, the tabular notation indicates that the default is closed. Character A, representing "initial encounter for closed fracture," listed in the box at the category level is the most appropriate option.

Step 8: Assign code S82.841A Displaced bimalleolar fracture of right lower leg, initial encounter for closed fracture.

Repeat steps 1 through 9 for any concomitant diagnoses.

Step 9: Review chapter-specific guideline I.C.19. and any other official conventions or guidelines to ensure appropriate code assignment.

Step 10: Additional codes can be applied to relate the specific cause of the injury, the place of occurrence, the activity of the patient at the time of the injury, and the patient's status, when this information is available in the record. However, coding this information is voluntary and reporting requirements depend on state mandates and/or facility-specific reporting requirements. If assigned, the external cause codes should be reported as secondary diagnoses only with the injury (fracture) sequenced first. Most codes in chapter 20, "External Causes of Morbidity," require a seventh character to identify the type of encounter. The seventh character assigned to an external cause code should match the seventh character of the code assigned for the associated injury or condition for the encounter.

2021 ICD-10-CM Official Guidelines for Coding and Reporting

Narrative changes appear in **bold** text

Items underlined have been moved within the guidelines since the FY 2020 version

Italics are used to indicate revisions to heading changes

The Centers for Medicare and Medicaid Services (CMS) and the National Center for Health Statistics (NCHS), two departments within the U.S. Federal Government's Department of Health and Human Services (DHHS) provide the following guidelines for coding and reporting using the International Classification of Diseases, 10th Revision, Clinical Modification (ICD-10-CM). These guidelines should be used as a companion document to the official version of the ICD-10-CM as published on the NCHS website. The ICD-10-CM is a morbidity classification published by the United States for classifying diagnoses and reason for visits in all health care settings. The ICD-10-CM is based on the ICD-10, the statistical classification of disease published by the World Health Organization (WHO).

These guidelines have been approved by the four organizations that make up the Cooperating Parties for the ICD-10-CM: the American Hospital Association (AHA), the American Health Information Management Association (AHIMA), CMS, and NCHS.

These guidelines are a set of rules that have been developed to accompany and complement the official conventions and instructions provided within the ICD-10-CM itself. The instructions and conventions of the classification take precedence over guidelines. These guidelines are based on the coding and sequencing instructions in the Tabular List and Alphabetic Index of ICD-10-CM, but provide additional instruction. Adherence to these guidelines when assigning ICD-10-CM diagnosis codes is required under the Health Insurance Portability and Accountability Act (HIPAA). The diagnosis codes (Tabular List and Alphabetic Index) have been adopted under HIPAA for all healthcare settings. A joint effort between the healthcare provider and the coder is essential to achieve complete and accurate documentation, code assignment, and reporting of diagnoses and procedures. These guidelines have been developed to assist both the healthcare provider and the coder in identifying those diagnoses that are to be reported. The importance of consistent, complete documentation in the medical record cannot be overemphasized. Without such documentation accurate coding cannot be achieved. The entire record should be reviewed to determine the specific reason for the encounter and the conditions treated.

The term encounter is used for all settings, including hospital admissions. In the context of these guidelines, the term provider is used throughout the guidelines to mean physician or any qualified health care practitioner who is legally accountable for establishing the patient's diagnosis. Only this set of guidelines, approved by the Cooperating Parties, is official.

The guidelines are organized into sections. Section I includes the structure and conventions of the classification and general guidelines that apply to the entire classification, and chapter-specific guidelines that correspond to the chapters as they are arranged in the classification. Section II includes guidelines for selection of principal diagnosis for non-outpatient settings. Section III includes guidelines for reporting additional diagnoses in non-outpatient settings. Section IV is for outpatient coding and reporting. It is necessary to review all sections of the guidelines to fully understand all of the rules and instructions needed to code properly.

Section I. Conventions, general coding guidelines and chapter specific guidelines

The conventions, general guidelines and chapter-specific guidelines are applicable to all health care settings unless otherwise indicated. The conventions and instructions of the classification take precedence over guidelines.

A. Conventions for the ICD-10-CM

The conventions for the ICD-10-CM are the general rules for use of the classification independent of the guidelines. These conventions are incorporated within the Alphabetic Index and Tabular List of the ICD-10-CM as instructional notes.

1. **The Alphabetic Index and Tabular List**
The ICD-10-CM is divided into the Alphabetic Index, an alphabetical list of terms and their corresponding code, and the Tabular List, a structured list of codes divided into chapters based on body system or condition. The Alphabetic Index consists of the following parts: the Index of Diseases and Injury, the Index of External Causes of Injury, the Table of Neoplasms and the Table of Drugs and Chemicals.
See Section I.C2. General guidelines
See Section I.C.19. Adverse effects, poisoning, underdosing and toxic effects

2. **Format and Structure:**
The ICD-10-CM Tabular List contains categories, subcategories and codes. Characters for categories, subcategories and codes may be either a letter or a number. All categories are 3 characters. A three-character category that has no further subdivision is equivalent to a code. Subcategories are either 4 or 5 characters. Codes may be 3, 4, 5, 6 or 7 characters. That is, each level of subdivision after a category is a subcategory. The final level of subdivision is a code. Codes that have applicable 7th characters are still referred to as codes, not subcategories. A code that has an applicable 7th character is considered invalid without the 7th character.
The ICD-10-CM uses an indented format for ease in reference.

3. **Use of codes for reporting purposes**
For reporting purposes only codes are permissible, not categories or subcategories, and any applicable 7th character is required.

4. **Placeholder character**
The ICD-10-CM utilizes a placeholder character "X". The "X" is used as a placeholder at certain codes to allow for future expansion. An example of this is at the poisoning, adverse effect and underdosing codes, categories T36-T5Ø.
Where a placeholder exists, the X must be used in order for the code to be considered a valid code.

5. **7th Characters**
Certain ICD-10-CM categories have applicable 7th characters. The applicable 7th character is required for all codes within the category, or as the notes in the Tabular List instruct. The 7th character must always be the 7th character in the data field. If a code that requires a 7th character is not 6 characters, a placeholder X must be used to fill in the empty characters.

6. **Abbreviations**
   a. **Alphabetic Index abbreviations**
   NEC "Not elsewhere classifiable"
   This abbreviation in the Alphabetic Index represents "other specified." When a specific code is not available for a condition, the Alphabetic Index directs the coder to the "other specified" code in the Tabular List.
   NOS "Not otherwise specified"
   This abbreviation is the equivalent of unspecified.
   b. **Tabular List abbreviations**
   NEC "Not elsewhere classifiable"
   This abbreviation in the Tabular List represents "other specified". When a specific code is not available for a condition, the Tabular List includes an NEC entry under a code to identify the code as the "other specified" code.
   NOS "Not otherwise specified"
   This abbreviation is the equivalent of unspecified.

7. **Punctuation**
[ ] Brackets are used in the Tabular List to enclose synonyms, alternative wording or explanatory phrases. Brackets are used in the Alphabetic Index to identify manifestation codes.
( ) Parentheses are used in both the Alphabetic Index and Tabular List to enclose supplementary words that may be present or absent in the statement of a disease or procedure without affecting the code number to which it is assigned. The terms within the parentheses are referred to as nonessential modifiers. The nonessential modifiers in the Alphabetic Index to Diseases apply to subterms following a main term except when a nonessential modifier and a subentry are mutually exclusive, the subentry takes precedence. For example, in the ICD-10-CM Alphabetic Index under the main term Enteritis, "acute" is a nonessential modifier and "chronic" is a subentry. In this case, the nonessential modifier "acute" does not apply to the subentry "chronic".
: Colons are used in the Tabular List after an incomplete term which needs one or more of the modifiers following the colon to make it assignable to a given category.

8. **Use of "and"**
See Section I.A.14. Use of the term "And"

9. **Other and Unspecified codes**
   a. **"Other" codes**
   Codes titled "other" or "other specified" are for use when the information in the medical record provides detail for which a specific code does not exist. Alphabetic Index entries with NEC in the line designate "other" codes in the Tabular List. These Alphabetic Index entries represent specific disease entities for which no specific code exists, so the term is included within an "other" code.
   b. **"Unspecified" codes**
   Codes titled "unspecified" are for use when the information in the medical record is insufficient to assign a more specific code. For those categories for which an unspecified code is not provided, the "other specified" code may represent both other and unspecified.
   See Section I.B.18 Use of Signs/Symptom/Unspecified Codes

10. **Includes Notes**
This note appears immediately under a three-character code title to further define, or give examples of, the content of the category.

11. **Inclusion terms**
List of terms is included under some codes. These terms are the conditions for which that code is to be used. The terms may be synonyms of the code title, or, in the case of "other specified" codes, the terms are a list of the various conditions assigned to that code. The inclusion terms are not necessarily exhaustive. Additional terms found only in the Alphabetic Index may also be assigned to a code.

12. **Excludes Notes**
The ICD-10-CM has two types of excludes notes. Each type of note has a different definition for use but they are all similar in that they indicate that codes excluded from each other are independent of each other.
   a. **Excludes1**
   A type 1 Excludes note is a pure excludes note. It means "NOT CODED HERE!" An Excludes1 note indicates that the code excluded should never be used at the same time as the code above the Excludes1 note. An Excludes1 is used when two conditions cannot occur together, such as a congenital form versus an acquired form of the same condition.
   An exception to the Excludes1 definition is the circumstance when the two conditions are unrelated to each other. If it is not clear whether the two conditions involving an Excludes1 note are related or not, query the provider. For example, code F45.8, Other somatoform disorders, has an Excludes1 note for "sleep related teeth grinding (G47.63)," because "teeth grinding" is an inclusion term under F45.8. Only one of these two codes should be assigned for teeth grinding. However psychogenic dysmenorrhea is also an inclusion term under F45.8, and a patient could have both this condition and sleep related teeth grinding. In this case, the two conditions are clearly unrelated to each other, and so it would be appropriate to report F45.8 and G47.63 together.
   b. **Excludes2**
   A type 2 Excludes note represents "Not included here." An excludes2 note indicates that the condition excluded is not part of the condition represented by the code, but a patient may have both conditions at the same time. When an Excludes2 note appears under a code, it is

acceptable to use both the code and the excluded code together, when appropriate.

13. **Etiology/manifestation convention ("code first", "use additional code" and "in diseases classified elsewhere" notes)**
Certain conditions have both an underlying etiology and multiple body system manifestations due to the underlying etiology. For such conditions, the ICD-10-CM has a coding convention that requires the underlying condition be sequenced first, if applicable, followed by the manifestation. Wherever such a combination exists, there is a "use additional code" note at the etiology code, and a "code first" note at the manifestation code. These instructional notes indicate the proper sequencing order of the codes, etiology followed by manifestation.

In most cases the manifestation codes will have in the code title, "in diseases classified elsewhere." Codes with this title are a component of the etiology/ manifestation convention. The code title indicates that it is a manifestation code. "In diseases classified elsewhere" codes are never permitted to be used as first listed or principal diagnosis codes. They must be used in conjunction with an underlying condition code and they must be listed following the underlying condition. See category FØ2, Dementia in other diseases classified elsewhere, for an example of this convention.

There are manifestation codes that do not have "in diseases classified elsewhere" in the title. For such codes, there is a "use additional code" note at the etiology code and a "code first" note at the manifestation code, and the rules for sequencing apply.

In addition to the notes in the Tabular List, these conditions also have a specific Alphabetic Index entry structure. In the Alphabetic Index both conditions are listed together with the etiology code first followed by the manifestation codes in brackets. The code in brackets is always to be sequenced second.

An example of the etiology/manifestation convention is dementia in Parkinson's disease. In the Alphabetic Index, code G2Ø is listed first, followed by code FØ2.8Ø or FØ2.81 in brackets. Code G2Ø represents the underlying etiology, Parkinson's disease, and must be sequenced first, whereas code FØ2.8Ø and FØ2.81 represent the manifestation of dementia in diseases classified elsewhere, with or without behavioral disturbance.

"Code first" and "Use additional code" notes are also used as sequencing rules in the classification for certain codes that are not part of an etiology/ manifestation combination.

See Section I.B.7. Multiple coding for a single condition.

14. **"And"**
The word "and" should be interpreted to mean either "and" or "or" when it appears in a title.

For example, cases of "tuberculosis of bones", "tuberculosis of joints" and "tuberculosis of bones and joints" are classified to subcategory A18.Ø, Tuberculosis of bones and joints.

15. **"With"**
The word "with" or "in" should be interpreted to mean "associated with" or "due to" when it appears in a code title, the Alphabetic Index (either under a main term or subterm), or an instructional note in the Tabular List. The classification presumes a causal relationship between the two conditions linked by these terms in the Alphabetic Index or Tabular List. These conditions should be coded as related even in the absence of provider documentation explicitly linking them, unless the documentation clearly states the conditions are unrelated or when another guideline exists that specifically requires a documented linkage between two conditions (e.g., sepsis guideline for "acute organ dysfunction that is not clearly associated with the sepsis").

For conditions not specifically linked by these relational terms in the classification or when a guideline requires that a linkage between two conditions be explicitly documented, provider documentation must link the conditions in order to code them as related.

The word "with" in the Alphabetic Index is sequenced immediately following the main term or subterm, not in alphabetical order.

16. **"See" and "See Also"**
The "see" instruction following a main term in the Alphabetic Index indicates that another term should be referenced. It is necessary to go to the main term referenced with the "see" note to locate the correct code.

A "see also" instruction following a main term in the Alphabetic Index instructs that there is another main term that may also be referenced that may provide additional Alphabetic Index entries that may be useful. It is not necessary to follow the "see also" note when the original main term provides the necessary code.

17. **"Code also" note**
A "code also" note instructs that two codes may be required to fully describe a condition, but this note does not provide sequencing direction. The sequencing depends on the circumstances of the encounter.

18. **Default codes**
A code listed next to a main term in the ICD-10-CM Alphabetic Index is referred to as a default code. The default code represents that condition that is most commonly associated with the main term, or is the unspecified code for the condition. If a condition is documented in a medical record (for example, appendicitis) without any additional information, such as acute or chronic, the default code should be assigned.

19. **Code assignment and Clinical Criteria**
The assignment of a diagnosis code is based on the provider's diagnostic statement that the condition exists. The provider's statement that the patient has a particular condition is sufficient. Code assignment is not based on clinical criteria used by the provider to establish the diagnosis.

B. General Coding Guidelines

1. **Locating a code in the ICD-10-CM**
To select a code in the classification that corresponds to a diagnosis or reason for visit documented in a medical record, first locate the term in the Alphabetic Index, and then verify the code in the Tabular List. Read and be guided by instructional notations that appear in both the Alphabetic Index and the Tabular List.

It is essential to use both the Alphabetic Index and Tabular List when locating and assigning a code. The Alphabetic Index does not always provide the full code. Selection of the full code, including laterality and any applicable 7th character can only be done in the Tabular List. A dash (-) at the end of an Alphabetic Index entry indicates that additional characters are required. Even if a dash is not included at the Alphabetic Index entry, it is necessary to refer to the Tabular List to verify that no 7th character is required.

2. **Level of Detail in Coding**
Diagnosis codes are to be used and reported at their highest number of characters available.

ICD-10-CM diagnosis codes are composed of codes with 3, 4, 5, 6 or 7 characters. Codes with three characters are included in ICD-10-CM as the heading of a category of codes that may be further subdivided by the use of fourth and/or fifth characters and/or sixth characters, which provide greater detail.

A three-character code is to be used only if it is not further subdivided. A code is invalid if it has not been coded to the full number of characters required for that code, including the 7th character, if applicable.

3. **Code or codes from AØØ.Ø through T88.9, ZØØ-Z99.8**
The appropriate code or codes from AØØ.Ø through T88.9, ZØØ-Z99.8 must be used to identify diagnoses, symptoms, conditions, problems, complaints or other reason(s) for the encounter/visit.

4. **Signs and symptoms**
Codes that describe symptoms and signs, as opposed to diagnoses, are acceptable for reporting purposes when a related definitive diagnosis has not been established (confirmed) by the provider. Chapter 18 of ICD-10-CM, Symptoms, Signs, and Abnormal Clinical and Laboratory Findings, Not Elsewhere Classified (codes RØØ.Ø - R99) contains many, but not all, codes for symptoms.

See Section I.B.18 Use of Signs/Symptom/Unspecified Codes

5. **Conditions that are an integral part of a disease process**
Signs and symptoms that are associated routinely with a disease process should not be assigned as additional codes, unless otherwise instructed by the classification.

6. **Conditions that are not an integral part of a disease process**
Additional signs and symptoms that may not be associated routinely with a disease process should be coded when present.

7. **Multiple coding for a single condition**
In addition to the etiology/manifestation convention that requires two codes to fully describe a single condition that affects multiple body systems, there are other single conditions that also require more than one code. "Use additional code" notes are found in the Tabular List at codes that are not part of an etiology/manifestation pair where a secondary code is useful to fully describe a condition. The sequencing rule is the same as the etiology/manifestation pair, "use additional code" indicates that a secondary code should be added, if known.

For example, for bacterial infections that are not included in chapter 1, a secondary code from category B95, Streptococcus, Staphylococcus, and Enterococcus, as the cause of diseases classified elsewhere, or B96, Other bacterial agents as the cause of diseases classified elsewhere, may be required to identify the bacterial organism causing the infection. A "use additional code" note will normally be found at the infectious disease code, indicating a need for the organism code to be added as a secondary code.

"Code first" notes are also under certain codes that are not specifically manifestation codes but may be due to an underlying cause. When there is a "code first" note and an underlying condition is present, the underlying condition should be sequenced first, if known.

"Code, if applicable, any causal condition first" notes indicate that this code may be assigned as a principal diagnosis when the causal condition is unknown or not applicable. If a causal condition is known, then the code for that condition should be sequenced as the principal or first-listed diagnosis.

Multiple codes may be needed for sequela, complication codes and obstetric codes to more fully describe a condition. See the specific guidelines for these conditions for further instruction.

8. **Acute and Chronic Conditions**

If the same condition is described as both acute (subacute) and chronic, and separate subentries exist in the Alphabetic Index at the same indentation level, code both and sequence the acute (subacute) code first.

9. **Combination Code**

A combination code is a single code used to classify:

Two diagnoses, or

A diagnosis with an associated secondary process (manifestation)

A diagnosis with an associated complication

Combination codes are identified by referring to subterm entries in the Alphabetic Index and by reading the inclusion and exclusion notes in the Tabular List.

Assign only the combination code when that code fully identifies the diagnostic conditions involved or when the Alphabetic Index so directs. Multiple coding should not be used when the classification provides a combination code that clearly identifies all of the elements documented in the diagnosis. When the combination code lacks necessary specificity in describing the manifestation or complication, an additional code should be used as a secondary code.

10. **Sequela (Late Effects)**

A sequela is the residual effect (condition produced) after the acute phase of an illness or injury has terminated. There is no time limit on when a sequela code can be used. The residual may be apparent early, such as in cerebral infarction, or it may occur months or years later, such as that due to a previous injury. Examples of sequela include: scar formation resulting from a burn, deviated septum due to a nasal fracture, and infertility due to tubal occlusion from old tuberculosis. Coding of sequela generally requires two codes sequenced in the following order: the condition or nature of the sequela is sequenced first. The sequela code is sequenced second.

An exception to the above guidelines are those instances where the code for the sequela is followed by a manifestation code identified in the Tabular List and title, or the sequela code has been expanded (at the fourth, fifth or sixth character levels) to include the manifestation(s). The code for the acute phase of an illness or injury that led to the sequela is never used with a code for the late effect.

See Section I.C.9. Sequelae of cerebrovascular disease

See Section I.C.15. Sequelae of complication of pregnancy, childbirth and the puerperium

See Section I.C.19. Application of 7th characters for Chapter 19

11. **Impending or Threatened Condition**

Code any condition described at the time of discharge as "impending" or "threatened" as follows:

If it did occur, code as confirmed diagnosis.

If it did not occur, reference the Alphabetic Index to determine if the condition has a subentry term for "impending" or "threatened" and also reference main term entries for "Impending" and for "Threatened."

If the subterms are listed, assign the given code.

If the subterms are not listed, code the existing underlying condition(s) and not the condition described as impending or threatened.

12. **Reporting Same Diagnosis Code More than Once**

Each unique ICD-10-CM diagnosis code may be reported only once for an encounter. This applies to bilateral conditions when there are no distinct codes identifying laterality or two different conditions classified to the same ICD-10-CM diagnosis code.

13. **Laterality**

Some ICD-10-CM codes indicate laterality, specifying whether the condition occurs on the left, right or is bilateral. If no bilateral code is provided and the condition is bilateral, assign separate codes for both the left and right side. If the side is not identified in the medical record, assign the code for the unspecified side.

When a patient has a bilateral condition and each side is treated during separate encounters, assign the "bilateral" code (as the condition still exists on both sides), including for the encounter to treat the first side. For the second encounter for treatment after one side has previously been treated and the condition no longer exists on that side, assign the appropriate unilateral code for the side where the condition still exists (e.g., cataract surgery performed on each eye in separate encounters). The bilateral code would not be assigned for the subsequent encounter, as the patient no longer has the condition in the previously-treated site. If the treatment on the first side did not completely resolve the condition, then the bilateral code would still be appropriate.

14. **Documentation by *Clinicians Other than the Patient's Provider***

Code assignment is based on the documentation by patient's provider (i.e., physician or other qualified healthcare practitioner legally accountable for establishing the patient's diagnosis). There are a few exceptions, such as codes for the Body Mass Index (BMI), depth of non-pressure chronic ulcers, pressure ulcer stage, coma scale, and NIH stroke scale (NIHSS) codes, code assignment may be based on medical record documentation from clinicians who are not the patient's provider (i.e., physician or other qualified healthcare practitioner legally accountable for establishing the patient's diagnosis), since this information is typically documented by other clinicians involved in the care of the patient (e.g., a dietitian often documents the BMI, a nurse often documents the pressure ulcer stages, and an emergency medical technician often documents the coma scale). However, the associated diagnosis (such as overweight, obesity, acute stroke, or pressure ulcer) must be documented by the patient's provider. If there is conflicting medical record documentation, either from the same clinician or different clinicians, the patient's attending provider should be queried for clarification.

For social determinants of health, such as information found in categories Z55-Z65, Persons with potential health hazards related to socioeconomic and psychosocial circumstances, code assignment may be based on medical record documentation from clinicians involved in the care of the patient who are not the patient's provider since this information represents social information, rather than medical diagnoses. **Patient self-reported documentation may also be used to assign codes for social determinants of health, as long as the patient self-reported information is signed-off by and incorporated into the health record by either a clinician or provider.**

The BMI, coma scale, NIHSS codes and categories Z55-Z65 should only be reported as secondary diagnoses.

15. **Syndromes**

Follow the Alphabetic Index guidance when coding syndromes. In the absence of Alphabetic Index guidance, assign codes for the documented manifestations of the syndrome. Additional codes for manifestations that are not an integral part of the disease process may also be assigned when the condition does not have a unique code.

16. **Documentation of Complications of Care**

Code assignment is based on the provider's documentation of the relationship between the condition and the care or procedure, unless otherwise instructed by the classification. The guideline extends to any complications of care, regardless of the chapter the code is located in. It is important to note that not all conditions that occur during or following medical care or surgery are classified as complications. There must be a cause-and-effect relationship between the care provided and the condition, and an indication in the documentation that it is a complication. Query the provider for clarification, if the complication is not clearly documented.

17. **Borderline Diagnosis**

If the provider documents a "borderline" diagnosis at the time of discharge, the diagnosis is coded as confirmed, unless the classification provides a specific entry (e.g., borderline diabetes). If a borderline condition has a specific index entry in ICD-10-CM, it should be coded as such. Since borderline conditions are not uncertain diagnoses, no distinction is made between the care setting (inpatient versus outpatient). Whenever the documentation is unclear regarding a borderline condition, coders are encouraged to query for clarification.

f Sign/Symptom/Unspecified Codes

/symptom and "unspecified" codes have acceptable, even necessary, s. While specific diagnosis codes should be reported when they are pported by the available medical record documentation and clinical knowledge of the patient's health condition, there are instances when signs/symptoms or unspecified codes are the best choices for accurately reflecting the healthcare encounter. Each healthcare encounter should be coded to the level of certainty known for that encounter.

If a definitive diagnosis has not been established by the end of the encounter, it is appropriate to report codes for sign(s) and/or symptom(s) in lieu of a definitive diagnosis. When sufficient clinical information isn't known or available about a particular health condition to assign a more specific code, it is acceptable to report the appropriate "unspecified" code (e.g., a diagnosis of pneumonia has been determined, but not the specific type). Unspecified codes should be reported when they are the codes that most accurately reflect what is known about the patient's condition at the time of that particular encounter. It would be inappropriate to select a specific code that is not supported by the medical record documentation or conduct medically unnecessary diagnostic testing in order to determine a more specific code.

19. Coding for Healthcare Encounters in Hurricane Aftermath

a. Use of External Cause of Morbidity Codes

An external cause of morbidity code should be assigned to identify the cause of the injury(ies) incurred as a result of the hurricane. The use of external cause of morbidity codes is supplemental to the application of ICD-10-CM codes. External cause of morbidity codes are never to be recorded as a principal diagnosis (first-listed in non-inpatient settings). The appropriate injury code should be sequenced before any external cause codes. The external cause of morbidity codes capture how the injury or health condition happened (cause), the intent (unintentional or accidental; or intentional, such as suicide or assault), the place where the event occurred, the activity of the patient at the time of the event, and the person's status (e.g., civilian, military). They should not be assigned for encounters to treat hurricane victims' medical conditions when no injury, adverse effect or poisoning is involved. External cause of morbidity codes should be assigned for each encounter for care and treatment of the injury. External cause of morbidity codes may be assigned in all health care settings. For the purpose of capturing complete and accurate ICD-10-CM data in the aftermath of the hurricane, a healthcare setting should be considered as any location where medical care is provided by licensed healthcare professionals.

b. Sequencing of External Causes of Morbidity Codes

Codes for cataclysmic events, such as a hurricane, take priority over all other external cause codes except child and adult abuse and terrorism and should be sequenced before other external cause of injury codes. Assign as many external cause of morbidity codes as necessary to fully explain each cause. For example, if an injury occurs as a result of a building collapse during the hurricane, external cause codes for both the hurricane and the building collapse should be assigned, with the external causes code for hurricane being sequenced as the first external cause code. For injuries incurred as a direct result of the hurricane, assign the appropriate code(s) for the injuries, followed by the code X37.0-, Hurricane (with the appropriate 7th character), and any other applicable external cause of injury codes. Code X37.0- also should be assigned when an injury is incurred as a result of flooding caused by a levee breaking related to the hurricane. Code X38.-, Flood (with the appropriate 7th character), should be assigned when an injury is from flooding resulting directly from the storm. Code X36.0.-, Collapse of dam or man-made structure, should not be assigned when the cause of the collapse is due to the hurricane. Use of code X36.0- is limited to collapses of man-made structures due to earth surface movements, not due to storm surges directly from a hurricane.

c. Other External Causes of Morbidity Code Issues

For injuries that are not a direct result of the hurricane, such as an evacuee that has incurred an injury as a result of a motor vehicle accident, assign the appropriate external cause of morbidity code(s) to describe the cause of the injury, but do not assign code X37.0-, Hurricane. If it is not clear whether the injury was a direct result of the hurricane, assume the injury is due to the hurricane and assign code X37.0-, Hurricane, as well as any other applicable external cause of morbidity codes. In addition to code X37.0-, Hurricane, other possible applicable external cause of morbidity codes include:

W54.0-, Bitten by dog
X30-, Exposure to excessive natural heat
X31-, Exposure to excessive natural cold
X38-, Flood

d. Use of Z codes

Z codes (other reasons for healthcare encounters) may be assigned as appropriate to further explain the reasons for presenting for healthcare services, including transfers between healthcare facilities. The ICD-10-CM Official Guidelines for Coding and Reporting identify which codes maybe assigned as principal or first-listed diagnosis only, secondary diagnosis only, or principal/first-listed or secondary (depending on the circumstances). Possible applicable Z codes include:

Z59.0, Homelessness
Z59.1, Inadequate housing
Z59.5, Extreme poverty
Z75.1, Person awaiting admission to adequate facility elsewhere
Z75.3, Unavailability and inaccessibility of health-care facilities
Z75.4, Unavailability and inaccessibility of other helping agencies
Z76.2, Encounter for health supervision and care of other healthy infant and child
Z99.12, Encounter for respirator [ventilator] dependence during power failure

The external cause of morbidity codes and the Z codes listed above are not an all-inclusive list. Other codes may be applicable to the encounter based upon the documentation. Assign as many codes as necessary to fully explain each healthcare encounter. Since patient history information may be very limited, use any available documentation to assign the appropriate external cause of morbidity and Z codes.

C. Chapter-Specific Coding Guidelines

In addition to general coding guidelines, there are guidelines for specific diagnoses and/or conditions in the classification. Unless otherwise indicated, these guidelines apply to all health care settings. Please refer to Section II for guidelines on the selection of principal diagnosis.

1. Chapter 1: Certain Infectious and Parasitic Diseases (A00-B99), ***U07.1***

a. Human Immunodeficiency Virus (HIV) Infections

1) Code only confirmed cases

Code only confirmed cases of HIV infection/illness. This is an exception to the hospital inpatient guideline Section II, H.

In this context, "confirmation" does not require documentation of positive serology or culture for HIV; the provider's diagnostic statement that the patient is HIV positive, or has an HIV-related illness is sufficient.

2) Selection and sequencing of HIV codes

(a) Patient admitted for HIV-related condition

If a patient is admitted for an HIV-related condition, the principal diagnosis should be B20, Human immunodeficiency virus [HIV] disease followed by additional diagnosis codes for all reported HIV-related conditions.

(b) Patient with HIV disease admitted for unrelated condition

If a patient with HIV disease is admitted for an unrelated condition (such as a traumatic injury), the code for the unrelated condition (e.g., the nature of injury code) should be the principal diagnosis. Other diagnoses would be B20 followed by additional diagnosis codes for all reported HIV-related conditions.

(c) Whether the patient is newly diagnosed

Whether the patient is newly diagnosed or has had previous admissions/encounters for HIV conditions is irrelevant to the sequencing decision.

(d) Asymptomatic human immunodeficiency virus

Z21, Asymptomatic human immunodeficiency virus [HIV] infection status, is to be applied when the patient without any documentation of symptoms is listed as being "HIV positive," "known HIV," "HIV test positive," or similar terminology. Do not use this code if the term "AIDS" is used or if the patient is treated for any HIV-related illness or is described as having any condition(s) resulting from his/her HIV positive status; use B20 in these cases.

(e) Patients with inconclusive HIV serology

Patients with inconclusive HIV serology, but no definitive diagnosis or manifestations of the illness, may be assigned code R75, Inconclusive laboratory evidence of human immunodeficiency virus [HIV].

(f) Previously diagnosed HIV-related illness

Patients with any known prior diagnosis of an HIV-related illness should be coded to B2Ø. Once a patient has developed an HIV-related illness, the patient should always be assigned code B2Ø on every subsequent admission/encounter. Patients previously diagnosed with any HIV illness (B2Ø) should never be assigned to R75 or Z21, Asymptomatic human immunodeficiency virus [HIV] infection status.

(g) HIV Infection in Pregnancy, Childbirth and the Puerperium

During pregnancy, childbirth or the puerperium, a patient admitted (or presenting for a health care encounter) because of an HIV-related illness should receive a principal diagnosis code of O98.7-, Human immunodeficiency [HIV] disease complicating pregnancy, childbirth and the puerperium, followed by B2Ø and the code(s) for the HIV-related illness(es). Codes from Chapter 15 always take sequencing priority.

Patients with asymptomatic HIV infection status admitted (or presenting for a health care encounter) during pregnancy, childbirth, or the puerperium should receive codes of O98.7- and Z21.

(h) Encounters for testing for HIV

If a patient is being seen to determine his/her HIV status, use code Z11.4, Encounter for screening for human immunodeficiency virus [HIV]. Use additional codes for any associated high-risk behavior.

If a patient with signs or symptoms is being seen for HIV testing, code the signs and symptoms. An additional counseling code Z71.7, Human immunodeficiency virus [HIV] counseling, may be used if counseling is provided during the encounter for the test.

When a patient returns to be informed of his/her HIV test results and the test result is negative, use code Z71.7, Human immunodeficiency virus [HIV] counseling.

If the results are positive, see previous guidelines and assign codes as appropriate.

b. Infectious agents as the cause of diseases classified to other chapters

Certain infections are classified in chapters other than Chapter 1 and no organism is identified as part of the infection code. In these instances, it is necessary to use an additional code from Chapter 1 to identify the organism. A code from category B95, Streptococcus, Staphylococcus, and Enterococcus as the cause of diseases classified to other chapters, B96, Other bacterial agents as the cause of diseases classified to other chapters, or B97, Viral agents as the cause of diseases classified to other chapters, is to be used as an additional code to identify the organism. An instructional note will be found at the infection code advising that an additional organism code is required.

c. Infections resistant to antibiotics

Many bacterial infections are resistant to current antibiotics. It is necessary to identify all infections documented as antibiotic resistant. Assign a code from category Z16, Resistance to antimicrobial drugs, following the infection code only if the infection code does not identify drug resistance.

d. Sepsis, Severe Sepsis, and Septic Shock

1) Coding of Sepsis and Severe Sepsis

(a) Sepsis

For a diagnosis of sepsis, assign the appropriate code for the underlying systemic infection. If the type of infection or causal organism is not further specified, assign code A41.9, Sepsis, unspecified organism.

A code from subcategory R65.2, Severe sepsis, should not be assigned unless severe sepsis or an associated acute organ dysfunction is documented.

(i) Negative or inconclusive blood cultures and sepsis

Negative or inconclusive blood cultures do not preclude a diagnosis of sepsis in patients with clinical evidence of the condition; however, the provider should be queried.

(ii) Urosepsis

The term urosepsis is a nonspecific term. It is not to be considered synonymous with sepsis. It has no default code in the Alphabetic Index. Should a provider use this term, he/she must be queried for clarification.

(iii) Sepsis with organ dysfunction

If a patient has sepsis and associated acute organ dysfunction or multiple organ dysfunction (MOD), follow the instructions for coding severe sepsis.

(iv) Acute organ dysfunction that is not clearly associated with the sepsis

If a patient has sepsis and an acute organ dysfunction, but the medical record documentation indicates that the acute organ dysfunction is related to a medical condition other than the sepsis, do not assign a code from subcategory R65.2, Severe sepsis. An acute organ dysfunction must be associated with the sepsis in order to assign the severe sepsis code. If the documentation is not clear as to whether an acute organ dysfunction is related to the sepsis or another medical condition, query the provider.

(b) Severe sepsis

The coding of severe sepsis requires a minimum of 2 codes: first a code for the underlying systemic infection, followed by a code from subcategory R65.2, Severe sepsis. If the causal organism is not documented, assign code A41.9, Sepsis, unspecified organism, for the infection. Additional code(s) for the associated acute organ dysfunction are also required.

Due to the complex nature of severe sepsis, some cases may require querying the provider prior to assignment of the codes.

2) Septic shock

(a) Septic shock generally refers to circulatory failure associated with severe sepsis, and therefore, it represents a type of acute organ dysfunction.

For cases of septic shock, the code for the systemic infection should be sequenced first, followed by code R65.21, Severe sepsis with septic shock or code T81.12, Postprocedural septic shock. Any additional codes for the other acute organ dysfunctions should also be assigned. As noted in the sequencing instructions in the Tabular List, the code for septic shock cannot be assigned as a principal diagnosis.

3) Sequencing of severe sepsis

If severe sepsis is present on admission, and meets the definition of principal diagnosis, the underlying systemic infection should be assigned as principal diagnosis followed by the appropriate code from subcategory R65.2 as required by the sequencing rules in the Tabular List. A code from subcategory R65.2 can never be assigned as a principal diagnosis.

When severe sepsis develops during an encounter (it was not present on admission), the underlying systemic infection and the appropriate code from subcategory R65.2 should be assigned as secondary diagnoses.

Severe sepsis may be present on admission, but the diagnosis may not be confirmed until sometime after admission. If the documentation is not clear whether severe sepsis was present on admission, the provider should be queried.

4) Sepsis or severe sepsis with a localized infection

If the reason for admission is sepsis or severe sepsis and a localized infection, such as pneumonia or cellulitis, a code(s) for the underlying systemic infection should be assigned first and the code for the localized infection should be assigned as a secondary diagnosis. If the patient has severe sepsis, a code from subcategory R65.2 should also be assigned as a secondary diagnosis. If the patient is admitted with a localized infection, such as pneumonia, and sepsis/severe sepsis doesn't develop until after admission, the localized infection should be assigned first, followed by the appropriate sepsis/severe sepsis codes.

Sepsis due to a postprocedural infection

(a) Documentation of causal relationship

As with all postprocedural complications, code assignment is based on the provider's documentation of the relationship between the infection and the procedure.

(b) Sepsis due to a postprocedural infection

For infections following a procedure, a code from T81.4Ø, to T81.43 Infection following a procedure, or a code from O86.ØØ to O86.Ø3, Infection of obstetric surgical wound, that identifies the site of the infection should be coded first, if known. Assign an additional code for sepsis following a procedure (T81.44) or sepsis following an obstetrical procedure (O86.Ø4). Use an additional code to identify the infectious agent. If the patient has severe sepsis, the appropriate code from subcategory R65.2 should also be assigned with the additional code(s) for any acute organ dysfunction.

For infections following infusion, transfusion, therapeutic injection, or immunization, a code from subcategory T8Ø.2, Infections following infusion, transfusion, and therapeutic injection, or code T88.Ø-, Infection following immunization, should be coded first, followed by the code for the specific infection. If the patient has severe sepsis, the appropriate code from subcategory R65.2 should also be assigned, with the additional codes(s) for any acute organ dysfunction.

(c) Postprocedural infection and postprocedural septic shock

If a postprocedural infection has resulted in postprocedural septic shock, assign the codes indicated above for sepsis due to a postprocedural infection, followed by code T81.12-, Postprocedural septic shock. Do not assign code R65.21, Severe sepsis with septic shock. Additional code(s) should be assigned for any acute organ dysfunction.

6) Sepsis and severe sepsis associated with a noninfectious process (condition)

In some cases, a noninfectious process (condition) such as trauma, may lead to an infection which can result in sepsis or severe sepsis. If sepsis or severe sepsis is documented as associated with a noninfectious condition, such as a burn or serious injury, and this condition meets the definition for principal diagnosis, the code for the noninfectious condition should be sequenced first, followed by the code for the resulting infection. If severe sepsis is present, a code from subcategory R65.2 should also be assigned with any associated organ dysfunction(s) codes. It is not necessary to assign a code from subcategory R65.1, Systemic inflammatory response syndrome (SIRS) of non-infectious origin, for these cases.

If the infection meets the definition of principal diagnosis, it should be sequenced before the non-infectious condition. When both the associated non-infectious condition and the infection meet the definition of principal diagnosis, either may be assigned as principal diagnosis.

Only one code from category R65, Symptoms and signs specifically associated with systemic inflammation and infection, should be assigned. Therefore, when a non-infectious condition leads to an infection resulting in severe sepsis, assign the appropriate code from subcategory R65.2, Severe sepsis. Do not additionally assign a code from subcategory R65.1, Systemic inflammatory response syndrome (SIRS) of non-infectious origin.

See Section I.C.18. SIRS due to non-infectious process

7) Sepsis and septic shock complicating abortion, pregnancy, childbirth, and the puerperium

See Section I.C.15. Sepsis and septic shock complicating abortion, pregnancy, childbirth and the puerperium

8) Newborn sepsis

See Section I.C.16. f. Bacterial sepsis of Newborn

e. Methicillin Resistant Staphylococcus aureus (MRSA) Conditions

1) Selection and sequencing of MRSA codes

(a) Combination codes for MRSA infection

When a patient is diagnosed with an infection that is due to methicillin resistant *Staphylococcus aureus* (MRSA), and that infection has a combination code that includes the causal organism (e.g., sepsis, pneumonia) assign the appropriate combination code for the condition (e.g., code A41.Ø2, Sepsis due to Methicillin resistant Staphylococcus aureus or code J15.212, Pneumonia due to Methicillin resistant Staphylococcus aureus). Do not assign code B95.62, Methicillin resistant Staphylococcus aureus infection as the cause of diseases classified elsewhere, as an additional code, because the combination code includes the type of infection and the MRSA organism. Do not assign a code from subcategory Z16.11, Resistance to penicillins, as an additional diagnosis.

See Section C.1. for instructions on coding and sequencing of sepsis and severe sepsis.

(b) Other codes for MRSA infection

When there is documentation of a current infection (e.g., wound infection, stitch abscess, urinary tract infection) due to MRSA, and that infection does not have a combination code that includes the causal organism, assign the appropriate code to identify the condition along with code B95.62, Methicillin resistant Staphylococcus aureus infection as the cause of diseases classified elsewhere for the MRSA infection. Do not assign a code from subcategory Z16.11, Resistance to penicillins.

(c) Methicillin susceptible Staphylococcus aureus (MSSA) and MRSA colonization

The condition or state of being colonized or carrying MSSA or MRSA is called colonization or carriage, while an individual person is described as being colonized or being a carrier. Colonization means that MSSA or MSRA is present on or in the body without necessarily causing illness. A positive MRSA colonization test might be documented by the provider as "MRSA screen positive" or "MRSA nasal swab positive".

Assign code Z22.322, Carrier or suspected carrier of Methicillin resistant Staphylococcus aureus, for patients documented as having MRSA colonization. Assign code Z22.321, Carrier or suspected carrier of Methicillin susceptible Staphylococcus aureus, for patients documented as having MSSA colonization. Colonization is not necessarily indicative of a disease process or as the cause of a specific condition the patient may have unless documented as such by the provider.

(d) MRSA colonization and infection

If a patient is documented as having both MRSA colonization and infection during a hospital admission, code Z22.322, Carrier or suspected carrier of Methicillin resistant Staphylococcus aureus, and a code for the MRSA infection may both be assigned.

f. Zika virus infections

1) Code only confirmed cases

Code only a confirmed diagnosis of Zika virus (A92.5, Zika virus disease) as documented by the provider. This is an exception to the hospital inpatient guideline Section II, H. In this context, "confirmation" does not require documentation of the type of test performed; the provider's diagnostic statement that the condition is confirmed is sufficient. This code should be assigned regardless of the stated mode of transmission.

If the provider documents "suspected", "possible" or "probable" Zika, do not assign code A92.5. Assign a code(s) explaining the reason for encounter (such as fever, rash, or joint pain) or Z2Ø.821, Contact with and (suspected) exposure to Zika virus.

g. Coronavirus infections

1) COVID-19 infections (Infections due to SARS-CoV-2)

a) Code only confirmed cases

Code only a confirmed diagnosis of the 2Ø19 novel coronavirus disease (COVID-19) as documented by the provider or documentation of a positive COVID-19 test result. For a confirmed diagnosis, assign code UØ7.1, COVID-19. This is an exception to the hospital inpatient guideline Section II, H. In this context, "confirmation" does not require documentation of a positive test result for COVID-19; the provider's documentation that the individual has COVID-19 is sufficient.

If the provider documents "suspected," "possible," "probable," or "inconclusive" COVID-19, do not assign code UØ7.1. Instead, code the signs and symptoms reported. See guideline I.C.1.g.1.g.

b) **Sequencing of codes**
When COVID-19 meets the definition of principal diagnosis, code UØ7.1, COVID-19, should be sequenced first, followed by the appropriate codes for associated manifestations, except when another guideline requires that certain codes be sequenced first, such as obstetrics, sepsis, or transplant complications.

For a COVID-19 infection that progresses to sepsis, see Section I.C.1.d. Sepsis, Severe Sepsis, and Septic Shock

See Section I.C.15.s. for COVID-19 infection in pregnancy, childbirth, and the puerperium

See Section I.C.16.h. for COVID-19 infection in newborn

For a COVID-19 infection in a lung transplant patient, see Section I.C.19.g.3.a. Transplant complications other than kidney.

c) **Acute respiratory manifestations of COVID-19**
When the reason for the encounter/admission is a respiratory manifestation of COVID-19, assign code UØ7.1, COVID-19, as the principal/first-listed diagnosis and assign code(s) for the respiratory manifestation(s) as additional diagnoses.

The following conditions are examples of common respiratory manifestations of COVID-19.

(i) **Pneumonia**
For a patient with pneumonia confirmed as due to COVID-19, assign codes UØ7.1, COVID-19, and J12.89, Other viral pneumonia.

(ii) **Acute bronchitis**
For a patient with acute bronchitis confirmed as due to COVID-19, assign codes UØ7.1, and J2Ø.8, Acute bronchitis due to other specified organisms.

Bronchitis not otherwise specified (NOS) due to COVID-19 should be coded using code UØ7.1 and J4Ø, Bronchitis, not specified as acute or chronic.

(iii) **Lower respiratory infection**
If the COVID-19 is documented as being associated with a lower respiratory infection, not otherwise specified (NOS), or an acute respiratory infection, NOS, codes UØ7.1 and J22, Unspecified acute lower respiratory infection, should be assigned.

If the COVID-19 is documented as being associated with a respiratory infection, NOS, codes UØ7.1 and J98.8, Other specified respiratory disorders, should be assigned.

(iv) **Acute respiratory distress syndrome**
For acute respiratory distress syndrome (ARDS) due to COVID-19, assign codes UØ7.1, and J8Ø, Acute respiratory distress syndrome.

(v) **Acute respiratory failure**
For acute respiratory failure due to COVID-19, assign code UØ7.1, and code J96.Ø-, Acute respiratory failure.

d) **Non-respiratory manifestations of COVID-19**
When the reason for the encounter/admission is a non-respiratory manifestation (e.g., viral enteritis) of COVID-19, assign code UØ7.1, COVID-19, as the principal/first-listed diagnosis and assign code(s) for the manifestation(s) as additional diagnoses.

e) **Exposure to COVID-19**
For asymptomatic individuals with actual or suspected exposure to COVID-19, assign code Z2Ø.828, Contact with and (suspected) exposure to other viral communicable diseases.

For symptomatic individuals with actual or suspected exposure to COVID-19 and the infection has been ruled out, or test results are inconclusive or unknown, assign code Z2Ø.828, Contact with and (suspected) exposure to other viral communicable diseases. See guideline I.C.21.c.1, Contact/Exposure, for additional guidance regarding the use of category Z2Ø codes.

If COVID-19 is confirmed, see guideline I.C.1.g.1.a.

f) **Screening for COVID-19**
During the COVID-19 pandemic, a screening code is generally not appropriate. For encounters for COVID-19 testing, including preoperative testing, code as exposure to COVID-19 (guideline I.C.1.g.1.e).

Coding guidance will be updated as new information concerning any changes in the pandemic status becomes available.

g) **Signs and symptoms without definitive diagnosis of COVID-19**
For patients presenting with any signs/symptoms associated with COVID-19 (such as fever, etc.) but a definitive diagnosis has not been established, assign the appropriate code(s) for each of the presenting signs and symptoms such as:

- **RØ5 Cough**
- **RØ6.Ø2 Shortness of breath**
- **R5Ø.9 Fever, unspecified**

If a patient with signs/symptoms associated with COVID-19 also has an actual or suspected contact with or exposure to COVID-19, assign Z2Ø.828, Contact with and (suspected) exposure to other viral communicable diseases, as an additional code.

h) **Asymptomatic individuals who test positive for COVID-19**
For asymptomatic individuals who test positive for COVID-19, see guideline I.C.1.g.1.a. Although the individual is asymptomatic, the individual has tested positive and is considered to have the COVID-19 infection.

(i) **Personal history of COVID-19**
For patients with a history of COVID-19, assign code Z86.19, Personal history of other infectious and parasitic diseases.

(j) **Follow-up visits after COVID-19 infection has resolved**
For individuals who previously had COVID-19 and are being seen for follow-up evaluation, and COVID-19 test results are negative, assign codes ZØ9, Encounter for follow-up examination after completed treatment for conditions other than malignant neoplasm, and Z86.19, Personal history of other infectious and parasitic diseases.

(k) **Encounter for antibody testing**
For an encounter for antibody testing that is not being performed to confirm a current COVID-19 infection, nor is a follow-up test after resolution of COVID-19, assign ZØ1.84, Encounter for antibody response examination.

Follow the applicable guidelines above if the individual is being tested to confirm a current COVID-19 infection.

For follow-up testing after a COVID-19 infection, see guideline I.C.1.g.1.j.

2. **Chapter 2: Neoplasms (CØØ-D49)**
General guidelines
Chapter 2 of the ICD-10-CM contains the codes for most benign and all malignant neoplasms. Certain benign neoplasms, such as prostatic adenomas, may be found in the specific body system chapters. To properly code a neoplasm, it is necessary to determine from the record if the neoplasm is benign, in-situ, malignant, or of uncertain histologic behavior. If malignant, any secondary (metastatic) sites should also be determined.

Primary malignant neoplasms overlapping site boundaries

A primary malignant neoplasm that overlaps two or more contiguous (next to each other) sites should be classified to the subcategory/code .8 ('overlapping lesion'), unless the combination is specifically indexed elsewhere. For multiple neoplasms of the same site that are not contiguous such as tumors in different quadrants of the same breast, codes for each site should be assigned.

Malignant neoplasm of ectopic tissue

Malignant neoplasms of ectopic tissue are to be coded to the site of origin mentioned, e.g., ectopic pancreatic malignant neoplasms involving the stomach are coded to malignant neoplasm of pancreas, unspecified (C25.9).

plasm table in the Alphabetic Index should be referenced first. ver, if the histological term is documented, that term should be enced first, rather than going immediately to the Neoplasm Table, in er to determine which column in the Neoplasm Table is appropriate. r example, if the documentation indicates "adenoma," refer to the term in the Alphabetic Index to review the entries under this term and the instructional note to "see also neoplasm, by site, benign." The table provides the proper code based on the type of neoplasm and the site. It is important to select the proper column in the table that corresponds to the type of neoplasm. The Tabular List should then be referenced to verify that the correct code has been selected from the table and that a more specific site code does not exist.

See Section I.C.21. Factors influencing health status and contact with health services, Status, for information regarding Z15.Ø, codes for genetic susceptibility to cancer.

a. Treatment directed at the malignancy

If the treatment is directed at the malignancy, designate the malignancy as the principal diagnosis.

The only exception to this guideline is if a patient admission/encounter is solely for the administration of chemotherapy, immunotherapy or external beam radiation therapy, assign the appropriate Z51.-- code as the first-listed or principal diagnosis, and the diagnosis or problem for which the service is being performed as a secondary diagnosis.

b. Treatment of secondary site

When a patient is admitted because of a primary neoplasm with metastasis and treatment is directed toward the secondary site only, the secondary neoplasm is designated as the principal diagnosis even though the primary malignancy is still present.

c. Coding and sequencing of complications

Coding and sequencing of complications associated with the malignancies or with the therapy thereof are subject to the following guidelines:

1) Anemia associated with malignancy

When admission/encounter is for management of an anemia associated with the malignancy, and the treatment is only for anemia, the appropriate code for the malignancy is sequenced as the principal or first-listed diagnosis followed by the appropriate code for the anemia (such as code D63.Ø, Anemia in neoplastic disease).

2) Anemia associated with chemotherapy, immunotherapy and radiation therapy

When the admission/encounter is for management of an anemia associated with an adverse effect of the administration of chemotherapy or immunotherapy and the only treatment is for the anemia, the anemia code is sequenced first followed by the appropriate codes for the neoplasm and the adverse effect (T45.1X5-, Adverse effect of antineoplastic and immunosuppressive drugs).

When the admission/encounter is for management of an anemia associated with an adverse effect of radiotherapy, the anemia code should be sequenced first, followed by the appropriate neoplasm code and code Y84.2, Radiological procedure and radiotherapy as the cause of abnormal reaction of the patient, or of later complication, without mention of misadventure at the time of the procedure.

3) Management of dehydration due to the malignancy

When the admission/encounter is for management of dehydration due to the malignancy and only the dehydration is being treated (intravenous rehydration), the dehydration is sequenced first, followed by the code(s) for the malignancy.

4) Treatment of a complication resulting from a surgical procedure

When the admission/encounter is for treatment of a complication resulting from a surgical procedure, designate the complication as the principal or first-listed diagnosis if treatment is directed at resolving the complication.

d. Primary malignancy previously excised

When a primary malignancy has been previously excised or eradicated from its site and there is no further treatment directed to that site and there is no evidence of any existing primary malignancy at that site, a code from category Z85, Personal history of malignant neoplasm, should be used to indicate the former site of the malignancy. Any mention of extension, invasion, or metastasis to another site is coded as a secondary malignant neoplasm to that site. The secondary site may be the principal or first-listed diagnosis with the Z85 code used as a secondary code.

e. Admissions/Encounters involving chemotherapy, immunotherapy and radiation therapy

1) Episode of care involves surgical removal of neoplasm

When an episode of care involves the surgical removal of a neoplasm, primary or secondary site, followed by adjunct chemotherapy or radiation treatment during the same episode of care, the code for the neoplasm should be assigned as principal or first-listed diagnosis.

2) Patient admission/encounter solely for administration of chemotherapy, immunotherapy and radiation therapy

If a patient admission/encounter is solely for the administration of chemotherapy, immunotherapy or external beam radiation therapy assign code Z51.Ø, Encounter for antineoplastic radiation therapy, or Z51.11, Encounter for antineoplastic chemotherapy, or Z51.12, Encounter for antineoplastic immunotherapy as the first-listed or principal diagnosis. If a patient receives more than one of these therapies during the same admission more than one of these codes may be assigned, in any sequence.

The malignancy for which the therapy is being administered should be assigned as a secondary diagnosis.

If a patient admission/encounter is for the insertion or implantation of radioactive elements (e.g., brachytherapy) the appropriate code for the malignancy is sequenced as the principal or first-listed diagnosis. Code Z51.Ø should not be assigned.

3) Patient admitted for radiation therapy, chemotherapy or immunotherapy and develops complications

When a patient is admitted for the purpose of external beam radiotherapy, immunotherapy or chemotherapy and develops complications such as uncontrolled nausea and vomiting or dehydration, the principal or first-listed diagnosis is Z51.Ø, Encounter for antineoplastic radiation therapy, or Z51.11, Encounter for antineoplastic chemotherapy, or Z51.12, Encounter for antineoplastic immunotherapy followed by any codes for the complications.

When a patient is admitted for the purpose of insertion or implantation of radioactive elements (e.g., brachytherapy) and develops complications such as uncontrolled nausea and vomiting or dehydration, the principal or first-listed diagnosis is the appropriate code for the malignancy followed by any codes for the complications.

f. Admission/encounter to determine extent of malignancy

When the reason for admission/encounter is to determine the extent of the malignancy, or for a procedure such as paracentesis or thoracentesis, the primary malignancy or appropriate metastatic site is designated as the principal or first-listed diagnosis, even though chemotherapy or radiotherapy is administered.

g. Symptoms, signs, and abnormal findings listed in Chapter 18 associated with neoplasms

Symptoms, signs, and ill-defined conditions listed in Chapter 18 characteristic of, or associated with, an existing primary or secondary site malignancy cannot be used to replace the malignancy as principal or first-listed diagnosis, regardless of the number of admissions or encounters for treatment and care of the neoplasm.

See section I.C.21. Factors influencing health status and contact with health services, Encounter for prophylactic organ removal.

h. Admission/encounter for pain control/management

See Section I.C.6. for information on coding admission/encounter for pain control/management.

i. Malignancy in two or more noncontiguous sites

A patient may have more than one malignant tumor in the same organ. These tumors may represent different primaries or metastatic disease, depending on the site. Should the documentation be unclear, the provider should be queried as to the status of each tumor so that the correct codes can be assigned.

j. Disseminated malignant neoplasm, unspecified

Code C80.Ø, Disseminated malignant neoplasm, unspecified, is for use only in those cases where the patient has advanced metastatic disease and no known primary or secondary sites are specified. It should not be used in place of assigning codes for the primary site and all known secondary sites.

k. Malignant neoplasm without specification of site

Code C8Ø.1, Malignant (primary) neoplasm, unspecified, equates to Cancer, unspecified. This code should only be used when no determination can be made as to the primary site of a malignancy. This code should rarely be used in the inpatient setting.

l. Sequencing of neoplasm codes

1) Encounter for treatment of primary malignancy

If the reason for the encounter is for treatment of a primary malignancy, assign the malignancy as the principal/first-listed diagnosis. The primary site is to be sequenced first, followed by any metastatic sites.

2) Encounter for treatment of secondary malignancy

When an encounter is for a primary malignancy with metastasis and treatment is directed toward the metastatic (secondary) site(s) only, the metastatic site(s) is designated as the principal/first-listed diagnosis. The primary malignancy is coded as an additional code.

3) Malignant neoplasm in a pregnant patient

When a pregnant woman has a malignant neoplasm, a code from subcategory O9A.1-, Malignant neoplasm complicating pregnancy, childbirth, and the puerperium, should be sequenced first, followed by the appropriate code from Chapter 2 to indicate the type of neoplasm.

4) Encounter for complication associated with a neoplasm

When an encounter is for management of a complication associated with a neoplasm, such as dehydration, and the treatment is only for the complication, the complication is coded first, followed by the appropriate code(s) for the neoplasm.

The exception to this guideline is anemia. When the admission/encounter is for management of an anemia associated with the malignancy, and the treatment is only for anemia, the appropriate code for the malignancy is sequenced as the principal or first-listed diagnosis followed by code D63.Ø, Anemia in neoplastic disease.

5) Complication from surgical procedure for treatment of a neoplasm

When an encounter is for treatment of a complication resulting from a surgical procedure performed for the treatment of the neoplasm, designate the complication as the principal/first-listed diagnosis. See the guideline regarding the coding of a current malignancy versus personal history to determine if the code for the neoplasm should also be assigned.

6) Pathologic fracture due to a neoplasm

When an encounter is for a pathological fracture due to a neoplasm, and the focus of treatment is the fracture, a code from subcategory M84.5, Pathological fracture in neoplastic disease, should be sequenced first, followed by the code for the neoplasm.

If the focus of treatment is the neoplasm with an associated pathological fracture, the neoplasm code should be sequenced first, followed by a code from M84.5 for the pathological fracture.

m. Current malignancy versus personal history of malignancy

When a primary malignancy has been excised but further treatment, such as an additional surgery for the malignancy, radiation therapy or chemotherapy is directed to that site, the primary malignancy code should be used until treatment is completed.

When a primary malignancy has been previously excised or eradicated from its site, there is no further treatment (of the malignancy) directed to that site, and there is no evidence of any existing primary malignancy at that site, a code from category Z85, Personal history of malignant neoplasm, should be used to indicate the former site of the malignancy.

Codes from subcategories Z85.Ø – Z85.85 should only be assigned for the former site of a primary malignancy, not the site of a secondary malignancy. **Code Z85.89** may be assigned for the former site(s) of either a primary or secondary malignancy.

See Section I.C.21. Factors influencing health status and contact with health services, History (of)

n. Leukemia, Multiple Myeloma, and Malignant Plasma Cell Neoplasms in remission versus personal history

The categories for leukemia, and category C9Ø, Multiple myeloma and malignant plasma cell neoplasms, have codes indicating whether or not the leukemia has achieved remission. There are also codes Z85.6, Personal history of leukemia, and Z85.79, Personal history of other malignant neoplasms of lymphoid, hematopoietic and related tissues. If the documentation is unclear as to whether the leukemia has achieved remission, the provider should be queried.

See Section I.C.21. Factors influencing health status and contact with health services, History (of)

o. Aftercare following surgery for neoplasm

See Section I.C.21. Factors influencing health status and contact with health services, Aftercare

p. Follow-up care for completed treatment of a malignancy

See Section I.C.21. Factors influencing health status and contact with health services, Follow-up

q. Prophylactic organ removal for prevention of malignancy

See Section I.C. 21, Factors influencing health status and contact with health services, Prophylactic organ removal

r. Malignant neoplasm associated with transplanted organ

A malignant neoplasm of a transplanted organ should be coded as a transplant complication. Assign first the appropriate code from category T86.-, Complications of transplanted organs and tissue, followed by code C8Ø.2, Malignant neoplasm associated with transplanted organ. Use an additional code for the specific malignancy.

3. Chapter 3: Disease of the blood and blood-forming organs and certain disorders involving the immune mechanism (D5Ø-D89)

Reserved for future guideline expansion

4. Chapter 4: Endocrine, Nutritional, and Metabolic Diseases (EØØ-E89)

a. Diabetes mellitus

The diabetes mellitus codes are combination codes that include the type of diabetes mellitus, the body system affected, and the complications affecting that body system. As many codes within a particular category as are necessary to describe all of the complications of the disease may be used. They should be sequenced based on the reason for a particular encounter. Assign as many codes from categories EØ8 – E13 as needed to identify all of the associated conditions that the patient has.

1) Type of diabetes

The age of a patient is not the sole determining factor, though most type 1 diabetics develop the condition before reaching puberty. For this reason type 1 diabetes mellitus is also referred to as juvenile diabetes.

2) Type of diabetes mellitus not documented

If the type of diabetes mellitus is not documented in the medical record the default is E11.-, Type 2 diabetes mellitus.

3) Diabetes mellitus and the use of insulin, oral hypoglycemics, and injectable non-insulin drugs

If the documentation in a medical record does not indicate the type of diabetes but does indicate that the patient uses insulin, code E11-, Type 2 diabetes mellitus, should be assigned. An additional code should be assigned from category Z79 to identify the long-term (current) use of insulin or oral hypoglycemic drugs. If the patient is treated with both oral medications and insulin, only the code for long-term (current) use of insulin should be assigned. **If the patient is treated with both insulin and an injectable non-insulin antidiabetic drug, assign codes Z79.4, Long-term (current) use of insulin, and Z79.899, Other long term (current) drug therapy. If the patient is treated with both oral hypoglycemic drugs and an injectable non-insulin antidiabetic drug, assign codes Z79.84, Long-term (current) use of oral hypoglycemic drugs, and Z79.899, Other long-term (current) drug therapy.** Code Z79.4 should not be assigned if insulin is given temporarily to bring a type 2 patient's blood sugar under control during an encounter.

4) Diabetes mellitus in pregnancy and gestational diabetes

See Section I.C.15. Diabetes mellitus in pregnancy.

See Section I.C.15. Gestational (pregnancy induced) diabetes

5) Complications due to insulin pump malfunction

(a) Underdose of insulin due to insulin pump failure

An underdose of insulin due to an insulin pump failure should be assigned to a code from subcategory T85.6, Mechanical complication of other specified internal and external prosthetic devices, implants and grafts, that specifies the type of pump malfunction, as the principal or first-listed code, followed by code T38.3X6-, Underdosing of insulin and oral hypoglycemic [antidiabetic] drugs.

Additional codes for the type of diabetes mellitus and any associated complications due to the underdosing should also be assigned.

(b) Overdose of insulin due to insulin pump failure

The principal or first-listed code for an encounter due to an insulin pump malfunction resulting in an overdose of insulin, should also be T85.6-, Mechanical complication of other specified internal and external prosthetic devices, implants and grafts, followed by code T38.3X1-, Poisoning by insulin and oral hypoglycemic [antidiabetic] drugs, accidental (unintentional).

6) Secondary diabetes mellitus

Codes under categories EØ8, Diabetes mellitus due to underlying condition, EØ9, Drug or chemical induced diabetes mellitus, and E13, Other specified diabetes mellitus, identify complications/manifestations associated with secondary diabetes mellitus. Secondary diabetes is always caused by another condition or event (e.g., cystic fibrosis, malignant neoplasm of pancreas, pancreatectomy, adverse effect of drug, or poisoning).

(a) Secondary diabetes mellitus and the use of insulin or oral hypoglycemic drugs

For patients with secondary diabetes mellitus who routinely use insulin or oral hypoglycemic drugs, an additional code from category Z79 should be assigned to identify the long-term (current) use of insulin or oral hypoglycemic drugs. If the patient is treated with both oral medications and insulin, only the code for long-term (current) use of insulin should be assigned. **If the patient is treated with both insulin and an injectable non-insulin antidiabetic drug, assign codes Z79.4, Long-term (current) use of insulin, and Z79.899, Other long term (current) drug therapy. If the patient is treated with both oral hypoglycemic drugs and an injectable non-insulin antidiabetic drug, assign codes Z79.84, Long-term (current) use of oral hypoglycemic drugs, and Z79.899, Other long-term (current) drug therapy.** Code Z79.4 should not be assigned if insulin is given temporarily to bring a secondary diabetic patient's blood sugar under control during an encounter.

(b) Assigning and sequencing secondary diabetes codes and its causes

The sequencing of the secondary diabetes codes in relationship to codes for the cause of the diabetes is based on the Tabular List instructions for categories EØ8, EØ9 and E13.

(i) Secondary diabetes mellitus due to pancreatectomy

For postpancreatectomy diabetes mellitus (lack of insulin due to the surgical removal of all or part of the pancreas), assign code E89.1, Postprocedural hypoinsulinemia. Assign a code from category E13 and a code from subcategory Z9Ø.41, Acquired absence of pancreas, as additional codes.

(ii) Secondary diabetes due to drugs

Secondary diabetes may be caused by an adverse effect of correctly administered medications, poisoning or sequela of poisoning.

See section I.C.19.e for coding of adverse effects and poisoning, and section I.C.20 for external cause code reporting.

5. Chapter 5: Mental, Behavioral and Neurodevelopmental disorders (FØ1-F99)

a. Pain disorders related to psychological factors

Assign code F45.41, for pain that is exclusively related to psychological disorders. As indicated by the Excludes 1 note under category G89, a code from category G89 should not be assigned with code F45.41.

Code F45.42, Pain disorders with related psychological factors, should be used with a code from category G89, Pain, not elsewhere classified, if there is documentation of a psychological component for a patient with acute or chronic pain.

See Section I.C.6. Pain

b. Mental and behavioral disorders due to psychoactive substance use

1) In Remission

Selection of codes for "in remission" for categories F1Ø-F19, Mental and behavioral disorders due to psychoactive substance use (categories F1Ø-F19 with -.11, -.21) requires the provider's clinical judgment. The appropriate codes for "in remission" are assigned only on the basis of provider documentation (as defined in the Official Guidelines for Coding and Reporting), unless otherwise instructed by the classification.

Mild substance use disorders in early or sustained remission are classified to the appropriate codes for substance abuse in remission, and moderate or severe substance use disorders in early or sustained remission are classified to the appropriate codes for substance dependence in remission.

2) Psychoactive Substance Use, Abuse and Dependence

When the provider documentation refers to use, abuse and dependence of the same substance (e.g. alcohol, opioid, cannabis, etc.), only one code should be assigned to identify the pattern of use based on the following hierarchy:

- If both use and abuse are documented, assign only the code for abuse
- If both abuse and dependence are documented, assign only the code for dependence
- If use, abuse and dependence are all documented, assign only the code for dependence
- If both use and dependence are documented, assign only the code for dependence.

3) Psychoactive Substance Use, Unspecified

As with all other unspecified diagnoses, the codes for unspecified psychoactive substance use (F1Ø.9-, F11.9-, F12.9-, F13.9-, F14.9-, F15.9-, F16.9-, F18.9-, F19.9-) should only be assigned based on provider documentation and when they meet the definition of a reportable diagnosis (see Section III, Reporting Additional Diagnoses). These codes are to be used only when the psychoactive substance use is associated with a physical **disorder included in chapter 5 (such as sexual dysfunction and sleep disorder), or a** mental or behavioral disorder, and such a relationship is documented by the provider.

c. Factitious Disorder

Factitious disorder imposed on self or Munchausen's syndrome is a disorder in which a person falsely reports or causes his or her own physical or psychological signs or symptoms. For patients with documented factitious disorder on self or Munchausen's syndrome, assign the appropriate code from subcategory F68.1-, Factitious disorder imposed on self.

Munchausen's syndrome by proxy (MSBP) is a disorder in which a caregiver (perpetrator) falsely reports or causes an illness or injury in another person (victim) under his or her care, such as a child, an elderly adult, or a person who has a disability. The condition is also referred to as "factitious disorder imposed on another" or "factitious disorder by proxy." The perpetrator, not the victim, receives this diagnosis. Assign code F68.A, Factitious disorder imposed on another, to the perpetrator's record. For the victim of a patient suffering from MSBP, assign the appropriate code from categories T74, Adult and child abuse, neglect and other maltreatment, confirmed, or T76, Adult and child abuse, neglect and other maltreatment, suspected.

See Section I.C.19.f. Adult and child abuse, neglect and other maltreatment

6. Chapter 6: Diseases of the Nervous System (GØØ-G99)

a. Dominant/nondominant side

Codes from category G81, Hemiplegia and hemiparesis, and subcategories G83.1, Monoplegia of lower limb, G83.2, Monoplegia of upper limb, and G83.3, Monoplegia, unspecified, identify whether the dominant or nondominant side is affected. Should the affected side be documented, but not specified as dominant or nondominant, and the classification system does not indicate a default, code selection is as follows:

- For ambidextrous patients, the default should be dominant.
- If the left side is affected, the default is non-dominant.
- If the right side is affected, the default is dominant.

b. Pain - Category G89

1) General coding information

Codes in category G89, Pain, not elsewhere classified, may be used in conjunction with codes from other categories and chapters to provide more detail about acute or chronic pain and neoplasm-related pain, unless otherwise indicated below.

If the pain is not specified as acute or chronic, post-thoracotomy, postprocedural, or neoplasm-related, do not assign codes from category G89.

A code from category G89 should not be assigned if the underlying (definitive) diagnosis is known, unless the reason for the encounter is pain control/ management and not management of the underlying condition.

When an admission or encounter is for a procedure aimed at treating the underlying condition (e.g., spinal fusion, kyphoplasty), a code for the underlying condition (e.g., vertebral fracture, spinal stenosis) should be assigned as the principal diagnosis. No code from category G89 should be assigned.

(a) Category G89 Codes as Principal or First-Listed Diagnosis

Category G89 codes are acceptable as principal diagnosis or the first-listed code:

- When pain control or pain management is the reason for the admission/encounter (e.g., a patient with displaced intervertebral disc, nerve impingement and severe back pain presents for injection of steroid into the spinal canal). The underlying cause of the pain should be reported as an additional diagnosis, if known.
- When a patient is admitted for the insertion of a neurostimulator for pain control, assign the appropriate pain code as the principal or first-listed diagnosis. When an admission or encounter is for a procedure aimed at treating the underlying condition and a neurostimulator is inserted for pain control during the same admission/encounter, a code for the underlying condition should be assigned as the principal diagnosis and the appropriate pain code should be assigned as a secondary diagnosis.

(b) Use of Category G89 Codes in Conjunction with Site Specific Pain Codes

(i) Assigning Category G89 and Site-Specific Pain Codes

Codes from category G89 may be used in conjunction with codes that identify the site of pain (including codes from chapter 18) if the category G89 code provides additional information. For example, if the code describes the site of the pain, but does not fully describe whether the pain is acute or chronic, then both codes should be assigned.

(ii) Sequencing of Category G89 Codes with Site-Specific Pain Codes

The sequencing of category G89 codes with site-specific pain codes (including chapter 18 codes), is dependent on the circumstances of the encounter/admission as follows:

- If the encounter is for pain control or pain management, assign the code from category G89 followed by the code identifying the specific site of pain (e.g., encounter for pain management for acute neck pain from trauma is assigned code G89.11, Acute pain due to trauma, followed by code M54.2, Cervicalgia, to identify the site of pain).
- If the encounter is for any other reason except pain control or pain management, and a related definitive diagnosis has not been established (confirmed) by the provider, assign the code for the specific site of pain first, followed by the appropriate code from category G89.

2) Pain due to devices, implants and grafts

See Section I.C.19. Pain due to medical devices

3) Postoperative Pain

The provider's documentation should be used to guide the coding of postoperative pain, as well as *Section III. Reporting Additional Diagnoses and Section IV. Diagnostic Coding and Reporting in the Outpatient Setting.*

The default for post-thoracotomy and other postoperative pain not specified as acute or chronic is the code for the acute form.

Routine or expected postoperative pain immediately after surgery should not be coded.

(a) Postoperative pain not associated with specific postoperative complication

Postoperative pain not associated with a specific postoperative complication is assigned to the appropriate postoperative pain code in category G89.

(b) Postoperative pain associated with specific postoperative complication

Postoperative pain associated with a specific postoperative complication (such as painful wire sutures) is assigned to the appropriate code(s) found in Chapter 19, Injury, poisoning, and certain other consequences of external causes. If appropriate, use additional code(s) from category G89 to identify acute or chronic pain (G89.18 or G89.28).

4) Chronic pain

Chronic pain is classified to subcategory G89.2. There is no time frame defining when pain becomes chronic pain. The provider's documentation should be used to guide use of these codes.

5) Neoplasm Related Pain

Code G89.3 is assigned to pain documented as being related, associated or due to cancer, primary or secondary malignancy, or tumor. This code is assigned regardless of whether the pain is acute or chronic.

This code may be assigned as the principal or first-listed code when the stated reason for the admission/encounter is documented as pain control/pain management. The underlying neoplasm should be reported as an additional diagnosis.

When the reason for the admission/encounter is management of the neoplasm and the pain associated with the neoplasm is also documented, code G89.3 may be assigned as an additional diagnosis. It is not necessary to assign an additional code for the site of the pain.

See Section I.C.2 for instructions on the sequencing of neoplasms for all other stated reasons for the admission/encounter (except for pain control/pain management).

6) Chronic pain syndrome

Central pain syndrome (G89.Ø) and chronic pain syndrome (G89.4) are different than the term "chronic pain," and therefore codes should only be used when the provider has specifically documented this condition.

See Section I.C.5. Pain disorders related to psychological factors

7. Chapter 7: Diseases of the Eye and Adnexa (HØØ-H59)

a. Glaucoma

1) Assigning Glaucoma Codes

Assign as many codes from category H4Ø, Glaucoma, as needed to identify the type of glaucoma, the affected eye, and the glaucoma stage.

2) Bilateral glaucoma with same type and stage

When a patient has bilateral glaucoma and both eyes are documented as being the same type and stage, and there is a code for bilateral glaucoma, report only the code for the type of glaucoma, bilateral, with the seventh character for the stage.

When a patient has bilateral glaucoma and both eyes are documented as being the same type and stage, and the classification does not provide a code for bilateral glaucoma (i.e. subcategories H4Ø.1Ø and H4Ø.2Ø) report only one code for the type of glaucoma with the appropriate seventh character for the stage.

3) Bilateral glaucoma stage with different types or stages

When a patient has bilateral glaucoma and each eye is documented as having a different type or stage, and the classification distinguishes laterality, assign the appropriate code for each eye rather than the code for bilateral glaucoma.

When a patient has bilateral glaucoma and each eye is documented as having a different type, and the classification does not distinguish laterality (i.e. subcategories H4Ø.1Ø and H4Ø.2Ø), assign one code for each type of glaucoma with the appropriate seventh character for the stage.

When a patient has bilateral glaucoma and each eye is documented as having the same type, but different stage, and the classification does not distinguish laterality (i.e. subcategories H40.10 and H40.20), assign a code for the type of glaucoma for each eye with the seventh character for the specific glaucoma stage documented for each eye.

4) Patient admitted with glaucoma and stage evolves during the admission

If a patient is admitted with glaucoma and the stage progresses during the admission, assign the code for highest stage documented.

5) Indeterminate stage glaucoma

Assignment of the seventh character "4" for "indeterminate stage" should be based on the clinical documentation. The seventh character "4" is used for glaucomas whose stage cannot be clinically determined. This seventh character should not be confused with the seventh character "0", unspecified, which should be assigned when there is no documentation regarding the stage of the glaucoma.

b. Blindness

If "blindness" or "low vision" of both eyes is documented but the visual impairment category is not documented, assign code H54.3, Unqualified visual loss, both eyes. If "blindness" or "low vision" in one eye is documented but the visual impairment category is not documented, assign a code from H54.6-, Unqualified visual loss, one eye. If "blindness" or "visual loss" is documented without any information about whether one or both eyes are affected, assign code H54.7, Unspecified visual loss.

8. Chapter 8: Diseases of the Ear and Mastoid Process (H60-H95)

Reserved for future guideline expansion

9. Chapter 9: Diseases of the Circulatory System (I00-I99)

a. Hypertension

The classification presumes a causal relationship between hypertension and heart involvement and between hypertension and kidney involvement, as the two conditions are linked by the term "with" in the Alphabetic Index. These conditions should be coded as related even in the absence of provider documentation explicitly linking them, unless the documentation clearly states the conditions are unrelated.

For hypertension and conditions not specifically linked by relational terms such as "with," "associated with" or "due to" in the classification, provider documentation must link the conditions in order to code them as related.

1) Hypertension with Heart Disease

Hypertension with heart conditions classified to I50.- or I51.4-I51.7, I51.89, I51.9, are assigned to a code from category I11, Hypertensive heart disease. Use additional code(s) from category I50, Heart failure, to identify the type(s) of heart failure in those patients with heart failure.

The same heart conditions (I50.-, I51.4-I51.7, I51.89, I51.9) with hypertension are coded separately if the provider has documented they are unrelated to the hypertension. Sequence according to the circumstances of the admission/encounter.

2) Hypertensive Chronic Kidney Disease

Assign codes from category I12, Hypertensive chronic kidney disease, when both hypertension and a condition classifiable to category N18, Chronic kidney disease (CKD), are present. CKD should not be coded as hypertensive if the provider indicates the CKD is not related to the hypertension.

The appropriate code from category N18 should be used as a secondary code with a code from category I12 to identify the stage of chronic kidney disease.

See Section I.C.14. Chronic kidney disease.

If a patient has hypertensive chronic kidney disease and acute renal failure, the acute renal failure should also be coded. Sequence according to the circumstances of the admission/encounter.

3) Hypertensive Heart and Chronic Kidney Disease

Assign codes from combination category I13, Hypertensive heart and chronic kidney disease, when there is hypertension with both heart and kidney involvement. If heart failure is present, assign an additional code from category I50 to identify the type of heart failure.

The appropriate code from category N18, Chronic kidney disease, should be used as a secondary code with a code from category I13 to identify the stage of chronic kidney disease.

See Section I.C.14. Chronic kidney disease.

The codes in category I13, Hypertensive heart and chronic kidney disease, are combination codes that include hypertension, heart disease and chronic kidney disease. The Includes note at I13 specifies that the conditions included at I11 and I12 are included together in I13. If a patient has hypertension, heart disease and chronic kidney disease, then a code from I13 should be used, not individual codes for hypertension, heart disease and chronic kidney disease, or codes from I11 or I12.

For patients with both acute renal failure and chronic kidney disease, **the** acute renal failure **should also be coded. Sequence according to the circumstances of the admission/encounter.**

4) Hypertensive Cerebrovascular Disease

For hypertensive cerebrovascular disease, first assign the appropriate code from categories I60-I69, followed by the appropriate hypertension code.

5) Hypertensive Retinopathy

Subcategory H35.0, Background retinopathy and retinal vascular changes, should be used with a code from category I10- I15, Hypertensive disease to include the systemic hypertension. The sequencing is based on the reason for the encounter.

6) Hypertension, Secondary

Secondary hypertension is due to an underlying condition. Two codes are required: one to identify the underlying etiology and one from category I15 to identify the hypertension. Sequencing of codes is determined by the reason for admission/encounter.

7) Hypertension, Transient

Assign code R03.0, Elevated blood pressure reading without diagnosis of hypertension, unless patient has an established diagnosis of hypertension. Assign code O13.-, Gestational [pregnancy-induced] hypertension without significant proteinuria, or O14.-, Pre-eclampsia, for transient hypertension of pregnancy.

8) Hypertension, Controlled

This diagnostic statement usually refers to an existing state of hypertension under control by therapy. Assign the appropriate code from categories I10-I15, Hypertensive diseases.

9) Hypertension, Uncontrolled

Uncontrolled hypertension may refer to untreated hypertension or hypertension not responding to current therapeutic regimen. In either case, assign the appropriate code from categories I10-I15, Hypertensive diseases.

10) Hypertensive Crisis

Assign a code from category I16, Hypertensive crisis, for documented hypertensive urgency, hypertensive emergency or unspecified hypertensive crisis. Code also any identified hypertensive disease (I10-I15). The sequencing is based on the reason for the encounter.

11) Pulmonary Hypertension

Pulmonary hypertension is classified to category I27, Other pulmonary heart diseases. For secondary pulmonary hypertension (I27.1, I27.2-), code also any associated conditions or adverse effects of drugs or toxins. The sequencing is based on the reason for the encounter, except for adverse effects of drugs (See Section I.C.19.e.).

b. Atherosclerotic Coronary Artery Disease and Angina

ICD-10-CM has combination codes for atherosclerotic heart disease with angina pectoris. The subcategories for these codes are I25.11, Atherosclerotic heart disease of native coronary artery with angina pectoris and I25.7, Atherosclerosis of coronary artery bypass graft(s) and coronary artery of transplanted heart with angina pectoris.

When using one of these combination codes it is not necessary to use an additional code for angina pectoris. A causal relationship can be assumed in a patient with both atherosclerosis and angina pectoris, unless the documentation indicates the angina is due to something other than the atherosclerosis.

If a patient with coronary artery disease is admitted due to an acute myocardial infarction (AMI), the AMI should be sequenced before the coronary artery disease.

See Section I.C.9. Acute myocardial infarction (AMI)

c. Intraoperative and Postprocedural Cerebrovascular Accident
Medical record documentation should clearly specify the cause-and-effect relationship between the medical intervention and the cerebrovascular accident in order to assign a code for intraoperative or postprocedural cerebrovascular accident.

Proper code assignment depends on whether it was an infarction or hemorrhage and whether it occurred intraoperatively or postoperatively. If it was a cerebral hemorrhage, code assignment depends on the type of procedure performed.

d. Sequelae of Cerebrovascular Disease

1) Category I69, Sequelae of Cerebrovascular disease
Category I69 is used to indicate conditions classifiable to categories I60-I67 as the causes of sequela (neurologic deficits), themselves classified elsewhere. These "late effects" include neurologic deficits that persist after initial onset of conditions classifiable to categories I60-I67. The neurologic deficits caused by cerebrovascular disease may be present from the onset or may arise at any time after the onset of the condition classifiable to categories I60-I67.

Codes from category I69, Sequelae of cerebrovascular disease, that specify hemiplegia, hemiparesis and monoplegia identify whether the dominant or nondominant side is affected. Should the affected side be documented, but not specified as dominant or nondominant, and the classification system does not indicate a default, code selection is as follows:

- For ambidextrous patients, the default should be dominant.
- If the left side is affected, the default is non-dominant.
- If the right side is affected, the default is dominant.

2) Codes from category I69 with codes from I60-I67
Codes from category I69 may be assigned on a health care record with codes from I60-I67, if the patient has a current cerebrovascular disease and deficits from an old cerebrovascular disease.

3) Codes from category I69 and Personal history of transient ischemic attack (TIA) and cerebral infarction (Z86.73)
Codes from category I69 should not be assigned if the patient does not have neurologic deficits.

See Section I.C.21. 4. History (of) for use of personal history codes

e. Acute myocardial infarction (AMI)

1) Type 1 ST elevation myocardial infarction (STEMI) and non-ST elevation myocardial infarction (NSTEMI)
The ICD-10-CM codes for type 1 acute myocardial infarction (AMI) identify the site, such as anterolateral wall or true posterior wall. Subcategories I21.0-I21.2 and code I21.3 are used for type 1 ST elevation myocardial infarction (STEMI). Code I21.4, Non-ST elevation (NSTEMI) myocardial infarction, is used for type 1 non-ST elevation myocardial infarction (NSTEMI) and nontransmural MIs.

If a type 1 NSTEMI evolves to STEMI, assign the STEMI code. If a type 1 STEMI converts to NSTEMI due to thrombolytic therapy, it is still coded as STEMI.

For encounters occurring while the myocardial infarction is equal to, or less than, four weeks old, including transfers to another acute setting or a postacute setting, and the myocardial infarction meets the definition for "other diagnoses" (see Section III, Reporting Additional Diagnoses), codes from category I21 may continue to be reported. For encounters after the 4 week time frame and the patient is still receiving care related to the myocardial infarction, the appropriate aftercare code should be assigned, rather than a code from category I21. For old or healed myocardial infarctions not requiring further care, code I25.2, Old myocardial infarction, may be assigned.

2) Acute myocardial infarction, unspecified
Code I21.9, Acute myocardial infarction, unspecified, is the default for unspecified acute myocardial infarction or unspecified type. If only type 1 STEMI or transmural MI without the site is documented, assign code I21.3, ST elevation (STEMI) myocardial infarction of unspecified site.

3) AMI documented as nontransmural or subendocardial but site provided
If an AMI is documented as nontransmural or subendocardial, but the site is provided, it is still coded as a subendocardial AMI.

See Section I.C.21.3 for information on coding status post administration of tPA in a different facility within the last 24 hours.

4) Subsequent acute myocardial infarction
A code from category I22, Subsequent ST elevation (STEMI) and non-ST elevation (NSTEMI) myocardial infarction, is to be used when a patient who has suffered a type 1 or unspecified AMI has a new AMI within the 4 week time frame of the initial AMI. A code from category I22 must be used in conjunction with a code from category I21. The sequencing of the I22 and I21 codes depends on the circumstances of the encounter.

Do not assign code I22 for subsequent myocardial infarctions other than type 1 or unspecified. For subsequent type 2 AMI assign only code I21.A1. For subsequent type 4 or type 5 AMI, assign only code I21.A9.

If a subsequent myocardial infarction of one type occurs within 4 weeks of a myocardial infarction of a different type, assign the appropriate codes from category I21 to identify each type. Do not assign a code from I22. Codes from category I22 should only be assigned if both the initial and subsequent myocardial infarctions are type 1 or unspecified.

5) Other Types of Myocardial Infarction
The ICD-10-CM provides codes for different types of myocardial infarction. Type 1 myocardial infarctions are assigned to codes I21.0-I21.4.

Type 2 myocardial infarction (myocardial infarction due to demand ischemia or secondary to ischemic imbalance), is assigned to code I21.A1, Myocardial infarction type 2 with the underlying cause coded first. Do not assign code I24.8, Other forms of acute ischemic heart disease, for the demand ischemia. If a type 2 AMI is described as NSTEMI or STEMI, only assign code I21.A1. Codes I21.01-I21.4 should only be assigned for type 1 AMIs.

Acute myocardial infarctions type 3, 4a, 4b, 4c and 5 are assigned to code I21.A9, Other myocardial infarction type.

The "Code also" and "Code first" notes should be followed related to complications, and for coding of postprocedural myocardial infarctions during or following cardiac surgery.

10. Chapter 10: Diseases of the Respiratory System (J00-J99), *U07.0*

a. Chronic Obstructive Pulmonary Disease [COPD] and Asthma

1) Acute exacerbation of chronic obstructive bronchitis and asthma
The codes in categories J44 and J45 distinguish between uncomplicated cases and those in acute exacerbation. An acute exacerbation is a worsening or a decompensation of a chronic condition. An acute exacerbation is not equivalent to an infection superimposed on a chronic condition, though an exacerbation may be triggered by an infection.

b. Acute Respiratory Failure

1) Acute respiratory failure as principal diagnosis
A code from subcategory J96.0, Acute respiratory failure, or subcategory J96.2, Acute and chronic respiratory failure, may be assigned as a principal diagnosis when it is the condition established after study to be chiefly responsible for occasioning the admission to the hospital, and the selection is supported by the Alphabetic Index and Tabular List. However, chapter-specific coding guidelines (such as obstetrics, poisoning, HIV, newborn) that provide sequencing direction take precedence.

2) Acute respiratory failure as secondary diagnosis
Respiratory failure may be listed as a secondary diagnosis if it occurs after admission, or if it is present on admission, but does not meet the definition of principal diagnosis.

3) Sequencing of acute respiratory failure and another acute condition
When a patient is admitted with respiratory failure and another acute condition, (e.g., myocardial infarction, cerebrovascular accident, aspiration pneumonia), the principal diagnosis will not be the same in every situation. This applies whether the other acute condition is a respiratory or nonrespiratory condition. Selection of the principal diagnosis will be dependent on the circumstances of admission. If both the respiratory failure and the other acute condition are equally responsible for occasioning the admission to the hospital, and there are no chapter-specific sequencing rules, the guideline regarding two or more diagnoses that equally meet the definition for principal diagnosis *(Section II, C.)* may be applied in these situations.

If the documentation is not clear as to whether acute respiratory failure and another condition are equally responsible for occasioning the admission, query the provider for clarification.

c. Influenza due to certain identified influenza viruses

Code only confirmed cases of influenza due to certain identified influenza viruses (category JØ9), and due to other identified influenza virus (category J1Ø). This is an exception to the hospital inpatient guideline Section II, H. (Uncertain Diagnosis).

In this context, "confirmation" does not require documentation of positive laboratory testing specific for avian or other novel influenza A or other identified influenza virus. However, coding should be based on the provider's diagnostic statement that the patient has avian influenza, or other novel influenza A, for category JØ9, or has another particular identified strain of influenza, such as H1N1 or H3N2, but not identified as novel or variant, for category J1Ø.

If the provider records "suspected" or "possible" or "probable" avian influenza, or novel influenza, or other identified influenza, then the appropriate influenza code from category J11, Influenza due to unidentified influenza virus, should be assigned. A code from category JØ9, Influenza due to certain identified influenza viruses, should not be assigned nor should a code from category J1Ø, Influenza due to other identified influenza virus.

d. Ventilator associated Pneumonia

1) Documentation of Ventilator associated Pneumonia

As with all procedural or postprocedural complications, code assignment is based on the provider's documentation of the relationship between the condition and the procedure.

Code J95.851, Ventilator associated pneumonia, should be assigned only when the provider has documented ventilator associated pneumonia (VAP). An additional code to identify the organism (e.g., Pseudomonas aeruginosa, code B96.5) should also be assigned. Do not assign an additional code from categories J12-J18 to identify the type of pneumonia.

Code J95.851 should not be assigned for cases where the patient has pneumonia and is on a mechanical ventilator and the provider has not specifically stated that the pneumonia is ventilator-associated pneumonia. If the documentation is unclear as to whether the patient has a pneumonia that is a complication attributable to the mechanical ventilator, query the provider.

2) Ventilator associated Pneumonia Develops after Admission

A patient may be admitted with one type of pneumonia (e.g., code J13, Pneumonia due to Streptococcus pneumonia) and subsequently develop VAP. In this instance, the principal diagnosis would be the appropriate code from categories J12-J18 for the pneumonia diagnosed at the time of admission. Code J95.851, Ventilator associated pneumonia, would be assigned as an additional diagnosis when the provider has also documented the presence of ventilator associated pneumonia.

e. Vaping-related disorders

For patients presenting with condition(s) related to vaping, assign code UØ7.Ø, Vaping-related disorder, as the principal diagnosis. For lung injury due to vaping, assign only code UØ7.Ø. Assign additional codes for other manifestations, such as acute respiratory failure (subcategory J96.Ø-) or pneumonitis (code J68.Ø).

Associated respiratory signs and symptoms due to vaping, such as cough, shortness of breath, etc., are not coded separately, when a definitive diagnosis has been established. However, it would be appropriate to code separately any gastrointestinal symptoms, such as diarrhea and abdominal pain.

11. Chapter 11: Diseases of the Digestive System (KØØ-K95)

Reserved for future guideline expansion

12. Chapter 12: Diseases of the Skin and Subcutaneous Tissue (LØØ-L99)

a. Pressure ulcer stage codes

1) Pressure ulcer stages

Codes in category L89, Pressure ulcer, identify the site and stage of the pressure ulcer.

The ICD-10-CM classifies pressure ulcer stages based on severity, which is designated by stages 1-4, deep tissue pressure injury, unspecified stage and unstageable.

Assign as many codes from category L89 as needed to identify all the pressure ulcers the patient has, if applicable.

See Section I.B.14 for pressure ulcer stage documentation by clinicians other than patient's provider

2) Unstageable pressure ulcers

Assignment of the code for unstageable pressure ulcer (L89.--Ø) should be based on the clinical documentation. These codes are used for pressure ulcers whose stage cannot be clinically determined (e.g., the ulcer is covered by eschar or has been treated with a skin or muscle graft). This code should not be confused with the codes for unspecified stage (L89.--9). When there is no documentation regarding the stage of the pressure ulcer, assign the appropriate code for unspecified stage (L89.--9).

3) Documented pressure ulcer stage

Assignment of the pressure ulcer stage code should be guided by clinical documentation of the stage or documentation of the terms found in the Alphabetic Index. For clinical terms describing the stage that are not found in the Alphabetic Index, and there is no documentation of the stage, the provider should be queried.

4) Patients admitted with pressure ulcers documented as healed

No code is assigned if the documentation states that the pressure ulcer is completely healed at the time of admission.

5) Pressure ulcers documented as healing

Pressure ulcers described as healing should be assigned the appropriate pressure ulcer stage code based on the documentation in the medical record. If the documentation does not provide information about the stage of the healing pressure ulcer, assign the appropriate code for unspecified stage.

If the documentation is unclear as to whether the patient has a current (new) pressure ulcer or if the patient is being treated for a healing pressure ulcer, query the provider.

For ulcers that were present on admission but healed at the time of discharge, assign the code for the site and stage of the pressure ulcer at the time of admission.

6) Patient admitted with pressure ulcer evolving into another stage during the admission

If a patient is admitted to an inpatient hospital with a pressure ulcer at one stage and it progresses to a higher stage, two separate codes should be assigned: one code for the site and stage of the ulcer on admission and a second code for the same ulcer site and the highest stage reported during the stay.

7) Pressure-induced deep tissue damage

For pressure-induced deep tissue damage or deep tissue pressure injury, assign only the appropriate code for pressure-induced deep tissue damage (L89.--6).

b. Non-Pressure Chronic Ulcers

1) Patients admitted with non-pressure ulcers documented as healed

No code is assigned if the documentation states that the non-pressure ulcer is completely healed at the time of admission.

2) Non-pressure ulcers documented as healing

Non-pressure ulcers described as healing should be assigned the appropriate non-pressure ulcer code based on the documentation in the medical record. If the documentation does not provide information about the severity of the healing non-pressure ulcer, assign the appropriate code for unspecified severity.

If the documentation is unclear as to whether the patient has a current (new) non-pressure ulcer or if the patient is being treated for a healing non-pressure ulcer, query the provider.

For ulcers that were present on admission but healed at the time of discharge, assign the code for the site and severity of the non-pressure ulcer at the time of admission.

3) Patient admitted with non-pressure ulcer that progresses to another severity level during the admission

If a patient is admitted to an inpatient hospital with a non-pressure ulcer at one severity level and it progresses to a higher severity level, two separate codes should be assigned: one code for the site and severity level of the ulcer on admission and a second code for the same ulcer site and the highest severity level reported during the stay.

See Section I.B.14 for pressure ulcer stage documentation by clinicians other than patient's provider

13. **Chapter 13: Diseases of the Musculoskeletal System and Connective Tissue (M00-M99)**

a. **Site and laterality**

Most of the codes within Chapter 13 have site and laterality designations. The site represents the bone, joint or the muscle involved. For some conditions where more than one bone, joint or muscle is usually involved, such as osteoarthritis, there is a "multiple sites" code available. For categories where no multiple site code is provided and more than one bone, joint or muscle is involved, multiple codes should be used to indicate the different sites involved.

1) **Bone versus joint**

For certain conditions, the bone may be affected at the upper or lower end, (e.g., avascular necrosis of bone, M87, Osteoporosis, M80, M81). Though the portion of the bone affected may be at the joint, the site designation will be the bone, not the joint.

b. **Acute traumatic versus chronic or recurrent musculoskeletal conditions**

Many musculoskeletal conditions are a result of previous injury or trauma to a site, or are recurrent conditions. Bone, joint or muscle conditions that are the result of a healed injury are usually found in chapter 13. Recurrent bone, joint or muscle conditions are also usually found in chapter 13. Any current, acute injury should be coded to the appropriate injury code from chapter 19. Chronic or recurrent conditions should generally be coded with a code from chapter 13. If it is difficult to determine from the documentation in the record which code is best to describe a condition, query the provider.

c. **Coding of Pathologic Fractures**

7th character A is for use as long as the patient is receiving active treatment for the fracture. While the patient may be seen by a new or different provider over the course of treatment for a pathological fracture, assignment of the 7th character is based on whether the patient is undergoing active treatment and not whether the provider is seeing the patient for the first time.

7th character D is to be used for encounters after the patient has completed active treatment for the fracture and is receiving routine care for the fracture during the healing or recovery phase. The other 7th characters, listed under each subcategory in the Tabular List, are to be used for subsequent encounters for treatment of problems associated with the healing, such as malunions, nonunions, and sequelae.

Care for complications of surgical treatment for fracture repairs during the healing or recovery phase should be coded with the appropriate complication codes.

See Section I.C.19. Coding of traumatic fractures.

d. **Osteoporosis**

Osteoporosis is a systemic condition, meaning that all bones of the musculoskeletal system are affected. Therefore, site is not a component of the codes under category M81, Osteoporosis without current pathological fracture. The site codes under category M80, Osteoporosis with current pathological fracture, identify the site of the fracture, not the osteoporosis.

1) **Osteoporosis without pathological fracture**

Category M81, Osteoporosis without current pathological fracture, is for use for patients with osteoporosis who do not currently have a pathologic fracture due to the osteoporosis, even if they have had a fracture in the past. For patients with a history of osteoporosis fractures, status code Z87.310, Personal history of (healed) osteoporosis fracture, should follow the code from M81.

2) **Osteoporosis with current pathological fracture**

Category M80, Osteoporosis with current pathological fracture, is for patients who have a current pathologic fracture at the time of an encounter. The codes under M80 identify the site of the fracture. A code from category M80, not a traumatic fracture code, should be used for any patient with known osteoporosis who suffers a fracture, even if the patient had a minor fall or trauma, if that fall or trauma would not usually break a normal, healthy bone.

14. **Chapter 14: Diseases of Genitourinary System (N00-N99)**

a. **Chronic kidney disease**

1) **Stages of chronic kidney disease (CKD)**

The ICD-10-CM classifies CKD based on severity. The severity of CKD is designated by stages 1-5. Stage 2, code N18.2, equates to mild CKD; stage 3, **codes N18.30-N18.32, equate** to moderate CKD; and stage 4, code N18.4, equates to severe CKD. Code N18.6, End stage renal disease (ESRD), is assigned when the provider has documented end-stage-renal disease (ESRD).

If both a stage of CKD and ESRD are documented, assign code N18.6 only.

2) **Chronic kidney disease and kidney transplant status**

Patients who have undergone kidney transplant may still have some form of chronic kidney disease (CKD) because the kidney transplant may not fully restore kidney function. Therefore, the presence of CKD alone does not constitute a transplant complication. Assign the appropriate N18 code for the patient's stage of CKD and code Z94.0, Kidney transplant status. If a transplant complication such as failure or rejection or other transplant complication is documented, see section I.C.19.g for information on coding complications of a kidney transplant. If the documentation is unclear as to whether the patient has a complication of the transplant, query the provider.

3) **Chronic kidney disease with other conditions**

Patients with CKD may also suffer from other serious conditions, most commonly diabetes mellitus and hypertension. The sequencing of the CKD code in relationship to codes for other contributing conditions is based on the conventions in the Tabular List.

See I.C.9. Hypertensive chronic kidney disease.

See I.C.19. Chronic kidney disease and kidney transplant complications.

15. **Chapter 15: Pregnancy, Childbirth, and the Puerperium (O00-O9A)**

a. **General Rules for Obstetric Cases**

1) **Codes from chapter 15 and sequencing priority**

Obstetric cases require codes from chapter 15, codes in the range O00-O9A, Pregnancy, Childbirth, and the Puerperium. Chapter 15 codes have sequencing priority over codes from other chapters. Additional codes from other chapters may be used in conjunction with chapter 15 codes to further specify conditions. Should the provider document that the pregnancy is incidental to the encounter, then code Z33.1, Pregnant state, incidental, should be used in place of any chapter 15 codes. It is the provider's responsibility to state that the condition being treated is not affecting the pregnancy.

2) **Chapter 15 codes used only on the maternal record**

Chapter 15 codes are to be used only on the maternal record, never on the record of the newborn.

3) **Final character for trimester**

The majority of codes in Chapter 15 have a final character indicating the trimester of pregnancy. The timeframes for the trimesters are indicated at the beginning of the chapter. If trimester is not a component of a code, it is because the condition always occurs in a specific trimester, or the concept of trimester of pregnancy is not applicable. Certain codes have characters for only certain trimesters because the condition does not occur in all trimesters, but it may occur in more than just one.

Assignment of the final character for trimester should be based on the provider's documentation of the trimester (or number of weeks) for the current admission/encounter. This applies to the assignment of trimester for pre-existing conditions as well as those that develop during or are due to the pregnancy. The provider's documentation of the number of weeks may be used to assign the appropriate code identifying the trimester.

Whenever delivery occurs during the current admission, and there is an "in childbirth" option for the obstetric complication being coded, the "in childbirth" code should be assigned.

4) **Selection of trimester for inpatient admissions that encompass more than one trimester**

In instances when a patient is admitted to a hospital for complications of pregnancy during one trimester and remains in the hospital into a subsequent trimester, the trimester character for the antepartum complication code should be assigned on the basis of the trimester when the complication developed, not the trimester of the discharge. If the condition developed prior to the current admission/encounter or represents a pre-existing condition, the trimester character for the trimester at the time of the admission/encounter should be assigned.

5) **Unspecified trimester**

Each category that includes codes for trimester has a code for "unspecified trimester." The "unspecified trimester" code should rarely be used, such as when the documentation in the record is insufficient to determine the trimester and it is not possible to obtain clarification.

6) **7th character for Fetus Identification**
Where applicable, a 7th character is to be assigned for certain categories (O31, O32, O33.3 - O33.6, O35, O36, O40, O41, O60.1, O60.2, O64, and O69) to identify the fetus for which the complication code applies.

Assign 7th character "0":

- For single gestations
- When the documentation in the record is insufficient to determine the fetus affected and it is not possible to obtain clarification.
- When it is not possible to clinically determine which fetus is affected.

b. Selection of OB Principal or First-listed Diagnosis

1) **Routine outpatient prenatal visits**
For routine outpatient prenatal visits when no complications are present, a code from category Z34, Encounter for supervision of normal pregnancy, should be used as the first-listed diagnosis. These codes should not be used in conjunction with chapter 15 codes.

2) **Supervision of High-Risk Pregnancy**
Codes from category O09, Supervision of high-risk pregnancy, are intended for use only during the prenatal period. For complications during the labor or delivery episode as a result of a high-risk pregnancy, assign the applicable complication codes from Chapter 15. If there are no complications during the labor or delivery episode, assign code O80, Encounter for full-term uncomplicated delivery.

For routine prenatal outpatient visits for patients with high-risk pregnancies, a code from category O09, Supervision of high-risk pregnancy, should be used as the first-listed diagnosis. Secondary chapter 15 codes may be used in conjunction with these codes if appropriate.

3) **Episodes when no delivery occurs**
In episodes when no delivery occurs, the principal diagnosis should correspond to the principal complication of the pregnancy which necessitated the encounter. Should more than one complication exist, all of which are treated or monitored, any of the complication codes may be sequenced first.

4) **When a delivery occurs**
When an obstetric patient is admitted and delivers during that admission, the condition that prompted the admission should be sequenced as the principal diagnosis. If multiple conditions prompted the admission, sequence the one most related to the delivery as the principal diagnosis. A code for any complication of the delivery should be assigned as an additional diagnosis. In cases of cesarean delivery, if the patient was admitted with a condition that resulted in the performance of a cesarean procedure, that condition should be selected as the principal diagnosis. If the reason for the admission was unrelated to the condition resulting in the cesarean delivery, the condition related to the reason for the admission should be selected as the principal diagnosis.

5) **Outcome of delivery**
A code from category Z37, Outcome of delivery, should be included on every maternal record when a delivery has occurred. These codes are not to be used on subsequent records or on the newborn record.

c. Pre-existing conditions versus conditions due to the pregnancy
Certain categories in Chapter 15 distinguish between conditions of the mother that existed prior to pregnancy (pre-existing) and those that are a direct result of pregnancy. When assigning codes from Chapter 15, it is important to assess if a condition was pre-existing prior to pregnancy or developed during or due to the pregnancy in order to assign the correct code.

Categories that do not distinguish between pre-existing and pregnancy-related conditions may be used for either. It is acceptable to use codes specifically for the puerperium with codes complicating pregnancy and childbirth if a condition arises postpartum during the delivery encounter.

d. Pre-existing hypertension in pregnancy
Category O10, Pre-existing hypertension complicating pregnancy, childbirth and the puerperium, includes codes for hypertensive heart and hypertensive chronic kidney disease. When assigning one of the O10 codes that includes hypertensive heart disease or hypertensive chronic kidney disease, it is necessary to add a secondary code from the appropriate hypertension category to specify the type of heart failure or chronic kidney disease.

See Section I.C.9. Hypertension.

e. Fetal Conditions Affecting the Management of the Mother

1) **Codes from categories O35 and O36**
Codes from categories O35, Maternal care for known or suspected fetal abnormality and damage, and O36, Maternal care for other fetal problems, are assigned only when the fetal condition is actually responsible for modifying the management of the mother, i.e., by requiring diagnostic studies, additional observation, special care, or termination of pregnancy. The fact that the fetal condition exists does not justify assigning a code from this series to the mother's record.

2) **In utero surgery**
In cases when surgery is performed on the fetus, a diagnosis code from category O35, Maternal care for known or suspected fetal abnormality and damage, should be assigned identifying the fetal condition. Assign the appropriate procedure code for the procedure performed.

No code from Chapter 16, the perinatal codes, should be used on the mother's record to identify fetal conditions. Surgery performed in utero on a fetus is still to be coded as an obstetric encounter.

f. HIV Infection in Pregnancy, Childbirth and the Puerperium
During pregnancy, childbirth or the puerperium, a patient admitted because of an HIV-related illness should receive a principal diagnosis from subcategory O98.7-, Human immunodeficiency [HIV] disease complicating pregnancy, childbirth and the puerperium, followed by the code(s) for the HIV-related illness(es).

Patients with asymptomatic HIV infection status admitted during pregnancy, childbirth, or the puerperium should receive codes of O98.7- and Z21, Asymptomatic human immunodeficiency virus [HIV] infection status.

g. Diabetes mellitus in pregnancy
Diabetes mellitus is a significant complicating factor in pregnancy. Pregnant women who are diabetic should be assigned a code from category O24, Diabetes mellitus in pregnancy, childbirth, and the puerperium, first, followed by the appropriate diabetes code(s) (E08-E13) from Chapter 4.

h. Long term use of insulin and oral hypoglycemics
See section I.C.4.a.3 for information on the long-term use of insulin and oral hypoglycemics.

i. Gestational (pregnancy induced) diabetes
Gestational (pregnancy induced) diabetes can occur during the second and third trimester of pregnancy in women who were not diabetic prior to pregnancy. Gestational diabetes can cause complications in the pregnancy similar to those of pre-existing diabetes mellitus. It also puts the woman at greater risk of developing diabetes after the pregnancy. Codes for gestational diabetes are in subcategory O24.4, Gestational diabetes mellitus. No other code from category O24, Diabetes mellitus in pregnancy, childbirth, and the puerperium, should be used with a code from O24.4.

The codes under subcategory O24.4 include diet controlled, insulin controlled, and controlled by oral hypoglycemic drugs. If a patient with gestational diabetes is treated with both diet and insulin, only the code for insulin-controlled is required. If a patient with gestational diabetes is treated with both diet and oral hypoglycemic medications, only the code for "controlled by oral hypoglycemic drugs" is required. Code Z79.4, Long-term (current) use of insulin or code Z79.84, Long-term (current) use of oral hypoglycemic drugs, should not be assigned with codes from subcategory O24.4.

An abnormal glucose tolerance in pregnancy is assigned a code from subcategory O99.81, Abnormal glucose complicating pregnancy, childbirth, and the puerperium.

j. Sepsis and septic shock complicating abortion, pregnancy, childbirth and the puerperium
When assigning a chapter 15 code for sepsis complicating abortion, pregnancy, childbirth, and the puerperium, a code for the specific type of infection should be assigned as an additional diagnosis. If severe sepsis is present, a code from subcategory R65.2, Severe sepsis, and code(s) for associated organ dysfunction(s) should also be assigned as additional diagnoses.

k. Puerperal sepsis

Code O85, Puerperal sepsis, should be assigned with a secondary code to identify the causal organism (e.g., for a bacterial infection, assign a code from category B95-B96, Bacterial infections in conditions classified elsewhere). A code from category A4Ø, Streptococcal sepsis, or A41, Other sepsis, should not be used for puerperal sepsis. If applicable, use additional codes to identify severe sepsis (R65.2-) and any associated acute organ dysfunction.

Code O85 should not be assigned for sepsis following an obstetrical procedure (See Section I.C.1.d.5.b., Sepsis due to a postprocedural infection).

l. Alcohol, tobacco and drug use during pregnancy, childbirth and the puerperium

1) Alcohol use during pregnancy, childbirth and the puerperium

Codes under subcategory O99.31, Alcohol use complicating pregnancy, childbirth, and the puerperium, should be assigned for any pregnancy case when a mother uses alcohol during the pregnancy or postpartum. A secondary code from category F1Ø, Alcohol related disorders, should also be assigned to identify manifestations of the alcohol use.

2) Tobacco use during pregnancy, childbirth and the puerperium

Codes under subcategory O99.33, Smoking (tobacco) complicating pregnancy, childbirth, and the puerperium, should be assigned for any pregnancy case when a mother uses any type of tobacco product during the pregnancy or postpartum. A secondary code from category F17, Nicotine dependence, should also be assigned to identify the type of nicotine dependence.

3) Drug use during pregnancy, childbirth and the puerperium

Codes under subcategory O99.32, Drug use complicating pregnancy, childbirth, and the puerperium, should be assigned for any pregnancy case when a mother uses drugs during the pregnancy or postpartum. This can involve illegal drugs, or inappropriate use or abuse of prescription drugs. Secondary code(s) from categories F11-F16 and F18-F19 should also be assigned to identify manifestations of the drug use.

m. Poisoning, toxic effects, adverse effects and underdosing in a pregnant patient

A code from subcategory O9A.2, Injury, poisoning and certain other consequences of external causes complicating pregnancy, childbirth, and the puerperium, should be sequenced first, followed by the appropriate injury, poisoning, toxic effect, adverse effect or underdosing code, and then the additional code(s) that specifies the condition caused by the poisoning, toxic effect, adverse effect or underdosing.

See Section I.C.19. Adverse effects, poisoning, underdosing and toxic effects.

n. Normal Delivery, Code O8Ø

1) Encounter for full term uncomplicated delivery

Code O8Ø should be assigned when a woman is admitted for a full-term normal delivery and delivers a single, healthy infant without any complications antepartum, during the delivery, or postpartum during the delivery episode. Code O8Ø is always a principal diagnosis. It is not to be used if any other code from chapter 15 is needed to describe a current complication of the antenatal, delivery, or postnatal period. Additional codes from other chapters may be used with code O8Ø if they are not related to or are in any way complicating the pregnancy.

2) Uncomplicated delivery with resolved antepartum complication

Code O8Ø may be used if the patient had a complication at some point during the pregnancy, but the complication is not present at the time of the admission for delivery.

3) Outcome of delivery for O8Ø

Z37.Ø, Single live birth, is the only outcome of delivery code appropriate for use with O8Ø.

o. The Peripartum and Postpartum Periods

1) Peripartum and Postpartum periods

The postpartum period begins immediately after delivery and continues for six weeks following delivery. The peripartum period is defined as the last month of pregnancy to five months postpartum.

2) Peripartum and postpartum complication

A postpartum complication is any complication occurring within the six-week period.

3) Pregnancy-related complications after 6-week period

Chapter 15 codes may also be used to describe pregnancy-related complications after the peripartum or postpartum period if the provider documents that a condition is pregnancy related.

4) Admission for routine postpartum care following delivery outside hospital

When the mother delivers outside the hospital prior to admission and is admitted for routine postpartum care and no complications are noted, code Z39.Ø, Encounter for care and examination of mother immediately after delivery, should be assigned as the principal diagnosis.

5) Pregnancy associated cardiomyopathy

Pregnancy associated cardiomyopathy, code O9Ø.3, is unique in that it may be diagnosed in the third trimester of pregnancy but may continue to progress months after delivery. For this reason, it is referred to as peripartum cardiomyopathy. Code O9Ø.3 is only for use when the cardiomyopathy develops as a result of pregnancy in a woman who did not have pre-existing heart disease.

p. Code O94, Sequelae of complication of pregnancy, childbirth, and the puerperium

1) Code O94

Code O94, Sequelae of complication of pregnancy, childbirth, and the puerperium, is for use in those cases when an initial complication of a pregnancy develops a sequelae requiring care or treatment at a future date.

2) After the initial postpartum period

This code may be used at any time after the initial postpartum period.

3) Sequencing of Code O94

This code, like all sequela codes, is to be sequenced following the code describing the sequelae of the complication.

q. Termination of Pregnancy and Spontaneous abortions

1) Abortion with Liveborn Fetus

When an attempted termination of pregnancy results in a liveborn fetus, assign code Z33.2, Encounter for elective termination of pregnancy and a code from category Z37, Outcome of Delivery.

2) Retained Products of Conception following an abortion

Subsequent encounters for retained products of conception following a spontaneous abortion or elective termination of pregnancy, without complications are assigned OØ3.4, Incomplete spontaneous abortion without complication, or code OØ7.4, Failed attempted termination of pregnancy without complication. This advice is appropriate even when the patient was discharged previously with a discharge diagnosis of complete abortion. If the patient has a specific complication associated with the spontaneous abortion or elective termination of pregnancy in addition to retained products of conception, assign the appropriate complication code (e.g., OØ3.-, OØ4.-, OØ7.-) instead of code OØ3.4 or OØ7.4

3) Complications leading to abortion

Codes from Chapter 15 may be used as additional codes to identify any documented complications of the pregnancy in conjunction with codes in categories in OØ4, OØ7 and OØ8.

r. Abuse in a pregnant patient

For suspected or confirmed cases of abuse of a pregnant patient, a code(s) from subcategories O9A.3, Physical abuse complicating pregnancy, childbirth, and the puerperium, O9A.4, Sexual abuse complicating pregnancy, childbirth, and the puerperium, and O9A.5, Psychological abuse complicating pregnancy, childbirth, and the puerperium, should be sequenced first, followed by the appropriate codes (if applicable) to identify any associated current injury due to physical abuse, sexual abuse, and the perpetrator of abuse.

See Section I.C.19. Adult and child abuse, neglect and other maltreatment.

s. **COVID-19 infection in pregnancy, childbirth, and the puerperium During pregnancy, childbirth or the puerperium, when COVID-19 is the reason for admission/encounter, code O98.5-, Other viral diseases complicating pregnancy, childbirth and the puerperium, should be sequenced as the principal/first-listed diagnosis, and code U07.1, COVID-19, and the appropriate codes for associated manifestation(s) should be assigned as additional diagnoses. Codes from Chapter 15 always take sequencing priority.**

If the reason for admission/encounter is unrelated to COVID-19 but the patient tests positive for COVID-19 during the admission/encounter, the appropriate code for the reason for admission/encounter should be sequenced as the principal/first-listed diagnosis, and codes O98.5- and U07.1, as well as the appropriate codes for associated COVID-19 manifestations, should be assigned as additional diagnoses.

16. **Chapter 16: Certain Conditions Originating in the Perinatal Period (P00-P96)**

For coding and reporting purposes the perinatal period is defined as before birth through the 28th day following birth. The following guidelines are provided for reporting purposes.

a. **General Perinatal Rules**

1) **Use of Chapter 16 Codes**

Codes in this chapter are <u>never</u> for use on the maternal record. Codes from Chapter 15, the obstetric chapter, are never permitted on the newborn record. Chapter 16 codes may be used throughout the life of the patient if the condition is still present.

2) **Principal Diagnosis for Birth Record**

When coding the birth episode in a newborn record, assign a code from category Z38, Liveborn infants according to place of birth and type of delivery, as the principal diagnosis. A code from category Z38 is assigned only once, to a newborn at the time of birth. If a newborn is transferred to another institution, a code from category Z38 should not be used at the receiving hospital.

A code from category Z38 is used only on the newborn record, not on the mother's record.

3) **Use of Codes from other Chapters with Codes from Chapter 16**

Codes from other chapters may be used with codes from chapter 16 if the codes from the other chapters provide more specific detail. Codes for signs and symptoms may be assigned when a definitive diagnosis has not been established. If the reason for the encounter is a perinatal condition, the code from chapter 16 should be sequenced first.

4) **Use of Chapter 16 Codes after the Perinatal Period**

Should a condition originate in the perinatal period, and continue throughout the life of the patient, the perinatal code should continue to be used regardless of the patient's age.

5) **Birth process or community acquired conditions**

If a newborn has a condition that may be either due to the birth process or community acquired and the documentation does not indicate which it is, the default is due to the birth process and the code from Chapter 16 should be used. If the condition is community-acquired, a code from Chapter 16 should not be assigned.

<u>**For COVID-19 infection in a newborn, see guideline I.C.16.h.**</u>

6) **Code all clinically significant conditions**

All clinically significant conditions noted on routine newborn examination should be coded. A condition is clinically significant if it requires:

- clinical evaluation; or
- therapeutic treatment; or
- diagnostic procedures; or
- extended length of hospital stay; or
- increased nursing care and/or monitoring; or
- has implications for future health care needs

Note: The perinatal guidelines listed above are the same as the general coding guidelines for "additional diagnoses," except for the final point regarding implications for future health care needs. Codes should be assigned for conditions that have been specified by the provider as having implications for future health care needs.

b. **Observation and Evaluation of Newborns for Suspected Conditions not Found**

1) **Use of Z05 codes**

Assign a code from category Z05, Observation and evaluation of newborns and infants for suspected conditions ruled out, to identify those instances when a healthy newborn is evaluated for a suspected condition that is determined after study not to be present. Do not use a code from category Z05 when the patient has identified signs or symptoms of a suspected problem; in such cases code the sign or symptom.

2) **Z05 on other than the birth record**

A code from category Z05 may also be assigned as a principal or first-listed code for readmissions or encounters when the code from category Z38 code no longer applies. Codes from category Z05 are for use only for healthy newborns and infants for which no condition after study is found to be present.

3) **Z05 on a birth record**

A code from category Z05 is to be used as a secondary code after the code from category Z38, Liveborn infants according to place of birth and type of delivery.

c. **Coding Additional Perinatal Diagnoses**

1) **Assigning codes for conditions that require treatment**

Assign codes for conditions that require treatment or further investigation, prolong the length of stay, or require resource utilization.

2) **Codes for conditions specified as having implications for future health care needs**

Assign codes for conditions that have been specified by the provider as having implications for future health care needs.

Note: This guideline should not be used for adult patients.

d. **Prematurity and Fetal Growth Retardation**

Providers utilize different criteria in determining prematurity. A code for prematurity should not be assigned unless it is documented. Assignment of codes in categories P05, Disorders of newborn related to slow fetal growth and fetal malnutrition, and P07, Disorders of newborn related to short gestation and low birth weight, not elsewhere classified, should be based on the recorded birth weight and estimated gestational age.

When both birth weight and gestational age are available, two codes from category P07 should be assigned, with the code for birth weight sequenced before the code for gestational age.

e. **Low birth weight and immaturity status**

Codes from category P07, Disorders of newborn related to short gestation and low birth weight, not elsewhere classified, are for use for a child or adult who was premature or had a low birth weight as a newborn and this is affecting the patient's current health status.

See Section I.C.21. Factors influencing health status and contact with health services, Status.

f. **Bacterial Sepsis of Newborn**

Category P36, Bacterial sepsis of newborn, includes congenital sepsis. If a perinate is documented as having sepsis without documentation of congenital or community acquired, the default is congenital and a code from category P36 should be assigned. If the P36 code includes the causal organism, an additional code from category B95, Streptococcus, Staphylococcus, and Enterococcus as the cause of diseases classified elsewhere, or B96, Other bacterial agents as the cause of diseases classified elsewhere, should not be assigned. If the P36 code does not include the causal organism, assign an additional code from category B96. If applicable, use additional codes to identify severe sepsis (R65.2-) and any associated acute organ dysfunction.

g. **Stillbirth**

Code P95, Stillbirth, is only for use in institutions that maintain separate records for stillbirths. No other code should be used with P95. Code P95 should not be used on the mother's record.

h. **COVID-19 Infection in Newborn**

For a newborn that tests positive for COVID-19, assign code U07.1, COVID-19, and the appropriate codes for associated manifestation(s) in neonates/newborns in the absence of documentation indicating a specific type of transmission. For a newborn that tests positive for COVID-19 and the provider documents the condition was contracted in utero or during the birth process, assign codes P35.8, Other congenital viral diseases, and U07.1, COVID-19. When coding the birth episode in a newborn record, the appropriate code from category Z38,

Liveborn infants according to place of birth and type of delivery, should be assigned as the principal diagnosis.

17. **Chapter 17: Congenital malformations, deformations, and chromosomal abnormalities (Q00-Q99)**
Assign an appropriate code(s) from categories Q00-Q99, Congenital malformations, deformations, and chromosomal abnormalities when a malformation/deformation or chromosomal abnormality is documented. A malformation/deformation/or chromosomal abnormality may be the principal/first-listed diagnosis on a record or a secondary diagnosis.

When a malformation/deformation or chromosomal abnormality does not have a unique code assignment, assign additional code(s) for any manifestations that may be present.

When the code assignment specifically identifies the malformation/deformation or chromosomal abnormality, manifestations that are an inherent component of the anomaly should not be coded separately. Additional codes should be assigned for manifestations that are not an inherent component.

Codes from Chapter 17 may be used throughout the life of the patient. If a congenital malformation or deformity has been corrected, a personal history code should be used to identify the history of the malformation or deformity. Although present at birth, a malformation/deformation/or chromosomal abnormality may not be identified until later in life. Whenever the condition is diagnosed by the provider, it is appropriate to assign a code from codes Q00-Q99. For the birth admission, the appropriate code from category Z38, Liveborn infants, according to place of birth and type of delivery, should be sequenced as the principal diagnosis, followed by any congenital anomaly codes, Q00- Q99.

18. **Chapter 18: Symptoms, signs, and abnormal clinical and laboratory findings, not elsewhere classified (R00-R99)**
Chapter 18 includes symptoms, signs, abnormal results of clinical or other investigative procedures, and ill-defined conditions regarding which no diagnosis classifiable elsewhere is recorded. Signs and symptoms that point to a specific diagnosis have been assigned to a category in other chapters of the classification.

a. **Use of symptom codes**
Codes that describe symptoms and signs are acceptable for reporting purposes when a related definitive diagnosis has not been established (confirmed) by the provider.

b. **Use of a symptom code with a definitive diagnosis code**
Codes for signs and symptoms may be reported in addition to a related definitive diagnosis when the sign or symptom is not routinely associated with that diagnosis, such as the various signs and symptoms associated with complex syndromes. The definitive diagnosis code should be sequenced before the symptom code.

Signs or symptoms that are associated routinely with a disease process should not be assigned as additional codes, unless otherwise instructed by the classification.

c. **Combination codes that include symptoms**
ICD-10-CM contains a number of combination codes that identify both the definitive diagnosis and common symptoms of that diagnosis.

When using one of these combination codes, an additional code should not be assigned for the symptom.

d. **Repeated falls**
Code R29.6, Repeated falls, is for use for encounters when a patient has recently fallen and the reason for the fall is being investigated.

Code Z91.81, History of falling, is for use when a patient has fallen in the past and is at risk for future falls. When appropriate, both codes R29.6 and Z91.81 may be assigned together.

e. **Coma scale**
The coma scale codes (R40.2-) can be used in conjunction with traumatic brain injury codes. These codes are primarily for use by trauma registries, but they may be used in any setting where this information is collected. The coma scale codes should be sequenced after the diagnosis code(s).

These codes, one from each subcategory, are needed to complete the scale. The 7th character indicates when the scale was recorded. The 7th character should match for all three codes.

At a minimum, report the initial score documented on presentation at your facility. This may be a score from the emergency medicine technician (EMT) or in the emergency department. If desired, a facility may choose to capture multiple coma scale scores.

Assign code R40.24, Glasgow coma scale, total score, when only the total score is documented in the medical record and not the individual score(s).

Do not report codes for individual or total Glasgow coma scale scores for a patient with a medically induced coma or a sedated patient.

See Section I.B.14 for coma scale documentation by clinicians other than patient's provider

f. **Functional quadriplegia**
GUIDELINE HAS BEEN DELETED EFFECTIVE OCTOBER 1, 2017

g. **SIRS due to Non-Infectious Process**
The systemic inflammatory response syndrome (SIRS) can develop as a result of certain non-infectious disease processes, such as trauma, malignant neoplasm, or pancreatitis. When SIRS is documented with a noninfectious condition, and no subsequent infection is documented, the code for the underlying condition, such as an injury, should be assigned, followed by code R65.10, Systemic inflammatory response syndrome (SIRS) of non-infectious origin without acute organ dysfunction, or code R65.11, Systemic inflammatory response syndrome (SIRS) of non-infectious origin with acute organ dysfunction. If an associated acute organ dysfunction is documented, the appropriate code(s) for the specific type of organ dysfunction(s) should be assigned in addition to code R65.11. If acute organ dysfunction is documented, but it cannot be determined if the acute organ dysfunction is associated with SIRS or due to another condition (e.g., directly due to the trauma), the provider should be queried.

h. **Death NOS**
Code R99, Ill-defined and unknown cause of mortality, is only for use in the very limited circumstance when a patient who has already died is brought into an emergency department or other healthcare facility and is pronounced dead upon arrival. It does not represent the discharge disposition of death.

i. **NIHSS Stroke Scale**
The NIH stroke scale (NIHSS) codes (R29.7- -) can be used in conjunction with acute stroke codes (I63) to identify the patient's neurological status and the severity of the stroke. The stroke scale codes should be sequenced after the acute stroke diagnosis code(s).

At a minimum, report the initial score documented. If desired, a facility may choose to capture multiple stroke scale scores.

See Section I.B.14 for NIHSS stroke scale documentation by clinicians other than patient's provider

19. **Chapter 19: Injury, poisoning, and certain other consequences of external causes (S00-T88)**

a. **Application of 7th Characters in Chapter 19**
Most categories in chapter 19 have a 7th character requirement for each applicable code. Most categories in this chapter have three 7th character values (with the exception of fractures): A, initial encounter, D, subsequent encounter and S, sequela. Categories for traumatic fractures have additional 7th character values. While the patient may be seen by a new or different provider over the course of treatment for an injury, assignment of the 7th character is based on whether the patient is undergoing active treatment and not whether the provider is seeing the patient for the first time.

For complication codes, active treatment refers to treatment for the condition described by the code, even though it may be related to an earlier precipitating problem. For example, code T84.50XA, Infection and inflammatory reaction due to unspecified internal joint prosthesis, initial encounter, is used when active treatment is provided for the infection, even though the condition relates to the prosthetic device, implant or graft that was placed at a previous encounter.

7th character "A", initial encounter is used for each encounter where the patient is receiving active treatment for the condition.

7th character "D" subsequent encounter is used for encounters after the patient has completed active treatment of the condition and is receiving routine care for the condition during the healing or recovery phase.

The aftercare Z codes should not be used for aftercare for conditions such as injuries or poisonings, where 7th characters are provided to identify subsequent care. For example, for aftercare of an injury, assign the acute injury code with the 7th character "D" (subsequent encounter).

7th character "S", sequela, is for use for complications or conditions that arise as a direct result of a condition, such as scar formation after a burn. The scars are sequelae of the burn. When using 7th character "S", it is necessary to use both the injury code that precipitated the sequela and the code for the sequela itself. The "S" is added only to the injury code, not the sequela code. The 7th character "S" identifies the injury responsible for the sequela. The specific type of sequela (e.g. scar) is sequenced first, followed by the injury code.

See Section I.B.10 Sequelae, (Late Effects)

b. Coding of Injuries

When coding injuries, assign separate codes for each injury unless a combination code is provided, in which case the combination code is assigned. Codes from category TØ7, Unspecified multiple injuries should not be assigned in the inpatient setting unless information for a more specific code is not available. Traumatic injury codes (SØØ-T14.9) are not to be used for normal, healing surgical wounds or to identify complications of surgical wounds.

The code for the most serious injury, as determined by the provider and the focus of treatment, is sequenced first.

1) Superficial injuries

Superficial injuries such as abrasions or contusions are not coded when associated with more severe injuries of the same site.

2) Primary injury with damage to nerves/blood vessels

When a primary injury results in minor damage to peripheral nerves or blood vessels, the primary injury is sequenced first with additional code(s) for injuries to nerves and spinal cord (such as category SØ4), and/or injury to blood vessels (such as category S15). When the primary injury is to the blood vessels or nerves, that injury should be sequenced first.

3) Iatrogenic injuries

Injury codes from Chapter 19 should not be assigned for injuries that occur during, or as a result of, a medical intervention. Assign the appropriate complication code(s).

c. Coding of Traumatic Fractures

The principles of multiple coding of injuries should be followed in coding fractures. Fractures of specified sites are coded individually by site in accordance with both the provisions within categories SØ2, S12, S22, S32, S42, S49, S52, S59, S62, S72, S79, S82, S89, S92 and the level of detail furnished by medical record content.

A fracture not indicated as open or closed should be coded to closed. A fracture not indicated whether displaced or not displaced should be coded to displaced.

More specific guidelines are as follows:

1) Initial vs. subsequent encounter for fractures

Traumatic fractures are coded using the appropriate 7th character for initial encounter (A, B, C) for each encounter where the patient is receiving active treatment for the fracture. The appropriate 7th character for initial encounter should also be assigned for a patient who delayed seeking treatment for the fracture or nonunion.

Fractures are coded using the appropriate 7th character for subsequent care for encounters after the patient has completed active treatment of the fracture and is receiving routine care for the fracture during the healing or recovery phase.

Care for complications of surgical treatment for fracture repairs during the healing or recovery phase should be coded with the appropriate complication codes.

Care of complications of fractures, such as malunion and nonunion, should be reported with the appropriate 7th character for subsequent care with nonunion (K, M, N,) or subsequent care with malunion (P, Q, R).

Malunion/nonunion: The appropriate 7th character for initial encounter should also be assigned for a patient who delayed seeking treatment for the fracture or nonunion.

The open fracture designations in the assignment of the 7th character for fractures of the forearm, femur and lower leg, including ankle are based on the Gustilo open fracture classification. When the Gustilo classification type is not specified for an open fracture, the 7th character for open fracture type I or II should be assigned (B, E, H, M, Q).

A code from category M8Ø, not a traumatic fracture code, should be used for any patient with known osteoporosis who suffers a fracture, even if the patient had a minor fall or trauma, if that fall or trauma would not usually break a normal, healthy bone.

See Section I.C.13. Osteoporosis.

The aftercare Z codes should not be used for aftercare for traumatic fractures. For aftercare of a traumatic fracture, assign the acute fracture code with the appropriate 7th character.

2) Multiple fractures sequencing

Multiple fractures are sequenced in accordance with the severity of the fracture.

3) Physeal fractures

For physeal fractures, assign only the code identifying the type of physeal fracture. Do not assign a separate code to identify the specific bone that is fractured.

d. Coding of Burns and Corrosions

The ICD-10-CM makes a distinction between burns and corrosions. The burn codes are for thermal burns, except sunburns, that come from a heat source, such as a fire or hot appliance. The burn codes are also for burns resulting from electricity and radiation. Corrosions are burns due to chemicals. The guidelines are the same for burns and corrosions.

Current burns (T2Ø-T25) are classified by depth, extent and by agent (X code). Burns are classified by depth as first degree (erythema), second degree (blistering), and third degree (full-thickness involvement). Burns of the eye and internal organs (T26-T28) are classified by site, but not by degree.

1) Sequencing of burn and related condition codes

Sequence first the code that reflects the highest degree of burn when more than one burn is present.

a. When the reason for the admission or encounter is for treatment of external multiple burns, sequence first the code that reflects the burn of the highest degree.

b. When a patient has both internal and external burns, the circumstances of admission govern the selection of the principal diagnosis or first-listed diagnosis.

c. When a patient is admitted for burn injuries and other related conditions such as smoke inhalation and/or respiratory failure, the circumstances of admission govern the selection of the principal or first-listed diagnosis.

2) Burns of the same anatomic site

Classify burns of the same anatomic site and on the same side but of different degrees to the subcategory identifying the highest degree recorded in the diagnosis (e.g., for second and third degree burns of right thigh, assign only code T24.311-).

3) Non-healing burns

Non-healing burns are coded as acute burns.

Necrosis of burned skin should be coded as a non-healed burn.

4) Infected burn

For any documented infected burn site, use an additional code for the infection.

5) Assign separate codes for each burn site

When coding burns, assign separate codes for each burn site. Category T3Ø, Burn and corrosion, body region unspecified is extremely vague and should rarely be used.

Codes for burns of "multiple sites" should only be assigned when the medical record documentation does not specify the individual sites.

6) Burns and corrosions classified according to extent of body surface involved

Assign codes from category T31, Burns classified according to extent of body surface involved, or T32, Corrosions classified according to extent of body surface involved, when the site of the burn is not specified or when there is a need for additional data. It is advisable to use category T31 as additional coding when needed to provide data for evaluating burn mortality, such as that needed by burn units. It is also advisable to use category T31 as an additional code for reporting purposes when there is mention of a third-degree burn involving 2Ø percent or more of the body surface.

Categories T31 and T32 are based on the classic "rule of nines" in estimating body surface involved: head and neck are assigned nine percent, each arm nine percent, each leg 18 percent, the anterior trunk 18 percent, posterior trunk 18 percent, and genitalia one percent. Providers may change these percentage assignments where necessary to accommodate infants and children who have proportionately larger heads than adults, and patients who have large buttocks, thighs, or abdomen that involve burns.

7) **Encounters for treatment of sequela of burns**
Encounters for the treatment of the late effects of burns or corrosions (i.e., scars or joint contractures) should be coded with a burn or corrosion code with the 7th character "S" for sequela.

8) **Sequelae with a late effect code and current burn**
When appropriate, both a code for a current burn or corrosion with 7th character "A" or "D" and a burn or corrosion code with 7th character "S" may be assigned on the same record (when both a current burn and sequelae of an old burn exist). Burns and corrosions do not heal at the same rate and a current healing wound may still exist with sequela of a healed burn or corrosion.

See Section I.B.10 Sequela (Late Effects)

9) **Use of an external cause code with burns and corrosions**
An external cause code should be used with burns and corrosions to identify the source and intent of the burn, as well as the place where it occurred.

e. **Adverse Effects, Poisoning, Underdosing and Toxic Effects**
Codes in categories T36-T65 are combination codes that include the substance that was taken as well as the intent. No additional external cause code is required for poisonings, toxic effects, adverse effects and underdosing codes.

1) **Do not code directly from the Table of Drugs**
Do not code directly from the Table of Drugs and Chemicals. Always refer back to the Tabular List.

2) **Use as many codes as necessary to describe**
Use as many codes as necessary to describe completely all drugs, medicinal or biological substances.

3) **If the same code would describe the causative agent**
If the same code would describe the causative agent for more than one adverse reaction, poisoning, toxic effect or underdosing, assign the code only once.

4) **If two or more drugs, medicinal or biological substances**
If two or more drugs, medicinal or biological substances are taken, code each individually unless a combination code is listed in the Table of Drugs and Chemicals.

If multiple unspecified drugs, medicinal or biological substances were taken, assign the appropriate code from subcategory T5Ø.91, Poisoning by, adverse effect of and underdosing of multiple unspecified drugs, medicaments and biological substances.

5) **The occurrence of drug toxicity is classified in ICD-10-CM as follows:**

(a) **Adverse Effect**
When coding an adverse effect of a drug that has been correctly prescribed and properly administered, assign the appropriate code for the nature of the adverse effect followed by the appropriate code for the adverse effect of the drug (T36-T5Ø). The code for the drug should have a 5th or 6th character "5" (for example T36.ØX5-) Examples of the nature of an adverse effect are tachycardia, delirium, gastrointestinal hemorrhaging, vomiting, hypokalemia, hepatitis, renal failure, or respiratory failure.

(b) **Poisoning**
When coding a poisoning or reaction to the improper use of a medication (e.g., overdose, wrong substance given or taken in error, wrong route of administration), first assign the appropriate code from categories T36-T5Ø. The poisoning codes have an associated intent as their 5th or 6th character (accidental, intentional self-harm, assault and undetermined. If the intent of the poisoning is unknown or unspecified, code the intent as accidental intent. The undetermined intent is only for use if the documentation in the record specifies that the intent cannot be determined. Use additional code(s) for all manifestations of poisonings.

If there is also a diagnosis of abuse or dependence of the substance, the abuse or dependence is assigned as an additional code.

Examples of poisoning include:

(i) Error was made in drug prescription
Errors made in drug prescription or in the administration of the drug by provider, nurse, patient, or other person.

(ii) Overdose of a drug intentionally taken
If an overdose of a drug was intentionally taken or administered and resulted in drug toxicity, it would be coded as a poisoning.

(iii) Nonprescribed drug taken with correctly prescribed and properly administered drug
If a nonprescribed drug or medicinal agent was taken in combination with a correctly prescribed and properly administered drug, any drug toxicity or other reaction resulting from the interaction of the two drugs would be classified as a poisoning.

(iv) Interaction of drug(s) and alcohol
When a reaction results from the interaction of a drug(s) and alcohol, this would be classified as poisoning.

See Section I.C.4. if poisoning is the result of insulin pump malfunctions.

(c) **Underdosing**
Underdosing refers to taking less of a medication than is prescribed by a provider or a manufacturer's instruction. Discontinuing the use of a prescribed medication on the patient's own initiative (not directed by the patient's provider) is also classified as an underdosing. For underdosing, assign the code from categories T36-T5Ø (fifth or sixth character "6").

Codes for underdosing should never be assigned as principal or first-listed codes. If a patient has a relapse or exacerbation of the medical condition for which the drug is prescribed because of the reduction in dose, then the medical condition itself should be coded.

Noncompliance (Z91.12-, Z91.13- and Z91.14-) or complication of care (Y63.6-Y63.9) codes are to be used with an underdosing code to indicate intent, if known.

(d) **Toxic Effects**
When a harmful substance is ingested or comes in contact with a person, this is classified as a toxic effect. The toxic effect codes are in categories T51-T65.

Toxic effect codes have an associated intent: accidental, intentional self-harm, assault and undetermined.

f. **Adult and child abuse, neglect and other maltreatment**
Sequence first the appropriate code from categories T74, Adult and child abuse, neglect and other maltreatment, confirmed) or T76, Adult and child abuse, neglect and other maltreatment, suspected) for abuse, neglect and other maltreatment, followed by any accompanying mental health or injury code(s).

If the documentation in the medical record states abuse or neglect it is coded as confirmed (T74.-). It is coded as suspected if it is documented as suspected (T76.-).

For cases of confirmed abuse or neglect an external cause code from the assault section (X92-YØ9) should be added to identify the cause of any physical injuries. A perpetrator code (YØ7) should be added when the perpetrator of the abuse is known. For suspected cases of abuse or neglect, do not report external cause or perpetrator code.

If a suspected case of abuse, neglect or mistreatment is ruled out during an encounter code ZØ4.71, Encounter for examination and observation following alleged physical adult abuse, ruled out, or code ZØ4.72, Encounter for examination and observation following alleged child physical abuse, ruled out, should be used, not a code from T76.

If a suspected case of alleged rape or sexual abuse is ruled out during an encounter code ZØ4.41, Encounter for examination and observation following alleged adult rape or code ZØ4.42, Encounter for examination and observation following alleged child rape, should be used, not a code from T76.

If a suspected case of forced sexual exploitation or forced labor exploitation is ruled out during an encounter, code ZØ4.81, Encounter for examination and observation of victim following forced sexual exploitation, or code ZØ4.82, Encounter for examination and observation of victim following forced labor exploitation, should be used, not a code from T76.

See Section I.C.15. Abuse in a pregnant patient.

g. **Complications of care**

1) **General guidelines for complications of care**

(a) **Documentation of complications of care**
See Section I.B.16. for information on documentation of complications of care.

2) **Pain due to medical devices**
Pain associated with devices, implants or grafts left in a surgical site (for example painful hip prosthesis) is assigned to the appropriate code(s) found in Chapter 19, Injury, poisoning, and certain other consequences of external causes. Specific codes for pain due to medical devices are found in the T code section of the ICD-10-CM. Use additional code(s) from category G89 to identify acute or chronic pain due to presence of the device, implant or graft (G89.18 or G89.28).

3) **Transplant complications**

(a) **Transplant complications other than kidney**
Codes under category T86, Complications of transplanted organs and tissues, are for use for both complications and rejection of transplanted organs. A transplant complication code is only assigned if the complication affects the function of the transplanted organ. Two codes are required to fully describe a transplant complication: the appropriate code from category T86 and a secondary code that identifies the complication.

Pre-existing conditions or conditions that develop after the transplant are not coded as complications unless they affect the function of the transplanted organs.

See I.C.21. for transplant organ removal status

See I.C.2. for malignant neoplasm associated with transplanted organ.

(b) **Kidney transplant complications**
Patients who have undergone kidney transplant may still have some form of chronic kidney disease (CKD) because the kidney transplant may not fully restore kidney function. Code T86.1- should be assigned for documented complications of a kidney transplant, such as transplant failure or rejection or other transplant complication. Code T86.1- should not be assigned for post kidney transplant patients who have chronic kidney (CKD) unless a transplant complication such as transplant failure or rejection is documented. If the documentation is unclear as to whether the patient has a complication of the transplant, query the provider.

Conditions that affect the function of the transplanted kidney, other than CKD, should be assigned a code from subcategory T86.1, Complications of transplanted organ, Kidney, and a secondary code that identifies the complication.

For patients with CKD following a kidney transplant, but who do not have a complication such as failure or rejection, *see section I.C.14. Chronic kidney disease and kidney transplant status.*

4) **Complication codes that include the external cause**
As with certain other T codes, some of the complications of care codes have the external cause included in the code. The code includes the nature of the complication as well as the type of procedure that caused the complication. No external cause code indicating the type of procedure is necessary for these codes.

5) **Complications of care codes within the body system chapters**
Intraoperative and postprocedural complication codes are found within the body system chapters with codes specific to the organs and structures of that body system. These codes should be sequenced first, followed by a code(s) for the specific complication, if applicable.

Complication codes from the body system chapters should be assigned for intraoperative and postprocedural complications (e.g., the appropriate complication code from chapter 9 would be assigned for a vascular intraoperative or postprocedural complication) unless the complication is specifically indexed to a T code in chapter 19.

20. Chapter 20: External Causes of Morbidity (VØØ-Y99)
The external causes of morbidity codes should never be sequenced as the first-listed or principal diagnosis.

External cause codes are intended to provide data for injury research and evaluation of injury prevention strategies. These codes capture how the injury or health condition happened (cause), the intent (unintentional or accidental; or intentional, such as suicide or assault), the place where the event occurred the activity of the patient at the time of the event, and the person's status (e.g., civilian, military).

There is no national requirement for mandatory ICD-10-CM external cause code reporting. Unless a provider is subject to a state-based external cause code reporting mandate or these codes are required by a particular payer, reporting of ICD-10-CM codes in Chapter 2Ø, External Causes of Morbidity, is not required. In the absence of a mandatory reporting requirement, providers are encouraged to voluntarily report external cause codes, as they provide valuable data for injury research and evaluation of injury prevention strategies.

a. **General External Cause Coding Guidelines**

1) **Used with any code in the range of AØØ.Ø-T88.9 ZØØ-Z99**
An external cause code may be used with any code in the range of AØØ.Ø-T88.9, ZØØ-Z99, classification that represents a health condition due to an external cause. Though they are most applicable to injuries, they are also valid for use with such things as infections or diseases due to an external source, and other health conditions, such as a heart attack that occurs during strenuous physical activity.

2) **External cause code used for length of treatment**
Assign the external cause code, with the appropriate 7th character (initial encounter, subsequent encounter or sequela) for each encounter for which the injury or condition is being treated.

Most categories in chapter 20 have a 7th character requirement for each applicable code. Most categories in this chapter have three 7th character values: A, initial encounter, D, subsequent encounter and S, sequela. While the patient may be seen by a new or different provider over the course of treatment for an injury or condition, assignment of the 7th character for external cause should match the 7th character of the code assigned for the associated injury or condition for the encounter.

3) **Use the full range of external cause codes**
Use the full range of external cause codes to completely describe the cause, the intent, the place of occurrence, and if applicable, the activity of the patient at the time of the event, and the patient's status, for all injuries, and other health conditions due to an external cause.

4) **Assign as many external cause codes as necessary**
Assign as many external cause codes as necessary to fully explain each cause. If only one external code can be recorded, assign the code most related to the principal diagnosis.

5) **The selection of the appropriate external cause code**
The selection of the appropriate external cause code is guided by the Alphabetic Index of External Causes and by Inclusion and Exclusion notes in the Tabular List.

6) **External cause code can never be a principal diagnosis**
An external cause code can never be a principal (first-listed) diagnosis.

7) **Combination external cause codes**
Certain of the external cause codes are combination codes that identify sequential events that result in an injury, such as a fall which results in striking against an object. The injury may be due to either event or both. The combination external cause code used should correspond to the sequence of events regardless of which caused the most serious injury.

8) **No external cause code needed in certain circumstances**
No external cause code from Chapter 20 is needed if the external cause and intent are included in a code from another chapter (e.g. T36.ØX1- Poisoning by penicillins, accidental (unintentional)).

b. **Place of Occurrence Guideline**
Codes from category Y92, Place of occurrence of the external cause, are secondary codes for use after other external cause codes to identify the location of the patient at the time of injury or other condition.

Generally, a place of occurrence code is assigned only once, at the initial encounter for treatment. However, in the rare instance that a new injury occurs during hospitalization, an additional place of occurrence code may be assigned. No 7th characters are used for Y92.

Do not use place of occurrence code Y92.9 if the place is not stated or is not applicable.

c. **Activity Code**
Assign a code from category Y93, Activity code, to describe the activity of the patient at the time the injury or other health condition occurred.

An activity code is used only once, at the initial encounter for treatment. Only one code from Y93 should be recorded on a medical record.

The activity codes are not applicable to poisonings, adverse effects, misadventures or sequela.

Do not assign Y93.9, Unspecified activity, if the activity is not stated.

A code from category Y93 is appropriate for use with external cause and intent codes if identifying the activity provides additional information about the event.

d. Place of Occurrence, Activity, and Status Codes Used with other External Cause Code

When applicable, place of occurrence, activity, and external cause status codes are sequenced after the main external cause code(s). Regardless of the number of external cause codes assigned, generally there should be only one place of occurrence code, one activity code, and one external cause status code assigned to an encounter. However, in the rare instance that a new injury occurs during hospitalization, an additional place of occurrence code may be assigned.

e. If the Reporting Format Limits the Number of External Cause Codes

If the reporting format limits the number of external cause codes that can be used in reporting clinical data, report the code for the cause/intent most related to the principal diagnosis. If the format permits capture of additional external cause codes, the cause/intent, including medical misadventures, of the additional events should be reported rather than the codes for place, activity, or external status.

f. Multiple External Cause Coding Guidelines

More than one external cause code is required to fully describe the external cause of an illness or injury. The assignment of external cause codes should be sequenced in the following priority:

If two or more events cause separate injuries, an external cause code should be assigned for each cause. The first-listed external cause code will be selected in the following order:

External codes for child and adult abuse take priority over all other external cause codes.

See Section I.C.19., Child and Adult abuse guidelines.

External cause codes for terrorism events take priority over all other external cause codes except child and adult abuse.

External cause codes for cataclysmic events take priority over all other external cause codes except child and adult abuse and terrorism.

External cause codes for transport accidents take priority over all other external cause codes except cataclysmic events, child and adult abuse and terrorism.

Activity and external cause status codes are assigned following all causal (intent) external cause codes.

The first-listed external cause code should correspond to the cause of the most serious diagnosis due to an assault, accident, or self-harm, following the order of hierarchy listed above.

g. Child and Adult Abuse Guideline

Adult and child abuse, neglect and maltreatment are classified as assault. Any of the assault codes may be used to indicate the external cause of any injury resulting from the confirmed abuse.

For confirmed cases of abuse, neglect and maltreatment, when the perpetrator is known, a code from Y07, Perpetrator of maltreatment and neglect, should accompany any other assault codes.

See Section I.C.19. Adult and child abuse, neglect and other maltreatment

h. Unknown or Undetermined Intent Guideline

If the intent (accident, self-harm, assault) of the cause of an injury or other condition is unknown or unspecified, code the intent as accidental intent. All transport accident categories assume accidental intent.

1) Use of undetermined intent

External cause codes for events of undetermined intent are only for use if the documentation in the record specifies that the intent cannot be determined.

i. Sequelae (Late Effects) of External Cause Guidelines

1) Sequelae external cause codes

Sequela are reported using the external cause code with the 7th character "S" for sequela. These codes should be used with any report of a late effect or sequela resulting from a previous injury.

See Section I.B.10 Sequela (Late Effects)

2) Sequela external cause code with a related current injury

A sequela external cause code should never be used with a related current nature of injury code.

3) Use of sequela external cause codes for subsequent visits

Use a late effect external cause code for subsequent visits when a late effect of the initial injury is being treated. Do not use a late effect external cause code for subsequent visits for follow-up care (e.g., to assess healing, to receive rehabilitative therapy) of the injury when no late effect of the injury has been documented.

j. Terrorism Guidelines

1) Cause of injury identified by the Federal Government (FBI) as terrorism

When the cause of an injury is identified by the Federal Government (FBI) as terrorism, the first-listed external cause code should be a code from category Y38, Terrorism. The definition of terrorism employed by the FBI is found at the inclusion note at the beginning of category Y38. Use additional code for place of occurrence (Y92.-). More than one Y38 code may be assigned if the injury is the result of more than one mechanism of terrorism.

2) Cause of an injury is suspected to be the result of terrorism

When the cause of an injury is suspected to be the result of terrorism a code from category Y38 should not be assigned. Suspected cases should be classified as assault.

3) Code Y38.9, Terrorism, secondary effects

Assign code Y38.9, Terrorism, secondary effects, for conditions occurring subsequent to the terrorist event. This code should not be assigned for conditions that are due to the initial terrorist act.

It is acceptable to assign code Y38.9 with another code from Y38 if there is an injury due to the initial terrorist event and an injury that is a subsequent result of the terrorist event.

k. External Cause Status

A code from category Y99, External cause status, should be assigned whenever any other external cause code is assigned for an encounter, including an Activity code, except for the events noted below. Assign a code from category Y99, External cause status, to indicate the work status of the person at the time the event occurred. The status code indicates whether the event occurred during military activity, whether a non-military person was at work, whether an individual including a student or volunteer was involved in a non-work activity at the time of the causal event.

A code from Y99, External cause status, should be assigned, when applicable, with other external cause codes, such as transport accidents and falls. The external cause status codes are not applicable to poisonings, adverse effects, misadventures or late effects.

Do not assign a code from category Y99 if no other external cause codes (cause, activity) are applicable for the encounter.

An external cause status code is used only once, at the initial encounter for treatment. Only one code from Y99 should be recorded on a medical record.

Do not assign code Y99.9, Unspecified external cause status, if the status is not stated.

21. Chapter 21: Factors influencing health status and contact with health services (Z00-Z99)

Note: The chapter specific guidelines provide additional information about the use of Z codes for specified encounters.

a. Use of Z Codes in Any Healthcare Setting

Z codes are for use in any healthcare setting. Z codes may be used as either a first-listed (principal diagnosis code in the inpatient setting) or secondary code, depending on the circumstances of the encounter. Certain Z codes may only be used as first-listed or principal diagnosis.

b. Z Codes Indicate a Reason for an Encounter

Z codes are not procedure codes. A corresponding procedure code must accompany a Z code to describe any procedure performed.

c. Categories of Z Codes

1) Contact/Exposure

Category Z20 indicates contact with, and suspected exposure to, communicable diseases. These codes are for patients who are suspected to have been exposed to **a disease** by close personal contact with an infected individual or are in an area where a disease is epidemic.

Category Z77, Other contact with and (suspected) exposures hazardous to health, indicates contact with and suspected exposures hazardous to health.

Contact/exposure codes may be used as a first-listed code to explain an encounter for testing, or, more commonly, as a secondary code to identify a potential risk.

2) Inoculations and vaccinations

Code Z23 is for encounters for inoculations and vaccinations. It indicates that a patient is being seen to receive a prophylactic inoculation against a disease. Procedure codes are required to identify the actual administration of the injection and the type(s) of immunizations given. Code Z23 may be used as a secondary code if the inoculation is given as a routine part of preventive health care, such as a well-baby visit.

3) Status

Status codes indicate that a patient is either a carrier of a disease or has the sequelae or residual of a past disease or condition. This includes such things as the presence of prosthetic or mechanical devices resulting from past treatment. A status code is informative, because the status may affect the course of treatment and its outcome. A status code is distinct from a history code. The history code indicates that the patient no longer has the condition.

A status code should not be used with a diagnosis code from one of the body system chapters, if the diagnosis code includes the information provided by the status code. For example, code Z94.1, Heart transplant status, should not be used with a code from subcategory T86.2, Complications of heart transplant. The status code does not provide additional information. The complication code indicates that the patient is a heart transplant patient.

For encounters for weaning from a mechanical ventilator, assign a code from subcategory J96.1, Chronic respiratory failure, followed by code Z99.11, Dependence on respirator [ventilator] status.

The status Z codes/categories are:

Z14 Genetic carrier

Genetic carrier status indicates that a person carries a gene, associated with a particular disease, which may be passed to offspring who may develop that disease. The person does not have the disease and is not at risk of developing the disease.

Z15 Genetic susceptibility to disease

Genetic susceptibility indicates that a person has a gene that increases the risk of that person developing the disease.

Codes from category Z15 should not be used as principal or first-listed codes. If the patient has the condition to which he/she is susceptible, and that condition is the reason for the encounter, the code for the current condition should be sequenced first. If the patient is being seen for follow-up after completed treatment for this condition, and the condition no longer exists, a follow-up code should be sequenced first, followed by the appropriate personal history and genetic susceptibility codes. If the purpose of the encounter is genetic counseling associated with procreative management, code Z31.5, Encounter for genetic counseling, should be assigned as the first-listed code, followed by a code from category Z15. Additional codes should be assigned for any applicable family or personal history.

Z16 Resistance to antimicrobial drugs

This code indicates that a patient has a condition that is resistant to antimicrobial drug treatment. Sequence the infection code first.

Z17 Estrogen receptor status

Z18 Retained foreign body fragments

Z19 Hormone sensitivity malignancy status

Z21 Asymptomatic HIV infection status

This code indicates that a patient has tested positive for HIV but has manifested no signs or symptoms of the disease.

Z22 Carrier of infectious disease

Carrier status indicates that a person harbors the specific organisms of a disease without manifest symptoms and is capable of transmitting the infection.

Z28.3 Underimmunization status

Z33.1 Pregnant state, incidental

This code is a secondary code only for use when the pregnancy is in no way complicating the reason for visit. Otherwise, a code from the obstetric chapter is required.

Z66 Do not resuscitate

This code may be used when it is documented by the provider that a patient is on do not resuscitate status at any time during the stay.

Z67 Blood type

Z68 Body mass index (BMI)

BMI codes should only be assigned when there is an associated, reportable diagnosis (such as obesity). Do not assign BMI codes during pregnancy.

See Section I.B.14 for BMI documentation by clinicians other than the patient's provider.

Z74.Ø1 Bed confinement status

Z76.82 Awaiting organ transplant status

Z78 Other specified health status

Code Z78.1, Physical restraint status, may be used when it is documented by the provider that a patient has been put in restraints during the current encounter. Please note that this code should not be reported when it is documented by the provider that a patient is temporarily restrained during a procedure.

Z79 Long-term (current) drug therapy

Codes from this category indicate a patient's continuous use of a prescribed drug (including such things as aspirin therapy) for the long-term treatment of a condition or for prophylactic use. It is not for use for patients who have addictions to drugs. This subcategory is not for use of medications for detoxification or maintenance programs to prevent withdrawal symptoms (e.g., methadone maintenance for opiate dependence). Assign the appropriate code for the drug **use, abuse, or** dependence instead.

Assign a code from Z79 if the patient is receiving a medication for an extended period as a prophylactic measure (such as for the prevention of deep vein thrombosis) or as treatment of a chronic condition (such as arthritis) or a disease requiring a lengthy course of treatment (such as cancer). Do not assign a code from category Z79 for medication being administered for a brief period of time to treat an acute illness or injury (such as a course of antibiotics to treat acute bronchitis).

Z88 Allergy status to drugs, medicaments and biological substances

Except: Z88.9, Allergy status to unspecified drugs, medicaments and biological substances status

Z89 Acquired absence of limb

Z9Ø Acquired absence of organs, not elsewhere classified

Z91.Ø- Allergy status, other than to drugs and biological substances

Z92.82 Status post administration of tPA (rtPA) in a different facility within the last 24 hours prior to admission to a current facility

Assign code Z92.82, Status post administration of tPA (rtPA) in a different facility within the last 24 hours prior to admission to current facility, as a secondary diagnosis when a patient is received by transfer into a facility and documentation indicates they were administered tissue plasminogen activator (tPA) within the last 24 hours prior to admission to the current facility.

This guideline applies even if the patient is still receiving the tPA at the time they are received into the current facility.

The appropriate code for the condition for which the tPA was administered (such as cerebrovascular disease or myocardial infarction) should be assigned first.

Code Z92.82 is only applicable to the receiving facility record and not to the transferring facility record.

Z93 Artificial opening status

Z94 Transplanted organ and tissue status

Z95 Presence of cardiac and vascular implants and grafts

Z96 Presence of other functional implants

Z97 Presence of other devices

Z98 Other postprocedural states

Assign code Z98.85, Transplanted organ removal status, to indicate that a transplanted organ has been previously removed. This code should not be assigned for the encounter in which the transplanted organ is removed. The complication necessitating removal of the transplant organ should be assigned for that encounter.

See section I.C19. for information on the coding of organ transplant complications.

Z99 Dependence on enabling machines and devices, not elsewhere classified

Note: Categories Z89-Z9Ø and Z93-Z99 are for use only if there are no complications or malfunctions of the organ or tissue replaced, the amputation site or the equipment on which the patient is dependent.

4) History (of)

There are two types of history Z codes, personal and family. Personal history codes explain a patient's past medical condition that no longer exists and is not receiving any treatment, but that has the potential for recurrence, and therefore may require continued monitoring.

Family history codes are for use when a patient has a family member(s) who has had a particular disease that causes the patient to be at higher risk of also contracting the disease.

Personal history codes may be used in conjunction with follow-up codes and family history codes may be used in conjunction with screening codes to explain the need for a test or procedure. History codes are also acceptable on any medical record regardless of the reason for visit. A history of an illness, even if no longer present, is important information that may alter the type of treatment ordered.

The history Z code categories are:

Z8Ø Family history of primary malignant neoplasm

Z81 Family history of mental and behavioral disorders

Z82 Family history of certain disabilities and chronic diseases (leading to disablement)

Z83 Family history of other specific disorders

Z84 Family history of other conditions

Z85 Personal history of malignant neoplasm

Z86 Personal history of certain other diseases

Z87 Personal history of other diseases and conditions

Z91.4- Personal history of psychological trauma, not elsewhere classified

Z91.5 Personal history of self-harm

Z91.81 History of falling

Z91.82 Personal history of military deployment

Z92 Personal history of medical treatment

Except: Z92.Ø, Personal history of contraception

Except: Z92.82, Status post administration of tPA (rtPA) in a different facility within the last 24 hours prior to admission to a current facility

5) Screening

Screening is the testing for disease or disease precursors in seemingly well individuals so that early detection and treatment can be provided for those who test positive for the disease (e.g., screening mammogram).

The testing of a person to rule out or confirm a suspected diagnosis because the patient has some sign or symptom is a diagnostic examination, not a screening. In these cases, the sign or symptom is used to explain the reason for the test.

A screening code may be a first-listed code if the reason for the visit is specifically the screening exam. It may also be used as an additional code if the screening is done during an office visit for other health problems. A screening code is not necessary if the screening is inherent to a routine examination, such as a pap smear done during a routine pelvic examination.

Should a condition be discovered during the screening then the code for the condition may be assigned as an additional diagnosis.

The Z code indicates that a screening exam is planned. A procedure code is required to confirm that the screening was performed.

The screening Z codes/categories:

Z11 Encounter for screening for infectious and parasitic diseases

Z12 Encounter for screening for malignant neoplasms

Z13 Encounter for screening for other diseases and disorders

Except: Z13.9, Encounter for screening, unspecified

Z36 Encounter for antenatal screening for mother

6) Observation

There are three observation Z code categories. They are for use in very limited circumstances when a person is being observed for a suspected condition that is ruled out. The observation codes are not for use if an injury or illness or any signs or symptoms related to the suspected condition are present. In such cases the diagnosis/symptom code is used with the corresponding external cause code.

The observation codes are **primarily** to be used as a principal/**first-listed** diagnosis. **An observation code may be assigned as a secondary diagnosis code when the patient is being observed for a condition that is ruled out and is unrelated to the principal/first-listed diagnosis (e.g., patient presents for treatment following injuries sustained in a motor vehicle accident and is also observed for suspected COVID-19 infection that is subsequently ruled out). Also,** when the principal diagnosis is required to be a code from category Z38, Liveborn infants according to place of birth and type of delivery, **then** a code from category Z05, Encounter for observation and evaluation of newborn for suspected diseases and conditions ruled out, is sequenced after the Z38 code. Additional codes may be used in addition to the observation code, but only if they are unrelated to the suspected condition being observed.

Codes from subcategory ZØ3.7, Encounter for suspected maternal and fetal conditions ruled out, may either be used as a first-listed or as an additional code assignment depending on the case. They are for use in very limited circumstances on a maternal record when an encounter is for a suspected maternal or fetal condition that is ruled out during that encounter (for example, a maternal or fetal condition may be suspected due to an abnormal test result). These codes should not be used when the condition is confirmed. In those cases, the confirmed condition should be coded. In addition, these codes are not for use if an illness or any signs or symptoms related to the suspected condition or problem are present. In such cases the diagnosis/symptom code is used.

Additional codes may be used in addition to the code from subcategory ZØ3.7, but only if they are unrelated to the suspected condition being evaluated.

Codes from subcategory ZØ3.7 may not be used for encounters for antenatal screening of mother. *See Section I.C.21. Screening.*

For encounters for suspected fetal condition that are inconclusive following testing and evaluation, assign the appropriate code from category O35, O36, O4Ø or O41.

The observation Z code categories:

ZØ3 Encounter for medical observation for suspected diseases and conditions ruled out

ZØ4 Encounter for examination and observation for other reasons

Except: ZØ4.9, Encounter for examination and observation for unspecified reason

ZØ5 Encounter for observation and evaluation of newborn for suspected diseases and conditions ruled out

7) Aftercare

Aftercare visit codes cover situations when the initial treatment of a disease has been performed and the patient requires continued care during the healing or recovery phase, or for the long-term consequences of the disease. The aftercare Z code should not be used if treatment is directed at a current, acute disease. The diagnosis code is to be used in these cases. Exceptions to this rule are codes Z51.Ø, Encounter for antineoplastic radiation therapy, and codes from subcategory Z51.1, Encounter for antineoplastic chemotherapy and immunotherapy. These codes are to be first listed, followed by the diagnosis code when a patient's encounter is solely to receive radiation therapy, chemotherapy, or immunotherapy for the treatment of a neoplasm. If the reason for the encounter is more than one type of antineoplastic therapy, code Z51.Ø and a code from subcategory Z51.1 may be assigned together, in which case one of these codes would be reported as a secondary diagnosis.

The aftercare Z codes should also not be used for aftercare for injuries. For aftercare of an injury, assign the acute injury code with the appropriate 7th character (for subsequent encounter).

The aftercare codes are generally first listed to explain the specific reason for the encounter. An aftercare code may be used as an additional code when some type of aftercare is provided in addition to the reason for admission and no diagnosis code is applicable. An example of this would be the closure of a colostomy during an encounter for treatment of another condition.

Aftercare codes should be used in conjunction with other aftercare codes or diagnosis codes to provide better detail on the specifics of an aftercare encounter visit, unless otherwise directed by the classification. The sequencing of multiple aftercare codes depends on the circumstances of the encounter.

Certain aftercare Z code categories need a secondary diagnosis code to describe the resolving condition or sequelae. For others, the condition is included in the code title.

Additional Z code aftercare category terms include fitting and adjustment, and attention to artificial openings.

Status Z codes may be used with aftercare Z codes to indicate the nature of the aftercare. For example, code Z95.1, Presence of aortocoronary bypass graft, may be used with code Z48.812, Encounter for surgical aftercare following surgery on the circulatory system, to indicate the surgery for which the aftercare is being performed. A status code should not be used when the aftercare code indicates the type of status, such as using Z43.Ø, Encounter for attention to tracheostomy, with Z93.Ø, Tracheostomy status.

The aftercare Z category/codes:

- Z42 Encounter for plastic and reconstructive surgery following medical procedure or healed injury
- Z43 Encounter for attention to artificial openings
- Z44 Encounter for fitting and adjustment of external prosthetic device
- Z45 Encounter for adjustment and management of implanted device
- Z46 Encounter for fitting and adjustment of other devices
- Z47 Orthopedic aftercare
- Z48 Encounter for other postprocedural aftercare
- Z49 Encounter for care involving renal dialysis
- Z51 Encounter for other aftercare and medical care

8) Follow-up

The follow-up codes are used to explain continuing surveillance following completed treatment of a disease, condition, or injury. They imply that the condition has been fully treated and no longer exists. They should not be confused with aftercare codes, or injury codes with a 7th character for subsequent encounter, that explain ongoing care of a healing condition or its sequelae. Follow-up codes may be used in conjunction with history codes to provide the full picture of the healed condition and its treatment. The follow-up code is sequenced first, followed by the history code.

A follow-up code may be used to explain multiple visits. Should a condition be found to have recurred on the follow-up visit, then the diagnosis code for the condition should be assigned in place of the follow-up code.

The follow-up Z code categories:

- ZØ8 Encounter for follow-up examination after completed treatment for malignant neoplasm
- ZØ9 Encounter for follow-up examination after completed treatment for conditions other than malignant neoplasm
- Z39 Encounter for maternal postpartum care and examination

9) Donor

Codes in category Z52, Donors of organs and tissues, are used for living individuals who are donating blood or other body tissue. These codes are only for individuals donating for others, not for self-donations. They are not used to identify cadaveric donations.

10) Counseling

Counseling Z codes are used when a patient or family member receives assistance in the aftermath of an illness or injury, or when support is required in coping with family or social problems.

The counseling Z codes/categories:

- Z3Ø.Ø- Encounter for general counseling and advice on contraception
- Z31.5 Encounter for procreative genetic counseling
- Z31.6- Encounter for general counseling and advice on procreation
- Z32.2 Encounter for childbirth instruction
- Z32.3 Encounter for childcare instruction
- Z69 Encounter for mental health services for victim and perpetrator of abuse
- Z7Ø Counseling related to sexual attitude, behavior and orientation
- Z71 Persons encountering health services for other counseling and medical advice, not elsewhere classified

  Note: Code Z71.84, Encounter for health counseling related to travel, is to be used for health risk and safety counseling for future travel purposes.
- Z76.81 Expectant mother prebirth pediatrician visit

11) Encounters for Obstetrical and Reproductive Services

See Section I.C.15. Pregnancy, Childbirth, and the Puerperium, for further instruction on the use of these codes.

Z codes for pregnancy are for use in those circumstances when none of the problems or complications included in the codes from the Obstetrics chapter exist (a routine prenatal visit or postpartum care). Codes in category Z34, Encounter for supervision of normal pregnancy, are always first listed and are not to be used with any other code from the OB chapter.

Codes in category Z3A, Weeks of gestation, may be assigned to provide additional information about the pregnancy. Category Z3A codes should not be assigned for pregnancies with abortive outcomes (categories OØØ-OØ8), elective termination of pregnancy (code Z33.2), nor for postpartum conditions, as category Z3A is not applicable to these conditions. The date of the admission should be used to determine weeks of gestation for inpatient admissions that encompass more than one gestational week.

The outcome of delivery, category Z37, should be included on all maternal delivery records. It is always a secondary code. Codes in category Z37 should not be used on the newborn record.

Z codes for family planning (contraceptive) or procreative management and counseling should be included on an obstetric record either during the pregnancy or the postpartum stage, if applicable.

Z codes/categories for obstetrical and reproductive services:

- Z3Ø Encounter for contraceptive management
- Z31 Encounter for procreative management
- Z32.2 Encounter for childbirth instruction
- Z32.3 Encounter for childcare instruction
- Z33 Pregnant state
- Z34 Encounter for supervision of normal pregnancy
- Z36 Encounter for antenatal screening of mother

Z3A Weeks of gestation
Z37 Outcome of delivery
Z39 Encounter for maternal postpartum care and examination
Z76.81 Expectant mother prebirth pediatrician visit

12) Newborns and Infants

See Section I.C.16. Newborn (Perinatal) Guidelines, for further instruction on the use of these codes.

Newborn Z codes/categories:

Z76.1 Encounter for health supervision and care of foundling
Z00.1- Encounter for routine child health examination
Z38 Liveborn infants according to place of birth and type of delivery

13) Routine and Administrative Examinations

The Z codes allow for the description of encounters for routine examinations, such as, a general check-up, or, examinations for administrative purposes, such as, a pre-employment physical. The codes are not to be used if the examination is for diagnosis of a suspected condition or for treatment purposes. In such cases the diagnosis code is used. During a routine exam, should a diagnosis or condition be discovered, it should be coded as an additional code. Pre-existing and chronic conditions and history codes may also be included as additional codes as long as the examination is for administrative purposes and not focused on any particular condition.

Some of the codes for routine health examinations distinguish between "with" and "without" abnormal findings. Code assignment depends on the information that is known at the time the encounter is being coded. For example, if no abnormal findings were found during the examination, but the encounter is being coded before test results are back, it is acceptable to assign the code for "without abnormal findings." When assigning a code for "with abnormal findings," additional code(s) should be assigned to identify the specific abnormal finding(s).

Pre-operative examination and pre-procedural laboratory examination Z codes are for use only in those situations when a patient is being cleared for a procedure or surgery and no treatment is given.

The Z codes/categories for routine and administrative examinations:

Z00 Encounter for general examination without complaint, suspected or reported diagnosis
Z01 Encounter for other special examination without complaint, suspected or reported diagnosis
Z02 Encounter for administrative examination
Except: Z02.9, Encounter for administrative examinations, unspecified
Z32.0- Encounter for pregnancy test

14) Miscellaneous Z Codes

The miscellaneous Z codes capture a number of other health care encounters that do not fall into one of the other categories. Certain of these codes identify the reason for the encounter; others are for use as additional codes that provide useful information on circumstances that may affect a patient's care and treatment.

Prophylactic Organ Removal

For encounters specifically for prophylactic removal of an organ (such as prophylactic removal of breasts due to a genetic susceptibility to cancer or a family history of cancer), the principal or first-listed code should be a code from category Z40, Encounter for prophylactic surgery, followed by the appropriate codes to identify the associated risk factor (such as genetic susceptibility or family history).

If the patient has a malignancy of one site and is having prophylactic removal at another site to prevent either a new primary malignancy or metastatic disease, a code for the malignancy should also be assigned in addition to a code from subcategory Z40.0, Encounter for prophylactic surgery for risk factors related to malignant neoplasms. A Z40.0 code should not be assigned if the patient is having organ removal for treatment of a malignancy, such as the removal of the testes for the treatment of prostate cancer.

Miscellaneous Z codes/categories:

Z28 Immunization not carried out
Except: Z28.3, Underimmunization status
Z29 Encounter for other prophylactic measures
Z40 Encounter for prophylactic surgery
Z41 Encounter for procedures for purposes other than remedying health state
Except: Z41.9, Encounter for procedure for purposes other than remedying health state, unspecified
Z53 Persons encountering health services for specific procedures and treatment, not carried out
Z55 Problems related to education and literacy
Z56 Problems related to employment and unemployment
Z57 Occupational exposure to risk factors
Z58 Problems related to physical environment
Z59 Problems related to housing and economic circumstances
Z60 Problems related to social environment
Z62 Problems related to upbringing
Z63 Other problems related to primary support group, including family circumstances
Z64 Problems related to certain psychosocial circumstances
Z65 Problems related to other psychosocial circumstances
Z72 Problems related to lifestyle
Note: These codes should be assigned only when the documentation specifies that the patient has an associated problem
Z73 Problems related to life management difficulty
Z74 Problems related to care provider dependency
Except: Z74.01, Bed confinement status
Z75 Problems related to medical facilities and other health care
Z76.0 Encounter for issue of repeat prescription
Z76.3 Healthy person accompanying sick person
Z76.4 Other boarder to healthcare facility
Z76.5 Malingerer [conscious simulation]
Z91.1- Patient's noncompliance with medical treatment and regimen
Z91.83 Wandering in diseases classified elsewhere
Z91.84- Oral health risk factors
Z91.89 Other specified personal risk factors, not elsewhere classified

See Section I.B.14 for Z55-Z65 Persons with potential health hazards related to socioeconomic and psychosocial circumstances, documentation by clinicians other than the patient's provider.

15) Nonspecific Z Codes

Certain Z codes are so non-specific, or potentially redundant with other codes in the classification, that there can be little justification for their use in the inpatient setting. Their use in the outpatient setting should be limited to those instances when there is no further documentation to permit more precise coding. Otherwise, any sign or symptom or any other reason for visit that is captured in another code should be used.

Nonspecific Z codes/categories:

Z02.9 Encounter for administrative examinations, unspecified
Z04.9 Encounter for examination and observation for unspecified reason
Z13.9 Encounter for screening, unspecified
Z41.9 Encounter for procedure for purposes other than remedying health state, unspecified
Z52.9 Donor of unspecified organ or tissue
Z86.59 Personal history of other mental and behavioral disorders
Z88.9 Allergy status to unspecified drugs, medicaments and biological substances status
Z92.0 Personal history of contraception

16) Z Codes That May Only be Principal/First-Listed Diagnosis

The following Z codes/categories may only be reported as the principal/first-listed diagnosis, except when there are multiple encounters on the same day and the medical records for the encounters are combined:

Z00 Encounter for general examination without complaint, suspected or reported diagnosis
Except: Z00.6
Z01 Encounter for other special examination without complaint, suspected or reported diagnosis
Z02 Encounter for administrative examination
Z04 Encounter for examination and observation for other reasons
Z33.2 Encounter for elective termination of pregnancy
Z31.81 Encounter for male factor infertility in female patient
Z31.83 Encounter for assisted reproductive fertility procedure cycle
Z31.84 Encounter for fertility preservation procedure
Z34 Encounter for supervision of normal pregnancy
Z39 Encounter for maternal postpartum care and examination
Z38 Liveborn infants according to place of birth and type of delivery
Z40 Encounter for prophylactic surgery
Z42 Encounter for plastic and reconstructive surgery following medical procedure or healed injury
Z51.0 Encounter for antineoplastic radiation therapy
Z51.1- Encounter for antineoplastic chemotherapy and immunotherapy
Z52 Donors of organs and tissues
Except: Z52.9, Donor of unspecified organ or tissue
Z76.1 Encounter for health supervision and care of foundling
Z76.2 Encounter for health supervision and care of other healthy infant and child
Z99.12 Encounter for respirator [ventilator] dependence during power failure

22. **Chapter 22: Codes for Special Purposes (U00-U85)**
U07.0 Vaping-related disorder (see Section I.C.10.e., Vaping-related disorders)
U07.1 COVID-19 (see Section I.C.1.g.1., COVID-19 infection)

Section II. Selection of Principal Diagnosis

The circumstances of inpatient admission always govern the selection of principal diagnosis. The principal diagnosis is defined in the Uniform Hospital Discharge Data Set (UHDDS) as "that condition established after study to be chiefly responsible for occasioning the admission of the patient to the hospital for care."

The UHDDS definitions are used by hospitals to report inpatient data elements in a standardized manner. These data elements and their definitions can be found in the July 31, 1985, Federal Register (Vol. 50, No, 147), pp. 31038-40.

Since that time, the application of the UHDDS definitions has been expanded to include all non-outpatient settings (acute care, short term, long term care and psychiatric hospitals; home health agencies; rehab facilities; nursing homes, etc.). The UHDDS definitions also apply to hospice services (all levels of care).

In determining principal diagnosis, coding conventions in the ICD-10-CM, the Tabular List and Alphabetic Index take precedence over these official coding guidelines.

(See Section I.A., Conventions for the ICD-10-CM)

The importance of consistent, complete documentation in the medical record cannot be overemphasized. Without such documentation the application of all coding guidelines is a difficult, if not impossible, task.

A. Codes for symptoms, signs, and ill-defined conditions
Codes for symptoms, signs, and ill-defined conditions from Chapter 18 are not to be used as principal diagnosis when a related definitive diagnosis has been established.

B. Two or more interrelated conditions, each potentially meeting the definition for principal diagnosis.
When there are two or more interrelated conditions (such as diseases in the same ICD-10-CM chapter or manifestations characteristically associated with a certain disease) potentially meeting the definition of principal diagnosis, either condition may be sequenced first, unless the circumstances of the admission, the therapy provided, the Tabular List, or the Alphabetic Index indicate otherwise.

C. Two or more diagnoses that equally meet the definition for principal diagnosis
In the unusual instance when two or more diagnoses equally meet the criteria for principal diagnosis as determined by the circumstances of admission, diagnostic workup and/or therapy provided, and the Alphabetic Index, Tabular List, or another coding guidelines does not provide sequencing direction, any one of the diagnoses may be sequenced first.

D. Two or more comparative or contrasting conditions
In those rare instances when two or more contrasting or comparative diagnoses are documented as "either/or" (or similar terminology), they are coded as if the diagnoses were confirmed and the diagnoses are sequenced according to the circumstances of the admission. If no further determination can be made as to which diagnosis should be principal, either diagnosis may be sequenced first.

E. A symptom(s) followed by contrasting/comparative diagnoses
GUIDELINE HAS BEEN DELETED EFFECTIVE OCTOBER 1, 2014

F. Original treatment plan not carried out
Sequence as the principal diagnosis the condition, which after study occasioned the admission to the hospital, even though treatment may not have been carried out due to unforeseen circumstances.

G. Complications of surgery and other medical care
When the admission is for treatment of a complication resulting from surgery or other medical care, the complication code is sequenced as the principal diagnosis. If the complication is classified to the T80-T88 series and the code lacks the necessary specificity in describing the complication, an additional code for the specific complication should be assigned.

H. Uncertain Diagnosis
If the diagnosis documented at the time of discharge is qualified as "probable," "suspected," "likely," "questionable," "possible," or "still to be ruled out," "compatible with," "consistent with," or other similar terms indicating uncertainty, code the condition as if it existed or was established. The bases for these guidelines are the diagnostic workup, arrangements for further workup or observation, and initial therapeutic approach that correspond most closely with the established diagnosis.

Note: This guideline is applicable only to inpatient admissions to short-term, acute, long-term care and psychiatric hospitals.

I. Admission from Observation Unit

1. **Admission Following Medical Observation**
When a patient is admitted to an observation unit for a medical condition, which either worsens or does not improve, and is subsequently admitted as an inpatient of the same hospital for this same medical condition, the principal diagnosis would be the medical condition which led to the hospital admission.
2. **Admission Following Post-Operative Observation**
When a patient is admitted to an observation unit to monitor a condition (or complication) that develops following outpatient surgery, and then is subsequently admitted as an inpatient of the same hospital, hospitals should apply the Uniform Hospital Discharge Data Set (UHDDS) definition of principal diagnosis as "that condition established after study to be chiefly responsible for occasioning the admission of the patient to the hospital for care."

J. Admission from Outpatient Surgery
When a patient receives surgery in the hospital's outpatient surgery department and is subsequently admitted for continuing inpatient care at the same hospital, the following guidelines should be followed in selecting the principal diagnosis for the inpatient admission:

- If the reason for the inpatient admission is a complication, assign the complication as the principal diagnosis.
- If no complication, or other condition, is documented as the reason for the inpatient admission, assign the reason for the outpatient surgery as the principal diagnosis.
- If the reason for the inpatient admission is another condition unrelated to the surgery, assign the unrelated condition as the principal diagnosis.

K. Admissions/Encounters for Rehabilitation
When the purpose for the admission/encounter is rehabilitation, sequence first the code for the condition for which the service is being performed. For example, for an admission/encounter for rehabilitation for right-sided dominant hemiplegia following a cerebrovascular infarction, report code I69.351, Hemiplegia and hemiparesis following cerebral infarction affecting right dominant side, as the first-listed or principal diagnosis.

If the condition for which the rehabilitation service is being provided is no longer present, report the appropriate aftercare code as the first-listed or principal diagnosis, unless the rehabilitation service is being provided following an injury. For rehabilitation services following active treatment of an injury, assign the injury code with the appropriate seventh character for subsequent encounter as the first-listed or principal diagnosis. For example, if a patient with severe degenerative osteoarthritis of the hip, underwent hip replacement and the current encounter/admission is for rehabilitation, report code Z47.1, Aftercare following joint replacement surgery, as the first-listed or principal diagnosis. If the patient requires rehabilitation post hip replacement for right intertrochanteric femur fracture, report code S72.141D, Displaced intertrochanteric fracture of right femur, subsequent encounter for closed fracture with routine healing, as the first-listed or principal diagnosis.

See Section I.C.21.c.7, Factors influencing health states and contact with health services, Aftercare.

See Section I.C.19.a, for additional information about the use of 7th characters for injury codes.

Section III. Reporting Additional Diagnoses

GENERAL RULES FOR OTHER (ADDITIONAL) DIAGNOSES

For reporting purposes, the definition for "other diagnoses" is interpreted as additional conditions that affect patient care in terms of requiring:

clinical evaluation; or
therapeutic treatment; or
diagnostic procedures; or
extended length of hospital stay; or
increased nursing care and/or monitoring.

The UHDDS item #11-b defines Other Diagnoses as "all conditions that coexist at the time of admission, that develop subsequently, or that affect the treatment received and/or the length of stay. Diagnoses that relate to an earlier episode which have no bearing on the current hospital stay are to be excluded." UHDDS definitions apply to inpatients in acute care, short-term, long term care and psychiatric hospital setting. The UHDDS definitions are used by acute care short-term hospitals to report inpatient data elements in a standardized manner. These data elements and their definitions can be found in the July 31, 1985, Federal Register (Vol. 50, No, 147), pp. 31038-40.

Since that time, the application of the UHDDS definitions has been expanded to include all non-outpatient settings (acute care, short term, long term care and psychiatric hospitals; home health agencies; rehab facilities; nursing homes, etc.). The UHDDS definitions also apply to hospice services (all levels of care).

The following guidelines are to be applied in designating "other diagnoses" when neither the Alphabetic Index nor the Tabular List in ICD-10-CM provide direction. The listing of the diagnoses in the patient record is the responsibility of the attending provider.

A. Previous conditions

If the provider has included a diagnosis in the final diagnostic statement, such as the discharge summary or the face sheet, it should ordinarily be coded. Some providers include in the diagnostic statement resolved conditions or diagnoses and status-post procedures from previous admissions that have no bearing on the current stay. Such conditions are not to be reported and are coded only if required by hospital policy.

However, history codes (categories Z80-Z87) may be used as secondary codes if the historical condition or family history has an impact on current care or influences treatment.

B. Abnormal findings

Abnormal findings (laboratory, x-ray, pathologic, and other diagnostic results) are not coded and reported unless the provider indicates their clinical significance. If the findings are outside the normal range and the attending provider has ordered other tests to evaluate the condition or prescribed treatment, it is appropriate to ask the provider whether the abnormal finding should be added.

Please note: This differs from the coding practices in the outpatient setting for coding encounters for diagnostic tests that have been interpreted by a provider.

C. Uncertain Diagnosis

If the diagnosis documented at the time of discharge is qualified as "probable," "suspected," "likely," "questionable," "possible," or "still to be ruled out," "compatible with," "consistent with," or other similar terms indicating uncertainty, code the condition as if it existed or was established. The bases for these guidelines are the diagnostic workup, arrangements for further workup or observation, and initial therapeutic approach that correspond most closely with the established diagnosis.

Note: This guideline is applicable only to inpatient admissions to short-term, acute, long-term care and psychiatric hospitals.

Section IV. Diagnostic Coding and Reporting Guidelines for Outpatient Services

These coding guidelines for outpatient diagnoses have been approved for use by hospitals/ providers in coding and reporting hospital-based outpatient services and provider-based office visits. Guidelines in Section I, Conventions, general coding guidelines and chapter-specific guidelines, should also be applied for outpatient services and office visits.

Information about the use of certain abbreviations, punctuation, symbols, and other conventions used in the ICD-10-CM Tabular List (code numbers and titles), can be found in Section IA of these guidelines, under "Conventions Used in the Tabular List." Section I.B. contains general guidelines that apply to the entire classification. Section I.C. contains chapter-specific guidelines that correspond to the chapters as they are arranged in the classification. Information about the correct sequence to use in finding a code is also described in Section I.

The terms encounter and visit are often used interchangeably in describing outpatient service contacts and, therefore, appear together in these guidelines without distinguishing one from the other.

Though the conventions and general guidelines apply to all settings, coding guidelines for outpatient and provider reporting of diagnoses will vary in a number of instances from those for inpatient diagnoses, recognizing that:

The Uniform Hospital Discharge Data Set (UHDDS) definition of principal diagnosis does not apply to hospital-based outpatient services and provider-based office visits.

Coding guidelines for inconclusive diagnoses (probable, suspected, rule out, etc.) were developed for inpatient reporting and do not apply to outpatients.

A. Selection of first-listed condition

In the outpatient setting, the term first-listed diagnosis is used in lieu of principal diagnosis.

In determining the first-listed diagnosis the coding conventions of ICD-10-CM, as well as the general and disease specific guidelines take precedence over the outpatient guidelines.

Diagnoses often are not established at the time of the initial encounter/visit. It may take two or more visits before the diagnosis is confirmed.

The most critical rule involves beginning the search for the correct code assignment through the Alphabetic Index. Never begin searching initially in the Tabular List as this will lead to coding errors.

1. Outpatient Surgery

When a patient presents for outpatient surgery (same day surgery), code the reason for the surgery as the first-listed diagnosis (reason for the encounter), even if the surgery is not performed due to a contraindication.

2. Observation Stay

When a patient is admitted for observation for a medical condition, assign a code for the medical condition as the first-listed diagnosis.

When a patient presents for outpatient surgery and develops complications requiring admission to observation, code the reason for the surgery as the first reported diagnosis (reason for the encounter), followed by codes for the complications as secondary diagnoses.

B. Codes from A00.0 through T88.9, Z00-Z99

The appropriate code(s) from A00.0 through T88.9, Z00-Z99 must be used to identify diagnoses, symptoms, conditions, problems, complaints, or other reason(s) for the encounter/visit.

C. Accurate reporting of ICD-10-CM diagnosis codes

For accurate reporting of ICD-10-CM diagnosis codes, the documentation should describe the patient's condition, using terminology which includes specific diagnoses as well as symptoms, problems, or reasons for the encounter. There are ICD-10-CM codes to describe all of these.

D. Codes that describe symptoms and signs

Codes that describe symptoms and signs, as opposed to diagnoses, are acceptable for reporting purposes when a diagnosis has not been established (confirmed) by the provider. Chapter 18 of ICD-10-CM, Symptoms, Signs, and Abnormal Clinical and Laboratory Findings Not Elsewhere Classified (codes R00-R99) contain many, but not all codes for symptoms.

E. Encounters for circumstances other than a disease or injury

ICD-10-CM provides codes to deal with encounters for circumstances other than a disease or injury. The Factors Influencing Health Status and Contact with Health Services codes (Z00-Z99) are provided to deal with occasions when circumstances other than a disease or injury are recorded as diagnosis or problems.

See Section I.C.21. Factors influencing health status and contact with health services.

F. Level of Detail in Coding

1. ICD-10-CM codes with 3, 4, 5, 6 or 7 characters

ICD-10-CM is composed of codes with 3, 4, 5, 6 or 7 characters. Codes with three characters are included in ICD-10-CM as the heading of a category of codes that may be further subdivided by the use of fourth, fifth, sixth or seventh characters to provide greater specificity.

2. Use of full number of characters required for a code

A three-character code is to be used only if it is not further subdivided. A code is invalid if it has not been coded to the full number of characters required for that code, including the 7th character, if applicable.

G. ICD-10-CM code for the diagnosis, condition, problem, or other reason for encounter/visit

List first the ICD-10-CM code for the diagnosis, condition, problem, or other reason for encounter/visit shown in the medical record to be chiefly responsible for the services provided. List additional codes that describe any coexisting conditions. In some cases the first-listed diagnosis may be a symptom when a diagnosis has not been established (confirmed) by the provider.

H. Uncertain diagnosis

Do not code diagnoses documented as "probable", "suspected," "questionable," "rule out," "compatible with," "consistent with," or "working diagnosis" or other similar terms indicating uncertainty. Rather, code the condition(s) to the highest degree of certainty for that encounter/visit, such as symptoms, signs, abnormal test results, or other reason for the visit.

Please note: This differs from the coding practices used by short-term, acute care, long-term care and psychiatric hospitals.

I. Chronic diseases

Chronic diseases treated on an ongoing basis may be coded and reported as many times as the patient receives treatment and care for the condition(s)

J. Code all documented conditions that coexist

Code all documented conditions that coexist at the time of the encounter/visit, and require or affect patient care treatment or management. Do not code conditions that were previously treated and no longer exist. However, history codes (categories Z80-Z87) may be used as secondary codes if the historical condition or family history has an impact on current care or influences treatment.

K. Patients receiving diagnostic services only

For patients receiving diagnostic services only during an encounter/visit, sequence first the diagnosis, condition, problem, or other reason for encounter/visit shown in the medical record to be chiefly responsible for the outpatient services provided during the encounter/visit. Codes for other diagnoses (e.g., chronic conditions) may be sequenced as additional diagnoses.

For encounters for routine laboratory/radiology testing in the absence of any signs, symptoms, or associated diagnosis, assign Z01.89, Encounter for other specified special examinations. If routine testing is performed during the same encounter as a test to evaluate a sign, symptom, or diagnosis, it is appropriate to assign both the Z code and the code describing the reason for the non-routine test.

For outpatient encounters for diagnostic tests that have been interpreted by a physician, and the final report is available at the time of coding, code any confirmed or definitive diagnosis(es) documented in the interpretation. Do not code related signs and symptoms as additional diagnoses.

Please note: This differs from the coding practice in the hospital inpatient setting regarding abnormal findings on test results.

L. Patients receiving therapeutic services only

For patients receiving therapeutic services only during an encounter/visit, sequence first the diagnosis, condition, problem, or other reason for encounter/visit shown in the medical record to be chiefly responsible for the outpatient services provided during the encounter/visit. Codes for other diagnoses (e.g., chronic conditions) may be sequenced as additional diagnoses.

The only exception to this rule is that when the primary reason for the admission/encounter is chemotherapy or radiation therapy, the appropriate Z code for the service is listed first, and the diagnosis or problem for which the service is being performed listed second.

M. Patients receiving preoperative evaluations only

For patients receiving preoperative evaluations only, sequence first a code from subcategory Z01.81, Encounter for pre-procedural examinations, to describe the pre-op consultations. Assign a code for the condition to describe the reason for the surgery as an additional diagnosis. Code also any findings related to the pre-op evaluation.

N. Ambulatory surgery

For ambulatory surgery, code the diagnosis for which the surgery was performed. If the postoperative diagnosis is known to be different from the preoperative diagnosis at the time the diagnosis is confirmed, select the postoperative diagnosis for coding, since it is the most definitive.

O. Routine outpatient prenatal visits

See Section I.C.15. Routine outpatient prenatal visits.

P. Encounters for general medical examinations with abnormal findings

The subcategories for encounters for general medical examinations, Z00.0- and encounter for routine child health examination, Z00.12-, provide codes for with and without abnormal findings. Should a general medical examination result in an abnormal finding, the code for general medical examination with abnormal finding should be assigned as the first-listed diagnosis. An examination with abnormal findings refers to a condition/diagnosis that is newly identified or a change in severity of a chronic condition (such as uncontrolled hypertension, or an acute exacerbation of chronic obstructive pulmonary disease) during a routine physical examination. A secondary code for the abnormal finding should also be coded.

Q. Encounters for routine health screenings

See Section I.C.21. Factors influencing health status and contact with health services, Screening

Appendix I. Present on Admission Reporting Guidelines

Introduction

These guidelines are to be used as a supplement to the *ICD-10-CM Official Guidelines for Coding and Reporting* to facilitate the assignment of the Present on Admission (POA) indicator for each diagnosis and external cause of injury code reported on claim forms (UB-04 and 837 Institutional).

These guidelines are not intended to replace any guidelines in the main body of the *ICD-10-CM Official Guidelines for Coding and Reporting*. The POA guidelines are not intended to provide guidance on when a condition should be coded, but rather, how to apply the POA indicator to the final set of diagnosis codes that have been assigned in accordance with Sections I, II, and III of the official coding guidelines. Subsequent to the assignment of the ICD-10-CM codes, the POA indicator should then be assigned to those conditions that have been coded.

As stated in the Introduction to the *ICD-10-CM Official Guidelines for Coding and Reporting*, a joint effort between the healthcare provider and the coder is essential to achieve complete and accurate documentation, code assignment, and reporting of diagnoses and procedures. The importance of consistent, complete documentation in the medical record cannot be overemphasized. Medical record documentation from any provider involved in the care and treatment of the patient may be used to support the determination of whether a condition was present on admission or not. In the context of the official coding guidelines, the term "provider" means a physician or any qualified healthcare practitioner who is legally accountable for establishing the patient's diagnosis.

These guidelines are not a substitute for the provider's clinical judgment as to the determination of whether a condition was/was not present on admission. The provider should be queried regarding issues related to the linking of signs/symptoms, timing of test results, and the timing of findings.

Please see the CDC website for the detailed list of ICD-10-CM codes that do not require the use of a POA indicator (https://www.cdc.gov/nchs/icd/icd10cm.htm). The codes and categories on this exempt list are for circumstances regarding the healthcare encounter or factors influencing health status that do not represent a current disease or injury or that describe conditions that are always present on admission.

General Reporting Requirements

All claims involving inpatient admissions to general acute care hospitals or other facilities that are subject to a law or regulation mandating collection of present on admission information.

Present on admission is defined as present at the time the order for inpatient admission occurs -- conditions that develop during an outpatient encounter, including emergency department, observation, or outpatient surgery, are considered as present on admission.

POA indicator is assigned to principal and secondary diagnoses (as defined in Section II of the Official Guidelines for Coding and Reporting) and the external cause of injury codes.

Issues related to inconsistent, missing, conflicting or unclear documentation must still be resolved by the provider.

If a condition would not be coded and reported based on UHDDS definitions and current official coding guidelines, then the POA indicator would not be reported.

Reporting Options

Y - Yes

N - No

U - Unknown

W – Clinically undetermined

Unreported/Not used – (Exempt from POA reporting)

Reporting Definitions

Y = present at the time of inpatient admission

N = not present at the time of inpatient admission

U = documentation is insufficient to determine if condition is present on admission

W = provider is unable to clinically determine whether condition was present on admission or not

Timeframe for POA Identification and Documentation

There is no required timeframe as to when a provider (per the definition of "provider" used in these guidelines) must identify or document a condition to be present on admission. In some clinical situations, it may not be possible for a provider to make a definitive diagnosis (or a condition may not be recognized or reported by the patient) for a period of time after admission. In some cases, it may be several days before the provider arrives at a definitive diagnosis. This does not mean that the condition was not present on admission. Determination of whether the condition was present on admission or not will be based on the applicable POA guideline as identified in this document, or on the provider's best clinical judgment.

If at the time of code assignment the documentation is unclear as to whether a condition was present on admission or not, it is appropriate to query the provider for clarification.

Assigning the POA Indicator

Condition is on the "Exempt from Reporting" list

Leave the "present on admission" field blank if the condition is on the list of ICD-10-CM codes for which this field is not applicable. This is the only circumstance in which the field may be left blank.

POA Explicitly Documented

Assign Y for any condition the provider explicitly documents as being present on admission.

Assign N for any condition the provider explicitly documents as not present at the time of admission.

Conditions diagnosed prior to inpatient admission

Assign "Y" for conditions that were diagnosed prior to admission (example: hypertension, diabetes mellitus, asthma)

Conditions diagnosed during the admission but clearly present before admission

Assign "Y" for conditions diagnosed during the admission that were clearly present but not diagnosed until after admission occurred.

Diagnoses subsequently confirmed after admission are considered present on admission if at the time of admission they are documented as suspected, possible, rule out, differential diagnosis, or constitute an underlying cause of a symptom that is present at the time of admission.

Condition develops during outpatient encounter prior to inpatient admission

Assign Y for any condition that develops during an outpatient encounter prior to a written order for inpatient admission.

Documentation does not indicate whether condition was present on admission

Assign "U" when the medical record documentation is unclear as to whether the condition was present on admission. "U" should not be routinely assigned and used only in very limited circumstances. Coders are encouraged to query the providers when the documentation is unclear.

Documentation states that it cannot be determined whether the condition was or was not present on admission

Assign "W" when the medical record documentation indicates that it cannot be clinically determined whether or not the condition was present on admission.

Chronic condition with acute exacerbation during the admission

If a single code identifies both the chronic condition and the acute exacerbation, see POA guidelines pertaining to codes that contain multiple clinical concepts.

If a single code only identifies the chronic condition and not the acute exacerbation (e.g., acute exacerbation of chronic leukemia), assign "Y."

Conditions documented as possible, probable, suspected, or rule out at the time of discharge

If the final diagnosis contains a possible, probable, suspected, or rule out diagnosis, and this diagnosis was based on signs, symptoms or clinical findings suspected at the time of inpatient admission, assign "Y."

If the final diagnosis contains a possible, probable, suspected, or rule out diagnosis, and this diagnosis was based on signs, symptoms or clinical findings that were not present on admission, assign "N".

Conditions documented as impending or threatened at the time of discharge

If the final diagnosis contains an impending or threatened diagnosis, and this diagnosis is based on symptoms or clinical findings that were present on admission, assign "Y".

If the final diagnosis contains an impending or threatened diagnosis, and this diagnosis is based on symptoms or clinical findings that were not present on admission, assign "N".

Acute and Chronic Conditions

Assign "Y" for acute conditions that are present at time of admission and N for acute conditions that are not present at time of admission.

Assign "Y" for chronic conditions, even though the condition may not be diagnosed until after admission.

If a single code identifies both an acute and chronic condition, see the POA guidelines for codes that contain multiple clinical concepts.

Codes That Contain Multiple Clinical Concepts

Assign "N" if at least one of the clinical concepts included in the code was not present on admission (e.g., COPD with acute exacerbation and the exacerbation was not present on admission; gastric ulcer that does not start bleeding until after admission; asthma patient develops status asthmaticus after admission).

Assign "Y" if all of the clinical concepts included in the code were present on admission (e.g., duodenal ulcer that perforates prior to admission).

For infection codes that include the causal organism, assign "Y" if the infection (or signs of the infection) were present on admission, even though the culture results may not be known until after admission (e.g., patient is admitted with pneumonia and the provider documents Pseudomonas as the causal organism a few days later).

Same Diagnosis Code for Two or More Conditions

When the same ICD-10-CM diagnosis code applies to two or more conditions during the same encounter (e.g. two separate conditions classified to the same ICD-10-CM diagnosis code):

Assign "Y" if all conditions represented by the single ICD-10-CM code were present on admission (e.g. bilateral unspecified age-related cataracts).

Assign "N" if any of the conditions represented by the single ICD-10-CM code was not present on admission (e.g. traumatic secondary and recurrent hemorrhage and seroma is assigned to a single code T79.2, but only one of the conditions was present on admission).

Obstetrical conditions

Whether or not the patient delivers during the current hospitalization does not affect assignment of the POA indicator. The determining factor for POA assignment is whether the pregnancy complication or obstetrical condition described by the code was present at the time of admission or not.

If the pregnancy complication or obstetrical condition was present on admission (e.g., patient admitted in preterm labor), assign "Y".

If the pregnancy complication or obstetrical condition was not present on admission (e.g., 2nd degree laceration during delivery, postpartum hemorrhage that occurred during current hospitalization, fetal distress develops after admission), assign "N".

If the obstetrical code includes more than one diagnosis and any of the diagnoses identified by the code were not present on admission assign "N". (e.g., Category O11, Pre-existing hypertension with pre-eclampsia)

Perinatal conditions

Newborns are not considered to be admitted until after birth. Therefore, any condition present at birth or that developed in utero is considered present at admission and should be assigned "Y". This includes conditions that occur during delivery (e.g., injury during delivery, meconium aspiration, exposure to streptococcus B in the vaginal canal).

Congenital conditions and anomalies

Assign "Y" for congenital conditions and anomalies except for categories QØØ-Q99, Congenital anomalies, which are on the exempt list. Congenital conditions are always considered present on admission.

External cause of injury codes

Assign "Y" for any external cause code representing an external cause of morbidity that occurred prior to inpatient admission (e.g., patient fell out of bed at home, patient fell out of bed in emergency room prior to admission)

Assign "N" for any external cause code representing an external cause of morbidity that occurred during inpatient hospitalization (e.g., patient fell out of hospital bed during hospital stay, patient experienced an adverse reaction to a medication administered after inpatient admission).

ICD-10-CM Index to Diseases and Injuries

A

- **Abrasion** — *continued*
  - chin S00.81 ☑
  - clitoris S30.814 ☑
  - cornea S05.0- ☑
  - costal region — *see* Abrasion, thorax
  - dental K03.1
  - digit(s)
    - foot — *see* Abrasion, toe
    - hand — *see* Abrasion, finger
  - ear S00.41- ☑
  - elbow S50.31- ☑
  - epididymis S30.813 ☑
  - epigastric region S30.811 ☑
  - epiglottis S10.11 ☑
  - esophagus (thoracic) S27.818 ☑
    - cervical S10.11 ☑
  - eyebrow — *see* Abrasion, eyelid
  - eyelid S00.21- ☑
  - face S00.81 ☑
  - finger(s) S60.41- ☑
    - index S60.41- ☑
    - little S60.41- ☑
    - middle S60.41- ☑
    - ring S60.41- ☑
  - flank S30.811 ☑
  - foot (except toe(s) alone) S90.81- ☑
    - toe — *see* Abrasion, toe
  - forearm S50.81- ☑
    - elbow only — *see* Abrasion, elbow
  - forehead S00.81 ☑
  - genital organs, external
    - female S30.816 ☑
    - male S30.815 ☑
  - groin S30.811 ☑
  - gum S00.512 ☑
  - hand S60.51- ☑
  - head S00.91 ☑
    - ear — *see* Abrasion, ear
    - eyelid — *see* Abrasion, eyelid
    - lip S00.511 ☑
    - nose S00.31 ☑
    - oral cavity S00.512 ☑
    - scalp S00.01 ☑
    - specified site NEC S00.81 ☑
  - heel — *see* Abrasion, foot
  - hip S70.21- ☑
  - inguinal region S30.811 ☑
  - interscapular region S20.419 ☑
  - jaw S00.81 ☑
  - knee S80.21- ☑
  - labium (majus) (minus) S30.814 ☑
  - larynx S10.11 ☑
  - leg (lower) S80.81- ☑
    - knee — *see* Abrasion, knee
    - upper — *see* Abrasion, thigh
  - lip S00.511 ☑
  - lower back S30.810 ☑
  - lumbar region S30.810 ☑
  - malar region S00.81 ☑
  - mammary — *see* Abrasion, breast
  - mastoid region S00.81 ☑
  - mouth S00.512 ☑
  - nail
    - finger — *see* Abrasion, finger
    - toe — *see* Abrasion, toe
  - nape S10.81 ☑
  - nasal S00.31 ☑
  - neck S10.91 ☑
    - specified site NEC S10.81 ☑
    - throat S10.11 ☑
  - nose S00.31 ☑
  - occipital region S00.01 ☑
  - oral cavity S00.512 ☑
  - orbital region — *see* Abrasion, eyelid
  - palate S00.512 ☑
  - palm — *see* Abrasion, hand
  - parietal region S00.01 ☑
  - pelvis S30.810 ☑
  - penis S30.812 ☑
  - perineum
    - female S30.814 ☑
    - male S30.810 ☑
  - periocular area — *see* Abrasion, eyelid
  - phalanges
    - finger — *see* Abrasion, finger
    - toe — *see* Abrasion, toe
  - pharynx S10.11 ☑
  - pinna — *see* Abrasion, ear
  - popliteal space — *see* Abrasion, knee
  - prepuce S30.812 ☑
  - pubic region S30.810 ☑
  - pudendum
    - female S30.816 ☑
    - male S30.815 ☑
  - sacral region S30.810 ☑
  - scalp S00.01 ☑
  - scapular region — *see* Abrasion, shoulder
  - scrotum S30.813 ☑
  - shin — *see* Abrasion, leg
  - shoulder S40.21- ☑
  - skin NEC T14.8 ☑
  - sternal region S20.319 ☑
  - submaxillary region S00.81 ☑
  - submental region S00.81 ☑
  - subungual
    - finger(s) — *see* Abrasion, finger
    - toe(s) — *see* Abrasion, toe
  - supraclavicular fossa S10.81 ☑
  - supraorbital S00.81 ☑
  - temple S00.81 ☑
  - temporal region S00.81 ☑
  - testis S30.813 ☑
  - thigh S70.31- ☑
  - thorax, thoracic (wall) S20.91 ☑
    - back S20.41- ☑
    - front S20.31- ☑
  - throat S10.11 ☑
  - thumb S60.31- ☑
  - toe(s) (lesser) S90.416 ☑
    - great S90.41- ☑
  - tongue S00.512 ☑
  - tooth, teeth (dentifrice) (habitual) (hard tissues) (occupational) (ritual) (traditional) K03.1
  - trachea S10.11 ☑
  - tunica vaginalis S30.813 ☑
  - tympanum, tympanic membrane — *see* Abrasion, ear
  - uvula S00.512 ☑
  - vagina S30.814 ☑
  - vocal cords S10.11 ☑
  - vulva S30.814 ☑
  - wrist S60.81- ☑
- **Abrism** — *see* Poisoning, food, noxious, plant
- **Abruptio placentae** O45.9- ☑
  - with
    - afibrinogenemia O45.01- ☑
    - coagulation defect O45.00- ☑
      - specified NEC O45.09- ☑
    - disseminated intravascular coagulation O45.02- ☑
    - hypofibrinogenemia O45.01- ☑
  - specified NEC O45.8- ☑
- **Abruption, placenta** — *see* Abruptio placentae
- **Abscess** (connective tissue) (embolic) (fistulous) (infective) (metastatic) (multiple) (pernicious) (pyogenic) (septic) L02.91
  - with
    - diverticular disease (intestine) K57.80
      - with bleeding K57.81
      - large intestine K57.20
        - with
          - bleeding K57.21
          - small intestine K57.40
            - with bleeding K57.41
      - small intestine K57.00
        - with
          - bleeding K57.01
          - large intestine K57.40
            - with bleeding K57.41
    - lymphangitis — *code by* site under Abscess
  - abdomen, abdominal
    - cavity K65.1
    - wall L02.211
  - abdominopelvic K65.1
  - accessory sinus — *see* Sinusitis
  - adrenal (capsule) (gland) E27.8
  - alveolar K04.7
    - with sinus K04.6
  - amebic A06.4
    - brain (and liver or lung abscess) A06.6
    - genitourinary tract A06.82
    - liver (without mention of brain or lung abscess) A06.4

- **Abscess** — *continued*
  - amebic — *continued*
    - lung (and liver) (without mention of brain abscess) A06.5
    - specified site NEC A06.89
    - spleen A06.89
  - anerobic A48.0
  - ankle — *see* Abscess, lower limb
  - anorectal K61.2
  - antecubital space — *see* Abscess, upper limb
  - antrum (chronic) (Highmore) — *see* Sinusitis, maxillary
  - anus K61.0
  - apical (tooth) K04.7
    - with sinus (alveolar) K04.6
  - appendix K35.33
  - areola (acute) (chronic) (nonpuerperal) N61.1
    - puerperal, postpartum or gestational — *see* Infection, nipple
  - arm (any part) — *see* Abscess, upper limb
  - artery (wall) I77.89
  - atheromatous I77.2
  - auricle, ear — *see* Abscess, ear, external
  - axilla (region) L02.41- ☑
    - lymph gland or node L04.2
  - back (any part, except buttock) L02.212
  - Bartholin's gland N75.1
    - with
      - abortion — *see* Abortion, by type complicated by, sepsis
      - ectopic or molar pregnancy O08.0
    - following ectopic or molar pregnancy O08.0
  - Bezold's — *see* Mastoiditis, acute
  - bilharziasis B65.1
  - bladder (wall) — *see* Cystitis, specified type NEC
  - bone (subperiosteal) — *see also* Osteomyelitis, specified type NEC
    - accessory sinus (chronic) — *see* Sinusitis
    - chronic or old — *see* Osteomyelitis, chronic
    - jaw (lower) (upper) M27.2
    - mastoid — *see* Mastoiditis, acute, subperiosteal
    - petrous — *see* Petrositis
    - spinal (tuberculous) A18.01
      - nontuberculous — *see* Osteomyelitis, vertebra
  - bowel K63.0
  - brain (any part) (cystic) (otogenic) G06.0
    - amebic (with abscess of any other site) A06.6
    - gonococcal A54.82
    - pheomycotic (chromomycotic) B43.1
    - tuberculous A17.81
  - breast (acute) (chronic) (nonpuerperal) N61.1
    - newborn P39.0
    - puerperal, postpartum, gestational — *see* Mastitis, obstetric, purulent
  - broad ligament N73.2
    - acute N73.0
    - chronic N73.1
  - Brodie's (localized) (chronic) M86.8X- ☑
  - bronchi J98.09
  - buccal cavity K12.2
  - bulbourethral gland N34.0
  - bursa M71.00
    - ankle M71.07- ☑
    - elbow M71.02- ☑
    - foot M71.07- ☑
    - hand M71.04- ☑
    - hip M71.05- ☑
    - knee M71.06- ☑
    - multiple sites M71.09
    - pharyngeal J39.1
    - shoulder M71.01- ☑
    - specified site NEC M71.08
    - wrist M71.03- ☑
  - buttock L02.31
  - canthus — *see* Blepharoconjunctivitis
  - cartilage — *see* Disorder, cartilage, specified type NEC
  - cecum K35.33
  - cerebellum, cerebellar G06.0
    - sequelae G09
  - cerebral (embolic) G06.0
    - sequelae G09
  - cervical (meaning neck) L02.11
    - lymph gland or node L04.0
  - cervix (stump) (uteri) — *see* Cervicitis
  - cheek (external) L02.01
    - inner K12.2
  - chest J86.9
    - with fistula J86.0
    - wall L02.213

Abscess — *continued*
- peritoneum, peritoneal — *continued*
  - pelvic — *continued*
    - male K65.1
  - postoperative T81.49 ☑
  - puerperal, postpartum, childbirth O85
  - tuberculous A18.31
- peritonsillar J36
- perityphlic K35.33
- periureteral N28.89
- periurethral N34.Ø
  - gonococcal (accessory gland) (periurethral) A54.1
- periuterine — *see also* Disease, pelvis, inflammatory N73.2
- perivesical — *see* Cystitis, specified type NEC
- petrous bone — *see* Petrositis
- phagedenic NOS LØ2.91
  - chancroid A57
- pharynx, pharyngeal (lateral) J39.1
- pilonidal LØ5.Ø1
- pituitary (gland) E23.6
- pleura J86.9
  - with fistula J86.Ø
- popliteal — *see* Abscess, lower limb
- postcecal K35.33
- postlaryngeal J38.7
- postnasal J34.Ø
- postoperative (any site) — *see also* Infection, postoperative wound T81.49 ☑
  - retroperitoneal K68.11
- postpharyngeal J39.Ø
- posttonsillar J36
- post-typhoid AØ1.Ø9
- pouch of Douglas — *see* Peritonitis, pelvic, female
- premammary — *see* Abscess, breast
- prepatellar — *see* Abscess, lower limb
- prostate N41.2
  - gonococcal (acute) (chronic) A54.22
- psoas muscle K68.12
- puerperal — *code by* site under Puerperal, abscess
- pulmonary — *see* Abscess, lung
- pulp, pulpal (dental) KØ4.Ø1
  - irreversible KØ4.Ø2
  - reversible KØ4.Ø1
- rectovaginal septum K63.Ø
- rectovesical — *see* Cystitis, specified type NEC
- rectum K61.1
- renal — *see* Abscess, kidney
- retina — *see* Inflammation, chorioretinal
- retrobulbar — *see* Abscess, orbit
- retrocecal K65.1
- retrolaryngeal J38.7
- retromammary — *see* Abscess, breast
- retroperitoneal NEC K68.19
  - postprocedural K68.11
- retropharyngeal J39.Ø
- retrouterine — *see* Peritonitis, pelvic, female
- retrovesical — *see* Cystitis, specified type NEC
- root, tooth KØ4.7
  - with sinus (alveolar) KØ4.6
- round ligament — *see also* Disease, pelvis, inflammatory N73.2
- rupture (spontaneous) NOS LØ2.91
- sacrum (tuberculous) A18.Ø1
  - nontuberculous M46.28
- salivary (duct) (gland) K11.3
- scalp (any part) LØ2.811
- scapular — *see* Osteomyelitis, specified type NEC
- sclera — *see* Scleritis
- scrofulous (tuberculous) A18.2
- scrotum N49.2
- seminal vesicle N49.Ø
- septal, dental KØ4.7
  - with sinus (alveolar) KØ4.6
- serous — *see* Periostitis
- shoulder (region) — *see* Abscess, upper limb
- sigmoid K63.Ø
- sinus (accessory) (chronic) (nasal) — *see also* Sinusitis
  - intracranial venous (any) GØ6.Ø
- Skene's duct or gland N34.Ø
- skin — *see* Abscess, by site
- specified site NEC LØ2.818
- spermatic cord N49.1
- sphenoidal (sinus) (chronic) J32.3
- spinal cord (any part) (staphylococcal) GØ6.1
  - tuberculous A17.81
- spine (column) (tuberculous) A18.Ø1
  - epidural GØ6.1

Abscess — *continued*
- spine — *continued*
  - nontuberculous — *see* Osteomyelitis, vertebra
- spleen D73.3
  - amebic AØ6.89
- stitch T81.41 ☑
  - following an obstetrical procedure O86.Ø1
- subarachnoid GØ6.2
  - brain GØ6.Ø
  - spinal cord GØ6.1
- subareolar — *see* Abscess, breast
- subcecal K35.33
- subcutaneous — *see also* Abscess, by site
  - following procedure T81.41 ☑
    - obstetrical O86.Ø1
  - pheomycotic (chromomycotic) B43.2
- subdiaphragmatic K65.1
- subdural GØ6.2
  - brain GØ6.Ø
    - sequelae GØ9
  - spinal cord GØ6.1
- sub-fascial, following an obstetrical procedure O86.Ø2
- subgaleal LØ2.811
- subhepatic K65.1
- sublingual K12.2
  - gland K11.3
- submammary — *see* Abscess, breast
- submandibular (region) (space) (triangle) K12.2
  - gland K11.3
- submaxillary (region) LØ2.Ø1
  - gland K11.3
- submental LØ2.Ø1
  - gland K11.3
- subperiosteal — *see* Osteomyelitis, specified type NEC
- subphrenic K65.1
  - following an obstetrical procedure O86.Ø3
  - postoperative T81.43 ☑
- suburethral N34.Ø
- sudoriparous L75.8
- supraclavicular (fossa) — *see* Abscess, upper limb
- supralevator K61.5
- suprapelvic, acute N73.Ø
- suprarenal (capsule) (gland) E27.8
- sweat gland L74.8
- tear duct — *see* Inflammation, lacrimal, passages, acute
- temple LØ2.Ø1
- temporal region LØ2.Ø1
- temporosphenoidal GØ6.Ø
- tendon (sheath) M65.ØØ
  - ankle M65.Ø7- ☑
  - foot M65.Ø7- ☑
  - forearm M65.Ø3- ☑
  - hand M65.Ø4- ☑
  - lower leg M65.Ø6- ☑
  - pelvic region M65.Ø5- ☑
  - shoulder region M65.Ø1- ☑
  - specified site NEC M65.Ø8
  - thigh M65.Ø5- ☑
  - upper arm M65.Ø2- ☑
- testis N45.4
- thigh — *see* Abscess, lower limb
- thorax J86.9
  - with fistula J86.Ø
- throat J39.1
- thumb — *see also* Abscess, hand
  - nail — *see* Cellulitis, finger
- thymus (gland) E32.1
- thyroid (gland) EØ6.Ø
- toe (any) — *see also* Abscess, foot
  - nail — *see* Cellulitis, toe
- tongue (staphylococcal) K14.Ø
- tonsil(s) (lingual) J36
- tonsillopharyngeal J36
- tooth, teeth (root) KØ4.7
  - with sinus (alveolar) KØ4.6
  - supporting structures NEC — *see* Periodontitis, aggressive, localized
- trachea J39.8
- trunk LØ2.219
  - abdominal wall LØ2.211
  - back LØ2.212
  - chest wall LØ2.213
  - groin LØ2.214
  - perineum LØ2.215
  - umbilicus LØ2.216
- tubal — *see* Salpingitis
- tuberculous — *see* Tuberculosis, abscess
- tubo-ovarian — *see* Salpingo-oophoritis

Abscess — *continued*
- tunica vaginalis N49.1
- umbilicus LØ2.216
- upper
  - limb LØ2.41- ☑
  - respiratory J39.8
- urethral (gland) N34.Ø
- urinary N34.Ø
- uterus, uterine (wall) — *see also* Endometritis
  - ligament — *see also* Disease, pelvis, inflammatory N73.2
  - neck — *see* Cervicitis
- uvula K12.2
- vagina (wall) — *see* Vaginitis
- vaginorectal — *see* Vaginitis
- vas deferens N49.1
- vermiform appendix K35.33
- vertebra (column) (tuberculous) A18.Ø1
  - nontuberculous — *see* Osteomyelitis, vertebra
- vesical — *see* Cystitis, specified type NEC
- vesico-uterine pouch — *see* Peritonitis, pelvic, female
- vitreous (humor) — *see* Endophthalmitis, purulent
- vocal cord J38.3
- von Bezold's — *see* Mastoiditis, acute
- vulva N76.4
- vulvovaginal gland N75.1
- web space — *see* Abscess, hand
- wound T81.49 ☑
- wrist — *see* Abscess, upper limb

Absence (of) (organ or part) (complete or partial)
- adrenal (gland) (congenital) Q89.1
  - acquired E89.6
- albumin in blood E88.Ø9
- alimentary tract (congenital) Q45.8
  - upper Q4Ø.8
- alveolar process (acquired) — *see* Anomaly, alveolar
- ankle (acquired) Z89.44- ☑
- anus (congenital) Q42.3
  - with fistula Q42.2
- aorta (congenital) Q25.41
- appendix, congenital Q42.8
- arm (acquired) Z89.2Ø- ☑
  - above elbow Z89.22- ☑
    - congenital (with hand present) — *see* Agenesis, arm, with hand present
      - and hand — *see* Agenesis, forearm, and hand
  - below elbow Z89.21- ☑
    - congenital (with hand present) — *see* Agenesis, arm, with hand present
      - and hand — *see* Agenesis, forearm, and hand
  - congenital — *see* Defect, reduction, upper limb
  - shoulder (following explantation of shoulder joint prosthesis) (joint) (with or without presence of antibiotic-impregnated cement spacer) Z89.23- ☑
    - congenital (with hand present) — *see* Agenesis, arm, with hand present
- artery (congenital) (peripheral) Q27.8
  - brain Q28.3
  - coronary Q24.5
  - pulmonary Q25.79
  - specified NEC Q27.8
  - umbilical Q27.Ø
- atrial septum (congenital) Q21.1
- auditory canal (congenital) (external) Q16.1
- auricle (ear), congenital Q16.Ø
- bile, biliary duct, congenital Q44.5
- bladder (acquired) Z9Ø.6
  - congenital Q64.5
- bowel sounds R19.11
- brain QØØ.Ø
  - part of QØ4.3
- breast(s) (and nipple(s)) (acquired) Z9Ø.1- ☑
  - congenital Q83.8
- broad ligament Q5Ø.6
- bronchus (congenital) Q32.4
- canaliculus lacrimalis, congenital Q1Ø.4
- cerebellum (vermis) QØ4.3
- cervix (acquired) (with uterus) Z9Ø.71Ø
  - with remaining uterus Z9Ø.712
  - congenital Q51.5
- chin, congenital Q18.8
- cilia (congenital) Q1Ø.3
  - acquired — *see* Madarosis
- clitoris (congenital) Q52.6
- coccyx, congenital Q76.49
- cold sense R2Ø.8

Absence — *continued*
- congenital
  - lumen — *see* Atresia
  - organ or site NEC — *see* Agenesis
  - septum — *see* Imperfect, closure
- corpus callosum QØ4.Ø
- cricoid cartilage, congenital Q31.8
- diaphragm (with hernia), congenital Q79.1
- digestive organ(s) or tract, congenital Q45.8
  - acquired NEC Z9Ø.49
  - upper Q4Ø.8
- ductus arteriosus Q28.8
- duodenum (acquired) Z9Ø.49
  - congenital Q41.Ø
- ear, congenital Q16.9
  - acquired H93.8- ☑
  - auricle Q16.Ø
  - external Q16.Ø
  - inner Q16.5
  - lobe, lobule Q17.8
  - middle, except ossicles Q16.4
    - ossicles Q16.3
  - ossicles Q16.3
- ejaculatory duct (congenital) Q55.4
- endocrine gland (congenital) NEC Q89.2
  - acquired E89.89
- epididymis (congenital) Q55.4
  - acquired Z9Ø.79
- epiglottis, congenital Q31.8
- esophagus (congenital) Q39.8
  - acquired (partial) Z9Ø.49
- eustachian tube (congenital) Q16.2
- extremity (acquired) Z89.9
  - congenital Q73.Ø
  - knee (following explantation of knee joint prosthesis) (joint) (with or without presence of antibiotic-impregnated cement spacer) Z89.52- ☑
  - lower (above knee) Z89.619
    - below knee Z89.51- ☑
  - upper — *see* Absence, arm
- eye (acquired) Z9Ø.Ø1
  - congenital Q11.1
  - muscle (congenital) Q1Ø.3
- eyeball (acquired) Z9Ø.Ø1
- eyelid (fold) (congenital) Q1Ø.3
  - acquired Z9Ø.Ø1
- face, specified part NEC Q18.8
- fallopian tube(s) (acquired) Z9Ø.79
  - congenital Q5Ø.6
- family member (causing problem in home) NEC — *see also* Disruption, family Z63.32
- femur, congenital — *see* Defect, reduction, lower limb, longitudinal, femur
- fibrinogen (congenital) D68.2
  - acquired D65
- finger(s) (acquired) Z89.Ø2- ☑
  - congenital — *see* Agenesis, hand
- foot (acquired) Z89.43- ☑
  - congenital — *see* Agenesis, foot
- forearm (acquired) — *see* Absence, arm, below elbow
- gallbladder (acquired) Z9Ø.49
  - congenital Q44.Ø
- gamma globulin in blood D8Ø.1
  - hereditary D8Ø.Ø
- genital organs
  - acquired (female) (male) Z9Ø.79
  - female, congenital Q52.8
    - external Q52.71
    - internal NEC Q52.8
  - male, congenital Q55.8
- genitourinary organs, congenital NEC
  - female Q52.8
  - male Q55.8
- globe (acquired) Z9Ø.Ø1
  - congenital Q11.1
- glottis, congenital Q31.8
- hand and wrist (acquired) Z89.11- ☑
  - congenital — *see* Agenesis, hand
- head, part (acquired) NEC Z9Ø.Ø9
- heat sense R2Ø.8
- hip (following explantation of hip joint prosthesis) (joint) (with or without presence of antibiotic-impregnated cement spacer) Z89.62- ☑
- hymen (congenital) Q52.4
- ileum (acquired) Z9Ø.49
  - congenital Q41.2
- immunoglobulin, isolated NEC D8Ø.3
  - IgA D8Ø.2

Absence — *continued*
- immunoglobulin, isolated — *continued*
  - IgG D8Ø.3
  - IgM D8Ø.4
- incus (acquired) — *see* Loss, ossicles, ear
  - congenital Q16.3
- inner ear, congenital Q16.5
- intestine (acquired) (small) Z9Ø.49
  - congenital Q41.9
    - specified NEC Q41.8
  - large Z9Ø.49
    - congenital Q42.9
      - specified NEC Q42.8
- iris, congenital Q13.1
- jejunum (acquired) Z9Ø.49
  - congenital Q41.1
- joint
  - acquired
    - hip (following explantation of hip joint prosthesis) (with or without presence of antibiotic-impregnated cement spacer) Z89.62- ☑
    - knee (following explantation of knee joint prosthesis) (with or without presence of antibiotic-impregnated cement spacer) Z89.52- ☑
    - shoulder (following explantation of shoulder joint prosthesis) (with or without presence of antibiotic-impregnated cement spacer) Z89.23- ☑
  - congenital NEC Q74.8
- kidney(s) (acquired) Z9Ø.5
  - congenital Q6Ø.2
    - bilateral Q6Ø.1
    - unilateral Q6Ø.Ø
- knee (following explantation of knee joint prosthesis) (joint) (with or without presence of antibiotic-impregnated cement spacer) Z89.52- ☑
- labyrinth, membranous Q16.5
- larynx (congenital) Q31.8
  - acquired Z9Ø.Ø2
- leg (acquired) (above knee) Z89.61- ☑
  - below knee (acquired) Z89.51- ☑
  - congenital — *see* Defect, reduction, lower limb
- lens (acquired) — *see also* Aphakia
  - congenital Q12.3
  - post cataract extraction Z98.4- ☑
- limb (acquired) — *see* Absence, extremity
- lip Q38.6
- liver (congenital) Q44.7
- lung (fissure) (lobe) (bilateral) (unilateral) (congenital) Q33.3
  - acquired (any part) Z9Ø.2
- menstruation — *see* Amenorrhea
- muscle (congenital) (pectoral) Q79.8
  - ocular Q1Ø.3
- neck, part Q18.8
- neutrophil — *see* Agranulocytosis
- nipple(s) (with breast(s)) (acquired) Z9Ø.1- ☑
  - congenital Q83.2
- nose (congenital) Q3Ø.1
  - acquired Z9Ø.Ø9
- organ
  - of Corti, congenital Q16.5
  - or site, congenital NEC Q89.8
    - acquired NEC Z9Ø.89
- osseous meatus (ear) Q16.4
- ovary (acquired)
  - bilateral Z9Ø.722
  - congenital
    - bilateral Q5Ø.Ø2
    - unilateral Q5Ø.Ø1
  - unilateral Z9Ø.721
- oviduct (acquired)
  - bilateral Z9Ø.722
  - congenital Q5Ø.6
  - unilateral Z9Ø.721
- pancreas (congenital) Q45.Ø
  - acquired Z9Ø.41Ø
    - complete Z9Ø.41Ø
    - partial Z9Ø.411
    - total Z9Ø.41Ø
- parathyroid gland (acquired) E89.2
  - congenital Q89.2
- patella, congenital Q74.1
- penis (congenital) Q55.5
  - acquired Z9Ø.79
- pericardium (congenital) Q24.8
- pituitary gland (congenital) Q89.2

Absence — *continued*
- pituitary gland — *continued*
  - acquired E89.3
- prostate (acquired) Z9Ø.79
  - congenital Q55.4
- pulmonary valve Q22.Ø
- punctum lacrimale (congenital) Q1Ø.4
- radius, congenital — *see* Defect, reduction, upper limb, longitudinal, radius
- rectum (congenital) Q42.1
  - with fistula Q42.Ø
  - acquired Z9Ø.49
- respiratory organ NOS Q34.9
- rib (acquired) Z9Ø.89
  - congenital Q76.6
- sacrum, congenital Q76.49
- salivary gland(s), congenital Q38.4
- scrotum, congenital Q55.29
- seminal vesicles (congenital) Q55.4
  - acquired Z9Ø.79
- septum
  - atrial (congenital) Q21.1
  - between aorta and pulmonary artery Q21.4
  - ventricular (congenital) Q2Ø.4
- sex chromosome
  - female phenotype Q97.8
  - male phenotype Q98.8
- skull bone (congenital) Q75.8
  - with
    - anencephaly QØØ.Ø
    - encephalocele — *see* Encephalocele
    - hydrocephalus QØ3.9
      - with spina bifida — *see* Spina bifida, by site, with hydrocephalus
    - microcephaly QØ2
- spermatic cord, congenital Q55.4
- spine, congenital Q76.49
- spleen (congenital) Q89.Ø1
  - acquired Z9Ø.81
- sternum, congenital Q76.7
- stomach (acquired) (partial) Z9Ø.3
  - congenital Q4Ø.2
- superior vena cava, congenital Q26.8
- teeth, tooth (congenital) KØØ.Ø
  - acquired (complete) KØ8.1Ø9
    - class I KØ8.1Ø1
    - class II KØ8.1Ø2
    - class III KØ8.1Ø3
    - class IV KØ8.1Ø4
    - due to
      - caries KØ8.139
        - class I KØ8.131
        - class II KØ8.132
        - class III KØ8.133
        - class IV KØ8.134
      - periodontal disease KØ8.129
        - class I KØ8.121
        - class II KØ8.122
        - class III KØ8.123
        - class IV KØ8.124
      - specified NEC KØ8.199
        - class I KØ8.191
        - class II KØ8.192
        - class III KØ8.193
        - class IV KØ8.194
      - trauma KØ8.119
        - class I KØ8.111
        - class II KØ8.112
        - class III KØ8.113
        - class IV KØ8.114
    - partial KØ8.4Ø9
      - class I KØ8.4Ø1
      - class II KØ8.4Ø2
      - class III KØ8.4Ø3
      - class IV KØ8.4Ø4
      - due to
        - caries KØ8.439
          - class I KØ8.431
          - class II KØ8.432
          - class III KØ8.433
          - class IV KØ8.434
        - periodontal disease KØ8.429
          - class I KØ8.421
          - class II KØ8.422
          - class III KØ8.423
          - class IV KØ8.424
        - specified NEC KØ8.499
          - class I KØ8.491
          - class II KØ8.492

- **Absence** — *continued*
  - teeth, tooth — *continued*
    - acquired — *continued*
      - partial — *continued*
        - due to — *continued*
          - specified — *continued*
            - class III KØ8.493
            - class IV KØ8.494
          - trauma KØ8.419
            - class I KØ8.411
            - class II KØ8.412
            - class III KØ8.413
            - class IV KØ8.414
  - tendon (congenital) Q79.8
  - testis (congenital) Q55.Ø
    - acquired Z9Ø.79
  - thumb (acquired) Z89.Ø1- ☑
    - congenital — *see* Agenesis, hand
  - thymus gland Q89.2
  - thyroid (gland) (acquired) E89.Ø
    - cartilage, congenital Q31.8
    - congenital EØ3.1
  - toe(s) (acquired) Z89.42- ☑
    - with foot — *see* Absence, foot and ankle
    - congenital — *see* Agenesis, foot
    - great Z89.41- ☑
  - tongue, congenital Q38.3
  - trachea (cartilage), congenital Q32.1
  - transverse aortic arch, congenital Q25.49
  - tricuspid valve Q22.4
  - umbilical artery, congenital Q27.Ø
  - upper arm and forearm with hand present, congenital — *see* Agenesis, arm, with hand present
  - ureter (congenital) Q62.4
    - acquired Z9Ø.6
  - urethra, congenital Q64.5
  - uterus (acquired) Z9Ø.71Ø
    - with cervix Z9Ø.71Ø
    - with remaining cervical stump Z9Ø.711
    - congenital Q51.Ø
  - uvula, congenital Q38.5
  - vagina, congenital Q52.Ø
  - vas deferens (congenital) Q55.4
    - acquired Z9Ø.79
  - vein (peripheral) congenital NEC Q27.8
    - cerebral Q28.3
    - digestive system Q27.8
    - great Q26.8
    - lower limb Q27.8
    - portal Q26.5
    - precerebral Q28.1
    - specified site NEC Q27.8
    - upper limb Q27.8
  - vena cava (inferior) (superior), congenital Q26.8
  - ventricular septum Q2Ø.4
  - vertebra, congenital Q76.49
  - vulva, congenital Q52.71
  - wrist (acquired) Z89.12- ☑
- **Absorbent system disease** I87.8
- **Absorption**
  - carbohydrate, disturbance K9Ø.49
  - chemical — *see* Table of Drugs and Chemicals
    - through placenta (newborn) PØ4.9
      - environmental substance PØ4.6
      - nutritional substance PØ4.5
      - obstetric anesthetic or analgesic drug PØ4.Ø
  - drug NEC — *see* Table of Drugs and Chemicals
    - addictive
      - through placenta (newborn) — *see also* Newborn, affected by, maternal, use of PØ4.4Ø
        - cocaine PØ4.41
        - hallucinogens PØ4.42
        - specified drug NEC PØ4.49
    - medicinal
      - through placenta (newborn) PØ4.19
    - through placenta (newborn) PØ4.19
      - obstetric anesthetic or analgesic drug PØ4.Ø
  - fat, disturbance K9Ø.49
    - pancreatic K9Ø.3
  - noxious substance — *see* Table of Drugs and Chemicals
  - protein, disturbance K9Ø.49
  - starch, disturbance K9Ø.49
  - toxic substance — *see* Table of Drugs and Chemicals
  - uremic — *see* Uremia
- **Abstinence symptoms, syndrome**
  - alcohol F1Ø.239
    - with delirium F1Ø.231
  - cocaine F14.23

- **Abstinence symptoms, syndrome** — *continued*
  - neonatal P96.1
  - nicotine — *see* Dependence, drug, nicotine, with, withdrawal
  - opioid F11.93
    - with dependence F11.23
  - psychoactive NEC F19.939
    - with
      - delirium F19.931
      - dependence F19.239
        - with
          - delirium F19.231
          - perceptual disturbance F19.232
        - uncomplicated F19.23Ø
      - perceptual disturbance F19.932
    - uncomplicated F19.93Ø
  - sedative F13.939
    - with
      - delirium F13.931
      - dependence F13.239
        - with
          - delirium F13.231
          - perceptual disturbance F13.232
        - uncomplicated F13.23Ø
      - perceptual disturbance F13.932
    - uncomplicated F13.93Ø
  - stimulant NEC F15.93
    - with dependence F15.23
- **Abulia** R68.89
- **Abulomania** F6Ø.7
- **Abuse**
  - adult — *see* Maltreatment, adult
    - as reason for
      - couple seeking advice (including offender) Z63.Ø
  - alcohol (non-dependent) F1Ø.1Ø
    - with
      - anxiety disorder F1Ø.18Ø
      - intoxication F1Ø.129
        - with delirium F1Ø.121
        - uncomplicated F1Ø.12Ø
      - mood disorder F1Ø.14
      - other specified disorder F1Ø.188
      - psychosis F1Ø.159
        - delusions F1Ø.15Ø
        - hallucinations F1Ø.151
      - sexual dysfunction F1Ø.181
      - sleep disorder F1Ø.182
      - unspecified disorder F1Ø.19
      - withdrawal F1Ø.139
        - with
          - perceptual disturbance F1Ø.132
        - delirium F1Ø.131
        - uncomplicated F1Ø.13Ø
    - counseling and surveillance Z71.41
    - in remission (early) (sustained) F1Ø.11
  - amphetamine (or related substance) — *see also* Abuse, drug, stimulant NEC
    - stimulant NEC F15.1Ø
      - with
        - anxiety disorder F15.18Ø
        - intoxication F15.129
          - with
            - delirium F15.121
            - perceptual disturbance F15.122
        - withdrawal F15.13
  - analgesics (non-prescribed) (over the counter) F55.8
  - antacids F55.Ø
  - antidepressants — *see* Abuse, drug, psychoactive NEC
  - anxiolytic — *see* Abuse, drug, sedative
  - barbiturates — *see* Abuse, drug, sedative
  - caffeine — *see* Abuse, drug, stimulant NEC
  - cannabis, cannabinoids — *see* Abuse, drug, cannabis
  - child — *see* Maltreatment, child
  - cocaine — *see* Abuse, drug, cocaine
  - drug NEC (non-dependent) F19.1Ø
    - with sleep disorder F19.182
    - amphetamine type — *see* Abuse, drug, stimulant NEC
    - analgesics (non-prescribed) (over the counter) F55.8
    - antacids F55.Ø
    - antidepressants — *see* Abuse, drug, psychoactive NEC
    - anxiolytics — *see* Abuse, drug, sedative
    - barbiturates — *see* Abuse, drug, sedative
    - caffeine — *see* Abuse, drug, stimulant NEC
    - cannabis F12.1Ø
      - with
        - anxiety disorder F12.18Ø

- **Abuse** — *continued*
  - drug — *continued*
    - cannabis — *continued*
      - with — *continued*
        - intoxication F12.129
          - with
            - delirium F12.121
            - perceptual disturbance F12.122
          - uncomplicated F12.12Ø
        - other specified disorder F12.188
        - psychosis F12.159
          - delusions F12.15Ø
          - hallucinations F12.151
        - unspecified disorder F12.19
        - withdrawal F12.13
      - in remission (early) (sustained) F12.11
    - cocaine F14.1Ø
      - with
        - anxiety disorder F14.18Ø
        - intoxication F14.129
          - with
            - delirium F14.121
            - perceptual disturbance F14.122
          - uncomplicated F14.12Ø
        - mood disorder F14.14
        - other specified disorder F14.188
        - psychosis F14.159
          - delusions F14.15Ø
          - hallucinations F14.151
        - sexual dysfunction F14.181
        - sleep disorder F14.182
        - unspecified disorder F14.19
        - withdrawal F14.13
      - in remission (early) (sustained) F14.11
    - counseling and surveillance Z71.51
    - hallucinogen F16.1Ø
      - with
        - anxiety disorder F16.18Ø
        - flashbacks F16.183
        - intoxication F16.129
          - with
            - delirium F16.121
            - perceptual disturbance F16.122
          - uncomplicated F16.12Ø
        - mood disorder F16.14
        - other specified disorder F16.188
        - perception disorder, persisting F16.183
        - psychosis F16.159
          - delusions F16.15Ø
          - hallucinations F16.151
        - unspecified disorder F16.19
      - in remission (early) (sustained) F16.11
    - hashish — *see* Abuse, drug, cannabis
    - herbal or folk remedies F55.1
    - hormones F55.3
    - hypnotics — *see* Abuse, drug, sedative
    - in remission (early) (sustained) F19.11
    - inhalant F18.1Ø
      - with
        - anxiety disorder F18.18Ø
        - dementia, persisting F18.17
        - intoxication F18.129
          - with delirium F18.121
          - uncomplicated F18.12Ø
        - mood disorder F18.14
        - other specified disorder F18.188
        - psychosis F18.159
          - delusions F18.15Ø
          - hallucinations F18.151
        - unspecified disorder F18.19
      - in remission (early) (sustained) F18.11
    - laxatives F55.2
    - LSD — *see* Abuse, drug, hallucinogen
    - marihuana — *see* Abuse, drug, cannabis
    - morphine type (opioids) — *see* Abuse, drug, opioid
    - opioid F11.1Ø
      - with
        - intoxication F11.129
          - with
            - delirium F11.121
            - perceptual disturbance F11.122
          - uncomplicated F11.12Ø
        - mood disorder F11.14
        - other specified disorder F11.188
        - psychosis F11.159
          - delusions F11.15Ø
          - hallucinations F11.151
        - sexual dysfunction F11.181
        - sleep disorder F11.182

- **Adenoma** — *continued*
  - apocrine
    - breast D24- ☑
    - specified site NEC — *see* Neoplasm, skin, benign, by site
    - unspecified site D23.9
  - basal cell D11.9
  - basophil
    - specified site — *see* Neoplasm, benign, by site
    - unspecified site D35.2
  - basophil-acidophil, mixed
    - specified site — *see* Neoplasm, benign, by site
    - unspecified site D35.2
  - beta-cell
    - pancreas D13.7
    - specified site NEC — *see* Neoplasm, benign, by site
    - unspecified site D13.7
  - bile duct D13.4
    - common D13.5
    - extrahepatic D13.5
    - intrahepatic D13.4
    - specified site NEC — *see* Neoplasm, benign, by site
    - unspecified site D13.4
  - black D35.00
  - bronchial D38.1
    - cylindroid type — *see* Neoplasm, lung, malignant
  - ceruminous D23.2- ☑
  - chief cell D35.1
  - chromophobe
    - specified site — *see* Neoplasm, benign, by site
    - unspecified site D35.2
  - colloid
    - specified site — *see* Neoplasm, benign, by site
    - unspecified site D34
  - duct
  - eccrine, papillary — *see* Neoplasm, skin, benign
  - endocrine, multiple
    - single specified site — *see* Neoplasm, uncertain behavior, by site
    - two or more specified sites D44- ☑
    - unspecified site D44.9
  - endometrioid — *see also* Neoplasm, benign
    - borderline malignancy — *see* Neoplasm, uncertain behavior, by site
  - eosinophil
    - specified site — *see* Neoplasm, benign, by site
    - unspecified site D35.2
  - fetal
    - specified site — *see* Neoplasm, benign, by site
    - unspecified site D34
  - follicular
    - specified site — *see* Neoplasm, benign, by site
    - unspecified site D34
  - hepatocellular D13.4
  - Hurthle cell D34
  - islet cell
    - pancreas D13.7
    - specified site NEC — *see* Neoplasm, benign, by site
    - unspecified site D13.7
  - liver cell D13.4
  - macrofollicular
    - specified site — *see* Neoplasm, benign, by site
    - unspecified site D34
  - malignant, malignum — *see* Neoplasm, malignant, by site
  - microcystic
    - pancreas D13.6
    - specified site NEC — *see* Neoplasm, benign, by site
    - unspecified site D13.6
  - microfollicular
    - specified site — *see* Neoplasm, benign, by site
    - unspecified site D34
  - mucoid cell
    - specified site — *see* Neoplasm, benign, by site
    - unspecified site D35.2
  - multiple endocrine
    - single specified site — *see* Neoplasm, uncertain behavior, by site
    - two or more specified sites D44- ☑
    - unspecified site D44.9
  - nipple D24- ☑
  - papillary — *see also* Neoplasm, benign, by site
    - eccrine — *see* Neoplasm, skin, benign, by site
  - Pick's tubular
    - specified site — *see* Neoplasm, benign, by site
    - unspecified site
      - female D27.9
      - male D29.20
- **Adenoma** — *continued*
  - pleomorphic
    - carcinoma in — *see* Neoplasm, salivary gland, malignant
      - specified site — *see* Neoplasm, malignant, by site
      - unspecified site C08.9
  - polypoid — *see also* Neoplasm, benign
    - adenocarcinoma in — *see* Neoplasm, malignant, by site
    - adenocarcinoma in situ — *see* Neoplasm, in situ, by site
  - prostate — *see* Neoplasm, benign, prostate
  - rete cell D29.20
  - sebaceous — *see* Neoplasm, skin, benign
  - Sertoli cell
    - specified site — *see* Neoplasm, benign, by site
    - unspecified site
      - female D27.9
      - male D29.20
  - skin appendage — *see* Neoplasm, skin, benign
  - sudoriferous gland — *see* Neoplasm, skin, benign
  - sweat gland — *see* Neoplasm, skin, benign
  - testicular
    - specified site — *see* Neoplasm, benign, by site
    - unspecified site
      - female D27.9
      - male D29.20
  - tubular — *see also* Neoplasm, benign, by site
    - adenocarcinoma in — *see* Neoplasm, malignant, by site
    - adenocarcinoma in situ — *see* Neoplasm, in situ, by site
    - Pick's
      - specified site — *see* Neoplasm, benign, by site
      - unspecified site
        - female D27.9
        - male D29.20
  - tubulovillous — *see also* Neoplasm, benign, by site
    - adenocarcinoma in — *see* Neoplasm, malignant, by site
    - adenocarcinoma in situ — *see* Neoplasm, in situ, by site
  - villous — *see* Neoplasm, uncertain behavior, by site
    - adenocarcinoma in — *see* Neoplasm, malignant, by site
    - adenocarcinoma in situ — *see* Neoplasm, in situ, by site
  - water-clear cell D35.1
- **Adenomatosis**
  - endocrine (multiple) E31.20
    - single specified site — *see* Neoplasm, uncertain behavior, by site
  - erosive of nipple D24- ☑
  - pluriendocrine — *see* Adenomatosis, endocrine
  - pulmonary D38.1
    - malignant — *see* Neoplasm, lung, malignant
  - specified site — *see* Neoplasm, benign, by site
  - unspecified site D12.6
- **Adenomatous**
  - goiter (nontoxic) E04.9
    - with hyperthyroidism — *see* Hyperthyroidism, with, goiter, nodular
    - toxic — *see* Hyperthyroidism, with, goiter, nodular
- **Adenomyoma** — *see also* Neoplasm, benign, by site
  - prostate — *see* Enlarged, prostate
- **Adenomyometritis** N80.0
- **Adenomyosis** N80.0
- **Adenopathy** (lymph gland) R59.9
  - generalized R59.1
  - inguinal R59.0
  - localized R59.0
  - mediastinal R59.0
  - mesentery R59.0
  - syphilitic (secondary) A51.49
  - tracheobronchial R59.0
    - tuberculous A15.4
      - primary (progressive) A15.7
  - tuberculous — *see also* Tuberculosis, lymph gland
    - tracheobronchial A15.4
      - primary (progressive) A15.7
- **Adenosalpingitis** — *see* Salpingitis
- **Adenosarcoma** — *see* Neoplasm, malignant, by site
- **Adenosclerosis** I88.8
- **Adenosis** (sclerosing) breast — *see* Fibroadenosis, breast
- **Adenovirus, as cause of disease classified elsewhere** B97.0
- **Adentia** (complete) (partial) — *see* Absence, teeth
- **Adherent** — *see also* Adhesions
  - labia (minora) N90.89
  - pericardium (nonrheumatic) I31.0
    - rheumatic I09.2
  - placenta (with hemorrhage) O72.0
    - without hemorrhage O73.0
  - prepuce, newborn N47.0
  - scar (skin) L90.5
  - tendon in scar L90.5
- **Adhesions, adhesive** (postinfective) K66.0
  - with intestinal obstruction K56.50
    - complete K56.52
    - incomplete K56.51
    - partial K56.51
  - abdominal (wall) — *see* Adhesions, peritoneum
  - appendix K38.8
  - bile duct (common) (hepatic) K83.8
  - bladder (sphincter) N32.89
  - bowel — *see* Adhesions, peritoneum
  - cardiac I31.0
    - rheumatic I09.2
  - cecum — *see* Adhesions, peritoneum
  - cervicovaginal N88.1
    - congenital Q52.8
    - postpartal O90.89
      - old N88.1
  - cervix N88.1
  - ciliary body NEC — *see* Adhesions, iris
  - clitoris N90.89
  - colon — *see* Adhesions, peritoneum
  - common duct K83.8
  - congenital — *see also* Anomaly, by site
    - fingers — *see* Syndactylism, complex, fingers
    - omental, anomalous Q43.3
    - peritoneal Q43.3
    - tongue (to gum or roof of mouth) Q38.3
  - conjunctiva (acquired) H11.21- ☑
    - congenital Q15.8
  - cystic duct K82.8
  - diaphragm — *see* Adhesions, peritoneum
  - due to foreign body — *see* Foreign body
  - duodenum — *see* Adhesions, peritoneum
  - ear
    - middle H74.1- ☑
  - epididymis N50.89
  - epidural — *see* Adhesions, meninges
  - epiglottis J38.7
  - eyelid H02.59
  - female pelvis N73.6
  - gallbladder K82.8
  - globe H44.89
  - heart I31.0
    - rheumatic I09.2
  - ileocecal (coil) — *see* Adhesions, peritoneum
  - ileum — *see* Adhesions, peritoneum
  - intestine — *see also* Adhesions, peritoneum
    - with obstruction K56.50
      - complete K56.52
      - incomplete K56.51
      - partial K56.51
  - intra-abdominal — *see* Adhesions, peritoneum
  - iris H21.50- ☑
    - anterior H21.51- ☑
    - goniosynechiae H21.52- ☑
    - posterior H21.54- ☑
    - to corneal graft T85.898 ☑
  - joint — *see* Ankylosis
    - knee M23.8X ☑
    - temporomandibular M26.61- ☑
  - labium (majus) (minus), congenital Q52.5
  - liver — *see* Adhesions, peritoneum
  - lung J98.4
  - mediastinum J98.59
  - meninges (cerebral) (spinal) G96.12
    - congenital Q07.8
    - tuberculous (cerebral) (spinal) A17.0
  - mesenteric — *see* Adhesions, peritoneum
  - nasal (septum) (to turbinates) J34.89
  - ocular muscle — *see* Strabismus, mechanical
  - omentum — *see* Adhesions, peritoneum
  - ovary N73.6
    - congenital (to cecum, kidney or omentum) Q50.39
  - paraovarian N73.6
  - pelvic (peritoneal)
    - female N73.6
      - postprocedural N99.4
    - male — *see* Adhesions, peritoneum

- **Adhesions, adhesive** — *continued*
  - pelvic — *continued*
    - postpartal (old) N73.6
    - tuberculous A18.17
  - penis to scrotum (congenital) Q55.8
  - periappendiceal — *see also* Adhesions, peritoneum
  - pericardium (nonrheumatic) I31.Ø
    - focal I31.8
    - rheumatic IØ9.2
    - tuberculous A18.84
  - pericholecystic K82.8
  - perigastric — *see* Adhesions, peritoneum
  - periovarian N73.6
  - periprostatic N42.89
  - perirectal — *see* Adhesions, peritoneum
  - perirenal N28.89
  - peritoneum, peritoneal (postinfective) K66.Ø
    - with obstruction (intestinal) K56.5Ø
      - complete K56.52
      - incomplete K56.51
      - partial K56.51
    - congenital Q43.3
    - pelvic, female N73.6
      - postprocedural N99.4
    - postpartal, pelvic N73.6
    - postprocedural K66.Ø
    - to uterus N73.6
  - peritubal N73.6
  - periureteral N28.89
  - periuterine N73.6
  - perivesical N32.89
  - perivesicular (seminal vesicle) N5Ø.89
  - pleura, pleuritic J94.8
    - tuberculous NEC A15.6
  - pleuropericardial J94.8
  - postoperative (gastrointestinal tract) K66.Ø
    - with obstruction — *see also* Obstruction, intestine, postoperative K91.3Ø
    - due to foreign body accidentally left in wound — *see* Foreign body, accidentally left during a procedure
    - pelvic peritoneal N99.4
    - urethra — *see* Stricture, urethra, postprocedural
    - vagina N99.2
  - postpartal, old (vulva or perineum) N9Ø.89
  - preputial, prepuce N47.5
  - pulmonary J98.4
  - pylorus — *see* Adhesions, peritoneum
  - sciatic nerve — *see* Lesion, nerve, sciatic
  - seminal vesicle N5Ø.89
  - shoulder (joint) — *see* Capsulitis, adhesive
  - sigmoid flexure — *see* Adhesions, peritoneum
  - spermatic cord (acquired) N5Ø.89
    - congenital Q55.4
  - spinal canal G96.12
  - stomach — *see* Adhesions, peritoneum
  - subscapular — *see* Capsulitis, adhesive
  - temporomandibular M26.61- ☑
  - tendinitis (*see also* Tenosynovitis, specified type NEC)
    - shoulder — *see* Capsulitis, adhesive
  - testis N44.8
  - tongue, congenital (to gum or roof of mouth) Q38.3
    - acquired K14.8
  - trachea J39.8
  - tubo-ovarian N73.6
  - tunica vaginalis N44.8
  - uterus N73.6
    - internal N85.6
    - to abdominal wall N73.6
  - vagina (chronic) N89.5
    - postoperative N99.2
  - vitreomacular H43.82- ☑
  - vitreous H43.89
  - vulva N9Ø.89
- **Adiaspiromycosis** B48.8
- **Adie** (-Holmes) **pupil or syndrome** — *see* Anomaly, pupil, function, tonic pupil
- **Adiponecrosis neonatorum** P83.88
- **Adiposis** — *see also* Obesity
  - cerebralis E23.6
  - dolorosa E88.2
- **Adiposity** — *see also* Obesity
  - heart — *see* Degeneration, myocardial
  - localized E65
- **Adiposogenital dystrophy** E23.6
- **Adjustment**
  - disorder — *see* Disorder, adjustment
- **Adjustment** — *continued*
  - implanted device — *see* Encounter (for), adjustment (of)
  - prosthesis, external — *see* Fitting
  - reaction — *see* Disorder, adjustment
- **Administration of tPA** (rtPA) in a different facility within the last 24 hours prior to admission to current facility Z92.82
- **Admission** (for) — *see also* Encounter (for)
  - adjustment (of)
    - artificial
      - arm Z44.ØØ- ☑
        - complete Z44.Ø1- ☑
        - partial Z44.Ø2- ☑
      - eye Z44.2 ☑
      - leg Z44.1Ø- ☑
        - complete Z44.11- ☑
        - partial Z44.12- ☑
    - brain neuropacemaker Z46.2
      - implanted Z45.42
    - breast
      - implant Z45.81 ☑
      - prosthesis (external) Z44.3 ☑
    - colostomy belt Z46.89
    - contact lenses Z46.Ø
    - cystostomy device Z46.6
    - dental prosthesis Z46.3
    - device NEC
      - abdominal Z46.89
      - implanted Z45.89
        - cardiac Z45.Ø9
          - defibrillator (with synchronous cardiac pacemaker) Z45.Ø2
          - pacemaker (cardiac resynchronization therapy (CRT-P)) Z45.Ø18
            - pulse generator Z45.Ø1Ø
          - resynchronization therapy defibrillator (CRT-D) Z45.Ø2
        - hearing device Z45.328
          - bone conduction Z45.32Ø
          - cochlear Z45.321
        - infusion pump Z45.1
        - nervous system Z45.49
          - CSF drainage Z45.41
          - hearing device — *see* Admission, adjustment, device, implanted, hearing device
          - neuropacemaker Z45.42
          - visual substitution Z45.31
        - specified NEC Z45.89
        - vascular access Z45.2
        - visual substitution Z45.31
      - nervous system Z46.2
        - implanted — *see* Admission, adjustment, device, implanted, nervous system
      - orthodontic Z46.4
      - prosthetic Z44.9
        - arm — *see* Admission, adjustment, artificial, arm
        - breast Z44.3 ☑
        - dental Z46.3
        - eye Z44.2 ☑
        - leg — *see* Admission, adjustment, artificial, leg
        - specified type NEC Z44.8
      - substitution
        - auditory Z46.2
          - implanted — *see* Admission, adjustment, device, implanted, hearing device
        - nervous system Z46.2
          - implanted — *see* Admission, adjustment, device, implanted, nervous system
        - visual Z46.2
          - implanted Z45.31
      - urinary Z46.6
    - hearing aid Z46.1
      - implanted — *see* Admission, adjustment, device, implanted, hearing device
    - ileostomy device Z46.89
    - intestinal appliance or device NEC Z46.89
    - neuropacemaker (brain) (peripheral nerve) (spinal cord) Z46.2
      - implanted Z45.42
    - orthodontic device Z46.4
    - orthopedic (brace) (cast) (device) (shoes) Z46.89
    - pacemaker (cardiac resynchronization therapy (CRT-P))
      - cardiac Z45.Ø18
- **Admission** — *continued*
  - adjustment — *continued*
    - pacemaker — *continued*
      - cardiac — *continued*
        - pulse generator Z45.Ø1Ø
      - nervous system Z46.2
        - implanted Z45.42
    - portacath (port-a-cath) Z45.2
    - prosthesis Z44.9
      - arm — *see* Admission, adjustment, artificial, arm
      - breast Z44.3 ☑
      - dental Z46.3
      - eye Z44.2 ☑
      - leg — *see* Admission, adjustment, artificial, leg
      - specified NEC Z44.8
    - spectacles Z46.Ø
  - aftercare — *see also* Aftercare Z51.89
    - postpartum
      - immediately after delivery Z39.Ø
      - routine follow-up Z39.2
    - radiation therapy (antineoplastic) Z51.Ø
  - attention to artificial opening (of) Z43.9
    - artificial vagina Z43.7
    - colostomy Z43.3
    - cystostomy Z43.5
    - enterostomy Z43.4
    - gastrostomy Z43.1
    - ileostomy Z43.2
    - jejunostomy Z43.4
    - nephrostomy Z43.6
    - specified site NEC Z43.8
      - intestinal tract Z43.4
      - urinary tract Z43.6
    - tracheostomy Z43.Ø
    - ureterostomy Z43.6
    - urethrostomy Z43.6
  - breast augmentation or reduction Z41.1
  - breast reconstruction following mastectomy Z42.1
  - change of
    - dressing (nonsurgical) Z48.ØØ
    - neuropacemaker device (brain) (peripheral nerve) (spinal cord) Z46.2
      - implanted Z45.42
    - surgical dressing Z48.Ø1
  - circumcision, ritual or routine (in absence of diagnosis) Z41.2
  - clinical research investigation (control) (normal comparison) (participant) ZØØ.6
  - contraceptive management Z3Ø.9
  - cosmetic surgery NEC Z41.1
  - counseling — *see also* Counseling
    - dietary Z71.3
    - gestational carrier Z31.7
    - HIV Z71.7
    - human immunodeficiency virus Z71.7
    - nonattending third party Z71.Ø
    - procreative management NEC Z31.69
  - delivery, full-term, uncomplicated O8Ø
    - cesarean, without indication O82
  - desensitization to allergens Z51.6
  - dietary surveillance and counseling Z71.3
  - ear piercing Z41.3
  - examination at health care facility (adult) — *see also* Examination ZØØ.ØØ
    - with abnormal findings ZØØ.Ø1
    - clinical research investigation (control) (normal comparison) (participant) ZØØ.6
    - dental ZØ1.2Ø
      - with abnormal findings ZØ1.21
    - donor (potential) ZØØ.5
    - ear ZØ1.1Ø
      - with abnormal findings NEC ZØ1.118
    - eye ZØ1.ØØ
      - with abnormal findings ZØ1.Ø1
      - following failed vision screening ZØ1.Ø2Ø
        - with abnormal findings ZØ1.Ø21
    - general, specified reason NEC ZØØ.8
    - hearing ZØ1.1Ø
      - with abnormal findings NEC ZØ1.118
      - infant or child (over 28 days old) ZØØ.129
        - with abnormal findings ZØØ.121
    - postpartum checkup Z39.2
    - psychiatric (general) ZØØ.8
      - requested by authority ZØ4.6
    - vision ZØ1.ØØ
      - with abnormal findings ZØ1.Ø1
      - following failed vision screening ZØ1.Ø2Ø
        - with abnormal findings ZØ1.Ø21

Admission — *continued*
- examination at health care facility — *see also* Examination — *continued*
  - vision — *continued*
    - infant or child (over 28 days old) Z00.129
      - with abnormal findings Z00.121
- fitting (of)
  - artificial
    - arm — *see* Admission, adjustment, artificial, arm
    - eye Z44.2 ☑
    - leg — *see* Admission, adjustment, artificial, leg
  - brain neuropacemaker Z46.2
    - implanted Z45.42
  - breast prosthesis (external) Z44.3 ☑
  - colostomy belt Z46.89
  - contact lenses Z46.0
  - cystostomy device Z46.6
  - dental prosthesis Z46.3
  - dentures Z46.3
  - device NEC
    - abdominal Z46.89
    - nervous system Z46.2
      - implanted — *see* Admission, adjustment, device, implanted, nervous system
    - orthodontic Z46.4
    - prosthetic Z44.9
      - breast Z44.3 ☑
      - dental Z46.3
      - eye Z44.2 ☑
    - substitution
      - auditory Z46.2
        - implanted — *see* Admission, adjustment, device, implanted, hearing device
      - nervous system Z46.2
        - implanted — *see* Admission, adjustment, device, implanted, nervous system
      - visual Z46.2
        - implanted Z45.31
  - hearing aid Z46.1
  - ileostomy device Z46.89
  - intestinal appliance or device NEC Z46.89
  - neuropacemaker (brain) (peripheral nerve) (spinal cord) Z46.2
    - implanted Z45.42
  - orthodontic device Z46.4
  - orthopedic device (brace) (cast) (shoes) Z46.89
  - prosthesis Z44.9
    - arm — *see* Admission, adjustment, artificial, arm
    - breast Z44.3 ☑
    - dental Z46.3
    - eye Z44.2 ☑
    - leg — *see* Admission, adjustment, artificial, leg
    - specified type NEC Z44.8
  - spectacles Z46.0
- follow-up examination Z09
- intrauterine device management Z30.431
  - initial prescription Z30.014
- mental health evaluation Z00.8
  - requested by authority Z04.6
- observation — *see* Observation
- Papanicolaou smear, cervix Z12.4
  - for suspected malignant neoplasm Z12.4
- plastic and reconstructive surgery following medical procedure or healed injury NEC Z42.8
- plastic surgery, cosmetic NEC Z41.1
- postpartum observation
  - immediately after delivery Z39.0
  - routine follow-up Z39.2
- poststerilization (for restoration) Z31.0
  - aftercare Z31.42
- procreative management Z31.9
- prophylactic (measure) — *see also* Encounter, prophylactic measures
  - organ removal Z40.00
    - breast Z40.01
    - fallopian tube(s) Z40.03
      - with ovary(s) Z40.02
    - ovary(s) Z40.02
    - specified organ NEC Z40.09
    - testes Z40.09
  - vaccination Z23
- psychiatric examination (general) Z00.8
  - requested by authority Z04.6
- radiation therapy (antineoplastic) Z51.0
- reconstructive surgery following medical procedure or healed injury NEC Z42.8
- removal of
  - cystostomy catheter Z43.5

Admission — *continued*
- removal of — *continued*
  - drains Z48.03
  - dressing (nonsurgical) Z48.00
  - implantable subdermal contraceptive Z30.46
  - intrauterine contraceptive device Z30.432
  - neuropacemaker (brain) (peripheral nerve) (spinal cord) Z46.2
    - implanted Z45.42
  - staples Z48.02
  - surgical dressing Z48.01
  - sutures Z48.02
  - ureteral stent Z46.6
- respirator [ventilator] use during power failure Z99.12
- restoration of organ continuity (poststerilization) Z31.0
  - aftercare Z31.42
- sensitivity test — *see also* Test, skin
  - allergy NEC Z01.82
  - Mantoux Z11.1
- tuboplasty following previous sterilization Z31.0
  - aftercare Z31.42
- vasoplasty following previous sterilization Z31.0
  - aftercare Z31.42
- vision examination Z01.00
  - with abnormal findings Z01.01
  - following failed vision screening Z01.020
    - with abnormal findings Z01.021
  - infant or child (over 28 days old) Z00.129
    - with abnormal findings Z00.121
- waiting period for admission to other facility Z75.1

Adnexitis (suppurative) — *see* Salpingo-oophoritis
Adolescent X-linked adrenoleukodystrophy E71.521
Adrenal (gland) — *see* condition
Adrenalism, tuberculous A18.7
Adrenalitis, adrenitis E27.8
- autoimmune E27.1
- meningococcal, hemorrhagic A39.1

Adrenarche, premature E27.0
Adrenocortical syndrome — *see* Cushing's, syndrome
Adrenogenital syndrome E25.9
- acquired E25.8
- congenital E25.0
- salt loss E25.0

Adrenogenitalism, congenital E25.0
Adrenoleukodystrophy E71.529
- neonatal E71.511
- X-linked E71.529
  - Addison only phenotype E71.528
  - Addison-Schilder E71.528
  - adolescent E71.521
  - adrenomyeloneuropathy E71.522
  - childhood cerebral E71.520
  - other specified E71.528

Adrenomyeloneuropathy E71.522
Adventitious bursa — *see* Bursopathy, specified type NEC
Adverse effect — *see* Table of Drugs and Chemicals, categories T36-T50, with 6th character 5
Advice — *see* Counseling
Adynamia (episodica) (hereditary) (periodic) G72.3
Aeration lung imperfect, newborn — *see* Atelectasis
Aerobullosis T70.3 ☑
Aerocele — *see* Embolism, air
Aerodermectasia
- subcutaneous (traumatic) T79.7 ☑

Aerodontalgia T70.29 ☑
Aeroembolism T70.3 ☑
Aerogenes capsulatus infection A48.0
Aero-otitis media T70.0 ☑
Aerophagy, aerophagia (psychogenic) F45.8
Aerophobia F40.228
Aerosinusitis T70.1 ☑
Aerotitis T70.0 ☑
Affection — *see* Disease
Afibrinogenemia — *see also* Defect, coagulation D68.8
- acquired D65
- congenital D68.2
- following ectopic or molar pregnancy O08.1
- in abortion — *see* Abortion, by type, complicated by, afibrinogenemia
- puerperal O72.3

African
- sleeping sickness B56.9
- tick fever A68.1
- trypanosomiasis B56.9
  - gambian B56.0
  - rhodesian B56.1

Aftercare — *see also* Care Z51.89

Aftercare — *continued*
- following surgery (for) (on)
  - amputation Z47.81
  - attention to
    - drains Z48.03
    - dressings (nonsurgical) Z48.00
      - surgical Z48.01
    - sutures Z48.02
  - circulatory system Z48.812
  - delayed (planned) wound closure Z48.1
  - digestive system Z48.815
  - explantation of joint prosthesis (staged procedure)
    - hip Z47.32
    - knee Z47.33
    - shoulder Z47.31
  - genitourinary system Z48.816
  - joint replacement Z47.1
  - neoplasm Z48.3
  - nervous system Z48.811
  - oral cavity Z48.814
  - organ transplant
    - bone marrow Z48.290
    - heart Z48.21
    - heart-lung Z48.280
    - kidney Z48.22
    - liver Z48.23
    - lung Z48.24
    - multiple organs NEC Z48.288
    - specified NEC Z48.298
  - orthopedic NEC Z47.89
  - planned wound closure Z48.1
  - removal of internal fixation device Z47.2
  - respiratory system Z48.813
  - scoliosis Z47.82
  - sense organs Z48.810
  - skin and subcutaneous tissue Z48.817
  - specified body system
    - circulatory Z48.812
    - digestive Z48.815
    - genitourinary Z48.816
    - nervous Z48.811
    - oral cavity Z48.814
    - respiratory Z48.813
    - sense organs Z48.810
    - skin and subcutaneous tissue Z48.817
    - teeth Z48.814
  - specified NEC Z48.89
  - spinal Z47.89
  - teeth Z48.814
- fracture — *code to* fracture with seventh character D
- involving
  - removal of
    - drains Z48.03
    - dressings (nonsurgical) Z48.00
    - staples Z48.02
    - surgical dressings Z48.01
    - sutures Z48.02
- neuropacemaker (brain) (peripheral nerve) (spinal cord) Z46.2
  - implanted Z45.42
- orthopedic NEC Z47.89
- postprocedural — *see* Aftercare, following surgery

After-cataract — *see* Cataract, secondary
Agalactia (primary) O92.3
- elective, secondary or therapeutic O92.5

Agammaglobulinemia (acquired (secondary)) (nonfamilial) D80.1
- with
  - immunoglobulin-bearing B-lymphocytes D80.1
  - lymphopenia D81.9
- autosomal recessive (Swiss type) D80.0
- Bruton's X-linked D80.0
- common variable (CVAgamma) D80.1
- congenital sex-linked D80.0
- hereditary D80.0
- lymphopenic D81.9
- Swiss type (autosomal recessive) D80.0
- X-linked (with growth hormone deficiency) (Bruton) D80.0

Aganglionosis (bowel) (colon) Q43.1
Age (old) — *see* Senility
Agenesis
- adrenal (gland) Q89.1
- alimentary tract (complete) (partial) NEC Q45.8
  - upper Q40.8
- anus, anal (canal) Q42.3
  - with fistula Q42.2
- aorta Q25.41

Agenesis — *continued*
- appendix Q42.8
- arm (complete) Q71.Ø- ☑
  - with hand present Q71.1- ☑
- artery (peripheral) Q27.9
  - brain Q28.3
  - coronary Q24.5
  - pulmonary Q25.79
  - specified NEC Q27.8
  - umbilical Q27.Ø
- auditory (canal) (external) Q16.1
- auricle (ear) Q16.Ø
- bile duct or passage Q44.5
- bladder Q64.5
- bone Q79.9
- brain QØØ.Ø
  - part of QØ4.3
- breast (with nipple present) Q83.8
  - with absent nipple Q83.Ø
- bronchus Q32.4
- canaliculus lacrimalis Q1Ø.4
- carpus — *see* Agenesis, hand
- cartilage Q79.9
- cecum Q42.8
- cerebellum QØ4.3
- cervix Q51.5
- chin Q18.8
- cilia Q1Ø.3
- circulatory system, part NOS Q28.9
- clavicle Q74.Ø
- clitoris Q52.6
- coccyx Q76.49
- colon Q42.9
  - specified NEC Q42.8
- corpus callosum QØ4.Ø
- cricoid cartilage Q31.8
- diaphragm (with hernia) Q79.1
- digestive organ(s) or tract (complete) (partial) NEC Q45.8
  - upper Q4Ø.8
- ductus arteriosus Q28.8
- duodenum Q41.Ø
- ear Q16.9
  - auricle Q16.Ø
  - lobe Q17.8
- ejaculatory duct Q55.4
- endocrine (gland) NEC Q89.2
- epiglottis Q31.8
- esophagus Q39.8
- eustachian tube Q16.2
- eye Q11.1
  - adnexa Q15.8
- eyelid (fold) Q1Ø.3
- face
  - bones NEC Q75.8
  - specified part NEC Q18.8
- fallopian tube Q5Ø.6
- femur — *see* Defect, reduction, lower limb, longitudinal, femur
- fibula — *see* Defect, reduction, lower limb, longitudinal, fibula
- finger (complete) (partial) — *see* Agenesis, hand
- foot (and toes) (complete) (partial) Q72.3- ☑
- forearm (with hand present) — *see* Agenesis, arm, with hand present
  - and hand Q71.2- ☑
- gallbladder Q44.Ø
- gastric Q4Ø.2
- genitalia, genital (organ(s))
  - female Q52.8
    - external Q52.71
    - internal NEC Q52.8
  - male Q55.8
- glottis Q31.8
- hair Q84.Ø
- hand (and fingers) (complete) (partial) Q71.3- ☑
- heart Q24.8
  - valve NEC Q24.8
    - pulmonary Q22.Ø
- hepatic Q44.7
- humerus — *see* Defect, reduction, upper limb
- hymen Q52.4
- ileum Q41.2
- incus Q16.3
- intestine (small) Q41.9
  - large Q42.9
    - specified NEC Q42.8
- iris (dilator fibers) Q13.1
- jaw M26.Ø9
- jejunum Q41.1
- kidney(s) (partial) Q6Ø.2
  - bilateral Q6Ø.1
  - unilateral Q6Ø.Ø
- labium (majus) (minus) Q52.71
- labyrinth, membranous Q16.5
- lacrimal apparatus Q1Ø.4
- larynx Q31.8
- leg (complete) Q72.Ø- ☑
  - with foot present Q72.1- ☑
  - lower leg (with foot present) — *see* Agenesis, leg, with foot present
    - and foot Q72.2- ☑
- lens Q12.3
- limb (complete) Q73.Ø
  - lower — *see* Agenesis, leg
  - upper — *see* Agenesis, arm
- lip Q38.Ø
- liver Q44.7
- lung (fissure) (lobe) (bilateral) (unilateral) Q33.3
- mandible, maxilla M26.Ø9
- metacarpus — *see* Agenesis, hand
- metatarsus — *see* Agenesis, foot
- muscle Q79.8
  - eyelid Q1Ø.3
  - ocular Q15.8
- musculoskeletal system NEC Q79.8
- nail(s) Q84.3
- neck, part Q18.8
- nerve QØ7.8
- nervous system, part NEC QØ7.8
- nipple Q83.2
- nose Q3Ø.1
- nuclear QØ7.8
- organ
  - of Corti Q16.5
  - or site not listed — *see* Anomaly, by site
- osseous meatus (ear) Q16.1
- ovary
  - bilateral Q5Ø.Ø2
  - unilateral Q5Ø.Ø1
- oviduct Q5Ø.6
- pancreas Q45.Ø
- parathyroid (gland) Q89.2
- parotid gland(s) Q38.4
- patella Q74.1
- pelvic girdle (complete) (partial) Q74.2
- penis Q55.5
- pericardium Q24.8
- pituitary (gland) Q89.2
- prostate Q55.4
- punctum lacrimale Q1Ø.4
- radioulnar — *see* Defect, reduction, upper limb
- radius — *see* Defect, reduction, upper limb, longitudinal, radius
- rectum Q42.1
  - with fistula Q42.Ø
- renal Q6Ø.2
  - bilateral Q6Ø.1
  - unilateral Q6Ø.Ø
- respiratory organ NEC Q34.8
- rib Q76.6
- roof of orbit Q75.8
- round ligament Q52.8
- sacrum Q76.49
- salivary gland Q38.4
- scapula Q74.Ø
- scrotum Q55.29
- seminal vesicles Q55.4
- septum
  - atrial Q21.1
  - between aorta and pulmonary artery Q21.4
  - ventricular Q2Ø.4
- shoulder girdle (complete) (partial) Q74.Ø
- skull (bone) Q75.8
  - with
    - anencephaly QØØ.Ø
    - encephalocele — *see* Encephalocele
    - hydrocephalus QØ3.9
      - with spina bifida — *see* Spina bifida, by site, with hydrocephalus
    - microcephaly QØ2
- spermatic cord Q55.4
- spinal cord QØ6.Ø
- spine Q76.49
- spleen Q89.Ø1
- sternum Q76.7
- stomach Q4Ø.2
- submaxillary gland(s) (congenital) Q38.4
- tarsus — *see* Agenesis, foot
- tendon Q79.8
- testicle Q55.Ø
- thymus (gland) Q89.2
- thyroid (gland) EØ3.1
  - cartilage Q31.8
- tibia — *see* Defect, reduction, lower limb, longitudinal, tibia
- tibiofibular — *see* Defect, reduction, lower limb, specified type NEC
- toe (and foot) (complete) (partial) — *see* Agenesis, foot
- tongue Q38.3
- trachea (cartilage) Q32.1
- ulna — *see* Defect, reduction, upper limb, longitudinal, ulna
- upper limb — *see* Agenesis, arm
- ureter Q62.4
- urethra Q64.5
- urinary tract NEC Q64.8
- uterus Q51.Ø
- uvula Q38.5
- vagina Q52.Ø
- vas deferens Q55.4
- vein(s) (peripheral) Q27.9
  - brain Q28.3
  - great NEC Q26.8
  - portal Q26.5
- vena cava (inferior) (superior) Q26.8
- vermis of cerebellum QØ4.3
- vertebra Q76.49
- vulva Q52.71

Ageusia R43.2

Agitated — *see* condition

Agitation R45.1

Aglossia (congenital) Q38.3

Aglossia-adactylia syndrome Q87.Ø

Aglycogenosis E74.ØØ

Agnosia (body image) (other senses) (tactile) R48.1
- developmental F88
- verbal R48.1
  - auditory R48.1
    - developmental F8Ø.2
  - developmental F8Ø.2
- visual (object) R48.3

Agoraphobia F4Ø.ØØ
- with panic disorder F4Ø.Ø1
- without panic disorder F4Ø.Ø2

Agrammatism R48.8

Agranulocytopenia — *see* Agranulocytosis

Agranulocytosis (chronic) (cyclical) (genetic) (infantile) (periodic) (pernicious) — *see also* Neutropenia D7Ø.9
- congenital D7Ø.Ø
- cytoreductive cancer chemotherapy sequela D7Ø.1
- drug-induced D7Ø.2
  - due to cytoreductive cancer chemotherapy D7Ø.1
- due to infection D7Ø.3
- secondary D7Ø.4
  - drug-induced D7Ø.2
    - due to cytoreductive cancer chemotherapy D7Ø.1

Agraphia (absolute) R48.8
- with alexia R48.Ø
- developmental F81.81

Ague (dumb) — *see* Malaria

Agyria QØ4.3

Ahumada-del Castillo syndrome E23.Ø

Aichomophobia F4Ø.298

AIDS (related complex) B2Ø

Ailment heart — *see* Disease, heart

Ailurophobia F4Ø.218

AIN — *see* Neoplasia, intraepithelial, anal

Ainhum (disease) L94.6

AIPHI (acute idiopathic pulmonary hemorrhage in infants (over 28 days old)) RØ4.81

Air
- anterior mediastinum J98.2
- compressed, disease T7Ø.3 ☑
- conditioner lung or pneumonitis J67.7
- embolism (artery) (cerebral) (any site) T79.Ø ☑
  - with ectopic or molar pregnancy OØ8.2
  - due to implanted device NEC — *see* Complications, by site and type, specified NEC

Air — *continued*
- embolism — *continued*
  - following
    - abortion — *see* Abortion by type, complicated by, embolism
    - ectopic or molar pregnancy O08.2
    - infusion, therapeutic injection or transfusion T80.0 ☑
  - in pregnancy, childbirth or puerperium — *see* Embolism, obstetric
  - traumatic T79.0 ☑
- hunger, psychogenic F45.8
- rarefied, effects of — *see* Effect, adverse, high altitude
- sickness T75.3 ☑

Airplane sickness T75.3 ☑

Akathisia (drug-induced) (treatment-induced) G25.71
- neuroleptic induced (acute) G25.71
- tardive G25.71

Akinesia R29.898

Akinetic mutism R41.89

Akureyri's disease G93.3

Alactasia, congenital E73.0

Alagille's syndrome Q44.7

Alastrim B03

Albers-Schönberg syndrome Q78.2

Albert's syndrome — *see* Tendinitis, Achilles

Albinism, albino E70.30
- with hematologic abnormality E70.339
  - Chédiak-Higashi syndrome E70.330
  - Hermansky-Pudlak syndrome E70.331
  - other specified E70.338
- I E70.320
- II E70.321
- ocular E70.319
  - autosomal recessive E70.311
  - other specified E70.318
  - X-linked E70.310
- oculocutaneous E70.329
  - other specified E70.328
  - tyrosinase (ty) negative E70.320
  - tyrosinase (ty) positive E70.321
- other specified E70.39

Albinismus E70.30

Albright (-McCune)(-Sternberg) syndrome Q78.1

Albuminous — *see* condition

Albuminuria, albuminuric (acute) (chronic) (subacute) — *see also* Proteinuria R80.9
- complicating pregnancy — *see* Proteinuria, gestational
  - with
    - gestational hypertension — *see* Pre-eclampsia
    - pre-existing hypertension — *see* Hypertension, complicating pregnancy, pre-existing, with, pre-eclampsia
- gestational — *see* Proteinuria, gestational
  - with
    - gestational hypertension — *see* Pre-eclampsia
    - pre-existing hypertension — *see* Hypertension, complicating pregnancy, pre-existing, with, pre-eclampsia
- orthostatic R80.2
- postural R80.2
- pre-eclamptic — *see* Pre-eclampsia
- scarlatinal A38.8

Albuminurophobia F40.298

Alcaptonuria E70.29

Alcohol, alcoholic, alcohol-induced
- addiction (without remission) F10.20
  - with remission F10.21
- amnestic disorder, persisting F10.96
  - with dependence F10.26
- anxiety disorder F10.980
- bipolar and related disorder F10.94
- brain syndrome, chronic F10.97
  - with dependence F10.27
- cardiopathy I42.6
- counseling and surveillance Z71.41
  - family member Z71.42
- delirium (acute) (tremens) (withdrawal) F10.231
  - with intoxication F10.921
    - in
      - abuse F10.121
      - dependence F10.221
- dementia F10.97
  - with dependence F10.27
- depressive disorder F10.94
- deterioration F10.97
  - with dependence F10.27
- hallucinosis (acute) F10.951

Alcohol, alcoholic, alcohol-induced — *continued*
- hallucinosis — *continued*
  - in
    - abuse F10.151
    - dependence F10.251
- insanity F10.959
- intoxication (acute) (without dependence) F10.129
  - with
    - delirium F10.121
    - dependence F10.229
      - with delirium F10.221
      - uncomplicated F10.220
  - uncomplicated F10.120
- jealousy F10.988
- Korsakoff's, Korsakov's, Korsakow's F10.26
- liver K70.9
  - acute — *see* Disease, liver, alcoholic, hepatitis
- major neurocognitive disorder, amnestic-confabulatory type F10.96
- major neurocognitive disorder, nonamnestic-confabulatory type F10.97
- mania (acute) (chronic) F10.959
- mild neurocognitive disorder F10.988
- paranoia, paranoid (type) psychosis F10.950
- pellagra E52
- poisoning, accidental (acute) NEC — *see* Table of Drugs and Chemicals, alcohol, poisoning
- psychosis — *see* Psychosis, alcoholic
- psychotic disorder F10.959
- sexual dysfunction F10.981
- sleep disorder F10.982
- withdrawal (without convulsions) F10.239
  - with delirium F10.231

Alcoholism (chronic) (without remission) F10.20
- with
  - psychosis — *see* Psychosis, alcoholic
  - remission F10.21
- Korsakov's F10.96
  - with dependence F10.26

Alder (-Reilly) **anomaly or syndrome** (leukocyte granulation) D72.0

Aldosteronism E26.9
- familial (type I) E26.02
- glucocorticoid-remediable E26.02
- primary (due to (bilateral) adrenal hyperplasia) E26.09
- primary NEC E26.09
- secondary E26.1
- specified NEC E26.89

Aldosteronoma D44.10

Aldrich (-Wiskott) **syndrome** (eczema-thrombocytopenia) D82.0

Alektorophobia F40.218

Aleppo boil B55.1

Aleukemic — *see* condition

Aleukia
- congenital D70.0
- hemorrhagica D61.9
  - congenital D61.09
- splenica D73.1

Alexia R48.0
- developmental F81.0
- secondary to organic lesion R48.0

Algoneurodystrophy M89.00
- ankle M89.07- ☑
- foot M89.07- ☑
- forearm M89.03- ☑
- hand M89.04- ☑
- lower leg M89.06- ☑
- multiple sites M89.0- ☑
- shoulder M89.01- ☑
- specified site NEC M89.08
- thigh M89.05- ☑
- upper arm M89.02- ☑

Algophobia F40.298

Alienation, mental — *see* Psychosis

Alkalemia E87.3

Alkalosis E87.3
- metabolic E87.3
  - with respiratory acidosis E87.4
  - of newborn P74.41
- respiratory E87.3

Alkaptonuria E70.29

Allen-Masters syndrome N83.8

Allergy, allergic (reaction) (to) T78.40 ☑
- air-borne substance NEC (rhinitis) J30.89
- alveolitis (extrinsic) J67.9
  - due to
    - Aspergillus clavatus J67.4

Allergy, allergic — *continued*
- alveolitis — *continued*
  - due to — *continued*
    - Cryptostroma corticale J67.6
    - organisms (fungal, thermophilic actinomycete) growing in ventilation (air conditioning) systems J67.7
  - specified type NEC J67.8
- anaphylactic reaction or shock T78.2 ☑
- angioneurotic edema T78.3 ☑
- animal (dander) (epidermal) (hair) (rhinitis) J30.81
- bee sting (anaphylactic shock) — *see* Toxicity, venom, arthropod, bee
- biological — *see* Allergy, drug
- colitis — *see also* Colitis, allergic K52.29
- dander (animal) (rhinitis) J30.81
- dandruff (rhinitis) J30.81
- dental restorative material (existing) K08.55
- dermatitis — *see* Dermatitis, contact, allergic
- diathesis — *see* History, allergy
- drug, medicament & biological (any) (external) (internal) T78.40 ☑
  - correct substance properly administered — *see* Table of Drugs and Chemicals, by drug, adverse effect
  - wrong substance given or taken NEC (by accident) — *see* Table of Drugs and Chemicals, by drug, poisoning
- due to pollen J30.1
- dust (house) (stock) (rhinitis) J30.89
  - with asthma — *see* Asthma, allergic extrinsic
- eczema — *see* Dermatitis, contact, allergic
- epidermal (animal) (rhinitis) J30.81
- feathers (rhinitis) J30.89
- food (any) (ingested) NEC T78.1 ☑
  - anaphylactic shock — *see* Shock, anaphylactic, due to food
  - dermatitis — *see* Dermatitis, due to, food
  - dietary counseling and surveillance Z71.3
  - in contact with skin L23.6
  - rhinitis J30.5
  - status (without reaction) Z91.018
    - eggs Z91.012
    - milk products Z91.011
    - peanuts Z91.010
    - seafood Z91.013
    - specified NEC Z91.018
- gastrointestinal — *see also* specific type of allergic reaction
  - meaning colitis — *see also* Colitis, allergic K52.29
  - meaning gastroenteritis — *see also* Gastroenteritis, allergic K52.29
  - meaning other adverse food reaction not elsewhere classified T78.1 ☑
- grain J30.1
- grass (hay fever) (pollen) J30.1
  - asthma — *see* Asthma, allergic extrinsic
- hair (animal) (rhinitis) J30.81
- history (of) — *see* History, allergy
- horse serum — *see* Allergy, serum
- inhalant (rhinitis) J30.89
  - pollen J30.1
- kapok (rhinitis) J30.89
- medicine — *see* Allergy, drug
- milk protein — *see also* Allergy, food Z91.011
  - anaphylactic reaction T78.07 ☑
  - dermatitis L27.2
  - enterocolitis syndrome K52.21
  - enteropathy K52.22
  - gastroenteritis K52.29
  - gastroesophageal reflux — *see also* Reaction, adverse, food K21.9
    - with esophagitis (without bleeding) K21.00
      - with bleeding K21.01
  - proctocolitis K52.82
- nasal, seasonal due to pollen J30.1
- pneumonia J82.89
- pollen (any) (hay fever) J30.1
  - asthma — *see* Asthma, allergic extrinsic
- primrose J30.1
- primula J30.1
- proctocolitis K52.82
- purpura D69.0
- ragweed (hay fever) (pollen) J30.1
  - asthma — *see* Asthma, allergic extrinsic
- rose (pollen) J30.1
- seasonal NEC J30.2
- Senecio jacobae (pollen) J30.1

Allergy, allergic — *continued*
serum — *see also* Reaction, serum T8Ø.69 ☑
anaphylactic shock T8Ø.59 ☑
shock (anaphylactic) T78.2 ☑
due to
administration of blood and blood products T8Ø.51 ☑
adverse effect of correct medicinal substance properly administered T88.6 ☑
immunization T8Ø.52 ☑
serum NEC T8Ø.59 ☑
vaccination T8Ø.52 ☑
specific NEC T78.49 ☑
tree (any) (hay fever) (pollen) J3Ø.1
asthma — *see* Asthma, allergic extrinsic
upper respiratory J3Ø.9
urticaria L5Ø.Ø
vaccine — *see* Allergy, serum
wheat — *see* Allergy, food
Allescheriasis B48.2
Alligator skin disease Q8Ø.9
Allocheiria, allochiria R2Ø.8
Almeida's disease — *see* Paracoccidioidomycosis
Alopecia (hereditaria) (seborrheica) L65.9
androgenic L64.9
drug-induced L64.Ø
specified NEC L64.8
areata L63.9
ophiasis L63.2
specified NEC L63.8
totalis L63.Ø
universalis L63.1
cicatricial L66.9
specified NEC L66.8
circumscripta L63.9
congenital, congenitalis Q84.Ø
due to cytotoxic drugs NEC L65.8
mucinosa L65.2
postinfective NEC L65.8
postpartum L65.Ø
premature L64.8
specific (syphilitic) A51.32
specified NEC L65.8
syphilitic (secondary) A51.32
totalis (capitis) L63.Ø
universalis (entire body) L63.1
X-ray L58.1
Alpers' disease G31.81
Alpine sickness T7Ø.29 ☑
Alport syndrome Q87.81
ALTE (apparent life threatening event) **in newborn and infant** R68.13
Alteration (of), **Altered**
awareness
transient R4Ø.4
unintended under general anesthesia, during procedure T88.53 ☑
mental status R41.82
pattern of family relationships affecting child Z62.898
sensation
following
cerebrovascular disease I69.998
cerebral infarction I69.398
intracerebral hemorrhage I69.198
nontraumatic intracranial hemorrhage NEC I69.298
specified disease NEC I69.898
subarachnoid hemorrhage I69.Ø98
Alternating — *see* condition
Altitude, high (effects) — *see* Effect, adverse, high altitude
Aluminosis (of lung) J63.Ø
Alveolitis
allergic (extrinsic) — *see* Pneumonitis, hypersensitivity
due to
Aspergillus clavatus J67.4
Cryptostroma corticale J67.6
fibrosing (cryptogenic) (idiopathic) J84.112
jaw M27.3
sicca dolorosa M27.3
Alveolus, alveolar — *see* condition
Alymphocytosis D72.81Ø
thymic (with immunodeficiency) D82.1
Alymphoplasia, thymic D82.1
Alzheimer's disease or sclerosis — *see* Disease, Alzheimer's
Amastia (with nipple present) Q83.8
with absent nipple Q83.Ø
Amathophobia F4Ø.228
Amaurosis (acquired) (congenital) — *see also* Blindness
fugax G45.3
hysterical F44.6
Leber's congenital H35.5Ø
uremic — *see* Uremia
Amaurotic idiocy (infantile) (juvenile) (late) E75.4
Amaxophobia F4Ø.248
Ambiguous genitalia Q56.4
Amblyopia (congenital) (ex anopsia) (partial) (suppression) H53.ØØ- ☑
anisometropic — *see* Amblyopia, refractive
deprivation H53.Ø1- ☑
hysterical F44.6
nocturnal — *see also* Blindness, night
vitamin A deficiency E5Ø.5
refractive H53.Ø2- ☑
strabismic H53.Ø3- ☑
suspect H53.Ø4- ☑
tobacco H53.8
toxic NEC H53.8
uremic — *see* Uremia
Ameba, amebic (histolytica) — *see also* Amebiasis
abscess (liver) AØ6.4
Amebiasis AØ6.9
with abscess — *see* Abscess, amebic
acute AØ6.Ø
chronic (intestine) AØ6.1
with abscess — *see* Abscess, amebic
cutaneous AØ6.7
cutis AØ6.7
cystitis AØ6.81
genitourinary tract NEC AØ6.82
hepatic — *see* Abscess, liver, amebic
intestine AØ6.Ø
nondysenteric colitis AØ6.2
skin AØ6.7
specified site NEC AØ6.89
Ameboma (of intestine) AØ6.3
Amelia Q73.Ø
lower limb — *see* Agenesis, leg
upper limb — *see* Agenesis, arm
Ameloblastoma — *see also* Cyst, calcifying odontogenic
long bones C4Ø.9- ☑
lower limb C4Ø.2- ☑
upper limb C4Ø.Ø- ☑
malignant C41.1
jaw (bone) (lower) C41.1
upper C41.Ø
tibial C4Ø.2- ☑
Amelogenesis imperfecta KØØ.5
nonhereditaria (segmentalis) KØØ.4
Amenorrhea N91.2
hyperhormonal E28.8
primary N91.Ø
secondary N91.1
Amentia — *see* Disability, intellectual
Meynert's (nonalcoholic) FØ4
American
leishmaniasis B55.2
mountain tick fever A93.2
Ametropia — *see* Disorder, refraction
AMH (asymptomatic microscopic hematuria) R31.21
Amianthosis J61
Amimia R48.8
Amino-acid disorder E72.9
anemia D53.Ø
Aminoacidopathy E72.9
Aminoaciduria E72.9
Amnesia R41.3
anterograde R41.1
auditory R48.8
dissociative F44.Ø
with dissociative fugue F44.1
hysterical F44.Ø
postictal in epilepsy — *see* Epilepsy
psychogenic F44.Ø
retrograde R41.2
transient global G45.4
Amnes(t)ic syndrome (post-traumatic) FØ4
induced by
alcohol F1Ø.96
with dependence F1Ø.26
psychoactive NEC F19.96
with
abuse F19.16
dependence F19.26
Amnes(t)ic syndrome — *continued*
induced by — *continued*
sedative F13.96
with dependence F13.26
Amnion, amniotic — *see* condition
Amnionitis — *see* Pregnancy, complicated by
Amok F68.8
Amoral traits F6Ø.89
Amphetamine (or other stimulant) **-induced**
anxiety disorder F15.98Ø
bipolar and related disorder F15.94
delirium F15.921
depressive disorder F15.94
obsessive-compulsive and related disorder F15.988
psychotic disorder F15.959
sexual dysfunction F15.981
sleep disorder F15.982
stimulant withdrawal F15.23
Ampulla
lower esophagus K22.8
phrenic K22.8
Amputation — *see also* Absence, by site, acquired
neuroma (postoperative) (traumatic) — *see* Complications, amputation stump, neuroma
stump (surgical)
abnormal, painful, or with complication (late) — *see* Complications, amputation stump
healed or old NOS Z89.9
traumatic (complete) (partial)
arm (upper) (complete) S48.91- ☑
at
elbow S58.Ø1- ☑
partial S58.Ø2- ☑
shoulder joint (complete) S48.Ø1- ☑
partial S48.Ø2- ☑
between
elbow and wrist (complete) S58.11- ☑
partial S58.12- ☑
shoulder and elbow (complete) S48.11- ☑
partial S48.12- ☑
partial S48.92- ☑
breast (complete) S28.21- ☑
partial S28.22- ☑
clitoris (complete) S38.211 ☑
partial S38.212 ☑
ear (complete) SØ8.11- ☑
partial SØ8.12- ☑
finger (complete) (metacarpophalangeal) S68.11- ☑
index S68.11- ☑
little S68.11- ☑
middle S68.11- ☑
partial S68.12- ☑
index S68.12- ☑
little S68.12- ☑
middle S68.12- ☑
ring S68.12- ☑
ring S68.11- ☑
thumb — *see* Amputation, traumatic, thumb
transphalangeal (complete) S68.61- ☑
index S68.61- ☑
little S68.61- ☑
middle S68.61- ☑
partial S68.62- ☑
index S68.62- ☑
little S68.62- ☑
middle S68.62- ☑
ring S68.62- ☑
ring S68.61- ☑
foot (complete) S98.91- ☑
at ankle level S98.Ø1- ☑
partial S98.Ø2- ☑
midfoot S98.31- ☑
partial S98.32- ☑
partial S98.92- ☑
forearm (complete) S58.91- ☑
at elbow level (complete) S58.Ø1- ☑
partial S58.Ø2- ☑
between elbow and wrist (complete) S58.11- ☑
partial S58.12- ☑
partial S58.92- ☑
genital organ(s) (external)
female (complete) S38.211 ☑
partial S38.212 ☑
male
penis (complete) S38.221 ☑
partial S38.222 ☑

- **Amputation** — *continued*
  - traumatic — *continued*
    - genital organ(s) — *continued*
      - male — *continued*
        - scrotum (complete) S38.231 ☑
          - partial S38.232 ☑
        - testes (complete) S38.231 ☑
          - partial S38.232 ☑
    - hand (complete) (wrist level) S68.41- ☑
      - finger(s) alone — *see* Amputation, traumatic, finger
      - partial S68.42- ☑
      - thumb alone — *see* Amputation, traumatic, thumb
      - transmetacarpal (complete) S68.71- ☑
        - partial S68.72- ☑
    - head
      - ear — *see* Amputation, traumatic, ear
      - nose (partial) SØ8.812 ☑
        - complete SØ8.811 ☑
      - part SØ8.89 ☑
        - scalp SØ8.Ø ☑
    - hip (and thigh) (complete) S78.91- ☑
      - at hip joint (complete) S78.Ø1- ☑
        - partial S78.Ø2- ☑
      - between hip and knee (complete) S78.11- ☑
        - partial S78.12- ☑
      - partial S78.92- ☑
    - labium (majus) (minus) (complete) S38.21- ☑
      - partial S38.21- ☑
    - leg (lower) S88.91- ☑
      - at knee level S88.Ø1- ☑
        - partial S88.Ø2- ☑
      - between knee and ankle S88.11- ☑
        - partial S88.12- ☑
      - partial S88.92- ☑
    - nose (partial) SØ8.812 ☑
      - complete SØ8.811 ☑
    - penis (complete) S38.221 ☑
      - partial S38.222 ☑
    - scrotum (complete) S38.231 ☑
      - partial S38.232 ☑
    - shoulder — *see* Amputation, traumatic, arm
      - at shoulder joint — *see* Amputation, traumatic, arm, at shoulder joint
    - testes (complete) S38.231 ☑
      - partial S38.232 ☑
    - thigh — *see* Amputation, traumatic, hip
    - thorax, part of S28.1 ☑
      - breast — *see* Amputation, traumatic, breast
    - thumb (complete) (metacarpophalangeal) S68.Ø1- ☑
      - partial S68.Ø2- ☑
      - transphalangeal (complete) S68.51- ☑
        - partial S68.52- ☑
    - toe (lesser) S98.13- ☑
      - great S98.11- ☑
        - partial S98.12- ☑
      - more than one S98.21- ☑
        - partial S98.22- ☑
      - partial S98.14- ☑
    - vulva (complete) S38.211 ☑
      - partial S38.212 ☑
- **Amputee** (bilateral) (old) Z89.9
- **Amsterdam dwarfism** Q87.19
- **Amusia** R48.8
  - developmental F8Ø.89
- **Amyelencephalus, amyelencephaly** QØØ.Ø
- **Amyelia** QØ6.Ø
- **Amygdalitis** — *see* Tonsillitis
- **Amygdalolith** J35.8
- **Amyloid heart** (disease) E85.4 *[I43]*
- **Amyloidosis** (generalized) (primary) E85.9
  - with lung involvement E85.4 *[J99]*
  - familial E85.2
  - genetic E85.2
  - heart E85.4 *[I43]*
  - hemodialysis-associated E85.3
  - light chain (AL) E85.81
  - liver E85.4 *[K77]*
  - localized E85.4
  - neuropathic heredofamilial E85.1
  - non-neuropathic heredofamilial E85.Ø
  - organ limited E85.4
  - Portuguese E85.1
  - pulmonary E85.4 *[J99]*
- **Amyloidosis** — *continued*
  - secondary systemic E85.3
  - senile systemic (SSA) E85.82
  - skin (lichen) (macular) E85.4 *[L99]*
  - specified NEC E85.89
  - subglottic E85.4 *[J99]*
  - wild-type transthyretin-related (ATTR) E85.82
- **Amylopectinosis** (brancher enzyme deficiency) E74.Ø3
- **Amylophagia** — *see* Pica
- **Amyoplasia congenita** Q79.8
- **Amyotonia** M62.89
  - congenita G7Ø.2
- **Amyotrophia, amyotrophy, amyotrophic** G71.8
  - congenita Q79.8
  - diabetic — *see* Diabetes, amyotrophy
  - lateral sclerosis G12.21
  - neuralgic G54.5
  - spinal progressive G12.25
- **Anacidity, gastric** K31.83
  - psychogenic F45.8
- **Anaerosis of newborn** P28.89
- **Analbuminemia** E88.Ø9
- **Analgesia** — *see* Anesthesia
- **Analphalipoproteinemia** E78.6
- **Anaphylactic**
  - purpura D69.Ø
  - shock or reaction — *see* Shock, anaphylactic
- **Anaphylactoid shock or reaction** — *see* Shock, anaphylactic
- **Anaphylactoid syndrome of pregnancy** O88.Ø1- ☑
- **Anaphylaxis** — *see* Shock, anaphylactic
- **Anaplasia cervix** — *see also* Dysplasia, cervix N87.9
- **Anaplasmosis, human** A77.49
- **Anarthria** R47.1
- **Anasarca** R6Ø.1
  - cardiac — *see* Failure, heart, congestive
  - lung J18.2
  - newborn P83.2
  - nutritional E43
  - pulmonary J18.2
  - renal NØ4.9
- **Anastomosis**
  - aneurysmal — *see* Aneurysm
  - arteriovenous ruptured brain I6Ø.8
    - intracerebral I61.8
    - intraparenchymal I61.8
    - intraventricular I61.5
    - subarachnoid I6Ø.8
  - intestinal K63.89
    - complicated NEC K91.89
      - involving urinary tract N99.89
  - retinal and choroidal vessels (congenital) Q14.8
- **Anatomical narrow angle** H4Ø.Ø3- ☑
- **Ancylostoma, ancylostomiasis** (braziliense) (caninum) (ceylanicum) (duodenale) B76.Ø
  - Necator americanus B76.1
- **Andersen's disease** (glycogen storage) E74.Ø9
- **Anderson-Fabry disease** E75.21
- **Andes disease** T7Ø.29 ☑
- **Andrews' disease** (bacterid) LØ8.89
- **Androblastoma**
  - benign
    - specified site — *see* Neoplasm, benign, by site
    - unspecified site
      - female D27.9
      - male D29.2Ø
  - malignant
    - specified site — *see* Neoplasm, malignant, by site
    - unspecified site
      - female C56.9
      - male C62.9Ø
  - specified site — *see* Neoplasm, uncertain behavior, by site
  - tubular
    - with lipid storage
      - specified site — *see* Neoplasm, benign, by site
      - unspecified site
        - female D27.9
        - male D29.2Ø
    - specified site — *see* Neoplasm, benign, by site
    - unspecified site
      - female D27.9
      - male D29.2Ø
  - unspecified site
    - female D39.1Ø
    - male D4Ø.1Ø
- **Androgen insensitivity syndrome** — *see also* Syndrome, androgen insensitivity E34.5Ø
- **Androgen resistance syndrome** — *see also* Syndrome, androgen insensitivity E34.5Ø
- **Android pelvis** Q74.2
  - with disproportion (fetopelvic) O33.3 ☑
    - causing obstructed labor O65.3
- **Androphobia** F4Ø.29Ø
- **Anectasis, pulmonary** (newborn) — *see* Atelectasis
- **Anemia** (essential) (general) (hemoglobin deficiency) (infantile) (primary) (profound) D64.9
  - with (due to) (in)
    - disorder of
      - anaerobic glycolysis D55.2
      - pentose phosphate pathway D55.1
    - koilonychia D5Ø.9
  - achlorhydric D5Ø.8
  - achrestic D53.1
  - Addison (-Biermer) (pernicious) D51.Ø
  - agranulocytic — *see* Agranulocytosis
  - amino-acid-deficiency D53.Ø
  - aplastic D61.9
    - congenital D61.Ø9
    - drug-induced D61.1
    - due to
      - drugs D61.1
      - external agents NEC D61.2
      - infection D61.2
      - radiation D61.2
    - idiopathic D61.3
    - red cell (pure) D6Ø.9
      - chronic D6Ø.Ø
      - congenital D61.Ø1
      - specified type NEC D6Ø.8
      - transient D6Ø.1
    - specified type NEC D61.89
    - toxic D61.2
  - aregenerative
    - congenital D61.Ø9
  - asiderotic D5Ø.9
  - atypical (primary) D64.9
  - Baghdad spring D55.Ø
  - Balantidium coli AØ7.Ø
  - Biermer's (pernicious) D51.Ø
  - blood loss (chronic) D5Ø.Ø
    - acute D62
  - bothriocephalus B7Ø.Ø *[D63.8]*
  - brickmaker's B76.9 *[D63.8]*
  - cerebral I67.89
  - childhood D58.9
  - chlorotic D5Ø.8
  - chronic
    - blood loss D5Ø.Ø
    - hemolytic D58.9
      - idiopathic D59.9
    - simple D53.9
  - chronica congenita aregenerativa D61.Ø9
  - combined system disease NEC D51.Ø *[G32.Ø]*
    - due to dietary vitamin B12 deficiency D51.3 *[G32.Ø]*
  - complicating pregnancy, childbirth or puerperium — *see* Pregnancy, complicated by (management affected by), anemia
  - congenital P61.4
    - aplastic D61.Ø9
    - due to isoimmunization NOS P55.9
    - dyserythropoietic, dyshematopoietic D64.4
    - following fetal blood loss P61.3
    - Heinz body D58.2
    - hereditary hemolytic NOS D58.9
    - pernicious D51.Ø
    - spherocytic D58.Ø
  - Cooley's (erythroblastic) D56.1
  - cytogenic D51.Ø
  - deficiency D53.9
    - 2, 3 diphosphoglycurate mutase D55.2
    - 2, 3 PG D55.2
    - 6 phosphogluconate dehydrogenase D55.1
    - 6-PGD D55.1
    - amino-acid D53.Ø
    - combined B12 and folate D53.1
    - enzyme D55.9
      - drug-induced (hemolytic) D59.2
      - glucose-6-phosphate dehydrogenase (G6PD) D55.Ø
      - glycolytic D55.2
      - nucleotide metabolism D55.3
      - related to hexose monophosphate (HMP) shunt pathway NEC D55.1

- **Anemia** — *continued*
  - nutritional — *continued*
    - with
      - poor iron absorption D5Ø.8
      - specified deficiency NEC D53.8
    - megaloblastic D52.Ø
  - of prematurity P61.2
  - orotaciduric (congenital) (hereditary) D53.Ø
  - osteosclerotic D64.89
  - ovalocytosis (hereditary) — *see* Elliptocytosis
  - paludal — *see also* Malaria B54 *[D63.8]*
  - pernicious (congenital) (malignant) (progressive) D51.Ø
  - pleochromic D64.89
    - of sprue D52.8
  - posthemorrhagic (chronic) D5Ø.Ø
    - acute D62
    - newborn P61.3
  - postoperative (postprocedural)
    - due to (acute) blood loss D62
      - chronic blood loss D5Ø.Ø
    - specified NEC D64.9
  - postpartum O9Ø.81
  - pressure D64.89
  - progressive D64.9
    - malignant D51.Ø
    - pernicious D51.Ø
  - protein-deficiency D53.Ø
  - pseudoleukemica infantum D64.89
  - pure red cell D6Ø.9
    - congenital D61.Ø1
  - pyridoxine-responsive D64.3
  - pyruvate kinase deficiency D55.2
  - refractory D46.4
    - with
      - excess of blasts D46.2Ø
        - 1 (RAEB 1) D46.21
        - 2 (RAEB 2) D46.22
        - in transformation (RAEB T) — *see* Leukemia, acute myeloblastic
      - hemochromatosis D46.1
      - sideroblasts (ring) (RARS) D46.1
    - megaloblastic D53.1
    - sideroblastic D46.1
    - sideropenic D5Ø.9
    - without ring sideroblasts, so stated D46.Ø
    - without sideroblasts without excess of blasts D46.Ø
  - Rietti-Greppi-Micheli D56.9
  - scorbutic D53.2
  - secondary to
    - blood loss (chronic) D5Ø.Ø
      - acute D62
    - hemorrhage (chronic) D5Ø.Ø
      - acute D62
  - semiplastic D61.89
  - sickle-cell — *see* Disease, sickle-cell
  - sideroblastic D64.3
    - hereditary D64.Ø
    - hypochromic, sex-linked D64.Ø
    - pyridoxine-responsive NEC D64.3
    - refractory D46.1
    - secondary (due to)
      - disease D64.1
      - drugs and toxins D64.2
    - specified type NEC D64.3
  - sideropenic (refractory) D5Ø.9
    - due to blood loss (chronic) D5Ø.Ø
      - acute D62
  - simple chronic D53.9
  - specified type NEC D64.89
  - spherocytic (hereditary) — *see* Spherocytosis
  - splenic D64.89
  - splenomegalic D64.89
  - stomatocytosis D58.8
  - syphilitic (acquired) (late) A52.79 *[D63.8]*
  - target cell D64.89
  - thalassemia D56.9
  - thrombocytopenic — *see* Thrombocytopenia
  - toxic D61.2
  - tropical B76.9 *[D63.8]*
    - macrocytic D52.8
  - tuberculous A18.89 *[D63.8]*
  - vegan D51.3
  - vitamin
    - B12 deficiency (dietary) pernicious D51.Ø
    - B6-responsive D64.3
  - von Jaksch's D64.89
  - Witts' (achlorhydric anemia) D5Ø.8
- **Anemophobia** F4Ø.228
- **Anencephalus, anencephaly** QØØ.Ø
- **Anergasia** — *see* Psychosis, organic
- **Anesthesia, anesthetic** R2Ø.Ø
  - complication or reaction NEC — *see also* Complications, anesthesia T88.59 ☑
    - due to
      - correct substance properly administered — *see* Table of Drugs and Chemicals, by drug, adverse effect
      - overdose or wrong substance given — *see* Table of Drugs and Chemicals, by drug, poisoning
    - unintended awareness under general anesthesia during procedure T88.53 ☑
      - personal history of Z92.84
  - cornea H18.81- ☑
  - dissociative F44.6
  - functional (hysterical) F44.6
  - hyperesthetic, thalamic G89.Ø
  - hysterical F44.6
  - local skin lesion R2Ø.Ø
  - sexual (psychogenic) F52.1
  - shock (due to) T88.2 ☑
  - skin R2Ø.Ø
  - testicular N5Ø.9
- **Anetoderma** (maculosum) (of) L9Ø.8
  - Jadassohn-Pellizzari L9Ø.2
  - Schweniger-Buzzi L9Ø.1
- **Aneurin deficiency** E51.9
- **Aneurysm** (anastomotic) (artery) (cirsoid) (diffuse) (false) (fusiform) (multiple) (saccular) I72.9
  - abdominal (aorta) I71.4
    - ruptured I71.3
    - syphilitic A52.Ø1
  - aorta, aortic (nonsyphilitic) I71.9
    - abdominal I71.4
      - ruptured I71.3
    - arch I71.2
      - ruptured I71.1
    - arteriosclerotic I71.9
      - ruptured I71.8
    - ascending I71.2
      - ruptured I71.1
    - congenital Q25.43
    - descending I71.9
      - abdominal I71.4
        - ruptured I71.3
      - ruptured I71.8
      - thoracic I71.2
        - ruptured I71.1
    - root Q25.43
    - ruptured I71.8
    - sinus, congenital Q25.43
    - syphilitic A52.Ø1
    - thoracic I71.2
      - ruptured I71.1
    - thoracoabdominal I71.6
      - ruptured I71.5
    - thorax, thoracic (arch) I71.2
      - ruptured I71.1
    - transverse I71.2
      - ruptured I71.1
    - valve (heart) — *see also* Endocarditis, aortic I35.8
  - arteriosclerotic I72.9
    - cerebral I67.1
      - ruptured — *see* Hemorrhage, intracranial, subarachnoid
  - arteriovenous (congenital) — *see also* Malformation, arteriovenous
    - acquired I77.Ø
      - brain I67.1
        - ruptured — *see* Aneurysm, arteriovenous, brain, ruptured
      - coronary I25.41
      - pulmonary I28.Ø
    - brain Q28.2
      - ruptured I6Ø.8
        - intracerebral I61.8
        - intraparenchymal I61.8
        - intraventricular I61.5
        - subarachnoid I6Ø.8
    - peripheral — *see* Malformation, arteriovenous, peripheral
    - precerebral vessels Q28.Ø
    - specified site NEC — *see also* Malformation, arteriovenous
      - acquired I77.Ø
  - basal — *see* Aneurysm, brain
- **Aneurysm** — *continued*
  - basilar (trunk) I72.5
  - berry (congenital) (nonruptured) I67.1
    - ruptured I6Ø.7
  - brain I67.1
    - arteriosclerotic I67.1
      - ruptured — *see* Hemorrhage, intracranial, subarachnoid
    - arteriovenous (congenital) (nonruptured) Q28.2
      - acquired I67.1
        - ruptured — *see* Aneurysm, arteriovenous, brain, ruptured I6Ø.8-
      - ruptured — *see* Aneurysm, arteriovenous, brain, ruptured I6Ø.8-
    - berry (congenital) (nonruptured) I67.1
      - ruptured — *see also* Hemorrhage, intracranial, subarachnoid I6Ø.7
    - congenital Q28.3
      - ruptured I6Ø.7
    - meninges I67.1
      - ruptured I6Ø.8
    - miliary (congenital) (nonruptured) I67.1
      - ruptured — *see also* Hemorrhage, intracranial, subarachnoid I6Ø.7
    - mycotic I33.Ø
    - ruptured — *see* Aneurysm, arteriovenous, brain, ruptured I6Ø.8
    - syphilitic (hemorrhage) A52.Ø5
  - cardiac (false) — *see also* Aneurysm, heart I25.3
  - carotid artery (common) (external) I72.Ø
    - internal (intracranial) I67.1
      - extracranial portion I72.Ø
    - ruptured into brain I6Ø.Ø- ☑
    - syphilitic A52.Ø9
      - intracranial A52.Ø5
  - cavernous sinus I67.1
    - arteriovenous (congenital) (nonruptured) Q28.3
      - ruptured I6Ø.8
  - celiac I72.8
  - central nervous system, syphilitic A52.Ø5
  - cerebral — *see* Aneurysm, brain
  - chest — *see* Aneurysm, thorax
  - circle of Willis I67.1
    - congenital Q28.3
      - ruptured I6Ø.6
    - ruptured I6Ø.6
  - common iliac artery I72.3
  - congenital (peripheral) Q27.8
    - aorta (root) (sinus) Q25.43
    - brain Q28.3
      - ruptured I6Ø.7
    - coronary Q24.5
    - digestive system Q27.8
    - lower limb Q27.8
    - pulmonary Q25.79
    - retina Q14.1
    - specified site NEC Q27.8
    - upper limb Q27.8
  - conjunctiva — *see* Abnormality, conjunctiva, vascular
  - conus arteriosus — *see* Aneurysm, heart
  - coronary (arteriosclerotic) (artery) I25.41
    - arteriovenous, congenital Q24.5
    - congenital Q24.5
    - ruptured — *see* Infarct, myocardium
    - syphilitic A52.Ø6
    - vein I25.89
  - cylindroid (aorta) I71.9
    - ruptured I71.8
    - syphilitic A52.Ø1
  - ductus arteriosus Q25.Ø
  - endocardial, infective (any valve) I33.Ø
  - femoral (artery) (ruptured) I72.4
  - gastroduodenal I72.8
  - gastroepiploic I72.8
  - heart (wall) (chronic or with a stated duration of over 4 weeks) I25.3
    - valve — *see* Endocarditis
  - hepatic I72.8
  - iliac (common) (artery) (ruptured) I72.3
  - infective I72.9
    - endocardial (any valve) I33.Ø
  - innominate (nonsyphilitic) I72.8
    - syphilitic A52.Ø9
  - interauricular septum — *see* Aneurysm, heart
  - interventricular septum — *see* Aneurysm, heart
  - intrathoracic (nonsyphilitic) I71.2
    - ruptured I71.1
    - syphilitic A52.Ø1

- **Aneurysm** — *continued*
  - lower limb I72.4
  - lung (pulmonary artery) I28.1
  - mediastinal (nonsyphilitic) I72.8
    - syphilitic A52.09
  - miliary (congenital) I67.1
    - ruptured — *see* Hemorrhage, intracerebral, subarachnoid, intracranial
  - mitral (heart) (valve) I34.8
  - mural — *see* Aneurysm, heart
  - mycotic I72.9
    - endocardial (any valve) I33.0
    - ruptured, brain — *see* Hemorrhage, intracerebral, subarachnoid
  - myocardium — *see* Aneurysm, heart
  - neck I72.0
  - pancreaticoduodenal I72.8
  - patent ductus arteriosus Q25.0
  - peripheral NEC I72.8
    - congenital Q27.8
      - digestive system Q27.8
      - lower limb Q27.8
      - specified site NEC Q27.8
      - upper limb Q27.8
  - popliteal (artery) (ruptured) I72.4
  - precerebral
    - congenital (nonruptured) Q28.1
    - specified site, NEC I72.5
  - pulmonary I28.1
    - arteriovenous Q25.72
      - acquired I28.0
    - syphilitic A52.09
    - valve (heart) — *see* Endocarditis, pulmonary
  - racemose (peripheral) I72.9
    - congenital — *see* Aneurysm, congenital
  - radial I72.1
  - Rasmussen NEC A15.0
  - renal (artery) I72.2
  - retina — *see also* Disorder, retina, microaneurysms
    - congenital Q14.1
    - diabetic — *see* E08-E13 with .3-
  - sinus of Valsalva Q25.49
  - specified NEC I72.8
  - spinal (cord) I72.8
    - syphilitic (hemorrhage) A52.09
  - splenic I72.8
  - subclavian (artery) (ruptured) I72.8
    - syphilitic A52.09
  - superior mesenteric I72.8
  - syphilitic (aorta) A52.01
    - central nervous system A52.05
    - congenital (late) A50.54 *[I79.0]*
    - spine, spinal A52.09
  - thoracoabdominal (aorta) I71.6
    - ruptured I71.5
    - syphilitic A52.01
  - thorax, thoracic (aorta) (arch) (nonsyphilitic) I71.2
    - ruptured I71.1
    - syphilitic A52.01
  - traumatic (complication) (early), specified site — *see* Injury, blood vessel
  - tricuspid (heart) (valve) I07.8
  - ulnar I72.1
  - upper limb (ruptured) I72.1
  - valve, valvular — *see* Endocarditis
  - venous — *see also* Varix I86.8
    - congenital Q27.8
      - digestive system Q27.8
      - lower limb Q27.8
      - specified site NEC Q27.8
      - upper limb Q27.8
  - ventricle — *see* Aneurysm, heart
  - vertebral artery I72.6
  - visceral NEC I72.8
- **Angelman syndrome** Q93.51
- **Anger** R45.4
- **Angiectasis, angiectopia** I99.8
- **Angiitis** I77.6
  - allergic granulomatous M30.1
  - hypersensitivity M31.0
  - necrotizing M31.9
    - specified NEC M31.8
  - nervous system, granulomatous I67.7
- **Angina** (attack) (cardiac) (chest) (heart) (pectoris) (syndrome) (vasomotor) I20.9
  - with
    - atherosclerotic heart disease — *see* Arteriosclerosis, coronary (artery),
- **Angina** — *continued*
  - with — *continued*
    - documented spasm I20.1
  - abdominal K55.1
  - accelerated — *see* Angina, unstable
  - agranulocytic — *see* Agranulocytosis
  - angiospastic — *see* Angina, with documented spasm
  - aphthous B08.5
  - crescendo — *see* Angina, unstable
  - croupous J05.0
  - cruris I73.9
  - de novo effort — *see* Angina, unstable
  - diphtheritic, membranous A36.0
  - equivalent I20.8
  - exudative, chronic J37.0
  - following acute myocardial infarction I23.7
  - gangrenous diphtheritic A36.0
  - intestinal K55.1
  - Ludovici K12.2
  - Ludwig's K12.2
  - malignant diphtheritic A36.0
  - membranous J05.0
    - diphtheritic A36.0
    - Vincent's A69.1
  - mesenteric K55.1
  - monocytic — *see* Mononucleosis, infectious
  - of effort — *see* Angina, specified NEC
  - phlegmonous J36
    - diphtheritic A36.0
  - post-infarctional I23.7
  - pre-infarctional — *see* Angina, unstable
  - Prinzmetal — *see* Angina, with documented spasm
  - progressive — *see* Angina, unstable
  - pseudomembranous A69.1
  - pultaceous, diphtheritic A36.0
  - spasm-induced — *see* Angina, with documented spasm
  - specified NEC I20.8
  - stable I20.8
  - stenocardia — *see* Angina, specified NEC
  - stridulous, diphtheritic A36.2
  - tonsil J36
  - trachealis J05.0
  - unstable I20.0
  - variant — *see* Angina, with documented spasm
  - Vincent's A69.1
  - worsening effort — *see* Angina, unstable
- **Angioblastoma** — *see* Neoplasm, connective tissue, uncertain behavior
- **Angiocholecystitis** — *see* Cholecystitis, acute
- **Angiocholitis** — *see also* Cholecystitis, acute K83.09
- **Angiodysgenesis spinalis** G95.19
- **Angiodysplasia** (cecum) (colon) K55.20
  - with bleeding K55.21
  - duodenum (and stomach) K31.819
    - with bleeding K31.811
  - stomach (and duodenum) K31.819
    - with bleeding K31.811
- **Angioedema** (allergic) (any site) (with urticaria) T78.3 ☑
  - episodic, with eosinophilia D72.118
  - hereditary D84.1
- **Angioendothelioma** — *see* Neoplasm, uncertain behavior, by site
  - benign D18.00
    - intra-abdominal D18.03
    - intracranial D18.02
    - skin D18.01
    - specified site NEC D18.09
  - bone — *see* Neoplasm, bone, malignant
  - Ewing's — *see* Neoplasm, bone, malignant
- **Angioendotheliomatosis** C85.8- ☑
- **Angiofibroma** — *see also* Neoplasm, benign, by site
  - juvenile
    - specified site — *see* Neoplasm, benign, by site
    - unspecified site D10.6
- **Angiohemophilia** (A) (B) D68.0
- **Angioid streaks** (choroid) (macula) (retina) H35.33
- **Angiokeratoma** — *see* Neoplasm, skin, benign
  - corporis diffusum E75.21
- **Angioleiomyoma** — *see* Neoplasm, connective tissue, benign
- **Angiolipoma** — *see also* Lipoma
  - infiltrating — *see* Lipoma
- **Angioma** — *see also* Hemangioma, by site
  - capillary I78.1
  - hemorrhagicum hereditaria I78.0
  - intra-abdominal D18.03
  - intracranial D18.02
- **Angioma** — *continued*
  - malignant — *see* Neoplasm, connective tissue, malignant
  - plexiform D18.00
    - intra-abdominal D18.03
    - intracranial D18.02
    - skin D18.01
    - specified site NEC D18.09
  - senile I78.1
  - serpiginosum L81.7
  - skin D18.01
  - specified site NEC D18.09
  - spider I78.1
  - stellate I78.1
  - venous Q28.3
- **Angiomatosis** Q82.8
  - bacillary A79.89
  - encephalotrigeminal Q85.8
  - hemorrhagic familial I78.0
  - hereditary familial I78.0
  - liver K76.4
- **Angiomyolipoma** — *see* Lipoma
- **Angiomyoliposarcoma** — *see* Neoplasm, connective tissue, malignant
- **Angiomyoma** — *see* Neoplasm, connective tissue, benign
- **Angiomyosarcoma** — *see* Neoplasm, connective tissue, malignant
- **Angiomyxoma** — *see* Neoplasm, connective tissue, uncertain behavior
- **Angioneurosis** F45.8
- **Angioneurotic edema** (allergic) (any site) (with urticaria) T78.3 ☑
  - hereditary D84.1
- **Angiopathia, angiopathy** I99.9
  - cerebral I67.9
    - amyloid E85.4 *[I68.0]*
  - diabetic (peripheral) — *see* Diabetes, angiopathy
  - peripheral I73.9
    - diabetic — *see* Diabetes, angiopathy
    - specified type NEC I73.89
  - retinae syphilitica A52.05
  - retinalis (juvenilis)
    - diabetic — *see* Diabetes, retinopathy
    - proliferative — *see* Retinopathy, proliferative
- **Angiosarcoma** — *see also* Neoplasm, connective tissue, malignant
  - liver C22.3
- **Angiosclerosis** — *see* Arteriosclerosis
- **Angiospasm** (peripheral) (traumatic) (vessel) I73.9
  - brachial plexus G54.0
  - cerebral G45.9
  - cervical plexus G54.2
  - nerve
    - arm — *see* Mononeuropathy, upper limb
      - axillary G54.0
      - median — *see* Lesion, nerve, median
      - ulnar — *see* Lesion, nerve, ulnar
    - axillary G54.0
    - leg — *see* Mononeuropathy, lower limb
    - median — *see* Lesion, nerve, median
    - plantar — *see* Lesion, nerve, plantar
    - ulnar — *see* Lesion, nerve, ulnar
- **Angiospastic disease or edema** I73.9
- **Angiostrongyliasis**
  - due to
    - Parastrongylus
      - cantonensis B83.2
      - costaricensis B81.3
  - intestinal B81.3
- **Anguillulosis** — *see* Strongyloidiasis
- **Angulation**
  - cecum — *see* Obstruction, intestine
  - coccyx (acquired) — *see also* subcategory M43.8 ☑
    - congenital NEC Q76.49
  - femur (acquired) — *see also* Deformity, limb, specified type NEC, thigh
    - congenital Q74.2
  - intestine (large) (small) — *see* Obstruction, intestine
  - sacrum (acquired) — *see also* subcategory M43.8 ☑
    - congenital NEC Q76.49
  - sigmoid (flexure) — *see* Obstruction, intestine
  - spine — *see* Dorsopathy, deforming, specified NEC
  - tibia (acquired) — *see also* Deformity, limb, specified type NEC, lower leg
    - congenital Q74.2
  - ureter N13.5
    - with infection N13.6

Angulation — *continued*
wrist (acquired) — *see also* Deformity, limb, specified type NEC, forearm
congenital Q74.Ø
Angulus infectiosus (lips) K13.Ø
Anhedonia R45.84
sexual F52.Ø
Anhidrosis L74.4
Anhydration E86.Ø
Anhydremia E86.Ø
Anidrosis L74.4
Aniridia (congenital) Q13.1
Anisakiasis (infection) (infestation) B81.Ø
Anisakis larvae infestation B81.Ø
Aniseikonia H52.32
Anisocoria (pupil) H57.Ø2
congenital Q13.2
Anisocytosis R71.8
Anisometropia (congenital) H52.31
Ankle — *see* condition
Ankyloblepharon (eyelid) (acquired) — *see also* Blepharophimosis
filiforme (adnatum) (congenital) Q1Ø.3
total Q1Ø.3
Ankyloglossia Q38.1
Ankylosis (fibrous) (osseous) (joint) M24.6Ø
ankle M24.67- ☑
arthrodesis status Z98.1
cricoarytenoid (cartilage) (joint) (larynx) J38.7
dental KØ3.5
ear ossicles H74.31- ☑
elbow M24.62- ☑
foot M24.67- ☑
hand M24.64- ☑
hip M24.65- ☑
incostapedial joint (infectional) — *see* Ankylosis, ear ossicles
jaw (temporomandibular) M26.61- ☑
knee M24.66- ☑
lumbosacral (joint) M43.27
postoperative (status) Z98.1
produced by surgical fusion, status Z98.1
sacro-iliac (joint) M43.28
shoulder M24.61- ☑
specified site NEC M24.69
spine (joint) — *see also* Fusion, spine
spondylitic — *see* Spondylitis, ankylosing
surgical Z98.1
temporomandibular M26.61- ☑
tooth, teeth (hard tissues) KØ3.5
wrist M24.63- ☑
Ankylostoma — *see* Ancylostoma
Ankylostomiasis — *see* Ancylostomiasis
Ankylurethria — *see* Stricture, urethra
Annular — *see also* condition
detachment, cervix N88.8
organ or site, congenital NEC — *see* Distortion
pancreas (congenital) Q45.1
Anodontia (complete) (partial) (vera) KØØ.Ø
acquired KØ8.1Ø ☑
Anomaly, anomalous (congenital) (unspecified type) Q89.9
abdominal wall NEC Q79.59
acoustic nerve QØ7.8
adrenal (gland) Q89.1
Alder (-Reilly) (leukocyte granulation) D72.Ø
alimentary tract Q45.9
upper Q4Ø.9
alveolar M26.7Ø
hyperplasia M26.79
mandibular M26.72
maxillary M26.71
hypoplasia M26.79
mandibular M26.74
maxillary M26.73
ridge (process) M26.79
specified NEC M26.79
ankle (joint) Q74.2
anus Q43.9
aorta (arch) NEC Q25.4Ø
coarctation (preductal) (postductal) Q25.1
aortic cusp or valve Q23.9
appendix Q43.8
apple peel syndrome Q41.1
aqueduct of Sylvius QØ3.Ø
with spina bifida — *see* Spina bifida, with hydrocephalus

Anomaly, anomalous — *continued*
arm Q74.Ø
arteriovenous NEC
coronary Q24.5
gastrointestinal Q27.33
acquired — *see* Angiodysplasia
artery (peripheral) Q27.9
basilar NEC Q28.1
cerebral Q28.3
coronary Q24.5
digestive system Q27.8
eye Q15.8
great Q25.9
specified NEC Q25.8
lower limb Q27.8
peripheral Q27.9
specified NEC Q27.8
pulmonary NEC Q25.79
renal Q27.2
retina Q14.1
specified site NEC Q27.8
subclavian Q27.8
origin Q25.48
umbilical Q27.Ø
upper limb Q27.8
vertebral NEC Q28.1
aryteno-epiglottic folds Q31.8
atrial
bands or folds Q2Ø.8
septa Q21.1
atrioventricular
excitation I45.6
septum Q21.Ø
auditory canal Q17.8
auricle
ear Q17.8
causing impairment of hearing Q16.9
heart Q2Ø.8
Axenfeld's Q15.Ø
back Q89.9
band
atrial Q2Ø.8
heart Q24.8
ventricular Q24.8
Bartholin's duct Q38.4
biliary duct or passage Q44.5
bladder Q64.7Ø
absence Q64.5
diverticulum Q64.6
exstrophy Q64.1Ø
cloacal Q64.12
extroversion Q64.19
specified type NEC Q64.19
supravesical fissure Q64.11
neck obstruction Q64.31
specified type NEC Q64.79
bone Q79.9
arm Q74.Ø
face Q75.9
leg Q74.2
pelvic girdle Q74.2
shoulder girdle Q74.Ø
skull Q75.9
with
anencephaly QØØ.Ø
encephalocele — *see* Encephalocele
hydrocephalus QØ3.9
with spina bifida — *see* Spina bifida, by site, with hydrocephalus
microcephaly QØ2
brain (multiple) QØ4.9
vessel Q28.3
breast Q83.9
broad ligament Q5Ø.6
bronchus Q32.4
bulbus cordis Q21.9
bursa Q79.9
canal of Nuck Q52.4
canthus Q1Ø.3
capillary Q27.9
cardiac Q24.9
chambers Q2Ø.9
specified NEC Q2Ø.8
septal closure Q21.9
specified NEC Q21.8
valve NEC Q24.8
pulmonary Q22.3
cardiovascular system Q28.8
carpus Q74.Ø

Anomaly, anomalous — *continued*
caruncle, lacrimal Q1Ø.6
cascade stomach Q4Ø.2
cauda equina QØ6.3
cecum Q43.9
cerebral QØ4.9
vessels Q28.3
cervix Q51.9
Chédiak-Higashi (-Steinbrinck) (congenital gigantism of peroxidase granules) E7Ø.33Ø
cheek Q18.9
chest wall Q67.8
bones Q76.9
chin Q18.9
chordae tendineae Q24.8
choroid Q14.3
plexus QØ7.8
chromosomes, chromosomal Q99.9
D (1) — *see* condition, chromosome 13
E (3) — *see* condition, chromosome 18
G — *see* condition, chromosome 21
sex
female phenotype Q97.8
gonadal dysgenesis (pure) Q99.1
Klinefelter's Q98.4
male phenotype Q98.9
Turner's Q96.9
specified NEC Q99.8
cilia Q1Ø.3
circulatory system Q28.9
clavicle Q74.Ø
clitoris Q52.6
coccyx Q76.49
colon Q43.9
common duct Q44.5
communication
coronary artery Q24.5
left ventricle with right atrium Q21.Ø
concha (ear) Q17.3
connection
portal vein Q26.5
pulmonary venous Q26.4
partial Q26.3
total Q26.2
renal artery with kidney Q27.2
cornea (shape) Q13.4
coronary artery or vein Q24.5
cranium — *see* Anomaly, skull
cricoid cartilage Q31.8
cystic duct Q44.5
dental
alveolar — *see* Anomaly, alveolar
arch relationship M26.2Ø
specified NEC M26.29
dentofacial M26.9
alveolar — *see* Anomaly, alveolar
dental arch relationship M26.2Ø
specified NEC M26.29
functional M26.5Ø
specified NEC M26.59
jaw size M26.ØØ
macrogenia M26.Ø5
mandibular
hyperplasia M26.Ø3
hypoplasia M26.Ø4
maxillary
hyperplasia M26.Ø1
hypoplasia M26.Ø2
microgenia M26.Ø6
specified type NEC M26.Ø9
jaw-cranial base relationship M26.1Ø
asymmetry M26.12
maxillary M26.11
specified type NEC M26.19
malocclusion M26.4
dental arch relationship NEC M26.29
jaw size — *see* Anomaly, dentofacial, jaw size
jaw-cranial base relationship — *see* Anomaly, dentofacial, jaw-cranial base relationship
specified type NEC M26.89
temporomandibular joint M26.6Ø- ☑
adhesions M26.61- ☑
ankylosis M26.61- ☑
arthralgia M26.62- ☑
articular disc M26.63- ☑
specified type NEC M26.69
tooth position, fully erupted M26.3Ø
specified NEC M26.39

Anomaly, anomalous — *continued*
- pigmentation — *continued*
  - congenital Q82.8
- pituitary (gland) Q89.2
- pleural (folds) Q34.Ø
- portal vein Q26.5
  - connection Q26.5
- position, tooth, teeth, fully erupted M26.3Ø
  - specified NEC M26.39
- precerebral vessel Q28.1
- prepuce Q55.69
- prostate Q55.4
- pulmonary Q33.9
  - artery NEC Q25.79
  - valve Q22.3
    - atresia Q22.Ø
    - insufficiency Q22.2
    - specified type NEC Q22.3
    - stenosis Q22.1
      - infundibular Q24.3
      - subvalvular Q24.3
  - venous connection Q26.4
    - partial Q26.3
    - total Q26.2
- pupil Q13.2
  - function H57.ØØ
    - anisocoria H57.Ø2
    - Argyll Robertson pupil H57.Ø1
    - miosis H57.Ø3
    - mydriasis H57.Ø4
    - specified type NEC H57.Ø9
    - tonic pupil H57.Ø5- ☑
- pylorus Q4Ø.3
- radius Q74.Ø
- rectum Q43.9
- reduction (extremity) (limb)
  - femur (longitudinal) — *see* Defect, reduction, lower limb, longitudinal, femur
  - fibula (longitudinal) — *see* Defect, reduction, lower limb, longitudinal, fibula
  - lower limb — *see* Defect, reduction, lower limb
  - radius (longitudinal) — *see* Defect, reduction, upper limb, longitudinal, radius
  - tibia (longitudinal) — *see* Defect, reduction, lower limb, longitudinal, tibia
  - ulna (longitudinal) — *see* Defect, reduction, upper limb, longitudinal, ulna
  - upper limb — *see* Defect, reduction, upper limb
- refraction — *see* Disorder, refraction
- renal Q63.9
  - artery Q27.2
  - pelvis Q63.9
    - specified NEC Q63.8
- respiratory system Q34.9
  - specified NEC Q34.8
- retina Q14.1
- rib Q76.6
  - cervical Q76.5
- Rieger's Q13.81
- rotation — *see* Malrotation
  - hip or thigh Q65.89
- round ligament Q52.8
- sacroiliac (joint) NEC Q74.2
- sacrum NEC Q76.49
  - kyphosis — *see* Kyphosis, congenital
  - lordosis — *see* Lordosis, congenital
- saddle nose, syphilitic A5Ø.57
- salivary duct or gland Q38.4
- scapula Q74.Ø
- scrotum — *see* Malformation, testis and scrotum
- sebaceous gland Q82.9
- seminal vesicles Q55.4
- sense organs NEC QØ7.8
- sex chromosomes NEC — *see also* Anomaly, chromosomes
  - female phenotype Q97.8
  - male phenotype Q98.9
- shoulder (girdle) (joint) Q74.Ø
- sigmoid (flexure) Q43.9
- simian crease Q82.8
- sinus of Valsalva Q25.49
- skeleton generalized Q78.9
- skin (appendage) Q82.9
- skull Q75.9
  - with
    - anencephaly QØØ.Ø
    - encephalocele — *see* Encephalocele
    - hydrocephalus QØ3.9

Anomaly, anomalous — *continued*
- skull — *continued*
  - with — *continued*
    - hydrocephalus — *continued*
      - with spina bifida — *see* Spina bifida, by site, with hydrocephalus
    - microcephaly QØ2
- specified organ or site NEC Q89.8
- spermatic cord Q55.4
- spine, spinal NEC Q76.49
  - column NEC Q76.49
    - kyphosis — *see* Kyphosis, congenital
    - lordosis — *see* Lordosis, congenital
  - cord QØ6.9
  - nerve root QØ7.8
- spleen Q89.Ø9
  - agenesis Q89.Ø1
- stenonian duct Q38.4
- sternum NEC Q76.7
- stomach Q4Ø.3
- submaxillary gland Q38.4
- tarsus NEC Q74.2
- tendon Q79.9
- testis — *see* Malformation, testis and scrotum
- thigh NEC Q74.2
- thorax (wall) Q67.8
  - bony Q76.9
- throat Q38.8
- thumb Q74.Ø
- thymus gland Q89.2
- thyroid (gland) Q89.2
  - cartilage Q31.8
- tibia NEC Q74.2
  - saber A5Ø.56
- toe Q74.2
- tongue Q38.3
- tooth, teeth KØØ.9
  - eruption KØØ.6
  - position, fully erupted M26.3Ø
  - spacing, fully erupted M26.3Ø
- trachea (cartilage) Q32.1
- tragus Q17.9
- tricuspid (leaflet) (valve) Q22.9
  - atresia or stenosis Q22.4
  - Ebstein's Q22.5
- Uhl's (hypoplasia of myocardium, right ventricle) Q24.8
- ulna Q74.Ø
- umbilical artery Q27.Ø
- union
  - cricoid cartilage and thyroid cartilage Q31.8
  - thyroid cartilage and hyoid bone Q31.8
  - trachea with larynx Q31.8
- upper limb Q74.Ø
- urachus Q64.4
- ureter Q62.8
  - obstructive NEC Q62.39
    - cecoureterocele Q62.32
    - orthotopic ureterocele Q62.31
- urethra Q64.7Ø
  - absence Q64.5
  - double Q64.74
  - fistula to rectum Q64.73
  - obstructive Q64.39
    - stricture Q64.32
  - prolapse Q64.71
  - specified type NEC Q64.79
- urinary tract Q64.9
- uterus Q51.9
  - with only one functioning horn Q51.4
- uvula Q38.5
- vagina Q52.4
- valleculae Q31.8
- valve (heart) NEC Q24.8
  - coronary sinus Q24.5
  - inferior vena cava Q24.8
  - pulmonary Q22.3
  - sinus coronario Q24.5
  - venae cavae inferioris Q24.8
- vas deferens Q55.4
- vascular Q27.9
  - brain Q28.3
  - ring Q25.45
- vein(s) (peripheral) Q27.9
  - brain Q28.3
  - cerebral Q28.3
  - coronary Q24.5
  - developmental Q28.3
  - great Q26.9
    - specified NEC Q26.8

Anomaly, anomalous — *continued*
- vena cava (inferior) (superior) Q26.9
- venous — *see* Anomaly, vein(s)
- venous return Q26.8
- ventricular
  - bands or folds Q24.8
  - septa Q21.Ø
- vertebra Q76.49
  - kyphosis — *see* Kyphosis, congenital
  - lordosis — *see* Lordosis, congenital
- vesicourethral orifice Q64.79
- vessel(s) Q27.9
  - optic papilla Q14.2
  - precerebral Q28.1
- vitelline duct Q43.Ø
- vitreous body or humor Q14.Ø
- vulva Q52.7Ø
- wrist (joint) Q74.Ø

Anomia R48.8

Anonychia (congenital) Q84.3
- acquired L6Ø.8

Anophthalmos, anophthalmus (congenital) (globe) Q11.1
- acquired Z9Ø.Ø1

Anopia, anopsia H53.46- ☑
- quadrant H53.46- ☑

Anorchia, anorchism, anorchidism Q55.Ø

Anorexia R63.Ø
- hysterical F44.89
- nervosa F5Ø.ØØ
  - atypical F5Ø.9
  - binge-eating type F5Ø.2
    - with purging F5Ø.Ø2
  - restricting type F5Ø.Ø1

Anorgasmy, psychogenic (female) F52.31
- male F52.32

Anosmia R43.Ø
- hysterical F44.6
- postinfectional J39.8

Anosognosia R41.89

Anosteoplasia Q78.9

Anovulatory cycle N97.Ø

Anoxemia RØ9.Ø2
- newborn P84

Anoxia (pathological) RØ9.Ø2
- altitude T7Ø.29 ☑
- cerebral G93.1
  - complicating
    - anesthesia (general) (local) or other sedation T88.59 ☑
      - in labor and delivery O74.3
      - in pregnancy O29.21- ☑
      - postpartum, puerperal O89.2
    - delivery (cesarean) (instrumental) O75.4
  - during a procedure G97.81
  - newborn P84
  - resulting from a procedure G97.82
- due to
  - drowning T75.1 ☑
  - high altitude T7Ø.29 ☑
- heart — *see* Insufficiency, coronary
- intrauterine P84
- myocardial — *see* Insufficiency, coronary
- newborn P84
- spinal cord G95.11
- systemic (by suffocation) (low content in atmosphere) — *see* Asphyxia, traumatic

Anteflexion — *see* Anteversion

Antenatal
- care (normal pregnancy) Z34.9Ø
- screening (encounter for) of mother — *see also* Encounter, antenatal screening Z36.9

Antepartum — *see* condition

Anterior — *see* condition

Antero-occlusion M26.22Ø

Anteversion
- cervix — *see* Anteversion, uterus
- femur (neck), congenital Q65.89
- uterus, uterine (cervix) (postinfectional) (postpartal, old) N85.4
  - congenital Q51.818
  - in pregnancy or childbirth — *see* Pregnancy, complicated by

Anthophobia F4Ø.228

Anthracosilicosis J6Ø

Anthracosis (lung) (occupational) J6Ø
- lingua K14.3

Anthrax A22.9
- with pneumonia A22.1
- cerebral A22.8
- colitis A22.2
- cutaneous A22.0
- gastrointestinal A22.2
- inhalation A22.1
- intestinal A22.2
- meningitis A22.8
- pulmonary A22.1
- respiratory A22.1
- sepsis A22.7
- specified manifestation NEC A22.8

Anthropoid pelvis Q74.2
- with disproportion (fetopelvic) O33.0

Anthropophobia F40.10
- generalized F40.11

Antibodies, maternal (blood group) — *see* Isoimmunization, affecting management of pregnancy
- anti-D — *see* Isoimmunization, affecting management of pregnancy, Rh
  - newborn P55.0

Antibody
- anticardiolipin R76.0
  - with
    - hemorrhagic disorder D68.312
    - hypercoagulable state D68.61
- antiphosphatidylglycerol R76.0
  - with
    - hemorrhagic disorder D68.312
    - hypercoagulable state D68.61
- antiphosphatidylinositol R76.0
  - with
    - hemorrhagic disorder D68.312
    - hypercoagulable state D68.61
- antiphosphatidylserine R76.0
  - with
    - hemorrhagic disorder D68.312
    - hypercoagulable state D68.61
- antiphospholipid R76.0
  - with
    - hemorrhagic disorder D68.312
    - hypercoagulable state D68.61

Anticardiolipin syndrome D68.61

Anticoagulant, circulating (intrinsic) — *see also* Disorder, hemorrhagic D68.318
- drug-induced (extrinsic) — *see also* Disorder, hemorrhagic D68.32
- iatrogenic D68.32

Antidiuretic hormone syndrome E22.2

Antimonial cholera — *see* Poisoning, antimony

Antiphospholipid
- antibody
  - with hemorrhagic disorder D68.312
  - syndrome D68.61

Antisocial personality F60.2

Antithrombinemia — *see* Circulating anticoagulants

Antithromboplastinemia D68.318

Antithromboplastinogenemia D68.318

Antitoxin complication or reaction — *see* Complications, vaccination

Antlophobia F40.228

Antritis J32.0
- maxilla J32.0
  - acute J01.00
    - recurrent J01.01
- stomach K29.60
  - with bleeding K29.61

Antrum, antral — *see* condition

Anuria R34
- calculous (impacted) (recurrent) — *see also* Calculus, urinary N20.9
- following
  - abortion — *see* Abortion by type complicated by, renal failure
  - ectopic or molar pregnancy O08.4
- newborn P96.0
- postprocedural N99.0
- postrenal N13.8
- traumatic (following crushing) T79.5 ☑

Anus, anal — *see* condition

Anusitis K62.89

Anxiety F41.9
- depression F41.8
- episodic paroxysmal F41.0
- generalized F41.1
- hysteria F41.8
- neurosis F41.1

Anxiety — *continued*
- panic type F41.0
- reaction F41.1
- separation, abnormal (of childhood) F93.0
- specified NEC F41.8
- state F41.1

Aorta, aortic — *see* condition

Aortectasia — *see* Ectasia, aorta
- with aneurysm — *see* Aneurysm, aorta

Aortitis (nonsyphilitic) (calcific) I77.6
- arteriosclerotic I70.0
- Doehle-Heller A52.02
- luetic A52.02
- rheumatic — *see* Endocarditis, acute, rheumatic
- specific (syphilitic) A52.02
- syphilitic A52.02
  - congenital A50.54 *[I79.1]*

Apathetic thyroid storm — *see* Thyrotoxicosis

Apathy R45.3

Apeirophobia F40.228

Apepsia K30
- psychogenic F45.8

Aperistalsis, esophagus K22.0

Apertognathia M26.29

Apert's syndrome Q87.0

Aphagia R13.0
- psychogenic F50.9

Aphakia (acquired) (postoperative) H27.0- ☑
- congenital Q12.3

Aphasia (amnestic) (global) (nominal) (semantic) (syntactic) R47.01
- acquired, with epilepsy (Landau-Kleffner syndrome) — *see* Epilepsy, specified NEC
- auditory (developmental) F80.2
- developmental (receptive type) F80.2
  - expressive type F80.1
  - Wernicke's F80.2
- following
  - cerebrovascular disease I69.920
    - cerebral infarction I69.320
    - intracerebral hemorrhage I69.120
    - nontraumatic intracranial hemorrhage NEC I69.220
    - specified disease NEC I69.820
    - subarachnoid hemorrhage I69.020
- primary progressive G31.01 *[F02.80]*
  - with behavioral disturbance G31.01 *[F02.81]*
- progressive isolated G31.01 *[F02.80]*
  - with behavioral disturbance G31.01 *[F02.81]*
- sensory F80.2
- syphilis, tertiary A52.19
- Wernicke's (developmental) F80.2

Aphonia (organic) R49.1
- hysterical F44.4
- psychogenic F44.4

Aphthae, aphthous — *see also* condition
- Bednar's K12.0
- cachectic K14.0
- epizootic B08.8
- fever B08.8
- oral (recurrent) K12.0
- stomatitis (major) (minor) K12.0
- thrush B37.0
- ulcer (oral) (recurrent) K12.0
  - genital organ(s) NEC
    - female N76.6
    - male N50.89
  - larynx J38.7

Apical — *see* condition

Apiphobia F40.218

Aplasia — *see also* Agenesis
- abdominal muscle syndrome Q79.4
- alveolar process (acquired) — *see* Anomaly, alveolar
  - congenital Q38.6
- aorta (congenital) Q25.41
- axialis extracorticalis (congenita) E75.29
- bone marrow (myeloid) D61.9
  - congenital D61.01
- brain Q00.0
  - part of Q04.3
- bronchus Q32.4
- cementum K00.4
- cerebellum Q04.3
- cervix (congenital) Q51.5
- congenital pure red cell D61.01
- corpus callosum Q04.0
- cutis congenita Q84.8
- erythrocyte congenital D61.01

Aplasia — *continued*
- extracortical axial E75.29
- eye Q11.1
- fovea centralis (congenital) Q14.1
- gallbladder, congenital Q44.0
- iris Q13.1
- labyrinth, membranous Q16.5
- limb (congenital) Q73.8
  - lower — *see* Defect, reduction, lower limb
  - upper — *see* Agenesis, arm
- lung, congenital (bilateral) (unilateral) Q33.3
- pancreas Q45.0
- parathyroid-thymic D82.1
- Pelizaeus-Merzbacher E75.29
- penis Q55.5
- prostate Q55.4
- red cell (with thymoma) D60.9
  - acquired D60.9
    - due to drugs D60.9
  - adult D60.9
  - chronic D60.0
  - congenital D61.01
  - constitutional D61.01
  - due to drugs D60.9
  - hereditary D61.01
  - of infants D61.01
  - primary D61.01
  - pure D61.01
    - due to drugs D60.9
  - specified type NEC D60.8
  - transient D60.1
- round ligament Q52.8
- skin Q84.8
- spermatic cord Q55.4
- spleen Q89.01
- testicle Q55.0
- thymic, with immunodeficiency D82.1
- thyroid (congenital) (with myxedema) E03.1
- uterus Q51.0
- ventral horn cell Q06.1

Apnea, apneic (of) (spells) R06.81
- newborn NEC P28.4
  - obstructive P28.4
  - sleep (central) (obstructive) (primary) P28.3
- prematurity P28.4
- sleep G47.30
  - central (primary) G47.31
    - idiopathic G47.31
    - in conditions classified elsewhere G47.37
  - obstructive (adult) (pediatric) G47.33
    - hypopnea G47.33
  - primary central G47.31
  - specified NEC G47.39

Apneumatosis, newborn P28.0

Apocrine metaplasia (breast) — *see* Dysplasia, mammary, specified type NEC

Apophysitis (bone) — *see also* Osteochondropathy
- calcaneus M92.8
- juvenile M92.9

Apoplectiform convulsions (cerebral ischemia) I67.82

Apoplexia, apoplexy, apoplectic
- adrenal A39.1
- heart (auricle) (ventricle) — *see* Infarct, myocardium
- heat T67.01 ☑
- hemorrhagic (stroke) — *see* Hemorrhage, intracranial
- meninges, hemorrhagic — *see* Hemorrhage, intracranial, subarachnoid
- uremic N18.9 *[I68.8]*

Appearance
- bizarre R46.1
- specified NEC R46.89
- very low level of personal hygiene R46.0

Appendage
- epididymal (organ of Morgagni) Q55.4
- intestine (epiploic) Q43.8
- preauricular Q17.0
- testicular (organ of Morgagni) Q55.29

Appendicitis (pneumococcal) (retrocecal) K37
- with
  - gangrene K35.891
  - perforation NOS K35.32
  - peritoneal abscess K35.33
  - peritonitis NEC K35.33
    - generalized (with perforation or rupture) K35.20
      - with abscess K35.21
    - localized K35.30
      - with
        - gangrene K35.31

- **Appendicitis** — *continued*
  - with — *continued*
    - peritonitis — *continued*
      - localized — *continued*
        - with — *continued*
          - perforation K35.32
            - and abscess K35.33
      - rupture (with localized peritonitis) K35.32
  - acute (catarrhal) (fulminating) (gangrenous) (obstructive) (retrocecal) (suppurative) K35.80
    - with
      - gangrene K35.891
      - peritoneal abscess K35.33
      - peritonitis NEC K35.33
        - generalized (with perforation or rupture) K35.20
          - with abscess K35.21
        - localized K35.30
          - with
            - gangrene K35.31
            - perforation K35.32
              - and abscess K35.33
    - specified NEC K35.890
      - with gangrene K35.891
  - amebic A06.89
  - chronic (recurrent) K36
  - exacerbation — *see* Appendicitis, acute
  - gangrenous — *see* Appendicitis, acute
  - healed (obliterative) K36
  - interval K36
  - neurogenic K36
  - obstructive K36
  - recurrent K36
  - relapsing K36
  - ruptured NOS (with localized peritonitis) K35.32
  - subacute (adhesive) K36
  - subsiding K36
  - suppurative — *see* Appendicitis, acute
  - tuberculous A18.32
- **Appendicopathia oxyurica** B80
- **Appendix, appendicular** — *see also* condition
  - epididymis Q55.4
  - Morgagni
    - female Q50.5
    - male (epididymal) Q55.4
      - testicular Q55.29
  - testis Q55.29
- **Appetite**
  - depraved — *see* Pica
  - excessive R63.2
  - lack or loss — *see also* Anorexia R63.0
    - nonorganic origin F50.89
    - psychogenic F50.89
  - perverted (hysterical) — *see* Pica
- **Apple peel syndrome** Q41.1
- **Apprehension state** F41.1
- **Apprehensiveness, abnormal** F41.9
- **Approximal wear** K03.0
- **Apraxia** (classic) (ideational) (ideokinetic) (ideomotor) (motor) (verbal) R48.2
  - following
    - cerebrovascular disease I69.990
      - cerebral infarction I69.390
      - intracerebral hemorrhage I69.190
      - nontraumatic intracranial hemorrhage NEC I69.290
      - specified disease NEC I69.890
      - subarachnoid hemorrhage I69.090
  - oculomotor, congenital H51.8
- **Aptyalism** K11.7
- **Apudoma** — *see* Neoplasm, uncertain behavior, by site
- **Aqueous misdirection** H40.83- ☑
- **Arabicum elephantiasis** — *see* Infestation, filarial
- **Arachnitis** — *see* Meningitis
- **Arachnodactyly** — *see* Syndrome, Marfan's
- **Arachnoiditis** (acute) (adhesive) (basal) (brain) (cerebrospinal) — *see* Meningitis
- **Arachnophobia** F40.210
- **Arboencephalitis, Australian** A83.4
- **Arborization block** (heart) I45.5
- **ARC** (AIDS-related complex) B20
- **Arch**
  - aortic Q25.49
  - bovine Q25.49
- **Arches** — *see* condition
- **Arcuate uterus** Q51.810
- **Arcuatus uterus** Q51.810
- **Arcus** (cornea) senilis — *see* Degeneration, cornea, senile
- **Arc-welder's lung** J63.4
- **Areflexia** R29.2
- **Areola** — *see* condition
- **Argentaffinoma** — *see also* Neoplasm, uncertain behavior, by site
  - malignant — *see* Neoplasm, malignant, by site
  - syndrome E34.0
- **Argininemia** E72.21
- **Arginosuccinic aciduria** E72.22
- **Argyll Robertson phenomenon, pupil or syndrome** (syphilitic) A52.19
  - atypical H57.09
  - nonsyphilitic H57.09
- **Argyria, argyriasis**
  - conjunctival H11.13- ☑
  - from drug or medicament — *see* Table of Drugs and Chemicals, by substance
- **Argyrosis, conjunctival** H11.13- ☑
- **Arhinencephaly** Q04.1
- **Ariboflavinosis** E53.0
- **Arm** — *see* condition
- **Arnold-Chiari disease, obstruction or syndrome** (type II) Q07.00
  - with
    - hydrocephalus Q07.02
      - with spina bifida Q07.03
    - spina bifida Q07.01
      - with hydrocephalus Q07.03
  - type III — *see* Encephalocele
  - type IV Q04.8
- **Aromatic amino-acid metabolism disorder** E70.9
  - specified NEC E70.89
- **Arousals, confusional** G47.51
- **Arrest, arrested**
  - cardiac I46.9
    - complicating
      - abortion — *see* Abortion, by type, complicated by, cardiac arrest
      - anesthesia (general) (local) or other sedation — *see* Table of Drugs and Chemicals, by drug
        - in labor and delivery O74.2
        - in pregnancy O29.11- ☑
        - postpartum, puerperal O89.1
      - delivery (cesarean) (instrumental) O75.4
    - due to
      - cardiac condition I46.2
      - specified condition NEC I46.8
    - intraoperative I97.71- ☑
    - newborn P29.81
    - personal history, successfully resuscitated Z86.74
    - postprocedural I97.12- ☑
      - obstetric procedure O75.4
  - cardiorespiratory — *see* Arrest, cardiac
  - circulatory — *see* Arrest, cardiac
  - deep transverse O64.0 ☑
  - development or growth
    - bone — *see* Disorder, bone, development or growth
    - child R62.50
    - tracheal rings Q32.1
  - epiphyseal
    - complete
      - femur M89.15- ☑
      - humerus M89.12- ☑
      - tibia M89.16- ☑
      - ulna M89.13- ☑
    - forearm M89.13- ☑
      - specified NEC M89.13- ☑
      - ulna — *see* Arrest, epiphyseal, by type, ulna
    - lower leg M89.16- ☑
      - specified NEC M89.168
      - tibia — *see* Arrest, epiphyseal, by type, tibia
    - partial
      - femur M89.15- ☑
      - humerus M89.12- ☑
      - tibia M89.16- ☑
      - ulna M89.13- ☑
    - specified NEC M89.18
  - granulopoiesis — *see* Agranulocytosis
  - growth plate — *see* Arrest, epiphyseal
  - heart — *see* Arrest, cardiac
  - legal, anxiety concerning Z65.3
  - physeal — *see* Arrest, epiphyseal
  - respiratory R09.2
    - newborn P28.81
  - sinus I45.5
  - spermatogenesis (complete) — *see* Azoospermia
    - incomplete — *see* Oligospermia
- **Arrest, arrested** — *continued*
  - transverse (deep) O64.0 ☑
- **Arrhenoblastoma**
  - benign
    - specified site — *see* Neoplasm, benign, by site
    - unspecified site
      - female D27.9
      - male D29.20
  - malignant
    - specified site — *see* Neoplasm, malignant, by site
    - unspecified site
      - female C56.9
      - male C62.90
  - specified site — *see* Neoplasm, uncertain behavior, by site
  - unspecified site
    - female D39.10
    - male D40.10
- **Arrhythmia** (auricle) (cardiac) (juvenile) (nodal) (reflex) (supraventricular) (transitory) (ventricle) I49.9
  - block I45.9
  - extrasystolic I49.49
  - newborn
    - bradycardia P29.12
    - occurring before birth P03.819
      - before onset of labor P03.810
      - during labor P03.811
    - tachycardia P29.11
  - psychogenic F45.8
  - sinus I49.8
  - specified NEC I49.8
  - vagal R55
  - ventricular re-entry I47.0
- **Arrillaga-Ayerza syndrome** (pulmonary sclerosis with pulmonary hypertension) I27.0
- **Arsenical pigmentation** L81.8
  - from drug or medicament — *see* Table of Drugs and Chemicals
- **Arsenism** — *see* Poisoning, arsenic
- **Arterial** — *see* condition
- **Arteriofibrosis** — *see* Arteriosclerosis
- **Arteriolar sclerosis** — *see* Arteriosclerosis
- **Arteriolith** — *see* Arteriosclerosis
- **Arteriolitis** I77.6
  - necrotizing, kidney I77.5
  - renal — *see* Hypertension, kidney
- **Arteriolosclerosis** — *see* Arteriosclerosis
- **Arterionephrosclerosis** — *see* Hypertension, kidney
- **Arteriopathy** I77.9
  - cerebral autosomal dominant, with subcortical infarcts and leukoencephalopathy (CADASIL) I67.850
- **Arteriosclerosis, arteriosclerotic** (diffuse) (obliterans) (of) (senile) (with calcification) I70.90
  - with
    - chronic limb-threatening ischemia — *see* Arteriosclerosis, with critical limb ischemia
    - critical limb ischemia
      - bypass graft I70.329
        - autologous vein graft I70.429
          - leg I70.429
            - with
              - gangrene (and intermittent claudication, rest pain, and ulcer) I70.469
              - rest pain (and intermittent claudication) I70.429
            - bilateral I70.423
              - with
                - gangrene (and intermittent claudication, rest pain, and ulcer) I70.463
                - rest pain (and intermittent claudication) I70.423
            - left I70.422
              - with
                - gangrene (and intermittent claudication, rest pain, and ulcer) I70.462
                - rest pain (and intermittent claudication) I70.422
                - ulceration (and intermittent claudication and rest pain) I70.449
                  - ankle I70.443
                  - calf I70.442
                  - foot site NEC I70.445
                  - heel I70.444
                  - lower leg NEC I70.448

Index
Arteriosclerosis, arteriosclerotic — Arteriosclerosis, arteriosclerotic

Arteriosclerosis, arteriosclerotic — *continued*
- with — *continued*
  - critical limb ischemia — *continued*
    - leg — *continued*
      - right — *continued*
        - with
          - gangrene (and intermittent claudication, rest pain, and ulcer) I7Ø.261
          - rest pain (and intermittent claudication) I7Ø.221
          - ulceration (and intermittent claudication and rest pain) I7Ø.239
            - ankle I7Ø.233
            - calf I7Ø.232
            - foot site NEC I7Ø.235
            - heel I7Ø.234
            - lower leg NEC I7Ø.238
            - midfoot I7Ø.234
            - thigh I7Ø.231
- aorta I7Ø.Ø
- arteries of extremities — *see* Arteriosclerosis, extremities
  - with
    - chronic limb-threatening ischemia — *see* Arteriosclerosis, with critical limb ischemia
    - critical limb ischemia — *see* Arteriosclerosis, with critical limb ischemia
- brain I67.2
- bypass graft
  - with
    - chronic limb-threatening ischemia — *see* Arteriosclerosis, with critical limb ischemia
    - critical limb ischemia — *see* Arteriosclerosis, with critical limb ischemia
  - coronary — *see* Arteriosclerosis, coronary, bypass graft
  - extremities — *see* Arteriosclerosis, extremities, bypass graft
- cardiac — *see* Disease, heart, ischemic, atherosclerotic
- cardiopathy — *see* Disease, heart, ischemic, atherosclerotic
- cardiorenal — *see* Hypertension, cardiorenal
- cardiovascular — *see* Disease, heart, ischemic, atherosclerotic
- carotid — *see also* Occlusion, artery, carotid I65.2- ☑
- central nervous system I67.2
- cerebral I67.2
- cerebrovascular I67.2
- coronary (artery)
  - due to
    - calcified coronary lesion (severely) I25.84
    - lipid rich plaque I25.83
  - bypass graft I25.81Ø
    - with
      - angina pectoris I25.7Ø9
        - with documented spasm I25.7Ø1
        - specified type NEC I25.7Ø8
        - unstable I25.7ØØ
      - ischemic chest pain I25.7Ø9
    - autologous artery I25.81Ø
      - with
        - angina pectoris I25.729
          - with documented spasm I25.721
          - specified type I25.728
          - unstable I25.72Ø
        - ischemic chest pain I25.729
    - autologous vein I25.81Ø
      - with
        - angina pectoris I25.719
          - with documented spasm I25.711
          - specified type I25.718
          - unstable I25.71Ø
        - ischemic chest pain I25.719
    - nonautologous biological I25.81Ø
      - with
        - angina pectoris I25.739
          - with documented spasm I25.731
          - specified type I25.738
          - unstable I25.73Ø
        - ischemic chest pain I25.739
    - specified type NEC I25.81Ø
      - with
        - angina pectoris I25.799
          - with documented spasm I25.791
          - specified type I25.798
          - unstable I25.79Ø
        - ischemic chest pain I25.799

Arteriosclerosis, arteriosclerotic — *continued*
- coronary — *continued*
  - native vessel
    - with
      - angina pectoris I25.119
        - with documented spasm I25.111
        - specified type NEC I25.118
        - unstable I25.11Ø
      - ischemic chest pain I25.119
  - transplanted heart I25.811
    - bypass graft I25.812
      - with
        - angina pectoris I25.769
          - with documented spasm I25.761
          - specified type I25.768
          - unstable I25.76Ø
        - ischemic chest pain I25.769
    - native coronary artery I25.811
      - with
        - angina pectoris I25.759
          - with documented spasm I25.751
          - specified type I25.758
          - unstable I25.75Ø
        - ischemic chest pain I25.759
- extremities (native arteries) I7Ø.2Ø9
  - with
    - chronic limb-threatening ischemia — *see* Arteriosclerosis, with critical limb ischemia
    - critical limb ischemia — *see* Arteriosclerosis, with critical limb ischemia
  - bypass graft I7Ø.3Ø9
    - with
      - chronic limb-threatening ischemia — *see* Arteriosclerosis, with critical limb ischemia
      - critical limb ischemia — *see* Arteriosclerosis, with critical limb ischemia
    - autologous vein graft I7Ø.4Ø9
      - leg I7Ø.4Ø9
        - with
          - gangrene (and intermittent claudication, rest pain and ulcer) I7Ø.469
          - intermittent claudication I7Ø.419
          - rest pain (and intermittent claudication) I7Ø.429
        - bilateral I7Ø.4Ø3
          - with
            - gangrene (and intermittent claudication, rest pain and ulcer) I7Ø.463
            - intermittent claudication I7Ø.463
            - rest pain (and intermittent claudication) I7Ø.423
          - specified type NEC I7Ø.493
        - left I7Ø.4Ø2
          - with
            - gangrene (and intermittent claudication, rest pain and ulcer) I7Ø.462
            - intermittent claudication I7Ø.412
            - rest pain (and intermittent claudication) I7Ø.422
            - ulceration (and intermittent claudication and rest pain) I7Ø.449
              - ankle I7Ø.443
              - calf I7Ø.442
              - foot site NEC I7Ø.445
              - heel I7Ø.444
              - lower leg NEC I7Ø.448
              - midfoot I7Ø.444
              - thigh I7Ø.441
          - specified type NEC I7Ø.492
        - right I7Ø.4Ø1
          - with
            - gangrene (and intermittent claudication, rest pain and ulcer) I7Ø.461
            - intermittent claudication I7Ø.411
            - rest pain (and intermittent claudication) I7Ø.421
            - ulceration (and intermittent claudication and rest pain) I7Ø.439
              - ankle I7Ø.433
              - calf I7Ø.432
              - foot site NEC I7Ø.435
              - heel I7Ø.434
              - lower leg NEC I7Ø.438
              - midfoot I7Ø.434
              - thigh I7Ø.431
          - specified type NEC I7Ø.491

Arteriosclerosis, arteriosclerotic — *continued*
- extremities — *continued*
  - bypass graft — *continued*
    - autologous vein graft — *continued*
      - leg — *continued*
        - specified type NEC I7Ø.499
      - specified NEC I7Ø.4Ø8
        - with
          - gangrene (and intermittent claudication, rest pain and ulcer) I7Ø.468
          - intermittent claudication I7Ø.418
          - rest pain (and intermittent claudication) I7Ø.428
          - ulceration (and intermittent claudication and rest pain) I7Ø.45
        - specified type NEC I7Ø.498
    - leg I7Ø.3Ø9
      - with
        - gangrene (and intermittent claudication, rest pain and ulcer) I7Ø.369
        - intermittent claudication I7Ø.319
        - rest pain (and intermittent claudication) I7Ø.329
      - bilateral I7Ø.3Ø3
        - with
          - gangrene (and intermittent claudication, rest pain and ulcer) I7Ø.363
          - intermittent claudication I7Ø.313
          - rest pain (and intermittent claudication) I7Ø.323
        - specified type NEC I7Ø.393
      - left I7Ø.3Ø2
        - with
          - gangrene (and intermittent claudication, rest pain and ulcer) I7Ø.362
          - intermittent claudication I7Ø.312
          - rest pain (and intermittent claudication) I7Ø.322
          - ulceration (and intermittent claudication and rest pain) I7Ø.349
            - ankle I7Ø.343
            - calf I7Ø.342
            - foot site NEC I7Ø.345
            - heel I7Ø.344
            - lower leg NEC I7Ø.348
            - midfoot I7Ø.344
            - thigh I7Ø.341
        - specified type NEC I7Ø.392
      - right I7Ø.3Ø1
        - with
          - gangrene (and intermittent claudication, rest pain and ulcer) I7Ø.361
          - intermittent claudication I7Ø.311
          - rest pain (and intermittent claudication) I7Ø.321
          - ulceration (and intermittent claudication and rest pain) I7Ø.339
            - ankle I7Ø.333
            - calf I7Ø.332
            - foot site NEC I7Ø.335
            - heel I7Ø.334
            - lower leg NEC I7Ø.338
            - midfoot I7Ø.334
            - thigh I7Ø.331
        - specified type NEC I7Ø.391
      - specified type NEC I7Ø.399
    - nonautologous biological graft I7Ø.5Ø9
      - leg I7Ø.5Ø9
        - with
          - gangrene (and intermittent claudication, rest pain and ulcer) I7Ø.569
          - intermittent claudication I7Ø.519
          - rest pain (and intermittent claudication) I7Ø.529
        - bilateral I7Ø.5Ø3
          - with
            - gangrene (and intermittent claudication, rest pain and ulcer) I7Ø.563
            - intermittent claudication I7Ø.513
            - rest pain (and intermittent claudication) I7Ø.523
          - specified type NEC I7Ø.593
        - left I7Ø.5Ø2
          - with
            - gangrene (and intermittent claudication, rest pain and ulcer) I7Ø.562
            - intermittent claudication I7Ø.512

- **Arteriosclerosis, arteriosclerotic** — *continued*
  - extremities — *continued*
    - bypass graft — *continued*
      - nonautologous biological graft — *continued*
        - leg — *continued*
          - left — *continued*
            - with — *continued*
              - rest pain (and intermittent claudication) I70.522
              - ulceration (and intermittent claudication and rest pain) I70.549
                - ankle I70.543
                - calf I70.542
                - foot site NEC I70.545
                - heel I70.544
                - lower leg NEC I70.548
                - midfoot I70.544
                - thigh I70.541
            - specified type NEC I70.592
          - right I70.501
            - with
              - gangrene (and intermittent claudication, rest pain and ulcer) I70.561
              - intermittent claudication I70.511
              - rest pain (and intermittent claudication) I70.521
              - ulceration (and intermittent claudication and rest pain) I70.539
                - ankle I70.533
                - calf I70.532
                - foot site NEC I70.535
                - heel I70.534
                - lower leg NEC I70.538
                - midfoot I70.534
                - thigh I70.531
            - specified type NEC I70.591
          - specified type NEC I70.599
        - specified NEC I70.508
          - with
            - gangrene (and intermittent claudication, rest pain and ulcer) I70.568
            - intermittent claudication I70.518
            - rest pain (and intermittent claudication) I70.528
            - ulceration (and intermittent claudication and rest pain) I70.55
          - specified type NEC I70.598
      - nonbiological graft I70.609
        - leg I70.609
          - with
            - gangrene (and intermittent claudication, rest pain and ulcer) I70.669
            - intermittent claudication I70.619
            - rest pain (and intermittent claudication) I70.629
          - bilateral I70.603
            - with
              - gangrene (and intermittent claudication, rest pain and ulcer) I70.663
              - intermittent claudication I70.613
              - rest pain (and intermittent claudication) I70.623
            - specified type NEC I70.693
          - left I70.602
            - with
              - gangrene (and intermittent claudication, rest pain and ulcer) I70.662
              - intermittent claudication I70.612
              - rest pain (and intermittent claudication) I70.622
              - ulceration (and intermittent claudication and rest pain) I70.649
                - ankle I70.643
                - calf I70.642
                - foot site NEC I70.645
                - heel I70.644
                - lower leg NEC I70.648
                - midfoot I70.644
                - thigh I70.641
            - specified type NEC I70.692
          - right I70.601
            - with
              - gangrene (and intermittent claudication, rest pain and ulcer) I70.661
              - intermittent claudication I70.611

- **Arteriosclerosis, arteriosclerotic** — *continued*
  - extremities — *continued*
    - bypass graft — *continued*
      - nonbiological graft — *continued*
        - leg — *continued*
          - right — *continued*
            - with — *continued*
              - rest pain (and intermittent claudication) I70.621
              - ulceration (and intermittent claudication and rest pain) I70.639
                - ankle I70.633
                - calf I70.632
                - foot site NEC I70.635
                - heel I70.634
                - lower leg NEC I70.638
                - midfoot I70.634
                - thigh I70.631
            - specified type NEC I70.691
          - specified type NEC I70.699
        - specified NEC I70.608
          - with
            - gangrene (and intermittent claudication, rest pain and ulcer) I70.668
            - intermittent claudication I70.618
            - rest pain (and intermittent claudication) I70.628
            - ulceration (and intermittent claudication and rest pain) I70.65
          - specified type NEC I70.698
      - specified graft NEC I70.709
        - leg I70.709
          - with
            - gangrene (and intermittent claudication, rest pain and ulcer) I70.769
            - intermittent claudication I70.719
            - rest pain (and intermittent claudication) I70.729
          - bilateral I70.703
            - with
              - gangrene (and intermittent claudication, rest pain and ulcer) I70.763
              - intermittent claudication I70.713
              - rest pain (and intermittent claudication) I70.723
            - specified type NEC I70.793
          - left I70.702
            - with
              - gangrene (and intermittent claudication, rest pain and ulcer) I70.762
              - intermittent claudication I70.712
              - rest pain (and intermittent claudication) I70.722
              - ulceration (and intermittent claudication and rest pain) I70.749
                - ankle I70.743
                - calf I70.742
                - foot site NEC I70.745
                - heel I70.744
                - lower leg NEC I70.748
                - midfoot I70.744
                - thigh I70.741
            - specified type NEC I70.792
          - right I70.701
            - with
              - gangrene (and intermittent claudication, rest pain and ulcer) I70.761
              - intermittent claudication I70.711
              - rest pain (and intermittent claudication) I70.721
              - ulceration (and intermittent claudication and rest pain) I70.739
                - ankle I70.733
                - calf I70.732
                - foot site NEC I70.735
                - heel I70.734
                - lower leg NEC I70.738
                - midfoot I70.734
                - thigh I70.731
            - specified type NEC I70.791
          - specified type NEC I70.799
        - specified NEC I70.708
          - with
            - gangrene (and intermittent claudication, rest pain and ulcer) I70.768
            - intermittent claudication I70.718

- **Arteriosclerosis, arteriosclerotic** — *continued*
  - extremities — *continued*
    - bypass graft — *continued*
      - specified graft — *continued*
        - specified — *continued*
          - with — *continued*
            - rest pain (and intermittent claudication) I70.728
            - ulceration (and intermittent claudication and rest pain) I70.75
          - specified type NEC I70.798
      - specified NEC I70.308
        - with
          - gangrene (and intermittent claudication, rest pain and ulcer) I70.368
          - intermittent claudication I70.318
          - rest pain (and intermittent claudication) I70.328
          - ulceration (and intermittent claudication and rest pain) I70.35
        - specifiec type NEC I70.398
    - leg I70.209
      - with
        - gangrene (and intermittent claudication, rest pain and ulcer) I70.269
        - intermittent claudication I70.219
        - rest pain (and intermittent claudication) I70.229
      - bilateral I70.203
        - with
          - gangrene (and intermittent claudication, rest pain and ulcer) I70.263
          - intermittent claudication I70.213
          - rest pain (and intermittent claudication) I70.223
        - specified type NEC I70.293
      - left I70.202
        - with
          - gangrene (and intermittent claudication, rest pain and ulcer) I70.262
          - intermittent claudication I70.212
          - rest pain (and intermittent claudication) I70.222
          - ulceration (and intermittent claudication and rest pain) I70.249
            - ankle I70.243
            - calf I70.242
            - foot site NEC I70.245
            - heel I70.244
            - lower leg NEC I70.248
            - midfoot I70.244
            - thigh I70.241
        - specified type NEC I70.292
      - right I70.201
        - with
          - gangrene (and intermittent claudication, rest pain and ulcer) I70.261
          - intermittent claudication I70.211
          - rest pain (and intermittent claudication) I70.221
          - ulceration (and intermittent claudication and rest pain) I70.239
            - ankle I70.233
            - calf I70.232
            - foot site NEC I70.235
            - heel I70.234
            - lower leg NEC I70.238
            - midfoot I70.234
            - thigh I70.231
        - specified type NEC I70.291
      - specified type NEC I70.299
    - specified site NEC I70.208
      - with
        - gangrene (and intermittent claudication, rest pain and ulcer) I70.268
        - intermittent claudication I70.218
        - rest pain (and intermittent claudication) I70.228
        - ulceration (and intermittent claudication and rest pain) I70.25
      - specified type NEC I70.298
  - generalized I70.91
  - heart (disease) — *see* Arteriosclerosis, coronary (artery),
  - kidney — *see* Hypertension, kidney
  - medial — *see* Arteriosclerosis, extremities
  - mesenteric (artery) K55.1
  - Mönckeberg's — *see* Arteriosclerosis, extremities
  - myocarditis I51.4

- **Arthropathy** — *continued*
  - in — *continued*
    - leukemia NEC C95.9- ☑ *[M36.1]*
    - malignant histiocytosis C96.A *[M36.1]*
    - metabolic disease NOS E88.9 *[M14.8-]* ☑
    - multiple myeloma C9Ø.Ø- ☑ *[M36.1]*
    - neoplastic disease NOS (*see also* Neoplasm) D49.9 *[M36.1]*
    - nutritional deficiency — *see also* subcategory M14.8- E63.9
    - psoriasis NOS L4Ø.5Ø
    - sarcoidosis D86.86
    - syphilis (late) A52.77
      - congenital A5Ø.55 *[M12.8Ø]*
    - thyrotoxicosis — *see also* subcategory M14.8- EØ5.9Ø
    - ulcerative colitis K51.9Ø *[MØ7.6Ø]*
    - viral hepatitis (postinfectious) NEC B19.9 *[M12.8Ø]*
    - Whipple's disease — *see also* subcategory M14.8- K9Ø.81
  - Jaccoud — *see* Arthropathy, postrheumatic, chronic
  - juvenile — *see* Arthritis, juvenile
    - psoriatic L4Ø.54
  - mutilans (psoriatic) L4Ø.52
  - neuropathic (Charcot) M14.6Ø
    - ankle M14.67- ☑
    - diabetic — *see* Diabetes, arthropathy, neuropathic
    - elbow M14.62- ☑
    - foot joint M14.67- ☑
    - hand joint M14.64- ☑
    - hip M14.65- ☑
    - knee M14.66- ☑
    - multiple site M14.69
    - nonsyphilitic NEC G98.Ø
    - shoulder M14.61- ☑
    - syringomyelic G95.Ø
    - vertebra M14.68
    - wrist M14.63- ☑
  - osteopulmonary — *see* Osteoarthropathy, hypertrophic, specified NEC
  - postdysenteric MØ2.1Ø
    - ankle MØ2.17- ☑
    - elbow MØ2.12- ☑
    - foot joint MØ2.17- ☑
    - hand joint MØ2.14- ☑
    - hip MØ2.15- ☑
    - knee MØ2.16- ☑
    - multiple site MØ2.19
    - shoulder MØ2.11- ☑
    - vertebra MØ2.18
    - wrist MØ2.13- ☑
  - postimmunization MØ2.2Ø
    - ankle MØ2.27- ☑
    - elbow MØ2.22- ☑
    - foot joint MØ2.27- ☑
    - hand joint MØ2.24- ☑
    - hip MØ2.25- ☑
    - knee MØ2.26- ☑
    - multiple site MØ2.29
    - shoulder MØ2.21- ☑
    - vertebra MØ2.28
    - wrist MØ2.23- ☑
  - postinfectious NEC B99 ☑ *[M12.8Ø]*
    - in (due to)
      - enteritis due to Yersinia enterocolitica AØ4.6 *[M12.8Ø]*
      - syphilis A52.77
      - viral hepatitis NEC B19.9 *[M12.8Ø]*
  - postrheumatic, chronic (Jaccoud) M12.ØØ
    - ankle M12.Ø7- ☑
    - elbow M12.Ø2- ☑
    - foot joint M12.Ø7- ☑
    - hand joint M12.Ø4- ☑
    - hip M12.Ø5- ☑
    - knee M12.Ø6- ☑
    - multiple site M12.Ø9
    - shoulder M12.Ø1- ☑
    - specified joint NEC M12.Ø8
    - vertebrae M12.Ø8
    - wrist M12.Ø3- ☑
  - psoriatic NEC L4Ø.59
    - interphalangeal, distal L4Ø.51
  - reactive MØ2.9
    - in (due to)
      - infective endocarditis I33.Ø *[MØ2.9]*
    - specified type NEC MØ2.8Ø
      - ankle MØ2.87- ☑

- **Arthropathy** — *continued*
  - reactive — *continued*
    - specified type — *continued*
      - elbow MØ2.82- ☑
      - foot joint MØ2.87- ☑
      - hand joint MØ2.84- ☑
      - hip MØ2.85- ☑
      - knee MØ2.86- ☑
      - multiple site MØ2.89
      - shoulder MØ2.81- ☑
      - vertebra MØ2.88
      - wrist MØ2.83- ☑
  - specified form NEC M12.8Ø
    - ankle M12.87- ☑
    - elbow M12.82- ☑
    - foot joint M12.87- ☑
    - hand joint M12.84- ☑
    - hip M12.85- ☑
    - knee M12.86- ☑
    - multiple site M12.89
    - shoulder M12.81- ☑
    - specified joint NEC M12.88
    - vertebrae M12.88
    - wrist M12.83- ☑
  - syringomyelic G95.Ø
  - tabes dorsalis A52.16
  - tabetic A52.16
  - temporomandibular joint M26.65- ☑
  - transient — *see* Arthropathy, specified form NEC
  - traumatic M12.5Ø
    - ankle M12.57- ☑
    - elbow M12.52- ☑
    - foot joint M12.57- ☑
    - hand joint M12.54- ☑
    - hip M12.55- ☑
    - knee M12.56- ☑
    - multiple site M12.59
    - shoulder M12.51- ☑
    - specified joint NEC M12.58
    - vertebrae M12.58
    - wrist M12.53- ☑
- **Arthropyosis** — *see* Arthritis, pyogenic or pyemic
- **Arthrosis** (deformans) (degenerative) (localized) — *see also* Osteoarthritis M19.9Ø
  - spine — *see* Spondylosis
- **Arthus' phenomenon or reaction** T78.41 ☑
  - due to
    - drug — *see* Table of Drugs and Chemicals, by drug
- **Articular** — *see* condition
- **Articulation, reverse** (teeth) M26.24
- **Artificial**
  - insemination complication — *see* Complications, artificial, fertilization
  - opening status (functioning) (without complication) Z93.9
    - anus (colostomy) Z93.3
    - colostomy Z93.3
    - cystostomy Z93.5Ø
      - appendico-vesicostomy Z93.52
      - cutaneous Z93.51
      - specified NEC Z93.59
    - enterostomy Z93.4
    - gastrostomy Z93.1
    - ileostomy Z93.2
    - intestinal tract NEC Z93.4
    - jejunostomy Z93.4
    - nephrostomy Z93.6
    - specified site NEC Z93.8
    - tracheostomy Z93.Ø
    - ureterostomy Z93.6
    - urethrostomy Z93.6
    - urinary tract NEC Z93.6
    - vagina Z93.8
  - vagina status Z93.8
- **Arytenoid** — *see* condition
- **Asbestosis** (occupational) J61
- **Ascariasis** B77.9
  - with
    - complications NEC B77.89
    - intestinal complications B77.Ø
    - pneumonia, pneumonitis B77.81
- **Ascaridosis, ascaridiasis** — *see* Ascariasis
- **Ascaris** (infection) (infestation) (lumbricoides) — *see* Ascariasis
- **Ascending** — *see* condition

- **ASC-H** (atypical squamous cells cannot exclude high grade squamous intraepithelial lesion on cytologic smear)
  - anus R85.611
  - cervix R87.611
  - vagina R87.621
- **Aschoff's bodies** — *see* Myocarditis, rheumatic
- **Ascites** (abdominal) R18.8
  - cardiac — *see also* Failure, heart, right I5Ø.81Ø
  - chylous (nonfilarial) I89.8
    - filarial — *see* Infestation, filarial
  - due to
    - cirrhosis, alcoholic K7Ø.31
    - hepatitis
      - alcoholic K7Ø.11
      - chronic active K71.51
    - S. japonicum B65.2
  - heart — *see also* Failure, heart, right I5Ø.81Ø
  - malignant R18.Ø
  - pseudochylous R18.8
  - syphilitic A52.74
  - tuberculous A18.31
- **ASC-US** (atypical squamous cells of undetermined significance on cytologic smear)
  - anus R85.61Ø
  - cervix R87.61Ø
  - vagina R87.62Ø
- **Aseptic** — *see* condition
- **Asherman's syndrome** N85.6
- **Asialia** K11.7
- **Asiatic cholera** — *see* Cholera
- **Asimultagnosia** (simultanagnosia) R48.3
- **Askin's tumor** — *see* Neoplasm, connective tissue, malignant
- **Asocial personality** F6Ø.2
- **Asomatognosia** R41.4
- **Aspartylglucosaminuria** E77.1
- **Asperger's disease or syndrome** F84.5
- **Aspergilloma** — *see* Aspergillosis
- **Aspergillosis** (with pneumonia) B44.9
  - bronchopulmonary, allergic B44.81
  - disseminated B44.7
  - generalized B44.7
  - pulmonary NEC B44.1
    - allergic B44.81
    - invasive B44.Ø
  - specified NEC B44.89
  - tonsillar B44.2
- **Aspergillus** (flavus) (fumigatus) (infection) (terreus) — *see* Aspergillosis
- **Aspermatogenesis** — *see* Azoospermia
- **Aspermia** (testis) — *see* Azoospermia
- **Asphyxia, asphyxiation** (by) RØ9.Ø1
  - antenatal P84
  - birth P84
  - bunny bag — *see* Asphyxia, due to, mechanical threat to breathing, trapped in bed clothes
  - crushing S28.Ø ☑
  - drowning T75.1 ☑
  - gas, fumes, or vapor — *see* Table of Drugs and Chemicals
  - inhalation — *see* Inhalation
  - intrauterine P84
  - local I73.ØØ
    - with gangrene I73.Ø1
  - mucus — *see also* Foreign body, respiratory tract, causing asphyxia
  - newborn P84
  - pathological RØ9.Ø1
  - postnatal P84
    - mechanical — *see* Asphyxia, due to, mechanical threat to breathing
  - prenatal P84
  - reticularis R23.1
  - strangulation — *see* Asphyxia, due to, mechanical threat to breathing
  - submersion T75.1 ☑
  - traumatic T71.9 ☑
    - due to
      - crushed chest S28.Ø ☑
      - foreign body (in) — *see* Foreign body, respiratory tract, causing asphyxia
      - low oxygen content of ambient air T71.2Ø ☑
        - due to
          - being trapped in
            - low oxygen environment T71.29 ☑
              - in car trunk T71.221 ☑

- **Asphyxia, asphyxiation** — *continued*
  - traumatic — *continued*
    - due to — *continued*
      - low oxygen content of ambient air — *continued*
        - due to — *continued*
          - being trapped in — *continued*
            - low oxygen environment — *continued*
              - in car trunk — *continued*
                - circumstances undetermined T71.224 ☑
                - done with intent to harm by
                  - another person T71.223 ☑
                  - self T71.222 ☑
              - in refrigerator T71.231 ☑
                - circumstances undetermined T71.234 ☑
                - done with intent to harm by
                  - another person T71.233 ☑
                  - self T71.232 ☑
          - cave-in T71.21 ☑
      - mechanical threat to breathing (accidental) T71.191 ☑
        - circumstances undetermined T71.194 ☑
        - done with intent to harm by
          - another person T71.193 ☑
          - self T71.192 ☑
        - hanging T71.161 ☑
          - circumstances undetermined T71.164 ☑
          - done with intent to harm by
            - another person T71.163 ☑
            - self T71.162 ☑
        - plastic bag T71.121 ☑
          - circumstances undetermined T71.124 ☑
          - done with intent to harm by
            - another person T71.123 ☑
            - self T71.122 ☑
        - smothering
          - in furniture T71.151 ☑
            - circumstances undetermined T71.154 ☑
            - done with intent to harm by
              - another person T71.153 ☑
              - self T71.152 ☑
          - under
            - another person's body T71.141 ☑
              - circumstances undetermined T71.144 ☑
              - done with intent to harm T71.143 ☑
            - pillow T71.111 ☑
              - circumstances undetermined T71.114 ☑
              - done with intent to harm by
                - another person T71.113 ☑
                - self T71.112 ☑
        - trapped in bed clothes T71.131 ☑
          - circumstances undetermined T71.134 ☑
          - done with intent to harm by
            - another person T71.133 ☑
            - self T71.132 ☑
  - vomiting, vomitus — *see* Foreign body, respiratory tract, causing asphyxia
- **Aspiration**
  - amniotic (clear) fluid (newborn) P24.10
    - with
      - pneumonia (pneumonitis) P24.11
      - respiratory symptoms P24.11
  - blood
    - newborn (without respiratory symptoms) P24.20
      - with
        - pneumonia (pneumonitis) P24.21
        - respiratory symptoms P24.21
    - specified age NEC — *see* Foreign body, respiratory tract
  - bronchitis J69.0
  - food or foreign body (with asphyxiation) — *see* Asphyxia, food
  - liquor (amnii) (newborn) P24.10
    - with
      - pneumonia (pneumonitis) P24.11
      - respiratory symptoms P24.11
  - meconium (newborn) (without respiratory symptoms) P24.00
    - with
      - pneumonitis (pneumonitis) P24.01
      - respiratory symptoms P24.01
- **Aspiration** — *continued*
  - milk (newborn) (without respiratory symptoms) P24.30
    - with
      - pneumonia (pneumonitis) P24.31
      - respiratory symptoms P24.31
    - specified age NEC — *see* Foreign body, respiratory tract
  - mucus — *see also* Foreign body, by site, causing asphyxia
    - newborn P24.10
      - with
        - pneumonia (pneumonitis) P24.11
        - respiratory symptoms P24.11
  - neonatal P24.9
    - specific NEC (without respiratory symptoms) P24.80
      - with
        - pneumonia (pneumonitis) P24.81
        - respiratory symptoms P24.81
  - newborn P24.9
    - specific NEC (without respiratory symptoms) P24.80
      - with
        - pneumonia (pneumonitis) P24.81
        - respiratory symptoms P24.81
  - pneumonia J69.0
  - pneumonitis J69.0
  - syndrome of newborn — *see* Aspiration, by substance, with pneumonia
  - vernix caseosa (newborn) P24.80
    - with
      - pneumonia (pneumonitis) P24.81
      - respiratory symptoms P24.81
  - vomitus — *see also* Foreign body, respiratory tract
    - newborn (without respiratory symptoms) P24.30
      - with
        - pneumonia (pneumonitis) P24.31
        - respiratory symptoms P24.31
- **Asplenia** (congenital) Q89.01
  - postsurgical Z90.81
- **Assam fever** B55.0
- **Assault, sexual** — *see* Maltreatment
- **Assmann's focus NEC** A15.0
- **Astasia** (-abasia) (hysterical) F44.4
- **Asteatosis cutis** L85.3
- **Astereognosia, astereognosis** R48.1
- **Asterixis** R27.8
  - in liver disease K71.3
- **Asteroid hyalitis** — *see* Deposit, crystalline
- **Asthenia, asthenic** R53.1
  - cardiac — *see also* Failure, heart I50.9
    - psychogenic F45.8
  - cardiovascular — *see also* Failure, heart I50.9
    - psychogenic F45.8
  - heart — *see also* Failure, heart I50.9
    - psychogenic F45.8
  - hysterical F44.4
  - myocardial — *see also* Failure, heart I50.9
    - psychogenic F45.8
  - nervous F48.8
  - neurocirculatory F45.8
  - neurotic F48.8
  - psychogenic F48.8
  - psychoneurotic F48.8
  - psychophysiologic F48.8
  - reaction (psychophysiologic) F48.8
  - senile R54
- **Asthenopia** — *see also* Discomfort, visual
  - hysterical F44.6
  - psychogenic F44.6
- **Asthenospermia** — *see* Abnormal, specimen, male genital organs
- **Asthma, asthmatic** (bronchial) (catarrh) (spasmodic) J45.909
  - with
    - chronic obstructive bronchitis J44.9
      - with
        - acute lower respiratory infection J44.0
        - exacerbation (acute) J44.1
    - chronic obstructive pulmonary disease J44.9
      - with
        - acute lower respiratory infection J44.0
        - exacerbation (acute) J44.1
    - exacerbation (acute) J45.901
    - hay fever — *see* Asthma, allergic extrinsic
    - rhinitis, allergic — *see* Asthma, allergic extrinsic
    - status asthmaticus J45.902
  - allergic extrinsic J45.909
    - with
      - exacerbation (acute) J45.901
- **Asthma, asthmatic** — *continued*
  - allergic extrinsic — *continued*
    - with — *continued*
      - status asthmaticus J45.902
  - atopic — *see* Asthma, allergic extrinsic
  - cardiac — *see* Failure, ventricular, left
  - cardiobronchial I50.1
  - childhood J45.909
    - with
      - exacerbation (acute) J45.901
      - status asthmaticus J45.902
  - chronic obstructive J44.9
    - with
      - acute lower respiratory infection J44.0
      - exacerbation (acute) J44.1
  - collier's J60
  - cough variant J45.991
  - detergent J69.8
  - due to
    - detergent J69.8
    - inhalation of fumes J68.3
  - eosinophilic J82.83
  - extrinsic, allergic — *see* Asthma, allergic extrinsic
  - grinder's J62.8
  - hay — *see* Asthma, allergic extrinsic
  - heart I50.1
  - idiosyncratic — *see* Asthma, nonallergic
  - intermittent (mild) J45.20
    - with
      - exacerbation (acute) J45.21
      - status asthmaticus J45.22
  - intrinsic, nonallergic — *see* Asthma, nonallergic
  - Kopp's E32.8
  - late-onset J45.909
    - with
      - exacerbation (acute) J45.901
      - status asthmaticus J45.902
  - mild intermittent J45.20
    - with
      - exacerbation (acute) J45.21
      - status asthmaticus J45.22
  - mild persistent J45.30
    - with
      - exacerbation (acute) J45.31
      - status asthmaticus J45.32
  - Millar's (laryngismus stridulus) J38.5
  - miner's J60
  - mixed J45.909
    - with
      - exacerbation (acute) J45.901
      - status asthmaticus J45.902
  - moderate persistent J45.40
    - with
      - exacerbation (acute) J45.41
      - status asthmaticus J45.42
  - nervous — *see* Asthma, nonallergic
  - nonallergic (intrinsic) J45.909
    - with
      - exacerbation (acute) J45.901
      - status asthmaticus J45.902
  - persistent
    - mild J45.30
      - with
        - exacerbation (acute) J45.31
        - status asthmaticus J45.32
    - moderate J45.40
      - with
        - exacerbation (acute) J45.41
        - status asthmaticus J45.42
    - severe J45.50
      - with
        - exacerbation (acute) J45.51
        - status asthmaticus J45.52
  - platinum J45.998
  - pneumoconiotic NEC J64
  - potter's J62.8
  - predominantly allergic J45.909
  - psychogenic F54
  - pulmonary eosinophilic J82.83
  - red cedar J67.8
  - Rostan's I50.1
  - sandblaster's J62.8
  - sequoiosis J67.8
  - severe persistent J45.50
    - with
      - exacerbation (acute) J45.51
      - status asthmaticus J45.52
  - specified NEC J45.998

Atresia, atretic — *continued*
- cystic duct — *continued*
  - acquired — *continued*
    - with obstruction K82.Ø
- digestive organs NEC Q45.8
- duodenum Q41.Ø
- ear canal Q16.1
- ejaculatory duct Q55.4
- epiglottis Q31.8
- esophagus Q39.Ø
  - with tracheoesophageal fistula Q39.1
- eustachian tube Q17.8
- fallopian tube (congenital) Q5Ø.6
  - acquired N97.1
- follicular cyst N83.Ø- ☑
- foramen of
  - Luschka QØ3.1
    - with spina bifida — *see* Spina bifida, with hydrocephalus
  - Magendie QØ3.1
    - with spina bifida — *see* Spina bifida, with hydrocephalus
- gallbladder Q44.1
- genital organ
  - external
    - female Q52.79
    - male Q55.8
  - internal
    - female Q52.8
    - male Q55.8
- glottis Q31.8
- gullet Q39.Ø
  - with tracheoesophageal fistula Q39.1
- heart valve NEC Q24.8
  - pulmonary Q22.Ø
  - tricuspid Q22.4
- hymen Q52.3
  - acquired (postinfective) N89.6
- ileum Q41.2
- intestine (small) Q41.9
  - large Q42.9
    - specified NEC Q42.8
- iris, filtration angle Q15.Ø
- jejunum Q41.1
- lacrimal apparatus Q1Ø.4
- larynx Q31.8
- meatus urinarius Q64.33
- mitral valve Q23.2
  - in hypoplastic left heart syndrome Q23.4
- nares (anterior) (posterior) Q3Ø.Ø
- nasopharynx Q34.8
- nose, nostril Q3Ø.Ø
  - acquired J34.89
- organ or site NEC Q89.8
- osseous meatus (ear) Q16.1
- oviduct (congenital) Q5Ø.6
  - acquired N97.1
- parotid duct Q38.4
  - acquired K11.8
- pulmonary (artery) Q25.5
  - valve Q22.Ø
- pulmonic Q22.Ø
- pupil Q13.2
- rectum Q42.1
  - with fistula Q42.Ø
- salivary duct Q38.4
  - acquired K11.8
- sublingual duct Q38.4
  - acquired K11.8
- submandibular duct Q38.4
  - acquired K11.8
- submaxillary duct Q38.4
  - acquired K11.8
- thyroid cartilage Q31.8
- trachea Q32.1
- tricuspid valve Q22.4
- ureter Q62.1Ø
  - pelvic junction Q62.11
  - vesical orifice Q62.12
- ureteropelvic junction Q62.11
- ureterovesical orifice Q62.12
- urethra (valvular) Q64.39
  - stricture Q64.32
- urinary tract NEC Q64.8
- uterus Q51.818
  - acquired N85.8
- vagina (congenital) Q52.4
  - acquired (postinfectional) (senile) N89.5
- vas deferens Q55.3

Atresia, atretic — *continued*
- vascular NEC Q27.8
  - cerebral Q28.3
  - digestive system Q27.8
  - lower limb Q27.8
  - specified site NEC Q27.8
  - upper limb Q27.8
- vein NEC Q27.8
  - digestive system Q27.8
  - great Q26.8
  - lower limb Q27.8
  - portal Q26.5
  - pulmonary Q26.4
    - partial Q26.3
    - total Q26.2
  - specified site NEC Q27.8
  - upper limb Q27.8
- vena cava (inferior) (superior) Q26.8
- vesicourethral orifice Q64.31
- vulva Q52.79
  - acquired N9Ø.5

Atrichia, atrichosis — *see* Alopecia

Atrophia — *see also* Atrophy
- cutis senilis L9Ø.8
  - due to radiation L57.8
- gyrata of choroid and retina H31.23
- senilis R54
  - dermatological L9Ø.8
    - due to radiation (nonionizing) (solar) L57.8
- unguium L6Ø.3
  - congenita Q84.6

Atrophie blanche (en plaque) (de Milian) L95.Ø

Atrophoderma, atrophodermia (of) L9Ø.9
- diffusum (idiopathic) L9Ø.4
- maculatum L9Ø.8
  - et striatum L9Ø.8
    - due to syphilis A52.79
  - syphilitic A51.39
- neuriticum L9Ø.8
- Pasini and Pierini L9Ø.3
- pigmentosum Q82.1
- reticulatum symmetricum faciei L66.4
- senile L9Ø.8
  - due to radiation (nonionizing) (solar) L57.8
- vermiculata (cheeks) L66.4

Atrophy, atrophic (of)
- adrenal (capsule) (gland) E27.49
  - primary (autoimmune) E27.1
- alveolar process or ridge (edentulous) KØ8.2Ø
- anal sphincter (disuse) N81.84
- appendix K38.8
- arteriosclerotic — *see* Arteriosclerosis
- bile duct (common) (hepatic) K83.8
- bladder N32.89
  - neurogenic N31.8
- blanche (en plaque) (of Milian) L95.Ø
- bone (senile) NEC — *see also* Disorder, bone, specified type NEC
  - due to
    - tabes dorsalis (neurogenic) A52.11
- brain (cortex) (progressive) G31.9
  - frontotemporal circumscribed G31.Ø1 *[FØ2.8Ø]*
    - with behavioral disturbance G31.Ø1 *[FØ2.81]*
  - senile NEC G31.1
- breast N64.2
  - obstetric — *see* Disorder, breast, specified type NEC
- buccal cavity K13.79
- cardiac — *see* Degeneration, myocardial
- cartilage (infectional) (joint) — *see* Disorder, cartilage, specified NEC
- cerebellar — *see* Atrophy, brain
- cerebral — *see* Atrophy, brain
- cervix (mucosa) (senile) (uteri) N88.8
  - menopausal N95.8
- Charcot-Marie-Tooth G6Ø.Ø
- choroid (central) (macular) (myopic) (retina) H31.1Ø- ☑
  - diffuse secondary H31.12- ☑
  - gyrate H31.23
  - senile H31.11- ☑
- ciliary body — *see* Atrophy, iris
- conjunctiva (senile) H11.89
- corpus cavernosum N48.89
- cortical — *see* Atrophy, brain
- cystic duct K82.8
- Déjérine-Thomas G23.8
- disuse NEC — *see* Atrophy, muscle
- Duchenne-Aran G12.21
- ear H93.8- ☑

Atrophy, atrophic — *continued*
- edentulous alveolar ridge KØ8.2Ø
- endometrium (senile) N85.8
  - cervix N88.8
- enteric K63.89
- epididymis N5Ø.89
- eyeball — *see* Disorder, globe, degenerated condition, atrophy
- eyelid (senile) — *see* Disorder, eyelid, degenerative
- facial (skin) L9Ø.9
- fallopian tube (senile) N83.32- ☑
  - with ovary N83.33- ☑
- fascioscapulohumeral (Landouzy- Déjérine) G71.Ø2
- fatty, thymus (gland) E32.8
- gallbladder K82.8
- gastric K29.4Ø
  - with bleeding K29.41
- gastrointestinal K63.89
- glandular I89.8
- globe H44.52- ☑
- gum — *see* Recession, gingival
- hair L67.8
- heart (brown) — *see* Degeneration, myocardial
- hemifacial Q67.4
  - Romberg G51.8
- infantile E41
  - paralysis, acute — *see* Poliomyelitis, paralytic
- intestine K63.89
- iris (essential) (progressive) H21.26- ☑
  - specified NEC H21.29
- kidney (senile) (terminal) — *see also* Sclerosis, renal N26.1
  - congenital or infantile Q6Ø.5
    - bilateral Q6Ø.4
    - unilateral Q6Ø.3
  - hydronephrotic — *see* Hydronephrosis
- lacrimal gland (primary) HØ4.14- ☑
  - secondary HØ4.15- ☑
- Landouzy-Déjérine G71.Ø2
- laryngitis, infective J37.Ø
- larynx J38.7
- Leber's optic (hereditary) H47.22
- lip K13.Ø
- liver (yellow) K72.9Ø
  - with coma K72.91
  - acute, subacute K72.ØØ
    - with coma K72.Ø1
  - chronic K72.1Ø
    - with coma K72.11
- lung (senile) J98.4
- macular (dermatological) L9Ø.8
  - syphilitic, skin A51.39
    - striated A52.79
- mandible (edentulous) KØ8.2Ø
  - minimal KØ8.21
  - moderate KØ8.22
  - severe KØ8.23
- maxilla KØ8.2Ø
  - minimal KØ8.24
  - moderate KØ8.25
  - severe KØ8.26
- muscle, muscular (diffuse) (general) (idiopathic) (primary) M62.5Ø
  - ankle M62.57- ☑
  - Duchenne-Aran G12.21
  - foot M62.57- ☑
  - forearm M62.53- ☑
  - hand M62.54- ☑
  - infantile spinal G12.Ø
  - lower leg M62.56- ☑
  - multiple sites M62.59
  - myelopathic — *see* Atrophy, muscle, spinal
  - myotonic G71.11
  - neuritic G58.9
  - neuropathic (peroneal) (progressive) G6Ø.Ø
  - pelvic (disuse) N81.84
  - peroneal G6Ø.Ø
  - progressive (bulbar) G12.21
    - adult G12.1
    - infantile (spinal) G12.Ø
    - spinal G12.25
      - adult G12.1
      - infantile G12.Ø
  - pseudohypertrophic G71.Ø2
  - shoulder region M62.51- ☑
  - specified site NEC M62.58
  - spinal G12.9
    - adult form G12.1

- **Atrophy, atrophic** — *continued*
  - muscle, muscular — *continued*
    - spinal — *continued*
      - Aran-Duchenne G12.21
      - childhood form, type II G12.1
      - distal G12.1
      - hereditary NEC G12.1
      - infantile, type I (Werdnig-Hoffmann) G12.Ø
      - juvenile form, type III (Kugelberg- Welander) G12.1
      - progressive G12.25
      - scapuloperoneal form G12.1
      - specified NEC G12.8
    - syphilitic A52.78
    - thigh M62.55- ☑
    - upper arm M62.52- ☑
  - myocardium — *see* Degeneration, myocardial
  - myometrium (senile) N85.8
    - cervix N88.8
  - myopathic NEC — *see* Atrophy, muscle
  - myotonia G71.11
  - nail L6Ø.3
  - nasopharynx J31.1
  - nerve — *see also* Disorder, nerve
    - abducens — *see* Strabismus, paralytic, sixth nerve
    - accessory G52.8
    - acoustic or auditory H93.3 ☑
    - cranial G52.9
      - eighth (auditory) H93.3 ☑
      - eleventh (accessory) G52.8
      - fifth (trigeminal) G5Ø.8
      - first (olfactory) G52.Ø
      - fourth (trochlear) — *see* Strabismus, paralytic, fourth nerve
      - second (optic) H47.2Ø
      - sixth (abducens) — *see* Strabismus, paralytic, sixth nerve
      - tenth (pneumogastric) (vagus) G52.2
      - third (oculomotor) — *see* Strabismus, paralytic, third nerve
      - twelfth (hypoglossal) G52.3
    - hypoglossal G52.3
    - oculomotor — *see* Strabismus, paralytic, third nerve
    - olfactory G52.Ø
    - optic (papillomacular bundle)
      - syphilitic (late) A52.15
        - congenital A5Ø.44
    - pneumogastric G52.2
    - trigeminal G5Ø.8
    - trochlear — *see* Strabismus, paralytic, fourth nerve
    - vagus (pneumogastric) G52.2
  - neurogenic, bone, tabetic A52.11
  - nutritional E41
  - old age R54
  - olivopontocerebellar G23.8
  - optic (nerve) H47.2Ø
    - glaucomatous H47.23- ☑
    - hereditary H47.22
    - primary H47.21- ☑
    - specified type NEC H47.29- ☑
    - syphilitic (late) A52.15
      - congenital A5Ø.44
  - orbit HØ5.31- ☑
  - ovary (senile) N83.31- ☑
    - with fallopian tube N83.33- ☑
  - oviduct (senile) — *see* Atrophy, fallopian tube
  - palsy, diffuse (progressive) G12.22
  - pancreas (duct) (senile) K86.89
  - parotid gland K11.Ø
  - pelvic muscle N81.84
  - penis N48.89
  - pharynx J39.2
  - pluriglandular E31.8
    - autoimmune E31.Ø
  - polyarthritis M15.9
  - prostate N42.89
  - pseudohypertrophic (muscle) G71.Ø2
  - renal — *see also* Sclerosis, renal N26.1
  - retina, retinal (postinfectional) H35.89
  - rhinitis J31.Ø
  - salivary gland K11.Ø
  - scar L9Ø.5
  - sclerosis, lobar (of brain) G31.Ø9 *[FØ2.8Ø]*
    - with behavioral disturbance G31.Ø9 *[FØ2.81]*
  - scrotum N5Ø.89
  - seminal vesicle N5Ø.89
  - senile R54
    - due to radiation (nonionizing) (solar) L57.8
- **Atrophy, atrophic** — *continued*
  - skin (patches) (spots) L9Ø.9
    - degenerative (senile) L9Ø.8
    - due to radiation (nonionizing) (solar) L57.8
    - senile L9Ø.8
  - spermatic cord N5Ø.89
  - spinal (acute) (cord) G95.89
    - muscular — *see* Atrophy, muscle, spinal
    - paralysis G12.2Ø
      - acute — *see* Poliomyelitis, paralytic
      - meaning progressive muscular atrophy G12.25
  - spine (column) — *see* Spondylopathy, specified NEC
  - spleen (senile) D73.Ø
  - stomach K29.4Ø
    - with bleeding K29.41
  - striate (skin) L9Ø.6
    - syphilitic A52.79
  - subcutaneous L9Ø.9
  - sublingual gland K11.Ø
  - submandibular gland K11.Ø
  - submaxillary gland K11.Ø
  - Sudeck's — *see* Algoneurodystrophy
  - suprarenal (capsule) (gland) E27.49
    - primary E27.1
  - systemic affecting central nervous system
    - in
      - myxedema EØ3.9 *[G13.2]*
      - neoplastic disease — *see also* Neoplasm D49.9 *[G13.1]*
      - specified disease NEC G13.8
  - tarso-orbital fascia, congenital Q1Ø.3
  - testis N5Ø.Ø
  - thenar, partial — *see* Syndrome, carpal tunnel
  - thymus (fatty) E32.8
  - thyroid (gland) (acquired) EØ3.4
    - with cretinism EØ3.1
    - congenital (with myxedema) EØ3.1
  - tongue (senile) K14.8
    - papillae K14.4
  - trachea J39.8
  - tunica vaginalis N5Ø.89
  - turbinate J34.89
  - tympanic membrane (nonflaccid) H73.82- ☑
    - flaccid H73.81- ☑
  - upper respiratory tract J39.8
  - uterus, uterine (senile) N85.8
    - cervix N88.8
    - due to radiation (intended effect) N85.8
      - adverse effect or misadventure N99.89
  - vagina (senile) N95.2
  - vas deferens N5Ø.89
  - vascular I99.8
  - vertebra (senile) — *see* Spondylopathy, specified NEC
  - vulva (senile) N9Ø.5
  - Werdnig-Hoffmann G12.Ø
  - yellow — *see* Failure, hepatic
- **Attack, attacks**
  - with alteration of consciousness (with automatisms) — *see* Epilepsy, localization-related, symptomatic, with complex partial seizures
  - Adams-Stokes I45.9
  - akinetic — *see* Epilepsy, generalized, specified NEC
  - angina — *see* Angina
  - atonic — *see* Epilepsy, generalized, specified NEC
  - benign shuddering G25.83
  - cataleptic — *see* Catalepsy
  - coronary — *see* Infarct, myocardium
  - cyanotic, newborn P28.2
  - drop NEC R55
  - epileptic — *see* Epilepsy
  - heart — *see* infarct, myocardium
  - hysterical F44.9
  - jacksonian — *see* Epilepsy, localization-related, symptomatic, with simple partial seizures
  - myocardium, myocardial — *see* Infarct, myocardium
  - myoclonic — *see* Epilepsy, generalized, specified NEC
  - panic F41.Ø
  - psychomotor — *see* Epilepsy, localization-related, symptomatic, with complex partial seizures
  - salaam — *see* Epilepsy, spasms
  - schizophreniform, brief F23
  - shuddering, benign G25.83
  - Stokes-Adams I45.9
  - syncope R55
  - transient ischemic (TIA) G45.9
    - specified NEC G45.8
  - unconsciousness R55
    - hysterical F44.89
- **Attack, attacks** — *continued*
  - vasomotor R55
  - vasovagal (paroxysmal) (idiopathic) R55
  - without alteration of consciousness — *see* Epilepsy, localization-related, symptomatic, with simple partial seizures
- **Attention** (to)
  - artificial
    - opening (of) Z43.9
      - digestive tract NEC Z43.4
        - colon Z43.3
        - ilium Z43.2
        - stomach Z43.1
      - specified NEC Z43.8
      - trachea Z43.Ø
      - urinary tract NEC Z43.6
        - cystostomy Z43.5
        - nephrostomy Z43.6
        - ureterostomy Z43.6
        - urethrostomy Z43.6
    - vagina Z43.7
  - colostomy Z43.3
  - cystostomy Z43.5
  - deficit disorder or syndrome F98.8
    - with hyperactivity — *see* Disorder, attention-deficit hyperactivity
  - gastrostomy Z43.1
  - ileostomy Z43.2
  - jejunostomy Z43.4
  - nephrostomy Z43.6
  - surgical dressings Z48.Ø1
  - sutures Z48.Ø2
  - tracheostomy Z43.Ø
  - ureterostomy Z43.6
  - urethrostomy Z43.6
- **Attrition**
  - gum — *see* Recession, gingival
  - tooth, teeth (excessive) (hard tissues) KØ3.Ø
- **Atypical, atypism** — *see also* condition
  - cells (on cytolgocial smear) (endocervical) (endometrial) (glandular)
    - cervix R87.619
    - vagina R87.629
  - cervical N87.9
  - endometrium N85.9
    - hyperplasia N85.ØØ
  - parenting situation Z62.9
- **Auditory** — *see* condition
- **Aujeszky's disease** B33.8
- **Aurantiasis, cutis** E67.1
- **Auricle, auricular** — *see also* condition
  - cervical Q18.2
- **Auriculotemporal syndrome** G5Ø.8
- **Austin Flint murmur** (aortic insufficiency) I35.1
- **Australian**
  - Q fever A78
  - X disease A83.4
- **Autism, autistic** (childhood) (infantile) F84.Ø
  - atypical F84.9
  - spectrum disorder F84.Ø
- **Autodigestion** R68.89
- **Autoerythrocyte sensitization** (syndrome) D69.2
- **Autographism** L5Ø.3
- **Autoimmune**
  - disease (systemic) M35.9
  - inhibitors to clotting factors D68.311
  - lymphoproliferative syndrome [ALPS] D89.82
  - thyroiditis EØ6.3
- **Autointoxication** R68.89
- **Automatism** G93.89
  - with temporal sclerosis G93.81
  - epileptic — *see* Epilepsy, localization-related, symptomatic, with complex partial seizures
  - paroxysmal, idiopathic — *see* Epilepsy, localization-related, symptomatic, with complex partial seizures
- **Autonomic, autonomous**
  - bladder (neurogenic) N31.2
  - hysteria seizure F44.5
- **Autosensitivity, erythrocyte** D69.2
- **Autosensitization, cutaneous** L3Ø.2
- **Autosome** — *see* condition by chromosome involved
- **Autotopagnosia** R48.1
- **Autotoxemia** R68.89
- **Autumn** — *see* condition
- **Avellis' syndrome** G46.8
- **Aversion**
  - oral R63.3

Aversion — *continued*
- oral — *continued*
  - newborn P92.- ☑
  - nonorganic origin F98.2 ☑
- sexual F52.1

Aviator's
- disease or sickness — *see* Effect, adverse, high altitude
- ear T70.0 ☑

Avitaminosis (multiple) — *see also* Deficiency, vitamin E56.9
- B E53.9
  - with
    - beriberi E51.11
    - pellagra E52
- B2 E53.0
- B6 E53.1
- B12 E53.8
- D E55.9
  - with rickets E55.0
- G E53.0
- K E56.1
- nicotinic acid E52

AVNRT (atrioventricular nodal re-entrant tachycardia) I47.1

AVRT (atrioventricular nodal re-entrant tachycardia) I47.1

Avulsion (traumatic)
- blood vessel — *see* Injury, blood vessel
- bone — *see* Fracture, by site
- cartilage — *see also* Dislocation, by site
  - symphyseal (inner), complicating delivery O71.6
- external site other than limb — *see* Wound, open, by site
- eye S05.7- ☑
- head (intracranial)
  - external site NEC S08.89 ☑
  - scalp S08.0 ☑
- internal organ or site — *see* Injury, by site
- joint — *see also* Dislocation, by site
  - capsule — *see* Sprain, by site
- kidney S37.06- ☑
- ligament — *see* Sprain, by site
- limb — *see also* Amputation, traumatic, by site
  - skin and subcutaneous tissue — *see* Wound, open, by site
- muscle — *see* Injury, muscle
- nerve (root) — *see* Injury, nerve
- scalp S08.0 ☑
- skin and subcutaneous tissue — *see* Wound, open, by site
- spleen S36.032 ☑
- symphyseal cartilage (inner), complicating delivery O71.6
- tendon — *see* Injury, muscle
- tooth S03.2 ☑

Awareness of heart beat R00.2

Axenfeld's
- anomaly or syndrome Q15.0
- degeneration (calcareous) Q13.4

Axilla, axillary — *see also* condition
- breast Q83.1

Axonotmesis — *see* Injury, nerve

Ayerza's disease or syndrome (pulmonary artery sclerosis with pulmonary hypertension) I27.0

Azoospermia (organic) N46.01
- due to
  - drug therapy N46.021
  - efferent duct obstruction N46.023
  - infection N46.022
  - radiation N46.024
  - specified cause NEC N46.029
  - systemic disease N46.025

Azotemia R79.89
- meaning uremia N19

Aztec ear Q17.3

Azygos
- continuation inferior vena cava Q26.8
- lobe (lung) Q33.1

B

Baastrup's disease — *see* Kissing spine

Babesiosis B60.00
- due to
  - Babesia
    - divergens B60.03
    - duncani B60.02
    - KO-1 B60.09
    - microti B60.01
    - MO-1 B60.03
    - species
      - unspecified B60.00
    - venatorum B60.09
  - specified NEC B60.09

Babington's disease (familial hemorrhagic telangiectasia) I78.0

Babinski's syndrome A52.79

Baby
- crying constantly R68.11
- floppy (syndrome) P94.2

Bacillary — *see* condition

Bacilluria R82.71

Bacillus — *see also* Infection, bacillus
- abortus infection A23.1
- anthracis infection A22.9
- coli infection — *see also* Escherichia coli B96.20
- Flexner's A03.1
- mallei infection A24.0
- Shiga's A03.0
- suipestifer infection — *see* Infection, salmonella

Back — *see* condition

Backache (postural) M54.9
- sacroiliac M53.3
- specified NEC M54.89

Backflow — *see* Reflux

Backward reading (dyslexia) F81.0

Bacteremia R78.81
- with sepsis — *see* Sepsis

Bactericholia — *see* Cholecystitis, acute

Bacterid, bacteride (pustular) L40.3

Bacterium, bacteria, bacterial
- agent NEC, as cause of disease classified elsewhere B96.89
- in blood — *see* Bacteremia
- in urine — *see* Bacteriuria

Bacteriuria, bacteruria R82.71
- asymptomatic R82.71

Bacteroides
- fragilis, as cause of disease classified elsewhere B96.6

Bad
- heart — *see* Disease, heart
- trip
  - due to drug abuse — *see* Abuse, drug, hallucinogen
  - due to drug dependence — *see* Dependence, drug, hallucinogen

Baelz's disease (cheilitis glandularis apostematosa) K13.0

Baerensprung's disease (eczema marginatum) B35.6

Bagasse disease or pneumonitis J67.1

Bagassosis J67.1

Baker's cyst — *see* Cyst, Baker's

Bakwin-Krida syndrome (metaphyseal dysplasia) Q78.5

Balancing side interference M26.56

Balanitis (circinata) (erosiva) (gangrenosa) (phagedenic) (vulgaris) N48.1
- amebic A06.82
- candidal B37.42
- due to Haemophilus ducreyi A57
- gonococcal (acute) (chronic) A54.23
- xerotica obliterans N48.0

Balanoposthitis N47.6
- gonococcal (acute) (chronic) A54.23
- ulcerative (specific) A63.8

Balanorrhagia — *see* Balanitis

Balantidiasis, balantidiosis A07.0

Bald tongue K14.4

Baldness — *see also* Alopecia
- male-pattern — *see* Alopecia, androgenic

Balkan grippe A78

Balloon disease — *see* Effect, adverse, high altitude

Balo's disease (concentric sclerosis) G37.5

Bamberger-Marie disease — *see* Osteoarthropathy, hypertrophic, specified type NEC

Bancroft's filariasis B74.0

Band(s)
- adhesive — *see* Adhesions, peritoneum
- anomalous or congenital — *see also* Anomaly, by site
  - heart (atrial) (ventricular) Q24.8
  - intestine Q43.3
  - omentum Q43.3
- cervix N88.1
- constricting, congenital Q79.8
- gallbladder (congenital) Q44.1
- intestinal (adhesive) — *see* Adhesions, peritoneum
- obstructive
  - intestine K56.50
    - complete K56.52
    - incomplete K56.51
    - partial K56.51
  - peritoneum K56.50
    - complete K56.52
    - incomplete K56.51
    - partial K56.51
- periappendiceal, congenital Q43.3
- peritoneal (adhesive) — *see* Adhesions, peritoneum
- uterus N73.6
  - internal N85.6
- vagina N89.5

Bandemia D72.825

Bandl's ring (contraction), complicating delivery O62.4

Bangkok hemorrhagic fever A91

Bang's disease (brucella abortus) A23.1

Bankruptcy, anxiety concerning Z59.8

Bannister's disease T78.3 ☑
- hereditary D84.1

Banti's disease or syndrome (with cirrhosis) (with portal hypertension) K76.6

Bar, median, prostate — *see* Enlargement, enlarged, prostate

Barcoo disease or rot — *see* Ulcer, skin

Barlow's disease E54

Barodontalgia T70.29 ☑

Baron Münchausen syndrome — *see* Disorder, factitious

Barosinusitis T70.1 ☑

Barotitis T70.0 ☑

Barotrauma T70.29 ☑
- odontalgia T70.29 ☑
- otitic T70.0 ☑
- sinus T70.1 ☑

Barraquer (-Simons) **disease or syndrome** (progressive lipodystrophy) E88.1

Barré-Guillain disease or syndrome G61.0

Barrel chest M95.4

Barré-Liéou syndrome (posterior cervical sympathetic) M53.0

Barrett's
- disease — *see* Barrett's, esophagus
- esophagus K22.70
  - with dysplasia K22.719
    - high grade K22.711
    - low grade K22.710
  - without dysplasia K22.70
- syndrome — *see* Barrett's, esophagus
- ulcer K22.10
  - with bleeding K22.11
  - without bleeding K22.10

Bársony (-Polgár) (-Teschendorf) **syndrome** (corkscrew esophagus) K22.4

Barth syndrome E78.71

Bartholinitis (suppurating) N75.8
- gonococcal (acute) (chronic) (with abscess) A54.1

Bartonellosis A44.9
- cutaneous A44.1
- mucocutaneous A44.1
- specified NEC A44.8
- systemic A44.0

Barton's fracture S52.56- ☑

Bartter's syndrome E26.81

Basal — *see* condition

Basan's (hidrotic) ectodermal dysplasia Q82.4

Baseball finger — *see* Dislocation, finger

Basedow's disease (exophthalmic goiter) — *see* Hyperthyroidism, with, goiter

Basic — *see* condition

Basilar — *see* condition

Bason's (hidrotic) ectodermal dysplasia Q82.4

Basopenia — *see* Agranulocytosis

Basophilia D72.824

Basophilism (cortico-adrenal) (Cushing's) (pituitary) E24.0

Bassen-Kornzweig disease or syndrome E78.6

Bat ear Q17.5

Bateman's
- disease B08.1
- purpura (senile) D69.2

Bathing cramp T75.1 ☑

Bathophobia F40.248

Batten (-Mayou) **disease** E75.4
- retina E75.4 *[H36]*

Batten-Steinert syndrome G71.11
Battered — *see* Maltreatment
Battey Mycobacterium infection A31.Ø
Battle exhaustion F43.Ø
Battledore placenta O43.19- ☑
Baumgarten-Cruveilhier cirrhosis, disease or syndrome K74.69
Bauxite fibrosis (of lung) J63.1
Bayle's disease (general paresis) A52.17
Bazin's disease (primary) (tuberculous) A18.4
Beach ear — *see* Swimmer's, ear
Beaded hair (congenital) Q84.1
Béal conjunctivitis or syndrome B3Ø.2
Beard's disease (neurasthenia) F48.8
Beat(s)
- atrial, premature I49.1
- ectopic I49.49
- elbow — *see* Bursitis, elbow
- escaped, heart I49.49
- hand — *see* Bursitis, hand
- knee — *see* Bursitis, knee
- premature I49.4Ø
  - atrial I49.1
  - auricular I49.1
  - supraventricular I49.1

Beau's
- disease or syndrome — *see* Degeneration, myocardial
- lines (transverse furrows on fingernails) L6Ø.4

Bechterev's syndrome — *see* Spondylitis, ankylosing
Becker's
- cardiomyopathy I42.8
- disease
  - idiopathic mural endomyocardial disease I42.3
  - myotonia congenita, recessive form G71.12
- dystrophy G71.Ø1
- pigmented hairy nevus D22.5

Beck's syndrome (anterior spinal artery occlusion) I65.8
Beckwith-Wiedemann syndrome Q87.3
Bed confinement status Z74.Ø1
Bed sore — *see* Ulcer, pressure, by site
Bedbug bite(s) — *see* Bite(s), by site, superficial, insect
Bedclothes, asphyxiation or suffocation by — *see* Asphyxia, traumatic, due to, mechanical, trapped
Bednar's
- aphthae K12.Ø
- tumor — *see* Neoplasm, malignant, by site

Bedridden Z74.Ø1
Bedsore — *see* Ulcer, pressure, by site
Bedwetting — *see* Enuresis
Bee sting (with allergic or anaphylactic shock) — *see* Toxicity, venom, arthropod, bee
Beer drinker's heart (disease) I42.6
Begbie's disease (exophthalmic goiter) — *see* Hyperthyroidism, with, goiter
Behavior
- antisocial
  - adult Z72.811
  - child or adolescent Z72.81Ø
- disorder, disturbance — *see* Disorder, conduct
- disruptive — *see* Disorder, conduct
- drug seeking Z76.5
- inexplicable R46.2
- marked evasiveness R46.5
- obsessive-compulsive R46.81
- overactivity R46.3
- poor responsiveness R46.4
- self-damaging (life-style) Z72.89
- sleep-incompatible Z72.821
- slowness R46.4
- specified NEC R46.89
- strange (and inexplicable) R46.2
- suspiciousness R46.5
- type A pattern Z73.1
- undue concern or preoccupation with stressful events R46.6
- verbosity and circumstantial detail obscuring reason for contact R46.7

Behçet's disease or syndrome M35.2
Behr's disease — *see* Degeneration, macula
Beigel's disease or morbus (white piedra) B36.2
Bejel A65
Bekhterev's syndrome — *see* Spondylitis, ankylosing
Belching — *see* Eructation
Bell's
- mania F3Ø.8
- palsy, paralysis G51.Ø
  - infant or newborn P11.3

Bell's — *continued*
- spasm G51.3- ☑

Bence Jones albuminuria or proteinuria NEC R8Ø.3
Bends T7Ø.3 ☑
Benedikt's paralysis or syndrome G46.3
Benign — *see also* condition
- prostatic hyperplasia — *see* Hyperplasia, prostate

Bennett's fracture (displaced) S62.21- ☑
Benson's disease — *see* Deposit, crystalline
Bent
- back (hysterical) F44.4
- nose M95.Ø
  - congenital Q67.4

Bereavement (uncomplicated) Z63.4
Bergeron's disease (hysterical chorea) F44.4
Berger's disease — *see* Nephropathy, IgA
Beriberi (dry) E51.11
- heart (disease) E51.12
- polyneuropathy E51.11
- wet E51.12
  - involving circulatory system E51.11

Berlin's disease or edema (traumatic) SØ5.8X- ☑
Berlock (berloque) **dermatitis** L56.2
Bernard-Horner syndrome G9Ø.2
Bernard-Soulier disease or thrombopathia D69.1
Bernhardt (-Roth) **disease** — *see* Mononeuropathy, lower limb, meralgia paresthetica
Bernheim's syndrome — *see* Failure, heart, right
Bertielliasis B71.8
Berylliosis (lung) J63.2
Besnier-Boeck (-Schaumann) **disease** — *see* Sarcoidosis
Besnier's
- lupus pernio D86.3
- prurigo L2Ø.Ø

Bestiality F65.89
Best's disease H35.5Ø
Betalipoproteinemia, broad or floating E78.2
Beta-mercaptolactate-cysteine disulfiduria E72.Ø9
Betting and gambling Z72.6
- pathological (compulsive) F63.Ø

Bezoar T18.9 ☑
- intestine T18.3 ☑
- stomach T18.2 ☑

Bezold's abscess — *see* Mastoiditis, acute
Bianchi's syndrome R48.8
Bicornate or bicornis uterus Q51.3
- in pregnancy or childbirth O34.ØØ
  - causing obstructed labor O65.5

Bicuspid aortic valve Q23.1
Biedl-Bardet syndrome Q87.89
Bielschowsky (-Jansky) disease E75.4
Biermer's (pernicious) anemia or disease D51.Ø
Biett's disease L93.Ø
Bifid (congenital)
- apex, heart Q24.8
- clitoris Q52.6
- kidney Q63.8
- nose Q3Ø.2
- patella Q74.1
- scrotum Q55.29
- toe NEC Q74.2
- tongue Q38.3
- ureter Q62.8
- uterus Q51.3
- uvula Q35.7

Biforis uterus (suprasimplex) Q51.3
Bifurcation (congenital)
- gallbladder Q44.1
- kidney pelvis Q63.8
- renal pelvis Q63.8
- rib Q76.6
- tongue, congenital Q38.3
- trachea Q32.1
- ureter Q62.8
- urethra Q64.74
- vertebra Q76.49

Big spleen syndrome D73.1
Bigeminal pulse RØØ.8
Bilateral — *see* condition
Bile
- duct — *see* condition
- pigments in urine R82.2

Bilharziasis — *see also* Schistosomiasis
- chyluria B65.Ø
- cutaneous B65.3
- galacturia B65.Ø
- hematochyluria B65.Ø

Bilharziasis — *continued*
- intestinal B65.1
- lipemia B65.9
- lipuria B65.Ø
- oriental B65.2
- piarhemia B65.9
- pulmonary NOS B65.9 *[J99]*
  - pneumonia B65.9 *[J17]*
- tropical hematuria B65.Ø
- vesical B65.Ø

Biliary — *see* condition
Bilirubin metabolism disorder E8Ø.7
- specified NEC E8Ø.6

Bilirubinemia, familial nonhemolytic E8Ø.4
Bilirubinuria R82.2
Biliuria R82.2
Bilocular stomach K31.2
Binswanger's disease I67.3
Biparta, bipartite
- carpal scaphoid Q74.Ø
- patella Q74.1
- vagina Q52.1Ø

Bird
- face Q75.8
- fancier's disease or lung J67.2

Birth
- complications in mother — *see* Delivery, complicated
- compression during NOS P15.9
- defect — *see* Anomaly
- immature (less than 37 completed weeks) — *see* Preterm, newborn
  - extremely (less than 28 completed weeks) — *see* Immaturity, extreme
- inattention, at or after — *see* Maltreatment, child, neglect
- injury NOS P15.9
  - basal ganglia P11.1
  - brachial plexus NEC P14.3
  - brain (compression) (pressure) P11.2
  - central nervous system NOS P11.9
  - cerebellum P11.1
  - cerebral hemorrhage P1Ø.1
  - external genitalia P15.5
  - eye P15.3
  - face P15.4
  - fracture
    - bone P13.9
      - specified NEC P13.8
    - clavicle P13.4
    - femur P13.2
    - humerus P13.3
    - long bone, except femur P13.3
    - radius and ulna P13.3
    - skull P13.Ø
    - spine P11.5
    - tibia and fibula P13.3
  - intracranial P11.2
    - laceration or hemorrhage P1Ø.9
      - specified NEC P1Ø.8
  - intraventricular hemorrhage P1Ø.2
  - laceration
    - brain P1Ø.1
    - by scalpel P15.8
    - peripheral nerve P14.9
  - liver P15.Ø
  - meninges
    - brain P11.1
    - spinal cord P11.5
  - nerve
    - brachial plexus P14.3
    - cranial NEC (except facial) P11.4
    - facial P11.3
    - peripheral P14.9
    - phrenic (paralysis) P14.2
  - paralysis
    - facial nerve P11.3
    - spinal P11.5
  - penis P15.5
  - rupture
    - spinal cord P11.5
  - scalp P12.9
  - scalpel wound P15.8
  - scrotum P15.5
  - skull NEC P13.1
    - fracture P13.Ø
  - specified type NEC P15.8
  - spinal cord P11.5
  - spine P11.5

- **Birth** — *continued*
  - injury — *continued*
    - spleen P15.1
    - sternomastoid (hematoma) P15.2
    - subarachnoid hemorrhage P10.3
    - subcutaneous fat necrosis P15.6
    - subdural hemorrhage P10.0
    - tentorial tear P10.4
    - testes P15.5
    - vulva P15.5
  - lack of care, at or after — *see* Maltreatment, child, neglect
  - neglect, at or after — *see* Maltreatment, child, neglect
  - palsy or paralysis, newborn, NOS (birth injury) P14.9
  - premature (infant) — *see* Preterm, newborn
  - shock, newborn P96.89
  - trauma — *see* Birth, injury
  - weight
    - low (2499 grams or less) — *see* Low, birthweight
      - extremely (999 grams or less) — *see* Low, birthweight, extreme
    - 4000 grams to 4499 grams P08.1
    - 4500 grams or more P08.0
- **Birthmark** Q82.5
- **Birt-Hogg-Dube syndrome** Q87.89
- **Bisalbuminemia** E88.09
- **Biskra's button** B55.1
- **Bite**(s) (animal) (human)
  - abdomen, abdominal
    - wall S31.159 ☑
      - with penetration into peritoneal cavity S31.659 ☑
      - epigastric region S31.152 ☑
        - with penetration into peritoneal cavity S31.652 ☑
      - left
        - lower quadrant S31.154 ☑
          - with penetration into peritoneal cavity S31.654 ☑
        - upper quadrant S31.151 ☑
          - with penetration into peritoneal cavity S31.651 ☑
      - periumbilic region S31.155 ☑
        - with penetration into peritoneal cavity S31.655 ☑
      - right
        - lower quadrant S31.153 ☑
          - with penetration into peritoneal cavity S31.653 ☑
        - upper quadrant S31.150 ☑
          - with penetration into peritoneal cavity S31.650 ☑
      - superficial NEC S30.871 ☑
        - insect S30.861 ☑
  - alveolar (process) — *see* Bite, oral cavity
  - amphibian (venomous) — *see* Venom, bite, amphibian
  - animal — *see also* Bite, by site
    - venomous — *see* Venom
  - ankle S91.05- ☑
    - superficial NEC S90.57- ☑
      - insect S90.56- ☑
  - antecubital space — *see* Bite, elbow
  - anus S31.835 ☑
    - superficial NEC S30.877 ☑
      - insect S30.867 ☑
  - arm (upper) S41.15- ☑
    - lower — *see* Bite, forearm
    - superficial NEC S40.87- ☑
      - insect S40.86- ☑
  - arthropod NEC — *see* Venom, bite, arthropod
  - auditory canal (external) (meatus) — *see* Bite, ear
  - auricle, ear — *see* Bite, ear
  - axilla — *see* Bite, arm
  - back — *see also* Bite, thorax, back
    - lower S31.050 ☑
      - with penetration into retroperitoneal space S31.051 ☑
      - superficial NEC S30.870 ☑
        - insect S30.860 ☑
  - bedbug — *see* Bite(s), by site, superficial, insect
  - breast S21.05- ☑
    - superficial NEC S20.17- ☑
      - insect S20.16- ☑
  - brow — *see* Bite, head, specified site NEC
  - buttock S31.805 ☑
    - left S31.825 ☑
    - right S31.815 ☑

- **Bite**(s) — *continued*
  - buttock — *continued*
    - superficial NEC S30.870 ☑
      - insect S30.860 ☑
  - calf — *see* Bite, leg
  - canaliculus lacrimalis — *see* Bite, eyelid
  - canthus, eye — *see* Bite, eyelid
  - centipede — *see* Toxicity, venom, arthropod, centipede
  - cheek (external) S01.45- ☑
    - internal — *see* Bite, oral cavity
    - superficial NEC S00.87 ☑
      - insect S00.86 ☑
  - chest wall — *see* Bite, thorax
  - chigger B88.0
  - chin — *see* Bite, head, specified site NEC
  - clitoris — *see* Bite, vulva
  - costal region — *see* Bite, thorax
  - digit(s)
    - hand — *see* Bite, finger
    - toe — *see* Bite, toe
  - ear (canal) (external) S01.35- ☑
    - superficial NEC S00.47- ☑
      - insect S00.46- ☑
  - elbow S51.05- ☑
    - superficial NEC S50.37- ☑
      - insect S50.36- ☑
  - epididymis — *see* Bite, testis
  - epigastric region — *see* Bite, abdomen
  - epiglottis — *see* Bite, neck, specified site NEC
  - esophagus, cervical S11.25 ☑
    - superficial NEC S10.17 ☑
      - insect S10.16 ☑
  - eyebrow — *see* Bite, eyelid
  - eyelid S01.15- ☑
    - superficial NEC S00.27- ☑
      - insect S00.26- ☑
  - face NEC — *see* Bite, head, specified site NEC
  - finger(s) S61.259 ☑
    - with
      - damage to nail S61.359 ☑
    - index S61.258 ☑
      - with
        - damage to nail S61.358 ☑
      - left S61.251 ☑
        - with
          - damage to nail S61.351 ☑
      - right S61.250 ☑
        - with
          - damage to nail S61.350 ☑
      - superficial NEC S60.478 ☑
        - insect S60.46- ☑
    - little S61.25- ☑
      - with
        - damage to nail S61.35- ☑
      - superficial NEC S60.47- ☑
        - insect S60.46- ☑
    - middle S61.25- ☑
      - with
        - damage to nail S61.35- ☑
      - superficial NEC S60.47- ☑
        - insect S60.46- ☑
    - ring S61.25- ☑
      - with
        - damage to nail S61.35- ☑
      - superficial NEC S60.47- ☑
        - insect S60.46- ☑
    - superficial NEC S60.479 ☑
      - insect S60.469 ☑
    - thumb — *see* Bite, thumb
  - flank — *see* Bite, abdomen, wall
  - flea — *see* Bite, by site, superficial, insect
  - foot (except toe(s) alone) S91.35- ☑
    - superficial NEC S90.87- ☑
      - insect S90.86- ☑
    - toe — *see* Bite, toe
  - forearm S51.85- ☑
    - elbow only — *see* Bite, elbow
    - superficial NEC S50.87- ☑
      - insect S50.86- ☑
  - forehead — *see* Bite, head, specified site NEC
  - genital organs, external
    - female S31.552 ☑
      - superficial NEC S30.876 ☑
        - insect S30.866 ☑
      - vagina and vulva — *see* Bite, vulva
    - male S31.551 ☑

- **Bite**(s) — *continued*
  - genital organs, external — *continued*
    - male — *continued*
      - penis — *see* Bite, penis
      - scrotum — *see* Bite, scrotum
      - superficial NEC S30.875 ☑
        - insect S30.865 ☑
      - testes — *see* Bite, testis
  - groin — *see* Bite, abdomen, wall
  - gum — *see* Bite, oral cavity
  - hand S61.45- ☑
    - finger — *see* Bite, finger
    - superficial NEC S60.57- ☑
      - insect S60.56- ☑
    - thumb — *see* Bite, thumb
  - head S01.95 ☑
    - cheek — *see* Bite, cheek
    - ear — *see* Bite, ear
    - eyelid — *see* Bite, eyelid
    - lip — *see* Bite, lip
    - nose — *see* Bite, nose
    - oral cavity — *see* Bite, oral cavity
    - scalp — *see* Bite, scalp
    - specified site NEC S01.85 ☑
      - superficial NEC S00.87 ☑
        - insect S00.86 ☑
    - superficial NEC S00.97 ☑
      - insect S00.96 ☑
    - temporomandibular area — *see* Bite, cheek
  - heel — *see* Bite, foot
  - hip S71.05- ☑
    - superficial NEC S70.27- ☑
      - insect S70.26- ☑
  - hymen S31.45 ☑
  - hypochondrium — *see* Bite, abdomen, wall
  - hypogastric region — *see* Bite, abdomen, wall
  - inguinal region — *see* Bite, abdomen, wall
  - insect — *see* Bite, by site, superficial, insect
  - instep — *see* Bite, foot
  - interscapular region — *see* Bite, thorax, back
  - jaw — *see* Bite, head, specified site NEC
  - knee S81.05- ☑
    - superficial NEC S80.27- ☑
      - insect S80.26- ☑
  - labium (majus) (minus) — *see* Bite, vulva
  - lacrimal duct — *see* Bite, eyelid
  - larynx S11.015 ☑
    - superficial NEC S10.17 ☑
      - insect S10.16 ☑
  - leg (lower) S81.85- ☑
    - ankle — *see* Bite, ankle
    - foot — *see* Bite, foot
    - knee — *see* Bite, knee
    - superficial NEC S80.87- ☑
      - insect S80.86- ☑
    - toe — *see* Bite, toe
    - upper — *see* Bite, thigh
  - lip S01.551 ☑
    - superficial NEC S00.571 ☑
      - insect S00.561 ☑
  - lizard (venomous) — *see* Venom, bite, reptile
  - loin — *see* Bite, abdomen, wall
  - lower back — *see* Bite, back, lower
  - lumbar region — *see* Bite, back, lower
  - malar region — *see* Bite, head, specified site NEC
  - mammary — *see* Bite, breast
  - marine animals (venomous) — *see* Toxicity, venom, marine animal
  - mastoid region — *see* Bite, head, specified site NEC
  - mouth — *see* Bite, oral cavity
  - nail
    - finger — *see* Bite, finger
    - toe — *see* Bite, toe
  - nape — *see* Bite, neck, specified site NEC
  - nasal (septum) (sinus) — *see* Bite, nose
  - nasopharynx — *see* Bite, head, specified site NEC
  - neck S11.95 ☑
    - involving
      - cervical esophagus — *see* Bite, esophagus, cervical
      - larynx — *see* Bite, larynx
      - pharynx — *see* Bite, pharynx
      - thyroid gland S11.15 ☑
      - trachea — *see* Bite, trachea
    - specified site NEC S11.85 ☑
      - superficial NEC S10.87 ☑

- **Bite**(s) — *continued*
  - neck — *continued*
    - specified site — *continued*
      - superficial — *continued*
        - insect S10.86 ☑
    - superficial NEC S10.97 ☑
      - insect S10.96 ☑
    - throat S11.85 ☑
      - superficial NEC S10.17 ☑
        - insect S10.16 ☑
  - nose (septum) (sinus) S01.25 ☑
    - superficial NEC S00.37 ☑
      - insect S00.36 ☑
  - occipital region — *see* Bite, scalp
  - oral cavity S01.552 ☑
    - superficial NEC S00.572 ☑
      - insect S00.562 ☑
  - orbital region — *see* Bite, eyelid
  - palate — *see* Bite, oral cavity
  - palm — *see* Bite, hand
  - parietal region — *see* Bite, scalp
  - pelvis S31.050 ☑
    - with penetration into retroperitoneal space S31.051 ☑
    - superficial NEC S30.870 ☑
      - insect S30.860 ☑
  - penis S31.25 ☑
    - superficial NEC S30.872 ☑
      - insect S30.862 ☑
  - perineum
    - female — *see* Bite, vulva
    - male — *see* Bite, pelvis
  - periocular area (with or without lacrimal passages) — *see* Bite, eyelid
  - phalanges
    - finger — *see* Bite, finger
    - toe — *see* Bite, toe
  - pharynx S11.25 ☑
    - superficial NEC S10.17 ☑
      - insect S10.16 ☑
  - pinna — *see* Bite, ear
  - poisonous — *see* Venom
  - popliteal space — *see* Bite, knee
  - prepuce — *see* Bite, penis
  - pubic region — *see* Bite, abdomen, wall
  - rectovaginal septum — *see* Bite, vulva
  - red bug B88.0
  - reptile NEC — *see also* Venom, bite, reptile
    - nonvenomous — *see* Bite, by site
    - snake — *see* Venom, bite, snake
  - sacral region — *see* Bite, back, lower
  - sacroiliac region — *see* Bite, back, lower
  - salivary gland — *see* Bite, oral cavity
  - scalp S01.05 ☑
    - superficial NEC S00.07 ☑
      - insect S00.06 ☑
  - scapular region — *see* Bite, shoulder
  - scrotum S31.35 ☑
    - superficial NEC S30.873 ☑
      - insect S30.863 ☑
  - sea-snake (venomous) — *see* Toxicity, venom, snake, sea snake
  - shin — *see* Bite, leg
  - shoulder S41.05- ☑
    - superficial NEC S40.27- ☑
      - insect S40.26- ☑
  - snake — *see also* Venom, bite, snake
    - nonvenomous — *see* Bite, by site
  - spermatic cord — *see* Bite, testis
  - spider (venomous) — *see* Toxicity, venom, spider
    - nonvenomous — *see* Bite, by site, superficial, insect
  - sternal region — *see* Bite, thorax, front
  - submaxillary region — *see* Bite, head, specified site NEC
  - submental region — *see* Bite, head, specified site NEC
  - subungual
    - finger(s) — *see* Bite, finger
    - toe — *see* Bite, toe
  - superficial — *see* Bite, by site, superficial
  - supraclavicular fossa S11.85 ☑
  - supraorbital — *see* Bite, head, specified site NEC
  - temple, temporal region — *see* Bite, head, specified site NEC
  - temporomandibular area — *see* Bite, cheek
  - testis S31.35 ☑
    - superficial NEC S30.873 ☑

- **Bite**(s) — *continued*
  - testis — *continued*
    - superficial — *continued*
      - insect S30.863 ☑
  - thigh S71.15- ☑
    - superficial NEC S70.37- ☑
      - insect S70.36- ☑
  - thorax, thoracic (wall) S21.95 ☑
    - back S21.25- ☑
      - with penetration into thoracic cavity S21.45- ☑
    - breast — *see* Bite, breast
    - front S21.15- ☑
      - with penetration into thoracic cavity S21.35- ☑
    - superficial NEC S20.97 ☑
      - back S20.47- ☑
      - front S20.37- ☑
      - insect S20.96 ☑
        - back S20.46- ☑
        - front S20.36- ☑
  - throat — *see* Bite, neck, throat
  - thumb S61.05- ☑
    - with
      - damage to nail S61.15- ☑
    - superficial NEC S60.37- ☑
      - insect S60.36- ☑
  - thyroid S11.15 ☑
    - superficial NEC S10.87 ☑
      - insect S10.86 ☑
  - toe(s) S91.15- ☑
    - with
      - damage to nail S91.25- ☑
    - great S91.15- ☑
      - with
        - damage to nail S91.25- ☑
    - lesser S91.15- ☑
      - with
        - damage to nail S91.25- ☑
    - superficial NEC S90.47- ☑
      - great S90.47- ☑
      - insect S90.46- ☑
        - great S90.46- ☑
  - tongue S01.552 ☑
  - trachea S11.025 ☑
    - superficial NEC S10.17 ☑
      - insect S10.16 ☑
  - tunica vaginalis — *see* Bite, testis
  - tympanum, tympanic membrane — *see* Bite, ear
  - umbilical region S31.155 ☑
  - uvula — *see* Bite, oral cavity
  - vagina — *see* Bite, vulva
  - venomous — *see* Venom
  - vocal cords S11.035 ☑
    - superficial NEC S10.17 ☑
      - insect S10.16 ☑
  - vulva S31.45 ☑
    - superficial NEC S30.874 ☑
      - insect S30.864 ☑
  - wrist S61.55- ☑
    - superficial NEC S60.87- ☑
      - insect S60.86- ☑
- **Biting, cheek or lip** K13.1
- **Biventricular failure** (heart) I50.82
- **Björck** (-Thorson) **syndrome** (malignant carcinoid) E34.0
- **Black**
  - death A20.9
  - eye S00.1- ☑
  - hairy tongue K14.3
  - heel (foot) S90.3- ☑
  - lung (disease) J60
  - palm (hand) S60.22- ☑
- **Blackfan-Diamond anemia or syndrome** (congenital hypoplastic anemia) D61.01
- **Blackhead** L70.0
- **Blackout** R55
- **Bladder** — *see* condition
- **Blast** (air) (hydraulic) (immersion) (underwater)
  - blindness S05.8X- ☑
  - injury
    - abdomen or thorax — *see* Injury, by site
    - ear (acoustic nerve trauma) — *see* Injury, nerve, acoustic, specified type NEC
  - syndrome NEC T70.8 ☑
- **Blastoma** — *see* Neoplasm, malignant, by site
  - pulmonary — *see* Neoplasm, lung, malignant
- **Blastomycosis, blastomycotic** B40.9
  - Brazilian — *see* Paracoccidioidomycosis

- **Blastomycosis, blastomycotic** — *continued*
  - cutaneous B40.3
  - disseminated B40.7
  - European — *see* Cryptococcosis
  - generalized B40.7
  - keloidal B48.0
  - North American B40.9
  - primary pulmonary B40.0
  - pulmonary B40.2
    - acute B40.0
    - chronic B40.1
  - skin B40.3
  - South American — *see* Paracoccidioidomycosis
  - specified NEC B40.89
- **Bleb**(s) R23.8
  - emphysematous (lung) (solitary) J43.9
  - endophthalmitis H59.43
  - filtering (vitreous), after glaucoma surgery Z98.83
  - inflammed (infected), postprocedural H59.40
    - stage 1 H59.41
    - stage 2 H59.42
    - stage 3 H59.43
  - lung (ruptured) J43.9
    - congenital — *see* Atelectasis
    - newborn P25.8
  - subpleural (emphysematous) J43.9
- **Blebitis, postprocedural** H59.40
  - stage 1 H59.41
  - stage 2 H59.42
  - stage 3 H59.43
- **Bleeder** (familial) (hereditary) — *see* Hemophilia
- **Bleeding** — *see also* Hemorrhage
  - anal K62.5
  - anovulatory N97.0
  - atonic, following delivery O72.1
  - capillary I78.8
    - puerperal O72.2
  - contact (postcoital) N93.0
  - due to uterine subinvolution N85.3
  - ear — *see* Otorrhagia
  - excessive, associated with menopausal onset N92.4
  - familial — *see* Defect, coagulation
  - following intercourse N93.0
  - gastrointestinal K92.2
  - hemorrhoids — *see* Hemorrhoids
  - intermenstrual (regular) N92.3
    - irregular N92.1
  - intraoperative — *see* Complication, intraoperative, hemorrhage
  - irregular N92.6
  - menopausal N92.4
  - newborn, intraventricular — *see* Newborn, affected by, hemorrhage, intraventricular
  - nipple N64.59
  - nose R04.0
  - ovulation N92.3
  - perimenopausal N92.4
  - postclimacteric N95.0
  - postcoital N93.0
  - postmenopausal N95.0
  - postoperative — *see* Complication, postprocedural, hemorrhage
  - preclimacteric N92.4
  - pre-pubertal vaginal N93.1
  - puberty (excessive, with onset of menstrual periods) N92.2
  - rectum, rectal K62.5
    - newborn P54.2
  - tendencies — *see* Defect, coagulation
  - throat R04.1
  - tooth socket (post-extraction) K91.840
  - umbilical stump P51.9
  - uterus, uterine NEC N93.9
    - climacteric N92.4
    - dysfunctional or functional N93.8
    - menopausal N92.4
    - preclimacteric or premenopausal N92.4
    - unrelated to menstrual cycle N93.9
  - vagina, vaginal (abnormal) N93.9
    - dysfunctional or functional N93.8
    - newborn P54.6
    - pre-pubertal N93.1
  - vicarious N94.89
- **Blennorrhagia, blennorrhagic** — *see* Gonorrhea
- **Blennorrhea** (acute) (chronic) — *see also* Gonorrhea
  - inclusion (neonatal) (newborn) P39.1
  - lower genitourinary tract (gonococcal) A54.00
  - neonatorum (gonococcal ophthalmia) A54.31

- **Block, blocked** — *continued*
  - bundle-branch — *continued*
    - bilateral I45.2
    - left I44.7
      - with right bundle branch block I45.2
      - hemiblock I44.60
        - anterior I44.4
        - posterior I44.5
      - incomplete I44.7
        - with right bundle branch block I45.2
    - right I45.10
      - with
        - left bundle branch block I45.2
        - left fascicular block I45.2
      - specified NEC I45.19
    - Wilson's type I45.19
  - cardiac I45.9
  - conduction I45.9
    - complete I44.2
  - fascicular (left) I44.60
    - anterior I44.4
    - posterior I44.5
    - right I45.0
    - specified NEC I44.69
  - foramen Magendie (acquired) G91.1
    - congenital Q03.1
      - with spina bifida — *see* Spina bifida, by site, with hydrocephalus
  - heart I45.9
    - bundle branch I45.4
      - bilateral I45.2
    - complete (atrioventricular) I44.2
    - congenital Q24.6
    - first degree (atrioventricular) I44.0
    - second degree (atrioventricular) I44.1
    - specified type NEC I45.5
    - third degree (atrioventricular) I44.2
  - hepatic vein I82.0
  - intraventricular (nonspecific) I45.4
    - bundle branch
      - bilateral I45.2
  - kidney N28.9
    - postcystoscopic or postprocedural N99.0
  - Mobitz (types I and II) I44.1
  - myocardial — *see* Block, heart
  - nodal I45.5
  - organ or site, congenital NEC — *see* Atresia, by site
  - portal (vein) I81
  - second degree (types I and II) I44.1
  - sinoatrial I45.5
  - sinoauricular I45.5
  - third degree I44.2
  - trifascicular I45.3
  - tubal N97.1
  - vein NOS I82.90
  - Wenckebach (types I and II) I44.1
- **Blockage** — *see* Obstruction
- **Blocq's disease** F44.4
- **Blood**
  - constituents, abnormal R78.9
  - disease D75.9
  - donor — *see* Donor, blood
  - dyscrasia D75.9
    - with
      - abortion — *see* Abortion, by type, complicated by, hemorrhage
      - ectopic pregnancy O08.1
      - molar pregnancy O08.1
    - following ectopic or molar pregnancy O08.1
    - newborn P61.9
    - puerperal, postpartum O72.3
  - flukes NEC — *see* Schistosomiasis
  - in
    - feces K92.1
      - occult R19.5
    - urine — *see* Hematuria
  - mole O02.0
  - occult in feces R19.5
  - pressure
    - decreased, due to shock following injury T79.4 ☑
    - examination only Z01.30
    - fluctuating I99.8
    - high — *see* Hypertension
      - borderline R03.0
      - incidental reading, without diagnosis of hypertension R03.0
    - low — *see also* Hypotension
      - incidental reading, without diagnosis of hypotension R03.1
  - spitting — *see* Hemoptysis
  - staining cornea — *see* Pigmentation, cornea, stromal
  - transfusion
    - reaction or complication — *see* Complications, transfusion
  - type
    - A (Rh positive) Z67.10
      - Rh negative Z67.11
    - AB (Rh positive) Z67.30
      - Rh negative Z67.31
    - B (Rh positive) Z67.20
      - Rh negative Z67.21
    - O (Rh positive) Z67.40
      - Rh negative Z67.41
    - Rh (positive) Z67.90
      - negative Z67.91
  - vessel rupture — *see* Hemorrhage
  - vomiting — *see* Hematemesis
- **Blood-forming organs, disease** D75.9
- **Bloodgood's disease** — *see* Mastopathy, cystic
- **Bloom** (-Machacek)(-Torre) **syndrome** Q82.8
- **Blount disease or osteochondrosis** M92.51- ☑
- **Blue**
  - baby Q24.9
  - diaper syndrome E72.09
  - dome cyst (breast) — *see* Cyst, breast
  - dot cataract Q12.0
  - nevus D22.9
  - sclera Q13.5
    - with fragility of bone and deafness Q78.0
  - toe syndrome I75.02- ☑
- **Blueness** — *see* Cyanosis
- **Blues, postpartal** O90.6
  - baby O90.6
- **Blurring, visual** H53.8
- **Blushing** (abnormal) (excessive) R23.2
- **BMI** — *see* Body, mass index
- **Boarder, hospital NEC** Z76.4
  - accompanying sick person Z76.3
  - healthy infant or child Z76.2
    - foundling Z76.1
- **Bockhart's impetigo** L01.02
- **Bodechtel-Guttman disease** (subacute sclerosing panencephalitis) A81.1
- **Boder-Sedgwick syndrome** (ataxia-telangiectasia) G11.3
- **Body, bodies**
  - Aschoff's — *see* Myocarditis, rheumatic
  - asteroid, vitreous — *see* Deposit, crystalline
  - cytoid (retina) — *see* Occlusion, artery, retina
  - drusen (degenerative) (macula) (retinal) — *see also* Degeneration, macula, drusen
    - optic disc — *see* Drusen, optic disc
  - foreign — *see* Foreign body
  - loose
    - joint, except knee — *see* Loose, body, joint
      - knee M23.4- ☑
    - sheath, tendon — *see* Disorder, tendon, specified type NEC
  - mass index (BMI)
    - adult
      - 19.9 or less Z68.1
      - 20.0-20.9 Z68.20
      - 21.0-21.9 Z68.21
      - 22.0-22.9 Z68.22
      - 23.0-23.9 Z68.23
      - 24.0-24.9 Z68.24
      - 25.0-25.9 Z68.25
      - 26.0-26.9 Z68.26
      - 27.0-27.9 Z68.27
      - 28.0-28.9 Z68.28
      - 29.0-29.9 Z68.29
      - 30.0-30.9 Z68.30
      - 31.0-31.9 Z68.31
      - 32.0-32.9 Z68.32
      - 33.0-33.9 Z68.33
      - 34.0-34.9 Z68.34
      - 35.0-35.9 Z68.35
      - 36.0-36.9 Z68.36
      - 37.0-37.9 Z68.37
      - 38.0-38.9 Z68.38
      - 39.0-39.9 Z68.39
      - 40.0-44.9 Z68.41
      - 45.0-49.9 Z68.42
      - 50.0-59.9 Z68.43
      - 60.0-69.9 Z68.44
      - 70 and over Z68.45
    - pediatric
      - 5th percentile to less than 85th percentile for age Z68.52
      - 85th percentile to less than 95th percentile for age Z68.53
      - greater than or equal to ninety-fifth percentile for age Z68.54
      - less than fifth percentile for age Z68.51
  - Mooser's A75.2
  - rice — *see also* Loose, body, joint
    - knee M23.4- ☑
  - rocking F98.4
- **Boeck's**
  - disease or sarcoid — *see* Sarcoidosis
  - lupoid (miliary) D86.3
- **Boerhaave's syndrome** (spontaneous esophageal rupture) K22.3
- **Boggy**
  - cervix N88.8
  - uterus N85.8
- **Boil** — *see also* Furuncle, by site
  - Aleppo B55.1
  - Baghdad B55.1
  - Delhi B55.1
  - lacrimal
    - gland — *see* Dacryoadenitis
    - passages (duct) (sac) — *see* Inflammation, lacrimal, passages, acute
  - Natal B55.1
  - orbit, orbital — *see* Abscess, orbit
  - tropical B55.1
- **Bold hives** — *see* Urticaria
- **Bombé, iris** — *see* Membrane, pupillary
- **Bone** — *see* condition
- **Bonnevie-Ullrich syndrome** — *see also* Turner's syndrome Q87.19
- **Bonnier's syndrome** H81.8 ☑
- **Bonvale dam fever** T73.3 ☑
- **Bony block of joint** — *see* Ankylosis
- **BOOP** (bronchiolitis obliterans organized pneumonia) J84.89
- **Borderline**
  - diabetes mellitus R73.03
  - hypertension R03.0
  - osteopenia M85.8- ☑
  - pelvis, with obstruction during labor O65.1
  - personality F60.3
- **Borna disease** A83.9
- **Bornholm disease** B33.0
- **Boston exanthem** A88.0
- **Botalli, ductus** (patent) (persistent) Q25.0
- **Bothriocephalus latus infestation** B70.0
- **Botulism** (foodborne intoxication) A05.1
  - infant A48.51
  - non-foodborne A48.52
  - wound A48.52
- **Bouba** — *see* Yaws
- **Bouchard's nodes** (with arthropathy) M15.2
- **Bouffée délirante** F23
- **Bouillaud's disease or syndrome** (rheumatic heart disease) I01.9
- **Bourneville's disease** Q85.1
- **Boutonniere deformity** (finger) — *see* Deformity, finger, boutonniere
- **Bouveret** (-Hoffmann) **syndrome** (paroxysmal tachycardia) I47.9
- **Bovine heart** — *see* Hypertrophy, cardiac
- **Bowel** — *see* condition
- **Bowen's**
  - dermatosis (precancerous) — *see* Neoplasm, skin, in situ
  - disease — *see* Neoplasm, skin, in situ
  - epithelioma — *see* Neoplasm, skin, in situ
  - type
    - epidermoid carcinoma-in-situ — *see* Neoplasm, skin, in situ
    - intraepidermal squamous cell carcinoma — *see* Neoplasm, skin, in situ
- **Bowing**
  - femur — *see also* Deformity, limb, specified type NEC, thigh

- **Bowing** — *continued*
  - femur — *see also* Deformity, limb, specified type, thigh — *continued*
    - congenital Q68.3
  - fibula — *see also* Deformity, limb, specified type NEC, lower leg
    - congenital Q68.4
  - forearm — *see* Deformity, limb, specified type NEC, forearm
  - leg(s), long bones, congenital Q68.5
  - radius — *see* Deformity, limb, specified type NEC, forearm
  - tibia — *see also* Deformity, limb, specified type NEC, lower leg
    - congenital Q68.4
- **Bowleg**(s) (acquired) M21.16- ☑
  - congenital Q68.5
  - rachitic E64.3
- **Boyd's dysentery** AØ3.2
- **Brachial** — *see* condition
- **Brachycardia** RØØ.1
- **Brachycephaly** Q75.Ø
- **Bradley's disease** AØ8.19
- **Bradyarrhythmia, cardiac** I49.8
- **Bradycardia** (sinoatrial) (sinus) (vagal) RØØ.1
  - neonatal P29.12
  - reflex G9Ø.Ø9
  - tachycardia syndrome I49.5
- **Bradykinesia** R25.8
- **Bradypnea** RØ6.89
- **Bradytachycardia** I49.5
- **Brailsford's disease or osteochondrosis** — *see* Osteochondrosis, juvenile, radius
- **Brain** — *see also* condition
  - death G93.82
  - syndrome — *see* Syndrome, brain
- **Branched-chain amino-acid disorder** E71.2
- **Branchial** — *see* condition
  - cartilage, congenital Q18.2
- **Branchiogenic remnant** (in neck) Q18.Ø
- **Brandt's syndrome** (acrodermatitis enteropathica) E83.2
- **Brash** (water) R12
- **Bravais-jacksonian epilepsy** — *see* Epilepsy, localization-related, symptomatic, with simple partial seizures
- **Braxton Hicks contractions** — *see* False, labor
- **Brazilian leishmaniasis** B55.2
- **BRBPR** K62.5
- **Break, retina** (without detachment) H33.3Ø- ☑
  - with retinal detachment — *see* Detachment, retina
  - horseshoe tear H33.31- ☑
  - multiple H33.33- ☑
  - round hole H33.32- ☑
- **Breakdown**
  - device, graft or implant — *see also* Complications, by site and type, mechanical T85.618 ☑
    - arterial graft NEC — *see* Complication, cardiovascular device, mechanical, vascular
    - breast (implant) T85.41 ☑
    - catheter NEC T85.618 ☑
      - cystostomy T83.Ø1Ø ☑
      - dialysis (renal) T82.41 ☑
        - intraperitoneal T85.611 ☑
      - Hopkins T83.Ø18 ☑
      - ileostomy T83.Ø18 ☑
      - infusion NEC T82.514 ☑
        - cranial T85.61Ø- ☑
        - epidural T85.61Ø ☑
        - intrathecal T85.61Ø ☑
        - spinal T85.61Ø ☑
        - subarachnoid T85.61Ø ☑
        - subdural T85.61Ø ☑
      - nephrostomy T83.Ø12 ☑
      - urethral indwelling T83.Ø11 ☑
      - urinary NEC T83.Ø18 ☑
      - urostomy T83.Ø18 ☑
    - electronic (electrode) (pulse generator) (stimulator)
      - bone T84.31Ø ☑
      - cardiac T82.119 ☑
        - electrode T82.11Ø ☑
        - pulse generator T82.111 ☑
        - specified type NEC T82.118 ☑
      - nervous system — *see* Complication, prosthetic device, mechanical, electronic nervous system stimulator
      - urinary — *see* Complication, genitourinary, device, urinary, mechanical

- **Breakdown** — *continued*
  - device, graft or implant — *see also* Complications, by site and type, mechanical — *continued*
    - fixation, internal (orthopedic) NEC — *see* Complication, fixation device, mechanical
    - gastrointestinal — *see* Complications, prosthetic device, mechanical, gastrointestinal device
    - genital NEC T83.418 ☑
      - intrauterine contraceptive device T83.31 ☑
      - penile prosthesis (cylinder) (implanted) (pump) (resevoir) T83.41Ø ☑
      - testicular prosthesis T83.411 ☑
    - heart NEC — *see* Complication, cardiovascular device, mechanical
    - intrathecal infusion pump T85.615 ☑
    - joint prosthesis — *see* Complications..., joint prosthesis,internal, mechanical, by site
    - nervous system, specified device NEC T85.615 ☑
    - ocular NEC — *see* Complications, prosthetic device, mechanical, ocular device
    - orthopedic NEC — *see* Complication, orthopedic, device, mechanical
    - specified NEC T85.618 ☑
    - subcutaneous device pocket
      - nervous system prosthetic device, implant, or graft T85.89Ø ☑
      - other internal prosthetic device, implant, or graft T85.898 ☑
    - sutures, permanent T85.612 ☑
      - used in bone repair — *see* Complications, fixation device, internal (orthopedic), mechanical
    - urinary NEC T83.118 ☑
      - graft T83.21 ☑
      - sphincter, implanted T83.111 ☑
      - stent (ileal conduit) (nephroureteral) T83.113 ☑
        - ureteral indwelling T83.112 ☑
    - vascular NEC — *see* Complication, cardiovascular device, mechanical
    - ventricular intracranial shunt T85.Ø1 ☑
  - nervous F48.8
  - perineum O9Ø.1
  - respirator J95.85Ø
    - specified NEC J95.859
  - ventilator J95.85Ø
    - specified NEC J95.859
- **Breast** — *see also* condition
  - buds E3Ø.1
    - in newborn P96.89
  - dense R92.2
  - nodule — *see also* Lump, breast N63.Ø
- **Breath**
  - foul R19.6
  - holder, child RØ6.89
  - holding spell RØ6.89
  - shortness RØ6.Ø2
- **Breathing**
  - labored — *see* Hyperventilation
  - mouth RØ6.5
    - causing malocclusion M26.5 ☑
  - periodic RØ6.3
    - high altitude G47.32
- **Breathlessness** RØ6.81
- **Breda's disease** — *see* Yaws
- **Breech presentation** (mother) O32.1 ☑
  - causing obstructed labor O64.1 ☑
  - footling O32.8 ☑
    - causing obstructed labor O64.8 ☑
  - incomplete O32.8 ☑
    - causing obstructed labor O64.8 ☑
- **Breisky's disease** N9Ø.4
- **Brennemann's syndrome** I88.Ø
- **Brenner**
  - tumor (benign) D27.9
    - borderline malignancy D39.1- ☑
    - malignant C56 ☑
    - proliferating D39.1- ☑
- **Bretonneau's disease or angina** A36.Ø
- **Breus' mole** OØ2.Ø
- **Brevicollis** Q76.49
- **Brickmakers' anemia** B76.9 *[D63.8]*
- **Bridge, myocardial** Q24.5
- **Bright red blood per rectum** (BRBPR) K62.5
- **Bright's disease** — *see also* Nephritis
  - arteriosclerotic — *see* Hypertension, kidney
- **Brill** (-Zinsser) **disease** (recrudescent typhus) A75.1
- **Brill-Symmers' disease** C82.9Ø
- **Brion-Kayser disease** — *see* Fever, parathyroid

- **Briquet's disorder or syndrome** F45.Ø
- **Brissaud's**
  - infantilism or dwarfism E23.Ø
  - motor-verbal tic F95.2
- **Brittle**
  - bones disease Q78.Ø
  - nails L6Ø.3
    - congenital Q84.6
- **Broad** — *see also* condition
  - beta disease E78.2
  - ligament laceration syndrome N83.8
- **Broad- or floating-betalipoproteinemia** E78.2
- **Brock's syndrome** (atelectasis due to enlarged lymph nodes) J98.19
- **Brocq-Duhring disease** (dermatitis herpetiformis) L13.Ø
- **Brodie's abscess or disease** M86.8X- ☑
- **Broken**
  - arches — *see also* Deformity, limb, flat foot
  - arm (meaning upper limb) — *see* Fracture, arm
  - back — *see* Fracture, vertebra
  - bone — *see* Fracture
  - implant or internal device — *see* Complications, by site and type, mechanical
  - leg (meaning lower limb) — *see* Fracture, leg
  - nose SØ2.2 ☑
  - tooth, teeth — *see* Fracture, tooth
- **Bromhidrosis, bromidrosis** L75.Ø
- **Bromidism, bromism** G92
  - due to
    - correct substance properly administered — *see* Table of Drugs and Chemicals, by drug, adverse effect
    - overdose or wrong substance given or taken — *see* Table of Drugs and Chemicals, by drug, poisoning
  - chronic (dependence) F13.2Ø
- **Bromidrosiphobia** F4Ø.298
- **Bronchi, bronchial** — *see* condition
- **Bronchiectasis** (cylindrical) (diffuse) (fusiform) (localized) (saccular) J47.9
  - with
    - acute
      - bronchitis J47.Ø
      - lower respiratory infection J47.Ø
    - exacerbation (acute) J47.1
  - congenital Q33.4
  - tuberculous NEC — *see* Tuberculosis, pulmonary
- **Bronchiolectasis** — *see* Bronchiectasis
- **Bronchiolitis** (acute) (infective) (subacute) J21.9
  - with
    - bronchospasm or obstruction J21.9
    - influenza, flu or grippe — *see* Influenza, with, respiratory manifestations NEC
  - chemical (chronic) J68.4
    - acute J68.Ø
  - chronic (fibrosing) (obliterative) J44.9
  - due to
    - external agent — *see* Bronchitis, acute, due to
    - human metapneumovirus J21.1
    - respiratory syncytial virus (RSV) J21.Ø
    - specified organism NEC J21.8
  - fibrosa obliterans J44.9
  - influenzal — *see* Influenza, with, respiratory manifestations NEC
  - obliterans J42
    - with organizing pneumonia (BOOP) J84.89
  - obliterative (chronic) (subacute) J44.9
    - due to fumes or vapors J68.4
    - due to chemicals, gases, fumes or vapors (inhalation) J68.4
  - respiratory, interstitial lung disease J84.115
- **Bronchitis** (diffuse) (fibrinous) (hypostatic) (infective) (membranous) J4Ø
  - with
    - influenza, flu or grippe — *see* Influenza, with, respiratory manifestations NEC
    - obstruction (airway) (lung) J44.9
    - tracheitis (15 years of age and above) J4Ø
      - acute or subacute J2Ø.9
      - chronic J42
      - under 15 years of age J2Ø.9
  - acute or subacute (with bronchospasm or obstruction) J2Ø.9
    - with
      - bronchiectasis J47.Ø
      - chronic obstructive pulmonary disease J44.Ø
    - chemical (due to gases, fumes or vapors) J68.Ø

Index

Bowing — Bronchitis

- **Bronchitis** — *continued*
  - acute or subacute — *continued*
    - due to
      - fumes or vapors J68.Ø
      - Haemophilus influenzae J2Ø.1
      - Mycoplasma pneumoniae J2Ø.Ø
      - radiation J7Ø.Ø
      - specified organism NEC J2Ø.8
      - Streptococcus J2Ø.2
      - virus
        - coxsackie J2Ø.3
        - echovirus J2Ø.7
        - parainfluenzae J2Ø.4
        - respiratory syncytial (RSV) J2Ø.5
        - rhinovirus J2Ø.6
    - viral NEC J2Ø.8
  - allergic (acute) J45.9Ø9
    - with
      - exacerbation (acute) J45.9Ø1
      - status asthmaticus J45.9Ø2
  - arachidic T17.528 ☑
  - aspiration (due to food and vomit) J69.Ø
  - asthmatic J45.9 ☑
    - chronic J44.9
      - with
        - acute lower respiratory infection J44.Ø
        - exacerbation (acute) J44.1
  - capillary — *see* Pneumonia, broncho
  - caseous (tuberculous) A15.5
  - Castellani's A69.8
  - catarrhal (15 years of age and above) J4Ø
    - acute — *see* Bronchitis, acute
    - chronic J41.Ø
    - under 15 years of age J2Ø.9
  - chemical (acute) (subacute) J68.Ø
    - chronic J68.4
    - due to fumes or vapors J68.Ø
      - chronic J68.4
  - chronic J42
    - with
      - airways obstruction J44.9
      - tracheitis (chronic) J42
    - asthmatic (obstructive) J44.9
    - catarrhal J41.Ø
    - chemical (due to fumes or vapors) J68.4
    - due to
      - chemicals, gases, fumes or vapors (inhalation) J68.4
      - radiation J7Ø.1
      - tobacco smoking J41.Ø
    - emphysematous J44.9
    - mucopurulent J41.1
    - non-obstructive J41.Ø
    - obliterans J44.9
    - obstructive J44.9
    - purulent J41.1
    - simple J41.Ø
  - croupous — *see* Bronchitis, acute
  - due to gases, fumes or vapors (chemical) J68.Ø
  - emphysematous (obstructive) J44.9
  - exudative — *see* Bronchitis, acute
  - fetid J41.1
  - grippal — *see* Influenza, with, respiratory manifestations NEC
  - in those under 15 years age — *see* Bronchitis, acute
    - chronic — *see* Bronchitis, chronic
  - influenzal — *see* Influenza, with, respiratory manifestations NEC
  - mixed simple and mucopurulent J41.8
  - moulder's J62.8
  - mucopurulent (chronic) (recurrent) J41.1
    - acute or subacute J2Ø.9
    - simple (mixed) J41.8
  - obliterans (chronic) J44.9
  - obstructive (chronic) (diffuse) J44.9
  - pituitous J41.1
  - pneumococcal, acute or subacute J2Ø.2
  - pseudomembranous, acute or subacute — *see* Bronchitis, acute
  - purulent (chronic) (recurrent) J41.1
    - acute or subacute — *see* Bronchitis, acute
  - putrid J41.1
  - senile (chronic) J42
  - simple and mucopurulent (mixed) J41.8
  - smokers' J41.Ø
  - spirochetal NEC A69.8
  - subacute — *see* Bronchitis, acute
  - suppurative (chronic) J41.1

- **Bronchitis** — *continued*
  - suppurative — *continued*
    - acute or subacute — *see* Bronchitis, acute
  - tuberculous A15.5
  - under 15 years of age — *see* Bronchitis, acute
    - chronic — *see* Bronchitis, chronic
  - viral NEC, acute or subacute — *see also* Bronchitis, acute J2Ø.8
- **Bronchoalveolitis** J18.Ø
- **Bronchoaspergillosis** B44.1
- **Bronchocele meaning goiter** EØ4.Ø
- **Broncholithiasis** J98.Ø9
  - tuberculous NEC A15.5
- **Bronchomalacia** J98.Ø9
  - congenital Q32.2
- **Bronchomycosis NOS** B49 *[J99]*
  - candidal B37.1
- **Bronchopleuropneumonia** — *see* Pneumonia, broncho
- **Bronchopneumonia** — *see* Pneumonia, broncho
- **Bronchopneumonitis** — *see* Pneumonia, broncho
- **Bronchopulmonary** — *see* condition
- **Bronchopulmonitis** — *see* Pneumonia, broncho
- **Bronchorrhagia** (see Hemoptysis)
- **Bronchorrhea** J98.Ø9
  - acute J2Ø.9
  - chronic (infective) (purulent) J42
- **Bronchospasm** (acute) J98.Ø1
  - with
    - bronchiolitis, acute J21.9
    - bronchitis, acute (conditions in J2Ø) — *see* Bronchitis, acute
  - due to external agent — *see* condition, respiratory, acute, due to
  - exercise induced J45.99Ø
- **Bronchospirochetosis** A69.8
  - Castellani A69.8
- **Bronchostenosis** J98.Ø9
- **Bronchus** — *see* condition
- **Brontophobia** F4Ø.22Ø
- **Bronze baby syndrome** P83.88
- **Brooke's tumor** — *see* Neoplasm, skin, benign
- **Brown enamel of teeth** (hereditary) KØØ.5
- **Brown's sheath syndrome** H5Ø.61- ☑
- **Brown-Séquard disease, paralysis or syndrome** G83.81
- **Bruce sepsis** A23.Ø
- **Brucellosis** (infection) A23.9
  - abortus A23.1
  - canis A23.3
  - dermatitis A23.9
  - melitensis A23.Ø
  - mixed A23.8
  - sepsis A23.9
    - melitensis A23.Ø
    - specified NEC A23.8
  - suis A23.2
- **Bruck-de Lange disease** Q87.19
- **Bruck's disease** — *see* Deformity, limb
- **BRUE** (brief resolved unexplained event) R68.13
- **Brugsch's syndrome** Q82.8
- **Bruise** (skin surface intact) — *see also* Contusion
  - with
    - open wound — *see* Wound, open
  - internal organ — *see* Injury, by site
  - newborn P54.5
  - scalp, due to birth injury, newborn P12.3
  - umbilical cord O69.5 ☑
- **Bruit** (arterial) RØ9.89
  - cardiac RØ1.1
- **Brush burn** — *see* Abrasion, by site
- **Bruton's X-linked agammaglobulinemia** D8Ø.Ø
- **Bruxism**
  - psychogenic F45.8
  - sleep related G47.63
- **Bubbly lung syndrome** P27.Ø
- **Bubo** I88.8
  - blennorrhagic (gonococcal) A54.89
  - chancroidal A57
  - climatic A55
  - due to Haemophilus ducreyi A57
  - gonococcal A54.89
  - indolent (nonspecific) I88.8
  - inguinal (nonspecific) I88.8
    - chancroidal A57
    - climatic A55
    - due to H. ducreyi A57
    - infective I88.8

- **Bubo** — *continued*
  - scrofulous (tuberculous) A18.2
  - soft chancre A57
  - suppurating — *see* Lymphadenitis, acute
  - syphilitic (primary) A51.Ø
    - congenital A5Ø.Ø7
  - tropical A55
  - virulent (chancroidal) A57
- **Bubonic plague** A2Ø.Ø
- **Bubonocele** — *see* Hernia, inguinal
- **Buccal** — *see* condition
- **Buchanan's disease or osteochondrosis** M91.Ø
- **Buchem's syndrome** (hyperostosis corticalis) M85.2
- **Bucket-handle fracture or tear** (semilunar cartilage) — *see* Tear, meniscus
- **Budd-Chiari syndrome** (hepatic vein thrombosis) I82.Ø
- **Budgerigar fancier's disease or lung** J67.2
- **Buds**
  - breast E3Ø.1
    - in newborn P96.89
- **Buerger's disease** (thromboangiitis obliterans) I73.1
- **Bulbar** — *see* condition
- **Bulbus cordis** (left ventricle) (persistent) Q21.8
- **Bulimia** (nervosa) F5Ø.2
  - atypical F5Ø.9
  - normal weight F5Ø.9
- **Bulky**
  - stools R19.5
  - uterus N85.2
- **Bulla** (e) R23.8
  - lung (emphysematous) (solitary) J43.9
    - newborn P25.8
- **Bullet wound** — *see also* Wound, open
  - fracture — *code as* Fracture, by site
  - internal organ — *see* Injury, by site
- **Bundle**
  - branch block (complete) (false) (incomplete) — *see* Block, bundle-branch
  - of His — *see* condition
- **Bunion** M21.61- ☑
  - tailor's M21.62- ☑
- **Bunionette** M21.62- ☑
- **Buphthalmia, buphthalmos** (congenital) Q15.Ø
- **Burdwan fever** B55.Ø
- **Bürger-Grütz disease or syndrome** E78.3
- **Buried**
  - penis (congenital) Q55.64
    - acquired N48.83
  - roots KØ8.3
- **Burke's syndrome** K86.89
- **Burkitt**
  - cell leukemia C91.Ø- ☑
  - lymphoma (malignant) C83.7- ☑
    - small noncleaved, diffuse C83.7- ☑
    - spleen C83.77
    - undifferentiated C83.7- ☑
  - tumor C83.7- ☑
  - type
    - acute lymphoblastic leukemia C91.Ø- ☑
    - undifferentiated C83.7- ☑
- **Burn** (electricity) (flame) (hot gas, liquid or hot object) (radiation) (steam) (thermal) T3Ø.Ø
  - abdomen, abdominal (muscle) (wall) T21.Ø2 ☑
    - first degree T21.12 ☑
    - second degree T21.22 ☑
    - third degree T21.32 ☑
  - above elbow T22.Ø39 ☑
    - first degree T22.139 ☑
    - left T22.Ø32 ☑
      - first degree T22.132 ☑
      - second degree T22.232 ☑
      - third degree T22.332 ☑
    - right T22.Ø31 ☑
      - first degree T22.131 ☑
      - second degree T22.231 ☑
      - third degree T22.331 ☑
    - second degree T22.239 ☑
    - third degree T22.339 ☑
  - acid (caustic) (external) (internal) — *see* Corrosion, by site
  - alimentary tract NEC T28.2 ☑
    - esophagus T28.1 ☑
    - mouth T28.Ø ☑
    - pharynx T28.Ø ☑
  - alkaline (caustic) (external) (internal) — *see* Corrosion, by site

- **Burn** — *continued*
  - thumb(s) — *continued*
    - left — *continued*
      - second degree T23.212 ☑
      - third degree T23.312 ☑
    - multiple sites with fingers T23.Ø49 ☑
      - first degree T23.149 ☑
      - left T23.Ø42 ☑
        - first degree T23.142 ☑
        - second degree T23.242 ☑
        - third degree T23.342 ☑
      - right T23.Ø41 ☑
        - first degree T23.141 ☑
        - second degree T23.241 ☑
        - third degree T23.341 ☑
      - second degree T23.249 ☑
      - third degree T23.349 ☑
    - right T23.Ø11 ☑
      - first degree T23.111 ☑
      - second degree T23.211 ☑
      - third degree T23.311 ☑
    - second degree T23.219 ☑
    - third degree T23.319 ☑
  - toe T25.Ø39 ☑
    - first degree T25.139 ☑
    - left T25.Ø32 ☑
      - first degree T25.132 ☑
      - second degree T25.232 ☑
      - third degree T25.332 ☑
    - right T25.Ø31 ☑
      - first degree T25.131 ☑
      - second degree T25.231 ☑
      - third degree T25.331 ☑
    - second degree T25.239 ☑
    - third degree T25.339 ☑
  - tongue T28.Ø ☑
  - tonsil(s) T28.Ø ☑
  - trachea T27.Ø ☑
    - with lung T27.1 ☑
  - trunk T21.ØØ ☑
    - abdominal wall — *see* Burn, abdominal wall
    - anus — *see* Burn, buttock
    - axilla — *see* Burn, upper limb
    - back — *see* Burn, back
    - breast — *see* Burn, chest wall
    - buttock — *see* Burn, buttock
    - chest wall — *see* Burn, chest wall
    - first degree T21.1Ø ☑
    - flank — *see* Burn, abdominal wall
    - genital
      - female — *see* Burn, genital organs, external, female
      - male — *see* Burn, genital organs, external, male
    - groin — *see* Burn, abdominal wall
    - interscapular region — *see* Burn, back, upper
    - labia — *see* Burn, genital organs, external, female
    - lower back — *see* Burn, back
    - penis — *see* Burn, genital organs, external, male
    - perineum
      - female — *see* Burn, genital organs, external, female
      - male — *see* Burn, genital organs, external, male
    - scapula region — *see* Burn, scapular region
    - scrotum — *see* Burn, genital organs, external, male
    - second degree T21.2Ø ☑
    - specified site NEC T21.Ø9 ☑
      - first degree T21.19 ☑
      - second degree T21.29 ☑
      - third degree T21.39 ☑
    - testes — *see* Burn, genital organs, external, male
    - third degree T21.3Ø ☑
    - upper back — *see* Burn, back, upper
    - vulva — *see* Burn, genital organs, external, female
  - unspecified site with extent of body surface involved specified
    - less than 1Ø percent T31.Ø
    - 1Ø-19 percent (Ø-9 percent third degree) T31.1Ø
      - with 1Ø-19 percent third degree T31.11
    - 2Ø-29 percent (Ø-9 percent third degree) T31.2Ø
      - with
        - 1Ø-19 percent third degree T31.21
        - 2Ø-29 percent third degree T31.22
    - 3Ø-39 percent (Ø-9 percent third degree) T31.3Ø
      - with
        - 1Ø-19 percent third degree T31.31
        - 2Ø-29 percent third degree T31.32

- **Burn** — *continued*
  - unspecified site with extent of body surface involved specified — *continued*
    - 3Ø-39 percent — *continued*
      - with — *continued*
        - 3Ø-39 percent third degree T31.33
    - 4Ø-49 percent (Ø-9 percent third degree) T31.4Ø
      - with
        - 1Ø-19 percent third degree T31.41
        - 2Ø-29 percent third degree T31.42
        - 3Ø-39 percent third degree T31.43
        - 4Ø-49 percent third degree T31.44
    - 5Ø-59 percent (Ø-9 percent third degree) T31.5Ø
      - with
        - 1Ø-19 percent third degree T31.51
        - 2Ø-29 percent third degree T31.52
        - 3Ø-39 percent third degree T31.53
        - 4Ø-49 percent third degree T31.54
        - 5Ø-59 percent third degree T31.55
    - 6Ø-69 percent (Ø-9 percent third degree) T31.6Ø
      - with
        - 1Ø-19 percent third degree T31.61
        - 2Ø-29 percent third degree T31.62
        - 3Ø-39 percent third degree T31.63
        - 4Ø-49 percent third degree T31.64
        - 5Ø-59 percent third degree T31.65
        - 6Ø-69 percent third degree T31.66
    - 7Ø-79 percent (Ø-9 percent third degree) T31.7Ø
      - with
        - 1Ø-19 percent third degree T31.71
        - 2Ø-29 percent third degree T31.72
        - 3Ø-39 percent third degree T31.73
        - 4Ø-49 percent third degree T31.74
        - 5Ø-59 percent third degree T31.75
        - 6Ø-69 percent third degree T31.76
        - 7Ø-79 percent third degree T31.77
    - 8Ø-89 percent (Ø-9 percent third degree) T31.8Ø
      - with
        - 1Ø-19 percent third degree T31.81
        - 2Ø-29 percent third degree T31.82
        - 3Ø-39 percent third degree T31.83
        - 4Ø-49 percent third degree T31.84
        - 5Ø-59 percent third degree T31.85
        - 6Ø-69 percent third degree T31.86
        - 7Ø-79 percent third degree T31.87
        - 8Ø-89 percent third degree T31.88
    - 9Ø percent or more (Ø-9 percent third degree) T31.9Ø
      - with
        - 1Ø-19 percent third degree T31.91
        - 2Ø-29 percent third degree T31.92
        - 3Ø-39 percent third degree T31.93
        - 4Ø-49 percent third degree T31.94
        - 5Ø-59 percent third degree T31.95
        - 6Ø-69 percent third degree T31.96
        - 7Ø-79 percent third degree T31.97
        - 8Ø-89 percent third degree T31.98
        - 9Ø-99 percent third degree T31.99
  - upper limb T22.ØØ ☑
    - above elbow — *see* Burn, above elbow
    - axilla — *see* Burn, axilla
    - elbow — *see* Burn, elbow
    - first degree T22.1Ø ☑
    - forearm — *see* Burn, forearm
    - hand — *see* Burn, hand
    - interscapular region — *see* Burn, back, upper
    - multiple sites T22.Ø99 ☑
      - first degree T22.199 ☑
      - left T22.Ø92 ☑
        - first degree T22.192 ☑
        - second degree T22.292 ☑
        - third degree T22.392 ☑
      - right T22.Ø91 ☑
        - first degree T22.191 ☑
        - second degree T22.291 ☑
        - third degree T22.391 ☑
      - second degree T22.299 ☑
      - third degree T22.399 ☑
    - scapular region — *see* Burn, scapular region
    - second degree T22.2Ø ☑
    - shoulder — *see* Burn, shoulder
    - third degree T22.3Ø ☑
    - wrist — *see* Burn, wrist
  - uterus T28.3 ☑
  - vagina T28.3 ☑
  - vulva — *see* Burn, genital organs, external, female
  - wrist T23.Ø79 ☑
    - first degree T23.179 ☑
    - left T23.Ø72 ☑

- **Burn** — *continued*
  - wrist — *continued*
    - left — *continued*
      - first degree T23.172 ☑
      - second degree T23.272 ☑
      - third degree T23.372 ☑
    - multiple sites with hand T23.Ø99 ☑
      - first degree T23.199 ☑
      - left T23.Ø92 ☑
        - first degree T23.192 ☑
        - second degree T23.292 ☑
        - third degree T23.392 ☑
      - right T23.Ø91 ☑
        - first degree T23.191 ☑
        - second degree T23.291 ☑
        - third degree T23.391 ☑
      - second degree T23.299 ☑
      - third degree T23.399 ☑
    - right T23.Ø71 ☑
      - first degree T23.171 ☑
      - second degree T23.271 ☑
      - third degree T23.371 ☑
    - second degree T23.279 ☑
    - third degree T23.379 ☑
- **Burnett's syndrome** E83.52
- **Burning**
  - feet syndrome E53.9
  - sensation R2Ø.8
  - tongue K14.6
- **Burn-out** (state) Z73.Ø
- **Burns' disease or osteochondrosis** — *see* Osteochondrosis, juvenile, ulna
- **Bursa** — *see* condition
- **Bursitis** M71.9
  - Achilles — *see* Tendinitis, Achilles
  - adhesive — *see* Bursitis, specified NEC
  - ankle — *see* Enthesopathy, lower limb, ankle, specified type NEC
  - calcaneal — *see* Enthesopathy, foot, specified type NEC
  - collateral ligament, tibial — *see* Bursitis, tibial collateral
  - due to use, overuse, pressure — *see also* Disorder, soft tissue, due to use, specified type NEC
    - specified NEC — *see* Disorder, soft tissue, due to use, specified NEC
  - Duplay's M75.Ø ☑
  - elbow NEC M7Ø.3- ☑
    - olecranon M7Ø.2- ☑
  - finger — *see* Disorder, soft tissue, due to use, specified type NEC, hand
  - foot — *see* Enthesopathy, foot, specified type NEC
  - gonococcal A54.49
  - gouty — *see* Gout
  - hand M7Ø.1- ☑
  - hip NEC M7Ø.7- ☑
    - trochanteric M7Ø.6- ☑
  - infective NEC M71.1Ø
    - abscess — *see* Abscess, bursa
    - ankle M71.17- ☑
    - elbow M71.12- ☑
    - foot M71.17- ☑
    - hand M71.14- ☑
    - hip M71.15- ☑
    - knee M71.16- ☑
    - multiple sites M71.19
    - shoulder M71.11- ☑
    - specified site NEC M71.18
    - wrist M71.13- ☑
  - ischial — *see* Bursitis, hip
  - knee NEC M7Ø.5- ☑
    - prepatellar M7Ø.4- ☑
  - occupational NEC — *see also* Disorder, soft tissue, due to, use
  - olecranon — *see* Bursitis, elbow, olecranon
  - pharyngeal J39.1
  - popliteal — *see* Bursitis, knee
  - prepatellar M7Ø.4- ☑
  - radiohumeral M77.8
  - rheumatoid MØ6.2Ø
    - ankle MØ6.27- ☑
    - elbow MØ6.22- ☑
    - foot joint MØ6.27- ☑
    - hand joint MØ6.24- ☑
    - hip MØ6.25- ☑
    - knee MØ6.26- ☑
    - multiple site MØ6.29
    - shoulder MØ6.21- ☑

C

- **Carbuncle** — *continued*
  - navel LØ2.236
  - neck LØ2.13
  - nose (external) (septum) J34.Ø
  - orbit, orbital — *see* Abscess, orbit
  - palmar (space) — *see* Carbuncle, hand
  - partes posteriores LØ2.33
  - pectoral region LØ2.233
  - penis N48.21
  - perineum LØ2.235
  - pinna — *see* Abscess, ear, external
  - popliteal — *see* Carbuncle, lower limb
  - scalp LØ2.831
  - seminal vesicle N49.Ø
  - shoulder — *see* Carbuncle, upper limb
  - specified site NEC LØ2.838
  - temple (region) LØ2.Ø3
  - thumb — *see* Carbuncle, hand
  - toe — *see* Carbuncle, foot
  - trunk LØ2.239
    - abdominal wall LØ2.231
    - back LØ2.232
    - chest wall LØ2.233
    - groin LØ2.234
    - perineum LØ2.235
    - umbilicus LØ2.236
  - umbilicus LØ2.236
  - upper limb LØ2.43- ☑
  - urethra N34.Ø
  - vulva N76.4
- **Carbunculus** — *see* Carbuncle
- **Carcinoid** (tumor) — *see* Tumor, carcinoid
- **Carcinoidosis** E34.Ø
- **Carcinoma** (malignant) — *see also* Neoplasm, by site, malignant
  - acidophil
    - specified site — *see* Neoplasm, malignant, by site
    - unspecified site C75.1
  - acidophil-basophil, mixed
    - specified site — *see* Neoplasm, malignant, by site
    - unspecified site C75.1
  - adnexal (skin) — *see* Neoplasm, skin, malignant
  - adrenal cortical C74.Ø- ☑
  - alveolar — *see* Neoplasm, lung, malignant
    - cell — *see* Neoplasm, lung, malignant
  - ameloblastic C41.1
    - upper jaw (bone) C41.Ø
  - apocrine
    - breast — *see* Neoplasm, breast, malignant
    - specified site NEC — *see* Neoplasm, skin, malignant
    - unspecified site C44.99
  - basal cell (pigmented) (*see also* Neoplasm, skin, malignant) C44.91
    - fibro-epithelial — *see* Neoplasm, skin, malignant
    - morphea — *see* Neoplasm, skin, malignant
    - multicentric — *see* Neoplasm, skin, malignant
  - basaloid
  - basal-squamous cell, mixed — *see* Neoplasm, skin, malignant
  - basophil
    - specified site — *see* Neoplasm, malignant, by site
    - unspecified site C75.1
  - basophil-acidophil, mixed
    - specified site — *see* Neoplasm, malignant, by site
    - unspecified site C75.1
  - basosquamous — *see* Neoplasm, skin, malignant
  - bile duct
    - with hepatocellular, mixed C22.Ø
    - liver C22.1
    - specified site NEC — *see* Neoplasm, malignant, by site
    - unspecified site C22.1
  - branchial or branchiogenic C1Ø.4
  - bronchial or bronchogenic — *see* Neoplasm, lung, malignant
  - bronchiolar — *see* Neoplasm, lung, malignant
  - bronchioloalveolar — *see* Neoplasm, lung, malignant
  - C cell
    - specified site — *see* Neoplasm, malignant, by site
    - unspecified site C73
  - ceruminous C44.29- ☑
  - cervix uteri
    - in situ DØ6.9
      - endocervix DØ6.Ø
      - exocervix DØ6.1
      - specified site NEC DØ6.7
  - chorionic
    - specified site — *see* Neoplasm, malignant, by site

- **Carcinoma** — *continued*
  - chorionic — *continued*
    - unspecified site
      - female C58
      - male C62.9Ø
  - chromophobe
    - specified site — *see* Neoplasm, malignant, by site
    - unspecified site C75.1
  - cloacogenic
    - specified site — *see* Neoplasm, malignant, by site
    - unspecified site C21.2
  - diffuse type
    - specified site — *see* Neoplasm, malignant, by site
    - unspecified site C16.9
  - duct (cell)
    - with Paget's disease — *see* Neoplasm, breast, malignant
    - infiltrating
      - with lobular carcinoma (in situ)
        - specified site — *see* Neoplasm, malignant, by site
        - unspecified site (female) C5Ø.91- ☑
          - male C5Ø.92- ☑
      - specified site — *see* Neoplasm, malignant, by site
        - unspecified site (female) C5Ø.91- ☑
          - male C5Ø.92- ☑
  - ductal
    - with lobular
      - specified site — *see* Neoplasm, malignant, by site
      - unspecified site (female) C5Ø.91- ☑
        - male C5Ø.92- ☑
  - ductular, infiltrating
    - specified site — *see* Neoplasm, malignant, by site
    - unspecified site (female) C5Ø.91- ☑
      - male C5Ø.92- ☑
  - embryonal
    - liver C22.7
  - endometrioid
    - specified site — *see* Neoplasm, malignant, by site
    - unspecified site
      - female C56.9
      - male C61
  - eosinophil
    - specified site — *see* Neoplasm, malignant, by site
    - unspecified site C75.1
  - epidermoid — *see also* Neoplasm, skin, malignant
    - in situ, Bowen's type — *see* Neoplasm, skin, in situ
  - fibroepithelial, basal cell — *see* Neoplasm, skin, malignant
  - follicular
    - with papillary (mixed) C73
    - moderately differentiated C73
    - pure follicle C73
    - specified site — *see* Neoplasm, malignant, by site
    - trabecular C73
    - unspecified site C73
    - well differentiated C73
  - generalized, with unspecified primary site C8Ø.Ø
  - glycogen-rich — *see* Neoplasm, breast, malignant
  - granulosa cell C56- ☑
  - hepatic cell C22.Ø
  - hepatocellular C22.Ø
    - with bile duct, mixed C22.Ø
    - fibrolamellar C22.Ø
  - hepatocholangiolitic C22.Ø
  - Hurthle cell C73
  - in
    - adenomatous
      - polyposis coli C18.9
    - pleomorphic adenoma — *see* Neoplasm, salivary glands, malignant
    - situ — *see* Carcinoma-in-situ
  - infiltrating
    - duct
      - with lobular
        - specified site — *see* Neoplasm, malignant, by site
        - unspecified site (female) C5Ø.91- ☑
          - male C5Ø.92- ☑
      - with Paget's disease — *see* Neoplasm, breast, malignant
      - specified site — *see* Neoplasm, malignant
      - unspecified site (female) C5Ø.91- ☑
        - male C5Ø.92- ☑
    - ductular
      - specified site — *see* Neoplasm, malignant

- **Carcinoma** — *continued*
  - infiltrating — *continued*
    - ductular — *continued*
      - unspecified site (female) C5Ø.91- ☑
        - male C5Ø.92- ☑
    - lobular
      - specified site — *see* Neoplasm, malignant
      - unspecified site (female) C5Ø.91- ☑
        - male C5Ø.92- ☑
  - inflammatory
    - specified site — *see* Neoplasm, malignant
    - unspecified site (female) C5Ø.91- ☑
      - male C5Ø.92- ☑
  - intestinal type
    - specified site — *see* Neoplasm, malignant, by site
    - unspecified site C16.9
  - intracystic
    - noninfiltrating — *see* Neoplasm, in situ, by site
  - intraductal (noninfiltrating)
    - with Paget's disease — *see* Neoplasm, breast, malignant
    - breast DØ5.1- ☑
    - papillary
      - with invasion
        - specified site — *see* Neoplasm, malignant, by site
        - unspecified site (female) C5Ø.91- ☑
          - male C5Ø.92- ☑
      - breast DØ5.1- ☑
      - specified site NEC — *see* Neoplasm, in situ, by site
      - unspecified site (female) DØ5.1- ☑
    - specified site NEC — *see* Neoplasm, in situ, by site
    - unspecified site (female) DØ5.1- ☑
  - intraepidermal — *see* Neoplasm, in situ
    - squamous cell, Bowen's type — *see* Neoplasm, skin, in situ
  - intraepithelial — *see* Neoplasm, in situ, by site
    - squamous cell — *see* Neoplasm, in situ, by site
  - intraosseous C41.1
    - upper jaw (bone) C41.Ø
  - islet cell
    - with exocrine, mixed
      - specified site — *see* Neoplasm, malignant, by site
      - unspecified site C25.9
    - pancreas C25.4
    - specified site NEC — *see* Neoplasm, malignant, by site
    - unspecified site C25.4
  - juvenile, breast — *see* Neoplasm, breast, malignant
  - large cell
    - small cell
      - specified site — *see* Neoplasm, malignant, by site
      - unspecified site C34.9Ø
  - Leydig cell (testis)
    - specified site — *see* Neoplasm, malignant, by site
    - unspecified site
      - female C56.9
      - male C62.9Ø
  - lipid-rich (female) C5Ø.91- ☑
    - male C5Ø.92- ☑
  - liver cell C22.Ø
  - liver NEC C22.7
  - lobular (infiltrating)
    - with intraductal
      - specified site — *see* Neoplasm, malignant, by site
      - unspecified site (female) C5Ø.91- ☑
        - male C5Ø.92- ☑
    - noninfiltrating
      - breast DØ5.Ø- ☑
      - specified site NEC — *see* Neoplasm, in situ, by site
      - unspecified site DØ5.Ø- ☑
    - specified site — *see* Neoplasm, malignant, by site
    - unspecified site (female) C5Ø.91- ☑
      - male C5Ø.92- ☑
  - medullary
    - with
      - amyloid stroma
        - specified site — *see* Neoplasm, malignant, by site
        - unspecified site C73

Carcinoma — *continued*
  medullary — *continued*
    with — *continued*
      lymphoid stroma
        specified site — *see* Neoplasm, malignant, by site
        unspecified site (female) C5Ø.91- ☑
          male C5Ø.92- ☑
  Merkel cell C4A.9 (*following* C43)
    anal margin C4A.51 (*following* C43)
    anal skin C4A.51 (*following* C43)
    canthus C4A.1- ☑ (*following* C43)
    ear and external auricular canal C4A.2- ☑ (*following* C43)
    external auricular canal C4A.2- ☑ (*following* C43)
    eyelid, including canthus C4A.1- ☑ (*following* C43)
    face C4A.3Ø (*following* C43)
      specified NEC C4A.39 (*following* C43)
    hip C4A.7- ☑ (*following* C43)
    lip C4A.Ø (*following* C43)
    lower limb, including hip C4A.7- ☑ (*following* C43)
    neck C4A.4 (*following* C43)
    nodal presentation C7B.1 (*following* C75)
    nose C4A.31 (*following* C43)
    overlapping sites C4A.8 (*following* C43)
    perianal skin C4A.51 (*following* C43)
    scalp C4A.4 (*following* C43)
    secondary C7B.1 (*following* C75)
    shoulder C4A.6- ☑ (*following* C43)
    skin of breast C4A.52 (*following* C43)
    trunk NEC C4A.59 (*following* C43)
    upper limb, including shoulder C4A.6- ☑ (*following* C43)
    visceral metastatic C7B.1 (*following* C75)
  metastatic — *see* Neoplasm, secondary, by site
  metatypical — *see* Neoplasm, skin, malignant
  morphea, basal cell — *see* Neoplasm, skin, malignant
  mucoid
    cell
      specified site — *see* Neoplasm, malignant, by site
      unspecified site C75.1
  neuroendocrine — *see also* Tumor, neuroendocrine
    high grade, any site C7A.1 (*following* C75)
    poorly differentiated, any site C7A.1 (*following* C75)
  nonencapsulated sclerosing C73
  noninfiltrating
    intracystic — *see* Neoplasm, in situ, by site
    intraductal
      breast DØ5.1- ☑
      papillary
        breast DØ5.1- ☑
        specified site NEC — *see* Neoplasm, in situ, by site
        unspecified site DØ5.1- ☑
      specified site — *see* Neoplasm, in situ, by site
      unspecified site DØ5.1- ☑
    lobular
      breast DØ5.Ø- ☑
      specified site NEC — *see* Neoplasm, in situ, by site
      unspecified site (female) DØ5.Ø- ☑
  oat cell
    specified site — *see* Neoplasm, malignant, by site
    unspecified site C34.9Ø
  odontogenic C41.1
    upper jaw (bone) C41.Ø
  papillary
    with follicular (mixed) C73
    follicular variant C73
    intraductal (noninfiltrating)
      with invasion
        specified site — *see* Neoplasm, malignant, by site
        unspecified site (female) C5Ø.91- ☑
          male C5Ø.92- ☑
      breast DØ5.1- ☑
      specified site NEC — *see* Neoplasm, in situ, by site
      unspecified site DØ5.1- ☑
    serous
      specified site — *see* Neoplasm, malignant, by site
      surface
        specified site — *see* Neoplasm, malignant, by site
        unspecified site C56.9

Carcinoma — *continued*
  papillary — *continued*
    serous — *continued*
      unspecified site C56.9
  papillocystic
    specified site — *see* Neoplasm, malignant, by site
    unspecified site C56.9
  parafollicular cell
    specified site — *see* Neoplasm, malignant, by site
    unspecified site C73
  pilomatrix — *see* Neoplasm, skin, malignant
  pseudomucinous
    specified site — *see* Neoplasm, malignant, by site
    unspecified site C56.9
  renal cell C64- ☑
  Schmincke — *see* Neoplasm, nasopharynx, malignant
  Schneiderian
    specified site — *see* Neoplasm, malignant, by site
    unspecified site C3Ø.Ø
  sebaceous — *see* Neoplasm, skin, malignant
  secondary — *see also* Neoplasm, secondary, by site
    Merkel cell C7B.1 (*following* C75)
  secretory, breast — *see* Neoplasm, breast, malignant
  serous
    papillary
      specified site — *see* Neoplasm, malignant, by site
      unspecified site C56.9
    surface, papillary
      specified site — *see* Neoplasm, malignant, by site
      unspecified site C56.9
  Sertoli cell
    specified site — *see* Neoplasm, malignant, by site
    unspecified site C62.9Ø
      female C56.9
      male C62.9Ø
  skin appendage — *see* Neoplasm, skin, malignant
  small cell
    fusiform cell
      specified site — *see* Neoplasm, malignant, by site
      unspecified site C34.9Ø
    intermediate cell
      specified site — *see* Neoplasm, malignant, by site
      unspecified site C34.9Ø
    large cell
      specified site — *see* Neoplasm, malignant, by site
      unspecified site C34.9Ø
  solid
    with amyloid stroma
      specified site — *see* Neoplasm, malignant, by site
      unspecified site C73
    microinvasive
      specified site — *see* Neoplasm, malignant, by site
      unspecified site C53.9
  sweat gland — *see* Neoplasm, skin, malignant
  theca cell C56.- ☑
  thymic C37
  unspecified site (primary) C8Ø.1
  water-clear cell C75.Ø

Carcinoma-in-situ — *see also* Neoplasm, in situ, by site
  breast NOS DØ5.9- ☑
    specified type NEC DØ5.8- ☑
  epidermoid — *see also* Neoplasm, in situ, by site
    with questionable stromal invasion
      cervix DØ6.9
      specified site NEC — *see* Neoplasm, in situ, by site
      unspecified site DØ6.9
    Bowen's type — *see* Neoplasm, skin, in situ
  intraductal
    breast DØ5.1- ☑
    specified site NEC — *see* Neoplasm, in situ, by site
    unspecified site DØ5.1- ☑
  lobular
    with
      infiltrating duct
        breast (female) C5Ø.91- ☑
          male C5Ø.92- ☑
        specified site NEC — *see* Neoplasm, malignant
        unspecified site (female) C5Ø.91- ☑
          male C5Ø.92- ☑

Carcinoma-in-situ — *continued*
  lobular — *continued*
    with — *continued*
      intraductal
        breast DØ5.8- ☑
        specified site NEC — *see* Neoplasm, in situ, by site
        unspecified site (female) DØ5.8- ☑
    breast DØ5.Ø- ☑
    specified site NEC — *see* Neoplasm, in situ, by site
    unspecified site DØ5.Ø- ☑
  squamous cell — *see also* Neoplasm, in situ, by site
    with questionable stromal invasion
      cervix DØ6.9
      specified site NEC — *see* Neoplasm, in situ, by site
      unspecified site DØ6.9

Carcinomaphobia F45.29
Carcinomatosis C8Ø.Ø
  peritonei C78.6
  unspecified site (primary) (secondary) C8Ø.Ø
Carcinosarcoma — *see* Neoplasm, malignant, by site
  embryonal — *see* Neoplasm, malignant, by site
Cardia, cardial — *see* condition
Cardiac — *see also* condition
  death, sudden — *see* Arrest, cardiac
  pacemaker
    in situ Z95.Ø
    management or adjustment Z45.Ø18
  tamponade I31.4
Cardialgia — *see* Pain, precordial
Cardiectasis — *see* Hypertrophy, cardiac
Cardiochalasia K21.9
Cardiomalacia I51.5
Cardiomegalia glycogenica diffusa E74.Ø2 *[I43]*
Cardiomegaly — *see also* Hypertrophy, cardiac
  congenital Q24.8
  glycogen E74.Ø2 *[I43]*
  idiopathic I51.7
Cardiomyoliposis I51.5
Cardiomyopathy (familial) (idiopathic) I42.9
  alcoholic I42.6
  amyloid E85.4 *[I43]*
    transthyretin-related (ATTR) familial E85.4 *[I43]*
  arteriosclerotic — *see* Disease, heart, ischemic, atherosclerotic
  beriberi E51.12
  cobalt-beer I42.6
  congenital I42.4
  congestive I42.Ø
  constrictive NOS I42.5
  dilated I42.Ø
  due to
    alcohol I42.6
    beriberi E51.12
    cardiac glycogenosis E74.Ø2 *[I43]*
    drugs I42.7
    external agents NEC I42.7
    Friedreich's ataxia G11.11
    myotonia atrophica G71.11 *[I43]*
    progressive muscular dystrophy G71.Ø9 *[I43]*
  glycogen storage E74.Ø2 *[I43]*
  hypertensive — *see* Hypertension, heart
  hypertrophic (nonobstructive) I42.2
    obstructive I42.1
      congenital Q24.8
  in
    Chagas' disease (chronic) B57.2
      acute B57.Ø
    sarcoidosis D86.85
  ischemic I25.5
  metabolic E88.9 *[I43]*
    thyrotoxic EØ5.9Ø *[I43]*
      with thyroid storm EØ5.91 *[I43]*
  newborn I42.8
    congenital I42.4
  non-ischemic — *see also* by cause I42.8
  nutritional E63.9 *[I43]*
    beriberi E51.12
  obscure of Africa I42.8
  peripartum O9Ø.3
  postpartum O9Ø.3
  restrictive NEC I42.5
  rheumatic IØ9.Ø
  secondary I42.9
  specified NEC I42.8
  stress induced I51.81
  takotsubo I51.81

- **Cardiomyopathy** — *continued*
  - thyrotoxic EØ5.9Ø *[I43]*
    - with thyroid storm EØ5.91 *[I43]*
  - toxic NEC I42.7
  - transthyretin-related (ATTR) familial amyloid E85.4
  - tuberculous A18.84
  - viral B33.24
- **Cardionephritis** — *see* Hypertension, cardiorenal
- **Cardionephropathy** — *see* Hypertension, cardiorenal
- **Cardionephrosis** — *see* Hypertension, cardiorenal
- **Cardiopathia nigra** I27.Ø
- **Cardiopathy** — *see also* Disease, heart I51.9
  - idiopathic I42.9
  - mucopolysaccharidosis E76.3 *[I52]*
- **Cardiopericarditis** — *see* Pericarditis
- **Cardiophobia** F45.29
- **Cardiorenal** — *see* condition
- **Cardiorrhexis** — *see* Infarct, myocardium
- **Cardiosclerosis** — *see* Disease, heart, ischemic, atherosclerotic
- **Cardiosis** — *see* Disease, heart
- **Cardiospasm** (esophagus) (reflex) (stomach) K22.Ø
  - congenital Q39.5
    - with megaesophagus Q39.5
- **Cardiostenosis** — *see* Disease, heart
- **Cardiosymphysis** I31.Ø
- **Cardiovascular** — *see* condition
- **Carditis** (acute) (bacterial) (chronic) (subacute) I51.89
  - meningococcal A39.5Ø
  - rheumatic — *see* Disease, heart, rheumatic
  - rheumatoid — *see* Rheumatoid, carditis
  - viral B33.2Ø
- **Care** (of) (for) (following)
  - child (routine) Z76.2
  - family member (handicapped) (sick)
    - creating problem for family Z63.6
    - provided away from home for holiday relief Z75.5
    - unavailable, due to
      - absence (person rendering care) (sufferer) Z74.2
      - inability (any reason) of person rendering care Z74.2
  - foundling Z76.1
  - holiday relief Z75.5
  - improper — *see* Maltreatment
  - lack of (at or after birth) (infant) — *see* Maltreatment, child, neglect
  - lactating mother Z39.1
  - palliative Z51.5
  - postpartum
    - immediately after delivery Z39.Ø
    - routine follow-up Z39.2
  - respite Z75.5
  - unavailable, due to
    - absence of person rendering care Z74.2
    - inability (any reason) of person rendering care Z74.2
  - well-baby Z76.2
- **Caries**
  - bone NEC A18.Ø3
  - dental (dentino enamel junction) (early childhood) (of dentine) (pre-eruptive) (recurrent) (to the pulp) KØ2.9
    - arrested (coronal) (root) KØ2.3
    - chewing surface
      - limited to enamel KØ2.51
      - penetrating into dentin KØ2.52
      - penetrating into pulp KØ2.53
    - coronal surface
      - chewing surface
        - limited to enamel KØ2.51
        - penetrating into dentin KØ2.52
        - penetrating into pulp KØ2.53
      - pit and fissure surface
        - limited to enamel KØ2.51
        - penetrating into dentin KØ2.52
        - penetrating into pulp KØ2.53
      - smooth surface
        - limited to enamel KØ2.61
        - penetrating into dentin KØ2.62
        - penetrating into pulp KØ2.63
    - pit and fissure surface
      - limited to enamel KØ2.51
      - penetrating into dentin KØ2.52
      - penetrating into pulp KØ2.53
    - primary, cervical origin KØ2.52
    - root KØ2.7
    - smooth surface
      - limited to enamel KØ2.61
      - penetrating into dentin KØ2.62

- **Caries** — *continued*
  - dental — *continued*
    - smooth surface — *continued*
      - penetrating into pulp KØ2.63
  - external meatus — *see* Disorder, ear, external, specified type NEC
  - hip (tuberculous) A18.Ø2
  - initial (tooth)
    - chewing surface KØ2.51
    - pit and fissure surface KØ2.51
    - smooth surface KØ2.61
  - knee (tuberculous) A18.Ø2
  - labyrinth H83.8 ☑
  - limb NEC (tuberculous) A18.Ø3
  - mastoid process (chronic) — *see* Mastoiditis, chronic
    - tuberculous A18.Ø3
  - middle ear H74.8 ☑
  - nose (tuberculous) A18.Ø3
  - orbit (tuberculous) A18.Ø3
  - ossicles, ear — *see* Abnormal, ear ossicles
  - petrous bone — *see* Petrositis
  - root (dental) (tooth) KØ2.7
  - sacrum (tuberculous) A18.Ø1
  - spine, spinal (column) (tuberculous) A18.Ø1
  - syphilitic A52.77
    - congenital (early) A5Ø.Ø2 *[M9Ø.8Ø]*
  - tooth, teeth — *see* Caries, dental
  - tuberculous A18.Ø3
  - vertebra (column) (tuberculous) A18.Ø1
- **Carious teeth** — *see* Caries, dental
- **Carneous mole** OØ2.Ø
- **Carnitine insufficiency** E71.4Ø
- **Carotenemia** (dietary) E67.1
- **Carotenosis** (cutis) (skin) E67.1
- **Carotid body or sinus syndrome** G9Ø.Ø1
- **Carotidynia** G9Ø.Ø1
- **Carpal tunnel syndrome** — *see* Syndrome, carpal tunnel
- **Carpenter's syndrome** Q87.Ø
- **Carpopedal spasm** — *see* Tetany
- **Carr-Barr-Plunkett syndrome** Q97.1
- **Carrier** (suspected) of
  - amebiasis Z22.1
  - bacterial disease NEC Z22.39
    - diphtheria Z22.2
    - intestinal infectious NEC Z22.1
      - typhoid Z22.Ø
    - meningococcal Z22.31
    - sexually transmitted Z22.4
    - specified NEC Z22.39
    - staphylococcal (Methicillin susceptible) Z22.321
      - Methicillin resistant Z22.322
    - streptococcal Z22.338
      - group B Z22.33Ø
        - complicating pregnancy or delivery O99.82- ☑
    - typhoid Z22.Ø
  - cholera Z22.1
  - diphtheria Z22.2
  - gastrointestinal pathogens NEC Z22.1
  - genetic Z14.8
    - cystic fibrosis Z14.1
    - hemophilia A (asymptomatic) Z14.Ø1
      - symptomatic Z14.Ø2
  - gestational, pregnant Z33.1
  - gonorrhea Z22.4
  - HAA (hepatitis Australian-antigen) B18.8
  - HB (c)(s)-AG B18.1
  - hepatitis (viral) B18.9
    - Australia-antigen (HAA) B18.8
    - B surface antigen (HBsAg) B18.1
      - with acute delta- (super)infection B17.Ø
    - C B18.2
    - specified NEC B18.8
  - human T-cell lymphotropic virus type-1 (HTLV-1) infection Z22.6
  - infectious organism Z22.9
    - specified NEC Z22.8
  - meningococci Z22.31
  - Salmonella typhosa Z22.Ø
  - serum hepatitis — *see* Carrier, hepatitis
  - staphylococci (Methicillin susceptible) Z22.321
    - Methicillin resistant Z22.322
  - streptococci Z22.338
    - group B Z22.33Ø
      - complicating pregnancy or delivery O99.82- ☑
  - syphilis Z22.4
  - typhoid Z22.Ø
  - venereal disease NEC Z22.4

- **Carrion's disease** A44.Ø
- **Carter's relapsing fever** (Asiatic) A68.1
- **Cartilage** — *see* condition
- **Caruncle** (inflamed)
  - conjunctiva (acute) — *see* Conjunctivitis, acute
  - labium (majus) (minus) N9Ø.89
  - lacrimal — *see* Inflammation, lacrimal, passages
  - myrtiform N89.8
  - urethral (benign) N36.2
- **Cascade stomach** K31.2
- **Caseation lymphatic gland** (tuberculous) A18.2
- **Cassidy** (-Scholte) syndrome (malignant carcinoid) E34.Ø
- **Castellani's disease** A69.8
- **Castration, traumatic, male** S38.231 ☑
- **Casts in urine** R82.998
- **Cat**
  - cry syndrome Q93.4
  - ear Q17.3
  - eye syndrome Q92.8
- **Catabolism, senile** R54
- **Catalepsy** (hysterical) F44.2
  - schizophrenic F2Ø.2
- **Cataplexy** (idiopathic) — *see* Narcolepsy
- **Cataract** (cortical) (immature) (incipient) H26.9
  - with
    - neovascularization — *see* Cataract, complicated
  - age-related — *see* Cataract, senile
  - anterior
    - and posterior axial embryonal Q12.Ø
    - pyramidal Q12.Ø
  - associated with
    - galactosemia E74.21 *[H28]*
    - myotonic disorders G71.19 *[H28]*
  - blue Q12.Ø
  - central Q12.Ø
  - cerulean Q12.Ø
  - complicated H26.2Ø
    - with
      - neovascularization H26.21- ☑
      - ocular disorder H26.22- ☑
    - glaucomatous flecks H26.23- ☑
  - congenital Q12.Ø
  - coraliform Q12.Ø
  - coronary Q12.Ø
  - crystalline Q12.Ø
  - diabetic — *see* Diabetes, cataract
  - drug-induced H26.3- ☑
  - due to
    - ocular disorder — *see* Cataract, complicated
    - radiation H26.8
  - electric H26.8
  - extraction status Z98.4- ☑
  - glass-blower's H26.8
  - heat ray H26.8
  - heterochromic — *see* Cataract, complicated
  - hypermature — *see* Cataract, senile, morgagnian type
  - in (due to)
    - chronic iridocyclitis — *see* Cataract, complicated
    - diabetes — *see* Diabetes, cataract
    - endocrine disease E34.9 *[H28]*
    - eye disease — *see* Cataract, complicated
    - hypoparathyroidism E2Ø.9 *[H28]*
    - malnutrition-dehydration E46 *[H28]*
    - metabolic disease E88.9 *[H28]*
    - myotonic disorders G71.19 *[H28]*
    - nutritional disease E63.9 *[H28]*
  - infantile — *see* Cataract, presenile
  - irradiational — *see* Cataract, specified NEC
  - juvenile — *see* Cataract, presenile
  - malnutrition-dehydration E46 *[H28]*
  - morgagnian — *see* Cataract, senile, morgagnian type
  - myotonic G71.19 *[H28]*
  - myxedema EØ3.9 *[H28]*
  - nuclear
    - embryonal Q12.Ø
    - sclerosis — *see* Cataract, senile, nuclear
  - presenile H26.ØØ- ☑
    - combined forms H26.Ø6- ☑
    - cortical H26.Ø1- ☑
    - lamellar — *see* Cataract, presenile, cortical
    - nuclear H26.Ø3- ☑
    - specified NEC H26.Ø9
    - subcapsular polar (anterior) H26.Ø4- ☑
      - posterior H26.Ø5- ☑
    - zonular — *see* Cataract, presenile, cortical
  - secondary H26.4Ø
    - Soemmering's ring H26.41- ☑

Cephalematocele, cephalhematocele — *continued*
  newborn — *continued*
    birth injury P1Ø.8
  traumatic — *see* Hematoma, brain
Cephalematoma, cephalhematoma (calcified)
  newborn (birth injury) P12.Ø
  traumatic — *see* Hematoma, brain
Cephalgia, cephalalgia — *see also* Headache
  histamine G44.ØØ9
    intractable G44.ØØ1
    not intractable G44.ØØ9
  trigeminal autonomic (TAC) NEC G44.Ø99
    intractable G44.Ø91
    not intractable G44.Ø99
Cephalic — *see* condition
Cephalitis — *see* Encephalitis
Cephalocele — *see* Encephalocele
Cephalomenia N94.89
Cephalopelvic — *see* condition
Cerclage (with cervical incompetence) in pregnancy — *see* Incompetence, cervix, in pregnancy
Cerebellitis — *see* Encephalitis
Cerebellum, cerebellar — *see* condition
Cerebral — *see* condition
Cerebritis — *see* Encephalitis
Cerebro-hepato-renal syndrome Q87.89
Cerebromalacia — *see* Softening, brain
  sequelae of cerebrovascular disease I69.398
Cerebroside lipidosis E75.22
Cerebrospasticity (congenital) G8Ø.1
Cerebrospinal — *see* condition
Cerebrum — *see* condition
Ceroid-lipofuscinosis, neuronal E75.4
Cerumen (accumulation) (impacted) H61.2- ☑
Cervical — *see also* condition
  auricle Q18.2
  dysplasia in pregnancy — *see* Abnormal, cervix, in pregnancy or childbirth
  erosion in pregnancy — *see* Abnormal, cervix, in pregnancy or childbirth
  fibrosis in pregnancy — *see* Abnormal, cervix, in pregnancy or childbirth
  fusion syndrome Q76.1
  rib Q76.5
  shortening (complicating pregnancy) O26.87- ☑
Cervicalgia M54.2
Cervicitis (acute) (chronic) (nonvenereal) (senile (atrophic)) (subacute) (with ulceration) N72
  with
    abortion — *see* Abortion, by type complicated by genital tract and pelvic infection
    ectopic pregnancy OØ8.Ø
    molar pregnancy OØ8.Ø
  chlamydial A56.Ø9
  gonococcal A54.Ø3
  herpesviral A6Ø.Ø3
  puerperal (postpartum) O86.11
  syphilitic A52.76
  trichomonal A59.Ø9
  tuberculous A18.16
Cervicocolpitis (emphysematosa) — *see also* Cervicitis N72
Cervix — *see* condition
Cesarean delivery, previous, affecting management of pregnancy O34.219
  classical (vertical) scar O34.212
  isthmocele O34.22
  low transverse scar O34.211
  mid-transverse T incision O34.218
  scar
    defect (isthmocele) O34.22
    specified type NEC O34.218
Céstan (-Chenais) paralysis or syndrome G46.3
Céstan-Raymond syndrome I65.8
Cestode infestation B71.9
  specified type NEC B71.8
Cestodiasis B71.9
Chabert's disease A22.9
Chacaleh E53.8
Chafing L3Ø.4
Chagas' (-Mazza) disease (chronic) B57.2
  with
    cardiovascular involvement NEC B57.2
    digestive system involvement B57.3Ø
      megacolon B57.32
      megaesophagus B57.31
      other specified B57.39
Chagas'disease — *continued*
  with — *continued*
    megacolon B57.32
    megaesophagus B57.31
    myocarditis B57.2
    nervous system involvement B57.4Ø
      meningitis B57.41
      meningoencephalitis B57.42
      other specified B57.49
    specified organ involvement NEC B57.5
  acute (with) B57.1
    cardiovascular NEC B57.Ø
    myocarditis B57.Ø
Chagres fever B5Ø.9
Chairridden Z74.Ø9
Chalasia (cardiac sphincter) K21.9
Chalazion HØØ.19
  left HØØ.16
    lower HØØ.15
    upper HØØ.14
  right HØØ.13
    lower HØØ.12
    upper HØØ.11
Chalcosis — *see also* Disorder, globe, degenerative, chalcosis
  cornea — *see* Deposit, cornea
  crystalline lens — *see* Cataract, complicated
  retina H35.89
Chalicosis (pulmonum) J62.8
Chancre (any genital site) (hard) (hunterian) (mixed) (primary) (seronegative) (seropositive) (syphilitic) A51.Ø
  congenital A5Ø.Ø7
  conjunctiva NEC A51.2
  Ducrey's A57
  extragenital A51.2
  eyelid A51.2
  lip A51.2
  nipple A51.2
  Nisbet's A57
  of
    carate A67.Ø
    pinta A67.Ø
    yaws A66.Ø
  palate, soft A51.2
  phagedenic A57
  simple A57
  soft A57
    bubo A57
    palate A51.2
  urethra A51.Ø
  yaws A66.Ø
Chancroid (anus) (genital) (penis) (perineum) (rectum) (urethra) (vulva) A57
Chandler's disease (osteochondritis dissecans, hip) — *see* Osteochondritis, dissecans, hip
Change(s) (in) (of) — *see also* Removal
  arteriosclerotic — *see* Arteriosclerosis
  bone — *see also* Disorder, bone
    diabetic — *see* Diabetes, bone change
  bowel habit R19.4
  cardiorenal (vascular) — *see* Hypertension, cardiorenal
  cardiovascular — *see* Disease, cardiovascular
  circulatory I99.9
  cognitive (mild) (organic) R41.89
  color, tooth, teeth
    during formation KØØ.8
    posteruptive KØ3.7
  contraceptive device Z3Ø.433
  corneal membrane H18.3Ø
    Bowman's membrane fold or rupture H18.31- ☑
    Descemet's membrane
      fold H18.32- ☑
      rupture H18.33- ☑
  coronary — *see* Disease, heart, ischemic
  degenerative, spine or vertebra — *see* Spondylosis
  dental pulp, regressive KØ4.2
  dressing (nonsurgical) Z48.ØØ
    surgical Z48.Ø1
  heart — *see* Disease, heart
  hip joint — *see* Derangement, joint, hip
  hyperplastic larynx J38.7
  hypertrophic
    nasal sinus J34.89
    turbinate, nasal J34.3
    upper respiratory tract J39.8
  indwelling catheter Z46.6
  inflammatory — *see also* Inflammation
Change(s) — *continued*
  inflammatory — *see also* Inflammation — *continued*
    sacroiliac M46.1
  job, anxiety concerning Z56.1
  joint — *see* Derangement, joint
  life — *see* Menopause
  mental status R41.82
  minimal (glomerular) — *see also* NØØ-NØ7 with fourth character .Ø NØ5.Ø
  myocardium, myocardial — *see* Degeneration, myocardial
  of life — *see* Menopause
  pacemaker Z45.Ø18
    pulse generator Z45.Ø1Ø
  personality (enduring) F68.8
    due to (secondary to)
      general medical condition FØ7.Ø
    secondary (nonspecific) F6Ø.89
  regressive, dental pulp KØ4.2
  renal — *see* Disease, renal
  retina H35.9
    myopic — *see also* Myopia, degenerative H44.2- ☑
  sacroiliac joint M53.3
  senile — *see also* condition R54
  sensory R2Ø.8
  skin R23.9
    acute, due to ultraviolet radiation L56.9
      specified NEC L56.8
    chronic, due to nonionizing radiation L57.9
      specified NEC L57.8
    cyanosis R23.Ø
    flushing R23.2
    pallor R23.1
    petechiae R23.3
    specified change NEC R23.8
    swelling — *see* Mass, localized
    texture R23.4
  trophic
    arm — *see* Mononeuropathy, upper limb
    leg — *see* Mononeuropathy, lower limb
  vascular I99.9
  vasomotor I73.9
  voice R49.9
    psychogenic F44.4
    specified NEC R49.8
Changing sleep-work schedule, affecting sleep G47.26
Changuinola fever A93.1
Chapping skin T69.8 ☑
Charcot-Marie-Tooth disease, paralysis or syndrome G6Ø.Ø
Charcot's
  arthropathy — *see* Arthropathy, neuropathic
  cirrhosis K74.3
  disease (tabetic arthropathy) A52.16
  joint (disease) (tabetic) A52.16
    diabetic — *see* Diabetes, with, arthropathy
    syringomyelic G95.Ø
  syndrome (intermittent claudication) I73.9
CHARGE association Q89.8
Charley-horse (quadriceps) M62.831
  traumatic (quadriceps) S76.11- ☑
Charlouis' disease — *see* Yaws
Cheadle's disease E54
Checking (of)
  cardiac pacemaker (battery) (electrode(s)) Z45.Ø18
    pulse generator Z45.Ø1Ø
  implantable subdermal contraceptive Z3Ø.46
  intrauterine contraceptive device Z3Ø.431
  wound Z48.Ø- ☑
    due to injury — code to Injury, by site, using appropriate seventh character for subsequent encounter
Check-up — *see* Examination
Chédiak-Higashi (-Steinbrinck) **syndrome** (congenital gigantism of peroxidase granules) E7Ø.33Ø
Cheek — *see* condition
Cheese itch B88.Ø
Cheese-washer's lung J67.8
Cheese-worker's lung J67.8
Cheilitis (acute) (angular) (catarrhal) (chronic) (exfoliative) (gangrenous) (glandular) (infectional) (suppurative) (ulcerative) (vesicular) K13.Ø
  actinic (due to sun) L56.8
    other than from sun L59.8
  candidal B37.83
Cheilodynia K13.Ø

- **Coccidioidomycosis** — *continued*
  - pulmonary B38.2
    - acute B38.Ø
    - chronic B38.1
  - skin B38.3
  - specified NEC B38.89
- **Coccidioidosis** — *see* Coccidioidomycosis
- **Coccidiosis** (intestinal) AØ7.3
- **Coccydynia, coccygodynia** M53.3
- **Coccyx** — *see* condition
- **Cochin-China diarrhea** K9Ø.1
- **Cockayne's syndrome** Q87.19
- **Cocked up toe** — *see* Deformity, toe, specified NEC
- **Cock's peculiar tumor** L72.3
- **Codman's tumor** — *see* Neoplasm, bone, benign
- **Coenurosis** B71.8
- **Coffee-worker's lung** J67.8
- **Cogan's syndrome** H16.32- ☑
  - oculomotor apraxia H51.8
- **Coitus, painful** (female) N94.1Ø
  - male N53.12
  - psychogenic F52.6
- **Cold** JØØ
  - with influenza, flu, or grippe — *see* Influenza, with, respiratory manifestations NEC
  - agglutinin disease or hemoglobinuria (chronic) D59.12
  - bronchial — *see* Bronchitis
  - chest — *see* Bronchitis
  - common (head) JØØ
  - effects of T69.9 ☑
    - specified effect NEC T69.8 ☑
  - excessive, effects of T69.9 ☑
    - specified effect NEC T69.8 ☑
  - exhaustion from T69.8 ☑
  - exposure to T69.9 ☑
    - specified effect NEC T69.8 ☑
  - head JØØ
  - injury syndrome (newborn) P8Ø.Ø
  - on lung — *see* Bronchitis
  - rose J3Ø.1
  - sensitivity, auto-immune D59.12
  - symptoms JØØ
  - virus JØØ
- **Coldsore** BØØ.1
- **Colibacillosis** A49.8
  - as the cause of other disease — *see also* Escherichia coli B96.2Ø
  - generalized A41.5Ø
- **Colic** (bilious) (infantile) (intestinal) (recurrent) (spasmodic) R1Ø.83
  - abdomen R1Ø.83
    - psychogenic F45.8
  - appendix, appendicular K38.8
  - bile duct — *see* Calculus, bile duct
  - biliary — *see* Calculus, bile duct
  - common duct — *see* Calculus, bile duct
  - cystic duct — *see* Calculus, gallbladder
  - Devonshire NEC — *see* Poisoning, lead
  - gallbladder — *see* Calculus, gallbladder
  - gallstone — *see* Calculus, gallbladder
    - gallbladder or cystic duct — *see* Calculus, gallbladder
  - hepatic (duct) — *see* Calculus, bile duct
  - hysterical F45.8
  - kidney N23
  - lead NEC — *see* Poisoning, lead
  - mucous K58.9
    - with diarrhea K58.Ø
    - psychogenic F54
  - nephritic N23
  - painter's NEC — *see* Poisoning, lead
  - pancreas K86.89
  - psychogenic F45.8
  - renal N23
  - saturnine NEC — *see* Poisoning, lead
  - ureter N23
  - urethral N36.8
    - due to calculus N21.1
  - uterus NEC N94.89
    - menstrual — *see* Dysmenorrhea
  - worm NOS B83.9
- **Colicystitis** — *see* Cystitis
- **Colitis** (acute) (catarrhal) (chronic) (noninfective) (hemorrhagic) — *see also* Enteritis K52.9
  - allergic K52.29

- **Colitis** — *continued*
  - allergic — *continued*
    - with
      - food protein-induced enterocolitis syndrome K52.21
      - proctocolitis K52.82
  - amebic (acute) — *see also* Amebiasis AØ6.Ø
    - nondysenteric AØ6.2
  - anthrax A22.2
  - bacillary — *see* Infection, Shigella
  - balantidial AØ7.Ø
  - Clostridium difficile
    - not specified as recurrent AØ4.72
    - recurrent AØ4.71
  - coccidial AØ7.3
  - collagenous K52.831
  - cystica superficialis K52.89
  - dietary counseling and surveillance (for) Z71.3
  - dietetic — *see also* Colitis, allergic K52.29
  - drug-induced K52.1
  - due to radiation K52.Ø
  - eosinophilic K52.82
  - food hypersensitivity — *see also* Colitis, allergic K52.29
  - giardial AØ7.1
  - granulomatous — *see* Enteritis, regional, large intestine
  - indeterminate, so stated K52.3
  - infectious — *see* Enteritis, infectious
  - ischemic K55.9
    - acute (subacute) — *see also* Ischemia, intestine, acute K55.Ø39
    - chronic K55.1
    - due to mesenteric artery insufficiency K55.1
    - fulminant (acute) — *see also* Ischemia, intestine, acute K55.Ø39
  - left sided K51.5Ø
    - with
      - abscess K51.514
      - complication K51.519
        - specified NEC K51.518
      - fistula K51.513
      - obstruction K51.512
      - rectal bleeding K51.511
  - lymphocytic K52.832
  - membranous
    - psychogenic F54
  - microscopic K52.839
    - specified NEC K52.838
  - mucous — *see* Syndrome, irritable, bowel
    - psychogenic F54
  - noninfective K52.9
    - specified NEC K52.89
  - polyposa — *see* Polyp, colon, inflammatory
  - protozoal AØ7.9
  - pseudomembranous
    - not specified as recurrent AØ4.72
    - recurrent AØ4.71
  - pseudomucinous — *see* Syndrome, irritable, bowel
  - regional — *see* Enteritis, regional, large intestine
    - infectious AØ9
  - segmental — *see* Enteritis, regional, large intestine
  - septic — *see* Enteritis, infectious
  - spastic K58.9
    - with diarrhea K58.Ø
    - psychogenic F54
  - staphylococcal AØ4.8
    - foodborne AØ5.Ø
  - subacute ischemic — *see also* Ischemia, intestine, acute K55.Ø39
  - thromboulcerative — *see also* Ischemia, intestine, acute K55.Ø39
  - toxic NEC K52.1
    - due to Clostridium difficile
      - not specified as recurrent AØ4.72
      - recurrent AØ4.71
  - transmural — *see* Enteritis, regional, large intestine
  - trichomonal AØ7.8
  - tuberculous (ulcerative) A18.32
  - ulcerative (chronic) K51.9Ø
    - with
      - complication K51.919
        - abscess K51.914
        - fistula K51.913
        - obstruction K51.912
        - rectal bleeding K51.911
        - specified complication NEC K51.918
    - enterocolitis — *see* Enterocolitis, ulcerative
    - ileocolitis — *see* Ileocolitis, ulcerative
    - mucosal proctocolitis — *see* Proctocolitis, mucosal

- **Colitis** — *continued*
  - ulcerative — *continued*
    - proctitis — *see* Proctitis, ulcerative
    - pseudopolyposis — *see* Polyp, colon, inflammatory
    - psychogenic F54
    - rectosigmoiditis — *see* Rectosigmoiditis, ulcerative
    - specified type NEC K51.8Ø
      - with
        - complication K51.819
          - abscess K51.814
          - fistula K51.813
          - obstruction K51.812
          - rectal bleeding K51.811
          - specified complication NEC K51.818
- **Collagenosis, collagen disease** (nonvascular) (vascular) M35.9
  - cardiovascular I42.8
  - reactive perforating L87.1
  - specified NEC M35.8
- **Collapse** R55
  - adrenal E27.2
  - cardiorespiratory R57.Ø
  - cardiovascular R57.Ø
    - newborn P29.89
  - circulatory (peripheral) R57.9
    - during or after labor and delivery O75.1
    - following ectopic or molar pregnancy OØ8.3
    - newborn P29.89
  - during or
    - after labor and delivery O75.1
    - resulting from a procedure, not elsewhere classified T81.1Ø ☑
  - external ear canal — *see* Stenosis, external ear canal
  - general R55
  - heart — *see* Disease, heart
  - heat T67.1 ☑
  - hysterical F44.89
  - labyrinth, membranous (congenital) Q16.5
  - lung (massive) — *see also* Atelectasis J98.19
    - pressure due to anesthesia (general) (local) or other sedation T88.2 ☑
      - during labor and delivery O74.1
      - in pregnancy O29.Ø2- ☑
      - postpartum, puerperal O89.Ø9
  - myocardial — *see* Disease, heart
  - nervous F48.8
  - neurocirculatory F45.8
  - nose M95.Ø
  - postoperative T81.1Ø ☑
  - pulmonary — *see also* Atelectasis J98.19
    - newborn — *see* Atelectasis
  - trachea J39.8
  - tracheobronchial J98.Ø9
  - valvular — *see* Endocarditis
  - vascular (peripheral) R57.9
    - during or after labor and delivery O75.1
    - following ectopic or molar pregnancy OØ8.3
    - newborn P29.89
  - vertebra M48.5Ø- ☑
    - cervical region M48.52- ☑
    - cervicothoracic region M48.53- ☑
    - in (due to)
      - metastasis — *see* Collapse, vertebra, in, specified disease NEC
      - osteoporosis — *see also* Osteoporosis M8Ø.88 ☑
        - cervical region M8Ø.88 ☑
        - cervicothoracic region M8Ø.88 ☑
        - lumbar region M8Ø.88 ☑
        - lumbosacral region M8Ø.88 ☑
        - multiple sites M8Ø.88 ☑
        - occipito-atlanto-axial region M8Ø.88 ☑
        - sacrococcygeal region M8Ø.88 ☑
        - thoracic region M8Ø.88 ☑
        - thoracolumbar region M8Ø.88 ☑
      - specified disease NEC M48.5Ø- ☑
        - cervical region M48.52- ☑
        - cervicothoracic region M48.53- ☑
        - lumbar region M48.56- ☑
        - lumbosacral region M48.57- ☑
        - occipito-atlanto-axial region M48.51- ☑
        - sacrococcygeal region M48.58- ☑
        - thoracic region M48.54- ☑
        - thoracolumbar region M48.55- ☑
    - lumbar region M48.56- ☑
    - lumbosacral region M48.57- ☑
    - occipito-atlanto-axial region M48.51- ☑
    - sacrococcygeal region M48.58- ☑

Complication(s) — *continued*
- anesthesia, anesthetic — *see also* Anesthesia, complication — *continued*
  - general, unintended awareness during procedure T88.53 ☑
  - hyperthermia, malignant T88.3 ☑
  - hypothermia T88.51 ☑
  - intubation failure T88.4 ☑
  - malignant hyperthermia T88.3 ☑
  - pulmonary
    - in
      - labor and delivery O74.1
      - pregnancy NEC O29.Ø9- ☑
    - postpartum, puerperal O89.Ø9
  - shock T88.2 ☑
  - spinal and epidural
    - in
      - labor and delivery NEC O74.6
        - headache O74.5
      - pregnancy NEC O29.5X- ☑
    - postpartum, puerperal NEC O89.5
      - headache O89.4
  - unintended awareness under general anesthesia during procedure T88.53 ☑
- anti-reflux device — *see* Complications, esophageal anti-reflux device
- aortic (bifurcation) graft — *see* Complications, graft, vascular
- aortocoronary (bypass) graft — *see* Complications, coronary artery (bypass) graft
- aortofemoral (bypass) graft — *see* Complications, extremity artery (bypass) graft
- arteriovenous
  - fistula, surgically created T82.9 ☑
    - embolism T82.818 ☑
    - fibrosis T82.828 ☑
    - hemorrhage T82.838 ☑
    - infection or inflammation T82.7 ☑
    - mechanical
      - breakdown T82.51Ø ☑
      - displacement T82.52Ø ☑
      - leakage T82.53Ø ☑
      - malposition T82.52Ø ☑
      - obstruction T82.59Ø ☑
      - perforation T82.59Ø ☑
      - protrusion T82.59Ø ☑
    - pain T82.848 ☑
    - specified type NEC T82.898 ☑
    - stenosis T82.858 ☑
    - thrombosis T82.868 ☑
  - shunt, surgically created T82.9 ☑
    - embolism T82.818 ☑
    - fibrosis T82.828 ☑
    - hemorrhage T82.838 ☑
    - infection or inflammation T82.7 ☑
    - mechanical
      - breakdown T82.511 ☑
      - displacement T82.521 ☑
      - leakage T82.531 ☑
      - malposition T82.521 ☑
      - obstruction T82.591 ☑
      - perforation T82.591 ☑
      - protrusion T82.591 ☑
    - pain T82.848 ☑
    - specified type NEC T82.898 ☑
    - stenosis T82.858 ☑
    - thrombosis T82.868 ☑
- arthroplasty — *see* Complications, joint prosthesis
- artificial
  - fertilization or insemination N98.9
    - attempted introduction (of)
      - embryo in embryo transfer N98.3
      - ovum following in vitro fertilization N98.2
    - hyperstimulation of ovaries N98.1
    - infection N98.Ø
    - specified NEC N98.8
  - heart T82.9 ☑
    - embolism T82.817 ☑
    - fibrosis T82.827 ☑
    - hemorrhage T82.837 ☑
    - infection or inflammation T82.7 ☑
    - mechanical
      - breakdown T82.512 ☑
      - displacement T82.522 ☑
      - leakage T82.532 ☑
      - malposition T82.522 ☑
      - obstruction T82.592 ☑

Complication(s) — *continued*
- artificial — *continued*
  - heart — *continued*
    - mechanical — *continued*
      - perforation T82.592 ☑
      - protrusion T82.592 ☑
    - pain T82.847 ☑
    - specified type NEC T82.897 ☑
    - stenosis T82.857 ☑
    - thrombosis T82.867 ☑
  - opening
    - cecostomy — *see* Complications, colostomy
    - colostomy — *see* Complications, colostomy
    - cystostomy — *see* Complications, cystostomy
    - enterostomy — *see* Complications, enterostomy
    - gastrostomy — *see* Complications, gastrostomy
    - ileostomy — *see* Complications, enterostomy
    - jejunostomy — *see* Complications, enterostomy
    - nephrostomy — *see* Complications, stoma, urinary tract
    - tracheostomy — *see* Complications, tracheostomy
    - ureterostomy — *see* Complications, stoma, urinary tract
    - urethrostomy — *see* Complications, stoma, urinary tract
- balloon implant or device
  - gastrointestinal T85.9 ☑
    - embolism T85.818 ☑
    - fibrosis T85.828 ☑
    - hemorrhage T85.838 ☑
    - infection and inflammation T85.79 ☑
    - pain T85.848 ☑
    - specified type NEC T85.898 ☑
    - stenosis T85.858 ☑
    - thrombosis T85.868 ☑
  - vascular (counterpulsation) T82.9 ☑
    - embolism T82.818 ☑
    - fibrosis T82.828 ☑
    - hemorrhage T82.838 ☑
    - infection or inflammation T82.7 ☑
    - mechanical
      - breakdown T82.513 ☑
      - displacement T82.523 ☑
      - leakage T82.533 ☑
      - malposition T82.523 ☑
      - obstruction T82.593 ☑
      - perforation T82.593 ☑
      - protrusion T82.593 ☑
    - pain T82.848 ☑
    - specified type NEC T82.898 ☑
    - stenosis T82.858 ☑
    - thrombosis T82.868 ☑
- bariatric procedure
  - gastric band procedure K95.Ø9
    - infection K95.Ø1
  - specified procedure NEC K95.89
    - infection K95.81
- bile duct implant (prosthetic) T85.9 ☑
  - embolism T85.818 ☑
  - fibrosis T85.828 ☑
  - hemorrhage T85.838 ☑
  - infection and inflammation T85.79 ☑
  - mechanical
    - breakdown T85.51Ø ☑
    - displacement T85.52Ø ☑
    - malfunction T85.51Ø ☑
    - malposition T85.52Ø ☑
    - obstruction T85.59Ø ☑
    - perforation T85.59Ø ☑
    - protrusion T85.59Ø ☑
    - specified NEC T85.59Ø ☑
  - pain T85.848 ☑
  - specified type NEC T85.898 ☑
  - stenosis T85.858 ☑
  - thrombosis T85.868 ☑
- bladder device (auxiliary) — *see* Complications, genitourinary, device or implant, urinary system
- bleeding (postoperative) — *see* Complication, postoperative, hemorrhage
  - intraoperative — *see* Complication, intraoperative, hemorrhage
- blood vessel graft — *see* Complications, graft, vascular
- bone
  - device NEC T84.9 ☑
    - embolism T84.81 ☑

Complication(s) — *continued*
- bone — *continued*
  - device — *continued*
    - fibrosis T84.82 ☑
    - hemorrhage T84.83 ☑
    - infection or inflammation T84.7 ☑
    - mechanical
      - breakdown T84.318 ☑
      - displacement T84.328 ☑
      - malposition T84.328 ☑
      - obstruction T84.398 ☑
      - perforation T84.398 ☑
      - protrusion T84.398 ☑
    - pain T84.84 ☑
    - specified type NEC T84.89 ☑
    - stenosis T84.85 ☑
    - thrombosis T84.86 ☑
  - graft — *see* Complications, graft, bone
  - growth stimulator (electrode) — *see* Complications, electronic stimulator device, bone
  - marrow transplant — *see* Complications, transplant, bone, marrow
- brain neurostimulator (electrode) — *see* Complications, electronic stimulator device, brain
- breast implant (prosthetic) T85.9 ☑
  - capsular contracture T85.44 ☑
  - embolism T85.818 ☑
  - fibrosis T85.828 ☑
  - hemorrhage T85.838 ☑
  - infection and inflammation T85.79 ☑
  - mechanical
    - breakdown T85.41 ☑
    - displacement T85.42 ☑
    - leakage T85.43 ☑
    - malposition T85.42 ☑
    - obstruction T85.49 ☑
    - perforation T85.49 ☑
    - protrusion T85.49 ☑
    - specified NEC T85.49 ☑
  - pain T85.848 ☑
  - specified type NEC T85.898 ☑
  - stenosis T85.858 ☑
  - thrombosis T85.868 ☑
- bypass — *see also* Complications, prosthetic device or implant
  - aortocoronary — *see* Complications, coronary artery (bypass) graft
  - arterial — *see also* Complications, graft, vascular
    - extremity — *see* Complications, extremity artery (bypass) graft
- cardiac — *see also* Disease, heart
  - device, implant or graft T82.9 ☑
    - embolism T82.817 ☑
    - fibrosis T82.827 ☑
    - hemorrhage T82.837 ☑
    - infection or inflammation T82.7 ☑
      - valve prosthesis T82.6 ☑
    - mechanical
      - breakdown T82.519 ☑
        - specified device NEC T82.518 ☑
      - displacement T82.529 ☑
        - specified device NEC T82.528 ☑
      - leakage T82.539 ☑
        - specified device NEC T82.538 ☑
      - malposition T82.529 ☑
        - specified device NEC T82.528 ☑
      - obstruction T82.599 ☑
        - specified device NEC T82.598 ☑
      - perforation T82.599 ☑
        - specified device NEC T82.598 ☑
      - protrusion T82.599 ☑
        - specified device NEC T82.598 ☑
    - pain T82.847 ☑
    - specified type NEC T82.897 ☑
    - stenosis T82.857 ☑
    - thrombosis T82.867 ☑
- cardiovascular device, graft or implant T82.9 ☑
  - aortic graft — *see* Complications, graft, vascular
  - arteriovenous
    - fistula, artificial — *see* Complication, arteriovenous, fistula, surgically created
    - shunt — *see* Complication, arteriovenous, shunt, surgically created
  - artificial heart — *see* Complication, artificial, heart
  - balloon (counterpulsation) device — *see* Complication, balloon implant, vascular

- **Complication**(s) — *continued*
  - catheter — *see also* Complications, prosthetic device or implant — *continued*
    - subdural infusion — *continued*
      - pain T85.84Ø ☑
      - specified type NEC T85.89Ø ☑
      - stenosis T85.85Ø ☑
      - thrombosis T85.86Ø ☑
    - urethral T83.9 ☑
      - displacement T83.Ø28 ☑
      - embolism T83.81 ☑
      - fibrosis T83.82 ☑
      - hemorrhage T83.83 ☑
      - indwelling
        - breakdown T83.Ø11 ☑
        - displacement T83.Ø21 ☑
        - infection and inflammation T83.511 ☑
        - leakage T83.Ø31 ☑
        - specified complication NEC T83.Ø91 ☑
      - infection and inflammation T83.511 ☑
      - leakage T83.Ø38 ☑
      - malposition T83.Ø28 ☑
      - mechanical
        - breakdown T83.Ø11 ☑
      - obstruction (mechanical) T83.Ø91 ☑
      - pain T83.84 ☑
      - perforation T83.Ø91 ☑
      - protrusion T83.Ø91 ☑
      - specified type NEC T83.Ø91 ☑
      - stenosis T83.85 ☑
      - thrombosis T83.86 ☑
    - urinary NEC
      - breakdown T83.Ø18 ☑
      - displacement T83.Ø28 ☑
      - infection and inflammation T83.518 ☑
      - leakage T83.Ø38 ☑
      - specified complication NEC T83.Ø98 ☑
  - cecostomy (stoma) — *see* Complications, colostomy
  - cesarean delivery wound NEC O9Ø.89
    - disruption O9Ø.Ø
    - hematoma O9Ø.2
    - infection (following delivery) O86.ØØ
  - chemotherapy (antineoplastic) NEC T88.7 ☑
  - chin implant (prosthetic) — *see* Complication, prosthetic device or implant, specified NEC
  - circulatory system I99.8
    - intraoperative I97.88
    - postprocedural I97.89
      - following cardiac surgery — *see also* Infarct, myocardium, associated with revascularization procedure I97.19- ☑
        - postcardiotomy syndrome I97.Ø
      - hypertension I97.3
      - lymphedema after mastectomy I97.2
      - postcardiotomy syndrome I97.Ø
      - specified NEC I97.89
  - colostomy (stoma) K94.ØØ
    - hemorrhage K94.Ø1
    - infection K94.Ø2
    - malfunction K94.Ø3
    - mechanical K94.Ø3
    - specified complication NEC K94.Ø9
  - contraceptive device, intrauterine — *see* Complications, intrauterine, contraceptive device
  - cord (umbilical) — *see* Complications, umbilical cord
  - corneal graft — *see* Complications, graft, cornea
  - coronary artery (bypass) graft T82.9 ☑
    - atherosclerosis — *see* Arteriosclerosis, coronary (artery),
    - embolism T82.818 ☑
    - fibrosis T82.828 ☑
    - hemorrhage T82.838 ☑
    - infection and inflammation T82.7 ☑
    - mechanical
      - breakdown T82.211 ☑
      - displacement T82.212 ☑
      - leakage T82.213 ☑
      - malposition T82.212 ☑
      - obstruction T82.218 ☑
      - perforation T82.218 ☑
      - protrusion T82.218 ☑
      - specified NEC T82.218 ☑
    - pain T82.848 ☑
    - specified type NEC T82.898 ☑
    - stenosis T82.858 ☑
    - thrombosis T82.868 ☑

- **Complication**(s) — *continued*
  - counterpulsation device (balloon), intra- aortic — *see* Complications, balloon implant, vascular
  - cystostomy (stoma) N99.518
    - catheter — *see* Complications, catheter, cystostomy
    - hemorrhage N99.51Ø
    - infection N99.511
    - malfunction N99.512
    - specified type NEC N99.518
  - delivery — *see also* Complications, obstetric O75.9
    - procedure (instrumental) (manual) (surgical) O75.4
    - specified NEC O75.89
  - dialysis (peritoneal) (renal) — *see also* Complications, infusion
    - catheter (vascular) — *see* Complication, catheter, dialysis
      - peritoneal, intraperitoneal — *see* Complications, catheter, intraperitoneal
  - dorsal column (spinal) neurostimulator — *see* Complications, electronic stimulator device, spinal cord
  - drug NEC T88.7 ☑
  - ear procedure — *see also* Disorder, ear
    - intraoperative H95.88
      - hematoma — *see* Complications, intraoperative, hemorrhage (hematoma) (of), ear
      - hemorrhage — *see* Complications, intraoperative, hemorrhage (hematoma) (of), ear
      - laceration — *see* Complications, intraoperative, puncture or laceration..., ear
      - specified NEC H95.88
    - postoperative H95.89
      - external ear canal stenosis H95.81- ☑
      - hematoma — *see* Complications, postprocedural, hematoma (of), ear
      - hemorrhage — *see* Complications, postprocedural, hemorrhage (of), ear
      - postmastoidectomy — *see* Complications, postmastoidectomy
      - seroma — *see* Complications, postprocedural, seroma (of), mastoid process
      - specified NEC H95.89
  - ectopic pregnancy OØ8.9
    - damage to pelvic organs OØ8.6
    - embolism OØ8.2
    - genital infection OØ8.Ø
    - hemorrhage (delayed) (excessive) OØ8.1
    - metabolic disorder OØ8.5
    - renal failure OØ8.4
    - shock OØ8.3
    - specified type NEC OØ8.Ø
    - venous complication NEC OØ8.7
  - electronic stimulator device
    - bladder (urinary) — *see* Complications, electronic stimulator device, urinary
    - bone T84.9 ☑
      - breakdown T84.31Ø ☑
      - displacement T84.32Ø ☑
      - embolism T84.81 ☑
      - fibrosis T84.82 ☑
      - hemorrhage T84.83 ☑
      - infection or inflammation T84.7 ☑
      - malfunction T84.31Ø ☑
      - malposition T84.32Ø ☑
      - mechanical NEC T84.39Ø ☑
      - obstruction T84.39Ø ☑
      - pain T84.84 ☑
      - perforation T84.39Ø ☑
      - protrusion T84.39Ø ☑
      - specified type NEC T84.89 ☑
      - stenosis T84.85 ☑
      - thrombosis T84.86 ☑
    - brain T85.9 ☑
      - embolism T85.81Ø ☑
      - fibrosis T85.82Ø ☑
      - hemorrhage T85.83Ø ☑
      - infection and inflammation T85.731 ☑
      - mechanical
        - breakdown T85.11Ø ☑
        - displacement T85.12Ø ☑
        - leakage T85.19Ø ☑
        - malposition T85.12Ø ☑
        - obstruction T85.19Ø ☑
        - perforation T85.19Ø ☑
        - protrusion T85.19Ø ☑
        - specified NEC T85.19Ø ☑
      - pain T85.84Ø ☑
      - specified type NEC T85.89Ø ☑

- **Complication**(s) — *continued*
  - electronic stimulator device — *continued*
    - brain — *continued*
      - stenosis T85.85Ø ☑
      - thrombosis T85.86Ø ☑
    - cardiac (defibrillator) (pacemaker) — *see* Complications, cardiovascular device or implant, electronic
    - generator (brain) (gastric) (peripheral) (sacral) (spinal)
      - breakdown T85.113 ☑
      - displacement T85.123 ☑
      - leakage T85.193 ☑
      - malposition T85.123 ☑
      - obstruction T85.193 ☑
      - perforation T85.193 ☑
      - protrusion T85.193 ☑
      - specified type NEC T85.193 ☑
    - muscle T84.9 ☑
      - breakdown T84.418 ☑
      - displacement T84.428 ☑
      - embolism T84.81 ☑
      - fibrosis T84.82 ☑
      - hemorrhage T84.83 ☑
      - infection or inflammation T84.7 ☑
      - mechanical NEC T84.498 ☑
      - pain T84.84 ☑
      - specified type NEC T84.89 ☑
      - stenosis T84.85 ☑
      - thrombosis T84.86 ☑
    - nervous system T85.9 ☑
      - brain — *see* Complications, electronic stimulator device, brain
      - cranial nerve — *see* Complications, electronic stimulator device, peripheral nerve
      - embolism T85.81Ø ☑
      - fibrosis T85.82Ø ☑
      - gastric nerve — *see* Complications, electronic stimulator device, peripheral nerve
      - hemorrhage T85.83Ø ☑
      - infection and inflammation T85.738 ☑
      - mechanical
        - breakdown T85.118 ☑
        - displacement T85.128 ☑
        - leakage T85.199 ☑
        - malposition T85.128 ☑
        - obstruction T85.199 ☑
        - perforation T85.199 ☑
        - protrusion T85.199 ☑
        - specified NEC T85.199 ☑
      - pain T85.84Ø ☑
      - peripheral nerve — *see* Complications, electronic stimulator device, peripheral nerve
      - sacral nerve — *see* Complications, electronic stimulator device, peripheral nerve
      - specified type NEC T85.89Ø ☑
      - spinal cord — *see* Complications, electronic stimulator device, spinal cord
      - stenosis T85.85Ø ☑
      - thrombosis T85.86Ø ☑
      - vagal nerve — *see* Complications, electronic stimulator device, peripheral nerve
    - peripheral nerve T85.9 ☑
      - embolism T85.81Ø ☑
      - fibrosis T85.82Ø ☑
      - hemorrhage T85.83Ø ☑
      - infection and inflammation T85.732 ☑
      - mechanical
        - breakdown T85.111 ☑
        - displacement T85.121 ☑
        - leakage T85.191 ☑
        - malposition T85.121 ☑
        - obstruction T85.191 ☑
        - perforation T85.191 ☑
        - protrusion T85.191 ☑
        - specified NEC T85.191 ☑
      - pain T85.84Ø ☑
      - specified type NEC T85.89Ø ☑
      - stenosis T85.85Ø ☑
      - thrombosis T85.86Ø ☑
    - spinal cord T85.9 ☑
      - embolism T85.81Ø ☑
      - fibrosis T85.82Ø ☑
      - hemorrhage T85.83Ø ☑
      - infection and inflammation T85.733 ☑

Index — Complication — Complication

Complication(s) — *continued*
- heart — *continued*
  - valve — *continued*
    - graft — *continued*
      - mechanical — *continued*
        - displacement T82.222 ☑
        - leakage T82.223 ☑
        - malposition T82.222 ☑
        - obstruction T82.228 ☑
        - perforation T82.228 ☑
        - protrusion T82.228 ☑
      - pain T82.847 ☑
      - specified type NEC T82.897 ☑
      - stenosis T82.857 ☑
      - thrombosis T82.867 ☑
    - prosthesis T82.9 ☑
      - embolism T82.817 ☑
      - fibrosis T82.827 ☑
      - hemorrhage T82.837 ☑
      - infection or inflammation T82.6 ☑
      - mechanical T82.09 ☑
        - breakdown T82.01 ☑
        - displacement T82.02 ☑
        - leakage T82.03 ☑
        - malposition T82.02 ☑
        - obstruction T82.09 ☑
        - perforation T82.09 ☑
        - protrusion T82.09 ☑
      - pain T82.847 ☑
      - specified type NEC T82.897 ☑
        - mechanical T82.09 ☑
      - stenosis T82.857 ☑
      - thrombosis T82.867 ☑
- hematoma
  - intraoperative — *see* Complication, intraoperative, hemorrhage
  - postprocedural — *see* Complication, postprocedural, hematoma
- hemodialysis — *see* Complications, dialysis
- hemorrhage
  - intraoperative — *see* Complication, intraoperative, hemorrhage
  - postprocedural — *see* Complication, postprocedural, hemorrhage
- ileostomy (stoma) — *see* Complications, enterostomy
- immunization (procedure) — *see* Complications, vaccination
- implant — *see also* Complications, by site and type
  - urinary sphincter T83.9 ☑
    - embolism T83.81 ☑
    - fibrosis T83.82 ☑
    - hemorrhage T83.83 ☑
    - infection and inflammation T83.591 ☑
    - mechanical
      - breakdown T83.111 ☑
      - displacement T83.121 ☑
      - leakage T83.191 ☑
      - malposition T83.121 ☑
      - obstruction T83.191 ☑
      - perforation T83.191 ☑
      - protrusion T83.191 ☑
      - specified NEC T83.191 ☑
    - pain T83.84 ☑
    - specified type NEC T83.89 ☑
    - stenosis T83.85 ☑
    - thrombosis T83.86 ☑
- infusion (procedure) T80.90 ☑
  - air embolism T80.0 ☑
  - blood — *see* Complications, transfusion
  - catheter — *see* Complications, catheter
  - infection T80.29 ☑
  - pump — *see* Complications, cardiovascular, device or implant
  - sepsis T80.29 ☑
  - serum reaction — *see also* Reaction, serum T80.69 ☑
    - anaphylactic shock — *see also* Shock, anaphylactic T80.59 ☑
  - specified type NEC T80.89 ☑
- inhalation therapy NEC T81.81 ☑
- injection (procedure) T80.90 ☑
  - drug reaction — *see* Reaction, drug
  - infection T80.29 ☑
  - sepsis T80.29 ☑
  - serum (prophylactic) (therapeutic) — *see* Complications, vaccination

Complication(s) — *continued*
- injection — *continued*
  - specified type NEC T80.89 ☑
  - vaccine (any) — *see* Complications, vaccination
- inoculation (any) — *see* Complications, vaccination
- insulin pump
  - infection and inflammation T85.72 ☑
  - mechanical
    - breakdown T85.614 ☑
    - displacement T85.624 ☑
    - leakage T85.633 ☑
    - malposition T85.624 ☑
    - obstruction T85.694 ☑
    - perforation T85.694 ☑
    - protrusion T85.694 ☑
    - specified NEC T85.694 ☑
- intestinal pouch NEC K91.858
- intraocular lens (prosthetic) T85.9 ☑
  - embolism T85.818 ☑
  - fibrosis T85.828 ☑
  - hemorrhage T85.838 ☑
  - infection and inflammation T85.79 ☑
  - mechanical
    - breakdown T85.21 ☑
    - displacement T85.22 ☑
    - malposition T85.22 ☑
    - obstruction T85.29 ☑
    - perforation T85.29 ☑
    - protrusion T85.29 ☑
    - specified NEC T85.29 ☑
  - pain T85.848 ☑
  - specified type NEC T85.898 ☑
  - stenosis T85.858 ☑
  - thrombosis T85.868 ☑
- intraoperative (intraprocedural)
  - cardiac arrest — *see also* Infarct, myocardium, associated with revascularization procedure
    - during cardiac surgery I97.710
    - during other surgery I97.711
  - cardiac functional disturbance NEC — *see also* Infarct, myocardium, associated with revascularization procedure
    - during cardiac surgery I97.790
    - during other surgery I97.791
  - hemorrhage (hematoma) (of)
    - circulatory system organ or structure
      - during cardiac bypass I97.411
      - during cardiac catheterization I97.410
      - during other circulatory system procedure I97.418
      - during other procedure I97.42
    - digestive system organ
      - during procedure on digestive system K91.61
      - during procedure on other organ K91.62
    - ear
      - during procedure on ear and mastoid process H95.21
      - during procedure on other organ H95.22
    - endocrine system organ or structure
      - during procedure on endocrine system organ or structure E36.01
      - during procedure on other organ E36.02
    - eye and adnexa
      - during ophthalmic procedure H59.11- ☑
      - during other procedure H59.12- ☑
    - genitourinary organ or structure
      - during procedure on genitourinary organ or structure N99.61
      - during procedure on other organ N99.62
    - mastoid process
      - during procedure on ear and mastoid process H95.21
      - during procedure on other organ H95.22
    - musculoskeletal structure
      - during musculoskeletal surgery M96.810
      - during non-orthopedic surgery M96.811
      - during orthopedic surgery M96.810
    - nervous system
      - during a nervous system procedure G97.31
      - during other procedure G97.32
    - respiratory system
      - during other procedure J95.62
      - during procedure on respiratory system organ or structure J95.61
    - skin and subcutaneous tissue
      - during a dermatologic procedure L76.01
      - during a procedure on other organ L76.02

Complication(s) — *continued*
- intraoperative — *continued*
  - hemorrhage — *continued*
    - spleen
      - during a procedure on other organ D78.02
      - during a procedure on the spleen D78.01
  - puncture or laceration (accidental) (unintentional) (of)
    - brain
      - during a nervous system procedure G97.48
      - during other procedure G97.49
    - circulatory system organ or structure
      - during circulatory system procedure I97.51
      - during other procedure I97.52
    - digestive system
      - during procedure on digestive system K91.71
      - during procedure on other organ K91.72
    - ear
      - during procedure on ear and mastoid process H95.31
      - during procedure on other organ H95.32
    - endocrine system organ or structure
      - during procedure on endocrine system organ or structure E36.11
      - during procedure on other organ E36.12
    - eye and adnexa
      - during ophthalmic procedure H59.21- ☑
      - during other procedure H59.22- ☑
    - genitourinary organ or structure
      - during procedure on genitourinary organ or structure N99.71
      - during procedure on other organ N99.72
    - mastoid process
      - during procedure on ear and mastoid process H95.31
      - during procedure on other organ H95.32
    - musculoskeletal structure
      - during musculoskeletal surgery M96.820
      - during non-orthopedic surgery M96.821
      - during orthopedic surgery M96.820
    - nervous system
      - during a nervous system procedure G97.48
      - during other procedure G97.49
    - respiratory system
      - during other procedure J95.72
      - during procedure on respiratory system organ or structure J95.71
    - skin and subcutaneous tissue
      - during a dermatologic procedure L76.11
      - during a procedure on other organ L76.12
    - spleen
      - during a procedure on other organ D78.12
      - during a procedure on the spleen D78.11
  - specified NEC
    - circulatory system I97.88
    - digestive system K91.81
    - ear H95.88
    - endocrine system E36.8
    - eye and adnexa H59.88
    - genitourinary system N99.81
    - mastoid process H95.88
    - musculoskeletal structure M96.89
    - nervous system G97.81
    - respiratory system J95.88
    - skin and subcutaneous tissue L76.81
    - spleen D78.81
- intraperitoneal catheter (dialysis) (infusion) — *see* Complications, catheter, intraperitoneal
- intrathecal infusion pump
  - infection and inflammation T85.738 ☑
  - mechanical
    - breakdown T85.615 ☑
    - displacement T85.625 ☑
    - leakage T85.635 ☑
    - malfunction T85.695 ☑
    - malposition T85.625 ☑
    - obstruction T85.695 ☑
    - perforation T85.695 ☑
    - protrusion T85.695 ☑
    - specified NEC T85.695 ☑
- intrauterine
  - contraceptive device
    - embolism T83.81 ☑
    - fibrosis T83.82 ☑
    - hemorrhage T83.83 ☑
    - infection and inflammation T83.69 ☑
    - mechanical
      - breakdown T83.31 ☑

Index

Complication — Complication

Compression — *continued*
- umbilical cord — *continued*
  - complicating delivery — *continued*
    - prolapse O69.0 ☑
    - specified NEC O69.2 ☑
- ureter N13.5
- vein I87.1
- vena cava (inferior) (superior) I87.1

Compulsion, compulsive
- gambling F63.0
- neurosis F42.8
- personality F60.5
- states F42.8
- swearing F42.8
  - in Gilles de la Tourette's syndrome F95.2
- tics and spasms F95.9

Concato's disease (pericardial polyserositis) A19.9
- nontubercular I31.1
- pleural — *see* Pleurisy, with effusion

Concavity chest wall M95.4

Concealed penis Q55.64

Concern (normal) **about sick person in family** Z63.6

Concrescence (teeth) K00.2

Concretio cordis I31.1
- rheumatic I09.2

Concretion — *see also* Calculus
- appendicular K38.1
- canaliculus — *see* Dacryolith
- clitoris N90.89
- conjunctiva H11.12- ☑
- eyelid — *see* Disorder, eyelid, specified type NEC
- lacrimal passages — *see* Dacryolith
- prepuce (male) N47.8
- salivary gland (any) K11.5
- seminal vesicle N50.89
- tonsil J35.8

Concussion (brain) (cerebral) (current) S06.0X9 ☑
- with
  - loss of consciousness of 30 minutes or less S06.0X1 ☑
  - loss of consciousness of unspecified duration S06.0X9 ☑
- blast (air) (hydraulic) (immersion) (underwater)
  - abdomen or thorax — *see* Injury, blast, by site
  - ear with acoustic nerve injury — *see* Injury, nerve, acoustic, specified type NEC
- cauda equina S34.3 ☑
- conus medullaris S34.02 ☑
- ocular S05.8X- ☑
- spinal (cord)
  - cervical S14.0 ☑
  - lumbar S34.01 ☑
  - sacral S34.02 ☑
  - thoracic S24.0 ☑
- syndrome F07.81
- without loss of consciousness S06.0X0 ☑

Condition — *see* Disease

Conditions arising in the perinatal period — *see* Newborn, affected by

Conduct disorder — *see* Disorder, conduct

Condyloma A63.0
- acuminatum A63.0
- gonorrheal A54.09
- latum A51.31
- syphilitic A51.31
  - congenital A50.07
- venereal, syphilitic A51.31

Conflagration — *see also* Burn
- asphyxia (by inhalation of gases, fumes or vapors) — *see also* Table of Drugs and Chemicals T59.9- ☑

Conflict (with) — *see also* Discord
- family Z73.9
- marital Z63.0
  - involving divorce or estrangement Z63.5
- parent-child Z62.820
  - parent-adopted child Z62.821
  - parent-biological child Z62.820
  - parent-foster child Z62.822
- social role NEC Z73.5

Confluent — *see* condition

Confusion, confused R41.0
- epileptic F05
- mental state (psychogenic) F44.89
- psychogenic F44.89
- reactive (from emotional stress, psychological trauma) F44.89

Confusional arousals G47.51

Congelation T69.9 ☑

Congenital — *see also* condition
- aortic septum Q25.49
- intrinsic factor deficiency D51.0
- malformation — *see* Anomaly

Congestion, congestive
- bladder N32.89
- bowel K63.89
- brain G93.89
- breast N64.59
- bronchial J98.09
- catarrhal J31.0
- chest R09.89
- chill, malarial — *see* Malaria
- circulatory NEC I99.8
- duodenum K31.89
- eye — *see* Hyperemia, conjunctiva
- facial, due to birth injury P15.4
- general R68.89
- glottis J37.0
- heart — *see* Failure, heart, congestive
- hepatic K76.1
- hypostatic (lung) — *see* Edema, lung
- intestine K63.89
- kidney N28.89
- labyrinth H83.8 ☑
- larynx J37.0
- liver K76.1
- lung R09.89
  - active or acute — *see* Pneumonia
- malaria, malarial — *see* Malaria
- nasal R09.81
- nose R09.81
- orbit, orbital — *see also* Exophthalmos
  - inflammatory (chronic) — *see* Inflammation, orbit
- ovary N83.8
- pancreas K86.89
- pelvic, female N94.89
- pleural J94.8
- prostate (active) N42.1
- pulmonary — *see* Congestion, lung
- renal N28.89
- retina H35.81
- seminal vesicle N50.1
- spinal cord G95.19
- spleen (chronic) D73.2
- stomach K31.89
- trachea — *see* Tracheitis
- urethra N36.8
- uterus N85.8
  - with subinvolution N85.3
- venous (passive) I87.8
- viscera R68.89

Congestive — *see* Congestion

Conical
- cervix (hypertrophic elongation) N88.4
- cornea — *see* Keratoconus
- teeth K00.2

Conjoined twins Q89.4

Conjugal maladjustment Z63.0
- involving divorce or estrangement Z63.5

Conjunctiva — *see* condition

Conjunctivitis (staphylococcal) (streptococcal) NOS H10.9
- Acanthamoeba B60.12
- acute H10.3- ☑
  - atopic H10.1- ☑
  - chemical — *see also* Corrosion, cornea H10.21- ☑
  - mucopurulent H10.02- ☑
    - follicular H10.01- ☑
  - pseudomembranous H10.22- ☑
  - serous except viral H10.23- ☑
    - viral — *see* Conjunctivitis, viral
  - toxic H10.21- ☑
- adenoviral (acute) (follicular) B30.1
- allergic (acute) — *see* Conjunctivitis, acute, atopic
  - chronic H10.45
    - vernal H10.44
- anaphylactic — *see* Conjunctivitis, acute, atopic
- Apollo B30.3
- atopic (acute) — *see* Conjunctivitis, acute, atopic
- Béal's B30.2
- blennorrhagic (gonococcal) (neonatorum) A54.31
- chemical (acute) — *see also* Corrosion, cornea H10.21- ☑
- chlamydial A74.0
  - due to trachoma A71.1
  - neonatal P39.1

Conjunctivitis — *continued*
- chronic (nodosa) (petrificans) (phlyctenular) H10.40- ☑
  - allergic H10.45
    - vernal H10.44
  - follicular H10.43- ☑
  - giant papillary H10.41- ☑
  - simple H10.42- ☑
  - vernal H10.44
- coxsackievirus 24 B30.3
- diphtheritic A36.86
- due to
  - dust — *see* Conjunctivitis, acute, atopic
  - filariasis B74.9
  - mucocutaneous leishmaniasis B55.2
- enterovirus type 70 (hemorrhagic) B30.3
- epidemic (viral) B30.9
  - hemorrhagic B30.3
- gonococcal (neonatorum) A54.31
- granular (trachomatous) A71.1
  - sequelae (late effect) B94.0
- hemorrhagic (acute) (epidemic) B30.3
- herpes zoster B02.31
- in (due to)
  - Acanthamoeba B60.12
  - adenovirus (acute) (follicular) B30.1
  - Chlamydia A74.0
  - coxsackievirus 24 B30.3
  - diphtheria A36.86
  - enterovirus type 70 (hemorrhagic) B30.3
  - filariasis B74.9
  - gonococci A54.31
  - herpes (simplex) virus B00.53
    - zoster B02.31
  - infectious disease NEC B99 ☑
  - meningococci A39.89
  - mucocutaneous leishmaniasis B55.2
  - rosacea H10.82- ☑
  - syphilis (late) A52.71
  - zoster B02.31
- inclusion A74.0
- infantile P39.1
  - gonococcal A54.31
- Koch-Weeks' — *see* Conjunctivitis, acute, mucopurulent
- light — *see* Conjunctivitis, acute, atopic
- ligneous — *see* Blepharoconjunctivitis, ligneous
- meningococcal A39.89
- mucopurulent — *see* Conjunctivitis, acute, mucopurulent
- neonatal P39.1
  - gonococcal A54.31
- Newcastle B30.8
- of Béal B30.2
- parasitic
  - filariasis B74.9
  - mucocutaneous leishmaniasis B55.2
- Parinaud's H10.89
- petrificans H10.89
- rosacea H10.82- ☑
- specified NEC H10.89
- swimming-pool B30.1
- trachomatous A71.1
  - acute A71.0
  - sequelae (late effect) B94.0
- traumatic NEC H10.89
- tuberculous A18.59
- tularemic A21.1
- tularensis A21.1
- viral B30.9
  - due to
    - adenovirus B30.1
    - enterovirus B30.3
  - specified NEC B30.8

Conjunctivochalasis H11.82- ☑

Connective tissue — *see* condition

Conn's syndrome E26.01

Conradi (-Hunermann) **disease** Q77.3

Consanguinity Z84.3
- counseling Z71.89

Conscious simulation (of illness) Z76.5

Consecutive — *see* condition

Consolidation lung (base) — *see* Pneumonia, lobar

Constipation (atonic) (neurogenic) (simple) (spastic) K59.00
- chronic K59.09
  - idiopathic K59.04
- drug-induced K59.03
- functional K59.04
- outlet dysfunction K59.02

- **Constipation** — *continued*
  - psychogenic F45.8
  - slow transit K59.Ø1
  - specified NEC K59.Ø9
- **Constitutional** — *see also* condition
  - substandard F6Ø.7
- **Constitutionally substandard** F6Ø.7
- **Constriction** — *see also* Stricture
  - auditory canal — *see* Stenosis, external ear canal
  - bronchial J98.Ø9
  - duodenum K31.5
  - esophagus K22.2
  - external
    - abdomen, abdominal (wall) S3Ø.841 ☑
    - alveolar process SØØ.542 ☑
    - ankle S9Ø.54- ☑
    - antecubital space — *see* Constriction, external, forearm
    - arm (upper) S4Ø.84- ☑
    - auricle — *see* Constriction, external, ear
    - axilla — *see* Constriction, external, arm
    - back, lower S3Ø.84Ø ☑
    - breast S2Ø.14- ☑
    - brow SØØ.84 ☑
    - buttock S3Ø.84Ø ☑
    - calf — *see* Constriction, external, leg
    - canthus — *see* Constriction, external, eyelid
    - cheek SØØ.84 ☑
      - internal SØØ.542 ☑
    - chest wall — *see* Constriction, external, thorax
    - chin SØØ.84 ☑
    - clitoris S3Ø.844 ☑
    - costal region — *see* Constriction, external, thorax
    - digit(s)
      - foot — *see* Constriction, external, toe
      - hand — *see* Constriction, external, finger
    - ear SØØ.44- ☑
    - elbow S5Ø.34- ☑
    - epididymis S3Ø.843 ☑
    - epigastric region S3Ø.841 ☑
    - esophagus, cervical S1Ø.14 ☑
    - eyebrow — *see* Constriction, external, eyelid
    - eyelid SØØ.24- ☑
    - face SØØ.84 ☑
    - finger(s) S6Ø.44- ☑
      - index S6Ø.44- ☑
      - little S6Ø.44- ☑
      - middle S6Ø.44- ☑
      - ring S6Ø.44- ☑
    - flank S3Ø.841 ☑
    - foot (except toe(s) alone) S9Ø.84- ☑
      - toe — *see* Constriction, external, toe
    - forearm S5Ø.84- ☑
      - elbow only — *see* Constriction, external, elbow
    - forehead SØØ.84 ☑
    - genital organs, external
      - female S3Ø.846 ☑
      - male S3Ø.845 ☑
    - groin S3Ø.841 ☑
    - gum SØØ.542 ☑
    - hand S6Ø.54- ☑
    - head SØØ.94 ☑
      - ear — *see* Constriction, external, ear
      - eyelid — *see* Constriction, external, eyelid
      - lip SØØ.541 ☑
      - nose SØØ.34 ☑
      - oral cavity SØØ.542 ☑
      - scalp SØØ.Ø4 ☑
      - specified site NEC SØØ.84 ☑
    - heel — *see* Constriction, external, foot
    - hip S7Ø.24- ☑
    - inguinal region S3Ø.841 ☑
    - interscapular region S2Ø.449 ☑
    - jaw SØØ.84 ☑
    - knee S8Ø.24- ☑
    - labium (majus) (minus) S3Ø.844 ☑
    - larynx S1Ø.14 ☑
    - leg (lower) S8Ø.84- ☑
      - knee — *see* Constriction, external, knee
      - upper — *see* Constriction, external, thigh
    - lip SØØ.541 ☑
    - lower back S3Ø.84Ø ☑
    - lumbar region S3Ø.84Ø ☑
    - malar region SØØ.84 ☑
    - mammary — *see* Constriction, external, breast
    - mastoid region SØØ.84 ☑

- **Constriction** — *continued*
  - external — *continued*
    - mouth SØØ.542 ☑
    - nail
      - finger — *see* Constriction, external, finger
      - toe — *see* Constriction, external, toe
    - nasal SØØ.34 ☑
    - neck S1Ø.94 ☑
      - specified site NEC S1Ø.84 ☑
      - throat S1Ø.14 ☑
    - nose SØØ.34 ☑
    - occipital region SØØ.Ø4 ☑
    - oral cavity SØØ.542 ☑
    - orbital region — *see* Constriction, external, eyelid
    - palate SØØ.542 ☑
    - palm — *see* Constriction, external, hand
    - parietal region SØØ.Ø4 ☑
    - pelvis S3Ø.84Ø ☑
    - penis S3Ø.842 ☑
    - perineum
      - female S3Ø.844 ☑
      - male S3Ø.84Ø ☑
    - periocular area — *see* Constriction, external, eyelid
    - phalanges
      - finger — *see* Constriction, external, finger
      - toe — *see* Constriction, external, toe
    - pharynx S1Ø.14 ☑
    - pinna — *see* Constriction, external, ear
    - popliteal space — *see* Constriction, external, knee
    - prepuce S3Ø.842 ☑
    - pubic region S3Ø.84Ø ☑
    - pudendum
      - female S3Ø.846 ☑
      - male S3Ø.845 ☑
    - sacral region S3Ø.84Ø ☑
    - scalp SØØ.Ø4 ☑
    - scapular region — *see* Constriction, external, shoulder
    - scrotum S3Ø.843 ☑
    - shin — *see* Constriction, external, leg
    - shoulder S4Ø.24- ☑
    - sternal region S2Ø.349 ☑
    - submaxillary region SØØ.84 ☑
    - submental region SØØ.84 ☑
    - subungual
      - finger(s) — *see* Constriction, external, finger
      - toe(s) — *see* Constriction, external, toe
    - supraclavicular fossa S1Ø.84 ☑
    - supraorbital SØØ.84 ☑
    - temple SØØ.84 ☑
    - temporal region SØØ.84 ☑
    - testis S3Ø.843 ☑
    - thigh S7Ø.34- ☑
    - thorax, thoracic (wall) S2Ø.94 ☑
      - back S2Ø.44- ☑
      - front S2Ø.34- ☑
    - throat S1Ø.14 ☑
    - thumb S6Ø.34- ☑
    - toe(s) (lesser) S9Ø.44- ☑
      - great S9Ø.44- ☑
    - tongue SØØ.542 ☑
    - trachea S1Ø.14 ☑
    - tunica vaginalis S3Ø.843 ☑
    - uvula SØØ.542 ☑
    - vagina S3Ø.844 ☑
    - vulva S3Ø.844 ☑
    - wrist S6Ø.84- ☑
  - gallbladder — *see* Obstruction, gallbladder
  - intestine — *see* Obstruction, intestine
  - larynx J38.6
    - congenital Q31.8
      - specified NEC Q31.8
      - subglottic Q31.1
  - organ or site, congenital NEC — *see* Atresia, by site
  - prepuce (acquired) (congenital) N47.1
  - pylorus (adult hypertrophic) K31.1
    - congenital or infantile Q4Ø.Ø
    - newborn Q4Ø.Ø
  - ring dystocia (uterus) O62.4
  - spastic — *see also* Spasm
    - ureter N13.5
  - ureter N13.5
    - with infection N13.6
  - urethra — *see* Stricture, urethra
  - visual field (peripheral) (functional) — *see* Defect, visual field

- **Constrictive** — *see* condition
- **Consultation**
  - medical — *see* Counseling, medical
  - religious Z71.81
  - specified reason NEC Z71.89
  - spiritual Z71.81
  - without complaint or sickness Z71.9
    - feared complaint unfounded Z71.1
    - specified reason NEC Z71.89
- **Consumption** — *see* Tuberculosis
- **Contact** (with) — *see also* Exposure (to)
  - acariasis Z2Ø.7
  - AIDS virus Z2Ø.6
  - air pollution Z77.11Ø
  - algae and algae toxins Z77.121
  - algae bloom Z77.121
  - anthrax Z2Ø.81Ø
  - aromatic amines Z77.Ø2Ø
  - aromatic (hazardous) compounds NEC Z77.Ø28
  - aromatic dyes NOS Z77.Ø28
  - arsenic Z77.Ø1Ø
  - asbestos Z77.Ø9Ø
  - bacterial disease NEC Z2Ø.818
  - benzene Z77.Ø21
  - blue-green algae bloom Z77.121
  - body fluids (potentially hazardous) Z77.21
  - brown tide Z77.121
  - chemicals (chiefly nonmedicinal) (hazardous) NEC Z77.Ø98
  - cholera Z2Ø.Ø9
  - chromium compounds Z77.Ø18
  - communicable disease Z2Ø.9
    - bacterial NEC Z2Ø.818
    - specified NEC Z2Ø.89
    - viral NEC Z2Ø.828
    - Zika virus Z2Ø.821
  - cyanobacteria bloom Z77.121
  - dyes Z77.Ø98
  - Escherichia coli (E. coli) Z2Ø.Ø1
  - fiberglass — *see* Table of Drugs and Chemicals, fiberglass
  - German measles Z2Ø.4
  - gonorrhea Z2Ø.2
  - hazardous metals NEC Z77.Ø18
  - hazardous substances NEC Z77.29
  - hazards in the physical environment NEC Z77.128
  - hazards to health NEC Z77.9
  - HIV Z2Ø.6
  - HTLV-III/LAV Z2Ø.6
  - human immunodeficiency virus (HIV) Z2Ø.6
  - infection Z2Ø.9
    - specified NEC Z2Ø.89
  - infestation (parasitic) NEC Z2Ø.7
  - intestinal infectious disease NEC Z2Ø.Ø9
    - Escherichia coli (E. coli) Z2Ø.Ø1
  - lead Z77.Ø11
  - meningococcus Z2Ø.811
  - mold (toxic) Z77.12Ø
  - nickel dust Z77.Ø18
  - noise Z77.122
  - parasitic disease Z2Ø.7
  - pediculosis Z2Ø.7
  - pfiesteria piscicida Z77.121
  - poliomyelitis Z2Ø.89
  - pollution
    - air Z77.11Ø
    - environmental NEC Z77.118
    - soil Z77.112
    - water Z77.111
  - polycyclic aromatic hydrocarbons Z77.Ø28
  - rabies Z2Ø.3
  - radiation, naturally occurring NEC Z77.123
  - radon Z77.123
  - red tide (Florida) Z77.121
  - rubella Z2Ø.4
  - sexually-transmitted disease Z2Ø.2
  - smallpox (laboratory) Z2Ø.89
  - syphilis Z2Ø.2
  - tuberculosis Z2Ø.1
  - uranium Z77.Ø12
  - varicella Z2Ø.82Ø
  - venereal disease Z2Ø.2
  - viral disease NEC Z2Ø.828
  - viral hepatitis Z2Ø.5
  - water pollution Z77.111
  - Zika virus Z2Ø.821
- **Contamination, food** — *see* Intoxication, foodborne

- **Contusion** — *continued*
  - costal region — *see* Contusion, thorax
  - cystic duct S36.13 ☑
  - diaphragm S27.8Ø2 ☑
  - duodenum S36.42Ø ☑
  - ear SØØ.43- ☑
  - elbow S5Ø.Ø- ☑
    - with forearm — *see* Contusion, forearm
  - epididymis S3Ø.22 ☑
  - epigastric region S3Ø.1 ☑
  - epiglottis S1Ø.Ø ☑
  - esophagus (thoracic) S27.812 ☑
    - cervical S1Ø.Ø ☑
  - eyeball SØ5.1- ☑
  - eyebrow SØØ.1- ☑
  - eyelid (and periocular area) SØØ.1- ☑
  - face NEC SØØ.83 ☑
  - fallopian tube S37.529 ☑
    - bilateral S37.522 ☑
    - unilateral S37.521 ☑
  - femoral triangle S3Ø.1 ☑
  - finger(s) S6Ø.ØØ ☑
    - with damage to nail (matrix) S6Ø.1Ø ☑
    - index S6Ø.Ø2- ☑
      - with damage to nail S6Ø.12- ☑
    - little S6Ø.Ø5- ☑
      - with damage to nail S6Ø.15- ☑
    - middle S6Ø.Ø3- ☑
      - with damage to nail S6Ø.13- ☑
    - ring S6Ø.Ø4- ☑
      - with damage to nail S6Ø.14- ☑
    - thumb — *see* Contusion, thumb
  - flank S3Ø.1 ☑
  - foot (except toe(s) alone) S9Ø.3- ☑
    - toe — *see* Contusion, toe
  - forearm S5Ø.1- ☑
    - elbow only — *see* Contusion, elbow
  - forehead SØØ.83 ☑
  - gallbladder S36.122 ☑
  - genital organs, external
    - female S3Ø.2Ø2 ☑
    - male S3Ø.2Ø1 ☑
  - globe (eye) — *see* Contusion, eyeball
  - groin S3Ø.1 ☑
  - gum SØØ.532 ☑
  - hand S6Ø.22- ☑
    - finger(s) — *see* Contusion, finger
    - wrist — *see* Contusion, wrist
  - head SØØ.93 ☑
    - ear — *see* Contusion, ear
    - eyelid — *see* Contusion, eyelid
    - lip SØØ.531 ☑
    - nose SØØ.33 ☑
    - oral cavity SØØ.532 ☑
    - scalp SØØ.Ø3 ☑
    - specified part NEC SØØ.83 ☑
  - heart — *see also* Injury, heart S26.91 ☑
  - heel — *see* Contusion, foot
  - hepatic duct S36.13 ☑
  - hip S7Ø.Ø- ☑
  - ileum S36.428 ☑
  - iliac region S3Ø.1 ☑
  - inguinal region S3Ø.1 ☑
  - interscapular region S2Ø.229 ☑
  - intra-abdominal organ S36.92 ☑
    - colon — *see* Injury, intestine, large, contusion
    - liver S36.112 ☑
    - pancreas — *see* Contusion, pancreas
    - rectum S36.62 ☑
    - small intestine — *see* Injury, intestine, small, contusion
    - specified organ NEC S36.892 ☑
    - spleen — *see* Contusion, spleen
    - stomach S36.32 ☑
  - iris (eye) — *see* Contusion, eyeball
  - jaw SØØ.83 ☑
  - jejunum S36.428 ☑
  - kidney S37.Ø1- ☑
    - major (greater than 2 cm) S37.Ø2- ☑
    - minor (less than 2 cm) S37.Ø1- ☑
  - knee S8Ø.Ø- ☑
  - labium (majus) (minus) S3Ø.23 ☑
  - lacrimal apparatus, gland or sac SØ5.8X- ☑
  - larynx S1Ø.Ø ☑
  - leg (lower) S8Ø.1- ☑
    - knee — *see* Contusion, knee

- **Contusion** — *continued*
  - lens — *see* Contusion, eyeball
  - lip SØØ.531 ☑
  - liver S36.112 ☑
  - lower back S3Ø.Ø ☑
  - lumbar region S3Ø.Ø ☑
  - lung S27.329 ☑
    - bilateral S27.322 ☑
    - unilateral S27.321 ☑
  - malar region SØØ.83 ☑
  - mastoid region SØØ.83 ☑
  - membrane, brain — *see* Injury, intracranial, diffuse
    - focal — *see* Injury, intracranial, focal
  - mesentery S36.892 ☑
  - mesosalpinx S37.892 ☑
  - mouth SØØ.532 ☑
  - muscle — *see* Contusion, by site
  - nail
    - finger — *see* Contusion, finger, with damage to nail
    - toe — *see* Contusion, toe, with damage to nail
  - nasal SØØ.33 ☑
  - neck S1Ø.93 ☑
    - specified site NEC S1Ø.83 ☑
    - throat S1Ø.Ø ☑
  - nerve — *see* Injury, nerve
  - newborn P54.5
  - nose SØØ.33 ☑
  - occipital
    - lobe (brain) — *see* Injury, intracranial, diffuse
      - focal — *see* Injury, intracranial, focal
    - region (scalp) SØØ.Ø3 ☑
  - orbit (region) (tissues) SØ5.1- ☑
  - ovary S37.429 ☑
    - bilateral S37.422 ☑
    - unilateral S37.421 ☑
  - palate SØØ.532 ☑
  - pancreas S36.229 ☑
    - body S36.221 ☑
    - head S36.22Ø ☑
    - tail S36.222 ☑
  - parietal
    - lobe (brain) — *see* Injury, intracranial, diffuse
      - focal — *see* Injury, intracranial, focal
    - region (scalp) SØØ.Ø3 ☑
  - pelvic organ S37.92 ☑
    - adrenal gland S37.812 ☑
    - bladder S37.22 ☑
    - fallopian tube — *see* Contusion, fallopian tube
    - kidney — *see* Contusion, kidney
    - ovary — *see* Contusion, ovary
    - prostate S37.822 ☑
    - specified organ NEC S37.892 ☑
    - ureter S37.12 ☑
    - urethra S37.32 ☑
    - uterus S37.62 ☑
  - pelvis S3Ø.Ø ☑
  - penis S3Ø.21 ☑
  - perineum
    - female S3Ø.23 ☑
    - male S3Ø.Ø ☑
  - periocular area SØØ.1- ☑
  - peritoneum S36.81 ☑
  - periurethral tissue — *see* Contusion, urethra
  - pharynx S1Ø.Ø ☑
  - pinna — *see* Contusion, ear
  - popliteal space — *see* Contusion, knee
  - prepuce S3Ø.21 ☑
  - prostate S37.822 ☑
  - pubic region S3Ø.1 ☑
  - pudendum
    - female S3Ø.2Ø2 ☑
    - male S3Ø.2Ø1 ☑
  - quadriceps femoris — *see* Contusion, thigh
  - rectum S36.62 ☑
  - retroperitoneum S36.892 ☑
  - round ligament S37.892 ☑
  - sacral region S3Ø.Ø ☑
  - scalp SØØ.Ø3 ☑
    - due to birth injury P12.3
  - scapular region — *see* Contusion, shoulder
  - sclera — *see* Contusion, eyeball
  - scrotum S3Ø.22 ☑
  - seminal vesicle S37.892 ☑
  - shoulder S4Ø.Ø1- ☑
  - skin NEC T14.8 ☑
  - small intestine — *see* Injury, intestine, small, contusion

- **Contusion** — *continued*
  - spermatic cord S3Ø.22 ☑
  - spinal cord — *see* Injury, spinal cord, by region
    - cauda equina S34.3 ☑
    - conus medullaris S34.139 ☑
  - spleen S36.Ø29 ☑
    - major S36.Ø21 ☑
    - minor S36.Ø2Ø ☑
  - sternal region S2Ø.219 ☑
  - stomach S36.32 ☑
  - subconjunctival SØ5.1- ☑
  - subcutaneous NEC T14.8 ☑
  - submaxillary region SØØ.83 ☑
  - submental region SØØ.83 ☑
  - subperiosteal NEC T14.8 ☑
  - subungual
    - finger — *see* Contusion, finger, with damage to nail
    - toe — *see* Contusion, toe, with damage to nail
  - supraclavicular fossa S1Ø.83 ☑
  - supraorbital SØØ.83 ☑
  - suprarenal gland S37.812 ☑
  - temple (region) SØØ.83 ☑
  - temporal
    - lobe (brain) — *see* Injury, intracranial, diffuse
      - focal — *see* Injury, intracranial, focal
    - region SØØ.83 ☑
  - testis S3Ø.22 ☑
  - thigh S7Ø.1- ☑
  - thorax (wall) S2Ø.2Ø ☑
    - back S2Ø.22- ☑
    - front S2Ø.21- ☑
  - throat S1Ø.Ø ☑
  - thumb S6Ø.Ø1- ☑
    - with damage to nail S6Ø.11- ☑
  - toe(s) (lesser) S9Ø.12- ☑
    - with damage to nail S9Ø.22- ☑
    - great S9Ø.11- ☑
      - with damage to nail S9Ø.21- ☑
  - tongue SØØ.532 ☑
  - trachea (cervical) S1Ø.Ø ☑
    - thoracic S27.52 ☑
  - tunica vaginalis S3Ø.22 ☑
  - tympanum, tympanic membrane — *see* Contusion, ear
  - ureter S37.12 ☑
  - urethra S37.32 ☑
  - urinary organ NEC S37.892 ☑
  - uterus S37.62 ☑
  - uvula SØØ.532 ☑
  - vagina S3Ø.23 ☑
  - vas deferens S37.892 ☑
  - vesical S37.22 ☑
  - vocal cord(s) S1Ø.Ø ☑
  - vulva S3Ø.23 ☑
  - wrist S6Ø.21- ☑
- **Conus** (congenital) (any type) Q14.8
  - cornea — *see* Keratoconus
  - medullaris syndrome G95.81
- **Conversion hysteria, neurosis or reaction** F44.9
- **Converter, tuberculosis** (test reaction) R76.11
- **Conviction** (legal), **anxiety concerning** Z65.Ø
  - with imprisonment Z65.1
- **Convulsions** (idiopathic) — *see also* Seizure(s) R56.9
  - apoplectiform (cerebral ischemia) I67.82
  - dissociative F44.5
  - epileptic — *see* Epilepsy
  - epileptiform, epileptoid — *see* Seizure, epileptiform
  - ether (anesthetic) — *see* Table of Drugs and Chemicals, by drug
  - febrile R56.ØØ
    - with status epilepticus G4Ø.9Ø1
    - complex R56.Ø1
      - with status epilepticus G4Ø.9Ø1
    - simple R56.ØØ
  - hysterical F44.5
  - infantile P9Ø
    - epilepsy — *see* Epilepsy
  - jacksonian — *see* Epilepsy, localization-related, symptomatic, with simple partial seizures
  - myoclonic G25.3
  - newborn P9Ø
  - obstetrical (nephritic) (uremic) — *see* Eclampsia
  - paretic A52.17
  - post traumatic R56.1
  - psychomotor — *see* Epilepsy, localization-related, symptomatic, with complex partial seizures

Convulsions — *continued*
- recurrent R56.9
- reflex R25.8
- scarlatinal A38.8
- tetanus, tetanic — *see* Tetanus
- thymic E32.8

Convulsive — *see also* Convulsions
Cooley's anemia D56.1
Coolie itch B76.9
Cooper's
- disease — *see* Mastopathy, cystic
- hernia — *see* Hernia, abdomen, specified site NEC

Copra itch B88.0
Coprophagy F50.89
Coprophobia F40.298
Coproporphyria, hereditary E80.29
Cor
- biloculare Q20.8
- bovis, bovinum — *see* Hypertrophy, cardiac
- pulmonale (chronic) I27.81
  - acute I26.09
- triatriatum, triatrium Q24.2
- triloculare Q20.8
  - biatrium Q20.4
  - biventriculare Q21.1

Corbus' disease (gangrenous balanitis) N48.1
Cord — *see also* condition
- around neck
  - complicating delivery O69.81 ☑
    - with compression O69.1 ☑
- bladder G95.89
  - tabetic A52.19

Cordis ectopia Q24.8
Corditis (spermatic) N49.1
Corectopia Q13.2
Cori's disease (glycogen storage) E74.03
Corkhandler's disease or lung J67.3
Corkscrew esophagus K22.4
Corkworker's disease or lung J67.3
Corn (infected) L84
Cornea — *see also* condition
- donor Z52.5
- plana Q13.4

Cornelia de Lange syndrome Q87.19
Cornu cutaneum L85.8
Cornual gestation or pregnancy O00.80
- with intrauterine pregnancy O00.81

Coronary (artery) — *see* condition
Coronavirus (infection)
- as cause of diseases classified elsewhere B97.29
- coronavirus-19 U07.1
- COVID-19 U07.1
- SARS-associated B97.21

Corpora — *see also* condition
- amylacea, prostate N42.89
- cavernosa — *see* condition

Corpulence — *see* Obesity
Corpus — *see* condition
Corrected transposition Q20.5
Corrosion (injury) (acid) (caustic) (chemical) (lime) (external) (internal) T30.4
- abdomen, abdominal (muscle) (wall) T21.42 ☑
  - first degree T21.52 ☑
  - second degree T21.62 ☑
  - third degree T21.72 ☑
- above elbow T22.439 ☑
  - first degree T22.539 ☑
  - left T22.432 ☑
    - first degree T22.532 ☑
    - second degree T22.632 ☑
    - third degree T22.732 ☑
  - right T22.431 ☑
    - first degree T22.531 ☑
    - second degree T22.631 ☑
    - third degree T22.731 ☑
  - second degree T22.639 ☑
  - third degree T22.739 ☑
- alimentary tract NEC T28.7 ☑
- ankle T25.419 ☑
  - first degree T25.519 ☑
  - left T25.412 ☑
    - first degree T25.512 ☑
    - second degree T25.612 ☑
    - third degree T25.712 ☑
  - multiple with foot — *see* Corrosion, lower, limb, multiple, ankle and foot
  - right T25.411 ☑

Corrosion — *continued*
- ankle — *continued*
  - right — *continued*
    - first degree T25.511 ☑
    - second degree T25.611 ☑
    - third degree T25.711 ☑
  - second degree T25.619 ☑
  - third degree T25.719 ☑
- anus — *see* Corrosion, buttock
- arm(s) (meaning upper limb(s)) — *see* Corrosion, upper limb
- axilla T22.449 ☑
  - first degree T22.549 ☑
  - left T22.442 ☑
    - first degree T22.542 ☑
    - second degree T22.642 ☑
    - third degree T22.742 ☑
  - right T22.441 ☑
    - first degree T22.541 ☑
    - second degree T22.641 ☑
    - third degree T22.741 ☑
  - second degree T22.649 ☑
  - third degree T22.749 ☑
- back (lower) T21.44 ☑
  - first degree T21.54 ☑
  - second degree T21.64 ☑
  - third degree T21.74 ☑
  - upper T21.43 ☑
    - first degree T21.53 ☑
    - second degree T21.63 ☑
    - third degree T21.73 ☑
- blisters — *code as* Corrosion, second degree, by site
- breast(s) — *see* Corrosion, chest wall
- buttock(s) T21.45 ☑
  - first degree T21.55 ☑
  - second degree T21.65 ☑
  - third degree T21.75 ☑
- calf T24.439 ☑
  - first degree T24.539 ☑
  - left T24.432 ☑
    - first degree T24.532 ☑
    - second degree T24.632 ☑
    - third degree T24.732 ☑
  - right T24.431 ☑
    - first degree T24.531 ☑
    - second degree T24.631 ☑
    - third degree T24.731 ☑
  - second degree T24.639 ☑
  - third degree T24.739 ☑
- canthus (eye) — *see* Corrosion, eyelid
- cervix T28.8 ☑
- cheek T20.46 ☑
  - first degree T20.56 ☑
  - second degree T20.66 ☑
  - third degree T20.76 ☑
- chest wall T21.41 ☑
  - first degree T21.51 ☑
  - second degree T21.61 ☑
  - third degree T21.71 ☑
- chin T20.43 ☑
  - first degree T20.53 ☑
  - second degree T20.63 ☑
  - third degree T20.73 ☑
- colon T28.7 ☑
- conjunctiva (and cornea) — *see* Corrosion, cornea
- cornea (and conjunctiva) T26.6- ☑
- deep necrosis of underlying tissue — *code as* Corrosion, third degree, by site
- dorsum of hand T23.469 ☑
  - first degree T23.569 ☑
  - left T23.462 ☑
    - first degree T23.562 ☑
    - second degree T23.662 ☑
    - third degree T23.762 ☑
  - right T23.461 ☑
    - first degree T23.561 ☑
    - second degree T23.661 ☑
    - third degree T23.761 ☑
  - second degree T23.669 ☑
  - third degree T23.769 ☑
- ear (auricle) (external) (canal) T20.41 ☑
  - drum T28.91 ☑
  - first degree T20.51 ☑
  - second degree T20.61 ☑
  - third degree T20.71 ☑
- elbow T22.429 ☑

Corrosion — *continued*
- elbow — *continued*
  - first degree T22.529 ☑
  - left T22.422 ☑
    - first degree T22.522 ☑
    - second degree T22.622 ☑
    - third degree T22.722 ☑
  - right T22.421 ☑
    - first degree T22.521 ☑
    - second degree T22.621 ☑
    - third degree T22.721 ☑
  - second degree T22.629 ☑
  - third degree T22.729 ☑
- entire body — *see* Corrosion, multiple body regions
- epidermal loss — *code as* Corrosion, second degree, by site
- epiglottis T27.4 ☑
- erythema, erythematous — *code as* Corrosion, first degree, by site
- esophagus T28.6 ☑
- extent (percentage of body surface)
  - less than 10 percent T32.0
  - 10-19 percent (0-9 percent third degree) T32.10
    - with 10-19 percent third degree T32.11
  - 20-29 percent (0-9 percent third degree) T32.20
    - with
      - 10-19 percent third degree T32.21
      - 20-29 percent third degree T32.22
  - 30-39 percent (0-9 percent third degree) T32.30
    - with
      - 10-19 percent third degree T32.31
      - 20-29 percent third degree T32.32
      - 30-39 percent third degree T32.33
  - 40-49 percent (0-9 percent third degree) T32.40
    - with
      - 10-19 percent third degree T32.41
      - 20-29 percent third degree T32.42
      - 30-39 percent third degree T32.43
      - 40-49 percent third degree T32.44
  - 50-59 percent (0-9 percent third degree) T32.50
    - with
      - 10-19 percent third degree T32.51
      - 20-29 percent third degree T32.52
      - 30-39 percent third degree T32.53
      - 40-49 percent third degree T32.54
      - 50-59 percent third degree T32.55
  - 60-69 percent (0-9 percent third degree) T32.60
    - with
      - 10-19 percent third degree T32.61
      - 20-29 percent third degree T32.62
      - 30-39 percent third degree T32.63
      - 40-49 percent third degree T32.64
      - 50-59 percent third degree T32.65
      - 60-69 percent third degree T32.66
  - 70-79 percent (0-9 percent third degree) T32.70
    - with
      - 10-19 percent third degree T32.71
      - 20-29 percent third degree T32.72
      - 30-39 percent third degree T32.73
      - 40-49 percent third degree T32.74
      - 50-59 percent third degree T32.75
      - 60-69 percent third degree T32.76
      - 70-79 percent third degree T32.77
  - 80-89 percent (0-9 percent third degree) T32.80
    - with
      - 10-19 percent third degree T32.81
      - 20-29 percent third degree T32.82
      - 30-39 percent third degree T32.83
      - 40-49 percent third degree T32.84
      - 50-59 percent third degree T32.85
      - 60-69 percent third degree T32.86
      - 70-79 percent third degree T32.87
      - 80-89 percent third degree T32.88
  - 90 percent or more (0-9 percent third degree) T32.90
    - with
      - 10-19 percent third degree T32.91
      - 20-29 percent third degree T32.92
      - 30-39 percent third degree T32.93
      - 40-49 percent third degree T32.94
      - 50-59 percent third degree T32.95
      - 60-69 percent third degree T32.96
      - 70-79 percent third degree T32.97
      - 80-89 percent third degree T32.98
      - 90-99 percent third degree T32.99
- extremity — *see* Corrosion, limb
- eye(s) and adnexa T26.9- ☑
  - with resulting rupture and destruction of eyeball T26.7- ☑

- **Corrosion** — *continued*
  - eye(s) and adnexa — *continued*
    - conjunctival sac — *see* Corrosion, cornea
    - cornea — *see* Corrosion, cornea
    - lid — *see* Corrosion, eyelid
    - periocular area — *see* Corrosion eyelid
    - specified site NEC T26.8- ☑
  - eyeball — *see* Corrosion, eye
  - eyelid(s) T26.5- ☑
  - face — *see* Corrosion, head
  - finger T23.429 ☑
    - first degree T23.529 ☑
    - left T23.422 ☑
      - first degree T23.522 ☑
      - second degree T23.622 ☑
      - third degree T23.722 ☑
    - multiple sites (without thumb) T23.439 ☑
      - with thumb T23.449 ☑
        - first degree T23.549 ☑
        - left T23.442 ☑
          - first degree T23.542 ☑
          - second degree T23.642 ☑
          - third degree T23.742 ☑
        - right T23.441 ☑
          - first degree T23.541 ☑
          - second degree T23.641 ☑
          - third degree T23.741 ☑
        - second degree T23.649 ☑
        - third degree T23.749 ☑
      - first degree T23.539 ☑
      - left T23.432 ☑
        - first degree T23.532 ☑
        - second degree T23.632 ☑
        - third degree T23.732 ☑
      - right T23.431 ☑
        - first degree T23.531 ☑
        - second degree T23.631 ☑
        - third degree T23.731 ☑
      - second degree T23.639 ☑
      - third degree T23.739 ☑
    - right T23.421 ☑
      - first degree T23.521 ☑
      - second degree T23.621 ☑
      - third degree T23.721 ☑
    - second degree T23.629 ☑
    - third degree T23.729 ☑
  - flank — *see* Corrosion, abdomen
  - foot T25.429 ☑
    - first degree T25.529 ☑
    - left T25.422 ☑
      - first degree T25.522 ☑
      - second degree T25.622 ☑
      - third degree T25.722 ☑
    - multiple with ankle — *see* Corrosion, lower, limb, multiple, ankle and foot
    - right T25.421 ☑
      - first degree T25.521 ☑
      - second degree T25.621 ☑
      - third degree T25.721 ☑
    - second degree T25.629 ☑
    - third degree T25.729 ☑
  - forearm T22.419 ☑
    - first degree T22.519 ☑
    - left T22.412 ☑
      - first degree T22.512 ☑
      - second degree T22.612 ☑
      - third degree T22.712 ☑
    - right T22.411 ☑
      - first degree T22.511 ☑
      - second degree T22.611 ☑
      - third degree T22.711 ☑
    - second degree T22.619 ☑
    - third degree T22.719 ☑
  - forehead T2Ø.46 ☑
    - first degree T2Ø.56 ☑
    - second degree T2Ø.66 ☑
    - third degree T2Ø.76 ☑
  - fourth degree — *code as* Corrosion, third degree, by site
  - full thickness skin loss — *code as* Corrosion, third degree, by site
  - gastrointestinal tract NEC T28.7 ☑
  - genital organs
    - external
      - female T21.47 ☑
        - first degree T21.57 ☑

- **Corrosion** — *continued*
  - genital organs — *continued*
    - external — *continued*
      - female — *continued*
        - second degree T21.67 ☑
        - third degree T21.77 ☑
      - male T21.46 ☑
        - first degree T21.56 ☑
        - second degree T21.66 ☑
        - third degree T21.76 ☑
    - internal T28.8 ☑
  - groin — *see* Corrosion, abdominal wall
  - hand(s) T23.4Ø9 ☑
    - back — *see* Corrosion, dorsum of hand
    - finger — *see* Corrosion, finger
    - first degree T23.5Ø9 ☑
    - left T23.4Ø2 ☑
      - first degree T23.5Ø2 ☑
      - second degree T23.6Ø2 ☑
      - third degree T23.7Ø2 ☑
    - multiple sites with wrist T23.499 ☑
      - first degree T23.599 ☑
      - left T23.492 ☑
        - first degree T23.592 ☑
        - second degree T23.692 ☑
        - third degree T23.792 ☑
      - right T23.491 ☑
        - first degree T23.591 ☑
        - second degree T23.691 ☑
        - third degree T23.791 ☑
      - second degree T23.699 ☑
      - third degree T23.799 ☑
    - palm — *see* Corrosion, palm
    - right T23.4Ø1 ☑
      - first degree T23.5Ø1 ☑
      - second degree T23.6Ø1 ☑
      - third degree T23.7Ø1 ☑
    - second degree T23.6Ø9 ☑
    - third degree T23.7Ø9 ☑
    - thumb — *see* Corrosion, thumb
  - head (and face) (and neck) T2Ø.4Ø ☑
    - cheek — *see* Corrosion, cheek
    - chin — *see* Corrosion, chin
    - ear — *see* Corrosion, ear
    - eye(s) only — *see* Corrosion, eye
    - first degree T2Ø.5Ø ☑
    - forehead — *see* Corrosion, forehead
    - lip — *see* Corrosion, lip
    - multiple sites T2Ø.49 ☑
      - first degree T2Ø.59 ☑
      - second degree T2Ø.69 ☑
      - third degree T2Ø.79 ☑
    - neck — *see* Corrosion, neck
    - nose — *see* Corrosion, nose
    - scalp — *see* Corrosion, scalp
    - second degree T2Ø.6Ø ☑
    - third degree T2Ø.7Ø ☑
  - hip(s) — *see* Corrosion, lower, limb
  - inhalation — *see* Corrosion, respiratory tract
  - internal organ(s) — *see also* Corrosion, by site T28.9Ø ☑
    - alimentary tract T28.7 ☑
      - esophagus T28.6 ☑
    - esophagus T28.6 ☑
    - genitourinary T28.8 ☑
    - mouth T28.5 ☑
    - pharynx T28.5 ☑
    - specified organ NEC T28.99 ☑
  - interscapular region — *see* Corrosion, back, upper
  - intestine (large) (small) T28.7 ☑
  - knee T24.429 ☑
    - first degree T24.529 ☑
    - left T24.422 ☑
      - first degree T24.522 ☑
      - second degree T24.622 ☑
      - third degree T24.722 ☑
    - right T24.421 ☑
      - first degree T24.521 ☑
      - second degree T24.621 ☑
      - third degree T24.721 ☑
    - second degree T24.629 ☑
    - third degree T24.729 ☑
  - labium (majus) (minus) — *see* Corrosion, genital organs, external, female
  - lacrimal apparatus, duct, gland or sac — *see* Corrosion, eye, specified site NEC

- **Corrosion** — *continued*
  - larynx T27.4 ☑
    - with lung T27.5 ☑
  - leg(s) (meaning lower limb(s)) — *see* Corrosion, lower limb
  - limb(s)
    - lower — *see* Corrosion, lower, limb
    - upper — *see* Corrosion, upper limb
  - lip(s) T2Ø.42 ☑
    - first degree T2Ø.52 ☑
    - second degree T2Ø.62 ☑
    - third degree T2Ø.72 ☑
  - lower
    - back — *see* Corrosion, back
    - limb T24.4Ø9 ☑
      - ankle — *see* Corrosion, ankle
      - calf — *see* Corrosion, calf
      - first degree T24.5Ø9 ☑
      - foot — *see* Corrosion, foot
      - knee — *see* Corrosion, knee
      - left T24.4Ø2 ☑
        - first degree T24.5Ø2 ☑
        - second degree T24.6Ø2 ☑
        - third degree T24.7Ø2 ☑
      - multiple sites, except ankle and foot T24.499 ☑
        - ankle and foot T25.499 ☑
          - first degree T25.599 ☑
          - left T25.492 ☑
            - first degree T25.592 ☑
            - second degree T25.692 ☑
            - third degree T25.792 ☑
          - right T25.491 ☑
            - first degree T25.591 ☑
            - second degree T25.691 ☑
            - third degree T25.791 ☑
          - second degree T25.699 ☑
          - third degree T25.799 ☑
        - first degree T24.599 ☑
        - left T24.492 ☑
          - first degree T24.592 ☑
          - second degree T24.692 ☑
          - third degree T24.792 ☑
        - right T24.491 ☑
          - first degree T24.591 ☑
          - second degree T24.691 ☑
          - third degree T24.791 ☑
        - second degree T24.699 ☑
        - third degree T24.799 ☑
      - right T24.4Ø1 ☑
        - first degree T24.5Ø1 ☑
        - second degree T24.6Ø1 ☑
        - third degree T24.7Ø1 ☑
      - second degree T24.6Ø9 ☑
      - thigh — *see* Corrosion, thigh
      - third degree T24.7Ø9 ☑
  - lung (with larynx and trachea) T27.5 ☑
  - mouth T28.5 ☑
  - neck T2Ø.47 ☑
    - first degree T2Ø.57 ☑
    - second degree T2Ø.67 ☑
    - third degree T2Ø.77 ☑
  - nose (septum) T2Ø.44 ☑
    - first degree T2Ø.54 ☑
    - second degree T2Ø.64 ☑
    - third degree T2Ø.74 ☑
  - ocular adnexa — *see* Corrosion, eye
  - orbit region — *see* Corrosion, eyelid
  - palm T23.459 ☑
    - first degree T23.559 ☑
    - left T23.452 ☑
      - first degree T23.552 ☑
      - second degree T23.652 ☑
      - third degree T23.752 ☑
    - right T23.451 ☑
      - first degree T23.551 ☑
      - second degree T23.651 ☑
      - third degree T23.751 ☑
    - second degree T23.659 ☑
    - third degree T23.759 ☑
  - partial thickness — *code as* Corrosion, unspecified degree, by site
  - pelvis — *see* Corrosion, trunk
  - penis — *see* Corrosion, genital organs, external, male
  - perineum
    - female — *see* Corrosion, genital organs, external, female

- **Crisis** — *continued*
  - Dietl's N13.8
  - emotional — *see also* Disorder, adjustment
    - acute reaction to stress F43.Ø
    - specific to childhood and adolescence F93.8
  - glaucomatocyclitic — *see* Glaucoma, secondary, inflammation
  - heart — *see* Failure, heart
  - nitritoid I95.2
    - correct substance properly administered — *see* Table of Drugs and Chemicals, by drug, adverse effect
    - overdose or wrong substance given or taken — *see* Table of Drugs and Chemicals, by drug, poisoning
  - oculogyric H51.8
    - psychogenic F45.8
  - Pel's (tabetic) A52.11
  - psychosexual identity F64.2
  - renal N28.Ø
  - sickle-cell D57.ØØ
    - with
      - acute chest syndrome D57.Ø1
      - cerebral vascular involvement D57.Ø3
      - crisis (painful) D57.ØØ
        - with complication specified NEC D57.Ø9
      - splenic sequestration D57.Ø2
      - vasoocclusive pain D57.ØØ
  - state (acute reaction) F43.Ø
  - tabetic A52.11
  - thyroid — *see* Thyrotoxicosis with thyroid storm
  - thyrotoxic — *see* Thyrotoxicosis with thyroid storm
- **Crocq's disease** (acrocyanosis) I73.89
- **Crohn's disease** — *see* Enteritis, regional
- **Crooked septum, nasal** J34.2
- **Cross syndrome** E7Ø.328
- **Crossbite** (anterior) (posterior) M26.24
- **Cross-eye** — *see* Strabismus, convergent concomitant
- **Croup, croupous** (catarrhal) (infectious) (inflammatory) (nondiphtheritic) JØ5.Ø
  - bronchial J2Ø.9
  - diphtheritic A36.2
  - false J38.5
  - spasmodic J38.5
    - diphtheritic A36.2
  - stridulous J38.5
    - diphtheritic A36.2
- **Crouzon's disease** Q75.1
- **Crowding, tooth, teeth, fully erupted** M26.31
- **CRST syndrome** M34.1
- **Cruchet's disease** A85.8
- **Cruelty in children** — *see also* Disorder, conduct
- **Crural ulcer** — *see* Ulcer, lower limb
- **Crush, crushed, crushing** T14.8 ☑
  - abdomen S38.1 ☑
  - ankle S97.Ø- ☑
  - arm (upper) (and shoulder) S47.- ☑
  - axilla — *see* Crush, arm
  - back, lower S38.1 ☑
  - buttock S38.1 ☑
  - cheek SØ7.Ø ☑
  - chest S28.Ø ☑
  - cranium SØ7.1 ☑
  - ear SØ7.Ø ☑
  - elbow S57.Ø- ☑
  - extremity
    - lower
      - ankle — *see* Crush, ankle
      - below knee — *see* Crush, leg
      - foot — *see* Crush, foot
      - hip — *see* Crush, hip
      - knee — *see* Crush, knee
      - thigh — *see* Crush, thigh
      - toe — *see* Crush, toe
    - upper
      - below elbow S67.9- ☑
      - elbow — *see* Crush, elbow
      - finger — *see* Crush, finger
      - forearm — *see* Crush, forearm
      - hand — *see* Crush, hand
      - thumb — *see* Crush, thumb
      - upper arm — *see* Crush, arm
      - wrist — *see* Crush, wrist
  - face SØ7.Ø ☑
  - finger(s) S67.1- ☑
    - with hand (and wrist) — *see* Crush, hand, specified site NEC

- **Crush, crushed, crushing** — *continued*
  - finger(s) — *continued*
    - index S67.19- ☑
    - little S67.19- ☑
    - middle S67.19- ☑
    - ring S67.19- ☑
    - thumb — *see* Crush, thumb
  - foot S97.8- ☑
    - toe — *see* Crush, toe
  - forearm S57.8- ☑
  - genitalia, external
    - female S38.ØØ2 ☑
      - vagina S38.Ø3 ☑
      - vulva S38.Ø3 ☑
    - male S38.ØØ1 ☑
      - penis S38.Ø1 ☑
      - scrotum S38.Ø2 ☑
      - testis S38.Ø2 ☑
  - hand (except fingers alone) S67.2- ☑
    - with wrist S67.4- ☑
  - head SØ7.9 ☑
    - specified NEC SØ7.8 ☑
  - heel — *see* Crush, foot
  - hip S77.Ø- ☑
    - with thigh S77.2- ☑
  - internal organ (abdomen, chest, or pelvis) NEC T14.8 ☑
  - knee S87.Ø- ☑
  - labium (majus) (minus) S38.Ø3 ☑
  - larynx S17.Ø ☑
  - leg (lower) S87.8- ☑
    - knee — *see* Crush, knee
  - lip SØ7.Ø ☑
  - lower
    - back S38.1 ☑
    - leg — *see* Crush, leg
  - neck S17.9 ☑
  - nerve — *see* Injury, nerve
  - nose SØ7.Ø ☑
  - pelvis S38.1 ☑
  - penis S38.Ø1 ☑
  - scalp SØ7.8 ☑
  - scapular region — *see* Crush, arm
  - scrotum S38.Ø2 ☑
  - severe, unspecified site T14.8 ☑
  - shoulder (and upper arm) — *see* Crush, arm
  - skull SØ7.1 ☑
  - syndrome (complication of trauma) T79.5 ☑
  - testis S38.Ø2 ☑
  - thigh S77.1- ☑
    - with hip S77.2- ☑
  - throat S17.8 ☑
  - thumb S67.Ø- ☑
    - with hand (and wrist) — *see* Crush, hand, specified site NEC
  - toe(s) S97.1Ø- ☑
    - great S97.11- ☑
    - lesser S97.12- ☑
  - trachea S17.Ø ☑
  - vagina S38.Ø3 ☑
  - vulva S38.Ø3 ☑
  - wrist S67.3- ☑
    - with hand S67.4- ☑
- **Crusta lactea** L21.Ø
- **Crusts** R23.4
- **Crutch paralysis** — *see* Injury, brachial plexus
- **Cruveilhier-Baumgarten cirrhosis, disease or syndrome** K74.69
- **Cruveilhier's atrophy or disease** G12.8
- **Crying** (constant) (continuous) (excessive)
  - child, adolescent, or adult R45.83
  - infant (baby) (newborn) R68.11
- **Cryofibrinogenemia** D89.2
- **Cryoglobulinemia** (essential) (idiopathic) (mixed) (primary) (purpura) (secondary) (vasculitis) D89.1
  - with lung involvement D89.1 *[J99]*
- **Cryptitis** (anal) (rectal) K62.89
- **Cryptococcosis, cryptococcus** (infection) (neoformans) B45.9
  - bone B45.3
  - cerebral B45.1
  - cutaneous B45.2
  - disseminated B45.7
  - generalized B45.7
  - meningitis B45.1
  - meningocerebralis B45.1
  - osseous B45.3

- **Cryptococcosis, cryptococcus** — *continued*
  - pulmonary B45.Ø
  - skin B45.2
  - specified NEC B45.8
- **Cryptopapillitis** (anus) K62.89
- **Cryptophthalmos** Q11.2
  - syndrome Q87.Ø
- **Cryptorchid, cryptorchism, cryptorchidism** Q53.9
  - bilateral Q53.2Ø
    - abdominal Q53.211
    - perineal Q53.22
  - unilateral Q53.1Ø
    - abdominal Q53.111
    - perineal Q53.12
- **Cryptosporidiosis** AØ7.2
  - hepatobiliary B88.8
  - respiratory B88.8
- **Cryptostromosis** J67.6
- **Crystalluria** R82.998
- **Cubitus**
  - congenital Q68.8
  - valgus (acquired) M21.Ø- ☑
    - congenital Q68.8
    - sequelae (late effect) of rickets E64.3
  - varus (acquired) M21.1- ☑
    - congenital Q68.8
    - sequelae (late effect) of rickets E64.3
- **Cultural deprivation or shock** Z6Ø.3
- **Curling esophagus** K22.4
- **Curling's ulcer** — *see* Ulcer, peptic, acute
- **Curschmann** (-Batten) (-Steinert) **disease or syndrome** G71.11
- **Curse, Ondine's** — *see* Apnea, sleep
- **Curvature**
  - organ or site, congenital NEC — *see* Distortion
  - penis (lateral) Q55.61
  - Pott's (spinal) A18.Ø1
  - radius, idiopathic, progressive (congenital) Q74.Ø
  - spine (acquired) (angular) (idiopathic) (incorrect) (postural) — *see* Dorsopathy, deforming
    - congenital Q67.5
    - due to or associated with
      - Charcot-Marie-Tooth disease — *see also* subcategory M49.8 G6Ø.Ø
      - osteitis
        - deformans M88.88
        - fibrosa cystica — *see also* subcategory M49.8 E21.Ø
      - tuberculosis (Pott's curvature) A18.Ø1
    - sequelae (late effect) of rickets E64.3
    - tuberculous A18.Ø1
- **Cushingoid due to steroid therapy** E24.2
  - correct substance properly administered — *see* Table of Drugs and Chemicals, by drug, adverse effect
  - overdose or wrong substance given or taken — *see* Table of Drugs and Chemicals, by drug, poisoning
- **Cushing's**
  - syndrome or disease E24.9
    - drug-induced E24.2
    - iatrogenic E24.2
    - pituitary-dependent E24.Ø
    - specified NEC E24.8
  - ulcer — *see* Ulcer, peptic, acute
- **Cusp, Carabelli** — *omit code*
- **Cut** (external) — *see also* Laceration
  - muscle — *see* Injury, muscle
- **Cutaneous** — *see also* condition
  - hemorrhage R23.3
  - larva migrans B76.9
- **Cutis** — *see also* condition
  - hyperelastica Q82.8
    - acquired L57.4
  - laxa (hyperelastica) — *see* Dermatolysis
  - marmorata R23.8
  - osteosis L94.2
  - pendula — *see* Dermatolysis
  - rhomboidalis nuchae L57.2
  - verticis gyrata Q82.8
    - acquired L91.8
- **Cyanosis** R23.Ø
  - due to
    - patent foramen botalli Q21.1
    - persistent foramen ovale Q21.1
  - enterogenous D74.8
  - paroxysmal digital — *see* Raynaud's disease
    - with gangrene I73.Ø1
  - retina, retinal H35.89
- **Cyanotic heart disease** I24.9

- **Cyanotic heart disease** — *continued*
  - congenital Q24.9
- **Cycle**
  - anovulatory N97.Ø
  - menstrual, irregular N92.6
- **Cyclencephaly** QØ4.9
- **Cyclical vomiting, in migraine** — *see also* Vomiting, cyclical G43.AØ (*following* G43.7)
  - psychogenic F5Ø.89
- **Cyclitis** — *see also* Iridocyclitis H2Ø.9
  - chronic — *see* Iridocyclitis, chronic
  - Fuchs' heterochromic H2Ø.81- ☑
  - granulomatous — *see* Iridocyclitis, chronic
  - lens-induced — *see* Iridocyclitis, lens-induced
  - posterior H3Ø.2- ☑
- **Cycloid personality** F34.Ø
- **Cyclophoria** H5Ø.54
- **Cyclopia, cyclops** Q87.Ø
- **Cyclopism** Q87.Ø
- **Cyclosporiasis** AØ7.4
- **Cyclothymia** F34.Ø
- **Cyclothymic personality** F34.Ø
- **Cyclotropia** H5Ø.41- ☑
- **Cylindroma** — *see also* Neoplasm, malignant, by site
  - eccrine dermal — *see* Neoplasm, skin, benign
  - skin — *see* Neoplasm, skin, benign
- **Cylindruria** R82.998
- **Cynanche**
  - diphtheritic A36.2
  - tonsillaris J36
- **Cynophobia** F4Ø.218
- **Cynorexia** R63.2
- **Cyphosis** — *see* Kyphosis
- **Cyprus fever** — *see* Brucellosis
- **Cyst** (colloid) (mucous) (simple) (retention)
  - adenoid (infected) J35.8
  - adrenal gland E27.8
    - congenital Q89.1
  - air, lung J98.4
  - allantoic Q64.4
  - alveolar process (jaw bone) M27.4Ø
  - amnion, amniotic O41.8X- ☑
  - aneurysmal M27.49
  - anterior
    - chamber (eye) — *see* Cyst, iris
    - nasopalatine KØ9.1
  - antrum J34.1
  - anus K62.89
  - apical (tooth) (periodontal) KØ4.8
  - appendix K38.8
  - arachnoid, brain (acquired) G93.Ø
    - congenital QØ4.6
  - arytenoid J38.7
  - Baker's M71.2- ☑
    - ruptured M66.Ø
    - tuberculous A18.Ø2
  - Bartholin's gland N75.Ø
  - bile duct (common) (hepatic) K83.5
  - bladder (multiple) (trigone) N32.89
  - blue dome (breast) — *see* Cyst, breast
  - bone (local) NEC M85.6Ø
    - aneurysmal M85.5Ø
      - ankle M85.57- ☑
      - foot M85.57- ☑
      - forearm M85.53- ☑
      - hand M85.54- ☑
      - jaw M27.49
      - lower leg M85.56- ☑
      - multiple site M85.59
      - neck M85.58
      - rib M85.58
      - shoulder M85.51- ☑
      - skull M85.58
      - specified site NEC M85.58
      - thigh M85.55- ☑
      - toe M85.57- ☑
      - upper arm M85.52- ☑
      - vertebra M85.58
    - solitary M85.4Ø
      - ankle M85.47- ☑
      - fibula M85.46- ☑
      - foot M85.47- ☑
      - hand M85.44- ☑
      - humerus M85.42- ☑
      - jaw M27.49
      - neck M85.48
      - pelvis M85.45- ☑

- **Cyst** — *continued*
  - bone — *continued*
    - solitary — *continued*
      - radius M85.43- ☑
      - rib M85.48
      - shoulder M85.41- ☑
      - skull M85.48
      - specified site NEC M85.48
      - tibia M85.46- ☑
      - toe M85.47- ☑
      - ulna M85.43- ☑
      - vertebra M85.48
    - specified type NEC M85.6Ø
      - ankle M85.67- ☑
      - foot M85.67- ☑
      - forearm M85.63- ☑
      - hand M85.64- ☑
      - jaw M27.4Ø
        - developmental (nonodontogenic) KØ9.1
          - odontogenic KØ9.Ø
        - latent M27.Ø
      - lower leg M85.66- ☑
      - multiple site M85.69
      - neck M85.68
      - rib M85.68
      - shoulder M85.61- ☑
      - skull M85.68
      - specified site NEC M85.68
      - thigh M85.65- ☑
      - toe M85.67- ☑
      - upper arm M85.62- ☑
      - vertebra M85.68
  - brain (acquired) G93.Ø
    - congenital QØ4.6
    - hydatid B67.99 *[G94]*
    - third ventricle (colloid), congenital QØ4.6
  - branchial (cleft) Q18.Ø
  - branchiogenic Q18.Ø
  - breast (benign) (blue dome) (pedunculated) (solitary) N6Ø.Ø- ☑
    - involution — *see* Dysplasia, mammary, specified type NEC
    - sebaceous — *see* Dysplasia, mammary, specified type NEC
  - broad ligament (benign) N83.8
  - bronchogenic (mediastinal) (sequestration) J98.4
    - congenital Q33.Ø
  - buccal KØ9.8
  - bulbourethral gland N36.8
  - bursa, bursal NEC M71.3Ø
    - with rupture — *see* Rupture, synovium
    - ankle M71.37- ☑
    - elbow M71.32- ☑
    - foot M71.37- ☑
    - hand M71.34- ☑
    - hip M71.35- ☑
    - multiple sites M71.39
    - pharyngeal J39.2
    - popliteal space — *see* Cyst, Baker's
    - shoulder M71.31- ☑
    - specified site NEC M71.38
    - wrist M71.33- ☑
  - calcifying odontogenic D16.5
    - upper jaw (bone) (maxilla) D16.4
  - canal of Nuck (female) N94.89
    - congenital Q52.4
  - canthus — *see* Cyst, conjunctiva
  - carcinomatous — *see* Neoplasm, malignant, by site
  - cauda equina G95.89
  - cavum septi pellucidi — *see* Cyst, brain
  - celomic (pericardium) Q24.8
  - cerebellopontine (angle) — *see* Cyst, brain
  - cerebellum — *see* Cyst, brain
  - cerebral — *see* Cyst, brain
  - cervical lateral Q18.Ø
  - cervix NEC N88.8
    - embryonic Q51.6
    - nabothian N88.8
  - chiasmal optic NEC — *see* Disorder, optic, chiasm
  - chocolate (ovary) N8Ø.1
  - choledochus, congenital Q44.4
  - chorion O41.8X- ☑
  - choroid plexus G93.Ø
    - congenital QØ4.6
  - ciliary body — *see* Cyst, iris
  - clitoris N9Ø.7
  - colon K63.89

- **Cyst** — *continued*
  - common (bile) duct K83.5
  - congenital NEC Q89.8
    - adrenal gland Q89.1
    - epiglottis Q31.8
    - esophagus Q39.8
    - fallopian tube Q5Ø.4
    - kidney Q61.ØØ
      - more than one (multiple) Q61.Ø2
        - specified as polycystic Q61.3
          - adult type Q61.2
          - infantile type NEC Q61.19
            - collecting duct dilation Q61.11
      - solitary Q61.Ø1
    - larynx Q31.8
    - liver Q44.6
    - lung Q33.Ø
    - mediastinum Q34.1
    - ovary Q5Ø.1
    - oviduct Q5Ø.4
    - periurethral (tissue) Q64.79
    - prepuce Q55.69
    - salivary gland (any) Q38.4
    - sublingual Q38.6
    - submaxillary gland Q38.6
    - thymus (gland) Q89.2
    - tongue Q38.3
    - ureterovesical orifice Q62.8
    - vulva Q52.79
  - conjunctiva H11.44- ☑
  - cornea H18.89- ☑
  - corpora quadrigemina G93.Ø
  - corpus
    - albicans N83.29- ☑
    - luteum (hemorrhagic) (ruptured) N83.1- ☑
  - Cowper's gland (benign) (infected) N36.8
  - cranial meninges G93.Ø
  - craniobuccal pouch E23.6
  - craniopharyngeal pouch E23.6
  - cystic duct K82.8
  - Cysticercus — *see* Cysticercosis
  - Dandy-Walker QØ3.1
    - with spina bifida — *see* Spina bifida
  - dental (root) KØ4.8
    - developmental KØ9.Ø
    - eruption KØ9.Ø
    - primordial KØ9.Ø
  - dentigerous (mandible) (maxilla) KØ9.Ø
  - dermoid — *see* Neoplasm, benign, by site
    - with malignant transformation C56.- ☑
    - implantation
      - external area or site (skin) NEC L72.Ø
      - iris — *see* Cyst, iris, implantation
      - vagina N89.8
      - vulva N9Ø.7
    - mouth KØ9.8
    - oral soft tissue KØ9.8
    - sacrococcygeal — *see* Cyst, pilonidal
  - developmental KØ9.1
    - odontogenic KØ9.Ø
    - oral region (nonodontogenic) KØ9.1
    - ovary, ovarian Q5Ø.1
  - dura (cerebral) G93.Ø
    - spinal G96.198
  - ear (external) Q18.1
  - echinococcal — *see* Echinococcus
  - embryonic
    - cervix uteri Q51.6
    - fallopian tube Q5Ø.4
    - vagina Q52.4
  - endometrium, endometrial (uterus) N85.8
    - ectopic — *see* Endometriosis
  - enterogenous Q43.8
  - epidermal, epidermoid (inclusion) (*see also* Cyst, skin) L72.Ø
    - mouth KØ9.8
    - oral soft tissue KØ9.8
  - epididymis N5Ø.3
  - epiglottis J38.7
  - epiphysis cerebri E34.8
  - epithelial (inclusion) L72.Ø
  - epoophoron Q5Ø.5
  - eruption KØ9.Ø
  - esophagus K22.8
  - ethmoid sinus J34.1
  - external female genital organs NEC N9Ø.7
  - eyelid (sebaceous) HØ2.829
    - infected — *see* Hordeolum

D

Da Costa's syndrome F45.8
Daae (-Finsen) **disease** (epidemic pleurodynia) B33.Ø
Dabney's grip B33.Ø
Dacryoadenitis, dacryadenitis HØ4.ØØ- ☑
- acute HØ4.Ø1- ☑
- chronic HØ4.Ø2- ☑

Dacryocystitis HØ4.3Ø- ☑
- acute HØ4.32- ☑
- chronic HØ4.41- ☑
- neonatal P39.1
- phlegmonous HØ4.31- ☑
- syphilitic A52.71
  - congenital (early) A5Ø.Ø1
- trachomatous, active A71.1
  - sequelae (late effect) B94.Ø

Dacryocystoblenorrhea — *see* Inflammation, lacrimal, passages, chronic
Dacryocystocele — *see* Disorder, lacrimal system, changes
Dacryolith, dacryolithiasis HØ4.51- ☑
Dacryoma — *see* Disorder, lacrimal system, changes
Dacryopericystitis — *see* Dacryocystitis
Dacryops HØ4.11- ☑
Dacryostenosis — *see also* Stenosis, lacrimal
- congenital Q1Ø.5

Dactylitis
- bone — *see* Osteomyelitis
- sickle-cell D57.ØØ
  - Hb C D57.219
  - Hb SS D57.ØØ
  - specified NEC D57.819
- skin LØ8.9
- syphilitic A52.77
- tuberculous A18.Ø3

Dactylolysis spontanea (ainhum) L94.6
Dactylosymphysis Q7Ø.9
- fingers — *see* Syndactylism, complex, fingers
- toes — *see* Syndactylism, complex, toes

Damage
- arteriosclerotic — *see* Arteriosclerosis
- brain (nontraumatic) G93.9
  - anoxic, hypoxic G93.1
    - resulting from a procedure G97.82
  - child NEC G8Ø.9
  - due to birth injury P11.2
- cardiorenal (vascular) — *see* Hypertension, cardiorenal
- cerebral NEC — *see* Damage, brain
- coccyx, complicating delivery O71.6
- coronary — *see* Disease, heart, ischemic
- deep tissue, pressure-induced — *see also* L89 with final character .6
- eye, birth injury P15.3
- liver (nontraumatic) K76.9
  - alcoholic K7Ø.9
  - due to drugs — *see* Disease, liver, toxic
  - toxic — *see* Disease, liver, toxic
- lung
  - dabbing (related) UØ7.Ø
  - electronic cigarette (related) UØ7.Ø
  - vaping (associated) (device) (product) (use) UØ7.Ø
- medication T88.7 ☑
- organ
  - dabbing (related) UØ7.Ø
  - electronic cigarette (related) UØ7.Ø
  - vaping (associated) (device) (product) (use) UØ7.Ø
- pelvic
  - joint or ligament, during delivery O71.6
  - organ NEC
    - during delivery O71.5
    - following ectopic or molar pregnancy OØ8.6
- renal — *see* Disease, renal
- subendocardium, subendocardial — *see* Degeneration, myocardial
- vascular I99.9

Dana-Putnam syndrome (subacute combined sclerosis with pernicious anemia) — *see* Degeneration, combined
Danbolt (-Cross) **syndrome** (acrodermatitis enteropathica) E83.2
Dandruff L21.Ø
Dandy-Walker syndrome QØ3.1
- with spina bifida — *see* Spina bifida

Danlos' syndrome — *see also* Syndrome, Ehlers-Danlos Q79.6Ø
Darier (-White) **disease** (congenital) Q82.8
- meaning erythema annulare centrifugum L53.1

Darier-Roussy sarcoid D86.3
Darling's disease or histoplasmosis B39.4
Darwin's tubercle Q17.8
Dawson's (inclusion body) **encephalitis** A81.1
De Beurmann (-Gougerot) **disease** B42.1
De la Tourette's syndrome F95.2
De Lange's syndrome Q87.19
De Morgan's spots (senile angiomas) I78.1
De Quervain's
- disease (tendon sheath) M65.4
- syndrome E34.51
- thyroiditis (subacute granulomatous thyroiditis) EØ6.1

De Toni-Fanconi (-Debré) **syndrome** E72.Ø9
- with cystinosis E72.Ø4

Dead
- fetus, retained (mother) O36.4 ☑
  - early pregnancy OØ2.1
- labyrinth H83.2 ☑
- ovum, retained OØ2.Ø

Deaf nonspeaking NEC H91.3
Deafmutism (acquired) (congenital) NEC H91.3
- hysterical F44.6
- syphilitic, congenital — *see also* subcategory H94.8 A5Ø.Ø9

Deafness (acquired) (complete) (hereditary) (partial) H91.9- ☑
- with blue sclera and fragility of bone Q78.Ø
- auditory fatigue — *see* Deafness, specified type NEC
- aviation T7Ø.Ø ☑
  - nerve injury — *see* Injury, nerve, acoustic, specified type NEC
- boilermaker's H83.3 ☑
- central — *see* Deafness, sensorineural
- conductive H9Ø.2
  - and sensorineural
    - mixed H9Ø.8
      - bilateral H9Ø.6
  - bilateral H9Ø.Ø
  - unilateral H9Ø.1- ☑
    - with restricted hearing on the contralateral side H9Ø.A- ☑
- congenital H9Ø.5
  - with blue sclera and fragility of bone Q78.Ø
- due to toxic agents — *see* Deafness, ototoxic
- emotional (hysterical) F44.6
- functional (hysterical) F44.6
- high frequency H91.9- ☑
- hysterical F44.6
- low frequency H91.9- ☑
- mental R48.8
- mixed conductive and sensorineural H9Ø.8
  - bilateral H9Ø.6
  - unilateral H9Ø.7- ☑
- nerve — *see* Deafness, sensorineural
- neural — *see* Deafness, sensorineural
- noise-induced — *see also* subcategory H83.3 ☑
  - nerve injury — *see* Injury, nerve, acoustic, specified type NEC
- nonspeaking H91.3
- ototoxic H91.Ø ☑
- perceptive — *see* Deafness, sensorineural
- psychogenic (hysterical) F44.6
- sensorineural H9Ø.5
  - and conductive
    - bilateral H9Ø.6
    - mixed H9Ø.8
      - bilateral H9Ø.6
  - bilateral H9Ø.3
  - unilateral H9Ø.4- ☑
    - with restricted hearing on the contralateral side H9Ø.A- ☑
- sensory — *see* Deafness, sensorineural
- specified type NEC H91.8 ☑
- sudden (idiopathic) H91.2- ☑
- syphilitic A52.15
- transient ischemic H93.Ø1- ☑
- traumatic — *see* Injury, nerve, acoustic, specified type NEC
- word (developmental) H93.25

Death (cause unknown) (of) (unexplained) (unspecified cause) R99
- brain G93.82
- cardiac (sudden) (with successful resuscitation) — *code to* underlying disease
  - family history of Z82.41

Death — *continued*
- cardiac — *code to* underlying disease — *continued*
  - personal history of Z86.74
- family member (assumed) Z63.4

Debility (chronic) (general) (nervous) R53.81
- congenital or neonatal NOS P96.9
- nervous R53.81
- old age R54
- senile R54

Débove's disease (splenomegaly) R16.1
Decalcification
- bone — *see* Osteoporosis
- teeth KØ3.89

Decapsulation, kidney N28.89
Decay
- dental — *see* Caries, dental
- senile R54
- tooth, teeth — *see* Caries, dental

Deciduitis (acute)
- following ectopic or molar pregnancy OØ8.Ø

Decline (general) — *see* Debility
- cognitive, age-associated R41.81

Decompensation
- cardiac (acute) (chronic) — *see* Disease, heart
- cardiovascular — *see* Disease, cardiovascular
- heart — *see* Disease, heart
- hepatic — *see* Failure, hepatic
- myocardial (acute) (chronic) — *see* Disease, heart
- respiratory J98.8

Decompression sickness T7Ø.3 ☑
Decrease (d)
- absolute neutrophile count — *see* Neutropenia
- blood
  - platelets — *see* Thrombocytopenia
  - pressure RØ3.1
    - due to shock following
      - injury T79.4 ☑
      - operation T81.19 ☑
- estrogen E28.39
  - postablative E89.4Ø
    - asymptomatic E89.4Ø
    - symptomatic E89.41
- fragility of erythrocytes D58.8
- function
  - lipase (pancreatic) K9Ø.3
  - ovary in hypopituitarism E23.Ø
  - parenchyma of pancreas K86.89
  - pituitary (gland) (anterior) (lobe) E23.Ø
    - posterior (lobe) E23.Ø
- functional activity R68.89
- glucose R73.Ø9
- hematocrit R71.Ø
- hemoglobin R71.Ø
- leukocytes D72.819
  - specified NEC D72.818
- libido R68.82
- lymphocytes D72.81Ø
- platelets D69.6
- respiration, due to shock following injury T79.4 ☑
- sexual desire R68.82
- tear secretion NEC — *see* Syndrome, dry eye
- tolerance
  - fat K9Ø.49
  - glucose R73.Ø9
  - pancreatic K9Ø.3
  - salt and water E87.8
- vision NEC H54.7
- white blood cell count D72.819
  - specified NEC D72.818

Decubitus (ulcer) — *see* Ulcer, pressure, by site
- cervix N86

Deepening acetabulum — *see* Derangement, joint, specified type NEC, hip
Defect, defective Q89.9
- 3-beta-hydroxysteroid dehydrogenase E25.Ø
- 11-hydroxylase E25.Ø
- 21-hydroxylase E25.Ø
- abdominal wall, congenital Q79.59
- antibody immunodeficiency D8Ø.9
- aorticopulmonary septum Q21.4
- atrial septal (ostium secundum type) Q21.1
  - following acute myocardial infarction (current complication) I23.1
  - ostium primum type Q21.2
- atrioventricular
  - canal Q21.2
  - septum Q21.2
- auricular septal Q21.1

- **Defect, defective** — *continued*
  - bilirubin excretion NEC E8Ø.6
  - biosynthesis, androgen (testicular) E29.1
  - bulbar septum Q21.Ø
  - catalase E8Ø.3
  - cell membrane receptor complex (CR3) D71
  - circulation I99.9
    - congenital Q28.9
    - newborn Q28.9
  - coagulation (factor) — *see also* Deficiency, factor D68.9
    - with
      - ectopic pregnancy OØ8.1
      - molar pregnancy OØ8.1
    - acquired D68.4
    - antepartum with hemorrhage — *see* Hemorrhage, antepartum, with coagulation defect
    - due to
      - liver disease D68.4
      - vitamin K deficiency D68.4
    - hereditary NEC D68.2
    - intrapartum O67.Ø
    - newborn, transient P61.6
    - postpartum O99.13
      - with hemorrhage O72.3
    - specified type NEC D68.8
  - complement system D84.1
  - conduction (heart) I45.9
    - bone — *see* Deafness, conductive
  - congenital, organ or site not listed — *see* Anomaly, by site
  - coronary sinus Q21.1
  - cushion, endocardial Q21.2
  - degradation, glycoprotein E77.1
  - dental bridge, crown, fillings — *see* Defect, dental restoration
  - dental restoration KØ8.5Ø
    - specified NEC KØ8.59
  - dentin (hereditary) KØØ.5
  - Descemet's membrane, congenital Q13.89
  - developmental — *see also* Anomaly
    - cauda equina QØ6.3
  - diaphragm
    - with elevation, eventration or hernia — *see* Hernia, diaphragm
    - congenital Q79.1
      - with hernia Q79.Ø
      - gross (with hernia) Q79.Ø
  - ectodermal, congenital Q82.9
  - Eisenmenger's Q21.8
  - enzyme
    - catalase E8Ø.3
    - peroxidase E8Ø.3
  - esophagus, congenital Q39.9
  - extensor retinaculum M62.89
  - fibrin polymerization D68.2
  - filling
    - bladder R93.41
    - kidney R93.42- ☑
    - renal pelvis R93.41
    - stomach R93.3
    - ureter R93.41
    - urinary organs, specified NEC R93.49
  - GABA (gamma aminobutyric acid) metabolic E72.81
  - Gerbode Q21.Ø
  - glucose transport, blood-brain barrier E74.81Ø
  - glycoprotein degradation E77.1
  - Hageman (factor) D68.2
  - hearing — *see* Deafness
  - high grade F7Ø
  - interatrial septal Q21.1
  - interauricular septal Q21.1
  - interventricular septal Q21.Ø
    - with dextroposition of aorta, pulmonary stenosis and hypertrophy of right ventricle Q21.3
    - in tetralogy of Fallot Q21.3
  - learning (specific) — *see* Disorder, learning
  - lymphocyte function antigen-1 (LFA-1) D84.Ø
  - lysosomal enzyme, post-translational modification E77.Ø
  - major osseous M89.7Ø
    - ankle M89.77- ☑
    - carpus M89.74- ☑
    - clavicle M89.71- ☑
    - femur M89.75- ☑
    - fibula M89.76- ☑
    - fingers M89.74- ☑
    - foot M89.77- ☑
    - forearm M89.73- ☑

- **Defect, defective** — *continued*
  - major osseous — *continued*
    - hand M89.74- ☑
    - humerus M89.72- ☑
    - lower leg M89.76- ☑
    - metacarpus M89.74- ☑
    - metatarsus M89.77- ☑
    - multiple sites M89.79
    - pelvic region M89.75- ☑
    - pelvis M89.75- ☑
    - radius M89.73- ☑
    - scapula M89.71- ☑
    - shoulder region M89.71- ☑
    - specified NEC M89.78
    - tarsus M89.77- ☑
    - thigh M89.75- ☑
    - tibia M89.76- ☑
    - toes M89.77- ☑
    - ulna M89.73- ☑
  - mental — *see* Disability, intellectual
  - modification, lysosomal enzymes, post-translational E77.Ø
  - obstructive, congenital
    - renal pelvis Q62.39
    - ureter Q62.39
      - atresia — *see* Atresia, ureter
      - cecoureterocele Q62.32
      - megaureter Q62.2
      - orthotopic ureterocele Q62.31
  - osseous, major M89.7Ø
    - ankle M89.77- ☑
    - carpus M89.74- ☑
    - clavicle M89.71- ☑
    - femur M89.75- ☑
    - fibula M89.76- ☑
    - fingers M89.74- ☑
    - foot M89.77- ☑
    - forearm M89.73- ☑
    - hand M89.74- ☑
    - humerus M89.72- ☑
    - lower leg M89.76- ☑
    - metacarpus M89.74- ☑
    - metatarsus M89.77- ☑
    - multiple sites M89.9
    - pelvic region M89.75- ☑
    - pelvis M89.75- ☑
    - radius M89.73- ☑
    - scapula M89.71- ☑
    - shoulder region M89.71- ☑
    - specified NEC M89.78
    - tarsus M89.77- ☑
    - thigh M89.75- ☑
    - tibia M89.76- ☑
    - toes M89.77- ☑
    - ulna M89.73- ☑
  - osteochondral NEC — *see also* Deformity M95.8
  - ostium
    - primum Q21.2
    - secundum Q21.1
  - peroxidase E8Ø.3
  - placental blood supply — *see* Insufficiency, placental
  - platelets, qualitative D69.1
    - constitutional D68.Ø
  - postural NEC, spine — *see* Dorsopathy, deforming
  - reduction
    - limb Q73.8
      - lower Q72.9- ☑
        - absence — *see* Agenesis, leg
          - foot — *see* Agenesis, foot
        - longitudinal
          - femur Q72.4- ☑
          - fibula Q72.6- ☑
          - tibia Q72.5- ☑
        - specified type NEC Q72.89- ☑
        - split foot Q72.7- ☑
      - specified type NEC Q73.8
      - upper Q71.9- ☑
        - absence — *see* Agenesis, arm
          - forearm — *see* Agenesis, forearm
          - hand — *see* Agenesis, hand
        - lobster-claw hand Q71.6- ☑
        - longitudinal
          - radius Q71.4- ☑
          - ulna Q71.5- ☑
        - specified type NEC Q71.89- ☑
  - renal pelvis Q63.8

- **Defect, defective** — *continued*
  - renal pelvis — *continued*
    - obstructive Q62.39
  - respiratory system, congenital Q34.9
  - restoration, dental KØ8.5Ø
    - specified NEC KØ8.59
  - retinal nerve bundle fibers H35.89
  - septal (heart) NOS Q21.9
    - acquired (atrial) (auricular) (ventricular) (old) I51.Ø
    - atrial Q21.1
      - concurrent with acute myocardial infarction — *see* Infarct, myocardium
      - following acute myocardial infarction (current complication) I23.1
    - ventricular — *see also* Defect, ventricular septal Q21.Ø
  - sinus venosus Q21.1
  - speech — *see* Disorder, speech
    - developmental F8Ø.9
    - specified NEC R47.89
  - Taussig-Bing (aortic transposition and overriding pulmonary artery) Q2Ø.1
  - teeth, wedge KØ3.1
  - vascular (local) I99.9
    - congenital Q27.9
  - ventricular septal Q21.Ø
    - concurrent with acute myocardial infarction — *see* Infarct, myocardium
    - following acute myocardial infarction (current complication) I23.2
    - in tetralogy of Fallot Q21.3
  - vision NEC H54.7
  - visual field H53.4Ø
    - bilateral
      - heteronymous H53.47
      - homonymous H53.46- ☑
    - generalized contraction H53.48- ☑
    - localized
      - arcuate H53.43- ☑
      - scotoma (central area) H53.41- ☑
        - blind spot area H53.42- ☑
      - sector H53.43- ☑
      - specified type NEC H53.45- ☑
  - voice R49.9
    - specified NEC R49.8
  - wedge, tooth, teeth (abrasion) KØ3.1
- **Deferentitis** N49.1
  - gonorrheal (acute) (chronic) A54.23
- **Defibrination** (syndrome) D65
  - antepartum — *see* Hemorrhage, antepartum, with coagulation defect, disseminated intravascular coagulation
  - following ectopic or molar pregnancy OØ8.1
  - intrapartum O67.Ø
  - newborn P6Ø
  - postpartum O72.3
- **Deficiency, deficient**
  - 3-beta hydroxysteroid dehydrogenase E25.Ø
  - 5-alpha reductase (with male pseudohermaphroditism) E29.1
  - 11-hydroxylase E25.Ø
  - 21-hydroxylase E25.Ø
  - AADC (aromatic L-amino acid decarboxylase) E7Ø.81
  - abdominal muscle syndrome Q79.4
  - AC globulin (congenital) (hereditary) D68.2
    - acquired D68.4
  - accelerator globulin (Ac G) (blood) D68.2
  - acid phosphatase E83.39
  - activating factor (blood) D68.2
  - ADA2 (adenosine deaminase 2) D81.32
  - adenosine deaminase (ADA) D81.3Ø
    - with severe combined immunodeficiency (SCID) D81.31
    - partial (type 1) D81.39
    - specified NEC D81.39
    - type 1 (without SCID) (without severe combined immunodeficiency) D81.39
    - type 2 D81.32
  - aldolase (hereditary) E74.19
  - alpha-1-antitrypsin E88.Ø1
  - amino-acids E72.9
  - anemia — *see* Anemia
  - aneurin E51.9
  - antibody with
    - hyperimmunoglobulinemia D8Ø.6
    - near-normal immunoglobins D8Ø.6
  - antidiuretic hormone E23.2

Deficiency, deficient — *continued*
- anti-hemophilic
  - factor (A) D66
    - B D67
    - C D68.1
  - globulin (AHG) NEC D66
- antithrombin (antithrombin III) D68.59
- aromatic L-amino acid decarboxylase (AADC) E7Ø.81
- ascorbic acid E54
- attention (disorder) (syndrome) F98.8
  - with hyperactivity — *see* Disorder, attention-deficit hyperactivity
- autoprothrombin
  - I D68.2
  - II D67
  - C D68.2
- beta-glucuronidase E76.29
- biotin E53.8
- biotin-dependent carboxylase D81.819
- biotinidase D81.81Ø
- brancher enzyme (amylopectinosis) E74.Ø3
- C1 esterase inhibitor (C1-INH) D84.1
- calciferol E55.9
  - with
    - adult osteomalacia M83.8
    - rickets — *see* Rickets
- calcium (dietary) E58
- calorie, severe E43
  - with marasmus E41
    - and kwashiorkor E42
- cardiac — *see* Insufficiency, myocardial
- carnitine E71.4Ø
  - due to
    - hemodialysis E71.43
    - inborn errors of metabolism E71.42
    - Valproic acid therapy E71.43
  - iatrogenic E71.43
  - muscle palmityltransferase E71.314
  - primary E71.41
  - secondary E71.448
- carotene E5Ø.9
- central nervous system G96.89
- ceruloplasmin (Wilson) E83.Ø1
- choline E53.8
- Christmas factor D67
- chromium E61.4
- clotting (blood) — *see also* Deficiency, coagulation factor D68.9
- clotting factor NEC (hereditary) — *see also* Deficiency, factor D68.2
- coagulation NOS D68.9
  - with
    - ectopic pregnancy OØ8.1
    - molar pregnancy OØ8.1
  - acquired (any) D68.4
  - antepartum hemorrhage — *see* Hemorrhage, antepartum, with coagulation defect
  - clotting factor NEC — *see also* Deficiency, factor D68.2
  - due to
    - hyperprothrombinemia D68.4
    - liver disease D68.4
    - vitamin K deficiency D68.4
  - newborn, transient P61.6
  - postpartum O72.3
  - specified NEC D68.8
- cognitive FØ9
- color vision H53.5Ø
  - achromatopsia H53.51
  - acquired H53.52
  - deuteranomaly H53.53
  - protanomaly H53.54
  - specified type NEC H53.59
  - tritanomaly H53.55
- combined glucocorticoid and mineralocorticoid E27.49
- contact factor D68.2
- copper (nutritional) E61.Ø
- corticoadrenal E27.4Ø
  - primary E27.1
- craniofacial axis Q75.Ø
- cyanocobalamin E53.8
- debrancher enzyme (limit dextrinosis) E74.Ø3
- dehydrogenase
  - long chain/very long chain acyl CoA E71.31Ø
  - medium chain acyl CoA E71.311
  - short chain acyl CoA E71.312
- diet E63.9
- dihydropyrimidine dehydrogenase (DPD) E88.89

Deficiency, deficient — *continued*
- disaccharidase E73.9
- edema — *see* Malnutrition, severe
- endocrine E34.9
- energy-supply — *see* Malnutrition
- enzymes, circulating NEC E88.Ø9
- ergosterol E55.9
  - with
    - adult osteomalacia M83.8
    - rickets — *see* Rickets
- essential fatty acid (EFA) E63.Ø
- eye movements
  - saccadic H55.81
  - smooth pursuit H55.82
- factor — *see also* Deficiency, coagulation
  - Hageman D68.2
  - I (congenital) (hereditary) D68.2
  - II (congenital) (hereditary) D68.2
  - IX (congenital) (functional) (hereditary) (with functional defect) D67
  - multiple (congenital) D68.8
    - acquired D68.4
  - V (congenital) (hereditary) D68.2
  - VII (congenital) (hereditary) D68.2
  - VIII (congenital) (functional) (hereditary) (with functional defect) D66
    - with vascular defect D68.Ø
  - X (congenital) (hereditary) D68.2
  - XI (congenital) (hereditary) D68.1
  - XII (congenital) (hereditary) D68.2
  - XIII (congenital) (hereditary) D68.2
- femoral, proximal focal (congenital) — *see* Defect, reduction, lower limb, longitudinal, femur
- fibrinase D68.2
- fibrinogen (congenital) (hereditary) D68.2
  - acquired D65
- fibrin-stabilizing factor (congenital) (hereditary) D68.2
  - acquired D68.4
- folate E53.8
- folic acid E53.8
- foreskin N47.3
- fructokinase E74.11
- fructose 1,6-diphosphatase E74.19
- fructose-1-phosphate aldolase E74.19
- GABA (gamma aminobutyric acid) transaminase E72.81
- GABA-T (gamma aminobutyric acid transaminase) E72.81
- galactokinase E74.29
- galactose-1-phosphate uridyl transferase E74.29
- gammaglobulin in blood D8Ø.1
  - hereditary D8Ø.Ø
- glass factor D68.2
- glucocorticoid E27.49
  - mineralocorticoid E27.49
- glucose transporter protein type 1 E74.81Ø
- glucose-6-phosphatase E74.Ø1
- glucose-6-phosphate dehydrogenase
  - anemia D55.Ø
  - without anemia D75.A
- glucuronyl transferase E8Ø.5
- Glut1 E74.81Ø
- glycogen synthetase E74.Ø9
- gonadotropin (isolated) E23.Ø
- growth hormone (idiopathic) (isolated) E23.Ø
- Hageman factor D68.2
- hemoglobin D64.9
- hepatophosphorylase E74.Ø9
- homogentisate 1,2-dioxygenase E7Ø.29
- hormone
  - anterior pituitary (partial) NEC E23.Ø
    - growth E23.Ø
  - growth (isolated) E23.Ø
  - pituitary E23.Ø
  - testicular E29.1
- hypoxanthine- (guanine)-phosphoribosyltransferase (HG- PRT) (total H-PRT) E79.1
- immunity D84.9
  - cell-mediated D84.89
    - with thrombocytopenia and eczema D82.Ø
  - combined D81.9
  - humoral D8Ø.9
  - IgA (secretory) D8Ø.2
  - IgG D8Ø.3
  - IgM D8Ø.4
- immuno — *see* Immunodeficiency
- immunoglobulin, selective
  - A (IgA) D8Ø.2
  - G (IgG) (subclasses) D8Ø.3
  - M (IgM) D8Ø.4

Deficiency, deficient — *continued*
- inositol (B complex) E53.8
- intrinsic
  - factor (congenital) D51.Ø
  - sphincter N36.42
    - with urethral hypermobility N36.43
- iodine E61.8
  - congenital syndrome — *see* Syndrome, iodine-deficiency, congenital
- iron E61.1
  - anemia D5Ø.9
- kalium E87.6
- kappa-light chain D8Ø.8
- labile factor (congenital) (hereditary) D68.2
  - acquired D68.4
- lacrimal fluid (acquired) — *see also* Syndrome, dry eye
  - congenital Q1Ø.6
- lactase
  - congenital E73.Ø
  - secondary E73.1
- Laki-Lorand factor D68.2
- lecithin cholesterol acyltransferase E78.6
- lipocaic K86.89
- lipoprotein (familial) (high density) E78.6
- liver phosphorylase E74.Ø9
- lysosomal alpha-1, 4 glucosidase E74.Ø2
- magnesium E61.2
- major histocompatibility complex
  - class I D81.6
  - class II D81.7
- manganese E61.3
- menadione (vitamin K) E56.1
  - newborn P53
- mental (familial) (hereditary) — *see* Disability, intellectual
- methylenetetrahydrofolate reductase (MTHFR) E72.12
- mevalonate kinase MØ4.1
- mineralocorticoid E27.49
  - with glucocorticoid E27.49
- mineral NEC E61.8
- molybdenum (nutritional) E61.5
- moral F6Ø.2
- multiple nutrient elements E61.7
- multiple sulfatase (MSD) E75.26
- muscle
  - carnitine (palmityltransferase) E71.314
  - phosphofructokinase E74.Ø9
- myoadenylate deaminase E79.2
- myocardial — *see* Insufficiency, myocardial
- myophosphorylase E74.Ø4
- NADH diaphorase or reductase (congenital) D74.Ø
- NADH-methemoglobin reductase (congenital) D74.Ø
- natrium E87.1
- niacin (amide) (-tryptophan) E52
- nicotinamide E52
- nicotinic acid E52
- number of teeth — *see* Anodontia
- nutrient element E61.9
  - multiple E61.7
  - specified NEC E61.8
- nutrition, nutritional E63.9
  - sequelae — *see* Sequelae, nutritional deficiency
  - specified NEC E63.8
- of interleukin 1 receptor antagonist [DIRA] MØ4.8
- ornithine transcarbamylase E72.4
- ovarian E28.39
- oxygen — *see* Anoxia
- pantothenic acid E53.8
- parathyroid (gland) E2Ø.9
- perineum (female) N81.89
- phenylalanine hydroxylase E7Ø.1
- phosphoenolpyruvate carboxykinase E74.4
- phosphofructokinase E74.19
- phosphomannomutuse E74.818
- phosphomannose isomerase E74.818
- phosphomannosyl mutase E74.818
- phosphorylase kinase, liver E74.Ø9
- pituitary hormone (isolated) E23.Ø
- plasma thromboplastin
  - antecedent (PTA) D68.1
  - component (PTC) D67
- plasminogen (type 1) (type 2) E88.Ø2
- platelet NEC D69.1
  - constitutional D68.Ø
- polyglandular E31.8
  - autoimmune E31.Ø
- potassium (K) E87.6
- prepuce N47.3

Deformity — *continued*
- limb — *continued*
  - foot — *continued*
    - drop M21.37- ☑
    - flat — *see* Deformity, limb, flat foot
    - specified NEC M21.6X- ☑
  - forearm M21.93- ☑
  - hand M21.94- ☑
  - lower leg M21.96- ☑
  - specified type NEC M21.8Ø
    - forearm M21.83- ☑
    - lower leg M21.86- ☑
    - thigh M21.85- ☑
    - upper arm M21.82- ☑
  - thigh M21.95- ☑
  - unequal length M21.7Ø
    - short site is
      - femur M21.75- ☑
      - fibula M21.76- ☑
      - humerus M21.72- ☑
      - radius M21.73- ☑
      - tibia M21.76- ☑
      - ulna M21.73- ☑
  - upper arm M21.92- ☑
  - valgus — *see* Deformity, valgus
  - varus — *see* Deformity, varus
  - wrist drop M21.33- ☑
- lip (acquired) NEC K13.Ø
  - congenital Q38.Ø
- liver (congenital) Q44.7
  - acquired K76.89
- lumbosacral (congenital) (joint) (region) Q76.49
  - acquired — *see* subcategory M43.8 ☑
  - kyphosis — *see* Kyphosis, congenital
  - lordosis — *see* Lordosis, congenital
- lung (congenital) Q33.9
  - acquired J98.4
- lymphatic system, congenital Q89.9
- Madelung's (radius) Q74.Ø
- mandible (acquired) (congenital) M26.9
- maxilla (acquired) (congenital) M26.9
- meninges or membrane (congenital) QØ7.9
  - cerebral QØ4.8
    - acquired G96.198
  - spinal cord (congenital) G96.198
    - acquired G96.198
- metacarpus (acquired) — *see* Deformity, limb, forearm
  - congenital Q74.Ø
- metatarsus (acquired) — *see* Deformity, foot
  - congenital Q66.9- ☑
- middle ear (congenital) Q16.4
  - ossicles Q16.3
- mitral (leaflets) (valve) IØ5.8
  - parachute Q23.2
  - stenosis, congenital Q23.2
- mouth (acquired) K13.79
  - congenital Q38.6
- multiple, congenital NEC Q89.7
- muscle (acquired) M62.89
  - congenital Q79.9
    - sternocleidomastoid Q68.Ø
- musculoskeletal system (acquired) M95.9
  - congenital Q79.9
  - specified NEC M95.8
- nail (acquired) L6Ø.8
  - congenital Q84.6
- nasal — *see* Deformity, nose
- neck (acquired) M95.3
  - congenital Q18.9
    - sternocleidomastoid Q68.Ø
- nervous system (congenital) QØ7.9
- nipple (congenital) Q83.9
  - acquired N64.89
- nose (acquired) (cartilage) M95.Ø
  - bone (turbinate) M95.Ø
  - congenital Q3Ø.9
    - bent or squashed Q67.4
  - saddle M95.Ø
    - syphilitic A5Ø.57
  - septum (acquired) J34.2
    - congenital Q3Ø.8
  - sinus (wall) (congenital) Q3Ø.8
    - acquired M95.Ø
  - syphilitic (congenital) A5Ø.57
    - late A52.73
- ocular muscle (congenital) Q1Ø.3
  - acquired — *see* Strabismus, mechanical
- opticociliary vessels (congenital) Q13.2

Deformity — *continued*
- orbit (eye) (acquired) HØ5.3Ø
  - atrophy — *see* Atrophy, orbit
  - congenital Q1Ø.7
  - due to
    - bone disease NEC HØ5.32- ☑
    - trauma or surgery HØ5.33- ☑
  - enlargement — *see* Enlargement, orbit
  - exostosis — *see* Exostosis, orbit
- organ of Corti (congenital) Q16.5
- ovary (congenital) Q5Ø.39
  - acquired N83.8
- oviduct, acquired N83.8
- palate (congenital) Q38.5
  - acquired M27.8
  - cleft (congenital) — *see* Cleft, palate
- pancreas (congenital) Q45.3
  - acquired K86.89
- parathyroid (gland) Q89.2
- parotid (gland) (congenital) Q38.4
  - acquired K11.8
- patella (acquired) — *see* Disorder, patella, specified NEC
- pelvis, pelvic (acquired) (bony) M95.5
  - with disproportion (fetopelvic) O33.Ø
    - causing obstructed labor O65.Ø
  - congenital Q74.2
  - rachitic sequelae (late effect) E64.3
- penis (glans) (congenital) Q55.69
  - acquired N48.89
- pericardium (congenital) Q24.8
  - acquired — *see* Pericarditis
- pharynx (congenital) Q38.8
  - acquired J39.2
- pinna, acquired — *see also* Disorder, pinna, deformity
  - congenital Q17.9
- pituitary (congenital) Q89.2
- posture — *see* Dorsopathy, deforming
- prepuce (congenital) Q55.69
  - acquired N47.8
- prostate (congenital) Q55.4
  - acquired N42.89
- pupil (congenital) Q13.2
  - acquired — *see* Abnormality, pupillary
- pylorus (congenital) Q4Ø.3
  - acquired K31.89
- rachitic (acquired), old or healed E64.3
- radius (acquired) — *see also* Deformity, limb, forearm
  - congenital Q68.8
- rectum (congenital) Q43.9
  - acquired K62.89
- reduction (extremity) (limb), congenital — *see also* condition and site Q73.8
  - brain QØ4.3
  - lower — *see* Defect, reduction, lower limb
  - upper — *see* Defect, reduction, upper limb
- renal — *see* Deformity, kidney
- respiratory system (congenital) Q34.9
- rib (acquired) M95.4
  - congenital Q76.6
    - cervical Q76.5
- rotation (joint) (acquired) — *see* Deformity, limb, specified site NEC
  - congenital Q74.9
  - hip — *see* Deformity, limb, specified type NEC, thigh
    - congenital Q65.89
- sacroiliac joint (congenital) — *see* subcategory Q74.2
  - acquired — *see* subcategory M43.8 ☑
- sacrum (acquired) — *see* subcategory M43.8 ☑
- saddle
  - back — *see* Lordosis
  - nose M95.Ø
    - syphilitic A5Ø.57
- salivary gland or duct (congenital) Q38.4
  - acquired K11.8
- scapula (acquired) M95.8
  - congenital Q68.8
- scrotum (congenital) — *see also* Malformation, testis and scrotum
  - acquired N5Ø.89
- seminal vesicles (congenital) Q55.4
  - acquired N5Ø.89
- septum, nasal (acquired) J34.2
- shoulder (joint) (acquired) — *see* Deformity, limb, upper arm
  - congenital Q74.Ø
  - contraction — *see* Contraction, joint, shoulder
- sigmoid (flexure) (congenital) Q43.9

Deformity — *continued*
- sigmoid — *continued*
  - acquired K63.89
- skin (congenital) Q82.9
- skull (acquired) M95.2
  - congenital Q75.8
    - with
      - anencephaly QØØ.Ø
      - encephalocele — *see* Encephalocele
      - hydrocephalus QØ3.9
        - with spina bifida — *see* Spina bifida, by site, with hydrocephalus
      - microcephaly QØ2
- soft parts, organs or tissues (of pelvis)
  - in pregnancy or childbirth NEC O34.8- ☑
    - causing obstructed labor O65.5
- spermatic cord (congenital) Q55.4
  - acquired N5Ø.89
    - torsion — *see* Torsion, spermatic cord
- spinal — *see* Dorsopathy, deforming
  - column (acquired) — *see* Dorsopathy, deforming
  - congenital Q67.5
  - cord (congenital) QØ6.9
    - acquired G95.89
  - nerve root (congenital) QØ7.9
- spine (acquired) — *see also* Dorsopathy, deforming
  - congenital Q67.5
  - rachitic E64.3
  - specified NEC — *see* Dorsopathy, deforming, specified NEC
- spleen
  - acquired D73.89
  - congenital Q89.Ø9
- Sprengel's (congenital) Q74.Ø
- sternocleidomastoid (muscle), congenital Q68.Ø
- sternum (acquired) M95.4
  - congenital NEC Q76.7
- stomach (congenital) Q4Ø.3
  - acquired K31.89
- submandibular gland (congenital) Q38.4
- submaxillary gland (congenital) Q38.4
  - acquired K11.8
- talipes — *see* Talipes
- testis (congenital) — *see also* Malformation, testis and scrotum
  - acquired N44.8
    - torsion — *see* Torsion, testis
- thigh (acquired) — *see also* Deformity, limb, thigh
  - congenital NEC Q68.8
- thorax (acquired) (wall) M95.4
  - congenital Q67.8
  - sequelae of rickets E64.3
- thumb (acquired) — *see also* Deformity, finger
  - congenital NEC Q68.1
- thymus (tissue) (congenital) Q89.2
- thyroid (gland) (congenital) Q89.2
  - cartilage Q31.8
    - acquired J38.7
- tibia (acquired) — *see also* Deformity, limb, specified type NEC, lower leg
  - congenital NEC Q68.8
  - saber (syphilitic) A5Ø.56
- toe (acquired) M2Ø.6- ☑
  - congenital Q66.9- ☑
  - hallux rigidus M2Ø.2- ☑
  - hallux valgus M2Ø.1- ☑
  - hallux varus M2Ø.3- ☑
  - hammer toe M2Ø.4- ☑
  - specified NEC M2Ø.5X- ☑
- tongue (congenital) Q38.3
  - acquired K14.8
- tooth, teeth KØØ.2
- trachea (rings) (congenital) Q32.1
  - acquired J39.8
- transverse aortic arch (congenital) Q25.49
- tricuspid (leaflets) (valve) IØ7.8
  - atresia or stenosis Q22.4
  - Ebstein's Q22.5
- trunk (acquired) M95.8
  - congenital Q89.9
- ulna (acquired) — *see also* Deformity, limb, forearm
  - congenital NEC Q68.8
- urachus, congenital Q64.4
- ureter (opening) (congenital) Q62.8
  - acquired N28.89
- urethra (congenital) Q64.79
  - acquired N36.8
- urinary tract (congenital) Q64.9

Delivery — *continued*
complicated — *continued*
by — *continued*
placenta, placental — *continued*
previa — *continued*
marginal — *continued*
with hemorrhage O44.3- ☑
partial O44.2- ☑
with hemorrhage O44.3- ☑
retained (with hemorrhage) O72.Ø
without hemorrhage O73.Ø
separation (premature) O45.9- ☑
specified NEC O45.8X- ☑
vicious insertion O44.1- ☑
precipitate labor O62.3
premature rupture, membranes — *see also* Pregnancy, complicated by, premature rupture of membranes O42.9Ø
prolapse
arm or hand O32.2 ☑
cord (umbilical) O69.Ø ☑
foot or leg O32.8 ☑
uterus O34.52- ☑
prolonged labor O63.9
first stage O63.Ø
second stage O63.1
protozoal disease (maternal) O98.62
respiratory disease NEC O99.52
retained membranes or portions of placenta O72.2
without hemorrhage O73.1
retarded birth O63.9
retention of secundines (with hemorrhage) O72.Ø
without hemorrhage O73.Ø
partial O72.2
without hemorrhage O73.1
rupture
bladder (urinary) O71.5
cervix O71.3
pelvic organ NEC O71.5
urethra O71.5
uterus (during or after labor) O71.1
before labor O71.Ø- ☑
separation, pubic bone (symphysis pubis) O71.6
shock O75.1
shoulder presentation O64.4 ☑
skin disorder NEC O99.72
spasm, cervix O62.4
stenosis or stricture, cervix O65.5
streptococcus group B (GBS) carrier state O99.824
subluxation of symphysis (pubis) O26.72
syphilis (maternal) O98.12
tear — *see* Delivery, complicated by, laceration
tetanic uterus O62.4
trauma (obstetrical) — *see also* Delivery, complicated, by, damage to O71.9
non-obstetric O9A.22 (*following* O99)
periurethral O71.82
specified NEC O71.89
tuberculosis (maternal) O98.Ø2
tumor, pelvic organs or tissues NEC O65.5
umbilical cord around neck
with compression O69.1 ☑
without compression O69.81 ☑
uterine inertia O62.2
during latent phase of labor O62.Ø
primary O62.Ø
secondary O62.1
vasa previa O69.4 ☑
velamentous insertion of cord O43.12- ☑
specified complication NEC O75.89
delayed NOS O63.9
following rupture of membranes
artificial O75.5
second twin, triplet, etc. O63.2
forceps, low following failed vacuum extraction O66.5
missed (at or near term) O36.4 ☑
normal O8Ø
obstructed — *see* Delivery, complicated by, obstructed labor
precipitate O62.3
preterm — *see also* Pregnancy, complicated by, preterm labor O6Ø.1Ø ☑
spontaneous O8Ø
term pregnancy NOS O8Ø
uncomplicated O8Ø
vaginal, following previous cesarean delivery O34.219
classical (vertical) scar O34.212

Delivery — *continued*
vaginal, following previous cesarean delivery — *continued*
low transverse scar O34.211
mid-transverse T incision O34.218
scar
defect (isthmocele) O34.22
specified type NEC O34.218
Delusions (paranoid) — *see* Disorder, delusional
Dementia (degenerative (primary)) (old age) (persisting) FØ3.9Ø
with
aggressive behavior FØ3.91
behavioral disturbance FØ3.91
combative behavior FØ3.91
Lewy bodies G31.83 *[FØ2.8Ø]*
with behavioral disturbance G31.83 *[FØ2.81]*
Parkinsonism G31.83 *[FØ2.8Ø]*
with behavioral disturbance G31.83 *[FØ2.81]*
Parkinson's disease G2Ø *[FØ2.8Ø]*
with behavioral disturbance G2Ø *[FØ2.81]*
violent behavior FØ3.91
alcoholic F1Ø.97
with dependence F1Ø.27
Alzheimer's type — *see* Disease, Alzheimer's
arteriosclerotic — *see* Dementia, vascular
atypical, Alzheimer's type — *see* Disease, Alzheimer's, specified NEC
congenital — *see* Disability, intellectual
frontal (lobe) G31.Ø9 *[FØ2.8Ø]*
with behavioral disturbance G31.Ø9 *[FØ2.81]*
frontotemporal G31.Ø9 *[FØ2.8Ø]*
with behavioral disturbance G31.Ø9 *[FØ2.81]*
specified NEC G31.Ø9 *[FØ2.8Ø]*
with behavioral disturbance G31.Ø9 *[FØ2.81]*
in (due to)
alcohol F1Ø.97
with dependence F1Ø.27
Alzheimer's disease — *see* Disease, Alzheimer's
arteriosclerotic brain disease — *see* Dementia, vascular
cerebral lipidoses E75.- ☑ *[FØ2.8Ø]*
with behavioral disturbance E75.- ☑ *[FØ2.81]*
Creutzfeldt-Jakob disease — *see also* Creutzfeldt-Jakob disease or syndrome (with dementia) A81.ØØ
epilepsy G4Ø.- ☑ *[FØ2.8Ø]*
with behavioral disturbance G4Ø.- ☑ *[FØ2.81]*
hepatolenticular degeneration E83.Ø1 *[FØ2.8Ø]*
with behavioral disturbance E83.Ø1 *[FØ2.81]*
human immunodeficiency virus (HIV) disease B2Ø *[FØ2.8Ø]*
with behavioral disturbance B2Ø *[FØ2.81]*
Huntington's disease or chorea G1Ø *[FØ2.8Ø]*
with behavioral disturbance G1Ø *[FØ2.81]*
hypercalcemia E83.52 *[FØ2.8Ø]*
with behavioral disturbance E83.52 *[FØ2.81]*
hypothyroidism, acquired EØ3.9 *[FØ2.8Ø]*
with behavioral disturbance EØ3.9 *[FØ2.81]*
due to iodine deficiency EØ1.8 *[FØ2.8Ø]*
with behavioral disturbance EØ1.8 *[FØ2.81]*
inhalants F18.97
with dependence F18.27
multiple
etiologies FØ3 ☑
sclerosis G35 *[FØ2.8Ø]*
with behavioral disturbance G35 *[FØ2.81]*
neurosyphilis A52.17 *[FØ2.8Ø]*
with behavioral disturbance A52.17 *[FØ2.81]*
juvenile A5Ø.49 *[FØ2.8Ø]*
with behavioral disturbance A5Ø.49 *[FØ2.81]*
niacin deficiency E52 *[FØ2.8Ø]*
with behavioral disturbance E52 *[FØ2.81]*
paralysis agitans G2Ø *[FØ2.8Ø]*
with behavioral disturbance G2Ø *[FØ2.81]*
Parkinson's disease G2Ø *[FØ2.8Ø]*
pellagra E52 *[FØ2.8Ø]*
with behavioral disturbance E52 *[FØ2.81]*
Pick's G31.Ø1 *[FØ2.8Ø]*
with behavioral disturbance G31.Ø1 *[FØ2.81]*
polyarteritis nodosa M3Ø.Ø *[FØ2.8Ø]*
with behavioral disturbance M3Ø.Ø *[FØ2.81]*
psychoactive drug F19.97
with dependence F19.27
inhalants F18.97
with dependence F18.27
sedatives, hypnotics or anxiolytics F13.97

Dementia — *continued*
in — *continued*
psychoactive drug — *continued*
sedatives, hypnotics or anxiolytics — *continued*
with dependence F13.27
sedatives, hypnotics or anxiolytics F13.97
with dependence F13.27
systemic lupus erythematosus M32.- ☑ *[FØ2.8Ø]*
with behavioral disturbance M32.- ☑ *[FØ2.81]*
trypanosomiasis
African B56.9 *[FØ2.8Ø]*
with behavioral disturbance B56.9 *[FØ2.81]*
unknown etiology FØ3 ☑
vitamin B12 deficiency E53.8 *[FØ2.8Ø]*
with behavioral disturbance E53.8 *[FØ2.81]*
volatile solvents F18.97
with dependence F18.27
with behavioral disturbance G31.83 *[FØ2.81]*
infantile, infantilis F84.3
Lewy body G31.83 *[FØ2.8Ø]*
with behavioral disturbance G31.83 *[FØ2.81]*
multi-infarct — *see* Dementia, vascular
paralytica, paralytic (syphilitic) A52.17 *[FØ2.8Ø]*
with behavioral disturbance A52.17 *[FØ2.81]*
juvenilis A5Ø.45
paretic A52.17
praecox — *see* Schizophrenia
presenile FØ3 ☑
Alzheimer's type — *see* Disease, Alzheimer's, early onset
primary degenerative FØ3 ☑
progressive, syphilitic A52.17
senile FØ3 ☑
with acute confusional state FØ5
Alzheimer's type — *see* Disease, Alzheimer's, late onset
depressed or paranoid type FØ3 ☑
vascular (acute onset) (mixed) (multi-infarct) (subcortical) FØ1.5Ø
with behavioral disturbance FØ1.51
Demineralization, bone — *see* Osteoporosis
Demodex folliculorum (infestation) B88.Ø
Demophobia F4Ø.248
Demoralization R45.3
Demyelination, demyelinization
central nervous system G37.9
specified NEC G37.8
corpus callosum (central) G37.1
disseminated, acute G36.9
specified NEC G36.8
global G35
in optic neuritis G36.Ø
Dengue (classical) (fever) A9Ø
hemorrhagic A91
sandfly A93.1
Dennie-Marfan syphilitic syndrome A5Ø.45
Dens evaginatus, in dente or invaginatus KØØ.2
Dense breasts R92.2
Density
increased, bone (disseminated) (generalized) (spotted) — *see* Disorder, bone, density and structure, specified type NEC
lung (nodular) J98.4
Dental — *see also* condition
examination ZØ1.2Ø
with abnormal findings ZØ1.21
restoration
aesthetically inadequate or displeasing KØ8.56
defective KØ8.5Ø
specified NEC KØ8.59
failure of marginal integrity KØ8.51
failure of periodontal anatomical integrity KØ8.54
Dentia praecox KØØ.6
Denticles (pulp) KØ4.2
Dentigerous cyst KØ9.Ø
Dentin
irregular (in pulp) KØ4.3
opalescent KØØ.5
secondary (in pulp) KØ4.3
sensitive KØ3.89
Dentinogenesis imperfecta KØØ.5
Dentinoma — *see* Cyst, calcifying odontogenic
Dentition (syndrome) KØØ.7
delayed KØØ.6
difficult KØØ.7
precocious KØØ.6

- **Dentition** — *continued*
  - premature K00.6
  - retarded K00.6
- **Dependence** (on) (syndrome) F19.20
  - with remission F19.21
  - alcohol (ethyl) (methyl) (without remission) F10.20
    - with
      - amnestic disorder, persisting F10.26
      - anxiety disorder F10.280
      - dementia, persisting F10.27
      - intoxication F10.229
        - with delirium F10.221
        - uncomplicated F10.220
      - mood disorder F10.24
      - psychotic disorder F10.259
        - with
          - delusions F10.250
          - hallucinations F10.251
      - remission F10.21
      - sexual dysfunction F10.281
      - sleep disorder F10.282
      - specified disorder NEC F10.288
      - withdrawal F10.239
        - with
          - delirium F10.231
          - perceptual disturbance F10.232
        - uncomplicated F10.230
    - counseling and surveillance Z71.41
  - amobarbital — *see* Dependence, drug, sedative
  - amphetamine(s) (type) — *see* Dependence, drug, stimulant NEC
  - amytal (sodium) — *see* Dependence, drug, sedative
  - analgesic NEC F55.8
  - anesthetic (agent) (gas) (general) (local) NEC — *see* Dependence, drug, psychoactive NEC
  - anxiolytic NEC — *see* Dependence, drug, sedative
  - barbital(s) — *see* Dependence, drug, sedative
  - barbiturate(s) (compounds) (drugs classifiable to T42) — *see* Dependence, drug, sedative
  - benzedrine — *see* Dependence, drug, stimulant NEC
  - bhang — *see* Dependence, drug, cannabis
  - bromide(s) NEC — *see* Dependence, drug, sedative
  - caffeine — *see* Dependence, drug, stimulant NEC
  - cannabis (sativa) (indica) (resin) (derivatives) (type) — *see* Dependence, drug, cannabis
  - chloral (betaine) (hydrate) — *see* Dependence, drug, sedative
  - chlordiazepoxide — *see* Dependence, drug, sedative
  - coca (leaf) (derivatives) — *see* Dependence, drug, cocaine
  - cocaine — *see* Dependence, drug, cocaine
  - codeine — *see* Dependence, drug, opioid
  - combinations of drugs F19.20
  - dagga — *see* Dependence, drug, cannabis
  - demerol — *see* Dependence, drug, opioid
  - dexamphetamine — *see* Dependence, drug, stimulant NEC
  - dexedrine — *see* Dependence, drug, stimulant NEC
  - dextromethorphan — *see* Dependence, drug, opioid
  - dextromoramide — *see* Dependence, drug, opioid
  - dextro-nor-pseudo-ephedrine — *see* Dependence, drug, stimulant NEC
  - dextrorphan — *see* Dependence, drug, opioid
  - diazepam — *see* Dependence, drug, sedative
  - dilaudid — *see* Dependence, drug, opioid
  - D-lysergic acid diethylamide — *see* Dependence, drug, hallucinogen
  - drug NEC F19.20
    - with sleep disorder F19.282
    - cannabis F12.20
      - with
        - anxiety disorder F12.280
        - intoxication F12.229
          - with
            - delirium F12.221
            - perceptual disturbance F12.222
          - uncomplicated F12.220
        - other specified disorder F12.288
        - psychosis F12.259
          - delusions F12.250
          - hallucinations F12.251
        - unspecified disorder F12.29
        - withdrawal F12.23
      - in remission F12.21
    - cocaine F14.20
      - with
        - anxiety disorder F14.280
        - intoxication F14.229

- **Dependence** — *continued*
  - drug — *continued*
    - cocaine — *continued*
      - with — *continued*
        - intoxication — *continued*
          - with
            - delirium F14.221
            - perceptual disturbance F14.222
          - uncomplicated F14.220
        - mood disorder F14.24
        - other specified disorder F14.288
        - psychosis F14.259
          - delusions F14.250
          - hallucinations F14.251
        - sexual dysfunction F14.281
        - sleep disorder F14.282
        - unspecified disorder F14.29
        - withdrawal F14.23
      - in remission F14.21
      - withdrawal symptoms in newborn P96.1
    - counseling and surveillance Z71.51
    - hallucinogen F16.20
      - with
        - anxiety disorder F16.280
        - flashbacks F16.283
        - intoxication F16.229
          - with delirium F16.221
          - uncomplicated F16.220
        - mood disorder F16.24
        - other specified disorder F16.288
        - perception disorder, persisting F16.283
        - psychosis F16.259
          - delusions F16.250
          - hallucinations F16.251
        - unspecified disorder F16.29
      - in remission F16.21
    - in remission F19.21
    - inhalant F18.20
      - with
        - anxiety disorder F18.280
        - dementia, persisting F18.27
        - intoxication F18.229
          - with delirium F18.221
          - uncomplicated F18.220
        - mood disorder F18.24
        - other specified disorder F18.288
        - psychosis F18.259
          - delusions F18.250
          - hallucinations F18.251
        - unspecified disorder F18.29
      - in remission F18.21
    - nicotine F17.200
      - with disorder F17.209
        - in remission F17.201
        - specified disorder NEC F17.208
        - withdrawal F17.203
      - chewing tobacco F17.220
        - with disorder F17.229
          - in remission F17.221
          - specified disorder NEC F17.228
          - withdrawal F17.223
      - cigarettes F17.210
        - with disorder F17.219
          - in remission F17.211
          - specified disorder NEC F17.218
          - withdrawal F17.213
      - specified product NEC F17.290
        - with disorder F17.299
          - remission F17.291
          - specified disorder NEC F17.298
          - withdrawal F17.293
    - opioid F11.20
      - with
        - intoxication F11.229
          - with
            - delirium F11.221
            - perceptual disturbance F11.222
          - uncomplicated F11.220
        - mood disorder F11.24
        - other specified disorder F11.288
        - psychosis F11.259
          - delusions F11.250
          - hallucinations F11.251
        - sexual dysfunction F11.281
        - sleep disorder F11.282
        - unspecified disorder F11.29
        - withdrawal F11.23
      - in remission F11.21
    - psychoactive NEC F19.20

- **Dependence** — *continued*
  - drug — *continued*
    - psychoactive — *continued*
      - with
        - amnestic disorder F19.26
        - anxiety disorder F19.280
        - dementia F19.27
        - intoxication F19.229
          - with
            - delirium F19.221
            - perceptual disturbance F19.222
          - uncomplicated F19.220
        - mood disorder F19.24
        - other specified disorder F19.288
        - psychosis F19.259
          - delusions F19.250
          - hallucinations F19.251
        - sexual dysfunction F19.281
        - sleep disorder F19.282
        - unspecified disorder F19.29
        - withdrawal F19.239
          - with
            - delirium F19.231
            - perceptual disturbance F19.232
          - uncomplicated F19.230
    - sedative, hypnotic or anxiolytic F13.20
      - with
        - amnestic disorder F13.26
        - anxiety disorder F13.280
        - dementia, persisting F13.27
        - intoxication F13.229
          - with delirium F13.221
          - uncomplicated F13.220
        - mood disorder F13.24
        - other specified disorder F13.288
        - psychosis F13.259
          - delusions F13.250
          - hallucinations F13.251
        - sexual dysfunction F13.281
        - sleep disorder F13.282
        - unspecified disorder F13.29
        - withdrawal F13.239
          - with
            - delirium F13.231
            - perceptual disturbance F13.232
          - uncomplicated F13.230
      - in remission F13.21
    - stimulant NEC F15.20
      - with
        - anxiety disorder F15.280
        - intoxication F15.229
          - with
            - delirium F15.221
            - perceptual disturbance F15.222
          - uncomplicated F15.220
        - mood disorder F15.24
        - other specified disorder F15.288
        - psychosis F15.259
          - delusions F15.250
          - hallucinations F15.251
        - sexual dysfunction F15.281
        - sleep disorder F15.282
        - unspecified disorder F15.29
        - withdrawal F15.23
      - in remission F15.21
  - ethyl
    - alcohol (without remission) F10.20
      - with remission F10.21
    - bromide — *see* Dependence, drug, sedative
    - carbamate F19.20
    - chloride F19.20
    - morphine — *see* Dependence, drug, opioid
  - ganja — *see* Dependence, drug, cannabis
  - glue (airplane) (sniffing) — *see* Dependence, drug, inhalant
  - glutethimide — *see* Dependence, drug, sedative
  - hallucinogenics — *see* Dependence, drug, hallucinogen
  - hashish — *see* Dependence, drug, cannabis
  - hemp — *see* Dependence, drug, cannabis
  - heroin (salt) (any) — *see* Dependence, drug, opioid
  - hypnotic NEC — *see* Dependence, drug, sedative
  - Indian hemp — *see* Dependence, drug, cannabis
  - inhalants — *see* Dependence, drug, inhalant
  - khat — *see* Dependence, drug, stimulant NEC
  - laudanum — *see* Dependence, drug, opioid
  - LSD (-25) (derivatives) — *see* Dependence, drug, hallucinogen
  - luminal — *see* Dependence, drug, sedative

Dermatitis — *continued*
- due to — *continued*
  - varicose veins — *see* Varix, leg, with, inflammation
  - X-rays L58.9
    - acute L58.Ø
    - chronic L58.1
- dyshydrotic L3Ø.1
- dysmenorrheica N94.6
- escharotica — *see* Burn
- exfoliative, exfoliativa (generalized) L26
  - neonatorum LØØ
- eyelid — *see also* Dermatosis, eyelid
  - allergic HØ1.119
    - left HØ1.116
      - lower HØ1.115
      - upper HØ1.114
    - right HØ1.113
      - lower HØ1.112
      - upper HØ1.111
  - contact — *see* Dermatitis, eyelid, allergic
  - due to
    - Demodex species B88.Ø
    - herpes (zoster) BØ2.39
      - simplex BØØ.59
  - eczematous HØ1.139
    - left HØ1.136
      - lower HØ1.135
      - upper HØ1.134
    - right HØ1.133
      - lower HØ1.132
      - upper HØ1.131
- facta, factitia, factitial L98.1
  - psychogenic F54
- flexural NEC L2Ø.82
- friction L3Ø.4
- fungus B36.9
  - specified type NEC B36.8
- gangrenosa, gangrenous infantum LØ8.Ø
- harvest mite B88.Ø
- heat L59.Ø
- herpesviral, vesicular (ear) (lip) BØØ.1
- herpetiformis (bullous) (erythematous) (pustular) (vesicular) L13.Ø
  - juvenile L12.2
  - senile L12.Ø
- hiemalis L3Ø.8
- hypostatic, hypostatica — *see* Varix, leg, with, inflammation
- infectious eczematoid L3Ø.3
- infective L3Ø.3
- irritant — *see* Dermatitis, contact, irritant
- Jacquet's (diaper dermatitis) L22
- Leptus B88.Ø
- lichenified NEC L28.Ø
- medicamentosa (generalized) (internal use) — *see* Dermatitis, due to drugs
- mite B88.Ø
- multiformis L13.Ø
  - juvenile L12.2
- napkin L22
- neurotica L13.Ø
- nummular L3Ø.Ø
- papillaris capillitii L73.Ø
- pellagrous E52
- perioral L71.Ø
- photocontact L56.2
- polymorpha dolorosa L13.Ø
- pruriginosa L13.Ø
- pruritic NEC L3Ø.8
- psychogenic F54
- purulent LØ8.Ø
- pustular
  - contagious BØ8.Ø2
  - subcorneal L13.1
- pyococcal LØ8.Ø
- pyogenica LØ8.Ø
- repens L4Ø.2
- Ritter's (exfoliativa) LØØ
- Schamberg's L81.7
- schistosome B65.3
- seasonal bullous L3Ø.8
- seborrheic L21.9
  - infantile L21.1
  - specified NEC L21.8
- sensitization NOS L23.9
- septic LØ8.Ø
- solare L57.8
- specified NEC L3Ø.8

Dermatitis — *continued*
- stasis I87.2
  - with
    - varicose ulcer — *see* Varix, leg, with ulcer, with inflammation
    - varicose veins — *see* Varix, leg, with, inflammation
  - due to postthrombotic syndrome — *see* Syndrome, postthrombotic
- suppurative LØ8.Ø
- traumatic NEC L3Ø.4
- trophoneurotica L13.Ø
- ultraviolet (sun) (chronic exposure) L57.8
  - acute L56.8
- varicose — *see* Varix, leg, with, inflammation
- vegetans L1Ø.1
- verrucosa B43.Ø
- vesicular, herpesviral BØØ.1

Dermatoarthritis, lipoid E78.81

Dermatochalasis, eyelid HØ2.839
- left HØ2.836
  - lower HØ2.835
  - upper HØ2.834
- right HØ2.833
  - lower HØ2.832
  - upper HØ2.831

Dermatofibroma (lenticulare) — *see* Neoplasm, skin, benign
- protuberans — *see* Neoplasm, skin, uncertain behavior

Dermatofibrosarcoma (pigmented) (protuberans) — *see* Neoplasm, skin, malignant

Dermatographia L5Ø.3

Dermatolysis (exfoliativa) (congenital) Q82.8
- acquired L57.4
- eyelids — *see* Blepharochalasis
- palpebrarum — *see* Blepharochalasis
- senile L57.4

Dermatomegaly NEC Q82.8

Dermatomucosomyositis M33.1Ø
- with
  - myopathy M33.12
  - respiratory involvement M33.11
  - specified organ involvement NEC M33.19

Dermatomycosis B36.9
- furfuracea B36.Ø
- specified type NEC B36.8

Dermatomyositis (acute) (chronic) — *see also* Dermatopolymyositis
- adult — *see also* Dermatomyositis, specified NEC M33.1Ø
- in (due to) neoplastic disease — *see also* Neoplasm D49.9 *[M36.Ø]*
- juvenile M33.ØØ
  - with
    - myopathy M33.Ø2
    - respiratory involvement M33.Ø1
    - specified organ involvement NEC M33.Ø9
  - without myopathy M33.Ø3
- specified NEC M33.1Ø
  - with
    - myopathy M33.12
    - respiratory involvement M33.11
    - specified organ involvement NEC M33.19
  - without myopathy M33.13

Dermatoneuritis of children — *see* Poisoning, mercury

Dermatophilosis A48.8

Dermatophytid L3Ø.2

Dermatophytide — *see* Dermatophytosis

Dermatophytosis (epidermophyton) (infection) (Microsporum) (tinea) (Trichophyton) B35.9
- beard B35.Ø
- body B35.4
- capitis B35.Ø
- corporis B35.4
- deep-seated B35.8
- disseminated B35.8
- foot B35.3
- granulomatous B35.8
- groin B35.6
- hand B35.2
- nail B35.1
- perianal (area) B35.6
- scalp B35.Ø
- specified NEC B35.8

Dermatopolymyositis M33.9Ø
- with
  - myopathy M33.92
  - respiratory involvement M33.91

Dermatopolymyositis — *continued*
- with — *continued*
  - specified organ involvement NEC M33.99
- in neoplastic disease — *see also* Neoplasm D49.9 *[M36.Ø]*
- juvenile M33.ØØ
  - with
    - myopathy M33.Ø2
    - respiratory involvement M33.Ø1
    - specified organ involvement NEC M33.Ø9
- specified NEC M33.1Ø
  - myopathy M33.12
  - respiratory involvement M33.11
  - specified organ involvement NEC M33.19
- without myopathy M33.93

Dermatopolyneuritis — *see* Poisoning, mercury

Dermatorrhexis — *see also* Syndrome, Ehlers-Danlos Q79.6Ø
- acquired L57.4

Dermatosclerosis — *see also* Scleroderma
- localized L94.Ø

Dermatosis L98.9
- Andrews' LØ8.89
- Bowen's — *see* Neoplasm, skin, in situ
- bullous L13.9
  - specified NEC L13.8
- exfoliativa L26
- eyelid (noninfectious)
  - dermatitis — *see* Dermatitis, eyelid
  - discoid lupus erythematosus — *see* Lupus, erythematosus, eyelid
  - xeroderma — *see* Xeroderma, acquired, eyelid
- factitial L98.1
- febrile neutrophilic L98.2
- gonococcal A54.89
- herpetiformis L13.Ø
  - juvenile L12.2
- linear IgA L13.8
- menstrual NEC L98.8
- neutrophilic, febrile L98.2
- occupational — *see* Dermatitis, contact
- papulosa nigra L82.1
- pigmentary L81.9
  - progressive L81.7
  - Schamberg's L81.7
- psychogenic F54
- purpuric, pigmented L81.7
- pustular, subcorneal L13.1
- transient acantholytic L11.1

Dermographia, dermographism L5Ø.3

Dermoid (cyst) — *see also* Neoplasm, benign, by site
- with malignant transformation C56- ☑
- due to radiation (nonionizing) L57.8

Dermopathy
- infiltrative with thyrotoxicosis — *see* Thyrotoxicosis
- nephrogenic fibrosing L9Ø.8

Dermophytosis — *see* Dermatophytosis

Descemetocele H18.73- ☑

Descemet's membrane — *see* condition

Descending — *see* condition

Descensus uteri — *see* Prolapse, uterus

Desert
- rheumatism B38.Ø
- sore — *see* Ulcer, skin

Desertion (newborn) — *see* Maltreatment

Desmoid (extra-abdominal) (tumor) — *see* Neoplasm, connective tissue, uncertain behavior
- abdominal D48.1

Despondency F32.9

Desquamation, skin R23.4

Destruction, destructive — *see also* Damage
- articular facet — *see also* Derangement, joint, specified type NEC
  - knee M23.8X- ☑
  - vertebra — *see* Spondylosis
- bone — *see also* Disorder, bone, specified type NEC
  - syphilitic A52.77
- joint — *see also* Derangement, joint, specified type NEC
  - sacroiliac M53.3
- rectal sphincter K62.89
- septum (nasal) J34.89
- tuberculous NEC — *see* Tuberculosis
- tympanum, tympanic membrane (nontraumatic) — *see* Disorder, tympanic membrane, specified NEC
- vertebral disc — *see* Degeneration, intervertebral disc

Destructiveness — *see also* Disorder, conduct

Destructiveness — *continued*
- adjustment reaction — *see* Disorder, adjustment

Desultory labor O62.2

Detachment
- cartilage — *see* Sprain
- cervix, annular N88.8
  - complicating delivery O71.3
- choroid (old) (postinfectional) (simple) (spontaneous) H31.4Ø- ☑
  - hemorrhagic H31.41- ☑
  - serous H31.42- ☑
- ligament — *see* Sprain
- meniscus (knee) — *see also* Derangement, knee, meniscus, specified NEC
  - current injury — *see* Tear, meniscus
  - due to old tear or injury — *see* Derangement, knee, meniscus, due to old tear
- retina (without retinal break) (serous) H33.2- ☑
  - with retinal:
    - break H33.ØØ- ☑
      - giant H33.Ø3- ☑
      - multiple H33.Ø2- ☑
      - single H33.Ø1- ☑
    - dialysis H33.Ø4- ☑
  - pigment epithelium — *see* Degeneration, retina, separation of layers, pigment epithelium detachment
  - rhegmatogenous — *see* Detachment, retina, with retinal, break
  - specified NEC H33.8
  - total H33.Ø5- ☑
  - traction H33.4- ☑
- vitreous (body) H43.81 ☑

Detergent asthma J69.8

Deterioration
- epileptic FØ6.8
- general physical R53.81
- heart, cardiac — *see* Degeneration, myocardial
- mental — *see* Psychosis
- myocardial, myocardium — *see* Degeneration, myocardial
- senile (simple) R54

Deuteranomaly (anomalous trichromat) H53.53

Deuteranopia (complete) (incomplete) H53.53

Development
- abnormal, bone Q79.9
- arrested R62.5Ø
  - bone — *see* Arrest, development or growth, bone
  - child R62.5Ø
  - due to malnutrition E45
- defective, congenital — *see also* Anomaly, by site
  - cauda equina QØ6.3
  - left ventricle Q24.8
    - in hypoplastic left heart syndrome Q23.4
  - valve Q24.8
    - pulmonary Q22.3
- delayed — *see also* Delay, development R62.5Ø
  - arithmetical skills F81.2
  - language (skills) (expressive) F8Ø.1
  - learning skill F81.9
  - mixed skills F88
  - motor coordination F82
  - reading F81.Ø
  - specified learning skill NEC F81.89
  - speech F8Ø.9
  - spelling F81.81
  - written expression F81.81
- imperfect, congenital — *see also* Anomaly, by site
  - heart Q24.9
  - lungs Q33.6
- incomplete
  - bronchial tree Q32.4
  - organ or site not listed — *see* Hypoplasia, by site
  - respiratory system Q34.9
- sexual, precocious NEC E3Ø.1
- tardy, mental — *see also* Disability, intellectual F79

Developmental — *see* condition
- testing, infant or child — *see* Examination, child

Devergie's disease (pityriasis rubra pilaris) L44.Ø

Deviation (in)
- conjugate palsy (eye) (spastic) H51.Ø
- esophagus (acquired) K22.8
- eye, skew H51.8
- midline (jaw) (teeth) (dental arch) M26.29
  - specified site NEC — *see* Malposition
- nasal septum J34.2
  - congenital Q67.4

Deviation — *continued*
- opening and closing of the mandible M26.53
- organ or site, congenital NEC — *see* Malposition, congenital
- septum (nasal) (acquired) J34.2
  - congenital Q67.4
- sexual F65.9
  - bestiality F65.89
  - erotomania F52.8
  - exhibitionism F65.2
  - fetishism, fetishistic F65.Ø
    - transvestism F65.1
  - frotteurism F65.81
  - masochism F65.51
  - multiple F65.89
  - necrophilia F65.89
  - nymphomania F52.8
  - pederosis F65.4
  - pedophilia F65.4
  - sadism, sadomasochism F65.52
  - satyriasis F52.8
  - specified type NEC F65.89
  - transvestism F64.1
  - voyeurism F65.3
- teeth, midline M26.29
- trachea J39.8
- ureter, congenital Q62.61

Device
- cerebral ventricle (communicating) in situ Z98.2
- contraceptive — *see* Contraceptive, device
- drainage, cerebrospinal fluid, in situ Z98.2

Devic's disease G36.Ø

Devil's
- grip B33.Ø
- pinches (purpura simplex) D69.2

Devitalized tooth KØ4.99

Devonshire colic — *see* Poisoning, lead

Dextraposition, aorta Q2Ø.3
- in tetralogy of Fallot Q21.3

Dextrinosis, limit (debrancher enzyme deficiency) E74.Ø3

Dextrocardia (true) Q24.Ø
- with
  - complete transposition of viscera Q89.3
  - situs inversus Q89.3

Dextrotransposition, aorta Q2Ø.3

d-glycericacidemia E72.59

Dhat syndrome F48.8

Dhobi itch B35.6

Di George's syndrome D82.1

Di Guglielmo's disease C94.Ø- ☑

Diabetes, diabetic (mellitus) (sugar) E11.9
- with
  - amyotrophy E11.44
  - arthropathy NEC E11.618
  - autonomic (poly)neuropathy E11.43
  - cataract E11.36
  - Charcot's joints E11.61Ø
  - chronic kidney disease E11.22
  - circulatory complication NEC E11.59
  - complication E11.8
    - specified NEC E11.69
  - dermatitis E11.62Ø
  - foot ulcer E11.621
  - gangrene E11.52
  - gastroparalysis E11.43
  - gastroparesis E11.43
  - glomerulonephrosis, intracapillary E11.21
  - glomerulosclerosis, intercapillary E11.21
  - hyperglycemia E11.65
  - hyperosmolarity E11.ØØ
    - with coma E11.Ø1
  - hypoglycemia E11.649
    - with coma E11.641
  - ketoacidosis E11.1Ø
    - with coma E11.11
  - kidney complications NEC E11.29
  - Kimmelsteil-Wilson disease E11.21
  - loss of protective sensation (LOPS) — *see* Diabetes, by type, with neuropathy
  - mononeuropathy E11.41
  - myasthenia E11.44
  - necrobiosis lipoidica E11.62Ø
  - nephropathy E11.21
  - neuralgia E11.42
  - neurologic complication NEC E11.49
  - neuropathic arthropathy E11.61Ø
  - neuropathy E11.4Ø
  - ophthalmic complication NEC E11.39

Diabetes, diabetic — *continued*
- with — *continued*
  - oral complication NEC E11.638
  - osteomyelitis E11.69
  - periodontal disease E11.63Ø
  - peripheral angiopathy E11.51
    - with gangrene E11.52
  - polyneuropathy E11.42
  - renal complication NEC E11.29
  - renal tubular degeneration E11.29
  - retinopathy E11.319
    - with macular edema E11.311
      - resolved following treatment E11.37- ☑
    - nonproliferative E11.329 ☑
      - with macular edema E11.321 ☑
      - mild E11.329 ☑
        - with macular edema E11.321 ☑
      - moderate E11.339 ☑
        - with macular edema E11.331 ☑
      - severe E11.349 ☑
        - with macular edema E11.341 ☑
    - proliferative E11.359 ☑
      - with
        - combined traction retinal detachment and rhegmatogenous retinal detachment E11.354 ☑
        - macular edema E11.351 ☑
        - stable proliferative diabetic retinopathy E11.355 ☑
        - traction retinal detachment involving the macula E11.352 ☑
        - traction retinal detachment not involving the macula E11.353 ☑
    - resolved following treatment EØ9.37 ☑
  - skin complication NEC E11.628
  - skin ulcer NEC E11.622
- brittle — *see* Diabetes, type 1
- bronzed E83.11Ø
- complicating pregnancy — *see* Pregnancy, complicated by, diabetes
- dietary counseling and surveillance Z71.3
- due to
  - autoimmune process — *see* Diabetes, type 1
  - immune mediated pancreatic islet beta-cell destruction — *see* Diabetes, type 1
- due to drug or chemical EØ9.9
  - with
    - amyotrophy EØ9.44
    - arthropathy NEC EØ9.618
    - autonomic (poly)neuropathy EØ9.43
    - cataract EØ9.36
    - Charcot's joints EØ9.61Ø
    - chronic kidney disease EØ9.22
    - circulatory complication NEC EØ9.59
    - complication EØ9.8
      - specified NEC EØ9.69
    - dermatitis EØ9.62Ø
    - foot ulcer EØ9.621
    - gangrene EØ9.52
    - gastroparalysis EØ9.43
    - gastroparesis EØ9.43
    - glomerulonephrosis, intracapillary EØ9.21
    - glomerulosclerosis, intercapillary EØ9.21
    - hyperglycemia EØ9.65
    - hyperosmolarity EØ9.ØØ
      - with coma EØ9.Ø1
    - hypoglycemia EØ9.649
      - with coma EØ9.641
    - ketoacidosis EØ9.1Ø
      - with coma EØ9.11
    - kidney complications NEC EØ9.29
    - Kimmelsteil-Wilson disease EØ9.21
    - mononeuropathy EØ9.41
    - myasthenia EØ9.44
    - necrobiosis lipoidica EØ9.62Ø
    - nephropathy EØ9.21
    - neuralgia EØ9.42
    - neurologic complication NEC EØ9.49
    - neuropathic arthropathy EØ9.61Ø
    - neuropathy EØ9.4Ø
    - ophthalmic complication NEC EØ9.39
    - oral complication NEC EØ9.638
    - periodontal disease EØ9.63Ø
    - peripheral angiopathy EØ9.51
      - with gangrene EØ9.52
    - polyneuropathy EØ9.42
    - renal complication NEC EØ9.29
    - renal tubular degeneration EØ9.29

Difficult, difficulty — *continued*
- feeding R63.3
  - newborn P92.9
    - breast P92.5
    - specified NEC P92.8
  - nonorganic (infant or child) F98.29
- intubation, in anesthesia T88.4 ☑
- mechanical, gastroduodenal stoma K91.89
  - causing obstruction — *see also* Obstruction, intestine, postoperative K91.3Ø
- micturition
  - need to immediately re-void R39.191
  - position dependent R39.192
  - specified NEC R39.198
- reading (developmental) F81.Ø
  - secondary to emotional disorders F93.9
- spelling (specific) F81.81
  - with reading disorder F81.89
  - due to inadequate teaching Z55.8
- swallowing — *see* Dysphagia
- walking R26.2
- work
  - conditions NEC Z56.5
  - schedule Z56.3

Diffuse — *see* condition

Digestive — *see* condition

Dihydropyrimidine dehydrogenase disease (DPD) E88.89

Diktyoma — *see* Neoplasm, malignant, by site

Dilaceration, tooth KØØ.4

Dilatation
- anus K59.89
  - venule — *see* Hemorrhoids
- aorta (focal) (general) — *see* Ectasia, aorta
  - with aneuysm — *see* Aneurysm, aorta
  - congenital Q25.44
- artery — *see* Aneurysm
- bladder (sphincter) N32.89
  - congenital Q64.79
- blood vessel I99.8
- bronchial J47.9
  - with
    - exacerbation (acute) J47.1
    - lower respiratory infection J47.Ø
- calyx (due to obstruction) — *see* Hydronephrosis
- capillaries I78.8
- cardiac (acute) (chronic) — *see also* Hypertrophy, cardiac
  - congenital Q24.8
    - valve NEC Q24.8
      - pulmonary Q22.3
  - valve — *see* Endocarditis
- cavum septi pellucidi QØ6.8
- cervix (uteri) — *see also* Incompetency, cervix
  - incomplete, poor, slow complicating delivery O62.Ø
- colon K59.39
  - congenital Q43.1
  - psychogenic F45.8
  - toxic K59.31
- common duct (acquired) K83.8
  - congenital Q44.5
- cystic duct (acquired) K82.8
  - congenital Q44.5
- duct, mammary — *see* Ectasia, mammary duct
- duodenum K59.89
- esophagus K22.8
  - congenital Q39.5
  - due to achalasia K22.Ø
- eustachian tube, congenital Q17.8
- gallbladder K82.8
- gastric — *see* Dilatation, stomach
- heart (acute) (chronic) — *see also* Hypertrophy, cardiac
  - congenital Q24.8
  - valve — *see* Endocarditis
- ileum K59.89
  - psychogenic F45.8
- jejunum K59.89
  - psychogenic F45.8
- kidney (calyx) (collecting structures) (cystic) (parenchyma) (pelvis) (idiopathic) N28.89
- lacrimal passages or duct — *see* Disorder, lacrimal system, changes
- lymphatic vessel I89.Ø
- mammary duct — *see* Ectasia, mammary duct
- Meckel's diverticulum (congenital) Q43.Ø
  - malignant — *see* Table of Neoplasms, small intestine, malignant

Dilatation — *continued*
- myocardium (acute) (chronic) — *see* Hypertrophy, cardiac
- organ or site, congenital NEC — *see* Distortion
- pancreatic duct K86.89
- pericardium — *see* Pericarditis
- pharynx J39.2
- prostate N42.89
- pulmonary
  - artery (idiopathic) I28.8
  - valve, congenital Q22.3
- pupil H57.Ø4
- rectum K59.39
- saccule, congenital Q16.5
- salivary gland (duct) K11.8
- sphincter ani K62.89
- stomach K31.89
  - acute K31.Ø
  - psychogenic F45.8
- submaxillary duct K11.8
- trachea, congenital Q32.1
- ureter (idiopathic) N28.82
  - congenital Q62.2
  - due to obstruction N13.4
- urethra (acquired) N36.8
- vasomotor I73.9
- vein I86.8
- ventricular, ventricle (acute) (chronic) — *see also* Hypertrophy, cardiac
  - cerebral, congenital QØ4.8
- venule NEC I86.8
- vesical orifice N32.89

Dilated, dilation — *see* Dilatation

Diminished, diminution
- hearing (acuity) — *see* Deafness
- sense or sensation (cold) (heat) (tactile) (vibratory) R2Ø.8
- vision NEC H54.7
- vital capacity R94.2

Diminuta taenia B71.Ø

Dimitri-Sturge-Weber disease Q85.8

Dimple
- congenital sacral Q82.6
- parasacral Q82.6
- pilonidal or postanal — *see* Cyst, pilonidal

Dioctophyme renalis (infection) (infestation) B83.8

Dipetalonemiasis B74.4

Diphallus Q55.69

Diphtheria, diphtheritic (gangrenous) (hemorrhagic) A36.9
- carrier (suspected) Z22.2
- cutaneous A36.3
- faucial A36.Ø
- infection of wound A36.3
- laryngeal A36.2
- myocarditis A36.81
- nasal, anterior A36.89
- nasopharyngeal A36.1
- neurological complication A36.89
- pharyngeal A36.Ø
- specified site NEC A36.89
- tonsillar A36.Ø

Diphyllobothriasis (intestine) B7Ø.Ø
- larval B7Ø.1

Diplacusis H93.22- ☑

Diplegia (upper limbs) G83.Ø
- congenital (cerebral) G8Ø.8
- facial G51.Ø
- lower limbs G82.2Ø
- spastic G8Ø.1

Diplococcus, diplococcal — *see* condition

Diplopia H53.2

Dipsomania F1Ø.2Ø
- with
  - psychosis — *see* Psychosis, alcoholic
- remission F1Ø.21

Dipylidiasis B71.1

DIRA (deficiency of interleukin 1 receptor antagonist) MØ4.8

Direction, teeth, abnormal, fully erupted M26.3Ø

Dirofilariasis B74.8

Dirt-eating child F98.3

Disability, disabilities
- heart — *see* Disease, heart
- intellectual F79
  - with
    - autistic features F84.9
  - mild (I.Q. 5Ø-69) F7Ø

Disability, disabilities — *continued*
- intellectual — *continued*
  - moderate (I.Q. 35-49) F71
  - profound (I.Q. under 2Ø) F73
  - severe (I.Q. 2Ø-34) F72
  - specified level NEC F78
- knowledge acquisition F81.9
- learning F81.9
- limiting activities Z73.6
- spelling, specific F81.81

Disappearance of family member Z63.4

Disarticulation — *see* Amputation
- meaning traumatic amputation — *see* Amputation, traumatic

Discharge (from)
- abnormal finding in — *see* Abnormal, specimen
- breast (female) (male) N64.52
- diencephalic autonomic idiopathic — *see* Epilepsy, specified NEC
- ear — *see also* Otorrhea
  - blood — *see* Otorrhagia
- excessive urine R35.8
- nipple N64.52
- penile R36.9
- postnasal RØ9.82
- prison, anxiety concerning Z65.2
- urethral R36.9
  - without blood R36.Ø
  - hematospermia R36.1
- vaginal N89.8

Discitis, diskitis M46.4Ø
- cervical region M46.42
- cervicothoracic region M46.43
- lumbar region M46.46
- lumbosacral region M46.47
- multiple sites M46.49
- occipito-atlanto-axial region M46.41
- pyogenic — *see* Infection, intervertebral disc, pyogenic
- sacrococcygeal region M46.48
- thoracic region M46.44
- thoracolumbar region M46.45

Discoid
- meniscus (congenital) Q68.6
- semilunar cartilage (congenital) — *see* Derangement, knee, meniscus, specified NEC

Discoloration
- nails L6Ø.8
- teeth (posteruptive) KØ3.7
  - during formation KØØ.8

Discomfort
- chest RØ7.89
- visual H53.14- ☑

Discontinuity, ossicles, ear H74.2- ☑

Discord (with)
- boss Z56.4
- classmates Z55.4
- counselor Z64.4
- employer Z56.4
- family Z63.8
- fellow employees Z56.4
- in-laws Z63.1
- landlord Z59.2
- lodgers Z59.2
- neighbors Z59.2
- probation officer Z64.4
- social worker Z64.4
- teachers Z55.4
- workmates Z56.4

Discordant connection
- atrioventricular (congenital) Q2Ø.5
- ventriculoarterial Q2Ø.3

Discrepancy
- centric occlusion maximum intercuspation M26.55
- leg length (acquired) — *see* Deformity, limb, unequal length
  - congenital — *see* Defect, reduction, lower limb
- uterine size date O26.84- ☑

Discrimination
- ethnic Z6Ø.5
- political Z6Ø.5
- racial Z6Ø.5
- religious Z6Ø.5
- sex Z6Ø.5

Disease, diseased — *see also* Syndrome
- absorbent system I87.8
- acid-peptic K3Ø
- Acosta's T7Ø.29 ☑

- **Disease, diseased** — *continued*
  - cerebrovascular — *continued*
    - acute — *continued*
      - thrombotic I63.3- ☑
    - arteriosclerotic I67.2
    - hereditary NEC I67.858
    - specified NEC I67.89
  - cervix (uteri) (noninflammatory) N88.9
    - inflammatory — *see* Cervicitis
    - specified NEC N88.8
  - Chabert's A22.9
  - Chandler's (osteochondritis dissecans, hip) — *see* Osteochondritis, dissecans, hip
  - Charlouis — *see* Yaws
  - Chédiak-Steinbrinck (-Higashi) (congenital gigantism of peroxidase granules) E7Ø.33Ø
  - chest J98.9
  - Chiari's (hepatic vein thrombosis) I82.Ø
  - Chicago B4Ø.9
  - Chignon B36.8
  - chigo, chigoe B88.1
  - childhood granulomatous D71
  - Chinese liver fluke B66.1
  - chlamydial A74.9
    - specified NEC A74.89
  - cholecystic K82.9
  - choroid H31.9
    - specified NEC H31.8
  - Christmas D67
  - chronic bullous of childhood L12.2
  - chylomicron retention E78.3
  - ciliary body H21.9
    - specified NEC H21.89
  - circulatory (system) NEC I99.8
    - newborn P29.9
    - syphilitic A52.ØØ
      - congenital A5Ø.54
  - coagulation factor deficiency (congenital) — *see* Defect, coagulation
  - coccidioidal — *see* Coccidioidomycosis
  - cold
    - agglutinin or hemoglobinuria D59.12
      - paroxysmal D59.6
    - hemagglutinin (chronic) D59.12
  - collagen NOS (nonvascular) (vascular) M35.9
    - specified NEC M35.8
  - colon K63.9
    - functional K59.9
      - congenital Q43.2
    - ischemic — *see also* Ischemia, intestine, acute K55.Ø39
  - colonic inflammatory bowel, unclassified (IBDU) K52.3
  - combined system — *see* Degeneration, combined
  - compressed air T7Ø.3 ☑
  - Concato's (pericardial polyserositis) A19.9
    - nontubercular I31.1
    - pleural — *see* Pleurisy, with effusion
  - conjunctiva H11.9
    - chlamydial A74.Ø
    - specified NEC H11.89
    - viral B3Ø.9
      - specified NEC B3Ø.8
  - connective tissue, systemic (diffuse) M35.9
    - in (due to)
      - hypogammaglobulinemia D8Ø.1 *[M36.8]*
      - ochronosis E7Ø.29 *[M36.8]*
    - specified NEC M35.8
  - Conor and Bruch's (boutonneuse fever) A77.1
  - Cooper's — *see* Mastopathy, cystic
  - Cori's (glycogenosis III) E74.Ø3
  - corkhandler's or corkworker's J67.3
  - cornea H18.9
    - specified NEC H18.89- ☑
  - coronary (artery) — *see* Disease, heart, ischemic, atherosclerotic
    - congenital Q24.5
    - ostial, syphilitic (aortic) (mitral) (pulmonary) A52.Ø3
  - corpus cavernosum N48.9
    - specified NEC N48.89
  - Cotugno's — *see* Sciatica
  - COVID-19 UØ7.1
  - coxsackie (virus) NEC B34.1
  - cranial nerve NOS G52.9
  - Creutzfeldt-Jakob — *see* Creutzfeldt-Jakob disease or syndrome
  - Crocq's (acrocyanosis) I73.89
  - Crohn's — *see* Enteritis, regional
  - Curschmann G71.11

- **Disease, diseased** — *continued*
  - cystic
    - breast (chronic) — *see* Mastopathy, cystic
    - kidney, congenital Q61.9
    - liver, congenital Q44.6
    - lung J98.4
      - congenital Q33.Ø
  - cytomegalic inclusion (generalized) B25.9
    - with pneumonia B25.Ø
    - congenital P35.1
  - cytomegaloviral B25.9
    - specified NEC B25.8
  - Czerny's (periodic hydrarthrosis of the knee) — *see* Effusion, joint, knee
  - Daae (-Finsen) (epidemic pleurodynia) B33.Ø
  - Darling's — *see* Histoplasmosis capsulati
  - de Quervain's (tendon sheath) M65.4
    - thyroid (subacute granulomatous thyroiditis) EØ6.1
  - Débove's (splenomegaly) R16.1
  - deer fly — *see* Tularemia
  - Degos' I77.89
  - demyelinating, demyelinizating (nervous system) G37.9
    - multiple sclerosis G35
    - specified NEC G37.8
  - dense deposit — *see also* NØØ-NØ7 with fourth character .6 NØ5.6
  - deposition, hydroxyapatite — *see* Disease, hydroxyapatite deposition
  - Devergie's (pityriasis rubra pilaris) L44.Ø
  - Devic's G36.Ø
  - diaphorase deficiency D74.Ø
  - diaphragm J98.6
  - diarrheal, infectious NEC AØ9
  - digestive system K92.9
    - specified NEC K92.89
  - disc, degenerative — *see* Degeneration, intervertebral disc
  - discogenic — *see also* Displacement, intervertebral disc NEC
    - with myelopathy — *see* Disorder, disc, with, myelopathy
  - diverticular — *see* Diverticula
  - Dubois (thymus) A5Ø.59 *[E35]*
  - Duchenne-Griesinger G71.Ø1
  - Duchenne's
    - muscular dystrophy G71.Ø1
    - pseudohypertrophy, muscles G71.Ø1
  - ductless glands E34.9
  - Duhring's (dermatitis herpetiformis) L13.Ø
  - duodenum K31.9
    - specified NEC K31.89
  - Dupré's (meningism) R29.1
  - Dupuytren's (muscle contracture) M72.Ø
  - Durand-Nicholas-Favre (climatic bubo) A55
  - Duroziez's (congenital mitral stenosis) Q23.2
  - ear — *see* Disorder, ear
  - Eberth's — *see* Fever, typhoid
  - Ebola (virus) A98.4
  - Ebstein's heart Q22.5
  - Echinococcus — *see* Echinococcus
  - echovirus NEC B34.1
  - Eddowes' (brittle bones and blue sclera) Q78.Ø
  - edentulous (alveolar) ridge KØ6.9
    - specified NEC KØ6.8
  - Edsall's T67.2 ☑
  - Eichstedt's (pityriasis versicolor) B36.Ø
  - Eisenmenger's (irreversible) I27.83
  - Ellis-van Creveld (chondroectodermal dysplasia) Q77.6
  - end stage renal (ESRD) N18.6
    - due to hypertension I12.Ø
  - endocrine glands or system NEC E34.9
  - endomyocardial (eosinophilic) I42.3
  - English (rickets) E55.Ø
  - enteroviral, enterovirus NEC B34.1
    - central nervous system NEC A88.8
  - epidemic B99.9
    - specified NEC B99.8
  - epididymis N5Ø.9
  - Erb (-Landouzy) G71.Ø2
  - Erdheim-Chester (ECD) E88.89
  - esophagus K22.9
    - functional K22.4
    - psychogenic F45.8
    - specified NEC K22.8
  - Eulenburg's (congenital paramyotonia) G71.19
  - eustachian tube — *see* Disorder, eustachian tube
  - external
    - auditory canal — *see* Disorder, ear, external

- **Disease, diseased** — *continued*
  - external — *continued*
    - ear — *see* Disorder, ear, external
  - extrapyramidal G25.9
    - specified NEC G25.89
  - eye H57.9
    - anterior chamber H21.9
    - inflammatory NEC H57.89
    - muscle (external) — *see* Strabismus
    - specified NEC H57.89
    - syphilitic — *see* Oculopathy, syphilitic
  - eyeball H44.9
    - specified NEC H44.89
  - eyelid — *see* Disorder, eyelid
    - specified NEC — *see* Disorder, eyelid, specified type NEC
  - eyeworm of Africa B74.3
  - facial nerve (seventh) G51.9
    - newborn (birth injury) P11.3
  - Fahr (of brain) G23.8
  - Fahr Volhard (of kidney) I12.- ☑
  - fallopian tube (noninflammatory) N83.9
    - inflammatory — *see* Salpingo-oophoritis
    - specified NEC N83.8
  - familial periodic paralysis G72.3
  - Fanconi's (congenital pancytopenia) D61.Ø9
  - fascia NEC — *see also* Disorder, muscle
    - inflammatory — *see* Myositis
    - specified NEC M62.89
  - Fauchard's (periodontitis) — *see* Periodontitis
  - Favre-Durand-Nicolas (climatic bubo) A55
  - Fede's K14.Ø
  - Feer's — *see* Poisoning, mercury
  - female pelvic inflammatory — *see also* Disease, pelvis, inflammatory N73.9
    - syphilitic (secondary) A51.42
    - tuberculous A18.17
  - Fernels' (aortic aneurysm) I71.9
  - fibrocaseous of lung — *see* Tuberculosis, pulmonary
  - fibrocystic — *see* Fibrocystic disease
  - Fiedler's (leptospiral jaundice) A27.Ø
  - fifth BØ8.3
  - file-cutter's — *see* Poisoning, lead
  - fish-skin Q8Ø.9
    - acquired L85.Ø
  - Flajani (-Basedow) (exophthalmic goiter) — *see* Hyperthyroidism, with, goiter (diffuse)
  - flax-dresser's J66.1
  - fluke — *see* Infestation, fluke
  - foot and mouth BØ8.8
  - foot process NØ4.9
  - Forbes' (glycogenosis III) E74.Ø3
  - Fordyce-Fox (apocrine miliaria) L75.2
  - Fordyce's (ectopic sebaceous glands) (mouth) Q38.6
  - Forestier's (rhizomelic pseudopolyarthritis) M35.3
    - meaning ankylosing hyperostosis — *see* Hyperostosis, ankylosing
  - Fothergill's
    - neuralgia — *see* Neuralgia, trigeminal
    - scarlatina anginosa A38.9
  - Fournier (gangrene) N49.3
    - female N76.89
  - fourth BØ8.8
  - Fox (-Fordyce) (apocrine miliaria) L75.2
  - Francis' — *see* Tularemia
  - Franklin C88.2
  - Frei's (climatic bubo) A55
  - Friedreich's
    - combined systemic or ataxia G11.11
    - myoclonia G25.3
  - frontal sinus — *see* Sinusitis, frontal
  - fungus NEC B49
  - Gaisböck's (polycythemia hypertonica) D75.1
  - gallbladder K82.9
    - calculus — *see* Calculus, gallbladder
    - cholecystitis — *see* Cholecystitis
    - cholesterolosis K82.4
    - fistula — *see* Fistula, gallbladder
    - hydrops K82.1
    - obstruction — *see* Obstruction, gallbladder
    - perforation K82.2
    - specified NEC K82.8
  - gamma heavy chain C88.2
  - Gamna's (siderotic splenomegaly) D73.2
  - Gamstorp's (adynamia episodica hereditaria) G72.3
  - Gandy-Nanta (siderotic splenomegaly) D73.2
  - ganister J62.8
  - gastric — *see* Disease, stomach

Disease, diseased — *continued*
Heubner-Herter (nontropical sprue) K9Ø.Ø
high fetal gene or hemoglobin thalassemia D56.9
Hildenbrand's — *see* Typhus
hip (joint) M25.9
congenital Q65.89
suppurative MØØ.9
tuberculous A18.Ø2
His (-Werner) (trench fever) A79.Ø
Hodgson's I71.2
ruptured I71.1
Holla — *see* Spherocytosis
hookworm B76.9
specified NEC B76.8
host-versus-graft D89.813
acute D89.81Ø
acute on chronic D89.812
chronic D89.811
human immunodeficiency virus (HIV) B2Ø
Huntington's G1Ø
with dementia G1Ø *[FØ2.8Ø]*
Hutchinson's (cheiropompholyx) — *see* Hutchinson's disease
hyaline (diffuse) (generalized)
membrane (lung) (newborn) P22.Ø
adult J8Ø
hydatid — *see* Echinococcus
hydroxyapatite deposition M11.ØØ
ankle M11.Ø7- ☑
elbow M11.Ø2- ☑
foot joint M11.Ø7- ☑
hand joint M11.Ø4- ☑
hip M11.Ø5- ☑
knee M11.Ø6- ☑
multiple site M11.Ø9
shoulder M11.Ø1- ☑
vertebra M11.Ø8
wrist M11.Ø3- ☑
hyperkinetic — *see* Hyperkinesia
hypertensive — *see* Hypertension
hypophysis E23.7
Iceland G93.3
I-cell E77.Ø
immune D89.9
immunoproliferative (malignant) C88.9
small intestinal C88.3
specified NEC C88.8
inclusion B25.9
salivary gland B25.9
infectious, infective B99.9
congenital P37.9
specified NEC P37.8
viral P35.9
specified type NEC P35.8
specified NEC B99.8
inflammatory
penis N48.29
abscess N48.21
cellulitis N48.22
prepuce N47.7
balanoposthitis N47.6
tubo-ovarian — *see* Salpingo-oophoritis
intervertebral disc — *see also* Disorder, disc
with myelopathy — *see* Disorder, disc, with, myelopathy
cervical, cervicothoracic — *see* Disorder, disc, cervical
with
myelopathy — *see* Disorder, disc, cervical, with myelopathy
neuritis, radiculitis or radiculopathy — *see* Disorder, disc, cervical, with neuritis
specified NEC — *see* Disorder, disc, cervical, specified type NEC
lumbar (with)
myelopathy M51.Ø6
neuritis, radiculitis, radiculopathy or sciatica M51.16
specified NEC M51.86
lumbosacral (with)
neuritis, radiculitis, radiculopathy or sciatica M51.17
specified NEC M51.87
specified NEC — *see* Disorder, disc, specified NEC
thoracic (with)
myelopathy M51.Ø4
neuritis, radiculitis or radiculopathy M51.14
specified NEC M51.84

Disease, diseased — *continued*
intervertebral disc — *see also* Disorder, disc — *continued*
thoracolumbar (with)
myelopathy M51.Ø5
neuritis, radiculitis or radiculopathy M51.15
specified NEC M51.85
intestine K63.9
functional K59.9
psychogenic F45.8
specified NEC K59.89
organic K63.9
protozoal AØ7.9
specified NEC K63.89
iris H21.9
specified NEC H21.89
iron metabolism or storage E83.1Ø
island (scrub typhus) A75.3
itai-itai — *see* Poisoning, cadmium
Jakob-Creutzfeldt — *see* Creutzfeldt-Jakob disease or syndrome
jaw M27.9
fibrocystic M27.49
specified NEC M27.8
jigger B88.1
joint — *see also* Disorder, joint
Charcot's — *see* Arthropathy, neuropathic (Charcot)
degenerative — *see* Osteoarthritis
multiple M15.9
spine — *see* Spondylosis
hypertrophic — *see* Osteoarthritis
sacroiliac M53.3
specified NEC — *see* Disorder, joint, specified type NEC
spine NEC — *see* Dorsopathy
suppurative — *see* Arthritis, pyogenic or pyemic
Jourdain's (acute gingivitis) KØ5.ØØ
nonplaque induced KØ5.Ø1
plaque induced KØ5.ØØ
Kaschin-Beck (endemic polyarthritis) M12.1Ø
ankle M12.17- ☑
elbow M12.12- ☑
foot joint M12.17- ☑
hand joint M12.14- ☑
hip M12.15- ☑
knee M12.16- ☑
multiple site M12.19
shoulder M12.11- ☑
vertebra M12.18
wrist M12.13- ☑
Katayama B65.2
Kedani (scrub typhus) A75.3
Keshan E59
kidney (functional) (pelvis) N28.9
chronic N18.9
hypertensive — *see* Hypertension, kidney
stage 1 N18.1
stage 2 (mild) N18.2
stage 3 (moderate) N18.3Ø
stage 3a N18.31
stage 3b N18.32
stage 4 (severe) N18.4
stage 5 N18.5
complicating pregnancy — *see* Pregnancy, complicated by, renal disease
cystic (congenital) Q61.9
fibrocystic (congenital) Q61.8
hypertensive — *see* Hypertension, kidney
in (due to)
schistosomiasis (bilharziasis) B65.9 *[N29]*
multicystic Q61.4
polycystic Q61.3
adult type Q61.2
childhood type NEC Q61.19
collecting duct dilatation Q61.11
Kimmelstiel (-Wilson) (intercapillary polycystic (congenital) glomerulosclerosis) — *see* EØ8-E13 with .21
Kinnier Wilson's (hepatolenticular degeneration) E83.Ø1
kissing — *see* Mononucleosis, infectious
Klebs' — *see also* Glomerulonephritis NØ5- ☑
Klippel-Feil (brevicollis) Q76.1
Köhler-Pellegrini-Stieda (calcification, knee joint) — *see* Bursitis, tibial collateral
Kok Q89.8
König's (osteochondritis dissecans) — *see* Osteochondritis, dissecans
Korsakoff's (nonalcoholic) FØ4
alcoholic F1Ø.96

Disease, diseased — *continued*
Korsakoff's — *continued*
alcoholic — *continued*
with dependence F1Ø.26
Kostmann's (infantile genetic agranulocytosis) D7Ø.Ø
kuru A81.81
Kyasanur Forest A98.2
labyrinth, ear — *see* Disorder, ear, inner
lacrimal system — *see* Disorder, lacrimal system
Lafora's — *see* Epilepsy, generalized, idiopathic
Lancereaux-Mathieu (leptospiral jaundice) A27.Ø
Landry's G61.Ø
Larrey-Weil (leptospiral jaundice) A27.Ø
larynx J38.7
legionnaires' A48.1
nonpneumonic A48.2
Lenegre's I44.2
lens H27.9
specified NEC H27.8
Lev's (acquired complete heart block) I44.2
Lewy body (dementia) G31.83 *[FØ2.8Ø]*
with behavioral disturbance G31.83 *[FØ2.81]*
Lichtheim's (subacute combined sclerosis with pernicious anemia) D51.Ø
Lightwood's (renal tubular acidosis) N25.89
Lignac's (cystinosis) E72.Ø4
lip K13.Ø
lipid-storage E75.6
specified NEC E75.5
Lipschütz's N76.6
liver (chronic) (organic) K76.9
alcoholic (chronic) K7Ø.9
acute — *see* Disease, liver, alcoholic, hepatitis
cirrhosis K7Ø.3Ø
with ascites K7Ø.31
failure K7Ø.4Ø
with coma K7Ø.41
fatty liver K7Ø.Ø
fibrosis K7Ø.2
hepatitis K7Ø.1Ø
with ascites K7Ø.11
sclerosis K7Ø.2
cystic, congenital Q44.6
drug-induced (idiosyncratic) (toxic) (predictable) (unpredictable) — *see* Disease, liver, toxic
end stage K72.9Ø
due to hepatitis — *see* Hepatitis
fatty, nonalcoholic (NAFLD) K76.Ø
alcoholic K7Ø.Ø
fibrocystic (congenital) Q44.6
fluke
Chinese B66.1
oriental B66.1
sheep B66.3
gestational alloimmune (GALD) P78.84
glycogen storage E74.Ø9 *[K77]*
in (due to)
schistosomiasis (bilharziasis) B65.9 *[K77]*
inflammatory K75.9
alcoholic K7Ø.1 ☑
specified NEC K75.89
polycystic (congenital) Q44.6
toxic K71.9
with
cholestasis K71.Ø
cirrhosis (liver) K71.7
fibrosis (liver) K71.7
focal nodular hyperplasia K71.8
hepatic granuloma K71.8
hepatic necrosis K71.1Ø
with coma K71.11
hepatitis NEC K71.6
acute K71.2
chronic
active K71.5Ø
with ascites K71.51
lobular K71.4
persistent K71.3
lupoid K71.5Ø
with ascites K71.51
peliosis hepatis K71.8
veno-occlusive disease (VOD) of liver K71.8
veno-occlusive K76.5
Lobo's (keloid blastomycosis) B48.Ø
Lobstein's (brittle bones and blue sclera) Q78.Ø
Ludwig's (submaxillary cellulitis) K12.2
lumbosacral region M53.87
lung J98.4

Disease, diseased — *continued*
- lung — *continued*
  - black J6Ø
  - congenital Q33.9
  - cystic J98.4
    - congenital Q33.Ø
  - dabbing (related) UØ7.Ø
  - electronic cigarette (related) UØ7.Ø
  - fibroid (chronic) — *see* Fibrosis, lung
  - fluke B66.4
    - oriental B66.4
  - in
    - amyloidosis E85.4 *[J99]*
    - sarcoidosis D86.Ø
    - Sjögren's syndrome M35.Ø2
    - systemic
      - lupus erythematosus M32.13
      - sclerosis M34.81
  - interstitial J84.9
    - of childhood, specified NEC J84.848
    - respiratory bronchiolitis J84.115
    - specified NEC J84.89
    - with progressive fibrotic phenotype, in diseases classified elsewhere J84.17Ø
  - obstructive (chronic) J44.9
    - with
      - acute
        - bronchitis J44.Ø
        - exacerbation NEC J44.1
        - lower respiratory infection J44.Ø
      - alveolitis, allergic J67.9
      - asthma J44.9
      - bronchiectasis J47.9
        - with
          - exacerbation (acute) J47.1
          - lower respiratory infection J47.Ø
      - bronchitis J44.9
        - with
          - exacerbation (acute) J44.1
          - lower respiratory infection J44.Ø
      - emphysema J43.9
      - hypersensitivity pneumonitis J67.9
    - decompensated J44.1
      - with
        - exacerbation (acute) J44.1
  - polycystic J98.4
    - congenital Q33.Ø
  - rheumatoid (diffuse) (interstitial) — *see* Rheumatoid, lung
  - vaping (associated) (device) (product) (use) UØ7.Ø
- Lutembacher's (atrial septal defect with mitral stenosis) Q21.1
- Lyme A69.2Ø
- lymphatic (gland) (system) (channel) (vessel) I89.9
- lymphoproliferative D47.9
  - specified NEC D47.Z9 (*following* D47.4)
  - T-gamma D47.Z9 (*following* D47.4)
  - X-linked D82.3
- Magitot's M27.2
- malarial — *see* Malaria
- malignant — *see also* Neoplasm, malignant, by site
- Manson's B65.1
- maple bark J67.6
- maple-syrup-urine E71.Ø
- Marburg (virus) A98.3
- Marion's (bladder neck obstruction) N32.Ø
- Marsh's (exophthalmic goiter) — *see* Hyperthyroidism, with, goiter (diffuse)
- mastoid (process) — *see* Disorder, ear, middle
- Mathieu's (leptospiral jaundice) A27.Ø
- Maxcy's A75.2
- McArdle (-Schmid-Pearson) (glycogenosis V) E74.Ø4
- mediastinum J98.59
- medullary center (idiopathic) (respiratory) G93.89
- Meige's (chronic hereditary edema) Q82.Ø
- meningococcal — *see* Infection, meningococcal
- mental F99
  - organic FØ9
- mesenchymal M35.9
- mesenteric embolic — *see also* Ischemia, intestine, acute K55.Ø39
- metabolic, metabolism E88.9
  - bilirubin E8Ø.7
- metal-polisher's J62.8
- metastatic — *see also* Neoplasm, secondary, by site C79.9
- microvascular - code to condition
- microvillus
  - atrophy Q43.8
  - inclusion (MVD) Q43.8
- middle ear — *see* Disorder, ear, middle
- Mikulicz' (dryness of mouth, absent or decreased lacrimation) K11.8
- Milroy's (chronic hereditary edema) Q82.Ø
- Minamata — *see* Poisoning, mercury
- minicore G71.29
- Minor's G95.19
- Minot's (hemorrhagic disease, newborn) P53
- Minot-von Willebrand-Jürgens (angiohemophilia) D68.Ø
- Mitchell's (erythromelalgia) I73.81
- mitral (valve) IØ5.9
  - nonrheumatic I34.9
- mixed connective tissue M35.1
- moldy hay J67.Ø
- Monge's T7Ø.29 ☑
- Morgagni-Adams-Stokes (syncope with heart block) I45.9
- Morgagni's (syndrome) (hyperostosis frontalis interna) M85.2
- Morton's (with metatarsalgia) — *see* Lesion, nerve, plantar
- Morvan's G6Ø.8
- motor neuron (bulbar) (mixed type) (spinal) G12.2Ø
  - amyotrophic lateral sclerosis G12.21
  - familial G12.24
  - progressive bulbar palsy G12.22
  - specified NEC G12.29
- moyamoya I67.5
- mu heavy chain disease C88.2
- multicore G71.29
- multiminicore G71.29
- muscle — *see also* Disorder, muscle
  - inflammatory — *see* Myositis
  - ocular (external) — *see* Strabismus
- musculoskeletal system, soft tissue — *see also* Disorder, soft tissue
  - specified NEC — *see* Disorder, soft tissue, specified type NEC
- mushroom workers' J67.5
- mycotic B49
- myelodysplastic, not classified C94.6
- myeloproliferative, not classified C94.6
  - chronic D47.1
- myocardium, myocardial — *see also* Degeneration, myocardial I51.5
  - primary (idiopathic) I42.9
- myoneural G7Ø.9
- Naegeli's D69.1
- nails L6Ø.9
  - specified NEC L6Ø.8
- Nairobi (sheep virus) A93.8
- nasal J34.9
- nemaline body G71.21
- nerve — *see* Disorder, nerve
- nervous system G98.8
  - autonomic G9Ø.9
  - central G96.9
    - specified NEC G96.89
  - congenital QØ7.9
  - parasympathetic G9Ø.9
  - specified NEC G98.8
  - sympathetic G9Ø.9
  - vegetative G9Ø.9
- neuromuscular system G7Ø.9
- Newcastle B3Ø.8
- Nicolas (-Durand)-Favre (climatic bubo) A55
- nipple N64.9
  - Paget's C5Ø.Ø1- ☑
    - female C5Ø.Ø1- ☑
    - male C5Ø.Ø2- ☑
- Nishimoto (-Takeuchi) I67.5
- nonarthropod-borne NOS (viral) B34.9
  - enterovirus NEC B34.1
- nonautoimmune hemolytic D59.4
  - drug-induced D59.2
- Nonne-Milroy-Meige (chronic hereditary edema) Q82.Ø
- nose J34.9
- nucleus pulposus — *see* Disorder, disc
- nutritional E63.9
- oast-house-urine E72.19
  - ocular
    - herpesviral BØØ.5Ø
    - zoster BØ2.3Ø
- obliterative vascular I77.1
- Ohara's — *see* Tularemia
- Opitz's (congestive splenomegaly) D73.2
- Oppenheim-Urbach (necrobiosis lipoidica diabeticorum) — *see* EØ8-E13 with .62Ø
- optic nerve NEC — *see* Disorder, nerve, optic
- orbit — *see* Disorder, orbit
- organ
  - dabbing (related) UØ7.Ø
  - electronic cigarette (related) UØ7.Ø
  - vaping (associated) (device) (product) (use) UØ7.Ø
- Oriental liver fluke B66.1
- Oriental lung fluke B66.4
- Ormond's N13.5
- Oropouche virus A93.Ø
- Osler-Rendu (familial hemorrhagic telangiectasia) I78.Ø
- osteofibrocystic E21.Ø
- Otto's M24.7
- outer ear — *see* Disorder, ear, external
- ovary (noninflammatory) N83.9
  - cystic N83.2Ø- ☑
  - inflammatory — *see* Salpingo-oophoritis
  - polycystic E28.2
  - specified NEC N83.8
- Owren's (congenital) — *see* Defect, coagulation
- pancreas K86.9
  - cystic K86.2
  - fibrocystic E84.9
  - specified NEC K86.89
- panvalvular IØ8.9
  - specified NEC IØ8.8
- parametrium (noninflammatory) N83.9
- parasitic B89
  - cerebral NEC B71.9 *[G94]*
  - intestinal NOS B82.9
  - mouth B37.Ø
  - skin NOS B88.9
  - specified type — *see* Infestation
  - tongue B37.Ø
- parathyroid (gland) E21.5
  - specified NEC E21.4
- Parkinson's G2Ø
- parodontal KØ5.6
- Parrot's (syphilitic osteochondritis) A5Ø.Ø2
- Parry's (exophthalmic goiter) — *see* Hyperthyroidism, with, goiter (diffuse)
- Parson's (exophthalmic goiter) — *see* Hyperthyroidism, with, goiter (diffuse)
- Paxton's (white piedra) B36.2
- pearl-worker's — *see* Osteomyelitis, specified type NEC
- Pellegrini-Stieda (calcification, knee joint) — *see* Bursitis, tibial collateral
- pelvis, pelvic
  - female NOS N94.9
    - specified NEC N94.89
  - gonococcal (acute) (chronic) A54.24
  - inflammatory (female) N73.9
    - acute N73.Ø
    - chlamydial A56.11
    - chronic N73.1
    - specified NEC N73.8
    - syphilitic (secondary) A51.42
      - late A52.76
    - tuberculous A18.17
  - organ, female N94.9
  - peritoneum, female NEC N94.89
- penis N48.9
  - inflammatory N48.29
    - abscess N48.21
    - cellulitis N48.22
  - specified NEC N48.89
- periapical tissues NOS KØ4.9Ø
- periodontal KØ5.6
  - specified NEC KØ5.5
- periosteum — *see* Disorder, bone, specified type NEC
- peripheral
  - arterial I73.9
  - autonomic nervous system G9Ø.9
  - nerves — *see* Polyneuropathy
  - vascular NOS I73.9
- peritoneum K66.9
  - pelvic, female NEC N94.89
  - specified NEC K66.8
- persistent mucosal (middle ear) H66.2Ø
  - left H66.22
    - with right H66.23
  - right H66.21

- **Disease, diseased** — *continued*
  - persistent mucosal — *continued*
    - right — *continued*
      - with left H66.23
  - Petit's — *see* Hernia, abdomen, specified site NEC
  - pharynx J39.2
    - specified NEC J39.2
  - Phocas' — *see* Mastopathy, cystic
  - photochromogenic (acid-fast bacilli) (pulmonary) A31.Ø
    - nonpulmonary A31.9
  - Pick's G31.Ø1 *[FØ2.8Ø]*
    - with behavioral disturbance G31.Ø1 *[FØ2.81]*
    - brain G31.Ø1 *[FØ2.8Ø]*
      - with behavioral disturbance G31.Ø1 *[FØ2.81]*
    - of pericardium (pericardial pseudocirrhosis of liver) I31.1
  - pigeon fancier's J67.2
  - pineal gland E34.8
  - pink — *see* Poisoning, mercury
  - Pinkus' (lichen nitidus) L44.1
  - pinworm B8Ø
  - Piry virus A93.8
  - pituitary (gland) E23.7
  - pituitary-snuff-taker's J67.8
  - pleura (cavity) J94.9
    - specified NEC J94.8
  - pneumatic drill (hammer) T75.21 ☑
  - Pollitzer's (hidradenitis suppurativa) L73.2
  - polycystic
    - kidney or renal Q61.3
      - adult type Q61.2
      - childhood type NEC Q61.19
        - collecting duct dilatation Q61.11
    - liver or hepatic Q44.6
    - lung or pulmonary J98.4
      - congenital Q33.Ø
    - ovary, ovaries E28.2
    - spleen Q89.Ø9
  - polyethylene T84.Ø5- ☑
  - Pompe's (glycogenosis II) E74.Ø2
  - Posadas-Wernicke B38.9
  - Potain's (pulmonary edema) — *see* Edema, lung
  - prepuce N47.8
    - inflammatory N47.7
      - balanoposthitis N47.6
  - Pringle's (tuberous sclerosis) Q85.1
  - prion, central nervous system A81.9
    - specified NEC A81.89
  - prostate N42.9
    - specified NEC N42.89
  - protozoal B64
    - acanthamebiasis — *see* Acanthamebiasis
    - African trypanosomiasis — *see* African trypanosomiasis
    - babesiosis — *see also* Babesiosis B6Ø.ØØ
    - Chagas disease — *see* Chagas disease
    - intestine, intestinal AØ7.9
    - leishmaniasis — *see* Leishmaniasis
    - malaria — *see* Malaria
    - naegleriasis B6Ø.2
    - pneumocystosis B59
    - specified organism NEC B6Ø.8
    - toxoplasmosis — *see* Toxoplasmosis
  - pseudo-Hurler's E77.Ø
  - psychiatric F99
  - psychotic — *see* Psychosis
  - Puente's (simple glandular cheilitis) K13.Ø
  - puerperal — *see also* Puerperal O9Ø.89
  - pulmonary — *see also* Disease, lung
    - artery I28.9
    - chronic obstructive J44.9
      - with
        - acute bronchitis J44.Ø
        - exacerbation (acute) J44.1
        - lower respiratory infection (acute) J44.Ø
      - decompensated J44.1
        - with
          - exacerbation (acute) J44.1
    - heart I27.9
      - specified NEC I27.89
    - hypertensive (vascular) — *see also* Hypertension, pulmonary I27.2Ø
      - NEC I27.2 ☑
      - primary (idiopathic) I27.Ø
    - valve I37.9
      - rheumatic IØ9.89
  - pulp (dental) NOS KØ4.9Ø
  - pulseless M31.4

- **Disease, diseased** — *continued*
  - Putnam's (subacute combined sclerosis with pernicious anemia) D51.Ø
  - Pyle (-Cohn) (metaphyseal dysplasia) Q78.5
  - ragpicker's or ragsorter's A22.1
  - Raynaud's — *see* Raynaud's disease
  - reactive airway — *see* Asthma
  - Reclus' (cystic) — *see* Mastopathy, cystic
  - rectum K62.9
    - specified NEC K62.89
  - Refsum's (heredopathia atactica polyneuritiformis) G6Ø.1
  - renal (functional) (pelvis) — *see also* Disease, kidney N28.9
    - with
      - edema — *see* Nephrosis
      - glomerular lesion — *see* Glomerulonephritis
        - with edema — *see* Nephrosis
      - interstitial nephritis N12
    - acute N28.9
    - chronic — *see also* Disease, kidney, chronic N18.9
    - cystic, congenital Q61.9
    - diabetic — *see* EØ8-E13 with .22
    - end-stage (failure) N18.6
      - due to hypertension I12.Ø
    - fibrocystic (congenital) Q61.8
    - hypertensive — *see* Hypertension, kidney
    - lupus M32.14
    - phosphate-losing (tubular) N25.Ø
    - polycystic (congenital) Q61.3
      - adult type Q61.2
      - childhood type NEC Q61.19
        - collecting duct dilatation Q61.11
    - rapidly progressive NØ1.9
    - subacute NØ1.9
  - Rendu-Osler-Weber (familial hemorrhagic telangiectasia) I78.Ø
  - renovascular (arteriosclerotic) — *see* Hypertension, kidney
  - respiratory (tract) J98.9
    - acute or subacute NOS JØ6.9
      - due to
        - chemicals, gases, fumes or vapors (inhalation) J68.3
        - external agent J7Ø.9
          - specified NEC J7Ø.8
        - radiation J7Ø.Ø
        - smoke inhalation J7Ø.5
      - noninfectious J39.8
    - chronic NOS J98.9
      - due to
        - chemicals, gases, fumes or vapors J68.4
        - external agent J7Ø.9
          - specified NEC J7Ø.8
        - radiation J7Ø.1
      - newborn P27.9
        - specified NEC P27.8
    - due to
      - chemicals, gases, fumes or vapors J68.9
        - acute or subacute NEC J68.3
        - chronic J68.4
      - external agent J7Ø.9
        - specified NEC J7Ø.8
    - newborn P28.9
      - specified type NEC P28.89
    - upper J39.9
      - acute or subacute JØ6.9
      - noninfectious NEC J39.8
      - specified NEC J39.8
      - streptococcal JØ6.9
  - retina, retinal H35.9
    - Batten's or Batten-Mayou E75.4 *[H36]*
    - specified NEC H35.89
  - rheumatoid — *see* Arthritis, rheumatoid
  - rickettsial NOS A79.9
    - specified type NEC A79.89
  - Riga (-Fede) (cachectic aphthae) K14.Ø
  - Riggs' (compound periodontitis) — *see* Periodontitis
  - Ritter's LØØ
  - Rivalta's (cervicofacial actinomycosis) A42.2
  - Robles' (onchocerciasis) B73.Ø1
  - rod body G71.21
  - Roger's (congenital interventricular septal defect) Q21.Ø
  - Rosenthal's (factor XI deficiency) D68.1
  - Ross River B33.1
  - Rossbach's (hyperchlorhydria) K31.89
    - psychogenic F45.8
  - Rotes Quérol — *see* Hyperostosis, ankylosing

- **Disease, diseased** — *continued*
  - Roth (-Bernhardt) — *see* Mononeuropathy, lower limb, meralgia paresthetica
  - Runeberg's (progressive pernicious anemia) D51.Ø
  - sacroiliac NEC M53.3
  - salivary gland or duct K11.9
    - inclusion B25.9
    - specified NEC K11.8
    - virus B25.9
  - sandworm B76.9
  - Schimmelbusch's — *see* Mastopathy, cystic
  - Schmorl's — *see* Schmorl's disease or nodes
  - Schönlein (-Henoch) (purpura rheumatica) D69.Ø
  - Schottmüller's — *see* Fever, paratyphoid
  - Schultz's (agranulocytosis) — *see* Agranulocytosis
  - Schwalbe-Ziehen-Oppenheim G24.1
  - Schwartz-Jampel G71.13
  - sclera H15.9
    - specified NEC H15.89
  - scrofulous (tuberculous) A18.2
  - scrotum N5Ø.9
  - sebaceous glands L73.9
  - semilunar cartilage, cystic — *see also* Derangement, knee, meniscus, cystic
  - seminal vesicle N5Ø.9
  - serum NEC — *see also* Reaction, serum T8Ø.69 ☑
  - sexually transmitted A64
    - anogenital
      - herpesviral infection — *see* Herpes, anogenital
      - warts A63.Ø
    - chancroid A57
    - chlamydial infection — *see* Chlamydia
    - gonorrhea — *see* Gonorrhea
    - granuloma inguinale A58
    - specified organism NEC A63.8
    - syphilis — *see* Syphilis
    - trichomoniasis — *see* Trichomoniasis
  - Sézary C84.1- ☑
  - shimamushi (scrub typhus) A75.3
  - shipyard B3Ø.Ø
  - sickle-cell D57.1
    - with
      - acute chest syndrome D57.Ø1
      - cerebral vascular involvement D57.Ø3
      - crisis (painful) D57.ØØ
        - with complication specified NEC D57.Ø9
      - splenic sequestration D57.Ø2
      - vasoocclusive pain D57.ØØ
    - elliptocytosis D57.8- ☑
    - Hb-C D57.2Ø
      - with
        - acute chest syndrome D57.211
        - cerebral vascular involvement D57.213
        - crisis D57.219
          - with specified complication NEC D57.218
        - splenic sequestration D57.212
        - vasoocclusive pain D57.219
      - without crisis D57.2Ø
    - Hb-SD D57.8Ø
      - with
        - acute chest syndrome D57.811
        - cerebral vascular involvement D57.813
        - crisis D57.819
          - with complication specified NEC D57.818
        - splenic sequestration D57.812
        - vasoocclusive pain D57.819
      - without crisis D57.8Ø
    - Hb-SE D57.8Ø
      - with
        - acute chest syndrome D57.811
        - cerebral vascular involvement D57.813
        - crisis D57.819
          - with complication specified NEC D57.818
        - splenic sequestration D57.812
        - vasoocclusive pain D57.819
      - without crisis D57.8Ø
    - specified NEC D57.8Ø
      - with
        - acute chest syndrome D57.811
        - cerebral vascular involvement D57.813
        - crisis D57.819
          - with complication specified NEC D57.818
        - splenic sequestration D57.812
        - vasoocclusive pain D57.819
      - without crisis D57.8Ø
    - spherocytosis D57.8Ø
      - with
        - acute chest syndrome D57.811

Disease, diseased — *continued*
- sickle-cell — *continued*
  - spherocytosis — *continued*
    - with — *continued*
      - cerebral vascular involvement D57.813
      - crisis D57.819
        - with complication specified NEC D57.818
      - splenic sequestration D57.812
      - vasoocclusive pain D57.819
    - without crisis D57.8Ø
  - thalassemia D57.4Ø
    - with
      - acute chest syndrome D57.411
      - cerebral vascular involvement D57.413
      - crisis (painful) D57.419
        - with specified complication NEC D57.418
      - splenic sequestration D57.412
      - vasoocclusive pain D57.419
    - beta plus D57.44
      - with
        - acute chest syndrome D57.451
        - cerebral vascular involvement D57.453
        - crisis D57.459
          - with specified complication NEC D57.458
        - splenic sequestration D57.452
        - vasoocclusive pain D57.459
      - without crisis D57.44
    - beta zero D57.42
      - with
        - acute chest syndrome D57.431
        - cerebral vascular involvement D57.433
        - crisis D57.439
          - with specified complication NEC D57.438
        - splenic sequestration D57.432
        - vasoocclusive pain D57.439
      - without crisis D57.42
- silo-filler's J68.8
  - bronchitis J68.Ø
  - pneumonitis J68.Ø
  - pulmonary edema J68.1
- simian B BØØ.4
- Simons' (progressive lipodystrophy) E88.1
- sin nombre virus B33.4
- sinus — *see* Sinusitis
- Sirkari's B55.Ø
- sixth BØ8.2Ø
  - due to human herpesvirus 6 BØ8.21
  - due to human herpesvirus 7 BØ8.22
- skin L98.9
  - due to metabolic disorder NEC E88.9 *[L99]*
  - specified NEC L98.8
- slim (HIV) B2Ø
- small vessel I73.9
- Sneddon-Wilkinson (subcorneal pustular dermatosis) L13.1
- South African creeping B88.Ø
- spinal (cord) G95.9
  - congenital QØ6.9
  - specified NEC G95.89
- spine — *see also* Spondylopathy
  - joint — *see* Dorsopathy
  - tuberculous A18.Ø1
- spinocerebellar (hereditary) G11.9
  - specified NEC G11.8
- spleen D73.9
  - amyloid E85.4 *[D77]*
  - organic D73.9
  - polycystic Q89.Ø9
  - postinfectional D73.89
- sponge-diver's — *see* Toxicity, venom, marine animal, sea anemone
- Startle Q89.8
- Steinert's G71.11
- Sticker's (erythema infectiosum) BØ8.3
- Stieda's (calcification, knee joint) — *see* Bursitis, tibial collateral
- Stokes' (exophthalmic goiter) — *see* Hyperthyroidism, with, goiter (diffuse)
- Stokes-Adams (syncope with heart block) I45.9
- stomach K31.9
  - functional, psychogenic F45.8
  - specified NEC K31.89
- stonemason's J62.8
- storage
  - glycogen — *see* Disease, glycogen storage
  - mucopolysaccharide — *see* Mucopolysaccharidosis

Disease, diseased — *continued*
- striatopallidal system NEC G25.89
- Stuart-Prower (congenital factor X deficiency) D68.2
- Stuart's (congenital factor X deficiency) D68.2
- subcutaneous tissue — *see* Disease, skin
- supporting structures of teeth KØ8.9
  - specified NEC KØ8.89
- suprarenal (capsule) (gland) E27.9
  - hyperfunction E27.Ø
  - specified NEC E27.8
- sweat glands L74.9
  - specified NEC L74.8
- Sweeley-Klionsky E75.21
- Swift (-Feer) — *see* Poisoning, mercury
- swimming-pool granuloma A31.1
- Sylvest's (epidemic pleurodynia) B33.Ø
- sympathetic nervous system G9Ø.9
- synovium — *see* Disorder, synovium
- syphilitic — *see* Syphilis
- systemic tissue mast cell D47.Ø2
- tanapox (virus) BØ8.71
- Tangier E78.6
- Tarral-Besnier (pityriasis rubra pilaris) L44.Ø
- Tauri's E74.Ø9
- tear duct — *see* Disorder, lacrimal system
- tendon, tendinous — *see also* Disorder, tendon
  - nodular — *see* Trigger finger
- terminal vessel I73.9
- testis N5Ø.9
- thalassemia Hb-S — *see* Disease, sickle-cell, thalassemia
- Thaysen-Gee (nontropical sprue) K9Ø.Ø
- Thomsen G71.12
- throat J39.2
  - septic JØ2.Ø
- thromboembolic — *see* Embolism
- thymus (gland) E32.9
  - specified NEC E32.8
- thyroid (gland) EØ7.9
  - heart — *see also* Hyperthyroidism EØ5.9Ø *[I43]*
    - with thyroid storm EØ5.91 *[I43]*
  - specified NEC EØ7.89
- Tietze's M94.Ø
- tongue K14.9
  - specified NEC K14.8
- tonsils, tonsillar (and adenoids) J35.9
- tooth, teeth KØ8.9
  - hard tissues KØ3.9
    - specified NEC KØ3.89
  - pulp NEC KØ4.99
  - specified NEC KØ8.89
- Tourette's F95.2
- trachea NEC J39.8
- tricuspid IØ7.9
  - nonrheumatic I36.9
- triglyceride-storage E75.5
- trophoblastic — *see* Mole, hydatidiform
- tsutsugamushi A75.3
- tube (fallopian) (noninflammatory) N83.9
  - inflammatory — *see* Salpingitis
  - specified NEC N83.8
- tuberculous NEC — *see* Tuberculosis
- tubo-ovarian (noninflammatory) N83.9
  - inflammatory — *see* Salpingo-oophoritis
  - specified NEC N83.8
- tubotympanic, chronic — *see* Otitis, media, suppurative, chronic, tubotympanic
- tubulo-interstitial N15.9
  - specified NEC N15.8
- tympanum — *see* Disorder, tympanic membrane
- Uhl's Q24.8
- Underwood's (sclerema neonatorum) P83.Ø
- Unverricht (-Lundborg) — *see* Epilepsy, generalized, idiopathic
- Urbach-Oppenheim (necrobiosis lipoidica diabeticorum) — *see* EØ8-E13 with .62Ø
- ureter N28.9
  - in (due to)
    - schistosomiasis (bilharziasis) B65.Ø *[N29]*
- urethra N36.9
  - specified NEC N36.8
- urinary (tract) N39.9
  - bladder N32.9
    - specified NEC N32.89
  - specified NEC N39.8
- uterus (noninflammatory) N85.9
  - infective — *see* Endometritis
  - inflammatory — *see* Endometritis
  - specified NEC N85.8

Disease, diseased — *continued*
- uveal tract (anterior) H21.9
  - posterior H31.9
- vagabond's B85.1
- vagina, vaginal (noninflammatory) N89.9
  - inflammatory NEC N76.89
  - specified NEC N89.8
- valve, valvular I38
  - multiple IØ8.9
    - specified NEC IØ8.8
- van Creveld-von Gierke (glycogenosis I) E74.Ø1
- vas deferens N5Ø.9
- vascular I99.9
  - arteriosclerotic — *see* Arteriosclerosis
  - ciliary body NEC — *see* Disorder, iris, vascular
  - hypertensive — *see* Hypertension
  - iris NEC — *see* Disorder, iris, vascular
  - obliterative I77.1
    - peripheral I73.9
  - occlusive I99.8
  - peripheral (occlusive) I73.9
    - in diabetes mellitus — *see* EØ8-E13 with .51
- vasomotor I73.9
- vasospastic I73.9
- vein I87.9
- venereal — *see also* Disease, sexually transmitted A64
  - chlamydial NEC A56.8
    - anus A56.3
    - genitourinary NOS A56.2
    - pharynx A56.4
    - rectum A56.3
  - fifth A55
  - sixth A55
  - specified nature or type NEC A63.8
- vertebra, vertebral — *see also* Spondylopathy
  - disc — *see* Disorder, disc
- vibration — *see* Vibration, adverse effects
- viral, virus — *see also* Disease, by type of virus B34.9
  - arbovirus NOS A94
  - arthropod-borne NOS A94
  - congenital P35.9
    - specified NEC P35.8
  - Hanta (with renal manifestations) (Dobrava) (Puumala) (Seoul) A98.5
    - with pulmonary manifestations (Andes) (Bayou) (Bermejo) (Black Creek Canal) (Choclo) (Juquitiba) (Laguna negra) (Lechiguanas) (New York) (Oran) (Sin nombre) B33.4
  - Hantaan (Korean hemorrhagic fever) A98.5
  - human immunodeficiency (HIV) B2Ø
  - Kunjin A83.4
  - nonarthropod-borne NOS B34.9
  - Powassan A84.81
  - Rocio (encephalitis) A83.6
  - Sin nombre (Hantavirus) (cardio)-pulmonary syndrome) B33.4
  - Tahyna B33.8
  - vesicular stomatitis A93.8
- vitreous H43.9
  - specified NEC H43.89
- vocal cord J38.3
- Volkmann's, acquired T79.6 ☑
- von Eulenburg's (congenital paramyotonia) G71.19
- von Gierke's (glycogenosis I) E74.Ø1
- von Graefe's — *see* Strabismus, paralytic, ophthalmoplegia, progressive
- von Willebrand (-Jürgens) (angiohemophilia) D68.Ø
- Vrolik's (osteogenesis imperfecta) Q78.Ø
- vulva (noninflammatory) N9Ø.9
  - inflammatory NEC N76.89
  - specified NEC N9Ø.89
- Wallgren's (obstruction of splenic vein with collateral circulation) I87.8
- Wassilieff's (leptospiral jaundice) A27.Ø
- wasting NEC R64
  - due to malnutrition E41
- Waterhouse-Friderichsen A39.1
- Wegner's (syphilitic osteochondritis) A5Ø.Ø2
- Weil's (leptospiral jaundice of lung) A27.Ø
- Weir Mitchell's (erythromelalgia) I73.81
- Werdnig-Hoffmann G12.Ø
- Wermer's E31.21
- Werner-His (trench fever) A79.Ø
- Werner-Schultz (neutropenic splenomegaly) D73.81
- Wernicke-Posadas B38.9
- whipworm B79
- white blood cells D72.9
  - specified NEC D72.89

Index Dislocation — Disorder

- **Disorder** — *continued*
  - bone — *continued*
    - development and growth — *continued*
      - radius M89.23- ☑
      - rib M89.28
      - scapula M89.21- ☑
      - skull M89.28
      - tarsus M89.27- ☑
      - tibia M89.26- ☑
      - toe M89.27- ☑
      - ulna M89.23- ☑
      - vertebra M89.28
    - specified type NEC M89.8X- ☑
  - brachial plexus G54.0
  - branched-chain amino-acid metabolism E71.2
    - specified NEC E71.19
  - breast N64.9
    - agalactia — *see* Agalactia
    - associated with
      - lactation O92.70
        - specified NEC O92.79
      - pregnancy O92.20
        - specified NEC O92.29
      - puerperium O92.20
        - specified NEC O92.29
    - cracked nipple — *see* Cracked nipple
    - galactorrhea — *see* Galactorrhea
    - hypogalactia O92.4
    - lactation disorder NEC O92.79
    - mastitis — *see* Mastitis
    - nipple infection — *see* Infection, nipple
    - retracted nipple — *see* Retraction, nipple
    - specified type NEC N64.89
  - Briquet's F45.0
  - bullous, in diseases classified elsewhere L14
  - caffeine use
    - mild
      - with
        - caffeine-induced
          - anxiety disorder F15.180
          - sleep disorder F15.182
    - moderate or severe
      - with
        - caffeine-induced
          - anxiety disorder F15.280
          - sleep disorder F15.282
  - cannabis use
    - mild F12.10
      - with
        - cannabis intoxication delirium F12.121
          - with perceptual disturbances F12.122
          - without perceptual disturbances F12.129
        - cannabis-induced
          - anxiety disorder F12.180
          - psychotic disorder F12.159
          - sleep disorder F12.188
      - in remission (early) (sustained) F12.11
    - moderate or severe F12.20
      - with
        - cannabis intoxication
          - with perceptual disturbances F12.222
          - without perceptual disturbances F12.229
        - cannabis-induced
          - anxiety disorder F12.280
          - psychotic disorder F12.259
          - sleep disorder F12.288
        - delirium F12.221
      - in remission (early) (sustained) F12.21
  - carbohydrate
    - absorption, intestinal NEC E74.39
    - metabolism (congenital) E74.9
      - specified NEC E74.89
  - cardiac, functional I51.89
  - carnitine metabolism E71.40
  - cartilage M94.9
    - articular NEC — *see* Derangement, joint, articular cartilage
      - chondrocalcinosis — *see* Chondrocalcinosis
    - specified type NEC M94.8X- ☑
      - articular — *see* Derangement, joint, articular cartilage
      - multiple sites M94.8X0
  - catatonia (due to known physiological condition) (with another mental disorder) F06.1
  - catatonic
    - due to (secondary to) known physiological condition F06.1
    - organic F06.1
  - central auditory processing H93.25
  - cervical
    - region NEC M53.82
    - root (nerve) NEC G54.2
  - character NOS F60.9
  - childhood disintegrative NEC F84.3
  - cholesterol and bile acid metabolism E78.70
    - Barth syndrome E78.71
    - other specified E78.79
    - Smith-Lemli-Opitz syndrome E78.72
  - choroid H31.9
    - atrophy — *see* Atrophy, choroid
    - degeneration — *see* Degeneration, choroid
    - detachment — *see* Detachment, choroid
    - dystrophy — *see* Dystrophy, choroid
    - hemorrhage — *see* Hemorrhage, choroid
    - rupture — *see* Rupture, choroid
    - scar — *see* Scar, chorioretinal
    - solar retinopathy — *see* Retinopathy, solar
    - specified type NEC H31.8
  - ciliary body — *see* Disorder, iris
    - degeneration — *see* Degeneration, ciliary body
  - coagulation (factor) — *see also* Defect, coagulation D68.9
    - newborn, transient P61.6
  - cocaine use
    - mild F14.10
      - with
        - amphetamine, cocaine, or other stimulant intoxication
          - with perceptual disturbances F14.122
          - without perceptual disturbances F14.129
        - cocaine intoxication delirium F14.121
        - cocaine-induced
          - anxiety disorder F14.180
          - bipolar and related disorder F14.14
          - depressive disorder F14.14
          - obsessive-compulsive and related disorder F14.188
          - psychotic disorder F14.159
          - sexual dysfunction F14.181
          - sleep disorder F14.182
      - in remission (early) (sustained) F14.11
    - moderate or severe F14.20
      - with
        - amphetamine, cocaine, or other stimulant intoxication
          - with perceptual disturbances F14.222
          - without perceptual disturbances F14.229
        - cocaine intoxication delirium F14.221
        - cocaine-induced
          - anxiety disorder F14.280
          - bipolar and related disorder F14.24
          - depressive disorder F14.24
          - obsessive-compulsive and related disorder F14.288
          - psychotic disorder F14.259
          - sexual dysfunction F14.281
          - sleep disorder F14.282
      - in remission (early) (sustained) F14.21
  - coccyx NEC M53.3
  - cognitive F09
    - due to (secondary to) general medical condition F09
    - persisting R41.89
      - due to
        - alcohol F10.97
          - with dependence F10.27
        - anxiolytics F13.97
          - with dependence F13.27
        - hypnotics F13.97
          - with dependence F13.27
        - sedatives F13.97
          - with dependence F13.27
        - specified substance NEC F19.97
          - with
            - abuse F19.17
            - dependence F19.27
  - communication F80.9
    - social pragmatic F80.82
  - conduct (childhood) F91.9
    - adjustment reaction — *see* Disorder, adjustment
    - adolescent onset type F91.2
    - childhood onset type F91.1
    - compulsive F63.9
    - confined to family context F91.0
    - depressive F91.8
    - group type F91.2
- **Disorder** — *continued*
  - conduct — *continued*
    - hyperkinetic — *see* Disorder, attention-deficit hyperactivity
    - oppositional defiance F91.3
    - socialized F91.2
    - solitary aggressive type F91.1
    - specified NEC F91.8
    - unsocialized (aggressive) F91.1
  - conduction, heart I45.9
  - congenital glycosylation (CDG) E74.89
  - conjunctiva H11.9
    - infection — *see* Conjunctivitis
  - connective tissue, localized L94.9
    - specified NEC L94.8
  - conversion (functional neurological symptom disorder)
    - with
      - abnormal movement F44.4
      - anesthesia or sensory loss F44.6
      - attacks or seizures F44.5
      - mixed symptoms F44.7
      - special sensory symptoms F44.6
      - speech symptoms F44.4
      - swallowing symptoms F44.4
      - weakness or paralysis F44.4
  - convulsive (secondary) — *see* Convulsions
  - cornea H18.9
    - deformity — *see* Deformity, cornea
    - degeneration — *see* Degeneration, cornea
    - deposits — *see* Deposit, cornea
    - due to contact lens H18.82- ☑
      - specified as edema — *see* Edema, cornea
    - edema — *see* Edema, cornea
    - keratitis — *see* Keratitis
    - keratoconjunctivitis — *see* Keratoconjunctivitis
    - membrane change — *see* Change, corneal membrane
    - neovascularization — *see* Neovascularization, cornea
    - scar — *see* Opacity, cornea
    - specified type NEC H18.89- ☑
    - ulcer — *see* Ulcer, cornea
  - corpus cavernosum N48.9
  - cranial nerve — *see* Disorder, nerve, cranial
  - Cyclin-Dependent Kinase-Like 5 Deficiency (CDKL5) G40.42
  - cyclothymic F34.0
  - defiant oppositional F91.3
  - delusional (persistent) (systematized) F22
    - induced F24
  - depersonalization F48.1
  - depressive F32.9
    - due to known physiological condition
      - with
        - depressive features F06.31
        - major depressive-like episode F06.32
        - mixed features F06.34
    - major F32.9
      - with psychotic symptoms F32.3
      - in remission (full) F32.5
        - partial F32.4
      - recurrent F33.9
        - with psychotic features F33.3
      - single episode F32.9
        - mild F32.0
        - moderate F32.1
        - severe (without psychotic symptoms) F32.2
          - with psychotic symptoms F32.3
    - organic F06.31
    - persistent F34.1
    - recurrent F33.9
      - current episode
        - mild F33.0
        - moderate F33.1
        - severe (without psychotic symptoms) F33.2
          - with psychotic symptoms F33.3
      - in remission F33.40
        - full F33.42
        - partial F33.41
      - specified NEC F33.8
    - single episode — *see* Episode, depressive
    - specified NEC F32.89
  - developmental F89
    - arithmetical skills F81.2
    - coordination (motor) F82
    - expressive writing F81.81
    - language F80.9
      - expressive F80.1

- **Disorder** — *continued*
  - developmental — *continued*
    - language — *continued*
      - mixed receptive and expressive F8Ø.2
      - receptive type F8Ø.2
      - specified NEC F8Ø.89
    - learning F81.9
      - arithmetical F81.2
      - reading F81.Ø
    - mixed F88
    - motor coordination or function F82
    - pervasive F84.9
      - specified NEC F84.8
    - phonological F8Ø.Ø
    - reading F81.Ø
    - scholastic skills — *see also* Disorder, learning
      - mixed F81.89
    - specified NEC F88
    - speech F8Ø.9
      - articulation F8Ø.Ø
      - specified NEC F8Ø.89
    - written expression F81.81
  - diaphragm J98.6
  - digestive (system) K92.9
    - newborn P78.9
      - specified NEC P78.89
    - postprocedural — *see* Complication, gastrointestinal
    - psychogenic F45.8
  - disc (intervertebral) M51.9
    - with
      - myelopathy
        - cervical region M5Ø.ØØ
        - cervicothoracic region M5Ø.Ø3
        - high cervical region M5Ø.Ø1
        - lumbar region M51.Ø6
        - mid-cervical region M5Ø.Ø2Ø
        - sacrococcygeal region M53.3
        - thoracic region M51.Ø4
        - thoracolumbar region M51.Ø5
      - radiculopathy
        - cervical region M5Ø.1Ø
        - cervicothoracic region M5Ø.13
        - high cervical region M5Ø.11
        - lumbar region M51.16
        - lumbosacral region M51.17
        - mid-cervical region M5Ø.12Ø
        - sacrococcygeal region M53.3
        - thoracic region M51.14
        - thoracolumbar region M51.15
    - cervical M5Ø.9Ø
      - with
        - myelopathy M5Ø.ØØ
          - C2-C3 M5Ø.Ø1
          - C3-C4 M5Ø.Ø1
          - C4-C5 M5Ø.Ø21
          - C5-C6 M5Ø.Ø22
          - C6-C7 M5Ø.Ø23
          - C7-T1 M5Ø.Ø3
          - cervicothoracic region M5Ø.Ø3
          - high cervical region M5Ø.Ø1
          - mid-cervical region M5Ø.Ø2Ø
        - neuritis, radiculitis or radiculopathy M5Ø.1Ø
          - C2-C3 M5Ø.11
          - C3-C4 M5Ø.11
          - C4-C5 M5Ø.121
          - C5-C6 M5Ø.122
          - C6-C7 M5Ø.123
          - C7-T1 M5Ø.13
          - cervicothoracic region M5Ø.13
          - high cervical region M5Ø.11
          - mid-cervical region M5Ø.12Ø
      - C2-C3 M5Ø.91
      - C3-C4 M5Ø.91
      - C4-C5 M5Ø.921
      - C5-C6 M5Ø.922
      - C6-C7 M5Ø.923
      - C7-T1 M5Ø.93
      - cervicothoracic region M5Ø.93
      - degeneration M5Ø.3Ø
        - C2-C3 M5Ø.31
        - C3-C4 M5Ø.31
        - C4-C5 M5Ø.321
        - C5-C6 M5Ø.322
        - C6-C7 M5Ø.323
        - C7-T1 M5Ø.33
        - cervicothoracic region M5Ø.33
        - high cervical region M5Ø.31
        - mid-cervical region M5Ø.32Ø
      - displacement M5Ø.2Ø

- **Disorder** — *continued*
  - disc — *continued*
    - cervical — *continued*
      - displacement — *continued*
        - C2-C3 M5Ø.21
        - C3-C4 M5Ø.21
        - C4-C5 M5Ø.221
        - C5-C6 M5Ø.222
        - C6-C7 M5Ø.223
        - C7-T1 M5Ø.23
        - cervicothoracic region M5Ø.23
        - high cervical region M5Ø.21
        - mid-cervical region M5Ø.22Ø
      - high cervical region M5Ø.91
      - mid-cervical region M5Ø.92Ø
      - specified type NEC M5Ø.8Ø
        - C2-C3 M5Ø.81
        - C3-C4 M5Ø.81
        - C4-C5 M5Ø.821
        - C5-C6 M5Ø.822
        - C6-C7 M5Ø.823
        - C7-T1 M5Ø.83
        - cervicothoracic region M5Ø.83
        - high cervical region M5Ø.81
        - mid-cervical region M5Ø.82Ø
    - specified NEC
      - lumbar region M51.86
      - lumbosacral region M51.87
      - sacrococcygeal region M53.3
      - thoracic region M51.84
      - thoracolumbar region M51.85
  - disinhibited attachment (childhood) F94.2
  - disintegrative, childhood NEC F84.3
  - disruptive F91.9
    - mood dysregulation F34.81
    - specified NEC F91.8
  - disruptive behavior — *see* Disorder, conduct
  - dissocial personality F6Ø.2
  - dissociative F44.9
    - affecting
      - motor function F44.4
        - and sensation F44.7
      - sensation F44.6
        - and motor function F44.7
    - brief reactive F43.Ø
    - due to (secondary to) general medical condition F Ø6.8
    - mixed F44.7
    - organic FØ6.8
    - other specified NEC F44.89
  - double heterozygous sickling — *see* Disease, sickle-cell
  - dream anxiety F51.5
  - drug induced hemorrhagic D68.32
  - drug related F19.99
    - abuse — *see* Abuse, drug
    - dependence — *see* Dependence, drug
  - dysmorphic body F45.22
  - dysthymic F34.1
  - ear H93.9- ☑
    - bleeding — *see* Otorrhagia
    - deafness — *see* Deafness
    - degenerative H93.Ø9- ☑
    - discharge — *see* Otorrhea
    - external H61.9- ☑
      - auditory canal stenosis — *see* Stenosis, external ear canal
      - exostosis — *see* Exostosis, external ear canal
      - impacted cerumen — *see* Impaction, cerumen
      - otitis — *see* Otitis, externa
      - perichondritis — *see* Perichondritis, ear
      - pinna — *see* Disorder, pinna
      - specified type NEC H61.89- ☑
    - inner H83.9- ☑
      - vestibular dysfunction — *see* Disorder, vestibular function
    - middle H74.9- ☑
      - adhesive H74.1- ☑
      - ossicle — *see* Abnormal, ear ossicles
      - polyp — *see* Polyp, ear (middle)
      - specified NEC, in diseases classified elsewhere H75.8- ☑
    - postprocedural — *see* Complications, ear, procedure
    - specified NEC, in diseases classified elsewhere H94.8- ☑
  - eating (adult) (psychogenic) F5Ø.9
    - anorexia — *see* Anorexia
    - binge F5Ø.81
    - bulimia F5Ø.2

- **Disorder** — *continued*
  - eating — *continued*
    - child F98.29
      - pica F98.3
      - rumination disorder F98.21
    - pica F5Ø.89
      - childhood F98.3
  - electrolyte (balance) NEC E87.8
    - with
      - abortion — *see* Abortion by type complicated by specified condition NEC
      - ectopic pregnancy OØ8.5
      - molar pregnancy OØ8.5
    - acidosis (metabolic) (respiratory) E87.2
    - alkalosis (metabolic) (respiratory) E87.3
  - elimination, transepidermal L87.9
    - specified NEC L87.8
  - emotional (persistent) F34.9
    - of childhood F93.9
      - specified NEC F93.8
  - endocrine E34.9
    - postprocedural E89.89
      - specified NEC E89.89
  - erectile (male) (organic) — *see also* Dysfunction, sexual, male, erectile N52.9
    - nonorganic F52.21
  - erythematous — *see* Erythema
  - esophagus K22.9
    - functional K22.4
    - psychogenic F45.8
  - eustachian tube H69.9- ☑
    - infection — *see* Salpingitis, eustachian
    - obstruction — *see* Obstruction, eustachian tube
    - patulous — *see* Patulous, eustachian tube
    - specified NEC H69.8- ☑
  - exhibitionistic F65.2
  - extrapyramidal G25.9
    - in deseases classified elsewhere — *see* category G26
    - specified type NEC G25.89
  - eye H57.9
    - postprocedural — *see* Complication, postprocedural, eye
  - eyelid HØ2.9
    - cyst — *see* Cyst, eyelid
    - degenerative HØ2.7Ø
      - chloasma — *see* Chloasma, eyelid
      - madarosis — *see* Madarosis
      - specified type NEC HØ2.79
      - vitiligo — *see* Vitiligo, eyelid
      - xanthelasma — *see* Xanthelasma
    - dermatochalasis — *see* Dermatochalasis
    - edema — *see* Edema, eyelid
    - elephantiasis — *see* Elephantiasis, eyelid
    - foreign body, retained — *see* Foreign body, retained, eyelid
    - function HØ2.59
      - abnormal innervation syndrome — *see* Syndrome, abnormal innervation
      - blepharochalasis — *see* Blepharochalasis
      - blepharoclonus — *see* Blepharoclonus
      - blepharophimosis — *see* Blepharophimosis
      - blepharoptosis — *see* Blepharoptosis
      - lagophthalmos — *see* Lagophthalmos
      - lid retraction — *see* Retraction, lid
    - hypertrichosis — *see* Hypertrichosis, eyelid
    - specified type NEC HØ2.89
    - vascular HØ2.879
      - left HØ2.876
        - lower HØ2.875
        - upper HØ2.874
      - right HØ2.873
        - lower HØ2.872
        - upper HØ2.871
  - factitious
    - by proxy F68.A
    - imposed on another F68.A
    - imposed on self F68.1Ø
      - with predominantly
        - psychological symptoms F68.11
          - with physical symptoms F68.13
        - physical symptoms F68.12
          - with psychological symptoms F68.13
  - factor, coagulation — *see* Defect, coagulation
  - fatty acid
    - metabolism E71.3Ø
      - specified NEC E71.39

- **Disorder** — *continued*
  - fatty acid — *continued*
    - oxidation
      - LCAD E71.310
      - MCAD E71.311
      - SCAD E71.312
      - specified deficiency NEC E71.318
  - feeding (infant or child) — *see also* Disorder, eating R63.3
    - or eating disorder F50.9
    - specified NEC F50.9
  - feigned (with obvious motivation) Z76.5
    - without obvious motivation — *see* Disorder, factitious
  - female
    - hypoactive sexual desire F52.0
    - orgasmic F52.31
    - sexual interest/arousal F52.22
  - fetishistic F65.0
  - fibroblastic M72.9
    - specified NEC M72.8
  - fluency
    - adult onset F98.5
    - childhood onset F80.81
    - following
      - cerebral infarction I69.323
      - cerebrovascular disease I69.923
        - specified disease NEC I69.823
      - intracerebral hemorrhage I69.123
      - nontraumatic intracranial hemorrhage NEC I69.223
      - subarachnoid hemorrhage I69.023
    - in conditions classified elsewhere R47.82
  - fluid balance E87.8
  - follicular (skin) L73.9
    - specified NEC L73.8
  - frotteuristic F65.81
  - fructose metabolism E74.10
    - essential fructosuria E74.11
    - fructokinase deficiency E74.11
    - fructose-1, 6-diphosphatase deficiency E74.19
    - hereditary fructose intolerance E74.12
    - other specified E74.19
  - functional polymorphonuclear neutrophils D71
  - gallbladder, biliary tract and pancreas in diseases classified elsewhere K87
  - gambling F63.0
  - gamma aminobutyric acid (GABA) metabolism E72.81
  - gamma-glutamyl cycle E72.89
  - gastric (functional) K31.9
    - motility K30
    - psychogenic F45.8
    - secretion K30
  - gastrointestinal (functional) NOS K92.9
    - newborn P78.9
    - psychogenic F45.8
  - gender-identity or -role F64.9
    - childhood F64.2
    - effect on relationship F66
    - of adolescence or adulthood F64.0
      - nontranssexual F64.8
    - specified NEC F64.8
    - uncertainty F66
  - genito-pelvic pain penetration F52.6
  - genitourinary system
    - female N94.9
    - male N50.9
    - psychogenic F45.8
  - globe H44.9
    - degenerated condition H44.50
      - absolute glaucoma H44.51- ☑
      - atrophy H44.52- ☑
      - leucocoria H44.53- ☑
    - degenerative H44.30
      - chalcosis H44.31- ☑
      - myopia — *see also* Myopia, degenerative H44.2- ☑
      - siderosis H44.32- ☑
      - specified type NEC H44.39- ☑
    - endophthalmitis — *see* Endophthalmitis
    - foreign body, retained — *see* Foreign body, intraocular, old, retained
    - hemophthalmos — *see* Hemophthalmos
    - hypotony H44.40
      - due to
        - ocular fistula H44.42- ☑
        - specified disorder NEC H44.43- ☑
      - flat anterior chamber H44.41- ☑

- **Disorder** — *continued*
  - globe — *continued*
    - hypotony — *continued*
      - primary H44.44- ☑
    - luxation — *see* Luxation, globe
    - specified type NEC H44.89
  - glomerular (in) N05.9
    - amyloidosis E85.4 *[N08]*
    - cryoglobulinemia D89.1 *[N08]*
    - disseminated intravascular coagulation D65 *[N08]*
    - Fabry's disease E75.21 *[N08]*
    - familial lecithin cholesterol acyltransferase deficiency E78.6 *[N08]*
    - Goodpasture's syndrome M31.0
    - hemolytic-uremic syndrome D59.3
    - Henoch (-Schönlein) purpura D69.0 *[N08]*
    - malariae malaria B52.0
    - microscopic polyangiitis M31.7 *[N08]*
    - multiple myeloma C90.0- ☑ *[N08]*
    - mumps B26.83
    - schistosomiasis B65.9 *[N08]*
    - sepsis NEC A41.- ☑ *[N08]*
      - streptococcal A40.- ☑ *[N08]*
    - sickle-cell disorders D57.- ☑ *[N08]*
    - strongyloidiasis B78.9 *[N08]*
    - subacute bacterial endocarditis I33.0 *[N08]*
    - syphilis A52.75
    - systemic lupus erythematosus M32.14
    - thrombotic thrombocytopenic purpura M31.1 *[N08]*
    - Waldenström macroglobulinemia C88.0 *[N08]*
    - Wegener's granulomatosis M31.31
  - gluconeogenesis E74.4
  - glucosaminoglycan metabolism — *see* Disorder, metabolism, glucosaminoglycan
  - gluecose transport E74.819
    - specified NEC E74.818
  - glycine metabolism E72.50
    - d-glycericacidemia E72.59
    - hyperhydroxyprolinemia E72.59
    - hyperoxaluria R82.992
      - primary E72.53
    - hyperprolinemia E72.59
    - non-ketotic hyperglycinemia E72.51
    - oxalosis E72.53
    - oxaluria E72.53
    - sarcosinemia E72.59
    - trimethylaminuria E72.52
  - glycoprotein metabolism E77.9
    - specified NEC E77.8
  - habit (and impulse) F63.9
    - involving sexual behavior NEC F65.9
    - specified NEC F63.89
  - hallucinogen use
    - mild F16.10
      - with
        - hallucinogen intoxication delirium F16.121
        - hallucinogen-induced
          - anxiety disorder F16.180
          - bipolar and related disorder F16.14
          - depressive disorder F16.14
          - psychotic disorder F16.159
        - other hallucinogen intoxication F16.129
      - in remission (early) (sustained) F16.11
    - moderate or severe F16.20
      - with
        - hallucinogen intoxication delirium F16.221
        - hallucinogen-induced
          - anxiety disorder F16.280
          - bipolar and related disorder F16.24
          - depressive disorder F16.24
          - psychotic disorder F16.259
        - other hallucinogen intoxication F16.229
      - in remission (early) (sustained) F16.21
  - heart action I49.9
  - hematological D75.9
    - newborn (transient) P61.9
      - specified NEC P61.8
  - hematopoietic organs D75.9
  - hemorrhagic NEC D69.9
    - drug-induced D68.32
    - due to
      - extrinsic circulating anticoagulants D68.32
      - increase in
        - anti-IIa D68.32
        - anti-Xa D68.32
      - intrinsic
        - circulating anticoagulants D68.318

- **Disorder** — *continued*
  - hemorrhagic — *continued*
    - due to — *continued*
      - intrinsic — *continued*
        - increase in
          - anti-IXa D68.318
          - antithrombin D68.318
          - anti-VIIIa D68.318
          - anti-XIa D68.318
    - following childbirth O72.3
  - hemostasis — *see* Defect, coagulation
  - histidine metabolism E70.40
    - histidinemia E70.41
    - other specified E70.49
  - hoarding F42.3
  - hyperkinetic — *see* Disorder, attention-deficit hyperactivity
  - hyperleucine-isoleucinemia E71.19
  - hypervalinemia E71.19
  - hypoactive sexual desire F52.0
  - hypochondriacal F45.20
    - body dysmorphic F45.22
    - neurosis F45.21
    - other specified F45.29
  - identity
    - dissociative F44.81
    - illness anxiety F45.21
    - of childhood F93.8
  - immune mechanism (immunity) D89.9
    - specified type NEC D89.89
  - impaired renal tubular function N25.9
    - specified NEC N25.89
  - impulse (control) F63.9
  - inflammatory
    - pelvic, in diseases classified elsewhere — *see* category N74
    - penis N48.29
      - abscess N48.21
      - cellulitis N48.22
  - inhalant use
    - mild F18.10
      - with
        - inhalant intoxication F18.129
        - inhalant intoxication delirium F18.121
        - inhalant-induced
          - anxiety disorder F18.180
          - depressive disorder F18.14
          - major neurocognitive disorder F18.17
          - mild neurocognitive disorder F18.188
          - psychotic disorder F18.159
      - in remission (early) (sustained) F18.11
    - moderate or severe F18.20
      - with
        - inhalant intoxication F18.229
        - inhalant intoxication delirium F18.221
        - inhalant-induced
          - anxiety disorder F18.280
          - depressive disorder F18.24
          - major neurocognitive disorder F18.27
          - mild neurocognitive disorder F18.288
          - psychotic disorder F18.259
      - in remission (early) (sustained) F18.21
  - integument, newborn P83.9
    - specified NEC P83.88
  - intermittent explosive F63.81
  - internal secretion pancreas — *see* Increased, secretion, pancreas, endocrine
  - intestine, intestinal
    - carbohydrate absorption NEC E74.39
      - postoperative K91.2
    - functional NEC K59.9
      - postoperative K91.89
    - psychogenic F45.8
    - vascular K55.9
      - chronic K55.1
      - specified NEC K55.8
  - intraoperative (intraprocedural) — *see* Complications, intraoperative
  - involuntary emotional expression (IEED) F07.89
  - iris H21.9
    - adhesions — *see* Adhesions, iris
    - atrophy — *see* Atrophy, iris
    - chamber angle recession — *see* Recession, chamber angle
    - cyst — *see* Cyst, iris
    - degeneration — *see* Degeneration, iris
    - in diseases classified elsewhere H22
    - iridodialysis — *see* Iridodialysis

- **Disorder** — *continued*
  - neurocognitive — *continued*
    - major — *continued*
      - due to vascular disease, with behavioral disturbance F01.51
      - in (due to) (other diseases classified elsewhere) — *see also* Dementia, in (due to) F02.80
        - with
          - aggressive behavior F02.81
          - combative behavior F02.81
          - violent behavior F02.81
      - without behavioral disturbance F01.50
    - mild G31.84
  - neurodevelopmental F89
    - specified NEC F88
  - neurohypophysis NEC E23.3
  - neurological NEC R29.818
  - neuromuscular G70.9
    - hereditary NEC G71.9
    - specified NEC G70.89
    - toxic G70.1
  - neurotic F48.9
    - specified NEC F48.8
  - neutrophil, polymorphonuclear D71
  - nicotine use — *see* Dependence, drug, nicotine
  - nightmare F51.5
  - non-rapid eye movement sleep arousal
    - sleep terror type F51.4
    - sleepwalking type F51.3
  - nose J34.9
    - specified NEC J34.89
  - obsessive-compulsive F42.9
    - and related disorder due to a known physiological condition F06.8
  - odontogenesis NOS K00.9
  - opioid use
    - with
      - opioid-induced psychotic disorder F11.959
        - with
          - delusions F11.950
          - hallucinations F11.951
    - due to drug abuse — *see* Abuse, drug, opioid
    - due to drug dependence — *see* Dependence, drug, opioid
    - mild F11.10
      - with
        - opioid-induced
          - anxiety disorder F11.188
          - depressive disorder F11.14
          - sexual dysfunction F11.181
        - opioid intoxication
          - with perceptual disturbances F11.122
          - delirium F11.121
          - without perceptual disturbances F11.129
      - in remission (early) (sustained) F11.11
    - moderate or severe F11.20
      - with
        - opioid-induced
          - anxiety disorder F11.288
          - anxiety disorder F11.988
          - depressive disorder F11.24
          - depressive disorder F11.94
          - sexual dysfunction F11.281
          - sexual dysfunction F11.981
        - opioid intoxication
          - with perceptual disturbances F11.222
          - delirium F11.221
          - without perceptual disturbances F11.229
      - in remission (early) (sustained) F11.21
  - oppositional defiant F91.3
  - optic
    - chiasm H47.49
      - due to
        - inflammatory disorder H47.41
        - neoplasm H47.42
        - vascular disorder H47.43
    - disc H47.39- ☑
      - coloboma — *see* Coloboma, optic disc
      - drusen — *see* Drusen, optic disc
      - pseudopapilledema — *see* Pseudopapilledema
    - radiations — *see* Disorder, visual, pathway
    - tracts — *see* Disorder, visual, pathway
  - orbit H05.9
    - cyst — *see* Cyst, orbit
    - deformity — *see* Deformity, orbit
    - edema — *see* Edema, orbit
    - enophthalmos — *see* Enophthalmos
    - exophthalmos — *see* Exophthalmos

- **Disorder** — *continued*
  - orbit — *continued*
    - hemorrhage — *see* Hemorrhage, orbit
    - inflammation — *see* Inflammation, orbit
    - myopathy — *see* Myopathy, extraocular muscles
    - retained foreign body — *see* Foreign body, orbit, old
    - specified type NEC H05.89
  - organic
    - anxiety F06.4
    - catatonic F06.1
    - delusional F06.2
    - dissociative F06.8
    - emotionally labile (asthenic) F06.8
    - mood (affective) F06.30
    - schizophrenia-like F06.2
  - orgasmic (female) F52.31
    - male F52.32
  - ornithine metabolism E72.4
  - overanxious F41.1
    - of childhood F93.8
  - pain
    - with related psychological factors F45.42
    - exclusively related to psychological factors F45.41
    - genito-pelvic penetration disorder F52.6
  - pancreatic internal secretion E16.9
    - specified NEC E16.8
  - panic F41.0
    - with agoraphobia F40.01
  - papulosquamous L44.9
    - in diseases classified elsewhere L45
    - specified NEC L44.8
  - paranoid F22
    - induced F24
    - shared F24
  - paraphilic F65.9
    - specified NEC F65.89
  - parathyroid (gland) E21.5
    - specified NEC E21.4
  - parietoalveolar NEC J84.09
  - paroxysmal, mixed R56.9
  - patella M22.9- ☑
    - chondromalacia — *see* Chondromalacia, patella
    - derangement NEC M22.3X- ☑
    - recurrent
      - dislocation — *see* Dislocation, patella, recurrent
      - subluxation — *see* Dislocation, patella, recurrent, incomplete
    - specified NEC M22.8X- ☑
  - patellofemoral M22.2X- ☑
  - pedophilic F65.4
  - pentose phosphate pathway with anemia D55.1
  - perception, due to hallucinogens F16.983
    - in
      - abuse F16.183
      - dependence F16.283
  - peripheral nervous system NEC G64
  - peroxisomal E71.50
    - biogenesis
      - neonatal adrenoleukodystrophy E71.511
      - specified disorder NEC E71.518
      - Zellweger syndrome E71.510
    - rhizomelic chondrodysplasia punctata E71.540
    - specified form NEC E71.548
      - group 1 E71.518
      - group 2 E71.53
      - group 3 E71.542
    - X-linked adrenoleukodystrophy E71.529
      - adolescent E71.521
      - adrenomyeloneuropathy E71.522
      - childhood E71.520
      - specified form NEC E71.528
    - Zellweger-like syndrome E71.541
  - persistent
    - (somatoform) pain F45.41
    - affective (mood) F34.9
  - personality — *see also* Personality F60.9
    - affective F34.0
    - aggressive F60.3
    - amoral F60.2
    - anankastic F60.5
    - antisocial F60.2
    - anxious F60.6
    - asocial F60.2
    - asthenic F60.7
    - avoidant F60.6
    - borderline F60.3

- **Disorder** — *continued*
  - personality — *see also* Personality — *continued*
    - change (secondary) due to general medical condition F07.0
    - compulsive F60.5
    - cyclothymic F34.0
    - dependent (passive) F60.7
    - depressive F34.1
    - dissocial F60.2
    - emotional instability F60.3
    - expansive paranoid F60.0
    - explosive F60.3
    - following organic brain damage F07.9
    - histrionic F60.4
    - hyperthymic F34.0
    - hypothymic F34.1
    - hysterical F60.4
    - immature F60.89
    - inadequate F60.7
    - labile F60.3
    - mixed (nonspecific) F60.89
    - moral deficiency F60.2
    - narcissistic F60.81
    - negativistic F60.89
    - obsessional F60.5
    - obsessive (-compulsive) F60.5
    - organic F07.9
    - overconscientious F60.5
    - paranoid F60.0
    - passive (-dependent) F60.7
    - passive-aggressive F60.89
    - pathological NEC F60.9
    - pseudosocial F60.2
    - psychopathic F60.2
    - schizoid F60.1
    - schizotypal F21
    - self-defeating F60.7
    - specified NEC F60.89
    - type A F60.5
    - unstable (emotional) F60.3
  - pervasive, developmental F84.9
  - phencyclidine use
    - mild F16.10
      - with
        - phencyclidine intoxication F16.129
        - phencyclidine intoxication delirium F16.121
        - phencyclidine-induced
          - anxiety disorder F16.180
          - bipolar and related disorder F16.14
          - depressive disorder F16.14
          - psychotic disorder F16.159
      - in remission (early) (sustained) F16.11
    - moderate or severe F16.20
      - with
        - phencyclidine intoxication F16.229
        - phencyclidine intoxication delirium F16.221
        - phencyclidine-induced
          - anxiety disorder F16.280
          - bipolar and related disorder F16.14
          - depressive disorder F16.24
          - psychotic disorder F16.259
      - in remission (early) (sustained) F16.21
  - phobic anxiety, childhood F40.8
  - phosphate-losing tubular N25.0
  - pigmentation L81.9
    - choroid, congenital Q14.3
    - diminished melanin formation L81.6
    - iron L81.8
    - specified NEC L81.8
  - pinna (noninfective) H61.10- ☑
    - deformity, acquired H61.11- ☑
    - hematoma H61.12- ☑
    - perichondritis — *see* Perichondritis, ear
    - specified type NEC H61.19- ☑
  - pituitary gland E23.7
    - iatrogenic (postprocedural) E89.3
    - specified NEC E23.6
  - platelets D69.1
  - plexus G54.9
    - specified NEC G54.8
  - polymorphonuclear neutrophils D71
  - porphyrin metabolism — *see* Porphyria
  - postconcussional F07.81
  - posthallucinogen perception F16.983
    - in
      - abuse F16.183
      - dependence F16.283
  - postmenopausal N95.9

Disorder — *continued*
tobacco use
chewing tobacco (mild) (moderate) (severe)
in remission (early) (sustained) F17.221
cigarettes (mild) (moderate) (severe)
in remission (early) (sustained) F17.211
mild F17.2ØØ
in remission (early) (sustained) F17.2Ø1
moderate F17.2ØØ
in remission (early) (sustained) F17.2Ø1
severe F17.2ØØ
in remission (early) (sustained) F17.2Ø1
specified product NEC (mild) (moderate) (severe)
in remission (early) (sustained) F17.291
tooth KØ8.9
development KØØ.9
specified NEC KØØ.8
eruption KØØ.6
Tourette's F95.2
trance and possession F44.89
transvestic F65.1
trauma and stressor-related F43.9
other specified F43.8
tricuspid (valve) — *see* Endocarditis, tricuspid
tryptophan metabolism E7Ø.5
tubular, phosphate-losing N25.Ø
tubulo-interstitial (in)
brucellosis A23.9 *[N16]*
cystinosis E72.Ø4
diphtheria A36.84
glycogen storage disease E74.ØØ *[N16]*
leukemia NEC C95.9- ☑ *[N16]*
lymphoma NEC C85.9- ☑ *[N16]*
mixed cryoglobulinemia D89.1 *[N16]*
multiple myeloma C9Ø.Ø- ☑ *[N16]*
Salmonella infection AØ2.25
sarcoidosis D86.84
sepsis A41.9 *[N16]*
streptococcal A4Ø.9 *[N16]*
systemic lupus erythematosus M32.15
toxoplasmosis B58.83
transplant rejection T86.91 *[N16]*
Wilson's disease E83.Ø1 *[N16]*
tubulo-renal function, impaired N25.9
specified NEC N25.89
tympanic membrane H73.9- ☑
atrophy — *see* Atrophy, tympanic membrane
infection — *see* Myringitis
perforation — *see* Perforation, tympanum
specified NEC H73.89- ☑
unsocialized aggressive F91.1
urea cycle metabolism E72.2Ø
argininemia E72.21
arginosuccinic aciduria E72.22
citrullinemia E72.23
ornithine transcarbamylase deficiency E72.4
other specified E72.29
ureter (in) N28.9
schistosomiasis B65.Ø *[N29]*
tuberculosis A18.11
urethra N36.9
specified NEC N36.8
urinary system N39.9
specified NEC N39.8
valve, heart
aortic — *see* Endocarditis, aortic
mitral — *see* Endocarditis, mitral
pulmonary — *see* Endocarditis, pulmonary
rheumatic
aortic — *see* Endocarditis, aortic, rheumatic
mitral — *see* Endocarditis, mitral
pulmonary — *see* Endocarditis, pulmonary, rheumatic
tricuspid — *see* Endocarditis, tricuspid
tricuspid — *see* Endocarditis, tricuspid
vestibular function H81.9- ☑
specified NEC — *see* subcategory H81.8 ☑
in diseases classified elsewhere H82.- ☑
vertigo — *see* Vertigo
vision, binocular H53.3Ø
abnormal retinal correspondence H53.31
diplopia H53.2
fusion with defective stereopsis H53.32
simultaneous perception H53.33
suppression H53.34
visual
cortex
blindness H47.619

Disorder — *continued*
visual — *continued*
cortex — *continued*
blindness — *continued*
left brain H47.612
right brain H47.611
due to
inflammatory disorder H47.629
left brain H47.622
right brain H47.621
neoplasm H47.639
left brain H47.632
right brain H47.631
vascular disorder H47.649
left brain H47.642
right brain H47.641
pathway H47.9
due to
inflammatory disorder H47.51- ☑
neoplasm H47.52- ☑
vascular disorder H47.53- ☑
optic chiasm — *see* Disorder, optic, chiasm
vitreous body H43.9
crystalline deposits — *see* Deposit, crystalline
degeneration — *see* Degeneration, vitreous
hemorrhage — *see* Hemorrhage, vitreous
opacities — *see* Opacity, vitreous
prolapse — *see* Prolapse, vitreous
specified type NEC H43.89
voice R49.9
specified type NEC R49.8
volatile solvent use
due to drug abuse — *see* Abuse, drug, inhalant
due to drug dependence — *see* Dependence, drug, inhalant
voyeuristic F65.3
white blood cells D72.9
specified NEC D72.89
withdrawing, child or adolescent F4Ø.1Ø
Disorientation R41.Ø
Displacement, displaced
acquired traumatic of bone, cartilage, joint, tendon NEC — *see* Dislocation
adrenal gland (congenital) Q89.1
appendix, retrocecal (congenital) Q43.8
auricle (congenital) Q17.4
bladder (acquired) N32.89
congenital Q64.19
brachial plexus (congenital) QØ7.8
brain stem, caudal (congenital) QØ4.8
canaliculus (lacrimalis), congenital Q1Ø.6
cardia through esophageal hiatus (congenital) Q4Ø.1
cerebellum, caudal (congenital) QØ4.8
cervix — *see* Malposition, uterus
colon (congenital) Q43.3
device, implant or graft — *see also* Complications, by site and type, mechanical T85.628 ☑
arterial graft NEC — *see* Complication, cardiovascular device, mechanical, vascular
breast (implant) T85.42 ☑
catheter NEC T85.628 ☑
dialysis (renal) T82.42 ☑
intraperitoneal T85.621 ☑
infusion NEC T82.524 ☑
spinal (epidural) (subdural) T85.62Ø ☑
urinary
cystostomy T83.Ø2Ø ☑
Hopkins T83.Ø28 ☑
ileostomy T83.Ø28 ☑
indwelling T83.Ø21 ☑
nephrostomy T83.Ø22 ☑
specified NEC T83.Ø28 ☑
urostomy T83.Ø28 ☑
electronic (electrode) (pulse generator) (stimulator) — *see* Complication, electronic stimulator
fixation, internal (orthopedic) NEC — *see* Complication, fixation device, mechanical
gastrointestinal — *see* Complications, prosthetic device, mechanical, gastrointestinal device
genital NEC T83.428 ☑
intrauterine contraceptive device (string) T83.32 ☑
penile prosthesis (cylinder) (implanted) (pump) (reservoir) T83.42Ø ☑
testicular prosthesis T83.421 ☑
heart NEC — *see* Complication, cardiovascular device, mechanical

Displacement, displaced — *continued*
device, implant or graft — *see also* Complications, by site and type, mechanical — *continued*
joint prosthesis — *see* Complications, joint prosthesis, mechanical
ocular — *see* Complications, prosthetic device, mechanical, ocular device
orthopedic NEC — *see* Complication, orthopedic, device or graft, mechanical
specified NEC T85.628 ☑
urinary NEC T83.128 ☑
graft T83.22 ☑
sphincter, implanted T83.121 ☑
stent (ileal conduit) (nephroureteral) T83.123 ☑
ureteral indwelling T83.122 ☑
vascular NEC — *see* Complication, cardiovascular device, mechanical
ventricular intracranial shunt T85.Ø2 ☑
electronic stimulator
bone T84.32Ø ☑
cardiac — *see* Complications, cardiac device, electronic
nervous system — *see* Complication, prosthetic device, mechanical, electronic nervous system stimulator
urinary — *see* Complications, electronic stimulator, urinary
esophageal mucosa into cardia of stomach, congenital Q39.8
esophagus (acquired) K22.8
congenital Q39.8
eyeball (acquired) (lateral) (old) — *see* Displacement, globe
congenital Q15.8
current — *see* Avulsion, eye
fallopian tube (acquired) N83.4- ☑
congenital Q5Ø.6
opening (congenital) Q5Ø.6
gallbladder (congenital) Q44.1
gastric mucosa (congenital) Q4Ø.2
globe (acquired) (old) (lateral) HØ5.21- ☑
current — *see* Avulsion, eye
heart (congenital) Q24.8
acquired I51.89
hymen (upward) (congenital) Q52.4
intervertebral disc NEC
with myelopathy — *see* Disorder, disc, with, myelopathy
cervical, cervicothoracic (with) M5Ø.2Ø
myelopathy — *see* Disorder, disc, cervical, with myelopathy
neuritis, radiculitis or radiculopathy — *see* Disorder, disc, cervical, with neuritis
due to trauma — *see* Dislocation, vertebra
lumbar region M51.26
with
myelopathy M51.Ø6
neuritis, radiculitis, radiculopathy or sciatica M51.16
lumbosacral region M51.27
with
neuritis, radiculitis, radiculopathy or sciatica M51.17
sacrococcygeal region M53.3
thoracic region M51.24
with
myelopathy M51.Ø4
neuritis, radiculitis, radiculopathy M51.14
thoracolumbar region M51.25
with
myelopathy M51.Ø5
neuritis, radiculitis, radiculopathy M51.15
intrauterine device (string) T83.32 ☑
kidney (acquired) N28.83
congenital Q63.2
lachrymal, lacrimal apparatus or duct (congenital) Q1Ø.6
lens, congenital Q12.1
macula (congenital) Q14.1
Meckel's diverticulum Q43.Ø
malignant — *see* Table of Neoplasms, small intestine, malignant
nail (congenital) Q84.6
acquired L6Ø.8
opening of Wharton's duct in mouth Q38.4
organ or site, congenital NEC — *see* Malposition, congenital
ovary (acquired) N83.4- ☑
congenital Q5Ø.39

Distress — *continued*
maternal, during labor and delivery O75.Ø
relationship, with spouse or intimate partner Z63.Ø
respiratory (adult) (child) RØ6.Ø3
newborn P22.9
specified NEC P22.8
orthopnea RØ6.Ø1
psychogenic F45.8
shortness of breath RØ6.Ø2
specified type NEC RØ6.Ø9
Distribution vessel, atypical Q27.9
coronary artery Q24.5
precerebral Q28.1
Districhiasis L68.8
Disturbance(s) — *see also* Disease
absorption K9Ø.9
calcium E58
carbohydrate K9Ø.49
fat K9Ø.49
pancreatic K9Ø.3
protein K9Ø.49
starch K9Ø.49
vitamin — *see* Deficiency, vitamin
acid-base equilibrium E87.8
mixed E87.4
activity and attention (with hyperkinesis) — *see* Disorder, attention-deficit hyperactivity
amino acid transport E72.ØØ
assimilation, food K9Ø.9
auditory nerve, except deafness — *see* subcategory H93.3 ☑
behavior — *see* Disorder, conduct
blood clotting (mechanism) — *see also* Defect, coagulation D68.9
cerebral
nerve — *see* Disorder, nerve, cranial
status, newborn P91.9
specified NEC P91.88
circulatory I99.9
conduct — *see also* Disorder, conduct F91.9
adjustment reaction — *see* Disorder, adjustment
compulsive F63.9
disruptive F91.9
hyperkinetic — *see* Disorder, attention-deficit hyperactivity
socialized F91.2
specified NEC F91.8
unsocialized F91.1
coordination R27.8
cranial nerve — *see* Disorder, nerve, cranial
deep sensibility — *see* Disturbance, sensation
digestive K3Ø
psychogenic F45.8
electrolyte — *see also* Imbalance, electrolyte
newborn, transitory P74.49
hyperammonemia P74.6
hyperchloremia P74.421
hyperchloremic metabolic acidosis P74.421
hypochloremia P74.422
potassium balance
hyperkalemia P74.31
hypokalemia P74.32
sodium balance
hypernatremia P74.21
hyponatremia P74.22
specified type NEC P74.49
emotions specific to childhood and adolescence F93.9
with
anxiety and fearfulness NEC F93.8
elective mutism F94.Ø
oppositional disorder F91.3
sensitivity (withdrawal) F4Ø.1Ø
shyness F4Ø.1Ø
social withdrawal F4Ø.1Ø
involving relationship problems F93.8
mixed F93.8
specified NEC F93.8
endocrine (gland) E34.9
neonatal, transitory P72.9
specified NEC P72.8
equilibrium R42
fructose metabolism E74.1Ø
gait — *see* Gait
hysterical F44.4
psychogenic F44.4
gastrointestinal (functional) K3Ø
psychogenic F45.8
habit, child F98.9

Disturbance(s) — *continued*
hearing, except deafness and tinnitus — *see* Abnormal, auditory perception
heart, functional (conditions in I44-I5Ø)
due to presence of (cardiac) prosthesis I97.19- ☑
postoperative I97.89
cardiac surgery — *see also* Infarct, myocardium, associated with revascularization procedure I97.19- ☑
hormones E34.9
innervation uterus (parasympathetic) (sympathetic) N85.8
keratinization NEC
gingiva KØ5.1Ø
nonplaque induced KØ5.11
plaque induced KØ5.1Ø
lip K13.Ø
oral (mucosa) (soft tissue) K13.29
tongue K13.29
learning (specific) — *see* Disorder, learning
memory — *see* Amnesia
mild, following organic brain damage FØ6.8
mental F99
associated with diseases classified elsewhere F54
metabolism E88.9
with
abortion — *see* Abortion, by type with other specified complication
ectopic pregnancy OØ8.5
molar pregnancy OØ8.5
amino-acid E72.9
aromatic E7Ø.9
branched-chain E71.2
straight-chain E72.89
sulfur-bearing E72.1Ø
ammonia E72.2Ø
arginine E72.21
arginosuccinic acid E72.22
carbohydrate E74.9
cholesterol E78.9
citrulline E72.23
cystathionine E72.19
general E88.9
glutamine E72.89
histidine E7Ø.4Ø
homocystine E72.19
hydroxylysine E72.3
in labor or delivery O75.89
iron E83.1Ø
lipoid E78.9
lysine E72.3
methionine E72.19
neonatal, transitory P74.9
calcium and magnesium P71.9
specified type NEC P71.8
carbohydrate metabolism P7Ø.9
specified type NEC P7Ø.8
specified NEC P74.8
ornithine E72.4
phosphate E83.39
sodium NEC E87.8
threonine E72.89
tryptophan E7Ø.5
tyrosine E7Ø.2Ø
urea cycle E72.2Ø
motor R29.2
nervous, functional R45.Ø
neuromuscular mechanism (eye), due to syphilis A52.15
nutritional E63.9
nail L6Ø.3
ocular motion H51.9
psychogenic F45.8
oculogyric H51.8
psychogenic F45.8
oculomotor H51.9
psychogenic F45.8
olfactory nerve R43.1
optic nerve NEC — *see* Disorder, nerve, optic
oral epithelium, including tongue NEC K13.29
perceptual due to
alcohol withdrawal F1Ø.232
amphetamine intoxication F15.922
in
abuse F15.122
dependence F15.222
anxiolytic withdrawal F13.232
cannabis intoxication (acute) F12.922

Disturbance(s) — *continued*
perceptual due to — *continued*
cannabis intoxication — *continued*
in
abuse F12.122
dependence F12.222
cocaine intoxication (acute) F14.922
in
abuse F14.122
dependence F14.222
hypnotic withdrawal F13.232
opioid intoxication (acute) F11.922
in
abuse F11.122
dependence F11.222
phencyclidine intoxication (acute) F16.122
sedative withdrawal F13.232
personality (pattern) (trait) — *see also* Disorder, personality F6Ø.9
following organic brain damage FØ7.9
polyglandular E31.9
specified NEC E31.8
potassium balance, newborn
hyperkalemia P74.31
hypokalemia P74.32
psychogenic F45.9
psychomotor F44.4
psychophysical visual H53.16
pupillary — *see* Anomaly, pupil, function
reflex R29.2
rhythm, heart I49.9
salivary secretion K11.7
sensation (cold) (heat) (localization) (tactile discrimination) (texture) (vibratory) NEC R2Ø.9
hysterical F44.6
skin R2Ø.9
anesthesia R2Ø.Ø
hyperesthesia R2Ø.3
hypoesthesia R2Ø.1
paresthesia R2Ø.2
specified type NEC R2Ø.8
smell R43.9
and taste (mixed) R43.8
anosmia R43.Ø
parosmia R43.1
specified NEC R43.8
taste R43.9
and smell (mixed) R43.8
parageusia R43.2
specified NEC R43.8
sensory — *see* Disturbance, sensation
situational (transient) — *see also* Disorder, adjustment
acute F43.Ø
sleep G47.9
nonorganic origin F51.9
smell — *see* Disturbance, sensation, smell
sociopathic F6Ø.2
sodium balance, newborn
hypernatremia P74.21
hyponatremia P74.22
speech R47.9
developmental F8Ø.9
specified NEC R47.89
stomach (functional) K31.9
sympathetic (nerve) G9Ø.9
taste — *see* Disturbance, sensation, taste
temperature
regulation, newborn P81.9
specified NEC P81.8
sense R2Ø.8
hysterical F44.6
tooth
eruption KØØ.6
formation KØØ.4
structure, hereditary NEC KØØ.5
touch — *see* Disturbance, sensation
vascular I99.9
arteriosclerotic — *see* Arteriosclerosis
vasomotor I73.9
vasospastic I73.9
vision, visual H53.9
following
cerebral infarction I69.398
cerebrovascular disease I69.998
specified NEC I69.898
intracerebral hemorrhage I69.198
nontraumatic intracranial hemorrhage NEC I69.298

Disturbance(s) — *continued*
  vision, visual — *continued*
    following — *continued*
      specified disease NEC I69.898
      subarachnoid hemorrhage I69.098
    psychophysical H53.16
    specified NEC H53.8
    subjective H53.10
      day blindness H53.11
      discomfort H53.14- ☑
      distortions of shape and size H53.15
      loss
        sudden H53.13- ☑
        transient H53.12- ☑
      specified type NEC H53.19
  voice R49.9
    psychogenic F44.4
    specified NEC R49.8
Diuresis R35.8
Diver's palsy, paralysis or squeeze T70.3 ☑
Diverticulitis (acute) K57.92
  bladder — *see* Cystitis
  ileum — *see* Diverticulitis, intestine, small
  intestine K57.92
    with
      abscess, perforation K57.80
        with bleeding K57.81
      bleeding K57.93
    congenital Q43.8
    large K57.32
      with
        abscess, perforation K57.20
          with bleeding K57.21
        bleeding K57.33
        small intestine K57.52
          with
            abscess, perforation K57.40
              with bleeding K57.41
            bleeding K57.53
    small K57.12
      with
        abscess, perforation K57.00
          with bleeding K57.01
        bleeding K57.13
        large intestine K57.52
          with
            abscess, perforation K57.40
              with bleeding K57.41
            bleeding K57.53
Diverticulosis K57.90
  with bleeding K57.91
  large intestine K57.30
    with
      bleeding K57.31
      small intestine K57.50
        with bleeding K57.51
  small intestine K57.10
    with
      bleeding K57.11
      large intestine K57.50
        with bleeding K57.51
Diverticulum, diverticula (multiple) K57.90
  appendix (noninflammatory) K38.2
  bladder (sphincter) N32.3
    congenital Q64.6
  bronchus (congenital) Q32.4
    acquired J98.09
  calyx, calyceal (kidney) N28.89
  cardia (stomach) K31.4
  cecum — *see* Diverticulosis, intestine, large
    congenital Q43.8
  colon — *see* Diverticulosis, intestine, large
    congenital Q43.8
  duodenum — *see* Diverticulosis, intestine, small
    congenital Q43.8
  epiphrenic (esophagus) K22.5
  esophagus (congenital) Q39.6
    acquired (epiphrenic) (pulsion) (traction) K22.5
  eustachian tube — *see* Disorder, eustachian tube, specified NEC
  fallopian tube N83.8
  gastric K31.4
  heart (congenital) Q24.8
  ileum — *see* Diverticulosis, intestine, small
  jejunum — *see* Diverticulosis, intestine, small
  kidney (pelvis) (calyces) N28.89
    with calculus — *see* Calculus, kidney
  Meckel's (displaced) (hypertrophic) Q43.0

Diverticulum, diverticula — *continued*
  Meckel's — *continued*
    malignant — *see* Table of Neoplasms, small intestine, malignant
  midthoracic K22.5
  organ or site, congenital NEC — *see* Distortion
  pericardium (congenital) (cyst) Q24.8
    acquired I31.8
  pharyngoesophageal (congenital) Q39.6
    acquired K22.5
  pharynx (congenital) Q38.7
  rectosigmoid — *see* Diverticulosis, intestine, large
    congenital Q43.8
  rectum — *see* Diverticulosis, intestine, large
  Rokitansky's K22.5
  seminal vesicle N50.89
  sigmoid — *see* Diverticulosis, intestine, large
    congenital Q43.8
  stomach (acquired) K31.4
    congenital Q40.2
  trachea (acquired) J39.8
  ureter (acquired) N28.89
    congenital Q62.8
  ureterovesical orifice N28.89
  urethra (acquired) N36.1
    congenital Q64.79
  ventricle, left (congenital) Q24.8
  vesical N32.3
    congenital Q64.6
  Zenker's (esophagus) K22.5
Division
  cervix uteri (acquired) N88.8
  glans penis Q55.69
  labia minora (congenital) Q52.79
  ligament (partial or complete) (current) — *see also* Sprain
    with open wound — *see* Wound, open
  muscle (partial or complete) (current) — *see also* Injury, muscle
    with open wound — *see* Wound, open
  nerve (traumatic) — *see* Injury, nerve
  spinal cord — *see* Injury, spinal cord, by region
  vein I87.8
Divorce, causing family disruption Z63.5
Dix-Hallpike neurolabyrinthitis — *see* Neuronitis, vestibular
Dizziness R42
  hysterical F44.89
  psychogenic F45.8
DMAC (disseminated mycobacterium avium-intracellulare complex) A31.2
DNR (do not resuscitate) Z66
Doan-Wiseman syndrome (primary splenic neutropenia) — *see* Agranulocytosis
Doehle-Heller aortitis A52.02
Dog bite — *see* Bite
Dohle body panmyelopathic syndrome D72.0
Dolichocephaly Q67.2
Dolichocolon Q43.8
Dolichostenomelia — *see* Syndrome, Marfan's
Donohue's syndrome E34.8
Donor (organ or tissue) Z52.9
  blood (whole) Z52.000
    autologous Z52.010
    specified component (lymphocytes) (platelets) NEC Z52.008
      autologous Z52.018
      specified donor NEC Z52.098
    specified donor NEC Z52.090
    stem cells Z52.001
      autologous Z52.011
      specified donor NEC Z52.091
  bone Z52.20
    autologous Z52.21
    marrow Z52.3
    specified type NEC Z52.29
  cornea Z52.5
  egg (Oocyte) Z52.819
    age 35 and over Z52.812
      anonymous recipient Z52.812
      designated recipient Z52.813
    under age 35 Z52.810
      anonymous recipient Z52.810
      designated recipient Z52.811
  kidney Z52.4
  liver Z52.6
  lung Z52.89

Donor — *continued*
  lymphocyte — *see* Donor, blood, specified components NEC
  Oocyte — *see* Donor, egg
  platelets Z52.008
  potential, examination of Z00.5
  semen Z52.89
  skin Z52.10
    autologous Z52.11
    specified type NEC Z52.19
  specified organ or tissue NEC Z52.89
  sperm Z52.89
Donovanosis A58
Dorsalgia M54.9
  psychogenic F45.41
  specified NEC M54.89
Dorsopathy M53.9
  deforming M43.9
    specified NEC — *see* subcategory M43.8 ☑
  specified NEC M53.80
    cervical region M53.82
    cervicothoracic region M53.83
    lumbar region M53.86
    lumbosacral region M53.87
    occipito-atlanto-axial region M53.81
    sacrococcygeal region M53.88
    thoracic region M53.84
    thoracolumbar region M53.85
Double
  albumin E88.09
  aortic arch Q25.45
  auditory canal Q17.8
  auricle (heart) Q20.8
  bladder Q64.79
  cervix Q51.820
    with doubling of uterus (and vagina) Q51.10
      with obstruction Q51.11
  inlet ventricle Q20.4
  kidney with double pelvis (renal) Q63.0
  meatus urinarius Q64.75
  monster Q89.4
  outlet
    left ventricle Q20.2
    right ventricle Q20.1
  pelvis (renal) with double ureter Q62.5
  tongue Q38.3
  ureter (one or both sides) Q62.5
    with double pelvis (renal) Q62.5
  urethra Q64.74
  urinary meatus Q64.75
  uterus Q51.28
    with
      doubling of cervix (and vagina) Q51.10
        with obstruction Q51.11
    complete Q51.21
    in pregnancy or childbirth O34.0- ☑
      causing obstructed labor O65.5
    partial Q51.22
    specified NEC Q51.28
  vagina Q52.10
    with doubling of uterus (and cervix) Q51.10
      with obstruction Q51.11
  vision H53.2
  vulva Q52.79
Douglas' pouch, cul-de-sac — *see* condition
Down syndrome Q90.9
  meiotic nondisjunction Q90.0
  mitotic nondisjunction Q90.1
  mosaicism Q90.1
  translocation Q90.2
DPD (dihydropyrimidine dehydrogenase deficiency) E88.89
Dracontiasis B72
Dracunculiasis, dracunculosis B72
Dream state, hysterical F44.89
Drepanocytic anemia — *see* Disease, sickle-cell
Dresbach's syndrome (elliptocytosis) D58.1
Dreschlera (hawaiiensis) (infection) B43.8
Dressler's syndrome I24.1
Drift, ulnar — *see* Deformity, limb, specified type NEC, forearm
Drinking (alcohol)
  excessive, to excess NEC (without dependence) F10.10
    habitual (continual) (without remission) F10.20
      with remission F10.21
Drip, postnasal (chronic) R09.82
  due to
    allergic rhinitis — *see* Rhinitis, allergic

Drip, postnasal — *continued*
- due to — *continued*
  - common cold J00
  - gastroesophageal reflux — *see* Reflux, gastroesophageal
  - nasopharyngitis — *see* Nasopharyngitis
  - other known condition — *code to* condition
  - sinusitis — *see* Sinusitis

Droop
- facial R29.810
  - cerebrovascular disease I69.992
    - cerebral infarction I69.392
    - intracerebral hemorrhage I69.192
    - nontraumatic intracranial hemorrhage NEC I69.292
    - specified disease NEC I69.892
    - subarachnoid hemorrhage I69.092

Drop (in)
- attack NEC R55
- finger — *see* Deformity, finger
- foot — *see* Deformity, limb, foot, drop
- hematocrit (precipitous) R71.0
- hemoglobin R71.0
- toe — *see* Deformity, toe, specified NEC
- wrist — *see* Deformity, limb, wrist drop

Dropped heart beats I45.9

Dropsy, dropsical — *see also* Hydrops
- abdomen R18.8
- brain — *see* Hydrocephalus
- cardiac, heart — *see* Failure, heart, congestive
- gangrenous — *see* Gangrene
- heart — *see* Failure, heart, congestive
- kidney — *see* Nephrosis
- lung — *see* Edema, lung
- newborn due to isoimmunization P56.0
- pericardium — *see* Pericarditis

Drowned, drowning (near) T75.1 ☑

Drowsiness R40.0

Drug
- abuse counseling and surveillance Z71.51
- addiction — *see* Dependence
- dependence — *see* Dependence
- habit — *see* Dependence
- harmful use — *see* Abuse, drug
- induced fever R50.2
- overdose — *see* Table of Drugs and Chemicals, by drug, poisoning
- poisoning — *see* Table of Drugs and Chemicals, by drug, poisoning
- resistant organism infection — *see also* Resistant, organism, to, drug Z16.30
- therapy
  - long term (current) (prophylactic) — *see* Therapy, drug long-term (current) (prophylactic)
  - short term — *omit code*
- wrong substance given or taken in error — *see* Table of Drugs and Chemicals, by drug, poisoning

Drunkenness (without dependence) F10.129
- acute in alcoholism F10.229
- chronic (without remission) F10.20
  - with remission F10.21
- pathological (without dependence) F10.129
  - with dependence F10.229
- sleep F51.9

Drusen
- macula (degenerative) (retina) — *see* Degeneration, macula, drusen
- optic disc H47.32- ☑

Dry, dryness — *see also* condition
- larynx J38.7
- mouth R68.2
  - due to dehydration E86.0
- nose J34.89
- socket (teeth) M27.3
- throat J39.2

DSAP L56.5

Duane's syndrome H50.81- ☑

Dubin-Johnson disease or syndrome E80.6

Dubois' disease (thymus gland) A50.59 *[E35]*

Dubowitz' syndrome Q87.19

Duchenne-Aran muscular atrophy G12.21

Duchenne-Griesinger disease G71.01

Duchenne's
- disease or syndrome
  - motor neuron disease G12.22
  - muscular dystrophy G71.01
- locomotor ataxia (syphilitic) A52.11

Duchenne's — *continued*
- paralysis
  - birth injury P14.0
  - due to or associated with
    - motor neuron disease G12.22
    - muscular dystrophy G71.01

Ducrey's chancre A57

Duct, ductus — *see* condition

Duhring's disease (dermatitis herpetiformis) L13.0

Dullness, cardiac (decreased) (increased) R01.2

Dumb ague — *see* Malaria

Dumbness — *see* Aphasia

Dumdum fever B55.0

Dumping syndrome (postgastrectomy) K91.1

Duodenitis (nonspecific) (peptic) K29.80
- with bleeding K29.81

Duodenocholangitis — *see* Cholangitis

Duodenum, duodenal — *see* condition

Duplay's bursitis or periarthritis — *see* Tendinitis, calcific, shoulder

Duplication, duplex — *see also* Accessory
- alimentary tract Q45.8
- anus Q43.4
- appendix (and cecum) Q43.4
- biliary duct (any) Q44.5
- bladder Q64.79
- cecum (and appendix) Q43.4
- cervix Q51.820
- chromosome NEC
  - with complex rearrangements NEC Q92.5
  - seen only at prometaphase Q92.8
- cystic duct Q44.5
- digestive organs Q45.8
- esophagus Q39.8
- frontonasal process Q75.8
- intestine (large) (small) Q43.4
- kidney Q63.0
- liver Q44.7
- pancreas Q45.3
- penis Q55.69
- respiratory organs NEC Q34.8
- salivary duct Q38.4
- spinal cord (incomplete) Q06.2
- stomach Q40.2

Dupré's disease (meningism) R29.1

Dupuytren's contraction or disease M72.0

Durand-Nicolas-Favre disease A55

Durotomy (inadvertent) (incidental) G97.41

Duroziez's disease (congenital mitral stenosis) Q23.2

Dutton's relapsing fever (West African) A68.1

Dwarfism E34.3
- achondroplastic Q77.4
- congenital E34.3
- constitutional E34.3
- hypochondroplastic Q77.4
- hypophyseal E23.0
- infantile E34.3
- Laron-type E34.3
- Lorain (-Levi) type E23.0
- metatropic Q77.8
- nephrotic-glycosuric (with hypophosphatemic rickets) E72.09
- nutritional E45
- pancreatic K86.89
- pituitary E23.0
- renal N25.0
- thanatophoric Q77.1

Dyke-Young anemia (secondary) (symptomatic) D59.19

Dysacusis — *see* Abnormal, auditory perception

Dysadrenocortism E27.9
- hyperfunction E27.0

Dysarthria R47.1
- following
  - cerebral infarction I69.322
  - cerebrovascular disease I69.922
    - specified disease NEC I69.822
  - intracerebral hemorrhage I69.122
  - nontraumatic intracranial hemorrhage NEC I69.222
  - subarachnoid hemorrhage I69.022

Dysautonomia (familial) G90.1

Dysbarism T70.3 ☑

Dysbasia R26.2
- angiosclerotica intermittens I73.9
- hysterical F44.4
- lordotica (progressiva) G24.1
- nonorganic origin F44.4
- psychogenic F44.4

Dysbetalipoproteinemia (familial) E78.2

Dyscalculia R48.8
- developmental F81.2

Dyschezia K59.00

Dyschondroplasia (with hemangiomata) Q78.4

Dyschromia (skin) L81.9

Dyscollagenosis M35.9

Dyscranio-pygo-phalangy Q87.0

Dyscrasia
- blood (with) D75.9
  - antepartum hemorrhage — *see* Hemorrhage, antepartum, with coagulation defect
  - intrapartum hemorrhage O67.0
  - newborn P61.9
    - specified type NEC P61.8
  - puerperal, postpartum O72.3
- polyglandular, pluriglandular E31.9

Dysendocrinism E34.9

Dysentery, dysenteric (catarrhal) (diarrhea) (epidemic) (hemorrhagic) (infectious) (sporadic) (tropical) A09
- abscess, liver A06.4
- amebic — *see also* Amebiasis A06.0
  - with abscess — *see* Abscess, amebic
  - acute A06.0
  - chronic A06.1
- arthritis — *see also* category M01 A09
  - bacillary (*see also* category M01) A03.9
- bacillary A03.9
  - arthritis — *see also* category M01 A03.9
  - Boyd A03.2
  - Flexner A03.1
  - Schmitz (-Stutzer) A03.0
  - Shiga (-Kruse) A03.0
  - Shigella A03.9
    - boydii A03.2
    - dysenteriae A03.0
    - flexneri A03.1
    - group A A03.0
    - group B A03.1
    - group C A03.2
    - group D A03.3
    - sonnei A03.3
    - specified type NEC A03.8
  - Sonne A03.3
  - specified type NEC A03.8
- balantidial A07.0
- Balantidium coli A07.0
- Boyd's A03.2
- candidal B37.82
- Chilomastix A07.8
- Chinese A03.9
- coccidial A07.3
- Dientamoeba (fragilis) A07.8
- Embadomonas A07.8
- Entamoeba, entamebic — *see* Dysentery, amebic
- Flexner-Boyd A03.2
- Flexner's A03.1
- Giardia lamblia A07.1
- Hiss-Russell A03.1
- Lamblia A07.1
- leishmanial B55.0
- malarial — *see* Malaria
- metazoal B82.0
- monilial B37.82
- protozoal A07.9
- Salmonella A02.0
- schistosomal B65.1
- Schmitz (-Stutzer) A03.0
- Shiga (-Kruse) A03.0
- Shigella NOS — *see* Dysentery, bacillary
- Sonne A03.3
- strongyloidiasis B78.0
- trichomonal A07.8
- viral — *see also* Enteritis, viral A08.4

Dysequilibrium R42

Dysesthesia R20.8
- hysterical F44.6

Dysfibrinogenemia (congenital) D68.2

Dysfunction
- adrenal E27.9
  - hyperfunction E27.0
- autonomic
  - due to alcohol G31.2
  - somatoform F45.8
- bladder N31.9
  - neurogenic NOS — *see* Dysfunction, bladder, neuromuscular
  - neuromuscular NOS N31.9
    - atonic (motor) (sensory) N31.2

Dyskinesia — *continued*
- intestinal K59.89
- nonorganic origin F44.4
- orofacial (idiopathic) G24.4
  - drug induced G24.01
- psychogenic F44.4
- subacute, drug induced G24.01
- tardive G24.01
  - neuroleptic induced G24.01
- trachea J39.8
- tracheobronchial J98.09

Dyslalia (developmental) F80.0
Dyslexia R48.0
- developmental F81.0

Dyslipidemia E78.5
- depressed HDL cholesterol E78.6
- elevated fasting triglycerides E78.1

Dysmaturity — *see also* Light for dates
- pulmonary (newborn) (Wilson-Mikity) P27.0

Dysmenorrhea (essential) (exfoliative) N94.6
- congestive (syndrome) N94.6
- primary N94.4
- psychogenic F45.8
- secondary N94.5

Dysmetabolic syndrome X E88.81
Dysmetria R27.8
Dysmorphism (due to)
- alcohol Q86.0
- exogenous cause NEC Q86.8
- hydantoin Q86.1
- warfarin Q86.2

Dysmorphophobia (nondelusional) F45.22
- delusional F22

Dysnomia R47.01
Dysorexia R63.0
- psychogenic F50.89

Dysostosis
- cleidocranial, cleidocranialis Q74.0
- craniofacial Q75.1
- Fairbank's (idiopathic familial generalized osteophytosis) Q78.9
- mandibulofacial (incomplete) Q75.4
- multiplex E76.01
- oculomandibular Q75.5

Dyspareunia (female) N94.10
- deep N94.12
- male N53.12
- nonorganic F52.6
- psychogenic F52.6
- secondary N94.19
- specified NEC N94.19
- superficial (introital) N94.11

Dyspepsia R10.13
- atonic K30
- functional (allergic) (congenital) (gastrointestinal) (occupational) (reflex) K30
- intestinal K59.89
- nervous F45.8
- neurotic F45.8
- psychogenic F45.8

Dysphagia R13.10
- cervical R13.19
- following
  - cerebral infarction I69.391
  - cerebrovascular disease I69.991
    - specified NEC I69.891
  - intracerebral hemorrhage I69.191
  - nontraumatic intracranial hemorrhage NEC I69.291
  - specified disease NEC I69.891
  - subarachnoid hemorrhage I69.091
- functional (hysterical) F45.8
- hysterical F45.8
- nervous (hysterical) F45.8
- neurogenic R13.19
- oral phase R13.11
- oropharyngeal phase R13.12
- pharyngeal phase R13.13
- pharyngoesophageal phase R13.14
- psychogenic F45.8
- sideropenic D50.1
- spastica K22.4
- specified NEC R13.19

Dysphagocytosis, congenital D71
Dysphasia R47.02
- developmental
  - expressive type F80.1
  - receptive type F80.2

Dysphasia — *continued*
- following
  - cerebrovascular disease I69.921
    - cerebral infarction I69.321
    - intracerebral hemorrhage I69.121
    - nontraumatic intracranial hemorrhage NEC I69.221
    - specified disease NEC I69.821
    - subarachnoid hemorrhage I69.021

Dysphonia R49.0
- functional F44.4
- hysterical F44.4
- psychogenic F44.4
- spastica J38.3

Dysphoria
- gender F64.9
  - in
    - adolescence and adulthood F64.0
    - children F64.2
  - specified NEC F64.8
- postpartal O90.6

Dyspituitarism E23.3
Dysplasia — *see also* Anomaly
- acetabular, congenital Q65.89
- alveolar capillary, with vein misalignment J84.843
- anus (histologically confirmed) (mild) (moderate) K62.82
  - severe D01.3
- arrhythmogenic right ventricular I42.8
- arterial, fibromuscular I77.3
- asphyxiating thoracic (congenital) Q77.2
- brain Q07.9
- bronchopulmonary, perinatal P27.1
- cervix (uteri) N87.9
  - mild N87.0
  - moderate N87.1
  - severe D06.9
- chondroectodermal Q77.6
- colon D12.6
- craniometaphyseal Q78.8
- dentinal K00.5
- diaphyseal, progressive Q78.3
- dystrophic Q77.5
- ectodermal (anhidrotic) (congenital) (hereditary) Q82.4
  - hydrotic Q82.8
- epithelial, uterine cervix — *see* Dysplasia, cervix
- eye (congenital) Q11.2
- fibrous
  - bone NEC (monostotic) M85.00
    - ankle M85.07- ☑
    - foot M85.07- ☑
    - forearm M85.03- ☑
    - hand M85.04- ☑
    - lower leg M85.06- ☑
    - multiple site M85.09
    - neck M85.08
    - rib M85.08
    - shoulder M85.01- ☑
    - skull M85.08
    - specified site NEC M85.08
    - thigh M85.05- ☑
    - toe M85.07- ☑
    - upper arm M85.02- ☑
    - vertebra M85.08
  - diaphyseal, progressive Q78.3
  - jaw M27.8
  - polyostotic Q78.1
- florid osseous — *see also* Cyst, calcifying odontogenic
- high grade, focal D12.6
- hip, congenital Q65.89
- joint, congenital Q74.8
- kidney Q61.4
  - multicystic Q61.4
- leg Q74.2
- lung, congenital (not associated with short gestation) Q33.6
- mammary (gland) (benign) N60.9- ☑
  - cyst (solitary) — *see* Cyst, breast
  - cystic — *see* Mastopathy, cystic
  - duct ectasia — *see* Ectasia, mammary duct
  - fibroadenosis — *see* Fibroadenosis, breast
  - fibrosclerosis — *see* Fibrosclerosis, breast
  - specified type NEC N60.8- ☑
- metaphyseal Q78.5
- muscle Q79.8
- oculodentodigital Q87.0
- periapical (cemental) (cemento-osseous) — *see* Cyst, calcifying odontogenic

Dysplasia — *continued*
- periosteum — *see* Disorder, bone, specified type NEC
- polyostotic fibrous Q78.1
- prostate — *see also* Neoplasia, intraepithelial, prostate N42.30
  - severe D07.5
  - specified NEC N42.39
- renal Q61.4
  - multicystic Q61.4
- retinal, congenital Q14.1
- right ventricular, arrhythmogenic I42.8
- septo-optic Q04.4
- skin L98.8
- spinal cord Q06.1
- spondyloepiphyseal Q77.7
- thymic, with immunodeficiency D82.1
- vagina N89.3
  - mild N89.0
  - moderate N89.1
  - severe NEC D07.2
- vulva N90.3
  - mild N90.0
  - moderate N90.1
  - severe NEC D07.1

Dysplasminogenemia E88.02
Dyspnea (nocturnal) (paroxysmal) R06.00
- asthmatic (bronchial) J45.909
  - with
    - bronchitis J45.909
      - with
        - exacerbation (acute) J45.901
        - status asthmaticus J45.902
      - chronic J44.9
    - exacerbation (acute) J45.901
    - status asthmaticus J45.902
  - cardiac — *see* Failure, ventricular, left
- cardiac — *see* Failure, ventricular, left
- functional F45.8
- hyperventilation R06.4
- hysterical F45.8
- newborn P28.89
- orthopnea R06.01
- psychogenic F45.8
- shortness of breath R06.02
- specified type NEC R06.09

Dyspraxia R27.8
- developmental (syndrome) F82

Dysproteinemia E88.09
Dysreflexia, autonomic G90.4
Dysrhythmia
- cardiac I49.9
  - newborn
    - bradycardia P29.12
    - occurring before birth P03.819
      - before onset of labor P03.810
      - during labor P03.811
    - tachycardia P29.11
  - postoperative I97.89
- cerebral or cortical — *see* Epilepsy

Dyssomnia — *see* Disorder, sleep
Dyssynergia
- biliary K83.8
- bladder sphincter N36.44
- cerebellaris myoclonica (Hunt's ataxia) G11.19

Dysthymia F34.1
Dysthyroidism E07.9
Dystocia O66.9
- affecting newborn P03.1
- cervical (hypotonic) O62.2
  - affecting newborn P03.6
  - primary O62.0
  - secondary O62.1
- contraction ring O62.4
- fetal O66.9
  - abnormality NEC O66.3
  - conjoined twins O66.3
  - oversize O66.2
- maternal O66.9
- positional O64.9 ☑
- shoulder (girdle) O66.0
  - causing obstructed labor O66.0
- uterine NEC O62.4

Dystonia G24.9
- cervical G24.3
- deformans progressiva G24.1
- drug induced NEC G24.09
  - acute G24.02
  - specified NEC G24.09

- **Effect, adverse** — *continued*
  - glue (airplane) sniffing
    - due to drug abuse — *see* Abuse, drug, inhalant
    - due to drug dependence — *see* Dependence, drug, inhalant
  - heat — *see* Heat
  - high altitude NEC T70.29 ☑
    - anoxia T70.29 ☑
    - on
      - ears T70.0 ☑
      - sinuses T70.1 ☑
    - polycythemia D75.1
  - high pressure fluids T70.4 ☑
  - hot weather — *see* Heat
  - hunger T73.0 ☑
  - immersion, foot — *see* Immersion
  - immunization — *see* Complications, vaccination
  - immunological agents — *see* Complications, vaccination
  - infrared (radiation) (rays) NOS T66 ☑
    - dermatitis or eczema L59.8
  - infusion — *see* Complications, infusion
  - lack of care of infants — *see* Maltreatment, child
  - lightning — *see* Lightning
  - medical care T88.9 ☑
    - specified NEC T88.8 ☑
  - medicinal substance, correct, properly administered — *see* Effect, adverse, drug
  - motion T75.3 ☑
  - noise, on inner ear — *see* subcategory H83.3 ☑
  - overheated places — *see* Heat
  - psychosocial, of work environment Z56.5
  - radiation (diagnostic) (infrared) (natural source) (therapeutic) (ultraviolet) (X-ray) NOS T66 ☑
    - dermatitis or eczema — *see* Dermatitis, due to, radiation
    - fibrosis of lung J70.1
    - pneumonitis J70.0
    - pulmonary manifestations
      - acute J70.0
      - chronic J70.1
    - skin L59.9
  - radioactive substance NOS
    - dermatitis or eczema — *see* Radiodermatitis
  - reduced temperature T69.9 ☑
    - immersion foot or hand — *see* Immersion
    - specified effect NEC T69.8 ☑
  - serum NEC — *see also* Reaction, serum T80.69 ☑
  - specified NEC T78.8 ☑
    - external cause NEC T75.89 ☑
  - strangulation — *see* Asphyxia, traumatic
  - submersion T75.1 ☑
  - thirst T73.1 ☑
  - toxic — *see* Toxicity
  - transfusion — *see* Complications, transfusion
  - ultraviolet (radiation) (rays) NOS T66 ☑
    - burn — *see* Burn
    - dermatitis or eczema — *see* Dermatitis, due to, ultraviolet rays
      - acute L56.8
  - vaccine (any) — *see* Complications, vaccination
  - vibration — *see* Vibration, adverse effects
  - water pressure NEC T70.9 ☑
    - specified NEC T70.8 ☑
  - weightlessness T75.82 ☑
  - whole blood — *see* Complications, transfusion
  - work environment Z56.5
- **Effects, late** — *see* Sequelae
- **Effluvium**
  - anagen L65.1
  - telogen L65.0
- **Effort syndrome** (psychogenic) F45.8
- **Effusion**
  - amniotic fluid — *see* Pregnancy, complicated by, prematue rupture of membranes
  - brain (serous) G93.6
  - bronchial — *see* Bronchitis
  - cerebral G93.6
  - cerebrospinal — *see also* Meningitis
    - vessel G93.6
  - chest — *see* Effusion, pleura
  - chylous, chyliform (pleura) J94.0
  - intracranial G93.6
  - joint M25.40
    - ankle M25.47- ☑
    - elbow M25.42- ☑
    - foot joint M25.47- ☑
- **Effusion** — *continued*
  - joint — *continued*
    - hand joint M25.44- ☑
    - hip M25.45- ☑
    - knee M25.46- ☑
    - shoulder M25.41- ☑
    - specified joint NEC M25.48
    - wrist M25.43- ☑
  - malignant pleural J91.0
  - meninges — *see* Meningitis
  - pericardium, pericardial (noninflammatory) I31.3
    - acute — *see* Pericarditis, acute
  - peritoneal (chronic) R18.8
  - pleura, pleurisy, pleuritic, pleuropericardial J90
    - chylous, chyliform J94.0
    - due to systemic lupus erythematosis M32.13
    - in conditions classified elsewhere J91.8
    - influenzal — *see* Influenza, with, respiratory manifestations NEC
    - malignant J91.0
    - newborn P28.89
    - tuberculous NEC A15.6
      - primary (progressive) A15.7
  - spinal — *see* Meningitis
  - thorax, thoracic — *see* Effusion, pleura
- **Egg shell nails** L60.3
  - congenital Q84.6
- **EGPA** (eosinophilic granulomatosis with polyangiitis) M30.1
- **Egyptian splenomegaly** B65.1
- **Ehlers-Danlos syndrome** — *see also* Syndrome, Ehlers-Danlos Q79.60
- **Ehrlichiosis** A77.40
  - due to
    - E. chafeensis A77.41
    - E. ewingii A77.49
    - E. muris euclairensis A77.49
    - E. sennetsu A79.81
    - specified organism NEC A77.49
- **Eichstedt's disease** B36.0
- **Eisenmenger's**
  - complex or syndrome I27.83
  - defect Q21.8
- **Ejaculation**
  - delayed F52.32
  - painful N53.12
  - premature F52.4
  - retarded N53.11
  - retrograde N53.14
  - semen, painful N53.12
    - psychogenic F52.6
- **Ekbom's syndrome** (restless legs) G25.81
- **Ekman's syndrome** (brittle bones and blue sclera) Q78.0
- **Elastic skin** Q82.8
  - acquired L57.4
- **Elastofibroma** — *see* Neoplasm, connective tissue, benign
- **Elastoma** (juvenile) Q82.8
  - Miescher's L87.2
- **Elastomyofibrosis** I42.4
- **Elastosis**
  - actinic, solar L57.8
  - atrophicans (senile) L57.4
  - perforans serpiginosa L87.2
  - senilis L57.4
- **Elbow** — *see* condition
- **Electric current, electricity, effects** (concussion) (fatal) (nonfatal) (shock) T75.4 ☑
  - burn — *see* Burn
- **Electric feet syndrome** E53.8
- **Electrocution** T75.4 ☑
  - from electroshock gun (taser) T75.4 ☑
- **Electrolyte imbalance** E87.8
  - with
    - abortion — *see* Abortion by type, complicated by, electrolyte imbalance
    - ectopic pregnancy O08.5
    - molar pregnancy O08.5
- **Elephantiasis** (nonfilarial) I89.0
  - arabicum — *see* Infestation, filarial
  - bancroftian B74.0
  - congenital (any site) (hereditary) Q82.0
  - due to
    - Brugia (malayi) B74.1
      - timori B74.2
    - mastectomy I97.2
    - Wuchereria (bancrofti) B74.0
  - eyelid H02.859
- **Elephantiasis** — *continued*
  - eyelid — *continued*
    - left H02.856
      - lower H02.855
      - upper H02.854
    - right H02.853
      - lower H02.852
      - upper H02.851
  - filarial, filariensis — *see* Infestation, filarial
  - glandular I89.0
  - graecorum A30.9
  - lymphangiectatic I89.0
  - lymphatic vessel I89.0
    - due to mastectomy I97.2
  - scrotum (nonfilarial) I89.0
  - streptococcal I89.0
  - surgical I97.89
    - postmastectomy I97.2
  - telangiectodes I89.0
  - vulva (nonfilarial) N90.89
- **Elevated, elevation**
  - alanine transaminase (ALT) R74.01
  - ALT (alanine transaminase) R74.01
  - antibody titer R76.0
  - aspartate transaminase (AST) R74.01
  - AST (aspartate transaminase) R74.01
  - basal metabolic rate R94.8
  - blood pressure — *see also* Hypertension
    - reading (incidental) (isolated) (nonspecific), no diagnosis of hypertension R03.0
  - blood sugar R73.9
  - body temperature (of unknown origin) R50.9
  - cancer antigen 125 [CA 125] R97.1
  - carcinoembryonic antigen [CEA] R97.0
  - cholesterol E78.00
    - with high triglycerides E78.2
  - conjugate, eye H51.0
  - C-reactive protein (CRP) R79.82
  - diaphragm, congenital Q79.1
  - erythrocyte sedimentation rate R70.0
  - fasting glucose R73.01
  - fasting triglycerides E78.1
  - finding on laboratory examination — *see* Findings, abnormal, inconclusive, without diagnosis, by type of exam
  - GFR (glomerular filtration rate) — *see* Findings, abnormal, inconclusive, without diagnosis, by type of exam
  - glucose tolerance (oral) R73.02
  - immunoglobulin level R76.8
  - indoleacetic acid R82.5
  - lactic acid dehydrogenase (LDH) level R74.02
  - leukocytes D72.829
  - lipoprotein a (Lp(a)) level E78.41
  - liver function
    - study R94.5
    - test R79.89
      - alkaline phosphatase R74.8
      - aminotransferase R74.01
      - bilirubin R17
      - hepatic enzyme R74.8
      - lactate dehydrogenase R74.02
  - Lp(a) (lipoprotein(a)) E78.41
  - lymphocytes D72.820
  - prostate specific antigen [PSA] R97.20
  - Rh titer — *see* Complication(s), transfusion, incompatibility reaction, Rh (factor)
  - scapula, congenital Q74.0
  - sedimentation rate R70.0
  - SGOT R74.01
  - SGPT R74.01
  - transaminase level R74.01
  - triglycerides E78.1
    - with high cholesterol E78.2
  - troponin R77.8
  - tumor associated antigens [TAA] NEC R97.8
  - tumor specific antigens [TSA] NEC R97.8
  - urine level of
    - 17-ketosteroids R82.5
    - catecholamine R82.5
    - indoleacetic acid R82.5
    - steroids R82.5
    - vanillylmandelic acid (VMA) R82.5
  - venous pressure I87.8
  - white blood cell count D72.829
    - specified NEC D72.828
- **Elliptocytosis** (congenital) (hereditary) D58.1
  - Hb C (disease) D58.1

- **Elliptocytosis** — *continued*
  - hemoglobin disease D58.1
  - sickle-cell (disease) D57.8- ☑
    - trait D57.3
- **Ellison-Zollinger syndrome** E16.4
- **Ellis-van Creveld syndrome** (chondroectodermal dysplasia) Q77.6
- **Elongated, elongation** (congenital) — *see also* Distortion
  - bone Q79.9
  - cervix (uteri) Q51.828
    - acquired N88.4
    - hypertrophic N88.4
  - colon Q43.8
  - common bile duct Q44.5
  - cystic duct Q44.5
  - frenulum, penis Q55.69
  - labia minora (acquired) N9Ø.69
  - ligamentum patellae Q74.1
  - petiolus (epiglottidis) Q31.8
  - tooth, teeth KØØ.2
  - uvula Q38.6
- **Eltor cholera** AØØ.1
- **Emaciation** (due to malnutrition) E43
- **Embadomoniasis** AØ7.8
- **Embedded tooth, teeth** KØ1.Ø
  - root only KØ8.3
- **Embolic** — *see* condition
- **Embolism** (multiple) (paradoxical) I74.9
  - air (any site) (traumatic) T79.Ø ☑
    - following
      - abortion — *see* Abortion by type complicated by embolism
      - ectopic pregnancy OØ8.2
      - infusion, therapeutic injection or transfusion T8Ø.Ø ☑
      - molar pregnancy OØ8.2
      - procedure NEC
        - artery T81.719 ☑
          - mesenteric T81.71Ø ☑
          - renal T81.711 ☑
          - specified NEC T81.718 ☑
        - vein T81.72 ☑
    - in pregnancy, childbirth or puerperium — *see* Embolism, obstetric
  - amniotic fluid (pulmonary) — *see also* Embolism, obstetric
    - following
      - abortion — *see* Abortion by type complicated by embolism
      - ectopic pregnancy OØ8.2
      - molar pregnancy OØ8.2
  - aorta, aortic I74.1Ø
    - abdominal I74.Ø9
      - saddle I74.Ø1
    - bifurcation I74.Ø9
    - saddle I74.Ø1
    - thoracic I74.11
  - artery I74.9
    - auditory, internal I65.8
    - basilar — *see* Occlusion, artery, basilar
    - carotid (common) (internal) — *see* Occlusion, artery, carotid
    - cerebellar (anterior inferior) (posterior inferior) (superior) I66.3
    - cerebral — *see* Occlusion, artery, cerebral
    - choroidal (anterior) I65.8
    - communicating posterior I65.8
    - coronary — *see also* Infarct, myocardium
      - not resulting in infarction I24.Ø
    - extremity I74.4
      - lower I74.3
      - upper I74.2
    - hypophyseal I65.8
    - iliac I74.5
    - limb I74.4
      - lower I74.3
      - upper I74.2
    - mesenteric (with gangrene) — *see also* Ischemia, intestine, acute K55.Ø59
    - ophthalmic — *see* Occlusion, artery, retina
    - peripheral I74.4
    - pontine I65.8
    - precerebral — *see* Occlusion, artery, precerebral
    - pulmonary — *see* Embolism, pulmonary
    - renal N28.Ø
    - retinal — *see* Occlusion, artery, retina
    - septic I76

- **Embolism** — *continued*
  - artery — *continued*
    - specified NEC I74.8
    - vertebral — *see* Occlusion, artery, vertebral
  - basilar (artery) I65.1
  - blood clot
    - following
      - abortion — *see* Abortion by type complicated by embolism
      - ectopic or molar pregnancy OØ8.2
    - in pregnancy, childbirth or puerperium — *see* Embolism, obstetric
  - brain — *see also* Occlusion, artery, cerebral
    - following
      - abortion — *see* Abortion by type complicated by embolism
      - ectopic or molar pregnancy OØ8.2
    - puerperal, postpartum, childbirth — *see* Embolism, obstetric
  - capillary I78.8
  - cardiac — *see also* Infarct, myocardium
    - not resulting in infarction I51.3
  - carotid (artery) (common) (internal) — *see* Occlusion, artery, carotid
  - cavernous sinus (venous) — *see* Embolism, intracranial venous sinus
  - cerebral — *see* Occlusion, artery, cerebral
  - cholesterol — *see* Atheroembolism
  - coronary (artery or vein) (systemic) — *see* Occlusion, coronary
  - due to device, implant or graft — *see also* Complications, by site and type, specified NEC
    - arterial graft NEC T82.818 ☑
    - breast (implant) T85.818 ☑
    - catheter NEC T85.818 ☑
      - dialysis (renal) T82.818 ☑
        - intraperitoneal T85.818 ☑
      - infusion NEC T82.818 ☑
        - spinal (epidural) (subdural) T85.81Ø ☑
      - urinary (indwelling) T83.81 ☑
    - electronic (electrode) (pulse generator) (stimulator)
      - bone T84.81 ☑
      - cardiac T82.817 ☑
      - nervous system (brain) (peripheral nerve) (spinal) T85.81Ø ☑
      - urinary T83.81 ☑
    - fixation, internal (orthopedic) NEC T84.81 ☑
    - gastrointestinal (bile duct) (esophagus) T85.818 ☑
    - genital NEC T83.81 ☑
    - heart (graft) (valve) T82.817 ☑
    - joint prosthesis T84.81 ☑
    - ocular (corneal graft) (orbital implant) T85.818 ☑
    - orthopedic (bone graft) NEC T86.838
    - specified NEC T85.818 ☑
    - urinary (graft) NEC T83.81 ☑
    - vascular NEC T82.818 ☑
    - ventricular intracranial shunt T85.81Ø ☑
  - extremities
    - lower — *see* Embolism, vein, lower extremity
      - arterial I74.3
    - upper I74.2
  - eye H34.9
  - fat (cerebral) (pulmonary) (systemic) T79.1 ☑
    - complicating delivery — *see* Embolism, obstetric
    - following
      - abortion — *see* Abortion by type complicated by embolism
      - ectopic or molar pregnancy OØ8.2
  - following
    - abortion — *see* Abortion by type complicated by embolism
    - ectopic or molar pregnancy OØ8.2
    - infusion, therapeutic injection or transfusion
      - air T8Ø.Ø ☑
  - heart (fatty) — *see also* Infarct, myocardium
    - not resulting in infarction I51.3
  - hepatic (vein) I82.Ø
  - in pregnancy, childbirth or puerperium — *see* Embolism, obstetric
  - intestine (artery) (vein) (with gangrene) — *see also* Ischemia, intestine, acute K55.Ø39
  - intracranial — *see also* Occlusion, artery, cerebral
    - venous sinus (any) GØ8
      - nonpyogenic I67.6
  - intraspinal venous sinuses or veins GØ8
    - nonpyogenic G95.19
  - kidney (artery) N28.Ø

- **Embolism** — *continued*
  - lateral sinus (venous) — *see* Embolism, intracranial, venous sinus
  - leg — *see* Embolism, vein, lower extremity
    - arterial I74.3
  - longitudinal sinus (venous) — *see* Embolism, intracranial, venous sinus
  - lung (massive) — *see* Embolism, pulmonary
  - meninges I66.8
  - mesenteric (artery) (vein) (with gangrene) — *see also* Ischemia, intestine, acute K55.Ø59
  - obstetric (in) (pulmonary)
    - childbirth O88.22
      - air O88.Ø2
      - amniotic fluid O88.12
      - blood clot O88.22
      - fat O88.82
      - pyemic O88.32
      - septic O88.32
      - specified type NEC O88.82
    - pregnancy O88.21- ☑
      - air O88.Ø1- ☑
      - amniotic fluid O88.11- ☑
      - blood clot O88.21- ☑
      - fat O88.81- ☑
      - pyemic O88.31- ☑
      - septic O88.31- ☑
      - specified type NEC O88.81- ☑
    - puerperal O88.23
      - air O88.Ø3
      - amniotic fluid O88.13
      - blood clot O88.23
      - fat O88.83
      - pyemic O88.33
      - septic O88.33
      - specified type NEC O88.83
  - ophthalmic — *see* Occlusion, artery, retina
  - penis N48.81
  - peripheral artery NOS I74.4
  - pituitary E23.6
  - popliteal (artery) I74.3
  - portal (vein) I81
  - postoperative, postprocedural
    - artery T81.719 ☑
      - mesenteric T81.71Ø ☑
      - renal T81.711 ☑
      - specified NEC T81.718 ☑
    - vein T81.72 ☑
  - precerebral artery — *see* Occlusion, artery, precerebral
  - puerperal — *see* Embolism, obstetric
  - pulmonary (acute) (artery) (vein) I26.99
    - with acute cor pulmonale I26.Ø9
    - chronic I27.82
    - following
      - abortion — *see* Abortion by type complicated by embolism
      - ectopic or molar pregnancy OØ8.2
    - healed or old Z86.711
    - in pregnancy, childbirth or puerperium — *see* Embolism, obstetric
    - multiple subsegmental without acute cor pulmonale I26.94
    - personal history of Z86.711
    - saddle I26.92
      - with acute cor pulmonale I26.Ø2
    - septic I26.9Ø
      - with acute cor pulmonale I26.Ø1
    - single subsegmental without acute cor pulmonale I26.93
    - subsegmental NOS I26.93
  - pyemic (multiple) I76
    - following
      - abortion — *see* Abortion by type complicated by embolism
      - ectopic or molar pregnancy OØ8.2
    - Hemophilus influenzae A41.3
    - pneumococcal A4Ø.3
      - with pneumonia J13
    - puerperal, postpartum, childbirth (any organism) — *see* Embolism, obstetric
    - specified organism NEC A41.89
    - staphylococcal A41.2
    - streptococcal A4Ø.9
  - renal (artery) N28.Ø
    - vein I82.3
  - retina, retinal — *see* Occlusion, artery, retina
  - saddle
    - abdominal aorta I74.Ø1

Encephalitis — *continued*
- periaxialis (concentrica) (diffuse) G37.5
- postchickenpox BØ1.11
- postexanthematous NEC BØ9
- postimmunization GØ4.Ø2
- postinfectious NEC GØ4.Ø1
- postmeasles BØ5.Ø
- postvaccinal GØ4.Ø2
- postvaricella BØ1.11
- postviral NEC A86
- Powassan A84.81
- Rasmussen GØ4.81
- Rio Bravo A85.8
- Russian
  - autumnal A83.Ø
  - spring-summer (taiga) A84.Ø
- saturnine — *see* Poisoning, lead
- specified NEC GØ4.81
- St. Louis A83.3
- subacute sclerosing A81.1
- summer A83.Ø
- suppurative GØ4.81
- tick-borne A84.9
- Torula, torular (cryptococcal) B45.1
- toxic NEC G92
- trichinosis B75 *[GØ5.3]*
- type
  - B A83.Ø
  - C A83.3
- van Bogaert's A81.1
- Venezuelan equine A92.2
- Vienna A85.8
- viral, virus A86
  - arthropod-borne NEC A85.2
    - mosquito-borne A83.9
      - Australian X disease A83.4
      - California virus A83.5
      - Eastern equine A83.2
      - Japanese (B type) A83.Ø
      - Murray Valley A83.4
      - specified NEC A83.8
      - St. Louis A83.3
      - type B A83.Ø
      - type C A83.3
      - Western equine A83.1
    - tick-borne A84.9
      - biundulant A84.1
      - central European A84.1
      - Czechoslovakian A84.1
      - diphasic meningoencephalitis A84.1
      - Far Eastern A84.Ø
      - Russian spring-summer (taiga) A84.Ø
      - specified NEC A84.89
  - specified type NEC A85.8
  - tick-borne, specified NEC A84.89
- Western equine A83.1

Encephalocele QØ1.9
- frontal QØ1.Ø
- nasofrontal QØ1.1
- occipital QØ1.2
- specified NEC QØ1.8

Encephalocystocele — *see* Encephalocele

Encephaloduroarteriomyosynangiosis (EDAMS) I67.5

Encephalomalacia (brain) (cerebellar) (cerebral) — *see* Softening, brain

Encephalomeningitis — *see* Meningoencephalitis

Encephalomeningocele — *see* Encephalocele

Encephalomeningomyelitis — *see* Meningoencephalitis

Encephalomyelitis — *see also* Encephalitis GØ4.9Ø
- acute disseminated GØ4.ØØ
  - infectious GØ4.Ø1
  - noninfectious GØ4.81
  - postimmunization GØ4.Ø2
  - postinfectious GØ4.Ø1
- acute necrotizing hemorrhagic GØ4.3Ø
  - postimmunization GØ4.32
  - postinfectious GØ4.31
  - specified NEC GØ4.39
- benign myalgic G93.3
- equine A83.9
  - Eastern A83.2
  - Venezuelan A92.2
  - Western A83.1
- in diseases classified elsewhere GØ5.3
- myalgic, benign G93.3
- postchickenpox BØ1.11
- postinfectious NEC GØ4.Ø1
- postmeasles BØ5.Ø

Encephalomyelitis — *continued*
- postvaccinal GØ4.Ø2
- postvaricella BØ1.11
- rubella BØ6.Ø1
- specified NEC GØ4.81
- Venezuelan equine A92.2

Encephalomyelocele — *see* Encephalocele

Encephalomyelomeningitis — *see* Meningoencephalitis

Encephalomyelopathy G96.9

Encephalomyeloradiculitis (acute) G61.Ø

Encephalomyeloradiculoneuritis (acute) (Guillain-Barré) G61.Ø

Encephalomyeloradiculopathy G96.9

Encephalopathia hyperbilirubinemica, newborn P57.9
- due to isoimmunization (conditions in P55) P57.Ø

Encephalopathy (acute) G93.4Ø
- acute necrotizing hemorrhagic GØ4.3Ø
  - postimmunization GØ4.32
  - postinfectious GØ4.31
  - specified NEC GØ4.39
- alcoholic G31.2
- anoxic — *see* Damage, brain, anoxic
- arteriosclerotic I67.2
- centrolobar progressive (Schilder) G37.Ø
- congenital QØ7.9
- degenerative, in specified disease NEC G32.89
- demyelinating callosal G37.1
- due to
  - drugs — *see also* Table of Drugs and Chemicals G92
- hepatic — *see* Failure, hepatic
- hyperbilirubinemic, newborn P57.9
  - due to isoimmunization (conditions in P55) P57.Ø
- hypertensive I67.4
- hypoglycemic E16.2
- hypoxic — *see* Damage, brain, anoxic
- hypoxic ischemic P91.6Ø
  - mild P91.61
  - moderate P91.62
  - severe P91.63
- in (due to) (with)
  - birth injury P11.1
  - hyperinsulinism E16.1 *[G94]*
  - influenza — *see* Influenza, with, encephalopathy
  - lack of vitamin — *see also* Deficiency, vitamin E56.9 *[G32.89]*
  - neoplastic disease — *see also* Neoplasm D49.9 *[G13.1]*
  - serum — *see also* Reaction, serum T8Ø.69 ☑
  - syphilis A52.17
  - trauma (postconcussional) FØ7.81
    - current injury — *see* Injury, intracranial
  - vaccination GØ4.Ø2
- lead — *see* Poisoning, lead
- metabolic G93.41
  - drug induced G92
  - toxic G92
- myoclonic, early, symptomatic — *see* Epilepsy, generalized, specified NEC
- necrotizing, subacute (Leigh) G31.82
- neonatal P91.819
  - in diseases classified elsewhere P91.811
- pellagrous E52 *[G32.89]*
- portosystemic — *see* Failure, hepatic
- postcontusional FØ7.81
  - current injury — *see* Injury, intracranial, diffuse
- posthypoglycemic (coma) E16.1 *[G94]*
- postradiation G93.89
- saturnine — *see* Poisoning, lead
- septic G93.41
- specified NEC G93.49
- spongioform, subacute (viral) A81.Ø9
- toxic G92
  - metabolic G92
- traumatic (postconcussional) FØ7.81
  - current injury — *see* Injury, intracranial
- vitamin B deficiency NEC E53.9 *[G32.89]*
  - vitamin B1 E51.2
- Wernicke's E51.2

Encephalorrhagia — *see* Hemorrhage, intracranial, intracerebral

Encephalosis, posttraumatic FØ7.81

Enchondroma — *see also* Neoplasm, bone, benign

Enchondromatosis (cartilaginous) (multiple) Q78.4

Encopresis R15.9
- functional F98.1
- nonorganic origin F98.1
- psychogenic F98.1

Encounter (with health service) (for) Z76.89
- adjustment and management (of)
  - breast implant Z45.81 ☑
  - implanted device NEC Z45.89
  - myringotomy device (stent) (tube) Z45.82
  - neurostimulator (brain) (gastric) (peripheral nerve) (sacral nerve) (spinal cord) (vagus nerve) Z45.42
- administrative purpose only ZØ2.9
  - examination for
    - adoption ZØ2.82
    - armed forces ZØ2.3
    - disability determination ZØ2.71
    - driving license ZØ2.4
    - employment ZØ2.1
    - insurance ZØ2.6
    - medical certificate NEC ZØ2.79
    - paternity testing ZØ2.81
    - residential institution admission ZØ2.2
    - school admission ZØ2.Ø
    - sports ZØ2.5
  - specified reason NEC ZØ2.89
- aftercare — *see* Aftercare
- antenatal screening Z36.9
  - cervical length Z36.86
  - chromosomal anomalies Z36.Ø
  - congenital cardiac abnormalities Z36.83
  - elevated maternal serum alphafetoprotein Z36.1
  - fetal growth retardation Z36.4
  - fetal lung maturity Z36.84
  - fetal macrosomia Z36.88
  - hydrops fetalis Z36.81
  - intrauterine growth restriction (IUGR) /small-for-dates Z36.4
  - isoimmunization Z36.5
  - large-for-dates Z36.88
  - malformations Z36.3
  - non-visualized anatomy on a previous scan Z36.2
  - nuchal translucency Z36.82
  - raised alphafetoprotein level Z36.1
  - risk of pre-term labor Z36.86
  - specified follow-up NEC Z36.2
  - specified genetic defects NEC Z36.8A
  - specified type NEC Z36.89
  - Streptococcus B Z36.85
  - suspected anomaly Z36.3
  - uncertain dates Z36.87
- assisted reproductive fertility procedure cycle Z31.83
- blood typing ZØ1.83
  - Rh typing ZØ1.83
- breast augmentation or reduction Z41.1
- breast implant exchange (different material) (different size) Z45.81 ☑
- breast reconstruction following mastectomy Z42.1
- check-up — *see* Examination
- chemotherapy for neoplasm Z51.11
- colonoscopy, screening Z12.11
- counseling — *see* Counseling
- delivery, full-term, uncomplicated O8Ø
  - cesarean, without indication O82
- desensitization to allergens Z51.6
- ear piercing Z41.3
- examination — *see* Examination
- expectant parent(s) (adoptive) pre-birth pediatrician visit Z76.81
- fertility preservation procedure (prior to cancer therapy) (prior to removal of gonads) Z31.84
- fitting (of) — *see* Fitting (and adjustment) (of)
- genetic
  - counseling
    - nonprocreative Z71.83
    - procreative Z31.5
  - testing — *see* Test, genetic
- hearing conservation and treatment ZØ1.12
- immunotherapy for neoplasm Z51.12
- in vitro fertilization cycle Z31.83
- instruction (in)
  - child care (postpartal) (prenatal) Z32.3
  - childbirth Z32.2
  - natural family planning
    - procreative Z31.61
    - to avoid pregnancy Z3Ø.Ø2
- insulin pump titration Z46.81
- joint prosthesis insertion following prior explantation of joint prosthesis (staged procedure)
  - hip Z47.32
  - knee Z47.33
  - shoulder Z47.31

Enthesopathy — *continued*
shoulder M77.8
shoulder region — *see* Lesion, shoulder
specified type NEC M77.8
spinal M46.ØØ
cervical region M46.Ø2
cervicothoracic region M46.Ø3
lumbar region M46.Ø6
lumbosacral region M46.Ø7
multiple sites M46.Ø9
occipito-atlanto-axial region M46.Ø1
sacrococcygeal region M46.Ø8
thoracic region M46.Ø4
thoracolumbar region M46.Ø5
tibial collateral bursitis — *see* Bursitis, tibial collateral
upper arm M77.8
wrist and carpus NEC M77.8
calcaneal spur — *see* Spur, bone, calcaneal
periarthritis of wrist — *see* Periarthritis, wrist
Entomophobia F4Ø.218
Entomophthoromycosis B46.8
Entrance, air into vein — *see* Embolism, air
Entrapment, nerve — *see* Neuropathy, entrapment
Entropion (eyelid) (paralytic) HØ2.ØØ9
cicatricial HØ2.Ø19
left HØ2.Ø16
lower HØ2.Ø15
upper HØ2.Ø14
right HØ2.Ø13
lower HØ2.Ø12
upper HØ2.Ø11
congenital Q1Ø.2
left HØ2.ØØ6
lower HØ2.ØØ5
upper HØ2.ØØ4
mechanical HØ2.Ø29
left HØ2.Ø26
lower HØ2.Ø25
upper HØ2.Ø24
right HØ2.Ø23
lower HØ2.Ø22
upper HØ2.Ø21
right HØ2.ØØ3
lower HØ2.ØØ2
upper HØ2.ØØ1
senile HØ2.Ø39
left HØ2.Ø36
lower HØ2.Ø35
upper HØ2.Ø34
right HØ2.Ø33
lower HØ2.Ø32
upper HØ2.Ø31
spastic HØ2.Ø49
left HØ2.Ø46
lower HØ2.Ø45
upper HØ2.Ø44
right HØ2.Ø43
lower HØ2.Ø42
upper HØ2.Ø41
Enucleated eye (traumatic, current) SØ5.7- ☑
Enuresis R32
functional F98.Ø
habit disturbance F98.Ø
nocturnal N39.44
psychogenic F98.Ø
nonorganic origin F98.Ø
psychogenic F98.Ø
Eosinopenia — *see* Agranulocytosis
Eosinophilia (allergic) (idiopathic) (secondary) D72.1Ø
with
angiolymphoid hyperplasia (ALHE) D18.Ø1
familial D72.19
hereditary D72.19
in disease classified elsewhere D72.18
infiltrative — *see* Eosinophilia, pulmonary
Löffler's J82.89
peritoneal — *see* Peritonitis, eosinophilic
pulmonary NEC J82.89
acute J82.82
asthmatic J82.83
chronic J82.81
specified NEC D72.19
tropical (pulmonary) J82.89
Eosinophilia-myalgia syndrome M35.8
Ependymitis (acute) (cerebral) (chronic) (granular) — *see* Encephalomyelitis
Ependymoblastoma
specified site — *see* Neoplasm, malignant, by site

Ependymoblastoma — *continued*
unspecified site C71.9
Ependymoma (epithelial) (malignant)
anaplastic
specified site — *see* Neoplasm, malignant, by site
unspecified site C71.9
benign
specified site — *see* Neoplasm, benign, by site
unspecified site D33.2
myxopapillary D43.2
specified site — *see* Neoplasm, uncertain behavior, by site
unspecified site D43.2
papillary D43.2
specified site — *see* Neoplasm, uncertain behavior, by site
unspecified site D43.2
specified site — *see* Neoplasm, malignant, by site
unspecified site C71.9
Ependymopathy G93.89
Ephelis, ephelides L81.2
Epiblepharon (congenital) Q1Ø.3
Epicanthus, epicanthic fold (eyelid) (congenital) Q1Ø.3
Epicondylitis (elbow)
lateral M77.1- ☑
medial M77.Ø- ☑
Epicystitis — *see* Cystitis
Epidemic — *see* condition
Epidermidalization, cervix — *see* Dysplasia, cervix
Epidermis, epidermal — *see* condition
Epidermodysplasia verruciformis BØ7.8
Epidermolysis
bullosa (congenital) Q81.9
acquired L12.3Ø
drug-induced L12.31
specified cause NEC L12.35
dystrophica Q81.2
letalis Q81.1
simplex Q81.Ø
specified NEC Q81.8
necroticans combustiformis L51.2
due to drug — *see* Table of Drugs and Chemicals, by drug
Epidermophytid — *see* Dermatophytosis
Epidermophytosis (infected) — *see* Dermatophytosis
Epididymis — *see* condition
Epididymitis (acute) (nonvenereal) (recurrent) (residual) N45.1
with orchitis N45.3
blennorrhagic (gonococcal) A54.23
caseous (tuberculous) A18.15
chlamydial A56.19
filarial — *see also* Infestation, filarial B74.9 *[N51]*
gonococcal A54.23
syphilitic A52.76
tuberculous A18.15
Epididymo-orchitis — *see also* Epididymitis N45.3
Epidural — *see* condition
Epigastrium, epigastric — *see* condition
Epigastrocele — *see* Hernia, ventral
Epiglottis — *see* condition
Epiglottitis, epiglottiditis (acute) JØ5.1Ø
with obstruction JØ5.11
chronic J37.Ø
Epignathus Q89.4
Epilepsia partialis continua — *see also* Kozhevnikof's epilepsy G4Ø.1- ☑
Epilepsy, epileptic, epilepsia (attack) (cerebral) (convulsion) (fit) (seizure) G4Ø.9Ø9

Note: the following terms are to be considered equivalent to intractable: pharmacoresistant (pharmacologically resistant), treatment resistant, refractory (medically) and poorly controlled

with
complex partial seizures — *see* Epilepsy, localization-related, symptomatic, with complex partial seizures
grand mal seizures on awakening — *see* Epilepsy, generalized, specified NEC
myoclonic absences — *see* Epilepsy, generalized, specified NEC
myoclonic-astatic seizures — *see* Epilepsy, generalized, specified NEC
simple partial seizures — *see* Epilepsy, localization-related, symptomatic, with simple partial seizures

Epilepsy, epileptic, epilepsia — *continued*
akinetic — *see* Epilepsy, generalized, specified NEC
benign childhood with centrotemporal EEG spikes — *see* Epilepsy, localization-related, idiopathic
benign myoclonic in infancy G4Ø.8Ø- ☑
Bravais-jacksonian — *see* Epilepsy, localization-related, symptomatic, with simple partial seizures
childhood
with occipital EEG paroxysms — *see* Epilepsy, localization-related, idiopathic
absence G4Ø.AØ9 (*following* G4Ø.3)
intractable G4Ø.A19 (*following* G4Ø.3)
with status epilepticus G4Ø.A11 (*following* G4Ø.3)
without status epilepticus G4Ø.A19 (*following* G4Ø.3)
not intractable G4Ø.AØ9 (*following* G4Ø.3)
with status epilepticus G4Ø.AØ1 (*following* G4Ø.3)
without status epilepticus G4Ø.AØ9 (*following* G4Ø.3)
climacteric — *see* Epilepsy, specified NEC
cysticercosis B69.Ø
deterioration (mental) FØ6.8
due to syphilis A52.19
focal — *see* Epilepsy, localization-related, symptomatic, with simple partial seizures
generalized
idiopathic G4Ø.3Ø9
intractable G4Ø.319
with status epilepticus G4Ø.311
without status epilepticus G4Ø.319
not intractable G4Ø.3Ø9
with status epilepticus G4Ø.3Ø1
without status epilepticus G4Ø.3Ø9
specified NEC G4Ø.4Ø9
intractable G4Ø.419
with status epilepticus G4Ø.411
without status epilepticus G4Ø.419
not intractable G4Ø.4Ø9
with status epilepticus G4Ø.4Ø1
without status epilepticus G4Ø.4Ø9
impulsive petit mal — *see* Epilepsy, juvenile myoclonic
intractable G4Ø.919
with status epilepticus G4Ø.911
without status epilepticus G4Ø.919
juvenile absence G4Ø.AØ9 (*following* G4Ø.3)
intractable G4Ø.A19 (*following* G4Ø.3)
with status epilepticus G4Ø.A11 (*following* G4Ø.3)
without status epilepticus G4Ø.A19 (*following* G4Ø.3)
not intractable G4Ø.AØ9 (*following* G4Ø.3)
with status epilepticus G4Ø.AØ1 (*following* G4Ø.3)
without status epilepticus G4Ø.AØ9 (*following* G4Ø.3)
juvenile myoclonic G4Ø.BØ9 (*following* G4Ø.3)
intractable G4Ø.B19 (*following* G4Ø.3)
with status epilepticus G4Ø.B11 (*following* G4Ø.3)
without status epilepticus G4Ø.B19 (*following* G4Ø.3)
not intractable G4Ø.BØ9 (*following* G4Ø.3)
with status epilepticus G4Ø.BØ1 (*following* G4Ø.3)
without status epilepticus G4Ø.BØ9 (*following* G4Ø.3)
localization-related (focal) (partial)
idiopathic G4Ø.ØØ9
with seizures of localized onset G4Ø.ØØ9
intractable G4Ø.Ø19
with status epilepticus G4Ø.Ø11
without status epilepticus G4Ø.Ø19
not intractable G4Ø.ØØ9
with status epilepticus G4Ø.ØØ1
without status epilepticus G4Ø.ØØ9
symptomatic
with complex partial seizures G4Ø.2Ø9
intractable G4Ø.219
with status epilepticus G4Ø.211
without status epilepticus G4Ø.219
not intractable G4Ø.2Ø9
with status epilepticus G4Ø.2Ø1
without status epilepticus G4Ø.2Ø9
with simple partial seizures G4Ø.1Ø9
intractable G4Ø.119
with status epilepticus G4Ø.111
without status epilepticus G4Ø.119
not intractable G4Ø.1Ø9
with status epilepticus G4Ø.1Ø1
without status epilepticus G4Ø.1Ø9

- **Erosion** — *continued*
  - uterus N85.8
- **Erotomania** F52.8
- **Error**
  - metabolism, inborn — *see* Disorder, metabolism
  - refractive — *see* Disorder, refraction
- **Eructation** R14.2
  - nervous or psychogenic F45.8
- **Eruption**
  - creeping B76.9
  - drug (generalized) (taken internally) L27.Ø
    - fixed L27.1
    - in contact with skin — *see* Dermatitis, due to drugs
    - localized L27.1
  - Hutchinson, summer L56.4
  - Kaposi's varicelliform BØØ.Ø
  - napkin L22
  - polymorphous light (sun) L56.4
  - recalcitrant pustular L13.8
  - ringed R23.8
  - skin (nonspecific) R21
    - creeping (meaning hookworm) B76.9
    - due to inoculation/vaccination (generalized) — *see also* Dermatitis, due to, vaccine L27.Ø
      - localized L27.1
    - erysipeloid A26.Ø
    - feigned L98.1
    - Kaposi's varicelliform BØØ.Ø
    - lichenoid L28.Ø
    - meaning dermatitis — *see* Dermatitis
    - toxic NEC L53.Ø
  - tooth, teeth, abnormal (incomplete) (late) (premature) (sequence) KØØ.6
  - vesicular R23.8
- **Erysipelas** (gangrenous) (infantile) (newborn) (phlegmonous) (suppurative) A46
  - external ear A46 *[H62.4Ø]*
  - puerperal, postpartum O86.89
- **Erysipeloid** A26.9
  - cutaneous (Rosenbach's) A26.Ø
  - disseminated A26.8
  - sepsis A26.7
  - specified NEC A26.8
- **Erythema, erythematous** (infectional) (inflammation) L53.9
  - ab igne L59.Ø
  - annulare (centrifugum) (rheumaticum) L53.1
  - arthriticum epidemicum A25.1
  - brucellum — *see* Brucellosis
  - chronic figurate NEC L53.3
  - chronicum migrans (Borrelia burgdorferi) A69.2Ø
  - diaper L22
  - due to
    - chemical NEC L53.Ø
      - in contact with skin L24.5
    - drug (internal use) — *see* Dermatitis, due to, drugs
  - elevatum diutinum L95.1
  - endemic E52
  - epidemic, arthritic A25.1
  - figuratum perstans L53.3
  - gluteal L22
  - heat — *code by site under* Burn, first degree
  - ichthyosiforme congenitum bullous Q8Ø.3
  - in diseases classified elsewhere L54
  - induratum (nontuberculous) L52
    - tuberculous A18.4
  - infectiosum BØ8.3
  - intertrigo L3Ø.4
  - iris L51.9
  - marginatum L53.2
    - in (due to) acute rheumatic fever IØØ
  - medicamentosum — *see* Dermatitis, due to, drugs
  - migrans A26.Ø
    - chronicum A69.2Ø
    - tongue K14.1
  - multiforme (major) (minor) L51.9
    - bullous, bullosum L51.1
    - conjunctiva L51.1
    - nonbullous L51.Ø
    - pemphigoides L12.Ø
    - specified NEC L51.8
  - napkin L22
  - neonatorum P83.88
    - toxic P83.1
  - nodosum L52
    - tuberculous A18.4
  - palmar L53.8
  - pernio T69.1 ☑
- **Erythema, erythematous** — *continued*
  - rash, newborn P83.88
  - scarlatiniform (recurrent) (exfoliative) L53.8
  - solare L55.Ø
  - specified NEC L53.8
  - toxic, toxicum NEC L53.Ø
    - newborn P83.1
  - tuberculous (primary) A18.4
- **Erythematous, erythematosus** — *see* condition
- **Erythermalgia** (primary) I73.81
- **Erythralgia** I73.81
- **Erythrasma** LØ8.1
- **Erythredema** (polyneuropathy) — *see* Poisoning, mercury
- **Erythremia** (acute) C94.Ø- ☑
  - chronic D45
  - secondary D75.1
- **Erythroblastopenia** — *see also* Aplasia, red cell D6Ø.9
  - congenital D61.Ø1
- **Erythroblastophthisis** D61.Ø9
- **Erythroblastosis** (fetalis) (newborn) P55.9
  - due to
    - ABO (antibodies) (incompatibility) (isoimmunization) P55.1
    - Rh (antibodies) (incompatibility) (isoimmunization) P55.Ø
- **Erythrocyanosis** (crurum) I73.89
- **Erythrocythemia** — *see* Erythremia
- **Erythrocytosis** (megalosplenic) (secondary) D75.1
  - familial D75.Ø
  - oval, hereditary — *see* Elliptocytosis
  - secondary D75.1
  - stress D75.1
- **Erythroderma** (secondary) — *see also* Erythema L53.9
  - bullous ichthyosiform, congenital Q8Ø.3
  - desquamativum L21.1
  - ichthyosiform, congenital (bullous) Q8Ø.3
  - neonatorum P83.88
  - psoriaticum L4Ø.8
- **Erythrodysesthesia, palmar plantar** (PPE) L27.1
- **Erythrogenesis imperfecta** D61.Ø9
- **Erythroleukemia** C94.Ø- ☑
- **Erythromelalgia** I73.81
- **Erythrophagocytosis** D75.89
- **Erythrophobia** F4Ø.298
- **Erythroplakia, oral epithelium, and tongue** K13.29
- **Erythroplasia** (Queyrat) DØ7.4
  - specified site — *see* Neoplasm, skin, in situ
  - unspecified site DØ7.4
- **Escherichia coli** (E. coli), **as cause of disease classified elsewhere** B96.2Ø
  - non-O157 Shiga toxin-producing (with known O group) B96.22
  - non-Shiga toxin-producing B96.29
  - O157 with confirmation of Shiga toxin when H antigen is unknown, or is not H7 B96.21
  - O157:H- (nonmotile) with confirmation of Shiga toxin B96.21
  - O157:H7 with or without confirmation of Shiga toxin-production B96.21
  - Shiga toxin-producing (with unspecified O group) (STEC) B96.23
  - O157 B96.21
  - specified NEC B96.29
- **Esophagismus** K22.4
- **Esophagitis** (acute) (alkaline) (chemical) (chronic) (infectional) (necrotic) (peptic) (postoperative) (without bleeding) K2Ø.9Ø
  - with bleeding K2Ø.91
  - candidal B37.81
  - due to gastrointestinal reflux disease (without bleeding) K21.ØØ
    - with bleeding K21.Ø1
  - eosinophilic K2Ø.Ø
  - reflux K21.ØØ
  - specified NEC (without bleeding) K2Ø.8Ø
    - with bleeding K2Ø.81
  - tuberculous A18.83
  - ulcerative K22.1Ø
    - with bleeding K22.11
- **Esophagocele** K22.5
- **Esophagomalacia** K22.8
- **Esophagospasm** K22.4
- **Esophagostenosis** K22.2
- **Esophagostomiasis** B81.8
- **Esophagotracheal** — *see* condition
- **Esophagus** — *see* condition
- **Esophoria** H5Ø.51
- **Esophoria** — *continued*
  - convergence, excess H51.12
  - divergence, insufficiency H51.8
- **Esotropia** — *see* Strabismus, convergent concomitant
- **Espundia** B55.2
- **Essential** — *see* condition
- **Esthesioneuroblastoma** C3Ø.Ø
- **Esthesioneurocytoma** C3Ø.Ø
- **Esthesioneuroepithelioma** C3Ø.Ø
- **Esthiomene** A55
- **Estivo-autumnal malaria** (fever) B5Ø.9
- **Estrangement** (marital) Z63.5
  - parent-child NEC Z62.89Ø
- **Estriasis** — *see* Myiasis
- **Ethanolism** — *see* Alcoholism
- **Etherism** — *see* Dependence, drug, inhalant
- **Ethmoid, ethmoidal** — *see* condition
- **Ethmoiditis** (chronic) (nonpurulent) (purulent) — *see also* Sinusitis, ethmoidal
  - influenzal — *see* Influenza, with, respiratory manifestations NEC
  - Woakes' J33.1
- **Ethylism** — *see* Alcoholism
- **Eulenburg's disease** (congenital paramyotonia) G71.19
- **Eumycetoma** B47.Ø
- **Eunuchoidism** E29.1
  - hypogonadotropic E23.Ø
- **European blastomycosis** — *see* Cryptococcosis
- **Eustachian** — *see* condition
- **Evaluation** (for) (of)
  - development state
    - adolescent ZØØ.3
    - period of
      - delayed growth in childhood ZØØ.7Ø
        - with abnormal findings ZØØ.71
      - rapid growth in childhood ZØØ.2
    - puberty ZØØ.3
  - growth and developmental state (period of rapid growth) ZØØ.2
    - delayed growth ZØØ.7Ø
      - with abnormal findings ZØØ.71
  - mental health (status) ZØØ.8
    - requested by authority ZØ4.6
  - period of
    - delayed growth in childhood ZØØ.7Ø
      - with abnormal findings ZØØ.71
    - rapid growth in childhood ZØØ.2
  - suspected condition — *see* Observation
- **Evans syndrome** D69.41
- **Event**
  - apparent life threatening in newborn and infant (ALTE) R68.13
  - brief resolved unexplained event (BRUE) R68.13
- **Eventration** — *see also* Hernia, ventral
  - colon into chest — *see* Hernia, diaphragm
  - diaphragm (congenital) Q79.1
- **Eversion**
  - bladder N32.89
  - cervix (uteri) N86
    - with cervicitis N72
  - foot NEC — *see also* Deformity, valgus, ankle
    - congenital Q66.6
  - punctum lacrimale (postinfectional) (senile) HØ4.52- ☑
  - ureter (meatus) N28.89
  - urethra (meatus) N36.8
  - uterus N81.4
- **Evidence**
  - cytologic
    - of malignancy on anal smear R85.614
    - of malignancy on cervical smear R87.614
    - of malignancy on vaginal smear R87.624
- **Evisceration**
  - birth injury P15.8
  - traumatic NEC
    - eye — *see* Enucleated eye
- **Evulsion** — *see* Avulsion
- **Ewing's sarcoma or tumor** — *see* Neoplasm, bone, malignant
- **Examination** (for) (following) (general) (of) (routine) ZØØ.ØØ
  - with abnormal findings ZØØ.Ø1
  - abuse, physical (alleged), ruled out
    - adult ZØ4.71
    - child ZØ4.72
  - adolescent (development state) ZØØ.3
  - alleged rape or sexual assault (victim), ruled out
    - adult ZØ4.41
    - child ZØ4.42

Examination — *continued*
  allergy Z01.82
  annual (adult) (periodic) (physical) Z00.00
    with abnormal findings Z00.01
    gynecological Z01.419
      with abnormal findings Z01.411
  antibody response Z01.84
  blood — *see* Examination, laboratory
  blood pressure Z01.30
    with abnormal findings Z01.31
  cancer staging — *see* Neoplasm, malignant, by site
  cervical Papanicolaou smear Z12.4
    as part of routine gynecological examination Z01.419
      with abnormal findings Z01.411
  child (over 28 days old) Z00.129
    with abnormal findings Z00.121
    under 28 days old — *see* Newborn, examination
  clinical research control or normal comparison (control) (participant) Z00.6
  contraceptive (drug) maintenance (routine) Z30.8
    device (intrauterine) Z30.431
  dental Z01.20
    with abnormal findings Z01.21
  developmental — *see* Examination, child
  donor (potential) Z00.5
  ear Z01.10
    with abnormal findings NEC Z01.118
  eye Z01.00
    with abnormal findings Z01.01
    following failed vision screening Z01.020
      with abnormal findings Z01.021
  follow-up (routine) (following) Z09
    chemotherapy NEC Z09
      malignant neoplasm Z08
    fracture Z09
    malignant neoplasm Z08
    postpartum Z39.2
    psychotherapy Z09
    radiotherapy NEC Z09
      malignant neoplasm Z08
    surgery NEC Z09
      malignant neoplasm Z08
  following
    accident NEC Z04.3
      transport Z04.1
      work Z04.2
    assault, alleged, ruled out
      adult Z04.71
      child Z04.72
    motor vehicle accident Z04.1
    treatment (for) Z09
      combined NEC Z09
        fracture Z09
        malignant neoplasm Z08
      malignant neoplasm Z08
      mental disorder Z09
      specified condition NEC Z09
  forced sexual exploitation Z04.81
  forced labor exploitation Z04.82
  gynecological Z01.419
    with abnormal findings Z01.411
    for contraceptive maintenance Z30.8
  health — *see* Examination, medical
  hearing Z01.10
    with abnormal findings NEC Z01.118
    following failed hearing screening Z01.110
    infant or child (over 28 days old) Z00.129
      with abnormal findings Z00.121
  immunity status testing Z01.84
  laboratory (as part of a general medical examination) Z00.00
    with abnormal findings Z00.01
    preprocedural Z01.812
  lactating mother Z39.1
  medical (adult) (for) (of) Z00.00
    with abnormal findings Z00.01
    administrative purpose only Z02.9
      specified NEC Z02.89
    admission to
      armed forces Z02.3
      old age home Z02.2
      prison Z02.89
      residential institution Z02.2
      school Z02.0
        following illness or medical treatment Z02.0
      summer camp Z02.89
    adoption Z02.82
    blood alcohol or drug level Z02.83

Examination — *continued*
  medical — *continued*
    camp (summer) Z02.89
    clinical research, normal subject (control) (participant) Z00.6
    control subject in clinical research (normal comparison) (participant) Z00.6
    donor (potential) Z00.5
    driving license Z02.4
    general (adult) Z00.00
      with abnormal findings Z00.01
    immigration Z02.89
    insurance purposes Z02.6
    marriage Z02.89
    medicolegal reasons NEC Z04.89
    naturalization Z02.89
    participation in sport Z02.5
    paternity testing Z02.81
    population survey Z00.8
    pre-employment Z02.1
    pre-operative — *see* Examination, pre-procedural
    pre-procedural
      cardiovascular Z01.810
      respiratory Z01.811
      specified NEC Z01.818
    preschool children
      for admission to school Z02.0
    prisoners
      for entrance into prison Z02.89
    recruitment for armed forces Z02.3
    specified NEC Z00.8
    sport competition Z02.5
  medicolegal reason NEC Z04.89
    following
      forced sexual exploitation Z04.81
      forced labor exploitation Z04.82
  newborn — *see* Newborn, examination
  pelvic (annual) (periodic) Z01.419
    with abnormal findings Z01.411
  period of rapid growth in childhood Z00.2
  periodic (adult) (annual) (routine) Z00.00
    with abnormal findings Z00.01
  physical (adult) — *see also* Examination, medical Z00.00
    sports Z02.5
  postpartum
    immediately after delivery Z39.0
    routine follow-up Z39.2
  pre-chemotherapy (antineoplastic) Z01.818
  prenatal (normal pregnancy) — *see also* Pregnancy, normal Z34.9- ☑
  pre-procedural (pre-operative)
    cardiovascular Z01.810
    laboratory Z01.812
    respiratory Z01.811
    specified NEC Z01.818
  prior to chemotherapy (antineoplastic) Z01.818
  psychiatric NEC Z00.8
    follow-up not needing further care Z09
    requested by authority Z04.6
  radiological (as part of a general medical examination) Z00.00
    with abnormal findings Z00.01
  repeat cervical smear to confirm findings of recent normal smear following initial abnormal smear Z01.42
  skin (hypersensitivity) Z01.82
  special — *see also* Examination, by type Z01.89
    specified type NEC Z01.89
  specified type or reason NEC Z04.89
  teeth Z01.20
    with abnormal findings Z01.21
  urine — *see* Examination, laboratory
  vision Z01.00
    with abnormal findings Z01.01
    following failed vision screening Z01.020
      with abnormal findings Z01.021
    infant or child (over 28 days old) Z00.129
      with abnormal findings Z00.121

Exanthem, exanthema — *see also* Rash
  with enteroviral vesicular stomatitis B08.4
  Boston A88.0
  epidemic with meningitis A88.0 *[G02]*
  subitum B08.20
    due to human herpesvirus 6 B08.21
    due to human herpesvirus 7 B08.22
  viral, virus B09
    specified type NEC B08.8

Excess, excessive, excessively
  alcohol level in blood R78.0
  androgen (ovarian) E28.1
  attrition, tooth, teeth K03.0
  carotene, carotin (dietary) E67.1
  cold, effects of T69.9 ☑
    specified effect NEC T69.8 ☑
  convergence H51.12
  crying
    in child, adolescent, or adult R45.83
    in infant R68.11
  development, breast N62
  divergence H51.8
  drinking (alcohol) NEC (without dependence) F10.10
    habitual (continual) (without remission) F10.20
  eating R63.2
  estrogen E28.0
  fat — *see also* Obesity
    in heart — *see* Degeneration, myocardial
    localized E65
  foreskin N47.8
  gas R14.0
  glucagon E16.3
  heat — *see* Heat
  intermaxillary vertical dimension of fully erupted teeth M26.37
  interocclusal distance of fully erupted teeth M26.37
  kalium E87.5
  large
    colon K59.39
      congenital Q43.8
    infant P08.0
    organ or site, congenital NEC — *see* Anomaly, by site
  long
    organ or site, congenital NEC — *see* Anomaly, by site
  menstruation (with regular cycle) N92.0
    with irregular cycle N92.1
  napping Z72.821
  natrium E87.0
  number of teeth K00.1
  nutrient (dietary) NEC R63.2
  potassium (K) E87.5
  salivation K11.7
  secretion — *see also* Hypersecretion
    milk O92.6
    sputum R09.3
    sweat R61
  sexual drive F52.8
  short
    organ or site, congenital NEC — *see* Anomaly, by site
    umbilical cord in labor or delivery O69.3 ☑
  skin L98.7
    and subcutaneous tissue L98.7
    eyelid (acquired) — *see* Blepharochalasis
      congenital Q10.3
  sodium (Na) E87.0
  spacing of fully erupted teeth M26.32
  sputum R09.3
  sweating R61
  thirst R63.1
    due to deprivation of water T73.1 ☑
  tuberosity of jaw M26.07
  vitamin
    A (dietary) E67.0
      administered as drug (prolonged intake) — *see* Table of Drugs and Chemicals, vitamins, adverse effect
      overdose or wrong substance given or taken — *see* Table of Drugs and Chemicals, vitamins, poisoning
    D (dietary) E67.3
      administered as drug (prolonged intake) — *see* Table of Drugs and Chemicals, vitamins, adverse effect
      overdose or wrong substance given or taken — *see* Table of Drugs and Chemicals, vitamins, poisoning
  weight
    gain R63.5
    loss R63.4

Excitability, abnormal, under minor stress (personality disorder) F60.3

Excitation
  anomalous atrioventricular I45.6
  psychogenic F30.8

Excitation — *continued*
- reactive (from emotional stress, psychological trauma) F3Ø.8

Excitement
- hypomanic F3Ø.8
- manic F3Ø.9
- mental, reactive (from emotional stress, psychological trauma) F3Ø.8
- state, reactive (from emotional stress, psychological trauma) F3Ø.8

Excoriation (traumatic) — *see also* Abrasion
- neurotic L98.1
- skin picking disorder F42.4

Exfoliation
- due to erythematous conditions according to extent of body surface involved L49.Ø
  - 1Ø-19 percent of body surface L49.1
  - 2Ø-29 percent of body surface L49.2
  - 3Ø-39 percent of body surface L49.3
  - 4Ø-49 percent of body surface L49.4
  - 5Ø-59 percent of body surface L49.5
  - 6Ø-69 percent of body surface L49.6
  - 7Ø-79 percent of body surface L49.7
  - 8Ø-89 percent of body surface L49.8
  - 9Ø-99 percent of body surface L49.9
  - less than 1Ø percent of body surface L49.Ø
- teeth, due to systemic causes KØ8.Ø

Exfoliative — *see* condition

Exhaustion, exhaustive (physical NEC) R53.83
- battle F43.Ø
- cardiac — *see* Failure, heart
- delirium F43.Ø
- due to
  - cold T69.8 ☑
  - excessive exertion T73.3 ☑
  - exposure T73.2 ☑
  - neurasthenia F48.8
- heart — *see* Failure, heart
- heat — *see also* Heat, exhaustion T67.5 ☑
  - due to
    - salt depletion T67.4 ☑
    - water depletion T67.3 ☑
- maternal, complicating delivery O75.81
- mental F48.8
- myocardium, myocardial — *see* Failure, heart
- nervous F48.8
- old age R54
- psychogenic F48.8
- psychosis F43.Ø
- senile R54
- vital NEC Z73.Ø

Exhibitionism F65.2

Exocervicitis — *see* Cervicitis

Exomphalos Q79.2
- meaning hernia — *see* Hernia, umbilicus

Exophoria H5Ø.52
- convergence, insufficiency H51.11
- divergence, excess H51.8

Exophthalmos HØ5.2- ☑
- congenital Q15.8
- constant NEC HØ5.24- ☑
- displacement, globe — *see* Displacement, globe
- due to thyrotoxicosis (hyperthyroidism) — *see* Hyperthyroidism, with, goiter (diffuse)
- dysthyroid — *see* Hyperthyroidism, with, goiter (diffuse)
- goiter — *see* Hyperthyroidism, with, goiter (diffuse)
- intermittent NEC HØ5.25- ☑
- malignant — *see* Hyperthyroidism, with, goiter (diffuse)
- orbital
  - edema — *see* Edema, orbit
  - hemorrhage — *see* Hemorrhage, orbit
- pulsating NEC HØ5.26- ☑
- thyrotoxic, thyrotropic — *see* Hyperthyroidism, with, goiter (diffuse)

Exostosis — *see also* Disorder, bone
- cartilaginous — *see* Neoplasm, bone, benign
- congenital (multiple) Q78.6
- external ear canal H61.81- ☑
- gonococcal A54.49
- jaw (bone) M27.8
- multiple, congenital Q78.6
- orbit HØ5.35- ☑
- osteocartilaginous — *see* Neoplasm, bone, benign
- syphilitic A52.77

Exotropia — *see* Strabismus, divergent concomitant

Explanation of
- investigation finding Z71.2
- medication Z71.89

Exposure (to) — *see also* Contact, with T75.89 ☑
- acariasis Z2Ø.7
- AIDS virus Z2Ø.6
- air pollution Z77.11Ø
- algae and algae toxins Z77.121
- algae bloom Z77.121
- anthrax Z2Ø.81Ø
- aromatic amines Z77.Ø2Ø
- aromatic (hazardous) compounds NEC Z77.Ø28
- aromatic dyes NOS Z77.Ø28
- arsenic Z77.Ø1Ø
- asbestos Z77.Ø9Ø
- bacterial disease NEC Z2Ø.818
- benzene Z77.Ø21
- blue-green algae bloom Z77.121
- body fluids (potentially hazardous) Z77.21
- brown tide Z77.121
- chemicals (chiefly nonmedicinal) (hazardous) NEC Z77.Ø98
- cholera Z2Ø.Ø9
- chromium compounds Z77.Ø18
- cold, effects of T69.9 ☑
  - specified effect NEC T69.8 ☑
- communicable disease Z2Ø.9
  - bacterial NEC Z2Ø.818
  - specified NEC Z2Ø.89
  - viral NEC Z2Ø.828
  - Zika virus Z2Ø.821
- cyanobacteria bloom Z77.121
- disaster Z65.5
- discrimination Z6Ø.5
- dyes Z77.Ø98
- effects of T73.9 ☑
- environmental tobacco smoke (acute) (chronic) Z77.22
- Escherichia coli (E. coli) Z2Ø.Ø1
- exhaustion due to T73.2 ☑
- fiberglass — *see* Table of Drugs and Chemicals, fiberglass
- German measles Z2Ø.4
- gonorrhea Z2Ø.2
- hazardous metals NEC Z77.Ø18
- hazardous substances NEC Z77.29
- hazards in the physical environment NEC Z77.128
- hazards to health NEC Z77.9
- human immunodeficiency virus (HIV) Z2Ø.6
- human T-lymphotropic virus type-1 (HTLV-1) Z2Ø.89
- implanted
  - mesh — *see* Complications, prosthetic devise or implant, mesh
  - prosthetic materials NEC — *see* Complications, prosthetic materials NEC
- infestation (parasitic) NEC Z2Ø.7
- intestinal infectious disease NEC Z2Ø.Ø9
  - Escherichia coli (E. coli) Z2Ø.Ø1
- lead Z77.Ø11
- meningococcus Z2Ø.811
- mold (toxic) Z77.12Ø
- nickel dust Z77.Ø18
- noise Z77.122
- occupational
  - air contaminants NEC Z57.39
  - dust Z57.2
  - environmental tobacco smoke Z57.31
  - extreme temperature Z57.6
  - noise Z57.Ø
  - radiation Z57.1
  - risk factors Z57.9
    - specified NEC Z57.8
  - toxic agents (gases) (liquids) (solids) (vapors) in agriculture Z57.4
  - toxic agents (gases) (liquids) (solids) (vapors) in industry NEC Z57.5
  - vibration Z57.7
- parasitic disease NEC Z2Ø.7
- pediculosis Z2Ø.7
- persecution Z6Ø.5
- pfiesteria piscicida Z77.121
- poliomyelitis Z2Ø.89
- pollution
  - air Z77.11Ø
  - environmental NEC Z77.118
  - soil Z77.112
  - water Z77.111
- polycyclic aromatic hydrocarbons Z77.Ø28

Exposure — *continued*
- prenatal (drugs) (toxic chemicals) — *see* Newborn, affected by, noxious substances transmitted via placenta or breast milk
- rabies Z2Ø.3
- radiation, naturally occurring NEC Z77.123
- radon Z77.123
- red tide (Florida) Z77.121
- rubella Z2Ø.4
- second hand tobacco smoke (acute) (chronic) Z77.22
  - in the perinatal period P96.81
- sexually-transmitted disease Z2Ø.2
- smallpox (laboratory) Z2Ø.89
- syphilis Z2Ø.2
- terrorism Z65.4
- torture Z65.4
- tuberculosis Z2Ø.1
- uranium Z77.Ø12
- varicella Z2Ø.82Ø
- venereal disease Z2Ø.2
- viral disease NEC Z2Ø.828
- war Z65.5
- water pollution Z77.111
- Zika virus Z2Ø.821

Exsanguination — *see* Hemorrhage

Exstrophy
- abdominal contents Q45.8
- bladder Q64.1Ø
  - cloacal Q64.12
  - specified type NEC Q64.19
  - supravesical fissure Q64.11

Extensive — *see* condition

Extra — *see also* Accessory
- marker chromosomes (normal individual) Q92.61
  - in abnormal individual Q92.62
- rib Q76.6
  - cervical Q76.5

Extrasystoles (supraventricular) I49.49
- atrial I49.1
- auricular I49.1
- junctional I49.2
- ventricular I49.3

Extrauterine gestation or pregnancy — *see* Pregnancy, by site

Extravasation
- blood R58
- chyle into mesentery I89.8
- pelvicalyceal N13.8
- pyelosinus N13.8
- urine (from ureter) R39.Ø
- vesicant agent
  - antineoplastic chemotherapy T8Ø.81Ø ☑
  - other agent NEC T8Ø.818 ☑

Extremity — *see* condition, limb

Extrophy — *see* Exstrophy

Extroversion
- bladder Q64.19
- uterus N81.4
  - complicating delivery O71.2
  - postpartal (old) N81.4

Extruded tooth (teeth) M26.34

Extrusion
- breast implant (prosthetic) T85.42 ☑
- eye implant (globe) (ball) T85.328 ☑
- intervertebral disc — *see* Displacement, intervertebral disc
- ocular lens implant (prosthetic) — *see* Complications, intraocular lens
- vitreous — *see* Prolapse, vitreous

Exudate
- pleural — *see* Effusion, pleura
- retina H35.89

Exudative — *see* condition

Eye, eyeball, eyelid — *see* condition

Eyestrain — *see* Disturbance, vision, subjective

Eyeworm disease of Africa B74.3

F

Faber's syndrome (achlorhydric anemia) D5Ø.9

Fabry (-Anderson) **disease** E75.21

Facet syndrome M47.89- ☑

Faciocephalalgia, autonomic — *see also* Neuropathy, peripheral, autonomic G9Ø.Ø9

Factor(s)
- psychic, associated with diseases classified elsewhere F54

- **Factor**(s) — *continued*
  - psychological
    - affecting physical conditions F54
    - or behavioral
      - affecting general medical condition F54
      - associated with disorders or diseases classified elsewhere F54
- **Fahr disease** (of brain) G23.8
- **Fahr Volhard disease** (of kidney) I12.- ☑
- **Failure, failed**
  - abortion — *see* Abortion, attempted
  - aortic (valve) I35.8
    - rheumatic IØ6.8
  - attempted abortion — *see* Abortion, attempted
  - biventricular I5Ø.82
    - due to left heart failure I5Ø.814
  - bone marrow — *see* Anemia, aplastic
  - cardiac — *see* Failure, heart
  - cardiorenal (chronic) — *see also* Failure, renal, and Failure, heart I5Ø.9
    - hypertensive I13.2
  - cardiorespiratory — *see also* Failure, heart RØ9.2
  - cardiovascular (chronic) — *see* Failure, heart
  - cerebrovascular I67.9
  - cervical dilatation in labor O62.Ø
  - circulation, circulatory (peripheral) R57.9
    - newborn P29.89
  - compensation — *see* Disease, heart
  - compliance with medical treatment or regimen — *see* Noncompliance
  - congestive — *see* Failure, heart, congestive
  - dental implant (endosseous) M27.69
    - due to
      - failure of dental prosthesis M27.63
      - lack of attached gingiva M27.62
      - occlusal trauma (poor prosthetic design) M27.62
      - parafunctional habits M27.62
      - periodontal infection (peri-implantitis) M27.62
      - poor oral hygiene M27.62
    - osseointegration M27.61
      - due to
        - complications of systemic disease M27.61
        - poor bone quality M27.61
      - iatrogenic M27.61
    - post-osseointegration
      - biological M27.62
      - due to complications of systemic disease M27.62
      - iatrogenic M27.62
      - mechanical M27.63
    - pre-integration M27.61
    - pre-osseointegration M27.61
    - specified NEC M27.69
  - descent of head (at term) of pregnancy (mother) O32.4 ☑
  - endosseous dental implant — *see* Failure, dental implant
  - engagement of head (term of pregnancy) (mother) O32.4 ☑
  - erection (penile) — *see also* Dysfunction, sexual, male, erectile N52.9
    - nonorganic F52.21
  - examination(s), anxiety concerning Z55.2
  - expansion terminal respiratory units (newborn) (primary) P28.Ø
  - forceps NOS (with subsequent cesarean delivery) O66.5
  - gain weight (child over 28 days old) R62.51
    - adult R62.7
    - newborn P92.6
  - genital response (male) F52.21
    - female F52.22
  - heart (acute) (senile) (sudden) I5Ø.9
    - with
      - acute pulmonary edema — *see* Failure, ventricular, left
      - decompensation — *see also* Failure, heart, by type as diastolic or systolic, acute and chronic I5Ø.9
      - dilatation — *see* Disease, heart
      - hypertension — *see* Hypertension, heart
      - normal ejection fraction — *see* Failure, heart, diastolic
      - preserved ejection fraction — *see* Failure, heart, diastolic
      - reduced ejection fraction — *see* Failure, heart, systolic
    - arteriosclerotic I7Ø.9Ø
    - biventricular I5Ø.82
      - due to left heart failure I5Ø.814

- **Failure, failed** — *continued*
  - heart — *continued*
    - combined left-right sided I5Ø.82
      - due to left heart failure I5Ø.814
    - compensated — *see also* Failure, heart, by type as diastolic or systolic, chronic I5Ø.9
    - complicating
      - anesthesia (general) (local) or other sedation
        - in labor and delivery O74.2
        - in pregnancy O29.12- ☑
        - postpartum, puerperal O89.1
      - delivery (cesarean) (instrumental) O75.4
    - congestive I5Ø.9
      - with rheumatic fever (conditions in IØØ)
        - active IØ1.8
        - inactive or quiescent (with chorea) IØ9.81
      - newborn P29.Ø
      - rheumatic (chronic) (inactive) (with chorea) IØ9.81
        - active or acute IØ1.8
          - with chorea IØ2.Ø
    - decompensated — *see also* Failure, heart, by type as diastolic or systolic, acute and chronic I5Ø.9
    - degenerative — *see* Degeneration, myocardial
    - diastolic (congestive) (left ventricular) I5Ø.3Ø
      - acute (congestive) I5Ø.31
        - and (on) chronic (congestive) I5Ø.33
      - chronic (congestive) I5Ø.32
        - and (on) acute (congestive) I5Ø.33
      - combined with systolic (congestive) I5Ø.4Ø
        - acute (congestive) I5Ø.41
          - and (on) chronic (congestive) I5Ø.43
        - chronic (congestive) I5Ø.42
          - and (on) acute (congestive) I5Ø.43
    - due to presence of cardiac prosthesis I97.13- ☑
    - end stage — *see also* Failure, heart, by type as diastolic or systolic, chronic I5Ø.84
    - following cardiac surgery I97.13- ☑
    - high output NOS I5Ø.83
    - hypertensive — *see* Hypertension, heart
    - left (ventricular) — *see also* Failure, ventricular, left
      - combined diastolic and systolic — *see* Failure, heart, diastolic, combined with systolic
      - diastolic — *see* Failure, heart, diastolic
      - systolic — *see* Failure, heart, systolic
    - low output (syndrome) NOS I5Ø.9
    - newborn P29.Ø
    - organic — *see* Disease, heart
    - peripartum O9Ø.3
    - postprocedural I97.13- ☑
    - rheumatic (chronic) (inactive) IØ9.9
    - right (isolated) (ventricular) I5Ø.81Ø
      - acute I5Ø.811
        - and (on) chronic I5Ø.813
      - chronic I5Ø.812
        - and acute I5Ø.813
      - secondary to left heart failure I5Ø.814
    - specified NEC I5Ø.89

> *Note: heart failure stages A, B, C, and D are based on the American College of Cardiology and American Heart Association stages of heart failure, which complement and should not be confused with the New York Heart Association Classification of Heart Failure, into Class I, Class II, Class III, and Class IV*

    - stage A Z91.89
    - stage B — *see also* Failure, heart, by type as diastolic or systolic I5Ø.9
    - stage C — *see also* Failure, heart, by type as diastolic or systolic I5Ø.9
    - stage D — *see also* Failure, heart, by type as diastolic or systolic, chronic I5Ø.84
    - systolic (congestive) (left ventricular) I5Ø.2Ø
      - acute (congestive) I5Ø.21
        - and (on) chronic (congestive) I5Ø.23
      - chronic (congestive) I5Ø.22
        - and (on) acute (congestive) I5Ø.23
      - combined with diastolic (congestive) I5Ø.4Ø
        - acute (congestive) I5Ø.41
          - and (on) chronic (congestive) I5Ø.43
        - chronic (congestive) I5Ø.42
          - and (on) acute (congestive) I5Ø.43
    - thyrotoxic — *see also* Thyrotoxicosis EØ5.9Ø *[I43]*
      - with
        - high output — *see also* Thyrotoxicosis I5Ø.83
        - thyroid storm EØ5.91 *[I43]*
          - high output — *see also* Thyrotoxicosis I5Ø.83

- **Failure, failed** — *continued*
  - heart — *continued*
    - valvular — *see* Endocarditis
  - hepatic K72.9Ø
    - with coma K72.91
    - acute or subacute K72.ØØ
      - with coma K72.Ø1
      - due to drugs K71.1Ø
        - with coma K71.11
    - alcoholic (acute) (chronic) (subacute) K7Ø.4Ø
      - with coma K7Ø.41
    - chronic K72.1Ø
      - with coma K72.11
      - due to drugs (acute) (subacute) (chronic) K71.1Ø
        - with coma K71.11
    - due to drugs (acute) (subacute) (chronic) K71.1Ø
      - with coma K71.11
    - postprocedural K91.82
  - hepatorenal K76.7
  - induction (of labor) O61.9
    - abortion — *see* Abortion, attempted
    - by
      - oxytocic drugs O61.Ø
      - prostaglandins O61.Ø
    - instrumental O61.1
    - mechanical O61.1
    - medical O61.Ø
    - specified NEC O61.8
    - surgical O61.1
  - intubation during anesthesia T88.4 ☑
    - in pregnancy O29.6- ☑
    - labor and delivery O74.7
    - postpartum, puerperal O89.6
  - involution, thymus (gland) E32.Ø
  - kidney — *see also* Disease, kidney, chronic N19
    - acute — *see also* Failure, renal, acute N17.9
  - lactation (complete) O92.3
    - partial O92.4
  - Leydig's cell, adult E29.1
  - liver — *see* Failure, hepatic
  - menstruation at puberty N91.Ø
  - mitral IØ5.8
  - myocardial, myocardium — *see also* Failure, heart I5Ø.9
    - chronic — *see also* Failure, heart, congestive I5Ø.9
    - congestive — *see also* Failure, heart, congestive I5Ø.9
  - orgasm (female) (psychogenic) F52.31
    - male F52.32
  - ovarian (primary) E28.39
    - iatrogenic E89.4Ø
      - asymptomatic E89.4Ø
      - symptomatic E89.41
    - postprocedural (postablative) (postirradiation) (postsurgical) E89.4Ø
      - asymptomatic E89.4Ø
      - symptomatic E89.41
  - ovulation causing infertility N97.Ø
  - polyglandular, autoimmune E31.Ø
  - prosthetic joint implant — *see* Complications, joint prosthesis, mechanical, breakdown, by site
  - renal N19
    - with
      - tubular necrosis (acute) N17.Ø
    - acute N17.9
      - with
        - cortical necrosis N17.1
        - medullary necrosis N17.2
        - tubular necrosis N17.Ø
      - specified NEC N17.8
    - chronic N18.9
      - hypertensive — *see* Hypertension, kidney
    - congenital P96.Ø
    - end stage (chronic) N18.6
      - due to hypertension I12.Ø
    - following
      - abortion — *see* Abortion by type complicated by specified condition NEC
      - crushing T79.5 ☑
      - ectopic or molar pregnancy OØ8.4
      - labor and delivery (acute) O9Ø.4
    - hypertensive — *see* Hypertension, kidney
    - postprocedural N99.Ø
  - respiration, respiratory J96.9Ø
    - with
      - hypercapnia J96.92
      - hypercarbia J96.92
      - hypoxia J96.91
    - acute J96.ØØ

Failure, failed — *continued*
- respiration, respiratory — *continued*
  - acute — *continued*
    - with
      - hypercapnia J96.Ø2
      - hypercarbia J96.Ø2
      - hypoxia J96.Ø1
  - center G93.89
  - acute and (on) chronic J96.2Ø
    - with
      - hypercapnia J96.22
      - hypercarbia J96.22
      - hypoxia J96.21
  - chronic J96.1Ø
    - with
      - hypercapnia J96.12
      - hypercarbia J96.12
      - hypoxia J96.11
  - newborn P28.5
  - postprocedural (acute) J95.821
    - acute and chronic J95.822
- rotation
  - cecum Q43.3
  - colon Q43.3
  - intestine Q43.3
  - kidney Q63.2
- sedation (conscious) (moderate) during procedure T88.52 ☑
  - history of Z92.83
- segmentation — *see also* Fusion
  - fingers — *see* Syndactylism, complex, fingers
  - vertebra Q76.49
    - with scoliosis Q76.3
- seminiferous tubule, adult E29.1
- senile (general) R54
- sexual arousal (male) F52.21
  - female F52.22
- testicular endocrine function E29.1
- to thrive (child over 28 days old) R62.51
  - adult R62.7
  - newborn P92.6
- transplant T86.92
  - bone T86.831
    - marrow T86.Ø2
  - cornea T86.841- ☑
  - heart T86.22
    - with lung(s) T86.32
  - intestine T86.851
  - kidney T86.12
  - liver T86.42
  - lung(s) T86.811
    - with heart T86.32
  - pancreas T86.891
  - skin (allograft) (autograft) T86.821
  - specified organ or tissue NEC T86.891
  - stem cell (peripheral blood) (umbilical cord) T86.5
- trial of labor (with subsequent cesarean delivery) O66.4Ø
  - following previous cesarean delivery O66.41
- tubal ligation N99.89
- urinary — *see* Disease, kidney, chronic
- vacuum extraction NOS (with subsequent cesarean delivery) O66.5
- vasectomy N99.89
- ventouse NOS (with subsequent cesarean delivery) O66.5
- ventricular — *see also* Failure, heart I5Ø.9
  - left — *see also* Failure, heart, left I5Ø.1
    - with rheumatic fever (conditions in IØØ)
      - active IØ1.8
        - with chorea IØ2.Ø
      - inactive or quiescent (with chorea) IØ9.81
    - rheumatic (chronic) (inactive) (with chorea) IØ9.81
      - active or acute IØ1.8
        - with chorea IØ2.Ø
  - right — *see* Failure, heart, right
- vital centers, newborn P91.88

Fainting (fit) R55

Fallen arches — *see* Deformity, limb, flat foot

Falling, falls (repeated) R29.6
- any organ or part — *see* Prolapse

Fallopian
- insufflation Z31.41
- tube — *see* condition

Fallot's
- pentalogy Q21.8
- tetrad or tetralogy Q21.3

Fallot's — *continued*
- triad or trilogy Q22.3

False — *see also* condition
- croup J38.5
- joint — *see* Nonunion, fracture
- labor (pains) O47.9
  - at or after 37 completed weeks of gestation O47.1
  - before 37 completed weeks of gestation O47.Ø- ☑
- passage, urethra (prostatic) N36.5
- pregnancy F45.8

Family, familial — *see also* condition
- disruption Z63.8
  - involving divorce or separation Z63.5
- Li-Fraumeni (syndrome) Z15.Ø1
- planning advice Z3Ø.Ø9
- problem Z63.9
  - specified NEC Z63.8
- retinoblastoma C69.2- ☑

Famine (effects of) T73.Ø ☑
- edema — *see* Malnutrition, severe

Fanconi (-de Toni)(-Debré) **syndrome** E72.Ø9
- with cystinosis E72.Ø4

Fanconi's anemia (congenital pancytopenia) D61.Ø9

Farber's disease or syndrome E75.29

Farcy A24.Ø

Farmer's
- lung J67.Ø
- skin L57.8

Farsightedness — *see* Hypermetropia

Fascia — *see* condition

Fasciculation R25.3

Fasciitis M72.9
- diffuse (eosinophilic) M35.4
- infective M72.8
  - necrotizing M72.6
- necrotizing M72.6
- nodular M72.4
- perirenal (with ureteral obstruction) N13.5
  - with infection N13.6
- plantar M72.2
- specified NEC M72.8
- traumatic (old) M72.8
  - current — *code by* site under Sprain

Fascioliasis B66.3

Fasciolopsis, fasciolopsiasis (intestinal) B66.5

Fascioscapulohumeral myopathy G71.Ø2

Fast pulse RØØ.Ø

Fat
- embolism — *see* Embolism, fat
- excessive — *see also* Obesity
  - in heart — *see* Degeneration, myocardial
- in stool R19.5
- localized (pad) E65
  - heart — *see* Degeneration, myocardial
  - knee M79.4
  - retropatellar M79.4
- necrosis
  - breast N64.1
  - mesentery K65.4
  - omentum K65.4
- pad E65
  - knee M79.4

Fatigue R53.83
- auditory deafness — *see* Deafness
- chronic R53.82
- combat F43.Ø
- general R53.83
  - psychogenic F48.8
- heat (transient) T67.6 ☑
- muscle M62.89
- myocardium — *see* Failure, heart
- neoplasm-related R53.Ø
- nervous, neurosis F48.8
- operational F48.8
- psychogenic (general) F48.8
- senile R54
- voice R49.8

Fatness — *see* Obesity

Fatty — *see also* condition
- apron E65
- degeneration — *see* Degeneration, fatty
- heart (enlarged) — *see* Degeneration, myocardial
- liver NEC K76.Ø
  - alcoholic K7Ø.Ø
  - nonalcoholic K76.Ø
- necrosis — *see* Degeneration, fatty

Fauces — *see* condition

Fauchard's disease (periodontitis) — *see* Periodontitis

Faucitis JØ2.9

Favism (anemia) D55.Ø

Favus — *see* Dermatophytosis

Fazio-Londe disease or syndrome G12.1

Fear complex or reaction F4Ø.9

Fear of — *see* Phobia

Feared complaint unfounded Z71.1

Febris, febrile — *see also* Fever
- flava — *see also* Fever, yellow A95.9
- melitensis A23.Ø
- pestis — *see* Plague
- recurrens — *see* Fever, relapsing
- rubra A38.9

Fecal
- incontinence R15.9
- smearing R15.1
- soiling R15.1
- urgency R15.2

Fecalith (impaction) K56.41
- appendix K38.1
- congenital P76.8

Fede's disease K14.Ø

Feeble rapid pulse due to shock following injury T79.4 ☑

Feeble-minded F7Ø

Feeding
- difficulties R63.3
- problem R63.3
  - newborn P92.9
    - specified NEC P92.8
  - nonorganic (adult) — *see* Disorder, eating

Feeling (of)
- foreign body in throat RØ9.89

Feer's disease — *see* Poisoning, mercury

Feet — *see* condition

Feigned illness Z76.5

Feil-Klippel syndrome (brevicollis) Q76.1

Feinmesser's (hidrotic) **ectodermal dysplasia** Q82.4

Felinophobia F4Ø.218

Felon — *see also* Cellulitis, digit
- with lymphangitis — *see* Lymphangitis, acute, digit

Felty's syndrome MØ5.ØØ
- ankle MØ5.Ø7- ☑
- elbow MØ5.Ø2- ☑
- foot joint MØ5.Ø7- ☑
- hand joint MØ5.Ø4- ☑
- hip MØ5.Ø5- ☑
- knee MØ5.Ø6- ☑
- multiple site MØ5.Ø9
- shoulder MØ5.Ø1- ☑
- vertebra — *see* Spondylitis, ankylosing
- wrist MØ5.Ø3- ☑

Female genital cutting status — *see* Female genital mutilation status (FGM)

Female genital mutilation status (FGM) N9Ø.81Ø
- specified NEC N9Ø.818
- type I (clitorectomy status) N9Ø.811
- type II (clitorectomy with excision of labia minora status) N9Ø.812
- type III (infibulation status) N9Ø.813
- type IV N9Ø.818

Femur, femoral — *see* condition

Fenestration, fenestrated — *see also* Imperfect, closure
- aortico-pulmonary Q21.4
- cusps, heart valve NEC Q24.8
  - pulmonary Q22.3
- pulmonic cusps Q22.3

Fernell's disease (aortic aneurysm) I71.9

Fertile eunuch syndrome E23.Ø

Fetid
- breath R19.6
- sweat L75.Ø

Fetishism F65.Ø
- transvestic F65.1

Fetus, fetal — *see also* condition
- alcohol syndrome (dysmorphic) Q86.Ø
- compressus O31.Ø- ☑
- hydantoin syndrome Q86.1
- lung tissue P28.Ø
- papyraceous O31.Ø- ☑

Fever (inanition) (of unknown origin) (persistent) (with chills) (with rigor) R5Ø.9
- abortus A23.1
- Aden (dengue) A9Ø
- African tick bite A77.8
- African tick-borne A68.1

- **Fever** — *continued*
  - American
    - mountain (tick) A93.2
    - spotted A77.Ø
  - aphthous BØ8.8
  - arbovirus, arboviral A94
    - hemorrhagic A94
    - specified NEC A93.8
  - Argentinian hemorrhagic A96.Ø
  - Assam B55.Ø
  - Australian Q A78
  - Bangkok hemorrhagic A91
  - Barmah forest A92.8
  - Bartonella A44.Ø
  - bilious, hemoglobinuric B5Ø.8
  - blackwater B5Ø.8
  - blister BØØ.1
  - Bolivian hemorrhagic A96.1
  - Bonvale dam T73.3 ☑
  - boutonneuse A77.1
  - brain — *see* Encephalitis
  - Brazilian purpuric A48.4
  - breakbone A9Ø
  - Bullis A77.Ø
  - Bunyamwera A92.8
  - Burdwan B55.Ø
  - Bwamba A92.8
  - Cameroon — *see* Malaria
  - Canton A75.9
  - catarrhal (acute) JØØ
    - chronic J31.Ø
  - cat-scratch A28.1
  - Central Asian hemorrhagic A98.Ø
  - cerebral — *see* Encephalitis
  - cerebrospinal meningococcal A39.Ø
  - Chagres B5Ø.9
  - Chandipura A92.8
  - Changuinola A93.1
  - Charcot's (biliary) (hepatic) (intermittent) — *see* Calculus, bile duct
  - Chikungunya (viral) (hemorrhagic) A92.Ø
  - Chitral A93.1
  - Colombo — *see* Fever, paratyphoid
  - Colorado tick (virus) A93.2
  - congestive (remittent) — *see* Malaria
  - Congo virus A98.Ø
  - continued malarial B5Ø.9
  - Corsican — *see* Malaria
  - Crimean-Congo hemorrhagic A98.Ø
  - Cyprus — *see* Brucellosis
  - dandy A9Ø
  - deer fly — *see* Tularemia
  - dengue (virus) A9Ø
    - hemorrhagic A91
    - sandfly A93.1
  - desert B38.Ø
  - drug induced R5Ø.2
  - due to
    - conditions classified elsewhere R5Ø.81
    - heat T67.Ø1 ☑
  - enteric AØ1.ØØ
  - enteroviral exanthematous (Boston exanthem) A88.Ø
  - ephemeral (of unknown origin) R5Ø.9
  - epidemic hemorrhagic A98.5
  - erysipelatous — *see* Erysipelas
  - estivo-autumnal (malarial) B5Ø.9
  - famine A75.Ø
  - five day A79.Ø
  - following delivery O86.4
  - Fort Bragg A27.89
  - gastroenteric AØ1.ØØ
  - gastromalarial — *see* Malaria
  - Gibraltar — *see* Brucellosis
  - glandular — *see* Mononucleosis, infectious
  - Guama (viral) A92.8
  - Haverhill A25.1
  - hay (allergic) J3Ø.1
    - with asthma (bronchial) J45.9Ø9
      - with
        - exacerbation (acute) J45.9Ø1
        - status asthmaticus J45.9Ø2
    - due to
      - allergen other than pollen J3Ø.89
      - pollen, any plant or tree J3Ø.1
  - heat (effects) T67.Ø1 ☑
  - hematuric, bilious B5Ø.8
  - hemoglobinuric (malarial) (bilious) B5Ø.8
  - hemorrhagic (arthropod-borne) NOS A94

- **Fever** — *continued*
  - hemorrhagic — *continued*
    - with renal syndrome A98.5
    - arenaviral A96.9
      - specified NEC A96.8
    - Argentinian A96.Ø
    - Bangkok A91
    - Bolivian A96.1
    - Central Asian A98.Ø
    - Chikungunya A92.Ø
    - Crimean-Congo A98.Ø
    - dengue (virus) A91
    - epidemic A98.5
    - Junin (virus) A96.Ø
    - Korean A98.5
    - Kyasanur forest A98.2
    - Machupo (virus) A96.1
    - mite-borne A93.8
    - mosquito-borne A92.8
    - Omsk A98.1
    - Philippine A91
    - Russian A98.5
    - Singapore A91
    - Southeast Asia A91
    - Thailand A91
    - tick-borne NEC A93.8
    - viral A99
      - specified NEC A98.8
  - hepatic — *see* Cholecystitis
  - herpetic — *see* Herpes
  - icterohemorrhagic A27.Ø
  - Indiana A93.8
  - infective B99.9
    - specified NEC B99.8
  - intermittent (bilious) — *see also* Malaria
    - of unknown origin R5Ø.9
    - pernicious B5Ø.9
  - iodide R5Ø.2
  - Japanese river A75.3
  - jungle — *see also* Malaria
    - yellow A95.Ø
  - Junin (virus) hemorrhagic A96.Ø
  - Katayama B65.2
  - kedani A75.3
  - Kenya (tick) A77.1
  - Kew Garden A79.1
  - Korean hemorrhagic A98.5
  - Lassa A96.2
  - Lone Star A77.Ø
  - Machupo (virus) hemorrhagic A96.1
  - malaria, malarial — *see* Malaria
  - Malta A23.9
  - Marseilles A77.1
  - marsh — *see* Malaria
  - Mayaro (viral) A92.8
  - Mediterranean — *see also* Brucellosis A23.9
    - familial MØ4.1
    - tick A77.1
  - meningeal — *see* Meningitis
  - Meuse A79.Ø
  - Mexican A75.2
  - mianeh A68.1
  - miasmatic — *see* Malaria
  - mosquito-borne (viral) A92.9
    - hemorrhagic A92.8
  - mountain — *see also* Brucellosis
    - meaning Rocky Mountain spotted fever A77.Ø
    - tick (American) (Colorado) (viral) A93.2
  - Mucambo (viral) A92.8
  - mud A27.9
  - Neapolitan — *see* Brucellosis
  - neutropenic D7Ø.9
  - newborn P81.9
    - environmental P81.Ø
  - Nine-Mile A78
  - non-exanthematous tick A93.2
  - North Asian tick-borne A77.2
  - Omsk hemorrhagic A98.1
  - O'nyong-nyong (viral) A92.1
  - Oropouche (viral) A93.Ø
  - Oroya A44.Ø
  - pacific coast tick A77.8
  - paludal — *see* Malaria
  - Panama (malarial) B5Ø.9
  - Pappataci A93.1
  - paratyphoid AØ1.4
    - A AØ1.1
    - B AØ1.2

- **Fever** — *continued*
  - paratyphoid — *continued*
    - C AØ1.3
  - parrot A7Ø
  - periodic (Mediterranean) MØ4.1
  - persistent (of unknown origin) R5Ø.9
  - petechial A39.Ø
  - pharyngoconjunctival B3Ø.2
  - Philippine hemorrhagic A91
  - phlebotomus A93.1
  - Piry (virus) A93.8
  - Pixuna (viral) A92.8
  - Plasmodium ovale B53.Ø
  - polioviral (nonparalytic) A8Ø.4
  - Pontiac A48.2
  - postimmunization R5Ø.83
  - postoperative R5Ø.82
    - due to infection T81.4Ø ☑
  - posttransfusion R5Ø.84
  - postvaccination R5Ø.83
  - presenting with conditions classified elsewhere R5Ø.81
  - pretibial A27.89
  - puerperal O86.4
  - Q A78
  - quadrilateral A78
  - quartan (malaria) B52.9
  - Queensland (coastal) (tick) A77.3
  - quintan A79.Ø
  - rabbit — *see* Tularemia
  - rat-bite A25.9
    - due to
      - Spirillum A25.Ø
      - Streptobacillus moniliformis A25.1
  - recurrent — *see* Fever, relapsing
  - relapsing (Borrelia) A68.9
    - Carter's (Asiatic) A68.1
    - Dutton's (West African) A68.1
    - Koch's A68.9
    - louse-borne A68.Ø
    - Novy's
      - louse-borne A68.Ø
      - tick-borne A68.1
    - Obermeyer's (European) A68.Ø
    - tick-borne A68.1
  - remittent (bilious) (congestive) (gastric) — *see* Malaria
  - rheumatic (active) (acute) (chronic) (subacute) IØØ
    - with central nervous system involvement IØ2.9
    - active with heart involvement — *see* category IØ1 ☑
    - inactive or quiescent with
      - cardiac hypertrophy IØ9.89
      - carditis IØ9.9
      - endocarditis IØ9.1
        - aortic (valve) IØ6.9
          - with mitral (valve) disease IØ8.Ø
        - mitral (valve) IØ5.9
          - with aortic (valve) disease IØ8.Ø
        - pulmonary (valve) IØ9.89
        - tricuspid (valve) IØ7.8
      - heart disease NEC IØ9.89
      - heart failure (congestive) (conditions in category I5Ø.) IØ9.81
      - left ventricular failure (conditions in I5Ø.1-I5Ø.4-) IØ9.81
      - myocarditis, myocardial degeneration (conditions in I51.4) IØ9.Ø
      - pancarditis IØ9.9
      - pericarditis IØ9.2
  - Rift Valley (viral) A92.4
  - Rocky Mountain spotted A77.Ø
  - rose J3Ø.1
  - Ross River B33.1
  - Russian hemorrhagic A98.5
  - San Joaquin (Valley) B38.Ø
  - sandfly A93.1
  - Sao Paulo A77.Ø
  - scarlet A38.9
  - seven day (leptospirosis) (autumnal) (Japanese) A27.89
    - dengue A9Ø
  - shin-bone A79.Ø
  - Singapore hemorrhagic A91
  - solar A9Ø
  - Songo A98.5
  - sore BØØ.1
  - South African tick-bite A68.1
  - Southeast Asia hemorrhagic A91
  - spinal — *see* Meningitis
  - spirillary A25.Ø
  - splenic — *see* Anthrax

Fever — *continued*
- spotted A77.9
  - American A77.Ø
  - Brazilian A77.Ø
  - cerebrospinal meningitis A39.Ø
  - Colombian A77.Ø
  - due to Rickettsia
    - africae (African tick bite fever) A77.8
    - australis A77.3
    - conorii A77.1
    - parkeri A77.8
    - rickettsii A77.Ø
    - sibirica A77.2
    - specified type NEC A77.8
  - Ehrlichiosis A77.40
    - due to
      - E. chafeensis A77.41
      - specified organism NEC A77.49
  - Rocky Mountain A77.Ø
- steroid R5Ø.2
- streptobacillary A25.1
- subtertian B5Ø.9
- Sumatran mite A75.3
- sun A9Ø
- swamp A27.9
- swine AØ2.8
- sylvatic, yellow A95.Ø
- Tahyna B33.8
- tertian — *see* Malaria, tertian
- Thailand hemorrhagic A91
- thermic T67.Ø1 ☑
- three-day A93.1
- tick
  - American mountain A93.2
  - Colorado A93.2
  - Kemerovo A93.8
  - Mediterranean A77.1
  - mountain A93.2
  - nonexanthematous A93.2
  - Quaranfil A93.8
- tick-bite NEC A93.8
- tick-borne (hemorrhagic) NEC A93.8
- trench A79.Ø
- tsutsugamushi A75.3
- typhogastric AØ1.ØØ
- typhoid (abortive) (hemorrhagic) (intermittent) (malignant) AØ1.ØØ
  - complicated by
    - arthritis AØ1.Ø4
    - heart involvement AØ1.Ø2
    - meningitis AØ1.Ø1
    - osteomyelitis AØ1.Ø5
    - pneumonia AØ1.Ø3
    - specified NEC AØ1.Ø9
- typhomalarial — *see* Malaria
- typhus — *see* Typhus (fever)
- undulant — *see* Brucellosis
- unknown origin R5Ø.9
- uveoparotid D86.89
- valley B38.Ø
- Venezuelan equine A92.2
- vesicular stomatitis A93.8
- viral hemorrhagic — *see* Fever, hemorrhagic, by type of virus
- Volhynian A79.Ø
- Wesselsbron (viral) A92.8
- West
  - African B5Ø.8
  - Nile (viral) A92.3Ø
    - with
      - complications NEC A92.39
      - cranial nerve disorders A92.32
      - encephalitis A92.31
      - encephalomyelitis A92.31
      - neurologic manifestation NEC A92.32
      - optic neuritis A92.32
      - polyradiculitis A92.32
- Whitmore's — *see* Melioidosis
- Wolhynian A79.Ø
- worm B83.9
- yellow A95.9
  - jungle A95.Ø
  - sylvatic A95.Ø
  - urban A95.1
- Zika virus A92.5

Fibrillation
- atrial or auricular (established) I48.91
  - chronic I48.2Ø

Fibrillation — *continued*
- atrial or auricular — *continued*
  - chronic — *continued*
    - persistent I48.19
  - paroxysmal I48.Ø
  - permanent I48.21
  - persistent (chronic) (NOS) (other) I48.19
    - longstanding I48.11
- cardiac I49.8
- heart I49.8
- muscular M62.89
- ventricular I49.Ø1

Fibrin
- ball or bodies, pleural (sac) J94.1
- chamber, anterior (eye) (gelatinous exudate) — *see* Iridocyclitis, acute

Fibrinogenolysis — *see* Fibrinolysis

Fibrinogenopenia D68.8
- acquired D65
- congenital D68.2

Fibrinolysis (hemorrhagic) (acquired) D65
- antepartum hemorrhage — *see* Hemorrhage, antepartum, with coagulation defect
- following
  - abortion — *see* Abortion by type complicated by hemorrhage
  - ectopic or molar pregnancy OØ8.1
- intrapartum O67.Ø
- newborn, transient P6Ø
- postpartum O72.3

Fibrinopenia (hereditary) D68.2
- acquired D68.4

Fibrinopurulent — *see* condition

Fibrinous — *see* condition

Fibroadenoma
- cellular intracanalicular D24- ☑
- giant D24- ☑
- intracanalicular
  - cellular D24- ☑
  - giant D24- ☑
  - specified site — *see* Neoplasm, benign, by site
  - unspecified site D24- ☑
- juvenile D24- ☑
- pericanalicular
  - specified site — *see* Neoplasm, benign, by site
  - unspecified site D24- ☑
- phyllodes D24- ☑
- prostate D29.1
- specified site NEC — *see* Neoplasm, benign, by site
- unspecified site D24- ☑

Fibroadenosis, breast (chronic) (cystic) (diffuse) (periodic) (segmental) N6Ø.2- ☑

Fibroangioma — *see also* Neoplasm, benign, by site
- juvenile
  - specified site — *see* Neoplasm, benign, by site
  - unspecified site D1Ø.6

Fibrochondrosarcoma — *see* Neoplasm, cartilage, malignant

Fibrocystic
- disease — *see also* Fibrosis, cystic
  - breast — *see* Mastopathy, cystic
  - jaw M27.49
  - kidney (congenital) Q61.8
  - liver Q44.6
  - pancreas E84.9
- kidney (congenital) Q61.8

Fibrodysplasia ossificans progressiva — *see* Myositis, ossificans, progressiva

Fibroelastosis (cordis) (endocardial) (endomyocardial) I42.4

Fibroid (tumor) — *see also* Neoplasm, connective tissue, benign
- disease, lung (chronic) — *see* Fibrosis, lung
- heart (disease) — *see* Myocarditis
- in pregnancy or childbirth O34.1- ☑
  - causing obstructed labor O65.5
- induration, lung (chronic) — *see* Fibrosis, lung
- lung — *see* Fibrosis, lung
- pneumonia (chronic) — *see* Fibrosis, lung
- uterus — *see also* Leiomyoma, uterus D25.9

Fibrolipoma — *see* Lipoma

Fibroliposarcoma — *see* Neoplasm, connective tissue, malignant

Fibroma — *see also* Neoplasm, connective tissue, benign
- ameloblastic — *see* Cyst, calcifying odontogenic
- bone (nonossifying) — *see* Disorder, bone, specified type NEC

Fibroma — *continued*
- bone — *see* Disorder, bone, specified type — *continued*
  - ossifying — *see* Neoplasm, bone, benign
- cementifying — *see* Neoplasm, bone, benign
- chondromyxoid — *see* Neoplasm, bone, benign
- desmoplastic — *see* Neoplasm, connective tissue, uncertain behavior
- durum — *see* Neoplasm, connective tissue, benign
- fascial — *see* Neoplasm, connective tissue, benign
- invasive — *see* Neoplasm, connective tissue, uncertain behavior
- molle — *see* Lipoma
- myxoid — *see* Neoplasm, connective tissue, benign
- nasopharynx, nasopharyngeal (juvenile) D1Ø.6
- nonosteogenic (nonossifying) — *see* Dysplasia, fibrous
- odontogenic (central) — *see* Cyst, calcifying odontogenic
- ossifying — *see* Neoplasm, bone, benign
- periosteal — *see* Neoplasm, bone, benign
- soft — *see* Lipoma

Fibromatosis M72.9
- abdominal — *see* Neoplasm, connective tissue, uncertain behavior
- aggressive — *see* Neoplasm, connective tissue, uncertain behavior
- congenital generalized — *see* Neoplasm, connective tissue, uncertain behavior
- Dupuytren's M72.Ø
- gingival KØ6.1
- palmar (fascial) M72.Ø
- plantar (fascial) M72.2
- pseudosarcomatous (proliferative) (subcutaneous) M72.4
- retroperitoneal D48.3
- specified NEC M72.8

Fibromyalgia M79.7

Fibromyoma — *see also* Neoplasm, connective tissue, benign
- uterus (corpus) — *see also* Leiomyoma, uterus
  - in pregnancy or childbirth — *see* Fibroid, in pregnancy or childbirth
    - causing obstructed labor O65.5

Fibromyositis M79.7

Fibromyxolipoma D17.9

Fibromyxoma — *see* Neoplasm, connective tissue, benign

Fibromyxosarcoma — *see* Neoplasm, connective tissue, malignant

Fibro-odontoma, ameloblastic — *see* Cyst, calcifying odontogenic

Fibro-osteoma — *see* Neoplasm, bone, benign

Fibroplasia, retrolental H35.17- ☑

Fibropurulent — *see* condition

Fibrosarcoma — *see also* Neoplasm, connective tissue, malignant
- ameloblastic C41.1
  - upper jaw (bone) C41.Ø
- congenital — *see* Neoplasm, connective tissue, malignant
- fascial — *see* Neoplasm, connective tissue, malignant
- infantile — *see* Neoplasm, connective tissue, malignant
- odontogenic C41.1
  - upper jaw (bone) C41.Ø
- periosteal — *see* Neoplasm, bone, malignant

Fibrosclerosis
- breast N6Ø.3- ☑
- multifocal M35.5
- penis (corpora cavernosa) N48.6

Fibrosis, fibrotic
- adrenal (gland) E27.8
- amnion O41.8X- ☑
- anal papillae K62.89
- arteriocapillary — *see* Arteriosclerosis
- bladder N32.89
  - interstitial — *see* Cystitis, chronic, interstitial
  - localized submucosal — *see* Cystitis, chronic, interstitial
  - panmural — *see* Cystitis, chronic, interstitial
- breast — *see* Fibrosclerosis, breast
- capillary — *see also* Arteriosclerosis I7Ø.9Ø
  - lung (chronic) — *see* Fibrosis, lung
- cardiac — *see* Myocarditis
- cervix N88.8
- chorion O41.8X- ☑
- corpus cavernosum (sclerosing) N48.6
- cystic (of pancreas) E84.9

Fistula — *continued*
- gastroesophageal K31.6
- gastrojejunal K31.6
- gastrojejunocolic K31.6
- genital tract (female) N82.9
  - specified NEC N82.8
  - to intestine NEC N82.4
  - to skin N82.5
- hepatic artery-portal vein, congenital Q26.6
- hepatopleural J86.Ø
- hepatopulmonary J86.Ø
- ileorectal or ileosigmoidal K63.2
- ileovaginal N82.2
- ileovesical N32.1
- ileum K63.2
- in ano K6Ø.3
  - tuberculous A18.32
- inner ear (labyrinth) — *see* subcategory H83.1 ☑
- intestine NEC K63.2
- intestinocolonic (abdominal) K63.2
- intestinoureteral N28.89
- intestinouterine N82.4
- intestinovaginal N82.4
  - large intestine N82.3
  - small intestine N82.2
- intestinovesical N32.1
- ischiorectal (fossa) K61.39
- jejunum K63.2
- joint M25.1Ø
  - ankle M25.17- ☑
  - elbow M25.12- ☑
  - foot joint M25.17- ☑
  - hand joint M25.14- ☑
  - hip M25.15- ☑
  - knee M25.16- ☑
  - shoulder M25.11- ☑
  - specified joint NEC M25.18
  - tuberculous — *see* Tuberculosis, joint
  - vertebrae M25.18
  - wrist M25.13- ☑
- kidney N28.89
- labium (majus) (minus) N82.8
- labyrinth — *see* subcategory H83.1 ☑
- lacrimal (gland) (sac) HØ4.61- ☑
- lacrimonasal duct — *see* Fistula, lacrimal
- laryngotracheal, congenital Q34.8
- larynx J38.7
- lip K13.Ø
  - congenital Q38.Ø
- lumbar, tuberculous A18.Ø1
- lung J86.Ø
- lymphatic I89.8
- mammary (gland) N61.Ø
- mastoid (process) (region) — *see* Mastoiditis, chronic
- maxillary J32.Ø
- medial, face and neck Q18.8
- mediastinal J86.Ø
- mediastinobronchial J86.Ø
- mediastinocutaneous J86.Ø
- middle ear — *see* subcategory H74.8 ☑
- mouth K12.2
- nasal J34.89
  - sinus — *see* Sinusitis
- nasopharynx J39.2
- nipple N64.Ø
- nose J34.89
- oral (cutaneous) K12.2
  - maxillary J32.Ø
  - nasal (with cleft palate) — *see* Cleft, palate
- orbit, orbital — *see* Disorder, orbit, specified type NEC
- oroantral J32.Ø
- oviduct, external N82.5
- palate (hard) M27.8
- pancreatic K86.89
- pancreaticoduodenal K86.89
- parotid (gland) K11.4
  - region K12.2
- penis N48.89
- perianal K6Ø.3
- pericardium (pleura) (sac) — *see* Pericarditis
- pericecal K63.2
- perineorectal K6Ø.4
- perineosigmoidal K63.2
- perineum, perineal (with urethral involvement) NEC N36.Ø
  - tuberculous A18.13
  - ureter N28.89
- perirectal K6Ø.4

Fistula — *continued*
- perirectal — *continued*
  - tuberculous A18.32
- peritoneum K65.9
- pharyngoesophageal J39.2
- pharynx J39.2
  - branchial cleft (congenital) Q18.Ø
- pilonidal (infected) (rectum) — *see* Sinus, pilonidal
- pleura, pleural, pleurocutaneous, pleuroperitoneal J86.Ø
  - tuberculous NEC A15.6
- pleuropericardial I31.8
- portal vein-hepatic artery, congenital Q26.6
- postauricular H7Ø.81- ☑
- postoperative, persistent T81.83 ☑
  - specified site — *see* Fistula, by site
- preauricular (congenital) Q18.1
- prostate N42.89
- pulmonary J86.Ø
  - arteriovenous I28.Ø
    - congenital Q25.72
  - tuberculous — *see* Tuberculosis, pulmonary
- pulmonoperitoneal J86.Ø
- rectolabial N82.4
- rectosigmoid (intercommunicating) K63.2
- rectoureteral N28.89
- rectourethral N36.Ø
  - congenital Q64.73
- rectouterine N82.4
  - congenital Q51.7
- rectovaginal N82.3
  - congenital Q52.2
  - tuberculous A18.18
- rectovesical N32.1
  - congenital Q64.79
- rectovesicovaginal N82.3
- rectovulval N82.4
  - congenital Q52.79
- rectum (to skin) K6Ø.4
  - congenital Q43.6
    - with absence, atresia and stenosis Q42.Ø
  - tuberculous A18.32
- renal N28.89
- retroauricular — *see* Fistula, postauricular
- salivary duct or gland (any) K11.4
  - congenital Q38.4
- scrotum (urinary) N5Ø.89
  - tuberculous A18.15
- semicircular canals — *see* subcategory H83.1 ☑
- sigmoid K63.2
  - to bladder N32.1
- sinus — *see* Sinusitis
- skin L98.8
  - to genital tract (female) N82.5
- splenocolic D73.89
- stercoral K63.2
- stomach K31.6
- sublingual gland K11.4
- submandibular gland K11.4
- submaxillary (gland) K11.4
  - region K12.2
- thoracic J86.Ø
  - duct I89.8
- thoracoabdominal J86.Ø
- thoracogastric J86.Ø
- thoracointestinal J86.Ø
- thorax J86.Ø
- thyroglossal duct Q89.2
- thyroid EØ7.89
- trachea, congenital (external) (internal) Q32.1
- tracheoesophageal J86.Ø
  - congenital Q39.2
    - with atresia of esophagus Q39.1
  - following tracheostomy J95.Ø4
- traumatic arteriovenous — *see* Injury, blood vessel, by site
- tuberculous — *code by* site under Tuberculosis
- typhoid AØ1.Ø9
- umbilicourinary Q64.8
- urachus, congenital Q64.4
- ureter (persistent) N28.89
- ureteroabdominal N28.89
- ureterorectal N28.89
- ureterosigmoido-abdominal N28.89
- ureterovaginal N82.1
- ureterovesical N32.2
- urethra N36.Ø
  - congenital Q64.79

Fistula — *continued*
- urethra — *continued*
  - tuberculous A18.13
- urethroperineal N36.Ø
- urethroperineovesical N32.2
- urethrorectal N36.Ø
  - congenital Q64.73
- urethroscrotal N5Ø.89
- urethrovaginal N82.1
- urethrovesical N32.2
- urinary (tract) (persistent) (recurrent) N36.Ø
- uteroabdominal N82.5
  - congenital Q51.7
- uteroenteric, uterointestinal N82.4
  - congenital Q51.7
- uterorectal N82.4
  - congenital Q51.7
- uteroureteric N82.1
- uterourethral Q51.7
- uterovaginal N82.8
- uterovesical N82.1
  - congenital Q51.7
- uterus N82.8
- vagina (postpartal) (wall) N82.8
- vaginocutaneous (postpartal) N82.5
- vaginointestinal NEC N82.4
  - large intestine N82.3
  - small intestine N82.2
- vaginoperineal N82.5
- vasocutaneous, congenital Q55.7
- vesical NEC N32.2
- vesicoabdominal N32.2
- vesicocervicovaginal N82.1
- vesicocolic N32.1
- vesicocutaneous N32.2
- vesicoenteric N32.1
- vesicointestinal N32.1
- vesicometrorectal N82.4
- vesicoperineal N32.2
- vesicorectal N32.1
  - congenital Q64.79
- vesicosigmoidal N32.1
- vesicosigmoidovaginal N82.3
- vesicoureteral N32.2
- vesicoureterovaginal N82.1
- vesicourethral N32.2
- vesicourethrorectal N32.1
- vesicouterine N82.1
  - congenital Q51.7
- vesicovaginal N82.Ø
- vulvorectal N82.4
  - congenital Q52.79

Fit R56.9
- epileptic — *see* Epilepsy
- fainting R55
- hysterical F44.5
- newborn P9Ø

Fitting (and adjustment) (of)
- artificial
  - arm — *see* Admission, adjustment, artificial, arm
  - breast Z44.3 ☑
  - eye Z44.2 ☑
  - leg — *see* Admission, adjustment, artificial, leg
- automatic implantable cardiac defibrillator (with synchronous cardiac pacemaker) Z45.Ø2
- brain neuropacemaker Z46.2
  - implanted Z45.42
- cardiac defibrillator — *see* Fitting (and adjustment) (of), automatic implantable cardiac defibrillator
- catheter, non-vascular Z46.82
- colostomy belt Z46.89
- contact lenses Z46.Ø
- CRT-D (resynchronization therapy defibrillator) Z45.Ø2
- CRT-P (cardiac resynchronization therapy pacemaker) Z45.Ø18
  - pulse generator Z45.Ø1Ø
- cystostomy device Z46.6
- defibrillator, cardiac — *see* Fitting (and adjustment) (of), automatic implantable cardiac defibrillator
- dentures Z46.3
- device NOS Z46.9
  - abdominal Z46.89
  - gastrointestinal NEC Z46.59
  - implanted NEC Z45.89
  - nervous system Z46.2
    - implanted — *see* Admission, adjustment, device, implanted, nervous system
  - orthodontic Z46.4

- **Fitting** — *continued*
  - device — *continued*
    - orthoptic Z46.0
    - orthotic Z46.89
    - prosthetic (external) Z44.9
      - breast Z44.3 ☑
      - dental Z46.3
      - eye Z44.2 ☑
      - specified NEC Z44.8
    - specified NEC Z46.89
    - substitution
      - auditory Z46.2
        - implanted — *see* Admission, adjustment, device, implanted, hearing device
      - nervous system Z46.2
        - implanted — *see* Admission, adjustment, device, implanted, nervous system
      - visual Z46.2
        - implanted Z45.31
    - urinary Z46.6
  - gastric lap band Z46.51
  - gastrointestinal appliance NEC Z46.59
  - glasses (reading) Z46.0
  - hearing aid Z46.1
  - ileostomy device Z46.89
  - insulin pump Z46.81
  - intestinal appliance NEC Z46.89
  - myringotomy device (stent) (tube) Z45.82
  - neuropacemaker Z46.2
    - implanted Z45.42
  - non-vascular catheter Z46.82
  - orthodontic device Z46.4
  - orthopedic device (brace) (cast) (corset) (shoes) Z46.89
  - pacemaker (cardiac) (cardiac resynchronization therapy (CRT-P)) Z45.018
    - nervous system (brain) (peripheral nerve) (spinal cord) Z46.2
      - implanted Z45.42
    - pulse generator Z45.010
  - portacath (port-a-cath) Z45.2
  - prosthesis (external) Z44.9
    - arm — *see* Admission, adjustment, artificial, arm
    - breast Z44.3 ☑
    - dental Z46.3
    - eye Z44.2 ☑
    - leg — *see* Admission, adjustment, artificial, leg
    - specified NEC Z44.8
  - spectacles Z46.0
  - wheelchair Z46.89
- **Fitzhugh-Curtis syndrome**
  - due to
    - Chlamydia trachomatis A74.81
    - Neisseria gonorrhorea (gonococcal peritonitis) A54.85
- **Fitz's syndrome** (acute hemorrhagic pancreatitis) — *see also* Pancreatitis, acute K85.80
- **Fixation**
  - joint — *see* Ankylosis
  - larynx J38.7
  - stapes — *see* Ankylosis, ear ossicles
    - deafness — *see* Deafness, conductive
  - uterus (acquired) — *see* Malposition, uterus
  - vocal cord J38.3
- **Flabby ridge** K06.8
- **Flaccid** — *see also* condition
  - palate, congenital Q38.5
- **Flail**
  - chest S22.5 ☑
    - newborn (birth injury) P13.8
  - joint (paralytic) M25.20
    - ankle M25.27- ☑
    - elbow M25.22- ☑
    - foot joint M25.27- ☑
    - hand joint M25.24- ☑
    - hip M25.25- ☑
    - knee M25.26- ☑
    - shoulder M25.21- ☑
    - specified joint NEC M25.28
    - wrist M25.23- ☑
- **Flajani's disease** — *see* Hyperthyroidism, with, goiter (diffuse)
- **Flap, liver** K71.3
- **Flashbacks** (residual to hallucinogen use) F16.283
- **Flat**
  - chamber (eye) — *see* Disorder, globe, hypotony, flat anterior chamber
  - chest, congenital Q67.8
- **Flat** — *continued*
  - foot (acquired) (fixed type) (painful) (postural) — *see also* Deformity, limb, flat foot
    - congenital (rigid) (spastic (everted)) Q66.5- ☑
    - rachitic sequelae (late effect) E64.3
  - organ or site, congenital NEC — *see* Anomaly, by site
  - pelvis M95.5
    - with disproportion (fetopelvic) O33.0
      - causing obstructed labor O65.0
    - congenital Q74.2
- **Flatau-Schilder disease** G37.0
- **Flatback syndrome** M40.30
  - lumbar region M40.36
  - lumbosacral region M40.37
  - thoracolumbar region M40.35
- **Flattening**
  - head, femur M89.8X5
  - hip — *see* Coxa, plana
  - lip (congenital) Q18.8
  - nose (congenital) Q67.4
    - acquired M95.0
- **Flatulence** R14.3
  - psychogenic F45.8
- **Flatus** R14.3
  - vaginalis N89.8
- **Flax-dresser's disease** J66.1
- **Flea bite** — *see* Injury, bite, by site, superficial, insect
- **Flecks, glaucomatous** (subcapsular) — *see* Cataract, complicated
- **Fleischer** (-Kayser) **ring** (cornea) H18.04- ☑
- **Fleshy mole** O02.0
- **Flexibilitas cerea** — *see* Catalepsy
- **Flexion**
  - amputation stump (surgical) T87.89
  - cervix — *see* Malposition, uterus
  - contracture, joint — *see* Contraction, joint
  - deformity, joint — *see also* Deformity, limb, flexion M21.20
    - hip, congenital Q65.89
  - uterus — *see also* Malposition, uterus
    - lateral — *see* Lateroversion, uterus
- **Flexner-Boyd dysentery** A03.2
- **Flexner's dysentery** A03.1
- **Flexure** — *see* Flexion
- **Flint murmur** (aortic insufficiency) I35.1
- **Floater, vitreous** — *see* Opacity, vitreous
- **Floating**
  - cartilage (joint) — *see also* Loose, body, joint
    - knee — *see* Derangement, knee, loose body
  - gallbladder, congenital Q44.1
  - kidney N28.89
    - congenital Q63.8
  - spleen D73.89
- **Flooding** N92.0
- **Floor** — *see* condition
- **Floppy**
  - baby syndrome (nonspecific) P94.2
  - iris syndrome (intraoperative) (IFIS) H21.81
  - nonrheumatic mitral valve syndrome I34.1
- **Flu** — *see also* Influenza
  - avian — *see also* Influenza, due to, identified novel influenza A virus J09.X2
  - bird — *see also* Influenza, due to, identified novel influenza A virus J09.X2
  - intestinal NEC A08.4
  - swine (viruses that normally cause infections in pigs) — *see also* Influenza, due to, identified novel influenza A virus J09.X2
- **Fluctuating blood pressure** I99.8
- **Fluid**
  - abdomen R18.8
  - chest J94.8
  - heart — *see* Failure, heart, congestive
  - joint — *see* Effusion, joint
  - loss (acute) E86.9
  - lung — *see* Edema, lung
  - overload E87.70
    - specified NEC E87.79
  - peritoneal cavity R18.8
  - pleural cavity J94.8
  - retention R60.9
- **Flukes NEC** — *see also* Infestation, fluke
  - blood NEC — *see* Schistosomiasis
  - liver B66.3
- **Fluor** (vaginalis) N89.8
  - trichomonal or due to Trichomonas (vaginalis) A59.00
- **Fluorosis**
  - dental K00.3
  - skeletal M85.10
    - ankle M85.17- ☑
    - foot M85.17- ☑
    - forearm M85.13- ☑
    - hand M85.14- ☑
    - lower leg M85.16- ☑
    - multiple site M85.19
    - neck M85.18
    - rib M85.18
    - shoulder M85.11- ☑
    - skull M85.18
    - specified site NEC M85.18
    - thigh M85.15- ☑
    - toe M85.17- ☑
    - upper arm M85.12- ☑
    - vertebra M85.18
- **Flush syndrome** E34.0
- **Flushing** R23.2
  - menopausal N95.1
- **Flutter**
  - atrial or auricular I48.92
    - atypical I48.4
    - type I I48.3
    - type II I48.4
    - typical I48.3
  - heart I49.8
    - atrial or auricular I48.92
      - atypical I48.4
      - type I I48.3
      - type II I48.4
      - typical I48.3
    - ventricular I49.02
  - ventricular I49.02
- **FNHTR** (febrile nonhemolytic transfusion reaction) R50.84
- **Fochier's abscess** — *code by* site under Abscess
- **Focus, Assmann's** — *see* Tuberculosis, pulmonary
- **Fogo selvagem** L10.3
- **Foix-Alajouanine syndrome** G95.19
- **Fold, folds** (anomalous) — *see also* Anomaly, by site
  - Descemet's membrane — *see* Change, corneal membrane, Descemet's, fold
  - epicanthic Q10.3
  - heart Q24.8
- **Folie à deux** F24
- **Follicle**
  - cervix (nabothian) (ruptured) N88.8
  - graafian, ruptured, with hemorrhage N83.0- ☑
  - nabothian N88.8
- **Follicular** — *see* condition
- **Folliculitis** (superficial) L73.9
  - abscedens et suffodiens L66.3
  - cyst N83.0- ☑
  - decalvans L66.2
  - deep — *see* Furuncle, by site
  - gonococcal (acute) (chronic) A54.01
  - keloid, keloidalis L73.0
  - pustular L01.02
  - ulerythematosa reticulata L66.4
- **Folliculome lipidique**
  - specified site — *see* Neoplasm, benign, by site
  - unspecified site
    - female D27.9
    - male D29.20
- **Følling's disease** E70.0
- **Follow-up** — *see* Examination, follow-up
- **Fong's syndrome** (hereditary osteo-onychodysplasia) Q87.2
- **Food**
  - allergy L27.2
  - asphyxia (from aspiration or inhalation) — *see* Foreign body, by site
  - choked on — *see* Foreign body, by site
  - deprivation T73.0 ☑
    - specified kind of food NEC E63.8
  - intoxication — *see* Poisoning, food
  - lack of T73.0 ☑
  - poisoning — *see* Poisoning, food
  - rejection NEC — *see* Disorder, eating
  - strangulation or suffocation — *see* Foreign body, by site
  - toxemia — *see* Poisoning, food
- **Foot** — *see* condition
- **Foramen ovale** (nonclosure) (patent) (persistent) Q21.1
- **Forbes' glycogen storage disease** E74.03
- **Fordyce-Fox disease** L75.2

- **Fracture, traumatic** — *continued*
  - ankle — *continued*
    - bimalleolar (displaced) S82.84- ☑
      - nondisplaced S82.84- ☑
    - lateral malleolus only (displaced) S82.6- ☑
      - nondisplaced S82.6- ☑
    - medial malleolus (displaced) S82.5- ☑
      - associated with Maisonneuve's fracture — *see* Fracture, Maisonneuve's
      - nondisplaced S82.5- ☑
    - talus — *see* Fracture, tarsal, talus
    - trimalleolar (displaced) S82.85- ☑
      - nondisplaced S82.85- ☑
  - arm (upper) — *see also* Fracture, humerus, shaft
    - humerus — *see* Fracture, humerus
    - radius — *see* Fracture, radius
    - ulna — *see* Fracture, ulna
  - astragalus — *see* Fracture, tarsal, talus
  - atlas — *see* Fracture, neck, cervical vertebra, first
  - axis — *see* Fracture, neck, cervical vertebra, second
  - back — *see* Fracture, vertebra
  - Barton's — *see* Barton's fracture
  - base of skull — *see* Fracture, skull, base
  - basicervical (basal) (femoral) S72.Ø ☑
  - Bennett's — *see* Bennett's fracture
  - bimalleolar — *see* Fracture, ankle, bimalleolar
  - blow-out SØ2.3- ☑
  - bone NEC T14.8 ☑
    - birth injury P13.9
    - following insertion of orthopedic implant, joint prosthesis or bone plate — *see* Fracture, following insertion of orthopedic implant, joint prosthesis or bone plate
    - in (due to) neoplastic disease NEC — *see* Fracture, pathological, due to, neoplastic disease
    - pathological (cause unknown) — *see* Fracture, pathological
  - breast bone — *see* Fracture, sternum
  - bucket handle (semilunar cartilage) — *see* Tear, meniscus
  - buckle — *see* Fracture, by site, torus
  - burst — *see* Fracture, traumatic, by site
  - calcaneus — *see* Fracture, tarsal, calcaneus
  - carpal bone(s) S62.1Ø- ☑
    - capitate (displaced) S62.13- ☑
      - nondisplaced S62.13- ☑
    - cuneiform — *see* Fracture, carpal bone, triquetrum
    - hamate (body) (displaced) S62.143 ☑
      - hook process (displaced) S62.15- ☑
        - nondisplaced S62.15- ☑
      - nondisplaced S62.14- ☑
    - larger multangular — *see* Fracture, carpal bones, trapezium
    - lunate (displaced) S62.12- ☑
      - nondisplaced S62.12- ☑
    - navicular S62.ØØ- ☑
      - distal pole (displaced) S62.Ø1- ☑
        - nondisplaced S62.Ø1- ☑
      - middle third (displaced) S62.Ø2- ☑
        - nondisplaced S62.Ø2- ☑
      - proximal third (displaced) S62.Ø3- ☑
        - nondisplaced S62.Ø3- ☑
      - volar tuberosity — *see* Fracture, carpal bones, navicular, distal pole
    - os magnum — *see* Fracture, carpal bones, capitate
    - pisiform (displaced) S62.16- ☑
      - nondisplaced S62.16- ☑
    - semilunar — *see* Fracture, carpal bones, lunate
    - smaller multangular — *see* Fracture, carpal bones, trapezoid
    - trapezium (displaced) S62.17- ☑
      - nondisplaced S62.17- ☑
    - trapezoid (displaced) S62.18- ☑
      - nondisplaced S62.18- ☑
    - triquetrum (displaced) S62.11- ☑
      - nondisplaced S62.11- ☑
    - unciform — *see* Fracture, carpal bones, hamate
  - cervical — *see* Fracture, vertebra, cervical
  - clavicle S42.ØØ- ☑
    - acromial end (displaced) S42.Ø3- ☑
      - nondisplaced S42.Ø3- ☑
    - birth injury P13.4
    - lateral end — *see* Fracture, clavicle, acromial end
    - shaft (displaced) S42.Ø2- ☑
      - nondisplaced S42.Ø2- ☑
    - sternal end (anterior) (displaced) S42.Ø1- ☑

- **Fracture, traumatic** — *continued*
  - clavicle — *continued*
    - sternal end — *continued*
      - nondisplaced S42.Ø1- ☑
      - posterior S42.Ø1- ☑
  - coccyx S32.2 ☑
  - collapsed — *see* Collapse, vertebra
  - collar bone — *see* Fracture, clavicle
  - Colles' — *see* Colles' fracture
  - coronoid process — *see* Fracture, ulna, upper end, coronoid process
  - corpus cavernosum penis S39.84Ø ☑
  - costochondral cartilage S23.41 ☑
  - costochondral, costosternal junction — *see* Fracture, rib
  - cranium — *see* Fracture, skull
  - cricoid cartilage S12.8 ☑
  - cuboid (ankle) — *see* Fracture, tarsal, cuboid
  - cuneiform
    - foot — *see* Fracture, tarsal, cuneiform
    - wrist — *see* Fracture, carpal, triquetrum
  - delayed union — *see* Delay, union, fracture
  - dental restorative material KØ8.539
    - with loss of material KØ8.531
    - without loss of material KØ8.53Ø
  - due to
    - birth injury — *see* Birth, injury, fracture
    - osteoporosis — *see* Osteoporosis, with fracture
  - Dupuytren's — *see* Fracture, ankle, lateral malleolus
  - elbow S42.4Ø- ☑
  - ethmoid (bone) (sinus) — *see* Fracture, skull, base
  - face bone SØ2.92 ☑
  - fatigue — *see also* Fracture, stress
    - vertebra M48.4Ø ☑
      - cervical region M48.42 ☑
      - cervicothoracic region M48.43 ☑
      - lumbar region M48.46 ☑
      - lumbosacral region M48.47 ☑
      - occipito-atlanto-axial region M48.41 ☑
      - sacrococcygeal region M48.48 ☑
      - thoracic region M48.44 ☑
      - thoracolumbar region M48.45 ☑
  - femur, femoral S72.9- ☑
    - basicervical (basal) S72.Ø ☑
    - birth injury P13.2
    - capital epiphyseal S79.Ø1- ☑
    - condyles, epicondyles — *see* Fracture, femur, lower end
    - distal end — *see* Fracture, femur, lower end
    - epiphysis
      - head — *see* Fracture, femur, upper end, epiphysis
      - lower — *see* Fracture, femur, lower end, epiphysis
      - upper — *see* Fracture, femur, upper end, epiphysis
    - following insertion of implant, prosthesis or plate M96.66- ☑
    - head — *see* Fracture, femur, upper end, head
    - intertrochanteric — *see* Fracture, femur, trochanteric
    - intratrochanteric — *see* Fracture, femur, trochanteric
    - lower end S72.4Ø- ☑
      - condyle (displaced) S72.41- ☑
        - lateral (displaced) S72.42- ☑
          - nondisplaced S72.42- ☑
        - medial (displaced) S72.43- ☑
          - nondisplaced S72.43- ☑
        - nondisplaced S72.41- ☑
      - epiphysis (displaced) S72.44- ☑
        - nondisplaced S72.44- ☑
      - physeal S79.1Ø- ☑
        - Salter-Harris
          - Type I S79.11- ☑
          - Type II S79.12- ☑
          - Type III S79.13- ☑
          - Type IV S79.14- ☑
        - specified NEC S79.19- ☑
      - specified NEC S72.49- ☑
      - supracondylar (displaced) S72.45- ☑
        - with intracondylar extension (displaced) S72.46- ☑
          - nondisplaced S72.46- ☑
        - nondisplaced S72.45- ☑
      - torus S72.47- ☑
    - neck — *see* Fracture, femur, upper end, neck

- **Fracture, traumatic** — *continued*
  - femur, femoral — *continued*
    - pertrochanteric — *see* Fracture, femur, trochanteric
    - shaft (lower third) (middle third) (upper third) S72.3Ø- ☑
      - comminuted (displaced) S72.35- ☑
        - nondisplaced S72.35- ☑
      - oblique (displaced) S72.33- ☑
        - nondisplaced S72.33- ☑
      - segmental (displaced) S72.36- ☑
        - nondisplaced S72.36- ☑
      - specified NEC S72.39- ☑
      - spiral (displaced) S72.34- ☑
        - nondisplaced S72.34- ☑
      - transverse (displaced) S72.32- ☑
        - nondisplaced S72.32- ☑
    - specified site NEC — *see* subcategory S72.8 ☑
    - subcapital (displaced) S72.Ø1- ☑
    - subtrochanteric (region) (section) (displaced) S72.2- ☑
      - nondisplaced S72.2- ☑
    - transcervical — *see* Fracture, femur, midcervical
    - transtrochanteric — *see* Fracture, femur, trochanteric
    - trochanteric S72.1Ø- ☑
      - apophyseal (displaced) S72.13- ☑
        - nondisplaced S72.13- ☑
      - greater trochanter (displaced) S72.11- ☑
        - nondisplaced S72.11- ☑
      - intertrochanteric (displaced) S72.14- ☑
        - nondisplaced S72.14- ☑
      - lesser trochanter (displaced) S72.12- ☑
        - nondisplaced S72.12- ☑
    - upper end S72.ØØ- ☑
      - apophyseal (displaced) S72.13- ☑
        - nondisplaced S72.13- ☑
      - cervicotrochanteric — *see* Fracture, femur, upper end, neck, base
      - epiphysis (displaced) S72.Ø2- ☑
        - nondisplaced S72.Ø2- ☑
      - head S72.Ø5- ☑
        - articular (displaced) S72.Ø6- ☑
          - nondisplaced S72.Ø6- ☑
        - specified NEC S72.Ø9- ☑
      - intertrochanteric (displaced) S72.14- ☑
        - nondisplaced S72.14- ☑
      - intracapsular S72.Ø1- ☑
      - midcervical (displaced) S72.Ø3- ☑
        - nondisplaced S72.Ø3- ☑
      - neck S72.ØØ- ☑
        - base (displaced) S72.Ø4- ☑
          - nondisplaced S72.Ø4- ☑
        - specified NEC S72.Ø9- ☑
      - pertrochanteric — *see* Fracture, femur, upper end, trochanteric
      - physeal S79.ØØ- ☑
        - Salter-Harris type I S79.Ø1- ☑
        - specified NEC S79.Ø9- ☑
      - subcapital (displaced) S72.Ø1- ☑
      - subtrochanteric (displaced) S72.2- ☑
        - nondisplaced S72.2- ☑
      - transcervical — *see* Fracture, femur, upper end, midcervical
      - trochanteric S72.1Ø- ☑
        - greater (displaced) S72.11- ☑
          - nondisplaced S72.11- ☑
        - lesser (displaced) S72.12- ☑
          - nondisplaced S72.12- ☑
  - fibula (shaft) (styloid) S82.4Ø- ☑
    - comminuted (displaced) S82.45- ☑
      - nondisplaced S82.45- ☑
    - following insertion of implant, prosthesis or plate M96.67- ☑
    - involving ankle or malleolus — *see* Fracture, fibula, lateral malleolus
    - lateral malleolus (displaced) S82.6- ☑
      - nondisplaced S82.6- ☑
    - lower end
      - physeal S89.3Ø- ☑
        - Salter-Harris
          - Type I S89.31- ☑
          - Type II S89.32- ☑
        - specified NEC S89.39- ☑
      - specified NEC S82.83- ☑
      - torus S82.82- ☑
    - oblique (displaced) S82.43- ☑

- Fracture, traumatic — *continued*
  - mandible — *continued*
    - coronoid process S02.63- ☑
    - ramus, unspecified S02.64- ☑
    - specified site NEC S02.69 ☑
    - subcondylar process S02.62- ☑
    - symphysis S02.66 ☑
  - manubrium (sterni) S22.21 ☑
    - dissociation from sternum S22.23 ☑
  - march — *see* Fracture, traumatic, stress, by site
  - maxilla, maxillary (bone) (sinus) (superior) (upper jaw) S02.401 ☑
    - alveolus S02.42 ☑
    - inferior — *see* Fracture, mandible
    - LeFort I S02.411 ☑
    - LeFort II S02.412 ☑
    - LeFort III S02.413 ☑
    - left side S02.40D ☑
    - right side S02.40C ☑
  - metacarpal S62.309 ☑
    - base (displaced) S62.319 ☑
      - nondisplaced S62.349 ☑
    - fifth S62.30- ☑
      - base (displaced) S62.31- ☑
        - nondisplaced S62.34- ☑
      - neck (displaced) S62.33- ☑
        - nondisplaced S62.36- ☑
      - shaft (displaced) S62.32- ☑
        - nondisplaced S62.35- ☑
      - specified NEC S62.398 ☑
    - first S62.20- ☑
      - base NEC (displaced) S62.23- ☑
        - nondisplaced S62.23- ☑
      - Bennett's — *see* Bennett's fracture
      - neck (displaced) S62.25- ☑
        - nondisplaced S62.25- ☑
      - shaft (displaced) S62.24- ☑
        - nondisplaced S62.24- ☑
      - specified NEC S62.29- ☑
    - fourth S62.30- ☑
      - base (displaced) S62.31- ☑
        - nondisplaced S62.34- ☑
      - neck (displaced) S62.33- ☑
        - nondisplaced S62.36- ☑
      - shaft (displaced) S62.32- ☑
        - nondisplaced S62.35- ☑
      - specified NEC S62.39- ☑
    - neck (displaced) S62.33- ☑
      - nondisplaced S62.36- ☑
    - Rolando's — *see* Rolando's fracture
    - second S62.30- ☑
      - base (displaced) S62.31- ☑
        - nondisplaced S62.34- ☑
      - neck (displaced) S62.33- ☑
        - nondisplaced S62.36- ☑
      - shaft (displaced) S62.32- ☑
        - nondisplaced S62.35- ☑
      - specified NEC S62.39- ☑
    - shaft (displaced) S62.32- ☑
      - nondisplaced S62.35- ☑
    - specified NEC S62.399 ☑
    - third S62.30- ☑
      - base (displaced) S62.31- ☑
        - nondisplaced S62.34- ☑
      - neck (displaced) S62.33- ☑
        - nondisplaced S62.36- ☑
      - shaft (displaced) S62.32- ☑
        - nondisplaced S62.35- ☑
      - specified NEC S62.39- ☑
  - metaphyseal — *see* Fracture, traumatic, by site, shaft
  - metastatic — *see* Fracture, pathological, due to, neoplastic disease — *see also* Neoplasm
  - metatarsal bone S92.30- ☑
    - fifth (displaced) S92.35- ☑
      - nondisplaced S92.35- ☑
    - first (displaced) S92.31- ☑
      - nondisplaced S92.31- ☑
    - fourth (displaced) S92.34- ☑
      - nondisplaced S92.34- ☑
    - physeal S99.10- ☑
      - Salter-Harris
        - Type I S99.11- ☑
        - Type II S99.12- ☑
        - Type III S99.13- ☑
        - Type IV S99.14- ☑
      - specified NEC S99.19- ☑

- Fracture, traumatic — *continued*
  - metatarsal bone — *continued*
    - second (displaced) S92.32- ☑
      - nondisplaced S92.32- ☑
    - third (displaced) S92.33- ☑
      - nondisplaced S92.33- ☑
  - Monteggia's — *see* Monteggia's fracture
  - multiple
    - hand (and wrist) NEC — *see* Fracture, by site
    - ribs — *see* Fracture, rib, multiple
  - nasal (bone(s)) S02.2 ☑
  - navicular (scaphoid) (foot) — *see also* Fracture, tarsal, navicular
    - hand — *see* Fracture, carpal, navicular
  - neck S12.9 ☑
    - cervical vertebra S12.9 ☑
      - fifth (displaced) S12.400 ☑
        - nondisplaced S12.401 ☑
        - specified type NEC (displaced) S12.490 ☑
          - nondisplaced S12.491 ☑
      - first (displaced) S12.000 ☑
        - burst (stable) S12.01 ☑
          - unstable S12.02 ☑
        - lateral mass (displaced) S12.040 ☑
          - nondisplaced S12.041 ☑
        - nondisplaced S12.001 ☑
        - posterior arch (displaced) S12.030 ☑
          - nondisplaced S12.031 ☑
        - specified type NEC (displaced) S12.090 ☑
          - nondisplaced S12.091 ☑
      - fourth (displaced) S12.300 ☑
        - nondisplaced S12.301 ☑
        - specified type NEC (displaced) S12.390 ☑
          - nondisplaced S12.391 ☑
      - second (displaced) S12.100 ☑
        - dens (anterior) (displaced) (type II) S12.110 ☑
          - nondisplaced S12.112 ☑
          - posterior S12.111 ☑
          - specified type NEC (displaced) S12.120 ☑
            - nondisplaced S12.121 ☑
        - nondisplaced S12.101 ☑
        - specified type NEC (displaced) S12.190 ☑
          - nondisplaced S12.191 ☑
      - seventh (displaced) S12.600 ☑
        - nondisplaced S12.601 ☑
        - specified type NEC (displaced) S12.690 ☑
          - nondisplaced S12.691 ☑
      - sixth (displaced) S12.500 ☑
        - nondisplaced S12.501 ☑
        - specified type NEC (displaced) S12.590 ☑
          - nondisplaced S12.591 ☑
      - third (displaced) S12.200 ☑
        - nondisplaced S12.201 ☑
        - specified type NEC (displaced) S12.290 ☑
          - nondisplaced S12.291 ☑
    - hyoid bone S12.8 ☑
    - larynx S12.8 ☑
    - specified site NEC S12.8 ☑
    - thyroid cartilage S12.8 ☑
    - trachea S12.8 ☑
  - neoplastic NEC — *see* Fracture, pathological, due to, neoplastic disease
  - neural arch — *see* Fracture, vertebra
  - newborn — *see* Birth, injury, fracture
  - nontraumatic — *see* Fracture, pathological
  - nonunion — *see* Nonunion, fracture
  - nose, nasal (bone) (septum) S02.2 ☑
  - occiput — *see* Fracture, skull, base, occiput
  - odontoid process — *see* Fracture, neck, cervical vertebra, second
  - olecranon (process) (ulna) — *see* Fracture, ulna, upper end, olecranon process
  - orbit, orbital (bone) (region) S02.85 ☑
    - floor (blow-out) S02.3- ☑
    - roof S02.12- ☑
    - wall S02.85 ☑
      - lateral S02.84- ☑
      - medial S02.83- ☑
  - os
    - calcis — *see* Fracture, tarsal, calcaneus
    - magnum — *see* Fracture, carpal, capitate
    - pubis — *see* Fracture, pubis
  - palate S02.8- ☑
  - parietal bone (skull) S02.0 ☑
  - patella S82.00- ☑
    - comminuted (displaced) S82.04- ☑

- Fracture, traumatic — *continued*
  - patella — *continued*
    - comminuted — *continued*
      - nondisplaced S82.04- ☑
    - longitudinal (displaced) S82.02- ☑
      - nondisplaced S82.02- ☑
    - osteochondral (displaced) S82.01- ☑
      - nondisplaced S82.01- ☑
    - specified NEC S82.09- ☑
    - transverse (displaced) S82.03- ☑
      - nondisplaced S82.03- ☑
  - pedicle (of vertebral arch) — *see* Fracture, vertebra
  - pelvis, pelvic (bone) S32.9 ☑
    - acetabulum — *see* Fracture, acetabulum
    - circle — *see* Disruption, pelvic ring
    - following insertion of implant, prosthesis or plate M96.65
    - ilium — *see* Fracture, ilium
    - ischium — *see* Fracture, ischium
    - multiple
      - with disruption of pelvic ring (circle) — *see* Disruption, pelvic ring
      - without disruption of pelvic ring (circle) S32.82 ☑
    - pubis — *see* Fracture, pubis
    - sacrum — *see* Fracture, sacrum
    - specified site NEC S32.89 ☑
  - periprosthetic, around internal prosthetic joint M97.9 ☑
    - ankle M97.2- ☑
    - elbow M97.4- ☑
    - finger M97.8 ☑
    - hip M97.0- ☑
    - knee M97.1- ☑
    - shoulder M97.3- ☑
    - specified joint NEC M97.8 ☑
    - spine M97.8 ☑
    - toe M97.8 ☑
    - wrist M97.8 ☑
  - phalanx
    - foot — *see* Fracture, toe
    - hand — *see* Fracture, finger
  - pisiform — *see* Fracture, carpal, pisiform
  - pond — *see* Fracture, skull
  - prosthetic device, internal — *see* Complications, prosthetic device, by site, mechanical
  - pubis S32.50- ☑
    - with disruption of pelvic ring — *see* Disruption, pelvic ring
    - specified site NEC S32.59- ☑
    - superior rim S32.51- ☑
  - radius S52.9- ☑
    - distal end — *see* Fracture, radius, lower end
    - following insertion of implant, prosthesis or plate M96.63- ☑
    - head — *see* Fracture, radius, upper end, head
    - lower end S52.50- ☑
      - Barton's — *see* Barton's fracture
      - Colles' — *see* Colles' fracture
      - extraarticular NEC S52.55- ☑
      - intraarticular NEC S52.57- ☑
      - physeal S59.20- ☑
        - Salter-Harris
          - Type I S59.21- ☑
          - Type II S59.22- ☑
          - Type III S59.23- ☑
          - Type IV S59.24- ☑
        - specified NEC S59.29- ☑
      - Smith's — *see* Smith's fracture
      - specified NEC S52.59- ☑
      - styloid process (displaced) S52.51- ☑
        - nondisplaced S52.51- ☑
      - torus S52.52- ☑
    - neck — *see* Fracture, radius, upper end
    - proximal end — *see* Fracture, radius, upper end
    - shaft S52.30- ☑
      - bent bone S52.38- ☑
      - comminuted (displaced) S52.35- ☑
        - nondisplaced S52.35- ☑
      - Galeazzi's — *see* Galeazzi's fracture
      - greenstick S52.31- ☑
      - oblique (displaced) S52.33- ☑
        - nondisplaced S52.33- ☑
      - segmental (displaced) S52.36- ☑
        - nondisplaced S52.36- ☑
      - specified NEC S52.39- ☑

G

Gain in weight (abnormal) (excessive) — *see also* Weight, gain
Gaisböck's disease (polycythemia hypertonica) D75.1
Gait abnormality R26.9
  ataxic R26.Ø
  falling R29.6
  hysterical (ataxic) (staggering) F44.4
  paralytic R26.1
  spastic R26.1
  specified type NEC R26.89
  staggering R26.Ø
  unsteadiness R26.81
  walking difficulty NEC R26.2
Galactocele (breast) N64.89
  puerperal, postpartum O92.79
Galactokinase deficiency E74.29
Galactophoritis N61.Ø
  gestational, puerperal, postpartum O91.2- ☑
Galactorrhea O92.6
  not associated with childbirth N64.3
Galactosemia (classic) (congenital) E74.21
Galactosuria E74.29
Galacturia R82.Ø
  schistosomiasis (bilharziasis) B65.Ø
GALD (gestational alloimmune liver disease) P78.84
Galeazzi's fracture S52.37- ☑
Galen's vein — *see* condition
Galeophobia F4Ø.218
Gall duct — *see* condition
Gallbladder — *see also* condition
  acute K81.Ø
Gallop rhythm RØØ.8
Gallstone (colic) (cystic duct) (gallbladder) (impacted) (multiple) — *see also* Calculus, gallbladder
  with
    cholecystitis — *see* Calculus, gallbladder, with cholecystitis
  bile duct (common) (hepatic) — *see* Calculus, bile duct
  causing intestinal obstruction K56.3
  specified NEC K8Ø.8Ø
    with obstruction K8Ø.81
Gambling Z72.6
  pathological (compulsive) F63.Ø
Gammopathy (of undetermined significance [MGUS]) D47.2
  associated with lymphoplasmacytic dyscrasia D47.2
  monoclonal D47.2
  polyclonal D89.Ø
Gamna's disease (siderotic splenomegaly) D73.1
Gamophobia F4Ø.298
Gampsodactylia (congenital) Q66.7- ☑
Gamstorp's disease (adynamia episodica hereditaria) G72.3
Gandy-Nanta disease (siderotic splenomegaly) D73.1
Gang
  membership offenses Z72.81Ø
Gangliocytoma D36.1Ø
Ganglioglioma — *see* Neoplasm, uncertain behavior, by site
Ganglion (compound) (diffuse) (joint) (tendon (sheath)) M67.4Ø
  ankle M67.47- ☑
  foot M67.47- ☑
  forearm M67.43- ☑
  hand M67.44- ☑
  lower leg M67.46- ☑
  multiple sites M67.49
  of yaws (early) (late) A66.6
  pelvic region M67.45- ☑
  periosteal — *see* Periostitis
  shoulder region M67.41- ☑
  specified site NEC M67.48
  thigh region M67.45- ☑
  tuberculous A18.Ø9
  upper arm M67.42- ☑
  wrist M67.43- ☑
Ganglioneuroblastoma — *see* Neoplasm, nerve, malignant
Ganglioneuroma D36.1Ø
  malignant — *see* Neoplasm, nerve, malignant
Ganglioneuromatosis D36.1Ø
Ganglionitis
  fifth nerve — *see* Neuralgia, trigeminal
  gasserian (postherpetic) (postzoster) BØ2.21

Ganglionitis — *continued*
  geniculate G51.1
    newborn (birth injury) P11.3
    postherpetic, postzoster BØ2.21
  herpes zoster BØ2.21
  postherpetic geniculate BØ2.21
Gangliosidosis E75.1Ø
  GM1 E75.19
  GM2 E75.ØØ
    other specified E75.Ø9
    Sandhoff disease E75.Ø1
    Tay-Sachs disease E75.Ø2
  GM3 E75.19
  mucolipidosis IV E75.11
Gangosa A66.5
Gangrene, gangrenous (connective tissue) (dropsical) (dry) (moist) (skin) (ulcer) — *see also* Necrosis I96
  with diabetes (mellitus) — *see* Diabetes, gangrene
  abdomen (wall) I96
  alveolar M27.3
  appendix K35.8Ø
    with
      peritonitis, localized — *see also* Appendicitis K35.31
  arteriosclerotic (general) (senile) — *see* Arteriosclerosis, extremities, with, gangrene
  auricle I96
  Bacillus welchii A48.Ø
  bladder (infectious) — *see* Cystitis, specified type NEC
  bowel, cecum, or colon — *see* Gangrene, intestine
  Clostridium perfringens or welchii A48.Ø
  cornea H18.89- ☑
  corpora cavernosa N48.29
    noninfective N48.89
  cutaneous, spreading I96
  decubital — *see* Ulcer, pressure, by site
  diabetic (any site) — *see* Diabetes, gangrene
  emphysematous — *see* Gangrene, gas
  epidemic — *see* Poisoning, food, noxious, plant
  epididymis (infectional) N45.1
  erysipelas — *see* Erysipelas
  extremity (lower) (upper) I96
  Fournier N49.3
    female N76.89
  fusospirochetal A69.Ø
  gallbladder — *see* Cholecystitis, acute
  gas (bacillus) A48.Ø
    following
      abortion — *see* Abortion by type complicated by infection
      ectopic or molar pregnancy OØ8.Ø
  glossitis K14.Ø
  hernia — *see* Hernia, by site, with gangrene
  intestine, intestinal (hemorrhagic) (massive) — *see also* Infarct, intestine K55.Ø69
    with
      mesenteric embolism — *see also* Infarct, intestine K55.Ø69
      obstruction — *see* Obstruction, intestine
  laryngitis JØ4.Ø
  limb (lower) (upper) I96
  lung J85.Ø
    spirochetal A69.8
  lymphangitis I89.1
  Meleney's (synergistic) — *see* Ulcer, skin
  mesentery — *see also* Infarct, intestine K55.Ø69
    with
      embolism — *see also* Infarct, intestine K55.Ø69
      intestinal obstruction — *see* Obstruction, intestine
  mouth A69.Ø
  ovary — *see* Oophoritis
  pancreas — *see* Pancreatitis, acute
  penis N48.29
    noninfective N48.89
  perineum I96
  pharynx — *see also* Pharyngitis
    Vincent's A69.1
  presenile I73.1
  progressive synergistic — *see* Ulcer, skin
  pulmonary J85.Ø
  pulpal (dental) KØ4.1
  quinsy J36
  Raynaud's (symmetric gangrene) I73.Ø1
  retropharyngeal J39.2
  scrotum N49.3
    noninfective N5Ø.89

Gangrene, gangrenous — *continued*
  senile (atherosclerotic) — *see* Arteriosclerosis, extremities, with, gangrene
  spermatic cord N49.1
    noninfective N5Ø.89
  spine I96
  spirochetal NEC A69.8
  spreading cutaneous I96
  stomatitis A69.Ø
  symmetrical I73.Ø1
  testis (infectional) N45.2
    noninfective N44.8
  throat — *see also* Pharyngitis
    diphtheritic A36.Ø
    Vincent's A69.1
  thyroid (gland) EØ7.89
  tooth (pulp) KØ4.1
  tuberculous NEC — *see* Tuberculosis
  tunica vaginalis N49.1
    noninfective N5Ø.89
  umbilicus I96
  uterus — *see* Endometritis
  uvulitis K12.2
  vas deferens N49.1
    noninfective N5Ø.89
  vulva N76.89
Ganister disease J62.8
Ganser's syndrome (hysterical) F44.89
Gardner-Diamond syndrome (autoerythrocyte sensitization) D69.2
Gargoylism E76.Ø1
Garré's disease, osteitis (sclerosing), osteomyelitis — *see* Osteomyelitis, specified type NEC
Garrod's pad, knuckle M72.1
Gartner's duct
  cyst Q52.4
  persistent Q5Ø.6
Gas R14.3
  asphyxiation, inhalation, poisoning, suffocation NEC — *see* Table of Drugs and Chemicals
  excessive R14.Ø
  gangrene A48.Ø
    following
      abortion — *see* Abortion by type complicated by infection
      ectopic or molar pregnancy OØ8.Ø
  on stomach R14.Ø
  pains R14.1
Gastralgia — *see also* Pain, abdominal
Gastrectasis K31.Ø
  psychogenic F45.8
Gastric — *see* condition
Gastrinoma
  malignant
    pancreas C25.4
    specified site NEC — *see* Neoplasm, malignant, by site
    unspecified site C25.4
  specified site — *see* Neoplasm, uncertain behavior
  unspecified site D37.9
Gastritis (simple) K29.7Ø
  with bleeding K29.71
  acute (erosive) K29.ØØ
    with bleeding K29.Ø1
  alcoholic K29.2Ø
    with bleeding K29.21
  allergic K29.6Ø
    with bleeding K29.61
  atrophic (chronic) K29.4Ø
    with bleeding K29.41
  chronic (antral) (fundal) K29.5Ø
    with bleeding K29.51
    atrophic K29.4Ø
      with bleeding K29.41
    superficial K29.3Ø
      with bleeding K29.31
  dietary counseling and surveillance Z71.3
  due to diet deficiency E63.9
  eosinophilic K52.81
  giant hypertrophic K29.6Ø
    with bleeding K29.61
  granulomatous K29.6Ø
    with bleeding K29.61
  hypertrophic (mucosa) K29.6Ø
    with bleeding K29.61
  nervous F54
  spastic K29.6Ø
    with bleeding K29.61

Gastritis — *continued*
  specified NEC K29.60
    with bleeding K29.61
  superficial chronic K29.30
    with bleeding K29.31
  tuberculous A18.83
  viral NEC A08.4
Gastrocarcinoma — *see* Neoplasm, malignant, stomach
Gastrocolic — *see* condition
Gastrodisciasis, gastrodiscoidiasis B66.8
Gastroduodenitis K29.90
  with bleeding K29.91
  virus, viral A08.4
    specified type NEC A08.39
Gastrodynia — *see* Pain, abdominal
Gastroenteritis (acute) (chronic) (noninfectious) — *see also* Enteritis K52.9
  allergic K52.29
    with
      eosinophilic gastritis or gastroenteritis K52.81
      food protein-induced enterocolitis syndrome K52.21
      food protein-induced enteropathy K52.22
  dietetic — *see also* Gastroenteritis, allergic K52.29
  drug-induced K52.1
  due to
    Cryptosporidium A07.2
    drugs K52.1
    food poisoning — *see* Intoxication, foodborne
    radiation K52.0
  eosinophilic K52.81
  epidemic (infectious) A09
  food hypersensitivity — *see also* Gastroenteritis, allergic K52.29
  infectious — *see* Enteritis, infectious
  influenzal — *see* Influenza, with gastroenteritis
  noninfectious K52.9
    specified NEC K52.89
  rotaviral A08.0
  Salmonella A02.0
  toxic K52.1
  viral NEC A08.4
    acute infectious A08.39
      type Norwalk A08.11
    infantile (acute) A08.39
    Norwalk agent A08.11
    rotaviral A08.0
    severe of infants A08.39
    specified type NEC A08.39
Gastroenteropathy — *see also* Gastroenteritis K52.9
  acute, due to Norovirus A08.11
  acute, due to Norwalk agent A08.11
  infectious A09
Gastroenteroptosis K63.4
Gastroesophageal laceration- hemorrhage syndrome K22.6
Gastrointestinal — *see* condition
Gastrojejunal — *see* condition
Gastrojejunitis — *see also* Enteritis K52.9
Gastrojejunocolic — *see* condition
Gastroliths K31.89
Gastromalacia K31.89
Gastroparalysis K31.84
  diabetic — *see* Diabetes, gastroparalysis
Gastroparesis K31.84
  diabetic — *see* Diabetes, by type, with gastroparesis
Gastropathy K31.9
  congestive portal K31.89
  erythematous K29.70
  exudative K90.89
  portal hypertensive K31.89
Gastroptosis K31.89
Gastrorrhagia K92.2
  psychogenic F45.8
Gastroschisis (congenital) Q79.3
Gastrospasm (neurogenic) (reflex) K31.89
  neurotic F45.8
  psychogenic F45.8
Gastrostaxis — *see* Gastritis, with bleeding
Gastrostenosis K31.89
Gastrostomy
  attention to Z43.1
  status Z93.1
Gastrosuccorrhea (continuous) (intermittent) K31.89
  neurotic F45.8
  psychogenic F45.8
Gatophobia F40.218
Gaucher's disease or splenomegaly (adult) (infantile) E75.22
Gee (-Herter)(-Thaysen) **disease** (nontropical sprue) K90.0
Gélineau's syndrome G47.419
  with cataplexy G47.411
Gemination, tooth, teeth K00.2
Gemistocytoma
  specified site — *see* Neoplasm, malignant, by site
  unspecified site C71.9
General, generalized — *see* condition
Genetic
  carrier (status)
    cystic fibrosis Z14.1
    hemophilia A (asymptomatic) Z14.01
      symptomatic Z14.02
    specified NEC Z14.8
  susceptibility to disease NEC Z15.89
    malignant neoplasm Z15.09
      breast Z15.01
      endometrium Z15.04
      ovary Z15.02
      prostate Z15.03
      specified NEC Z15.09
    multiple endocrine neoplasia Z15.81
Genital — *see* condition
Genito-anorectal syndrome A55
Genitourinary system — *see* condition
Genu
  congenital Q74.1
  extrorsum (acquired) — *see also* Deformity, varus, knee
    congenital Q74.1
    sequelae (late effect) of rickets E64.3
  introrsum (acquired) — *see also* Deformity, valgus, knee
    congenital Q74.1
    sequelae (late effect) of rickets E64.3
  rachitic (old) E64.3
  recurvatum (acquired) — *see also* Deformity, limb, specified type NEC, lower leg
    congenital Q68.2
    sequelae (late effect) of rickets E64.3
  valgum (acquired) (knock-knee) M21.06- ☑
    congenital Q74.1
    sequelae (late effect) of rickets E64.3
  varum (acquired) (bowleg) M21.16- ☑
    congenital Q74.1
    sequelae (late effect) of rickets E64.3
Geographic tongue K14.1
Geophagia — *see* Pica
Geotrichosis B48.3
  stomatitis B48.3
Gephyrophobia F40.242
Gerbode defect Q21.0
GERD (gastroesophageal reflux disease) K21.9
Gerhardt's
  disease (erythromelalgia) I73.81
  syndrome (vocal cord paralysis) J38.00
    bilateral J38.02
    unilateral J38.01
German measles — *see also* Rubella
  exposure to Z20.4
Germinoblastoma (diffuse) C85.9- ☑
  follicular C82.9- ☑
Germinoma — *see* Neoplasm, malignant, by site
Gerontoxon — *see* Degeneration, cornea, senile
Gerstmann's syndrome R48.8
  developmental F81.2
Gerstmann-Sträussler-Scheinker syndrome (GSS) A81.82
Gestation (period) — *see also* Pregnancy
  ectopic — *see* Pregnancy, by site
  multiple O30.9- ☑
    greater than quadruplets — *see* Pregnancy, multiple (gestation), specified NEC
    specified NEC — *see* Pregnancy, multiple (gestation), specified NEC
Gestational
  mammary abscess O91.11- ☑
  purulent mastitis O91.11- ☑
  subareolar abscess O91.11- ☑
Ghon tubercle, primary infection A15.7
Ghost
  teeth K00.4
  vessels (cornea) H16.41- ☑
Ghoul hand A66.3
Gianotti-Crosti disease L44.4
Giant
  cell
    epulis K06.8
    peripheral granuloma K06.8
  esophagus, congenital Q39.5
  kidney, congenital Q63.3
  urticaria T78.3 ☑
    hereditary D84.1
Giardiasis A07.1
Gibert's disease or pityriasis L42
Giddiness R42
  hysterical F44.89
  psychogenic F45.8
Gierke's disease (glycogenosis I) E74.01
Gigantism (cerebral) (hypophyseal) (pituitary) E22.0
  constitutional E34.4
Gilbert's disease or syndrome E80.4
Gilchrist's disease B40.9
Gilford-Hutchinson disease E34.8
Gilles de la Tourette's disease or syndrome (motor-verbal tic) F95.2
Gingivitis K05.10
  acute (catarrhal) K05.00
    necrotizing A69.1
    nonplaque induced K05.01
    plaque induced K05.00
  chronic (desquamative) (hyperplastic) (simple marginal) (pregnancy associated) (ulcerative) K05.10
    nonplaque induced K05.11
    plaque induced K05.10
  expulsiva — *see* Periodontitis
  necrotizing ulcerative (acute) A69.1
  pellagrous E52
    acute necrotizing A69.1
  Vincent's A69.1
Gingivoglossitis K14.0
Gingivopericementitis — *see* Periodontitis
Gingivosis — *see* Gingivitis, chronic
Gingivostomatitis K05.10
  herpesviral B00.2
  necrotizing ulcerative (acute) A69.1
Gland, glandular — *see* condition
Glanders A24.0
Glanzmann (-Naegeli) **disease or thrombasthenia** D69.1
Glasgow coma scale
  total score
    3-8 R40.243 ☑
    9-12 R40.242 ☑
    13-15 R40.241 ☑
Glass-blower's disease (cataract) — *see* Cataract, specified NEC
Glaucoma H40.9
  with
    increased episcleral venous pressure H40.81- ☑
    pseudoexfoliation of lens — *see* Glaucoma, open angle, primary, capsular
  absolute H44.51- ☑
  angle-closure (primary) H40.20- ☑
    acute (attack) (crisis) H40.21- ☑
    chronic H40.22- ☑
    intermittent H40.23- ☑
    residual stage H40.24- ☑
  borderline H40.00- ☑
  capsular (with pseudoexfoliation of lens) — *see* Glaucoma, open angle, primary, capsular
  childhood Q15.0
  closed angle — *see* Glaucoma, angle-closure
  congenital Q15.0
  corticosteroid-induced — *see* Glaucoma, secondary, drugs
  hypersecretion H40.82- ☑
  in (due to)
    amyloidosis E85.4 *[H42]*
    aniridia Q13.1 *[H42]*
    concussion of globe — *see* Glaucoma, secondary, trauma
    dislocation of lens — *see* Glaucoma, secondary
    disorder of lens NEC — *see* Glaucoma, secondary
    drugs — *see* Glaucoma, secondary, drugs
    endocrine disease NOS E34.9 *[H42]*
    eye
      inflammation — *see* Glaucoma, secondary, inflammation
      trauma — *see* Glaucoma, secondary, trauma
    hypermature cataract — *see* Glaucoma, secondary

Index

Gastritis — Glaucoma

- **Glycogen**
  - infiltration — *see* Disease, glycogen storage
  - storage disease — *see* Disease, glycogen storage
- **Glycogenosis** (diffuse) (generalized) — *see also* Disease, glycogen storage
  - cardiac E74.Ø2 *[I43]*
  - diabetic, secondary — *see* Diabetes, glycogenosis, secondary
  - pulmonary interstitial J84.842
- **Glycopenia** E16.2
- **Glycosuria** R81
  - renal E74.818
- **Gnathostoma spinigerum** (infection) (infestation), **gnathostomiasis** (wandering swelling) B83.1
- **Goiter** (plunging) (substernal) EØ4.9
  - with
    - hyperthyroidism (recurrent) — *see* Hyperthyroidism, with, goiter
    - thyrotoxicosis — *see* Hyperthyroidism, with, goiter
  - adenomatous — *see* Goiter, nodular
  - cancerous C73
  - congenital (nontoxic) EØ3.Ø
    - diffuse EØ3.Ø
    - parenchymatous EØ3.Ø
    - transitory, with normal functioning P72.Ø
  - cystic EØ4.2
    - due to iodine-deficiency EØ1.1
  - due to
    - enzyme defect in synthesis of thyroid hormone EØ7.1
    - iodine-deficiency (endemic) EØ1.2
  - dyshormonogenetic (familial) EØ7.1
  - endemic (iodine-deficiency) EØ1.2
    - diffuse EØ1.Ø
    - multinodular EØ1.1
  - exophthalmic — *see* Hyperthyroidism, with, goiter
  - iodine-deficiency (endemic) EØ1.2
    - diffuse EØ1.Ø
    - multinodular EØ1.1
    - nodular EØ1.1
  - lingual Q89.2
  - lymphadenoid EØ6.3
  - malignant C73
  - multinodular (cystic) (nontoxic) EØ4.2
    - toxic or with hyperthyroidism EØ5.2Ø
      - with thyroid storm EØ5.21
  - neonatal NEC P72.Ø
  - nodular (nontoxic) (due to) EØ4.9
    - with
      - hyperthyroidism EØ5.2Ø
        - with thyroid storm EØ5.21
      - thyrotoxicosis EØ5.2Ø
        - with thyroid storm EØ5.21
    - endemic EØ1.1
    - iodine-deficiency EØ1.1
    - sporadic EØ4.9
    - toxic EØ5.2Ø
      - with thyroid storm EØ5.21
  - nontoxic EØ4.9
    - diffuse (colloid) EØ4.Ø
    - multinodular EØ4.2
    - simple EØ4.Ø
    - specified NEC EØ4.8
    - uninodular EØ4.1
  - simple EØ4.Ø
  - toxic — *see* Hyperthyroidism, with, goiter
  - uninodular (nontoxic) EØ4.1
    - toxic or with hyperthyroidism EØ5.1Ø
      - with thyroid storm EØ5.11
- **Goiter-deafness syndrome** EØ7.1
- **Goldberg syndrome** Q89.8
- **Goldberg-Maxwell syndrome** E34.51
- **Goldblatt's hypertension or kidney** I7Ø.1
- **Goldenhar** (-Gorlin) **syndrome** Q87.Ø
- **Goldflam-Erb disease or syndrome** G7Ø.ØØ
  - with exacerbation (acute) G7Ø.Ø1
  - in crisis G7Ø.Ø1
- **Goldscheider's disease** Q81.8
- **Goldstein's disease** (familial hemorrhagic telangiectasia) I78.Ø
- **Golfer's elbow** — *see* Epicondylitis, medial
- **Gonadoblastoma**
  - specified site — *see* Neoplasm, uncertain behavior, by site
  - unspecified site
    - female D39.1Ø
    - male D4Ø.1Ø
- **Gonecystitis** — *see* Vesiculitis
- **Gongylonemiasis** B83.8
- **Goniosynechiae** — *see* Adhesions, iris, goniosynechiae
- **Gonococcemia** A54.86
- **Gonococcus, gonococcal** (disease) (infection) — *see also* condition A54.9
  - anus A54.6
  - bursa, bursitis A54.49
  - conjunctiva, conjunctivitis (neonatorum) A54.31
  - endocardium A54.83
  - eye A54.3Ø
    - conjunctivitis A54.31
    - iridocyclitis A54.32
    - keratitis A54.33
    - newborn A54.31
    - other specified A54.39
  - fallopian tubes (acute) (chronic) A54.24
  - genitourinary (organ) (system) (tract) (acute)
    - lower A54.ØØ
      - with abscess (accessory gland) (periurethral) A54.1
    - upper — *see also* condition A54.29
  - heart A54.83
  - iridocyclitis A54.32
  - joint A54.42
  - lymphatic (gland) (node) A54.89
  - meninges, meningitis A54.81
  - musculoskeletal A54.4Ø
    - arthritis A54.42
    - osteomyelitis A54.43
    - other specified A54.49
    - spondylopathy A54.41
  - pelviperitonitis A54.24
  - pelvis (acute) (chronic) A54.24
  - pharynx A54.5
  - proctitis A54.6
  - pyosalpinx (acute) (chronic) A54.24
  - rectum A54.6
  - skin A54.89
  - specified site NEC A54.89
  - tendon sheath A54.49
  - throat A54.5
  - urethra (acute) (chronic) A54.Ø1
    - with abscess (accessory gland) (periurethral) A54.1
  - vulva (acute) (chronic) A54.Ø2
- **Gonocytoma**
  - specified site — *see* Neoplasm, uncertain behavior, by site
  - unspecified site
    - female D39.1Ø
    - male D4Ø.1Ø
- **Gonorrhea** (acute) (chronic) A54.9
  - Bartholin's gland (acute) (chronic) (purulent) A54.Ø2
    - with abscess (accessory gland) (periurethral) A54.1
  - bladder A54.Ø1
  - cervix A54.Ø3
  - conjunctiva, conjunctivitis (neonatorum) A54.31
  - contact Z2Ø.2
  - Cowper's gland (with abscess) A54.1
  - exposure to Z2Ø.2
  - fallopian tube (acute) (chronic) A54.24
  - kidney (acute) (chronic) A54.21
  - lower genitourinary tract A54.ØØ
    - with abscess (accessory gland) (periurethral) A54.1
  - ovary (acute) (chronic) A54.24
  - pelvis (acute) (chronic) A54.24
    - female pelvic inflammatory disease A54.24
  - penis A54.Ø9
  - prostate (acute) (chronic) A54.22
  - seminal vesicle (acute) (chronic) A54.23
  - specified site not listed — *see also* Gonococcus A54.89
  - spermatic cord (acute) (chronic) A54.23
  - urethra A54.Ø1
    - with abscess (accessory gland) (periurethral) A54.1
  - vagina A54.Ø2
  - vas deferens (acute) (chronic) A54.23
  - vulva A54.Ø2
- **Goodall's disease** AØ8.19
- **Goodpasture's syndrome** M31.Ø
- **Gopalan's syndrome** (burning feet) E53.Ø
- **Gorlin-Chaudry-Moss syndrome** Q87.Ø
- **Gottron's papules** L94.4
- **Gougerot-Blum syndrome** (pigmented purpuric lichenoid dermatitis) L81.7
- **Gougerot-Carteaud disease or syndrome** (confluent reticulate papillomatosis) L83
- **Gougerot's syndrome** (trisymptomatic) L81.7
- **Gouley's syndrome** (constrictive pericarditis) I31.1
- **Goundou** A66.6
- **Gout, chronic** — *see also* Gout, gouty M1A.9 ☑ *(following* MØ8)
  - drug-induced M1A.2Ø ☑ *(following* MØ8)
    - ankle M1A.27- ☑ *(following* MØ8)
    - elbow M1A.22- ☑ *(following* MØ8)
    - foot joint M1A.27- ☑ *(following* MØ8)
    - hand joint M1A.24- ☑ *(following* MØ8)
    - hip M1A.25- ☑ *(following* MØ8)
    - knee M1A.26- ☑ *(following* MØ8)
    - multiple site M1A.29- ☑ *(following* MØ8)
    - shoulder M1A.21- ☑ *(following* MØ8)
    - vertebrae M1A.28 ☑ *(following* MØ8)
    - wrist M1A.23- ☑ *(following* MØ8)
  - idiopathic M1A.ØØ ☑ *(following* MØ8)
    - ankle M1A.Ø7- ☑ *(following* MØ8)
    - elbow M1A.Ø2- ☑ *(following* MØ8)
    - foot joint M1A.Ø7- ☑ *(following* MØ8)
    - hand joint M1A.Ø4- ☑ *(following* MØ8)
    - hip M1A.Ø5- ☑ *(following* MØ8)
    - knee M1A.Ø6- ☑ *(following* MØ8)
    - multiple site M1A.Ø9 ☑ *(following* MØ8)
    - shoulder M1A.Ø1- ☑ *(following* MØ8)
    - vertebrae M1A.Ø8 ☑ *(following* MØ8)
    - wrist M1A.Ø3- ☑ *(following* MØ8)
  - in (due to) renal impairment M1A.3Ø ☑ *(following* MØ8)
    - ankle M1A.37- ☑ *(following* MØ8)
    - elbow M1A.32- ☑ *(following* MØ8)
    - foot joint M1A.37- ☑ *(following* MØ8)
    - hand joint M1A.34- ☑ *(following* MØ8)
    - hip M1A.35- ☑ *(following* MØ8)
    - knee M1A.36- ☑ *(following* MØ8)
    - multiple site M1A.39 ☑ *(following* MØ8)
    - shoulder M1A.31- ☑ *(following* MØ8)
    - vertebrae M1A.38 ☑ *(following* MØ8)
    - wrist M1A.33- ☑ *(following* MØ8)
  - lead-induced M1A.1Ø ☑ *(following* MØ8)
    - ankle M1A.17- ☑ *(following* MØ8)
    - elbow M1A.12- ☑ *(following* MØ8)
    - foot joint M1A.17- ☑ *(following* MØ8)
    - hand joint M1A.14- ☑ *(following* MØ8)
    - hip M1A.15- ☑ *(following* MØ8)
    - knee M1A.16- ☑ *(following* MØ8)
    - multiple site M1A.19 ☑ *(following* MØ8)
    - shoulder M1A.11- ☑ *(following* MØ8)
    - vertebrae M1A.18 ☑ *(following* MØ8)
    - wrist M1A.13- ☑ *(following* MØ8)
  - primary — *see* Gout, chronic, idiopathic
  - saturnine — *see* Gout, chronic, lead-induced
  - secondary NEC M1A.4Ø ☑ *(following* MØ8)
    - ankle M1A.47- ☑ *(following* MØ8)
    - elbow M1A.42- ☑ *(following* MØ8)
    - foot joint M1A.47- ☑ *(following* MØ8)
    - hand joint M1A.44- ☑ *(following* MØ8)
    - hip M1A.45- ☑ *(following* MØ8)
    - knee M1A.46- ☑ *(following* MØ8)
    - multiple site M1A.49 ☑ *(following* MØ8)
    - shoulder M1A.41- ☑ *(following* MØ8)
    - vertebrae M1A.48 ☑ *(following* MØ8)
    - wrist M1A.43- ☑ *(following* MØ8)
  - syphilitic — *see also* subcategory M14.8- A52.77
  - tophi M1A.9 ☑ *(following* MØ8)
- **Gout, gouty** (acute) (attack) (flare) — *see also* Gout, chronic M1Ø.9
  - drug-induced M1Ø.2Ø
    - ankle M1Ø.27- ☑
    - elbow M1Ø.22- ☑
    - foot joint M1Ø.27- ☑
    - hand joint M1Ø.24- ☑
    - hip M1Ø.25- ☑
    - knee M1Ø.26- ☑
    - multiple site M1Ø.29
    - shoulder M1Ø.21- ☑
    - vertebrae M1Ø.28
    - wrist M1Ø.23- ☑
  - idiopathic M1Ø.ØØ
    - ankle M1Ø.Ø7- ☑
    - elbow M1Ø.Ø2- ☑
    - foot joint M1Ø.Ø7- ☑
    - hand joint M1Ø.Ø4- ☑
    - hip M1Ø.Ø5- ☑
    - knee M1Ø.Ø6- ☑
    - multiple site M1Ø.Ø9
    - shoulder M1Ø.Ø1- ☑
    - vertebrae M1Ø.Ø8
    - wrist M1Ø.Ø3- ☑
  - in (due to) renal impairment M1Ø.3Ø

Gout, gouty — *continued*
- in renal impairment — *continued*
  - ankle M1Ø.37- ☑
  - elbow M1Ø.32- ☑
  - foot joint M1Ø.37- ☑
  - hand joint M1Ø.34- ☑
  - hip M1Ø.35- ☑
  - knee M1Ø.36- ☑
  - multiple site M1Ø.39
  - shoulder M1Ø.31- ☑
  - vertebrae M1Ø.38
  - wrist M1Ø.33- ☑
- lead-induced M1Ø.1Ø
  - ankle M1Ø.17- ☑
  - elbow M1Ø.12- ☑
  - foot joint M1Ø.17- ☑
  - hand joint M1Ø.14- ☑
  - hip M1Ø.15- ☑
  - knee M1Ø.16- ☑
  - multiple site M1Ø.19
  - shoulder M1Ø.11- ☑
  - vertebrae M1Ø.18
  - wrist M1Ø.13- ☑
- primary — *see* Gout, idiopathic
- saturnine — *see* Gout, lead-induced
- secondary NEC M1Ø.4Ø
  - ankle M1Ø.47- ☑
  - elbow M1Ø.42- ☑
  - foot joint M1Ø.47- ☑
  - hand joint M1Ø.44- ☑
  - hip M1Ø.45- ☑
  - knee M1Ø.46- ☑
  - multiple site M1Ø.49
  - shoulder M1Ø.41- ☑
  - vertebrae M1Ø.48
  - wrist M1Ø.43- ☑
- syphilitic — *see also* subcategory M14.8- A52.77
- tophi — *see* Gout, chronic

Gower's
- muscular dystrophy G71.Ø1
- syndrome (vasovagal attack) R55

Gradenigo's syndrome — *see* Otitis, media, suppurative, acute

Graefe's disease — *see* Strabismus, paralytic, ophthalmoplegia, progressive

Graft-versus-host disease D89.813
- acute D89.81Ø
- acute on chronic D89.812
- chronic D89.811

Grain mite (itch) B88.Ø

Grainhandler's disease or lung J67.8

Grand mal — *see* Epilepsy, generalized, specified NEC

Grand multipara status only (not pregnant) Z64.1
- pregnant — *see* Pregnancy, complicated by, grand multiparity

Granite worker's lung J62.8

Granular — *see also* condition
- inflammation, pharynx J31.2
- kidney (contracting) — *see* Sclerosis, renal
- liver K74.69

Granulation tissue (abnormal) (excessive) L92.9
- postmastoidectomy cavity — *see* Complications, postmastoidectomy, granulation

Granulocytopenia (primary) (malignant) — *see* Agranulocytosis

Granuloma L92.9
- abdomen K66.8
  - from residual foreign body L92.3
  - pyogenicum L98.Ø
- actinic L57.5
- annulare (perforating) L92.Ø
- apical KØ4.5
- aural — *see* Otitis, externa, specified NEC
- beryllium (skin) L92.3
- bone
  - eosinophilic C96.6
  - from residual foreign body — *see* Osteomyelitis, specified type NEC
  - lung C96.6
- brain (any site) GØ6.Ø
  - schistosomiasis B65.9 *[GØ7]*
- canaliculus lacrimalis — *see* Granuloma, lacrimal
- candidal (cutaneous) B37.2
- cerebral (any site) GØ6.Ø
- coccidioidal (primary) (progressive) B38.7
  - lung B38.1
  - meninges B38.4

Granuloma — *continued*
- colon K63.89
- conjunctiva H11.22- ☑
- dental KØ4.5
- ear, middle — *see* Cholesteatoma
- eosinophilic C96.6
  - bone C96.6
  - lung C96.6
  - oral mucosa K13.4
  - skin L92.2
- eyelid HØ1.8
- facial (e) L92.2
- foreign body (in soft tissue) NEC M6Ø.2Ø
  - ankle M6Ø.27- ☑
  - foot M6Ø.27- ☑
  - forearm M6Ø.23- ☑
  - hand M6Ø.24- ☑
  - in operation wound — *see* Foreign body, accidentally left during a procedure
  - lower leg M6Ø.26- ☑
  - pelvic region M6Ø.25- ☑
  - shoulder region M6Ø.21- ☑
  - skin L92.3
  - specified site NEC M6Ø.28
  - subcutaneous tissue L92.3
  - thigh M6Ø.25- ☑
  - upper arm M6Ø.22- ☑
- gangraenescens M31.2
- genito-inguinale A58
- giant cell (central) (reparative) (jaw) M27.1
  - gingiva (peripheral) KØ6.8
- gland (lymph) I88.8
- hepatic NEC K75.3
  - in (due to)
    - berylliosis J63.2 *[K77]*
    - sarcoidosis D86.89
- Hodgkin C81.9 ☑
- ileum K63.89
- infectious B99.9
  - specified NEC B99.8
- inguinale (Donovan) (venereal) A58
- intestine NEC K63.89
- intracranial (any site) GØ6.Ø
- intraspinal (any part) GØ6.1
- iridocyclitis — *see* Iridocyclitis, chronic
- jaw (bone) (central) M27.1
  - reparative giant cell M27.1
- kidney — *see also* Infection, kidney N15.8
- lacrimal HØ4.81- ☑
- larynx J38.7
- lethal midline (faciale(e)) M31.2
- liver NEC — *see* Granuloma, hepatic
- lung (infectious) — *see also* Fibrosis, lung
  - coccidioidal B38.1
  - eosinophilic C96.6
- Majocchi's B35.8
- malignant (facial(e)) M31.2
- mandible (central) M27.1
- midline (lethal) M31.2
- monilial (cutaneous) B37.2
- nasal sinus — *see* Sinusitis
- operation wound T81.89 ☑
  - foreign body — *see* Foreign body, accidentally left during a procedure
  - stitch T81.89 ☑
  - talc — *see* Foreign body, accidentally left during a procedure
- oral mucosa K13.4
- orbit, orbital HØ5.11- ☑
- paracoccidioidal B41.8
- penis, venereal A58
- periapical KØ4.5
- peritoneum K66.8
  - due to ova of helminths NOS — *see also* Helminthiasis B83.9 *[K67]*
- postmastoidectomy cavity — *see* Complications, postmastoidectomy, recurrent cholesteatoma
- prostate N42.89
- pudendi (ulcerating) A58
- pulp, internal (tooth) KØ3.3
- pyogenic, pyogenicum (of) (skin) L98.Ø
  - gingiva KØ6.8
  - maxillary alveolar ridge KØ4.5
  - oral mucosa K13.4
- rectum K62.89
- reticulohistiocytic D76.3
- rubrum nasi L74.8
- Schistosoma — *see* Schistosomiasis

Granuloma — *continued*
- septic (skin) L98.Ø
- silica (skin) L92.3
- sinus (accessory) (infective) (nasal) — *see* Sinusitis
- skin L92.9
  - from residual foreign body L92.3
  - pyogenicum L98.Ø
- spine
  - syphilitic (epidural) A52.19
  - tuberculous A18.Ø1
- stitch (postoperative) T81.89 ☑
- suppurative (skin) L98.Ø
- swimming pool A31.1
- talc — *see also* Granuloma, foreign body
  - in operation wound — *see* Foreign body, accidentally left during a procedure
- telangiectaticum (skin) L98.Ø
- tracheostomy J95.Ø9
- trichophyticum B35.8
- tropicum A66.4
- umbilical P83.81
- umbilicus P83.81
- urethra N36.8
- uveitis — *see* Iridocyclitis, chronic
- vagina A58
- venereum A58
- vocal cord J38.3

Granulomatosis L92.9
- with polyangiitis M31.3 ☑
- eosinophilic, with polyangiitis [EGPA] M3Ø.1
- lymphoid C83.8- ☑
- miliary (listerial) A32.89
- necrotizing, respiratory M31.3Ø
- progressive septic D71
- specified NEC L92.8
- Wegener's M31.3Ø
  - with renal involvement M31.31

Granulomatous tissue (abnormal) (excessive) L92.9

Granulosis rubra nasi L74.8

Graphite fibrosis (of lung) J63.3

Graphospasm F48.8
- organic G25.89

Grating scapula M89.8X1

Gravel (urinary) — *see* Calculus, urinary

Graves' disease — *see* Hyperthyroidism, with, goiter

Gravis — *see* condition

Grawitz tumor C64.- ☑

Gray syndrome (newborn) P93.Ø

Grayness, hair (premature) L67.1
- congenital Q84.2

Green sickness D5Ø.8

Greenfield's disease
- meaning
  - concentric sclerosis (encephalitis periaxialis concentrica) G37.5
  - metachromatic leukodystrophy E75.25

Greenstick fracture — *code as* Fracture, by site

Grey syndrome (newborn) P93.Ø

Grief F43.21
- prolonged F43.29
- reaction — *see also* Disorder, adjustment F43.2Ø

Griesinger's disease B76.Ø

Grinder's lung or pneumoconiosis J62.8

Grinding, teeth
- psychogenic F45.8
- sleep related G47.63

Grip
- Dabney's B33.Ø
- devil's B33.Ø

Grippe, grippal — *see also* Influenza
- Balkan A78
- summer, of Italy A93.1

Grisel's disease M43.6

Groin — *see* condition

Grooved tongue K14.5

Ground itch B76.9

Grover's disease or syndrome L11.1

Growing pains, children R29.898

Growth (fungoid) (neoplastic) (new) — *see also* Neoplasm
- adenoid (vegetative) J35.8
- benign — *see* Neoplasm, benign, by site
- malignant — *see* Neoplasm, malignant, by site
- rapid, childhood ZØØ.2
- secondary — *see* Neoplasm, secondary, by site

Gruby's disease B35.Ø

Gubler-Millard paralysis or syndrome G46.3

Guerin-Stern syndrome Q74.3

- **Guidance, insufficient anterior** (occlusal) M26.54
- **Guillain-Barré disease or syndrome** G61.Ø
  - sequelae G65.Ø
- **Guinea worms** (infection) (infestation) B72
- **Guinon's disease** (motor-verbal tic) F95.2
- **Gull's disease** EØ3.4
- **Gum** — *see* condition
- **Gumboil** KØ4.7
  - with sinus KØ4.6
- **Gumma** (syphilitic) A52.79
  - artery A52.Ø9
    - cerebral A52.Ø4
  - bone A52.77
    - of yaws (late) A66.6
  - brain A52.19
  - cauda equina A52.19
  - central nervous system A52.3
  - ciliary body A52.71
  - congenital A5Ø.59
  - eyelid A52.71
  - heart A52.Ø6
  - intracranial A52.19
  - iris A52.71
  - kidney A52.75
  - larynx A52.73
  - leptomeninges A52.19
  - liver A52.74
  - meninges A52.19
  - myocardium A52.Ø6
  - nasopharynx A52.73
  - neurosyphilitic A52.3
  - nose A52.73
  - orbit A52.71
  - palate (soft) A52.79
  - penis A52.76
  - pericardium A52.Ø6
  - pharynx A52.73
  - pituitary A52.79
  - scrofulous (tuberculous) A18.4
  - skin A52.79
  - specified site NEC A52.79
  - spinal cord A52.19
  - tongue A52.79
  - tonsil A52.73
  - trachea A52.73
  - tuberculous A18.4
  - ulcerative due to yaws A66.4
  - ureter A52.75
  - yaws A66.4
    - bone A66.6
- **Gunn's syndrome** QØ7.8
- **Gunshot wound** — *see also* Puncture, open
  - fracture — *code as* Fracture, by site
  - internal organs — *see* Injury, by site
- **Gynandrism** Q56.Ø
- **Gynandroblastoma**
  - specified site — *see* Neoplasm, uncertain behavior, by site
  - unspecified site
    - female D39.1Ø
    - male D4Ø.1Ø
- **Gynecological examination** (periodic) (routine) ZØ1.419
  - with abnormal findings ZØ1.411
- **Gynecomastia** N62
- **Gynephobia** F4Ø.291
- **Gyrate scalp** Q82.8

H

- H (Hartnup's) **disease** E72.Ø2
- **Haas' disease or osteochondrosis** (juvenile) (head of humerus) — *see* Osteochondrosis, juvenile, humerus
- **Habit, habituation**
  - bad sleep Z72.821
  - chorea F95.8
  - disturbance, child F98.9
  - drug — *see* Dependence, drug
  - irregular sleep Z72.821
  - laxative F55.2
  - spasm — *see* Tic
  - tic — *see* Tic
- **Haemophilus** (H.) **influenzae, as cause of disease classified elsewhere** B96.3
- **Haff disease** — *see* Poisoning, mercury
- **Hageman's factor defect, deficiency or disease** D68.2
- **Haglund's disease or osteochondrosis** (juvenile) (os tibiale externum) — *see* Osteochondrosis, juvenile, tarsus
- **Hailey-Hailey disease** Q82.8
- **Hair** — *see also* condition
  - plucking F63.3
    - in stereotyped movement disorder F98.4
  - tourniquet syndrome — *see also* Constriction, external, by site
    - finger S6Ø.44- ☑
    - penis S3Ø.842 ☑
    - thumb S6Ø.34- ☑
    - toe S9Ø.44- ☑
- **Hairball in stomach** T18.2 ☑
- **Hair-pulling, pathological** (compulsive) F63.3
- **Hairy black tongue** K14.3
- **Half vertebra** Q76.49
- **Halitosis** R19.6
- **Hallerman-Streiff syndrome** Q87.Ø
- **Hallervorden-Spatz disease** G23.Ø
- **Hallopeau's acrodermatitis or disease** L4Ø.2
- **Hallucination** R44.3
  - auditory R44.Ø
  - gustatory R44.2
  - olfactory R44.2
  - specified NEC R44.2
  - tactile R44.2
  - visual R44.1
- **Hallucinosis** (chronic) F28
  - alcoholic (acute) F1Ø.951
    - in
      - abuse F1Ø.151
      - dependence F1Ø.251
  - drug-induced F19.951
    - cannabis F12.951
    - cocaine F14.951
    - hallucinogen F16.151
    - in
      - abuse F19.151
        - cannabis F12.151
        - cocaine F14.151
        - hallucinogen F16.151
        - inhalant F18.151
        - opioid F11.151
        - sedative, anxiolytic or hypnotic F13.151
        - stimulant NEC F15.151
      - dependence F19.251
        - cannabis F12.251
        - cocaine F14.251
        - hallucinogen F16.251
        - inhalant F18.251
        - opioid F11.251
        - sedative, anxiolytic or hypnotic F13.251
        - stimulant NEC F15.251
    - inhalant F18.951
    - opioid F11.951
    - sedative, anxiolytic or hypnotic F13.951
    - stimulant NEC F15.951
  - organic FØ6.Ø
- **Hallux**
  - deformity (acquired) NEC M2Ø.5X- ☑
  - limitus M2Ø.5X- ☑
  - malleus (acquired) NEC M2Ø.3- ☑
  - rigidus (acquired) M2Ø.2- ☑
    - congenital Q74.2
    - sequelae (late effect) of rickets E64.3
  - valgus (acquired) M2Ø.1- ☑
    - congenital Q66.6
  - varus (acquired) M2Ø.3- ☑
    - congenital Q66.3- ☑
- **Halo, visual** H53.19
- **Hamartoma, hamartoblastoma** Q85.9
  - epithelial (gingival), odontogenic, central or peripheral — *see* Cyst, calcifying odontogenic
- **Hamartosis** Q85.9
- **Hamman-Rich syndrome** J84.114
- **Hammer toe** (acquired) NEC — *see also* Deformity, toe, hammer toe
  - congenital Q66.89
  - sequelae (late effect) of rickets E64.3
- **Hand** — *see* condition
- **Hand-foot syndrome** L27.1
- **Handicap, handicapped**
  - educational Z55.9
    - specified NEC Z55.8
- **Hand-Schüller-Christian disease or syndrome** C96.5
- **Hanging** (asphyxia) (strangulation) (suffocation) — *see* Asphyxia, traumatic, due to mechanical threat
- **Hangnail** — *see also* Cellulitis, digit
  - with lymphangitis — *see* Lymphangitis, acute, digit
- **Hangover** (alcohol) F1Ø.129
- **Hanhart's syndrome** Q87.Ø
- **Hanot-Chauffard** (-Troisier) **syndrome** E83.19
- **Hanot's cirrhosis or disease** K74.3
- **Hansen's disease** — *see* Leprosy
- **Hantaan virus disease** (Korean hemorrhagic fever) A98.5
- **Hantavirus disease** (with renal manifestations) (Dobrava) (Puumala) (Seoul) A98.5
  - with pulmonary manifestations (Andes) (Bayou) (Bermejo) (Black Creek Canal) (Choclo) (Juquitiba) (Laguna negra) (Lechiguanas) (New York) (Oran) (Sin nombre) B33.4
- **Happy puppet syndrome** Q93.51
- **Harada's disease or syndrome** H3Ø.81- ☑
- **Hardening**
  - artery — *see* Arteriosclerosis
  - brain G93.89
- **Harelip** (complete) (incomplete) — *see* Cleft, lip
- **Harlequin** (newborn) Q8Ø.4
- **Harley's disease** D59.6
- **Harmful use** (of)
  - alcohol F1Ø.1Ø
  - anxiolytics — *see* Abuse, drug, sedative
  - cannabinoids — *see* Abuse, drug, cannabis
  - cocaine — *see* Abuse, drug, cocaine
  - drug — *see* Abuse, drug
  - hallucinogens — *see* Abuse, drug, hallucinogen
  - hypnotics — *see* Abuse, drug, sedative
  - opioids — *see* Abuse, drug, opioid
  - PCP (phencyclidine) — *see* Abuse, drug, hallucinogen
  - sedatives — *see* Abuse, drug, sedative
  - stimulants NEC — *see* Abuse, drug, stimulant
- **Harris' lines** — *see* Arrest, epiphyseal
- **Hartnup's disease** E72.Ø2
- **Harvester's lung** J67.Ø
- **Harvesting ovum for in vitro fertilization** Z31.83
- **Hashimoto's disease or thyroiditis** EØ6.3
- **Hashitoxicosis** (transient) EØ6.3
- **Hassal-Henle bodies or warts** (cornea) H18.49
- **Haut mal** — *see* Epilepsy, generalized, specified NEC
- **Haverhill fever** A25.1
- **Hay fever** — *see also* Fever, hay J3Ø.1
- **Hayem-Widal syndrome** D59.8
- **Haygarth's nodes** M15.8
- **Haymaker's lung** J67.Ø
- **Hb** (abnormal)
  - Bart's disease D56.Ø
  - disease — *see* Disease, hemoglobin
  - trait — *see* Trait
- **Head** — *see* condition
- **Headache** R51.9
  - with
    - orthostatic component NEC R51.Ø
    - positional component NEC R51.Ø
  - allergic NEC G44.89
  - associated with sexual activity G44.82
  - chronic daily R51.9
  - cluster G44.ØØ9
    - chronic G44.Ø29
      - intractable G44.Ø21
      - not intractable G44.Ø29
    - episodic G44.Ø19
      - intractable G44.Ø11
      - not intractable G44.Ø19
    - intractable G44.ØØ1
    - not intractable G44.ØØ9
  - cough (primary) G44.83
  - daily chronic R51.9
  - drug-induced NEC G44.4Ø
    - intractable G44.41
    - not intractable G44.4Ø
  - exertional (primary) G44.84
  - histamine G44.ØØ9
    - intractable G44.ØØ1
    - not intractable G44.ØØ9
  - hypnic G44.81
  - lumbar puncture G97.1
  - medication overuse G44.4Ø
    - intractable G44.41
    - not intractable G44.4Ø
  - menstrual — *see* Migraine, menstrual
  - migraine (type) — *see also* Migraine G43.9Ø9
  - nasal septum R51.9
  - neuralgiform, short lasting unilateral, with conjunctival injection and tearing (SUNCT) G44.Ø59
    - intractable G44.Ø51
    - not intractable G44.Ø59

Headache — *continued*
- new daily persistent (NDPH) G44.52
- orgasmic G44.82
- periodic syndromes in adults and children G43.CØ (*following* G43.7)
  - with refractory migraine G43.C1 (*following* G43.7)
  - intractable G43.C1 (*following* G43.7)
  - not intractable G43.CØ (*following* G43.7)
  - without refractory migraine G43.CØ (*following* G43.7)
- postspinal puncture G97.1
- post-traumatic G44.3Ø9
  - acute G44.319
    - intractable G44.311
    - not intractable G44.319
  - chronic G44.329
    - intractable G44.321
    - not intractable G44.329
  - intractable G44.3Ø1
  - not intractable G44.3Ø9
- pre-menstrual — *see* Migraine, menstrual
- preorgasmic G44.82
- primary
  - cough G44.83
  - exertional G44.84
  - stabbing G44.85
  - thunderclap G44.53
- rebound G44.4Ø
  - intractable G44.41
  - not intractable G44.4Ø
- short lasting unilateral neuralgiform, with conjunctival injection and tearing (SUNCT) G44.Ø59
  - intractable G44.Ø51
  - not intractable G44.Ø59
- specified syndrome NEC G44.89
- spinal and epidural anesthesia - induced T88.59 ☑
  - in labor and delivery O74.5
  - in pregnancy O29.4- ☑
  - postpartum, puerperal O89.4
- spinal fluid loss (from puncture) G97.1
- stabbing (primary) G44.85
- tension (-type) G44.2Ø9
  - chronic G44.229
    - intractable G44.221
    - not intractable G44.229
  - episodic G44.219
    - intractable G44.211
    - not intractable G44.219
  - intractable G44.2Ø1
  - not intractable G44.2Ø9
- thunderclap (primary) G44.53
- vascular NEC G44.1

Healthy
- infant
  - accompanying sick mother Z76.3
  - receiving care Z76.2
- person accompanying sick person Z76.3

Hearing examination ZØ1.1Ø
- with abnormal findings NEC ZØ1.118
- following failed hearing screening ZØ1.11Ø
- for hearing conservation and treatment ZØ1.12
- infant or child (over 28 days old) ZØØ.129
  - with abnormal findings ZØØ.121

Heart — *see* condition

Heart beat
- abnormality RØØ.9
  - specified NEC RØØ.8
- awareness RØØ.2
- rapid RØØ.Ø
- slow RØØ.1

Heartburn R12
- psychogenic F45.8

Heartland virus disease A93.8

Heat (effects) T67.9 ☑
- apoplexy T67.Ø1 ☑
- burn — *see also* Burn L55.9
- collapse T67.1 ☑
- cramps T67.2 ☑
- dermatitis or eczema L59.Ø
- edema T67.7 ☑
- erythema — *code by site under* Burn, first degree
- excessive T67.9 ☑
  - specified effect NEC T67.8 ☑
- exhaustion T67.5 ☑
  - anhydrotic T67.3 ☑
  - due to
    - salt (and water) depletion T67.4 ☑
    - water depletion T67.3 ☑
      - with salt depletion T67.4 ☑

Heat — *continued*
- fatigue (transient) T67.6 ☑
- fever T67.Ø1 ☑
- hyperpyrexia T67.Ø1 ☑
- prickly L74.Ø
- prostration — *see* Heat, exhaustion
- pyrexia T67.Ø1 ☑
- rash L74.Ø
- specified effect NEC T67.8 ☑
- stroke T67.Ø1 ☑
  - exertional T67.Ø2 ☑
  - specified NEC T67.Ø9 ☑
- sunburn — *see* Sunburn
- syncope T67.1 ☑

Heavy-for-dates NEC (infant) (4ØØØg to 4499g) PØ8.1
- exceptionally (45ØØg or more) PØ8.Ø

Hebephrenia, hebephrenic (schizophrenia) F2Ø.1

Heberden's disease or nodes (with arthropathy) M15.1

Hebra's
- pityriasis L26
- prurigo L28.2

Heel — *see* condition

Heerfordt's disease D86.89

Hegglin's anomaly or syndrome D72.Ø

Heilmeyer-Schoner disease D45

Heine-Medin disease A8Ø.9

Heinz body anemia, congenital D58.2

Heliophobia F4Ø.228

Heller's disease or syndrome F84.3

HELLP syndrome (hemolysis, elevated liver enzymes and low platelet count) O14.2- ☑
- complicating
  - childbirth O14.24
  - puerperium O14.25

Helminthiasis — *see also* Infestation, helminth
- Ancylostoma B76.Ø
- intestinal B82.Ø
  - mixed types (types classifiable to more than one of the titles B65.Ø-B81.3 and B81.8) B81.4
  - specified type NEC B81.8
- mixed types (intestinal) (types classifiable to more than one of the titles B65.Ø-B81.3 and B81.8) B81.4
- Necator (americanus) B76.1
- specified type NEC B83.8

Heloma L84

Hemangioblastoma — *see* Neoplasm, connective tissue, uncertain behavior
- malignant — *see* Neoplasm, connective tissue, malignant

Hemangioendothelioma — *see also* Neoplasm, uncertain behavior, by site
- benign D18.ØØ
  - intra-abdominal D18.Ø3
  - intracranial D18.Ø2
  - skin D18.Ø1
  - specified site NEC D18.Ø9
- bone (diffuse) — *see* Neoplasm, bone, malignant
- epithelioid — *see also* Neoplasm, uncertain behavior, by site
  - malignant — *see* Neoplasm, malignant, by site
- malignant — *see* Neoplasm, connective tissue, malignant

Hemangiofibroma — *see* Neoplasm, benign, by site

Hemangiolipoma — *see* Lipoma

Hemangioma D18.ØØ
- arteriovenous D18.ØØ
  - intra-abdominal D18.Ø3
  - intracranial D18.Ø2
  - skin D18.Ø1
  - specified site NEC D18.Ø9
- capillary I78.1
  - intra-abdominal D18.Ø3
  - intracranial D18.Ø2
  - skin D18.Ø1
  - specified site NEC D18.Ø9
- cavernous D18.ØØ
  - intra-abdominal D18.Ø3
  - intracranial D18.Ø2
  - skin D18.Ø1
  - specified site NEC D18.Ø9
- epithelioid D18.ØØ
  - intra-abdominal D18.Ø3
  - intracranial D18.Ø2
  - skin D18.Ø1
  - specified site NEC D18.Ø9
- histiocytoid D18.ØØ
  - intra-abdominal D18.Ø3

Hemangioma — *continued*
- histiocytoid — *continued*
  - intracranial D18.Ø2
  - skin D18.Ø1
  - specified site NEC D18.Ø9
- infantile D18.ØØ
  - intra-abdominal D18.Ø3
  - intracranial D18.Ø2
  - skin D18.Ø1
  - specified site NEC D18.Ø9
- intra-abdominal D18.Ø3
- intracranial D18.Ø2
- intramuscular D18.ØØ
  - intra-abdominal D18.Ø3
  - intracranial D18.Ø2
  - skin D18.Ø1
  - specified site NEC D18.Ø9
- intrathoracic structures D18.Ø9
- juvenile D18.ØØ
- malignant — *see* Neoplasm,connective tissue, malignant
- plexiform D18.ØØ
  - intra-abdominal D18.Ø3
  - intracranial D18.Ø2
  - skin D18.Ø1
  - specified site NEC D18.Ø9
- racemose D18.ØØ
  - intra-abdominal D18.Ø3
  - intracranial D18.Ø2
  - skin D18.Ø1
  - specified site NEC D18.Ø9
- sclerosing — *see* Neoplasm, skin, benign
- simplex D18.ØØ
  - intra-abdominal D18.Ø3
  - intracranial D18.Ø2
  - skin D18.Ø1
  - specified site NEC D18.Ø9
- skin D18.Ø1
- specified site NEC D18.Ø9
- venous D18.ØØ
  - intra-abdominal D18.Ø3
  - intracranial D18.Ø2
  - skin D18.Ø1
  - specified site NEC D18.Ø9
- verrucous keratotic D18.ØØ
  - intra-abdominal D18.Ø3
  - intracranial D18.Ø2
  - skin D18.Ø1
  - specified site NEC D18.Ø9

Hemangiomatosis (systemic) I78.8
- involving single site — *see* Hemangioma

Hemangiopericytoma — *see also* Neoplasm, connective tissue, uncertain behavior
- benign — *see* Neoplasm, connective tissue, benign
- malignant — *see* Neoplasm, connective tissue, malignant

Hemangiosarcoma — *see* Neoplasm, connective tissue, malignant

Hemarthrosis (nontraumatic) M25.ØØ
- ankle M25.Ø7- ☑
- elbow M25.Ø2- ☑
- foot joint M25.Ø7- ☑
- hand joint M25.Ø4- ☑
- hip M25.Ø5- ☑
- in hemophilic arthropathy — *see* Arthropathy, hemophilic
- knee M25.Ø6- ☑
- shoulder M25.Ø1- ☑
- specified joint NEC M25.Ø8
- traumatic — *see* Sprain, by site
- vertebrae M25.Ø8
- wrist M25.Ø3- ☑

Hematemesis K92.Ø
- with ulcer — *code by site under* Ulcer, with hemorrhage K27.4
- newborn, neonatal P54.Ø
  - due to swallowed maternal blood P78.2

Hematidrosis L74.8

Hematinuria — *see also* Hemoglobinuria
- malarial B5Ø.8

Hematobilia K83.8

Hematocele
- female NEC N94.89
  - with ectopic pregnancy OØØ.9Ø
    - with intrauterine pregnancy OØØ.91
  - ovary N83.8
- male N5Ø.1

Hematochezia — *see also* Melena K92.1

Hernia, hernial — *continued*
- abdomen, abdominal — *continued*
  - incisional — *see* Hernia, incisional
  - inguinal — *see* Hernia, inguinal
  - specified site NEC K45.8
    - with
      - gangrene (and obstruction) K45.1
      - obstruction K45.0
  - umbilical — *see* Hernia, umbilical
  - wall — *see* Hernia, ventral
- appendix — *see* Hernia, abdomen
- bladder (mucosa) (sphincter)
  - congenital (female) (male) Q79.51
  - female — *see* Cystocele
  - male N32.89
- brain, congenital — *see* Encephalocele
- cartilage, vertebra — *see* Displacement, intervertebral disc
- cerebral, congenital — *see also* Encephalocele
  - endaural Q01.8
- ciliary body (traumatic) S05.2- ☑
- colon — *see* Hernia, abdomen
- Cooper's — *see* Hernia, abdomen, specified site NEC
- crural — *see* Hernia, femoral
- diaphragm, diaphragmatic K44.9
  - with
    - gangrene (and obstruction) K44.1
    - obstruction K44.0
  - congenital Q79.0
- direct (inguinal) — *see* Hernia, inguinal
- diverticulum, intestine — *see* Hernia, abdomen
- double (inguinal) — *see* Hernia, inguinal, bilateral
- due to adhesions (with obstruction) K56.50
- epigastric — *see also* Hernia, ventral K43.9
- esophageal hiatus — *see* Hernia, hiatal
- external (inguinal) — *see* Hernia, inguinal
- fallopian tube N83.4- ☑
- fascia M62.89
- femoral K41.90
  - with
    - gangrene (and obstruction) K41.40
      - not specified as recurrent K41.40
      - recurrent K41.41
    - obstruction K41.30
      - not specified as recurrent K41.30
      - recurrent K41.31
  - not specified as recurrent K41.90
  - recurrent K41.91
  - bilateral K41.20
    - with
      - gangrene (and obstruction) K41.10
        - not specified as recurrent K41.10
        - recurrent K41.11
      - obstruction K41.00
        - not specified as recurrent K41.00
        - recurrent K41.01
    - not specified as recurrent K41.20
    - recurrent K41.21
  - unilateral K41.90
    - with
      - gangrene (and obstruction) K41.40
        - not specified as recurrent K41.40
        - recurrent K41.41
      - obstruction K41.30
        - not specified as recurrent K41.30
        - recurrent K41.31
    - not specified as recurrent K41.90
    - recurrent K41.91
- foramen magnum G93.5
  - congenital Q01.8
- funicular (umbilical) — *see also* Hernia, umbilicus
  - spermatic (cord) — *see* Hernia, inguinal
- gastrointestinal tract — *see* Hernia, abdomen
- Hesselbach's — *see* Hernia, femoral, specified site NEC
- hiatal (esophageal) (sliding) K44.9
  - with
    - gangrene (and obstruction) K44.1
    - obstruction K44.0
  - congenital Q40.1
- hypogastric — *see* Hernia, ventral
- incarcerated — *see also* Hernia, by site, with obstruction
  - with gangrene — *see* Hernia, by site, with gangrene
- incisional K43.2
  - with
    - gangrene (and obstruction) K43.1
    - obstruction K43.0
- indirect (inguinal) — *see* Hernia, inguinal

Hernia, hernial — *continued*
- inguinal (direct) (external) (funicular) (indirect) (internal) (oblique) (scrotal) (sliding) K40.90
  - with
    - gangrene (and obstruction) K40.40
      - not specified as recurrent K40.40
      - recurrent K40.41
    - obstruction K40.30
      - not specified as recurrent K40.30
      - recurrent K40.31
  - not specified as recurrent K40.90
  - recurrent K40.91
  - bilateral K40.20
    - with
      - gangrene (and obstruction) K40.10
        - not specified as recurrent K40.10
        - recurrent K40.11
      - obstruction K40.00
        - not specified as recurrent K40.00
        - recurrent K40.01
    - not specified as recurrent K40.20
    - recurrent K40.21
  - unilateral K40.90
    - with
      - gangrene (and obstruction) K40.40
        - not specified as recurrent K40.40
        - recurrent K40.41
      - obstruction K40.30
        - not specified as recurrent K40.30
        - recurrent K40.31
    - not specified as recurrent K40.90
    - recurrent K40.91
- internal — *see also* Hernia, abdomen
  - inguinal — *see* Hernia, inguinal
- interstitial — *see* Hernia, abdomen
- intervertebral cartilage or disc — *see* Displacement, intervertebral disc
- intestine, intestinal — *see* Hernia, by site
- intra-abdominal — *see* Hernia, abdomen
- iris (traumatic) S05.2- ☑
- irreducible — *see also* Hernia, by site, with obstruction
  - with gangrene — *see* Hernia, by site, with gangrene
- ischiatic — *see* Hernia, abdomen, specified site NEC
- ischiorectal — *see* Hernia, abdomen, specified site NEC
- lens (traumatic) S05.2- ☑
- linea (alba) (semilunaris) — *see* Hernia, ventral
- Littre's — *see* Hernia, abdomen
- lumbar — *see* Hernia, abdomen, specified site NEC
- lung (subcutaneous) J98.4
- mediastinum J98.59
- mesenteric (internal) — *see* Hernia, abdomen
- midline — *see* Hernia, ventral
- muscle (sheath) M62.89
- nucleus pulposus — *see* Displacement, intervertebral disc
- oblique (inguinal) — *see* Hernia, inguinal
- obstructive — *see also* Hernia, by site, with obstruction
  - with gangrene — *see* Hernia, by site, with gangrene
- obturator — *see* Hernia, abdomen, specified site NEC
- omental — *see* Hernia, abdomen
- ovary N83.4- ☑
- oviduct N83.4- ☑
- paraesophageal — *see also* Hernia, diaphragm
  - congenital Q40.1
- parastomal K43.5
  - with
    - gangrene (and obstruction) K43.4
    - obstruction K43.3
- paraumbilical — *see* Hernia, umbilicus
- perineal — *see* Hernia, abdomen, specified site NEC
- Petit's — *see* Hernia, abdomen, specified site NEC
- postoperative — *see* Hernia, incisional
- pregnant uterus — *see* Abnormal, uterus in pregnancy or childbirth
- prevesical N32.89
- properitoneal — *see* Hernia, abdomen, specified site NEC
- pudendal — *see* Hernia, abdomen, specified site NEC
- rectovaginal N81.6
- retroperitoneal — *see* Hernia, abdomen, specified site NEC
- Richter's — *see* Hernia, abdomen, with obstruction
- Rieux's, Riex's — *see* Hernia, abdomen, specified site NEC

Hernia, hernial — *continued*
- sac condition (adhesion) (dropsy) (inflammation) (laceration) (suppuration) — *code by site under* Hernia
- sciatic — *see* Hernia, abdomen, specified site NEC
- scrotum, scrotal — *see* Hernia, inguinal
- sliding (inguinal) — *see also* Hernia, inguinal
  - hiatus — *see* Hernia, hiatal
- spigelian — *see* Hernia, ventral
- spinal — *see* Spina bifida
- strangulated — *see also* Hernia, by site, with obstruction
  - with gangrene — *see* Hernia, by site, with gangrene
- subxiphoid — *see* Hernia, ventral
- supra-umbilicus — *see* Hernia, ventral
- tendon — *see* Disorder, tendon, specified type NEC
- Treitz's (fossa) — *see* Hernia, abdomen, specified site NEC
- tunica vaginalis Q55.29
- umbilicus, umbilical K42.9
  - with
    - gangrene (and obstruction) K42.1
    - obstruction K42.0
- ureter N28.89
- urethra, congenital Q64.79
- urinary meatus, congenital Q64.79
- uterus N81.4
  - pregnant — *see* Abnormal, uterus in pregnancy or childbirth
- vaginal (anterior) (wall) — *see* Cystocele
- Velpeau's — *see* Hernia, femoral
- ventral K43.9
  - with
    - gangrene (and obstruction) K43.7
    - obstruction K43.6
  - incisional K43.2
    - with
      - gangrene (and obstruction) K43.1
      - obstruction K43.0
  - recurrent — *see* Hernia, incisional
  - specified NEC K43.9
    - with
      - gangrene (and obstruction) K43.7
      - obstruction K43.6
- vesical
  - congenital (female) (male) Q79.51
  - female — *see* Cystocele
  - male N32.89
- vitreous (into wound) S05.2- ☑
  - into anterior chamber — *see* Prolapse, vitreous

Herniation — *see also* Hernia
- brain (stem) G93.5
- cerebral G93.5
- mediastinum J98.59
- nucleus pulposus — *see* Displacement, intervertebral disc

Herpangina B08.5

Herpes, herpesvirus, herpetic B00.9
- anogenital A60.9
  - perianal skin A60.1
  - rectum A60.1
  - urogenital tract A60.00
    - cervix A60.03
    - male genital organ NEC A60.02
    - penis A60.01
    - specified site NEC A60.09
    - vagina A60.04
    - vulva A60.04
- blepharitis (zoster) B02.39
  - simplex B00.59
- circinatus B35.4
  - bullosus L12.0
- conjunctivitis (simplex) B00.53
  - zoster B02.31
- cornea B02.33
- encephalitis B00.4
  - due to herpesvirus 6 B10.01
  - due to herpesvirus 7 B10.09
  - specified NEC B10.09
- eye (zoster) B02.30
  - simplex B00.50
- eyelid (zoster) B02.39
  - simplex B00.59
- facialis B00.1
- febrilis B00.1
- geniculate ganglionitis B02.21
- genital, genitalis A60.00
  - female A60.09

- **History** — *continued*
  - personal — *see also* History, family — *continued*
    - in situ neoplasm — *continued*
      - specified NEC Z86.ØØ8
      - stomach Z86.ØØ3
    - in utero procedure during pregnancy Z98.87Ø
    - in utero procedure while a fetus Z98.871
    - infection NEC Z86.19
      - central nervous system Z86.61
      - latent tuberculosis Z86.15
      - Methicillin resistant Staphylococcus aureus (MRSA) Z86.14
      - urinary (recurrent) (tract) Z87.44Ø
    - injury NEC Z87.828
    - irradiation Z92.3
    - kidney stones Z87.442
    - latent tuberculosis infection Z86.15
    - leukemia Z85.6
    - lymphoma (non-Hodgkin) Z85.72
    - malignant melanoma (skin) Z85.82Ø
    - malignant neoplasm (of) Z85.9
      - accessory sinuses Z85.22
      - anus NEC Z85.Ø48
        - carcinoid Z85.Ø4Ø
      - bladder Z85.51
      - bone Z85.83Ø
      - brain Z85.841
      - breast Z85.3
      - bronchus NEC Z85.118
        - carcinoid Z85.11Ø
      - carcinoid — *see* History, personal (of), malignant neoplasm, by site, carcinioid
      - cervix Z85.41
      - colon NEC Z85.Ø38
        - carcinoid Z85.Ø3Ø
      - digestive organ Z85.ØØ
        - specified NEC Z85.Ø9
      - endocrine gland NEC Z85.858
      - epididymis Z85.48
      - esophagus Z85.Ø1
      - eye Z85.84Ø
      - gastrointestinal tract — *see* History, malignant neoplasm, digestive organ
      - genital organ
        - female Z85.4Ø
          - specified NEC Z85.44
        - male Z85.45
          - specified NEC Z85.49
      - hematopoietic NEC Z85.79
      - intrathoracic organ Z85.2Ø
      - kidney NEC Z85.528
        - carcinoid Z85.52Ø
      - large intestine NEC Z85.Ø38
        - carcinoid Z85.Ø3Ø
      - larynx Z85.21
      - liver Z85.Ø5
      - lung NEC Z85.118
        - carcinoid Z85.11Ø
      - mediastinum Z85.29
      - Merkel cell Z85.821
      - middle ear Z85.22
      - nasal cavities Z85.22
      - nervous system NEC Z85.848
      - oral cavity Z85.819
        - specified site NEC Z85.818
      - ovary Z85.43
      - pancreas Z85.Ø7
      - pelvis Z85.53
      - pharynx Z85.819
        - specified site NEC Z85.818
      - pleura Z85.29
      - prostate Z85.46
      - rectosigmoid junction NEC Z85.Ø48
        - carcinoid Z85.Ø4Ø
      - rectum NEC Z85.Ø48
        - carcinoid Z85.Ø4Ø
      - respiratory organ Z85.2Ø
      - sinuses, accessory Z85.22
      - skin NEC Z85.828
        - melanoma Z85.82Ø
        - Merkel cell Z85.821
      - small intestine NEC Z85.Ø68
        - carcinoid Z85.Ø6Ø
      - soft tissue Z85.831
      - specified site NEC Z85.89
      - stomach NEC Z85.Ø28
        - carcinoid Z85.Ø2Ø
      - testis Z85.47
      - thymus NEC Z85.238

- **History** — *continued*
  - personal — *see also* History, family — *continued*
    - malignant neoplasm — *continued*
      - thymus — *continued*
        - carcinoid Z85.23Ø
      - thyroid Z85.85Ø
      - tongue Z85.81Ø
      - trachea Z85.12
      - urinary organ or tract Z85.5Ø
        - specified NEC Z85.59
      - uterus Z85.42
    - maltreatment Z91.89
    - medical treatment NEC Z92.89
    - melanoma Z85.82Ø
      - in situ Z86.ØØ6
      - malignant (skin) Z85.82Ø
    - meningitis Z86.61
    - mental disorder Z86.59
    - Merkel cell carcinoma (skin) Z85.821
    - Methicillin resistant Staphylococcus aureus (MRSA) Z86.14
    - military deployment Z91.82
    - military war, peacekeeping and humanitarian deployment (current or past conflict) Z91.82
    - myocardial infarction (old) I25.2
    - neglect (in)
      - adult Z91.412
      - childhood Z62.812
    - neoplasia
      - anal intraepithelial, III [AIN III] Z86.ØØ4
      - high-grade prostatic intraepithelial, III [HGPIN III] Z86.ØØ2
      - vaginal intraepithelial, III [VAIN III] Z86.ØØ2
      - vulvar intraepithelial, III [VIN III] Z86.ØØ2
    - neoplasm
      - benign Z86.Ø18
        - brain Z86.Ø11
        - colon polyp Z86.Ø1Ø
      - in situ
        - breast Z86.ØØØ
        - cervix uteri Z86.ØØ1
        - digestive organs, specified NEC Z86.ØØ4
        - esophagus Z86.ØØ3
        - genital organs, specified NEC Z86.ØØ2
        - melanoma Z86.ØØ6
        - middle ear Z86.ØØ5
        - oral cavity Z86.ØØ3
        - respiratory system Z86.ØØ5
        - skin Z86.ØØ7
        - specified NEC Z86.ØØ8
        - stomach Z86.ØØ3
      - malignant — *see* History of, malignant neoplasm
      - uncertain behavior Z86.Ø3
    - nephrotic syndrome Z87.441
    - nicotine dependence Z87.891
    - noncompliance with medical treatment or regimen — *see* Noncompliance
    - nutritional deficiency Z86.39
    - obstetric complications Z87.59
      - childbirth Z87.59
      - pregnancy Z87.59
      - pre-term labor Z87.51
      - puerperium Z87.59
    - osteoporosis fractures Z87.31 ☑
    - parasuicide (attempt) Z91.5
    - physical trauma NEC Z87.828
      - self-harm or suicide attempt Z91.5
    - pneumonia (recurrent) Z87.Ø1
    - poisoning NEC Z91.89
      - self-harm or suicide attempt Z91.5
    - poor personal hygiene Z91.89
    - preterm labor Z87.51
    - procedure during pregnancy Z98.87Ø
    - procedure while a fetus Z98.871
    - prolonged reversible ischemic neurologic deficit (PRIND) Z86.73
    - prostatic dysplasia Z87.43Ø
    - psychological
      - abuse
        - adult Z91.411
        - child Z62.811
      - trauma, specified NEC Z91.49
    - radiation therapy Z92.3
    - removal
      - implant
        - breast Z98.86
    - renal calculi Z87.442
    - respiratory condition NEC Z87.Ø9
    - retained foreign body fully removed Z87.821

- **History** — *continued*
  - personal — *see also* History, family — *continued*
    - risk factors NEC Z91.89
    - self-harm Z91.5
    - self-poisoning attempt Z91.5
    - sex reassignment Z87.89Ø
    - sleep-wake cycle problem Z72.821
    - specified NEC Z87.898
    - steroid therapy (systemic) Z92.241
      - inhaled Z92.24Ø
    - stroke without residual deficits Z86.73
    - substance abuse NEC F1Ø-F19
    - sudden cardiac arrest Z86.74
    - sudden cardiac death successfully resuscitated Z86.74
    - suicide attempt Z91.5
    - surgery NEC Z98.89Ø
      - with uterine scar Z98.891
      - sex reassignment Z87.89Ø
      - transplant — *see* Transplant
    - thrombophlebitis Z86.72
    - thrombosis (venous) Z86.718
      - pulmonary Z86.711
    - tobacco dependence Z87.891
    - transient ischemic attack (TIA) without residual deficits Z86.73
    - trauma (physical) NEC Z87.828
      - psychological NEC Z91.49
      - self-harm Z91.5
    - traumatic brain injury Z87.82Ø
    - tuberculosis, latent infection Z86.15
    - unhealthy sleep-wake cycle Z72.821
    - unintended awareness under general anesthesia Z92.84
    - urinary calculi Z87.442
    - urinary (recurrent) (tract) infection(s) Z87.44Ø
    - uterine scar from previous surgery Z98.891
    - vaginal dysplasia Z87.411
    - venous thrombosis or embolism Z86.718
      - pulmonary Z86.711
    - vulvar dysplasia Z87.412
- **His-Werner disease** A79.Ø
- **HIV** — *see also* Human, immunodeficiency virus B2Ø
  - laboratory evidence (nonconclusive) R75
  - nonconclusive test (in infants) R75
  - positive, seropositive Z21
- **Hives** (bold) — *see* Urticaria
- **Hoarseness** R49.Ø
- **Hobo** Z59.Ø
- **Hodgkin disease** — *see* Lymphoma, Hodgkin
- **Hodgson's disease** I71.2
  - ruptured I71.1
- **Hoffa-Kastert disease** E88.89
- **Hoffa's disease** E88.89
- **Hoffmann-Bouveret syndrome** I47.9
- **Hoffmann's syndrome** EØ3.9 *[G73.7]*
- **Hole** (round)
  - macula H35.34- ☑
  - retina (without detachment) — *see* Break, retina, round hole
    - with detachment — *see* Detachment, retina, with retinal, break
- **Holiday relief care** Z75.5
- **Hollenhorst's plaque** — *see* Occlusion, artery, retina
- **Hollow foot** (congenital) Q66.7- ☑
  - acquired — *see* Deformity, limb, foot, specified NEC
- **Holoprosencephaly** QØ4.2
- **Holt-Oram syndrome** Q87.2
- **Homelessness** Z59.Ø
- **Homesickness** — *see* Disorder, adjustment
- **Homocystinemia, homocystinuria** E72.11
- **Homogentisate 1,2-dioxygenase deficiency** E7Ø.29
- **Homologous serum hepatitis** (prophylactic) (therapeutic) — *see* Hepatitis, viral, type B
- **Honeycomb lung** J98.4
  - congenital Q33.Ø
- **Hooded**
  - clitoris Q52.6
  - penis Q55.69
- **Hookworm** (disease) (infection) (infestation) B76.9
  - with anemia B76.9 *[D63.8]*
  - specified NEC B76.8
- **Hordeolum** (eyelid) (externum) (recurrent) HØØ.Ø19
  - internum HØØ.Ø29
    - left HØØ.Ø26
      - lower HØØ.Ø25
      - upper HØØ.Ø24
    - right HØØ.Ø23

- **Hydropneumothorax** — *continued*
  - tuberculous NEC A15.6
- **Hydrops** R6Ø.9
  - abdominis R18.8
  - articulorum intermittens — *see* Hydrarthrosis, intermittent
  - cardiac — *see* Failure, heart, congestive
  - causing obstructed labor (mother) O66.3
  - endolymphatic H81.Ø- ☑
  - fetal — *see* Pregnancy, complicated by, hydrops, fetalis
  - fetalis P83.2
    - due to
      - ABO isoimmunization P56.Ø
      - alpha thalassemia D56.Ø
      - hemolytic disease P56.9Ø
        - specified NEC P56.99
      - isoimmunization (ABO) (Rh) P56.Ø
      - other specified nonhemolytic disease NEC P83.2
      - Rh incompatibility P56.Ø
    - during pregnancy — *see* Pregnancy, complicated by, hydrops, fetalis
  - gallbladder K82.1
  - joint — *see* Effusion, joint
  - labyrinth H81.Ø- ☑
  - newborn (idiopathic) P83.2
    - due to
      - ABO isoimmunization P56.Ø
      - alpha thalassemia D56.Ø
      - hemolytic disease P56.9Ø
        - specified NEC P56.99
      - isoimmunization (ABO) (Rh) P56.Ø
      - Rh incompatibility P56.Ø
  - nutritional — *see* Malnutrition, severe
  - pericardium — *see* Pericarditis
  - pleura — *see* Hydrothorax
  - spermatic cord — *see* Hydrocele
- **Hydropyonephrosis** N13.6
- **Hydrorachis** QØ6.4
- **Hydrorrhea** (nasal) J34.89
  - pregnancy — *see* Rupture, membranes, premature
- **Hydrosadenitis** (axillaris) (suppurative) L73.2
- **Hydrosalpinx** (fallopian tube) (follicularis) N7Ø.11
- **Hydrothorax** (double) (pleura) J94.8
  - chylous (nonfilarial) I89.8
    - filarial — *see also* Infestation, filarial B74.9 *[J91.8]*
  - traumatic — *see* Injury, intrathoracic
  - tuberculous NEC (non primary) A15.6
- **Hydroureter** — *see also* Hydronephrosis N13.4
  - with infection N13.6
  - congenital Q62.39
- **Hydroureteronephrosis** — *see* Hydronephrosis
- **Hydrourethra** N36.8
- **Hydroxykynureninuria** E7Ø.89
- **Hydroxylysinemia** E72.3
- **Hydroxyprolinemia** E72.59
- **Hygiene, sleep**
  - abuse Z72.821
  - inadequate Z72.821
  - poor Z72.821
- **Hygroma** (congenital) (cystic) D18.1
  - praepatellare, prepatellar — *see* Bursitis, prepatellar
- **Hymen** — *see* condition
- **Hymenolepis, hymenolepiasis** (diminuta) (infection) (infestation) (nana) B71.Ø
- **Hypalgesia** R2Ø.8
- **Hyperacidity** (gastric) K31.89
  - psychogenic F45.8
- **Hyperactive, hyperactivity** F9Ø.9
  - basal cell, uterine cervix — *see* Dysplasia, cervix
  - bowel sounds R19.12
  - cervix epithelial (basal) — *see* Dysplasia, cervix
  - child F9Ø.9
    - attention deficit — *see* Disorder, attention-deficit hyperactivity
  - detrusor muscle N32.81
  - gastrointestinal K31.89
    - psychogenic F45.8
  - nasal mucous membrane J34.3
  - stomach K31.89
  - thyroid (gland) — *see* Hyperthyroidism
- **Hyperacusis** H93.23- ☑
- **Hyperadrenalism** E27.5
- **Hyperadrenocorticism** E24.9
  - congenital E25.Ø
  - iatrogenic E24.2
- **Hyperadrenocorticism** — *continued*
  - iatrogenic — *continued*
    - correct substance properly administered — *see* Table of Drugs and Chemicals, by drug, adverse effect
    - overdose or wrong substance given or taken — *see* Table of Drugs and Chemicals, by drug, poisoning
  - not associated with Cushing's syndrome E27.Ø
  - pituitary-dependent E24.Ø
- **Hyperaldosteronism** E26.9
  - familial (type I) E26.Ø2
  - glucocorticoid-remediable E26.Ø2
  - primary (due to (bilateral) adrenal hyperplasia) E26.Ø9
  - primary NEC E26.Ø9
  - secondary E26.1
  - specified NEC E26.89
- **Hyperalgesia** R2Ø.8
- **Hyperalimentation** R63.2
  - carotene, carotin E67.1
  - specified NEC E67.8
  - vitamin
    - A E67.Ø
    - D E67.3
- **Hyperaminoaciduria**
  - arginine E72.21
  - cystine E72.Ø1
  - lysine E72.3
  - ornithine E72.4
- **Hyperammonemia** (congenital) E72.2Ø
- **Hyperazotemia** — *see* Uremia
- **Hyperbetalipoproteinemia** (familial) E78.ØØ
  - with prebetalipoproteinemia E78.2
- **Hyperbicarbonatemia** P74.41
- **Hyperbilirubinemia**
  - constitutional E8Ø.6
  - familial conjugated E8Ø.6
  - neonatal (transient) — *see* Jaundice, newborn
- **Hypercalcemia, hypocalciuric, familial** E83.52
- **Hypercalciuria, idiopathic** R82.994
- **Hypercapnia** RØ6.89
  - newborn P84
- **Hypercarotenemia** (dietary) E67.1
- **Hypercementosis** KØ3.4
- **Hyperchloremia** E87.8
- **Hyperchlorhydria** K31.89
  - neurotic F45.8
  - psychogenic F45.8
- **Hypercholesterinemia** — *see* Hypercholesterolemia
- **Hypercholesterolemia** (essential) (primary) (pure) E78.ØØ
  - with hyperglyceridemia, endogenous E78.2
  - dietary counseling and surveillance Z71.3
  - familial E78.Ø1
  - hereditary E78.Ø1
- **Hyperchylia gastrica, psychogenic** F45.8
- **Hyperchylomicronemia** (familial) (primary) E78.3
  - with hyperbetalipoproteinemia E78.3
- **Hypercoagulable** (state) D68.59
  - activated protein C resistance D68.51
  - antithrombin (III) deficiency D68.59
  - factor V Leiden mutation D68.51
  - primary NEC D68.59
  - protein C deficiency D68.59
  - protein S deficiency D68.59
  - prothrombin gene mutation D68.52
  - secondary D68.69
  - specified NEC D68.69
- **Hypercoagulation** (state) D68.59
- **Hypercorticalism, pituitary-dependent** E24.Ø
- **Hypercorticosolism** — *see* Cushing's, syndrome
- **Hypercorticosteronism** E24.2
  - correct substance properly administered — *see* Table of Drugs and Chemicals, by drug, adverse effect
  - overdose or wrong substance given or taken — *see* Table of Drugs and Chemicals, by drug, poisoning
- **Hypercortisonism** E24.2
  - correct substance properly administered — *see* Table of Drugs and Chemicals, by drug, adverse effect
  - overdose or wrong substance given or taken — *see* Table of Drugs and Chemicals, by drug, poisoning
- **Hyperekplexia** Q89.8
- **Hyperelectrolytemia** E87.8
- **Hyperemesis** R11.1Ø
  - with nausea R11.2
  - gravidarum (mild) O21.Ø
    - with
      - carbohydrate depletion O21.1
      - dehydration O21.1
- **Hyperemesis** — *continued*
  - gravidarum — *continued*
    - with — *continued*
      - electrolyte imbalance O21.1
      - metabolic disturbance O21.1
    - severe (with metabolic disturbance) O21.1
  - projectile R11.12
  - psychogenic F45.8
- **Hyperemia** (acute) (passive) R68.89
  - anal mucosa K62.89
  - bladder N32.89
  - cerebral I67.89
  - conjunctiva H11.43- ☑
  - ear internal, acute — *see* subcategory H83.Ø ☑
  - enteric K59.89
  - eye — *see* Hyperemia, conjunctiva
  - eyelid (active) (passive) — *see* Disorder, eyelid, specified type NEC
  - intestine K59.89
  - iris — *see* Disorder, iris, vascular
  - kidney N28.89
  - labyrinth — *see* subcategory H83.Ø ☑
  - liver (active) K76.89
  - lung (passive) — *see* Edema, lung
  - pulmonary (passive) — *see* Edema, lung
  - renal N28.89
  - retina H35.89
  - stomach K31.89
- **Hyperesthesia** (body surface) R2Ø.3
  - larynx (reflex) J38.7
    - hysterical F44.89
  - pharynx (reflex) J39.2
    - hysterical F44.89
- **Hyperestrogenism** (drug-induced) (iatrogenic) E28.Ø
- **Hyperexplexia** Q89.8
- **Hyperfibrinolysis** — *see* Fibrinolysis
- **Hyperfructosemia** E74.19
- **Hyperfunction**
  - adrenal cortex, not associated with Cushing's syndrome E27.Ø
    - medulla E27.5
      - adrenomedullary E27.5
    - virilism E25.9
      - congenital E25.Ø
  - ovarian E28.8
  - pancreas K86.89
  - parathyroid (gland) E21.3
  - pituitary (gland) (anterior) E22.9
    - specified NEC E22.8
  - polyglandular E31.1
  - testicular E29.Ø
- **Hypergammaglobulinemia** D89.2
  - polyclonal D89.Ø
  - Waldenström D89.Ø
- **Hypergastrinemia** E16.4
- **Hyperglobulinemia** R77.1
- **Hyperglycemia, hyperglycemic** (transient) R73.9
  - coma — *see* Diabetes, by type, with coma
  - postpancreatectomy E89.1
- **Hyperglyceridemia** (endogenous) (essential) (familial) (hereditary) (pure) E78.1
  - mixed E78.3
- **Hyperglycinemia** (non-ketotic) E72.51
- **Hypergonadism**
  - ovarian E28.8
  - testicular (primary) (infantile) E29.Ø
- **Hyperheparinemia** D68.32
- **Hyperhidrosis, hyperidrosis** R61
  - focal
    - primary L74.519
      - axilla L74.51Ø
      - face L74.511
      - palms L74.512
      - soles L74.513
    - secondary L74.52
  - generalized R61
  - localized
    - primary L74.519
      - axilla L74.51Ø
      - face L74.511
      - palms L74.512
      - soles L74.513
    - secondary L74.52
  - psychogenic F45.8
  - secondary R61
    - focal L74.52
- **Hyperhistidinemia** E7Ø.41
- **Hyperhomocysteinemia** E72.11

Hypoplasia, hypoplastic — *continued*
- hair Q84.2
- hand (congenital) — *see* Defect, reduction, upper limb, specified type NEC
- heart Q24.8
- humerus (congenital) — *see* Defect, reduction, upper limb, specified type NEC
- intestine (small) Q41.9
  - large Q42.9
    - specified NEC Q42.8
- jaw M26.Ø9
  - alveolar M26.79
  - lower M26.Ø4
    - alveolar M26.74
  - upper M26.Ø2
    - alveolar M26.73
- kidney(s) Q6Ø.5
  - bilateral Q6Ø.4
  - unilateral Q6Ø.3
- labium (majus) (minus), congenital Q52.79
- larynx Q31.2
- left heart syndrome Q23.4
- leg (congenital) — *see* Defect, reduction, lower limb
- limb Q73.8
  - lower (congenital) — *see* Defect, reduction, lower limb
  - upper (congenital) — *see* Defect, reduction, upper limb
- liver Q44.7
- lung (lobe) (not associated with short gestation) Q33.6
  - associated with immaturity, low birth weight, prematurity, or short gestation P28.Ø
- mammary (areola), congenital Q83.8
- mandible, mandibular M26.Ø4
  - alveolar M26.74
  - unilateral condylar M27.8
- maxillary M26.Ø2
  - alveolar M26.73
- medullary D61.9
- megakaryocytic D69.49
- metacarpus — *see* Defect, reduction, upper limb, specified type NEC
- metatarsus — *see* Defect, reduction, lower limb, specified type NEC
- muscle Q79.8
- nail(s) Q84.6
- nose, nasal Q3Ø.1
- optic nerve H47.Ø3- ☑
- osseous meatus (ear) Q17.8
- ovary, congenital Q5Ø.39
- pancreas Q45.Ø
- parathyroid (gland) Q89.2
- parotid gland Q38.4
- patella Q74.1
- pelvis, pelvic girdle Q74.2
- penis (congenital) Q55.62
- peripheral vascular system Q27.8
  - digestive system Q27.8
  - lower limb Q27.8
  - specified site NEC Q27.8
  - upper limb Q27.8
- pituitary (gland) (congenital) Q89.2
- pulmonary (not associated with short gestation) Q33.6
  - artery, functional J43.Ø
  - associated with short gestation P28.Ø
- radioulnar — *see* Defect, reduction, upper limb, specified type NEC
- radius — *see* Defect, reduction, upper limb
- rectum Q42.1
  - with fistula Q42.Ø
- respiratory system NEC Q34.8
- rib Q76.6
- right heart syndrome Q22.6
- sacrum Q76.49
- scapula Q74.Ø
- scrotum Q55.1
- shoulder girdle Q74.Ø
- skin Q82.8
- skull (bone) Q75.8
  - with
    - anencephaly QØØ.Ø
    - encephalocele — *see* Encephalocele
    - hydrocephalus QØ3.9
      - with spina bifida — *see* Spina bifida, by site, with hydrocephalus
    - microcephaly QØ2
- spinal (cord) (ventral horn cell) QØ6.1
- spine Q76.49

Hypoplasia, hypoplastic — *continued*
- sternum Q76.7
- tarsus — *see* Defect, reduction, lower limb, specified type NEC
- testis Q55.1
- thymic, with immunodeficiency D82.1
- thymus (gland) Q89.2
  - with immunodeficiency D82.1
- thyroid (gland) EØ3.1
  - cartilage Q31.2
- tibiofibular (congenital) — *see* Defect, reduction, lower limb, specified type NEC
- toe — *see* Defect, reduction, lower limb, specified type NEC
- tongue Q38.3
- Turner's KØØ.4
- ulna (congenital) — *see* Defect, reduction, upper limb
- umbilical artery Q27.Ø
- unilateral condylar M27.8
- ureter Q62.8
- uterus, congenital Q51.811
- vagina Q52.4
- vascular NEC peripheral Q27.8
  - brain Q28.3
  - digestive system Q27.8
  - lower limb Q27.8
  - specified site NEC Q27.8
  - upper limb Q27.8
- vein(s) (peripheral) Q27.8
  - brain Q28.3
  - digestive system Q27.8
  - great Q26.8
  - lower limb Q27.8
  - specified site NEC Q27.8
  - upper limb Q27.8
- vena cava (inferior) (superior) Q26.8
- vertebra Q76.49
- vulva, congenital Q52.79
- zonule (ciliary) Q12.8

Hypoplasminogenemia E88.Ø2

Hypopnea, obstructive sleep apnea G47.33

Hypopotassemia E87.6

Hypoproconvertinemia, congenital (hereditary) D68.2

Hypoproteinemia E77.8

Hypoprothrombinemia (congenital) (hereditary) (idiopathic) D68.2
- acquired D68.4
- newborn, transient P61.6

Hypoptyalism K11.7

Hypopyon (eye) (anterior chamber) — *see* Iridocyclitis, acute, hypopyon

Hypopyrexia R68.Ø

Hyporeflexia R29.2

Hyposecretion
- ACTH E23.Ø
- antidiuretic hormone E23.2
- ovary E28.39
- salivary gland (any) K11.7
- vasopressin E23.2

Hyposegmentation, leukocytic, hereditary D72.Ø

Hyposiderinemia D5Ø.9

Hypospadias Q54.9
- balanic Q54.Ø
- coronal Q54.Ø
- glandular Q54.Ø
- penile Q54.1
- penoscrotal Q54.2
- perineal Q54.3
- specified NEC Q54.8

Hypospermatogenesis — *see* Oligospermia

Hyposplenism D73.Ø

Hypostasis pulmonary, passive — *see* Edema, lung

Hypostatic — *see* condition

Hyposthenuria N28.89

Hypotension (arterial) (constitutional) I95.9
- chronic I95.89
- due to (of) hemodialysis I95.3
- drug-induced I95.2
- iatrogenic I95.89
- idiopathic (permanent) I95.Ø
- intracranial G96.81Ø
  - following
    - lumbar cerebrospinal fluid shunting G97.83
    - specified procedure NEC G97.84
    - ventricular shunting (ventriculostomy) G97.2
  - specified NEC G96.819
  - spontaneous G96.811
- intra-dialytic I95.3

Hypotension — *continued*
- maternal, syndrome (following labor and delivery) O26.5- ☑
- neurogenic, orthostatic G9Ø.3
- orthostatic (chronic) I95.1
  - due to drugs I95.2
  - neurogenic G9Ø.3
- postoperative I95.81
- postural I95.1
- specified NEC I95.89

Hypothermia (accidental) T68 ☑
- due to anesthesia, anesthetic T88.51 ☑
- low environmental temperature T68 ☑
- neonatal P8Ø.9
  - environmental (mild) NEC P8Ø.8
  - mild P8Ø.8
  - severe (chronic) (cold injury syndrome) P8Ø.Ø
  - specified NEC P8Ø.8
- not associated with low environmental temperature R68.Ø

Hypothyroidism (acquired) EØ3.9
- autoimmune — *see* Thyroiditis, autoimmune
- congenital (without goiter) EØ3.1
  - with goiter (diffuse) EØ3.Ø
- due to
  - exogenous substance NEC EØ3.2
  - iodine-deficiency, acquired EØ1.8
    - subclinical EØ2
  - irradiation therapy E89.Ø
  - medicament NEC EØ3.2
  - P-aminosalicylic acid (PAS) EØ3.2
  - phenylbutazone EØ3.2
  - resorcinol EØ3.2
  - sulfonamide EØ3.2
  - surgery E89.Ø
  - thiourea group drugs EØ3.2
- iatrogenic NEC EØ3.2
- iodine-deficiency (acquired) EØ1.8
  - congenital — *see* Syndrome, iodine- deficiency, congenital
  - subclinical EØ2
- neonatal, transitory P72.2
- postinfectious EØ3.3
- postirradiation E89.Ø
- postprocedural E89.Ø
- postsurgical E89.Ø
- specified NEC EØ3.8
- subclinical, iodine-deficiency related EØ2

Hypotonia, hypotonicity, hypotony
- bladder N31.2
- congenital (benign) P94.2
- eye — *see* Disorder, globe, hypotony

Hypotrichosis — *see* Alopecia

Hypotropia H5Ø.2- ☑

Hypoventilation RØ6.89
- congenital central alveolar G47.35
- sleep related
  - idiopathic nonobstructive alveolar G47.34
  - in conditions classified elsewhere G47.36

Hypovitaminosis — *see* Deficiency, vitamin

Hypovolemia E86.1
- surgical shock T81.19 ☑
- traumatic (shock) T79.4 ☑

Hypoxemia RØ9.Ø2
- newborn P84
- sleep related, in conditions classified elsewhere G47.36

Hypoxia — *see also* Anoxia RØ9.Ø2
- cerebral, during a procedure NEC G97.81
  - postprocedural NEC G97.82
- intrauterine P84
- myocardial — *see* Insufficiency, coronary
- newborn P84
- sleep-related G47.34

Hypsarhythmia — *see* Epilepsy, generalized, specified NEC

Hysteralgia, pregnant uterus O26.89- ☑

Hysteria, hysterical (conversion) (dissociative state) F44.9
- anxiety F41.8
- convulsions F44.5
- psychosis, acute F44.9

Hysteroepilepsy F44.5

I

IBDU (colonic inflammatory bowel dissease unclassified) K52.3

Ichthyoparasitism due to Vandellia cirrhosa B88.8

- **Ichthyosis** (congenital) Q8Ø.9
  - acquired L85.Ø
  - fetalis Q8Ø.4
  - hystrix Q8Ø.8
  - lamellar Q8Ø.2
  - lingual K13.29
  - palmaris and plantaris Q82.8
  - simplex Q8Ø.Ø
  - vera Q8Ø.8
  - vulgaris Q8Ø.Ø
  - X-linked Q8Ø.1
- **Ichthyotoxism** — *see* Poisoning, fish
  - bacterial — *see* Intoxication, foodborne
- **Icteroanemia, hemolytic** (acquired) D59.9
  - congenital — *see* Spherocytosis
- **Icterus** — *see also* Jaundice
  - conjunctiva R17
  - gravis, newborn P55.Ø
  - hematogenous (acquired) D59.9
  - hemolytic (acquired) D59.9
    - congenital — *see* Spherocytosis
  - hemorrhagic (acute) (leptospiral) (spirochetal) A27.Ø
    - newborn P53
  - infectious B15.9
    - with hepatic coma B15.Ø
    - leptospiral A27.Ø
    - spirochetal A27.Ø
  - neonatorum — *see* Jaundice, newborn
  - newborn P59.9
  - spirochetal A27.Ø
- **Ictus solaris, solis** T67.Ø1 ☑
- **Id reaction** (due to bacteria) L3Ø.2
- **Ideation**
  - homicidal R45.85Ø
  - suicidal R45.851
- **Identity disorder** (child) F64.9
  - gender role F64.2
  - psychosexual F64.2
- **Idioglossia** F8Ø.Ø
- **Idiopathic** — *see* condition
- **Idiot, idiocy** (congenital) F73
  - amaurotic (Bielschowsky(-Jansky)) (family) (infantile (late)) (juvenile (late)) (Vogt-Spielmeyer) E75.4
  - microcephalic QØ2
- **IgE asthma** J45.9Ø9
- **IIAC** (idiopathic infantile arterial calcification) Q28.8
- **Ileitis** (chronic) (noninfectious) — *see also* Enteritis K52.9
  - backwash — *see* Pancolitis, ulcerative (chronic)
  - infectious AØ9
  - regional (ulcerative) — *see* Enteritis, regional, small intestine
  - segmental — *see* Enteritis, regional
  - terminal (ulcerative) — *see* Enteritis, regional, small intestine
- **Ileocolitis** — *see also* Enteritis K52.9
  - infectious AØ9
  - regional — *see* Enteritis, regional
  - ulcerative K51.Ø- ☑
- **Ileostomy**
  - attention to Z43.2
  - malfunctioning K94.13
  - status Z93.2
    - with complication — *see* Complications, enterostomy
- **Ileotyphus** — *see* Typhoid
- **Ileum** — *see* condition
- **Ileus** (bowel) (colon) (inhibitory) (intestine) K56.7
  - adynamic K56.Ø
  - due to gallstone (in intestine) K56.3
  - duodenal (chronic) K31.5
  - gallstone K56.3
  - mechanical NEC — *see also* Obstruction, intestine, specified NEC K56.699
  - meconium P76.Ø
    - in cystic fibrosis E84.11
    - meaning meconium plug (without cystic fibrosis) P76.Ø
  - myxedema K59.89
  - neurogenic K56.Ø
    - Hirschsprung's disease or megacolon Q43.1
  - newborn
    - due to meconium P76.Ø
      - in cystic fibrosis E84.11
      - meaning meconium plug (without cystic fibrosis) P76.Ø
    - transitory P76.1
  - obstructive — *see also* Obstruction, intestine, specified NEC K56.699

- **Ileus** — *continued*
  - paralytic K56.Ø
  - postoperative K91.89
- **Iliac** — *see* condition
- **Iliotibial band syndrome** M76.3- ☑
- **Illiteracy** Z55.Ø
- **Illness** — *see also* Disease R69
  - manic-depressive — *see* Disorder, bipolar
- **Imbalance** R26.89
  - autonomic G9Ø.8
  - constituents of food intake E63.1
  - electrolyte E87.8
    - with
      - abortion — *see* Abortion by type, complicated by, electrolyte imbalance
      - molar pregnancy OØ8.5
    - due to hyperemesis gravidarum O21.1
    - following ectopic or molar pregnancy OØ8.5
    - neonatal, transitory NEC P74.49
      - potassium
        - hyperkalemia P74.31
        - hypokalemia P74.32
      - sodium
        - hypernatremia P74.21
        - hyponatremia P74.22
  - endocrine E34.9
  - eye muscle NOS H5Ø.9
  - hormone E34.9
  - hysterical F44.4
  - labyrinth — *see* subcategory H83.2 ☑
  - posture R29.3
  - protein-energy — *see* Malnutrition
  - sympathetic G9Ø.8
- **Imbecile, imbecility** (I.Q. 35-49) F71
- **Imbedding, intrauterine device** T83.39 ☑
- **Imbibition, cholesterol** (gallbladder) K82.4
- **Imbrication, teeth,, fully erupted** M26.3Ø
- **Imerslund** (-Gräsbeck) **syndrome** D51.1
- **Immature** — *see also* Immaturity
  - birth (less than 37 completed weeks) — *see* Preterm, newborn
    - extremely (less than 28 completed weeks) — *see* Immaturity, extreme
  - personality F6Ø.89
- **Immaturity** (less than 37 completed weeks) — *see also* Preterm, newborn
  - extreme of newborn (less than 28 completed weeks of gestation) (less than 196 completed days of gestation) (unspecified weeks of gestation) PØ7.2Ø
    - gestational age
      - 23 completed weeks (23 weeks, Ø days through 23 weeks, 6 days) PØ7.22
      - 24 completed weeks (24 weeks, Ø days through 24 weeks, 6 days) PØ7.23
      - 25 completed weeks (25 weeks, Ø days through 25 weeks, 6 days) PØ7.24
      - 26 completed weeks (26 weeks, Ø days through 26 weeks, 6 days) PØ7.25
      - 27 completed weeks (27 weeks, Ø days through 27 weeks, 6 days) PØ7.26
      - less than 23 completed weeks PØ7.21
  - fetus or infant light-for-dates — *see* Light-for-dates
  - lung, newborn P28.Ø
  - organ or site NEC — *see* Hypoplasia
  - pulmonary, newborn P28.Ø
  - reaction F6Ø.89
  - sexual (female) (male), after puberty E3Ø.Ø
- **Immersion** T75.1 ☑
  - foot T69.Ø2- ☑
  - hand T69.Ø1- ☑
- **Immobile, immobility**
  - complete, due to severe physical disability or frailty R53.2
  - intestine K59.89
  - syndrome (paraplegic) M62.3
- **Immune reconstitution** (inflammatory) syndrome [IRIS] D89.3
- **Immunization** — *see also* Vaccination
  - ABO — *see* Incompatibility, ABO
    - in newborn P55.1
  - appropriate for age
    - child (over 28 days old) ZØØ.129
      - with abnormal findings ZØØ.121
  - complication — *see* Complications, vaccination
  - encounter for Z23
  - not done (not carried out) Z28.9
    - because (of)

- **Immunization** — *continued*
  - not done — *continued*
    - because — *continued*
      - acute illness of patient Z28.Ø1
      - allergy to vaccine (or component) Z28.Ø4
      - caregiver refusal Z28.82
      - chronic illness of patient Z28.Ø2
      - contraindication NEC Z28.Ø9
      - delay in delivery of vaccine Z28.83
      - group pressure Z28.1
      - guardian refusal Z28.82
      - immune compromised state of patient Z28.Ø3
      - lack of availability of vaccine Z28.83
      - manufacturer delay of vaccine Z28.83
      - parent refusal Z28.82
      - patient had disease being vaccinated against Z28.81
      - patient refusal Z28.21
      - patient's belief Z28.1
      - religious beliefs of patient Z28.1
      - specified reason NEC Z28.89
        - of patient Z28.29
      - unavailability of vaccine Z28.83
      - unspecified patient reason Z28.2Ø
  - Rh factor
    - affecting management of pregnancy NEC O36.Ø9- ☑
      - anti-D antibody O36.Ø1- ☑
    - from transfusion — *see* Complication(s), transfusion, incompatibility reaction, Rh (factor)
- **Immunocompromised NOS** D84.9
- **Immunocytoma** C83.Ø- ☑
- **Immunodeficiency** D84.9
  - with
    - adenosine-deaminase deficiency — *see also* Deficiency, adenosine deaminase D81.3Ø
    - antibody defects D8Ø.9
      - specified type NEC D8Ø.8
    - hyperimmunoglobulinemia D8Ø.6
    - increased immunoglobulin M (IgM) D8Ø.5
    - major defect D82.9
      - specified type NEC D82.8
    - partial albinism D82.8
    - short-limbed stature D82.2
    - thrombocytopenia and eczema D82.Ø
  - antibody with
    - hyperimmunoglobulinemia D8Ø.6
    - near-normal immunoglobulins D8Ø.6
  - autosomal recessive, Swiss type D8Ø.Ø
  - combined D81.9
    - biotin-dependent carboxylase D81.819
      - biotinidase D81.81Ø
      - holocarboxylase synthetase D81.818
      - specified type NEC D81.818
    - severe (SCID) D81.9
      - with
        - low or normal B-cell numbers D81.2
        - low T- and B-cell numbers D81.1
        - reticular dysgenesis D81.Ø
    - specified type NEC D81.89
  - common variable D83.9
    - with
      - abnormalities of B-cell numbers and function D83.Ø
      - autoantibodies to B- or T-cells D83.2
      - immunoregulatory T-cell disorders D83.1
    - specified type NEC D83.8
  - due to
    - conditions classified elsewhere D84.81
    - drugs D84.821
    - external causes D84.822
    - medication (current or past) D84.821
  - following hereditary defective response to Epstein-Barr virus (EBV) D82.3
  - selective, immunoglobulin
    - A (IgA) D8Ø.2
    - G (IgG) (subclasses) D8Ø.3
    - M (IgM) D8Ø.4
  - severe combined (SCID) D81.9
    - due to adenosine deaminase deficiency D81.31
  - specified type NEC D84.89
  - X-linked, with increased IgM D8Ø.5
- **Immunodeficient NOS** D84.9
- **Immunosuppressed NOS** D84.9
- **Immunotherapy** (encounter for)
  - antineoplastic Z51.12
- **Impaction, impacted**
  - bowel, colon, rectum — *see also* Impaction, fecal K56.49

Index

Impaction, impacted — Inadequate, inadequacy

- **Inadequate, inadequacy** — *continued*
  - pulmonary
    - function RØ6.89
      - newborn P28.5
    - ventilation, newborn P28.5
  - sample of cytologic smear
    - anus R85.615
    - cervix R87.615
    - vagina R87.625
  - social F6Ø.7
    - insurance Z59.7
    - skills NEC Z73.4
  - supervision of child by parent Z62.Ø
  - teaching affecting education Z55.8
  - welfare support Z59.7
- **Inanition** R64
  - with edema — *see* Malnutrition, severe
  - due to
    - deprivation of food T73.Ø ☑
    - malnutrition — *see* Malnutrition
  - fever R5Ø.9
- **Inappropriate**
  - change in quantitative human chorionic gonadotropin (hCG) in early pregnancy OØ2.81
  - diet or eating habits Z72.4
  - level of quantitative human chorionic gonadotropin (hCG) for gestational age in early pregnancy OØ2.81
  - secretion
    - antidiuretic hormone (ADH) (excessive) E22.2
      - deficiency E23.2
    - pituitary (posterior) E22.2
- **Inattention at or after birth** — *see* Neglect
- **Incarceration, incarcerated**
  - enterocele K46.Ø
    - gangrenous K46.1
  - epiplocele K46.Ø
    - gangrenous K46.1
  - exomphalos K42.Ø
    - gangrenous K42.1
  - hernia — *see also* Hernia, by site, with obstruction
    - with gangrene — *see* Hernia, by site, with gangrene
  - iris, in wound — *see* Injury, eye, laceration, with prolapse
  - lens, in wound — *see* Injury, eye, laceration, with prolapse
  - omphalocele K42.Ø
  - prison, anxiety concerning Z65.1
  - rupture — *see* Hernia, by site
  - sarcoepiplocele K46.Ø
    - gangrenous K46.1
  - sarcoepiplomphalocele K42.Ø
    - with gangrene K42.1
  - uterus N85.8
    - gravid O34.51- ☑
      - causing obstructed labor O65.5
- **Incised wound**
  - external — *see* Laceration
  - internal organs — *see* Injury, by site
- **Incision, incisional**
  - hernia K43.2
    - with
      - gangrene (and obstruction) K43.1
      - obstruction K43.Ø
  - surgical, complication — *see* Complications, surgical procedure
  - traumatic
    - external — *see* Laceration
    - internal organs — *see* Injury, by site
- **Inclusion**
  - azurophilic leukocytic D72.Ø
  - blennorrhea (neonatal) (newborn) P39.1
  - gallbladder in liver (congenital) Q44.1
- **Incompatibility**
  - ABO
    - affecting management of pregnancy O36.11- ☑
      - anti-A sensitization O36.11- ☑
      - anti-B sensitization O36.19- ☑
      - specified NEC O36.19- ☑
    - infusion or transfusion reaction — *see* Complication(s), transfusion, incompatibility reaction, ABO
    - newborn P55.1
  - blood (group) (Duffy) (K) (Kell) (Kidd) (Lewis) (M) (S) NEC
    - affecting management of pregnancy O36.11- ☑
      - anti-A sensitization O36.11- ☑
      - anti-B sensitization O36.19- ☑

- **Incompatibility** — *continued*
  - blood (S) — *continued*
    - infusion or transfusion reaction T8Ø.89 ☑
    - newborn P55.8
  - divorce or estrangement Z63.5
  - Rh (blood group) (factor) Z31.82
    - affecting management of pregnancy NEC O36.Ø9- ☑
      - anti-D antibody O36.Ø1- ☑
    - infusion or transfusion reaction — *see* Complication(s), transfusion, incompatibility reaction, Rh (factor)
    - newborn P55.Ø
  - rhesus — *see* Incompatibility, Rh
- **Incompetency, incompetent, incompetence**
  - annular
    - aortic (valve) — *see* Insufficiency, aortic
    - mitral (valve) I34.Ø
    - pulmonary valve (heart) I37.1
  - aortic (valve) — *see* Insufficiency, aortic
  - cardiac valve — *see* Endocarditis
  - cervix, cervical (os) N88.3
    - in pregnancy O34.3- ☑
  - chronotropic I45.89
    - with
      - autonomic dysfunction G9Ø.8
      - ischemic heart disease I25.89
      - left ventricular dysfunction I51.89
      - sinus node dysfunction I49.8
  - esophagogastric (junction) (sphincter) K22.Ø
  - mitral (valve) — *see* Insufficiency, mitral
  - pelvic fundus N81.89
  - pubocervical tissue N81.82
  - pulmonary valve (heart) I37.1
    - congenital Q22.3
  - rectovaginal tissue N81.83
  - tricuspid (annular) (valve) — *see* Insufficiency, tricuspid
  - valvular — *see* Endocarditis
    - congenital Q24.8
  - vein, venous (saphenous) (varicose) — *see* Varix, leg
- **Incomplete** — *see also* condition
  - bladder, emptying R33.9
  - defecation R15.Ø
  - expansion lungs (newborn) NEC — *see* Atelectasis
  - rotation, intestine Q43.3
- **Inconclusive**
  - diagnostic imaging due to excess body fat of patient R93.9
  - findings on diagnostic imaging of breast NEC R92.8
  - mammogram (due to dense breasts) R92.2
- **Incontinence** R32
  - anal sphincter R15.9
  - coital N39.491
  - feces R15.9
    - nonorganic origin F98.1
  - insensible (urinary) N39.42
  - overflow N39.49Ø
  - postural (urinary) N39.492
  - psychogenic F45.8
  - rectal R15.9
  - reflex N39.498
  - stress (female) (male) N39.3
    - and urge N39.46
  - urethral sphincter R32
  - urge N39.41
    - and stress (female) (male) N39.46
  - urine (urinary) R32
    - continuous N39.45
    - due to cognitive impairment, or severe physical disability or immobility R39.81
    - functional R39.81
    - insensible N39.42
    - mixed (stress and urge) N39.46
    - nocturnal N39.44
    - nonorganic origin F98.Ø
    - overflow N39.49Ø
    - post dribbling N39.43
    - postural N39.492
    - reflex N39.498
    - specified NEC N39.498
    - stress (female) (male) N39.3
      - and urge N39.46
    - total N39.498
    - unaware N39.42
    - urge N39.41
      - and stress (female) (male) N39.46
- **Incontinentia pigmenti** Q82.3
- **Incoordinate, incoordination**
  - esophageal-pharyngeal (newborn) — *see* Dysphagia

- **Incoordinate, incoordination** — *continued*
  - muscular R27.8
  - uterus (action) (contractions) (complicating delivery) O62.4
- **Increase, increased**
  - abnormal, in development R63.8
  - androgens (ovarian) E28.1
  - anticoagulants (antithrombin) (anti-VIIIa) (anti-IXa) (anti-Xa) (anti-XIa) — *see* Circulating anticoagulants
  - cold sense R2Ø.8
  - estrogen E28.Ø
  - function
    - adrenal
      - cortex — *see* Cushing's, syndrome
      - medulla E27.5
    - pituitary (gland) (anterior) (lobe) E22.9
      - posterior E22.2
  - heat sense R2Ø.8
  - intracranial pressure (benign) G93.2
  - permeability, capillaries I78.8
  - pressure, intracranial G93.2
  - secretion
    - gastrin E16.4
    - glucagon E16.3
    - pancreas, endocrine E16.9
      - growth hormone-releasing hormone E16.8
      - pancreatic polypeptide E16.8
      - somatostatin E16.8
      - vasoactive-intestinal polypeptide E16.8
  - sphericity, lens Q12.4
  - splenic activity D73.1
  - venous pressure I87.8
    - portal K76.6
- **Increta placenta** O43.22- ☑
- **Incrustation, cornea, foreign body** (lead)(zinc) — *see* Foreign body, cornea
- **Incyclophoria** H5Ø.54
- **Incyclotropia** — *see* Cyclotropia
- **Indeterminate sex** Q56.4
- **India rubber skin** Q82.8
- **Indigestion** (acid) (bilious) (functional) K3Ø
  - catarrhal K31.89
  - due to decomposed food NOS AØ5.9
  - nervous F45.8
  - psychogenic F45.8
- **Indirect** — *see* condition
- **Induratio penis plastica** N48.6
- **Induration, indurated**
  - brain G93.89
  - breast (fibrous) N64.51
    - puerperal, postpartum O92.29
  - broad ligament N83.8
  - chancre
    - anus A51.1
    - congenital A5Ø.Ø7
    - extragenital NEC A51.2
  - corpora cavernosa (penis) (plastic) N48.6
  - liver (chronic) K76.89
  - lung (black) (chronic) (fibroid) — *see also* Fibrosis, lung J84.1Ø
    - essential brown J84.Ø3
  - penile (plastic) N48.6
  - phlebitic — *see* Phlebitis
  - skin R23.4
- **Inebriety** (without dependence) — *see* Alcohol, intoxication
- **Inefficiency, kidney** N28.9
- **Inelasticity, skin** R23.4
- **Inequality, leg** (length) (acquired) — *see also* Deformity, limb, unequal length
  - congenital — *see* Defect, reduction, lower limb
  - lower leg — *see* Deformity, limb, unequal length
- **Inertia**
  - bladder (neurogenic) N31.2
  - stomach K31.89
    - psychogenic F45.8
  - uterus, uterine during labor O62.2
    - during latent phase of labor O62.Ø
    - primary O62.Ø
    - secondary O62.1
  - vesical (neurogenic) N31.2
- **Infancy, infantile, infantilism** — *see also* condition
  - celiac K9Ø.Ø
  - genitalia, genitals (after puberty) E3Ø.Ø
  - Herter's (nontropical sprue) K9Ø.Ø
  - intestinal K9Ø.Ø
  - Lorain E23.Ø

Infection, infected, infective — *continued*
- coxsackie — *see* Coxsackie
- Cryptococcus neoformans — *see* Cryptococcosis
- Cryptosporidium AØ7.2
- Cunninghamella — *see* Mucormycosis
- cyst — *see* Cyst
- cystic duct — *see also* Cholecystitis K81.9
- Cysticercus cellulosae — *see* Cysticercosis
- cytomegalovirus, cytomegaloviral B25.9
  - congenital P35.1
  - maternal, maternal care for (suspected) damage to fetus O35.3 ☑
  - mononucleosis B27.1Ø
    - with
      - complication NEC B27.19
      - meningitis B27.12
      - polyneuropathy B27.11
- delta-agent (acute), in hepatitis B carrier B17.Ø
- dental (pulpal origin) KØ4.7
- Deuteromycetes B47.Ø
- Dicrocoelium dendriticum B66.2
- Dipetalonema (perstans) (streptocerca) B74.4
- diphtherial — *see* Diphtheria
- Diphyllobothrium (adult) (latum) (pacificum) B7Ø.Ø
  - larval B7Ø.1
- Diplogonoporus (grandis) B71.8
- Dipylidium caninum B67.4
- Dirofilaria B74.8
- Dracunculus medinensis B72
- Drechslera (hawaiiensis) B43.8
- Ducrey Haemophilus (any location) A57
- due to or resulting from
  - artificial insemination N98.Ø
  - Babesia
    - divergens (-like) strain B6Ø.Ø3
    - duncani (-type) species B6Ø.Ø2
    - microti B6Ø.Ø1
    - species
      - specified NEC B6Ø.Ø9
  - central venous catheter T8Ø.219 ☑
    - bloodstream T8Ø.211 ☑
    - exit or insertion site T8Ø.212 ☑
    - localized T8Ø.212 ☑
    - port or reservoir T8Ø.212 ☑
    - specified NEC T8Ø.218 ☑
    - tunnel T8Ø.212 ☑
  - device, implant or graft — *see also* Complications, by site and type, infection or inflammation T85.79 ☑
    - arterial graft NEC T82.7 ☑
    - breast (implant) T85.79 ☑
    - catheter NEC T85.79 ☑
      - dialysis (renal) T82.7 ☑
        - central line T8Ø.211 ☑
        - intraperitoneal T85.71 ☑
      - infusion NEC T82.7 ☑
        - cranial T85.735 ☑
        - intrathecal T85.735 ☑
        - spinal (epidural) (subdural) T85.735 ☑
        - subarachnoid T85.735 ☑
      - urinary T83.518 ☑
        - cystostomy T83.51Ø ☑
        - Hopkins T83.518 ☑
        - ileostomy T83.518 ☑
        - nephrostomy T83.512 ☑
        - specified NEC T83.518 ☑
        - urethral indwelling T83.511 ☑
        - urostomy T83.518 ☑
    - electronic (electrode) (pulse generator) (stimulator)
      - bone T84.7 ☑
      - cardiac T82.7 ☑
      - nervous system T85.738 ☑
        - brain T85.731 ☑
        - cranial nerve T85.732 ☑
        - gastric nerve T85.732 ☑
        - generator pocket T85.734 ☑
        - neurostimulator generator T85.734 ☑
        - peripheral nerve T85.732 ☑
        - sacral nerve T85.732 ☑
        - spinal cord T85.733 ☑
        - vagal nerve T85.732 ☑
      - urinary (indwelling) T83.51 ☑
    - fixation, internal (orthopedic) NEC — *see* Complication, fixation device, infection
    - gastrointestinal (bile duct) (esophagus) T85.79 ☑
      - neurostimulator electrode (lead) T85.732 ☑

Infection, infected, infective — *continued*
- due to or resulting from — *continued*
  - device, implant or graft — *see also* Complications, by site and type, infection or inflammation — *continued*
    - genital NEC T83.69 ☑
    - heart NEC T82.7 ☑
      - valve (prosthesis) T82.6 ☑
        - graft T82.7 ☑
    - joint prosthesis — *see* Complication, joint prosthesis, infection
    - ocular (corneal graft) (orbital implant) NEC T85.79 ☑
    - orthopedic NEC T84.7 ☑
    - penile (cylinder) (pump) (resevoir) T83.61 ☑
    - specified NEC T85.79 ☑
    - testicular T83.62 ☑
    - urinary NEC T83.598 ☑
      - ileal conduit stent T83.593 ☑
      - implanted neurostimulation T83.59Ø ☑
      - implanted sphincter T83.591 ☑
      - indwelling ureteral stent T83.592 ☑
      - nephroureteral stent T83.593 ☑
      - specified stent NEC T83.593 ☑
    - vascular NEC T82.7 ☑
    - ventricular intracranial (communicating) shunt T85.73Ø ☑
  - Hickman catheter T8Ø.219 ☑
    - bloodstream T8Ø.211 ☑
    - localized T8Ø.212 ☑
    - specified NEC T8Ø.218 ☑
  - immunization or vaccination T88.Ø ☑
  - infusion, injection or transfusion NEC T8Ø.29 ☑
  - injury NEC — *code by* site under Wound, open
  - peripherally inserted central catheter (PICC) T8Ø.219 ☑
    - bloodstream T8Ø.211 ☑
    - localized T8Ø.212 ☑
    - specified NEC T8Ø.218 ☑
  - portacath (port-a-cath) T8Ø.219 ☑
    - bloodstream T8Ø.211 ☑
    - localized T8Ø.212 ☑
    - specified NEC T8Ø.218 ☑
  - protozoa of the order Piroplasmida NEC B6Ø.Ø9
  - pulmonary artery catheter — *see* Infection, due to or resulting from, central venous catheter
  - surgery T81.4Ø ☑
  - Swan Ganz catheter — *see* Infection, due to or resulting from, central venous catheter
  - triple lumen catheter T8Ø.219 ☑
    - bloodstream T8Ø.211 ☑
    - localized T8Ø.212 ☑
    - specified NEC T8Ø.218 ☑
  - umbilical venous catheter T8Ø.219 ☑
    - bloodstream T8Ø.211 ☑
    - localized T8Ø.212 ☑
    - specified NEC T8Ø.218 ☑
- during labor NEC O75.3
- ear (middle) — *see also* Otitis media
  - external — *see* Otitis, externa, infective
  - inner — *see* subcategory H83.Ø ☑
- Eberthella typhosa AØ1.ØØ
- Echinococcus — *see* Echinococcus
- echovirus
  - as cause of disease classified elsewhere B97.12
  - unspecified nature or site B34.1
- endocardium I33.Ø
- endocervix — *see* Cervicitis
- Entamoeba — *see* Amebiasis
- enteric — *see* Enteritis, infectious
- Enterobacter sakazakii B96.89
- Enterobius vermicularis B8Ø
- enterostomy K94.12
- enterovirus B34.1
  - as cause of disease classified elsewhere B97.1Ø
    - coxsackievirus B97.11
    - echovirus B97.12
    - specified NEC B97.19
- Entomophthora B46.8
- Epidermophyton — *see* Dermatophytosis
- epididymis — *see* Epididymitis
- episiotomy (puerperal) O86.Ø9
- Erysipelothrix (insidiosa) (rhusiopathiae) — *see* Erysipeloid
- erythema infectiosum BØ8.3
- Escherichia (E.) coli NEC A49.8

Infection, infected, infective — *continued*
- Escherichia coli — *continued*
  - as cause of disease classified elsewhere — *see also* Escherichia coli B96.2Ø
  - congenital P39.8
    - sepsis P36.4
  - generalized A41.51
  - intestinal — *see* Enteritis, infectious, due to, Escherichia coli
- ethmoidal (chronic) (sinus) — *see* Sinusitis, ethmoidal
- eustachian tube (ear) — *see* Salpingitis, eustachian
- external auditory canal (meatus) NEC — *see* Otitis, externa, infective
- eye (purulent) — *see* Endophthalmitis, purulent
- eyelid — *see* Inflammation, eyelid
- fallopian tube — *see* Salpingo-oophoritis
- Fasciola (gigantica) (hepatica) (indica) B66.3
- Fasciolopsis (buski) B66.5
- filarial — *see* Infestation, filarial
- finger (skin) LØ8.9
  - nail LØ3.Ø1- ☑
    - fungus B35.1
- fish tapeworm B7Ø.Ø
  - larval B7Ø.1
- flagellate, intestinal AØ7.9
- fluke — *see* Infestation, fluke
- focal
  - teeth (pulpal origin) KØ4.7
  - tonsils J35.Ø1
- Fonsecaea (compactum) (pedrosoi) B43.Ø
- food — *see* Intoxication, foodborne
- foot (skin) LØ8.9
  - dermatophytic fungus B35.3
- Francisella tularensis — *see* Tularemia
- frontal (sinus) (chronic) — *see* Sinusitis, frontal
- fungus NOS B49
  - beard B35.Ø
  - dermatophytic — *see* Dermatophytosis
  - foot B35.3
  - groin B35.6
  - hand B35.2
  - nail B35.1
  - pathogenic to compromised host only B48.8
  - perianal (area) B35.6
  - scalp B35.Ø
  - skin B36.9
    - foot B35.3
    - hand B35.2
    - toenails B35.1
- Fusarium B48.8
- gallbladder — *see* Cholecystitis
- gas bacillus — *see* Gangrene, gas
- gastrointestinal — *see* Enteritis, infectious
- generalized NEC — *see* Sepsis
- generator pocket, implanted electronic neurostimulator T85.734 ☑
- genital organ or tract
  - female — *see* Disease, pelvis, inflammatory
  - male N49.9
    - multiple sites N49.8
    - specified NEC N49.8
- Ghon tubercle, primary A15.7
- Giardia lamblia AØ7.1
- gingiva (chronic) KØ5.1Ø
  - acute KØ5.ØØ
    - nonplaque induced KØ5.Ø1
    - plaque induced KØ5.ØØ
  - nonplaque induced KØ5.11
  - plaque induced KØ5.1Ø
- glanders A24.Ø
- glenosporopsis B48.Ø
- Gnathostoma (spinigerum) B83.1
- Gongylonema B83.8
- gonococcal — *see* Gonococcus
- gram-negative bacilli NOS A49.9
- guinea worm B72
- gum (chronic) KØ5.1Ø
  - acute KØ5.ØØ
    - nonplaque induced KØ5.Ø1
    - plaque induced KØ5.ØØ
  - nonplaque induced KØ5.11
  - plaque induced KØ5.1Ø
- Haemophilus — *see* Infection, Hemophilus
- heart — *see* Carditis
- Helicobacter pylori AØ4.8
  - as cause of disease classified elsewhere B96.81
- helminths B83.9
  - intestinal B82.Ø

- **Infection, infected, infective** — *continued*
  - helminths — *continued*
    - intestinal — *continued*
      - mixed (types classifiable to more than one of the titles B65.Ø-B81.3 and B81.8) B81.4
      - specified type NEC B81.8
    - specified type NEC B83.8
  - Hemophilus
    - aegyptius, systemic A48.4
    - ducrey (any location) A57
    - generalized A41.3
    - influenzae NEC A49.2
      - as cause of disease classified elsewhere B96.3
  - herpes (simplex) — *see also* Herpes
    - congenital P35.2
    - disseminated BØØ.7
    - zoster BØ2.9
  - herpesvirus, herpesviral — *see* Herpes
  - Heterophyes (heterophyes) B66.8
  - hip (joint) NEC MØØ.9
    - due to internal joint prosthesis
      - left T84.52 ☑
      - right T84.51 ☑
    - skin NEC LØ8.9
  - Histoplasma — *see* Histoplasmosis
    - American B39.4
    - capsulatum B39.4
  - hookworm B76.9
  - human
    - papilloma virus A63.Ø
    - T-cell lymphotropic virus type-1 (HTLV-1) B33.3
  - hydrocele N43.Ø
  - Hymenolepis B71.Ø
  - hypopharynx — *see* Pharyngitis
  - inguinal (lymph) glands LØ4.1
    - due to soft chancre A57
  - intervertebral disc, pyogenic M46.3Ø
    - cervical region M46.32
    - cervicothoracic region M46.33
    - lumbar region M46.36
    - lumbosacral region M46.37
    - multiple sites M46.39
    - occipito-atlanto-axial region M46.31
    - sacrococcygeal region M46.38
    - thoracic region M46.34
    - thoracolumbar region M46.35
  - intestine, intestinal — *see* Enteritis, infectious
    - specified NEC AØ8.8
  - intra-amniotic affecting newborn NEC P39.2
  - intrauterine inflammation O41.12- ☑
  - Isospora belli or hominis AØ7.3
  - Japanese B encephalitis A83.Ø
  - jaw (bone) (lower) (upper) M27.2
  - joint NEC MØØ.9
    - due to internal joint prosthesis T84.5Ø ☑
  - kidney (cortex) (hematogenous) N15.9
    - with calculus N2Ø.Ø
      - with hydronephrosis N13.6
    - following ectopic gestation OØ8.83
    - pelvis and ureter (cystic) N28.85
    - puerperal (postpartum) O86.21
    - specified NEC N15.8
  - Klebsiella (K.) pneumoniae NEC A49.8
    - as cause of disease classified elsewhere B96.1
  - knee (joint) NEC MØØ.9
    - joint MØØ.9
    - due to internal joint prosthesis
      - left T84.54 ☑
      - right T84.53 ☑
    - skin LØ8.9
  - Koch's — *see* Tuberculosis
  - labia (majora) (minora) (acute) — *see* Vulvitis
  - lacrimal
    - gland — *see* Dacryoadenitis
    - passages (duct) (sac) — *see* Inflammation, lacrimal, passages
  - lancet fluke B66.2
  - larynx NEC J38.7
  - leg (skin) NOS LØ8.9
  - Legionella pneumophila A48.1
    - nonpneumonic A48.2
  - Leishmania — *see also* Leishmaniasis
    - aethiopica B55.1
    - braziliensis B55.2
    - chagasi B55.Ø
    - donovani B55.Ø
    - infantum B55.Ø
    - major B55.1

- **Infection, infected, infective** — *continued*
  - Leishmania — *see also* Leishmaniasis — *continued*
    - mexicana B55.1
    - tropica B55.1
  - lentivirus, as cause of disease classified elsewhere B97.31
  - Leptosphaeria senegalensis B47.Ø
  - Leptospira interrogans A27.9
    - autumnalis A27.89
    - canicola A27.89
    - hebdomadis A27.89
    - icterohaemorrhagiae A27.Ø
    - pomona A27.89
    - specified type NEC A27.89
  - leptospirochetal NEC — *see* Leptospirosis
  - Listeria monocytogenes — *see also* Listeriosis
    - congenital P37.2
  - Loa loa B74.3
    - with conjunctival infestation B74.3
    - eyelid B74.3
  - Loboa loboi B48.Ø
  - local, skin (staphylococcal) (streptococcal) LØ8.9
    - abscess — *code by* site under Abscess
    - cellulitis — *code by* site under Cellulitis
    - specified NEC LØ8.89
    - ulcer — *see* Ulcer, skin
  - Loefflerella mallei A24.Ø
  - lung — *see also* Pneumonia J18.9
    - atypical Mycobacterium A31.Ø
    - spirochetal A69.8
    - tuberculous — *see* Tuberculosis, pulmonary
    - virus — *see* Pneumonia, viral
  - lymph gland — *see also* Lymphadenitis, acute
    - mesenteric I88.Ø
  - lymphoid tissue, base of tongue or posterior pharynx, NEC (chronic) J35.Ø3
  - Madurella (grisea) (mycetomii) B47.Ø
  - major
    - following ectopic or molar pregnancy OØ8.Ø
    - puerperal, postpartum, childbirth O85
  - Malassezia furfur B36.Ø
  - Malleomyces
    - mallei A24.Ø
    - pseudomallei (whitmori) — *see* Melioidosis
  - mammary gland N61.Ø
  - Mansonella (ozzardi) (perstans) (streptocerca) B74.4
  - mastoid — *see* Mastoiditis
  - maxilla, maxillary M27.2
    - sinus (chronic) — *see* Sinusitis, maxillary
  - mediastinum J98.51
  - Medina (worm) B72
  - meibomian cyst or gland — *see* Hordeolum
  - meninges — *see* Meningitis, bacterial
  - meningococcal — *see also* condition A39.9
    - adrenals A39.1
    - brain A39.81
    - cerebrospinal A39.Ø
    - conjunctiva A39.89
    - endocardium A39.51
    - heart A39.5Ø
      - endocardium A39.51
      - myocardium A39.52
      - pericardium A39.53
    - joint A39.83
    - meninges A39.Ø
    - meningococcemia A39.4
      - acute A39.2
      - chronic A39.3
    - myocardium A39.52
    - pericardium A39.53
    - retrobulbar neuritis A39.82
    - specified site NEC A39.89
  - mesenteric lymph nodes or glands NEC I88.Ø
  - Metagonimus B66.8
  - metatarsophalangeal MØØ.9
  - methicillin
    - resistant Staphylococcus aureus (MRSA) A49.Ø2
    - susceptible Staphylococcus aureus (MSSA) A49.Ø1
  - Microsporum, microsporic — *see* Dermatophytosis
  - mixed flora (bacterial) NEC A49.8
  - Monilia — *see* Candidiasis
  - Monosporium apiospermum B48.2
  - mouth, parasitic B37.Ø
  - Mucor — *see* Mucormycosis
  - muscle NEC — *see* Myositis, infective
  - mycelium NOS B49
  - mycetoma B47.9
    - actinomycotic NEC B47.1

- **Infection, infected, infective** — *continued*
  - mycetoma — *continued*
    - mycotic NEC B47.Ø
  - Mycobacterium, mycobacterial — *see* Mycobacterium
  - Mycoplasma NEC A49.3
    - pneumoniae, as cause of disease classified elsewhere B96.Ø
  - mycotic NOS B49
    - pathogenic to compromised host only B48.8
    - skin NOS B36.9
  - myocardium NEC I4Ø.Ø
  - nail (chronic)
    - with lymphangitis — *see* Lymphangitis, acute, digit
    - finger LØ3.Ø1- ☑
      - fungus B35.1
    - ingrowing L6Ø.Ø
    - toe LØ3.Ø3- ☑
      - fungus B35.1
  - nasal sinus (chronic) — *see* Sinusitis
  - nasopharynx — *see* Nasopharyngitis
  - navel LØ8.82
  - Necator americanus B76.1
  - Neisseria — *see* Gonococcus
  - Neotestudina rosatii B47.Ø
  - newborn P39.9
    - intra-amniotic NEC P39.2
    - skin P39.4
    - specified type NEC P39.8
  - nipple N61.Ø
    - associated with
      - lactation O91.Ø3
      - pregnancy O91.Ø1- ☑
      - puerperium O91.Ø2
  - Nocardia — *see* Nocardiosis
  - obstetrical surgical wound (puerperal) O86.ØØ
    - incisional site
      - deep O86.Ø2
      - superficial O86.Ø1
    - organ and space site O86.Ø3
    - surgical site specified NEC O86.Ø9
  - Oesophagostomum (apiostomum) B81.8
  - Oestrus ovis — *see* Myiasis
  - Oidium albicans B37.9
  - Onchocerca (volvulus) — *see* Onchocerciasis
  - oncovirus, as cause of disease classified elsewhere B97.32
  - operation wound T81.49 ☑
  - Opisthorchis (felineus) (viverrini) B66.Ø
  - orbit, orbital — *see* Inflammation, orbit
  - orthopoxvirus NEC BØ8.Ø9
  - ovary — *see* Salpingo-oophoritis
  - Oxyuris vermicularis B8Ø
  - pancreas (acute) — *see* Pancreatitis, acute
    - abscess — *see* Pancreatitis, acute
    - specified NEC — *see also* Pancreatitis, acute K85.8Ø
  - papillomavirus, as cause of disease classified elsewhere B97.7
  - papovavirus NEC B34.4
  - Paracoccidioides brasiliensis — *see* Paracoccidioidomycosis
  - Paragonimus (westermani) B66.4
  - parainfluenza virus B34.8
  - parameningococcus NOS A39.9
  - parapoxvirus BØ8.6Ø
    - specified NEC BØ8.69
  - parasitic B89
  - Parastrongylus
    - cantonensis B83.2
    - costaricensis B81.3
    - paratyphoid AØ1.4
      - Type A AØ1.1
      - Type B AØ1.2
      - Type C AØ1.3
  - paraurethral ducts N34.2
  - parotid gland — *see* Sialoadenitis
  - parvovirus NEC B34.3
    - as cause of disease classified elsewhere B97.6
  - Pasteurella NEC A28.Ø
    - multocida A28.Ø
    - pestis — *see* Plague
    - pseudotuberculosis A28.Ø
    - septica (cat bite) (dog bite) A28.Ø
    - tularensis — *see* Tularemia
  - pelvic, female — *see* Disease, pelvis, inflammatory
  - Penicillium (marneffei) B48.4
  - penis (glans) (retention) NEC N48.29
  - periapical KØ4.5
  - peridental, periodontal KØ5.2Ø

- **Inflammation, inflamed, inflammatory** — *continued*
  - parotid region LØ8.9
  - pelvis, female — *see* Disease, pelvis, inflammatory
  - penis (corpora cavernosa) N48.29
  - perianal K62.89
  - pericardium — *see* Pericarditis
  - perineum (female) (male) LØ8.9
  - perirectal K62.89
  - peritoneum — *see* Peritonitis
  - periuterine — *see* Disease, pelvis, inflammatory
  - perivesical — *see* Cystitis
  - petrous bone (acute) (chronic) — *see* Petrositis
  - pharynx (acute) — *see* Pharyngitis
  - pia mater — *see* Meningitis
  - pleura — *see* Pleurisy
  - polyp, colon — *see also* Polyp, colon, inflammatory K51.4Ø
  - prostate — *see also* Prostatitis
    - specified type NEC N41.8
  - rectosigmoid — *see* Rectosigmoiditis
  - rectum — *see also* Proctitis K62.89
  - respiratory, upper — *see also* Infection, respiratory, upper JØ6.9
    - acute, due to radiation J7Ø.Ø
    - chronic, due to external agent — *see* condition, respiratory, chronic, due to
    - due to
      - chemicals, gases, fumes or vapors (inhalation) J68.2
      - radiation J7Ø.1
  - retina — *see* Chorioretinitis
  - retrocecal — *see* Appendicitis
  - retroperitoneal — *see* Peritonitis
  - salivary duct or gland (any) (suppurative) — *see* Sialoadenitis
  - scorbutic, alveoli, teeth E54
  - scrotum N49.2
  - seminal vesicle — *see* Vesiculitis
  - sigmoid — *see* Enteritis
  - sinus — *see* Sinusitis
  - Skene's duct or gland — *see* Urethritis
  - skin LØ8.9
  - spermatic cord N49.1
  - sphenoidal (sinus) — *see* Sinusitis, sphenoidal
  - spinal
    - cord — *see* Encephalitis
    - membrane — *see* Meningitis
    - nerve — *see* Disorder, nerve
  - spine — *see* Spondylopathy, inflammatory
  - spleen (capsule) D73.89
  - stomach — *see* Gastritis
  - subcutaneous tissue LØ8.9
  - suprarenal (gland) E27.8
  - synovial — *see* Tenosynovitis
  - tendon (sheath) NEC — *see* Tenosynovitis
  - testis — *see* Orchitis
  - throat (acute) — *see* Pharyngitis
  - thymus (gland) E32.8
  - thyroid (gland) — *see* Thyroiditis
  - tongue K14.Ø
  - tonsil — *see* Tonsillitis
  - trachea — *see* Tracheitis
  - trochlear (nerve) — *see* Strabismus, paralytic, fourth nerve
  - tubal — *see* Salpingo-oophoritis
  - tuberculous NEC — *see* Tuberculosis
  - tubo-ovarian — *see* Salpingo-oophoritis
  - tunica vaginalis N49.1
  - tympanic membrane — *see* Tympanitis
  - umbilicus, umbilical LØ8.82
  - uterine ligament — *see* Disease, pelvis, inflammatory
  - uterus (catarrhal) — *see* Endometritis
  - uveal tract (anterior) NOS — *see also* Iridocyclitis
    - posterior — *see* Chorioretinitis
  - vagina — *see* Vaginitis
  - vas deferens N49.1
  - vein — *see also* Phlebitis
    - intracranial or intraspinal (septic) GØ8
    - thrombotic I8Ø.9
      - leg — *see* Phlebitis, leg
      - lower extremity — *see* Phlebitis, leg
  - vocal cord J38.3
  - vulva — *see* Vulvitis
  - Wharton's duct (suppurative) — *see* Sialoadenitis
- **Inflation, lung, imperfect** (newborn) — *see* Atelectasis
- **Influenza** (bronchial) (epidemic) (respiratory (upper)) (unidentified influenza virus) J11.1
  - with
    - digestive manifestations J11.2
    - encephalopathy J11.81
    - enteritis J11.2
    - gastroenteritis J11.2
    - gastrointestinal manifestations J11.2
    - laryngitis J11.1
    - myocarditis J11.82
    - otitis media J11.83
    - pharyngitis J11.1
    - pneumonia J11.ØØ
      - specified type J11.Ø8
    - respiratory manifestations NEC J11.1
    - specified manifestation NEC J11.89
  - A (non-novel) J1Ø- ☑
  - A/H5N1 — *see also* Influenza, due to, identified novel influenza A virus JØ9.X2
  - avian — *see also* Influenza, due to, identified novel influenza A virus JØ9.X2
  - B J1Ø- ☑
  - bird — *see also* Influenza, due to, identified novel influenza A virus JØ9.X2
  - C J1Ø- ☑
  - due to
    - avian — *see also* Influenza, due to, identified novel influenza A virus JØ9.X2
    - identified influenza virus NEC J1Ø.1
      - with
        - digestive manifestations J1Ø.2
        - encephalopathy J1Ø.81
        - enteritis J1Ø.2
        - gastroenteritis J1Ø.2
        - gastrointestinal manifestations J1Ø.2
        - laryngitis J1Ø.1
        - myocarditis J1Ø.82
        - otitis media J1Ø.83
        - pharyngitis J1Ø.1
        - pneumonia (unspecified type) J1Ø.ØØ
          - with same identified influenza virus J1Ø.Ø1
          - specified type NEC J1Ø.Ø8
        - respiratory manifestations NEC J1Ø.1
        - specified manifestation NEC J1Ø.89
    - identified novel influenza A virus JØ9.X2
      - with
        - digestive manifestations JØ9.X3
        - encephalopathy JØ9.X9
        - enteritis JØ9.X3
        - gastroenteritis JØ9.X3
        - gastrointestinal manifestations JØ9.X3
        - laryngitis JØ9.X2
        - myocarditis JØ9.X9
        - otitis media JØ9.X9
        - pharyngitis JØ9.X2
        - pneumonia JØ9.X1
        - respiratory manifestations NEC JØ9.X2
        - specified manifestation NEC JØ9.X9
        - upper respiratory symptoms JØ9.X2
  - novel (2ØØ9) H1N1 influenza — *see also* Influenza, due to, identified influenza virus NEC J1Ø.1
  - novel influenza A/H1N1 — *see also* Influenza, due to, identified influenza virus NEC J1Ø.1
  - of other animal origin, not bird or swine — *see also* Influenza, due to, identified novel influenza A virus JØ9.X2
  - swine (viruses that normally cause infections in pigs) — *see also* Influenza, due to, identified novel influenza A virus JØ9.X2
- **Influenzal** — *see* Influenza
- **Influenza-like disease** — *see* Influenza
- **Infraction, Freiberg's** (metatarsal head) — *see* Osteochondrosis, juvenile, metatarsus
- **Infraeruption of tooth** (teeth) M26.34
- **Infusion complication, misadventure, or reaction** — *see* Complications, infusion
- **Ingestion**
  - chemical — *see* Table of Drugs and Chemicals, by substance, poisoning
  - drug or medicament
    - correct substance properly administered — *see* Table of Drugs and Chemicals, by drug, adverse effect
    - overdose or wrong substance given or taken — *see* Table of Drugs and Chemicals, by drug, poisoning
  - foreign body — *see* Foreign body, alimentary tract
- **Ingestion** — *continued*
  - multiple drug — *see* Table of Drugs and Chemicals, multiple
  - tularemia A21.3
- **Ingrowing**
  - hair (beard) L73.1
  - nail (finger) (toe) L6Ø.Ø
- **Inguinal** — *see also* condition
  - testicle Q53.9
    - bilateral Q53.212
    - unilateral Q53.112
- **Inhalant-induced**
  - anxiety disorder F18.98Ø
  - depressive disorder F18.94
  - major neurocognitive disorder F18.97
  - mild neurocognitive disorder F18.988
  - psychotic disorder F18.959
- **Inhalation**
  - anthrax A22.1
  - flame T27.3 ☑
  - food or foreign body — *see* Foreign body, by site
  - gases, fumes, or vapors T59.9- ☑
    - specified agent NEC — *see* Table of Drugs and Chemicals, by substance T59.89- ☑
  - liquid or vomitus — *see* Asphyxia
  - meconium (newborn) P24.ØØ
    - with
      - with respiratory symptoms P24.Ø1
      - pneumonia (pneumonitis) P24.Ø1
  - mucus — *see* Asphyxia, mucus
  - oil or gasoline (causing suffocation) — *see* Foreign body, by site
  - smoke T59.81- ☑
    - with respiratory conditions J7Ø.5
      - due to chemicals, gases, fumes and vapors J68.9
  - steam T59.9- ☑
  - stomach contents or secretions — *see* Foreign body, by site
    - due to anesthesia (general) (local) or other sedation T88.59 ☑
      - in labor and delivery O74.Ø
      - in pregnancy O29.Ø1- ☑
      - postpartum, puerperal O89.Ø1
- **Inhibition, orgasm**
  - female F52.31
  - male F52.32
- **Inhibitor, systemic lupus erythematosus** (presence of) D68.62
- **Iniencephalus, iniencephaly** QØØ.2
- **Injection, traumatic jet** (air) (industrial) (water) (paint or dye) T7Ø.4 ☑
- **Injury** — *see also* specified injury type T14.9Ø ☑
  - abdomen, abdominal S39.91 ☑
    - blood vessel — *see* Injury, blood vessel, abdomen
    - cavity — *see* Injury, intra-abdominal
    - contusion S3Ø.1 ☑
    - internal — *see* Injury, intra-abdominal
    - intra-abdominal organ — *see* Injury, intra-abdominal
    - nerve — *see* Injury, nerve, abdomen
    - open — *see* Wound, open, abdomen
    - specified NEC S39.81 ☑
    - superficial — *see* Injury, superficial, abdomen
  - Achilles tendon S86.ØØ- ☑
    - laceration S86.Ø2- ☑
    - specified type NEC S86.Ø9- ☑
    - strain S86.Ø1- ☑
  - acoustic, resulting in deafness — *see* Injury, nerve, acoustic
  - adrenal (gland) S37.819 ☑
    - contusion S37.812 ☑
    - laceration S37.813 ☑
    - specified type NEC S37.818 ☑
  - alveolar (process) SØ9.93 ☑
  - ankle S99.91- ☑
    - contusion — *see* Contusion, ankle
    - dislocation — *see* Dislocation, ankle
    - fracture — *see* Fracture, ankle
    - nerve — *see* Injury, nerve, ankle
    - open — *see* Wound, open, ankle
    - specified type NEC S99.81- ☑
    - sprain — *see* Sprain, ankle
    - superficial — *see* Injury, superficial, ankle
  - anterior chamber, eye — *see* Injury, eye, specified site NEC
  - anus — *see* Injury, abdomen
  - aorta (thoracic) S25.ØØ ☑

- **Injury** — *continued*
  - blood vessel — *continued*
    - leg — *continued*
      - popliteal — *continued*
        - vein — *see* Injury, blood vessel, popliteal, vein
      - specified
        - site NEC S85.80- ☑
          - laceration S85.81- ☑
          - specified type NEC S85.89- ☑
        - type NEC S85.99- ☑
      - thigh — *see* Injury, blood vessel, hip
      - tibial artery — *see* Injury, blood vessel, tibial artery
    - lesser saphenous vein (lower leg level) S85.40- ☑
      - laceration S85.41- ☑
      - specified type NEC S85.49- ☑
    - limb
      - lower — *see* Injury, blood vessel, leg
      - upper — *see* Injury, blood vessel, arm
    - lower back — *see* Injury, blood vessel, abdomen
      - specified NEC — *see* Injury, blood vessel, abdomen, specified, site NEC
    - mammary (artery) (vein) — *see* Injury, blood vessel, thoracic, specified site NEC
    - mesenteric (inferior) (superior)
      - artery — *see* Injury, mesenteric, artery
      - vein — *see* Injury, blood vessel, mesenteric, vein
    - neck S15.9 ☑
      - specified site NEC S15.8 ☑
    - ovarian (artery) (vein) — *see* subcategory S35.8 ☑
    - palmar arch (superficial) S65.20- ☑
      - deep S65.30- ☑
        - laceration S65.31- ☑
        - specified type NEC S65.39- ☑
      - laceration S65.21- ☑
      - specified type NEC S65.29- ☑
    - pelvis — *see* Injury, blood vessel, abdomen
      - specified NEC — *see* Injury, blood vessel, abdomen, specified, site NEC
    - peroneal artery S85.20- ☑
      - laceration S85.21- ☑
      - specified type NEC S85.29- ☑
    - plantar artery (deep) (foot) S95.10- ☑
      - laceration S95.11- ☑
      - specified type NEC S95.19- ☑
    - popliteal
      - artery S85.00- ☑
        - laceration S85.01- ☑
        - specified type NEC S85.09- ☑
      - vein S85.50- ☑
        - laceration S85.51- ☑
        - specified type NEC S85.59- ☑
    - portal vein S35.319 ☑
      - laceration S35.311 ☑
      - specified type NEC S35.318 ☑
    - precerebral — *see* Injury, blood vessel, neck
    - pulmonary (artery) (vein) — *see* Injury, blood vessel, thoracic, pulmonary
    - radial artery (forearm level) S55.10- ☑
      - hand and wrist (level) S65.10- ☑
        - laceration S65.11- ☑
        - specified type NEC S65.19- ☑
      - laceration S55.11- ☑
      - specified type NEC S55.19- ☑
    - renal
      - artery S35.40- ☑
        - laceration S35.41- ☑
        - specified NEC S35.49- ☑
      - vein S35.40- ☑
        - laceration S35.41- ☑
        - specified NEC S35.49- ☑
    - saphenous vein (greater) (lower leg level) — *see* Injury, blood vessel, greater saphenous
      - hip and thigh level — *see* Injury, blood vessel, greater saphenous, hip level
      - lesser — *see* Injury, blood vessel, lesser saphenous
    - shoulder
      - specified NEC — *see* Injury, blood vessel, arm, specified site NEC
      - superficial vein — *see* Injury, blood vessel, arm, superficial vein
    - specified NEC T14.8 ☑
    - splenic
      - artery — *see* Injury, blood vessel, celiac artery, branch

- **Injury** — *continued*
  - blood vessel — *continued*
    - splenic — *continued*
      - vein S35.329 ☑
        - laceration S35.321 ☑
        - specified NEC S35.328 ☑
    - subclavian — *see* Injury, blood vessel, thoracic, innominate
    - thigh — *see* Injury, blood vessel, hip
    - thoracic S25.90 ☑
      - aorta S25.00 ☑
        - laceration (minor) (superficial) S25.01 ☑
          - major S25.02 ☑
        - specified type NEC S25.09 ☑
      - azygos vein — *see* Injury, blood vessel, thoracic, specified, site NEC
      - innominate
        - artery S25.10- ☑
          - laceration (minor) (superficial) S25.11- ☑
            - major S25.12- ☑
          - specified type NEC S25.19- ☑
        - vein S25.30- ☑
          - laceration (minor) (superficial) S25.31- ☑
            - major S25.32- ☑
          - specified type NEC S25.39- ☑
      - intercostal S25.50- ☑
        - laceration S25.51- ☑
        - specified type NEC S25.59- ☑
      - laceration S25.91 ☑
      - mammary vessel — *see* Injury, blood vessel, thoracic, specified, site NEC
      - pulmonary S25.40- ☑
        - laceration (minor) (superficial) S25.41- ☑
          - major S25.42- ☑
        - specified type NEC S25.49- ☑
      - specified
        - site NEC S25.80- ☑
          - laceration S25.81 ☑
          - specified type NEC S25.89 ☑
        - type NEC S25.99 ☑
      - subclavian — *see* Injury, blood vessel, thoracic, innominate
      - vena cava (superior) S25.20 ☑
        - laceration (minor) (superficial) S25.21 ☑
          - major S25.22 ☑
        - specified type NEC S25.29 ☑
    - thumb S65.40- ☑
      - laceration S65.41- ☑
      - specified type NEC S65.49- ☑
    - tibial artery S85.10- ☑
      - anterior S85.13- ☑
        - laceration S85.14- ☑
        - specified injury NEC S85.15- ☑
      - laceration S85.11- ☑
      - posterior S85.16- ☑
        - laceration S85.17- ☑
        - specified injury NEC S85.18- ☑
      - specified injury NEC S85.12- ☑
    - ulnar artery (forearm level) S55.00- ☑
      - hand and wrist (level) S65.00- ☑
        - laceration S65.01- ☑
        - specified type NEC S65.09- ☑
      - laceration S55.01- ☑
      - specified type NEC S55.09- ☑
    - upper arm (level) — *see* Injury, blood vessel, arm
      - superficial vein — *see* Injury, blood vessel, arm, superficial vein
    - uterine S35.5- ☑
      - artery S35.53- ☑
      - vein S35.53- ☑
    - vena cava — *see* Injury, vena cava
    - vertebral artery S15.10- ☑
      - laceration (minor) (superficial) S15.11- ☑
        - major S15.12- ☑
      - specified type NEC S15.19- ☑
    - wrist (level) — *see* Injury, blood vessel, hand
  - brachial plexus S14.3 ☑
    - newborn P14.3
  - brain (traumatic) S06.9- ☑
    - diffuse (axonal) S06.2X- ☑
    - focal S06.30- ☑
  - brainstem S06.38- ☑
  - breast NOS S29.9 ☑
  - broad ligament — *see* Injury, pelvic organ, specified site NEC
  - bronchus, bronchi — *see* Injury, intrathoracic, bronchus

- **Injury** — *continued*
  - brow S09.90 ☑
  - buttock S39.92 ☑
  - canthus, eye S05.90 ☑
  - cardiac plexus — *see* Injury, nerve, thorax, sympathetic
  - cauda equina S34.3 ☑
  - cavernous sinus — *see* Injury, intracranial
  - cecum — *see* Injury, colon
  - celiac ganglion or plexus — *see* Injury, nerve, lumbosacral, sympathetic
  - cerebellum — *see* Injury, intracranial
  - cerebral — *see* Injury, intracranial
  - cervix (uteri) — *see* Injury, uterus
  - cheek (wall) S09.93 ☑
  - chest — *see* Injury, thorax
  - childbirth (newborn) — *see also* Birth, injury
    - maternal NEC O71.9
  - chin S09.93 ☑
  - choroid (eye) — *see* Injury, eye, specified site NEC
  - clitoris S39.94 ☑
  - coccyx — *see also* Injury, back, lower
    - complicating delivery O71.6
  - colon — *see* Injury, intestine, large
  - common bile duct — *see* Injury, liver
  - conjunctiva (superficial) — *see* Injury, eye, conjunctiva
  - conus medullaris — *see* Injury, spinal, sacral
  - cord
    - spermatic (pelvic region) S37.898 ☑
      - scrotal region S39.848 ☑
    - spinal — *see* Injury, spinal cord, by region
  - cornea — *see* Injury, eye, specified site NEC
    - abrasion — *see* Injury, eye, cornea, abrasion
  - cortex (cerebral) — *see also* Injury, intracranial
    - visual — *see* Injury, nerve, optic
  - costal region NEC S29.9 ☑
  - costochondral NEC S29.9 ☑
  - cranial
    - cavity — *see* Injury, intracranial
    - nerve — *see* Injury, nerve, cranial
  - crushing — *see* Crush
  - cutaneous sensory nerve
  - cystic duct — *see* Injury, liver
  - deep tissue — *see* Contusion, by site
    - meaning pressure ulcer — *see* Ulcer, pressure L89 with final character .6
  - delivery (newborn) P15.9
    - maternal NEC O71.9
  - Descemet's membrane — *see* Injury, eyeball, penetrating
  - diaphragm — *see* Injury, intrathoracic, diaphragm
  - duodenum — *see* Injury, intestine, small, duodenum
  - ear (auricle) (external) (canal) S09.91 ☑
    - abrasion — *see* Abrasion, ear
    - bite — *see* Bite, ear
    - blister — *see* Blister, ear
    - bruise — *see* Contusion, ear
    - contusion — *see* Contusion, ear
    - external constriction — *see* Constriction, external, ear
    - hematoma — *see* Hematoma, ear
    - inner — *see* Injury, ear, middle
    - laceration — *see* Laceration, ear
    - middle S09.30- ☑
      - blast — *see* Injury, blast, ear
      - specified NEC S09.39- ☑
    - puncture — *see* Puncture, ear
    - superficial — *see* Injury, superficial, ear
  - eighth cranial nerve (acoustic or auditory) — *see* Injury, nerve, acoustic
  - elbow S59.90- ☑
    - contusion — *see* Contusion, elbow
    - dislocation — *see* Dislocation, elbow
    - fracture — *see* Fracture, ulna, upper end
    - open — *see* Wound, open, elbow
    - specified NEC S59.80- ☑
    - sprain — *see* Sprain, elbow
    - superficial — *see* Injury, superficial, elbow
  - eleventh cranial nerve (accessory) — *see* Injury, nerve, accessory
  - epididymis S39.94 ☑
  - epigastric region S39.91 ☑
  - epiglottis NEC S19.89 ☑
  - esophageal plexus — *see* Injury, nerve, thorax, sympathetic
  - esophagus (thoracic part) — *see also* Injury, intrathoracic, esophagus

- **Injury** — *continued*
  - intestine — *continued*
    - large — *continued*
      - blast injury — *continued*
        - rectum S36.61 ☑
        - sigmoid S36.513 ☑
        - specified site NEC S36.518 ☑
        - transverse S36.511 ☑
      - contusion S36.529 ☑
        - ascending (right) S36.52Ø ☑
        - descending (left) S36.522 ☑
        - rectum S36.62 ☑
        - sigmoid S36.523 ☑
        - specified site NEC S36.528 ☑
        - transverse S36.521 ☑
      - descending (left) S36.5Ø2 ☑
        - blast injury (primary) S36.512 ☑
          - secondary S36.592 ☑
        - contusion S36.522 ☑
        - laceration S36.532 ☑
        - specified type NEC S36.592 ☑
      - laceration S36.539 ☑
        - ascending (right) S36.53Ø ☑
        - descending (left) S36.532 ☑
        - rectum S36.63 ☑
        - sigmoid S36.533 ☑
        - specified site NEC S36.538 ☑
        - transverse S36.531 ☑
      - rectum S36.6Ø ☑
        - blast injury (primary) S36.61 ☑
          - secondary S36.69 ☑
        - contusion S36.62 ☑
        - laceration S36.63 ☑
        - specified type NEC S36.69 ☑
      - sigmoid S36.5Ø3 ☑
        - blast injury (primary) S36.513 ☑
          - secondary S36.593 ☑
        - contusion S36.523 ☑
        - laceration S36.533 ☑
        - specified type NEC S36.593 ☑
      - specified
        - site NEC S36.5Ø8 ☑
          - blast injury (primary) S36.518 ☑
            - secondary S36.598 ☑
          - contusion S36.528 ☑
          - laceration S36.538 ☑
          - specified type NEC S36.598 ☑
        - type NEC S36.599 ☑
          - ascending (right) S36.59Ø ☑
          - descending (left) S36.592 ☑
          - rectum S36.69 ☑
          - sigmoid S36.593 ☑
          - specified site NEC S36.598 ☑
          - transverse S36.591 ☑
      - transverse S36.5Ø1 ☑
        - blast injury (primary) S36.511 ☑
          - secondary S36.591 ☑
        - contusion S36.521 ☑
        - laceration S36.531 ☑
        - specified type NEC S36.591 ☑
    - small S36.4Ø9 ☑
      - blast injury (primary) S36.419 ☑
        - duodenum S36.41Ø ☑
        - secondary S36.499 ☑
          - duodenum S36.49Ø ☑
          - specified site NEC S36.498 ☑
        - specified site NEC S36.418 ☑
      - contusion S36.429 ☑
        - duodenum S36.42Ø ☑
        - specified site NEC S36.428 ☑
      - duodenum S36.4ØØ ☑
        - blast injury (primary) S36.41Ø ☑
          - secondary S36.49Ø ☑
        - contusion S36.42Ø ☑
        - laceration S36.43Ø ☑
        - specified NEC S36.49Ø ☑
      - laceration S36.439 ☑
        - duodenum S36.43Ø ☑
        - specified site NEC S36.438 ☑
      - specified
        - site NEC S36.4Ø8 ☑
        - type NEC S36.499 ☑
          - duodenum S36.49Ø ☑
          - specified site NEC S36.498 ☑
  - intra-abdominal S36.9Ø ☑
    - adrenal gland — *see* Injury, adrenal gland

- **Injury** — *continued*
  - intra-abdominal — *continued*
    - bladder — *see* Injury, bladder
    - colon — *see* Injury, intestine, large
    - contusion S36.92 ☑
    - fallopian tube — *see* Injury, fallopian tube
    - gallbladder — *see* Injury, gallbladder
    - intestine — *see* Injury, intestine
    - kidney — *see* Injury, kidney
    - laceration S36.93 ☑
    - liver — *see* Injury, liver
    - ovary — *see* Injury, ovary
    - pancreas — *see* Injury, pancreas
    - pelvic NOS S37.9Ø ☑
    - peritoneum — *see* Injury, intra-abdominal, specified, site NEC
    - prostate — *see* Injury, prostate
    - rectum — *see* Injury, intestine, large, rectum
    - retroperitoneum — *see* Injury, intra-abdominal, specified, site NEC
    - seminal vesicle — *see* Injury, pelvis, organ, specified site NEC
    - small intestine — *see* Injury, intestine, small
    - specified
      - pelvic S37.9Ø ☑
        - specified
          - site NEC S37.899 ☑
            - specified type NEC S37.898 ☑
          - type NEC S37.99 ☑
      - site NEC S36.899 ☑
        - contusion S36.892 ☑
        - laceration S36.893 ☑
        - specified type NEC S36.898 ☑
      - type NEC S36.99 ☑
    - spleen — *see* Injury, spleen
    - stomach — *see* Injury, stomach
    - ureter — *see* Injury, ureter
    - urethra — *see* Injury, urethra
    - uterus — *see* Injury, uterus
    - vas deferens — *see* Injury, pelvis, organ, specified site NEC
  - intracranial (traumatic) SØ6.9- ☑
    - cerebellar hemorrhage, traumatic — *see* Injury, intracranial, focal
    - cerebral edema, traumatic SØ6.1X- ☑
      - diffuse SØ6.1X- ☑
      - focal SØ6.1X- ☑
    - diffuse (axonal) SØ6.2X- ☑
    - epidural hemorrhage (traumatic) SØ6.4X- ☑
    - focal brain injury SØ6.3Ø- ☑
      - contusion — *see* Contusion, cerebral
      - laceration — *see* Laceration, cerebral
    - intracerebral hemorrhage, traumatic SØ6.36- ☑
      - left side SØ6.35- ☑
      - right side SØ6.34- ☑
    - subarachnoid hemorrhage, traumatic SØ6.6X- ☑
    - subdural hemorrhage, traumatic SØ6.5X- ☑
  - intraocular — *see* Injury, eyeball, penetrating
  - intrathoracic S27.9 ☑
    - bronchus S27.4Ø9 ☑
      - bilateral S27.4Ø2 ☑
      - blast injury (primary) S27.419 ☑
        - bilateral S27.412 ☑
        - secondary — *see* Injury, intrathoracic, bronchus, specified type NEC
        - unilateral S27.411 ☑
      - contusion S27.429 ☑
        - bilateral S27.422 ☑
        - unilateral S27.421 ☑
      - laceration S27.439 ☑
        - bilateral S27.432 ☑
        - unilateral S27.431 ☑
      - specified type NEC S27.499 ☑
        - bilateral S27.492 ☑
        - unilateral S27.491 ☑
      - unilateral S27.4Ø1 ☑
    - diaphragm S27.8Ø9 ☑
      - contusion S27.8Ø2 ☑
      - laceration S27.8Ø3 ☑
      - specified type NEC S27.8Ø8 ☑
    - esophagus (thoracic) S27.819 ☑
      - contusion S27.812 ☑
      - laceration S27.813 ☑
      - specified type NEC S27.818 ☑
    - heart — *see* Injury, heart
    - hemopneumothorax S27.2 ☑

- **Injury** — *continued*
  - intrathoracic — *continued*
    - hemothorax S27.1 ☑
    - lung S27.3Ø9 ☑
      - aspiration J69.Ø
      - bilateral S27.3Ø2 ☑
      - blast injury (primary) S27.319 ☑
        - bilateral S27.312 ☑
        - secondary — *see* Injury, intrathoracic, lung, specified type NEC
        - unilateral S27.311 ☑
      - contusion S27.329 ☑
        - bilateral S27.322 ☑
        - unilateral S27.321 ☑
      - laceration S27.339 ☑
        - bilateral S27.332 ☑
        - unilateral S27.331 ☑
      - specified type NEC S27.399 ☑
        - bilateral S27.392 ☑
        - unilateral S27.391 ☑
      - unilateral S27.3Ø1 ☑
    - pleura S27.6Ø ☑
      - laceration S27.63 ☑
      - specified type NEC S27.69 ☑
    - pneumothorax S27.Ø ☑
    - specified organ NEC S27.899 ☑
      - contusion S27.892 ☑
      - laceration S27.893 ☑
      - specified type NEC S27.898 ☑
    - thoracic duct — *see* Injury, intrathoracic, specified organ NEC
    - thymus gland — *see* Injury, intrathoracic, specified organ NEC
    - trachea, thoracic S27.5Ø ☑
      - blast (primary) S27.51 ☑
      - contusion S27.52 ☑
      - laceration S27.53 ☑
      - specified type NEC S27.59 ☑
  - iris — *see* Injury, eye, specified site NEC
    - penetrating — *see* Injury, eyeball, penetrating
  - jaw SØ9.93 ☑
  - jejunum — *see* Injury, intestine, small
  - joint NOS T14.8 ☑
    - old or residual — *see* Disorder, joint, specified type NEC
  - kidney S37.ØØ- ☑
    - acute (nontraumatic) N17.9
    - contusion — *see* Contusion, kidney
    - laceration — *see* Laceration, kidney
    - specified NEC S37.Ø9- ☑
  - knee S89.9- ☑
    - contusion — *see* Contusion, knee
    - dislocation — *see* Dislocation, knee
    - meniscus (lateral) (medial) — *see* Sprain, knee, specified site NEC
      - old injury or tear — *see* Derangement, knee, meniscus, due to old injury
    - open — *see* Wound, open, knee
    - specified NEC S89.8- ☑
    - sprain — *see* Sprain, knee
    - superficial — *see* Injury, superficial, knee
  - labium (majus) (minus) S39.94 ☑
  - labyrinth, ear SØ9.3Ø- ☑
  - lacrimal apparatus, duct, gland, or sac — *see* Injury, eye, specified site NEC
  - larynx NEC S19.81 ☑
  - leg (lower) S89.9- ☑
    - blood vessel — *see* Injury, blood vessel, leg
    - contusion — *see* Contusion, leg
    - fracture — *see* Fracture, leg
    - muscle — *see* Injury, muscle, leg
    - nerve — *see* Injury, nerve, leg
    - open — *see* Wound, open, leg
    - specified NEC S89.8- ☑
    - superficial — *see* Injury, superficial, leg
  - lens, eye — *see* Injury, eye, specified site NEC
    - penetrating — *see* Injury, eyeball, penetrating
  - limb NEC T14.8 ☑
  - lip SØ9.93 ☑
  - liver S36.119 ☑
    - contusion S36.112 ☑
    - laceration S36.113 ☑
      - major (stellate) S36.116 ☑
      - minor S36.114 ☑
      - moderate S36.115 ☑
    - specified NEC S36.118 ☑

- **Injury** — *continued*
  - muscle — *continued*
    - intrinsic
      - ankle and foot level — *see* Injury, muscle, foot, intrinsic
      - finger (other than thumb) — *see* Injury, muscle, finger by site, intrinsic
      - foot (level) — *see* Injury, muscle, foot, intrinsic
      - thumb — *see* Injury, muscle, thumb, intrinsic
    - leg (level) (lower) S86.9Ø- ☑
      - Achilles tendon — *see* Injury, Achilles tendon
      - anterior muscle group — *see* Injury, muscle, anterior muscle group
      - laceration S86.92- ☑
      - peroneal muscle group — *see* Injury, muscle, peroneal muscle group
      - posterior muscle group — *see* Injury, muscle, posterior muscle group, leg level
      - specified
        - site NEC S86.8Ø- ☑
          - laceration S86.82- ☑
          - specified type NEC S86.89- ☑
          - strain S86.81- ☑
        - type NEC S86.99- ☑
      - strain S86.91- ☑
    - long
      - extensor toe, at ankle and foot level — *see* Injury, muscle, toe, extensor
      - flexor, toe, at ankle and foot level — *see* Injury, muscle, toe, flexor
      - head, biceps — *see* Injury, muscle, biceps, long head
    - lower back S39.ØØ2 ☑
      - laceration S39.Ø22 ☑
      - specified type NEC S39.Ø92 ☑
      - strain S39.Ø12 ☑
    - neck (level) S16.9 ☑
      - laceration S16.2 ☑
      - specified type NEC S16.8 ☑
      - strain S16.1 ☑
    - pelvis S39.ØØ3 ☑
      - laceration S39.Ø23 ☑
      - specified type NEC S39.Ø93 ☑
      - strain S39.Ø13 ☑
    - peroneal muscle group, at leg level (lower) S86.3Ø- ☑
      - laceration S86.32- ☑
      - specified type NEC S86.39- ☑
      - strain S86.31- ☑
    - posterior muscle (group)
      - leg level (lower) S86.1Ø- ☑
        - laceration S86.12- ☑
        - specified type NEC S86.19- ☑
        - strain S86.11- ☑
      - thigh level S76.3Ø- ☑
        - laceration S76.32- ☑
        - specified type NEC S76.39- ☑
        - strain S76.31- ☑
    - quadriceps (thigh) S76.1Ø- ☑
      - laceration S76.12- ☑
      - specified type NEC S76.19- ☑
      - strain S76.11- ☑
    - shoulder S46.9Ø- ☑
      - laceration S46.92- ☑
      - rotator cuff — *see* Injury, rotator cuff
      - specified site NEC S46.8Ø- ☑
        - laceration S46.82- ☑
        - specified type NEC S46.89- ☑
        - strain S46.81- ☑
      - specified type NEC S46.99- ☑
      - strain S46.91- ☑
    - thigh NEC (level) S76.9Ø- ☑
      - adductor — *see* Injury, muscle, adductor, thigh
      - laceration S76.92- ☑
      - posterior muscle (group) — *see* Injury, muscle, posterior muscle, thigh level
      - quadriceps — *see* Injury, muscle, quadriceps
      - specified
        - site NEC S76.8Ø- ☑
          - laceration S76.82- ☑
          - specified type NEC S76.89- ☑
          - strain S76.81- ☑
        - type NEC S76.99- ☑
      - strain S76.91- ☑
    - thorax (level) S29.ØØ9 ☑
      - back wall S29.ØØ2 ☑

- **Injury** — *continued*
  - muscle — *continued*
    - thorax — *continued*
      - front wall S29.ØØ1 ☑
      - laceration S29.Ø29 ☑
        - back wall S29.Ø22 ☑
        - front wall S29.Ø21 ☑
      - specified type NEC S29.Ø99 ☑
        - back wall S29.Ø92 ☑
        - front wall S29.Ø91 ☑
      - strain S29.Ø19 ☑
        - back wall S29.Ø12 ☑
        - front wall S29.Ø11 ☑
    - thumb
      - abductor (forearm level) S56.3Ø- ☑
        - laceration S56.32- ☑
        - specified type NEC S56.39- ☑
        - strain S56.31- ☑
      - extensor (forearm level) S56.3Ø- ☑
        - hand level S66.2Ø- ☑
          - laceration S66.22- ☑
          - specified type NEC S66.29- ☑
          - strain S66.21- ☑
        - laceration S56.32- ☑
        - specified type NEC S56.39- ☑
        - strain S56.31- ☑
      - flexor (forearm level) S56.ØØ- ☑
        - hand level S66.ØØ- ☑
          - laceration S66.Ø2- ☑
          - specified type NEC S66.Ø9- ☑
          - strain S66.Ø1- ☑
        - laceration S56.Ø2- ☑
        - specified type NEC S56.Ø9- ☑
        - strain S56.Ø1- ☑
        - wrist level — *see* Injury, muscle, thumb, flexor, hand level
      - intrinsic S66.4Ø- ☑
        - laceration S66.42- ☑
        - specified type NEC S66.49- ☑
        - strain S66.41- ☑
    - toe — *see also* Injury, muscle, foot
      - extensor, long S96.1Ø- ☑
        - laceration S96.12- ☑
        - specified type NEC S96.19- ☑
        - strain S96.11- ☑
      - flexor, long S96.ØØ- ☑
        - laceration S96.Ø2- ☑
        - specified type NEC S96.Ø9- ☑
        - strain S96.Ø1- ☑
    - triceps S46.3Ø- ☑
      - laceration S46.32- ☑
      - specified type NEC S46.39- ☑
      - strain S46.31- ☑
    - wrist (and hand) level — *see* Injury, muscle, hand
  - musculocutaneous nerve — *see* Injury, nerve, musculocutaneous
  - myocardium — *see* Injury, heart
  - nape — *see* Injury, neck
  - nasal (septum) (sinus) SØ9.92 ☑
  - nasopharynx SØ9.92 ☑
  - neck S19.9 ☑
    - specified NEC S19.8Ø ☑
      - specified site NEC S19.89 ☑
  - nerve NEC T14.8 ☑
    - abdomen S34.9 ☑
      - peripheral S34.6 ☑
      - specified site NEC S34.8 ☑
    - abducens SØ4.4- ☑
      - contusion SØ4.4- ☑
      - laceration SØ4.4- ☑
      - specified type NEC SØ4.4- ☑
    - abducent — *see* Injury, nerve, abducens
    - accessory SØ4.7- ☑
      - contusion SØ4.7- ☑
      - laceration SØ4.7- ☑
      - specified type NEC SØ4.7- ☑
    - acoustic SØ4.6- ☑
      - contusion SØ4.6- ☑
      - laceration SØ4.6- ☑
      - specified type NEC SØ4.6- ☑
    - ankle S94.9- ☑
      - cutaneous sensory S94.3- ☑
      - specified site NEC — *see* subcategory S94.8 ☑
    - anterior crural, femoral — *see* Injury, nerve, femoral
    - arm (upper) S44.9- ☑
      - axillary — *see* Injury, nerve, axillary

- **Injury** — *continued*
  - nerve — *continued*
    - arm — *continued*
      - cutaneous — *see* Injury, nerve, cutaneous, arm
      - median — *see* Injury, nerve, median, upper arm
      - musculocutaneous — *see* Injury, nerve, musculocutaneous
      - radial — *see* Injury, nerve, radial, upper arm
      - specified site NEC — *see* subcategory S44.8 ☑
      - ulnar — *see* Injury, nerve, ulnar, arm
    - auditory — *see* Injury, nerve, acoustic
    - axillary S44.3- ☑
    - brachial plexus — *see* Injury, brachial plexus
    - cervical sympathetic S14.5 ☑
    - cranial SØ4.9 ☑
      - contusion SØ4.9 ☑
      - eighth (acoustic or auditory) — *see* Injury, nerve, acoustic
      - eleventh (accessory) — *see* Injury, nerve, accessory
      - fifth (trigeminal) — *see* Injury, nerve, trigeminal
      - first (olfactory) — *see* Injury, nerve, olfactory
      - fourth (trochlear) — *see* Injury, nerve, trochlear
      - laceration SØ4.9 ☑
      - ninth (glossopharyngeal) — *see* Injury, nerve, glossopharyngeal
      - second (optic) — *see* Injury, nerve, optic
      - seventh (facial) — *see* Injury, nerve, facial
      - sixth (abducent) — *see* Injury, nerve, abducens
      - specified
        - nerve NEC SØ4.89- ☑
          - contusion SØ4.89- ☑
          - laceration SØ4.89- ☑
          - specified type NEC SØ4.89- ☑
        - type NEC SØ4.9 ☑
      - tenth (pneumogastric or vagus) — *see* Injury, nerve, vagus
      - third (oculomotor) — *see* Injury, nerve, oculomotor
      - twelfth (hypoglossal) — *see* Injury, nerve, hypoglossal
    - cutaneous sensory
      - ankle (level) S94.3- ☑
      - arm (upper) (level) S44.5- ☑
      - foot (level) — *see* Injury, nerve, cutaneous sensory, ankle
      - forearm (level) S54.3- ☑
      - hip (level) S74.2- ☑
      - leg (lower level) S84.2- ☑
      - shoulder (level) — *see* Injury, nerve, cutaneous sensory, arm
      - thigh (level) — *see* Injury, nerve, cutaneous sensory, hip
    - deep peroneal — *see* Injury, nerve, peroneal, foot
    - digital
      - finger S64.4- ☑
        - index S64.49- ☑
        - little S64.49- ☑
        - middle S64.49- ☑
        - ring S64.49- ☑
      - thumb S64.3- ☑
      - toe — *see* Injury, nerve, ankle, specified site NEC
    - eighth cranial (acoustic or auditory) — *see* Injury, nerve, acoustic
    - eleventh cranial (accessory) — *see* Injury, nerve, accessory
    - facial SØ4.5- ☑
      - contusion SØ4.5- ☑
      - laceration SØ4.5- ☑
      - newborn P11.3
      - specified type NEC SØ4.5- ☑
    - femoral (hip level) (thigh level) S74.1- ☑
    - fifth cranial (trigeminal) — *see* Injury, nerve, trigeminal
    - finger (digital) — *see* Injury, nerve, digital, finger
    - first cranial (olfactory) — *see* Injury, nerve, olfactory
    - foot S94.9- ☑
      - cutaneous sensory S94.3- ☑
      - deep peroneal S94.2- ☑
      - lateral plantar S94.Ø- ☑
      - medial plantar S94.1- ☑
      - specified site NEC — *see* subcategory S94.8 ☑
    - forearm (level) S54.9- ☑
      - cutaneous sensory — *see* Injury, nerve, cutaneous sensory, forearm
      - median — *see* Injury, nerve, median

- **Injury** — *continued*
  - nerve — *continued*
    - forearm — *continued*
      - radial — *see* Injury, nerve, radial
      - specified site NEC — *see* subcategory S54.8 ☑
      - ulnar — *see* Injury, nerve, ulnar
    - fourth cranial (trochlear) — *see* Injury, nerve, trochlear
    - glossopharyngeal SØ4.89- ☑
      - specified type NEC SØ4.89- ☑
    - hand S64.9- ☑
      - median — *see* Injury, nerve, median, hand
      - radial — *see* Injury, nerve, radial, hand
      - specified NEC — *see* subcategory S64.8 ☑
      - ulnar — *see* Injury, nerve, ulnar, hand
    - hip (level) S74.9- ☑
      - cutaneous sensory — *see* Injury, nerve, cutaneous sensory, hip
      - femoral — *see* Injury, nerve, femoral
      - sciatic — *see* Injury, nerve, sciatic
      - specified site NEC — *see* subcategory S74.8 ☑
    - hypoglossal SØ4.89- ☑
      - specified type NEC SØ4.89- ☑
    - lateral plantar S94.Ø- ☑
    - leg (lower) S84.9- ☑
      - cutaneous sensory — *see* Injury, nerve, cutaneous sensory, leg
      - peroneal — *see* Injury, nerve, peroneal
      - specified site NEC — *see* subcategory S84.8 ☑
      - tibial — *see* Injury, nerve, tibial
      - upper — *see* Injury, nerve, thigh
    - lower
      - back — *see* Injury, nerve, abdomen, specified site NEC
        - peripheral — *see* Injury, nerve, abdomen, peripheral
      - limb — *see* Injury, nerve, leg
    - lumbar plexus — *see* Injury, nerve, lumbosacral, sympathetic
    - lumbar spinal — *see* Injury, nerve, spinal, lumbar
    - lumbosacral
      - plexus — *see* Injury, nerve, lumbosacral, sympathetic
      - sympathetic S34.5 ☑
    - medial plantar S94.1- ☑
    - median (forearm level) S54.1- ☑
      - hand (level) S64.1- ☑
      - upper arm (level) S44.1- ☑
      - wrist (level) — *see* Injury, nerve, median, hand
    - musculocutaneous S44.4- ☑
    - musculospiral (upper arm level) — *see* Injury, nerve, radial, upper arm
    - neck S14.9 ☑
      - peripheral S14.4 ☑
      - specified site NEC S14.8 ☑
      - sympathetic S14.5 ☑
    - ninth cranial (glossopharyngeal) — *see* Injury, nerve, glossopharyngeal
    - oculomotor SØ4.1- ☑
      - contusion SØ4.1- ☑
      - laceration SØ4.1- ☑
      - specified type NEC SØ4.1- ☑
    - olfactory SØ4.81- ☑
      - specified type NEC SØ4.81- ☑
    - optic SØ4.Ø1- ☑
      - contusion SØ4.Ø1- ☑
      - laceration SØ4.Ø1- ☑
      - specified type NEC SØ4.Ø1- ☑
    - pelvic girdle — *see* Injury, nerve, hip
    - pelvis — *see* Injury, nerve, abdomen, specified site NEC
      - peripheral — *see* Injury, nerve, abdomen, peripheral
    - peripheral NEC T14.8 ☑
      - abdomen — *see* Injury, nerve, abdomen, peripheral
      - lower back — *see* Injury, nerve, abdomen, peripheral
      - neck — *see* Injury, nerve, neck, peripheral
      - pelvis — *see* Injury, nerve, abdomen, peripheral
      - specified NEC T14.8 ☑
    - peroneal (lower leg level) S84.1- ☑
      - foot S94.2- ☑
    - plexus
      - brachial — *see* Injury, brachial plexus

- **Injury** — *continued*
  - nerve — *continued*
    - plexus — *continued*
      - celiac, coeliac — *see* Injury, nerve, lumbosacral, sympathetic
      - mesenteric, inferior — *see* Injury, nerve, lumbosacral, sympathetic
      - sacral — *see* Injury, lumbosacral plexus
      - spinal
        - brachial — *see* Injury, brachial plexus
        - lumbosacral — *see* Injury, lumbosacral plexus
    - pneumogastric — *see* Injury, nerve, vagus
    - radial (forearm level) S54.2- ☑
      - hand (level) S64.2- ☑
      - upper arm (level) S44.2- ☑
      - wrist (level) — *see* Injury, nerve, radial, hand
    - root — *see* Injury, nerve, spinal, root
    - sacral plexus — *see* Injury, lumbosacral plexus
    - sacral spinal — *see* Injury, nerve, spinal, sacral
    - sciatic (hip level) (thigh level) S74.Ø- ☑
    - second cranial (optic) — *see* Injury, nerve, optic
    - seventh cranial (facial) — *see* Injury, nerve, facial
    - shoulder — *see* Injury, nerve, arm
    - sixth cranial (abducent) — *see* Injury, nerve, abducens
    - spinal
      - plexus — *see* Injury, nerve, plexus, spinal
      - root
        - cervical S14.2 ☑
        - dorsal S24.2 ☑
        - lumbar S34.21 ☑
        - sacral S34.22 ☑
        - thoracic — *see* Injury, nerve, spinal, root, dorsal
    - splanchnic — *see* Injury, nerve, lumbosacral, sympathetic
    - sympathetic NEC — *see* Injury, nerve, lumbosacral, sympathetic
      - cervical — *see* Injury, nerve, cervical sympathetic
    - tenth cranial (pneumogastric or vagus) — *see* Injury, nerve, vagus
    - thigh (level) — *see* Injury, nerve, hip
      - cutaneous sensory — *see* Injury, nerve, cutaneous sensory, hip
      - femoral — *see* Injury, nerve, femoral
      - sciatic — *see* Injury, nerve, sciatic
      - specified NEC — *see* Injury, nerve, hip
    - third cranial (oculomotor) — *see* Injury, nerve, oculomotor
    - thorax S24.9 ☑
      - peripheral S24.3 ☑
      - specified site NEC S24.8 ☑
      - sympathetic S24.4 ☑
    - thumb, digital — *see* Injury, nerve, digital, thumb
    - tibial (lower leg level) (posterior) S84.Ø- ☑
    - toe — *see* Injury, nerve, ankle
    - trigeminal SØ4.3- ☑
      - contusion SØ4.3- ☑
      - laceration SØ4.3- ☑
      - specified type NEC SØ4.3- ☑
    - trochlear SØ4.2- ☑
      - contusion SØ4.2- ☑
      - laceration SØ4.2- ☑
      - specified type NEC SØ4.2- ☑
    - twelfth cranial (hypoglossal) — *see* Injury, nerve, hypoglossal
    - ulnar (forearm level) S54.Ø- ☑
      - arm (upper) (level) S44.Ø- ☑
      - hand (level) S64.Ø- ☑
      - wrist (level) — *see* Injury, nerve, ulnar, hand
    - vagus SØ4.89- ☑
      - specified type NEC SØ4.89- ☑
    - wrist (level) — *see* Injury, nerve, hand
  - ninth cranial nerve (glossopharyngeal) — *see* Injury, nerve, glossopharyngeal
  - nose (septum) SØ9.92 ☑
  - obstetrical O71.9
    - specified NEC O71.89
  - occipital (region) (scalp) SØ9.9Ø ☑
    - lobe — *see* Injury, intracranial
  - optic chiasm SØ4.Ø2 ☑
  - optic radiation SØ4.Ø3- ☑
  - optic tract and pathways SØ4.Ø3- ☑
  - orbit, orbital (region) — *see* Injury, eye
    - penetrating (with foreign body) — *see* Injury, eye, orbit, penetrating

- **Injury** — *continued*
  - orbit, orbital — *see* Injury, eye — *continued*
    - specified NEC — *see* Injury, eye, specified site NEC
  - ovary, ovarian S37.4Ø9 ☑
    - bilateral S37.4Ø2 ☑
      - contusion S37.422 ☑
      - laceration S37.432 ☑
      - specified type NEC S37.492 ☑
    - blood vessel — *see* Injury, blood vessel, ovarian
    - contusion S37.429 ☑
      - bilateral S37.422 ☑
      - unilateral S37.421 ☑
    - laceration S37.439 ☑
      - bilateral S37.432 ☑
      - unilateral S37.431 ☑
    - specified type NEC S37.499 ☑
      - bilateral S37.492 ☑
      - unilateral S37.491 ☑
    - unilateral S37.4Ø1 ☑
      - contusion S37.421 ☑
      - laceration S37.431 ☑
      - specified type NEC S37.491 ☑
  - palate (hard) (soft) SØ9.93 ☑
  - pancreas S36.2Ø9 ☑
    - body S36.2Ø1 ☑
      - contusion S36.221 ☑
      - laceration S36.231 ☑
        - major S36.261 ☑
        - minor S36.241 ☑
        - moderate S36.251 ☑
      - specified type NEC S36.291 ☑
    - contusion S36.229 ☑
    - head S36.2ØØ ☑
      - contusion S36.22Ø ☑
      - laceration S36.23Ø ☑
        - major S36.26Ø ☑
        - minor S36.24Ø ☑
        - moderate S36.25Ø ☑
      - specified type NEC S36.29Ø ☑
    - laceration S36.239 ☑
      - major S36.269 ☑
      - minor S36.249 ☑
      - moderate S36.259 ☑
    - specified type NEC S36.299 ☑
    - tail S36.2Ø2 ☑
      - contusion S36.222 ☑
      - laceration S36.232 ☑
        - major S36.262 ☑
        - minor S36.242 ☑
        - moderate S36.252 ☑
      - specified type NEC S36.292 ☑
  - parietal (region) (scalp) SØ9.9Ø ☑
    - lobe — *see* Injury, intracranial
  - patellar ligament (tendon) S76.1Ø- ☑
    - laceration S76.12- ☑
    - specified NEC S76.19- ☑
    - strain S76.11- ☑
  - pelvis, pelvic (floor) S39.93 ☑
    - complicating delivery O7Ø.1
    - joint or ligament, complicating delivery O71.6
    - organ S37.9Ø ☑
      - with ectopic or molar pregnancy OØ8.6
      - complication of abortion — *see* Abortion
      - contusion S37.92 ☑
      - following ectopic or molar pregnancy OØ8.6
      - laceration S37.93 ☑
      - obstetrical trauma NEC O71.5
      - specified
        - site NEC S37.899 ☑
          - contusion S37.892 ☑
          - laceration S37.893 ☑
          - specified type NEC S37.898 ☑
        - type NEC S37.99 ☑
    - specified NEC S39.83 ☑
  - penis S39.94 ☑
  - perineum S39.94 ☑
  - peritoneum S36.81 ☑
    - laceration S36.893 ☑
  - periurethral tissue — *see* Injury, urethra
    - complicating delivery O71.82
  - phalanges
    - foot — *see* Injury, foot
    - hand — *see* Injury, hand
  - pharynx NEC S19.85 ☑
  - pleura — *see* Injury, intrathoracic, pleura

Insufficiency, insufficient — *continued*
- pulmonary — *continued*
  - following
    - shock J98.4
    - trauma J98.4
  - newborn P28.89
  - valve I37.1
    - with stenosis I37.2
    - congenital Q22.2
    - rheumatic IØ9.89
      - with aortic, mitral or tricuspid (valve) disease IØ8.8
- pyloric K31.89
- renal (acute) N28.9
  - chronic N18.9
- respiratory RØ6.89
  - newborn P28.5
- rotation — *see* Malrotation
- sleep syndrome F51.12
- social insurance Z59.7
- suprarenal E27.4Ø
  - primary E27.1
- tarso-orbital fascia, congenital Q1Ø.3
- testis E29.1
- thyroid (gland) (acquired) EØ3.9
  - congenital EØ3.1
- tricuspid (valve) (rheumatic) IØ7.1
  - with
    - aortic (valve) disease IØ8.2
      - with mitral (valve) disease IØ8.3
    - mitral (valve) disease IØ8.1
      - with aortic (valve) disease IØ8.3
    - obstruction or stenosis IØ7.2
      - with aortic (valve) disease IØ8.2
        - with mitral (valve) disease IØ8.3
  - congenital Q22.8
  - nonrheumatic I36.1
    - with stenosis I36.2
- urethral sphincter R32
- valve, valvular (heart) I38
  - aortic — *see* Insufficiency, aortic (valve)
  - congenital Q24.8
  - mitral — *see* Insufficiency, mitral (valve)
  - pulmonary — *see* Insufficiency, pulmonary, valve
  - tricuspid — *see* Insufficiency, tricuspid (valve)
- vascular I99.8
  - intestine K55.9
    - acute — *see also* Ischemia, intestine, acute K55.Ø59
  - mesenteric K55.1
  - peripheral I73.9
  - renal — *see* Hypertension, kidney
- velopharyngeal
  - acquired K13.79
  - congenital Q38.8
- venous (chronic) (peripheral) I87.2
- ventricular — *see* Insufficiency, myocardial
- welfare support Z59.7

Insufflation, fallopian Z31.41

Insular — *see* condition

Insulinoma
- pancreas
  - benign D13.7
  - malignant C25.4
  - uncertain behavior D37.8
- specified site
  - benign — *see* Neoplasm, by site, benign
  - malignant — *see* Neoplasm, by site, malignant
  - uncertain behavior — *see* Neoplasm, by site, uncertain behavior
- unspecified site
  - benign D13.7
  - malignant C25.4
  - uncertain behavior D37.8

Insuloma — *see* Insulinoma

Interference
- balancing side M26.56
- non-working side M26.56

Intermenstrual — *see* condition

Intermittent — *see* condition

Internal — *see* condition

Interrogation
- cardiac defibrillator (automatic) (implantable) Z45.Ø2
- cardiac pacemaker Z45.Ø18
- cardiac (event) (loop) recorder Z45.Ø9
- infusion pump (implanted) (intrathecal) Z45.1
- neurostimulator Z46.2

Interruption
- aortic arch Q25.21
- bundle of His I44.3Ø
- phase-shift, sleep cycle — *see* Disorder, sleep, circadian rhythm
- sleep phase-shift, or 24 hour sleep-wake cycle — *see* Disorder, sleep, circadian rhythm

Interstitial — *see* condition

Intertrigo L3Ø.4
- labialis K13.Ø

Intervertebral disc — *see* condition

Intestine, intestinal — *see* condition

Intolerance
- carbohydrate K9Ø.49
- disaccharide, hereditary E73.Ø
- fat NEC K9Ø.49
  - pancreatic K9Ø.3
- food K9Ø.49
  - dietary counseling and surveillance Z71.3
- fructose E74.1Ø
  - hereditary E74.12
- glucose (-galactose) E74.39
- gluten K9Ø.41
- lactose E73.9
  - specified NEC E73.8
- lysine E72.3
- milk NEC K9Ø.49
  - lactose E73.9
- protein K9Ø.49
- starch NEC K9Ø.49
- sucrose (-isomaltose) E74.31

Intoxicated NEC (without dependence) — *see* Alcohol, intoxication

Intoxication
- acid E87.2
- alcoholic (acute) (without dependence) — *see* Alcohol, intoxication
- alimentary canal K52.1
- amphetamine (without dependence) — *see also* Abuse, drug, stimulant, with intoxication
  - with dependence — *see* Dependence, drug, stimulant, with intoxication
  - stimulant NEC F15.1Ø
    - with
      - anxiety disorder F15.18Ø
      - intoxication F15.129
        - with
          - delirium F15.121
          - perceptual disturbance F15.122
- anxiolytic (acute) (without dependence) — *see* Abuse, drug, sedative, with intoxication
  - with dependence — *see* Dependence, drug, sedative, with intoxication
- caffeine F15.929
  - with dependence — *see* Dependence, drug, stimulant, with intoxication
- cannabinoids (acute) (without dependence) — *see* Use, cannabis, with intoxication
  - with
    - abuse — *see* Abuse, drug, cannabis, with intoxication
    - dependence — *see* Dependence, drug, cannabis, with intoxication
- chemical — *see* Table of Drugs and Chemicals
  - via placenta or breast milk — *see* - Absorption, chemical, through placenta
- cocaine (acute) (without dependence) — *see* Abuse, drug, cocaine, with intoxication
  - with dependence — *see* Dependence, drug, cocaine, with intoxication
- drug
  - acute (without dependence) — *see* Abuse, drug, by type with intoxication
    - with dependence — *see* Dependence, drug, by type with intoxication
  - addictive
    - via placenta or breast milk — *see* Absorption, drug, addictive, through placenta
  - newborn P93.8
    - gray baby syndrome P93.Ø
  - overdose or wrong substance given or taken — *see* Table of Drugs and Chemicals, by drug, poisoning
- enteric K52.1
- foodborne AØ5.9
  - bacterial AØ5.9
  - classical (Clostridium botulinum) AØ5.1
  - due to
    - Bacillus cereus AØ5.4
    - bacterium AØ5.9
      - specified NEC AØ5.8
    - Clostridium
      - botulinum AØ5.1
      - perfringens AØ5.2
      - welchii AØ5.2
    - Salmonella AØ2.9
      - with
        - (gastro)enteritis AØ2.Ø
        - localized infection(s) AØ2.2Ø
          - arthritis AØ2.23
          - meningitis AØ2.21
          - osteomyelitis AØ2.24
          - pneumonia AØ2.22
          - pyelonephritis AØ2.25
          - specified NEC AØ2.29
        - sepsis AØ2.1
        - specified manifestation NEC AØ2.8
    - Staphylococcus AØ5.Ø
    - Vibrio
      - parahaemolyticus AØ5.3
      - vulnificus AØ5.5
  - enterotoxin, staphylococcal AØ5.Ø
  - noxious — *see* Poisoning, food, noxious
- gastrointestinal K52.1
- hallucinogenic (without dependence) — *see* Abuse, drug, hallucinogen, with intoxication
  - with dependence — *see* Dependence, drug, hallucinogen, with intoxication
- hypnotic (acute) (without dependence) — *see* Abuse, drug, sedative, with intoxication
  - with dependence — *see* Dependence, drug, sedative, with intoxication
- inhalant (acute) (without dependence) — *see* Abuse, drug, inhalant, with intoxication
  - with dependence — *see* Dependence, drug, inhalant, with intoxication
- meaning
  - inebriation — *see* category F1Ø ☑
  - poisoning — *see* Table of Drugs and Chemicals
- methyl alcohol (acute) (without dependence) — *see* Alcohol, intoxication
- opioid (acute) (without dependence) — *see* Abuse, drug, opioid, with intoxication
  - with dependence — *see* Dependence, drug, opioid, with intoxication
- pathologic NEC (without dependence) — *see* Alcohol, intoxication
- phencyclidine (without dependence) — *see* Abuse, drug, hallucinogen, with intoxication
  - with dependence — *see* Dependence, drug, hallucinogen, with intoxication
- potassium (K) E87.5
- psychoactive substance NEC (without dependence) — *see* Abuse, drug, psychoactive NEC, with intoxication
  - with dependence — *see* Dependence, drug, psychoactive NEC, with intoxication
- sedative (acute) (without dependence) — *see* Abuse, drug, sedative, with intoxication
  - with dependence — *see* Dependence, drug, sedative, with intoxication
- serum — *see also* Reaction, serum T8Ø.69 ☑
- uremic — *see* Uremia
- volatile solvents (acute) (without dependence) — *see* Abuse, drug, inhalant, with intoxication
  - with dependence — *see* Dependence, drug, inhalant, with intoxication
- water E87.79

Intraabdominal testis, testes
- bilateral Q53.211
- unilateral Q53.111

Intracranial — *see* condition

Intrahepatic gallbladder Q44.1

Intraligamentous — *see* condition

Intrathoracic — *see also* condition
- kidney Q63.2

Intrauterine contraceptive device
- checking Z3Ø.431
- in situ Z97.5
- insertion Z3Ø.43Ø
  - immediately following removal Z3Ø.433
- management Z3Ø.431
- reinsertion Z3Ø.433

- **Kaposi's**
  - dermatosis (xeroderma pigmentosum) Q82.1
  - lichen ruber L44.Ø
    - acuminatus L44.Ø
  - sarcoma
    - colon C46.4
    - connective tissue C46.1
    - gastrointestinal organ C46.4
    - lung C46.5- ☑
    - lymph node (multiple) C46.3
    - palate (hard) (soft) C46.2
    - rectum C46.4
    - skin (multiple sites) C46.Ø
    - specified site NEC C46.7
    - stomach C46.4
    - unspecified site C46.9
  - varicelliform eruption BØØ.Ø
    - vaccinia T88.1 ☑
- **Kartagener's syndrome or triad** (sinusitis, bronchiectasis, situs inversus) Q89.3
- **Karyotype**
  - with abnormality except iso (Xq) Q96.2
  - 45,X Q96.Ø
  - 46,X
    - iso (Xq) Q96.1
  - 46,XX Q98.3
    - with streak gonads Q5Ø.32
    - hermaphrodite (true) Q99.1
    - male Q98.3
  - 46,XY
    - with streak gonads Q56.1
    - female Q97.3
    - hermaphrodite (true) Q99.1
  - 47,XXX Q97.Ø
  - 47,XXY Q98.Ø
  - 47,XYY Q98.5
- **Kaschin-Beck disease** — *see* Disease, Kaschin-Beck
- **Katayama's disease or fever** B65.2
- **Kawasaki's syndrome** M3Ø.3
- **Kayser-Fleischer ring** (cornea) (pseudosclerosis) H18.Ø4- ☑
- **Kaznelson's syndrome** (congenital hypoplastic anemia) D61.Ø1
- **Kearns-Sayre syndrome** H49.81- ☑
- **Kedani fever** A75.3
- **Kelis** L91.Ø
- **Kelly** (-Patterson) **syndrome** (sideropenic dysphagia) D5Ø.1
- **Keloid, cheloid** L91.Ø
  - acne L73.Ø
  - Addison's L94.Ø
  - cornea — *see* Opacity, cornea
  - Hawkin's L91.Ø
  - scar L91.Ø
- **Keloma** L91.Ø
- **Kenya fever** A77.1
- **Keratectasia** — *see also* Ectasia, cornea
  - congenital Q13.4
- **Keratinization of alveolar ridge mucosa**
  - excessive K13.23
  - minimal K13.22
- **Keratinized residual ridge mucosa**
  - excessive K13.23
  - minimal K13.22
- **Keratitis** (nodular) (nonulcerative) (simple) (zonular) H16.9
  - with ulceration (central) (marginal) (perforated) (ring) — *see* Ulcer, cornea
  - actinic — *see* Photokeratitis
  - arborescens (herpes simplex) BØØ.52
  - areolar H16.11- ☑
  - bullosa H16.8
  - deep H16.3Ø9
    - specified type NEC H16.399
  - dendritic (a) (herpes simplex) BØØ.52
  - disciform (is) (herpes simplex) BØØ.52
    - varicella BØ1.81
  - filamentary H16.12- ☑
  - gonococcal (congenital or prenatal) A54.33
  - herpes, herpetic (simplex) BØØ.52
    - zoster BØ2.33
  - in (due to)
    - acanthamebiasis B6Ø.13
    - adenovirus B3Ø.Ø
    - exanthema — *see also* Exanthem BØ9
    - herpes (simplex) virus BØØ.52
    - measles BØ5.81
    - syphilis A5Ø.31

- **Keratitis** — *continued*
  - in — *continued*
    - tuberculosis A18.52
    - zoster BØ2.33
  - interstitial (nonsyphilitic) H16.3Ø- ☑
    - diffuse H16.32- ☑
    - herpes, herpetic (simplex) BØØ.52
      - zoster BØ2.33
    - sclerosing H16.33- ☑
    - specified type NEC H16.39- ☑
    - syphilitic (congenital) (late) A5Ø.31
    - tuberculous A18.52
  - macular H16.11- ☑
  - nummular H16.11- ☑
  - oyster shuckers' H16.8
  - parenchymatous — *see* Keratitis, interstitial
  - petrificans H16.8
  - postmeasles BØ5.81
  - punctata
    - leprosa A3Ø.9 *[H16.14-]* ☑
    - syphilitic (profunda) A5Ø.31
  - punctate H16.14- ☑
  - purulent H16.8
  - rosacea L71.8
  - sclerosing H16.33- ☑
  - specified type NEC H16.8
  - stellate H16.11- ☑
  - striate H16.11- ☑
  - superficial H16.1Ø- ☑
    - with conjunctivitis — *see* Keratoconjunctivitis
    - due to light — *see* Photokeratitis
  - suppurative H16.8
  - syphilitic (congenital) (prenatal) A5Ø.31
  - trachomatous A71.1
    - sequelae B94.Ø
  - tuberculous A18.52
  - vesicular H16.8
  - xerotic — *see also* Keratomalacia H16.8
    - vitamin A deficiency E5Ø.4
- **Keratoacanthoma** L85.8
- **Keratocele** — *see* Descemetocele
- **Keratoconjunctivitis** H16.2Ø- ☑
  - Acanthamoeba B6Ø.13
  - adenoviral B3Ø.Ø
  - epidemic B3Ø.Ø
  - exposure H16.21- ☑
  - herpes, herpetic (simplex) BØØ.52
    - zoster BØ2.33
  - in exanthema — *see also* Exanthem BØ9
  - infectious B3Ø.Ø
  - lagophthalmic — *see* Keratoconjunctivitis, specified type NEC
  - neurotrophic H16.23- ☑
  - phlyctenular H16.25- ☑
  - postmeasles BØ5.81
  - shipyard B3Ø.Ø
  - sicca (Sjogren's) M35.Ø- ☑
    - not Sjogren's H16.22- ☑
  - specified type NEC H16.29- ☑
  - tuberculous (phlyctenular) A18.52
  - vernal H16.26- ☑
- **Keratoconus** H18.6Ø- ☑
  - congenital Q13.4
  - stable H18.61- ☑
  - unstable H18.62- ☑
- **Keratocyst** (dental) (odontogenic) — *see* Cyst, calcifying odontogenic
- **Keratoderma, keratodermia** (congenital) (palmaris et plantaris) (symmetrical) Q82.8
  - acquired L85.1
    - in diseases classified elsewhere L86
  - climactericum L85.1
  - gonococcal A54.89
  - gonorrheal A54.89
  - punctata L85.2
  - Reiter's — *see* Reiter's disease
- **Keratodermatocele** — *see* Descemetocele
- **Keratoglobus** H18.79 ☑
  - congenital Q15.8
    - with glaucoma Q15.Ø
- **Keratohemia** — *see* Pigmentation, cornea, stromal
- **Keratoiritis** — *see also* Iridocyclitis
  - syphilitic A5Ø.39
  - tuberculous A18.54
- **Keratoma** L57.Ø
  - palmaris and plantaris hereditarium Q82.8
  - senile L57.Ø

- **Keratomalacia** H18.44- ☑
  - vitamin A deficiency E5Ø.4
- **Keratomegaly** Q13.4
- **Keratomycosis** B49
  - nigrans, nigricans (palmaris) B36.1
- **Keratopathy** H18.9
  - band H18.42- ☑
  - bullous (aphakic), following cataract surgery H59.Ø1- ☑
  - bullous H18.1- ☑
- **Keratoscleritis, tuberculous** A18.52
- **Keratosis** L57.Ø
  - actinic L57.Ø
  - arsenical L85.8
  - congenital, specified NEC Q8Ø.8
  - female genital NEC N94.89
  - follicularis Q82.8
    - acquired L11.Ø
    - congenita Q82.8
    - et parafollicularis in cutem penetrans L87.Ø
    - spinulosa (decalvans) Q82.8
    - vitamin A deficiency E5Ø.8
  - gonococcal A54.89
  - male genital (external) N5Ø.89
  - nigricans L83
  - obturans, external ear (canal) — *see* Cholesteatoma, external ear
  - palmaris et plantaris (inherited) (symmetrical) Q82.8
    - acquired L85.1
  - penile N48.89
  - pharynx J39.2
  - pilaris, acquired L85.8
  - punctata (palmaris et plantaris) L85.2
  - scrotal N5Ø.89
  - seborrheic L82.1
    - inflamed L82.Ø
  - senile L57.Ø
  - solar L57.Ø
  - tonsillaris J35.8
  - vagina N89.4
  - vegetans Q82.8
  - vitamin A deficiency E5Ø.8
  - vocal cord J38.3
- **Kerato-uveitis** — *see* Iridocyclitis
- **Kerion** (celsi) B35.Ø
- **Kernicterus of newborn** (not due to isoimmunization) P57.9
  - due to isoimmunization (conditions in P55.Ø-P55.9) P57.Ø
  - specified type NEC P57.8
- **Kerunoparalysis** T75.Ø9 ☑
- **Keshan disease** E59
- **Ketoacidosis** E87.2
  - diabetic — *see* Diabetes, by type, with ketoacidosis
- **Ketonuria** R82.4
- **Ketosis NEC** E88.89
  - diabetic — *see* Diabetes, by type, with ketoacidosis
- **Kew Garden fever** A79.1
- **Kidney** — *see* condition
- **Kienböck's disease** — *see also* Osteochondrosis, juvenile, hand, carpal lunate
  - adult M93.1
- **Kimmelstiel** (-Wilson) **disease** — *see* Diabetes, Kimmelstiel (-Wilson) disease
- **Kink, kinking**
  - artery I77.1
  - hair (acquired) L67.8
  - ileum or intestine — *see* Obstruction, intestine
  - Lane's — *see* Obstruction, intestine
  - organ or site, congenital NEC — *see* Anomaly, by site
  - ureter (pelvic junction) N13.5
    - with
      - hydronephrosis N13.1
        - with infection N13.6
      - pyelonephritis (chronic) N11.1
    - congenital Q62.39
  - vein(s) I87.8
    - caval I87.1
      - peripheral I87.1
- **Kinnier Wilson's disease** (hepatolenticular degeneration) E83.Ø1
- **Kissing spine** M48.2Ø
  - cervical region M48.22
  - cervicothoracic region M48.23
  - lumbar region M48.26
  - lumbosacral region M48.27
  - occipito-atlanto-axial region M48.21
  - thoracic region M48.24
  - thoracolumbar region M48.25

Klatskin's tumor C22.1
Klauder's disease A26.8
Klebs' disease — *see also* Glomerulonephritis N05- ☑
Klebsiella (K.) **pneumoniae, as cause of disease classified elsewhere** B96.1
Klein (e)-**Levin syndrome** G47.13
Kleptomania F63.2
Klinefelter's syndrome Q98.4
  karyotype 47,XXY Q98.0
  male with more than two X chromosomes Q98.1
Klippel-Feil deficiency, disease, or syndrome (brevicollis) Q76.1
Klippel's disease I67.2
Klippel-Trenaunay (-Weber) **syndrome** Q87.2
Klumpke (-Déjerine) **palsy, paralysis** (birth) (newborn) P14.1
Knee — *see* condition
Knock knee (acquired) M21.06- ☑
  congenital Q74.1
Knot(s)
  intestinal, syndrome (volvulus) K56.2
  surfer S89.8- ☑
  umbilical cord (true) O69.2 ☑
Knotting (of)
  hair L67.8
  intestine K56.2
Knuckle pad (Garrod's) M72.1
Koch's
  infection — *see* Tuberculosis
  relapsing fever A68.9
Koch-Weeks' conjunctivitis — *see* Conjunctivitis, acute, mucopurulent
Köebner's syndrome Q81.8
Köenig's disease (osteochondritis dissecans) — *see* Osteochondritis, dissecans
Köhler-Pellegrini-Steida disease or syndrome (calcification, knee joint) — *see* Bursitis, tibial collateral
Köhler's disease
  patellar — *see* Osteochondrosis, juvenile, patella
  tarsal navicular — *see* Osteochondrosis, juvenile, tarsus
Koilonychia L60.3
  congenital Q84.6
Kojevnikov's, epilepsy — *see* Kozhevnikof's epilepsy
Koplik's spots B05.9
Kopp's asthma E32.8
Korsakoff's (Wernicke) **disease, psychosis or syndrome** (alcoholic) F10.96
  with dependence F10.26
  drug-induced
    due to drug abuse — *see* Abuse, drug, by type, with amnestic disorder
    due to drug dependence — *see* Dependence, drug, by type, with amnestic disorder
  nonalcoholic F04
Korsakov's disease, psychosis or syndrome — *see* Korsakoff's disease
Korsakow's disease, psychosis or syndrome — *see* Korsakoff's disease
Kostmann's disease or syndrome (infantile genetic agranulocytosis) — *see* Agranulocytosis
Kozhevnikof's epilepsy G40.109
  intractable G40.119
    with status epilepticus G40.111
    without status epilepticus G40.119
  not intractable G40.109
    with status epilepticus G40.101
    without status epilepticus G40.109
Krabbe's
  disease E75.23
  syndrome, congenital muscle hypoplasia Q79.8
Kraepelin-Morel disease — *see* Schizophrenia
Kraft-Weber-Dimitri disease Q85.8
Kraurosis
  ani K62.89
  penis N48.0
  vagina N89.8
  vulva N90.4
Kreotoxism A05.9
Krukenberg's
  spindle — *see* Pigmentation, cornea, posterior
  tumor C79.6- ☑
Kufs' disease E75.4
Kugelberg-Welander disease G12.1
Kuhnt-Junius degeneration — *see also* Degeneration, macula H35.32- ☑
Kümmell's disease or spondylitis — *see* Spondylopathy, traumatic
Kupffer cell sarcoma C22.3
Kuru A81.81
Kussmaul's
  disease M30.0
  respiration E87.2
    in diabetic acidosis — *see* Diabetes, by type, with ketoacidosis
Kwashiorkor E40
  marasmic, marasmus type E42
Kyasanur Forest disease A98.2
Kyphoscoliosis, kyphoscoliotic (acquired) — *see also* Scoliosis M41.9
  congenital Q67.5
  heart (disease) I27.1
  sequelae of rickets E64.3
  tuberculous A18.01
Kyphosis, kyphotic (acquired) M40.209
  cervical region M40.202
  cervicothoracic region M40.203
  congenital Q76.419
    cervical region Q76.412
    cervicothoracic region Q76.413
    occipito-atlanto-axial region Q76.411
    thoracic region Q76.414
    thoracolumbar region Q76.415
  Morquio-Brailsford type (spinal) — *see also* subcategory M49.8 E76.219
  postlaminectomy M96.3
  postradiation therapy M96.2
  postural (adolescent) M40.00
    cervicothoracic region M40.03
    thoracic region M40.04
    thoracolumbar region M40.05
  secondary NEC M40.10
    cervical region M40.12
    cervicothoracic region M40.13
    thoracic region M40.14
    thoracolumbar region M40.15
  sequelae of rickets E64.3
  specified type NEC M40.299
    cervical region M40.292
    cervicothoracic region M40.293
    thoracic region M40.294
    thoracolumbar region M40.295
  syphilitic, congenital A50.56
  thoracic region M40.204
  thoracolumbar region M40.205
  tuberculous A18.01
Kyrle disease L87.0

L

Labia, labium — *see* condition
Labile
  blood pressure R09.89
  vasomotor system I73.9
Labioglossal paralysis G12.29
Labium leporinum — *see* Cleft, lip
Labor — *see* Delivery
Labored breathing — *see* Hyperventilation
Labyrinthitis (circumscribed) (destructive) (diffuse) (inner ear) (latent) (purulent) (suppurative) — *see also* subcategory H83.0 ☑
  syphilitic A52.79
Laceration
  with abortion — *see* Abortion, by type, complicated by laceration of pelvic organs
  abdomen, abdominal
    wall S31.119 ☑
      with
        foreign body S31.129 ☑
        penetration into peritoneal cavity S31.619 ☑
          with foreign body S31.629 ☑
      epigastric region S31.112 ☑
        with
          foreign body S31.122 ☑
          penetration into peritoneal cavity S31.612 ☑
            with foreign body S31.622 ☑
      left
        lower quadrant S31.114 ☑
          with
            foreign body S31.124 ☑
            penetration into peritoneal cavity S31.614 ☑
              with foreign body S31.624 ☑
        upper quadrant S31.111 ☑

Laceration — *continued*
  abdomen, abdominal — *continued*
    wall — *continued*
      left — *continued*
        upper quadrant — *continued*
          with
            foreign body S31.121 ☑
            penetration into peritoneal cavity S31.611 ☑
              with foreign body S31.621 ☑
      periumbilic region S31.115 ☑
        with
          foreign body S31.125 ☑
          penetration into peritoneal cavity S31.615 ☑
            with foreign body S31.625 ☑
      right
        lower quadrant S31.113 ☑
          with
            foreign body S31.123 ☑
            penetration into peritoneal cavity S31.613 ☑
              with foreign body S31.623 ☑
        upper quadrant S31.110 ☑
          with
            foreign body S31.120 ☑
            penetration into peritoneal cavity S31.610 ☑
              with foreign body S31.620 ☑
  accidental, complicating surgery — *see* Complications, surgical, accidental puncture or laceration
  Achilles tendon S86.02- ☑
  adrenal gland S37.813 ☑
  alveolar (process) — *see* Laceration, oral cavity
  ankle S91.01- ☑
    with
      foreign body S91.02- ☑
  antecubital space — *see* Laceration, elbow
  anus (sphincter) S31.831 ☑
    with
      ectopic or molar pregnancy O08.6
      foreign body S31.832 ☑
    complicating delivery — *see* Delivery, complicated, by, laceration, anus (sphincter)
    following ectopic or molar pregnancy O08.6
    nontraumatic, nonpuerperal — *see* Fissure, anus
  arm (upper) S41.11- ☑
    with foreign body S41.12- ☑
    lower — *see* Laceration, forearm
  auditory canal (external) (meatus) — *see* Laceration, ear
  auricle, ear — *see* Laceration, ear
  axilla — *see* Laceration, arm
  back — *see also* Laceration, thorax, back
    lower S31.010 ☑
      with
        foreign body S31.020 ☑
          with penetration into retroperitoneal space S31.021 ☑
        penetration into retroperitoneal space S31.011 ☑
  bile duct S36.13 ☑
  bladder S37.23 ☑
    with ectopic or molar pregnancy O08.6
    following ectopic or molar pregnancy O08.6
    obstetrical trauma O71.5
  blood vessel — *see* Injury, blood vessel
  bowel — *see also* Laceration, intestine
    with ectopic or molar pregnancy O08.6
    complicating abortion — *see* Abortion, by type, complicated by, specified condition NEC
    following ectopic or molar pregnancy O08.6
    obstetrical trauma O71.5
  brain (any part) (cortex) (diffuse) (membrane) — *see also* Injury, intracranial, diffuse
    during birth P10.8
      with hemorrhage P10.1
    focal — *see* Injury, intracranial, focal brain injury
  brainstem S06.38- ☑
  breast S21.01- ☑
    with foreign body S21.02- ☑
  broad ligament S37.893 ☑
    with ectopic or molar pregnancy O08.6
    following ectopic or molar pregnancy O08.6
    laceration syndrome N83.8
    obstetrical trauma O71.6
    syndrome (laceration) N83.8

Laceration — *continued*
- toe(s) — *continued*
  - lesser — *continued*
    - with — *continued*
      - foreign body S91.126 ☑
    - left S91.115 ☑
      - with
        - damage to nail S91.215 ☑
          - with
            - foreign body S91.225 ☑
        - foreign body S91.125 ☑
    - right S91.114 ☑
      - with
        - damage to nail S91.214 ☑
          - with
            - foreign body S91.224 ☑
        - foreign body S91.124 ☑
- tongue — *see* Laceration, oral cavity
- trachea S11.Ø21 ☑
  - with foreign body S11.Ø22 ☑
- tunica vaginalis — *see* Laceration, testis
- tympanum, tympanic membrane — *see* Laceration, ear, drum
- umbilical region S31.115 ☑
  - with foreign body S31.125 ☑
- ureter S37.13 ☑
- urethra S37.33 ☑
  - with or following ectopic or molar pregnancy OØ8.6
  - obstetrical trauma O71.5
- urinary organ NEC S37.893 ☑
- uterus S37.63 ☑
  - with ectopic or molar pregnancy OØ8.6
  - following ectopic or molar pregnancy OØ8.6
  - nonpuerperal, nontraumatic N85.8
  - obstetrical trauma NEC O71.81
  - old (postpartal) N85.8
- uvula — *see* Laceration, oral cavity
- vagina S31.41 ☑
  - with
    - ectopic or molar pregnancy OØ8.6
    - foreign body S31.42 ☑
  - during delivery O71.4
    - with perineal laceration — *see* Laceration, perineum, female, during delivery
  - following ectopic or molar pregnancy OØ8.6
  - nonpuerperal, nontraumatic N89.8
  - old (postpartal) N89.8
- vas deferens S37.893 ☑
- vesical — *see* Laceration, bladder
- vocal cords S11.Ø31 ☑
  - with foreign body S11.Ø32 ☑
- vulva S31.41 ☑
  - with
    - ectopic or molar pregnancy OØ8.6
    - foreign body S31.42 ☑
  - complicating delivery O7Ø.Ø
  - following ectopic or molar pregnancy OØ8.6
  - nonpuerperal, nontraumatic N9Ø.89
  - old (postpartal) N9Ø.89
- wrist S61.519 ☑
  - with
    - foreign body S61.529 ☑
  - left S61.512 ☑
    - with
      - foreign body S61.522 ☑
  - right S61.511 ☑
    - with
      - foreign body S61.521 ☑

Lack of
- achievement in school Z55.3
- adequate
  - food Z59.4
  - intermaxillary vertical dimension of fully erupted teeth M26.36
  - sleep Z72.82Ø
- appetite (see Anorexia) R63.Ø
- awareness R41.9
- care
  - in home Z74.2
  - of infant (at or after birth) T76.Ø2 ☑
    - confirmed T74.Ø2 ☑
- cognitive functions R41.9
- coordination R27.9
  - ataxia R27.Ø
  - specified type NEC R27.8
- development (physiological) R62.5Ø
  - failure to thrive (child over 28 days old) R62.51

Lack of — *continued*
- development — *continued*
  - failure to thrive — *continued*
    - adult R62.7
    - newborn P92.6
  - short stature R62.52
  - specified type NEC R62.59
- energy R53.83
- financial resources Z59.6
- food T73.Ø ☑
- growth R62.52
- heating Z59.1
- housing (permanent) (temporary) Z59.Ø
  - adequate Z59.1
- learning experiences in childhood Z62.898
- leisure time (affecting life-style) Z73.2
- material resources Z59.9
- memory — *see also* Amnesia
  - mild, following organic brain damage FØ6.8
- ovulation N97.Ø
- parental supervision or control of child Z62.Ø
- person able to render necessary care Z74.2
- physical exercise Z72.3
- play experience in childhood Z62.898
- posterior occlusal support M26.57
- relaxation (affecting life-style) Z73.2
- sexual
  - desire F52.Ø
  - enjoyment F52.1
- shelter Z59.Ø
- sleep (adequate) Z72.82Ø
- supervision of child by parent Z62.Ø
- support, posterior occlusal M26.57
- water T73.1 ☑

Lacrimal — *see* condition

Lacrimation, abnormal — *see* Epiphora

Lacrimonasal duct — *see* condition

Lactation, lactating (breast) (puerperal, postpartum)
- associated
  - cracked nipple O92.13
  - retracted nipple O92.Ø3
- defective O92.4
- disorder NEC O92.79
- excessive O92.6
- failed (complete) O92.3
  - partial O92.4
- mastitis NEC — *see* Mastitis, obstetric
- mother (care and/or examination) Z39.1
- nonpuerperal N64.3

Lacticemia, excessive E87.2

Lacunar skull Q75.8

Laennec's cirrhosis K7Ø.3Ø
- with ascites K7Ø.31
- nonalcoholic K74.69

Lafora's disease — *see* Epilepsy, generalized, idiopathic

Lag, lid (nervous) — *see* Retraction, lid

Lagophthalmos (eyelid) (nervous) HØ2.2Ø9
- bilateral, upper and lower eyelids HØ2.2ØC
- cicatricial HØ2.219
  - bilateral, upper and lower eyelids HØ2.21C
  - left HØ2.216
    - lower HØ2.215
    - upper HØ2.214
    - upper and lower eyelids HØ2.21B
  - right HØ2.213
    - lower HØ2.212
    - upper HØ2.211
    - upper and lower eyelids HØ2.21A
- keratoconjunctivitis — *see* Keratoconjunctivitis
- left HØ2.2Ø6
  - lower HØ2.2Ø5
  - upper HØ2.2Ø4
  - upper and lower eyelids HØ2.2ØB
- mechanical HØ2.229
  - bilateral, upper and lower eyelids HØ2.22C
  - left HØ2.226
    - lower HØ2.225
    - upper HØ2.224
    - upper and lower eyelids HØ2.22B
  - right HØ2.223
    - lower HØ2.222
    - upper HØ2.221
    - upper and lower eyelids HØ2.22A
- paralytic HØ2.239
  - bilateral, upper and lower eyelids HØ2.23C
  - left HØ2.236
    - lower HØ2.235
    - upper HØ2.234

Lagophthalmos — *continued*
- paralytic — *continued*
  - left — *continued*
    - upper and lower eyelids HØ2.23B
  - right HØ2.233
    - lower HØ2.232
    - upper HØ2.231
    - upper and lower eyelids HØ2.23A
- right HØ2.2Ø3
  - lower HØ2.2Ø2
  - upper HØ2.2Ø1
  - upper and lower eyelids HØ2.2ØA

Laki-Lorand factor deficiency — *see* Defect, coagulation, specified type NEC

Lalling F8Ø.Ø

Lambert-Eaton syndrome — *see* Syndrome, Lambert-Eaton

Lambliasis, lambliosis AØ7.1

Landau-Kleffner syndrome — *see* Epilepsy, specified NEC

Landouzy-Déjérine dystrophy or facioscapulohumeral atrophy G71.Ø2

Landouzy's disease (icterohemorrhagic leptospirosis) A27.Ø

Landry-Guillain-Barré, syndrome or paralysis G61.Ø

Landry's disease or paralysis G61.Ø

Lane's
- band Q43.3
- kink — *see* Obstruction, intestine
- syndrome K9Ø.2

Langdon Down syndrome — *see* Trisomy, 21

Lapsed immunization schedule status Z28.3

Large
- baby (regardless of gestational age) (4ØØØg to 4499g) PØ8.1
- ear, congenital Q17.1
- physiological cup Q14.2
- stature R68.89

Large-for-dates NEC (infant) (4ØØØg to 4499g) PØ8.1
- affecting management of pregnancy O36.6- ☑
- exceptionally (45ØØg or more) PØ8.Ø

Larsen-Johansson disease orosteochondrosis — *see* Osteochondrosis, juvenile, patella

Larsen's syndrome (flattened facies and multiple congenital dislocations) Q74.8

Larva migrans
- cutaneous B76.9
  - Ancylostoma B76.Ø
- visceral B83.Ø

Laryngeal — *see* condition

Laryngismus (stridulus) J38.5
- congenital P28.89
- diphtheritic A36.2

Laryngitis (acute) (edematous) (fibrinous) (infective) (infiltrative) (malignant) (membranous) (phlegmonous) (pneumococcal) (pseudomembranous) (septic) (subglottic) (suppurative) (ulcerative) JØ4.Ø
- with
  - influenza, flu, or grippe — *see* Influenza, with, laryngitis
  - tracheitis (acute) — *see* Laryngotracheitis
- atrophic J37.Ø
- catarrhal J37.Ø
- chronic J37.Ø
  - with tracheitis (chronic) J37.1
- diphtheritic A36.2
- due to external agent — *see* Inflammation, respiratory, upper, due to
- H. influenzae JØ4.Ø
- Hemophilus influenzae JØ4.Ø
- hypertrophic J37.Ø
- influenzal — *see* Influenza, with, respiratory manifestations NEC
- obstructive JØ5.Ø
- sicca J37.Ø
- spasmodic JØ5.Ø
  - acute JØ4.Ø
- streptococcal JØ4.Ø
- stridulous JØ5.Ø
- syphilitic (late) A52.73
  - congenital A5Ø.59 *[J99]*
    - early A5Ø.Ø3 *[J99]*
- tuberculous A15.5
- Vincent's A69.1

Laryngocele (congenital) (ventricular) Q31.3

Laryngofissure J38.7
- congenital Q31.8

Laryngomalacia (congenital) Q31.5

Laryngopharyngitis (acute) J06.0
- chronic J37.0
- due to external agent — *see* Inflammation, respiratory, upper, due to

Laryngoplegia J38.00
- bilateral J38.02
- unilateral J38.01

Laryngoptosis J38.7

Laryngospasm J38.5

Laryngostenosis J38.6

Laryngotracheitis (acute) (Infectional) (infective) (viral) J04.2
- atrophic J37.1
- catarrhal J37.1
- chronic J37.1
- diphtheritic A36.2
- due to external agent — *see* Inflammation, respiratory, upper, due to
- Hemophilus influenzae J04.2
- hypertrophic J37.1
- influenzal — *see* Influenza, with, respiratory manifestations NEC
- pachydermic J38.7
- sicca J37.1
- spasmodic J38.5
  - acute J05.0
- streptococcal J04.2
- stridulous J38.5
- syphilitic (late) A52.73
  - congenital A50.59 *[J99]*
    - early A50.03 *[J99]*
- tuberculous A15.5
- Vincent's A69.1

Laryngotracheobronchitis — *see* Bronchitis

Larynx, laryngeal — *see* condition

Lassa fever A96.2

Lassitude — *see* Weakness

Late
- talker R62.0
- walker R62.0

Late effect(s) — *see* Sequelae

Latent — *see* condition

Laterocession — *see* Lateroversion

Lateroflexion — *see* Lateroversion

Lateroversion
- cervix — *see* Lateroversion, uterus
- uterus, uterine (cervix) (postinfectional) (postpartal, old) N85.4
  - congenital Q51.818
  - in pregnancy or childbirth O34.59- ☑

Lathyrism — *see* Poisoning, food, noxious, plant

Launois' syndrome (pituitary gigantism) E22.0

Launois-Bensaude adenolipomatosis E88.89

Laurence-Moon (-Bardet)-**Biedl syndrome** Q87.89

Lax, laxity — *see also* Relaxation
- ligament (ous) — *see also* Disorder, ligament
  - familial M35.7
  - knee — *see* Derangement, knee
- skin (acquired) L57.4
  - congenital Q82.8

Laxative habit F55.2

Lazy leukocyte syndrome D70.8

Lead miner's lung J63.6

Leak, leakage
- air NEC J93.82
  - postprocedural J95.812
- amniotic fluid — *see* Rupture, membranes, premature
- blood (microscopic), fetal, into maternal circulation affecting management of pregnancy — *see* Pregnancy, complicated by
- cerebrospinal fluid G96.00
  - cranial
    - postoperative G96.08
    - specified NEC G96.08
    - spontaneous G96.01
    - traumatic G96.08
  - from spinal (lumbar) puncture G97.0
  - spinal
    - postoperative G96.09
    - post-traumatic G96.09
    - specified NEC G96.09
    - spontaneous G96.02
  - spontaneous
    - from
      - skull base G96.01
      - spine G96.02
- CSF — *see* Leak, cerebrospinal fluid

Leak, leakage — *continued*
- device, implant or graft — *see also* Complications, by site and type, mechanical
  - arterial graft NEC — *see* Complication, cardiovascular device, mechanical, vascular
  - breast (implant) T85.43 ☑
  - catheter NEC T85.638 ☑
    - dialysis (renal) T82.43 ☑
      - intraperitoneal T85.631 ☑
    - infusion NEC T82.534 ☑
      - spinal (epidural) (subdural) T85.630 ☑
    - urinary T83.038 ☑
      - cystostomy T83.030 ☑
      - Hopkins T83.038 ☑
      - ileostomy T83.038 ☑
      - indwelling T83.031 ☑
      - nephrostomy T83.032 ☑
      - specified T83.038 ☑
      - urostomy T83.038 ☑
  - gastrointestinal — *see* Complications, prosthetic device, mechanical, gastrointestinal device
  - genital NEC T83.498 ☑
    - penile prosthesis (cylinder) (implanted) (pump) (reservoir) T83.490 ☑
    - testicular prosthesis T83.491 ☑
  - heart NEC — *see* Complication, cardiovascular device, mechanical
  - joint prosthesis — *see* Complications, joint prosthesis, mechanical, specified NEC, by site
  - ocular NEC — *see* Complications, prosthetic device, mechanical, ocular device
  - orthopedic NEC — *see* Complication, orthopedic, device, mechanical
  - persistent air J93.82
  - specified NEC T85.638 ☑
  - urinary NEC — *see also* Complication, genitourinary, device, urinary, mechanical
    - graft T83.23 ☑
  - vascular NEC — *see* Complication, cardiovascular device, mechanical
  - ventricular intracranial shunt T85.03 ☑
- urine — *see* Incontinence

Leaky heart — *see* Endocarditis

Learning defect (specific) F81.9

Leather bottle stomach C16.9

Leber's
- congenital amaurosis H35.50
- optic atrophy (hereditary) H47.22

Lederer's anemia D59.19

Leeches (external) — *see* Hirudiniasis

Leg — *see* condition

Legg (-Calvé)-**Perthes disease, syndrome or osteochondrosis** M91.1- ☑

Legionellosis A48.1
- nonpneumonic A48.2

Legionnaires'
- disease A48.1
  - nonpneumonic A48.2
- pneumonia A48.1

Leigh's disease G31.82

Leiner's disease L21.1

Leiofibromyoma — *see* Leiomyoma

Leiomyoblastoma — *see* Neoplasm, connective tissue, benign

Leiomyofibroma — *see also* Neoplasm, connective tissue, benign
- uterus (cervix) (corpus) D25.9

Leiomyoma — *see also* Neoplasm, connective tissue, benign
- bizarre — *see* Neoplasm, connective tissue, benign
- cellular — *see* Neoplasm, connective tissue, benign
- epithelioid — *see* Neoplasm, connective tissue, benign
- uterus (cervix) (corpus) D25.9
  - intramural D25.1
  - submucous D25.0
  - subserosal D25.2
- vascular — *see* Neoplasm, connective tissue, benign

Leiomyoma, leiomyomatosis (intravascular) — *see* Neoplasm, connective tissue, uncertain behavior

Leiomyosarcoma — *see also* Neoplasm, connective tissue, malignant
- epithelioid — *see* Neoplasm, connective tissue, malignant
- myxoid — *see* Neoplasm, connective tissue, malignant

Leishmaniasis B55.9
- American (mucocutaneous) B55.2
  - cutaneous B55.1

Leishmaniasis — *continued*
- Asian Desert B55.1
- Brazilian B55.2
- cutaneous (any type) B55.1
- dermal — *see also* Leishmaniasis, cutaneous
  - post-kala-azar B55.0
- eyelid B55.1
- infantile B55.0
- Mediterranean B55.0
- mucocutaneous (American) (New World) B55.2
- naso-oral B55.2
- nasopharyngeal B55.2
- old world B55.1
- tegumentaria diffusa B55.1
- visceral B55.0

Leishmanoid, dermal — *see also* Leishmaniasis, cutaneous
- post-kala-azar B55.0

Lenegre's disease I44.2

Lengthening, leg — *see* Deformity, limb, unequal length

Lennert's lymphoma — *see* Lymphoma, Lennert's

Lennox-Gastaut syndrome G40.812
- intractable G40.814
  - with status epilepticus G40.813
  - without status epilepticus G40.814
- not intractable G40.812
  - with status epilepticus G40.811
  - without status epilepticus G40.812

Lens — *see* condition

Lenticonus (anterior) (posterior) (congenital) Q12.8

Lenticular degeneration, progressive E83.01

Lentiglobus (posterior) (congenital) Q12.8

Lentigo (congenital) L81.4
- maligna — *see also* Melanoma, in situ
  - melanoma — *see* Melanoma

Lentivirus, as cause of disease classified elsewhere B97.31

Leontiasis
- ossium M85.2
- syphilitic (late) A52.78
  - congenital A50.59

Lepothrix A48.8

Lepra — *see* Leprosy

Leprechaunism E34.8

Leprosy A30.- ☑
- with muscle disorder A30.9 *[M63.80]*
  - ankle A30.9 *[M63.87-]* ☑
  - foot A30.9 *[M63.87-]* ☑
  - forearm A30.9 *[M63.83-]* ☑
  - hand A30.9 *[M63.84-]* ☑
  - lower leg A30.9 *[M63.86-]* ☑
  - multiple sites A30.9 *[M63.89]*
  - pelvic region A30.9 *[M63.85-]* ☑
  - shoulder region A30.9 *[M63.81-]* ☑
  - specified site NEC A30.9 *[M63.88]*
  - thigh A30.9 *[M63.85-]* ☑
  - upper arm A30.9 *[M63.82-]* ☑
- anesthetic A30.9
- BB A30.3
- BL A30.4
- borderline (infiltrated) (neuritic) A30.3
  - lepromatous A30.4
  - tuberculoid A30.2
- BT A30.2
- dimorphous (infiltrated) (neuritic) A30.3
- I A30.0
- indeterminate (macular) (neuritic) A30.0
- lepromatous (diffuse) (infiltrated) (macular) (neuritic) (nodular) A30.5
- LL A30.5
- macular (early) (neuritic) (simple) A30.9
- maculoanesthetic A30.9
- mixed A30.3
- neural A30.9
- nodular A30.5
- primary neuritic A30.3
- specified type NEC A30.8
- TT A30.1
- tuberculoid (major) (minor) A30.1

Leptocytosis, hereditary D56.9

Leptomeningitis (chronic) (circumscribed) (hemorrhagic) (nonsuppurative) — *see* Meningitis

Leptomeningopathy G96.198

Leptospiral — *see* condition

Leptospirochetal — *see* condition

Leptospirosis A27.9
- canicola A27.89

Leukemia, leukemic — *continued*
- biphenotypic acute C95.Ø- ☑
- blast cell C95.Ø- ☑
- Burkitt-type, mature B-cell C91.A- ☑ *(following* C91.6)
- chronic eosinophilic — *see also* Syndrome, hypereosinophilic, myeloid C94.8- ☑
- chronic lymphocytic, of B-cell type C91.1- ☑
- chronic monocytic C93.1- ☑
- chronic myelogenous (Philadelphia chromosome (Ph1) positive) (t(9;22)) (q34;q11) (with crisis of blast cells) C92.1- ☑
- chronic myeloid, BCR/ABL-positive C92.1- ☑
  - atypical, BCR/ABL-negative C92.2- ☑
- chronic myelomonocytic C93.1- ☑
- chronic neutrophilic D47.1
- CMML (-1) (-2) (with eosinophilia) C93.1- ☑
- granulocytic — *see also* Category C92 C92.9- ☑
- hairy cell C91.4- ☑
- juvenile myelomonocytic C93.3- ☑
- lymphoid C91.9- ☑
  - specified NEC C91.Z- ☑ *(following* C91.6)
- mast cell C94.3- ☑
- mature B-cell, Burkitt-type C91.A- ☑ *(following* C91.6)
- monocytic (subacute) C93.9- ☑
  - specified NEC C93.Z- ☑ *(following* C93.3)
- myelogenous — *see also* Category C92 C92.9- ☑
- myeloid C92.9- ☑
  - specified NEC C92.Z- ☑ *(following* C92.6)
- plasma cell C9Ø.1- ☑
- plasmacytic C9Ø.1- ☑
- prolymphocytic
  - of B-cell type C91.3- ☑
  - of T-cell type C91.6- ☑
- specified NEC C94.8- ☑
- stem cell, of unclear lineage C95.Ø- ☑
- subacute lymphocytic C91.9- ☑
- T-cell large granular lymphocytic C91.Z- ☑ *(following* C91.6)
- unspecified cell type C95.9- ☑
  - acute C95.Ø- ☑
  - chronic C95.1- ☑

Leukemoid reaction — *see also* Reaction, leukemoid D72.823

Leukoaraiosis (hypertensive) I67.81

Leukoariosis — *see* Leukoaraiosis

Leukocoria — *see* Disorder, globe, degenerated condition, leucocoria

Leukocytopenia D72.819

Leukocytosis D72.829
- eosinophilic D72.19

Leukoderma, leukodermia NEC L81.5
- syphilitic A51.39
  - late A52.79

Leukodystrophy E75.29

Leukoedema, oral epithelium K13.29

Leukoencephalitis GØ4.81
- acute (subacute) hemorrhagic G36.1
  - postimmunization or postvaccinal GØ4.Ø2
- postinfectious GØ4.Ø1
- subacute sclerosing A81.1
- van Bogaert's (sclerosing) A81.1

Leukoencephalopathy — *see also* Encephalopathy G93.49
- Binswanger's I67.3
- heroin vapor G92
- metachromatic E75.25
- multifocal (progressive) A81.2
- postimmunization and postvaccinal GØ4.Ø2
- progressive multifocal A81.2
- reversible, posterior G93.6
- van Bogaert's (sclerosing) A81.1
- vascular, progressive I67.3

Leukoerythroblastosis D75.9

Leukokeratosis — *see also* Leukoplakia
- mouth K13.21
- nicotina palati K13.24
- oral mucosa K13.21
- tongue K13.21
- vocal cord J38.3

Leukokraurosis vulva (e) N9Ø.4

Leukoma (cornea) — *see also* Opacity, cornea
- adherent H17.Ø- ☑
- interfering with central vision — *see* Opacity, cornea, central

Leukomalacia, cerebral, newborn P91.2
- periventricular P91.2

Leukomelanopathy, hereditary D72.Ø

Leukonychia (punctata) (striata) L6Ø.8
- congenital Q84.4

Leukopathia unguium L6Ø.8
- congenital Q84.4

Leukopenia D72.819
- basophilic D72.818
- chemotherapy (cancer) induced D7Ø.1
- congenital D7Ø.Ø
- cyclic D7Ø.Ø
- drug induced NEC D7Ø.2
  - due to cytoreductive cancer chemotherapy D7Ø.1
- eosinophilic D72.818
- familial D7Ø.Ø
- infantile genetic D7Ø.Ø
- malignant D7Ø.9
- periodic D7Ø.Ø
- transitory neonatal P61.5

Leukopenic — *see* condition

Leukoplakia
- anus K62.89
- bladder (postinfectional) N32.89
- buccal K13.21
- cervix (uteri) N88.Ø
- esophagus K22.8
- gingiva K13.21
- hairy (oral mucosa) (tongue) K13.3
- kidney (pelvis) N28.89
- larynx J38.7
- lip K13.21
- mouth K13.21
- oral epithelium, including tongue (mucosa) K13.21
- palate K13.21
- pelvis (kidney) N28.89
- penis (infectional) N48.Ø
- rectum K62.89
- syphilitic (late) A52.79
- tongue K13.21
- ureter (postinfectional) N28.89
- urethra (postinfectional) N36.8
- uterus N85.8
- vagina N89.4
- vocal cord J38.3
- vulva N9Ø.4

Leukorrhea N89.8
- due to Trichomonas (vaginalis) A59.ØØ
- trichomonal A59.ØØ

Leukosarcoma C85.9- ☑

Levocardia (isolated) Q24.1
- with situs inversus Q89.3

Levotransposition Q2Ø.5

Lev's disease or syndrome (acquired complete heart block) I44.2

Levulosuria — *see* Fructosuria

Levurid L3Ø.2

Lewy body (ies) (dementia) (disease) G31.83

Leyden-Moebius dystrophy G71.Ø9

Leydig cell
- carcinoma
  - specified site — *see* Neoplasm, malignant, by site
  - unspecified site
    - female C56.9
    - male C62.9- ☑
- tumor
  - benign
    - specified site — *see* Neoplasm, benign, by site
    - unspecified site
      - female D27.- ☑
      - male D29.2- ☑
  - malignant
    - specified site — *see* Neoplasm, malignant, by site
    - unspecified site
      - female C56.- ☑
      - male C62.9- ☑
  - specified site — *see* Neoplasm, uncertain behavior, by site
  - unspecified site
    - female D39.1- ☑
    - male D4Ø.1- ☑

Leydig-Sertoli cell tumor
- specified site — *see* Neoplasm, benign, by site
- unspecified site
  - female D27.- ☑
  - male D29.2- ☑

LGSIL (Low grade squamous intraepithelial lesion on cytologic smear of)
- anus R85.612
- cervix R87.612

LGSIL — *continued*
- vagina R87.622

Liar, pathologic F6Ø.2

Libido
- decreased R68.82

Libman-Sacks disease M32.11

Lice (infestation) B85.2
- body (Pediculus corporis) B85.1
- crab B85.3
- head (Pediculus capitis) B85.Ø
- mixed (classifiable to more than one of the titles B85.Ø-B85.3) B85.4
- pubic (Phthirus pubis) B85.3

Lichen L28.Ø
- albus L9Ø.Ø
  - penis N48.Ø
  - vulva N9Ø.4
- amyloidosis E85.4 *[L99]*
- atrophicus L9Ø.Ø
  - penis N48.Ø
  - vulva N9Ø.4
- congenital Q82.8
- myxedematosus L98.5
- nitidus L44.1
- pilaris Q82.8
  - acquired L85.8
- planopilaris L66.1
- planus (chronicus) L43.9
  - annularis L43.8
  - bullous L43.1
  - follicular L66.1
  - hypertrophic L43.Ø
  - moniliformis L44.3
  - of Wilson L43.9
  - specified NEC L43.8
  - subacute (active) L43.3
  - tropicus L43.3
- ruber
  - acuminatus L44.Ø
  - moniliformis L44.3
  - planus L43.9
- sclerosus (et atrophicus) L9Ø.Ø
  - penis N48.Ø
  - vulva N9Ø.4
- scrofulosus (primary) (tuberculous) A18.4
- simplex (chronicus) (circumscriptus) L28.Ø
- striatus L44.2
- urticatus L28.2

Lichenification L28.Ø

Lichenoides tuberculosis (primary) A18.4

Lichtheim's disease or syndrome D51.Ø

Lien migrans D73.89

Ligament — *see* condition

Light
- for gestational age — *see* Light for dates
- headedness R42

Light-for-dates (infant) PØ5.ØØ
- with weight of
  - 499 grams or less PØ5.Ø1
  - 5ØØ-749 grams PØ5.Ø2
  - 75Ø-999 grams PØ5.Ø3
  - 1ØØØ-1249 grams PØ5.Ø4
  - 125Ø-1499 grams PØ5.Ø5
  - 15ØØ-1749 grams PØ5.Ø6
  - 175Ø-1999 grams PØ5.Ø7
  - 2ØØØ-2499 grams PØ5.Ø8
  - 25ØØ grams and over PØ5.Ø9
- affecting management of pregnancy O36.59- ☑
- and small-for-dates — *see* Small for dates
- specified NEC PØ5.Ø9

Lightning (effects) (stroke) (struck by) T75.ØØ ☑
- burn — *see* Burn
- foot E53.8
- shock T75.Ø1 ☑
- specified effect NEC T75.Ø9 ☑

Lightwood-Albright syndrome N25.89

Lightwood's disease or syndrome (renal tubular acidosis) N25.89

Lignac (-de Toni) (-Fanconi) (-Debré) **disease or syndrome** E72.Ø9
- with cystinosis E72.Ø4

Ligneous thyroiditis EØ6.5

Likoff's syndrome I2Ø.8

Limb — *see* condition

Limbic epilepsy personality syndrome FØ7.Ø

Limitation, limited
- activities due to disability Z73.6
- cardiac reserve — *see* Disease, heart

Limitation, limited — *continued*
eye muscle duction, traumatic — *see* Strabismus, mechanical
mandibular range of motion M26.52
Lindau (-von Hippel) **disease** Q85.8
Line(s)
Beau's L6Ø.4
Harris' — *see* Arrest, epiphyseal
Hudson's (cornea) — *see* Pigmentation, cornea, anterior
Stähli's (cornea) — *see* Pigmentation, cornea, anterior
Linea corneae senilis — *see* Change, cornea, senile
Lingua
geographica K14.1
nigra (villosa) K14.3
plicata K14.5
tylosis K13.29
Lingual — *see* condition
Linguatulosis B88.8
Linitis (gastric) **plastica** C16.9
Lip — *see* condition
Lipedema — *see* Edema
Lipemia — *see also* Hyperlipidemia
retina, retinalis E78.3
Lipidosis E75.6
cerebral (infantile) (juvenile) (late) E75.4
cerebroretinal E75.4
cerebroside E75.22
cholesterol (cerebral) E75.5
glycolipid E75.21
hepatosplenomegalic E78.3
sphingomyelin — *see* Niemann-Pick disease or syndrome
sulfatide E75.29
Lipoadenoma — *see* Neoplasm, benign, by site
Lipoblastoma — *see* Lipoma
Lipoblastomatosis — *see* Lipoma
Lipochondrodystrophy E76.Ø1
Lipochrome histiocytosis (familial) D71
Lipodermatosclerosis — *see* Varix, leg, with, inflammation
ulcerated — *see* Varix, leg, with, ulcer, with inflammation by site
Lipodystrophia progressiva E88.1
Lipodystrophy (progressive) E88.1
insulin E88.1
intestinal K9Ø.81
mesenteric K65.4
Lipofibroma — *see* Lipoma
Lipofuscinosis, neuronal (with ceroidosis) E75.4
Lipogranuloma, sclerosing L92.8
Lipogranulomatosis E78.89
Lipoid — *see also* condition
histiocytosis D76.3
essential E75.29
nephrosis NØ4.9
proteinosis of Urbach E78.89
Lipoidemia — *see* Hyperlipidemia
Lipoidosis — *see* Lipidosis
Lipoma D17.9
fetal D17.9
fat cell D17.9
infiltrating D17.9
intramuscular D17.9
pleomorphic D17.9
site classification
arms (skin) (subcutaneous) D17.2- ☑
connective tissue D17.3Ø
intra-abdominal D17.5
intrathoracic D17.4
peritoneum D17.79
retroperitoneum D17.79
specified site NEC D17.39
spermatic cord D17.6
face (skin) (subcutaneous) D17.Ø
genitourinary organ NEC D17.72
head (skin) (subcutaneous) D17.Ø
intra-abdominal D17.5
intrathoracic D17.4
kidney D17.71
legs (skin) (subcutaneous) D17.2- ☑
neck (skin) (subcutaneous) D17.Ø
peritoneum D17.79
retroperitoneum D17.79
skin D17.3Ø
specified site NEC D17.39
specified site NEC D17.79
spermatic cord D17.6
subcutaneous D17.3Ø

Lipoma — *continued*
site classification — *continued*
subcutaneous — *continued*
specified site NEC D17.39
trunk (skin) (subcutaneous) D17.1
unspecified D17.9
spindle cell D17.9
Lipomatosis E88.2
dolorosa (Dercum) E88.2
fetal — *see* Lipoma
Launois-Bensaude E88.89
Lipomyoma — *see* Lipoma
Lipomyxoma — *see* Lipoma
Lipomyxosarcoma — *see* Neoplasm, connective tissue, malignant
Lipoprotein metabolism disorder E78.9
Lipoproteinemia E78.5
broad-beta E78.2
floating-beta E78.2
hyper-pre-beta E78.1
Liposarcoma — *see also* Neoplasm, connective tissue, malignant
dedifferentiated — *see* Neoplasm, connective tissue, malignant
differentiated type — *see* Neoplasm, connective tissue, malignant
embryonal — *see* Neoplasm, connective tissue, malignant
mixed type — *see* Neoplasm, connective tissue, malignant
myxoid — *see* Neoplasm, connective tissue, malignant
pleomorphic — *see* Neoplasm, connective tissue, malignant
round cell — *see* Neoplasm, connective tissue, malignant
well differentiated type — *see* Neoplasm, connective tissue, malignant
Liposynovitis prepatellaris E88.89
Lipping, cervix N86
Lipschütz disease or ulcer N76.6
Lipuria R82.Ø
schistosomiasis (bilharziasis) B65.Ø
Lisping F8Ø.Ø
Lissauer's paralysis A52.17
Lissencephalia, lissencephaly QØ4.3
Listeriosis, listerellosis A32.9
congenital (disseminated) P37.2
cutaneous A32.Ø
neonatal, newborn (disseminated) P37.2
oculoglandular A32.81
specified NEC A32.89
Lithemia E79.Ø
Lithiasis — *see* Calculus
Lithosis J62.8
Lithuria R82.998
Litigation, anxiety concerning Z65.3
Little leaguer's elbow — *see* Epicondylitis, medial
Little's disease G8Ø.9
Littre's
gland — *see* condition
hernia — *see* Hernia, abdomen
Littritis — *see* Urethritis
Livedo (annularis) (racemosa) (reticularis) R23.1
Liver — *see* condition
Living alone (problems with) Z6Ø.2
with handicapped person Z74.2
Lloyd's syndrome — *see* Adenomatosis, endocrine
Loa loa, loaiasis, loasis B74.3
Lobar — *see* condition
Lobomycosis B48.Ø
Lobo's disease B48.Ø
Lobotomy syndrome FØ7.Ø
Lobstein (-Ekman) **disease or syndrome** Q78.Ø
Lobster-claw hand Q71.6- ☑
Lobulation (congenital) — *see also* Anomaly, by site
kidney, Q63.1
liver, abnormal Q44.7
spleen Q89.Ø9
Lobule, lobular — *see* condition
Local, localized — *see* condition
Locked twins causing obstructed labor O66.1
Locked-in state G83.5
Locking
joint — *see* Derangement, joint, specified type NEC
knee — *see* Derangement, knee
Lockjaw — *see* Tetanus

Löffler's
endocarditis I42.3
eosinophilia J82.89
pneumonia J82.89
syndrome (eosinophilic pneumonitis) J82.89
Loiasis (with conjunctival infestation) (eyelid) B74.3
Lone Star fever A77.Ø
Long
labor O63.9
first stage O63.Ø
second stage O63.1
QT syndrome I45.81
Longitudinal stripes or grooves, nails L6Ø.8
congenital Q84.6
Long-term (current) (prophylactic) **drug therapy** (use of)
agents affecting estrogen receptors and estrogen levels NEC Z79.818
anastrozole (Arimidex) Z79.811
antibiotics Z79.2
short-term use — *omit code*
anticoagulants Z79.Ø1
anti-inflammatory, non-steroidal (NSAID) Z79.1
antiplatelet Z79.Ø2
antithrombotics Z79.Ø2
aromatase inhibitors Z79.811
aspirin Z79.82
birth control pill or patch Z79.3
bisphosphonates Z79.83
contraceptive, oral Z79.3
drug, specified NEC Z79.899
estrogen receptor downregulators Z79.818
Evista Z79.81Ø
exemestane (Aromasin) Z79.811
Fareston Z79.81Ø
fulvestrant (Faslodex) Z79.818
gonadotropin-releasing hormone (GnRH) agonist Z79.818
goserelin acetate (Zoladex) Z79.818
hormone replacement Z79.89Ø
insulin Z79.4
letrozole (Femara) Z79.811
leuprolide acetate (leuprorelin) (Lupron) Z79.818
megestrol acetate (Megace) Z79.818
methadone for pain management Z79.891
Nolvadex Z79.81Ø
non-steroidal anti-inflammatories (NSAID) Z79.1
opiate analgesic Z79.891
oral
antidiabetic Z79.84
contraceptive Z79.3
hypoglycemic Z79.84
raloxifene (Evista) Z79.81Ø
selective estrogen receptor modulators (SERMs) Z79.81Ø
steroids
inhaled Z79.51
systemic Z79.52
tamoxifen (Nolvadex) Z79.81Ø
toremifene (Fareston) Z79.81Ø
Loop
intestine — *see* Volvulus
vascular on papilla (optic) Q14.2
Loose — *see also* condition
body
joint M24.ØØ
ankle M24.Ø7- ☑
elbow M24.Ø2- ☑
hand M24.Ø4- ☑
hip M24.Ø5- ☑
knee M23.4- ☑
shoulder (region) M24.Ø1- ☑
specified site NEC M24.Ø8
toe M24.Ø7- ☑
vertebra M24.Ø8
wrist M24.Ø3- ☑
knee M23.4- ☑
sheath, tendon — *see* Disorder, tendon, specified type NEC
cartilage — *see* Loose, body, joint
skin and subcutaneous tissue (following bariatric surgery weight loss) (following dietary weight loss) L98.7
tooth, teeth KØ8.89
Loosening
aseptic
joint prosthesis — *see* Complications, joint prosthesis, mechanical, loosening, by site

Loosening — *continued*
- epiphysis — *see* Osteochondropathy
- mechanical
  - joint prosthesis — *see* Complications, joint prosthesis, mechanical, loosening, by site

Looser-Milkman (-Debray) **syndrome** M83.8
Lop ear (deformity) Q17.3
Lorain (-Levi) **short stature syndrome** E23.0
Lordosis M40.50
- acquired — *see* Lordosis, specified type NEC
- congenital Q76.429
  - lumbar region Q76.426
  - lumbosacral region Q76.427
  - sacral region Q76.428
  - sacrococcygeal region Q76.428
  - thoracolumbar region Q76.425
- lumbar region M40.56
- lumbosacral region M40.57
- postsurgical M96.4
- postural — *see* Lordosis, specified type NEC
- rachitic (late effect) (sequelae) E64.3
- sequelae of rickets E64.3
- specified type NEC M40.40
  - lumbar region M40.46
  - lumbosacral region M40.47
  - thoracolumbar region M40.45
- thoracolumbar region M40.55
- tuberculous A18.01

Loss (of)
- appetite — *see also* Anorexia R63.0
  - hysterical F50.89
  - nonorganic origin F50.89
  - psychogenic F50.89
- blood — *see* Hemorrhage
- bone —*see* Loss, substance of, bone
- consciousness, transient R55
  - traumatic — *see* Injury, intracranial
- control, sphincter, rectum R15.9
  - nonorganic origin F98.1
- elasticity, skin R23.4
- family (member) in childhood Z62.898
- fluid (acute) E86.9
- function of labyrinth — *see* subcategory H83.2 ☑
- hair, nonscarring — *see* Alopecia
- hearing — *see also* Deafness
  - central NOS H90.5
  - conductive H90.2
    - bilateral H90.0
    - unilateral
      - with
        - restricted hearing on the contralateral side H90.A1- ☑
        - unrestricted hearing on the contralateral side H90.1- ☑
  - mixed conductive and sensorineural hearing loss H90.8
    - bilateral H90.6
    - unilateral
      - with
        - restricted hearing on the contralateral side H90.A3- ☑
        - unrestricted hearing on the contralateral side H90.7- ☑
  - neural NOS H90.5
  - perceptive NOS H90.5
  - sensorineural NOS H90.5
    - bilateral H90.3
    - unilateral
      - with
        - restricted hearing onthe contralateral side H90.A2- ☑
        - unrestricted hearing on the contralateral side H90.4- ☑
  - sensory NOS H90.5
- height R29.890
- limb or member, traumatic, current — *see* Amputation, traumatic
- love relationship in childhood Z62.898
- memory — *see also* Amnesia
  - mild, following organic brain damage F06.8
- mind — *see* Psychosis
- occlusal vertical dimension of fully erupted teeth M26.37
- organ or part — *see* Absence, by site, acquired
- ossicles, ear (partial) H74.32- ☑
- parent in childhood Z63.4
- pregnancy, recurrent N96
  - care in current pregnancy O26.2- ☑

Loss — *continued*
- pregnancy, recurrent — *continued*
  - without current pregnancy N96
- recurrent pregnancy — *see* Loss, pregnancy, recurrent
- self-esteem, in childhood Z62.898
- sense of
  - smell — *see* Disturbance, sensation, smell
  - taste — *see* Disturbance, sensation, taste
  - touch R20.8
- sensory R44.9
  - dissociative F44.6
- sexual desire F52.0
- sight (acquired) (complete) (congenital) — *see* Blindness
- substance of
  - bone — *see* Disorder, bone, density and structure, specified NEC
    - horizontal alveolar K06.3
  - cartilage — *see* Disorder, cartilage, specified type NEC
    - auricle (ear) — *see* Disorder, pinna, specified type NEC
  - vitreous (humor) H15.89
- tooth, teeth — *see* Absence, teeth, acquired
- vision, visual H54.7
  - both eyes H54.3
  - one eye H54.60
    - left (normal vision on right) H54.62
    - right (normal vision on left) H54.61
  - specified as blindness — *see* Blindness
  - subjective
    - sudden H53.13- ☑
    - transient H53.12- ☑
- vitreous — *see* Prolapse, vitreous
- voice — *see* Aphonia
- weight (abnormal) (cause unknown) R63.4

Louis-Bar syndrome (ataxia-telangiectasia) G11.3
Louping ill (encephalitis) A84.89
Louse, lousiness — *see* Lice
Low
- achiever, school Z55.3
- back syndrome M54.5
- basal metabolic rate R94.8
- birthweight (2499 grams or less) P07.10
  - with weight of
    - 1000-1249 grams P07.14
    - 1250-1499 grams P07.15
    - 1500-1749 grams P07.16
    - 1750-1999 grams P07.17
    - 2000-2499 grams P07.18
  - extreme (999 grams or less) P07.00
    - with weight of
      - 499 grams or less P07.01
      - 500-749 grams P07.02
      - 750-999 grams P07.03
  - for gestational age — *see* Light for dates
- blood pressure — *see also* Hypotension
  - reading (incidental) (isolated) (nonspecific) R03.1
- cardiac reserve — *see* Disease, heart
- function — *see also* Hypofunction
  - kidney N28.9
- hematocrit D64.9
- hemoglobin D64.9
- income Z59.6
- level of literacy Z55.0
- lying
  - kidney N28.89
  - organ or site, congenital — *see* Malposition, congenital
- output syndrome (cardiac) — *see* Failure, heart
- platelets (blood) — *see* Thrombocytopenia
- reserve, kidney N28.89
- salt syndrome E87.1
- self esteem R45.81
- set ears Q17.4
- vision H54.2X- ☑
  - one eye (other eye normal) H54.50
    - left (normal vision on right) H54.52A- ☑
    - other eye blind — *see* Blindness
    - right (normal vision on left) H54.511- ☑

Low-density-lipoprotein-type (LDL) **hyperlipoproteinemia** E78.00
Lowe's syndrome E72.03
Lown-Ganong-Levine syndrome I45.6
LSD reaction (acute) (without dependence) F16.90
- with dependence F16.20

L-shaped kidney Q63.8
LTBI (latent tuberculosis infection) Z22.7

Ludwig's angina or disease K12.2
Lues (venerea), **luetic** — *see* Syphilis
Luetscher's syndrome (dehydration) E86.0
Lumbago, lumbalgia M54.5
- with sciatica M54.4- ☑
  - due to intervertebral disc disorder M51.17
- due to displacement, intervertebral disc M51.27
  - with sciatica M51.17

Lumbar — *see* condition
Lumbarization, vertebra, congenital Q76.49
Lumbermen's itch B88.0
Lump — *see also* Mass
- breast N63.0
  - axillary tail
    - left N63.32
    - right N63.31
  - left
    - lower inner quadrant N63.24
    - lower outer quadrant N63.23
    - overlapping quadrants N63.25
    - unspecified quadrant N63.20
    - upper inner quadrant N63.22
    - upper outer quadrant N63.21
  - right
    - lower inner quadrant N63.14
    - lower outer quadrant N63.13
    - overlapping quadrants N63.15
    - unspecified quadrant N63.10
    - upper inner quadrant N63.12
    - upper outer quadrant N63.11
  - subareolar
    - left N63.42
    - right N63.41

Lunacy — *see* Psychosis
Lung — *see* condition
Lupoid (miliary) **of Boeck** D86.3
Lupus
- anticoagulant D68.62
  - with
    - hemorrhagic disorder D68.312
    - hypercoagulable state D68.62
  - finding without diagnosis R76.0
- discoid (local) L93.0
- erythematosus (discoid) (local) L93.0
  - disseminated — *see* Lupus, erythematosus, systemic
  - eyelid H01.129
    - left H01.126
      - lower H01.125
      - upper H01.124
    - right H01.123
      - lower H01.122
      - upper H01.121
  - profundus L93.2
  - specified NEC L93.2
  - subacute cutaneous L93.1
  - systemic M32.9
    - with organ or system involvement M32.10
      - endocarditis M32.11
      - lung M32.13
      - pericarditis M32.12
      - renal (glomerular) M32.14
        - tubulo-interstitial M32.15
      - specified organ or system NEC M32.19
    - drug-induced M32.0
    - inhibitor (presence of) D68.62
      - with
        - hemorrhagic disorder D68.312
        - hypercoagulable state D68.62
      - finding without diagnosis R76.0
    - specified NEC M32.8
- exedens A18.4
- hydralazine M32.0
  - correct substance properly administered — *see* Table of Drugs and Chemicals, by drug, adverse effect
  - overdose or wrong substance given or taken — *see* Table of Drugs and Chemicals, by drug, poisoning
- nephritis (chronic) M32.14
- nontuberculous, not disseminated L93.0
- panniculitis L93.2
- pernio (Besnier) D86.3
- systemic — *see* Lupus, erythematosus, systemic
- tuberculous A18.4
  - eyelid A18.4
- vulgaris A18.4
  - eyelid A18.4

Luteinoma D27.- ☑

Lutembacher's disease or syndrome (atrial septal defect with mitral stenosis) Q21.1
Luteoma D27.- ☑
Lutz (-Splendore-de Almeida) **disease** — *see* Paracoccidioidomycosis
Luxation — *see also* Dislocation
  eyeball (nontraumatic) — *see* Luxation, globe
    birth injury P15.3
  globe, nontraumatic H44.82- ☑
  lacrimal gland — *see* Dislocation, lacrimal gland
  lens (old) (partial) (spontaneous)
    congenital Q12.1
      syphilitic A5Ø.39
Lycanthropy F22
Lyell's syndrome L51.2
  due to drug L51.2
    correct substance properly administered — *see* Table of Drugs and Chemicals, by drug, adverse effect
    overdose or wrong substance given or taken — *see* Table of Drugs and Chemicals, by drug, poisoning
Lyme disease A69.2Ø
Lymph
  gland or node — *see* condition
  scrotum — *see* Infestation, filarial
Lymphadenitis I88.9
  with ectopic or molar pregnancy OØ8.Ø
  acute LØ4.9
    axilla LØ4.2
    face LØ4.Ø
    head LØ4.Ø
    hip LØ4.3
    limb
      lower LØ4.3
      upper LØ4.2
    neck LØ4.Ø
    shoulder LØ4.2
    specified site NEC LØ4.8
    trunk LØ4.1
  anthracosis (occupational) J6Ø
  any site, except mesenteric I88.9
    chronic I88.1
    subacute I88.1
  breast
    gestational — *see* Mastitis, obstetric
    puerperal, postpartum (nonpurulent) O91.22
  chancroidal (congenital) A57
  chronic I88.1
    mesenteric I88.Ø
  due to
    Brugia (malayi) B74.1
      timori B74.2
    chlamydial lymphogranuloma A55
    diphtheria (toxin) A36.89
    lymphogranuloma venereum A55
    Wuchereria bancrofti B74.Ø
  following ectopic or molar pregnancy OØ8.Ø
  gonorrheal A54.89
  infective — *see* Lymphadenitis, acute
  mesenteric (acute) (chronic) (nonspecific) (subacute) I88.Ø
    due to Salmonella typhi AØ1.Ø9
    tuberculous A18.39
  mycobacterial A31.8
  purulent — *see* Lymphadenitis, acute
  pyogenic — *see* Lymphadenitis, acute
  regional, nonbacterial I88.8
  septic — *see* Lymphadenitis, acute
  subacute, unspecified site I88.1
  suppurative — *see* Lymphadenitis, acute
  syphilitic (early) (secondary) A51.49
    late A52.79
  tuberculous — *see* Tuberculosis, lymph gland
  venereal (chlamydial) A55
Lymphadenoid goiter EØ6.3
Lymphadenopathy (generalized) R59.1
  angioimmunoblastic, with dysproteinemia (AILD) C86.5
  due to toxoplasmosis (acquired) B58.89
    congenital (acute) (subacute) (chronic) P37.1
  localized R59.Ø
  syphilitic (early) (secondary) A51.49
Lymphadenosis R59.1
Lymphangiectasis I89.Ø
  conjunctiva H11.89
  postinfectional I89.Ø
  scrotum I89.Ø
Lymphangiectatic elephantiasis, nonfilarial I89.Ø
Lymphangioendothelioma D18.1
  malignant — *see* Neoplasm, connective tissue, malignant
Lymphangioleiomyomatosis J84.81
Lymphangioma D18.1
  capillary D18.1
  cavernous D18.1
  cystic D18.1
  malignant — *see* Neoplasm, connective tissue, malignant
Lymphangiomyoma D18.1
Lymphangiomyomatosis J84.81
Lymphangiosarcoma — *see* Neoplasm, connective tissue, malignant
Lymphangitis I89.1
  with
    abscess — *code by* site under Abscess
    cellulitis — *code by* site under Cellulitis
    ectopic or molar pregnancy OØ8.Ø
  acute LØ3.91
    abdominal wall LØ3.321
    ankle — *see* Lymphangitis, acute, lower limb
    arm — *see* Lymphangitis, acute, upper limb
    auricle (ear) — *see* Lymphangitis, acute, ear
    axilla LØ3.12- ☑
    back (any part) LØ3.322
    buttock LØ3.327
    cervical (meaning neck) LØ3.222
    cheek (external) LØ3.212
    chest wall LØ3.323
    digit
      finger — *see* Lymphangitis, acute, finger
      toe — *see* Lymphangitis, acute, toe
    ear (external) H6Ø.1- ☑
    external auditory canal — *see* Lymphangitis, acute, ear
    eyelid — *see* Abscess, eyelid
    face NEC LØ3.212
    finger (intrathecal) (periosteal) (subcutaneous) (subcuticular) LØ3.Ø2- ☑
    foot — *see* Lymphangitis, acute, lower limb
    gluteal (region) LØ3.327
    groin LØ3.324
    hand — *see* Lymphangitis, acute, upper limb
    head NEC LØ3.891
      face (any part, except ear, eye and nose) LØ3.212
    heel — *see* Lymphangitis, acute, lower limb
    hip — *see* Lymphangitis, acute, lower limb
    jaw (region) LØ3.212
    knee — *see* Lymphangitis, acute, lower limb
    leg — *see* Lymphangitis, acute, lower limb
    lower limb LØ3.12- ☑
      toe — *see* Lymphangitis, acute, toe
    navel LØ3.326
    neck (region) LØ3.222
    orbit, orbital — *see* Cellulitis, orbit
    pectoral (region) LØ3.323
    perineal, perineum LØ3.325
    scalp (any part) LØ3.891
    shoulder — *see* Lymphangitis, acute, upper limb
    specified site NEC LØ3.898
    thigh — *see* Lymphangitis, acute, lower limb
    thumb (intrathecal) (periosteal) (subcutaneous) (subcuticular) — *see* Lymphangitis, acute, finger
    toe (intrathecal) (periosteal) (subcutaneous) (subcuticular) LØ3.Ø4- ☑
    trunk LØ3.329
      abdominal wall LØ3.321
      back (any part) LØ3.322
      buttock LØ3.327
      chest wall LØ3.323
      groin LØ3.324
      perineal, perineum LØ3.325
      umbilicus LØ3.326
    umbilicus LØ3.326
    upper limb LØ3.12- ☑
      axilla — *see* Lymphangitis, acute, axilla
      finger — *see* Lymphangitis, acute, finger
      thumb — *see* Lymphangitis, acute, finger
    wrist — *see* Lymphangitis, acute, upper limb
  breast
    gestational — *see* Mastitis, obstetric
  chancroidal A57
  chronic (any site) I89.1
  due to
    Brugia (malayi) B74.1
Lymphangitis — *continued*
  due to — *continued*
    Brugia — *continued*
      timori B74.2
    Wuchereria bancrofti B74.Ø
  following ectopic or molar pregnancy OØ8.89
  penis
    acute N48.29
    gonococcal (acute) (chronic) A54.Ø9
  puerperal, postpartum, childbirth O86.89
  strumous, tuberculous A18.2
  subacute (any site) I89.1
  tuberculous — *see* Tuberculosis, lymph gland
Lymphatic (vessel) — *see* condition
Lymphatism E32.8
Lymphectasia I89.Ø
Lymphedema (acquired) — *see also* Elephantiasis
  congenital Q82.Ø
  hereditary (chronic) (idiopathic) Q82.Ø
  postmastectomy I97.2
  praecox I89.Ø
  secondary I89.Ø
  surgical NEC I97.89
    postmastectomy (syndrome) I97.2
Lymphoblastic — *see* condition
Lymphoblastoma (diffuse) — *see* Lymphoma, lymphoblastic (diffuse)
  giant follicular — *see* Lymphoma, lymphoblastic (diffuse)
  macrofollicular — *see* Lymphoma, lymphoblastic (diffuse)
Lymphocele I89.8
Lymphocytic
  chorioencephalitis (acute) (serous) A87.2
  choriomeningitis (acute) (serous) A87.2
  meningoencephalitis A87.2
Lymphocytoma, benign cutis L98.8
Lymphocytopenia D72.81Ø
Lymphocytosis (symptomatic) D72.82Ø
  infectious (acute) B33.8
Lymphoepithelioma — *see* Neoplasm, malignant, by site
Lymphogranuloma (malignant) — *see also* Lymphoma, Hodgkin
  chlamydial A55
  inguinale A55
  venereum (any site) (chlamydial) (with stricture of rectum) A55
Lymphogranulomatosis (malignant) — *see also* Lymphoma, Hodgkin
  benign (Boeck's sarcoid) (Schaumann's) D86.1
Lymphohistiocytosis, hemophagocytic (familial) D76.1
Lymphoid — *see* condition
Lymphoma (of) (malignant) C85.9Ø
  adult T-cell (HTLV-1-associated) (acute variant) (chronic variant) (lymphomatoid variant) (smouldering variant) C91.5- ☑
  anaplastic large cell
    ALK-negative C84.7- ☑
    ALK-positive C84.6- ☑
    CD3Ø-positive C84.6- ☑
    primary cutaneous C86.6
  angioimmunoblastic T-cell C86.5
  BALT C88.4
  B-cell C85.1- ☑
  blastic NK-cell C86.4
  blastic plasmacytoid dendritic cell neoplasm (BPDCN) C86.4
  B-precursor C83.5- ☑
  bronchial-associated lymphoid tissue [BALT-lymphoma] C88.4
  Burkitt (atypical) C83.7- ☑
  Burkitt-like C83.7- ☑
  centrocytic C83.1- ☑
  cutaneous follicle center C82.6- ☑
  cutaneous T-cell C84.A- ☑ (*following* C84.7)
  diffuse follicle center C82.5- ☑
  diffuse large cell C83.3- ☑
    anaplastic C83.3- ☑
    B-cell C83.3- ☑
    CD3Ø-positive C83.3- ☑
    centroblastic C83.3- ☑
    immunoblastic C83.3- ☑
    plasmablastic C83.3- ☑
    subtype not specified C83.3- ☑
    T-cell rich C83.3- ☑
  enteropathy-type (associated) (intestinal) T-cell C86.2

Lymphoma — *continued*
- extranodal marginal zone B-cell lymphoma of mucosa-associated lymphoid tissue [MALT-lymphoma] C88.4
- extranodal NK/T-cell, nasal type C86.Ø
- follicular C82.9- ☑
  - grade
    - I C82.Ø- ☑
    - II C82.1- ☑
    - III C82.2- ☑
    - IIIa C82.3- ☑
    - IIIb C82.4- ☑
  - specified NEC C82.8- ☑
- hepatosplenic T-cell (alpha-beta) (gamma-delta) C86.1
- histiocytic C85.9- ☑
  - true C96.A (*following* C96.6)
- Hodgkin C81.9 ☑
  - lymphocyte depleted (classical) C81.3- ☑
  - lymphocyte-rich (classical) C81.4- ☑
  - mixed cellularity (classical) C81.2- ☑
  - nodular
    - lymphocyte predominant C81.Ø- ☑
    - sclerosis (classical) C81.1- ☑
  - nodular sclerosis (classical) C81.1- ☑
  - specified NEC (classical) C81.7- ☑
- intravascular large B-cell C83.8- ☑
- Lennert's C84.4- ☑
- lymphoblastic (diffuse) C83.5- ☑
- lymphoblastic B-cell C83.5- ☑
- lymphoblastic T-cell C83.5- ☑
- lymphoepithelioid C84.4- ☑
- lymphoplasmacytic C83.Ø- ☑
  - with IgM-production C88.Ø
- MALT C88.4
- mantle cell C83.1- ☑
- mature T-cell NEC C84.4- ☑
- mature T/NK-cell C84.9- ☑
  - specified NEC C84.Z- ☑ (*following* C84.7)
- mediastinal (thymic) large B-cell C85.2- ☑
- Mediterranean C88.3
- mucosa-associated lymphoid tissue [MALT-lymphoma] C88.4
- NK/T cell C84.9- ☑
- nodal marginal zone C83.Ø- ☑
- non-follicular (diffuse) C83.9- ☑
  - specified NEC C83.8- ☑
- non-Hodgkin — *see also* Lymphoma, by type C85.9- ☑
  - specified NEC C85.8- ☑
- non-leukemic variant of B-CLL C83.Ø- ☑
- peripheral T-cell, not classified C84.4- ☑
- primary cutaneous
  - anaplastic large cell C86.6
  - CD3Ø-positive large T-cell C86.6
- primary effusion B-cell C83.8- ☑
- SALT C88.4
- skin-associated lymphoid tissue [SALT-lymphoma] C88.4
- small cell B-cell C83.Ø- ☑
- splenic marginal zone C83.Ø- ☑
- subcutaneous panniculitis-like T-cell C86.3
- T-precursor C83.5- ☑
- true histiocytic C96.A (*following* C96.6)

Lymphomatosis — *see* Lymphoma
Lymphopathia venereum, veneris A55
Lymphopenia D72.81Ø
Lymphoplasmacytic leukemia — *see* Leukemia, chronic lymphocytic, B-cell type
Lymphoproliferation, X-linked disease D82.3
Lymphoreticulosis, benign (of inoculation) A28.1
Lymphorrhea I89.8
Lymphosarcoma (diffuse) — *see also* Lymphoma C85.9- ☑
Lymphostasis I89.8
Lypemania — *see* Melancholia
Lysine and hydroxylysine metabolism disorder E72.3
Lyssa — *see* Rabies

M

Macacus ear Q17.3
Maceration, wet feet, tropical (syndrome) T69.Ø2- ☑
MacLeod's syndrome J43.Ø
Macrocephalia, macrocephaly Q75.3
Macrocheilia, macrochilia (congenital) Q18.6
Macrocolon — *see also* Megacolon Q43.1
Macrocornea Q15.8

Macrocornea — *continued*
- with glaucoma Q15.Ø

Macrocytic — *see* condition
Macrocytosis D75.89
Macrodactylia, macrodactylism (fingers) (thumbs) Q74.Ø
- toes Q74.2

Macrodontia KØØ.2
Macrogenia M26.Ø5
Macrogenitosomia (adrenal) (male) (praecox) E25.9
- congenital E25.Ø

Macroglobulinemia (idiopathic) (primary) C88.Ø
- monoclonal (essential) D47.2
- Waldenström C88.Ø

Macroglossia (congenital) Q38.2
- acquired K14.8

Macrognathia, macrognathism (congenital) (mandibular) (maxillary) M26.Ø9
Macrogyria (congenital) QØ4.8
Macrohydrocephalus — *see* Hydrocephalus
Macromastia — *see* Hypertrophy, breast
Macrophthalmos Q11.3
- in congenital glaucoma Q15.Ø

Macropsia H53.15
Macrosigmoid K59.39
- congenital Q43.2

Macrospondylitis , acromegalic E22.Ø
Macrostomia (congenital) Q18.4
Macrotia (external ear) (congenital) Q17.1
Macula
- cornea, corneal — *see* Opacity, cornea
- degeneration (atrophic) (exudative) (senile) — *see also* Degeneration, macula
  - hereditary — *see* Dystrophy, retina

Maculae ceruleae B85.1
Maculopathy, toxic — *see* Degeneration, macula, toxic
Madarosis (eyelid) HØ2.729
- left HØ2.726
  - lower HØ2.725
  - upper HØ2.724
- right HØ2.723
  - lower HØ2.722
  - upper HØ2.721

Madelung's
- deformity (radius) Q74.Ø
- disease
  - radial deformity Q74.Ø
  - symmetrical lipomas, neck E88.89

Madness — *see* Psychosis
Madura
- foot B47.9
  - actinomycotic B47.1
  - mycotic B47.Ø

Maduromycosis B47.Ø
Maffucci's syndrome Q78.4
Magnesium metabolism disorder — *see* Disorder, metabolism, magnesium
Main en griffe (acquired) — *see also* Deformity, limb, clawhand
- congenital Q74.Ø

Maintenance (encounter for)
- antineoplastic chemotherapy Z51.11
- antineoplastic radiation therapy Z51.Ø
- methadone F11.2Ø

Majocchi's
- disease L81.7
- granuloma B35.8

Major — *see* condition
Mal de los pintos — *see* Pinta
Mal de mer T75.3 ☑
Malabar itch (any site) B35.5
Malabsorption K9Ø.9
- calcium K9Ø.89
- carbohydrate K9Ø.49
- disaccharide E73.9
- fat K9Ø.49
- galactose E74.2Ø
- glucose (-galactose) E74.39
- intestinal K9Ø.9
  - specified NEC K9Ø.89
- isomaltose E74.31
- lactose E73.9
- methionine E72.19
- monosaccharide E74.39
- postgastrectomy K91.2
- postsurgical K91.2
- protein K9Ø.49

Malabsorption — *continued*
- starch K9Ø.49
- sucrose E74.39
- syndrome K9Ø.9
  - postsurgical K91.2

Malacia, bone (adult) M83.9
- juvenile — *see* Rickets

Malacoplakia
- bladder N32.89
- pelvis (kidney) N28.89
- ureter N28.89
- urethra N36.8

Malacosteon, juvenile — *see* Rickets
Maladaptation — *see* Maladjustment
Maladie de Roger Q21.Ø
Maladjustment
- conjugal Z63.Ø
  - involving divorce or estrangement Z63.5
- educational Z55.4
- family Z63.9
- marital Z63.Ø
  - involving divorce or estrangement Z63.5
- occupational NEC Z56.89
- simple, adult — *see* Disorder, adjustment
- situational — *see* Disorder, adjustment
- social Z6Ø.9
  - due to
    - acculturation difficulty Z6Ø.3
    - discrimination and persecution (perceived) Z6Ø.5
    - exclusion and isolation Z6Ø.4
    - life-cycle (phase of life) transition Z6Ø.Ø
    - rejection Z6Ø.4
    - specified reason NEC Z6Ø.8

Malaise R53.81
Malakoplakia — *see* Malacoplakia
Malaria, malarial (fever) B54
- with
  - blackwater fever B5Ø.8
    - hemoglobinuric (bilious) B5Ø.8
  - hemoglobinuria B5Ø.8
- accidentally induced (therapeutically) — *code by* type under Malaria
- algid B5Ø.9
- cerebral B5Ø.Ø *[G94]*
- clinically diagnosed (without parasitological confirmation) B54
- congenital NEC P37.4
  - falciparum P37.3
- congestion, congestive B54
- continued (fever) B5Ø.9
- estivo-autumnal B5Ø.9
- falciparum B5Ø.9
  - with complications NEC B5Ø.8
    - cerebral B5Ø.Ø *[G94]*
  - severe B5Ø.8
- hemorrhagic B54
- malariae B52.9
  - with
    - complications NEC B52.8
    - glomerular disorder B52.Ø
- malignant (tertian) — *see* Malaria, falciparum
- mixed infections — *code to* first listed type in B5Ø-B53
- ovale B53.Ø
- parasitologically confirmed NEC B53.8
- pernicious, acute — *see* Malaria, falciparum
- Plasmodium (P.)
  - falciparum NEC — *see* Malaria, falciparum
  - malariae NEC B52.9
    - with Plasmodium
      - falciparum (and or vivax) — *see* Malaria, falciparum
      - vivax — *see also* Malaria, vivax
        - and falciparum — *see* Malaria, falciparum
  - ovale B53.Ø
    - with Plasmodium malariae — *see also* Malaria, malariae
      - and vivax — *see also* Malaria, vivax
        - and falciparum — *see* Malaria, falciparum
  - simian B53.1
    - with Plasmodium malariae — *see also* Malaria, malariae
      - and vivax — *see also* Malaria, vivax
        - and falciparum — *see* Malaria, falciparum
  - vivax NEC B51.9
    - with Plasmodium falciparum — *see* Malaria, falciparum
- quartan — *see* Malaria, malariae
- quotidian — *see* Malaria, falciparum

- **Mass** — *continued*
  - localized — *continued*
    - head R22.0
    - limb
      - lower R22.4- ☑
      - upper R22.3- ☑
    - neck R22.1
    - trunk R22.2
  - lung R91.8
  - malignant — *see* Neoplasm, malignant, by site
  - neck R22.1
  - pelvic (diffuse) (generalized) — *see* Mass, abdominal
  - specified organ NEC — *see* Disease, by site
  - splenic R16.1
  - substernal thyroid — *see* Goiter
  - superficial (localized) R22.9
  - umbilical (diffuse) (generalized) R19.09
- **Massive** — *see* condition
- **Mast cell**
  - disease, systemic tissue D47.02
  - leukemia C94.3- ☑
  - neoplasm
    - malignant C96.20
      - specified type NEC C96.29
    - of uncertain behavior NEC D47.09
  - sarcoma C96.22
  - tumor D47.09
- **Mastalgia** N64.4
- **Masters-Allen syndrome** N83.8
- **Mastitis** (acute) (diffuse) (nonpuerperal) (subacute) N61.0
  - with abscess N61.1
  - chronic (cystic) — *see* Mastopathy, cystic
  - cystic (Schimmelbusch's type) — *see* Mastopathy, cystic
  - fibrocystic — *see* Mastopathy, cystic
  - granulomatous N61.2- ☑
  - infective N61.0
    - newborn P39.0
  - interstitial, gestational or puerperal — *see* Mastitis, obstetric
  - neonatal (noninfective) P83.4
    - infective P39.0
  - obstetric (interstitial) (nonpurulent)
    - associated with
      - lactation O91.23
      - pregnancy O91.21- ☑
      - puerperium O91.22
    - purulent
      - associated with
        - lactation O91.13
        - pregnancy O91.11- ☑
        - puerperium O91.12
  - periductal — *see* Ectasia, mammary duct
  - phlegmonous — *see* Mastopathy, cystic
  - plasma cell — *see* Ectasia, mammary duct
  - without abscess N61.0
- **Mastocytoma** (extracutaneous) D47.09
  - malignant C96.29
  - solitary D47.01
- **Mastocytosis** D47.09
  - aggressive systemic C96.21
  - cutaneous (diffuse) (maculopapular) D47.01
    - congenital Q82.2
    - of neonatal onset Q82.2
    - of newborn onset Q82.2
  - indolent systemic D47.02
  - isolated bone marrow D47.02
  - malignant C96.29
  - systemic (indolent) (smoldering)
    - with an associated hematological non-mast cell lineage disease (SM-AHNMD) D47.02
- **Mastodynia** N64.4
- **Mastoid** — *see* condition
- **Mastoidalgia** — *see* subcategory H92.0 ☑
- **Mastoiditis** (coalescent) (hemorrhagic) (suppurative) H70.9- ☑
  - acute, subacute H70.00- ☑
    - complicated NEC H70.09- ☑
    - subperiosteal H70.01- ☑
  - chronic (necrotic) (recurrent) H70.1- ☑
  - in (due to)
    - infectious disease NEC B99 ☑ *[H75.0-]* ☑
    - parasitic disease NEC B89 *[H75.0-]* ☑
    - tuberculosis A18.03
  - petrositis — *see* Petrositis
  - postauricular fistula — *see* Fistula, postauricular
  - specified NEC H70.89- ☑
  - tuberculous A18.03
- **Mastopathy, mastopathia** N64.9
  - chronica cystica — *see* Mastopathy, cystic
  - cystic (chronic) (diffuse) N60.1- ☑
    - with epithelial proliferation N60.3- ☑
  - diffuse cystic — *see* Mastopathy, cystic
  - estrogenic, oestrogenica N64.89
  - ovarian origin N64.89
- **Mastoplasia, mastoplastia** N62
- **Masturbation** (excessive) F98.8
- **Maternal care** (for) — *see* Pregnancy (complicated by) (management affected by)
- **Matheiu's disease** (leptospiral jaundice) A27.0
- **Mauclaire's disease or osteochondrosis** — *see* Osteochondrosis, juvenile, hand, metacarpal
- **Maxcy's disease** A75.2
- **Maxilla, maxillary** — *see* condition
- **May** (-Hegglin) **anomaly or syndrome** D72.0
- **McArdle** (-Schmid)(-Pearson) **disease** (glycogen storage) E74.04
- **McCune-Albright syndrome** Q78.1
- **McQuarrie's syndrome** (idiopathic familial hypoglycemia) E16.2
- **Meadow's syndrome** Q86.1
- **Measles** (black) (hemorrhagic) (suppressed) B05.9
  - with
    - complications NEC B05.89
    - encephalitis B05.0
    - intestinal complications B05.4
    - keratitis (keratoconjunctivitis) B05.81
    - meningitis B05.1
    - otitis media B05.3
    - pneumonia B05.2
  - French — *see* Rubella
  - German — *see* Rubella
  - Liberty — *see* Rubella
- **Meatitis, urethral** — *see* Urethritis
- **Meatus, meatal** — *see* condition
- **Meat-wrappers' asthma** J68.9
- **Meckel-Gruber syndrome** Q61.9
- **Meckel's diverticulitis, diverticulum** (displaced) (hypertrophic) Q43.0
  - malignant — *see* Table of Neoplasms, small intestine, malignant
- **Meconium**
  - ileus, newborn P76.0
    - in cystic fibrosis E84.11
    - meaning meconium plug (without cystic fibrosis) P76.0
  - obstruction, newborn P76.0
    - due to fecaliths P76.0
    - in mucoviscidosis E84.11
  - peritonitis P78.0
  - plug syndrome (newborn) NEC P76.0
- **Median** — *see also* condition
  - arcuate ligament syndrome I77.4
  - bar (prostate) (vesical orifice) — *see* Hyperplasia, prostate
  - rhomboid glossitis K14.2
- **Mediastinal shift** R93.89
- **Mediastinitis** (acute) (chronic) J98.51
  - syphilitic A52.73
  - tuberculous A15.8
- **Mediastinopericarditis** — *see also* Pericarditis
  - acute I30.9
  - adhesive I31.0
  - chronic I31.8
    - rheumatic I09.2
- **Mediastinum, mediastinal** — *see* condition
- **Medicine poisoning** — *see* Table of Drugs and Chemicals, by drug, poisoning
- **Mediterranean**
  - fever — *see* Brucellosis
    - familial M04.1
    - tick A77.1
  - kala-azar B55.0
  - leishmaniasis B55.0
  - tick fever A77.1
- **Medulla** — *see* condition
- **Medullary cystic kidney** Q61.5
- **Medullated fibers**
  - optic (nerve) Q14.8
  - retina Q14.1
- **Medulloblastoma**
  - desmoplastic C71.6
  - specified site — *see* Neoplasm, malignant, by site
  - unspecified site C71.6
- **Medulloepithelioma** — *see also* Neoplasm, malignant, by site
  - teratoid — *see* Neoplasm, malignant, by site
- **Medullomyoblastoma**
  - specified site — *see* Neoplasm, malignant, by site
  - unspecified site C71.6
- **Meekeren-Ehlers-Danlos syndrome** — *see also* Syndrome, Ehlers-Danlos Q79.69
- **Megacolon** (acquired) (functional) (not Hirschsprung's disease) (in) K59.39
  - Chagas' disease B57.32
  - congenital, congenitum (aganglionic) Q43.1
  - Hirschsprung's (disease) Q43.1
  - toxic NEC K59.31
    - due to Clostridium difficile
      - not specified as recurrent A04.72
      - recurrent A04.71
- **Megaesophagus** (functional) K22.0
  - congenital Q39.5
  - in (due to) Chagas' disease B57.31
- **Megalencephaly** Q04.5
- **Megalerythema** (epidemic) B08.3
- **Megaloappendix** Q43.8
- **Megalocephalus, megalocephaly NEC** Q75.3
- **Megalocornea** Q15.8
  - with glaucoma Q15.0
- **Megalocytic anemia** D53.1
- **Megalodactylia** (fingers) (thumbs) (congenital) Q74.0
  - toes Q74.2
- **Megaloduodenum** Q43.8
- **Megaloesophagus** (functional) K22.0
  - congenital Q39.5
- **Megalogastria** (acquired) K31.89
  - congenital Q40.2
- **Megalophthalmos** Q11.3
- **Megalopsia** H53.15
- **Megalosplenia** — *see* Splenomegaly
- **Megaloureter** N28.82
  - congenital Q62.2
- **Megarectum** K62.89
- **Megasigmoid** K59.39
  - congenital Q43.2
- **Megaureter** N28.82
  - congenital Q62.2
- **Megavitamin-B6 syndrome** E67.2
- **Megrim** — *see* Migraine
- **Meibomian**
  - cyst, infected — *see* Hordeolum
  - gland — *see* condition
  - sty, stye — *see* Hordeolum
- **Meibomitis** — *see* Hordeolum
- **Meige-Milroy disease** (chronic hereditary edema) Q82.0
- **Meige's syndrome** Q82.0
- **Melalgia, nutritional** E53.8
- **Melancholia** F32.9
  - climacteric (single episode) F32.89
    - recurrent episode F33.8
  - hypochondriac F45.29
  - intermittent (single episode) F32.89
    - recurrent episode F33.8
  - involutional (single episode) F32.89
    - recurrent episode F33.8
  - menopausal (single episode) F32.89
    - recurrent episode F33.8
  - puerperal F32.89
  - reactive (emotional stress or trauma) F32.3
  - recurrent F33.9
  - senile F03 ☑
  - stuporous (single episode) F32.89
    - recurrent episode F33.8
- **Melanemia** R79.89
- **Melanoameloblastoma** — *see* Neoplasm, bone, benign
- **Melanoblastoma** — *see* Melanoma
- **Melanocarcinoma** — *see* Melanoma
- **Melanocytoma, eyeball** D31.9- ☑
- **Melanocytosis, neurocutaneous** Q82.8
- **Melanoderma, melanodermia** L81.4
- **Melanodontia, infantile** K03.89
- **Melanodontoclasia** K03.89
- **Melanoepithelioma** — *see* Melanoma
- **Melanoma** (malignant) C43.9
  - acral lentiginous, malignant — *see* Melanoma, skin, by site
  - amelanotic — *see* Melanoma, skin, by site
  - balloon cell — *see* Melanoma, skin, by site
  - benign — *see* Nevus

- **Melanoma** — *continued*
  - desmoplastic, malignant — *see* Melanoma, skin, by site
  - epithelioid cell — *see* Melanoma, skin, by site
    - with spindle cell, mixed — *see* Melanoma, skin, by site
  - in
    - giant pigmented nevus — *see* Melanoma, skin, by site
    - Hutchinson's melanotic freckle — *see* Melanoma, skin, by site
    - junctional nevus — *see* Melanoma, skin, by site
    - precancerous melanosis — *see* Melanoma, skin, by site
  - in situ DØ3.9
    - abdominal wall DØ3.59
    - ala nasi DØ3.39
    - ankle DØ3.7- ☑
    - anus, anal (margin) (skin) DØ3.51
    - arm DØ3.6- ☑
    - auditory canal DØ3.2- ☑
    - auricle (ear) DØ3.2- ☑
    - auricular canal (external) DØ3.2- ☑
    - axilla, axillary fold DØ3.59
    - back DØ3.59
    - breast DØ3.52
    - brow DØ3.39
    - buttock DØ3.59
    - canthus (eye) DØ3.1- ☑
    - cheek (external) DØ3.39
    - chest wall DØ3.59
    - chin DØ3.39
    - choroid DØ3.8
    - conjunctiva DØ3.8
    - ear (external) DØ3.2- ☑
    - external meatus (ear) DØ3.2- ☑
    - eye DØ3.8
    - eyebrow DØ3.39
    - eyelid (lower) (upper) DØ3.1- ☑
    - face DØ3.3Ø
      - specified NEC DØ3.39
    - female genital organ (external) NEC DØ3.8
    - finger DØ3.6- ☑
    - flank DØ3.59
    - foot DØ3.7- ☑
    - forearm DØ3.6- ☑
    - forehead DØ3.39
    - foreskin DØ3.8
    - gluteal region DØ3.59
    - groin DØ3.59
    - hand DØ3.6- ☑
    - heel DØ3.7- ☑
    - helix DØ3.2- ☑
    - hip DØ3.7- ☑
    - interscapular region DØ3.59
    - iris DØ3.8
    - jaw DØ3.39
    - knee DØ3.7- ☑
    - labium (majus) (minus) DØ3.8
    - lacrimal gland DØ3.8
    - leg DØ3.7- ☑
    - lip (lower) (upper) DØ3.Ø
    - lower limb NEC DØ3.7- ☑
    - male genital organ (external) NEC DØ3.8
    - nail DØ3.9
      - finger DØ3.6- ☑
      - toe DØ3.7- ☑
    - neck DØ3.4
    - nose (external) DØ3.39
    - orbit DØ3.8
    - penis DØ3.8
    - perianal skin DØ3.51
    - perineum DØ3.51
    - pinna DØ3.2- ☑
    - popliteal fossa or space DØ3.7- ☑
    - prepuce DØ3.8
    - pudendum DØ3.8
    - retina DØ3.8
    - retrobulbar DØ3.8
    - scalp DØ3.4
    - scrotum DØ3.8
    - shoulder DØ3.6- ☑
    - specified site NEC DØ3.8
    - submammary fold DØ3.52
    - temple DØ3.39
    - thigh DØ3.7- ☑
    - toe DØ3.7- ☑

- **Melanoma** — *continued*
  - in situ — *continued*
    - trunk NEC DØ3.59
    - umbilicus DØ3.59
    - upper limb NEC DØ3.6- ☑
    - vulva DØ3.8
  - juvenile — *see* Nevus
  - malignant, of soft parts except skin — *see* Neoplasm, connective tissue, malignant
  - metastatic
    - breast C79.81
    - genital organ C79.82
    - specified site NEC C79.89
  - neurotropic, malignant — *see* Melanoma, skin, by site
  - nodular — *see* Melanoma, skin, by site
  - regressing, malignant — *see* Melanoma, skin, by site
  - skin C43.9
    - abdominal wall C43.59
    - ala nasi C43.31
    - ankle C43.7- ☑
    - anus, anal (skin) C43.51
    - arm C43.6- ☑
    - auditory canal (external) C43.2- ☑
    - auricle (ear) C43.2- ☑
    - auricular canal (external) C43.2- ☑
    - axilla, axillary fold C43.59
    - back C43.59
    - breast (female) (male) C43.52
    - brow C43.39
    - buttock C43.59
    - canthus (eye) C43.1- ☑
    - cheek (external) C43.39
    - chest wall C43.59
    - chin C43.39
    - ear (external) C43.2- ☑
    - elbow C43.6- ☑
    - external meatus (ear) C43.2- ☑
    - eyebrow C43.39
    - eyelid (lower) (upper) C43.1- ☑
    - face C43.3Ø
      - specified NEC C43.39
    - female genital organ (external) NEC C51.9
    - finger C43.6- ☑
    - flank C43.59
    - foot C43.7- ☑
    - forearm C43.6- ☑
    - forehead C43.39
    - foreskin C6Ø.Ø
    - glabella C43.39
    - gluteal region C43.59
    - groin C43.59
    - hand C43.6- ☑
    - heel C43.7- ☑
    - helix C43.2- ☑
    - hip C43.7- ☑
    - interscapular region C43.59
    - jaw (external) C43.39
    - knee C43.7- ☑
    - labium C51.9
      - majus C51.Ø
      - minus C51.1
    - leg C43.7- ☑
    - lip (lower) (upper) C43.Ø
    - lower limb NEC C43.7- ☑
    - male genital organ (external) NEC C63.9
    - nail
      - finger C43.6- ☑
      - toe C43.7- ☑
    - nasolabial groove C43.39
    - nates C43.59
    - neck C43.4
    - nose (external) C43.31
    - overlapping site C43.8
    - palpebra C43.1- ☑
    - penis C6Ø.9
    - perianal skin C43.51
    - perineum C43.51
    - pinna C43.2- ☑
    - popliteal fossa or space C43.7- ☑
    - prepuce C6Ø.Ø
    - pudendum C51.9
    - scalp C43.4
    - scrotum C63.2
    - shoulder C43.6- ☑
    - skin NEC C43.9
    - submammary fold C43.52
    - temple C43.39

- **Melanoma** — *continued*
  - skin — *continued*
    - thigh C43.7- ☑
    - toe C43.7- ☑
    - trunk NEC C43.59
    - umbilicus C43.59
    - upper limb NEC C43.6- ☑
    - vulva C51.9
      - overlapping sites C51.8
  - spindle cell
    - with epithelioid, mixed — *see* Melanoma, skin, by site
    - type A C69.4- ☑
    - type B C69.4- ☑
  - superficial spreading — *see* Melanoma, skin, by site
- **Melanosarcoma** — *see also* Melanoma
  - epithelioid cell — *see* Melanoma
- **Melanosis** L81.4
  - addisonian E27.1
    - tuberculous A18.7
  - adrenal E27.1
  - colon K63.89
  - conjunctiva — *see* Pigmentation, conjunctiva
    - congenital Q13.89
  - cornea (presenile) (senile) — *see also* Pigmentation, cornea
    - congenital Q13.4
  - eye NEC H57.89
    - congenital Q15.8
  - lenticularis progressiva Q82.1
  - liver K76.89
  - precancerous — *see also* Melanoma, in situ
    - malignant melanoma in — *see* Melanoma
  - Riehl's L81.4
  - sclera H15.89
    - congenital Q13.89
  - suprarenal E27.1
  - tar L81.4
  - toxic L81.4
- **Melanuria** R82.998
- **MELAS syndrome** E88.41
- **Melasma** L81.1
  - adrenal (gland) E27.1
  - suprarenal (gland) E27.1
- **Melena** K92.1
  - with ulcer — *code by* site under Ulcer, with hemorrhage K27.4
  - due to swallowed maternal blood P78.2
  - newborn, neonatal P54.1
    - due to swallowed maternal blood P78.2
- **Meleney's**
  - gangrene (cutaneous) — *see* Ulcer, skin
  - ulcer (chronic undermining) — *see* Ulcer, skin
- **Melioidosis** A24.9
  - acute A24.1
  - chronic A24.2
  - fulminating A24.1
  - pneumonia A24.1
  - pulmonary (chronic) A24.2
    - acute A24.1
    - subacute A24.2
  - sepsis A24.1
  - specified NEC A24.3
  - subacute A24.2
- **Melitensis, febris** A23.Ø
- **Melkersson** (-Rosenthal) **syndrome** G51.2
- **Mellitus, diabetes** — *see* Diabetes
- **Melorheostosis** (bone) — *see* Disorder, bone, density and structure, specified NEC
- **Meloschisis** Q18.4
- **Melotia** Q17.4
- **Membrana**
  - capsularis lentis posterior Q13.89
  - epipapillaris Q14.2
- **Membranacea placenta** O43.19- ☑
- **Membranaceous uterus** N85.8
- **Membrane**(s), membranous — *see also* condition
  - cyclitic — *see* Membrane, pupillary
  - folds, congenital — *see* Web
  - Jackson's Q43.3
  - over face of newborn P28.9
  - premature rupture — *see* Rupture, membranes, premature
  - pupillary H21.4- ☑
    - persistent Q13.89
  - retained (with hemorrhage) (complicating delivery) O72.2

- **Meningovascular** — *see* condition
- **Menkes' disease or syndrome** E83.Ø9
  - meaning maple-syrup-urine disease E71.Ø
- **Menometrorrhagia** N92.1
- **Menopause, menopausal** (asymptomatic) (state) Z78.Ø
  - arthritis (any site) NEC — *see* Arthritis, specified form NEC
  - bleeding N92.4
  - depression (single episode) F32.89
    - agitated (single episode) F32.2
      - recurrent episode F33.9
    - psychotic (single episode) F32.89
      - recurrent episode F33.9
    - recurrent episode F33.8
  - melancholia (single episode) F32.89
    - recurrent episode F33.8
  - paranoid state F22
  - premature E28.319
    - asymptomatic E28.319
      - postirradiation E89.4Ø
      - postsurgical E89.4Ø
    - symptomatic E28.31Ø
      - postirradiation E89.41
      - postsurgical E89.41
  - psychosis NEC F28
  - symptomatic N95.1
  - toxic polyarthritis NEC — *see* Arthritis, specified form NEC
- **Menorrhagia** (primary) N92.Ø
  - climacteric N92.4
    - menopausal N92.4
  - menopausal N92.4
  - perimenopausal N92.4
  - postclimacteric N95.Ø
  - postmenopausal N95.Ø
  - preclimacteric or premenopausal N92.4
  - pubertal (menses retained) N92.2
- **Menostaxis** N92.Ø
- **Menses, retention** N94.89
- **Menstrual** — *see* Menstruation
- **Menstruation**
  - absent — *see* Amenorrhea
  - anovulatory N97.Ø
  - cycle, irregular N92.6
  - delayed N91.Ø
  - disorder N93.9
    - psychogenic F45.8
  - during pregnancy O2Ø.8
  - excessive (with regular cycle) N92.Ø
    - with irregular cycle N92.1
    - at puberty N92.2
  - frequent N92.Ø
  - infrequent — *see* Oligomenorrhea
  - irregular N92.6
    - specified NEC N92.5
  - latent N92.5
  - membranous N92.5
  - painful — *see also* Dysmenorrhea N94.6
    - primary N94.4
    - psychogenic F45.8
    - secondary N94.5
  - passage of clots N92.Ø
  - precocious E3Ø.1
  - protracted N92.5
  - rare — *see* Oligomenorrhea
  - retained N94.89
  - retrograde N92.5
  - scanty — *see* Oligomenorrhea
  - suppression N94.89
  - vicarious (nasal) N94.89
- **Mental** — *see also* condition
  - deficiency — *see* Disability, intellectual
  - deterioration — *see* Psychosis
  - disorder — *see* Disorder, mental
  - exhaustion F48.8
  - insufficiency (congenital) — *see* Disability, intellectual
  - observation without need for further medical care Z03.89
  - retardation — *see* Disability, intellectual
  - subnormality — *see* Disability, intellectuall
  - upset — *see* Disorder, mental
- **Meralgia paresthetica** G57.1- ☑
- **Mercurial** — *see* condition
- **Mercurialism** — *see* subcategory T56.1 ☑
- **Merkel cell tumor** — *see* Carcinoma, Merkel cell
- **Merocele** — *see* Hernia, femoral
- **Meromelia**
  - lower limb — *see* Defect, reduction, lower limb
- **Meromelia** — *continued*
  - lower limb — *see* Defect, reduction, lower limb — *continued*
    - intercalary
      - femur — *see* Defect, reduction, lower limb, specified type NEC
        - tibiofibular (complete) (incomplete) — *see* Defect, reduction, lower limb
  - upper limb — *see* Defect, reduction, upper limb
    - intercalary, humeral, radioulnar — *see* Agenesis, arm, with hand present
- **MERRF syndrome** (myoclonic epilepsy associated with ragged-red fiber) E88.42
- **Merzbacher-Pelizaeus disease** E75.29
- **Mesaortitis** — *see* Aortitis
- **Mesarteritis** — *see* Arteritis
- **Mesencephalitis** — *see* Encephalitis
- **Mesenchymoma** — *see also* Neoplasm, connective tissue, uncertain behavior
  - benign — *see* Neoplasm, connective tissue, benign
  - malignant — *see* Neoplasm, connective tissue, malignant
- **Mesenteritis**
  - retractile K65.4
  - sclerosing K65.4
- **Mesentery, mesenteric** — *see* condition
- **Mesiodens, mesiodentes** KØØ.1
- **Mesio-occlusion** M26.213
- **Mesocolon** — *see* condition
- **Mesonephroma** (malignant) — *see* Neoplasm, malignant, by site
  - benign — *see* Neoplasm, benign, by site
- **Mesophlebitis** — *see* Phlebitis
- **Mesostromal dysgenesia** Q13.89
- **Mesothelioma** (malignant) C45.9
  - benign
    - mesentery D19.1
    - mesocolon D19.1
    - omentum D19.1
    - peritoneum D19.1
    - pleura D19.Ø
    - specified site NEC D19.7
    - unspecified site D19.9
  - biphasic C45.9
    - benign
      - mesentery D19.1
      - mesocolon D19.1
      - omentum D19.1
      - peritoneum D19.1
      - pleura D19.Ø
      - specified site NEC D19.7
      - unspecified site D19.9
  - cystic D48.4
  - epithelioid C45.9
    - benign
      - mesentery D19.1
      - mesocolon D19.1
      - omentum D19.1
      - peritoneum D19.1
      - pleura D19.Ø
      - specified site NEC D19.7
      - unspecified site D19.9
  - fibrous C45.9
    - benign
      - mesentery D19.1
      - mesocolon D19.1
      - omentum D19.1
      - peritoneum D19.1
      - pleura D19.Ø
      - specified site NEC D19.7
      - unspecified site D19.9
  - site classification
    - liver C45.7
    - lung C45.7
    - mediastinum C45.7
    - mesentery C45.1
    - mesocolon C45.1
    - omentum C45.1
    - pericardium C45.2
    - peritoneum C45.1
    - pleura C45.Ø
      - parietal C45.Ø
    - retroperitoneum C45.7
    - specified site NEC C45.7
    - unspecified C45.9
- **Metabolic syndrome** E88.81
- **Metagonimiasis** B66.8
- **Metagonimus infestation** (intestine) B66.8
- **Metal**
  - pigmentation L81.8
  - polisher's disease J62.8
- **Metamorphopsia** H53.15
- **Metaplasia**
  - apocrine (breast) — *see* Dysplasia, mammary, specified type NEC
  - cervix (squamous) — *see* Dysplasia, cervix
  - endometrium (squamous) (uterus) N85.8
  - esophagus K22.7- ☑
  - kidney (pelvis) (squamous) N28.89
  - myelogenous D73.1
  - myeloid (agnogenic) (megakaryocytic) D73.1
  - spleen D73.1
  - squamous cell, bladder N32.89
- **Metastasis, metastatic**
  - abscess — *see* Abscess
  - calcification E83.59
  - cancer
    - from specified site — *see* Neoplasm, malignant, by site
    - to specified site — *see* Neoplasm, secondary, by site
  - deposits (in) — *see* Neoplasm, secondary, by site
  - disease — *see also* Neoplasm, secondary, by site C79.9
  - spread (to) — *see* Neoplasm, secondary, by site
- **Metastrongyliasis** B83.8
- **Metatarsalgia** M77.4- ☑
  - anterior G57.6- ☑
  - Morton's G57.6- ☑
- **Metatarsus, metatarsal** — *see also* condition
  - adductus, congenital Q66.22- ☑
  - valgus (abductus), congenital Q66.6
  - varus (congenital) Q66.22- ☑
    - primus Q66.21- ☑
- **Methadone use** — *see* Use, opioid
- **Methemoglobinemia** D74.9
  - acquired (with sulfhemoglobinemia) D74.8
  - congenital D74.Ø
  - enzymatic (congenital) D74.Ø
  - Hb M disease D74.Ø
  - hereditary D74.Ø
  - toxic D74.8
- **Methemoglobinuria** — *see* Hemoglobinuria
- **Methioninemia** E72.19
- **Methylmalonic acidemia** E71.12Ø
- **Metritis** (catarrhal) (hemorrhagic) (septic) (suppurative) — *see also* Endometritis
  - cervical — *see* Cervicitis
- **Metropathia hemorrhagica** N93.8
- **Metroperitonitis** — *see* Peritonitis, pelvic, female
- **Metrorrhagia** N92.1
  - climacteric N92.4
  - menopausal N92.4
  - perimenopausal N92.4
  - postpartum NEC (atonic) (following delivery of placenta) O72.1
    - delayed or secondary O72.2
  - preclimacteric or premenopausal N92.4
  - psychogenic F45.8
- **Metrorrhexis** — *see* Rupture, uterus
- **Metrosalpingitis** N7Ø.91
- **Metrostaxis** N93.8
- **Metrovaginitis** — *see* Endometritis
- **Meyer-Schwickerath and Weyers syndrome** Q87.Ø
- **Meynert's amentia** (nonalcoholic) FØ4
  - alcoholic F1Ø.96
    - with dependence F1Ø.26
- **Mibelli's disease** (porokeratosis) Q82.8
- **Mice, joint** — *see* Loose, body, joint
  - knee M23.4- ☑
- **Micrencephalon, micrencephaly** QØ2
- **Microalbuminuria** R8Ø.9
- **Microaneurysm, retinal** — *see also* Disorder, retina, microaneurysms
  - diabetic — *see* EØ8-E13 with .31
- **Microangiopathy** (peripheral) I73.9
  - thrombotic M31.1
- **Microcalcifications, breast** R92.Ø
- **Microcephalus, microcephalic, microcephaly** QØ2
  - due to toxoplasmosis (congenital) P37.1
- **Microcheilia** Q18.7
- **Microcolon** (congenital) Q43.8
- **Microcornea** (congenital) Q13.4
- **Microcytic** — *see* condition
- **Microdeletions NEC** Q93.88
- **Microdontia** KØØ.2
- **Microdrepanocytosis** D57.4Ø

Mirror writing F81.Ø
Misadventure (of) (prophylactic) (therapeutic) — *see also* Complications T88.9 ☑
  administration of insulin (by accident) — *see* subcategory T38.3 ☑
  infusion — *see* Complications, infusion
  local applications (of fomentations, plasters, etc.) T88.9 ☑
    burn or scald — *see* Burn
    specified NEC T88.8 ☑
  medical care (early) (late) T88.9 ☑
    adverse effect of drugs or chemicals — *see* Table of Drugs and Chemicals
    burn or scald — *see* Burn
    specified NEC T88.8 ☑
  specified NEC T88.8 ☑
  surgical procedure (early) (late) — *see* Complications, surgical procedure
  transfusion — *see* Complications, transfusion
  vaccination or other immunological procedure — *see* Complications, vaccination
Miscarriage OØ3.9
Misdirection, aqueous H4Ø.83- ☑
Misperception, sleep state F51.Ø2
Misplaced, misplacement
  ear Q17.4
  kidney (acquired) N28.89
    congenital Q63.2
  organ or site, congenital NEC — *see* Malposition, congenital
Missed
  abortion OØ2.1
  delivery O36.4 ☑
Missing — *see also* Absence
  string of intrauterine contraceptive device T83.32- ☑
Misuse of drugs F19.99
Mitchell's disease (erythromelalgia) I73.81
Mite(s) (infestation) B88.9
  diarrhea B88.Ø
  grain (itch) B88.Ø
  hair follicle (itch) B88.Ø
  in sputum B88.Ø
Mitral — *see* condition
Mittelschmerz N94.Ø
Mixed — *see* condition
MMN (multifocal motor neuropathy) G61.82
MNGIE (Mitochondrial Neurogastrointestinal Encephalopathy) **syndrome** E88.49
Mobile, mobility
  cecum Q43.3
  excessive — *see* Hypermobility
  gallbladder, congenital Q44.1
  kidney N28.89
  organ or site, congenital NEC — *see* Malposition, congenital
Mobitz heart block (atrioventricular) I44.1
Moebius, Möbius
  disease (ophthalmoplegic migraine) — *see* Migraine, ophthalmoplegic
  syndrome Q87.Ø
    congenital oculofacial paralysis (with other anomalies) Q87.Ø
    ophthalmoplegic migraine — *see* Migraine, ophthalmoplegic
Moeller's glossitis K14.Ø
Mohr's syndrome (Types I and II) Q87.Ø
Mola destruens D39.2
Molar pregnancy OØ2.Ø
Molarization of premolars KØØ.2
Molding, head (during birth) — *omit code*
Mole (pigmented) — *see also* Nevus
  blood OØ2.Ø
  Breus' OØ2.Ø
  cancerous — *see* Melanoma
  carneous OØ2.Ø
  destructive D39.2
  fleshy OØ2.Ø
  hydatid, hydatidiform (benign) (complicating pregnancy) (delivered) (undelivered) OØ1.9
    classical OØ1.Ø
    complete OØ1.Ø
    incomplete OØ1.1
    invasive D39.2
    malignant D39.2
    partial OØ1.1
  intrauterine OØ2.Ø
  invasive (hydatidiform) D39.2

Mole — *continued*
  malignant
    meaning
      malignant hydatidiform mole D39.2
      melanoma — *see* Melanoma
  nonhydatidiform OØ2.Ø
  nonpigmented — *see* Nevus
  pregnancy NEC OØ2.Ø
  skin — *see* Nevus
  tubal OØØ.1Ø- ☑
    with intrauterine pregnancy OØØ.11- ☑
  vesicular — *see* Mole, hydatidiform
Molimen, molimina (menstrual) N94.3
Molluscum contagiosum (epitheliale) BØ8.1
Mönckeberg's arteriosclerosis, disease, or sclerosis — *see* Arteriosclerosis, extremities
Mondini's malformation (cochlea) Q16.5
Mondor's disease I8Ø.8
Monge's disease T7Ø.29 ☑
Monilethrix (congenital) Q84.1
Moniliasis — *see also* Candidiasis B37.9
  neonatal P37.5
Monitoring (encounter for)
  therapeutic drug level Z51.81
Monkey malaria B53.1
Monkeypox BØ4
Monoarthritis M13.1Ø
  ankle M13.17- ☑
  elbow M13.12- ☑
  foot joint M13.17- ☑
  hand joint M13.14- ☑
  hip M13.15- ☑
  knee M13.16- ☑
  shoulder M13.11- ☑
  wrist M13.13- ☑
Monoblastic — *see* condition
Monochromat (ism), monochromatopsia (acquired) (congenital) H53.51
Monocytic — *see* condition
Monocytopenia D72.818
Monocytosis (symptomatic) D72.821
Monomania — *see* Psychosis
Mononeuritis G58.9
  cranial nerve — *see* Disorder, nerve, cranial
  femoral nerve G57.2- ☑
  lateral
    cutaneous nerve of thigh G57.1- ☑
    popliteal nerve G57.3- ☑
  lower limb G57.9- ☑
    specified nerve NEC G57.8- ☑
  medial popliteal nerve G57.4- ☑
  median nerve G56.1- ☑
  multiplex G58.7
  plantar nerve G57.6- ☑
  posterior tibial nerve G57.5- ☑
  radial nerve G56.3- ☑
  sciatic nerve G57.Ø- ☑
  specified NEC G58.8
  tibial nerve G57.4- ☑
  ulnar nerve G56.2- ☑
  upper limb G56.9- ☑
    specified nerve NEC G56.8- ☑
  vestibular — *see* subcategory H93.3 ☑
Mononeuropathy G58.9
  carpal tunnel syndrome — *see* Syndrome, carpal tunnel
  diabetic NEC — *see* EØ8-E13 with .41
  femoral nerve — *see* Lesion, nerve, femoral
  ilioinguinal nerve G57.8- ☑
  in diseases classified elsewhere — *see* category G59
  intercostal G58.Ø
  lower limb G57.9- ☑
    causalgia — *see* Causalgia, lower limb
    femoral nerve — *see* Lesion, nerve, femoral
    meralgia paresthetica G57.1- ☑
    plantar nerve — *see* Lesion, nerve, plantar
    popliteal nerve — *see* Lesion, nerve, popliteal
    sciatic nerve — *see* Lesion, nerve, sciatic
    specified NEC G57.8- ☑
    tarsal tunnel syndrome — *see* Syndrome, tarsal tunnel
  median nerve — *see* Lesion, nerve, median
  multiplex G58.7
  obturator nerve G57.8- ☑
  popliteal nerve — *see* Lesion, nerve, popliteal
  radial nerve — *see* Lesion, nerve, radial
  saphenous nerve G57.8- ☑

Mononeuropathy — *continued*
  specified NEC G58.8
  tarsal tunnel syndrome — *see* Syndrome, tarsal tunnel
  tuberculous A17.83
  ulnar nerve — *see* Lesion, nerve, ulnar
  upper limb G56.9- ☑
    carpal tunnel syndrome — *see* Syndrome, carpal tunnel
    causalgia — *see* Causalgia
    median nerve — *see* Lesion, nerve, median
    radial nerve — *see* Lesion, nerve, radial
    specified site NEC G56.8- ☑
    ulnar nerve — *see* Lesion, nerve, ulnar
Mononucleosis, infectious B27.9Ø
  with
    complication NEC B27.99
    meningitis B27.92
    polyneuropathy B27.91
  cytomegaloviral B27.1Ø
    with
      complication NEC B27.19
      meningitis B27.12
      polyneuropathy B27.11
  Epstein-Barr (virus) B27.ØØ
    with
      complication NEC B27.Ø9
      meningitis B27.Ø2
      polyneuropathy B27.Ø1
  gammaherpesviral B27.ØØ
    with
      complication NEC B27.Ø9
      meningitis B27.Ø2
      polyneuropathy B27.Ø1
  specified NEC B27.8Ø
    with
      complication NEC B27.89
      meningitis B27.82
      polyneuropathy B27.81
Monoplegia G83.3- ☑
  congenital (cerebral) G8Ø.8
    spastic G8Ø.1
  embolic (current episode) I63.4- ☑
  following
    cerebrovascular disease
      cerebral infarction
        lower limb I69.34- ☑
        upper limb I69.33- ☑
      intracerebral hemorrhage
        lower limb I69.14- ☑
        upper limb I69.13- ☑
      lower limb I69.94- ☑
      nontraumatic intracranial hemorrhage NEC
        lower limb I69.24- ☑
        upper limb I69.23- ☑
      specified disease NEC
        lower limb I69.84- ☑
        upper limb I69.83- ☑
      stroke NOS
        lower limb I69.34- ☑
        upper limb I69.33- ☑
      subarachnoid hemorrhage
        lower limb I69.Ø4- ☑
        upper limb I69.Ø3- ☑
      upper limb I69.93- ☑
  hysterical (transient) F44.4
  lower limb G83.1- ☑
  psychogenic (conversion reaction) F44.4
  thrombotic (current episode) I63.3- ☑
  transient R29.818
  upper limb G83.2- ☑
Monorchism, monorchidism Q55.Ø
Monosomy — *see also* Deletion, chromosome Q93.9
  specified NEC Q93.89
  whole chromosome
    meiotic nondisjunction Q93.Ø
    mitotic nondisjunction Q93.1
    mosaicism Q93.1
  X Q96.9
Monster, monstrosity (single) Q89.7
  acephalic QØØ.Ø
  twin Q89.4
Monteggia's fracture (-dislocation) S52.27- ☑
Mooren's ulcer (cornea) — *see* Ulcer, cornea, Mooren's
Moore's syndrome — *see* Epilepsy, specified NEC
Mooser-Neill reaction A75.2
Mooser's bodies A75.2
Morbidity not stated or unknown R69

N

Nephropathy — *continued*
- hereditary — *continued*
  - with — *continued*
    - diffuse — *continued*
      - endocapillary proliferative glomerulonephritis NØ7.4
      - membranous glomerulonephritis NØ7.2
      - mesangial proliferative glomerulonephritis NØ7.3
      - mesangiocapillary glomerulonephritis NØ7.5
    - focal and segmental glomerular lesions NØ7.1
    - minor glomerular abnormality NØ7.Ø
    - specified morphological changes NEC NØ7.8
- hypercalcemic N25.89
- hypertensive — *see* Hypertension, kidney
- hypokalemic (vacuolar) N25.89
- IgA NØ2.8
  - with glomerular lesion NØ2.9
    - focal and segmental hyalinosis or sclerosis NØ2.1
    - membranoproliferative (diffuse) NØ2.5
    - membranous (diffuse) NØ2.2
    - mesangial proliferative (diffuse) NØ2.3
    - mesangiocapillary (diffuse) NØ2.5
    - proliferative NEC NØ2.8
    - specified pathology NEC NØ2.8
- lead N14.3
- membranoproliferative (diffuse) NØ2.5
- membranous (diffuse) NØ2.2
- mesangial (IgA/IgG) — *see* Nephropathy, IgA
  - proliferative (diffuse) NØ2.3
- mesangiocapillary (diffuse) NØ2.5
- obstructive N13.8
- phenacetin N17.2
- phosphate-losing N25.Ø
- potassium depletion N25.89
- pregnancy-related O26.83- ☑
- proliferative NEC — *see also* NØØ-NØ7 with fourth character .8 NØ5.8
- protein-losing N25.89
- saturnine N14.3
- sickle-cell D57.- ☑ *[NØ8]*
- toxic NEC N14.4
  - due to
    - drugs N14.2
      - analgesic N14.Ø
      - specified NEC N14.1
    - heavy metals N14.3
- vasomotor N17.Ø
- water-losing N25.89

Nephroptosis N28.83

Nephropyosis — *see* Abscess, kidney

Nephrorrhagia N28.89

Nephrosclerosis (arteriolar)(arteriosclerotic) (chronic) (hyaline) — *see also* Hypertension, kidney
- hyperplastic — *see* Hypertension, kidney
- senile N26.9

Nephrosis, nephrotic (Epstein's) (syndrome) (congenital) NØ4.9
- with
  - foot process disease NØ4.9
  - glomerular lesion NØ4.1
  - hypocomplementemic NØ4.5
- acute NØ4.9
- anoxic — *see* Nephrosis, tubular
- chemical — *see* Nephrosis, tubular
- cholemic K76.7
- diabetic — *see* EØ8-E13 with .21
- Finnish type (congenital) Q89.8
- hemoglobin N1Ø
- hemoglobinuric — *see* Nephrosis, tubular
- in
  - amyloidosis E85.4 *[NØ8]*
  - diabetes mellitus — *see* EØ8-E13 with .21
  - epidemic hemorrhagic fever A98.5
  - malaria (malariae) B52.Ø
- ischemic — *see* Nephrosis, tubular
- lipoid NØ4.9
- lower nephron — *see* Nephrosis, tubular
- malarial (malariae) B52.Ø
- minimal change NØ4.Ø
- myoglobin N1Ø
- necrotizing — *see* Nephrosis, tubular
- osmotic (sucrose) N25.89
- radiation NØ4.9
- syphilitic (late) A52.75
- toxic — *see* Nephrosis, tubular
- tubular (acute) N17.Ø
  - postprocedural N99.Ø

Nephrosis, nephrotic — *continued*
- tubular — *continued*
  - radiation NØ4.9

Nephrosonephritis, hemorrhagic (endemic) A98.5

Nephrostomy
- attention to Z43.6
- status Z93.6

Nerve — *see also* condition
- injury — *see* Injury, nerve, by body site

Nerves R45.Ø

Nervous — *see also* condition R45.Ø
- heart F45.8
- stomach F45.8
- tension R45.Ø

Nervousness R45.Ø

Nesidioblastoma
- pancreas D13.7
- specified site NEC — *see* Neoplasm, benign, by site
- unspecified site D13.7

Nettleship's syndrome — *see* Urticaria pigmentosa

Neumann's disease or syndrome L1Ø.1

Neuralgia, neuralgic (acute) M79.2
- accessory (nerve) G52.8
- acoustic (nerve) — *see* subcategory H93.3 ☑
- auditory (nerve) — *see* subcategory H93.3 ☑
- ciliary G44.ØØ9
  - intractable G44.ØØ1
  - not intractable G44.ØØ9
- cranial
  - nerve — *see also* Disorder, nerve, cranial
    - fifth or trigeminal — *see* Neuralgia, trigeminal
  - postherpetic, postzoster BØ2.29
- ear — *see* subcategory H92.Ø ☑
- facialis vera G51.1
- Fothergill's — *see* Neuralgia, trigeminal
- glossopharyngeal (nerve) G52.1
- Horton's G44.Ø99
  - intractable G44.Ø91
  - not intractable G44.Ø99
- Hunt's BØ2.21
- hypoglossal (nerve) G52.3
- infraorbital — *see* Neuralgia, trigeminal
- malarial — *see* Malaria
- migrainous G44.ØØ9
  - intractable G44.ØØ1
  - not intractable G44.ØØ9
- Morton's G57.6- ☑
- nerve, cranial — *see* Disorder, nerve, cranial
- nose G52.Ø
- occipital M54.81
- olfactory G52.Ø
- penis N48.9
- perineum R1Ø.2
- postherpetic NEC BØ2.29
  - trigeminal BØ2.22
- pubic region R1Ø.2
- scrotum R1Ø.2
- Sluder's G44.89
- specified nerve NEC G58.8
- spermatic cord R1Ø.2
- sphenopalatine (ganglion) G9Ø.Ø9
- trifacial — *see* Neuralgia, trigeminal
- trigeminal G5Ø.Ø
  - postherpetic, postzoster BØ2.22
- vagus (nerve) G52.2
- writer's F48.8
  - organic G25.89

Neurapraxia — *see* Injury, nerve

Neurasthenia F48.8
- cardiac F45.8
- gastric F45.8
- heart F45.8

Neurilemmoma — *see also* Neoplasm, nerve, benign
- acoustic (nerve) D33.3
- malignant — *see also* Neoplasm, nerve, malignant
  - acoustic (nerve) C72.4- ☑

Neurilemmosarcoma — *see* Neoplasm, nerve, malignant

Neurinoma — *see* Neoplasm, nerve, benign

Neurinomatosis — *see* Neoplasm, nerve, uncertain behavior

Neuritis (rheumatoid) M79.2
- abducens (nerve) — *see* Strabismus, paralytic, sixth nerve
- accessory (nerve) G52.8
- acoustic (nerve) — *see also* subcategory H93.3 ☑
  - in (due to)
    - infectious disease NEC B99 ☑ *[H94.Ø-]* ☑

Neuritis — *continued*
- acoustic — *see also* subcategory — *continued*
  - in — *continued*
    - parasitic disease NEC B89 *[H94.Ø-]* ☑
  - syphilitic A52.15
- alcoholic G62.1
  - with psychosis — *see* Psychosis, alcoholic
- amyloid, any site E85.4 *[G63]*
- auditory (nerve) — *see* subcategory H93.3 ☑
- brachial — *see* Radiculopathy
  - due to displacement, intervertebral disc — *see* Disorder, disc, cervical, with neuritis
- cranial nerve
  - due to Lyme disease A69.22
  - eighth or acoustic or auditory — *see* subcategory H93.3 ☑
  - eleventh or accessory G52.8
  - fifth or trigeminal G51.Ø
  - first or olfactory G52.Ø
  - fourth or trochlear — *see* Strabismus, paralytic, fourth nerve
  - second or optic — *see* Neuritis, optic
  - seventh or facial G51.8
    - newborn (birth injury) P11.3
  - sixth or abducent — *see* Strabismus, paralytic, sixth nerve
  - tenth or vagus G52.2
  - third or oculomotor — *see* Strabismus, paralytic, third nerve
  - twelfth or hypoglossal G52.3
- Déjérine-Sottas G6Ø.Ø
- diabetic (mononeuropathy) — *see* EØ8-E13 with .41
  - polyneuropathy — *see* EØ8-E13 with .42
- due to
  - beriberi E51.11
  - displacement, prolapse or rupture, intervertebral disc — *see* Disorder, disc, with, radiculopathy
  - herniation, nucleus pulposus M51.9 *[G55]*
- endemic E51.11
- facial G51.8
  - newborn (birth injury) P11.3
- general — *see* Polyneuropathy
- geniculate ganglion G51.1
  - due to herpes (zoster) BØ2.21
- gouty — *see also* Gout, by type M1Ø.9 *[G63]*
- hypoglossal (nerve) G52.3
- ilioinguinal (nerve) G57.9- ☑
- infectious (multiple) NEC G61.Ø
- interstitial hypertrophic progressive G6Ø.Ø
- lumbar M54.16
- lumbosacral M54.17
- multiple — *see also* Polyneuropathy
  - endemic E51.11
  - infective, acute G61.Ø
- multiplex endemica E51.11
- nerve root — *see* Radiculopathy
- oculomotor (nerve) — *see* Strabismus, paralytic, third nerve
- olfactory nerve G52.Ø
- optic (nerve) (hereditary) (sympathetic) H46.9
  - with demyelination G36.Ø
  - in myelitis G36.Ø
  - nutritional H46.2
  - papillitis — *see* Papillitis, optic
  - retrobulbar H46.1- ☑
  - specified type NEC H46.8
  - toxic H46.3
- peripheral (nerve) G62.9
  - multiple — *see* Polyneuropathy
  - single — *see* Mononeuritis
- pneumogastric (nerve) G52.2
- postherpetic, postzoster BØ2.29
- progressive hypertrophic interstitial G6Ø.Ø
- retrobulbar — *see also* Neuritis, optic, retrobulbar
  - in (due to)
    - late syphilis A52.15
    - meningococcal infection A39.82
  - meningococcal A39.82
  - syphilitic A52.15
- sciatic (nerve) — *see also* Sciatica
  - due to displacement of intervertebral disc — *see* Disorder, disc, with, radiculopathy
- serum — *see also* Reaction, serum T8Ø.69 ☑
- shoulder-girdle G54.5
- specified nerve NEC G58.8
- spinal (nerve) root — *see* Radiculopathy
- syphilitic A52.15
- thenar (median) G56.1- ☑

- **Neuritis** — *continued*
  - thoracic M54.14
  - toxic NEC G62.2
  - trochlear (nerve) — *see* Strabismus, paralytic, fourth nerve
  - vagus (nerve) G52.2
- **Neuroastrocytoma** — *see* Neoplasm, uncertain behavior, by site
- **Neuroavitaminosis** E56.9 *[G99.8]*
- **Neuroblastoma**
  - olfactory C3Ø.Ø
  - specified site — *see* Neoplasm, malignant, by site
  - unspecified site C74.9Ø
- **Neurochorioretinitis** — *see* Chorioretinitis
- **Neurocirculatory asthenia** F45.8
- **Neurocysticercosis** B69.Ø
- **Neurocytoma** — *see* Neoplasm, benign, by site
- **Neurodermatitis** (circumscribed) (circumscripta) (local) L28.Ø
  - atopic L2Ø.81
  - diffuse (Brocq) L2Ø.81
  - disseminated L2Ø.81
- **Neuroencephalomyelopathy, optic** G36.Ø
- **Neuroepithelioma** — *see also* Neoplasm, malignant, by site
  - olfactory C3Ø.Ø
- **Neurofibroma** — *see also* Neoplasm, nerve, benign
  - melanotic — *see* Neoplasm, nerve, benign
  - multiple — *see* Neurofibromatosis
  - plexiform — *see* Neoplasm, nerve, benign
- **Neurofibromatosis** (multiple) (nonmalignant) Q85.ØØ
  - acoustic Q85.Ø2
  - malignant — *see* Neoplasm, nerve, malignant
  - specified NEC Q85.Ø9
  - type 1 (von Recklinghausen) Q85.Ø1
  - type 2 Q85.Ø2
- **Neurofibrosarcoma** — *see* Neoplasm, nerve, malignant
- **Neurogenic** — *see also* condition
  - bladder — *see also* Dysfunction, bladder, neuromuscular N31.9
    - cauda equina syndrome G83.4
  - bowel NEC K59.2
  - heart F45.8
- **Neuroglioma** — *see* Neoplasm, uncertain behavior, by site
- **Neurolabyrinthitis** (of Dix and Hallpike) — *see* Neuronitis, vestibular
- **Neurolathyrism** — *see* Poisoning, food, noxious, plant
- **Neuroleprosy** A3Ø.9
- **Neuroma** — *see also* Neoplasm, nerve, benign
  - acoustic (nerve) D33.3
  - amputation (stump) (traumatic) (surgical complication) (late) T87.3- ☑
    - arm T87.3- ☑
    - leg T87.3- ☑
  - digital (toe) G57.6- ☑
  - interdigital G58.8
    - lower limb (toe) G57.8- ☑
    - upper limb G56.8- ☑
  - intermetatarsal G57.8- ☑
  - Morton's G57.6- ☑
  - nonneoplastic
    - arm G56.9- ☑
    - leg G57.9- ☑
    - lower extremity G57.9- ☑
    - upper extremity G56.9- ☑
  - optic (nerve) D33.3
  - plantar G57.6- ☑
  - plexiform — *see* Neoplasm, nerve, benign
  - surgical (nonneoplastic)
    - arm G56.9- ☑
    - leg G57.9- ☑
    - lower extremity G57.9- ☑
    - upper extremity G56.9- ☑
- **Neuromyalgia** — *see* Neuralgia
- **Neuromyasthenia** (epidemic) (postinfectious) G93.3
- **Neuromyelitis** G36.9
  - ascending G61.Ø
  - optica G36.Ø
- **Neuromyopathy** G7Ø.9
  - paraneoplastic D49.9 *[G13.Ø]*
- **Neuromyotonia** (Isaacs) G71.19
- **Neuronevus** — *see* Nevus
- **Neuronitis** G58.9
  - ascending (acute) G57.2- ☑
  - vestibular H81.2- ☑
- **Neuroparalytic** — *see* condition
- **Neuropathy, neuropathic** G62.9
  - acute motor G62.81
  - alcoholic G62.1
    - with psychosis — *see* Psychosis, alcoholic
  - arm G56.9- ☑
  - autonomic, peripheral — *see* Neuropathy, peripheral, autonomic
  - axillary G56.9- ☑
  - bladder N31.9
    - atonic (motor) (sensory) N31.2
    - autonomous N31.2
    - flaccid N31.2
    - nonreflex N31.2
    - reflex N31.1
    - uninhibited N31.Ø
  - brachial plexus G54.Ø
  - cervical plexus G54.2
  - chronic
    - progressive segmentally demyelinating G62.89
    - relapsing demyelinating G62.89
  - Déjérine-Sottas G6Ø.Ø
  - diabetic — *see* EØ8-E13 with .4Ø
    - mononeuropathy — *see* EØ8-E13 with .41
    - polyneuropathy — *see* EØ8-E13 with .42
  - entrapment G58.9
    - iliohypogastric nerve G57.8- ☑
    - ilioinguinal nerve G57.8- ☑
    - lateral cutaneous nerve of thigh G57.1- ☑
    - median nerve G56.Ø- ☑
    - obturator nerve G57.8- ☑
    - peroneal nerve G57.3- ☑
    - posterior tibial nerve G57.5- ☑
    - saphenous nerve G57.8- ☑
    - ulnar nerve G56.2- ☑
  - facial nerve G51.9
  - hereditary G6Ø.9
    - motor and sensory (types I-IV) G6Ø.Ø
    - sensory G6Ø.8
    - specified NEC G6Ø.8
  - hypertrophic G6Ø.Ø
    - Charcot-Marie-Tooth G6Ø.Ø
    - Déjérine-Sottas G6Ø.Ø
    - interstitial progressive G6Ø.Ø
    - of infancy G6Ø.Ø
    - Refsum G6Ø.1
  - idiopathic G6Ø.9
    - progressive G6Ø.3
    - specified NEC G6Ø.8
  - in association with hereditary ataxia G6Ø.2
  - intercostal G58.Ø
  - ischemic — *see* Disorder, nerve
  - Jamaica (ginger) G62.2
  - leg NEC G57.9- ☑
  - lower extremity G57.9- ☑
  - lumbar plexus G54.1
  - median nerve G56.1- ☑
  - motor and sensory — *see also* Polyneuropathy
    - hereditary (types I-IV) G6Ø.Ø
  - multifocal motor (MMN) G61.82
  - multiple (acute) (chronic) — *see* Polyneuropathy
  - optic (nerve) — *see also* Neuritis, optic
    - ischemic H47.Ø1- ☑
  - paraneoplastic (sensorial) (Denny Brown) D49.9 *[G13.Ø]*
  - peripheral (nerve) — *see also* Polyneuropathy G62.9
    - autonomic G9Ø.9
      - idiopathic G9Ø.Ø9
      - in (due to)
        - amyloidosis E85.4 *[G99.Ø]*
        - diabetes mellitus — *see* EØ8-E13 with .43
        - endocrine disease NEC E34.9 *[G99.Ø]*
        - gout M1Ø.ØØ *[G99.Ø]*
        - hyperthyroidism EØ5.9Ø *[G99.Ø]*
          - with thyroid storm EØ5.91 *[G99.Ø]*
        - metabolic disease NEC E88.9 *[G99.Ø]*
    - idiopathic G6Ø.9
      - progressive G6Ø.3
    - in (due to)
      - antitetanus serum G62.Ø
      - arsenic G62.2
      - drugs NEC G62.Ø
      - lead G62.2
      - organophosphate compounds G62.2
      - toxic agent NEC G62.2
  - plantar nerves G57.6- ☑
  - progressive
    - hypertrophic interstitial G6Ø.Ø
    - inflammatory G62.81
- **Neuropathy, neuropathic** — *continued*
  - radicular NEC — *see* Radiculopathy
  - sacral plexus G54.1
  - sciatic G57.Ø- ☑
  - serum G61.1
  - toxic NEC G62.2
  - trigeminal sensory G5Ø.8
  - ulnar nerve G56.2- ☑
  - uremic N18.9 *[G63]*
  - vitamin B12 E53.8 *[G63]*
    - with anemia (pernicious) D51.Ø *[G63]*
      - due to dietary deficiency D51.3 *[G63]*
- **Neurophthisis** — *see also* Disorder, nerve
  - peripheral, diabetic — *see* EØ8-E13 with .42
- **Neuroretinitis** — *see* Chorioretinitis
- **Neuroretinopathy, hereditary optic** H47.22
- **Neurosarcoma** — *see* Neoplasm, nerve, malignant
- **Neurosclerosis** — *see* Disorder, nerve
- **Neurosis, neurotic** F48.9
  - anankastic F42.8
  - anxiety (state) F41.1
    - panic type F41.Ø
  - asthenic F48.8
  - bladder F45.8
  - cardiac (reflex) F45.8
  - cardiovascular F45.8
  - character F6Ø.9
  - colon F45.8
  - compensation F68.1Ø
  - compulsive, compulsion F42.8
  - conversion F44.9
  - craft F48.8
  - cutaneous F45.8
  - depersonalization F48.1
  - depressive (reaction) (type) F34.1
  - environmental F48.8
  - excoriation L98.1
  - fatigue F48.8
  - functional — *see* Disorder, somatoform
  - gastric F45.8
  - gastrointestinal F45.8
  - heart F45.8
  - hypochondriacal F45.21
  - hysterical F44.9
  - incoordination F45.8
    - larynx F45.8
    - vocal cord F45.8
  - intestine F45.8
  - larynx (sensory) F45.8
    - hysterical F44.4
  - mixed NEC F48.8
  - musculoskeletal F45.8
  - obsessional F42.8
  - obsessive-compulsive F42.8
  - occupational F48.8
  - ocular NEC F45.8
  - organ — *see* Disorder, somatoform
  - pharynx F45.8
  - phobic F4Ø.9
  - posttraumatic (situational) F43.1Ø
    - acute F43.11
    - chronic F43.12
  - psychasthenic (type) F48.8
  - railroad F48.8
  - rectum F45.8
  - respiratory F45.8
  - rumination F45.8
  - sexual F65.9
  - situational F48.8
  - social F4Ø.1Ø
    - generalized F4Ø.11
  - specified type NEC F48.8
  - state F48.9
    - with depersonalization episode F48.1
  - stomach F45.8
  - traumatic F43.1Ø
    - acute F43.11
    - chronic F43.12
  - vasomotor F45.8
  - visceral F45.8
  - war F48.8
- **Neurospongioblastosis diffusa** Q85.1
- **Neurosyphilis** (arrested) (early) (gumma) (late) (latent) (recurrent) (relapse) A52.3
  - with ataxia (cerebellar) (locomotor) (spastic) (spinal) A52.19
  - aneurysm (cerebral) A52.Ø5
  - arachnoid (adhesive) A52.13

Nodule(s), **nodular** — *continued*
- Haygarth's M15.8
- inflammatory — *see* Inflammation
- juxta-articular
  - syphilitic A52.77
  - yaws A66.7
- larynx J38.7
- lung, solitary (subsegmental branch of the bronchial tree) R91.1
  - multiple R91.8
- milker's BØ8.Ø3
- prostate N4Ø.2
  - with lower urinary tract symptoms (LUTS) N4Ø.3
  - without lower urinary tract symtpoms (LUTS) N4Ø.2
- pulmonary, solitary (subsegmental branch of the bronchial tree) R91.1
- retrocardiac RØ9.89
- rheumatoid MØ6.3Ø
  - ankle MØ6.37- ☑
  - elbow MØ6.32- ☑
  - foot joint MØ6.37- ☑
  - hand joint MØ6.34- ☑
  - hip MØ6.35- ☑
  - knee MØ6.36- ☑
  - multiple site MØ6.39
  - shoulder MØ6.31- ☑
  - vertebra MØ6.38
  - wrist MØ6.33- ☑
- scrotum (inflammatory) N49.2
- singer's J38.2
- solitary, lung (subsegmental branch of the bronchial tree) R91.1
  - multiple R91.8
- subcutaneous — *see* Swelling, localized
- teacher's J38.2
- thyroid (cold) (gland) (nontoxic) EØ4.1
  - with thyrotoxicosis EØ5.2Ø
    - with thyroid storm EØ5.21
  - toxic or with hyperthyroidism EØ5.2Ø
    - with thyroid storm EØ5.21
- vocal cord J38.2

Noma (gangrenous) (hospital) (infective) A69.Ø
- auricle I96
- mouth A69.Ø
- pudendi N76.89
- vulvae N76.89

Nomad, nomadism Z59.Ø

NOMID (neonatal onset multisystemic inflammatory disorder) MØ4.2

Nonadherence to medical treatment Z91.19

Nonautoimmune hemolytic anemia D59.4
- drug-induced D59.2

Nonclosure — *see also* Imperfect, closure
- ductus arteriosus (Botallo's) Q25.Ø
- foramen
  - botalli Q21.1
  - ovale Q21.1

Noncompliance Z91.19
- with
  - dialysis Z91.15
  - dietary regimen Z91.11
  - medical treatment Z91.19
  - medication regimen NEC Z91.14
    - underdosing — *see also* Table of Drugs and Chemicals, categories T36-T5Ø, with final character 6 Z91.14
      - intentional NEC Z91.128
        - due to financial hardship of patient Z91.12Ø
      - unintentional NEC Z91.138
        - due to patient's age related debility Z91.13Ø
  - renal dialysis Z91.15

Nondescent (congenital) — *see also* Malposition, congenital
- cecum Q43.3
- colon Q43.3
- testicle Q53.9
  - bilateral Q53.2Ø
    - abdominal Q53.211
    - perineal Q53.22
  - unilateral Q53.1Ø
    - abdominal Q53.111
    - perineal Q53.12

Nondevelopment
- brain QØ2
  - part of QØ4.3
- heart Q24.8

Nondevelopment — *continued*
- organ or site, congenital NEC — *see* Hypoplasia

Nonengagement
- head NEC O32.4 ☑
  - in labor, causing obstructed labor O64.8 ☑

Nonexanthematous tick fever A93.2

Nonexpansion, lung (newborn) P28.Ø

Nonfunctioning
- cystic duct — *see also* Disease, gallbladder K82.8
- gallbladder — *see also* Disease, gallbladder K82.8
- kidney N28.9
- labyrinth — *see* subcategory H83.2 ☑

Non-Hodgkin lymphoma NEC — *see* Lymphoma, non-Hodgkin

Nonimplantation, ovum N97.2

Noninsufflation, fallopian tube N97.1

Non-ketotic hyperglycinemia E72.51

Nonne-Milroy syndrome Q82.Ø

Nonovulation N97.Ø

Non-palpable testicle(s)
- bilateral R39.84
- unilateral R39.83

Nonpatent fallopian tube N97.1

Nonpneumatization, lung NEC P28.Ø

Nonrotation — *see* Malrotation

Nonsecretion, urine — *see* Anuria

Nonunion
- fracture — *see* Fracture, by site
- joint, following fusion or arthrodesis M96.Ø
- organ or site, congenital NEC — *see* Imperfect, closure
- symphysis pubis, congenital Q74.2

Nonvisualization, gallbladder R93.2

Nonvital, nonvitalized tooth KØ4.99

Non-working side interference M26.56

Noonan's syndrome Q87.19

Normocytic anemia (infectional) due to blood loss (chronic) D5Ø.Ø
- acute D62

Norrie's disease (congenital) Q15.8

North American blastomycosis B4Ø.9

Norwegian itch B86

Nose, nasal — *see* condition

Nosebleed RØ4.Ø

Nose-picking F98.8

Nosomania F45.21

Nosophobia F45.22

Nostalgia F43.2Ø

Notch of iris Q13.2

Notching nose, congenital (tip) Q3Ø.2

Nothnagel's
- syndrome — *see* Strabismus, paralytic, third nerve
- vasomotor acroparesthesia I73.89

Novy's relapsing fever A68.9
- louse-borne A68.Ø
- tick-borne A68.1

Noxious
- foodstuffs, poisoning by — *see* Poisoning, food, noxious, plant
- substances transmitted through placenta or breast milk PØ4.9

Nucleus pulposus — *see* condition

Numbness R2Ø.Ø

Nuns' knee — *see* Bursitis, prepatellar

Nursemaid's elbow S53.Ø3- ☑

Nutcracker esophagus K22.4

Nutmeg liver K76.1

Nutrient element deficiency E61.9
- specified NEC E61.8

Nutrition deficient or insufficient — *see also* Malnutrition E46
- due to
  - insufficient food T73.Ø ☑
  - lack of
    - care (child) T76.Ø2 ☑
      - adult T76.Ø1 ☑
    - food T73.Ø ☑

Nutritional stunting E45

Nyctalopia (night blindness) — *see* Blindness, night

Nycturia R35.1
- psychogenic F45.8

Nymphomania F52.8

Nystagmus H55.ØØ
- benign paroxysmal — *see* Vertigo, benign paroxysmal
- central positional H81.4
- congenital H55.Ø1
- dissociated H55.Ø4
- latent H55.Ø2

Nystagmus — *continued*
- miners' H55.Ø9
- positional
  - benign paroxysmal H81.4
  - central H81.4
- specified form NEC H55.Ø9
- visual deprivation H55.Ø3

O

Obermeyer's relapsing fever (European) A68.Ø

Obesity E66.9
- with alveolar hypoventilation E66.2
- adrenal E27.8
- complicating
  - childbirth O99.214
  - pregnancy O99.21- ☑
  - puerperium O99.215
- constitutional E66.8
- dietary counseling and surveillance Z71.3
- drug-induced E66.1
- due to
  - drug E66.1
  - excess calories E66.Ø9
    - morbid E66.Ø1
    - severe E66.Ø1
- endocrine E66.8
- endogenous E66.8
- exogenous E66.Ø9
- familial E66.8
- glandular E66.8
- hypothyroid — *see* Hypothyroidism
- hypoventilation syndrome (OHS) E66.2
- morbid E66.Ø1
  - with
    - alveolar hypoventilation E66.2
    - obesity hypoventilation syndrome (OHS) E66.2
  - due to excess calories E66.Ø1
- nutritional E66.Ø9
- pituitary E23.6
- severe E66.Ø1
- specified type NEC E66.8

Oblique — *see* condition

Obliteration
- appendix (lumen) K38.8
- artery I77.1
- bile duct (noncalculous) K83.1
- common duct (noncalculous) K83.1
- cystic duct — *see* Obstruction, gallbladder
- disease, arteriolar I77.1
- endometrium N85.8
- eye, anterior chamber — *see* Disorder, globe, hypotony
- fallopian tube N97.1
- lymphatic vessel I89.Ø
  - due to mastectomy I97.2
- organ or site, congenital NEC — *see* Atresia, by site
- ureter N13.5
  - with infection N13.6
- urethra — *see* Stricture, urethra
- vein I87.8
- vestibule (oral) KØ8.89

Observation (following) (for) (without need for further medical care) ZØ4.9
- accident NEC ZØ4.3
  - at work ZØ4.2
  - transport ZØ4.1
- adverse effect of drug ZØ3.6
- alleged rape or sexual assault (victim), ruled out
  - adult ZØ4.41
  - child ZØ4.42
- criminal assault ZØ4.89
- development state
  - adolescent ZØØ.3
  - period of rapid growth in childhood ZØØ.2
  - puberty ZØØ.3
- disease, specified NEC ZØ3.89
- following work accident ZØ4.2
- forced sexual exploitation ZØ4.81
- forced labor exploitation ZØ4.82
- growth and development state — *see* Observation, development state
- injuries (accidental) NEC — *see also* Observation, accident
- newborn (for)
  - suspected condition, related to exposure from the mother or birth process — *see* Newborn, affected by, maternal
    - ruled out ZØ5.9

- **Obstruction, obstructed, obstructive** — *continued*
  - parotid duct or gland K11.8
  - pelviureteral junction N13.5
    - with hydronephrosis N13.0
    - congenital Q62.39
  - pharynx J39.2
  - portal (circulation) (vein) I81
  - prostate — *see also* Hyperplasia, prostate
    - valve (urinary) N32.0
  - pulmonary valve (heart) I37.0
  - pyelonephritis (chronic) N11.1
  - pylorus
    - adult K31.1
    - congenital or infantile Q40.0
  - rectosigmoid — *see* Obstruction, intestine
  - rectum K62.4
  - renal N28.89
    - outflow N13.8
    - pelvis, congenital Q62.39
  - respiratory J98.8
    - chronic J44.9
  - retinal (vessels) H34.9
  - salivary duct (any) K11.8
    - with calculus K11.5
  - sigmoid — *see* Obstruction, intestine
  - sinus (accessory) (nasal) J34.89
  - Stensen's duct K11.8
  - stomach NEC K31.89
    - acute K31.0
    - congenital Q40.2
    - due to pylorospasm K31.3
  - submandibular duct K11.8
  - submaxillary gland K11.8
    - with calculus K11.5
  - thoracic duct I89.0
  - thrombotic — *see* Thrombosis
  - trachea J39.8
  - tracheostomy airway J95.03
  - tricuspid (valve) — *see* Stenosis, tricuspid
  - upper respiratory, congenital Q34.8
  - ureter (functional) (pelvic junction) NEC N13.5
    - with
      - hydronephrosis N13.1
        - with infection N13.6
      - pyelonephritis (chronic) N11.1
    - congenital Q62.39
    - due to calculus — *see* Calculus, ureter
  - urethra NEC N36.8
    - congenital Q64.39
  - urinary (moderate) N13.9
    - due to hyperplasia (hypertrophy) of prostate — *see* Hyperplasia, prostate
    - organ or tract (lower) N13.9
    - prostatic valve N32.0
    - specified NEC N13.8
  - uropathy N13.9
  - uterus N85.8
  - vagina N89.5
  - valvular — *see* Endocarditis
  - vein, venous I87.1
    - caval (inferior) (superior) I87.1
    - thrombotic — *see* Thrombosis
  - vena cava (inferior) (superior) I87.1
  - vesical NEC N32.0
  - vesicourethral orifice N32.0
    - congenital Q64.31
  - vessel NEC I99.8
    - stent — *see* Restenosis, stent
- **Obturator** — *see* condition
- **Occlusal wear, teeth** K03.0
- **Occlusio pupillae** — *see* Membrane, pupillary
- **Occlusion, occluded**
  - anus K62.4
    - congenital Q42.3
      - with fistula Q42.2
  - aortoiliac (chronic) I74.09
  - aqueduct of Sylvius G91.1
    - congenital Q03.0
      - with spina bifida — *see* Spina bifida, by site, with hydrocephalus
  - artery — *see also* Atherosclerosis, artery I70.9 ☑
    - auditory, internal I65.8
    - basilar I65.1
      - with
        - infarction I63.22
          - due to
            - embolism I63.12
            - thrombosis I63.02

- **Occlusion, occluded** — *continued*
  - artery — *see also* Atherosclerosis, artery — *continued*
    - brain or cerebral I66.9
      - with infarction (due to) I63.5- ☑
        - embolism I63.4- ☑
        - thrombosis I63.3- ☑
    - carotid I65.2- ☑
      - with
        - infarction I63.23- ☑
          - due to
            - embolism I63.13- ☑
            - thrombosis I63.03- ☑
    - cerebellar (anterior inferior) (posterior inferior) (superior) I66.3
      - with infarction I63.54- ☑
        - due to
          - embolism I63.44- ☑
          - thrombosis I63.34- ☑
    - cerebral I66.9
      - with infarction I63.50
        - due to
          - embolism I63.40
            - specified NEC I63.49
          - thrombosis I63.30
            - specified NEC I63.39
      - anterior I66.1- ☑
        - with infarction I63.52- ☑
          - due to
            - embolism I63.42- ☑
            - thrombosis I63.32- ☑
      - middle I66.0- ☑
        - with infarction I63.51- ☑
          - due to
            - embolism I63.41- ☑
            - thrombosis I63.31- ☑
      - posterior I66.2- ☑
        - with infarction I63.53- ☑
          - due to
            - embolism I63.43- ☑
            - thrombosis I63.33- ☑
      - specified NEC I66.8
        - with infarction I63.59
          - due to
            - embolism I63.4- ☑
            - thrombosis I63.3- ☑
    - choroidal (anterior) — *see* Occlusion, artery, precerebral, specified NEC
    - communicating posterior — *see* Occlusion, artery, precerebral, specified NEC
    - complete
      - coronary I25.82
      - extremities I70.92
    - coronary (acute) (thrombotic) (without myocardial infarction) I24.0
      - with myocardial infarction — *see* Infarction, myocardium
      - chronic total I25.82
      - complete I25.82
      - healed or old I25.2
      - total (chronic) I25.82
    - hypophyseal — *see* Occlusion, artery, precerebral, specified NEC
    - iliac I74.5
    - lower extremities due to stenosis or stricture I77.1
    - mesenteric (embolic) (thrombotic) — *see also* Infarct, intestine K55.069
    - perforating — *see* Occlusion, artery, cerebral, specified NEC
    - peripheral I77.9
      - thrombotic or embolic I74.4
    - pontine — *see* Occlusion, artery, precerebral, specified NEC
    - precerebral I65.9
      - with infarction I63.20
        - specified NEC I63.29
        - due to
          - embolism I63.10
            - specified NEC I63.19
          - thrombosis I63.00
            - specified NEC I63.09
      - basilar — *see* Occlusion, artery, basilar
      - carotid — *see* Occlusion, artery, carotid
      - puerperal O88.23
      - specified NEC I65.8
        - with infarction I63.29

- **Occlusion, occluded** — *continued*
  - artery — *see also* Atherosclerosis, artery — *continued*
    - precerebral — *continued*
      - specified — *continued*
        - with infarction — *continued*
          - due to
            - embolism I63.19
            - thrombosis I63.09
      - vertebral — *see* Occlusion, artery, vertebral
    - renal N28.0
    - retinal
      - branch H34.23- ☑
      - central H34.1- ☑
      - partial H34.21- ☑
      - transient H34.0- ☑
    - spinal — *see* Occlusion, artery, precerebral, vertebral
    - total (chronic)
      - coronary I25.82
      - extremities I70.92
    - vertebral I65.0- ☑
      - with
        - infarction I63.21- ☑
          - due to
            - embolism I63.11- ☑
            - thrombosis I63.01- ☑
  - basilar artery — *see* Occlusion, artery, basilar
  - bile duct (common) (hepatic) (noncalculous) K83.1
  - bowel — *see* Obstruction, intestine
  - carotid (artery) (common) (internal) — *see* Occlusion, artery, carotid
  - centric (of teeth) M26.59
    - maximum intercuspation discrepancy M26.55
  - cerebellar (artery) — *see* Occlusion, artery, cerebellar
  - cerebral (artery) — *see* Occlusion, artery, cerebral
  - cerebrovascular — *see also* Occlusion, artery, cerebral
    - with infarction I63.5- ☑
  - cervical canal — *see* Stricture, cervix
  - cervix (uteri) — *see* Stricture, cervix
  - choanal Q30.0
  - choroidal (artery) — *see* Occlusion, artery, precerebral, specified NEC
  - colon — *see* Obstruction, intestine
  - communicating posterior artery — *see* Occlusion, artery, precerebral, specified NEC
  - coronary (artery) (vein) (thrombotic) — *see also* Infarct, myocardium
    - chronic total I25.82
    - healed or old I25.2
    - not resulting in infarction I24.0
    - total (chronic) I25.82
  - cystic duct — *see* Obstruction, gallbladder
  - embolic — *see* Embolism
  - fallopian tube N97.1
    - congenital Q50.6
  - gallbladder — *see also* Obstruction, gallbladder
    - congenital (causing jaundice) Q44.1
  - gingiva, traumatic K06.2
  - hymen N89.6
    - congenital Q52.3
  - hypophyseal (artery) — *see* Occlusion, artery, precerebral, specified NEC
  - iliac artery I74.5
  - intestine — *see* Obstruction, intestine
  - lacrimal passages — *see* Obstruction, lacrimal
  - lung J98.4
  - lymph or lymphatic channel I89.0
  - mammary duct N64.89
  - mesenteric artery (embolic) (thrombotic) — *see also* Infarct, intestine K55.069
  - nose J34.89
    - congenital Q30.0
  - organ or site, congenital NEC — *see* Atresia, by site
  - oviduct N97.1
    - congenital Q50.6
  - peripheral arteries
    - due to stricture or stenosis I77.1
    - upper extremity I74.2
  - pontine (artery) — *see* Occlusion, artery, precerebral, specified NEC
  - posterior lingual, of mandibular teeth M26.29
  - precerebral artery — *see* Occlusion, artery, precerebral
  - punctum lacrimale — *see* Obstruction, lacrimal
  - pupil — *see* Membrane, pupillary
  - pylorus, adult — *see also* Stricture, pylorus K31.1
  - renal artery N28.0

Occlusion, occluded — *continued*
retina, retinal
artery — *see* Occlusion, artery, retinal
vein (central) H34.81- ☑
engorgement H34.82- ☑
tributary H34.83- ☑
vessels H34.9
spinal artery — *see* Occlusion, artery, precerebral, vertebral
teeth (mandibular) (posterior lingual) M26.29
thoracic duct I89.Ø
thrombotic — *see* Thrombosis, artery
traumatic
edentulous (alveolar) ridge KØ6.2
gingiva KØ6.2
periodontal KØ5.5
tubal N97.1
ureter (complete) (partial) N13.5
congenital Q62.1Ø
ureteropelvic junction N13.5
congenital Q62.11
ureterovesical orifice N13.5
congenital Q62.12
urethra — *see* Stricture, urethra
uterus N85.8
vagina N89.5
vascular NEC I99.8
vein — *see* Thrombosis
retinal — *see* Occlusion, retinal, vein
vena cava (inferior) (superior) — *see* Embolism, vena cava
ventricle (brain) NEC G91.1
vertebral (artery) — *see* Occlusion, artery, vertebral
vessel (blood) I99.8
vulva N9Ø.5
Occult
blood in feces (stools) R19.5
Occupational
problems NEC Z56.89
Ochlophobia — *see* Agoraphobia
Ochronosis (endogenous) E7Ø.29
Ocular muscle — *see* condition
Oculogyric crisis or disturbance H51.8
psychogenic F45.8
Oculomotor syndrome H51.9
Oculopathy
syphilitic NEC A52.71
congenital
early A5Ø.Ø1
late A5Ø.3Ø
early (secondary) A51.43
late A52.71
Oddi's sphincter spasm K83.4
Odontalgia KØ8.89
Odontoameloblastoma — *see* Cyst, calcifying odontogenic
Odontoclasia KØ3.89
Odontodysplasia, regional KØØ.4
Odontogenesis imperfecta KØØ.5
Odontoma (ameloblastic) (complex) (compound) (fibroameloblastic) — *see* Cyst, calcifying odontogenic
Odontomyelitis (closed) (open) KØ4.Ø1
irreversible KØ4.Ø2
reversible KØ4.Ø1
Odontorrhagia KØ8.89
Odontosarcoma, ameloblastic C41.1
upper jaw (bone) C41.Ø
Oestriasis — *see* Myiasis
Oguchi's disease H53.63
Ohara's disease — *see* Tularemia
OHS (obesity hypoventilation syndrome) E66.2
Oidiomycosis — *see* Candidiasis
Oidium albicans infection — *see* Candidiasis
Old age (without mention of debility) R54
dementia FØ3 ☑
Old (previous) **myocardial infarction** I25.2
Olfactory — *see* condition
Oligemia — *see* Anemia
Oligoastrocytoma
specified site — *see* Neoplasm, malignant, by site
unspecified site C71.9
Oligocythemia D64.9
Oligodendroblastoma
specified site — *see* Neoplasm, malignant
unspecified site C71.9
Oligodendroglioma
anaplastic type
specified site — *see* Neoplasm, malignant, by site
unspecified site C71.9
specified site — *see* Neoplasm, malignant, by site
unspecified site C71.9
Oligodontia — *see* Anodontia
Oligoencephalon QØ2
Oligohidrosis L74.4
Oligohydramnios O41.Ø- ☑
Oligohydrosis L74.4
Oligomenorrhea N91.5
primary N91.3
secondary N91.4
Oligophrenia — *see also* Disability, intellectual
phenylpyruvic E7Ø.Ø
Oligospermia N46.11
due to
drug therapy N46.121
efferent duct obstruction N46.123
infection N46.122
radiation N46.124
specified cause NEC N46.129
systemic disease N46.125
Oligotrichia — *see* Alopecia
Oliguria R34
with, complicating or following ectopic or molar pregnancy OØ8.4
postprocedural N99.Ø
Ollier's disease Q78.4
Omenotocele — *see* Hernia, abdomen, specified site NEC
Omentitis — *see* Peritonitis
Omentum, omental — *see* condition
Omphalitis (congenital) (newborn) P38.9
with mild hemorrhage P38.1
without hemorrhage P38.9
not of newborn LØ8.82
tetanus A33
Omphalocele Q79.2
Omphalomesenteric duct, persistent Q43.Ø
Omphalorrhagia, newborn P51.9
Omsk hemorrhagic fever A98.1
Onanism (excessive) F98.8
Onchocerciasis, onchocercosis B73.1
with
eye disease B73.ØØ
endophthalmitis B73.Ø1
eyelid B73.Ø9
glaucoma B73.Ø2
specified NEC B73.Ø9
eyelid B73.Ø9
eye NEC B73.ØØ
Oncocytoma — *see* Neoplasm, benign, by site
Oncovirus, as cause of disease classified elsewhere B97.32
Ondine's curse — *see* Apnea, sleep
Oneirophrenia F23
Onychauxis L6Ø.2
congenital Q84.5
Onychia — *see also* Cellulitis, digit
with lymphangitis — *see* Lymphangitis, acute, digit
candidal B37.2
dermatophytic B35.1
Onychitis — *see also* Cellulitis, digit
with lymphangitis — *see* Lymphangitis, acute, digit
Onychocryptosis L6Ø.Ø
Onychodystrophy L6Ø.3
congenital Q84.6
Onychogryphosis, onychogryposis L6Ø.2
Onycholysis L6Ø.1
Onychomadesis L6Ø.8
Onychomalacia L6Ø.3
Onychomycosis (finger) (toe) B35.1
Onycho-osteodysplasia Q87.2
Onychophagia F98.8
Onychophosis L6Ø.8
Onychoptosis L6Ø.8
Onychorrhexis L6Ø.3
congenital Q84.6
Onychoschizia L6Ø.3
Onyxis (finger) (toe) L6Ø.Ø
Onyxitis — *see also* Cellulitis, digit
with lymphangitis — *see* Lymphangitis, acute, digit
Oophoritis (cystic) (infectional) (interstitial) N7Ø.92
with salpingitis N7Ø.93
acute N7Ø.Ø2
with salpingitis N7Ø.Ø3
Oophoritis — *continued*
chronic N7Ø.12
with salpingitis N7Ø.13
complicating abortion — *see* Abortion, by type, complicated by, oophoritis
Oophorocele N83.4- ☑
Opacity, opacities
cornea H17.- ☑
central H17.1- ☑
congenital Q13.3
degenerative — *see* Degeneration, cornea
hereditary — *see* Dystrophy, cornea
inflammatory — *see* Keratitis
minor H17.81- ☑
peripheral H17.82- ☑
sequelae of trachoma (healed) B94.Ø
specified NEC H17.89
enamel (teeth) (fluoride) (nonfluoride) KØØ.3
lens — *see* Cataract
snowball — *see* Deposit, crystalline
vitreous (humor) NEC H43.39- ☑
congenital Q14.Ø
membranes and strands H43.31- ☑
Opalescent dentin (hereditary) KØØ.5
Open, opening
abnormal, organ or site, congenital — *see* Imperfect, closure
angle with
borderline
findings
high risk H4Ø.Ø2- ☑
low risk H4Ø.Ø1- ☑
intraocular pressure H4Ø.ØØ- ☑
cupping of discs H4Ø.Ø1- ☑
glaucoma (primary) — *see* Glaucoma, open angle
bite
anterior M26.22Ø
posterior M26.221
false — *see* Imperfect, closure
margin on tooth restoration KØ8.51
restoration margins of tooth KØ8.51
wound — *see* Wound, open
Operational fatigue F48.8
Operative — *see* condition
Operculitis — *see* Periodontitis
Operculum — *see* Break, retina
Ophiasis L63.2
Ophthalmia — *see also* Conjunctivitis H1Ø.9
actinic rays — *see* Photokeratitis
allergic (acute) — *see* Conjunctivitis, acute, atopic
blennorrhagic (gonococcal) (neonatorum) A54.31
diphtheritic A36.86
Egyptian A71.1
electrica — *see* Photokeratitis
gonococcal (neonatorum) A54.31
metastatic — *see* Endophthalmitis, purulent
migraine — *see* Migraine, ophthalmoplegic
neonatorum, newborn P39.1
gonococcal A54.31
nodosa H16.24- ☑
purulent — *see* Conjunctivitis, acute, mucopurulent
spring — *see* Conjunctivitis, acute, atopic
sympathetic — *see* Uveitis, sympathetic
Ophthalmitis — *see* Ophthalmia
Ophthalmocele (congenital) Q15.8
Ophthalmoneuromyelitis G36.Ø
Ophthalmoplegia — *see also* Strabismus, paralytic
anterior internuclear — *see* Ophthalmoplegia, internuclear
ataxia-areflexia G61.Ø
diabetic — *see* EØ8-E13 with .39
exophthalmic EØ5.ØØ
with thyroid storm EØ5.Ø1
external H49.88- ☑
progressive H49.4- ☑
with pigmentary retinopathy — *see* Kearns-Sayre syndrome
total H49.3- ☑
internal (complete) (total) H52.51- ☑
internuclear H51.2- ☑
migraine — *see* Migraine, ophthalmoplegic
Parinaud's H49.88- ☑
progressive external — *see* Ophthalmoplegia, external, progressive
supranuclear, progressive G23.1
total (external) — *see* Ophthalmoplegia, external, total

Opioid(s)
- abuse — *see* Abuse, drug, opioids
- dependence — *see* Dependence, drug, opioids
- induced, without use disorder
  - anxiety disorder F11.988
  - delirium F11.921
  - depressive disorder F11.94
  - sexual dysfunction F11.981
  - sleep disorder F11.982

Opisthognathism M26.Ø9
Opisthorchiasis (felineus) (viverrini) B66.Ø
Opitz' disease D73.2
Opiumism — *see* Dependence, drug, opioid
Oppenheim's disease G7Ø.2
Oppenheim-Urbach disease (necrobiosis lipoidica diabeticorum) — *see* EØ8-E13 with .62Ø
Optic nerve — *see* condition
Orbit — *see* condition
Orchioblastoma C62.9- ☑
Orchitis (gangrenous) (nonspecific) (septic) (suppurative) N45.2
- blennorrhagic (gonococcal) (acute) (chronic) A54.23
- chlamydial A56.19
- filarial — *see also* Infestation, filarial B74.9 *[N51]*
- gonococcal (acute) (chronic) A54.23
- mumps B26.Ø
- syphilitic A52.76
- tuberculous A18.15

Orf (virus disease) BØ8.Ø2
Organic — *see also* condition
- brain syndrome FØ9
- heart — *see* Disease, heart
- mental disorder FØ9
- psychosis FØ9

Orgasm
- anejaculatory N53.13

Oriental
- bilharziasis B65.2
- schistosomiasis B65.2

Orifice — *see* condition
Origin of both great vessels from right ventricle Q2Ø.1
Ormond's disease (with ureteral obstruction) N13.5
- with infection N13.6

Ornithine metabolism disorder E72.4
Ornithinemia (Type I) (Type II) E72.4
Ornithosis A7Ø
Orotaciduria, oroticaciduria (congenital) (hereditary) (pyrimidine deficiency) E79.8
- anemia D53.Ø

Orthodontics
- adjustment Z46.4
- fitting Z46.4

Orthopnea RØ6.Ø1
Orthopoxvirus BØ8.Ø9
Os, uterus — *see* condition
Osgood-Schlatter disease or osteochondrosis M92.52- ☑
Osler (-Weber)-**Rendu disease** I78.Ø
Osler's nodes I33.Ø
Osmidrosis L75.Ø
Osseous — *see* condition
Ossification
- artery — *see* Arteriosclerosis
- auricle (ear) — *see* Disorder, pinna, specified type NEC
- bronchial J98.Ø9
- cardiac — *see* Degeneration, myocardial
- cartilage (senile) — *see* Disorder, cartilage, specified type NEC
- coronary (artery) — *see* Disease, heart, ischemic, atherosclerotic
- diaphragm J98.6
- ear, middle — *see* Otosclerosis
- falx cerebri G96.198
- fontanel, premature Q75.Ø
- heart — *see also* Degeneration, myocardial
  - valve — *see* Endocarditis
- larynx J38.7
- ligament — *see* Disorder, tendon, specified type NEC
  - posterior longitudinal — *see* Spondylopathy, specified NEC
- meninges (cerebral) (spinal) G96.198
- multiple, eccentric centers — *see* Disorder, bone, development or growth
- muscle — *see also* Calcification, muscle
  - due to burns — *see* Myositis, ossificans, in, burns
  - paralytic — *see* Myositis, ossificans, in, quadriplegia

Ossification — *continued*
- muscle — *see also* Calcification, muscle — *continued*
  - progressive — *see* Myositis, ossificans, progressiva
  - specified NEC M61.5Ø
    - ankle M61.57- ☑
    - foot M61.57- ☑
    - forearm M61.53- ☑
    - hand M61.54- ☑
    - lower leg M61.56- ☑
    - multiple sites M61.59
    - pelvic region M61.55- ☑
    - shoulder region M61.51- ☑
    - specified site NEC M61.58
    - thigh M61.55- ☑
    - upper arm M61.52- ☑
  - traumatic — *see* Myositis, ossificans, traumatica
- myocardium, myocardial — *see* Degeneration, myocardial
- penis N48.89
- periarticular — *see* Disorder, joint, specified type NEC
- pinna — *see* Disorder, pinna, specified type NEC
- rider's bone — *see* Ossification, muscle, specified NEC
- sclera H15.89
- subperiosteal, post-traumatic M89.8X- ☑
- tendon — *see* Disorder, tendon, specified type NEC
- trachea J39.8
- tympanic membrane — *see* Disorder, tympanic membrane, specified NEC
- vitreous (humor) — *see* Deposit, crystalline

Osteitis — *see also* Osteomyelitis
- alveolar M27.3
- condensans M85.3Ø
  - ankle M85.37- ☑
  - foot M85.37- ☑
  - forearm M85.33- ☑
  - hand M85.34- ☑
  - lower leg M85.36- ☑
  - multiple site M85.39
  - neck M85.38
  - rib M85.38
  - shoulder M85.31- ☑
  - skull M85.38
  - specified site NEC M85.38
  - thigh M85.35- ☑
  - toe M85.37- ☑
  - upper arm M85.32- ☑
  - vertebra M85.38
- deformans M88.9
  - in (due to)
    - malignant neoplasm of bone C41.9 *[M9Ø.6Ø]*
    - neoplastic disease — *see also* Neoplasm D49.9 *[M9Ø.6Ø]*
      - carpus D49.9 *[M9Ø.64-]* ☑
      - clavicle D49.9 *[M9Ø.61-]* ☑
      - femur D49.9 *[M9Ø.65-]* ☑
      - fibula D49.9 *[M9Ø.66-]* ☑
      - finger D49.9 *[M9Ø.64-]* ☑
      - humerus D49.9 *[M9Ø.62-]* ☑
      - ilium D49.9 *[M9Ø.65-]* ☑
      - ischium D49.9 *[M9Ø.65-]* ☑
      - metacarpus D49.9 *[M9Ø.64-]* ☑
      - metatarsus D49.9 *[M9Ø.67-]* ☑
      - multiple sites D49.9 *[M9Ø.69]*
      - neck D49.9 *[M9Ø.68]*
      - radius D49.9 *[M9Ø.63-]* ☑
      - rib D49.9 *[M9Ø.68]*
      - scapula D49.9 *[M9Ø.61-]* ☑
      - skull D49.9 *[M9Ø.68]*
      - tarsus D49.9 *[M9Ø.67-]* ☑
      - tibia D49.9 *[M9Ø.66-]* ☑
      - toe D49.9 *[M9Ø.67-]* ☑
      - ulna D49.9 *[M9Ø.63-]* ☑
      - vertebra D49.9 *[M9Ø.68]*
  - skull M88.Ø
  - specified NEC — *see* Paget's disease, bone, by site
  - vertebra M88.1
- due to yaws A66.6
- fibrosa NEC — *see* Cyst, bone, by site
  - circumscripta — *see* Dysplasia, fibrous, bone NEC
  - cystica (generalisata) E21.Ø
  - disseminata Q78.1
  - osteoplastica E21.Ø
- fragilitans Q78.Ø
- Garr's (sclerosing) — *see* Osteomyelitis, specified type NEC

Osteitis — *continued*
- jaw (acute) (chronic) (lower) (suppurative) (upper) M27.2
- parathyroid E21.Ø
- petrous bone (acute) (chronic) — *see* Petrositis
- sclerotic, nonsuppurative — *see* Osteomyelitis, specified type NEC
- tuberculosa A18.Ø9
  - cystica D86.89
  - multiplex cystoides D86.89

Osteoarthritis M19.9Ø
- ankle M19.Ø7- ☑
- elbow M19.Ø2- ☑
- foot joint M19.Ø7- ☑
- generalized M15.9
  - erosive M15.4
  - primary M15.Ø
  - specified NEC M15.8
- hand joint M19.Ø4- ☑
  - first carpometacarpal joint M18.9
- hip M16.1- ☑
  - bilateral M16.Ø
  - due to hip dysplasia (unilateral) M16.3- ☑
    - bilateral M16.2
- interphalangeal
  - distal (Heberden) M15.1
  - proximal (Bouchard) M15.2
- knee M17.1- ☑
  - bilateral M17.Ø
- post-traumatic NEC M19.92
  - ankle M19.17- ☑
  - elbow M19.12- ☑
  - foot joint M19.17- ☑
  - hand joint M19.14- ☑
    - first carpometacarpal joint M18.3- ☑
      - bilateral M18.2
  - hip M16.5- ☑
    - bilateral M16.4
  - knee M17.3- ☑
    - bilateral M17.2
  - shoulder M19.11- ☑
  - specified site NEC M19.19
  - wrist M19.13- ☑
- primary M19.91
  - ankle M19.Ø7- ☑
  - elbow M19.Ø2- ☑
  - foot joint M19.Ø7- ☑
  - hand joint M19.Ø4- ☑
    - first carpometacarpal joint M18.1- ☑
      - bilateral M18.Ø
  - hip M16.1- ☑
    - bilateral M16.Ø
  - knee M17.1- ☑
    - bilateral M17.Ø
  - multiple sites M89.49
  - shoulder M19.Ø1- ☑
  - spine — *see* Spondylosis
  - wrist M19.Ø3- ☑
- secondary M19.93
  - ankle M19.27- ☑
  - elbow M19.22- ☑
  - foot joint M19.27- ☑
  - hand joint M19.24- ☑
    - first carpometacarpal joint M18.5- ☑
      - bilateral M18.4
  - hip M16.7
    - bilateral M16.6
  - knee M17.5
    - bilateral M17.4
  - multiple M15.3
  - shoulder M19.21- ☑
  - specified site NEC M19.29
  - spine — *see* Spondylosis
  - wrist M19.23- ☑
- shoulder M19.Ø1- ☑
- specified site NEC M19.Ø9
- spine — *see* Spondylosis
- wrist M19.Ø3- ☑

Osteoarthropathy (hypertrophic) M19.9Ø
- ankle — *see* Osteoarthritis, primary, ankle
- elbow — *see* Osteoarthritis, primary, elbow
- foot joint — *see* Osteoarthritis, primary, foot
- hand joint — *see* Osteoarthritis, primary, hand joint
- knee joint — *see* Osteoarthritis, primary, knee
- multiple site — *see* Osteoarthritis, primary, multiple joint

Osteomyelitis — *continued*
- chronic — *continued*
  - vertebra — *see* Osteomyelitis, vertebra
- echinococcal B67.2
- Garr's — *see* Osteomyelitis, specified type NEC
- in diabetes mellitus — *see* EØ8-E13 with .69
- jaw (acute) (chronic) (lower) (neonatal) (suppurative) (upper) M27.2
- nonsuppurating — *see* Osteomyelitis, specified type NEC
- orbit HØ5.Ø2- ☑
- petrous bone — *see* Petrositis
- Salmonella (arizonae) (cholerae-suis) (enteritidis) (typhimurium) AØ2.24
- sclerosing, nonsuppurative — *see* Osteomyelitis, specified type NEC
- specified type NEC — *see also* subcategory M86.8X- ☑
  - mandible M27.2
  - orbit HØ5.Ø2- ☑
  - petrous bone — *see* Petrositis
  - vertebra — *see* Osteomyelitis, vertebra
- subacute M86.2Ø
  - carpus M86.24- ☑
  - clavicle M86.21- ☑
  - femur M86.25- ☑
  - fibula M86.26- ☑
  - finger M86.24- ☑
  - humerus M86.22- ☑
  - mandible M27.2
  - metacarpus M86.24- ☑
  - metatarsus M86.27- ☑
  - multiple sites M86.29
  - neck M86.28
  - orbit HØ5.Ø2- ☑
  - petrous bone — *see* Petrositis
  - radius M86.23- ☑
  - rib M86.28
  - scapula M86.21- ☑
  - skull M86.28
  - tarsus M86.27- ☑
  - tibia M86.26- ☑
  - toe M86.27- ☑
  - ulna M86.23- ☑
  - vertebra — *see* Osteomyelitis, vertebra
- syphilitic A52.77
  - congenital (early) A5Ø.Ø2 *[M9Ø.8Ø]*
- tuberculous — *see* Tuberculosis, bone
- typhoid AØ1.Ø5
- vertebra M46.2Ø
  - cervical region M46.22
  - cervicothoracic region M46.23
  - lumbar region M46.26
  - lumbosacral region M46.27
  - occipito-atlanto-axial region M46.21
  - sacrococcygeal region M46.28
  - thoracic region M46.24
  - thoracolumbar region M46.25

Osteomyelofibrosis D47.4

Osteomyelosclerosis D75.89

Osteonecrosis M87.9
- due to
  - drugs — *see* Osteonecrosis, secondary, due to, drugs
  - trauma — *see* Osteonecrosis, secondary, due to, trauma
- idiopathic aseptic M87.ØØ
  - ankle M87.Ø7- ☑
  - carpus M87.Ø3- ☑
  - clavicle M87.Ø1- ☑
  - femur M87.Ø5- ☑
  - fibula M87.Ø6- ☑
  - finger M87.Ø4- ☑
  - humerus M87.Ø2- ☑
  - ilium M87.Ø5Ø
  - ischium M87.Ø5Ø
  - metacarpus M87.Ø4- ☑
  - metatarsus M87.Ø7- ☑
  - multiple sites M87.Ø9
  - neck M87.Ø8
  - pelvis M87.Ø5Ø
  - radius M87.Ø3- ☑
  - rib M87.Ø8
  - scapula M87.Ø1- ☑
  - skull M87.Ø8
  - tarsus M87.Ø7- ☑
  - tibia M87.Ø6- ☑
  - toe M87.Ø7- ☑
  - ulna M87.Ø3- ☑

Osteonecrosis — *continued*
- idiopathic aseptic — *continued*
  - vertebra M87.Ø8
- secondary NEC M87.3Ø
  - carpus M87.33- ☑
  - clavicle M87.31- ☑
  - due to
    - drugs M87.1Ø
      - carpus M87.13- ☑
      - clavicle M87.11- ☑
      - femur M87.15- ☑
      - fibula M87.16- ☑
      - finger M87.14- ☑
      - humerus M87.12- ☑
      - ilium M87.159
      - ischium M87.159
      - jaw M87.18Ø
      - metacarpus M87.14- ☑
      - metatarsus M87.17- ☑
      - multiple sites M87.19
      - neck M87.18 ☑
      - radius M87.13- ☑
      - rib M87.18 ☑
      - scapula M87.11- ☑
      - skull M87.18 ☑
      - tarsus M87.17- ☑
      - tibia M87.16- ☑
      - toe M87.17- ☑
      - ulna M87.13- ☑
      - vertebra M87.18 ☑
    - hemoglobinopathy NEC D58.2 *[M9Ø.5Ø]*
      - carpus D58.2 *[M9Ø.54-]* ☑
      - clavicle D58.2 *[M9Ø.51-]* ☑
      - femur D58.2 *[M9Ø.55-]* ☑
      - fibula D58.2 *[M9Ø.56-]* ☑
      - finger D58.2 *[M9Ø.54-]* ☑
      - humerus D58.2 *[M9Ø.52-]* ☑
      - ilium D58.2 *[M9Ø.55-]* ☑
      - ischium D58.2 *[M9Ø.55-]* ☑
      - metacarpus D58.2 *[M9Ø.54-]* ☑
      - metatarsus D58.2 *[M9Ø.57-]* ☑
      - multiple sites D58.2 *[M9Ø.58]*
      - neck D58.2 *[M9Ø.58]*
      - radius D58.2 *[M9Ø.53-]* ☑
      - rib D58.2 *[M9Ø.58]*
      - scapula D58.2 *[M9Ø.51-]* ☑
      - skull D58.2 *[M9Ø.58]*
      - tarsus D58.2 *[M9Ø.57-]* ☑
      - tibia D58.2 *[M9Ø.56-]* ☑
      - toe D58.2 *[M9Ø.57-]* ☑
      - ulna D58.2 *[M9Ø.53-]* ☑
      - vertebra D58.2 *[M9Ø.58]*
    - trauma (previous) M87.2Ø
      - carpus M87.23- ☑
      - clavicle M87.21- ☑
      - femur M87.25- ☑
      - fibula M87.26- ☑
      - finger M87.24- ☑
      - humerus M87.22- ☑
      - ilium M87.25- ☑
      - ischium M87.25- ☑
      - metacarpus M87.24- ☑
      - metatarsus M87.27- ☑
      - multiple sites M87.29
      - neck M87.28
      - radius M87.23- ☑
      - rib M87.28
      - scapula M87.21- ☑
      - skull M87.28
      - tarsus M87.27- ☑
      - tibia M87.26- ☑
      - toe M87.27- ☑
      - ulna M87.23- ☑
      - vertebra M87.28
  - femur M87.35- ☑
  - fibula M87.36- ☑
  - finger M87.34- ☑
  - humerus M87.32- ☑
  - ilium M87.35Ø
  - in
    - caisson disease T7Ø.3 ☑ *[M9Ø.5Ø]*
      - carpus T7Ø.3 ☑ *[M9Ø.54-]* ☑
      - clavicle T7Ø.3 ☑ *[M9Ø.51-]* ☑
      - femur T7Ø.3 ☑ *[M9Ø.55-]* ☑
      - fibula T7Ø.3 ☑ *[M9Ø.56-]* ☑
      - finger T7Ø.3 ☑ *[M9Ø.54-]* ☑

Osteonecrosis — *continued*
- secondary — *continued*
  - in — *continued*
    - caisson disease — *continued*
      - humerus T7Ø.3 ☑ *[M9Ø.52-]* ☑
      - ilium T7Ø.3 ☑ *[M9Ø.55-]* ☑
      - ischium T7Ø.3 ☑ *[M9Ø.55-]* ☑
      - metacarpus T7Ø.3 ☑ *[M9Ø.54-]* ☑
      - metatarsus T7Ø.3 ☑ *[M9Ø.57-]* ☑
      - multiple sites T7Ø.3 ☑ *[M9Ø.59]*
      - neck T7Ø.3 ☑ *[M9Ø.58]*
      - radius T7Ø.3 ☑ *[M9Ø.53-]* ☑
      - rib T7Ø.3 ☑ *[M9Ø.58]*
      - scapula T7Ø.3 ☑ *[M9Ø.51-]* ☑
      - skull T7Ø.3 ☑ *[M9Ø.58]*
      - tarsus T7Ø.3 ☑ *[M9Ø.57-]* ☑
      - tibia T7Ø.3 ☑ *[M9Ø.56-]* ☑
      - toe T7Ø.3 ☑ *[M9Ø.57-]* ☑
      - ulna T7Ø.3 ☑ *[M9Ø.53-]* ☑
      - vertebra T7Ø.3 ☑ *[M9Ø.58]*
  - ischium M87.35Ø
  - metacarpus M87.34- ☑
  - metatarsus M87.37- ☑
  - multiple site M87.39
  - neck M87.38
  - radius M87.33- ☑
  - rib M87.38
  - scapula M87.319
  - skull M87.38
  - tarsus M87.379
  - tibia M87.366
  - toe M87.379
  - ulna M87.33- ☑
  - vertebra M87.38
- specified type NEC M87.8Ø
  - carpus M87.83- ☑
  - clavicle M87.81- ☑
  - femur M87.85- ☑
  - fibula M87.86- ☑
  - finger M87.84- ☑
  - humerus M87.82- ☑
  - ilium M87.85- ☑
  - ischium M87.85- ☑
  - metacarpus M87.84- ☑
  - metatarsus M87.87- ☑
  - multiple sites M87.89
  - neck M87.88
  - radius M87.83- ☑
  - rib M87.88
  - scapula M87.81- ☑
  - skull M87.88
  - tarsus M87.87- ☑
  - tibia M87.86- ☑
  - toe M87.87- ☑
  - ulna M87.83- ☑
  - vertebra M87.88

Osteo-onycho-arthro-dysplasia Q87.2

Osteo-onychodysplasia, hereditary Q87.2

Osteopathia condensans disseminata Q78.8

Osteopathy — *see also* Osteomyelitis, Osteonecrosis, Osteoporosis
- after poliomyelitis M89.6Ø
  - carpus M89.64- ☑
  - clavicle M89.61- ☑
  - femur M89.65- ☑
  - fibula M89.66- ☑
  - finger M89.64- ☑
  - humerus M89.62- ☑
  - ilium M89.659
  - ischium M89.659
  - metacarpus M89.64- ☑
  - metatarsus M89.67- ☑
  - multiple sites M89.69
  - neck M89.68
  - radius M89.63- ☑
  - rib M89.68
  - scapula M89.61- ☑
  - skull M89.68
  - tarsus M89.67- ☑
  - tibia M89.66- ☑
  - toe M89.67- ☑
  - ulna M89.63- ☑
  - vertebra M89.68
- in (due to)
  - renal osteodystrophy N25.Ø

P

Palsy — *continued*
cerebral — *continued*
dyskinetic — *continued*
athetoid G8Ø.3
choreathetoid G8Ø.3
distonic G8Ø.3
dystonic G8Ø.3
hemiplegic G8Ø.8
spastic G8Ø.2
mixed G8Ø.8
monoplegic G8Ø.8
spastic G8Ø.1
paraplegic G8Ø.8
spastic G8Ø.1
quadriplegic G8Ø.8
spastic G8Ø.Ø
spastic G8Ø.1
diplegic G8Ø.1
hemiplegic G8Ø.2
monoplegic G8Ø.1
quadriplegic G8Ø.Ø
specified NEC G8Ø.1
tetrapelgic G8Ø.Ø
specified NEC G8Ø.8
syphilitic A52.12
congenital A5Ø.49
tetraplegic G8Ø.8
spastic G8Ø.Ø
cranial nerve — *see also* Disorder, nerve, cranial
multiple G52.7
in
infectious disease B99 ☑ *[G53]*
neoplastic disease — *see also* Neoplasm D49.9 *[G53]*
parasitic disease B89 *[G53]*
sarcoidosis D86.82
creeping G12.22
diver's T7Ø.3 ☑
Erb's P14.Ø
facial G51.Ø
newborn (birth injury) P11.3
glossopharyngeal G52.1
Klumpke (-Déjérine) P14.1
lead — *see* subcategory T56.Ø ☑
median nerve (tardy) G56.1- ☑
nerve G58.9
specified NEC G58.8
peroneal nerve (acute) (tardy) G57.3- ☑
progressive supranuclear G23.1
pseudobulbar NEC G12.29
radial nerve (acute) G56.3- ☑
seventh nerve — *see also* Palsy, facial
newborn P11.3
shaking — *see* Parkinsonism
spastic (cerebral) (spinal) G8Ø.1
ulnar nerve (tardy) G56.2- ☑
wasting G12.29
Paludism — *see* Malaria
Panangiitis M3Ø.Ø
Panaris, panaritium — *see also* Cellulitis, digit
with lymphangitis — *see* Lymphangitis, acute, digit
Panarteritis nodosa M3Ø.Ø
brain or cerebral I67.7
Pancake heart R93.1
with cor pulmonale (chronic) I27.81
Pancarditis (acute) (chronic) I51.89
rheumatic IØ9.89
active or acute IØ1.8
Pancoast's syndrome or tumor C34.1- ☑
Pancolitis, ulcerative (chronic) K51.ØØ
with
abscess K51.Ø14
complication K51.Ø19
fistula K51.Ø13
obstruction K51.Ø12
rectal bleeding K51.Ø11
specified complication NEC K51.Ø18
Pancreas, pancreatic — *see* condition
Pancreatitis (annular) (apoplectic) (calcareous) (edematous) (hemorrhagic) (malignant) (subacute) (suppurative) K85.9Ø
with necrosis (uninfected) K85.91
infected K85.92
acute (without necrosis or infection) K85.9Ø
with necrosis (uninfected) K85.91
infected K85.92
alcohol induced (without necrosis or infection) K85.2Ø
Pancreatitis — *continued*
acute — *continued*
alcohol induced — *continued*
with necrosis (uninfected) K85.21
infected K85.22
biliary (without necrosis or infection) K85.1Ø
with necrosis (uninfected) K85.11
infected K85.12
drug induced (without necrosis or infection) K85.3Ø
with necrosis (uninfected) K85.31
infected K85.32
gallstone (without necrosis or infection) K85.1Ø
with necrosis (uninfected) K85.11
infected K85.12
idiopathic (without necrosis or infection) K85.ØØ
with necrosis (uninfected) K85.Ø1
infected K85.Ø2
specified NEC (without necrosis or infection) K85.8Ø
with necrosis (uninfected) K85.81
infected K85.82
chronic (infectious) K86.1
alcohol-induced K86.Ø
recurrent K86.1
relapsing K86.1
cystic (chronic) K86.1
cytomegaloviral B25.2
fibrous (chronic) K86.1
gallstone (without necrosis or infection) K85.1Ø
with necrosis (uninfected) K85.11
infected K85.12
gangrenous — *see* Pancreatitis, acute
interstitial (chronic) K86.1
acute — *see also* Pancreatitis, acute K85.8Ø
mumps B26.3
recurrent
acute K85.- ☑
chronic K86.1
relapsing, chronic K86.1
syphilitic A52.74
Pancreatoblastoma — *see* Neoplasm, pancreas, malignant
Pancreolithiasis K86.89
Pancytolysis D75.89
Pancytopenia (acquired) D61.818
with
malformations D61.Ø9
myelodysplastic syndrome — *see* Syndrome, myelodysplastic
antineoplastic chemotherapy induced D61.81Ø
congenital D61.Ø9
drug-induced NEC D61.811
PANDAS (pediatric autoimmune neuropsychiatric disorders associated with streptococcal infections syndrome) D89.89
Panencephalitis, subacute, sclerosing A81.1
Panhematopenia D61.9
congenital D61.Ø9
constitutional D61.Ø9
splenic, primary D73.1
Panhemocytopenia D61.9
congenital D61.Ø9
constitutional D61.Ø9
Panhypogonadism E29.1
Panhypopituitarism E23.Ø
prepubertal E23.Ø
Panic (attack) (state) F41.Ø
reaction to exceptional stress (transient) F43.Ø
Panmyelopathy, familial, constitutional D61.Ø9
Panmyelophthisis D61.82
congenital D61.Ø9
Panmyelosis (acute) (with myelofibrosis) C94.4- ☑
Panner's disease — *see* Osteochondrosis, juvenile, humerus
Panneuritis endemica E51.11
Panniculitis (nodular) (nonsuppurative) M79.3
back M54.ØØ
cervical region M54.Ø2
cervicothoracic region M54.Ø3
lumbar region M54.Ø6
lumbosacral region M54.Ø7
multiple sites M54.Ø9
occipito-atlanto-axial region M54.Ø1
sacrococcygeal region M54.Ø8
thoracic region M54.Ø4
thoracolumbar region M54.Ø5
lupus L93.2
mesenteric K65.4
neck M54.Ø2
Panniculitis — *continued*
neck — *continued*
cervicothoracic region M54.Ø3
occipito-atlanto-axial region M54.Ø1
relapsing M35.6
Panniculus adiposus (abdominal) E65
Pannus (allergic) (cornea) (degenerativus) (keratic) H16.42- ☑
abdominal (symptomatic) E65
trachomatosus, trachomatous (active) A71.1
Panophthalmitis H44.Ø1- ☑
Pansinusitis (chronic) (hyperplastic) (nonpurulent) (purulent) J32.4
acute JØ1.4Ø
recurrent JØ1.41
tuberculous A15.8
Panuveitis (sympathetic) H44.11- ☑
Panvalvular disease IØ8.9
specified NEC IØ8.8
PAPA (pyogenic arthritis, pyoderma gangrenosum, and acne syndrome) MØ4.8
Papanicolaou smear, cervix Z12.4
as part of routine gynecological examination ZØ1.419
with abnormal findings ZØ1.411
for suspected neoplasm Z12.4
nonspecific abnormal finding R87.619
routine ZØ1.419
with abnormal findings ZØ1.411
Papilledema (choked disc) H47.1Ø
associated with
decreased ocular pressure H47.12
increased intracranial pressure H47.11
retinal disorder H47.13
Foster-Kennedy syndrome H47.14- ☑
Papillitis H46.ØØ
anus K62.89
chronic lingual K14.4
necrotizing, kidney N17.2
optic H46.Ø- ☑
rectum K62.89
renal, necrotizing N17.2
tongue K14.Ø
Papilloma — *see also* Neoplasm, benign, by site
acuminatum (female) (male) (anogenital) A63.Ø
basal cell L82.1
inflamed L82.Ø
benign pinta (primary) A67.Ø
bladder (urinary) (transitional cell) D41.4
choroid plexus (lateral ventricle) (third ventricle) D33.Ø
anaplastic C71.5
fourth ventricle D33.1
malignant C71.5
renal pelvis (transitional cell) D41.1- ☑
benign D3Ø.1- ☑
Schneiderian
specified site — *see* Neoplasm, benign, by site
unspecified site D14.Ø
serous surface
borderline malignancy
specified site — *see* Neoplasm, uncertain behavior, by site
unspecified site D39.1Ø
specified site — *see* Neoplasm, benign, by site
unspecified site D27.9
transitional (cell)
bladder (urinary) D41.4
inverted type — *see* Neoplasm, uncertain behavior, by site
renal pelvis D41.1- ☑
ureter D41.2- ☑
ureter (transitional cell) D41.2- ☑
benign D3Ø.2- ☑
urothelial — *see* Neoplasm, uncertain behavior, by site
villous — *see* Neoplasm, uncertain behavior, by site
adenocarcinoma in — *see* Neoplasm, malignant, by site
in situ — *see* Neoplasm, in situ
yaws, plantar or palmar A66.1
Papillomata, multiple, of yaws A66.1
Papillomatosis — *see also* Neoplasm, benign, by site
confluent and reticulated L83
cystic, breast — *see* Mastopathy, cystic
ductal, breast — *see* Mastopathy, cystic
intraductal (diffuse) — *see* Neoplasm, benign, by site
subareolar duct D24- ☑
Papillomavirus, as cause of disease classified elsewhere B97.7

- **Papillon-Léage and Psaume syndrome** Q87.Ø
- **Papule(s)** R23.8
  - carate (primary) A67.Ø
  - fibrous, of nose D22.39
  - Gottron's L94.4
  - pinta (primary) A67.Ø
- **Papulosis**
  - lymphomatoid C86.6
  - malignant I77.89
- **Papyraceous fetus** O31.Ø- ☑
- **Para-albuminemia** E88.Ø9
- **Paracephalus** Q89.7
- **Parachute mitral valve** Q23.2
- **Paracoccidioidomycosis** B41.9
  - disseminated B41.7
  - generalized B41.7
  - mucocutaneous-lymphangitic B41.8
  - pulmonary B41.Ø
  - specified NEC B41.8
  - visceral B41.8
- **Paradentosis** KØ5.4
- **Paraffinoma** T88.8 ☑
- **Paraganglioma** D44.7
  - adrenal D35.Ø- ☑
    - malignant C74.1- ☑
  - aortic body D44.7
    - malignant C75.5
  - carotid body D44.6
    - malignant C75.4
  - chromaffin — *see also* Neoplasm, benign, by site
    - malignant — *see* Neoplasm, malignant, by site
  - extra-adrenal D44.7
    - malignant C75.5
      - specified site — *see* Neoplasm, malignant, by site
      - unspecified site C75.5
    - specified site — *see* Neoplasm, uncertain behavior, by site
    - unspecified site D44.7
  - gangliocytic D13.2
    - specified site — *see* Neoplasm, benign, by site
    - unspecified site D13.2
  - glomus jugulare D44.7
    - malignant C75.5
  - jugular D44.7
  - malignant C75.5
    - specified site — *see* Neoplasm, malignant, by site
    - unspecified site C75.5
  - nonchromaffin D44.7
    - malignant C75.5
      - specified site — *see* Neoplasm, malignant, by site
      - unspecified site C75.5
    - specified site — *see* Neoplasm, uncertain behavior, by site
    - unspecified site D44.7
  - parasympathetic D44.7
    - specified site — *see* Neoplasm, uncertain behavior, by site
    - unspecified site D44.7
  - specified site — *see* Neoplasm, uncertain behavior, by site
  - sympathetic D44.7
    - specified site — *see* Neoplasm, uncertain behavior, by site
    - unspecified site D44.7
  - unspecified site D44.7
- **Parageusia** R43.2
  - psychogenic F45.8
- **Paragonimiasis** B66.4
- **Paragranuloma, Hodgkin** — *see* Lymphoma, Hodgkin, specified NEC
- **Parahemophilia** — *see also* Defect, coagulation D68.2
- **Parakeratosis** R23.4
  - variegata L41.Ø
- **Paralysis, paralytic** (complete) (incomplete) G83.9
  - with
    - syphilis A52.17
  - abducens, abducent (nerve) — *see* Strabismus, paralytic, sixth nerve
  - abductor, lower extremity G57.9- ☑
  - accessory nerve G52.8
  - accommodation — *see also* Paresis, of accommodation
    - hysterical F44.89
  - acoustic nerve (except Deafness) H93.3 ☑
  - agitans — *see also* Parkinsonism G2Ø
    - arteriosclerotic G21.4
  - alternating (oculomotor) G83.89

Paralysis, paralytic — *continued*

  - amyotrophic G12.21
  - ankle G57.9- ☑
  - anus (sphincter) K62.89
  - arm — *see* Monoplegia, upper limb
  - ascending (spinal), acute G61.Ø
  - association G12.29
  - asthenic bulbar G7Ø.ØØ
    - with exacerbation (acute) G7Ø.Ø1
    - in crisis G7Ø.Ø1
  - ataxic (hereditary) G11.9
    - general (syphilitic) A52.17
  - atrophic G58.9
    - infantile, acute — *see* Poliomyelitis, paralytic
    - progressive G12.22
    - spinal (acute) — *see* Poliomyelitis, paralytic
  - axillary G54.Ø
  - Babinski-Nageotte's G83.89
  - Bell's G51.Ø
    - newborn P11.3
  - Benedikt's G46.3
  - birth injury P14.9
    - spinal cord P11.5
  - bladder (neurogenic) (sphincter) N31.2
  - bowel, colon or intestine K56.Ø
  - brachial plexus G54.Ø
    - birth injury P14.3
    - newborn (birth injury) P14.3
  - brain G83.9
    - diplegia G83.Ø
    - triplegia G83.89
  - bronchial J98.Ø9
  - Brown-Séquard G83.81
  - bulbar (chronic) (progressive) G12.22
    - infantile — *see* Poliomyelitis, paralytic
    - poliomyelitic — *see* Poliomyelitis, paralytic
    - pseudo G12.29
  - bulbospinal G7Ø.ØØ
    - with exacerbation (acute) G7Ø.Ø1
    - in crisis G7Ø.Ø1
  - cardiac — *see also* Failure, heart I5Ø.9
  - cerebrocerebellar, diplegic G8Ø.1
  - cervical
    - plexus G54.2
    - sympathetic G9Ø.Ø9
  - Céstan-Chenais G46.3
  - Charcot-Marie-Tooth type G6Ø.Ø
  - Clark's G8Ø.9
  - colon K56.Ø
  - compressed air T7Ø.3 ☑
  - compression
    - arm G56.9- ☑
    - leg G57.9- ☑
    - lower extremity G57.9- ☑
    - upper extremity G56.9- ☑
  - congenital (cerebral) — *see* Palsy, cerebral
  - conjugate movement (gaze) (of eye) H51.Ø
    - cortical (nuclear) (supranuclear) H51.Ø
  - cordis — *see* Failure, heart
  - cranial or cerebral nerve G52.9
  - creeping G12.22
  - crossed leg G83.89
  - crutch — *see* Injury, brachial plexus
  - deglutition R13.Ø
    - hysterical F44.4
  - dementia A52.17
  - descending (spinal) NEC G12.29
  - diaphragm (flaccid) J98.6
    - due to accidental dissection of phrenic nerve during procedure — *see* Puncture, accidental complicating surgery
  - digestive organs NEC K59.89
  - diplegic — *see* Diplegia
  - divergence (nuclear) H51.8
  - diver's T7Ø.3 ☑
  - Duchenne's
    - birth injury P14.Ø
    - due to or associated with
      - motor neuron disease G12.22
      - muscular dystrophy G71.Ø1
  - due to intracranial or spinal birth injury — *see* Palsy, cerebral
  - embolic (current episode) I63.4- ☑
  - Erb (-Duchenne) (birth) (newborn) P14.Ø
  - Erb's syphilitic spastic spinal A52.17
  - esophagus K22.8
  - eye muscle (extrinsic) H49.9
    - intrinsic — *see also* Paresis, of accommodation

Paralysis, paralytic — *continued*

  - facial (nerve) G51.Ø
    - birth injury P11.3
    - congenital P11.3
    - following operation NEC — *see* Puncture, accidental complicating surgery
    - newborn (birth injury) P11.3
  - familial (recurrent) (periodic) G72.3
    - spastic G11.4
  - fauces J39.2
  - finger G56.9- ☑
  - gait R26.1
  - gastric nerve (nondiabetic) G52.2
  - gaze, conjugate H51.Ø
  - general (progressive) (syphilitic) A52.17
    - juvenile A5Ø.45
  - glottis J38.ØØ
    - bilateral J38.Ø2
    - unilateral J38.Ø1
  - gluteal G54.1
  - Gubler (-Millard) G46.3
  - hand — *see* Monoplegia, upper limb
  - heart — *see* Arrest, cardiac
  - hemiplegic — *see* Hemiplegia
  - hyperkalemic periodic (familial) G72.3
  - hypoglossal (nerve) G52.3
  - hypokalemic periodic G72.3
  - hysterical F44.4
  - ileus K56.Ø
  - infantile — *see also* Poliomyelitis, paralytic A8Ø.3Ø
    - bulbar — *see* Poliomyelitis, paralytic
    - cerebral — *see* Palsy, cerebral
    - spastic — *see* Palsy, cerebral, spastic
  - infective — *see* Poliomyelitis, paralytic
  - inferior nuclear G83.9
  - internuclear — *see* Ophthalmoplegia, internuclear
  - intestine K56.Ø
  - iris H57.Ø9
    - due to diphtheria (toxin) A36.89
  - ischemic, Volkmann's (complicating trauma) T79.6 ☑
  - Jackson's G83.89
  - jake — *see* Poisoning, food, noxious, plant
  - Jamaica ginger (jake) G62.2
  - juvenile general A5Ø.45
  - Klumpke (-Déjérine) (birth) (newborn) P14.1
  - labioglossal (laryngeal) (pharyngeal) G12.29
  - Landry's G61.Ø
  - laryngeal nerve (recurrent) (superior) (unilateral) J38.ØØ
    - bilateral J38.Ø2
    - unilateral J38.Ø1
  - larynx J38.ØØ
    - bilateral J38.Ø2
    - due to diphtheria (toxin) A36.2
    - unilateral J38.Ø1
  - lateral G12.23
  - lead T56.Ø ☑
  - left side — *see* Hemiplegia
  - leg G83.1- ☑
    - both — *see* Paraplegia
    - crossed G83.89
    - hysterical F44.4
    - psychogenic F44.4
    - transient or transitory R29.818
      - traumatic NEC — *see* Injury, nerve, leg
  - levator palpebrae superioris — *see* Blepharoptosis, paralytic
  - limb — *see* Monoplegia
  - lip K13.Ø
  - Lissauer's A52.17
  - lower limb — *see* Monoplegia, lower limb
    - both — *see* Paraplegia
  - lung J98.4
  - median nerve G56.1- ☑
  - medullary (tegmental) G83.89
  - mesencephalic NEC G83.89
    - tegmental G83.89
  - middle alternating G83.89
  - Millard-Gubler-Foville G46.3
  - monoplegic — *see* Monoplegia
  - motor G83.9
  - muscle, muscular NEC G72.89
    - due to nerve lesion G58.9
    - eye (extrinsic) H49.9
      - intrinsic — *see* Paresis, of accommodation
      - oblique — *see* Strabismus, paralytic, fourth nerve
    - iris sphincter H21.9
    - ischemic (Volkmann's) (complicating trauma) T79.6 ☑

Penetrating wound — *continued*
with internal injury — *see* Injury, by site
eyeball — *see* Puncture, eyeball
orbit (with or without foreign body) — *see* Puncture, orbit
uterus by instrument with or following ectopic or molar pregnancy O08.6
Penicillosis B48.4
Penis — *see* condition
Penitis N48.29
Pentalogy of Fallot Q21.8
Pentasomy X syndrome Q97.1
Pentosuria (essential) E74.89
Percreta placenta - O43.23 ☑
Peregrinating patient — *see* Disorder, factitious
Perforation, perforated (nontraumatic) (of)
accidental during procedure (blood vessel) (nerve) (organ) — *see* Complication, accidental puncture or laceration
antrum — *see* Sinusitis, maxillary
appendix K35.32
with localized peritonitis K35.32
atrial septum, multiple Q21.1
attic, ear — *see* Perforation, tympanum, attic
bile duct (common) (hepatic) K83.2
cystic K82.2
bladder (urinary)
with or following ectopic or molar pregnancy O08.6
obstetrical trauma O71.5
traumatic S37.29 ☑
at delivery O71.5
bowel K63.1
with or following ectopic or molar pregnancy O08.6
newborn P78.0
obstetrical trauma O71.5
traumatic — *see* Laceration, intestine
broad ligament N83.8
with or following ectopic or molar pregnancy O08.6
obstetrical trauma O71.6
by
device, implant or graft — *see also* Complications, by site and type, mechanical T85.628 ☑
arterial graft NEC — *see* Complication, cardiovascular device, mechanical, vascular
breast (implant) T85.49 ☑
catheter NEC T85.698 ☑
cystostomy T83.090 ☑
dialysis (renal) T82.49 ☑
intraperitoneal T85.691 ☑
infusion NEC T82.594 ☑
spinal (epidural) (subdural) T85.690 ☑
urinary — *see also* Complications, catheter, urinary T83.098 ☑
electronic (electrode) (pulse generator) (stimulator)
bone T84.390 ☑
cardiac T82.199 ☑
electrode T82.190 ☑
pulse generator T82.191 ☑
specified type NEC T82.198 ☑
nervous system — *see* Complication, prosthetic device, mechanical, electronic nervous system stimulator
urinary — *see* Complication, genitourinary, device, urinary, mechanical
fixation, internal (orthopedic) NEC — *see* Complication, fixation device, mechanical
gastrointestinal — *see* Complications, prosthetic device, mechanical, gastrointestinal device
genital NEC T83.498 ☑
intrauterine contraceptive device T83.39 ☑
penile prosthesis T83.490 ☑
heart NEC — *see* Complication, cardiovascular device, mechanical
joint prosthesis — *see* Complications, joint prosthesis, mechanical, specified NEC, by site
ocular NEC — *see* Complications, prosthetic device, mechanical, ocular device
orthopedic NEC — *see* Complication, orthopedic, device, mechanical
specified NEC T85.628 ☑
urinary NEC — *see also* Complication, genitourinary, device, urinary, mechanical
graft T83.29 ☑
vascular NEC — *see* Complication, cardiovascular device, mechanical

Perforation, perforated — *continued*
by — *continued*
device, implant or graft — *see also* Complications, by site and type, mechanical — *continued*
ventricular intracranial shunt T85.09 ☑
foreign body left accidentally in operative wound T81.539 ☑
instrument (any) during a procedure, accidental — *see* Puncture, accidental complicating surgery
cecum K35.32
with localized peritonitis K35.32
cervix (uteri) N88.8
with or following ectopic or molar pregnancy O08.6
obstetrical trauma O71.3
colon K63.1
newborn P78.0
obstetrical trauma O71.5
traumatic — *see* Laceration, intestine, large
common duct (bile) K83.2
cornea (due to ulceration) — *see* Ulcer, cornea, perforated
cystic duct K82.2
diverticulum (intestine) K57.80
with bleeding K57.81
large intestine K57.20
with
bleeding K57.21
small intestine K57.40
with bleeding K57.41
small intestine K57.00
with
bleeding K57.01
large intestine K57.40
with bleeding K57.41
ear drum — *see* Perforation, tympanum
esophagus K22.3
ethmoidal sinus — *see* Sinusitis, ethmoidal
frontal sinus — *see* Sinusitis, frontal
gallbladder K82.2
heart valve — *see* Endocarditis
ileum K63.1
newborn P78.0
obstetrical trauma O71.5
traumatic — *see* Laceration, intestine, small
instrumental, surgical (accidental) (blood vessel) (nerve) (organ) — *see* Puncture, accidental complicating surgery
intestine NEC K63.1
with ectopic or molar pregnancy O08.6
newborn P78.0
obstetrical trauma O71.5
traumatic — *see* Laceration, intestine
ulcerative NEC K63.1
newborn P78.0
jejunum, jejunal K63.1
obstetrical trauma O71.5
traumatic — *see* Laceration, intestine, small
ulcer — *see* Ulcer, gastrojejunal, with perforation
joint prosthesis — *see* Complications, joint prosthesis, mechanical, specified NEC, by site
mastoid (antrum) (cell) — *see* Disorder, mastoid, specified NEC
maxillary sinus — *see* Sinusitis, maxillary
membrana tympani — *see* Perforation, tympanum
nasal
septum J34.89
congenital Q30.3
syphilitic A52.73
sinus J34.89
congenital Q30.8
due to sinusitis — *see* Sinusitis
palate — *see also* Cleft, palate Q35.9
syphilitic A52.79
palatine vault — *see also* Cleft, palate, hard Q35.1
syphilitic A52.79
congenital A50.59
pars flaccida (ear drum) — *see* Perforation, tympanum, attic
pelvic
floor S31.030 ☑
with
ectopic or molar pregnancy O08.6
penetration into retroperitoneal space S31.031 ☑
retained foreign body S31.040 ☑
with penetration into retroperitoneal space S31.041 ☑
following ectopic or molar pregnancy O08.6

Perforation, perforated — *continued*
pelvic — *continued*
floor — *continued*
obstetrical trauma O70.1
organ S37.99 ☑
adrenal gland S37.818 ☑
bladder — *see* Perforation, bladder
fallopian tube S37.599 ☑
bilateral S37.592 ☑
unilateral S37.591 ☑
kidney S37.09- ☑
obstetrical trauma O71.5
ovary S37.499 ☑
bilateral S37.492 ☑
unilateral S37.491 ☑
prostate S37.828 ☑
specified organ NEC S37.898 ☑
ureter — *see* Perforation, ureter
urethra — *see* Perforation, urethra
uterus — *see* Perforation, uterus
perineum — *see* Laceration, perineum
pharynx J39.2
rectum K63.1
newborn P78.0
obstetrical trauma O71.5
traumatic S36.63 ☑
root canal space due to endodontic treatment M27.51
sigmoid K63.1
newborn P78.0
obstetrical trauma O71.5
traumatic S36.533 ☑
sinus (accessory) (chronic) (nasal) J34.89
sphenoidal sinus — *see* Sinusitis, sphenoidal
surgical (accidental) (by instrument) (blood vessel) (nerve) (organ) — *see* Puncture, accidental complicating surgery
traumatic
external — *see* Puncture
eye — *see* Puncture, eyeball
internal organ — *see* Injury, by site
tympanum, tympanic (membrane) (persistent post-traumatic) (postinflammatory) H72.9- ☑
attic H72.1- ☑
multiple — *see* Perforation, tympanum, multiple
total — *see* Perforation, tympanum, total
central H72.0- ☑
multiple — *see* Perforation, tympanum, multiple
total — *see* Perforation, tympanum, total
marginal NEC — *see* subcategory H72.2 ☑
multiple H72.81- ☑
pars flaccida — *see* Perforation, tympanum, attic
total H72.82- ☑
traumatic, current episode S09.2- ☑
typhoid, gastrointestinal — *see* Typhoid
ulcer — *see* Ulcer, by site, with perforation
ureter N28.89
traumatic S37.19 ☑
urethra N36.8
with ectopic or molar pregnancy O08.6
following ectopic or molar pregnancy O08.6
obstetrical trauma O71.5
traumatic S37.39 ☑
at delivery O71.5
uterus
with ectopic or molar pregnancy O08.6
by intrauterine contraceptive device T83.39 ☑
following ectopic or molar pregnancy O08.6
obstetrical trauma O71.1
traumatic S37.69 ☑
obstetric O71.1
uvula K13.79
syphilitic A52.79
vagina O71.4
obstetrical trauma O71.4
other trauma — *see* Puncture, vagina
Periadenitis mucosa necrotica recurrens K12.0
Periappendicitis (acute) — *see* Appendicitis
Periarteritis nodosa (disseminated) (infectious) (necrotizing) M30.0
Periarthritis (joint) — *see also* Enthesopathy
Duplay's M75.0- ☑
gonococcal A54.42
humeroscapularis — *see* Capsulitis, adhesive
scapulohumeral — *see* Capsulitis, adhesive
shoulder — *see* Capsulitis, adhesive
wrist M77.2- ☑
Periarthrosis (angioneural) — *see* Enthesopathy

Pericapsulitis, adhesive (shoulder) — *see* Capsulitis, adhesive
Pericarditis (with decompensation) (with effusion) I31.9
- with rheumatic fever (conditions in IØØ)
  - active — *see* Pericarditis, rheumatic
  - inactive or quiescent IØ9.2
- acute (hemorrhagic) (nonrheumatic) (Sicca) I3Ø.9
  - with chorea (acute) (rheumatic) (Sydenham's) IØ2.Ø
  - benign I3Ø.8
  - nonspecific I3Ø.Ø
  - rheumatic IØ1.Ø
    - with chorea (acute) (Sydenham's) IØ2.Ø
- adhesive or adherent (chronic) (external) (internal) I31.Ø
  - acute — *see* Pericarditis, acute
  - rheumatic IØ9.2
- bacterial (acute) (subacute) (with serous or seropurulent effusion) I3Ø.1
- calcareous I31.1
- cholesterol (chronic) I31.8
  - acute I3Ø.9
- chronic (nonrheumatic) I31.9
  - rheumatic IØ9.2
- constrictive (chronic) I31.1
- coxsackie B33.23
- fibrinocaseous (tuberculous) A18.84
- fibrinopurulent I3Ø.1
- fibrinous I3Ø.8
- fibrous I31.Ø
- gonococcal A54.83
- idiopathic I3Ø.Ø
- in systemic lupus erythematosus M32.12
- infective I3Ø.1
- meningococcal A39.53
- neoplastic (chronic) I31.8
  - acute I3Ø.9
- obliterans, obliterating I31.Ø
- plastic I31.Ø
- pneumococcal I3Ø.1
- postinfarction I24.1
- purulent I3Ø.1
- rheumatic (active) (acute) (with effusion) (with pneumonia) IØ1.Ø
  - with chorea (acute) (rheumatic) (Sydenham's) IØ2.Ø
  - chronic or inactive (with chorea) IØ9.2
- rheumatoid — *see* Rheumatoid, carditis
- septic I3Ø.1
- serofibrinous I3Ø.8
- staphylococcal I3Ø.1
- streptococcal I3Ø.1
- suppurative I3Ø.1
- syphilitic A52.Ø6
- tuberculous A18.84
- uremic N18.9 *[I32]*
- viral I3Ø.1

Pericardium, pericardial — *see* condition
Pericellulitis — *see* Cellulitis
Pericementitis (chronic) (suppurative) — *see also* Periodontitis
- acute KØ5.2Ø
  - generalized — *see* Periodontitis, aggressive, generalized
  - localized — *see* Periodontitis, aggressive, localized

Perichondritis
- auricle — *see* Perichondritis, ear
- bronchus J98.Ø9
- ear (external) H61.ØØ- ☑
  - acute H61.Ø1- ☑
  - chronic H61.Ø2- ☑
- external auditory canal — *see* Perichondritis, ear
- larynx J38.7
  - syphilitic A52.73
  - typhoid AØ1.Ø9
- nose J34.89
- pinna — *see* Perichondritis, ear
- trachea J39.8

Periclasia KØ5.4
Pericoronitis — *see* Periodontitis
Pericystitis N3Ø.9Ø
- with hematuria N3Ø.91

Peridiverticulitis (intestine) K57.92
- cecum — *see* Diverticulitis, intestine, large
- colon — *see* Diverticulitis, intestine, large
- duodenum — *see* Diverticulitis, intestine, small
- intestine — *see* Diverticulitis, intestine
- jejunum — *see* Diverticulitis, intestine, small
- rectosigmoid — *see* Diverticulitis, intestine, large
- rectum — *see* Diverticulitis, intestine, large
- sigmoid — *see* Diverticulitis, intestine, large

Periendocarditis — *see* Endocarditis
Periepididymitis N45.1
Perifolliculitis LØ1.Ø2
- abscedens, caput, scalp L66.3
- capitis, abscedens (et suffodiens) L66.3
- superficial pustular LØ1.Ø2

Perihepatitis K65.8
Perilabyrinthitis (acute) — *see* subcategory H83.Ø ☑
Perimeningitis — *see* Meningitis
Perimetritis — *see* Endometritis
Perimetrosalpingitis — *see* Salpingo-oophoritis
Perineocele N81.81
Perinephric, perinephritic — *see* condition
Perinephritis — *see also* Infection, kidney
- purulent — *see* Abscess, kidney

Perineum, perineal — *see* condition
Perineuritis NEC — *see* Neuralgia
Periodic — *see* condition
Periodontitis (chronic) (complex) (compound) (local) (simplex) KØ5.3Ø
- acute KØ5.2Ø
  - generalized KØ5.229
    - moderate KØ5.222
    - severe KØ5.223
    - slight KØ5.221
  - localized KØ5.219
    - moderate KØ5.212
    - severe KØ5.213
    - slight KØ5.211
- apical KØ4.5
  - acute (pulpal origin) KØ4.4
- generalized KØ5.329
  - moderate KØ5.322
  - severe KØ5.323
  - slight KØ5.321
- localized KØ5.319
  - moderate KØ5.312
  - severe KØ5.313
  - slight KØ5.311

Periodontoclasia KØ5.4
Periodontosis (juvenile) KØ5.4
Periods — *see also* Menstruation
- heavy N92.Ø
- irregular N92.6
- shortened intervals (irregular) N92.1

Perionychia — *see also* Cellulitis, digit
- with lymphangitis — *see* Lymphangitis, acute, digit

Perioophoritis — *see* Salpingo-oophoritis
Periorchitis N45.2
Periosteum, periosteal — *see* condition
Periostitis (albuminosa) (circumscribed) (diffuse) (infective) (monomelic) — *see also* Osteomyelitis
- alveolar M27.3
- alveolodental M27.3
- dental M27.3
- gonorrheal A54.43
- jaw (lower) (upper) M27.2
- orbit HØ5.Ø3- ☑
- syphilitic A52.77
  - congenital (early) A5Ø.Ø2 *[M9Ø.8Ø]*
  - secondary A51.46
- tuberculous — *see* Tuberculosis, bone
- yaws (hypertrophic) (early) (late) A66.6 *[M9Ø.8Ø]*

Periostosis (hyperplastic) — *see also* Disorder, bone, specified type NEC
- with osteomyelitis — *see* Osteomyelitis, specified type NEC

Peripartum
- cardiomyopathy O9Ø.3

Periphlebitis — *see* Phlebitis
Periproctitis K62.89
Periprostatitis — *see* Prostatitis
Perirectal — *see* condition
Perirenal — *see* condition
Perisalpingitis — *see* Salpingo-oophoritis
Perisplenitis (infectional) D73.89
Peristalsis, visible or reversed R19.2
Peritendinitis — *see* Enthesopathy
Peritoneum, peritoneal — *see* condition
Peritonitis (adhesive) (bacterial) (fibrinous) (hemorrhagic) (idiopathic) (localized) (perforative) (primary) (with adhesions) (with effusion) K65.9
- with or following
  - abscess K65.1
  - appendicitis
    - with perforation or rupture K35.32
    - generalized — *see also* Appendicitis K35.2Ø
    - localized — *see also* Appendicitis K35.3Ø
  - diverticular disease (intestine) K57.8Ø
    - with bleeding K57.81
    - ectopic or molar pregnancy OØ8.Ø
    - large intestine K57.2Ø
      - with
        - bleeding K57.21
        - small intestine K57.4Ø
          - with bleeding K57.41
    - small intestine K57.ØØ
      - with
        - bleeding K57.Ø1
        - large intestine K57.4Ø
          - with bleeding K57.41
- acute (generalized) K65.Ø
- aseptic T81.61 ☑
- bile, biliary K65.3
- chemical T81.61 ☑
- chlamydial A74.81
- chronic proliferative K65.8
- complicating abortion — *see* Abortion, by type, complicated by, pelvic peritonitis
- congenital P78.1
- diaphragmatic K65.Ø
- diffuse K65.Ø
- diphtheritic A36.89
- disseminated K65.Ø
- due to
  - bile K65.3
  - foreign
    - body or object accidentally left during a procedure (instrument) (sponge) (swab) T81.599 ☑
    - substance accidentally left during a procedure (chemical) (powder) (talc) T81.61 ☑
  - talc T81.61 ☑
  - urine K65.8
- eosinophilic K65.8
  - acute K65.Ø
- fibrocaseous (tuberculous) A18.31
- fibropurulent K65.Ø
- following ectopic or molar pregnancy OØ8.Ø
- general (ized) K65.Ø
- gonococcal A54.85
- meconium (newborn) P78.Ø
- neonatal P78.1
  - meconium P78.Ø
- pancreatic K65.Ø
- paroxysmal, familial E85.Ø
  - benign E85.Ø
- pelvic
  - female N73.5
    - acute N73.3
    - chronic N73.4
      - with adhesions N73.6
  - male K65.Ø
- periodic, familial E85.Ø
- proliferative, chronic K65.8
- puerperal, postpartum, childbirth O85
- purulent K65.Ø
- septic K65.Ø
- specified NEC K65.8
- spontaneous bacterial K65.2
- subdiaphragmatic K65.Ø
- subphrenic K65.Ø
- suppurative K65.Ø
- syphilitic A52.74
  - congenital (early) A5Ø.Ø8 *[K67]*
- talc T81.61 ☑
- tuberculous A18.31
- urine K65.8

Peritonsillar — *see* condition
Peritonsillitis J36
Perityphlitis K37
Periureteritis N28.89
Periurethral — *see* condition
Periurethritis (gangrenous) — *see* Urethritis
Periuterine — *see* condition
Perivaginitis — *see* Vaginitis
Perivasculitis, retinal H35.Ø6- ☑
Perivasitis (chronic) N49.1
Perivesiculitis (seminal) — *see* Vesiculitis
Perlèche NEC K13.Ø
- due to
  - candidiasis B37.83

- **Perlèche** — *continued*
  - due to — *continued*
    - moniliasis B37.83
    - riboflavin deficiency E53.0
    - vitamin B2 (riboflavin) deficiency E53.0
- **Pernicious** — *see* condition
- **Pernio, perniosis** T69.1 ☑
- **Perpetrator** (of abuse) — *see* Index to External Causes of Injury, Perpetrator
- **Persecution**
  - delusion F22
  - social Z60.5
- **Perseveration** (tonic) R48.8
- **Persistence, persistent** (congenital)
  - anal membrane Q42.3
    - with fistula Q42.2
  - arteria stapedia Q16.3
  - atrioventricular canal Q21.2
  - branchial cleft NOS Q18.2
    - cyst Q18.0
    - fistula Q18.0
    - sinus Q18.0
  - bulbus cordis in left ventricle Q21.8
  - canal of Cloquet Q14.0
  - capsule (opaque) Q12.8
  - cilioretinal artery or vein Q14.8
  - cloaca Q43.7
  - communication — *see* Fistula, congenital
  - convolutions
    - aortic arch Q25.46
    - fallopian tube Q50.6
    - oviduct Q50.6
    - uterine tube Q50.6
  - double aortic arch Q25.45
  - ductus arteriosus (Botalli) Q25.0
  - fetal
    - circulation P29.38
    - form of cervix (uteri) Q51.828
    - hemoglobin, hereditary (HPFH) D56.4
  - foramen
    - Botalli Q21.1
    - ovale Q21.1
  - Gartner's duct Q52.4
  - hemoglobin, fetal (hereditary) (HPFH) D56.4
  - hyaloid
    - artery (generally incomplete) Q14.0
    - system Q14.8
  - hymen, in pregnancy or childbirth — *see* Pregnancy, complicated by, abnormal, vulva
  - lanugo Q84.2
  - left
    - posterior cardinal vein Q26.8
    - root with right arch of aorta Q25.49
    - superior vena cava Q26.1
  - Meckel's diverticulum Q43.0
    - malignant — *see* Table of Neoplasms, small intestine, malignant
  - mucosal disease (middle ear) — *see* Otitis, media, suppurative, chronic, tubotympanic
  - nail(s), anomalous Q84.6
  - omphalomesenteric duct Q43.0
  - organ or site not listed — *see* Anomaly, by site
  - ostium
    - atrioventriculare commune Q21.2
    - primum Q21.2
    - secundum Q21.1
  - ovarian rests in fallopian tube Q50.6
  - pancreatic tissue in intestinal tract Q43.8
  - primary (deciduous)
    - teeth K00.6
    - vitreous hyperplasia Q14.0
  - pupillary membrane Q13.89
  - rhesus (Rh) titer — *see* Complication(s), transfusion, incompatibility reaction, Rh (factor)
  - right aortic arch Q25.47
  - sinus
    - urogenitalis
      - female Q52.8
      - male Q55.8
    - venosus with imperfect incorporation in right auricle Q26.8
  - thymus (gland) (hyperplasia) E32.0
  - thyroglossal duct Q89.2
  - thyrolingual duct Q89.2
  - truncus arteriosus or communis Q20.0
  - tunica vasculosa lentis Q12.2
  - umbilical sinus Q64.4
  - urachus Q64.4
- **Persistence, persistent** — *continued*
  - vitelline duct Q43.0
- **Person** (with)
  - admitted for clinical research, as a control subject (normal comparison) (participant) Z00.6
  - awaiting admission to adequate facility elsewhere Z75.1
  - concern (normal) about sick person in family Z63.6
  - consulting on behalf of another Z71.0
  - feigning illness Z76.5
  - living (in)
    - alone Z60.2
    - boarding school Z59.3
    - residential institution Z59.3
    - without
      - adequate housing (heating) (space) Z59.1
      - housing (permanent) (temporary) Z59.0
      - person able to render necessary care Z74.2
      - shelter Z59.0
  - on waiting list Z75.1
  - sick or handicapped in family Z63.6
- **Personality** (disorder) F60.9
  - accentuation of traits (type A pattern) Z73.1
  - affective F34.0
  - aggressive F60.3
  - amoral F60.2
  - anacastic, anankastic F60.5
  - antisocial F60.2
  - anxious F60.6
  - asocial F60.2
  - asthenic F60.7
  - avoidant F60.6
  - borderline F60.3
  - change due to organic condition (enduring) F07.0
  - compulsive F60.5
  - cycloid F34.0
  - cyclothymic F34.0
  - dependent F60.7
  - depressive F34.1
  - dissocial F60.2
  - dual F44.81
  - eccentric F60.89
  - emotionally unstable F60.3
  - expansive paranoid F60.0
  - explosive F60.3
  - fanatic F60.0
  - haltlose type F60.89
  - histrionic F60.4
  - hyperthymic F34.0
  - hypothymic F34.1
  - hysterical F60.4
  - immature F60.89
  - inadequate F60.7
  - labile (emotional) F60.3
  - mixed (nonspecific) F60.89
  - morally defective F60.2
  - multiple F44.81
  - narcissistic F60.81
  - obsessional F60.5
  - obsessive (-compulsive) F60.5
  - organic F07.0
  - overconscientious F60.5
  - paranoid F60.0
  - passive (-dependent) F60.7
  - passive-aggressive F60.89
  - pathologic F60.9
  - pattern defect or disturbance F60.9
  - pseudopsychopathic (organic) F07.0
  - pseudoretarded (organic) F07.0
  - psychoinfantile F60.4
  - psychoneurotic NEC F60.89
  - psychopathic F60.2
  - querulant F60.0
  - sadistic F60.89
  - schizoid F60.1
  - self-defeating F60.89
  - sensitive paranoid F60.0
  - sociopathic (amoral) (antisocial) (asocial) (dissocial) F60.2
  - specified NEC F60.89
  - type A Z73.1
  - unstable (emotional) F60.3
- **Perthes' disease** — *see* Legg-Calvé-Perthes disease
- **Pertussis** — *see also* Whooping cough A37.90
- **Perversion, perverted**
  - appetite F50.89
    - psychogenic F50.89
  - function
    - pituitary gland E23.2
- **Perversion, perverted** — *continued*
  - function — *continued*
    - pituitary gland — *continued*
      - posterior lobe E22.2
  - sense of smell and taste R43.8
    - psychogenic F45.8
  - sexual — *see* Deviation, sexual
- **Pervious, congenital** — *see also* Imperfect, closure
  - ductus arteriosus Q25.0
- **Pes** (congenital) — *see also* Talipes
  - acquired — *see also* Deformity, limb, foot, specified NEC
    - planus — *see* Deformity, limb, flat foot
  - adductus Q66.89
  - cavus Q66.7- ☑
  - deformity NEC, acquired — *see* Deformity, limb, foot, specified NEC
  - planus (acquired) (any degree) — *see also* Deformity, limb, flat foot
    - rachitic sequelae (late effect) E64.3
  - valgus Q66.6
- **Pest, pestis** — *see* Plague
- **Petechia, petechiae** R23.3
  - newborn P54.5
- **Petechial typhus** A75.9
- **Peter's anomaly** Q13.4
- **Petit mal seizure** — *see* Epilepsy, childhood, absence
- **Petit's hernia** — *see* Hernia, abdomen, specified site NEC
- **Petrellidosis** B48.2
- **Petrositis** H70.20- ☑
  - acute H70.21- ☑
  - chronic H70.22- ☑
- **Peutz-Jeghers disease or syndrome** Q85.8
- **Peyronie's disease** N48.6
- **PFAPA** (periodic fever, aphthous stomatitis, pharyngitis, and adenopathy syndrome) M04.8
- **Pfeiffer's disease** — *see* Mononucleosis, infectious
- **Phagedena** (dry) (moist) (sloughing) — *see also* Gangrene
  - geometric L88
  - penis N48.29
  - tropical — *see* Ulcer, skin
  - vulva N76.6
- **Phagedenic** — *see* condition
- **Phakoma** H35.89
- **Phakomatosis** — *see also* specific eponymous syndromes Q85.9
  - Bourneville's Q85.1
  - specified NEC Q85.8
- **Phantom limb syndrome** (without pain) G54.7
  - with pain G54.6
- **Pharyngeal pouch syndrome** D82.1
- **Pharyngitis** (acute) (catarrhal)(gangrenous) (infective) (malignant) (membranous) (phlegmonous) (pseudomembranous) (simple) (subacute) (suppurative) (ulcerative) (viral) J02.9
  - with influenza, flu, or grippe — *see* Influenza, with, pharyngitis
  - aphthous B08.5
  - atrophic J31.2
  - chlamydial A56.4
  - chronic (atrophic) (granular) (hypertrophic) J31.2
  - coxsackievirus B08.5
  - diphtheritic A36.0
  - enteroviral vesicular B08.5
  - follicular (chronic) J31.2
  - fusospirochetal A69.1
  - gonococcal A54.5
  - granular (chronic) J31.2
  - herpesviral B00.2
  - hypertrophic J31.2
  - infectional, chronic J31.2
  - influenzal — *see* Influenza, with, respiratory manifestations NEC
  - lymphonodular, acute (enteroviral) B08.8
  - pneumococcal J02.8
  - purulent J02.9
  - putrid J02.9
  - septic J02.0
  - sicca J31.2
  - specified organism NEC J02.8
  - staphylococcal J02.8
  - streptococcal J02.0
  - syphilitic, congenital (early) A50.03
  - tuberculous A15.8
  - vesicular, enteroviral B08.5
  - viral NEC J02.8
- **Pharyngoconjunctivitis, viral** B30.2

- **Pharyngolaryngitis** (acute) J06.Ø
  - chronic J37.Ø
- **Pharyngoplegia** J39.2
- **Pharyngotonsillitis, herpesviral** BØØ.2
- **Pharyngotracheitis, chronic** J42
- **Pharynx, pharyngeal** — *see* condition
- **Phencyclidine-induced**
  - anxiety disorder F16.98Ø
  - bipolar and related disorder F16.94
  - depressive disorder F16.94
  - psychotic disorder F16.959
- **Phenomenon**
  - Arthus' — *see* Arthus' phenomenon
  - jaw-winking QØ7.8
  - lupus erythematosus (LE) cell M32.9
  - Raynaud's (secondary) I73.ØØ
    - with gangrene I73.Ø1
  - vasomotor R55
  - vasospastic I73.9
  - vasovagal R55
  - Wenckebach's I44.1
- **Phenylketonuria** E7Ø.1
  - classical E7Ø.Ø
  - maternal E7Ø.1
- **Pheochromoblastoma**
  - specified site — *see* Neoplasm, malignant, by site
  - unspecified site C74.1Ø
- **Pheochromocytoma**
  - malignant
    - specified site — *see* Neoplasm, malignant, by site
    - unspecified site C74.1Ø
  - specified site — *see* Neoplasm, benign, by site
  - unspecified site D35.ØØ
- **Pheohyphomycosis** — *see* Chromomycosis
- **Pheomycosis** — *see* Chromomycosis
- **Phimosis** (congenital) (due to infection) N47.1
  - chancroidal A57
- **Phlebectasia** — *see also* Varix
  - congenital Q27.4
- **Phlebitis** (infective) (pyemic) (septic) (suppurative) I8Ø.9
  - antepartum — *see* Thrombophlebitis, antepartum
  - blue — *see* Phlebitis, leg, deep
  - breast, superficial I8Ø.8
  - calf muscular vein (NOS) I8Ø.25- ☑
  - cavernous (venous) sinus — *see* Phlebitis, intracranial (venous) sinus
  - cerebral (venous) sinus — *see* Phlebitis, intracranial (venous) sinus
  - chest wall, superficial I8Ø.8
  - cranial (venous) sinus — *see* Phlebitis, intracranial (venous) sinus
  - deep (vessels) — *see* Phlebitis, leg, deep
  - due to implanted device — *see* Complications, by site and type, specified NEC
  - during or resulting from a procedure T81.72 ☑
  - femoral vein (superficial) I8Ø.1- ☑
  - femoropopliteal vein I8Ø.Ø- ☑
  - gastrocnemial vein I8Ø.25- ☑
  - gestational — *see* Phlebopathy, gestational
  - hepatic veins I8Ø.8
  - iliac vein (common) (external) (internal) I8Ø.21- ☑
  - iliofemoral — *see* Phlebitis, femoral vein
  - intracranial (venous) sinus (any) GØ8
    - nonpyogenic I67.6
  - intraspinal venous sinuses and veins GØ8
    - nonpyogenic G95.19
  - lateral (venous) sinus — *see* Phlebitis, intracranial (venous) sinus
  - leg I8Ø.3
    - antepartum — *see* Thrombophlebitis, antepartum
    - deep (vessels) NEC I8Ø.2Ø- ☑
      - iliac I8Ø.21- ☑
      - popliteal vein I8Ø.22- ☑
      - specified vessel NEC I8Ø.29- ☑
      - tibial vein (anterior) (posterior) I8Ø.23- ☑
    - femoral vein (superficial) I8Ø.1- ☑
    - superficial (vessels) I8Ø.Ø- ☑
  - longitudinal sinus — *see* Phlebitis, intracranial (venous) sinus
  - lower limb — *see* Phlebitis, leg
  - migrans, migrating (superficial) I82.1
  - pelvic
    - with ectopic or molar pregnancy OØ8.Ø
    - following ectopic or molar pregnancy OØ8.Ø
    - puerperal, postpartum O87.1
  - peroneal vein I8Ø.24- ☑
  - popliteal vein — *see* Phlebitis, leg, deep, popliteal
- **Phlebitis** — *continued*
  - portal (vein) K75.1
  - postoperative T81.72 ☑
  - pregnancy — *see* Thrombophlebitis, antepartum
  - puerperal, postpartum, childbirth O87.Ø
    - deep O87.1
    - pelvic O87.1
    - superficial O87.Ø
  - retina — *see* Vasculitis, retina
  - saphenous (accessory) (great) (long) (small) — *see* Phlebitis, leg, superficial
  - sinus (meninges) — *see* Phlebitis, intracranial (venous) sinus
  - soleal vein I8Ø.25- ☑
  - specified site NEC I8Ø.8
  - syphilitic A52.Ø9
  - tibial vein — *see* Phlebitis, leg, deep, tibial
  - ulcerative I8Ø.9
    - leg — *see* Phlebitis, leg
  - umbilicus I8Ø.8
  - uterus (septic) — *see* Endometritis
  - varicose (leg) (lower limb) — *see* Varix, leg, with, inflammation
- **Phlebofibrosis** I87.8
- **Phleboliths** I87.8
- **Phlebopathy,**
  - gestational O22.9- ☑
  - puerperal O87.9
- **Phlebosclerosis** I87.8
- **Phlebothrombosis** — *see also* Thrombosis
  - antepartum — *see* Thrombophlebitis, antepartum
  - pregnancy — *see* Thrombophlebitis, antepartum
  - puerperal — *see* Thrombophlebitis, puerperal
- **Phlebotomus fever** A93.1
- **Phlegmasia**
  - alba dolens O87.1
    - nonpuerperal — *see* Phlebitis, femoral vein
  - cerulea dolens — *see* Phlebitis, leg, deep
- **Phlegmon** — *see* Abscess
- **Phlegmonous** — *see* condition
- **Phlyctenulosis** (allergic) (keratoconjunctivitis) (nontuberculous) — *see also* Keratoconjunctivitis
  - cornea — *see* Keratoconjunctivitis
  - tuberculous A18.52
- **Phobia, phobic** F4Ø.9
  - animal F4Ø.218
    - spiders F4Ø.21Ø
  - examination F4Ø.298
  - reaction F4Ø.9
  - simple F4Ø.298
  - social F4Ø.1Ø
    - generalized F4Ø.11
  - specific (isolated) F4Ø.298
    - animal F4Ø.218
      - spiders F4Ø.21Ø
    - blood F4Ø.23Ø
    - injection F4Ø.231
    - injury F4Ø.233
    - men F4Ø.29Ø
    - natural environment F4Ø.228
      - thunderstorms F4Ø.22Ø
    - situational F4Ø.248
      - bridges F4Ø.242
      - closed in spaces F4Ø.24Ø
      - flying F4Ø.243
      - heights F4Ø.241
    - specified focus NEC F4Ø.298
    - transfusion F4Ø.231
    - women F4Ø.291
  - specified NEC F4Ø.8
    - medical care NEC F4Ø.232
  - state F4Ø.9
- **Phocas' disease** — *see* Mastopathy, cystic
- **Phocomelia** Q73.1
  - lower limb — *see* Agenesis, leg, with foot present
  - upper limb — *see* Agenesis, arm, with hand present
- **Phoria** H5Ø.5Ø
- **Phosphate-losing tubular disorder** N25.Ø
- **Phosphatemia** E83.39
- **Phosphaturia** E83.39
- **Photodermatitis** (sun) L56.8
  - chronic L57.8
  - due to drug L56.8
  - light other than sun L59.8
- **Photokeratitis** H16.13- ☑
- **Photophobia** H53.14- ☑
- **Photophthalmia** — *see* Photokeratitis
- **Photopsia** H53.19
- **Photoretinitis** — *see* Retinopathy, solar
- **Photosensitivity, photosensitization** (sun) skin L56.8
  - light other than sun L59.8
- **Phrenitis** — *see* Encephalitis
- **Phrynoderma** (vitamin A deficiency) E5Ø.8
- **Phthiriasis** (pubis) B85.3
  - with any infestation classifiable to B85.Ø-B85.2 B85.4
- **Phthirus infestation** — *see* Phthiriasis
- **Phthisis** — *see also* Tuberculosis
  - bulbi (infectional) — *see* Disorder, globe, degenerated condition, atrophy
  - eyeball (due to infection) — *see* Disorder, globe, degenerated condition, atrophy
- **Phycomycosis** — *see* Zygomycosis
- **Physalopteriasis** B81.8
- **Physical restraint status** Z78.1
- **Phytobezoar** T18.9 ☑
  - intestine T18.3 ☑
  - stomach T18.2 ☑
- **Pian** — *see* Yaws
- **Pianoma** A66.1
- **Pica** F5Ø.89
  - in adults F5Ø.89
  - infant or child F98.3
- **Picking, nose** F98.8
- **Pick-Niemann disease** — *see* Niemann-Pick disease or syndrome
- **Pick's**
  - cerebral atrophy G31.Ø1 *[FØ2.8Ø]*
    - with behavioral disturbance G31.Ø1 *[FØ2.81]*
  - disease or syndrome (brain) G31.Ø1 *[FØ2.8Ø]*
    - with behavioral disturbance G31.Ø1 *[FØ2.81]*
    - brain G31.Ø1 *[FØ2.8Ø]*
      - with behavioral disturbance G31.Ø1 *[FØ2.81]*
    - pericardium (pericardial pseudocirrhosis of liver) I31.1
  - syndrome
    - brain G31.Ø1 *[FØ2.8Ø]*
      - with behavioral disturbance G31.Ø1 *[FØ2.81]*
    - of heart (pericardial pseudocirrhosis of liver) I31.1
- **Pickwickian syndrome** E66.2
- **Piebaldism** E7Ø.39
- **Piedra** (beard) (scalp) B36.8
  - black B36.3
  - white B36.2
- **Pierre Robin deformity or syndrome** Q87.Ø
- **Pierson's disease or osteochondrosis** M91.Ø
- **Pig-bel** AØ5.2
- **Pigeon**
  - breast or chest (acquired) M95.4
    - congenital Q67.7
    - rachitic sequelae (late effect) E64.3
  - breeder's disease or lung J67.2
  - fancier's disease or lung J67.2
  - toe — *see* Deformity, toe, specified NEC
- **Pigmentation** (abnormal) (anomaly) L81.9
  - conjunctiva H11.13- ☑
  - cornea (anterior) H18.Ø1- ☑
    - posterior H18.Ø5- ☑
    - stromal H18.Ø6- ☑
  - diminished melanin formation NEC L81.6
  - iron L81.8
  - lids, congenital Q82.8
  - limbus corneae — *see* Pigmentation, cornea
  - metals L81.8
  - optic papilla, congenital Q14.2
  - retina, congenital (grouped) (nevoid) Q14.1
  - scrotum, congenital Q82.8
  - tattoo L81.8
- **Piles** — *see also* Hemorrhoids K64.9
- **Pili**
  - annulati or torti (congenital) Q84.1
  - incarnati L73.1
- **Pill roller hand** (intrinsic) — *see* Parkinsonism
- **Pilomatrixoma** — *see* Neoplasm, skin, benign
  - malignant — *see* Neoplasm, skin, malignant
- **Pilonidal** — *see* condition
- **Pimple** R23.8
- **PIN** — *see* Neoplasia, intraepithelial, prostate
- **Pinched nerve** — *see* Neuropathy, entrapment
- **Pindborg tumor** — *see* Cyst, calcifying odontogenic
- **Pineal body or gland** — *see* condition
- **Pinealoblastoma** C75.3
- **Pinealoma** D44.5
  - malignant C75.3
- **Pineoblastoma** C75.3

- **Polyosteoarthritis** — *see also* Osteoarthritis, generalized M15.9
  - post-traumatic M15.3
  - specified NEC M15.8
- **Polyostotic fibrous dysplasia** Q78.1
- **Polyotia** Q17.Ø
- **Polyp, polypus**
  - accessory sinus J33.8
  - adenocarcinoma in — *see* Neoplasm, malignant, by site
  - adenocarcinoma in situ in — *see* Neoplasm, in situ, by site
  - adenoid tissue J33.Ø
  - adenomatous — *see also* Neoplasm, benign, by site
    - adenocarcinoma in — *see* Neoplasm, malignant, by site
    - adenocarcinoma in situ in — *see* Neoplasm, in situ, by site
    - carcinoma in — *see* Neoplasm, malignant, by site
    - carcinoma in situ in — *see* Neoplasm, in situ, by site
    - multiple — *see* Neoplasm, benign
      - adenocarcinoma in — *see* Neoplasm, malignant, by site
      - adenocarcinoma in situ in — *see* Neoplasm, in situ, by site
  - antrum J33.8
  - anus, anal (canal) K62.Ø
  - Bartholin's gland N84.3
  - bladder D41.4
  - carcinoma in — *see* Neoplasm, malignant, by site
  - carcinoma in situ in — *see* Neoplasm, in situ, by site
  - cecum D12.Ø
  - cervix (uteri) N84.1
    - in pregnancy or childbirth — *see* Pregnancy, complicated by, abnormal, cervix
    - mucous N84.1
    - nonneoplastic N84.1
  - choanal J33.Ø
  - cholesterol K82.4
  - clitoris N84.3
  - colon K63.5
    - adenomatous D12.6
      - ascending D12.2
      - cecum D12.Ø
      - descending D12.4
    - hyperplastic, (any site) K63.5
    - inflammatory K51.4Ø
      - with
        - abscess K51.414
        - complication K51.419
          - specified NEC K51.418
        - fistula K51.413
        - intestinal obstruction K51.412
        - rectal bleeding K51.411
    - sigmoid D12.5
    - transverse D12.3
  - corpus uteri N84.Ø
  - dental KØ4.Ø1
    - irreversible KØ4.Ø2
    - reversible KØ4.Ø1
  - duodenum K31.7
  - ear (middle) H74.4- ☑
  - endometrium N84.Ø
  - ethmoidal (sinus) J33.8
  - fallopian tube N84.8
  - female genital tract N84.9
    - specified NEC N84.8
  - frontal (sinus) J33.8
  - gallbladder K82.4
  - gingiva, gum KØ6.8
  - labia, labium (majus) (minus) N84.3
  - larynx (mucous) J38.1
    - adenomatous D14.1
  - malignant — *see* Neoplasm, malignant, by site
  - maxillary (sinus) J33.8
  - middle ear — *see* Polyp, ear (middle)
  - myometrium N84.Ø
  - nares
    - anterior J33.9
    - posterior J33.Ø
  - nasal (mucous) J33.9
    - cavity J33.Ø
    - septum J33.Ø
  - nasopharyngeal J33.Ø
  - nose (mucous) J33.9
  - oviduct N84.8
  - pharynx J39.2
  - placenta O9Ø.89

Polyp, polypus — *continued*
  - prostate — *see* Enlargement, enlarged, prostate
  - pudenda, pudendum N84.3
  - pulpal (dental) KØ4.Ø1
    - irreversible KØ4.Ø2
    - reversible KØ4.Ø1
  - rectum (nonadenomatous) K62.1
    - adenomatous — *see* Polyp, adenomatous
  - septum (nasal) J33.Ø
  - sinus (accessory) (ethmoidal) (frontal) (maxillary) (sphenoidal) J33.8
  - sphenoidal (sinus) J33.8
  - stomach K31.7
    - adenomatous D13.1
  - tube, fallopian N84.8
  - turbinate, mucous membrane J33.8
  - umbilical, newborn P83.6
  - ureter N28.89
  - urethra N36.2
  - uterus (body) (corpus) (mucous) N84.Ø
    - cervix N84.1
    - in pregnancy or childbirth — *see* Pregnancy, complicated by, tumor, uterus
  - vagina N84.2
  - vocal cord (mucous) J38.1
  - vulva N84.3
- **Polyphagia** R63.2
- **Polyploidy** Q92.7
- **Polypoid** — *see* condition
- **Polyposis** — *see also* Polyp
  - coli (adenomatous) D12.6
    - adenocarcinoma in C18.9
    - adenocarcinoma in situ in — *see* Neoplasm, in situ, by site
    - carcinoma in C18.9
  - colon (adenomatous) D12.6
  - familial D12.6
    - adenocarcinoma in situ in — *see* Neoplasm, in situ, by site
  - intestinal (adenomatous) D12.6
  - malignant lymphomatous C83.1- ☑
  - multiple, adenomatous — *see also* Neoplasm, benign D36.9
- **Polyradiculitis** — *see* Polyneuropathy
- **Polyradiculoneuropathy** (acute) (postinfective) (segmentally demyelinating) G61.Ø
- **Polyserositis**
  - due to pericarditis I31.1
  - pericardial I31.1
  - periodic, familial E85.Ø
  - tuberculous A19.9
    - acute A19.1
    - chronic A19.8
- **Polysplenia syndrome** Q89.Ø9
- **Polysyndactyly** — *see also* Syndactylism, syndactyly Q7Ø.4
- **Polytrichia** L68.3
- **Polyunguia** Q84.6
- **Polyuria** R35.8
  - nocturnal R35.1
  - psychogenic F45.8
- **Pompe's disease** (glycogen storage) E74.Ø2
- **Pompholyx** L3Ø.1
- **Poncet's disease** (tuberculous rheumatism) A18.Ø9
- **Pond fracture** — *see* Fracture, skull
- **Ponos** B55.Ø
- **Pons, pontine** — *see* condition
- **Poor**
  - aesthetic of existing restoration of tooth KØ8.56
  - contractions, labor O62.2
  - gingival margin to tooth restoration KØ8.51
  - personal hygiene R46.Ø
  - prenatal care, affecting management of pregnancy — *see* Pregnancy, complicated by, insufficient, prenatal care
  - sucking reflex (newborn) R29.2
  - urinary stream R39.12
  - vision NEC H54.7
- **Poradenitis, nostras inguinalis or venerea** A55
- **Porencephaly** (congenital) (developmental) (true) QØ4.6
  - acquired G93.Ø
  - nondevelopmental G93.Ø
  - traumatic (post) FØ7.89
- **Porocephaliasis** B88.8
- **Porokeratosis** Q82.8
- **Poroma, eccrine** — *see* Neoplasm, skin, benign
- **Porphyria** (South African) E8Ø.2Ø
  - acquired E8Ø.2Ø

Porphyria — *continued*
  - acute intermittent (hepatic) (Swedish) E8Ø.21
  - cutanea tarda (hereditary) (symptomatic) E8Ø.1
  - due to drugs E8Ø.2Ø
    - correct substance properly administered — *see* Table of Drugs and Chemicals, by drug, adverse effect
    - overdose or wrong substance given or taken — *see* Table of Drugs and Chemicals, by drug, poisoning
  - erythropoietic (congenital) (hereditary) E8Ø.Ø
  - hepatocutaneous type E8Ø.1
  - secondary E8Ø.2Ø
  - toxic NEC E8Ø.2Ø
  - variegata E8Ø.2Ø
- **Porphyrinuria** — *see* Porphyria
- **Porphyruria** — *see* Porphyria
- **Port wine nevus, mark, or stain** Q82.5
- **Portal** — *see* condition
- **Posadas-Wernicke disease** B38.9
- **Positive**
  - culture (nonspecific)
    - blood R78.81
    - bronchial washings R84.5
    - cerebrospinal fluid R83.5
    - cervix uteri R87.5
    - nasal secretions R84.5
    - nipple discharge R89.5
    - nose R84.5
      - staphylococcus (Methicillin susceptible) Z22.321
        - Methicillin resistant Z22.322
    - peritoneal fluid R85.5
    - pleural fluid R84.5
    - prostatic secretions R86.5
    - saliva R85.5
    - seminal fluid R86.5
    - sputum R84.5
    - synovial fluid R89.5
    - throat scrapings R84.5
    - urine R82.79
    - vagina R87.5
    - vulva R87.5
    - wound secretions R89.5
  - PPD (skin test) R76.11
  - serology for syphilis A53.Ø
    - false R76.8
    - with signs or symptoms — *code as* Syphilis, by site and stage
  - skin test, tuberculin (without active tuberculosis) R76.11
  - test, human immunodeficiency virus (HIV) R75
  - VDRL A53.Ø
    - with signs or symptoms — *code by* site and stage under Syphilis A53.9
  - Wassermann reaction A53.Ø
- **Postcardiotomy syndrome** I97.Ø
- **Postcaval ureter** Q62.62
- **Postcholecystectomy syndrome** K91.5
- **Postclimacteric bleeding** N95.Ø
- **Postcommissurotomy syndrome** I97.Ø
- **Postconcussional syndrome** FØ7.81
- **Postcontusional syndrome** FØ7.81
- **Postcricoid region** — *see* condition
- **Post-dates** (4Ø-42 weeks) (pregnancy) (mother) O48.Ø
  - more than 42 weeks gestation O48.1
- **Postencephalitic syndrome** FØ7.89
- **Posterior** — *see* condition
- **Posterolateral sclerosis** (spinal cord) — *see* Degeneration, combined
- **Postexanthematous** — *see* condition
- **Postfebrile** — *see* condition
- **Postgastrectomy dumping syndrome** K91.1
- **Posthemiplegic chorea** — *see* Monoplegia
- **Posthemorrhagic anemia** (chronic) D5Ø.Ø
  - acute D62
  - newborn P61.3
- **Postherpetic neuralgia** (zoster) BØ2.29
  - trigeminal BØ2.22
- **Posthitis** N47.7
- **Postimmunization complication or reaction** — *see* Complications, vaccination
- **Postinfectious** — *see* condition
- **Postlaminectomy syndrome NEC** M96.1
- **Postleukotomy syndrome** FØ7.Ø
- **Postmastectomy lymphedema** (syndrome) I97.2
- **Postmaturity, postmature** (over 42 weeks)
  - maternal (over 42 weeks gestation) O48.1
  - newborn PØ8.22

- **Postmeasles complication NEC** — *see also* condition BØ5.89
- **Postmenopausal**
  - endometrium (atrophic) N95.8
    - suppurative — *see also* Endometritis N71.9
  - osteoporosis — *see* Osteoporosis, postmenopausal
- **Postnasal drip** RØ9.82
  - due to
    - allergic rhinitis — *see* Rhinitis, allergic
    - common cold JØØ
    - gastroesophageal reflux — *see* Reflux, gastroesophageal
    - nasopharyngitis — *see* Nasopharyngitis
    - other known condition — *code to* condition
    - sinusitis — *see* Sinusitis
- **Postnatal** — *see* condition
- **Postoperative** (postprocedural) — *see* Complication, postoperative
  - pneumothorax, therapeutic Z98.3
  - state NEC Z98.89Ø
- **Postpancreatectomy hyperglycemia** E89.1
- **Postpartum** — *see* Puerperal
- **Postphlebitic syndrome** — *see* Syndrome, postthrombotic
- **Postpolio** (myelitic) **syndrome** G14
- **Postpoliomyelitic** — *see also* condition
  - osteopathy — *see* Osteopathy, after poliomyelitis
- **Postprocedural** — *see also* Postoperative
  - hypoinsulinemia E89.1
- **Postschizophrenic depression** F32.89
- **Postsurgery status** — *see also* Status (post)
  - pneumothorax, therapeutic Z98.3
- **Post-term** (4Ø-42 weeks) (pregnancy) (mother) O48.Ø
  - infant PØ8.21
  - more than 42 weeks gestation (mother) O48.1
- **Post-traumatic brain syndrome, nonpsychotic** FØ7.81
- **Post-typhoid abscess** AØ1.Ø9
- **Postures, hysterical** F44.2
- **Postvaccinal reaction or complication** — *see* Complications, vaccination
- **Postvalvulotomy syndrome** I97.Ø
- **Potain's**
  - disease (pulmonary edema) — *see* Edema, lung
  - syndrome (gastrectasis with dyspepsia) K31.Ø
- **Potter's**
  - asthma J62.8
  - facies Q6Ø.6
  - lung J62.8
  - syndrome (with renal agenesis) Q6Ø.6
- **Pott's**
  - curvature (spinal) A18.Ø1
  - disease or paraplegia A18.Ø1
  - spinal curvature A18.Ø1
  - tumor, puffy — *see* Osteomyelitis, specified type NEC
- **Pouch**
  - bronchus Q32.4
  - Douglas' — *see* condition
  - esophagus, esophageal, congenital Q39.6
    - acquired K22.5
  - gastric K31.4
  - Hartmann's K82.8
  - pharynx, pharyngeal (congenital) Q38.7
- **Pouchitis** K91.85Ø
- **Poultrymen's itch** B88.Ø
- **Poverty NEC** Z59.6
  - extreme Z59.5
- **Poxvirus NEC** BØ8.8
- **Prader-Willi syndrome** Q87.11
- **Prader-Willi-like syndrome** Q87.19
- **Preauricular appendage or tag** Q17.Ø
- **Prebetalipoproteinemia** (acquired) (essential) (familial) (hereditary) (primary) (secondary) E78.1
  - with chylomicronemia E78.3
- **Precipitate labor or delivery** O62.3
- **Preclimacteric bleeding** (menorrhagia) N92.4
- **Precocious**
  - adrenarche E3Ø.1
  - menarche E3Ø.1
  - menstruation E3Ø.1
  - pubarche E3Ø.1
  - puberty E3Ø.1
    - central E22.8
  - sexual development NEC E3Ø.1
  - thelarche E3Ø.8
- **Precocity, sexual** (constitutional) (cryptogenic) (female) (idiopathic) (male) E3Ø.1
  - with adrenal hyperplasia E25.9
- **Precocity, sexual** — *continued*
  - with adrenal hyperplasia — *continued*
    - congenital E25.Ø
- **Precordial pain** RØ7.2
- **Predeciduous teeth** KØØ.2
- **Prediabetes, prediabetic** R73.Ø3
  - complicating
    - pregnancy — *see* Pregnancy, complicated by, diseases of, specified type or system NEC
    - puerperium O99.893
- **Predislocation status of hip at birth** Q65.6
- **Pre-eclampsia** O14.9- ☑
  - with pre-existing hypertension — *see* Hypertension, complicating pregnancy, pre-existing, with, pre-eclampsia
  - complicating
    - childbirth O14.94
    - puerperium O14.95
  - mild O14.Ø- ☑
    - complicating
      - childbirth O14.Ø4
      - puerperium O14.Ø5
  - moderate O14.Ø- ☑
    - complicating
      - childbirth O14.Ø4
      - puerperium O14.Ø5
  - severe O14.1- ☑
    - with hemolysis, elevated liver enzymes and low platelet count (HELLP) O14.2- ☑
      - complicating
        - childbirth O14.24
        - puerperium O14.25
    - complicating
      - childbirth O14.14
      - puerperium O14.15
- **Pre-eruptive color change, teeth, tooth** KØØ.8
- **Pre-excitation atrioventricular conduction** I45.6
- **Preglaucoma** H4Ø.ØØ- ☑
- **Pregnancy** (single) (uterine) — *see also* Delivery and Puerperal Z33.1

> *Note: The Tabular must be reviewed for assignment of appropriate seventh character for multiple gestation codes in Chapter 15*

> *Note: The Tabular must be reviewed for assignment of the appropriate character indicating the trimester of the pregnancy*

  - abdominal (ectopic) OØØ.ØØ
    - with intrauterine pregnancy OØØ.Ø1
    - with viable fetus O36.7- ☑
  - ampullar OØØ.1Ø- ☑
    - with intrauterine pregnancy OØØ.11- ☑
  - biochemical OØ2.81
  - broad ligament OØØ.8Ø
    - with intrauterine pregnancy OØØ.81
  - cervical OØØ.8
    - with intrauterine pregnancy OØØ.81
  - chemical OØ2.81
  - complicated by (care of) (management affected by)
    - abnormal, abnormality
      - cervix O34.4- ☑
        - causing obstructed labor O65.5
      - cord (umbilical) O69.9 ☑
      - fetal heart rate or rhythm O36.83- ☑
      - findings on antenatal screening of mother O28.9
        - biochemical O28.1
        - chromosomal O28.5
        - cytological O28.2
        - genetic O28.5
        - hematological O28.Ø
        - radiological O28.4
        - specified NEC O28.8
        - ultrasonic O28.3
      - glucose (tolerance) NEC O99.81Ø
      - pelvic organs O34.9- ☑
        - specified NEC O34.8- ☑
          - causing obstructed labor O65.5
      - pelvis (bony) (major) NEC O33.Ø
      - perineum O34.7- ☑
      - position
        - placenta O44.Ø- ☑
          - with hemorrhage O44.1- ☑
        - uterus O34.59- ☑
      - uterus O34.59- ☑
        - causing obstructed labor O65.5
        - congenital O34.Ø- ☑
- **Pregnancy** — *continued*
  - complicated by — *continued*
    - abnormal, abnormality — *continued*
      - vagina O34.6- ☑
        - causing obstructed labor O65.5
      - vulva O34.7- ☑
        - causing obstructed labor O65.5
    - abruptio placentae — *see* Abruptio placentae
    - abscess or cellulitis
      - bladder O23.1- ☑
      - breast O91.11- ☑
      - genital organ or tract O23.9- ☑
    - abuse
      - physical O9A.31 ☑ (*following* O99)
      - psychological O9A.51 ☑ (*following* O99)
      - sexual O9A.41 ☑ (*following* O99)
    - adverse effect anesthesia O29.9- ☑
      - aspiration pneumonitis O29.Ø1- ☑
      - cardiac arrest O29.11- ☑
      - cardiac complication NEC O29.19- ☑
      - cardiac failure O29.12- ☑
      - central nervous system complication NEC O29.29- ☑
      - cerebral anoxia O29.21- ☑
      - failed or difficult intubation O29.6- ☑
      - inhalation of stomach contents or secretions NOS O29.Ø1- ☑
      - local, toxic reaction O29.3X ☑
      - Mendelson's syndrome O29.Ø1- ☑
      - pressure collapse of lung O29.Ø2- ☑
      - pulmonary complications NEC O29.Ø9- ☑
      - specified NEC O29.8X- ☑
      - spinal and epidural type NEC O29.5X ☑
        - induced headache O29.4- ☑
    - albuminuria — *see also* Proteinuria, gestational O12.1- ☑
    - alcohol use O99.31- ☑
    - amnionitis O41.12- ☑
    - anaphylactoid syndrome of pregnancy O88.Ø1- ☑
    - anemia (conditions in D5Ø-D64) (pre-existing) O99.Ø1- ☑
      - complicating the puerperium O99.Ø3
    - antepartum hemorrhage O46.9- ☑
      - with coagulation defect — *see* Hemorrhage, antepartum, with coagulation defect
      - specified NEC O46.8X- ☑
    - appendicitis O99.61- ☑
    - atrophy (yellow) (acute) liver (subacute) O26.61- ☑
    - bariatric surgery status O99.84- ☑
    - bicornis or bicornuate uterus O34.Ø- ☑
    - biliary tract problems O26.61- ☑
    - breech presentation O32.1 ☑
    - cardiovascular diseases (conditions in IØØ-IØ9, I2Ø-I52, I7Ø-I99) O99.41- ☑
    - cerebrovascular disorders (conditions in I6Ø-I69) O99.41- ☑
    - cervical shortening O26.87- ☑
    - cervicitis O23.51- ☑
    - cesarean scar defect (isthmocele) O34.22
    - chloasma (gravidarum) O26.89- ☑
    - cholecystitis O99.61- ☑
    - cholestasis (intrahepatic) O26.61- ☑
    - chorioamnionitis O41.12- ☑
    - circulatory system disorder (conditions in IØØ-IØ9, I2Ø-I99, O99.41-)
    - compound presentation O32.6 ☑
    - conjoined twins O3Ø.Ø2- ☑
    - connective system disorders (conditions in MØØ-M99) O99.891
    - contracted pelvis (general) O33.1
      - inlet O33.2
      - outlet O33.3 ☑
    - convulsions (eclamptic) (uremic) — *see also* Eclampsia O15.9
    - cracked nipple O92.11- ☑
    - cystitis O23.1- ☑
    - cystocele O34.8- ☑
    - death of fetus (near term) O36.4 ☑
      - early pregnancy OØ2.1
      - of one fetus or more in multiple gestation O31.2- ☑
    - deciduitis O41.14- ☑
    - decreased fetal movement O36.81- ☑
    - dental problems O99.61- ☑
    - diabetes (mellitus) O24.91- ☑

- **Pregnancy** — *continued*
  - complicated by — *continued*
    - diabetes — *continued*
      - gestational (pregnancy induced) — *see* Diabetes, gestational
      - pre-existing O24.31- ☑
        - specified NEC O24.81- ☑
        - type 1 O24.Ø1- ☑
        - type 2 O24.11- ☑
    - digestive system disorders (conditions in KØØ-K93) O99.61- ☑
    - diseases of — *see* Pregnancy, complicated by, specified body system disease
      - biliary tract O26.61- ☑
      - blood NEC (conditions in D65-D77) O99.11- ☑
      - liver O26.61- ☑
      - specified NEC O99.891
    - disorders of — *see* Pregnancy, complicated by, specified body system disorder
      - amniotic fluid and membranes O41.9- ☑
        - specified NEC O41.8X- ☑
      - biliary tract O26.61- ☑
      - ear and mastoid process (conditions in H6Ø-H95) O99.891
      - eye and adnexa (conditions in HØØ-H59) O99.891
      - liver O26.61- ☑
      - skin (conditions in LØØ-L99) O99.71- ☑
      - specified NEC O99.891
    - displacement, uterus NEC O34.59- ☑
      - causing obstructed labor O65.5
    - disproportion (due to) O33.9
      - fetal (ascites) (hydrops) (meningomyelocele) (sacral teratoma) (tumor) deformities NEC O33.7 ☑
      - generally contracted pelvis O33.1
      - hydrocephalic fetus O33.6 ☑
      - inlet contraction of pelvis O33.2
      - mixed maternal and fetal origin O33.4 ☑
      - specified NEC O33.8
    - double uterus O34.Ø- ☑
      - causing obstructed labor O65.5
    - drug use (conditions in F11-F19) O99.32- ☑
    - eclampsia, eclamptic (coma) (convulsions) (delirium) (nephritis) (uremia) — *see also* Eclampsia O15.- ☑
    - ectopic pregnancy — *see* Pregnancy, ectopic
    - edema O12.Ø- ☑
      - with
        - gestational hypertension, mild — *see also* Pre-eclampsia O14.Ø- ☑
        - proteinuria O12.2- ☑
    - effusion, amniotic fluid — *see* Pregnancy, complicated by, premature rupture of membranes
    - elderly
      - multigravida OØ9.52- ☑
      - primigravida OØ9.51- ☑
    - embolism — *see also* Embolism, obstetric, pregnancy O88.- ☑
    - endocrine diseases NEC O99.28- ☑
    - endometritis O86.12
    - excessive weight gain O26.Ø- ☑
    - exhaustion O26.81- ☑
      - during labor and delivery O75.81
    - face presentation O32.3 ☑
    - failed induction of labor O61.9
      - instrumental O61.1
      - mechanical O61.1
      - medical O61.Ø
      - specified NEC O61.8
      - surgical O61.1
    - failed or difficult intubation for anesthesia O29.6- ☑
    - false labor (pains) O47.9
      - at or after 37 completed weeks of pregnancy O47.1
      - before 37 completed weeks of pregnancy O47.Ø- ☑
    - fatigue O26.81- ☑
      - during labor and delivery O75.81
    - fatty metamorphosis of liver O26.61- ☑
    - female genital mutilation O34.8- ☑ *[N9Ø.81-]* ☑
    - fetal (maternal care for)
      - abnormality or damage O35.9 ☑
        - acid-base balance O68
        - specified type NEC O35.8 ☑
      - acidemia O68
      - acidosis O68
      - alkalosis O68

- **Pregnancy** — *continued*
  - complicated by — *continued*
    - fetal — *continued*
      - anemia and thrombocytopenia O36.82- ☑
      - anencephaly O35.Ø ☑
      - bradycardia O36.83- ☑
      - chromosomal abnormality (conditions in Q9Ø-Q99) O35.1 ☑
      - conjoined twins O3Ø.Ø2- ☑
      - damage from
        - amniocentesis O35.7 ☑
        - biopsy procedures O35.7 ☑
        - drug addiction O35.5 ☑
        - hematological investigation O35.7 ☑
        - intrauterine contraceptive device O35.7 ☑
        - maternal
          - alcohol addiction O35.4 ☑
          - cytomegalovirus infection O35.3 ☑
          - disease NEC O35.8 ☑
          - drug addiction O35.5 ☑
          - listeriosis O35.8 ☑
          - rubella O35.3 ☑
          - toxoplasmosis O35.8 ☑
          - viral infection O35.3 ☑
        - medical procedure NEC O35.7 ☑
        - radiation O35.6 ☑
      - death (near term) O36.4 ☑
        - early pregnancy OØ2.1
      - decreased movement O36.81- ☑
      - depressed heart rate tones O36.83- ☑
      - disproportion due to deformity (fetal) O33.7 ☑
      - excessive growth (large for dates) O36.6- ☑
      - growth retardation O36.59- ☑
        - light for dates O36.59- ☑
        - small for dates O36.59- ☑
      - heart rate irregularity (abnormal variability) (bradycardia) (decelerations) (tachycardia) O36.83- ☑
      - hereditary disease O35.2 ☑
      - hydrocephalus O35.Ø ☑
      - intrauterine death O36.4 ☑
      - non-reassuring heart rate or rhythm O36.83- ☑
      - poor growth O36.59- ☑
        - light for dates O36.59- ☑
        - small for dates O36.59- ☑
      - problem O36.9- ☑
        - specified NEC O36.89- ☑
      - reduction (elective) O31.3- ☑
      - selective termination O31.3- ☑
      - spina bifida O35.Ø ☑
      - thrombocytopenia O36.82- ☑
    - fibroid (tumor) (uterus) O34.1- ☑
    - fissure of nipple O92.11- ☑
    - gallstones O99.61- ☑
    - gastric banding status O99.84- ☑
    - gastric bypass status O99.84- ☑
    - genital herpes (asymptomatic) (history of) (inactive) O98.3- ☑
    - genital tract infection O23.9- ☑
    - glomerular diseases (conditions in NØØ-NØ7) O26.83- ☑
      - with hypertension, pre-existing — *see* Hypertension, complicating, pregnancy, pre-existing, with, renal disease
    - gonorrhea O98.21- ☑
    - grand multiparity OØ9.4 ☑
    - habitual aborter — *see* Pregnancy, complicated by, recurrent pregnancy loss
    - HELLP syndrome (hemolysis, elevated liver enzymes and low platelet count) O14.2- ☑
    - hemorrhage
      - antepartum — *see* Hemorrhage, antepartum
      - before 2Ø completed weeks gestation O2Ø.9
        - specified NEC O2Ø.8
      - due to premature separation, placenta — *see also* Abruptio placentae O45.9- ☑
      - early O2Ø.9
        - specified NEC O2Ø.8
      - threatened abortion O2Ø.Ø
    - hemorrhoids O22.4- ☑
    - hepatitis (viral) O98.41- ☑
    - herniation of uterus O34.59- ☑
    - high
      - head at term O32.4 ☑
      - risk — *see* Supervision (of) (for), high-risk

- **Pregnancy** — *continued*
  - complicated by — *continued*
    - history of in utero procedure during previous pregnancy OØ9.82- ☑
    - HIV O98.71- ☑
    - human immunodeficiency virus (HIV) disease O98.71- ☑
    - hydatidiform mole — *see also* Mole, hydatidiform OØ1.9
    - hydramnios O4Ø.- ☑
    - hydrocephalic fetus (disproportion) O33.6 ☑
    - hydrops
      - amnii O4Ø.- ☑
      - fetalis O36.2- ☑
        - associated with isoimmunization — *see also* Pregnancy, complicated by, isoimmunization O36.11- ☑
    - hydrorrhea O42.9Ø
    - hyperemesis (gravidarum) (mild) — *see also* Hyperemesis, gravidarum O21.Ø
    - hypertension — *see* Hypertension, complicating pregnancy
    - hypertensive
      - heart and renal disease, pre-existing — *see* Hypertension, complicating, pregnancy, pre-existing, with, heart disease, with renal disease
      - heart disease, pre-existing — *see* Hypertension, complicating, pregnancy, pre-existing, with, heart disease
      - renal disease, pre-existing — *see* Hypertension, complicating, pregnancy, pre-existing, with, renal disease
    - hypotension O26.5- ☑
    - immune disorders NEC (conditions in D8Ø-D89) O99.11- ☑
    - incarceration, uterus O34.51- ☑
    - incompetent cervix O34.3- ☑
    - inconclusive fetal viability O36.8Ø ☑
    - infection(s) O98.91- ☑
      - amniotic fluid or sac O41.1Ø- ☑
      - bladder O23.1- ☑
      - carrier state NEC O99.83Ø
        - streptococcus B O99.82Ø
      - genital organ or tract O23.9- ☑
        - specified NEC O23.59- ☑
      - genitourinary tract O23.9- ☑
      - gonorrhea O98.21- ☑
      - hepatitis (viral) O98.41- ☑
      - HIV O98.71- ☑
      - human immunodeficiency virus (HIV) O98.71- ☑
      - kidney O23.Ø- ☑
      - nipple O91.Ø1- ☑
      - parasitic disease O98.91- ☑
        - specified NEC O98.81- ☑
      - protozoal disease O98.61- ☑
      - sexually transmitted NEC O98.31- ☑
      - specified type NEC O98.81- ☑
      - syphilis O98.11- ☑
      - tuberculosis O98.Ø1- ☑
      - urethra O23.2- ☑
      - urinary (tract) O23.4- ☑
        - specified NEC O23.3- ☑
      - viral disease O98.51- ☑
    - injury or poisoning (conditions in SØØ-T88) O9A.21- ☑ (*following* O99)
      - due to abuse
        - physical O9A.31- ☑ (*following* O99)
        - psychological O9A.51- ☑ (*following* O99)
        - sexual O9A.41- ☑ (*following* O99)
    - insufficient
      - prenatal care OØ9.3- ☑
      - weight gain O26.1- ☑
    - insulin resistance O26.89 ☑
    - intrauterine fetal death (near term) O36.4 ☑
      - early pregnancy OØ2.1
      - multiple gestation (one fetus or more) O31.2- ☑
    - isoimmunization O36.11- ☑
      - anti-A sensitization O36.11- ☑
      - anti-B sensitization O36.19- ☑
      - Rh O36.Ø9- ☑
        - anti-D antibody O36.Ø1- ☑
      - specified NEC O36.19- ☑
    - laceration of uterus NEC O71.81
    - malformation
      - placenta, placental (vessel) O43.1Ø- ☑

- **Presentation, fetal** — *see* Delivery, complicated by, malposition
- **Prespondylolisthesis** (congenital) Q76.2
- **Pressure**
  - area, skin — *see* Ulcer, pressure, by site
  - brachial plexus G54.Ø
  - brain G93.5
    - injury at birth NEC P11.1
  - cerebral — *see* Pressure, brain
  - chest RØ7.89
  - cone, tentorial G93.5
  - hyposystolic — *see also* Hypotension
    - incidental reading, without diagnosis of hypotension RØ3.1
  - increased
    - intracranial benign G93.2
      - injury at birth P11.Ø
    - intraocular H4Ø.Ø5- ☑
  - injury — *see* Ulcer, pressure, by site
  - lumbosacral plexus G54.1
  - mediastinum J98.59
  - necrosis (chronic) — *see* Ulcer, pressure, by site
  - parental, inappropriate (excessive) Z62.6
  - sore (chronic) — *see* Ulcer, pressure, by site
  - spinal cord G95.2Ø
  - ulcer (chronic) — *see* Ulcer, pressure, by site
  - venous, increased I87.8
- **Pre-syncope** R55
- **Preterm**
  - delivery — *see also* Pregnancy, complicated by, preterm labor O6Ø.1Ø ☑
  - labor — *see* Pregnancy, complicated by, preterm labor
  - newborn (infant) PØ7.3Ø
    - gestational age
      - 28 completed weeks (28 weeks, Ø days through 28 weeks, 6 days) PØ7.31
      - 29 completed weeks (29 weeks, Ø days through 29 weeks, 6 days) PØ7.32
      - 3Ø completed weeks (3Ø weeks, Ø days through 3Ø weeks, 6 days) PØ7.33
      - 31 completed weeks (31 weeks, Ø days through 31 weeks, 6 days) PØ7.34
      - 32 completed weeks (32 weeks, Ø days through 32 weeks, 6 days) PØ7.35
      - 33 completed weeks (33 weeks, Ø days through 33 weeks, 6 days) PØ7.36
      - 34 completed weeks (34 weeks, Ø days through 34 weeks, 6 days) PØ7.37
      - 35 completed weeks (35 weeks, Ø days through 35 weeks, 6 days) PØ7.38
      - 36 completed weeks (36 weeks, Ø days through 36 weeks, 6 days) PØ7.39
- **Previa**
  - placenta (total) (without hemorrhage) O44.Ø- ☑
    - with hemorrhage O44.1- ☑
    - complete O44.Ø- ☑
      - with hemorrhage O44.1- ☑
    - low — *see also* Delivery, complicated, by, placenta, low O44.4- ☑
      - with hemorrhage O44.5- ☑
    - marginal O44.2- ☑
      - with hemorrhage O44.3- ☑
    - partial O44.2- ☑
      - with hemorrhage O44.3- ☑
  - vasa O69.4 ☑
- **Priapism** N48.3Ø
  - due to
    - disease classified elsewhere N48.32
    - drug N48.33
    - specified cause NEC N48.39
    - trauma N48.31
- **Prickling sensation** (skin) R2Ø.2
- **Prickly heat** L74.Ø
- **Primary** — *see* condition
- **Primigravida**
  - elderly, affecting management of pregnancy, labor and delivery (supervision only) — *see* Pregnancy, complicated by, elderly, primigravida
  - older, affecting management of pregnancy, labor and delivery (supervision only) — *see* Pregnancy, complicated by, elderly, primigravida
  - very young, affecting management of pregnancy, labor and delivery (supervision only) — *see* Pregnancy, complicated by, young mother, primigravida
- **Primipara**
  - elderly, affecting management of pregnancy, labor and delivery (supervision only) — *see* Pregnancy, complicated by, elderly, primigravida
  - older, affecting management of pregnancy, labor and delivery (supervision only) — *see* Pregnancy, complicated by, elderly, primigravida
  - very young, affecting management of pregnancy, labor and delivery (supervision only) — *see* Pregnancy, complicated by, young mother, primigravida
- **Primus varus** Q66.21- ☑
- **PRIND** (Prolonged reversible ischemic neurologic deficit) I63.9
- **Pringle's disease** (tuberous sclerosis) Q85.1
- **Prinzmetal angina** I2Ø.1
- **Prizefighter ear** — *see* Cauliflower ear
- **Problem** (with) (related to)
  - academic Z55.8
  - acculturation Z6Ø.3
  - adjustment (to)
    - change of job Z56.1
    - life-cycle transition Z6Ø.Ø
    - pension Z6Ø.Ø
    - retirement Z6Ø.Ø
  - adopted child Z62.821
  - alcoholism in family Z63.72
  - atypical parenting situation Z62.9
  - bankruptcy Z59.8
  - behavioral (adult) F69
    - drug seeking Z76.5
  - birth of sibling affecting child Z62.898
  - care (of)
    - provider dependency Z74.9
      - specified NEC Z74.8
    - sick or handicapped person in family or household Z63.6
  - child
    - abuse (affecting the child) — *see* Maltreatment, child
    - custody or support proceedings Z65.3
    - in care of non-parental family member Z62.21
    - in foster care Z62.21
    - in welfare custody Z62.21
    - living in orphanage or group home Z62.22
  - child-rearing Z62.9
    - specified NEC Z62.898
  - communication (developmental) F8Ø.9
  - conflict or discord (with)
    - boss Z56.4
    - classmates Z55.4
    - counselor Z64.4
    - employer Z56.4
    - family Z63.9
      - specified NEC Z63.8
    - probation officer Z64.4
    - social worker Z64.4
    - teachers Z55.4
    - workmates Z56.4
  - conviction in legal proceedings Z65.Ø
    - with imprisonment Z65.1
  - counselor Z64.4
  - creditors Z59.8
  - digestive K92.9
  - drug addict in family Z63.72
  - ear — *see* Disorder, ear
  - economic Z59.9
    - affecting care Z59.9
    - specified NEC Z59.8
  - education Z55.9
    - specified NEC Z55.8
  - employment Z56.9
    - change of job Z56.1
    - discord Z56.4
    - environment Z56.5
    - sexual harassment Z56.81
    - specified NEC Z56.89
    - stressful schedule Z56.3
    - stress NEC Z56.6
    - threat of job loss Z56.2
    - unemployment Z56.Ø
  - enuresis, child F98.Ø
  - eye H57.9
  - failed examinations (school) Z55.2
  - falling Z91.81
  - family — *see also* Disruption, family Z63.9
    - specified NEC Z63.8
  - feeding (elderly) (infant) R63.3
    - newborn P92.9

Problem — *continued*
  - feeding — *continued*
    - newborn — *continued*
      - breast P92.5
      - overfeeding P92.4
      - slow P92.2
      - specified NEC P92.8
      - underfeeding P92.3
    - nonorganic F5Ø.89
  - finance Z59.9
    - specified NEC Z59.8
  - foreclosure on loan Z59.8
  - foster child Z62.822
  - frightening experience(s) in childhood Z62.898
  - genital NEC
    - female N94.9
    - male N5Ø.9
  - health care Z75.9
    - specified NEC Z75.8
  - hearing — *see* Deafness
  - homelessness Z59.Ø
  - housing Z59.9
    - inadequate Z59.1
    - isolated Z59.8
    - specified NEC Z59.8
  - identity (of childhood) F93.8
  - illegitimate pregnancy (unwanted) Z64.Ø
  - illiteracy Z55.Ø
  - impaired mobility Z74.Ø9
  - imprisonment or incarceration Z65.1
  - inadequate teaching affecting education Z55.8
  - inappropriate (excessive) parental pressure Z62.6
  - influencing health status NEC Z78.9
  - in-law Z63.1
  - institutionalization, affecting child Z62.22
  - intrafamilial communication Z63.8
  - jealousy, child F93.8
  - landlord Z59.2
  - language (developmental) F8Ø.9
  - learning (developmental) F81.9
  - legal Z65.3
    - conviction without imprisonment Z65.Ø
    - imprisonment Z65.1
    - release from prison Z65.2
  - life-management Z73.9
    - specified NEC Z73.89
  - life-style Z72.9
    - gambling Z72.6
    - high-risk sexual behavior (heterosexual) Z72.51
      - bisexual Z72.53
      - homosexual Z72.52
    - inappropriate eating habits Z72.4
    - self-damaging behavior NEC Z72.89
    - specified NEC Z72.89
    - tobacco use Z72.Ø
  - literacy Z55.9
    - low level Z55.Ø
    - specified NEC Z55.8
  - living alone Z6Ø.2
  - lodgers Z59.2
  - loss of love relationship in childhood Z62.898
  - marital Z63.Ø
    - involving
      - divorce Z63.5
      - estrangement Z63.5
      - gender identity F66
  - mastication KØ8.89
  - medical
    - care, within family Z63.6
    - facilities Z75.9
      - specified NEC Z75.8
  - mental F48.9
  - multiparity Z64.1
  - negative life events in childhood Z62.9
    - altered pattern of family relationships Z62.898
    - frightening experience Z62.898
    - loss of
      - love relationship Z62.898
      - self-esteem Z62.898
    - physical abuse (alleged) — *see* Maltreatment, child
    - removal from home Z62.29
    - specified event NEC Z62.898
  - neighbor Z59.2
  - neurological NEC R29.818
  - new step-parent affecting child Z62.898
  - none (feared complaint unfounded) Z71.1
  - occupational NEC Z56.89
  - parent-child — *see* Conflict, parent-child
  - personal hygiene Z91.89

Problem — *continued*
- personality F69
- phase-of-life transition, adjustment Z6Ø.Ø
- presence of sick or disabled person in family or household Z63.79
  - needing care Z63.6
- primary support group (family) Z63.9
  - specified NEC Z63.8
- probation officer Z64.4
- psychiatric F99
- psychosexual (development) F66
- psychosocial Z65.9
  - religious or spiritual Z65.8
  - specified NEC Z65.8
- relationship Z63.9
  - childhood F93.8
- release from prison Z65.2
  - religious or spiritual Z65.8
- removal from home affecting child Z62.29
- seeking and accepting known hazardous and harmful
  - behavioral or psychological interventions Z65.8
  - chemical, nutritional or physical interventions Z65.8
- sexual function (nonorganic) F52.9
- sight H54.7
- sleep disorder, child F51.9
- smell — *see* Disturbance, sensation, smell
- social
  - environment Z6Ø.9
    - specified NEC Z6Ø.8
  - exclusion and rejection Z6Ø.4
  - worker Z64.4
- speech R47.9
  - developmental F8Ø.9
  - specified NEC R47.89
- swallowing — *see* Dysphagia
- taste — *see* Disturbance, sensation, taste
- tic, child F95.Ø
- underachievement in school Z55.3
- unemployment Z56.Ø
  - threatened Z56.2
- unwanted pregnancy Z64.Ø
- upbringing Z62.9
  - specified NEC Z62.898
- urinary N39.9
- voice production R47.89
- work schedule (stressful) Z56.3

Procedure (surgical)
- converted
  - arthroscopic to open Z53.33
  - laparoscopic to open Z53.31
  - specified procedure NEC to open Z53.39
  - thoracoscopic to open Z53.32
- for purpose other than remedying health state Z41.9
  - specified NEC Z41.8
- not done Z53.9
  - because of
    - administrative reasons Z53.8
    - contraindication Z53.Ø9
      - smoking Z53.Ø1
    - patient's decision Z53.2Ø
      - for reasons of belief or group pressure Z53.1
      - left against medical advice (AMA) Z53.21
      - specified reason NEC Z53.29
    - specified reason NEC Z53.8

Procidentia (uteri) N81.3

Proctalgia K62.89
- fugax K59.4
- spasmodic K59.4

Proctitis K62.89
- amebic (acute) AØ6.Ø
- chlamydial A56.3
- gonococcal A54.6
- granulomatous — *see* Enteritis, regional, large intestine
- herpetic A6Ø.1
- radiation K62.7
- tuberculous A18.32
- ulcerative (chronic) K51.2Ø
  - with
    - complication K51.219
      - abscess K51.214
      - fistula K51.213
      - obstruction K51.212
      - rectal bleeding K51.211
      - specified NEC K51.218

Proctocele
- female (without uterine prolapse) N81.6
  - with uterine prolapse N81.2
    - complete N81.3

Proctocele — *continued*
- male K62.3

Proctocolitis
- food protein-induced K52.82
- food-induced eosinophilic K52.82
- milk protein-induced K52.82
- mucosal — *see* Rectosigmoiditis, ulcerative

Proctoptosis K62.3

Proctorrhagia K62.5

Proctosigmoiditis K63.89
- ulcerative (chronic) — *see* Rectosigmoiditis, ulcerative

Proctospasm K59.4
- psychogenic F45.8

Proficher's disease — *see* Disorder, soft tissue, specified type NEC

Progeria E34.8

Prognathism (mandibular) (maxillary) M26.19

Progonoma (melanotic) — *see* Neoplasm, benign, by site

Progressive — *see* condition

Prolactinoma
- specified site — *see* Neoplasm, benign, by site
- unspecified site D35.2

Prolapse, prolapsed
- anus, anal (canal) (sphincter) K62.2
- arm or hand O32.2 ☑
  - causing obstructed labor O64.4 ☑
- bladder (mucosa) (sphincter) (acquired)
  - congenital Q79.4
  - female — *see* Cystocele
  - male N32.89
- breast implant (prosthetic) T85.49 ☑
- cecostomy K94.Ø9
- cecum K63.4
- cervix, cervical (hypertrophied) N81.2
  - anterior lip, obstructing labor O65.5
  - congenital Q51.828
  - postpartal, old N81.2
  - stump N81.85
- ciliary body (traumatic) — *see* Laceration, eye(ball), with prolapse or loss of interocular tissue
- colon (pedunculated) K63.4
- colostomy K94.Ø9
- disc (intervertebral) — *see* Displacement, intervertebral disc
- eye implant (orbital) T85.398 ☑
  - lens (ocular) — *see* Complications, intraocular lens
- fallopian tube N83.4- ☑
- gastric (mucosa) K31.89
- genital, female N81.9
  - specified NEC N81.89
- globe, nontraumatic — *see* Luxation, globe
- ileostomy bud K94.19
- intervertebral disc — *see* Displacement, intervertebral disc
- intestine (small) K63.4
- iris (traumatic) — *see* Laceration, eye(ball), with prolapse or loss of interocular tissue
  - nontraumatic H21.89
- kidney N28.83
  - congenital Q63.2
- laryngeal muscles or ventricle J38.7
- liver K76.89
- meatus urinarius N36.8
- mitral (valve) I34.1
- ocular lens implant — *see* Complications, intraocular lens
- organ or site, congenital NEC — *see* Malposition, congenital
- ovary N83.4- ☑
- pelvic floor, female N81.89
- perineum, female N81.89
- rectum (mucosa) (sphincter) K62.3
  - due to trichuris trichuria B79
- spleen D73.89
- stomach K31.89
- umbilical cord
  - complicating delivery O69.Ø ☑
- urachus, congenital Q64.4
- ureter N28.89
  - with obstruction N13.5
    - with infection N13.6
- ureterovesical orifice N28.89
- urethra (acquired) (infected) (mucosa) N36.8
  - congenital Q64.71
- urinary meatus N36.8
  - congenital Q64.72
- uterovaginal N81.4

Prolapse, prolapsed — *continued*
- uterovaginal — *continued*
  - complete N81.3
  - incomplete N81.2
- uterus (with prolapse of vagina) N81.4
  - complete N81.3
  - congenital Q51.818
  - first degree N81.2
  - in pregnancy or childbirth — *see* Pregnancy, complicated by, abnormal, uterus
  - incomplete N81.2
  - postpartal (old) N81.4
  - second degree N81.2
  - third degree N81.3
- uveal (traumatic) — *see* Laceration, eye(ball), with prolapse or loss of interocular tissue
- vagina (anterior) (wall) — *see* Cystocele
  - with prolapse of uterus N81.4
    - complete N81.3
    - incomplete N81.2
  - posterior wall N81.6
  - posthysterectomy N99.3
- vitreous (humor) H43.Ø- ☑
  - in wound — *see* Laceration, eye(ball), with prolapse or loss of interocular tissue
- womb — *see* Prolapse, uterus

Prolapsus, female N81.9
- specified NEC N81.89

Proliferation(s)
- primary cutaneous CD3Ø-positive large T-cell C86.6
- prostate, atypical small acinar N42.32

Proliferative — *see* condition

Prolonged, prolongation (of)
- bleeding (time) (idiopathic) R79.1
- coagulation (time) R79.1
- gestation (over 42 completed weeks)
  - mother O48.1
  - newborn PØ8.22
- interval I44.Ø
- labor O63.9
  - first stage O63.Ø
  - second stage O63.1
- partial thromboplastin time (PTT) R79.1
- pregnancy (more than 42 weeks gestation) O48.1
- prothrombin time R79.1
- QT interval R94.31
- uterine contractions in labor O62.4

Prominence, prominent
- auricle (congenital) (ear) Q17.5
- ischial spine or sacral promontory with disproportion (fetopelvic) O33.Ø
  - causing obstructed labor O65.Ø
- nose (congenital) acquired M95.Ø

Promiscuity — *see* High, risk, sexual behavior

Pronation
- ankle — *see* Deformity, limb, foot, specified NEC
- foot — *see also* Deformity, limb, foot, specified NEC
  - congenital Q74.2

Prophylactic
- administration of
  - antibiotics, long-term Z79.2
    - short-term use — *omit code*
  - drug — *see also* Long-term (current) drug therapy (use of) Z79.899
- medication Z79.899
- organ removal (for neoplasia management) Z4Ø.ØØ
  - breast Z4Ø.Ø1
  - fallopian tube(s) Z4Ø.Ø3
    - with ovary(s) Z4Ø.Ø2
  - ovary(s) Z4Ø.Ø2
  - specified site NEC Z4Ø.Ø9
- surgery Z4Ø.9
  - for risk factors related to malignant neoplasm — *see* Prophylactic, organ removal
  - specified NEC Z4Ø.8
- vaccination Z23

Propionic acidemia E71.121

Proptosis (ocular) — *see also* Exophthalmos
- thyroid — *see* Hyperthyroidism, with goiter

Prosecution, anxiety concerning Z65.3

Prosopagnosia R48.3

Prostadynia N42.81

Prostate, prostatic — *see* condition

Prostatism — *see* Hyperplasia, prostate

Prostatitis (congestive) (suppurative) (with cystitis) N41.9
- acute N41.Ø
- cavitary N41.8
- chronic N41.1

☑ Additional Character Required — Refer to the Tabular List for Character Selection
Subterms under main terms may continue to next column or page

Pseudotuberculosis A28.2
- enterocolitis AØ4.8
- pasteurella (infection) A28.Ø

Pseudotumor G93.2
- cerebri G93.2
- orbital HØ5.11 ☑

Pseudoxanthoma elasticum Q82.8

Psilosis (sprue) (tropical) K9Ø.1
- nontropical K9Ø.Ø

Psittacosis A7Ø

Psoitis M6Ø.88

Psoriasis L4Ø.9
- arthropathic L4Ø.5Ø
  - arthritis mutilans L4Ø.52
  - distal interphalangeal L4Ø.51
  - juvenile L4Ø.54
  - other specified L4Ø.59
  - spondylitis L4Ø.53
- buccal K13.29
- flexural L4Ø.8
- guttate L4Ø.4
- mouth K13.29
- nummular L4Ø.Ø
- plaque L4Ø.Ø
- psychogenic F54
- pustular (generalized) L4Ø.1
  - palmaris et plantaris L4Ø.3
- specified NEC L4Ø.8
- vulgaris L4Ø.Ø

Psychasthenia F48.8

Psychiatric disorder or problem F99

Psychogenic — *see also* condition
- factors associated with physical conditions F54

Psychological and behavioral factors affecting medical condition F59

Psychoneurosis, psychoneurotic — *see also* Neurosis
- anxiety (state) F41.1
- depersonalization F48.1
- hypochondriacal F45.21
- hysteria F44.9
- neurasthenic F48.8
- personality NEC F6Ø.89

Psychopathy, psychopathic
- affectionless F94.2
- autistic F84.5
- constitution, post-traumatic FØ7.81
- personality — *see* Disorder, personality
- sexual — *see* Deviation, sexual
- state F6Ø.2

Psychosexual identity disorder of childhood F64.2

Psychosis, psychotic F29
- acute (transient) F23
  - hysterical F44.9
- affective — *see* Disorder, mood
- alcoholic F1Ø.959
  - with
    - abuse F1Ø.159
    - anxiety disorder F1Ø.98Ø
      - with
        - abuse F1Ø.18Ø
        - dependence F1Ø.28Ø
    - delirium tremens F1Ø.231
    - delusions F1Ø.95Ø
      - with
        - abuse F1Ø.15Ø
        - dependence F1Ø.25Ø
    - dementia F1Ø.97
      - with dependence F1Ø.27
    - dependence F1Ø.259
    - hallucinosis F1Ø.951
      - with
        - abuse F1Ø.151
        - dependence F1Ø.251
    - mood disorder F1Ø.94
      - with
        - abuse F1Ø.14
        - dependence F1Ø.24
    - paranoia F1Ø.95Ø
      - with
        - abuse F1Ø.15Ø
        - dependence F1Ø.25Ø
    - persisting amnesia F1Ø.96
      - with dependence F1Ø.26
  - amnestic confabulatory F1Ø.96
    - with dependence F1Ø.26
  - delirium tremens F1Ø.231
  - Korsakoff's, Korsakov's, Korsakow's F1Ø.26
  - paranoid type F1Ø.95Ø

Psychosis, psychotic — *continued*
- alcoholic — *continued*
  - paranoid type — *continued*
    - with
      - abuse F1Ø.15Ø
      - dependence F1Ø.25Ø
- anergastic — *see* Psychosis, organic
- arteriosclerotic (simple type) (uncomplicated) FØ1.5Ø
  - with behavioral disturbance FØ1.51
- childhood F84.Ø
  - atypical F84.8
- climacteric — *see* Psychosis, involutional
- confusional F29
  - acute or subacute FØ5
  - reactive F23
- cycloid F23
- depressive — *see* Disorder, depressive
- disintegrative (childhood) F84.3
- drug-induced — *see* F11-F19 with .X59
  - paranoid and hallucinatory states — *see* F11-F19 with .X5Ø or .X51
- due to or associated with
  - addiction, drug — *see* F11-F19 with .X59
  - dependence
    - alcohol F1Ø.259
    - drug — *see* F11-F19 with .X59
  - epilepsy FØ6.8
  - Huntington's chorea FØ6.8
  - ischemia, cerebrovascular (generalized) FØ6.8
  - multiple sclerosis FØ6.8
  - physical disease FØ6.8
  - presenile dementia FØ3 ☑
  - senile dementia FØ3 ☑
  - vascular disease (arteriosclerotic) (cerebral) FØ1.5Ø
    - with behavioral disturbance FØ1.51
- epileptic FØ6.8
- episode F23
  - due to or associated with physical condition FØ6.8
- exhaustive F43.Ø
- hallucinatory, chronic F28
- hypomanic F3Ø.8
- hysterical (acute) F44.9
- induced F24
- infantile F84.Ø
  - atypical F84.8
- infective (acute) (subacute) FØ5
- involutional F28
  - depressive — *see* Disorder, depressive
  - melancholic — *see* Disorder, depressive
  - paranoid (state) F22
- Korsakoff's, Korsakov's, Korsakow's (nonalcoholic) FØ4
  - alcoholic F1Ø.96
    - in dependence F1Ø.26
  - induced by other psychoactive substance — *see* categories F11-F19 with .X5X
- mania, manic (single episode) F3Ø.2
  - recurrent type F31.89
- manic-depressive — *see* Disorder, bipolar
- menopausal — *see* Psychosis, involutional
- mixed schizophrenic and affective F25.8
- multi-infarct (cerebrovascular) FØ1.5Ø
  - with behavioral disturbance FØ1.51
- nonorganic F29
  - specified NEC F28
- organic FØ9
  - due to or associated with
    - arteriosclerosis (cerebral) — *see* Psychosis, arteriosclerotic
    - cerebrovascular disease, arteriosclerotic — *see* Psychosis, arteriosclerotic
    - childbirth — *see* Psychosis, puerperal
    - Creutzfeldt-Jakob disease or syndrome — *see* Creutzfeldt-Jakob disease or syndrome
    - dependence, alcohol F1Ø.259
    - disease
      - alcoholic liver F1Ø.259
      - brain, arteriosclerotic — *see* Psychosis, arteriosclerotic
      - cerebrovascular FØ1.5Ø
        - with behavioral disturbance FØ1.51
      - Creutzfeldt-Jakob — *see* Creutzfeldt-Jakob disease or syndrome
      - endocrine or metabolic FØ6.8
        - acute or subacute FØ5
      - liver, alcoholic F1Ø.259
    - epilepsy transient (acute) FØ5
    - infection
      - brain (intracranial) FØ6.8

Psychosis, psychotic — *continued*
- organic — *continued*
  - due to or associated with — *continued*
    - infection — *continued*
      - brain — *continued*
        - acute or subacute FØ5
    - intoxication
      - alcoholic (acute) F1Ø.259
      - drug F11-F19 with .x59
    - ischemia, cerebrovascular (generalized) — *see* Psychosis, arteriosclerotic
    - puerperium — *see* Psychosis, puerperal
    - trauma, brain (birth) (from electric current) (surgical) FØ6.8
      - acute or subacute FØ5
  - infective FØ6.8
    - acute or subacute FØ5
  - post-traumatic FØ6.8
    - acute or subacute FØ5
- paranoiac F22
- paranoid (climacteric) (involutional) (menopausal) F22
  - psychogenic (acute) F23
  - schizophrenic F2Ø.Ø
  - senile FØ3 ☑
- postpartum (NOS) F53.1
- presbyophrenic (type) FØ3 ☑
- presenile FØ3 ☑
- psychogenic (paranoid) F23
  - depressive F32.3
- puerperal (NOS) F53.1
  - specified type — *see* Psychosis, by type
- reactive (brief) (transient) (emotional stress) (psychological trauma) F23
  - depressive F32.3
    - recurrent F33.3
  - excitative type F3Ø.8
- schizoaffective F25.9
  - depressive type F25.1
  - manic type F25.Ø
- schizophrenia, schizophrenic — *see* Schizophrenia
- schizophrenia-like, in epilepsy FØ6.2
- schizophreniform F2Ø.81
  - affective type F25.9
  - brief F23
  - confusional type F23
  - mixed type F25.Ø
- senile NEC FØ3 ☑
  - depressed or paranoid type FØ3 ☑
  - simple deterioration FØ3 ☑
  - specified type — *code to* condition
- shared F24
- situational (reactive) F23
- symbiotic (childhood) F84.3
- symptomatic FØ9

Psychosomatic — *see* Disorder, psychosomatic

Psychosyndrome, organic FØ7.9

Psychotic episode due to or associated with physical condition FØ6.8

Pterygium (eye) H11.ØØ- ☑
- amyloid H11.Ø1- ☑
- central H11.Ø2- ☑
- colli Q18.3
- double H11.Ø3- ☑
- peripheral
  - progressive H11.Ø5- ☑
  - stationary H11.Ø4- ☑
- recurrent H11.Ø6- ☑

Ptilosis (eyelid) — *see* Madarosis

Ptomaine (poisoning) — *see* Poisoning, food

Ptosis — *see also* Blepharoptosis
- adiposa (false) — *see* Blepharoptosis
- breast N64.81-
- brow H57.81- ☑
- cecum K63.4
- colon K63.4
- congenital (eyelid) Q1Ø.Ø
  - specified site NEC — *see* Anomaly, by site
- eyebrow H57.81- ☑
- eyelid — *see* Blepharoptosis
  - congenital Q1Ø.Ø
- gastric K31.89
- intestine K63.4
- kidney N28.83
- liver K76.89
- renal N28.83
- splanchnic K63.4
- spleen D73.89
- stomach K31.89

- **Ptosis** — *continued*
  - viscera K63.4
- **PTP** D69.51
- **Ptyalism** (periodic) K11.7
  - hysterical F45.8
  - pregnancy — *see* Pregnancy, complicated by, specified pregnancy-related condition NEC
  - psychogenic F45.8
- **Ptyalolithiasis** K11.5
- **Pubarche, precocious** E3Ø.1
- **Pubertas praecox** E3Ø.1
- **Puberty** (development state) ZØØ.3
  - bleeding (excessive) N92.2
  - delayed E3Ø.Ø
  - precocious (constitutional) (cryptogenic) (idiopathic) E3Ø.1
    - central E22.8
    - due to
      - ovarian hyperfunction E28.1
        - estrogen E28.Ø
      - testicular hyperfunction E29.Ø
  - premature E3Ø.1
    - due to
      - adrenal cortical hyperfunction E25.8
      - pineal tumor E34.8
      - pituitary (anterior) hyperfunction E22.8
- **Puckering, macula** — *see* Degeneration, macula, puckering
- **Pudenda, pudendum** — *see* condition
- **Puente's disease** (simple glandular cheilitis) K13.Ø
- **Puerperal, puerperium** (complicated by, complications)
  - abnormal glucose (tolerance test) O99.815
  - abscess
    - areola O91.Ø2
      - associated with lactation O91.Ø3
    - Bartholin's gland O86.19
    - breast O91.12
      - associated with lactation O91.13
    - cervix (uteri) O86.11
    - genital organ NEC O86.19
    - kidney O86.21
    - mammary O91.12
      - associated with lactation O91.13
    - nipple O91.Ø2
      - associated with lactation O91.Ø3
    - peritoneum O85
    - subareolar O91.12
      - associated with lactation O91.13
    - urinary tract — *see* Puerperal, infection, urinary
    - uterus O86.12
    - vagina (wall) O86.13
    - vaginorectal O86.13
    - vulvovaginal gland O86.13
  - adnexitis O86.19
  - afibrinogenemia, or other coagulation defect O72.3
  - albuminuria (acute) (subacute) — *see* Proteinuria, gestational
  - alcohol use O99.315
  - anemia O9Ø.81
    - pre-existing (pre-pregnancy) O99.Ø3
  - anesthetic death O89.8
  - apoplexy O99.43
  - bariatric surgery status O99.845
  - blood disorder NEC O99.13
  - blood dyscrasia O72.3
  - cardiomyopathy O9Ø.3
  - cerebrovascular disorder (conditions in I6Ø-I69) O99.43
  - cervicitis O86.11
  - circulatory system disorder O99.43
  - coagulopathy (any) O99.13
    - with hemorrhage O72.3
  - complications O9Ø.9
    - specified NEC O9Ø.89
  - convulsions — *see* Eclampsia
  - cystitis O86.22
  - cystopyelitis O86.29
  - delirium NEC FØ5
  - diabetes O24.93
    - gestational — *see* Puerperal, gestational diabetes
    - pre-existing O24.33
      - specified NEC O24.83
      - type 1 O24.Ø3
      - type 2 O24.13
  - digestive system disorder O99.63
  - disease O9Ø.9
    - breast NEC O92.29
    - cerebrovascular (acute) O99.43
    - nonobstetric NEC O99.893

- **Puerperal, puerperium** — *continued*
  - disease — *continued*
    - tubo-ovarian O86.19
    - Valsuani's O99.Ø3
  - disorder O9Ø.9
    - biliary tract O26.63
    - lactation O92.7Ø
    - liver O26.63
    - nonobstetric NEC O99.893
  - disruption
    - cesarean wound O9Ø.Ø
    - episiotomy wound O9Ø.1
    - perineal laceration wound O9Ø.1
  - drug use O99.325
  - eclampsia (with pre-existing hypertension) O15.2
  - embolism (pulmonary) (blood clot) — *see* Embolism, obstetric, puerperal
  - endocrine, nutritional or metabolic disease NEC O99.285
  - endophlebitis — *see* Puerperal, phlebitis
  - endotrachelitis O86.11
  - failure
    - lactation (complete) O92.3
      - partial O92.4
    - renal, acute O9Ø.4
  - fever (of unknown origin) O86.4
    - septic O85
  - fissure, nipple O92.12
    - associated with lactation O92.13
  - fistula
    - breast (due to mastitis) O91.12
      - associated with lactation O91.13
    - nipple O91.Ø2
      - associated with lactation O91.Ø3
  - galactophoritis O91.22
    - associated with lactation O91.23
  - galactorrhea O92.6
  - gastric banding status O99.845
  - gastric bypass status O99.845
  - gastrointestinal disease NEC O99.63
  - gestational
    - diabetes O24.439
      - diet controlled O24.43Ø
      - insulin (and diet) controlled O24.434
      - oral drug controlled (antidiabetic) (hypoglycemic) O24.435
    - edema O12.Ø5
      - with proteinuria O12.25
    - proteinuria O12.15
  - gonorrhea O98.23
  - hematoma, subdural O99.43
  - hemiplegia, cerebral O99.355
    - due to cerbrovascular disorder O99.43
  - hemorrhage O72.1
    - brain O99.43
    - bulbar O99.43
    - cerebellar O99.43
    - cerebral O99.43
    - cortical O99.43
    - delayed or secondary O72.2
    - extradural O99.43
    - internal capsule O99.43
    - intracranial O99.43
    - intrapontine O99.43
    - meningeal O99.43
    - pontine O99.43
    - retained placenta O72.Ø
    - subarachnoid O99.43
    - subcortical O99.43
    - subdural O99.43
    - third stage O72.Ø
    - uterine, delayed O72.2
    - ventricular O99.43
  - hemorrhoids O87.2
  - hepatorenal syndrome O9Ø.4
  - hypertension — *see* Hypertension, complicating, puerperium
  - hypertrophy, breast O92.29
  - induration breast (fibrous) O92.29
  - infection O86.4
    - cervix O86.11
    - generalized O85
    - genital tract NEC O86.19
      - obstetric surgical wound O86.Ø9
    - kidney (bacillus coli) O86.21
    - maternal O98.93
      - carrier state NEC O99.835
      - gonorrhea O98.23
      - human immunodeficiency virus (HIV) O98.73

- **Puerperal, puerperium** — *continued*
  - infection — *continued*
    - maternal — *continued*
      - protozoal O98.63
      - sexually transmitted NEC O98.33
      - specified NEC O98.83
      - streptococcus group B (GBS) carrier state O99.825
      - syphilis O98.13
      - tuberculosis O98.Ø3
      - viral hepatitis O98.43
      - viral NEC O98.53
    - nipple O91.Ø2
      - associated with lactation O91.Ø3
    - peritoneum O85
    - renal O86.21
    - specified NEC O86.89
    - urinary (asymptomatic) (tract) NEC O86.2Ø
      - bladder O86.22
      - kidney O86.21
      - specified site NEC O86.29
      - urethra O86.22
    - vagina O86.13
    - vein — *see* Puerperal, phlebitis
  - ischemia, cerebral O99.43
  - lymphangitis O86.89
    - breast O91.22
      - associated with lactation O91.23
  - malignancy O9A.13 (*following* O99)
  - malnutrition O25.3
  - mammillitis O91.Ø2
    - associated with lactation O91.Ø3
  - mammitis O91.22
    - associated with lactation O91.23
  - mania F3Ø.8
  - mastitis O91.22
    - associated with lactation O91.23
    - purulent O91.12
      - associated with lactation O91.13
  - melancholia — *see* Disorder, depressive
  - mental disorder NEC O99.345
  - metroperitonitis O85
  - metrorrhagia — *see* Hemorrhage, postpartum
  - metrosalpingitis O86.19
  - metrovaginitis O86.13
  - milk leg O87.1
  - monoplegia, cerebral O99.43
  - mood disturbance O9Ø.6
  - necrosis, liver (acute) (subacute) (conditions in subcategory K72.Ø) O26.63
    - with renal failure O9Ø.4
  - nervous system disorder O99.355
  - obesity (pre-existing prior to pregnancy) O99.215
  - obesity surgery status O99.845
  - occlusion, precerebral artery O99.43
  - paralysis
    - bladder (sphincter) O9Ø.89
    - cerebral O99.43
  - paralytic stroke O99.43
  - parametritis O85
  - paravaginitis O86.13
  - pelviperitonitis O85
  - perimetritis O86.12
  - perimetrosalpingitis O86.19
  - perinephritis O86.21
  - periphlebitis — *see* Puerperal phlebitis
  - peritoneal infection O85
  - peritonitis (pelvic) O85
  - perivaginitis O86.13
  - phlebitis O87.Ø
    - deep O87.1
    - pelvic O87.1
    - superficial O87.Ø
  - phlebothrombosis, deep O87.1
  - phlegmasia alba dolens O87.1
  - placental polyp O9Ø.89
  - pneumonia, embolic — *see* Embolism, obstetric, puerperal
  - pre-eclampsia — *see* Pre-eclampsia
  - psychosis (NOS) F53.1
  - pyelitis O86.21
  - pyelocystitis O86.29
  - pyelonephritis O86.21
  - pyelonephrosis O86.21
  - pyemia O85
  - pyocystitis O86.29
  - pyohemia O85
  - pyometra O86.12
  - pyonephritis O86.21
  - pyosalpingitis O86.19

- **Puerperal, puerperium** — *continued*
  - pyrexia (of unknown origin) O86.4
  - renal
    - disease NEC O90.89
    - failure O90.4
  - respiratory disease NEC O99.53
  - retention
    - decidua — *see* Retention, decidua
    - placenta O72.0
    - secundines — *see* Retention, secundines
  - retracted nipple O92.02
  - salpingo-ovaritis O86.19
  - salpingoperitonitis O85
  - secondary perineal tear O90.1
  - sepsis (pelvic) O85
  - sepsis O85
  - septic thrombophlebitis O86.81
  - skin disorder NEC O99.73
  - specified condition NEC O99.893
  - stroke O99.43
  - subinvolution (uterus) O90.89
  - subluxation of symphysis (pubis) O26.73
  - suppuration — *see* Puerperal, abscess
  - tetanus A34
  - thelitis O91.02
    - associated with lactation O91.03
  - thrombocytopenia O72.3
  - thrombophlebitis (superficial) O87.0
    - deep O87.1
    - pelvic O87.1
    - septic O86.81
  - thrombosis (venous) — *see* Thrombosis, puerperal
  - thyroiditis O90.5
  - toxemia (eclamptic) (pre-eclamptic) (with convulsions) O15.2
  - trauma, non-obstetric O9A.23 (*following* O99)
    - caused by abuse (physical) (suspected) O9A.33 (*following* O99)
      - confirmed O9A.33 (*following* O99)
      - psychological (suspected) O9A.53 (*following* O99)
        - confirmed O9A.53 (*following* O99)
      - sexual (suspected) O9A.43 (*following* O99)
        - confirmed O9A.43 (*following* O99)
  - uremia (due to renal failure) O90.4
  - urethritis O86.22
  - vaginitis O86.13
  - varicose veins (legs) O87.4
    - vulva or perineum O87.8
  - venous O87.9
  - vulvitis O86.19
  - vulvovaginitis O86.13
  - white leg O87.1
- **Puerperium** — *see* Puerperal
- **Pulmolithiasis** J98.4
- **Pulmonary** — *see* condition
- **Pulpitis** (acute) (anachoretic) (chronic) (hyperplastic) (putrescent) (suppurative) (ulcerative) K04.01
  - irreversible K04.02
  - reversible K04.01
- **Pulpless tooth** K04.99
- **Pulse**
  - alternating R00.8
  - bigeminal R00.8
  - fast R00.0
  - feeble, rapid due to shock following injury T79.4 ☑
  - rapid R00.0
  - weak R09.89
- **Pulsus alternans or trigeminus** R00.8
- **Punch drunk** F07.81
- **Punctum lacrimale occlusion** — *see* Obstruction, lacrimal
- **Puncture**
  - abdomen, abdominal
    - wall S31.139 ☑
      - with
        - foreign body S31.149 ☑
        - penetration into peritoneal cavity S31.639 ☑
          - with foreign body S31.649 ☑
      - epigastric region S31.132 ☑
        - with
          - foreign body S31.142 ☑
          - penetration into peritoneal cavity S31.632 ☑
            - with foreign body S31.642 ☑
      - left
        - lower quadrant S31.134 ☑
          - with
            - foreign body S31.144 ☑

- **Puncture** — *continued*
  - abdomen, abdominal — *continued*
    - wall — *continued*
      - left — *continued*
        - lower quadrant — *continued*
          - with — *continued*
            - penetration into peritoneal cavity S31.634 ☑
              - with foreign body S31.644 ☑
        - upper quadrant S31.131 ☑
          - with
            - foreign body S31.141 ☑
            - penetration into peritoneal cavity S31.631 ☑
              - with foreign body S31.641 ☑
      - periumbilic region S31.135 ☑
        - with
          - foreign body S31.145 ☑
          - penetration into peritoneal cavity S31.635 ☑
            - with foreign body S31.645 ☑
      - right
        - lower quadrant S31.133 ☑
          - with
            - foreign body S31.143 ☑
            - penetration into peritoneal cavity S31.633 ☑
              - with foreign body S31.643 ☑
        - upper quadrant S31.130 ☑
          - with
            - foreign body S31.140 ☑
            - penetration into peritoneal cavity S31.630 ☑
              - with foreign body S31.640 ☑
  - accidental, complicating surgery — *see* Complication, accidental puncture or laceration
  - alveolar (process) — *see* Puncture, oral cavity
  - ankle S91.039 ☑
    - with
      - foreign body S91.049 ☑
    - left S91.032 ☑
      - with
        - foreign body S91.042 ☑
    - right S91.031 ☑
      - with
        - foreign body S91.041 ☑
  - anus S31.833 ☑
    - with foreign body S31.834 ☑
  - arm (upper) S41.139 ☑
    - with foreign body S41.149 ☑
    - left S41.132 ☑
      - with foreign body S41.142 ☑
    - lower — *see* Puncture, forearm
    - right S41.131 ☑
      - with foreign body S41.141 ☑
  - auditory canal (external) (meatus) — *see* Puncture, ear
  - auricle, ear — *see* Puncture, ear
  - axilla — *see* Puncture, arm
  - back — *see also* Puncture, thorax, back
    - lower S31.030 ☑
      - with
        - foreign body S31.040 ☑
          - with penetration into retroperitoneal space S31.041 ☑
        - penetration into retroperitoneal space S31.031 ☑
  - bladder (traumatic) S37.29 ☑
    - nontraumatic N32.89
  - breast S21.039 ☑
    - with foreign body S21.049 ☑
    - left S21.032 ☑
      - with foreign body S21.042 ☑
    - right S21.031 ☑
      - with foreign body S21.041 ☑
  - buttock S31.803 ☑
    - with foreign body S31.804 ☑
    - left S31.823 ☑
      - with foreign body S31.824 ☑
    - right S31.813 ☑
      - with foreign body S31.814 ☑
  - by
    - device, implant or graft — *see* Complications, by site and type, mechanical
    - foreign body left accidentally in operative wound T81.539 ☑

- **Puncture** — *continued*
  - by — *continued*
    - instrument (any) during a procedure, accidental — *see* Puncture, accidental complicating surgery
  - calf — *see* Puncture, leg
  - canaliculus lacrimalis — *see* Puncture, eyelid
  - canthus, eye — *see* Puncture, eyelid
  - cervical esophagus S11.23 ☑
    - with foreign body S11.24 ☑
  - cheek (external) S01.439 ☑
    - with foreign body S01.449 ☑
    - internal — *see* Puncture, oral cavity
    - left S01.432 ☑
      - with foreign body S01.442 ☑
    - right S01.431 ☑
      - with foreign body S01.441 ☑
  - chest wall — *see* Puncture, thorax
  - chin — *see* Puncture, head, specified site NEC
  - clitoris — *see* Puncture, vulva
  - costal region — *see* Puncture, thorax
  - digit(s)
    - foot — *see* Puncture, toe
    - hand — *see* Puncture, finger
  - ear (canal) (external) S01.339 ☑
    - with foreign body S01.349 ☑
    - drum S09.2- ☑
    - left S01.332 ☑
      - with foreign body S01.342 ☑
    - right S01.331 ☑
      - with foreign body S01.341 ☑
  - elbow S51.039 ☑
    - with
      - foreign body S51.049 ☑
    - left S51.032 ☑
      - with
        - foreign body S51.042 ☑
    - right S51.031 ☑
      - with
        - foreign body S51.041 ☑
  - epididymis — *see* Puncture, testis
  - epigastric region — *see* Puncture, abdomen, wall, epigastric
  - epiglottis S11.83 ☑
    - with foreign body S11.84 ☑
  - esophagus
    - cervical S11.23 ☑
      - with foreign body S11.24 ☑
    - thoracic S27.818 ☑
  - eyeball S05.6- ☑
    - with foreign body S05.5- ☑
  - eyebrow — *see* Puncture, eyelid
  - eyelid S01.13- ☑
    - with foreign body S01.14- ☑
    - left S01.132 ☑
      - with foreign body S01.142 ☑
    - right S01.131 ☑
      - with foreign body S01.141 ☑
  - face NEC — *see* Puncture, head, specified site NEC
  - finger(s) S61.239 ☑
    - with
      - damage to nail S61.339 ☑
        - with
          - foreign body S61.349 ☑
      - foreign body S61.249 ☑
    - index S61.238 ☑
      - with
        - damage to nail S61.338 ☑
          - with
            - foreign body S61.348 ☑
        - foreign body S61.248 ☑
      - left S61.231 ☑
        - with
          - damage to nail S61.331 ☑
            - with
              - foreign body S61.341 ☑
          - foreign body S61.241 ☑
      - right S61.230 ☑
        - with
          - damage to nail S61.330 ☑
            - with
              - foreign body S61.340 ☑
          - foreign body S61.240 ☑
    - little S61.238 ☑
      - with
        - damage to nail S61.338 ☑

Puncture — *continued*
- supraclavicular fossa — *see* Puncture, neck, specified site NEC
- temple, temporal region — *see* Puncture, head, specified site NEC
- temporomandibular area — *see* Puncture, cheek
- testis S31.33 ☑
  - with foreign body S31.34 ☑
- thigh S71.139 ☑
  - with foreign body S71.149 ☑
  - left S71.132 ☑
    - with foreign body S71.142 ☑
  - right S71.131 ☑
    - with foreign body S71.141 ☑
- thorax, thoracic (wall) S21.93 ☑
  - with foreign body S21.94 ☑
  - back S21.23- ☑
    - with
      - foreign body S21.24- ☑
        - with penetration S21.44 ☑
      - penetration S21.43 ☑
  - breast — *see* Puncture, breast
  - front S21.13- ☑
    - with
      - foreign body S21.14- ☑
        - with penetration S21.34 ☑
      - penetration S21.33 ☑
- throat — *see* Puncture, neck
- thumb S61.Ø39 ☑
  - with
    - damage to nail S61.139 ☑
      - with
        - foreign body S61.149 ☑
    - foreign body S61.Ø49 ☑
  - left S61.Ø32 ☑
    - with
      - damage to nail S61.132 ☑
        - with
          - foreign body S61.142 ☑
      - foreign body S61.Ø42 ☑
  - right S61.Ø31 ☑
    - with
      - damage to nail S61.131 ☑
        - with
          - foreign body S61.141 ☑
      - foreign body S61.Ø41 ☑
- thyroid gland S11.13 ☑
  - with foreign body S11.14 ☑
- toe(s) S91.139 ☑
  - with
    - damage to nail S91.239 ☑
      - with
        - foreign body S91.249 ☑
    - foreign body S91.149 ☑
  - great S91.133 ☑
    - with
      - damage to nail S91.233 ☑
        - with
          - foreign body S91.243 ☑
      - foreign body S91.143 ☑
    - left S91.132 ☑
      - with
        - damage to nail S91.232 ☑
          - with
            - foreign body S91.242 ☑
        - foreign body S91.142 ☑
    - right S91.131 ☑
      - with
        - damage to nail S91.231 ☑
          - with
            - foreign body S91.241 ☑
        - foreign body S91.141 ☑
  - lesser S91.136 ☑
    - with
      - damage to nail S91.236 ☑
        - with
          - foreign body S91.246 ☑
      - foreign body S91.146 ☑
    - left S91.135 ☑
      - with
        - damage to nail S91.235 ☑
          - with
            - foreign body S91.245 ☑
        - foreign body S91.145 ☑
    - right S91.134 ☑

Puncture — *continued*
- toe(s) — *continued*
  - lesser — *continued*
    - right — *continued*
      - with
        - damage to nail S91.234 ☑
          - with
            - foreign body S91.244 ☑
        - foreign body S91.144 ☑
- tongue — *see* Puncture, oral cavity
- trachea S11.Ø23 ☑
  - with foreign body S11.Ø24 ☑
- tunica vaginalis — *see* Puncture, testis
- tympanum, tympanic membrane SØ9.2- ☑
- umbilical region S31.135 ☑
  - with foreign body S31.145 ☑
- uvula — *see* Puncture, oral cavity
- vagina S31.43 ☑
  - with foreign body S31.44 ☑
- vocal cords S11.Ø33 ☑
  - with foreign body S11.Ø34 ☑
- vulva S31.43 ☑
  - with foreign body S31.44 ☑
- wrist S61.539 ☑
  - with
    - foreign body S61.549 ☑
  - left S61.532 ☑
    - with
      - foreign body S61.542 ☑
  - right S61.531 ☑
    - with
      - foreign body S61.541 ☑

PUO (pyrexia of unknown origin) R5Ø.9

Pupillary membrane (persistent) Q13.89

Pupillotonia — *see* Anomaly, pupil, function, tonic pupil

Purpura D69.2
- abdominal D69.Ø
- allergic D69.Ø
- anaphylactoid D69.Ø
- annularis telangiectodes L81.7
- arthritic D69.Ø
- autoerythrocyte sensitization D69.2
- autoimmune D69.Ø
- bacterial D69.Ø
- Bateman's (senile) D69.2
- capillary fragility (hereditary) (idiopathic) D69.8
- cryoglobulinemic D89.1
- Devil's pinches D69.2
- fibrinolytic — *see* Fibrinolysis
- fulminans, fulminous D65
- gangrenous D65
- hemorrhagic, hemorrhagica D69.3
  - not due to thrombocytopenia D69.Ø
- Henoch (-Schönlein) (allergic) D69.Ø
- hypergammaglobulinemic (benign) (Waldenström) D89.Ø
- idiopathic (thrombocytopenic) D69.3
  - nonthrombocytopenic D69.Ø
- immune thrombocytopenic D69.3
- infectious D69.Ø
- malignant D69.Ø
- neonatorum P54.5
- nervosa D69.Ø
- newborn P54.5
- nonthrombocytopenic D69.2
  - hemorrhagic D69.Ø
  - idiopathic D69.Ø
- nonthrombopenic D69.2
- peliosis rheumatica D69.Ø
- posttransfusion (post-transfusion) (from (fresh) whole blood or blood products) D69.51
- primary D69.49
- red cell membrane sensitivity D69.2
- rheumatica D69.Ø
- Schönlein (-Henoch) (allergic) D69.Ø
- scorbutic E54 *[D77]*
- senile D69.2
- simplex D69.2
- symptomatica D69.Ø
- telangiectasia annularis L81.7
- thrombocytopenic D69.49
  - congenital D69.42
  - hemorrhagic D69.3
  - hereditary D69.42
  - idiopathic D69.3
  - immune D69.3
  - neonatal, transitory P61.Ø
  - thrombotic M31.1

Purpura — *continued*
- thrombohemolytic — *see* Fibrinolysis
- thrombolytic — *see* Fibrinolysis
- thrombopenic D69.49
- thrombotic, thrombocytopenic M31.1
- toxic D69.Ø
- vascular D69.Ø
- visceral symptoms D69.Ø

Purpuric spots R23.3

Purulent — *see* condition

Pus
- in
  - stool R19.5
  - urine N39.Ø
- tube (rupture) — *see* Salpingo-oophoritis

Pustular rash LØ8.Ø

Pustule (nonmalignant) LØ8.9
- malignant A22.Ø

Pustulosis palmaris et plantaris L4Ø.3

Putnam (-Dana) **disease or syndrome** — *see* Degeneration, combined

Putrescent pulp (dental) KØ4.1

Pyarthritis, pyarthrosis — *see* Arthritis, pyogenic or pyemic
- tuberculous — *see* Tuberculosis, joint

Pyelectasis — *see* Hydronephrosis

Pyelitis (congenital) (uremic) — *see also* Pyelonephritis
- with
  - calculus — *see* category N2Ø ☑
    - with hydronephrosis N13.6
  - contracted kidney N11.9
- acute N1Ø
- chronic N11.9
  - with calculus — *see* category N2Ø ☑
    - with hydronephrosis N13.6
- cystica N28.84
- puerperal (postpartum) O86.21
- tuberculous A18.11

Pyelocystitis — *see* Pyelonephritis

Pyelonephritis — *see also* Nephritis, tubulo-interstitial
- with
  - calculus — *see* category N2Ø ☑
    - with hydronephrosis N13.6
  - contracted kidney N11.9
- acute N1Ø
- calculous — *see* category N2Ø ☑
  - with hydronephrosis N13.6
- chronic N11.9
  - with calculus — *see* category N2Ø ☑
    - with hydronephrosis N13.6
  - associated with ureteral obstruction or stricture N11.1
  - nonobstructive N11.8
    - with reflux (vesicoureteral) N11.Ø
  - obstructive N11.1
  - specified NEC N11.8
- in (due to)
  - brucellosis A23.9 *[N16]*
  - cryoglobulinemia (mixed) D89.1 *[N16]*
  - cystinosis E72.Ø4
  - diphtheria A36.84
  - glycogen storage disease E74.Ø9 *[N16]*
  - leukemia NEC C95.9- ☑ *[N16]*
  - lymphoma NEC C85.9Ø *[N16]*
  - multiple myeloma C9Ø.Ø- ☑ *[N16]*
  - obstruction N11.1
  - Salmonella infection AØ2.25
  - sarcoidosis D86.84
  - sepsis A41.9 *[N16]*
  - Sjögren's disease M35.Ø4
  - toxoplasmosis B58.83
  - transplant rejection T86.91 *[N16]*
  - Wilson's disease E83.Ø1 *[N16]*
- nonobstructive N12
  - with reflux (vesicoureteral) N11.Ø
  - chronic N11.8
- syphilitic A52.75

Pyelonephrosis (obstructive) N11.1
- chronic N11.9

Pyelophlebitis I8Ø.8

Pyeloureteritis cystica N28.85

Pyemia, pyemic (fever) (infection) (purulent) — *see also* Sepsis
- joint — *see* Arthritis, pyogenic or pyemic
- liver K75.1
- pneumococcal A4Ø.3
- portal K75.1

Pyemia, pyemic — *continued*
- postvaccinal T88.Ø ☑
- puerperal, postpartum, childbirth O85
- specified organism NEC A41.89
- tuberculous — *see* Tuberculosis, miliary

Pygopagus Q89.4
Pyknoepilepsy (idiopathic) — *see* Pyknolepsy
Pyknolepsy G4Ø.AØ9 (*following* G4Ø.3)
- intractable G4Ø.A19 (*following* G4Ø.3)
  - with status epilepticus G4Ø.A11 (*following* G4Ø.3)
  - without status epilepticus G4Ø.A19 (*following* G4Ø.3)
- not intractable G4Ø.AØ9 (*following* G4Ø.3)
  - with status epilepticus G4Ø.AØ1 (*following* G4Ø.3)
  - without status epilepticus G4Ø.AØ9 (*following* G4Ø.3)

Pylephlebitis K75.1
Pyle's syndrome Q78.5
Pylethrombophlebitis K75.1
Pylethrombosis K75.1
Pyloritis K29.9Ø
- with bleeding K29.91

Pylorospasm (reflex) **NEC** K31.3
- congenital or infantile Q4Ø.Ø
- neurotic F45.8
- newborn Q4Ø.Ø
- psychogenic F45.8

Pylorus, pyloric — *see* condition
Pyoarthrosis — *see* Arthritis, pyogenic or pyemic
Pyocele
- mastoid — *see* Mastoiditis, acute
- sinus (accessory) — *see* Sinusitis
- turbinate (bone) J32.9
- urethra — *see also* Urethritis N34.Ø

Pyocolpos — *see* Vaginitis
Pyocystitis N3Ø.8Ø
- with hematuria N3Ø.81

Pyoderma, pyodermia LØ8.Ø
- gangrenosum L88
- newborn P39.4
- phagedenic L88
- vegetans LØ8.81

Pyodermatitis LØ8.Ø
- vegetans LØ8.81

Pyogenic — *see* condition
Pyohydronephrosis N13.6
Pyometra, pyometrium, pyometritis — *see* Endometritis
Pyomyositis (tropical) — *see* Myositis, infective
Pyonephritis N12
Pyonephrosis N13.6
- tuberculous A18.11

Pyo-oophoritis — *see* Salpingo-oophoritis
Pyo-ovarium — *see* Salpingo-oophoritis
Pyopericarditis, pyopericardium I3Ø.1
Pyophlebitis — *see* Phlebitis
Pyopneumopericardium I3Ø.1
Pyopneumothorax (infective) J86.9
- with fistula J86.Ø
- tuberculous NEC A15.6

Pyosalpinx, pyosalpingitis — *see also* Salpingo-oophoritis
Pyothorax J86.9
- with fistula J86.Ø
- tuberculous NEC A15.6

Pyoureter N28.89
- tuberculous A18.11

Pyramidopallidonigral syndrome G2Ø
Pyrexia (of unknown origin) R5Ø.9
- atmospheric T67.Ø1 ☑
- during labor NEC O75.2
- heat T67.Ø1 ☑
- newborn P81.9
  - environmentally-induced P81.Ø
- persistent R5Ø.9
- puerperal O86.4

Pyroglobulinemia NEC E88.Ø9
Pyromania F63.1
Pyrosis R12
Pyuria (bacterial) (sterile) R82.81

Q

Q fever A78
- with pneumonia A78

Quadricuspid aortic valve Q23.8
Quadrilateral fever A78
Quadriparesis — *see* Quadriplegia
- meaning muscle weakness M62.81

Quadriplegia G82.5Ø
- complete
  - C1-C4 level G82.51
  - C5-C7 level G82.53
- congenital (cerebral) (spinal) G8Ø.8
  - spastic G8Ø.Ø
- embolic (current episode) I63.4- ☑
- functional R53.2
- incomplete
  - C1-C4 level G82.52
  - C5-C7 level G82.54
- thrombotic (current episode) I63.3- ☑
- traumatic — *code to* injury with seventh character S
  - current episode — *see* Injury, spinal (cord), cervical

Quadruplet, pregnancy — *see* Pregnancy, quadruplet
Quarrelsomeness F6Ø.3
Queensland fever A77.3
Quervain's disease M65.4
- thyroid EØ6.1

Queyrat's erythroplasia DØ7.4
- penis DØ7.4
- specified site — *see* Neoplasm, skin, in situ
- unspecified site DØ7.4

Quincke's disease or edema T78.3 ☑
- hereditary D84.1

Quinsy (gangrenous) J36
Quintan fever A79.Ø
Quintuplet, pregnancy — *see* Pregnancy, quintuplet

R

Rabbit fever — *see* Tularemia
Rabies A82.9
- contact Z2Ø.3
- exposure to Z2Ø.3
- inoculation reaction — *see* Complications, vaccination
- sylvatic A82.Ø
- urban A82.1

Rachischisis — *see* Spina bifida
Rachitic — *see also* condition
- deformities of spine (late effect) (sequelae) E64.3
- pelvis (late effect) (sequelae) E64.3
  - with disproportion (fetopelvic) O33.Ø
    - causing obstructed labor O65.Ø

Rachitis, rachitism (acute) (tarda) — *see also* Rickets
- renalis N25.Ø
- sequelae E64.3

Radial nerve — *see* condition
Radiation
- burn — *see* Burn
- effects NOS T66 ☑
- sickness NOS T66 ☑
- therapy, encounter for Z51.Ø

Radiculitis (pressure) (vertebrogenic) — *see* Radiculopathy
Radiculomyelitis — *see also* Encephalitis
- toxic, due to
  - Clostridium tetani A35
  - Corynebacterium diphtheriae A36.82

Radiculopathy M54.1Ø
- cervical region M54.12
- cervicothoracic region M54.13
- due to
  - disc disorder
    - C3 M5Ø.11
    - C4 M5Ø.11
    - C5 M5Ø.121
    - C6 M5Ø.122
    - C7 M5Ø.123
  - displacement of intervertebral disc — *see* Disorder, disc, with, radiculopathy
- leg M54.1- ☑
- lumbar region M54.16
- lumbosacral region M54.17
- occipito-atlanto-axial region M54.11
- postherpetic BØ2.29
- sacrococcygeal region M54.18
- syphilitic A52.11
- thoracic region (with visceral pain) M54.14
- thoracolumbar region M54.15

Radiodermal burns (acute, chronic, or occupational) — *see* Burn
Radiodermatitis L58.9
- acute L58.Ø
- chronic L58.1

Radiotherapy session Z51.Ø
RAEB (refractory anemia with excess blasts) D46.2- ☑
Rage, meaning rabies — *see* Rabies
Ragpicker's disease A22.1
Ragsorter's disease A22.1
Raillietiniasis B71.8
Railroad neurosis F48.8
Railway spine F48.8
Raised — *see also* Elevated
- antibody titer R76.Ø

Rake teeth, tooth M26.39
Rales RØ9.89
Ramifying renal pelvis Q63.8
Ramsay-Hunt disease or syndrome — *see also* Hunt's disease BØ2.21
- meaning dyssynergia cerebellaris myoclonica G11.19

Ranula K11.6
- congenital Q38.4

Rape
- adult
  - confirmed T74.21 ☑
  - suspected T76.21 ☑
- alleged, observation or examination, ruled out
  - adult ZØ4.41
  - child ZØ4.42
- child
  - confirmed T74.22 ☑
  - suspected T76.22 ☑

Rapid
- feeble pulse, due to shock, following injury T79.4 ☑
- heart (beat) RØØ.Ø
  - psychogenic F45.8
- second stage (delivery) O62.3
- time-zone change syndrome G47.25

Rarefaction, bone — *see* Disorder, bone, density and structure, specified NEC
Rash (toxic) R21
- canker A38.9
- diaper L22
- drug (internal use) L27.Ø
  - contact — *see also* Dermatitis, due to, drugs, external L25.1
- following immunization T88.1 ☑
- food — *see* Dermatitis, due to, food
- heat L74.Ø
- napkin (psoriasiform) L22
- nettle — *see* Urticaria
- pustular LØ8.Ø
- rose R21
  - epidemic BØ6.9
- scarlet A38.9
- serum — *see also* Reaction, serum T8Ø.69 ☑
- wandering tongue K14.1

Rasmussen aneurysm — *see* Tuberculosis, pulmonary
Rasmussen encephalitis GØ4.81
Rat-bite fever A25.9
- due to Streptobacillus moniliformis A25.1
- spirochetal (morsus muris) A25.Ø

Rathke's pouch tumor D44.3
Raymond (-Céstan) **syndrome** I65.8
Raynaud's disease, phenomenon or syndrome (secondary) I73.ØØ
- with gangrene (symmetric) I73.Ø1

RDS (newborn) (type I) P22.Ø
- type II P22.1

Reaction — *see also* Disorder
- withdrawing, child or adolescent F93.8
- adaptation — *see* Disorder, adjustment
- adjustment (anxiety) (conduct disorder) (depressiveness) (distress) — *see* Disorder, adjustment
  - with
    - mutism, elective (child) (adolescent) F94.Ø
- adverse
  - food (any) (ingested) NEC T78.1 ☑
    - anaphylactic — *see* Shock, anaphylactic, due to food
- affective — *see* Disorder, mood
- allergic — *see* Allergy
- anaphylactic — *see* Shock, anaphylactic
- anaphylactoid — *see* Shock, anaphylactic
- anesthesia — *see* Anesthesia, complication
- antitoxin (prophylactic) (therapeutic) — *see* Complications, vaccination
- anxiety F41.1
- Arthus — *see* Arthus' phenomenon
- asthenic F48.8
- combat and operational stress F43.Ø
- compulsive F42.8
- conversion F44.9

☑ Additional Character Required — Refer to the Tabular List for Character Selection

Subterms under main terms may continue to next column or page

Reflux — *continued*
- vesicoureteral — *continued*
  - with — *continued*
    - nephropathy — *continued*
      - bilateral N13.722
      - unilateral N13.721
      - without hydroureter N13.729
        - bilateral N13.722
        - unilateral N13.721
    - pyelonephritis (chronic) N11.Ø
  - congenital Q62.7
  - without nephropathy N13.71

Reforming, artificial openings — *see* Attention to, artificial, opening

Refractive error — *see* Disorder, refraction

Refsum's disease or syndrome G6Ø.1

Refusal of
- food, psychogenic F5Ø.89
- treatment (because of) Z53.2Ø
  - left against medical advice (AMA) Z53.21
  - patient's decision NEC Z53.29
  - reasons of belief or group pressure Z53.1

Regional — *see* condition

Regurgitation R11.1Ø
- aortic (valve) — *see* Insufficiency, aortic
- food — *see also* Vomiting
  - with reswallowing — *see* Rumination
  - newborn P92.1
- gastric contents — *see* Vomiting
- heart — *see* Endocarditis
- mitral (valve) — *see* Insufficiency, mitral
  - congenital Q23.3
- myocardial — *see* Endocarditis
- pulmonary (valve) (heart) I37.1
  - congenital Q22.2
  - syphilitic A52.Ø3
- tricuspid — *see* Insufficiency, tricuspid
- valve, valvular — *see* Endocarditis
  - congenital Q24.8
- vesicoureteral — *see* Reflux, vesicoureteral

Reichmann's disease or syndrome K31.89

Reifenstein syndrome E34.52

Reinsertion
- implantable subdermal contraceptive Z3Ø.46
- intrauterine contraceptive device Z3Ø.433

Reiter's disease, syndrome, or urethritis MØ2.3Ø
- ankle MØ2.37- ☑
- elbow MØ2.32- ☑
- foot joint MØ2.37- ☑
- hand joint MØ2.34- ☑
- hip MØ2.35- ☑
- knee MØ2.36- ☑
- multiple site MØ2.39
- shoulder MØ2.31- ☑
- vertebra MØ2.38
- wrist MØ2.33- ☑

Rejection
- food, psychogenic F5Ø.89
- transplant T86.91
  - bone T86.83Ø
    - marrow T86.Ø1
  - cornea T86.84Ø- ☑
  - heart T86.21
    - with lung(s) T86.31
  - intestine T86.85Ø
  - kidney T86.11
  - liver T86.41
  - lung(s) T86.81Ø
    - with heart T86.31
  - organ (immune or nonimmune cause) T86.91
  - pancreas T86.89Ø
  - skin (allograft) (autograft) T86.82Ø
  - specified NEC T86.89Ø
  - stem cell (peripheral blood) (umbilical cord) T86.5

Relapsing fever A68.9
- Carter's (Asiatic) A68.1
- Dutton's (West African) A68.1
- Koch's A68.9
- louse-borne (epidemic) A68.Ø
- Novy's (American) A68.1
- Obermeyers's (European) A68.Ø
- Spirillum A68.9
- tick-borne (endemic) A68.1

Relationship
- occlusal
  - open anterior M26.22Ø
  - open posterior M26.221

Relaxation
- anus (sphincter) K62.89
  - psychogenic F45.8
- arch (foot) — *see also* Deformity, limb, flat foot
- back ligaments — *see* Instability, joint, spine
- bladder (sphincter) N31.2
- cardioesophageal K21.9
- cervix — *see* Incompetency, cervix
- diaphragm J98.6
- joint (capsule) (ligament) (paralytic) — *see* Flail, joint
  - congenital NEC Q74.8
- lumbosacral (joint) — *see* subcategory M53.2 ☑
- pelvic floor N81.89
- perineum N81.89
- posture R29.3
- rectum (sphincter) K62.89
- sacroiliac (joint) — *see* subcategory M53.2 ☑
- scrotum N5Ø.89
- urethra (sphincter) N36.44
- vesical N31.2

Release from prison, anxiety concerning Z65.2

Remains
- canal of Cloquet Q14.Ø
- capsule (opaque) Q14.8

Remittent fever (malarial) B54

Remnant
- canal of Cloquet Q14.Ø
- capsule (opaque) Q14.8
- cervix, cervical stump (acquired) (postoperative) N88.8
- cystic duct, postcholecystectomy K91.5
- fingernail L6Ø.8
  - congenital Q84.6
- meniscus, knee — *see* Derangement, knee, meniscus, specified NEC
- thyroglossal duct Q89.2
- tonsil J35.8
  - infected (chronic) J35.Ø1
- urachus Q64.4

Removal (from) (of)
- artificial
  - arm Z44.ØØ- ☑
    - complete Z44.Ø1- ☑
    - partial Z44.Ø2- ☑
  - eye Z44.2- ☑
  - leg Z44.1Ø- ☑
    - complete Z44.11- ☑
    - partial Z44.12- ☑
- breast implant Z45.81 ☑
- cardiac pulse generator (battery) (end-of-life) Z45.Ø1Ø
- catheter (urinary) (indwelling) Z46.6
  - from artificial opening — *see* Attention to, artificial, opening
  - non-vascular Z46.82
  - vascular NEC Z45.2
- device Z46.9
  - contraceptive Z3Ø.432
    - implantable subdermal Z3Ø.46
  - implanted NEC Z45.89
  - specified NEC Z46.89
- drains Z48.Ø3
- dressing (nonsurgical) Z48.ØØ
  - surgical Z48.Ø1
- external
  - fixation device — *code to* fracture with seventh character D
  - prosthesis, prosthetic device Z44.9
    - breast Z44.3- ☑
    - specified NEC Z44.8
- home in childhood (to foster home or institution) Z62.29
- ileostomy Z43.2
- insulin pump Z46.81
- myringotomy device (stent) (tube) Z45.82
- nervous system device NEC Z46.2
  - brain neuropacemaker Z46.2
  - visual substitution device Z46.2
    - implanted Z45.31
- non-vascular catheter Z46.82
- organ, prophylactic (for neoplasia management) — *see* Prophylactic, organ removal
- orthodontic device Z46.4
- staples Z48.Ø2
- stent
  - ureteral Z46.6
- suture Z48.Ø2
- urinary device Z46.6
- vascular access device or catheter Z45.2

Ren
- arcuatus Q63.1
- mobile, mobilis N28.89
  - congenital Q63.8
- unguliformis Q63.1

Renal — *see* condition

Rendu-Osler-Weber disease or syndrome I78.Ø

Reninoma D41.Ø- ☑

Renon-Delille syndrome E23.3

Reovirus, as cause of disease classified elsewhere B97.5

Repeated falls NEC R29.6

Replaced chromosome by dicentric ring Q93.2

Replacement by artificial or mechanical device or prosthesis of
- bladder Z96.Ø
- blood vessel NEC Z95.828
- bone NEC Z96.7
- cochlea Z96.21
- coronary artery Z95.5
- eustachian tube Z96.29
- eye globe Z97.Ø
- heart Z95.812
  - valve Z95.2
    - prosthetic Z95.2
    - specified NEC Z95.4
    - xenogenic Z95.3
- intestine Z96.89
- joint Z96.6Ø
  - hip — *see* Presence, hip joint implant
  - knee — *see* Presence, knee joint implant
  - specified site NEC Z96.698
- larynx Z96.3
- lens Z96.1
- limb(s) — *see* Presence, artificial, limb
- mandible NEC (for tooth root implant(s)) Z96.5
- organ NEC Z96.89
- peripheral vessel NEC Z95.828
- stapes Z96.29
- teeth Z97.2
- tendon Z96.7
- tissue NEC Z96.89
- tooth root(s) Z96.5
- vessel NEC Z95.828
  - coronary (artery) Z95.5

Request for expert evidence ZØ4.89

Reserve, decreased or low
- cardiac — *see* Disease, heart
- kidney N28.89

Residual — *see also* condition
- ovary syndrome N99.83
- state, schizophrenic F2Ø.5
- urine R39.198

Resistance, resistant (to)
- activated protein C D68.51
- complicating pregnancy O26.89 ☑
- insulin E88.81
- organism(s)
  - to
    - drug Z16.3Ø
      - aminoglycosides Z16.29
      - amoxicillin Z16.11
      - ampicillin Z16.11
      - antibiotic(s) Z16.2Ø
        - multiple Z16.24
        - specified NEC Z16.29
      - antifungal Z16.32
      - antimicrobial (single) Z16.3Ø
        - multiple Z16.35
        - specified NEC Z16.39
      - antimycobacterial (single) Z16.341
        - multiple Z16.342
      - antiparasitic Z16.31
      - antiviral Z16.33
      - beta lactam antibiotics Z16.1Ø
        - specified NEC Z16.19
      - cephalosporins Z16.19
      - extended beta lactamase (ESBL) Z16.12
      - fluoroquinolones Z16.23
      - macrolides Z16.29
      - methicillin — *see* MRSA
      - multiple drugs (MDRO)
        - antibiotics Z16.24
        - antimicrobial Z16.35
        - antimycobacterials Z16.342
      - penicillins Z16.11
      - quinine (and related compounds) Z16.31
      - quinolones Z16.23

Rhinorrhea J34.89
- cerebrospinal (fluid) G96.Ø1
  - postoperative G96.Ø8
  - specified NEC G96.Ø8
  - spontaneous G96.Ø1
  - traumatic G96.Ø8
- paroxysmal — *see* Rhinitis, allergic
- spasmodic — *see* Rhinitis, allergic

Rhinosalpingitis — *see* Salpingitis, eustachian
Rhinoscleroma A48.8
Rhinosporidiosis B48.1
Rhinovirus infection NEC B34.8
Rhizomelic chondrodysplasia punctata E71.54Ø
Rhythm
- atrioventricular nodal I49.8
- disorder I49.9
  - coronary sinus I49.8
  - ectopic I49.8
  - nodal I49.8
- escape I49.9
- heart, abnormal I49.9
- idioventricular I44.2
- nodal I49.8
- sleep, inversion G47.2- ☑
  - nonorganic origin — *see* Disorder, sleep, circadian rhythm, psychogenic

Rhytidosis facialis L98.8
Rib — *see also* condition
- cervical Q76.5

Riboflavin deficiency E53.Ø
Rice bodies — *see also* Loose, body, joint
- knee M23.4- ☑

Richter syndrome — *see* Leukemia, chronic lymphocytic, B-cell type
Richter's hernia — *see* Hernia, abdomen, with obstruction
Ricinism — *see* Poisoning, food, noxious, plant
Rickets (active) (acute) (adolescent) (chest wall) (congenital) (current) (infantile) (intestinal) E55.Ø
- adult — *see* Osteomalacia
- celiac K9Ø.Ø
- hypophosphatemic with nephrotic-glycosuric dwarfism E72.Ø9
- inactive E64.3
- kidney N25.Ø
- renal N25.Ø
- sequelae, any E64.3
- vitamin-D-resistant E83.31 *[M9Ø.8Ø]*

Rickettsia 364D/R. philipii (Pacific Coast tick fever) A77.8
Rickettsial disease A79.9
- specified type NEC A79.89

Rickettsialpox (Rickettsia akari) A79.1
Rickettsiosis A79.9
- due to
  - Ehrlichia sennetsu A79.81
  - Neorickettsia sennetsu A79.81
  - Rickettsia akari (rickettsialpox) A79.1
- specified type NEC A79.89
- tick-borne A77.9
- vesicular A79.1

Rider's bone — *see* Ossification, muscle, specified NEC
Ridge, alveolus — *see also* condition
- flabby KØ6.8

Ridged ear, congenital Q17.3
Riedel's
- lobe, liver Q44.7
- struma, thyroiditis or disease EØ6.5

Rieger's anomaly or syndrome Q13.81
Riehl's melanosis L81.4
Rietti-Greppi-Micheli anemia D56.9
Rieux's hernia — *see* Hernia, abdomen, specified site NEC
Riga (-Fede) **disease** K14.Ø
Riggs' disease — *see* Periodontitis
Right aortic arch Q25.47
Right middle lobe syndrome J98.11
Rigid, rigidity — *see also* condition
- abdominal R19.3Ø
  - with severe abdominal pain R1Ø.Ø
  - epigastric R19.36
  - generalized R19.37
  - left lower quadrant R19.34
  - left upper quadrant R19.32
  - periumbilic R19.35
  - right lower quadrant R19.33
  - right upper quadrant R19.31

Rigid, rigidity — *continued*
- articular, multiple, congenital Q68.8
- cervix (uteri) in pregnancy — *see* Pregnancy, complicated by, abnormal, cervix
- hymen (acquired) (congenital) N89.6
- nuchal R29.1
- pelvic floor in pregnancy — *see* Pregnancy, complicated by, abnormal, pelvic organs or tissues NEC
- perineum or vulva in pregnancy — *see* Pregnancy, complicated by, abnormal, vulva
- spine — *see* Dorsopathy, specified NEC
- vagina in pregnancy — *see* Pregnancy, complicated by, abnormal, vagina

Rigors R68.89
- with fever R5Ø.9

Riley-Day syndrome G9Ø.1
RIND (reversible ischemic neurologic deficit) I63.9
Ring(s)
- aorta (vascular) Q25.45
- Bandl's O62.4
- contraction, complicating delivery O62.4
- esophageal, lower (muscular) K22.2
- Fleischer's (cornea) H18.Ø4- ☑
- hymenal, tight (acquired) (congenital) N89.6
- Kayser-Fleischer (cornea) H18.Ø4- ☑
- retraction, uterus, pathological O62.4
- Schatzki's (esophagus) (lower) K22.2
  - congenital Q39.3
- Soemmerring's — *see* Cataract, secondary
- vascular (congenital) Q25.8
  - aorta Q25.45

Ringed hair (congenital) Q84.1
Ringworm B35.9
- beard B35.Ø
- black dot B35.Ø
- body B35.4
- Burmese B35.5
- corporeal B35.4
- foot B35.3
- groin B35.6
- hand B35.2
- honeycomb B35.Ø
- nails B35.1
- perianal (area) B35.6
- scalp B35.Ø
- specified NEC B35.8
- Tokelau B35.5

Rise, venous pressure I87.8
Rising, PSA following treatment for malignant neoplasm of prostate R97.21
Risk
- for
  - dental caries Z91.849
    - high Z91.843
    - low Z91.841
    - moderate Z91.842
- suicidal
  - meaning personal history of attempted suicide Z91.5
  - meaning suicidal ideation — *see* Ideation, suicidal

Ritter's disease LØØ
Rivalry, sibling Z62.891
Rivalta's disease A42.2
River blindness B73.Ø1
Robert's pelvis Q74.2
- with disproportion (fetopelvic) O33.Ø
  - causing obstructed labor O65.Ø

Robin (-Pierre) **syndrome** Q87.Ø
Robinow-Silvermann-Smith syndrome Q87.19
Robinson's (hidrotic) **ectodermal dysplasia or syndrome** Q82.4
Robles' disease B73.Ø1
Rocky Mountain (spotted) **fever** A77.Ø
Roetheln — *see* Rubella
Roger's disease Q21.Ø
Rokitansky-Aschoff sinuses (gallbladder) K82.8
Rolando's fracture (displaced) S62.22- ☑
- nondisplaced S62.22- ☑

Romano-Ward (prolonged QT interval) **syndrome** I45.81
Romberg's disease or syndrome G51.8
Roof, mouth — *see* condition
Rosacea L71.9
- acne L71.9
- keratitis L71.8
- specified NEC L71.8

Rosary, rachitic E55.Ø
Rose
- cold J3Ø.1

Rose — *continued*
- fever J3Ø.1
- rash R21
  - epidemic BØ6.9

Rosenbach's erysipeloid A26.Ø
Rosenthal's disease or syndrome D68.1
Roseola BØ9
- infantum BØ8.2Ø
  - due to human herpesvirus 6 BØ8.21
  - due to human herpesvirus 7 BØ8.22

Ross River disease or fever B33.1
Rossbach's disease K31.89
- psychogenic F45.8

Rostan's asthma (cardiac) — *see* Failure, ventricular, left
Rotation
- anomalous, incomplete or insufficient, intestine Q43.3
- cecum (congenital) Q43.3
- colon (congenital) Q43.3
- spine, incomplete or insufficient — *see* Dorsopathy, deforming, specified NEC
- tooth, teeth, fully erupted M26.35
- vertebra, incomplete or insufficient — *see* Dorsopathy, deforming, specified NEC

Rotes Quérol disease or syndrome — *see* Hyperostosis, ankylosing
Roth (-Bernhardt) **disease or syndrome** — *see* Meralgia paraesthetica
Rothmund (-Thomson) **syndrome** Q82.8
Rotor's disease or syndrome E8Ø.6
Round
- back (with wedging of vertebrae) — *see* Kyphosis
  - sequelae (late effect) of rickets E64.3
- worms (large) (infestation) NEC B82.Ø
  - Ascariasis — *see also* Ascariasis B77.9

Roussy-Lévy syndrome G6Ø.Ø
Rubella (German measles) BØ6.9
- complication NEC BØ6.Ø9
  - neurological BØ6.ØØ
- congenital P35.Ø
- contact Z2Ø.4
- exposure to Z2Ø.4
- maternal
  - care for (suspected) damage to fetus O35.3 ☑
  - manifest rubella in infant P35.Ø
  - suspected damage to fetus affecting management of pregnancy O35.3 ☑
- specified complications NEC BØ6.89

Rubeola (meaning measles) — *see* Measles
- meaning rubella — *see* Rubella

Rubeosis, iris — *see* Disorder, iris, vascular
Rubinstein-Taybi syndrome Q87.2
Rudimentary (congenital) — *see also* Agenesis
- arm — *see* Defect, reduction, upper limb
- bone Q79.9
- cervix uteri Q51.828
- eye Q11.2
- lobule of ear Q17.3
- patella Q74.1
- respiratory organs in thoracopagus Q89.4
- tracheal bronchus Q32.4
- uterus Q51.818
  - in male Q56.1
- vagina Q52.Ø

Ruled out condition — *see* Observation, suspected
Rumination R11.1Ø
- with nausea R11.2
- disorder of infancy F98.21
- neurotic F42.8
- newborn P92.1
- obsessional F42.8
- psychogenic F42.8

Runeberg's disease D51.Ø
Runny nose RØ9.89
Rupia (syphilitic) A51.39
- congenital A5Ø.Ø6
- tertiary A52.79

Rupture, ruptured
- abscess (spontaneous) — *code by* site under Abscess
- aneurysm — *see* Aneurysm
- anus (sphincter) — *see* Laceration, anus
- aorta, aortic I71.8
  - abdominal I71.3
  - arch I71.1
  - ascending I71.1
  - descending I71.8
    - abdominal I71.3
    - thoracic I71.1
  - syphilitic A52.Ø1

Rupture, ruptured — *continued*
tendon — *see* Strain — *continued*
nontraumatic — *continued*
extensor — *continued*
specified site NEC M66.28
thigh M66.25- ☑
upper arm M66.22- ☑
flexor M66.3Ø
ankle M66.37- ☑
foot M66.37- ☑
forearm M66.33- ☑
hand M66.34- ☑
lower leg M66.36- ☑
multiple sites M66.39
pelvic region M66.35- ☑
shoulder region M66.31- ☑
specified site NEC M66.38
thigh M66.35- ☑
upper arm M66.32- ☑
foot M66.87- ☑
forearm M66.83- ☑
hand M66.84- ☑
lower leg M66.86- ☑
multiple sites M66.89
pelvic region M66.85- ☑
shoulder region M66.81- ☑
specified
site NEC M66.88
tendon M66.8Ø
thigh M66.85- ☑
upper arm M66.82- ☑
thoracic duct I89.8
tonsil J35.8
traumatic
aorta — *see* Injury, aorta, laceration, major
diaphragm — *see* Injury, intrathoracic, diaphragm
external site — *see* Wound, open, by site
eye — *see* Injury, eye, laceration
internal organ — *see* Injury, by site
intervertebral disc
cervical S13.Ø ☑
lumbar S33.Ø ☑
thoracic S23.Ø ☑
kidney S37.Ø6- ☑
ligament — *see also* Sprain
ankle — *see* Sprain, ankle
carpus — *see* Rupture, traumatic, ligament, wrist
collateral (hand) — *see* Rupture, traumatic, ligament, finger, collateral
finger (metacarpophalangeal) (interphalangeal) S63.4Ø- ☑
collateral S63.41- ☑
index S63.41- ☑
little S63.41- ☑
middle S63.41- ☑
ring S63.41- ☑
index S63.4Ø- ☑
little S63.4Ø- ☑
middle S63.4Ø- ☑
palmar S63.42- ☑
index S63.42- ☑
little S63.42- ☑
middle S63.42- ☑
ring S63.42- ☑
ring S63.4Ø- ☑
specified site NEC S63.499 ☑
index S63.49- ☑
little S63.49- ☑
middle S63.49- ☑
ring S63.49- ☑
volar plate S63.43- ☑
index S63.43- ☑
little S63.43- ☑
middle S63.43- ☑
ring S63.43- ☑
foot — *see* Sprain, foot
radial collateral S53.2- ☑
radiocarpal — *see* Rupture, traumatic, ligament, wrist, radiocarpal
ulnar collateral S53.3- ☑
ulnocarpal — *see* Rupture, traumatic, ligament, wrist, ulnocarpal
wrist S63.3Ø- ☑
collateral S63.31- ☑
radiocarpal S63.32- ☑
specified site NEC S63.39- ☑

Rupture, ruptured — *continued*
traumatic — *continued*
ligament — *see also* Sprain — *continued*
wrist — *continued*
ulnocarpal (palmar) S63.33- ☑
liver S36.116 ☑
membrana tympani — *see* Rupture, ear drum, traumatic
muscle or tendon — *see* Strain
myocardium — *see* Injury, heart
pancreas S36.299 ☑
rectum S36.69 ☑
sigmoid S36.593 ☑
spleen S36.Ø9 ☑
stomach S36.39 ☑
symphysis pubis S33.4 ☑
tympanum, tympanic (membrane) — *see* Rupture, ear drum, traumatic
ureter S37.19 ☑
uterus S37.69 ☑
vagina — *see* Injury, vagina
vena cava — *see* Injury, vena cava, laceration, major
tricuspid (heart) (valve) IØ7.8
tube, tubal (nonobstetric) (nontraumatic) N83.8
abscess — *see* Salpingitis
due to pregnancy OØØ.1Ø- ☑
with intrauterine pregnancy OØØ.11- ☑
tympanum, tympanic (membrane) (nontraumatic) — *see also* Perforation, tympanic membrane H72.9- ☑
traumatic — *see* Rupture, ear drum, traumatic
umbilical cord, complicating delivery O69.89 ☑
ureter (traumatic) S37.19 ☑
nontraumatic N28.89
urethra (nontraumatic) N36.8
with ectopic or molar pregnancy OØ8.6
following ectopic or molar pregnancy OØ8.6
obstetrical trauma O71.5
traumatic S37.39 ☑
uterosacral ligament (nonobstetric) (nontraumatic) N83.8
uterus (traumatic) S37.69 ☑
before labor O71.Ø- ☑
during or after labor O71.1
nonpuerperal, nontraumatic N85.8
pregnant (during labor) O71.1
before labor O71.Ø- ☑
vagina — *see* Injury, vagina
valve, valvular (heart) — *see* Endocarditis
varicose vein — *see* Varix
varix — *see* Varix
vena cava R58
traumatic — *see* Injury, vena cava, laceration, major
vesical (urinary) N32.89
vessel (blood) R58
pulmonary I28.8
traumatic — *see* Injury, blood vessel
viscus R19.8
vulva complicating delivery O7Ø.Ø
Russell-Silver syndrome Q87.19
Russian spring-summer type encephalitis A84.Ø
Rust's disease (tuberculous cervical spondylitis) A18.Ø1
Ruvalcaba-Myhre-Smith syndrome E71.44Ø
Rytand-Lipsitch syndrome I44.2

S

Saber, sabre shin or tibia (syphilitic) A5Ø.56 *[M9Ø.8-]* ☑
Sac lacrimal — *see* condition
Saccharomyces infection B37.9
Saccharopinuria E72.3
Saccular — *see* condition
Sacculation
aorta (nonsyphilitic) — *see* Aneurysm, aorta
bladder N32.3
intralaryngeal (congenital) (ventricular) Q31.3
larynx (congenital) (ventricular) Q31.3
organ or site, congenital — *see* Distortion
pregnant uterus — *see* Pregnancy, complicated by, abnormal, uterus
ureter N28.89
urethra N36.1
vesical N32.3
Sachs' amaurotic familial idiocy or disease E75.Ø2
Sachs-Tay disease E75.Ø2
Sacks-Libman disease M32.11
Sacralgia M53.3
Sacralization Q76.49
Sacrodynia M53.3
Sacroiliac joint — *see* condition
Sacroiliitis NEC M46.1
Sacrum — *see* condition
Saddle
back — *see* Lordosis
embolus
abdominal aorta I74.Ø1
pulmonary artery I26.92
with acute cor pulmonale I26.Ø2
injury — *code to* condition
nose M95.Ø
due to syphilis A5Ø.57
Sadism (sexual) F65.52
Sadness, postpartal O9Ø.6
Sadomasochism F65.5Ø
Saemisch's ulcer (cornea) — *see* Ulcer, cornea, central
Sagging
skin and subcutaneous tissue (following bariatric surgery weight loss) (following dietary weight loss) L98.7
Sahib disease B55.Ø
Sailors' skin L57.8
Saint
Anthony's fire — *see* Erysipelas
triad — *see* Hernia, diaphragm
Vitus' dance — *see* Chorea, Sydenham's
Salaam
attack(s) — *see* Epilepsy, spasms
tic R25.8
Salicylism
abuse F55.8
overdose or wrong substance given — *see* Table of Drugs and Chemicals, by drug, poisoning
Salivary duct or gland — *see* condition
Salivation, excessive K11.7
Salmonella — *see* Infection, Salmonella
Salmonellosis AØ2.Ø
Salpingitis (catarrhal) (fallopian tube) (nodular) (pseudofollicular) (purulent) (septic) N7Ø.91
with oophoritis N7Ø.93
acute N7Ø.Ø1
with oophoritis N7Ø.Ø3
chlamydial A56.11
chronic N7Ø.11
with oophoritis N7Ø.13
complicating abortion — *see* Abortion, by type, complicated by, salpingitis
ear — *see* Salpingitis, eustachian
eustachian (tube) H68.ØØ- ☑
acute H68.Ø1- ☑
chronic H68.Ø2- ☑
follicularis N7Ø.11
with oophoritis N7Ø.13
gonococcal (acute) (chronic) A54.24
interstitial, chronic N7Ø.11
with oophoritis N7Ø.13
isthmica nodosa N7Ø.11
with oophoritis N7Ø.13
specific (gonococcal) (acute) (chronic) A54.24
tuberculous (acute) (chronic) A18.17
venereal (gonococcal) (acute) (chronic) A54.24
Salpingocele N83.4- ☑
Salpingo-oophoritis (catarrhal) (purulent) (ruptured) (septic) (suppurative) N7Ø.93
acute N7Ø.Ø3
with ectopic or molar pregnancy OØ8.Ø
following ectopic or molar pregnancy OØ8.Ø
gonococcal A54.24
chronic N7Ø.13
following ectopic or molar pregnancy OØ8.Ø
gonococcal (acute) (chronic) A54.24
puerperal O86.19
specific (gonococcal) (acute) (chronic) A54.24
subacute N7Ø.Ø3
tuberculous (acute) (chronic) A18.17
venereal (gonococcal) (acute) (chronic) A54.24
Salpingo-ovaritis — *see* Salpingo-oophoritis
Salpingoperitonitis — *see* Salpingo-oophoritis
Salzmann's nodular dystrophy — *see* Degeneration, cornea, nodular
Sampson's cyst or tumor N8Ø.1
San Joaquin (Valley) **fever** B38.Ø
Sandblaster's asthma, lung or pneumoconiosis J62.8
Sander's disease (paranoia) F22
Sandfly fever A93.1

- **Sandhoff's disease** E75.Ø1
- **Sanfilippo** (Type B) (Type C) (Type D) **syndrome** E76.22
- **Sanger-Brown ataxia** G11.2
- **Sao Paulo fever or typhus** A77.Ø
- **Saponification, mesenteric** K65.8
- **Sarcocele** (benign)
  - syphilitic A52.76
    - congenital A5Ø.59
- **Sarcocystosis** AØ7.8
- **Sarcoepiplocele** — *see* Hernia
- **Sarcoepiplomphalocele** Q79.2
- **Sarcoid** — *see also* Sarcoidosis
  - arthropathy D86.86
  - Boeck's D86.9
  - Darier-Roussy D86.3
  - iridocyclitis D86.83
  - meningitis D86.81
  - myocarditis D86.85
  - myositis D86.87
  - pyelonephritis D86.84
  - Spiegler-Fendt LØ8.89
- **Sarcoidosis** D86.9
  - with
    - cranial nerve palsies D86.82
    - hepatic granuloma D86.89
    - polyarthritis D86.86
    - tubulo-interstitial nephropathy D86.84
  - combined sites NEC D86.89
  - lung D86.Ø
    - and lymph nodes D86.2
  - lymph nodes D86.1
    - and lung D86.2
  - meninges D86.81
  - skin D86.3
  - specified type NEC D86.89
- **Sarcoma** (of) — *see also* Neoplasm, connective tissue, malignant
  - alveolar soft part — *see* Neoplasm, connective tissue, malignant
  - ameloblastic C41.1
    - upper jaw (bone) C41.Ø
  - botryoid — *see* Neoplasm, connective tissue, malignant
  - botryoides — *see* Neoplasm, connective tissue, malignant
  - cerebellar C71.6
    - circumscribed (arachnoidal) C71.6
  - circumscribed (arachnoidal) cerebellar C71.6
  - clear cell — *see also* Neoplasm, connective tissue, malignant
    - kidney C64.- ☑
  - dendritic cells (accessory cells) C96.4
  - embryonal — *see* Neoplasm, connective tissue, malignant
  - endometrial (stromal) C54.1
    - isthmus C54.Ø
  - epithelioid (cell) — *see* Neoplasm, connective tissue, malignant
  - Ewing's — *see* Neoplasm, bone, malignant
  - follicular dendritic cell C96.4
  - germinoblastic (diffuse) — *see* Lymphoma, diffuse large cell
    - follicular — *see* Lymphoma, follicular, specified NEC
  - giant cell (except of bone) — *see also* Neoplasm, connective tissue, malignant
    - bone — *see* Neoplasm, bone, malignant
  - glomoid — *see* Neoplasm, connective tissue, malignant
  - granulocytic C92.3- ☑
  - hemangioendothelial — *see* Neoplasm, connective tissue, malignant
  - hemorrhagic, multiple — *see* Sarcoma, Kaposi's
  - histiocytic C96.A (*following* C96.6)
  - Hodgkin — *see* Lymphoma, Hodgkin
  - immunoblastic (diffuse) — *see* Lymphoma, diffuse large cell
  - interdigitating dendritic cell C96.4
  - Kaposi's
    - colon C46.4
    - connective tissue C46.1
    - gastrointestinal organ C46.4
    - lung C46.5- ☑
    - lymph node(s) C46.3
    - palate (hard) (soft) C46.2
    - rectum C46.4
    - skin C46.Ø
    - specified site NEC C46.7
    - stomach C46.4
    - unspecified site C46.9
  - Kupffer cell C22.3

Sarcoma — *continued*

  - Langerhans cell C96.4
  - leptomeningeal — *see* Neoplasm, meninges, malignant
  - liver NEC C22.4
  - lymphangioendothelial — *see* Neoplasm, connective tissue, malignant
  - lymphoblastic — *see* Lymphoma, lymphoblastic (diffuse)
  - lymphocytic — *see* Lymphoma, small cell B-cell
  - mast cell C96.22
  - melanotic — *see* Melanoma
  - meningeal — *see* Neoplasm, meninges, malignant
  - meningothelial — *see* Neoplasm, meninges, malignant
  - mesenchymal — *see also* Neoplasm, connective tissue, malignant
    - mixed — *see* Neoplasm, connective tissue, malignant
  - mesothelial — *see* Mesothelioma
  - monstrocellular
    - specified site — *see* Neoplasm, malignant, by site
    - unspecified site C71.9
  - myeloid C92.3- ☑
  - neurogenic — *see* Neoplasm, nerve, malignant
  - odontogenic C41.1
    - upper jaw (bone) C41.Ø
  - osteoblastic — *see* Neoplasm, bone, malignant
  - osteogenic — *see also* Neoplasm, bone, malignant
    - juxtacortical — *see* Neoplasm, bone, malignant
    - periosteal — *see* Neoplasm, bone, malignant
  - periosteal — *see also* Neoplasm, bone, malignant
    - osteogenic — *see* Neoplasm, bone, malignant
  - pleomorphic cell — *see* Neoplasm, connective tissue, malignant
  - reticulum cell (diffuse) — *see* Lymphoma, diffuse large cell
    - nodular — *see* Lymphoma, follicular
    - pleomorphic cell type — *see* Lymphoma, diffuse large cell
  - rhabdoid — *see* Neoplasm, malignant, by site
  - round cell — *see* Neoplasm, connective tissue, malignant
  - small cell — *see* Neoplasm, connective tissue, malignant
  - soft tissue — *see* Neoplasm, connective tissue, malignant
  - spindle cell — *see* Neoplasm, connective tissue, malignant
  - stromal (endometrial) C54.1
    - isthmus C54.Ø
  - synovial — *see also* Neoplasm, connective tissue, malignant
    - biphasic — *see* Neoplasm, connective tissue, malignant
    - epithelioid cell — *see* Neoplasm, connective tissue, malignant
    - spindle cell — *see* Neoplasm, connective tissue, malignant
- **Sarcomatosis**
  - meningeal — *see* Neoplasm, meninges, malignant
  - specified site NEC — *see* Neoplasm, connective tissue, malignant
  - unspecified site C8Ø.1
- **Sarcopenia** (age-related) M62.84
- **Sarcosinemia** E72.59
- **Sarcosporidiosis** (intestinal) AØ7.8
- **Satiety, early** R68.81
- **Saturnine** — *see* condition
- **Saturnism**
  - overdose or wrong substance given or taken — *see* Table of Drugs and Chemicals, by drug, poisoning
- **Satyriasis** F52.8
- **Sauriasis** — *see* Ichthyosis
- **SBE** (subacute bacterial endocarditis) I33.Ø
- **Scabies** (any site) B86
- **Scabs** R23.4
- **Scaglietti-Dagnini syndrome** E22.Ø
- **Scald** — *see* Burn
- **Scalenus anticus** (anterior) **syndrome** G54.Ø
- **Scales** R23.4
- **Scaling, skin** R23.4
- **Scalp** — *see* condition
- **Scapegoating affecting child** Z62.3
- **Scaphocephaly** Q75.Ø
- **Scapulalgia** M89.8X1
- **Scapulohumeral myopathy** G71.Ø2
- **Scar, scarring** — *see also* Cicatrix L9Ø.5
  - adherent L9Ø.5

Scar, scarring — *continued*

  - atrophic L9Ø.5
  - cervix
    - in pregnancy or childbirth — *see* Pregnancy, complicated by, abnormal cervix
  - cheloid L91.Ø
  - chorioretinal H31.ØØ- ☑
    - posterior pole macula H31.Ø1- ☑
    - postsurgical H59.81- ☑
    - solar retinopathy H31.Ø2- ☑
    - specified type NEC H31.Ø9- ☑
  - choroid — *see* Scar, chorioretinal
  - conjunctiva H11.24- ☑
  - cornea H17.9
    - xerophthalmic — *see also* Opacity, cornea
      - vitamin A deficiency E5Ø.6
  - defect (isthmocele) O34.22
  - duodenum, obstructive K31.5
  - hypertrophic L91.Ø
  - keloid L91.Ø
  - labia N9Ø.89
  - lung (base) J98.4
  - macula — *see* Scar, chorioretinal, posterior pole
  - muscle M62.89
  - myocardium, myocardial I25.2
  - painful L9Ø.5
  - posterior pole (eye) — *see* Scar, chorioretinal, posterior pole
  - retina — *see* Scar, chorioretinal
  - trachea J39.8
  - transmural uterine, in pregnancy O34.29
  - uterus N85.8
    - in pregnancy O34.29
  - vagina N89.8
    - postoperative N99.2
  - vulva N9Ø.89
- **Scarabiasis** B88.2
- **Scarlatina** (anginosa) (maligna) A38.9
  - myocarditis (acute) A38.1
    - old — *see* Myocarditis
  - otitis media A38.Ø
  - ulcerosa A38.8
- **Scarlet fever** (albuminuria) (angina) A38.9
- **Schamberg's disease** (progressive pigmentary dermatosis) L81.7
- **Schatzki's ring** (acquired) (esophagus) (lower) K22.2
  - congenital Q39.3
- **Schaufenster krankheit** I2Ø.8
- **Schaumann's**
  - benign lymphogranulomatosis D86.1
  - disease or syndrome — *see* Sarcoidosis
- **Scheie's syndrome** E76.Ø3
- **Schenck's disease** B42.1
- **Scheuermann's disease or osteochondrosis** — *see* Osteochondrosis, juvenile, spine
- **Schilder** (-Flatau) **disease** G37.Ø
- **Schilling-type monocytic leukemia** C93.Ø- ☑
- **Schimmelbusch's disease, cystic mastitis, or hyperplasia** — *see* Mastopathy, cystic
- **Schistosoma infestation** — *see* Infestation, Schistosoma
- **Schistosomiasis** B65.9
  - with muscle disorder B65.9 *[M63.8Ø]*
    - ankle B65.9 *[M63.87-]* ☑
    - foot B65.9 *[M63.87-]* ☑
    - forearm B65.9 *[M63.83-]* ☑
    - hand B65.9 *[M63.84-]* ☑
    - lower leg B65.9 *[M63.86-]* ☑
    - multiple sites B65.9 *[M63.89]*
    - pelvic region B65.9 *[M63.85-]* ☑
    - shoulder region B65.9 *[M63.81-]* ☑
    - specified site NEC B65.9 *[M63.88]*
    - thigh B65.9 *[M63.85-]* ☑
    - upper arm B65.9 *[M63.82-]* ☑
  - Asiatic B65.2
  - bladder B65.Ø
  - chestermani B65.8
  - colon B65.1
  - cutaneous B65.3
  - due to
    - S. haematobium B65.Ø
    - S. japonicum B65.2
    - S. mansoni B65.1
    - S. mattheii B65.8
  - Eastern B65.2
  - genitourinary tract B65.Ø
  - intestinal B65.1
  - lung NEC B65.9 *[J99]*

Schistosomiasis — *continued*
lung — *continued*
pneumonia B65.9 *[J17]*
Manson's (intestinal) B65.1
oriental B65.2
pulmonary NEC B65.9 *[J99]*
pneumonia B65.9
Schistosoma
haematobium B65.0
japonicum B65.2
mansoni B65.1
specified type NEC B65.8
urinary B65.0
vesical B65.0
Schizencephaly Q04.6
Schizoaffective psychosis F25.9
Schizodontia K00.2
Schizoid personality F60.1
Schizophrenia, schizophrenic F20.9
acute (brief) (undifferentiated) F23
atypical (form) F20.3
borderline F21
catalepsy F20.2
catatonic (type) (excited) (withdrawn) F20.2
cenesthopathic, cenesthesiopathic F20.89
childhood type F84.5
chronic undifferentiated F20.9
cyclic F25.0
disorganized (type) F20.1
flexibilitas cerea F20.2
hebephrenic (type) F20.1
incipient F21
latent F21
negative type F20.5
paranoid (type) F20.0
paraphrenic F20.0
post-psychotic depression F32.89
prepsychotic F21
prodromal F21
pseudoneurotic F21
pseudopsychopathic F21
reaction F23
residual (state) (type) F20.5
restzustand F20.5
schizoaffective (type) — *see* Psychosis, schizoaffective
simple (type) F20.89
simplex F20.89
specified type NEC F20.89
spectrum and other psychotic disorder F29
specified NEC F28
stupor F20.2
syndrome of childhood F84.5
undifferentiated (type) F20.3
chronic F20.5
Schizothymia (persistent) F60.1
Schlatter-Osgood disease or osteochondrosis M92.52- ☑
Schlatter's tibia — *see* Osteochondrosis, juvenile, tibia
Schmidt's syndrome (polyglandular, autoimmune) E31.0
Schmincke's carcinoma or tumor — *see* Neoplasm, nasopharynx, malignant
Schmitz (-Stutzer) **dysentery** A03.0
Schmorl's disease or nodes
lumbar region M51.46
lumbosacral region M51.47
sacrococcygeal region M53.3
thoracic region M51.44
thoracolumbar region M51.45
Schneiderian
papilloma — *see* Neoplasm, nasopharynx, benign
specified site — *see* Neoplasm, benign, by site
unspecified site D14.0
specified site — *see* Neoplasm, malignant, by site
unspecified site C30.0
Scholte's syndrome (malignant carcinoid) E34.0
Scholz (-Bielchowsky-Henneberg) **disease or syndrome** E75.25
Schönlein (-Henoch) disease or purpura (primary) (rheumatic) D69.0
Schottmuller's disease A01.4
Schroeder's syndrome (endocrine hypertensive) E27.0
Schüller-Christian disease or syndrome C96.5
Schultze's type acroparesthesia, simple I73.89
Schultz's disease or syndrome — *see* Agranulocytosis
Schwalbe-Ziehen-Oppenheim disease G24.1
Schwannoma — *see also* Neoplasm, nerve, benign
malignant — *see also* Neoplasm, nerve, malignant

Schwannoma — *continued*
malignant — *see also* Neoplasm, nerve, malignant — *continued*
with rhabdomyoblastic differentiation — *see* Neoplasm, nerve, malignant
melanocytic — *see* Neoplasm, nerve, benign
pigmented — *see* Neoplasm, nerve, benign
Schwannomatosis Q85.03
Schwartz (-Jampel) **syndrome** G71.13
Schwartz-Bartter syndrome E22.2
Schweniger-Buzzi anetoderma L90.1
Sciatic — *see* condition
Sciatica (infective)
with lumbago M54.4- ☑
due to intervertebral disc disorder — *see* Disorder, disc, with, radiculopathy
due to displacement of intervertebral disc (with lumbago) — *see* Disorder, disc, with, radiculopathy
wallet M54.3- ☑
Scimitar syndrome Q26.8
Sclera — *see* condition
Sclerectasia H15.84- ☑
Scleredema
adultorum — *see* Sclerosis, systemic
Buschke's — *see* Sclerosis, systemic
newborn P83.0
Sclerema (adiposum) (edematosum) (neonatorum) (newborn) P83.0
adultorum — *see* Sclerosis, systemic
Scleriasis — *see* Scleroderma
Scleritis H15.00- ☑
with corneal involvement H15.04- ☑
anterior H15.01- ☑
brawny H15.02- ☑
in (due to) zoster B02.34
posterior H15.03- ☑
specified type NEC H15.09- ☑
syphilitic A52.71
tuberculous (nodular) A18.51
Sclerochoroiditis H31.8
Scleroconjunctivitis — *see* Scleritis
Sclerocystic ovary syndrome E28.2
Sclerodactyly, sclerodactylia L94.3
Scleroderma, sclerodermia (acrosclerotic) (diffuse) (generalized) (progressive) (pulmonary) — *see also* Sclerosis, systemic M34.9
circumscribed L94.0
linear L94.1
localized L94.0
newborn P83.88
systemic M34.9
Sclerokeratitis H16.8
tuberculous A18.52
Scleroma nasi A48.8
Scleromalacia (perforans) H15.05- ☑
Scleromyxedema L98.5
Sclérose en plaques G35
Sclerosis, sclerotic
adrenal (gland) E27.8
Alzheimer's — *see* Disease, Alzheimer's
amyotrophic (lateral) G12.21
aorta, aortic I70.0
valve — *see* Endocarditis, aortic
artery, arterial, arteriolar, arteriovascular — *see* Arteriosclerosis
ascending multiple G35
brain (generalized) (lobular) G37.9
artery, arterial I67.2
diffuse G37.0
disseminated G35
insular G35
Krabbe's E75.23
miliary G35
multiple G35
presenile (Alzheimer's) — *see* Disease, Alzheimer's, early onset
senile (arteriosclerotic) I67.2
stem, multiple G35
tuberous Q85.1
bulbar, multiple G35
bundle of His I44.39
cardiac — *see* Disease, heart, ischemic, atherosclerotic
cardiorenal — *see* Hypertension, cardiorenal
cardiovascular — *see also* Disease, cardiovascular
renal — *see* Hypertension, cardiorenal
cerebellar — *see* Sclerosis, brain
cerebral — *see* Sclerosis, brain

Sclerosis, sclerotic — *continued*
cerebrospinal (disseminated) (multiple) G35
cerebrovascular I67.2
choroid — *see* Degeneration, choroid
combined (spinal cord) — *see also* Degeneration, combined
multiple G35
concentric (Balo) G37.5
cornea — *see* Opacity, cornea
coronary (artery) I25.10
with angina pectoris — *see* Arteriosclerosis, coronary (artery),
corpus cavernosum
female N90.89
male N48.6
diffuse (brain) (spinal cord) G37.0
disseminated G35
dorsal G35
dorsolateral (spinal cord) — *see* Degeneration, combined
endometrium N85.5
extrapyramidal G25.9
eye, nuclear (senile) — *see* Cataract, senile, nuclear
focal and segmental (glomerular) — *see also* N00-N07 with fourth character .1 N05.1
Friedreich's (spinal cord) G11.11
funicular (spermatic cord) N50.89
general (vascular) — *see* Arteriosclerosis
gland (lymphatic) I89.8
hepatic K74.1
alcoholic K70.2
hereditary
cerebellar G11.9
spinal (Friedreich's ataxia) G11.11
hippocampal G93.81
insular G35
kidney — *see* Sclerosis, renal
larynx J38.7
lateral (amyotrophic) (descending) (spinal) G12.21
primary G12.23
lens, senile nuclear — *see* Cataract, senile, nuclear
liver K74.1
with fibrosis K74.2
alcoholic K70.2
alcoholic K70.2
cardiac K76.1
lung — *see* Fibrosis, lung
mastoid — *see* Mastoiditis, chronic
mesial temporal G93.81
mitral I05.8
Mönckeberg's (medial) — *see* Arteriosclerosis, extremities
multiple (brain stem) (cerebral) (generalized) (spinal cord) G35
myocardium, myocardial — *see* Disease, heart, ischemic, atherosclerotic
nuclear (senile), eye — *see* Cataract, senile, nuclear
ovary N83.8
pancreas K86.89
penis N48.6
peripheral arteries — *see* Arteriosclerosis, extremities
plaques G35
pluriglandular E31.8
polyglandular E31.8
posterolateral (spinal cord) — *see* Degeneration, combined
presenile (Alzheimer's) — *see* Disease, Alzheimer's, early onset
primary, lateral G12.23
progressive, systemic M34.0
pulmonary — *see* Fibrosis, lung
artery I27.0
valve (heart) — *see* Endocarditis, pulmonary
renal N26.9
with
cystine storage disease E72.09
hypertensive heart disease (conditions in I11) — *see* Hypertension, cardiorenal
arteriolar (hyaline) (hyperplastic) — *see* Hypertension, kidney
retina (senile) (vascular) H35.00
senile (vascular) — *see* Arteriosclerosis
spinal (cord) (progressive) G95.89
ascending G61.0
combined — *see also* Degeneration, combined
multiple G35
syphilitic A52.11
disseminated G35

Sequelae — *continued*
- disease — *continued*
  - cerebrovascular — *continued*
    - specified type NEC I69.8Ø
      - alteration of sensation I69.898
      - aphasia I69.82Ø
      - apraxia I69.89Ø
      - ataxia I69.893
      - cognitive deficits I69.81 ☑
      - disturbance of vision I69.898
      - dysarthria I69.822
      - dysphagia I69.891
      - dysphasia I69.821
      - facial droop I69.892
      - facial weakness I69.892
      - fluency disorder I69.823
      - hemiplegia I69.85- ☑
      - language deficit I69.828
      - monoplegia
        - lower limb I69.84- ☑
        - upper limb I69.83- ☑
      - paralytic syndrome I69.86- ☑
      - specified effect NEC I69.898
    - speech deficit I69.928
      - speech deficit I69.828
    - stroke NOS — *see* Sequelae, stroke NOS
- dislocation — *code to* injury with seventh character S
- encephalitis or encephalomyelitis (conditions in GØ4) GØ9
  - in infectious disease NEC B94.8
  - viral B94.1
- external cause — *code to* injury with seventh character S
- foreign body entering natural orifice — *code to* injury with seventh character S
- fracture — *code to* injury with seventh character S
- frostbite — *code to* injury with seventh character S
- Hansen's disease B92
- hemorrhage
  - intracerebral I69.1Ø
    - alteration of sensation I69.198
    - aphasia I69.12Ø
    - apraxia I69.19Ø
    - ataxia I69.193
    - cognitive deficits I69.11 ☑
    - disturbance of vision I69.198
    - dysarthria I69.122
    - dysphagia I69.191
    - dysphasia I69.121
    - facial droop I69.192
    - facial weakness I69.192
    - fluency disorder I69.123
    - hemiplegia I69.15- ☑
    - language deficit NEC I69.128
    - monoplegia
      - lower limb I69.14- ☑
      - upper limb I69.13- ☑
    - paralytic syndrome I69.16- ☑
    - specified effect NEC I69.198
    - speech deficit NEC I69.128
  - intracranial, nontraumatic NEC I69.2Ø
    - alteration of sensation I69.298
    - aphasia I69.22Ø
    - apraxia I69.29Ø
    - ataxia I69.293
    - cognitive deficits I69.21 ☑
    - disturbance of vision I69.298
    - dysarthria I69.222
    - dysphagia I69.291
    - dysphasia I69.221
    - facial droop I69.292
    - facial weakness I69.292
    - fluency disorder I69.223
    - hemiplegia I69.25- ☑
    - language deficit NEC I69.228
    - monoplegia
      - lower limb I69.24- ☑
      - upper limb I69.23- ☑
    - paralytic syndrome I69.26- ☑
    - specified effect NEC I69.298
    - speech deficit NEC I69.228
  - subarachnoid I69.ØØ
    - alteration of sensation I69.Ø98
    - aphasia I69.Ø2Ø
    - apraxia I69.Ø9Ø
    - ataxia I69.Ø93
    - cognitive deficits — *see* subcategory I69.Ø1- ☑
    - disturbance of vision I69.Ø98

Sequelae — *continued*
- hemorrhage — *continued*
  - subarachnoid — *continued*
    - dysarthria I69.Ø22
    - dysphagia I69.Ø91
    - dysphasia I69.Ø21
    - facial droop I69.Ø92
    - facial weakness I69.Ø92
    - fluency disorder I69.Ø23
    - hemiplegia I69.Ø5- ☑
    - language deficit NEC I69.Ø28
    - monoplegia
      - lower limb I69.Ø4- ☑
      - upper limb I69.Ø3- ☑
    - paralytic syndrome I69.Ø6- ☑
    - specified effect NEC I69.Ø98
    - speech deficit NEC I69.Ø28
- hepatitis, viral B94.2
- hyperalimentation E68
- infarction
  - cerebral I69.3Ø
    - alteration of sensation I69.398
    - aphasia I69.32Ø
    - apraxia I69.39Ø
    - ataxia I69.393
    - cognitive deficits I69.31 ☑
    - disturbance of vision I69.398
    - dysarthria I69.322
    - dysphagia I69.391
    - dysphasia I69.321
    - facial droop I69.392
    - facial weakness I69.392
    - fluency disorder I69.323
    - hemiplegia I69.35- ☑
    - language deficit NEC I69.328
    - monoplegia
      - lower limb I69.34- ☑
      - upper limb I69.33- ☑
    - paralytic syndrome I69.36- ☑
    - specified effect NEC I69.398
    - speech deficit NEC I69.328
- infection, pyogenic, intracranial or intraspinal GØ9
- infectious disease B94.9
  - specified NEC B94.8
- injury — *code to* injury with seventh character S
- leprosy B92
- meningitis
  - bacterial (conditions in GØØ) GØ9
  - other or unspecified cause (conditions in GØ3) GØ9
- muscle (and tendon) injury — *code to* injury with seventh character S
- myelitis — *see* Sequelae, encephalitis
- niacin deficiency E64.8
- nutritional deficiency E64.9
  - specified NEC E64.8
- obstetrical condition O94
- parasitic disease B94.9
- phlebitis or thrombophlebitis of intracranial or intraspinal venous sinuses and veins (conditions in GØ8) GØ9
- poisoning — *code to* poisoning with seventh character S
  - nonmedicinal substance — *see* Sequelae, toxic effect, nonmedicinal substance
- poliomyelitis (acute) B91
- pregnancy O94
- protein-energy malnutrition E64.Ø
- puerperium O94
- rickets E64.3
- selenium deficiency E64.8
- sprain and strain — *code to* injury with seventh character S
- stroke NOS I69.3Ø
  - alteration in sensation I69.398
  - aphasia I69.32Ø
  - apraxia I69.39Ø
  - ataxia I69.393
  - cognitive deficits I69.31 ☑
  - disturbance of vision I69.398
  - dysarthria I69.322
  - dysphagia I69.391
  - dysphasia I69.321
  - facial droop I69.392
  - facial weakness I69.392
  - hemiplegia I69.35- ☑
  - language deficit NEC I69.328
  - monoplegia
    - lower limb I69.34- ☑

Sequelae — *continued*
- stroke — *continued*
  - monoplegia — *continued*
    - upper limb I69.33- ☑
  - paralytic syndrome I69.36- ☑
  - specified effect NEC I69.398
  - speech deficit NEC I69.328
- tendon and muscle injury — *code to* injury with seventh character S
- thiamine deficiency E64.8
- trachoma B94.Ø
- tuberculosis B9Ø.9
  - bones and joints B9Ø.2
  - central nervous system B9Ø.Ø
  - genitourinary B9Ø.1
  - pulmonary (respiratory) B9Ø.9
  - specified organs NEC B9Ø.8
- viral
  - encephalitis B94.1
  - hepatitis B94.2
- vitamin deficiency NEC E64.8
  - A E64.1
  - B E64.8
  - C E64.2
- wound, open — *code to* injury with seventh character S

Sequestration — *see also* Sequestrum
- disc — *see* Displacement, intervertebral disc
- lung, congenital Q33.2

Sequestrum
- bone — *see* Osteomyelitis, chronic
- dental M27.2
- jaw bone M27.2
- orbit — *see* Osteomyelitis, orbit
- sinus (accessory) (nasal) — *see* Sinusitis

Sequoiosis lung or pneumonitis J67.8

Serology for syphilis
- doubtful
  - with signs or symptoms — *code by* site and stage under Syphilis
  - follow-up of latent syphilis — *see* Syphilis, latent
- negative, with signs or symptoms — *code by* site and stage under Syphilis
- positive A53.Ø
  - with signs or symptoms — *code by* site and stage under Syphilis
- reactivated A53.Ø

Seroma — *see also* Hematoma
- postprocedural — *see* Complication, postprocedural, seroma
- traumatic, secondary and recurrent T79.2 ☑

Seropurulent — *see* condition

Serositis, multiple K65.8
- pericardial I31.1
- peritoneal K65.8

Serous — *see* condition

Sertoli cell
- adenoma
  - specified site — *see* Neoplasm, benign, by site
  - unspecified site
    - female D27.9
    - male D29.2Ø
- carcinoma
  - specified site — *see* Neoplasm, malignant, by site
  - unspecified site (male) C62.9- ☑
    - female C56.9
- tumor
  - with lipid storage
    - specified site — *see* Neoplasm, benign, by site
    - unspecified site
      - female D27.9
      - male D29.2Ø
  - specified site — *see* Neoplasm, benign, by site
  - unspecified site
    - female D27.9
    - male D29.2Ø

Sertoli-Leydig cell tumor — *see* Neoplasm, benign, by site
- specified site — *see* Neoplasm, benign, by site
- unspecified site
  - female D27.9
  - male D29.2Ø

Serum
- allergy, allergic reaction — *see also* Reaction, serum T8Ø.69 ☑
  - shock — *see also* Shock, anaphylactic T8Ø.59 ☑
- arthritis — *see also* Reaction, serum T8Ø.69 ☑

Serum — *continued*
- complication or reaction NEC — *see also* Reaction, serum T8Ø.69 ☑
- disease NEC — *see also* Reaction, serum T8Ø.69 ☑
- hepatitis — *see also* Hepatitis, viral, type B
  - carrier (suspected) of B18.1
- intoxication — *see also* Reaction, serum T8Ø.69 ☑
- neuritis — *see also* Reaction, serum T8Ø.69 ☑
- neuropathy G61.1
- poisoning NEC — *see also* Reaction, serum T8Ø.69 ☑
- rash NEC — *see also* Reaction, serum T8Ø.69 ☑
- reaction NEC — *see also* Reaction, serum T8Ø.69 ☑
- sickness NEC — *see also* Reaction, serum T8Ø.69 ☑
- urticaria — *see also* Reaction, serum T8Ø.69 ☑

Sesamoiditis M25.8- ☑

Severe sepsis R65.2Ø
- with septic shock R65.21

Sever's disease or osteochondrosis — *see* Osteochondrosis, juvenile, tarsus

Sex
- chromosome mosaics Q97.8
  - lines with various numbers of X chromosomes Q97.2
- education Z7Ø.8
- reassignment surgery status Z87.89Ø

Sextuplet pregnancy — *see* Pregnancy, sextuplet

Sexual
- function, disorder of (psychogenic) F52.9
- immaturity (female) (male) E3Ø.Ø
- impotence (psychogenic) organic origin NEC — *see* Dysfunction, sexual, male
- precocity (constitutional) (cryptogenic)(female) (idiopathic) (male) E3Ø.1

Sexuality, pathologic — *see* Deviation, sexual

Sézary disease C84.1- ☑

Shadow, lung R91.8

Shaking palsy or paralysis — *see* Parkinsonism

Shallowness, acetabulum — *see* Derangement, joint, specified type NEC, hip

Shaver's disease J63.1

Sheath (tendon) — *see* condition

Sheathing, retinal vessels H35.Ø1- ☑

Shedding
- nail L6Ø.8
- premature, primary (deciduous) teeth KØØ.6

Sheehan's disease or syndrome E23.Ø

Shelf, rectal K62.89

Shell teeth KØØ.5

Shellshock (current) F43.Ø
- lasting state — *see* Disorder, post-traumatic stress

Shield kidney Q63.1

Shift
- auditory threshold (temporary) H93.24- ☑
- mediastinal R93.89

Shifting sleep-work schedule (affecting sleep) G47.26

Shiga (-Kruse) **dysentery** AØ3.Ø

Shiga's bacillus AØ3.Ø

Shigella (dysentery) — *see* Dysentery, bacillary

Shigellosis AØ3.9
- Group A AØ3.Ø
- Group B AØ3.1
- Group C AØ3.2
- Group D AØ3.3

Shin splints S86.89- ☑

Shingles — *see* Herpes, zoster

Shipyard disease or eye B3Ø.Ø

Shirodkar suture, in pregnancy — *see* Pregnancy, complicated by, incompetent cervix

Shock R57.9
- with ectopic or molar pregnancy OØ8.3
- adrenal (cortical) (Addisonian) E27.2
- adverse food reaction (anaphylactic) — *see* Shock, anaphylactic, due to food
- allergic — *see* Shock, anaphylactic
- anaphylactic T78.2 ☑
  - chemical — *see* Table of Drugs and Chemicals
  - due to drug or medicinal substance
    - correct substance properly administered T88.6 ☑
    - overdose or wrong substance given or taken (by accident) — *see* Table of Drugs and Chemicals, by drug, poisoning
  - due to food (nonpoisonous) T78.ØØ ☑
    - additives T78.Ø6 ☑
    - dairy products T78.Ø7 ☑
    - eggs T78.Ø8 ☑
    - fish T78.Ø3 ☑
      - shellfish T78.Ø2 ☑
    - fruit T78.Ø4 ☑

Shock — *continued*
- anaphylactic — *continued*
  - due to food — *continued*
    - milk T78.Ø7 ☑
    - nuts T78.Ø5 ☑
      - multiple types T78.Ø5 ☑
      - peanuts T78.Ø1 ☑
    - peanuts T78.Ø1 ☑
    - seeds T78.Ø5 ☑
    - specified type NEC T78.Ø9 ☑
    - vegetable T78.Ø4 ☑
  - following sting(s) — *see* Venom
  - immunization T8Ø.52 ☑
  - serum T8Ø.59 ☑
    - blood and blood products T8Ø.51 ☑
    - immunization T8Ø.52 ☑
    - specified NEC T8Ø.59 ☑
    - vaccination T8Ø.52 ☑
- anaphylactoid — *see* Shock, anaphylactic
- anesthetic
  - correct substance properly administered T88.2 ☑
  - overdose or wrong substance given or taken — *see* Table of Drugs and Chemicals, by drug, poisoning
    - specified anesthetic — *see* Table of Drugs and Chemicals, by drug, poisoning
- cardiogenic R57.Ø
- chemical substance — *see* Table of Drugs and Chemicals
- complicating ectopic or molar pregnancy OØ8.3
- culture — *see* Disorder, adjustment
- drug
  - due to correct substance properly administered T88.6 ☑
  - overdose or wrong substance given or taken (by accident) — *see* Table of Drugs and Chemicals, by drug, poisoning
- during or after labor and delivery O75.1
- electric T75.4 ☑
  - (taser) T75.4 ☑
- endotoxic R65.21
  - postprocedural (resulting from a procedure, not elsewhere classified) T81.12 ☑
- following
  - ectopic or molar pregnancy OØ8.3
  - injury (immediate) (delayed) T79.4 ☑
  - labor and delivery O75.1
- food (anaphylactic) — *see* Shock, anaphylactic, due to food
- from electroshock gun (taser) T75.4 ☑
- gram-negative R65.21
  - postprocedural (resulting from a procedure, not elsewhere classified) T81.12 ☑
- hematologic R57.8
- hemorrhagic R57.8
  - surgery (intraoperative) (postoperative) T81.19 ☑
  - trauma T79.4 ☑
- hypovolemic R57.1
  - surgical T81.19 ☑
  - traumatic T79.4 ☑
- insulin E15
  - therapeutic misadventure — *see* subcategory T38.3 ☑
- kidney N17.Ø
  - traumatic (following crushing) T79.5 ☑
- lightning T75.Ø1 ☑
- liver K72.ØØ
- lung J8Ø
- obstetric O75.1
  - with ectopic or molar pregnancy OØ8.3
  - following ectopic or molar pregnancy OØ8.3
- pleural (surgical) T81.19 ☑
  - due to trauma T79.4 ☑
- postprocedural (postoperative) T81.1Ø ☑
  - with ectopic or molar pregnancy OØ8.3
  - cardiogenic T81.11 ☑
  - endotoxic T81.12 ☑
  - following ectopic or molar pregnancy OØ8.3
  - gram-negative T81.12 ☑
  - hypovolemic T81.19 ☑
  - septic T81.12 ☑
  - specified type NEC T81.19 ☑
- psychic F43.Ø
- septic (due to severe sepsis) R65.21
- specified NEC R57.8
- surgical T81.1Ø ☑
- taser gun (taser) T75.4 ☑

Shock — *continued*
- therapeutic misadventure NEC T81.1Ø ☑
- thyroxin
  - overdose or wrong substance given or taken — *see* Table of Drugs and Chemicals, by drug, poisoning
- toxic, syndrome A48.3
- transfusion — *see* Complications, transfusion
- traumatic (immediate) (delayed) T79.4 ☑

Shoemaker's chest M95.4

Short, shortening, shortness
- arm (acquired) — *see also* Deformity, limb, unequal length
  - congenital Q71.81- ☑
  - forearm — *see* Deformity, limb, unequal length
- bowel syndrome K91.2
- breath RØ6.Ø2
- cervical (complicating pregnancy) O26.87- ☑
  - non-gravid uterus N88.3
- common bile duct, congenital Q44.5
- cord (umbilical), complicating delivery O69.3 ☑
- cystic duct, congenital Q44.5
- esophagus (congenital) Q39.8
- femur (acquired) — *see* Deformity, limb, unequal length, femur
  - congenital — *see* Defect, reduction, lower limb, longitudinal, femur
- frenum, frenulum, linguae (congenital) Q38.1
- hip (acquired) — *see also* Deformity, limb, unequal length
  - congenital Q65.89
- leg (acquired) — *see also* Deformity, limb, unequal length
  - congenital Q72.81- ☑
  - lower leg — *see also* Deformity, limb, unequal length
- limbed stature, with immunodeficiency D82.2
- lower limb (acquired) — *see also* Deformity, limb, unequal length
  - congenital Q72.81- ☑
- organ or site, congenital NEC — *see* Distortion
- palate, congenital Q38.5
- radius (acquired) — *see also* Deformity, limb, unequal length
  - congenital — *see* Defect, reduction, upper limb, longitudinal, radius
- rib syndrome Q77.2
- stature (child) (hereditary) (idiopathic) NEC R62.52
  - constitutional E34.3
  - due to endocrine disorder E34.3
  - Laron-type E34.3
- tendon — *see also* Contraction, tendon
  - with contracture of joint — *see* Contraction, joint
  - Achilles (acquired) M67.Ø- ☑
    - congenital Q66.89
  - congenital Q79.8
- thigh (acquired) — *see also* Deformity, limb, unequal length, femur
  - congenital — *see* Defect, reduction, lower limb, longitudinal, femur
- tibialis anterior (tendon) — *see* Contraction, tendon
- umbilical cord
  - complicating delivery O69.3 ☑
- upper limb, congenital — *see* Defect, reduction, upper limb, specified type NEC
- urethra N36.8
- uvula, congenital Q38.5
- vagina (congenital) Q52.4

Shortsightedness — *see* Myopia

Shoshin (acute fulminating beriberi) E51.11

Shoulder — *see* condition

Shovel-shaped incisors KØØ.2

Shower, thromboembolic — *see* Embolism

Shunt
- arterial-venous (dialysis) Z99.2
- arteriovenous, pulmonary (acquired) I28.Ø
  - congenital Q25.72
- cerebral ventricle (communicating) in situ Z98.2
- surgical, prosthetic, with complications — *see* Complications, cardiovascular, device or implant

Shutdown, renal N28.9

Shy-Drager syndrome G9Ø.3

Sialadenitis, sialadenosis (any gland) (chronic) (periodic) (suppurative) — *see* Sialoadenitis

Sialectasia K11.8

Sialidosis E77.1

Slipped, slipping — *continued*
- vertebra NEC — *see* Spondylolisthesis

Slocumb's syndrome E27.Ø
Sloughing (multiple) (phagedena) (skin) — *see also* Gangrene
- abscess — *see* Abscess
- appendix K38.8
- fascia — *see* Disorder, soft tissue, specified type NEC
- scrotum N5Ø.89
- tendon — *see* Disorder, tendon
- transplanted organ — *see* Rejection, transplant
- ulcer — *see* Ulcer, skin

Slow
- feeding, newborn P92.2
- flow syndrome, coronary I2Ø.8
- heart (beat) RØØ.1

Slowing, urinary stream R39.198
Sluder's neuralgia (syndrome) G44.89
Slurred, slurring speech R47.81
Small (ness)
- for gestational age — *see* Small for dates
- introitus, vagina N89.6
- kidney (unknown cause) N27.9
  - bilateral N27.1
  - unilateral N27.Ø
- ovary (congenital) Q5Ø.39
- pelvis
  - with disproportion (fetopelvic) O33.1
    - causing obstructed labor O65.1
- uterus N85.8
- white kidney NØ3.9

Small-and-light-for-dates — *see* Small for dates
Small-for-dates (infant) PØ5.1Ø
- with weight of
  - 499 grams or less PØ5.11
  - 5ØØ-749 grams PØ5.12
  - 75Ø-999 grams PØ5.13
  - 1ØØØ-1249 grams PØ5.14
  - 125Ø-1499 grams PØ5.15
  - 15ØØ-1749 grams PØ5.16
  - 175Ø-1999 grams PØ5.17
  - 2ØØØ-2499 grams PØ5.18
  - 25ØØ grams and over PØ5.19
- specified NEC PØ5.19

Smallpox BØ3
Smearing, fecal R15.1
SMEI (severe myoclonic epilepsy in infancy) G4Ø.83- ☑
Smith-Lemli-Opitz syndrome E78.72
Smith's fracture S52.54- ☑
Smoker — *see* Dependence, drug, nicotine
Smoker's
- bronchitis J41.Ø
- cough J41.Ø
- palate K13.24
- throat J31.2
- tongue K13.24

Smoking
- passive Z77.22

Smothering spells RØ6.81
Snaggle teeth, tooth M26.39
Snapping
- finger — *see* Trigger finger
- hip — *see* Derangement, joint, specified type NEC, hip
  - involving the iliotiblial band M76.3- ☑
- knee — *see* Derangement, knee
  - involving the iliotiblial band M76.3- ☑

Sneddon-Wilkinson disease or syndrome (sub-corneal pustular dermatosis) L13.1
Sneezing (intractable) RØ6.7
Sniffing
- cocaine
  - abuse — *see* Abuse, drug, cocaine
  - dependence — *see* Dependence, drug, cocaine
- gasoline
  - abuse — *see* Abuse, drug, inhalant
  - dependence — *see* Dependence, drug, inhalant
- glue (airplane)
  - abuse — *see* Abuse, drug, inhalant
  - drug dependence — *see* Dependence, drug, inhalant

Sniffles
- newborn P28.89

Snoring RØ6.83
Snow blindness — *see* Photokeratitis
Snuffles (non-syphilitic) RØ6.5
- newborn P28.89
- syphilitic (infant) A5Ø.Ø5 *[J99]*

Social
- exclusion Z6Ø.4
  - due to discrimination or persecution (perceived) Z6Ø.5
- migrant Z59.Ø
  - acculturation difficulty Z6Ø.3
- rejection Z6Ø.4
  - due to discrimination or persecution Z6Ø.5
- role conflict NEC Z73.5
- skills inadequacy NEC Z73.4
- transplantation Z6Ø.3

Sodoku A25.Ø
Soemmerring's ring — *see* Cataract, secondary
Soft — *see also* condition
- nails L6Ø.3

Softening
- bone — *see* Osteomalacia
- brain (necrotic) (progressive) G93.89
  - congenital QØ4.8
  - embolic I63.4- ☑
  - hemorrhagic — *see* Hemorrhage, intracranial, intracerebral
  - occlusive I63.5- ☑
  - thrombotic I63.3- ☑
- cartilage M94.2- ☑
  - patella M22.4- ☑
- cerebellar — *see* Softening, brain
- cerebral — *see* Softening, brain
- cerebrospinal — *see* Softening, brain
- myocardial, heart — *see* Degeneration, myocardial
- spinal cord G95.89
- stomach K31.89

Soldier's
- heart F45.8
- patches I31.Ø

Solitary
- cyst, kidney N28.1
- kidney, congenital Q6Ø.Ø

Solvent abuse — *see* Abuse, drug, inhalant
- dependence — *see* Dependence, drug, inhalant

Somatization reaction, somatic reaction — *see* Disorder, somatoform
Somnambulism F51.3
- hysterical F44.89

Somnolence R4Ø.Ø
- nonorganic origin F51.11

Sonne dysentery AØ3.3
Soor B37.Ø
Sore
- bed — *see* Ulcer, pressure, by site
- chiclero B55.1
- Delhi B55.1
- desert — *see* Ulcer, skin
- eye H57.1- ☑
- Lahore B55.1
- mouth K13.79
  - canker K12.Ø
- muscle M79.1Ø
- Naga — *see* Ulcer, skin
- of skin — *see* Ulcer, skin
- oriental B55.1
- pressure — *see* Ulcer, pressure, by site
- skin L98.9
- soft A57
- throat (acute) — *see also* Pharyngitis
  - with influenza, flu, or grippe — *see* Influenza, with, respiratory manifestations NEC
  - chronic J31.2
  - coxsackie (virus) BØ8.5
  - diphtheritic A36.Ø
  - herpesviral BØØ.2
  - influenzal — *see* Influenza, with, respiratory manifestations NEC
  - septic JØ2.Ø
  - streptococcal (ulcerative) JØ2.Ø
  - viral NEC JØ2.8
    - coxsackie BØ8.5
- tropical — *see* Ulcer, skin
- veldt — *see* Ulcer, skin

Soto's syndrome (cerebral gigantism) Q87.3
South African cardiomyopathy syndrome I42.8
Southeast Asian hemorrhagic fever A91
Spacing
- abnormal, tooth, teeth, fully erupted M26.3Ø
- excessive, tooth, fully erupted M26.32

Spade-like hand (congenital) Q68.1
Spading nail L6Ø.8

Spading nail — *continued*
- congenital Q84.6

Spanish collar N47.1
Sparganosis B7Ø.1
Spasm(s), spastic, spasticity — *see also* condition R25.2
- accommodation — *see* Spasm, of accommodation
- ampulla of Vater K83.4
- anus, ani (sphincter) (reflex) K59.4
  - psychogenic F45.8
- artery I73.9
  - cerebral G45.9
- Bell's G51.3- ☑
- bladder (sphincter, external or internal) N32.89
  - psychogenic F45.8
- bronchus, bronchiole J98.Ø1
- cardia K22.Ø
- cardiac I2Ø.1
- carpopedal — *see* Tetany
- cerebral (arteries) (vascular) G45.9
- cervix, complicating delivery O62.4
- ciliary body (of accommodation) — *see* Spasm, of accommodation
- colon — *see also* Irritable, bowel K58.9
  - with diarrhea K58.Ø
  - psychogenic F45.8
- common duct K83.8
- compulsive — *see* Tic
- conjugate H51.8
- coronary (artery) I2Ø.1
- diaphragm (reflex) RØ6.6
  - epidemic B33.Ø
  - psychogenic F45.8
- duodenum K59.89
- epidemic diaphragmatic (transient) B33.Ø
- esophagus (diffuse) K22.4
  - psychogenic F45.8
- facial G51.3- ☑
- fallopian tube N83.8
- gastrointestinal (tract) K31.89
  - psychogenic F45.8
- glottis J38.5
  - hysterical F44.4
  - psychogenic F45.8
    - conversion reaction F44.4
  - reflex through recurrent laryngeal nerve J38.5
- habit — *see* Tic
- heart I2Ø.1
- hemifacial (clonic) G51.3- ☑
- hourglass — *see* Contraction, hourglass
- hysterical F44.4
- infantile — *see* Epilepsy, spasms
- inferior oblique, eye H51.8
- intestinal — *see also* Syndrome, irritable bowel K58.9
  - psychogenic F45.8
- larynx, laryngeal J38.5
  - hysterical F44.4
  - psychogenic F45.8
    - conversion reaction F44.4
- levator palpebrae superioris — *see* Disorder, eyelid function
- muscle NEC M62.838
  - back M62.83Ø
- nerve, trigeminal G51.Ø
- nervous F45.8
- nodding F98.4
- occupational F48.8
- oculogyric H51.8
  - psychogenic F45.8
- of accommodation H52.53- ☑
- ophthalmic artery — *see* Occlusion, artery, retina
- perineal, female N94.89
- peroneo-extensor — *see also* Deformity, limb, flat foot
- pharynx (reflex) J39.2
  - hysterical F45.8
  - psychogenic F45.8
- psychogenic F45.8
- pylorus NEC K31.3
  - adult hypertrophic K31.89
  - congenital or infantile Q4Ø.Ø
  - psychogenic F45.8
- rectum (sphincter) K59.4
  - psychogenic F45.8
- retinal (artery) — *see* Occlusion, artery, retina
- sigmoid — *see also* Syndrome, irritable bowel K58.9
  - psychogenic F45.8
- sphincter of Oddi K83.4
- stomach K31.89
  - neurotic F45.8

Spondylopathy — *continued*
- infective — *continued*
  - cervical region M46.52
  - cervicothoracic region M46.53
  - lumbar region M46.56
  - lumbosacral region M46.57
  - multiple sites M46.59
  - occipito-atlanto-axial region M46.51
  - sacrococcygeal region M46.58
  - thoracic region M46.54
  - thoracolumbar region M46.55
- inflammatory M46.9Ø
  - cervical region M46.92
  - cervicothoracic region M46.93
  - lumbar region M46.96
  - lumbosacral region M46.97
  - multiple sites M46.99
  - occipito-atlanto-axial region M46.91
  - sacrococcygeal region M46.98
  - specified type NEC M46.8Ø
    - cervical region M46.82
    - cervicothoracic region M46.83
    - lumbar region M46.86
    - lumbosacral region M46.87
    - multiple sites M46.89
    - occipito-atlanto-axial region M46.81
    - sacrococcygeal region M46.88
    - thoracic region M46.84
    - thoracolumbar region M46.85
  - thoracic region M46.94
  - thoracolumbar region M46.95
- neuropathic, in
  - syringomyelia and syringobulbia G95.Ø
  - tabes dorsalis A52.11
- specified NEC — *see* subcategory M48.8 ☑
- traumatic M48.3Ø
  - cervical region M48.32
  - cervicothoracic region M48.33
  - lumbar region M48.36
  - lumbosacral region M48.37
  - occipito-atlanto-axial region M48.31
  - sacrococcygeal region M48.38
  - thoracic region M48.34
  - thoracolumbar region M48.35

Spondylosis M47.9
- with
  - disproportion (fetopelvic) O33.Ø
    - causing obstructed labor O65.Ø
  - myelopathy NEC M47.1Ø
    - cervical region M47.12
    - cervicothoracic region M47.13
    - lumbar region M47.16
    - occipito-atlanto-axial region M47.11
    - thoracic region M47.14
    - thoracolumbar region M47.15
  - radiculopathy M47.2Ø
    - cervical region M47.22
    - cervicothoracic region M47.23
    - lumbar region M47.26
    - lumbosacral region M47.27
    - occipito-atlanto-axial region M47.21
    - sacrococcygeal region M47.28
    - thoracic region M47.24
    - thoracolumbar region M47.25
- specified NEC M47.899
  - cervical region M47.892
  - cervicothoracic region M47.893
  - lumbar region M47.896
  - lumbosacral region M47.897
  - occipito-atlanto-axial region M47.891
  - sacrococcygeal region M47.898
  - thoracic region M47.894
  - thoracolumbar region M47.895
- traumatic — *see* Spondylopathy, traumatic
- without myelopathy or radiculopathy M47.819
  - cervical region M47.812
  - cervicothoracic region M47.813
  - lumbar region M47.816
  - lumbosacral region M47.817
  - occipito-atlanto-axial region M47.811
  - sacrococcygeal region M47.818
  - thoracic region M47.814
  - thoracolumbar region M47.815

Sponge
- inadvertently left in operation wound — *see* Foreign body, accidentally left during a procedure
- kidney (medullary) Q61.5

Sponge-diver's disease — *see* Toxicity, venom, marine animal, sea anemone

Spongioblastoma (any type) — *see* Neoplasm, malignant, by site
- specified site — *see* Neoplasm, malignant, by site
- unspecified site C71.9

Spongioneuroblastoma — *see* Neoplasm, malignant, by site

Spontaneous — *see also* condition
- fracture (cause unknown) — *see* Fracture, pathological

Spoon nail L6Ø.3
- congenital Q84.6

Sporadic — *see* condition

Sporothrix schenckii infection — *see* Sporotrichosis

Sporotrichosis B42.9
- arthritis B42.82
- disseminated B42.7
- generalized B42.7
- lymphocutaneous (fixed) (progressive) B42.1
- pulmonary B42.Ø
- specified NEC B42.89

Spots, spotting (in) (of)
- Bitot's — *see also* Pigmentation, conjunctiva
  - in the young child E5Ø.1
  - vitamin A deficiency E5Ø.1
- café, au lait L81.3
- Cayenne pepper I78.1
- cotton wool, retina — *see* Occlusion, artery, retina
- de Morgan's (senile angiomas) I78.1
- Fuchs' black (myopic) — *see also* Myopia, degenerative H44.2- ☑
- intermenstrual (regular) N92.Ø
  - irregular N92.1
- Koplik's BØ5.9
- liver L81.4
- pregnancy O26.85- ☑
- purpuric R23.3
- ruby I78.1

Spotted fever — *see* Fever, spotted A77.9

Sprain (joint) (ligament)
- acromioclavicular joint or ligament S43.5- ☑
- ankle S93.4Ø- ☑
  - calcaneofibular ligament S93.41- ☑
  - deltoid ligament S93.42- ☑
  - internal collateral ligament — *see* Sprain, ankle, specified ligament NEC
  - specified ligament NEC S93.49- ☑
  - talofibular ligament — *see* Sprain, ankle, specified ligament NEC
  - tibiofibular ligament S93.43- ☑
- anterior longitudinal, cervical S13.4 ☑
- atlas, atlanto-axial, atlanto-occipital S13.4 ☑
- breast bone — *see* Sprain, sternum
- calcaneofibular — *see* Sprain, ankle
- carpal — *see* Sprain, wrist
- carpometacarpal — *see* Sprain, hand, specified site NEC
- cartilage
  - costal S23.41 ☑
  - semilunar (knee) — *see* Sprain, knee, specified site NEC
    - with current tear — *see* Tear, meniscus
  - thyroid region S13.5 ☑
  - xiphoid — *see* Sprain, sternum
- cervical, cervicodorsal, cervicothoracic S13.4 ☑
- chondrosternal S23.421 ☑
- coracoclavicular S43.8- ☑
- coracohumeral S43.41- ☑
- coronary, knee — *see* Sprain, knee, specified site NEC
- costal cartilage S23.41 ☑
- cricoarytenoid articulation or ligament S13.5 ☑
- cricothyroid articulation S13.5 ☑
- cruciate, knee — *see* Sprain, knee, cruciate
- deltoid, ankle — *see* Sprain, ankle
- dorsal (spine) S23.3 ☑
- elbow S53.4Ø- ☑
  - radial collateral ligament S53.43- ☑
  - radiohumeral S53.41- ☑
  - rupture
    - radial collateral ligament — *see* Rupture, traumatic, ligament, radial collateral
    - ulnar collateral ligament — *see* Rupture, traumatic, ligament, ulnar collateral
  - specified type NEC S53.49- ☑
  - ulnar collateral ligament S53.44- ☑
  - ulnohumeral S53.42- ☑
- femur, head — *see* Sprain, hip

Sprain — *continued*
- fibular collateral, knee — *see* Sprain, knee, collateral
- fibulocalcaneal — *see* Sprain, ankle
- finger(s) S63.61- ☑
  - index S63.61- ☑
  - interphalangeal (joint) S63.63- ☑
    - index S63.63- ☑
    - little S63.63- ☑
    - middle S63.63- ☑
    - ring S63.63- ☑
  - little S63.61- ☑
  - metacarpophalangeal (joint) S63.65- ☑
  - middle S63.61- ☑
  - ring S63.61- ☑
  - specified site NEC S63.69- ☑
    - index S63.69- ☑
    - little S63.69- ☑
    - middle S63.69- ☑
    - ring S63.69- ☑
- foot S93.6Ø- ☑
  - specified ligament NEC S93.69- ☑
  - tarsal ligament S93.61- ☑
  - tarsometatarsal ligament S93.62- ☑
  - toe — *see* Sprain, toe
- hand S63.9- ☑
  - finger — *see* Sprain, finger
  - specified site NEC — *see* subcategory S63.8 ☑
  - thumb — *see* Sprain, thumb
- head SØ3.9 ☑
- hip S73.1Ø- ☑
  - iliofemoral ligament S73.11- ☑
  - ischiocapsular (ligament) S73.12- ☑
  - specified NEC S73.19- ☑
- iliofemoral — *see* Sprain, hip
- innominate
  - acetabulum — *see* Sprain, hip
  - sacral junction S33.6 ☑
- internal
  - collateral, ankle — *see* Sprain, ankle
  - semilunar cartilage — *see* Sprain, knee, specified site NEC
- interphalangeal
  - finger — *see* Sprain, finger, interphalangeal (joint)
  - toe — *see* Sprain, toe, interphalangeal joint
- ischiocapsular — *see* Sprain, hip
- ischiofemoral — *see* Sprain, hip
- jaw (articular disc) (cartilage) (meniscus) SØ3.4- ☑
  - old M26.69
- knee S83.9- ☑
  - collateral ligament S83.4Ø- ☑
    - lateral (fibular) S83.42- ☑
    - medial (tibial) S83.41- ☑
  - cruciate ligament S83.5Ø- ☑
    - anterior S83.51- ☑
    - posterior S83.52- ☑
  - lateral (fibular) collateral ligament S83.42- ☑
  - medial (tibial) collateral ligament S83.41- ☑
  - patellar ligament S76.11- ☑
  - specified site NEC S83.8X- ☑
  - superior tibiofibular joint (ligament) S83.6- ☑
- lateral collateral, knee — *see* Sprain, knee, collateral
- lumbar (spine) S33.5 ☑
- lumbosacral S33.9 ☑
- mandible (articular disc) SØ3.4- ☑
  - old M26.69
- medial collateral, knee — *see* Sprain, knee, collateral
- meniscus
  - jaw SØ3.4- ☑
    - old M26.69
  - knee — *see* Sprain, knee, specified site NEC
    - with current tear — *see* Tear, meniscus
      - old — *see* Derangement, knee, meniscus, due to old tear
  - mandible SØ3.4- ☑
    - old M26.69
- metacarpal (distal) (proximal) — *see* Sprain, hand, specified site NEC
- metacarpophalangeal — *see* Sprain, finger, metacarpophalangeal (joint)
- metatarsophalangeal — *see* Sprain, toe, metatarsophalangeal joint
- midcarpal — *see* Sprain, hand, specified site NEC
- midtarsal — *see* Sprain, foot, specified site NEC
- neck S13.9 ☑
  - anterior longitudinal cervical ligament S13.4 ☑
  - atlanto-axial joint S13.4 ☑

- **Sprain** — *continued*
  - neck — *continued*
    - atlanto-occipital joint S13.4 ☑
    - cervical spine S13.4 ☑
    - cricoarytenoid ligament S13.5 ☑
    - cricothyroid ligament S13.5 ☑
    - specified site NEC S13.8 ☑
    - thyroid region (cartilage) S13.5 ☑
  - nose SØ3.8 ☑
  - orbicular, hip — *see* Sprain, hip
  - patella — *see* Sprain, knee, specified site NEC
  - patellar ligament S76.11- ☑
  - pelvis NEC S33.8 ☑
  - phalanx
    - finger — *see* Sprain, finger
    - toe — *see* Sprain, toe
  - pubofemoral — *see* Sprain, hip
  - radiocarpal — *see* Sprain, wrist
  - radiohumeral — *see* Sprain, elbow
  - radius, collateral — *see* Rupture, traumatic, ligament, radial collateral
  - rib (cage) S23.41 ☑
  - rotator cuff (capsule) S43.42- ☑
  - sacroiliac (region)
    - chronic or old — *see* subcategory M53.2 ☑
    - joint S33.6 ☑
  - scaphoid (hand) — *see* Sprain, hand, specified site NEC
  - scapula (r) — *see* Sprain, shoulder girdle, specified site NEC
  - semilunar cartilage (knee) — *see* Sprain, knee, specified site NEC
    - with current tear — *see* Tear, meniscus
      - old — *see* Derangement, knee, meniscus, due to old tear
  - shoulder joint S43.4Ø- ☑
    - acromioclavicular joint (ligament) — *see* Sprain, acromioclavicular joint
    - blade — *see* Sprain, shoulder, girdle, specified site NEC
    - coracoclavicular joint (ligament) — *see* Sprain, coracoclavicular joint
    - coracohumeral ligament — *see* Sprain, coracohumeral joint
    - girdle S43.9- ☑
      - specified site NEC S43.8- ☑
    - rotator cuff — *see* Sprain, rotator cuff
    - specified site NEC S43.49- ☑
    - sternoclavicular joint (ligament) — *see* Sprain, sternoclavicular joint
  - spine
    - cervical S13.4 ☑
    - lumbar S33.5 ☑
    - thoracic S23.3 ☑
  - sternoclavicular joint S43.6- ☑
  - sternum S23.429 ☑
    - chondrosternal joint S23.421 ☑
    - specified site NEC S23.428 ☑
    - sternoclavicular (joint) (ligament) S23.42Ø ☑
  - symphysis
    - jaw SØ3.4- ☑
      - old M26.69
    - mandibular SØ3.4- ☑
      - old M26.69
  - talofibular — *see* Sprain, ankle
  - tarsal — *see* Sprain, foot, specified site NEC
  - tarsometatarsal — *see* Sprain, foot, specified site NEC
  - temporomandibular SØ3.4- ☑
    - old M26.69
  - thorax S23.9 ☑
    - ribs S23.41 ☑
    - specified site NEC S23.8 ☑
    - spine S23.3 ☑
    - sternum — *see* Sprain, sternum
  - thumb S63.6Ø- ☑
    - interphalangeal (joint) S63.62- ☑
    - metacarpophalangeal (joint) S63.64- ☑
    - specified site NEC S63.68- ☑
  - thyroid cartilage or region S13.5 ☑
  - tibia (proximal end) — *see* Sprain, knee, specified site NEC
  - tibial collateral, knee — *see* Sprain, knee, collateral
  - tibiofibular
    - distal — *see* Sprain, ankle
    - superior — *see* Sprain, knee, specified site NEC
  - toe(s) S93.5Ø- ☑
    - great S93.5Ø- ☑

- **Sprain** — *continued*
  - toe(s) — *continued*
    - interphalangeal joint S93.51- ☑
      - great S93.51- ☑
      - lesser S93.51- ☑
    - lesser S93.5Ø- ☑
    - metatarsophalangeal joint S93.52- ☑
      - great S93.52- ☑
      - lesser S93.52- ☑
  - ulna, collateral — *see* Rupture, traumatic, ligament, ulnar collateral
  - ulnohumeral — *see* Sprain, elbow
  - wrist S63.5Ø- ☑
    - carpal S63.51- ☑
    - radiocarpal S63.52- ☑
    - specified site NEC S63.59- ☑
  - xiphoid cartilage — *see* Sprain, sternum
- **Sprengel's deformity** (congenital) Q74.Ø
- **Sprue** (tropical) K9Ø.1
  - celiac K9Ø.Ø
  - idiopathic K9Ø.49
  - meaning thrush B37.Ø
  - nontropical K9Ø.Ø
- **Spur, bone** — *see also* Enthesopathy
  - calcaneal M77.3- ☑
  - iliac crest M76.2- ☑
  - nose (septum) J34.89
- **Spurway's syndrome** Q78.Ø
- **Sputum**
  - abnormal (amount) (color) (odor) (purulent) RØ9.3
  - blood-stained RØ4.2
  - excessive (cause unknown) RØ9.3
- **Squamous** — *see also* condition
  - epithelium in
    - cervical canal (congenital) Q51.828
    - uterine mucosa (congenital) Q51.818
- **Squashed nose** M95.Ø
  - congenital Q67.4
- **Squeeze, diver's** T7Ø.3 ☑
- **Squint** — *see also* Strabismus
  - accommodative — *see* Strabismus, convergent concomitant
- **SSADHD** (succinic semialdehyde dehydrogenase deficiency) E72.81
- **St. Hubert's disease** A82.9
- **Stab** — *see also* Laceration
  - internal organs — *see* Injury, by site
- **Stafne's cyst or cavity** M27.Ø
- **Staggering gait** R26.Ø
  - hysterical F44.4
- **Staghorn calculus** — *see* Calculus, kidney
- **Stähli's line** (cornea) (pigment) — *see* Pigmentation, cornea, anterior
- **Stain, staining**
  - meconium (newborn) P96.83
  - port wine Q82.5
  - tooth, teeth (hard tissues) (extrinsic) KØ3.6
    - due to
      - accretions KØ3.6
      - deposits (betel) (black) (green) (materia alba) (orange) (soft) (tobacco) KØ3.6
      - metals (copper) (silver) KØ3.7
      - nicotine KØ3.6
      - pulpal bleeding KØ3.7
      - tobacco KØ3.6
    - intrinsic KØØ.8
- **Stammering** — *see also* Disorder, fluency F8Ø.81
- **Standstill**
  - auricular I45.5
  - cardiac — *see* Arrest, cardiac
  - sinoatrial I45.5
  - ventricular — *see* Arrest, cardiac
- **Stannosis** J63.5
- **Stanton's disease** — *see* Melioidosis
- **Staphylitis** (acute) (catarrhal) (chronic) (gangrenous) (membranous) (suppurative) (ulcerative) K12.2
- **Staphylococcal scalded skin syndrome** LØØ
- **Staphylococcemia** A41.2
- **Staphylococcus, staphylococcal** — *see also* condition
  - as cause of disease classified elsewhere B95.8
    - aureus (methicillin susceptible) (MSSA) B95.61
      - methicillin resistant (MRSA) B95.62
  - specified NEC, as cause of disease classified elsewhere B95.7
- **Staphyloma** (sclera)
  - cornea H18.72- ☑
  - equatorial H15.81- ☑

- **Staphyloma** — *continued*
  - localized (anterior) H15.82- ☑
  - posticum H15.83- ☑
  - ring H15.85- ☑
- **Stargardt's disease** — *see* Dystrophy, retina
- **Starvation** (inanition) (due to lack of food) T73.Ø ☑
  - edema — *see* Malnutrition, severe
- **Stasis**
  - bile (noncalculous) K83.1
  - bronchus J98.Ø9
    - with infection — *see* Bronchitis
  - cardiac — *see* Failure, heart, congestive
  - cecum K59.89
  - colon K59.89
  - dermatitis I87.2
    - with
      - varicose ulcer — *see* Varix, leg, with ulcer, with inflammation
      - varicose veins — *see* Varix, leg, with, inflammation
    - due to postthrombotic syndrome — *see* Syndrome, postthrombotic
  - duodenal K31.5
  - eczema — *see* Varix, leg, with, inflammation
  - edema — *see* Hypertension, venous (chronic), idiopathic
  - foot T69.Ø- ☑
  - ileocecal coil K59.89
  - ileum K59.89
  - intestinal K59.89
  - jejunum K59.89
  - kidney N19
  - liver (cirrhotic) K76.1
  - lymphatic I89.8
  - pneumonia J18.2
  - pulmonary — *see* Edema, lung
  - rectal K59.89
  - renal N19
    - tubular N17.Ø
  - ulcer — *see* Varix, leg, with, ulcer
    - without varicose veins I87.2
  - urine — *see* Retention, urine
  - venous I87.8
- **State** (of)
  - affective and paranoid, mixed, organic psychotic FØ6.8
  - agitated R45.1
    - acute reaction to stress F43.Ø
  - anxiety (neurotic) F41.1
  - apprehension F41.1
  - burn-out Z73.Ø
  - climacteric, female Z78.Ø
    - symptomatic N95.1
  - compulsive F42.8
    - mixed with obsessional thoughts F42.2
  - confusional (psychogenic) F44.89
    - acute — *see also* Delirium
      - with
        - arteriosclerotic dementia FØ1.5Ø
          - with behavioral disturbance FØ1.51
        - senility or dementia FØ5
      - alcoholic F1Ø.231
    - epileptic FØ5
    - reactive (from emotional stress, psychological trauma) F44.89
    - subacute — *see* Delirium
  - convulsive — *see* Convulsions
  - crisis F43.Ø
  - depressive F32.9
    - neurotic F34.1
  - dissociative F44.9
  - emotional shock (stress) R45.7
  - hypercoagulation — *see* Hypercoagulable
  - locked-in G83.5
  - menopausal Z78.Ø
    - symptomatic N95.1
  - neurotic F48.9
    - with depersonalization F48.1
  - obsessional F42.8
  - oneiroid (schizophrenia-like) F23
  - organic
    - hallucinatory (nonalcoholic) FØ6.Ø
    - paranoid (-hallucinatory) FØ6.2
  - panic F41.Ø
  - paranoid F22
    - climacteric F22
    - involutional F22
    - menopausal F22
    - organic FØ6.2

Index

Stenosis, stenotic — Stenosis, stenotic

- **Stenosis, stenotic** — *continued*
  - neural canal — *see also* Lesion, biomechanical, specified — *continued*
    - osseous — *continued*
      - abdomen M99.39
      - cervical region M99.31
      - cervicothoracic M99.31
      - head region M99.30
      - lower extremity M99.36
      - lumbar region M99.33
      - lumbosacral M99.33
      - occipitocervical M99.30
      - pelvic M99.35
      - rib cage M99.38
      - sacral region M99.34
      - sacrococcygeal M99.34
      - sacroiliac M99.34
      - specified NEC M99.39
      - thoracic region M99.32
      - thoracolumbar M99.32
      - upper extremity M99.37
    - subluxation M99.29
      - cervical region M99.21
      - cervicothoracic M99.21
      - head region M99.20
      - lower extremity M99.26
      - lumbar region M99.23
      - lumbosacral M99.23
      - occipitocervical M99.20
      - pelvic M99.25
      - rib cage M99.28
      - sacral region M99.24
      - sacrococcygeal M99.24
      - sacroiliac M99.24
      - specified NEC M99.29
      - thoracic region M99.22
      - thoracolumbar M99.22
      - upper extremity M99.27
  - organ or site, congenital NEC — *see* Atresia, by site
  - papilla of Vater K83.1
  - pulmonary (artery) (congenital) Q25.6
    - with ventricular septal defect, transposition of aorta, and hypertrophy of right ventricle Q21.3
    - acquired I28.8
    - in tetralogy of Fallot Q21.3
    - infundibular Q24.3
    - subvalvular Q24.3
    - supravalvular Q25.6
    - valve I37.0
      - with insufficiency I37.2
      - congenital Q22.1
      - rheumatic I09.89
        - with aortic, mitral or tricuspid (valve) disease I08.8
    - vein, acquired I28.8
    - vessel NEC I28.8
  - pulmonic (congenital) Q22.1
    - infundibular Q24.3
    - subvalvular Q24.3
  - pylorus (hypertrophic) (acquired) K31.1
    - adult K31.1
    - congenital Q40.0
    - infantile Q40.0
  - rectum (sphincter) — *see* Stricture, rectum
  - renal artery I70.1
    - congenital Q27.1
  - salivary duct (any) K11.8
  - sphincter of Oddi K83.1
  - spinal M48.00
    - cervical region M48.02
    - cervicothoracic region M48.03
    - lumbar region (NOS) (without neurogenic claudication) M48.061
      - with neurogenic claudication M48.062
    - lumbosacral region M48.07
    - occipito-atlanto-axial region M48.01
    - sacrococcygeal region M48.08
    - thoracic region M48.04
    - thoracolumbar region M48.05
  - stomach, hourglass K31.2
  - subaortic (congenital) Q24.4
    - hypertrophic (idiopathic) I42.1
  - subglottic J38.6
    - congenital Q31.1
    - postprocedural J95.5
  - trachea J39.8
    - congenital Q32.1
    - syphilitic A52.73
    - tuberculous NEC A15.5

- **Stenosis, stenotic** — *continued*
  - tracheostomy J95.03
  - tricuspid (valve) I07.0
    - with
      - aortic (valve) disease I08.2
      - incompetency, insufficiency or regurgitation I07.2
        - with aortic (valve) disease I08.2
          - with mitral (valve) disease I08.3
      - mitral (valve) disease I08.1
        - with aortic (valve) disease I08.3
    - congenital Q22.4
    - nonrheumatic I36.0
      - with insufficiency I36.2
  - tubal N97.1
  - ureter — *see* Atresia, ureter
  - ureteropelvic junction, congenital Q62.11
  - ureterovesical orifice, congenital Q62.12
  - urethra (valve) *see also* Stricture, urethra
    - congenital Q64.32
  - urinary meatus, congenital Q64.33
  - vagina N89.5
    - congenital Q52.4
    - in pregnancy — *see* Pregnancy, complicated by, abnormal vagina
      - causing obstructed labor O65.5
  - valve (cardiac) (heart) — *see also* Endocarditis I38
    - congenital Q24.8
      - aortic Q23.0
      - mitral Q23.2
      - pulmonary Q22.1
      - tricuspid Q22.4
  - vena cava (inferior) (superior) I87.1
    - congenital Q26.0
  - vesicourethral orifice Q64.31
  - vulva N90.5
- **Stent jail** T82.897 ☑
- **Stercolith** (impaction) K56.41
  - appendix K38.1
- **Stercoraceous, stercoral ulcer** K63.3
  - anus or rectum K62.6
- **Stereotypies NEC** F98.4
- **Sterility** — *see* Infertility
- **Sterilization** — *see* Encounter (for), sterilization
- **Sternalgia** — *see* Angina
- **Sternopagus** Q89.4
- **Sternum bifidum** Q76.7
- **Steroid**
  - effects (adverse) (adrenocortical) (iatrogenic)
    - cushingoid E24.2
      - correct substance properly administered — *see* Table of Drugs and Chemicals, by drug, adverse effect
      - overdose or wrong substance given or taken — *see* Table of Drugs and Chemicals, by drug, poisoning
    - diabetes — *see* subcategory E09 ☑
      - correct substance properly administered — *see* Table of Drugs and Chemicals, by drug, adverse effect
      - overdose or wrong substance given or taken — *see* Table of Drugs and Chemicals, by drug, poisoning
    - fever R50.2
    - insufficiency E27.3
      - correct substance properly administered — *see* Table of Drugs and Chemicals, by drug, adverse effect
      - overdose or wrong substance given or taken — *see* Table of Drugs and Chemicals, by drug, poisoning
  - responder H40.04- ☑
- **Stevens-Johnson disease or syndrome** L51.1
  - toxic epidermal necrolysis overlap L51.3
- **Stewart-Morel syndrome** M85.2
- **Sticker's disease** B08.3
- **Sticky eye** — *see* Conjunctivitis, acute, mucopurulent
- **Stieda's disease** — *see* Bursitis, tibial collateral
- **Stiff neck** — *see* Torticollis
- **Stiff-man syndrome** G25.82
- **Stiffness, joint NEC** M25.60
  - ankle M25.67- ☑
  - ankylosis — *see* Ankylosis, joint
  - contracture — *see* Contraction, joint
  - elbow M25.62- ☑
  - foot M25.67- ☑
  - hand M25.64- ☑

- **Stiffness, joint** — *continued*
  - hip M25.65- ☑
  - knee M25.66- ☑
  - shoulder M25.61- ☑
  - specified site NEC M25.69
  - wrist M25.63- ☑
- **Stigmata congenital syphilis** A50.59
- **Stillbirth** P95
- **Still-Felty syndrome** — *see* Felty's syndrome
- **Still's disease or syndrome** (juvenile) M08.20
  - adult-onset M06.1
  - ankle M08.27- ☑
  - elbow M08.22- ☑
  - foot joint M08.27- ☑
  - hand joint M08.24- ☑
  - hip M08.25- ☑
  - knee M08.26- ☑
  - multiple site M08.29
  - shoulder M08.21- ☑
  - specified site NEC M08.2A
  - vertebra M08.28
  - wrist M08.23- ☑
- **Stimulation, ovary** E28.1
- **Sting** (venomous) (with allergic or anaphylactic shock) — *see* Table of Drugs and Chemicals, by animal or substance, poisoning
- **Stippled epiphyses** Q78.8
- **Stitch**
  - abscess T81.41 ☑
  - burst (in operation wound) — *see* Disruption, wound, operation
- **Stokes' disease** E05.00
  - with thyroid storm E05.01
- **Stokes-Adams disease or syndrome** I45.9
- **Stokvis** (-Talma) **disease** D74.8
- **Stoma malfunction**
  - colostomy K94.03
  - enterostomy K94.13
  - gastrostomy K94.23
  - ileostomy K94.13
  - tracheostomy J95.03
- **Stomach** — *see* condition
- **Stomatitis** (denture) (ulcerative) K12.1
  - angular K13.0
    - due to dietary or vitamin deficiency E53.0
  - aphthous K12.0
  - bovine B08.61
  - candidal B37.0
  - catarrhal K12.1
  - diphtheritic A36.89
  - due to
    - dietary deficiency E53.0
    - thrush B37.0
    - vitamin deficiency
      - B group NEC E53.9
      - B2 (riboflavin) E53.0
  - epidemic B08.8
  - epizootic B08.8
  - follicular K12.1
  - gangrenous A69.0
  - Geotrichum B48.3
  - herpesviral, herpetic B00.2
  - herpetiformis K12.0
  - malignant K12.1
  - membranous acute K12.1
  - monilial B37.0
  - mycotic B37.0
  - necrotizing ulcerative A69.0
  - parasitic B37.0
  - septic K12.1
  - spirochetal A69.1
  - suppurative (acute) K12.2
  - ulceromembranous A69.1
  - vesicular K12.1
    - with exanthem (enteroviral) B08.4
    - virus disease A93.8
  - Vincent's A69.1
- **Stomatocytosis** D58.8
- **Stomatomycosis** B37.0
- **Stomatorrhagia** K13.79
- **Stone(s)** — *see also* Calculus
  - bladder (diverticulum) N21.0
  - cystine E72.09
  - heart syndrome I50.1
  - kidney N20.0
  - prostate N42.0
  - pulpal (dental) K04.2
  - renal N20.0

Stone(s) — *continued*
- salivary gland or duct (any) K11.5
- urethra (impacted) N21.1
- urinary (duct) (impacted) (passage) N20.9
  - bladder (diverticulum) N21.0
  - lower tract N21.9
  - specified NEC N21.8
- xanthine E79.8 *[N22]*

Stonecutter's lung J62.8
Stonemason's asthma, disease, lung or pneumoconiosis J62.8
Stoppage
- heart — *see* Arrest, cardiac
- urine — *see* Retention, urine

Storm, thyroid — *see* Thyrotoxicosis
Strabismus (congenital) (nonparalytic) H50.9
- concomitant H50.40
  - convergent — *see* Strabismus, convergent concomitant
  - divergent — *see* Strabismus, divergent concomitant
- convergent concomitant H50.00
  - accommodative component H50.43
  - alternating H50.05
    - with
      - A pattern H50.06
      - specified nonconcomitances NEC H50.08
      - V pattern H50.07
  - monocular H50.01- ☑
    - with
      - A pattern H50.02- ☑
      - specified nonconcomitances NEC H50.04- ☑
      - V pattern H50.03- ☑
    - intermittent H50.31- ☑
      - alternating H50.32
- cyclotropia H50.41 ☑
- divergent concomitant H50.10
  - alternating H50.15
    - with
      - A pattern H50.16
      - specified noncomitances NEC H50.18
      - V pattern H50.17
  - monocular H50.11- ☑
    - with
      - A pattern H50.12- ☑
      - specified noncomitances NEC H50.14- ☑
      - V pattern H50.13- ☑
    - intermittent H50.33 ☑
      - alternating H50.34
- Duane's syndrome H50.81- ☑
- due to adhesions, scars H50.69
- heterophoria H50.50
  - alternating H50.55
  - cyclophoria H50.54
  - esophoria H50.51
  - exophoria H50.52
  - vertical H50.53
- heterotropia H50.40
  - intermittent H50.30
- hypertropia H50.2- ☑
- hypotropia — *see* Hypertropia
- latent H50.50
- mechanical H50.60
  - Brown's sheath syndrome H50.61- ☑
  - specified type NEC H50.69
- monofixation syndrome H50.42
- paralytic H49.9
  - abducens nerve H49.2- ☑
  - fourth nerve H49.1- ☑
  - Kearns-Sayre syndrome H49.81- ☑
  - ophthalmoplegia (external)
    - progressive H49.4- ☑
      - with pigmentary retinopathy H49.81- ☑
    - total H49.3- ☑
  - sixth nerve H49.2- ☑
  - specified type NEC H49.88- ☑
  - third nerve H49.0- ☑
  - trochlear nerve H49.1- ☑
- specified type NEC H50.89
- vertical H50.2- ☑

Strain
- back S39.012 ☑
- cervical S16.1 ☑
- eye NEC — *see* Disturbance, vision, subjective
- heart — *see* Disease, heart
- low back S39.012 ☑
- mental NOS Z73.3
  - work-related Z56.6
- muscle (tendon) — *see* Injury, muscle, by site, strain
- neck S16.1 ☑
- physical NOS Z73.3
  - work-related Z56.6
- postural — *see also* Disorder, soft tissue, due to use
- psychological NEC Z73.3
- tendon — *see* Injury, muscle, by site, strain

Straining, on urination R39.16
Strand, vitreous — *see* Opacity, vitreous, membranes and strands
Strangulation, strangulated — *see also* Asphyxia, traumatic
- appendix K38.8
- bladder-neck N32.0
- bowel or colon K56.2
- food or foreign body — *see* Foreign body, by site
- hemorrhoids — *see* Hemorrhoids, with complication
- hernia — *see also* Hernia, by site, with obstruction
  - with gangrene — *see* Hernia, by site, with gangrene
- intestine (large) (small) K56.2
  - with hernia — *see also* Hernia, by site, with obstruction
    - with gangrene — *see* Hernia, by site, with gangrene
- mesentery K56.2
- mucus — *see* Asphyxia, mucus
- omentum K56.2
- organ or site, congenital NEC — *see* Atresia, by site
- ovary — *see* Torsion, ovary
- penis N48.89
  - foreign body T19.4 ☑
- rupture — *see* Hernia, by site, with obstruction
- stomach due to hernia — *see also* Hernia, by site, with obstruction
  - with gangrene — *see* Hernia, by site, with gangrene
- vesicourethral orifice N32.0

Strangury R30.0
Straw itch B88.0
Strawberry
- gallbladder K82.4
- mark Q82.5
- tongue (red) (white) K14.3

Streak(s)
- macula, angioid H35.33
- ovarian Q50.32

Strephosymbolia F81.0
- secondary to organic lesion R48.8

Streptobacillary fever A25.1
Streptobacillosis A25.1
Streptobacillus moniliformis A25.1
Streptococcus, streptococcal — *see also* condition
- as cause of disease classified elsewhere B95.5
- group
  - A, as cause of disease classified elsewhere B95.0
  - B, as cause of disease classified elsewhere B95.1
  - D, as cause of disease classified elsewhere B95.2
- pneumoniae, as cause of disease classified elsewhere B95.3
- specified NEC, as cause of disease classified elsewhere B95.4

Streptomycosis B47.1
Streptotrichosis A48.8
Stress F43.9
- family — *see* Disruption, family
- fetal P84
  - complicating pregnancy O77.9
    - due to drug administration O77.1
- mental NEC Z73.3
  - work-related Z56.6
- physical NEC Z73.3
  - work-related Z56.6
- polycythemia D75.1
- reaction — *see also* Reaction, stress F43.9
- work schedule Z56.3

Stretching, nerve — *see* Injury, nerve
Striae albicantes, atrophicae or distensae (cutis) L90.6
Stricture — *see also* Stenosis
- ampulla of Vater K83.1
- anus (sphincter) K62.4
  - congenital Q42.3
    - with fistula Q42.2
  - infantile Q42.3
    - with fistula Q42.2
- aorta (ascending) (congenital) Q25.1
  - arteriosclerotic I70.0
  - calcified I70.0
  - supravalvular, congenital Q25.3
- aortic (valve) — *see* Stenosis, aortic
- aqueduct of Sylvius (congenital) Q03.0
  - with spina bifida — *see* Spina bifida, by site, with hydrocephalus
  - acquired G91.1
- artery I77.1
  - basilar — *see* Occlusion, artery, basilar
  - carotid — *see* Occlusion, artery, carotid
  - celiac I77.4
  - congenital (peripheral) Q27.8
    - cerebral Q28.3
    - coronary Q24.5
    - digestive system Q27.8
    - lower limb Q27.8
    - retinal Q14.1
    - specified site NEC Q27.8
    - umbilical Q27.0
    - upper limb Q27.8
  - coronary — *see* Disease, heart, ischemic, atherosclerotic
    - congenital Q24.5
  - precerebral — *see* Occlusion, artery, precerebral
  - pulmonary (congenital) Q25.6
    - acquired I28.8
  - renal I70.1
  - vertebral — *see* Occlusion, artery, vertebral
- auditory canal (external) (congenital)
  - acquired — *see* Stenosis, external ear canal
- bile duct (common) (hepatic) K83.1
  - congenital Q44.3
  - postoperative K91.89
- bladder N32.89
  - neck N32.0
- bowel — *see* Obstruction, intestine
- brain G93.89
- bronchus J98.09
  - congenital Q32.3
  - syphilitic A52.72
- cardia (stomach) K22.2
  - congenital Q39.3
- cardiac — *see also* Disease, heart
  - orifice (stomach) K22.2
- cecum — *see* Obstruction, intestine
- cervix, cervical (canal) N88.2
  - congenital Q51.828
  - in pregnancy — *see* Pregnancy, complicated by, abnormal cervix
    - causing obstructed labor O65.5
- colon — *see also* Obstruction, intestine
  - congenital Q42.9
    - specified NEC Q42.8
- colostomy K94.03
- common (bile) duct K83.1
- coronary (artery) — *see* Disease, heart, ischemic, atherosclerotic
- cystic duct — *see* Obstruction, gallbladder
- digestive organs NEC, congenital Q45.8
- duodenum K31.5
  - congenital Q41.0
- ear canal (external) (congenital) Q16.1
  - acquired — *see* Stricture, auditory canal, acquired
- ejaculatory duct N50.89
- enterostomy K94.13
- esophagus K22.2
  - congenital Q39.3
  - syphilitic A52.79
    - congenital A50.59 *[K23]*
- eustachian tube — *see also* Obstruction, eustachian tube
  - congenital Q17.8
- fallopian tube N97.1
  - gonococcal A54.24
  - tuberculous A18.17
- gallbladder — *see* Obstruction, gallbladder
- glottis J38.6
- heart — *see also* Disease, heart
  - valve — *see also* Endocarditis I38
    - aortic Q23.0
    - mitral Q23.2
    - pulmonary Q22.1
    - tricuspid Q22.4
- hepatic duct K83.1
- hourglass, of stomach K31.2
- hymen N89.6
- hypopharynx J39.2
- ileum — *see also* Obstruction, intestine, specified NEC K56.699

Struma — *continued*
- ovarii D27.- ☑
- Riedel's E06.5

Strumipriva cachexia E03.4
Strümpell-Marie spine — *see* Spondylitis, ankylosing
Strümpell-Westphal pseudosclerosis E83.01
Stuart deficiency disease (factor X) D68.2
Stuart-Prower factor deficiency (factor X) D68.2
Student's elbow — *see* Bursitis, elbow, olecranon
Stump — *see* Amputation
Stunting, nutritional E45
Stupor (catatonic) R40.1
- depressive (single episode) F32.89
  - recurrent episode F33.8
- dissociative F44.2
- manic F30.2
- manic-depressive F31.89
- psychogenic (anergic) F44.2
- reaction to exceptional stress (transient) F43.0

Sturge (-Weber) (-Dimitri) (-Kalischer) **disease or syndrome** Q85.8
Stuttering F80.81
- adult onset F98.5
- childhood onset F80.81
- following cerebrovascular disease — *see* Disorder, fluency. following cerebrovascular disease
- in conditions classified elsewhere R47.82

Sty, stye (external) (internal) (meibomian) (zeisian) — *see* Hordeolum
Subacidity, gastric K31.89
- psychogenic F45.8

Subacute — *see* condition
Subarachnoid — *see* condition
Subcortical — *see* condition
Subcostal syndrome, nerve compression — *see* Mononeuropathy, upper limb, specified site NEC
Subcutaneous, subcuticular — *see* condition
Subdural — *see* condition
Subendocardium — *see* condition
Subependymoma
- specified site — *see* Neoplasm, uncertain behavior, by site
- unspecified site D43.2

Suberosis J67.3
Subglossitis — *see* Glossitis
Subhemophilia D66
Subinvolution
- breast (postlactational) (postpuerperal) N64.89
- puerperal O90.89
- uterus (chronic) (nonpuerperal) N85.3
  - puerperal O90.89

Sublingual — *see* condition
Sublinguitis — *see* Sialoadenitis
Subluxatable hip Q65.6
Subluxation — *see also* Dislocation
- acromioclavicular S43.11- ☑
- ankle S93.0- ☑
- atlantoaxial, recurrent M43.4
  - with myelopathy M43.3
- carpometacarpal (joint) NEC S63.05- ☑
  - thumb S63.04- ☑
- complex, vertebral — *see* Complex, subluxation
- congenital — *see also* Malposition, congenital
  - hip — *see* Dislocation, hip, congenital, partial
  - joint (excluding hip)
    - lower limb Q68.8
    - shoulder Q68.8
    - upper limb Q68.8
- elbow (traumatic) S53.10- ☑
  - anterior S53.11- ☑
  - lateral S53.14- ☑
  - medial S53.13- ☑
  - posterior S53.12- ☑
  - specified type NEC S53.19- ☑
- finger S63.20- ☑
  - index S63.20- ☑
  - interphalangeal S63.22- ☑
    - distal S63.24- ☑
      - index S63.24- ☑
      - little S63.24- ☑
      - middle S63.24- ☑
      - ring S63.24- ☑
    - index S63.22- ☑
    - little S63.22- ☑
    - middle S63.22- ☑
    - proximal S63.23- ☑
      - index S63.23- ☑

Subluxation — *continued*
- finger — *continued*
  - interphalangeal — *continued*
    - proximal — *continued*
      - little S63.23- ☑
      - middle S63.23- ☑
      - ring S63.23- ☑
    - ring S63.22- ☑
  - little S63.20- ☑
  - metacarpophalangeal S63.21- ☑
    - index S63.21- ☑
    - little S63.21- ☑
    - middle S63.21- ☑
    - ring S63.21- ☑
  - middle S63.20- ☑
  - ring S63.20- ☑
- foot S93.30- ☑
  - specified site NEC S93.33- ☑
  - tarsal joint S93.31- ☑
  - tarsometatarsal joint S93.32- ☑
  - toe — *see* Subluxation, toe
- hip S73.00- ☑
  - anterior S73.03- ☑
    - obturator S73.02- ☑
  - central S73.04- ☑
  - posterior S73.01- ☑
- interphalangeal (joint)
  - finger S63.22- ☑
    - distal joint S63.24- ☑
      - index S63.24- ☑
      - little S63.24- ☑
      - middle S63.24- ☑
      - ring S63.24- ☑
    - index S63.22- ☑
    - little S63.22- ☑
    - middle S63.22- ☑
    - proximal joint S63.23- ☑
      - index S63.23- ☑
      - little S63.23- ☑
      - middle S63.23- ☑
      - ring S63.23- ☑
    - ring S63.22- ☑
  - thumb S63.12- ☑
  - toe S93.13- ☑
    - great S93.13- ☑
    - lesser S93.13- ☑
- joint prosthesis — *see* Complications, joint prosthesis, mechanical, displacement, by site
- knee S83.10- ☑
  - cap — *see* Subluxation, patella
  - patella — *see* Subluxation, patella
  - proximal tibia
    - anteriorly S83.11- ☑
    - laterally S83.14- ☑
    - medially S83.13- ☑
    - posteriorly S83.12- ☑
  - specified type NEC S83.19- ☑
- lens — *see* Dislocation, lens, partial
- ligament, traumatic — *see* Sprain, by site
- metacarpal (bone)
  - proximal end S63.06- ☑
- metacarpophalangeal (joint)
  - finger S63.21- ☑
    - index S63.21- ☑
    - little S63.21- ☑
    - middle S63.21- ☑
    - ring S63.21- ☑
  - thumb S63.11- ☑
- metatarsophalangeal joint S93.14- ☑
  - great toe S93.14- ☑
  - lesser toe S93.14- ☑
- midcarpal (joint) S63.03- ☑
- patella S83.00- ☑
  - lateral S83.01- ☑
  - recurrent (nontraumatic) — *see* Dislocation, patella, recurrent, incomplete
  - specified type NEC S83.09- ☑
- pathological — *see* Dislocation, pathological
- radial head S53.00- ☑
  - anterior S53.01- ☑
  - nursemaid's elbow S53.03- ☑
  - posterior S53.02- ☑
  - specified type NEC S53.09- ☑
- radiocarpal (joint) S63.02- ☑
- radioulnar (joint)
  - distal S63.01- ☑

Subluxation — *continued*
- radioulnar — *continued*
  - proximal — *see* Subluxation, elbow
- shoulder
  - congenital Q68.8
  - girdle S43.30- ☑
    - scapula S43.31- ☑
    - specified site NEC S43.39- ☑
  - traumatic S43.00- ☑
    - anterior S43.01- ☑
    - inferior S43.03- ☑
    - posterior S43.02- ☑
    - specified type NEC S43.08- ☑
- sternoclavicular (joint) S43.20- ☑
  - anterior S43.21- ☑
  - posterior S43.22- ☑
- symphysis (pubis)
- thumb S63.103 ☑
  - interphalangeal joint — *see* Subluxation, interphalangeal (joint), thumb
  - metacarpophalangeal joint — *see* Subluxation, metacarpophalangeal (joint), thumb
- toe(s) S93.10- ☑
  - great S93.10- ☑
    - interphalangeal joint S93.13- ☑
    - metatarsophalangeal joint S93.14- ☑
  - interphalangeal joint S93.13- ☑
  - lesser S93.10- ☑
    - interphalangeal joint S93.13- ☑
    - metatarsophalangeal joint S93.14- ☑
  - metatarsophalangeal joint S93.149 ☑
- ulna
  - distal end S63.07- ☑
  - proximal end — *see* Subluxation, elbow
- ulnohumeral joint — *see* Subluxation, elbow
- vertebral
  - recurrent NEC — *see* subcategory M43.5 ☑
  - traumatic
    - cervical S13.100 ☑
      - atlantoaxial joint S13.120 ☑
      - atlantooccipital joint S13.110 ☑
      - atloidooccipital joint S13.110 ☑
      - joint between
        - C0 and C1 S13.110 ☑
        - C1 and C2 S13.120 ☑
        - C2 and C3 S13.130 ☑
        - C3 and C4 S13.140 ☑
        - C4 and C5 S13.150 ☑
        - C5 and C6 S13.160 ☑
        - C6 and C7 S13.170 ☑
        - C7 and T1 S13.180 ☑
      - occipitoatloid joint S13.110 ☑
    - lumbar S33.100 ☑
      - joint between
        - L1 and L2 S33.110 ☑
        - L2 and L3 S33.120 ☑
        - L3 and L4 S33.130 ☑
        - L4 and L5 S33.140 ☑
    - thoracic S23.100 ☑
      - joint between
        - T1 and T2 S23.110 ☑
        - T2 and T3 S23.120 ☑
        - T3 and T4 S23.122 ☑
        - T4 and T5 S23.130 ☑
        - T5 and T6 S23.132 ☑
        - T6 and T7 S23.140 ☑
        - T7 and T8 S23.142 ☑
        - T8 and T9 S23.150 ☑
        - T9 and T10 S23.152 ☑
        - T10 and T11 S23.160 ☑
        - T11 and T12 S23.162 ☑
        - T12 and L1 S23.170 ☑
- wrist (carpal bone) S63.00- ☑
  - carpometacarpal joint — *see* Subluxation, carpometacarpal (joint)
  - distal radioulnar joint — *see* Subluxation, radioulnar (joint), distal
  - metacarpal bone, proximal — *see* Subluxation, metacarpal (bone), proximal end
  - midcarpal — *see* Subluxation, midcarpal (joint)
  - radiocarpal joint — *see* Subluxation, radiocarpal (joint)
  - recurrent — *see* Dislocation, recurrent, wrist
  - specified site NEC S63.09- ☑
  - ulna — *see* Subluxation, ulna, distal end

Submaxillary — *see* condition

Submersion (fatal) (nonfatal) T75.1 ☑

Submucous — *see* condition

Subnormal, subnormality
- accommodation (old age) H52.4
- mental — *see* Disability, intellectual
- temperature (accidental) T68 ☑

Subphrenic — *see* condition

Subscapular nerve — *see* condition

Subseptus uterus Q51.28

Subsiding appendicitis K36

Substance (other psychoactive) **-induced**
- anxiety disorder F19.980
- bipolar and related disorder F19.94
- delirium F19.921
- depressive disorder F19.94
- major neurocognitive disorder F19.97
- mild neurocognitive disorder F19.988
- obsessive-compulsive and related disorder F19.988
- psychotic disorder F19.959
- sexual dysfunction F19.981
- sleep disorder F19.982

Substernal thyroid E04.9
- congenital Q89.2

Substitution disorder F44.9

Subtentorial — *see* condition

Subthyroidism (acquired) — *see also* Hypothyroidism
- congenital E03.1

Succenturiate placenta O43.19- ☑

Sucking thumb, child (excessive) F98.8

Sudamen, sudamina L74.1

Sudanese kala-azar B55.0

Sudden
- hearing loss — *see* Deafness, sudden
- heart failure — *see* Failure, heart

Sudeck's atrophy, disease, or syndrome — *see* Algoneurodystrophy

Suffocation — *see* Asphyxia, traumatic

Sugar
- blood
  - high (transient) R73.9
  - low (transient) E16.2
- in urine R81

Suicide, suicidal (attempted) T14.91 ☑
- by poisoning — *see* Table of Drugs and Chemicals
- history of (personal) Z91.5
  - in family Z81.8
- ideation — *see* Ideation, suicidal
- risk
  - meaning personal history of attempted suicide Z91.5
  - meaning suicidal ideation — *see* Ideation, suicidal
- tendencies
  - meaning personal history of attempted suicide Z91.5
  - meaning suicidal ideation — *see* Ideation, suicidal
- trauma — *see* nature of injury by site

Suipestifer infection — *see* Infection, salmonella

Sulfhemoglobinemia, sulphemoglobinemia (acquired) (with methemoglobinemia) D74.8

Sumatran mite fever A75.3

Summer — *see* condition

Sunburn L55.9
- due to
  - tanning bed (acute) L56.8
    - chronic L57.8
  - ultraviolet radiation (acute) L56.8
    - chronic L57.8
- first degree L55.0
- second degree L55.1
- third degree L55.2

SUNCT (short lasting unilateral neuralgiform headache with conjunctival injection and tearing) G44.059
- intractable G44.051
- not intractable G44.059

Sundowning F05

Sunken acetabulum — *see* Derangement, joint, specified type NEC, hip

Sunstroke T67.01 ☑
- specified NEC T67.09 ☑

Superfecundation — *see* Pregnancy, multiple

Superfetation — *see* Pregnancy, multiple

Superinvolution (uterus) N85.8

Supernumerary (congenital)
- aortic cusps Q23.8
- auditory ossicles Q16.3
- bone Q79.8
- breast Q83.1
- carpal bones Q74.0
- cusps, heart valve NEC Q24.8

Supernumerary — *continued*
- cusps, heart valve — *continued*
  - aortic Q23.8
  - mitral Q23.2
  - pulmonary Q22.3
- digit(s) Q69.9
- ear (lobule) Q17.0
- fallopian tube Q50.6
- finger Q69.0
- hymen Q52.4
- kidney Q63.0
- lacrimonasal duct Q10.6
- lobule (ear) Q17.0
- mitral cusps Q23.2
- muscle Q79.8
- nipple(s) Q83.3
- organ or site not listed — *see* Accessory
- ossicles, auditory Q16.3
- ovary Q50.31
- oviduct Q50.6
- pulmonary, pulmonic cusps Q22.3
- rib Q76.6
  - cervical or first (syndrome) Q76.5
- roots (of teeth) K00.2
- spleen Q89.09
- tarsal bones Q74.2
- teeth K00.1
- testis Q55.29
- thumb Q69.1
- toe Q69.2
- uterus Q51.28
- vagina Q52.1 ☑
- vertebra Q76.49

Supervision (of)
- contraceptive — *see* Prescription, contraceptives
- dietary (for) Z71.3
  - allergy (food) Z71.3
  - colitis Z71.3
  - diabetes mellitus Z71.3
  - food allergy or intolerance Z71.3
  - gastritis Z71.3
  - hypercholesterolemia Z71.3
  - hypoglycemia Z71.3
  - intolerance (food) Z71.3
  - obesity Z71.3
  - specified NEC Z71.3
- healthy infant or child Z76.2
  - foundling Z76.1
- high-risk pregnancy — *see* Pregnancy, complicated by, high, risk
- lactation Z39.1
- pregnancy — *see* Pregnancy, supervision of

Supplemental teeth K00.1

Suppression
- binocular vision H53.34
- lactation O92.5
- menstruation N94.89
- ovarian secretion E28.39
- renal N28.9
- urine, urinary secretion R34

Suppuration, suppurative — *see also* condition
- accessory sinus (chronic) — *see* Sinusitis
- adrenal gland
- antrum (chronic) — *see* Sinusitis, maxillary
- bladder — *see* Cystitis
- brain G06.0
  - sequelae G09
- breast N61.1
  - puerperal, postpartum or gestational — *see* Mastitis, obstetric, purulent
- dental periosteum M27.3
- ear (middle) — *see also* Otitis, media
  - external NEC — *see* Otitis, externa, infective
  - internal — *see* subcategory H83.0 ☑
- ethmoidal (chronic) (sinus) — *see* Sinusitis, ethmoidal
- fallopian tube — *see* Salpingo-oophoritis
- frontal (chronic) (sinus) — *see* Sinusitis, frontal
- gallbladder (acute) K81.0
- gum K05.20
  - generalized — *see* Periodontitis, aggressive, generalized
  - localized — *see* Periodontitis, aggressive, localized
- intracranial G06.0
- joint — *see* Arthritis, pyogenic or pyemic
- labyrinthine — *see* subcategory H83.0 ☑
- lung — *see* Abscess, lung
- mammary gland N61.1
  - puerperal, postpartum O91.12

Suppuration, suppurative — *continued*
- mammary gland — *continued*
  - puerperal, postpartum — *continued*
    - associated with lactation O91.13
- maxilla, maxillary M27.2
  - sinus (chronic) — *see* Sinusitis, maxillary
- muscle — *see* Myositis, infective
- nasal sinus (chronic) — *see* Sinusitis
- pancreas, acute — *see also* Pancreatitis, acute K85.80
- parotid gland — *see* Sialoadenitis
- pelvis, pelvic
  - female — *see* Disease, pelvis, inflammatory
  - male K65.0
- pericranial — *see* Osteomyelitis
- salivary duct or gland (any) — *see* Sialoadenitis
- sinus (accessory) (chronic) (nasal) — *see* Sinusitis
- sphenoidal sinus (chronic) — *see* Sinusitis, sphenoidal
- thymus (gland) E32.1
- thyroid (gland) E06.0
- tonsil — *see* Tonsillitis
- uterus — *see* Endometritis

Supraeruption of tooth (teeth) M26.34

Supraglottitis J04.30
- with obstruction J04.31

Suprarenal (gland) — *see* condition

Suprascapular nerve — *see* condition

Suprasellar — *see* condition

Surfer's knots or nodules S89.8- ☑

Surgical
- emphysema T81.82 ☑
- procedures, complication or misadventure — *see* Complications, surgical procedures
- shock T81.10 ☑

Surveillance (of) (for) — *see also* Observation
- alcohol abuse Z71.41
- contraceptive — *see* Prescription, contraceptives
- dietary Z71.3
- drug abuse Z71.51

Susceptibility to disease, genetic Z15.89
- malignant neoplasm Z15.09
  - breast Z15.01
  - endometrium Z15.04
  - ovary Z15.02
  - prostate Z15.03
  - specified NEC Z15.09
- multiple endocrine neoplasia Z15.81

Suspected condition, ruled out — *see also* Observation, suspected
- amniotic cavity and membrane Z03.71
- cervical shortening Z03.75
- fetal anomaly Z03.73
- fetal growth Z03.74
- maternal and fetal conditions NEC Z03.79
- newborn — *see also* Observation, newborn, suspected condition ruled out Z05.9
- oligohydramnios Z03.71
- placental problem Z03.72
- polyhydramnios Z03.71

Suspended uterus
- in pregnancy or childbirth — *see* Pregnancy, complicated by, abnormal uterus

Sutton's nevus D22.9

Suture
- burst (in operation wound) T81.31 ☑
  - external operation wound T81.31 ☑
  - internal operation wound T81.32 ☑
- inadvertently left in operation wound — *see* Foreign body, accidentally left during a procedure
- removal Z48.02

Swab inadvertently left in operation wound — *see* Foreign body, accidentally left during a procedure

Swallowed, swallowing
- difficulty — *see* Dysphagia
- foreign body — *see* Foreign body, alimentary tract

Swan-neck deformity (finger) — *see* Deformity, finger, swan-neck

Swearing, compulsive F42.8
- in Gilles de la Tourette's syndrome F95.2

Sweat, sweats
- fetid L75.0
- night R61

Sweating, excessive R61

Sweeley-Klionsky disease E75.21

Sweet's disease or dermatosis L98.2

Swelling (of) R60.9
- abdomen, abdominal (not referable to any particular organ) — *see* Mass, abdominal

Syndrome — *continued*
- diabetic amyotrophy — *see* Diabetes, amyotrophy
- dialysis associated steal T82.898- ☑
- Diamond-Blackfan D61.Ø1
- Diamond-Gardener D69.2
- DIC (diffuse or disseminated intravascular coagulopathy) D65
- Dighton's Q78.Ø
- disequilibrium E87.8
- Döhle body-panmyelopathic D72.Ø
- dorsolateral medullary G46.4
- double athetosis G8Ø.3
- Down — *see also* Down syndrome Q9Ø.9
- Dravet (intractable) G4Ø.834
  - with status epilepticus G4Ø.833
  - without status epilepticus G4Ø.834
- Dresbach's (elliptocytosis) D58.1
- DRESS (drug rash with eosinophilia and systemic symptoms) D72.12
- Dressler's (postmyocardial infarction) I24.1
  - postcardiotomy I97.Ø
- drug rash with eosinophilia and systemic symptoms (DRESS) D72.12
- drug withdrawal, infant of dependent mother P96.1
- dry eye HØ4.12- ☑
- due to abnormality
  - chromosomal Q99.9
    - sex
      - female phenotype Q97.9
      - male phenotype Q98.9
    - specified NEC Q99.8
- dumping (postgastrectomy) K91.1
  - nonsurgical K31.89
- Dupré's (meningism) R29.1
- dysmetabolic X E88.81
- dyspraxia, developmental F82
- Eagle-Barrett Q79.4
- Eaton-Lambert — *see* Syndrome, Lambert-Eaton
- Ebstein's Q22.5
- ectopic ACTH E24.3
- eczema-thrombocytopenia D82.Ø
- Eddowes' Q78.Ø
- effort (psychogenic) F45.8
- Ehlers-Danlos Q79.6Ø
  - classical (cEDS) (classical EDS) Q79.61
  - hypermobile (hEDS) (hypermobile EDS) Q79.62
  - specified NEC Q79.69
  - vascular (vascular EDS) (vEDS) Q79.63
- Eisenmenger's I27.83
- Ekman's Q78.Ø
- electric feet E53.8
- Ellis-van Creveld Q77.6
- empty nest Z6Ø.Ø
- endocrine-hypertensive E27.Ø
- entrapment — *see* Neuropathy, entrapment
- eosinophilia-myalgia M35.8
- epileptic — *see also* Epilepsy, by type
  - absence G4Ø.AØ9 (*following* G4Ø.3)
    - intractable G4Ø.A19 (*following* G4Ø.3)
      - with status epilepticus G4Ø.A11 (*following* G4Ø.3)
      - without status epilepticus G4Ø.A19 (*following* G4Ø.3)
    - not intractable G4Ø.AØ9 (*following* G4Ø.3)
      - with status epilepticus G4Ø.AØ1 (*following* G4Ø.3)
      - without status epilepticus G4Ø.AØ9 (*following* G4Ø.3)
- Erdheim-Chester (ECD) E88.89
- Erdheim's E22.Ø
- erythrocyte fragmentation D59.4
- Evans D69.41
- exhaustion F48.8
- extrapyramidal G25.9
  - specified NEC G25.89
- eye retraction — *see* Strabismus
- eyelid-malar-mandible Q87.Ø
- Faber's D5Ø.9
- facet M47.89- ☑
- facial pain, paroxysmal G5Ø.Ø
- Fallot's Q21.3
- familial cold autoinflammatory MØ4.2
- familial eczema-thrombocytopenia (Wiskott-Aldrich) D82.Ø
- Fanconi (-de Toni) (-Debré) E72.Ø9
  - with cystinosis E72.Ø4
- Fanconi's (anemia) (congenital pancytopenia) D61.Ø9

Syndrome — *continued*
- fatigue
  - chronic R53.82
  - psychogenic F48.8
- faulty bowel habit K59.39
- Feil-Klippel (brevicollis) Q76.1
- Felty's — *see* Felty's syndrome
- fertile eunuch E23.Ø
- fetal
  - alcohol (dysmorphic) Q86.Ø
  - hydantoin Q86.1
- Fiedler's I4Ø.1
- first arch Q87.Ø
- fish odor E72.89
- Fisher's G61.Ø
- Fitzhugh-Curtis
  - due to
    - Chlamydia trachomatis A74.81
    - Neisseria gonorrhorea (gonococcal peritonitis) A54.85
- Fitz's — *see also* Pancreatitis, acute K85.8Ø
- Flajani (-Basedow) EØ5.ØØ
  - with thyroid storm EØ5.Ø1
- flatback — *see* Flatback syndrome
- floppy
  - baby P94.2
  - iris (intraoeprative) (IFIS) H21.81
  - mitral valve I34.1
- flush E34.Ø
- Foix-Alajouanine G95.19
- Fong's Q87.2
- food protein-induced enterocolitis (FPIES) K52.21
- foramen magnum G93.5
- Foster-Kennedy H47.14- ☑
- Foville's (peduncular) G46.3
- fragile X Q99.2
- Franceschetti Q75.4
- Frey's
  - auriculotemporal G5Ø.8
  - hyperhidrosis L74.52
- Friderichsen-Waterhouse A39.1
- Froin's G95.89
- frontal lobe FØ7.Ø
- Fukuhara E88.49
- functional
  - bowel K59.9
  - prepubertal castrate E29.1
- Gaisböck's D75.1
- ganglion (basal ganglia brain) G25.9
  - geniculi G51.1
- Gardner-Diamond D69.2
- gastroesophageal
  - junction K22.Ø
  - laceration-hemorrhage K22.6
- gastrojejunal loop obstruction K91.89
- Gee-Herter-Heubner K9Ø.Ø
- Gelineau's G47.419
  - with cataplexy G47.411
- genito-anorectal A55
- Gerstmann-Sträussler-Scheinker (GSS) A81.82
- Gianotti-Crosti L44.4
- giant platelet (Bernard-Soulier) D69.1
- Gilles de la Tourette's F95.2
- Glass Q87.89
- Gleich's D72.118
- goiter-deafness EØ7.1
- Goldberg Q89.8
- Goldberg-Maxwell E34.51
- Good's D83.8
- Gopalan' (burning feet) E53.8
- Gorlin's Q87.89
- Gougerot-Blum L81.7
- Gouley's I31.1
- Gower's R55
- gray or grey (newborn) P93.Ø
  - platelet D69.1
- Gubler-Millard G46.3
- Guillain-Barré (-Strohl) G61.Ø
- gustatory sweating G5Ø.8
- Hadfield-Clarke K86.89
- hair tourniquet — *see* Constriction, external, by site
- Hamman's J98.19
- hand-foot L27.1
- hand-shoulder G9Ø.8
- hantavirus (cardio)-pulmonary (HPS) (HCPS) B33.4
- happy puppet Q93.51
- Harada's H3Ø.81- ☑
- Hayem-Faber D5Ø.9
- headache NEC G44.89

Syndrome — *continued*
- headache — *continued*
  - complicated NEC G44.59
- Heberden's I2Ø.8
- Hedinger's E34.Ø
- Hegglin's D72.Ø
- HELLP (hemolysis, elevated liver enzymes and low platelet count) O14.2- ☑
  - complicating
    - childbirth O14.24
    - puerperium O14.25
- hemolytic-uremic D59.3
- hemophagocytic, infection-associated D76.2
- Henoch-Schönlein D69.Ø
- hepatic flexure K59.89
- hepatopulmonary K76.81
- hepatorenal K76.7
  - following delivery O9Ø.4
  - postoperative or postprocedural K91.83
  - postpartum, puerperal O9Ø.4
- hepatourologic K76.7
- Herter (-Gee) (nontropical sprue) K9Ø.Ø
- Heubner-Herter K9Ø.Ø
- Heyd's K76.7
- Hilger's G9Ø.Ø9
- histamine-like (fish poisoning) — *see* Poisoning, fish
- histiocytic D76.3
- histiocytosis NEC D76.3
- HIV infection, acute B2Ø
- Hoffmann-Werdnig G12.Ø
- Hollander-Simons E88.1
- Hoppe-Goldflam G7Ø.ØØ
  - with exacerbation (acute) G7Ø.Ø1
  - in crisis G7Ø.Ø1
- Horner's G9Ø.2
- hungry bone E83.81
- hunterian glossitis D51.Ø
- Hutchinson's triad A5Ø.53
- hyperabduction G54.Ø
- hyperammonemia-hyperornithinemia-homocitrullinemia E72.4
- hypereosinophilic (HES) D72.119
  - idiopathic (IHES) D72.11Ø
  - lymphocytic variant (LHES) D72.111
  - specified NEC D72.118
- hyperimmunoglobulin D MØ4.1
- hyperimmunoglobulin E (IgE) D82.4
- hyperkalemic E87.5
- hyperkinetic — *see* Hyperkinesia
- hypermobility M35.7
- hypernatremia E87.Ø
- hyperosmolarity E87.Ø
- hyperperfusion G97.82
- hypersplenic D73.1
- hypertransfusion, newborn P61.1
- hyperventilation F45.8
- hyperviscosity (of serum)
  - polycythemic D75.1
  - sclerothymic D58.8
- hypoglycemic (familial) (neonatal) E16.2
- hypokalemic E87.6
- hyponatremic E87.1
- hypopituitarism E23.Ø
- hypoplastic left-heart Q23.4
- hypopotassemia E87.6
- hyposmolality E87.1
- hypotension, maternal O26.5- ☑
- hypothenar hammer I73.89
- hypoventilation, obesity (OHS) E66.2
- ICF (intravascular coagulation-fibrinolysis) D65
- idiopathic
  - cardiorespiratory distress, newborn P22.Ø
  - nephrotic (infantile) NØ4.9
- iliotibial band M76.3- ☑
- immobility, immobilization (paraplegic) M62.3
- immune reconstitution D89.3
- immune reconstitution inflammatory [IRIS] D89.3
- immunity deficiency, combined D81.9
- immunodeficiency
  - acquired — *see* Human, immunodeficiency virus (HIV) disease
  - combined D81.9
- impending coronary I2Ø.Ø
- impingement, shoulder M75.4- ☑
- inappropriate secretion of antidiuretic hormone E22.2
- infant
  - gestational diabetes P7Ø.Ø
  - of diabetic mother P7Ø.1

Syndrome — *continued*
- os trigonum Q68.8
- Osler-Weber-Rendu I78.Ø
- osteoporosis-osteomalacia M83.8
- Osterreicher-Turner Q87.2
- otolith — *see* subcategory H81.8 ☑
- oto-palatal-digital Q87.Ø
- outlet (thoracic) G54.Ø
- ovary
  - polycystic E28.2
  - resistant E28.39
  - sclerocystic E28.2
- Owren's D68.2
- Paget-Schroetter I82.89Ø
- pain — *see also* Pain
  - complex regional I G9Ø.5Ø
    - lower limb G9Ø.52- ☑
    - specified site NEC G9Ø.59
    - upper limb G9Ø.51- ☑
  - complex regional II — *see* Causalgia
- painful
  - bruising D69.2
  - feet E53.8
  - prostate N42.81
- paralysis agitans — *see* Parkinsonism
- paralytic G83.9
  - specified NEC G83.89
- Parinaud's H51.Ø
- parkinsonian — *see* Parkinsonism
- Parkinson's — *see* Parkinsonism
- paroxysmal facial pain G5Ø.Ø
- Parry's EØ5.ØØ
  - with thyroid storm EØ5.Ø1
- Parsonage (-Aldren)-Turner G54.5
- patella clunk M25.86- ☑
- Paterson (-Brown) (-Kelly) D5Ø.1
- pectoral girdle I77.89
- pectoralis minor I77.89
- pediatric autoimmune neuropsychiatric disorders associated with streptococcal infections (PANDAS) D89.89
- Pelger-Huet D72.Ø
- pellagra-cerebellar ataxia-renal aminoaciduria E72.Ø2
- pellagroid E52
- Pellegrini-Stieda — *see* Bursitis, tibial collateral
- pelvic congestion-fibrosis, female N94.89
- penta X Q97.1
- peptic ulcer — *see* Ulcer, peptic
- perabduction I77.89
- periodic fever MØ4.1
- periodic fever, aphthous stomatitis, pharyngitis, and adenopathy [PFAPA] MØ4.8
- periodic headache, in adults and children — *see* Headache, periodic syndromes in adults and children
- periurethral fibrosis N13.5
- phantom limb (without pain) G54.7
  - with pain G54.6
- pharyngeal pouch D82.1
- Pick's — *see* Disease, Pick's
- Pickwickian E66.2
- PIE (pulmonary infiltration with eosinophilia) — *see also* Eosinophilia, pulmonary J82.89
- pigmentary pallidal degeneration (progressive) G23.Ø
- pineal E34.8
- pituitary E22.Ø
- placental transfusion — *see* Pregnancy, complicated by, placental transfusion syndromes
- plantar fascia M72.2
- plateau iris (post-iridectomy) (postprocedural) H21.82
- Plummer-Vinson D5Ø.1
- pluricarential of infancy E4Ø
- plurideficiency E4Ø
- pluriglandular (compensatory) E31.8
  - autoimmune E31.Ø
- pneumatic hammer T75.21 ☑
- polyangiitis overlap M3Ø.8
- polycarential of infancy E4Ø
- polyglandular E31.8
  - autoimmune E31.Ø
- polysplenia Q89.Ø9
- pontine NEC G93.89
- popliteal
  - artery entrapment I77.89
  - web Q87.89
- post chemoembolization — *code to* associated conditions
- post endometrial ablation N99.85

Syndrome — *continued*
- postcardiac injury
  - postcardiotomy I97.Ø
  - postmyocardial infarction I24.1
- postcardiotomy I97.Ø
- postcholecystectomy K91.5
- postcommissurotomy I97.Ø
- postconcussional FØ7.81
- postcontusional FØ7.81
- postencephalitic FØ7.89
- posterior
  - cervical sympathetic M53.Ø
  - cord G83.83
  - fossa compression G93.5
  - reversible encephalopathy (PRES) I67.83
- postgastrectomy (dumping) K91.1
- postgastric surgery K91.1
- postinfarction I24.1
- postlaminectomy NEC M96.1
- postleukotomy FØ7.Ø
- postmastectomy lymphedema I97.2
- postmyocardial infarction I24.1
- postoperative NEC T81.9 ☑
  - blind loop K9Ø.2
- postpartum panhypopituitary (Sheehan) E23.Ø
- postpolio (myelitic) G14
- postthrombotic I87.ØØ9
  - with
    - inflammation I87.Ø2- ☑
      - with ulcer I87.Ø3- ☑
    - specified complication NEC I87.Ø9- ☑
    - ulcer I87.Ø1- ☑
      - with inflammation I87.Ø3- ☑
  - asymptomatic I87.ØØ- ☑
- postvagotomy K91.1
- postvalvulotomy I97.Ø
- postviral NEC G93.3
  - fatigue G93.3
- Potain's K31.Ø
- potassium intoxication E87.5
- Prader-Willi Q87.11
- Prader-Willi-like Q87.19
- precerebral artery (multiple) (bilateral) G45.2
- preinfarction I2Ø.Ø
- preleukemic D46.9
- premature senility E34.8
- premenstrual dysphoric F32.81
- premenstrual tension N94.3
- Prinzmetal-Massumi RØ7.1
- prune belly Q79.4
- pseudo -Turner's Q87.19
- pseudocarpal tunnel (sublimis) — *see* Syndrome, carpal tunnel
- pseudoparalytica G7Ø.ØØ
  - with exacerbation (acute) G7Ø.Ø1
  - in crisis G7Ø.Ø1
- psycho-organic (nonpsychotic severity) FØ7.9
  - acute or subacute FØ5
  - depressive type FØ6.31
  - hallucinatory type FØ6.Ø
  - nonpsychotic severity FØ7.Ø
  - specified NEC FØ7.89
- pulmonary
  - arteriosclerosis I27.Ø
  - dysmaturity (Wilson-Mikity) P27.Ø
  - hypoperfusion (idiopathic) P22.Ø
  - renal (hemorrhagic) (Goodpasture's) M31.Ø
- pure
  - motor lacunar G46.5
  - sensory lacunar G46.6
- Putnam-Dana D51.Ø
- pyogenic arthritis, pyoderma gangrenosum, and acne [PAPA] MØ4.8
- pyramidopallidonigral G2Ø
- pyriformis — *see* Lesion, nerve, sciatic
- QT interval prolongation I45.81
- radicular NEC — *see* Radiculopathy
  - upper limbs, newborn (birth injury) P14.3
- rapid time-zone change G47.25
- Rasmussen GØ4.81
- Raymond (-Céstan) I65.8
- Raynaud's I73.ØØ
  - with gangrene I73.Ø1
- RDS (respiratory distress syndrome, newborn) P22.Ø
- reactive airways dysfunction J68.3
- Refsum's G6Ø.1
- Reifenstein E34.52

Syndrome — *continued*
- renal glomerulohyalinosis-diabetic — *see* Diabetes, nephrosis
- Rendu-Osler-Weber I78.Ø
- residual ovary N99.83
- resistant ovary E28.39
- respiratory
  - distress
    - acute J8Ø
      - adult J8Ø
      - child J8Ø
      - idiopathic J84.114
    - newborn (idiopathic) (type I) P22.Ø
      - type II P22.1
- restless legs G25.81
- retinoblastoma (familial) C69.2 ☑
- retroperitoneal fibrosis N13.5
- retroviral seroconversion (acute) Z21
- Reye's G93.7
- Richter — *see* Leukemia, chronic lymphocytic, B-cell type
- Ridley's I5Ø.1
- right
  - heart, hypoplastic Q22.6
  - ventricular obstruction — *see* Failure, heart, right
- Romano-Ward (prolonged QT interval) I45.81
- rotator cuff, shoulder — *see also* Tear, rotator cuff M75.1Ø- ☑
- Rotes Quérol — *see* Hyperostosis, ankylosing
- Roth — *see* Meralgia paresthetica
- rubella (congenital) P35.Ø
- Ruvalcaba-Myhre-Smith E71.44Ø
- Rytand-Lipsitch I44.2
- salt
  - depletion E87.1
    - due to heat NEC T67.8 ☑
      - causing heat exhaustion or prostration T67.4 ☑
  - low E87.1
- salt-losing N28.89
- SATB2-associated Q87.89
- Scaglietti-Dagnini E22.Ø
- scalenus anticus (anterior) G54.Ø
- scapulocostal — *see* Mononeuropathy, upper limb, specified site NEC
- scapuloperoneal G71.Ø9
- schizophrenic, of childhood NEC F84.5
- Schnitzler D47.2
- Scholte's E34.Ø
- Schroeder's E27.Ø
- Schüller-Christian C96.5
- Schwachman's — *see* Syndrome, Shwachman's
- Schwartz (-Jampel) G71.13
- Schwartz-Bartter E22.2
- scimitar Q26.8
- sclerocystic ovary E28.2
- Seitelberger's G31.89
- septicemic adrenal hemorrhage A39.1
- seroconversion, retroviral (acute) Z21
- serous meningitis G93.2
- severe acute respiratory (SARS) J12.81
- shaken infant T74.4 ☑
- shock (traumatic) T79.4 ☑
  - kidney N17.Ø
    - following crush injury T79.5 ☑
  - toxic A48.3
- shock-lung J8Ø
- Shone's — *code to* specific anomalies
- short
  - bowel K91.2
  - rib Q77.2
- shoulder-hand — *see* Algoneurodystrophy
- Shwachman's D7Ø.4
- sicca — *see* Sicca syndrome
- sick
  - cell E87.1
  - sinus I49.5
- sick-euthyroid EØ7.81
- sideropenic D5Ø.1
- Siemens' ectodermal dysplasia Q82.4
- Silfversköld's Q78.9
- Simons' E88.1
- sinus tarsi M25.57- ☑
- sinusitis-bronchiectasis-situs inversus Q89.3
- Sipple's E31.22
- sirenomelia Q87.2
- Slocumb's E27.Ø
- slow flow, coronary I2Ø.8

Index
Syndrome — Syndrome

- **Syndrome** — *continued*
  - Sluder's G44.89
  - Smith-Magenis Q93.88
  - Sneddon-Wilkinson L13.1
  - Sotos' Q87.3
  - South African cardiomyopathy I42.8
  - spasmodic
    - upward movement, eyes H51.8
    - winking F95.8
  - Spen's I45.9
  - splenic
    - agenesis Q89.Ø1
    - flexure K59.89
    - neutropenia D73.81
  - Spurway's Q78.Ø
  - staphylococcal scalded skin LØØ
  - steal
    - arteriovenous T82.898- ☑
    - ischemic T82.898- ☑
    - subclavian G45.8
  - Stein-Leventhal E28.2
  - Stein's E28.2
  - Stevens-Johnson syndrome L51.1
    - toxic epidermal necrolysis overlap L51.3
  - Stewart-Morel M85.2
  - Stickler Q89.8
  - stiff baby Q89.8
  - stiff man G25.82
  - Still-Felty — *see* Felty's syndrome
  - Stokes (-Adams) I45.9
  - stone heart I5Ø.1
  - straight back, congenital Q76.49
  - subclavian steal G45.8
  - subcoracoid-pectoralis minor G54.Ø
  - subcostal nerve compression I77.89
  - subphrenic interposition Q43.3
  - superior
    - cerebellar artery I63.89
    - mesenteric artery K55.1
    - semi-circular canal dehiscence H83.8X- ☑
    - vena cava I87.1
  - supine hypotensive (maternal) — *see* Syndrome, hypotension, maternal
  - suprarenal cortical E27.Ø
  - supraspinatus — *see also* Tear, rotator cuff M75.1Ø- ☑
  - Susac G93.49
  - swallowed blood P78.2
  - sweat retention L74.Ø
  - Swyer Q99.1
  - Symond's G93.2
  - sympathetic
    - cervical paralysis G9Ø.2
    - pelvic, female N94.89
  - systemic inflammatory response (SIRS), of non-infectious origin (without organ dysfunction) R65.1Ø
    - with acute organ dysfunction R65.11
  - tachycardia-bradycardia I49.5
  - takotsubo I51.81
  - TAR (thrombocytopenia with absent radius) Q87.2
  - tarsal tunnel G57.5- ☑
  - teething KØØ.7
  - tegmental G93.89
  - telangiectasic-pigmentation-cataract Q82.8
  - temporal pyramidal apex — *see* Otitis, media, suppurative, acute
  - temporomandibular joint-pain-dysfunction M26.62- ☑
  - Terry's — *see also* Myopia, degenerative H44.2- ☑
  - testicular feminization — *see also* Syndrome, androgen insensitivity E34.51
  - thalamic pain (hyperesthetic) G89.Ø
  - thoracic outlet (compression) G54.Ø
  - Thorson-Björck E34.Ø
  - thrombocytopenia with absent radius (TAR) Q87.2
  - thyroid-adrenocortical insufficiency E31.Ø
  - tibial
    - anterior M76.81- ☑
    - posterior M76.82- ☑
  - Tietze's M94.Ø
  - time-zone (rapid) G47.25
  - Toni-Fanconi E72.Ø9
    - with cystinosis E72.Ø4
  - Touraine's Q79.8
  - tourniquet — *see* Constriction, external, by site
  - toxic shock A48.3
  - transient left ventricular apical ballooning I51.81
  - traumatic vasospastic T75.22 ☑
  - Treacher Collins Q75.4
  - triple X, female Q97.Ø

- **Syndrome** — *continued*
  - trisomy Q92.9
    - 13 Q91.7
      - meiotic nondisjunction Q91.4
      - mitotic nondisjunction Q91.5
      - mosaicism Q91.5
      - translocation Q91.6
    - 18 Q91.3
      - meiotic nondisjunction Q91.Ø
      - mitotic nondisjunction Q91.1
      - mosaicism Q91.1
      - translocation Q91.2
    - 2Ø (q)(p) Q92.8
    - 21 Q9Ø.9
      - meiotic nondisjunction Q9Ø.Ø
      - mitotic nondisjunction Q9Ø.1
      - mosaicism Q9Ø.1
      - translocation Q9Ø.2
    - 22 Q92.8
  - tropical wet feet T69.Ø- ☑
  - Trousseau's I82.1
  - tumor lysis (following antineoplastic chemotherapy) (spontaneous) NEC E88.3
  - tumor necrosis factor receptor associated periodic (TRAPS) MØ4.1
  - Twiddler's (due to)
    - automatic implantable defibrillator T82.198 ☑
    - cardiac pacemaker T82.198 ☑
  - Unverricht (-Lundborg) — *see* Epilepsy, generalized, idiopathic
  - upward gaze H51.8
  - uremia, chronic — *see also* Disease, kidney, chronic N18.9
  - urethral N34.3
  - urethro-oculo-articular — *see* Reiter's disease
  - urohepatic K76.7
  - vago-hypoglossal G52.7
  - van Buchem's M85.2
  - van der Hoeve's Q78.Ø
  - vascular NEC in cerebrovascular disease G46.8
  - vasoconstriction, reversible cerebrovascular I67.841
  - vasomotor I73.9
  - vasospastic (traumatic) T75.22 ☑
  - vasovagal R55
  - VATER Q87.2
  - velo-cardio-facial Q93.81
  - vena cava (inferior) (superior) (obstruction) I87.1
  - vertebral
    - artery G45.Ø
      - compression — *see* Syndrome, anterior, spinal artery, compression
    - steal G45.Ø
  - vertebro-basilar artery G45.Ø
  - vertebrogenic (pain) M54.89
  - vertiginous — *see* Disorder, vestibular function
  - Vinson-Plummer D5Ø.1
  - virus B34.9
  - visceral larva migrans B83.Ø
  - visual disorientation H53.8
  - vitamin B6 deficiency E53.1
  - vitreal corneal H59.Ø1- ☑
  - vitreous (touch) H59.Ø1- ☑
  - Vogt-Koyanagi H2Ø.82- ☑
  - Volkmann's T79.6 ☑
  - von Schroetter's I82.89Ø
  - von Willebrand (-Jürgen) D68.Ø
  - Waldenström-Kjellberg D5Ø.1
  - Wallenberg's G46.3
  - water retention E87.79
  - Waterhouse (-Friderichsen) A39.1
  - Weber-Gubler G46.3
  - Weber-Leyden G46.3
  - Weber's G46.3
  - Wegener's M31.3Ø
    - with
      - kidney involvement M31.31
      - lung involvement M31.3Ø
        - with kidney involvement M31.31
  - Weingarten's (tropical eosinophilia) J82.89
  - Weiss-Baker G9Ø.Ø9
  - Werdnig-Hoffman G12.Ø
  - Wermer's E31.21
  - Werner's E34.8
  - Wernicke-Korsakoff (nonalcoholic) FØ4
    - alcoholic F1Ø.26
  - Westphal-Strümpell E83.Ø1
  - West's — *see* Epilepsy, spasms

- **Syndrome** — *continued*
  - wet
    - feet (maceration) (tropical) T69.Ø- ☑
    - lung, newborn P22.1
  - whiplash S13.4 ☑
  - whistling face Q87.Ø
  - Wilkie's K55.1
  - Wilkinson-Sneddon L13.1
  - Willebrand (-Jürgens) D68.Ø
  - Williams Q93.82
  - Wilson's (hepatolenticular degeneration) E83.Ø1
  - Wiskott-Aldrich D82.Ø
  - withdrawal — *see* Withdrawal, state
    - drug
      - infant of dependent mother P96.1
      - therapeutic use, newborn P96.2
  - Woakes' (ethmoiditis) J33.1
  - Wright's (hyperabduction) G54.Ø
  - X I2Ø.9
  - XXXX Q97.1
  - XXXXX Q97.1
  - XXXXY Q98.1
  - XXY Q98.Ø
  - Yao MØ4.8
  - yellow nail L6Ø.5
  - Zahorsky's BØ8.5
  - Zellweger syndrome E71.51Ø
  - Zellweger-like syndrome E71.541
- **Synechia** (anterior) (iris) (posterior) (pupil) — *see also* Adhesions, iris
  - intra-uterine (traumatic) N85.6
- **Synesthesia** R2Ø.8
- **Syngamiasis, syngamosis** B83.3
- **Synodontia** KØØ.2
- **Synorchidism, synorchism** Q55.1
- **Synostosis** (congenital) Q78.8
  - astragalo-scaphoid Q74.2
  - radioulnar Q74.Ø
- **Synovial sarcoma** — *see* Neoplasm, connective tissue, malignant
- **Synovioma** (malignant) — *see also* Neoplasm, connective tissue, malignant
  - benign — *see* Neoplasm, connective tissue, benign
- **Synoviosarcoma** — *see* Neoplasm, connective tissue, malignant
- **Synovitis** — *see also* Tenosynovitis M65.9
  - crepitant
    - hand M7Ø.Ø- ☑
    - wrist M7Ø.Ø3- ☑
  - gonococcal A54.49
  - gouty — *see* Gout
  - in (due to)
    - crystals M65.8- ☑
    - gonorrhea A54.49
    - syphilis (late) A52.78
    - use, overuse, pressure — *see* Disorder, soft tissue, due to use
  - infective NEC — *see* Tenosynovitis, infective NEC
  - specified NEC — *see* Tenosynovitis, specified type NEC
  - syphilitic A52.78
    - congenital (early) A5Ø.Ø2
  - toxic — *see* Synovitis, transient
  - transient M67.3- ☑
    - ankle M67.37- ☑
    - elbow M67.32- ☑
    - foot joint M67.37- ☑
    - hand joint M67.34- ☑
    - hip M67.35- ☑
    - knee M67.36- ☑
    - multiple site M67.39
    - pelvic region M67.35- ☑
    - shoulder M67.31- ☑
    - specified joint NEC M67.38
    - wrist M67.33- ☑
  - traumatic, current — *see* Sprain
  - tuberculous — *see* Tuberculosis, synovitis
  - villonodular (pigmented) M12.2- ☑
    - ankle M12.27- ☑
    - elbow M12.22- ☑
    - foot joint M12.27- ☑
    - hand joint M12.24- ☑
    - hip M12.25- ☑
    - knee M12.26- ☑
    - multiple site M12.29
    - pelvic region M12.25- ☑
    - shoulder M12.21- ☑
    - specified joint NEC M12.28

T

- **Tabacism, tabacosis, tabagism** — *see also* Poisoning, tobacco
  - meaning dependence (without remission) F17.200
    - with
      - disorder F17.299
        - in remission F17.211
        - specified disorder NEC F17.298
        - withdrawal F17.203
- **Tabardillo** A75.9
  - flea-borne A75.2
  - louse-borne A75.0
- **Tabes, tabetic** A52.10
  - with
    - central nervous system syphilis A52.10
    - Charcot's joint A52.16
    - cord bladder A52.19
    - crisis, viscera (any) A52.19
    - paralysis, general A52.17
    - paresis (general) A52.17
    - perforating ulcer (foot) A52.19
  - arthropathy (Charcot) A52.16
  - bladder A52.19
  - bone A52.11
  - cerebrospinal A52.12
  - congenital A50.45
  - conjugal A52.10
  - dorsalis A52.11
    - juvenile A50.49
  - juvenile A50.49
  - latent A52.19
  - mesenterica A18.39
  - paralysis, insane, general A52.17
  - spasmodic A52.17
  - syphilis (cerebrospinal) A52.12
- **Taboparalysis** A52.17
- **Taboparesis** (remission) A52.17
  - juvenile A50.45
- **TAC** (trigeminal autonomic cephalgia) **NEC** G44.099
  - intractable G44.091
  - not intractable G44.099
- **Tache noir** S60.22- ☑
- **Tachyalimentation** K91.2
- **Tachyarrhythmia, tachyrhythmia** — *see* Tachycardia
- **Tachycardia** R00.0
  - atrial (paroxysmal) I47.1
  - auricular I47.1
  - AV nodal re-entry (re-entrant) I47.1
  - junctional (paroxysmal) I47.1
  - newborn P29.11
  - nodal (paroxysmal) I47.1
  - non-paroxysmal AV nodal I45.89
  - paroxysmal (sustained) (nonsustained) I47.9
    - with sinus bradycardia I49.5
    - atrial (PAT) I47.1
    - atrioventricular (AV) (re-entrant) I47.1
      - psychogenic F54
    - junctional I47.1
      - ectopic I47.1
    - nodal I47.1
    - psychogenic (atrial) (supraventricular) (ventricular) F54
    - supraventricular (sustained) I47.1
      - psychogenic F54
    - ventricular I47.2
      - psychogenic F54
  - psychogenic F45.8
  - sick sinus I49.5
  - sinoauricular NOS R00.0
    - paroxysmal I47.1
  - sinus [sinusal] NOS R00.0
    - paroxysmal I47.1
  - supraventricular I47.1
  - ventricular (paroxysmal) (sustained) I47.2
    - psychogenic F54
- **Tachygastria** K31.89
- **Tachypnea** R06.82
  - hysterical F45.8
  - newborn (idiopathic) (transitory) P22.1
  - psychogenic F45.8
  - transitory, of newborn P22.1
- **TACO** (transfusion associated circulatory overload) E87.71
- **Taenia** (infection) (infestation) B68.9
  - diminuta B71.0
  - echinococcal infestation B67.90
  - mediocanellata B68.1
- **Taenia** — *continued*
  - nana B71.0
  - saginata B68.1
  - solium (intestinal form) B68.0
    - larval form — *see* Cysticercosis
- **Taeniasis** (intestine) — *see* Taenia
- **Tag** (hypertrophied skin) (infected) L91.8
  - adenoid J35.8
  - anus K64.4
  - hemorrhoidal K64.4
  - hymen N89.8
  - perineal N90.89
  - preauricular Q17.0
  - sentinel K64.4
  - skin L91.8
    - accessory (congenital) Q82.8
    - anus K64.4
    - congenital Q82.8
      - preauricular Q17.0
  - tonsil J35.8
  - urethra, urethral N36.8
  - vulva N90.89
- **Tahyna fever** B33.8
- **Takahara's disease** E80.3
- **Takayasu's disease or syndrome** M31.4
- **Talaromycosis** B48.4
- **Talcosis** (pulmonary) J62.0
- **Talipes** (congenital) Q66.89
  - acquired, planus — *see* Deformity, limb, flat foot
  - asymmetric Q66.89
  - calcaneovalgus Q66.4- ☑
  - calcaneovarus Q66.1- ☑
  - calcaneus Q66.89
  - cavus Q66.7- ☑
  - equinovalgus Q66.6
  - equinovarus Q66.0- ☑
  - equinus Q66.89
  - percavus Q66.7- ☑
  - planovalgus Q66.6
  - planus (acquired) (any degree) — *see also* Deformity, limb, flat foot
    - congenital Q66.5- ☑
    - due to rickets (sequelae) E64.3
  - valgus Q66.6
  - varus Q66.3- ☑
- **Tall stature, constitutional** E34.4
- **Talma's disease** M62.89
- **Talon noir** S90.3- ☑
  - hand S60.22- ☑
  - heel S90.3- ☑
  - toe S90.1- ☑
- **Tamponade, heart** I31.4
- **Tanapox** (virus disease) B08.71
- **Tangier disease** E78.6
- **Tantrum, child problem** F91.8
- **Tapeworm** (infection) (infestation) — *see* Infestation, tapeworm
- **Tapia's syndrome** G52.7
- **TAR** (thrombocytopenia with absent radius) **syndrome** Q87.2
- **Tarral-Besnier disease** L44.0
- **Tarsal tunnel syndrome** — *see* Syndrome, tarsal tunnel
- **Tarsalgia** — *see* Pain, limb, lower
- **Tarsitis** (eyelid) H01.8
  - syphilitic A52.71
  - tuberculous A18.4
- **Tartar** (teeth) (dental calculus) K03.6
- **Tattoo** (mark) L81.8
- **Tauri's disease** E74.09
- **Taurodontism** K00.2
- **Taussig-Bing syndrome** Q20.1
- **Taybi's syndrome** Q87.2
- **Tay-Sachs amaurotic familial idiocy or disease** E75.02
- **TBI** (traumatic brain injury) S06.9 ☑
- **Teacher's node or nodule** J38.2
- **Tear, torn** (traumatic) — *see also* Laceration
  - with abortion — *see* Abortion
  - annular fibrosis M51.35
  - anus, anal (sphincter) S31.831 ☑
    - complicating delivery
      - with third degree perineal laceration — *see also* Delivery, complicated, by, laceration, perineum, third degree O70.20
        - with mucosa O70.3
      - without third degree perineal laceration O70.4
    - nontraumatic (healed) (old) K62.81
- **Tear, torn** — *continued*
  - articular cartilage, old — *see* Derangement, joint, articular cartilage, by site
  - bladder
    - with ectopic or molar pregnancy O08.6
    - following ectopic or molar pregnancy O08.6
    - obstetrical O71.5
    - traumatic — *see* Injury, bladder
  - bowel
    - with ectopic or molar pregnancy O08.6
    - following ectopic or molar pregnancy O08.6
    - obstetrical trauma O71.5
  - broad ligament
    - with ectopic or molar pregnancy O08.6
    - following ectopic or molar pregnancy O08.6
    - obstetrical trauma O71.6
  - bucket handle (knee) (meniscus) — *see* Tear, meniscus
  - capsule, joint — *see* Sprain
  - cartilage — *see also* Sprain
    - articular, old — *see* Derangement, joint, articular cartilage, by site
  - cervix
    - with ectopic or molar pregnancy O08.6
    - following ectopic or molar pregnancy O08.6
    - obstetrical trauma (current) O71.3
    - old N88.1
    - traumatic — *see* Injury, uterus
  - dural G97.41
    - nontraumatic G96.11
  - internal organ — *see* Injury, by site
  - knee cartilage
    - articular (current) S83.3- ☑
    - old — *see* Derangement, knee, meniscus, due to old tear
  - ligament — *see* Sprain
  - meniscus (knee) (current injury) S83.209 ☑
    - bucket-handle S83.20- ☑
    - lateral
      - bucket-handle S83.25- ☑
      - complex S83.27- ☑
      - peripheral S83.26- ☑
      - specified type NEC S83.28- ☑
    - medial
      - bucket-handle S83.21- ☑
      - complex S83.23- ☑
      - peripheral S83.22- ☑
      - specified type NEC S83.24- ☑
    - old — *see* Derangement, knee, meniscus, due to old tear
    - site other than knee — *code as* Sprain
    - specified type NEC S83.20- ☑
  - muscle — *see* Strain
  - pelvic
    - floor, complicating delivery O70.1
    - organ NEC, obstetrical trauma O71.5
      - with ectopic or molar pregnancy O08.6
      - following ectopic or molar pregnancy O08.6
  - perineal, secondary O90.1
  - periurethral tissue, obstetrical trauma O71.82
    - with ectopic or molar pregnancy O08.6
    - following ectopic or molar pregnancy O08.6
  - rectovaginal septum — *see* Laceration, vagina
  - retina, retinal (without detachment) (horseshoe) — *see also* Break, retina, horseshoe
    - with detachment — *see* Detachment, retina, with retinal, break
  - rotator cuff (nontraumatic) M75.10- ☑
    - complete M75.12- ☑
    - incomplete M75.11- ☑
    - traumatic S46.01- ☑
      - capsule S43.42- ☑
  - semilunar cartilage, knee — *see* Tear, meniscus
  - supraspinatus (complete) (incomplete) (nontraumatic) — *see also* Tear, rotator cuff M75.10- ☑
  - tendon — *see* Strain
  - tentorial, at birth P10.4
  - umbilical cord
    - complicating delivery O69.89 ☑
  - urethra
    - with ectopic or molar pregnancy O08.6
    - following ectopic or molar pregnancy O08.6
    - obstetrical trauma O71.5
  - uterus — *see* Injury, uterus
  - vagina — *see* Laceration, vagina
  - vessel, from catheter — *see* Puncture, accidental complicating surgery
  - vulva, complicating delivery O70.0

- **Thrombophlebitis** — *continued*
  - intraspinal venous sinuses and veins — *continued*
    - nonpyogenic G95.19
  - lateral (venous) sinus GØ8
    - nonpyogenic I67.6
  - leg I8Ø.3
    - superficial I8Ø.Ø- ☑
  - longitudinal (venous) sinus GØ8
    - nonpyogenic I67.6
  - lower extremity I8Ø.299
  - migrans, migrating I82.1
  - pelvic
    - with ectopic or molar pregnancy OØ8.Ø
    - following ectopic or molar pregnancy OØ8.Ø
    - puerperal O87.1
  - peroneal vein I8Ø.24- ☑
  - popliteal vein — *see* Phlebitis, leg, deep, popliteal
  - portal (vein) K75.1
  - postoperative T81.72 ☑
  - pregnancy — *see* Thrombophlebitis, antepartum
  - puerperal, postpartum, childbirth O87.Ø
    - deep O87.1
    - pelvic O87.1
    - septic O86.81
    - superficial O87.Ø
  - saphenous (greater) (lesser) I8Ø.Ø- ☑
  - sinus (intracranial) GØ8
    - nonpyogenic I67.6
  - soleal vein I8Ø.25- ☑
  - specified site NEC I8Ø.8
  - tibial vein (anterior) (posterior) I8Ø.23- ☑
- **Thrombosis, thrombotic** (bland) (multiple) (progressive) (silent) (vessel) I82.9Ø
  - anal K64.5
  - antepartum — *see* Thrombophlebitis, antepartum
  - aorta, aortic I74.1Ø
    - abdominal I74.Ø9
      - saddle I74.Ø1
    - bifurcation I74.Ø9
    - saddle I74.Ø1
    - specified site NEC I74.19
    - terminal I74.Ø9
    - thoracic I74.11
    - valve — *see* Endocarditis, aortic
  - apoplexy I63.3- ☑
  - artery, arteries (postinfectional) I74.9
    - auditory, internal — *see* Occlusion, artery, precerebral, specified NEC
    - basilar — *see* Occlusion, artery, basilar
    - carotid (common) (internal) — *see* Occlusion, artery, carotid
    - cerebellar (anterior inferior) (posterior inferior) (superior) — *see* Occlusion, artery, cerebellar
    - cerebral — *see* Occlusion, artery, cerebral
    - choroidal (anterior) — *see* Occlusion, artery, precerebral, specified NEC
    - communicating, posterior — *see* Occlusion, artery, precerebral, specified NEC
    - coronary — *see also* Infarct, myocardium
      - not resulting in infarction I24.Ø
    - hepatic I74.8
    - hypophyseal — *see* Occlusion, artery, precerebral, specified NEC
    - iliac I74.5
    - limb I74.4
      - lower I74.3
      - upper I74.2
    - meningeal, anterior or posterior — *see* Occlusion, artery, cerebral, specified NEC
    - mesenteric (with gangrene) — *see also* Infarct, intestine K55.Ø69
    - ophthalmic — *see* Occlusion, artery, retina
    - pontine — *see* Occlusion, artery, precerebral, specified NEC
    - precerebral — *see* Occlusion, artery, precerebral
    - pulmonary (iatrogenic) — *see* Embolism, pulmonary
    - renal N28.Ø
    - retinal — *see* Occlusion, artery, retina
    - spinal, anterior or posterior G95.11
    - traumatic NEC T14.8 ☑
    - vertebral — *see* Occlusion, artery, vertebral
  - atrium, auricular — *see also* Infarct, myocardium
    - following acute myocardial infarction (current complication) I23.6
    - not resulting in infarction I51.3
    - old I51.3
  - basilar (artery) — *see* Occlusion, artery, basilar
  - brain (artery) (stem) — *see also* Occlusion, artery, cerebral
    - due to syphilis A52.Ø5
    - puerperal O99.43
    - sinus — *see* Thrombosis, intracranial venous sinus
  - capillary I78.8
  - cardiac — *see also* Infarct, myocardium
    - not resulting in infarction I51.3
    - old I51.3
    - valve — *see* Endocarditis
  - carotid (artery) (common) (internal) — *see* Occlusion, artery, carotid
  - cavernous (venous) sinus — *see* Thrombosis, intracranial venous sinus
  - cerebellar artery (anterior inferior) (posterior inferior) (superior) I66.3
  - cerebral (artery) — *see* Occlusion, artery, cerebral
  - cerebrovenous sinus — *see also* Thrombosis, intracranial venous sinus
    - puerperium O87.3
  - chronic I82.91
  - coronary (artery) (vein) — *see also* Infarct, myocardium
    - not resulting in infarction I24.Ø
  - corpus cavernosum N48.89
  - cortical I66.9
  - deep — *see* Embolism, vein, lower extremity
  - due to device, implant or graft — *see also* Complications, by site and type, specified NEC T85.868 ☑
    - arterial graft NEC T82.868 ☑
    - breast (implant) T85.868 ☑
    - catheter NEC T85.868 ☑
      - dialysis (renal) T82.868 ☑
        - intraperitoneal T85.868 ☑
      - infusion NEC T82.868 ☑
        - spinal (epidural) (subdural) T85.86Ø ☑
      - urinary (indwelling) T83.86 ☑
    - electronic (electrode) (pulse generator) (stimulator)
      - bone T84.86 ☑
      - cardiac T82.867 ☑
      - nervous system (brain) (peripheral nerve) (spinal) T85.86Ø ☑
      - urinary T83.86 ☑
    - fixation, internal (orthopedic) NEC T84.86 ☑
    - gastrointestinal (bile duct) (esophagus) T85.868 ☑
    - genital NEC T83.86 ☑
    - heart T82.867 ☑
    - joint prosthesis T84.86 ☑
    - ocular (corneal graft) (orbital implant) NEC T85.868 ☑
    - orthopedic NEC T84.86 ☑
    - specified NEC T85.868 ☑
    - urinary NEC T83.86 ☑
    - vascular NEC T82.868 ☑
    - ventricular intracranial shunt T85.86Ø ☑
  - during the puerperium — *see* Thrombosis, puerperal
  - endocardial — *see also* Infarct, myocardium
    - not resulting in infarction I51.3
  - eye — *see* Occlusion, retina
  - genital organ
    - female NEC N94.89
      - pregnancy — *see* Thrombophlebitis, antepartum
    - male N5Ø.1
  - gestational — *see* Phlebopathy, gestational
  - heart (chamber) — *see also* Infarct, myocardium
    - not resulting in infarction I51.3
    - old I51.3
  - hepatic (vein) I82.Ø
    - artery I74.8
  - history (of) Z86.718
  - intestine (with gangrene) — *see also* Infarct, intestine K55.Ø69
  - intracardiac NEC (apical) (atrial) (auricular) (ventricular) (old) I51.3
  - intracranial (arterial) I66.9
    - venous sinus (any) GØ8
      - nonpyogenic origin I67.6
      - puerperium O87.3
  - intramural — *see also* Infarct, myocardium
    - not resulting in infarction I51.3
    - old I51.3
  - intraspinal venous sinuses and veins GØ8
    - nonpyogenic G95.19
  - kidney (artery) N28.Ø
  - lateral (venous) sinus — *see* Thrombosis, intracranial venous sinus
  - leg — *see* Thrombosis, vein, lower extremity
- **Thrombosis, thrombotic** — *continued*
  - leg — *see* Thrombosis, vein, lower extremity — *continued*
    - arterial I74.3
  - liver (venous) I82.Ø
    - artery I74.8
    - portal vein I81
  - longitudinal (venous) sinus — *see* Thrombosis, intracranial venous sinus
  - lower limb — *see* Thrombosis, vein, lower extremity
  - lung (iatrogenic) (postoperative) — *see* Embolism, pulmonary
  - meninges (brain) (arterial) I66.8
  - mesenteric (artery) (with gangrene) — *see also* Infarct, intestine K55.Ø69
    - vein (inferior) (superior) K55.Ø- ☑
  - mitral I34.8
  - mural — *see also* Infarct, myocardium
    - due to syphilis A52.Ø6
    - not resulting in infarction I51.3
    - old I51.3
  - omentum (with gangrene) — *see also* Infarct, intestine K55.Ø69
  - ophthalmic — *see* Occlusion, retina
  - pampiniform plexus (male) N5Ø.1
  - parietal — *see also* Infarct, myocardium
    - not resulting in infarction I24.Ø
  - penis, superficial vein N48.81
  - perianal venous K64.5
  - peripheral arteries I74.4
    - upper I74.2
  - personal history (of) Z86.718
  - portal I81
    - due to syphilis A52.Ø9
  - precerebral artery — *see* Occlusion, artery, precerebral
  - puerperal, postpartum O87.Ø
    - brain (artery) O99.43
      - venous (sinus) O87.3
    - cardiac O99.43
    - cerebral (artery) O99.43
      - venous (sinus) O87.3
    - superficial O87.Ø
  - pulmonary (artery) (iatrogenic) (postoperative) (vein) — *see* Embolism, pulmonary
  - renal (artery) N28.Ø
    - vein I82.3
  - resulting from presence of device, implant or graft — *see* Complications, by site and type, specified NEC
  - retina, retinal — *see* Occlusion, retina
  - scrotum N5Ø.1
  - seminal vesicle N5Ø.1
  - sigmoid (venous) sinus — *see* Thrombosis, intracranial venous sinus
  - sinus, intracranial (any) — *see* Thrombosis, intracranial venous sinus
  - specified site NEC I82.89Ø
    - chronic I82.891
  - spermatic cord N5Ø.1
  - spinal cord (arterial) G95.11
    - due to syphilis A52.Ø9
    - pyogenic origin GØ6.1
  - spleen, splenic D73.5
    - artery I74.8
  - testis N5Ø.1
  - traumatic NEC T14.8 ☑
  - tricuspid IØ7.8
  - tumor — *see* Neoplasm, unspecified behavior, by site
  - tunica vaginalis N5Ø.1
  - umbilical cord (vessels), complicating delivery O69.5 ☑
  - vas deferens N5Ø.1
  - vein (acute) I82.9Ø
    - antecubital I82.61- ☑
      - chronic I82.71- ☑
    - axillary I82.A1- ☑ (*following* I82.7)
      - chronic I82.A2- ☑ (*following* I82.7)
    - basilic I82.61- ☑
      - chronic I82.71- ☑
    - brachial I82.62- ☑
      - chronic I82.72- ☑
    - brachiocephalic (innominate) I82.29Ø
      - chronic I82.291
    - cephalic I82.61- ☑
      - chronic I82.71- ☑
    - cerebral, nonpyogenic I67.6
    - chronic I82.91
    - deep (DVT) I82.4Ø- ☑
      - calf I82.4Z- ☑

Tobacco (nicotine)
- abuse — *see* Tobacco, use
- dependence — *see* Dependence, drug, nicotine
- harmful use Z72.Ø
- heart — *see* Tobacco, toxic effect
- maternal use, affecting newborn PØ4.2
- toxic effect — *see* Table of Drugs and Chemicals, by substance, poisoning
  - chewing tobacco — *see* Table of Drugs and Chemicals, by substance, poisoning
  - cigarettes — *see* Table of Drugs and Chemicals, by substance, poisoning
- use Z72.Ø
  - complicating
    - childbirth O99.334
    - pregnancy O99.33- ☑
    - puerperium O99.335
  - counseling and surveillance Z71.6
  - history Z87.891
- withdrawal state — *see also* Dependence, drug, nicotine F17.2Ø3

Tocopherol deficiency E56.Ø

Todd's
- cirrhosis K74.3
- paralysis (postepileptic) (transitory) G83.84

Toe — *see* condition

Toilet, artificial opening — *see* Attention to, artificial, opening

Tokelau (ringworm) B35.5

Tollwut — *see* Rabies

Tommaselli's disease R31.9
- correct substance properly administered — *see* Table of Drugs and Chemicals, by drug, adverse effect
- overdose or wrong substance given or taken — *see* Table of Drugs and Chemicals, by drug, poisoning

Tongue — *see also* condition
- tie Q38.1

Tonic pupil — *see* Anomaly, pupil, function, tonic pupil

Toni-Fanconi syndrome (cystinosis) E72.Ø9
- with cystinosis E72.Ø4

Tonsil — *see* condition

Tonsillitis (acute) (catarrhal) (croupous) (follicular) (gangrenous) (infective) (lacunar) (lingual) (malignant) (membranous) (parenchymatous) (phlegmonous) (pseudomembranous) (purulent) (septic) (subacute) (suppurative) (toxic) (ulcerative) (vesicular) (viral) JØ3.9Ø
- chronic J35.Ø1
  - with adenoiditis J35.Ø3
- diphtheritic A36.Ø
- hypertrophic J35.Ø1
  - with adenoiditis J35.Ø3
- recurrent JØ3.91
- specified organism NEC JØ3.8Ø
  - recurrent JØ3.81
- staphylococcal JØ3.8Ø
  - recurrent JØ3.81
- streptococcal JØ3.ØØ
  - recurrent JØ3.Ø1
- tuberculous A15.8
- Vincent's A69.1

Tooth, teeth — *see* condition

Toothache KØ8.89

Topagnosis R2Ø.8

Tophi — *see* Gout, chronic

TORCH infection — *see* Infection, congenital
- without active infection PØØ.2

Torn — *see* Tear

Tornwaldt's cyst or disease J39.2

Torsion
- accessory tube — *see* Torsion, fallopian tube
- adnexa (female) — *see* Torsion, fallopian tube
- aorta, acquired I77.1
- appendix epididymis N44.Ø4
- appendix testis N44.Ø3
- bile duct (common) (hepatic) K83.8
  - congenital Q44.5
- bowel, colon or intestine K56.2
- cervix — *see* Malposition, uterus
- cystic duct K82.8
- dystonia — *see* Dystonia, torsion
- epididymis (appendix) N44.Ø4
- fallopian tube N83.52- ☑
  - with ovary N83.53
- gallbladder K82.8
  - congenital Q44.1
- hydatid of Morgagni
  - female N83.52- ☑

Torsion — *continued*
- hydatid of Morgagni — *continued*
  - male N44.Ø3
- kidney (pedicle) (leading to infarction) N28.Ø
- Meckel's diverticulum (congenital) Q43.Ø
  - malignant — *see* Table of Neoplasms, small intestine, malignant
- mesentery K56.2
- omentum K56.2
- organ or site, congenital NEC — *see* Anomaly, by site
- ovary (pedicle) N83.51- ☑
  - with fallopian tube N83.53
  - congenital Q5Ø.2
- oviduct — *see* Torsion, fallopian tube
- penis (acquired) N48.82
  - congenital Q55.63
- spasm — *see* Dystonia, torsion
- spermatic cord N44.Ø2
  - extravaginal N44.Ø1
  - intravaginal N44.Ø2
- spleen D73.5
- testis, testicle N44.ØØ
  - appendix N44.Ø3
- tibia — *see* Deformity, limb, specified type NEC, lower leg
- uterus — *see* Malposition, uterus

Torticollis (intermittent) (spastic) M43.6
- congenital (sternomastoid) Q68.Ø
- due to birth injury P15.8
- hysterical F44.4
- ocular R29.891
- psychogenic F45.8
  - conversion reaction F44.4
- rheumatic M43.6
- rheumatoid MØ6.88
- spasmodic G24.3
- traumatic, current S13.4 ☑

Tortipelvis G24.1

Tortuous
- aortic arch Q25.46
- artery I77.1
- organ or site, congenital NEC — *see* Distortion
- retinal vessel, congenital Q14.1
- ureter N13.8
- urethra N36.8
- vein — *see* Varix

Torture, victim of Z65.4

Torula, torular (histolytica) (infection) — *see* Cryptococcosis

Torulosis — *see* Cryptococcosis

Torus (mandibularis) (palatinus) M27.Ø
- fracture — *see* Fracture, by site, torus

Touraine's syndrome Q79.8

Tourette's syndrome F95.2

Tourniquet syndrome — *see* Constriction, external, by site

Tower skull Q75.Ø
- with exophthalmos Q87.Ø

Toxemia R68.89
- bacterial — *see* Sepsis
- burn — *see* Burn
- eclamptic (with pre-existing hypertension) — *see* Eclampsia
- erysipelatous — *see* Erysipelas
- fatigue R68.89
- food — *see* Poisoning, food
- gastrointestinal K52.1
- intestinal K52.1
- kidney — *see* Uremia
- malarial — *see* Malaria
- myocardial — *see* Myocarditis, toxic
- of pregnancy — *see* Pre-eclampsia
- pre-eclamptic — *see* Pre-eclampsia
- small intestine K52.1
- staphylococcal, due to food AØ5.Ø
- stasis R68.89
- uremic — *see* Uremia
- urinary — *see* Uremia

Toxemica cerebropathia psychica (nonalcoholic) FØ4
- alcoholic — *see* Alcohol, amnestic disorder

Toxic (poisoning) — *see also* condition T65.91 ☑
- effect — *see* Table of Drugs and Chemicals, by substance, poisoning
- shock syndrome A48.3
- thyroid (gland) — *see* Thyrotoxicosis

Toxicemia — *see* Toxemia

Toxicity — *see* Table of Drugs and Chemicals, by substance, poisoning
- fava bean D55.Ø
- food, noxious — *see* Poisoning, food
- from drug or nonmedicinal substance — *see* Table of Drugs and Chemicals, by drug

Toxicosis — *see also* Toxemia
- capillary, hemorrhagic D69.Ø

Toxinfection, gastrointestinal K52.1

Toxocariasis B83.Ø

Toxoplasma, toxoplasmosis (acquired) B58.9
- with
  - hepatitis B58.1
  - meningoencephalitis B58.2
  - ocular involvement B58.ØØ
  - other organ involvement B58.89
  - pneumonia, pneumonitis B58.3
- congenital (acute) (subacute) (chronic) P37.1
- maternal, manifest toxoplasmosis in infant (acute) (subacute) (chronic) P37.1

tPA (rtPA) **administation in a different facility within the last 24 hours prior to admission to current facility** Z92.82

Trabeculation, bladder N32.89

Trachea — *see* condition

Tracheitis (catarrhal) (infantile) (membranous) (plastic) (septal) (suppurative) (viral) JØ4.1Ø
- with
  - bronchitis (15 years of age and above) J4Ø
    - acute or subacute — *see* Bronchitis, acute
    - chronic J42
    - tuberculous NEC A15.5
    - under 15 years of age J2Ø.9
  - laryngitis (acute) JØ4.2
    - chronic J37.1
    - tuberculous NEC A15.5
- acute JØ4.1Ø
  - with obstruction JØ4.11
- chronic J42
  - with
    - bronchitis (chronic) J42
    - laryngitis (chronic) J37.1
- diphtheritic (membranous) A36.89
- due to external agent — *see* Inflammation, respiratory, upper, due to
- syphilitic A52.73
- tuberculous A15.5

Trachelitis (nonvenereal) — *see* Cervicitis

Tracheobronchial — *see* condition

Tracheobronchitis (15 years of age and above) — *see also* Bronchitis
- due to
  - Bordetella bronchiseptica A37.8Ø
    - with pneumonia A37.81
  - Francisella tularensis A21.8

Tracheobronchomegaly Q32.4
- with bronchiectasis J47.9
  - with
    - exacerbation (acute) J47.1
    - lower respiratory infection J47.Ø
- acquired J98.Ø9
  - with bronchiectasis J47.9
    - with
      - exacerbation (acute) J47.1
      - lower respiratory infection J47.Ø

Tracheobronchopneumonitis — *see* Pneumonia, broncho-

Tracheocele (external) (internal) J39.8
- congenital Q32.1

Tracheomalacia J39.8
- congenital Q32.Ø

Tracheopharyngitis (acute) JØ6.9
- chronic J42
- due to external agent — *see* Inflammation, respiratory, upper, due to

Tracheostenosis J39.8

Tracheostomy
- complication — *see* Complication, tracheostomy
- status Z93.Ø
  - attention to Z43.Ø
  - malfunctioning J95.Ø3

Trachoma, trachomatous A71.9
- active (stage) A71.1
- contraction of conjunctiva A71.1
- dubium A71.Ø
- healed or sequelae B94.Ø
- initial (stage) A71.Ø
- pannus A71.1

Trachoma, trachomatous — *continued*
- Türck's J37.Ø

Traction, vitreomacular H43.82- ☑
Train sickness T75.3 ☑
Trait(s)
- Hb-S D57.3
- hemoglobin
  - abnormal NEC D58.2
    - with thalassemia D56.3
  - C — *see* Disease, hemoglobin C
  - S (Hb-S) D57.3
- Lepore D56.3
- personality, accentuated Z73.1
- sickle-cell D57.3
  - with elliptocytosis or spherocytosis D57.3
- type A personality Z73.1

Tramp Z59.Ø
Trance R41.89
- hysterical F44.89

Transaminasemia R74.Ø1
Transection
- abdomen (partial) S38.3 ☑
- aorta (incomplete) — *see also* Injury, aorta
  - complete — *see* Injury, aorta, laceration, major
- carotid artery (incomplete) — *see also* Injury, blood vessel, carotid, laceration
  - complete — *see* Injury, blood vessel, carotid, laceration, major
- celiac artery (incomplete) S35.211 ☑
  - branch (incomplete) S35.291 ☑
    - complete S35.292 ☑
  - complete S35.212 ☑
- innominate
  - artery (incomplete) — *see also* Injury, blood vessel, thoracic, innominate, artery, laceration
    - complete — *see* Injury, blood vessel, thoracic, innominate, artery, laceration, major
  - vein (incomplete) — *see also* Injury, blood vessel, thoracic, innominate, vein, laceration
    - complete — *see* Injury, blood vessel, thoracic, innominate, vein, laceration, major
- jugular vein (external) (incomplete) — *see also* Injury, blood vessel, jugular vein, laceration
  - complete — *see* Injury, blood vessel, jugular vein, laceration, major
  - internal (incomplete) — *see also* Injury, blood vessel, jugular vein, internal, laceration
    - complete — *see* Injury, blood vessel, jugular vein, internal, laceration, major
- mesenteric artery (incomplete) — *see also* Injury, mesenteric, artery, laceration
  - complete — *see* Injury, mesenteric artery, laceration, major
- pulmonary vessel (incomplete) — *see also* Injury, blood vessel, thoracic, pulmonary, laceration
  - complete — *see* Injury, blood vessel, thoracic, pulmonary, laceration, major
- subclavian — *see* Transection, innominate
- vena cava (incomplete) — *see also* Injury, vena cava
  - complete — *see* Injury, vena cava, laceration, major
- vertebral artery (incomplete) — *see also* Injury, blood vessel, vertebral, laceration
  - complete — *see* Injury, blood vessel, vertebral, laceration, major

Transfusion
- associated (red blood cell) hemochromatosis E83.111
- blood
  - ABO incompatible — *see* Complication(s), transfusion, incompatibility reaction, ABO
  - minor blood group (Duffy) (E) (K) (Kell) (Kidd) (Lewis) (M) (N) (P) (S) T80.89 ☑
  - reaction or complication — *see* Complications, transfusion
- fetomaternal (mother) — *see* Pregnancy, complicated by, placenta, transfusion syndrome
- maternofetal (mother) — *see* Pregnancy, complicated by, placenta, transfusion syndrome
- placental (syndrome) (mother) — *see* Pregnancy, complicated by, placenta, transfusion syndrome
- reaction (adverse) — *see* Complications, transfusion
- related acute lung injury (TRALI) J95.84
- twin-to-twin — *see* Pregnancy, complicated by, placenta, transfusion syndrome, fetus to fetus

Transient (meaning homeless) — *see also* condition Z59.Ø
Translocation
- balanced autosomal Q95.9
  - in normal individual Q95.Ø

Translocation — *continued*
- chromosomes NEC Q99.8
  - balanced and insertion in normal individual Q95.Ø
- Down syndrome Q9Ø.2
- trisomy
  - 13 Q91.6
  - 18 Q91.2
  - 21 Q9Ø.2

Translucency, iris — *see* Degeneration, iris
Transmission of chemical substances through the placenta — *see* Absorption, chemical, through placenta
Transparency, lung, unilateral J43.Ø
Transplant (ed) (status) Z94.9
- awaiting organ Z76.82
- bone Z94.6
  - marrow Z94.81
- candidate Z76.82
- complication — *see* Complication, transplant
- cornea Z94.7
- heart Z94.1
  - and lung(s) Z94.3
  - valve Z95.2
    - prosthetic Z95.2
    - specified NEC Z95.4
    - xenogenic Z95.3
- intestine Z94.82
- kidney Z94.Ø
- liver Z94.4
- lung(s) Z94.2
  - and heart Z94.3
- organ (failure) (infection) (rejection) Z94.9
  - removal status Z98.85
- pancreas Z94.83
- skin Z94.5
- social Z6Ø.3
- specified organ or tissue NEC Z94.89
- stem cells Z94.84
- tissue Z94.9

Transplants, ovarian, endometrial N8Ø.1
Transposed — *see* Transposition
Transposition (congenital) — *see also* Malposition, congenital
- abdominal viscera Q89.3
- aorta (dextra) Q2Ø.3
- appendix Q43.8
- colon Q43.8
- corrected Q2Ø.5
- great vessels (complete) (partial) Q2Ø.3
- heart Q24.Ø
  - with complete transposition of viscera Q89.3
- intestine (large) (small) Q43.8
- reversed jejunal (for bypass) (status) Z98.Ø
- scrotum Q55.23
- stomach Q4Ø.2
  - with general transposition of viscera Q89.3
- tooth, teeth, fully erupted M26.3Ø
- vessels, great (complete) (partial) Q2Ø.3
- viscera (abdominal) (thoracic) Q89.3

Transsexualism F64.Ø
Transverse — *see also* condition
- arrest (deep), in labor O64.Ø ☑
- lie (mother) O32.2 ☑
  - causing obstructed labor O64.8 ☑

Transvestism, transvestitism (dual-role) F64.1
- fetishistic F65.1

Trapped placenta (with hemorrhage) O72.Ø
- without hemorrhage O73.Ø

TRAPS (tumor necrosis factor receptor associated periodic syndrome) MØ4.1
Trauma, traumatism — *see also* Injury
- acoustic — *see* subcategory H83.3 ☑
- birth — *see* Birth, injury
- complicating ectopic or molar pregnancy OØ8.6
- during delivery O71.9
- following ectopic or molar pregnancy OØ8.6
- obstetric O71.9
  - specified NEC O71.89
- occusal
  - primary KØ8.81
  - secondary KØ8.82

Traumatic — *see also* condition
- brain injury SØ6.9 ☑

Treacher Collins syndrome Q75.4
Treitz's hernia — *see* Hernia, abdomen, specified site NEC
Trematode infestation — *see* Infestation, fluke
Trematodiasis — *see* Infestation, fluke
Trembling paralysis — *see* Parkinsonism
Tremor(s) R25.1
- drug induced G25.1
- essential (benign) G25.Ø
- familial G25.Ø
- hereditary G25.Ø
- hysterical F44.4
- intention G25.2
- medication induced postural G25.1
- mercurial — *see* subcategory T56.1 ☑
- Parkinson's — *see* Parkinsonism
- psychogenic (conversion reaction) F44.4
- senilis R54
- specified type NEC G25.2

Trench
- fever A79.Ø
- foot — *see* Immersion, foot
- mouth A69.1

Treponema pallidum infection — *see* Syphilis
Treponematosis
- due to
  - T. pallidum — *see* Syphilis
  - T. pertenue — *see* Yaws

Triad
- Hutchinson's (congenital syphilis) A5Ø.53
- Kartagener's Q89.3
- Saint's — *see* Hernia, diaphragm

Trichiasis (eyelid) HØ2.Ø59
- with entropion — *see* Entropion
- left HØ2.Ø56
  - lower HØ2.Ø55
  - upper HØ2.Ø54
- right HØ2.Ø53
  - lower HØ2.Ø52
  - upper HØ2.Ø51

Trichinella spiralis (infection) (infestation) B75
Trichinellosis, trichiniasis, trichinelliasis, trichinosis B75
- with muscle disorder B75 *[M63.8Ø]*
  - ankle B75 *[M63.87-]* ☑
  - foot B75 *[M63.87-]* ☑
  - forearm B75 *[M63.83-]* ☑
  - hand B75 *[M63.84-]* ☑
  - lower leg B75 *[M63.86-]* ☑
  - multiple sites B75 *[M63.89]*
  - pelvic region B75 *[M63.85-]* ☑
  - shoulder region B75 *[M63.81-]* ☑
  - specified site NEC B75 *[M63.88]*
  - thigh B75 *[M63.85-]* ☑
  - upper arm B75 *[M63.82-]* ☑

Trichobezoar T18.9 ☑
- intestine T18.3 ☑
- stomach T18.2 ☑

Trichocephaliasis, trichocephalosis B79
Trichocephalus infestation B79
Trichoclasis L67.8
Trichoepithelioma — *see also* Neoplasm, skin, benign
- malignant — *see* Neoplasm, skin, malignant

Trichofolliculoma — *see* Neoplasm, skin, benign
Tricholemmoma — *see* Neoplasm, skin, benign
Trichomoniasis A59.9
- bladder A59.Ø3
- cervix A59.Ø9
- intestinal AØ7.8
- prostate A59.Ø2
- seminal vesicles A59.Ø9
- specified site NEC A59.8
- urethra A59.Ø3
- urogenitalis A59.ØØ
- vagina A59.Ø1
- vulva A59.Ø1

Trichomycosis
- axillaris A48.8
- nodosa, nodularis B36.8

Trichonodosis L67.8
Trichophytid, trichophyton infection — *see* Dermatophytosis
Trichophytobezoar T18.9 ☑
- intestine T18.3 ☑
- stomach T18.2 ☑

Trichophytosis — *see* Dermatophytosis
Trichoptilosis L67.8
Trichorrhexis (nodosa) (invaginata) L67.Ø
Trichosis axillaris A48.8
Trichosporosis nodosa B36.2
Trichostasis spinulosa (congenital) Q84.1

Tumor — *continued*
- germ cell — *see also* Neoplasm, malignant, by site
  - mixed — *see* Neoplasm, malignant, by site
- ghost cell, odontogenic — *see* Cyst, calcifying odontogenic
- giant cell — *see also* Neoplasm, uncertain behavior, by site
  - bone D48.Ø
    - malignant — *see* Neoplasm, bone, malignant
  - chondromatous — *see* Neoplasm, bone, benign
  - malignant — *see* Neoplasm, malignant, by site
  - soft parts — *see* Neoplasm, connective tissue, uncertain behavior
    - malignant — *see* Neoplasm, connective tissue, malignant
- glomus D18.ØØ
  - intra-abdominal D18.Ø3
  - intracranial D18.Ø2
  - jugulare D44.7
    - malignant C75.5
  - skin D18.Ø1
  - specified site NEC D18.Ø9
- gonadal stromal — *see* Neoplasm, uncertain behavior, by site
- granular cell — *see also* Neoplasm, connective tissue, benign
  - malignant — *see* Neoplasm, connective tissue, malignant
- granulosa cell D39.1- ☑
  - juvenile D39.1- ☑
  - malignant C56- ☑
- granulosa cell-theca cell D39.1- ☑
  - malignant C56- ☑
- Grawitz's C64- ☑
- hemorrhoidal — *see* Hemorrhoids
- hilar cell D27- ☑
- hilus cell D27- ☑
- Hurthle cell (benign) D34
  - malignant C73
- hydatid — *see* Echinococcus
- hypernephroid — *see also* Neoplasm, uncertain behavior, by site
- interstitial cell — *see also* Neoplasm, uncertain behavior, by site
  - benign — *see* Neoplasm, benign, by site
  - malignant — *see* Neoplasm, malignant, by site
- intravascular bronchial alveolar D38.1
- islet cell — *see* Neoplasm, benign, by site
  - malignant — *see* Neoplasm, malignant, by site
    - pancreas C25.4
    - specified site NEC — *see* Neoplasm, malignant, by site
    - unspecified site C25.4
  - pancreas D13.7
  - specified site NEC — *see* Neoplasm, benign, by site
  - unspecified site D13.7
- juxtaglomerular D41.Ø- ☑
- Klatskin's C22.1
- Krukenberg's C79.6- ☑
- Leydig cell — *see* Neoplasm, uncertain behavior, by site
  - benign — *see* Neoplasm, benign, by site
    - specified site — *see* Neoplasm, benign, by site
    - unspecified site
      - female D27.9
      - male D29.2Ø
  - malignant — *see* Neoplasm, malignant, by site
    - specified site — *see* Neoplasm, malignant, by site
    - unspecified site
      - female C56.9
      - male C62.9Ø
  - specified site — *see* Neoplasm, uncertain behavior, by site
  - unspecified site
    - female D39.1Ø
    - male D4Ø.1Ø
- lipid cell, ovary D27- ☑
- lipoid cell, ovary D27- ☑
- malignant — *see also* Neoplasm, malignant, by site C8Ø.1
  - fusiform cell (type) C8Ø.1
  - giant cell (type) C8Ø.1
  - localized, plasma cell — *see* Plasmacytoma, solitary
  - mixed NEC C8Ø.1
  - small cell (type) C8Ø.1
  - spindle cell (type) C8Ø.1

Tumor — *continued*
- malignant — *see also* Neoplasm, malignant, by site — *continued*
  - unclassified C8Ø.1
- mast cell D47.Ø9
- melanotic, neuroectodermal — *see* Neoplasm, benign, by site
- Merkel cell — *see* Carcinoma, Merkel cell
- mesenchymal
  - malignant — *see* Neoplasm, connective tissue, malignant
  - mixed — *see* Neoplasm, connective tissue, uncertain behavior
- mesodermal, mixed — *see also* Neoplasm, malignant, by site
  - liver C22.4
- mesonephric — *see also* Neoplasm, uncertain behavior, by site
  - malignant — *see* Neoplasm, malignant, by site
- metastatic
  - from specified site — *see* Neoplasm, malignant, by site
  - of specified site — *see* Neoplasm, malignant, by site
  - to specified site — *see* Neoplasm, secondary, by site
- mixed NEC — *see also* Neoplasm, benign, by site
  - malignant — *see* Neoplasm, malignant, by site
- mucinous of low malignant potential
  - specified site — *see* Neoplasm, malignant, by site
  - unspecified site C56.9
- mucocarcinoid
  - specified site — *see* Neoplasm, malignant, by site
  - unspecified site C18.1
- mucoepidermoid — *see* Neoplasm, uncertain behavior, by site
- Müllerian, mixed
  - specified site — *see* Neoplasm, malignant, by site
  - unspecified site C54.9
- myoepithelial — *see* Neoplasm, benign, by site
- neuroectodermal (peripheral) — *see* Neoplasm, malignant, by site
  - primitive
    - specified site — *see* Neoplasm, malignant, by site
    - unspecified site C71.9
- neuroendocrine D3A.8 (*following* D36)
  - malignant poorly differentiated C7A.1 (*following* C75)
  - secondary NEC C7B.8 (*following* C75)
  - specified NEC C7A.8 (*following* C75)
- neurogenic olfactory C3Ø.Ø
- nonencapsulated sclerosing C73
- odontogenic (adenomatoid) (benign) (calcifying epithelial) (keratocystic) (squamous) — *see* Cyst, calcifying odontogenic
  - malignant C41.1
    - upper jaw (bone) C41.Ø
- ovarian stromal D39.1- ☑
- ovary, in pregnancy — *see* Pregnancy, complicated by
- pacinian — *see* Neoplasm, skin, benign
- Pancoast's — *see* Pancoast's syndrome
- papillary — *see also* Papilloma
  - cystic D37.9
  - mucinous of low malignant potential C56- ☑
    - specified site — *see* Neoplasm, malignant, by site
    - unspecified site C56.9
  - serous of low malignant potential
    - specified site — *see* Neoplasm, malignant, by site
    - unspecified site C56.9
- pelvic, in pregnancy or childbirth — *see* Pregnancy, complicated by
- phantom F45.8
- phyllodes D48.6- ☑
  - benign D24- ☑
  - malignant — *see* Neoplasm, breast, malignant
- Pindborg — *see* Cyst, calcifying odontogenic
- placental site trophoblastic D39.2
- plasma cell (malignant) (localized) — *see* Plasmacytoma, solitary
- polyvesicular vitelline
  - specified site — *see* Neoplasm, malignant, by site
  - unspecified site
    - female C56.9
    - male C62.9Ø
- Pott's puffy — *see* Osteomyelitis, specified NEC
- Rathke's pouch D44.3
- retinal anlage — *see* Neoplasm, benign, by site

Tumor — *continued*
- salivary gland type, mixed — *see* Neoplasm, salivary gland, benign
  - malignant — *see* Neoplasm, salivary gland, malignant
- Sampson's N8Ø.1
- Schmincke's — *see* Neoplasm, nasopharynx, malignant
- sclerosing stromal D27- ☑
- sebaceous — *see* Cyst, sebaceous
- secondary — *see* Neoplasm, secondary, by site
  - carcinoid C7B.ØØ (*following* C75)
    - bone C7B.Ø3 (*following* C75)
    - distant lymph nodes C7B.Ø1 (*following* C75)
    - liver C7B.Ø2 (*following* C75)
    - peritoneum C7B.Ø4 (*following* C75)
    - specified NEC C7B.Ø9 (*following* C75)
  - neuroendocrine NEC C7B.8 (*following* C75)
- serous of low malignant potential
  - specified site — *see* Neoplasm, malignant, by site
  - unspecified site C56.9
- Sertoli cell — *see* Neoplasm, benign, by site
  - with lipid storage
    - specified site — *see* Neoplasm, benign, by site
    - unspecified site
      - female D27.9
      - male D29.2Ø
  - specified site — *see* Neoplasm, benign, by site
  - unspecified site
    - female D27.9
    - male D29.2Ø
- Sertoli-Leydig cell — *see* Neoplasm, benign, by site
  - specified site — *see* Neoplasm, benign, by site
  - unspecified site
    - female D27.9
    - male D29.2Ø
- sex cord (-stromal) — *see* Neoplasm, uncertain behavior, by site
  - with annular tubules D39.1- ☑
- skin appendage — *see* Neoplasm, skin, benign
- smooth muscle — *see* Neoplasm, connective tissue, uncertain behavior
- soft tissue
  - benign — *see* Neoplasm, connective tissue, benign
  - malignant — *see* Neoplasm, connective tissue, malignant
- sternomastoid (congenital) Q68.Ø
- stromal
  - endometrial D39.Ø
  - gastric D48.1
    - benign D21.4
    - malignant C16.9
    - uncertain behavior D48.1
  - gastrointestinal C49.A- ☑
    - benign D21.4
    - esophagus C49.A1
    - malignant C49.AØ
      - colon C49.A4
      - duodenum C49.A3
      - esophagus C49.A1
      - ileum C49.A3
      - jejunum C49.A3
      - large intestine C49.A4
      - Meckel diverticulum C49.A3
      - omentum C49.A9
      - peritoneum C49.A9
      - rectum C49.A5
      - small intestine C49.A3
      - specified site NEC C49.A9
      - stomach C49.A2
    - rectum C49.A5
    - small intestine C49.A3
    - specified site NEC C49.A9
    - stomach C49.A2
    - uncertain behavior D48.1
  - intestine
    - benign D21.4
    - malignant
      - large C49.A4
      - small C49.A3
    - uncertain behavior D48.1
  - ovarian D39.1- ☑
  - stomach C49.A2
    - benign D21.4
    - malignant C49.A2
    - uncertain behavior D48.1
- sweat gland — *see also* Neoplasm, skin, uncertain behavior
  - benign — *see* Neoplasm, skin, benign

Index

Tumor — Tumor

- **Tumor** — *continued*
  - sweat gland — *see also* Neoplasm, skin, uncertain behavior — *continued*
    - malignant — *see* Neoplasm, skin, malignant
  - syphilitic, brain A52.17
  - testicular D4Ø.1Ø
  - testicular stromal D4Ø.1- ☑
  - theca cell D27.- ☑
  - theca cell-granulosa cell D39.1- ☑
  - Triton, malignant — *see* Neoplasm, nerve, malignant
  - trophoblastic, placental site D39.2
  - turban D23.4
  - uterus (body), in pregnancy or childbirth — *see* Pregnancy, complicated by, tumor, uterus
  - vagina, in pregnancy or childbirth — *see* Pregnancy, complicated by
  - varicose — *see* Varix
  - von Recklinghausen's — *see* Neurofibromatosis
  - vulva or perineum, in pregnancy or childbirth — *see* Pregnancy, complicated by
    - causing obstructed labor O65.5
  - Warthin's — *see* Neoplasm, salivary gland, benign
  - Wilms' C64- ☑
  - yolk sac — *see* Neoplasm, malignant, by site
    - specified site — *see* Neoplasm, malignant, by site
    - unspecified site
      - female C56.9
      - male C62.9Ø
- **Tumor lysis syndrome** (following antineoplastic chemotherapy) (spontaneous) NEC E88.3
- **Tumorlet** — *see* Neoplasm, uncertain behavior, by site
- **Tungiasis** B88.1
- **Tunica vasculosa lentis** Q12.2
- **Turban tumor** D23.4
- **Türck's trachoma** J37.Ø
- **Turner-Kieser syndrome** Q87.2
- **Turner-like syndrome** Q87.19
- **Turner's**
  - hypoplasia (tooth) KØØ.4
  - syndrome Q96.9
    - specified NEC Q96.8
  - tooth KØØ.4
- **Turner-Ullrich syndrome** Q96.9
- **Tussis convulsiva** — *see* Whooping cough
- **Twiddler's syndrome** (due to)
  - automatic implantable defibrillatorT82.198
  - cardiac pacemaker T82.198 ☑
- **Twilight state**
  - epileptic FØ5
  - psychogenic F44.89
- **Twin** (newborn) — *see also* Newborn, twin
  - conjoined Q89.4
  - pregnancy — *see* Pregnancy, twin
- **Twinning, teeth** KØØ.2
- **Twist, twisted**
  - bowel, colon or intestine K56.2
  - hair (congenital) Q84.1
  - mesentery K56.2
  - omentum K56.2
  - organ or site, congenital NEC — *see* Anomaly, by site
  - ovarian pedicle — *see* Torsion, ovary
- **Twitching** R25.3
- **Tylosis** (acquired) L84
  - buccalis K13.29
  - linguae K13.29
  - palmaris et plantaris (congenital) (inherited) Q82.8
    - acquired L85.1
- **Tympanism** R14.Ø
- **Tympanites** (abdominal) (intestinal) R14.Ø
- **Tympanitis** — *see* Myringitis
- **Tympanosclerosis** H74.Ø ☑
- **Tympanum** — *see* condition
- **Tympany**
  - abdomen R14.Ø
  - chest RØ9.89
- **Type A behavior pattern** Z73.1
- **Typhlitis** — *see* Appendicitis
- **Typhoenteritis** — *see* Typhoid
- **Typhoid** (abortive) (ambulant) (any site) (clinical) (fever) (hemorrhagic) (infection) (intermittent) (malignant) (rheumatic) (Widal negative) AØ1.ØØ
  - with pneumonia AØ1.Ø3
  - abdominal AØ1.Ø9
  - arthritis AØ1.Ø4
  - carrier (suspected) of Z22.Ø
  - cholecystitis (current) AØ1.Ø9
  - endocarditis AØ1.Ø2
- **Typhoid** — *continued*
  - heart involvement AØ1.Ø2
  - inoculation reaction — *see* Complications, vaccination
  - meningitis AØ1.Ø1
  - mesenteric lymph nodes AØ1.Ø9
  - myocarditis AØ1.Ø2
  - osteomyelitis AØ1.Ø5
  - perichondritis, larynx AØ1.Ø9
  - pneumonia AØ1.Ø3
  - specified NEC AØ1.Ø9
  - spine AØ1.Ø5
  - ulcer (perforating) AØ1.Ø9
- **Typhomalaria** (fever) — *see* Malaria
- **Typhomania** AØ1.ØØ
- **Typhoperitonitis** AØ1.Ø9
- **Typhus** (fever) A75.9
  - abdominal, abdominalis — *see* Typhoid
  - African tick A77.1
  - amarillic A95.9
  - brain A75.9 *[G94]*
  - cerebral A75.9 *[G94]*
  - classical A75.Ø
  - due to Rickettsia
    - prowazekii A75.Ø
      - recrudescent A75.1
    - tsutsugamushi A75.3
    - typhi A75.2
  - endemic (flea-borne) A75.2
  - epidemic (louse-borne) A75.Ø
  - exanthematicus SAI A75.Ø
    - brillii SAI A75.1
    - mexicanus SAI A75.2
    - typhus murinus A75.2
  - exanthematic NEC A75.Ø
  - flea-borne A75.2
  - India tick A77.1
  - Kenya (tick) A77.1
  - louse-borne A75.Ø
  - Mexican A75.2
  - mite-borne A75.3
  - murine A75.2
  - North Asian tick-borne A77.2
  - Orientia Tsutsugamushi (scrub typhus) A75.3
  - petechial A75.9
  - Queensland tick A77.3
  - rat A75.2
  - recrudescent A75.1
  - recurrens — *see* Fever, relapsing
  - Sao Paulo A77.Ø
  - scrub (China) (India) (Malaysia) (New Guinea) A75.3
  - shop (of Malaysia) A75.2
  - Siberian tick A77.2
  - tick-borne A77.9
  - tropical (mite-borne) A75.3
- **Tyrosinemia** E7Ø.21
  - newborn, transitory P74.5
- **Tyrosinosis** E7Ø.21
- **Tyrosinuria** E7Ø.29

U

- **Uhl's anomaly or disease** Q24.8
- **Ulcer, ulcerated, ulcerating, ulceration, ulcerative**
  - alveolar process M27.3
  - amebic (intestine) AØ6.1
    - skin AØ6.7
  - anastomotic — *see* Ulcer, gastrojejunal
  - anorectal K62.6
  - antral — *see* Ulcer, stomach
  - anus (sphincter) (solitary) K62.6
  - aorta — *see* Aneurysm
  - aphthous (oral) (recurrent) K12.Ø
    - genital organ(s)
      - female N76.6
      - male N5Ø.89
  - artery I77.2
  - atrophic — *see* Ulcer, skin
    - decubitus — *see* Ulcer, pressure, by site
  - back L98.429
    - with
      - bone involvement without evidence of necrosis L98.426
      - bone necrosis L98.424
      - exposed fat layer L98.422
      - muscle involvement without evidence of necrosis L98.425
      - muscle necrosis L98.423
      - skin breakdown only L98.421
- **Ulcer, ulcerated, ulcerating, ulceration, ulcerative** — *continued*
  - back — *continued*
    - with — *continued*
      - specified severity NEC L98.428
  - Barrett's (esophagus) K22.1Ø
    - with bleeding K22.11
  - bile duct (common) (hepatic) K83.8
  - bladder (solitary) (sphincter) NEC N32.89
    - bilharzial B65.9 *[N33]*
    - in schistosomiasis (bilharzial) B65.9 *[N33]*
    - submucosal — *see* Cystitis, interstitial
    - tuberculous A18.12
  - bleeding K27.4
  - bone — *see* Osteomyelitis, specified type NEC
  - bowel — *see* Ulcer, intestine
  - breast N61.1
  - bronchus J98.Ø9
  - buccal (cavity) (traumatic) K12.1
  - Buruli A31.1
  - buttock L98.419
    - with
      - bone involvement without evidence of necrosis L98.416
      - bone necrosis L98.414
      - exposed fat layer L98.412
      - muscle involvement without evidence of necrosis L98.415
      - muscle necrosis L98.413
      - skin breakdown only L98.411
      - specified severity NEC L98.418
  - cancerous — *see* Neoplasm, malignant, by site
  - cardia K22.1Ø
    - with bleeding K22.11
  - cardioesophageal (peptic) K22.1Ø
    - with bleeding K22.11
  - cecum — *see* Ulcer, intestine
  - cervix (uteri) (decubitus) (trophic) N86
    - with cervicitis N72
  - chancroidal A57
  - chiclero B55.1
  - chronic (cause unknown) — *see* Ulcer, skin
  - Cochin-China B55.1
  - colon — *see* Ulcer, intestine
  - conjunctiva H1Ø.89
  - cornea H16.ØØ- ☑
    - with hypopyon H16.Ø3- ☑
    - central H16.Ø1- ☑
    - dendritic (herpes simplex) BØØ.52
    - marginal H16.Ø4- ☑
    - Mooren's H16.Ø5- ☑
    - mycotic H16.Ø6- ☑
    - perforated H16.Ø7- ☑
    - ring H16.Ø2- ☑
    - tuberculous (phlyctenular) A18.52
  - corpus cavernosum (chronic) N48.5
  - crural — *see* Ulcer, lower limb
  - Curling's — *see* Ulcer, peptic, acute
  - Cushing's — *see* Ulcer, peptic, acute
  - cystic duct K82.8
  - cystitis (interstitial) — *see* Cystitis, interstitial
  - decubitus — *see* Ulcer, pressure, by site
  - dendritic, cornea (herpes simplex) BØØ.52
  - diabetes, diabetic — *see* Diabetes, ulcer
  - Dieulafoy's K25.Ø
  - due to
    - infection NEC — *see* Ulcer, skin
    - radiation NEC L59.8
    - trophic disturbance (any region) — *see* Ulcer, skin
    - X-ray L58.1
  - duodenum, duodenal (eroded) (peptic) K26.9
    - with
      - hemorrhage K26.4
        - and perforation K26.6
      - perforation K26.5
    - acute K26.3
      - with
        - hemorrhage K26.Ø
          - and perforation K26.2
        - perforation K26.1
    - chronic K26.7
      - with
        - hemorrhage K26.4
          - and perforation K26.6
        - perforation K26.5
  - dysenteric AØ9
  - elusive — *see* Cystitis, interstitial
  - endocarditis (acute) (chronic) (subacute) I28.8

Ulcer, ulcerated, ulcerating, ulceration, ulcerative — *continued*

- epiglottis J38.7
- esophagus (peptic) K22.1Ø
  - with bleeding K22.11
  - due to
    - aspirin K22.1Ø
      - with bleeding K22.11
    - gastrointestinal reflux disease (without bleeding) K21.ØØ
      - with bleeding K21.Ø1
    - ingestion of chemical or medicament K22.1Ø
      - with bleeding K22.11
  - fungal K22.1Ø
    - with bleeding K22.11
  - infective K22.1Ø
    - with bleeding K22.11
  - varicose — *see* Varix, esophagus
- eyelid (region) HØ1.8
- fauces J39.2
- Fenwick (-Hunner) (solitary) — *see* Cystitis, interstitial
- fistulous — *see* Ulcer, skin
- foot (indolent) (trophic) — *see* Ulcer, lower limb
- frambesial, initial A66.Ø
- frenum (tongue) K14.Ø
- gallbladder or duct K82.8
- gangrenous — *see* Gangrene
- gastric — *see* Ulcer, stomach
- gastrocolic — *see* Ulcer, gastrojejunal
- gastroduodenal — *see* Ulcer, peptic
- gastroesophageal — *see* Ulcer, stomach
- gastrointestinal — *see* Ulcer, gastrojejunal
- gastrojejunal (peptic) K28.9
  - with
    - hemorrhage K28.4
      - and perforation K28.6
    - perforation K28.5
  - acute K28.3
    - with
      - hemorrhage K28.Ø
        - and perforation K28.2
      - perforation K28.1
  - chronic K28.7
    - with
      - hemorrhage K28.4
        - and perforation K28.6
      - perforation K28.5
- gastrojejunocolic — *see* Ulcer, gastrojejunal
- gingiva KØ6.8
- gingivitis KØ5.1Ø
  - nonplaque induced KØ5.11
  - plaque induced KØ5.1Ø
- glottis J38.7
- granuloma of pudenda A58
- gum KØ6.8
- gumma, due to yaws A66.4
- heel — *see* Ulcer, lower limb
- hemorrhoid — *see also* Hemorrhoids, by degree K64.8
- Hunner's — *see* Cystitis, interstitial
- hypopharynx J39.2
- hypopyon (chronic) (subacute) — *see* Ulcer, cornea, with hypopyon
- hypostaticum — *see* Ulcer, varicose
- ileum — *see* Ulcer, intestine
- intestine, intestinal K63.3
  - with perforation K63.1
  - amebic AØ6.1
  - duodenal — *see* Ulcer, duodenum
  - granulocytopenic (with hemorrhage) — *see* Neutropenia
  - marginal — *see* Ulcer, gastrojejunal
  - perforating K63.1
    - newborn P78.Ø
  - primary, small intestine K63.3
  - rectum K62.6
  - stercoraceous, stercoral K63.3
  - tuberculous A18.32
  - typhoid (fever) — *see* Typhoid
  - varicose I86.8
- jejunum, jejunal — *see* Ulcer, gastrojejunal
- keratitis — *see* Ulcer, cornea
- knee — *see* Ulcer, lower limb
- labium (majus) (minus) N76.6
- laryngitis — *see* Laryngitis
- larynx (aphthous) (contact) J38.7
  - diphtheritic A36.2
- leg — *see* Ulcer, lower limb
- lip K13.Ø

Ulcer, ulcerated, ulcerating, ulceration, ulcerative — *continued*

- Lipschütz's N76.6
- lower limb (atrophic) (chronic) (neurogenic) (perforating) (pyogenic) (trophic) (tropical) L97.9Ø9
  - with
    - bone involvement without evidence of necrosis L97.9Ø6
    - bone necrosis L97.9Ø4
    - exposed fat layer L97.9Ø2
    - muscle involvement without evidence of necrosis L97.9Ø5
    - muscle necrosis L97.9Ø3
    - skin breakdown only L97.9Ø1
    - specified severity NEC L97.9Ø8
  - ankle L97.3Ø9
    - with
      - bone involvement without evidence of necrosis L97.3Ø6
      - bone necrosis L97.3Ø4
      - exposed fat layer L97.3Ø2
      - muscle involvement without evidence of necrosis L97.3Ø5
      - muscle necrosis L97.3Ø3
      - skin breakdown only L97.3Ø1
      - specified severity NEC L97.3Ø8
    - left L97.329
      - with
        - bone involvement without evidence of necrosis L97.326
        - bone necrosis L97.324
        - exposed fat layer L97.322
        - muscle involvement without evidence of necrosis L97.325
        - muscle necrosis L97.323
        - skin breakdown only L97.321
        - specified severity NEC L97.328
    - right L97.319
      - with
        - bone involvement without evidence of necrosis L97.316
        - bone necrosis L97.314
        - exposed fat layer L97.312
        - muscle involvement without evidence of necrosis L97.315
        - muscle necrosis L97.313
        - skin breakdown only L97.311
        - specified severity NEC L97.318
  - calf L97.2Ø9
    - with
      - bone involvement without evidence of necrosis L97.2Ø6
      - bone necrosis L97.2Ø4
      - exposed fat layer L97.2Ø2
      - muscle involvement without evidence of necrosis L97.2Ø5
      - muscle necrosis L97.2Ø3
      - skin breakdown only L97.2Ø1
      - specified severity NEC L97.2Ø8
    - left L97.229
      - with
        - bone involvement without evidence of necrosis L97.226
        - bone necrosis L97.224
        - exposed fat layer L97.222
        - muscle involvement without evidence of necrosis L97.225
        - muscle necrosis L97.223
        - skin breakdown only L97.221
        - specified severity NEC L97.228
    - right L97.219
      - with
        - bone involvement without evidence of necrosis L97.216
        - bone necrosis L97.214
        - exposed fat layer L97.212
        - muscle involvement without evidence of necrosis L97.215
        - muscle necrosis L97.213
        - skin breakdown only L97.211
        - specified severity NEC L97.218
  - decubitus — *see* Ulcer, pressure, by site
  - foot specified NEC L97.5Ø9
    - with
      - bone involvement without evidence of necrosis L97.5Ø6
      - bone necrosis L97.5Ø4
      - exposed fat layer L97.5Ø2

Ulcer, ulcerated, ulcerating, ulceration, ulcerative — *continued*

- lower limb — *continued*
  - foot specified — *continued*
    - with — *continued*
      - muscle involvement without evidence of necrosis L97.5Ø5
      - muscle necrosis L97.5Ø3
      - skin breakdown only L97.5Ø1
      - specified severity NEC L97.5Ø8
    - left L97.529
      - with
        - bone involvement without evidence of necrosis L97.526
        - bone necrosis L97.524
        - exposed fat layer L97.522
        - muscle involvement without evidence of necrosis L97.525
        - muscle necrosis L97.523
        - skin breakdown only L97.521
        - specified severity NEC L97.528
    - right L97.519
      - with
        - bone involvement without evidence of necrosis L97.516
        - bone necrosis L97.514
        - exposed fat layer L97.512
        - muscle involvement without evidence of necrosis L97.515
        - muscle necrosis L97.513
        - skin breakdown only L97.511
        - specified severity NEC L97.518
  - heel L97.4Ø9
    - with
      - bone involvement without evidence of necrosis L97.4Ø6
      - bone necrosis L97.4Ø4
      - exposed fat layer L97.4Ø2
      - muscle involvement without evidence of necrosis L97.4Ø5
      - muscle necrosis L97.4Ø3
      - skin breakdown only L97.4Ø1
      - specified severity NEC L97.4Ø8
    - left L97.429
      - with
        - bone involvement without evidence of necrosis L97.426
        - bone necrosis L97.424
        - exposed fat layer L97.422
        - muscle involvement without evidence of necrosis L97.425
        - muscle necrosis L97.423
        - skin breakdown only L97.421
        - specified severity NEC L97.428
    - right L97.419
      - with
        - bone involvement without evidence of necrosis L97.416
        - bone necrosis L97.414
        - exposed fat layer L97.412
        - muscle involvement without evidence of necrosis L97.415
        - muscle necrosis L97.413
        - skin breakdown only L97.411
        - specified severity NEC L97.418
  - left L97.929
    - with
      - bone involvement without evidence of necrosis L97.926
      - bone necrosis L97.924
      - exposed fat layer L97.922
      - muscle involvement without evidence of necrosis L97.925
      - muscle necrosis L97.923
      - skin breakdown only L97.921
      - specified severity NEC L97.928
  - leprous A3Ø.1
  - lower leg NOS L97.9Ø9
    - with
      - bone involvement without evidence of necrosis L97.9Ø6
      - bone necrosis L97.9Ø4
      - exposed fat layer L97.9Ø2
      - muscle involvement without evidence of necrosis L97.9Ø5
      - muscle necrosis L97.9Ø3
      - skin breakdown only L97.9Ø1
      - specified severity NEC L97.9Ø8
    - left L97.929

Undeveloped, undevelopment — *continued*
- heart Q24.8
- lung Q33.6
- testis E29.1
- uterus E30.0

Undiagnosed (disease) R69
Undulant fever — *see* Brucellosis
Unemployment, anxiety concerning Z56.0
- threatened Z56.2

Unequal length (acquired) (limb) — *see also* Deformity, limb, unequal length
- leg — *see also* Deformity, limb, unequal length
  - congenital Q72.9- ☑

Unextracted dental root K08.3
Unguis incarnatus L60.0
Unhappiness R45.2
Unicornate uterus Q51.4
- in pregnancy or childbirth O34.00

Unilateral — *see also* condition
- development, breast N64.89
- organ or site, congenital NEC — *see* Agenesis, by site

Unilocular heart Q20.8
Union, abnormal — *see also* Fusion
- larynx and trachea Q34.8

Universal mesentery Q43.3
Unrepairable overhanging of dental restorative materials K08.52
Unsatisfactory
- restoration of tooth K08.50
  - specified NEC K08.59
- sample of cytologic smear
  - anus R85.615
  - cervix R87.615
  - vagina R87.625
- surroundings Z59.1
  - work Z56.5

Unsoundness of mind — *see* Psychosis
Unstable
- back NEC — *see* Instability, joint, spine
- hip (congenital) Q65.6
  - acquired — *see* Derangement, joint, specified type NEC, hip
- joint — *see* Instability, joint
  - secondary to removal of joint prosthesis M96.89
- lie (mother) O32.0 ☑
- lumbosacral joint (congenital) — *see* subcategory M53.2
- sacroiliac — *see* subcategory M53.2 ☑
- spine NEC — *see* Instability, joint, spine

Unsteadiness on feet R26.81
Untruthfulness, child problem F91.8
Unverricht (-Lundborg) **disease or epilepsy** — *see* Epilepsy, generalized, idiopathic
Unwanted pregnancy Z64.0
Upbringing, institutional Z62.22
- away from parents NEC Z62.29
- in care of non-parental family member Z62.21
- in foster care Z62.21
- in orphanage or group home Z62.22
- in welfare custody Z62.21

Upper respiratory — *see* condition
Upset
- gastric K30
- gastrointestinal K30
  - psychogenic F45.8
- intestinal (large) (small) K59.9
  - psychogenic F45.8
- menstruation N93.9
- mental F48.9
- stomach K30
  - psychogenic F45.8

Urachus — *see also* condition
- patent or persistent Q64.4

Urbach-Oppenheim disease (necrobiosis lipoidica diabeticorum) — *see* E08-E13 with .620
Urbach's lipoid proteinosis E78.89
Urbach-Wiethe disease E78.89
Urban yellow fever A95.1
Urea
- blood, high — *see* Uremia
- cycle metabolism disorder — *see* Disorder, urea cycle metabolism

Uremia, uremic N19
- with
  - ectopic or molar pregnancy O08.4
  - polyneuropathy N18.9 *[G63]*
- chronic NOS — *see also* Disease, kidney, chronic N18.9

Uremia, uremic — *continued*
- chronic — *see also* Disease, kidney, chronic — *continued*
  - due to hypertension — *see* Hypertensive, kidney
- complicating
  - ectopic or molar pregnancy O08.4
- congenital P96.0
- extrarenal R39.2
- following ectopic or molar pregnancy O08.4
- newborn P96.0
- prerenal R39.2

Ureter, ureteral — *see* condition
Ureteralgia N23
Ureterectasis — *see* Hydroureter
Ureteritis N28.89
- cystica N28.86
- due to calculus N20.1
  - with calculus, kidney N20.2
    - with hydronephrosis N13.2
- gonococcal (acute) (chronic) A54.21
- nonspecific N28.89

Ureterocele N28.89
- congenital (orthotopic) Q62.31
  - ectopic Q62.32

Ureterolith, ureterolithiasis — *see* Calculus, ureter
Ureterostomy
- attention to Z43.6
- status Z93.6

Urethra, urethral — *see* condition
Urethralgia R39.89
Urethritis (anterior) (posterior) N34.2
- calculous N21.1
- candidal B37.41
- chlamydial A56.01
- diplococcal (gonococcal) A54.01
  - with abscess (accessory gland) (periurethral) A54.1
- gonococcal A54.01
  - with abscess (accessory gland) (periurethral) A54.1
- nongonococcal N34.1
  - Reiter's — *see* Reiter's disease
- nonspecific N34.1
- nonvenereal N34.1
- postmenopausal N34.2
- puerperal O86.22
- Reiter's — *see* Reiter's disease
- specified NEC N34.2
- trichomonal or due to Trichomonas (vaginalis) A59.03

Urethrocele N81.0
- with
  - cystocele — *see* Cystocele
  - prolapse of uterus — *see* Prolapse, uterus

Urethrolithiasis (with colic or infection) N21.1
Urethrorectal — *see* condition
Urethrorrhagia N36.8
Urethrorrhea R36.9
Urethrostomy
- attention to Z43.6
- status Z93.6

Urethrotrigonitis — *see* Trigonitis
Urethrovaginal — *see* condition
Urgency
- fecal R15.2
- hypertensive — *see* Hypertension
- urinary R39.15

Urhidrosis, uridrosis L74.8
Uric acid in blood (increased) E79.0
Uricacidemia (asymptomatic) E79.0
Uricemia (asymptomatic) E79.0
Uricosuria R82.998
Urinary — *see* condition
Urination
- frequent R35.0
- painful R30.9

Urine
- blood in — *see* Hematuria
- discharge, excessive R35.8
- enuresis, nonorganic origin F98.0
- extravasation R39.0
- frequency R35.0
- incontinence R32
  - nonorganic origin F98.0
- intermittent stream R39.198
- pus in N39.0
- retention or stasis R33.9
  - organic R33.8
    - drug-induced R33.0
  - psychogenic F45.8

Urine — *continued*
- secretion
  - deficient R34
  - excessive R35.8
  - frequency R35.0
- stream
  - intermittent R39.198
  - slowing R39.198
  - splitting R39.13
  - weak R39.12

Urinemia — *see* Uremia
Urinoma, urethra N36.8
Uroarthritis, infectious (Reiter's) — *see* Reiter's disease
Urodialysis R34
Urolithiasis — *see* Calculus, urinary
Uronephrosis — *see* Hydronephrosis
Uropathy N39.9
- obstructive N13.9
  - specified NEC N13.8
- reflux N13.9
  - specified NEC N13.8
- vesicoureteral reflux-associated — *see* Reflux, vesicoureteral

Urosepsis — *code to* condition
Urticaria L50.9
- with angioneurotic edema T78.3 ☑
  - hereditary D84.1
- allergic L50.0
- cholinergic L50.5
- chronic L50.8
- cold, familial L50.2
- contact L50.6
- dermatographic L50.3
- due to
  - cold or heat L50.2
  - drugs L50.0
  - food L50.0
  - inhalants L50.0
  - plants L50.6
  - serum — *see also* Reaction, serum T80.69 ☑
- factitial L50.3
- familial cold M04.2
- giant T78.3 ☑
  - hereditary D84.1
- gigantea T78.3 ☑
- idiopathic L50.1
- larynx T78.3 ☑
  - hereditary D84.1
- neonatorum P83.88
- nonallergic L50.1
- papulosa (Hebra) L28.2
- pigmentosa D47.01
  - congenital Q82.2
  - of neonatal onset Q82.2
  - of newborn onset Q82.2
- recurrent periodic L50.8
- serum — *see also* Reaction, serum T80.69 ☑
- solar L56.3
- specified type NEC L50.8
- thermal (cold) (heat) L50.2
- vibratory L50.4
- xanthelasmoidea — *see* Urticaria pigmentosa

Use (of)
- alcohol Z72.89
  - with
    - intoxication F10.929
    - sleep disorder F10.982
    - withdrawal F10.939
      - with
        - perceptual disturbance F10.932
      - delirium F10.931
      - uncomplicated F10.930
  - harmful — *see* Abuse, alcohol
- amphetamines — *see* Use, stimulant NEC
- caffeine — *see* Use, stimulant NEC
- cannabis F12.90
  - with
    - anxiety disorder F12.980
    - intoxication F12.929
      - with
        - delirium F12.921
        - perceptual disturbance F12.922
      - uncomplicated F12.920
    - other specified disorder F12.988
    - psychosis F12.959
      - delusions F12.950
      - hallucinations F12.951
    - unspecified disorder F12.99

Use — *continued*
  cannabis — *continued*
    with — *continued*
      withdrawal F12.93
  cocaine F14.90
    with
      anxiety disorder F14.980
      intoxication F14.929
        with
          delirium F14.921
          perceptual disturbance F14.922
        uncomplicated F14.920
      other specified disorder F14.988
      psychosis F14.959
        delusions F14.950
        hallucinations F14.951
      sexual dysfunction F14.981
      sleep disorder F14.982
      unspecified disorder F14.99
      withdrawal F14.93
    harmful — *see* Abuse, drug, cocaine
  drug(s) NEC F19.90
    with sleep disorder F19.982
    harmful — *see* Abuse, drug, by type
  hallucinogen NEC F16.90
    with
      anxiety disorder F16.980
      intoxication F16.929
        with
          delirium F16.921
        uncomplicated F16.920
      mood disorder F16.94
      other specified disorder F16.988
      perception disorder (flashbacks) F16.983
      psychosis F16.959
        delusions F16.950
        hallucinations F16.951
      unspecified disorder F16.99
    harmful — *see* Abuse, drug, hallucinogen NEC
  inhalants F18.90
    with
      anxiety disorder F18.980
      intoxication F18.929
        with delirium F18.921
        uncomplicated F18.920
      mood disorder F18.94
      other specified disorder F18.988
      persisting dementia F18.97
      psychosis F18.959
        delusions F18.950
        hallucinations F18.951
      unspecified disorder F18.99
    harmful — *see* Abuse, drug, inhalant
  methadone — *see* Use, opioid
  nonprescribed drugs F19.90
    harmful — *see* Abuse, non-psychoactive substance
  opioid F11.90
    with
      disorder F11.99
        mood F11.94
        sleep F11.982
        specified type NEC F11.988
      intoxication F11.929
        with
          delirium F11.921
          perceptual disturbance F11.922
        uncomplicated F11.920
      withdrawal F11.93
    harmful — *see* Abuse, drug, opioid
  patent medicines F19.90
    harmful — *see* Abuse, non-psychoactive substance
  psychoactive drug NEC F19.90
    with
      anxiety disorder F19.980
      intoxication F19.929
        with
          delirium F19.921
          perceptual disturbance F19.922
        uncomplicated F19.920
      mood disorder F19.94
      other specified disorder F19.988
      persisting
        amnestic disorder F19.96
        dementia F19.97
      psychosis F19.959
        delusions F19.950
        hallucinations F19.951
      sexual dysfunction F19.981

Use — *continued*
  psychoactive drug — *continued*
    with — *continued*
      sleep disorder F19.982
      unspecified disorder F19.99
      withdrawal F19.939
        with
          delirium F19.931
          perceptual disturbance F19.932
        uncomplicated F19.930
    harmful — *see* Abuse, drug NEC, psychoactive NEC
  sedative, hypnotic, or anxiolytic F13.90
    with
      anxiety disorder F13.980
      intoxication F13.929
        with
          delirium F13.921
        uncomplicated F13.920
      other specified disorder F13.988
      persisting
        amnestic disorder F13.96
        dementia F13.97
      psychosis F13.959
        delusions F13.950
        hallucinations F13.951
      sexual dysfunction F13.981
      sleep disorder F13.982
      unspecified disorder F13.99
    harmful — *see* Abuse, drug, sedative, hypnotic, or anxiolytic
  stimulant NEC F15.90
    with
      anxiety disorder F15.980
      intoxication F15.929
        with
          delirium F15.921
          perceptual disturbance F15.922
        uncomplicated F15.920
      mood disorder F15.94
      other specified disorder F15.988
      psychosis F15.959
        delusions F15.950
        hallucinations F15.951
      sexual dysfunction F15.981
      sleep disorder F15.982
      unspecified disorder F15.99
      withdrawal F15.93
    harmful — *see* Abuse, drug, stimulant NEC
  tobacco Z72.0
    with dependence — *see* Dependence, drug, nicotine
  volatile solvents — *see also* Use, inhalant F18.90
    harmful — *see* Abuse, drug, inhalant
Usher-Senear disease or syndrome L10.4
Uta B55.1
Uteromegaly N85.2
Uterovaginal — *see* condition
Uterovesical — *see* condition
Uveal — *see* condition
Uveitis (anterior) — *see also* Iridocyclitis
  acute — *see* Iridocyclitis, acute
  chronic — *see* Iridocyclitis, chronic
  due to toxoplasmosis (acquired) B58.09
    congenital P37.1
  granulomatous — *see* Iridocyclitis, chronic
  heterochromic — *see* Cyclitis, Fuchs' heterochromic
  lens-induced — *see* Iridocyclitis, lens-induced
  posterior — *see* Chorioretinitis
  sympathetic H44.13- ☑
  syphilitic (secondary) A51.43
    congenital (early) A50.01
    late A52.71
  tuberculous A18.54
Uveoencephalitis — *see* Inflammation, chorioretinal
Uveokeratitis — *see* Iridocyclitis
Uveoparotitis D86.89
Uvula — *see* condition
Uvulitis (acute) (catarrhal) (chronic) (membranous) (suppurative) (ulcerative) K12.2

V

Vaccination (prophylactic)
  complication or reaction — *see* Complications, vaccination
  delayed Z28.9
  encounter for Z23
  not done — *see* Immunization, not done, because (of)
Vaccinia (generalized) (localized) T88.1 ☑

Vaccinia — *continued*
  congenital P35.8
  without vaccination B08.011
Vacuum, in sinus (accessory) (nasal) J34.89
Vagabond, vagabondage Z59.0
Vagabond's disease B85.1
Vagina, vaginal — *see* condition
Vaginalitis (tunica) (testis) N49.1
Vaginismus (reflex) N94.2
  functional F52.5
  nonorganic F52.5
  psychogenic F52.5
  secondary N94.2
Vaginitis (acute) (circumscribed) (diffuse) (emphysematous) (nonvenereal) (ulcerative) N76.0
  with ectopic or molar pregnancy O08.0
  amebic A06.82
  atrophic, postmenopausal N95.2
  bacterial N76.0
  blennorrhagic (gonococcal) A54.02
  candidal B37.3
  chlamydial A56.02
  chronic N76.1
  due to Trichomonas (vaginalis) A59.01
  following ectopic or molar pregnancy O08.0
  gonococcal A54.02
    with abscess (accessory gland) (periurethral) A54.1
  granuloma A58
  in (due to)
    candidiasis B37.3
    herpesviral (herpes simplex) infection A60.04
    pinworm infection B80 *[N77.1]*
  monilial B37.3
  mycotic (candidal) B37.3
  postmenopausal atrophic N95.2
  puerperal (postpartum) O86.13
  senile (atrophic) N95.2
  subacute or chronic N76.1
  syphilitic (early) A51.0
    late A52.76
  trichomonal A59.01
  tuberculous A18.18
Vaginosis — *see* Vaginitis
Vagotonia G52.2
Vagrancy Z59.0
VAIN — *see* Neoplasia, intraepithelial, vagina
Vallecula — *see* condition
Valley fever B38.0
Valsuani's disease — *see* Anemia, obstetric
Valve, valvular (formation) — *see also* condition
  cerebral ventricle (communicating) in situ Z98.2
  cervix, internal os Q51.828
  congenital NEC — *see* Atresia, by site
  ureter (pelvic junction) (vesical orifice) Q62.39
  urethra (congenital) (posterior) Q64.2
Valvulitis (chronic) — *see* Endocarditis
Valvulopathy — *see* Endocarditis
Van Bogaert's leukoencephalopathy (sclerosing) (subacute) A81.1
Van Bogaert-Scherer-Epstein disease or syndrome E75.5
Van Buchem's syndrome M85.2
Van Creveld-von Gierke disease E74.01
Van der Hoeve (-de Kleyn) **syndrome** Q78.0
Van der Woude's syndrome Q38.0
Van Neck's disease or osteochondrosis M91.0
Vanishing lung J44.9
Vapor asphyxia or suffocation T59.9 ☑
  specified agent — *see* Table of Drugs and Chemicals
Variance, lethal ball, prosthetic heart valve T82.09 ☑
Variants, thalassemic D56.8
Variations in hair color L67.1
Varicella B01.9
  with
    complications NEC B01.89
    encephalitis B01.11
    encephalomyelitis B01.11
    meningitis B01.0
    myelitis B01.12
    pneumonia B01.2
  congenital P35.8
Varices — *see* Varix
Varicocele (scrotum) (thrombosed) I86.1
  ovary I86.2
  perineum I86.3
  spermatic cord (ulcerated) I86.1
Varicose
  aneurysm (ruptured) I77.0

Wound, open — *continued*
- shin — *see* Wound, open, leg
- shoulder S41.ØØ- ☑
  - with amputation — *see* Amputation, traumatic, arm
  - bite — *see* Bite, shoulder
  - laceration — *see* Laceration, shoulder
  - puncture — *see* Puncture, shoulder
- skin NOS T14.8 ☑
- spermatic cord — *see* Wound, open, testis
- sternal region — *see* Wound, open, thorax, front wall
- submaxillary region — *see* Wound, open, head, specified site NEC
- submental region — *see* Wound, open, head, specified site NEC
- subungual
  - finger(s) — *see* Wound, open, finger
  - toe(s) — *see* Wound, open, toe
- supraclavicular region — *see* Wound, open, neck, specified site NEC
- temple, temporal region — *see* Wound, open, head, specified site NEC
- temporomandibular area — *see* Wound, open, cheek
- testis S31.3Ø ☑
  - with amputation — *see* Amputation, traumatic, testes
  - bite S31.35 ☑
  - laceration — *see* Laceration, testis
  - puncture — *see* Puncture, testis
- thigh S71.1Ø- ☑
  - with amputation — *see* Amputation, traumatic, hip
  - bite — *see* Bite, thigh
  - laceration — *see* Laceration, thigh
  - puncture — *see* Puncture, thigh
- thorax, thoracic (wall) S21.9Ø ☑
  - back S21.2Ø- ☑
    - with penetration S21.4Ø ☑
  - bite — *see* Bite, thorax
  - breast — *see* Wound, open, breast
  - front S21.1Ø- ☑
    - with penetration S21.3Ø ☑
  - laceration — *see* Laceration, thorax
  - puncture — *see* Puncture, thorax
- throat — *see* Wound, open, neck
- thumb S61.ØØ9 ☑
  - with
    - amputation — *see* Amputation, traumatic, thumb
    - damage to nail S61.1Ø9 ☑
  - bite — *see* Bite, thumb
  - laceration — *see* Laceration, thumb
  - left S61.ØØ2 ☑
    - with
      - damage to nail S61.1Ø2 ☑
  - puncture — *see* Puncture, thumb
  - right S61.ØØ1 ☑
    - with
      - damage to nail S61.1Ø1 ☑
- thyroid (gland) — *see* Wound, open, neck, thyroid
- toe(s) S91.1Ø9 ☑
  - with
    - amputation — *see* Amputation, traumatic, toe
    - damage to nail S91.2Ø9 ☑
  - bite — *see* Bite, toe
  - great S91.1Ø3 ☑
    - with
      - damage to nail S91.2Ø3 ☑
    - left S91.1Ø2 ☑
      - with
        - damage to nail S91.2Ø2 ☑
    - right S91.1Ø1 ☑
      - with
        - damage to nail S91.2Ø1 ☑
  - laceration — *see* Laceration, toe
  - lesser S91.1Ø6 ☑
    - with
      - damage to nail S91.2Ø6 ☑
    - left S91.1Ø5 ☑
      - with
        - damage to nail S91.2Ø5 ☑
    - right S91.1Ø4 ☑
      - with
        - damage to nail S91.2Ø4 ☑
  - puncture — *see* Puncture, toe
- tongue — *see* Wound, open, oral cavity
- trachea (cervical region) — *see* Wound, open, neck, trachea

Wound, open — *continued*
- tunica vaginalis — *see* Wound, open, testis
- tympanum, tympanic membrane SØ9.2- ☑
  - laceration — *see* Laceration, ear, drum
  - puncture — *see* Puncture, tympanum
- umbilical region — *see* Wound, open, abdomen, wall, periumbilic region
- uvula — *see* Wound, open, oral cavity
- vagina S31.4Ø ☑
  - bite S31.45 ☑
  - laceration — *see* Laceration, vagina
  - puncture — *see* Puncture, vagina
- vitreous (humor) — *see* Wound, open, ocular
- vocal cord S11.Ø39 ☑
  - bite — *see* Bite, vocal cord
  - laceration S11.Ø31 ☑
    - with foreign body S11.Ø32 ☑
  - puncture S11.Ø33 ☑
    - with foreign body S11.Ø34 ☑
- vulva S31.4Ø ☑
  - with amputation — *see* Amputation, traumatic, vulva
  - bite S31.45 ☑
  - laceration — *see* Laceration, vulva
  - puncture — *see* Puncture, vulva
- wrist S61.5Ø- ☑
  - bite — *see* Bite, wrist
  - laceration — *see* Laceration, wrist
  - puncture — *see* Puncture, wrist

Wound, superficial — *see* Injury — *see also* specified injury type

Wright's syndrome G54.Ø

Wrist — *see* condition

Wrong drug (by accident) (given in error) — *see* Table of Drugs and Chemicals, by drug, poisoning

Wry neck — *see* Torticollis

Wuchereria (bancrofti) **infestation** B74.Ø

Wuchereriasis B74.Ø

Wuchernde Struma Langhans C73

X

Xanthelasma (eyelid) (palpebrarum) HØ2.6Ø
- left HØ2.66
  - lower HØ2.65
  - upper HØ2.64
- right HØ2.63
  - lower HØ2.62
  - upper HØ2.61

Xanthelasmatosis (essential) E78.2

Xanthinuria, hereditary E79.8

Xanthoastrocytoma
- specified site — *see* Neoplasm, malignant, by site
- unspecified site C71.9

Xanthofibroma — *see* Neoplasm, connective tissue, benign

Xanthogranuloma D76.3

Xanthoma(s), xanthomatosis (primary) (familial) (hereditary) E75.5
- with
  - hyperlipoproteinemia
    - Type I E78.3
    - Type III E78.2
    - Type IV E78.1
    - Type V E78.3
- bone (generalisata) C96.5
- cerebrotendinous E75.5
- cutaneotendinous E75.5
- disseminatum (skin) E78.2
- eruptive E78.2
- hypercholesterinemic E78.ØØ
- hypercholesterolemic E78.ØØ
- hyperlipidemic E78.5
- joint E75.5
- multiple (skin) E78.2
- tendon (sheath) E75.5
- tuberosum E78.2
- tuberous E78.2
- tubo-eruptive E78.2
- verrucous, oral mucosa K13.4

Xanthosis R23.8

Xenophobia F4Ø.1Ø

Xeroderma — *see also* Ichthyosis
- acquired L85.Ø
  - eyelid HØ1.149
    - left HØ1.146
      - lower HØ1.145

Xeroderma — *continued*
- acquired — *continued*
  - eyelid — *continued*
    - left — *continued*
      - upper HØ1.144
    - right HØ1.143
      - lower HØ1.142
      - upper HØ1.141
- pigmentosum Q82.1
- vitamin A deficiency E5Ø.8

Xerophthalmia (vitamin A deficiency) E5Ø.7
- unrelated to vitamin A deficiency — *see* Keratoconjunctivitis

Xerosis
- conjunctiva H11.14- ☑
  - with Bitot's spots — *see also* Pigmentation, conjunctiva
    - vitamin A deficiency E5Ø.1
  - vitamin A deficiency E5Ø.Ø
- cornea H18.89- ☑
  - with ulceration — *see* Ulcer, cornea
    - vitamin A deficiency E5Ø.3
  - vitamin A deficiency E5Ø.2
- cutis L85.3
- skin L85.3

Xerostomia K11.7

Xiphopagus Q89.4

XO syndrome Q96.9

X-ray (of)
- abnormal findings — *see* Abnormal, diagnostic imaging
- breast (mammogram) (routine) Z12.31
- chest
  - routine (as part of a general medical examination) ZØØ.ØØ
    - with abnormal findings ZØØ.Ø1
- routine (as part of a general medical examination) ZØØ.ØØ
  - with abnormal findings ZØØ.Ø1

XXXXY syndrome Q98.1

XXY syndrome Q98.Ø

Y

Yaba pox (virus disease) BØ8.72

Yatapoxvirus BØ8.7Ø
- specified NEC BØ8.79

Yawning RØ6.89
- psychogenic F45.8

Yaws A66.9
- bone lesions A66.6
- butter A66.1
- chancre A66.Ø
- cutaneous, less than five years after infection A66.2
- early (cutaneous) (macular) (maculopapular) (micropapular) (papular) A66.2
  - frambeside A66.2
  - skin lesions NEC A66.2
- eyelid A66.2
- ganglion A66.6
- gangosis, gangosa A66.5
- gumma, gummata A66.4
  - bone A66.6
- gummatous
  - frambeside A66.4
  - osteitis A66.6
  - periostitis A66.6
- hydrarthrosis — *see also* subcategory M14.8- A66.6
- hyperkeratosis (early) (late) A66.3
- initial lesions A66.Ø
- joint lesions — *see also* subcategory M14.8- A66.6
- juxta-articular nodules A66.7
- late nodular (ulcerated) A66.4
- latent (without clinical manifestations) (with positive serology) A66.8
- mother A66.Ø
- mucosal A66.7
- multiple papillomata A66.1
- nodular, late (ulcerated) A66.4
- osteitis A66.6
- papilloma, plantar or palmar A66.1
- periostitis (hypertrophic) A66.6
- specified NEC A66.7
- ulcers A66.4
- wet crab A66.1

Yeast infection — *see also* Candidiasis B37.9

Yellow
- atrophy (liver) — *see* Failure, hepatic
- fever — *see* Fever, yellow

Note: The list below gives the code number for neoplasms by anatomical site. For each site there are six possible code numbers according to whether the neoplasm in question is malignant, benign, in situ, of uncertain behavior, or of unspecified nature. The description of the neoplasm will often indicate which of the six columns is appropriate; e.g., malignant melanoma of skin, benign fibroadenoma of breast, carcinoma in situ of cervix uteri. Where such descriptors are not present, the remainder of the Index should be consulted where guidance is given to the appropriate column for each morphological (histological) variety listed; e.g., Mesonephroma – see Neoplasm, malignant; Embryoma — see also Neoplasm, uncertain behavior; Disease, Bowen's – see Neoplasm, skin, in situ. However, the guidance in the Index can be overridden if one of the descriptors mentioned above is present; e.g., malignant adenoma of colon is coded to C18.9 and not to D12.6 as the adjective "malignant" overrides the Index entry "Adenoma — *see also* Neoplasm, benign, by site." Codes listed with a dash -, following the code have a required additional character for laterality. The tabular list must be reviewed for the complete code.

	Malignant Primary	Malignant Secondary	Ca in situ	Benign	Uncertain Behavior	Unspecified Behavior
Neoplasm, neoplastic	C80.1	C79.9	D09.9	D36.9	D48.9	D49.9
abdomen, abdominal	C76.2	C79.8-☑	D09.8	D36.7	D48.7	D49.89
cavity	C76.2	C79.8-☑	D09.8	D36.7	D48.7	D49.89
organ	C76.2	C79.8-☑	D09.8	D36.7	D48.7	D49.89
viscera	C76.2	C79.8-☑	D09.8	D36.7	D48.7	D49.89
wall — *see also* Neoplasm, abdomen, wall, skin	C44.509	C79.2	D04.5	D23.5	D48.5	D49.2
connective tissue	C49.4	C79.8-☑	—	D21.4	D48.1	D49.2
skin	C44.509	—	—	—	—	—
basal cell carcinoma	C44.519	—	—	—	—	—
specified type NEC	C44.599	—	—	—	—	—
squamous cell carcinoma	C44.529	—	—	—	—	—
abdominopelvic	C76.8	C79.8-☑	—	D36.7	D48.7	D49.89
accessory sinus — *see* Neoplasm, sinus						
acoustic nerve	C72.4-☑	C79.49	—	D33.3	D43.3	D49.7
adenoid (pharynx) (tissue)	C11.1	C79.89	D00.08	D10.6	D37.05	D49.0
adipose tissue — *see also* Neoplasm, connective tissue	C49.4	C79.89	—	D21.9	D48.1	D49.2
adnexa (uterine)	C57.4	C79.89	D07.39	D28.7	D39.8	D49.59
adrenal	C74.9-☑	C79.7-☑	D09.3	D35.0-☑	D44.1-☑	D49.7
capsule	C74.9-☑	C79.7-☑	D09.3	D35.0-☑	D44.1-☑	D49.7
cortex	C74.0-☑	C79.7-☑	D09.3	D35.0-☑	D44.1-☑	D49.7
gland	C74.9-☑	C79.7-☑	D09.3	D35.0-☑	D44.1-☑	D49.7
medulla	C74.1-☑	C79.7-☑	D09.3	D35.0-☑	D44.1-☑	D49.7
ala nasi (external) — *see also* Neoplasm, skin, nose	C44.301	C79.2	D04.39	D23.39	D48.5	D49.2
alimentary canal or tract NEC	C26.9	C78.80	D01.9	D13.9	D37.9	D49.0
alveolar	C03.9	C79.89	D00.03	D10.39	D37.09	D49.0
mucosa	C03.9	C79.89	D00.03	D10.39	D37.09	D49.0
lower	C03.1	C79.89	D00.03	D10.39	D37.09	D49.0
upper	C03.0	C79.89	D00.03	D10.39	D37.09	D49.0
ridge or process	C41.1	C79.51	—	D16.5	D48.0	D49.2
carcinoma	C03.9	C79.8-☑	—	—	—	—
lower	C03.1	C79.8-☑	—	—	—	—
upper	C03.0	C79.8-☑	—	—	—	—
lower	C41.1	C79.51	—	D16.5	D48.0	D49.2
mucosa	C03.9	C79.89	D00.03	D10.39	D37.09	D49.0
lower	C03.1	C79.89	D00.03	D10.39	D37.09	D49.0
upper	C03.0	C79.89	D00.03	D10.39	D37.09	D49.0
upper	C41.0	C79.51	—	D16.4	D48.0	D49.2
sulcus	C06.1	C79.89	D00.02	D10.39	D37.09	D49.0
alveolus	C03.9	C79.89	D00.03	D10.39	D37.09	D49.0
lower	C03.1	C79.89	D00.03	D10.39	D37.09	D49.0
upper	C03.0	C79.89	D00.03	D10.39	D37.09	D49.0
ampulla of Vater	C24.1	C78.89	D01.5	D13.5	D37.6	D49.0
ankle NEC	C76.5-☑	C79.89	D04.7-☑	D36.7	D48.7	D49.89
anorectum, anorectal (junction)	C21.8	C78.5	D01.3	D12.9	D37.8	D49.0
antecubital fossa or space	C76.4-☑	C79.89	D04.6-☑	D36.7	D48.7	D49.89

	Malignant Primary	Malignant Secondary	Ca in situ	Benign	Uncertain Behavior	Unspecified Behavior
Neoplasm, neoplastic — *continued*						
antrum (Highmore) (maxillary)	C31.0	C78.39	D02.3	D14.0	D38.5	D49.1
pyloric	C16.3	C78.89	D00.2	D13.1	D37.1	D49.0
tympanicum	C30.1	C78.39	D02.3	D14.0	D38.5	D49.1
anus, anal	C21.0	C78.5	D01.3	D12.9	D37.8	D49.0
canal	C21.1	C78.5	D01.3	D12.9	D37.8	D49.0
cloacogenic zone	C21.2	C78.5	D01.3	D12.9	D37.8	D49.0
margin — *see also* Neoplasm, anus, skin	C44.500	C79.2	D04.5	D23.5	D48.5	D49.2
overlapping lesion with rectosigmoid junction or rectum	C21.8	—	—	—	—	—
skin	C44.500	C79.2	D04.5	D23.5	D48.5	D49.2
basal cell carcinoma	C44.510	—	—	—	—	—
specified type NEC	C44.590	—	—	—	—	—
squamous cell carcinoma	C44.520	—	—	—	—	—
sphincter	C21.1	C78.5	D01.3	D12.9	D37.8	D49.0
aorta (thoracic)	C49.3	C79.89	—	D21.3	D48.1	D49.2
abdominal	C49.4	C79.89	—	D21.4	D48.1	D49.2
aortic body	C75.5	C79.89	—	D35.6	D44.7	D49.7
aponeurosis	C49.9	C79.89	—	D21.9	D48.1	D49.2
palmar	C49.1-☑	C79.89	—	D21.1-☑	D48.1	D49.2
plantar	C49.2-☑	C79.89	—	D21.2-☑	D48.1	D49.2
appendix	C18.1	C78.5	D01.0	D12.1	D37.3	D49.0
arachnoid	C70.9	C79.49	—	D32.9	D42.9	D49.7
cerebral	C70.0	C79.32	—	D32.0	D42.0	D49.7
spinal	C70.1	C79.49	—	D32.1	D42.1	D49.7
areola	C50.0-☑	C79.81	D05-☑	D24-☑	D48.6-☑	D49.3
arm NEC	C76.4-☑	C79.89	D04.6-☑	D36.7	D48.7	D49.89
artery — *see* Neoplasm, connective tissue						
aryepiglottic fold	C13.1	C79.89	D00.08	D10.7	D37.05	D49.0
hypopharyngeal aspect	C13.1	C79.89	D00.08	D10.7	D37.05	D49.0
laryngeal aspect	C32.1	C78.39	D02.0	D14.1	D38.0	D49.1
marginal zone	C13.1	C79.89	D00.08	D10.7	D37.05	D49.0
arytenoid (cartilage)	C32.3	C78.39	D02.0	D14.1	D38.0	D49.1
fold — *see* Neoplasm, aryepiglottic						
associated with transplanted organ	C80.2	—	—	—	—	—
atlas	C41.2	C79.51	—	D16.6	D48.0	D49.2
atrium, cardiac	C38.0	C79.89	—	D15.1	D48.7	D49.89
auditory						
canal (external) (skin)	C44.20-☑	C79.2	D04.2-☑	D23.2-☑	D48.5	D49.2
internal	C30.1	C78.39	D02.3	D14.0	D38.5	D49.1
nerve	C72.4-☑	C79.49	—	D33.3	D43.3	D49.7
tube	C30.1	C78.39	D02.3	D14.0	D38.5	D49.1
opening	C11.2	C79.89	D00.08	D10.6	D37.05	D49.0
auricle, ear — *see also* Neoplasm, skin, ear	C44.20-☑	C79.2	D04.2-☑	D23.2-☑	D48.5	D49.2
auricular canal (external) — *see also* Neoplasm, skin, ear	C44.20-☑	C79.2	D04.2-☑	D23.2-☑	D48.5	D49.2
internal	C30.1	C78.39	D02.3	D14.0	D38.5	D49.2
autonomic nerve or nervous system NEC (see Neoplasm, nerve, peripheral)						
axilla, axillary	C76.1	C79.89	D09.8	D36.7	D48.7	D49.89
fold — *see also* Neoplasm, skin, trunk	C44.509	C79.2	D04.5	D23.5	D48.5	D49.2
back NEC	C76.8	C79.89	D04.5	D36.7	D48.7	D49.89
Bartholin's gland	C51.0	C79.82	D07.1	D28.0	D39.8	D49.59
basal ganglia	C71.0	C79.31	—	D33.0	D43.0	D49.6
basis pedunculi	C71.7	C79.31	—	D33.1	D43.1	D49.6
bile or biliary (tract)	C24.9	C78.89	D01.5	D13.5	D37.6	D49.0

	Malignant Primary	Malignant Secondary	Ca in situ	Benign	Uncertain Behavior	Unspecified Behavior
Neoplasm, neoplastic — *continued*						
bile or biliary — *continued*						
canaliculi (biliferi) (intrahepatic)	C22.1	C78.7	DØ1.5	D13.4	D37.6	D49.Ø
canals, interlobular	C22.1	C78.89	DØ1.5	D13.4	D37.6	D49.Ø
duct or passage (common) (cystic) (extrahepatic)	C24.Ø	C78.89	DØ1.5	D13.5	D37.6	D49.Ø
interlobular	C22.1	C78.89	DØ1.5	D13.4	D37.6	D49.Ø
intrahepatic	C22.1	C78.7	DØ1.5	D13.4	D37.6	D49.Ø
and extrahepatic	C24.8	C78.89	DØ1.5	D13.5	D37.6	D49.Ø
bladder (urinary)	C67.9	C79.11	DØ9.Ø	D3Ø.3	D41.4	D49.4
dome	C67.1	C79.11	DØ9.Ø	D3Ø.3	D41.4	D49.4
neck	C67.5	C79.11	DØ9.Ø	D3Ø.3	D41.4	D49.4
orifice	C67.9	C79.11	DØ9.Ø	D3Ø.3	D41.4	D49.4
ureteric	C67.6	C79.11	DØ9.Ø	D3Ø.3	D41.4	D49.4
urethral	C67.5	C79.11	DØ9.Ø	D3Ø.3	D41.4	D49.4
overlapping lesion	C67.8	—	—	—	—	—
sphincter	C67.8	C79.11	DØ9.Ø	D3Ø.3	D41.4	D49.4
trigone	C67.Ø	C79.11	DØ9.Ø	D3Ø.3	D41.4	D49.4
urachus	C67.7	C79.11	DØ9.Ø	D3Ø.3	D41.4	D49.4
wall	C67.9	C79.11	DØ9.Ø	D3Ø.3	D41.4	D49.4
anterior	C67.3	C79.11	DØ9.Ø	D3Ø.3	D41.4	D49.4
lateral	C67.2	C79.11	DØ9.Ø	D3Ø.3	D41.4	D49.4
posterior	C67.4	C79.11	DØ9.Ø	D3Ø.3	D41.4	D49.4
blood vessel — *see* Neoplasm, connective tissue						
bone (periosteum)	C41.9	C79.51	—	D16.9-	D48.Ø	D49.2
acetabulum						
ankle	C4Ø.3-☑	C79.51	—	D16.3-☑	—	—
arm NEC	C4Ø.Ø-☑	C79.51	—	D16.Ø-☑	—	—
astragalus	C4Ø.3-☑	C79.51	—	D16.3-☑	—	—
atlas	C41.2	C79.51	—	D16.6	D48.Ø	D49.2
axis	C41.2	C79.51	—	D16.6	D48.Ø	D49.2
back NEC	C41.2	C79.51	—	D16.6	D48.Ø	D49.2
calcaneus	C4Ø.3-☑	C79.51	—	D16.3-☑	—	—
calvarium	C41.Ø	C79.51	—	D16.4	D48.Ø	D49.2
carpus (any)	C4Ø.1-☑	C79.51	—	D16.1-☑	—	—
cartilage NEC	C41.9	C79.51	—	D16.9	D48.Ø	D49.2
clavicle	C41.3	C79.51	—	D16.7	D48.Ø	D49.2
clivus	C41.Ø	C79.51	—	D16.4	D48.Ø	D49.2
coccygeal vertebra	C41.4	C79.51	—	D16.8	D48.Ø	D49.2
coccyx	C41.4	C79.51	—	D16.8	D48.Ø	D49.2
costal cartilage	C41.3	C79.51	—	D16.7	D48.Ø	D49.2
costovertebral joint	C41.3	C79.51	—	D16.7	D48.Ø	D49.2
cranial	C41.Ø	C79.51	—	D16.4	D48.Ø	D49.2
cuboid	C4Ø.3-☑	C79.51	—	D16.3-☑	—	—
cuneiform	C41.9	C79.51	—	D16.9	D48.Ø	D49.2
elbow	C4Ø.Ø-☑	C79.51	—	D16.Ø-☑	—	—
ethmoid (labyrinth)	C41.Ø	C79.51	—	D16.4	D48.Ø	D49.2
face	C41.Ø	C79.51	—	D16.4	D48.Ø	D49.2
femur (any part)	C4Ø.2-☑	C79.51	—	D16.2-☑	—	—
fibula (any part)	C4Ø.2-☑	C79.51	—	D16.2-☑	—	—
finger (any)	C4Ø.1-☑	C79.51	—	D16.1-☑	—	—
foot	C4Ø.3-☑	C79.51	—	D16.3-☑	—	—
forearm	C4Ø.Ø-☑	C79.51	—	D16.Ø-☑	—	—
frontal	C41.Ø	C79.51	—	D16.4	D48.Ø	D49.2
hand	C4Ø.1-☑	C79.51	—	D16.1-☑	—	—
heel	C4Ø.3-☑	C79.51	—	D16.3-☑	—	—
hip	C41.4	C79.51	—	D16.8	D48.Ø	D49.2
humerus (any part)	C4Ø.Ø-☑	C79.51	—	D16.Ø-☑	—	—
hyoid	C41.Ø	C79.51	—	D16.4	D48.Ø	D49.2
ilium	C41.4	C79.51	—	D16.8	D48.Ø	D49.2
innominate	C41.4	C79.51	—	D16.8	D48.Ø	D49.2
intervertebral cartilage or disc	C41.2	C79.51	—	D16.6	D48.Ø	D49.2
ischium	C41.4	C79.51	—	D16.8	D48.Ø	D49.2
jaw (lower)	C41.1	C79.51	—	D16.5	D48.Ø	D49.2
knee	C4Ø.2-☑	C79.51	—	D16.2-☑	—	—
leg NEC	C4Ø.2-☑	C79.51	—	D16.2-☑	—	—
limb NEC	C4Ø.9-☑	C79.51	—	D16.9	—	—

	Malignant Primary	Malignant Secondary	Ca in situ	Benign	Uncertain Behavior	Unspecified Behavior
Neoplasm, neoplastic — *continued*						
bone — *continued*						
limb — *continued*						
lower (long bones)	C4Ø.2-☑	C79.51	—	D16.2-☑	—	—
short bones	C4Ø.3-☑	C79.51	—	D16.3-☑	—	—
upper (long bones)	C4Ø.Ø-☑	C79.51	—	D16.Ø-☑	—	—
short bones	C4Ø.1-☑	C79.51	—	D16.1-☑	—	—
malar	C41.Ø	C79.51	—	D16.4	D48.Ø	D49.2
mandible	C41.1	C79.51	—	D16.5	D48.Ø	D49.2
marrow NEC (any bone)	C96.9	C79.52	—	—	D47.9	D49.89
mastoid	C41.Ø	C79.51	—	D16.4	D48.Ø	D49.2
maxilla, maxillary (superior)	C41.Ø	C79.51	—	D16.4	D48.Ø	D49.2
inferior	C41.1	C79.51	—	D16.5	D48.Ø	D49.2
metacarpus (any)	C4Ø.1-☑	C79.51	—	D16.1-☑	—	—
metatarsus (any)	C4Ø.3-☑	C79.51	—	D16.3-☑	—	—
navicular						
ankle	C4Ø.3-☑	C79.51	—	—	—	—
hand	C4Ø.1-☑	C79.51	—	—	—	—
nose, nasal	C41.Ø	C79.51	—	D16.4	D48.Ø	D49.2
occipital	C41.Ø	C79.51	—	D16.4	D48.Ø	D49.2
orbit	C41.Ø	C79.51	—	D16.4	D48.Ø	D49.2
overlapping sites	C4Ø.8-☑	—	—	—	—	—
parietal	C41.Ø	C79.51	—	D16.4	D48.Ø	D49.2
patella	C4Ø.2-☑	C79.51	—	—	—	—
pelvic	C41.4	C79.51	—	D16.8	D48.Ø	D49.2
phalanges						
foot	C4Ø.3-☑	C79.51	—	—	—	—
hand	C4Ø.1-☑	C79.51	—	—	—	—
pubic	C41.4	C79.51	—	D16.8	D48.Ø	D49.2
radius (any part)	C4Ø.Ø-☑	C79.51	—	D16.Ø-☑	—	—
rib	C41.3	C79.51	—	D16.7	D48.Ø	D49.2
sacral vertebra	C41.4	C79.51	—	D16.8	D48.Ø	D49.2
sacrum	C41.4	C79.51	—	D16.8	D48.Ø	D49.2
scaphoid						
of ankle	C4Ø.3-☑	C79.51	—	—	—	—
of hand	C4Ø.1-☑	C79.51	—	—	—	—
scapula (any part)	C4Ø.Ø-☑	C79.51	—	D16.Ø-☑	—	—
sella turcica	C41.Ø	C79.51	—	D16.4	D48.Ø	D49.2
shoulder	C4Ø.Ø-☑	C79.51	—	D16.Ø-☑	—	—
skull	C41.Ø	C79.51	—	D16.4	D48.Ø	D49.2
sphenoid	C41.Ø	C79.51	—	D16.4	D48.Ø	D49.2
spine, spinal (column)	C41.2	C79.51	—	D16.6	D48.Ø	D49.2
coccyx	C41.4	C79.51	—	D16.8	D48.Ø	D49.2
sacrum	C41.4	C79.51	—	D16.8	D48.Ø	D49.2
sternum	C41.3	C79.51	—	D16.7	D48.Ø	D49.2
tarsus (any)	C4Ø.3-☑	C79.51	—	—	—	—
temporal	C41.Ø	C79.51	—	D16.4	D48.Ø	D49.2
thumb	C4Ø.1-☑	C79.51	—	—	—	—
tibia (any part)	C4Ø.2-☑	C79.51	—	—	—	—
toe (any)	C4Ø.3-☑	C79.51	—	—	—	—
trapezium	C4Ø.1-☑	C79.51	—	—	—	—
trapezoid	C4Ø.1-☑	C79.51	—	—	—	—
turbinate	C41.Ø	C79.51	—	D16.4	D48.Ø	D49.2
ulna (any part)	C4Ø.Ø-☑	C79.51	—	D16.Ø-☑	—	—
unciform	C4Ø.1-☑	C79.51	—	—	—	—
vertebra (column)	C41.2	C79.51	—	D16.6	D48.Ø	D49.2
coccyx	C41.4	C79.51	—	D16.8	D48.Ø	D49.2
sacrum	C41.4	C79.51	—	D16.8	D48.Ø	D49.2
vomer	C41.Ø	C79.51	—	D16.4	D48.Ø	D49.2
wrist	C4Ø.1-☑	C79.51	—	—	—	—
xiphoid process	C41.3	C79.51	—	D16.7	D48.Ø	D49.2
zygomatic	C41.Ø	C79.51	—	D16.4	D48.Ø	D49.2
book-leaf (mouth) — *ventral surface of tongue and floor of mouth*	CØ6.89	C79.89	DØØ.ØØ	D1Ø.39	D37.Ø9	D49.Ø
bowel — *see* Neoplasm, intestine						
brachial plexus	C47.1-☑	C79.89	—	D36.12	D48.2	D49.2
brain NEC	C71.9	C79.31	—	D33.2	D43.2	D49.6

	Malignant Primary	Malignant Secondary	Ca in situ	Benign	Uncertain Behavior	Unspecified Behavior
Neoplasm, neoplastic — *continued*						
brain — *continued*						
basal ganglia	C71.Ø	C79.31	—	D33.Ø	D43.Ø	D49.6
cerebellopontine angle	C71.6	C79.31	—	D33.1	D43.1	D49.6
cerebellum NOS	C71.6	C79.31	—	D33.1	D43.1	D49.6
cerebrum	C71.Ø	C79.31	—	D33.Ø	D43.Ø	D49.6
choroid plexus	C71.7	C79.31	—	D33.1	D43.1	D49.6
corpus callosum	C71.8	C79.31	—	D33.2	D43.2	D49.6
corpus striatum	C71.Ø	C79.31	—	D33.Ø	D43.Ø	D49.6
cortex (cerebral)	C71.Ø	C79.31	—	D33.Ø	D43.Ø	D49.6
frontal lobe	C71.1	C79.31	—	D33.Ø	D43.Ø	D49.6
globus pallidus	C71.Ø	C79.31	—	D33.Ø	D43.Ø	D49.6
hippocampus	C71.2	C79.31	—	D33.Ø	D43.Ø	D49.6
hypothalamus	C71.Ø	C79.31	—	D33.Ø	D43.Ø	D49.6
internal capsule	C71.Ø	C79.31	—	D33.Ø	D43.Ø	D49.6
medulla oblongata	C71.7	C79.31	—	D33.1	D43.1	D49.6
meninges	C7Ø.Ø	C79.32	—	D32.Ø	D42.Ø	D49.7
midbrain	C71.7	C79.31	—	D33.1	D43.1	D49.6
occipital lobe	C71.4	C79.31	—	D33.Ø	D43.Ø	D49.6
overlapping lesion	C71.8	C79.31	—	—	—	—
parietal lobe	C71.3	C79.31	—	D33.Ø	D43.Ø	D49.6
peduncle	C71.7	C79.31	—	D33.1	D43.1	D49.6
pons	C71.7	C79.31	—	D33.1	D43.1	D49.6
stem	C71.7	C79.31	—	D33.1	D43.1	D49.6
tapetum	C71.8	C79.31	—	D33.2	D43.2	D49.6
temporal lobe	C71.2	C79.31	—	D33.Ø	D43.Ø	D49.6
thalamus	C71.Ø	C79.31	—	D33.Ø	D43.Ø	D49.6
uncus	C71.2	C79.31	—	D33.Ø	D43.Ø	D49.6
ventricle (floor)	C71.5	C79.31	—	D33.Ø	D43.Ø	D49.6
fourth	C71.7	C79.31	—	D33.1	D43.1	D49.6
branchial (cleft) (cyst) (vestiges)	C1Ø.4	C79.89	DØØ.Ø8	D1Ø.5	D37.Ø5	D49.Ø
breast (connective tissue) (glandular tissue) (soft parts)	C5Ø.9-☑	C79.81	DØ5.-☑	D24.-☑	D48.6-☑	D49.3
areola	C5Ø.Ø-☑	C79.81	DØ5.-☑	D24.-☑	D48.6-☑	D49.3
axillary tail	C5Ø.6-☑	C79.81	DØ5.-☑	D24.-☑	D48.6-☑	D49.3
central portion	C5Ø.1-☑	C79.81	DØ5.-☑	D24.-☑	D48.6-☑	D49.3
inner	C5Ø.8-☑	C79.81	DØ5.-☑	D24.-☑	D48.6-☑	D49.3
lower	C5Ø.8-☑	C79.81	DØ5.-☑	D24.-☑	D48.6-☑	D49.3
lower-inner quadrant	C5Ø.3-☑	C79.81	DØ5.-☑	D24.-☑	D48.6-☑	D49.3
lower-outer quadrant	C5Ø.5-☑	C79.81	DØ5.-☑	D24.-☑	D48.6-☑	D49.3
mastectomy site (skin) — *see also* Neoplasm, breast, skin	C44.5Ø1	C79.2	—	—	—	—
specified as breast tissue	C5Ø.8-☑	C79.81	—	—	—	—
midline	C5Ø.8-☑	C79.81	DØ5.-☑	D24.-☑	D48.6-☑	D49.3
nipple	C5Ø.Ø-☑	C79.81	DØ5.-☑	D24.-☑	D48.6-☑	D49.3
outer	C5Ø.8-☑	C79.81	DØ5.-☑	D24.-☑	D48.6-☑	D49.3
overlapping lesion	C5Ø.8-☑	—	—	—	—	—
skin	C44.5Ø1	C79.2	DØ4.5	D23.5	D48.5	D49.2
basal cell carcinoma	C44.511	—	—	—	—	—
specified type NEC	C44.591	—	—	—	—	—
squamous cell carcinoma	C44.521	—	—	—	—	—
tail (axillary)	C5Ø.6-☑	C79.81	DØ5.-☑	D24.-☑	D48.6-☑	D49.3
upper	C5Ø.8-☑	C79.81	DØ5.-☑	D24.-☑	D48.6-☑	D49.3
upper-inner quadrant	C5Ø.2-☑	C79.81	DØ5.-☑	D24.-☑	D48.6-☑	D49.3
upper-outer quadrant	C5Ø.4-☑	C79.81	DØ5.-☑	D24.-☑	D48.6-☑	D49.3
broad ligament	C57.1-☑	C79.82	DØ7.39	D28.2	D39.8	D49.59
bronchiogenic, bronchogenic (lung)	C34.9-☑	C78.Ø-☑	DØ2.2-☑	D14.3-☑	D38.1	D49.1
bronchiole	C34.9-☑	C78.Ø-☑	DØ2.2-☑	D14.3-☑	D38.1	D49.1
bronchus	C34.9-☑	C78.Ø-☑	DØ2.2-☑	D14.3-☑	D38.1	D49.1
carina	C34.Ø-☑	C78.Ø-☑	DØ2.2-☑	D14.3-☑	D38.1	D49.1
lower lobe of lung	C34.3-☑	C78.Ø-☑	DØ2.2-☑	D14.3-☑	D38.1	D49.1

	Malignant Primary	Malignant Secondary	Ca in situ	Benign	Uncertain Behavior	Unspecified Behavior
Neoplasm, neoplastic — *continued*						
bronchus — *continued*						
main	C34.Ø-☑	C78.Ø-☑	DØ2.2-☑	D14.3-☑	D38.1	D49.1
middle lobe of lung	C34.2	C78.Ø-☑	DØ2.21	D14.31	D38.1	D49.1
overlapping lesion	C34.8-☑	—	—	—	—	—
upper lobe of lung	C34.1-☑	C78.Ø-☑	DØ2.2-☑	D14.3-☑	D38.1	D49.1
brow	C44.3Ø9	C79.2	DØ4.39	D23.39	D48.5	D49.2
basal cell carcinoma	C44.319	—	—	—	—	—
specified type NEC	C44.399	—	—	—	—	—
squamous cell carcinoma	C44.329	—	—	—	—	—
buccal (cavity)	CØ6.9	C79.89	DØØ.ØØ	D1Ø.39	D37.Ø9	D49.Ø
commissure	CØ6.Ø	C79.89	DØØ.Ø2	D1Ø.39	D37.Ø9	D49.Ø
groove (lower) (upper)	CØ6.1	C79.89	DØØ.Ø2	D1Ø.39	D37.Ø9	D49.Ø
mucosa	CØ6.Ø	C79.89	DØØ.Ø2	D1Ø.39	D37.Ø9	D49.Ø
sulcus (lower) (upper)	CØ6.1	C79.89	DØØ.Ø2	D1Ø.39	D37.Ø9	D49.Ø
bulbourethral gland	C68.Ø	C79.19	DØ9.19	D3Ø.4	D41.3	D49.59
bursa — *see* Neoplasm, connective tissue						
buttock NEC	C76.3	C79.89	DØ4.5	D36.7	D48.7	D49.89
calf	C76.5-☑	C79.89	DØ4.7-☑	D36.7	D48.7	D49.89
calvarium	C41.Ø	C79.51	—	D16.4	D48.Ø	D49.2
calyx, renal	C65.-☑	C79.Ø-☑	DØ9.19	D3Ø.1-☑	D41.1-☑	D49.51-☑
canal						
anal	C21.1	C78.5	DØ1.3	D12.9	D37.8	D49.Ø
auditory (external) — *see also* Neoplasm, skin, ear	C44.2Ø-☑	C79.2	DØ4.2-☑	D23.2-☑	D48.5	D49.2
auricular (external) — *see also* Neoplasm, skin, ear	C44.2Ø-☑	C79.2	DØ4.2-☑	D23.2-☑	D48.5	D49.2
canaliculi, biliary (biliferi) (intrahepatic)	C22.1	C78.7	DØ1.5	D13.4	D37.6	D49.Ø
canthus (eye) (inner) (outer)	C44.1Ø-☑	C79.2	DØ4.1-☑	D23.1-☑	D48.5	D49.2
basal cell carcinoma	C44.11-☑	—	—	—	—	—
sebaceous cell	C44.13-☑	—	—	—	—	—
specified type NEC	C44.19-☑	—	—	—	—	—
squamous cell carcinoma	C44.12-☑	—	—	—	—	—
capillary — *see* Neoplasm, connective tissue						
caput coli	C18.Ø	C78.5	DØ1.Ø	D12.Ø	D37.4	D49.Ø
carcinoid — *see* Tumor, carcinoid						
cardia (gastric)	C16.Ø	C78.89	DØØ.2	D13.1	D37.1	D49.Ø
cardiac orifice (stomach)	C16.Ø	C78.89	DØØ.2	D13.1	D37.1	D49.Ø
cardio-esophageal junction	C16.Ø	C78.89	DØØ.2	D13.1	D37.1	D49.Ø
cardio-esophagus	C16.Ø	C78.89	DØØ.2	D13.1	D37.1	D49.Ø
carina (bronchus)	C34.Ø-☑	C78.Ø-☑	DØ2.2-☑	D14.3-☑	D38.1	D49.1
carotid (artery)	C49.Ø	C79.89	—	D21.Ø	D48.1	D49.2
body	C75.4	C79.89	—	D35.5	D44.6	D49.7
carpus (any bone)	C4Ø.1-☑	C79.51	—	D16.1-☑	—	—
cartilage (articular) (joint) NEC — *see also* Neoplasm, bone	C41.9	C79.51	—	D16.9	D48.Ø	D49.2
arytenoid	C32.3	C78.39	DØ2.Ø	D14.1	D38.Ø	D49.1
auricular	C49.Ø	C79.89	—	D21.Ø	D48.1	D49.2
bronchi	C34.Ø-☑	C78.39	—	D14.3-☑	D38.1	D49.1
costal	C41.3	C79.51	—	D16.7	D48.Ø	D49.2
cricoid	C32.3	C78.39	DØ2.Ø	D14.1	D38.Ø	D49.1
cuneiform	C32.3	C78.39	DØ2.Ø	D14.1	D38.Ø	D49.1
ear (external)	C49.Ø	C79.89	—	D21.Ø	D48.1	D49.2
ensiform	C41.3	C79.51	—	D16.7	D48.Ø	D49.2
epiglottis	C32.1	C78.39	DØ2.Ø	D14.1	D38.Ø	D49.1

	Malignant Primary	Malignant Secondary	Ca in situ	Benign	Uncertain Behavior	Unspecified Behavior
Neoplasm, neoplastic — *continued*						
cartilage — *see also* Neoplasm, bone — *continued*						
epiglottis — *continued*						
anterior surface	C1Ø.1	C79.89	DØØ.Ø8	D1Ø.5	D37.Ø5	D49.Ø
eyelid	C49.Ø	C79.89	—	D21.Ø	D48.1	D49.2
intervertebral	C41.2	C79.51	—	D16.6	D48.Ø	D49.2
larynx, laryngeal	C32.3	C78.39	DØ2.Ø	D14.1	D38.Ø	D49.1
nose, nasal	C3Ø.Ø	C78.39	DØ2.3	D14.Ø	D38.5	D49.1
pinna	C49.Ø	C79.89	—	D21.Ø	D48.1	D49.2
rib	C41.3	C79.51	—	D16.7	D48.Ø	D49.2
semilunar (knee)	C4Ø.2-☑	C79.51	—	D16.2-☑	D48.Ø	D49.2
thyroid	C32.3	C78.39	DØ2.Ø	D14.1	D38.Ø	D49.1
trachea	C33	C78.39	DØ2.1	D14.2	D38.1	D49.1
cauda equina	C72.1	C79.49	—	D33.4	D43.4	D49.7
cavity						
buccal	CØ6.9	C79.89	DØØ.ØØ	D1Ø.3Ø	D37.Ø9	D49.Ø
nasal	C3Ø.Ø	C78.39	DØ2.3	D14.Ø	D38.5	D49.1
oral	CØ6.9	C79.89	DØØ.ØØ	D1Ø.3Ø	D37.Ø9	D49.Ø
peritoneal	C48.2	C78.6	—	D2Ø.1	D48.4	D49.Ø
tympanic	C3Ø.1	C78.39	DØ2.3	D14.Ø	D38.5	D49.1
cecum	C18.Ø	C78.5	DØ1.Ø	D12.Ø	D37.4	D49.Ø
central nervous system	C72.9	C79.4Ø	—	—	—	—
cerebellopontine (angle)	C71.6	C79.31	—	D33.1	D43.1	D49.6
cerebellum, cerebellar	C71.6	C79.31	—	D33.1	D43.1	D49.6
cerebrum, cerebra (cortex) (hemisphere) (white matter)	C71.Ø	C79.31	—	D33.Ø	D43.Ø	D49.6
meninges	C7Ø.Ø	C79.32	—	D32.Ø	D42.Ø	D49.7
peduncle	C71.7	C79.31	—	D33.1	D43.1	D49.6
ventricle	C71.5	C79.31	—	D33.Ø	D43.Ø	D49.6
fourth	C71.7	C79.31	—	D33.1	D43.1	D49.6
cervical region	C76.Ø	C79.89	DØ9.8	D36.7	D48.7	D49.89
cervix (cervical) (uteri) (uterus)	C53.9	C79.82	DØ6.9	D26.Ø	D39.Ø	D49.59
canal	C53.Ø	C79.82	DØ6.Ø	D26.Ø	D39.Ø	D49.59
endocervix (canal) (gland)	C53.Ø	C79.82	DØ6.Ø	D26.Ø	D39.Ø	D49.59
exocervix	C53.1	C79.82	DØ6.1	D26.Ø	D39.Ø	D49.59
external os	C53.1	C79.82	DØ6.1	D26.Ø	D39.Ø	D49.59
internal os	C53.Ø	C79.82	DØ6.Ø	D26.Ø	D39.Ø	D49.59
nabothian gland	C53.Ø	C79.82	DØ6.Ø	D26.Ø	D39.Ø	D49.59
overlapping lesion	C53.8	—	—	—	—	—
squamocolumnar junction	C53.8	C79.82	DØ6.7	D26.Ø	D39.Ø	D49.59
stump	C53.8	C79.82	DØ6.7	D26.Ø	D39.Ø	D49.59
cheek	C76.Ø	C79.89	DØ9.8	D36.7	D48.7	D49.89
external	C44.3Ø9	C79.2	DØ4.39	D23.39	D48.5	D49.2
basal cell carcinoma	C44.319	—	—	—	—	—
specified type NEC	C44.399	—	—	—	—	—
squamous cell carcinoma	C44.329	—	—	—	—	—
inner aspect	CØ6.Ø	C79.89	DØØ.Ø2	D1Ø.39	D37.Ø9	D49.Ø
internal	CØ6.Ø	C79.89	DØØ.Ø2	D1Ø.39	D37.Ø9	D49.Ø
mucosa	CØ6.Ø	C79.89	DØØ.Ø2	D1Ø.39	D37.Ø9	D49.Ø
chest (wall) NEC	C76.1	C79.89	DØ9.8	D36.7	D48.7	D49.89
chiasma opticum	C72.3-☑	C79.49	—	D33.3	D43.3	D49.7
chin	C44.3Ø9	C79.2	DØ4.39	D23.39	D48.5	D49.2
basal cell carcinoma	C44.319	—	—	—	—	—
specified type NEC	C44.399	—	—	—	—	—
squamous cell carcinoma	C44.329	—	—	—	—	—
choana	C11.3	C79.89	DØØ.Ø8	D1Ø.6	D37.Ø5	D49.Ø
cholangiole	C22.1	C78.89	DØ1.5	D13.4	D37.6	D49.Ø
choledochal duct	C24.Ø	C78.89	DØ1.5	D13.5	D37.6	D49.Ø
choroid	C69.3-☑	C79.49	DØ9.2-☑	D31.3-☑	D48.7	D49.81
plexus	C71.5	C79.31	—	D33.Ø	D43.Ø	D49.6
ciliary body	C69.4-☑	C79.49	DØ9.2-☑	D31.4-☑	D48.7	D49.89
clavicle	C41.3	C79.51	—	D16.7	D48.Ø	D49.2

	Malignant Primary	Malignant Secondary	Ca in situ	Benign	Uncertain Behavior	Unspecified Behavior
Neoplasm, neoplastic — *continued*						
clitoris	C51.2	C79.82	DØ7.1	D28.Ø	D39.8	D49.59
clivus	C41.Ø	C79.51	—	D16.4	D48.Ø	D49.2
cloacogenic zone	C21.2	C78.5	DØ1.3	D12.9	D37.8	D49.Ø
coccygeal						
body or glomus	C49.5	C79.89	—	D21.5	D48.1	D49.2
vertebra	C41.4	C79.51	—	D16.8	D48.Ø	D49.2
coccyx	C41.4	C79.51	—	D16.8	D48.Ø	D49.2
colon — *see also* Neoplasm, intestine, large	C18.9	C78.5	—	—	—	—
with rectum	C19	C78.5	DØ1.1	D12.7	D37.5	D49.Ø
columnella — *see also* Neoplasm, skin, face	C44.39Ø	C79.2	DØ4.39	D23.39	D48.5	D49.2
column, spinal — *see* Neoplasm, spine						
commissure						
labial, lip	CØØ.6	C79.89	DØØ.Ø1	D1Ø.39	D37.Ø1	D49.Ø
laryngeal	C32.Ø	C78.39	DØ2.Ø	D14.1	D38.Ø	D49.1
common (bile) duct	C24.Ø	C78.89	DØ1.5	D13.5	D37.6	D49.Ø
concha — *see also* Neoplasm, skin, ear	C44.2Ø-☑	C79.2	DØ4.2-☑	D23.2-☑	D48.5	D49.2
nose	C3Ø.Ø	C78.39	DØ2.3	D14.Ø	D38.5	D49.1
conjunctiva	C69.Ø-☑	C79.49	DØ9.2-☑	D31.Ø-☑	D48.7	D49.89
connective tissue NEC	C49.9	C79.89	—	D21.9	D48.1	D49.2

Note: For neoplasms of connective tissue (blood vessel, bursa, fascia, ligament, muscle, peripheral nerves, sympathetic and parasympathetic nerves and ganglia, synovia, tendon, etc.) or of morphological types that indicate connective tissue, code according to the list under "Neoplasm, connective tissue". For sites that do not appear in this list, code to neoplasm of that site; e.g., fibrosarcoma, pancreas (C25.9)

Note: Morphological types that indicate connective tissue appear in their proper place in the alphabetic index with the instruction "see Neoplasm, connective tissue ...."

	Malignant Primary	Malignant Secondary	Ca in situ	Benign	Uncertain Behavior	Unspecified Behavior
abdomen	C49.4	C79.89	—	D21.4	D48.1	D49.2
abdominal wall	C49.4	C79.89	—	D21.4	D48.1	D49.2
ankle	C49.2-☑	C79.89	—	D21.2-☑	D48.1	D49.2
antecubital fossa or space	C49.1-☑	C79.89	—	D21.1-☑	D48.1	D49.2
arm	C49.1-☑	C79.89	—	D21.1-☑	D48.1	D49.2
auricle (ear)	C49.Ø	C79.89	—	D21.Ø	D48.1	D49.2
axilla	C49.3	C79.89	—	D21.3	D48.1	D49.2
back	C49.6	C79.89	—	D21.6	D48.1	D49.2
breast — *see* Neoplasm, breast						
buttock	C49.5	C79.89	—	D21.5	D48.1	D49.2
calf	C49.2-☑	C79.89	—	D21.2-☑	D48.1	D49.2
cervical region	C49.Ø	C79.89	—	D21.Ø	D48.1	D49.2
cheek	C49.Ø	C79.89	—	D21.Ø	D48.1	D49.2
chest (wall)	C49.3	C79.89	—	D21.3	D48.1	D49.2
chin	C49.Ø	C79.89	—	D21.Ø	D48.1	D49.2
diaphragm	C49.3	C79.89	—	D21.3	D48.1	D49.2
ear (external)	C49.Ø	C79.89	—	D21.Ø	D48.1	D49.2
elbow	C49.1-☑	C79.89	—	D21.1-☑	D48.1	D49.2
extrarectal	C49.5	C79.89	—	D21.5	D48.1	D49.2
extremity	C49.9	C79.89	—	D21.9	D48.1	D49.2
lower	C49.2-☑	C79.89	—	D21.2-☑	D48.1	D49.2
upper	C49.1-☑	C79.89	—	D21.1-☑	D48.1	D49.2
eyelid	C49.Ø	C79.89	—	D21.Ø	D48.1	D49.2
face	C49.Ø	C79.89	—	D21.Ø	D48.1	D49.2
finger	C49.1-☑	C79.89	—	D21.1-☑	D48.1	D49.2
flank	C49.6	C79.89	—	D21.6	D48.1	D49.2
foot	C49.2-☑	C79.89	—	D21.2-☑	D48.1	D49.2
forearm	C49.1-☑	C79.89	—	D21.1-☑	D48.1	D49.2
forehead	C49.Ø	C79.89	—	D21.Ø	D48.1	D49.2
gastric	C49.4	C79.89	—	D21.4	D48.1	D49.2
gastrointestinal	C49.4	C79.89	—	D21.4	D48.1	D49.2
gluteal region	C49.5	C79.89	—	D21.5	D48.1	D49.2
great vessels NEC	C49.3	C79.89	—	D21.3	D48.1	D49.2
groin	C49.5	C79.89	—	D21.5	D48.1	D49.2
hand	C49.1-☑	C79.89	—	D21.1-☑	D48.1	D49.2
head	C49.Ø	C79.89	—	D21.Ø	D48.1	D49.2

Neoplasm, neoplastic — continued	Malignant Primary	Malignant Secondary	Ca in situ	Benign	Uncertain Behavior	Unspecified Behavior
connective tissue — continued						
heel	C49.2-☑	C79.89	—	D21.2-☑	D48.1	D49.2
hip	C49.2-☑	C79.89	—	D21.2-☑	D48.1	D49.2
hypochondrium	C49.4	C79.89	—	D21.4	D48.1	D49.2
iliopsoas muscle	C49.5	C79.89	—	D21.5	D48.1	D49.2
infraclavicular region	C49.3	C79.89	—	D21.3	D48.1	D49.2
inguinal (canal) (region)	C49.5	C79.89	—	D21.5	D48.1	D49.2
intestinal	C49.4	C79.89	—	D21.4	D48.1	D49.2
intrathoracic	C49.3	C79.89	—	D21.3	D48.1	D49.2
ischiorectal fossa	C49.5	C79.89	—	D21.5	D48.1	D49.2
jaw	CØ3.9	C79.89	DØØ.Ø3	D1Ø.39	D48.1	D49.Ø
knee	C49.2-☑	C79.89	—	D21.2-☑	D48.1	D49.2
leg	C49.2-☑	C79.89	—	D21.2-☑	D48.1	D49.2
limb NEC	C49.9	C79.89	—	D21.9	D48.1	D49.2
lower	C49.2-☑	C79.89	—	D21.2-☑	D48.1	D49.2
upper	C49.1-☑	C79.89	—	D21.1-☑	D48.1	D49.2
nates	C49.5	C79.89	—	D21.5	D48.1	D49.2
neck	C49.Ø	C79.89	—	D21.Ø	D48.1	D49.2
orbit	C69.6-☑	C79.49	DØ9.2-☑	D31.6-☑	D48.1	D49.89
overlapping lesion	C49.8	—	—	—	—	—
pararectal	C49.5	C79.89	—	D21.5	D48.1	D49.2
para-urethral	C49.5	C79.89	—	D21.5	D48.1	D49.2
paravaginal	C49.5	C79.89	—	D21.5	D48.1	D49.2
pelvis (floor)	C49.5	C79.89	—	D21.5	D48.1	D49.2
pelvo-abdominal	C49.8	C79.89	—	D21.6	D48.1	D49.2
perineum	C49.5	C79.89	—	D21.5	D48.1	D49.2
perirectal (tissue)	C49.5	C79.89	—	D21.5	D48.1	D49.2
periurethral (tissue)	C49.5	C79.89	—	D21.5	D48.1	D49.2
popliteal fossa or space	C49.2-☑	C79.89	—	D21.2-☑	D48.1	D49.2
presacral	C49.5	C79.89	—	D21.5	D48.1	D49.2
psoas muscle	C49.4	C79.89	—	D21.4	D48.1	D49.2
pterygoid fossa	C49.Ø	C79.89	—	D21.Ø	D48.1	D49.2
rectovaginal septum or wall	C49.5	C79.89	—	D21.5	D48.1	D49.2
rectovesical	C49.5	C79.89	—	D21.5	D48.1	D49.2
retroperitoneum	C48.Ø	C78.6	—	D2Ø.Ø	D48.3	D49.Ø
sacrococcygeal region	C49.5	C79.89	—	D21.5	D48.1	D49.2
scalp	C49.Ø	C79.89	—	D21.Ø	D48.1	D49.2
scapular region	C49.3	C79.89	—	D21.3	D48.1	D49.2
shoulder	C49.1-☑	C79.89	—	D21.1-☑	D48.1	D49.2
skin (dermis) NEC — *see also* Neoplasm, skin, by site	C44.90	C79.2	DØ4.9	D23.9	D48.5	D49.2
stomach	C49.4	C79.89	—	D21.4	D48.1	D49.2
submental	C49.Ø	C79.89	—	D21.Ø	D48.1	D49.2
supraclavicular region	C49.Ø	C79.89	—	D21.Ø	D48.1	D49.2
temple	C49.Ø	C79.89	—	D21.Ø	D48.1	D49.2
temporal region	C49.Ø	C79.89	—	D21.Ø	D48.1	D49.2
thigh	C49.2-☑	C79.89	—	D21.2-☑	D48.1	D49.2
thoracic (duct) (wall)	C49.3	C79.89	—	D21.3	D48.1	D49.2
thorax	C49.3	C79.89	—	D21.3	D48.1	D49.2
thumb	C49.1-☑	C79.89	—	D21.1-☑	D48.1	D49.2
toe	C49.2-☑	C79.89	—	D21.2-☑	D48.1	D49.2
trunk	C49.6	C79.89	—	D21.6	D48.1	D49.2
umbilicus	C49.4	C79.89	—	D21.4	D48.1	D49.2
vesicorectal	C49.5	C79.89	—	D21.5	D48.1	D49.2
wrist	C49.1-☑	C79.89	—	D21.1-☑	D48.1	D49.2
conus medullaris	C72.Ø	C79.49	—	D33.4	D43.4	D49.7
cord (true) (vocal)	C32.Ø	C78.39	DØ2.Ø	D14.1	D38.Ø	D49.1
false	C32.1	C78.39	DØ2.Ø	D14.1	D38.Ø	D49.1
spermatic	C63.1-☑	C79.82	DØ7.69	D29.8	D4Ø.8	D49.59
spinal (cervical) (lumbar) (thoracic)	C72.Ø	C79.49	—	D33.4	D43.4	D49.7
cornea (limbus)	C69.1-☑	C79.49	DØ9.2-☑	D31.1-☑	D48.7	D49.89
corpus						
albicans	C56.-☑	C79.6-☑	DØ7.39	D27.-☑	D39.1-☑	D49.59
callosum, brain	C71.Ø	C79.31	—	D33.2	D43.2	D49.6

Neoplasm, neoplastic — continued	Malignant Primary	Malignant Secondary	Ca in situ	Benign	Uncertain Behavior	Unspecified Behavior
corpus — continued						
cavernosum	C6Ø.2	C79.82	DØ7.4	D29.Ø	D4Ø.8	D49.59
gastric	C16.2	C78.89	DØØ.2	D13.1	D37.1	D49.Ø
overlapping sites	C54.8	—	—	—	—	—
penis	C6Ø.2	C79.82	DØ7.4	D29.Ø	D4Ø.8	D49.59
striatum, cerebrum	C71.Ø	C79.31	—	D33.Ø	D43.Ø	D49.6
uteri	C54.9	C79.82	DØ7.Ø	D26.1	D39.Ø	D49.59
isthmus	C54.Ø	C79.82	DØ7.Ø	D26.1	D39.Ø	D49.59
cortex						
adrenal	C74.Ø-☑	C79.7-☑	DØ9.3	D35.Ø-☑	D44.1-☑	D49.7
cerebral	C71.Ø	C79.31	—	D33.Ø	D43.Ø	D49.6
costal cartilage	C41.3	C79.51	—	D16.7	D48.Ø	D49.2
costovertebral joint	C41.3	C79.51	—	D16.7	D48.Ø	D49.2
Cowper's gland	C68.Ø	C79.19	DØ9.19	D3Ø.4	D41.3	D49.59
cranial (fossa, any)	C71.9	C79.31	—	D33.2	D43.2	D49.6
meninges	C7Ø.Ø	C79.32	—	D32.Ø	D42.Ø	D49.7
nerve	C72.5Ø	C79.49	—	D33.3	D43.3	D49.7
specified NEC	C72.59	C79.49	—	D33.3	D43.3	D49.7
craniobuccal pouch	C75.2	C79.89	DØ9.3	D35.2	D44.3	D49.7
craniopharyngeal (duct) (pouch)	C75.2	C79.89	DØ9.3	D35.3	D44.4	D49.7
cricoid	C13.Ø	C79.89	DØØ.Ø8	D1Ø.7	D37.Ø5	D49.Ø
cartilage	C32.3	C78.39	DØ2.Ø	D14.1	D38.Ø	D49.1
cricopharynx	C13.Ø	C79.89	DØØ.Ø8	D1Ø.7	D37.Ø5	D49.Ø
crypt of Morgagni	C21.8	C78.5	DØ1.3	D12.9	D37.8	D49.Ø
crystalline lens	C69.4-☑	C79.49	DØ9.2-☑	D31.4-☑	D48.7	D49.89
cul-de-sac (Douglas')	C48.1	C78.6	—	D2Ø.1	D48.4	D49.Ø
cuneiform cartilage	C32.3	C78.39	DØ2.Ø	D14.1	D38.Ø	D49.1
cutaneous — *see* Neoplasm, skin						
cutis — *see* Neoplasm, skin						
cystic (bile) duct (common)	C24.Ø	C78.89	DØ1.5	D13.5	D37.6	D49.Ø
dermis — *see* Neoplasm, skin						
diaphragm	C49.3	C79.89	—	D21.3	D48.1	D49.2
digestive organs, system, tube, or tract NEC	C26.9	C78.89	DØ1.9	D13.9	D37.9	D49.Ø
disc, intervertebral	C41.2	C79.51	—	D16.6	D48.Ø	D49.2
disease, generalized	C8Ø.Ø	—	—	—	—	—
disseminated	C8Ø.Ø	—	—	—	—	—
Douglas' cul-de-sac or pouch	C48.1	C78.6	—	D2Ø.1	D48.4	D49.Ø
duodenojejunal junction	C17.8	C78.4	DØ1.49	D13.39	D37.2	D49.Ø
duodenum	C17.Ø	C78.4	DØ1.49	D13.2	D37.2	D49.Ø
dura (cranial) (mater)	C7Ø.9	C79.49	—	D32.9	D42.9	D49.7
cerebral	C7Ø.Ø	C79.32	—	D32.Ø	D42.Ø	D49.7
spinal	C7Ø.1	C79.49	—	D32.1	D42.1	D49.7
ear (external) — *see also* Neoplasm, skin, ear	C44.2Ø-☑	C79.2	DØ4.2-☑	D23.2-☑	D48.5	D49.2
auricle or auris — *see also* Neoplasm, skin, ear	C44.2Ø-☑	C79.2	DØ4.2-☑	D23.2-☑	D48.5	D49.2
canal, external — *see also* Neoplasm, skin, ear	C44.2Ø-☑	C79.2	DØ4.2-☑	D23.2-☑	D48.5	D49.2
cartilage	C49.Ø	C79.89	—	D21.Ø	D48.1	D49.2
external meatus — *see also* Neoplasm, skin, ear	C44.2Ø-☑	C79.2	DØ4.2-☑	D23.2-☑	D48.5	D49.2
inner	C3Ø.1	C78.39	DØ2.3	D14.Ø	D38.5	D49.1
lobule — *see also* Neoplasm, skin, ear	C44.2Ø-☑	C79.2	DØ4.2-☑	D23.2-☑	D48.5	D49.2
middle	C3Ø.1	C78.39	DØ2.3	D14.Ø	D38.5	D49.1
overlapping lesion with accessory sinuses	C31.8	—	—	—	—	—

	Malignant Primary	Malignant Secondary	Ca in situ	Benign	Uncertain Behavior	Unspecified Behavior
Neoplasm, neoplastic — *continued*						
ear — *see also* Neoplasm, skin, ear — *continued*						
skin	C44.2Ø-☑	C79.2	DØ4.2-☑	D23.2-☑	D48.5	D49.2
basal cell carcinoma	C44.21-☑	—	—	—	—	—
specified type NEC	C44.29-☑	—	—	—	—	—
squamous cell carcinoma	C44.22-☑	—	—	—	—	—
earlobe	C44.2Ø-☑	C79.2	DØ4.2-☑	D23.2-☑	D48.5	D49.2
basal cell carcinoma	C44.21-☑	—	—	—	—	—
specified type NEC	C44.29-☑	—	—	—	—	—
squamous cell carcinoma	C44.22-☑	—	—	—	—	—
ejaculatory duct	C63.7	C79.82	DØ7.69	D29.8	D4Ø.8	D49.59
elbow NEC	C76.4-☑	C79.89	DØ4.6-☑	D36.7	D48.7	D49.89
endocardium	C38.Ø	C79.89	—	D15.1	D48.7	D49.89
endocervix (canal) (gland)	C53.Ø	C79.82	DØ6.Ø	D26.Ø	D39.Ø	D49.59
endocrine gland NEC	C75.9	C79.89	DØ9.3	D35.9	D44.9	D49.7
pluriglandular	C75.8	C79.89	DØ9.3	D35.7	D44.9	D49.7
endometrium (gland) (stroma)	C54.1	C79.82	DØ7.Ø	D26.1	D39.Ø	D49.59
ensiform cartilage	C41.3	C79.51	—	D16.7	D48.Ø	D49.2
enteric — *see* Neoplasm, intestine						
ependyma (brain)	C71.5	C79.31	—	D33.Ø	D43.Ø	D49.6
fourth ventricle	C71.7	C79.31	—	D33.1	D43.1	D49.6
epicardium	C38.Ø	C79.89	—	D15.1	D48.7	D49.89
epididymis	C63.Ø-☑	C79.82	DØ7.69	D29.3-☑	D4Ø.8	D49.59
epidural	C72.9	C79.49	—	D33.9	D43.9	D49.7
epiglottis	C32.1	C78.39	DØ2.Ø	D14.1	D38.Ø	D49.1
anterior aspect or surface	C1Ø.1	C79.89	DØØ.Ø8	D1Ø.5	D37.Ø5	D49.Ø
cartilage	C32.3	C78.39	DØ2.Ø	D14.1	D38.Ø	D49.1
free border (margin)	C1Ø.1	C79.89	DØØ.Ø8	D1Ø.5	D37.Ø5	D49.Ø
junctional region	C1Ø.8	C79.89	DØØ.Ø8	D1Ø.5	D37.Ø5	D49.Ø
posterior (laryngeal) surface	C32.1	C78.39	DØ2.Ø	D14.1	D38.Ø	D49.1
suprahyoid portion	C32.1	C78.39	DØ2.Ø	D14.1	D38.Ø	D49.1
esophagogastric junction	C16.Ø	C78.89	DØØ.2	D13.1	D37.1	D49.Ø
esophagus	C15.9	C78.89	DØØ.1	D13.Ø	D37.8	D49.Ø
abdominal	C15.5	C78.89	DØØ.1	D13.Ø	D37.8	D49.Ø
cervical	C15.3	C78.89	DØØ.1	D13.Ø	D37.8	D49.Ø
distal (third)	C15.5	C78.89	DØØ.1	D13.Ø	D37.8	D49.Ø
lower (third)	C15.5	C78.89	DØØ.1	D13.Ø	D37.8	D49.Ø
middle (third)	C15.4	C78.89	DØØ.1	D13.Ø	D37.8	D49.Ø
overlapping lesion	C15.8	—	—	—	—	—
proximal (third)	C15.3	C78.89	DØØ.1	D13.Ø	D37.8	D49.Ø
thoracic	C15.4	C78.89	DØØ.1	D13.Ø	D37.8	D49.Ø
upper (third)	C15.3	C78.89	DØØ.1	D13.Ø	D37.8	D49.Ø
ethmoid (sinus)	C31.1	C78.39	DØ2.3	D14.Ø	D38.5	D49.1
bone or labyrinth	C41.Ø	C79.51	—	D16.4	D48.Ø	D49.2
eustachian tube	C3Ø.1	C78.39	DØ2.3	D14.Ø	D38.5	D49.1
exocervix	C53.1	C79.82	DØ6.1	D26.Ø	D39.Ø	D49.59
external						
meatus (ear) — *see also* Neoplasm, skin, ear	C44.2Ø-☑	C79.2	DØ4.2-☑	D23.2-☑	D48.5	D49.2
os, cervix uteri	C53.1	C79.82	DØ6.1	D26.Ø	D39.Ø	D49.59
extradural	C72.9	C79.49	—	D33.9	D43.9	D49.7
extrahepatic (bile) duct	C24.Ø	C78.89	DØ1.5	D13.5	D37.6	D49.Ø
overlapping lesion with gallbladder	C24.8	—	—	—	—	—
extraocular muscle	C69.6-☑	C79.49	DØ9.2-☑	D31.6-☑	D48.7	D49.89
extrarectal	C76.3	C79.89	DØ9.8	D36.7	D48.7	D49.89
extremity	C76.8	C79.89	DØ4.8	D36.7	D48.7	D49.89

	Malignant Primary	Malignant Secondary	Ca in situ	Benign	Uncertain Behavior	Unspecified Behavior
Neoplasm, neoplastic — *continued*						
extremity — *continued*						
lower	C76.5-☑	C79.89	DØ4.7-☑	D36.7	D48.7	D49.89
upper	C76.4-☑	C79.89	DØ4.6-☑	D36.7	D48.7	D49.89
eyeball	C69.9-☑	C79.49	DØ9.2-☑	D31.9-☑	D48.7	D49.89
eyebrow	C44.3Ø9	C79.2	DØ4.39	D23.39	D48.5	D49.2
basal cell carcinoma	C44.319	—	—	—	—	—
specified type NEC	C44.399	—	—	—	—	—
squamous cell carcinoma	C44.329	—	—	—	—	—
eyelid (lower) (skin) (upper)	C44.1Ø-☑	—	—	—	—	—
basal cell carcinoma	C44.11-☑	—	—	—	—	—
cartilage	C49.Ø	C79.89	—	D21.Ø	D48.1	D49.2
sebaceous cell	C44.13-☑	—	—	—	—	—
specified type NEC	C44.19-☑	—	—	—	—	—
squamous cell carcinoma	C44.12-☑	—	—	—	—	—
eye NEC	C69.9-☑	C79.49	DØ9.2-☑	D31.9-☑	D48.7	D49.89
overlapping sites	C69.8-☑	—	—	—	—	—
face NEC	C76.Ø	C79.89	DØ4.39	D36.7	D48.7	D49.89
fallopian tube (accessory)	C57.Ø-☑	C79.82	DØ7.39	D28.2	D39.8	D49.59
falx (cerebella) (cerebri)	C7Ø.Ø	C79.32	—	D32.Ø	D42.Ø	D49.7
fascia — *see also* Neoplasm, connective tissue						
palmar	C49.1-☑	C79.89	—	D21.1-☑	D48.1	D49.2
plantar	C49.2-☑	C79.89	—	D21.2-☑	D48.1	D49.2
fatty tissue — *see* Neoplasm, connective tissue						
fauces, faucial NEC	C1Ø.9	C79.89	DØØ.Ø8	D1Ø.5	D37.Ø5	D49.Ø
pillars	CØ9.1	C79.89	DØØ.Ø8	D1Ø.5	D37.Ø5	D49.Ø
tonsil	CØ9.9	C79.89	DØØ.Ø8	D1Ø.4	D37.Ø5	D49.Ø
femur (any part)	C4Ø.2-☑	—	—	D16.2-☑	—	—
fetal membrane	C58	C79.82	DØ7.Ø	D26.7	D39.2	D49.59
fibrous tissue — *see* Neoplasm, connective tissue						
fibula (any part)	C4Ø.2-☑	C79.51	—	D16.2-☑	—	—
filum terminale	C72.Ø	C79.49	—	D33.4	D43.4	D49.7
finger NEC	C76.4-☑	C79.89	DØ4.6-☑	D36.7	D48.7	D49.89
flank NEC	C76.8	C79.89	DØ4.5	D36.7	D48.7	D49.89
follicle, nabothian	C53.Ø	C79.82	DØ6.Ø	D26.Ø	D39.Ø	D49.59
foot NEC	C76.5-☑	C79.89	DØ4.7-☑	D36.7	D48.7	D49.89
forearm NEC	C76.4-☑	C79.89	DØ4.6-☑	D36.7	D48.7	D49.89
forehead (skin)	C44.3Ø9	C79.2	DØ4.39	D23.39	D48.5	D49.2
basal cell carcinoma	C44.319	—	—	—	—	—
specified type NEC	C44.399	—	—	—	—	—
squamous cell carcinoma	C44.329	—	—	—	—	—
foreskin	C6Ø.Ø	C79.82	DØ7.4	D29.Ø	D4Ø.8	D49.59
fornix						
pharyngeal	C11.3	C79.89	DØØ.Ø8	D1Ø.6	D37.Ø5	D49.Ø
vagina	C52	C79.82	DØ7.2	D28.1	D39.8	D49.59
fossa (of)						
anterior (cranial)	C71.9	C79.31	—	D33.2	D43.2	D49.6
cranial	C71.9	C79.31	—	D33.2	D43.2	D49.6
ischiorectal	C76.3	C79.89	DØ9.8	D36.7	D48.7	D49.89
middle (cranial)	C71.9	C79.31	—	D33.2	D43.2	D49.6
piriform	C12	C79.89	DØØ.Ø8	D1Ø.7	D37.Ø5	D49.Ø
pituitary	C75.1	C79.89	DØ9.3	D35.2	D44.3	D49.7
posterior (cranial)	C71.9	C79.31	—	D33.2	D43.2	D49.6
pterygoid	C49.Ø	C79.89	—	D21.Ø	D48.1	D49.2
pyriform	C12	C79.89	DØØ.Ø8	D1Ø.7	D37.Ø5	D49.Ø
Rosenmuller	C11.2	C79.89	DØØ.Ø8	D1Ø.6	D37.Ø5	D49.Ø
tonsillar	CØ9.Ø	C79.89	DØØ.Ø8	D1Ø.5	D37.Ø5	D49.Ø
fourchette	C51.9	C79.82	DØ7.1	D28.Ø	D39.8	D49.59
frenulum						
labii — *see* Neoplasm, lip, internal						

	Malignant Primary	Malignant Secondary	Ca in situ	Benign	Uncertain Behavior	Unspecified Behavior
Neoplasm, neoplastic — *continued*						
frenulum — *continued*						
linguae	CØ2.2	C79.89	DØØ.Ø7	D1Ø.1	D37.Ø2	D49.Ø
frontal						
bone	C41.Ø	C79.51	—	D16.4	D48.Ø	D49.2
lobe, brain	C71.1	C79.31	—	D33.Ø	D43.Ø	D49.6
pole	C71.1	C79.31	—	D33.Ø	D43.Ø	D49.6
sinus	C31.2	C78.39	DØ2.3	D14.Ø	D38.5	D49.1
fundus						
stomach	C16.1	C78.89	DØØ.2	D13.1	D37.1	D49.Ø
uterus	C54.3	C79.82	DØ7.Ø	D26.1	D39.Ø	D49.59
gallbladder	C23	C78.89	DØ1.5	D13.5	D37.6	D49.Ø
overlapping lesion with extrahepatic bile ducts	C24.8	—	—	—	—	—
gall duct (extrahepatic)	C24.Ø	C78.89	DØ1.5	D13.5	D37.6	D49.Ø
intrahepatic	C22.1	C78.7	DØ1.5	D13.4	D37.6	D49.Ø
ganglia — *see also* Neoplasm, nerve, peripheral	C47.9	C79.89	—	D36.1Ø	D48.2	D49.2
basal	C71.Ø	C79.31	—	D33.Ø	D43.Ø	D49.6
cranial nerve	C72.5Ø	C79.49	—	D33.3	D43.3	D49.7
Gartner's duct	C52	C79.82	DØ7.2	D28.1	D39.8	D49.59
gastric — *see* Neoplasm, stomach						
gastrocolic	C26.9	C78.89	DØ1.9	D13.9	D37.9	D49.Ø
gastroesophageal junction	C16.Ø	C78.89	DØØ.2	D13.1	D37.1	D49.Ø
gastrointestinal (tract) NEC	C26.9	C78.89	DØ1.9	D13.9	D37.9	D49.Ø
generalized	C8Ø.Ø	—	—	—	—	—
genital organ or tract						
female NEC	C57.9	C79.82	DØ7.3Ø	D28.9	D39.9	D49.59
overlapping lesion	C57.8	—	—	—	—	—
specified site NEC	C57.7	C79.82	DØ7.39	D28.7	D39.8	D49.59
male NEC	C63.9	C79.82	DØ7.6Ø	D29.9	D4Ø.9	D49.59
overlapping lesion	C63.8	—	—	—	—	—
specified site NEC	C63.7	C79.82	DØ7.69	D29.8	D4Ø.8	D49.59
genitourinary tract						
female	C57.9	C79.82	DØ7.3Ø	D28.9	D39.9	D49.59
male	C63.9	C79.82	DØ7.6Ø	D29.9	D4Ø.9	D49.59
gingiva (alveolar) (marginal)	CØ3.9	C79.89	DØØ.Ø3	D1Ø.39	D37.Ø9	D49.Ø
lower	CØ3.1	C79.89	DØØ.Ø3	D1Ø.39	D37.Ø9	D49.Ø
mandibular	CØ3.1	C79.89	DØØ.Ø3	D1Ø.39	D37.Ø9	D49.Ø
maxillary	CØ3.Ø	C79.89	DØØ.Ø3	D1Ø.39	D37.Ø9	D49.Ø
upper	CØ3.Ø	C79.89	DØØ.Ø3	D1Ø.39	D37.Ø9	D49.Ø
gland, glandular (lymphatic) (system) — *see also* Neoplasm, lymph gland						
endocrine NEC	C75.9	C79.89	DØ9.3	D35.9	D44.9	D49.7
salivary — *see* Neoplasm, salivary gland						
glans penis	C6Ø.1	C79.82	DØ7.4	D29.Ø	D4Ø.8	D49.59
globus pallidus	C71.Ø	C79.31	—	D33.Ø	D43.Ø	D49.6
glomus						
coccygeal	C49.5	C79.89	—	D21.5	D48.1	D49.2
jugularis	C75.5	C79.89	—	D35.6	D44.7	D49.7
glosso-epiglottic fold(s)	C1Ø.1	C79.89	DØØ.Ø8	D1Ø.5	D37.Ø5	D49.Ø
glossopalatine fold	CØ9.1	C79.89	DØØ.Ø8	D1Ø.5	D37.Ø5	D49.Ø
glossopharyngeal sulcus	CØ9.Ø	C79.89	DØØ.Ø8	D1Ø.5	D37.Ø5	D49.Ø
glottis	C32.Ø	C78.39	DØ2.Ø	D14.1	D38.Ø	D49.1
gluteal region	C76.3	C79.89	DØ4.5	D36.7	D48.7	D49.89
great vessels NEC	C49.3	C79.89	—	D21.3	D48.1	D49.2
groin NEC	C76.3	C79.89	DØ4.5	D36.7	D48.7	D49.89
gum	CØ3.9	C79.89	DØØ.Ø3	D1Ø.39	D37.Ø9	D49.Ø
lower	CØ3.1	C79.89	DØØ.Ø3	D1Ø.39	D37.Ø9	D49.Ø
upper	CØ3.Ø	C79.89	DØØ.Ø3	D1Ø.39	D37.Ø9	D49.Ø
hand NEC	C76.4-☑	C79.89	DØ4.6-☑	D36.7	D48.7	D49.89
head NEC	C76.Ø	C79.89	DØ4.4	D36.7	D48.7	D49.89
heart	C38.Ø	C79.89	—	D15.1	D48.7	D49.89

	Malignant Primary	Malignant Secondary	Ca in situ	Benign	Uncertain Behavior	Unspecified Behavior
Neoplasm, neoplastic — *continued*						
heel NEC	C76.5-☑	C79.89	DØ4.7-☑	D36.7	D48.7	D49.89
helix — *see also* Neoplasm, skin, ear	C44.2Ø-☑	C79.2	DØ4.2-☑	D23.2-☑	D48.5	D49.2
hematopoietic, hemopoietic tissue NEC	C96.9	—	—	—	—	—
specified NEC	C96.Z	—	—	—	—	—
hemisphere, cerebral	C71.Ø	C79.31	—	D33.Ø	D43.Ø	D49.6
hemorrhoidal zone	C21.1	C78.5	DØ1.3	D12.9	D37.8	D49.Ø
hepatic — *see also* Index to disease, by histology	C22.9	C78.7	DØ1.5	D13.4	D37.6	D49.Ø
duct (bile)	C24.Ø	C78.89	DØ1.5	D13.5	D37.6	D49.Ø
flexure (colon)	C18.3	C78.5	DØ1.Ø	D12.3	D37.4	D49.Ø
primary	C22.8	C78.7	DØ1.5	D13.4	D37.6	D49.Ø
hepatobiliary	C24.9	C78.89	DØ1.5	D13.5	D37.6	D49.Ø
hepatoblastoma	C22.2	C78.7	DØ1.5	D13.4	D37.6	D49.Ø
hepatoma	C22.Ø	C78.7	DØ1.5	D13.4	D37.6	D49.Ø
hilus of lung	C34.Ø-☑	C78.Ø-☑	DØ2.2-☑	D14.3-☑	D38.1	D49.1
hippocampus, brain	C71.2	C79.31	—	D33.Ø	D43.Ø	D49.6
hip NEC	C76.5-☑	C79.89	DØ4.7-☑	D36.7	D48.7	D49.89
humerus (any part)	C4Ø.Ø-☑	C79.51	—	D16.Ø-☑	—	—
hymen	C52	C79.82	DØ7.2	D28.1	D39.8	D49.59
hypopharynx, hypopharyngeal NEC	C13.9	C79.89	DØØ.Ø8	D1Ø.7	D37.Ø5	D49.Ø
overlapping lesion	C13.8	—	—	—	—	—
postcricoid region	C13.Ø	C79.89	DØØ.Ø8	D1Ø.7	D37.Ø5	D49.Ø
posterior wall	C13.2	C79.89	DØØ.Ø8	D1Ø.7	D37.Ø5	D49.Ø
pyriform fossa (sinus)	C12	C79.89	DØØ.Ø8	D1Ø.7	D37.Ø5	D49.Ø
hypophysis	C75.1	C79.89	DØ9.3	D35.2	D44.3	D49.7
hypothalamus	C71.Ø	C79.31	—	D33.Ø	D43.Ø	D49.6
ileocecum, ileocecal (coil) (junction) (valve)	C18.Ø	C78.5	DØ1.Ø	D12.Ø	D37.4	D49.Ø
ileum	C17.2	C78.4	DØ1.49	D13.39	D37.2	D49.Ø
ilium	C41.4	C79.51	—	D16.8	D48.Ø	D49.2
immunoproliferative NEC	C88.9	—	—	—	—	—
infraclavicular (region)	C76.1	C79.89	DØ4.5	D36.7	D48.7	D49.89
inguinal (region)	C76.3	C79.89	DØ4.5	D36.7	D48.7	D49.89
insula	C71.Ø	C79.31	—	D33.Ø	D43.Ø	D49.6
insular tissue (pancreas)	C25.4	C78.89	DØ1.7	D13.7	D37.8	D49.Ø
brain	C71.Ø	C79.31	—	D33.Ø	D43.Ø	D49.6
interarytenoid fold	C13.1	C78.39	DØØ.Ø8	D1Ø.7	D37.Ø5	D49.Ø
hypopharyngeal aspect	C13.1	C79.89	DØØ.Ø8	D1Ø.7	D37.Ø5	D49.Ø
laryngeal aspect	C32.1	C78.39	DØ2.Ø	D14.1	D38.Ø	D49.1
marginal zone	C13.1	C79.89	DØØ.Ø8	D1Ø.7	D37.Ø5	D49.Ø
interdental papillae	CØ3.9	C79.89	DØØ.Ø3	D1Ø.39	D37.Ø9	D49.Ø
lower	CØ3.1	C79.89	DØØ.Ø3	D1Ø.39	D37.Ø9	D49.Ø
upper	CØ3.Ø	C79.89	DØØ.Ø3	D1Ø.39	D37.Ø9	D49.Ø
internal						
capsule	C71.Ø	C79.31	—	D33.Ø	D43.Ø	D49.6
os (cervix)	C53.Ø	C79.82	DØ6.Ø	D26.Ø	D39.Ø	D49.59
intervertebral cartilage or disc	C41.2	C79.51	—	D16.6	D48.Ø	D49.2
intestine, intestinal	C26.Ø	C78.8Ø	DØ1.4Ø	D13.9	D37.8	D49.Ø
large	C18.9	C78.5	DØ1.Ø	D12.6	D37.4	D49.Ø
appendix	C18.1	C78.5	DØ1.Ø	D12.1	D37.3	D49.Ø
caput coli	C18.Ø	C78.5	DØ1.Ø	D12.Ø	D37.4	D49.Ø
cecum	C18.Ø	C78.5	DØ1.Ø	D12.Ø	D37.4	D49.Ø
colon	C18.9	C78.5	DØ1.Ø	D12.6	D37.4	D49.Ø
and rectum	C19	C78.5	DØ1.1	D12.7	D37.5	D49.Ø
ascending	C18.2	C78.5	DØ1.Ø	D12.2	D37.4	D49.Ø
caput	C18.Ø	C78.5	DØ1.Ø	D12.Ø	D37.4	D49.Ø
descending	C18.6	C78.5	DØ1.Ø	D12.4	D37.4	D49.Ø
distal	C18.6	C78.5	DØ1.Ø	D12.4	D37.4	D49.Ø

	Malignant Primary	Malignant Secondary	Ca in situ	Benign	Uncertain Behavior	Unspecified Behavior
Neoplasm, neoplastic — *continued*						
intestine, intestinal — *continued*						
large — *continued*						
colon — *continued*						
left	C18.6	C78.5	DØ1.Ø	D12.4	D37.4	D49.Ø
overlapping lesion	C18.8	—	—	—	—	—
pelvic	C18.7	C78.5	DØ1.Ø	D12.5	D37.4	D49.Ø
right	C18.2	C78.5	DØ1.Ø	D12.2	D37.4	D49.Ø
sigmoid (flexure)	C18.7	C78.5	DØ1.Ø	D12.5	D37.4	D49.Ø
transverse	C18.4	C78.5	DØ1.Ø	D12.3	D37.4	D49.Ø
hepatic flexure	C18.3	C78.5	DØ1.Ø	D12.3	D37.4	D49.Ø
ileocecum, ileocecal (coil) (valve)	C18.Ø	C78.5	DØ1.Ø	D12.Ø	D37.4	D49.Ø
overlapping lesion	C18.8	—	—	—	—	—
sigmoid flexure (lower) (upper)	C18.7	C78.5	DØ1.Ø	D12.5	D37.4	D49.Ø
splenic flexure	C18.5	C78.5	DØ1.Ø	D12.3	D37.4	D49.Ø
small	C17.9	C78.4	DØ1.4Ø	D13.3Ø	D37.2	D49.Ø
duodenum	C17.Ø	C78.4	DØ1.49	D13.2	D37.2	D49.Ø
ileum	C17.2	C78.4	DØ1.49	D13.39	D37.2	D49.Ø
jejunum	C17.1	C78.4	DØ1.49	D13.39	D37.2	D49.Ø
overlapping lesion	C17.8	—	—	—	—	—
tract NEC	C26.Ø	C78.89	DØ1.4Ø	D13.9	D37.8	D49.Ø
intra-abdominal	C76.2	C79.89	DØ9.8	D36.7	D48.7	D49.89
intracranial NEC	C71.9	C79.31	—	D33.2	D43.2	D49.6
intrahepatic (bile) duct	C22.1	C78.7	DØ1.5	D13.4	D37.6	D49.Ø
intraocular	C69.9-☑	C79.49	DØ9.2-☑	D31.9-☑	D48.7	D49.89
intraorbital	C69.6-☑	C79.49	DØ9.2-☑	D31.6-☑	D48.7	D49.89
intrasellar	C75.1	C79.89	DØ9.3	D35.2	D44.3	D49.7
intrathoracic (cavity) (organs)	C76.1	C79.89	DØ9.8	D15.9	D48.7	D49.89
specified NEC	C76.1	C79.89	DØ9.8	D15.7	—	—
iris	C69.4-☑	C79.49	DØ9.2-☑	D31.4-☑	D48.7	D49.89
ischiorectal (fossa)	C76.3	C79.89	DØ9.8	D36.7	D48.7	D49.89
ischium	C41.4	C79.51	—	D16.8	D48.Ø	D49.2
island of Reil	C71.Ø	C79.31	—	D33.Ø	D43.Ø	D49.6
islands or islets of Langerhans	C25.4	C78.89	DØ1.7	D13.7	D37.8	D49.Ø
isthmus uteri	C54.Ø	C79.82	DØ7.Ø	D26.1	D39.Ø	D49.59
jaw	C76.Ø	C79.89	DØ9.8	D36.7	D48.7	D49.89
bone	C41.1	C79.51	—	D16.5	D48.Ø	D49.2
lower	C41.1	C79.51	—	D16.5	—	—
upper	C41.Ø	C79.51	—	D16.4	—	—
carcinoma (any type) (lower) (upper)	C76.Ø	C79.89	—	—	—	—
skin — *see also* Neoplasm, skin, face	C44.3Ø9	C79.2	DØ4.39	D23.39	D48.5	D49.2
soft tissues	CØ3.9	C79.89	DØØ.Ø3	D1Ø.39	D37.Ø9	D49.Ø
lower	CØ3.1	C79.89	DØØ.Ø3	D1Ø.39	D37.Ø9	D49.Ø
upper	CØ3.Ø	C79.89	DØØ.Ø3	D1Ø.39	D37.Ø9	D49.Ø
jejunum	C17.1	C78.4	DØ1.49	D13.39	D37.2	D49.Ø
joint NEC — *see also* Neoplasm, bone	C41.9	C79.51	—	D16.9	D48.Ø	D49.2
acromioclavicular	C4Ø.Ø-☑	C79.51	—	D16.Ø-☑	—	—
bursa or synovial membrane — *see* Neoplasm, connective tissue						
costovertebral	C41.3	C79.51	—	D16.7	D48.Ø	D49.2
sternocostal	C41.3	C79.51	—	D16.7	D48.Ø	D49.2
temporomandibular	C41.1	C79.51	—	D16.5	D48.Ø	D49.2
junction						
anorectal	C21.8	C78.5	DØ1.3	D12.9	D37.8	D49.Ø
cardioesophageal	C16.Ø	C78.89	DØØ.2	D13.1	D37.1	D49.Ø
esophagogastric	C16.Ø	C78.89	DØØ.2	D13.1	D37.1	D49.Ø
gastroesophageal	C16.Ø	C78.89	DØØ.2	D13.1	D37.1	D49.Ø
hard and soft palate	CØ5.9	C79.89	DØØ.ØØ	D1Ø.39	D37.Ø9	D49.Ø
ileocecal	C18.Ø	C78.5	DØ1.Ø	D12.Ø	D37.4	D49.Ø

	Malignant Primary	Malignant Secondary	Ca in situ	Benign	Uncertain Behavior	Unspecified Behavior
Neoplasm, neoplastic — *continued*						
junction — *continued*						
pelvirectal	C19	C78.5	DØ1.1	D12.7	D37.5	D49.Ø
pelviureteric	C65.-☑	C79.Ø-☑	DØ9.19	D3Ø.1-☑	D41.1-☑	D49.59
rectosigmoid	C19	C78.5	DØ1.1	D12.7	D37.5	D49.Ø
squamocolumnar, of cervix	C53.8	C79.82	DØ6.7	D26.Ø	D39.Ø	D49.59
Kaposi's sarcoma — *see* Kaposi's, sarcoma						
kidney (parenchymal)	C64.-☑	C79.Ø-☑	DØ9.19	D3Ø.Ø-☑	D41.Ø-☑	D49.51-☑
calyx	C65.-☑	C79.Ø-☑	DØ9.19	D3Ø.1-☑	D41.1-☑	D49.51-☑
hilus	C65.-☑	C79.Ø-☑	DØ9.19	D3Ø.1-☑	D41.1-☑	D49.51-☑
pelvis	C65.-☑	C79.Ø-☑	DØ9.19	D3Ø.1-☑	D41.1-☑	D49.51-☑
knee NEC	C76.5-☑	C79.89	DØ4.7-☑	D36.7	D48.7	D49.89
labia (skin)	C51.9	C79.82	DØ7.1	D28.Ø	D39.8	D49.59
majora	C51.Ø	C79.82	DØ7.1	D28.Ø	D39.8	D49.59
minora	C51.1	C79.82	DØ7.1	D28.Ø	D39.8	D49.59
labial — *see also* Neoplasm, lip	CØØ.9	C79.89	DØØ.Ø1	D1Ø.Ø	D37.Ø1	D49.Ø
sulcus (lower) (upper)	CØ6.1	C79.89	DØØ.Ø2	D1Ø.39	D37.Ø9	D49.Ø
labium (skin)	C51.9	C79.82	DØ7.1	D28.Ø	D39.8	D49.59
majus	C51.Ø	C79.82	DØ7.1	D28.Ø	D39.8	D49.59
minus	C51.1	C79.82	DØ7.1	D28.Ø	D39.8	D49.59
lacrimal						
canaliculi	C69.5-☑	C79.49	DØ9.2-☑	D31.5-☑	D48.7	D49.89
duct (nasal)	C69.5-☑	C79.49	DØ9.2-☑	D31.5-☑	D48.7	D49.89
gland	C69.5-☑	C79.49	DØ9.2-☑	D31.5-☑	D48.7	D49.89
punctum	C69.5-☑	C79.49	DØ9.2-☑	D31.5-☑	D48.7	D49.89
sac	C69.5-☑	C79.49	DØ9.2-☑	D31.5-☑	D48.7	D49.89
Langerhans, islands or islets	C25.4	C78.89	DØ1.7	D13.7	D37.8	D49.Ø
laryngopharynx	C13.9	C79.89	DØØ.Ø8	D1Ø.7	D37.Ø5	D49.Ø
larynx, laryngeal NEC	C32.9	C78.39	DØ2.Ø	D14.1	D38.Ø	D49.1
aryepiglottic fold	C32.1	C78.39	DØ2.Ø	D14.1	D38.Ø	D49.1
cartilage (arytenoid) (cricoid) (cuneiform) (thyroid)	C32.3	C78.39	DØ2.Ø	D14.1	D38.Ø	D49.1
commissure (anterior) (posterior)	C32.Ø	C78.39	DØ2.Ø	D14.1	D38.Ø	D49.1
extrinsic NEC	C32.1	C78.39	DØ2.Ø	D14.1	D38.Ø	D49.1
meaning hypopharynx	C13.9	C79.89	DØØ.Ø8	D1Ø.7	D37.Ø5	D49.Ø
interarytenoid fold	C32.1	C78.39	DØ2.Ø	D14.1	D38.Ø	D49.1
intrinsic	C32.Ø	C78.39	DØ2.Ø	D14.1	D38.Ø	D49.1
overlapping lesion	C32.8	—	—	—	—	—
ventricular band	C32.1	C78.39	DØ2.Ø	D14.1	D38.Ø	D49.1
leg NEC	C76.5-☑	C79.89	DØ4.7-☑	D36.7	D48.7	D49.89
lens, crystalline	C69.4-☑	C79.49	DØ9.2-☑	D31.4-☑	D48.7	D49.89
lid (lower) (upper)	C44.1Ø-☑	C79.2	DØ4.1-☑	D23.1-☑	D48.5	D49.2
basal cell carcinoma	C44.11-☑	—	—	—	—	—
sebaceous cell	C44.13-☑	—	—	—	—	—
specified type NEC	C44.19-☑	—	—	—	—	—
squamous cell carcinoma	C44.12-☑	—	—	—	—	—
ligament — *see also* Neoplasm, connective tissue						
broad	C57.1-☑	C79.82	DØ7.39	D28.2	D39.8	D49.59
Mackenrodt's	C57.7	C79.82	DØ7.39	D28.7	D39.8	D49.59
non-uterine — *see* Neoplasm, connective tissue						
round	C57.2-☑	C79.82	—	D28.2	D39.8	D49.59
sacro-uterine	C57.3	C79.82	—	D28.2	D39.8	D49.59
uterine	C57.3	C79.82	—	D28.2	D39.8	D49.59
utero-ovarian	C57.7	C79.82	DØ7.39	D28.2	D39.8	D49.59
uterosacral	C57.3	C79.82	—	D28.2	D39.8	D49.59
limb	C76.8	C79.89	DØ4.8	D36.7	D48.7	D49.89
lower	C76.5-☑	C79.89	DØ4.7-☑	D36.7	D48.7	D49.89
upper	C76.4-☑	C79.89	DØ4.6-☑	D36.7	D48.7	D49.89
limbus of cornea	C69.1-☑	C79.49	DØ9.2-☑	D31.1-☑	D48.7	D49.89

	Malignant Primary	Malignant Secondary	Ca in situ	Benign	Uncertain Behavior	Unspecified Behavior
Neoplasm, neoplastic — *continued*						
lingual NEC — *see also* Neoplasm, tongue	CØ2.9	C79.89	DØØ.07	D1Ø.1	D37.Ø2	D49.Ø
lingula, lung	C34.1-☑	C78.Ø-☑	DØ2.2-☑	D14.3-☑	D38.1	D49.1
lip	CØØ.9	C79.89	DØØ.Ø1	D1Ø.Ø	D37.Ø1	D49.Ø
buccal aspect — *see* Neoplasm, lip, internal						
commissure	CØØ.6	C79.89	DØØ.Ø1	D1Ø.Ø	D37.Ø1	D49.Ø
external	CØØ.2	C79.89	DØØ.Ø1	D1Ø.Ø	D37.Ø1	D49.Ø
lower	CØØ.1	C79.89	DØØ.Ø1	D1Ø.Ø	D37.Ø1	D49.Ø
upper	CØØ.Ø	C79.89	DØØ.Ø1	D1Ø.Ø	D37.Ø1	D49.Ø
frenulum — *see* Neoplasm, lip, internal						
inner aspect — *see* Neoplasm, lip, internal						
internal	CØØ.5	C79.89	DØØ.Ø1	D1Ø.Ø	D37.Ø1	D49.Ø
lower	CØØ.4	C79.89	DØØ.Ø1	D1Ø.Ø	D37.Ø1	D49.Ø
upper	CØØ.3	C79.89	DØØ.Ø1	D1Ø.Ø	D37.Ø1	D49.Ø
lipstick area	CØØ.2	C79.89	DØØ.Ø1	D1Ø.Ø	D37.Ø1	D49.Ø
lower	CØØ.1	C79.89	DØØ.Ø1	D1Ø.Ø	D37.Ø1	D49.Ø
upper	CØØ.Ø	C79.89	DØØ.Ø1	D1Ø.Ø	D37.Ø1	D49.Ø
lower	CØØ.1	C79.89	DØØ.Ø1	D1Ø.Ø	D37.Ø1	D49.Ø
internal	CØØ.4	C79.89	DØØ.Ø1	D1Ø.Ø	D37.Ø1	D49.Ø
mucosa — *see* Neoplasm, lip, internal						
oral aspect — *see* Neoplasm, lip, internal						
overlapping lesion	CØØ.8	—	—	—	—	—
with oral cavity or pharynx	C14.8	—	—	—	—	—
skin (commissure) (lower) (upper)	C44.ØØ	C79.2	DØ4.Ø	D23.Ø	D48.5	D49.2
basal cell carcinoma	C44.Ø1	—	—	—	—	—
specified type NEC	C44.Ø9	—	—	—	—	—
squamous cell carcinoma	C44.Ø2	—	—	—	—	—
upper	CØØ.Ø	C79.89	DØØ.Ø1	D1Ø.Ø	D37.Ø1	D49.Ø
internal	CØØ.3	C79.89	DØØ.Ø1	D1Ø.Ø	D37.Ø1	D49.Ø
vermilion border	CØØ.2	C79.89	DØØ.Ø1	D1Ø.Ø	D37.Ø1	D49.Ø
lower	CØØ.1	C79.89	DØØ.Ø1	D1Ø.Ø	D37.Ø1	D49.Ø
upper	CØØ.Ø	C79.89	DØØ.Ø1	D1Ø.Ø	D37.Ø1	D49.Ø
lipomatous — *see* Lipoma, by site						
liver — *see also* Index to disease, by histology	C22.9	C78.7	DØ1.5	D13.4	D37.6	D49.Ø
primary	C22.8	C78.7	DØ1.5	D13.4	D37.6	D49.Ø
lumbosacral plexus	C47.5	C79.89	—	D36.16	D48.2	D49.2
lung	C34.9-☑	C78.Ø-☑	DØ2.2-☑	D14.3-☑	D38.1	D49.1
azygos lobe	C34.1-☑	C78.Ø-☑	DØ2.2-☑	D14.3-☑	D38.1	D49.1
carina	C34.Ø-☑	C78.Ø-☑	DØ2.2-☑	D14.3-☑	D38.1	D49.1
hilus	C34.Ø-☑	C78.Ø-☑	DØ2.2-☑	D14.3-☑	D38.1	D49.1
linqula	C34.1-☑	C78.Ø-☑	DØ2.2-☑	D14.3-☑	D38.1	D49.1
lobe NEC	C34.9-☑	C78.Ø-☑	DØ2.2-☑	D14.3-☑	D38.1	D49.1
lower lobe	C34.3-☑	C78.Ø-☑	DØ2.2-☑	D14.3-☑	D38.1	D49.1
main bronchus	C34.Ø-☑	C78.Ø-☑	DØ2.2-☑	D14.3-☑	D38.1	D49.1
mesothelioma — *see* Mesothelioma						
middle lobe	C34.2	C78.Ø-☑	DØ2.21	D14.31	D38.1	D49.1
overlapping lesion	C34.8-☑	—	—	—	—	—
upper lobe	C34.1-☑	C78.Ø-☑	DØ2.2-☑	D14.3-☑	D38.1	D49.1
lymph, lymphatic channel NEC	C49.9	C79.89	—	D21.9	D48.1	D49.2
gland (secondary)	—	C77.9	—	D36.Ø	D48.7	D49.89
abdominal	—	C77.2	—	D36.Ø	D48.7	D49.89
aortic	—	C77.2	—	D36.Ø	D48.7	D49.89
arm	—	C77.3	—	D36.Ø	D48.7	D49.89

	Malignant Primary	Malignant Secondary	Ca in situ	Benign	Uncertain Behavior	Unspecified Behavior
Neoplasm, neoplastic — *continued*						
lymph, lymphatic channel — *continued*						
gland — *continued*						
auricular (anterior) (posterior)	—	C77.Ø	—	D36.Ø	D48.7	D49.89
axilla, axillary	—	C77.3	—	D36.Ø	D48.7	D49.89
brachial	—	C77.3	—	D36.Ø	D48.7	D49.89
bronchial	—	C77.1	—	D36.Ø	D48.7	D49.89
bronchopulmonary	—	C77.1	—	D36.Ø	D48.7	D49.89
celiac	—	C77.2	—	D36.Ø	D48.7	D49.89
cervical	—	C77.Ø	—	D36.Ø	D48.7	D49.89
cervicofacial	—	C77.Ø	—	D36.Ø	D48.7	D49.89
Cloquet	—	C77.4	—	D36.Ø	D48.7	D49.89
colic	—	C77.2	—	D36.Ø	D48.7	D49.89
common duct	—	C77.2	—	D36.Ø	D48.7	D49.89
cubital	—	C77.3	—	D36.Ø	D48.7	D49.89
diaphragmatic	—	C77.1	—	D36.Ø	D48.7	D49.89
epigastric, inferior	—	C77.1	—	D36.Ø	D48.7	D49.89
epitrochlear	—	C77.3	—	D36.Ø	D48.7	D49.89
esophageal	—	C77.1	—	D36.Ø	D48.7	D49.89
face	—	C77.Ø	—	D36.Ø	D48.7	D49.89
femoral	—	C77.4	—	D36.Ø	D48.7	D49.89
gastric	—	C77.2	—	D36.Ø	D48.7	D49.89
groin	—	C77.4	—	D36.Ø	D48.7	D49.89
head	—	C77.Ø	—	D36.Ø	D48.7	D49.89
hepatic	—	C77.2	—	D36.Ø	D48.7	D49.89
hilar (pulmonary)	—	C77.1	—	D36.Ø	D48.7	D49.89
splenic	—	C77.2	—	D36.Ø	D48.7	D49.89
hypogastric	—	C77.5	—	D36.Ø	D48.7	D49.89
ileocolic	—	C77.2	—	D36.Ø	D48.7	D49.89
iliac	—	C77.5	—	D36.Ø	D48.7	D49.89
infraclavicular	—	C77.3	—	D36.Ø	D48.7	D49.89
inguina, inguinal	—	C77.4	—	D36.Ø	D48.7	D49.89
innominate	—	C77.1	—	D36.Ø	D48.7	D49.89
intercostal	—	C77.1	—	D36.Ø	D48.7	D49.89
intestinal	—	C77.2	—	D36.Ø	D48.7	D49.89
intrabdominal	—	C77.2	—	D36.Ø	D48.7	D49.89
intrapelvic	—	C77.5	—	D36.Ø	D48.7	D49.89
intrathoracic	—	C77.1	—	D36.Ø	D48.7	D49.89
jugular	—	C77.Ø	—	D36.Ø	D48.7	D49.89
leg	—	C77.4	—	D36.Ø	D48.7	D49.89
limb						
lower	—	C77.4	—	D36.Ø	D48.7	D49.89
upper	—	C77.3	—	D36.Ø	D48.7	D49.89
lower limb	—	C77.4	—	D36.Ø	D48.7	D49.89
lumbar	—	C77.2	—	D36.Ø	D48.7	D49.89
mandibular	—	C77.Ø	—	D36.Ø	D48.7	D49.89
mediastinal	—	C77.1	—	D36.Ø	D48.7	D49.89
mesenteric (inferior) (superior)	—	C77.2	—	D36.Ø	D48.7	D49.89
midcolic	—	C77.2	—	D36.Ø	D48.7	D49.89
multiple sites in categories C77.0 - C77.5	—	C77.8	—	D36.Ø	D48.7	D49.89
neck	—	C77.Ø	—	D36.Ø	D48.7	D49.89
obturator	—	C77.5	—	D36.Ø	D48.7	D49.89
occipital	—	C77.Ø	—	D36.Ø	D48.7	D49.89
pancreatic	—	C77.2	—	D36.Ø	D48.7	D49.89
para-aortic	—	C77.2	—	D36.Ø	D48.7	D49.89
paracervical	—	C77.5	—	D36.Ø	D48.7	D49.89
parametrial	—	C77.5	—	D36.Ø	D48.7	D49.89
parasternal	—	C77.1	—	D36.Ø	D48.7	D49.89
parotid	—	C77.Ø	—	D36.Ø	D48.7	D49.89
pectoral	—	C77.3	—	D36.Ø	D48.7	D49.89
pelvic	—	C77.5	—	D36.Ø	D48.7	D49.89
peri-aortic	—	C77.2	—	D36.Ø	D48.7	D49.89
peripancreatic	—	C77.2	—	D36.Ø	D48.7	D49.89
popliteal	—	C77.4	—	D36.Ø	D48.7	D49.89
porta hepatis	—	C77.2	—	D36.Ø	D48.7	D49.89
portal	—	C77.2	—	D36.Ø	D48.7	D49.89
preauricular	—	C77.Ø	—	D36.Ø	D48.7	D49.89
prelaryngeal	—	C77.Ø	—	D36.Ø	D48.7	D49.89
presymphysial	—	C77.5	—	D36.Ø	D48.7	D49.89
pretracheal	—	C77.Ø	—	D36.Ø	D48.7	D49.89
primary (any site) NEC	C96.9	—	—	—	—	—

	Malignant Primary	Malignant Secondary	Ca in situ	Benign	Uncertain Behavior	Unspecified Behavior
Neoplasm, neoplastic — *continued*						
lymph, lymphatic channel — *continued*						
gland — *continued*						
pulmonary (hiler)	—	C77.1	—	D36.Ø	D48.7	D49.89
pyloric	—	C77.2	—	D36.Ø	D48.7	D49.89
retroperitoneal	—	C77.2	—	D36.Ø	D48.7	D49.89
retropharyngeal	—	C77.Ø	—	D36.Ø	D48.7	D49.89
Rosenmuller's	—	C77.4	—	D36.Ø	D48.7	D49.89
sacral	—	C77.5	—	D36.Ø	D48.7	D49.89
scalene	—	C77.Ø	—	D36.Ø	D48.7	D49.89
site NEC	—	C77.9	—	D36.Ø	D48.7	D49.89
splenic (hilar)	—	C77.2	—	D36.Ø	D48.7	D49.89
subclavicular	—	C77.3	—	D36.Ø	D48.7	D49.89
subinguinal	—	C77.4	—	D36.Ø	D48.7	D49.89
sublingual	—	C77.Ø	—	D36.Ø	D48.7	D49.89
submandibular	—	C77.Ø	—	D36.Ø	D48.7	D49.89
submaxillary	—	C77.Ø	—	D36.Ø	D48.7	D49.89
submental	—	C77.Ø	—	D36.Ø	D48.7	D49.89
subscapular	—	C77.3	—	D36.Ø	D48.7	D49.89
supraclavicular	—	C77.Ø	—	D36.Ø	D48.7	D49.89
thoracic	—	C77.1	—	D36.Ø	D48.7	D49.89
tibial	—	C77.4	—	D36.Ø	D48.7	D49.89
tracheal	—	C77.1	—	D36.Ø	D48.7	D49.89
tracheobronchial	—	C77.1	—	D36.Ø	D48.7	D49.89
upper limb	—	C77.3	—	D36.Ø	D48.7	D49.89
Virchow's	—	C77.Ø	—	D36.Ø	D48.7	D49.89
node — *see also* Neoplasm, lymph gland						
primary NEC	C96.9	—	—	—	—	—
vessel — *see also* Neoplasm, connective tissue	C49.9	C79.89	—	D21.9	D48.1	D49.2
Mackenrodt's ligament	C57.7	C79.82	DØ7.39	D28.7	D39.8	D49.59
malar	C41.Ø	C79.51	—	D16.4	D48.Ø	D49.2
region — *see* Neoplasm, cheek						
mammary gland — *see* Neoplasm, breast						
mandible	C41.1	C79.51	—	D16.5	D48.Ø	D49.2
alveolar						
mucosa (carcinoma)	CØ3.1	C79.89	DØØ.Ø3	D1Ø.39	D37.Ø9	D49.Ø
ridge or process	C41.1	C79.51	—	D16.5	D48.Ø	D49.2
marrow (bone)						
NEC	C96.9	C79.52	—	—	D47.9	D49.89
mastectomy site (skin) — *see also* Neoplasm, breast, skin	C44.5Ø1	C79.2	—	—	—	—
specified as breast tissue	C5Ø.8-☑	C79.81	—	—	—	—
mastoid (air cells) (antrum) (cavity)	C3Ø.1	C78.39	DØ2.3	D14.Ø	D38.5	D49.1
bone or process	C41.Ø	C79.51	—	D16.4	D48.Ø	D49.2
maxilla, maxillary (superior)	C41.Ø	C79.51	—	D16.4	D48.Ø	D49.2
alveolar						
mucosa	CØ3.Ø	C79.89	DØØ.Ø3	D1Ø.39	D37.Ø9	D49.Ø
ridge or process (carcinoma)	C41.Ø	C79.51	—	D16.4	D48.Ø	D49.2
antrum	C31.Ø	C78.39	DØ2.3	D14.Ø	D38.5	D49.1
carcinoma	CØ3.Ø	C79.51	—	—	—	—
inferior — *see* Neoplasm, mandible						
sinus	C31.Ø	C78.39	DØ2.3	D14.Ø	D38.5	D49.1
meatus external (ear) — *see also* Neoplasm, skin, ear	C44.2Ø-☑	C79.2	DØ4.2-☑	D23.2-☑	D48.5	D49.2
Meckel diverticulum, malignant	C17.3	C78.4	DØ1.49	D13.39	D37.2	D49.Ø
mediastinum, mediastinal	C38.3	C78.1	—	D15.2	D38.3	D49.89
anterior	C38.1	C78.1	—	D15.2	D38.3	D49.89

	Malignant Primary	Malignant Secondary	Ca in situ	Benign	Uncertain Behavior	Unspecified Behavior
Neoplasm, neoplastic — *continued*						
mediastinum, mediastinal — *continued*						
posterior	C38.2	C78.1	—	D15.2	D38.3	D49.89
medulla						
adrenal	C74.1-☑	C79.7-☑	DØ9.3	D35.Ø-☑	D44.1-☑	D49.7
oblongata	C71.7	C79.31	—	D33.1	D43.1	D49.6
meibomian gland	C44.1Ø-☑	C79.2	DØ4.1-☑	D23.1-☑	D48.5	D49.2
basal cell carcinoma	C44.11-☑	—	—	—	—	—
sebaceous cell	C44.13-☑	—	—	—	—	—
specified type NEC	C44.19-☑	—	—	—	—	—
squamous cell carcinoma	C44.12-☑	—	—	—	—	—
melanoma — *see* Melanoma						
meninges	C7Ø.9	C79.49	—	D32.9	D42.9	D49.7
brain	C7Ø.Ø	C79.32	—	D32.Ø	D42.Ø	D49.7
cerebral	C7Ø.Ø	C79.32	—	D32.Ø	D42.Ø	D49.7
crainial	C7Ø.Ø	C79.32	—	D32.Ø	D42.Ø	D49.7
intracranial	C7Ø.Ø	C79.32	—	D32.Ø	D42.Ø	D49.7
spinal (cord)	C7Ø.1	C79.49	—	D32.1	D42.1	D49.7
meniscus, knee joint (lateral) (medial)	C4Ø.2-☑	C79.51	—	D16.2-☑	D48.Ø	D49.2
Merkel cell — *see* Carcinoma, Merkel cell						
mesentery, mesenteric	C48.1	C78.6	—	D2Ø.1	D48.4	D49.Ø
mesoappendix	C48.1	C78.6	—	D2Ø.1	D48.4	D49.Ø
mesocolon	C48.1	C78.6	—	D2Ø.1	D48.4	D49.Ø
mesopharynx — *see* Neoplasm, oropharynx						
mesosalpinx	C57.1-☑	C79.82	DØ7.39	D28.2	D39.8	D49.59
mesothelial tissue — *see* Mesothelioma						
mesothelioma — *see* Mesothelioma						
mesovarium	C57.1-☑	C79.82	DØ7.39	D28.2	D39.8	D49.59
metacarpus (any bone)	C4Ø.1-☑	C79.51	—	D16.1-☑	—	—
metastatic NEC — *see also* Neoplasm, by site, secondary	—	C79.9	—	—	—	—
metatarsus (any bone)	C4Ø.3-☑	C79.51	—	D16.3-☑	—	—
midbrain	C71.7	C79.31	—	D33.1	D43.1	D49.6
milk duct — *see* Neoplasm, breast						
mons						
pubis	C51.9	C79.82	DØ7.1	D28.Ø	D39.8	D49.59
veneris	C51.9	C79.82	DØ7.1	D28.Ø	D39.8	D49.59
motor tract	C72.9	C79.49	—	D33.9	D43.9	D49.7
brain	C71.9	C79.31	—	D33.2	D43.2	D49.6
cauda equina	C72.1	C79.49	—	D33.4	D43.4	D49.7
spinal	C72.Ø	C79.49	—	D33.4	D43.4	D49.7
mouth	CØ6.9	C79.89	DØØ.ØØ	D1Ø.3Ø	D37.Ø9	D49.Ø
book-leaf	CØ6.89	C79.89	—	—	—	—
floor	CØ4.9	C79.89	DØØ.Ø6	D1Ø.2	D37.Ø9	D49.Ø
anterior portion	CØ4.Ø	C79.89	DØØ.Ø6	D1Ø.2	D37.Ø9	D49.Ø
lateral portion	CØ4.1	C79.89	DØØ.Ø6	D1Ø.2	D37.Ø9	D49.Ø
overlapping lesion	CØ4.8	—	—	—	—	—
overlapping NEC	CØ6.8Ø	—	—	—	—	—
roof	CØ5.9	C79.89	DØØ.ØØ	D1Ø.39	D37.Ø9	D49.Ø
specified part NEC	CØ6.89	C79.89	DØØ.ØØ	D1Ø.39	D37.Ø9	D49.Ø
vestibule	CØ6.1	C79.89	DØØ.ØØ	D1Ø.39	D37.Ø9	D49.Ø
mucosa						
alveolar (ridge or process)	CØ3.9	C79.89	DØØ.Ø3	D1Ø.39	D37.Ø9	D49.Ø
lower	CØ3.1	C79.89	DØØ.Ø3	D1Ø.39	D37.Ø9	D49.Ø
upper	CØ3.Ø	C79.89	DØØ.Ø3	D1Ø.39	D37.Ø9	D49.Ø
buccal	CØ6.Ø	C79.89	DØØ.Ø2	D1Ø.39	D37.Ø9	D49.Ø
cheek	CØ6.Ø	C79.89	DØØ.Ø2	D1Ø.39	D37.Ø9	D49.Ø

	Malignant Primary	Malignant Secondary	Ca in situ	Benign	Uncertain Behavior	Unspecified Behavior
Neoplasm, neoplastic — *continued*						
mucosa — *continued*						
lip — *see* Neoplasm, lip, internal						
nasal	C30.0	C78.39	D02.3	D14.0	D38.5	D49.1
oral	C06.0	C79.89	D00.02	D10.39	D37.09	D49.0
Mullerian duct						
female	C57.7	C79.82	D07.39	D28.7	D39.8	D49.59
male	C63.7	C79.82	D07.69	D29.8	D40.8	D49.59
muscle — *see also* Neoplasm, connective tissue						
extraocular	C69.6-☑	C79.49	D09.2-☑	D31.6-☑	D48.7	D49.89
myocardium	C38.0	C79.89	—	D15.1	D48.7	D49.89
myometrium	C54.2	C79.82	D07.0	D26.1	D39.0	D49.59
myopericardium	C38.0	C79.89	—	D15.1	D48.7	D49.89
nabothian gland (follicle)	C53.0	C79.82	D06.0	D26.0	D39.0	D49.59
nail — *see also* Neoplasm, skin, limb	C44.90	C79.2	D04.9	D23.9	D48.5	D49.2
finger — *see also* Neoplasm, skin, limb, upper	C44.60-☑	C79.2	D04.6-☑	D23.6-☑	D48.5	D49.2
toe — *see also* Neoplasm, skin, limb, lower	C44.70-☑	C79.2	D04.7-☑	D23.7-☑	D48.5	D49.2
nares, naris (anterior) (posterior)	C30.0	C78.39	D02.3	D14.0	D38.5	D49.1
nasal — *see* Neoplasm, nose						
nasolabial groove — *see also* Neoplasm, skin, face	C44.309	C79.2	D04.39	D23.39	D48.5	D49.2
nasolacrimal duct	C69.5-☑	C79.49	D09.2-☑	D31.5-☑	D48.7	D49.89
nasopharynx, nasopharyngeal	C11.9	C79.89	D00.08	D10.6	D37.05	D49.0
floor	C11.3	C79.89	D00.08	D10.6	D37.05	D49.0
overlapping lesion	C11.8	—	—	—	—	—
roof	C11.0	C79.89	D00.08	D10.6	D37.05	D49.0
wall	C11.9	C79.89	D00.08	D10.6	D37.05	D49.0
anterior	C11.3	C79.89	D00.08	D10.6	D37.05	D49.0
lateral	C11.2	C79.89	D00.08	D10.6	D37.05	D49.0
posterior	C11.1	C79.89	D00.08	D10.6	D37.05	D49.0
superior	C11.0	C79.89	D00.08	D10.6	D37.05	D49.0
nates — *see also* Neoplasm, skin, trunk	C44.509	C79.2	D04.5	D23.5	D48.5	D49.2
neck NEC	C76.0	C79.89	D09.8	D36.7	D48.7	D49.89
skin	C44.40	—	—	—	—	—
basal cell carcinoma	C44.41	—	—	—	—	—
specified type NEC	C44.49	—	—	—	—	—
squamous cell carcinoma	C44.42	—	—	—	—	—
nerve (ganglion)	C47.9	C79.89	—	D36.10	D48.2	D49.2
abducens	C72.59	C79.49	—	D33.3	D43.3	D49.7
accessory (spinal)	C72.59	C79.49	—	D33.3	D43.3	D49.7
acoustic	C72.4-☑	C79.49	—	D33.3	D43.3	D49.7
auditory	C72.4-☑	C79.49	—	D33.3	D43.3	D49.7
autonomic NEC — *see also* Neoplasm, nerve, peripheral	C47.9	C79.89	—	D36.10	D48.2	D49.2
brachial	C47.1-☑	C79.89	—	D36.12	D48.2	D49.2
cranial	C72.50	C79.49	—	D33.3	D43.3	D49.7
specified NEC	C72.59	C79.49	—	D33.3	D43.3	D49.7
facial	C72.59	C79.49	—	D33.3	D43.3	D49.7
femoral	C47.2-☑	C79.89	—	D36.13	D48.2	D49.2
ganglion NEC — *see also* Neoplasm, nerve, peripheral	C47.9	C79.89	—	D36.10	D48.2	D49.2
glossopharyngeal	C72.59	C79.49	—	D33.3	D43.3	D49.7
hypoglossal	C72.59	C79.49	—	D33.3	D43.3	D49.7
intercostal	C47.3	C79.89	—	D36.14	D48.2	D49.2
lumbar	C47.6	C79.89	—	D36.17	D48.2	D49.2
median	C47.1-☑	C79.89	—	D36.12	D48.2	D49.2
obturator	C47.2-☑	C79.89	—	D36.13	D48.2	D49.2

	Malignant Primary	Malignant Secondary	Ca in situ	Benign	Uncertain Behavior	Unspecified Behavior
Neoplasm, neoplastic — *continued*						
nerve — *continued*						
oculomotor	C72.59	C79.49	—	D33.3	D43.3	D49.7
olfactory	C47.2-☑	C79.49	—	D33.3	D43.3	D49.7
optic	C72.3-☑	C79.49	—	D33.3	D43.3	D49.7
parasympathetic NEC	C47.9	C79.89	—	D36.10	D48.2	D49.2
peripheral NEC	C47.9	C79.89	—	D36.10	D48.2	D49.2
abdomen	C47.4	C79.89	—	D36.15	D48.2	D49.2
abdominal wall	C47.4	C79.89	—	D36.15	D48.2	D49.2
ankle	C47.2-☑	C79.89	—	D36.13	D48.2	D49.2
antecubital fossa or space	C47.1-☑	C79.89	—	D36.12	D48.2	D49.2
arm	C47.1-☑	C79.89	—	D36.12	D48.2	D49.2
auricle (ear)	C47.0	C79.89	—	D36.11	D48.2	D49.2
axilla	C47.3	C79.89	—	D36.12	D48.2	D49.2
back	C47.6	C79.89	—	D36.17	D48.2	D49.2
buttock	C47.5	C79.89	—	D36.16	D48.2	D49.2
calf	C47.2-☑	C79.89	—	D36.13	D48.2	D49.2
cervical region	C47.0	C79.89	—	D36.11	D48.2	D49.2
cheek	C47.0	C79.89	—	D36.11	D48.2	D49.2
chest (wall)	C47.3	C79.89	—	D36.14	D48.2	D49.2
chin	C47.0	C79.89	—	D36.11	D48.2	D49.2
ear (external)	C47.0	C79.89	—	D36.11	D48.2	D49.2
elbow	C47.1-☑	C79.89	—	D36.12	D48.2	D49.2
extrarectal	C47.5	C79.89	—	D36.16	D48.2	D49.2
extremity	C47.9	C79.89	—	D36.10	D48.2	D49.2
lower	C47.2-☑	C79.89	—	D36.13	D48.2	D49.2
upper	C47.1-☑	C79.89	—	D36.12	D48.2	D49.2
eyelid	C47.0	C79.89	—	D36.11	D48.2	D49.2
face	C47.0	C79.89	—	D36.11	D48.2	D49.2
finger	C47.1-☑	C79.89	—	D36.12	D48.2	D49.2
flank	C47.6	C79.89	—	D36.17	D48.2	D49.2
foot	C47.2-☑	C79.89	—	D36.13	D48.2	D49.2
forearm	C47.1-☑	C79.89	—	D36.12	D48.2	D49.2
forehead	C47.0	C79.89	—	D36.11	D48.2	D49.2
gluteal region	C47.5	C79.89	—	D36.16	D48.2	D49.2
groin	C47.5	C79.89	—	D36.16	D48.2	D49.2
hand	C47.1-☑	C79.89	—	D36.12	D48.2	D49.2
head	C47.0	C79.89	—	D36.11	D48.2	D49.2
heel	C47.2-☑	C79.89	—	D36.13	D48.2	D49.2
hip	C47.2-☑	C79.89	—	D36.13	D48.2	D49.2
infraclavicular region	C47.3	C79.89	—	D36.14	D48.2	D49.2
inguinal (canal) (region)	C47.5	C79.89	—	D36.16	D48.2	D49.2
intrathoracic	C47.3	C79.89	—	D36.14	D48.2	D49.2
ischiorectal fossa	C47.5	C79.89	—	D36.16	D48.2	D49.2
knee	C47.2-☑	C79.89	—	D36.13	D48.2	D49.2
leg	C47.2-☑	C79.89	—	D36.13	D48.2	D49.2
limb NEC	C47.9	C79.89	—	D36.10	D48.2	D49.2
lower	C47.2-☑	C79.89	—	D36.13	D48.2	D49.2
upper	C47.1-☑	C79.89	—	D36.12	D48.2	D49.2
nates	C47.5	C79.89	—	D36.16	D48.2	D49.2
neck	C47.0	C79.89	—	D36.11	D48.2	D49.2
orbit	C69.6-☑	C79.49	—	D31.6-☑	D48.7	D49.2
pararectal	C47.5	C79.89	—	D36.16	D48.2	D49.2
paraurethral	C47.5	C79.89	—	D36.16	D48.2	D49.2
paravaginal	C47.5	C79.89	—	D36.16	D48.2	D49.2
pelvis (floor)	C47.5	C79.89	—	D36.16	D48.2	D49.2
pelvoabdominal	C47.8	C79.89	—	D36.17	D48.2	D49.2
perineum	C47.5	C79.89	—	D36.16	D48.2	D49.2
perirectal (tissue)	C47.5	C79.89	—	D36.16	D48.2	D49.2
periurethral (tissue)	C47.5	C79.89	—	D36.16	D48.2	D49.2
popliteal fossa or space	C47.2-☑	C79.89	—	D36.13	D48.2	D49.2
presacral	C47.5	C79.89	—	D36.16	D48.2	D49.2
pterygoid fossa	C47.0	C79.89	—	D36.11	D48.2	D49.2
rectovaginal septum or wall	C47.5	C79.89	—	D36.16	D48.2	D49.2
rectovesical	C47.5	C79.89	—	D36.16	D48.2	D49.2
sacrococcygeal region	C47.5	C79.89	—	D36.16	D48.2	D49.2
scalp	C47.0	C79.89	—	D36.11	D48.2	D49.2

	Malignant Primary	Malignant Secondary	Ca in situ	Benign	Uncertain Behavior	Unspecified Behavior
Neoplasm, neoplastic — *continued*						
nerve — *continued*						
peripheral — *continued*						
scapular region	C47.3	C79.89	—	D36.14	D48.2	D49.2
shoulder	C47.1-☑	C79.89	—	D36.12	D48.2	D49.2
submental	C47.Ø	C79.89	—	D36.11	D48.2	D49.2
supraclavicular region	C47.Ø	C79.89	—	D36.11	D48.2	D49.2
temple	C47.Ø	C79.89	—	D36.11	D48.2	D49.2
temporal region	C47.Ø	C79.89	—	D36.11	D48.2	D49.2
thigh	C47.2-☑	C79.89	—	D36.13	D48.2	D49.2
thoracic (duct) (wall)	C47.3	C79.89	—	D36.14	D48.2	D49.2
thorax	C47.3	C79.89	—	D36.14	D48.2	D49.2
thumb	C47.1-☑	C79.89	—	D36.12	D48.2	D49.2
toe	C47.2-☑	C79.89	—	D36.13	D48.2	D49.2
trunk	C47.6	C79.89	—	D36.17	D48.2	D49.2
umbilicus	C47.4	C79.89	—	D36.15	D48.2	D49.2
vesicorectal	C47.5	C79.89	—	D36.16	D48.2	D49.2
wrist	C47.1-☑	C79.89	—	D36.12	D48.2	D49.2
radial	C47.1-☑	C79.89	—	D36.12	D48.2	D49.2
sacral	C47.5	C79.89	—	D36.16	D48.2	D49.2
sciatic	C47.2-☑	C79.89	—	D36.13	D48.2	D49.2
spinal NEC	C47.9	C79.89	—	D36.1Ø	D48.2	D49.2
accessory	C72.59	C79.49	—	D33.3	D43.3	D49.7
sympathetic NEC — *see also* Neoplasm, nerve, peripheral	C47.9	C79.89	—	D36.1Ø	D48.2	D49.2
trigeminal	C72.59	C79.49	—	D33.3	D43.3	D49.7
trochlear	C72.59	C79.49	—	D33.3	D43.3	D49.7
ulnar	C47.1-☑	C79.89	—	D36.12	D48.2	D49.2
vagus	C72.59	C79.49	—	D33.3	D43.3	D49.7
nervous system (central)	C72.9	C79.4Ø	—	D33.9	D43.9	D49.7
autonomic — *see* Neoplasm, nerve, peripheral						
parasympathetic — *see* Neoplasm, nerve, peripheral						
specified site NEC	—	C79.49	—	D33.7	D43.8	—
sympathetic — *see* Neoplasm, nerve, peripheral						
nevus — *see* Nevus						
nipple	C5Ø.Ø-☑	C79.81	DØ5.-☑	D24.-☑	—	—
nose, nasal	C76.Ø	C79.89	DØ9.8	D36.7	D48.7	D49.89
ala (external) (nasi) — *see also* Neoplasm, nose, skin	C44.3Ø1	C79.2	DØ4.39	D23.39	D48.5	D49.2
bone	C41.Ø	C79.51	—	D16.4	D48.Ø	D49.2
cartilage	C3Ø.Ø	C78.39	DØ2.3	D14.Ø	D38.5	D49.1
cavity	C3Ø.Ø	C78.39	DØ2.3	D14.Ø	D38.5	D49.1
choana	C11.3	C79.89	DØØ.Ø8	D1Ø.6	D37.Ø5	D49.Ø
external (skin) — *see also* Neoplasm, nose, skin	C44.3Ø1	C79.2	DØ4.39	D23.39	D48.5	D49.2
fossa	C3Ø.Ø	C78.39	DØ2.3	D14.Ø	D38.5	D49.1
internal	C3Ø.Ø	C78.39	DØ2.3	D14.Ø	D38.5	D49.1
mucosa	C3Ø.Ø	C78.39	DØ2.3	D14.Ø	D38.5	D49.1
septum	C3Ø.Ø	C78.39	DØ2.3	D14.Ø	D38.5	D49.1
posterior margin	C11.3	C79.89	DØØ.Ø8	D1Ø.6	D37.Ø5	D49.Ø
sinus — *see* Neoplasm, sinus						
skin	C44.3Ø1	C79.2	DØ4.39	D23.39	D48.5	D49.2
basal cell carcinoma	C44.311	—	—	—	—	—
specified type NEC	C44.391	—	—	—	—	—
squamous cell carcinoma	C44.321	—	—	—	—	—
turbinate (mucosa)	C3Ø.Ø	C78.39	DØ2.3	D14.Ø	D38.5	D49.1
bone	C41.Ø	C79.51	—	D16.4	D48.Ø	D49.2
vestibule	C3Ø.Ø	C78.39	DØ2.3	D14.Ø	D38.5	D49.1
Neoplasm, neoplastic — *continued*						
nostril	C3Ø.Ø	C78.39	DØ2.3	D14.Ø	D38.5	D49.1
nucleus pulposus	C41.2	C79.51	—	D16.6	D48.Ø	D49.2
occipital						
bone	C41.Ø	C79.51	—	D16.4	D48.Ø	D49.2
lobe or pole, brain	C71.4	C79.31	—	D33.Ø	D43.Ø	D49.6
odontogenic — *see* Neoplasm, jaw bone						
olfactory nerve or bulb	C72.2-☑	C79.49	—	D33.3	D43.3	D49.7
olive (brain)	C71.7	C79.31	—	D33.1	D43.1	D49.6
omentum	C48.1	C78.6	—	D2Ø.1	D48.4	D49.Ø
operculum (brain)	C71.Ø	C79.31	—	D33.Ø	D43.Ø	D49.6
optic nerve, chiasm, or tract	C72.3-☑	C79.49	—	D33.3	D43.3	D49.7
oral (cavity)	CØ6.9	C79.89	DØØ.ØØ	D1Ø.3Ø	D37.Ø9	D49.Ø
ill-defined	C14.8	C79.89	DØØ.ØØ	D1Ø.3Ø	D37.Ø9	D49.Ø
mucosa	CØ6.Ø	C79.89	DØØ.Ø2	D1Ø.39	D37.Ø9	D49.Ø
orbit	C69.6-☑	C79.49	DØ9.2-☑	D31.6-☑	D48.7	D49.89
autonomic nerve	C69.6-☑	C79.49	—	D31.6-☑	D48.7	D49.2
bone	C41.Ø	C79.51	—	D16.4	D48.Ø	D49.2
eye	C69.6-☑	C79.49	DØ9.2-☑	D31.6-☑	D48.7	D49.89
peripheral nerves	C69.6-☑	C79.49	—	D31.6-☑	D48.7	D49.2
soft parts	C69.6-☑	C79.49	DØ9.2-☑	D31.6-☑	D48.7	D49.89
organ of Zuckerkandl	C75.5	C79.89	—	D35.6	D44.7	D49.7
oropharynx	C1Ø.9	C79.89	DØØ.Ø8	D1Ø.5	D37.Ø5	D49.Ø
branchial cleft (vestige)	C1Ø.4	C79.89	DØØ.Ø8	D1Ø.5	D37.Ø5	D49.Ø
junctional region	C1Ø.8	C79.89	DØØ.Ø8	D1Ø.5	D37.Ø5	D49.Ø
lateral wall	C1Ø.2	C79.89	DØØ.Ø8	D1Ø.5	D37.Ø5	D49.Ø
overlapping lesion	C1Ø.8	—	—	—	—	—
pillars or fauces	CØ9.1	C79.89	DØØ.Ø8	D1Ø.5	D37.Ø5	D49.Ø
posterior wall	C1Ø.3	C79.89	DØØ.Ø8	D1Ø.5	D37.Ø5	D49.Ø
vallecula	C1Ø.Ø	C79.89	DØØ.Ø8	D1Ø.5	D37.Ø5	D49.Ø
os						
external	C53.1	C79.82	DØ6.1	D26.Ø	D39.Ø	D49.59
internal	C53.Ø	C79.82	DØ6.Ø	D26.Ø	D39.Ø	D49.59
ovary	C56.-☑	C79.6-☑	DØ7.39	D27.-☑	D39.1-☑	D49.59
oviduct	C57.Ø-☑	C79.82	DØ7.39	D28.2	D39.8	D49.59
palate	CØ5.9	C79.89	DØØ.ØØ	D1Ø.39	D37.Ø9	D49.Ø
hard	CØ5.Ø	C79.89	DØØ.Ø5	D1Ø.39	D37.Ø9	D49.Ø
junction of hard and soft palate	CØ5.9	C79.89	DØØ.ØØ	D1Ø.39	D37.Ø9	D49.Ø
overlapping lesions	CØ5.8	—	—	—	—	—
soft	CØ5.1	C79.89	DØØ.Ø4	D1Ø.39	D37.Ø9	D49.Ø
nasopharyngeal surface	C11.3	C79.89	DØØ.Ø8	D1Ø.6	D37.Ø5	D49.Ø
posterior surface	C11.3	C79.89	DØØ.Ø8	D1Ø.6	D37.Ø5	D49.Ø
superior surface	C11.3	C79.89	DØØ.Ø8	D1Ø.6	D37.Ø5	D49.Ø
palatoglossal arch	CØ9.1	C79.89	DØØ.ØØ	D1Ø.5	D37.Ø9	D49.Ø
palatopharyngeal arch	CØ9.1	C79.89	DØØ.ØØ	D1Ø.5	D37.Ø9	D49.Ø
pallium	C71.Ø	C79.31	—	D33.Ø	D43.Ø	D49.6
palpebra	C44.1Ø-☑	C79.2	DØ4.1-☑	D23.1-☑	D48.5	D49.2
basal cell carcinoma	C44.11-☑	—	—	—	—	—
sebaceous cell	C44.13-☑	—	—	—	—	—
specified type NEC	C44.19-☑	—	—	—	—	—
squamous cell carcinoma	C44.12-☑	—	—	—	—	—
pancreas	C25.9	C78.89	DØ1.7	D13.6	D37.8	D49.Ø
body	C25.1	C78.89	DØ1.7	D13.6	D37.8	D49.Ø
duct (of Santorini) (of Wirsung)	C25.3	C78.89	DØ1.7	D13.6	D37.8	D49.Ø
ectopic tissue	C25.7	C78.89	—	D13.6	D37.8	D49.Ø
head	C25.Ø	C78.89	DØ1.7	D13.6	D37.8	D49.Ø
islet cells	C25.4	C78.89	DØ1.7	D13.7	D37.8	D49.Ø
neck	C25.7	C78.89	DØ1.7	D13.6	D37.8	D49.Ø
overlapping lesion	C25.8	—	—	—	—	—
tail	C25.2	C78.89	DØ1.7	D13.6	D37.8	D49.Ø

	Malignant Primary	Malignant Secondary	Ca in situ	Benign	Uncertain Behavior	Unspecified Behavior
Neoplasm, neoplastic — *continued*						
para-aortic body	C75.5	C79.89	—	D35.6	D44.7	D49.7
paraganglion NEC	C75.5	C79.89	—	D35.6	D44.7	D49.7
parametrium	C57.3	C79.82	—	D28.2	D39.8	D49.59
paranephric	C48.0	C78.6	—	D20.0	D48.3	D49.0
pararectal	C76.3	C79.89	—	D36.7	D48.7	D49.89
parasagittal (region)	C76.0	C79.89	D09.8	D36.7	D48.7	D49.89
parasellar	C72.9	C79.49	—	D33.9	D43.8	D49.7
parathyroid (gland)	C75.0	C79.89	D09.3	D35.1	D44.2	D49.7
paraurethral	C76.3	C79.89	—	D36.7	D48.7	D49.89
gland	C68.1	C79.19	D09.19	D30.8	D41.8	D49.59
paravaginal	C76.3	C79.89	—	D36.7	D48.7	D49.89
parenchyma, kidney	C64.-☑	C79.0-☑	D09.19	D30.0-☑	D41.0-☑	D49.51-☑
parietal						
bone	C41.0	C79.51	—	D16.4	D48.0	D49.2
lobe, brain	C71.3	C79.31	—	D33.0	D43.0	D49.6
paroophoron	C57.1-☑	C79.82	D07.39	D28.2	D39.8	D49.59
parotid (duct) (gland)	C07	C79.89	D00.00	D11.0	D37.030	D49.0
parovarium	C57.1-☑	C79.82	D07.39	D28.2	D39.8	D49.59
patella	C40.20	C79.51	—	—	—	—
peduncle, cerebral	C71.7	C79.31	—	D33.1	D43.1	D49.6
pelvirectal junction	C19	C78.5	D01.1	D12.7	D37.5	D49.0
pelvis, pelvic	C76.3	C79.89	D09.8	D36.7	D48.7	D49.89
bone	C41.4	C79.51	—	D16.8	D48.0	D49.2
floor	C76.3	C79.89	D09.8	D36.7	D48.7	D49.89
renal	C65.-☑	C79.0-☑	D09.19	D30.1-☑	D41.1-☑	D49.51-☑
viscera	C76.3	C79.89	D09.8	D36.7	D48.7	D49.89
wall	C76.3	C79.89	D09.8	D36.7	D48.7	D49.89
pelvo-abdominal	C76.8	C79.89	D09.8	D36.7	D48.7	D49.89
penis	C60.9	C79.82	D07.4	D29.0	D40.8	D49.59
body	C60.2	C79.82	D07.4	D29.0	D40.8	D49.59
corpus (cavernosum)	C60.2	C79.82	D07.4	D29.0	D40.8	D49.59
glans	C60.1	C79.82	D07.4	D29.0	D40.8	D49.59
overlapping sites	C60.8	—	—	—	—	—
skin NEC	C60.9	C79.82	D07.4	D29.0	D40.8	D49.59
periadrenal (tissue)	C48.0	C78.6	—	D20.0	D48.3	D49.0
perianal (skin) — *see also* Neoplasm, anus, skin	C44.500	C79.2	D04.5	D23.5	D48.5	D49.2
pericardium	C38.0	C79.89	—	D15.1	D48.7	D49.89
perinephric	C48.0	C78.6	—	D20.0	D48.3	D49.0
perineum	C76.3	C79.89	D09.8	D36.7	D48.7	D49.89
periodontal tissue NEC	C03.9	C79.89	D00.03	D10.39	D37.09	D49.0
periosteum — *see* Neoplasm, bone						
peripancreatic	C48.0	C78.6	—	D20.0	D48.3	D49.0
peripheral nerve NEC	C47.9	C79.89	—	D36.10	D48.2	D49.2
perirectal (tissue)	C76.3	C79.89	—	D36.7	D48.7	D49.89
perirenal (tissue)	C48.0	C78.6	—	D20.0	D48.3	D49.0
peritoneum, peritoneal (cavity)	C48.2	C78.6	—	D20.1	D48.4	D49.0
benign mesothelial tissue — *see* Mesothelioma, benign						
overlapping lesion	C48.8	—	—	—	—	—
with digestive organs	C26.9	—	—	—	—	—
parietal	C48.1	C78.6	—	D20.1	D48.4	D49.0
pelvic	C48.1	C78.6	—	D20.1	D48.4	D49.0
specified part NEC	C48.1	C78.6	—	D20.1	D48.4	D49.0
peritonsillar (tissue)	C76.0	C79.89	D09.8	D36.7	D48.7	D49.89
periurethral tissue	C76.3	C79.89	—	D36.7	D48.7	D49.89
phalanges						
foot	C40.3-☑	C79.51	—	D16.3-☑	—	—
hand	C40.1-☑	C79.51	—	D16.1-☑	—	—
pharynx, pharyngeal	C14.0	C79.89	D00.08	D10.9	D37.05	D49.0
bursa	C11.1	C79.89	D00.08	D10.6	D37.05	D49.0

	Malignant Primary	Malignant Secondary	Ca in situ	Benign	Uncertain Behavior	Unspecified Behavior
Neoplasm, neoplastic — *continued*						
pharynx, pharyngeal — *continued*						
fornix	C11.3	C79.89	D00.08	D10.6	D37.05	D49.0
recess	C11.2	C79.89	D00.08	D10.6	D37.05	D49.0
region	C14.0	C79.89	D00.08	D10.9	D37.05	D49.0
tonsil	C11.1	C79.89	D00.08	D10.6	D37.05	D49.0
wall (lateral) (posterior)	C14.0	C79.89	D00.08	D10.9	D37.05	D49.0
pia mater	C70.9	C79.40	—	D32.9	D42.9	D49.7
cerebral	C70.0	C79.32	—	D32.0	D42.0	D49.7
cranial	C70.0	C79.32	—	D32.0	D42.0	D49.7
spinal	C70.1	C79.49	—	D32.1	D42.1	D49.7
pillars of fauces	C09.1	C79.89	D00.08	D10.5	D37.05	D49.0
pineal (body) (gland)	C75.3	C79.89	D09.3	D35.4	D44.5	D49.7
pinna (ear) NEC — *see also* Neoplasm, skin, ear	C44.20-☑	C79.2	D04.2-☑	D23.2-☑	D48.5	D49.2
piriform fossa or sinus	C12	C79.89	D00.08	D10.7	D37.05	D49.0
pituitary (body) (fossa) (gland) (lobe)	C75.1	C79.89	D09.3	D35.2	D44.3	D49.7
placenta	C58	C79.82	D07.0	D26.7	D39.2	D49.59
pleura, pleural (cavity)	C38.4	C78.2	—	D19.0	D38.2	D49.1
overlapping lesion with heart or mediastinum	C38.8	—	—	—	—	—
parietal	C38.4	C78.2	—	D19.0	D38.2	D49.1
visceral	C38.4	C78.2	—	D19.0	D38.2	D49.1
plexus						
brachial	C47.1-☑	C79.89	—	D36.12	D48.2	D49.2
cervical	C47.0	C79.89	—	D36.11	D48.2	D49.2
choroid	C71.5	C79.31	—	D33.0	D43.0	D49.6
lumbosacral	C47.5	C79.89	—	D36.16	D48.2	D49.2
sacral	C47.5	C79.89	—	D36.16	D48.2	D49.2
pluriendocrine	C75.8	C79.89	D09.3	D35.7	D44.9	D49.7
pole						
frontal	C71.1	C79.31	—	D33.0	D43.0	D49.6
occipital	C71.4	C79.31	—	D33.0	D43.0	D49.6
pons (varolii)	C71.7	C79.31	—	D33.1	D43.1	D49.6
popliteal fossa or space	C76.5-☑	C79.89	D04.7-☑	D36.7	D48.7	D49.89
postcricoid (region)	C13.0	C79.89	D00.08	D10.7	D37.05	D49.0
posterior fossa (cranial)	C71.9	C79.31	—	D33.2	D43.2	D49.6
postnasal space	C11.9	C79.89	D00.08	D10.6	D37.05	D49.0
prepuce	C60.0	C79.82	D07.4	D29.0	D40.8	D49.59
prepylorus	C16.4	C78.89	D00.2	D13.1	D37.1	D49.0
presacral (region)	C76.3	C79.89	—	D36.7	D48.7	D49.89
prostate (gland)	C61	C79.82	D07.5	D29.1	D40.0	D49.59
utricle	C68.0	C79.19	D09.19	D30.4	D41.3	D49.59
pterygoid fossa	C49.0	C79.89	—	D21.0	D48.1	D49.2
pubic bone	C41.4	C79.51	—	D16.8	D48.0	D49.2
pudenda, pudendum (female)	C51.9	C79.82	D07.1	D28.0	D39.8	D49.59
pulmonary — *see also* Neoplasm, lung	C34.9-☑	C78.0-☑	D02.2-☑	D14.3-☑	D38.1	D49.1
putamen	C71.0	C79.31	—	D33.0	D43.0	D49.6
pyloric						
antrum	C16.3	C78.89	D00.2	D13.1	D37.1	D49.0
canal	C16.4	C78.89	D00.2	D13.1	D37.1	D49.0
pylorus	C16.4	C78.89	D00.2	D13.1	D37.1	D49.0
pyramid (brain)	C71.7	C79.31	—	D33.1	D43.1	D49.6
pyriform fossa or sinus	C12	C79.89	D00.08	D10.7	D37.05	D49.0
radius (any part)	C40.0-☑	C79.51	—	D16.0-☑	—	—
Rathke's pouch	C75.1	C79.89	D09.3	D35.2	D44.3	D49.7
rectosigmoid (junction)	C19	C78.5	D01.1	D12.7	D37.5	D49.0
overlapping lesion with anus or rectum	C21.8	—	—	—	—	—
rectouterine pouch	C48.1	C78.6	—	D20.1	D48.4	D49.0
rectovaginal septum or wall	C76.3	C79.89	D09.8	D36.7	D48.7	D49.89
rectovesical septum	C76.3	C79.89	D09.8	D36.7	D48.7	D49.89
rectum (ampulla)	C20	C78.5	D01.2	D12.8	D37.5	D49.0

	Malignant Primary	Malignant Secondary	Ca in situ	Benign	Uncertain Behavior	Unspecified Behavior
Neoplasm, neoplastic — *continued*						
rectum — *continued*						
and colon	C19	C78.5	D01.1	D12.7	D37.5	D49.0
overlapping lesion						
with anus or rectosigmoid junction	C21.8	—	—	—	—	—
renal	C64.-☑	C79.0-☑	D09.19	D30.0-☑	D41.0-☑	D49.51-☑
calyx	C65.-☑	C79.0-☑	D09.19	D30.1-☑	D41.1-☑	D49.51-☑
hilus	C65.-☑	C79.0-☑	D09.19	D30.1-☑	D41.1-☑	D49.51-☑
parenchyma	C64.-☑	C79.0-☑	D09.19	D30.0-☑	D41.0-☑	D49.51-☑
pelvis	C65.-☑	C79.0-☑	D09.19	D30.1-☑	D41.1-☑	D49.51-☑
respiratory						
organs or system NEC	C39.9	C78.30	D02.4	D14.4	D38.6	D49.1
tract NEC	C39.9	C78.30	D02.4	D14.4	D38.5	D49.1
upper	C39.0	C78.30	D02.4	D14.4	D38.5	D49.1
retina	C69.2-☑	C79.49	D09.2-☑	D31.2-☑	D48.7	D49.81
retrobulbar	C69.6-☑	C79.49	—	D31.6-☑	D48.7	D49.89
retrocecal	C48.0	C78.6	—	D20.0	D48.3	D49.0
retromolar (area) (triangle) (trigone)	C06.2	C79.89	D00.00	D10.39	D37.09	D49.0
retro-orbital	C76.0	C79.89	D09.8	D36.7	D48.7	D49.89
retroperitoneal (space) (tissue)	C48.0	C78.6	—	D20.0	D48.3	D49.0
retroperitoneum	C48.0	C78.6	—	D20.0	D48.3	D49.0
retropharyngeal	C14.0	C79.89	D00.08	D10.9	D37.05	D49.0
retrovesical (septum)	C76.3	C79.89	D09.8	D36.7	D48.7	D49.89
rhinencephalon	C71.0	C79.31	—	D33.0	D43.0	D49.6
rib	C41.3	C79.51	—	D16.7	D48.0	D49.2
Rosenmuller's fossa	C11.2	C79.89	D00.08	D10.6	D37.05	D49.0
round ligament	C57.2-☑	C79.82	—	D28.2	D39.8	D49.59
sacrococcyx, sacrococcygeal	C41.4	C79.51	—	D16.8	D48.0	D49.2
region	C76.3	C79.89	D09.8	D36.7	D48.7	D49.89
sacrouterine ligament	C57.3	C79.82	—	D28.2	D39.8	D49.59
sacrum, sacral (vertebra)	C41.4	C79.51	—	D16.8	D48.0	D49.2
salivary gland or duct (major)	C08.9	C79.89	D00.00	D11.9	D37.039	D49.0
minor NEC	C06.9	C79.89	D00.00	D10.39	D37.04	D49.0
overlapping lesion	C08.9	—	—	—	—	—
parotid	C07	C79.89	D00.00	D11.0	D37.030	D49.0
pluriglandular	C08.9	C79.89	D00.00	D11.9	D37.039	D49.0
sublingual	C08.1	C79.89	D00.00	D11.7	D37.031	D49.0
submandibular	C08.0	C79.89	D00.00	D11.7	D37.032	D49.0
submaxillary	C08.0	C79.89	D00.00	D11.7	D37.032	D49.0
salpinx (uterine)	C57.0-☑	C79.82	D07.39	D28.2	D39.8	D49.59
Santorini's duct	C25.3	C78.89	D01.7	D13.6	D37.8	D49.0
scalp	C44.40	C79.2	D04.4	D23.4	D48.5	D49.2
basal cell carcinoma	C44.41	—	—	—	—	—
specified type NEC	C44.49	—	—	—	—	—
squamous cell carcinoma	C44.42	—	—	—	—	—
scapula (any part)	C40.0-☑	C79.51	—	D16.0-☑	—	—
scapular region	C76.1	C79.89	D09.8	D36.7	D48.7	D49.89
scar NEC — *see also* Neoplasm, skin, by site	C44.90	C79.2	D04.9	D23.9	D48.5	D49.2
sciatic nerve	C47.2-☑	C79.89	—	D36.13	D48.2	D49.2
sclera	C69.4-☑	C79.49	D09.2-☑	D31.4-☑	D48.7	D49.89
scrotum (skin)	C63.2	C79.82	D07.61	D29.4	D40.8	D49.59
sebaceous gland — *see* Neoplasm, skin						
sella turcica	C75.1	C79.89	D09.3	D35.2	D44.3	D49.7
bone	C41.0	C79.51	—	D16.4	D48.0	D49.2
semilunar cartilage (knee)	C40.2-☑	C79.51	—	D16.2-☑	D48.0	D49.2
seminal vesicle	C63.7	C79.82	D07.69	D29.8	D40.8	D49.59
septum						
nasal	C30.0	C78.39	D02.3	D14.0	D38.5	D49.1
posterior margin	C11.3	C79.89	D00.08	D10.6	D37.05	D49.0
rectovaginal	C76.3	C79.89	D09.8	D36.7	D48.7	D49.89
rectovesical	C76.3	C79.89	D09.8	D36.7	D48.7	D49.89

	Malignant Primary	Malignant Secondary	Ca in situ	Benign	Uncertain Behavior	Unspecified Behavior
Neoplasm, neoplastic — *continued*						
septum — *continued*						
urethrovaginal	C57.9	C79.82	D07.30	D28.9	D39.9	D49.59
vesicovaginal	C57.9	C79.82	D07.30	D28.9	D39.9	D49.59
shoulder NEC	C76.4-☑	C79.89	D04.6-☑	D36.7	D48.7	D49.89
sigmoid flexure (lower) (upper)	C18.7	C78.5	D01.0	D12.5	D37.4	D49.0
sinus (accessory)	C31.9	C78.39	D02.3	D14.0	D38.5	D49.1
bone (any)	C41.0	C79.51	—	D16.4	D48.0	D49.2
ethmoidal	C31.1	C78.39	D02.3	D14.0	D38.5	D49.1
frontal	C31.2	C78.39	D02.3	D14.0	D38.5	D49.1
maxillary	C31.0	C78.39	D02.3	D14.0	D38.5	D49.1
nasal, paranasal NEC	C31.9	C78.39	D02.3	D14.0	D38.5	D49.1
overlapping lesion	C31.8	—	—	—	—	—
pyriform	C12	C79.89	D00.08	D10.7	D37.05	D49.0
sphenoid	C31.3	C78.39	D02.3	D14.0	D38.5	D49.1
skeleton, skeletal NEC	C41.9	C79.51	—	D16.9	D48.0	D49.2
Skene's gland	C68.1	C79.19	D09.19	D30.8	D41.8	D49.59
skin NOS	C44.90	C79.2	D04.9	D23.9	D48.5	D49.2
abdominal wall	C44.509	C79.2	D04.5	D23.5	D48.5	D49.2
basal cell carcinoma	C44.519	—	—	—	—	—
specified type NEC	C44.599	—	—	—	—	—
squamous cell carcinoma	C44.529	—	—	—	—	—
ala nasi — *see also* Neoplasm, nose, skin	C44.301	C79.2	D04.39	D23.39	D48.5	D49.2
ankle — *see also* Neoplasm, skin, limb, lower	C44.70-☑	C79.2	D04.7-☑	D23.7-☑	D48.5	D49.2
antecubital space — *see also* Neoplasm, skin, limb, upper	C44.60-☑	C79.2	D04.6-☑	D23.6-☑	D48.5	D49.2
anus	C44.500	C79.2	D04.5	D23.5	D48.5	D49.2
basal cell carcinoma	C44.510	—	—	—	—	—
specified type NEC	C44.590	—	—	—	—	—
squamous cell carcinoma	C44.520	—	—	—	—	—
arm — *see also* Neoplasm, skin, limb, upper	C44.60-☑	C79.2	D04.6-☑	D23.6-☑	D48.5	D49.2
auditory canal (external) — *see also* Neoplasm, skin, ear	C44.20-☑	C79.2	D04.2-☑	D23.2-☑	D48.5	D49.2
auricle (ear) — *see also* Neoplasm, skin, ear	C44.20-☑	C79.2	D04.2-☑	D23.2-☑	D48.5	D49.2
auricular canal (external) — *see also* Neoplasm, skin, ear	C44.20-☑	C79.2	D04.2-☑	D23.2-☑	D48.5	D49.2
axilla, axillary fold — *see also* Neoplasm, skin, trunk	C44.509	C79.2	D04.5	D23.5	D48.5	D49.2
back — *see also* Neoplasm, skin, trunk	C44.509	C79.2	D04.5	D23.5	D48.5	D49.2
basal cell carcinoma	C44.91	—	—	—	—	—
breast	C44.501	C79.2	D04.5	D23.5	D48.5	D49.2
basal cell carcinoma	C44.511	—	—	—	—	—
specified type NEC	C44.591	—	—	—	—	—
squamous cell carcinoma	C44.521	—	—	—	—	—
brow — *see also* Neoplasm, skin, face	C44.309	C79.2	D04.39	D23.39	D48.5	D49.2
buttock — *see also* Neoplasm, skin, trunk	C44.509	C79.2	D04.5	D23.5	D48.5	D49.2

	Malignant Primary	Malignant Secondary	Ca in situ	Benign	Uncertain Behavior	Unspecified Behavior
Neoplasm, neoplastic — *continued*						
skin — *continued*						
calf — *see also* Neoplasm, skin, limb, lower	C44.70-☑	C79.2	D04.7-☑	D23.7-☑	D48.5	D49.2
canthus (eye) (inner) (outer)	C44.10-☑	C79.2	D04.1-☑	D23.1-☑	D48.5	D49.2
basal cell carcinoma	C44.11-☑	—	—	—	—	—
sebaceous cell	C44.13-☑	—	—	—	—	—
specified type NEC	C44.19-☑	—	—	—	—	—
squamous cell carcinoma	C44.12-☑	—	—	—	—	—
cervical region — *see also* Neoplasm, skin, neck	C44.40	C79.2	D04.4	D23.4	D48.5	D49.2
cheek (external) — *see also* Neoplasm, skin, face	C44.309	C79.2	D04.39	D23.39	D48.5	D49.2
chest (wall) — *see also* Neoplasm, skin, trunk	C44.509	C79.2	D04.5	D23.5	D48.5	D49.2
chin — *see also* Neoplasm, skin, face	C44.309	C79.2	D04.39	D23.39	D48.5	D49.2
clavicular area — *see also* Neoplasm, skin, trunk	C44.509	C79.2	D04.5	D23.5	D48.5	D49.2
clitoris	C51.2	C79.82	D07.1	D28.0	D39.8	D49.59
columnella — *see also* Neoplasm, skin, face	C44.309	C79.2	D04.39	D23.39	D48.5	D49.2
concha — *see also* Neoplasm, skin, ear	C44.20-☑	C79.2	D04.2-☑	D23.2-☑	D48.5	D49.2
ear (external)	C44.20-☑	C79.2	D04.2-☑	D23.2-☑	D48.5	D49.2
basal cell carcinoma	C44.21-☑	—	—	—	—	—
specified type NEC	C44.29-☑	—	—	—	—	—
squamous cell carcinoma	C44.22-☑	—	—	—	—	—
elbow — *see also* Neoplasm, skin, limb, upper	C44.60-☑	C79.2	D04.6-☑	D23.6-☑	D48.5	D49.2
eyebrow — *see also* Neoplasm, skin, face	C44.309	C79.2	D04.39	D23.39	D48.5	D49.2
eyelid	C44.10-☑	C79.2	D04.1-☑	D23.1-☑	D48.5	D49.2
basal cell carcinoma	C44.11-☑	—	—	—	—	—
sebaceous cell	C44.13-☑	—	—	—	—	—
specified type NEC	C44.19-☑	—	—	—	—	—
squamous cell carcinoma	C44.12-☑	—	—	—	—	—
face NOS	C44.300	C79.2	D04.30	D23.30	D48.5	D49.2
basal cell carcinoma	C44.310	—	—	—	—	—
specified type NEC	C44.390	—	—	—	—	—
squamous cell carcinoma	C44.320	—	—	—	—	—
female genital organs (external)	C51.9	C79.82	D07.1	D28.0	D39.8	D49.59
clitoris	C51.2	C79.82	D07.1	D28.0	D39.8	D49.59
labium NEC	C51.9	C79.82	D07.1	D28.0	D39.8	D49.59
majus	C51.0	C79.82	D07.1	D28.0	D39.8	D49.59
minus	C51.1	C79.82	D07.1	D28.0	D39.8	D49.59
pudendum	C51.9	C79.82	D07.1	D28.0	D39.8	D49.59
vulva	C51.9	C79.82	D07.1	D28.0	D39.8	D49.59
finger — *see also* Neoplasm, skin, limb, upper	C44.60-☑	C79.2	D04.6-☑	D23.6-☑	D48.5	D49.2
flank — *see also* Neoplasm, skin, trunk	C44.509	C79.2	D04.5	D23.5	D48.5	D49.2
foot — *see also* Neoplasm, skin, limb, lower	C44.70-☑	C79.2	D04.7-☑	D23.7-☑	D48.5	D49.2

	Malignant Primary	Malignant Secondary	Ca in situ	Benign	Uncertain Behavior	Unspecified Behavior
Neoplasm, neoplastic — *continued*						
skin — *continued*						
forearm — *see also* Neoplasm, skin, limb, upper	C44.60-☑	C79.2	D04.6-☑	D23.6-☑	D48.5	D49.2
forehead — *see also* Neoplasm, skin, face	C44.309	C79.2	D04.39	D23.39	D48.5	D49.2
glabella — *see also* Neoplasm, skin, face	C44.309	C79.2	D04.39	D23.39	D48.5	D49.2
gluteal region — *see also* Neoplasm, skin, trunk	C44.509	C79.2	D04.5	D23.5	D48.5	D49.2
groin — *see also* Neoplasm, skin, trunk	C44.509	C79.2	D04.5	D23.5	D48.5	D49.2
hand — *see also* Neoplasm, skin, limb, upper	C44.60-☑	C79.2	D04.6-☑	D23.6-☑	D48.5	D49.2
head NEC — *see also* Neoplasm, skin, scalp	C44.40	C79.2	D04.4	D23.4	D48.5	D49.2
heel — *see also* Neoplasm, skin, limb, lower	C44.70-☑	C79.2	D04.7-☑	D23.7-☑	D48.5	D49.2
helix — *see also* Neoplasm, skin, ear	C44.20-☑	C79.2	D04.2-☑	D23.2-☑	D48.5	D49.2
hip — *see also* Neoplasm, skin, limb, lower	C44.70-☑	C79.2	D04.7-☑	D23.7-☑	D48.5	D49.2
infraclavicular region — *see also* Neoplasm, skin, trunk	C44.509	C79.2	D04.5	D23.5	D48.5	D49.2
inguinal region — *see also* Neoplasm, skin, trunk	C44.509	C79.2	D04.5	D23.5	D48.5	D49.2
jaw — *see also* Neoplasm, skin, face	C44.309	C79.2	D04.39	D23.39	D48.5	D49.2
Kaposi's sarcoma — *see* Kaposi's, sarcoma, skin						
knee — *see also* Neoplasm, skin, limb, lower	C44.70-☑	C79.2	D04.7-☑	D23.7-☑	D48.5	D49.2
labia						
majora	C51.0	C79.82	D07.1	D28.0	D39.8	D49.59
minora	C51.1	C79.82	D07.1	D28.0	D39.8	D49.59
leg — *see also* Neoplasm, skin, limb, lower	C44.70-☑	C79.2	D04.7-☑	D23.7-☑	D48.5	D49.2
lid (lower) (upper)	C44.10-☑	C79.2	D04.1-☑	D23.1-☑	D48.5	D49.2
basal cell carcinoma	C44.11-☑	—	—	—	—	—
sebaceous cell	C44.13-☑	—	—	—	—	—
specified type NEC	C44.19-☑	—	—	—	—	—
squamous cell carcinoma	C44.12-☑	—	—	—	—	—
limb NEC	C44.90	C79.2	D04.9	D23.9	D48.5	D49.2
basal cell carcinoma	C44.91	—	—	—	—	—
lower	C44.70-☑	C79.2	D04.7-☑	D23.7-☑	D48.5	D49.2
basal cell carcinoma	C44.71-☑	—	—	—	—	—
specified type NEC	C44.79-☑	—	—	—	—	—
squamous cell carcinoma	C44.72-☑	—	—	—	—	—
upper	C44.60-☑	C79.2	D04.6-☑	D23.6-☑	D48.5	D49.2
basal cell carcinoma	C44.61-☑	—	—	—	—	—
specified type NEC	C44.69-☑	—	—	—	—	—
squamous cell carcinoma	C44.62-☑	—	—	—	—	—
lip (lower) (upper)	C44.00	C79.2	D04.0	D23.0	D48.5	D49.2

	Malignant Primary	Malignant Secondary	Ca in situ	Benign	Uncertain Behavior	Unspecified Behavior
Neoplasm, neoplastic — *continued*						
skin — *continued*						
lip — *continued*						
basal cell carcinoma	C44.Ø1	—	—	—	—	—
specified type NEC	C44.Ø9	—	—	—	—	—
squamous cell carcinoma	C44.Ø2	—	—	—	—	—
male genital organs	C63.9	C79.82	DØ7.6Ø	D29.9	D4Ø.8	D49.59
penis	C6Ø.9	C79.82	DØ7.4	D29.Ø	D4Ø.8	D49.59
prepuce	C6Ø.Ø	C79.82	DØ7.4	D29.Ø	D4Ø.8	D49.59
scrotum	C63.2	C79.82	DØ7.61	D29.4	D4Ø.8	D49.59
mastectomy site (skin) — *see also* Neoplasm, skin, breast	C44.5Ø1	C79.2	—	—	—	—
specified as breast tissue	C5Ø.8-☑	C79.81	—	—	—	—
meatus, acoustic (external) — *see also* Neoplasm, skin, ear	C44.2Ø-☑	C79.2	DØ4.2-☑	D23.2-☑	D48.5	D49.2
melanotic — *see* Melanoma						
Merkel cell — *see* Carcinoma, Merkel cell						
nates — *see also* Neoplasm, skin, trunk	C44.5Ø9	C79.2	DØ4.5	D23.5	D48.5	D49.2
neck	C44.4Ø	C79.2	DØ4.4	D23.4	D48.5	D49.2
basal cell carcinoma	C44.41	—	—	—	—	—
specified type NEC	C44.49	—	—	—	—	—
squamous cell carcinoma	C44.42	—	—	—	—	—
nevus — *see* Nevus, skin						
nose (external) — *see also* Neoplasm, nose, skin	C44.3Ø1	C79.2	DØ4.39	D23.39	D48.5	D49.2
overlapping lesion	C44.8Ø	—	—	—	—	—
basal cell carcinoma	C44.81	—	—	—	—	—
specified type NEC	C44.89	—	—	—	—	—
squamous cell carcinoma	C44.82	—	—	—	—	—
palm — *see also* Neoplasm, skin, limb, upper	C44.6Ø-☑	C79.2	DØ4.6-☑	D23.6-☑	D48.5	D49.2
palpebra	C44.1Ø-☑	C79.2	DØ4.1-☑	D23.1-☑	D48.5	D49.2
basal cell carcinoma	C44.11-☑	—	—	—	—	—
sebaceous cell	C44.13-☑	—	—	—	—	—
specified type NEC	C44.19-☑	—	—	—	—	—
squamous cell carcinoma	C44.12-☑	—	—	—	—	—
penis NEC	C6Ø.9	C79.82	DØ7.4	D29.Ø	D4Ø.8	D49.59
perianal — *see also* Neoplasm, skin, anus	C44.5ØØ	C79.2	DØ4.5	D23.5	D48.5	D49.2
perineum — *see also* Neoplasm, skin, anus	C44.5ØØ	C79.2	DØ4.5	D23.5	D48.5	D49.2
pinna — *see also* Neoplasm, skin, ear	C44.2Ø-☑	C79.2	DØ4.2-☑	D23.2-☑	D48.5	D49.2
plantar — *see also* Neoplasm, skin, limb, lower	C44.7Ø-☑	C79.2	DØ4.7-☑	D23.7-☑	D48.5	D49.2
popliteal fossa or space — *see also* Neoplasm, skin, limb, lower	C44.7Ø-☑	C79.2	DØ4.7-☑	D23.7-☑	D48.5	D49.2
prepuce	C6Ø.Ø	C79.82	DØ7.4	D29.Ø	D4Ø.8	D49.59
Neoplasm, neoplastic — *continued*						
skin — *continued*						
pubes — *see also* Neoplasm, skin, trunk	C44.5Ø9	C79.2	DØ4.5	D23.5	D48.5	D49.2
sacrococcygeal region — *see also* Neoplasm, skin, trunk	C44.5Ø9	C79.2	DØ4.5	D23.5	D48.5	D49.2
scalp	C44.4Ø	C79.2	DØ4.4	D23.4	D48.5	D49.2
basal cell carcinoma	C44.41	—	—	—	—	—
specified type NEC	C44.49	—	—	—	—	—
squamous cell carcinoma	C44.42	—	—	—	—	—
scapular region — *see also* Neoplasm, skin, trunk	C44.5Ø9	C79.2	DØ4.5	D23.5	D48.5	D49.2
scrotum	C63.2	C79.82	DØ7.61	D29.4	D4Ø.8	D49.59
shoulder — *see also* Neoplasm, skin, limb, upper	C44.6Ø-☑	C79.2	DØ4.6-☑	D23.6-☑	D48.5	D49.2
sole (foot) — *see also* Neoplasm, skin, limb, lower	C44.7Ø-☑	C79.2	DØ4.7-☑	D23.7-☑	D48.5	D49.2
specified sites NEC	C44.8Ø	C79.2	DØ4.8	D23.9	D48.5	D49.2
basal cell carcinoma	C44.81	—	—	—	—	—
specified type NEC	C44.89	—	—	—	—	—
squamous cell carcinoma	C44.82	—	—	—	—	—
specified type NEC	C44.99	—	—	—	—	—
squamous cell carcinoma	C44.92	—	—	—	—	—
submammary fold — *see also* Neoplasm, skin, trunk	C44.5Ø9	C79.2	DØ4.5	D23.5	D48.5	D49.2
supraclavicular region — *see also* Neoplasm, skin, neck	C44.4Ø	C79.2	DØ4.4	D23.4	D48.5	D49.2
temple — *see also* Neoplasm, skin, face	C44.3Ø9	C79.2	DØ4.39	D23.39	D48.5	D49.2
thigh — *see also* Neoplasm, skin, limb, lower	C44.7Ø-☑	C79.2	DØ4.7-☑	D23.7-☑	D48.5	D49.2
thoracic wall — *see also* Neoplasm, skin, trunk	C44.5Ø9	C79.2	DØ4.5	D23.5	D48.5	D49.2
thumb — *see also* Neoplasm, skin, limb, upper	C44.6Ø-☑	C79.2	DØ4.6-☑	D23.6-☑	D48.5	D49.2
toe — *see also* Neoplasm, skin, limb, lower	C44.7Ø-☑	C79.2	DØ4.7-☑	D23.7-☑	D48.5	D49.2
tragus — *see also* Neoplasm, skin, ear	C44.2Ø-☑	C79.2	DØ4.2-☑	D23.2-☑	D48.5	D49.2
trunk	C44.5Ø9	C79.2	DØ4.5	D23.5	D48.5	D49.2
basal cell carcinoma	C44.519	—	—	—	—	—
specified type NEC	C44.599	—	—	—	—	—
squamous cell carcinoma	C44.529	—	—	—	—	—
umbilicus — *see also* Neoplasm, skin, trunk	C44.5Ø9	C79.2	DØ4.5	D23.5	D48.5	D49.2
vulva	C51.9	C79.82	DØ7.1	D28.Ø	D39.8	D49.59
overlapping lesion	C51.8	—	—	—	—	—
wrist — *see also* Neoplasm, skin, limb, upper	C44.6Ø-☑	C79.2	DØ4.6-☑	D23.6-☑	D48.5	D49.2
skull	C41.Ø	C79.51	—	D16.4	D48.Ø	D49.2

	Malignant Primary	Malignant Secondary	Ca in situ	Benign	Uncertain Behavior	Unspecified Behavior
Neoplasm, neoplastic — *continued*						
soft parts or tissues — *see* Neoplasm, connective tissue						
specified site NEC	C76.8	C79.89	D09.8	D36.7	D48.7	D49.89
spermatic cord	C63.1-☑	C79.82	D07.69	D29.8	D40.8	D49.59
sphenoid	C31.3	C78.39	D02.3	D14.0	D38.5	D49.1
bone	C41.0	C79.51	—	D16.4	D48.0	D49.2
sinus	C31.3	C78.39	D02.3	D14.0	D38.5	D49.1
sphincter						
anal	C21.1	C78.5	D01.3	D12.9	D37.8	D49.0
of Oddi	C24.0	C78.89	D01.5	D13.5	D37.6	D49.0
spine, spinal (column)	C41.2	C79.51	—	D16.6	D48.0	D49.2
bulb	C71.7	C79.31	—	D33.1	D43.1	D49.6
coccyx	C41.4	C79.51	—	D16.8	D48.0	D49.2
cord (cervical) (lumbar) (sacral) (thoracic)	C72.0	C79.49	—	D33.4	D43.4	D49.7
dura mater	C70.1	C79.49	—	D32.1	D42.1	D49.7
lumbosacral	C41.2	C79.51	—	D16.6	D48.0	D49.2
marrow NEC	C96.9	C79.52	—	—	D47.9	D49.89
membrane	C70.1	C79.49	—	D32.1	D42.1	D49.7
meninges	C70.1	C79.49	—	D32.1	D42.1	D49.7
nerve (root)	C47.9	C79.89	—	D36.10	D48.2	D49.2
pia mater	C70.1	C79.49	—	D32.1	D42.1	D49.7
root	C47.9	C79.89	—	D36.10	D48.2	D49.2
sacrum	C41.4	C79.51	—	D16.8	D48.0	D49.2
spleen, splenic NEC	C26.1	C78.89	D01.7	D13.9	D37.8	D49.0
flexure (colon)	C18.5	C78.5	D01.0	D12.3	D37.4	D49.0
stem, brain	C71.7	C79.31	—	D33.1	D43.1	D49.6
Stensen's duct	C07	C79.89	D00.00	D11.0	D37.030	D49.0
sternum	C41.3	C79.51	—	D16.7	D48.0	D49.2
stomach	C16.9	C78.89	D00.2	D13.1	D37.1	D49.0
antrum (pyloric)	C16.3	C78.89	D00.2	D13.1	D37.1	D49.0
body	C16.2	C78.89	D00.2	D13.1	D37.1	D49.0
cardia	C16.0	C78.89	D00.2	D13.1	D37.1	D49.0
cardiac orifice	C16.0	C78.89	D00.2	D13.1	D37.1	D49.0
corpus	C16.2	C78.89	D00.2	D13.1	D37.1	D49.0
fundus	C16.1	C78.89	D00.2	D13.1	D37.1	D49.0
greater curvature NEC	C16.6	C78.89	D00.2	D13.1	D37.1	D49.0
lesser curvature NEC	C16.5	C78.89	D00.2	D13.1	D37.1	D49.0
overlapping lesion	C16.8	—	—	—	—	—
prepylorus	C16.4	C78.89	D00.2	D13.1	D37.1	D49.0
pylorus	C16.4	C78.89	D00.2	D13.1	D37.1	D49.0
wall NEC	C16.9	C78.89	D00.2	D13.1	D37.1	D49.0
anterior NEC	C16.8	C78.89	D00.2	D13.1	D37.1	D49.0
posterior NEC	C16.8	C78.89	D00.2	D13.1	D37.1	D49.0
stroma, endometrial	C54.1	C79.82	D07.0	D26.1	D39.0	D49.59
stump, cervical	C53.8	C79.82	D06.7	D26.0	D39.0	D49.59
subcutaneous (nodule) (tissue) NEC — *see* Neoplasm, connective tissue						
subdural	C70.9	C79.32	—	D32.9	D42.9	D49.7
subglottis, subglottic	C32.2	C78.39	D02.0	D14.1	D38.0	D49.1
sublingual	C04.9	C79.89	D00.06	D10.2	D37.09	D49.0
gland or duct	C08.1	C79.89	D00.00	D11.7	D37.031	D49.0
submandibular gland	C08.0	C79.89	D00.00	D11.7	D37.032	D49.0
submaxillary gland or duct	C08.0	C79.89	D00.00	D11.7	D37.032	D49.0
submental	C76.0	C79.89	D09.8	D36.7	D48.7	D49.89
subpleural	C34.9-☑	C78.0-☑	D02.2-☑	D14.3-☑	D38.1	D49.1
substernal	C38.1	C78.1	—	D15.2	D38.3	D49.89
sudoriferous, sudoriparous gland, site unspecified	C44.90	C79.2	D04.9	D23.9	D48.5	D49.2
specified site — *see* Neoplasm, skin						
supraclavicular region	C76.0	C79.89	D09.8	D36.7	D48.7	D49.89
supraglottis	C32.1	C78.39	D02.0	D14.1	D38.0	D49.1
suprarenal	C74.9-☑	C79.7-☑	D09.3	D35.0-☑	D44.1-☑	D49.7
capsule	C74.9-☑	C79.7-☑	D09.3	D35.0-☑	D44.1-☑	D49.7

	Malignant Primary	Malignant Secondary	Ca in situ	Benign	Uncertain Behavior	Unspecified Behavior
Neoplasm, neoplastic — *continued*						
suprarenal — *continued*						
cortex	C74.0-☑	C79.7-☑	D09.3	D35.0-☑	D44.1-☑	D49.7
gland	C74.9-☑	C79.7-☑	D09.3	D35.0-☑	D44.1-☑	D49.7
medulla	C74.1-☑	C79.7-☑	D09.3	D35.0-☑	D44.1-☑	D49.7
suprasellar (region)	C71.9	C79.31	—	D33.2	D43.2	D49.6
supratentorial (brain) NEC	C71.0	C79.31	—	D33.0	D43.0	D49.6
sweat gland (apocrine) (eccrine), site unspecified	C44.90	C79.2	D04.9	D23.9	D48.5	D49.2
specified site — *see* Neoplasm, skin						
sympathetic nerve or nervous system NEC	C47.9	C79.89	—	D36.10	D48.2	D49.2
symphysis pubis	C41.4	C79.51	—	D16.8	D48.0	D49.2
synovial membrane — *see* Neoplasm, connective tissue						
tapetum, brain	C71.8	C79.31	—	D33.2	D43.2	D49.6
tarsus (any bone)	C40.3-☑	C79.51	—	D16.3-☑	—	—
temple (skin) — *see also* Neoplasm, skin, face	C44.309	C79.2	D04.39	D23.39	D48.5	D49.2
temporal						
bone	C41.0	C79.51	—	D16.4	D48.0	D49.2
lobe or pole	C71.2	C79.31	—	D33.0	D43.0	D49.6
region	C76.0	C79.89	D09.8	D36.7	D48.7	D49.89
skin — *see also* Neoplasm, skin, face	C44.309	C79.2	D04.39	D23.39	D48.5	D49.2
tendon (sheath) — *see* Neoplasm, connective tissue						
tentorium (cerebelli)	C70.0	C79.32	—	D32.0	D42.0	D49.7
testis, testes	C62.9-☑	C79.82	D07.69	D29.2-☑	D40.1-☑	D49.59
descended	C62.1-☑	C79.82	D07.69	D29.2-☑	D40.1-☑	D49.59
ectopic	C62.0-☑	C79.82	D07.69	D29.2-☑	D40.1-☑	D49.59
retained	C62.0-☑	C79.82	D07.69	D29.2-☑	D40.1-☑	D49.59
scrotal	C62.1-☑	C79.82	D07.69	D29.2-☑	D40.1-☑	D49.59
undescended	C62.0-☑	C79.82	D07.69	D29.2-☑	D40.1-☑	D49.59
unspecified whether descended or undescended	C62.9-☑	C79.82	D07.69	D29.2-☑	D40.1-☑	D49.59
thalamus	C71.0	C79.31	—	D33.0	D43.0	D49.6
thigh NEC	C76.5-☑	C79.89	D04.7-☑	D36.7	D48.7	D49.89
thorax, thoracic (cavity) (organs NEC)	C76.1	C79.89	D09.8	D36.7	D48.7	D49.89
duct	C49.3	C79.89	—	D21.3	D48.1	D49.2
wall NEC	C76.1	C79.89	D09.8	D36.7	D48.7	D49.89
throat	C14.0	C79.89	D00.08	D10.9	D37.05	D49.0
thumb NEC	C76.4-☑	C79.89	D04.6-☑	D36.7	D48.7	D49.89
thymus (gland)	C37	C79.89	D09.3	D15.0	D38.4	D49.89
thyroglossal duct	C73	C79.89	D09.3	D34	D44.0	D49.7
thyroid (gland)	C73	C79.89	D09.3	D34	D44.0	D49.7
cartilage	C32.3	C78.39	D02.0	D14.1	D38.0	D49.1
tibia (any part)	C40.2-☑	C79.51	—	D16.2-☑	—	—
toe NEC	C76.5-☑	C79.89	D04.7-☑	D36.7	D48.7	D49.89
tongue	C02.9	C79.89	D00.07	D10.1	D37.02	D49.0
anterior (two-thirds) NEC	C02.3	C79.89	D00.07	D10.1	D37.02	D49.0
dorsal surface	C02.0	C79.89	D00.07	D10.1	D37.02	D49.0
ventral surface	C02.2	C79.89	D00.07	D10.1	D37.02	D49.0
base (dorsal surface)	C01	C79.89	D00.07	D10.1	D37.02	D49.0
border (lateral)	C02.1	C79.89	D00.07	D10.1	D37.02	D49.0
dorsal surface NEC	C02.0	C79.89	D00.07	D10.1	D37.02	D49.0
fixed part NEC	C01	C79.89	D00.07	D10.1	D37.02	D49.0
foreamen cecum	C02.0	C79.89	D00.07	D10.1	D37.02	D49.0
frenulum linguae	C02.2	C79.89	D00.07	D10.1	D37.02	D49.0
junctional zone	C02.8	C79.89	D00.07	D10.1	D37.02	D49.0
margin (lateral)	C02.1	C79.89	D00.07	D10.1	D37.02	D49.0
midline NEC	C02.0	C79.89	D00.07	D10.1	D37.02	D49.0
mobile part NEC	C02.3	C79.89	D00.07	D10.1	D37.02	D49.0

	Malignant Primary	Malignant Secondary	Ca in situ	Benign	Uncertain Behavior	Unspecified Behavior
Neoplasm, neoplastic — *continued*						
tongue — *continued*						
overlapping lesion	CØ2.8	—	—	—	—	—
posterior (third)	CØ1	C79.89	DØØ.Ø7	D1Ø.1	D37.Ø2	D49.Ø
root	CØ1	C79.89	DØØ.Ø7	D1Ø.1	D37.Ø2	D49.Ø
surface (dorsal)	CØ2.Ø	C79.89	DØØ.Ø7	D1Ø.1	D37.Ø2	D49.Ø
base	CØ1	C79.89	DØØ.Ø7	D1Ø.1	D37.Ø2	D49.Ø
ventral	CØ2.2	C79.89	DØØ.Ø7	D1Ø.1	D37.Ø2	D49.Ø
tip	CØ2.1	C79.89	DØØ.Ø7	D1Ø.1	D37.Ø2	D49.Ø
tonsil	CØ2.4	C79.89	DØØ.Ø7	D1Ø.1	D37.Ø2	D49.Ø
tonsil	CØ9.9	C79.89	DØØ.Ø8	D1Ø.4	D37.Ø5	D49.Ø
fauces, faucial	CØ9.9	C79.89	DØØ.Ø8	D1Ø.4	D37.Ø5	D49.Ø
lingual	CØ2.4	C79.89	DØØ.Ø7	D1Ø.1	D37.Ø2	D49.Ø
overlapping sites	CØ9.8	—	—	—	—	—
palatine	CØ9.9	C79.89	DØØ.Ø8	D1Ø.4	D37.Ø5	D49.Ø
pharyngeal	C11.1	C79.89	DØØ.Ø8	D1Ø.6	D37.Ø5	D49.Ø
pillar (anterior) (posterior)	CØ9.1	C79.89	DØØ.Ø8	D1Ø.5	D37.Ø5	D49.Ø
tonsillar fossa	CØ9.Ø	C79.89	DØØ.Ø8	D1Ø.5	D37.Ø5	D49.Ø
tooth socket NEC	CØ3.9	C79.89	DØØ.Ø3	D1Ø.39	D37.Ø9	D49.Ø
trachea (cartilage) (mucosa)	C33	C78.39	DØ2.1	D14.2	D38.1	D49.1
overlapping lesion with bronchus or lung	C34.8-☑	—	—	—	—	—
tracheobronchial	C34.8-☑	C78.39	DØ2.1	D14.2	D38.1	D49.1
overlapping lesion with lung	C34.8-☑	—	—	—	—	—
tragus — *see also* Neoplasm, skin, ear	C44.2Ø-☑	C79.2	DØ4.2-☑	D23.2-☑	D48.5	D49.2
trunk NEC	C76.8	C79.89	DØ4.5	D36.7	D48.7	D49.89
tubo-ovarian	C57.8	C79.82	DØ7.39	D28.7	D39.8	D49.59
tunica vaginalis	C63.7	C79.82	DØ7.69	D29.8	D4Ø.8	D49.59
turbinate (bone)	C41.Ø	C79.51	—	D16.4	D48.Ø	D49.2
nasal	C3Ø.Ø	C78.39	DØ2.3	D14.Ø	D38.5	D49.1
tympanic cavity	C3Ø.1	C78.39	DØ2.3	D14.Ø	D38.5	D49.1
ulna (any part)	C4Ø.Ø-☑	C79.51	—	D16.Ø-☑	—	—
umbilicus, umbilical — *see also* Neoplasm, skin, trunk	C44.5Ø9	C79.2	DØ4.5	D23.5	D48.5	D49.2
uncus, brain	C71.2	C79.31	—	D33.Ø	D43.Ø	D49.6
unknown site or unspecified	C8Ø.1	C79.9	DØ9.9	D36.9	D48.9	D49.9
urachus	C67.7	C79.11	DØ9.Ø	D3Ø.3	D41.4	D49.4
ureter-bladder (junction)	C67.6	C79.11	DØ9.Ø	D3Ø.3	D41.4	D49.4
ureter, ureteral	C66.-☑	C79.19	DØ9.19	D3Ø.2-☑	D41.2-☑	D49.59
orifice (bladder)	C67.6	C79.11	DØ9.Ø	D3Ø.3	D41.4	D49.4
urethra, urethral (gland)	C68.Ø	C79.19	DØ9.19	D3Ø.4	D41.3	D49.59
orifice, internal	C67.5	C79.11	DØ9.Ø	D3Ø.3	D41.4	D49.4
urethrovaginal (septum)	C57.9	C79.82	DØ7.3Ø	D28.9	D39.8	D49.59
urinary organ or system	C68.9	C79.1Ø	DØ9.1Ø	D3Ø.9	D41.9	D49.59
bladder — *see* Neoplasm, bladder						
overlapping lesion	C68.8	—	—	—	—	—
specified sites NEC	C68.8	C79.19	DØ9.19	D3Ø.8	D41.8	D49.59
utero-ovarian	C57.8	C79.82	DØ7.39	D28.7	D39.8	D49.59
ligament	C57.1-☑	C79.82	DØ7.39	D28.2	D39.8	D49.59
uterosacral ligament	C57.3	C79.82	—	D28.2	D39.8	D49.59
uterus, uteri, uterine	C55	C79.82	DØ7.Ø	D26.9	D39.Ø	D49.59
adnexa NEC	C57.4	C79.82	DØ7.39	D28.7	D39.8	D49.59
body	C54.9	C79.82	DØ7.Ø	D26.1	D39.Ø	D49.59
cervix	C53.9	C79.82	DØ6.9	D26.Ø	D39.Ø	D49.59
cornu	C54.9	C79.82	DØ7.Ø	D26.1	D39.Ø	D49.59
corpus	C54.9	C79.82	DØ7.Ø	D26.1	D39.Ø	D49.59
endocervix (canal) (gland)	C53.Ø	C79.82	DØ6.Ø	D26.Ø	D39.Ø	D49.59
endometrium	C54.1	C79.82	DØ7.Ø	D26.1	D39.Ø	D49.59
exocervix	C53.1	C79.82	DØ6.1	D26.Ø	D39.Ø	D49.59
external os	C53.1	C79.82	DØ6.1	D26.Ø	D39.Ø	D49.59
fundus	C54.3	C79.82	DØ7.Ø	D26.1	D39.Ø	D49.59

	Malignant Primary	Malignant Secondary	Ca in situ	Benign	Uncertain Behavior	Unspecified Behavior
Neoplasm, neoplastic — *continued*						
uterus, uteri, uterine — *continued*						
internal os	C53.Ø	C79.82	DØ6.Ø	D26.Ø	D39.Ø	D49.59
isthmus	C54.Ø	C79.82	DØ7.Ø	D26.1	D39.Ø	D49.59
ligament	C57.3	C79.82	—	D28.2	D39.8	D49.59
broad	C57.1-☑	C79.82	DØ7.39	D28.2	D39.8	D49.59
round	C57.2-☑	C79.82	—	D28.2	D39.8	D49.59
lower segment	C54.Ø	C79.82	DØ7.Ø	D26.1	D39.Ø	D49.59
myometrium	C54.2	C79.82	DØ7.Ø	D26.1	D39.Ø	D49.59
overlapping sites	C54.8	—	—	—	—	—
squamocolumnar junction	C53.8	C79.82	DØ6.7	D26.Ø	D39.Ø	D49.59
tube	C57.Ø-☑	C79.82	DØ7.39	D28.2	D39.8	D49.59
utricle, prostatic	C68.Ø	C79.19	DØ9.19	D3Ø.4	D41.3	D49.59
uveal tract	C69.4-☑	C79.49	DØ9.2-☑	D31.4-☑	D48.7	D49.89
uvula	CØ5.2	C79.89	DØØ.Ø4	D1Ø.39	D37.Ø9	D49.Ø
vagina, vaginal (fornix) (vault) (wall)	C52	C79.82	DØ7.2	D28.1	D39.8	D49.59
vaginovesical	C57.9	C79.82	DØ7.3Ø	D28.9	D39.9	D49.59
septum	C57.9	C79.82	DØ7.3Ø	D28.9	D39.9	D49.59
vallecula (epigiottis)	C1Ø.Ø	C79.89	DØØ.Ø8	D1Ø.5	D37.Ø5	D49.Ø
vascular — *see* Neoplasm, connective tissue						
vas deferens	C63.1-☑	C79.82	DØ7.69	D29.8	D4Ø.8	D49.59
Vater's ampulla	C24.1	C78.89	DØ1.5	D13.5	D37.6	D49.Ø
vein, venous — *see* Neoplasm, connective tissue						
vena cava (abdominal) (inferior)	C49.4	C79.89	—	D21.4	D48.1	D49.2
superior	C49.3	C79.89	—	D21.3	D48.1	D49.2
ventricle (cerebral) (floor) (lateral) (third)	C71.5	C79.31	—	D33.Ø	D43.Ø	D49.6
cardiac (left) (right)	C38.Ø	C79.89	—	D15.1	D48.7	D49.89
fourth	C71.7	C79.31	—	D33.1	D43.1	D49.6
ventricular band of larynx	C32.1	C78.39	DØ2.Ø	D14.1	D38.Ø	D49.1
ventriculus — *see* Neoplasm, stomach						
vermillion border — *see* Neoplasm, lip						
vermis, cerebellum	C71.6	C79.31	—	D33.1	D43.1	D49.6
vertebra (column)	C41.2	C79.51	—	D16.6	D48.Ø	D49.2
coccyx	C41.4	C79.51	—	D16.8	D48.Ø	D49.2
marrow NEC	C96.9	C79.52	—	—	D47.9	D49.89
sacrum	C41.4	C79.51	—	D16.8	D48.Ø	D49.2
vesical — *see* Neoplasm, bladder						
vesicle, seminal	C63.7	C79.82	DØ7.69	D29.8	D4Ø.8	D49.59
vesicocervical tissue	C57.9	C79.82	DØ7.3Ø	D28.9	D39.9	D49.59
vesicorectal	C76.3	C79.82	DØ9.8	D36.7	D48.7	D49.89
vesicovaginal	C57.9	C79.82	DØ7.3Ø	D28.9	D39.9	D49.59
septum	C57.9	C79.82	DØ7.3Ø	D28.9	D39.8	D49.59
vessel (blood) — *see* Neoplasm, connective tissue						
vestibular gland, greater	C51.Ø	C79.82	DØ7.1	D28.Ø	D39.8	D49.59
vestibule						
mouth	CØ6.1	C79.89	DØØ.ØØ	D1Ø.39	D37.Ø9	D49.Ø
nose	C3Ø.Ø	C78.39	DØ2.3	D14.Ø	D38.5	D49.1
Virchow's gland	C77.Ø	C77.Ø	—	D36.Ø	D48.7	D49.89
viscera NEC	C76.8	C79.89	DØ9.8	D36.7	D48.7	D49.89
vocal cords (true)	C32.Ø	C78.39	DØ2.Ø	D14.1	D38.Ø	D49.1
false	C32.1	C78.39	DØ2.Ø	D14.1	D38.Ø	D49.1
vomer	C41.Ø	C79.51	—	D16.4	D48.Ø	D49.2
vulva	C51.9	C79.82	DØ7.1	D28.Ø	D39.8	D49.59
vulvovaginal gland	C51.Ø	C79.82	DØ7.1	D28.Ø	D39.8	D49.59
Waldeyer's ring	C14.2	C79.89	DØØ.Ø8	D1Ø.9	D37.Ø5	D49.Ø
Wharton's duct	CØ8.Ø	C79.89	DØØ.ØØ	D11.7	D37.Ø32	D49.Ø
white matter (central) (cerebral)	C71.Ø	C79.31	—	D33.Ø	D43.Ø	D49.6

	Malignant Primary	Malignant Secondary	Ca in situ	Benign	Uncertain Behavior	Unspecified Behavior
Neoplasm, neoplastic — *continued*						
windpipe	C33	C78.39	DØ2.1	D14.2	D38.1	D49.1
Wirsung's duct	C25.3	C78.89	DØ1.7	D13.6	D37.8	D49.Ø
wolffian (body) (duct)						
female	C57.7	C79.82	DØ7.39	D28.7	D39.8	D49.59
male	C63.7	C79.82	DØ7.69	D29.8	D4Ø.8	D49.59
womb — *see* Neoplasm, uterus						
wrist NEC	C76.4-☑	C79.89	DØ4.6-☑	D36.7	D48.7	D49.89
xiphoid process	C41.3	C79.51	—	D16.7	D48.Ø	D49.2
Zuckerkandl organ	C75.5	C79.89	—	D35.6	D44.7	D49.7

Substance	Poisoning, Accidental (unintentional)	Poisoning, Intentional Self-harm	Poisoning, Assault	Poisoning, Undetermined	Adverse Effect	Under-dosing
14-hydroxydihydro-morphinone	T40.2X1	T40.2X2	T40.2X3	T40.2X4	T40.2X5	T40.2X6
1-Propanol	T51.3X1	T51.3X2	T51.3X3	T51.3X4	—	—
2,3,7,8-Tetrachlorodibenzo-p-dioxin	T53.7X1	T53.7X2	T53.7X3	T53.7X4	—	—
2,4,5-T (trichloro-phenoxyacetic acid)	T60.1X1	T60.1X2	T60.1X3	T60.1X4	—	—
2,4,5-Trichlorophen-oxyacetic acid	T60.3X1	T60.3X2	T60.3X3	T60.3X4	—	—
2,4-D (dichlorophen-oxyacetic acid)	T60.3X1	T60.3X2	T60.3X3	T60.3X4	—	—
2,4-Toluene diisocyanate	T65.0X1	T65.0X2	T65.0X3	T65.0X4	—	—
2-Deoxy-5-fluorouridine	T45.1X1	T45.1X2	T45.1X3	T45.1X4	T45.1X5	T45.1X6
2-Ethoxyethanol	T52.3X1	T52.3X2	T52.3X3	T52.3X4	—	—
2-Methoxyethanol	T52.3X1	T52.3X2	T52.3X3	T52.3X4	—	—
2-Propanol	T51.2X1	T51.2X2	T51.2X3	T51.2X4	—	—
3,4-methylenedioxymeth-amphetamine	T43.641	T43.642	T43.643	T43.644	—	—
4-Aminobutyric acid	T43.8X1	T43.8X2	T43.8X3	T43.8X4	T43.8X5	T43.8X6
4-Aminophenol derivatives	T39.1X1	T39.1X2	T39.1X3	T39.1X4	T39.1X5	T39.1X6
5-Deoxy-5-fluorouridine	T45.1X1	T45.1X2	T45.1X3	T45.1X4	T45.1X5	T45.1X6
5-Methoxypsoralen (5-MOP)	T50.991	T50.992	T50.993	T50.994	T50.995	T50.996
8-Aminoquinoline drugs	T37.2X1	T37.2X2	T37.2X3	T37.2X4	T37.2X5	T37.2X6
8-Methoxypsoralen (8-MOP)	T50.991	T50.992	T50.993	T50.994	T50.995	T50.996
ABOB	T37.5X1	T37.5X2	T37.5X3	T37.5X4	T37.5X5	T37.5X6
Abrine	T62.2X1	T62.2X2	T62.2X3	T62.2X4	—	—
Abrus (seed)	T62.2X1	T62.2X2	T62.2X3	T62.2X4	—	—
Absinthe	T51.0X1	T51.0X2	T51.0X3	T51.0X4	—	—
beverage	T51.0X1	T51.0X2	T51.0X3	T51.0X4	—	—
Acaricide	T60.8X1	T60.8X2	T60.8X3	T60.8X4	—	—
Acebutolol	T44.7X1	T44.7X2	T44.7X3	T44.7X4	T44.7X5	T44.7X6
Acecarbromal	T42.6X1	T42.6X2	T42.6X3	T42.6X4	T42.6X5	T42.6X6
Aceclidine	T44.1X1	T44.1X2	T44.1X3	T44.1X4	T44.1X5	T44.1X6
Acedapsone	T37.0X1	T37.0X2	T37.0X3	T37.0X4	T37.0X5	T37.0X6
Acefylline piperazine	T48.6X1	T48.6X2	T48.6X3	T48.6X4	T48.6X5	T48.6X6
Acemorphan	T40.2X1	T40.2X2	T40.2X3	T40.2X4	T40.2X5	T40.2X6
Acenocoumarin	T45.511	T45.512	T45.513	T45.514	T45.515	T45.516
Acenocoumarol	T45.511	T45.512	T45.513	T45.514	T45.515	T45.516
Acepifylline	T48.6X1	T48.6X2	T48.6X3	T48.6X4	T48.6X5	T48.6X6
Acepromazine	T43.3X1	T43.3X2	T43.3X3	T43.3X4	T43.3X5	T43.3X6
Acesulfamethoxypyridazine	T37.0X1	T37.0X2	T37.0X3	T37.0X4	T37.0X5	T37.0X6
Acetal	T52.8X1	T52.8X2	T52.8X3	T52.8X4	—	—
Acetaldehyde (vapor)	T52.8X1	T52.8X2	T52.8X3	T52.8X4	—	—
liquid	T65.891	T65.892	T65.893	T65.894	—	—
Acetaminophen	T39.1X1	T39.1X2	T39.1X3	T39.1X4	T39.1X5	T39.1X6
Acetaminosalol	T39.1X1	T39.1X2	T39.1X3	T39.1X4	T39.1X5	T39.1X6
Acetanilide	T39.1X1	T39.1X2	T39.1X3	T39.1X4	T39.1X5	T39.1X6
Acetarsol	T37.3X1	T37.3X2	T37.3X3	T37.3X4	T37.3X5	T37.3X6
Acetazolamide	T50.2X1	T50.2X2	T50.2X3	T50.2X4	T50.2X5	T50.2X6
Acetiamine	T45.2X1	T45.2X2	T45.2X3	T45.2X4	T45.2X5	T45.2X6
Acetic						
acid	T54.2X1	T54.2X2	T54.2X3	T54.2X4	—	—
with sodium acetate (ointment)	T49.3X1	T49.3X2	T49.3X3	T49.3X4	T49.3X5	T49.3X6
ester (solvent)(vapor)	T52.8X1	T52.8X2	T52.8X3	T52.8X4	—	—
irrigating solution	T50.3X1	T50.3X2	T50.3X3	T50.3X4	T50.3X5	T50.3X6
medicinal (lotion)	T49.2X1	T49.2X2	T49.2X3	T49.2X4	T49.2X5	T49.2X6
anhydride	T65.891	T65.892	T65.893	T65.894	—	—
ether (vapor)	T52.8X1	T52.8X2	T52.8X3	T52.8X4	—	—
Acetohexamide	T38.3X1	T38.3X2	T38.3X3	T38.3X4	T38.3X5	T38.3X6
Acetohydroxamic acid	T50.991	T50.992	T50.993	T50.994	T50.995	T50.996
Acetomenaphthone	T45.7X1	T45.7X2	T45.7X3	T45.7X4	T45.7X5	T45.7X6
Acetomorphine	T40.1X1	T40.1X2	T40.1X3	T40.1X4	—	—
Acetone (oils)	T52.4X1	T52.4X2	T52.4X3	T52.4X4	—	—
chlorinated	T52.4X1	T52.4X2	T52.4X3	T52.4X4	—	—
vapor	T52.4X1	T52.4X2	T52.4X3	T52.4X4	—	—
Acetonitrile	T52.8X1	T52.8X2	T52.8X3	T52.8X4	—	—
Acetophenazine	T43.3X1	T43.3X2	T43.3X3	T43.3X4	T43.3X5	T43.3X6
Acetophenetedin	T39.1X1	T39.1X2	T39.1X3	T39.1X4	T39.1X5	T39.1X6
Acetophenone	T52.4X1	T52.4X2	T52.4X3	T52.4X4	—	—
Acetorphine	T40.2X1	T40.2X2	T40.2X3	T40.2X4	—	—
Acetosulfone (sodium)	T37.1X1	T37.1X2	T37.1X3	T37.1X4	T37.1X5	T37.1X6
Acetrizoate (sodium)	T50.8X1	T50.8X2	T50.8X3	T50.8X4	T50.8X5	T50.8X6
Acetrizoic acid	T50.8X1	T50.8X2	T50.8X3	T50.8X4	T50.8X5	T50.8X6
Acetyl						
bromide	T53.6X1	T53.6X2	T53.6X3	T53.6X4	—	—
chloride	T53.6X1	T53.6X2	T53.6X3	T53.6X4	—	—
Acetylcarbromal	T42.6X1	T42.6X2	T42.6X3	T42.6X4	T42.6X5	T42.6X6
Acetylcholine						
chloride	T44.1X1	T44.1X2	T44.1X3	T44.1X4	T44.1X5	T44.1X6
derivative	T44.1X1	T44.1X2	T44.1X3	T44.1X4	T44.1X5	T44.1X6

Substance	Poisoning, Accidental (unintentional)	Poisoning, Intentional Self-harm	Poisoning, Assault	Poisoning, Undetermined	Adverse Effect	Under-dosing
Acetylcysteine	T48.4X1	T48.4X2	T48.4X3	T48.4X4	T48.4X5	T48.4X6
Acetyldigitoxin	T46.0X1	T46.0X2	T46.0X3	T46.0X4	T46.0X5	T46.0X6
Acetyldigoxin	T46.0X1	T46.0X2	T46.0X3	T46.0X4	T46.0X5	T46.0X6
Acetyldihydrocodeine	T40.2X1	T40.2X2	T40.2X3	T40.2X4	—	—
Acetyldihydrocodeinone	T40.2X1	T40.2X2	T40.2X3	T40.2X4	—	—
Acetylene (gas)	T59.891	T59.892	T59.893	T59.894	—	—
dichloride	T53.6X1	T53.6X2	T53.6X3	T53.6X4	—	—
incomplete combustion of	T58.11	T58.12	T58.13	T58.14	—	—
industrial	T59.891	T59.892	T59.893	T59.894	—	—
tetrachloride	T53.6X1	T53.6X2	T53.6X3	T53.6X4	—	—
vapor	T53.6X1	T53.6X2	T53.6X3	T53.6X4	—	—
Acetylpheneturide	T42.6X1	T42.6X2	T42.6X3	T42.6X4	T42.6X5	T42.6X6
Acetylphenylhydrazine	T39.8X1	T39.8X2	T39.8X3	T39.8X4	T39.8X5	T39.8X6
Acetylsalicylic acid (salts)	T39.011	T39.012	T39.013	T39.014	T39.015	T39.016
enteric coated	T39.011	T39.012	T39.013	T39.014	T39.015	T39.016
Acetylsulfamethoxypyridazine	T37.0X1	T37.0X2	T37.0X3	T37.0X4	T37.0X5	T37.0X6
Achromycin	T36.4X1	T36.4X2	T36.4X3	T36.4X4	T36.4X5	T36.4X6
ophthalmic preparation	T49.5X1	T49.5X2	T49.5X3	T49.5X4	T49.5X5	T49.5X6
topical NEC	T49.0X1	T49.0X2	T49.0X3	T49.0X4	T49.0X5	T49.0X6
Aciclovir	T37.5X1	T37.5X2	T37.5X3	T37.5X4	T37.5X5	T37.5X6
Acidifying agent NEC	T50.901	T50.902	T50.903	T50.904	T50.905	T50.906
Acid (corrosive) **NEC**	T54.2X1	T54.2X2	T54.2X3	T54.2X4	—	—
Acipimox	T46.6X1	T46.6X2	T46.6X3	T46.6X4	T46.6X5	T46.6X6
Acitretin	T50.991	T50.992	T50.993	T50.994	T50.995	T50.996
Aclarubicin	T45.1X1	T45.1X2	T45.1X3	T45.1X4	T45.1X5	T45.1X6
Aclatonium napadisilate	T48.1X1	T48.1X2	T48.1X3	T48.1X4	T48.1X5	T48.1X6
Aconite (wild)	T46.991	T46.992	T46.993	T46.994	T46.995	T46.996
Aconitine	T46.991	T46.992	T46.993	T46.994	T46.995	T46.996
Aconitum ferox	T46.991	T46.992	T46.993	T46.994	T46.995	T46.996
Acridine	T65.6X1	T65.6X2	T65.6X3	T65.6X4	—	—
vapor	T59.891	T59.892	T59.893	T59.894	—	—
Acriflavine	T37.91	T37.92	T37.93	T37.94	T37.95	T37.96
Acriflavinium chloride	T49.0X1	T49.0X2	T49.0X3	T49.0X4	T49.0X5	T49.0X6
Acrinol	T49.0X1	T49.0X2	T49.0X3	T49.0X4	T49.0X5	T49.0X6
Acrisorcin	T49.0X1	T49.0X2	T49.0X3	T49.0X4	T49.0X5	T49.0X6
Acrivastine	T45.0X1	T45.0X2	T45.0X3	T45.0X4	T45.0X5	T45.0X6
Acrolein (gas)	T59.891	T59.892	T59.893	T59.894	—	—
liquid	T54.1X1	T54.1X2	T54.1X3	T54.1X4	—	—
Acrylamide	T65.891	T65.892	T65.893	T65.894	—	—
Acrylic resin	T49.3X1	T49.3X2	T49.3X3	T49.3X4	T49.3X5	T49.3X6
Acrylonitrile	T65.891	T65.892	T65.893	T65.894	—	—
Actaea spicata	T62.2X1	T62.2X2	T62.2X3	T62.2X4	—	—
berry	T62.1X1	T62.1X2	T62.1X3	T62.1X4	—	—
Acterol	T37.3X1	T37.3X2	T37.3X3	T37.3X4	T37.3X5	T37.3X6
ACTH	T38.811	T38.812	T38.813	T38.814	T38.815	T38.816
Actinomycin C	T45.1X1	T45.1X2	T45.1X3	T45.1X4	T45.1X5	T45.1X6
Actinomycin D	T45.1X1	T45.1X2	T45.1X3	T45.1X4	T45.1X5	T45.1X6
Activated charcoal — *see also* Charcoal, medicinal	T47.6X1	T47.6X2	T47.6X3	T47.6X4	T47.6X5	T47.6X6
Acyclovir	T37.5X1	T37.5X2	T37.5X3	T37.5X4	T37.5X5	T37.5X6
Adenine	T45.2X1	T45.2X2	T45.2X3	T45.2X4	T45.2X5	T45.2X6
arabinoside	T37.5X1	T37.5X2	T37.5X3	T37.5X4	T37.5X5	T37.5X6
Adenosine (phosphate)	T46.2X1	T46.2X2	T46.2X3	T46.2X4	T46.2X5	T46.2X6
ADH	T38.891	T38.892	T38.893	T38.894	T38.895	T38.896
Adhesive NEC	T65.891	T65.892	T65.893	T65.894	—	—
Adicillin	T36.0X1	T36.0X2	T36.0X3	T36.0X4	T36.0X5	T36.0X6
Adiphenine	T44.3X1	T44.3X2	T44.3X3	T44.3X4	T44.3X5	T44.3X6
Adipiodone	T50.8X1	T50.8X2	T50.8X3	T50.8X4	T50.8X5	T50.8X6
Adjunct, pharmaceutical	T50.901	T50.902	T50.903	T50.904	T50.905	T50.906
Adrenal (extract, cortex or medulla) (glucocorticoids) (hormones) (mineralocorticoids)	T38.0X1	T38.0X2	T38.0X3	T38.0X4	T38.0X5	T38.0X6
ENT agent	T49.6X1	T49.6X2	T49.6X3	T49.6X4	T49.6X5	T49.6X6
ophthalmic preparation	T49.5X1	T49.5X2	T49.5X3	T49.5X4	T49.5X5	T49.5X6
topical NEC	T49.0X1	T49.0X2	T49.0X3	T49.0X4	T49.0X5	T49.0X6
Adrenalin — *see* Adrenaline						
Adrenaline	T44.5X1	T44.5X2	T44.5X3	T44.5X4	T44.5X5	T44.5X6
Adrenergic NEC	T44.901	T44.902	T44.903	T44.904	T44.905	T44.906
blocking agent NEC	T44.8X1	T44.8X2	T44.8X3	T44.8X4	T44.8X5	T44.8X6
beta, heart	T44.7X1	T44.7X2	T44.7X3	T44.7X4	T44.7X5	T44.7X6
specified NEC	T44.991	T44.992	T44.993	T44.994	T44.995	T44.996
Adrenochrome						
derivative	T46.991	T46.992	T46.993	T46.994	T46.995	T46.996
(mono) semicarbazone	T46.991	T46.992	T46.993	T46.994	T46.995	T46.996
Adrenocorticotrophic hormone	T38.811	T38.812	T38.813	T38.814	T38.815	T38.816
Adrenocorticotrophin	T38.811	T38.812	T38.813	T38.814	T38.815	T38.816
Adriamycin	T45.1X1	T45.1X2	T45.1X3	T45.1X4	T45.1X5	T45.1X6
Aerosol spray NEC	T65.91	T65.92	T65.93	T65.94	—	—
Aerosporin	T36.8X1	T36.8X2	T36.8X3	T36.8X4	T36.8X5	T36.8X6
ENT agent	T49.6X1	T49.6X2	T49.6X3	T49.6X4	T49.6X5	T49.6X6
ophthalmic preparation	T49.5X1	T49.5X2	T49.5X3	T49.5X4	T49.5X5	T49.5X6

Substance	Poisoning, Accidental (unintentional)	Poisoning, Intentional Self-harm	Poisoning, Assault	Poisoning, Undetermined	Adverse Effect	Under-dosing
Aerosporin — *continued*						
topical NEC	T49.ØX1	T49.ØX2	T49.ØX3	T49.ØX4	T49.ØX5	T49.ØX6
Aethusa cynapium	T62.2X1	T62.2X2	T62.2X3	T62.2X4	—	—
Afghanistan black	T4Ø.7X1	T4Ø.7X2	T4Ø.7X3	T4Ø.7X4	T4Ø.7X5	T4Ø.7X6
Aflatoxin	T64.Ø1	T64.Ø2	T64.Ø3	T64.Ø4	—	—
Afloqualone	T42.8X1	T42.8X2	T42.8X3	T42.8X4	T42.8X5	T42.8X6
African boxwood	T62.2X1	T62.2X2	T62.2X3	T62.2X4	—	—
Agar	T47.4X1	T47.4X2	T47.4X3	T47.4X4	T47.4X5	T47.4X6
Agonist						
predominantly						
alpha-adrenoreceptor	T44.4X1	T44.4X2	T44.4X3	T44.4X4	T44.4X5	T44.4X6
beta-adrenoreceptor	T44.5X1	T44.5X2	T44.5X3	T44.5X4	T44.5X5	T44.5X6
Agricultural agent NEC	T65.91	T65.92	T65.93	T65.94	—	—
Agrypnal	T42.3X1	T42.3X2	T42.3X3	T42.3X4	T42.3X5	T42.3X6
AHLG	T5Ø.Z11	T5Ø.Z12	T5Ø.Z13	T5Ø.Z14	T5Ø.Z15	T5Ø.Z16
Air contaminant(s), **source/type NOS**	T65.91	T65.92	T65.93	T65.94	—	—
Ajmaline	T46.2X1	T46.2X2	T46.2X3	T46.2X4	T46.2X5	T46.2X6
Akee	T62.1X1	T62.1X2	T62.1X3	T62.1X4	—	—
Akrinol	T49.ØX1	T49.ØX2	T49.ØX3	T49.ØX4	T49.ØX5	T49.ØX6
Akritoin	T37.8X1	T37.8X2	T37.8X3	T37.8X4	T37.8X5	T37.8X6
Alacepril	T46.4X1	T46.4X2	T46.4X3	T46.4X4	T46.4X5	T46.4X6
Alantolactone	T37.4X1	T37.4X2	T37.4X3	T37.4X4	T37.4X5	T37.4X6
Albamycin	T36.8X1	T36.8X2	T36.8X3	T36.8X4	T36.8X5	T36.8X6
Albendazole	T37.4X1	T37.4X2	T37.4X3	T37.4X4	T37.4X5	T37.4X6
Albumin						
bovine	T45.8X1	T45.8X2	T45.8X3	T45.8X4	T45.8X5	T45.8X6
human serum	T45.8X1	T45.8X2	T45.8X3	T45.8X4	T45.8X5	T45.8X6
salt-poor	T45.8X1	T45.8X2	T45.8X3	T45.8X4	T45.8X5	T45.8X6
normal human serum	T45.8X1	T45.8X2	T45.8X3	T45.8X4	T45.8X5	T45.8X6
Albuterol	T48.6X1	T48.6X2	T48.6X3	T48.6X4	T48.6X5	T48.6X6
Albutoin	T42.ØX1	T42.ØX2	T42.ØX3	T42.ØX4	T42.ØX5	T42.ØX6
Alclometasone	T49.ØX1	T49.ØX2	T49.ØX3	T49.ØX4	T49.ØX5	T49.ØX6
Alcohol	T51.91	T51.92	T51.93	T51.94	—	—
absolute	T51.ØX1	T51.ØX2	T51.ØX3	T51.ØX4	—	—
beverage	T51.ØX1	T51.ØX2	T51.ØX3	T51.ØX4	—	—
allyl	T51.8X1	T51.8X2	T51.8X3	T51.8X4	—	—
amyl	T51.3X1	T51.3X2	T51.3X3	T51.3X4	—	—
antifreeze	T51.1X1	T51.1X2	T51.1X3	T51.1X4	—	—
beverage	T51.ØX1	T51.ØX2	T51.ØX3	T51.ØX4	—	—
butyl	T51.3X1	T51.3X2	T51.3X3	T51.3X4	—	—
dehydrated	T51.ØX1	T51.ØX2	T51.ØX3	T51.ØX4	—	—
beverage	T51.ØX1	T51.ØX2	T51.ØX3	T51.ØX4	—	—
denatured	T51.ØX1	T51.ØX2	T51.ØX3	T51.ØX4	—	—
deterrent NEC	T5Ø.6X1	T5Ø.6X2	T5Ø.6X3	T5Ø.6X4	T5Ø.6X5	T5Ø.6X6
diagnostic (gastric function)	T5Ø.8X1	T5Ø.8X2	T5Ø.8X3	T5Ø.8X4	T5Ø.8X5	T5Ø.8X6
ethyl	T51.ØX1	T51.ØX2	T51.ØX3	T51.ØX4	—	—
beverage	T51.ØX1	T51.ØX2	T51.ØX3	T51.ØX4	—	—
grain	T51.ØX1	T51.ØX2	T51.ØX3	T51.ØX4	—	—
beverage	T51.ØX1	T51.ØX2	T51.ØX3	T51.ØX4	—	—
industrial	T51.ØX1	T51.ØX2	T51.ØX3	T51.ØX4	—	—
isopropyl	T51.2X1	T51.2X2	T51.2X3	T51.2X4	—	—
methyl	T51.1X1	T51.1X2	T51.1X3	T51.1X4	—	—
preparation for consumption	T51.ØX1	T51.ØX2	T51.ØX3	T51.ØX4	—	—
propyl	T51.3X1	T51.3X2	T51.3X3	T51.3X4	—	—
secondary	T51.2X1	T51.2X2	T51.2X3	T51.2X4	—	—
radiator	T51.1X1	T51.1X2	T51.1X3	T51.1X4	—	—
rubbing	T51.2X1	T51.2X2	T51.2X3	T51.2X4	—	—
specified type NEC	T51.8X1	T51.8X2	T51.8X3	T51.8X4	—	—
surgical	T51.ØX1	T51.ØX2	T51.ØX3	T51.ØX4	—	—
vapor (from any type of Alcohol)	T59.891	T59.892	T59.893	T59.894	—	—
wood	T51.1X1	T51.1X2	T51.1X3	T51.1X4	—	—
Alcuronium (chloride)	T48.1X1	T48.1X2	T48.1X3	T48.1X4	T48.1X5	T48.1X6
Aldactone	T5Ø.ØX1	T5Ø.ØX2	T5Ø.ØX3	T5Ø.ØX4	T5Ø.ØX5	T5Ø.ØX6
Aldesulfone sodium	T37.1X1	T37.1X2	T37.1X3	T37.1X4	T37.1X5	T37.1X6
Aldicarb	T6Ø.ØX1	T6Ø.ØX2	T6Ø.ØX3	T6Ø.ØX4	—	—
Aldomet	T46.5X1	T46.5X2	T46.5X3	T46.5X4	T46.5X5	T46.5X6
Aldosterone	T5Ø.ØX1	T5Ø.ØX2	T5Ø.ØX3	T5Ø.ØX4	T5Ø.ØX5	T5Ø.ØX6
Aldrin (dust)	T6Ø.1X1	T6Ø.1X2	T6Ø.1X3	T6Ø.1X4	—	—
Aleve — *see* Naproxen						
Alexitol sodium	T47.1X1	T47.1X2	T47.1X3	T47.1X4	T47.1X5	T47.1X6
Alfacalcidol	T45.2X1	T45.2X2	T45.2X3	T45.2X4	T45.2X5	T45.2X6
Alfadolone	T41.1X1	T41.1X2	T41.1X3	T41.1X4	T41.1X5	T41.1X6
Alfaxalone	T41.1X1	T41.1X2	T41.1X3	T41.1X4	T41.1X5	T41.1X6
Alfentanil	T4Ø.411	T4Ø.412	T4Ø.413	T4Ø.414	T4Ø.415	T4Ø.416
Alfuzosin (hydrochloride)	T44.8X1	T44.8X2	T44.8X3	T44.8X4	T44.8X5	T44.8X6
Algae (harmful) (toxin)	T65.821	T65.822	T65.823	T65.824	—	—
Algeldrate	T47.1X1	T47.1X2	T47.1X3	T47.1X4	T47.1X5	T47.1X6
Algin	T47.8X1	T47.8X2	T47.8X3	T47.8X4	T47.8X5	T47.8X6
Alglucerase	T45.3X1	T45.3X2	T45.3X3	T45.3X4	T45.3X5	T45.3X6

Substance	Poisoning, Accidental (unintentional)	Poisoning, Intentional Self-harm	Poisoning, Assault	Poisoning, Undetermined	Adverse Effect	Under-dosing
Alidase	T45.3X1	T45.3X2	T45.3X3	T45.3X4	T45.3X5	T45.3X6
Alimemazine	T43.3X1	T43.3X2	T43.3X3	T43.3X4	T43.3X5	T43.3X6
Aliphatic thiocyanates	T65.ØX1	T65.ØX2	T65.ØX3	T65.ØX4	—	—
Alizapride	T45.ØX1	T45.ØX2	T45.ØX3	T45.ØX4	T45.ØX5	T45.ØX6
Alkali (caustic)	T54.3X1	T54.3X2	T54.3X3	T54.3X4	—	—
Alkaline antiseptic solution (aromatic)	T49.6X1	T49.6X2	T49.6X3	T49.6X4	T49.6X5	T49.6X6
Alkalinizing agents (medicinal)	T5Ø.9Ø1	T5Ø.9Ø2	T5Ø.9Ø3	T5Ø.9Ø4	T5Ø.9Ø5	T5Ø.9Ø6
Alkalizing agent NEC	T5Ø.9Ø1	T5Ø.9Ø2	T5Ø.9Ø3	T5Ø.9Ø4	T5Ø.9Ø5	T5Ø.9Ø6
Alka-seltzer	T39.Ø11	T39.Ø12	T39.Ø13	T39.Ø14	T39.Ø15	T39.Ø16
Alkavervir	T46.5X1	T46.5X2	T46.5X3	T46.5X4	T46.5X5	T46.5X6
Alkonium (bromide)	T49.ØX1	T49.ØX2	T49.ØX3	T49.ØX4	T49.ØX5	T49.ØX6
Alkylating drug NEC	T45.1X1	T45.1X2	T45.1X3	T45.1X4	T45.1X5	T45.1X6
antimyeloproliferative	T45.1X1	T45.1X2	T45.1X3	T45.1X4	T45.1X5	T45.1X6
lymphatic	T45.1X1	T45.1X2	T45.1X3	T45.1X4	T45.1X5	T45.1X6
Alkylisocyanate	T65.ØX1	T65.ØX2	T65.ØX3	T65.ØX4	—	—
Allantoin	T49.4X1	T49.4X2	T49.4X3	T49.4X4	T49.4X5	T49.4X6
Allegron	T43.Ø11	T43.Ø12	T43.Ø13	T43.Ø14	T43.Ø15	T43.Ø16
Allethrin	T49.ØX1	T49.ØX2	T49.ØX3	T49.ØX4	T49.ØX5	T49.ØX6
Allobarbital	T42.3X1	T42.3X2	T42.3X3	T42.3X4	T42.3X5	T42.3X6
Allopurinol	T5Ø.4X1	T5Ø.4X2	T5Ø.4X3	T5Ø.4X4	T5Ø.4X5	T5Ø.4X6
Allyl						
alcohol	T51.8X1	T51.8X2	T51.8X3	T51.8X4	—	—
disulfide	T46.6X1	T46.6X2	T46.6X3	T46.6X4	T46.6X5	T46.6X6
Allylestrenol	T38.5X1	T38.5X2	T38.5X3	T38.5X4	T38.5X5	T38.5X6
Allylisopropylacetylurea	T42.6X1	T42.6X2	T42.6X3	T42.6X4	T42.6X5	T42.6X6
Allylisopropylmalonylurea	T42.3X1	T42.3X2	T42.3X3	T42.3X4	T42.3X5	T42.3X6
Allylthiourea	T49.3X1	T49.3X2	T49.3X3	T49.3X4	T49.3X5	T49.3X6
Allyltribromide	T42.6X1	T42.6X2	T42.6X3	T42.6X4	T42.6X5	T42.6X6
Allypropymal	T42.3X1	T42.3X2	T42.3X3	T42.3X4	T42.3X5	T42.3X6
Almagate	T47.1X1	T47.1X2	T47.1X3	T47.1X4	T47.1X5	T47.1X6
Almasilate	T47.1X1	T47.1X2	T47.1X3	T47.1X4	T47.1X5	T47.1X6
Almitrine	T5Ø.7X1	T5Ø.7X2	T5Ø.7X3	T5Ø.7X4	T5Ø.7X5	T5Ø.7X6
Aloes	T47.2X1	T47.2X2	T47.2X3	T47.2X4	T47.2X5	T47.2X6
Aloglutamol	T47.1X1	T47.1X2	T47.1X3	T47.1X4	T47.1X5	T47.1X6
Aloin	T47.2X1	T47.2X2	T47.2X3	T47.2X4	T47.2X5	T47.2X6
Aloxidone	T42.2X1	T42.2X2	T42.2X3	T42.2X4	T42.2X5	T42.2X6
Alpha						
acetyldigoxin	T46.ØX1	T46.ØX2	T46.ØX3	T46.ØX4	T46.ØX5	T46.ØX6
adrenergic blocking drug	T44.6X1	T44.6X2	T44.6X3	T44.6X4	T44.6X5	T44.6X6
amylase	T45.3X1	T45.3X2	T45.3X3	T45.3X4	T45.3X5	T45.3X6
tocoferol (acetate)	T45.2X1	T45.2X2	T45.2X3	T45.2X4	T45.2X5	T45.2X6
tocopherol	T45.2X1	T45.2X2	T45.2X3	T45.2X4	T45.2X5	T45.2X6
Alphadolone	T41.1X1	T41.1X2	T41.1X3	T41.1X4	T41.1X5	T41.1X6
Alphaprodine	T4Ø.491	T4Ø.492	T4Ø.493	T4Ø.494	T4Ø.495	T4Ø.496
Alphaxalone	T41.1X1	T41.1X2	T41.1X3	T41.1X4	T41.1X5	T41.1X6
Alprazolam	T42.4X1	T42.4X2	T42.4X3	T42.4X4	T42.4X5	T42.4X6
Alprenolol	T44.7X1	T44.7X2	T44.7X3	T44.7X4	T44.7X5	T44.7X6
Alprostadil	T46.7X1	T46.7X2	T46.7X3	T46.7X4	T46.7X5	T46.7X6
Alsactide	T38.811	T38.812	T38.813	T38.814	T38.815	T38.816
Alseroxylon	T46.5X1	T46.5X2	T46.5X3	T46.5X4	T46.5X5	T46.5X6
Alteplase	T45.611	T45.612	T45.613	T45.614	T45.615	T45.616
Altizide	T5Ø.2X1	T5Ø.2X2	T5Ø.2X3	T5Ø.2X4	T5Ø.2X5	T5Ø.2X6
Altretamine	T45.1X1	T45.1X2	T45.1X3	T45.1X4	T45.1X5	T45.1X6
Alum (medicinal)	T49.4X1	T49.4X2	T49.4X3	T49.4X4	T49.4X5	T49.4X6
nonmedicinal (ammonium) (potassium)	T56.891	T56.892	T56.893	T56.894	—	—
Aluminium, aluminum						
acetate	T49.2X1	T49.2X2	T49.2X3	T49.2X4	T49.2X5	T49.2X6
solution	T49.ØX1	T49.ØX2	T49.ØX3	T49.ØX4	T49.ØX5	T49.ØX6
aspirin	T39.Ø11	T39.Ø12	T39.Ø13	T39.Ø14	T39.Ø15	T39.Ø16
bis (acetylsalicylate)	T39.Ø11	T39.Ø12	T39.Ø13	T39.Ø14	T39.Ø15	T39.Ø16
carbonate (gel, basic)	T47.1X1	T47.1X2	T47.1X3	T47.1X4	T47.1X5	T47.1X6
chlorhydroxide-complex	T47.1X1	T47.1X2	T47.1X3	T47.1X4	T47.1X5	T47.1X6
chloride	T49.2X1	T49.2X2	T49.2X3	T49.2X4	T49.2X5	T49.2X6
clofibrate	T46.6X1	T46.6X2	T46.6X3	T46.6X4	T46.6X5	T46.6X6
diacetate	T49.2X1	T49.2X2	T49.2X3	T49.2X4	T49.2X5	T49.2X6
glycinate	T47.1X1	T47.1X2	T47.1X3	T47.1X4	T47.1X5	T47.1X6
hydroxide (gel)	T47.1X1	T47.1X2	T47.1X3	T47.1X4	T47.1X5	T47.1X6
hydroxide-magnesium carb. gel	T47.1X1	T47.1X2	T47.1X3	T47.1X4	T47.1X5	T47.1X6
magnesium silicate	T47.1X1	T47.1X2	T47.1X3	T47.1X4	T47.1X5	T47.1X6
nicotinate	T46.7X1	T46.7X2	T46.7X3	T46.7X4	T46.7X5	T46.7X6
ointment (surgical) (topical)	T49.3X1	T49.3X2	T49.3X3	T49.3X4	T49.3X5	T49.3X6
phosphate	T47.1X1	T47.1X2	T47.1X3	T47.1X4	T47.1X5	T47.1X6
salicylate	T39.Ø91	T39.Ø92	T39.Ø93	T39.Ø94	T39.Ø95	T39.Ø96
silicate	T47.1X1	T47.1X2	T47.1X3	T47.1X4	T47.1X5	T47.1X6
sodium silicate	T47.1X1	T47.1X2	T47.1X3	T47.1X4	T47.1X5	T47.1X6
subacetate	T49.2X1	T49.2X2	T49.2X3	T49.2X4	T49.2X5	T49.2X6
sulfate	T49.ØX1	T49.ØX2	T49.ØX3	T49.ØX4	T49.ØX5	T49.ØX6
tannate	T47.6X1	T47.6X2	T47.6X3	T47.6X4	T47.6X5	T47.6X6

Substance	Poisoning, Accidental (unintentional)	Poisoning, Intentional Self-harm	Poisoning, Assault	Poisoning, Undetermined	Adverse Effect	Under-dosing
Aluminium, aluminum — *continued*						
topical NEC	T49.3X1	T49.3X2	T49.3X3	T49.3X4	T49.3X5	T49.3X6
Alurate	T42.3X1	T42.3X2	T42.3X3	T42.3X4	T42.3X5	T42.3X6
Alverine	T44.3X1	T44.3X2	T44.3X3	T44.3X4	T44.3X5	T44.3X6
Alvodine	T4Ø.2X1	T4Ø.2X2	T4Ø.2X3	T4Ø.2X4	T4Ø.2X5	T4Ø.2X6
Amanita phalloides	T62.ØX1	T62.ØX2	T62.ØX3	T62.ØX4	—	—
Amanitine	T62.ØX1	T62.ØX2	T62.ØX3	T62.ØX4	—	—
Amantadine	T42.8X1	T42.8X2	T42.8X3	T42.8X4	T42.8X5	T42.8X6
Ambazone	T49.6X1	T49.6X2	T49.6X3	T49.6X4	T49.6X5	T49.6X6
Ambenonium (chloride)	T44.ØX1	T44.ØX2	T44.ØX3	T44.ØX4	T44.ØX5	T44.ØX6
Ambroxol	T48.4X1	T48.4X2	T48.4X3	T48.4X4	T48.4X5	T48.4X6
Ambuphylline	T48.6X1	T48.6X2	T48.6X3	T48.6X4	T48.6X5	T48.6X6
Ambutonium bromide	T44.3X1	T44.3X2	T44.3X3	T44.3X4	T44.3X5	T44.3X6
Amcinonide	T49.ØX1	T49.ØX2	T49.ØX3	T49.ØX4	T49.ØX5	T49.ØX6
Amdinocilline	T36.ØX1	T36.ØX2	T36.ØX3	T36.ØX4	T36.ØX5	T36.ØX6
Ametazole	T5Ø.8X1	T5Ø.8X2	T5Ø.8X3	T5Ø.8X4	T5Ø.8X5	T5Ø.8X6
Amethocaine	T41.3X1	T41.3X2	T41.3X3	T41.3X4	T41.3X5	T41.3X6
regional	T41.3X1	T41.3X2	T41.3X3	T41.3X4	T41.3X5	T41.3X6
spinal	T41.3X1	T41.3X2	T41.3X3	T41.3X4	T41.3X5	T41.3X6
Amethopterin	T45.1X1	T45.1X2	T45.1X3	T45.1X4	T45.1X5	T45.1X6
Amezinium metilsulfate	T44.991	T44.992	T44.993	T44.994	T44.995	T44.996
Amfebutamone	T43.291	T43.292	T43.293	T43.294	T43.295	T43.296
Amfepramone	T5Ø.5X1	T5Ø.5X2	T5Ø.5X3	T5Ø.5X4	T5Ø.5X5	T5Ø.5X6
Amfetamine	T43.621	T43.622	T43.623	T43.624	T43.625	T43.626
Amfetaminil	T43.621	T43.622	T43.623	T43.624	T43.625	T43.626
Amfomycin	T36.8X1	T36.8X2	T36.8X3	T36.8X4	T36.8X5	T36.8X6
Amidefrine mesilate	T48.5X1	T48.5X2	T48.5X3	T48.5X4	T48.5X5	T48.5X6
Amidone	T4Ø.3X1	T4Ø.3X2	T4Ø.3X3	T4Ø.3X4	T4Ø.3X5	T4Ø.3X6
Amidopyrine	T39.2X1	T39.2X2	T39.2X3	T39.2X4	T39.2X5	T39.2X6
Amidotrizoate	T5Ø.8X1	T5Ø.8X2	T5Ø.8X3	T5Ø.8X4	T5Ø.8X5	T5Ø.8X6
Amiflamine	T43.1X1	T43.1X2	T43.1X3	T43.1X4	T43.1X5	T43.1X6
Amikacin	T36.5X1	T36.5X2	T36.5X3	T36.5X4	T36.5X5	T36.5X6
Amikhelline	T46.3X1	T46.3X2	T46.3X3	T46.3X4	T46.3X5	T46.3X6
Amiloride	T5Ø.2X1	T5Ø.2X2	T5Ø.2X3	T5Ø.2X4	T5Ø.2X5	T5Ø.2X6
Aminacrine	T49.ØX1	T49.ØX2	T49.ØX3	T49.ØX4	T49.ØX5	T49.ØX6
Amineptine	T43.Ø11	T43.Ø12	T43.Ø13	T43.Ø14	T43.Ø15	T43.Ø16
Aminitrozole	T37.3X1	T37.3X2	T37.3X3	T37.3X4	T37.3X5	T37.3X6
Aminoacetic acid (derivatives)	T5Ø.3X1	T5Ø.3X2	T5Ø.3X3	T5Ø.3X4	T5Ø.3X5	T5Ø.3X6
Amino acids	T5Ø.3X1	T5Ø.3X2	T5Ø.3X3	T5Ø.3X4	T5Ø.3X5	T5Ø.3X6
Aminoacridine	T49.ØX1	T49.ØX2	T49.ØX3	T49.ØX4	T49.ØX5	T49.ØX6
Aminobenzoic acid (-p)	T49.3X1	T49.3X2	T49.3X3	T49.3X4	T49.3X5	T49.3X6
Aminocaproic acid	T45.621	T45.622	T45.623	T45.624	T45.625	T45.626
Aminoethylisothiourium	T45.8X1	T45.8X2	T45.8X3	T45.8X4	T45.8X5	T45.8X6
Aminofenazone	T39.2X1	T39.2X2	T39.2X3	T39.2X4	T39.2X5	T39.2X6
Aminoglutethimide	T45.1X1	T45.1X2	T45.1X3	T45.1X4	T45.1X5	T45.1X6
Aminohippuric acid	T5Ø.8X1	T5Ø.8X2	T5Ø.8X3	T5Ø.8X4	T5Ø.8X5	T5Ø.8X6
Aminomethylbenzoic acid	T45.691	T45.692	T45.693	T45.694	T45.695	T45.696
Aminometradine	T5Ø.2X1	T5Ø.2X2	T5Ø.2X3	T5Ø.2X4	T5Ø.2X5	T5Ø.2X6
Aminopentamide	T44.3X1	T44.3X2	T44.3X3	T44.3X4	T44.3X5	T44.3X6
Aminophenazone	T39.2X1	T39.2X2	T39.2X3	T39.2X4	T39.2X5	T39.2X6
Aminophenol	T54.ØX1	T54.ØX2	T54.ØX3	T54.ØX4	—	—
Aminophenylpyridone	T43.591	T43.592	T43.593	T43.594	T43.595	T43.596
Aminophylline	T48.6X1	T48.6X2	T48.6X3	T48.6X4	T48.6X5	T48.6X6
Aminopterin sodium	T45.1X1	T45.1X2	T45.1X3	T45.1X4	T45.1X5	T45.1X6
Aminopyrine	T39.2X1	T39.2X2	T39.2X3	T39.2X4	T39.2X5	T39.2X6
Aminorex	T5Ø.5X1	T5Ø.5X2	T5Ø.5X3	T5Ø.5X4	T5Ø.5X5	T5Ø.5X6
Aminosalicylic acid	T37.1X1	T37.1X2	T37.1X3	T37.1X4	T37.1X5	T37.1X6
Aminosalylum	T37.1X1	T37.1X2	T37.1X3	T37.1X4	T37.1X5	T37.1X6
Amiodarone	T46.2X1	T46.2X2	T46.2X3	T46.2X4	T46.2X5	T46.2X6
Amiphenazole	T5Ø.7X1	T5Ø.7X2	T5Ø.7X3	T5Ø.7X4	T5Ø.7X5	T5Ø.7X6
Amiquinsin	T46.5X1	T46.5X2	T46.5X3	T46.5X4	T46.5X5	T46.5X6
Amisometradine	T5Ø.2X1	T5Ø.2X2	T5Ø.2X3	T5Ø.2X4	T5Ø.2X5	T5Ø.2X6
Amisulpride	T43.591	T43.592	T43.593	T43.594	T43.595	T43.596
Amitriptyline	T43.Ø11	T43.Ø12	T43.Ø13	T43.Ø14	T43.Ø15	T43.Ø16
Amitriptylinoxide	T43.Ø11	T43.Ø12	T43.Ø13	T43.Ø14	T43.Ø15	T43.Ø16
Amlexanox	T48.6X1	T48.6X2	T48.6X3	T48.6X4	T48.6X5	T48.6X6
Ammonia (fumes) (gas) (vapor)	T59.891	T59.892	T59.893	T59.894	—	—
aromatic spirit	T48.991	T48.992	T48.993	T48.994	T48.995	T48.996
liquid (household)	T54.3X1	T54.3X2	T54.3X3	T54.3X4	—	—
Ammoniated mercury	T49.ØX1	T49.ØX2	T49.ØX3	T49.ØX4	T49.ØX5	T49.ØX6
Ammonium						
acid tartrate	T49.5X1	T49.5X2	T49.5X3	T49.5X4	T49.5X5	T49.5X6
bromide	T42.6X1	T42.6X2	T42.6X3	T42.6X4	T42.6X5	T42.6X6
carbonate	T54.3X1	T54.3X2	T54.3X3	T54.3X4	—	—
chloride	T5Ø.991	T5Ø.992	T5Ø.993	T5Ø.994	T5Ø.995	T5Ø.996
expectorant	T48.4X1	T48.4X2	T48.4X3	T48.4X4	T48.4X5	T48.4X6
compounds (household) NEC	T54.3X1	T54.3X2	T54.3X3	T54.3X4	—	—
fumes (any usage)	T59.891	T59.892	T59.893	T59.894	—	—
industrial	T54.3X1	T54.3X2	T54.3X3	T54.3X4	—	—

Substance	Poisoning, Accidental (unintentional)	Poisoning, Intentional Self-harm	Poisoning, Assault	Poisoning, Undetermined	Adverse Effect	Under-dosing
Ammonium — *continued*						
ichthyosulronate	T49.4X1	T49.4X2	T49.4X3	T49.4X4	T49.4X5	T49.4X6
mandelate	T37.91	T37.92	T37.93	T37.94	T37.95	T37.96
sulfamate	T6Ø.3X1	T6Ø.3X2	T6Ø.3X3	T6Ø.3X4	—	—
sulfonate resin	T47.8X1	T47.8X2	T47.8X3	T47.8X4	T47.8X5	T47.8X6
Amobarbital (sodium)	T42.3X1	T42.3X2	T42.3X3	T42.3X4	T42.3X5	T42.3X6
Amodiaquine	T37.2X1	T37.2X2	T37.2X3	T37.2X4	T37.2X5	T37.2X6
Amopyroquin (e)	T37.2X1	T37.2X2	T37.2X3	T37.2X4	T37.2X5	T37.2X6
Amoxapine	T43.Ø11	T43.Ø12	T43.Ø13	T43.Ø14	T43.Ø15	T43.Ø16
Amoxicillin	T36.ØX1	T36.ØX2	T36.ØX3	T36.ØX4	T36.ØX5	T36.ØX6
Amperozide	T43.591	T43.592	T43.593	T43.594	T43.595	T43.596
Amphenidone	T43.591	T43.592	T43.593	T43.594	T43.595	T43.596
Amphetamine NEC	T43.621	T43.622	T43.623	T43.624	T43.625	T43.626
Amphomycin	T36.8X1	T36.8X2	T36.8X3	T36.8X4	T36.8X5	T36.8X6
Amphotalide	T37.4X1	T37.4X2	T37.4X3	T37.4X4	T37.4X5	T37.4X6
Amphotericin B	T36.7X1	T36.7X2	T36.7X3	T36.7X4	T36.7X5	T36.7X6
topical	T49.ØX1	T49.ØX2	T49.ØX3	T49.ØX4	T49.ØX5	T49.ØX6
Ampicillin	T36.ØX1	T36.ØX2	T36.ØX3	T36.ØX4	T36.ØX5	T36.ØX6
Amprotropine	T44.3X1	T44.3X2	T44.3X3	T44.3X4	T44.3X5	T44.3X6
Amsacrine	T45.1X1	T45.1X2	T45.1X3	T45.1X4	T45.1X5	T45.1X6
Amygdaline	T62.2X1	T62.2X2	T62.2X3	T62.2X4	—	—
Amyl						
acetate	T52.8X1	T52.8X2	T52.8X3	T52.8X4	—	—
vapor	T59.891	T59.892	T59.893	T59.894	—	—
alcohol	T51.3X1	T51.3X2	T51.3X3	T51.3X4	—	—
chloride	T53.6X1	T53.6X2	T53.6X3	T53.6X4	—	—
formate	T52.8X1	T52.8X2	T52.8X3	T52.8X4	—	—
nitrite	T46.3X1	T46.3X2	T46.3X3	T46.3X4	T46.3X5	T46.3X6
propionate	T65.891	T65.892	T65.893	T65.894	—	—
Amylase	T47.5X1	T47.5X2	T47.5X3	T47.5X4	T47.5X5	T47.5X6
Amyleine, regional	T41.3X1	T41.3X2	T41.3X3	T41.3X4	T41.3X5	T41.3X6
Amylene						
dichloride	T53.6X1	T53.6X2	T53.6X3	T53.6X4	—	—
hydrate	T51.3X1	T51.3X2	T51.3X3	T51.3X4	—	—
Amylmetacresol	T49.6X1	T49.6X2	T49.6X3	T49.6X4	T49.6X5	T49.6X6
Amylobarbitone	T42.3X1	T42.3X2	T42.3X3	T42.3X4	T42.3X5	T42.3X6
Amylocaine, regional	T41.3X1	T41.3X2	T41.3X3	T41.3X4	T41.3X5	T41.3X6
infiltration (subcutaneous)	T41.3X1	T41.3X2	T41.3X3	T41.3X4	T41.3X5	T41.3X6
nerve block (peripheral) (plexus)	T41.3X1	T41.3X2	T41.3X3	T41.3X4	T41.3X5	T41.3X6
spinal	T41.3X1	T41.3X2	T41.3X3	T41.3X4	T41.3X5	T41.3X6
topical (surface)	T41.3X1	T41.3X2	T41.3X3	T41.3X4	T41.3X5	T41.3X6
Amylopectin	T47.6X1	T47.6X2	T47.6X3	T47.6X4	T47.6X5	T47.6X6
Amytal (sodium)	T42.3X1	T42.3X2	T42.3X3	T42.3X4	T42.3X5	T42.3X6
Anabolic steroid	T38.7X1	T38.7X2	T38.7X3	T38.7X4	T38.7X5	T38.7X6
Analeptic NEC	T5Ø.7X1	T5Ø.7X2	T5Ø.7X3	T5Ø.7X4	T5Ø.7X5	T5Ø.7X6
Analgesic	T39.91	T39.92	T39.93	T39.94	T39.95	T39.96
anti-inflammatory NEC	T39.91	T39.92	T39.93	T39.94	T39.95	T39.96
propionic acid derivative	T39.311	T39.312	T39.313	T39.314	T39.315	T39.316
antirheumatic NEC	T39.4X1	T39.4X2	T39.4X3	T39.4X4	T39.4X5	T39.4X6
aromatic NEC	T39.1X1	T39.1X2	T39.1X3	T39.1X4	T39.1X5	T39.1X6
narcotic NEC	T4Ø.6Ø1	T4Ø.6Ø2	T4Ø.6Ø3	T4Ø.6Ø4	T4Ø.6Ø5	T4Ø.6Ø6
combination	T4Ø.6Ø1	T4Ø.6Ø2	T4Ø.6Ø3	T4Ø.6Ø4	T4Ø.6Ø5	T4Ø.6Ø6
obstetric	T4Ø.6Ø1	T4Ø.6Ø2	T4Ø.6Ø3	T4Ø.6Ø4	T4Ø.6Ø5	T4Ø.6Ø6
non-narcotic NEC	T39.91	T39.92	T39.93	T39.94	T39.95	T39.96
combination	T39.91	T39.92	T39.93	T39.94	T39.95	T39.96
pyrazole	T39.2X1	T39.2X2	T39.2X3	T39.2X4	T39.2X5	T39.2X6
specified NEC	T39.8X1	T39.8X2	T39.8X3	T39.8X4	T39.8X5	T39.8X6
Analgin	T39.2X1	T39.2X2	T39.2X3	T39.2X4	T39.2X5	T39.2X6
Anamirta cocculus	T62.1X1	T62.1X2	T62.1X3	T62.1X4	—	—
Ancillin	T36.ØX1	T36.ØX2	T36.ØX3	T36.ØX4	T36.ØX5	T36.ØX6
Ancrod	T45.691	T45.692	T45.693	T45.694	T45.695	T45.696
Androgen	T38.7X1	T38.7X2	T38.7X3	T38.7X4	T38.7X5	T38.7X6
Androgen-estrogen mixture	T38.7X1	T38.7X2	T38.7X3	T38.7X4	T38.7X5	T38.7X6
Androstalone	T38.7X1	T38.7X2	T38.7X3	T38.7X4	T38.7X5	T38.7X6
Androstanolone	T38.7X1	T38.7X2	T38.7X3	T38.7X4	T38.7X5	T38.7X6
Androsterone	T38.7X1	T38.7X2	T38.7X3	T38.7X4	T38.7X5	T38.7X6
Anemone pulsatilla	T62.2X1	T62.2X2	T62.2X3	T62.2X4	—	—
Anesthesia						
caudal	T41.3X1	T41.3X2	T41.3X3	T41.3X4	T41.3X5	T41.3X6
endotracheal	T41.ØX1	T41.ØX2	T41.ØX3	T41.ØX4	T41.ØX5	T41.ØX6
epidural	T41.3X1	T41.3X2	T41.3X3	T41.3X4	T41.3X5	T41.3X6
inhalation	T41.ØX1	T41.ØX2	T41.ØX3	T41.ØX4	T41.ØX5	T41.ØX6
local	T41.3X1	T41.3X2	T41.3X3	T41.3X4	T41.3X5	T41.3X6
mucosal	T41.3X1	T41.3X2	T41.3X3	T41.3X4	T41.3X5	T41.3X6
muscle relaxation	T48.1X1	T48.1X2	T48.1X3	T48.1X4	T48.1X5	T48.1X6
nerve blocking	T41.3X1	T41.3X2	T41.3X3	T41.3X4	T41.3X5	T41.3X6
plexus blocking	T41.3X1	T41.3X2	T41.3X3	T41.3X4	T41.3X5	T41.3X6
potentiated	T41.2Ø1	T41.2Ø2	T41.2Ø3	T41.2Ø4	T41.2Ø5	T41.2Ø6
rectal	T41.2Ø1	T41.2Ø2	T41.2Ø3	T41.2Ø4	T41.2Ø5	T41.2Ø6
general	T41.2Ø1	T41.2Ø2	T41.2Ø3	T41.2Ø4	T41.2Ø5	T41.2Ø6
local	T41.3X1	T41.3X2	T41.3X3	T41.3X4	T41.3X5	T41.3X6

Substance	Poisoning, Accidental (unintentional)	Poisoning, Intentional Self-harm	Poisoning, Assault	Poisoning, Undetermined	Adverse Effect	Under-dosing
Anesthesia — *continued*						
regional	T41.3X1	T41.3X2	T41.3X3	T41.3X4	T41.3X5	T41.3X6
surface	T41.3X1	T41.3X2	T41.3X3	T41.3X4	T41.3X5	T41.3X6
Anesthetic NEC — *see also* Anesthesia	T41.41	T41.42	T41.43	T41.44	T41.45	T41.46
with muscle relaxant	T41.2Ø1	T41.2Ø2	T41.2Ø3	T41.2Ø4	T41.2Ø5	T41.2Ø6
general	T41.2Ø1	T41.2Ø2	T41.2Ø3	T41.2Ø4	T41.2Ø5	T41.2Ø6
local	T41.3X1	T41.3X2	T41.3X3	T41.3X4	T41.3X5	T41.3X6
gaseous NEC	T41.ØX1	T41.ØX2	T41.ØX3	T41.ØX4	T41.ØX5	T41.ØX6
general NEC	T41.2Ø1	T41.2Ø2	T41.2Ø3	T41.2Ø4	T41.2Ø5	T41.2Ø6
halogenated hydrocarbon derivatives NEC	T41.ØX1	T41.ØX2	T41.ØX3	T41.ØX4	T41.ØX5	T41.ØX6
infiltration NEC	T41.3X1	T41.3X2	T41.3X3	T41.3X4	T41.3X5	T41.3X6
intravenous NEC	T41.1X1	T41.1X2	T41.1X3	T41.1X4	T41.1X5	T41.1X6
local NEC	T41.3X1	T41.3X2	T41.3X3	T41.3X4	T41.3X5	T41.3X6
rectal	T41.2Ø1	T41.2Ø2	T41.2Ø3	T41.2Ø4	T41.2Ø5	T41.2Ø6
general	T41.2Ø1	T41.2Ø2	T41.2Ø3	T41.2Ø4	T41.2Ø5	T41.2Ø6
local	T41.3X1	T41.3X2	T41.3X3	T41.3X4	T41.3X5	T41.3X6
regional NEC	T41.3X1	T41.3X2	T41.3X3	T41.3X4	T41.3X5	T41.3X6
spinal NEC	T41.3X1	T41.3X2	T41.3X3	T41.3X4	T41.3X5	T41.3X6
thiobarbiturate	T41.1X1	T41.1X2	T41.1X3	T41.1X4	T41.1X5	T41.1X6
topical	T41.3X1	T41.3X2	T41.3X3	T41.3X4	T41.3X5	T41.3X6
Aneurine	T45.2X1	T45.2X2	T45.2X3	T45.2X4	T45.2X5	T45.2X6
Angio-Conray	T5Ø.8X1	T5Ø.8X2	T5Ø.8X3	T5Ø.8X4	T5Ø.8X5	T5Ø.8X6
Angiotensin	T44.5X1	T44.5X2	T44.5X3	T44.5X4	T44.5X5	T44.5X6
Angiotensinamide	T44.991	T44.992	T44.993	T44.994	T44.995	T44.996
Anhydrohydroxy-progesterone	T38.5X1	T38.5X2	T38.5X3	T38.5X4	T38.5X5	T38.5X6
Anhydron	T5Ø.2X1	T5Ø.2X2	T5Ø.2X3	T5Ø.2X4	T5Ø.2X5	T5Ø.2X6
Anileridine	T4Ø.491	T4Ø.492	T4Ø.493	T4Ø.494	T4Ø.495	T4Ø.496
Aniline (dye) (liquid)	T65.3X1	T65.3X2	T65.3X3	T65.3X4	—	—
analgesic	T39.1X1	T39.1X2	T39.1X3	T39.1X4	T39.1X5	T39.1X6
derivatives, therapeutic NEC	T39.1X1	T39.1X2	T39.1X3	T39.1X4	T39.1X5	T39.1X6
vapor	T65.3X1	T65.3X2	T65.3X3	T65.3X4	—	—
Aniscoropine	T44.3X1	T44.3X2	T44.3X3	T44.3X4	T44.3X5	T44.3X6
Anise oil	T47.5X1	T47.5X2	T47.5X3	T47.5X4	T47.5X5	T47.5X6
Anisidine	T65.3X1	T65.3X2	T65.3X3	T65.3X4	—	—
Anisindione	T45.511	T45.512	T45.513	T45.514	T45.515	T45.516
Anisotropine methyl-bromide	T44.3X1	T44.3X2	T44.3X3	T44.3X4	T44.3X5	T44.3X6
Anistreplase	T45.611	T45.612	T45.613	T45.614	T45.615	T45.616
Anorexiant (central)	T5Ø.5X1	T5Ø.5X2	T5Ø.5X3	T5Ø.5X4	T5Ø.5X5	T5Ø.5X6
Anorexic agents	T5Ø.5X1	T5Ø.5X2	T5Ø.5X3	T5Ø.5X4	T5Ø.5X5	T5Ø.5X6
Ansamycin	T36.6X1	T36.6X2	T36.6X3	T36.6X4	T36.6X5	T36.6X6
Ant (bite) (sting)	T63.421	T63.422	T63.423	T63.424	—	—
Antabuse	T5Ø.6X1	T5Ø.6X2	T5Ø.6X3	T5Ø.6X4	T5Ø.6X5	T5Ø.6X6
Antacid NEC	T47.1X1	T47.1X2	T47.1X3	T47.1X4	T47.1X5	T47.1X6
Antagonist						
Aldosterone	T5Ø.ØX1	T5Ø.ØX2	T5Ø.ØX3	T5Ø.ØX4	T5Ø.ØX5	T5Ø.ØX6
alpha-adrenoreceptor	T44.6X1	T44.6X2	T44.6X3	T44.6X4	T44.6X5	T44.6X6
anticoagulant	T45.7X1	T45.7X2	T45.7X3	T45.7X4	T45.7X5	T45.7X6
beta-adrenoreceptor	T44.7X1	T44.7X2	T44.7X3	T44.7X4	T44.7X5	T44.7X6
extrapyramidal NEC	T44.3X1	T44.3X2	T44.3X3	T44.3X4	T44.3X5	T44.3X6
folic acid	T45.1X1	T45.1X2	T45.1X3	T45.1X4	T45.1X5	T45.1X6
H2 receptor	T47.ØX1	T47.ØX2	T47.ØX3	T47.ØX4	T47.ØX5	T47.ØX6
heavy metal	T45.8X1	T45.8X2	T45.8X3	T45.8X4	T45.8X5	T45.8X6
narcotic analgesic	T5Ø.7X1	T5Ø.7X2	T5Ø.7X3	T5Ø.7X4	T5Ø.7X5	T5Ø.7X6
opiate	T5Ø.7X1	T5Ø.7X2	T5Ø.7X3	T5Ø.7X4	T5Ø.7X5	T5Ø.7X6
pyrimidine	T45.1X1	T45.1X2	T45.1X3	T45.1X4	T45.1X5	T45.1X6
serotonin	T46.5X1	T46.5X2	T46.5X3	T46.5X4	T46.5X5	T46.5X6
Antazolin (e)	T45.ØX1	T45.ØX2	T45.ØX3	T45.ØX4	T45.ØX5	T45.ØX6
Anterior pituitary hormone NEC	T38.811	T38.812	T38.813	T38.814	T38.815	T38.816
Anthelmintic NEC	T37.4X1	T37.4X2	T37.4X3	T37.4X4	T37.4X5	T37.4X6
Anthiolimine	T37.4X1	T37.4X2	T37.4X3	T37.4X4	T37.4X5	T37.4X6
Anthralin	T49.4X1	T49.4X2	T49.4X3	T49.4X4	T49.4X5	T49.4X6
Anthramycin	T45.1X1	T45.1X2	T45.1X3	T45.1X4	T45.1X5	T45.1X6
Antiadrenergic NEC	T44.8X1	T44.8X2	T44.8X3	T44.8X4	T44.8X5	T44.8X6
Antiallergic NEC	T45.ØX1	T45.ØX2	T45.ØX3	T45.ØX4	T45.ØX5	T45.ØX6
Antiandrogen NEC	T38.6X1	T38.6X2	T38.6X3	T38.6X4	T38.6X5	T38.6X6
Anti-anemic (drug) (preparation)	T45.8X1	T45.8X2	T45.8X3	T45.8X4	T45.8X5	T45.8X6
Antianxiety drug NEC	T43.5Ø1	T43.5Ø2	T43.5Ø3	T43.5Ø4	T43.5Ø5	T43.5Ø6
Antiaris toxicaria	T65.891	T65.892	T65.893	T65.894	—	—
Antiarteriosclerotic drug	T46.6X1	T46.6X2	T46.6X3	T46.6X4	T46.6X5	T46.6X6
Antiasthmatic drug NEC	T48.6X1	T48.6X2	T48.6X3	T48.6X4	T48.6X5	T48.6X6
Antibiotic NEC	T36.91	T36.92	T36.93	T36.94	T36.95	T36.96
aminoglycoside	T36.5X1	T36.5X2	T36.5X3	T36.5X4	T36.5X5	T36.5X6
anticancer	T45.1X1	T45.1X2	T45.1X3	T45.1X4	T45.1X5	T45.1X6
antifungal	T36.7X1	T36.7X2	T36.7X3	T36.7X4	T36.7X5	T36.7X6
antimycobacterial	T36.5X1	T36.5X2	T36.5X3	T36.5X4	T36.5X5	T36.5X6
antineoplastic	T45.1X1	T45.1X2	T45.1X3	T45.1X4	T45.1X5	T45.1X6
b-lactam NEC	T36.1X1	T36.1X2	T36.1X3	T36.1X4	T36.1X5	T36.1X6

Substance	Poisoning, Accidental (unintentional)	Poisoning, Intentional Self-harm	Poisoning, Assault	Poisoning, Undetermined	Adverse Effect	Under-dosing
Antibiotic — *continued*						
cephalosporin (group)	T36.1X1	T36.1X2	T36.1X3	T36.1X4	T36.1X5	T36.1X6
chloramphenicol (group)	T36.2X1	T36.2X2	T36.2X3	T36.2X4	T36.2X5	T36.2X6
ENT	T49.6X1	T49.6X2	T49.6X3	T49.6X4	T49.6X5	T49.6X6
eye	T49.5X1	T49.5X2	T49.5X3	T49.5X4	T49.5X5	T49.5X6
fungicidal (local)	T49.ØX1	T49.ØX2	T49.ØX3	T49.ØX4	T49.ØX5	T49.ØX6
intestinal	T36.8X1	T36.8X2	T36.8X3	T36.8X4	T36.8X5	T36.8X6
local	T49.ØX1	T49.ØX2	T49.ØX3	T49.ØX4	T49.ØX5	T49.ØX6
macrolides	T36.3X1	T36.3X2	T36.3X3	T36.3X4	T36.3X5	T36.3X6
polypeptide	T36.8X1	T36.8X2	T36.8X3	T36.8X4	T36.8X5	T36.8X6
specified NEC	T36.8X1	T36.8X2	T36.8X3	T36.8X4	T36.8X5	T36.8X6
tetracycline (group)	T36.4X1	T36.4X2	T36.4X3	T36.4X4	T36.4X5	T36.4X6
throat	T49.6X1	T49.6X2	T49.6X3	T49.6X4	T49.6X5	T49.6X6
Anticancer agents NEC	T45.1X1	T45.1X2	T45.1X3	T45.1X4	T45.1X5	T45.1X6
Anticholesterolemic drug NEC	T46.6X1	T46.6X2	T46.6X3	T46.6X4	T46.6X5	T46.6X6
Anticholinergic NEC	T44.3X1	T44.3X2	T44.3X3	T44.3X4	T44.3X5	T44.3X6
Anticholinesterase	T44.ØX1	T44.ØX2	T44.ØX3	T44.ØX4	T44.ØX5	T44.ØX6
organophosphorus	T44.ØX1	T44.ØX2	T44.ØX3	T44.ØX4	T44.ØX5	T44.ØX6
insecticide	T6Ø.ØX1	T6Ø.ØX2	T6Ø.ØX3	T6Ø.ØX4	—	—
nerve gas	T59.891	T59.892	T59.893	T59.894	—	—
reversible	T44.ØX1	T44.ØX2	T44.ØX3	T44.ØX4	T44.ØX5	T44.ØX6
ophthalmological	T49.5X1	T49.5X2	T49.5X3	T49.5X4	T49.5X5	T49.5X6
Anticoagulant NEC	T45.511	T45.512	T45.513	T45.514	T45.515	T45.516
Antagonist	T45.7X1	T45.7X2	T45.7X3	T45.7X4	T45.7X5	T45.7X6
Anti-common-cold drug NEC	T48.5X1	T48.5X2	T48.5X3	T48.5X4	T48.5X5	T48.5X6
Anticonvulsant	T42.71	T42.72	T42.73	T42.74	T42.75	T42.76
barbiturate	T42.3X1	T42.3X2	T42.3X3	T42.3X4	T42.3X5	T42.3X6
combination (with barbiturate)	T42.3X1	T42.3X2	T42.3X3	T42.3X4	T42.3X5	T42.3X6
hydantoin	T42.ØX1	T42.ØX2	T42.ØX3	T42.ØX4	T42.ØX5	T42.ØX6
hypnotic NEC	T42.6X1	T42.6X2	T42.6X3	T42.6X4	T42.6X5	T42.6X6
oxazolidinedione	T42.2X1	T42.2X2	T42.2X3	T42.2X4	T42.2X5	T42.2X6
pyrimidinedione	T42.6X1	T42.6X2	T42.6X3	T42.6X4	T42.6X5	T42.6X6
specified NEC	T42.6X1	T42.6X2	T42.6X3	T42.6X4	T42.6X5	T42.6X6
succinimide	T42.2X1	T42.2X2	T42.2X3	T42.2X4	T42.2X5	T42.2X6
Antidepressant	T43.2Ø1	T43.2Ø2	T43.2Ø3	T43.2Ø4	T43.2Ø5	T43.2Ø6
monoamine oxidase inhibitor	T43.1X1	T43.1X2	T43.1X3	T43.1X4	T43.1X5	T43.1X6
selective serotonin norepinephrine reuptake inhibitor	T43.211	T43.212	T43.213	T43.214	T43.215	T43.216
selective serotonin reuptake inhibitor	T43.221	T43.222	T43.223	T43.224	T43.225	T43.226
specified NEC	T43.291	T43.292	T43.293	T43.294	T43.295	T43.296
tetracyclic	T43.Ø21	T43.Ø22	T43.Ø23	T43.Ø24	T43.Ø25	T43.Ø26
triazolopyridine	T43.211	T43.212	T43.213	T43.214	T43.215	T43.216
tricyclic	T43.Ø11	T43.Ø12	T43.Ø13	T43.Ø14	T43.Ø15	T43.Ø16
Antidiabetic NEC	T38.3X1	T38.3X2	T38.3X3	T38.3X4	T38.3X5	T38.3X6
biguanide	T38.3X1	T38.3X2	T38.3X3	T38.3X4	T38.3X5	T38.3X6
and sulfonyl combined	T38.3X1	T38.3X2	T38.3X3	T38.3X4	T38.3X5	T38.3X6
combined	T38.3X1	T38.3X2	T38.3X3	T38.3X4	T38.3X5	T38.3X6
sulfonylurea	T38.3X1	T38.3X2	T38.3X3	T38.3X4	T38.3X5	T38.3X6
Antidiarrheal drug NEC	T47.6X1	T47.6X2	T47.6X3	T47.6X4	T47.6X5	T47.6X6
absorbent	T47.6X1	T47.6X2	T47.6X3	T47.6X4	T47.6X5	T47.6X6
Anti-D immunoglobulin (human)	T5Ø.Z11	T5Ø.Z12	T5Ø.Z13	T5Ø.Z14	T5Ø.Z15	T5Ø.Z16
Antidiphtheria serum	T5Ø.Z11	T5Ø.Z12	T5Ø.Z13	T5Ø.Z14	T5Ø.Z15	T5Ø.Z16
Antidiuretic hormone	T38.891	T38.892	T38.893	T38.894	T38.895	T38.896
Antidote NEC	T5Ø.6X1	T5Ø.6X2	T5Ø.6X3	T5Ø.6X4	T5Ø.6X5	T5Ø.6X6
heavy metal	T45.8X1	T45.8X2	T45.8X3	T45.8X4	T45.8X5	T45.8X6
Antidysrhythmic NEC	T46.2X1	T46.2X2	T46.2X3	T46.2X4	T46.2X5	T46.2X6
Antiemetic drug	T45.ØX1	T45.ØX2	T45.ØX3	T45.ØX4	T45.ØX5	T45.ØX6
Antiepilepsy agent	T42.71	T42.72	T42.73	T42.74	T42.75	T42.76
combination	T42.5X1	T42.5X2	T42.5X3	T42.5X4	T42.5X5	T42.5X6
mixed	T42.5X1	T42.5X2	T42.5X3	T42.5X4	T42.5X5	T42.5X6
specified, NEC	T42.6X1	T42.6X2	T42.6X3	T42.6X4	T42.6X5	T42.6X6
Antiestrogen NEC	T38.6X1	T38.6X2	T38.6X3	T38.6X4	T38.6X5	T38.6X6
Antifertility pill	T38.4X1	T38.4X2	T38.4X3	T38.4X4	T38.4X5	T38.4X6
Antifibrinolytic drug	T45.621	T45.622	T45.623	T45.624	T45.625	T45.626
Antifilarial drug	T37.4X1	T37.4X2	T37.4X3	T37.4X4	T37.4X5	T37.4X6
Antiflatulent	T47.5X1	T47.5X2	T47.5X3	T47.5X4	T47.5X5	T47.5X6
Antifreeze	T65.91	T65.92	T65.93	T65.94	—	—
alcohol	T51.1X1	T51.1X2	T51.1X3	T51.1X4	—	—
ethylene glycol	T51.8X1	T51.8X2	T51.8X3	T51.8X4	—	—
Antifungal						
antibiotic (systemic)	T36.7X1	T36.7X2	T36.7X3	T36.7X4	T36.7X5	T36.7X6
anti-infective NEC	T37.91	T37.92	T37.93	T37.94	T37.95	T37.96
disinfectant, local	T49.ØX1	T49.ØX2	T49.ØX3	T49.ØX4	T49.ØX5	T49.ØX6
nonmedicinal (spray)	T6Ø.3X1	T6Ø.3X2	T6Ø.3X3	T6Ø.3X4	—	—
topical	T49.ØX1	T49.ØX2	T49.ØX3	T49.ØX4	T49.ØX5	T49.ØX6

Substance	Poisoning, Accidental (unintentional)	Poisoning, Intentional Self-harm	Poisoning, Assault	Poisoning, Undetermined	Adverse Effect	Under-dosing
Anti-gastric-secretion drug NEC	T47.1X1	T47.1X2	T47.1X3	T47.1X4	T47.1X5	T47.1X6
Antigonadotrophin NEC	T38.6X1	T38.6X2	T38.6X3	T38.6X4	T38.6X5	T38.6X6
Antihallucinogen	T43.5Ø1	T43.5Ø2	T43.5Ø3	T43.5Ø4	T43.5Ø5	T43.5Ø6
Antihelmintics	T37.4X1	T37.4X2	T37.4X3	T37.4X4	T37.4X5	T37.4X6
Antihemophilic						
factor	T45.8X1	T45.8X2	T45.8X3	T45.8X4	T45.8X5	T45.8X6
fraction	T45.8X1	T45.8X2	T45.8X3	T45.8X4	T45.8X5	T45.8X6
globulin concentrate	T45.7X1	T45.7X2	T45.7X3	T45.7X4	T45.7X5	T45.7X6
human plasma	T45.8X1	T45.8X2	T45.8X3	T45.8X4	T45.8X5	T45.8X6
plasma, dried	T45.7X1	T45.7X2	T45.7X3	T45.7X4	T45.7X5	T45.7X6
Antihemorrhoidal preparation	T49.2X1	T49.2X2	T49.2X3	T49.2X4	T49.2X5	T49.2X6
Antiheparin drug	T45.7X1	T45.7X2	T45.7X3	T45.7X4	T45.7X5	T45.7X6
Antihistamine	T45.ØX1	T45.ØX2	T45.ØX3	T45.ØX4	T45.ØX5	T45.ØX6
Antihookworm drug	T37.4X1	T37.4X2	T37.4X3	T37.4X4	T37.4X5	T37.4X6
Anti-human lymphocytic globulin	T5Ø.Z11	T5Ø.Z12	T5Ø.Z13	T5Ø.Z14	T5Ø.Z15	T5Ø.Z16
Antihyperlipidemic drug	T46.6X1	T46.6X2	T46.6X3	T46.6X4	T46.6X5	T46.6X6
Antihypertensive drug NEC	T46.5X1	T46.5X2	T46.5X3	T46.5X4	T46.5X5	T46.5X6
Anti-infective NEC	T37.91	T37.92	T37.93	T37.94	T37.95	T37.96
anthelmintic	T37.4X1	T37.4X2	T37.4X3	T37.4X4	T37.4X5	T37.4X6
antibiotics	T36.91	T36.92	T36.93	T36.94	T36.95	T36.96
specified NEC	T36.8X1	T36.8X2	T36.8X3	T36.8X4	T36.8X5	T36.8X6
antimalarial	T37.2X1	T37.2X2	T37.2X3	T37.2X4	T37.2X5	T37.2X6
antimycobacterial NEC	T37.1X1	T37.1X2	T37.1X3	T37.1X4	T37.1X5	T37.1X6
antibiotics	T36.5X1	T36.5X2	T36.5X3	T36.5X4	T36.5X5	T36.5X6
antiprotozoal NEC	T37.3X1	T37.3X2	T37.3X3	T37.3X4	T37.3X5	T37.3X6
blood	T37.2X1	T37.2X2	T37.2X3	T37.2X4	T37.2X5	T37.2X6
antiviral	T37.5X1	T37.5X2	T37.5X3	T37.5X4	T37.5X5	T37.5X6
arsenical	T37.8X1	T37.8X2	T37.8X3	T37.8X4	T37.8X5	T37.8X6
bismuth, local	T49.ØX1	T49.ØX2	T49.ØX3	T49.ØX4	T49.ØX5	T49.ØX6
ENT	T49.6X1	T49.6X2	T49.6X3	T49.6X4	T49.6X5	T49.6X6
eye NEC	T49.5X1	T49.5X2	T49.5X3	T49.5X4	T49.5X5	T49.5X6
heavy metals NEC	T37.8X1	T37.8X2	T37.8X3	T37.8X4	T37.8X5	T37.8X6
local NEC	T49.ØX1	T49.ØX2	T49.ØX3	T49.ØX4	T49.ØX5	T49.ØX6
specified NEC	T49.ØX1	T49.ØX2	T49.ØX3	T49.ØX4	T49.ØX5	T49.ØX6
mixed	T37.91	T37.92	T37.93	T37.94	T37.95	T37.96
ophthalmic preparation	T49.5X1	T49.5X2	T49.5X3	T49.5X4	T49.5X5	T49.5X6
topical NEC	T49.ØX1	T49.ØX2	T49.ØX3	T49.ØX4	T49.ØX5	T49.ØX6
Anti-inflammatory drug NEC	T39.391	T39.392	T39.393	T39.394	T39.395	T39.396
local	T49.ØX1	T49.ØX2	T49.ØX3	T49.ØX4	T49.ØX5	T49.ØX6
nonsteroidal NEC	T39.391	T39.392	T39.393	T39.394	T39.395	T39.396
propionic acid derivative	T39.311	T39.312	T39.313	T39.314	T39.315	T39.316
specified NEC	T39.391	T39.392	T39.393	T39.394	T39.395	T39.396
Antikaluretic	T5Ø.3X1	T5Ø.3X2	T5Ø.3X3	T5Ø.3X4	T5Ø.3X5	T5Ø.3X6
Antiknock (tetraethyl lead)	T56.ØX1	T56.ØX2	T56.ØX3	T56.ØX4	—	—
Antilipemic drug NEC	T46.6X1	T46.6X2	T46.6X3	T46.6X4	T46.6X5	T46.6X6
Antimalarial	T37.2X1	T37.2X2	T37.2X3	T37.2X4	T37.2X5	T37.2X6
prophylactic NEC	T37.2X1	T37.2X2	T37.2X3	T37.2X4	T37.2X5	T37.2X6
pyrimidine derivative	T37.2X1	T37.2X2	T37.2X3	T37.2X4	T37.2X5	T37.2X6
Antimetabolite	T45.1X1	T45.1X2	T45.1X3	T45.1X4	T45.1X5	T45.1X6
Antimitotic agent	T45.1X1	T45.1X2	T45.1X3	T45.1X4	T45.1X5	T45.1X6
Antimony (compounds) (vapor) **NEC**	T56.891	T56.892	T56.893	T56.894	—	—
anti-infectives	T37.8X1	T37.8X2	T37.8X3	T37.8X4	T37.8X5	T37.8X6
dimercaptosuccinate	T37.3X1	T37.3X2	T37.3X3	T37.3X4	T37.3X5	T37.3X6
hydride	T56.891	T56.892	T56.893	T56.894	—	—
pesticide (vapor)	T6Ø.8X1	T6Ø.8X2	T6Ø.8X3	T6Ø.8X4	—	—
potassium (sodium) tartrate	T37.8X1	T37.8X2	T37.8X3	T37.8X4	T37.8X5	T37.8X6
sodium dimercaptosuccinate	T37.3X1	T37.3X2	T37.3X3	T37.3X4	T37.3X5	T37.3X6
tartrated	T37.8X1	T37.8X2	T37.8X3	T37.8X4	T37.8X5	T37.8X6
Antimuscarinic NEC	T44.3X1	T44.3X2	T44.3X3	T44.3X4	T44.3X5	T44.3X6
Antimycobacterial drug NEC	T37.1X1	T37.1X2	T37.1X3	T37.1X4	T37.1X5	T37.1X6
antibiotics	T36.5X1	T36.5X2	T36.5X3	T36.5X4	T36.5X5	T36.5X6
combination	T37.1X1	T37.1X2	T37.1X3	T37.1X4	T37.1X5	T37.1X6
Antinausea drug	T45.ØX1	T45.ØX2	T45.ØX3	T45.ØX4	T45.ØX5	T45.ØX6
Antinematode drug	T37.4X1	T37.4X2	T37.4X3	T37.4X4	T37.4X5	T37.4X6
Antineoplastic NEC	T45.1X1	T45.1X2	T45.1X3	T45.1X4	T45.1X5	T45.1X6
alkaloidal	T45.1X1	T45.1X2	T45.1X3	T45.1X4	T45.1X5	T45.1X6
antibiotics	T45.1X1	T45.1X2	T45.1X3	T45.1X4	T45.1X5	T45.1X6
combination	T45.1X1	T45.1X2	T45.1X3	T45.1X4	T45.1X5	T45.1X6
estrogen	T38.5X1	T38.5X2	T38.5X3	T38.5X4	T38.5X5	T38.5X6
steroid	T38.7X1	T38.7X2	T38.7X3	T38.7X4	T38.7X5	T38.7X6
Antiparasitic drug (systemic)	T37.91	T37.92	T37.93	T37.94	T37.95	T37.96
local	T49.ØX1	T49.ØX2	T49.ØX3	T49.ØX4	T49.ØX5	T49.ØX6
specified NEC	T37.8X1	T37.8X2	T37.8X3	T37.8X4	T37.8X5	T37.8X6
Antiparkinsonism drug NEC	T42.8X1	T42.8X2	T42.8X3	T42.8X4	T42.8X5	T42.8X6
Antiperspirant NEC	T49.2X1	T49.2X2	T49.2X3	T49.2X4	T49.2X5	T49.2X6
Antiphlogistic NEC	T39.4X1	T39.4X2	T39.4X3	T39.4X4	T39.4X5	T39.4X6
Antiplatyhelmintic drug	T37.4X1	T37.4X2	T37.4X3	T37.4X4	T37.4X5	T37.4X6
Antiprotozoal drug NEC	T37.3X1	T37.3X2	T37.3X3	T37.3X4	T37.3X5	T37.3X6
blood	T37.2X1	T37.2X2	T37.2X3	T37.2X4	T37.2X5	T37.2X6
local	T49.ØX1	T49.ØX2	T49.ØX3	T49.ØX4	T49.ØX5	T49.ØX6
Antipruritic drug NEC	T49.1X1	T49.1X2	T49.1X3	T49.1X4	T49.1X5	T49.1X6
Antipsychotic drug	T43.5Ø1	T43.5Ø2	T43.5Ø3	T43.5Ø4	T43.5Ø5	T43.5Ø6
specified NEC	T43.591	T43.592	T43.593	T43.594	T43.595	T43.596
Antipyretic	T39.91	T39.92	T39.93	T39.94	T39.95	T39.96
specified NEC	T39.8X1	T39.8X2	T39.8X3	T39.8X4	T39.8X5	T39.8X6
Antipyrine	T39.2X1	T39.2X2	T39.2X3	T39.2X4	T39.2X5	T39.2X6
Antirabies hyperimmune serum	T5Ø.Z11	T5Ø.Z12	T5Ø.Z13	T5Ø.Z14	T5Ø.Z15	T5Ø.Z16
Antirheumatic NEC	T39.4X1	T39.4X2	T39.4X3	T39.4X4	T39.4X5	T39.4X6
Antirigidity drug NEC	T42.8X1	T42.8X2	T42.8X3	T42.8X4	T42.8X5	T42.8X6
Antischistosomal drug	T37.4X1	T37.4X2	T37.4X3	T37.4X4	T37.4X5	T37.4X6
Antiscorpion sera	T5Ø.Z11	T5Ø.Z12	T5Ø.Z13	T5Ø.Z14	T5Ø.Z15	T5Ø.Z16
Antiseborrheics	T49.4X1	T49.4X2	T49.4X3	T49.4X4	T49.4X5	T49.4X6
Antiseptics (external) (medicinal)	T49.ØX1	T49.ØX2	T49.ØX3	T49.ØX4	T49.ØX5	T49.ØX6
Antistine	T45.ØX1	T45.ØX2	T45.ØX3	T45.ØX4	T45.ØX5	T45.ØX6
Antitapeworm drug	T37.4X1	T37.4X2	T37.4X3	T37.4X4	T37.4X5	T37.4X6
Antitetanus immunoglobulin	T5Ø.Z11	T5Ø.Z12	T5Ø.Z13	T5Ø.Z14	T5Ø.Z15	T5Ø.Z16
Antithrombotic	T45.521	T45.522	T45.523	T45.524	T45.525	T45.526
Antithyroid drug NEC	T38.2X1	T38.2X2	T38.2X3	T38.2X4	T38.2X5	T38.2X6
Antitoxin	T5Ø.Z11	T5Ø.Z12	T5Ø.Z13	T5Ø.Z14	T5Ø.Z15	T5Ø.Z16
diphtheria	T5Ø.Z11	T5Ø.Z12	T5Ø.Z13	T5Ø.Z14	T5Ø.Z15	T5Ø.Z16
gas gangrene	T5Ø.Z11	T5Ø.Z12	T5Ø.Z13	T5Ø.Z14	T5Ø.Z15	T5Ø.Z16
tetanus	T5Ø.Z11	T5Ø.Z12	T5Ø.Z13	T5Ø.Z14	T5Ø.Z15	T5Ø.Z16
Antitrichomonal drug	T37.3X1	T37.3X2	T37.3X3	T37.3X4	T37.3X5	T37.3X6
Antituberculars	T37.1X1	T37.1X2	T37.1X3	T37.1X4	T37.1X5	T37.1X6
antibiotics	T36.5X1	T36.5X2	T36.5X3	T36.5X4	T36.5X5	T36.5X6
Antitussive NEC	T48.3X1	T48.3X2	T48.3X3	T48.3X4	T48.3X5	T48.3X6
codeine mixture	T4Ø.2X1	T4Ø.2X2	T4Ø.2X3	T4Ø.2X4	T4Ø.2X5	T4Ø.2X6
opiate	T4Ø.2X1	T4Ø.2X2	T4Ø.2X3	T4Ø.2X4	T4Ø.2X5	T4Ø.2X6
Antivaricose drug	T46.8X1	T46.8X2	T46.8X3	T46.8X4	T46.8X5	T46.8X6
Antivenin, antivenom (sera)	T5Ø.Z11	T5Ø.Z12	T5Ø.Z13	T5Ø.Z14	T5Ø.Z15	T5Ø.Z16
crotaline	T5Ø.Z11	T5Ø.Z12	T5Ø.Z13	T5Ø.Z14	T5Ø.Z15	T5Ø.Z16
spider bite	T5Ø.Z11	T5Ø.Z12	T5Ø.Z13	T5Ø.Z14	T5Ø.Z15	T5Ø.Z16
Antivertigo drug	T45.ØX1	T45.ØX2	T45.ØX3	T45.ØX4	T45.ØX5	T45.ØX6
Antiviral drug NEC	T37.5X1	T37.5X2	T37.5X3	T37.5X4	T37.5X5	T37.5X6
eye	T49.5X1	T49.5X2	T49.5X3	T49.5X4	T49.5X5	T49.5X6
Antiwhipworm drug	T37.4X1	T37.4X2	T37.4X3	T37.4X4	T37.4X5	T37.4X6
Ant poison — *see* Insecticide						
Antrol — *see also* by specific chemical substance	T6Ø.91	T6Ø.92	T6Ø.93	T6Ø.94	—	—
fungicide	T6Ø.91	T6Ø.92	T6Ø.93	T6Ø.94	—	—
ANTU (alpha naphthylthiourea)	T6Ø.4X1	T6Ø.4X2	T6Ø.4X3	T6Ø.4X4	—	—
Apalcillin	T36.ØX1	T36.ØX2	T36.ØX3	T36.ØX4	T36.ØX5	T36.ØX6
APC	T48.5X1	T48.5X2	T48.5X3	T48.5X4	T48.5X5	T48.5X6
Aplonidine	T44.4X1	T44.4X2	T44.4X3	T44.4X4	T44.4X5	T44.4X6
Apomorphine	T47.7X1	T47.7X2	T47.7X3	T47.7X4	T47.7X5	T47.7X6
Appetite depressants, central	T5Ø.5X1	T5Ø.5X2	T5Ø.5X3	T5Ø.5X4	T5Ø.5X5	T5Ø.5X6
Apraclonidine (hydrochloride)	T44.4X1	T44.4X2	T44.4X3	T44.4X4	T44.4X5	T44.4X6
Apresoline	T46.5X1	T46.5X2	T46.5X3	T46.5X4	T46.5X5	T46.5X6
Aprindine	T46.2X1	T46.2X2	T46.2X3	T46.2X4	T46.2X5	T46.2X6
Aprobarbital	T42.3X1	T42.3X2	T42.3X3	T42.3X4	T42.3X5	T42.3X6
Apronalide	T42.6X1	T42.6X2	T42.6X3	T42.6X4	T42.6X5	T42.6X6
Aprotinin	T45.621	T45.622	T45.623	T45.624	T45.625	T45.626
Aptocaine	T41.3X1	T41.3X2	T41.3X3	T41.3X4	T41.3X5	T41.3X6
Aqua fortis	T54.2X1	T54.2X2	T54.2X3	T54.2X4	—	—
Ara-A	T37.5X1	T37.5X2	T37.5X3	T37.5X4	T37.5X5	T37.5X6
Ara-C	T45.1X1	T45.1X2	T45.1X3	T45.1X4	T45.1X5	T45.1X6
Arachis oil	T49.3X1	T49.3X2	T49.3X3	T49.3X4	T49.3X5	T49.3X6
cathartic	T47.4X1	T47.4X2	T47.4X3	T47.4X4	T47.4X5	T47.4X6
Aralen	T37.2X1	T37.2X2	T37.2X3	T37.2X4	T37.2X5	T37.2X6
Arecoline	T44.1X1	T44.1X2	T44.1X3	T44.1X4	T44.1X5	T44.1X6
Arginine	T5Ø.991	T5Ø.992	T5Ø.993	T5Ø.994	T5Ø.995	T5Ø.996
glutamate	T5Ø.991	T5Ø.992	T5Ø.993	T5Ø.994	T5Ø.995	T5Ø.996
Argyrol	T49.ØX1	T49.ØX2	T49.ØX3	T49.ØX4	T49.ØX5	T49.ØX6
ENT agent	T49.6X1	T49.6X2	T49.6X3	T49.6X4	T49.6X5	T49.6X6
ophthalmic preparation	T49.5X1	T49.5X2	T49.5X3	T49.5X4	T49.5X5	T49.5X6
Aristocort	T38.ØX1	T38.ØX2	T38.ØX3	T38.ØX4	T38.ØX5	T38.ØX6
ENT agent	T49.6X1	T49.6X2	T49.6X3	T49.6X4	T49.6X5	T49.6X6
ophthalmic preparation	T49.5X1	T49.5X2	T49.5X3	T49.5X4	T49.5X5	T49.5X6

Substance	Poisoning, Accidental (unintentional)	Poisoning, Intentional Self-harm	Poisoning, Assault	Poisoning, Undetermined	Adverse Effect	Under-dosing
Aristocort — *continued*						
topical NEC	T49.ØX1	T49.ØX2	T49.ØX3	T49.ØX4	T49.ØX5	T49.ØX6
Aromatics, corrosive	T54.1X1	T54.1X2	T54.1X3	T54.1X4	—	—
disinfectants	T54.1X1	T54.1X2	T54.1X3	T54.1X4	—	—
Arsenate of lead	T57.ØX1	T57.ØX2	T57.ØX3	T57.ØX4	—	—
herbicide	T57.ØX1	T57.ØX2	T57.ØX3	T57.ØX4	—	—
Arsenic, arsenicals (compounds) (dust) (vapor) **NEC**	T57.ØX1	T57.ØX2	T57.ØX3	T57.ØX4	—	—
anti-infectives	T37.8X1	T37.8X2	T37.8X3	T37.8X4	T37.8X5	T37.8X6
pesticide (dust) (fumes)	T57.ØX1	T57.ØX2	T57.ØX3	T57.ØX4	—	—
Arsine (gas)	T57.ØX1	T57.ØX2	T57.ØX3	T57.ØX4	—	—
Arsphenamine (silver)	T37.8X1	T37.8X2	T37.8X3	T37.8X4	T37.8X5	T37.8X6
Arsthinol	T37.3X1	T37.3X2	T37.3X3	T37.3X4	T37.3X5	T37.3X6
Artane	T44.3X1	T44.3X2	T44.3X3	T44.3X4	T44.3X5	T44.3X6
Arthropod (venomous) **NEC**	T63.481	T63.482	T63.483	T63.484	—	—
Articaine	T41.3X1	T41.3X2	T41.3X3	T41.3X4	T41.3X5	T41.3X6
Asbestos	T57.8X1	T57.8X2	T57.8X3	T57.8X4	—	—
Ascaridole	T37.4X1	T37.4X2	T37.4X3	T37.4X4	T37.4X5	T37.4X6
Ascorbic acid	T45.2X1	T45.2X2	T45.2X3	T45.2X4	T45.2X5	T45.2X6
Asiaticoside	T49.ØX1	T49.ØX2	T49.ØX3	T49.ØX4	T49.ØX5	T49.ØX6
Asparaginase	T45.1X1	T45.1X2	T45.1X3	T45.1X4	T45.1X5	T45.1X6
Aspidium (oleoresin)	T37.4X1	T37.4X2	T37.4X3	T37.4X4	T37.4X5	T37.4X6
Aspirin (aluminum) (soluble)	T39.Ø11	T39.Ø12	T39.Ø13	T39.Ø14	T39.Ø15	T39.Ø16
Aspoxicillin	T36.ØX1	T36.ØX2	T36.ØX3	T36.ØX4	T36.ØX5	T36.ØX6
Astemizole	T45.ØX1	T45.ØX2	T45.ØX3	T45.ØX4	T45.ØX5	T45.ØX6
Astringent (local)	T49.2X1	T49.2X2	T49.2X3	T49.2X4	T49.2X5	T49.2X6
specified NEC	T49.2X1	T49.2X2	T49.2X3	T49.2X4	T49.2X5	T49.2X6
Astromicin	T36.5X1	T36.5X2	T36.5X3	T36.5X4	T36.5X5	T36.5X6
Ataractic drug NEC	T43.5Ø1	T43.5Ø2	T43.5Ø3	T43.5Ø4	T43.5Ø5	T43.5Ø6
Atenolol	T44.7X1	T44.7X2	T44.7X3	T44.7X4	T44.7X5	T44.7X6
Atonia drug, intestinal	T47.4X1	T47.4X2	T47.4X3	T47.4X4	T47.4X5	T47.4X6
Atophan	T5Ø.4X1	T5Ø.4X2	T5Ø.4X3	T5Ø.4X4	T5Ø.4X5	T5Ø.4X6
Atracurium besilate	T48.1X1	T48.1X2	T48.1X3	T48.1X4	T48.1X5	T48.1X6
Atropine	T44.3X1	T44.3X2	T44.3X3	T44.3X4	T44.3X5	T44.3X6
derivative	T44.3X1	T44.3X2	T44.3X3	T44.3X4	T44.3X5	T44.3X6
methonitrate	T44.3X1	T44.3X2	T44.3X3	T44.3X4	T44.3X5	T44.3X6
Attapulgite	T47.6X1	T47.6X2	T47.6X3	T47.6X4	T47.6X5	T47.6X6
Auramine	T65.891	T65.892	T65.893	T65.894	—	—
dye	T65.6X1	T65.6X2	T65.6X3	T65.6X4	—	—
fungicide	T6Ø.3X1	T6Ø.3X2	T6Ø.3X3	T6Ø.3X4	—	—
Auranofin	T39.4X1	T39.4X2	T39.4X3	T39.4X4	T39.4X5	T39.4X6
Aurantiin	T46.991	T46.992	T46.993	T46.994	T46.995	T46.996
Aureomycin	T36.4X1	T36.4X2	T36.4X3	T36.4X4	T36.4X5	T36.4X6
ophthalmic preparation	T49.5X1	T49.5X2	T49.5X3	T49.5X4	T49.5X5	T49.5X6
topical NEC	T49.ØX1	T49.ØX2	T49.ØX3	T49.ØX4	T49.ØX5	T49.ØX6
Aurothioglucose	T39.4X1	T39.4X2	T39.4X3	T39.4X4	T39.4X5	T39.4X6
Aurothioglycanide	T39.4X1	T39.4X2	T39.4X3	T39.4X4	T39.4X5	T39.4X6
Aurothiomalate sodium	T39.4X1	T39.4X2	T39.4X3	T39.4X4	T39.4X5	T39.4X6
Aurotioprol	T39.4X1	T39.4X2	T39.4X3	T39.4X4	T39.4X5	T39.4X6
Automobile fuel	T52.ØX1	T52.ØX2	T52.ØX3	T52.ØX4	—	—
Autonomic nervous system agent NEC	T44.9Ø1	T44.9Ø2	T44.9Ø3	T44.9Ø4	T44.9Ø5	T44.9Ø6
Avlosulfon	T37.1X1	T37.1X2	T37.1X3	T37.1X4	T37.1X5	T37.1X6
Avomine	T42.6X1	T42.6X2	T42.6X3	T42.6X4	T42.6X5	T42.6X6
Axerophthol	T45.2X1	T45.2X2	T45.2X3	T45.2X4	T45.2X5	T45.2X6
Azacitidine	T45.1X1	T45.1X2	T45.1X3	T45.1X4	T45.1X5	T45.1X6
Azacyclonol	T43.591	T43.592	T43.593	T43.594	T43.595	T43.596
Azadirachta	T6Ø.2X1	T6Ø.2X2	T6Ø.2X3	T6Ø.2X4	—	—
Azanidazole	T37.3X1	T37.3X2	T37.3X3	T37.3X4	T37.3X5	T37.3X6
Azapetine	T46.7X1	T46.7X2	T46.7X3	T46.7X4	T46.7X5	T46.7X6
Azapropazone	T39.2X1	T39.2X2	T39.2X3	T39.2X4	T39.2X5	T39.2X6
Azaribine	T45.1X1	T45.1X2	T45.1X3	T45.1X4	T45.1X5	T45.1X6
Azaserine	T45.1X1	T45.1X2	T45.1X3	T45.1X4	T45.1X5	T45.1X6
Azatadine	T45.ØX1	T45.ØX2	T45.ØX3	T45.ØX4	T45.ØX5	T45.ØX6
Azatepa	T45.1X1	T45.1X2	T45.1X3	T45.1X4	T45.1X5	T45.1X6
Azathioprine	T45.1X1	T45.1X2	T45.1X3	T45.1X4	T45.1X5	T45.1X6
Azelaic acid	T49.ØX1	T49.ØX2	T49.ØX3	T49.ØX4	T49.ØX5	T49.ØX6
Azelastine	T45.ØX1	T45.ØX2	T45.ØX3	T45.ØX4	T45.ØX5	T45.ØX6
Azidocillin	T36.ØX1	T36.ØX2	T36.ØX3	T36.ØX4	T36.ØX5	T36.ØX6
Azidothymidine	T37.5X1	T37.5X2	T37.5X3	T37.5X4	T37.5X5	T37.5X6
Azinphos (ethyl) (methyl)	T6Ø.ØX1	T6Ø.ØX2	T6Ø.ØX3	T6Ø.ØX4	—	—
Aziridine (chelating)	T54.1X1	T54.1X2	T54.1X3	T54.1X4	—	—
Azithromycin	T36.3X1	T36.3X2	T36.3X3	T36.3X4	T36.3X5	T36.3X6
Azlocillin	T36.ØX1	T36.ØX2	T36.ØX3	T36.ØX4	T36.ØX5	T36.ØX6
Azobenzene smoke	T65.3X1	T65.3X2	T65.3X3	T65.3X4	—	—
acaricide	T6Ø.8X1	T6Ø.8X2	T6Ø.8X3	T6Ø.8X4	—	—
Azosulfamide	T37.ØX1	T37.ØX2	T37.ØX3	T37.ØX4	T37.ØX5	T37.ØX6
AZT	T37.5X1	T37.5X2	T37.5X3	T37.5X4	T37.5X5	T37.5X6
Aztreonam	T36.1X1	T36.1X2	T36.1X3	T36.1X4	T36.1X5	T36.1X6
Azulfidine	T37.ØX1	T37.ØX2	T37.ØX3	T37.ØX4	T37.ØX5	T37.ØX6
Azuresin	T5Ø.8X1	T5Ø.8X2	T5Ø.8X3	T5Ø.8X4	T5Ø.8X5	T5Ø.8X6
b-acetyldigoxin	T46.ØX1	T46.ØX2	T46.ØX3	T46.ØX4	T46.ØX5	T46.ØX6

Substance	Poisoning, Accidental (unintentional)	Poisoning, Intentional Self-harm	Poisoning, Assault	Poisoning, Undetermined	Adverse Effect	Under-dosing
P-Acetamidophenol	T39.1X1	T39.1X2	T39.1X3	T39.1X4	T39.1X5	T39.1X6
Bacampicillin	T36.ØX1	T36.ØX2	T36.ØX3	T36.ØX4	T36.ØX5	T36.ØX6
Bacillus						
lactobacillus	T47.8X1	T47.8X2	T47.8X3	T47.8X4	T47.8X5	T47.8X6
subtilis	T47.6X1	T47.6X2	T47.6X3	T47.6X4	T47.6X5	T47.6X6
Bacimycin	T49.ØX1	T49.ØX2	T49.ØX3	T49.ØX4	T49.ØX5	T49.ØX6
ophthalmic preparation	T49.5X1	T49.5X2	T49.5X3	T49.5X4	T49.5X5	T49.5X6
Bacitracin zinc	T49.ØX1	T49.ØX2	T49.ØX3	T49.ØX4	T49.ØX5	T49.ØX6
with neomycin	T49.ØX1	T49.ØX2	T49.ØX3	T49.ØX4	T49.ØX5	T49.ØX6
ENT agent	T49.6X1	T49.6X2	T49.6X3	T49.6X4	T49.6X5	T49.6X6
ophthalmic preparation	T49.5X1	T49.5X2	T49.5X3	T49.5X4	T49.5X5	T49.5X6
topical NEC	T49.ØX1	T49.ØX2	T49.ØX3	T49.ØX4	T49.ØX5	T49.ØX6
Baclofen	T42.8X1	T42.8X2	T42.8X3	T42.8X4	T42.8X5	T42.8X6
Baking soda	T5Ø.991	T5Ø.992	T5Ø.993	T5Ø.994	T5Ø.995	T5Ø.996
BAL	T45.8X1	T45.8X2	T45.8X3	T45.8X4	T45.8X5	T45.8X6
Bambuterol	T48.6X1	T48.6X2	T48.6X3	T48.6X4	T48.6X5	T48.6X6
Bamethan (sulfate)	T46.7X1	T46.7X2	T46.7X3	T46.7X4	T46.7X5	T46.7X6
Bamifylline	T48.6X1	T48.6X2	T48.6X3	T48.6X4	T48.6X5	T48.6X6
Bamipine	T45.ØX1	T45.ØX2	T45.ØX3	T45.ØX4	T45.ØX5	T45.ØX6
Baneberry — *see* Actaea spicata						
Banewort — *see* Belladonna						
Barbenyl	T42.3X1	T42.3X2	T42.3X3	T42.3X4	T42.3X5	T42.3X6
Barbexaclone	T42.6X1	T42.6X2	T42.6X3	T42.6X4	T42.6X5	T42.6X6
Barbital	T42.3X1	T42.3X2	T42.3X3	T42.3X4	T42.3X5	T42.3X6
sodium	T42.3X1	T42.3X2	T42.3X3	T42.3X4	T42.3X5	T42.3X6
Barbitone	T42.3X1	T42.3X2	T42.3X3	T42.3X4	T42.3X5	T42.3X6
Barbiturate NEC	T42.3X1	T42.3X2	T42.3X3	T42.3X4	T42.3X5	T42.3X6
with tranquilizer	T42.3X1	T42.3X2	T42.3X3	T42.3X4	T42.3X5	T42.3X6
anesthetic (intravenous)	T41.1X1	T41.1X2	T41.1X3	T41.1X4	T41.1X5	T41.1X6
Barium (carbonate) (chloride) (sulfite)	T57.8X1	T57.8X2	T57.8X3	T57.8X4	—	—
diagnostic agent	T5Ø.8X1	T5Ø.8X2	T5Ø.8X3	T5Ø.8X4	T5Ø.8X5	T5Ø.8X6
pesticide	T6Ø.4X1	T6Ø.4X2	T6Ø.4X3	T6Ø.4X4	—	—
rodenticide	T6Ø.4X1	T6Ø.4X2	T6Ø.4X3	T6Ø.4X4	—	—
sulfate (medicinal)	T5Ø.8X1	T5Ø.8X2	T5Ø.8X3	T5Ø.8X4	T5Ø.8X5	T5Ø.8X6
Barrier cream	T49.3X1	T49.3X2	T49.3X3	T49.3X4	T49.3X5	T49.3X6
Basic fuchsin	T49.ØX1	T49.ØX2	T49.ØX3	T49.ØX4	T49.ØX5	T49.ØX6
Battery acid or fluid	T54.2X1	T54.2X2	T54.2X3	T54.2X4	—	—
Bay rum	T51.8X1	T51.8X2	T51.8X3	T51.8X4	—	—
b-benzalbutyramide	T46.6X1	T46.6X2	T46.6X3	T46.6X4	T46.6X5	T46.6X6
BCG (vaccine)	T5Ø.A91	T5Ø.A92	T5Ø.A93	T5Ø.A94	T5Ø.A95	T5Ø.A96
BCNU	T45.1X1	T45.1X2	T45.1X3	T45.1X4	T45.1X5	T45.1X6
Bearsfoot	T62.2X1	T62.2X2	T62.2X3	T62.2X4	—	—
Beclamide	T42.6X1	T42.6X2	T42.6X3	T42.6X4	T42.6X5	T42.6X6
Beclomethasone	T44.5X1	T44.5X2	T44.5X3	T44.5X4	T44.5X5	T44.5X6
Bee (sting) (venom)	T63.441	T63.442	T63.443	T63.444	—	—
Befunolol	T49.5X1	T49.5X2	T49.5X3	T49.5X4	T49.5X5	T49.5X6
Bekanamycin	T36.5X1	T36.5X2	T36.5X3	T36.5X4	T36.5X5	T36.5X6
Belladonna — *see also* Nightshade						
alkaloids	T44.3X1	T44.3X2	T44.3X3	T44.3X4	T44.3X5	T44.3X6
extract	T44.3X1	T44.3X2	T44.3X3	T44.3X4	T44.3X5	T44.3X6
herb	T44.3X1	T44.3X2	T44.3X3	T44.3X4	T44.3X5	T44.3X6
Bemegride	T5Ø.7X1	T5Ø.7X2	T5Ø.7X3	T5Ø.7X4	T5Ø.7X5	T5Ø.7X6
Benactyzine	T44.3X1	T44.3X2	T44.3X3	T44.3X4	T44.3X5	T44.3X6
Benadryl	T45.ØX1	T45.ØX2	T45.ØX3	T45.ØX4	T45.ØX5	T45.ØX6
Benaprizine	T44.3X1	T44.3X2	T44.3X3	T44.3X4	T44.3X5	T44.3X6
Benazepril	T46.4X1	T46.4X2	T46.4X3	T46.4X4	T46.4X5	T46.4X6
Bencyclane	T46.7X1	T46.7X2	T46.7X3	T46.7X4	T46.7X5	T46.7X6
Bendazol	T46.3X1	T46.3X2	T46.3X3	T46.3X4	T46.3X5	T46.3X6
Bendrofluazide	T5Ø.2X1	T5Ø.2X2	T5Ø.2X3	T5Ø.2X4	T5Ø.2X5	T5Ø.2X6
Bendroflumethiazide	T5Ø.2X1	T5Ø.2X2	T5Ø.2X3	T5Ø.2X4	T5Ø.2X5	T5Ø.2X6
Benemid	T5Ø.4X1	T5Ø.4X2	T5Ø.4X3	T5Ø.4X4	T5Ø.4X5	T5Ø.4X6
Benethamine penicillin	T36.ØX1	T36.ØX2	T36.ØX3	T36.ØX4	T36.ØX5	T36.ØX6
Benexate	T47.1X1	T47.1X2	T47.1X3	T47.1X4	T47.1X5	T47.1X6
Benfluorex	T46.6X1	T46.6X2	T46.6X3	T46.6X4	T46.6X5	T46.6X6
Benfotiamine	T45.2X1	T45.2X2	T45.2X3	T45.2X4	T45.2X5	T45.2X6
Benisone	T49.ØX1	T49.ØX2	T49.ØX3	T49.ØX4	T49.ØX5	T49.ØX6
Benomyl	T6Ø.ØX1	T6Ø.ØX2	T6Ø.ØX3	T6Ø.ØX4	—	—
Benoquin	T49.8X1	T49.8X2	T49.8X3	T49.8X4	T49.8X5	T49.8X6
Benoxinate	T41.3X1	T41.3X2	T41.3X3	T41.3X4	T41.3X5	T41.3X6
Benperidol	T43.4X1	T43.4X2	T43.4X3	T43.4X4	T43.4X5	T43.4X6
Benproperine	T48.3X1	T48.3X2	T48.3X3	T48.3X4	T48.3X5	T48.3X6
Benserazide	T42.8X1	T42.8X2	T42.8X3	T42.8X4	T42.8X5	T42.8X6
Bentazepam	T42.4X1	T42.4X2	T42.4X3	T42.4X4	T42.4X5	T42.4X6
Bentiromide	T5Ø.8X1	T5Ø.8X2	T5Ø.8X3	T5Ø.8X4	T5Ø.8X5	T5Ø.8X6
Bentonite	T49.3X1	T49.3X2	T49.3X3	T49.3X4	T49.3X5	T49.3X6
Benzalbutyramide	T46.6X1	T46.6X2	T46.6X3	T46.6X4	T46.6X5	T46.6X6
Benzalkonium (chloride)	T49.ØX1	T49.ØX2	T49.ØX3	T49.ØX4	T49.ØX5	T49.ØX6
ophthalmic preparation	T49.5X1	T49.5X2	T49.5X3	T49.5X4	T49.5X5	T49.5X6
Benzamidosalicylate (calcium)	T37.1X1	T37.1X2	T37.1X3	T37.1X4	T37.1X5	T37.1X6
Benzamine	T41.3X1	T41.3X2	T41.3X3	T41.3X4	T41.3X5	T41.3X6

Substance	Poisoning, Accidental (unintentional)	Poisoning, Intentional Self-harm	Poisoning, Assault	Poisoning, Undetermined	Adverse Effect	Under-dosing
Benzamine — *continued*						
lactate	T49.1X1	T49.1X2	T49.1X3	T49.1X4	T49.1X5	T49.1X6
Benzamphetamine	T5Ø.5X1	T5Ø.5X2	T5Ø.5X3	T5Ø.5X4	T5Ø.5X5	T5Ø.5X6
Benzapril hydrochloride	T46.5X1	T46.5X2	T46.5X3	T46.5X4	T46.5X5	T46.5X6
Benzathine benzylpenicillin	T36.ØX1	T36.ØX2	T36.ØX3	T36.ØX4	T36.ØX5	T36.ØX6
Benzathine penicillin	T36.ØX1	T36.ØX2	T36.ØX3	T36.ØX4	T36.ØX5	T36.ØX6
Benzatropine	T42.8X1	T42.8X2	T42.8X3	T42.8X4	T42.8X5	T42.8X6
Benzbromarone	T5Ø.4X1	T5Ø.4X2	T5Ø.4X3	T5Ø.4X4	T5Ø.4X5	T5Ø.4X6
Benzcarbimine	T45.1X1	T45.1X2	T45.1X3	T45.1X4	T45.1X5	T45.1X6
Benzedrex	T44.991	T44.992	T44.993	T44.994	T44.995	T44.996
Benzedrine (amphetamine)	T43.621	T43.622	T43.623	T43.624	T43.625	T43.626
Benzenamine	T65.3X1	T65.3X2	T65.3X3	T65.3X4	—	—
Benzene	T52.1X1	T52.1X2	T52.1X3	T52.1X4	—	—
homologues (acetyl) (dimethyl) (methyl) (solvent)	T52.2X1	T52.2X2	T52.2X3	T52.2X4	—	—
Benzethonium (chloride)	T49.ØX1	T49.ØX2	T49.ØX3	T49.ØX4	T49.ØX5	T49.ØX6
Benzfetamine	T5Ø.5X1	T5Ø.5X2	T5Ø.5X3	T5Ø.5X4	T5Ø.5X5	T5Ø.5X6
Benzhexol	T44.3X1	T44.3X2	T44.3X3	T44.3X4	T44.3X5	T44.3X6
Benzhydramine (chloride)	T45.ØX1	T45.ØX2	T45.ØX3	T45.ØX4	T45.ØX5	T45.ØX6
Benzidine	T65.891	T65.892	T65.893	T65.894	—	—
Benzilonium bromide	T44.3X1	T44.3X2	T44.3X3	T44.3X4	T44.3X5	T44.3X6
Benzimidazole	T6Ø.3X1	T6Ø.3X2	T6Ø.3X3	T6Ø.3X4	—	—
Benzin (e) — *see* Ligroin						
Benziodarone	T46.3X1	T46.3X2	T46.3X3	T46.3X4	T46.3X5	T46.3X6
Benznidazole	T37.3X1	T37.3X2	T37.3X3	T37.3X4	T37.3X5	T37.3X6
Benzocaine	T41.3X1	T41.3X2	T41.3X3	T41.3X4	T41.3X5	T41.3X6
Benzodiapin	T42.4X1	T42.4X2	T42.4X3	T42.4X4	T42.4X5	T42.4X6
Benzodiazepine NEC	T42.4X1	T42.4X2	T42.4X3	T42.4X4	T42.4X5	T42.4X6
Benzoic acid	T49.ØX1	T49.ØX2	T49.ØX3	T49.ØX4	T49.ØX5	T49.ØX6
with salicylic acid	T49.ØX1	T49.ØX2	T49.ØX3	T49.ØX4	T49.ØX5	T49.ØX6
Benzoin (tincture)	T48.5X1	T48.5X2	T48.5X3	T48.5X4	T48.5X5	T48.5X6
Benzol (benzene)	T52.1X1	T52.1X2	T52.1X3	T52.1X4	—	—
vapor	T52.ØX1	T52.ØX2	T52.ØX3	T52.ØX4	—	—
Benzomorphan	T4Ø.2X1	T4Ø.2X2	T4Ø.2X3	T4Ø.2X4	T4Ø.2X5	T4Ø.2X6
Benzonatate	T48.3X1	T48.3X2	T48.3X3	T48.3X4	T48.3X5	T48.3X6
Benzophenones	T49.3X1	T49.3X2	T49.3X3	T49.3X4	T49.3X5	T49.3X6
Benzopyrone	T46.991	T46.992	T46.993	T46.994	T46.995	T46.996
Benzothiadiazides	T5Ø.2X1	T5Ø.2X2	T5Ø.2X3	T5Ø.2X4	T5Ø.2X5	T5Ø.2X6
Benzoxonium chloride	T49.ØX1	T49.ØX2	T49.ØX3	T49.ØX4	T49.ØX5	T49.ØX6
Benzoylpas calcium	T37.1X1	T37.1X2	T37.1X3	T37.1X4	T37.1X5	T37.1X6
Benzoyl peroxide	T49.ØX1	T49.ØX2	T49.ØX3	T49.ØX4	T49.ØX5	T49.ØX6
Benzperidin	T43.591	T43.592	T43.593	T43.594	T43.595	T43.596
Benzperidol	T43.591	T43.592	T43.593	T43.594	T43.595	T43.596
Benzphetamine	T5Ø.5X1	T5Ø.5X2	T5Ø.5X3	T5Ø.5X4	T5Ø.5X5	T5Ø.5X6
Benzpyrinium bromide	T44.1X1	T44.1X2	T44.1X3	T44.1X4	T44.1X5	T44.1X6
Benzquinamide	T45.ØX1	T45.ØX2	T45.ØX3	T45.ØX4	T45.ØX5	T45.ØX6
Benzthiazide	T5Ø.2X1	T5Ø.2X2	T5Ø.2X3	T5Ø.2X4	T5Ø.2X5	T5Ø.2X6
Benztropine						
anticholinergic	T44.3X1	T44.3X2	T44.3X3	T44.3X4	T44.3X5	T44.3X6
antiparkinson	T42.8X1	T42.8X2	T42.8X3	T42.8X4	T42.8X5	T42.8X6
Benzydamine	T49.ØX1	T49.ØX2	T49.ØX3	T49.ØX4	T49.ØX5	T49.ØX6
Benzyl						
acetate	T52.8X1	T52.8X2	T52.8X3	T52.8X4	—	—
alcohol	T49.ØX1	T49.ØX2	T49.ØX3	T49.ØX4	T49.ØX5	T49.ØX6
benzoate	T49.ØX1	T49.ØX2	T49.ØX3	T49.ØX4	T49.ØX5	T49.ØX6
Benzoic acid	T49.ØX1	T49.ØX2	T49.ØX3	T49.ØX4	T49.ØX5	T49.ØX6
morphine	T4Ø.2X1	T4Ø.2X2	T4Ø.2X3	T4Ø.2X4	—	—
nicotinate	T46.6X1	T46.6X2	T46.6X3	T46.6X4	T46.6X5	T46.6X6
penicillin	T36.ØX1	T36.ØX2	T36.ØX3	T36.ØX4	T36.ØX5	T36.ØX6
Benzylhydrochlorthiazide	T5Ø.2X1	T5Ø.2X2	T5Ø.2X3	T5Ø.2X4	T5Ø.2X5	T5Ø.2X6
Benzylpenicillin	T36.ØX1	T36.ØX2	T36.ØX3	T36.ØX4	T36.ØX5	T36.ØX6
Benzylthiouracil	T38.2X1	T38.2X2	T38.2X3	T38.2X4	T38.2X5	T38.2X6
Bephenium hydroxynaphthoate	T37.4X1	T37.4X2	T37.4X3	T37.4X4	T37.4X5	T37.4X6
Bepridil	T46.1X1	T46.1X2	T46.1X3	T46.1X4	T46.1X5	T46.1X6
Bergamot oil	T65.891	T65.892	T65.893	T65.894	—	—
Bergapten	T5Ø.991	T5Ø.992	T5Ø.993	T5Ø.994	T5Ø.995	T5Ø.996
Berries, poisonous	T62.1X1	T62.1X2	T62.1X3	T62.1X4	—	—
Beryllium (compounds)	T56.7X1	T56.7X2	T56.7X3	T56.7X4	—	—
beta adrenergic blocking agent, heart	T44.7X1	T44.7X2	T44.7X3	T44.7X4	T44.7X5	T44.7X6
Betacarotene	T45.2X1	T45.2X2	T45.2X3	T45.2X4	T45.2X5	T45.2X6
Beta-Chlor	T42.6X1	T42.6X2	T42.6X3	T42.6X4	T42.6X5	T42.6X6
Betahistine	T46.7X1	T46.7X2	T46.7X3	T46.7X4	T46.7X5	T46.7X6
Betaine	T47.5X1	T47.5X2	T47.5X3	T47.5X4	T47.5X5	T47.5X6
Betamethasone	T49.ØX1	T49.ØX2	T49.ØX3	T49.ØX4	T49.ØX5	T49.ØX6
topical	T49.ØX1	T49.ØX2	T49.ØX3	T49.ØX4	T49.ØX5	T49.ØX6
Betamicin	T36.8X1	T36.8X2	T36.8X3	T36.8X4	T36.8X5	T36.8X6
Betanidine	T46.5X1	T46.5X2	T46.5X3	T46.5X4	T46.5X5	T46.5X6
Betaxolol	T44.7X1	T44.7X2	T44.7X3	T44.7X4	T44.7X5	T44.7X6
Betazole	T5Ø.8X1	T5Ø.8X2	T5Ø.8X3	T5Ø.8X4	T5Ø.8X5	T5Ø.8X6
Bethanechol	T44.1X1	T44.1X2	T44.1X3	T44.1X4	T44.1X5	T44.1X6

Substance	Poisoning, Accidental (unintentional)	Poisoning, Intentional Self-harm	Poisoning, Assault	Poisoning, Undetermined	Adverse Effect	Under-dosing
Bethanechol — *continued*						
chloride	T44.1X1	T44.1X2	T44.1X3	T44.1X4	T44.1X5	T44.1X6
Bethanidine	T46.5X1	T46.5X2	T46.5X3	T46.5X4	T46.5X5	T46.5X6
Betoxycaine	T41.3X1	T41.3X2	T41.3X3	T41.3X4	T41.3X5	T41.3X6
Betula oil	T49.3X1	T49.3X2	T49.3X3	T49.3X4	T49.3X5	T49.3X6
Bevantolol	T44.7X1	T44.7X2	T44.7X3	T44.7X4	T44.7X5	T44.7X6
Bevonium metilsulfate	T44.3X1	T44.3X2	T44.3X3	T44.3X4	T44.3X5	T44.3X6
Bezafibrate	T46.6X1	T46.6X2	T46.6X3	T46.6X4	T46.6X5	T46.6X6
Bezitramide	T4Ø.491	T4Ø.492	T4Ø.493	T4Ø.494	T4Ø.495	T4Ø.496
BHA	T5Ø.991	T5Ø.992	T5Ø.993	T5Ø.994	T5Ø.995	T5Ø.996
Bhang	T4Ø.7X1	T4Ø.7X2	T4Ø.7X3	T4Ø.7X4	T4Ø.7X5	T4Ø.7X6
BHC (medicinal)	T49.ØX1	T49.ØX2	T49.ØX3	T49.ØX4	T49.ØX5	T49.ØX6
nonmedicinal (vapor)	T53.6X1	T53.6X2	T53.6X3	T53.6X4	—	—
Bialamicol	T37.3X1	T37.3X2	T37.3X3	T37.3X4	T37.3X5	T37.3X6
Bibenzonium bromide	T48.3X1	T48.3X2	T48.3X3	T48.3X4	T48.3X5	T48.3X6
Bibrocathol	T49.5X1	T49.5X2	T49.5X3	T49.5X4	T49.5X5	T49.5X6
Bichloride of mercury — *see* Mercury, chloride						
Bichromates (calcium) (potassium)(sodium) (crystals)	T57.8X1	T57.8X2	T57.8X3	T57.8X4	—	—
fumes	T56.2X1	T56.2X2	T56.2X3	T56.2X4	—	—
Biclotymol	T49.6X1	T49.6X2	T49.6X3	T49.6X4	T49.6X5	T49.6X6
Bicucculine	T5Ø.7X1	T5Ø.7X2	T5Ø.7X3	T5Ø.7X4	T5Ø.7X5	T5Ø.7X6
Bifemelane	T43.291	T43.292	T43.293	T43.294	T43.295	T43.296
Biguanide derivatives, oral	T38.3X1	T38.3X2	T38.3X3	T38.3X4	T38.3X5	T38.3X6
Bile salts	T47.5X1	T47.5X2	T47.5X3	T47.5X4	T47.5X5	T47.5X6
Biligrafin	T5Ø.8X1	T5Ø.8X2	T5Ø.8X3	T5Ø.8X4	T5Ø.8X5	T5Ø.8X6
Bilopaque	T5Ø.8X1	T5Ø.8X2	T5Ø.8X3	T5Ø.8X4	T5Ø.8X5	T5Ø.8X6
Binifibrate	T46.6X1	T46.6X2	T46.6X3	T46.6X4	T46.6X5	T46.6X6
Binitrobenzol	T65.3X1	T65.3X2	T65.3X3	T65.3X4	—	—
Bioflavonoid(s)	T46.991	T46.992	T46.993	T46.994	T46.995	T46.996
Biological substance NEC	T5Ø.9Ø1	T5Ø.9Ø2	T5Ø.9Ø3	T5Ø.9Ø4	T5Ø.9Ø5	T5Ø.9Ø6
Biotin	T45.2X1	T45.2X2	T45.2X3	T45.2X4	T45.2X5	T45.2X6
Biperiden	T44.3X1	T44.3X2	T44.3X3	T44.3X4	T44.3X5	T44.3X6
Bisacodyl	T47.2X1	T47.2X2	T47.2X3	T47.2X4	T47.2X5	T47.2X6
Bisbentiamine	T45.2X1	T45.2X2	T45.2X3	T45.2X4	T45.2X5	T45.2X6
Bisbutiamine	T45.2X1	T45.2X2	T45.2X3	T45.2X4	T45.2X5	T45.2X6
Bisdequalinium (salts) (diacetate)	T49.6X1	T49.6X2	T49.6X3	T49.6X4	T49.6X5	T49.6X6
Bishydroxycoumarin	T45.511	T45.512	T45.513	T45.514	T45.515	T45.516
Bismarsen	T37.8X1	T37.8X2	T37.8X3	T37.8X4	T37.8X5	T37.8X6
Bismuth salts	T47.6X1	T47.6X2	T47.6X3	T47.6X4	T47.6X5	T47.6X6
aluminate	T47.1X1	T47.1X2	T47.1X3	T47.1X4	T47.1X5	T47.1X6
anti-infectives	T37.8X1	T37.8X2	T37.8X3	T37.8X4	T37.8X5	T37.8X6
formic iodide	T49.ØX1	T49.ØX2	T49.ØX3	T49.ØX4	T49.ØX5	T49.ØX6
glycolylarsenate	T49.ØX1	T49.ØX2	T49.ØX3	T49.ØX4	T49.ØX5	T49.ØX6
nonmedicinal (compounds) NEC	T65.91	T65.92	T65.93	T65.94	—	—
subcarbonate	T47.6X1	T47.6X2	T47.6X3	T47.6X4	T47.6X5	T47.6X6
subsalicylate	T37.8X1	T37.8X2	T37.8X3	T37.8X4	T37.8X5	T37.8X6
sulfarsphenamine	T37.8X1	T37.8X2	T37.8X3	T37.8X4	T37.8X5	T37.8X6
Bisoprolol	T44.7X1	T44.7X2	T44.7X3	T44.7X4	T44.7X5	T44.7X6
Bisoxatin	T47.2X1	T47.2X2	T47.2X3	T47.2X4	T47.2X5	T47.2X6
Bisulepin (hydrochloride)	T45.ØX1	T45.ØX2	T45.ØX3	T45.ØX4	T45.ØX5	T45.ØX6
Bithionol	T37.8X1	T37.8X2	T37.8X3	T37.8X4	T37.8X5	T37.8X6
anthelminthic	T37.4X1	T37.4X2	T37.4X3	T37.4X4	T37.4X5	T37.4X6
Bitolterol	T48.6X1	T48.6X2	T48.6X3	T48.6X4	T48.6X5	T48.6X6
Bitoscanate	T37.4X1	T37.4X2	T37.4X3	T37.4X4	T37.4X5	T37.4X6
Bitter almond oil	T62.8X1	T62.8X2	T62.8X3	T62.8X4	—	—
Bittersweet	T62.2X1	T62.2X2	T62.2X3	T62.2X4	—	—
Black						
flag	T6Ø.91	T6Ø.92	T6Ø.93	T6Ø.94	—	—
henbane	T62.2X1	T62.2X2	T62.2X3	T62.2X4	—	—
leaf (40)	T6Ø.91	T6Ø.92	T6Ø.93	T6Ø.94	—	—
widow spider (bite)	T63.311	T63.312	T63.313	T63.314	—	—
antivenin	T5Ø.Z11	T5Ø.Z12	T5Ø.Z13	T5Ø.Z14	T5Ø.Z15	T5Ø.Z16
Blast furnace gas (carbon monoxide from)	T58.8X1	T58.8X2	T58.8X3	T58.8X4	—	—
Bleach	T54.91	T54.92	T54.93	T54.94	—	—
Bleaching agent (medicinal)	T49.4X1	T49.4X2	T49.4X3	T49.4X4	T49.4X5	T49.4X6
Bleomycin	T45.1X1	T45.1X2	T45.1X3	T45.1X4	T45.1X5	T45.1X6
Blockain	T41.3X1	T41.3X2	T41.3X3	T41.3X4	T41.3X5	T41.3X6
infiltration (subcutaneous)	T41.3X1	T41.3X2	T41.3X3	T41.3X4	T41.3X5	T41.3X6
nerve block (peripheral) (plexus)	T41.3X1	T41.3X2	T41.3X3	T41.3X4	T41.3X5	T41.3X6
topical (surface)	T41.3X1	T41.3X2	T41.3X3	T41.3X4	T41.3X5	T41.3X6
Blockers, calcium channel	T46.1X1	T46.1X2	T46.1X3	T46.1X4	T46.1X5	T46.1X6
Blood (derivatives) (natural) (plasma) (whole)	T45.8X1	T45.8X2	T45.8X3	T45.8X4	T45.8X5	T45.8X6
dried	T45.8X1	T45.8X2	T45.8X3	T45.8X4	T45.8X5	T45.8X6

Subterms under main terms may continue to next column or page

Substance	Poisoning, Accidental (unintentional)	Poisoning, Intentional Self-harm	Poisoning, Assault	Poisoning, Undetermined	Adverse Effect	Under-dosing
Blood — *continued*						
drug affecting NEC	T45.91	T45.92	T45.93	T45.94	T45.95	T45.96
expander NEC	T45.8X1	T45.8X2	T45.8X3	T45.8X4	T45.8X5	T45.8X6
fraction NEC	T45.8X1	T45.8X2	T45.8X3	T45.8X4	T45.8X5	T45.8X6
substitute (macromolecular)	T45.8X1	T45.8X2	T45.8X3	T45.8X4	T45.8X5	T45.8X6
Blue velvet	T4Ø.2X1	T4Ø.2X2	T4Ø.2X3	T4Ø.2X4	—	—
Bone meal	T62.8X1	T62.8X2	T62.8X3	T62.8X4	—	—
Bonine	T45.ØX1	T45.ØX2	T45.ØX3	T45.ØX4	T45.ØX5	T45.ØX6
Bopindolol	T44.7X1	T44.7X2	T44.7X3	T44.7X4	T44.7X5	T44.7X6
Boracic acid	T49.ØX1	T49.ØX2	T49.ØX3	T49.ØX4	T49.ØX5	T49.ØX6
ENT agent	T49.6X1	T49.6X2	T49.6X3	T49.6X4	T49.6X5	T49.6X6
ophthalmic preparation	T49.5X1	T49.5X2	T49.5X3	T49.5X4	T49.5X5	T49.5X6
Borane complex	T57.8X1	T57.8X2	T57.8X3	T57.8X4	—	—
Borate(s)	T57.8X1	T57.8X2	T57.8X3	T57.8X4	—	—
buffer	T5Ø.991	T5Ø.992	T5Ø.993	T5Ø.994	T5Ø.995	T5Ø.996
cleanser	T54.91	T54.92	T54.93	T54.94	—	—
sodium	T57.8X1	T57.8X2	T57.8X3	T57.8X4	—	—
Borax (cleanser)	T54.91	T54.92	T54.93	T54.94	—	—
Bordeaux mixture	T6Ø.3X1	T6Ø.3X2	T6Ø.3X3	T6Ø.3X4	—	—
Boric acid	T49.ØX1	T49.ØX2	T49.ØX3	T49.ØX4	T49.ØX5	T49.ØX6
ENT agent	T49.6X1	T49.6X2	T49.6X3	T49.6X4	T49.6X5	T49.6X6
ophthalmic preparation	T49.5X1	T49.5X2	T49.5X3	T49.5X4	T49.5X5	T49.5X6
Bornaprine	T44.3X1	T44.3X2	T44.3X3	T44.3X4	T44.3X5	T44.3X6
Boron	T57.8X1	T57.8X2	T57.8X3	T57.8X4	—	—
hydride NEC	T57.8X1	T57.8X2	T57.8X3	T57.8X4	—	—
fumes or gas	T57.8X1	T57.8X2	T57.8X3	T57.8X4	—	—
trifluoride	T59.891	T59.892	T59.893	T59.894	—	—
Botox	T48.291	T48.292	T48.293	T48.294	T48.295	T48.296
Botulinus anti-toxin (type A, B)	T5Ø.Z11	T5Ø.Z12	T5Ø.Z13	T5Ø.Z14	T5Ø.Z15	T5Ø.Z16
Brake fluid vapor	T59.891	T59.892	T59.893	T59.894	—	—
Brallobarbital	T42.3X1	T42.3X2	T42.3X3	T42.3X4	T42.3X5	T42.3X6
Bran (wheat)	T47.4X1	T47.4X2	T47.4X3	T47.4X4	T47.4X5	T47.4X6
Brass (fumes)	T56.891	T56.892	T56.893	T56.894	—	—
Brasso	T52.ØX1	T52.ØX2	T52.ØX3	T52.ØX4	—	—
Bretylium tosilate	T46.2X1	T46.2X2	T46.2X3	T46.2X4	T46.2X5	T46.2X6
Brevital (sodium)	T41.1X1	T41.1X2	T41.1X3	T41.1X4	T41.1X5	T41.1X6
Brinase	T45.3X1	T45.3X2	T45.3X3	T45.3X4	T45.3X5	T45.3X6
British antilewisite	T45.8X1	T45.8X2	T45.8X3	T45.8X4	T45.8X5	T45.8X6
Brodifacoum	T6Ø.4X1	T6Ø.4X2	T6Ø.4X3	T6Ø.4X4	—	—
Bromal (hydrate)	T42.6X1	T42.6X2	T42.6X3	T42.6X4	T42.6X5	T42.6X6
Bromazepam	T42.4X1	T42.4X2	T42.4X3	T42.4X4	T42.4X5	T42.4X6
Bromazine	T45.ØX1	T45.ØX2	T45.ØX3	T45.ØX4	T45.ØX5	T45.ØX6
Brombenzylcyanide	T59.3X1	T59.3X2	T59.3X3	T59.3X4	—	—
Bromelains	T45.3X1	T45.3X2	T45.3X3	T45.3X4	T45.3X5	T45.3X6
Bromethalin	T6Ø.4X1	T6Ø.4X2	T6Ø.4X3	T6Ø.4X4	—	—
Bromhexine	T48.4X1	T48.4X2	T48.4X3	T48.4X4	T48.4X5	T48.4X6
Bromide salts	T42.6X1	T42.6X2	T42.6X3	T42.6X4	T42.6X5	T42.6X6
Bromindione	T45.511	T45.512	T45.513	T45.514	T45.515	T45.516
Bromine						
compounds (medicinal)	T42.6X1	T42.6X2	T42.6X3	T42.6X4	T42.6X5	T42.6X6
sedative	T42.6X1	T42.6X2	T42.6X3	T42.6X4	T42.6X5	T42.6X6
vapor	T59.891	T59.892	T59.893	T59.894	—	—
Bromisoval	T42.6X1	T42.6X2	T42.6X3	T42.6X4	T42.6X5	T42.6X6
Bromisovalum	T42.6X1	T42.6X2	T42.6X3	T42.6X4	T42.6X5	T42.6X6
Bromobenzylcyanide	T59.3X1	T59.3X2	T59.3X3	T59.3X4	—	—
Bromochlorosalicylani-lide	T49.ØX1	T49.ØX2	T49.ØX3	T49.ØX4	T49.ØX5	T49.ØX6
Bromocriptine	T42.8X1	T42.8X2	T42.8X3	T42.8X4	T42.8X5	T42.8X6
Bromodiphenhydramine	T45.ØX1	T45.ØX2	T45.ØX3	T45.ØX4	T45.ØX5	T45.ØX6
Bromoform	T42.6X1	T42.6X2	T42.6X3	T42.6X4	T42.6X5	T42.6X6
Bromophenol blue reagent	T5Ø.991	T5Ø.992	T5Ø.993	T5Ø.994	T5Ø.995	T5Ø.996
Bromopride	T47.8X1	T47.8X2	T47.8X3	T47.8X4	T47.8X5	T47.8X6
Bromosalicylchloranitide	T49.ØX1	T49.ØX2	T49.ØX3	T49.ØX4	T49.ØX5	T49.ØX6
Bromosalicylhydroxamic acid	T37.1X1	T37.1X2	T37.1X3	T37.1X4	T37.1X5	T37.1X6
Bromo-seltzer	T39.1X1	T39.1X2	T39.1X3	T39.1X4	T39.1X5	T39.1X6
Bromoxynil	T6Ø.3X1	T6Ø.3X2	T6Ø.3X3	T6Ø.3X4	—	—
Bromperidol	T43.4X1	T43.4X2	T43.4X3	T43.4X4	T43.4X5	T43.4X6
Brompheniramine	T45.ØX1	T45.ØX2	T45.ØX3	T45.ØX4	T45.ØX5	T45.ØX6
Bromsulfophthalein	T5Ø.8X1	T5Ø.8X2	T5Ø.8X3	T5Ø.8X4	T5Ø.8X5	T5Ø.8X6
Bromural	T42.6X1	T42.6X2	T42.6X3	T42.6X4	T42.6X5	T42.6X6
Bromvaletone	T42.6X1	T42.6X2	T42.6X3	T42.6X4	T42.6X5	T42.6X6
Bronchodilator NEC	T48.6X1	T48.6X2	T48.6X3	T48.6X4	T48.6X5	T48.6X6
Brotizolam	T42.4X1	T42.4X2	T42.4X3	T42.4X4	T42.4X5	T42.4X6
Brovincamine	T46.7X1	T46.7X2	T46.7X3	T46.7X4	T46.7X5	T46.7X6
Brown recluse spider (bite) (venom)	T63.331	T63.332	T63.333	T63.334	—	—
Brown spider (bite) (venom)	T63.391	T63.392	T63.393	T63.394	—	—
Broxaterol	T48.6X1	T48.6X2	T48.6X3	T48.6X4	T48.6X5	T48.6X6
Broxuridine	T45.1X1	T45.1X2	T45.1X3	T45.1X4	T45.1X5	T45.1X6

Substance	Poisoning, Accidental (unintentional)	Poisoning, Intentional Self-harm	Poisoning, Assault	Poisoning, Undetermined	Adverse Effect	Under-dosing
Broxyquinoline	T37.8X1	T37.8X2	T37.8X3	T37.8X4	T37.8X5	T37.8X6
Bruceine	T48.291	T48.292	T48.293	T48.294	T48.295	T48.296
Brucia	T62.2X1	T62.2X2	T62.2X3	T62.2X4	—	—
Brucine	T65.1X1	T65.1X2	T65.1X3	T65.1X4	—	—
Brunswick green — *see* Copper						
Bruten — *see* Ibuprofen						
Bryonia	T47.2X1	T47.2X2	T47.2X3	T47.2X4	T47.2X5	T47.2X6
Buclizine	T45.ØX1	T45.ØX2	T45.ØX3	T45.ØX4	T45.ØX5	T45.ØX6
Buclosamide	T49.ØX1	T49.ØX2	T49.ØX3	T49.ØX4	T49.ØX5	T49.ØX6
Budesonide	T44.5X1	T44.5X2	T44.5X3	T44.5X4	T44.5X5	T44.5X6
Budralazine	T46.5X1	T46.5X2	T46.5X3	T46.5X4	T46.5X5	T46.5X6
Bufferin	T39.Ø11	T39.Ø12	T39.Ø13	T39.Ø14	T39.Ø15	T39.Ø16
Buflomedil	T46.7X1	T46.7X2	T46.7X3	T46.7X4	T46.7X5	T46.7X6
Buformin	T38.3X1	T38.3X2	T38.3X3	T38.3X4	T38.3X5	T38.3X6
Bufotenine	T4Ø.991	T4Ø.992	T4Ø.993	T4Ø.994	—	—
Bufrolin	T48.6X1	T48.6X2	T48.6X3	T48.6X4	T48.6X5	T48.6X6
Bufylline	T48.6X1	T48.6X2	T48.6X3	T48.6X4	T48.6X5	T48.6X6
Bulk filler	T5Ø.5X1	T5Ø.5X2	T5Ø.5X3	T5Ø.5X4	T5Ø.5X5	T5Ø.5X6
cathartic	T47.4X1	T47.4X2	T47.4X3	T47.4X4	T47.4X5	T47.4X6
Bumetanide	T5Ø.1X1	T5Ø.1X2	T5Ø.1X3	T5Ø.1X4	T5Ø.1X5	T5Ø.1X6
Bunaftine	T46.2X1	T46.2X2	T46.2X3	T46.2X4	T46.2X5	T46.2X6
Bunamiodyl	T5Ø.8X1	T5Ø.8X2	T5Ø.8X3	T5Ø.8X4	T5Ø.8X5	T5Ø.8X6
Bunazosin	T44.6X1	T44.6X2	T44.6X3	T44.6X4	T44.6X5	T44.6X6
Bunitrolol	T44.7X1	T44.7X2	T44.7X3	T44.7X4	T44.7X5	T44.7X6
Buphenine	T46.7X1	T46.7X2	T46.7X3	T46.7X4	T46.7X5	T46.7X6
Bupivacaine	T41.3X1	T41.3X2	T41.3X3	T41.3X4	T41.3X5	T41.3X6
infiltration (subcutaneous)	T41.3X1	T41.3X2	T41.3X3	T41.3X4	T41.3X5	T41.3X6
nerve block (peripheral) (plexus)	T41.3X1	T41.3X2	T41.3X3	T41.3X4	T41.3X5	T41.3X6
spinal	T41.3X1	T41.3X2	T41.3X3	T41.3X4	T41.3X5	T41.3X6
Bupranolol	T44.7X1	T44.7X2	T44.7X3	T44.7X4	T44.7X5	T44.7X6
Buprenorphine	T4Ø.491	T4Ø.492	T4Ø.493	T4Ø.494	T4Ø.495	T4Ø.496
Bupropion	T43.291	T43.292	T43.293	T43.294	T43.295	T43.296
Burimamide	T47.1X1	T47.1X2	T47.1X3	T47.1X4	T47.1X5	T47.1X6
Buserelin	T38.891	T38.892	T38.893	T38.894	T38.895	T38.896
Buspirone	T43.591	T43.592	T43.593	T43.594	T43.595	T43.596
Busulfan, busulphan	T45.1X1	T45.1X2	T45.1X3	T45.1X4	T45.1X5	T45.1X6
Butabarbital (sodium)	T42.3X1	T42.3X2	T42.3X3	T42.3X4	T42.3X5	T42.3X6
Butabarbitone	T42.3X1	T42.3X2	T42.3X3	T42.3X4	T42.3X5	T42.3X6
Butabarpal	T42.3X1	T42.3X2	T42.3X3	T42.3X4	T42.3X5	T42.3X6
Butacaine	T41.3X1	T41.3X2	T41.3X3	T41.3X4	T41.3X5	T41.3X6
Butalamine	T46.7X1	T46.7X2	T46.7X3	T46.7X4	T46.7X5	T46.7X6
Butalbital	T42.3X1	T42.3X2	T42.3X3	T42.3X4	T42.3X5	T42.3X6
Butallylonal	T42.3X1	T42.3X2	T42.3X3	T42.3X4	T42.3X5	T42.3X6
Butamben	T41.3X1	T41.3X2	T41.3X3	T41.3X4	T41.3X5	T41.3X6
Butamirate	T48.3X1	T48.3X2	T48.3X3	T48.3X4	T48.3X5	T48.3X6
Butane (distributed in mobile container)	T59.891	T59.892	T59.893	T59.894	—	—
distributed through pipes	T59.891	T59.892	T59.893	T59.894	—	—
incomplete combustion	T58.11	T58.12	T58.13	T58.14	—	—
Butanilicaine	T41.3X1	T41.3X2	T41.3X3	T41.3X4	T41.3X5	T41.3X6
Butanol	T51.3X1	T51.3X2	T51.3X3	T51.3X4	—	—
Butanone, 2-butanone	T52.4X1	T52.4X2	T52.4X3	T52.4X4	—	—
Butantrone	T49.4X1	T49.4X2	T49.4X3	T49.4X4	T49.4X5	T49.4X6
Butaperazine	T43.3X1	T43.3X2	T43.3X3	T43.3X4	T43.3X5	T43.3X6
Butazolidin	T39.2X1	T39.2X2	T39.2X3	T39.2X4	T39.2X5	T39.2X6
Butetamate	T48.6X1	T48.6X2	T48.6X3	T48.6X4	T48.6X5	T48.6X6
Butethal	T42.3X1	T42.3X2	T42.3X3	T42.3X4	T42.3X5	T42.3X6
Butethamate	T44.3X1	T44.3X2	T44.3X3	T44.3X4	T44.3X5	T44.3X6
Buthalitone (sodium)	T41.1X1	T41.1X2	T41.1X3	T41.1X4	T41.1X5	T41.1X6
Butisol (sodium)	T42.3X1	T42.3X2	T42.3X3	T42.3X4	T42.3X5	T42.3X6
Butizide	T5Ø.2X1	T5Ø.2X2	T5Ø.2X3	T5Ø.2X4	T5Ø.2X5	T5Ø.2X6
Butobarbital	T42.3X1	T42.3X2	T42.3X3	T42.3X4	T42.3X5	T42.3X6
sodium	T42.3X1	T42.3X2	T42.3X3	T42.3X4	T42.3X5	T42.3X6
Butobarbitone	T42.3X1	T42.3X2	T42.3X3	T42.3X4	T42.3X5	T42.3X6
Butoconazole (nitrate)	T49.ØX1	T49.ØX2	T49.ØX3	T49.ØX4	T49.ØX5	T49.ØX6
Butorphanol	T4Ø.491	T4Ø.492	T4Ø.493	T4Ø.494	T4Ø.495	T4Ø.496
Butriptyline	T43.Ø11	T43.Ø12	T43.Ø13	T43.Ø14	T43.Ø15	T43.Ø16
Butropium bromide	T44.3X1	T44.3X2	T44.3X3	T44.3X4	T44.3X5	T44.3X6
Buttercups	T62.2X1	T62.2X2	T62.2X3	T62.2X4	—	—
Butter of antimony — *see* Antimony						
Butyl						
acetate (secondary)	T52.8X1	T52.8X2	T52.8X3	T52.8X4	—	—
alcohol	T51.3X1	T51.3X2	T51.3X3	T51.3X4	—	—
aminobenzoate	T41.3X1	T41.3X2	T41.3X3	T41.3X4	T41.3X5	T41.3X6
butyrate	T52.8X1	T52.8X2	T52.8X3	T52.8X4	—	—
carbinol	T51.3X1	T51.3X2	T51.3X3	T51.3X4	—	—
carbitol	T52.3X1	T52.3X2	T52.3X3	T52.3X4	—	—
cellosolve	T52.3X1	T52.3X2	T52.3X3	T52.3X4	—	—
chloral (hydrate)	T42.6X1	T42.6X2	T42.6X3	T42.6X4	T42.6X5	T42.6X6
formate	T52.8X1	T52.8X2	T52.8X3	T52.8X4	—	—
lactate	T52.8X1	T52.8X2	T52.8X3	T52.8X4	—	—

Substance	Poisoning, Accidental (unintentional)	Poisoning, Intentional Self-harm	Poisoning, Assault	Poisoning, Undetermined	Adverse Effect	Under-dosing
Butyl — *continued*						
propionate	T52.8X1	T52.8X2	T52.8X3	T52.8X4	—	—
scopolamine bromide	T44.3X1	T44.3X2	T44.3X3	T44.3X4	T44.3X5	T44.3X6
thiobarbital sodium	T41.1X1	T41.1X2	T41.1X3	T41.1X4	T41.1X5	T41.1X6
Butylated hydroxyanisole	T50.991	T50.992	T50.993	T50.994	T50.995	T50.996
Butylchloral hydrate	T42.6X1	T42.6X2	T42.6X3	T42.6X4	T42.6X5	T42.6X6
Butyltoluene	T52.2X1	T52.2X2	T52.2X3	T52.2X4	—	—
Butyn	T41.3X1	T41.3X2	T41.3X3	T41.3X4	T41.3X5	T41.3X6
Butyrophenone (-based tranquilizers)	T43.4X1	T43.4X2	T43.4X3	T43.4X4	T43.4X5	T43.4X6
Cabergoline	T42.8X1	T42.8X2	T42.8X3	T42.8X4	T42.8X5	T42.8X6
Cacodyl, cacodylic acid	T57.ØX1	T57.ØX2	T57.ØX3	T57.ØX4	—	—
Cactinomycin	T45.1X1	T45.1X2	T45.1X3	T45.1X4	T45.1X5	T45.1X6
Cade oil	T49.4X1	T49.4X2	T49.4X3	T49.4X4	T49.4X5	T49.4X6
Cadexomer iodine	T49.ØX1	T49.ØX2	T49.ØX3	T49.ØX4	T49.ØX5	T49.ØX6
Cadmium (chloride) (fumes) (oxide)	T56.3X1	T56.3X2	T56.3X3	T56.3X4	—	—
sulfide (medicinal) NEC	T49.4X1	T49.4X2	T49.4X3	T49.4X4	T49.4X5	T49.4X6
Cadralazine	T46.5X1	T46.5X2	T46.5X3	T46.5X4	T46.5X5	T46.5X6
Caffeine	T43.611	T43.612	T43.613	T43.614	T43.615	T43.616
Calabar bean	T62.2X1	T62.2X2	T62.2X3	T62.2X4	—	—
Caladium seguinum	T62.2X1	T62.2X2	T62.2X3	T62.2X4	—	—
Calamine (lotion)	T49.3X1	T49.3X2	T49.3X3	T49.3X4	T49.3X5	T49.3X6
Calcifediol	T45.2X1	T45.2X2	T45.2X3	T45.2X4	T45.2X5	T45.2X6
Calciferol	T45.2X1	T45.2X2	T45.2X3	T45.2X4	T45.2X5	T45.2X6
Calcitonin	T50.991	T50.992	T50.993	T50.994	T50.995	T50.996
Calcitriol	T45.2X1	T45.2X2	T45.2X3	T45.2X4	T45.2X5	T45.2X6
Calcium	T50.3X1	T50.3X2	T50.3X3	T50.3X4	T50.3X5	T50.3X6
actylsalicylate	T39.Ø11	T39.Ø12	T39.Ø13	T39.Ø14	T39.Ø15	T39.Ø16
benzamidosalicylate	T37.1X1	T37.1X2	T37.1X3	T37.1X4	T37.1X5	T37.1X6
bromide	T42.6X1	T42.6X2	T42.6X3	T42.6X4	T42.6X5	T42.6X6
bromolactobionate	T42.6X1	T42.6X2	T42.6X3	T42.6X4	T42.6X5	T42.6X6
carbaspirin	T39.Ø11	T39.Ø12	T39.Ø13	T39.Ø14	T39.Ø15	T39.Ø16
carbimide	T50.6X1	T50.6X2	T50.6X3	T50.6X4	T50.6X5	T50.6X6
carbonate	T47.1X1	T47.1X2	T47.1X3	T47.1X4	T47.1X5	T47.1X6
chloride	T50.991	T50.992	T50.993	T50.994	T50.995	T50.996
anhydrous	T50.991	T50.992	T50.993	T50.994	T50.995	T50.996
cyanide	T57.8X1	T57.8X2	T57.8X3	T57.8X4	—	—
dioctyl sulfosuccinate	T47.4X1	T47.4X2	T47.4X3	T47.4X4	T47.4X5	T47.4X6
disodium edathamil	T45.8X1	T45.8X2	T45.8X3	T45.8X4	T45.8X5	T45.8X6
disodium edetate	T45.8X1	T45.8X2	T45.8X3	T45.8X4	T45.8X5	T45.8X6
dobesilate	T46.991	T46.992	T46.993	T46.994	T46.995	T46.996
EDTA	T45.8X1	T45.8X2	T45.8X3	T45.8X4	T45.8X5	T45.8X6
ferrous citrate	T45.4X1	T45.4X2	T45.4X3	T45.4X4	T45.4X5	T45.4X6
folinate	T45.8X1	T45.8X2	T45.8X3	T45.8X4	T45.8X5	T45.8X6
glubionate	T50.3X1	T50.3X2	T50.3X3	T50.3X4	T50.3X5	T50.3X6
gluconate	T50.3X1	T50.3X2	T50.3X3	T50.3X4	T50.3X5	T50.3X6
gluconogalactogluconate	T50.3X1	T50.3X2	T50.3X3	T50.3X4	T50.3X5	T50.3X6
hydrate, hydroxide	T54.3X1	T54.3X2	T54.3X3	T54.3X4	—	—
hypochlorite	T54.3X1	T54.3X2	T54.3X3	T54.3X4	—	—
iodide	T48.4X1	T48.4X2	T48.4X3	T48.4X4	T48.4X5	T48.4X6
ipodate	T50.8X1	T50.8X2	T50.8X3	T50.8X4	T50.8X5	T50.8X6
lactate	T50.3X1	T50.3X2	T50.3X3	T50.3X4	T50.3X5	T50.3X6
leucovorin	T45.8X1	T45.8X2	T45.8X3	T45.8X4	T45.8X5	T45.8X6
mandelate	T37.91	T37.92	T37.93	T37.94	T37.95	T37.96
oxide	T54.3X1	T54.3X2	T54.3X3	T54.3X4	—	—
pantothenate	T45.2X1	T45.2X2	T45.2X3	T45.2X4	T45.2X5	T45.2X6
phosphate	T50.3X1	T50.3X2	T50.3X3	T50.3X4	T50.3X5	T50.3X6
salicylate	T39.Ø91	T39.Ø92	T39.Ø93	T39.Ø94	T39.Ø95	T39.Ø96
salts	T50.3X1	T50.3X2	T50.3X3	T50.3X4	T50.3X5	T50.3X6
Calculus-dissolving drug	T50.991	T50.992	T50.993	T50.994	T50.995	T50.996
Calomel	T49.ØX1	T49.ØX2	T49.ØX3	T49.ØX4	T49.ØX5	T49.ØX6
Caloric agent	T50.3X1	T50.3X2	T50.3X3	T50.3X4	T50.3X5	T50.3X6
Calusterone	T38.7X1	T38.7X2	T38.7X3	T38.7X4	T38.7X5	T38.7X6
Camazepam	T42.4X1	T42.4X2	T42.4X3	T42.4X4	T42.4X5	T42.4X6
Camomile	T49.ØX1	T49.ØX2	T49.ØX3	T49.ØX4	T49.ØX5	T49.ØX6
Camoquin	T37.2X1	T37.2X2	T37.2X3	T37.2X4	T37.2X5	T37.2X6
Camphor						
insecticide	T60.2X1	T60.2X2	T60.2X3	T60.2X4	—	—
medicinal	T49.8X1	T49.8X2	T49.8X3	T49.8X4	T49.8X5	T49.8X6
Camylofin	T44.3X1	T44.3X2	T44.3X3	T44.3X4	T44.3X5	T44.3X6
Cancer chemotherapy drug regimen	T45.1X1	T45.1X2	T45.1X3	T45.1X4	T45.1X5	T45.1X6
Candeptin	T49.ØX1	T49.ØX2	T49.ØX3	T49.ØX4	T49.ØX5	T49.ØX6
Candicidin	T49.ØX1	T49.ØX2	T49.ØX3	T49.ØX4	T49.ØX5	T49.ØX6
Cannabinol	T40.7X1	T40.7X2	T40.7X3	T40.7X4	T40.7X5	T40.7X6
Cannabis (derivatives)	T40.7X1	T40.7X2	T40.7X3	T40.7X4	T40.7X5	T40.7X6
Canned heat	T51.1X1	T51.1X2	T51.1X3	T51.1X4	—	—
Canrenoic acid	T50.ØX1	T50.ØX2	T50.ØX3	T50.ØX4	T50.ØX5	T50.ØX6
Canrenone	T50.ØX1	T50.ØX2	T50.ØX3	T50.ØX4	T50.ØX5	T50.ØX6
Cantharides, cantharidin, cantharis	T49.8X1	T49.8X2	T49.8X3	T49.8X4	T49.8X5	T49.8X6
Canthaxanthin	T50.991	T50.992	T50.993	T50.994	T50.995	T50.996
Capillary-active drug NEC	T46.901	T46.902	T46.903	T46.904	T46.905	T46.906
Capreomycin	T36.8X1	T36.8X2	T36.8X3	T36.8X4	T36.8X5	T36.8X6
Capsicum	T49.4X1	T49.4X2	T49.4X3	T49.4X4	T49.4X5	T49.4X6
Captafol	T60.3X1	T60.3X2	T60.3X3	T60.3X4	—	—
Captan	T60.3X1	T60.3X2	T60.3X3	T60.3X4	—	—
Captodiame, captodiamine	T43.591	T43.592	T43.593	T43.594	T43.595	T43.596
Captopril	T46.4X1	T46.4X2	T46.4X3	T46.4X4	T46.4X5	T46.4X6
Caramiphen	T44.3X1	T44.3X2	T44.3X3	T44.3X4	T44.3X5	T44.3X6
Carazolol	T44.7X1	T44.7X2	T44.7X3	T44.7X4	T44.7X5	T44.7X6
Carbachol	T44.1X1	T44.1X2	T44.1X3	T44.1X4	T44.1X5	T44.1X6
Carbacrylamine (resin)	T50.3X1	T50.3X2	T50.3X3	T50.3X4	T50.3X5	T50.3X6
Carbamate (insecticide)	T60.ØX1	T60.ØX2	T60.ØX3	T60.ØX4	—	—
Carbamate (sedative)	T42.6X1	T42.6X2	T42.6X3	T42.6X4	T42.6X5	T42.6X6
herbicide	T60.ØX1	T60.ØX2	T60.ØX3	T60.ØX4	—	—
insecticide	T60.ØX1	T60.ØX2	T60.ØX3	T60.ØX4	—	—
Carbamazepine	T42.1X1	T42.1X2	T42.1X3	T42.1X4	T42.1X5	T42.1X6
Carbamide	T47.3X1	T47.3X2	T47.3X3	T47.3X4	T47.3X5	T47.3X6
peroxide	T49.ØX1	T49.ØX2	T49.ØX3	T49.ØX4	T49.ØX5	T49.ØX6
topical	T49.8X1	T49.8X2	T49.8X3	T49.8X4	T49.8X5	T49.8X6
Carbamylcholine chloride	T44.1X1	T44.1X2	T44.1X3	T44.1X4	T44.1X5	T44.1X6
Carbaril	T60.ØX1	T60.ØX2	T60.ØX3	T60.ØX4	—	—
Carbarsone	T37.3X1	T37.3X2	T37.3X3	T37.3X4	T37.3X5	T37.3X6
Carbaryl	T60.ØX1	T60.ØX2	T60.ØX3	T60.ØX4	—	—
Carbaspirin	T39.Ø11	T39.Ø12	T39.Ø13	T39.Ø14	T39.Ø15	T39.Ø16
Carbazochrome (salicylate) (sodium sulfonate)	T49.4X1	T49.4X2	T49.4X3	T49.4X4	T49.4X5	T49.4X6
Carbenicillin	T36.ØX1	T36.ØX2	T36.ØX3	T36.ØX4	T36.ØX5	T36.ØX6
Carbenoxolone	T47.1X1	T47.1X2	T47.1X3	T47.1X4	T47.1X5	T47.1X6
Carbetapentane	T48.3X1	T48.3X2	T48.3X3	T48.3X4	T48.3X5	T48.3X6
Carbethyl salicylate	T39.Ø91	T39.Ø92	T39.Ø93	T39.Ø94	T39.Ø95	T39.Ø96
Carbidopa (with levodopa)	T42.8X1	T42.8X2	T42.8X3	T42.8X4	T42.8X5	T42.8X6
Carbimazole	T38.2X1	T38.2X2	T38.2X3	T38.2X4	T38.2X5	T38.2X6
Carbinol	T51.1X1	T51.1X2	T51.1X3	T51.1X4	—	—
Carbinoxamine	T45.ØX1	T45.ØX2	T45.ØX3	T45.ØX4	T45.ØX5	T45.ØX6
Carbiphene	T39.8X1	T39.8X2	T39.8X3	T39.8X4	T39.8X5	T39.8X6
Carbitol	T52.3X1	T52.3X2	T52.3X3	T52.3X4	—	—
Carbocaine	T41.3X1	T41.3X2	T41.3X3	T41.3X4	T41.3X5	T41.3X6
infiltration (subcutaneous)	T41.3X1	T41.3X2	T41.3X3	T41.3X4	T41.3X5	T41.3X6
nerve block (peripheral) (plexus)	T41.3X1	T41.3X2	T41.3X3	T41.3X4	T41.3X5	T41.3X6
topical (surface)	T41.3X1	T41.3X2	T41.3X3	T41.3X4	T41.3X5	T41.3X6
Carbocisteine	T48.4X1	T48.4X2	T48.4X3	T48.4X4	T48.4X5	T48.4X6
Carbocromen	T46.3X1	T46.3X2	T46.3X3	T46.3X4	T46.3X5	T46.3X6
Carbol fuchsin	T49.ØX1	T49.ØX2	T49.ØX3	T49.ØX4	T49.ØX5	T49.ØX6
Carbolic acid — *see also* Phenol	T54.ØX1	T54.ØX2	T54.ØX3	T54.ØX4	—	—
Carbolonium (bromide)	T48.1X1	T48.1X2	T48.1X3	T48.1X4	T48.1X5	T48.1X6
Carbo medicinalis	T47.6X1	T47.6X2	T47.6X3	T47.6X4	T47.6X5	T47.6X6
Carbomycin	T36.8X1	T36.8X2	T36.8X3	T36.8X4	T36.8X5	T36.8X6
Carbon						
bisulfide (liquid)	T65.4X1	T65.4X2	T65.4X3	T65.4X4	—	—
vapor	T65.4X1	T65.4X2	T65.4X3	T65.4X4	—	—
dioxide (gas)	T59.7X1	T59.7X2	T59.7X3	T59.7X4	—	—
medicinal	T41.5X1	T41.5X2	T41.5X3	T41.5X4	T41.5X5	T41.5X6
nonmedicinal	T59.7X1	T59.7X2	T59.7X3	T59.7X4	—	—
snow	T49.4X1	T49.4X2	T49.4X3	T49.4X4	T49.4X5	T49.4X6
disulfide (liquid)	T65.4X1	T65.4X2	T65.4X3	T65.4X4	—	—
vapor	T65.4X1	T65.4X2	T65.4X3	T65.4X4	—	—
monoxide (from incomplete combustion)	T58.91	T58.92	T58.93	T58.94	—	—
blast furnace gas	T58.8X1	T58.8X2	T58.8X3	T58.8X4	—	—
butane (distributed in mobile container)	T58.11	T58.12	T58.13	T58.14	—	—
distributed through pipes	T58.11	T58.12	T58.13	T58.14	—	—
charcoal fumes	T58.2X1	T58.2X2	T58.2X3	T58.2X4	—	—
coal	T58.2X1	T58.2X2	T58.2X3	T58.2X4	—	—
coke (in domestic stoves, fireplaces)	T58.2X1	T58.2X2	T58.2X3	T58.2X4	—	—
exhaust gas (motor) not in transit	T58.Ø1	T58.Ø2	T58.Ø3	T58.Ø4	—	—
combustion engine, any not in watercraft	T58.Ø1	T58.Ø2	T58.Ø3	T58.Ø4	—	—
farm tractor, not in transit	T58.Ø1	T58.Ø2	T58.Ø3	T58.Ø4	—	—
gas engine	T58.Ø1	T58.Ø2	T58.Ø3	T58.Ø4	—	—
motor pump	T58.Ø1	T58.Ø2	T58.Ø3	T58.Ø4	—	—
motor vehicle, not in transit	T58.Ø1	T58.Ø2	T58.Ø3	T58.Ø4	—	—
fuel (in domestic use)	T58.2X1	T58.2X2	T58.2X3	T58.2X4	—	—
gas (piped)	T58.11	T58.12	T58.13	T58.14	—	—
in mobile container	T58.11	T58.12	T58.13	T58.14	—	—

Substance	Poisoning, Accidental (unintentional)	Poisoning, Intentional Self-harm	Poisoning, Assault	Poisoning, Undetermined	Adverse Effect	Under-dosing
Carbon — *continued*						
monoxide — *continued*						
fuel — *continued*						
piped (natural)	T58.11	T58.12	T58.13	T58.14	—	—
utility	T58.11	T58.12	T58.13	T58.14	—	—
in mobile container	T58.11	T58.12	T58.13	T58.14	—	—
gas (piped)	T58.11	T58.12	T58.13	T58.14	—	—
illuminating gas	T58.11	T58.12	T58.13	T58.14	—	—
industrial fuels or gases, any	T58.8X1	T58.8X2	T58.8X3	T58.8X4	—	—
kerosene (in domestic stoves, fireplaces)	T58.2X1	T58.2X2	T58.2X3	T58.2X4	—	—
kiln gas or vapor	T58.8X1	T58.8X2	T58.8X3	T58.8X4	—	—
motor exhaust gas, not in transit	T58.Ø1	T58.Ø2	T58.Ø3	T58.Ø4	—	—
piped gas (manufactured) (natural)	T58.11	T58.12	T58.13	T58.14	—	—
producer gas	T58.8X1	T58.8X2	T58.8X3	T58.8X4	—	—
propane (distributed in mobile container)	T58.11	T58.12	T58.13	T58.14	—	—
distributed through pipes	T58.11	T58.12	T58.13	T58.14	—	—
solid (in domestic stoves, fireplaces)	T58.2X1	T58.2X2	T58.2X3	T58.2X4	—	—
specified source NEC	T58.8X1	T58.8X2	T58.8X3	T58.8X4	—	—
stove gas	T58.11	T58.12	T58.13	T58.14	—	—
piped	T58.11	T58.12	T58.13	T58.14	—	—
utility gas	T58.11	T58.12	T58.13	T58.14	—	—
piped	T58.11	T58.12	T58.13	T58.14	—	—
water gas	T58.11	T58.12	T58.13	T58.14	—	—
wood (in domestic stoves, fireplaces)	T58.2X1	T58.2X2	T58.2X3	T58.2X4	—	—
tetrachloride (vapor) NEC	T53.ØX1	T53.ØX2	T53.ØX3	T53.ØX4	—	—
liquid (cleansing agent) NEC	T53.ØX1	T53.ØX2	T53.ØX3	T53.ØX4	—	—
solvent	T53.ØX1	T53.ØX2	T53.ØX3	T53.ØX4	—	—
Carbonic acid gas	T59.7X1	T59.7X2	T59.7X3	T59.7X4	—	—
anhydrase inhibitor NEC	T5Ø.2X1	T5Ø.2X2	T5Ø.2X3	T5Ø.2X4	T5Ø.2X5	T5Ø.2X6
Carbophenothion	T6Ø.ØX1	T6Ø.ØX2	T6Ø.ØX3	T6Ø.ØX4	—	—
Carboplatin	T45.1X1	T45.1X2	T45.1X3	T45.1X4	T45.1X5	T45.1X6
Carboprost	T48.ØX1	T48.ØX2	T48.ØX3	T48.ØX4	T48.ØX5	T48.ØX6
Carboquone	T45.1X1	T45.1X2	T45.1X3	T45.1X4	T45.1X5	T45.1X6
Carbowax	T49.3X1	T49.3X2	T49.3X3	T49.3X4	T49.3X5	T49.3X6
Carboxymethylcellulose	T47.4X1	T47.4X2	T47.4X3	T47.4X4	T47.4X5	T47.4X6
Carbrital	T42.3X1	T42.3X2	T42.3X3	T42.3X4	T42.3X5	T42.3X6
Carbromal	T42.6X1	T42.6X2	T42.6X3	T42.6X4	T42.6X5	T42.6X6
Carbutamide	T38.3X1	T38.3X2	T38.3X3	T38.3X4	T38.3X5	T38.3X6
Carbuterol	T48.6X1	T48.6X2	T48.6X3	T48.6X4	T48.6X5	T48.6X6
Cardiac						
depressants	T46.2X1	T46.2X2	T46.2X3	T46.2X4	T46.2X5	T46.2X6
rhythm regulator	T46.2X1	T46.2X2	T46.2X3	T46.2X4	T46.2X5	T46.2X6
specified NEC	T46.2X1	T46.2X2	T46.2X3	T46.2X4	T46.2X5	T46.2X6
Cardiografin	T5Ø.8X1	T5Ø.8X2	T5Ø.8X3	T5Ø.8X4	T5Ø.8X5	T5Ø.8X6
Cardiogreen	T5Ø.8X1	T5Ø.8X2	T5Ø.8X3	T5Ø.8X4	T5Ø.8X5	T5Ø.8X6
Cardiotonic (glycoside) **NEC**	T46.ØX1	T46.ØX2	T46.ØX3	T46.ØX4	T46.ØX5	T46.ØX6
Cardiovascular drug NEC	T46.9Ø1	T46.9Ø2	T46.9Ø3	T46.9Ø4	T46.9Ø5	T46.9Ø6
Cardrase	T5Ø.2X1	T5Ø.2X2	T5Ø.2X3	T5Ø.2X4	T5Ø.2X5	T5Ø.2X6
Carfecillin	T36.ØX1	T36.ØX2	T36.ØX3	T36.ØX4	T36.ØX5	T36.ØX6
Carfenazine	T43.3X1	T43.3X2	T43.3X3	T43.3X4	T43.3X5	T43.3X6
Carfusin	T49.ØX1	T49.ØX2	T49.ØX3	T49.ØX4	T49.ØX5	T49.ØX6
Carindacillin	T36.ØX1	T36.ØX2	T36.ØX3	T36.ØX4	T36.ØX5	T36.ØX6
Carisoprodol	T42.8X1	T42.8X2	T42.8X3	T42.8X4	T42.8X5	T42.8X6
Carmellose	T47.4X1	T47.4X2	T47.4X3	T47.4X4	T47.4X5	T47.4X6
Carminative	T47.5X1	T47.5X2	T47.5X3	T47.5X4	T47.5X5	T47.5X6
Carmofur	T45.1X1	T45.1X2	T45.1X3	T45.1X4	T45.1X5	T45.1X6
Carmustine	T45.1X1	T45.1X2	T45.1X3	T45.1X4	T45.1X5	T45.1X6
Carotene	T45.2X1	T45.2X2	T45.2X3	T45.2X4	T45.2X5	T45.2X6
Carphenazine	T43.3X1	T43.3X2	T43.3X3	T43.3X4	T43.3X5	T43.3X6
Carpipramine	T42.4X1	T42.4X2	T42.4X3	T42.4X4	T42.4X5	T42.4X6
Carprofen	T39.311	T39.312	T39.313	T39.314	T39.315	T39.316
Carpronium chloride	T44.3X1	T44.3X2	T44.3X3	T44.3X4	T44.3X5	T44.3X6
Carrageenan	T47.8X1	T47.8X2	T47.8X3	T47.8X4	T47.8X5	T47.8X6
Carteolol	T44.7X1	T44.7X2	T44.7X3	T44.7X4	T44.7X5	T44.7X6
Carter's Little Pills	T47.2X1	T47.2X2	T47.2X3	T47.2X4	T47.2X5	T47.2X6
Cascara (sagrada)	T47.2X1	T47.2X2	T47.2X3	T47.2X4	T47.2X5	T47.2X6
Cassava	T62.2X1	T62.2X2	T62.2X3	T62.2X4	—	—
Castellani's paint	T49.ØX1	T49.ØX2	T49.ØX3	T49.ØX4	T49.ØX5	T49.ØX6
Castor						
bean	T62.2X1	T62.2X2	T62.2X3	T62.2X4	—	—
oil	T47.2X1	T47.2X2	T47.2X3	T47.2X4	T47.2X5	T47.2X6
Catalase	T45.3X1	T45.3X2	T45.3X3	T45.3X4	T45.3X5	T45.3X6
Caterpillar (sting)	T63.431	T63.432	T63.433	T63.434	—	—
Catha (edulis) (tea)	T43.691	T43.692	T43.693	T43.694	—	—

Substance	Poisoning, Accidental (unintentional)	Poisoning, Intentional Self-harm	Poisoning, Assault	Poisoning, Undetermined	Adverse Effect	Under-dosing
Cathartic NEC	T47.4X1	T47.4X2	T47.4X3	T47.4X4	T47.4X5	T47.4X6
anthacene derivative	T47.2X1	T47.2X2	T47.2X3	T47.2X4	T47.2X5	T47.2X6
bulk	T47.4X1	T47.4X2	T47.4X3	T47.4X4	T47.4X5	T47.4X6
contact	T47.2X1	T47.2X2	T47.2X3	T47.2X4	T47.2X5	T47.2X6
emollient NEC	T47.4X1	T47.4X2	T47.4X3	T47.4X4	T47.4X5	T47.4X6
irritant NEC	T47.2X1	T47.2X2	T47.2X3	T47.2X4	T47.2X5	T47.2X6
mucilage	T47.4X1	T47.4X2	T47.4X3	T47.4X4	T47.4X5	T47.4X6
saline	T47.3X1	T47.3X2	T47.3X3	T47.3X4	T47.3X5	T47.3X6
vegetable	T47.2X1	T47.2X2	T47.2X3	T47.2X4	T47.2X5	T47.2X6
Cathine	T5Ø.5X1	T5Ø.5X2	T5Ø.5X3	T5Ø.5X4	T5Ø.5X5	T5Ø.5X6
Cathomycin	T36.8X1	T36.8X2	T36.8X3	T36.8X4	T36.8X5	T36.8X6
Cation exchange resin	T5Ø.3X1	T5Ø.3X2	T5Ø.3X3	T5Ø.3X4	T5Ø.3X5	T5Ø.3X6
Caustic(s) **NEC**	T54.91	T54.92	T54.93	T54.94	—	—
alkali	T54.3X1	T54.3X2	T54.3X3	T54.3X4	—	—
hydroxide	T54.3X1	T54.3X2	T54.3X3	T54.3X4	—	—
potash	T54.3X1	T54.3X2	T54.3X3	T54.3X4	—	—
soda	T54.3X1	T54.3X2	T54.3X3	T54.3X4	—	—
specified NEC	T54.91	T54.92	T54.93	T54.94	—	—
Ceepryn	T49.ØX1	T49.ØX2	T49.ØX3	T49.ØX4	T49.ØX5	T49.ØX6
ENT agent	T49.6X1	T49.6X2	T49.6X3	T49.6X4	T49.6X5	T49.6X6
lozenges	T49.6X1	T49.6X2	T49.6X3	T49.6X4	T49.6X5	T49.6X6
Cefacetrile	T36.1X1	T36.1X2	T36.1X3	T36.1X4	T36.1X5	T36.1X6
Cefaclor	T36.1X1	T36.1X2	T36.1X3	T36.1X4	T36.1X5	T36.1X6
Cefadroxil	T36.1X1	T36.1X2	T36.1X3	T36.1X4	T36.1X5	T36.1X6
Cefalexin	T36.1X1	T36.1X2	T36.1X3	T36.1X4	T36.1X5	T36.1X6
Cefaloglycin	T36.1X1	T36.1X2	T36.1X3	T36.1X4	T36.1X5	T36.1X6
Cefaloridine	T36.1X1	T36.1X2	T36.1X3	T36.1X4	T36.1X5	T36.1X6
Cefalosporins	T36.1X1	T36.1X2	T36.1X3	T36.1X4	T36.1X5	T36.1X6
Cefalotin	T36.1X1	T36.1X2	T36.1X3	T36.1X4	T36.1X5	T36.1X6
Cefamandole	T36.1X1	T36.1X2	T36.1X3	T36.1X4	T36.1X5	T36.1X6
Cefamycin antibiotic	T36.1X1	T36.1X2	T36.1X3	T36.1X4	T36.1X5	T36.1X6
Cefapirin	T36.1X1	T36.1X2	T36.1X3	T36.1X4	T36.1X5	T36.1X6
Cefatrizine	T36.1X1	T36.1X2	T36.1X3	T36.1X4	T36.1X5	T36.1X6
Cefazedone	T36.1X1	T36.1X2	T36.1X3	T36.1X4	T36.1X5	T36.1X6
Cefazolin	T36.1X1	T36.1X2	T36.1X3	T36.1X4	T36.1X5	T36.1X6
Cefbuperazone	T36.1X1	T36.1X2	T36.1X3	T36.1X4	T36.1X5	T36.1X6
Cefetamet	T36.1X1	T36.1X2	T36.1X3	T36.1X4	T36.1X5	T36.1X6
Cefixime	T36.1X1	T36.1X2	T36.1X3	T36.1X4	T36.1X5	T36.1X6
Cefmenoxime	T36.1X1	T36.1X2	T36.1X3	T36.1X4	T36.1X5	T36.1X6
Cefmetazole	T36.1X1	T36.1X2	T36.1X3	T36.1X4	T36.1X5	T36.1X6
Cefminox	T36.1X1	T36.1X2	T36.1X3	T36.1X4	T36.1X5	T36.1X6
Cefonicid	T36.1X1	T36.1X2	T36.1X3	T36.1X4	T36.1X5	T36.1X6
Cefoperazone	T36.1X1	T36.1X2	T36.1X3	T36.1X4	T36.1X5	T36.1X6
Ceforanide	T36.1X1	T36.1X2	T36.1X3	T36.1X4	T36.1X5	T36.1X6
Cefotaxime	T36.1X1	T36.1X2	T36.1X3	T36.1X4	T36.1X5	T36.1X6
Cefotetan	T36.1X1	T36.1X2	T36.1X3	T36.1X4	T36.1X5	T36.1X6
Cefotiam	T36.1X1	T36.1X2	T36.1X3	T36.1X4	T36.1X5	T36.1X6
Cefoxitin	T36.1X1	T36.1X2	T36.1X3	T36.1X4	T36.1X5	T36.1X6
Cefpimizole	T36.1X1	T36.1X2	T36.1X3	T36.1X4	T36.1X5	T36.1X6
Cefpiramide	T36.1X1	T36.1X2	T36.1X3	T36.1X4	T36.1X5	T36.1X6
Cefradine	T36.1X1	T36.1X2	T36.1X3	T36.1X4	T36.1X5	T36.1X6
Cefroxadine	T36.1X1	T36.1X2	T36.1X3	T36.1X4	T36.1X5	T36.1X6
Cefsulodin	T36.1X1	T36.1X2	T36.1X3	T36.1X4	T36.1X5	T36.1X6
Ceftazidime	T36.1X1	T36.1X2	T36.1X3	T36.1X4	T36.1X5	T36.1X6
Cefteram	T36.1X1	T36.1X2	T36.1X3	T36.1X4	T36.1X5	T36.1X6
Ceftezole	T36.1X1	T36.1X2	T36.1X3	T36.1X4	T36.1X5	T36.1X6
Ceftizoxime	T36.1X1	T36.1X2	T36.1X3	T36.1X4	T36.1X5	T36.1X6
Ceftriaxone	T36.1X1	T36.1X2	T36.1X3	T36.1X4	T36.1X5	T36.1X6
Cefuroxime	T36.1X1	T36.1X2	T36.1X3	T36.1X4	T36.1X5	T36.1X6
Cefuzonam	T36.1X1	T36.1X2	T36.1X3	T36.1X4	T36.1X5	T36.1X6
Celestone	T38.ØX1	T38.ØX2	T38.ØX3	T38.ØX4	T38.ØX5	T38.ØX6
topical	T49.ØX1	T49.ØX2	T49.ØX3	T49.ØX4	T49.ØX5	T49.ØX6
Celiprolol	T44.7X1	T44.7X2	T44.7X3	T44.7X4	T44.7X5	T44.7X6
Cellosolve	T52.91	T52.92	T52.93	T52.94	—	—
Cell stimulants and proliferants	T49.8X1	T49.8X2	T49.8X3	T49.8X4	T49.8X5	T49.8X6
Cellulose						
cathartic	T47.4X1	T47.4X2	T47.4X3	T47.4X4	T47.4X5	T47.4X6
hydroxyethyl	T47.4X1	T47.4X2	T47.4X3	T47.4X4	T47.4X5	T47.4X6
nitrates (topical)	T49.3X1	T49.3X2	T49.3X3	T49.3X4	T49.3X5	T49.3X6
oxidized	T49.4X1	T49.4X2	T49.4X3	T49.4X4	T49.4X5	T49.4X6
Centipede (bite)	T63.411	T63.412	T63.413	T63.414	—	—
Central nervous system						
depressants	T42.71	T42.72	T42.73	T42.74	T42.75	T42.76
anesthetic (general) NEC	T41.2Ø1	T41.2Ø2	T41.2Ø3	T41.2Ø4	T41.2Ø5	T41.2Ø6
gases NEC	T41.ØX1	T41.ØX2	T41.ØX3	T41.ØX4	T41.ØX5	T41.ØX6
intravenous	T41.1X1	T41.1X2	T41.1X3	T41.1X4	T41.1X5	T41.1X6
barbiturates	T42.3X1	T42.3X2	T42.3X3	T42.3X4	T42.3X5	T42.3X6
benzodiazepines	T42.4X1	T42.4X2	T42.4X3	T42.4X4	T42.4X5	T42.4X6
bromides	T42.6X1	T42.6X2	T42.6X3	T42.6X4	T42.6X5	T42.6X6
cannabis sativa	T4Ø.7X1	T4Ø.7X2	T4Ø.7X3	T4Ø.7X4	T4Ø.7X5	T4Ø.7X6
chloral hydrate	T42.6X1	T42.6X2	T42.6X3	T42.6X4	T42.6X5	T42.6X6
ethanol	T51.ØX1	T51.ØX2	T51.ØX3	T51.ØX4	—	—

Substance	Poisoning, Accidental (unintentional)	Poisoning, Intentional Self-harm	Poisoning, Assault	Poisoning, Undetermined	Adverse Effect	Under-dosing
Central nervous system — *continued*						
depressants — *continued*						
hallucinogenics	T4Ø.9Ø1	T4Ø.9Ø2	T4Ø.9Ø3	T4Ø.9Ø4	T4Ø.9Ø5	T4Ø.9Ø6
hypnotics	T42.71	T42.72	T42.73	T42.74	T42.75	T42.76
specified NEC	T42.6X1	T42.6X2	T42.6X3	T42.6X4	T42.6X5	T42.6X6
muscle relaxants	T42.8X1	T42.8X2	T42.8X3	T42.8X4	T42.8X5	T42.8X6
paraldehyde	T42.6X1	T42.6X2	T42.6X3	T42.6X4	T42.6X5	T42.6X6
sedatives; sedative-hypnotics	T42.71	T42.72	T42.73	T42.74	T42.75	T42.76
mixed NEC	T42.6X1	T42.6X2	T42.6X3	T42.6X4	T42.6X5	T42.6X6
specified NEC	T42.6X1	T42.6X2	T42.6X3	T42.6X4	T42.6X5	T42.6X6
muscle-tone depressants	T42.8X1	T42.8X2	T42.8X3	T42.8X4	T42.8X5	T42.8X6
stimulants	T43.6Ø1	T43.6Ø2	T43.6Ø3	T43.6Ø4	T43.6Ø5	T43.6Ø6
amphetamines	T43.621	T43.622	T43.623	T43.624	T43.625	T43.626
analeptics	T5Ø.7X1	T5Ø.7X2	T5Ø.7X3	T5Ø.7X4	T5Ø.7X5	T5Ø.7X6
antidepressants	T43.2Ø1	T43.2Ø2	T43.2Ø3	T43.2Ø4	T43.2Ø5	T43.2Ø6
opiate antagonists	T5Ø.7X1	T5Ø.7X2	T5Ø.7X3	T5Ø.7X4	T5Ø.7X5	T5Ø.7X6
specified NEC	T43.691	T43.692	T43.693	T43.694	T43.695	T43.696
Cephalexin	T36.1X1	T36.1X2	T36.1X3	T36.1X4	T36.1X5	T36.1X6
Cephaloglycin	T36.1X1	T36.1X2	T36.1X3	T36.1X4	T36.1X5	T36.1X6
Cephaloridine	T36.1X1	T36.1X2	T36.1X3	T36.1X4	T36.1X5	T36.1X6
Cephalosporins	T36.1X1	T36.1X2	T36.1X3	T36.1X4	T36.1X5	T36.1X6
N (adicillin)	T36.ØX1	T36.ØX2	T36.ØX3	T36.ØX4	T36.ØX5	T36.ØX6
Cephalothin	T36.1X1	T36.1X2	T36.1X3	T36.1X4	T36.1X5	T36.1X6
Cephalotin	T36.1X1	T36.1X2	T36.1X3	T36.1X4	T36.1X5	T36.1X6
Cephradine	T36.1X1	T36.1X2	T36.1X3	T36.1X4	T36.1X5	T36.1X6
Cerbera (odallam)	T62.2X1	T62.2X2	T62.2X3	T62.2X4	—	—
Cerberin	T46.ØX1	T46.ØX2	T46.ØX3	T46.ØX4	T46.ØX5	T46.ØX6
Cerebral stimulants	T43.6Ø1	T43.6Ø2	T43.6Ø3	T43.6Ø4	T43.6Ø5	T43.6Ø6
psychotherapeutic	T43.6Ø1	T43.6Ø2	T43.6Ø3	T43.6Ø4	T43.6Ø5	T43.6Ø6
specified NEC	T43.691	T43.692	T43.693	T43.694	T43.695	T43.696
Cerium oxalate	T45.ØX1	T45.ØX2	T45.ØX3	T45.ØX4	T45.ØX5	T45.ØX6
Cerous oxalate	T45.ØX1	T45.ØX2	T45.ØX3	T45.ØX4	T45.ØX5	T45.ØX6
Ceruletide	T5Ø.8X1	T5Ø.8X2	T5Ø.8X3	T5Ø.8X4	T5Ø.8X5	T5Ø.8X6
Cetalkonium (chloride)	T49.ØX1	T49.ØX2	T49.ØX3	T49.ØX4	T49.ØX5	T49.ØX6
Cethexonium chloride	T49.ØX1	T49.ØX2	T49.ØX3	T49.ØX4	T49.ØX5	T49.ØX6
Cetiedil	T46.7X1	T46.7X2	T46.7X3	T46.7X4	T46.7X5	T46.7X6
Cetirizine	T45.ØX1	T45.ØX2	T45.ØX3	T45.ØX4	T45.ØX5	T45.ØX6
Cetomacrogol	T5Ø.991	T5Ø.992	T5Ø.993	T5Ø.994	T5Ø.995	T5Ø.996
Cetotiamine	T45.2X1	T45.2X2	T45.2X3	T45.2X4	T45.2X5	T45.2X6
Cetoxime	T45.ØX1	T45.ØX2	T45.ØX3	T45.ØX4	T45.ØX5	T45.ØX6
Cetraxate	T47.1X1	T47.1X2	T47.1X3	T47.1X4	T47.1X5	T47.1X6
Cetrimide	T49.ØX1	T49.ØX2	T49.ØX3	T49.ØX4	T49.ØX5	T49.ØX6
Cetrimonium (bromide)	T49.ØX1	T49.ØX2	T49.ØX3	T49.ØX4	T49.ØX5	T49.ØX6
Cetylpyridinium chloride	T49.ØX1	T49.ØX2	T49.ØX3	T49.ØX4	T49.ØX5	T49.ØX6
ENT agent	T49.6X1	T49.6X2	T49.6X3	T49.6X4	T49.6X5	T49.6X6
lozenges	T49.6X1	T49.6X2	T49.6X3	T49.6X4	T49.6X5	T49.6X6
Cevadilla — *see* Sabadilla						
Cevitamic acid	T45.2X1	T45.2X2	T45.2X3	T45.2X4	T45.2X5	T45.2X6
Chalk, precipitated	T47.1X1	T47.1X2	T47.1X3	T47.1X4	T47.1X5	T47.1X6
Chamomile	T49.ØX1	T49.ØX2	T49.ØX3	T49.ØX4	T49.ØX5	T49.ØX6
Ch'an su	T46.ØX1	T46.ØX2	T46.ØX3	T46.ØX4	T46.ØX5	T46.ØX6
Charcoal	T47.6X1	T47.6X2	T47.6X3	T47.6X4	T47.6X5	T47.6X6
activated — *see also* Charcoal, medicinal	T47.6X1	T47.6X2	T47.6X3	T47.6X4	T47.6X5	T47.6X6
fumes (Carbon monoxide)	T58.2X1	T58.2X2	T58.2X3	T58.2X4	—	—
industrial	T58.8X1	T58.8X2	T58.8X3	T58.8X4	—	—
medicinal (activated)	T47.6X1	T47.6X2	T47.6X3	T47.6X4	T47.6X5	T47.6X6
antidiarrheal	T47.6X1	T47.6X2	T47.6X3	T47.6X4	T47.6X5	T47.6X6
poison control	T47.8X1	T47.8X2	T47.8X3	T47.8X4	T47.8X5	T47.8X6
specified use other than for diarrhea	T47.8X1	T47.8X2	T47.8X3	T47.8X4	T47.8X5	T47.8X6
topical	T49.8X1	T49.8X2	T49.8X3	T49.8X4	T49.8X5	T49.8X6
Chaulmosulfone	T37.1X1	T37.1X2	T37.1X3	T37.1X4	T37.1X5	T37.1X6
Chelating agent NEC	T5Ø.6X1	T5Ø.6X2	T5Ø.6X3	T5Ø.6X4	T5Ø.6X5	T5Ø.6X6
Chelidonium majus	T62.2X1	T62.2X2	T62.2X3	T62.2X4	—	—
Chemical substance NEC	T65.91	T65.92	T65.93	T65.94	—	—
Chenodeoxycholic acid	T47.5X1	T47.5X2	T47.5X3	T47.5X4	T47.5X5	T47.5X6
Chenodiol	T47.5X1	T47.5X2	T47.5X3	T47.5X4	T47.5X5	T47.5X6
Chenopodium	T37.4X1	T37.4X2	T37.4X3	T37.4X4	T37.4X5	T37.4X6
Cherry laurel	T62.2X1	T62.2X2	T62.2X3	T62.2X4	—	—
Chinidin (e)	T46.2X1	T46.2X2	T46.2X3	T46.2X4	T46.2X5	T46.2X6
Chiniofon	T37.8X1	T37.8X2	T37.8X3	T37.8X4	T37.8X5	T37.8X6
Chlophedianol	T48.3X1	T48.3X2	T48.3X3	T48.3X4	T48.3X5	T48.3X6
Chloral	T42.6X1	T42.6X2	T42.6X3	T42.6X4	T42.6X5	T42.6X6
derivative	T42.6X1	T42.6X2	T42.6X3	T42.6X4	T42.6X5	T42.6X6
hydrate	T42.6X1	T42.6X2	T42.6X3	T42.6X4	T42.6X5	T42.6X6
Chloralamide	T42.6X1	T42.6X2	T42.6X3	T42.6X4	T42.6X5	T42.6X6
Chloralodol	T42.6X1	T42.6X2	T42.6X3	T42.6X4	T42.6X5	T42.6X6
Chloralose	T6Ø.4X1	T6Ø.4X2	T6Ø.4X3	T6Ø.4X4	—	—
Chlorambucil	T45.1X1	T45.1X2	T45.1X3	T45.1X4	T45.1X5	T45.1X6
Chloramine	T57.8X1	T57.8X2	T57.8X3	T57.8X4	—	—
Chloramine — *continued*						
T	T49.ØX1	T49.ØX2	T49.ØX3	T49.ØX4	T49.ØX5	T49.ØX6
topical	T49.ØX1	T49.ØX2	T49.ØX3	T49.ØX4	T49.ØX5	T49.ØX6
Chloramphenicol	T36.2X1	T36.2X2	T36.2X3	T36.2X4	T36.2X5	T36.2X6
ENT agent	T49.6X1	T49.6X2	T49.6X3	T49.6X4	T49.6X5	T49.6X6
ophthalmic preparation	T49.5X1	T49.5X2	T49.5X3	T49.5X4	T49.5X5	T49.5X6
topical NEC	T49.ØX1	T49.ØX2	T49.ØX3	T49.ØX4	T49.ØX5	T49.ØX6
Chlorate (potassium) (sodium) **NEC**	T6Ø.3X1	T6Ø.3X2	T6Ø.3X3	T6Ø.3X4	—	—
herbicide	T6Ø.3X1	T6Ø.3X2	T6Ø.3X3	T6Ø.3X4	—	—
Chlorazanil	T5Ø.2X1	T5Ø.2X2	T5Ø.2X3	T5Ø.2X4	T5Ø.2X5	T5Ø.2X6
Chlorbenzene, chlorbenzol	T53.7X1	T53.7X2	T53.7X3	T53.7X4	—	—
Chlorbenzoxamine	T44.3X1	T44.3X2	T44.3X3	T44.3X4	T44.3X5	T44.3X6
Chlorbutol	T42.6X1	T42.6X2	T42.6X3	T42.6X4	T42.6X5	T42.6X6
Chlorcyclizine	T45.ØX1	T45.ØX2	T45.ØX3	T45.ØX4	T45.ØX5	T45.ØX6
Chlordan (e) (dust)	T6Ø.1X1	T6Ø.1X2	T6Ø.1X3	T6Ø.1X4	—	—
Chlordantoin	T49.ØX1	T49.ØX2	T49.ØX3	T49.ØX4	T49.ØX5	T49.ØX6
Chlordiazepoxide	T42.4X1	T42.4X2	T42.4X3	T42.4X4	T42.4X5	T42.4X6
Chlordiethyl benzamide	T49.3X1	T49.3X2	T49.3X3	T49.3X4	T49.3X5	T49.3X6
Chloresium	T49.8X1	T49.8X2	T49.8X3	T49.8X4	T49.8X5	T49.8X6
Chlorethiazol	T42.6X1	T42.6X2	T42.6X3	T42.6X4	T42.6X5	T42.6X6
Chlorethyl — *see* Ethyl chloride						
Chloretone	T42.6X1	T42.6X2	T42.6X3	T42.6X4	T42.6X5	T42.6X6
Chlorex	T53.6X1	T53.6X2	T53.6X3	T53.6X4	—	—
insecticide	T6Ø.1X1	T6Ø.1X2	T6Ø.1X3	T6Ø.1X4	—	—
Chlorfenvinphos	T6Ø.ØX1	T6Ø.ØX2	T6Ø.ØX3	T6Ø.ØX4	—	—
Chlorhexadol	T42.6X1	T42.6X2	T42.6X3	T42.6X4	T42.6X5	T42.6X6
Chlorhexamide	T45.1X1	T45.1X2	T45.1X3	T45.1X4	T45.1X5	T45.1X6
Chlorhexidine	T49.ØX1	T49.ØX2	T49.ØX3	T49.ØX4	T49.ØX5	T49.ØX6
Chlorhydroxyquinolin	T49.ØX1	T49.ØX2	T49.ØX3	T49.ØX4	T49.ØX5	T49.ØX6
Chloride of lime (bleach)	T54.3X1	T54.3X2	T54.3X3	T54.3X4	—	—
Chlorimipramine	T43.Ø11	T43.Ø12	T43.Ø13	T43.Ø14	T43.Ø15	T43.Ø16
Chlorinated						
camphene	T53.6X1	T53.6X2	T53.6X3	T53.6X4	—	—
diphenyl	T53.7X1	T53.7X2	T53.7X3	T53.7X4	—	—
hydrocarbons NEC	T53.91	T53.92	T53.93	T53.94	—	—
solvents	T53.91	T53.92	T53.93	T53.94	—	—
lime (bleach)	T54.3X1	T54.3X2	T54.3X3	T54.3X4	—	—
and boric acid solution	T49.ØX1	T49.ØX2	T49.ØX3	T49.ØX4	T49.ØX5	T49.ØX6
naphthalene (insecticide)	T6Ø.1X1	T6Ø.1X2	T6Ø.1X3	T6Ø.1X4	—	—
industrial (non-pesticide)	T53.7X1	T53.7X2	T53.7X3	T53.7X4	—	—
pesticide NEC	T6Ø.8X1	T6Ø.8X2	T6Ø.8X3	T6Ø.8X4	—	—
soda — *see also* sodium hypochlorite						
solution	T49.ØX1	T49.ØX2	T49.ØX3	T49.ØX4	T49.ØX5	T49.ØX6
Chlorine (fumes) (gas)	T59.4X1	T59.4X2	T59.4X3	T59.4X4	—	—
bleach	T54.3X1	T54.3X2	T54.3X3	T54.3X4	—	—
compound gas NEC	T59.4X1	T59.4X2	T59.4X3	T59.4X4	—	—
disinfectant	T59.4X1	T59.4X2	T59.4X3	T59.4X4	—	—
releasing agents NEC	T59.4X1	T59.4X2	T59.4X3	T59.4X4	—	—
Chlorisondamine chloride	T46.991	T46.992	T46.993	T46.994	T46.995	T46.996
Chlormadinone	T38.5X1	T38.5X2	T38.5X3	T38.5X4	T38.5X5	T38.5X6
Chlormephos	T6Ø.ØX1	T6Ø.ØX2	T6Ø.ØX3	T6Ø.ØX4	—	—
Chlormerodrin	T5Ø.2X1	T5Ø.2X2	T5Ø.2X3	T5Ø.2X4	T5Ø.2X5	T5Ø.2X6
Chlormethiazole	T42.6X1	T42.6X2	T42.6X3	T42.6X4	T42.6X5	T42.6X6
Chlormethine	T45.1X1	T45.1X2	T45.1X3	T45.1X4	T45.1X5	T45.1X6
Chlormethylenecycline	T36.4X1	T36.4X2	T36.4X3	T36.4X4	T36.4X5	T36.4X6
Chlormezanone	T42.6X1	T42.6X2	T42.6X3	T42.6X4	T42.6X5	T42.6X6
Chloroacetic acid	T6Ø.3X1	T6Ø.3X2	T6Ø.3X3	T6Ø.3X4	—	—
Chloroacetone	T59.3X1	T59.3X2	T59.3X3	T59.3X4	—	—
Chloroacetophenone	T59.3X1	T59.3X2	T59.3X3	T59.3X4	—	—
Chloroaniline	T53.7X1	T53.7X2	T53.7X3	T53.7X4	—	—
Chlorobenzene, chlorobenzol	T53.7X1	T53.7X2	T53.7X3	T53.7X4	—	—
Chlorobromomethane (fire extinguisher)	T53.6X1	T53.6X2	T53.6X3	T53.6X4	—	—
Chlorobutanol	T49.ØX1	T49.ØX2	T49.ØX3	T49.ØX4	T49.ØX5	T49.ØX6
Chlorocresol	T49.ØX1	T49.ØX2	T49.ØX3	T49.ØX4	T49.ØX5	T49.ØX6
Chlorodehydromethyltestosterone	T38.7X1	T38.7X2	T38.7X3	T38.7X4	T38.7X5	T38.7X6
Chlorodinitrobenzene	T53.7X1	T53.7X2	T53.7X3	T53.7X4	—	—
dust or vapor	T53.7X1	T53.7X2	T53.7X3	T53.7X4	—	—
Chlorodiphenyl	T53.7X1	T53.7X2	T53.7X3	T53.7X4	—	—
Chloroethane — *see* Ethyl chloride						
Chloroethylene	T53.6X1	T53.6X2	T53.6X3	T53.6X4	—	—
Chlorofluorocarbons	T53.5X1	T53.5X2	T53.5X3	T53.5X4	—	—
Chloroform (fumes) (vapor)	T53.1X1	T53.1X2	T53.1X3	T53.1X4	—	—
anesthetic	T41.ØX1	T41.ØX2	T41.ØX3	T41.ØX4	T41.ØX5	T41.ØX6
solvent	T53.1X1	T53.1X2	T53.1X3	T53.1X4	—	—
water, concentrated	T41.ØX1	T41.ØX2	T41.ØX3	T41.ØX4	T41.ØX5	T41.ØX6
Chloroguanide	T37.2X1	T37.2X2	T37.2X3	T37.2X4	T37.2X5	T37.2X6

Substance	Poisoning, Accidental (unintentional)	Poisoning, Intentional Self-harm	Poisoning, Assault	Poisoning, Undetermined	Adverse Effect	Under-dosing
Chloromycetin	T36.2X1	T36.2X2	T36.2X3	T36.2X4	T36.2X5	T36.2X6
ENT agent	T49.6X1	T49.6X2	T49.6X3	T49.6X4	T49.6X5	T49.6X6
ophthalmic preparation	T49.5X1	T49.5X2	T49.5X3	T49.5X4	T49.5X5	T49.5X6
otic solution	T49.6X1	T49.6X2	T49.6X3	T49.6X4	T49.6X5	T49.6X6
topical NEC	T49.ØX1	T49.ØX2	T49.ØX3	T49.ØX4	T49.ØX5	T49.ØX6
Chloronitrobenzene	T53.7X1	T53.7X2	T53.7X3	T53.7X4	—	—
dust or vapor	T53.7X1	T53.7X2	T53.7X3	T53.7X4	—	—
Chlorophacinone	T6Ø.4X1	T6Ø.4X2	T6Ø.4X3	T6Ø.4X4	—	—
Chlorophenol	T53.7X1	T53.7X2	T53.7X3	T53.7X4	—	—
Chlorophenothane	T6Ø.1X1	T6Ø.1X2	T6Ø.1X3	T6Ø.1X4	—	—
Chlorophyll	T5Ø.991	T5Ø.992	T5Ø.993	T5Ø.994	T5Ø.995	T5Ø.996
Chloropicrin (fumes)	T53.6X1	T53.6X2	T53.6X3	T53.6X4	—	—
fumigant	T6Ø.8X1	T6Ø.8X2	T6Ø.8X3	T6Ø.8X4	—	—
fungicide	T6Ø.3X1	T6Ø.3X2	T6Ø.3X3	T6Ø.3X4	—	—
pesticide	T6Ø.8X1	T6Ø.8X2	T6Ø.8X3	T6Ø.8X4	—	—
Chloroprocaine	T41.3X1	T41.3X2	T41.3X3	T41.3X4	T41.3X5	T41.3X6
infiltration (subcutaneous)	T41.3X1	T41.3X2	T41.3X3	T41.3X4	T41.3X5	T41.3X6
nerve block (peripheral) (plexus)	T41.3X1	T41.3X2	T41.3X3	T41.3X4	T41.3X5	T41.3X6
spinal	T41.3X1	T41.3X2	T41.3X3	T41.3X4	T41.3X5	T41.3X6
Chloroptic	T49.5X1	T49.5X2	T49.5X3	T49.5X4	T49.5X5	T49.5X6
Chloropurine	T45.1X1	T45.1X2	T45.1X3	T45.1X4	T45.1X5	T45.1X6
Chloropyramine	T45.ØX1	T45.ØX2	T45.ØX3	T45.ØX4	T45.ØX5	T45.ØX6
Chloropyrifos	T6Ø.ØX1	T6Ø.ØX2	T6Ø.ØX3	T6Ø.ØX4	—	—
Chloropyrilene	T45.ØX1	T45.ØX2	T45.ØX3	T45.ØX4	T45.ØX5	T45.ØX6
Chloroquine	T37.2X1	T37.2X2	T37.2X3	T37.2X4	T37.2X5	T37.2X6
Chlorothalonil	T6Ø.3X1	T6Ø.3X2	T6Ø.3X3	T6Ø.3X4	—	—
Chlorothen	T45.ØX1	T45.ØX2	T45.ØX3	T45.ØX4	T45.ØX5	T45.ØX6
Chlorothiazide	T5Ø.2X1	T5Ø.2X2	T5Ø.2X3	T5Ø.2X4	T5Ø.2X5	T5Ø.2X6
Chlorothymol	T49.4X1	T49.4X2	T49.4X3	T49.4X4	T49.4X5	T49.4X6
Chlorotrianisene	T38.5X1	T38.5X2	T38.5X3	T38.5X4	T38.5X5	T38.5X6
Chlorovinyldichloroarsine, not in war	T57.ØX1	T57.ØX2	T57.ØX3	T57.ØX4	—	—
Chloroxine	T49.4X1	T49.4X2	T49.4X3	T49.4X4	T49.4X5	T49.4X6
Chloroxylenol	T49.ØX1	T49.ØX2	T49.ØX3	T49.ØX4	T49.ØX5	T49.ØX6
Chlorphenamine	T45.ØX1	T45.ØX2	T45.ØX3	T45.ØX4	T45.ØX5	T45.ØX6
Chlorphenesin	T42.8X1	T42.8X2	T42.8X3	T42.8X4	T42.8X5	T42.8X6
topical (antifungal)	T49.ØX1	T49.ØX2	T49.ØX3	T49.ØX4	T49.ØX5	T49.ØX6
Chlorpheniramine	T45.ØX1	T45.ØX2	T45.ØX3	T45.ØX4	T45.ØX5	T45.ØX6
Chlorphenoxamine	T45.ØX1	T45.ØX2	T45.ØX3	T45.ØX4	T45.ØX5	T45.ØX6
Chlorphentermine	T5Ø.5X1	T5Ø.5X2	T5Ø.5X3	T5Ø.5X4	T5Ø.5X5	T5Ø.5X6
Chlorprocaine — *see* Chloroprocaine						
Chlorproguanil	T37.2X1	T37.2X2	T37.2X3	T37.2X4	T37.2X5	T37.2X6
Chlorpromazine	T43.3X1	T43.3X2	T43.3X3	T43.3X4	T43.3X5	T43.3X6
Chlorpropamide	T38.3X1	T38.3X2	T38.3X3	T38.3X4	T38.3X5	T38.3X6
Chlorprothixene	T43.4X1	T43.4X2	T43.4X3	T43.4X4	T43.4X5	T43.4X6
Chlorquinaldol	T49.ØX1	T49.ØX2	T49.ØX3	T49.ØX4	T49.ØX5	T49.ØX6
Chlorquinol	T49.ØX1	T49.ØX2	T49.ØX3	T49.ØX4	T49.ØX5	T49.ØX6
Chlortalidone	T5Ø.2X1	T5Ø.2X2	T5Ø.2X3	T5Ø.2X4	T5Ø.2X5	T5Ø.2X6
Chlortetracycline	T36.4X1	T36.4X2	T36.4X3	T36.4X4	T36.4X5	T36.4X6
Chlorthalidone	T5Ø.2X1	T5Ø.2X2	T5Ø.2X3	T5Ø.2X4	T5Ø.2X5	T5Ø.2X6
Chlorthion	T6Ø.ØX1	T6Ø.ØX2	T6Ø.ØX3	T6Ø.ØX4	—	—
Chlorthiophos	T6Ø.ØX1	T6Ø.ØX2	T6Ø.ØX3	T6Ø.ØX4	—	—
Chlortrianisene	T38.5X1	T38.5X2	T38.5X3	T38.5X4	T38.5X5	T38.5X6
Chlor-Trimeton	T45.ØX1	T45.ØX2	T45.ØX3	T45.ØX4	T45.ØX5	T45.ØX6
Chlorzoxazone	T42.8X1	T42.8X2	T42.8X3	T42.8X4	T42.8X5	T42.8X6
Choke damp	T59.7X1	T59.7X2	T59.7X3	T59.7X4	—	—
Cholagogues	T47.5X1	T47.5X2	T47.5X3	T47.5X4	T47.5X5	T47.5X6
Cholebrine	T5Ø.8X1	T5Ø.8X2	T5Ø.8X3	T5Ø.8X4	T5Ø.8X5	T5Ø.8X6
Cholecalciferol	T45.2X1	T45.2X2	T45.2X3	T45.2X4	T45.2X5	T45.2X6
Cholecystokinin	T5Ø.8X1	T5Ø.8X2	T5Ø.8X3	T5Ø.8X4	T5Ø.8X5	T5Ø.8X6
Cholera vaccine	T5Ø.A91	T5Ø.A92	T5Ø.A93	T5Ø.A94	T5Ø.A95	T5Ø.A96
Choleretic	T47.5X1	T47.5X2	T47.5X3	T47.5X4	T47.5X5	T47.5X6
Cholesterol-lowering agents	T46.6X1	T46.6X2	T46.6X3	T46.6X4	T46.6X5	T46.6X6
Cholestyramine (resin)	T46.6X1	T46.6X2	T46.6X3	T46.6X4	T46.6X5	T46.6X6
Cholic acid	T47.5X1	T47.5X2	T47.5X3	T47.5X4	T47.5X5	T47.5X6
Choline	T48.6X1	T48.6X2	T48.6X3	T48.6X4	T48.6X5	T48.6X6
chloride	T5Ø.991	T5Ø.992	T5Ø.993	T5Ø.994	T5Ø.995	T5Ø.996
dihydrogen citrate	T5Ø.991	T5Ø.992	T5Ø.993	T5Ø.994	T5Ø.995	T5Ø.996
salicylate	T39.Ø91	T39.Ø92	T39.Ø93	T39.Ø94	T39.Ø95	T39.Ø96
theophyllinate	T48.6X1	T48.6X2	T48.6X3	T48.6X4	T48.6X5	T48.6X6
Cholinergic (drug) **NEC**	T44.1X1	T44.1X2	T44.1X3	T44.1X4	T44.1X5	T44.1X6
muscle tone enhancer	T44.1X1	T44.1X2	T44.1X3	T44.1X4	T44.1X5	T44.1X6
organophosphorus	T44.ØX1	T44.ØX2	T44.ØX3	T44.ØX4	T44.ØX5	T44.ØX6
insecticide	T6Ø.ØX1	T6Ø.ØX2	T6Ø.ØX3	T6Ø.ØX4	—	—
nerve gas	T59.891	T59.892	T59.893	T59.894	—	—
trimethyl ammonium propanediol	T44.1X1	T44.1X2	T44.1X3	T44.1X4	T44.1X5	T44.1X6
Cholinesterase reactivator	T5Ø.6X1	T5Ø.6X2	T5Ø.6X3	T5Ø.6X4	T5Ø.6X5	T5Ø.6X6
Chholografin	T5Ø.8X1	T5Ø.8X2	T5Ø.8X3	T5Ø.8X4	T5Ø.8X5	T5Ø.8X6
Chorionic gonadotropin	T38.891	T38.892	T38.893	T38.894	T38.895	T38.896

Substance	Poisoning, Accidental (unintentional)	Poisoning, Intentional Self-harm	Poisoning, Assault	Poisoning, Undetermined	Adverse Effect	Under-dosing
Chromate	T56.2X1	T56.2X2	T56.2X3	T56.2X4	—	—
dust or mist	T56.2X1	T56.2X2	T56.2X3	T56.2X4	—	—
lead — *see also* lead	T56.ØX1	T56.ØX2	T56.ØX3	T56.ØX4	—	—
paint	T56.ØX1	T56.ØX2	T56.ØX3	T56.ØX4	—	—
Chromic						
acid	T56.2X1	T56.2X2	T56.2X3	T56.2X4	—	—
dust or mist	T56.2X1	T56.2X2	T56.2X3	T56.2X4	—	—
phosphate 32P	T45.1X1	T45.1X2	T45.1X3	T45.1X4	T45.1X5	T45.1X6
Chromium	T56.2X1	T56.2X2	T56.2X3	T56.2X4	—	—
compounds — *see* Chromate						
sesquioxide	T5Ø.8X1	T5Ø.8X2	T5Ø.8X3	T5Ø.8X4	T5Ø.8X5	T5Ø.8X6
Chromomycin A3	T45.1X1	T45.1X2	T45.1X3	T45.1X4	T45.1X5	T45.1X6
Chromonar	T46.3X1	T46.3X2	T46.3X3	T46.3X4	T46.3X5	T46.3X6
Chromyl chloride	T56.2X1	T56.2X2	T56.2X3	T56.2X4	—	—
Chrysarobin	T49.4X1	T49.4X2	T49.4X3	T49.4X4	T49.4X5	T49.4X6
Chrysazin	T47.2X1	T47.2X2	T47.2X3	T47.2X4	T47.2X5	T47.2X6
Chymar	T45.3X1	T45.3X2	T45.3X3	T45.3X4	T45.3X5	T45.3X6
ophthalmic preparation	T49.5X1	T49.5X2	T49.5X3	T49.5X4	T49.5X5	T49.5X6
Chymopapain	T45.3X1	T45.3X2	T45.3X3	T45.3X4	T45.3X5	T45.3X6
Chymotrypsin	T45.3X1	T45.3X2	T45.3X3	T45.3X4	T45.3X5	T45.3X6
ophthalmic preparation	T49.5X1	T49.5X2	T49.5X3	T49.5X4	T49.5X5	T49.5X6
Cianidanol	T5Ø.991	T5Ø.992	T5Ø.993	T5Ø.994	T5Ø.995	T5Ø.996
Cianopramine	T43.Ø11	T43.Ø12	T43.Ø13	T43.Ø14	T43.Ø15	T43.Ø16
Cibenzoline	T46.2X1	T46.2X2	T46.2X3	T46.2X4	T46.2X5	T46.2X6
Ciclacillin	T36.ØX1	T36.ØX2	T36.ØX3	T36.ØX4	T36.ØX5	T36.ØX6
Ciclobarbital — *see* Hexobarbital						
Ciclonicate	T46.7X1	T46.7X2	T46.7X3	T46.7X4	T46.7X5	T46.7X6
Ciclopirox (olamine)	T49.ØX1	T49.ØX2	T49.ØX3	T49.ØX4	T49.ØX5	T49.ØX6
Ciclosporin	T45.1X1	T45.1X2	T45.1X3	T45.1X4	T45.1X5	T45.1X6
Cicuta maculata or virosa	T62.2X1	T62.2X2	T62.2X3	T62.2X4	—	—
Cicutoxin	T62.2X1	T62.2X2	T62.2X3	T62.2X4	—	—
Cigarette lighter fluid	T52.ØX1	T52.ØX2	T52.ØX3	T52.ØX4	—	—
Cigarettes (tobacco)	T65.221	T65.222	T65.223	T65.224	—	—
Ciguatoxin	T61.Ø1	T61.Ø2	T61.Ø3	T61.Ø4	—	—
Cilazapril	T46.4X1	T46.4X2	T46.4X3	T46.4X4	T46.4X5	T46.4X6
Cimetidine	T47.ØX1	T47.ØX2	T47.ØX3	T47.ØX4	T47.ØX5	T47.ØX6
Cimetropium bromide	T44.3X1	T44.3X2	T44.3X3	T44.3X4	T44.3X5	T44.3X6
Cinchocaine	T41.3X1	T41.3X2	T41.3X3	T41.3X4	T41.3X5	T41.3X6
topical (surface)	T41.3X1	T41.3X2	T41.3X3	T41.3X4	T41.3X5	T41.3X6
Cinchona	T37.2X1	T37.2X2	T37.2X3	T37.2X4	T37.2X5	T37.2X6
Cinchonine alkaloids	T37.2X1	T37.2X2	T37.2X3	T37.2X4	T37.2X5	T37.2X6
Cinchophen	T5Ø.4X1	T5Ø.4X2	T5Ø.4X3	T5Ø.4X4	T5Ø.4X5	T5Ø.4X6
Cinepazide	T46.7X1	T46.7X2	T46.7X3	T46.7X4	T46.7X5	T46.7X6
Cinnamedrine	T48.5X1	T48.5X2	T48.5X3	T48.5X4	T48.5X5	T48.5X6
Cinnarizine	T45.ØX1	T45.ØX2	T45.ØX3	T45.ØX4	T45.ØX5	T45.ØX6
Cinoxacin	T37.8X1	T37.8X2	T37.8X3	T37.8X4	T37.8X5	T37.8X6
Ciprofibrate	T46.6X1	T46.6X2	T46.6X3	T46.6X4	T46.6X5	T46.6X6
Ciprofloxacin	T36.8X1	T36.8X2	T36.8X3	T36.8X4	T36.8X5	T36.8X6
Cisapride	T47.8X1	T47.8X2	T47.8X3	T47.8X4	T47.8X5	T47.8X6
Cisplatin	T45.1X1	T45.1X2	T45.1X3	T45.1X4	T45.1X5	T45.1X6
Citalopram	T43.221	T43.222	T43.223	T43.224	T43.225	T43.226
Citanest	T41.3X1	T41.3X2	T41.3X3	T41.3X4	T41.3X5	T41.3X6
infiltration (subcutaneous)	T41.3X1	T41.3X2	T41.3X3	T41.3X4	T41.3X5	T41.3X6
nerve block (peripheral) (plexus)	T41.3X1	T41.3X2	T41.3X3	T41.3X4	T41.3X5	T41.3X6
Citric acid	T47.5X1	T47.5X2	T47.5X3	T47.5X4	T47.5X5	T47.5X6
Citrovorum (factor)	T45.8X1	T45.8X2	T45.8X3	T45.8X4	T45.8X5	T45.8X6
Claviceps purpurea	T62.2X1	T62.2X2	T62.2X3	T62.2X4	—	—
Clavulanic acid	T36.1X1	T36.1X2	T36.1X3	T36.1X4	T36.1X5	T36.1X6
Cleaner, cleansing agent, type not specified	T65.891	T65.892	T65.893	T65.894	—	—
of paint or varnish	T52.91	T52.92	T52.93	T52.94	—	—
specified type NEC	T65.891	T65.892	T65.893	T65.894	—	—
Clebopride	T47.8X1	T47.8X2	T47.8X3	T47.8X4	T47.8X5	T47.8X6
Clefamide	T37.3X1	T37.3X2	T37.3X3	T37.3X4	T37.3X5	T37.3X6
Clemastine	T45.ØX1	T45.ØX2	T45.ØX3	T45.ØX4	T45.ØX5	T45.ØX6
Clematis vitalba	T62.2X1	T62.2X2	T62.2X3	T62.2X4	—	—
Clemizole	T45.ØX1	T45.ØX2	T45.ØX3	T45.ØX4	T45.ØX5	T45.ØX6
penicillin	T36.ØX1	T36.ØX2	T36.ØX3	T36.ØX4	T36.ØX5	T36.ØX6
Clenbuterol	T48.6X1	T48.6X2	T48.6X3	T48.6X4	T48.6X5	T48.6X6
Clidinium bromide	T44.3X1	T44.3X2	T44.3X3	T44.3X4	T44.3X5	T44.3X6
Clindamycin	T36.8X1	T36.8X2	T36.8X3	T36.8X4	T36.8X5	T36.8X6
Clinofibrate	T46.6X1	T46.6X2	T46.6X3	T46.6X4	T46.6X5	T46.6X6
Clioquinol	T37.8X1	T37.8X2	T37.8X3	T37.8X4	T37.8X5	T37.8X6
Cliradon	T4Ø.2X1	T4Ø.2X2	T4Ø.2X3	T4Ø.2X4	—	—
Clobazam	T42.4X1	T42.4X2	T42.4X3	T42.4X4	T42.4X5	T42.4X6
Clobenzorex	T5Ø.5X1	T5Ø.5X2	T5Ø.5X3	T5Ø.5X4	T5Ø.5X5	T5Ø.5X6
Clobetasol	T49.ØX1	T49.ØX2	T49.ØX3	T49.ØX4	T49.ØX5	T49.ØX6
Clobetasone	T49.ØX1	T49.ØX2	T49.ØX3	T49.ØX4	T49.ØX5	T49.ØX6
Clobutinol	T48.3X1	T48.3X2	T48.3X3	T48.3X4	T48.3X5	T48.3X6
Clocortolone	T38.ØX1	T38.ØX2	T38.ØX3	T38.ØX4	T38.ØX5	T38.ØX6
Clodantoin	T49.ØX1	T49.ØX2	T49.ØX3	T49.ØX4	T49.ØX5	T49.ØX6

Substance	Poisoning, Accidental (unintentional)	Poisoning, Intentional Self-harm	Poisoning, Assault	Poisoning, Undetermined	Adverse Effect	Under-dosing
Clodronic acid	T50.991	T50.992	T50.993	T50.994	T50.995	T50.996
Clofazimine	T37.1X1	T37.1X2	T37.1X3	T37.1X4	T37.1X5	T37.1X6
Clofedanol	T48.3X1	T48.3X2	T48.3X3	T48.3X4	T48.3X5	T48.3X6
Clofenamide	T50.2X1	T50.2X2	T50.2X3	T50.2X4	T50.2X5	T50.2X6
Clofenotane	T49.0X1	T49.0X2	T49.0X3	T49.0X4	T49.0X5	T49.0X6
Clofezone	T39.2X1	T39.2X2	T39.2X3	T39.2X4	T39.2X5	T39.2X6
Clofibrate	T46.6X1	T46.6X2	T46.6X3	T46.6X4	T46.6X5	T46.6X6
Clofibride	T46.6X1	T46.6X2	T46.6X3	T46.6X4	T46.6X5	T46.6X6
Cloforex	T50.5X1	T50.5X2	T50.5X3	T50.5X4	T50.5X5	T50.5X6
Clomethiazole	T42.6X1	T42.6X2	T42.6X3	T42.6X4	T42.6X5	T42.6X6
Clometocillin	T36.0X1	T36.0X2	T36.0X3	T36.0X4	T36.0X5	T36.0X6
Clomifene	T38.5X1	T38.5X2	T38.5X3	T38.5X4	T38.5X5	T38.5X6
Clomiphene	T38.5X1	T38.5X2	T38.5X3	T38.5X4	T38.5X5	T38.5X6
Clomipramine	T43.011	T43.012	T43.013	T43.014	T43.015	T43.016
Clomocycline	T36.4X1	T36.4X2	T36.4X3	T36.4X4	T36.4X5	T36.4X6
Clonazepam	T42.4X1	T42.4X2	T42.4X3	T42.4X4	T42.4X5	T42.4X6
Clonidine	T46.5X1	T46.5X2	T46.5X3	T46.5X4	T46.5X5	T46.5X6
Clonixin	T39.8X1	T39.8X2	T39.8X3	T39.8X4	T39.8X5	T39.8X6
Clopamide	T50.2X1	T50.2X2	T50.2X3	T50.2X4	T50.2X5	T50.2X6
Clopenthixol	T43.4X1	T43.4X2	T43.4X3	T43.4X4	T43.4X5	T43.4X6
Cloperastine	T48.3X1	T48.3X2	T48.3X3	T48.3X4	T48.3X5	T48.3X6
Clophedianol	T48.3X1	T48.3X2	T48.3X3	T48.3X4	T48.3X5	T48.3X6
Cloponone	T36.2X1	T36.2X2	T36.2X3	T36.2X4	T36.2X5	T36.2X6
Cloprednol	T38.0X1	T38.0X2	T38.0X3	T38.0X4	T38.0X5	T38.0X6
Cloral betaine	T42.6X1	T42.6X2	T42.6X3	T42.6X4	T42.6X5	T42.6X6
Cloramfenicol	T36.2X1	T36.2X2	T36.2X3	T36.2X4	T36.2X5	T36.2X6
Clorazepate (dipotassium)	T42.4X1	T42.4X2	T42.4X3	T42.4X4	T42.4X5	T42.4X6
Clorexolone	T50.2X1	T50.2X2	T50.2X3	T50.2X4	T50.2X5	T50.2X6
Clorfenamine	T45.0X1	T45.0X2	T45.0X3	T45.0X4	T45.0X5	T45.0X6
Clorgiline	T43.1X1	T43.1X2	T43.1X3	T43.1X4	T43.1X5	T43.1X6
Clorotepine	T44.3X1	T44.3X2	T44.3X3	T44.3X4	T44.3X5	T44.3X6
Clorox (bleach)	T54.91	T54.92	T54.93	T54.94	—	—
Clorprenaline	T48.6X1	T48.6X2	T48.6X3	T48.6X4	T48.6X5	T48.6X6
Clortermine	T50.5X1	T50.5X2	T50.5X3	T50.5X4	T50.5X5	T50.5X6
Clotiapine	T43.591	T43.592	T43.593	T43.594	T43.595	T43.596
Clotiazepam	T42.4X1	T42.4X2	T42.4X3	T42.4X4	T42.4X5	T42.4X6
Clotibric acid	T46.6X1	T46.6X2	T46.6X3	T46.6X4	T46.6X5	T46.6X6
Clotrimazole	T49.0X1	T49.0X2	T49.0X3	T49.0X4	T49.0X5	T49.0X6
Cloxacillin	T36.0X1	T36.0X2	T36.0X3	T36.0X4	T36.0X5	T36.0X6
Cloxazolam	T42.4X1	T42.4X2	T42.4X3	T42.4X4	T42.4X5	T42.4X6
Cloxiquine	T49.0X1	T49.0X2	T49.0X3	T49.0X4	T49.0X5	T49.0X6
Clozapine	T42.4X1	T42.4X2	T42.4X3	T42.4X4	T42.4X5	T42.4X6
Coagulant NEC	T45.7X1	T45.7X2	T45.7X3	T45.7X4	T45.7X5	T45.7X6
Coal (carbon monoxide from) — *see also* Carbon, monoxide, coal	T58.2X1	T58.2X2	T58.2X3	T58.2X4	—	—
oil — *see* Kerosene						
tar	T49.1X1	T49.1X2	T49.1X3	T49.1X4	T49.1X5	T49.1X6
fumes	T59.891	T59.892	T59.893	T59.894	—	—
medicinal (ointment)	T49.4X1	T49.4X2	T49.4X3	T49.4X4	T49.4X5	T49.4X6
analgesics NEC	T39.2X1	T39.2X2	T39.2X3	T39.2X4	T39.2X5	T39.2X6
naphtha (solvent)	T52.0X1	T52.0X2	T52.0X3	T52.0X4	—	—
Cobalamine	T45.2X1	T45.2X2	T45.2X3	T45.2X4	T45.2X5	T45.2X6
Cobalt (nonmedicinal) (fumes) (industrial)	T56.891	T56.892	T56.893	T56.894	—	—
medicinal (trace) (chloride)	T45.8X1	T45.8X2	T45.8X3	T45.8X4	T45.8X5	T45.8X6
Cobra (venom)	T63.041	T63.042	T63.043	T63.044	—	—
Coca (leaf)	T40.5X1	T40.5X2	T40.5X3	T40.5X4	T40.5X5	T40.5X6
Cocaine	T40.5X1	T40.5X2	T40.5X3	T40.5X4	T40.5X5	T40.5X6
topical anesthetic	T41.3X1	T41.3X2	T41.3X3	T41.3X4	T41.3X5	T41.3X6
Cocarboxylase	T45.3X1	T45.3X2	T45.3X3	T45.3X4	T45.3X5	T45.3X6
Coccidioidin	T50.8X1	T50.8X2	T50.8X3	T50.8X4	T50.8X5	T50.8X6
Cocculus indicus	T62.1X1	T62.1X2	T62.1X3	T62.1X4	—	—
Cochineal	T65.6X1	T65.6X2	T65.6X3	T65.6X4	—	—
medicinal products	T50.991	T50.992	T50.993	T50.994	T50.995	T50.996
Codeine	T40.2X1	T40.2X2	T40.2X3	T40.2X4	T40.2X5	T40.2X6
Cod-liver oil	T45.2X1	T45.2X2	T45.2X3	T45.2X4	T45.2X5	T45.2X6
Coenzyme A	T50.991	T50.992	T50.993	T50.994	T50.995	T50.996
Coffee	T62.8X1	T62.8X2	T62.8X3	T62.8X4	—	—
Cogalactoisomerase	T50.991	T50.992	T50.993	T50.994	T50.995	T50.996
Cogentin	T44.3X1	T44.3X2	T44.3X3	T44.3X4	T44.3X5	T44.3X6
Coke fumes or gas (carbon monoxide)	T58.2X1	T58.2X2	T58.2X3	T58.2X4	—	—
industrial use	T58.8X1	T58.8X2	T58.8X3	T58.8X4	—	—
Colace	T47.4X1	T47.4X2	T47.4X3	T47.4X4	T47.4X5	T47.4X6
Colaspase	T45.1X1	T45.1X2	T45.1X3	T45.1X4	T45.1X5	T45.1X6
Colchicine	T50.4X1	T50.4X2	T50.4X3	T50.4X4	T50.4X5	T50.4X6
Colchicum	T62.2X1	T62.2X2	T62.2X3	T62.2X4	—	—
Cold cream	T49.3X1	T49.3X2	T49.3X3	T49.3X4	T49.3X5	T49.3X6
Colecalciferol	T45.2X1	T45.2X2	T45.2X3	T45.2X4	T45.2X5	T45.2X6
Colestipol	T46.6X1	T46.6X2	T46.6X3	T46.6X4	T46.6X5	T46.6X6
Colestyramine	T46.6X1	T46.6X2	T46.6X3	T46.6X4	T46.6X5	T46.6X6
Colimycin	T36.8X1	T36.8X2	T36.8X3	T36.8X4	T36.8X5	T36.8X6

Substance	Poisoning, Accidental (unintentional)	Poisoning, Intentional Self-harm	Poisoning, Assault	Poisoning, Undetermined	Adverse Effect	Under-dosing
Colistimethate	T36.8X1	T36.8X2	T36.8X3	T36.8X4	T36.8X5	T36.8X6
Colistin	T36.8X1	T36.8X2	T36.8X3	T36.8X4	T36.8X5	T36.8X6
sulfate (eye preparation)	T49.5X1	T49.5X2	T49.5X3	T49.5X4	T49.5X5	T49.5X6
Collagen	T50.991	T50.992	T50.993	T50.994	T50.995	T50.996
Collagenase	T49.4X1	T49.4X2	T49.4X3	T49.4X4	T49.4X5	T49.4X6
Collodion	T49.3X1	T49.3X2	T49.3X3	T49.3X4	T49.3X5	T49.3X6
Colocynth	T47.2X1	T47.2X2	T47.2X3	T47.2X4	T47.2X5	T47.2X6
Colophony adhesive	T49.3X1	T49.3X2	T49.3X3	T49.3X4	T49.3X5	T49.3X6
Colorant — *see also* Dye	T50.991	T50.992	T50.993	T50.994	T50.995	T50.996
Coloring matter — *see* Dye(s)						
Combustion gas (after combustion) — *see* Carbon, monoxide						
prior to combustion	T59.891	T59.892	T59.893	T59.894	—	—
Compazine	T43.3X1	T43.3X2	T43.3X3	T43.3X4	T43.3X5	T43.3X6
Compound						
1080 (sodium fluoroacetate)	T60.4X1	T60.4X2	T60.4X3	T60.4X4	—	—
269 (endrin)	T60.1X1	T60.1X2	T60.1X3	T60.1X4	—	—
3422 (parathion)	T60.0X1	T60.0X2	T60.0X3	T60.0X4	—	—
3911 (phorate)	T60.0X1	T60.0X2	T60.0X3	T60.0X4	—	—
3956 (toxaphene)	T60.1X1	T60.1X2	T60.1X3	T60.1X4	—	—
4049 (malathion)	T60.0X1	T60.0X2	T60.0X3	T60.0X4	—	—
4069 (malathion)	T60.0X1	T60.0X2	T60.0X3	T60.0X4	—	—
4124 (dicapthon)	T60.0X1	T60.0X2	T60.0X3	T60.0X4	—	—
42 (warfarin)	T60.4X1	T60.4X2	T60.4X3	T60.4X4	—	—
497 (dieldrin)	T60.1X1	T60.1X2	T60.1X3	T60.1X4	—	—
E (cortisone)	T38.0X1	T38.0X2	T38.0X3	T38.0X4	T38.0X5	T38.0X6
F (hydrocortisone)	T38.0X1	T38.0X2	T38.0X3	T38.0X4	T38.0X5	T38.0X6
Congener, anabolic	T38.7X1	T38.7X2	T38.7X3	T38.7X4	T38.7X5	T38.7X6
Congo red	T50.8X1	T50.8X2	T50.8X3	T50.8X4	T50.8X5	T50.8X6
Coniine, conine	T62.2X1	T62.2X2	T62.2X3	T62.2X4	—	—
Conium (maculatum)	T62.2X1	T62.2X2	T62.2X3	T62.2X4	—	—
Conjugated estrogenic substances	T38.5X1	T38.5X2	T38.5X3	T38.5X4	T38.5X5	T38.5X6
Contac	T48.5X1	T48.5X2	T48.5X3	T48.5X4	T48.5X5	T48.5X6
Contact lens solution	T49.5X1	T49.5X2	T49.5X3	T49.5X4	T49.5X5	T49.5X6
Contraceptive (oral)	T38.4X1	T38.4X2	T38.4X3	T38.4X4	T38.4X5	T38.4X6
vaginal	T49.8X1	T49.8X2	T49.8X3	T49.8X4	T49.8X5	T49.8X6
Contrast medium, radiography	T50.8X1	T50.8X2	T50.8X3	T50.8X4	T50.8X5	T50.8X6
Convallaria glycosides	T46.0X1	T46.0X2	T46.0X3	T46.0X4	T46.0X5	T46.0X6
Convallaria majalis	T62.2X1	T62.2X2	T62.2X3	T62.2X4	—	—
berry	T62.1X1	T62.1X2	T62.1X3	T62.1X4	—	—
Copperhead snake (bite) (venom)	T63.061	T63.062	T63.063	T63.064	—	—
Copper (dust) (fumes) (nonmedicinal) **NEC**	T56.4X1	T56.4X2	T56.4X3	T56.4X4	—	—
arsenate, arsenite	T57.0X1	T57.0X2	T57.0X3	T57.0X4	—	—
insecticide	T60.2X1	T60.2X2	T60.2X3	T60.2X4	—	—
emetic	T47.7X1	T47.7X2	T47.7X3	T47.7X4	T47.7X5	T47.7X6
fungicide	T60.3X1	T60.3X2	T60.3X3	T60.3X4	—	—
gluconate	T49.0X1	T49.0X2	T49.0X3	T49.0X4	T49.0X5	T49.0X6
insecticide	T60.2X1	T60.2X2	T60.2X3	T60.2X4	—	—
medicinal (trace)	T45.8X1	T45.8X2	T45.8X3	T45.8X4	T45.8X5	T45.8X6
oleate	T49.0X1	T49.0X2	T49.0X3	T49.0X4	T49.0X5	T49.0X6
sulfate	T56.4X1	T56.4X2	T56.4X3	T56.4X4	—	—
cupric	T56.4X1	T56.4X2	T56.4X3	T56.4X4	—	—
fungicide	T60.3X1	T60.3X2	T60.3X3	T60.3X4	—	—
medicinal						
ear	T49.6X1	T49.6X2	T49.6X3	T49.6X4	T49.6X5	T49.6X6
emetic	T47.7X1	T47.7X2	T47.7X3	T47.7X4	T47.7X5	T47.7X6
eye	T49.5X1	T49.5X2	T49.5X3	T49.5X4	T49.5X5	T49.5X6
cuprous	T56.4X1	T56.4X2	T56.4X3	T56.4X4	—	—
fungicide	T60.3X1	T60.3X2	T60.3X3	T60.3X4	—	—
medicinal						
ear	T49.6X1	T49.6X2	T49.6X3	T49.6X4	T49.6X5	T49.6X6
emetic	T47.7X1	T47.7X2	T47.7X3	T47.7X4	T47.7X5	T47.7X6
eye	T49.5X1	T49.5X2	T49.5X3	T49.5X4	T49.5X5	T49.5X6
Coral (sting)	T63.691	T63.692	T63.693	T63.694	—	—
snake (bite) (venom)	T63.021	T63.022	T63.023	T63.024	—	—
Corbadrine	T49.6X1	T49.6X2	T49.6X3	T49.6X4	T49.6X5	T49.6X6
Cordite	T65.891	T65.892	T65.893	T65.894	—	—
vapor	T59.891	T59.892	T59.893	T59.894	—	—
Cordran	T49.0X1	T49.0X2	T49.0X3	T49.0X4	T49.0X5	T49.0X6
Corn cures	T49.4X1	T49.4X2	T49.4X3	T49.4X4	T49.4X5	T49.4X6
Cornhusker's lotion	T49.3X1	T49.3X2	T49.3X3	T49.3X4	T49.3X5	T49.3X6
Corn starch	T49.3X1	T49.3X2	T49.3X3	T49.3X4	T49.3X5	T49.3X6
Coronary vasodilator NEC	T46.3X1	T46.3X2	T46.3X3	T46.3X4	T46.3X5	T46.3X6
Corrosive NEC	T54.91	T54.92	T54.93	T54.94	—	—
acid NEC	T54.2X1	T54.2X2	T54.2X3	T54.2X4	—	—
aromatics	T54.1X1	T54.1X2	T54.1X3	T54.1X4	—	—
disinfectant	T54.1X1	T54.1X2	T54.1X3	T54.1X4	—	—

Substance	Poisoning, Accidental (unintentional)	Poisoning, Intentional Self-harm	Poisoning, Assault	Poisoning, Undetermined	Adverse Effect	Under-dosing
Corrosive — *continued*						
fumes NEC	T54.91	T54.92	T54.93	T54.94	—	—
specified NEC	T54.91	T54.92	T54.93	T54.94	—	—
sublimate	T56.1X1	T56.1X2	T56.1X3	T56.1X4	—	—
Cortate	T38.0X1	T38.0X2	T38.0X3	T38.0X4	T38.0X5	T38.0X6
Cort-Dome	T38.0X1	T38.0X2	T38.0X3	T38.0X4	T38.0X5	T38.0X6
ENT agent	T49.6X1	T49.6X2	T49.6X3	T49.6X4	T49.6X5	T49.6X6
ophthalmic preparation	T49.5X1	T49.5X2	T49.5X3	T49.5X4	T49.5X5	T49.5X6
topical NEC	T49.0X1	T49.0X2	T49.0X3	T49.0X4	T49.0X5	T49.0X6
Cortef	T38.0X1	T38.0X2	T38.0X3	T38.0X4	T38.0X5	T38.0X6
ENT agent	T49.6X1	T49.6X2	T49.6X3	T49.6X4	T49.6X5	T49.6X6
ophthalmic preparation	T49.5X1	T49.5X2	T49.5X3	T49.5X4	T49.5X5	T49.5X6
topical NEC	T49.0X1	T49.0X2	T49.0X3	T49.0X4	T49.0X5	T49.0X6
Corticosteroid	T38.0X1	T38.0X2	T38.0X3	T38.0X4	T38.0X5	T38.0X6
ENT agent	T49.6X1	T49.6X2	T49.6X3	T49.6X4	T49.6X5	T49.6X6
mineral	T50.0X1	T50.0X2	T50.0X3	T50.0X4	T50.0X5	T50.0X6
ophthalmic	T49.5X1	T49.5X2	T49.5X3	T49.5X4	T49.5X5	T49.5X6
topical NEC	T49.0X1	T49.0X2	T49.0X3	T49.0X4	T49.0X5	T49.0X6
Corticotropin	T38.811	T38.812	T38.813	T38.814	T38.815	T38.816
Cortisol	T49.0X1	T49.0X2	T49.0X3	T49.0X4	T49.0X5	T49.0X6
ENT agent	T49.6X1	T49.6X2	T49.6X3	T49.6X4	T49.6X5	T49.6X6
ophthalmic preparation	T49.5X1	T49.5X2	T49.5X3	T49.5X4	T49.5X5	T49.5X6
topical NEC	T49.0X1	T49.0X2	T49.0X3	T49.0X4	T49.0X5	T49.0X6
Cortisone (acetate)	T38.0X1	T38.0X2	T38.0X3	T38.0X4	T38.0X5	T38.0X6
ENT agent	T49.6X1	T49.6X2	T49.6X3	T49.6X4	T49.6X5	T49.6X6
ophthalmic preparation	T49.5X1	T49.5X2	T49.5X3	T49.5X4	T49.5X5	T49.5X6
topical NEC	T49.0X1	T49.0X2	T49.0X3	T49.0X4	T49.0X5	T49.0X6
Cortivazol	T38.0X1	T38.0X2	T38.0X3	T38.0X4	T38.0X5	T38.0X6
Cortogen	T38.0X1	T38.0X2	T38.0X3	T38.0X4	T38.0X5	T38.0X6
ENT agent	T49.6X1	T49.6X2	T49.6X3	T49.6X4	T49.6X5	T49.6X6
ophthalmic preparation	T49.5X1	T49.5X2	T49.5X3	T49.5X4	T49.5X5	T49.5X6
Cortone	T38.0X1	T38.0X2	T38.0X3	T38.0X4	T38.0X5	T38.0X6
ENT agent	T49.6X1	T49.6X2	T49.6X3	T49.6X4	T49.6X5	T49.6X6
ophthalmic preparation	T49.5X1	T49.5X2	T49.5X3	T49.5X4	T49.5X5	T49.5X6
Cortril	T38.0X1	T38.0X2	T38.0X3	T38.0X4	T38.0X5	T38.0X6
ENT agent	T49.6X1	T49.6X2	T49.6X3	T49.6X4	T49.6X5	T49.6X6
ophthalmic preparation	T49.5X1	T49.5X2	T49.5X3	T49.5X4	T49.5X5	T49.5X6
topical NEC	T49.0X1	T49.0X2	T49.0X3	T49.0X4	T49.0X5	T49.0X6
Corynebacterium parvum	T45.1X1	T45.1X2	T45.1X3	T45.1X4	T45.1X5	T45.1X6
Cosmetic preparation	T49.8X1	T49.8X2	T49.8X3	T49.8X4	T49.8X5	T49.8X6
Cosmetics	T49.8X1	T49.8X2	T49.8X3	T49.8X4	T49.8X5	T49.8X6
Cosyntropin	T38.811	T38.812	T38.813	T38.814	T38.815	T38.816
Cotarnine	T45.7X1	T45.7X2	T45.7X3	T45.7X4	T45.7X5	T45.7X6
Co-trimoxazole	T36.8X1	T36.8X2	T36.8X3	T36.8X4	T36.8X5	T36.8X6
Cottonseed oil	T49.3X1	T49.3X2	T49.3X3	T49.3X4	T49.3X5	T49.3X6
Cough mixture (syrup)	T48.4X1	T48.4X2	T48.4X3	T48.4X4	T48.4X5	T48.4X6
containing opiates	T40.2X1	T40.2X2	T40.2X3	T40.2X4	T40.2X5	T40.2X6
expectorants	T48.4X1	T48.4X2	T48.4X3	T48.4X4	T48.4X5	T48.4X6
Coumadin	T45.511	T45.512	T45.513	T45.514	T45.515	T45.516
rodenticide	T60.4X1	T60.4X2	T60.4X3	T60.4X4	—	—
Coumaphos	T60.0X1	T60.0X2	T60.0X3	T60.0X4	—	—
Coumarin	T45.511	T45.512	T45.513	T45.514	T45.515	T45.516
Coumetarol	T45.511	T45.512	T45.513	T45.514	T45.515	T45.516
Cowbane	T62.2X1	T62.2X2	T62.2X3	T62.2X4	—	—
Cozyme	T45.2X1	T45.2X2	T45.2X3	T45.2X4	T45.2X5	T45.2X6
Crack	T40.5X1	T40.5X2	T40.5X3	T40.5X4	—	—
Crataegus extract	T46.0X1	T46.0X2	T46.0X3	T46.0X4	T46.0X5	T46.0X6
Creolin	T54.1X1	T54.1X2	T54.1X3	T54.1X4	—	—
disinfectant	T54.1X1	T54.1X2	T54.1X3	T54.1X4	—	—
Creosol (compound)	T49.0X1	T49.0X2	T49.0X3	T49.0X4	T49.0X5	T49.0X6
Creosote (coal tar) (beechwood)	T49.0X1	T49.0X2	T49.0X3	T49.0X4	T49.0X5	T49.0X6
medicinal (expectorant)	T48.4X1	T48.4X2	T48.4X3	T48.4X4	T48.4X5	T48.4X6
syrup	T48.4X1	T48.4X2	T48.4X3	T48.4X4	T48.4X5	T48.4X6
Cresol(s)	T49.0X1	T49.0X2	T49.0X3	T49.0X4	T49.0X5	T49.0X6
and soap solution	T49.0X1	T49.0X2	T49.0X3	T49.0X4	T49.0X5	T49.0X6
Cresyl acetate	T49.0X1	T49.0X2	T49.0X3	T49.0X4	T49.0X5	T49.0X6
Cresylic acid	T49.0X1	T49.0X2	T49.0X3	T49.0X4	T49.0X5	T49.0X6
Crimidine	T60.4X1	T60.4X2	T60.4X3	T60.4X4	—	—
Croconazole	T37.8X1	T37.8X2	T37.8X3	T37.8X4	T37.8X5	T37.8X6
Cromoglicic acid	T48.6X1	T48.6X2	T48.6X3	T48.6X4	T48.6X5	T48.6X6
Cromolyn	T48.6X1	T48.6X2	T48.6X3	T48.6X4	T48.6X5	T48.6X6
Cromonar	T46.3X1	T46.3X2	T46.3X3	T46.3X4	T46.3X5	T46.3X6
Cropropamide	T39.8X1	T39.8X2	T39.8X3	T39.8X4	T39.8X5	T39.8X6
with crotethamide	T50.7X1	T50.7X2	T50.7X3	T50.7X4	T50.7X5	T50.7X6
Crotamiton	T49.0X1	T49.0X2	T49.0X3	T49.0X4	T49.0X5	T49.0X6
Crotethamide	T39.8X1	T39.8X2	T39.8X3	T39.8X4	T39.8X5	T39.8X6
with cropropamide	T50.7X1	T50.7X2	T50.7X3	T50.7X4	T50.7X5	T50.7X6
Croton (oil)	T47.2X1	T47.2X2	T47.2X3	T47.2X4	T47.2X5	T47.2X6
chloral	T42.6X1	T42.6X2	T42.6X3	T42.6X4	T42.6X5	T42.6X6
Crude oil	T52.0X1	T52.0X2	T52.0X3	T52.0X4	—	—
Cryogenine	T39.8X1	T39.8X2	T39.8X3	T39.8X4	T39.8X5	T39.8X6
Cryolite (vapor)	T60.1X1	T60.1X2	T60.1X3	T60.1X4	—	—

Substance	Poisoning, Accidental (unintentional)	Poisoning, Intentional Self-harm	Poisoning, Assault	Poisoning, Undetermined	Adverse Effect	Under-dosing
Cryolite — *continued*						
insecticide	T60.1X1	T60.1X2	T60.1X3	T60.1X4	—	—
Cryptenamine (tannates)	T46.5X1	T46.5X2	T46.5X3	T46.5X4	T46.5X5	T46.5X6
Crystal violet	T49.0X1	T49.0X2	T49.0X3	T49.0X4	T49.0X5	T49.0X6
Cuckoopint	T62.2X1	T62.2X2	T62.2X3	T62.2X4	—	—
Cumetharol	T45.511	T45.512	T45.513	T45.514	T45.515	T45.516
Cupric						
acetate	T60.3X1	T60.3X2	T60.3X3	T60.3X4	—	—
acetoarsenite	T57.0X1	T57.0X2	T57.0X3	T57.0X4	—	—
arsenate	T57.0X1	T57.0X2	T57.0X3	T57.0X4	—	—
gluconate	T49.0X1	T49.0X2	T49.0X3	T49.0X4	T49.0X5	T49.0X6
oleate	T49.0X1	T49.0X2	T49.0X3	T49.0X4	T49.0X5	T49.0X6
sulfate	T56.4X1	T56.4X2	T56.4X3	T56.4X4	—	—
Cuprous sulfate — *see also* Copper sulfate	T56.4X1	T56.4X2	T56.4X3	T56.4X4	—	—
Curare, curarine	T48.1X1	T48.1X2	T48.1X3	T48.1X4	T48.1X5	T48.1X6
Cyamemazine	T43.3X1	T43.3X2	T43.3X3	T43.3X4	T43.3X5	T43.3X6
Cyamopsis tetragonoloba	T46.6X1	T46.6X2	T46.6X3	T46.6X4	T46.6X5	T46.6X6
Cyanacetyl hydrazide	T37.1X1	T37.1X2	T37.1X3	T37.1X4	T37.1X5	T37.1X6
Cyanic acid (gas)	T59.891	T59.892	T59.893	T59.894	—	—
Cyanide(s) (compounds) (potassium) (sodium) **NEC**	T65.0X1	T65.0X2	T65.0X3	T65.0X4	—	—
dust or gas (inhalation) NEC	T57.3X1	T57.3X2	T57.3X3	T57.3X4	—	—
fumigant	T65.0X1	T65.0X2	T65.0X3	T65.0X4	—	—
hydrogen	T57.3X1	T57.3X2	T57.3X3	T57.3X4	—	—
mercuric — *see* Mercury						
pesticide (dust) (fumes)	T65.0X1	T65.0X2	T65.0X3	T65.0X4	—	—
Cyanoacrylate adhesive	T49.3X1	T49.3X2	T49.3X3	T49.3X4	T49.3X5	T49.3X6
Cyanocobalamin	T45.8X1	T45.8X2	T45.8X3	T45.8X4	T45.8X5	T45.8X6
Cyanogen (chloride) (gas) **NEC**	T59.891	T59.892	T59.893	T59.894	—	—
Cyclacillin	T36.0X1	T36.0X2	T36.0X3	T36.0X4	T36.0X5	T36.0X6
Cyclaine	T41.3X1	T41.3X2	T41.3X3	T41.3X4	T41.3X5	T41.3X6
Cyclamate	T50.991	T50.992	T50.993	T50.994	T50.995	T50.996
Cyclamen europaeum	T62.2X1	T62.2X2	T62.2X3	T62.2X4	—	—
Cyclandelate	T46.7X1	T46.7X2	T46.7X3	T46.7X4	T46.7X5	T46.7X6
Cyclazocine	T50.7X1	T50.7X2	T50.7X3	T50.7X4	T50.7X5	T50.7X6
Cyclizine	T45.0X1	T45.0X2	T45.0X3	T45.0X4	T45.0X5	T45.0X6
Cyclobarbital	T42.3X1	T42.3X2	T42.3X3	T42.3X4	T42.3X5	T42.3X6
Cyclobarbitone	T42.3X1	T42.3X2	T42.3X3	T42.3X4	T42.3X5	T42.3X6
Cyclobenzaprine	T48.1X1	T48.1X2	T48.1X3	T48.1X4	T48.1X5	T48.1X6
Cyclodrine	T44.3X1	T44.3X2	T44.3X3	T44.3X4	T44.3X5	T44.3X6
Cycloguanil embonate	T37.2X1	T37.2X2	T37.2X3	T37.2X4	T37.2X5	T37.2X6
Cyclohexane	T52.8X1	T52.8X2	T52.8X3	T52.8X4	—	—
Cyclohexanol	T51.8X1	T51.8X2	T51.8X3	T51.8X4	—	—
Cyclohexanone	T52.4X1	T52.4X2	T52.4X3	T52.4X4	—	—
Cycloheximide	T60.3X1	T60.3X2	T60.3X3	T60.3X4	—	—
Cyclohexyl acetate	T52.8X1	T52.8X2	T52.8X3	T52.8X4	—	—
Cycloleucin	T45.1X1	T45.1X2	T45.1X3	T45.1X4	T45.1X5	T45.1X6
Cyclomethycaine	T41.3X1	T41.3X2	T41.3X3	T41.3X4	T41.3X5	T41.3X6
Cyclopentamine	T44.4X1	T44.4X2	T44.4X3	T44.4X4	T44.4X5	T44.4X6
Cyclopenthiazide	T50.2X1	T50.2X2	T50.2X3	T50.2X4	T50.2X5	T50.2X6
Cyclopentolate	T44.3X1	T44.3X2	T44.3X3	T44.3X4	T44.3X5	T44.3X6
Cyclophosphamide	T45.1X1	T45.1X2	T45.1X3	T45.1X4	T45.1X5	T45.1X6
Cycloplegic drug	T49.5X1	T49.5X2	T49.5X3	T49.5X4	T49.5X5	T49.5X6
Cyclopropane	T41.291	T41.292	T41.293	T41.294	T41.295	T41.296
Cyclopyrabital	T39.8X1	T39.8X2	T39.8X3	T39.8X4	T39.8X5	T39.8X6
Cycloserine	T37.1X1	T37.1X2	T37.1X3	T37.1X4	T37.1X5	T37.1X6
Cyclosporin	T45.1X1	T45.1X2	T45.1X3	T45.1X4	T45.1X5	T45.1X6
Cyclothiazide	T50.2X1	T50.2X2	T50.2X3	T50.2X4	T50.2X5	T50.2X6
Cycrimine	T44.3X1	T44.3X2	T44.3X3	T44.3X4	T44.3X5	T44.3X6
Cyhalothrin	T60.1X1	T60.1X2	T60.1X3	T60.1X4	—	—
Cymarin	T46.0X1	T46.0X2	T46.0X3	T46.0X4	T46.0X5	T46.0X6
Cypermethrin	T60.1X1	T60.1X2	T60.1X3	T60.1X4	—	—
Cyphenothrin	T60.2X1	T60.2X2	T60.2X3	T60.2X4	—	—
Cyproheptadine	T45.0X1	T45.0X2	T45.0X3	T45.0X4	T45.0X5	T45.0X6
Cyproterone	T38.6X1	T38.6X2	T38.6X3	T38.6X4	T38.6X5	T38.6X6
Cysteamine	T50.6X1	T50.6X2	T50.6X3	T50.6X4	T50.6X5	T50.6X6
Cytarabine	T45.1X1	T45.1X2	T45.1X3	T45.1X4	T45.1X5	T45.1X6
Cytisus						
laburnum	T62.2X1	T62.2X2	T62.2X3	T62.2X4	—	—
scoparius	T62.2X1	T62.2X2	T62.2X3	T62.2X4	—	—
Cytochrome C	T47.5X1	T47.5X2	T47.5X3	T47.5X4	T47.5X5	T47.5X6
Cytomel	T38.1X1	T38.1X2	T38.1X3	T38.1X4	T38.1X5	T38.1X6
Cytosine arabinoside	T45.1X1	T45.1X2	T45.1X3	T45.1X4	T45.1X5	T45.1X6
Cytoxan	T45.1X1	T45.1X2	T45.1X3	T45.1X4	T45.1X5	T45.1X6
Cytozyme	T45.7X1	T45.7X2	T45.7X3	T45.7X4	T45.7X5	T45.7X6
S-Carboxymethylcysteine	T48.4X1	T48.4X2	T48.4X3	T48.4X4	T48.4X5	T48.4X6
Dacarbazine	T45.1X1	T45.1X2	T45.1X3	T45.1X4	T45.1X5	T45.1X6
Dactinomycin	T45.1X1	T45.1X2	T45.1X3	T45.1X4	T45.1X5	T45.1X6
DADPS	T37.1X1	T37.1X2	T37.1X3	T37.1X4	T37.1X5	T37.1X6

Substance	Poisoning, Accidental (unintentional)	Poisoning, Intentional Self-harm	Poisoning, Assault	Poisoning, Undetermined	Adverse Effect	Under-dosing
Dakin's solution	T49.0X1	T49.0X2	T49.0X3	T49.0X4	T49.0X5	T49.0X6
Dalapon (sodium)	T60.3X1	T60.3X2	T60.3X3	T60.3X4	—	—
Dalmane	T42.4X1	T42.4X2	T42.4X3	T42.4X4	T42.4X5	T42.4X6
Danazol	T38.6X1	T38.6X2	T38.6X3	T38.6X4	T38.6X5	T38.6X6
Danilone	T45.511	T45.512	T45.513	T45.514	T45.515	T45.516
Danthron	T47.2X1	T47.2X2	T47.2X3	T47.2X4	T47.2X5	T47.2X6
Dantrolene	T42.8X1	T42.8X2	T42.8X3	T42.8X4	T42.8X5	T42.8X6
Dantron	T47.2X1	T47.2X2	T47.2X3	T47.2X4	T47.2X5	T47.2X6
Daphne (gnidium) (mezereum)	T62.2X1	T62.2X2	T62.2X3	T62.2X4	—	—
berry	T62.1X1	T62.1X2	T62.1X3	T62.1X4	—	—
Dapsone	T37.1X1	T37.1X2	T37.1X3	T37.1X4	T37.1X5	T37.1X6
Daraprim	T37.2X1	T37.2X2	T37.2X3	T37.2X4	T37.2X5	T37.2X6
Darnel	T62.2X1	T62.2X2	T62.2X3	T62.2X4	—	—
Darvon	T39.8X1	T39.8X2	T39.8X3	T39.8X4	T39.8X5	T39.8X6
Daunomycin	T45.1X1	T45.1X2	T45.1X3	T45.1X4	T45.1X5	T45.1X6
Daunorubicin	T45.1X1	T45.1X2	T45.1X3	T45.1X4	T45.1X5	T45.1X6
DBI	T38.3X1	T38.3X2	T38.3X3	T38.3X4	T38.3X5	T38.3X6
D-Con	T60.91	T60.92	T60.93	T60.94	—	—
insecticide	T60.2X1	T60.2X2	T60.2X3	T60.2X4	—	—
rodenticide	T60.4X1	T60.4X2	T60.4X3	T60.4X4	—	—
DDAVP	T38.891	T38.892	T38.893	T38.894	T38.895	T38.896
DDE (bis(chlorophenyl)-dichloroethylene)	T60.2X1	T60.2X2	T60.2X3	T60.2X4	—	—
DDS	T37.1X1	T37.1X2	T37.1X3	T37.1X4	T37.1X5	T37.1X6
DDT (dust)	T60.1X1	T60.1X2	T60.1X3	T60.1X4	—	—
Deadly nightshade — *see also* Belladonna	T62.2X1	T62.2X2	T62.2X3	T62.2X4	—	—
berry	T62.1X1	T62.1X2	T62.1X3	T62.1X4	—	—
Deamino-D-arginine vasopressin	T38.891	T38.892	T38.893	T38.894	T38.895	T38.896
Deanol (aceglumate)	T50.991	T50.992	T50.993	T50.994	T50.995	T50.996
Debrisoquine	T46.5X1	T46.5X2	T46.5X3	T46.5X4	T46.5X5	T46.5X6
Decaborane	T57.8X1	T57.8X2	T57.8X3	T57.8X4	—	—
fumes	T59.891	T59.892	T59.893	T59.894	—	—
Decadron	T38.0X1	T38.0X2	T38.0X3	T38.0X4	T38.0X5	T38.0X6
ENT agent	T49.6X1	T49.6X2	T49.6X3	T49.6X4	T49.6X5	T49.6X6
ophthalmic preparation	T49.5X1	T49.5X2	T49.5X3	T49.5X4	T49.5X5	T49.5X6
topical NEC	T49.0X1	T49.0X2	T49.0X3	T49.0X4	T49.0X5	T49.0X6
Decahydronaphthalene	T52.8X1	T52.8X2	T52.8X3	T52.8X4	—	—
Decalin	T52.8X1	T52.8X2	T52.8X3	T52.8X4	—	—
Decamethonium (bromide)	T48.1X1	T48.1X2	T48.1X3	T48.1X4	T48.1X5	T48.1X6
Decholin	T47.5X1	T47.5X2	T47.5X3	T47.5X4	T47.5X5	T47.5X6
Declomycin	T36.4X1	T36.4X2	T36.4X3	T36.4X4	T36.4X5	T36.4X6
Decongestant, nasal (mucosa)	T48.5X1	T48.5X2	T48.5X3	T48.5X4	T48.5X5	T48.5X6
combination	T48.5X1	T48.5X2	T48.5X3	T48.5X4	T48.5X5	T48.5X6
Deet	T60.8X1	T60.8X2	T60.8X3	T60.8X4	—	—
Deferoxamine	T45.8X1	T45.8X2	T45.8X3	T45.8X4	T45.8X5	T45.8X6
Deflazacort	T38.0X1	T38.0X2	T38.0X3	T38.0X4	T38.0X5	T38.0X6
Deglycyrrhizinized extract of licorice	T48.4X1	T48.4X2	T48.4X3	T48.4X4	T48.4X5	T48.4X6
Dehydrocholic acid	T47.5X1	T47.5X2	T47.5X3	T47.5X4	T47.5X5	T47.5X6
Dehydroemetine	T37.3X1	T37.3X2	T37.3X3	T37.3X4	T37.3X5	T37.3X6
Dekalin	T52.8X1	T52.8X2	T52.8X3	T52.8X4	—	—
Delalutin	T38.5X1	T38.5X2	T38.5X3	T38.5X4	T38.5X5	T38.5X6
Delorazepam	T42.4X1	T42.4X2	T42.4X3	T42.4X4	T42.4X5	T42.4X6
Delphinium	T62.2X1	T62.2X2	T62.2X3	T62.2X4	—	—
Deltamethrin	T60.1X1	T60.1X2	T60.1X3	T60.1X4	—	—
Deltasone	T38.0X1	T38.0X2	T38.0X3	T38.0X4	T38.0X5	T38.0X6
Deltra	T38.0X1	T38.0X2	T38.0X3	T38.0X4	T38.0X5	T38.0X6
Delvinal	T42.3X1	T42.3X2	T42.3X3	T42.3X4	T42.3X5	T42.3X6
Demecarium (bromide)	T49.5X1	T49.5X2	T49.5X3	T49.5X4	T49.5X5	T49.5X6
Demeclocycline	T36.4X1	T36.4X2	T36.4X3	T36.4X4	T36.4X5	T36.4X6
Demecolcine	T45.1X1	T45.1X2	T45.1X3	T45.1X4	T45.1X5	T45.1X6
Demegestone	T38.5X1	T38.5X2	T38.5X3	T38.5X4	T38.5X5	T38.5X6
Demelanizing agents	T49.8X1	T49.8X2	T49.8X3	T49.8X4	T49.8X5	T49.8X6
Demephion -O and -S	T60.0X1	T60.0X2	T60.0X3	T60.0X4	—	—
Demerol	T40.2X1	T40.2X2	T40.2X3	T40.2X4	T40.2X5	T40.2X6
Demethylchlortetracycline	T36.4X1	T36.4X2	T36.4X3	T36.4X4	T36.4X5	T36.4X6
Demethyltetracycline	T36.4X1	T36.4X2	T36.4X3	T36.4X4	T36.4X5	T36.4X6
Demeton -O and -S	T60.0X1	T60.0X2	T60.0X3	T60.0X4	—	—
Demulcent (external)	T49.3X1	T49.3X2	T49.3X3	T49.3X4	T49.3X5	T49.3X6
specified NEC	T49.3X1	T49.3X2	T49.3X3	T49.3X4	T49.3X5	T49.3X6
Demulen	T38.4X1	T38.4X2	T38.4X3	T38.4X4	T38.4X5	T38.4X6
Denatured alcohol	T51.0X1	T51.0X2	T51.0X3	T51.0X4	—	—
Dendrid	T49.5X1	T49.5X2	T49.5X3	T49.5X4	T49.5X5	T49.5X6
Dental drug, topical application NEC	T49.7X1	T49.7X2	T49.7X3	T49.7X4	T49.7X5	T49.7X6
Dentifrice	T49.7X1	T49.7X2	T49.7X3	T49.7X4	T49.7X5	T49.7X6
Deodorant spray (feminine hygiene)	T49.8X1	T49.8X2	T49.8X3	T49.8X4	T49.8X5	T49.8X6
Deoxycortone	T50.0X1	T50.0X2	T50.0X3	T50.0X4	T50.0X5	T50.0X6

Substance	Poisoning, Accidental (unintentional)	Poisoning, Intentional Self-harm	Poisoning, Assault	Poisoning, Undetermined	Adverse Effect	Under-dosing
Deoxyribonuclease (pancreatic)	T45.3X1	T45.3X2	T45.3X3	T45.3X4	T45.3X5	T45.3X6
Depilatory	T49.4X1	T49.4X2	T49.4X3	T49.4X4	T49.4X5	T49.4X6
Deprenalin	T42.8X1	T42.8X2	T42.8X3	T42.8X4	T42.8X5	T42.8X6
Deprenyl	T42.8X1	T42.8X2	T42.8X3	T42.8X4	T42.8X5	T42.8X6
Depressant						
appetite (central)	T50.5X1	T50.5X2	T50.5X3	T50.5X4	T50.5X5	T50.5X6
cardiac	T46.2X1	T46.2X2	T46.2X3	T46.2X4	T46.2X5	T46.2X6
central nervous system (anesthetic) — *see also* Central nervous system, depressants	T42.71	T42.72	T42.73	T42.74	T42.75	T42.76
general anesthetic	T41.201	T41.202	T41.203	T41.204	T41.205	T41.206
muscle tone	T42.8X1	T42.8X2	T42.8X3	T42.8X4	T42.8X5	T42.8X6
muscle tone, central	T42.8X1	T42.8X2	T42.8X3	T42.8X4	T42.8X5	T42.8X6
psychotherapeutic	T43.501	T43.502	T43.503	T43.504	T43.505	T43.506
Depressant, appetite	T50.5X1	T50.5X2	T50.5X3	T50.5X4	T50.5X5	T50.5X6
Deptropine	T45.0X1	T45.0X2	T45.0X3	T45.0X4	T45.0X5	T45.0X6
Dequalinium (chloride)	T49.0X1	T49.0X2	T49.0X3	T49.0X4	T49.0X5	T49.0X6
Derris root	T60.2X1	T60.2X2	T60.2X3	T60.2X4	—	—
Deserpidine	T46.5X1	T46.5X2	T46.5X3	T46.5X4	T46.5X5	T46.5X6
Desferrioxamine	T45.8X1	T45.8X2	T45.8X3	T45.8X4	T45.8X5	T45.8X6
Desipramine	T43.011	T43.012	T43.013	T43.014	T43.015	T43.016
Deslanoside	T46.0X1	T46.0X2	T46.0X3	T46.0X4	T46.0X5	T46.0X6
Desloughing agent	T49.4X1	T49.4X2	T49.4X3	T49.4X4	T49.4X5	T49.4X6
Desmethylimipramine	T43.011	T43.012	T43.013	T43.014	T43.015	T43.016
Desmopressin	T38.891	T38.892	T38.893	T38.894	T38.895	T38.896
Desocodeine	T40.2X1	T40.2X2	T40.2X3	T40.2X4	T40.2X5	T40.2X6
Desogestrel	T38.5X1	T38.5X2	T38.5X3	T38.5X4	T38.5X5	T38.5X6
Desomorphine	T40.2X1	T40.2X2	T40.2X3	T40.2X4	—	—
Desonide	T49.0X1	T49.0X2	T49.0X3	T49.0X4	T49.0X5	T49.0X6
Desoximetasone	T49.0X1	T49.0X2	T49.0X3	T49.0X4	T49.0X5	T49.0X6
Desoxycorticosteroid	T50.0X1	T50.0X2	T50.0X3	T50.0X4	T50.0X5	T50.0X6
Desoxycortone	T50.0X1	T50.0X2	T50.0X3	T50.0X4	T50.0X5	T50.0X6
Desoxyephedrine	T43.621	T43.622	T43.623	T43.624	T43.625	T43.626
Detaxtran	T46.6X1	T46.6X2	T46.6X3	T46.6X4	T46.6X5	T46.6X6
Detergent	T49.2X1	T49.2X2	T49.2X3	T49.2X4	T49.2X5	T49.2X6
external medication	T49.2X1	T49.2X2	T49.2X3	T49.2X4	T49.2X5	T49.2X6
local	T49.2X1	T49.2X2	T49.2X3	T49.2X4	T49.2X5	T49.2X6
medicinal	T49.2X1	T49.2X2	T49.2X3	T49.2X4	T49.2X5	T49.2X6
nonmedicinal	T55.1X1	T55.1X2	T55.1X3	T55.1X4	—	—
specified NEC	T55.1X1	T55.1X2	T55.1X3	T55.1X4	—	—
Deterrent, alcohol	T50.6X1	T50.6X2	T50.6X3	T50.6X4	T50.6X5	T50.6X6
Detoxifying agent	T50.6X1	T50.6X2	T50.6X3	T50.6X4	T50.6X5	T50.6X6
Detrothyronine	T38.1X1	T38.1X2	T38.1X3	T38.1X4	T38.1X5	T38.1X6
Dettol (external medication)	T49.0X1	T49.0X2	T49.0X3	T49.0X4	T49.0X5	T49.0X6
Dexamethasone	T38.0X1	T38.0X2	T38.0X3	T38.0X4	T38.0X5	T38.0X6
ENT agent	T49.6X1	T49.6X2	T49.6X3	T49.6X4	T49.6X5	T49.6X6
ophthalmic preparation	T49.5X1	T49.5X2	T49.5X3	T49.5X4	T49.5X5	T49.5X6
topical NEC	T49.0X1	T49.0X2	T49.0X3	T49.0X4	T49.0X5	T49.0X6
Dexamfetamine	T43.621	T43.622	T43.623	T43.624	T43.625	T43.626
Dexamphetamine	T43.621	T43.622	T43.623	T43.624	T43.625	T43.626
Dexbrompheniramine	T45.0X1	T45.0X2	T45.0X3	T45.0X4	T45.0X5	T45.0X6
Dexchlorpheniramine	T45.0X1	T45.0X2	T45.0X3	T45.0X4	T45.0X5	T45.0X6
Dexedrine	T43.621	T43.622	T43.623	T43.624	T43.625	T43.626
Dexetimide	T44.3X1	T44.3X2	T44.3X3	T44.3X4	T44.3X5	T44.3X6
Dexfenfluramine	T50.5X1	T50.5X2	T50.5X3	T50.5X4	T50.5X5	T50.5X6
Dexpanthenol	T45.2X1	T45.2X2	T45.2X3	T45.2X4	T45.2X5	T45.2X6
Dextran (40) (70) (150)	T45.8X1	T45.8X2	T45.8X3	T45.8X4	T45.8X5	T45.8X6
Dextriferron	T45.4X1	T45.4X2	T45.4X3	T45.4X4	T45.4X5	T45.4X6
Dextroamphetamine	T43.621	T43.622	T43.623	T43.624	T43.625	T43.626
Dextro calcium pantothenate	T45.2X1	T45.2X2	T45.2X3	T45.2X4	T45.2X5	T45.2X6
Dextromethorphan	T48.3X1	T48.3X2	T48.3X3	T48.3X4	T48.3X5	T48.3X6
Dextromoramide	T40.491	T40.492	T40.493	T40.494	—	—
topical	T49.8X1	T49.8X2	T49.8X3	T49.8X4	T49.8X5	T49.8X6
Dextro pantothenyl alcohol	T45.2X1	T45.2X2	T45.2X3	T45.2X4	T45.2X5	T45.2X6
Dextropropoxyphene	T40.491	T40.492	T40.493	T40.494	T40.495	T40.496
Dextrorphan	T40.2X1	T40.2X2	T40.2X3	T40.2X4	T40.2X5	T40.2X6
Dextrose	T50.3X1	T50.3X2	T50.3X3	T50.3X4	T50.3X5	T50.3X6
concentrated solution, intravenous	T46.8X1	T46.8X2	T46.8X3	T46.8X4	T46.8X5	T46.8X6
Dextrothyroxin	T38.1X1	T38.1X2	T38.1X3	T38.1X4	T38.1X5	T38.1X6
Dextrothyroxine sodium	T38.1X1	T38.1X2	T38.1X3	T38.1X4	T38.1X5	T38.1X6
DFP	T44.0X1	T44.0X2	T44.0X3	T44.0X4	T44.0X5	T44.0X6
DHE	T37.3X1	T37.3X2	T37.3X3	T37.3X4	T37.3X5	T37.3X6
45	T46.5X1	T46.5X2	T46.5X3	T46.5X4	T46.5X5	T46.5X6
Diabinese	T38.3X1	T38.3X2	T38.3X3	T38.3X4	T38.3X5	T38.3X6
Diacetone alcohol	T52.4X1	T52.4X2	T52.4X3	T52.4X4	—	—
Diacetyl monoxime	T50.991	T50.992	T50.993	T50.994	—	—
Diacetylmorphine	T40.1X1	T40.1X2	T40.1X3	T40.1X4	—	—
Diachylon plaster	T49.4X1	T49.4X2	T49.4X3	T49.4X4	T49.4X5	T49.4X6

Substance	Poisoning, Accidental (unintentional)	Poisoning, Intentional Self-harm	Poisoning, Assault	Poisoning, Undetermined	Adverse Effect	Under-dosing
Diaethylstilboestrolum	T38.5X1	T38.5X2	T38.5X3	T38.5X4	T38.5X5	T38.5X6
Diagnostic agent NEC	T5Ø.8X1	T5Ø.8X2	T5Ø.8X3	T5Ø.8X4	T5Ø.8X5	T5Ø.8X6
Dial (soap)	T49.2X1	T49.2X2	T49.2X3	T49.2X4	T49.2X5	T49.2X6
sedative	T42.3X1	T42.3X2	T42.3X3	T42.3X4	T42.3X5	T42.3X6
Dialkyl carbonate	T52.91	T52.92	T52.93	T52.94	—	—
Diallylbarbituric acid	T42.3X1	T42.3X2	T42.3X3	T42.3X4	T42.3X5	T42.3X6
Diallymal	T42.3X1	T42.3X2	T42.3X3	T42.3X4	T42.3X5	T42.3X6
Dialysis solution (intraperitoneal)	T5Ø.3X1	T5Ø.3X2	T5Ø.3X3	T5Ø.3X4	T5Ø.3X5	T5Ø.3X6
Diaminodiphenylsulfone	T37.1X1	T37.1X2	T37.1X3	T37.1X4	T37.1X5	T37.1X6
Diamorphine	T4Ø.1X1	T4Ø.1X2	T4Ø.1X3	T4Ø.1X4	—	—
Diamox	T5Ø.2X1	T5Ø.2X2	T5Ø.2X3	T5Ø.2X4	T5Ø.2X5	T5Ø.2X6
Diamthazole	T49.ØX1	T49.ØX2	T49.ØX3	T49.ØX4	T49.ØX5	T49.ØX6
Dianthone	T47.2X1	T47.2X2	T47.2X3	T47.2X4	T47.2X5	T47.2X6
Diaphenylsulfone	T37.ØX1	T37.ØX2	T37.ØX3	T37.ØX4	T37.ØX5	T37.ØX6
Diasone (sodium)	T37.1X1	T37.1X2	T37.1X3	T37.1X4	T37.1X5	T37.1X6
Diastase	T47.5X1	T47.5X2	T47.5X3	T47.5X4	T47.5X5	T47.5X6
Diatrizoate	T5Ø.8X1	T5Ø.8X2	T5Ø.8X3	T5Ø.8X4	T5Ø.8X5	T5Ø.8X6
Diazepam	T42.4X1	T42.4X2	T42.4X3	T42.4X4	T42.4X5	T42.4X6
Diazinon	T6Ø.ØX1	T6Ø.ØX2	T6Ø.ØX3	T6Ø.ØX4	—	—
Diazomethane (gas)	T59.891	T59.892	T59.893	T59.894	—	—
Diazoxide	T46.5X1	T46.5X2	T46.5X3	T46.5X4	T46.5X5	T46.5X6
Dibekacin	T36.5X1	T36.5X2	T36.5X3	T36.5X4	T36.5X5	T36.5X6
Dibenamine	T44.6X1	T44.6X2	T44.6X3	T44.6X4	T44.6X5	T44.6X6
Dibenzepin	T43.Ø11	T43.Ø12	T43.Ø13	T43.Ø14	T43.Ø15	T43.Ø16
Dibenzheptropine	T45.ØX1	T45.ØX2	T45.ØX3	T45.ØX4	T45.ØX5	T45.ØX6
Dibenzyline	T44.6X1	T44.6X2	T44.6X3	T44.6X4	T44.6X5	T44.6X6
Diborane (gas)	T59.891	T59.892	T59.893	T59.894	—	—
Dibromochloropropane	T6Ø.8X1	T6Ø.8X2	T6Ø.8X3	T6Ø.8X4	—	—
Dibromodulcitol	T45.1X1	T45.1X2	T45.1X3	T45.1X4	T45.1X5	T45.1X6
Dibromoethane	T53.6X1	T53.6X2	T53.6X3	T53.6X4	—	—
Dibromomannitol	T45.1X1	T45.1X2	T45.1X3	T45.1X4	T45.1X5	T45.1X6
Dibromopropamidine isethionate	T49.ØX1	T49.ØX2	T49.ØX3	T49.ØX4	T49.ØX5	T49.ØX6
Dibrompropamidine	T49.ØX1	T49.ØX2	T49.ØX3	T49.ØX4	T49.ØX5	T49.ØX6
Dibucaine	T41.3X1	T41.3X2	T41.3X3	T41.3X4	T41.3X5	T41.3X6
topical (surface)	T41.3X1	T41.3X2	T41.3X3	T41.3X4	T41.3X5	T41.3X6
Dibunate sodium	T48.3X1	T48.3X2	T48.3X3	T48.3X4	T48.3X5	T48.3X6
Dibutoline sulfate	T44.3X1	T44.3X2	T44.3X3	T44.3X4	T44.3X5	T44.3X6
Dicamba	T6Ø.3X1	T6Ø.3X2	T6Ø.3X3	T6Ø.3X4	—	—
Dicapthon	T6Ø.ØX1	T6Ø.ØX2	T6Ø.ØX3	T6Ø.ØX4	—	—
Dichlobenil	T6Ø.3X1	T6Ø.3X2	T6Ø.3X3	T6Ø.3X4	—	—
Dichlone	T6Ø.3X1	T6Ø.3X2	T6Ø.3X3	T6Ø.3X4	—	—
Dichloralphenozone	T42.6X1	T42.6X2	T42.6X3	T42.6X4	T42.6X5	T42.6X6
Dichlorbenzidine	T65.3X1	T65.3X2	T65.3X3	T65.3X4	—	—
Dichlorhydrin	T52.8X1	T52.8X2	T52.8X3	T52.8X4	—	—
Dichlorhydroxyquinoline	T37.8X1	T37.8X2	T37.8X3	T37.8X4	T37.8X5	T37.8X6
Dichlorobenzene	T53.7X1	T53.7X2	T53.7X3	T53.7X4	—	—
Dichlorobenzyl alcohol	T49.6X1	T49.6X2	T49.6X3	T49.6X4	T49.6X5	T49.6X6
Dichlorodifluoromethane	T53.5X1	T53.5X2	T53.5X3	T53.5X4	—	—
Dichloroethane	T52.8X1	T52.8X2	T52.8X3	T52.8X4	—	—
Dichloroethylene	T53.6X1	T53.6X2	T53.6X3	T53.6X4	—	—
Dichloroethyl sulfide, not in war	T59.891	T59.892	T59.893	T59.894	—	—
Dichloroformoxine, not in war	T59.891	T59.892	T59.893	T59.894	—	—
Dichlorohydrin, alpha-dichlorohydrin	T52.8X1	T52.8X2	T52.8X3	T52.8X4	—	—
Dichloromethane (solvent)	T53.4X1	T53.4X2	T53.4X3	T53.4X4	—	—
vapor	T53.4X1	T53.4X2	T53.4X3	T53.4X4	—	—
Dichloronaphthoquinone	T6Ø.3X1	T6Ø.3X2	T6Ø.3X3	T6Ø.3X4	—	—
Dichlorophen	T37.4X1	T37.4X2	T37.4X3	T37.4X4	T37.4X5	T37.4X6
Dichloropropene	T6Ø.3X1	T6Ø.3X2	T6Ø.3X3	T6Ø.3X4	—	—
Dichloropropionic acid	T6Ø.3X1	T6Ø.3X2	T6Ø.3X3	T6Ø.3X4	—	—
Dichlorphenamide	T5Ø.2X1	T5Ø.2X2	T5Ø.2X3	T5Ø.2X4	T5Ø.2X5	T5Ø.2X6
Dichlorvos	T6Ø.ØX1	T6Ø.ØX2	T6Ø.ØX3	T6Ø.ØX4	—	—
Diclofenac	T39.391	T39.392	T39.393	T39.394	T39.395	T39.396
Diclofenamide	T5Ø.2X1	T5Ø.2X2	T5Ø.2X3	T5Ø.2X4	T5Ø.2X5	T5Ø.2X6
Diclofensine	T43.291	T43.292	T43.293	T43.294	T43.295	T43.296
Diclonixine	T39.8X1	T39.8X2	T39.8X3	T39.8X4	T39.8X5	T39.8X6
Dicloxacillin	T36.ØX1	T36.ØX2	T36.ØX3	T36.ØX4	T36.ØX5	T36.ØX6
Dicophane	T49.ØX1	T49.ØX2	T49.ØX3	T49.ØX4	T49.ØX5	T49.ØX6
Dicoumarol, dicoumarin, dicumarol	T45.511	T45.512	T45.513	T45.514	T45.515	T45.516
Dicrotophos	T6Ø.ØX1	T6Ø.ØX2	T6Ø.ØX3	T6Ø.ØX4	—	—
Dicyanogen (gas)	T65.ØX1	T65.ØX2	T65.ØX3	T65.ØX4	—	—
Dicyclomine	T44.3X1	T44.3X2	T44.3X3	T44.3X4	T44.3X5	T44.3X6
Dicycloverine	T44.3X1	T44.3X2	T44.3X3	T44.3X4	T44.3X5	T44.3X6
Dideoxycytidine	T37.5X1	T37.5X2	T37.5X3	T37.5X4	T37.5X5	T37.5X6
Dideoxyinosine	T37.5X1	T37.5X2	T37.5X3	T37.5X4	T37.5X5	T37.5X6
Dieldrin (vapor)	T6Ø.1X1	T6Ø.1X2	T6Ø.1X3	T6Ø.1X4	—	—
Diemal	T42.3X1	T42.3X2	T42.3X3	T42.3X4	T42.3X5	T42.3X6
Dienestrol	T38.5X1	T38.5X2	T38.5X3	T38.5X4	T38.5X5	T38.5X6

Substance	Poisoning, Accidental (unintentional)	Poisoning, Intentional Self-harm	Poisoning, Assault	Poisoning, Undetermined	Adverse Effect	Under-dosing
Dienoestrol	T38.5X1	T38.5X2	T38.5X3	T38.5X4	T38.5X5	T38.5X6
Dietetic drug NEC	T5Ø.9Ø1	T5Ø.9Ø2	T5Ø.9Ø3	T5Ø.9Ø4	T5Ø.9Ø5	T5Ø.9Ø6
Diethazine	T42.8X1	T42.8X2	T42.8X3	T42.8X4	T42.8X5	T42.8X6
Diethyl						
barbituric acid	T42.3X1	T42.3X2	T42.3X3	T42.3X4	T42.3X5	T42.3X6
carbamazine	T37.4X1	T37.4X2	T37.4X3	T37.4X4	T37.4X5	T37.4X6
carbinol	T51.3X1	T51.3X2	T51.3X3	T51.3X4	—	—
carbonate	T52.8X1	T52.8X2	T52.8X3	T52.8X4	—	—
ether (vapor) — *see also* ether	T41.ØX1	T41.ØX2	T41.ØX3	T41.ØX4	T41.ØX5	T41.ØX6
oxide	T52.8X1	T52.8X2	T52.8X3	T52.8X4	—	—
propion	T5Ø.5X1	T5Ø.5X2	T5Ø.5X3	T5Ø.5X4	T5Ø.5X5	T5Ø.5X6
stilbestrol	T38.5X1	T38.5X2	T38.5X3	T38.5X4	T38.5X5	T38.5X6
toluamide (nonmedicinal)	T6Ø.8X1	T6Ø.8X2	T6Ø.8X3	T6Ø.8X4	—	—
medicinal	T49.3X1	T49.3X2	T49.3X3	T49.3X4	T49.3X5	T49.3X6
Diethylcarbamazine	T37.4X1	T37.4X2	T37.4X3	T37.4X4	T37.4X5	T37.4X6
Diethylene						
dioxide	T52.8X1	T52.8X2	T52.8X3	T52.8X4	—	—
glycol (monoacetate) (monobutyl ether) (monoethyl ether)	T52.3X1	T52.3X2	T52.3X3	T52.3X4	—	—
Diethylhexylphthalate	T65.891	T65.892	T65.893	T65.894	—	—
Diethylpropion	T5Ø.5X1	T5Ø.5X2	T5Ø.5X3	T5Ø.5X4	T5Ø.5X5	T5Ø.5X6
Diethylstilbestrol	T38.5X1	T38.5X2	T38.5X3	T38.5X4	T38.5X5	T38.5X6
Diethylstilboestrol	T38.5X1	T38.5X2	T38.5X3	T38.5X4	T38.5X5	T38.5X6
Diethylsulfone-diethylmethane	T42.6X1	T42.6X2	T42.6X3	T42.6X4	T42.6X5	T42.6X6
Diethyltoluamide	T49.ØX1	T49.ØX2	T49.ØX3	T49.ØX4	T49.ØX5	T49.ØX6
Diethyltryptamine (DET)	T4Ø.991	T4Ø.992	T4Ø.993	T4Ø.994	—	—
Difebarbamate	T42.3X1	T42.3X2	T42.3X3	T42.3X4	T42.3X5	T42.3X6
Difencloxazine	T4Ø.2X1	T4Ø.2X2	T4Ø.2X3	T4Ø.2X4	T4Ø.2X5	T4Ø.2X6
Difenidol	T45.ØX1	T45.ØX2	T45.ØX3	T45.ØX4	T45.ØX5	T45.ØX6
Difenoxin	T47.6X1	T47.6X2	T47.6X3	T47.6X4	T47.6X5	T47.6X6
Difetarsone	T37.3X1	T37.3X2	T37.3X3	T37.3X4	T37.3X5	T37.3X6
Diffusin	T45.3X1	T45.3X2	T45.3X3	T45.3X4	T45.3X5	T45.3X6
Diflorasone	T49.ØX1	T49.ØX2	T49.ØX3	T49.ØX4	T49.ØX5	T49.ØX6
Diflos	T44.ØX1	T44.ØX2	T44.ØX3	T44.ØX4	T44.ØX5	T44.ØX6
Diflubenzuron	T6Ø.1X1	T6Ø.1X2	T6Ø.1X3	T6Ø.1X4	—	—
Diflucortolone	T49.ØX1	T49.ØX2	T49.ØX3	T49.ØX4	T49.ØX5	T49.ØX6
Diflunisal	T39.Ø91	T39.Ø92	T39.Ø93	T39.Ø94	T39.Ø95	T39.Ø96
Difluoromethyldopa	T42.8X1	T42.8X2	T42.8X3	T42.8X4	T42.8X5	T42.8X6
Difluorophate	T44.ØX1	T44.ØX2	T44.ØX3	T44.ØX4	T44.ØX5	T44.ØX6
Digestant NEC	T47.5X1	T47.5X2	T47.5X3	T47.5X4	T47.5X5	T47.5X6
Digitalin (e)	T46.ØX1	T46.ØX2	T46.ØX3	T46.ØX4	T46.ØX5	T46.ØX6
Digitalis (leaf)(glycoside)	T46.ØX1	T46.ØX2	T46.ØX3	T46.ØX4	T46.ØX5	T46.ØX6
lanata	T46.ØX1	T46.ØX2	T46.ØX3	T46.ØX4	T46.ØX5	T46.ØX6
purpurea	T46.ØX1	T46.ØX2	T46.ØX3	T46.ØX4	T46.ØX5	T46.ØX6
Digitoxin	T46.ØX1	T46.ØX2	T46.ØX3	T46.ØX4	T46.ØX5	T46.ØX6
Digitoxose	T46.ØX1	T46.ØX2	T46.ØX3	T46.ØX4	T46.ØX5	T46.ØX6
Digoxin	T46.ØX1	T46.ØX2	T46.ØX3	T46.ØX4	T46.ØX5	T46.ØX6
Digoxine	T46.ØX1	T46.ØX2	T46.ØX3	T46.ØX4	T46.ØX5	T46.ØX6
Dihydralazine	T46.5X1	T46.5X2	T46.5X3	T46.5X4	T46.5X5	T46.5X6
Dihydrazine	T46.5X1	T46.5X2	T46.5X3	T46.5X4	T46.5X5	T46.5X6
Dihydrocodeine	T4Ø.2X1	T4Ø.2X2	T4Ø.2X3	T4Ø.2X4	T4Ø.2X5	T4Ø.2X6
Dihydrocodeinone	T4Ø.2X1	T4Ø.2X2	T4Ø.2X3	T4Ø.2X4	T4Ø.2X5	T4Ø.2X6
Dihydroergocornine	T46.7X1	T46.7X2	T46.7X3	T46.7X4	T46.7X5	T46.7X6
Dihydroergocristine (mesilate)	T46.7X1	T46.7X2	T46.7X3	T46.7X4	T46.7X5	T46.7X6
Dihydroergokryptine	T46.7X1	T46.7X2	T46.7X3	T46.7X4	T46.7X5	T46.7X6
Dihydroergotamine	T46.5X1	T46.5X2	T46.5X3	T46.5X4	T46.5X5	T46.5X6
Dihydroergotoxine	T46.7X1	T46.7X2	T46.7X3	T46.7X4	T46.7X5	T46.7X6
mesilate	T46.7X1	T46.7X2	T46.7X3	T46.7X4	T46.7X5	T46.7X6
Dihydrohydroxycodeinone	T4Ø.2X1	T4Ø.2X2	T4Ø.2X3	T4Ø.2X4	T4Ø.2X5	T4Ø.2X6
Dihydrohydroxymorphinone	T4Ø.2X1	T4Ø.2X2	T4Ø.2X3	T4Ø.2X4	T4Ø.2X5	T4Ø.2X6
Dihydroisocodeine	T4Ø.2X1	T4Ø.2X2	T4Ø.2X3	T4Ø.2X4	T4Ø.2X5	T4Ø.2X6
Dihydromorphine	T4Ø.2X1	T4Ø.2X2	T4Ø.2X3	T4Ø.2X4	—	—
Dihydromorphinone	T4Ø.2X1	T4Ø.2X2	T4Ø.2X3	T4Ø.2X4	T4Ø.2X5	T4Ø.2X6
Dihydrostreptomycin	T36.5X1	T36.5X2	T36.5X3	T36.5X4	T36.5X5	T36.5X6
Dihydrotachysterol	T45.2X1	T45.2X2	T45.2X3	T45.2X4	T45.2X5	T45.2X6
Dihydroxyaluminum aminoacetate	T47.1X1	T47.1X2	T47.1X3	T47.1X4	T47.1X5	T47.1X6
Dihydroxyaluminum sodium carbonate	T47.1X1	T47.1X2	T47.1X3	T47.1X4	T47.1X5	T47.1X6
Dihydroxyanthraquinone	T47.2X1	T47.2X2	T47.2X3	T47.2X4	T47.2X5	T47.2X6
Dihydroxycodeinone	T4Ø.2X1	T4Ø.2X2	T4Ø.2X3	T4Ø.2X4	T4Ø.2X5	T4Ø.2X6
Dihydroxypropyl theophylline	T5Ø.2X1	T5Ø.2X2	T5Ø.2X3	T5Ø.2X4	T5Ø.2X5	T5Ø.2X6
Diiodohydroxyquin	T37.8X1	T37.8X2	T37.8X3	T37.8X4	T37.8X5	T37.8X6
topical	T49.ØX1	T49.ØX2	T49.ØX3	T49.ØX4	T49.ØX5	T49.ØX6
Diiodohydroxyquinoline	T37.8X1	T37.8X2	T37.8X3	T37.8X4	T37.8X5	T37.8X6
Diiodotyrosine	T38.2X1	T38.2X2	T38.2X3	T38.2X4	T38.2X5	T38.2X6
Diisopromine	T44.3X1	T44.3X2	T44.3X3	T44.3X4	T44.3X5	T44.3X6
Diisopropylamine	T46.3X1	T46.3X2	T46.3X3	T46.3X4	T46.3X5	T46.3X6
Diisopropylfluorophosphonate	T44.ØX1	T44.ØX2	T44.ØX3	T44.ØX4	T44.ØX5	T44.ØX6

Substance	Poisoning, Accidental (unintentional)	Poisoning, Intentional Self-harm	Poisoning, Assault	Poisoning, Undetermined	Adverse Effect	Under-dosing
Dilantin	T42.ØX1	T42.ØX2	T42.ØX3	T42.ØX4	T42.ØX5	T42.ØX6
Dilaudid	T4Ø.2X1	T4Ø.2X2	T4Ø.2X3	T4Ø.2X4	T4Ø.2X5	T4Ø.2X6
Dilazep	T46.3X1	T46.3X2	T46.3X3	T46.3X4	T46.3X5	T46.3X6
Dill	T47.5X1	T47.5X2	T47.5X3	T47.5X4	T47.5X5	T47.5X6
Diloxanide	T37.3X1	T37.3X2	T37.3X3	T37.3X4	T37.3X5	T37.3X6
Diltiazem	T46.1X1	T46.1X2	T46.1X3	T46.1X4	T46.1X5	T46.1X6
Dimazole	T49.ØX1	T49.ØX2	T49.ØX3	T49.ØX4	T49.ØX5	T49.ØX6
Dimefline	T5Ø.7X1	T5Ø.7X2	T5Ø.7X3	T5Ø.7X4	T5Ø.7X5	T5Ø.7X6
Dimefox	T6Ø.ØX1	T6Ø.ØX2	T6Ø.ØX3	T6Ø.ØX4	—	—
Dimemorfan	T48.3X1	T48.3X2	T48.3X3	T48.3X4	T48.3X5	T48.3X6
Dimenhydrinate	T45.ØX1	T45.ØX2	T45.ØX3	T45.ØX4	T45.ØX5	T45.ØX6
Dimercaprol (British anti-lewisite)	T45.8X1	T45.8X2	T45.8X3	T45.8X4	T45.8X5	T45.8X6
Dimercaptopropanol	T45.8X1	T45.8X2	T45.8X3	T45.8X4	T45.8X5	T45.8X6
Dimestrol	T38.5X1	T38.5X2	T38.5X3	T38.5X4	T38.5X5	T38.5X6
Dimetane	T45.ØX1	T45.ØX2	T45.ØX3	T45.ØX4	T45.ØX5	T45.ØX6
Dimethicone	T47.1X1	T47.1X2	T47.1X3	T47.1X4	T47.1X5	T47.1X6
Dimethindene	T45.ØX1	T45.ØX2	T45.ØX3	T45.ØX4	T45.ØX5	T45.ØX6
Dimethisoquin	T49.1X1	T49.1X2	T49.1X3	T49.1X4	T49.1X5	T49.1X6
Dimethisterone	T38.5X1	T38.5X2	T38.5X3	T38.5X4	T38.5X5	T38.5X6
Dimethoate	T6Ø.ØX1	T6Ø.ØX2	T6Ø.ØX3	T6Ø.ØX4	—	—
Dimethocaine	T41.3X1	T41.3X2	T41.3X3	T41.3X4	T41.3X5	T41.3X6
Dimethoxanate	T48.3X1	T48.3X2	T48.3X3	T48.3X4	T48.3X5	T48.3X6
Dimethyl						
arsine, arsinic acid	T57.ØX1	T57.ØX2	T57.ØX3	T57.ØX4	—	—
carbinol	T51.2X1	T51.2X2	T51.2X3	T51.2X4	—	—
carbonate	T52.8X1	T52.8X2	T52.8X3	T52.8X4	—	—
diguanide	T38.3X1	T38.3X2	T38.3X3	T38.3X4	T38.3X5	T38.3X6
ketone	T52.4X1	T52.4X2	T52.4X3	T52.4X4	—	—
vapor	T52.4X1	T52.4X2	T52.4X3	T52.4X4	—	—
meperidine	T4Ø.2X1	T4Ø.2X2	T4Ø.2X3	T4Ø.2X4	T4Ø.2X5	T4Ø.2X6
parathion	T6Ø.ØX1	T6Ø.ØX2	T6Ø.ØX3	T6Ø.ØX4	—	—
phthlate	T49.3X1	T49.3X2	T49.3X3	T49.3X4	T49.3X5	T49.3X6
polysiloxane	T47.8X1	T47.8X2	T47.8X3	T47.8X4	T47.8X5	T47.8X6
sulfate (fumes)	T59.891	T59.892	T59.893	T59.894	—	—
liquid	T65.891	T65.892	T65.893	T65.894	—	—
sulfoxide (nonmedicinal)	T52.8X1	T52.8X2	T52.8X3	T52.8X4	—	—
medicinal	T49.4X1	T49.4X2	T49.4X3	T49.4X4	T49.4X5	T49.4X6
tryptamine	T4Ø.991	T4Ø.992	T4Ø.993	T4Ø.994	—	—
tubocurarine	T48.1X1	T48.1X2	T48.1X3	T48.1X4	T48.1X5	T48.1X6
Dimethylamine sulfate	T49.4X1	T49.4X2	T49.4X3	T49.4X4	T49.4X5	T49.4X6
Dimethylformamide	T52.8X1	T52.8X2	T52.8X3	T52.8X4	—	—
Dimethyltubocurarinium chloride	T48.1X1	T48.1X2	T48.1X3	T48.1X4	T48.1X5	T48.1X6
Dimeticone	T47.1X1	T47.1X2	T47.1X3	T47.1X4	T47.1X5	T47.1X6
Dimetilan	T6Ø.ØX1	T6Ø.ØX2	T6Ø.ØX3	T6Ø.ØX4	—	—
Dimetindene	T45.ØX1	T45.ØX2	T45.ØX3	T45.ØX4	T45.ØX5	T45.ØX6
Dimetotiazine	T43.3X1	T43.3X2	T43.3X3	T43.3X4	T43.3X5	T43.3X6
Dimorpholamine	T5Ø.7X1	T5Ø.7X2	T5Ø.7X3	T5Ø.7X4	T5Ø.7X5	T5Ø.7X6
Dimoxyline	T46.3X1	T46.3X2	T46.3X3	T46.3X4	T46.3X5	T46.3X6
Dinitrobenzene	T65.3X1	T65.3X2	T65.3X3	T65.3X4	—	—
vapor	T59.891	T59.892	T59.893	T59.894	—	—
Dinitrobenzol	T65.3X1	T65.3X2	T65.3X3	T65.3X4	—	—
vapor	T59.891	T59.892	T59.893	T59.894	—	—
Dinitrobutylphenol	T65.3X1	T65.3X2	T65.3X3	T65.3X4	—	—
Dinitro (-ortho-)cresol (pesticide) (spray)	T65.3X1	T65.3X2	T65.3X3	T65.3X4	—	—
Dinitrocyclohexylphenol	T65.3X1	T65.3X2	T65.3X3	T65.3X4	—	—
Dinitrophenol	T65.3X1	T65.3X2	T65.3X3	T65.3X4	—	—
Dinoprost	T48.ØX1	T48.ØX2	T48.ØX3	T48.ØX4	T48.ØX5	T48.ØX6
Dinoprostone	T48.ØX1	T48.ØX2	T48.ØX3	T48.ØX4	T48.ØX5	T48.ØX6
Dinoseb	T6Ø.3X1	T6Ø.3X2	T6Ø.3X3	T6Ø.3X4	—	—
Dioctyl sulfosuccinate (calcium) (sodium)	T47.4X1	T47.4X2	T47.4X3	T47.4X4	T47.4X5	T47.4X6
Diodone	T5Ø.8X1	T5Ø.8X2	T5Ø.8X3	T5Ø.8X4	T5Ø.8X5	T5Ø.8X6
Diodoquin	T37.8X1	T37.8X2	T37.8X3	T37.8X4	T37.8X5	T37.8X6
Dionin	T4Ø.2X1	T4Ø.2X2	T4Ø.2X3	T4Ø.2X4	T4Ø.2X5	T4Ø.2X6
Diosmin	T46.991	T46.992	T46.993	T46.994	T46.995	T46.996
Dioxane	T52.8X1	T52.8X2	T52.8X3	T52.8X4	—	—
Dioxathion	T6Ø.ØX1	T6Ø.ØX2	T6Ø.ØX3	T6Ø.ØX4	—	—
Dioxin	T53.7X1	T53.7X2	T53.7X3	T53.7X4	—	—
Dioxopromethazine	T43.3X1	T43.3X2	T43.3X3	T43.3X4	T43.3X5	T43.3X6
Dioxyline	T46.3X1	T46.3X2	T46.3X3	T46.3X4	T46.3X5	T46.3X6
Dipentene	T52.8X1	T52.8X2	T52.8X3	T52.8X4	—	—
Diperodon	T41.3X1	T41.3X2	T41.3X3	T41.3X4	T41.3X5	T41.3X6
Diphacinone	T6Ø.4X1	T6Ø.4X2	T6Ø.4X3	T6Ø.4X4	—	—
Diphemanil	T44.3X1	T44.3X2	T44.3X3	T44.3X4	T44.3X5	T44.3X6
metilsulfate	T44.3X1	T44.3X2	T44.3X3	T44.3X4	T44.3X5	T44.3X6
Diphenadione	T45.511	T45.512	T45.513	T45.514	T45.515	T45.516
rodenticide	T6Ø.4X1	T6Ø.4X2	T6Ø.4X3	T6Ø.4X4	—	—
Diphenhydramine	T45.ØX1	T45.ØX2	T45.ØX3	T45.ØX4	T45.ØX5	T45.ØX6
Diphenidol	T45.ØX1	T45.ØX2	T45.ØX3	T45.ØX4	T45.ØX5	T45.ØX6
Diphenoxylate	T47.6X1	T47.6X2	T47.6X3	T47.6X4	T47.6X5	T47.6X6

Substance	Poisoning, Accidental (unintentional)	Poisoning, Intentional Self-harm	Poisoning, Assault	Poisoning, Undetermined	Adverse Effect	Under-dosing
Diphenylamine	T65.3X1	T65.3X2	T65.3X3	T65.3X4	—	—
Diphenylbutazone	T39.2X1	T39.2X2	T39.2X3	T39.2X4	T39.2X5	T39.2X6
Diphenylchloroarsine, not in war	T57.ØX1	T57.ØX2	T57.ØX3	T57.ØX4	—	—
Diphenylhydantoin	T42.ØX1	T42.ØX2	T42.ØX3	T42.ØX4	T42.ØX5	T42.ØX6
Diphenylmethane dye	T52.1X1	T52.1X2	T52.1X3	T52.1X4	—	—
Diphenylpyraline	T45.ØX1	T45.ØX2	T45.ØX3	T45.ØX4	T45.ØX5	T45.ØX6
Diphtheria						
antitoxin	T5Ø.Z11	T5Ø.Z12	T5Ø.Z13	T5Ø.Z14	T5Ø.Z15	T5Ø.Z16
toxoid	T5Ø.A91	T5Ø.A92	T5Ø.A93	T5Ø.A94	T5Ø.A95	T5Ø.A96
with tetanus toxoid	T5Ø.A21	T5Ø.A22	T5Ø.A23	T5Ø.A24	T5Ø.A25	T5Ø.A26
with pertussis component	T5Ø.A11	T5Ø.A12	T5Ø.A13	T5Ø.A14	T5Ø.A15	T5Ø.A16
vaccine	T5Ø.A91	T5Ø.A92	T5Ø.A93	T5Ø.A94	T5Ø.A95	T5Ø.A96
combination						
without pertussis	T5Ø.A21	T5Ø.A22	T5Ø.A23	T5Ø.A24	T5Ø.A25	T5Ø.A26
including pertussis	T5Ø.A11	T5Ø.A12	T5Ø.A13	T5Ø.A14	T5Ø.A15	T5Ø.A16
Diphylline	T5Ø.2X1	T5Ø.2X2	T5Ø.2X3	T5Ø.2X4	T5Ø.2X5	T5Ø.2X6
Dipipanone	T4Ø.491	T4Ø.492	T4Ø.493	T4Ø.494	—	—
Dipivefrine	T49.5X1	T49.5X2	T49.5X3	T49.5X4	T49.5X5	T49.5X6
Diplovax	T5Ø.B91	T5Ø.B92	T5Ø.B93	T5Ø.B94	T5Ø.B95	T5Ø.B96
Diprophylline	T5Ø.2X1	T5Ø.2X2	T5Ø.2X3	T5Ø.2X4	T5Ø.2X5	T5Ø.2X6
Dipropyline	T48.291	T48.292	T48.293	T48.294	T48.295	T48.296
Dipyridamole	T46.3X1	T46.3X2	T46.3X3	T46.3X4	T46.3X5	T46.3X6
Dipyrone	T39.2X1	T39.2X2	T39.2X3	T39.2X4	T39.2X5	T39.2X6
Diquat (dibromide)	T6Ø.3X1	T6Ø.3X2	T6Ø.3X3	T6Ø.3X4	—	—
Disinfectant	T65.891	T65.892	T65.893	T65.894	—	—
alkaline	T54.3X1	T54.3X2	T54.3X3	T54.3X4	—	—
aromatic	T54.1X1	T54.1X2	T54.1X3	T54.1X4	—	—
intestinal	T37.8X1	T37.8X2	T37.8X3	T37.8X4	T37.8X5	T37.8X6
Disipal	T42.8X1	T42.8X2	T42.8X3	T42.8X4	T42.8X5	T42.8X6
Disodium edetate	T5Ø.6X1	T5Ø.6X2	T5Ø.6X3	T5Ø.6X4	T5Ø.6X5	T5Ø.6X6
Disoprofol	T41.291	T41.292	T41.293	T41.294	T41.295	T41.296
Disopyramide	T46.2X1	T46.2X2	T46.2X3	T46.2X4	T46.2X5	T46.2X6
Distigmine (bromide)	T44.ØX1	T44.ØX2	T44.ØX3	T44.ØX4	T44.ØX5	T44.ØX6
Disulfamide	T5Ø.2X1	T5Ø.2X2	T5Ø.2X3	T5Ø.2X4	T5Ø.2X5	T5Ø.2X6
Disulfanilamide	T37.ØX1	T37.ØX2	T37.ØX3	T37.ØX4	T37.ØX5	T37.ØX6
Disulfiram	T5Ø.6X1	T5Ø.6X2	T5Ø.6X3	T5Ø.6X4	T5Ø.6X5	T5Ø.6X6
Disulfoton	T6Ø.ØX1	T6Ø.ØX2	T6Ø.ØX3	T6Ø.ØX4	—	—
Dithiazanine iodide	T37.4X1	T37.4X2	T37.4X3	T37.4X4	T37.4X5	T37.4X6
Dithiocarbamate	T6Ø.ØX1	T6Ø.ØX2	T6Ø.ØX3	T6Ø.ØX4	—	—
Dithranol	T49.4X1	T49.4X2	T49.4X3	T49.4X4	T49.4X5	T49.4X6
Diucardin	T5Ø.2X1	T5Ø.2X2	T5Ø.2X3	T5Ø.2X4	T5Ø.2X5	T5Ø.2X6
Diupres	T5Ø.2X1	T5Ø.2X2	T5Ø.2X3	T5Ø.2X4	T5Ø.2X5	T5Ø.2X6
Diuretic NEC	T5Ø.2X1	T5Ø.2X2	T5Ø.2X3	T5Ø.2X4	T5Ø.2X5	T5Ø.2X6
benzothiadiazine	T5Ø.2X1	T5Ø.2X2	T5Ø.2X3	T5Ø.2X4	T5Ø.2X5	T5Ø.2X6
carbonic acid anhydrase inhibitors	T5Ø.2X1	T5Ø.2X2	T5Ø.2X3	T5Ø.2X4	T5Ø.2X5	T5Ø.2X6
furfuryl NEC	T5Ø.2X1	T5Ø.2X2	T5Ø.2X3	T5Ø.2X4	T5Ø.2X5	T5Ø.2X6
loop (high-ceiling)	T5Ø.1X1	T5Ø.1X2	T5Ø.1X3	T5Ø.1X4	T5Ø.1X5	T5Ø.1X6
mercurial NEC	T5Ø.2X1	T5Ø.2X2	T5Ø.2X3	T5Ø.2X4	T5Ø.2X5	T5Ø.2X6
osmotic	T5Ø.2X1	T5Ø.2X2	T5Ø.2X3	T5Ø.2X4	T5Ø.2X5	T5Ø.2X6
purine NEC	T5Ø.2X1	T5Ø.2X2	T5Ø.2X3	T5Ø.2X4	T5Ø.2X5	T5Ø.2X6
saluretic NEC	T5Ø.2X1	T5Ø.2X2	T5Ø.2X3	T5Ø.2X4	T5Ø.2X5	T5Ø.2X6
sulfonamide	T5Ø.2X1	T5Ø.2X2	T5Ø.2X3	T5Ø.2X4	T5Ø.2X5	T5Ø.2X6
thiazide NEC	T5Ø.2X1	T5Ø.2X2	T5Ø.2X3	T5Ø.2X4	T5Ø.2X5	T5Ø.2X6
xanthine	T5Ø.2X1	T5Ø.2X2	T5Ø.2X3	T5Ø.2X4	T5Ø.2X5	T5Ø.2X6
Diurgin	T5Ø.2X1	T5Ø.2X2	T5Ø.2X3	T5Ø.2X4	T5Ø.2X5	T5Ø.2X6
Diuril	T5Ø.2X1	T5Ø.2X2	T5Ø.2X3	T5Ø.2X4	T5Ø.2X5	T5Ø.2X6
Diuron	T6Ø.3X1	T6Ø.3X2	T6Ø.3X3	T6Ø.3X4	—	—
Divalproex	T42.6X1	T42.6X2	T42.6X3	T42.6X4	T42.6X5	T42.6X6
Divinyl ether	T41.ØX1	T41.ØX2	T41.ØX3	T41.ØX4	T41.ØX5	T41.ØX6
Dixanthogen	T49.ØX1	T49.ØX2	T49.ØX3	T49.ØX4	T49.ØX5	T49.ØX6
Dixyrazine	T43.3X1	T43.3X2	T43.3X3	T43.3X4	T43.3X5	T43.3X6
D-lysergic acid diethylamide	T4Ø.8X1	T4Ø.8X2	T4Ø.8X3	T4Ø.8X4	—	—
DMCT	T36.4X1	T36.4X2	T36.4X3	T36.4X4	T36.4X5	T36.4X6
DMSO — *see* Dimethyl sulfoxide						
DNBP	T6Ø.3X1	T6Ø.3X2	T6Ø.3X3	T6Ø.3X4	—	—
DNOC	T65.3X1	T65.3X2	T65.3X3	T65.3X4	—	—
Dobutamine	T44.5X1	T44.5X2	T44.5X3	T44.5X4	T44.5X5	T44.5X6
DOCA	T38.ØX1	T38.ØX2	T38.ØX3	T38.ØX4	T38.ØX5	T38.ØX6
Docusate sodium	T47.4X1	T47.4X2	T47.4X3	T47.4X4	T47.4X5	T47.4X6
Dodicin	T49.ØX1	T49.ØX2	T49.ØX3	T49.ØX4	T49.ØX5	T49.ØX6
Dofamium chloride	T49.ØX1	T49.ØX2	T49.ØX3	T49.ØX4	T49.ØX5	T49.ØX6
Dolophine	T4Ø.3X1	T4Ø.3X2	T4Ø.3X3	T4Ø.3X4	T4Ø.3X5	T4Ø.3X6
Doloxene	T39.8X1	T39.8X2	T39.8X3	T39.8X4	T39.8X5	T39.8X6
Domestic gas (after combustion) — *see* Gas, utility						
prior to combustion	T59.891	T59.892	T59.893	T59.894	—	—
Domiodol	T48.4X1	T48.4X2	T48.4X3	T48.4X4	T48.4X5	T48.4X6
Domiphen (bromide)	T49.ØX1	T49.ØX2	T49.ØX3	T49.ØX4	T49.ØX5	T49.ØX6
Domperidone	T45.ØX1	T45.ØX2	T45.ØX3	T45.ØX4	T45.ØX5	T45.ØX6

Substance	Poisoning, Accidental (unintentional)	Poisoning, Intentional Self-harm	Poisoning, Assault	Poisoning, Undetermined	Adverse Effect	Under-dosing
Dopa	T42.8X1	T42.8X2	T42.8X3	T42.8X4	T42.8X5	T42.8X6
Dopamine	T44.991	T44.992	T44.993	T44.994	T44.995	T44.996
Doriden	T42.6X1	T42.6X2	T42.6X3	T42.6X4	T42.6X5	T42.6X6
Dormiral	T42.3X1	T42.3X2	T42.3X3	T42.3X4	T42.3X5	T42.3X6
Dormison	T42.6X1	T42.6X2	T42.6X3	T42.6X4	T42.6X5	T42.6X6
Dornase	T48.4X1	T48.4X2	T48.4X3	T48.4X4	T48.4X5	T48.4X6
Dorsacaine	T41.3X1	T41.3X2	T41.3X3	T41.3X4	T41.3X5	T41.3X6
Dosulepin	T43.Ø11	T43.Ø12	T43.Ø13	T43.Ø14	T43.Ø15	T43.Ø16
Dothiepin	T43.Ø11	T43.Ø12	T43.Ø13	T43.Ø14	T43.Ø15	T43.Ø16
Doxantrazole	T48.6X1	T48.6X2	T48.6X3	T48.6X4	T48.6X5	T48.6X6
Doxapram	T5Ø.7X1	T5Ø.7X2	T5Ø.7X3	T5Ø.7X4	T5Ø.7X5	T5Ø.7X6
Doxazosin	T44.6X1	T44.6X2	T44.6X3	T44.6X4	T44.6X5	T44.6X6
Doxepin	T43.Ø11	T43.Ø12	T43.Ø13	T43.Ø14	T43.Ø15	T43.Ø16
Doxifluridine	T45.1X1	T45.1X2	T45.1X3	T45.1X4	T45.1X5	T45.1X6
Doxorubicin	T45.1X1	T45.1X2	T45.1X3	T45.1X4	T45.1X5	T45.1X6
Doxycycline	T36.4X1	T36.4X2	T36.4X3	T36.4X4	T36.4X5	T36.4X6
Doxylamine	T45.ØX1	T45.ØX2	T45.ØX3	T45.ØX4	T45.ØX5	T45.ØX6
Dramamine	T45.ØX1	T45.ØX2	T45.ØX3	T45.ØX4	T45.ØX5	T45.ØX6
Drano (drain cleaner)	T54.3X1	T54.3X2	T54.3X3	T54.3X4	—	—
Dressing, live pulp	T49.7X1	T49.7X2	T49.7X3	T49.7X4	T49.7X5	T49.7X6
Drocode	T4Ø.2X1	T4Ø.2X2	T4Ø.2X3	T4Ø.2X4	T4Ø.2X5	T4Ø.2X6
Dromoran	T4Ø.2X1	T4Ø.2X2	T4Ø.2X3	T4Ø.2X4	T4Ø.2X5	T4Ø.2X6
Dromostanolone	T38.7X1	T38.7X2	T38.7X3	T38.7X4	T38.7X5	T38.7X6
Dronabinol	T4Ø.7X1	T4Ø.7X2	T4Ø.7X3	T4Ø.7X4	T4Ø.7X5	T4Ø.7X6
Droperidol	T43.591	T43.592	T43.593	T43.594	T43.595	T43.596
Dropropizine	T48.3X1	T48.3X2	T48.3X3	T48.3X4	T48.3X5	T48.3X6
Drostanolone	T38.7X1	T38.7X2	T38.7X3	T38.7X4	T38.7X5	T38.7X6
Drotaverine	T44.3X1	T44.3X2	T44.3X3	T44.3X4	T44.3X5	T44.3X6
Drotrecogin alfa	T45.511	T45.512	T45.513	T45.514	T45.515	T45.516
Drug NEC	T5Ø.9Ø1	T5Ø.9Ø2	T5Ø.9Ø3	T5Ø.9Ø4	T5Ø.9Ø5	T5Ø.9Ø6
specified NEC	T5Ø.991	T5Ø.992	T5Ø.993	T5Ø.994	T5Ø.995	T5Ø.996
DTIC	T45.1X1	T45.1X2	T45.1X3	T45.1X4	T45.1X5	T45.1X6
Duboisine	T44.3X1	T44.3X2	T44.3X3	T44.3X4	T44.3X5	T44.3X6
Dulcolax	T47.2X1	T47.2X2	T47.2X3	T47.2X4	T47.2X5	T47.2X6
Duponol (C) (EP)	T49.2X1	T49.2X2	T49.2X3	T49.2X4	T49.2X5	T49.2X6
Durabolin	T38.7X1	T38.7X2	T38.7X3	T38.7X4	T38.7X5	T38.7X6
Dyclone	T41.3X1	T41.3X2	T41.3X3	T41.3X4	T41.3X5	T41.3X6
Dyclonine	T41.3X1	T41.3X2	T41.3X3	T41.3X4	T41.3X5	T41.3X6
Dydrogesterone	T38.5X1	T38.5X2	T38.5X3	T38.5X4	T38.5X5	T38.5X6
Dye NEC	T65.6X1	T65.6X2	T65.6X3	T65.6X4	—	—
antiseptic	T49.ØX1	T49.ØX2	T49.ØX3	T49.ØX4	T49.ØX5	T49.ØX6
diagnostic agents	T5Ø.8X1	T5Ø.8X2	T5Ø.8X3	T5Ø.8X4	T5Ø.8X5	T5Ø.8X6
pharmaceutical NEC	T5Ø.9Ø1	T5Ø.9Ø2	T5Ø.9Ø3	T5Ø.9Ø4	T5Ø.9Ø5	T5Ø.9Ø6
Dyflos	T44.ØX1	T44.ØX2	T44.ØX3	T44.ØX4	T44.ØX5	T44.ØX6
Dymelor	T38.3X1	T38.3X2	T38.3X3	T38.3X4	T38.3X5	T38.3X6
Dynamite	T65.3X1	T65.3X2	T65.3X3	T65.3X4	—	—
fumes	T59.891	T59.892	T59.893	T59.894	—	—
Dyphylline	T44.3X1	T44.3X2	T44.3X3	T44.3X4	T44.3X5	T44.3X6
b-eucaine	T49.1X1	T49.1X2	T49.1X3	T49.1X4	T49.1X5	T49.1X6
Ear drug NEC	T49.6X1	T49.6X2	T49.6X3	T49.6X4	T49.6X5	T49.6X6
Ear preparations	T49.6X1	T49.6X2	T49.6X3	T49.6X4	T49.6X5	T49.6X6
Echothiophate, echothiopate, ecothiopate	T49.5X1	T49.5X2	T49.5X3	T49.5X4	T49.5X5	T49.5X6
Econazole	T49.ØX1	T49.ØX2	T49.ØX3	T49.ØX4	T49.ØX5	T49.ØX6
Ecothiopate iodide	T49.5X1	T49.5X2	T49.5X3	T49.5X4	T49.5X5	T49.5X6
Ecstasy	T43.641	T43.642	T43.643	T43.644	—	—
Ectylurea	T42.6X1	T42.6X2	T42.6X3	T42.6X4	T42.6X5	T42.6X6
Edathamil disodium	T45.8X1	T45.8X2	T45.8X3	T45.8X4	T45.8X5	T45.8X6
Edecrin	T5Ø.1X1	T5Ø.1X2	T5Ø.1X3	T5Ø.1X4	T5Ø.1X5	T5Ø.1X6
Edetate, disodium (calcium)	T45.8X1	T45.8X2	T45.8X3	T45.8X4	T45.8X5	T45.8X6
Edoxudine	T49.5X1	T49.5X2	T49.5X3	T49.5X4	T49.5X5	T49.5X6
Edrophonium	T44.ØX1	T44.ØX2	T44.ØX3	T44.ØX4	T44.ØX5	T44.ØX6
chloride	T44.ØX1	T44.ØX2	T44.ØX3	T44.ØX4	T44.ØX5	T44.ØX6
EDTA	T5Ø.6X1	T5Ø.6X2	T5Ø.6X3	T5Ø.6X4	T5Ø.6X5	T5Ø.6X6
Eflornithine	T37.2X1	T37.2X2	T37.2X3	T37.2X4	T37.2X5	T37.2X6
Efloxate	T46.3X1	T46.3X2	T46.3X3	T46.3X4	T46.3X5	T46.3X6
Elase	T49.8X1	T49.8X2	T49.8X3	T49.8X4	T49.8X5	T49.8X6
Elastase	T47.5X1	T47.5X2	T47.5X3	T47.5X4	T47.5X5	T47.5X6
Elaterium	T47.2X1	T47.2X2	T47.2X3	T47.2X4	T47.2X5	T47.2X6
Elcatonin	T5Ø.991	T5Ø.992	T5Ø.993	T5Ø.994	T5Ø.995	T5Ø.996
Elder	T62.2X1	T62.2X2	T62.2X3	T62.2X4	—	—
berry, (unripe)	T62.1X1	T62.1X2	T62.1X3	T62.1X4	—	—
Electrolyte balance drug	T5Ø.3X1	T5Ø.3X2	T5Ø.3X3	T5Ø.3X4	T5Ø.3X5	T5Ø.3X6
Electrolytes NEC	T5Ø.3X1	T5Ø.3X2	T5Ø.3X3	T5Ø.3X4	T5Ø.3X5	T5Ø.3X6
Electrolytic agent NEC	T5Ø.3X1	T5Ø.3X2	T5Ø.3X3	T5Ø.3X4	T5Ø.3X5	T5Ø.3X6
Elemental diet	T5Ø.9Ø1	T5Ø.9Ø2	T5Ø.9Ø3	T5Ø.9Ø4	T5Ø.9Ø5	T5Ø.9Ø6
Elliptinium acetate	T45.1X1	T45.1X2	T45.1X3	T45.1X4	T45.1X5	T45.1X6
Embramine	T45.ØX1	T45.ØX2	T45.ØX3	T45.ØX4	T45.ØX5	T45.ØX6
Emepronium (salts)	T44.3X1	T44.3X2	T44.3X3	T44.3X4	T44.3X5	T44.3X6
bromide	T44.3X1	T44.3X2	T44.3X3	T44.3X4	T44.3X5	T44.3X6
Emetic NEC	T47.7X1	T47.7X2	T47.7X3	T47.7X4	T47.7X5	T47.7X6
Emetine	T37.3X1	T37.3X2	T37.3X3	T37.3X4	T37.3X5	T37.3X6
Emollient NEC	T49.3X1	T49.3X2	T49.3X3	T49.3X4	T49.3X5	T49.3X6
Emorfazone	T39.8X1	T39.8X2	T39.8X3	T39.8X4	T39.8X5	T39.8X6
Emylcamate	T43.591	T43.592	T43.593	T43.594	T43.595	T43.596
Enalapril	T46.4X1	T46.4X2	T46.4X3	T46.4X4	T46.4X5	T46.4X6
Enalaprilat	T46.4X1	T46.4X2	T46.4X3	T46.4X4	T46.4X5	T46.4X6
Encainide	T46.2X1	T46.2X2	T46.2X3	T46.2X4	T46.2X5	T46.2X6
Endocaine	T41.3X1	T41.3X2	T41.3X3	T41.3X4	T41.3X5	T41.3X6
Endosulfan	T6Ø.2X1	T6Ø.2X2	T6Ø.2X3	T6Ø.2X4	—	—
Endothall	T6Ø.3X1	T6Ø.3X2	T6Ø.3X3	T6Ø.3X4	—	—
Endralazine	T46.5X1	T46.5X2	T46.5X3	T46.5X4	T46.5X5	T46.5X6
Endrin	T6Ø.1X1	T6Ø.1X2	T6Ø.1X3	T6Ø.1X4	—	—
Enflurane	T41.ØX1	T41.ØX2	T41.ØX3	T41.ØX4	T41.ØX5	T41.ØX6
Enhexymal	T42.3X1	T42.3X2	T42.3X3	T42.3X4	T42.3X5	T42.3X6
Enocitabine	T45.1X1	T45.1X2	T45.1X3	T45.1X4	T45.1X5	T45.1X6
Enovid	T38.4X1	T38.4X2	T38.4X3	T38.4X4	T38.4X5	T38.4X6
Enoxacin	T36.8X1	T36.8X2	T36.8X3	T36.8X4	T36.8X5	T36.8X6
Enoxaparin (sodium)	T45.511	T45.512	T45.513	T45.514	T45.515	T45.516
Enpiprazole	T43.591	T43.592	T43.593	T43.594	T43.595	T43.596
Enprofylline	T48.6X1	T48.6X2	T48.6X3	T48.6X4	T48.6X5	T48.6X6
Enprostil	T47.1X1	T47.1X2	T47.1X3	T47.1X4	T47.1X5	T47.1X6
Enterogastrone	T38.891	T38.892	T38.893	T38.894	T38.895	T38.896
ENT preparations (anti-infectives)	T49.6X1	T49.6X2	T49.6X3	T49.6X4	T49.6X5	T49.6X6
Enviomycin	T36.8X1	T36.8X2	T36.8X3	T36.8X4	T36.8X5	T36.8X6
Enzodase	T45.3X1	T45.3X2	T45.3X3	T45.3X4	T45.3X5	T45.3X6
Enzyme NEC	T45.3X1	T45.3X2	T45.3X3	T45.3X4	T45.3X5	T45.3X6
depolymerizing	T49.8X1	T49.8X2	T49.8X3	T49.8X4	T49.8X5	T49.8X6
fibrolytic	T45.3X1	T45.3X2	T45.3X3	T45.3X4	T45.3X5	T45.3X6
gastric	T47.5X1	T47.5X2	T47.5X3	T47.5X4	T47.5X5	T47.5X6
intestinal	T47.5X1	T47.5X2	T47.5X3	T47.5X4	T47.5X5	T47.5X6
local action	T49.4X1	T49.4X2	T49.4X3	T49.4X4	T49.4X5	T49.4X6
proteolytic	T49.4X1	T49.4X2	T49.4X3	T49.4X4	T49.4X5	T49.4X6
thrombolytic	T45.3X1	T45.3X2	T45.3X3	T45.3X4	T45.3X5	T45.3X6
EPAB	T41.3X1	T41.3X2	T41.3X3	T41.3X4	T41.3X5	T41.3X6
Epanutin	T42.ØX1	T42.ØX2	T42.ØX3	T42.ØX4	T42.ØX5	T42.ØX6
Ephedra	T44.991	T44.992	T44.993	T44.994	T44.995	T44.996
Ephedrine	T44.991	T44.992	T44.993	T44.994	T44.995	T44.996
Epichlorhydrin, epichlorohydrin	T52.8X1	T52.8X2	T52.8X3	T52.8X4	—	—
Epicillin	T36.ØX1	T36.ØX2	T36.ØX3	T36.ØX4	T36.ØX5	T36.ØX6
Epiestriol	T38.5X1	T38.5X2	T38.5X3	T38.5X4	T38.5X5	T38.5X6
Epilim — *see* Sodium valproate						
Epimestrol	T38.5X1	T38.5X2	T38.5X3	T38.5X4	T38.5X5	T38.5X6
Epinephrine	T44.5X1	T44.5X2	T44.5X3	T44.5X4	T44.5X5	T44.5X6
Epirubicin	T45.1X1	T45.1X2	T45.1X3	T45.1X4	T45.1X5	T45.1X6
Epitiostanol	T38.7X1	T38.7X2	T38.7X3	T38.7X4	T38.7X5	T38.7X6
Epitizide	T5Ø.2X1	T5Ø.2X2	T5Ø.2X3	T5Ø.2X4	T5Ø.2X5	T5Ø.2X6
EPN	T6Ø.ØX1	T6Ø.ØX2	T6Ø.ØX3	T6Ø.ØX4	—	—
EPO	T45.8X1	T45.8X2	T45.8X3	T45.8X4	T45.8X5	T45.8X6
Epoetin alpha	T45.8X1	T45.8X2	T45.8X3	T45.8X4	T45.8X5	T45.8X6
Epomediol	T5Ø.991	T5Ø.992	T5Ø.993	T5Ø.994	T5Ø.995	T5Ø.996
Epoprostenol	T45.521	T45.522	T45.523	T45.524	T45.525	T45.526
Epoxy resin	T65.891	T65.892	T65.893	T65.894	—	—
Eprazinone	T48.4X1	T48.4X2	T48.4X3	T48.4X4	T48.4X5	T48.4X6
Epsilon aminocaproic acid	T45.621	T45.622	T45.623	T45.624	T45.625	T45.626
Epsom salt	T47.3X1	T47.3X2	T47.3X3	T47.3X4	T47.3X5	T47.3X6
Eptazocine	T4Ø.491	T4Ø.492	T4Ø.493	T4Ø.494	T4Ø.495	T4Ø.496
Equanil	T43.591	T43.592	T43.593	T43.594	T43.595	T43.596
Equisetum	T62.2X1	T62.2X2	T62.2X3	T62.2X4	—	—
diuretic	T5Ø.2X1	T5Ø.2X2	T5Ø.2X3	T5Ø.2X4	T5Ø.2X5	T5Ø.2X6
Ergobasine	T48.ØX1	T48.ØX2	T48.ØX3	T48.ØX4	T48.ØX5	T48.ØX6
Ergocalciferol	T45.2X1	T45.2X2	T45.2X3	T45.2X4	T45.2X5	T45.2X6
Ergoloid mesylates	T46.7X1	T46.7X2	T46.7X3	T46.7X4	T46.7X5	T46.7X6
Ergometrine	T48.ØX1	T48.ØX2	T48.ØX3	T48.ØX4	T48.ØX5	T48.ØX6
Ergonovine	T48.ØX1	T48.ØX2	T48.ØX3	T48.ØX4	T48.ØX5	T48.ØX6
Ergotamine	T46.5X1	T46.5X2	T46.5X3	T46.5X4	T46.5X5	T46.5X6
Ergotocine	T48.ØX1	T48.ØX2	T48.ØX3	T48.ØX4	T48.ØX5	T48.ØX6
Ergotrate	T48.ØX1	T48.ØX2	T48.ØX3	T48.ØX4	T48.ØX5	T48.ØX6
Ergot NEC	T64.81	T64.82	T64.83	T64.84	—	—
derivative	T48.ØX1	T48.ØX2	T48.ØX3	T48.ØX4	T48.ØX5	T48.ØX6
medicinal (alkaloids)	T48.ØX1	T48.ØX2	T48.ØX3	T48.ØX4	T48.ØX5	T48.ØX6
prepared	T48.ØX1	T48.ØX2	T48.ØX3	T48.ØX4	T48.ØX5	T48.ØX6
Eritrityl tetranitrate	T46.3X1	T46.3X2	T46.3X3	T46.3X4	T46.3X5	T46.3X6
Erythrityl tetranitrate	T46.3X1	T46.3X2	T46.3X3	T46.3X4	T46.3X5	T46.3X6
Erythrol tetranitrate	T46.3X1	T46.3X2	T46.3X3	T46.3X4	T46.3X5	T46.3X6
Erythromycin (salts)	T36.3X1	T36.3X2	T36.3X3	T36.3X4	T36.3X5	T36.3X6
ophthalmic preparation	T49.5X1	T49.5X2	T49.5X3	T49.5X4	T49.5X5	T49.5X6
topical NEC	T49.ØX1	T49.ØX2	T49.ØX3	T49.ØX4	T49.ØX5	T49.ØX6
Erythropoietin	T45.8X1	T45.8X2	T45.8X3	T45.8X4	T45.8X5	T45.8X6
human	T45.8X1	T45.8X2	T45.8X3	T45.8X4	T45.8X5	T45.8X6
Escin	T46.991	T46.992	T46.993	T46.994	T46.995	T46.996
Esculin	T45.2X1	T45.2X2	T45.2X3	T45.2X4	T45.2X5	T45.2X6
Esculoside	T45.2X1	T45.2X2	T45.2X3	T45.2X4	T45.2X5	T45.2X6

Substance	Poisoning, Accidental (unintentional)	Poisoning, Intentional Self-harm	Poisoning, Assault	Poisoning, Undetermined	Adverse Effect	Under-dosing
ESDT (ether-soluble tar distillate)	T49.1X1	T49.1X2	T49.1X3	T49.1X4	T49.1X5	T49.1X6
Eserine	T49.5X1	T49.5X2	T49.5X3	T49.5X4	T49.5X5	T49.5X6
Esflurbiprofen	T39.311	T39.312	T39.313	T39.314	T39.315	T39.316
Eskabarb	T42.3X1	T42.3X2	T42.3X3	T42.3X4	T42.3X5	T42.3X6
Eskalith	T43.8X1	T43.8X2	T43.8X3	T43.8X4	T43.8X5	T43.8X6
Esmolol	T44.7X1	T44.7X2	T44.7X3	T44.7X4	T44.7X5	T44.7X6
Estanozolol	T38.7X1	T38.7X2	T38.7X3	T38.7X4	T38.7X5	T38.7X6
Estazolam	T42.4X1	T42.4X2	T42.4X3	T42.4X4	T42.4X5	T42.4X6
Estradiol	T38.5X1	T38.5X2	T38.5X3	T38.5X4	T38.5X5	T38.5X6
with testosterone	T38.7X1	T38.7X2	T38.7X3	T38.7X4	T38.7X5	T38.7X6
benzoate	T38.5X1	T38.5X2	T38.5X3	T38.5X4	T38.5X5	T38.5X6
Estramustine	T45.1X1	T45.1X2	T45.1X3	T45.1X4	T45.1X5	T45.1X6
Estriol	T38.5X1	T38.5X2	T38.5X3	T38.5X4	T38.5X5	T38.5X6
Estrogen	T38.5X1	T38.5X2	T38.5X3	T38.5X4	T38.5X5	T38.5X6
with progesterone	T38.5X1	T38.5X2	T38.5X3	T38.5X4	T38.5X5	T38.5X6
conjugated	T38.5X1	T38.5X2	T38.5X3	T38.5X4	T38.5X5	T38.5X6
Estrone	T38.5X1	T38.5X2	T38.5X3	T38.5X4	T38.5X5	T38.5X6
Estropipate	T38.5X1	T38.5X2	T38.5X3	T38.5X4	T38.5X5	T38.5X6
Etacrynate sodium	T5Ø.1X1	T5Ø.1X2	T5Ø.1X3	T5Ø.1X4	T5Ø.1X5	T5Ø.1X6
Etacrynic acid	T5Ø.1X1	T5Ø.1X2	T5Ø.1X3	T5Ø.1X4	T5Ø.1X5	T5Ø.1X6
Etafedrine	T48.6X1	T48.6X2	T48.6X3	T48.6X4	T48.6X5	T48.6X6
Etafenone	T46.3X1	T46.3X2	T46.3X3	T46.3X4	T46.3X5	T46.3X6
Etambutol	T37.1X1	T37.1X2	T37.1X3	T37.1X4	T37.1X5	T37.1X6
Etamiphyllin	T48.6X1	T48.6X2	T48.6X3	T48.6X4	T48.6X5	T48.6X6
Etamivan	T5Ø.7X1	T5Ø.7X2	T5Ø.7X3	T5Ø.7X4	T5Ø.7X5	T5Ø.7X6
Etamsylate	T45.7X1	T45.7X2	T45.7X3	T45.7X4	T45.7X5	T45.7X6
Etebenecid	T5Ø.4X1	T5Ø.4X2	T5Ø.4X3	T5Ø.4X4	T5Ø.4X5	T5Ø.4X6
Ethacridine	T49.ØX1	T49.ØX2	T49.ØX3	T49.ØX4	T49.ØX5	T49.ØX6
Ethacrynic acid	T5Ø.1X1	T5Ø.1X2	T5Ø.1X3	T5Ø.1X4	T5Ø.1X5	T5Ø.1X6
Ethadione	T42.2X1	T42.2X2	T42.2X3	T42.2X4	T42.2X5	T42.2X6
Ethambutol	T37.1X1	T37.1X2	T37.1X3	T37.1X4	T37.1X5	T37.1X6
Ethamide	T5Ø.2X1	T5Ø.2X2	T5Ø.2X3	T5Ø.2X4	T5Ø.2X5	T5Ø.2X6
Ethamivan	T5Ø.7X1	T5Ø.7X2	T5Ø.7X3	T5Ø.7X4	T5Ø.7X5	T5Ø.7X6
Ethamsylate	T45.7X1	T45.7X2	T45.7X3	T45.7X4	T45.7X5	T45.7X6
Ethanol	T51.ØX1	T51.ØX2	T51.ØX3	T51.ØX4	—	—
beverage	T51.ØX1	T51.ØX2	T51.ØX3	T51.ØX4	—	—
Ethanolamine oleate	T46.8X1	T46.8X2	T46.8X3	T46.8X4	T46.8X5	T46.8X6
Ethaverine	T44.3X1	T44.3X2	T44.3X3	T44.3X4	T44.3X5	T44.3X6
Ethchlorvynol	T42.6X1	T42.6X2	T42.6X3	T42.6X4	T42.6X5	T42.6X6
Ethebenecid	T5Ø.4X1	T5Ø.4X2	T5Ø.4X3	T5Ø.4X4	T5Ø.4X5	T5Ø.4X6
Ether (vapor)	T41.ØX1	T41.ØX2	T41.ØX3	T41.ØX4	T41.ØX5	T41.ØX6
anesthetic	T41.ØX1	T41.ØX2	T41.ØX3	T41.ØX4	T41.ØX5	T41.ØX6
divinyl	T41.ØX1	T41.ØX2	T41.ØX3	T41.ØX4	T41.ØX5	T41.ØX6
ethyl (medicinal)	T41.ØX1	T41.ØX2	T41.ØX3	T41.ØX4	T41.ØX5	T41.ØX6
nonmedicinal	T52.8X1	T52.8X2	T52.8X3	T52.8X4	—	—
petroleum — *see* Ligroin						
solvent	T52.8X1	T52.8X2	T52.8X3	T52.8X4	—	—
Ethiazide	T5Ø.2X1	T5Ø.2X2	T5Ø.2X3	T5Ø.2X4	T5Ø.2X5	T5Ø.2X6
Ethidium chloride (vapor)	T59.891	T59.892	T59.893	T59.894	—	—
Ethinamate	T42.6X1	T42.6X2	T42.6X3	T42.6X4	T42.6X5	T42.6X6
Ethinylestradiol, ethinyloestradiol	T38.5X1	T38.5X2	T38.5X3	T38.5X4	T38.5X5	T38.5X6
with						
levonorgestrel	T38.4X1	T38.4X2	T38.4X3	T38.4X4	T38.4X5	T38.4X6
norethisterone	T38.4X1	T38.4X2	T38.4X3	T38.4X4	T38.4X5	T38.4X6
Ethiodized oil (131 I)	T5Ø.8X1	T5Ø.8X2	T5Ø.8X3	T5Ø.8X4	T5Ø.8X5	T5Ø.8X6
Ethion	T6Ø.ØX1	T6Ø.ØX2	T6Ø.ØX3	T6Ø.ØX4	—	—
Ethionamide	T37.1X1	T37.1X2	T37.1X3	T37.1X4	T37.1X5	T37.1X6
Ethioniamide	T37.1X1	T37.1X2	T37.1X3	T37.1X4	T37.1X5	T37.1X6
Ethisterone	T38.5X1	T38.5X2	T38.5X3	T38.5X4	T38.5X5	T38.5X6
Ethobral	T42.3X1	T42.3X2	T42.3X3	T42.3X4	T42.3X5	T42.3X6
Ethocaine (infiltration) (topical)	T41.3X1	T41.3X2	T41.3X3	T41.3X4	T41.3X5	T41.3X6
nerve block (peripheral) (plexus)	T41.3X1	T41.3X2	T41.3X3	T41.3X4	T41.3X5	T41.3X6
spinal	T41.3X1	T41.3X2	T41.3X3	T41.3X4	T41.3X5	T41.3X6
Ethoheptazine	T4Ø.491	T4Ø.492	T4Ø.493	T4Ø.494	T4Ø.495	T4Ø.496
Ethopropazine	T44.3X1	T44.3X2	T44.3X3	T44.3X4	T44.3X5	T44.3X6
Ethosuximide	T42.2X1	T42.2X2	T42.2X3	T42.2X4	T42.2X5	T42.2X6
Ethotoin	T42.ØX1	T42.ØX2	T42.ØX3	T42.ØX4	T42.ØX5	T42.ØX6
Ethoxazene	T37.91	T37.92	T37.93	T37.94	T37.95	T37.96
Ethoxazorutoside	T46.991	T46.992	T46.993	T46.994	T46.995	T46.996
Ethoxzolamide	T5Ø.2X1	T5Ø.2X2	T5Ø.2X3	T5Ø.2X4	T5Ø.2X5	T5Ø.2X6
Ethyl						
acetate	T52.8X1	T52.8X2	T52.8X3	T52.8X4	—	—
alcohol	T51.ØX1	T51.ØX2	T51.ØX3	T51.ØX4	—	—
beverage	T51.ØX1	T51.ØX2	T51.ØX3	T51.ØX4	—	—
aldehyde (vapor)	T59.891	T59.892	T59.893	T59.894	—	—
liquid	T52.8X1	T52.8X2	T52.8X3	T52.8X4	—	—
aminobenzoate	T41.3X1	T41.3X2	T41.3X3	T41.3X4	T41.3X5	T41.3X6
aminophenothiazine	T43.3X1	T43.3X2	T43.3X3	T43.3X4	T43.3X5	T43.3X6
benzoate	T52.8X1	T52.8X2	T52.8X3	T52.8X4	—	—

Substance	Poisoning, Accidental (unintentional)	Poisoning, Intentional Self-harm	Poisoning, Assault	Poisoning, Undetermined	Adverse Effect	Under-dosing
Ethyl — *continued*						
biscoumacetate	T45.511	T45.512	T45.513	T45.514	T45.515	T45.516
bromide (anesthetic)	T41.ØX1	T41.ØX2	T41.ØX3	T41.ØX4	T41.ØX5	T41.ØX6
carbamate	T45.1X1	T45.1X2	T45.1X3	T45.1X4	T45.1X5	T45.1X6
carbinol	T51.3X1	T51.3X2	T51.3X3	T51.3X4	—	—
carbonate	T52.8X1	T52.8X2	T52.8X3	T52.8X4	—	—
chaulmoograte	T37.1X1	T37.1X2	T37.1X3	T37.1X4	T37.1X5	T37.1X6
chloride (anesthetic)	T41.ØX1	T41.ØX2	T41.ØX3	T41.ØX4	T41.ØX5	T41.ØX6
anesthetic (local)	T41.3X1	T41.3X2	T41.3X3	T41.3X4	T41.3X5	T41.3X6
inhaled	T41.ØX1	T41.ØX2	T41.ØX3	T41.ØX4	T41.ØX5	T41.ØX6
local	T49.4X1	T49.4X2	T49.4X3	T49.4X4	T49.4X5	T49.4X6
solvent	T53.6X1	T53.6X2	T53.6X3	T53.6X4	—	—
dibunate	T48.3X1	T48.3X2	T48.3X3	T48.3X4	T48.3X5	T48.3X6
dichloroarsine (vapor)	T57.ØX1	T57.ØX2	T57.ØX3	T57.ØX4	—	—
estranol	T38.7X1	T38.7X2	T38.7X3	T38.7X4	T38.7X5	T38.7X6
ether — *see also* ether	T52.8X1	T52.8X2	T52.8X3	T52.8X4	—	—
formate NEC (solvent)	T52.ØX1	T52.ØX2	T52.ØX3	T52.ØX4	—	—
fumarate	T49.4X1	T49.4X2	T49.4X3	T49.4X4	T49.4X5	T49.4X6
hydroxyisobutyrate NEC (solvent)	T52.8X1	T52.8X2	T52.8X3	T52.8X4	—	—
iodoacetate	T59.3X1	T59.3X2	T59.3X3	T59.3X4	—	—
lactate NEC (solvent)	T52.8X1	T52.8X2	T52.8X3	T52.8X4	—	—
loflazepate	T42.4X1	T42.4X2	T42.4X3	T42.4X4	T42.4X5	T42.4X6
mercuric chloride	T56.1X1	T56.1X2	T56.1X3	T56.1X4	—	—
methylcarbinol	T51.8X1	T51.8X2	T51.8X3	T51.8X4	—	—
morphine	T4Ø.2X1	T4Ø.2X2	T4Ø.2X3	T4Ø.2X4	T4Ø.2X5	T4Ø.2X6
noradrenaline	T48.6X1	T48.6X2	T48.6X3	T48.6X4	T48.6X5	T48.6X6
oxybutyrate NEC (solvent)	T52.8X1	T52.8X2	T52.8X3	T52.8X4	—	—
Ethylene (gas)	T59.891	T59.892	T59.893	T59.894	—	—
anesthetic (general)	T41.ØX1	T41.ØX2	T41.ØX3	T41.ØX4	T41.ØX5	T41.ØX6
chlorohydrin	T52.8X1	T52.8X2	T52.8X3	T52.8X4	—	—
vapor	T53.6X1	T53.6X2	T53.6X3	T53.6X4	—	—
dichloride	T52.8X1	T52.8X2	T52.8X3	T52.8X4	—	—
vapor	T53.6X1	T53.6X2	T53.6X3	T53.6X4	—	—
dinitrate	T52.3X1	T52.3X2	T52.3X3	T52.3X4	—	—
glycol(s)	T52.8X1	T52.8X2	T52.8X3	T52.8X4	—	—
dinitrate	T52.3X1	T52.3X2	T52.3X3	T52.3X4	—	—
monobutyl ether	T52.3X1	T52.3X2	T52.3X3	T52.3X4	—	—
imine	T54.1X1	T54.1X2	T54.1X3	T54.1X4	—	—
oxide (fumigant) (nonmedicinal)	T59.891	T59.892	T59.893	T59.894	—	—
medicinal	T49.ØX1	T49.ØX2	T49.ØX3	T49.ØX4	T49.ØX5	T49.ØX6
Ethylenediaminetetra-acetic acid	T5Ø.6X1	T5Ø.6X2	T5Ø.6X3	T5Ø.6X4	T5Ø.6X5	T5Ø.6X6
Ethylenediamine theophylline	T48.6X1	T48.6X2	T48.6X3	T48.6X4	T48.6X5	T48.6X6
Ethylenedinitrilotetra-acetate	T5Ø.6X1	T5Ø.6X2	T5Ø.6X3	T5Ø.6X4	T5Ø.6X5	T5Ø.6X6
Ethylestrenol	T38.7X1	T38.7X2	T38.7X3	T38.7X4	T38.7X5	T38.7X6
Ethylhydroxycellulose	T47.4X1	T47.4X2	T47.4X3	T47.4X4	T47.4X5	T47.4X6
Ethylidene						
chloride NEC	T53.6X1	T53.6X2	T53.6X3	T53.6X4	—	—
diacetate	T6Ø.3X1	T6Ø.3X2	T6Ø.3X3	T6Ø.3X4	—	—
dicoumarin	T45.511	T45.512	T45.513	T45.514	T45.515	T45.516
dicoumarol	T45.511	T45.512	T45.513	T45.514	T45.515	T45.516
diethyl ether	T52.ØX1	T52.ØX2	T52.ØX3	T52.ØX4	—	—
Ethylmorphine	T4Ø.2X1	T4Ø.2X2	T4Ø.2X3	T4Ø.2X4	T4Ø.2X5	T4Ø.2X6
Ethylnorepinephrine	T48.6X1	T48.6X2	T48.6X3	T48.6X4	T48.6X5	T48.6X6
Ethylparachlorophen-oxyisobutyrate	T46.6X1	T46.6X2	T46.6X3	T46.6X4	T46.6X5	T46.6X6
Ethynodiol	T38.4X1	T38.4X2	T38.4X3	T38.4X4	T38.4X5	T38.4X6
with mestranol diacetate	T38.4X1	T38.4X2	T38.4X3	T38.4X4	T38.4X5	T38.4X6
Etidocaine	T41.3X1	T41.3X2	T41.3X3	T41.3X4	T41.3X5	T41.3X6
infiltration (subcutaneous)	T41.3X1	T41.3X2	T41.3X3	T41.3X4	T41.3X5	T41.3X6
nerve (peripheral) (plexus)	T41.3X1	T41.3X2	T41.3X3	T41.3X4	T41.3X5	T41.3X6
Etidronate	T5Ø.991	T5Ø.992	T5Ø.993	T5Ø.994	T5Ø.995	T5Ø.996
Etidronic acid (disodium salt)	T5Ø.991	T5Ø.992	T5Ø.993	T5Ø.994	T5Ø.995	T5Ø.996
Etifoxine	T42.6X1	T42.6X2	T42.6X3	T42.6X4	T42.6X5	T42.6X6
Etilefrine	T44.4X1	T44.4X2	T44.4X3	T44.4X4	T44.4X5	T44.4X6
Etilfen	T42.3X1	T42.3X2	T42.3X3	T42.3X4	T42.3X5	T42.3X6
Etinodiol	T38.4X1	T38.4X2	T38.4X3	T38.4X4	T38.4X5	T38.4X6
Etiroxate	T46.6X1	T46.6X2	T46.6X3	T46.6X4	T46.6X5	T46.6X6
Etizolam	T42.4X1	T42.4X2	T42.4X3	T42.4X4	T42.4X5	T42.4X6
Etodolac	T39.391	T39.392	T39.393	T39.394	T39.395	T39.396
Etofamide	T37.3X1	T37.3X2	T37.3X3	T37.3X4	T37.3X5	T37.3X6
Etofibrate	T46.6X1	T46.6X2	T46.6X3	T46.6X4	T46.6X5	T46.6X6
Etofylline	T46.7X1	T46.7X2	T46.7X3	T46.7X4	T46.7X5	T46.7X6
clofibrate	T46.6X1	T46.6X2	T46.6X3	T46.6X4	T46.6X5	T46.6X6
Etoglucid	T45.1X1	T45.1X2	T45.1X3	T45.1X4	T45.1X5	T45.1X6
Etomidate	T41.1X1	T41.1X2	T41.1X3	T41.1X4	T41.1X5	T41.1X6
Etomide	T39.8X1	T39.8X2	T39.8X3	T39.8X4	T39.8X5	T39.8X6
Etomidoline	T44.3X1	T44.3X2	T44.3X3	T44.3X4	T44.3X5	T44.3X6
Etoposide	T45.1X1	T45.1X2	T45.1X3	T45.1X4	T45.1X5	T45.1X6

Substance	Poisoning, Accidental (unintentional)	Poisoning, Intentional Self-harm	Poisoning, Assault	Poisoning, Undetermined	Adverse Effect	Under-dosing
Etorphine	T40.2X1	T40.2X2	T40.2X3	T40.2X4	T40.2X5	T40.2X6
Etoval	T42.3X1	T42.3X2	T42.3X3	T42.3X4	T42.3X5	T42.3X6
Etozolin	T50.1X1	T50.1X2	T50.1X3	T50.1X4	T50.1X5	T50.1X6
Etretinate	T50.991	T50.992	T50.993	T50.994	T50.995	T50.996
Etryptamine	T43.691	T43.692	T43.693	T43.694	T43.695	T43.696
Etybenzatropine	T44.3X1	T44.3X2	T44.3X3	T44.3X4	T44.3X5	T44.3X6
Etynodiol	T38.4X1	T38.4X2	T38.4X3	T38.4X4	T38.4X5	T38.4X6
Eucaine	T41.3X1	T41.3X2	T41.3X3	T41.3X4	T41.3X5	T41.3X6
Eucalyptus oil	T49.7X1	T49.7X2	T49.7X3	T49.7X4	T49.7X5	T49.7X6
Eucatropine	T49.5X1	T49.5X2	T49.5X3	T49.5X4	T49.5X5	T49.5X6
Eucodal	T40.2X1	T40.2X2	T40.2X3	T40.2X4	T40.2X5	T40.2X6
Euneryl	T42.3X1	T42.3X2	T42.3X3	T42.3X4	T42.3X5	T42.3X6
Euphthalmine	T44.3X1	T44.3X2	T44.3X3	T44.3X4	T44.3X5	T44.3X6
Eurax	T49.0X1	T49.0X2	T49.0X3	T49.0X4	T49.0X5	T49.0X6
Euresol	T49.4X1	T49.4X2	T49.4X3	T49.4X4	T49.4X5	T49.4X6
Euthroid	T38.1X1	T38.1X2	T38.1X3	T38.1X4	T38.1X5	T38.1X6
Evans blue	T50.8X1	T50.8X2	T50.8X3	T50.8X4	T50.8X5	T50.8X6
Evipal	T42.3X1	T42.3X2	T42.3X3	T42.3X4	T42.3X5	T42.3X6
sodium	T41.1X1	T41.1X2	T41.1X3	T41.1X4	T41.1X5	T41.1X6
Evipan	T42.3X1	T42.3X2	T42.3X3	T42.3X4	T42.3X5	T42.3X6
sodium	T41.1X1	T41.1X2	T41.1X3	T41.1X4	T41.1X5	T41.1X6
Exalamide	T49.0X1	T49.0X2	T49.0X3	T49.0X4	T49.0X5	T49.0X6
Exalgin	T39.1X1	T39.1X2	T39.1X3	T39.1X4	T39.1X5	T39.1X6
Excipients, pharmaceutical	T50.901	T50.902	T50.903	T50.904	T50.905	T50.906
Exhaust gas (engine) (motor vehicle)	T58.01	T58.02	T58.03	T58.04	—	—
Ex-Lax (phenolphthalein)	T47.2X1	T47.2X2	T47.2X3	T47.2X4	T47.2X5	T47.2X6
Expectorant NEC	T48.4X1	T48.4X2	T48.4X3	T48.4X4	T48.4X5	T48.4X6
Extended insulin zinc suspension	T38.3X1	T38.3X2	T38.3X3	T38.3X4	T38.3X5	T38.3X6
External medications (skin) (mucous membrane)	T49.91	T49.92	T49.93	T49.94	T49.95	T49.96
dental agent	T49.7X1	T49.7X2	T49.7X3	T49.7X4	T49.7X5	T49.7X6
ENT agent	T49.6X1	T49.6X2	T49.6X3	T49.6X4	T49.6X5	T49.6X6
ophthalmic preparation	T49.5X1	T49.5X2	T49.5X3	T49.5X4	T49.5X5	T49.5X6
specified NEC	T49.8X1	T49.8X2	T49.8X3	T49.8X4	T49.8X5	T49.8X6
Extrapyramidal antagonist NEC	T44.3X1	T44.3X2	T44.3X3	T44.3X4	T44.3X5	T44.3X6
Eye agents (anti-infective)	T49.5X1	T49.5X2	T49.5X3	T49.5X4	T49.5X5	T49.5X6
Eye drug NEC	T49.5X1	T49.5X2	T49.5X3	T49.5X4	T49.5X5	T49.5X6
FAC (fluorouracil + doxorubicin + cyclophosphamide)	T45.1X1	T45.1X2	T45.1X3	T45.1X4	T45.1X5	T45.1X6
Factor						
I (fibrinogen)	T45.8X1	T45.8X2	T45.8X3	T45.8X4	T45.8X5	T45.8X6
III (thromboplastin)	T45.8X1	T45.8X2	T45.8X3	T45.8X4	T45.8X5	T45.8X6
IX complex	T45.7X1	T45.7X2	T45.7X3	T45.7X4	T45.7X5	T45.7X6
human	T45.8X1	T45.8X2	T45.8X3	T45.8X4	T45.8X5	T45.8X6
VIII (antihemophilic Factor) (concentrate)	T45.8X1	T45.8X2	T45.8X3	T45.8X4	T45.8X5	T45.8X6
Famotidine	T47.0X1	T47.0X2	T47.0X3	T47.0X4	T47.0X5	T47.0X6
Fat suspension, intravenous	T50.991	T50.992	T50.993	T50.994	T50.995	T50.996
Fazadinium bromide	T48.1X1	T48.1X2	T48.1X3	T48.1X4	T48.1X5	T48.1X6
Febarbamate	T42.3X1	T42.3X2	T42.3X3	T42.3X4	T42.3X5	T42.3X6
Fecal softener	T47.4X1	T47.4X2	T47.4X3	T47.4X4	T47.4X5	T47.4X6
Fedrilate	T48.3X1	T48.3X2	T48.3X3	T48.3X4	T48.3X5	T48.3X6
Felodipine	T46.1X1	T46.1X2	T46.1X3	T46.1X4	T46.1X5	T46.1X6
Felypressin	T38.891	T38.892	T38.893	T38.894	T38.895	T38.896
Femoxetine	T43.221	T43.222	T43.223	T43.224	T43.225	T43.226
Fenalcomine	T46.3X1	T46.3X2	T46.3X3	T46.3X4	T46.3X5	T46.3X6
Fenamisal	T37.1X1	T37.1X2	T37.1X3	T37.1X4	T37.1X5	T37.1X6
Fenazone	T39.2X1	T39.2X2	T39.2X3	T39.2X4	T39.2X5	T39.2X6
Fenbendazole	T37.4X1	T37.4X2	T37.4X3	T37.4X4	T37.4X5	T37.4X6
Fenbutrazate	T50.5X1	T50.5X2	T50.5X3	T50.5X4	T50.5X5	T50.5X6
Fencamfamine	T43.691	T43.692	T43.693	T43.694	T43.695	T43.696
Fendiline	T46.1X1	T46.1X2	T46.1X3	T46.1X4	T46.1X5	T46.1X6
Fenetylline	T43.691	T43.692	T43.693	T43.694	T43.695	T43.696
Fenflumizole	T39.391	T39.392	T39.393	T39.394	T39.395	T39.396
Fenfluramine	T50.5X1	T50.5X2	T50.5X3	T50.5X4	T50.5X5	T50.5X6
Fenobarbital	T42.3X1	T42.3X2	T42.3X3	T42.3X4	T42.3X5	T42.3X6
Fenofibrate	T46.6X1	T46.6X2	T46.6X3	T46.6X4	T46.6X5	T46.6X6
Fenoprofen	T39.311	T39.312	T39.313	T39.314	T39.315	T39.316
Fenoterol	T48.6X1	T48.6X2	T48.6X3	T48.6X4	T48.6X5	T48.6X6
Fenoverine	T44.3X1	T44.3X2	T44.3X3	T44.3X4	T44.3X5	T44.3X6
Fenoxazoline	T48.5X1	T48.5X2	T48.5X3	T48.5X4	T48.5X5	T48.5X6
Fenproporex	T50.5X1	T50.5X2	T50.5X3	T50.5X4	T50.5X5	T50.5X6
Fenquizone	T50.2X1	T50.2X2	T50.2X3	T50.2X4	T50.2X5	T50.2X6
Fentanyl (analogs)	T40.411	T40.412	T40.413	T40.414	T40.415	T40.416
Fentazin	T43.3X1	T43.3X2	T43.3X3	T43.3X4	T43.3X5	T43.3X6
Fenthion	T60.0X1	T60.0X2	T60.0X3	T60.0X4	—	—
Fenticlor	T49.0X1	T49.0X2	T49.0X3	T49.0X4	T49.0X5	T49.0X6
Fenylbutazone	T39.2X1	T39.2X2	T39.2X3	T39.2X4	T39.2X5	T39.2X6

Substance	Poisoning, Accidental (unintentional)	Poisoning, Intentional Self-harm	Poisoning, Assault	Poisoning, Undetermined	Adverse Effect	Under-dosing
Feprazone	T39.2X1	T39.2X2	T39.2X3	T39.2X4	T39.2X5	T39.2X6
Fer de lance (bite) (venom)	T63.061	T63.062	T63.063	T63.064	—	—
Ferric — *see also* Iron						
chloride	T45.4X1	T45.4X2	T45.4X3	T45.4X4	T45.4X5	T45.4X6
citrate	T45.4X1	T45.4X2	T45.4X3	T45.4X4	T45.4X5	T45.4X6
hydroxide						
colloidal	T45.4X1	T45.4X2	T45.4X3	T45.4X4	T45.4X5	T45.4X6
polymaltose	T45.4X1	T45.4X2	T45.4X3	T45.4X4	T45.4X5	T45.4X6
pyrophosphate	T45.4X1	T45.4X2	T45.4X3	T45.4X4	T45.4X5	T45.4X6
Ferritin	T45.4X1	T45.4X2	T45.4X3	T45.4X4	T45.4X5	T45.4X6
Ferrocholinate	T45.4X1	T45.4X2	T45.4X3	T45.4X4	T45.4X5	T45.4X6
Ferrodextrane	T45.4X1	T45.4X2	T45.4X3	T45.4X4	T45.4X5	T45.4X6
Ferropolimaler	T45.4X1	T45.4X2	T45.4X3	T45.4X4	T45.4X5	T45.4X6
Ferrous — *see also* Iron						
phosphate	T45.4X1	T45.4X2	T45.4X3	T45.4X4	T45.4X5	T45.4X6
salt	T45.4X1	T45.4X2	T45.4X3	T45.4X4	T45.4X5	T45.4X6
with folic acid	T45.4X1	T45.4X2	T45.4X3	T45.4X4	T45.4X5	T45.4X6
Ferrous fumerate, gluconate, lactate, salt NEC, sulfate (medicinal)	T45.4X1	T45.4X2	T45.4X3	T45.4X4	T45.4X5	T45.4X6
Ferrovanadium (fumes)	T59.891	T59.892	T59.893	T59.894	—	—
Ferrum — *see* Iron						
Fertilizers NEC	T65.891	T65.892	T65.893	T65.894	—	—
with herbicide mixture	T60.3X1	T60.3X2	T60.3X3	T60.3X4	—	—
Fetoxilate	T47.6X1	T47.6X2	T47.6X3	T47.6X4	T47.6X5	T47.6X6
Fiber, dietary	T47.4X1	T47.4X2	T47.4X3	T47.4X4	T47.4X5	T47.4X6
Fiberglass	T65.831	T65.832	T65.833	T65.834	—	—
Fibrinogen (human)	T45.8X1	T45.8X2	T45.8X3	T45.8X4	T45.8X5	T45.8X6
Fibrinolysin (human)	T45.691	T45.692	T45.693	T45.694	T45.695	T45.696
Fibrinolysis						
affecting drug	T45.601	T45.602	T45.603	T45.604	T45.605	T45.606
inhibitor NEC	T45.621	T45.622	T45.623	T45.624	T45.625	T45.626
Fibrinolytic drug	T45.611	T45.612	T45.613	T45.614	T45.615	T45.616
Filix mas	T37.4X1	T37.4X2	T37.4X3	T37.4X4	T37.4X5	T37.4X6
Filtering cream	T49.3X1	T49.3X2	T49.3X3	T49.3X4	T49.3X5	T49.3X6
Fiorinal	T39.011	T39.012	T39.013	T39.014	T39.015	T39.016
Firedamp	T59.891	T59.892	T59.893	T59.894	—	—
Fish, noxious, nonbacterial	T61.91	T61.92	T61.93	T61.94	—	—
ciguatera	T61.01	T61.02	T61.03	T61.04	—	—
scombroid	T61.11	T61.12	T61.13	T61.14	—	—
shell	T61.781	T61.782	T61.783	T61.784	—	—
specified NEC	T61.771	T61.772	T61.773	T61.774	—	—
Flagyl	T37.3X1	T37.3X2	T37.3X3	T37.3X4	T37.3X5	T37.3X6
Flavine adenine dinucleotide	T45.2X1	T45.2X2	T45.2X3	T45.2X4	T45.2X5	T45.2X6
Flavodic acid	T46.991	T46.992	T46.993	T46.994	T46.995	T46.996
Flavoxate	T44.3X1	T44.3X2	T44.3X3	T44.3X4	T44.3X5	T44.3X6
Flaxedil	T48.1X1	T48.1X2	T48.1X3	T48.1X4	T48.1X5	T48.1X6
Flaxseed (medicinal)	T49.3X1	T49.3X2	T49.3X3	T49.3X4	T49.3X5	T49.3X6
Flecainide	T46.2X1	T46.2X2	T46.2X3	T46.2X4	T46.2X5	T46.2X6
Fleroxacin	T36.8X1	T36.8X2	T36.8X3	T36.8X4	T36.8X5	T36.8X6
Floctafenine	T39.8X1	T39.8X2	T39.8X3	T39.8X4	T39.8X5	T39.8X6
Flomax	T44.6X1	T44.6X2	T44.6X3	T44.6X4	T44.6X5	T44.6X6
Flomoxef	T36.1X1	T36.1X2	T36.1X3	T36.1X4	T36.1X5	T36.1X6
Flopropione	T44.3X1	T44.3X2	T44.3X3	T44.3X4	T44.3X5	T44.3X6
Florantyrone	T47.5X1	T47.5X2	T47.5X3	T47.5X4	T47.5X5	T47.5X6
Floraquin	T37.8X1	T37.8X2	T37.8X3	T37.8X4	T37.8X5	T37.8X6
Florinef	T38.0X1	T38.0X2	T38.0X3	T38.0X4	T38.0X5	T38.0X6
ENT agent	T49.6X1	T49.6X2	T49.6X3	T49.6X4	T49.6X5	T49.6X6
ophthalmic preparation	T49.5X1	T49.5X2	T49.5X3	T49.5X4	T49.5X5	T49.5X6
topical NEC	T49.0X1	T49.0X2	T49.0X3	T49.0X4	T49.0X5	T49.0X6
Flowers of sulfur	T49.4X1	T49.4X2	T49.4X3	T49.4X4	T49.4X5	T49.4X6
Floxuridine	T45.1X1	T45.1X2	T45.1X3	T45.1X4	T45.1X5	T45.1X6
Fluanisone	T43.4X1	T43.4X2	T43.4X3	T43.4X4	T43.4X5	T43.4X6
Flubendazole	T37.4X1	T37.4X2	T37.4X3	T37.4X4	T37.4X5	T37.4X6
Fluclorolone acetonide	T49.0X1	T49.0X2	T49.0X3	T49.0X4	T49.0X5	T49.0X6
Flucloxacillin	T36.0X1	T36.0X2	T36.0X3	T36.0X4	T36.0X5	T36.0X6
Fluconazole	T37.8X1	T37.8X2	T37.8X3	T37.8X4	T37.8X5	T37.8X6
Flucytosine	T37.8X1	T37.8X2	T37.8X3	T37.8X4	T37.8X5	T37.8X6
Fludeoxyglucose (18F)	T50.8X1	T50.8X2	T50.8X3	T50.8X4	T50.8X5	T50.8X6
Fludiazepam	T42.4X1	T42.4X2	T42.4X3	T42.4X4	T42.4X5	T42.4X6
Fludrocortisone	T50.0X1	T50.0X2	T50.0X3	T50.0X4	T50.0X5	T50.0X6
ENT agent	T49.6X1	T49.6X2	T49.6X3	T49.6X4	T49.6X5	T49.6X6
ophthalmic preparation	T49.5X1	T49.5X2	T49.5X3	T49.5X4	T49.5X5	T49.5X6
topical NEC	T49.0X1	T49.0X2	T49.0X3	T49.0X4	T49.0X5	T49.0X6
Fludroxycortide	T49.0X1	T49.0X2	T49.0X3	T49.0X4	T49.0X5	T49.0X6
Flufenamic acid	T39.391	T39.392	T39.393	T39.394	T39.395	T39.396
Fluindione	T45.511	T45.512	T45.513	T45.514	T45.515	T45.516
Flumequine	T37.8X1	T37.8X2	T37.8X3	T37.8X4	T37.8X5	T37.8X6
Flumethasone	T49.0X1	T49.0X2	T49.0X3	T49.0X4	T49.0X5	T49.0X6
Flumethiazide	T50.2X1	T50.2X2	T50.2X3	T50.2X4	T50.2X5	T50.2X6
Flumidin	T37.5X1	T37.5X2	T37.5X3	T37.5X4	T37.5X5	T37.5X6

Substance	Poisoning, Accidental (unintentional)	Poisoning, Intentional Self-harm	Poisoning, Assault	Poisoning, Undetermined	Adverse Effect	Under-dosing
Flunarizine	T46.7X1	T46.7X2	T46.7X3	T46.7X4	T46.7X5	T46.7X6
Flunidazole	T37.8X1	T37.8X2	T37.8X3	T37.8X4	T37.8X5	T37.8X6
Flunisolide	T48.6X1	T48.6X2	T48.6X3	T48.6X4	T48.6X5	T48.6X6
Flunitrazepam	T42.4X1	T42.4X2	T42.4X3	T42.4X4	T42.4X5	T42.4X6
Fluocinolone (acetonide)	T49.ØX1	T49.ØX2	T49.ØX3	T49.ØX4	T49.ØX5	T49.ØX6
Fluocinonide	T49.ØX1	T49.ØX2	T49.ØX3	T49.ØX4	T49.ØX5	T49.ØX6
Fluocortin (butyl)	T49.ØX1	T49.ØX2	T49.ØX3	T49.ØX4	T49.ØX5	T49.ØX6
Fluocortolone	T49.ØX1	T49.ØX2	T49.ØX3	T49.ØX4	T49.ØX5	T49.ØX6
Fluohydrocortisone	T38.ØX1	T38.ØX2	T38.ØX3	T38.ØX4	T38.ØX5	T38.ØX6
ENT agent	T49.6X1	T49.6X2	T49.6X3	T49.6X4	T49.6X5	T49.6X6
ophthalmic preparation	T49.5X1	T49.5X2	T49.5X3	T49.5X4	T49.5X5	T49.5X6
topical NEC	T49.ØX1	T49.ØX2	T49.ØX3	T49.ØX4	T49.ØX5	T49.ØX6
Fluonid	T49.ØX1	T49.ØX2	T49.ØX3	T49.ØX4	T49.ØX5	T49.ØX6
Fluopromazine	T43.3X1	T43.3X2	T43.3X3	T43.3X4	T43.3X5	T43.3X6
Fluoracetate	T6Ø.8X1	T6Ø.8X2	T6Ø.8X3	T6Ø.8X4	—	—
Fluorescein	T5Ø.8X1	T5Ø.8X2	T5Ø.8X3	T5Ø.8X4	T5Ø.8X5	T5Ø.8X6
Fluorhydrocortisone	T5Ø.ØX1	T5Ø.ØX2	T5Ø.ØX3	T5Ø.ØX4	T5Ø.ØX5	T5Ø.ØX6
Fluoride (nonmedicinal) (pesticide) (sodium) **NEC**	T6Ø.8X1	T6Ø.8X2	T6Ø.8X3	T6Ø.8X4	—	—
hydrogen — *see* Hydrofluoric acid						
medicinal NEC	T5Ø.991	T5Ø.992	T5Ø.993	T5Ø.994	T5Ø.995	T5Ø.996
dental use	T49.7X1	T49.7X2	T49.7X3	T49.7X4	T49.7X5	T49.7X6
not pesticide NEC	T54.91	T54.92	T54.93	T54.94	—	—
stannous	T49.7X1	T49.7X2	T49.7X3	T49.7X4	T49.7X5	T49.7X6
Fluorinated corticosteroids	T38.ØX1	T38.ØX2	T38.ØX3	T38.ØX4	T38.ØX5	T38.ØX6
Fluorine (gas)	T59.5X1	T59.5X2	T59.5X3	T59.5X4	—	—
salt — *see* Fluoride(s)						
Fluoristan	T49.7X1	T49.7X2	T49.7X3	T49.7X4	T49.7X5	T49.7X6
Fluormetholone	T49.ØX1	T49.ØX2	T49.ØX3	T49.ØX4	T49.ØX5	T49.ØX6
Fluoroacetate	T6Ø.8X1	T6Ø.8X2	T6Ø.8X3	T6Ø.8X4	—	—
Fluorocarbon monomer	T53.6X1	T53.6X2	T53.6X3	T53.6X4	—	—
Fluorocytosine	T37.8X1	T37.8X2	T37.8X3	T37.8X4	T37.8X5	T37.8X6
Fluorodeoxyuridine	T45.1X1	T45.1X2	T45.1X3	T45.1X4	T45.1X5	T45.1X6
Fluorometholone	T49.ØX1	T49.ØX2	T49.ØX3	T49.ØX4	T49.ØX5	T49.ØX6
ophthalmic preparation	T49.5X1	T49.5X2	T49.5X3	T49.5X4	T49.5X5	T49.5X6
Fluorophosphate insecticide	T6Ø.ØX1	T6Ø.ØX2	T6Ø.ØX3	T6Ø.ØX4	—	—
Fluorosol	T46.3X1	T46.3X2	T46.3X3	T46.3X4	T46.3X5	T46.3X6
Fluorouracil	T45.1X1	T45.1X2	T45.1X3	T45.1X4	T45.1X5	T45.1X6
Fluorphenylalanine	T49.5X1	T49.5X2	T49.5X3	T49.5X4	T49.5X5	T49.5X6
Fluothane	T41.ØX1	T41.ØX2	T41.ØX3	T41.ØX4	T41.ØX5	T41.ØX6
Fluoxetine	T43.221	T43.222	T43.223	T43.224	T43.225	T43.226
Fluoxymesterone	T38.7X1	T38.7X2	T38.7X3	T38.7X4	T38.7X5	T38.7X6
Flupenthixol	T43.4X1	T43.4X2	T43.4X3	T43.4X4	T43.4X5	T43.4X6
Flupentixol	T43.4X1	T43.4X2	T43.4X3	T43.4X4	T43.4X5	T43.4X6
Fluphenazine	T43.3X1	T43.3X2	T43.3X3	T43.3X4	T43.3X5	T43.3X6
Fluprednidene	T49.ØX1	T49.ØX2	T49.ØX3	T49.ØX4	T49.ØX5	T49.ØX6
Fluprednisolone	T38.ØX1	T38.ØX2	T38.ØX3	T38.ØX4	T38.ØX5	T38.ØX6
Fluradoline	T39.8X1	T39.8X2	T39.8X3	T39.8X4	T39.8X5	T39.8X6
Flurandrenolide	T49.ØX1	T49.ØX2	T49.ØX3	T49.ØX4	T49.ØX5	T49.ØX6
Flurandrenolone	T49.ØX1	T49.ØX2	T49.ØX3	T49.ØX4	T49.ØX5	T49.ØX6
Flurazepam	T42.4X1	T42.4X2	T42.4X3	T42.4X4	T42.4X5	T42.4X6
Flurbiprofen	T39.311	T39.312	T39.313	T39.314	T39.315	T39.316
Flurobate	T49.ØX1	T49.ØX2	T49.ØX3	T49.ØX4	T49.ØX5	T49.ØX6
Fluroxene	T41.ØX1	T41.ØX2	T41.ØX3	T41.ØX4	T41.ØX5	T41.ØX6
Fluspirilene	T43.591	T43.592	T43.593	T43.594	T43.595	T43.596
Flutamide	T38.6X1	T38.6X2	T38.6X3	T38.6X4	T38.6X5	T38.6X6
Flutazolam	T38.ØX1	T38.ØX2	T38.ØX3	T38.ØX4	T38.ØX5	T38.ØX6
Fluticasone propionate	T38.ØX1	T38.ØX2	T38.ØX3	T38.ØX4	T38.ØX5	T38.ØX6
Flutoprazepam	T42.4X1	T42.4X2	T42.4X3	T42.4X4	T42.4X5	T42.4X6
Flutropium bromide	T48.6X1	T48.6X2	T48.6X3	T48.6X4	T48.6X5	T48.6X6
Fluvoxamine	T43.221	T43.222	T43.223	T43.224	T43.225	T43.226
Folacin	T45.8X1	T45.8X2	T45.8X3	T45.8X4	T45.8X5	T45.8X6
Folic acid	T45.8X1	T45.8X2	T45.8X3	T45.8X4	T45.8X5	T45.8X6
with ferrous salt	T45.2X1	T45.2X2	T45.2X3	T45.2X4	T45.2X5	T45.2X6
antagonist	T45.1X1	T45.1X2	T45.1X3	T45.1X4	T45.1X5	T45.1X6
Folinic acid	T45.8X1	T45.8X2	T45.8X3	T45.8X4	T45.8X5	T45.8X6
Folium stramoniae	T48.6X1	T48.6X2	T48.6X3	T48.6X4	T48.6X5	T48.6X6
Follicle-stimulating hormone, human	T38.811	T38.812	T38.813	T38.814	T38.815	T38.816
Folpet	T6Ø.3X1	T6Ø.3X2	T6Ø.3X3	T6Ø.3X4	—	—
Fominoben	T48.3X1	T48.3X2	T48.3X3	T48.3X4	T48.3X5	T48.3X6
Food, foodstuffs, noxious, nonbacterial, NEC	T62.91	T62.92	T62.93	T62.94	—	—
berries	T62.1X1	T62.1X2	T62.1X3	T62.1X4	—	—
fish — *see also* Fish	T61.91	T61.92	T61.93	T61.94	—	—
mushrooms	T62.ØX1	T62.ØX2	T62.ØX3	T62.ØX4	—	—
plants	T62.2X1	T62.2X2	T62.2X3	T62.2X4	—	—
seafood	T61.91	T61.92	T61.93	T61.94	—	—
specified NEC	T61.8X1	T61.8X2	T61.8X3	T61.8X4	—	—
seeds	T62.2X1	T62.2X2	T62.2X3	T62.2X4	—	—

Substance	Poisoning, Accidental (unintentional)	Poisoning, Intentional Self-harm	Poisoning, Assault	Poisoning, Undetermined	Adverse Effect	Under-dosing
Food, foodstuffs, noxious, nonbacterial, — *continued*						
shellfish	T61.781	T61.782	T61.783	T61.784	—	—
specified NEC	T62.8X1	T62.8X2	T62.8X3	T62.8X4	—	—
Fool's parsley	T62.2X1	T62.2X2	T62.2X3	T62.2X4	—	—
Formaldehyde (solution), gas or vapor	T59.2X1	T59.2X2	T59.2X3	T59.2X4	—	—
fungicide	T6Ø.3X1	T6Ø.3X2	T6Ø.3X3	T6Ø.3X4	—	—
Formalin	T59.2X1	T59.2X2	T59.2X3	T59.2X4	—	—
fungicide	T6Ø.3X1	T6Ø.3X2	T6Ø.3X3	T6Ø.3X4	—	—
vapor	T59.2X1	T59.2X2	T59.2X3	T59.2X4	—	—
Formic acid	T54.2X1	T54.2X2	T54.2X3	T54.2X4	—	—
vapor	T59.891	T59.892	T59.893	T59.894	—	—
Foscarnet sodium	T37.5X1	T37.5X2	T37.5X3	T37.5X4	T37.5X5	T37.5X6
Fosfestrol	T38.5X1	T38.5X2	T38.5X3	T38.5X4	T38.5X5	T38.5X6
Fosfomycin	T36.8X1	T36.8X2	T36.8X3	T36.8X4	T36.8X5	T36.8X6
Fosfonet sodium	T37.5X1	T37.5X2	T37.5X3	T37.5X4	T37.5X5	T37.5X6
Fosinopril	T46.4X1	T46.4X2	T46.4X3	T46.4X4	T46.4X5	T46.4X6
sodium	T46.4X1	T46.4X2	T46.4X3	T46.4X4	T46.4X5	T46.4X6
Fowler's solution	T57.ØX1	T57.ØX2	T57.ØX3	T57.ØX4	—	—
Foxglove	T62.2X1	T62.2X2	T62.2X3	T62.2X4	—	—
Framycetin	T36.5X1	T36.5X2	T36.5X3	T36.5X4	T36.5X5	T36.5X6
Frangula	T47.2X1	T47.2X2	T47.2X3	T47.2X4	T47.2X5	T47.2X6
extract	T47.2X1	T47.2X2	T47.2X3	T47.2X4	T47.2X5	T47.2X6
Frei antigen	T5Ø.8X1	T5Ø.8X2	T5Ø.8X3	T5Ø.8X4	T5Ø.8X5	T5Ø.8X6
Freon	T53.5X1	T53.5X2	T53.5X3	T53.5X4	—	—
Fructose	T5Ø.3X1	T5Ø.3X2	T5Ø.3X3	T5Ø.3X4	T5Ø.3X5	T5Ø.3X6
Frusemide	T5Ø.1X1	T5Ø.1X2	T5Ø.1X3	T5Ø.1X4	T5Ø.1X5	T5Ø.1X6
FSH	T38.811	T38.812	T38.813	T38.814	T38.815	T38.816
Ftorafur	T45.1X1	T45.1X2	T45.1X3	T45.1X4	T45.1X5	T45.1X6
Fuel						
automobile	T52.ØX1	T52.ØX2	T52.ØX3	T52.ØX4	—	—
exhaust gas, not in transit	T58.Ø1	T58.Ø2	T58.Ø3	T58.Ø4	—	—
vapor NEC	T52.ØX1	T52.ØX2	T52.ØX3	T52.ØX4	—	—
gas (domestic use) — *see also* Carbon, monoxide, fuel, utility	T59.891	T59.892	T59.893	T59.894	—	—
utility	T59.891	T59.892	T59.893	T59.894	—	—
incomplete combustion of — *see* Carbon, monoxide, fuel, utility						
in mobile container	T59.891	T59.892	T59.893	T59.894	—	—
piped (natural)	T59.891	T59.892	T59.893	T59.894	—	—
industrial, incomplete combustion	T58.8X1	T58.8X2	T58.8X3	T58.8X4	—	—
Fugillin	T36.8X1	T36.8X2	T36.8X3	T36.8X4	T36.8X5	T36.8X6
Fulminate of mercury	T56.1X1	T56.1X2	T56.1X3	T56.1X4	—	—
Fulvicin	T36.7X1	T36.7X2	T36.7X3	T36.7X4	T36.7X5	T36.7X6
Fumadil	T36.8X1	T36.8X2	T36.8X3	T36.8X4	T36.8X5	T36.8X6
Fumagillin	T36.8X1	T36.8X2	T36.8X3	T36.8X4	T36.8X5	T36.8X6
Fumaric acid	T49.4X1	T49.4X2	T49.4X3	T49.4X4	T49.4X5	T49.4X6
Fumes (from)	T59.91	T59.92	T59.93	T59.94	—	—
carbon monoxide — *see* Carbon, monoxide						
charcoal (domestic use) — *see* Charcoal, fumes						
chloroform — *see* Chloroform						
coke (in domestic stoves, fireplaces) — *see* Coke fumes						
corrosive NEC	T54.91	T54.92	T54.93	T54.94	—	—
ether — *see* ether						
freons	T53.5X1	T53.5X2	T53.5X3	T53.5X4	—	—
hydrocarbons	T59.891	T59.892	T59.893	T59.894	—	—
petroleum (liquefied)	T59.891	T59.892	T59.893	T59.894	—	—
distributed through pipes (pure or mixed with air)	T59.891	T59.892	T59.893	T59.894	—	—
lead — *see* lead						
metal — *see* Metals, or the specified metal						
nitrogen dioxide	T59.ØX1	T59.ØX2	T59.ØX3	T59.ØX4	—	—
pesticides — *see* Pesticides						
petroleum (liquefied)	T59.891	T59.892	T59.893	T59.894	—	—
distributed through pipes (pure or mixed with air)	T59.891	T59.892	T59.893	T59.894	—	—
polyester	T59.891	T59.892	T59.893	T59.894	—	—
specified source NEC — *see also* substance specified	T59.891	T59.892	T59.893	T59.894	—	—
sulfur dioxide	T59.1X1	T59.1X2	T59.1X3	T59.1X4	—	—
Fumigant NEC	T6Ø.91	T6Ø.92	T6Ø.93	T6Ø.94	—	—

Substance	Poisoning, Accidental (unintentional)	Poisoning, Intentional Self-harm	Poisoning, Assault	Poisoning, Undetermined	Adverse Effect	Under-dosing
Fungicide NEC (nonmedicinal)	T6Ø.3X1	T6Ø.3X2	T6Ø.3X3	T6Ø.3X4	—	—
Fungi, noxious, used as food	T62.ØX1	T62.ØX2	T62.ØX3	T62.ØX4	—	—
Fungizone	T36.7X1	T36.7X2	T36.7X3	T36.7X4	T36.7X5	T36.7X6
topical	T49.ØX1	T49.ØX2	T49.ØX3	T49.ØX4	T49.ØX5	T49.ØX6
Furacin	T49.ØX1	T49.ØX2	T49.ØX3	T49.ØX4	T49.ØX5	T49.ØX6
Furadantin	T37.91	T37.92	T37.93	T37.94	T37.95	T37.96
Furazolidone	T37.8X1	T37.8X2	T37.8X3	T37.8X4	T37.8X5	T37.8X6
Furazolium chloride	T49.ØX1	T49.ØX2	T49.ØX3	T49.ØX4	T49.ØX5	T49.ØX6
Furfural	T52.8X1	T52.8X2	T52.8X3	T52.8X4	—	—
Furnace (coal burning) (domestic), gas from	T58.2X1	T58.2X2	T58.2X3	T58.2X4	—	—
industrial	T58.8X1	T58.8X2	T58.8X3	T58.8X4	—	—
Furniture polish	T65.891	T65.892	T65.893	T65.894	—	—
Furosemide	T5Ø.1X1	T5Ø.1X2	T5Ø.1X3	T5Ø.1X4	T5Ø.1X5	T5Ø.1X6
Furoxone	T37.91	T37.92	T37.93	T37.94	T37.95	T37.96
Fursultiamine	T45.2X1	T45.2X2	T45.2X3	T45.2X4	T45.2X5	T45.2X6
Fusafungine	T36.8X1	T36.8X2	T36.8X3	T36.8X4	T36.8X5	T36.8X6
Fusel oil (any) (amyl) (butyl) (propyl), vapor	T51.3X1	T51.3X2	T51.3X3	T51.3X4	—	—
Fusidate (ethanolamine) (sodium)	T36.8X1	T36.8X2	T36.8X3	T36.8X4	T36.8X5	T36.8X6
Fusidic acid	T36.8X1	T36.8X2	T36.8X3	T36.8X4	T36.8X5	T36.8X6
Fytic acid, nonasodium	T5Ø.6X1	T5Ø.6X2	T5Ø.6X3	T5Ø.6X4	T5Ø.6X5	T5Ø.6X6
b-Galactosidase	T47.5X1	T47.5X2	T47.5X3	T47.5X4	T47.5X5	T47.5X6
GABA	T43.8X1	T43.8X2	T43.8X3	T43.8X4	T43.8X5	T43.8X6
Gadopentetic acid	T5Ø.8X1	T5Ø.8X2	T5Ø.8X3	T5Ø.8X4	T5Ø.8X5	T5Ø.8X6
Galactose	T5Ø.3X1	T5Ø.3X2	T5Ø.3X3	T5Ø.3X4	T5Ø.3X5	T5Ø.3X6
Galantamine	T44.ØX1	T44.ØX2	T44.ØX3	T44.ØX4	T44.ØX5	T44.ØX6
Gallamine (triethiodide)	T48.1X1	T48.1X2	T48.1X3	T48.1X4	T48.1X5	T48.1X6
Gallium citrate	T5Ø.991	T5Ø.992	T5Ø.993	T5Ø.994	T5Ø.995	T5Ø.996
Gallopamil	T46.1X1	T46.1X2	T46.1X3	T46.1X4	T46.1X5	T46.1X6
Gamboge	T47.2X1	T47.2X2	T47.2X3	T47.2X4	T47.2X5	T47.2X6
Gamimune	T5Ø.Z11	T5Ø.Z12	T5Ø.Z13	T5Ø.Z14	T5Ø.Z15	T5Ø.Z16
Gamma-aminobutyric acid	T43.8X1	T43.8X2	T43.8X3	T43.8X4	T43.8X5	T43.8X6
Gamma-benzene hexachloride (medicinal)	T49.ØX1	T49.ØX2	T49.ØX3	T49.ØX4	T49.ØX5	T49.ØX6
nonmedicinal, vapor	T53.6X1	T53.6X2	T53.6X3	T53.6X4	—	—
Gamma-BHC (medicinal) — *see also* Gamma-benzene hexachloride	T49.ØX1	T49.ØX2	T49.ØX3	T49.ØX4	T49.ØX5	T49.ØX6
Gamma globulin	T5Ø.Z11	T5Ø.Z12	T5Ø.Z13	T5Ø.Z14	T5Ø.Z15	T5Ø.Z16
Gamulin	T5Ø.Z11	T5Ø.Z12	T5Ø.Z13	T5Ø.Z14	T5Ø.Z15	T5Ø.Z16
Ganciclovir (sodium)	T37.5X1	T37.5X2	T37.5X3	T37.5X4	T37.5X5	T37.5X6
Ganglionic blocking drug NEC	T44.2X1	T44.2X2	T44.2X3	T44.2X4	T44.2X5	T44.2X6
specified NEC	T44.2X1	T44.2X2	T44.2X3	T44.2X4	T44.2X5	T44.2X6
Ganja	T4Ø.7X1	T4Ø.7X2	T4Ø.7X3	T4Ø.7X4	T4Ø.7X5	T4Ø.7X6
Garamycin	T36.5X1	T36.5X2	T36.5X3	T36.5X4	T36.5X5	T36.5X6
ophthalmic preparation	T49.5X1	T49.5X2	T49.5X3	T49.5X4	T49.5X5	T49.5X6
topical NEC	T49.ØX1	T49.ØX2	T49.ØX3	T49.ØX4	T49.ØX5	T49.ØX6
Gardenal	T42.3X1	T42.3X2	T42.3X3	T42.3X4	T42.3X5	T42.3X6
Gardepanyl	T42.3X1	T42.3X2	T42.3X3	T42.3X4	T42.3X5	T42.3X6
Gaseous substance — *see* Gas						
Gasoline	T52.ØX1	T52.ØX2	T52.ØX3	T52.ØX4	—	—
vapor	T52.ØX1	T52.ØX2	T52.ØX3	T52.ØX4	—	—
Gastric enzymes	T47.5X1	T47.5X2	T47.5X3	T47.5X4	T47.5X5	T47.5X6
Gastrografin	T5Ø.8X1	T5Ø.8X2	T5Ø.8X3	T5Ø.8X4	T5Ø.8X5	T5Ø.8X6
Gastrointestinal drug	T47.91	T47.92	T47.93	T47.94	T47.95	T47.96
biological	T47.8X1	T47.8X2	T47.8X3	T47.8X4	T47.8X5	T47.8X6
specified NEC	T47.8X1	T47.8X2	T47.8X3	T47.8X4	T47.8X5	T47.8X6
Gas NEC	T59.91	T59.92	T59.93	T59.94	—	—
acetylene	T59.891	T59.892	T59.893	T59.894	—	—
incomplete combustion of	T58.11	T58.12	T58.13	T58.14	—	—
air contaminants, source or type not specified	T59.91	T59.92	T59.93	T59.94	—	—
anesthetic	T41.ØX1	T41.ØX2	T41.ØX3	T41.ØX4	T41.ØX5	T41.ØX6
blast furnace	T58.8X1	T58.8X2	T58.8X3	T58.8X4	—	—
butane — *see* butane						
carbon monoxide — *see* Carbon, monoxide						
chlorine	T59.4X1	T59.4X2	T59.4X3	T59.4X4	—	—
coal	T58.2X1	T58.2X2	T58.2X3	T58.2X4	—	—
cyanide	T57.3X1	T57.3X2	T57.3X3	T57.3X4	—	—
dicyanogen	T65.ØX1	T65.ØX2	T65.ØX3	T65.ØX4	—	—
domestic — *see* Domestic gas						
exhaust	T58.Ø1	T58.Ø2	T58.Ø3	T58.Ø4	—	—
from utility (for cooking, heating, or lighting) (after combustion) — *see* Carbon, monoxide, fuel, utility						

Substance	Poisoning, Accidental (unintentional)	Poisoning, Intentional Self-harm	Poisoning, Assault	Poisoning, Undetermined	Adverse Effect	Under-dosing
Gas — *continued*						
from utility — *see* Carbon, monoxide, fuel, utility — *continued*						
prior to combustion	T59.891	T59.892	T59.893	T59.894	—	—
from wood- or coal-burning stove or fireplace	T58.2X1	T58.2X2	T58.2X3	T58.2X4	—	—
fuel (domestic use) (after combustion) — *see also* Carbon, monoxide, fuel						
industrial use	T58.8X1	T58.8X2	T58.8X3	T58.8X4	—	—
prior to combustion	T59.891	T59.892	T59.893	T59.894	—	—
utility	T59.891	T59.892	T59.893	T59.894	—	—
incomplete combustion of — *see* Carbon, monoxide, fuel, utility						
in mobile container	T59.891	T59.892	T59.893	T59.894	—	—
piped (natural)	T59.891	T59.892	T59.893	T59.894	—	—
garage	T58.Ø1	T58.Ø2	T58.Ø3	T58.Ø4	—	—
hydrocarbon NEC	T59.891	T59.892	T59.893	T59.894	—	—
incomplete combustion of — *see* Carbon, monoxide, fuel, utility						
liquefied — *see* butane						
piped	T59.891	T59.892	T59.893	T59.894	—	—
hydrocyanic acid	T65.ØX1	T65.ØX2	T65.ØX3	T65.ØX4	—	—
illuminating (after combustion)	T58.11	T58.12	T58.13	T58.14	—	—
prior to combustion	T59.891	T59.892	T59.893	T59.894	—	—
incomplete combustion, any — *see* Carbon, monoxide						
kiln	T58.8X1	T58.8X2	T58.8X3	T58.8X4	—	—
lacrimogenic	T59.3X1	T59.3X2	T59.3X3	T59.3X4	—	—
liquefied petroleum — *see* butane						
marsh	T59.891	T59.892	T59.893	T59.894	—	—
motor exhaust, not in transit	T58.Ø1	T58.Ø2	T58.Ø3	T58.Ø4	—	—
mustard, not in war	T59.891	T59.892	T59.893	T59.894	—	—
natural	T59.891	T59.892	T59.893	T59.894	—	—
nerve, not in war	T59.91	T59.92	T59.93	T59.94	—	—
oil	T52.ØX1	T52.ØX2	T52.ØX3	T52.ØX4	—	—
petroleum (liquefied) (distributed in mobile containers)	T59.891	T59.892	T59.893	T59.894	—	—
piped (pure or mixed with air)	T59.891	T59.892	T59.893	T59.894	—	—
piped (manufactured) (natural) NEC	T59.891	T59.892	T59.893	T59.894	—	—
producer	T58.8X1	T58.8X2	T58.8X3	T58.8X4	—	—
propane — *see* propane						
refrigerant (chlorofluoro-carbon)	T53.5X1	T53.5X2	T53.5X3	T53.5X4	—	—
not chlorofluoro-carbon	T59.891	T59.892	T59.893	T59.894	—	—
sewer	T59.91	T59.92	T59.93	T59.94	—	—
specified source NEC	T59.91	T59.92	T59.93	T59.94	—	—
stove (after combustion)	T58.11	T58.12	T58.13	T58.14	—	—
prior to combustion	T59.891	T59.892	T59.893	T59.894	—	—
tear	T59.3X1	T59.3X2	T59.3X3	T59.3X4	—	—
therapeutic	T41.5X1	T41.5X2	T41.5X3	T41.5X4	T41.5X5	T41.5X6
utility (for cooking, heating, or lighting) (piped) NEC	T59.891	T59.892	T59.893	T59.894	—	—
incomplete combustion of — *see* Carbon, monoxide, fuel, utilty						
in mobile container	T59.891	T59.892	T59.893	T59.894	—	—
piped (natural)	T59.891	T59.892	T59.893	T59.894	—	—
water	T58.11	T58.12	T58.13	T58.14	—	—
incomplete combustion of — *see* Carbon, monoxide, fuel, utility						
Gaultheria procumbens	T62.2X1	T62.2X2	T62.2X3	T62.2X4	—	—
Gefarnate	T44.3X1	T44.3X2	T44.3X3	T44.3X4	T44.3X5	T44.3X6
Gelatin (intravenous)	T45.8X1	T45.8X2	T45.8X3	T45.8X4	T45.8X5	T45.8X6
absorbable (sponge)	T45.7X1	T45.7X2	T45.7X3	T45.7X4	T45.7X5	T45.7X6
Gelfilm	T49.8X1	T49.8X2	T49.8X3	T49.8X4	T49.8X5	T49.8X6
Gelfoam	T45.7X1	T45.7X2	T45.7X3	T45.7X4	T45.7X5	T45.7X6
Gelsemine	T5Ø.991	T5Ø.992	T5Ø.993	T5Ø.994	T5Ø.995	T5Ø.996
Gelsemium (sempervirens)	T62.2X1	T62.2X2	T62.2X3	T62.2X4	—	—
Gemeprost	T48.ØX1	T48.ØX2	T48.ØX3	T48.ØX4	T48.ØX5	T48.ØX6
Gemfibrozil	T46.6X1	T46.6X2	T46.6X3	T46.6X4	T46.6X5	T46.6X6
Gemonil	T42.3X1	T42.3X2	T42.3X3	T42.3X4	T42.3X5	T42.3X6
Gentamicin	T36.5X1	T36.5X2	T36.5X3	T36.5X4	T36.5X5	T36.5X6

Substance	Poisoning, Accidental (unintentional)	Poisoning, Intentional Self-harm	Poisoning, Assault	Poisoning, Undetermined	Adverse Effect	Under-dosing
Gentamicin — *continued*						
ophthalmic preparation	T49.5X1	T49.5X2	T49.5X3	T49.5X4	T49.5X5	T49.5X6
topical NEC	T49.ØX1	T49.ØX2	T49.ØX3	T49.ØX4	T49.ØX5	T49.ØX6
Gentian	T47.5X1	T47.5X2	T47.5X3	T47.5X4	T47.5X5	T47.5X6
violet	T49.ØX1	T49.ØX2	T49.ØX3	T49.ØX4	T49.ØX5	T49.ØX6
Gepefrine	T44.4X1	T44.4X2	T44.4X3	T44.4X4	T44.4X5	T44.4X6
Gestonorone caproate	T38.5X1	T38.5X2	T38.5X3	T38.5X4	T38.5X5	T38.5X6
Gexane	T49.ØX1	T49.ØX2	T49.ØX3	T49.ØX4	T49.ØX5	T49.ØX6
Gila monster (venom)	T63.111	T63.112	T63.113	T63.114	—	—
Ginger	T47.5X1	T47.5X2	T47.5X3	T47.5X4	T47.5X5	T47.5X6
Jamaica — *see* Jamaica, ginger						
Gitalin	T46.ØX1	T46.ØX2	T46.ØX3	T46.ØX4	T46.ØX5	T46.ØX6
amorphous	T46.ØX1	T46.ØX2	T46.ØX3	T46.ØX4	T46.ØX5	T46.ØX6
Gitaloxin	T46.ØX1	T46.ØX2	T46.ØX3	T46.ØX4	T46.ØX5	T46.ØX6
Gitoxin	T46.ØX1	T46.ØX2	T46.ØX3	T46.ØX4	T46.ØX5	T46.ØX6
Glafenine	T39.8X1	T39.8X2	T39.8X3	T39.8X4	T39.8X5	T39.8X6
Glandular extract (medicinal) **NEC**	T5Ø.Z91	T5Ø.Z92	T5Ø.Z93	T5Ø.Z94	T5Ø.Z95	T5Ø.Z96
Glaucarubin	T37.3X1	T37.3X2	T37.3X3	T37.3X4	T37.3X5	T37.3X6
Glibenclamide	T38.3X1	T38.3X2	T38.3X3	T38.3X4	T38.3X5	T38.3X6
Glibornuride	T38.3X1	T38.3X2	T38.3X3	T38.3X4	T38.3X5	T38.3X6
Gliclazide	T38.3X1	T38.3X2	T38.3X3	T38.3X4	T38.3X5	T38.3X6
Glimidine	T38.3X1	T38.3X2	T38.3X3	T38.3X4	T38.3X5	T38.3X6
Glipizide	T38.3X1	T38.3X2	T38.3X3	T38.3X4	T38.3X5	T38.3X6
Gliquidone	T38.3X1	T38.3X2	T38.3X3	T38.3X4	T38.3X5	T38.3X6
Glisolamide	T38.3X1	T38.3X2	T38.3X3	T38.3X4	T38.3X5	T38.3X6
Glisoxepide	T38.3X1	T38.3X2	T38.3X3	T38.3X4	T38.3X5	T38.3X6
Globin zinc insulin	T38.3X1	T38.3X2	T38.3X3	T38.3X4	T38.3X5	T38.3X6
Globulin						
antilymphocytic	T5Ø.Z11	T5Ø.Z12	T5Ø.Z13	T5Ø.Z14	T5Ø.Z15	T5Ø.Z16
antirhesus	T5Ø.Z11	T5Ø.Z12	T5Ø.Z13	T5Ø.Z14	T5Ø.Z15	T5Ø.Z16
antivenin	T5Ø.Z11	T5Ø.Z12	T5Ø.Z13	T5Ø.Z14	T5Ø.Z15	T5Ø.Z16
antiviral	T5Ø.Z11	T5Ø.Z12	T5Ø.Z13	T5Ø.Z14	T5Ø.Z15	T5Ø.Z16
Glucagon	T38.3X1	T38.3X2	T38.3X3	T38.3X4	T38.3X5	T38.3X6
Glucocorticoids	T38.ØX1	T38.ØX2	T38.ØX3	T38.ØX4	T38.ØX5	T38.ØX6
Glucocorticosteroid	T38.ØX1	T38.ØX2	T38.ØX3	T38.ØX4	T38.ØX5	T38.ØX6
Gluconic acid	T5Ø.991	T5Ø.992	T5Ø.993	T5Ø.994	T5Ø.995	T5Ø.996
Glucosamine sulfate	T39.4X1	T39.4X2	T39.4X3	T39.4X4	T39.4X5	T39.4X6
Glucose	T5Ø.3X1	T5Ø.3X2	T5Ø.3X3	T5Ø.3X4	T5Ø.3X5	T5Ø.3X6
with sodium chloride	T5Ø.3X1	T5Ø.3X2	T5Ø.3X3	T5Ø.3X4	T5Ø.3X5	T5Ø.3X6
Glucosulfone sodium	T37.1X1	T37.1X2	T37.1X3	T37.1X4	T37.1X5	T37.1X6
Glucurolactone	T47.8X1	T47.8X2	T47.8X3	T47.8X4	T47.8X5	T47.8X6
Glue NEC	T52.8X1	T52.8X2	T52.8X3	T52.8X4	—	—
Glutamic acid	T47.5X1	T47.5X2	T47.5X3	T47.5X4	T47.5X5	T47.5X6
Glutaral (medicinal)	T49.ØX1	T49.ØX2	T49.ØX3	T49.ØX4	T49.ØX5	T49.ØX6
nonmedicinal	T65.891	T65.892	T65.893	T65.894	—	—
Glutaraldehyde (nonmedicinal)	T65.891	T65.892	T65.893	T65.894	—	—
medicinal	T49.ØX1	T49.ØX2	T49.ØX3	T49.ØX4	T49.ØX5	T49.ØX6
Glutathione	T5Ø.6X1	T5Ø.6X2	T5Ø.6X3	T5Ø.6X4	T5Ø.6X5	T5Ø.6X6
Glutethimide	T42.6X1	T42.6X2	T42.6X3	T42.6X4	T42.6X5	T42.6X6
Glyburide	T38.3X1	T38.3X2	T38.3X3	T38.3X4	T38.3X5	T38.3X6
Glycerin	T47.4X1	T47.4X2	T47.4X3	T47.4X4	T47.4X5	T47.4X6
Glycerol	T47.4X1	T47.4X2	T47.4X3	T47.4X4	T47.4X5	T47.4X6
borax	T49.6X1	T49.6X2	T49.6X3	T49.6X4	T49.6X5	T49.6X6
intravenous	T5Ø.3X1	T5Ø.3X2	T5Ø.3X3	T5Ø.3X4	T5Ø.3X5	T5Ø.3X6
iodinated	T48.4X1	T48.4X2	T48.4X3	T48.4X4	T48.4X5	T48.4X6
Glycerophosphate	T5Ø.991	T5Ø.992	T5Ø.993	T5Ø.994	T5Ø.995	T5Ø.996
Glyceryl						
gualacolate	T48.4X1	T48.4X2	T48.4X3	T48.4X4	T48.4X5	T48.4X6
nitrate	T46.3X1	T46.3X2	T46.3X3	T46.3X4	T46.3X5	T46.3X6
triacetate (topical)	T49.ØX1	T49.ØX2	T49.ØX3	T49.ØX4	T49.ØX5	T49.ØX6
trinitrate	T46.3X1	T46.3X2	T46.3X3	T46.3X4	T46.3X5	T46.3X6
Glycine	T5Ø.3X1	T5Ø.3X2	T5Ø.3X3	T5Ø.3X4	T5Ø.3X5	T5Ø.3X6
Glyclopyramide	T38.3X1	T38.3X2	T38.3X3	T38.3X4	T38.3X5	T38.3X6
Glycobiarsol	T37.3X1	T37.3X2	T37.3X3	T37.3X4	T37.3X5	T37.3X6
Glycols (ether)	T52.3X1	T52.3X2	T52.3X3	T52.3X4	—	—
Glyconiazide	T37.1X1	T37.1X2	T37.1X3	T37.1X4	T37.1X5	T37.1X6
Glycopyrrolate	T44.3X1	T44.3X2	T44.3X3	T44.3X4	T44.3X5	T44.3X6
Glycopyrronium	T44.3X1	T44.3X2	T44.3X3	T44.3X4	T44.3X5	T44.3X6
bromide	T44.3X1	T44.3X2	T44.3X3	T44.3X4	T44.3X5	T44.3X6
Glycoside, cardiac (stimulant)	T46.ØX1	T46.ØX2	T46.ØX3	T46.ØX4	T46.ØX5	T46.ØX6
Glycyclamide	T38.3X1	T38.3X2	T38.3X3	T38.3X4	T38.3X5	T38.3X6
Glycyrrhiza extract	T48.4X1	T48.4X2	T48.4X3	T48.4X4	T48.4X5	T48.4X6
Glycyrrhizic acid	T48.4X1	T48.4X2	T48.4X3	T48.4X4	T48.4X5	T48.4X6
Glycyrrhizinate potassium	T48.4X1	T48.4X2	T48.4X3	T48.4X4	T48.4X5	T48.4X6
Glymidine sodium	T38.3X1	T38.3X2	T38.3X3	T38.3X4	T38.3X5	T38.3X6
Glyphosate	T6Ø.3X1	T6Ø.3X2	T6Ø.3X3	T6Ø.3X4	—	—
Glyphylline	T48.6X1	T48.6X2	T48.6X3	T48.6X4	T48.6X5	T48.6X6
Gold						
colloidal (I98Au)	T45.1X1	T45.1X2	T45.1X3	T45.1X4	T45.1X5	T45.1X6
salts	T39.4X1	T39.4X2	T39.4X3	T39.4X4	T39.4X5	T39.4X6

Substance	Poisoning, Accidental (unintentional)	Poisoning, Intentional Self-harm	Poisoning, Assault	Poisoning, Undetermined	Adverse Effect	Under-dosing
Golden sulfide of antimony	T56.891	T56.892	T56.893	T56.894	—	—
Goldylocks	T62.2X1	T62.2X2	T62.2X3	T62.2X4	—	—
Gonadal tissue extract	T38.9Ø1	T38.9Ø2	T38.9Ø3	T38.9Ø4	T38.9Ø5	T38.9Ø6
female	T38.5X1	T38.5X2	T38.5X3	T38.5X4	T38.5X5	T38.5X6
male	T38.7X1	T38.7X2	T38.7X3	T38.7X4	T38.7X5	T38.7X6
Gonadorelin	T38.891	T38.892	T38.893	T38.894	T38.895	T38.896
Gonadotropin	T38.891	T38.892	T38.893	T38.894	T38.895	T38.896
chorionic	T38.891	T38.892	T38.893	T38.894	T38.895	T38.896
pituitary	T38.811	T38.812	T38.813	T38.814	T38.815	T38.816
Goserelin	T45.1X1	T45.1X2	T45.1X3	T45.1X4	T45.1X5	T45.1X6
Grain alcohol	T51.ØX1	T51.ØX2	T51.ØX3	T51.ØX4	—	—
Gramicidin	T49.ØX1	T49.ØX2	T49.ØX3	T49.ØX4	T49.ØX5	T49.ØX6
Granisetron	T45.ØX1	T45.ØX2	T45.ØX3	T45.ØX4	T45.ØX5	T45.ØX6
Gratiola officinalis	T62.2X1	T62.2X2	T62.2X3	T62.2X4	—	—
Grease	T65.891	T65.892	T65.893	T65.894	—	—
Green hellebore	T62.2X1	T62.2X2	T62.2X3	T62.2X4	—	—
Green soap	T49.2X1	T49.2X2	T49.2X3	T49.2X4	T49.2X5	T49.2X6
Grifulvin	T36.7X1	T36.7X2	T36.7X3	T36.7X4	T36.7X5	T36.7X6
Griseofulvin	T36.7X1	T36.7X2	T36.7X3	T36.7X4	T36.7X5	T36.7X6
Growth hormone	T38.811	T38.812	T38.813	T38.814	T38.815	T38.816
Guaiacol derivatives	T48.4X1	T48.4X2	T48.4X3	T48.4X4	T48.4X5	T48.4X6
Guaiac reagent	T5Ø.991	T5Ø.992	T5Ø.993	T5Ø.994	T5Ø.995	T5Ø.996
Guaifenesin	T48.4X1	T48.4X2	T48.4X3	T48.4X4	T48.4X5	T48.4X6
Guaimesal	T48.4X1	T48.4X2	T48.4X3	T48.4X4	T48.4X5	T48.4X6
Guaiphenesin	T48.4X1	T48.4X2	T48.4X3	T48.4X4	T48.4X5	T48.4X6
Guamecycline	T36.4X1	T36.4X2	T36.4X3	T36.4X4	T36.4X5	T36.4X6
Guanabenz	T46.5X1	T46.5X2	T46.5X3	T46.5X4	T46.5X5	T46.5X6
Guanacline	T46.5X1	T46.5X2	T46.5X3	T46.5X4	T46.5X5	T46.5X6
Guanadrel	T46.5X1	T46.5X2	T46.5X3	T46.5X4	T46.5X5	T46.5X6
Guanatol	T37.2X1	T37.2X2	T37.2X3	T37.2X4	T37.2X5	T37.2X6
Guanethidine	T46.5X1	T46.5X2	T46.5X3	T46.5X4	T46.5X5	T46.5X6
Guanfacine	T46.5X1	T46.5X2	T46.5X3	T46.5X4	T46.5X5	T46.5X6
Guano	T65.891	T65.892	T65.893	T65.894	—	—
Guanochlor	T46.5X1	T46.5X2	T46.5X3	T46.5X4	T46.5X5	T46.5X6
Guanoclor	T46.5X1	T46.5X2	T46.5X3	T46.5X4	T46.5X5	T46.5X6
Guanoctine	T46.5X1	T46.5X2	T46.5X3	T46.5X4	T46.5X5	T46.5X6
Guanoxabenz	T46.5X1	T46.5X2	T46.5X3	T46.5X4	T46.5X5	T46.5X6
Guanoxan	T46.5X1	T46.5X2	T46.5X3	T46.5X4	T46.5X5	T46.5X6
Guar gum (medicinal)	T46.6X1	T46.6X2	T46.6X3	T46.6X4	T46.6X5	T46.6X6
Hachimycin	T36.7X1	T36.7X2	T36.7X3	T36.7X4	T36.7X5	T36.7X6
Hair						
dye	T49.4X1	T49.4X2	T49.4X3	T49.4X4	T49.4X5	T49.4X6
preparation NEC	T49.4X1	T49.4X2	T49.4X3	T49.4X4	T49.4X5	T49.4X6
Halazepam	T42.4X1	T42.4X2	T42.4X3	T42.4X4	T42.4X5	T42.4X6
Halcinolone	T49.ØX1	T49.ØX2	T49.ØX3	T49.ØX4	T49.ØX5	T49.ØX6
Halcinonide	T49.ØX1	T49.ØX2	T49.ØX3	T49.ØX4	T49.ØX5	T49.ØX6
Halethazole	T49.ØX1	T49.ØX2	T49.ØX3	T49.ØX4	T49.ØX5	T49.ØX6
Hallucinogen NOS	T4Ø.9Ø1	T4Ø.9Ø2	T4Ø.9Ø3	T4Ø.9Ø4	T4Ø.9Ø5	T4Ø.9Ø6
specified NEC	T4Ø.991	T4Ø.992	T4Ø.993	T4Ø.994	T4Ø.995	T4Ø.996
Halofantrine	T37.2X1	T37.2X2	T37.2X3	T37.2X4	T37.2X5	T37.2X6
Halofenate	T46.6X1	T46.6X2	T46.6X3	T46.6X4	T46.6X5	T46.6X6
Halometasone	T49.ØX1	T49.ØX2	T49.ØX3	T49.ØX4	T49.ØX5	T49.ØX6
Haloperidol	T43.4X1	T43.4X2	T43.4X3	T43.4X4	T43.4X5	T43.4X6
Haloprogin	T49.ØX1	T49.ØX2	T49.ØX3	T49.ØX4	T49.ØX5	T49.ØX6
Halotex	T49.ØX1	T49.ØX2	T49.ØX3	T49.ØX4	T49.ØX5	T49.ØX6
Halothane	T41.ØX1	T41.ØX2	T41.ØX3	T41.ØX4	T41.ØX5	T41.ØX6
Haloxazolam	T42.4X1	T42.4X2	T42.4X3	T42.4X4	T42.4X5	T42.4X6
Halquinols	T49.ØX1	T49.ØX2	T49.ØX3	T49.ØX4	T49.ØX5	T49.ØX6
Hamamelis	T49.2X1	T49.2X2	T49.2X3	T49.2X4	T49.2X5	T49.2X6
Haptendextran	T45.8X1	T45.8X2	T45.8X3	T45.8X4	T45.8X5	T45.8X6
Harmonyl	T46.5X1	T46.5X2	T46.5X3	T46.5X4	T46.5X5	T46.5X6
Hartmann's solution	T5Ø.3X1	T5Ø.3X2	T5Ø.3X3	T5Ø.3X4	T5Ø.3X5	T5Ø.3X6
Hashish	T4Ø.7X1	T4Ø.7X2	T4Ø.7X3	T4Ø.7X4	T4Ø.7X5	T4Ø.7X6
Hawaiian Woodrose seeds	T4Ø.991	T4Ø.992	T4Ø.993	T4Ø.994	—	—
HCB	T6Ø.3X1	T6Ø.3X2	T6Ø.3X3	T6Ø.3X4	—	—
HCH	T53.6X1	T53.6X2	T53.6X3	T53.6X4	—	—
medicinal	T49.ØX1	T49.ØX2	T49.ØX3	T49.ØX4	T49.ØX5	T49.ØX6
HCN	T57.3X1	T57.3X2	T57.3X3	T57.3X4	—	—
Headache cures, drugs, powders NEC	T5Ø.9Ø1	T5Ø.9Ø2	T5Ø.9Ø3	T5Ø.9Ø4	T5Ø.9Ø5	T5Ø.9Ø6
Heavenly Blue (morning glory)	T4Ø.991	T4Ø.992	T4Ø.993	T4Ø.994	—	—
Heavy metal antidote	T45.8X1	T45.8X2	T45.8X3	T45.8X4	T45.8X5	T45.8X6
Hedaquinium	T49.ØX1	T49.ØX2	T49.ØX3	T49.ØX4	T49.ØX5	T49.ØX6
Hedge hyssop	T62.2X1	T62.2X2	T62.2X3	T62.2X4	—	—
Heet	T49.8X1	T49.8X2	T49.8X3	T49.8X4	T49.8X5	T49.8X6
Helenin	T37.4X1	T37.4X2	T37.4X3	T37.4X4	T37.4X5	T37.4X6
Helium (nonmedicinal) **NEC**	T59.891	T59.892	T59.893	T59.894	—	—
medicinal	T48.991	T48.992	T48.993	T48.994	T48.995	T48.996
Hellebore (black) (green) (white)	T62.2X1	T62.2X2	T62.2X3	T62.2X4	—	—
Hematin	T45.8X1	T45.8X2	T45.8X3	T45.8X4	T45.8X5	T45.8X6

Substance	Poisoning, Accidental (unintentional)	Poisoning, Intentional Self-harm	Poisoning, Assault	Poisoning, Undetermined	Adverse Effect	Under-dosing
Hematinic preparation	T45.8X1	T45.8X2	T45.8X3	T45.8X4	T45.8X5	T45.8X6
Hematological agent	T45.91	T45.92	T45.93	T45.94	T45.95	T45.96
specified NEC	T45.8X1	T45.8X2	T45.8X3	T45.8X4	T45.8X5	T45.8X6
Hemlock	T62.2X1	T62.2X2	T62.2X3	T62.2X4	—	—
Hemostatic	T45.621	T45.622	T45.623	T45.624	T45.625	T45.626
drug, systemic	T45.621	T45.622	T45.623	T45.624	T45.625	T45.626
Hemostyptic	T49.4X1	T49.4X2	T49.4X3	T49.4X4	T49.4X5	T49.4X6
Henbane	T62.2X1	T62.2X2	T62.2X3	T62.2X4	—	—
Heparin (sodium)	T45.511	T45.512	T45.513	T45.514	T45.515	T45.516
action reverser	T45.7X1	T45.7X2	T45.7X3	T45.7X4	T45.7X5	T45.7X6
Heparin-fraction	T45.511	T45.512	T45.513	T45.514	T45.515	T45.516
Heparinoid (systemic)	T45.511	T45.512	T45.513	T45.514	T45.515	T45.516
Hepatic secretion stimulant	T47.8X1	T47.8X2	T47.8X3	T47.8X4	T47.8X5	T47.8X6
Hepatitis B						
immune globulin	T5Ø.Z11	T5Ø.Z12	T5Ø.Z13	T5Ø.Z14	T5Ø.Z15	T5Ø.Z16
vaccine	T5Ø.B91	T5Ø.B92	T5Ø.B93	T5Ø.B94	T5Ø.B95	T5Ø.B96
Hepronicate	T46.7X1	T46.7X2	T46.7X3	T46.7X4	T46.7X5	T46.7X6
Heptabarb	T42.3X1	T42.3X2	T42.3X3	T42.3X4	T42.3X5	T42.3X6
Heptabarbital	T42.3X1	T42.3X2	T42.3X3	T42.3X4	T42.3X5	T42.3X6
Heptabarbitone	T42.3X1	T42.3X2	T42.3X3	T42.3X4	T42.3X5	T42.3X6
Heptachlor	T6Ø.1X1	T6Ø.1X2	T6Ø.1X3	T6Ø.1X4	—	—
Heptalgin	T4Ø.2X1	T4Ø.2X2	T4Ø.2X3	T4Ø.2X4	T4Ø.2X5	T4Ø.2X6
Heptaminol	T46.3X1	T46.3X2	T46.3X3	T46.3X4	T46.3X5	T46.3X6
Herbicide NEC	T6Ø.3X1	T6Ø.3X2	T6Ø.3X3	T6Ø.3X4	—	—
Heroin	T4Ø.1X1	T4Ø.1X2	T4Ø.1X3	T4Ø.1X4	—	—
Herplex	T49.5X1	T49.5X2	T49.5X3	T49.5X4	T49.5X5	T49.5X6
HES	T45.8X1	T45.8X2	T45.8X3	T45.8X4	T45.8X5	T45.8X6
Hesperidin	T46.991	T46.992	T46.993	T46.994	T46.995	T46.996
Hetacillin	T36.ØX1	T36.ØX2	T36.ØX3	T36.ØX4	T36.ØX5	T36.ØX6
Hetastarch	T45.8X1	T45.8X2	T45.8X3	T45.8X4	T45.8X5	T45.8X6
HETP	T6Ø.ØX1	T6Ø.ØX2	T6Ø.ØX3	T6Ø.ØX4	—	—
Hexachlorobenzene (vapor)	T6Ø.3X1	T6Ø.3X2	T6Ø.3X3	T6Ø.3X4	—	—
Hexachlorocyclohexane	T53.6X1	T53.6X2	T53.6X3	T53.6X4	—	—
Hexachlorophene	T49.ØX1	T49.ØX2	T49.ØX3	T49.ØX4	T49.ØX5	T49.ØX6
Hexadiline	T46.3X1	T46.3X2	T46.3X3	T46.3X4	T46.3X5	T46.3X6
Hexadimethrine (bromide)	T45.7X1	T45.7X2	T45.7X3	T45.7X4	T45.7X5	T45.7X6
Hexadylamine	T46.3X1	T46.3X2	T46.3X3	T46.3X4	T46.3X5	T46.3X6
Hexaethyl tetraphosphate	T6Ø.ØX1	T6Ø.ØX2	T6Ø.ØX3	T6Ø.ØX4	—	—
Hexafluorenium bromide	T48.1X1	T48.1X2	T48.1X3	T48.1X4	T48.1X5	T48.1X6
Hexafluronium (bromide)	T48.1X1	T48.1X2	T48.1X3	T48.1X4	T48.1X5	T48.1X6
Hexa-germ	T49.2X1	T49.2X2	T49.2X3	T49.2X4	T49.2X5	T49.2X6
Hexahydrobenzol	T52.8X1	T52.8X2	T52.8X3	T52.8X4	—	—
Hexahydrocresol(s)	T51.8X1	T51.8X2	T51.8X3	T51.8X4	—	—
arsenide	T57.ØX1	T57.ØX2	T57.ØX3	T57.ØX4	—	—
arseniurated	T57.ØX1	T57.ØX2	T57.ØX3	T57.ØX4	—	—
cyanide	T57.3X1	T57.3X2	T57.3X3	T57.3X4	—	—
gas	T59.891	T59.892	T59.893	T59.894	—	—
Fluoride (liquid)	T57.8X1	T57.8X2	T57.8X3	T57.8X4	—	—
vapor	T59.891	T59.892	T59.893	T59.894	—	—
phophorated	T6Ø.ØX1	T6Ø.ØX2	T6Ø.ØX3	T6Ø.ØX4	—	—
sulfate	T57.8X1	T57.8X2	T57.8X3	T57.8X4	—	—
sulfide (gas)	T59.6X1	T59.6X2	T59.6X3	T59.6X4	—	—
arseniurated	T57.ØX1	T57.ØX2	T57.ØX3	T57.ØX4	—	—
sulfurated	T57.8X1	T57.8X2	T57.8X3	T57.8X4	—	—
Hexahydrophenol	T51.8X1	T51.8X2	T51.8X3	T51.8X4	—	—
Hexalen	T51.8X1	T51.8X2	T51.8X3	T51.8X4	—	—
Hexamethonium bromide	T44.2X1	T44.2X2	T44.2X3	T44.2X4	T44.2X5	T44.2X6
Hexamethylene	T52.8X1	T52.8X2	T52.8X3	T52.8X4	—	—
Hexamethylmelamine	T45.1X1	T45.1X2	T45.1X3	T45.1X4	T45.1X5	T45.1X6
Hexamidine	T49.ØX1	T49.ØX2	T49.ØX3	T49.ØX4	T49.ØX5	T49.ØX6
Hexamine (mandelate)	T37.8X1	T37.8X2	T37.8X3	T37.8X4	T37.8X5	T37.8X6
Hexanone, 2-hexanone	T52.4X1	T52.4X2	T52.4X3	T52.4X4	—	—
Hexanuorenium	T48.1X1	T48.1X2	T48.1X3	T48.1X4	T48.1X5	T48.1X6
Hexapropymate	T42.6X1	T42.6X2	T42.6X3	T42.6X4	T42.6X5	T42.6X6
Hexasonium iodide	T44.3X1	T44.3X2	T44.3X3	T44.3X4	T44.3X5	T44.3X6
Hexcarbacholine bromide	T48.1X1	T48.1X2	T48.1X3	T48.1X4	T48.1X5	T48.1X6
Hexemal	T42.3X1	T42.3X2	T42.3X3	T42.3X4	T42.3X5	T42.3X6
Hexestrol	T38.5X1	T38.5X2	T38.5X3	T38.5X4	T38.5X5	T38.5X6
Hexethal (sodium)	T42.3X1	T42.3X2	T42.3X3	T42.3X4	T42.3X5	T42.3X6
Hexetidine	T37.8X1	T37.8X2	T37.8X3	T37.8X4	T37.8X5	T37.8X6
Hexobarbital	T42.3X1	T42.3X2	T42.3X3	T42.3X4	T42.3X5	T42.3X6
rectal	T41.291	T41.292	T41.293	T41.294	T41.295	T41.296
sodium	T41.1X1	T41.1X2	T41.1X3	T41.1X4	T41.1X5	T41.1X6
Hexobendine	T46.3X1	T46.3X2	T46.3X3	T46.3X4	T46.3X5	T46.3X6
Hexocyclium	T44.3X1	T44.3X2	T44.3X3	T44.3X4	T44.3X5	T44.3X6
metilsulfate	T44.3X1	T44.3X2	T44.3X3	T44.3X4	T44.3X5	T44.3X6
Hexoestrol	T38.5X1	T38.5X2	T38.5X3	T38.5X4	T38.5X5	T38.5X6
Hexone	T52.4X1	T52.4X2	T52.4X3	T52.4X4	—	—
Hexoprenaline	T48.6X1	T48.6X2	T48.6X3	T48.6X4	T48.6X5	T48.6X6
Hexylcaine	T41.3X1	T41.3X2	T41.3X3	T41.3X4	T41.3X5	T41.3X6
Hexylresorcinol	T52.2X1	T52.2X2	T52.2X3	T52.2X4	—	—

Substance	Poisoning, Accidental (unintentional)	Poisoning, Intentional Self-harm	Poisoning, Assault	Poisoning, Undetermined	Adverse Effect	Under-dosing
HGH (human growth hormone)	T38.811	T38.812	T38.813	T38.814	T38.815	T38.816
Hinkle's pills	T47.2X1	T47.2X2	T47.2X3	T47.2X4	T47.2X5	T47.2X6
Histalog	T5Ø.8X1	T5Ø.8X2	T5Ø.8X3	T5Ø.8X4	T5Ø.8X5	T5Ø.8X6
Histamine (phosphate)	T5Ø.8X1	T5Ø.8X2	T5Ø.8X3	T5Ø.8X4	T5Ø.8X5	T5Ø.8X6
Histoplasmin	T5Ø.8X1	T5Ø.8X2	T5Ø.8X3	T5Ø.8X4	T5Ø.8X5	T5Ø.8X6
Holly berries	T62.2X1	T62.2X2	T62.2X3	T62.2X4	—	—
Homatropine	T44.3X1	T44.3X2	T44.3X3	T44.3X4	T44.3X5	T44.3X6
methylbromide	T44.3X1	T44.3X2	T44.3X3	T44.3X4	T44.3X5	T44.3X6
Homochlorcyclizine	T45.ØX1	T45.ØX2	T45.ØX3	T45.ØX4	T45.ØX5	T45.ØX6
Homosalate	T49.3X1	T49.3X2	T49.3X3	T49.3X4	T49.3X5	T49.3X6
Homo-tet	T5Ø.Z11	T5Ø.Z12	T5Ø.Z13	T5Ø.Z14	T5Ø.Z15	T5Ø.Z16
Hormone	T38.8Ø1	T38.8Ø2	T38.8Ø3	T38.8Ø4	T38.8Ø5	T38.8Ø6
adrenal cortical steroids	T38.ØX1	T38.ØX2	T38.ØX3	T38.ØX4	T38.ØX5	T38.ØX6
androgenic	T38.7X1	T38.7X2	T38.7X3	T38.7X4	T38.7X5	T38.7X6
anterior pituitary NEC	T38.811	T38.812	T38.813	T38.814	T38.815	T38.816
antidiabetic agents	T38.3X1	T38.3X2	T38.3X3	T38.3X4	T38.3X5	T38.3X6
antidiuretic	T38.891	T38.892	T38.893	T38.894	T38.895	T38.896
cancer therapy	T45.1X1	T45.1X2	T45.1X3	T45.1X4	T45.1X5	T45.1X6
follicle stimulating	T38.811	T38.812	T38.813	T38.814	T38.815	T38.816
gonadotropic	T38.891	T38.892	T38.893	T38.894	T38.895	T38.896
pituitary	T38.811	T38.812	T38.813	T38.814	T38.815	T38.816
growth	T38.811	T38.812	T38.813	T38.814	T38.815	T38.816
luteinizing	T38.811	T38.812	T38.813	T38.814	T38.815	T38.816
ovarian	T38.5X1	T38.5X2	T38.5X3	T38.5X4	T38.5X5	T38.5X6
oxytocic	T48.ØX1	T48.ØX2	T48.ØX3	T48.ØX4	T48.ØX5	T48.ØX6
parathyroid (derivatives)	T5Ø.991	T5Ø.992	T5Ø.993	T5Ø.994	T5Ø.995	T5Ø.996
pituitary (posterior) NEC	T38.891	T38.892	T38.893	T38.894	T38.895	T38.896
anterior	T38.811	T38.812	T38.813	T38.814	T38.815	T38.816
specified, NEC	T38.891	T38.892	T38.893	T38.894	T38.895	T38.896
thyroid	T38.1X1	T38.1X2	T38.1X3	T38.1X4	T38.1X5	T38.1X6
Hornet (sting)	T63.451	T63.452	T63.453	T63.454	—	—
Horse anti-human lymphocytic serum	T5Ø.Z11	T5Ø.Z12	T5Ø.Z13	T5Ø.Z14	T5Ø.Z15	T5Ø.Z16
Horticulture agent NEC	T65.91	T65.92	T65.93	T65.94	—	—
with pesticide	T6Ø.91	T6Ø.92	T6Ø.93	T6Ø.94	—	—
Human						
albumin	T45.8X1	T45.8X2	T45.8X3	T45.8X4	T45.8X5	T45.8X6
growth hormone (HGH)	T38.811	T38.812	T38.813	T38.814	T38.815	T38.816
immune serum	T5Ø.Z11	T5Ø.Z12	T5Ø.Z13	T5Ø.Z14	T5Ø.Z15	T5Ø.Z16
Hyaluronidase	T45.3X1	T45.3X2	T45.3X3	T45.3X4	T45.3X5	T45.3X6
Hyazyme	T45.3X1	T45.3X2	T45.3X3	T45.3X4	T45.3X5	T45.3X6
Hycodan	T4Ø.2X1	T4Ø.2X2	T4Ø.2X3	T4Ø.2X4	T4Ø.2X5	T4Ø.2X6
Hydantoin derivative NEC	T42.ØX1	T42.ØX2	T42.ØX3	T42.ØX4	T42.ØX5	T42.ØX6
Hydeltra	T38.ØX1	T38.ØX2	T38.ØX3	T38.ØX4	T38.ØX5	T38.ØX6
Hydergine	T44.6X1	T44.6X2	T44.6X3	T44.6X4	T44.6X5	T44.6X6
Hydrabamine penicillin	T36.ØX1	T36.ØX2	T36.ØX3	T36.ØX4	T36.ØX5	T36.ØX6
Hydralazine	T46.5X1	T46.5X2	T46.5X3	T46.5X4	T46.5X5	T46.5X6
Hydrargaphen	T49.ØX1	T49.ØX2	T49.ØX3	T49.ØX4	T49.ØX5	T49.ØX6
Hydrargyri aminochloridum	T49.ØX1	T49.ØX2	T49.ØX3	T49.ØX4	T49.ØX5	T49.ØX6
Hydrastine	T48.291	T48.292	T48.293	T48.294	T48.295	T48.296
Hydrazine	T54.1X1	T54.1X2	T54.1X3	T54.1X4	—	—
monoamine oxidase inhibitors	T43.1X1	T43.1X2	T43.1X3	T43.1X4	T43.1X5	T43.1X6
Hydrazoic acid, azides	T54.2X1	T54.2X2	T54.2X3	T54.2X4	—	—
Hydriodic acid	T48.4X1	T48.4X2	T48.4X3	T48.4X4	T48.4X5	T48.4X6
Hydrocarbon gas	T59.891	T59.892	T59.893	T59.894	—	—
incomplete combustion of — *see* Carbon, monoxide, fuel, utility						
liquefied (mobile container)	T59.891	T59.892	T59.893	T59.894	—	—
piped (natural)	T59.891	T59.892	T59.893	T59.894	—	—
Hydrochloric acid (liquid)	T54.2X1	T54.2X2	T54.2X3	T54.2X4	—	—
medicinal (digestant)	T47.5X1	T47.5X2	T47.5X3	T47.5X4	T47.5X5	T47.5X6
vapor	T59.891	T59.892	T59.893	T59.894	—	—
Hydrochlorothiazide	T5Ø.2X1	T5Ø.2X2	T5Ø.2X3	T5Ø.2X4	T5Ø.2X5	T5Ø.2X6
Hydrocodone	T4Ø.2X1	T4Ø.2X2	T4Ø.2X3	T4Ø.2X4	T4Ø.2X5	T4Ø.2X6
Hydrocortisone (derivatives)	T38.ØX1	T38.ØX2	T38.ØX3	T38.ØX4	T38.ØX5	T38.ØX6
aceponate	T49.ØX1	T49.ØX2	T49.ØX3	T49.ØX4	T49.ØX5	T49.ØX6
ENT agent	T49.6X1	T49.6X2	T49.6X3	T49.6X4	T49.6X5	T49.6X6
ophthalmic preparation	T49.5X1	T49.5X2	T49.5X3	T49.5X4	T49.5X5	T49.5X6
topical NEC	T49.ØX1	T49.ØX2	T49.ØX3	T49.ØX4	T49.ØX5	T49.ØX6
Hydrocortone	T38.ØX1	T38.ØX2	T38.ØX3	T38.ØX4	T38.ØX5	T38.ØX6
ENT agent	T49.6X1	T49.6X2	T49.6X3	T49.6X4	T49.6X5	T49.6X6
ophthalmic preparation	T49.5X1	T49.5X2	T49.5X3	T49.5X4	T49.5X5	T49.5X6
topical NEC	T49.ØX1	T49.ØX2	T49.ØX3	T49.ØX4	T49.ØX5	T49.ØX6
Hydrocyanic acid (liquid)	T57.3X1	T57.3X2	T57.3X3	T57.3X4	—	—
gas	T65.ØX1	T65.ØX2	T65.ØX3	T65.ØX4	—	—
Hydroflumethiazide	T5Ø.2X1	T5Ø.2X2	T5Ø.2X3	T5Ø.2X4	T5Ø.2X5	T5Ø.2X6
Hydrofluoric acid (liquid)	T54.2X1	T54.2X2	T54.2X3	T54.2X4	—	—

Substance	Poisoning, Accidental (unintentional)	Poisoning, Intentional Self-harm	Poisoning, Assault	Poisoning, Undetermined	Adverse Effect	Under-dosing
Hydrofluoric acid — *continued*						
vapor	T59.891	T59.892	T59.893	T59.894	—	—
Hydrogen	T59.891	T59.892	T59.893	T59.894	—	—
arsenide	T57.ØX1	T57.ØX2	T57.ØX3	T57.ØX4	—	—
arseniureted	T57.ØX1	T57.ØX2	T57.ØX3	T57.ØX4	—	—
chloride	T57.8X1	T57.8X2	T57.8X3	T57.8X4	—	—
cyanide (salts)	T57.3X1	T57.3X2	T57.3X3	T57.3X4	—	—
gas	T57.3X1	T57.3X2	T57.3X3	T57.3X4	—	—
Fluoride	T59.5X1	T59.5X2	T59.5X3	T59.5X4	—	—
vapor	T59.5X1	T59.5X2	T59.5X3	T59.5X4	—	—
peroxide	T49.ØX1	T49.ØX2	T49.ØX3	T49.ØX4	T49.ØX5	T49.ØX6
phosphureted	T57.1X1	T57.1X2	T57.1X3	T57.1X4	—	—
sulfide	T59.6X1	T59.6X2	T59.6X3	T59.6X4	—	—
arseniureted	T57.ØX1	T57.ØX2	T57.ØX3	T57.ØX4	—	—
sulfureted	T59.6X1	T59.6X2	T59.6X3	T59.6X4	—	—
Hydromethylpyridine	T46.7X1	T46.7X2	T46.7X3	T46.7X4	T46.7X5	T46.7X6
Hydromorphinol	T4Ø.2X1	T4Ø.2X2	T4Ø.2X3	T4Ø.2X4	—	—
Hydromorphinone	T4Ø.2X1	T4Ø.2X2	T4Ø.2X3	T4Ø.2X4	T4Ø.2X5	T4Ø.2X6
Hydromorphone	T4Ø.2X1	T4Ø.2X2	T4Ø.2X3	T4Ø.2X4	T4Ø.2X5	T4Ø.2X6
Hydromox	T5Ø.2X1	T5Ø.2X2	T5Ø.2X3	T5Ø.2X4	T5Ø.2X5	T5Ø.2X6
Hydrophilic lotion	T49.3X1	T49.3X2	T49.3X3	T49.3X4	T49.3X5	T49.3X6
Hydroquinidine	T46.2X1	T46.2X2	T46.2X3	T46.2X4	T46.2X5	T46.2X6
Hydroquinone	T52.2X1	T52.2X2	T52.2X3	T52.2X4	—	—
vapor	T59.891	T59.892	T59.893	T59.894	—	—
Hydrosulfuric acid (gas)	T59.6X1	T59.6X2	T59.6X3	T59.6X4	—	—
Hydrotalcite	T47.1X1	T47.1X2	T47.1X3	T47.1X4	T47.1X5	T47.1X6
Hydrous wool fat	T49.3X1	T49.3X2	T49.3X3	T49.3X4	T49.3X5	T49.3X6
Hydroxide, caustic	T54.3X1	T54.3X2	T54.3X3	T54.3X4	—	—
Hydroxocobalamin	T45.8X1	T45.8X2	T45.8X3	T45.8X4	T45.8X5	T45.8X6
Hydroxyamphetamine	T49.5X1	T49.5X2	T49.5X3	T49.5X4	T49.5X5	T49.5X6
Hydroxycarbamide	T45.1X1	T45.1X2	T45.1X3	T45.1X4	T45.1X5	T45.1X6
Hydroxychloroquine	T37.8X1	T37.8X2	T37.8X3	T37.8X4	T37.8X5	T37.8X6
Hydroxydihydrocodeinone	T4Ø.2X1	T4Ø.2X2	T4Ø.2X3	T4Ø.2X4	T4Ø.2X5	T4Ø.2X6
Hydroxyestrone	T38.5X1	T38.5X2	T38.5X3	T38.5X4	T38.5X5	T38.5X6
Hydroxyethyl starch	T45.8X1	T45.8X2	T45.8X3	T45.8X4	T45.8X5	T45.8X6
Hydroxymethylpentanone	T52.4X1	T52.4X2	T52.4X3	T52.4X4	—	—
Hydroxyphenamate	T43.591	T43.592	T43.593	T43.594	T43.595	T43.596
Hydroxyphenylbutazone	T39.2X1	T39.2X2	T39.2X3	T39.2X4	T39.2X5	T39.2X6
Hydroxyprogesterone	T38.5X1	T38.5X2	T38.5X3	T38.5X4	T38.5X5	T38.5X6
caproate	T38.5X1	T38.5X2	T38.5X3	T38.5X4	T38.5X5	T38.5X6
Hydroxyquinoline (derivatives) **NEC**	T37.8X1	T37.8X2	T37.8X3	T37.8X4	T37.8X5	T37.8X6
Hydroxystilbamidine	T37.3X1	T37.3X2	T37.3X3	T37.3X4	T37.3X5	T37.3X6
Hydroxytoluene (nonmedicinal)	T54.ØX1	T54.ØX2	T54.ØX3	T54.ØX4	—	—
medicinal	T49.ØX1	T49.ØX2	T49.ØX3	T49.ØX4	T49.ØX5	T49.ØX6
Hydroxyurea	T45.1X1	T45.1X2	T45.1X3	T45.1X4	T45.1X5	T45.1X6
Hydroxyzine	T43.591	T43.592	T43.593	T43.594	T43.595	T43.596
Hyoscine	T44.3X1	T44.3X2	T44.3X3	T44.3X4	T44.3X5	T44.3X6
Hyoscyamine	T44.3X1	T44.3X2	T44.3X3	T44.3X4	T44.3X5	T44.3X6
Hyoscyamus	T44.3X1	T44.3X2	T44.3X3	T44.3X4	T44.3X5	T44.3X6
dry extract	T44.3X1	T44.3X2	T44.3X3	T44.3X4	T44.3X5	T44.3X6
Hypaque	T5Ø.8X1	T5Ø.8X2	T5Ø.8X3	T5Ø.8X4	T5Ø.8X5	T5Ø.8X6
Hypertussis	T5Ø.Z11	T5Ø.Z12	T5Ø.Z13	T5Ø.Z14	T5Ø.Z15	T5Ø.Z16
Hypnotic	T42.71	T42.72	T42.73	T42.74	T42.75	T42.76
anticonvulsant	T42.71	T42.72	T42.73	T42.74	T42.75	T42.76
specified NEC	T42.6X1	T42.6X2	T42.6X3	T42.6X4	T42.6X5	T42.6X6
Hypochlorite	T49.ØX1	T49.ØX2	T49.ØX3	T49.ØX4	T49.ØX5	T49.ØX6
Hypophysis, posterior	T38.891	T38.892	T38.893	T38.894	T38.895	T38.896
Hypotensive NEC	T46.5X1	T46.5X2	T46.5X3	T46.5X4	T46.5X5	T46.5X6
Hypromellose	T49.5X1	T49.5X2	T49.5X3	T49.5X4	T49.5X5	T49.5X6
Ibacitabine	T37.5X1	T37.5X2	T37.5X3	T37.5X4	T37.5X5	T37.5X6
Ibopamine	T44.991	T44.992	T44.993	T44.994	T44.995	T44.996
Ibufenac	T39.311	T39.312	T39.313	T39.314	T39.315	T39.316
Ibuprofen	T39.311	T39.312	T39.313	T39.314	T39.315	T39.316
Ibuproxam	T39.311	T39.312	T39.313	T39.314	T39.315	T39.316
Ibuterol	T48.6X1	T48.6X2	T48.6X3	T48.6X4	T48.6X5	T48.6X6
Ichthammol	T49.ØX1	T49.ØX2	T49.ØX3	T49.ØX4	T49.ØX5	T49.ØX6
Ichthyol	T49.4X1	T49.4X2	T49.4X3	T49.4X4	T49.4X5	T49.4X6
Idarubicin	T45.1X1	T45.1X2	T45.1X3	T45.1X4	T45.1X5	T45.1X6
Idrocilamide	T42.8X1	T42.8X2	T42.8X3	T42.8X4	T42.8X5	T42.8X6
Ifenprodil	T46.7X1	T46.7X2	T46.7X3	T46.7X4	T46.7X5	T46.7X6
Ifosfamide	T45.1X1	T45.1X2	T45.1X3	T45.1X4	T45.1X5	T45.1X6
Iletin	T38.3X1	T38.3X2	T38.3X3	T38.3X4	T38.3X5	T38.3X6
Ilex	T62.2X1	T62.2X2	T62.2X3	T62.2X4	—	—
Illuminating gas (after combustion)	T58.11	T58.12	T58.13	T58.14	—	—
prior to combustion	T59.891	T59.892	T59.893	T59.894	—	—
Ilopan	T45.2X1	T45.2X2	T45.2X3	T45.2X4	T45.2X5	T45.2X6
Iloprost	T46.7X1	T46.7X2	T46.7X3	T46.7X4	T46.7X5	T46.7X6
Ilotycin	T36.3X1	T36.3X2	T36.3X3	T36.3X4	T36.3X5	T36.3X6
ophthalmic preparation	T49.5X1	T49.5X2	T49.5X3	T49.5X4	T49.5X5	T49.5X6
topical NEC	T49.ØX1	T49.ØX2	T49.ØX3	T49.ØX4	T49.ØX5	T49.ØX6

Substance	Poisoning, Accidental (unintentional)	Poisoning, Intentional Self-harm	Poisoning, Assault	Poisoning, Undetermined	Adverse Effect	Under-dosing
Imidazole-4-carboxamide	T45.1X1	T45.1X2	T45.1X3	T45.1X4	T45.1X5	T45.1X6
Iminostilbene	T42.1X1	T42.1X2	T42.1X3	T42.1X4	T42.1X5	T42.1X6
Imipenem	T36.ØX1	T36.ØX2	T36.ØX3	T36.ØX4	T36.ØX5	T36.ØX6
Imipramine	T43.Ø11	T43.Ø12	T43.Ø13	T43.Ø14	T43.Ø15	T43.Ø16
Immu-G	T5Ø.Z11	T5Ø.Z12	T5Ø.Z13	T5Ø.Z14	T5Ø.Z15	T5Ø.Z16
Immuglobin	T5Ø.Z11	T5Ø.Z12	T5Ø.Z13	T5Ø.Z14	T5Ø.Z15	T5Ø.Z16
Immune						
globulin	T5Ø.Z11	T5Ø.Z12	T5Ø.Z13	T5Ø.Z14	T5Ø.Z15	T5Ø.Z16
serum globulin	T5Ø.Z11	T5Ø.Z12	T5Ø.Z13	T5Ø.Z14	T5Ø.Z15	T5Ø.Z16
Immunoglobin human (intravenous) (normal)	T5Ø.Z11	T5Ø.Z12	T5Ø.Z13	T5Ø.Z14	T5Ø.Z15	T5Ø.Z16
unmodified	T5Ø.Z11	T5Ø.Z12	T5Ø.Z13	T5Ø.Z14	T5Ø.Z15	T5Ø.Z16
Immunosuppressive drug	T45.1X1	T45.1X2	T45.1X3	T45.1X4	T45.1X5	T45.1X6
Immu-tetanus	T5Ø.Z11	T5Ø.Z12	T5Ø.Z13	T5Ø.Z14	T5Ø.Z15	T5Ø.Z16
Indalpine	T43.221	T43.222	T43.223	T43.224	T43.225	T43.226
Indanazoline	T48.5X1	T48.5X2	T48.5X3	T48.5X4	T48.5X5	T48.5X6
Indandione (derivatives)	T45.511	T45.512	T45.513	T45.514	T45.515	T45.516
Indapamide	T46.5X1	T46.5X2	T46.5X3	T46.5X4	T46.5X5	T46.5X6
Indendione (derivatives)	T45.511	T45.512	T45.513	T45.514	T45.515	T45.516
Indenolol	T44.7X1	T44.7X2	T44.7X3	T44.7X4	T44.7X5	T44.7X6
Inderal	T44.7X1	T44.7X2	T44.7X3	T44.7X4	T44.7X5	T44.7X6
Indian						
hemp	T4Ø.7X1	T4Ø.7X2	T4Ø.7X3	T4Ø.7X4	T4Ø.7X5	T4Ø.7X6
tobacco	T62.2X1	T62.2X2	T62.2X3	T62.2X4	—	—
Indigo carmine	T5Ø.8X1	T5Ø.8X2	T5Ø.8X3	T5Ø.8X4	T5Ø.8X5	T5Ø.8X6
Indobufen	T45.521	T45.522	T45.523	T45.524	T45.525	T45.526
Indocin	T39.2X1	T39.2X2	T39.2X3	T39.2X4	T39.2X5	T39.2X6
Indocyanine green	T5Ø.8X1	T5Ø.8X2	T5Ø.8X3	T5Ø.8X4	T5Ø.8X5	T5Ø.8X6
Indometacin	T39.391	T39.392	T39.393	T39.394	T39.395	T39.396
Indomethacin	T39.391	T39.392	T39.393	T39.394	T39.395	T39.396
farnesil	T39.4X1	T39.4X2	T39.4X3	T39.4X4	T39.4X5	T39.4X6
Indoramin	T44.6X1	T44.6X2	T44.6X3	T44.6X4	T44.6X5	T44.6X6
Industrial						
alcohol	T51.ØX1	T51.ØX2	T51.ØX3	T51.ØX4	—	—
fumes	T59.891	T59.892	T59.893	T59.894	—	—
solvents (fumes) (vapors)	T52.91	T52.92	T52.93	T52.94	—	—
Influenza vaccine	T5Ø.B91	T5Ø.B92	T5Ø.B93	T5Ø.B94	T5Ø.B95	T5Ø.B96
Ingested substance NEC	T65.91	T65.92	T65.93	T65.94	—	—
INH	T37.1X1	T37.1X2	T37.1X3	T37.1X4	T37.1X5	T37.1X6
Inhalation, gas (noxious) — *see* Gas						
Inhibitor						
angiotensin-converting enzyme	T46.4X1	T46.4X2	T46.4X3	T46.4X4	T46.4X5	T46.4X6
carbonic anhydrase	T5Ø.2X1	T5Ø.2X2	T5Ø.2X3	T5Ø.2X4	T5Ø.2X5	T5Ø.2X6
fibrinolysis	T45.621	T45.622	T45.623	T45.624	T45.625	T45.626
monoamine oxidase NEC	T43.1X1	T43.1X2	T43.1X3	T43.1X4	T43.1X5	T43.1X6
hydrazine	T43.1X1	T43.1X2	T43.1X3	T43.1X4	T43.1X5	T43.1X6
postsynaptic	T43.8X1	T43.8X2	T43.8X3	T43.8X4	T43.8X5	T43.8X6
prothrombin synthesis	T45.511	T45.512	T45.513	T45.514	T45.515	T45.516
Ink	T65.891	T65.892	T65.893	T65.894	—	—
Inorganic substance NEC	T57.91	T57.92	T57.93	T57.94	—	—
Inosine pranobex	T37.5X1	T37.5X2	T37.5X3	T37.5X4	T37.5X5	T37.5X6
Inositol	T5Ø.991	T5Ø.992	T5Ø.993	T5Ø.994	T5Ø.995	T5Ø.996
nicotinate	T46.7X1	T46.7X2	T46.7X3	T46.7X4	T46.7X5	T46.7X6
Inproquone	T45.1X1	T45.1X2	T45.1X3	T45.1X4	T45.1X5	T45.1X6
Insecticide NEC	T6Ø.91	T6Ø.92	T6Ø.93	T6Ø.94	—	—
carbamate	T6Ø.ØX1	T6Ø.ØX2	T6Ø.ØX3	T6Ø.ØX4	—	—
chlorinated	T6Ø.1X1	T6Ø.1X2	T6Ø.1X3	T6Ø.1X4	—	—
mixed	T6Ø.91	T6Ø.92	T6Ø.93	T6Ø.94	—	—
organochlorine	T6Ø.1X1	T6Ø.1X2	T6Ø.1X3	T6Ø.1X4	—	—
organophosphorus	T6Ø.ØX1	T6Ø.ØX2	T6Ø.ØX3	T6Ø.ØX4	—	—
Insect (sting), venomous	T63.481	T63.482	T63.483	T63.484	—	—
ant	T63.421	T63.422	T63.423	T63.424	—	—
bee	T63.441	T63.442	T63.443	T63.444	—	—
caterpillar	T63.431	T63.432	T63.433	T63.434	—	—
hornet	T63.451	T63.452	T63.453	T63.454	—	—
wasp	T63.461	T63.462	T63.463	T63.464	—	—
Insular tissue extract	T38.3X1	T38.3X2	T38.3X3	T38.3X4	T38.3X5	T38.3X6
Insulin (amorphous) (globin) (isophane) (Lente) (NPH) (Semilente) (Ultralente)	T38.3X1	T38.3X2	T38.3X3	T38.3X4	T38.3X5	T38.3X6
defalan	T38.3X1	T38.3X2	T38.3X3	T38.3X4	T38.3X5	T38.3X6
human	T38.3X1	T38.3X2	T38.3X3	T38.3X4	T38.3X5	T38.3X6
injection, soluble	T38.3X1	T38.3X2	T38.3X3	T38.3X4	T38.3X5	T38.3X6
biphasic	T38.3X1	T38.3X2	T38.3X3	T38.3X4	T38.3X5	T38.3X6
intermediate acting	T38.3X1	T38.3X2	T38.3X3	T38.3X4	T38.3X5	T38.3X6
protamine zinc	T38.3X1	T38.3X2	T38.3X3	T38.3X4	T38.3X5	T38.3X6
slow acting	T38.3X1	T38.3X2	T38.3X3	T38.3X4	T38.3X5	T38.3X6
zinc						
protamine injection	T38.3X1	T38.3X2	T38.3X3	T38.3X4	T38.3X5	T38.3X6
suspension (amorphous) (crystalline)	T38.3X1	T38.3X2	T38.3X3	T38.3X4	T38.3X5	T38.3X6

Substance	Poisoning, Accidental (unintentional)	Poisoning, Intentional Self-harm	Poisoning, Assault	Poisoning, Undetermined	Adverse Effect	Under-dosing
Interferon (alpha) (beta) (gamma)	T37.5X1	T37.5X2	T37.5X3	T37.5X4	T37.5X5	T37.5X6
Intestinal motility control drug	T47.6X1	T47.6X2	T47.6X3	T47.6X4	T47.6X5	T47.6X6
biological	T47.8X1	T47.8X2	T47.8X3	T47.8X4	T47.8X5	T47.8X6
Intranarcon	T41.1X1	T41.1X2	T41.1X3	T41.1X4	T41.1X5	T41.1X6
Intravenous						
amino acids	T5Ø.991	T5Ø.992	T5Ø.993	T5Ø.994	T5Ø.995	T5Ø.996
fat suspension	T5Ø.991	T5Ø.992	T5Ø.993	T5Ø.994	T5Ø.995	T5Ø.996
Inulin	T5Ø.8X1	T5Ø.8X2	T5Ø.8X3	T5Ø.8X4	T5Ø.8X5	T5Ø.8X6
Invert sugar	T5Ø.3X1	T5Ø.3X2	T5Ø.3X3	T5Ø.3X4	T5Ø.3X5	T5Ø.3X6
Inza — *see* Naproxen						
Iobenzamic acid	T5Ø.8X1	T5Ø.8X2	T5Ø.8X3	T5Ø.8X4	T5Ø.8X5	T5Ø.8X6
Iocarmic acid	T5Ø.8X1	T5Ø.8X2	T5Ø.8X3	T5Ø.8X4	T5Ø.8X5	T5Ø.8X6
Iocetamic acid	T5Ø.8X1	T5Ø.8X2	T5Ø.8X3	T5Ø.8X4	T5Ø.8X5	T5Ø.8X6
Iodamide	T5Ø.8X1	T5Ø.8X2	T5Ø.8X3	T5Ø.8X4	T5Ø.8X5	T5Ø.8X6
Iodide NEC — *see also* Iodine	T49.ØX1	T49.ØX2	T49.ØX3	T49.ØX4	T49.ØX5	T49.ØX6
mercury (ointment)	T49.ØX1	T49.ØX2	T49.ØX3	T49.ØX4	T49.ØX5	T49.ØX6
methylate	T49.ØX1	T49.ØX2	T49.ØX3	T49.ØX4	T49.ØX5	T49.ØX6
potassium (expectorant) NEC	T48.4X1	T48.4X2	T48.4X3	T48.4X4	T48.4X5	T48.4X6
Iodinated						
contrast medium	T5Ø.8X1	T5Ø.8X2	T5Ø.8X3	T5Ø.8X4	T5Ø.8X5	T5Ø.8X6
glycerol	T48.4X1	T48.4X2	T48.4X3	T48.4X4	T48.4X5	T48.4X6
human serum albumin (131I)	T5Ø.8X1	T5Ø.8X2	T5Ø.8X3	T5Ø.8X4	T5Ø.8X5	T5Ø.8X6
Iodine (antiseptic, external) (tincture) **NEC**	T49.ØX1	T49.ØX2	T49.ØX3	T49.ØX4	T49.ØX5	T49.ØX6
125 — *see also* Radiation sickness, and Exposure to radioactivce isotopes	T5Ø.8X1	T5Ø.8X2	T5Ø.8X3	T5Ø.8X4	T5Ø.8X5	T5Ø.8X6
therapeutic	T5Ø.991	T5Ø.992	T5Ø.993	T5Ø.994	T5Ø.995	T5Ø.996
131 — *see also* Radiation sickness, and Exposure to radioactivce isotopes	T5Ø.8X1	T5Ø.8X2	T5Ø.8X3	T5Ø.8X4	T5Ø.8X5	T5Ø.8X6
therapeutic	T38.2X1	T38.2X2	T38.2X3	T38.2X4	T38.2X5	T38.2X6
diagnostic	T5Ø.8X1	T5Ø.8X2	T5Ø.8X3	T5Ø.8X4	T5Ø.8X5	T5Ø.8X6
for thyroid conditions (antithyroid)	T38.2X1	T38.2X2	T38.2X3	T38.2X4	T38.2X5	T38.2X6
solution	T49.ØX1	T49.ØX2	T49.ØX3	T49.ØX4	T49.ØX5	T49.ØX6
vapor	T59.891	T59.892	T59.893	T59.894	—	—
Iodipamide	T5Ø.8X1	T5Ø.8X2	T5Ø.8X3	T5Ø.8X4	T5Ø.8X5	T5Ø.8X6
Iodized (poppy seed) oil	T5Ø.8X1	T5Ø.8X2	T5Ø.8X3	T5Ø.8X4	T5Ø.8X5	T5Ø.8X6
Iodobismitol	T37.8X1	T37.8X2	T37.8X3	T37.8X4	T37.8X5	T37.8X6
Iodochlorhydroxyquin	T37.8X1	T37.8X2	T37.8X3	T37.8X4	T37.8X5	T37.8X6
topical	T49.ØX1	T49.ØX2	T49.ØX3	T49.ØX4	T49.ØX5	T49.ØX6
Iodochlorhydroxyquinoline	T37.8X1	T37.8X2	T37.8X3	T37.8X4	T37.8X5	T37.8X6
Iodocholesterol (131I)	T5Ø.8X1	T5Ø.8X2	T5Ø.8X3	T5Ø.8X4	T5Ø.8X5	T5Ø.8X6
Iodoform	T49.ØX1	T49.ØX2	T49.ØX3	T49.ØX4	T49.ØX5	T49.ØX6
Iodohippuric acid	T5Ø.8X1	T5Ø.8X2	T5Ø.8X3	T5Ø.8X4	T5Ø.8X5	T5Ø.8X6
Iodopanoic acid	T5Ø.8X1	T5Ø.8X2	T5Ø.8X3	T5Ø.8X4	T5Ø.8X5	T5Ø.8X6
Iodophthalein (sodium)	T5Ø.8X1	T5Ø.8X2	T5Ø.8X3	T5Ø.8X4	T5Ø.8X5	T5Ø.8X6
Iodopyracet	T5Ø.8X1	T5Ø.8X2	T5Ø.8X3	T5Ø.8X4	T5Ø.8X5	T5Ø.8X6
Iodoquinol	T37.8X1	T37.8X2	T37.8X3	T37.8X4	T37.8X5	T37.8X6
Iodoxamic acid	T5Ø.8X1	T5Ø.8X2	T5Ø.8X3	T5Ø.8X4	T5Ø.8X5	T5Ø.8X6
Iofendylate	T5Ø.8X1	T5Ø.8X2	T5Ø.8X3	T5Ø.8X4	T5Ø.8X5	T5Ø.8X6
Ioglycamic acid	T5Ø.8X1	T5Ø.8X2	T5Ø.8X3	T5Ø.8X4	T5Ø.8X5	T5Ø.8X6
Iohexol	T5Ø.8X1	T5Ø.8X2	T5Ø.8X3	T5Ø.8X4	T5Ø.8X5	T5Ø.8X6
Ion exchange resin						
anion	T47.8X1	T47.8X2	T47.8X3	T47.8X4	T47.8X5	T47.8X6
cation	T5Ø.3X1	T5Ø.3X2	T5Ø.3X3	T5Ø.3X4	T5Ø.3X5	T5Ø.3X6
cholestyramine	T46.6X1	T46.6X2	T46.6X3	T46.6X4	T46.6X5	T46.6X6
intestinal	T47.8X1	T47.8X2	T47.8X3	T47.8X4	T47.8X5	T47.8X6
Iopamidol	T5Ø.8X1	T5Ø.8X2	T5Ø.8X3	T5Ø.8X4	T5Ø.8X5	T5Ø.8X6
Iopanoic acid	T5Ø.8X1	T5Ø.8X2	T5Ø.8X3	T5Ø.8X4	T5Ø.8X5	T5Ø.8X6
Iophenoic acid	T5Ø.8X1	T5Ø.8X2	T5Ø.8X3	T5Ø.8X4	T5Ø.8X5	T5Ø.8X6
Iopodate, sodium	T5Ø.8X1	T5Ø.8X2	T5Ø.8X3	T5Ø.8X4	T5Ø.8X5	T5Ø.8X6
Iopodic acid	T5Ø.8X1	T5Ø.8X2	T5Ø.8X3	T5Ø.8X4	T5Ø.8X5	T5Ø.8X6
Iopromide	T5Ø.8X1	T5Ø.8X2	T5Ø.8X3	T5Ø.8X4	T5Ø.8X5	T5Ø.8X6
Iopydol	T5Ø.8X1	T5Ø.8X2	T5Ø.8X3	T5Ø.8X4	T5Ø.8X5	T5Ø.8X6
Iotalamic acid	T5Ø.8X1	T5Ø.8X2	T5Ø.8X3	T5Ø.8X4	T5Ø.8X5	T5Ø.8X6
Iothalamate	T5Ø.8X1	T5Ø.8X2	T5Ø.8X3	T5Ø.8X4	T5Ø.8X5	T5Ø.8X6
Iothiouracil	T38.2X1	T38.2X2	T38.2X3	T38.2X4	T38.2X5	T38.2X6
Iotrol	T5Ø.8X1	T5Ø.8X2	T5Ø.8X3	T5Ø.8X4	T5Ø.8X5	T5Ø.8X6
Iotrolan	T5Ø.8X1	T5Ø.8X2	T5Ø.8X3	T5Ø.8X4	T5Ø.8X5	T5Ø.8X6
Iotroxate	T5Ø.8X1	T5Ø.8X2	T5Ø.8X3	T5Ø.8X4	T5Ø.8X5	T5Ø.8X6
Iotroxic acid	T5Ø.8X1	T5Ø.8X2	T5Ø.8X3	T5Ø.8X4	T5Ø.8X5	T5Ø.8X6
Ioversol	T5Ø.8X1	T5Ø.8X2	T5Ø.8X3	T5Ø.8X4	T5Ø.8X5	T5Ø.8X6
Ioxaglate	T5Ø.8X1	T5Ø.8X2	T5Ø.8X3	T5Ø.8X4	T5Ø.8X5	T5Ø.8X6
Ioxaglic acid	T5Ø.8X1	T5Ø.8X2	T5Ø.8X3	T5Ø.8X4	T5Ø.8X5	T5Ø.8X6
Ioxitalamic acid	T5Ø.8X1	T5Ø.8X2	T5Ø.8X3	T5Ø.8X4	T5Ø.8X5	T5Ø.8X6
Ipecac	T47.7X1	T47.7X2	T47.7X3	T47.7X4	T47.7X5	T47.7X6

Substance	Poisoning, Accidental (unintentional)	Poisoning, Intentional Self-harm	Poisoning, Assault	Poisoning, Undetermined	Adverse Effect	Under-dosing
Ipecacuanha	T48.4X1	T48.4X2	T48.4X3	T48.4X4	T48.4X5	T48.4X6
Ipodate, calcium	T5Ø.8X1	T5Ø.8X2	T5Ø.8X3	T5Ø.8X4	T5Ø.8X5	T5Ø.8X6
Ipral	T42.3X1	T42.3X2	T42.3X3	T42.3X4	T42.3X5	T42.3X6
Ipratropium (bromide)	T48.6X1	T48.6X2	T48.6X3	T48.6X4	T48.6X5	T48.6X6
Ipriflavone	T46.3X1	T46.3X2	T46.3X3	T46.3X4	T46.3X5	T46.3X6
Iprindole	T43.Ø11	T43.Ø12	T43.Ø13	T43.Ø14	T43.Ø15	T43.Ø16
Iproclozide	T43.1X1	T43.1X2	T43.1X3	T43.1X4	T43.1X5	T43.1X6
Iprofenin	T5Ø.8X1	T5Ø.8X2	T5Ø.8X3	T5Ø.8X4	T5Ø.8X5	T5Ø.8X6
Iproheptine	T49.2X1	T49.2X2	T49.2X3	T49.2X4	T49.2X5	T49.2X6
Iproniazid	T43.1X1	T43.1X2	T43.1X3	T43.1X4	T43.1X5	T43.1X6
Iproplatin	T45.1X1	T45.1X2	T45.1X3	T45.1X4	T45.1X5	T45.1X6
Iproveratril	T46.1X1	T46.1X2	T46.1X3	T46.1X4	T46.1X5	T46.1X6
Iron (compounds) (medicinal) **NEC**	T45.4X1	T45.4X2	T45.4X3	T45.4X4	T45.4X5	T45.4X6
ammonium	T45.4X1	T45.4X2	T45.4X3	T45.4X4	T45.4X5	T45.4X6
dextran injection	T45.4X1	T45.4X2	T45.4X3	T45.4X4	T45.4X5	T45.4X6
nonmedicinal	T56.891	T56.892	T56.893	T56.894	—	—
salts	T45.4X1	T45.4X2	T45.4X3	T45.4X4	T45.4X5	T45.4X6
sorbitex	T45.4X1	T45.4X2	T45.4X3	T45.4X4	T45.4X5	T45.4X6
sorbitol citric acid complex	T45.4X1	T45.4X2	T45.4X3	T45.4X4	T45.4X5	T45.4X6
Irrigating fluid (vaginal)	T49.8X1	T49.8X2	T49.8X3	T49.8X4	T49.8X5	T49.8X6
eye	T49.5X1	T49.5X2	T49.5X3	T49.5X4	T49.5X5	T49.5X6
Isepamicin	T36.5X1	T36.5X2	T36.5X3	T36.5X4	T36.5X5	T36.5X6
Isoaminile (citrate)	T48.3X1	T48.3X2	T48.3X3	T48.3X4	T48.3X5	T48.3X6
Isoamyl nitrite	T46.3X1	T46.3X2	T46.3X3	T46.3X4	T46.3X5	T46.3X6
Isobenzan	T6Ø.1X1	T6Ø.1X2	T6Ø.1X3	T6Ø.1X4	—	—
Isobutyl acetate	T52.8X1	T52.8X2	T52.8X3	T52.8X4	—	—
Isocarboxazid	T43.1X1	T43.1X2	T43.1X3	T43.1X4	T43.1X5	T43.1X6
Isoconazole	T49.ØX1	T49.ØX2	T49.ØX3	T49.ØX4	T49.ØX5	T49.ØX6
Isocyanate	T65.ØX1	T65.ØX2	T65.ØX3	T65.ØX4	—	—
Isoephedrine	T44.991	T44.992	T44.993	T44.994	T44.995	T44.996
Isoetarine	T48.6X1	T48.6X2	T48.6X3	T48.6X4	T48.6X5	T48.6X6
Isoethadione	T42.2X1	T42.2X2	T42.2X3	T42.2X4	T42.2X5	T42.2X6
Isoetharine	T44.5X1	T44.5X2	T44.5X3	T44.5X4	T44.5X5	T44.5X6
Isoflurane	T41.ØX1	T41.ØX2	T41.ØX3	T41.ØX4	T41.ØX5	T41.ØX6
Isoflurophate	T44.ØX1	T44.ØX2	T44.ØX3	T44.ØX4	T44.ØX5	T44.ØX6
Isomaltose, ferric complex	T45.4X1	T45.4X2	T45.4X3	T45.4X4	T45.4X5	T45.4X6
Isometheptene	T44.3X1	T44.3X2	T44.3X3	T44.3X4	T44.3X5	T44.3X6
Isoniazid	T37.1X1	T37.1X2	T37.1X3	T37.1X4	T37.1X5	T37.1X6
with						
rifampicin	T36.6X1	T36.6X2	T36.6X3	T36.6X4	T36.6X5	T36.6X6
thioacetazone	T37.1X1	T37.1X2	T37.1X3	T37.1X4	T37.1X5	T37.1X6
Isonicotinic acid hydrazide	T37.1X1	T37.1X2	T37.1X3	T37.1X4	T37.1X5	T37.1X6
Isonipecaine	T4Ø.491	T4Ø.492	T4Ø.493	T4Ø.494	T4Ø.495	T4Ø.496
Isopentaquine	T37.2X1	T37.2X2	T37.2X3	T37.2X4	T37.2X5	T37.2X6
Isophane insulin	T38.3X1	T38.3X2	T38.3X3	T38.3X4	T38.3X5	T38.3X6
Isophorone	T65.891	T65.892	T65.893	T65.894	—	—
Isophosphamide	T45.1X1	T45.1X2	T45.1X3	T45.1X4	T45.1X5	T45.1X6
Isopregnenone	T38.5X1	T38.5X2	T38.5X3	T38.5X4	T38.5X5	T38.5X6
Isoprenaline	T48.6X1	T48.6X2	T48.6X3	T48.6X4	T48.6X5	T48.6X6
Isopromethazine	T43.3X1	T43.3X2	T43.3X3	T43.3X4	T43.3X5	T43.3X6
Isopropamide	T44.3X1	T44.3X2	T44.3X3	T44.3X4	T44.3X5	T44.3X6
iodide	T44.3X1	T44.3X2	T44.3X3	T44.3X4	T44.3X5	T44.3X6
Isopropanol	T51.2X1	T51.2X2	T51.2X3	T51.2X4	—	—
Isopropyl						
acetate	T52.8X1	T52.8X2	T52.8X3	T52.8X4	—	—
alcohol	T51.2X1	T51.2X2	T51.2X3	T51.2X4	—	—
medicinal	T49.4X1	T49.4X2	T49.4X3	T49.4X4	T49.4X5	T49.4X6
ether	T52.8X1	T52.8X2	T52.8X3	T52.8X4	—	—
Isopropylaminophenazone	T39.2X1	T39.2X2	T39.2X3	T39.2X4	T39.2X5	T39.2X6
Isoproterenol	T48.6X1	T48.6X2	T48.6X3	T48.6X4	T48.6X5	T48.6X6
Isosorbide dinitrate	T46.3X1	T46.3X2	T46.3X3	T46.3X4	T46.3X5	T46.3X6
Isothipendyl	T45.ØX1	T45.ØX2	T45.ØX3	T45.ØX4	T45.ØX5	T45.ØX6
Isotretinoin	T5Ø.991	T5Ø.992	T5Ø.993	T5Ø.994	T5Ø.995	T5Ø.996
Isoxazolyl penicillin	T36.ØX1	T36.ØX2	T36.ØX3	T36.ØX4	T36.ØX5	T36.ØX6
Isoxicam	T39.391	T39.392	T39.393	T39.394	T39.395	T39.396
Isoxsuprine	T46.7X1	T46.7X2	T46.7X3	T46.7X4	T46.7X5	T46.7X6
Ispagula	T47.4X1	T47.4X2	T47.4X3	T47.4X4	T47.4X5	T47.4X6
husk	T47.4X1	T47.4X2	T47.4X3	T47.4X4	T47.4X5	T47.4X6
Isradipine	T46.1X1	T46.1X2	T46.1X3	T46.1X4	T46.1X5	T46.1X6
I-thyroxine sodium	T38.1X1	T38.1X2	T38.1X3	T38.1X4	T38.1X5	T38.1X6
Itraconazole	T37.8X1	T37.8X2	T37.8X3	T37.8X4	T37.8X5	T37.8X6
Itramin tosilate	T46.3X1	T46.3X2	T46.3X3	T46.3X4	T46.3X5	T46.3X6
Ivermectin	T37.4X1	T37.4X2	T37.4X3	T37.4X4	T37.4X5	T37.4X6
Izoniazid	T37.1X1	T37.1X2	T37.1X3	T37.1X4	T37.1X5	T37.1X6
with thioacetazone	T37.1X1	T37.1X2	T37.1X3	T37.1X4	T37.1X5	T37.1X6
Jalap	T47.2X1	T47.2X2	T47.2X3	T47.2X4	T47.2X5	T47.2X6
Jamaica						
dogwood (bark)	T39.8X1	T39.8X2	T39.8X3	T39.8X4	T39.8X5	T39.8X6
ginger	T65.891	T65.892	T65.893	T65.894	—	—
root	T62.2X1	T62.2X2	T62.2X3	T62.2X4	—	—
Jatropha	T62.2X1	T62.2X2	T62.2X3	T62.2X4	—	—
curcas	T62.2X1	T62.2X2	T62.2X3	T62.2X4	—	—

Substance	Poisoning, Accidental (unintentional)	Poisoning, Intentional Self-harm	Poisoning, Assault	Poisoning, Undetermined	Adverse Effect	Under-dosing
Jectofer	T45.4X1	T45.4X2	T45.4X3	T45.4X4	T45.4X5	T45.4X6
Jellyfish (sting)	T63.621	T63.622	T63.623	T63.624	—	—
Jequirity (bean)	T62.2X1	T62.2X2	T62.2X3	T62.2X4	—	—
Jimson weed (stramonium)	T62.2X1	T62.2X2	T62.2X3	T62.2X4	—	—
seeds	T62.2X1	T62.2X2	T62.2X3	T62.2X4	—	—
Josamycin	T36.3X1	T36.3X2	T36.3X3	T36.3X4	T36.3X5	T36.3X6
Juniper tar	T49.1X1	T49.1X2	T49.1X3	T49.1X4	T49.1X5	T49.1X6
Kallidinogenase	T46.7X1	T46.7X2	T46.7X3	T46.7X4	T46.7X5	T46.7X6
Kallikrein	T46.7X1	T46.7X2	T46.7X3	T46.7X4	T46.7X5	T46.7X6
Kanamycin	T36.5X1	T36.5X2	T36.5X3	T36.5X4	T36.5X5	T36.5X6
Kantrex	T36.5X1	T36.5X2	T36.5X3	T36.5X4	T36.5X5	T36.5X6
Kaolin	T47.6X1	T47.6X2	T47.6X3	T47.6X4	T47.6X5	T47.6X6
light	T47.6X1	T47.6X2	T47.6X3	T47.6X4	T47.6X5	T47.6X6
Karaya (gum)	T47.4X1	T47.4X2	T47.4X3	T47.4X4	T47.4X5	T47.4X6
Kebuzone	T39.2X1	T39.2X2	T39.2X3	T39.2X4	T39.2X5	T39.2X6
Kelevan	T6Ø.1X1	T6Ø.1X2	T6Ø.1X3	T6Ø.1X4	—	—
Kemithal	T41.1X1	T41.1X2	T41.1X3	T41.1X4	T41.1X5	T41.1X6
Kenacort	T38.ØX1	T38.ØX2	T38.ØX3	T38.ØX4	T38.ØX5	T38.ØX6
Keratolytic drug NEC	T49.4X1	T49.4X2	T49.4X3	T49.4X4	T49.4X5	T49.4X6
anthracene	T49.4X1	T49.4X2	T49.4X3	T49.4X4	T49.4X5	T49.4X6
Keratoplastic NEC	T49.4X1	T49.4X2	T49.4X3	T49.4X4	T49.4X5	T49.4X6
Kerosene, kerosine (fuel) (solvent) **NEC**	T52.ØX1	T52.ØX2	T52.ØX3	T52.ØX4	—	—
insecticide	T52.ØX1	T52.ØX2	T52.ØX3	T52.ØX4	—	—
vapor	T52.ØX1	T52.ØX2	T52.ØX3	T52.ØX4	—	—
Ketamine	T41.291	T41.292	T41.293	T41.294	T41.295	T41.296
Ketazolam	T42.4X1	T42.4X2	T42.4X3	T42.4X4	T42.4X5	T42.4X6
Ketazon	T39.2X1	T39.2X2	T39.2X3	T39.2X4	T39.2X5	T39.2X6
Ketobemidone	T4Ø.491	T4Ø.492	T4Ø.493	T4Ø.494	—	—
Ketoconazole	T49.ØX1	T49.ØX2	T49.ØX3	T49.ØX4	T49.ØX5	T49.ØX6
Ketols	T52.4X1	T52.4X2	T52.4X3	T52.4X4	—	—
Ketone oils	T52.4X1	T52.4X2	T52.4X3	T52.4X4	—	—
Ketoprofen	T39.311	T39.312	T39.313	T39.314	T39.315	T39.316
Ketorolac	T39.8X1	T39.8X2	T39.8X3	T39.8X4	T39.8X5	T39.8X6
Ketotifen	T45.ØX1	T45.ØX2	T45.ØX3	T45.ØX4	T45.ØX5	T45.ØX6
Khat	T43.691	T43.692	T43.693	T43.694	—	—
Khellin	T46.3X1	T46.3X2	T46.3X3	T46.3X4	T46.3X5	T46.3X6
Khelloside	T46.3X1	T46.3X2	T46.3X3	T46.3X4	T46.3X5	T46.3X6
Kiln gas or vapor (carbon monoxide)	T58.8X1	T58.8X2	T58.8X3	T58.8X4	—	—
Kitasamycin	T36.3X1	T36.3X2	T36.3X3	T36.3X4	T36.3X5	T36.3X6
Konsyl	T47.4X1	T47.4X2	T47.4X3	T47.4X4	T47.4X5	T47.4X6
Kosam seed	T62.2X1	T62.2X2	T62.2X3	T62.2X4	—	—
Krait (venom)	T63.Ø91	T63.Ø92	T63.Ø93	T63.Ø94	—	—
Kwell (insecticide)	T6Ø.1X1	T6Ø.1X2	T6Ø.1X3	T6Ø.1X4	—	—
anti-infective (topical)	T49.ØX1	T49.ØX2	T49.ØX3	T49.ØX4	T49.ØX5	T49.ØX6
Labetalol	T44.8X1	T44.8X2	T44.8X3	T44.8X4	T44.8X5	T44.8X6
Laburnum (seeds)	T62.2X1	T62.2X2	T62.2X3	T62.2X4	—	—
leaves	T62.2X1	T62.2X2	T62.2X3	T62.2X4	—	—
Lachesine	T49.5X1	T49.5X2	T49.5X3	T49.5X4	T49.5X5	T49.5X6
Lacidipine	T46.5X1	T46.5X2	T46.5X3	T46.5X4	T46.5X5	T46.5X6
Lacquer	T65.6X1	T65.6X2	T65.6X3	T65.6X4	—	—
Lacrimogenic gas	T59.3X1	T59.3X2	T59.3X3	T59.3X4	—	—
Lactated potassic saline	T5Ø.3X1	T5Ø.3X2	T5Ø.3X3	T5Ø.3X4	T5Ø.3X5	T5Ø.3X6
Lactic acid	T49.8X1	T49.8X2	T49.8X3	T49.8X4	T49.8X5	T49.8X6
Lactobacillus						
acidophilus	T47.6X1	T47.6X2	T47.6X3	T47.6X4	T47.6X5	T47.6X6
compound	T47.6X1	T47.6X2	T47.6X3	T47.6X4	T47.6X5	T47.6X6
bifidus, lyophilized	T47.6X1	T47.6X2	T47.6X3	T47.6X4	T47.6X5	T47.6X6
bulgaricus	T47.6X1	T47.6X2	T47.6X3	T47.6X4	T47.6X5	T47.6X6
sporogenes	T47.6X1	T47.6X2	T47.6X3	T47.6X4	T47.6X5	T47.6X6
Lactoflavin	T45.2X1	T45.2X2	T45.2X3	T45.2X4	T45.2X5	T45.2X6
Lactose (as excipient)	T5Ø.9Ø1	T5Ø.9Ø2	T5Ø.9Ø3	T5Ø.9Ø4	T5Ø.9Ø5	T5Ø.9Ø6
Lactuca (virosa) (extract)	T42.6X1	T42.6X2	T42.6X3	T42.6X4	T42.6X5	T42.6X6
Lactucarium	T42.6X1	T42.6X2	T42.6X3	T42.6X4	T42.6X5	T42.6X6
Lactulose	T47.3X1	T47.3X2	T47.3X3	T47.3X4	T47.3X5	T47.3X6
Laevo — *see* Levo-						
Lanatosides	T46.ØX1	T46.ØX2	T46.ØX3	T46.ØX4	T46.ØX5	T46.ØX6
Lanolin	T49.3X1	T49.3X2	T49.3X3	T49.3X4	T49.3X5	T49.3X6
Largactil	T43.3X1	T43.3X2	T43.3X3	T43.3X4	T43.3X5	T43.3X6
Larkspur	T62.2X1	T62.2X2	T62.2X3	T62.2X4	—	—
Laroxyl	T43.Ø11	T43.Ø12	T43.Ø13	T43.Ø14	T43.Ø15	T43.Ø16
Lasix	T5Ø.1X1	T5Ø.1X2	T5Ø.1X3	T5Ø.1X4	T5Ø.1X5	T5Ø.1X6
Lassar's paste	T49.4X1	T49.4X2	T49.4X3	T49.4X4	T49.4X5	T49.4X6
Latamoxef	T36.1X1	T36.1X2	T36.1X3	T36.1X4	T36.1X5	T36.1X6
Latex	T65.811	T65.812	T65.813	T65.814	—	—
Lathyrus (seed)	T62.2X1	T62.2X2	T62.2X3	T62.2X4	—	—
Laudanum	T4Ø.ØX1	T4Ø.ØX2	T4Ø.ØX3	T4Ø.ØX4	T4Ø.ØX5	T4Ø.ØX6
Laudexium	T48.1X1	T48.1X2	T48.1X3	T48.1X4	T48.1X5	T48.1X6
Laughing gas	T41.ØX1	T41.ØX2	T41.ØX3	T41.ØX4	T41.ØX5	T41.ØX6
Laurel, black or cherry	T62.2X1	T62.2X2	T62.2X3	T62.2X4	—	—
Laurolinium	T49.ØX1	T49.ØX2	T49.ØX3	T49.ØX4	T49.ØX5	T49.ØX6
Lauryl sulfoacetate	T49.2X1	T49.2X2	T49.2X3	T49.2X4	T49.2X5	T49.2X6

Substance	Poisoning, Accidental (unintentional)	Poisoning, Intentional Self-harm	Poisoning, Assault	Poisoning, Undetermined	Adverse Effect	Under-dosing
Laxative NEC	T47.4X1	T47.4X2	T47.4X3	T47.4X4	T47.4X5	T47.4X6
osmotic	T47.3X1	T47.3X2	T47.3X3	T47.3X4	T47.3X5	T47.3X6
saline	T47.3X1	T47.3X2	T47.3X3	T47.3X4	T47.3X5	T47.3X6
stimulant	T47.2X1	T47.2X2	T47.2X3	T47.2X4	T47.2X5	T47.2X6
L-dopa	T42.8X1	T42.8X2	T42.8X3	T42.8X4	T42.8X5	T42.8X6
Lead (dust) (fumes) (vapor) **NEC**	T56.ØX1	T56.ØX2	T56.ØX3	T56.ØX4	—	—
acetate	T49.2X1	T49.2X2	T49.2X3	T49.2X4	T49.2X5	T49.2X6
alkyl (fuel additive)	T56.ØX1	T56.ØX2	T56.ØX3	T56.ØX4	—	—
anti-infectives	T37.8X1	T37.8X2	T37.8X3	T37.8X4	T37.8X5	T37.8X6
antiknock compound (tetraethyl)	T56.ØX1	T56.ØX2	T56.ØX3	T56.ØX4	—	—
arsenate, arsenite (dust)(herbicide) (insecticide) (vapor)	T57.ØX1	T57.ØX2	T57.ØX3	T57.ØX4	—	—
carbonate	T56.ØX1	T56.ØX2	T56.ØX3	T56.ØX4	—	—
paint	T56.ØX1	T56.ØX2	T56.ØX3	T56.ØX4	—	—
chromate	T56.ØX1	T56.ØX2	T56.ØX3	T56.ØX4	—	—
paint	T56.ØX1	T56.ØX2	T56.ØX3	T56.ØX4	—	—
dioxide	T56.ØX1	T56.ØX2	T56.ØX3	T56.ØX4	—	—
inorganic	T56.ØX1	T56.ØX2	T56.ØX3	T56.ØX4	—	—
iodide	T56.ØX1	T56.ØX2	T56.ØX3	T56.ØX4	—	—
pigment (paint)	T56.ØX1	T56.ØX2	T56.ØX3	T56.ØX4	—	—
monoxide (dust)	T56.ØX1	T56.ØX2	T56.ØX3	T56.ØX4	—	—
paint	T56.ØX1	T56.ØX2	T56.ØX3	T56.ØX4	—	—
organic	T56.ØX1	T56.ØX2	T56.ØX3	T56.ØX4	—	—
oxide	T56.ØX1	T56.ØX2	T56.ØX3	T56.ØX4	—	—
paint	T56.ØX1	T56.ØX2	T56.ØX3	T56.ØX4	—	—
paint	T56.ØX1	T56.ØX2	T56.ØX3	T56.ØX4	—	—
salts	T56.ØX1	T56.ØX2	T56.ØX3	T56.ØX4	—	—
specified compound NEC	T56.ØX1	T56.ØX2	T56.ØX3	T56.ØX4	—	—
tetra-ethyl	T56.ØX1	T56.ØX2	T56.ØX3	T56.ØX4	—	—
Lebanese red	T4Ø.7X1	T4Ø.7X2	T4Ø.7X3	T4Ø.7X4	T4Ø.7X5	T4Ø.7X6
Lefetamine	T39.8X1	T39.8X2	T39.8X3	T39.8X4	T39.8X5	T39.8X6
Lenperone	T43.4X1	T43.4X2	T43.4X3	T43.4X4	T43.4X5	T43.4X6
Lente lietin (insulin)	T38.3X1	T38.3X2	T38.3X3	T38.3X4	T38.3X5	T38.3X6
Leptazol	T5Ø.7X1	T5Ø.7X2	T5Ø.7X3	T5Ø.7X4	T5Ø.7X5	T5Ø.7X6
Leptophos	T6Ø.ØX1	T6Ø.ØX2	T6Ø.ØX3	T6Ø.ØX4	—	—
Leritine	T4Ø.2X1	T4Ø.2X2	T4Ø.2X3	T4Ø.2X4	T4Ø.2X5	T4Ø.2X6
Letosteine	T48.4X1	T48.4X2	T48.4X3	T48.4X4	T48.4X5	T48.4X6
Letter	T38.1X1	T38.1X2	T38.1X3	T38.1X4	T38.1X5	T38.1X6
Lettuce opium	T42.6X1	T42.6X2	T42.6X3	T42.6X4	T42.6X5	T42.6X6
Leucinocaine	T41.3X1	T41.3X2	T41.3X3	T41.3X4	T41.3X5	T41.3X6
Leucocianidol	T46.991	T46.992	T46.993	T46.994	T46.995	T46.996
Leucovorin (factor)	T45.8X1	T45.8X2	T45.8X3	T45.8X4	T45.8X5	T45.8X6
Leukeran	T45.1X1	T45.1X2	T45.1X3	T45.1X4	T45.1X5	T45.1X6
Leuprolide	T38.891	T38.892	T38.893	T38.894	T38.895	T38.896
Levalbuterol	T48.6X1	T48.6X2	T48.6X3	T48.6X4	T48.6X5	T48.6X6
Levallorphan	T5Ø.7X1	T5Ø.7X2	T5Ø.7X3	T5Ø.7X4	T5Ø.7X5	T5Ø.7X6
Levamisole	T37.4X1	T37.4X2	T37.4X3	T37.4X4	T37.4X5	T37.4X6
Levanil	T42.6X1	T42.6X2	T42.6X3	T42.6X4	T42.6X5	T42.6X6
Levarterenol	T44.4X1	T44.4X2	T44.4X3	T44.4X4	T44.4X5	T44.4X6
Levdropropizine	T48.3X1	T48.3X2	T48.3X3	T48.3X4	T48.3X5	T48.3X6
Levobunolol	T49.5X1	T49.5X2	T49.5X3	T49.5X4	T49.5X5	T49.5X6
Levocabastine (hydrochloride)	T45.ØX1	T45.ØX2	T45.ØX3	T45.ØX4	T45.ØX5	T45.ØX6
Levocarnitine	T5Ø.991	T5Ø.992	T5Ø.993	T5Ø.994	T5Ø.995	T5Ø.996
Levodopa	T42.8X1	T42.8X2	T42.8X3	T42.8X4	T42.8X5	T42.8X6
with carbidopa	T42.8X1	T42.8X2	T42.8X3	T42.8X4	T42.8X5	T42.8X6
Levo-dromoran	T4Ø.2X1	T4Ø.2X2	T4Ø.2X3	T4Ø.2X4	T4Ø.2X5	T4Ø.2X6
Levoglutamide	T5Ø.991	T5Ø.992	T5Ø.993	T5Ø.994	T5Ø.995	T5Ø.996
Levoid	T38.1X1	T38.1X2	T38.1X3	T38.1X4	T38.1X5	T38.1X6
Levo-isomethadone	T4Ø.3X1	T4Ø.3X2	T4Ø.3X3	T4Ø.3X4	T4Ø.3X5	T4Ø.3X6
Levomepromazine	T43.3X1	T43.3X2	T43.3X3	T43.3X4	T43.3X5	T43.3X6
Levonordefrin	T49.6X1	T49.6X2	T49.6X3	T49.6X4	T49.6X5	T49.6X6
Levonorgestrel	T38.4X1	T38.4X2	T38.4X3	T38.4X4	T38.4X5	T38.4X6
with ethinylestradiol	T38.5X1	T38.5X2	T38.5X3	T38.5X4	T38.5X5	T38.5X6
Levopromazine	T43.3X1	T43.3X2	T43.3X3	T43.3X4	T43.3X5	T43.3X6
Levoprome	T42.6X1	T42.6X2	T42.6X3	T42.6X4	T42.6X5	T42.6X6
Levopropoxyphene	T4Ø.491	T4Ø.492	T4Ø.493	T4Ø.494	T4Ø.495	T4Ø.496
Levopropylhexedrine	T5Ø.5X1	T5Ø.5X2	T5Ø.5X3	T5Ø.5X4	T5Ø.5X5	T5Ø.5X6
Levoproxyphylline	T48.6X1	T48.6X2	T48.6X3	T48.6X4	T48.6X5	T48.6X6
Levorphanol	T4Ø.491	T4Ø.492	T4Ø.493	T4Ø.494	T4Ø.495	T4Ø.496
Levothyroxine	T38.1X1	T38.1X2	T38.1X3	T38.1X4	T38.1X5	T38.1X6
sodium	T38.1X1	T38.1X2	T38.1X3	T38.1X4	T38.1X5	T38.1X6
Levsin	T44.3X1	T44.3X2	T44.3X3	T44.3X4	T44.3X5	T44.3X6
Levulose	T5Ø.3X1	T5Ø.3X2	T5Ø.3X3	T5Ø.3X4	T5Ø.3X5	T5Ø.3X6
Lewisite (gas), not in war	T57.ØX1	T57.ØX2	T57.ØX3	T57.ØX4	—	—
Librium	T42.4X1	T42.4X2	T42.4X3	T42.4X4	T42.4X5	T42.4X6
Lidex	T49.ØX1	T49.ØX2	T49.ØX3	T49.ØX4	T49.ØX5	T49.ØX6
Lidocaine	T41.3X1	T41.3X2	T41.3X3	T41.3X4	T41.3X5	T41.3X6
regional	T41.3X1	T41.3X2	T41.3X3	T41.3X4	T41.3X5	T41.3X6
spinal	T41.3X1	T41.3X2	T41.3X3	T41.3X4	T41.3X5	T41.3X6

Substance	Poisoning, Accidental (unintentional)	Poisoning, Intentional Self-harm	Poisoning, Assault	Poisoning, Undetermined	Adverse Effect	Under-dosing
Lidofenin	T5Ø.8X1	T5Ø.8X2	T5Ø.8X3	T5Ø.8X4	T5Ø.8X5	T5Ø.8X6
Lidoflazine	T46.1X1	T46.1X2	T46.1X3	T46.1X4	T46.1X5	T46.1X6
Lighter fluid	T52.ØX1	T52.ØX2	T52.ØX3	T52.ØX4	—	—
Lignin hemicellulose	T47.6X1	T47.6X2	T47.6X3	T47.6X4	T47.6X5	T47.6X6
Lignocaine	T41.3X1	T41.3X2	T41.3X3	T41.3X4	T41.3X5	T41.3X6
regional	T41.3X1	T41.3X2	T41.3X3	T41.3X4	T41.3X5	T41.3X6
spinal	T41.3X1	T41.3X2	T41.3X3	T41.3X4	T41.3X5	T41.3X6
Ligroin (e) (solvent)	T52.ØX1	T52.ØX2	T52.ØX3	T52.ØX4	—	—
vapor	T59.891	T59.892	T59.893	T59.894	—	—
Ligustrum vulgare	T62.2X1	T62.2X2	T62.2X3	T62.2X4	—	—
Lily of the valley	T62.2X1	T62.2X2	T62.2X3	T62.2X4	—	—
Lime (chloride)	T54.3X1	T54.3X2	T54.3X3	T54.3X4	—	—
Limonene	T52.8X1	T52.8X2	T52.8X3	T52.8X4	—	—
Lincomycin	T36.8X1	T36.8X2	T36.8X3	T36.8X4	T36.8X5	T36.8X6
Lindane (insecticide) (nonmedicinal) (vapor)	T53.6X1	T53.6X2	T53.6X3	T53.6X4	—	—
medicinal	T49.ØX1	T49.ØX2	T49.ØX3	T49.ØX4	T49.ØX5	T49.ØX6
Liniments NEC	T49.91	T49.92	T49.93	T49.94	T49.95	T49.96
Linoleic acid	T46.6X1	T46.6X2	T46.6X3	T46.6X4	T46.6X5	T46.6X6
Linolenic acid	T46.6X1	T46.6X2	T46.6X3	T46.6X4	T46.6X5	T46.6X6
Linseed	T47.4X1	T47.4X2	T47.4X3	T47.4X4	T47.4X5	T47.4X6
Liothyronine	T38.1X1	T38.1X2	T38.1X3	T38.1X4	T38.1X5	T38.1X6
Liotrix	T38.1X1	T38.1X2	T38.1X3	T38.1X4	T38.1X5	T38.1X6
Lipancreatin	T47.5X1	T47.5X2	T47.5X3	T47.5X4	T47.5X5	T47.5X6
Lipo-alprostadil	T46.7X1	T46.7X2	T46.7X3	T46.7X4	T46.7X5	T46.7X6
Lipo-Lutin	T38.5X1	T38.5X2	T38.5X3	T38.5X4	T38.5X5	T38.5X6
Lipotropic drug NEC	T5Ø.9Ø1	T5Ø.9Ø2	T5Ø.9Ø3	T5Ø.9Ø4	T5Ø.9Ø5	T5Ø.9Ø6
Liquefied petroleum gases	T59.891	T59.892	T59.893	T59.894	—	—
piped (pure or mixed with air)	T59.891	T59.892	T59.893	T59.894	—	—
Liquid						
paraffin	T47.4X1	T47.4X2	T47.4X3	T47.4X4	T47.4X5	T47.4X6
petrolatum	T47.4X1	T47.4X2	T47.4X3	T47.4X4	T47.4X5	T47.4X6
topical	T49.3X1	T49.3X2	T49.3X3	T49.3X4	T49.3X5	T49.3X6
specified NEC	T65.891	T65.892	T65.893	T65.894	—	—
substance	T65.91	T65.92	T65.93	T65.94	—	—
Liquor creosolis compositus	T65.891	T65.892	T65.893	T65.894	—	—
Liquorice	T48.4X1	T48.4X2	T48.4X3	T48.4X4	T48.4X5	T48.4X6
extract	T47.8X1	T47.8X2	T47.8X3	T47.8X4	T47.8X5	T47.8X6
Lisinopril	T46.4X1	T46.4X2	T46.4X3	T46.4X4	T46.4X5	T46.4X6
Lisuride	T42.8X1	T42.8X2	T42.8X3	T42.8X4	T42.8X5	T42.8X6
Lithane	T43.8X1	T43.8X2	T43.8X3	T43.8X4	T43.8X5	T43.8X6
Lithium	T56.891	T56.892	T56.893	T56.894	—	—
gluconate	T43.591	T43.592	T43.593	T43.594	T43.595	T43.596
salts (carbonate)	T43.591	T43.592	T43.593	T43.594	T43.595	T43.596
Lithonate	T43.8X1	T43.8X2	T43.8X3	T43.8X4	T43.8X5	T43.8X6
Liver						
extract	T45.8X1	T45.8X2	T45.8X3	T45.8X4	T45.8X5	T45.8X6
for parenteral use	T45.8X1	T45.8X2	T45.8X3	T45.8X4	T45.8X5	T45.8X6
fraction 1	T45.8X1	T45.8X2	T45.8X3	T45.8X4	T45.8X5	T45.8X6
hydrolysate	T45.8X1	T45.8X2	T45.8X3	T45.8X4	T45.8X5	T45.8X6
Lizard (bite) (venom)	T63.121	T63.122	T63.123	T63.124	—	—
LMD	T45.8X1	T45.8X2	T45.8X3	T45.8X4	T45.8X5	T45.8X6
Lobelia	T62.2X1	T62.2X2	T62.2X3	T62.2X4	—	—
Lobeline	T5Ø.7X1	T5Ø.7X2	T5Ø.7X3	T5Ø.7X4	T5Ø.7X5	T5Ø.7X6
Local action drug NEC	T49.8X1	T49.8X2	T49.8X3	T49.8X4	T49.8X5	T49.8X6
Locorten	T49.ØX1	T49.ØX2	T49.ØX3	T49.ØX4	T49.ØX5	T49.ØX6
Lofepramine	T43.Ø11	T43.Ø12	T43.Ø13	T43.Ø14	T43.Ø15	T43.Ø16
Lolium temulentum	T62.2X1	T62.2X2	T62.2X3	T62.2X4	—	—
Lomotil	T47.6X1	T47.6X2	T47.6X3	T47.6X4	T47.6X5	T47.6X6
Lomustine	T45.1X1	T45.1X2	T45.1X3	T45.1X4	T45.1X5	T45.1X6
Lonidamine	T45.1X1	T45.1X2	T45.1X3	T45.1X4	T45.1X5	T45.1X6
Loperamide	T47.6X1	T47.6X2	T47.6X3	T47.6X4	T47.6X5	T47.6X6
Loprazolam	T42.4X1	T42.4X2	T42.4X3	T42.4X4	T42.4X5	T42.4X6
Lorajmine	T46.2X1	T46.2X2	T46.2X3	T46.2X4	T46.2X5	T46.2X6
Loratidine	T45.ØX1	T45.ØX2	T45.ØX3	T45.ØX4	T45.ØX5	T45.ØX6
Lorazepam	T42.4X1	T42.4X2	T42.4X3	T42.4X4	T42.4X5	T42.4X6
Lorcainide	T46.2X1	T46.2X2	T46.2X3	T46.2X4	T46.2X5	T46.2X6
Lormetazepam	T42.4X1	T42.4X2	T42.4X3	T42.4X4	T42.4X5	T42.4X6
Lotions NEC	T49.91	T49.92	T49.93	T49.94	T49.95	T49.96
Lotusate	T42.3X1	T42.3X2	T42.3X3	T42.3X4	T42.3X5	T42.3X6
Lovastatin	T46.6X1	T46.6X2	T46.6X3	T46.6X4	T46.6X5	T46.6X6
Lowila	T49.2X1	T49.2X2	T49.2X3	T49.2X4	T49.2X5	T49.2X6
Loxapine	T43.591	T43.592	T43.593	T43.594	T43.595	T43.596
Lozenges (throat)	T49.6X1	T49.6X2	T49.6X3	T49.6X4	T49.6X5	T49.6X6
LSD	T4Ø.8X1	T4Ø.8X2	T4Ø.8X3	T4Ø.8X4	—	—
L-Tryptophan — *see* amino acid						
Lubricant, eye	T49.5X1	T49.5X2	T49.5X3	T49.5X4	T49.5X5	T49.5X6
Lubricating oil NEC	T52.ØX1	T52.ØX2	T52.ØX3	T52.ØX4	—	—
Lucanthone	T37.4X1	T37.4X2	T37.4X3	T37.4X4	T37.4X5	T37.4X6
Luminal	T42.3X1	T42.3X2	T42.3X3	T42.3X4	T42.3X5	T42.3X6
Lung irritant (gas) **NEC**	T59.91	T59.92	T59.93	T59.94	—	—

Substance	Poisoning, Accidental (unintentional)	Poisoning, Intentional Self-harm	Poisoning, Assault	Poisoning, Undetermined	Adverse Effect	Under-dosing
Luteinizing hormone	T38.811	T38.812	T38.813	T38.814	T38.815	T38.816
Lutocylol	T38.5X1	T38.5X2	T38.5X3	T38.5X4	T38.5X5	T38.5X6
Lutromone	T38.5X1	T38.5X2	T38.5X3	T38.5X4	T38.5X5	T38.5X6
Lututrin	T48.291	T48.292	T48.293	T48.294	T48.295	T48.296
Lye (concentrated)	T54.3X1	T54.3X2	T54.3X3	T54.3X4	—	—
Lygranum (skin test)	T5Ø.8X1	T5Ø.8X2	T5Ø.8X3	T5Ø.8X4	T5Ø.8X5	T5Ø.8X6
Lymecycline	T36.4X1	T36.4X2	T36.4X3	T36.4X4	T36.4X5	T36.4X6
Lymphogranuloma venereum antigen	T5Ø.8X1	T5Ø.8X2	T5Ø.8X3	T5Ø.8X4	T5Ø.8X5	T5Ø.8X6
Lynestrenol	T38.4X1	T38.4X2	T38.4X3	T38.4X4	T38.4X5	T38.4X6
Lyovac Sodium Edecrin	T5Ø.1X1	T5Ø.1X2	T5Ø.1X3	T5Ø.1X4	T5Ø.1X5	T5Ø.1X6
Lypressin	T38.891	T38.892	T38.893	T38.894	T38.895	T38.896
Lysergic acid diethylamide	T4Ø.8X1	T4Ø.8X2	T4Ø.8X3	T4Ø.8X4	—	—
Lysergide	T4Ø.8X1	T4Ø.8X2	T4Ø.8X3	T4Ø.8X4	—	—
Lysine vasopressin	T38.891	T38.892	T38.893	T38.894	T38.895	T38.896
Lysol	T54.1X1	T54.1X2	T54.1X3	T54.1X4	—	—
Lysozyme	T49.ØX1	T49.ØX2	T49.ØX3	T49.ØX4	T49.ØX5	T49.ØX6
Lytta (vitatta)	T49.8X1	T49.8X2	T49.8X3	T49.8X4	T49.8X5	T49.8X6
Mace	T59.3X1	T59.3X2	T59.3X3	T59.3X4	—	—
Macrogol	T5Ø.991	T5Ø.992	T5Ø.993	T5Ø.994	T5Ø.995	T5Ø.996
Macrolide						
anabolic drug	T38.7X1	T38.7X2	T38.7X3	T38.7X4	T38.7X5	T38.7X6
antibiotic	T36.3X1	T36.3X2	T36.3X3	T36.3X4	T36.3X5	T36.3X6
Mafenide	T49.ØX1	T49.ØX2	T49.ØX3	T49.ØX4	T49.ØX5	T49.ØX6
Magaldrate	T47.1X1	T47.1X2	T47.1X3	T47.1X4	T47.1X5	T47.1X6
Magic mushroom	T4Ø.991	T4Ø.992	T4Ø.993	T4Ø.994	—	—
Magnamycin	T36.8X1	T36.8X2	T36.8X3	T36.8X4	T36.8X5	T36.8X6
Magnesia magma	T47.1X1	T47.1X2	T47.1X3	T47.1X4	T47.1X5	T47.1X6
Magnesium NEC	T56.891	T56.892	T56.893	T56.894	—	—
carbonate	T47.1X1	T47.1X2	T47.1X3	T47.1X4	T47.1X5	T47.1X6
citrate	T47.4X1	T47.4X2	T47.4X3	T47.4X4	T47.4X5	T47.4X6
hydroxide	T47.1X1	T47.1X2	T47.1X3	T47.1X4	T47.1X5	T47.1X6
oxide	T47.1X1	T47.1X2	T47.1X3	T47.1X4	T47.1X5	T47.1X6
peroxide	T49.ØX1	T49.ØX2	T49.ØX3	T49.ØX4	T49.ØX5	T49.ØX6
salicylate	T39.Ø91	T39.Ø92	T39.Ø93	T39.Ø94	T39.Ø95	T39.Ø96
silicofluoride	T5Ø.3X1	T5Ø.3X2	T5Ø.3X3	T5Ø.3X4	T5Ø.3X5	T5Ø.3X6
sulfate	T47.4X1	T47.4X2	T47.4X3	T47.4X4	T47.4X5	T47.4X6
thiosulfate	T45.ØX1	T45.ØX2	T45.ØX3	T45.ØX4	T45.ØX5	T45.ØX6
trisilicate	T47.1X1	T47.1X2	T47.1X3	T47.1X4	T47.1X5	T47.1X6
Malathion (medicinal)	T49.ØX1	T49.ØX2	T49.ØX3	T49.ØX4	T49.ØX5	T49.ØX6
insecticide	T6Ø.ØX1	T6Ø.ØX2	T6Ø.ØX3	T6Ø.ØX4	—	—
Male fern extract	T37.4X1	T37.4X2	T37.4X3	T37.4X4	T37.4X5	T37.4X6
M-AMSA	T45.1X1	T45.1X2	T45.1X3	T45.1X4	T45.1X5	T45.1X6
Mandelic acid	T37.8X1	T37.8X2	T37.8X3	T37.8X4	T37.8X5	T37.8X6
Manganese (dioxide) (salts)	T57.2X1	T57.2X2	T57.2X3	T57.2X4	—	—
medicinal	T5Ø.991	T5Ø.992	T5Ø.993	T5Ø.994	T5Ø.995	T5Ø.996
Mannitol	T47.3X1	T47.3X2	T47.3X3	T47.3X4	T47.3X5	T47.3X6
hexanitrate	T46.3X1	T46.3X2	T46.3X3	T46.3X4	T46.3X5	T46.3X6
Mannomustine	T45.1X1	T45.1X2	T45.1X3	T45.1X4	T45.1X5	T45.1X6
MAO inhibitors	T43.1X1	T43.1X2	T43.1X3	T43.1X4	T43.1X5	T43.1X6
Mapharsen	T37.8X1	T37.8X2	T37.8X3	T37.8X4	T37.8X5	T37.8X6
Maphenide	T49.ØX1	T49.ØX2	T49.ØX3	T49.ØX4	T49.ØX5	T49.ØX6
Maprotiline	T43.Ø21	T43.Ø22	T43.Ø23	T43.Ø24	T43.Ø25	T43.Ø26
Marcaine	T41.3X1	T41.3X2	T41.3X3	T41.3X4	T41.3X5	T41.3X6
infiltration (subcutaneous)	T41.3X1	T41.3X2	T41.3X3	T41.3X4	T41.3X5	T41.3X6
nerve block (peripheral) (plexus)	T41.3X1	T41.3X2	T41.3X3	T41.3X4	T41.3X5	T41.3X6
Marezine	T45.ØX1	T45.ØX2	T45.ØX3	T45.ØX4	T45.ØX5	T45.ØX6
Marihuana	T4Ø.7X1	T4Ø.7X2	T4Ø.7X3	T4Ø.7X4	T4Ø.7X5	T4Ø.7X6
Marijuana	T4Ø.7X1	T4Ø.7X2	T4Ø.7X3	T4Ø.7X4	T4Ø.7X5	T4Ø.7X6
Marine (sting)	T63.691	T63.692	T63.693	T63.694	—	—
animals (sting)	T63.691	T63.692	T63.693	T63.694	—	—
plants (sting)	T63.711	T63.712	T63.713	T63.714	—	—
Marplan	T43.1X1	T43.1X2	T43.1X3	T43.1X4	T43.1X5	T43.1X6
Marsh gas	T59.891	T59.892	T59.893	T59.894	—	—
Marsilid	T43.1X1	T43.1X2	T43.1X3	T43.1X4	T43.1X5	T43.1X6
Matulane	T45.1X1	T45.1X2	T45.1X3	T45.1X4	T45.1X5	T45.1X6
Mazindol	T5Ø.5X1	T5Ø.5X2	T5Ø.5X3	T5Ø.5X4	T5Ø.5X5	T5Ø.5X6
MCPA	T6Ø.3X1	T6Ø.3X2	T6Ø.3X3	T6Ø.3X4	—	—
MDMA	T43.641	T43.642	T43.643	T43.644	—	—
Meadow saffron	T62.2X1	T62.2X2	T62.2X3	T62.2X4	—	—
Measles virus vaccine (attenuated)	T5Ø.B91	T5Ø.B92	T5Ø.B93	T5Ø.B94	T5Ø.B95	T5Ø.B96
Meat, noxious	T62.8X1	T62.8X2	T62.8X3	T62.8X4	—	—
Meballymal	T42.3X1	T42.3X2	T42.3X3	T42.3X4	T42.3X5	T42.3X6
Mebanazine	T43.1X1	T43.1X2	T43.1X3	T43.1X4	T43.1X5	T43.1X6
Mebaral	T42.3X1	T42.3X2	T42.3X3	T42.3X4	T42.3X5	T42.3X6
Mebendazole	T37.4X1	T37.4X2	T37.4X3	T37.4X4	T37.4X5	T37.4X6
Mebeverine	T44.3X1	T44.3X2	T44.3X3	T44.3X4	T44.3X5	T44.3X6
Mebhydrolin	T45.ØX1	T45.ØX2	T45.ØX3	T45.ØX4	T45.ØX5	T45.ØX6
Mebumal	T42.3X1	T42.3X2	T42.3X3	T42.3X4	T42.3X5	T42.3X6
Mebutamate	T43.591	T43.592	T43.593	T43.594	T43.595	T43.596
Mecamylamine	T44.2X1	T44.2X2	T44.2X3	T44.2X4	T44.2X5	T44.2X6

Substance	Poisoning, Accidental (unintentional)	Poisoning, Intentional Self-harm	Poisoning, Assault	Poisoning, Undetermined	Adverse Effect	Under-dosing
Mechlorethamine	T45.1X1	T45.1X2	T45.1X3	T45.1X4	T45.1X5	T45.1X6
Mecillinam	T36.ØX1	T36.ØX2	T36.ØX3	T36.ØX4	T36.ØX5	T36.ØX6
Meclizine (hydrochloride)	T45.ØX1	T45.ØX2	T45.ØX3	T45.ØX4	T45.ØX5	T45.ØX6
Meclocycline	T36.4X1	T36.4X2	T36.4X3	T36.4X4	T36.4X5	T36.4X6
Meclofenamate	T39.391	T39.392	T39.393	T39.394	T39.395	T39.396
Meclofenamic acid	T39.391	T39.392	T39.393	T39.394	T39.395	T39.396
Meclofenoxate	T43.691	T43.692	T43.693	T43.694	T43.695	T43.696
Meclozine	T45.ØX1	T45.ØX2	T45.ØX3	T45.ØX4	T45.ØX5	T45.ØX6
Mecobalamin	T45.8X1	T45.8X2	T45.8X3	T45.8X4	T45.8X5	T45.8X6
Mecoprop	T6Ø.3X1	T6Ø.3X2	T6Ø.3X3	T6Ø.3X4	—	—
Mecrilate	T49.3X1	T49.3X2	T49.3X3	T49.3X4	T49.3X5	T49.3X6
Mecysteine	T48.4X1	T48.4X2	T48.4X3	T48.4X4	T48.4X5	T48.4X6
Medazepam	T42.4X1	T42.4X2	T42.4X3	T42.4X4	T42.4X5	T42.4X6
Medicament NEC	T5Ø.9Ø1	T5Ø.9Ø2	T5Ø.9Ø3	T5Ø.9Ø4	T5Ø.9Ø5	T5Ø.9Ø6
Medinal	T42.3X1	T42.3X2	T42.3X3	T42.3X4	T42.3X5	T42.3X6
Medomin	T42.3X1	T42.3X2	T42.3X3	T42.3X4	T42.3X5	T42.3X6
Medrogestone	T38.5X1	T38.5X2	T38.5X3	T38.5X4	T38.5X5	T38.5X6
Medroxalol	T44.8X1	T44.8X2	T44.8X3	T44.8X4	T44.8X5	T44.8X6
Medroxyprogesterone acetate (depot)	T38.5X1	T38.5X2	T38.5X3	T38.5X4	T38.5X5	T38.5X6
Medrysone	T49.ØX1	T49.ØX2	T49.ØX3	T49.ØX4	T49.ØX5	T49.ØX6
Mefenamic acid	T39.391	T39.392	T39.393	T39.394	T39.395	T39.396
Mefenorex	T5Ø.5X1	T5Ø.5X2	T5Ø.5X3	T5Ø.5X4	T5Ø.5X5	T5Ø.5X6
Mefloquine	T37.2X1	T37.2X2	T37.2X3	T37.2X4	T37.2X5	T37.2X6
Mefruside	T5Ø.2X1	T5Ø.2X2	T5Ø.2X3	T5Ø.2X4	T5Ø.2X5	T5Ø.2X6
Megahallucinogen	T4Ø.9Ø1	T4Ø.9Ø2	T4Ø.9Ø3	T4Ø.9Ø4	T4Ø.9Ø5	T4Ø.9Ø6
Megestrol	T38.5X1	T38.5X2	T38.5X3	T38.5X4	T38.5X5	T38.5X6
Meglumine						
antimoniate	T37.8X1	T37.8X2	T37.8X3	T37.8X4	T37.8X5	T37.8X6
diatrizoate	T5Ø.8X1	T5Ø.8X2	T5Ø.8X3	T5Ø.8X4	T5Ø.8X5	T5Ø.8X6
iodipamide	T5Ø.8X1	T5Ø.8X2	T5Ø.8X3	T5Ø.8X4	T5Ø.8X5	T5Ø.8X6
iotroxate	T5Ø.8X1	T5Ø.8X2	T5Ø.8X3	T5Ø.8X4	T5Ø.8X5	T5Ø.8X6
MEK (methyl ethyl ketone)	T52.4X1	T52.4X2	T52.4X3	T52.4X4	—	—
Meladinin	T49.3X1	T49.3X2	T49.3X3	T49.3X4	T49.3X5	T49.3X6
Meladrazine	T44.3X1	T44.3X2	T44.3X3	T44.3X4	T44.3X5	T44.3X6
Melaleuca alternifolia oil	T49.ØX1	T49.ØX2	T49.ØX3	T49.ØX4	T49.ØX5	T49.ØX6
Melanizing agents	T49.3X1	T49.3X2	T49.3X3	T49.3X4	T49.3X5	T49.3X6
Melanocyte-stimulating hormone	T38.891	T38.892	T38.893	T38.894	T38.895	T38.896
Melarsonyl potassium	T37.3X1	T37.3X2	T37.3X3	T37.3X4	T37.3X5	T37.3X6
Melarsoprol	T37.3X1	T37.3X2	T37.3X3	T37.3X4	T37.3X5	T37.3X6
Melia azedarach	T62.2X1	T62.2X2	T62.2X3	T62.2X4	—	—
Melitracen	T43.Ø11	T43.Ø12	T43.Ø13	T43.Ø14	T43.Ø15	T43.Ø16
Mellaril	T43.3X1	T43.3X2	T43.3X3	T43.3X4	T43.3X5	T43.3X6
Meloxine	T49.3X1	T49.3X2	T49.3X3	T49.3X4	T49.3X5	T49.3X6
Melperone	T43.4X1	T43.4X2	T43.4X3	T43.4X4	T43.4X5	T43.4X6
Melphalan	T45.1X1	T45.1X2	T45.1X3	T45.1X4	T45.1X5	T45.1X6
Memantine	T43.8X1	T43.8X2	T43.8X3	T43.8X4	T43.8X5	T43.8X6
Menadiol	T45.7X1	T45.7X2	T45.7X3	T45.7X4	T45.7X5	T45.7X6
sodium sulfate	T45.7X1	T45.7X2	T45.7X3	T45.7X4	T45.7X5	T45.7X6
Menadione	T45.7X1	T45.7X2	T45.7X3	T45.7X4	T45.7X5	T45.7X6
sodium bisulfite	T45.7X1	T45.7X2	T45.7X3	T45.7X4	T45.7X5	T45.7X6
Menaphthone	T45.7X1	T45.7X2	T45.7X3	T45.7X4	T45.7X5	T45.7X6
Menaquinone	T45.7X1	T45.7X2	T45.7X3	T45.7X4	T45.7X5	T45.7X6
Menatetrenone	T45.7X1	T45.7X2	T45.7X3	T45.7X4	T45.7X5	T45.7X6
Meningococcal vaccine	T5Ø.A91	T5Ø.A92	T5Ø.A93	T5Ø.A94	T5Ø.A95	T5Ø.A96
Menningovax (-AC) (-C)	T5Ø.A91	T5Ø.A92	T5Ø.A93	T5Ø.A94	T5Ø.A95	T5Ø.A96
Menotropins	T38.811	T38.812	T38.813	T38.814	T38.815	T38.816
Menthol	T48.5X1	T48.5X2	T48.5X3	T48.5X4	T48.5X5	T48.5X6
Mepacrine	T37.2X1	T37.2X2	T37.2X3	T37.2X4	T37.2X5	T37.2X6
Meparfynol	T42.6X1	T42.6X2	T42.6X3	T42.6X4	T42.6X5	T42.6X6
Mepartricin	T36.7X1	T36.7X2	T36.7X3	T36.7X4	T36.7X5	T36.7X6
Mepazine	T43.3X1	T43.3X2	T43.3X3	T43.3X4	T43.3X5	T43.3X6
Mepenzolate	T44.3X1	T44.3X2	T44.3X3	T44.3X4	T44.3X5	T44.3X6
bromide	T44.3X1	T44.3X2	T44.3X3	T44.3X4	T44.3X5	T44.3X6
Meperidine	T4Ø.491	T4Ø.492	T4Ø.493	T4Ø.494	T4Ø.495	T4Ø.496
Mephebarbital	T42.3X1	T42.3X2	T42.3X3	T42.3X4	T42.3X5	T42.3X6
Mephenamin (e)	T42.8X1	T42.8X2	T42.8X3	T42.8X4	T42.8X5	T42.8X6
Mephenesin	T42.8X1	T42.8X2	T42.8X3	T42.8X4	T42.8X5	T42.8X6
Mephenhydramine	T45.ØX1	T45.ØX2	T45.ØX3	T45.ØX4	T45.ØX5	T45.ØX6
Mephenoxalone	T42.8X1	T42.8X2	T42.8X3	T42.8X4	T42.8X5	T42.8X6
Mephentermine	T44.991	T44.992	T44.993	T44.994	T44.995	T44.996
Mephenytoin	T42.ØX1	T42.ØX2	T42.ØX3	T42.ØX4	T42.ØX5	T42.ØX6
with phenobarbital	T42.3X1	T42.3X2	T42.3X3	T42.3X4	T42.3X5	T42.3X6
Mephobarbital	T42.3X1	T42.3X2	T42.3X3	T42.3X4	T42.3X5	T42.3X6
Mephosfolan	T6Ø.ØX1	T6Ø.ØX2	T6Ø.ØX3	T6Ø.ØX4	—	—
Mepindolol	T44.7X1	T44.7X2	T44.7X3	T44.7X4	T44.7X5	T44.7X6
Mepiperphenidol	T44.3X1	T44.3X2	T44.3X3	T44.3X4	T44.3X5	T44.3X6
Mepitiostane	T38.7X1	T38.7X2	T38.7X3	T38.7X4	T38.7X5	T38.7X6
Mepivacaine	T41.3X1	T41.3X2	T41.3X3	T41.3X4	T41.3X5	T41.3X6
epidural	T41.3X1	T41.3X2	T41.3X3	T41.3X4	T41.3X5	T41.3X6
Meprednisone	T38.ØX1	T38.ØX2	T38.ØX3	T38.ØX4	T38.ØX5	T38.ØX6
Meprobam	T43.591	T43.592	T43.593	T43.594	T43.595	T43.596
Meprobamate	T43.591	T43.592	T43.593	T43.594	T43.595	T43.596
Meproscillarin	T46.ØX1	T46.ØX2	T46.ØX3	T46.ØX4	T46.ØX5	T46.ØX6
Meprylcaine	T41.3X1	T41.3X2	T41.3X3	T41.3X4	T41.3X5	T41.3X6
Meptazinol	T39.8X1	T39.8X2	T39.8X3	T39.8X4	T39.8X5	T39.8X6
Mepyramine	T45.ØX1	T45.ØX2	T45.ØX3	T45.ØX4	T45.ØX5	T45.ØX6
Mequitazine	T43.3X1	T43.3X2	T43.3X3	T43.3X4	T43.3X5	T43.3X6
Meralluride	T5Ø.2X1	T5Ø.2X2	T5Ø.2X3	T5Ø.2X4	T5Ø.2X5	T5Ø.2X6
Merbaphen	T5Ø.2X1	T5Ø.2X2	T5Ø.2X3	T5Ø.2X4	T5Ø.2X5	T5Ø.2X6
Merbromin	T49.ØX1	T49.ØX2	T49.ØX3	T49.ØX4	T49.ØX5	T49.ØX6
Mercaptobenzothiazole salts	T49.ØX1	T49.ØX2	T49.ØX3	T49.ØX4	T49.ØX5	T49.ØX6
Mercaptomerin	T5Ø.2X1	T5Ø.2X2	T5Ø.2X3	T5Ø.2X4	T5Ø.2X5	T5Ø.2X6
Mercaptopurine	T45.1X1	T45.1X2	T45.1X3	T45.1X4	T45.1X5	T45.1X6
Mercumatilin	T5Ø.2X1	T5Ø.2X2	T5Ø.2X3	T5Ø.2X4	T5Ø.2X5	T5Ø.2X6
Mercuramide	T5Ø.2X1	T5Ø.2X2	T5Ø.2X3	T5Ø.2X4	T5Ø.2X5	T5Ø.2X6
Mercurochrome	T49.ØX1	T49.ØX2	T49.ØX3	T49.ØX4	T49.ØX5	T49.ØX6
Mercurophylline	T5Ø.2X1	T5Ø.2X2	T5Ø.2X3	T5Ø.2X4	T5Ø.2X5	T5Ø.2X6
Mercury, mercurial, mercuric, mercurous (compounds) (cyanide) (fumes) (nonmedicinal) (vapor) **NEC**	T56.1X1	T56.1X2	T56.1X3	T56.1X4	—	—
ammoniated	T49.ØX1	T49.ØX2	T49.ØX3	T49.ØX4	T49.ØX5	T49.ØX6
anti-infective						
local	T49.ØX1	T49.ØX2	T49.ØX3	T49.ØX4	T49.ØX5	T49.ØX6
systemic	T37.8X1	T37.8X2	T37.8X3	T37.8X4	T37.8X5	T37.8X6
topical	T49.ØX1	T49.ØX2	T49.ØX3	T49.ØX4	T49.ØX5	T49.ØX6
chloride (ammoniated)	T49.ØX1	T49.ØX2	T49.ØX3	T49.ØX4	T49.ØX5	T49.ØX6
fungicide	T56.1X1	T56.1X2	T56.1X3	T56.1X4	—	—
diuretic NEC	T5Ø.2X1	T5Ø.2X2	T5Ø.2X3	T5Ø.2X4	T5Ø.2X5	T5Ø.2X6
fungicide	T56.1X1	T56.1X2	T56.1X3	T56.1X4	—	—
organic (fungicide)	T56.1X1	T56.1X2	T56.1X3	T56.1X4	—	—
oxide, yellow	T49.ØX1	T49.ØX2	T49.ØX3	T49.ØX4	T49.ØX5	T49.ØX6
Mersalyl	T5Ø.2X1	T5Ø.2X2	T5Ø.2X3	T5Ø.2X4	T5Ø.2X5	T5Ø.2X6
Merthiolate	T49.ØX1	T49.ØX2	T49.ØX3	T49.ØX4	T49.ØX5	T49.ØX6
ophthalmic preparation	T49.5X1	T49.5X2	T49.5X3	T49.5X4	T49.5X5	T49.5X6
Meruvax	T5Ø.B91	T5Ø.B92	T5Ø.B93	T5Ø.B94	T5Ø.B95	T5Ø.B96
Mesalazine	T47.8X1	T47.8X2	T47.8X3	T47.8X4	T47.8X5	T47.8X6
Mescal buttons	T4Ø.991	T4Ø.992	T4Ø.993	T4Ø.994	—	—
Mescaline	T4Ø.991	T4Ø.992	T4Ø.993	T4Ø.994	—	—
Mesna	T48.4X1	T48.4X2	T48.4X3	T48.4X4	T48.4X5	T48.4X6
Mesoglycan	T46.6X1	T46.6X2	T46.6X3	T46.6X4	T46.6X5	T46.6X6
Mesoridazine	T43.3X1	T43.3X2	T43.3X3	T43.3X4	T43.3X5	T43.3X6
Mestanolone	T38.7X1	T38.7X2	T38.7X3	T38.7X4	T38.7X5	T38.7X6
Mesterolone	T38.7X1	T38.7X2	T38.7X3	T38.7X4	T38.7X5	T38.7X6
Mestranol	T38.5X1	T38.5X2	T38.5X3	T38.5X4	T38.5X5	T38.5X6
Mesulergine	T42.8X1	T42.8X2	T42.8X3	T42.8X4	T42.8X5	T42.8X6
Mesulfen	T49.ØX1	T49.ØX2	T49.ØX3	T49.ØX4	T49.ØX5	T49.ØX6
Mesuximide	T42.2X1	T42.2X2	T42.2X3	T42.2X4	T42.2X5	T42.2X6
Metabutethamine	T41.3X1	T41.3X2	T41.3X3	T41.3X4	T41.3X5	T41.3X6
Metactesylacetate	T49.ØX1	T49.ØX2	T49.ØX3	T49.ØX4	T49.ØX5	T49.ØX6
Metacycline	T36.4X1	T36.4X2	T36.4X3	T36.4X4	T36.4X5	T36.4X6
Metaldehyde (snail killer) **NEC**	T6Ø.8X1	T6Ø.8X2	T6Ø.8X3	T6Ø.8X4	—	—
Metals (heavy) (nonmedicinal)	T56.91	T56.92	T56.93	T56.94	—	—
dust, fumes, or vapor NEC	T56.91	T56.92	T56.93	T56.94	—	—
light NEC	T56.91	T56.92	T56.93	T56.94	—	—
dust, fumes, or vapor NEC	T56.91	T56.92	T56.93	T56.94	—	—
specified NEC	T56.891	T56.892	T56.893	T56.894	—	—
thallium	T56.811	T56.812	T56.813	T56.814	—	—
Metamfetamine	T43.621	T43.622	T43.623	T43.624	T43.625	T43.626
Metamizole sodium	T39.2X1	T39.2X2	T39.2X3	T39.2X4	T39.2X5	T39.2X6
Metampicillin	T36.ØX1	T36.ØX2	T36.ØX3	T36.ØX4	T36.ØX5	T36.ØX6
Metamucil	T47.4X1	T47.4X2	T47.4X3	T47.4X4	T47.4X5	T47.4X6
Metandienone	T38.7X1	T38.7X2	T38.7X3	T38.7X4	T38.7X5	T38.7X6
Metandrostenolone	T38.7X1	T38.7X2	T38.7X3	T38.7X4	T38.7X5	T38.7X6
Metaphen	T49.ØX1	T49.ØX2	T49.ØX3	T49.ØX4	T49.ØX5	T49.ØX6
Metaphos	T6Ø.ØX1	T6Ø.ØX2	T6Ø.ØX3	T6Ø.ØX4	—	—
Metapramine	T43.Ø11	T43.Ø12	T43.Ø13	T43.Ø14	T43.Ø15	T43.Ø16
Metaproterenol	T48.291	T48.292	T48.293	T48.294	T48.295	T48.296
Metaraminol	T44.4X1	T44.4X2	T44.4X3	T44.4X4	T44.4X5	T44.4X6
Metaxalone	T42.8X1	T42.8X2	T42.8X3	T42.8X4	T42.8X5	T42.8X6
Metenolone	T38.7X1	T38.7X2	T38.7X3	T38.7X4	T38.7X5	T38.7X6
Metergoline	T42.8X1	T42.8X2	T42.8X3	T42.8X4	T42.8X5	T42.8X6
Metescufylline	T46.991	T46.992	T46.993	T46.994	T46.995	T46.996
Metetoin	T42.ØX1	T42.ØX2	T42.ØX3	T42.ØX4	T42.ØX5	T42.ØX6
Metformin	T38.3X1	T38.3X2	T38.3X3	T38.3X4	T38.3X5	T38.3X6
Methacholine	T44.1X1	T44.1X2	T44.1X3	T44.1X4	T44.1X5	T44.1X6
Methacycline	T36.4X1	T36.4X2	T36.4X3	T36.4X4	T36.4X5	T36.4X6
Methadone	T4Ø.3X1	T4Ø.3X2	T4Ø.3X3	T4Ø.3X4	T4Ø.3X5	T4Ø.3X6
Methallenestril	T38.5X1	T38.5X2	T38.5X3	T38.5X4	T38.5X5	T38.5X6

Substance	Poisoning, Accidental (unintentional)	Poisoning, Intentional Self-harm	Poisoning, Assault	Poisoning, Undetermined	Adverse Effect	Under-dosing
Methallenoestril	T38.5X1	T38.5X2	T38.5X3	T38.5X4	T38.5X5	T38.5X6
Methamphetamine	T43.621	T43.622	T43.623	T43.624	T43.625	T43.626
Methampyrone	T39.2X1	T39.2X2	T39.2X3	T39.2X4	T39.2X5	T39.2X6
Methandienone	T38.7X1	T38.7X2	T38.7X3	T38.7X4	T38.7X5	T38.7X6
Methandriol	T38.7X1	T38.7X2	T38.7X3	T38.7X4	T38.7X5	T38.7X6
Methandrostenolone	T38.7X1	T38.7X2	T38.7X3	T38.7X4	T38.7X5	T38.7X6
Methane	T59.891	T59.892	T59.893	T59.894	—	—
Methanethiol	T59.891	T59.892	T59.893	T59.894	—	—
Methaniazide	T37.1X1	T37.1X2	T37.1X3	T37.1X4	T37.1X5	T37.1X6
Methanol (vapor)	T51.1X1	T51.1X2	T51.1X3	T51.1X4	—	—
Methantheline	T44.3X1	T44.3X2	T44.3X3	T44.3X4	T44.3X5	T44.3X6
Methanthelinium bromide	T44.3X1	T44.3X2	T44.3X3	T44.3X4	T44.3X5	T44.3X6
Methaphenilene	T45.ØX1	T45.ØX2	T45.ØX3	T45.ØX4	T45.ØX5	T45.ØX6
Methapyrilene	T45.ØX1	T45.ØX2	T45.ØX3	T45.ØX4	T45.ØX5	T45.ØX6
Methaqualone (compound)	T42.6X1	T42.6X2	T42.6X3	T42.6X4	T42.6X5	T42.6X6
Metharbital	T42.3X1	T42.3X2	T42.3X3	T42.3X4	T42.3X5	T42.3X6
Methazolamide	T5Ø.2X1	T5Ø.2X2	T5Ø.2X3	T5Ø.2X4	T5Ø.2X5	T5Ø.2X6
Methdilazine	T43.3X1	T43.3X2	T43.3X3	T43.3X4	T43.3X5	T43.3X6
Methedrine	T43.621	T43.622	T43.623	T43.624	T43.625	T43.626
Methenamine (mandelate)	T37.8X1	T37.8X2	T37.8X3	T37.8X4	T37.8X5	T37.8X6
Methenolone	T38.7X1	T38.7X2	T38.7X3	T38.7X4	T38.7X5	T38.7X6
Methergine	T48.ØX1	T48.ØX2	T48.ØX3	T48.ØX4	T48.ØX5	T48.ØX6
Methetoin	T42.ØX1	T42.ØX2	T42.ØX3	T42.ØX4	T42.ØX5	T42.ØX6
Methiacil	T38.2X1	T38.2X2	T38.2X3	T38.2X4	T38.2X5	T38.2X6
Methicillin	T36.ØX1	T36.ØX2	T36.ØX3	T36.ØX4	T36.ØX5	T36.ØX6
Methimazole	T38.2X1	T38.2X2	T38.2X3	T38.2X4	T38.2X5	T38.2X6
Methiodal sodium	T5Ø.8X1	T5Ø.8X2	T5Ø.8X3	T5Ø.8X4	T5Ø.8X5	T5Ø.8X6
Methionine	T5Ø.991	T5Ø.992	T5Ø.993	T5Ø.994	T5Ø.995	T5Ø.996
Methisazone	T37.5X1	T37.5X2	T37.5X3	T37.5X4	T37.5X5	T37.5X6
Methisoprinol	T37.5X1	T37.5X2	T37.5X3	T37.5X4	T37.5X5	T37.5X6
Methitural	T42.3X1	T42.3X2	T42.3X3	T42.3X4	T42.3X5	T42.3X6
Methixene	T44.3X1	T44.3X2	T44.3X3	T44.3X4	T44.3X5	T44.3X6
Methobarbital, methobarbitone	T42.3X1	T42.3X2	T42.3X3	T42.3X4	T42.3X5	T42.3X6
Methocarbamol	T42.8X1	T42.8X2	T42.8X3	T42.8X4	T42.8X5	T42.8X6
skeletal muscle relaxant	T48.1X1	T48.1X2	T48.1X3	T48.1X4	T48.1X5	T48.1X6
Methohexital	T41.1X1	T41.1X2	T41.1X3	T41.1X4	T41.1X5	T41.1X6
Methohexitone	T41.1X1	T41.1X2	T41.1X3	T41.1X4	T41.1X5	T41.1X6
Methoin	T42.ØX1	T42.ØX2	T42.ØX3	T42.ØX4	T42.ØX5	T42.ØX6
Methopholine	T39.8X1	T39.8X2	T39.8X3	T39.8X4	T39.8X5	T39.8X6
Methopromazine	T43.3X1	T43.3X2	T43.3X3	T43.3X4	T43.3X5	T43.3X6
Methorate	T48.3X1	T48.3X2	T48.3X3	T48.3X4	T48.3X5	T48.3X6
Methoserpidine	T46.5X1	T46.5X2	T46.5X3	T46.5X4	T46.5X5	T46.5X6
Methotrexate	T45.1X1	T45.1X2	T45.1X3	T45.1X4	T45.1X5	T45.1X6
Methotrimeprazine	T43.3X1	T43.3X2	T43.3X3	T43.3X4	T43.3X5	T43.3X6
Methoxa-Dome	T49.3X1	T49.3X2	T49.3X3	T49.3X4	T49.3X5	T49.3X6
Methoxamine	T44.4X1	T44.4X2	T44.4X3	T44.4X4	T44.4X5	T44.4X6
Methoxsalen	T5Ø.991	T5Ø.992	T5Ø.993	T5Ø.994	T5Ø.995	T5Ø.996
Methoxyaniline	T65.3X1	T65.3X2	T65.3X3	T65.3X4	—	—
Methoxybenzyl penicillin	T36.ØX1	T36.ØX2	T36.ØX3	T36.ØX4	T36.ØX5	T36.ØX6
Methoxychlor	T53.7X1	T53.7X2	T53.7X3	T53.7X4	—	—
Methoxy-DDT	T53.7X1	T53.7X2	T53.7X3	T53.7X4	—	—
Methoxyflurane	T41.ØX1	T41.ØX2	T41.ØX3	T41.ØX4	T41.ØX5	T41.ØX6
Methoxyphenamine	T48.6X1	T48.6X2	T48.6X3	T48.6X4	T48.6X5	T48.6X6
Methoxypromazine	T43.3X1	T43.3X2	T43.3X3	T43.3X4	T43.3X5	T43.3X6
Methscopolamine bromide	T44.3X1	T44.3X2	T44.3X3	T44.3X4	T44.3X5	T44.3X6
Methsuximide	T42.2X1	T42.2X2	T42.2X3	T42.2X4	T42.2X5	T42.2X6
Methyclothiazide	T5Ø.2X1	T5Ø.2X2	T5Ø.2X3	T5Ø.2X4	T5Ø.2X5	T5Ø.2X6
Methyl						
acetate	T52.4X1	T52.4X2	T52.4X3	T52.4X4	—	—
acetone	T52.4X1	T52.4X2	T52.4X3	T52.4X4	—	—
acrylate	T65.891	T65.892	T65.893	T65.894	—	—
alcohol	T51.1X1	T51.1X2	T51.1X3	T51.1X4	—	—
aminophenol	T65.3X1	T65.3X2	T65.3X3	T65.3X4	—	—
amphetamine	T43.621	T43.622	T43.623	T43.624	T43.625	T43.626
androstanolone	T38.7X1	T38.7X2	T38.7X3	T38.7X4	T38.7X5	T38.7X6
atropine	T44.3X1	T44.3X2	T44.3X3	T44.3X4	T44.3X5	T44.3X6
benzene	T52.2X1	T52.2X2	T52.2X3	T52.2X4	—	—
benzoate	T52.8X1	T52.8X2	T52.8X3	T52.8X4	—	—
benzol	T52.2X1	T52.2X2	T52.2X3	T52.2X4	—	—
bromide (gas)	T59.891	T59.892	T59.893	T59.894	—	—
fumigant	T6Ø.8X1	T6Ø.8X2	T6Ø.8X3	T6Ø.8X4	—	—
butanol	T51.3X1	T51.3X2	T51.3X3	T51.3X4	—	—
carbinol	T51.1X1	T51.1X2	T51.1X3	T51.1X4	—	—
carbonate	T52.8X1	T52.8X2	T52.8X3	T52.8X4	—	—
CCNU	T45.1X1	T45.1X2	T45.1X3	T45.1X4	T45.1X5	T45.1X6
cellosolve	T52.91	T52.92	T52.93	T52.94	—	—
cellulose	T47.4X1	T47.4X2	T47.4X3	T47.4X4	T47.4X5	T47.4X6
chloride (gas)	T59.891	T59.892	T59.893	T59.894	—	—
chloroformate	T59.3X1	T59.3X2	T59.3X3	T59.3X4	—	—
cyclohexane	T52.8X1	T52.8X2	T52.8X3	T52.8X4	—	—
cyclohexanol	T51.8X1	T51.8X2	T51.8X3	T51.8X4	—	—

Substance	Poisoning, Accidental (unintentional)	Poisoning, Intentional Self-harm	Poisoning, Assault	Poisoning, Undetermined	Adverse Effect	Under-dosing
Methyl — *continued*						
cyclohexanone	T52.8X1	T52.8X2	T52.8X3	T52.8X4	—	—
cyclohexyl acetate	T52.8X1	T52.8X2	T52.8X3	T52.8X4	—	—
demeton	T6Ø.ØX1	T6Ø.ØX2	T6Ø.ØX3	T6Ø.ØX4	—	—
dihydromorphinone	T4Ø.2X1	T4Ø.2X2	T4Ø.2X3	T4Ø.2X4	T4Ø.2X5	T4Ø.2X6
ergometrine	T48.ØX1	T48.ØX2	T48.ØX3	T48.ØX4	T48.ØX5	T48.ØX6
ergonovine	T48.ØX1	T48.ØX2	T48.ØX3	T48.ØX4	T48.ØX5	T48.ØX6
ethyl ketone	T52.4X1	T52.4X2	T52.4X3	T52.4X4	—	—
glucamine antimonate	T37.8X1	T37.8X2	T37.8X3	T37.8X4	T37.8X5	T37.8X6
hydrazine	T65.891	T65.892	T65.893	T65.894	—	—
iodide	T65.891	T65.892	T65.893	T65.894	—	—
isobutyl ketone	T52.4X1	T52.4X2	T52.4X3	T52.4X4	—	—
isothiocyanate	T6Ø.3X1	T6Ø.3X2	T6Ø.3X3	T6Ø.3X4	—	—
mercaptan	T59.891	T59.892	T59.893	T59.894	—	—
morphine NEC	T4Ø.2X1	T4Ø.2X2	T4Ø.2X3	T4Ø.2X4	T4Ø.2X5	T4Ø.2X6
nicotinate	T49.4X1	T49.4X2	T49.4X3	T49.4X4	T49.4X5	T49.4X6
paraben	T49.ØX1	T49.ØX2	T49.ØX3	T49.ØX4	T49.ØX5	T49.ØX6
parafynol	T42.6X1	T42.6X2	T42.6X3	T42.6X4	T42.6X5	T42.6X6
parathion	T6Ø.ØX1	T6Ø.ØX2	T6Ø.ØX3	T6Ø.ØX4	—	—
peridol	T43.4X1	T43.4X2	T43.4X3	T43.4X4	T43.4X5	T43.4X6
phenidate	T43.631	T43.632	T43.633	T43.634	T43.635	T43.636
prednisolone	T38.ØX1	T38.ØX2	T38.ØX3	T38.ØX4	T38.ØX5	T38.ØX6
ENT agent	T49.6X1	T49.6X2	T49.6X3	T49.6X4	T49.6X5	T49.6X6
ophthalmic preparation	T49.5X1	T49.5X2	T49.5X3	T49.5X4	T49.5X5	T49.5X6
topical NEC	T49.ØX1	T49.ØX2	T49.ØX3	T49.ØX4	T49.ØX5	T49.ØX6
propylcarbinol	T51.3X1	T51.3X2	T51.3X3	T51.3X4	—	—
rosaniline NEC	T49.ØX1	T49.ØX2	T49.ØX3	T49.ØX4	T49.ØX5	T49.ØX6
salicylate	T49.2X1	T49.2X2	T49.2X3	T49.2X4	T49.2X5	T49.2X6
sulfate (fumes)	T59.891	T59.892	T59.893	T59.894	—	—
liquid	T52.8X1	T52.8X2	T52.8X3	T52.8X4	—	—
sulfonal	T42.6X1	T42.6X2	T42.6X3	T42.6X4	T42.6X5	T42.6X6
testosterone	T38.7X1	T38.7X2	T38.7X3	T38.7X4	T38.7X5	T38.7X6
thiouracil	T38.2X1	T38.2X2	T38.2X3	T38.2X4	T38.2X5	T38.2X6
Methylamphetamine	T43.621	T43.622	T43.623	T43.624	T43.625	T43.626
Methylated spirit	T51.1X1	T51.1X2	T51.1X3	T51.1X4	—	—
Methylatropine nitrate	T44.3X1	T44.3X2	T44.3X3	T44.3X4	T44.3X5	T44.3X6
Methylbenactyzium bromide	T44.3X1	T44.3X2	T44.3X3	T44.3X4	T44.3X5	T44.3X6
Methylbenzethonium chloride	T49.ØX1	T49.ØX2	T49.ØX3	T49.ØX4	T49.ØX5	T49.ØX6
Methylcellulose	T47.4X1	T47.4X2	T47.4X3	T47.4X4	T47.4X5	T47.4X6
laxative	T47.4X1	T47.4X2	T47.4X3	T47.4X4	T47.4X5	T47.4X6
Methylchlorophenoxyacetic acid	T6Ø.3X1	T6Ø.3X2	T6Ø.3X3	T6Ø.3X4	—	—
Methyldopa	T46.5X1	T46.5X2	T46.5X3	T46.5X4	T46.5X5	T46.5X6
Methyldopate	T46.5X1	T46.5X2	T46.5X3	T46.5X4	T46.5X5	T46.5X6
Methylene						
blue	T5Ø.6X1	T5Ø.6X2	T5Ø.6X3	T5Ø.6X4	T5Ø.6X5	T5Ø.6X6
chloride or dichloride (solvent) NEC	T53.4X1	T53.4X2	T53.4X3	T53.4X4	—	—
Methylenedioxyamphetamine	T43.621	T43.622	T43.623	T43.624	T43.625	T43.626
Methylenedioxymeth-amphetamine	T43.641	T43.642	T43.643	T43.644	—	—
Methylergometrine	T48.ØX1	T48.ØX2	T48.ØX3	T48.ØX4	T48.ØX5	T48.ØX6
Methylergonovine	T48.ØX1	T48.ØX2	T48.ØX3	T48.ØX4	T48.ØX5	T48.ØX6
Methylestrenolone	T38.5X1	T38.5X2	T38.5X3	T38.5X4	T38.5X5	T38.5X6
Methylethyl cellulose	T5Ø.991	T5Ø.992	T5Ø.993	T5Ø.994	T5Ø.995	T5Ø.996
Methylhexabital	T42.3X1	T42.3X2	T42.3X3	T42.3X4	T42.3X5	T42.3X6
Methylmorphine	T4Ø.2X1	T4Ø.2X2	T4Ø.2X3	T4Ø.2X4	T4Ø.2X5	T4Ø.2X6
Methylparaben (ophthalmic)	T49.5X1	T49.5X2	T49.5X3	T49.5X4	T49.5X5	T49.5X6
Methylparafynol	T42.6X1	T42.6X2	T42.6X3	T42.6X4	T42.6X5	T42.6X6
Methylpentynol, methylpenthynol	T42.6X1	T42.6X2	T42.6X3	T42.6X4	T42.6X5	T42.6X6
Methylphenidate	T43.631	T43.632	T43.633	T43.634	T43.635	T43.636
Methylphenobarbital	T42.3X1	T42.3X2	T42.3X3	T42.3X4	T42.3X5	T42.3X6
Methylpolysiloxane	T47.1X1	T47.1X2	T47.1X3	T47.1X4	T47.1X5	T47.1X6
Methylprednisolone — *see* Methyl, prednisolone						
Methylrosaniline	T49.ØX1	T49.ØX2	T49.ØX3	T49.ØX4	T49.ØX5	T49.ØX6
Methylrosanilinium chloride	T49.ØX1	T49.ØX2	T49.ØX3	T49.ØX4	T49.ØX5	T49.ØX6
Methyltestosterone	T38.7X1	T38.7X2	T38.7X3	T38.7X4	T38.7X5	T38.7X6
Methylthionine chloride	T5Ø.6X1	T5Ø.6X2	T5Ø.6X3	T5Ø.6X4	T5Ø.6X5	T5Ø.6X6
Methylthioninium chloride	T5Ø.6X1	T5Ø.6X2	T5Ø.6X3	T5Ø.6X4	T5Ø.6X5	T5Ø.6X6
Methylthiouracil	T38.2X1	T38.2X2	T38.2X3	T38.2X4	T38.2X5	T38.2X6
Methyprylon	T42.6X1	T42.6X2	T42.6X3	T42.6X4	T42.6X5	T42.6X6
Methysergide	T46.5X1	T46.5X2	T46.5X3	T46.5X4	T46.5X5	T46.5X6
Metiamide	T47.1X1	T47.1X2	T47.1X3	T47.1X4	T47.1X5	T47.1X6
Meticillin	T36.ØX1	T36.ØX2	T36.ØX3	T36.ØX4	T36.ØX5	T36.ØX6
Meticrane	T5Ø.2X1	T5Ø.2X2	T5Ø.2X3	T5Ø.2X4	T5Ø.2X5	T5Ø.2X6
Metildigoxin	T46.ØX1	T46.ØX2	T46.ØX3	T46.ØX4	T46.ØX5	T46.ØX6

Substance	Poisoning, Accidental (unintentional)	Poisoning, Intentional Self-harm	Poisoning, Assault	Poisoning, Undetermined	Adverse Effect	Under-dosing
Metipranolol	T49.5X1	T49.5X2	T49.5X3	T49.5X4	T49.5X5	T49.5X6
Metirosine	T46.5X1	T46.5X2	T46.5X3	T46.5X4	T46.5X5	T46.5X6
Metisazone	T37.5X1	T37.5X2	T37.5X3	T37.5X4	T37.5X5	T37.5X6
Metixene	T44.3X1	T44.3X2	T44.3X3	T44.3X4	T44.3X5	T44.3X6
Metizoline	T48.5X1	T48.5X2	T48.5X3	T48.5X4	T48.5X5	T48.5X6
Metoclopramide	T45.ØX1	T45.ØX2	T45.ØX3	T45.ØX4	T45.ØX5	T45.ØX6
Metofenazate	T43.3X1	T43.3X2	T43.3X3	T43.3X4	T43.3X5	T43.3X6
Metofoline	T39.8X1	T39.8X2	T39.8X3	T39.8X4	T39.8X5	T39.8X6
Metolazone	T5Ø.2X1	T5Ø.2X2	T5Ø.2X3	T5Ø.2X4	T5Ø.2X5	T5Ø.2X6
Metopon	T4Ø.2X1	T4Ø.2X2	T4Ø.2X3	T4Ø.2X4	T4Ø.2X5	T4Ø.2X6
Metoprine	T45.1X1	T45.1X2	T45.1X3	T45.1X4	T45.1X5	T45.1X6
Metoprolol	T44.7X1	T44.7X2	T44.7X3	T44.7X4	T44.7X5	T44.7X6
Metrifonate	T6Ø.ØX1	T6Ø.ØX2	T6Ø.ØX3	T6Ø.ØX4	—	—
Metrizamide	T5Ø.8X1	T5Ø.8X2	T5Ø.8X3	T5Ø.8X4	T5Ø.8X5	T5Ø.8X6
Metrizoic acid	T5Ø.8X1	T5Ø.8X2	T5Ø.8X3	T5Ø.8X4	T5Ø.8X5	T5Ø.8X6
Metronidazole	T37.8X1	T37.8X2	T37.8X3	T37.8X4	T37.8X5	T37.8X6
Metycaine	T41.3X1	T41.3X2	T41.3X3	T41.3X4	T41.3X5	T41.3X6
infiltration (subcutaneous)	T41.3X1	T41.3X2	T41.3X3	T41.3X4	T41.3X5	T41.3X6
nerve block (peripheral) (plexus)	T41.3X1	T41.3X2	T41.3X3	T41.3X4	T41.3X5	T41.3X6
topical (surface)	T41.3X1	T41.3X2	T41.3X3	T41.3X4	T41.3X5	T41.3X6
Metyrapone	T5Ø.8X1	T5Ø.8X2	T5Ø.8X3	T5Ø.8X4	T5Ø.8X5	T5Ø.8X6
Mevinphos	T6Ø.ØX1	T6Ø.ØX2	T6Ø.ØX3	T6Ø.ØX4	—	—
Mexazolam	T42.4X1	T42.4X2	T42.4X3	T42.4X4	T42.4X5	T42.4X6
Mexenone	T49.3X1	T49.3X2	T49.3X3	T49.3X4	T49.3X5	T49.3X6
Mexiletine	T46.2X1	T46.2X2	T46.2X3	T46.2X4	T46.2X5	T46.2X6
Mezereon	T62.2X1	T62.2X2	T62.2X3	T62.2X4	—	—
berries	T62.1X1	T62.1X2	T62.1X3	T62.1X4	—	—
Mezlocillin	T36.ØX1	T36.ØX2	T36.ØX3	T36.ØX4	T36.ØX5	T36.ØX6
Mianserin	T43.Ø21	T43.Ø22	T43.Ø23	T43.Ø24	T43.Ø25	T43.Ø26
Micatin	T49.ØX1	T49.ØX2	T49.ØX3	T49.ØX4	T49.ØX5	T49.ØX6
Miconazole	T49.ØX1	T49.ØX2	T49.ØX3	T49.ØX4	T49.ØX5	T49.ØX6
Micronomicin	T36.5X1	T36.5X2	T36.5X3	T36.5X4	T36.5X5	T36.5X6
Midazolam	T42.4X1	T42.4X2	T42.4X3	T42.4X4	T42.4X5	T42.4X6
Midecamycin	T36.3X1	T36.3X2	T36.3X3	T36.3X4	T36.3X5	T36.3X6
Mifepristone	T38.6X1	T38.6X2	T38.6X3	T38.6X4	T38.6X5	T38.6X6
Milk of magnesia	T47.1X1	T47.1X2	T47.1X3	T47.1X4	T47.1X5	T47.1X6
Millipede (tropical) (venomous)	T63.411	T63.412	T63.413	T63.414	—	—
Miltown	T43.591	T43.592	T43.593	T43.594	T43.595	T43.596
Milverine	T44.3X1	T44.3X2	T44.3X3	T44.3X4	T44.3X5	T44.3X6
Minaprine	T43.291	T43.292	T43.293	T43.294	T43.295	T43.296
Minaxolone	T41.291	T41.292	T41.293	T41.294	T41.295	T41.296
Mineral						
acids	T54.2X1	T54.2X2	T54.2X3	T54.2X4	—	—
oil (laxative)(medicinal)	T47.4X1	T47.4X2	T47.4X3	T47.4X4	T47.4X5	T47.4X6
emulsion	T47.2X1	T47.2X2	T47.2X3	T47.2X4	T47.2X5	T47.2X6
nonmedicinal	T52.ØX1	T52.ØX2	T52.ØX3	T52.ØX4	—	—
topical	T49.3X1	T49.3X2	T49.3X3	T49.3X4	T49.3X5	T49.3X6
salt NEC	T5Ø.3X1	T5Ø.3X2	T5Ø.3X3	T5Ø.3X4	T5Ø.3X5	T5Ø.3X6
spirits	T52.ØX1	T52.ØX2	T52.ØX3	T52.ØX4	—	—
Mineralocorticosteroid	T5Ø.ØX1	T5Ø.ØX2	T5Ø.ØX3	T5Ø.ØX4	T5Ø.ØX5	T5Ø.ØX6
Minocycline	T36.4X1	T36.4X2	T36.4X3	T36.4X4	T36.4X5	T36.4X6
Minoxidil	T46.7X1	T46.7X2	T46.7X3	T46.7X4	T46.7X5	T46.7X6
Miokamycin	T36.3X1	T36.3X2	T36.3X3	T36.3X4	T36.3X5	T36.3X6
Miotic drug	T49.5X1	T49.5X2	T49.5X3	T49.5X4	T49.5X5	T49.5X6
Mipafox	T6Ø.ØX1	T6Ø.ØX2	T6Ø.ØX3	T6Ø.ØX4	—	—
Mirex	T6Ø.1X1	T6Ø.1X2	T6Ø.1X3	T6Ø.1X4	—	—
Mirtazapine	T43.Ø21	T43.Ø22	T43.Ø23	T43.Ø24	T43.Ø25	T43.Ø26
Misonidazole	T37.3X1	T37.3X2	T37.3X3	T37.3X4	T37.3X5	T37.3X6
Misoprostol	T47.1X1	T47.1X2	T47.1X3	T47.1X4	T47.1X5	T47.1X6
Mithramycin	T45.1X1	T45.1X2	T45.1X3	T45.1X4	T45.1X5	T45.1X6
Mitobronitol	T45.1X1	T45.1X2	T45.1X3	T45.1X4	T45.1X5	T45.1X6
Mitoguazone	T45.1X1	T45.1X2	T45.1X3	T45.1X4	T45.1X5	T45.1X6
Mitolactol	T45.1X1	T45.1X2	T45.1X3	T45.1X4	T45.1X5	T45.1X6
Mitomycin	T45.1X1	T45.1X2	T45.1X3	T45.1X4	T45.1X5	T45.1X6
Mitopodozide	T45.1X1	T45.1X2	T45.1X3	T45.1X4	T45.1X5	T45.1X6
Mitotane	T45.1X1	T45.1X2	T45.1X3	T45.1X4	T45.1X5	T45.1X6
Mitoxantrone	T45.1X1	T45.1X2	T45.1X3	T45.1X4	T45.1X5	T45.1X6
Mivacurium chloride	T48.1X1	T48.1X2	T48.1X3	T48.1X4	T48.1X5	T48.1X6
Miyari bacteria	T47.6X1	T47.6X2	T47.6X3	T47.6X4	T47.6X5	T47.6X6
Moclobemide	T43.1X1	T43.1X2	T43.1X3	T43.1X4	T43.1X5	T43.1X6
Moderil	T46.5X1	T46.5X2	T46.5X3	T46.5X4	T46.5X5	T46.5X6
Mofebutazone	T39.2X1	T39.2X2	T39.2X3	T39.2X4	T39.2X5	T39.2X6
Mogadon — *see* Nitrazepam						
Molindone	T43.591	T43.592	T43.593	T43.594	T43.595	T43.596
Molsidomine	T46.3X1	T46.3X2	T46.3X3	T46.3X4	T46.3X5	T46.3X6
Mometasone	T49.ØX1	T49.ØX2	T49.ØX3	T49.ØX4	T49.ØX5	T49.ØX6
Monistat	T49.ØX1	T49.ØX2	T49.ØX3	T49.ØX4	T49.ØX5	T49.ØX6
Monkshood	T62.2X1	T62.2X2	T62.2X3	T62.2X4	—	—
Monoamine oxidase inhibitor NEC	T43.1X1	T43.1X2	T43.1X3	T43.1X4	T43.1X5	T43.1X6
hydrazine	T43.1X1	T43.1X2	T43.1X3	T43.1X4	T43.1X5	T43.1X6

Substance	Poisoning, Accidental (unintentional)	Poisoning, Intentional Self-harm	Poisoning, Assault	Poisoning, Undetermined	Adverse Effect	Under-dosing
Monobenzone	T49.4X1	T49.4X2	T49.4X3	T49.4X4	T49.4X5	T49.4X6
Monochloroacetic acid	T6Ø.3X1	T6Ø.3X2	T6Ø.3X3	T6Ø.3X4	—	—
Monochlorobenzene	T53.7X1	T53.7X2	T53.7X3	T53.7X4	—	—
Monoethanolamine	T46.8X1	T46.8X2	T46.8X3	T46.8X4	T46.8X5	T46.8X6
oleate	T46.8X1	T46.8X2	T46.8X3	T46.8X4	T46.8X5	T46.8X6
Monooctanoin	T5Ø.991	T5Ø.992	T5Ø.993	T5Ø.994	T5Ø.995	T5Ø.996
Monophenylbutazone	T39.2X1	T39.2X2	T39.2X3	T39.2X4	T39.2X5	T39.2X6
Monosodium glutamate	T65.891	T65.892	T65.893	T65.894	—	—
Monosulfiram	T49.ØX1	T49.ØX2	T49.ØX3	T49.ØX4	T49.ØX5	T49.ØX6
Monoxide, carbon — *see* Carbon, monoxide						
Monoxidine hydrochloride	T46.1X1	T46.1X2	T46.1X3	T46.1X4	T46.1X5	T46.1X6
Monuron	T6Ø.3X1	T6Ø.3X2	T6Ø.3X3	T6Ø.3X4	—	—
Moperone	T43.4X1	T43.4X2	T43.4X3	T43.4X4	T43.4X5	T43.4X6
Mopidamol	T45.1X1	T45.1X2	T45.1X3	T45.1X4	T45.1X5	T45.1X6
MOPP (mechloreth-amine + vincristine + prednisone + procarba-zine)	T45.1X1	T45.1X2	T45.1X3	T45.1X4	T45.1X5	T45.1X6
Morfin	T4Ø.2X1	T4Ø.2X2	T4Ø.2X3	T4Ø.2X4	T4Ø.2X5	T4Ø.2X6
Morinamide	T37.1X1	T37.1X2	T37.1X3	T37.1X4	T37.1X5	T37.1X6
Morning glory seeds	T4Ø.991	T4Ø.992	T4Ø.993	T4Ø.994	—	—
Moroxydine	T37.5X1	T37.5X2	T37.5X3	T37.5X4	T37.5X5	T37.5X6
Morphazinamide	T37.1X1	T37.1X2	T37.1X3	T37.1X4	T37.1X5	T37.1X6
Morphine	T4Ø.2X1	T4Ø.2X2	T4Ø.2X3	T4Ø.2X4	T4Ø.2X5	T4Ø.2X6
antagonist	T5Ø.7X1	T5Ø.7X2	T5Ø.7X3	T5Ø.7X4	T5Ø.7X5	T5Ø.7X6
Morpholinylethylmorphine	T4Ø.2X1	T4Ø.2X2	T4Ø.2X3	T4Ø.2X4	—	—
Morsuximide	T42.2X1	T42.2X2	T42.2X3	T42.2X4	T42.2X5	T42.2X6
Mosapramine	T43.591	T43.592	T43.593	T43.594	T43.595	T43.596
Moth balls — *see also* Pesticides	T6Ø.2X1	T6Ø.2X2	T6Ø.2X3	T6Ø.2X4	—	—
naphthalene	T6Ø.2X1	T6Ø.2X2	T6Ø.2X3	T6Ø.2X4	—	—
paradichlorobenzene	T6Ø.1X1	T6Ø.1X2	T6Ø.1X3	T6Ø.1X4	—	—
Motor exhaust gas	T58.Ø1	T58.Ø2	T58.Ø3	T58.Ø4	—	—
Mouthwash (antiseptic) (zinc chloride)	T49.6X1	T49.6X2	T49.6X3	T49.6X4	T49.6X5	T49.6X6
Moxastine	T45.ØX1	T45.ØX2	T45.ØX3	T45.ØX4	T45.ØX5	T45.ØX6
Moxaverine	T44.3X1	T44.3X2	T44.3X3	T44.3X4	T44.3X5	T44.3X6
Moxisylyte	T46.7X1	T46.7X2	T46.7X3	T46.7X4	T46.7X5	T46.7X6
Mucilage, plant	T47.4X1	T47.4X2	T47.4X3	T47.4X4	T47.4X5	T47.4X6
Mucolytic drug	T48.4X1	T48.4X2	T48.4X3	T48.4X4	T48.4X5	T48.4X6
Mucomyst	T48.4X1	T48.4X2	T48.4X3	T48.4X4	T48.4X5	T48.4X6
Mucous membrane agents (external)	T49.91	T49.92	T49.93	T49.94	T49.95	T49.96
specified NEC	T49.8X1	T49.8X2	T49.8X3	T49.8X4	T49.8X5	T49.8X6
Multiple unspecified drugs, medicaments and biological substances	T5Ø.911	T5Ø.912	T5Ø.913	T5Ø.914	T5Ø.915	T5Ø.916
Mumps						
immune globulin (human)	T5Ø.Z11	T5Ø.Z12	T5Ø.Z13	T5Ø.Z14	T5Ø.Z15	T5Ø.Z16
skin test antigen	T5Ø.8X1	T5Ø.8X2	T5Ø.8X3	T5Ø.8X4	T5Ø.8X5	T5Ø.8X6
vaccine	T5Ø.B91	T5Ø.B92	T5Ø.B93	T5Ø.B94	T5Ø.B95	T5Ø.B96
Mumpsvax	T5Ø.B91	T5Ø.B92	T5Ø.B93	T5Ø.B94	T5Ø.B95	T5Ø.B96
Mupirocin	T49.ØX1	T49.ØX2	T49.ØX3	T49.ØX4	T49.ØX5	T49.ØX6
Muriatic acid — *see* Hydrochloric acid						
Muromonab-CD3	T45.1X1	T45.1X2	T45.1X3	T45.1X4	T45.1X5	T45.1X6
Muscle-action drug NEC	T48.2Ø1	T48.2Ø2	T48.2Ø3	T48.2Ø4	T48.2Ø5	T48.2Ø6
Muscle affecting agents NEC	T48.2Ø1	T48.2Ø2	T48.2Ø3	T48.2Ø4	T48.2Ø5	T48.2Ø6
oxytocic	T48.ØX1	T48.ØX2	T48.ØX3	T48.ØX4	T48.ØX5	T48.ØX6
relaxants	T48.2Ø1	T48.2Ø2	T48.2Ø3	T48.2Ø4	T48.2Ø5	T48.2Ø6
central nervous system	T42.8X1	T42.8X2	T42.8X3	T42.8X4	T42.8X5	T42.8X6
skeletal	T48.1X1	T48.1X2	T48.1X3	T48.1X4	T48.1X5	T48.1X6
smooth	T44.3X1	T44.3X2	T44.3X3	T44.3X4	T44.3X5	T44.3X6
Muscle relaxant — *see* Relaxant, muscle						
Muscle-tone depressant, central NEC	T42.8X1	T42.8X2	T42.8X3	T42.8X4	T42.8X5	T42.8X6
specified NEC	T42.8X1	T42.8X2	T42.8X3	T42.8X4	T42.8X5	T42.8X6
Mushroom, noxious	T62.ØX1	T62.ØX2	T62.ØX3	T62.ØX4	—	—
Mussel, noxious	T61.781	T61.782	T61.783	T61.784	—	—
Mustard (emetic)	T47.7X1	T47.7X2	T47.7X3	T47.7X4	T47.7X5	T47.7X6
black	T47.7X1	T47.7X2	T47.7X3	T47.7X4	T47.7X5	T47.7X6
gas, not in war	T59.91	T59.92	T59.93	T59.94	—	—
nitrogen	T45.1X1	T45.1X2	T45.1X3	T45.1X4	T45.1X5	T45.1X6
Mustine	T45.1X1	T45.1X2	T45.1X3	T45.1X4	T45.1X5	T45.1X6
M-vac	T45.1X1	T45.1X2	T45.1X3	T45.1X4	T45.1X5	T45.1X6
Mycifradin	T36.5X1	T36.5X2	T36.5X3	T36.5X4	T36.5X5	T36.5X6
topical	T49.ØX1	T49.ØX2	T49.ØX3	T49.ØX4	T49.ØX5	T49.ØX6
Mycitracin	T36.8X1	T36.8X2	T36.8X3	T36.8X4	T36.8X5	T36.8X6
ophthalmic preparation	T49.5X1	T49.5X2	T49.5X3	T49.5X4	T49.5X5	T49.5X6
Mycostatin	T36.7X1	T36.7X2	T36.7X3	T36.7X4	T36.7X5	T36.7X6
topical	T49.ØX1	T49.ØX2	T49.ØX3	T49.ØX4	T49.ØX5	T49.ØX6

Substance	Poisoning, Accidental (unintentional)	Poisoning, Intentional Self-harm	Poisoning, Assault	Poisoning, Undetermined	Adverse Effect	Under-dosing
Mycotoxins	T64.81	T64.82	T64.83	T64.84	—	—
aflatoxin	T64.01	T64.02	T64.03	T64.04	—	—
specified NEC	T64.81	T64.82	T64.83	T64.84	—	—
Mydriacyl	T44.3X1	T44.3X2	T44.3X3	T44.3X4	T44.3X5	T44.3X6
Mydriatic drug	T49.5X1	T49.5X2	T49.5X3	T49.5X4	T49.5X5	T49.5X6
Myelobromal	T45.1X1	T45.1X2	T45.1X3	T45.1X4	T45.1X5	T45.1X6
Myleran	T45.1X1	T45.1X2	T45.1X3	T45.1X4	T45.1X5	T45.1X6
Myochrysin (e)	T39.2X1	T39.2X2	T39.2X3	T39.2X4	T39.2X5	T39.2X6
Myoneural blocking agents	T48.1X1	T48.1X2	T48.1X3	T48.1X4	T48.1X5	T48.1X6
Myralact	T49.0X1	T49.0X2	T49.0X3	T49.0X4	T49.0X5	T49.0X6
Myristica fragrans	T62.2X1	T62.2X2	T62.2X3	T62.2X4	—	—
Myristicin	T65.891	T65.892	T65.893	T65.894	—	—
Mysoline	T42.3X1	T42.3X2	T42.3X3	T42.3X4	T42.3X5	T42.3X6
Nabilone	T40.7X1	T40.7X2	T40.7X3	T40.7X4	T40.7X5	T40.7X6
Nabumetone	T39.391	T39.392	T39.393	T39.394	T39.395	T39.396
Nadolol	T44.7X1	T44.7X2	T44.7X3	T44.7X4	T44.7X5	T44.7X6
Nafcillin	T36.0X1	T36.0X2	T36.0X3	T36.0X4	T36.0X5	T36.0X6
Nafoxidine	T38.6X1	T38.6X2	T38.6X3	T38.6X4	T38.6X5	T38.6X6
Naftazone	T46.991	T46.992	T46.993	T46.994	T46.995	T46.996
Naftidrofuryl (oxalate)	T46.7X1	T46.7X2	T46.7X3	T46.7X4	T46.7X5	T46.7X6
Naftifine	T49.0X1	T49.0X2	T49.0X3	T49.0X4	T49.0X5	T49.0X6
Nail polish remover	T52.91	T52.92	T52.93	T52.94	—	—
Nalbuphine	T40.491	T40.492	T40.493	T40.494	T40.495	T40.496
Naled	T60.0X1	T60.0X2	T60.0X3	T60.0X4	—	—
Nalidixic acid	T37.8X1	T37.8X2	T37.8X3	T37.8X4	T37.8X5	T37.8X6
Nalorphine	T50.7X1	T50.7X2	T50.7X3	T50.7X4	T50.7X5	T50.7X6
Naloxone	T50.7X1	T50.7X2	T50.7X3	T50.7X4	T50.7X5	T50.7X6
Naltrexone	T50.7X1	T50.7X2	T50.7X3	T50.7X4	T50.7X5	T50.7X6
Namenda	T43.8X1	T43.8X2	T43.8X3	T43.8X4	T43.8X5	T43.8X6
Nandrolone	T38.7X1	T38.7X2	T38.7X3	T38.7X4	T38.7X5	T38.7X6
Naphazoline	T48.5X1	T48.5X2	T48.5X3	T48.5X4	T48.5X5	T48.5X6
Naphtha (painters') (petroleum)	T52.0X1	T52.0X2	T52.0X3	T52.0X4	—	—
solvent	T52.0X1	T52.0X2	T52.0X3	T52.0X4	—	—
vapor	T52.0X1	T52.0X2	T52.0X3	T52.0X4	—	—
Naphthalene (non-chlorinated)	T60.2X1	T60.2X2	T60.2X3	T60.2X4	—	—
chlorinated	T60.1X1	T60.1X2	T60.1X3	T60.1X4	—	—
vapor	T60.1X1	T60.1X2	T60.1X3	T60.1X4	—	—
insecticide or moth repellent	T60.2X1	T60.2X2	T60.2X3	T60.2X4	—	—
chlorinated	T60.1X1	T60.1X2	T60.1X3	T60.1X4	—	—
vapor	T60.2X1	T60.2X2	T60.2X3	T60.2X4	—	—
chlorinated	T60.1X1	T60.1X2	T60.1X3	T60.1X4	—	—
Naphthol	T65.891	T65.892	T65.893	T65.894	—	—
Naphthylamine	T65.891	T65.892	T65.893	T65.894	—	—
Naphthylthiourea (ANTU)	T60.4X1	T60.4X2	T60.4X3	T60.4X4	—	—
Naprosyn — *see* Naproxen						
Naproxen	T39.311	T39.312	T39.313	T39.314	T39.315	T39.316
Narcotic (drug)	T40.601	T40.602	T40.603	T40.604	T40.605	T40.606
analgesic NEC	T40.601	T40.602	T40.603	T40.604	T40.605	T40.606
antagonist	T50.7X1	T50.7X2	T50.7X3	T50.7X4	T50.7X5	T50.7X6
specified NEC	T40.691	T40.692	T40.693	T40.694	T40.695	T40.696
synthetic	T40.491	T40.492	T40.493	T40.494	T40.495	T40.496
Narcotine	T48.3X1	T48.3X2	T48.3X3	T48.3X4	T48.3X5	T48.3X6
Nardil	T43.1X1	T43.1X2	T43.1X3	T43.1X4	T43.1X5	T43.1X6
Nasal drug NEC	T49.6X1	T49.6X2	T49.6X3	T49.6X4	T49.6X5	T49.6X6
Natamycin	T49.0X1	T49.0X2	T49.0X3	T49.0X4	T49.0X5	T49.0X6
Natrium cyanide — *see* Cyanide(s)						
Natural						
blood (product)	T45.8X1	T45.8X2	T45.8X3	T45.8X4	T45.8X5	T45.8X6
gas (piped)	T59.891	T59.892	T59.893	T59.894	—	—
incomplete combustion	T58.11	T58.12	T58.13	T58.14	—	—
Nealbarbital	T42.3X1	T42.3X2	T42.3X3	T42.3X4	T42.3X5	T42.3X6
Nectadon	T48.3X1	T48.3X2	T48.3X3	T48.3X4	T48.3X5	T48.3X6
Nedocromil	T48.6X1	T48.6X2	T48.6X3	T48.6X4	T48.6X5	T48.6X6
Nefopam	T39.8X1	T39.8X2	T39.8X3	T39.8X4	T39.8X5	T39.8X6
Nematocyst (sting)	T63.691	T63.692	T63.693	T63.694	—	—
Nembutal	T42.3X1	T42.3X2	T42.3X3	T42.3X4	T42.3X5	T42.3X6
Nemonapride	T43.591	T43.592	T43.593	T43.594	T43.595	T43.596
Neoarsphenamine	T37.8X1	T37.8X2	T37.8X3	T37.8X4	T37.8X5	T37.8X6
Neocinchophen	T50.4X1	T50.4X2	T50.4X3	T50.4X4	T50.4X5	T50.4X6
Neomycin (derivatives)	T36.5X1	T36.5X2	T36.5X3	T36.5X4	T36.5X5	T36.5X6
with						
bacitracin	T49.0X1	T49.0X2	T49.0X3	T49.0X4	T49.0X5	T49.0X6
neostigmine	T44.0X1	T44.0X2	T44.0X3	T44.0X4	T44.0X5	T44.0X6
ENT agent	T49.6X1	T49.6X2	T49.6X3	T49.6X4	T49.6X5	T49.6X6
ophthalmic preparation	T49.5X1	T49.5X2	T49.5X3	T49.5X4	T49.5X5	T49.5X6
topical NEC	T49.0X1	T49.0X2	T49.0X3	T49.0X4	T49.0X5	T49.0X6
Neonal	T42.3X1	T42.3X2	T42.3X3	T42.3X4	T42.3X5	T42.3X6
Neoprontosil	T37.0X1	T37.0X2	T37.0X3	T37.0X4	T37.0X5	T37.0X6

Substance	Poisoning, Accidental (unintentional)	Poisoning, Intentional Self-harm	Poisoning, Assault	Poisoning, Undetermined	Adverse Effect	Under-dosing
Neosalvarsan	T37.8X1	T37.8X2	T37.8X3	T37.8X4	T37.8X5	T37.8X6
Neosilversalvarsan	T37.8X1	T37.8X2	T37.8X3	T37.8X4	T37.8X5	T37.8X6
Neosporin	T36.8X1	T36.8X2	T36.8X3	T36.8X4	T36.8X5	T36.8X6
ENT agent	T49.6X1	T49.6X2	T49.6X3	T49.6X4	T49.6X5	T49.6X6
opthalmic preparation	T49.5X1	T49.5X2	T49.5X3	T49.5X4	T49.5X5	T49.5X6
topical NEC	T49.0X1	T49.0X2	T49.0X3	T49.0X4	T49.0X5	T49.0X6
Neostigmine bromide	T44.0X1	T44.0X2	T44.0X3	T44.0X4	T44.0X5	T44.0X6
Neraval	T42.3X1	T42.3X2	T42.3X3	T42.3X4	T42.3X5	T42.3X6
Neravan	T42.3X1	T42.3X2	T42.3X3	T42.3X4	T42.3X5	T42.3X6
Nerium oleander	T62.2X1	T62.2X2	T62.2X3	T62.2X4	—	—
Nerve gas, not in war	T59.91	T59.92	T59.93	T59.94	—	—
Nesacaine	T41.3X1	T41.3X2	T41.3X3	T41.3X4	T41.3X5	T41.3X6
infiltration (subcutaneous)	T41.3X1	T41.3X2	T41.3X3	T41.3X4	T41.3X5	T41.3X6
nerve block (peripheral) (plexus)	T41.3X1	T41.3X2	T41.3X3	T41.3X4	T41.3X5	T41.3X6
Netilmicin	T36.5X1	T36.5X2	T36.5X3	T36.5X4	T36.5X5	T36.5X6
Neurobarb	T42.3X1	T42.3X2	T42.3X3	T42.3X4	T42.3X5	T42.3X6
Neuroleptic drug NEC	T43.501	T43.502	T43.503	T43.504	T43.505	T43.506
Neuromuscular blocking drug	T48.1X1	T48.1X2	T48.1X3	T48.1X4	T48.1X5	T48.1X6
Neutral insulin injection	T38.3X1	T38.3X2	T38.3X3	T38.3X4	T38.3X5	T38.3X6
Neutral spirits	T51.0X1	T51.0X2	T51.0X3	T51.0X4	—	—
beverage	T51.0X1	T51.0X2	T51.0X3	T51.0X4	—	—
Niacin	T46.7X1	T46.7X2	T46.7X3	T46.7X4	T46.7X5	T46.7X6
Niacinamide	T45.2X1	T45.2X2	T45.2X3	T45.2X4	T45.2X5	T45.2X6
Nialamide	T43.1X1	T43.1X2	T43.1X3	T43.1X4	T43.1X5	T43.1X6
Niaprazine	T42.6X1	T42.6X2	T42.6X3	T42.6X4	T42.6X5	T42.6X6
Nicametate	T46.7X1	T46.7X2	T46.7X3	T46.7X4	T46.7X5	T46.7X6
Nicardipine	T46.1X1	T46.1X2	T46.1X3	T46.1X4	T46.1X5	T46.1X6
Nicergoline	T46.7X1	T46.7X2	T46.7X3	T46.7X4	T46.7X5	T46.7X6
Nickel (carbonyl) (tetra-carbonyl) (fumes) (vapor)	T56.891	T56.892	T56.893	T56.894	—	—
Nickelocene	T56.891	T56.892	T56.893	T56.894	—	—
Niclosamide	T37.4X1	T37.4X2	T37.4X3	T37.4X4	T37.4X5	T37.4X6
Nicofuranose	T46.7X1	T46.7X2	T46.7X3	T46.7X4	T46.7X5	T46.7X6
Nicomorphine	T40.2X1	T40.2X2	T40.2X3	T40.2X4	—	—
Nicorandil	T46.3X1	T46.3X2	T46.3X3	T46.3X4	T46.3X5	T46.3X6
Nicotiana (plant)	T62.2X1	T62.2X2	T62.2X3	T62.2X4	—	—
Nicotinamide	T45.2X1	T45.2X2	T45.2X3	T45.2X4	T45.2X5	T45.2X6
Nicotine (insecticide) (spray) (sulfate) **NEC**	T60.2X1	T60.2X2	T60.2X3	T60.2X4	—	—
from tobacco	T65.291	T65.292	T65.293	T65.294	—	—
cigarettes	T65.221	T65.222	T65.223	T65.224	—	—
not insecticide	T65.291	T65.292	T65.293	T65.294	—	—
Nicotinic acid	T46.7X1	T46.7X2	T46.7X3	T46.7X4	T46.7X5	T46.7X6
Nicotinyl alcohol	T46.7X1	T46.7X2	T46.7X3	T46.7X4	T46.7X5	T46.7X6
Nicoumalone	T45.511	T45.512	T45.513	T45.514	T45.515	T45.516
Nifedipine	T46.1X1	T46.1X2	T46.1X3	T46.1X4	T46.1X5	T46.1X6
Nifenazone	T39.2X1	T39.2X2	T39.2X3	T39.2X4	T39.2X5	T39.2X6
Nifuraldezone	T37.91	T37.92	T37.93	T37.94	T37.95	T37.96
Nifuratel	T37.8X1	T37.8X2	T37.8X3	T37.8X4	T37.8X5	T37.8X6
Nifurtimox	T37.3X1	T37.3X2	T37.3X3	T37.3X4	T37.3X5	T37.3X6
Nifurtoinol	T37.8X1	T37.8X2	T37.8X3	T37.8X4	T37.8X5	T37.8X6
Nightshade, deadly (solanum) — *see also* Belladonna	T62.2X1	T62.2X2	T62.2X3	T62.2X4	—	—
berry	T62.1X1	T62.1X2	T62.1X3	T62.1X4	—	—
Nikethamide	T50.7X1	T50.7X2	T50.7X3	T50.7X4	T50.7X5	T50.7X6
Nilstat	T36.7X1	T36.7X2	T36.7X3	T36.7X4	T36.7X5	T36.7X6
topical	T49.0X1	T49.0X2	T49.0X3	T49.0X4	T49.0X5	T49.0X6
Nilutamide	T38.6X1	T38.6X2	T38.6X3	T38.6X4	T38.6X5	T38.6X6
Nimesulide	T39.391	T39.392	T39.393	T39.394	T39.395	T39.396
Nimetazepam	T42.4X1	T42.4X2	T42.4X3	T42.4X4	T42.4X5	T42.4X6
Nimodipine	T46.1X1	T46.1X2	T46.1X3	T46.1X4	T46.1X5	T46.1X6
Nimorazole	T37.3X1	T37.3X2	T37.3X3	T37.3X4	T37.3X5	T37.3X6
Nimustine	T45.1X1	T45.1X2	T45.1X3	T45.1X4	T45.1X5	T45.1X6
Niridazole	T37.4X1	T37.4X2	T37.4X3	T37.4X4	T37.4X5	T37.4X6
Nisentil	T40.2X1	T40.2X2	T40.2X3	T40.2X4	T40.2X5	T40.2X6
Nisoldipine	T46.1X1	T46.1X2	T46.1X3	T46.1X4	T46.1X5	T46.1X6
Nitramine	T65.3X1	T65.3X2	T65.3X3	T65.3X4	—	—
Nitrate, organic	T46.3X1	T46.3X2	T46.3X3	T46.3X4	T46.3X5	T46.3X6
Nitrazepam	T42.4X1	T42.4X2	T42.4X3	T42.4X4	T42.4X5	T42.4X6
Nitrefazole	T50.6X1	T50.6X2	T50.6X3	T50.6X4	T50.6X5	T50.6X6
Nitrendipine	T46.1X1	T46.1X2	T46.1X3	T46.1X4	T46.1X5	T46.1X6
Nitric						
acid (liquid)	T54.2X1	T54.2X2	T54.2X3	T54.2X4	—	—
vapor	T59.891	T59.892	T59.893	T59.894	—	—
oxide (gas)	T59.0X1	T59.0X2	T59.0X3	T59.0X4	—	—
Nitrimidazine	T37.3X1	T37.3X2	T37.3X3	T37.3X4	T37.3X5	T37.3X6
Nitrite, amyl (medicinal) (vapor)	T46.3X1	T46.3X2	T46.3X3	T46.3X4	T46.3X5	T46.3X6
Nitroaniline	T65.3X1	T65.3X2	T65.3X3	T65.3X4	—	—
vapor	T59.891	T59.892	T59.893	T59.894	—	—
Nitrobenzene, nitrobenzol	T65.3X1	T65.3X2	T65.3X3	T65.3X4	—	—

Substance	Poisoning, Accidental (unintentional)	Poisoning, Intentional Self-harm	Poisoning, Assault	Poisoning, Undetermined	Adverse Effect	Under-dosing
Nitrobenzene, nitrobenzol — *continued*						
vapor	T65.3X1	T65.3X2	T65.3X3	T65.3X4	—	—
Nitrocellulose	T65.891	T65.892	T65.893	T65.894	—	—
lacquer	T65.891	T65.892	T65.893	T65.894	—	—
Nitrodiphenyl	T65.3X1	T65.3X2	T65.3X3	T65.3X4	—	—
Nitrofural	T49.ØX1	T49.ØX2	T49.ØX3	T49.ØX4	T49.ØX5	T49.ØX6
Nitrofurantoin	T37.8X1	T37.8X2	T37.8X3	T37.8X4	T37.8X5	T37.8X6
Nitrofurazone	T49.ØX1	T49.ØX2	T49.ØX3	T49.ØX4	T49.ØX5	T49.ØX6
Nitrogen	T59.ØX1	T59.ØX2	T59.ØX3	T59.ØX4	—	—
mustard	T45.1X1	T45.1X2	T45.1X3	T45.1X4	T45.1X5	T45.1X6
Nitroglycerin, nitroglycerol (medicinal)	T46.3X1	T46.3X2	T46.3X3	T46.3X4	T46.3X5	T46.3X6
nonmedicinal	T65.5X1	T65.5X2	T65.5X3	T65.5X4	—	—
fumes	T65.5X1	T65.5X2	T65.5X3	T65.5X4	—	—
Nitroglycol	T52.3X1	T52.3X2	T52.3X3	T52.3X4	—	—
Nitrohydrochloric acid	T54.2X1	T54.2X2	T54.2X3	T54.2X4	—	—
Nitromersol	T49.ØX1	T49.ØX2	T49.ØX3	T49.ØX4	T49.ØX5	T49.ØX6
Nitronaphthalene	T65.891	T65.892	T65.893	T65.894	—	—
Nitrophenol	T54.ØX1	T54.ØX2	T54.ØX3	T54.ØX4	—	—
Nitropropane	T52.8X1	T52.8X2	T52.8X3	T52.8X4	—	—
Nitroprusside	T46.5X1	T46.5X2	T46.5X3	T46.5X4	T46.5X5	T46.5X6
Nitrosodimethylamine	T65.3X1	T65.3X2	T65.3X3	T65.3X4	—	—
Nitrothiazol	T37.4X1	T37.4X2	T37.4X3	T37.4X4	T37.4X5	T37.4X6
Nitrotoluene, nitrotoluol	T65.3X1	T65.3X2	T65.3X3	T65.3X4	—	—
vapor	T65.3X1	T65.3X2	T65.3X3	T65.3X4	—	—
Nitrous						
acid (liquid)	T54.2X1	T54.2X2	T54.2X3	T54.2X4	—	—
fumes	T59.891	T59.892	T59.893	T59.894	—	—
ether spirit	T46.3X1	T46.3X2	T46.3X3	T46.3X4	T46.3X5	T46.3X6
oxide	T41.ØX1	T41.ØX2	T41.ØX3	T41.ØX4	T41.ØX5	T41.ØX6
Nitroxoline	T37.8X1	T37.8X2	T37.8X3	T37.8X4	T37.8X5	T37.8X6
Nitrozone	T49.ØX1	T49.ØX2	T49.ØX3	T49.ØX4	T49.ØX5	T49.ØX6
Nizatidine	T47.ØX1	T47.ØX2	T47.ØX3	T47.ØX4	T47.ØX5	T47.ØX6
Nizofenone	T43.8X1	T43.8X2	T43.8X3	T43.8X4	T43.8X5	T43.8X6
Noctec	T42.6X1	T42.6X2	T42.6X3	T42.6X4	T42.6X5	T42.6X6
Noludar	T42.6X1	T42.6X2	T42.6X3	T42.6X4	T42.6X5	T42.6X6
Nomegestrol	T38.5X1	T38.5X2	T38.5X3	T38.5X4	T38.5X5	T38.5X6
Nomifensine	T43.291	T43.292	T43.293	T43.294	T43.295	T43.296
Nonoxinol	T49.8X1	T49.8X2	T49.8X3	T49.8X4	T49.8X5	T49.8X6
Nonylphenoxy (polyethoxyethanol)	T49.8X1	T49.8X2	T49.8X3	T49.8X4	T49.8X5	T49.8X6
Noptil	T42.3X1	T42.3X2	T42.3X3	T42.3X4	T42.3X5	T42.3X6
Noradrenaline	T44.4X1	T44.4X2	T44.4X3	T44.4X4	T44.4X5	T44.4X6
Noramidopyrine	T39.2X1	T39.2X2	T39.2X3	T39.2X4	T39.2X5	T39.2X6
methanesulfonate sodium	T39.2X1	T39.2X2	T39.2X3	T39.2X4	T39.2X5	T39.2X6
Norbormide	T60.4X1	T60.4X2	T60.4X3	T60.4X4	—	—
Nordazepam	T42.4X1	T42.4X2	T42.4X3	T42.4X4	T42.4X5	T42.4X6
Norepinephrine	T44.4X1	T44.4X2	T44.4X3	T44.4X4	T44.4X5	T44.4X6
Norethandrolone	T38.7X1	T38.7X2	T38.7X3	T38.7X4	T38.7X5	T38.7X6
Norethindrone	T38.4X1	T38.4X2	T38.4X3	T38.4X4	T38.4X5	T38.4X6
Norethisterone (acetate) (enantate)	T38.4X1	T38.4X2	T38.4X3	T38.4X4	T38.4X5	T38.4X6
with ethinylestradiol	T38.5X1	T38.5X2	T38.5X3	T38.5X4	T38.5X5	T38.5X6
Noretynodrel	T38.5X1	T38.5X2	T38.5X3	T38.5X4	T38.5X5	T38.5X6
Norfenefrine	T44.4X1	T44.4X2	T44.4X3	T44.4X4	T44.4X5	T44.4X6
Norfloxacin	T36.8X1	T36.8X2	T36.8X3	T36.8X4	T36.8X5	T36.8X6
Norgestrel	T38.4X1	T38.4X2	T38.4X3	T38.4X4	T38.4X5	T38.4X6
Norgestrienone	T38.4X1	T38.4X2	T38.4X3	T38.4X4	T38.4X5	T38.4X6
Norlestrin	T38.4X1	T38.4X2	T38.4X3	T38.4X4	T38.4X5	T38.4X6
Norlutin	T38.4X1	T38.4X2	T38.4X3	T38.4X4	T38.4X5	T38.4X6
Normal serum albumin (human), salt-poor	T45.8X1	T45.8X2	T45.8X3	T45.8X4	T45.8X5	T45.8X6
Normethandrone	T38.5X1	T38.5X2	T38.5X3	T38.5X4	T38.5X5	T38.5X6
Normison — *see* Benzodiazepines						
Normorphine	T40.2X1	T40.2X2	T40.2X3	T40.2X4	—	—
Norpseudoephedrine	T50.5X1	T50.5X2	T50.5X3	T50.5X4	T50.5X5	T50.5X6
Nortestosterone (furanpropionate)	T38.7X1	T38.7X2	T38.7X3	T38.7X4	T38.7X5	T38.7X6
Nortriptyline	T43.Ø11	T43.Ø12	T43.Ø13	T43.Ø14	T43.Ø15	T43.Ø16
Noscapine	T48.3X1	T48.3X2	T48.3X3	T48.3X4	T48.3X5	T48.3X6
Nose preparations	T49.6X1	T49.6X2	T49.6X3	T49.6X4	T49.6X5	T49.6X6
Novobiocin	T36.5X1	T36.5X2	T36.5X3	T36.5X4	T36.5X5	T36.5X6
Novocain (infiltration) (topical)	T41.3X1	T41.3X2	T41.3X3	T41.3X4	T41.3X5	T41.3X6
nerve block (peripheral) (plexus)	T41.3X1	T41.3X2	T41.3X3	T41.3X4	T41.3X5	T41.3X6
spinal	T41.3X1	T41.3X2	T41.3X3	T41.3X4	T41.3X5	T41.3X6
Noxious foodstuff	T62.91	T62.92	T62.93	T62.94	—	—
specified NEC	T62.8X1	T62.8X2	T62.8X3	T62.8X4	—	—
Noxiptiline	T43.Ø11	T43.Ø12	T43.Ø13	T43.Ø14	T43.Ø15	T43.Ø16
Noxytiolin	T49.ØX1	T49.ØX2	T49.ØX3	T49.ØX4	T49.ØX5	T49.ØX6

Substance	Poisoning, Accidental (unintentional)	Poisoning, Intentional Self-harm	Poisoning, Assault	Poisoning, Undetermined	Adverse Effect	Under-dosing
NPH Iletin (insulin)	T38.3X1	T38.3X2	T38.3X3	T38.3X4	T38.3X5	T38.3X6
Numorphan	T40.2X1	T40.2X2	T40.2X3	T40.2X4	T40.2X5	T40.2X6
Nunol	T42.3X1	T42.3X2	T42.3X3	T42.3X4	T42.3X5	T42.3X6
Nupercaine (spinal anesthetic)	T41.3X1	T41.3X2	T41.3X3	T41.3X4	T41.3X5	T41.3X6
topical (surface)	T41.3X1	T41.3X2	T41.3X3	T41.3X4	T41.3X5	T41.3X6
Nutmeg oil (liniment)	T49.3X1	T49.3X2	T49.3X3	T49.3X4	T49.3X5	T49.3X6
Nutritional supplement	T50.901	T50.902	T50.903	T50.904	T50.905	T50.906
Nux vomica	T65.1X1	T65.1X2	T65.1X3	T65.1X4	—	—
Nydrazid	T37.1X1	T37.1X2	T37.1X3	T37.1X4	T37.1X5	T37.1X6
Nylidrin	T46.7X1	T46.7X2	T46.7X3	T46.7X4	T46.7X5	T46.7X6
Nystatin	T36.7X1	T36.7X2	T36.7X3	T36.7X4	T36.7X5	T36.7X6
topical	T49.ØX1	T49.ØX2	T49.ØX3	T49.ØX4	T49.ØX5	T49.ØX6
Nytol	T45.ØX1	T45.ØX2	T45.ØX3	T45.ØX4	T45.ØX5	T45.ØX6
Obidoxime chloride	T50.6X1	T50.6X2	T50.6X3	T50.6X4	T50.6X5	T50.6X6
Octafonium (chloride)	T49.3X1	T49.3X2	T49.3X3	T49.3X4	T49.3X5	T49.3X6
Octamethyl pyrophosphoramide	T60.ØX1	T60.ØX2	T60.ØX3	T60.ØX4	—	—
Octanoin	T50.991	T50.992	T50.993	T50.994	T50.995	T50.996
Octatropine methylbromide	T44.3X1	T44.3X2	T44.3X3	T44.3X4	T44.3X5	T44.3X6
Octotiamine	T45.2X1	T45.2X2	T45.2X3	T45.2X4	T45.2X5	T45.2X6
Octoxinol (9)	T49.8X1	T49.8X2	T49.8X3	T49.8X4	T49.8X5	T49.8X6
Octreotide	T38.991	T38.992	T38.993	T38.994	T38.995	T38.996
Octyl nitrite	T46.3X1	T46.3X2	T46.3X3	T46.3X4	T46.3X5	T46.3X6
Oestradiol	T38.5X1	T38.5X2	T38.5X3	T38.5X4	T38.5X5	T38.5X6
Oestriol	T38.5X1	T38.5X2	T38.5X3	T38.5X4	T38.5X5	T38.5X6
Oestrogen	T38.5X1	T38.5X2	T38.5X3	T38.5X4	T38.5X5	T38.5X6
Oestrone	T38.5X1	T38.5X2	T38.5X3	T38.5X4	T38.5X5	T38.5X6
Ofloxacin	T36.8X1	T36.8X2	T36.8X3	T36.8X4	T36.8X5	T36.8X6
Oil (of)	T65.891	T65.892	T65.893	T65.894	—	—
bitter almond	T62.8X1	T62.8X2	T62.8X3	T62.8X4	—	—
cloves	T49.7X1	T49.7X2	T49.7X3	T49.7X4	T49.7X5	T49.7X6
colors	T65.6X1	T65.6X2	T65.6X3	T65.6X4	—	—
fumes	T59.891	T59.892	T59.893	T59.894	—	—
lubricating	T52.ØX1	T52.ØX2	T52.ØX3	T52.ØX4	—	—
Niobe	T52.8X1	T52.8X2	T52.8X3	T52.8X4	—	—
vitriol (liquid)	T54.2X1	T54.2X2	T54.2X3	T54.2X4	—	—
fumes	T54.2X1	T54.2X2	T54.2X3	T54.2X4	—	—
wintergreen (bitter) NEC	T49.3X1	T49.3X2	T49.3X3	T49.3X4	T49.3X5	T49.3X6
Oily preparation (for skin)	T49.3X1	T49.3X2	T49.3X3	T49.3X4	T49.3X5	T49.3X6
Ointment NEC	T49.3X1	T49.3X2	T49.3X3	T49.3X4	T49.3X5	T49.3X6
Olanzapine	T43.591	T43.592	T43.593	T43.594	T43.595	T43.596
Oleander	T62.2X1	T62.2X2	T62.2X3	T62.2X4	—	—
Oleandomycin	T36.3X1	T36.3X2	T36.3X3	T36.3X4	T36.3X5	T36.3X6
Oleandrin	T46.ØX1	T46.ØX2	T46.ØX3	T46.ØX4	T46.ØX5	T46.ØX6
Oleic acid	T46.6X1	T46.6X2	T46.6X3	T46.6X4	T46.6X5	T46.6X6
Oleovitamin A	T45.2X1	T45.2X2	T45.2X3	T45.2X4	T45.2X5	T45.2X6
Oleum ricini	T47.2X1	T47.2X2	T47.2X3	T47.2X4	T47.2X5	T47.2X6
Olive oil (medicinal) **NEC**	T47.4X1	T47.4X2	T47.4X3	T47.4X4	T47.4X5	T47.4X6
Olivomycin	T45.1X1	T45.1X2	T45.1X3	T45.1X4	T45.1X5	T45.1X6
Olsalazine	T47.8X1	T47.8X2	T47.8X3	T47.8X4	T47.8X5	T47.8X6
Omeprazole	T47.1X1	T47.1X2	T47.1X3	T47.1X4	T47.1X5	T47.1X6
OMPA	T60.ØX1	T60.ØX2	T60.ØX3	T60.ØX4	—	—
Oncovin	T45.1X1	T45.1X2	T45.1X3	T45.1X4	T45.1X5	T45.1X6
Ondansetron	T45.ØX1	T45.ØX2	T45.ØX3	T45.ØX4	T45.ØX5	T45.ØX6
Ophthaine	T41.3X1	T41.3X2	T41.3X3	T41.3X4	T41.3X5	T41.3X6
Ophthetic	T41.3X1	T41.3X2	T41.3X3	T41.3X4	T41.3X5	T41.3X6
Opiate NEC	T40.601	T40.602	T40.603	T40.604	T40.605	T40.606
antagonists	T50.7X1	T50.7X2	T50.7X3	T50.7X4	T50.7X5	T50.7X6
Opioid NEC	T40.2X1	T40.2X2	T40.2X3	T40.2X4	T40.2X5	T40.2X6
Opipramol	T43.Ø11	T43.Ø12	T43.Ø13	T43.Ø14	T43.Ø15	T43.Ø16
Opium alkaloids (total)	T40.ØX1	T40.ØX2	T40.ØX3	T40.ØX4	T40.ØX5	T40.ØX6
standardized powdered	T40.ØX1	T40.ØX2	T40.ØX3	T40.ØX4	T40.ØX5	T40.ØX6
tincture (camphorated)	T40.ØX1	T40.ØX2	T40.ØX3	T40.ØX4	T40.ØX5	T40.ØX6
Oracon	T38.4X1	T38.4X2	T38.4X3	T38.4X4	T38.4X5	T38.4X6
Oragrafin	T50.8X1	T50.8X2	T50.8X3	T50.8X4	T50.8X5	T50.8X6
Oral contraceptives	T38.4X1	T38.4X2	T38.4X3	T38.4X4	T38.4X5	T38.4X6
Oral rehydration salts	T50.3X1	T50.3X2	T50.3X3	T50.3X4	T50.3X5	T50.3X6
Orazamide	T50.991	T50.992	T50.993	T50.994	T50.995	T50.996
Orciprenaline	T48.291	T48.292	T48.293	T48.294	T48.295	T48.296
Organidin	T48.4X1	T48.4X2	T48.4X3	T48.4X4	T48.4X5	T48.4X6
Organonitrate NEC	T46.3X1	T46.3X2	T46.3X3	T46.3X4	T46.3X5	T46.3X6
Organophosphates	T60.ØX1	T60.ØX2	T60.ØX3	T60.ØX4	—	—
Orimune	T50.B91	T50.B92	T50.B93	T50.B94	T50.B95	T50.B96
Orinase	T38.3X1	T38.3X2	T38.3X3	T38.3X4	T38.3X5	T38.3X6
Ormeloxifene	T38.6X1	T38.6X2	T38.6X3	T38.6X4	T38.6X5	T38.6X6
Ornidazole	T37.3X1	T37.3X2	T37.3X3	T37.3X4	T37.3X5	T37.3X6
Ornithine aspartate	T50.991	T50.992	T50.993	T50.994	T50.995	T50.996
Ornoprostil	T47.1X1	T47.1X2	T47.1X3	T47.1X4	T47.1X5	T47.1X6
Orphenadrine (hydrochloride)	T42.8X1	T42.8X2	T42.8X3	T42.8X4	T42.8X5	T42.8X6
Ortal (sodium)	T42.3X1	T42.3X2	T42.3X3	T42.3X4	T42.3X5	T42.3X6

Substance	Poisoning, Accidental (unintentional)	Poisoning, Intentional Self-harm	Poisoning, Assault	Poisoning, Undetermined	Adverse Effect	Under-dosing
Orthoboric acid	T49.ØX1	T49.ØX2	T49.ØX3	T49.ØX4	T49.ØX5	T49.ØX6
ENT agent	T49.6X1	T49.6X2	T49.6X3	T49.6X4	T49.6X5	T49.6X6
ophthalmic preparation	T49.5X1	T49.5X2	T49.5X3	T49.5X4	T49.5X5	T49.5X6
Orthocaine	T41.3X1	T41.3X2	T41.3X3	T41.3X4	T41.3X5	T41.3X6
Orthodichlorobenzene	T53.7X1	T53.7X2	T53.7X3	T53.7X4	—	—
Ortho-Novum	T38.4X1	T38.4X2	T38.4X3	T38.4X4	T38.4X5	T38.4X6
Orthotolidine (reagent)	T54.2X1	T54.2X2	T54.2X3	T54.2X4	—	—
Osmic acid (liquid)	T54.2X1	T54.2X2	T54.2X3	T54.2X4	—	—
fumes	T54.2X1	T54.2X2	T54.2X3	T54.2X4	—	—
Osmotic diuretics	T5Ø.2X1	T5Ø.2X2	T5Ø.2X3	T5Ø.2X4	T5Ø.2X5	T5Ø.2X6
Otilonium bromide	T44.3X1	T44.3X2	T44.3X3	T44.3X4	T44.3X5	T44.3X6
Otorhinolaryngological drug NEC	T49.6X1	T49.6X2	T49.6X3	T49.6X4	T49.6X5	T49.6X6
Ouabain (e)	T46.ØX1	T46.ØX2	T46.ØX3	T46.ØX4	T46.ØX5	T46.ØX6
Ovarian						
hormone	T38.5X1	T38.5X2	T38.5X3	T38.5X4	T38.5X5	T38.5X6
stimulant	T38.5X1	T38.5X2	T38.5X3	T38.5X4	T38.5X5	T38.5X6
Ovral	T38.4X1	T38.4X2	T38.4X3	T38.4X4	T38.4X5	T38.4X6
Ovulen	T38.4X1	T38.4X2	T38.4X3	T38.4X4	T38.4X5	T38.4X6
Oxacillin	T36.ØX1	T36.ØX2	T36.ØX3	T36.ØX4	T36.ØX5	T36.ØX6
Oxalic acid	T54.2X1	T54.2X2	T54.2X3	T54.2X4	—	—
ammonium salt	T5Ø.991	T5Ø.992	T5Ø.993	T5Ø.994	T5Ø.995	T5Ø.996
Oxamniquine	T37.4X1	T37.4X2	T37.4X3	T37.4X4	T37.4X5	T37.4X6
Oxanamide	T43.591	T43.592	T43.593	T43.594	T43.595	T43.596
Oxandrolone	T38.7X1	T38.7X2	T38.7X3	T38.7X4	T38.7X5	T38.7X6
Oxantel	T37.4X1	T37.4X2	T37.4X3	T37.4X4	T37.4X5	T37.4X6
Oxapium iodide	T44.3X1	T44.3X2	T44.3X3	T44.3X4	T44.3X5	T44.3X6
Oxaprotiline	T43.Ø21	T43.Ø22	T43.Ø23	T43.Ø24	T43.Ø25	T43.Ø26
Oxaprozin	T39.311	T39.312	T39.313	T39.314	T39.315	T39.316
Oxatomide	T45.ØX1	T45.ØX2	T45.ØX3	T45.ØX4	T45.ØX5	T45.ØX6
Oxazepam	T42.4X1	T42.4X2	T42.4X3	T42.4X4	T42.4X5	T42.4X6
Oxazimedrine	T5Ø.5X1	T5Ø.5X2	T5Ø.5X3	T5Ø.5X4	T5Ø.5X5	T5Ø.5X6
Oxazolam	T42.4X1	T42.4X2	T42.4X3	T42.4X4	T42.4X5	T42.4X6
Oxazolidine derivatives	T42.2X1	T42.2X2	T42.2X3	T42.2X4	T42.2X5	T42.2X6
Oxazolidinedione (derivative)	T42.2X1	T42.2X2	T42.2X3	T42.2X4	T42.2X5	T42.2X6
Ox bile extract	T47.5X1	T47.5X2	T47.5X3	T47.5X4	T47.5X5	T47.5X6
Oxcarbazepine	T42.1X1	T42.1X2	T42.1X3	T42.1X4	T42.1X5	T42.1X6
Oxedrine	T44.4X1	T44.4X2	T44.4X3	T44.4X4	T44.4X5	T44.4X6
Oxeladin (citrate)	T48.3X1	T48.3X2	T48.3X3	T48.3X4	T48.3X5	T48.3X6
Oxendolone	T38.5X1	T38.5X2	T38.5X3	T38.5X4	T38.5X5	T38.5X6
Oxetacaine	T41.3X1	T41.3X2	T41.3X3	T41.3X4	T41.3X5	T41.3X6
Oxethazine	T41.3X1	T41.3X2	T41.3X3	T41.3X4	T41.3X5	T41.3X6
Oxetorone	T39.8X1	T39.8X2	T39.8X3	T39.8X4	T39.8X5	T39.8X6
Oxiconazole	T49.ØX1	T49.ØX2	T49.ØX3	T49.ØX4	T49.ØX5	T49.ØX6
Oxidizing agent NEC	T54.91	T54.92	T54.93	T54.94	—	—
Oxipurinol	T5Ø.4X1	T5Ø.4X2	T5Ø.4X3	T5Ø.4X4	T5Ø.4X5	T5Ø.4X6
Oxitriptan	T43.291	T43.292	T43.293	T43.294	T43.295	T43.296
Oxitropium bromide	T48.6X1	T48.6X2	T48.6X3	T48.6X4	T48.6X5	T48.6X6
Oxodipine	T46.1X1	T46.1X2	T46.1X3	T46.1X4	T46.1X5	T46.1X6
Oxolamine	T48.3X1	T48.3X2	T48.3X3	T48.3X4	T48.3X5	T48.3X6
Oxolinic acid	T37.8X1	T37.8X2	T37.8X3	T37.8X4	T37.8X5	T37.8X6
Oxomemazine	T43.3X1	T43.3X2	T43.3X3	T43.3X4	T43.3X5	T43.3X6
Oxophenarsine	T37.3X1	T37.3X2	T37.3X3	T37.3X4	T37.3X5	T37.3X6
Oxprenolol	T44.7X1	T44.7X2	T44.7X3	T44.7X4	T44.7X5	T44.7X6
Oxsoralen	T49.3X1	T49.3X2	T49.3X3	T49.3X4	T49.3X5	T49.3X6
Oxtriphylline	T48.6X1	T48.6X2	T48.6X3	T48.6X4	T48.6X5	T48.6X6
Oxybate sodium	T41.291	T41.292	T41.293	T41.294	T41.295	T41.296
Oxybuprocaine	T41.3X1	T41.3X2	T41.3X3	T41.3X4	T41.3X5	T41.3X6
Oxybutynin	T44.3X1	T44.3X2	T44.3X3	T44.3X4	T44.3X5	T44.3X6
Oxychlorosene	T49.ØX1	T49.ØX2	T49.ØX3	T49.ØX4	T49.ØX5	T49.ØX6
Oxycodone	T4Ø.2X1	T4Ø.2X2	T4Ø.2X3	T4Ø.2X4	T4Ø.2X5	T4Ø.2X6
Oxyfedrine	T46.3X1	T46.3X2	T46.3X3	T46.3X4	T46.3X5	T46.3X6
Oxygen	T41.5X1	T41.5X2	T41.5X3	T41.5X4	T41.5X5	T41.5X6
Oxylone	T49.ØX1	T49.ØX2	T49.ØX3	T49.ØX4	T49.ØX5	T49.ØX6
ophthalmic preparation	T49.5X1	T49.5X2	T49.5X3	T49.5X4	T49.5X5	T49.5X6
Oxymesterone	T38.7X1	T38.7X2	T38.7X3	T38.7X4	T38.7X5	T38.7X6
Oxymetazoline	T48.5X1	T48.5X2	T48.5X3	T48.5X4	T48.5X5	T48.5X6
Oxymetholone	T38.7X1	T38.7X2	T38.7X3	T38.7X4	T38.7X5	T38.7X6
Oxymorphone	T4Ø.2X1	T4Ø.2X2	T4Ø.2X3	T4Ø.2X4	T4Ø.2X5	T4Ø.2X6
Oxypertine	T43.591	T43.592	T43.593	T43.594	T43.595	T43.596
Oxyphenbutazone	T39.2X1	T39.2X2	T39.2X3	T39.2X4	T39.2X5	T39.2X6
Oxyphencyclimine	T44.3X1	T44.3X2	T44.3X3	T44.3X4	T44.3X5	T44.3X6
Oxyphenisatine	T47.2X1	T47.2X2	T47.2X3	T47.2X4	T47.2X5	T47.2X6
Oxyphenonium bromide	T44.3X1	T44.3X2	T44.3X3	T44.3X4	T44.3X5	T44.3X6
Oxypolygelatin	T45.8X1	T45.8X2	T45.8X3	T45.8X4	T45.8X5	T45.8X6
Oxyquinoline (derivatives)	T37.8X1	T37.8X2	T37.8X3	T37.8X4	T37.8X5	T37.8X6
Oxytetracycline	T36.4X1	T36.4X2	T36.4X3	T36.4X4	T36.4X5	T36.4X6
Oxytocic drug NEC	T48.ØX1	T48.ØX2	T48.ØX3	T48.ØX4	T48.ØX5	T48.ØX6
Oxytocin (synthetic)	T48.ØX1	T48.ØX2	T48.ØX3	T48.ØX4	T48.ØX5	T48.ØX6
Ozone	T59.891	T59.892	T59.893	T59.894	—	—
PABA	T49.3X1	T49.3X2	T49.3X3	T49.3X4	T49.3X5	T49.3X6
Packed red cells	T45.8X1	T45.8X2	T45.8X3	T45.8X4	T45.8X5	T45.8X6
Padimate	T49.3X1	T49.3X2	T49.3X3	T49.3X4	T49.3X5	T49.3X6
Paint NEC	T65.6X1	T65.6X2	T65.6X3	T65.6X4	—	—
cleaner	T52.91	T52.92	T52.93	T52.94	—	—
fumes NEC	T59.891	T59.892	T59.893	T59.894	—	—
lead (fumes)	T56.ØX1	T56.ØX2	T56.ØX3	T56.ØX4	—	—
solvent NEC	T52.8X1	T52.8X2	T52.8X3	T52.8X4	—	—
stripper	T52.8X1	T52.8X2	T52.8X3	T52.8X4	—	—
Palfium	T4Ø.2X1	T4Ø.2X2	T4Ø.2X3	T4Ø.2X4	—	—
Palm kernel oil	T5Ø.991	T5Ø.992	T5Ø.993	T5Ø.994	T5Ø.995	T5Ø.996
Paludrine	T37.2X1	T37.2X2	T37.2X3	T37.2X4	T37.2X5	T37.2X6
PAM (pralidoxime)	T5Ø.6X1	T5Ø.6X2	T5Ø.6X3	T5Ø.6X4	T5Ø.6X5	T5Ø.6X6
Pamaquine (naphthoute)	T37.2X1	T37.2X2	T37.2X3	T37.2X4	T37.2X5	T37.2X6
Panadol	T39.1X1	T39.1X2	T39.1X3	T39.1X4	T39.1X5	T39.1X6
Pancreatic						
digestive secretion stimulant	T47.8X1	T47.8X2	T47.8X3	T47.8X4	T47.8X5	T47.8X6
dornase	T45.3X1	T45.3X2	T45.3X3	T45.3X4	T45.3X5	T45.3X6
Pancreatin	T47.5X1	T47.5X2	T47.5X3	T47.5X4	T47.5X5	T47.5X6
Pancrelipase	T47.5X1	T47.5X2	T47.5X3	T47.5X4	T47.5X5	T47.5X6
Pancuronium (bromide)	T48.1X1	T48.1X2	T48.1X3	T48.1X4	T48.1X5	T48.1X6
Pangamic acid	T45.2X1	T45.2X2	T45.2X3	T45.2X4	T45.2X5	T45.2X6
Panthenol	T45.2X1	T45.2X2	T45.2X3	T45.2X4	T45.2X5	T45.2X6
topical	T49.8X1	T49.8X2	T49.8X3	T49.8X4	T49.8X5	T49.8X6
Pantopon	T4Ø.ØX1	T4Ø.ØX2	T4Ø.ØX3	T4Ø.ØX4	T4Ø.ØX5	T4Ø.ØX6
Pantothenic acid	T45.2X1	T45.2X2	T45.2X3	T45.2X4	T45.2X5	T45.2X6
Panwarfin	T45.511	T45.512	T45.513	T45.514	T45.515	T45.516
Papain	T47.5X1	T47.5X2	T47.5X3	T47.5X4	T47.5X5	T47.5X6
digestant	T47.5X1	T47.5X2	T47.5X3	T47.5X4	T47.5X5	T47.5X6
Papaveretum	T4Ø.ØX1	T4Ø.ØX2	T4Ø.ØX3	T4Ø.ØX4	T4Ø.ØX5	T4Ø.ØX6
Papaverine	T44.3X1	T44.3X2	T44.3X3	T44.3X4	T44.3X5	T44.3X6
Para-acetamidophenol	T39.1X1	T39.1X2	T39.1X3	T39.1X4	T39.1X5	T39.1X6
Para-aminobenzoic acid	T49.3X1	T49.3X2	T49.3X3	T49.3X4	T49.3X5	T49.3X6
Para-aminophenol derivatives	T39.1X1	T39.1X2	T39.1X3	T39.1X4	T39.1X5	T39.1X6
Para-aminosalicylic acid	T37.1X1	T37.1X2	T37.1X3	T37.1X4	T37.1X5	T37.1X6
Paracetaldehyde	T42.6X1	T42.6X2	T42.6X3	T42.6X4	T42.6X5	T42.6X6
Paracetamol	T39.1X1	T39.1X2	T39.1X3	T39.1X4	T39.1X5	T39.1X6
Parachlorophenol (camphorated)	T49.ØX1	T49.ØX2	T49.ØX3	T49.ØX4	T49.ØX5	T49.ØX6
Paracodin	T4Ø.2X1	T4Ø.2X2	T4Ø.2X3	T4Ø.2X4	T4Ø.2X5	T4Ø.2X6
Paradione	T42.2X1	T42.2X2	T42.2X3	T42.2X4	T42.2X5	T42.2X6
Paraffin(s) (wax)	T52.ØX1	T52.ØX2	T52.ØX3	T52.ØX4	—	—
liquid (medicinal)	T47.4X1	T47.4X2	T47.4X3	T47.4X4	T47.4X5	T47.4X6
nonmedicinal	T52.ØX1	T52.ØX2	T52.ØX3	T52.ØX4	—	—
Paraformaldehyde	T6Ø.3X1	T6Ø.3X2	T6Ø.3X3	T6Ø.3X4	—	—
Paraldehyde	T42.6X1	T42.6X2	T42.6X3	T42.6X4	T42.6X5	T42.6X6
Paramethadione	T42.2X1	T42.2X2	T42.2X3	T42.2X4	T42.2X5	T42.2X6
Paramethasone	T38.ØX1	T38.ØX2	T38.ØX3	T38.ØX4	T38.ØX5	T38.ØX6
acetate	T49.ØX1	T49.ØX2	T49.ØX3	T49.ØX4	T49.ØX5	T49.ØX6
Paraoxon	T6Ø.ØX1	T6Ø.ØX2	T6Ø.ØX3	T6Ø.ØX4	—	—
Paraquat	T6Ø.3X1	T6Ø.3X2	T6Ø.3X3	T6Ø.3X4	—	—
Parasympatholytic NEC	T44.3X1	T44.3X2	T44.3X3	T44.3X4	T44.3X5	T44.3X6
Parasympathomimetic drug NEC	T44.1X1	T44.1X2	T44.1X3	T44.1X4	T44.1X5	T44.1X6
Parathion	T6Ø.ØX1	T6Ø.ØX2	T6Ø.ØX3	T6Ø.ØX4	—	—
Parathormone	T5Ø.991	T5Ø.992	T5Ø.993	T5Ø.994	T5Ø.995	T5Ø.996
Parathyroid extract	T5Ø.991	T5Ø.992	T5Ø.993	T5Ø.994	T5Ø.995	T5Ø.996
Paratyphoid vaccine	T5Ø.A91	T5Ø.A92	T5Ø.A93	T5Ø.A94	T5Ø.A95	T5Ø.A96
Paredrine	T44.4X1	T44.4X2	T44.4X3	T44.4X4	T44.4X5	T44.4X6
Paregoric	T4Ø.ØX1	T4Ø.ØX2	T4Ø.ØX3	T4Ø.ØX4	T4Ø.ØX5	T4Ø.ØX6
Pargyline	T46.5X1	T46.5X2	T46.5X3	T46.5X4	T46.5X5	T46.5X6
Paris green	T57.ØX1	T57.ØX2	T57.ØX3	T57.ØX4	—	—
insecticide	T57.ØX1	T57.ØX2	T57.ØX3	T57.ØX4	—	—
Parnate	T43.1X1	T43.1X2	T43.1X3	T43.1X4	T43.1X5	T43.1X6
Paromomycin	T36.5X1	T36.5X2	T36.5X3	T36.5X4	T36.5X5	T36.5X6
Paroxypropione	T45.1X1	T45.1X2	T45.1X3	T45.1X4	T45.1X5	T45.1X6
Parzone	T4Ø.2X1	T4Ø.2X2	T4Ø.2X3	T4Ø.2X4	T4Ø.2X5	T4Ø.2X6
PAS	T37.1X1	T37.1X2	T37.1X3	T37.1X4	T37.1X5	T37.1X6
Pasiniazid	T37.1X1	T37.1X2	T37.1X3	T37.1X4	T37.1X5	T37.1X6
PBB (polybrominated biphenyls)	T65.891	T65.892	T65.893	T65.894	—	—
PCB	T65.891	T65.892	T65.893	T65.894	—	—
PCP						
meaning pentachlorophenol	T6Ø.1X1	T6Ø.1X2	T6Ø.1X3	T6Ø.1X4	—	—
fungicide	T6Ø.3X1	T6Ø.3X2	T6Ø.3X3	T6Ø.3X4	—	—
herbicide	T6Ø.3X1	T6Ø.3X2	T6Ø.3X3	T6Ø.3X4	—	—
insecticide	T6Ø.1X1	T6Ø.1X2	T6Ø.1X3	T6Ø.1X4	—	—
meaning phencyclidine	T4Ø.991	T4Ø.992	T4Ø.993	T4Ø.994	—	—
Peach kernel oil (emulsion)	T47.4X1	T47.4X2	T47.4X3	T47.4X4	T47.4X5	T47.4X6
Peanut oil (emulsion) **NEC**	T47.4X1	T47.4X2	T47.4X3	T47.4X4	T47.4X5	T47.4X6
topical	T49.3X1	T49.3X2	T49.3X3	T49.3X4	T49.3X5	T49.3X6

Substance	Poisoning, Accidental (unintentional)	Poisoning, Intentional Self-harm	Poisoning, Assault	Poisoning, Undetermined	Adverse Effect	Under-dosing
Pearly Gates (morning glory seeds)	T40.991	T40.992	T40.993	T40.994	—	—
Pecazine	T43.3X1	T43.3X2	T43.3X3	T43.3X4	T43.3X5	T43.3X6
Pectin	T47.6X1	T47.6X2	T47.6X3	T47.6X4	T47.6X5	T47.6X6
Pefloxacin	T37.8X1	T37.8X2	T37.8X3	T37.8X4	T37.8X5	T37.8X6
Pegademase, bovine	T5Ø.Z91	T5Ø.Z92	T5Ø.Z93	T5Ø.Z94	T5Ø.Z95	T5Ø.Z96
Pelletierine tannate	T37.4X1	T37.4X2	T37.4X3	T37.4X4	T37.4X5	T37.4X6
Pemirolast (potassium)	T48.6X1	T48.6X2	T48.6X3	T48.6X4	T48.6X5	T48.6X6
Pemoline	T5Ø.7X1	T5Ø.7X2	T5Ø.7X3	T5Ø.7X4	T5Ø.7X5	T5Ø.7X6
Pempidine	T44.2X1	T44.2X2	T44.2X3	T44.2X4	T44.2X5	T44.2X6
Penamecillin	T36.ØX1	T36.ØX2	T36.ØX3	T36.ØX4	T36.ØX5	T36.ØX6
Penbutolol	T44.7X1	T44.7X2	T44.7X3	T44.7X4	T44.7X5	T44.7X6
Penethamate	T36.ØX1	T36.ØX2	T36.ØX3	T36.ØX4	T36.ØX5	T36.ØX6
Penfluridol	T43.591	T43.592	T43.593	T43.594	T43.595	T43.596
Penflutizide	T5Ø.2X1	T5Ø.2X2	T5Ø.2X3	T5Ø.2X4	T5Ø.2X5	T5Ø.2X6
Pengitoxin	T46.ØX1	T46.ØX2	T46.ØX3	T46.ØX4	T46.ØX5	T46.ØX6
Penicillamine	T5Ø.6X1	T5Ø.6X2	T5Ø.6X3	T5Ø.6X4	T5Ø.6X5	T5Ø.6X6
Penicillin (any)	T36.ØX1	T36.ØX2	T36.ØX3	T36.ØX4	T36.ØX5	T36.ØX6
Penicillinase	T45.3X1	T45.3X2	T45.3X3	T45.3X4	T45.3X5	T45.3X6
Penicilloyl polylysine	T5Ø.8X1	T5Ø.8X2	T5Ø.8X3	T5Ø.8X4	T5Ø.8X5	T5Ø.8X6
Penimepicycline	T36.4X1	T36.4X2	T36.4X3	T36.4X4	T36.4X5	T36.4X6
Pentachloroethane	T53.6X1	T53.6X2	T53.6X3	T53.6X4	—	—
Pentachloronaphthalene	T53.7X1	T53.7X2	T53.7X3	T53.7X4	—	—
Pentachlorophenol (pesticide)	T6Ø.1X1	T6Ø.1X2	T6Ø.1X3	T6Ø.1X4	—	—
fungicide	T6Ø.3X1	T6Ø.3X2	T6Ø.3X3	T6Ø.3X4	—	—
herbicide	T6Ø.3X1	T6Ø.3X2	T6Ø.3X3	T6Ø.3X4	—	—
insecticide	T6Ø.1X1	T6Ø.1X2	T6Ø.1X3	T6Ø.1X4	—	—
Pentaerythritol	T46.3X1	T46.3X2	T46.3X3	T46.3X4	T46.3X5	T46.3X6
chloral	T42.6X1	T42.6X2	T42.6X3	T42.6X4	T42.6X5	T42.6X6
tetranitrate NEC	T46.3X1	T46.3X2	T46.3X3	T46.3X4	T46.3X5	T46.3X6
Pentaerythrityl tetranitrate	T46.3X1	T46.3X2	T46.3X3	T46.3X4	T46.3X5	T46.3X6
Pentagastrin	T5Ø.8X1	T5Ø.8X2	T5Ø.8X3	T5Ø.8X4	T5Ø.8X5	T5Ø.8X6
Pentalin	T53.6X1	T53.6X2	T53.6X3	T53.6X4	—	—
Pentamethonium bromide	T44.2X1	T44.2X2	T44.2X3	T44.2X4	T44.2X5	T44.2X6
Pentamidine	T37.3X1	T37.3X2	T37.3X3	T37.3X4	T37.3X5	T37.3X6
Pentanol	T51.3X1	T51.3X2	T51.3X3	T51.3X4	—	—
Pentapyrrolinium (bitartrate)	T44.2X1	T44.2X2	T44.2X3	T44.2X4	T44.2X5	T44.2X6
Pentaquine	T37.2X1	T37.2X2	T37.2X3	T37.2X4	T37.2X5	T37.2X6
Pentazocine	T4Ø.491	T4Ø.492	T4Ø.493	T4Ø.494	T4Ø.495	T4Ø.496
Pentetrazole	T5Ø.7X1	T5Ø.7X2	T5Ø.7X3	T5Ø.7X4	T5Ø.7X5	T5Ø.7X6
Penthienate bromide	T44.3X1	T44.3X2	T44.3X3	T44.3X4	T44.3X5	T44.3X6
Pentifylline	T46.7X1	T46.7X2	T46.7X3	T46.7X4	T46.7X5	T46.7X6
Pentobarbital	T42.3X1	T42.3X2	T42.3X3	T42.3X4	T42.3X5	T42.3X6
sodium	T42.3X1	T42.3X2	T42.3X3	T42.3X4	T42.3X5	T42.3X6
Pentobarbitone	T42.3X1	T42.3X2	T42.3X3	T42.3X4	T42.3X5	T42.3X6
Pentolonium tartrate	T44.2X1	T44.2X2	T44.2X3	T44.2X4	T44.2X5	T44.2X6
Pentosan polysulfate (sodium)	T39.8X1	T39.8X2	T39.8X3	T39.8X4	T39.8X5	T39.8X6
Pentostatin	T45.1X1	T45.1X2	T45.1X3	T45.1X4	T45.1X5	T45.1X6
Pentothal	T41.1X1	T41.1X2	T41.1X3	T41.1X4	T41.1X5	T41.1X6
Pentoxifylline	T46.7X1	T46.7X2	T46.7X3	T46.7X4	T46.7X5	T46.7X6
Pentoxyverine	T48.3X1	T48.3X2	T48.3X3	T48.3X4	T48.3X5	T48.3X6
Pentrinat	T46.3X1	T46.3X2	T46.3X3	T46.3X4	T46.3X5	T46.3X6
Pentylenetetrazole	T5Ø.7X1	T5Ø.7X2	T5Ø.7X3	T5Ø.7X4	T5Ø.7X5	T5Ø.7X6
Pentylsalicylamide	T37.1X1	T37.1X2	T37.1X3	T37.1X4	T37.1X5	T37.1X6
Pentymal	T42.3X1	T42.3X2	T42.3X3	T42.3X4	T42.3X5	T42.3X6
Peplomycin	T45.1X1	T45.1X2	T45.1X3	T45.1X4	T45.1X5	T45.1X6
Peppermint (oil)	T47.5X1	T47.5X2	T47.5X3	T47.5X4	T47.5X5	T47.5X6
Pepsin	T47.5X1	T47.5X2	T47.5X3	T47.5X4	T47.5X5	T47.5X6
digestant	T47.5X1	T47.5X2	T47.5X3	T47.5X4	T47.5X5	T47.5X6
Pepstatin	T47.1X1	T47.1X2	T47.1X3	T47.1X4	T47.1X5	T47.1X6
Peptavlon	T5Ø.8X1	T5Ø.8X2	T5Ø.8X3	T5Ø.8X4	T5Ø.8X5	T5Ø.8X6
Perazine	T43.3X1	T43.3X2	T43.3X3	T43.3X4	T43.3X5	T43.3X6
Percaine (spinal)	T41.3X1	T41.3X2	T41.3X3	T41.3X4	T41.3X5	T41.3X6
topical (surface)	T41.3X1	T41.3X2	T41.3X3	T41.3X4	T41.3X5	T41.3X6
Perchloroethylene	T53.3X1	T53.3X2	T53.3X3	T53.3X4	—	—
medicinal	T37.4X1	T37.4X2	T37.4X3	T37.4X4	T37.4X5	T37.4X6
vapor	T53.3X1	T53.3X2	T53.3X3	T53.3X4	—	—
Percodan	T4Ø.2X1	T4Ø.2X2	T4Ø.2X3	T4Ø.2X4	T4Ø.2X5	T4Ø.2X6
Percogesic — *see also* acetaminophen	T45.ØX1	T45.ØX2	T45.ØX3	T45.ØX4	T45.ØX5	T45.ØX6
Percorten	T38.ØX1	T38.ØX2	T38.ØX3	T38.ØX4	T38.ØX5	T38.ØX6
Pergolide	T42.8X1	T42.8X2	T42.8X3	T42.8X4	T42.8X5	T42.8X6
Pergonal	T38.811	T38.812	T38.813	T38.814	T38.815	T38.816
Perhexilene	T46.3X1	T46.3X2	T46.3X3	T46.3X4	T46.3X5	T46.3X6
Perhexiline (maleate)	T46.3X1	T46.3X2	T46.3X3	T46.3X4	T46.3X5	T46.3X6
Periactin	T45.ØX1	T45.ØX2	T45.ØX3	T45.ØX4	T45.ØX5	T45.ØX6
Periciazine	T43.3X1	T43.3X2	T43.3X3	T43.3X4	T43.3X5	T43.3X6
Periclor	T42.6X1	T42.6X2	T42.6X3	T42.6X4	T42.6X5	T42.6X6
Perindopril	T46.4X1	T46.4X2	T46.4X3	T46.4X4	T46.4X5	T46.4X6

Substance	Poisoning, Accidental (unintentional)	Poisoning, Intentional Self-harm	Poisoning, Assault	Poisoning, Undetermined	Adverse Effect	Under-dosing
Perisoxal	T39.8X1	T39.8X2	T39.8X3	T39.8X4	T39.8X5	T39.8X
Peritoneal dialysis solution	T5Ø.3X1	T5Ø.3X2	T5Ø.3X3	T5Ø.3X4	T5Ø.3X5	T5Ø.3X
Peritrate	T46.3X1	T46.3X2	T46.3X3	T46.3X4	T46.3X5	T46.3X
Perlapine	T42.4X1	T42.4X2	T42.4X3	T42.4X4	T42.4X5	T42.4X
Permanganate	T65.891	T65.892	T65.893	T65.894	—	—
Permethrin	T6Ø.1X1	T6Ø.1X2	T6Ø.1X3	T6Ø.1X4	—	—
Pernocton	T42.3X1	T42.3X2	T42.3X3	T42.3X4	T42.3X5	T42.3X
Pernoston	T42.3X1	T42.3X2	T42.3X3	T42.3X4	T42.3X5	T42.3X
Peronine	T4Ø.2X1	T4Ø.2X2	T4Ø.2X3	T4Ø.2X4	—	—
Perphenazine	T43.3X1	T43.3X2	T43.3X3	T43.3X4	T43.3X5	T43.3X
Pertofrane	T43.Ø11	T43.Ø12	T43.Ø13	T43.Ø14	T43.Ø15	T43.Ø1
Pertussis						
immune serum (human)	T5Ø.Z11	T5Ø.Z12	T5Ø.Z13	T5Ø.Z14	T5Ø.Z15	T5Ø.Z1
vaccine (with diphtheria toxoid) (with tetanus toxoid)	T5Ø.A11	T5Ø.A12	T5Ø.A13	T5Ø.A14	T5Ø.A15	T5Ø.A1
Peruvian balsam	T49.ØX1	T49.ØX2	T49.ØX3	T49.ØX4	T49.ØX5	T49.ØX
Peruvoside	T46.ØX1	T46.ØX2	T46.ØX3	T46.ØX4	T46.ØX5	T46.ØX
Pesticide (dust) (fumes) (vapor) **NEC**	T6Ø.91	T6Ø.92	T6Ø.93	T6Ø.94	—	—
arsenic	T57.ØX1	T57.ØX2	T57.ØX3	T57.ØX4	—	—
chlorinated	T6Ø.1X1	T6Ø.1X2	T6Ø.1X3	T6Ø.1X4	—	—
cyanide	T65.ØX1	T65.ØX2	T65.ØX3	T65.ØX4	—	—
kerosene	T52.ØX1	T52.ØX2	T52.ØX3	T52.ØX4	—	—
mixture (of compounds)	T6Ø.91	T6Ø.92	T6Ø.93	T6Ø.94	—	—
naphthalene	T6Ø.2X1	T6Ø.2X2	T6Ø.2X3	T6Ø.2X4	—	—
organochlorine (compounds)	T6Ø.1X1	T6Ø.1X2	T6Ø.1X3	T6Ø.1X4	—	—
petroleum (distillate) (products) NEC	T6Ø.8X1	T6Ø.8X2	T6Ø.8X3	T6Ø.8X4	—	—
specified ingredient NEC	T6Ø.8X1	T6Ø.8X2	T6Ø.8X3	T6Ø.8X4	—	—
strychnine	T65.1X1	T65.1X2	T65.1X3	T65.1X4	—	—
thallium	T6Ø.4X1	T6Ø.4X2	T6Ø.4X3	T6Ø.4X4	—	—
Pethidine	T4Ø.491	T4Ø.492	T4Ø.493	T4Ø.494	T4Ø.495	T4Ø.49
Petrichloral	T42.6X1	T42.6X2	T42.6X3	T42.6X4	T42.6X5	T42.6X
Petrol	T52.ØX1	T52.ØX2	T52.ØX3	T52.ØX4	—	—
vapor	T52.ØX1	T52.ØX2	T52.ØX3	T52.ØX4	—	—
Petrolatum	T49.3X1	T49.3X2	T49.3X3	T49.3X4	T49.3X5	T49.3X
hydrophilic	T49.3X1	T49.3X2	T49.3X3	T49.3X4	T49.3X5	T49.3X
liquid	T47.4X1	T47.4X2	T47.4X3	T47.4X4	T47.4X5	T47.4X
topical	T49.3X1	T49.3X2	T49.3X3	T49.3X4	T49.3X5	T49.3X
nonmedicinal	T52.ØX1	T52.ØX2	T52.ØX3	T52.ØX4	—	—
red veterinary	T49.3X1	T49.3X2	T49.3X3	T49.3X4	T49.3X5	T49.3X
white	T49.3X1	T49.3X2	T49.3X3	T49.3X4	T49.3X5	T49.3X
Petroleum (products) **NEC**	T52.ØX1	T52.ØX2	T52.ØX3	T52.ØX4	—	—
benzine(s) — *see* Ligroin						
ether — *see* Ligroin						
jelly — *see* Petrolatum						
naphtha — *see* Ligroin						
pesticide	T6Ø.8X1	T6Ø.8X2	T6Ø.8X3	T6Ø.8X4	—	—
solids	T52.ØX1	T52.ØX2	T52.ØX3	T52.ØX4	—	—
solvents	T52.ØX1	T52.ØX2	T52.ØX3	T52.ØX4	—	—
vapor	T52.ØX1	T52.ØX2	T52.ØX3	T52.ØX4	—	—
Peyote	T4Ø.991	T4Ø.992	T4Ø.993	T4Ø.994	—	—
Phanodorm, phanodorn	T42.3X1	T42.3X2	T42.3X3	T42.3X4	T42.3X5	T42.3X
Phanquinone	T37.3X1	T37.3X2	T37.3X3	T37.3X4	T37.3X5	T37.3X
Phanquone	T37.3X1	T37.3X2	T37.3X3	T37.3X4	T37.3X5	T37.3X
Pharmaceutical						
adjunct NEC	T5Ø.9Ø1	T5Ø.9Ø2	T5Ø.9Ø3	T5Ø.9Ø4	T5Ø.9Ø5	T5Ø.9Ø
excipient NEC	T5Ø.9Ø1	T5Ø.9Ø2	T5Ø.9Ø3	T5Ø.9Ø4	T5Ø.9Ø5	T5Ø.9Ø
sweetener	T5Ø.9Ø1	T5Ø.9Ø2	T5Ø.9Ø3	T5Ø.9Ø4	T5Ø.9Ø5	T5Ø.9Ø
viscous agent	T5Ø.9Ø1	T5Ø.9Ø2	T5Ø.9Ø3	T5Ø.9Ø4	T5Ø.9Ø5	T5Ø.9Ø
Phemitone	T42.3X1	T42.3X2	T42.3X3	T42.3X4	T42.3X5	T42.3X
Phenacaine	T41.3X1	T41.3X2	T41.3X3	T41.3X4.	T41.3X5	T41.3X
Phenacemide	T42.6X1	T42.6X2	T42.6X3	T42.6X4	T42.6X5	T42.6X
Phenacetin	T39.1X1	T39.1X2	T39.1X3	T39.1X4	T39.1X5	T39.1X
Phenadoxone	T4Ø.2X1	T4Ø.2X2	T4Ø.2X3	T4Ø.2X4	—	—
Phenaglycodol	T43.591	T43.592	T43.593	T43.594	T43.595	T43.59
Phenantoin	T42.ØX1	T42.ØX2	T42.ØX3	T42.ØX4	T42.ØX5	T42.ØX
Phenaphthazine reagent	T5Ø.991	T5Ø.992	T5Ø.993	T5Ø.994	T5Ø.995	T5Ø.99
Phenazocine	T4Ø.491	T4Ø.492	T4Ø.493	T4Ø.494	T4Ø.495	T4Ø.49
Phenazone	T39.2X1	T39.2X2	T39.2X3	T39.2X4	T39.2X5	T39.2X
Phenazopyridine	T39.8X1	T39.8X2	T39.8X3	T39.8X4	T39.8X5	T39.8X
Phenbenicillin	T36.ØX1	T36.ØX2	T36.ØX3	T36.ØX4	T36.ØX5	T36.ØX
Phenbutrazate	T5Ø.5X1	T5Ø.5X2	T5Ø.5X3	T5Ø.5X4	T5Ø.5X5	T5Ø.5X
Phencyclidine	T4Ø.991	T4Ø.992	T4Ø.993	T4Ø.994	T4Ø.995	T4Ø.99
Phendimetrazine	T5Ø.5X1	T5Ø.5X2	T5Ø.5X3	T5Ø.5X4	T5Ø.5X5	T5Ø.5X
Phenelzine	T43.1X1	T43.1X2	T43.1X3	T43.1X4	T43.1X5	T43.1X
Phenemal	T42.3X1	T42.3X2	T42.3X3	T42.3X4	T42.3X5	T42.3X
Phenergan	T42.6X1	T42.6X2	T42.6X3	T42.6X4	T42.6X5	T42.6X
Pheneticillin	T36.ØX1	T36.ØX2	T36.ØX3	T36.ØX4	T36.ØX5	T36.ØX
Pheneturide	T42.6X1	T42.6X2	T42.6X3	T42.6X4	T42.6X5	T42.6X
Phenformin	T38.3X1	T38.3X2	T38.3X3	T38.3X4	T38.3X5	T38.3X

Substance	Poisoning, Accidental (unintentional)	Poisoning, Intentional Self-harm	Poisoning, Assault	Poisoning, Undetermined	Adverse Effect	Under-dosing
Phenglutarimide	T44.3X1	T44.3X2	T44.3X3	T44.3X4	T44.3X5	T44.3X6
Phenicarbazide	T39.8X1	T39.8X2	T39.8X3	T39.8X4	T39.8X5	T39.8X6
Phenindamine	T45.ØX1	T45.ØX2	T45.ØX3	T45.ØX4	T45.ØX5	T45.ØX6
Phenindione	T45.511	T45.512	T45.513	T45.514	T45.515	T45.516
Pheniprazine	T43.1X1	T43.1X2	T43.1X3	T43.1X4	T43.1X5	T43.1X6
Pheniramine	T45.ØX1	T45.ØX2	T45.ØX3	T45.ØX4	T45.ØX5	T45.ØX6
Phenisatin	T47.2X1	T47.2X2	T47.2X3	T47.2X4	T47.2X5	T47.2X6
Phenmetrazine	T5Ø.5X1	T5Ø.5X2	T5Ø.5X3	T5Ø.5X4	T5Ø.5X5	T5Ø.5X6
Phenobal	T42.3X1	T42.3X2	T42.3X3	T42.3X4	T42.3X5	T42.3X6
Phenobarbital	T42.3X1	T42.3X2	T42.3X3	T42.3X4	T42.3X5	T42.3X6
with						
mephenytoin	T42.3X1	T42.3X2	T42.3X3	T42.3X4	T42.3X5	T42.3X6
phenytoin	T42.3X1	T42.3X2	T42.3X3	T42.3X4	T42.3X5	T42.3X6
sodium	T42.3X1	T42.3X2	T42.3X3	T42.3X4	T42.3X5	T42.3X6
Phenobarbitone	T42.3X1	T42.3X2	T42.3X3	T42.3X4	T42.3X5	T42.3X6
Phenobutiodil	T5Ø.8X1	T5Ø.8X2	T5Ø.8X3	T5Ø.8X4	T5Ø.8X5	T5Ø.8X6
Phenoctide	T49.ØX1	T49.ØX2	T49.ØX3	T49.ØX4	T49.ØX5	T49.ØX6
Phenol	T49.ØX1	T49.ØX2	T49.ØX3	T49.ØX4	T49.ØX5	T49.ØX6
disinfectant	T54.ØX1	T54.ØX2	T54.ØX3	T54.ØX4	—	—
in oil injection	T46.8X1	T46.8X2	T46.8X3	T46.8X4	T46.8X5	T46.8X6
medicinal	T49.1X1	T49.1X2	T49.1X3	T49.1X4	T49.1X5	T49.1X6
nonmedicinal NEC	T54.ØX1	T54.ØX2	T54.ØX3	T54.ØX4	—	—
pesticide	T6Ø.8X1	T6Ø.8X2	T6Ø.8X3	T6Ø.8X4	—	—
red	T5Ø.8X1	T5Ø.8X2	T5Ø.8X3	T5Ø.8X4	T5Ø.8X5	T5Ø.8X6
Phenolic preparation	T49.1X1	T49.1X2	T49.1X3	T49.1X4	T49.1X5	T49.1X6
Phenolphthalein	T47.2X1	T47.2X2	T47.2X3	T47.2X4	T47.2X5	T47.2X6
Phenolsulfonphthalein	T5Ø.8X1	T5Ø.8X2	T5Ø.8X3	T5Ø.8X4	T5Ø.8X5	T5Ø.8X6
Phenomorphan	T4Ø.2X1	T4Ø.2X2	T4Ø.2X3	T4Ø.2X4	—	—
Phenonyl	T42.3X1	T42.3X2	T42.3X3	T42.3X4	T42.3X5	T42.3X6
Phenoperidine	T4Ø.491	T4Ø.492	T4Ø.493	T4Ø.494	—	—
Phenopyrazone	T46.991	T46.992	T46.993	T46.994	T46.995	T46.996
Phenoquin	T5Ø.4X1	T5Ø.4X2	T5Ø.4X3	T5Ø.4X4	T5Ø.4X5	T5Ø.4X6
Phenothiazine (psychotropic) **NEC**	T43.3X1	T43.3X2	T43.3X3	T43.3X4	T43.3X5	T43.3X6
insecticide	T6Ø.2X1	T6Ø.2X2	T6Ø.2X3	T6Ø.2X4	—	—
Phenothrin	T49.ØX1	T49.ØX2	T49.ØX3	T49.ØX4	T49.ØX5	T49.ØX6
Phenoxybenzamine	T46.7X1	T46.7X2	T46.7X3	T46.7X4	T46.7X5	T46.7X6
Phenoxyethanol	T49.ØX1	T49.ØX2	T49.ØX3	T49.ØX4	T49.ØX5	T49.ØX6
Phenoxymethyl penicillin	T36.ØX1	T36.ØX2	T36.ØX3	T36.ØX4	T36.ØX5	T36.ØX6
Phenprobamate	T42.8X1	T42.8X2	T42.8X3	T42.8X4	T42.8X5	T42.8X6
Phenprocoumon	T45.511	T45.512	T45.513	T45.514	T45.515	T45.516
Phensuximide	T42.2X1	T42.2X2	T42.2X3	T42.2X4	T42.2X5	T42.2X6
Phentermine	T5Ø.5X1	T5Ø.5X2	T5Ø.5X3	T5Ø.5X4	T5Ø.5X5	T5Ø.5X6
Phenthicillin	T36.ØX1	T36.ØX2	T36.ØX3	T36.ØX4	T36.ØX5	T36.ØX6
Phentolamine	T46.7X1	T46.7X2	T46.7X3	T46.7X4	T46.7X5	T46.7X6
Phenyl						
butazone	T39.2X1	T39.2X2	T39.2X3	T39.2X4	T39.2X5	T39.2X6
enediamine	T65.3X1	T65.3X2	T65.3X3	T65.3X4	—	—
hydrazine	T65.3X1	T65.3X2	T65.3X3	T65.3X4	—	—
antineoplastic	T45.1X1	T45.1X2	T45.1X3	T45.1X4	T45.1X5	T45.1X6
mercuric compounds — *see* Mercury						
salicylate	T49.3X1	T49.3X2	T49.3X3	T49.3X4	T49.3X5	T49.3X6
Phenylalanine mustard	T45.1X1	T45.1X2	T45.1X3	T45.1X4	T45.1X5	T45.1X6
Phenylbutazone	T39.2X1	T39.2X2	T39.2X3	T39.2X4	T39.2X5	T39.2X6
Phenylenediamine	T65.3X1	T65.3X2	T65.3X3	T65.3X4	—	—
Phenylephrine	T44.4X1	T44.4X2	T44.4X3	T44.4X4	T44.4X5	T44.4X6
Phenylethylbiguanide	T38.3X1	T38.3X2	T38.3X3	T38.3X4	T38.3X5	T38.3X6
Phenylmercuric						
acetate	T49.ØX1	T49.ØX2	T49.ØX3	T49.ØX4	T49.ØX5	T49.ØX6
borate	T49.ØX1	T49.ØX2	T49.ØX3	T49.ØX4	T49.ØX5	T49.ØX6
nitrate	T49.ØX1	T49.ØX2	T49.ØX3	T49.ØX4	T49.ØX5	T49.ØX6
Phenylmethylbarbitone	T42.3X1	T42.3X2	T42.3X3	T42.3X4	T42.3X5	T42.3X6
Phenylpropanol	T47.5X1	T47.5X2	T47.5X3	T47.5X4	T47.5X5	T47.5X6
Phenylpropanolamine	T44.991	T44.992	T44.993	T44.994	T44.995	T44.996
Phenylsulfthion	T6Ø.ØX1	T6Ø.ØX2	T6Ø.ØX3	T6Ø.ØX4	—	—
Phenyltoloxamine	T45.ØX1	T45.ØX2	T45.ØX3	T45.ØX4	T45.ØX5	T45.ØX6
Phenyramidol, phenyramidon	T39.8X1	T39.8X2	T39.8X3	T39.8X4	T39.8X5	T39.8X6
Phenytoin	T42.ØX1	T42.ØX2	T42.ØX3	T42.ØX4	T42.ØX5	T42.ØX6
with Phenobarbital	T42.3X1	T42.3X2	T42.3X3	T42.3X4	T42.3X5	T42.3X6
pHisoHex	T49.2X1	T49.2X2	T49.2X3	T49.2X4	T49.2X5	T49.2X6
Pholcodine	T48.3X1	T48.3X2	T48.3X3	T48.3X4	T48.3X5	T48.3X6
Pholedrine	T46.991	T46.992	T46.993	T46.994	T46.995	T46.996
Phorate	T6Ø.ØX1	T6Ø.ØX2	T6Ø.ØX3	T6Ø.ØX4	—	—
Phosdrin	T6Ø.ØX1	T6Ø.ØX2	T6Ø.ØX3	T6Ø.ØX4	—	—
Phosfolan	T6Ø.ØX1	T6Ø.ØX2	T6Ø.ØX3	T6Ø.ØX4	—	—
Phosgene (gas)	T59.891	T59.892	T59.893	T59.894	—	—
Phosphamidon	T6Ø.ØX1	T6Ø.ØX2	T6Ø.ØX3	T6Ø.ØX4	—	—
Phosphate	T65.891	T65.892	T65.893	T65.894	—	—
laxative	T47.4X1	T47.4X2	T47.4X3	T47.4X4	T47.4X5	T47.4X6
organic	T6Ø.ØX1	T6Ø.ØX2	T6Ø.ØX3	T6Ø.ØX4	—	—
solvent	T52.91	T52.92	T52.93	T52.94	—	—
Phosphate — *continued*						
tricresyl	T65.891	T65.892	T65.893	T65.894	—	—
Phosphine	T57.1X1	T57.1X2	T57.1X3	T57.1X4	—	—
fumigant	T57.1X1	T57.1X2	T57.1X3	T57.1X4	—	—
Phospholine	T49.5X1	T49.5X2	T49.5X3	T49.5X4	T49.5X5	T49.5X6
Phosphoric acid	T54.2X1	T54.2X2	T54.2X3	T54.2X4	—	—
Phosphorus (compound) **NEC**	T57.1X1	T57.1X2	T57.1X3	T57.1X4	—	—
pesticide	T6Ø.ØX1	T6Ø.ØX2	T6Ø.ØX3	T6Ø.ØX4	—	—
Phthalates	T65.891	T65.892	T65.893	T65.894	—	—
Phthalic anhydride	T65.891	T65.892	T65.893	T65.894	—	—
Phthalimidoglutarimide	T42.6X1	T42.6X2	T42.6X3	T42.6X4	T42.6X5	T42.6X6
Phthalylsulfathiazole	T37.ØX1	T37.ØX2	T37.ØX3	T37.ØX4	T37.ØX5	T37.ØX6
Phylloquinone	T45.7X1	T45.7X2	T45.7X3	T45.7X4	T45.7X5	T45.7X6
Physeptone	T4Ø.3X1	T4Ø.3X2	T4Ø.3X3	T4Ø.3X4	T4Ø.3X5	T4Ø.3X6
Physostigma venenosum	T62.2X1	T62.2X2	T62.2X3	T62.2X4	—	—
Physostigmine	T49.5X1	T49.5X2	T49.5X3	T49.5X4	T49.5X5	T49.5X6
Phytolacca decandra	T62.2X1	T62.2X2	T62.2X3	T62.2X4	—	—
berries	T62.1X1	T62.1X2	T62.1X3	T62.1X4	—	—
Phytomenadione	T45.7X1	T45.7X2	T45.7X3	T45.7X4	T45.7X5	T45.7X6
Phytonadione	T45.7X1	T45.7X2	T45.7X3	T45.7X4	T45.7X5	T45.7X6
Picoperine	T48.3X1	T48.3X2	T48.3X3	T48.3X4	T48.3X5	T48.3X6
Picosulfate (sodium)	T47.2X1	T47.2X2	T47.2X3	T47.2X4	T47.2X5	T47.2X6
Picric (acid)	T54.2X1	T54.2X2	T54.2X3	T54.2X4	—	—
Picrotoxin	T5Ø.7X1	T5Ø.7X2	T5Ø.7X3	T5Ø.7X4	T5Ø.7X5	T5Ø.7X6
Piketoprofen	T49.ØX1	T49.ØX2	T49.ØX3	T49.ØX4	T49.ØX5	T49.ØX6
Pilocarpine	T44.1X1	T44.1X2	T44.1X3	T44.1X4	T44.1X5	T44.1X6
Pilocarpus (jaborandi) extract	T44.1X1	T44.1X2	T44.1X3	T44.1X4	T44.1X5	T44.1X6
Pilsicainide (hydrochloride)	T46.2X1	T46.2X2	T46.2X3	T46.2X4	T46.2X5	T46.2X6
Pimaricin	T36.7X1	T36.7X2	T36.7X3	T36.7X4	T36.7X5	T36.7X6
Pimeclone	T5Ø.7X1	T5Ø.7X2	T5Ø.7X3	T5Ø.7X4	T5Ø.7X5	T5Ø.7X6
Pimelic ketone	T52.8X1	T52.8X2	T52.8X3	T52.8X4	—	—
Pimethixene	T45.ØX1	T45.ØX2	T45.ØX3	T45.ØX4	T45.ØX5	T45.ØX6
Piminodine	T4Ø.2X1	T4Ø.2X2	T4Ø.2X3	T4Ø.2X4	T4Ø.2X5	T4Ø.2X6
Pimozide	T43.591	T43.592	T43.593	T43.594	T43.595	T43.596
Pinacidil	T46.5X1	T46.5X2	T46.5X3	T46.5X4	T46.5X5	T46.5X6
Pinaverium bromide	T44.3X1	T44.3X2	T44.3X3	T44.3X4	T44.3X5	T44.3X6
Pinazepam	T42.4X1	T42.4X2	T42.4X3	T42.4X4	T42.4X5	T42.4X6
Pindolol	T44.7X1	T44.7X2	T44.7X3	T44.7X4	T44.7X5	T44.7X6
Pindone	T6Ø.4X1	T6Ø.4X2	T6Ø.4X3	T6Ø.4X4	—	—
Pine oil (disinfectant)	T65.891	T65.892	T65.893	T65.894	—	—
Pinkroot	T37.4X1	T37.4X2	T37.4X3	T37.4X4	T37.4X5	T37.4X6
Pipadone	T4Ø.2X1	T4Ø.2X2	T4Ø.2X3	T4Ø.2X4	—	—
Pipamazine	T45.ØX1	T45.ØX2	T45.ØX3	T45.ØX4	T45.ØX5	T45.ØX6
Pipamperone	T43.4X1	T43.4X2	T43.4X3	T43.4X4	T43.4X5	T43.4X6
Pipazetate	T48.3X1	T48.3X2	T48.3X3	T48.3X4	T48.3X5	T48.3X6
Pipemidic acid	T37.8X1	T37.8X2	T37.8X3	T37.8X4	T37.8X5	T37.8X6
Pipenzolate bromide	T44.3X1	T44.3X2	T44.3X3	T44.3X4	T44.3X5	T44.3X6
Piperacetazine	T43.3X1	T43.3X2	T43.3X3	T43.3X4	T43.3X5	T43.3X6
Piperacillin	T36.ØX1	T36.ØX2	T36.ØX3	T36.ØX4	T36.ØX5	T36.ØX6
Piperazine	T37.4X1	T37.4X2	T37.4X3	T37.4X4	T37.4X5	T37.4X6
estrone sulfate	T38.5X1	T38.5X2	T38.5X3	T38.5X4	T38.5X5	T38.5X6
Piper cubeba	T62.2X1	T62.2X2	T62.2X3	T62.2X4	—	—
Piperidione	T48.3X1	T48.3X2	T48.3X3	T48.3X4	T48.3X5	T48.3X6
Piperidolate	T44.3X1	T44.3X2	T44.3X3	T44.3X4	T44.3X5	T44.3X6
Piperocaine	T41.3X1	T41.3X2	T41.3X3	T41.3X4	T41.3X5	T41.3X6
infiltration (subcutaneous)	T41.3X1	T41.3X2	T41.3X3	T41.3X4	T41.3X5	T41.3X6
nerve block (peripheral) (plexus)	T41.3X1	T41.3X2	T41.3X3	T41.3X4	T41.3X5	T41.3X6
topical (surface)	T41.3X1	T41.3X2	T41.3X3	T41.3X4	T41.3X5	T41.3X6
Piperonyl butoxide	T6Ø.8X1	T6Ø.8X2	T6Ø.8X3	T6Ø.8X4	—	—
Pipethanate	T44.3X1	T44.3X2	T44.3X3	T44.3X4	T44.3X5	T44.3X6
Pipobroman	T45.1X1	T45.1X2	T45.1X3	T45.1X4	T45.1X5	T45.1X6
Pipotiazine	T43.3X1	T43.3X2	T43.3X3	T43.3X4	T43.3X5	T43.3X6
Pipoxizine	T45.ØX1	T45.ØX2	T45.ØX3	T45.ØX4	T45.ØX5	T45.ØX6
Pipradrol	T43.691	T43.692	T43.693	T43.694	T43.695	T43.696
Piprinhydrinate	T45.ØX1	T45.ØX2	T45.ØX3	T45.ØX4	T45.ØX5	T45.ØX6
Pirarubicin	T45.1X1	T45.1X2	T45.1X3	T45.1X4	T45.1X5	T45.1X6
Pirazinamide	T37.1X1	T37.1X2	T37.1X3	T37.1X4	T37.1X5	T37.1X6
Pirbuterol	T48.6X1	T48.6X2	T48.6X3	T48.6X4	T48.6X5	T48.6X6
Pirenzepine	T47.1X1	T47.1X2	T47.1X3	T47.1X4	T47.1X5	T47.1X6
Piretanide	T5Ø.1X1	T5Ø.1X2	T5Ø.1X3	T5Ø.1X4	T5Ø.1X5	T5Ø.1X6
Piribedil	T42.8X1	T42.8X2	T42.8X3	T42.8X4	T42.8X5	T42.8X6
Piridoxilate	T46.3X1	T46.3X2	T46.3X3	T46.3X4	T46.3X5	T46.3X6
Piritramide	T4Ø.491	T4Ø.492	T4Ø.493	T4Ø.494	—	—
Piromidic acid	T37.8X1	T37.8X2	T37.8X3	T37.8X4	T37.8X5	T37.8X6
Piroxicam	T39.391	T39.392	T39.393	T39.394	T39.395	T39.396
beta-cyclodextrin complex	T39.8X1	T39.8X2	T39.8X3	T39.8X4	T39.8X5	T39.8X6
Pirozadil	T46.6X1	T46.6X2	T46.6X3	T46.6X4	T46.6X5	T46.6X6
Piscidia (bark) (erythrina)	T39.8X1	T39.8X2	T39.8X3	T39.8X4	T39.8X5	T39.8X6
Pitch	T65.891	T65.892	T65.893	T65.894	—	—
Pitkin's solution	T41.3X1	T41.3X2	T41.3X3	T41.3X4	T41.3X5	T41.3X6

Substance	Poisoning, Accidental (unintentional)	Poisoning, Intentional Self-harm	Poisoning, Assault	Poisoning, Undetermined	Adverse Effect	Under-dosing
Pitocin	T48.ØX1	T48.ØX2	T48.ØX3	T48.ØX4	T48.ØX5	T48.ØX6
Pitressin (tannate)	T38.891	T38.892	T38.893	T38.894	T38.895	T38.896
Pituitary extracts (posterior)	T38.891	T38.892	T38.893	T38.894	T38.895	T38.896
anterior	T38.811	T38.812	T38.813	T38.814	T38.815	T38.816
Pituitrin	T38.891	T38.892	T38.893	T38.894	T38.895	T38.896
Pivampicillin	T36.ØX1	T36.ØX2	T36.ØX3	T36.ØX4	T36.ØX5	T36.ØX6
Pivmecillinam	T36.ØX1	T36.ØX2	T36.ØX3	T36.ØX4	T36.ØX5	T36.ØX6
Placental hormone	T38.891	T38.892	T38.893	T38.894	T38.895	T38.896
Placidyl	T42.6X1	T42.6X2	T42.6X3	T42.6X4	T42.6X5	T42.6X6
Plague vaccine	T5Ø.A91	T5Ø.A92	T5Ø.A93	T5Ø.A94	T5Ø.A95	T5Ø.A96
Plant						
food or fertilizer NEC	T65.891	T65.892	T65.893	T65.894	—	—
containing herbicide	T6Ø.3X1	T6Ø.3X2	T6Ø.3X3	T6Ø.3X4	—	—
noxious, used as food	T62.2X1	T62.2X2	T62.2X3	T62.2X4	—	—
berries	T62.1X1	T62.1X2	T62.1X3	T62.1X4	—	—
seeds	T62.2X1	T62.2X2	T62.2X3	T62.2X4	—	—
specified type NEC	T62.2X1	T62.2X2	T62.2X3	T62.2X4	—	—
Plasma	T45.8X1	T45.8X2	T45.8X3	T45.8X4	T45.8X5	T45.8X6
expander NEC	T45.8X1	T45.8X2	T45.8X3	T45.8X4	T45.8X5	T45.8X6
protein fraction (human)	T45.8X1	T45.8X2	T45.8X3	T45.8X4	T45.8X5	T45.8X6
Plasmanate	T45.8X1	T45.8X2	T45.8X3	T45.8X4	T45.8X5	T45.8X6
Plasminogen (tissue) activator	T45.611	T45.612	T45.613	T45.614	T45.615	T45.616
Plaster dressing	T49.3X1	T49.3X2	T49.3X3	T49.3X4	T49.3X5	T49.3X6
Plastic dressing	T49.3X1	T49.3X2	T49.3X3	T49.3X4	T49.3X5	T49.3X6
Plegicil	T43.3X1	T43.3X2	T43.3X3	T43.3X4	T43.3X5	T43.3X6
Plicamycin	T45.1X1	T45.1X2	T45.1X3	T45.1X4	T45.1X5	T45.1X6
Podophyllotoxin	T49.8X1	T49.8X2	T49.8X3	T49.8X4	T49.8X5	T49.8X6
Podophyllum (resin)	T49.4X1	T49.4X2	T49.4X3	T49.4X4	T49.4X5	T49.4X6
Poisonous berries	T62.1X1	T62.1X2	T62.1X3	T62.1X4	—	—
Poison NEC	T65.91	T65.92	T65.93	T65.94	—	—
Pokeweed (any part)	T62.2X1	T62.2X2	T62.2X3	T62.2X4	—	—
Poldine metilsulfate	T44.3X1	T44.3X2	T44.3X3	T44.3X4	T44.3X5	T44.3X6
Polidexide (sulfate)	T46.6X1	T46.6X2	T46.6X3	T46.6X4	T46.6X5	T46.6X6
Polidocanol	T46.8X1	T46.8X2	T46.8X3	T46.8X4	T46.8X5	T46.8X6
Poliomyelitis vaccine	T5Ø.B91	T5Ø.B92	T5Ø.B93	T5Ø.B94	T5Ø.B95	T5Ø.B96
Polish (car) (floor) (furniture) (metal) (porcelain) (silver)	T65.891	T65.892	T65.893	T65.894	—	—
abrasive	T65.891	T65.892	T65.893	T65.894	—	—
porcelain	T65.891	T65.892	T65.893	T65.894	—	—
Poloxalkol	T47.4X1	T47.4X2	T47.4X3	T47.4X4	T47.4X5	T47.4X6
Poloxamer	T47.4X1	T47.4X2	T47.4X3	T47.4X4	T47.4X5	T47.4X6
Polyaminostyrene resins	T5Ø.3X1	T5Ø.3X2	T5Ø.3X3	T5Ø.3X4	T5Ø.3X5	T5Ø.3X6
Polycarbophil	T47.4X1	T47.4X2	T47.4X3	T47.4X4	T47.4X5	T47.4X6
Polychlorinated biphenyl	T65.891	T65.892	T65.893	T65.894	—	—
Polycycline	T36.4X1	T36.4X2	T36.4X3	T36.4X4	T36.4X5	T36.4X6
Polyester fumes	T59.891	T59.892	T59.893	T59.894	—	—
Polyester resin hardener	T52.91	T52.92	T52.93	T52.94	—	—
fumes	T59.891	T59.892	T59.893	T59.894	—	—
Polyestradiol phosphate	T38.5X1	T38.5X2	T38.5X3	T38.5X4	T38.5X5	T38.5X6
Polyethanolamine alkyl sulfate	T49.2X1	T49.2X2	T49.2X3	T49.2X4	T49.2X5	T49.2X6
Polyethylene adhesive	T49.3X1	T49.3X2	T49.3X3	T49.3X4	T49.3X5	T49.3X6
Polyferose	T45.4X1	T45.4X2	T45.4X3	T45.4X4	T45.4X5	T45.4X6
Polygeline	T45.8X1	T45.8X2	T45.8X3	T45.8X4	T45.8X5	T45.8X6
Polymyxin	T36.8X1	T36.8X2	T36.8X3	T36.8X4	T36.8X5	T36.8X6
B	T36.8X1	T36.8X2	T36.8X3	T36.8X4	T36.8X5	T36.8X6
ENT agent	T49.6X1	T49.6X2	T49.6X3	T49.6X4	T49.6X5	T49.6X6
ophthalmic preparation	T49.5X1	T49.5X2	T49.5X3	T49.5X4	T49.5X5	T49.5X6
topical NEC	T49.ØX1	T49.ØX2	T49.ØX3	T49.ØX4	T49.ØX5	T49.ØX6
E sulfate (eye preparation)	T49.5X1	T49.5X2	T49.5X3	T49.5X4	T49.5X5	T49.5X6
Polynoxylin	T49.ØX1	T49.ØX2	T49.ØX3	T49.ØX4	T49.ØX5	T49.ØX6
Polyoestradiol phosphate	T38.5X1	T38.5X2	T38.5X3	T38.5X4	T38.5X5	T38.5X6
Polyoxymethyleneurea	T49.ØX1	T49.ØX2	T49.ØX3	T49.ØX4	T49.ØX5	T49.ØX6
Polysilane	T47.8X1	T47.8X2	T47.8X3	T47.8X4	T47.8X5	T47.8X6
Polytetrafluoroethylene (inhaled)	T59.891	T59.892	T59.893	T59.894	—	—
Polythiazide	T5Ø.2X1	T5Ø.2X2	T5Ø.2X3	T5Ø.2X4	T5Ø.2X5	T5Ø.2X6
Polyvidone	T45.8X1	T45.8X2	T45.8X3	T45.8X4	T45.8X5	T45.8X6
Polyvinylpyrrolidone	T45.8X1	T45.8X2	T45.8X3	T45.8X4	T45.8X5	T45.8X6
Pontocaine (hydrochloride) (infiltration) (topical)	T41.3X1	T41.3X2	T41.3X3	T41.3X4	T41.3X5	T41.3X6
nerve block (peripheral) (plexus)	T41.3X1	T41.3X2	T41.3X3	T41.3X4	T41.3X5	T41.3X6
spinal	T41.3X1	T41.3X2	T41.3X3	T41.3X4	T41.3X5	T41.3X6
Porfiromycin	T45.1X1	T45.1X2	T45.1X3	T45.1X4	T45.1X5	T45.1X6
Posterior pituitary hormone NEC	T38.891	T38.892	T38.893	T38.894	T38.895	T38.896
Pot	T4Ø.7X1	T4Ø.7X2	T4Ø.7X3	T4Ø.7X4	T4Ø.7X5	T4Ø.7X6
Potash (caustic)	T54.3X1	T54.3X2	T54.3X3	T54.3X4	—	—

Substance	Poisoning, Accidental (unintentional)	Poisoning, Intentional Self-harm	Poisoning, Assault	Poisoning, Undetermined	Adverse Effect	Under-dosing
Potassic saline injection (lactated)	T5Ø.3X1	T5Ø.3X2	T5Ø.3X3	T5Ø.3X4	T5Ø.3X5	T5Ø.3X6
Potassium (salts) **NEC**	T5Ø.3X1	T5Ø.3X2	T5Ø.3X3	T5Ø.3X4	T5Ø.3X5	T5Ø.3X6
aminobenzoate	T45.8X1	T45.8X2	T45.8X3	T45.8X4	T45.8X5	T45.8X6
aminosalicylate	T37.1X1	T37.1X2	T37.1X3	T37.1X4	T37.1X5	T37.1X6
antimony 'tartrate'	T37.8X1	T37.8X2	T37.8X3	T37.8X4	T37.8X5	T37.8X6
arsenite (solution)	T57.ØX1	T57.ØX2	T57.ØX3	T57.ØX4	—	—
bichromate	T56.2X1	T56.2X2	T56.2X3	T56.2X4	—	—
bisulfate	T47.3X1	T47.3X2	T47.3X3	T47.3X4	T47.3X5	T47.3X6
bromide	T42.6X1	T42.6X2	T42.6X3	T42.6X4	T42.6X5	T42.6X6
canrenoate	T5Ø.ØX1	T5Ø.ØX2	T5Ø.ØX3	T5Ø.ØX4	T5Ø.ØX5	T5Ø.ØX6
carbonate	T54.3X1	T54.3X2	T54.3X3	T54.3X4	—	—
chlorate NEC	T65.891	T65.892	T65.893	T65.894	—	—
chloride	T5Ø.3X1	T5Ø.3X2	T5Ø.3X3	T5Ø.3X4	T5Ø.3X5	T5Ø.3X6
citrate	T5Ø.991	T5Ø.992	T5Ø.993	T5Ø.994	T5Ø.995	T5Ø.996
cyanide	T65.ØX1	T65.ØX2	T65.ØX3	T65.ØX4	—	—
ferric hexacyanoferrate (medicinal)	T5Ø.6X1	T5Ø.6X2	T5Ø.6X3	T5Ø.6X4	T5Ø.6X5	T5Ø.6X6
nonmedicinal	T65.891	T65.892	T65.893	T65.894	—	—
Fluoride	T57.8X1	T57.8X2	T57.8X3	T57.8X4	—	—
glucaldrate	T47.1X1	T47.1X2	T47.1X3	T47.1X4	T47.1X5	T47.1X6
hydroxide	T54.3X1	T54.3X2	T54.3X3	T54.3X4	—	—
iodate	T49.ØX1	T49.ØX2	T49.ØX3	T49.ØX4	T49.ØX5	T49.ØX6
iodide	T48.4X1	T48.4X2	T48.4X3	T48.4X4	T48.4X5	T48.4X6
nitrate	T57.8X1	T57.8X2	T57.8X3	T57.8X4	—	—
oxalate	T65.891	T65.892	T65.893	T65.894	—	—
perchlorate (nonmedicinal) NEC	T65.891	T65.892	T65.893	T65.894	—	—
antithyroid	T38.2X1	T38.2X2	T38.2X3	T38.2X4	T38.2X5	T38.2X6
medicinal	T38.2X1	T38.2X2	T38.2X3	T38.2X4	T38.2X5	T38.2X6
Permanganate (nonmedicinal)	T65.891	T65.892	T65.893	T65.894	—	—
medicinal	T49.ØX1	T49.ØX2	T49.ØX3	T49.ØX4	T49.ØX5	T49.ØX6
sulfate	T47.2X1	T47.2X2	T47.2X3	T47.2X4	T47.2X5	T47.2X6
Potassium-removing resin	T5Ø.3X1	T5Ø.3X2	T5Ø.3X3	T5Ø.3X4	T5Ø.3X5	T5Ø.3X6
Potassium-retaining drug	T5Ø.3X1	T5Ø.3X2	T5Ø.3X3	T5Ø.3X4	T5Ø.3X5	T5Ø.3X6
Povidone	T45.8X1	T45.8X2	T45.8X3	T45.8X4	T45.8X5	T45.8X6
iodine	T49.ØX1	T49.ØX2	T49.ØX3	T49.ØX4	T49.ØX5	T49.ØX6
Practolol	T44.7X1	T44.7X2	T44.7X3	T44.7X4	T44.7X5	T44.7X6
Prajmalium bitartrate	T46.2X1	T46.2X2	T46.2X3	T46.2X4	T46.2X5	T46.2X6
Pralidoxime (iodide)	T5Ø.6X1	T5Ø.6X2	T5Ø.6X3	T5Ø.6X4	T5Ø.6X5	T5Ø.6X6
chloride	T5Ø.6X1	T5Ø.6X2	T5Ø.6X3	T5Ø.6X4	T5Ø.6X5	T5Ø.6X6
Pramiverine	T44.3X1	T44.3X2	T44.3X3	T44.3X4	T44.3X5	T44.3X6
Pramocaine	T49.1X1	T49.1X2	T49.1X3	T49.1X4	T49.1X5	T49.1X6
Pramoxine	T49.1X1	T49.1X2	T49.1X3	T49.1X4	T49.1X5	T49.1X6
Prasterone	T38.7X1	T38.7X2	T38.7X3	T38.7X4	T38.7X5	T38.7X6
Pravastatin	T46.6X1	T46.6X2	T46.6X3	T46.6X4	T46.6X5	T46.6X6
Prazepam	T42.4X1	T42.4X2	T42.4X3	T42.4X4	T42.4X5	T42.4X6
Praziquantel	T37.4X1	T37.4X2	T37.4X3	T37.4X4	T37.4X5	T37.4X6
Prazitone	T43.291	T43.292	T43.293	T43.294	T43.295	T43.296
Prazosin	T44.6X1	T44.6X2	T44.6X3	T44.6X4	T44.6X5	T44.6X6
Prednicarbate	T49.ØX1	T49.ØX2	T49.ØX3	T49.ØX4	T49.ØX5	T49.ØX6
Prednimustine	T45.1X1	T45.1X2	T45.1X3	T45.1X4	T45.1X5	T45.1X6
Prednisolone	T38.ØX1	T38.ØX2	T38.ØX3	T38.ØX4	T38.ØX5	T38.ØX6
ENT agent	T49.6X1	T49.6X2	T49.6X3	T49.6X4	T49.6X5	T49.6X6
ophthalmic preparation	T49.5X1	T49.5X2	T49.5X3	T49.5X4	T49.5X5	T49.5X6
steaglate	T49.ØX1	T49.ØX2	T49.ØX3	T49.ØX4	T49.ØX5	T49.ØX6
topical NEC	T49.ØX1	T49.ØX2	T49.ØX3	T49.ØX4	T49.ØX5	T49.ØX6
Prednisone	T38.ØX1	T38.ØX2	T38.ØX3	T38.ØX4	T38.ØX5	T38.ØX6
Prednylidene	T38.ØX1	T38.ØX2	T38.ØX3	T38.ØX4	T38.ØX5	T38.ØX6
Pregnandiol	T38.5X1	T38.5X2	T38.5X3	T38.5X4	T38.5X5	T38.5X6
Pregneninolone	T38.5X1	T38.5X2	T38.5X3	T38.5X4	T38.5X5	T38.5X6
Preludin	T43.691	T43.692	T43.693	T43.694	T43.695	T43.696
Premarin	T38.5X1	T38.5X2	T38.5X3	T38.5X4	T38.5X5	T38.5X6
Premedication anesthetic	T41.2Ø1	T41.2Ø2	T41.2Ø3	T41.2Ø4	T41.2Ø5	T41.2Ø6
Prenalterol	T44.5X1	T44.5X2	T44.5X3	T44.5X4	T44.5X5	T44.5X6
Prenoxdiazine	T48.3X1	T48.3X2	T48.3X3	T48.3X4	T48.3X5	T48.3X6
Prenylamine	T46.3X1	T46.3X2	T46.3X3	T46.3X4	T46.3X5	T46.3X6
Preparation H	T49.8X1	T49.8X2	T49.8X3	T49.8X4	T49.8X5	T49.8X6
Preparation, local	T49.4X1	T49.4X2	T49.4X3	T49.4X4	T49.4X5	T49.4X6
Preservative (nonmedicinal)	T65.891	T65.892	T65.893	T65.894	—	—
medicinal	T5Ø.9Ø1	T5Ø.9Ø2	T5Ø.9Ø3	T5Ø.9Ø4	T5Ø.9Ø5	T5Ø.9Ø6
wood	T6Ø.91	T6Ø.92	T6Ø.93	T6Ø.94	—	—
Prethcamide	T5Ø.7X1	T5Ø.7X2	T5Ø.7X3	T5Ø.7X4	T5Ø.7X5	T5Ø.7X6
Pride of China	T62.2X1	T62.2X2	T62.2X3	T62.2X4	—	—
Pridinol	T44.3X1	T44.3X2	T44.3X3	T44.3X4	T44.3X5	T44.3X6
Prifinium bromide	T44.3X1	T44.3X2	T44.3X3	T44.3X4	T44.3X5	T44.3X6
Prilocaine	T41.3X1	T41.3X2	T41.3X3	T41.3X4	T41.3X5	T41.3X6
infiltration (subcutaneous)	T41.3X1	T41.3X2	T41.3X3	T41.3X4	T41.3X5	T41.3X6
nerve block (peripheral) (plexus)	T41.3X1	T41.3X2	T41.3X3	T41.3X4	T41.3X5	T41.3X6
regional	T41.3X1	T41.3X2	T41.3X3	T41.3X4	T41.3X5	T41.3X6

Substance	Poisoning, Accidental (unintentional)	Poisoning, Intentional Self-harm	Poisoning, Assault	Poisoning, Undetermined	Adverse Effect	Under-dosing
Primaquine	T37.2X1	T37.2X2	T37.2X3	T37.2X4	T37.2X5	T37.2X6
Primidone	T42.6X1	T42.6X2	T42.6X3	T42.6X4	T42.6X5	T42.6X6
Primula (veris)	T62.2X1	T62.2X2	T62.2X3	T62.2X4	—	—
Prinadol	T40.2X1	T40.2X2	T40.2X3	T40.2X4	T40.2X5	T40.2X6
Priscol, Priscoline	T44.6X1	T44.6X2	T44.6X3	T44.6X4	T44.6X5	T44.6X6
Pristinamycin	T36.3X1	T36.3X2	T36.3X3	T36.3X4	T36.3X5	T36.3X6
Privet	T62.2X1	T62.2X2	T62.2X3	T62.2X4	—	—
berries	T62.1X1	T62.1X2	T62.1X3	T62.1X4	—	—
Privine	T44.4X1	T44.4X2	T44.4X3	T44.4X4	T44.4X5	T44.4X6
Pro-Banthine	T44.3X1	T44.3X2	T44.3X3	T44.3X4	T44.3X5	T44.3X6
Probarbital	T42.3X1	T42.3X2	T42.3X3	T42.3X4	T42.3X5	T42.3X6
Probenecid	T50.4X1	T50.4X2	T50.4X3	T50.4X4	T50.4X5	T50.4X6
Probucol	T46.6X1	T46.6X2	T46.6X3	T46.6X4	T46.6X5	T46.6X6
Procainamide	T46.2X1	T46.2X2	T46.2X3	T46.2X4	T46.2X5	T46.2X6
Procaine	T41.3X1	T41.3X2	T41.3X3	T41.3X4	T41.3X5	T41.3X6
benzylpenicillin	T36.0X1	T36.0X2	T36.0X3	T36.0X4	T36.0X5	T36.0X6
nerve block (periphreal) (plexus)	T41.3X1	T41.3X2	T41.3X3	T41.3X4	T41.3X5	T41.3X6
penicillin G	T36.0X1	T36.0X2	T36.0X3	T36.0X4	T36.0X5	T36.0X6
regional	T41.3X1	T41.3X2	T41.3X3	T41.3X4	T41.3X5	T41.3X6
spinal	T41.3X1	T41.3X2	T41.3X3	T41.3X4	T41.3X5	T41.3X6
Procalmidol	T43.591	T43.592	T43.593	T43.594	T43.595	T43.596
Procarbazine	T45.1X1	T45.1X2	T45.1X3	T45.1X4	T45.1X5	T45.1X6
Procaterol	T44.5X1	T44.5X2	T44.5X3	T44.5X4	T44.5X5	T44.5X6
Prochlorperazine	T43.3X1	T43.3X2	T43.3X3	T43.3X4	T43.3X5	T43.3X6
Procyclidine	T44.3X1	T44.3X2	T44.3X3	T44.3X4	T44.3X5	T44.3X6
Producer gas	T58.8X1	T58.8X2	T58.8X3	T58.8X4	—	—
Profadol	T40.491	T40.492	T40.493	T40.494	T40.495	T40.496
Profenamine	T44.3X1	T44.3X2	T44.3X3	T44.3X4	T44.3X5	T44.3X6
Profenil	T44.3X1	T44.3X2	T44.3X3	T44.3X4	T44.3X5	T44.3X6
Proflavine	T49.0X1	T49.0X2	T49.0X3	T49.0X4	T49.0X5	T49.0X6
Progabide	T42.6X1	T42.6X2	T42.6X3	T42.6X4	T42.6X5	T42.6X6
Progesterone	T38.5X1	T38.5X2	T38.5X3	T38.5X4	T38.5X5	T38.5X6
Progestin	T38.5X1	T38.5X2	T38.5X3	T38.5X4	T38.5X5	T38.5X6
oral contraceptive	T38.4X1	T38.4X2	T38.4X3	T38.4X4	T38.4X5	T38.4X6
Progestogen NEC	T38.5X1	T38.5X2	T38.5X3	T38.5X4	T38.5X5	T38.5X6
Progestone	T38.5X1	T38.5X2	T38.5X3	T38.5X4	T38.5X5	T38.5X6
Proglumide	T47.1X1	T47.1X2	T47.1X3	T47.1X4	T47.1X5	T47.1X6
Proguanil	T37.2X1	T37.2X2	T37.2X3	T37.2X4	T37.2X5	T37.2X6
Prolactin	T38.811	T38.812	T38.813	T38.814	T38.815	T38.816
Prolintane	T43.691	T43.692	T43.693	T43.694	T43.695	T43.696
Proloid	T38.1X1	T38.1X2	T38.1X3	T38.1X4	T38.1X5	T38.1X6
Proluton	T38.5X1	T38.5X2	T38.5X3	T38.5X4	T38.5X5	T38.5X6
Promacetin	T37.1X1	T37.1X2	T37.1X3	T37.1X4	T37.1X5	T37.1X6
Promazine	T43.3X1	T43.3X2	T43.3X3	T43.3X4	T43.3X5	T43.3X6
Promedol	T40.2X1	T40.2X2	T40.2X3	T40.2X4	—	—
Promegestone	T38.5X1	T38.5X2	T38.5X3	T38.5X4	T38.5X5	T38.5X6
Promethazine (teoclate)	T43.3X1	T43.3X2	T43.3X3	T43.3X4	T43.3X5	T43.3X6
Promin	T37.1X1	T37.1X2	T37.1X3	T37.1X4	T37.1X5	T37.1X6
Pronase	T45.3X1	T45.3X2	T45.3X3	T45.3X4	T45.3X5	T45.3X6
Pronestyl (hydrochloride)	T46.2X1	T46.2X2	T46.2X3	T46.2X4	T46.2X5	T46.2X6
Pronetalol	T44.7X1	T44.7X2	T44.7X3	T44.7X4	T44.7X5	T44.7X6
Prontosil	T37.0X1	T37.0X2	T37.0X3	T37.0X4	T37.0X5	T37.0X6
Propachlor	T60.3X1	T60.3X2	T60.3X3	T60.3X4	—	—
Propafenone	T46.2X1	T46.2X2	T46.2X3	T46.2X4	T46.2X5	T46.2X6
Propallylonal	T42.3X1	T42.3X2	T42.3X3	T42.3X4	T42.3X5	T42.3X6
Propamidine	T49.0X1	T49.0X2	T49.0X3	T49.0X4	T49.0X5	T49.0X6
Propane (distributed in mobile container)	T59.891	T59.892	T59.893	T59.894	—	—
distributed through pipes	T59.891	T59.892	T59.893	T59.894	—	—
incomplete combustion	T58.11	T58.12	T58.13	T58.14	—	—
Propanidid	T41.291	T41.292	T41.293	T41.294	T41.295	T41.296
Propanil	T60.3X1	T60.3X2	T60.3X3	T60.3X4	—	—
Propantheline	T44.3X1	T44.3X2	T44.3X3	T44.3X4	T44.3X5	T44.3X6
bromide	T44.3X1	T44.3X2	T44.3X3	T44.3X4	T44.3X5	T44.3X6
Proparacaine	T41.3X1	T41.3X2	T41.3X3	T41.3X4	T41.3X5	T41.3X6
Propatylnitrate	T46.3X1	T46.3X2	T46.3X3	T46.3X4	T46.3X5	T46.3X6
Propicillin	T36.0X1	T36.0X2	T36.0X3	T36.0X4	T36.0X5	T36.0X6
Propiolactone	T49.0X1	T49.0X2	T49.0X3	T49.0X4	T49.0X5	T49.0X6
Propiomazine	T45.0X1	T45.0X2	T45.0X3	T45.0X4	T45.0X5	T45.0X6
Propionaldehyde (medicinal)	T42.6X1	T42.6X2	T42.6X3	T42.6X4	T42.6X5	T42.6X6
Propionate (calcium) (sodium)	T49.0X1	T49.0X2	T49.0X3	T49.0X4	T49.0X5	T49.0X6
Propion gel	T49.0X1	T49.0X2	T49.0X3	T49.0X4	T49.0X5	T49.0X6
Propitocaine	T41.3X1	T41.3X2	T41.3X3	T41.3X4	T41.3X5	T41.3X6
infiltration (subcutaneous)	T41.3X1	T41.3X2	T41.3X3	T41.3X4	T41.3X5	T41.3X6
nerve block (peripheral) (plexus)	T41.3X1	T41.3X2	T41.3X3	T41.3X4	T41.3X5	T41.3X6
Propofol	T41.291	T41.292	T41.293	T41.294	T41.295	T41.296
Propoxur	T60.0X1	T60.0X2	T60.0X3	T60.0X4	—	—
Propoxycaine	T41.3X1	T41.3X2	T41.3X3	T41.3X4	T41.3X5	T41.3X6
infiltration (subcutaneous)	T41.3X1	T41.3X2	T41.3X3	T41.3X4	T41.3X5	T41.3X6

Substance	Poisoning, Accidental (unintentional)	Poisoning, Intentional Self-harm	Poisoning, Assault	Poisoning, Undetermined	Adverse Effect	Under-dosing
Propoxycaine — *continued*						
nerve block (peripheral) (plexus)	T41.3X1	T41.3X2	T41.3X3	T41.3X4	T41.3X5	T41.3X6
topical (surface)	T41.3X1	T41.3X2	T41.3X3	T41.3X4	T41.3X5	T41.3X6
Propoxyphene	T40.491	T40.492	T40.493	T40.494	T40.495	T40.496
Propranolol	T44.7X1	T44.7X2	T44.7X3	T44.7X4	T44.7X5	T44.7X6
Propyl						
alcohol	T51.3X1	T51.3X2	T51.3X3	T51.3X4	—	—
carbinol	T51.3X1	T51.3X2	T51.3X3	T51.3X4	—	—
hexadrine	T44.4X1	T44.4X2	T44.4X3	T44.4X4	T44.4X5	T44.4X6
iodone	T50.8X1	T50.8X2	T50.8X3	T50.8X4	T50.8X5	T50.8X6
thiouracil	T38.2X1	T38.2X2	T38.2X3	T38.2X4	T38.2X5	T38.2X6
Propylaminophenothiazine	T43.3X1	T43.3X2	T43.3X3	T43.3X4	T43.3X5	T43.3X6
Propylene	T59.891	T59.892	T59.893	T59.894	—	—
Propylhexedrine	T48.5X1	T48.5X2	T48.5X3	T48.5X4	T48.5X5	T48.5X6
Propyliodone	T50.8X1	T50.8X2	T50.8X3	T50.8X4	T50.8X5	T50.8X6
Propylparaben (ophthalmic)	T49.5X1	T49.5X2	T49.5X3	T49.5X4	T49.5X5	T49.5X6
Propylthiouracil	T38.2X1	T38.2X2	T38.2X3	T38.2X4	T38.2X5	T38.2X6
Propyphenazone	T39.2X1	T39.2X2	T39.2X3	T39.2X4	T39.2X5	T39.2X6
Proquazone	T39.391	T39.392	T39.393	T39.394	T39.395	T39.396
Proscillaridin	T46.0X1	T46.0X2	T46.0X3	T46.0X4	T46.0X5	T46.0X6
Prostacyclin	T45.521	T45.522	T45.523	T45.524	T45.525	T45.526
Prostaglandin (I2)	T45.521	T45.522	T45.523	T45.524	T45.525	T45.526
E1	T46.7X1	T46.7X2	T46.7X3	T46.7X4	T46.7X5	T46.7X6
E2	T48.0X1	T48.0X2	T48.0X3	T48.0X4	T48.0X5	T48.0X6
F2 alpha	T48.0X1	T48.0X2	T48.0X3	T48.0X4	T48.0X5	T48.0X6
Prostigmin	T44.0X1	T44.0X2	T44.0X3	T44.0X4	T44.0X5	T44.0X6
Prosultiamine	T45.2X1	T45.2X2	T45.2X3	T45.2X4	T45.2X5	T45.2X6
Protamine sulfate	T45.7X1	T45.7X2	T45.7X3	T45.7X4	T45.7X5	T45.7X6
zinc insulin	T38.3X1	T38.3X2	T38.3X3	T38.3X4	T38.3X5	T38.3X6
Protease	T47.5X1	T47.5X2	T47.5X3	T47.5X4	T47.5X5	T47.5X6
Protectant, skin NEC	T49.3X1	T49.3X2	T49.3X3	T49.3X4	T49.3X5	T49.3X6
Protein hydrolysate	T50.991	T50.992	T50.993	T50.994	T50.995	T50.996
Prothiaden — *see* Dothiepin hydrochloride						
Prothionamide	T37.1X1	T37.1X2	T37.1X3	T37.1X4	T37.1X5	T37.1X6
Prothipendyl	T43.591	T43.592	T43.593	T43.594	T43.595	T43.596
Prothoate	T60.0X1	T60.0X2	T60.0X3	T60.0X4	—	—
Prothrombin						
activator	T45.7X1	T45.7X2	T45.7X3	T45.7X4	T45.7X5	T45.7X6
synthesis inhibitor	T45.511	T45.512	T45.513	T45.514	T45.515	T45.516
Protionamide	T37.1X1	T37.1X2	T37.1X3	T37.1X4	T37.1X5	T37.1X6
Protirelin	T38.891	T38.892	T38.893	T38.894	T38.895	T38.896
Protokylol	T48.6X1	T48.6X2	T48.6X3	T48.6X4	T48.6X5	T48.6X6
Protopam	T50.6X1	T50.6X2	T50.6X3	T50.6X4	T50.6X5	T50.6X6
Protoveratrine(s) (A) (B)	T46.5X1	T46.5X2	T46.5X3	T46.5X4	T46.5X5	T46.5X6
Protriptyline	T43.011	T43.012	T43.013	T43.014	T43.015	T43.016
Provera	T38.5X1	T38.5X2	T38.5X3	T38.5X4	T38.5X5	T38.5X6
Provitamin A	T45.2X1	T45.2X2	T45.2X3	T45.2X4	T45.2X5	T45.2X6
Proxibarbal	T42.3X1	T42.3X2	T42.3X3	T42.3X4	T42.3X5	T42.3X6
Proxymetacaine	T41.3X1	T41.3X2	T41.3X3	T41.3X4	T41.3X5	T41.3X6
Proxyphylline	T48.6X1	T48.6X2	T48.6X3	T48.6X4	T48.6X5	T48.6X6
Prozac — *see* Fluoxetine hydrochloride						
Prunus						
laurocerasus	T62.2X1	T62.2X2	T62.2X3	T62.2X4	—	—
virginiana	T62.2X1	T62.2X2	T62.2X3	T62.2X4	—	—
Prussian blue						
commercial	T65.891	T65.892	T65.893	T65.894	—	—
therapeutic	T50.6X1	T50.6X2	T50.6X3	T50.6X4	T50.6X5	T50.6X6
Prussic acid	T65.0X1	T65.0X2	T65.0X3	T65.0X4	—	—
vapor	T57.3X1	T57.3X2	T57.3X3	T57.3X4	—	—
Pseudoephedrine	T44.991	T44.992	T44.993	T44.994	T44.995	T44.996
Psilocin	T40.991	T40.992	T40.993	T40.994	—	—
Psilocybin	T40.991	T40.992	T40.993	T40.994	—	—
Psilocybine	T40.991	T40.992	T40.993	T40.994	—	—
Psoralene (nonmedicinal)	T65.891	T65.892	T65.893	T65.894	—	—
Psoralens (medicinal)	T50.991	T50.992	T50.993	T50.994	T50.995	T50.996
PSP (phenolsulfonphthalein)	T50.8X1	T50.8X2	T50.8X3	T50.8X4	T50.8X5	T50.8X6
Psychodysleptic drug NOS	T40.901	T40.902	T40.903	T40.904	T40.905	T40.906
specified NEC	T40.991	T40.992	T40.993	T40.994	T40.995	T40.996
Psychostimulant	T43.601	T43.602	T43.603	T43.604	T43.605	T43.606
amphetamine	T43.621	T43.622	T43.623	T43.624	T43.625	T43.626
caffeine	T43.611	T43.612	T43.613	T43.614	T43.615	T43.616
methylphenidate	T43.631	T43.632	T43.633	T43.634	T43.635	T43.636
specified NEC	T43.691	T43.692	T43.693	T43.694	T43.695	T43.696
Psychotherapeutic drug NEC	T43.91	T43.92	T43.93	T43.94	T43.95	T43.96
antidepressants — *see also* Antidepressant	T43.201	T43.202	T43.203	T43.204	T43.205	T43.206
specified NEC	T43.8X1	T43.8X2	T43.8X3	T43.8X4	T43.8X5	T43.8X6

Substance	Poisoning, Accidental (unintentional)	Poisoning, Intentional Self-harm	Poisoning, Assault	Poisoning, Undetermined	Adverse Effect	Under-dosing
Psychotherapeutic drug — *continued*						
tranquilizers NEC	T43.5Ø1	T43.5Ø2	T43.5Ø3	T43.5Ø4	T43.5Ø5	T43.5Ø6
Psychotomimetic agents	T4Ø.9Ø1	T4Ø.9Ø2	T4Ø.9Ø3	T4Ø.9Ø4	T4Ø.9Ø5	T4Ø.9Ø6
Psychotropic drug NEC	T43.91	T43.92	T43.93	T43.94	T43.95	T43.96
specified NEC	T43.8X1	T43.8X2	T43.8X3	T43.8X4	T43.8X5	T43.8X6
Psyllium hydrophilic mucilloid	T47.4X1	T47.4X2	T47.4X3	T47.4X4	T47.4X5	T47.4X6
Pteroylglutamic acid	T45.8X1	T45.8X2	T45.8X3	T45.8X4	T45.8X5	T45.8X6
Pteroyltriglutamate	T45.1X1	T45.1X2	T45.1X3	T45.1X4	T45.1X5	T45.1X6
PTFE — *see* Polytetrafluoroethylene						
Pulp						
devitalizing paste	T49.7X1	T49.7X2	T49.7X3	T49.7X4	T49.7X5	T49.7X6
dressing	T49.7X1	T49.7X2	T49.7X3	T49.7X4	T49.7X5	T49.7X6
Pulsatilla	T62.2X1	T62.2X2	T62.2X3	T62.2X4	—	—
Pumpkin seed extract	T37.4X1	T37.4X2	T37.4X3	T37.4X4	T37.4X5	T37.4X6
Purex (bleach)	T54.91	T54.92	T54.93	T54.94	—	—
Purgative NEC — *see also* Cathartic	T47.4X1	T47.4X2	T47.4X3	T47.4X4	T47.4X5	T47.4X6
Purine analogue (antineoplastic)	T45.1X1	T45.1X2	T45.1X3	T45.1X4	T45.1X5	T45.1X6
Purine diuretics	T5Ø.2X1	T5Ø.2X2	T5Ø.2X3	T5Ø.2X4	T5Ø.2X5	T5Ø.2X6
Purinethol	T45.1X1	T45.1X2	T45.1X3	T45.1X4	T45.1X5	T45.1X6
PVP	T45.8X1	T45.8X2	T45.8X3	T45.8X4	T45.8X5	T45.8X6
Pyrabital	T39.8X1	T39.8X2	T39.8X3	T39.8X4	T39.8X5	T39.8X6
Pyramidon	T39.2X1	T39.2X2	T39.2X3	T39.2X4	T39.2X5	T39.2X6
Pyrantel	T37.4X1	T37.4X2	T37.4X3	T37.4X4	T37.4X5	T37.4X6
Pyrathiazine	T45.ØX1	T45.ØX2	T45.ØX3	T45.ØX4	T45.ØX5	T45.ØX6
Pyrazinamide	T37.1X1	T37.1X2	T37.1X3	T37.1X4	T37.1X5	T37.1X6
Pyrazinoic acid (amide)	T37.1X1	T37.1X2	T37.1X3	T37.1X4	T37.1X5	T37.1X6
Pyrazole (derivatives)	T39.2X1	T39.2X2	T39.2X3	T39.2X4	T39.2X5	T39.2X6
Pyrazolone analgesic NEC	T39.2X1	T39.2X2	T39.2X3	T39.2X4	T39.2X5	T39.2X6
Pyrethrin, pyrethrum (nonmedicinal)	T6Ø.2X1	T6Ø.2X2	T6Ø.2X3	T6Ø.2X4	—	—
Pyrethrum extract	T49.ØX1	T49.ØX2	T49.ØX3	T49.ØX4	T49.ØX5	T49.ØX6
Pyribenzamine	T45.ØX1	T45.ØX2	T45.ØX3	T45.ØX4	T45.ØX5	T45.ØX6
Pyridine	T52.8X1	T52.8X2	T52.8X3	T52.8X4	—	—
aldoxime methiodide	T5Ø.6X1	T5Ø.6X2	T5Ø.6X3	T5Ø.6X4	T5Ø.6X5	T5Ø.6X6
aldoxime methyl chloride	T5Ø.6X1	T5Ø.6X2	T5Ø.6X3	T5Ø.6X4	T5Ø.6X5	T5Ø.6X6
vapor	T59.891	T59.892	T59.893	T59.894	—	—
Pyridium	T39.8X1	T39.8X2	T39.8X3	T39.8X4	T39.8X5	T39.8X6
Pyridostigmine bromide	T44.ØX1	T44.ØX2	T44.ØX3	T44.ØX4	T44.ØX5	T44.ØX6
Pyridoxal phosphate	T45.2X1	T45.2X2	T45.2X3	T45.2X4	T45.2X5	T45.2X6
Pyridoxine	T45.2X1	T45.2X2	T45.2X3	T45.2X4	T45.2X5	T45.2X6
Pyrilamine	T45.ØX1	T45.ØX2	T45.ØX3	T45.ØX4	T45.ØX5	T45.ØX6
Pyrimethamine	T37.2X1	T37.2X2	T37.2X3	T37.2X4	T37.2X5	T37.2X6
with sulfadoxine	T37.2X1	T37.2X2	T37.2X3	T37.2X4	T37.2X5	T37.2X6
Pyrimidine antagonist	T45.1X1	T45.1X2	T45.1X3	T45.1X4	T45.1X5	T45.1X6
Pyriminil	T6Ø.4X1	T6Ø.4X2	T6Ø.4X3	T6Ø.4X4	—	—
Pyrithione zinc	T49.4X1	T49.4X2	T49.4X3	T49.4X4	T49.4X5	T49.4X6
Pyrithyldione	T42.6X1	T42.6X2	T42.6X3	T42.6X4	T42.6X5	T42.6X6
Pyrogallic acid	T49.ØX1	T49.ØX2	T49.ØX3	T49.ØX4	T49.ØX5	T49.ØX6
Pyrogallol	T49.ØX1	T49.ØX2	T49.ØX3	T49.ØX4	T49.ØX5	T49.ØX6
Pyroxylin	T49.3X1	T49.3X2	T49.3X3	T49.3X4	T49.3X5	T49.3X6
Pyrrobutamine	T45.ØX1	T45.ØX2	T45.ØX3	T45.ØX4	T45.ØX5	T45.ØX6
Pyrrolizidine alkaloids	T62.8X1	T62.8X2	T62.8X3	T62.8X4	—	—
Pyrvinium chloride	T37.4X1	T37.4X2	T37.4X3	T37.4X4	T37.4X5	T37.4X6
PZI	T38.3X1	T38.3X2	T38.3X3	T38.3X4	T38.3X5	T38.3X6
Quaalude	T42.6X1	T42.6X2	T42.6X3	T42.6X4	T42.6X5	T42.6X6
Quarternary ammonium						
anti-infective	T49.ØX1	T49.ØX2	T49.ØX3	T49.ØX4	T49.ØX5	T49.ØX6
ganglion blocking	T44.2X1	T44.2X2	T44.2X3	T44.2X4	T44.2X5	T44.2X6
parasympatholytic	T44.3X1	T44.3X2	T44.3X3	T44.3X4	T44.3X5	T44.3X6
Quazepam	T42.4X1	T42.4X2	T42.4X3	T42.4X4	T42.4X5	T42.4X6
Quicklime	T54.3X1	T54.3X2	T54.3X3	T54.3X4	—	—
Quillaja extract	T48.4X1	T48.4X2	T48.4X3	T48.4X4	T48.4X5	T48.4X6
Quinacrine	T37.2X1	T37.2X2	T37.2X3	T37.2X4	T37.2X5	T37.2X6
Quinaglute	T46.2X1	T46.2X2	T46.2X3	T46.2X4	T46.2X5	T46.2X6
Quinalbarbital	T42.3X1	T42.3X2	T42.3X3	T42.3X4	T42.3X5	T42.3X6
Quinalbarbitone sodium	T42.3X1	T42.3X2	T42.3X3	T42.3X4	T42.3X5	T42.3X6
Quinalphos	T6Ø.ØX1	T6Ø.ØX2	T6Ø.ØX3	T6Ø.ØX4	—	—
Quinapril	T46.4X1	T46.4X2	T46.4X3	T46.4X4	T46.4X5	T46.4X6
Quinestradiol	T38.5X1	T38.5X2	T38.5X3	T38.5X4	T38.5X5	T38.5X6
Quinestradol	T38.5X1	T38.5X2	T38.5X3	T38.5X4	T38.5X5	T38.5X6
Quinestrol	T38.5X1	T38.5X2	T38.5X3	T38.5X4	T38.5X5	T38.5X6
Quinethazone	T5Ø.2X1	T5Ø.2X2	T5Ø.2X3	T5Ø.2X4	T5Ø.2X5	T5Ø.2X6
Quingestanol	T38.4X1	T38.4X2	T38.4X3	T38.4X4	T38.4X5	T38.4X6
Quinidine	T46.2X1	T46.2X2	T46.2X3	T46.2X4	T46.2X5	T46.2X6
Quinine	T37.2X1	T37.2X2	T37.2X3	T37.2X4	T37.2X5	T37.2X6
Quiniobine	T37.8X1	T37.8X2	T37.8X3	T37.8X4	T37.8X5	T37.8X6
Quinisocaine	T49.1X1	T49.1X2	T49.1X3	T49.1X4	T49.1X5	T49.1X6
Quinocide	T37.2X1	T37.2X2	T37.2X3	T37.2X4	T37.2X5	T37.2X6

Substance	Poisoning, Accidental (unintentional)	Poisoning, Intentional Self-harm	Poisoning, Assault	Poisoning, Undetermined	Adverse Effect	Under-dosing
Quinoline (derivatives) **NEC**	T37.8X1	T37.8X2	T37.8X3	T37.8X4	T37.8X5	T37.8X6
Quinupramine	T43.Ø11	T43.Ø12	T43.Ø13	T43.Ø14	T43.Ø15	T43.Ø16
Quotane	T41.3X1	T41.3X2	T41.3X3	T41.3X4	T41.3X5	T41.3X6
Rabies						
immune globulin (human)	T5Ø.Z11	T5Ø.Z12	T5Ø.Z13	T5Ø.Z14	T5Ø.Z15	T5Ø.Z16
vaccine	T5Ø.B91	T5Ø.B92	T5Ø.B93	T5Ø.B94	T5Ø.B95	T5Ø.B96
Racemoramide	T4Ø.2X1	T4Ø.2X2	T4Ø.2X3	T4Ø.2X4	—	—
Racemorphan	T4Ø.2X1	T4Ø.2X2	T4Ø.2X3	T4Ø.2X4	T4Ø.2X5	T4Ø.2X6
Racepinefrin	T44.5X1	T44.5X2	T44.5X3	T44.5X4	T44.5X5	T44.5X6
Raclopride	T43.591	T43.592	T43.593	T43.594	T43.595	T43.596
Radiator alcohol	T51.1X1	T51.1X2	T51.1X3	T51.1X4	—	—
Radioactive drug NEC	T5Ø.8X1	T5Ø.8X2	T5Ø.8X3	T5Ø.8X4	T5Ø.8X5	T5Ø.8X6
Radio-opaque (drugs) (materials)	T5Ø.8X1	T5Ø.8X2	T5Ø.8X3	T5Ø.8X4	T5Ø.8X5	T5Ø.8X6
Ramifenazone	T39.2X1	T39.2X2	T39.2X3	T39.2X4	T39.2X5	T39.2X6
Ramipril	T46.4X1	T46.4X2	T46.4X3	T46.4X4	T46.4X5	T46.4X6
Ranitidine	T47.ØX1	T47.ØX2	T47.ØX3	T47.ØX4	T47.ØX5	T47.ØX6
Ranunculus	T62.2X1	T62.2X2	T62.2X3	T62.2X4	—	—
Rat poison NEC	T6Ø.4X1	T6Ø.4X2	T6Ø.4X3	T6Ø.4X4	—	—
Rattlesnake (venom)	T63.Ø11	T63.Ø12	T63.Ø13	T63.Ø14	—	—
Raubasine	T46.7X1	T46.7X2	T46.7X3	T46.7X4	T46.7X5	T46.7X6
Raudixin	T46.5X1	T46.5X2	T46.5X3	T46.5X4	T46.5X5	T46.5X6
Rautensin	T46.5X1	T46.5X2	T46.5X3	T46.5X4	T46.5X5	T46.5X6
Rautina	T46.5X1	T46.5X2	T46.5X3	T46.5X4	T46.5X5	T46.5X6
Rautotal	T46.5X1	T46.5X2	T46.5X3	T46.5X4	T46.5X5	T46.5X6
Rauwiloid	T46.5X1	T46.5X2	T46.5X3	T46.5X4	T46.5X5	T46.5X6
Rauwoldin	T46.5X1	T46.5X2	T46.5X3	T46.5X4	T46.5X5	T46.5X6
Rauwolfia (alkaloids)	T46.5X1	T46.5X2	T46.5X3	T46.5X4	T46.5X5	T46.5X6
Razoxane	T45.1X1	T45.1X2	T45.1X3	T45.1X4	T45.1X5	T45.1X6
Realgar	T57.ØX1	T57.ØX2	T57.ØX3	T57.ØX4	—	—
Recombinant (R) — *see* specific protein						
Red blood cells, packed	T45.8X1	T45.8X2	T45.8X3	T45.8X4	T45.8X5	T45.8X6
Red squill (scilliroside)	T6Ø.4X1	T6Ø.4X2	T6Ø.4X3	T6Ø.4X4	—	—
Reducing agent, industrial NEC	T65.891	T65.892	T65.893	T65.894	—	—
Refrigerant gas (chlorofluorocarbon)	T53.5X1	T53.5X2	T53.5X3	T53.5X4	—	—
not chlorofluorocarbon	T59.891	T59.892	T59.893	T59.894	—	—
Regroton	T5Ø.2X1	T5Ø.2X2	T5Ø.2X3	T5Ø.2X4	T5Ø.2X5	T5Ø.2X6
Rehydration salts (oral)	T5Ø.3X1	T5Ø.3X2	T5Ø.3X3	T5Ø.3X4	T5Ø.3X5	T5Ø.3X6
Rela	T42.8X1	T42.8X2	T42.8X3	T42.8X4	T42.8X5	T42.8X6
Relaxant, muscle						
anesthetic	T48.1X1	T48.1X2	T48.1X3	T48.1X4	T48.1X5	T48.1X6
central nervous system	T42.8X1	T42.8X2	T42.8X3	T42.8X4	T42.8X5	T42.8X6
skeletal NEC	T48.1X1	T48.1X2	T48.1X3	T48.1X4	T48.1X5	T48.1X6
smooth NEC	T44.3X1	T44.3X2	T44.3X3	T44.3X4	T44.3X5	T44.3X6
Remoxipride	T43.591	T43.592	T43.593	T43.594	T43.595	T43.596
Renese	T5Ø.2X1	T5Ø.2X2	T5Ø.2X3	T5Ø.2X4	T5Ø.2X5	T5Ø.2X6
Renografin	T5Ø.8X1	T5Ø.8X2	T5Ø.8X3	T5Ø.8X4	T5Ø.8X5	T5Ø.8X6
Replacement solution	T5Ø.3X1	T5Ø.3X2	T5Ø.3X3	T5Ø.3X4	T5Ø.3X5	T5Ø.3X6
Reproterol	T48.6X1	T48.6X2	T48.6X3	T48.6X4	T48.6X5	T48.6X6
Rescinnamine	T46.5X1	T46.5X2	T46.5X3	T46.5X4	T46.5X5	T46.5X6
Reserpin (e)	T46.5X1	T46.5X2	T46.5X3	T46.5X4	T46.5X5	T46.5X6
Resorcin, resorcinol (nonmedicinal)	T65.891	T65.892	T65.893	T65.894	—	—
medicinal	T49.4X1	T49.4X2	T49.4X3	T49.4X4	T49.4X5	T49.4X6
Respaire	T48.4X1	T48.4X2	T48.4X3	T48.4X4	T48.4X5	T48.4X6
Respiratory drug NEC	T48.9Ø1	T48.9Ø2	T48.9Ø3	T48.9Ø4	T48.9Ø5	T48.9Ø6
antiasthmatic NEC	T48.6X1	T48.6X2	T48.6X3	T48.6X4	T48.6X5	T48.6X6
anti-common-cold NEC	T48.5X1	T48.5X2	T48.5X3	T48.5X4	T48.5X5	T48.5X6
expectorant NEC	T48.4X1	T48.4X2	T48.4X3	T48.4X4	T48.4X5	T48.4X6
stimulant	T48.9Ø1	T48.9Ø2	T48.9Ø3	T48.9Ø4	T48.9Ø5	T48.9Ø6
Retinoic acid	T49.ØX1	T49.ØX2	T49.ØX3	T49.ØX4	T49.ØX5	T49.ØX6
Retinol	T45.2X1	T45.2X2	T45.2X3	T45.2X4	T45.2X5	T45.2X6
Rh (D) **immune globulin** (human)	T5Ø.Z11	T5Ø.Z12	T5Ø.Z13	T5Ø.Z14	T5Ø.Z15	T5Ø.Z16
Rhodine	T39.Ø11	T39.Ø12	T39.Ø13	T39.Ø14	T39.Ø15	T39.Ø16
RhoGAM	T5Ø.Z11	T5Ø.Z12	T5Ø.Z13	T5Ø.Z14	T5Ø.Z15	T5Ø.Z16
Rhubarb						
dry extract	T47.2X1	T47.2X2	T47.2X3	T47.2X4	T47.2X5	T47.2X6
tincture, compound	T47.2X1	T47.2X2	T47.2X3	T47.2X4	T47.2X5	T47.2X6
Ribavirin	T37.5X1	T37.5X2	T37.5X3	T37.5X4	T37.5X5	T37.5X6
Riboflavin	T45.2X1	T45.2X2	T45.2X3	T45.2X4	T45.2X5	T45.2X6
Ribostamycin	T36.5X1	T36.5X2	T36.5X3	T36.5X4	T36.5X5	T36.5X6
Ricin	T62.2X1	T62.2X2	T62.2X3	T62.2X4	—	—
Ricinus communis	T62.2X1	T62.2X2	T62.2X3	T62.2X4	—	—
Rickettsial vaccine NEC	T5Ø.A91	T5Ø.A92	T5Ø.A93	T5Ø.A94	T5Ø.A95	T5Ø.A96
Rifabutin	T36.6X1	T36.6X2	T36.6X3	T36.6X4	T36.6X5	T36.6X6
Rifamide	T36.6X1	T36.6X2	T36.6X3	T36.6X4	T36.6X5	T36.6X6
Rifampicin	T36.6X1	T36.6X2	T36.6X3	T36.6X4	T36.6X5	T36.6X6
with isoniazid	T37.1X1	T37.1X2	T37.1X3	T37.1X4	T37.1X5	T37.1X6
Rifampin	T36.6X1	T36.6X2	T36.6X3	T36.6X4	T36.6X5	T36.6X6

Substance	Poisoning, Accidental (unintentional)	Poisoning, Intentional Self-harm	Poisoning, Assault	Poisoning, Undetermined	Adverse Effect	Under-dosing
Rifamycin	T36.6X1	T36.6X2	T36.6X3	T36.6X4	T36.6X5	T36.6X6
Rifaximin	T36.6X1	T36.6X2	T36.6X3	T36.6X4	T36.6X5	T36.6X6
Rimantadine	T37.5X1	T37.5X2	T37.5X3	T37.5X4	T37.5X5	T37.5X6
Rimazolium metilsulfate	T39.8X1	T39.8X2	T39.8X3	T39.8X4	T39.8X5	T39.8X6
Rimifon	T37.1X1	T37.1X2	T37.1X3	T37.1X4	T37.1X5	T37.1X6
Rimiterol	T48.6X1	T48.6X2	T48.6X3	T48.6X4	T48.6X5	T48.6X6
Ringer (lactate) **solution**	T5Ø.3X1	T5Ø.3X2	T5Ø.3X3	T5Ø.3X4	T5Ø.3X5	T5Ø.3X6
Ristocetin	T36.8X1	T36.8X2	T36.8X3	T36.8X4	T36.8X5	T36.8X6
Ritalin	T43.631	T43.632	T43.633	T43.634	T43.635	T43.636
Ritodrine	T44.5X1	T44.5X2	T44.5X3	T44.5X4	T44.5X5	T44.5X6
Roach killer — *see* Insecticide						
Rociverine	T44.3X1	T44.3X2	T44.3X3	T44.3X4	T44.3X5	T44.3X6
Rocky Mountain spotted fever vaccine	T5Ø.A91	T5Ø.A92	T5Ø.A93	T5Ø.A94	T5Ø.A95	T5Ø.A96
Rodenticide NEC	T6Ø.4X1	T6Ø.4X2	T6Ø.4X3	T6Ø.4X4	—	—
Rohypnol	T42.4X1	T42.4X2	T42.4X3	T42.4X4	T42.4X5	T42.4X6
Rokitamycin	T36.3X1	T36.3X2	T36.3X3	T36.3X4	T36.3X5	T36.3X6
Rolaids	T47.1X1	T47.1X2	T47.1X3	T47.1X4	T47.1X5	T47.1X6
Rolitetracycline	T36.4X1	T36.4X2	T36.4X3	T36.4X4	T36.4X5	T36.4X6
Romilar	T48.3X1	T48.3X2	T48.3X3	T48.3X4	T48.3X5	T48.3X6
Ronifibrate	T46.6X1	T46.6X2	T46.6X3	T46.6X4	T46.6X5	T46.6X6
Rosaprostol	T47.1X1	T47.1X2	T47.1X3	T47.1X4	T47.1X5	T47.1X6
Rose bengal sodium (131I)	T5Ø.8X1	T5Ø.8X2	T5Ø.8X3	T5Ø.8X4	T5Ø.8X5	T5Ø.8X6
Rose water ointment	T49.3X1	T49.3X2	T49.3X3	T49.3X4	T49.3X5	T49.3X6
Rosoxacin	T37.8X1	T37.8X2	T37.8X3	T37.8X4	T37.8X5	T37.8X6
Rotenone	T6Ø.2X1	T6Ø.2X2	T6Ø.2X3	T6Ø.2X4	—	—
Rotoxamine	T45.ØX1	T45.ØX2	T45.ØX3	T45.ØX4	T45.ØX5	T45.ØX6
Rough-on-rats	T6Ø.4X1	T6Ø.4X2	T6Ø.4X3	T6Ø.4X4	—	—
Roxatidine	T47.ØX1	T47.ØX2	T47.ØX3	T47.ØX4	T47.ØX5	T47.ØX6
Roxithromycin	T36.3X1	T36.3X2	T36.3X3	T36.3X4	T36.3X5	T36.3X6
Rt-PA	T45.611	T45.612	T45.613	T45.614	T45.615	T45.616
Rubbing alcohol	T51.2X1	T51.2X2	T51.2X3	T51.2X4	—	—
Rubefacient	T49.4X1	T49.4X2	T49.4X3	T49.4X4	T49.4X5	T49.4X6
Rubella vaccine	T5Ø.B91	T5Ø.B92	T5Ø.B93	T5Ø.B94	T5Ø.B95	T5Ø.B96
Rubeola vaccine	T5Ø.B91	T5Ø.B92	T5Ø.B93	T5Ø.B94	T5Ø.B95	T5Ø.B96
Rubidium chloride Rb82	T5Ø.8X1	T5Ø.8X2	T5Ø.8X3	T5Ø.8X4	T5Ø.8X5	T5Ø.8X6
Rubidomycin	T45.1X1	T45.1X2	T45.1X3	T45.1X4	T45.1X5	T45.1X6
Rue	T62.2X1	T62.2X2	T62.2X3	T62.2X4	—	—
Rufocromomycin	T45.1X1	T45.1X2	T45.1X3	T45.1X4	T45.1X5	T45.1X6
Russel's viper venin	T45.7X1	T45.7X2	T45.7X3	T45.7X4	T45.7X5	T45.7X6
Ruta (graveolens)	T62.2X1	T62.2X2	T62.2X3	T62.2X4	—	—
Rutinum	T46.991	T46.992	T46.993	T46.994	T46.995	T46.996
Rutoside	T46.991	T46.992	T46.993	T46.994	T46.995	T46.996
b-sitosterol(s)	T46.6X1	T46.6X2	T46.6X3	T46.6X4	T46.6X5	T46.6X6
Sabadilla (plant)	T62.2X1	T62.2X2	T62.2X3	T62.2X4	—	—
pesticide	T6Ø.2X1	T6Ø.2X2	T6Ø.2X3	T6Ø.2X4	—	—
Saccharated iron oxide	T45.8X1	T45.8X2	T45.8X3	T45.8X4	T45.8X5	T45.8X6
Saccharin	T5Ø.9Ø1	T5Ø.9Ø2	T5Ø.9Ø3	T5Ø.9Ø4	T5Ø.9Ø5	T5Ø.9Ø6
Saccharomyces boulardii	T47.6X1	T47.6X2	T47.6X3	T47.6X4	T47.6X5	T47.6X6
Safflower oil	T46.6X1	T46.6X2	T46.6X3	T46.6X4	T46.6X5	T46.6X6
Safrazine	T43.1X1	T43.1X2	T43.1X3	T43.1X4	T43.1X5	T43.1X6
Salazosulfapyridine	T37.ØX1	T37.ØX2	T37.ØX3	T37.ØX4	T37.ØX5	T37.ØX6
Salbutamol	T48.6X1	T48.6X2	T48.6X3	T48.6X4	T48.6X5	T48.6X6
Salicylamide	T39.Ø91	T39.Ø92	T39.Ø93	T39.Ø94	T39.Ø95	T39.Ø96
Salicylate NEC	T39.Ø91	T39.Ø92	T39.Ø93	T39.Ø94	T39.Ø95	T39.Ø96
methyl	T49.3X1	T49.3X2	T49.3X3	T49.3X4	T49.3X5	T49.3X6
theobromine calcium	T5Ø.2X1	T5Ø.2X2	T5Ø.2X3	T5Ø.2X4	T5Ø.2X5	T5Ø.2X6
Salicylazosulfapyridine	T37.ØX1	T37.ØX2	T37.ØX3	T37.ØX4	T37.ØX5	T37.ØX6
Salicylhydroxamic acid	T49.ØX1	T49.ØX2	T49.ØX3	T49.ØX4	T49.ØX5	T49.ØX6
Salicylic acid	T49.4X1	T49.4X2	T49.4X3	T49.4X4	T49.4X5	T49.4X6
with benzoic acid	T49.4X1	T49.4X2	T49.4X3	T49.4X4	T49.4X5	T49.4X6
congeners	T39.Ø91	T39.Ø92	T39.Ø93	T39.Ø94	T39.Ø95	T39.Ø96
derivative	T39.Ø91	T39.Ø92	T39.Ø93	T39.Ø94	T39.Ø95	T39.Ø96
salts	T39.Ø91	T39.Ø92	T39.Ø93	T39.Ø94	T39.Ø95	T39.Ø96
Salinazid	T37.1X1	T37.1X2	T37.1X3	T37.1X4	T37.1X5	T37.1X6
Salmeterol	T48.6X1	T48.6X2	T48.6X3	T48.6X4	T48.6X5	T48.6X6
Salol	T49.3X1	T49.3X2	T49.3X3	T49.3X4	T49.3X5	T49.3X6
Salsalate	T39.Ø91	T39.Ø92	T39.Ø93	T39.Ø94	T39.Ø95	T39.Ø96
Salt-replacing drug	T5Ø.9Ø1	T5Ø.9Ø2	T5Ø.9Ø3	T5Ø.9Ø4	T5Ø.9Ø5	T5Ø.9Ø6
Salt-retaining mineralocorticoid	T5Ø.ØX1	T5Ø.ØX2	T5Ø.ØX3	T5Ø.ØX4	T5Ø.ØX5	T5Ø.ØX6
Salt substitute	T5Ø.9Ø1	T5Ø.9Ø2	T5Ø.9Ø3	T5Ø.9Ø4	T5Ø.9Ø5	T5Ø.9Ø6
Saluretic NEC	T5Ø.2X1	T5Ø.2X2	T5Ø.2X3	T5Ø.2X4	T5Ø.2X5	T5Ø.2X6
Saluron	T5Ø.2X1	T5Ø.2X2	T5Ø.2X3	T5Ø.2X4	T5Ø.2X5	T5Ø.2X6
Salvarsan 606 (neosilver) (silver)	T37.8X1	T37.8X2	T37.8X3	T37.8X4	T37.8X5	T37.8X6
Sambucus canadensis	T62.2X1	T62.2X2	T62.2X3	T62.2X4	—	—
berry	T62.1X1	T62.1X2	T62.1X3	T62.1X4	—	—
Sandril	T46.5X1	T46.5X2	T46.5X3	T46.5X4	T46.5X5	T46.5X6
Sanguinaria canadensis	T62.2X1	T62.2X2	T62.2X3	T62.2X4	—	—
Saniflush (cleaner)	T54.2X1	T54.2X2	T54.2X3	T54.2X4	—	—
Santonin	T37.4X1	T37.4X2	T37.4X3	T37.4X4	T37.4X5	T37.4X6
Santyl	T49.8X1	T49.8X2	T49.8X3	T49.8X4	T49.8X5	T49.8X6

Substance	Poisoning, Accidental (unintentional)	Poisoning, Intentional Self-harm	Poisoning, Assault	Poisoning, Undetermined	Adverse Effect	Under-dosing
Saralasin	T46.5X1	T46.5X2	T46.5X3	T46.5X4	T46.5X5	T46.5X6
Sarcolysin	T45.1X1	T45.1X2	T45.1X3	T45.1X4	T45.1X5	T45.1X6
Sarkomycin	T45.1X1	T45.1X2	T45.1X3	T45.1X4	T45.1X5	T45.1X6
Saroten	T43.Ø11	T43.Ø12	T43.Ø13	T43.Ø14	T43.Ø15	T43.Ø16
Saturnine — *see* Lead						
Savin (oil)	T49.4X1	T49.4X2	T49.4X3	T49.4X4	T49.4X5	T49.4X6
Scammony	T47.2X1	T47.2X2	T47.2X3	T47.2X4	T47.2X5	T47.2X6
Scarlet red	T49.8X1	T49.8X2	T49.8X3	T49.8X4	T49.8X5	T49.8X6
Scheele's green	T57.ØX1	T57.ØX2	T57.ØX3	T57.ØX4	—	—
insecticide	T57.ØX1	T57.ØX2	T57.ØX3	T57.ØX4	—	—
Schizontozide (blood) (tissue)	T37.2X1	T37.2X2	T37.2X3	T37.2X4	T37.2X5	T37.2X6
Schradan	T6Ø.ØX1	T6Ø.ØX2	T6Ø.ØX3	T6Ø.ØX4	—	—
Schweinfurth green	T57.ØX1	T57.ØX2	T57.ØX3	T57.ØX4	—	—
insecticide	T57.ØX1	T57.ØX2	T57.ØX3	T57.ØX4	—	—
Scilla, rat poison	T6Ø.4X1	T6Ø.4X2	T6Ø.4X3	T6Ø.4X4	—	—
Scillaren	T6Ø.4X1	T6Ø.4X2	T6Ø.4X3	T6Ø.4X4	—	—
Sclerosing agent	T46.8X1	T46.8X2	T46.8X3	T46.8X4	T46.8X5	T46.8X6
Scombrotoxin	T61.11	T61.12	T61.13	T61.14	—	—
Scopolamine	T44.3X1	T44.3X2	T44.3X3	T44.3X4	T44.3X5	T44.3X6
Scopolia extract	T44.3X1	T44.3X2	T44.3X3	T44.3X4	T44.3X5	T44.3X6
Scouring powder	T65.891	T65.892	T65.893	T65.894	—	—
Sea						
anemone (sting)	T63.631	T63.632	T63.633	T63.634	—	—
cucumber (sting)	T63.691	T63.692	T63.693	T63.694	—	—
snake (bite) (venom)	T63.Ø91	T63.Ø92	T63.Ø93	T63.Ø94	—	—
urchin spine (puncture)	T63.691	T63.692	T63.693	T63.694	—	—
Seafood	T61.91	T61.92	T61.93	T61.94	—	—
specified NEC	T61.8X1	T61.8X2	T61.8X3	T61.8X4	—	—
Secbutabarbital	T42.3X1	T42.3X2	T42.3X3	T42.3X4	T42.3X5	T42.3X6
Secbutabarbitone	T42.3X1	T42.3X2	T42.3X3	T42.3X4	T42.3X5	T42.3X6
Secnidazole	T37.3X1	T37.3X2	T37.3X3	T37.3X4	T37.3X5	T37.3X6
Secobarbital	T42.3X1	T42.3X2	T42.3X3	T42.3X4	T42.3X5	T42.3X6
Seconal	T42.3X1	T42.3X2	T42.3X3	T42.3X4	T42.3X5	T42.3X6
Secretin	T5Ø.8X1	T5Ø.8X2	T5Ø.8X3	T5Ø.8X4	T5Ø.8X5	T5Ø.8X6
Sedative NEC	T42.71	T42.72	T42.73	T42.74	T42.75	T42.76
mixed NEC	T42.6X1	T42.6X2	T42.6X3	T42.6X4	T42.6X5	T42.6X6
Sedormid	T42.6X1	T42.6X2	T42.6X3	T42.6X4	T42.6X5	T42.6X6
Seed disinfectant or dressing	T6Ø.8X1	T6Ø.8X2	T6Ø.8X3	T6Ø.8X4	—	—
Seeds (poisonous)	T62.2X1	T62.2X2	T62.2X3	T62.2X4	—	—
Selegiline	T42.8X1	T42.8X2	T42.8X3	T42.8X4	T42.8X5	T42.8X6
Selenium NEC	T56.891	T56.892	T56.893	T56.894	—	—
disulfide or sulfide	T49.4X1	T49.4X2	T49.4X3	T49.4X4	T49.4X5	T49.4X6
fumes	T59.891	T59.892	T59.893	T59.894	—	—
sulfide	T49.4X1	T49.4X2	T49.4X3	T49.4X4	T49.4X5	T49.4X6
Selenomethionine (75Se)	T5Ø.8X1	T5Ø.8X2	T5Ø.8X3	T5Ø.8X4	T5Ø.8X5	T5Ø.8X6
Selsun	T49.4X1	T49.4X2	T49.4X3	T49.4X4	T49.4X5	T49.4X6
Semustine	T45.1X1	T45.1X2	T45.1X3	T45.1X4	T45.1X5	T45.1X6
Senega syrup	T48.4X1	T48.4X2	T48.4X3	T48.4X4	T48.4X5	T48.4X6
Senna	T47.2X1	T47.2X2	T47.2X3	T47.2X4	T47.2X5	T47.2X6
Sennoside A+B	T47.2X1	T47.2X2	T47.2X3	T47.2X4	T47.2X5	T47.2X6
Septisol	T49.2X1	T49.2X2	T49.2X3	T49.2X4	T49.2X5	T49.2X6
Seractide	T38.811	T38.812	T38.813	T38.814	T38.815	T38.816
Serax	T42.4X1	T42.4X2	T42.4X3	T42.4X4	T42.4X5	T42.4X6
Serenesil	T42.6X1	T42.6X2	T42.6X3	T42.6X4	T42.6X5	T42.6X6
Serenium (hydrochloride)	T37.91	T37.92	T37.93	T37.94	T37.95	T37.96
Serepax — *see* Oxazepam						
Sermorelin	T38.891	T38.892	T38.893	T38.894	T38.895	T38.896
Sernyl	T41.1X1	T41.1X2	T41.1X3	T41.1X4	T41.1X5	T41.1X6
Serotonin	T5Ø.991	T5Ø.992	T5Ø.993	T5Ø.994	T5Ø.995	T5Ø.996
Serpasil	T46.5X1	T46.5X2	T46.5X3	T46.5X4	T46.5X5	T46.5X6
Serrapeptase	T45.3X1	T45.3X2	T45.3X3	T45.3X4	T45.3X5	T45.3X6
Serum						
antibotulinus	T5Ø.Z11	T5Ø.Z12	T5Ø.Z13	T5Ø.Z14	T5Ø.Z15	T5Ø.Z16
anticytotoxic	T5Ø.Z11	T5Ø.Z12	T5Ø.Z13	T5Ø.Z14	T5Ø.Z15	T5Ø.Z16
antidiphtheria	T5Ø.Z11	T5Ø.Z12	T5Ø.Z13	T5Ø.Z14	T5Ø.Z15	T5Ø.Z16
antimeningococcus	T5Ø.Z11	T5Ø.Z12	T5Ø.Z13	T5Ø.Z14	T5Ø.Z15	T5Ø.Z16
anti-Rh	T5Ø.Z11	T5Ø.Z12	T5Ø.Z13	T5Ø.Z14	T5Ø.Z15	T5Ø.Z16
anti-snake-bite	T5Ø.Z11	T5Ø.Z12	T5Ø.Z13	T5Ø.Z14	T5Ø.Z15	T5Ø.Z16
antitetanic	T5Ø.Z11	T5Ø.Z12	T5Ø.Z13	T5Ø.Z14	T5Ø.Z15	T5Ø.Z16
antitoxic	T5Ø.Z11	T5Ø.Z12	T5Ø.Z13	T5Ø.Z14	T5Ø.Z15	T5Ø.Z16
complement (inhibitor)	T45.8X1	T45.8X2	T45.8X3	T45.8X4	T45.8X5	T45.8X6
convalescent	T5Ø.Z11	T5Ø.Z12	T5Ø.Z13	T5Ø.Z14	T5Ø.Z15	T5Ø.Z16
hemolytic complement	T45.8X1	T45.8X2	T45.8X3	T45.8X4	T45.8X5	T45.8X6
immune (human)	T5Ø.Z11	T5Ø.Z12	T5Ø.Z13	T5Ø.Z14	T5Ø.Z15	T5Ø.Z16
protective NEC	T5Ø.Z11	T5Ø.Z12	T5Ø.Z13	T5Ø.Z14	T5Ø.Z15	T5Ø.Z16
Setastine	T45.ØX1	T45.ØX2	T45.ØX3	T45.ØX4	T45.ØX5	T45.ØX6
Setoperone	T43.591	T43.592	T43.593	T43.594	T43.595	T43.596
Sewer gas	T59.91	T59.92	T59.93	T59.94	—	—
Shampoo	T55.ØX1	T55.ØX2	T55.ØX3	T55.ØX4	—	—
Shellfish, noxious, nonbacterial	T61.781	T61.782	T61.783	T61.784	—	—

Substance	Poisoning, Accidental (unintentional)	Poisoning, Intentional Self-harm	Poisoning, Assault	Poisoning, Undetermined	Adverse Effect	Under-dosing
Sildenafil	T46.7X1	T46.7X2	T46.7X3	T46.7X4	T46.7X5	T46.7X6
Silibinin	T5Ø.991	T5Ø.992	T5Ø.993	T5Ø.994	T5Ø.995	T5Ø.996
Silicone NEC	T65.891	T65.892	T65.893	T65.894	—	—
medicinal	T49.3X1	T49.3X2	T49.3X3	T49.3X4	T49.3X5	T49.3X6
Silvadene	T49.ØX1	T49.ØX2	T49.ØX3	T49.ØX4	T49.ØX5	T49.ØX6
Silver	T49.ØX1	T49.ØX2	T49.ØX3	T49.ØX4	T49.ØX5	T49.ØX6
anti-infectives	T49.ØX1	T49.ØX2	T49.ØX3	T49.ØX4	T49.ØX5	T49.ØX6
arsphenamine	T37.8X1	T37.8X2	T37.8X3	T37.8X4	T37.8X5	T37.8X6
colloidal	T49.ØX1	T49.ØX2	T49.ØX3	T49.ØX4	T49.ØX5	T49.ØX6
nitrate	T49.ØX1	T49.ØX2	T49.ØX3	T49.ØX4	T49.ØX5	T49.ØX6
ophthalmic preparation	T49.5X1	T49.5X2	T49.5X3	T49.5X4	T49.5X5	T49.5X6
toughened (keratolytic)	T49.4X1	T49.4X2	T49.4X3	T49.4X4	T49.4X5	T49.4X6
nonmedicinal (dust)	T56.891	T56.892	T56.893	T56.894	—	—
protein	T49.5X1	T49.5X2	T49.5X3	T49.5X4	T49.5X5	T49.5X6
salvarsan	T37.8X1	T37.8X2	T37.8X3	T37.8X4	T37.8X5	T37.8X6
sulfadiazine	T49.4X1	T49.4X2	T49.4X3	T49.4X4	T49.4X5	T49.4X6
Silymarin	T5Ø.991	T5Ø.992	T5Ø.993	T5Ø.994	T5Ø.995	T5Ø.996
Simaldrate	T47.1X1	T47.1X2	T47.1X3	T47.1X4	T47.1X5	T47.1X6
Simazine	T6Ø.3X1	T6Ø.3X2	T6Ø.3X3	T6Ø.3X4	—	—
Simethicone	T47.1X1	T47.1X2	T47.1X3	T47.1X4	T47.1X5	T47.1X6
Simfibrate	T46.6X1	T46.6X2	T46.6X3	T46.6X4	T46.6X5	T46.6X6
Simvastatin	T46.6X1	T46.6X2	T46.6X3	T46.6X4	T46.6X5	T46.6X6
Sincalide	T5Ø.8X1	T5Ø.8X2	T5Ø.8X3	T5Ø.8X4	T5Ø.8X5	T5Ø.8X6
Sinequan	T43.Ø11	T43.Ø12	T43.Ø13	T43.Ø14	T43.Ø15	T43.Ø16
Singoserp	T46.5X1	T46.5X2	T46.5X3	T46.5X4	T46.5X5	T46.5X6
Sintrom	T45.511	T45.512	T45.513	T45.514	T45.515	T45.516
Sisomicin	T36.5X1	T36.5X2	T36.5X3	T36.5X4	T36.5X5	T36.5X6
Sitosterols	T46.6X1	T46.6X2	T46.6X3	T46.6X4	T46.6X5	T46.6X6
Skeletal muscle relaxants	T48.1X1	T48.1X2	T48.1X3	T48.1X4	T48.1X5	T48.1X6
Skin						
agents (external)	T49.91	T49.92	T49.93	T49.94	T49.95	T49.96
specified NEC	T49.8X1	T49.8X2	T49.8X3	T49.8X4	T49.8X5	T49.8X6
test antigen	T5Ø.8X1	T5Ø.8X2	T5Ø.8X3	T5Ø.8X4	T5Ø.8X5	T5Ø.8X6
Sleep-eze	T45.ØX1	T45.ØX2	T45.ØX3	T45.ØX4	T45.ØX5	T45.ØX6
Sleeping draught, pill	T42.71	T42.72	T42.73	T42.74	T42.75	T42.76
Smallpox vaccine	T5Ø.B11	T5Ø.B12	T5Ø.B13	T5Ø.B14	T5Ø.B15	T5Ø.B16
Smelter fumes NEC	T56.91	T56.92	T56.93	T56.94	—	—
Smog	T59.1X1	T59.1X2	T59.1X3	T59.1X4	—	—
Smoke NEC	T59.811	T59.812	T59.813	T59.814	—	—
Smooth muscle relaxant	T44.3X1	T44.3X2	T44.3X3	T44.3X4	T44.3X5	T44.3X6
Snail killer NEC	T6Ø.8X1	T6Ø.8X2	T6Ø.8X3	T6Ø.8X4	—	—
Snake venom or bite	T63.ØØ1	T63.ØØ2	T63.ØØ3	T63.ØØ4	—	—
hemocoagulase	T45.7X1	T45.7X2	T45.7X3	T45.7X4	T45.7X5	T45.7X6
Snuff	T65.211	T65.212	T65.213	T65.214	—	—
Soap (powder) (product)	T55.ØX1	T55.ØX2	T55.ØX3	T55.ØX4	—	—
enema	T47.4X1	T47.4X2	T47.4X3	T47.4X4	T47.4X5	T47.4X6
medicinal, soft	T49.2X1	T49.2X2	T49.2X3	T49.2X4	T49.2X5	T49.2X6
superfatted	T49.2X1	T49.2X2	T49.2X3	T49.2X4	T49.2X5	T49.2X6
Sobrerol	T48.4X1	T48.4X2	T48.4X3	T48.4X4	T48.4X5	T48.4X6
Soda (caustic)	T54.3X1	T54.3X2	T54.3X3	T54.3X4	—	—
bicarb	T47.1X1	T47.1X2	T47.1X3	T47.1X4	T47.1X5	T47.1X6
chlorinated — *see* Sodium, hypochlorite						
Sodium						
acetosulfone	T37.1X1	T37.1X2	T37.1X3	T37.1X4	T37.1X5	T37.1X6
acetrizoate	T5Ø.8X1	T5Ø.8X2	T5Ø.8X3	T5Ø.8X4	T5Ø.8X5	T5Ø.8X6
acid phosphate	T5Ø.3X1	T5Ø.3X2	T5Ø.3X3	T5Ø.3X4	T5Ø.3X5	T5Ø.3X6
alginate	T47.8X1	T47.8X2	T47.8X3	T47.8X4	T47.8X5	T47.8X6
amidotrizoate	T5Ø.8X1	T5Ø.8X2	T5Ø.8X3	T5Ø.8X4	T5Ø.8X5	T5Ø.8X6
aminopterin	T45.1X1	T45.1X2	T45.1X3	T45.1X4	T45.1X5	T45.1X6
amylosulfate	T47.8X1	T47.8X2	T47.8X3	T47.8X4	T47.8X5	T47.8X6
amytal	T42.3X1	T42.3X2	T42.3X3	T42.3X4	T42.3X5	T42.3X6
antimony gluconate	T37.3X1	T37.3X2	T37.3X3	T37.3X4	T37.3X5	T37.3X6
arsenate	T57.ØX1	T57.ØX2	T57.ØX3	T57.ØX4	—	—
aurothiomalate	T39.4X1	T39.4X2	T39.4X3	T39.4X4	T39.4X5	T39.4X6
aurothiosulfate	T39.4X1	T39.4X2	T39.4X3	T39.4X4	T39.4X5	T39.4X6
barbiturate	T42.3X1	T42.3X2	T42.3X3	T42.3X4	T42.3X5	T42.3X6
basic phosphate	T47.4X1	T47.4X2	T47.4X3	T47.4X4	T47.4X5	T47.4X6
bicarbonate	T47.1X1	T47.1X2	T47.1X3	T47.1X4	T47.1X5	T47.1X6
bichromate	T57.8X1	T57.8X2	T57.8X3	T57.8X4	—	—
biphosphate	T5Ø.3X1	T5Ø.3X2	T5Ø.3X3	T5Ø.3X4	T5Ø.3X5	T5Ø.3X6
bisulfate	T65.891	T65.892	T65.893	T65.894	—	—
borate						
cleanser	T57.8X1	T57.8X2	T57.8X3	T57.8X4	—	—
eye	T49.5X1	T49.5X2	T49.5X3	T49.5X4	T49.5X5	T49.5X6
therapeutic	T49.8X1	T49.8X2	T49.8X3	T49.8X4	T49.8X5	T49.8X6
bromide	T42.6X1	T42.6X2	T42.6X3	T42.6X4	T42.6X5	T42.6X6
cacodylate (nonmedicinal) NEC	T5Ø.8X1	T5Ø.8X2	T5Ø.8X3	T5Ø.8X4	T5Ø.8X5	T5Ø.8X6
anti-infective	T37.8X1	T37.8X2	T37.8X3	T37.8X4	T37.8X5	T37.8X6
herbicide	T6Ø.3X1	T6Ø.3X2	T6Ø.3X3	T6Ø.3X4	—	—
calcium edetate	T45.8X1	T45.8X2	T45.8X3	T45.8X4	T45.8X5	T45.8X6
carbonate NEC	T54.3X1	T54.3X2	T54.3X3	T54.3X4	—	—

Substance	Poisoning, Accidental (unintentional)	Poisoning, Intentional Self-harm	Poisoning, Assault	Poisoning, Undetermined	Adverse Effect	Under-dosing
Sodium — *continued*						
chlorate NEC	T65.891	T65.892	T65.893	T65.894	—	—
herbicide	T54.91	T54.92	T54.93	T54.94	—	—
chloride	T5Ø.3X1	T5Ø.3X2	T5Ø.3X3	T5Ø.3X4	T5Ø.3X5	T5Ø.3X6
with glucose	T5Ø.3X1	T5Ø.3X2	T5Ø.3X3	T5Ø.3X4	T5Ø.3X5	T5Ø.3X6
chromate	T65.891	T65.892	T65.893	T65.894	—	—
citrate	T5Ø.991	T5Ø.992	T5Ø.993	T5Ø.994	T5Ø.995	T5Ø.996
cromoglicate	T48.6X1	T48.6X2	T48.6X3	T48.6X4	T48.6X5	T48.6X6
cyanide	T65.ØX1	T65.ØX2	T65.ØX3	T65.ØX4	—	—
cyclamate	T5Ø.3X1	T5Ø.3X2	T5Ø.3X3	T5Ø.3X4	T5Ø.3X5	T5Ø.3X6
dehydrocholate	T45.8X1	T45.8X2	T45.8X3	T45.8X4	T45.8X5	T45.8X6
diatrizoate	T5Ø.8X1	T5Ø.8X2	T5Ø.8X3	T5Ø.8X4	T5Ø.8X5	T5Ø.8X6
dibunate	T48.4X1	T48.4X2	T48.4X3	T48.4X4	T48.4X5	T48.4X6
dioctyl sulfosuccinate	T47.4X1	T47.4X2	T47.4X3	T47.4X4	T47.4X5	T47.4X6
dipantoyl ferrate	T45.8X1	T45.8X2	T45.8X3	T45.8X4	T45.8X5	T45.8X6
edetate	T45.8X1	T45.8X2	T45.8X3	T45.8X4	T45.8X5	T45.8X6
ethacrynate	T5Ø.1X1	T5Ø.1X2	T5Ø.1X3	T5Ø.1X4	T5Ø.1X5	T5Ø.1X6
feredetate	T45.8X1	T45.8X2	T45.8X3	T45.8X4	T45.8X5	T45.8X6
Fluoride — *see* Fluoride						
fluoroacetate (dust) (pesticide)	T6Ø.4X1	T6Ø.4X2	T6Ø.4X3	T6Ø.4X4	—	—
free salt	T5Ø.3X1	T5Ø.3X2	T5Ø.3X3	T5Ø.3X4	T5Ø.3X5	T5Ø.3X6
fusidate	T36.8X1	T36.8X2	T36.8X3	T36.8X4	T36.8X5	T36.8X6
glucaldrate	T47.1X1	T47.1X2	T47.1X3	T47.1X4	T47.1X5	T47.1X6
glucosulfone	T37.1X1	T37.1X2	T37.1X3	T37.1X4	T37.1X5	T37.1X6
glutamate	T45.8X1	T45.8X2	T45.8X3	T45.8X4	T45.8X5	T45.8X6
hydrogen carbonate	T5Ø.3X1	T5Ø.3X2	T5Ø.3X3	T5Ø.3X4	T5Ø.3X5	T5Ø.3X6
hydroxide	T54.3X1	T54.3X2	T54.3X3	T54.3X4	—	—
hypochlorite (bleach) NEC	T54.3X1	T54.3X2	T54.3X3	T54.3X4	—	—
disinfectant	T54.3X1	T54.3X2	T54.3X3	T54.3X4	—	—
medicinal (anti-infective) (external)	T49.ØX1	T49.ØX2	T49.ØX3	T49.ØX4	T49.ØX5	T49.ØX6
vapor	T54.3X1	T54.3X2	T54.3X3	T54.3X4	—	—
hyposulfite	T49.ØX1	T49.ØX2	T49.ØX3	T49.ØX4	T49.ØX5	T49.ØX6
indigotin disulfonate	T5Ø.8X1	T5Ø.8X2	T5Ø.8X3	T5Ø.8X4	T5Ø.8X5	T5Ø.8X6
iodide	T5Ø.991	T5Ø.992	T5Ø.993	T5Ø.994	T5Ø.995	T5Ø.996
I-131	T5Ø.8X1	T5Ø.8X2	T5Ø.8X3	T5Ø.8X4	T5Ø.8X5	T5Ø.8X6
therapeutic	T38.2X1	T38.2X2	T38.2X3	T38.2X4	T38.2X5	T38.2X6
iodohippurate (131I)	T5Ø.8X1	T5Ø.8X2	T5Ø.8X3	T5Ø.8X4	T5Ø.8X5	T5Ø.8X6
iopodate	T5Ø.8X1	T5Ø.8X2	T5Ø.8X3	T5Ø.8X4	T5Ø.8X5	T5Ø.8X6
iothalamate	T5Ø.8X1	T5Ø.8X2	T5Ø.8X3	T5Ø.8X4	T5Ø.8X5	T5Ø.8X6
iron edetate	T45.4X1	T45.4X2	T45.4X3	T45.4X4	T45.4X5	T45.4X6
lactate (compound solution)	T45.8X1	T45.8X2	T45.8X3	T45.8X4	T45.8X5	T45.8X6
lauryl (sulfate)	T49.2X1	T49.2X2	T49.2X3	T49.2X4	T49.2X5	T49.2X6
L-triiodothyronine	T38.1X1	T38.1X2	T38.1X3	T38.1X4	T38.1X5	T38.1X6
magnesium citrate	T5Ø.991	T5Ø.992	T5Ø.993	T5Ø.994	T5Ø.995	T5Ø.996
mersalate	T5Ø.2X1	T5Ø.2X2	T5Ø.2X3	T5Ø.2X4	T5Ø.2X5	T5Ø.2X6
metasilicate	T65.891	T65.892	T65.893	T65.894	—	—
metrizoate	T5Ø.8X1	T5Ø.8X2	T5Ø.8X3	T5Ø.8X4	T5Ø.8X5	T5Ø.8X6
monofluoroacetate (pesticide)	T6Ø.1X1	T6Ø.1X2	T6Ø.1X3	T6Ø.1X4	—	—
morrhuate	T46.8X1	T46.8X2	T46.8X3	T46.8X4	T46.8X5	T46.8X6
nafcillin	T36.ØX1	T36.ØX2	T36.ØX3	T36.ØX4	T36.ØX5	T36.ØX6
nitrate (oxidizing agent)	T65.891	T65.892	T65.893	T65.894	—	—
nitrite	T5Ø.6X1	T5Ø.6X2	T5Ø.6X3	T5Ø.6X4	T5Ø.6X5	T5Ø.6X6
nitroferricyanide	T46.5X1	T46.5X2	T46.5X3	T46.5X4	T46.5X5	T46.5X6
nitroprusside	T46.5X1	T46.5X2	T46.5X3	T46.5X4	T46.5X5	T46.5X6
oxalate	T65.891	T65.892	T65.893	T65.894	—	—
oxide/peroxide	T65.891	T65.892	T65.893	T65.894	—	—
oxybate	T41.291	T41.292	T41.293	T41.294	T41.295	T41.296
para-aminohippurate	T5Ø.8X1	T5Ø.8X2	T5Ø.8X3	T5Ø.8X4	T5Ø.8X5	T5Ø.8X6
perborate (nonmedicinal) NEC	T65.891	T65.892	T65.893	T65.894	—	—
medicinal	T49.ØX1	T49.ØX2	T49.ØX3	T49.ØX4	T49.ØX5	T49.ØX6
soap	T55.ØX1	T55.ØX2	T55.ØX3	T55.ØX4	—	—
percarbonate — *see* Sodium, perborate						
pertechnetate Tc99m	T5Ø.8X1	T5Ø.8X2	T5Ø.8X3	T5Ø.8X4	T5Ø.8X5	T5Ø.8X6
phosphate						
cellulose	T45.8X1	T45.8X2	T45.8X3	T45.8X4	T45.8X5	T45.8X6
dibasic	T47.2X1	T47.2X2	T47.2X3	T47.2X4	T47.2X5	T47.2X6
monobasic	T47.2X1	T47.2X2	T47.2X3	T47.2X4	T47.2X5	T47.2X6
phytate	T5Ø.6X1	T5Ø.6X2	T5Ø.6X3	T5Ø.6X4	T5Ø.6X5	T5Ø.6X6
picosulfate	T47.2X1	T47.2X2	T47.2X3	T47.2X4	T47.2X5	T47.2X6
polyhydroxyaluminium monocarbonate	T47.1X1	T47.1X2	T47.1X3	T47.1X4	T47.1X5	T47.1X6
polystyrene sulfonate	T5Ø.3X1	T5Ø.3X2	T5Ø.3X3	T5Ø.3X4	T5Ø.3X5	T5Ø.3X6
propionate	T49.ØX1	T49.ØX2	T49.ØX3	T49.ØX4	T49.ØX5	T49.ØX6
propyl hydroxybenzoate	T5Ø.991	T5Ø.992	T5Ø.993	T5Ø.994	T5Ø.995	T5Ø.996
psylliate	T46.8X1	T46.8X2	T46.8X3	T46.8X4	T46.8X5	T46.8X6
removing resins	T5Ø.3X1	T5Ø.3X2	T5Ø.3X3	T5Ø.3X4	T5Ø.3X5	T5Ø.3X6
salicylate	T39.Ø91	T39.Ø92	T39.Ø93	T39.Ø94	T39.Ø95	T39.Ø96

Substance	Poisoning, Accidental (unintentional)	Poisoning, Intentional Self-harm	Poisoning, Assault	Poisoning, Undetermined	Adverse Effect	Under-dosing
Sodium — *continued*						
salt NEC	T5Ø.3X1	T5Ø.3X2	T5Ø.3X3	T5Ø.3X4	T5Ø.3X5	T5Ø.3X6
selenate	T6Ø.2X1	T6Ø.2X2	T6Ø.2X3	T6Ø.2X4	—	—
stibogluconate	T37.3X1	T37.3X2	T37.3X3	T37.3X4	T37.3X5	T37.3X6
sulfate	T47.4X1	T47.4X2	T47.4X3	T47.4X4	T47.4X5	T47.4X6
sulfoxone	T37.1X1	T37.1X2	T37.1X3	T37.1X4	T37.1X5	T37.1X6
tetradecyl sulfate	T46.8X1	T46.8X2	T46.8X3	T46.8X4	T46.8X5	T46.8X6
thiopental	T41.1X1	T41.1X2	T41.1X3	T41.1X4	T41.1X5	T41.1X6
thiosalicylate	T39.Ø91	T39.Ø92	T39.Ø93	T39.Ø94	T39.Ø95	T39.Ø96
thiosulfate	T5Ø.6X1	T5Ø.6X2	T5Ø.6X3	T5Ø.6X4	T5Ø.6X5	T5Ø.6X6
tolbutamide	T38.3X1	T38.3X2	T38.3X3	T38.3X4	T38.3X5	T38.3X6
(L)-triiodothyronine	T38.1X1	T38.1X2	T38.1X3	T38.1X4	T38.1X5	T38.1X6
tyropanoate	T5Ø.8X1	T5Ø.8X2	T5Ø.8X3	T5Ø.8X4	T5Ø.8X5	T5Ø.8X6
valproate	T42.6X1	T42.6X2	T42.6X3	T42.6X4	T42.6X5	T42.6X6
versenate	T5Ø.6X1	T5Ø.6X2	T5Ø.6X3	T5Ø.6X4	T5Ø.6X5	T5Ø.6X6
Sodium-free salt	T5Ø.9Ø1	T5Ø.9Ø2	T5Ø.9Ø3	T5Ø.9Ø4	T5Ø.9Ø5	T5Ø.9Ø6
Sodium-removing resin	T5Ø.3X1	T5Ø.3X2	T5Ø.3X3	T5Ø.3X4	T5Ø.3X5	T5Ø.3X6
Soft soap	T55.ØX1	T55.ØX2	T55.ØX3	T55.ØX4	—	—
Solanine	T62.2X1	T62.2X2	T62.2X3	T62.2X4	—	—
berries	T62.1X1	T62.1X2	T62.1X3	T62.1X4	—	—
Solanum dulcamara	T62.2X1	T62.2X2	T62.2X3	T62.2X4	—	—
berries	T62.1X1	T62.1X2	T62.1X3	T62.1X4	—	—
Solapsone	T37.1X1	T37.1X2	T37.1X3	T37.1X4	T37.1X5	T37.1X6
Solar lotion	T49.3X1	T49.3X2	T49.3X3	T49.3X4	T49.3X5	T49.3X6
Solasulfone	T37.1X1	T37.1X2	T37.1X3	T37.1X4	T37.1X5	T37.1X6
Soldering fluid	T65.891	T65.892	T65.893	T65.894	—	—
Solid substance	T65.91	T65.92	T65.93	T65.94	—	—
specified NEC	T65.891	T65.892	T65.893	T65.894	—	—
Solvent, industrial NEC	T52.91	T52.92	T52.93	T52.94	—	—
naphtha	T52.ØX1	T52.ØX2	T52.ØX3	T52.ØX4	—	—
petroleum	T52.ØX1	T52.ØX2	T52.ØX3	T52.ØX4	—	—
specified NEC	T52.8X1	T52.8X2	T52.8X3	T52.8X4	—	—
Soma	T42.8X1	T42.8X2	T42.8X3	T42.8X4	T42.8X5	T42.8X6
Somatorelin	T38.891	T38.892	T38.893	T38.894	T38.895	T38.896
Somatostatin	T38.991	T38.992	T38.993	T38.994	T38.995	T38.996
Somatotropin	T38.811	T38.812	T38.813	T38.814	T38.815	T38.816
Somatrem	T38.811	T38.812	T38.813	T38.814	T38.815	T38.816
Somatropin	T38.811	T38.812	T38.813	T38.814	T38.815	T38.816
Sominex	T45.ØX1	T45.ØX2	T45.ØX3	T45.ØX4	T45.ØX5	T45.ØX6
Somnos	T42.6X1	T42.6X2	T42.6X3	T42.6X4	T42.6X5	T42.6X6
Somonal	T42.3X1	T42.3X2	T42.3X3	T42.3X4	T42.3X5	T42.3X6
Soneryl	T42.3X1	T42.3X2	T42.3X3	T42.3X4	T42.3X5	T42.3X6
Soothing syrup	T5Ø.9Ø1	T5Ø.9Ø2	T5Ø.9Ø3	T5Ø.9Ø4	T5Ø.9Ø5	T5Ø.9Ø6
Sopor	T42.6X1	T42.6X2	T42.6X3	T42.6X4	T42.6X5	T42.6X6
Soporific	T42.71	T42.72	T42.73	T42.74	T42.75	T42.76
Soporific drug	T42.71	T42.72	T42.73	T42.74	T42.75	T42.76
specified type NEC	T42.6X1	T42.6X2	T42.6X3	T42.6X4	T42.6X5	T42.6X6
Sorbide nitrate	T46.3X1	T46.3X2	T46.3X3	T46.3X4	T46.3X5	T46.3X6
Sorbitol	T47.4X1	T47.4X2	T47.4X3	T47.4X4	T47.4X5	T47.4X6
Sotalol	T44.7X1	T44.7X2	T44.7X3	T44.7X4	T44.7X5	T44.7X6
Sotradecol	T46.8X1	T46.8X2	T46.8X3	T46.8X4	T46.8X5	T46.8X6
Soysterol	T46.6X1	T46.6X2	T46.6X3	T46.6X4	T46.6X5	T46.6X6
Spacoline	T44.3X1	T44.3X2	T44.3X3	T44.3X4	T44.3X5	T44.3X6
Spanish fly	T49.8X1	T49.8X2	T49.8X3	T49.8X4	T49.8X5	T49.8X6
Sparine	T43.3X1	T43.3X2	T43.3X3	T43.3X4	T43.3X5	T43.3X6
Sparteine	T48.ØX1	T48.ØX2	T48.ØX3	T48.ØX4	T48.ØX5	T48.ØX6
Spasmolytic						
anticholinergics	T44.3X1	T44.3X2	T44.3X3	T44.3X4	T44.3X5	T44.3X6
autonomic	T44.3X1	T44.3X2	T44.3X3	T44.3X4	T44.3X5	T44.3X6
bronchial NEC	T48.6X1	T48.6X2	T48.6X3	T48.6X4	T48.6X5	T48.6X6
quaternary ammonium	T44.3X1	T44.3X2	T44.3X3	T44.3X4	T44.3X5	T44.3X6
skeletal muscle NEC	T48.1X1	T48.1X2	T48.1X3	T48.1X4	T48.1X5	T48.1X6
Spectinomycin	T36.5X1	T36.5X2	T36.5X3	T36.5X4	T36.5X5	T36.5X6
Speed	T43.621	T43.622	T43.623	T43.624	T43.625	T43.626
Spermicide	T49.8X1	T49.8X2	T49.8X3	T49.8X4	T49.8X5	T49.8X6
Spider (bite) (venom)	T63.391	T63.392	T63.393	T63.394	—	—
antivenin	T5Ø.Z11	T5Ø.Z12	T5Ø.Z13	T5Ø.Z14	T5Ø.Z15	T5Ø.Z16
Spigelia (root)	T37.4X1	T37.4X2	T37.4X3	T37.4X4	T37.4X5	T37.4X6
Spindle inactivator	T5Ø.4X1	T5Ø.4X2	T5Ø.4X3	T5Ø.4X4	T5Ø.4X5	T5Ø.4X6
Spiperone	T43.4X1	T43.4X2	T43.4X3	T43.4X4	T43.4X5	T43.4X6
Spiramycin	T36.3X1	T36.3X2	T36.3X3	T36.3X4	T36.3X5	T36.3X6
Spirapril	T46.4X1	T46.4X2	T46.4X3	T46.4X4	T46.4X5	T46.4X6
Spirilene	T43.591	T43.592	T43.593	T43.594	T43.595	T43.596
Spirit(s) (neutral) **NEC**	T51.ØX1	T51.ØX2	T51.ØX3	T51.ØX4	—	—
beverage	T51.ØX1	T51.ØX2	T51.ØX3	T51.ØX4	—	—
industrial	T51.ØX1	T51.ØX2	T51.ØX3	T51.ØX4	—	—
mineral	T52.ØX1	T52.ØX2	T52.ØX3	T52.ØX4	—	—
of salt — *see* Hydrochloric acid						
surgical	T51.ØX1	T51.ØX2	T51.ØX3	T51.ØX4	—	—
Spironolactone	T5Ø.ØX1	T5Ø.ØX2	T5Ø.ØX3	T5Ø.ØX4	T5Ø.ØX5	T5Ø.ØX6
Spiroperidol	T43.4X1	T43.4X2	T43.4X3	T43.4X4	T43.4X5	T43.4X6
Sponge, absorbable (gelatin)	T45.7X1	T45.7X2	T45.7X3	T45.7X4	T45.7X5	T45.7X6

Substance	Poisoning, Accidental (unintentional)	Poisoning, Intentional Self-harm	Poisoning, Assault	Poisoning, Undetermined	Adverse Effect	Under-dosing
Sporostacin	T49.ØX1	T49.ØX2	T49.ØX3	T49.ØX4	T49.ØX5	T49.ØX6
Spray (aerosol)	T65.91	T65.92	T65.93	T65.94	—	—
cosmetic	T65.891	T65.892	T65.893	T65.894	—	—
medicinal NEC	T5Ø.9Ø1	T5Ø.9Ø2	T5Ø.9Ø3	T5Ø.9Ø4	T5Ø.9Ø5	T5Ø.9Ø6
pesticides — *see* Pesticides						
specified content — *see* specific substance						
Spurge flax	T62.2X1	T62.2X2	T62.2X3	T62.2X4	—	—
Spurges	T62.2X1	T62.2X2	T62.2X3	T62.2X4	—	—
Sputum viscosity-lowering drug	T48.4X1	T48.4X2	T48.4X3	T48.4X4	T48.4X5	T48.4X6
Squill	T46.ØX1	T46.ØX2	T46.ØX3	T46.ØX4	T46.ØX5	T46.ØX6
rat poison	T6Ø.4X1	T6Ø.4X2	T6Ø.4X3	T6Ø.4X4	—	—
Squirting cucumber (cathartic)	T47.2X1	T47.2X2	T47.2X3	T47.2X4	T47.2X5	T47.2X6
Stains	T65.6X1	T65.6X2	T65.6X3	T65.6X4	—	—
Stannous fluoride	T49.7X1	T49.7X2	T49.7X3	T49.7X4	T49.7X5	T49.7X6
Stanolone	T38.7X1	T38.7X2	T38.7X3	T38.7X4	T38.7X5	T38.7X6
Stanozolol	T38.7X1	T38.7X2	T38.7X3	T38.7X4	T38.7X5	T38.7X6
Staphisagria or stavesacre (pediculicide)	T49.ØX1	T49.ØX2	T49.ØX3	T49.ØX4	T49.ØX5	T49.ØX6
Starch	T5Ø.9Ø1	T5Ø.9Ø2	T5Ø.9Ø3	T5Ø.9Ø4	T5Ø.9Ø5	T5Ø.9Ø6
Stelazine	T43.3X1	T43.3X2	T43.3X3	T43.3X4	T43.3X5	T43.3X6
Stemetil	T43.3X1	T43.3X2	T43.3X3	T43.3X4	T43.3X5	T43.3X6
Stepronin	T48.4X1	T48.4X2	T48.4X3	T48.4X4	T48.4X5	T48.4X6
Sterculia	T47.4X1	T47.4X2	T47.4X3	T47.4X4	T47.4X5	T47.4X6
Sternutator gas	T59.891	T59.892	T59.893	T59.894	—	—
Steroid	T38.ØX1	T38.ØX2	T38.ØX3	T38.ØX4	T38.ØX5	T38.ØX6
anabolic	T38.7X1	T38.7X2	T38.7X3	T38.7X4	T38.7X5	T38.7X6
androgenic	T38.7X1	T38.7X2	T38.7X3	T38.7X4	T38.7X5	T38.7X6
antineoplastic, hormone	T38.7X1	T38.7X2	T38.7X3	T38.7X4	T38.7X5	T38.7X6
estrogen	T38.5X1	T38.5X2	T38.5X3	T38.5X4	T38.5X5	T38.5X6
ENT agent	T49.6X1	T49.6X2	T49.6X3	T49.6X4	T49.6X5	T49.6X6
ophthalmic preparation	T49.5X1	T49.5X2	T49.5X3	T49.5X4	T49.5X5	T49.5X6
topical NEC	T49.ØX1	T49.ØX2	T49.ØX3	T49.ØX4	T49.ØX5	T49.ØX6
Stibine	T56.891	T56.892	T56.893	T56.894	—	—
Stibogluconate	T37.3X1	T37.3X2	T37.3X3	T37.3X4	T37.3X5	T37.3X6
Stibophen	T37.4X1	T37.4X2	T37.4X3	T37.4X4	T37.4X5	T37.4X6
Stilbamidine (isetionate)	T37.3X1	T37.3X2	T37.3X3	T37.3X4	T37.3X5	T37.3X6
Stilbestrol	T38.5X1	T38.5X2	T38.5X3	T38.5X4	T38.5X5	T38.5X6
Stilboestrol	T38.5X1	T38.5X2	T38.5X3	T38.5X4	T38.5X5	T38.5X6
Stimulant						
central nervous system — *see also* Psychostimulant	T43.6Ø1	T43.6Ø2	T43.6Ø3	T43.6Ø4	T43.6Ø5	T43.6Ø6
analeptics	T5Ø.7X1	T5Ø.7X2	T5Ø.7X3	T5Ø.7X4	T5Ø.7X5	T5Ø.7X6
opiate antagonist	T5Ø.7X1	T5Ø.7X2	T5Ø.7X3	T5Ø.7X4	T5Ø.7X5	T5Ø.7X6
psychotherapeutic NEC — *see also* Psychotherapeutic drug	T43.6Ø1	T43.6Ø2	T43.6Ø3	T43.6Ø4	T43.6Ø5	T43.6Ø6
specified NEC	T43.691	T43.692	T43.693	T43.694	T43.695	T43.696
respiratory	T48.9Ø1	T48.9Ø2	T48.9Ø3	T48.9Ø4	T48.9Ø5	T48.9Ø6
Stone-dissolving drug	T5Ø.9Ø1	T5Ø.9Ø2	T5Ø.9Ø3	T5Ø.9Ø4	T5Ø.9Ø5	T5Ø.9Ø6
Storage battery (cells) (acid)	T54.2X1	T54.2X2	T54.2X3	T54.2X4	—	—
Stovaine	T41.3X1	T41.3X2	T41.3X3	T41.3X4	T41.3X5	T41.3X6
infiltration (subcutaneous)	T41.3X1	T41.3X2	T41.3X3	T41.3X4	T41.3X5	T41.3X6
nerve block (peripheral) (plexus)	T41.3X1	T41.3X2	T41.3X3	T41.3X4	T41.3X5	T41.3X6
spinal	T41.3X1	T41.3X2	T41.3X3	T41.3X4	T41.3X5	T41.3X6
topical (surface)	T41.3X1	T41.3X2	T41.3X3	T41.3X4	T41.3X5	T41.3X6
Stovarsal	T37.8X1	T37.8X2	T37.8X3	T37.8X4	T37.8X5	T37.8X6
Stove gas — *see* Gas, stove						
Stoxil	T49.5X1	T49.5X2	T49.5X3	T49.5X4	T49.5X5	T49.5X6
Stramonium	T48.6X1	T48.6X2	T48.6X3	T48.6X4	T48.6X5	T48.6X6
natural state	T62.2X1	T62.2X2	T62.2X3	T62.2X4	—	—
Streptodornase	T45.3X1	T45.3X2	T45.3X3	T45.3X4	T45.3X5	T45.3X6
Streptoduocin	T36.5X1	T36.5X2	T36.5X3	T36.5X4	T36.5X5	T36.5X6
Streptokinase	T45.611	T45.612	T45.613	T45.614	T45.615	T45.616
Streptomycin (derivative)	T36.5X1	T36.5X2	T36.5X3	T36.5X4	T36.5X5	T36.5X6
Streptonivicin	T36.5X1	T36.5X2	T36.5X3	T36.5X4	T36.5X5	T36.5X6
Streptovarycin	T36.5X1	T36.5X2	T36.5X3	T36.5X4	T36.5X5	T36.5X6
Streptozocin	T45.1X1	T45.1X2	T45.1X3	T45.1X4	T45.1X5	T45.1X6
Streptozotocin	T45.1X1	T45.1X2	T45.1X3	T45.1X4	T45.1X5	T45.1X6
Stripper (paint) (solvent)	T52.8X1	T52.8X2	T52.8X3	T52.8X4	—	—
Strobane	T6Ø.1X1	T6Ø.1X2	T6Ø.1X3	T6Ø.1X4	—	—
Strofantina	T46.ØX1	T46.ØX2	T46.ØX3	T46.ØX4	T46.ØX5	T46.ØX6
Strophanthin (g) (k)	T46.ØX1	T46.ØX2	T46.ØX3	T46.ØX4	T46.ØX5	T46.ØX6
Strophanthus	T46.ØX1	T46.ØX2	T46.ØX3	T46.ØX4	T46.ØX5	T46.ØX6
Strophantin	T46.ØX1	T46.ØX2	T46.ØX3	T46.ØX4	T46.ØX5	T46.ØX6
Strophantin-g	T46.ØX1	T46.ØX2	T46.ØX3	T46.ØX4	T46.ØX5	T46.ØX6
Strychnine (nonmedicinal) (pesticide) (salts)	T65.1X1	T65.1X2	T65.1X3	T65.1X4	—	—
medicinal	T48.291	T48.292	T48.293	T48.294	T48.295	T48.296

Substance	Poisoning, Accidental (unintentional)	Poisoning, Intentional Self-harm	Poisoning, Assault	Poisoning, Undetermined	Adverse Effect	Under-dosing
Strychnos (ignatii) — *see* Strychnine						
Styramate	T42.8X1	T42.8X2	T42.8X3	T42.8X4	T42.8X5	T42.8X6
Styrene	T65.891	T65.892	T65.893	T65.894	—	—
Succinimide, antiepileptic or anticonvulsant	T42.2X1	T42.2X2	T42.2X3	T42.2X4	T42.2X5	T42.2X6
mercuric — *see* Mercury						
Succinylcholine	T48.1X1	T48.1X2	T48.1X3	T48.1X4	T48.1X5	T48.1X6
Succinylsulfathiazole	T37.0X1	T37.0X2	T37.0X3	T37.0X4	T37.0X5	T37.0X6
Sucralfate	T47.1X1	T47.1X2	T47.1X3	T47.1X4	T47.1X5	T47.1X6
Sucrose	T50.3X1	T50.3X2	T50.3X3	T50.3X4	T50.3X5	T50.3X6
Sufentanil	T40.411	T40.412	T40.413	T40.414	T40.415	T40.416
Sulbactam	T36.0X1	T36.0X2	T36.0X3	T36.0X4	T36.0X5	T36.0X6
Sulbenicillin	T36.0X1	T36.0X2	T36.0X3	T36.0X4	T36.0X5	T36.0X6
Sulbentine	T49.0X1	T49.0X2	T49.0X3	T49.0X4	T49.0X5	T49.0X6
Sulfacetamide	T49.0X1	T49.0X2	T49.0X3	T49.0X4	T49.0X5	T49.0X6
ophthalmic preparation	T49.5X1	T49.5X2	T49.5X3	T49.5X4	T49.5X5	T49.5X6
Sulfachlorpyridazine	T37.0X1	T37.0X2	T37.0X3	T37.0X4	T37.0X5	T37.0X6
Sulfacitine	T37.0X1	T37.0X2	T37.0X3	T37.0X4	T37.0X5	T37.0X6
Sulfadiasulfone sodium	T37.0X1	T37.0X2	T37.0X3	T37.0X4	T37.0X5	T37.0X6
Sulfadiazine	T37.0X1	T37.0X2	T37.0X3	T37.0X4	T37.0X5	T37.0X6
silver (topical)	T49.0X1	T49.0X2	T49.0X3	T49.0X4	T49.0X5	T49.0X6
Sulfadimethoxine	T37.0X1	T37.0X2	T37.0X3	T37.0X4	T37.0X5	T37.0X6
Sulfadimidine	T37.0X1	T37.0X2	T37.0X3	T37.0X4	T37.0X5	T37.0X6
Sulfadoxine	T37.0X1	T37.0X2	T37.0X3	T37.0X4	T37.0X5	T37.0X6
with pyrimethamine	T37.2X1	T37.2X2	T37.2X3	T37.2X4	T37.2X5	T37.2X6
Sulfaethidole	T37.0X1	T37.0X2	T37.0X3	T37.0X4	T37.0X5	T37.0X6
Sulfafurazole	T37.0X1	T37.0X2	T37.0X3	T37.0X4	T37.0X5	T37.0X6
Sulfaguanidine	T37.0X1	T37.0X2	T37.0X3	T37.0X4	T37.0X5	T37.0X6
Sulfalene	T37.0X1	T37.0X2	T37.0X3	T37.0X4	T37.0X5	T37.0X6
Sulfaloxate	T37.0X1	T37.0X2	T37.0X3	T37.0X4	T37.0X5	T37.0X6
Sulfaloxic acid	T37.0X1	T37.0X2	T37.0X3	T37.0X4	T37.0X5	T37.0X6
Sulfamazone	T39.2X1	T39.2X2	T39.2X3	T39.2X4	T39.2X5	T39.2X6
Sulfamerazine	T37.0X1	T37.0X2	T37.0X3	T37.0X4	T37.0X5	T37.0X6
Sulfameter	T37.0X1	T37.0X2	T37.0X3	T37.0X4	T37.0X5	T37.0X6
Sulfamethazine	T37.0X1	T37.0X2	T37.0X3	T37.0X4	T37.0X5	T37.0X6
Sulfamethizole	T37.0X1	T37.0X2	T37.0X3	T37.0X4	T37.0X5	T37.0X6
Sulfamethoxazole	T37.0X1	T37.0X2	T37.0X3	T37.0X4	T37.0X5	T37.0X6
with trimethoprim	T36.8X1	T36.8X2	T36.8X3	T36.8X4	T36.8X5	T36.8X6
Sulfamethoxydiazine	T37.0X1	T37.0X2	T37.0X3	T37.0X4	T37.0X5	T37.0X6
Sulfamethoxypyridazine	T37.0X1	T37.0X2	T37.0X3	T37.0X4	T37.0X5	T37.0X6
Sulfamethylthiazole	T37.0X1	T37.0X2	T37.0X3	T37.0X4	T37.0X5	T37.0X6
Sulfametoxydiazine	T37.0X1	T37.0X2	T37.0X3	T37.0X4	T37.0X5	T37.0X6
Sulfamidopyrine	T39.2X1	T39.2X2	T39.2X3	T39.2X4	T39.2X5	T39.2X6
Sulfamonomethoxine	T37.0X1	T37.0X2	T37.0X3	T37.0X4	T37.0X5	T37.0X6
Sulfamoxole	T37.0X1	T37.0X2	T37.0X3	T37.0X4	T37.0X5	T37.0X6
Sulfamylon	T49.0X1	T49.0X2	T49.0X3	T49.0X4	T49.0X5	T49.0X6
Sulfan blue (diagnostic dye)	T50.8X1	T50.8X2	T50.8X3	T50.8X4	T50.8X5	T50.8X6
Sulfanilamide	T37.0X1	T37.0X2	T37.0X3	T37.0X4	T37.0X5	T37.0X6
Sulfanilylguanidine	T37.0X1	T37.0X2	T37.0X3	T37.0X4	T37.0X5	T37.0X6
Sulfaperin	T37.0X1	T37.0X2	T37.0X3	T37.0X4	T37.0X5	T37.0X6
Sulfaphenazole	T37.0X1	T37.0X2	T37.0X3	T37.0X4	T37.0X5	T37.0X6
Sulfaphenylthiazole	T37.0X1	T37.0X2	T37.0X3	T37.0X4	T37.0X5	T37.0X6
Sulfaproxyline	T37.0X1	T37.0X2	T37.0X3	T37.0X4	T37.0X5	T37.0X6
Sulfapyridine	T37.0X1	T37.0X2	T37.0X3	T37.0X4	T37.0X5	T37.0X6
Sulfapyrimidine	T37.0X1	T37.0X2	T37.0X3	T37.0X4	T37.0X5	T37.0X6
Sulfarsphenamine	T37.8X1	T37.8X2	T37.8X3	T37.8X4	T37.8X5	T37.8X6
Sulfasalazine	T37.0X1	T37.0X2	T37.0X3	T37.0X4	T37.0X5	T37.0X6
Sulfasuxidine	T37.0X1	T37.0X2	T37.0X3	T37.0X4	T37.0X5	T37.0X6
Sulfasymazine	T37.0X1	T37.0X2	T37.0X3	T37.0X4	T37.0X5	T37.0X6
Sulfated amylopectin	T47.8X1	T47.8X2	T47.8X3	T47.8X4	T47.8X5	T47.8X6
Sulfathiazole	T37.0X1	T37.0X2	T37.0X3	T37.0X4	T37.0X5	T37.0X6
Sulfatostearate	T49.2X1	T49.2X2	T49.2X3	T49.2X4	T49.2X5	T49.2X6
Sulfinpyrazone	T50.4X1	T50.4X2	T50.4X3	T50.4X4	T50.4X5	T50.4X6
Sulfiram	T49.0X1	T49.0X2	T49.0X3	T49.0X4	T49.0X5	T49.0X6
Sulfisomidine	T37.0X1	T37.0X2	T37.0X3	T37.0X4	T37.0X5	T37.0X6
Sulfisoxazole	T37.0X1	T37.0X2	T37.0X3	T37.0X4	T37.0X5	T37.0X6
ophthalmic preparation	T49.5X1	T49.5X2	T49.5X3	T49.5X4	T49.5X5	T49.5X6
Sulfobromophthalein (sodium)	T50.8X1	T50.8X2	T50.8X3	T50.8X4	T50.8X5	T50.8X6
Sulfobromphthalein	T50.8X1	T50.8X2	T50.8X3	T50.8X4	T50.8X5	T50.8X6
Sulfogaiacol	T48.4X1	T48.4X2	T48.4X3	T48.4X4	T48.4X5	T48.4X6
Sulfomyxin	T36.8X1	T36.8X2	T36.8X3	T36.8X4	T36.8X5	T36.8X6
Sulfonal	T42.6X1	T42.6X2	T42.6X3	T42.6X4	T42.6X5	T42.6X6
Sulfonamide NEC	T37.0X1	T37.0X2	T37.0X3	T37.0X4	T37.0X5	T37.0X6
eye	T49.5X1	T49.5X2	T49.5X3	T49.5X4	T49.5X5	T49.5X6
Sulfonazide	T37.1X1	T37.1X2	T37.1X3	T37.1X4	T37.1X5	T37.1X6
Sulfones	T37.1X1	T37.1X2	T37.1X3	T37.1X4	T37.1X5	T37.1X6
Sulfonethylmethane	T42.6X1	T42.6X2	T42.6X3	T42.6X4	T42.6X5	T42.6X6
Sulfonmethane	T42.6X1	T42.6X2	T42.6X3	T42.6X4	T42.6X5	T42.6X6
Sulfonphthal, sulfonphthol	T50.8X1	T50.8X2	T50.8X3	T50.8X4	T50.8X5	T50.8X6

Substance	Poisoning, Accidental (unintentional)	Poisoning, Intentional Self-harm	Poisoning, Assault	Poisoning, Undetermined	Adverse Effect	Under-dosing
Sulfonylurea derivatives, oral	T38.3X1	T38.3X2	T38.3X3	T38.3X4	T38.3X5	T38.3X6
Sulforidazine	T43.3X1	T43.3X2	T43.3X3	T43.3X4	T43.3X5	T43.3X6
Sulfoxone	T37.1X1	T37.1X2	T37.1X3	T37.1X4	T37.1X5	T37.1X6
Sulfuric acid	T54.2X1	T54.2X2	T54.2X3	T54.2X4	—	—
Sulfur, sulfurated, sulfuric, sulfurous, sulfuryl (compounds NEC) (medicinal)	T49.4X1	T49.4X2	T49.4X3	T49.4X4	T49.4X5	T49.4X6
acid	T54.2X1	T54.2X2	T54.2X3	T54.2X4	—	—
dioxide (gas)	T59.1X1	T59.1X2	T59.1X3	T59.1X4	—	—
ether — *see* Ether(s)						
hydrogen	T59.6X1	T59.6X2	T59.6X3	T59.6X4	—	—
medicinal (keratolytic) (ointment) NEC	T49.4X1	T49.4X2	T49.4X3	T49.4X4	T49.4X5	T49.4X6
ointment	T49.0X1	T49.0X2	T49.0X3	T49.0X4	T49.0X5	T49.0X6
pesticide (vapor)	T60.91	T60.92	T60.93	T60.94	—	—
vapor NEC	T59.891	T59.892	T59.893	T59.894	—	—
Sulglicotide	T47.1X1	T47.1X2	T47.1X3	T47.1X4	T47.1X5	T47.1X6
Sulindac	T39.391	T39.392	T39.393	T39.394	T39.395	T39.396
Sulisatin	T47.2X1	T47.2X2	T47.2X3	T47.2X4	T47.2X5	T47.2X6
Sulisobenzone	T49.3X1	T49.3X2	T49.3X3	T49.3X4	T49.3X5	T49.3X6
Sulkowitch's reagent	T50.8X1	T50.8X2	T50.8X3	T50.8X4	T50.8X5	T50.8X6
Sulmetozine	T44.3X1	T44.3X2	T44.3X3	T44.3X4	T44.3X5	T44.3X6
Suloctidil	T46.7X1	T46.7X2	T46.7X3	T46.7X4	T46.7X5	T46.7X6
Sulph- — *see also* Sulf-						
Sulphadiazine	T37.0X1	T37.0X2	T37.0X3	T37.0X4	T37.0X5	T37.0X6
Sulphadimethoxine	T37.0X1	T37.0X2	T37.0X3	T37.0X4	T37.0X5	T37.0X6
Sulphadimidine	T37.0X1	T37.0X2	T37.0X3	T37.0X4	T37.0X5	T37.0X6
Sulphadione	T37.1X1	T37.1X2	T37.1X3	T37.1X4	T37.1X5	T37.1X6
Sulphafurazole	T37.0X1	T37.0X2	T37.0X3	T37.0X4	T37.0X5	T37.0X6
Sulphamethizole	T37.0X1	T37.0X2	T37.0X3	T37.0X4	T37.0X5	T37.0X6
Sulphamethoxazole	T37.0X1	T37.0X2	T37.0X3	T37.0X4	T37.0X5	T37.0X6
Sulphan blue	T50.8X1	T50.8X2	T50.8X3	T50.8X4	T50.8X5	T50.8X6
Sulphaphenazole	T37.0X1	T37.0X2	T37.0X3	T37.0X4	T37.0X5	T37.0X6
Sulphapyridine	T37.0X1	T37.0X2	T37.0X3	T37.0X4	T37.0X5	T37.0X6
Sulphasalazine	T37.0X1	T37.0X2	T37.0X3	T37.0X4	T37.0X5	T37.0X6
Sulphinpyrazone	T50.4X1	T50.4X2	T50.4X3	T50.4X4	T50.4X5	T50.4X6
Sulpiride	T43.591	T43.592	T43.593	T43.594	T43.595	T43.596
Sulprostone	T48.0X1	T48.0X2	T48.0X3	T48.0X4	T48.0X5	T48.0X6
Sulpyrine	T39.2X1	T39.2X2	T39.2X3	T39.2X4	T39.2X5	T39.2X6
Sultamicillin	T36.0X1	T36.0X2	T36.0X3	T36.0X4	T36.0X5	T36.0X6
Sulthiame	T42.6X1	T42.6X2	T42.6X3	T42.6X4	T42.6X5	T42.6X6
Sultiame	T42.6X1	T42.6X2	T42.6X3	T42.6X4	T42.6X5	T42.6X6
Sultopride	T43.591	T43.592	T43.593	T43.594	T43.595	T43.596
Sumatriptan	T39.8X1	T39.8X2	T39.8X3	T39.8X4	T39.8X5	T39.8X6
Sunflower seed oil	T46.6X1	T46.6X2	T46.6X3	T46.6X4	T46.6X5	T46.6X6
Superinone	T48.4X1	T48.4X2	T48.4X3	T48.4X4	T48.4X5	T48.4X6
Suprofen	T39.311	T39.312	T39.313	T39.314	T39.315	T39.316
Suramin (sodium)	T37.4X1	T37.4X2	T37.4X3	T37.4X4	T37.4X5	T37.4X6
Surfacaine	T41.3X1	T41.3X2	T41.3X3	T41.3X4	T41.3X5	T41.3X6
Surital	T41.1X1	T41.1X2	T41.1X3	T41.1X4	T41.1X5	T41.1X6
Sutilains	T45.3X1	T45.3X2	T45.3X3	T45.3X4	T45.3X5	T45.3X6
Suxamethonium (chloride)	T48.1X1	T48.1X2	T48.1X3	T48.1X4	T48.1X5	T48.1X6
Suxethonium (chloride)	T48.1X1	T48.1X2	T48.1X3	T48.1X4	T48.1X5	T48.1X6
Suxibuzone	T39.2X1	T39.2X2	T39.2X3	T39.2X4	T39.2X5	T39.2X6
Sweetener	T50.901	T50.902	T50.903	T50.904	T50.905	T50.906
Sweet niter spirit	T46.3X1	T46.3X2	T46.3X3	T46.3X4	T46.3X5	T46.3X6
Sweet oil (birch)	T49.3X1	T49.3X2	T49.3X3	T49.3X4	T49.3X5	T49.3X6
Sym-dichloroethyl ether	T53.6X1	T53.6X2	T53.6X3	T53.6X4	—	—
Sympatholytic NEC	T44.8X1	T44.8X2	T44.8X3	T44.8X4	T44.8X5	T44.8X6
haloalkylamine	T44.8X1	T44.8X2	T44.8X3	T44.8X4	T44.8X5	T44.8X6
Sympathomimetic NEC	T44.901	T44.902	T44.903	T44.904	T44.905	T44.906
anti-common-cold	T48.5X1	T48.5X2	T48.5X3	T48.5X4	T48.5X5	T48.5X6
bronchodilator	T48.6X1	T48.6X2	T48.6X3	T48.6X4	T48.6X5	T48.6X6
specified NEC	T44.991	T44.992	T44.993	T44.994	T44.995	T44.996
Synagis	T50.B91	T50.B92	T50.B93	T50.B94	T50.B95	T50.B96
Synalar	T49.0X1	T49.0X2	T49.0X3	T49.0X4	T49.0X5	T49.0X6
Synthroid	T38.1X1	T38.1X2	T38.1X3	T38.1X4	T38.1X5	T38.1X6
Syntocinon	T48.0X1	T48.0X2	T48.0X3	T48.0X4	T48.0X5	T48.0X6
Syrosingopine	T46.5X1	T46.5X2	T46.5X3	T46.5X4	T46.5X5	T46.5X6
Systemic drug	T45.91	T45.92	T45.93	T45.94	T45.95	T45.96
specified NEC	T45.8X1	T45.8X2	T45.8X3	T45.8X4	T45.8X5	T45.8X6
Tablets — *see also* specified substance	T50.901	T50.902	T50.903	T50.904	T50.905	T50.906
Tace	T38.5X1	T38.5X2	T38.5X3	T38.5X4	T38.5X5	T38.5X6
Tacrine	T44.0X1	T44.0X2	T44.0X3	T44.0X4	T44.0X5	T44.0X6
Tadalafil	T46.7X1	T46.7X2	T46.7X3	T46.7X4	T46.7X5	T46.7X6
Talampicillin	T36.0X1	T36.0X2	T36.0X3	T36.0X4	T36.0X5	T36.0X6
Talbutal	T42.3X1	T42.3X2	T42.3X3	T42.3X4	T42.3X5	T42.3X6
Talc powder	T49.3X1	T49.3X2	T49.3X3	T49.3X4	T49.3X5	T49.3X6
Talcum	T49.3X1	T49.3X2	T49.3X3	T49.3X4	T49.3X5	T49.3X6
Taleranol	T38.6X1	T38.6X2	T38.6X3	T38.6X4	T38.6X5	T38.6X6

Substance	Poisoning, Accidental (unintentional)	Poisoning, Intentional Self-harm	Poisoning, Assault	Poisoning, Undetermined	Adverse Effect	Under-dosing
Tamoxifen	T38.6X1	T38.6X2	T38.6X3	T38.6X4	T38.6X5	T38.6X6
Tamsulosin	T44.6X1	T44.6X2	T44.6X3	T44.6X4	T44.6X5	T44.6X6
Tandearil, tanderil	T39.2X1	T39.2X2	T39.2X3	T39.2X4	T39.2X5	T39.2X6
Tannic acid	T49.2X1	T49.2X2	T49.2X3	T49.2X4	T49.2X5	T49.2X6
medicinal (astringent)	T49.2X1	T49.2X2	T49.2X3	T49.2X4	T49.2X5	T49.2X6
Tannin — *see* Tannic acid						
Tansy	T62.2X1	T62.2X2	T62.2X3	T62.2X4	—	—
TAO	T36.3X1	T36.3X2	T36.3X3	T36.3X4	T36.3X5	T36.3X6
Tapazole	T38.2X1	T38.2X2	T38.2X3	T38.2X4	T38.2X5	T38.2X6
Taractan	T43.591	T43.592	T43.593	T43.594	T43.595	T43.596
Tarantula (venomous)	T63.321	T63.322	T63.323	T63.324	—	—
Tartar emetic	T37.8X1	T37.8X2	T37.8X3	T37.8X4	T37.8X5	T37.8X6
Tartaric acid	T65.891	T65.892	T65.893	T65.894	—	—
Tartrated antimony (anti-infective)	T37.8X1	T37.8X2	T37.8X3	T37.8X4	T37.8X5	T37.8X6
Tartrate, laxative	T47.4X1	T47.4X2	T47.4X3	T47.4X4	T47.4X5	T47.4X6
Tar NEC	T52.ØX1	T52.ØX2	T52.ØX3	T52.ØX4	—	—
camphor	T6Ø.1X1	T6Ø.1X2	T6Ø.1X3	T6Ø.1X4	—	—
distillate	T49.1X1	T49.1X2	T49.1X3	T49.1X4	T49.1X5	T49.1X6
fumes	T59.891	T59.892	T59.893	T59.894	—	—
medicinal	T49.1X1	T49.1X2	T49.1X3	T49.1X4	T49.1X5	T49.1X6
ointment	T49.1X1	T49.1X2	T49.1X3	T49.1X4	T49.1X5	T49.1X6
Tauromustine	T45.1X1	T45.1X2	T45.1X3	T45.1X4	T45.1X5	T45.1X6
TCA — *see* Trichloroacetic acid						
TCDD	T53.7X1	T53.7X2	T53.7X3	T53.7X4	—	—
TDI (vapor)	T65.ØX1	T65.ØX2	T65.ØX3	T65.ØX4	—	—
Tear						
gas	T59.3X1	T59.3X2	T59.3X3	T59.3X4	—	—
solution	T49.5X1	T49.5X2	T49.5X3	T49.5X4	T49.5X5	T49.5X6
Teclothiazide	T5Ø.2X1	T5Ø.2X2	T5Ø.2X3	T5Ø.2X4	T5Ø.2X5	T5Ø.2X6
Teclozan	T37.3X1	T37.3X2	T37.3X3	T37.3X4	T37.3X5	T37.3X6
Tegafur	T45.1X1	T45.1X2	T45.1X3	T45.1X4	T45.1X5	T45.1X6
Tegretol	T42.1X1	T42.1X2	T42.1X3	T42.1X4	T42.1X5	T42.1X6
Teicoplanin	T36.8X1	T36.8X2	T36.8X3	T36.8X4	T36.8X5	T36.8X6
Telepaque	T5Ø.8X1	T5Ø.8X2	T5Ø.8X3	T5Ø.8X4	T5Ø.8X5	T5Ø.8X6
Tellurium	T56.891	T56.892	T56.893	T56.894	—	—
fumes	T56.891	T56.892	T56.893	T56.894	—	—
TEM	T45.1X1	T45.1X2	T45.1X3	T45.1X4	T45.1X5	T45.1X6
Temazepam	T42.4X1	T42.4X2	T42.4X3	T42.4X4	T42.4X5	T42.4X6
Temocillin	T36.ØX1	T36.ØX2	T36.ØX3	T36.ØX4	T36.ØX5	T36.ØX6
Tenamfetamine	T43.621	T43.622	T43.623	T43.624	T43.625	T43.626
Teniposide	T45.1X1	T45.1X2	T45.1X3	T45.1X4	T45.1X5	T45.1X6
Tenitramine	T46.3X1	T46.3X2	T46.3X3	T46.3X4	T46.3X5	T46.3X6
Tenoglicin	T48.4X1	T48.4X2	T48.4X3	T48.4X4	T48.4X5	T48.4X6
Tenonitrozole	T37.3X1	T37.3X2	T37.3X3	T37.3X4	T37.3X5	T37.3X6
Tenoxicam	T39.391	T39.392	T39.393	T39.394	T39.395	T39.396
TEPA	T45.1X1	T45.1X2	T45.1X3	T45.1X4	T45.1X5	T45.1X6
TEPP	T6Ø.ØX1	T6Ø.ØX2	T6Ø.ØX3	T6Ø.ØX4	—	—
Teprotide	T46.5X1	T46.5X2	T46.5X3	T46.5X4	T46.5X5	T46.5X6
Terazosin	T44.6X1	T44.6X2	T44.6X3	T44.6X4	T44.6X5	T44.6X6
Terbufos	T6Ø.ØX1	T6Ø.ØX2	T6Ø.ØX3	T6Ø.ØX4	—	—
Terbutaline	T48.6X1	T48.6X2	T48.6X3	T48.6X4	T48.6X5	T48.6X6
Terconazole	T49.ØX1	T49.ØX2	T49.ØX3	T49.ØX4	T49.ØX5	T49.ØX6
Terfenadine	T45.ØX1	T45.ØX2	T45.ØX3	T45.ØX4	T45.ØX5	T45.ØX6
Teriparatide (acetate)	T5Ø.991	T5Ø.992	T5Ø.993	T5Ø.994	T5Ø.995	T5Ø.996
Terizidone	T37.1X1	T37.1X2	T37.1X3	T37.1X4	T37.1X5	T37.1X6
Terlipressin	T38.891	T38.892	T38.893	T38.894	T38.895	T38.896
Terodiline	T46.3X1	T46.3X2	T46.3X3	T46.3X4	T46.3X5	T46.3X6
Teroxalene	T37.4X1	T37.4X2	T37.4X3	T37.4X4	T37.4X5	T37.4X6
Terpin (cis) **hydrate**	T48.4X1	T48.4X2	T48.4X3	T48.4X4	T48.4X5	T48.4X6
Terramycin	T36.4X1	T36.4X2	T36.4X3	T36.4X4	T36.4X5	T36.4X6
Tertatolol	T44.7X1	T44.7X2	T44.7X3	T44.7X4	T44.7X5	T44.7X6
Tessalon	T48.3X1	T48.3X2	T48.3X3	T48.3X4	T48.3X5	T48.3X6
Testolactone	T38.7X1	T38.7X2	T38.7X3	T38.7X4	T38.7X5	T38.7X6
Testosterone	T38.7X1	T38.7X2	T38.7X3	T38.7X4	T38.7X5	T38.7X6
Tetanus toxoid or vaccine	T5Ø.A91	T5Ø.A92	T5Ø.A93	T5Ø.A94	T5Ø.A95	T5Ø.A96
antitoxin	T5Ø.Z11	T5Ø.Z12	T5Ø.Z13	T5Ø.Z14	T5Ø.Z15	T5Ø.Z16
immune globulin (human)	T5Ø.Z11	T5Ø.Z12	T5Ø.Z13	T5Ø.Z14	T5Ø.Z15	T5Ø.Z16
toxoid	T5Ø.A91	T5Ø.A92	T5Ø.A93	T5Ø.A94	T5Ø.A95	T5Ø.A96
with diphtheria toxoid	T5Ø.A21	T5Ø.A22	T5Ø.A23	T5Ø.A24	T5Ø.A25	T5Ø.A26
with pertussis	T5Ø.A11	T5Ø.A12	T5Ø.A13	T5Ø.A14	T5Ø.A15	T5Ø.A16
Tetrabenazine	T43.591	T43.592	T43.593	T43.594	T43.595	T43.596
Tetracaine	T41.3X1	T41.3X2	T41.3X3	T41.3X4	T41.3X5	T41.3X6
nerve block (peripheral) (plexus)	T41.3X1	T41.3X2	T41.3X3	T41.3X4	T41.3X5	T41.3X6
regional	T41.3X1	T41.3X2	T41.3X3	T41.3X4	T41.3X5	T41.3X6
spinal	T41.3X1	T41.3X2	T41.3X3	T41.3X4	T41.3X5	T41.3X6
Tetrachlorethylene — *see* Tetrachloroethylene						
Tetrachlormethiazide	T5Ø.2X1	T5Ø.2X2	T5Ø.2X3	T5Ø.2X4	T5Ø.2X5	T5Ø.2X6
Tetrachloroethane	T53.6X1	T53.6X2	T53.6X3	T53.6X4	—	—
vapor	T53.6X1	T53.6X2	T53.6X3	T53.6X4	—	—
paint or varnish	T53.6X1	T53.6X2	T53.6X3	T53.6X4	—	—
Tetrachloroethylene (liquid)	T53.3X1	T53.3X2	T53.3X3	T53.3X4	—	—
medicinal	T37.4X1	T37.4X2	T37.4X3	T37.4X4	T37.4X5	T37.4X6
vapor	T53.3X1	T53.3X2	T53.3X3	T53.3X4	—	—
Tetrachloromethane — *see* Carbon tetrachloride						
Tetracosactide	T38.811	T38.812	T38.813	T38.814	T38.815	T38.816
Tetracosactrin	T38.811	T38.812	T38.813	T38.814	T38.815	T38.816
Tetracycline	T36.4X1	T36.4X2	T36.4X3	T36.4X4	T36.4X5	T36.4X6
ophthalmic preparation	T49.5X1	T49.5X2	T49.5X3	T49.5X4	T49.5X5	T49.5X6
topical NEC	T49.ØX1	T49.ØX2	T49.ØX3	T49.ØX4	T49.ØX5	T49.ØX6
Tetradifon	T6Ø.8X1	T6Ø.8X2	T6Ø.8X3	T6Ø.8X4	—	—
Tetradotoxin	T61.771	T61.772	T61.773	T61.774	—	—
Tetraethyl						
lead	T56.ØX1	T56.ØX2	T56.ØX3	T56.ØX4	—	—
pyrophosphate	T6Ø.ØX1	T6Ø.ØX2	T6Ø.ØX3	T6Ø.ØX4	—	—
Tetraethylammonium chloride	T44.2X1	T44.2X2	T44.2X3	T44.2X4	T44.2X5	T44.2X6
Tetraethylthiuram disulfide	T5Ø.6X1	T5Ø.6X2	T5Ø.6X3	T5Ø.6X4	T5Ø.6X5	T5Ø.6X6
Tetrahydroaminoacridine	T44.ØX1	T44.ØX2	T44.ØX3	T44.ØX4	T44.ØX5	T44.ØX6
Tetrahydrocannabinol	T4Ø.7X1	T4Ø.7X2	T4Ø.7X3	T4Ø.7X4	T4Ø.7X5	T4Ø.7X6
Tetrahydrofuran	T52.8X1	T52.8X2	T52.8X3	T52.8X4	—	—
Tetrahydronaphthalene	T52.8X1	T52.8X2	T52.8X3	T52.8X4	—	—
Tetrahydrozoline	T49.5X1	T49.5X2	T49.5X3	T49.5X4	T49.5X5	T49.5X6
Tetralin	T52.8X1	T52.8X2	T52.8X3	T52.8X4	—	—
Tetramethrin	T6Ø.2X1	T6Ø.2X2	T6Ø.2X3	T6Ø.2X4	—	—
Tetramethylthiuram (disulfide) **NEC**	T6Ø.3X1	T6Ø.3X2	T6Ø.3X3	T6Ø.3X4	—	—
medicinal	T49.ØX1	T49.ØX2	T49.ØX3	T49.ØX4	T49.ØX5	T49.ØX6
Tetramisole	T37.4X1	T37.4X2	T37.4X3	T37.4X4	T37.4X5	T37.4X6
Tetranicotinoyl fructose	T46.7X1	T46.7X2	T46.7X3	T46.7X4	T46.7X5	T46.7X6
Tetrazepam	T42.4X1	T42.4X2	T42.4X3	T42.4X4	T42.4X5	T42.4X6
Tetronal	T42.6X1	T42.6X2	T42.6X3	T42.6X4	T42.6X5	T42.6X6
Tetryl	T65.3X1	T65.3X2	T65.3X3	T65.3X4	—	—
Tetrylammonium chloride	T44.2X1	T44.2X2	T44.2X3	T44.2X4	T44.2X5	T44.2X6
Tetryzoline	T49.5X1	T49.5X2	T49.5X3	T49.5X4	T49.5X5	T49.5X6
Thalidomide	T45.1X1	T45.1X2	T45.1X3	T45.1X4	T45.1X5	T45.1X6
Thallium (compounds) (dust) **NEC**	T56.811	T56.812	T56.813	T56.814	—	—
pesticide	T6Ø.4X1	T6Ø.4X2	T6Ø.4X3	T6Ø.4X4	—	—
THC	T4Ø.7X1	T4Ø.7X2	T4Ø.7X3	T4Ø.7X4	T4Ø.7X5	T4Ø.7X6
Thebacon	T48.3X1	T48.3X2	T48.3X3	T48.3X4	T48.3X5	T48.3X6
Thebaine	T4Ø.2X1	T4Ø.2X2	T4Ø.2X3	T4Ø.2X4	T4Ø.2X5	T4Ø.2X6
Thenoic acid	T49.6X1	T49.6X2	T49.6X3	T49.6X4	T49.6X5	T49.6X6
Thenyldiamine	T45.ØX1	T45.ØX2	T45.ØX3	T45.ØX4	T45.ØX5	T45.ØX6
Theobromine (calcium salicylate)	T48.6X1	T48.6X2	T48.6X3	T48.6X4	T48.6X5	T48.6X6
sodium salicylate	T48.6X1	T48.6X2	T48.6X3	T48.6X4	T48.6X5	T48.6X6
Theophyllamine	T48.6X1	T48.6X2	T48.6X3	T48.6X4	T48.6X5	T48.6X6
Theophylline	T48.6X1	T48.6X2	T48.6X3	T48.6X4	T48.6X5	T48.6X6
aminobenzoic acid	T48.6X1	T48.6X2	T48.6X3	T48.6X4	T48.6X5	T48.6X6
ethylenediamine	T48.6X1	T48.6X2	T48.6X3	T48.6X4	T48.6X5	T48.6X6
piperazine p-amino-benzoate	T48.6X1	T48.6X2	T48.6X3	T48.6X4	T48.6X5	T48.6X6
Thiabendazole	T37.4X1	T37.4X2	T37.4X3	T37.4X4	T37.4X5	T37.4X6
Thialbarbital	T41.1X1	T41.1X2	T41.1X3	T41.1X4	T41.1X5	T41.1X6
Thiamazole	T38.2X1	T38.2X2	T38.2X3	T38.2X4	T38.2X5	T38.2X6
Thiambutosine	T37.1X1	T37.1X2	T37.1X3	T37.1X4	T37.1X5	T37.1X6
Thiamine	T45.2X1	T45.2X2	T45.2X3	T45.2X4	T45.2X5	T45.2X6
Thiamphenicol	T36.2X1	T36.2X2	T36.2X3	T36.2X4	T36.2X5	T36.2X6
Thiamylal	T41.1X1	T41.1X2	T41.1X3	T41.1X4	T41.1X5	T41.1X6
sodium	T41.1X1	T41.1X2	T41.1X3	T41.1X4	T41.1X5	T41.1X6
Thiazesim	T43.291	T43.292	T43.293	T43.294	T43.295	T43.296
Thiazides (diuretics)	T5Ø.2X1	T5Ø.2X2	T5Ø.2X3	T5Ø.2X4	T5Ø.2X5	T5Ø.2X6
Thiazinamium metilsulfate	T43.3X1	T43.3X2	T43.3X3	T43.3X4	T43.3X5	T43.3X6
Thiethylperazine	T43.3X1	T43.3X2	T43.3X3	T43.3X4	T43.3X5	T43.3X6
Thimerosal	T49.ØX1	T49.ØX2	T49.ØX3	T49.ØX4	T49.ØX5	T49.ØX6
ophthalmic preparation	T49.5X1	T49.5X2	T49.5X3	T49.5X4	T49.5X5	T49.5X6
Thioacetazone	T37.1X1	T37.1X2	T37.1X3	T37.1X4	T37.1X5	T37.1X6
with isoniazid	T37.1X1	T37.1X2	T37.1X3	T37.1X4	T37.1X5	T37.1X6
Thiobarbital sodium	T41.1X1	T41.1X2	T41.1X3	T41.1X4	T41.1X5	T41.1X6
Thiobarbiturate anesthetic	T41.1X1	T41.1X2	T41.1X3	T41.1X4	T41.1X5	T41.1X6
Thiobismol	T37.8X1	T37.8X2	T37.8X3	T37.8X4	T37.8X5	T37.8X6
Thiobutabarbital sodium	T41.1X1	T41.1X2	T41.1X3	T41.1X4	T41.1X5	T41.1X6
Thiocarbamate (insecticide)	T6Ø.ØX1	T6Ø.ØX2	T6Ø.ØX3	T6Ø.ØX4	—	—
Thiocarbamide	T38.2X1	T38.2X2	T38.2X3	T38.2X4	T38.2X5	T38.2X6
Thiocarbarsone	T37.8X1	T37.8X2	T37.8X3	T37.8X4	T37.8X5	T37.8X6
Thiocarlide	T37.1X1	T37.1X2	T37.1X3	T37.1X4	T37.1X5	T37.1X6
Thioctamide	T5Ø.991	T5Ø.992	T5Ø.993	T5Ø.994	T5Ø.995	T5Ø.996

Substance	Poisoning, Accidental (unintentional)	Poisoning, Intentional Self-harm	Poisoning, Assault	Poisoning, Undetermined	Adverse Effect	Under-dosing
Thioctic acid	T50.991	T50.992	T50.993	T50.994	T50.995	T50.996
Thiofos	T60.0X1	T60.0X2	T60.0X3	T60.0X4	—	—
Thioglycolate	T49.4X1	T49.4X2	T49.4X3	T49.4X4	T49.4X5	T49.4X6
Thioglycolic acid	T65.891	T65.892	T65.893	T65.894	—	—
Thioguanine	T45.1X1	T45.1X2	T45.1X3	T45.1X4	T45.1X5	T45.1X6
Thiomercaptomerin	T50.2X1	T50.2X2	T50.2X3	T50.2X4	T50.2X5	T50.2X6
Thiomerin	T50.2X1	T50.2X2	T50.2X3	T50.2X4	T50.2X5	T50.2X6
Thiomersal	T49.0X1	T49.0X2	T49.0X3	T49.0X4	T49.0X5	T49.0X6
Thionazin	T60.0X1	T60.0X2	T60.0X3	T60.0X4	—	—
Thiopental (sodium)	T41.1X1	T41.1X2	T41.1X3	T41.1X4	T41.1X5	T41.1X6
Thiopentone (sodium)	T41.1X1	T41.1X2	T41.1X3	T41.1X4	T41.1X5	T41.1X6
Thiopropazate	T43.3X1	T43.3X2	T43.3X3	T43.3X4	T43.3X5	T43.3X6
Thioproperazine	T43.3X1	T43.3X2	T43.3X3	T43.3X4	T43.3X5	T43.3X6
Thioridazine	T43.3X1	T43.3X2	T43.3X3	T43.3X4	T43.3X5	T43.3X6
Thiosinamine	T49.3X1	T49.3X2	T49.3X3	T49.3X4	T49.3X5	T49.3X6
Thiotepa	T45.1X1	T45.1X2	T45.1X3	T45.1X4	T45.1X5	T45.1X6
Thiothixene	T43.4X1	T43.4X2	T43.4X3	T43.4X4	T43.4X5	T43.4X6
Thiouracil (benzyl) (methyl) (propyl)	T38.2X1	T38.2X2	T38.2X3	T38.2X4	T38.2X5	T38.2X6
Thiourea	T38.2X1	T38.2X2	T38.2X3	T38.2X4	T38.2X5	T38.2X6
Thiphenamil	T44.3X1	T44.3X2	T44.3X3	T44.3X4	T44.3X5	T44.3X6
Thiram	T60.3X1	T60.3X2	T60.3X3	T60.3X4	—	—
medicinal	T49.2X1	T49.2X2	T49.2X3	T49.2X4	T49.2X5	T49.2X6
Thonzylamine (systemic)	T45.0X1	T45.0X2	T45.0X3	T45.0X4	T45.0X5	T45.0X6
mucosal decongestant	T48.5X1	T48.5X2	T48.5X3	T48.5X4	T48.5X5	T48.5X6
Thorazine	T43.3X1	T43.3X2	T43.3X3	T43.3X4	T43.3X5	T43.3X6
Thorium dioxide suspension	T50.8X1	T50.8X2	T50.8X3	T50.8X4	T50.8X5	T50.8X6
Thornapple	T62.2X1	T62.2X2	T62.2X3	T62.2X4	—	—
Throat drug NEC	T49.6X1	T49.6X2	T49.6X3	T49.6X4	T49.6X5	T49.6X6
Thrombin	T45.7X1	T45.7X2	T45.7X3	T45.7X4	T45.7X5	T45.7X6
Thrombolysin	T45.611	T45.612	T45.613	T45.614	T45.615	T45.616
Thromboplastin	T45.7X1	T45.7X2	T45.7X3	T45.7X4	T45.7X5	T45.7X6
Thurfyl nicotinate	T46.7X1	T46.7X2	T46.7X3	T46.7X4	T46.7X5	T46.7X6
Thymol	T49.0X1	T49.0X2	T49.0X3	T49.0X4	T49.0X5	T49.0X6
Thymopentin	T37.5X1	T37.5X2	T37.5X3	T37.5X4	T37.5X5	T37.5X6
Thymoxamine	T46.7X1	T46.7X2	T46.7X3	T46.7X4	T46.7X5	T46.7X6
Thymus extract	T38.891	T38.892	T38.893	T38.894	T38.895	T38.896
Thyreotrophic hormone	T38.811	T38.812	T38.813	T38.814	T38.815	T38.816
Thyroglobulin	T38.1X1	T38.1X2	T38.1X3	T38.1X4	T38.1X5	T38.1X6
Thyroid (hormone)	T38.1X1	T38.1X2	T38.1X3	T38.1X4	T38.1X5	T38.1X6
Thyrolar	T38.1X1	T38.1X2	T38.1X3	T38.1X4	T38.1X5	T38.1X6
Thyrotrophin	T38.811	T38.812	T38.813	T38.814	T38.815	T38.816
Thyrotropic hormone	T38.811	T38.812	T38.813	T38.814	T38.815	T38.816
Thyroxine	T38.1X1	T38.1X2	T38.1X3	T38.1X4	T38.1X5	T38.1X6
Tiabendazole	T37.4X1	T37.4X2	T37.4X3	T37.4X4	T37.4X5	T37.4X6
Tiamizide	T50.2X1	T50.2X2	T50.2X3	T50.2X4	T50.2X5	T50.2X6
Tianeptine	T43.291	T43.292	T43.293	T43.294	T43.295	T43.296
Tiapamil	T46.1X1	T46.1X2	T46.1X3	T46.1X4	T46.1X5	T46.1X6
Tiapride	T43.591	T43.592	T43.593	T43.594	T43.595	T43.596
Tiaprofenic acid	T39.311	T39.312	T39.313	T39.314	T39.315	T39.316
Tiaramide	T39.8X1	T39.8X2	T39.8X3	T39.8X4	T39.8X5	T39.8X6
Ticarcillin	T36.0X1	T36.0X2	T36.0X3	T36.0X4	T36.0X5	T36.0X6
Ticlatone	T49.0X1	T49.0X2	T49.0X3	T49.0X4	T49.0X5	T49.0X6
Ticlopidine	T45.521	T45.522	T45.523	T45.524	T45.525	T45.526
Ticrynafen	T50.1X1	T50.1X2	T50.1X3	T50.1X4	T50.1X5	T50.1X6
Tidiacic	T50.991	T50.992	T50.993	T50.994	T50.995	T50.996
Tiemonium	T44.3X1	T44.3X2	T44.3X3	T44.3X4	T44.3X5	T44.3X6
iodide	T44.3X1	T44.3X2	T44.3X3	T44.3X4	T44.3X5	T44.3X6
Tienilic acid	T50.1X1	T50.1X2	T50.1X3	T50.1X4	T50.1X5	T50.1X6
Tifenamil	T44.3X1	T44.3X2	T44.3X3	T44.3X4	T44.3X5	T44.3X6
Tigan	T45.0X1	T45.0X2	T45.0X3	T45.0X4	T45.0X5	T45.0X6
Tigloidine	T44.3X1	T44.3X2	T44.3X3	T44.3X4	T44.3X5	T44.3X6
Tilactase	T47.5X1	T47.5X2	T47.5X3	T47.5X4	T47.5X5	T47.5X6
Tiletamine	T41.291	T41.292	T41.293	T41.294	T41.295	T41.296
Tilidine	T40.491	T40.492	T40.493	T40.494	—	—
Timepidium bromide	T44.3X1	T44.3X2	T44.3X3	T44.3X4	T44.3X5	T44.3X6
Timiperone	T43.4X1	T43.4X2	T43.4X3	T43.4X4	T43.4X5	T43.4X6
Timolol	T44.7X1	T44.7X2	T44.7X3	T44.7X4	T44.7X5	T44.7X6
Tincture, iodine — *see* Iodine						
Tindal	T43.3X1	T43.3X2	T43.3X3	T43.3X4	T43.3X5	T43.3X6
Tinidazole	T37.3X1	T37.3X2	T37.3X3	T37.3X4	T37.3X5	T37.3X6
Tin (chloride) (dust) (oxide) **NEC**	T56.6X1	T56.6X2	T56.6X3	T56.6X4	—	—
anti-infectives	T37.8X1	T37.8X2	T37.8X3	T37.8X4	T37.8X5	T37.8X6
Tinoridine	T39.8X1	T39.8X2	T39.8X3	T39.8X4	T39.8X5	T39.8X6
Tiocarlide	T37.1X1	T37.1X2	T37.1X3	T37.1X4	T37.1X5	T37.1X6
Tioclomarol	T45.511	T45.512	T45.513	T45.514	T45.515	T45.516
Tioconazole	T49.0X1	T49.0X2	T49.0X3	T49.0X4	T49.0X5	T49.0X6
Tioguanine	T45.1X1	T45.1X2	T45.1X3	T45.1X4	T45.1X5	T45.1X6
Tiopronin	T50.991	T50.992	T50.993	T50.994	T50.995	T50.996
Tiotixene	T43.4X1	T43.4X2	T43.4X3	T43.4X4	T43.4X5	T43.4X6
Tioxolone	T49.4X1	T49.4X2	T49.4X3	T49.4X4	T49.4X5	T49.4X6
Tipepidine	T48.3X1	T48.3X2	T48.3X3	T48.3X4	T48.3X5	T48.3X6
Tiquizium bromide	T44.3X1	T44.3X2	T44.3X3	T44.3X4	T44.3X5	T44.3X6
Tiratricol	T38.1X1	T38.1X2	T38.1X3	T38.1X4	T38.1X5	T38.1X6
Tisopurine	T50.4X1	T50.4X2	T50.4X3	T50.4X4	T50.4X5	T50.4X6
Titanium (compounds) (vapor)	T56.891	T56.892	T56.893	T56.894	—	—
dioxide	T49.3X1	T49.3X2	T49.3X3	T49.3X4	T49.3X5	T49.3X6
ointment	T49.3X1	T49.3X2	T49.3X3	T49.3X4	T49.3X5	T49.3X6
oxide	T49.3X1	T49.3X2	T49.3X3	T49.3X4	T49.3X5	T49.3X6
tetrachloride	T56.891	T56.892	T56.893	T56.894	—	—
Titanocene	T56.891	T56.892	T56.893	T56.894	—	—
Titroid	T38.1X1	T38.1X2	T38.1X3	T38.1X4	T38.1X5	T38.1X6
Tizanidine	T42.8X1	T42.8X2	T42.8X3	T42.8X4	T42.8X5	T42.8X6
TMTD	T60.3X1	T60.3X2	T60.3X3	T60.3X4	—	—
TNT (fumes)	T65.3X1	T65.3X2	T65.3X3	T65.3X4	—	—
Toadstool	T62.0X1	T62.0X2	T62.0X3	T62.0X4	—	—
Tobacco NEC	T65.291	T65.292	T65.293	T65.294	—	—
cigarettes	T65.221	T65.222	T65.223	T65.224	—	—
Indian	T62.2X1	T62.2X2	T62.2X3	T62.2X4	—	—
smoke, second-hand	T65.221	T65.222	T65.223	T65.224	—	—
Tobramycin	T36.5X1	T36.5X2	T36.5X3	T36.5X4	T36.5X5	T36.5X6
Tocainide	T46.2X1	T46.2X2	T46.2X3	T46.2X4	T46.2X5	T46.2X6
Tocoferol	T45.2X1	T45.2X2	T45.2X3	T45.2X4	T45.2X5	T45.2X6
Tocopherol	T45.2X1	T45.2X2	T45.2X3	T45.2X4	T45.2X5	T45.2X6
acetate	T45.2X1	T45.2X2	T45.2X3	T45.2X4	T45.2X5	T45.2X6
Tocosamine	T48.0X1	T48.0X2	T48.0X3	T48.0X4	T48.0X5	T48.0X6
Todralazine	T46.5X1	T46.5X2	T46.5X3	T46.5X4	T46.5X5	T46.5X6
Tofisopam	T42.4X1	T42.4X2	T42.4X3	T42.4X4	T42.4X5	T42.4X6
Tofranil	T43.011	T43.012	T43.013	T43.014	T43.015	T43.016
Toilet deodorizer	T65.891	T65.892	T65.893	T65.894	—	—
Tolamolol	T44.7X1	T44.7X2	T44.7X3	T44.7X4	T44.7X5	T44.7X6
Tolazamide	T38.3X1	T38.3X2	T38.3X3	T38.3X4	T38.3X5	T38.3X6
Tolazoline	T46.7X1	T46.7X2	T46.7X3	T46.7X4	T46.7X5	T46.7X6
Tolbutamide (sodium)	T38.3X1	T38.3X2	T38.3X3	T38.3X4	T38.3X5	T38.3X6
Tolciclate	T49.0X1	T49.0X2	T49.0X3	T49.0X4	T49.0X5	T49.0X6
Tolmetin	T39.391	T39.392	T39.393	T39.394	T39.395	T39.396
Tolnaftate	T49.0X1	T49.0X2	T49.0X3	T49.0X4	T49.0X5	T49.0X6
Tolonidine	T46.5X1	T46.5X2	T46.5X3	T46.5X4	T46.5X5	T46.5X6
Toloxatone	T42.6X1	T42.6X2	T42.6X3	T42.6X4	T42.6X5	T42.6X6
Tolperisone	T44.3X1	T44.3X2	T44.3X3	T44.3X4	T44.3X5	T44.3X6
Tolserol	T42.8X1	T42.8X2	T42.8X3	T42.8X4	T42.8X5	T42.8X6
Toluene (liquid)	T52.2X1	T52.2X2	T52.2X3	T52.2X4	—	—
diisocyanate	T65.0X1	T65.0X2	T65.0X3	T65.0X4	—	—
Toluidine	T65.891	T65.892	T65.893	T65.894	—	—
vapor	T59.891	T59.892	T59.893	T59.894	—	—
Toluol (liquid)	T52.2X1	T52.2X2	T52.2X3	T52.2X4	—	—
vapor	T52.2X1	T52.2X2	T52.2X3	T52.2X4	—	—
Toluylenediamine	T65.3X1	T65.3X2	T65.3X3	T65.3X4	—	—
Tolylene-2,4-diisocyanate	T65.0X1	T65.0X2	T65.0X3	T65.0X4	—	—
Tonic NEC	T50.901	T50.902	T50.903	T50.904	T50.905	T50.906
Topical action drug NEC	T49.91	T49.92	T49.93	T49.94	T49.95	T49.96
ear, nose or throat	T49.6X1	T49.6X2	T49.6X3	T49.6X4	T49.6X5	T49.6X6
eye	T49.5X1	T49.5X2	T49.5X3	T49.5X4	T49.5X5	T49.5X6
skin	T49.91	T49.92	T49.93	T49.94	T49.95	T49.96
specified NEC	T49.8X1	T49.8X2	T49.8X3	T49.8X4	T49.8X5	T49.8X6
Toquizine	T44.3X1	T44.3X2	T44.3X3	T44.3X4	T44.3X5	T44.3X6
Toremifene	T38.6X1	T38.6X2	T38.6X3	T38.6X4	T38.6X5	T38.6X6
Tosylchloramide sodium	T49.8X1	T49.8X2	T49.8X3	T49.8X4	T49.8X5	T49.8X6
Toxaphene (dust) (spray)	T60.1X1	T60.1X2	T60.1X3	T60.1X4	—	—
Toxin, diphtheria (Schick Test)	T50.8X1	T50.8X2	T50.8X3	T50.8X4	T50.8X5	T50.8X6
Toxoid						
combined	T50.A21	T50.A22	T50.A23	T50.A24	T50.A25	T50.A26
diphtheria	T50.A91	T50.A92	T50.A93	T50.A94	T50.A95	T50.A96
tetanus	T50.A91	T50.A92	T50.A93	T50.A94	T50.A95	T50.A96
Trace element NEC	T45.8X1	T45.8X2	T45.8X3	T45.8X4	T45.8X5	T45.8X6
Tractor fuel NEC	T52.0X1	T52.0X2	T52.0X3	T52.0X4	—	—
Tragacanth	T50.991	T50.992	T50.993	T50.994	T50.995	T50.996
Tramadol	T40.421	T40.422	T40.423	T40.424	T40.425	T40.426
Tramazoline	T48.5X1	T48.5X2	T48.5X3	T48.5X4	T48.5X5	T48.5X6
Tranexamic acid	T45.621	T45.622	T45.623	T45.624	T45.625	T45.626
Tranilast	T45.0X1	T45.0X2	T45.0X3	T45.0X4	T45.0X5	T45.0X6
Tranquilizer NEC	T43.501	T43.502	T43.503	T43.504	T43.505	T43.506
with hypnotic or sedative	T42.6X1	T42.6X2	T42.6X3	T42.6X4	T42.6X5	T42.6X6
benzodiazepine NEC	T42.4X1	T42.4X2	T42.4X3	T42.4X4	T42.4X5	T42.4X6
butyrophenone NEC	T43.4X1	T43.4X2	T43.4X3	T43.4X4	T43.4X5	T43.4X6
carbamate	T43.591	T43.592	T43.593	T43.594	T43.595	T43.596
dimethylamine	T43.3X1	T43.3X2	T43.3X3	T43.3X4	T43.3X5	T43.3X6
ethylamine	T43.3X1	T43.3X2	T43.3X3	T43.3X4	T43.3X5	T43.3X6
hydroxyzine	T43.591	T43.592	T43.593	T43.594	T43.595	T43.596
major NEC	T43.501	T43.502	T43.503	T43.504	T43.505	T43.506
penothiazine NEC	T43.3X1	T43.3X2	T43.3X3	T43.3X4	T43.3X5	T43.3X6
phenothiazine-based	T43.3X1	T43.3X2	T43.3X3	T43.3X4	T43.3X5	T43.3X6

Substance	Poisoning, Accidental (unintentional)	Poisoning, Intentional Self-harm	Poisoning, Assault	Poisoning, Undetermined	Adverse Effect	Under-dosing
Tranquilizer — *continued*						
piperazine NEC	T43.3X1	T43.3X2	T43.3X3	T43.3X4	T43.3X5	T43.3X6
piperidine	T43.3X1	T43.3X2	T43.3X3	T43.3X4	T43.3X5	T43.3X6
propylamine	T43.3X1	T43.3X2	T43.3X3	T43.3X4	T43.3X5	T43.3X6
specified NEC	T43.591	T43.592	T43.593	T43.594	T43.595	T43.596
thioxanthene NEC	T43.591	T43.592	T43.593	T43.594	T43.595	T43.596
Tranxene	T42.4X1	T42.4X2	T42.4X3	T42.4X4	T42.4X5	T42.4X6
Tranylcypromine	T43.1X1	T43.1X2	T43.1X3	T43.1X4	T43.1X5	T43.1X6
Trapidil	T46.3X1	T46.3X2	T46.3X3	T46.3X4	T46.3X5	T46.3X6
Trasentine	T44.3X1	T44.3X2	T44.3X3	T44.3X4	T44.3X5	T44.3X6
Travert	T5Ø.3X1	T5Ø.3X2	T5Ø.3X3	T5Ø.3X4	T5Ø.3X5	T5Ø.3X6
Trazodone	T43.211	T43.212	T43.213	T43.214	T43.215	T43.216
Trecator	T37.1X1	T37.1X2	T37.1X3	T37.1X4	T37.1X5	T37.1X6
Treosulfan	T45.1X1	T45.1X2	T45.1X3	T45.1X4	T45.1X5	T45.1X6
Tretamine	T45.1X1	T45.1X2	T45.1X3	T45.1X4	T45.1X5	T45.1X6
Tretinoin	T49.ØX1	T49.ØX2	T49.ØX3	T49.ØX4	T49.ØX5	T49.ØX6
Tretoquinol	T48.6X1	T48.6X2	T48.6X3	T48.6X4	T48.6X5	T48.6X6
Triacetin	T49.ØX1	T49.ØX2	T49.ØX3	T49.ØX4	T49.ØX5	T49.ØX6
Triacetoxyanthracene	T49.4X1	T49.4X2	T49.4X3	T49.4X4	T49.4X5	T49.4X6
Triacetyloleandomycin	T36.3X1	T36.3X2	T36.3X3	T36.3X4	T36.3X5	T36.3X6
Triamcinolone	T38.ØX1	T38.ØX2	T38.ØX3	T38.ØX4	T38.ØX5	T38.ØX6
ENT agent	T49.6X1	T49.6X2	T49.6X3	T49.6X4	T49.6X5	T49.6X6
hexacetonide	T49.ØX1	T49.ØX2	T49.ØX3	T49.ØX4	T49.ØX5	T49.ØX6
ophthalmic preparation	T49.5X1	T49.5X2	T49.5X3	T49.5X4	T49.5X5	T49.5X6
topical NEC	T49.ØX1	T49.ØX2	T49.ØX3	T49.ØX4	T49.ØX5	T49.ØX6
Triampyzine	T44.3X1	T44.3X2	T44.3X3	T44.3X4	T44.3X5	T44.3X6
Triamterene	T5Ø.2X1	T5Ø.2X2	T5Ø.2X3	T5Ø.2X4	T5Ø.2X5	T5Ø.2X6
Triazine (herbicide)	T6Ø.3X1	T6Ø.3X2	T6Ø.3X3	T6Ø.3X4	—	—
Triaziquone	T45.1X1	T45.1X2	T45.1X3	T45.1X4	T45.1X5	T45.1X6
Triazolam	T42.4X1	T42.4X2	T42.4X3	T42.4X4	T42.4X5	T42.4X6
Triazole (herbicide)	T6Ø.3X1	T6Ø.3X2	T6Ø.3X3	T6Ø.3X4	—	—
Tribenoside	T46.991	T46.992	T46.993	T46.994	T46.995	T46.996
Tribromacetaldehyde	T42.6X1	T42.6X2	T42.6X3	T42.6X4	T42.6X5	T42.6X6
Tribromoethanol, rectal	T41.291	T41.292	T41.293	T41.294	T41.295	T41.296
Tribromomethane	T42.6X1	T42.6X2	T42.6X3	T42.6X4	T42.6X5	T42.6X6
Trichlorethane	T53.2X1	T53.2X2	T53.2X3	T53.2X4	—	—
Trichlorethylene	T53.2X1	T53.2X2	T53.2X3	T53.2X4	—	—
Trichlorfon	T6Ø.ØX1	T6Ø.ØX2	T6Ø.ØX3	T6Ø.ØX4	—	—
Trichlormethiazide	T5Ø.2X1	T5Ø.2X2	T5Ø.2X3	T5Ø.2X4	T5Ø.2X5	T5Ø.2X6
Trichlormethine	T45.1X1	T45.1X2	T45.1X3	T45.1X4	T45.1X5	T45.1X6
Trichloroacetic acid, Trichloracetic acid	T54.2X1	T54.2X2	T54.2X3	T54.2X4	—	—
medicinal	T49.4X1	T49.4X2	T49.4X3	T49.4X4	T49.4X5	T49.4X6
Trichloroethane	T53.2X1	T53.2X2	T53.2X3	T53.2X4	—	—
Trichloroethanol	T42.6X1	T42.6X2	T42.6X3	T42.6X4	T42.6X5	T42.6X6
Trichloroethylene (liquid) (vapor)	T53.2X1	T53.2X2	T53.2X3	T53.2X4	—	—
anesthetic (gas)	T41.ØX1	T41.ØX2	T41.ØX3	T41.ØX4	T41.ØX5	T41.ØX6
vapor NEC	T53.2X1	T53.2X2	T53.2X3	T53.2X4	—	—
Trichloroethyl phosphate	T42.6X1	T42.6X2	T42.6X3	T42.6X4	T42.6X5	T42.6X6
Trichlorofluoromethane NEC	T53.5X1	T53.5X2	T53.5X3	T53.5X4	—	—
Trichloronate	T6Ø.ØX1	T6Ø.ØX2	T6Ø.ØX3	T6Ø.ØX4	—	—
Trichloropropane	T53.6X1	T53.6X2	T53.6X3	T53.6X4	—	—
Trichlorotriethylamine	T45.1X1	T45.1X2	T45.1X3	T45.1X4	T45.1X5	T45.1X6
Trichomonacides NEC	T37.3X1	T37.3X2	T37.3X3	T37.3X4	T37.3X5	T37.3X6
Trichomycin	T36.7X1	T36.7X2	T36.7X3	T36.7X4	T36.7X5	T36.7X6
Triclobisonium chloride	T49.ØX1	T49.ØX2	T49.ØX3	T49.ØX4	T49.ØX5	T49.ØX6
Triclocarban	T49.ØX1	T49.ØX2	T49.ØX3	T49.ØX4	T49.ØX5	T49.ØX6
Triclofos	T42.6X1	T42.6X2	T42.6X3	T42.6X4	T42.6X5	T42.6X6
Triclosan	T49.ØX1	T49.ØX2	T49.ØX3	T49.ØX4	T49.ØX5	T49.ØX6
Tricresyl phosphate	T65.891	T65.892	T65.893	T65.894	—	—
solvent	T52.91	T52.92	T52.93	T52.94	—	—
Tricyclamol chloride	T44.3X1	T44.3X2	T44.3X3	T44.3X4	T44.3X5	T44.3X6
Tridesilon	T49.ØX1	T49.ØX2	T49.ØX3	T49.ØX4	T49.ØX5	T49.ØX6
Tridihexethyl iodide	T44.3X1	T44.3X2	T44.3X3	T44.3X4	T44.3X5	T44.3X6
Tridione	T42.2X1	T42.2X2	T42.2X3	T42.2X4	T42.2X5	T42.2X6
Trientine	T45.8X1	T45.8X2	T45.8X3	T45.8X4	T45.8X5	T45.8X6
Triethanolamine NEC	T54.3X1	T54.3X2	T54.3X3	T54.3X4	—	—
detergent	T54.3X1	T54.3X2	T54.3X3	T54.3X4	—	—
trinitrate (biphosphate)	T46.3X1	T46.3X2	T46.3X3	T46.3X4	T46.3X5	T46.3X6
Triethanomelamine	T45.1X1	T45.1X2	T45.1X3	T45.1X4	T45.1X5	T45.1X6
Triethylenemelamine	T45.1X1	T45.1X2	T45.1X3	T45.1X4	T45.1X5	T45.1X6
Triethylenephosphoramide	T45.1X1	T45.1X2	T45.1X3	T45.1X4	T45.1X5	T45.1X6
Triethylenethiophosphoramide	T45.1X1	T45.1X2	T45.1X3	T45.1X4	T45.1X5	T45.1X6
Trifluoperazine	T43.3X1	T43.3X2	T43.3X3	T43.3X4	T43.3X5	T43.3X6
Trifluoroethyl vinyl ether	T41.ØX1	T41.ØX2	T41.ØX3	T41.ØX4	T41.ØX5	T41.ØX6
Trifluperidol	T43.4X1	T43.4X2	T43.4X3	T43.4X4	T43.4X5	T43.4X6
Triflupromazine	T43.3X1	T43.3X2	T43.3X3	T43.3X4	T43.3X5	T43.3X6
Trifluridine	T37.5X1	T37.5X2	T37.5X3	T37.5X4	T37.5X5	T37.5X6
Triflusal	T45.521	T45.522	T45.523	T45.524	T45.525	T45.526
Trihexyphenidyl	T44.3X1	T44.3X2	T44.3X3	T44.3X4	T44.3X5	T44.3X6
Triiodothyronine	T38.1X1	T38.1X2	T38.1X3	T38.1X4	T38.1X5	T38.1X6

Substance	Poisoning, Accidental (unintentional)	Poisoning, Intentional Self-harm	Poisoning, Assault	Poisoning, Undetermined	Adverse Effect	Under-dosing
Trilene	T41.ØX1	T41.ØX2	T41.ØX3	T41.ØX4	T41.ØX5	T41.ØX6
Trilostane	T38.991	T38.992	T38.993	T38.994	T38.995	T38.996
Trimebutine	T44.3X1	T44.3X2	T44.3X3	T44.3X4	T44.3X5	T44.3X6
Trimecaine	T41.3X1	T41.3X2	T41.3X3	T41.3X4	T41.3X5	T41.3X6
Trimeprazine (tartrate)	T44.3X1	T44.3X2	T44.3X3	T44.3X4	T44.3X5	T44.3X6
Trimetaphan camsilate	T44.2X1	T44.2X2	T44.2X3	T44.2X4	T44.2X5	T44.2X6
Trimetazidine	T46.7X1	T46.7X2	T46.7X3	T46.7X4	T46.7X5	T46.7X6
Trimethadione	T42.2X1	T42.2X2	T42.2X3	T42.2X4	T42.2X5	T42.2X6
Trimethaphan	T44.2X1	T44.2X2	T44.2X3	T44.2X4	T44.2X5	T44.2X6
Trimethidinium	T44.2X1	T44.2X2	T44.2X3	T44.2X4	T44.2X5	T44.2X6
Trimethobenzamide	T45.ØX1	T45.ØX2	T45.ØX3	T45.ØX4	T45.ØX5	T45.ØX6
Trimethoprim	T37.8X1	T37.8X2	T37.8X3	T37.8X4	T37.8X5	T37.8X6
with sulfamethoxazole	T36.8X1	T36.8X2	T36.8X3	T36.8X4	T36.8X5	T36.8X6
Trimethylcarbinol	T51.3X1	T51.3X2	T51.3X3	T51.3X4	—	—
Trimethylpsoralen	T49.3X1	T49.3X2	T49.3X3	T49.3X4	T49.3X5	T49.3X6
Trimeton	T45.ØX1	T45.ØX2	T45.ØX3	T45.ØX4	T45.ØX5	T45.ØX6
Trimetrexate	T45.1X1	T45.1X2	T45.1X3	T45.1X4	T45.1X5	T45.1X6
Trimipramine	T43.Ø11	T43.Ø12	T43.Ø13	T43.Ø14	T43.Ø15	T43.Ø16
Trimustine	T45.1X1	T45.1X2	T45.1X3	T45.1X4	T45.1X5	T45.1X6
Trinitrine	T46.3X1	T46.3X2	T46.3X3	T46.3X4	T46.3X5	T46.3X6
Trinitrobenzol	T65.3X1	T65.3X2	T65.3X3	T65.3X4	—	—
Trinitrophenol	T65.3X1	T65.3X2	T65.3X3	T65.3X4	—	—
Trinitrotoluene (fumes)	T65.3X1	T65.3X2	T65.3X3	T65.3X4	—	—
Trional	T42.6X1	T42.6X2	T42.6X3	T42.6X4	T42.6X5	T42.6X6
Triorthocresyl phosphate	T65.891	T65.892	T65.893	T65.894	—	—
Trioxide of arsenic	T57.ØX1	T57.ØX2	T57.ØX3	T57.ØX4	—	—
Trioxysalen	T49.4X1	T49.4X2	T49.4X3	T49.4X4	T49.4X5	T49.4X6
Tripamide	T5Ø.2X1	T5Ø.2X2	T5Ø.2X3	T5Ø.2X4	T5Ø.2X5	T5Ø.2X6
Triparanol	T46.6X1	T46.6X2	T46.6X3	T46.6X4	T46.6X5	T46.6X6
Tripelennamine	T45.ØX1	T45.ØX2	T45.ØX3	T45.ØX4	T45.ØX5	T45.ØX6
Triperiden	T44.3X1	T44.3X2	T44.3X3	T44.3X4	T44.3X5	T44.3X6
Triperidol	T43.4X1	T43.4X2	T43.4X3	T43.4X4	T43.4X5	T43.4X6
Triphenylphosphate	T65.891	T65.892	T65.893	T65.894	—	—
Triple						
bromides	T42.6X1	T42.6X2	T42.6X3	T42.6X4	T42.6X5	T42.6X6
carbonate	T47.1X1	T47.1X2	T47.1X3	T47.1X4	T47.1X5	T47.1X6
vaccine						
DPT	T5Ø.A11	T5Ø.A12	T5Ø.A13	T5Ø.A14	T5Ø.A15	T5Ø.A16
including pertussis	T5Ø.A11	T5Ø.A12	T5Ø.A13	T5Ø.A14	T5Ø.A15	T5Ø.A16
MMR	T5Ø.B91	T5Ø.B92	T5Ø.B93	T5Ø.B94	T5Ø.B95	T5Ø.B96
Triprolidine	T45.ØX1	T45.ØX2	T45.ØX3	T45.ØX4	T45.ØX5	T45.ØX6
Trisodium hydrogen edetate	T5Ø.6X1	T5Ø.6X2	T5Ø.6X3	T5Ø.6X4	T5Ø.6X5	T5Ø.6X6
Trisoralen	T49.3X1	T49.3X2	T49.3X3	T49.3X4	T49.3X5	T49.3X6
Trisulfapyrimidines	T37.ØX1	T37.ØX2	T37.ØX3	T37.ØX4	T37.ØX5	T37.ØX6
Trithiozine	T44.3X1	T44.3X2	T44.3X3	T44.3X4	T44.3X5	T44.3X6
Tritiozine	T44.3X1	T44.3X2	T44.3X3	T44.3X4	T44.3X5	T44.3X6
Tritoqualine	T45.ØX1	T45.ØX2	T45.ØX3	T45.ØX4	T45.ØX5	T45.ØX6
Trofosfamide	T45.1X1	T45.1X2	T45.1X3	T45.1X4	T45.1X5	T45.1X6
Troleandomycin	T36.3X1	T36.3X2	T36.3X3	T36.3X4	T36.3X5	T36.3X6
Trolnitrate (phosphate)	T46.3X1	T46.3X2	T46.3X3	T46.3X4	T46.3X5	T46.3X6
Tromantadine	T37.5X1	T37.5X2	T37.5X3	T37.5X4	T37.5X5	T37.5X6
Trometamol	T5Ø.2X1	T5Ø.2X2	T5Ø.2X3	T5Ø.2X4	T5Ø.2X5	T5Ø.2X6
Tromethamine	T5Ø.2X1	T5Ø.2X2	T5Ø.2X3	T5Ø.2X4	T5Ø.2X5	T5Ø.2X6
Tronothane	T41.3X1	T41.3X2	T41.3X3	T41.3X4	T41.3X5	T41.3X6
Tropacine	T44.3X1	T44.3X2	T44.3X3	T44.3X4	T44.3X5	T44.3X6
Tropatepine	T44.3X1	T44.3X2	T44.3X3	T44.3X4	T44.3X5	T44.3X6
Tropicamide	T44.3X1	T44.3X2	T44.3X3	T44.3X4	T44.3X5	T44.3X6
Trospium chloride	T44.3X1	T44.3X2	T44.3X3	T44.3X4	T44.3X5	T44.3X6
Troxerutin	T46.991	T46.992	T46.993	T46.994	T46.995	T46.996
Troxidone	T42.2X1	T42.2X2	T42.2X3	T42.2X4	T42.2X5	T42.2X6
Tryparsamide	T37.3X1	T37.3X2	T37.3X3	T37.3X4	T37.3X5	T37.3X6
Trypsin	T45.3X1	T45.3X2	T45.3X3	T45.3X4	T45.3X5	T45.3X6
Tryptizol	T43.Ø11	T43.Ø12	T43.Ø13	T43.Ø14	T43.Ø15	T43.Ø16
TSH	T38.811	T38.812	T38.813	T38.814	T38.815	T38.816
Tuaminoheptane	T48.5X1	T48.5X2	T48.5X3	T48.5X4	T48.5X5	T48.5X6
Tuberculin, purified protein derivative (PPD)	T5Ø.8X1	T5Ø.8X2	T5Ø.8X3	T5Ø.8X4	T5Ø.8X5	T5Ø.8X6
Tubocurare	T48.1X1	T48.1X2	T48.1X3	T48.1X4	T48.1X5	T48.1X6
Tubocurarine (chloride)	T48.1X1	T48.1X2	T48.1X3	T48.1X4	T48.1X5	T48.1X6
Tulobuterol	T48.6X1	T48.6X2	T48.6X3	T48.6X4	T48.6X5	T48.6X6
Turpentine (spirits of)	T52.8X1	T52.8X2	T52.8X3	T52.8X4	—	—
vapor	T52.8X1	T52.8X2	T52.8X3	T52.8X4	—	—
Tybamate	T43.591	T43.592	T43.593	T43.594	T43.595	T43.596
Tyloxapol	T48.4X1	T48.4X2	T48.4X3	T48.4X4	T48.4X5	T48.4X6
Tymazoline	T48.5X1	T48.5X2	T48.5X3	T48.5X4	T48.5X5	T48.5X6
Typhoid-paratyphoid vaccine	T5Ø.A91	T5Ø.A92	T5Ø.A93	T5Ø.A94	T5Ø.A95	T5Ø.A96
Typhus vaccine	T5Ø.A91	T5Ø.A92	T5Ø.A93	T5Ø.A94	T5Ø.A95	T5Ø.A96
Tyropanoate	T5Ø.8X1	T5Ø.8X2	T5Ø.8X3	T5Ø.8X4	T5Ø.8X5	T5Ø.8X6
Tyrothricin	T49.6X1	T49.6X2	T49.6X3	T49.6X4	T49.6X5	T49.6X6
ENT agent	T49.6X1	T49.6X2	T49.6X3	T49.6X4	T49.6X5	T49.6X6
ophthalmic preparation	T49.5X1	T49.5X2	T49.5X3	T49.5X4	T49.5X5	T49.5X6

Substance	Poisoning, Accidental (unintentional)	Poisoning, Intentional Self-harm	Poisoning, Assault	Poisoning, Undetermined	Adverse Effect	Under-dosing
Ufenamate	T39.391	T39.392	T39.393	T39.394	T39.395	T39.396
Ultraviolet light protectant	T49.3X1	T49.3X2	T49.3X3	T49.3X4	T49.3X5	T49.3X6
Undecenoic acid	T49.ØX1	T49.ØX2	T49.ØX3	T49.ØX4	T49.ØX5	T49.ØX6
Undecoylium	T49.ØX1	T49.ØX2	T49.ØX3	T49.ØX4	T49.ØX5	T49.ØX6
Undecylenic acid (derivatives)	T49.ØX1	T49.ØX2	T49.ØX3	T49.ØX4	T49.ØX5	T49.ØX6
Unna's boot	T49.3X1	T49.3X2	T49.3X3	T49.3X4	T49.3X5	T49.3X6
Unsaturated fatty acid	T46.6X1	T46.6X2	T46.6X3	T46.6X4	T46.6X5	T46.6X6
Uracil mustard	T45.1X1	T45.1X2	T45.1X3	T45.1X4	T45.1X5	T45.1X6
Uramustine	T45.1X1	T45.1X2	T45.1X3	T45.1X4	T45.1X5	T45.1X6
Urapidil	T46.5X1	T46.5X2	T46.5X3	T46.5X4	T46.5X5	T46.5X6
Urari	T48.1X1	T48.1X2	T48.1X3	T48.1X4	T48.1X5	T48.1X6
Urate oxidase	T5Ø.4X1	T5Ø.4X2	T5Ø.4X3	T5Ø.4X4	T5Ø.4X5	T5Ø.4X6
Urea	T47.3X1	T47.3X2	T47.3X3	T47.3X4	T47.3X5	T47.3X6
peroxide	T49.ØX1	T49.ØX2	T49.ØX3	T49.ØX4	T49.ØX5	T49.ØX6
stibamine	T37.4X1	T37.4X2	T37.4X3	T37.4X4	T37.4X5	T37.4X6
topical	T49.8X1	T49.8X2	T49.8X3	T49.8X4	T49.8X5	T49.8X6
Urethane	T45.1X1	T45.1X2	T45.1X3	T45.1X4	T45.1X5	T45.1X6
Urginea (maritima) (scilla) — *see* Squill						
Uric acid metabolism drug NEC	T5Ø.4X1	T5Ø.4X2	T5Ø.4X3	T5Ø.4X4	T5Ø.4X5	T5Ø.4X6
Uricosuric agent	T5Ø.4X1	T5Ø.4X2	T5Ø.4X3	T5Ø.4X4	T5Ø.4X5	T5Ø.4X6
Urinary anti-infective	T37.8X1	T37.8X2	T37.8X3	T37.8X4	T37.8X5	T37.8X6
Urofollitropin	T38.811	T38.812	T38.813	T38.814	T38.815	T38.816
Urokinase	T45.611	T45.612	T45.613	T45.614	T45.615	T45.616
Urokon	T5Ø.8X1	T5Ø.8X2	T5Ø.8X3	T5Ø.8X4	T5Ø.8X5	T5Ø.8X6
Ursodeoxycholic acid	T5Ø.991	T5Ø.992	T5Ø.993	T5Ø.994	T5Ø.995	T5Ø.996
Ursodiol	T5Ø.991	T5Ø.992	T5Ø.993	T5Ø.994	T5Ø.995	T5Ø.996
Urtica	T62.2X1	T62.2X2	T62.2X3	T62.2X4	—	—
Utility gas — *see* Gas, utility						
Vaccine NEC	T5Ø.Z91	T5Ø.Z92	T5Ø.Z93	T5Ø.Z94	T5Ø.Z95	T5Ø.Z96
antineoplastic	T5Ø.Z91	T5Ø.Z92	T5Ø.Z93	T5Ø.Z94	T5Ø.Z95	T5Ø.Z96
bacterial NEC	T5Ø.A91	T5Ø.A92	T5Ø.A93	T5Ø.A94	T5Ø.A95	T5Ø.A96
with						
other bacterial component	T5Ø.A21	T5Ø.A22	T5Ø.A23	T5Ø.A24	T5Ø.A25	T5Ø.A26
pertussis component	T5Ø.A11	T5Ø.A12	T5Ø.A13	T5Ø.A14	T5Ø.A15	T5Ø.A16
viral-rickettsial component	T5Ø.A21	T5Ø.A22	T5Ø.A23	T5Ø.A24	T5Ø.A25	T5Ø.A26
mixed NEC	T5Ø.A21	T5Ø.A22	T5Ø.A23	T5Ø.A24	T5Ø.A25	T5Ø.A26
BCG	T5Ø.A91	T5Ø.A92	T5Ø.A93	T5Ø.A94	T5Ø.A95	T5Ø.A96
cholera	T5Ø.A91	T5Ø.A92	T5Ø.A93	T5Ø.A94	T5Ø.A95	T5Ø.A96
diphtheria	T5Ø.A91	T5Ø.A92	T5Ø.A93	T5Ø.A94	T5Ø.A95	T5Ø.A96
with tetanus	T5Ø.A21	T5Ø.A22	T5Ø.A23	T5Ø.A24	T5Ø.A25	T5Ø.A26
and pertussis	T5Ø.A11	T5Ø.A12	T5Ø.A13	T5Ø.A14	T5Ø.A15	T5Ø.A16
influenza	T5Ø.B91	T5Ø.B92	T5Ø.B93	T5Ø.B94	T5Ø.B95	T5Ø.B96
measles	T5Ø.B91	T5Ø.B92	T5Ø.B93	T5Ø.B94	T5Ø.B95	T5Ø.B96
with mumps and rubella	T5Ø.B91	T5Ø.B92	T5Ø.B93	T5Ø.B94	T5Ø.B95	T5Ø.B96
meningococcal	T5Ø.A91	T5Ø.A92	T5Ø.A93	T5Ø.A94	T5Ø.A95	T5Ø.A96
mumps	T5Ø.B91	T5Ø.B92	T5Ø.B93	T5Ø.B94	T5Ø.B95	T5Ø.B96
paratyphoid	T5Ø.A91	T5Ø.A92	T5Ø.A93	T5Ø.A94	T5Ø.A95	T5Ø.A96
pertussis	T5Ø.A11	T5Ø.A12	T5Ø.A13	T5Ø.A14	T5Ø.A15	T5Ø.A16
with diphtheria	T5Ø.A11	T5Ø.A12	T5Ø.A13	T5Ø.A14	T5Ø.A15	T5Ø.A16
and tetanus	T5Ø.A11	T5Ø.A12	T5Ø.A13	T5Ø.A14	T5Ø.A15	T5Ø.A16
with other component	T5Ø.A11	T5Ø.A12	T5Ø.A13	T5Ø.A14	T5Ø.A15	T5Ø.A16
plague	T5Ø.A91	T5Ø.A92	T5Ø.A93	T5Ø.A94	T5Ø.A95	T5Ø.A96
poliomyelitis	T5Ø.B91	T5Ø.B92	T5Ø.B93	T5Ø.B94	T5Ø.B95	T5Ø.B96
poliovirus	T5Ø.B91	T5Ø.B92	T5Ø.B93	T5Ø.B94	T5Ø.B95	T5Ø.B96
rabies	T5Ø.B91	T5Ø.B92	T5Ø.B93	T5Ø.B94	T5Ø.B95	T5Ø.B96
respiratory syncytial virus	T5Ø.B91	T5Ø.B92	T5Ø.B93	T5Ø.B94	T5Ø.B95	T5Ø.B96
rickettsial NEC	T5Ø.A91	T5Ø.A92	T5Ø.A93	T5Ø.A94	T5Ø.A95	T5Ø.A96
with						
bacterial component	T5Ø.A21	T5Ø.A22	T5Ø.A23	T5Ø.A24	T5Ø.A25	T5Ø.A26
Rocky Mountain spotted fever	T5Ø.A91	T5Ø.A92	T5Ø.A93	T5Ø.A94	T5Ø.A95	T5Ø.A96
rubella	T5Ø.B91	T5Ø.B92	T5Ø.B93	T5Ø.B94	T5Ø.B95	T5Ø.B96
sabin oral	T5Ø.B91	T5Ø.B92	T5Ø.B93	T5Ø.B94	T5Ø.B95	T5Ø.B96
smallpox	T5Ø.B11	T5Ø.B12	T5Ø.B13	T5Ø.B14	T5Ø.B15	T5Ø.B16
TAB	T5Ø.A91	T5Ø.A92	T5Ø.A93	T5Ø.A94	T5Ø.A95	T5Ø.A96
tetanus	T5Ø.A91	T5Ø.A92	T5Ø.A93	T5Ø.A94	T5Ø.A95	T5Ø.A96
typhoid	T5Ø.A91	T5Ø.A92	T5Ø.A93	T5Ø.A94	T5Ø.A95	T5Ø.A96
typhus	T5Ø.A91	T5Ø.A92	T5Ø.A93	T5Ø.A94	T5Ø.A95	T5Ø.A96
viral NEC	T5Ø.B91	T5Ø.B92	T5Ø.B93	T5Ø.B94	T5Ø.B95	T5Ø.B96
yellow fever	T5Ø.B91	T5Ø.B92	T5Ø.B93	T5Ø.B94	T5Ø.B95	T5Ø.B96
Vaccinia immune globulin	T5Ø.Z11	T5Ø.Z12	T5Ø.Z13	T5Ø.Z14	T5Ø.Z15	T5Ø.Z16
Vaginal contraceptives	T49.8X1	T49.8X2	T49.8X3	T49.8X4	T49.8X5	T49.8X6
Valerian						
root	T42.6X1	T42.6X2	T42.6X3	T42.6X4	T42.6X5	T42.6X6
tincture	T42.6X1	T42.6X2	T42.6X3	T42.6X4	T42.6X5	T42.6X6
Valethamate bromide	T44.3X1	T44.3X2	T44.3X3	T44.3X4	T44.3X5	T44.3X6
Valisone	T49.ØX1	T49.ØX2	T49.ØX3	T49.ØX4	T49.ØX5	T49.ØX6
Valium	T42.4X1	T42.4X2	T42.4X3	T42.4X4	T42.4X5	T42.4X6
Valmid	T42.6X1	T42.6X2	T42.6X3	T42.6X4	T42.6X5	T42.6X6
Valnoctamide	T42.6X1	T42.6X2	T42.6X3	T42.6X4	T42.6X5	T42.6X6
Valproate (sodium)	T42.6X1	T42.6X2	T42.6X3	T42.6X4	T42.6X5	T42.6X6
Valproic acid	T42.6X1	T42.6X2	T42.6X3	T42.6X4	T42.6X5	T42.6X6
Valpromide	T42.6X1	T42.6X2	T42.6X3	T42.6X4	T42.6X5	T42.6X6
Vanadium	T56.891	T56.892	T56.893	T56.894	—	—
Vancomycin	T36.8X1	T36.8X2	T36.8X3	T36.8X4	T36.8X5	T36.8X6
Vapor — *see also* Gas	T59.91	T59.92	T59.93	T59.94	—	—
kiln (carbon monoxide)	T58.8X1	T58.8X2	T58.8X3	T58.8X4	—	—
lead — *see* lead						
specified source NEC	T59.891	T59.892	T59.893	T59.894	—	—
Vardenafil	T46.7X1	T46.7X2	T46.7X3	T46.7X4	T46.7X5	T46.7X6
Varicose reduction drug	T46.8X1	T46.8X2	T46.8X3	T46.8X4	T46.8X5	T46.8X6
Varnish	T65.4X1	T65.4X2	T65.4X3	T65.4X4	—	—
cleaner	T52.91	T52.92	T52.93	T52.94	—	—
Vaseline	T49.3X1	T49.3X2	T49.3X3	T49.3X4	T49.3X5	T49.3X6
Vasodilan	T46.7X1	T46.7X2	T46.7X3	T46.7X4	T46.7X5	T46.7X6
Vasodilator						
coronary NEC	T46.3X1	T46.3X2	T46.3X3	T46.3X4	T46.3X5	T46.3X6
peripheral NEC	T46.7X1	T46.7X2	T46.7X3	T46.7X4	T46.7X5	T46.7X6
Vasopressin	T38.891	T38.892	T38.893	T38.894	T38.895	T38.896
Vasopressor drugs	T38.891	T38.892	T38.893	T38.894	T38.895	T38.896
Vecuronium bromide	T48.1X1	T48.1X2	T48.1X3	T48.1X4	T48.1X5	T48.1X6
Vegetable extract, astringent	T49.2X1	T49.2X2	T49.2X3	T49.2X4	T49.2X5	T49.2X6
Venlafaxine	T43.211	T43.212	T43.213	T43.214	T43.215	T43.216
Venom, venomous (bite) (sting)	T63.91	T63.92	T63.93	T63.94	—	—
amphibian NEC	T63.831	T63.832	T63.833	T63.834	—	—
animal NEC	T63.891	T63.892	T63.893	T63.894	—	—
ant	T63.421	T63.422	T63.423	T63.424	—	—
arthropod NEC	T63.481	T63.482	T63.483	T63.484	—	—
bee	T63.441	T63.442	T63.443	T63.444	—	—
centipede	T63.411	T63.412	T63.413	T63.414	—	—
fish	T63.591	T63.592	T63.593	T63.594	—	—
frog	T63.811	T63.812	T63.813	T63.814	—	—
hornet	T63.451	T63.452	T63.453	T63.454	—	—
insect NEC	T63.481	T63.482	T63.483	T63.484	—	—
lizard	T63.121	T63.122	T63.123	T63.124	—	—
marine						
animals	T63.691	T63.692	T63.693	T63.694	—	—
bluebottle	T63.611	T63.612	T63.613	T63.614	—	—
jellyfish NEC	T63.621	T63.622	T63.623	T63.624	—	—
Portugese Man-o-war	T63.611	T63.612	T63.613	T63.614	—	—
sea anemone	T63.631	T63.632	T63.633	T63.634	—	—
specified NEC	T63.691	T63.692	T63.693	T63.694	—	—
fish	T63.591	T63.592	T63.593	T63.594	—	—
plants	T63.711	T63.712	T63.713	T63.714	—	—
sting ray	T63.511	T63.512	T63.513	T63.514	—	—
millipede (tropical)	T63.411	T63.412	T63.413	T63.414	—	—
plant NEC	T63.791	T63.792	T63.793	T63.794	—	—
marine	T63.711	T63.712	T63.713	T63.714	—	—
reptile	T63.191	T63.192	T63.193	T63.194	—	—
gila monster	T63.111	T63.112	T63.113	T63.114	—	—
lizard NEC	T63.121	T63.122	T63.123	T63.124	—	—
scorpion	T63.2X1	T63.2X2	T63.2X3	T63.2X4	—	—
snake	T63.ØØ1	T63.ØØ2	T63.ØØ3	T63.ØØ4	—	—
African NEC	T63.Ø81	T63.Ø82	T63.Ø83	T63.Ø84	—	—
American (North) (South) NEC	T63.Ø61	T63.Ø62	T63.Ø63	T63.Ø64	—	—
Asian	T63.Ø81	T63.Ø82	T63.Ø83	T63.Ø84	—	—
Australian	T63.Ø71	T63.Ø72	T63.Ø73	T63.Ø74	—	—
cobra	T63.Ø41	T63.Ø42	T63.Ø43	T63.Ø44	—	—
coral snake	T63.Ø21	T63.Ø22	T63.Ø23	T63.Ø24	—	—
rattlesnake	T63.Ø11	T63.Ø12	T63.Ø13	T63.Ø14	—	—
specified NEC	T63.Ø91	T63.Ø92	T63.Ø93	T63.Ø94	—	—
taipan	T63.Ø31	T63.Ø32	T63.Ø33	T63.Ø34	—	—
specified NEC	T63.891	T63.892	T63.893	T63.894	—	—
spider	T63.3Ø1	T63.3Ø2	T63.3Ø3	T63.3Ø4	—	—
black widow	T63.311	T63.312	T63.313	T63.314	—	—
brown recluse	T63.331	T63.332	T63.333	T63.334	—	—
specified NEC	T63.391	T63.392	T63.393	T63.394	—	—
tarantula	T63.321	T63.322	T63.323	T63.324	—	—
sting ray	T63.511	T63.512	T63.513	T63.514	—	—
toad	T63.821	T63.822	T63.823	T63.824	—	—
wasp	T63.461	T63.462	T63.463	T63.464	—	—
Venous sclerosing drug NEC	T46.8X1	T46.8X2	T46.8X3	T46.8X4	T46.8X5	T46.8X6
Ventolin — *see* Albuterol						
Veramon	T42.3X1	T42.3X2	T42.3X3	T42.3X4	T42.3X5	T42.3X6
Verapamil	T46.1X1	T46.1X2	T46.1X3	T46.1X4	T46.1X5	T46.1X6
Veratrine	T46.5X1	T46.5X2	T46.5X3	T46.5X4	T46.5X5	T46.5X6

Substance	Poisoning, Accidental (unintentional)	Poisoning, Intentional Self-harm	Poisoning, Assault	Poisoning, Undetermined	Adverse Effect	Under-dosing
Veratrum						
album	T62.2X1	T62.2X2	T62.2X3	T62.2X4	—	—
alkaloids	T46.5X1	T46.5X2	T46.5X3	T46.5X4	T46.5X5	T46.5X6
viride	T62.2X1	T62.2X2	T62.2X3	T62.2X4	—	—
Verdigris	T60.3X1	T60.3X2	T60.3X3	T60.3X4	—	—
Veronal	T42.3X1	T42.3X2	T42.3X3	T42.3X4	T42.3X5	T42.3X6
Veroxil	T37.4X1	T37.4X2	T37.4X3	T37.4X4	T37.4X5	T37.4X6
Versenate	T50.6X1	T50.6X2	T50.6X3	T50.6X4	T50.6X5	T50.6X6
Versidyne	T39.8X1	T39.8X2	T39.8X3	T39.8X4	T39.8X5	T39.8X6
Vetrabutine	T48.0X1	T48.0X2	T48.0X3	T48.0X4	T48.0X5	T48.0X6
Vidarabine	T37.5X1	T37.5X2	T37.5X3	T37.5X4	T37.5X5	T37.5X6
Vienna						
green	T57.0X1	T57.0X2	T57.0X3	T57.0X4	—	—
insecticide	T60.2X1	T60.2X2	T60.2X3	T60.2X4	—	—
red	T57.0X1	T57.0X2	T57.0X3	T57.0X4	—	—
pharmaceutical dye	T50.991	T50.992	T50.993	T50.994	T50.995	T50.996
Vigabatrin	T42.6X1	T42.6X2	T42.6X3	T42.6X4	T42.6X5	T42.6X6
Viloxazine	T43.291	T43.292	T43.293	T43.294	T43.295	T43.296
Viminol	T39.8X1	T39.8X2	T39.8X3	T39.8X4	T39.8X5	T39.8X6
Vinbarbital, vinbarbitone	T42.3X1	T42.3X2	T42.3X3	T42.3X4	T42.3X5	T42.3X6
Vinblastine	T45.1X1	T45.1X2	T45.1X3	T45.1X4	T45.1X5	T45.1X6
Vinburnine	T46.7X1	T46.7X2	T46.7X3	T46.7X4	T46.7X5	T46.7X6
Vincamine	T45.1X1	T45.1X2	T45.1X3	T45.1X4	T45.1X5	T45.1X6
Vincristine	T45.1X1	T45.1X2	T45.1X3	T45.1X4	T45.1X5	T45.1X6
Vindesine	T45.1X1	T45.1X2	T45.1X3	T45.1X4	T45.1X5	T45.1X6
Vinesthene, vinethene	T41.0X1	T41.0X2	T41.0X3	T41.0X4	T41.0X5	T41.0X6
Vinorelbine tartrate	T45.1X1	T45.1X2	T45.1X3	T45.1X4	T45.1X5	T45.1X6
Vinpocetine	T46.7X1	T46.7X2	T46.7X3	T46.7X4	T46.7X5	T46.7X6
Vinyl						
acetate	T65.891	T65.892	T65.893	T65.894	—	—
bital	T42.3X1	T42.3X2	T42.3X3	T42.3X4	T42.3X5	T42.3X6
bromide	T65.891	T65.892	T65.893	T65.894	—	—
chloride	T59.891	T59.892	T59.893	T59.894	—	—
ether	T41.0X1	T41.0X2	T41.0X3	T41.0X4	T41.0X5	T41.0X6
Vinylbital	T42.3X1	T42.3X2	T42.3X3	T42.3X4	T42.3X5	T42.3X6
Vinylidene chloride	T65.891	T65.892	T65.893	T65.894	—	—
Vioform	T37.8X1	T37.8X2	T37.8X3	T37.8X4	T37.8X5	T37.8X6
topical	T49.0X1	T49.0X2	T49.0X3	T49.0X4	T49.0X5	T49.0X6
Viomycin	T36.8X1	T36.8X2	T36.8X3	T36.8X4	T36.8X5	T36.8X6
Viosterol	T45.2X1	T45.2X2	T45.2X3	T45.2X4	T45.2X5	T45.2X6
Viper (venom)	T63.091	T63.092	T63.093	T63.094	—	—
Viprynium	T37.4X1	T37.4X2	T37.4X3	T37.4X4	T37.4X5	T37.4X6
Viquidil	T46.7X1	T46.7X2	T46.7X3	T46.7X4	T46.7X5	T46.7X6
Viral vaccine NEC	T50.B91	T50.B92	T50.B93	T50.B94	T50.B95	T50.B96
Virginiamycin	T36.8X1	T36.8X2	T36.8X3	T36.8X4	T36.8X5	T36.8X6
Virugon	T37.5X1	T37.5X2	T37.5X3	T37.5X4	T37.5X5	T37.5X6
Viscous agent	T50.901	T50.902	T50.903	T50.904	T50.905	T50.906
Visine	T49.5X1	T49.5X2	T49.5X3	T49.5X4	T49.5X5	T49.5X6
Visnadine	T46.3X1	T46.3X2	T46.3X3	T46.3X4	T46.3X5	T46.3X6
Vitamin NEC	T45.2X1	T45.2X2	T45.2X3	T45.2X4	T45.2X5	T45.2X6
A	T45.2X1	T45.2X2	T45.2X3	T45.2X4	T45.2X5	T45.2X6
B1	T45.2X1	T45.2X2	T45.2X3	T45.2X4	T45.2X5	T45.2X6
B2	T45.2X1	T45.2X2	T45.2X3	T45.2X4	T45.2X5	T45.2X6
B6	T45.2X1	T45.2X2	T45.2X3	T45.2X4	T45.2X5	T45.2X6
B12	T45.2X1	T45.2X2	T45.2X3	T45.2X4	T45.2X5	T45.2X6
B15	T45.2X1	T45.2X2	T45.2X3	T45.2X4	T45.2X5	T45.2X6
B NEC	T45.2X1	T45.2X2	T45.2X3	T45.2X4	T45.2X5	T45.2X6
nicotinic acid	T46.7X1	T46.7X2	T46.7X3	T46.7X4	T46.7X5	T46.7X6
C	T45.2X1	T45.2X2	T45.2X3	T45.2X4	T45.2X5	T45.2X6
D	T45.2X1	T45.2X2	T45.2X3	T45.2X4	T45.2X5	T45.2X6
D2	T45.2X1	T45.2X2	T45.2X3	T45.2X4	T45.2X5	T45.2X6
D3	T45.2X1	T45.2X2	T45.2X3	T45.2X4	T45.2X5	T45.2X6
E	T45.2X1	T45.2X2	T45.2X3	T45.2X4	T45.2X5	T45.2X6
E acetate	T45.2X1	T45.2X2	T45.2X3	T45.2X4	T45.2X5	T45.2X6
hematopoietic	T45.8X1	T45.8X2	T45.8X3	T45.8X4	T45.8X5	T45.8X6
K1	T45.7X1	T45.7X2	T45.7X3	T45.7X4	T45.7X5	T45.7X6
K2	T45.7X1	T45.7X2	T45.7X3	T45.7X4	T45.7X5	T45.7X6
K NEC	T45.7X1	T45.7X2	T45.7X3	T45.7X4	T45.7X5	T45.7X6
PP	T45.2X1	T45.2X2	T45.2X3	T45.2X4	T45.2X5	T45.2X6
ulceroprotectant	T47.1X1	T47.1X2	T47.1X3	T47.1X4	T47.1X5	T47.1X6
Vleminckx's solution	T49.4X1	T49.4X2	T49.4X3	T49.4X4	T49.4X5	T49.4X6
Voltaren — *see* Diclofenac sodium						
Warfarin	T45.511	T45.512	T45.513	T45.514	T45.515	T45.516
rodenticide	T60.4X1-	T60.4X2-	T60.4X3-	T60.4X4-	—	—
sodium	T45.511	T45.512	T45.513	T45.514	T45.515	T45.516
Wasp (sting)	T63.461	T63.462	T63.463	T63.464	—	—
Water						
balance drug	T50.3X1	T50.3X2	T50.3X3	T50.3X4	T50.3X5	T50.3X6
distilled	T50.3X1	T50.3X2	T50.3X3	T50.3X4	T50.3X5	T50.3X6
gas — *see* Gas, water						

Substance	Poisoning, Accidental (unintentional)	Poisoning, Intentional Self-harm	Poisoning, Assault	Poisoning, Undetermined	Adverse Effect	Under-dosing
Water — *continued*						
gas — *see* Gas, water — *continued*						
incomplete combustion of — *see* Carbon, monoxide, fuel, utility						
hemlock	T62.2X1	T62.2X2	T62.2X3	T62.2X4	—	—
moccasin (venom)	T63.061	T63.062	T63.063	T63.064	—	—
purified	T50.3X1	T50.3X2	T50.3X3	T50.3X4	T50.3X5	T50.3X6
Wax (paraffin) (petroleum)	T52.0X1	T52.0X2	T52.0X3	T52.0X4	—	—
automobile	T65.891	T65.892	T65.893	T65.894	—	—
floor	T52.0X1	T52.0X2	T52.0X3	T52.0X4	—	—
Weed killers NEC	T60.3X1	T60.3X2	T60.3X3	T60.3X4	—	—
Welldorm	T42.6X1	T42.6X2	T42.6X3	T42.6X4	T42.6X5	T42.6X6
White						
arsenic	T57.0X1	T57.0X2	T57.0X3	T57.0X4	—	—
hellebore	T62.2X1	T62.2X2	T62.2X3	T62.2X4	—	—
lotion (keratolytic)	T49.4X1	T49.4X2	T49.4X3	T49.4X4	T49.4X5	T49.4X6
spirit	T52.0X1	T52.0X2	T52.0X3	T52.0X4	—	—
Whitewash	T65.891	T65.892	T65.893	T65.894	—	—
Whole blood (human)	T45.8X1	T45.8X2	T45.8X3	T45.8X4	T45.8X5	T45.8X6
Wild						
black cherry	T62.2X1	T62.2X2	T62.2X3	T62.2X4	—	—
poisonous plants NEC	T62.2X1	T62.2X2	T62.2X3	T62.2X4	—	—
Window cleaning fluid	T65.891	T65.892	T65.893	T65.894	—	—
Wintergreen (oil)	T49.3X1	T49.3X2	T49.3X3	T49.3X4	T49.3X5	T49.3X6
Wisterine	T62.2X1	T62.2X2	T62.2X3	T62.2X4	—	—
Witch hazel	T49.2X1	T49.2X2	T49.2X3	T49.2X4	T49.2X5	T49.2X6
Wood alcohol or spirit	T51.1X1	T51.1X2	T51.1X3	T51.1X4	—	—
Wool fat (hydrous)	T49.3X1	T49.3X2	T49.3X3	T49.3X4	T49.3X5	T49.3X6
Woorali	T48.1X1	T48.1X2	T48.1X3	T48.1X4	T48.1X5	T48.1X6
Wormseed, American	T37.4X1	T37.4X2	T37.4X3	T37.4X4	T37.4X5	T37.4X6
Xamoterol	T44.5X1	T44.5X2	T44.5X3	T44.5X4	T44.5X5	T44.5X6
Xanthine diuretics	T50.2X1	T50.2X2	T50.2X3	T50.2X4	T50.2X5	T50.2X6
Xanthinol nicotinate	T46.7X1	T46.7X2	T46.7X3	T46.7X4	T46.7X5	T46.7X6
Xanthotoxin	T49.3X1	T49.3X2	T49.3X3	T49.3X4	T49.3X5	T49.3X6
Xantinol nicotinate	T46.7X1	T46.7X2	T46.7X3	T46.7X4	T46.7X5	T46.7X6
Xantocillin	T36.0X1	T36.0X2	T36.0X3	T36.0X4	T36.0X5	T36.0X6
Xenon (127Xe) (133Xe)	T50.8X1	T50.8X2	T50.8X3	T50.8X4	T50.8X5	T50.8X6
Xenysalate	T49.4X1	T49.4X2	T49.4X3	T49.4X4	T49.4X5	T49.4X6
Xibornol	T37.8X1	T37.8X2	T37.8X3	T37.8X4	T37.8X5	T37.8X6
Xigris	T45.511	T45.512	T45.513	T45.514	T45.515	T45.516
Xipamide	T50.2X1	T50.2X2	T50.2X3	T50.2X4	T50.2X5	T50.2X6
Xylene (vapor)	T52.2X1	T52.2X2	T52.2X3	T52.2X4	—	—
Xylocaine (infiltration) (topical)	T41.3X1	T41.3X2	T41.3X3	T41.3X4	T41.3X5	T41.3X6
nerve block (peripheral) (plexus)	T41.3X1	T41.3X2	T41.3X3	T41.3X4	T41.3X5	T41.3X6
spinal	T41.3X1	T41.3X2	T41.3X3	T41.3X4	T41.3X5	T41.3X6
Xylol (vapor)	T52.2X1	T52.2X2	T52.2X3	T52.2X4	—	—
Xylometazoline	T48.5X1	T48.5X2	T48.5X3	T48.5X4	T48.5X5	T48.5X6
Yeast	T45.2X1	T45.2X2	T45.2X3	T45.2X4	T45.2X5	T45.2X6
dried	T45.2X1	T45.2X2	T45.2X3	T45.2X4	T45.2X5	T45.2X6
Yellow						
fever vaccine	T50.B91	T50.B92	T50.B93	T50.B94	T50.B95	T50.B96
jasmine	T62.2X1	T62.2X2	T62.2X3	T62.2X4	—	—
phenolphthalein	T47.2X1	T47.2X2	T47.2X3	T47.2X4	T47.2X5	T47.2X6
Yew	T62.2X1	T62.2X2	T62.2X3	T62.2X4	—	—
Yohimbic acid	T40.991	T40.992	T40.993	T40.994	T40.995	T40.996
Zactane	T39.8X1	T39.8X2	T39.8X3	T39.8X4	T39.8X5	T39.8X6
Zalcitabine	T37.5X1	T37.5X2	T37.5X3	T37.5X4	T37.5X5	T37.5X6
Zaroxolyn	T50.2X1	T50.2X2	T50.2X3	T50.2X4	T50.2X5	T50.2X6
Zephiran (topical)	T49.0X1	T49.0X2	T49.0X3	T49.0X4	T49.0X5	T49.0X6
ophthalmic preparation	T49.5X1	T49.5X2	T49.5X3	T49.5X4	T49.5X5	T49.5X6
Zeranol	T38.7X1	T38.7X2	T38.7X3	T38.7X4	T38.7X5	T38.7X6
Zerone	T51.1X1	T51.1X2	T51.1X3	T51.1X4	—	—
Zidovudine	T37.5X1	T37.5X2	T37.5X3	T37.5X4	T37.5X5	T37.5X6
Zimeldine	T43.221	T43.222	T43.223	T43.224	T43.225	T43.226
Zinc (compounds) (fumes) (vapor) **NEC**	T56.5X1	T56.5X2	T56.5X3	T56.5X4	—	—
anti-infectives	T49.0X1	T49.0X2	T49.0X3	T49.0X4	T49.0X5	T49.0X6
antivaricose	T46.8X1	T46.8X2	T46.8X3	T46.8X4	T46.8X5	T46.8X6
bacitracin	T49.0X1	T49.0X2	T49.0X3	T49.0X4	T49.0X5	T49.0X6
chloride (mouthwash)	T49.6X1	T49.6X2	T49.6X3	T49.6X4	T49.6X5	T49.6X6
chromate	T56.5X1	T56.5X2	T56.5X3	T56.5X4	—	—
gelatin	T49.3X1	T49.3X2	T49.3X3	T49.3X4	T49.3X5	T49.3X6
oxide	T49.3X1	T49.3X2	T49.3X3	T49.3X4	T49.3X5	T49.3X6
plaster	T49.3X1	T49.3X2	T49.3X3	T49.3X4	T49.3X5	T49.3X6
peroxide	T49.0X1	T49.0X2	T49.0X3	T49.0X4	T49.0X5	T49.0X6
pesticides	T56.5X1	T56.5X2	T56.5X3	T56.5X4	—	—
phosphide	T60.4X1	T60.4X2	T60.4X3	T60.4X4	—	—
pyrithionate	T49.4X1	T49.4X2	T49.4X3	T49.4X4	T49.4X5	T49.4X6
stearate	T49.3X1	T49.3X2	T49.3X3	T49.3X4	T49.3X5	T49.3X6

Substance	Poisoning, Accidental (unintentional)	Poisoning, Intentional Self-harm	Poisoning, Assault	Poisoning, Undetermined	Adverse Effect	Under-dosing
Zinc (compounds) (fumes) (vapor) **NEC** — *continued*						
sulfate	T49.5X1	T49.5X2	T49.5X3	T49.5X4	T49.5X5	T49.5X6
ENT agent	T49.6X1	T49.6X2	T49.6X3	T49.6X4	T49.6X5	T49.6X6
ophthalmic solution	T49.5X1	T49.5X2	T49.5X3	T49.5X4	T49.5X5	T49.5X6
topical NEC	T49.ØX1	T49.ØX2	T49.ØX3	T49.ØX4	T49.ØX5	T49.ØX6
undecylenate	T49.ØX1	T49.ØX2	T49.ØX3	T49.ØX4	T49.ØX5	T49.ØX6
Zineb	T6Ø.ØX1	T6Ø.ØX2	T6Ø.ØX3	T6Ø.ØX4	—	—
Zinostatin	T45.1X1	T45.1X2	T45.1X3	T45.1X4	T45.1X5	T45.1X6
Zipeprol	T48.3X1	T48.3X2	T48.3X3	T48.3X4	T48.3X5	T48.3X6
Zofenopril	T46.4X1	T46.4X2	T46.4X3	T46.4X4	T46.4X5	T46.4X6
Zolpidem	T42.6X1	T42.6X2	T42.6X3	T42.6X4	T42.6X5	T42.6X6
Zomepirac	T39.391	T39.392	T39.393	T39.394	T39.395	T39.396
Zopiclone	T42.6X1	T42.6X2	T42.6X3	T42.6X4	T42.6X5	T42.6X6
Zorubicin	T45.1X1	T45.1X2	T45.1X3	T45.1X4	T45.1X5	T45.1X6
Zotepine	T43.591	T43.592	T43.593	T43.594	T43.595	T43.596
Zovant	T45.511	T45.512	T45.513	T45.514	T45.515	T45.516
Zoxazolamine	T42.8X1	T42.8X2	T42.8X3	T42.8X4	T42.8X5	T42.8X6
Zuclopenthixol	T43.4X1	T43.4X2	T43.4X3	T43.4X4	T43.4X5	T43.4X6
Zygadenus (venenosus)	T62.2X1	T62.2X2	T62.2X3	T62.2X4	—	—
Zyprexa	T43.591	T43.592	T43.593	T43.594	T43.595	T43.596

A

- **Abandonment** (causing exposure to weather conditions) (with intent to injure or kill) NEC X58 ☑
- **Abuse** (adult) (child) (mental) (physical) (sexual) X58 ☑
- **Accident** (to) X58 ☑
  - aircraft (in transit) (powered) — *see also* Accident, transport, aircraft
    - due to, caused by cataclysm — *see* Forces of nature, by type
  - animal-drawn vehicle — *see* Accident, transport, animal-drawn vehicle occupant
  - animal-rider — *see* Accident, transport, animal-rider
  - automobile — *see* Accident, transport, car occupant
  - bare foot water skier V94.4 ☑
  - boat, boating — *see also* Accident, watercraft
    - striking swimmer
      - powered V94.11 ☑
      - unpowered V94.12 ☑
  - bus — *see* Accident, transport, bus occupant
  - cable car, not on rails V98.0 ☑
    - on rails — *see* Accident, transport, streetcar occupant
  - car — *see* Accident, transport, car occupant
  - caused by, due to
    - animal NEC W64 ☑
    - chain hoist W24.0 ☑
    - cold (excessive) — *see* Exposure, cold
    - corrosive liquid, substance — *see* Table of Drugs and Chemicals
    - cutting or piercing instrument — *see* Contact, with, by type of instrument
    - drive belt W24.0 ☑
    - electric
      - current — *see* Exposure, electric current
      - motor — *see also* Contact, with, by type of machine W31.3 ☑
        - current (of) W86.8 ☑
    - environmental factor NEC X58 ☑
    - explosive material — *see* Explosion
    - fire, flames — *see* Exposure, fire
    - firearm missile — *see* Discharge, firearm by type
    - heat (excessive) — *see* Heat
    - hot — *see* Contact, with, hot
    - ignition — *see* Ignition
    - lifting device W24.0 ☑
    - lightning — *see* subcategory T75.0 ☑
      - causing fire — *see* Exposure, fire
    - machine, machinery — *see* Contact, with, by type of machine
    - natural factor NEC X58 ☑
    - pulley (block) W24.0 ☑
    - radiation — *see* Radiation
    - steam X13.1 ☑
      - inhalation X13.0 ☑
      - pipe X16 ☑
    - thunderbolt — *see* subcategory T75.0 ☑
      - causing fire — *see* Exposure, fire
    - transmission device W24.1 ☑
  - coach — *see* Accident, transport, bus occupant
  - coal car — *see* Accident, transport, industrial vehicle occupant
  - diving — *see also* Fall, into, water
    - with
      - drowning or submersion — *see* Drowning
  - forklift — *see* Accident, transport, industrial vehicle occupant
  - heavy transport vehicle NOS — *see* Accident, transport, truck occupant
  - ice yacht V98.2 ☑
  - in
    - medical, surgical procedure
      - as, or due to misadventure — *see* Misadventure
      - causing an abnormal reaction or later complication without mention of misadventure — *see also* Complication of or following, by type of procedure Y84.9
  - land yacht V98.1 ☑
  - late effect of — *see* W00-X58 with 7th character S
  - logging car — *see* Accident, transport, industrial vehicle occupant
  - machine, machinery — *see also* Contact, with, by type of machine
    - on board watercraft V93.69 ☑
      - explosion — *see* Explosion, in, watercraft

Accident — *continued*
  - machine, machinery — *see also* Contact, with, by type of machine — *continued*
    - on board watercraft — *continued*
      - fire — *see* Burn, on board watercraft
      - powered craft V93.63 ☑
        - ferry boat V93.61 ☑
        - fishing boat V93.62 ☑
        - jetskis V93.63 ☑
        - liner V93.61 ☑
        - merchant ship V93.60 ☑
        - passenger ship V93.61 ☑
        - sailboat V93.64 ☑
  - mine tram — *see* Accident, transport, industrial vehicle occupant
  - mobility scooter (motorized) — *see* Accident, transport, pedestrian, conveyance, specified type NEC
  - motor scooter — *see* Accident, transport, motorcyclist
  - motor vehicle NOS (traffic) — *see also* Accident, transport V89.2 ☑
    - nontraffic V89.0 ☑
    - three-wheeled NOS — *see* Accident, transport, three-wheeled motor vehicle occupant
  - motorcycle NOS — *see* Accident, transport, motorcyclist
  - nonmotor vehicle NOS (nontraffic) — *see also* Accident, transport V89.1 ☑
    - traffic NOS V89.3 ☑
  - nontraffic (victim's mode of transport NOS) V88.9 ☑
    - collision (between) V88.7 ☑
      - bus and truck V88.5 ☑
      - car and:
        - bus V88.3 ☑
        - pickup V88.2 ☑
        - three-wheeled motor vehicle V88.0 ☑
        - train V88.6 ☑
        - truck V88.4 ☑
        - two-wheeled motor vehicle V88.0 ☑
        - van V88.2 ☑
      - specified vehicle NEC and:
        - three-wheeled motor vehicle V88.1 ☑
        - two-wheeled motor vehicle V88.1 ☑
    - known mode of transport — *see* Accident, transport, by type of vehicle
    - noncollision V88.8 ☑
  - on board watercraft V93.89 ☑
    - powered craft V93.83 ☑
      - ferry boat V93.81 ☑
      - fishing boat V93.82 ☑
      - jetskis V93.83 ☑
      - liner V93.81 ☑
      - merchant ship V93.80 ☑
      - passenger ship V93.81 ☑
    - unpowered craft V93.88 ☑
      - canoe V93.85 ☑
      - inflatable V93.86 ☑
        - in tow
          - recreational V94.31 ☑
          - specified NEC V94.32 ☑
      - kayak V93.85 ☑
      - sailboat V93.84 ☑
      - surf-board V93.88 ☑
      - water skis V93.87 ☑
      - windsurfer V93.88 ☑
  - parachutist V97.29 ☑
    - entangled in object V97.21 ☑
    - injured on landing V97.22 ☑
  - pedal cycle — *see* Accident, transport, pedal cyclist
  - pedestrian (on foot)
    - with
      - another pedestrian W51 ☑
        - on pedestrian conveyance NEC V00.09 ☑
        - with fall W03 ☑
          - due to ice or snow W00.0 ☑
      - rider of
        - hoverboard V00.038 ☑
        - Segway V00.038 ☑
        - standing
          - electric scooter V00.031 ☑
          - micro-mobility pedestrian conveyance NEC V00.038 ☑
      - roller skater (in-line) V00.01 ☑
      - skate boarder V00.02 ☑
      - transport vehicle — *see* Accident, transport
    - on pedestrian conveyance — *see* Accident, transport, pedestrian, conveyance

Accident — *continued*
  - pick-up truck or van — *see* Accident, transport, pickup truck occupant
  - quarry truck — *see* Accident, transport, industrial vehicle occupant
  - railway vehicle (any) (in motion) — *see* Accident, transport, railway vehicle occupant
    - due to cataclysm — *see* Forces of nature, by type
  - scooter (non-motorized) — *see* Accident, transport, pedestrian, conveyance, scooter
  - sequelae of — *see* categories W00-X58 with 7th character S
  - skateboard — *see* Accident, transport, pedestrian, conveyance, skateboard
  - ski(ing) — *see* Accident, transport, pedestrian, conveyance
    - lift V98.3 ☑
  - specified cause NEC X58 ☑
  - streetcar — *see* Accident, transport, streetcar occupant
  - traffic (victim's mode of transport NOS) V87.9 ☑
    - collision (between) V87.7 ☑
      - bus and truck V87.5 ☑
      - car and:
        - bus V87.3 ☑
        - pickup V87.2 ☑
        - three-wheeled motor vehicle V87.0 ☑
        - train V87.6 ☑
        - truck V87.4 ☑
        - two-wheeled motor vehicle V87.0 ☑
        - van V87.2 ☑
      - specified vehicle NEC V86.39 ☑
        - and
          - three-wheeled motor vehicle V87.1 ☑
          - two-wheeled motor vehicle V87.1 ☑
        - driver V86.09 ☑
        - passenger V86.19 ☑
        - person on outside V86.29 ☑
        - while boarding or alighting V86.49 ☑
    - known mode of transport — *see* Accident, transport, by type of vehicle
    - noncollision V87.8 ☑
  - transport (involving injury to) V99 ☑
    - 18 wheeler — *see* Accident, transport, truck occupant
    - agricultural vehicle occupant (nontraffic) V84.9 ☑
      - driver V84.5 ☑
      - hanger-on V84.7 ☑
      - passenger V84.6 ☑
      - traffic V84.3 ☑
        - driver V84.0 ☑
        - hanger-on V84.2 ☑
        - passenger V84.1 ☑
      - while boarding or alighting V84.4 ☑
    - aircraft NEC V97.89 ☑
      - military NEC V97.818 ☑
        - civilian injured by V97.811 ☑
        - with civilian aircraft V97.810 ☑
      - occupant injured (in)
        - nonpowered craft accident V96.9 ☑
          - balloon V96.00 ☑
            - collision V96.03 ☑
            - crash V96.01 ☑
            - explosion V96.05 ☑
            - fire V96.04 ☑
            - forced landing V96.02 ☑
            - specified type NEC V96.09 ☑
          - glider V96.20 ☑
            - collision V96.23 ☑
            - crash V96.21 ☑
            - explosion V96.25 ☑
            - fire V96.24 ☑
            - forced landing V96.22 ☑
            - specified type NEC V96.29 ☑
          - hang glider V96.10 ☑
            - collision V96.13 ☑
            - crash V96.11 ☑
            - explosion V96.15 ☑
            - fire V96.14 ☑
            - forced landing V96.12 ☑
            - specified type NEC V96.19 ☑
          - specified craft NEC V96.8 ☑
        - powered craft accident V95.9 ☑
          - fixed wing NEC
            - commercial V95.30 ☑
              - collision V95.33 ☑
              - crash V95.31 ☑

- **Accident** — *continued*
  - transport — *continued*
    - aircraft — *continued*
      - occupant injured — *continued*
        - powered craft accident — *continued*
          - fixed wing — *continued*
            - commercial — *continued*
              - explosion V95.35 ☑
              - fire V95.34 ☑
              - forced landing V95.32 ☑
              - specified type NEC V95.39 ☑
            - private V95.2Ø ☑
              - collision V95.23 ☑
              - crash V95.21 ☑
              - explosion V95.25 ☑
              - fire V95.24 ☑
              - forced landing V95.22 ☑
              - specified type NEC V95.29 ☑
          - glider V95.1Ø ☑
            - collision V95.13 ☑
            - crash V95.11 ☑
            - explosion V95.15 ☑
            - fire V95.14 ☑
            - forced landing V95.12 ☑
            - specified type NEC V95.19 ☑
          - helicopter V95.ØØ ☑
            - collision V95.Ø3 ☑
            - crash V95.Ø1 ☑
            - explosion V95.Ø5 ☑
            - fire V95.Ø4 ☑
            - forced landing V95.Ø2 ☑
            - specified type NEC V95.Ø9 ☑
          - spacecraft V95.4Ø ☑
            - collision V95.43 ☑
            - crash V95.41 ☑
            - explosion V95.45 ☑
            - fire V95.44 ☑
            - forced landing V95.42 ☑
            - specified type NEC V95.49 ☑
          - specified craft NEC V95.8 ☑
          - ultralight V95.1Ø ☑
            - collision V95.13 ☑
            - crash V95.11 ☑
            - explosion V95.15 ☑
            - fire V95.14 ☑
            - forced landing V95.12 ☑
            - specified type NEC V95.19 ☑
        - specified accident NEC V97.Ø ☑
        - while boarding or alighting V97.1 ☑
      - person (injured by)
        - falling from, in or on aircraft V97.Ø ☑
        - machinery on aircraft V97.89 ☑
        - on ground with aircraft involvement V97.39 ☑
        - rotating propeller V97.32 ☑
        - struck by object falling from aircraft V97.31 ☑
        - sucked into aircraft jet V97.33 ☑
        - while boarding or alighting aircraft V97.1 ☑
    - airport (battery-powered) passenger vehicle — *see* Accident, transport, industrial vehicle occupant
    - all-terrain vehicle occupant (nontraffic) V86.95 ☑
      - driver V86.55 ☑
      - dune buggy — *see* Accident, transport, dune buggy occupant
      - hanger-on V86.75 ☑
      - passenger V86.65 ☑
      - snowmobile — *see* Accident, transport, snowmobile occupant
      - specified type NEC V86.99 ☑
        - driver V86.59 ☑
        - passenger V86.69 ☑
        - person on outside V86.79 ☑
      - traffic V86.35 ☑
        - driver V86.Ø5 ☑
        - hanger-on V86.25 ☑
        - passenger V86.15 ☑
      - while boarding or alighting V86.45 ☑
    - ambulance occupant (traffic) V86.31 ☑
      - driver V86.Ø1 ☑
      - hanger-on V86.21 ☑
      - nontraffic V86.91 ☑
        - driver V86.51 ☑
        - hanger-on V86.71 ☑
        - passenger V86.61 ☑
      - passenger V86.11 ☑

- **Accident** — *continued*
  - transport — *continued*
    - ambulance occupant — *continued*
      - while boarding or alighting V86.41 ☑
    - animal-drawn vehicle occupant (in) V8Ø.929 ☑
      - collision (with)
        - animal V8Ø.12 ☑
          - being ridden V8Ø.711 ☑
        - animal-drawn vehicle V8Ø.721 ☑
        - bus V8Ø.42 ☑
        - car V8Ø.42 ☑
        - fixed or stationary object V8Ø.82 ☑
        - military vehicle V8Ø.92Ø ☑
        - nonmotor vehicle V8Ø.791 ☑
        - pedal cycle V8Ø.22 ☑
        - pedestrian V8Ø.12 ☑
        - pickup V8Ø.42 ☑
        - railway train or vehicle V8Ø.62 ☑
        - specified motor vehicle NEC V8Ø.52 ☑
        - streetcar V8Ø.731 ☑
        - truck V8Ø.42 ☑
        - two- or three-wheeled motor vehicle V8Ø.32 ☑
        - van V8Ø.42 ☑
      - noncollision V8Ø.Ø2 ☑
      - specified circumstance NEC V8Ø.928 ☑
    - animal-rider V8Ø.919 ☑
      - collision (with)
        - animal V8Ø.11 ☑
          - being ridden V8Ø.71Ø ☑
        - animal-drawn vehicle V8Ø.72Ø ☑
        - bus V8Ø.41 ☑
        - car V8Ø.41 ☑
        - fixed or stationary object V8Ø.81 ☑
        - military vehicle V8Ø.91Ø ☑
        - nonmotor vehicle V8Ø.79Ø ☑
        - pedal cycle V8Ø.21 ☑
        - pedestrian V8Ø.11 ☑
        - pickup V8Ø.41 ☑
        - railway train or vehicle V8Ø.61 ☑
        - specified motor vehicle NEC V8Ø.51 ☑
        - streetcar V8Ø.73Ø ☑
        - truck V8Ø.41 ☑
        - two- or three-wheeled motor vehicle V8Ø.31 ☑
        - van V8Ø.41 ☑
      - noncollision V8Ø.Ø18 ☑
        - specified as horse rider V8Ø.Ø1Ø ☑
      - specified circumstance NEC V8Ø.918 ☑
    - armored car — *see* Accident, transport, truck occupant
    - battery-powered truck (baggage) (mail) — *see* Accident, transport, industrial vehicle occupant
    - bus occupant V79.9 ☑
      - collision (with)
        - animal (traffic) V7Ø.9 ☑
          - being ridden (traffic) V76.9 ☑
            - nontraffic V76.3 ☑
            - while boarding or alighting V76.4 ☑
          - nontraffic V7Ø.3 ☑
          - while boarding or alighting V7Ø.4 ☑
        - animal-drawn vehicle (traffic) V76.9 ☑
          - nontraffic V76.3 ☑
          - while boarding or alighting V76.4 ☑
        - bus (traffic) V74.9 ☑
          - nontraffic V74.3 ☑
          - while boarding or alighting V74.4 ☑
        - car (traffic) V73.9 ☑
          - nontraffic V73.3 ☑
          - while boarding or alighting V73.4 ☑
        - motor vehicle NOS (traffic) V79.6Ø ☑
          - nontraffic V79.2Ø ☑
          - specified type NEC (traffic) V79.69 ☑
            - nontraffic V79.29 ☑
        - pedal cycle (traffic) V71.9 ☑
          - nontraffic V71.3 ☑
          - while boarding or alighting V71.4 ☑
        - pickup truck (traffic) V73.9 ☑
          - nontraffic V73.3 ☑
          - while boarding or alighting V73.4 ☑
        - railway vehicle (traffic) V75.9 ☑
          - nontraffic V75.3 ☑
          - while boarding or alighting V75.4 ☑
        - specified vehicle NEC (traffic) V76.9 ☑
          - nontraffic V76.3 ☑
          - while boarding or alighting V76.4 ☑

- **Accident** — *continued*
  - transport — *continued*
    - bus occupant — *continued*
      - collision — *continued*
        - stationary object (traffic) V77.9 ☑
          - nontraffic V77.3 ☑
          - while boarding or alighting V77.4 ☑
        - streetcar (traffic) V76.9 ☑
          - nontraffic V76.3 ☑
          - while boarding or alighting V76.4 ☑
        - three wheeled motor vehicle (traffic) V72.9 ☑
          - nontraffic V72.3 ☑
          - while boarding or alighting V72.4 ☑
        - truck (traffic) V74.9 ☑
          - nontraffic V74.3 ☑
          - while boarding or alighting V74.4 ☑
        - two wheeled motor vehicle (traffic) V72.9 ☑
          - nontraffic V72.3 ☑
          - while boarding or alighting V72.4 ☑
        - van (traffic) V73.9 ☑
          - nontraffic V73.3 ☑
          - while boarding or alighting V73.4 ☑
      - driver
        - collision (with)
          - animal (traffic) V7Ø.5 ☑
            - being ridden (traffic) V76.5 ☑
              - nontraffic V76.Ø ☑
            - nontraffic V7Ø.Ø ☑
          - animal-drawn vehicle (traffic) V76.5 ☑
            - nontraffic V76.Ø ☑
          - bus (traffic) V74.5 ☑
            - nontraffic V74.Ø ☑
          - car (traffic) V73.5 ☑
            - nontraffic V73.Ø ☑
          - motor vehicle NOS (traffic) V79.4Ø ☑
            - nontraffic V79.ØØ ☑
            - specified type NEC (traffic) V79.49 ☑
              - nontraffic V79.Ø9 ☑
          - pedal cycle (traffic) V71.5 ☑
            - nontraffic V71.Ø ☑
          - pickup truck (traffic) V73.5 ☑
            - nontraffic V73.Ø ☑
          - railway vehicle (traffic) V75.5 ☑
            - nontraffic V75.Ø ☑
          - specified vehicle NEC (traffic) V76.5 ☑
            - nontraffic V76.Ø ☑
          - stationary object (traffic) V77.5 ☑
            - nontraffic V77.Ø ☑
          - streetcar (traffic) V76.5 ☑
            - nontraffic V76.Ø ☑
          - three wheeled motor vehicle (traffic) V72.5 ☑
            - nontraffic V72.Ø ☑
          - truck (traffic) V74.5 ☑
            - nontraffic V74.Ø ☑
          - two wheeled motor vehicle (traffic) V72.5 ☑
            - nontraffic V72.Ø ☑
          - van (traffic) V73.5 ☑
            - nontraffic V73.Ø ☑
        - noncollision accident (traffic) V78.5 ☑
          - nontraffic V78.Ø ☑
      - hanger-on
        - collision (with)
          - animal (traffic) V7Ø.7 ☑
            - being ridden (traffic) V76.7 ☑
              - nontraffic V76.2 ☑
            - nontraffic V7Ø.2 ☑
          - animal-drawn vehicle (traffic) V76.7 ☑
            - nontraffic V76.2 ☑
          - bus (traffic) V74.7 ☑
            - nontraffic V74.2 ☑
          - car (traffic) V73.7 ☑
            - nontraffic V73.2 ☑
          - pedal cycle (traffic) V71.7 ☑
            - nontraffic V71.2 ☑
          - pickup truck (traffic) V73.7 ☑
            - nontraffic V73.2 ☑
          - railway vehicle (traffic) V75.7 ☑
            - nontraffic V75.2 ☑
          - specified vehicle NEC (traffic) V76.7 ☑
            - nontraffic V76.2 ☑
          - stationary object (traffic) V77.7 ☑
            - nontraffic V77.2 ☑
          - streetcar (traffic) V76.7 ☑
            - nontraffic V76.2 ☑

- **Accident** — *continued*
  - transport — *continued*
    - bus occupant — *continued*
      - hanger-on — *continued*
        - collision — *continued*
          - three wheeled motor vehicle (traffic) V72.7 ☑
            - nontraffic V72.2 ☑
          - truck (traffic) V74.7 ☑
            - nontraffic V74.2 ☑
          - two wheeled motor vehicle (traffic) V72.7 ☑
            - nontraffic V72.2 ☑
          - van (traffic) V73.7 ☑
            - nontraffic V73.2 ☑
        - noncollision accident (traffic) V78.7 ☑
          - nontraffic V78.2 ☑
      - noncollision accident (traffic) V78.9 ☑
        - nontraffic V78.3 ☑
        - while boarding or alighting V78.4 ☑
      - nontraffic V79.3 ☑
      - passenger
        - collision (with)
          - animal (traffic) V70.6 ☑
            - being ridden (traffic) V76.6 ☑
              - nontraffic V76.1 ☑
            - nontraffic V70.1 ☑
          - animal-drawn vehicle (traffic) V76.6 ☑
            - nontraffic V76.1 ☑
          - bus (traffic) V74.6 ☑
            - nontraffic V74.1 ☑
          - car (traffic) V73.6 ☑
            - nontraffic V73.1 ☑
          - motor vehicle NOS (traffic) V79.50 ☑
            - nontraffic V79.10 ☑
            - specified type NEC (traffic) V79.59 ☑
              - nontraffic V79.19 ☑
          - pedal cycle (traffic) V71.6 ☑
            - nontraffic V71.1 ☑
          - pickup truck (traffic) V73.6 ☑
            - nontraffic V73.1 ☑
          - railway vehicle (traffic) V75.6 ☑
            - nontraffic V75.1 ☑
          - specified vehicle NEC (traffic) V76.6 ☑
            - nontraffic V76.1 ☑
          - stationary object (traffic) V77.6 ☑
            - nontraffic V77.1 ☑
          - streetcar (traffic) V76.6 ☑
            - nontraffic V76.1 ☑
          - three wheeled motor vehicle (traffic) V72.6 ☑
            - nontraffic V72.1 ☑
          - truck (traffic) V74.6 ☑
            - nontraffic V74.1 ☑
          - two wheeled motor vehicle (traffic) V72.6 ☑
            - nontraffic V72.1 ☑
          - van (traffic) V73.6 ☑
            - nontraffic V73.1 ☑
        - noncollision accident (traffic) V78.6 ☑
          - nontraffic V78.1 ☑
      - specified type NEC V79.88 ☑
        - military vehicle V79.81 ☑
    - cable car, not on rails V98.0 ☑
      - on rails — *see* Accident, transport, streetcar occupant
    - car occupant V49.9 ☑
      - ambulance occupant — *see* Accident, transport, ambulance occupant
      - collision (with)
        - animal (traffic) V40.9 ☑
          - being ridden (traffic) V46.9 ☑
            - nontraffic V46.3 ☑
            - while boarding or alighting V46.4 ☑
          - nontraffic V40.3 ☑
          - while boarding or alighting V40.4 ☑
        - animal-drawn vehicle (traffic) V46.9 ☑
          - nontraffic V46.3 ☑
          - while boarding or alighting V46.4 ☑
        - bus (traffic) V44.9 ☑
          - nontraffic V44.3 ☑
          - while boarding or alighting V44.4 ☑
        - car (traffic) V43.92 ☑
          - nontraffic V43.32 ☑
          - while boarding or alighting V43.42 ☑
        - motor vehicle NOS (traffic) V49.60 ☑

- **Accident** — *continued*
  - transport — *continued*
    - car occupant — *continued*
      - collision — *continued*
        - motor vehicle — *continued*
          - nontraffic V49.20 ☑
          - specified type NEC (traffic) V49.69 ☑
            - nontraffic V49.29 ☑
        - pedal cycle (traffic) V41.9 ☑
          - nontraffic V41.3 ☑
          - while boarding or alighting V41.4 ☑
        - pickup truck (traffic) V43.93 ☑
          - nontraffic V43.33 ☑
          - while boarding or alighting V43.43 ☑
        - railway vehicle (traffic) V45.9 ☑
          - nontraffic V45.3 ☑
          - while boarding or alighting V45.4 ☑
        - specified vehicle NEC (traffic) V46.9 ☑
          - nontraffic V46.3 ☑
          - while boarding or alighting V46.4 ☑
        - sport utility vehicle (traffic) V43.91 ☑
          - nontraffic V43.31 ☑
          - while boarding or alighting V43.41 ☑
        - stationary object (traffic) V47.9 ☑
          - nontraffic V47.3 ☑
          - while boarding or alighting V47.4 ☑
        - streetcar (traffic) V46.9 ☑
          - nontraffic V46.3 ☑
          - while boarding or alighting V46.4 ☑
        - three wheeled motor vehicle (traffic) V42.9 ☑
          - nontraffic V42.3 ☑
          - while boarding or alighting V42.4 ☑
        - truck (traffic) V44.9 ☑
          - nontraffic V44.3 ☑
          - while boarding or alighting V44.4 ☑
        - two wheeled motor vehicle (traffic) V42.9 ☑
          - nontraffic V42.3 ☑
          - while boarding or alighting V42.4 ☑
        - van (traffic) V43.94 ☑
          - nontraffic V43.34 ☑
          - while boarding or alighting V43.44 ☑
      - driver
        - collision (with)
          - animal (traffic) V40.5 ☑
            - being ridden (traffic) V46.5 ☑
              - nontraffic V46.0 ☑
            - nontraffic V40.0 ☑
          - animal-drawn vehicle (traffic) V46.5 ☑
            - nontraffic V46.0 ☑
          - bus (traffic) V44.5 ☑
            - nontraffic V44.0 ☑
          - car (traffic) V43.52 ☑
            - nontraffic V43.02 ☑
          - motor vehicle NOS (traffic) V49.40 ☑
            - nontraffic V49.00 ☑
            - specified type NEC (traffic) V49.49 ☑
              - nontraffic V49.09 ☑
          - pedal cycle (traffic) V41.5 ☑
            - nontraffic V41.0 ☑
          - pickup truck (traffic) V43.53 ☑
            - nontraffic V43.03 ☑
          - railway vehicle (traffic) V45.5 ☑
            - nontraffic V45.0 ☑
          - specified vehicle NEC (traffic) V46.5 ☑
            - nontraffic V46.0 ☑
          - sport utility vehicle (traffic) V43.51 ☑
            - nontraffic V43.01 ☑
          - stationary object (traffic) V47.5 ☑
            - nontraffic V47.0 ☑
          - streetcar (traffic) V46.5 ☑
            - nontraffic V46.0 ☑
          - three wheeled motor vehicle (traffic) V42.5 ☑
            - nontraffic V42.0 ☑
          - truck (traffic) V44.5 ☑
            - nontraffic V44.0 ☑
          - two wheeled motor vehicle (traffic) V42.5 ☑
            - nontraffic V42.0 ☑
          - van (traffic) V43.54 ☑
            - nontraffic V43.04 ☑
        - noncollision accident (traffic) V48.5 ☑
          - nontraffic V48.0 ☑
      - hanger-on
        - collision (with)
          - animal (traffic) V40.7 ☑

- **Accident** — *continued*
  - transport — *continued*
    - car occupant — *continued*
      - hanger-on — *continued*
        - collision — *continued*
          - animal — *continued*
            - being ridden (traffic) V46.7 ☑
              - nontraffic V46.2 ☑
            - nontraffic V40.2 ☑
          - animal-drawn vehicle (traffic) V46.7 ☑
            - nontraffic V46.2 ☑
          - bus (traffic) V44.7 ☑
            - nontraffic V44.2 ☑
          - car (traffic) V43.72 ☑
            - nontraffic V43.22 ☑
          - pedal cycle (traffic) V41.7 ☑
            - nontraffic V41.2 ☑
          - pickup truck (traffic) V43.73 ☑
            - nontraffic V43.23 ☑
          - railway vehicle (traffic) V45.7 ☑
            - nontraffic V45.2 ☑
          - specified vehicle NEC (traffic) V46.7 ☑
            - nontraffic V46.2 ☑
          - sport utility vehicle (traffic) V43.71 ☑
            - nontraffic V43.21 ☑
          - stationary object (traffic) V47.7 ☑
            - nontraffic V47.2 ☑
          - streetcar (traffic) V46.7 ☑
            - nontraffic V46.2 ☑
          - three wheeled motor vehicle (traffic) V42.7 ☑
            - nontraffic V42.2 ☑
          - truck (traffic) V44.7 ☑
            - nontraffic V44.2 ☑
          - two wheeled motor vehicle (traffic) V42.7 ☑
            - nontraffic V42.2 ☑
          - van (traffic) V43.74 ☑
            - nontraffic V43.24 ☑
        - noncollision accident (traffic) V48.7 ☑
          - nontraffic V48.2 ☑
      - noncollision accident (traffic) V48.9 ☑
        - nontraffic V48.3 ☑
        - while boarding or alighting V48.4 ☑
      - nontraffic V49.3 ☑
      - passenger
        - collision (with)
          - animal (traffic) V40.6 ☑
            - being ridden (traffic) V46.6 ☑
              - nontraffic V46.1 ☑
            - nontraffic V40.1 ☑
          - animal-drawn vehicle (traffic) V46.6 ☑
            - nontraffic V46.1 ☑
          - bus (traffic) V44.6 ☑
            - nontraffic V44.1 ☑
          - car (traffic) V43.62 ☑
            - nontraffic V43.12 ☑
          - motor vehicle NOS (traffic) V49.50 ☑
            - nontraffic V49.10 ☑
            - specified type NEC (traffic) V49.59 ☑
              - nontraffic V49.19 ☑
          - pedal cycle (traffic) V41.6 ☑
            - nontraffic V41.1 ☑
          - pickup truck (traffic) V43.63 ☑
            - nontraffic V43.13 ☑
          - railway vehicle (traffic) V45.6 ☑
            - nontraffic V45.1 ☑
          - specified vehicle NEC (traffic) V46.6 ☑
            - nontraffic V46.1 ☑
          - sport utility vehicle (traffic) V43.61 ☑
            - nontraffic V43.11 ☑
          - stationary object (traffic) V47.6 ☑
            - nontraffic V47.1 ☑
          - streetcar (traffic) V46.6 ☑
            - nontraffic V46.1 ☑
          - three wheeled motor vehicle (traffic) V42.6 ☑
            - nontraffic V42.1 ☑
          - truck (traffic) V44.6 ☑
            - nontraffic V44.1 ☑
          - two wheeled motor vehicle (traffic) V42.6 ☑
            - nontraffic V42.1 ☑
          - van (traffic) V43.64 ☑
            - nontraffic V43.14 ☑
        - noncollision accident (traffic) V48.6 ☑

- **Accident** — *continued*
  - transport — *continued*
    - occupant — *continued*
      - car — *see also* Accident, transport, car occupant — *continued*
        - cable (on rails) — *see also* Accident, transport, streetcar occupant
          - not on rails V98.Ø ☑
      - coach — *see* Accident, transport, bus occupant
      - coal-car — *see* Accident, transport, industrial vehicle occupant
      - digger — *see* Accident, transport, construction vehicle occupant
      - dump truck — *see* Accident, transport, construction vehicle occupant
      - earth-leveler — *see* Accident, transport, construction vehicle occupant
      - farm machinery (self-propelled) — *see* Accident, transport, agricultural vehicle occupant
      - forklift — *see* Accident, transport, industrial vehicle occupant
      - glider (unpowered) V96.2Ø ☑
        - hang V96.1Ø ☑
        - powered (microlight) (ultralight) — *see* Accident, transport, aircraft, occupant, powered, glider
      - glider (unpowered) NEC V96.2Ø ☑
      - hang-glider V96.1Ø ☑
      - harvester — *see* Accident, transport, agricultural vehicle occupant
      - heavy (transport) vehicle — *see* Accident, transport, truck occupant
      - helicopter — *see* Accident, transport, aircraft, occupant, helicopter
      - ice-yacht V98.2 ☑
      - kite (carrying person) V96.8 ☑
      - land-yacht V98.1 ☑
      - logging car — *see* Accident, transport, industrial vehicle occupant
      - mechanical shovel — *see* Accident, transport, construction vehicle occupant
      - microlight — *see* Accident, transport, aircraft, occupant, powered, glider
      - minibus — *see* Accident, transport, pickup truck occupant
      - minivan — *see* Accident, transport, pickup truck occupant
      - moped — *see* Accident, transport, motorcycle
      - motor scooter — *see* Accident, transport, motorcycle
      - motorcycle (with sidecar) — *see* Accident, transport, motorcycle
      - off-road motor-vehicle — *see also* Accident, transport, all-terrain vehicle occupant V86.99 ☑
      - pedal cycle — *see also* Accident, transport, pedal cyclist
      - pick-up (truck) — *see* Accident, transport, pickup truck occupant
      - railway (train) (vehicle) (subterranean) (elevated) — *see* Accident, transport, railway vehicle occupant
      - rickshaw — *see* Accident, transport, pedal cycle
        - motorized — *see* Accident, transport, three-wheeled motor vehicle
        - pedal driven — *see* Accident, transport, pedal cyclist
      - road-roller — *see* Accident, transport, construction vehicle occupant
      - ship NOS V94.9 ☑
      - ski-lift (chair) (gondola) V98.3 ☑
      - snowmobile — *see* Accident, transport, snowmobile occupant
      - spacecraft, spaceship — *see* Accident, transport, aircraft, occupant, spacecraft
      - sport utility vehicle — *see* Accident, transport, pickup truck occupant
      - streetcar (interurban) (operating on public street or highway) — *see* Accident, transport, streetcar occupant
      - SUV — *see* Accident, transport, pickup truck occupant
      - téléférique V98.Ø ☑
      - three-wheeled vehicle (motorized) — *see also* Accident, transport, three-wheeled motor vehicle occupant

- **Accident** — *continued*
  - transport — *continued*
    - occupant — *continued*
      - three-wheeled vehicle — *see also* Accident, transport, three-wheeled motor vehicle occupant — *continued*
        - nonmotorized — *see* Accident, transport, pedal cycle
      - tractor (farm) (and trailer) — *see* Accident, transport, agricultural vehicle occupant
      - train — *see* Accident, transport, railway vehicle occupant
      - tram — *see* Accident, transport, streetcar occupant
        - in mine or quarry — *see* Accident, transport, industrial vehicle occupant
      - tricycle — *see* Accident, transport, pedal cycle
        - motorized — *see* Accident, transport, three-wheeled motor vehicle
      - trolley — *see* Accident, transport, streetcar occupant
        - in mine or quarry — *see* Accident, transport, industrial vehicle occupant
      - tub, in mine or quarry — *see* Accident, transport, industrial vehicle occupant
      - ultralight — *see* Accident, transport, aircraft, occupant, powered, glider
      - van — *see* Accident, transport, van occupant
      - vehicle NEC V89.9 ☑
        - heavy transport — *see* Accident, transport, truck occupant
        - motor (traffic) NEC V89.2 ☑
          - nontraffic NEC V89.Ø ☑
      - watercraft NOS V94.9 ☑
        - causing drowning — *see* Drowning, resulting from accident to boat
    - off-road motor-vehicle — *see also* Accident, transport, all-terrain vehicle occupant V86.99 ☑
    - parachutist V97.29 ☑
      - after accident to aircraft — *see* Accident, transport, aircraft
      - entangled in object V97.21 ☑
      - injured on landing V97.22 ☑
    - pedal cyclist V19.9 ☑
      - collision (with)
        - animal (traffic) V1Ø.9 ☑
          - being ridden (traffic) V16.9 ☑
            - nontraffic V16.2 ☑
            - while boarding or alighting V16.3 ☑
          - nontraffic V1Ø.2 ☑
          - while boarding or alighting V1Ø.3 ☑
        - animal-drawn vehicle (traffic) V16.9 ☑
          - nontraffic V16.2 ☑
          - while boarding or alighting V16.3 ☑
        - bus (traffic) V14.9 ☑
          - nontraffic V14.2 ☑
          - while boarding or alighting V14.3 ☑
        - car (traffic) V13.9 ☑
          - nontraffic V13.2 ☑
          - while boarding or alighting V13.3 ☑
        - motor vehicle NOS (traffic) V19.6Ø ☑
          - nontraffic V19.2Ø ☑
          - specified type NEC (traffic) V19.69 ☑
            - nontraffic V19.29 ☑
        - pedal cycle (traffic) V11.9 ☑
          - nontraffic V11.2 ☑
          - while boarding or alighting V11.3 ☑
        - pickup truck (traffic) V13.9 ☑
          - nontraffic V13.2 ☑
          - while boarding or alighting V13.3 ☑
        - railway vehicle (traffic) V15.9 ☑
          - nontraffic V15.2 ☑
          - while boarding or alighting V15.3 ☑
        - specified vehicle NEC (traffic) V16.9 ☑
          - nontraffic V16.2 ☑
          - while boarding or alighting V16.3 ☑
        - stationary object (traffic) V17.9 ☑
          - nontraffic V17.2 ☑
          - while boarding or alighting V17.3 ☑
        - streetcar (traffic) V16.9 ☑
          - nontraffic V16.2 ☑
          - while boarding or alighting V16.3 ☑
        - three wheeled motor vehicle (traffic) V12.9 ☑
          - nontraffic V12.2 ☑
          - while boarding or alighting V12.3 ☑
        - truck (traffic) V14.9 ☑

- **Accident** — *continued*
  - transport — *continued*
    - pedal cyclist — *continued*
      - collision — *continued*
        - truck — *continued*
          - nontraffic V14.2 ☑
          - while boarding or alighting V14.3 ☑
        - two wheeled motor vehicle (traffic) V12.9 ☑
          - nontraffic V12.2 ☑
          - while boarding or alighting V12.3 ☑
        - van (traffic) V13.9 ☑
          - nontraffic V13.2 ☑
          - while boarding or alighting V13.3 ☑
      - driver
        - collision (with)
          - animal (traffic) V1Ø.4 ☑
            - being ridden (traffic) V16.4 ☑
              - nontraffic V16.Ø ☑
            - nontraffic V1Ø.Ø ☑
          - animal-drawn vehicle (traffic) V16.4 ☑
            - nontraffic V16.Ø ☑
          - bus (traffic) V14.4 ☑
            - nontraffic V14.Ø ☑
          - car (traffic) V13.4 ☑
            - nontraffic V13.Ø ☑
          - motor vehicle NOS (traffic) V19.4Ø ☑
            - nontraffic V19.ØØ ☑
            - specified type NEC (traffic) V19.49 ☑
              - nontraffic V19.Ø9 ☑
          - pedal cycle (traffic) V11.4 ☑
            - nontraffic V11.Ø ☑
          - pickup truck (traffic) V13.4 ☑
            - nontraffic V13.Ø ☑
          - railway vehicle (traffic) V15.4 ☑
            - nontraffic V15.Ø ☑
          - specified vehicle NEC (traffic) V16.4 ☑
            - nontraffic V16.Ø ☑
          - stationary object (traffic) V17.4 ☑
            - nontraffic V17.Ø ☑
          - streetcar (traffic) V16.4 ☑
            - nontraffic V16.Ø ☑
          - three wheeled motor vehicle (traffic) V12.4 ☑
            - nontraffic V12.Ø ☑
          - truck (traffic) V14.4 ☑
            - nontraffic V14.Ø ☑
          - two wheeled motor vehicle (traffic) V12.4 ☑
            - nontraffic V12.Ø ☑
          - van (traffic) V13.4 ☑
            - nontraffic V13.Ø ☑
        - noncollision accident (traffic) V18.4 ☑
          - nontraffic V18.Ø ☑
      - noncollision accident (traffic) V18.9 ☑
        - nontraffic V18.2 ☑
        - while boarding or alighting V18.3 ☑
      - nontraffic V19.3 ☑
      - passenger
        - collision (with)
          - animal (traffic) V1Ø.5 ☑
            - being ridden (traffic) V16.5 ☑
              - nontraffic V16.1 ☑
            - nontraffic V1Ø.1 ☑
          - animal-drawn vehicle (traffic) V16.5 ☑
            - nontraffic V16.1 ☑
          - bus (traffic) V14.5 ☑
            - nontraffic V14.1 ☑
          - car (traffic) V13.5 ☑
            - nontraffic V13.1 ☑
          - motor vehicle NOS (traffic) V19.5Ø ☑
            - nontraffic V19.1Ø ☑
            - specified type NEC (traffic) V19.59 ☑
              - nontraffic V19.19 ☑
          - pedal cycle (traffic) V11.5 ☑
            - nontraffic V11.1 ☑
          - pickup truck (traffic) V13.5 ☑
            - nontraffic V13.1 ☑
          - railway vehicle (traffic) V15.5 ☑
            - nontraffic V15.1 ☑
          - specified vehicle NEC (traffic) V16.5 ☑
            - nontraffic V16.1 ☑
          - stationary object (traffic) V17.5 ☑
            - nontraffic V17.1 ☑
          - streetcar (traffic) V16.5 ☑
            - nontraffic V16.1 ☑

- **Accident** — *continued*
  - transport — *continued*
    - pedestrian — *continued*
      - conveyance — *continued*
        - skis — *continued*
          - collision — *continued*
            - pedal cycle — *continued*
              - traffic V01.19 ☑
            - pick-up truck or van V03.99 ☑
              - nontraffic V03.09 ☑
              - traffic V03.19 ☑
            - railway (train) (vehicle) V05.99 ☑
              - nontraffic V05.09 ☑
              - traffic V05.19 ☑
            - stationary object V00.322 ☑
            - streetcar V06.99 ☑
              - nontraffic V06.09 ☑
              - traffic V06.19 ☑
            - two- or three-wheeled motor vehicle V02.99 ☑
              - nontraffic V02.09 ☑
              - traffic V02.19 ☑
            - vehicle V09.9 ☑
              - animal-drawn V06.99 ☑
                - nontraffic V06.09 ☑
                - traffic V06.19 ☑
              - motor
                - nontraffic V09.00 ☑
                - traffic V09.20 ☑
          - fall V00.321 ☑
          - nontraffic V09.1 ☑
            - involving motor vehicle NEC V09.00 ☑
          - traffic V09.3 ☑
            - involving motor vehicle NEC V09.20 ☑
        - sled V00.228 ☑
          - collision (with) V09.9 ☑
            - animal being ridden or animal drawn vehicle V06.99 ☑
              - nontraffic V06.09 ☑
              - traffic V06.19 ☑
            - bus or heavy transport V04.99 ☑
              - nontraffic V04.09 ☑
              - traffic V04.19 ☑
            - car V03.99 ☑
              - nontraffic V03.09 ☑
              - traffic V03.19 ☑
            - pedal cycle V01.99 ☑
              - nontraffic V01.09 ☑
              - traffic V01.19 ☑
            - pick-up truck or van V03.99 ☑
              - nontraffic V03.09 ☑
              - traffic V03.19 ☑
            - railway (train) (vehicle) V05.99 ☑
              - nontraffic V05.09 ☑
              - traffic V05.19 ☑
            - stationary object V00.222 ☑
            - streetcar V06.99 ☑
              - nontraffic V06.09 ☑
              - traffic V06.19 ☑
            - two- or three-wheeled motor vehicle V02.99 ☑
              - nontraffic V02.09 ☑
              - traffic V02.19 ☑
            - vehicle V09.9 ☑
              - animal-drawn V06.99 ☑
                - nontraffic V06.09 ☑
                - traffic V06.19 ☑
              - motor
                - nontraffic V09.00 ☑
                - traffic V09.20 ☑
          - fall V00.221 ☑
          - nontraffic V09.1 ☑
            - involving motor vehicle NEC V09.00 ☑
          - traffic V09.3 ☑
            - involving motor vehicle NEC V09.20 ☑
        - snow board V00.318 ☑
          - collision (with) V09.9 ☑
            - animal being ridden or animal drawn vehicle V06.99 ☑
              - nontraffic V06.09 ☑
              - traffic V06.19 ☑
            - bus or heavy transport V04.99 ☑
              - nontraffic V04.09 ☑
              - traffic V04.19 ☑
            - car V03.99 ☑
              - nontraffic V03.09 ☑

- **Accident** — *continued*
  - transport — *continued*
    - pedestrian — *continued*
      - conveyance — *continued*
        - snow board — *continued*
          - collision — *continued*
            - car — *continued*
              - traffic V03.19 ☑
            - pedal cycle V01.99 ☑
              - nontraffic V01.09 ☑
              - traffic V01.19 ☑
            - pick-up truck or van V03.99 ☑
              - nontraffic V03.09 ☑
              - traffic V03.19 ☑
            - railway (train) (vehicle) V05.99 ☑
              - nontraffic V05.09 ☑
              - traffic V05.19 ☑
            - stationary object V00.312 ☑
            - streetcar V06.99 ☑
              - nontraffic V06.09 ☑
              - traffic V06.19 ☑
            - two- or three-wheeled motor vehicle V02.99 ☑
              - nontraffic V02.09 ☑
              - traffic V02.19 ☑
            - vehicle V09.9 ☑
              - animal-drawn V06.99 ☑
                - nontraffic V06.09 ☑
                - traffic V06.19 ☑
              - motor
                - nontraffic V09.00 ☑
                - traffic V09.20 ☑
          - fall V00.311 ☑
          - nontraffic V09.1 ☑
            - involving motor vehicle NEC V09.00 ☑
          - traffic V09.3 ☑
            - involving motor vehicle NEC V09.20 ☑
        - specified type NEC V00.898 ☑
          - collision (with) V09.9 ☑
            - animal being ridden or animal drawn vehicle V06.99 ☑
              - nontraffic V06.09 ☑
              - traffic V06.19 ☑
            - bus or heavy transport V04.99 ☑
              - nontraffic V04.09 ☑
              - traffic V04.19 ☑
            - car V03.99 ☑
              - nontraffic V03.09 ☑
              - traffic V03.19 ☑
            - pedal cycle V01.99 ☑
              - nontraffic V01.09 ☑
              - traffic V01.19 ☑
            - pick-up truck or van V03.99 ☑
              - nontraffic V03.09 ☑
              - traffic V03.19 ☑
            - railway (train) (vehicle) V05.99 ☑
              - nontraffic V05.09 ☑
              - traffic V05.19 ☑
            - stationary object V00.892 ☑
            - streetcar V06.99 ☑
              - nontraffic V06.09 ☑
              - traffic V06.19 ☑
            - two- or three-wheeled motor vehicle V02.99 ☑
              - nontraffic V02.09 ☑
              - traffic V02.19 ☑
            - vehicle V09.9 ☑
              - animal-drawn V06.99 ☑
                - nontraffic V06.09 ☑
                - traffic V06.19 ☑
              - motor
                - nontraffic V09.00 ☑
                - traffic V09.20 ☑
          - fall V00.891 ☑
          - nontraffic V09.1 ☑
            - involving motor vehicle NEC V09.00 ☑
          - traffic V09.3 ☑
            - involving motor vehicle NEC V09.20 ☑
        - standing
          - electric scooter
            - collsion with
              - animal being ridden or animal drawn vehicle V06.931 ☑
                - nontraffic V06.031 ☑
                - traffic V06.131 ☑
              - bus or heavy transport V04.931 ☑

- **Accident** — *continued*
  - transport — *continued*
    - pedestrian — *continued*
      - conveyance — *continued*
        - standing — *continued*
          - electric scooter — *continued*
            - collsion with — *continued*
              - bus or heavy transport — *continued*
                - nontraffic V04.031 ☑
                - traffic V04.131 ☑
              - car V03.931 ☑
                - nontraffic V04.031 ☑
                - traffic V04.131 ☑
              - pedal cycle V01.931 ☑
                - nontraffic V01.031 ☑
                - traffic V01.131 ☑
              - pick-up or van V03.931 ☑
                - nontraffic V03.031 ☑
                - traffic V03.131 ☑
              - railway (train) (vehicle) V05.931 ☑
                - nontraffic V05.031 ☑
                - traffic V05.131 ☑
              - streetcar V06.931 ☑
                - nontraffic V06.031 ☑
                - traffic V06.131 ☑
              - three-wheeled motor vehicle V02.931 ☑
                - nontraffic V02.031 ☑
                - traffic V02.131 ☑
              - two-wheeled motor vehicle V02.931 ☑
                - nontraffic V02.031 ☑
                - traffic V02.131 ☑
              - vehicle, nonmotor, specified NEC V06.931 ☑
                - nontraffic V06.031 ☑
                - traffic V06.131 ☑
            - fall V00.841 ☑
          - micro-mobility pedestrian conveyance
            - collision with
              - animal being ridden or animal drawn vehicle V06.938 ☑
                - nontraffic V06.038 ☑
                - traffic V06.138 ☑
              - bus or heavy transport V04.938 ☑
                - nontraffic V04.038 ☑
                - traffic V04.138 ☑
              - car V03.938 ☑
                - nontraffic V03.038 ☑
                - traffic V03.138 ☑
              - pedal cycle V01.938 ☑
                - nontraffic V01.038 ☑
                - traffic V01.138 ☑
              - pick-up or van V03.938 ☑
                - nontraffic V03.038 ☑
                - traffic V03.138 ☑
              - railway (train) (vehicle) V05.938 ☑
                - nontraffic V05.038 ☑
                - traffic V05.138 ☑
              - stationary object V00.842 ☑
              - streetcar V06.938 ☑
                - nontraffic V06.038 ☑
                - traffic V06.138 ☑
              - three-wheeled motor vehicle V02.938 ☑
                - nontraffic V02.038 ☑
                - traffic V02.138 ☑
              - two-wheeled motor vehicle V02.938 ☑
                - nontraffic V02.038 ☑
                - traffic V02.138 ☑
              - vehicle, nonmotor, specified NEC V06.938 ☑
                - nontraffic V06.038 ☑
                - traffic V06.138 ☑
            - fall V00.848 ☑
        - traffic V09.3 ☑
          - involving motor vehicle V09.20 ☑
            - military V09.21 ☑
            - specified type NEC V09.29 ☑
        - wheelchair (powered) V00.818 ☑
          - collision (with) V09.9 ☑
            - animal being ridden or animal drawn vehicle V06.99 ☑
              - nontraffic V06.09 ☑

- **Accident** — *continued*
  - transport — *continued*
    - pickup truck occupant — *continued*
      - passenger — *continued*
        - collision — *continued*
          - animal — *continued*
            - being ridden (traffic) V56.6 ☑
              - nontraffic V56.1 ☑
            - nontraffic V5Ø.1 ☑
          - animal-drawn vehicle (traffic) V56.6 ☑
            - nontraffic V56.1 ☑
          - bus (traffic) V54.6 ☑
            - nontraffic V54.1 ☑
          - car (traffic) V53.6 ☑
            - nontraffic V53.1 ☑
          - motor vehicle NOS (traffic) V59.5Ø ☑
            - nontraffic V59.1Ø ☑
            - specified type NEC (traffic) V59.59 ☑
              - nontraffic V59.19 ☑
          - pedal cycle (traffic) V51.6 ☑
            - nontraffic V51.1 ☑
          - pickup truck (traffic) V53.6 ☑
            - nontraffic V53.1 ☑
          - railway vehicle (traffic) V55.6 ☑
            - nontraffic V55.1 ☑
          - specified vehicle NEC (traffic) V56.6 ☑
            - nontraffic V56.1 ☑
          - stationary object (traffic) V57.6 ☑
            - nontraffic V57.1 ☑
          - streetcar (traffic) V56.6 ☑
            - nontraffic V56.1 ☑
          - three wheeled motor vehicle (traffic) V52.6 ☑
            - nontraffic V52.1 ☑
          - truck (traffic) V54.6 ☑
            - nontraffic V54.1 ☑
          - two wheeled motor vehicle (traffic) V52.6 ☑
            - nontraffic V52.1 ☑
          - van (traffic) V53.6 ☑
            - nontraffic V53.1 ☑
        - noncollision accident (traffic) V58.6 ☑
          - nontraffic V58.1 ☑
      - specified type NEC V59.88 ☑
        - military vehicle V59.81 ☑
    - quarry truck — *see* Accident, transport, industrial vehicle occupant
    - race car — *see* Accident, transport, motor vehicle NEC occupant
    - railway vehicle occupant V81.9 ☑
      - collision (with) V81.3 ☑
        - motor vehicle (non-military) (traffic) V81.1 ☑
          - military V81.83 ☑
          - nontraffic V81.Ø ☑
        - rolling stock V81.2 ☑
        - specified object NEC V81.3 ☑
      - during derailment V81.7 ☑
        - with antecedent collision — *see* Accident, transport, railway vehicle occupant, collision
      - explosion V81.81 ☑
      - fall (in railway vehicle) V81.5 ☑
        - during derailment V81.7 ☑
          - with antecedent collision — *see* Accident, transport, railway vehicle occupant, collision
        - from railway vehicle V81.6 ☑
          - during derailment V81.7 ☑
            - with antecedent collision — *see* Accident, transport, railway vehicle occupant, collision
        - while boarding or alighting V81.4 ☑
      - fire V81.81 ☑
      - object falling onto train V81.82 ☑
      - specified type NEC V81.89 ☑
      - while boarding or alighting V81.4 ☑
    - Segway VØØ.848 ☑
    - ski lift V98.3 ☑
    - snowmobile occupant (nontraffic) V86.92 ☑
      - driver V86.52 ☑
      - hanger-on V86.72 ☑
      - passenger V86.62 ☑
      - traffic V86.32 ☑
        - driver V86.Ø2 ☑
        - hanger-on V86.22 ☑
        - passenger V86.12 ☑

- **Accident** — *continued*
  - transport — *continued*
    - snowmobile occupant — *continued*
      - while boarding or alighting V86.42 ☑
    - specified NEC V98.8 ☑
    - sport utility vehicle occupant — *see also* Accident, transport, pickup truck occupant
    - streetcar occupant V82.9 ☑
      - collision (with) V82.3 ☑
        - motor vehicle (traffic) V82.1 ☑
          - nontraffic V82.Ø ☑
        - rolling stock V82.2 ☑
      - during derailment V82.7 ☑
        - with antecedent collision — *see* Accident, transport, streetcar occupant, collision
      - fall (in streetcar) V82.5 ☑
        - during derailment V82.7 ☑
          - with antecedent collision — *see* Accident, transport, streetcar occupant, collision
        - from streetcar V82.6 ☑
          - during derailment V82.7 ☑
            - with antecedent collision — *see* Accident, transport, streetcar occupant, collision
          - while boarding or alighting V82.4 ☑
        - while boarding or alighting V82.4 ☑
      - specified type NEC V82.8 ☑
      - while boarding or alighting V82.4 ☑
    - three-wheeled motor vehicle occupant V39.9 ☑
      - collision (with)
        - animal (traffic) V3Ø.9 ☑
          - being ridden (traffic) V36.9 ☑
            - nontraffic V36.3 ☑
            - while boarding or alighting V36.4 ☑
          - nontraffic V3Ø.3 ☑
          - while boarding or alighting V3Ø.4 ☑
        - animal-drawn vehicle (traffic) V36.9 ☑
          - nontraffic V36.3 ☑
          - while boarding or alighting V36.4 ☑
        - bus (traffic) V34.9 ☑
          - nontraffic V34.3 ☑
          - while boarding or alighting V34.4 ☑
        - car (traffic) V33.9 ☑
          - nontraffic V33.3 ☑
          - while boarding or alighting V33.4 ☑
        - motor vehicle NOS (traffic) V39.6Ø ☑
          - nontraffic V39.2Ø ☑
          - specified type NEC (traffic) V39.69 ☑
            - nontraffic V39.29 ☑
        - pedal cycle (traffic) V31.9 ☑
          - nontraffic V31.3 ☑
          - while boarding or alighting V31.4 ☑
        - pickup truck (traffic) V33.9 ☑
          - nontraffic V33.3 ☑
          - while boarding or alighting V33.4 ☑
        - railway vehicle (traffic) V35.9 ☑
          - nontraffic V35.3 ☑
          - while boarding or alighting V35.4 ☑
        - specified vehicle NEC (traffic) V36.9 ☑
          - nontraffic V36.3 ☑
          - while boarding or alighting V36.4 ☑
        - stationary object (traffic) V37.9 ☑
          - nontraffic V37.3 ☑
          - while boarding or alighting V37.4 ☑
        - streetcar (traffic) V36.9 ☑
          - nontraffic V36.3 ☑
          - while boarding or alighting V36.4 ☑
        - three wheeled motor vehicle (traffic) V32.9 ☑
          - nontraffic V32.3 ☑
          - while boarding or alighting V32.4 ☑
        - truck (traffic) V34.9 ☑
          - nontraffic V34.3 ☑
          - while boarding or alighting V34.4 ☑
        - two wheeled motor vehicle (traffic) V32.9 ☑
          - nontraffic V32.3 ☑
          - while boarding or alighting V32.4 ☑
        - van (traffic) V33.9 ☑
          - nontraffic V33.3 ☑
          - while boarding or alighting V33.4 ☑
      - driver
        - collision (with)
          - animal (traffic) V3Ø.5 ☑
            - being ridden (traffic) V36.5 ☑
              - nontraffic V36.Ø ☑
            - nontraffic V3Ø.Ø ☑

- **Accident** — *continued*
  - transport — *continued*
    - three-wheeled motor vehicle occupant — *continued*
      - driver — *continued*
        - collision — *continued*
          - animal-drawn vehicle (traffic) V36.5 ☑
            - nontraffic V36.Ø ☑
          - bus (traffic) V34.5 ☑
            - nontraffic V34.Ø ☑
          - car (traffic) V33.5 ☑
            - nontraffic V33.Ø ☑
          - motor vehicle NOS (traffic) V39.4Ø ☑
            - nontraffic V39.ØØ ☑
            - specified type NEC (traffic) V39.49 ☑
              - nontraffic V39.Ø9 ☑
          - pedal cycle (traffic) V31.5 ☑
            - nontraffic V31.Ø ☑
          - pickup truck (traffic) V33.5 ☑
            - nontraffic V33.Ø ☑
          - railway vehicle (traffic) V35.5 ☑
            - nontraffic V35.Ø ☑
          - specified vehicle NEC (traffic) V36.5 ☑
            - nontraffic V36.Ø ☑
          - stationary object (traffic) V37.5 ☑
            - nontraffic V37.Ø ☑
          - streetcar (traffic) V36.5 ☑
            - nontraffic V36.Ø ☑
          - three wheeled motor vehicle (traffic) V32.5 ☑
            - nontraffic V32.Ø ☑
          - truck (traffic) V34.5 ☑
            - nontraffic V34.Ø ☑
          - two wheeled motor vehicle (traffic) V32.5 ☑
            - nontraffic V32.Ø ☑
          - van (traffic) V33.5 ☑
            - nontraffic V33.Ø ☑
        - noncollision accident (traffic) V38.5 ☑
          - nontraffic V38.Ø ☑
      - hanger-on
        - collision (with)
          - animal (traffic) V3Ø.7 ☑
            - being ridden (traffic) V36.7 ☑
              - nontraffic V36.2 ☑
            - nontraffic V3Ø.2 ☑
          - animal-drawn vehicle (traffic) V36.7 ☑
            - nontraffic V36.2 ☑
          - bus (traffic) V34.7 ☑
            - nontraffic V34.2 ☑
          - car (traffic) V33.7 ☑
            - nontraffic V33.2 ☑
          - pedal cycle (traffic) V31.7 ☑
            - nontraffic V31.2 ☑
          - pickup truck (traffic) V33.7 ☑
            - nontraffic V33.2 ☑
          - railway vehicle (traffic) V35.7 ☑
            - nontraffic V35.2 ☑
          - specified vehicle NEC (traffic) V36.7 ☑
            - nontraffic V36.2 ☑
          - stationary object (traffic) V37.7 ☑
            - nontraffic V37.2 ☑
          - streetcar (traffic) V36.7 ☑
            - nontraffic V36.2 ☑
          - three wheeled motor vehicle (traffic) V32.7 ☑
            - nontraffic V32.2 ☑
          - truck (traffic) V34.7 ☑
            - nontraffic V34.2 ☑
          - two wheeled motor vehicle (traffic) V32.7 ☑
            - nontraffic V32.2 ☑
          - van (traffic) V33.7 ☑
            - nontraffic V33.2 ☑
        - noncollision accident (traffic) V38.7 ☑
          - nontraffic V38.2 ☑
      - noncollision accident (traffic) V38.9 ☑
        - nontraffic V38.3 ☑
        - while boarding or alighting V38.4 ☑
      - nontraffic V39.3 ☑
      - passenger
        - collision (with)
          - animal (traffic) V3Ø.6 ☑
            - being ridden (traffic) V36.6 ☑
              - nontraffic V36.1 ☑
            - nontraffic V3Ø.1 ☑

- **Accident** — *continued*
  - transport — *continued*
    - three-wheeled motor vehicle occupant — *continued*
      - passenger — *continued*
        - collision — *continued*
          - animal-drawn vehicle (traffic) V36.6 ☑
            - nontraffic V36.1 ☑
          - bus (traffic) V34.6 ☑
            - nontraffic V34.1 ☑
          - car (traffic) V33.6 ☑
            - nontraffic V33.1 ☑
          - motor vehicle NOS (traffic) V39.5Ø ☑
            - nontraffic V39.1Ø ☑
            - specified type NEC (traffic) V39.59 ☑
              - nontraffic V39.19 ☑
          - pedal cycle (traffic) V31.6 ☑
            - nontraffic V31.1 ☑
          - pickup truck (traffic) V33.6 ☑
            - nontraffic V33.1 ☑
          - railway vehicle (traffic) V35.6 ☑
            - nontraffic V35.1 ☑
          - specified vehicle NEC (traffic) V36.6 ☑
            - nontraffic V36.1 ☑
          - stationary object (traffic) V37.6 ☑
            - nontraffic V37.1 ☑
          - streetcar (traffic) V36.6 ☑
            - nontraffic V36.1 ☑
          - three wheeled motor vehicle (traffic) V32.6 ☑
            - nontraffic V32.1 ☑
          - truck (traffic) V34.6 ☑
            - nontraffic V34.1 ☑
          - two wheeled motor vehicle (traffic) V32.6 ☑
            - nontraffic V32.1 ☑
          - van (traffic) V33.6 ☑
            - nontraffic V33.1 ☑
        - noncollision accident (traffic) V38.6 ☑
          - nontraffic V38.1 ☑
      - specified type NEC V39.89 ☑
        - military vehicle V39.81 ☑
    - tractor (farm) (and trailer) — *see* Accident, transport, agricultural vehicle occupant
    - tram — *see* Accident, transport, streetcar
      - in mine or quarry — *see* Accident, transport, industrial vehicle occupant
    - trolley — *see* Accident, transport, streetcar
      - in mine or quarry — *see* Accident, transport, industrial vehicle occupant
    - truck (heavy) occupant V69.9 ☑
      - collision (with)
        - animal (traffic) V6Ø.9 ☑
          - being ridden (traffic) V66.9 ☑
            - nontraffic V66.3 ☑
              - while boarding or alighting V66.4 ☑
          - nontraffic V6Ø.3 ☑
          - while boarding or alighting V6Ø.4 ☑
        - animal-drawn vehicle (traffic) V66.9 ☑
          - nontraffic V66.3 ☑
          - while boarding or alighting V66.4 ☑
        - bus (traffic) V64.9 ☑
          - nontraffic V64.3 ☑
          - while boarding or alighting V64.4 ☑
        - car (traffic) V63.9 ☑
          - nontraffic V63.3 ☑
          - while boarding or alighting V63.4 ☑
        - motor vehicle NOS (traffic) V69.6Ø ☑
          - nontraffic V69.2Ø ☑
          - specified type NEC (traffic) V69.69 ☑
            - nontraffic V69.29 ☑
        - pedal cycle (traffic) V61.9 ☑
          - nontraffic V61.3 ☑
          - while boarding or alighting V61.4 ☑
        - pickup truck (traffic) V63.9 ☑
          - nontraffic V63.3 ☑
          - while boarding or alighting V63.4 ☑
        - railway vehicle (traffic) V65.9 ☑
          - nontraffic V65.3 ☑
          - while boarding or alighting V65.4 ☑
        - specified vehicle NEC (traffic) V66.9 ☑
          - nontraffic V66.3 ☑
          - while boarding or alighting V66.4 ☑
        - stationary object (traffic) V67.9 ☑
          - nontraffic V67.3 ☑
          - while boarding or alighting V67.4 ☑

- **Accident** — *continued*
  - transport — *continued*
    - truck occupant — *continued*
      - collision — *continued*
        - streetcar (traffic) V66.9 ☑
          - nontraffic V66.3 ☑
          - while boarding or alighting V66.4 ☑
        - three wheeled motor vehicle (traffic) V62.9 ☑
          - nontraffic V62.3 ☑
          - while boarding or alighting V62.4 ☑
        - truck (traffic) V64.9 ☑
          - nontraffic V64.3 ☑
          - while boarding or alighting V64.4 ☑
        - two wheeled motor vehicle (traffic) V62.9 ☑
          - nontraffic V62.3 ☑
          - while boarding or alighting V62.4 ☑
        - van (traffic) V63.9 ☑
          - nontraffic V63.3 ☑
          - while boarding or alighting V63.4 ☑
      - driver
        - collision (with)
          - animal (traffic) V6Ø.5 ☑
            - being ridden (traffic) V66.5 ☑
              - nontraffic V66.Ø ☑
            - nontraffic V6Ø.Ø ☑
          - animal-drawn vehicle (traffic) V66.5 ☑
            - nontraffic V66.Ø ☑
          - bus (traffic) V64.5 ☑
            - nontraffic V64.Ø ☑
          - car (traffic) V63.5 ☑
            - nontraffic V63.Ø ☑
          - motor vehicle NOS (traffic) V69.4Ø ☑
            - nontraffic V69.ØØ ☑
            - specified type NEC (traffic) V69.49 ☑
              - nontraffic V69.Ø9 ☑
          - pedal cycle (traffic) V61.5 ☑
            - nontraffic V61.Ø ☑
          - pickup truck (traffic) V63.5 ☑
            - nontraffic V63.Ø ☑
          - railway vehicle (traffic) V65.5 ☑
            - nontraffic V65.Ø ☑
          - specified vehicle NEC (traffic) V66.5 ☑
            - nontraffic V66.Ø ☑
          - stationary object (traffic) V67.5 ☑
            - nontraffic V67.Ø ☑
          - streetcar (traffic) V66.5 ☑
            - nontraffic V66.Ø ☑
          - three wheeled motor vehicle (traffic) V62.5 ☑
            - nontraffic V62.Ø ☑
          - truck (traffic) V64.5 ☑
            - nontraffic V64.Ø ☑
          - two wheeled motor vehicle (traffic) V62.5 ☑
            - nontraffic V62.Ø ☑
          - van (traffic) V63.5 ☑
            - nontraffic V63.Ø ☑
        - noncollision accident (traffic) V68.5 ☑
          - nontraffic V68.Ø ☑
      - dump — *see* Accident, transport, construction vehicle occupant
      - hanger-on
        - collision (with)
          - animal (traffic) V6Ø.7 ☑
            - being ridden (traffic) V66.7 ☑
              - nontraffic V66.2 ☑
            - nontraffic V6Ø.2 ☑
          - animal-drawn vehicle (traffic) V66.7 ☑
            - nontraffic V66.2 ☑
          - bus (traffic) V64.7 ☑
            - nontraffic V64.2 ☑
          - car (traffic) V63.7 ☑
            - nontraffic V63.2 ☑
          - pedal cycle (traffic) V61.7 ☑
            - nontraffic V61.2 ☑
          - pickup truck (traffic) V63.7 ☑
            - nontraffic V63.2 ☑
          - railway vehicle (traffic) V65.7 ☑
            - nontraffic V65.2 ☑
          - specified vehicle NEC (traffic) V66.7 ☑
            - nontraffic V66.2 ☑
          - stationary object (traffic) V67.7 ☑
            - nontraffic V67.2 ☑
          - streetcar (traffic) V66.7 ☑
            - nontraffic V66.2 ☑

- **Accident** — *continued*
  - transport — *continued*
    - truck occupant — *continued*
      - hanger-on — *continued*
        - collision — *continued*
          - three wheeled motor vehicle (traffic) V62.7 ☑
            - nontraffic V62.2 ☑
          - truck (traffic) V64.7 ☑
            - nontraffic V64.2 ☑
          - two wheeled motor vehicle (traffic) V62.7 ☑
            - nontraffic V62.2 ☑
          - van (traffic) V63.7 ☑
            - nontraffic V63.2 ☑
        - noncollision accident (traffic) V68.7 ☑
          - nontraffic V68.2 ☑
      - noncollision accident (traffic) V68.9 ☑
        - nontraffic V68.3 ☑
        - while boarding or alighting V68.4 ☑
      - nontraffic V69.3 ☑
      - passenger
        - collision (with)
          - animal (traffic) V6Ø.6 ☑
            - being ridden (traffic) V66.6 ☑
              - nontraffic V66.1- ☑
            - nontraffic V6Ø.1 ☑
          - animal-drawn vehicle (traffic) V66.6 ☑
            - nontraffic V66.1 ☑
          - bus (traffic) V64.6 ☑
            - nontraffic V64.1 ☑
          - car (traffic) V63.6 ☑
            - nontraffic V63.1 ☑
          - motor vehicle NOS (traffic) V69.5Ø ☑
            - nontraffic V69.1Ø ☑
            - specified type NEC (traffic) V69.59 ☑
              - nontraffic V69.19 ☑
          - pedal cycle (traffic) V61.6 ☑
            - nontraffic V61.1 ☑
          - pickup truck (traffic) V63.6 ☑
            - nontraffic V63.1 ☑
          - railway vehicle (traffic) V65.6 ☑
            - nontraffic V65.1 ☑
          - specified vehicle NEC (traffic) V66.6 ☑
            - nontraffic V66.1 ☑
          - stationary object (traffic) V67.6 ☑
            - nontraffic V67.1 ☑
          - streetcar (traffic) V66.6 ☑
            - nontraffic V66.1 ☑
          - three wheeled motor vehicle (traffic) V62.6 ☑
            - nontraffic V62.1 ☑
          - truck (traffic) V64.6 ☑
            - nontraffic V64.1 ☑
          - two wheeled motor vehicle (traffic) V62.6 ☑
            - nontraffic V62.1 ☑
          - van (traffic) V63.6 ☑
            - nontraffic V63.1 ☑
        - noncollision accident (traffic) V68.6 ☑
          - nontraffic V68.1 ☑
      - pickup — *see* Accident, transport, pickup truck occupant
      - specified type NEC V69.88 ☑
        - military vehicle V69.81 ☑
    - van occupant V59.9 ☑
      - collision (with)
        - animal (traffic) V5Ø.9 ☑
          - being ridden (traffic) V56.9 ☑
            - nontraffic V56.3 ☑
              - while boarding or alighting V56.4 ☑
          - nontraffic V5Ø.3 ☑
          - while boarding or alighting V5Ø.4 ☑
        - animal-drawn vehicle (traffic) V56.9 ☑
          - nontraffic V56.3 ☑
          - while boarding or alighting V56.4 ☑
        - bus (traffic) V54.9 ☑
          - nontraffic V54.3 ☑
          - while boarding or alighting V54.4 ☑
        - car (traffic) V53.9 ☑
          - nontraffic V53.3 ☑
          - while boarding or alighting V53.4 ☑
        - motor vehicle NOS (traffic) V59.6Ø ☑
          - nontraffic V59.2Ø ☑
          - specified type NEC (traffic) V59.69 ☑
            - nontraffic V59.29 ☑

- **Accident** — *continued*
  - watercraft — *continued*
    - due to, caused by cataclysm — *see* Forces of nature, by type
    - military NEC V94.818 ☑
      - civilian in water injured by V94.811 ☑
      - with civilian watercraft V94.81Ø ☑
    - nonpowered, struck by
      - nonpowered vessel V94.22 ☑
      - powered vessel V94.21 ☑
    - specified type NEC V94.89 ☑
    - striking swimmer
      - powered V94.11 ☑
      - unpowered V94.12 ☑
- **Acid throwing** (assault) YØ8.89 ☑
- **Activity** (involving) (of victim at time of event) Y93.9
  - aerobic and step exercise (class) Y93.A3 (*following* Y93.7)
  - alpine skiing Y93.23
  - animal care NEC Y93.K9 (*following* Y93.7)
  - arts and handcrafts NEC Y93.D9 (*following* Y93.7)
  - athletics played as a team or group NEC Y93.69
  - athletics played individually NEC Y93.59
  - athletics NEC Y93.79
  - baking Y93.G3 (*following* Y93.7)
  - ballet Y93.41
  - barbells Y93.B3 (*following* Y93.7)
  - BASE (Building, Antenna, Span, Earth) jumping Y93.33
  - baseball Y93.64
  - basketball Y93.67
  - bathing (personal) Y93.E1 (*following* Y93.7)
  - beach volleyball Y93.68
  - bike riding Y93.55
  - blackout game Y93.85
  - boogie boarding Y93.18
  - bowling Y93.54
  - boxing Y93.71
  - brass instrument playing Y93.J4 (*following* Y93.7)
  - building construction Y93.H3 (*following* Y93.7)
  - bungee jumping Y93.34
  - calisthenics Y93.A2 (*following* Y93.7)
  - canoeing (in calm and turbulent water) Y93.16
  - capture the flag Y93.6A
  - cardiorespiratory exercise NEC Y93.A9 (*following* Y93.7)
  - caregiving (providing) NEC Y93.F9 (*following* Y93.7)
    - bathing Y93.F1 (*following* Y93.7)
    - lifting Y93.F2 (*following* Y93.7)
  - cellular
    - communication device Y93.C2 (*following* Y93.7)
    - telephone Y93.C2 (*following* Y93.7)
  - challenge course Y93.A5 (*following* Y93.7)
  - cheerleading Y93.45
  - choking game Y93.85
  - circuit training Y93.A4 (*following* Y93.7)
  - cleaning
    - floor Y93.E5 (*following* Y93.7)
  - climbing NEC Y93.39
    - mountain Y93.31
    - rock Y93.31
    - wall Y93.31
  - clothing care and maintenance NEC Y93.E9 (*following* Y93.7)
  - combatives Y93.75
  - computer
    - keyboarding Y93.C1 (*following* Y93.7)
    - technology NEC Y93.C9 (*following* Y93.7)
  - confidence course Y93.A5 (*following* Y93.7)
  - construction (building) Y93.H3 (*following* Y93.7)
  - cooking and baking Y93.G3 (*following* Y93.7)
  - cool down exercises Y93.A2 (*following* Y93.7)
  - cricket Y93.69
  - crocheting Y93.D1 (*following* Y93.7)
  - cross country skiing Y93.24
  - dancing (all types) Y93.41
  - digging
    - dirt Y93.H1 (*following* Y93.7)
  - dirt digging Y93.H1 (*following* Y93.7)
  - dishwashing Y93.G1 (*following* Y93.7)
  - diving (platform) (springboard) Y93.12
    - underwater Y93.15
  - dodge ball Y93.6A
  - downhill skiing Y93.23
  - drum playing Y93.J2 (*following* Y93.7)
  - dumbbells Y93.B3 (*following* Y93.7)
  - electronic
    - devices NEC Y93.C9 (*following* Y93.7)
      - hand held interactive Y93.C2 (*following* Y93.7)

- **Activity** — *continued*
  - electronic — *continued*
    - game playing (using) (with)
      - interactive device Y93.C2 (*following* Y93.7)
      - keyboard or other stationary device Y93.C1 (*following* Y93.7)
  - elliptical machine Y93.A1 (*following* Y93.7)
  - exercise(s)
    - machines ((primarily) for)
      - cardiorespiratory conditioning Y93.A1 (*following* Y93.7)
      - muscle strengthening Y93.B1 (*following* Y93.7)
    - muscle strengthening (non-machine) NEC Y93.B9 (*following* Y93.7)
  - external motion NEC Y93.I9 (*following* Y93.7)
    - rollercoaster Y93.I1 (*following* Y93.7)
  - fainting game Y93.85
  - field hockey Y93.65
  - figure skating (pairs) (singles) Y93.21
  - flag football Y93.62
  - floor mopping and cleaning Y93.E5 (*following* Y93.7)
  - food preparation and clean up Y93.G1 (*following* Y93.7)
  - football (American) NOS Y93.61
    - flag Y93.62
    - tackle Y93.61
    - touch Y93.62
  - four square Y93.6A
  - free weights Y93.B3 (*following* Y93.7)
  - frisbee (ultimate) Y93.74
  - furniture
    - building Y93.D3 (*following* Y93.7)
    - finishing Y93.D3 (*following* Y93.7)
    - repair Y93.D3 (*following* Y93.7)
  - game playing (electronic)
    - using interactive device Y93.C2 (*following* Y93.7)
    - using keyboard or other stationary device Y93.C1 (*following* Y93.7)
  - gardening Y93.H2 (*following* Y93.7)
  - golf Y93.53
  - grass drills Y93.A6 (*following* Y93.7)
  - grilling and smoking food Y93.G2 (*following* Y93.7)
  - grooming and shearing an animal Y93.K3 (*following* Y93.7)
  - guerilla drills Y93.A6 (*following* Y93.7)
  - gymnastics (rhythmic) Y93.43
  - hand held interactive electronic device Y93.C2 (*following* Y93.7)
  - handball Y93.73
  - handcrafts NEC Y93.D9 (*following* Y93.7)
  - hang gliding Y93.35
  - hiking (on level or elevated terrain) Y93.Ø1
  - hockey (ice) Y93.22
    - field Y93.65
  - horseback riding Y93.52
  - household (interior) maintenance NEC Y93.E9 (*following* Y93.7)
  - ice NEC Y93.29
    - dancing Y93.21
    - hockey Y93.22
    - skating Y93.21
  - inline roller skating Y93.51
  - ironing Y93.E4 (*following* Y93.7)
  - judo Y93.75
  - jumping jacks Y93.A2 (*following* Y93.7)
  - jumping rope Y93.56
  - jumping (off) NEC Y93.39
    - BASE (Building, Antenna, Span, Earth) Y93.33
    - bungee Y93.34
    - jacks Y93.A2 (*following* Y93.7)
    - rope Y93.56
  - karate Y93.75
  - kayaking (in calm and turbulent water) Y93.16
  - keyboarding (computer) Y93.C1 (*following* Y93.7)
  - kickball Y93.6A
  - knitting Y93.D1 (*following* Y93.7)
  - lacrosse Y93.65
  - land maintenance NEC Y93.H9 (*following* Y93.7)
  - landscaping Y93.H2 (*following* Y93.7)
  - laundry Y93.E2 (*following* Y93.7)
  - machines (exercise)
    - primarily for cardiorespiratory conditioning Y93.A1 (*following* Y93.7)
    - primarily for muscle strengthening Y93.B1 (*following* Y93.7)
  - maintenance
    - exterior building NEC Y93.H9 (*following* Y93.7)
    - household (interior) NEC Y93.E9 (*following* Y93.7)
    - land Y93.H9 (*following* Y93.7)
    - property Y93.H9 (*following* Y93.7)

- **Activity** — *continued*
  - marching (on level or elevated terrain) Y93.Ø1
  - martial arts Y93.75
  - microwave oven Y93.G3 (*following* Y93.7)
  - milking an animal Y93.K2 (*following* Y93.7)
  - mopping (floor) Y93.E5 (*following* Y93.7)
  - mountain climbing Y93.31
  - muscle strengthening
    - exercises (non-machine) NEC Y93.B9 (*following* Y93.7)
    - machines Y93.B1 (*following* Y93.7)
  - musical keyboard (electronic) playing Y93.J1 (*following* Y93.7)
  - nordic skiing Y93.24
  - obstacle course Y93.A5 (*following* Y93.7)
  - oven (microwave) Y93.G3 (*following* Y93.7)
  - packing up and unpacking in moving to a new residence Y93.E6 (*following* Y93.7)
  - parasailing Y93.19
  - pass out game Y93.85
  - percussion instrument playing NEC Y93.J2 (*following* Y93.7)
  - personal
    - bathing and showering Y93.E1 (*following* Y93.7)
    - hygiene NEC Y93.E8 (*following* Y93.7)
    - showering Y93.E1 (*following* Y93.7)
  - physical games generally associated with school recess, summer camp and children Y93.6A
  - physical training NEC Y93.A9 (*following* Y93.7)
  - piano playing Y93.J1 (*following* Y93.7)
  - pilates Y93.B4 (*following* Y93.7)
  - platform diving Y93.12
  - playing musical instrument
    - brass instrument Y93.J4 (*following* Y93.7)
    - drum Y93.J2 (*following* Y93.7)
    - musical keyboard (electronic) Y93.J1 (*following* Y93.7)
    - percussion instrument NEC Y93.J2 (*following* Y93.7)
    - piano Y93.J1 (*following* Y93.7)
    - string instrument Y93.J3 (*following* Y93.7)
    - winds instrument Y93.J4 (*following* Y93.7)
  - property maintenance
    - exterior NEC Y93.H9 (*following* Y93.7)
    - interior NEC Y93.E9 (*following* Y93.7)
  - pruning (garden and lawn) Y93.H2 (*following* Y93.7)
  - pull-ups Y93.B2 (*following* Y93.7)
  - push-ups Y93.B2 (*following* Y93.7)
  - racquetball Y93.73
  - rafting (in calm and turbulent water) Y93.16
  - raking (leaves) Y93.H1 (*following* Y93.7)
  - rappelling Y93.32
  - refereeing a sports activity Y93.81
  - residential relocation Y93.E6 (*following* Y93.7)
  - rhythmic gymnastics Y93.43
  - rhythmic movement NEC Y93.49
  - riding
    - horseback Y93.52
    - rollercoaster Y93.I1 (*following* Y93.7)
  - rock climbing Y93.31
  - roller skating (inline) Y93.51
  - rollercoaster riding Y93.I1 (*following* Y93.7)
  - rough housing and horseplay Y93.83
  - rowing (in calm and turbulent water) Y93.16
  - rugby Y93.63
  - running Y93.Ø2
  - SCUBA diving Y93.15
  - sewing Y93.D2 (*following* Y93.7)
  - shoveling Y93.H1 (*following* Y93.7)
    - dirt Y93.H1 (*following* Y93.7)
    - snow Y93.H1 (*following* Y93.7)
  - showering (personal) Y93.E1 (*following* Y93.7)
  - sit-ups Y93.B2 (*following* Y93.7)
  - skateboarding Y93.51
  - skating (ice) Y93.21
    - roller Y93.51
  - skiing (alpine) (downhill) Y93.23
    - cross country Y93.24
    - nordic Y93.24
    - water Y93.17
  - sledding (snow) Y93.23
  - sleeping (sleep) Y93.84
  - smoking and grilling food Y93.G2 (*following* Y93.7)
  - snorkeling Y93.15
  - snow NEC Y93.29
    - boarding Y93.23
    - shoveling Y93.H1 (*following* Y93.7)
    - sledding Y93.23
    - tubing Y93.23
  - soccer Y93.66

Activity — *continued*
- softball Y93.64
- specified NEC Y93.89
- spectator at an event Y93.82
- sports NEC Y93.79
  - sports played as a team or group NEC Y93.69
  - sports played individually NEC Y93.59
- springboard diving Y93.12
- squash Y93.73
- stationary bike Y93.A1 (*following* Y93.7)
- step (stepping) exercise (class) Y93.A3 (*following* Y93.7)
- stepper machine Y93.A1 (*following* Y93.7)
- stove Y93.G3 (*following* Y93.7)
- string instrument playing Y93.J3 (*following* Y93.7)
- surfing Y93.18
  - wind Y93.18
- swimming Y93.11
- tackle football Y93.61
- tap dancing Y93.41
- tennis Y93.73
- tobogganing Y93.23
- touch football Y93.62
- track and field events (non-running) Y93.57
  - running Y93.Ø2
- trampoline Y93.44
- treadmill Y93.A1 (*following* Y93.7)
- trimming shrubs Y93.H2 (*following* Y93.7)
- tubing (in calm and turbulent water) Y93.16
  - snow Y93.23
- ultimate frisbee Y93.74
- underwater diving Y93.15
- unpacking in moving to a new residence Y93.E6 (*following* Y93.7)
- use of stove, oven and microwave oven Y93.G3 (*following* Y93.7)
- vacuuming Y93.E3 (*following* Y93.7)
- volleyball (beach) (court) Y93.68
- wake boarding Y93.17
- walking (on level or elevated terrain) Y93.Ø1
  - an animal Y93.K1 (*following* Y93.7)
- walking an animal Y93.K1 (*following* Y93.7)
- wall climbing Y93.31
- warm up and cool down exercises Y93.A2 (*following* Y93.7)
- water NEC Y93.19
  - aerobics Y93.14
  - craft NEC Y93.19
  - exercise Y93.14
  - polo Y93.13
  - skiing Y93.17
  - sliding Y93.18
  - survival training and testing Y93.19
- weeding (garden and lawn) Y93.H2 (*following* Y93.7)
- wind instrument playing Y93.J4 (*following* Y93.7)
- windsurfing Y93.18
- wrestling Y93.72
- yoga Y93.42

Adverse effect of drugs — *see* Table of Drugs and Chemicals

Aerosinusitis — *see* Air, pressure

After-effect, late — *see* Sequelae

Air
- blast in war operations — *see* War operations, air blast
- pressure
  - change, rapid
    - during
      - ascent W94.29 ☑
        - while (in) (surfacing from)
          - aircraft W94.23 ☑
          - deep water diving W94.21 ☑
          - underground W94.22 ☑
      - descent W94.39 ☑
        - in
          - aircraft W94.31 ☑
          - water W94.32 ☑
  - high, prolonged W94.Ø ☑
  - low, prolonged W94.12 ☑
    - due to residence or long visit at high altitude W94.11 ☑

Alpine sickness W94.11 ☑

Altitude sickness W94.11 ☑

Anaphylactic shock, anaphylaxis — *see* Table of Drugs and Chemicals

Andes disease W94.11 ☑

Arachnidism, arachnoidism X58 ☑

Arson (with intent to injure or kill) X97 ☑

Asphyxia, asphyxiation
- by
  - food (bone) (seed) — *see* categories T17 and T18 ☑
  - gas — *see also* Table of Drugs and Chemicals
    - legal
      - execution — *see* Legal, intervention, gas
      - intervention — *see* Legal, intervention, gas
- from
  - fire — *see also* Exposure, fire
    - in war operations — *see* War operations, fire
  - ignition — *see* Ignition
  - vomitus T17.81 ☑
- in war operations — *see* War operations, restriction of airway

Aspiration
- food (any type) (into respiratory tract) (with asphyxia, obstruction respiratory tract, suffocation) — *see* categories T17 and T18 ☑
- foreign body — *see* Foreign body, aspiration
- vomitus (with asphyxia, obstruction respiratory tract, suffocation) T17.81 ☑

Assassination (attempt) — *see* Assault

Assault (homicidal) (by) (in) YØ9
- arson X97 ☑
- bite (of human being) YØ4.1 ☑
- bodily force YØ4.8 ☑
  - bite YØ4.1 ☑
  - bumping into YØ4.2 ☑
  - sexual — *see* subcategories T74.Ø, T76.Ø ☑
  - unarmed fight YØ4.Ø ☑
- bomb X96.9 ☑
  - antipersonnel X96.Ø ☑
  - fertilizer X96.3 ☑
  - gasoline X96.1 ☑
  - letter X96.2 ☑
  - petrol X96.1 ☑
  - pipe X96.3 ☑
  - specified NEC X96.8 ☑
- brawl (hand) (fists) (foot) (unarmed) YØ4.Ø ☑
- burning, burns (by fire) NEC X97 ☑
  - acid YØ8.89 ☑
  - caustic, corrosive substance YØ8.89 ☑
  - chemical from swallowing caustic, corrosive substance — *see* Table of Drugs and Chemicals
  - cigarette(s) X97 ☑
  - hot object X98.9 ☑
    - fluid NEC X98.2 ☑
    - household appliance X98.3 ☑
    - specified NEC X98.8 ☑
    - steam X98.Ø ☑
    - tap water X98.1 ☑
    - vapors X98.Ø ☑
  - scalding — *see* Assault, burning
  - steam X98.Ø ☑
  - vitriol YØ8.89 ☑
- caustic, corrosive substance (gas) YØ8.89 ☑
- crashing of
  - aircraft YØ8.81 ☑
  - motor vehicle YØ3.8 ☑
    - pushed in front of YØ2.Ø ☑
    - run over YØ3.Ø ☑
    - specified NEC YØ3.8 ☑
- cutting or piercing instrument X99.9 ☑
  - dagger X99.2 ☑
  - glass X99.Ø ☑
  - knife X99.1 ☑
  - specified NEC X99.8 ☑
  - sword X99.2 ☑
- dagger X99.2 ☑
- drowning (in) X92.9 ☑
  - bathtub X92.Ø ☑
  - natural water X92.3 ☑
  - specified NEC X92.8 ☑
  - swimming pool X92.1 ☑
    - following fall X92.2 ☑
- dynamite X96.8 ☑
- explosive(s) (material) X96.9 ☑
- fight (hand) (fists) (foot) (unarmed) YØ4.Ø ☑
  - with weapon — *see* Assault, by type of weapon
- fire X97 ☑
- firearm X95.9 ☑
  - airgun X95.Ø1 ☑
  - handgun X93 ☑
  - hunting rifle X94.1 ☑
  - larger X94.9 ☑
    - specified NEC X94.8 ☑

Assault — *continued*
- firearm — *continued*
  - machine gun X94.2 ☑
  - shotgun X94.Ø ☑
  - specified NEC X95.8 ☑
- from high place YØ1 ☑
- gunshot (wound) NEC — *see* Assault, firearm, by type
- incendiary device X97 ☑
- injury YØ9
  - to child due to criminal abortion attempt NEC YØ8.89 ☑
- knife X99.1 ☑
- late effect of — *see* categories X92-YØ8 with 7th character S
- placing before moving object NEC YØ2.8 ☑
  - motor vehicle YØ2.Ø ☑
- poisoning — *see* categories T36-T65 with 7th character S
- puncture, any part of body — *see* Assault, cutting or piercing instrument
- pushing
  - before moving object NEC YØ2.8 ☑
    - motor vehicle YØ2.Ø ☑
    - subway train YØ2.1 ☑
    - train YØ2.1 ☑
  - from high place YØ1 ☑
- rape T74.2- ☑
- scalding — *see* Assault, burning
- sequelae of — *see* categories X92-YØ8 with 7th character S
- sexual (by bodily force) T74.2- ☑
- shooting — *see* Assault, firearm
- specified means NEC YØ8.89 ☑
- stab, any part of body — *see* Assault, cutting or piercing instrument
- steam X98.Ø ☑
- striking against
  - other person YØ4.2 ☑
  - sports equipment YØ8.Ø9 ☑
    - baseball bat YØ8.Ø2 ☑
    - hockey stick YØ8.Ø1 ☑
- struck by
  - sports equipment YØ8.Ø9 ☑
    - baseball bat YØ8.Ø2 ☑
    - hockey stick YØ8.Ø1 ☑
- submersion — *see* Assault, drowning
- violence YØ9
- weapon YØ9
  - blunt YØØ ☑
  - cutting or piercing — *see* Assault, cutting or piercing instrument
  - firearm — *see* Assault, firearm
- wound YØ9
  - cutting — *see* Assault, cutting or piercing instrument
  - gunshot — *see* Assault, firearm
  - knife X99.1 ☑
  - piercing — *see* Assault, cutting or piercing instrument
  - puncture — *see* Assault, cutting or piercing instrument
  - stab — *see* Assault, cutting or piercing instrument

Attack by mammals NEC W55.89 ☑

Avalanche — *see* Landslide

Aviator's disease — *see* Air, pressure

B

Barotitis, barodontalgia, barosinusitis, barotrauma (otitic) (sinus) — *see* Air, pressure

Battered (baby) (child) (person) (syndrome) X58 ☑

Bayonet wound W26.1 ☑
- in
  - legal intervention — *see* Legal, intervention, sharp object, bayonet
  - war operations — *see* War operations, combat
- stated as undetermined whether accidental or intentional Y28.8 ☑
- suicide (attempt) X78.2 ☑

Bean in nose — *see* categories T17 and T18 ☑

Bed set on fire NEC — *see* Exposure, fire, uncontrolled, building, bed

Beheading (by guillotine)
- homicide X99.9 ☑
- legal execution — *see* Legal, intervention

Bending, injury in (prolonged) (static) X5Ø.1 ☑

- **Bends** — *see* Air, pressure, change
- **Bite, bitten by**
  - alligator W58.Ø1 ☑
  - arthropod (nonvenomous) NEC W57 ☑
  - bull W55.21 ☑
  - cat W55.Ø1 ☑
  - cow W55.21 ☑
  - crocodile W58.11 ☑
  - dog W54.Ø ☑
  - goat W55.31 ☑
  - hoof stock NEC W55.31 ☑
  - horse W55.11 ☑
  - human being (accidentally) W5Ø.3 ☑
    - with intent to injure or kill YØ4.1 ☑
    - as, or caused by, a crowd or human stampede (with fall) W52 ☑
    - assault YØ4.1 ☑
    - homicide (attempt) YØ4.1 ☑
    - in
      - fight YØ4.1 ☑
  - insect (nonvenomous) W57 ☑
  - lizard (nonvenomous) W59.Ø1 ☑
  - mammal NEC W55.81 ☑
    - marine W56.31 ☑
  - marine animal (nonvenomous) W56.81 ☑
  - millipede W57 ☑
  - moray eel W56.51 ☑
  - mouse W53.Ø1 ☑
  - person(s) (accidentally) W5Ø.3 ☑
    - with intent to injure or kill YØ4.1 ☑
    - as, or caused by, a crowd or human stampede (with fall) W52 ☑
    - assault YØ4.1 ☑
    - homicide (attempt) YØ4.1 ☑
    - in
      - fight YØ4.1 ☑
  - pig W55.41 ☑
  - raccoon W55.51 ☑
  - rat W53.11 ☑
  - reptile W59.81 ☑
    - lizard W59.Ø1 ☑
    - snake W59.11 ☑
    - turtle W59.21 ☑
      - terrestrial W59.81 ☑
  - rodent W53.81 ☑
    - mouse W53.Ø1 ☑
    - rat W53.11 ☑
    - specified NEC W53.81 ☑
    - squirrel W53.21 ☑
  - shark W56.41 ☑
  - sheep W55.31 ☑
  - snake (nonvenomous) W59.11 ☑
  - spider (nonvenomous) W57 ☑
  - squirrel W53.21 ☑
- **Blast** (air) in war operations — *see* War operations, blast
- **Blizzard** X37.2 ☑
- **Blood alcohol level** Y9Ø.9
  - less than 2Ømg/1ØØml Y9Ø.Ø
  - presence in blood, level not specified Y9Ø.9
  - 2Ø-39mg/1ØØml Y9Ø.1
  - 4Ø-59mg/1ØØml Y9Ø.2
  - 6Ø-79mg/1ØØml Y9Ø.3
  - 8Ø-99mg/1ØØml Y9Ø.4
  - 1ØØ-119mg/1ØØml Y9Ø.5
  - 12Ø-199mg/1ØØml Y9Ø.6
  - 2ØØ-239mg/1ØØml Y9Ø.7
- **Blow** X58 ☑
  - by law-enforcing agent, police (on duty) — *see* Legal, intervention, manhandling
    - blunt object — *see* Legal, intervention, blunt object
- **Blowing up** — *see* Explosion
- **Brawl** (hand) (fists) (foot) YØ4.Ø ☑
- **Breakage** (accidental) (part of)
  - ladder (causing fall) W11 ☑
  - scaffolding (causing fall) W12 ☑
- **Broken**
  - glass, contact with — *see* Contact, with, glass
  - power line (causing electric shock) W85 ☑
- **Bumping against, into** (accidentally)
  - object NEC W22.8 ☑
    - caused by crowd or human stampede (with fall) W52 ☑
    - sports equipment W21.9 ☑
    - with fall — *see* Fall, due to, bumping against, object
  - person(s) W51 ☑
    - with fall WØ3 ☑
- **Bumping against, into** — *continued*
  - person(s) — *continued*
    - with fall — *continued*
      - due to ice or snow WØØ.Ø ☑
    - assault YØ4.2 ☑
    - caused by, a crowd or human stampede (with fall) W52 ☑
    - homicide (attempt) YØ4.2 ☑
  - sports equipment W21.9 ☑
- **Burn, burned, burning** (accidental) (by) (from) (on)
  - acid NEC — *see* Table of Drugs and Chemicals
  - bed linen — *see* Exposure, fire, uncontrolled, in building, bed
  - blowtorch XØ8.8 ☑
    - with ignition of clothing NEC XØ6.2 ☑
      - nightwear XØ5 ☑
  - bonfire, campfire (controlled) — *see also* Exposure, fire, controlled, not in building)
    - uncontrolled — *see* Exposure, fire, uncontrolled, not in building
  - candle XØ8.8 ☑
    - with ignition of clothing NEC XØ6.2 ☑
      - nightwear XØ5 ☑
  - caustic liquid, substance (external) (internal) NEC — *see* Table of Drugs and Chemicals
  - chemical (external) (internal) — *see also* Table of Drugs and Chemicals
    - in war operations — *see* War operations. fire
  - cigar(s) or cigarette(s) XØ8.8 ☑
    - with ignition of clothing NEC XØ6.2 ☑
      - nightwear XØ5 ☑
  - clothes, clothing NEC (from controlled fire) XØ6.2 ☑
    - with conflagration — *see* Exposure, fire, uncontrolled, building
      - not in building or structure — *see* Exposure, fire, uncontrolled, not in building
  - cooker (hot) X15.8 ☑
    - stated as undetermined whether accidental or intentional Y27.3 ☑
    - suicide (attempt) X77.3 ☑
  - electric blanket X16 ☑
  - engine (hot) X17 ☑
  - fire, flames — *see* Exposure, fire
  - flare, Very pistol — *see* Discharge, firearm NEC
  - heat
    - from appliance (electrical) (household) X15.8 ☑
      - cooker X15.8 ☑
      - hotplate X15.2 ☑
      - kettle X15.8 ☑
      - light bulb X15.8 ☑
      - saucepan X15.3 ☑
      - skillet X15.3 ☑
      - stated as undetermined whether accidental or intentional Y27.3 ☑
      - stove X15.Ø ☑
      - suicide (attempt) X77.3 ☑
      - toaster X15.1 ☑
    - in local application or packing during medical or surgical procedure Y63.5
  - heating
    - appliance, radiator or pipe X16 ☑
  - homicide (attempt) — *see* Assault, burning
  - hot
    - air X14.1 ☑
    - cooker X15.8 ☑
    - drink X1Ø.Ø ☑
    - engine X17 ☑
    - fat X1Ø.2 ☑
    - fluid NEC X12 ☑
    - food X1Ø.1 ☑
    - gases X14.1 ☑
    - heating appliance X16 ☑
    - household appliance NEC X15.8 ☑
    - kettle X15.8 ☑
    - liquid NEC X12 ☑
    - machinery X17 ☑
    - metal (molten) (liquid) NEC X18 ☑
    - object (not producing fire or flames) NEC X19 ☑
    - oil (cooking) X1Ø.2 ☑
    - pipe(s) X16 ☑
    - radiator X16 ☑
    - saucepan (glass) (metal) X15.3 ☑
    - stove (kitchen) X15.Ø ☑
    - substance NEC X19 ☑
      - caustic or corrosive NEC — *see* Table of Drugs and Chemicals
- **Burn, burned, burning** — *continued*
  - hot — *continued*
    - toaster X15.1 ☑
    - tool X17 ☑
    - vapor X13.1 ☑
    - water (tap) — *see* Contact, with, hot, tap water
  - hotplate X15.2 ☑
    - suicide (attempt) X77.3 ☑
  - ignition — *see* Ignition
  - in war operations — *see* War operations, fire
  - inflicted by other person X97 ☑
    - by hot objects, hot vapor, and steam — *see* Assault, burning, hot object
  - internal, from swallowed caustic, corrosive liquid, substance — *see* Table of Drugs and Chemicals
  - iron (hot) X15.8 ☑
    - stated as undetermined whether accidental or intentional Y27.3 ☑
    - suicide (attempt) X77.3 ☑
  - kettle (hot) X15.8 ☑
    - stated as undetermined whether accidental or intentional Y27.3 ☑
    - suicide (attempt) X77.3 ☑
  - lamp (flame) XØ8.8 ☑
    - with ignition of clothing NEC XØ6.2 ☑
      - nightwear XØ5 ☑
  - lighter (cigar) (cigarette) XØ8.8 ☑
    - with ignition of clothing NEC XØ6.2 ☑
      - nightwear XØ5 ☑
  - lightning — *see* subcategory T75.Ø ☑
    - causing fire — *see* Exposure, fire
  - liquid (boiling) (hot) NEC X12 ☑
    - stated as undetermined whether accidental or intentional Y27.2 ☑
    - suicide (attempt) X77.2 ☑
  - local application of externally applied substance in medical or surgical care Y63.5
  - machinery (hot) X17 ☑
  - matches XØ8.8 ☑
    - with ignition of clothing NEC XØ6.2 ☑
      - nightwear XØ5 ☑
  - mattress — *see* Exposure, fire, uncontrolled, building, bed
  - medicament, externally applied Y63.5
  - metal (hot) (liquid) (molten) NEC X18 ☑
  - nightwear (nightclothes, nightdress, gown, pajamas, robe) XØ5 ☑
  - object (hot) NEC X19 ☑
  - on board watercraft
    - due to
      - accident to watercraft V91.Ø9 ☑
        - powered craft V91.Ø3 ☑
          - ferry boat V91.Ø1 ☑
          - fishing boat V91.Ø2 ☑
          - jetskis V91.Ø3 ☑
          - liner V91.Ø1 ☑
          - merchant ship V91.ØØ ☑
          - passenger ship V91.Ø1 ☑
        - unpowered craft V91.Ø8 ☑
          - canoe V91.Ø5 ☑
          - inflatable V91.Ø6 ☑
          - kayak V91.Ø5 ☑
          - sailboat V91.Ø4 ☑
          - surf-board V91.Ø8 ☑
          - water skis V91.Ø7 ☑
          - windsurfer V91.Ø8 ☑
      - fire on board V93.Ø9 ☑
        - ferry boat V93.Ø1 ☑
        - fishing boat V93.Ø2 ☑
        - jetskis V93.Ø3 ☑
        - liner V93.Ø1 ☑
        - merchant ship V93.ØØ ☑
        - passenger ship V93.Ø1 ☑
        - powered craft NEC V93.Ø3 ☑
        - sailboat V93.Ø4 ☑
      - specified heat source NEC on board V93.19 ☑
        - ferry boat V93.11 ☑
        - fishing boat V93.12 ☑
        - jetskis V93.13 ☑
        - liner V93.11 ☑
        - merchant ship V93.1Ø ☑
        - passenger ship V93.11 ☑
        - powered craft NEC V93.13 ☑
        - sailboat V93.14 ☑
  - pipe (hot) X16 ☑
    - smoking XØ8.8 ☑

Burn, burned, burning — *continued*
- pipe — *continued*
  - smoking — *continued*
    - with ignition of clothing NEC XØ6.2 ☑
      - nightwear XØ5 ☑
- powder — *see* Powder burn
- radiator (hot) X16 ☑
- saucepan (hot) (glass) (metal) X15.3 ☑
  - stated as undetermined whether accidental or intentional Y27.3 ☑
  - suicide (attempt) X77.3 ☑
- self-inflicted X76 ☑
  - stated as undetermined whether accidental or intentional Y26 ☑
- stated as undetermined whether accidental or intentional Y27.Ø ☑
- steam X13.1 ☑
  - pipe X16 ☑
    - stated as undetermined whether accidental or intentional Y27.8 ☑
  - stated as undetermined whether accidental or intentional Y27.Ø ☑
  - suicide (attempt) X77.Ø ☑
- stove (hot) (kitchen) X15.Ø ☑
  - stated as undetermined whether accidental or intentional Y27.3 ☑
  - suicide (attempt) X77.3 ☑
- substance (hot) NEC X19 ☑
  - boiling X12 ☑
    - stated as undetermined whether accidental or intentional Y27.2 ☑
    - suicide (attempt) X77.2 ☑
  - molten (metal) X18 ☑
- suicide (attempt) NEC X76 ☑
  - hot
    - household appliance X77.3 ☑
    - object X77.9 ☑
- therapeutic misadventure
  - heat in local application or packing during medical or surgical procedure Y63.5
  - overdose of radiation Y63.2
- toaster (hot) X15.1 ☑
  - stated as undetermined whether accidental or intentional Y27.3 ☑
  - suicide (attempt) X77.3 ☑
- tool (hot) X17 ☑
- torch, welding XØ8.8 ☑
  - with ignition of clothing NEC XØ6.2 ☑
    - nightwear XØ5 ☑
- trash fire (controlled) — *see* Exposure, fire, controlled, not in building
  - uncontrolled — *see* Exposure, fire, uncontrolled, not in building
- vapor (hot) X13.1 ☑
  - stated as undetermined whether accidental or intentional Y27.Ø ☑
  - suicide (attempt) X77.Ø ☑
- Very pistol — *see* Discharge, firearm NEC

Butted by animal W55.82 ☑
- bull W55.22 ☑
- cow W55.22 ☑
- goat W55.32 ☑
- horse W55.12 ☑
- pig W55.42 ☑
- sheep W55.32 ☑

C

Caisson disease — *see* Air, pressure, change

Campfire (exposure to) (controlled) — *see also* Exposure, fire, controlled, not in building
- uncontrolled — *see* Exposure, fire, uncontrolled, not in building

Capital punishment (any means) — *see* Legal, intervention

Car sickness T75.3 ☑

Casualty (not due to war) NEC X58 ☑
- war — *see* War operations

Cat
- bite W55.Ø1 ☑
- scratch W55.Ø3 ☑

Cataclysm, cataclysmic (any injury) NEC — *see* Forces of nature

Catching fire — *see* Exposure, fire

Caught
- between
  - folding object W23.Ø ☑
  - objects (moving) (stationary and moving) W23.Ø ☑
    - and machinery — *see* Contact, with, by type of machine
    - stationary W23.1 ☑
  - sliding door and door frame W23.Ø ☑
- by, in
  - machinery (moving parts of) — *see* Contact, with, by type of machine
  - washing-machine wringer W23.Ø ☑
- under packing crate (due to losing grip) W23.1 ☑

Cave-in caused by cataclysmic earth surface movement or eruption — *see* Landslide

Change(s) in air pressure — *see* Air, pressure, change

Choked, choking (on) (any object except food or vomitus)
- food (bone) (seed) — *see* categories T17 and T18 ☑
- vomitus T17.81- ☑

Civil insurrection — *see* War operations

Cloudburst (any injury) X37.8 ☑

Cold, exposure to (accidental) (excessive) (extreme) (natural) (place) NEC — *see* Exposure, cold

Collapse
- building W2Ø.1 ☑
  - burning (uncontrolled fire) XØØ.2 ☑
- dam or man-made structure (causing earth movement) X36.Ø ☑
- machinery — *see* Contact, with, by type of machine
- structure W2Ø.1 ☑
  - burning (uncontrolled fire) XØØ.2 ☑

Collision (accidental) NEC — *see also* Accident, transport V89.9 ☑
- pedestrian W51 ☑
  - with fall WØ3 ☑
    - due to ice or snow WØØ.Ø ☑
    - involving pedestrian conveyance — *see* Accident, transport, pedestrian, conveyance
  - and
    - crowd or human stampede (with fall) W52 ☑
    - object W22.8 ☑
      - with fall — *see* Fall, due to, bumping against, object
- person(s) — *see* Collision, pedestrian
- transport vehicle NEC V89.9 ☑
  - and
    - avalanche, fallen or not moving — *see* Accident, transport
      - falling or moving — *see* Landslide
    - landslide, fallen or not moving — *see* Accident, transport
      - falling or moving — *see* Landslide
  - due to cataclysm — *see* Forces of nature, by type
  - intentional, purposeful suicide (attempt) — *see* Suicide, collision

Combustion, spontaneous — *see* Ignition

Complication (delayed) **of or following** (medical or surgical procedure) Y84.9
- with misadventure — *see* Misadventure
- amputation of limb(s) Y83.5
- anastomosis (arteriovenous) (blood vessel) (gastrojejunal) (tendon) (natural or artificial material) Y83.2
- aspiration (of fluid) Y84.4
  - tissue Y84.8
- biopsy Y84.8
- blood
  - sampling Y84.7
  - transfusion
    - procedure Y84.8
- bypass Y83.2
- catheterization (urinary) Y84.6
  - cardiac Y84.Ø
- colostomy Y83.3
- cystostomy Y83.3
- dialysis (kidney) Y84.1
- drug — *see* Table of Drugs and Chemicals
- due to misadventure — *see* Misadventure
- duodenostomy Y83.3
- electroshock therapy Y84.3
- external stoma, creation of Y83.3
- formation of external stoma Y83.3
- gastrostomy Y83.3
- graft Y83.2
- hypothermia (medically-induced) Y84.8

Complication (delayed) **of or following** — *continued*
- implant, implantation (of)
  - artificial
    - internal device (cardiac pacemaker) (electrodes in brain) (heart valve prosthesis) (orthopedic) Y83.1
    - material or tissue (for anastomosis or bypass) Y83.2
      - with creation of external stoma Y83.3
  - natural tissues (for anastomosis or bypass) Y83.2
    - with creation of external stoma Y83.3
- infusion
  - procedure Y84.8
- injection — *see* Table of Drugs and Chemicals
  - procedure Y84.8
- insertion of gastric or duodenal sound Y84.5
- insulin-shock therapy Y84.3
- paracentesis (abdominal) (thoracic) (aspirative) Y84.4
- procedures other than surgical operation — *see* Complication of or following, by type of procedure
- radiological procedure or therapy Y84.2
- removal of organ (partial) (total) NEC Y83.6
- sampling
  - blood Y84.7
  - fluid NEC Y84.4
  - tissue Y84.8
- shock therapy Y84.3
- surgical operation NEC — *see also* Complication of or following, by type of operation Y83.9
  - reconstructive NEC Y83.4
    - with
      - anastomosis, bypass or graft Y83.2
      - formation of external stoma Y83.3
  - specified NEC Y83.8
- transfusion — *see also* Table of Drugs and Chemicals
  - procedure Y84.8
- transplant, transplantation (heart) (kidney) (liver) (whole organ, any) Y83.Ø
  - partial organ Y83.4
- ureterostomy Y83.3
- vaccination — *see also* Table of Drugs and Chemicals
  - procedure Y84.8

Compression
- divers' squeeze — *see* Air, pressure, change
- trachea by
  - food (lodged in esophagus) — *see* categories T17 and T18 ☑
  - vomitus (lodged in esophagus) T17.81- ☑

Conflagration — *see* Exposure, fire, uncontrolled

Constriction (external)
- hair W49.Ø1 ☑
- jewelry W49.Ø4 ☑
- ring W49.Ø4 ☑
- rubber band W49.Ø3 ☑
- specified item NEC W49.Ø9 ☑
- string W49.Ø2 ☑
- thread W49.Ø2 ☑

Contact (accidental)
- with
  - abrasive wheel (metalworking) W31.1 ☑
  - alligator W58.Ø9 ☑
    - bite W58.Ø1 ☑
    - crushing W58.Ø3 ☑
    - strike W58.Ø2 ☑
  - amphibian W62.9 ☑
    - frog W62.Ø ☑
    - toad W62.1 ☑
  - animal (nonvenomous) NEC W64 ☑
    - marine W56.89 ☑
      - bite W56.81 ☑
      - dolphin — *see* Contact, with, dolphin
      - fish NEC — *see* Contact, with, fish
      - mammal — *see* Contact, with, mammal, marine
      - orca — *see* Contact, with, orca
      - sea lion — *see* Contact, with, sea lion
      - shark — *see* Contact, with, shark
      - strike W56.82 ☑
  - animate mechanical force NEC W64 ☑
  - arrow W21.89 ☑
    - not thrown, projected or falling W45.8 ☑
  - arthropods (nonvenomous) W57 ☑
  - axe W27.Ø ☑
  - band-saw (industrial) W31.2 ☑
  - bayonet — *see* Bayonet wound
  - bee(s) X58 ☑

- **Contact** — *continued*
  - with — *continued*
    - bench-saw (industrial) W31.2 ☑
    - bird W61.99 ☑
      - bite W61.91 ☑
      - chicken — *see* Contact, with, chicken
      - duck — *see* Contact, with, duck
      - goose — *see* Contact, with, goose
      - macaw — *see* Contact, with, macaw
      - parrot — *see* Contact, with, parrot
      - psittacine — *see* Contact, with, psittacine
      - strike W61.92 ☑
      - turkey — *see* Contact, with, turkey
    - blender W29.Ø ☑
    - boiling water X12 ☑
      - stated as undetermined whether accidental or intentional Y27.2 ☑
      - suicide (attempt) X77.2 ☑
    - bore, earth-drilling or mining (land) (seabed) W31.Ø ☑
    - buffalo — *see* Contact, with, hoof stock NEC
    - bull W55.29 ☑
      - bite W55.21 ☑
      - gored W55.22 ☑
      - strike W55.22 ☑
    - bumper cars W31.81 ☑
    - camel — *see* Contact, with, hoof stock NEC
    - can
      - lid W26.8 ☑
      - opener W27.4 ☑
        - powered W29.Ø ☑
    - cat W55.Ø9 ☑
      - bite W55.Ø1 ☑
      - scratch W55.Ø3 ☑
    - caterpillar (venomous) X58 ☑
    - centipede (venomous) X58 ☑
    - chain
      - hoist W24.Ø ☑
        - agricultural operations W3Ø.89 ☑
      - saw W29.3 ☑
    - chicken W61.39 ☑
      - peck W61.33 ☑
      - strike W61.32 ☑
    - chisel W27.Ø ☑
    - circular saw W31.2 ☑
    - cobra X58 ☑
    - combine (harvester) W3Ø.Ø ☑
    - conveyer belt W24.1 ☑
    - cooker (hot) X15.8 ☑
      - stated as undetermined whether accidental or intentional Y27.3 ☑
      - suicide (attempt) X77.3 ☑
    - coral X58 ☑
    - cotton gin W31.82 ☑
    - cow W55.29 ☑
      - bite W55.21 ☑
      - strike W55.22 ☑
    - crane W24.Ø ☑
      - agricultural operations W3Ø.89 ☑
    - crocodile W58.19 ☑
      - bite W58.11 ☑
      - crushing W58.13 ☑
      - strike W58.12 ☑
    - dagger W26.1 ☑
      - stated as undetermined whether accidental or intentional Y28.2 ☑
      - suicide (attempt) X78.2 ☑
    - dairy equipment W31.82 ☑
    - dart W21.89 ☑
      - not thrown, projected or falling W45.8 ☑
    - deer — *see* Contact, with, hoof stock NEC
    - derrick W24.Ø ☑
      - agricultural operations W3Ø.89 ☑
        - hay W3Ø.2 ☑
    - dog W54.8 ☑
      - bite W54.Ø ☑
      - strike W54.1 ☑
    - dolphin W56.Ø9 ☑
      - bite W56.Ø1 ☑
      - strike W56.Ø2 ☑
    - donkey — *see* Contact, with, hoof stock NEC
    - drill (powered) W29.8 ☑
      - earth (land) (seabed) W31.Ø ☑
      - nonpowered W27.8 ☑
    - drive belt W24.Ø ☑
      - agricultural operations W3Ø.89 ☑

- **Contact** — *continued*
  - with — *continued*
    - dry ice — *see* Exposure, cold, man-made
    - dryer (clothes) (powered) (spin) W29.2 ☑
    - duck W61.69 ☑
      - bite W61.61 ☑
      - strike W61.62 ☑
    - earth (-)
      - drilling machine (industrial) W31.Ø ☑
      - scraping machine in stationary use W31.83 ☑
    - edge of stiff paper W26.2 ☑
    - electric
      - beater W29.Ø ☑
      - blanket X16 ☑
      - fan W29.2 ☑
        - commercial W31.82 ☑
      - knife W29.1 ☑
      - mixer W29.Ø ☑
    - elevator (building) W24.Ø ☑
      - agricultural operations W3Ø.89 ☑
        - grain W3Ø.3 ☑
    - engine(s), hot NEC X17 ☑
    - excavating machine W31.Ø ☑
    - farm machine W3Ø.9 ☑
    - feces — *see* Contact, with, by type of animal
    - fer de lance X58 ☑
    - fish W56.59 ☑
      - bite W56.51 ☑
      - shark — *see* Contact, with, shark
      - strike W56.52 ☑
    - flying horses W31.81 ☑
    - forging (metalworking) machine W31.1 ☑
    - fork W27.4 ☑
    - forklift (truck) W24.Ø ☑
      - agricultural operations W3Ø.89 ☑
    - frog W62.Ø ☑
    - garden
      - cultivator (powered) W29.3 ☑
        - riding W3Ø.89 ☑
      - fork W27.1 ☑
    - gas turbine W31.3 ☑
    - Gila monster X58 ☑
    - giraffe — *see* Contact, with, hoof stock NEC
    - glass (sharp) (broken) W25 ☑
      - assault X99.Ø ☑
      - due to fall — *see* Fall, by type
      - stated as undetermined whether accidental or intentional Y28.Ø ☑
      - suicide (attempt) X78.Ø ☑
      - with subsequent fall W18.Ø2 ☑
    - goat W55.39 ☑
      - bite W55.31 ☑
      - strike W55.32 ☑
    - goose W61.59 ☑
      - bite W61.51 ☑
      - strike W61.52 ☑
    - hand
      - saw W27.Ø ☑
      - tool (not powered) NEC W27.8 ☑
        - powered W29.8 ☑
    - harvester W3Ø.Ø ☑
    - hay-derrick W3Ø.2 ☑
    - heating
      - appliance (hot) X16 ☑
      - pad (electric) X16 ☑
    - heat NEC X19 ☑
      - from appliance (electrical) (household) — *see* Contact, with, hot, household appliance
        - heating appliance X16 ☑
    - hedge-trimmer (powered) W29.3 ☑
    - hoe W27.1 ☑
    - hoist (chain) (shaft) NEC W24.Ø ☑
      - agricultural W3Ø.89 ☑
    - hoof stock NEC W55.39 ☑
      - bite W55.31 ☑
      - strike W55.32 ☑
    - hornet(s) X58 ☑
    - horse W55.19 ☑
      - bite W55.11 ☑
      - strike W55.12 ☑
    - hot
      - air X14.1 ☑
        - inhalation X14.Ø ☑
      - cooker X15.8 ☑
      - drinks X1Ø.Ø ☑
      - engine X17 ☑

- **Contact** — *continued*
  - with — *continued*
    - hot — *continued*
      - fats X1Ø.2 ☑
      - fluids NEC X12 ☑
        - assault X98.2 ☑
        - suicide (attempt) X77.2 ☑
        - undetermined whether accidental or intentional Y27.2 ☑
      - food X1Ø.1 ☑
      - gases X14.1 ☑
        - inhalation X14.Ø ☑
      - heating appliance X16 ☑
      - household appliance X15.8 ☑
        - assault X98.3 ☑
        - cooker X15.8 ☑
        - hotplate X15.2 ☑
        - kettle X15.8 ☑
        - light bulb X15.8 ☑
        - object NEC X19 ☑
          - assault X98.8 ☑
          - stated as undetermined whether accidental or intentional Y27.9 ☑
          - suicide (attempt) X77.8 ☑
        - saucepan X15.3 ☑
        - skillet X15.3 ☑
        - stated as undetermined whether accidental or intentional Y27.3 ☑
        - stove X15.Ø ☑
        - suicide (attempt) X77.3 ☑
        - toaster X15.1 ☑
      - kettle X15.8 ☑
      - light bulb X15.8 ☑
      - liquid NEC — *see also* Burn X12 ☑
        - drinks X1Ø.Ø ☑
        - stated as undetermined whether accidental or intentional Y27.2 ☑
        - suicide (attempt) X77.2 ☑
        - tap water X11.8 ☑
          - stated as undetermined whether accidental or intentional Y27.1 ☑
          - suicide (attempt) X77.1 ☑
      - machinery X17 ☑
      - metal (molten) (liquid) NEC X18 ☑
      - object (not producing fire or flames) NEC X19 ☑
      - oil (cooking) X1Ø.2 ☑
      - pipe X16 ☑
      - plate X15.2 ☑
      - radiator X16 ☑
      - saucepan (glass) (metal) X15.3 ☑
      - skillet X15.3 ☑
      - stove (kitchen) X15.Ø ☑
      - substance NEC X19 ☑
      - tap-water X11.8 ☑
        - assault X98.1 ☑
        - heated on stove X12 ☑
          - stated as undetermined whether accidental or intentional Y27.2 ☑
          - suicide (attempt) X77.2 ☑
        - in bathtub X11.Ø ☑
        - running X11.1 ☑
          - stated as undetermined whether accidental or intentional Y27.1 ☑
          - suicide (attempt) X77.1 ☑
      - toaster X15.1 ☑
      - tool X17 ☑
      - vapors X13.1 ☑
        - inhalation X13.Ø ☑
      - water (tap) X11.8 ☑
        - boiling X12 ☑
          - stated as undetermined whether accidental or intentional Y27.2 ☑
          - suicide (attempt) X77.2 ☑
        - heated on stove X12 ☑
          - stated as undetermined whether accidental or intentional Y27.2 ☑
          - suicide (attempt) X77.2 ☑
        - in bathtub X11.Ø ☑
        - running X11.1 ☑
          - stated as undetermined whether accidental or intentional Y27.1 ☑
          - suicide (attempt) X77.1 ☑
    - hotplate X15.2 ☑
    - ice-pick W27.4 ☑
    - insect (nonvenomous) NEC W57 ☑
    - kettle (hot) X15.8 ☑

Contact — *continued*
- with — *continued*
  - steam — *continued*
    - engine W31.3 ☑
    - inhalation X13.Ø ☑
    - pipe X16 ☑
    - shovel W31.89 ☑
  - stove (hot) (kitchen) X15.Ø ☑
  - substance, hot NEC X19 ☑
    - molten (metal) X18 ☑
  - sword W26.1 ☑
    - assault X99.2 ☑
    - stated as undetermined whether accidental or intentional Y28.2 ☑
    - suicide (attempt) X78.2 ☑
  - tarantula X58 ☑
  - thresher W3Ø.Ø ☑
  - tin can lid W26.8 ☑
  - toad W62.1 ☑
  - toaster (hot) X15.1 ☑
  - tool W27.8 ☑
    - hand (not powered) W27.8 ☑
      - auger W27.Ø ☑
      - axe W27.Ø ☑
      - can opener W27.4 ☑
      - chisel W27.Ø ☑
      - fork W27.4 ☑
      - garden W27.1 ☑
      - handsaw W27.Ø ☑
      - hoe W27.1 ☑
      - ice-pick W27.4 ☑
      - kitchen utensil W27.4 ☑
      - manual
        - lawn mower W27.1 ☑
        - sewing machine W27.8 ☑
      - meat grinder W27.4 ☑
      - needle (sewing) W27.3 ☑
        - hypodermic W46.Ø ☑
          - contaminated W46.1 ☑
      - paper cutter W27.5 ☑
      - pitchfork W27.1 ☑
      - rake W27.1 ☑
      - scissors W27.2 ☑
      - screwdriver W27.Ø ☑
      - specified NEC W27.8 ☑
      - workbench W27.Ø ☑
    - hot X17 ☑
    - powered W29.8 ☑
      - blender W29.Ø ☑
        - commercial W31.82 ☑
      - can opener W29.Ø ☑
        - commercial W31.82 ☑
      - chainsaw W29.3 ☑
      - clothes dryer W29.2 ☑
        - commercial W31.82 ☑
      - dishwasher W29.2 ☑
        - commercial W31.82 ☑
      - edger W29.3 ☑
      - electric fan W29.2 ☑
        - commercial W31.82 ☑
      - electric knife W29.1 ☑
      - food processor W29.Ø ☑
        - commercial W31.82 ☑
      - garbage disposal W29.Ø ☑
        - commercial W31.82 ☑
      - garden tool W29.3 ☑
      - hedge trimmer W29.3 ☑
      - ice maker W29.Ø ☑
        - commercial W31.82 ☑
      - kitchen appliance W29.Ø ☑
        - commercial W31.82 ☑
      - lawn mower W28 ☑
      - meat grinder W29.Ø ☑
        - commercial W31.82 ☑
      - mixer W29.Ø ☑
        - commercial W31.82 ☑
      - rototiller W29.3 ☑
      - sewing machine W29.2 ☑
        - commercial W31.82 ☑
      - washing machine W29.2 ☑
        - commercial W31.82 ☑
  - transmission device (belt, cable, chain, gear, pinion, shaft) W24.1 ☑
    - agricultural operations W3Ø.89 ☑
  - turbine (gas) (water-driven) W31.3 ☑
  - turkey W61.49 ☑

Contact — *continued*
- with — *continued*
  - turkey — *continued*
    - peck W61.43 ☑
    - strike W61.42 ☑
  - turtle (nonvenomous) W59.29 ☑
    - bite W59.21 ☑
    - strike W59.22 ☑
    - terrestrial W59.89 ☑
      - bite W59.81 ☑
      - crushing W59.83 ☑
      - strike W59.82 ☑
  - under-cutter W31.Ø ☑
  - urine — *see* Contact, with, by type of animal
  - vehicle
    - agricultural use (transport) — *see* Accident, transport, agricultural vehicle
      - not on public highway W3Ø.81 ☑
    - industrial use (transport) — *see* Accident, transport, industrial vehicle
      - not on public highway W31.83 ☑
    - off-road use (transport) — *see* Accident, transport, all-terrain or off-road vehicle
      - not on public highway W31.83 ☑
    - special construction use (transport) — *see* Accident, transport, construction vehicle
      - not on public highway W31.83 ☑
  - venomous
    - animal X58 ☑
    - arthropods X58 ☑
    - lizard X58 ☑
    - marine animal NEC X58 ☑
    - marine plant NEC X58 ☑
    - millipedes (tropical) X58 ☑
    - plant(s) X58 ☑
    - snake X58 ☑
    - spider X58 ☑
  - viper X58 ☑
  - washing-machine (powered) W29.2 ☑
  - wasp X58 ☑
  - weaving-machine W31.89 ☑
  - winch W24.Ø ☑
    - agricultural operations W3Ø.89 ☑
  - wire NEC W24.Ø ☑
    - agricultural operations W3Ø.89 ☑
  - wood slivers W45.8 ☑
  - yellow jacket X58 ☑
  - zebra — *see* Contact, with, hoof stock NEC
- pressure X5Ø.9 ☑
- stress X5Ø.9 ☑

Coup de soleil X32 ☑

Crash
- aircraft (in transit) (powered) V95.9 ☑
  - balloon V96.Ø1 ☑
  - fixed wing NEC (private) V95.21 ☑
    - commercial V95.31 ☑
  - glider V96.21 ☑
    - hang V96.11 ☑
    - powered V95.11 ☑
  - helicopter V95.Ø1 ☑
  - in war operations — *see* War operations, destruction of aircraft
  - microlight V95.11 ☑
  - nonpowered V96.9 ☑
    - specified NEC V96.8 ☑
  - powered NEC V95.8 ☑
  - stated as
    - homicide (attempt) YØ8.81 ☑
    - suicide (attempt) X83.Ø ☑
  - ultralight V95.11 ☑
- spacecraft V95.41 ☑
- transport vehicle NEC — *see also* Accident, transport V89.9 ☑
  - homicide (attempt) YØ3.8 ☑
  - motor NEC (traffic) V89.2 ☑
    - homicide (attempt) YØ3.8 ☑
    - suicide (attempt) — *see* Suicide, collision

Cruelty (mental) (physical) (sexual) X58 ☑

Crushed (accidentally) X58 ☑
- between objects (moving) (stationary and moving) W23.Ø ☑
  - stationary W23.1 ☑
- by
  - alligator W58.Ø3 ☑
  - avalanche NEC — *see* Landslide
  - cave-in W2Ø.Ø ☑

Crushed — *continued*
- by — *continued*
  - cave-in — *continued*
    - caused by cataclysmic earth surface movement — *see* Landslide
  - crocodile W58.13 ☑
  - crowd or human stampede W52 ☑
  - falling
    - aircraft V97.39 ☑
      - in war operations — *see* War operations, destruction of aircraft
    - earth, material W2Ø.Ø ☑
      - caused by cataclysmic earth surface movement — *see* Landslide
    - object NEC W2Ø.8 ☑
  - landslide NEC — *see* Landslide
  - lizard (nonvenomous) W59.Ø9 ☑
  - machinery — *see* Contact, with, by type of machine
  - reptile NEC W59.89 ☑
  - snake (nonvenomous) W59.13 ☑
- in
  - machinery — *see* Contact, with, by type of machine

Cut, cutting (any part of body) (accidental) — *see also* Contact, with, by object or machine
- during medical or surgical treatment as misadventure — *see* Index to Diseases and Injuries, Complications
- homicide (attempt) — *see* Assault, cutting or piercing instrument
- inflicted by other person — *see* Assault, cutting or piercing instrument
- legal
  - execution — *see* Legal, intervention
  - intervention — *see* Legal, intervention, sharp object
- machine NEC — *see also* Contact, with, by type of machine W31.9 ☑
- self-inflicted — *see* Suicide, cutting or piercing instrument
- suicide (attempt) — *see* Suicide, cutting or piercing instrument

Cyclone (any injury) X37.1 ☑

D

Decapitation (accidental circumstances) NEC X58 ☑
- homicide X99.9 ☑
- legal execution — *see* Legal, intervention

Dehydration from lack of water X58 ☑

Deprivation X58 ☑

Derailment (accidental)
- railway (rolling stock) (train) (vehicle) (without antecedent collision) V81.7 ☑
  - with antecedent collision — *see* Accident, transport, railway vehicle occupant
- streetcar (without antecedent collision) V82.7 ☑
  - with antecedent collision — *see* Accident, transport, streetcar occupant

Descent
- parachute (voluntary) (without accident to aircraft) V97.29 ☑
  - due to accident to aircraft — *see* Accident, transport, aircraft

Desertion X58 ☑

Destitution X58 ☑

Disability, late effect or sequela of injury — *see* Sequelae

Discharge (accidental)
- airgun W34.Ø1Ø ☑
  - assault X95.Ø1 ☑
  - homicide (attempt) X95.Ø1 ☑
  - stated as undetermined whether accidental or intentional Y24.Ø ☑
  - suicide (attempt) X74.Ø1 ☑
- BB gun — *see* Discharge, airgun
- firearm (accidental) W34.ØØ ☑
  - assault X95.9 ☑
  - handgun (pistol) (revolver) W32.Ø ☑
    - assault X93 ☑
    - homicide (attempt) X93 ☑
    - legal intervention — *see* Legal, intervention, firearm, handgun
    - stated as undetermined whether accidental or intentional Y22 ☑
    - suicide (attempt) X72 ☑
  - homicide (attempt) X95.9 ☑
  - hunting rifle W33.Ø2 ☑

E

Explosion — *continued*
- explosive — *continued*
  - specified — *continued*
    - in — *continued*
      - suicide (attempt) X75 ☑
- factory (munitions) W40.8 ☑
- fertilizer bomb W40.8 ☑
  - assault X96.3 ☑
  - homicide (attempt) X96.3 ☑
  - suicide (attempt) X75 ☑
- firearm (parts) NEC W34.19 ☑
  - airgun W34.110 ☑
  - BB gun W34.110 ☑
  - gas, air or spring-operated gun NEC W34.118 ☑
  - hangun W32.1 ☑
  - hunting rifle W33.12 ☑
  - larger firearm W33.10 ☑
    - specified NEC W33.19 ☑
  - machine gun W33.13 ☑
  - paintball gun W34.111 ☑
  - pellet gun W34.110 ☑
  - shotgun W33.11 ☑
  - Very pistol [flare] W34.19 ☑
- fire-damp W40.1 ☑
- fireworks W39 ☑
- gas (coal) (explosive) W40.1 ☑
  - cylinder W36.9 ☑
    - aerosol can W36.1 ☑
    - air tank W36.2 ☑
    - pressurized W36.3 ☑
    - specified NEC W36.8 ☑
- gasoline (fumes) (tank) not in moving motor vehicle W40.1 ☑
  - bomb W40.8 ☑
    - assault X96.1 ☑
    - homicide (attempt) X96.1 ☑
    - suicide (attempt) X75 ☑
  - in motor vehicle — *see* Accident, transport, by type of vehicle
- grain store W40.8 ☑
- grenade W40.8 ☑
  - in
    - assault X96.8 ☑
    - homicide (attempt) X96.8 ☑
    - legal intervention
      - injuring
        - bystander Y35.192 ☑
        - law enforcement personnel Y35.191 ☑
        - suspect Y35.193 ☑
        - unspecified person Y35.199 ☑
    - suicide (attempt) X75 ☑
- handgun (parts) — *see* Explosion, firearm, hangun (parts)
- homicide (attempt) X96.9 ☑
  - antipersonnel bomb — *see* Explosion, antipersonnel bomb
  - fertilizer bomb — *see* Explosion, fertilizer bomb
  - gasoline bomb — *see* Explosion, gasoline bomb
  - letter bomb — *see* Explosion, letter bomb
  - pipe bomb — *see* Explosion, pipe bomb
  - specified NEC X96.8 ☑
- hose, pressurized W37.8 ☑
- hot water heater, tank (in machinery) W35 ☑
  - on watercraft — *see* Explosion, in, watercraft
- in, on
  - dump W40.8 ☑
  - factory W40.8 ☑
  - mine (of explosive gases) NEC W40.1 ☑
  - watercraft V93.59 ☑
    - powered craft V93.53 ☑
      - ferry boat V93.51 ☑
      - fishing boat V93.52 ☑
      - jetskis V93.53 ☑
      - liner V93.51 ☑
      - merchant ship V93.50 ☑
      - passenger ship V93.51 ☑
      - sailboat V93.54 ☑
- letter bomb W40.8 ☑
  - assault X96.2 ☑
  - homicide (attempt) X96.2 ☑
  - suicide (attempt) X75 ☑
- machinery — *see also* Contact, with, by type of machine
  - on board watercraft — *see* Explosion, in, watercraft
  - pressure vessel — *see* Explosion, by type of vessel
- methane W40.1 ☑

Explosion — *continued*
- mine W40.1 ☑
- missile NEC W40.8 ☑
- mortar bomb W40.8 ☑
  - in
    - assault X96.8 ☑
    - homicide (attempt) X96.8 ☑
    - legal intervention
      - injuring
        - bystander Y35.192 ☑
        - law enforcement personnel Y35.191 ☑
        - suspect Y35.193 ☑
        - unspecified person Y35.199 ☑
    - suicide (attempt) X75 ☑
- munitions (dump) (factory) W40.8 ☑
- pipe, pressurized W37.8 ☑
  - bomb W40.8 ☑
    - assault X96.4 ☑
    - homicide (attempt) X96.4 ☑
    - suicide (attempt) X75 ☑
- pressure, pressurized
  - cooker W38 ☑
  - gas tank (in machinery) W36.3 ☑
  - hose W37.8 ☑
  - pipe W37.8 ☑
  - specified device NEC W38 ☑
  - tire W37.8 ☑
    - bicycle W37.0 ☑
  - vessel (in machinery) W38 ☑
- propane W40.1 ☑
- self-inflicted X75 ☑
- shell (artillery) NEC W40.8 ☑
  - during war operations — *see* War operations, explosion
  - in
    - legal intervention
      - injuring
        - bystander Y35.122 ☑
        - law enforcement personnel Y35.121 ☑
        - suspect Y35.123 ☑
        - unspecified person Y35.129 ☑
    - war — *see* War operations, explosion
- spacecraft V95.45 ☑
- stated as undetermined whether accidental or intentional Y25 ☑
- steam or water lines (in machinery) W37.8 ☑
- stove W40.9 ☑
- suicide (attempt) X75 ☑
- tire, pressurized W37.8 ☑
  - bicycle W37.0 ☑
- undetermined whether accidental or intentional Y25 ☑
- vehicle tire NEC W37.8 ☑
  - bicycle W37.0 ☑
- war operations — *see* War operations, explosion

Exposure (to) X58 ☑
- air pressure change — *see* Air, pressure
- cold (accidental) (excessive) (extreme) (natural) (place) X31 ☑
  - assault Y08.89 ☑
  - due to
    - man-made conditions W93.8 ☑
      - dry ice (contact) W93.01 ☑
        - inhalation W93.02 ☑
      - liquid air (contact) (hydrogen) (nitrogen) W93.11 ☑
        - inhalation W93.12 ☑
      - refrigeration unit (deep freeze) W93.2 ☑
      - suicide (attempt) X83.2 ☑
    - weather (conditions) X31 ☑
  - homicide (attempt) Y08.89 ☑
  - self-inflicted X83.2 ☑
- due to abandonment or neglect X58 ☑
- electric current W86.8 ☑
  - appliance (faulty) W86.8 ☑
    - domestic W86.0 ☑
  - caused by other person Y08.89 ☑
  - conductor (faulty) W86.1 ☑
  - control apparatus (faulty) W86.1 ☑
  - electric power generating plant, distribution station W86.1 ☑
  - electroshock gun — *see* Exposure, electric current, taser
  - high-voltage cable W85 ☑
  - homicide (attempt) Y08.89 ☑
  - legal execution — *see* Legal, intervention, specified means NEC

Exposure — *continued*
- electric current — *continued*
  - lightning — *see* subcategory T75.0 ☑
  - live rail W86.8 ☑
  - misadventure in medical or surgical procedure in electroshock therapy Y63.4
  - motor (electric) (faulty) W86.8 ☑
    - domestic W86.0 ☑
  - self-inflicted X83.1 ☑
  - specified NEC W86.8 ☑
    - domestic W86.0 ☑
  - stun gun — *see* Exposure, electric current, taser
  - suicide (attempt) X83.1 ☑
  - taser W86.8 ☑
    - assault Y08.89 ☑
    - legal intervention — *see* category Y35 ☑
    - self-harm (intentional) X83.8 ☑
    - undeterned intent Y33 ☑
  - third rail W86.8 ☑
  - transformer (faulty) W86.1 ☑
  - transmission lines W85 ☑
- environmental tobacco smoke X58 ☑
- excessive
  - cold — *see* Exposure, cold
  - heat (natural) NEC X30 ☑
    - man-made W92 ☑
- factor(s) NOS X58 ☑
  - environmental NEC X58 ☑
    - man-made NEC W99 ☑
    - natural NEC — *see* Forces of nature
  - specified NEC X58 ☑
- fire, flames (accidental) X08.8 ☑
  - assault X97 ☑
  - campfire — *see* Exposure, fire, controlled, not in building
  - controlled (in)
    - with ignition (of) clothing — *see also* Ignition, clothes X06.2 ☑
      - nightwear X05 ☑
    - bonfire — *see* Exposure, fire, controlled, not in building
    - brazier (in building or structure) — *see also* Exposure, fire, controlled, building
      - not in building or structure — *see* Exposure, fire, controlled, not in building
    - building or structure X02.0 ☑
      - with
        - fall from building X02.3 ☑
        - from building X02.5 ☑
        - injury due to building collapse X02.2 ☑
        - smoke inhalation X02.1 ☑
      - hit by object from building X02.4 ☑
      - specified mode of injury NEC X02.8 ☑
    - fireplace, furnace or stove — *see* Exposure, fire, controlled, building
    - not in building or structure X03.0 ☑
      - with
        - fall X03.3 ☑
        - smoke inhalation X03.1 ☑
      - hit by object X03.4 ☑
      - specified mode of injury NEC X03.8 ☑
    - trash — *see* Exposure, fire, controlled, not in building
  - fireplace — *see* Exposure, fire, controlled, building
  - fittings or furniture (in building or structure) (uncontrolled) — *see* Exposure, fire, uncontrolled, building
  - forest (uncontrolled) — *see* Exposure, fire, uncontrolled, not in building
  - grass (uncontrolled) — *see* Exposure, fire, uncontrolled, not in building
  - hay (uncontrolled) — *see* Exposure, fire, uncontrolled, not in building
  - homicide (attempt) X97 ☑
  - ignition of highly flammable material X04 ☑
  - in, of, on, starting in
    - machinery — *see* Contact, with, by type of machine
    - motor vehicle (in motion) — *see also* Accident, transport, occupant by type of vehicle V87.8 ☑
      - with collision — *see* Collision
    - railway rolling stock, train, vehicle V81.81 ☑
      - with collision — *see* Accident, transport, railway vehicle occupant
    - street car (in motion) V82.8 ☑

Exposure — *continued*
- fire, flames — *continued*
  - in, of, on, starting in — *continued*
    - street car — *continued*
      - with collision — *see* Accident, transport, streetcar occupant
    - transport vehicle NEC — *see also* Accident, transport
      - with collision — *see* Collision
    - war operations — *see also* War operations, fire
      - from nuclear explosion — *see* War operations, nuclear weapons
    - watercraft (in transit) (not in transit) V91.09 ☑
      - localized — *see* Burn, on board watercraft, due to, fire on board
      - powered craft V91.03 ☑
        - ferry boat V91.01 ☑
        - fishing boat V91.02 ☑
        - jet skis V91.03 ☑
        - liner V91.01 ☑
        - merchant ship V91.00 ☑
        - passenger ship V91.01 ☑
      - unpowered craft V91.08 ☑
        - canoe V91.05 ☑
        - inflatable V91.06 ☑
        - kayak V91.05 ☑
        - sailboat V91.04 ☑
        - surf-board V91.08 ☑
        - waterskis V91.07 ☑
        - windsurfer V91.08 ☑
  - lumber (uncontrolled) — *see* Exposure, fire, uncontrolled, not in building
  - mine (uncontrolled) — *see* Exposure, fire, uncontrolled, not in building
  - prairie (uncontrolled) — *see* Exposure, fire, uncontrolled, not in building
  - resulting from
    - explosion — *see* Explosion
    - lightning X08.8 ☑
  - self-inflicted X76 ☑
  - specified NEC X08.8 ☑
  - started by other person X97 ☑
  - stated as undetermined whether accidental or intentional Y26 ☑
  - stove — *see* Exposure, fire, controlled, building
  - suicide (attempt) X76 ☑
  - tunnel (uncontrolled) — *see* Exposure, fire, uncontrolled, not in building
  - uncontrolled
    - in building or structure X00.0 ☑
      - with
        - fall from building X00.3 ☑
        - injury due to building collapse X00.2 ☑
        - jump from building X00.5 ☑
        - smoke inhalation X00.1 ☑
      - bed X08.00 ☑
        - due to
          - cigarette X08.01 ☑
          - specified material NEC X08.09 ☑
      - furniture NEC X08.20 ☑
        - due to
          - cigarette X08.21 ☑
          - specified material NEC X08.29 ☑
      - hit by object from building X00.4 ☑
      - sofa X08.10 ☑
        - due to
          - cigarette X08.11 ☑
          - specified material NEC X08.19 ☑
      - specified mode of injury NEC X00.8 ☑
    - not in building or structure (any) X01.0 ☑
      - with
        - fall X01.3 ☑
        - smoke inhalation X01.1 ☑
      - hit by object X01.4 ☑
      - specified mode of injury NEC X01.8 ☑
  - undetermined whether accidental or intentional Y26 ☑
- forces of nature NEC — *see* Forces of nature
- G-forces (abnormal) W49.9 ☑
- gravitational forces (abnormal) W49.9 ☑
- heat (natural) NEC — *see* Heat
- high-pressure jet (hydraulic) (pneumatic) W49.9 ☑
- hydraulic jet W49.9 ☑
- inanimate mechanical force W49.9 ☑
- jet, high-pressure (hydraulic) (pneumatic) W49.9 ☑
- lightning — *see* subcategory T75.0 ☑

Exposure — *continued*
- lightning — *see* subcategory — *continued*
  - causing fire — *see* Exposure, fire
- mechanical forces NEC W49.9 ☑
  - animate NEC W64 ☑
  - inanimate NEC W49.9 ☑
- noise W42.9 ☑
  - supersonic W42.0 ☑
- noxious substance — *see* Table of Drugs and Chemicals
- pneumatic jet W49.9 ☑
- prolonged in deep-freeze unit or refrigerator W93.2 ☑
- radiation — *see* Radiation
- smoke — *see also* Exposure, fire
  - tobacco, second hand Z77.22
- specified factors NEC X58 ☑
- sunlight X32 ☑
  - man-made (sun lamp) W89.8 ☑
    - tanning bed W89.1 ☑
- supersonic waves W42.0 ☑
- transmission line(s), electric W85 ☑
- vibration W49.9 ☑
- waves
  - infrasound W49.9 ☑
  - sound W42.9 ☑
  - supersonic W42.0 ☑
- weather NEC — *see* Forces of nature

External cause status Y99.9
- child assisting in compensated work for family Y99.8
- civilian activity done for financial or other compensation Y99.0
- civilian activity done for income or pay Y99.0
- family member assisting in compensated work for other family member Y99.8
- hobby not done for income Y99.8
- leisure activity Y99.8
- military activity Y99.1
- off-duty activity of military personnel Y99.8
- recreation or sport not for income or while a student Y99.8
- specified NEC Y99.8
- student activity Y99.8
- volunteer activity Y99.2

F

Factors, supplemental
- alcohol
  - blood level
    - less than 20mg/100ml Y90.0
    - presence in blood, level not specified Y90.9
    - 20-39mg/100ml Y90.1
    - 40-59mg/100ml Y90.2
    - 60-79mg/100ml Y90.3
    - 80-99mg/100ml Y90.4
    - 100-119mg/100ml Y90.5
    - 120-199mg/100ml Y90.6
    - 200-239mg/100ml Y90.7
    - 240mg/100ml or more Y90.8
  - presence in blood, but level not specified Y90.9
- environmental-pollution-related condition- see Z57 ☑
- nosocomial condition Y95
- work-related condition Y99.0

Failure
- in suture or ligature during surgical procedure Y65.2
- mechanical, of instrument or apparatus (any) (during any medical or surgical procedure) Y65.8
- sterile precautions (during medical and surgical care) — *see* Misadventure, failure, sterile precautions, by type of procedure
- to
  - introduce tube or instrument Y65.4
    - endotracheal tube during anesthesia Y65.3
  - make curve (transport vehicle) NEC — *see* Accident, transport
  - remove tube or instrument Y65.4

Fall, falling (accidental) W19 ☑
- building W20.1 ☑
  - burning (uncontrolled fire) X00.3 ☑
- down
  - embankment W17.81 ☑
  - escalator W10.0 ☑
  - hill W17.81 ☑
  - ladder W11 ☑
  - ramp W10.2 ☑
  - stairs, steps W10.9 ☑

Fall, falling — *continued*
- due to
  - bumping against
    - object W18.00 ☑
      - sharp glass W18.02 ☑
      - specified NEC W18.09 ☑
      - sports equipment W18.01 ☑
    - person W03 ☑
      - due to ice or snow W00.0 ☑
      - on pedestrian conveyance — *see* Accident, transport, pedestrian, conveyance
  - collision with another person W03 ☑
    - due to ice or snow W00.0 ☑
    - involving pedestrian conveyance — *see* Accident, transport, pedestrian, conveyance
  - grocery cart tipping over W17.82 ☑
  - ice or snow W00.9 ☑
    - from one level to another W00.2 ☑
      - on stairs or steps W00.1 ☑
    - involving pedestrian conveyance — *see* Accident, transport, pedestrian, conveyance
    - on same level W00.0 ☑
  - slipping (on moving sidewalk) W01.0 ☑
    - with subsequent striking against object W01.10 ☑
      - furniture W01.190 ☑
      - sharp object W01.119 ☑
        - glass W01.110 ☑
        - power tool or machine W01.111 ☑
        - specified NEC W01.118 ☑
      - specified NEC W01.198 ☑
  - striking against
    - object W18.00 ☑
      - sharp glass W18.02 ☑
      - specified NEC W18.09 ☑
      - sports equipment W18.01 ☑
    - person W03 ☑
      - due to ice or snow W00.0 ☑
      - on pedestrian conveyance — *see* Accident, transport, pedestrian, conveyance
- earth (with asphyxia or suffocation (by pressure)) — *see* Earth, falling
- from, off, out of
  - aircraft NEC (with accident to aircraft NEC) V97.0 ☑
    - while boarding or alighting V97.1 ☑
  - balcony W13.0 ☑
  - bed W06 ☑
  - boat, ship, watercraft NEC (with drowning or submersion) — *see* Drowning, due to, fall overboard
    - with hitting bottom or object V94.0 ☑
  - bridge W13.1 ☑
  - building W13.9 ☑
    - burning (uncontrolled fire) X00.3 ☑
  - cavity W17.2 ☑
  - chair W07 ☑
  - cherry picker W17.89 ☑
  - cliff W15 ☑
  - dock W17.4 ☑
  - embankment W17.81 ☑
  - escalator W10.0 ☑
  - flagpole W13.8 ☑
  - furniture NEC W08 ☑
  - grocery cart W17.82 ☑
  - haystack W17.89 ☑
  - high place NEC W17.89 ☑
    - stated as undetermined whether accidental or intentional Y30 ☑
  - hole W17.2 ☑
  - incline W10.2 ☑
  - ladder W11 ☑
  - lifting device W17.89 ☑
  - machine, machinery — *see also* Contact, with, by type of machine
    - not in operation W17.89 ☑
  - manhole W17.1 ☑
  - mobile elevated work platform [MEWP] W17.89 ☑
  - motorized mobility scooter W05.2 ☑
  - one level to another NEC W17.89 ☑
    - intentional, purposeful, suicide (attempt) X80 ☑
    - stated as undetermined whether accidental or intentional Y30 ☑
  - pit W17.2 ☑
  - playground equipment W09.8 ☑
    - jungle gym W09.2 ☑
    - slide W09.0 ☑

- **Fall, falling** — *continued*
  - structure — *continued*
    - burning (uncontrolled fire) XØØ.3 ☑
  - through
    - bridge W13.1 ☑
    - floor W13.3 ☑
    - roof W13.2 ☑
    - wall W13.8 ☑
    - window W13.4 ☑
  - timber W2Ø.8 ☑
  - tree (caused by lightning) W2Ø.8 ☑
  - while being carried or supported by other person(s) WØ4 ☑
- **Fallen on by**
  - animal (not being ridden) NEC W55.89 ☑
- **Felo-de-se** — *see* Suicide
- **Fight** (hand) (fists) (foot) — *see* Assault, fight
- **Fire** (accidental) — *see* Exposure, fire
- **Firearm discharge** — *see* Discharge, firearm
- **Fireball effects from nuclear explosion in war operations** — *see* War operations, nuclear weapons
- **Fireworks** (explosion) W39 ☑
- **Flash burns from explosion** — *see* Explosion
- **Flood** (any injury) (caused by) X38 ☑
  - collapse of man-made structure causing earth movement X36.Ø ☑
  - tidal wave — *see* Forces of nature, tidal wave
- **Food** (any type) **in**
  - air passages (with asphyxia, obstruction, or suffocation) — *see* categories T17 and T18 ☑
  - alimentary tract causing asphyxia (due to compression of trachea) — *see* categories T17 and T18 ☑
- **Forces of nature** X39.8 ☑
  - avalanche X36.1 ☑
    - causing transport accident — *see* Accident, transport, by type of vehicle
  - blizzard X37.2 ☑
  - cataclysmic storm X37.9 ☑
    - with flood X38 ☑
    - blizzard X37.2 ☑
    - cloudburst X37.8 ☑
    - cyclone X37.1 ☑
    - dust storm X37.3 ☑
    - hurricane X37.Ø ☑
    - specified storm NEC X37.8 ☑
    - storm surge X37.Ø ☑
    - tornado X37.1 ☑
    - twister X37.1 ☑
    - typhoon X37.Ø ☑
  - cloudburst X37.8 ☑
  - cold (natural) X31 ☑
  - cyclone X37.1 ☑
  - dam collapse causing earth movement X36.Ø ☑
  - dust storm X37.3 ☑
  - earth movement X36.1 ☑
    - caused by dam or structure collapse X36.Ø ☑
    - earthquake X34 ☑
  - earthquake X34 ☑
  - flood (caused by) X38 ☑
    - dam collapse X36.Ø ☑
    - tidal wave — *see* Forces of nature, tidal wave
  - heat (natural) X3Ø ☑
  - hurricane X37.Ø ☑
  - landslide X36.1 ☑
    - causing transport accident — *see* Accident, transport, by type of vehicle
  - lightning — *see* subcategory T75.Ø ☑
    - causing fire — *see* Exposure, fire
  - mudslide X36.1 ☑
    - causing transport accident — *see* Accident, transport, by type of vehicle
  - radiation (natural) X39.Ø8 ☑
    - radon X39.Ø1 ☑
  - radon X39.Ø1 ☑
  - specified force NEC X39.8 ☑
  - storm surge X37.Ø ☑
  - structure collapse causing earth movement X36.Ø ☑
  - sunlight X32 ☑
  - tidal wave X37.41 ☑
    - due to
      - earthquake X37.41 ☑
      - landslide X37.43 ☑
      - storm X37.42 ☑
      - volcanic eruption X37.41 ☑
  - tornado X37.1 ☑
  - tsunami X37.41 ☑
- **Forces of nature** — *continued*
  - twister X37.1 ☑
  - typhoon X37.Ø ☑
  - volcanic eruption X35 ☑
- **Foreign body**
  - aspiration — *see* Index to Diseases and Injuries, Foreign body, respiratory tract
  - embedded in skin W45 ☑
  - entering through skin W45.8 ☑
    - can lid W26.8 ☑
    - nail W45.Ø ☑
    - paper W26.2 ☑
    - specified NEC W45.8 ☑
    - splinter W45.8 ☑
- **Forest fire** (exposure to) — *see* Exposure, fire, uncontrolled, not in building
- **Found injured** X58 ☑
  - from exposure (to) — *see* Exposure
  - on
    - highway, road(way), street V89.9 ☑
    - railway right of way V81.9 ☑
- **Fracture** (circumstances unknown or unspecified) X58 ☑
  - due to specified cause NEC X58 ☑
- **Freezing** — *see* Exposure, cold
- **Frostbite** X31 ☑
  - due to man-made conditions — *see* Exposure, cold, man-made
- **Frozen** — *see* Exposure, cold

G

- **Gored by bull** W55.22 ☑
- **Gunshot wound** W34.ØØ ☑

H

- **Hailstones, injured by** X39.8 ☑
- **Hanged herself or himself** — *see* Hanging, self-inflicted
- **Hanging** (accidental) — *see also* category T71 ☑
  - legal execution — *see* Legal, intervention, specified means NEC
- **Heat** (effects of) (excessive) X3Ø ☑
  - due to
    - man-made conditions W92 ☑
      - on board watercraft V93.29 ☑
        - fishing boat V93.22 ☑
        - merchant ship V93.2Ø ☑
        - passenger ship V93.21 ☑
        - sailboat V93.24 ☑
        - specified powered craft NEC V93.23 ☑
    - weather (conditions) X3Ø ☑
  - from
    - electric heating apparatus causing burning X16 ☑
    - nuclear explosion in war operations — *see* War operations, nuclear weapons
  - inappropriate in local application or packing in medical or surgical procedure Y63.5
- **Hemorrhage**
  - delayed following medical or surgical treatment without mention of misadventure — *see* Index to Diseases and Injuries, Complication(s)
  - during medical or surgical treatment as misadventure — *see* Index to Diseases and Injuries, Complication(s)
- **High**
  - altitude (effects) — *see* Air, pressure, low
  - level of radioactivity, effects — *see* Radiation
  - pressure (effects) — *see* Air, pressure, high
  - temperature, effects — *see* Heat
- **Hit, hitting** (accidental) by — *see* Struck by
- **Hitting against** — *see* Striking against
- **Homicide** (attempt) (justifiable) — *see* Assault
- **Hot**
  - place, effects — *see also* Heat
  - weather, effects X3Ø ☑
- **House fire** (uncontrolled) — *see* Exposure, fire, uncontrolled, building
- **Humidity, causing problem** X39.8 ☑
- **Hunger** X58 ☑
- **Hurricane** (any injury) X37.Ø ☑
- **Hypobarism, hypobaropathy** — *see* Air, pressure, low

I

- **Ictus**
  - caloris — *see also* Heat
- **Ictus** — *continued*
  - solaris X3Ø ☑
- **Ignition** (accidental) — *see also* Exposure, fire XØ8.8 ☑
  - anesthetic gas in operating room W4Ø.1 ☑
  - apparel XØ6.2 ☑
    - from highly flammable material XØ4 ☑
    - nightwear XØ5 ☑
  - bed linen (sheets) (spreads) (pillows) (mattress) — *see* Exposure, fire, uncontrolled, building, bed
  - benzine XØ4 ☑
  - clothes, clothing NEC (from controlled fire) XØ6.2 ☑
    - from
      - highly flammable material XØ4 ☑
  - ether XØ4 ☑
    - in operating room W4Ø.1 ☑
  - explosive material — *see* Explosion
  - gasoline XØ4 ☑
  - jewelry (plastic) (any) XØ6.Ø ☑
  - kerosene XØ4 ☑
  - material
    - explosive — *see* Explosion
    - highly flammable with secondary explosion XØ4 ☑
  - nightwear XØ5 ☑
  - paraffin XØ4 ☑
  - petrol XØ4 ☑
- **Immersion** (accidental) — *see also* Drowning
  - hand or foot due to cold (excessive) X31 ☑
- **Implantation of quills of porcupine** W55.89 ☑
- **Inanition** (from) (hunger) X58 ☑
  - thirst X58 ☑
- **Inappropriate operation performed**
  - correct operation on wrong side or body part (wrong side) (wrong site) Y65.53
  - operation intended for another patient done on wrong patient Y65.52
  - wrong operation performed on correct patient Y65.51
- **Inattention after, at birth** (homicidal intent) (infanticidal intent) X58 ☑
- **Incident, adverse**
  - device
    - anesthesiology Y7Ø.8
      - accessory Y7Ø.2
      - diagnostic Y7Ø.Ø
      - miscellaneous Y7Ø.8
      - monitoring Y7Ø.Ø
      - prosthetic Y7Ø.2
      - rehabilitative Y7Ø.1
      - surgical Y7Ø.3
      - therapeutic Y7Ø.1
    - cardiovascular Y71.8
      - accessory Y71.2
      - diagnostic Y71.Ø
      - miscellaneous Y71.8
      - monitoring Y71.Ø
      - prosthetic Y71.2
      - rehabilitative Y71.1
      - surgical Y71.3
      - therapeutic Y71.1
    - gastroenterology Y73.8
      - accessory Y73.2
      - diagnostic Y73.Ø
      - miscellaneous Y73.8
      - monitoring Y73.Ø
      - prosthetic Y73.2
      - rehabilitative Y73.1
      - surgical Y73.3
      - therapeutic Y73.1
    - general
      - hospital Y74.8
        - accessory Y74.2
        - diagnostic Y74.Ø
        - miscellaneous Y74.8
        - monitoring Y74.Ø
        - prosthetic Y74.2
        - rehabilitative Y74.1
        - surgical Y74.3
        - therapeutic Y74.1
      - surgical Y81.8
        - accessory Y81.2
        - diagnostic Y81.Ø
        - miscellaneous Y81.8
        - monitoring Y81.Ø
        - prosthetic Y81.2
        - rehabilitative Y81.1
        - surgical Y81.3
        - therapeutic Y81.1
    - gynecological Y76.8
      - accessory Y76.2

- **Incident, adverse** — *continued*
  - device — *continued*
    - gynecological — *continued*
      - diagnostic Y76.Ø
      - miscellaneous Y76.8
      - monitoring Y76.Ø
      - prosthetic Y76.2
      - rehabilitative Y76.1
      - surgical Y76.3
      - therapeutic Y76.1
    - medical Y82.9
      - specified type NEC Y82.8
    - neurological Y75.8
      - accessory Y75.2
      - diagnostic Y75.Ø
      - miscellaneous Y75.8
      - monitoring Y75.Ø
      - prosthetic Y75.2
      - rehabilitative Y75.1
      - surgical Y75.3
      - therapeutic Y75.1
    - obstetrical Y76.8
      - accessory Y76.2
      - diagnostic Y76.Ø
      - miscellaneous Y76.8
      - monitoring Y76.Ø
      - prosthetic Y76.2
      - rehabilitative Y76.1
      - surgical Y76.3
      - therapeutic Y76.1
    - ophthalmic Y77.8
      - accessory Y77.2
      - contact lens (rigid gas permeable) (soft (hydrophilic)) Y77.11
      - diagnostic Y77.Ø
      - miscellaneous Y77.8
      - monitoring Y77.Ø
      - prosthetic Y77.2
      - rehabilitative Y77.19
      - surgical Y77.3
      - therapeutic Y77.19
    - orthopedic Y79.8
      - accessory Y79.2
      - diagnostic Y79.Ø
      - miscellaneous Y79.8
      - monitoring Y79.Ø
      - prosthetic Y79.2
      - rehabilitative Y79.1
      - surgical Y79.3
      - therapeutic Y79.1
    - otorhinolaryngological Y72.8
      - accessory Y72.2
      - diagnostic Y72.Ø
      - miscellaneous Y72.8
      - monitoring Y72.Ø
      - prosthetic Y72.2
      - rehabilitative Y72.1
      - surgical Y72.3
      - therapeutic Y72.1
    - personal use Y74.8
      - accessory Y74.2
      - diagnostic Y74.Ø
      - miscellaneous Y74.8
      - monitoring Y74.Ø
      - prosthetic Y74.2
      - rehabilitative Y74.1
      - surgical Y74.3
      - therapeutic Y74.1
    - physical medicine Y8Ø.8
      - accessory Y8Ø.2
      - diagnostic Y8Ø.Ø
      - miscellaneous Y8Ø.8
      - monitoring Y8Ø.Ø
      - prosthetic Y8Ø.2
      - rehabilitative Y8Ø.1
      - surgical Y8Ø.3
      - therapeutic Y8Ø.1
    - plastic surgical Y81.8
      - accessory Y81.2
      - diagnostic Y81.Ø
      - miscellaneous Y81.8
      - monitoring Y81.Ø
      - prosthetic Y81.2
      - rehabilitative Y81.1
      - surgical Y81.3
      - therapeutic Y81.1
    - radiological Y78.8
      - accessory Y78.2
      - diagnostic Y78.Ø

- **Incident, adverse** — *continued*
  - device — *continued*
    - radiological — *continued*
      - miscellaneous Y78.8
      - monitoring Y78.Ø
      - prosthetic Y78.2
      - rehabilitative Y78.1
      - surgical Y78.3
      - therapeutic Y78.1
    - urology Y73.8
      - accessory Y73.2
      - diagnostic Y73.Ø
      - miscellaneous Y73.8
      - monitoring Y73.Ø
      - prosthetic Y73.2
      - rehabilitative Y73.1
      - surgical Y73.3
      - therapeutic Y73.1
- **Incineration** (accidental) — *see* Exposure, fire
- **Infanticide** — *see* Assault
- **Infrasound waves** (causing injury) W49.9 ☑
- **Ingestion**
  - foreign body (causing injury) (with obstruction) — *see* Foreign body, alimentary canal
  - poisonous
    - plant(s) X58 ☑
    - substance NEC — *see* Table of Drugs and Chemicals
- **Inhalation**
  - excessively cold substance, man-made — *see* Exposure, cold, man-made
  - food (any type) (into respiratory tract) (with asphyxia, obstruction respiratory tract, suffocation) — *see* categories T17 and T18 ☑
  - foreign body — *see* Foreign body, aspiration
  - gastric contents (with asphyxia, obstruction respiratory passage, suffocation) T17.81- ☑
  - hot air or gases X14.Ø ☑
  - liquid air, hydrogen, nitrogen W93.12 ☑
    - suicide (attempt) X83.2 ☑
  - steam X13.Ø ☑
    - assault X98.Ø ☑
    - stated as undetermined whether accidental or intentional Y27.Ø ☑
    - suicide (attempt) X77.Ø ☑
  - toxic gas — *see* Table of Drugs and Chemicals
  - vomitus (with asphyxia, obstruction respiratory passage, suffocation) T17.81- ☑
- **Injury, injured** (accidental(ly)) NOS X58 ☑
  - by, caused by, from
    - assault — *see* Assault
    - law-enforcing agent, police, in course of legal intervention — *see* Legal intervention
    - suicide (attempt) X83.8 ☑
  - due to, in
    - civil insurrection — *see* War operations
    - fight — *see also* Assault, fight YØ4.Ø ☑
    - war operations — *see* War operations
  - homicide — *see also* Assault YØ9
  - inflicted (by)
    - in course of arrest (attempted), suppression of disturbance, maintenance of order, by law-enforcing agents — *see* Legal intervention
    - other person
      - stated as
        - accidental X58 ☑
        - intentional, homicide (attempt) — *see* Assault
        - undetermined whether accidental or intentional Y33 ☑
  - purposely (inflicted) by other person(s) — *see* Assault
  - self-inflicted X83.8 ☑
    - stated as accidental X58 ☑
  - specified cause NEC X58 ☑
  - undetermined whether accidental or intentional Y33 ☑
- **Insolation, effects** X3Ø ☑
- **Insufficient nourishment** X58 ☑
- **Interruption of respiration** (by)
  - food (lodged in esophagus) — *see* categories T17 and T18 ☑
  - vomitus (lodged in esophagus) T17.81- ☑
- **Intervention, legal** — *see* Legal intervention
- **Intoxication**
  - drug — *see* Table of Drugs and Chemicals
  - poison — *see* Table of Drugs and Chemicals

J

- **Jammed** (accidentally)
  - between objects (moving) (stationary and moving) W23.Ø ☑
    - stationary W23.1 ☑
- **Jumped, jumping**
  - before moving object NEC X81.8 ☑
    - motor vehicle X81.Ø ☑
    - subway train X81.1 ☑
    - train X81.1 ☑
    - undetermined whether accidental or intentional Y31 ☑
  - from
    - boat (into water) voluntarily, without accident (to or on boat) W16.712 ☑
      - striking bottom W16.722 ☑
        - causing drowning W16.721 ☑
      - with
        - accident to or on boat — *see* Accident, watercraft
        - drowning or submersion W16.711 ☑
          - suicide (attempt) X71.3 ☑
    - building — *see also* Jumped, from, high place W13.9 ☑
      - burning (uncontrolled fire) XØØ.5 ☑
    - high place NEC W17.89 ☑
      - suicide (attempt) X8Ø ☑
      - undetermined whether accidental or intentional Y3Ø ☑
    - structure — *see also* Jumped, from, high place W13.9 ☑
      - burning (uncontrolled fire) XØØ.5 ☑
  - into water W16.92 ☑
    - causing drowning W16.91 ☑
    - from, off watercraft — *see* Jumped, from, boat
    - in
      - natural body W16.612 ☑
        - causing drowning W16.611 ☑
        - striking bottom W16.622 ☑
          - causing drowning W16.621 ☑
      - specified place NEC W16.812 ☑
        - causing drowning W16.811 ☑
        - striking
          - bottom W16.822 ☑
            - causing drowning W16.821 ☑
          - wall W16.832 ☑
            - causing drowning W16.831 ☑
      - swimming pool W16.512 ☑
        - causing drowning W16.511 ☑
        - striking
          - bottom W16.522 ☑
            - causing drowning W16.521 ☑
          - wall W16.532 ☑
            - causing drowning W16.531 ☑
    - suicide (attempt) X71.3 ☑

K

- **Kicked by**
  - animal NEC W55.82 ☑
  - person(s) (accidentally) W5Ø.1 ☑
    - with intent to injure or kill YØ4.Ø ☑
    - as, or caused by, a crowd or human stampede (with fall) W52 ☑
    - assault YØ4.Ø ☑
    - homicide (attempt) YØ4.Ø ☑
    - in
      - fight YØ4.Ø ☑
      - legal intervention
        - injuring
          - bystander Y35.812 ☑
          - law enforcement personnel Y35.811 ☑
          - suspect Y35.813 ☑
          - unspecified person Y35.819 ☑
- **Kicking**
  - against
    - object W22.8 ☑
      - sports equipment W21.9 ☑
      - stationary W22.Ø9 ☑
        - sports equipment W21.89 ☑
    - person — *see* Striking against, person
    - sports equipment W21.9 ☑
  - carpet stretcher with knee X5Ø.3 ☑
- **Killed, killing** (accidentally) NOS — *see also* Injury X58 ☑

- **Killed, killing** — *continued*
  - in
    - action — *see* War operations
    - brawl, fight (hand) (fists) (foot) Y04.Ø ☑
      - by weapon — *see also* Assault
        - cutting, piercing — *see* Assault, cutting or piercing instrument
        - firearm — *see* Discharge, firearm, by type, homicide
  - self
    - stated as
      - accident NOS X58 ☑
      - suicide — *see* Suicide
      - undetermined whether accidental or intentional Y33 ☑
- **Kneeling** (prolonged (static) X5Ø.1 ☑
- **Knocked down** (accidentally) (by) NOS X58 ☑
  - animal (not being ridden) NEC — *see also* Struck by, by type of animal
  - crowd or human stampede W52 ☑
  - person W51 ☑
    - in brawl, fight Y04.Ø ☑
  - transport vehicle NEC — *see also* Accident, transport VØ9.9 ☑

L

- **Laceration NEC** — *see* Injury
- **Lack of**
  - care (helpless person) (infant) (newborn) X58 ☑
  - food except as result of abandonment or neglect X58 ☑
    - due to abandonment or neglect X58 ☑
  - water except as result of transport accident X58 ☑
    - due to transport accident — *see* Accident, transport, by type
    - helpless person, infant, newborn X58 ☑
- **Landslide** (falling on transport vehicle) X36.1 ☑
  - caused by collapse of man-made structure X36.Ø ☑
- **Late effect** — *see* Sequelae
- **Legal**
  - execution (any method) — *see* Legal, intervention
  - intervention (by)
    - baton — *see* Legal, intervention, blunt object, baton
    - bayonet — *see* Legal, intervention, sharp object, bayonet
    - blow — *see* Legal, intervention, manhandling
    - blunt object
      - baton
        - injuring
          - bystander Y35.312 ☑
          - law enforcement personnel Y35.311 ☑
          - suspect Y35.313 ☑
          - unspecified person Y35.319 ☑
      - injuring
        - bystander Y35.3Ø2 ☑
        - law enforcement personnel Y35.3Ø1 ☑
        - suspect Y35.3Ø3 ☑
        - unspecified person Y35.3Ø9 ☑
      - specified NEC
        - injuring
          - bystander Y35.392 ☑
          - law enforcement personnel Y35.391 ☑
          - suspect Y35.393 ☑
          - unspecified person Y35.399 ☑
      - stave
        - injuring
          - bystander Y35.392 ☑
          - law enforcement personnel Y35.391 ☑
          - suspect Y35.393 ☑
          - unspecified person Y35.399 ☑
    - bomb — *see* Legal, intervention, explosive
    - conducted energy device
      - injuring
        - bystander Y35.832 ☑
        - law enforcement personnel Y35.831 ☑
        - suspect Y35.833 ☑
        - unspecified person Y35.839 ☑
    - cutting or piercing instrument — *see* Legal, intervention, sharp object
    - dynamite — *see* Legal, intervention, explosive, dynamite
    - electroshock device (taser)
      - injuring
        - bystander Y35.832 ☑
        - law enforcement personnel Y35.831 ☑

- **Legal** — *continued*
  - intervention — *continued*
    - electroshock device — *continued*
      - injuring — *continued*
        - suspect Y35.833 ☑
        - unspecified person Y35.839 ☑
    - explosive(s)
      - dynamite
        - injuring
          - bystander Y35.112 ☑
          - law enforcement personnel Y35.111 ☑
          - suspect Y35.113 ☑
          - unspecified person Y35.119 ☑
      - grenade
        - injuring
          - bystander Y35.192 ☑
          - law enforcement personnel Y35.191 ☑
          - suspect Y35.193 ☑
          - unspecified person Y35.199 ☑
      - injuring
        - bystander Y35.1Ø2 ☑
        - law enforcement personnel Y35.1Ø1 ☑
        - suspect Y35.1Ø3 ☑
        - unspecified person Y35.1Ø9 ☑
      - mortar bomb
        - injuring
          - bystander Y35.192 ☑
          - law enforcement personnel Y35.191 ☑
          - suspect Y35.193 ☑
          - unspecified person Y35.199 ☑
      - shell
        - injuring
          - bystander Y35.122 ☑
          - law enforcement personnel Y35.121 ☑
          - suspect Y35.123 ☑
          - unspecified person Y35.129 ☑
      - specified NEC
        - injuring
          - bystander Y35.192 ☑
          - law enforcement personnel Y35.191 ☑
          - suspect Y35.193 ☑
          - unspecified person Y35.199 ☑
    - firearm(s) (discharge)
      - handgun
        - injuring
          - bystander Y35.Ø22 ☑
          - law enforcement personnel Y35.Ø21 ☑
          - suspect Y35.Ø23 ☑
          - unspecified person Y35.Ø29 ☑
      - injuring
        - bystander Y35.ØØ2 ☑
        - law enforcement personnel Y35.ØØ1 ☑
        - suspect Y35.ØØ3 ☑
        - unspecified person Y35.ØØ9 ☑
      - machine gun
        - injuring
          - bystander Y35.Ø12 ☑
          - law enforcement personnel Y35.Ø11 ☑
          - suspect Y35.Ø13 ☑
          - unspecified person Y35.Ø19 ☑
      - rifle pellet
        - injuring
          - bystander Y35.Ø32 ☑
          - law enforcement personnel Y35.Ø31 ☑
          - suspect Y35.Ø33 ☑
          - unspecified person Y35.Ø39 ☑
      - rubber bullet
        - injuring
          - bystander Y35.Ø42 ☑
          - law enforcement personnel Y35.Ø41 ☑
          - suspect Y35.Ø43 ☑
          - unspecified person Y35.Ø49 ☑
      - shotgun — *see* Legal, intervention, firearm, specified NEC
      - specified NEC
        - injuring
          - bystander Y35.Ø92 ☑
          - law enforcement personnel Y35.Ø91 ☑
          - suspect Y35.Ø93 ☑
          - unspecified person Y35.Ø99 ☑
    - gas (asphyxiation) (poisoning)
      - injuring
        - bystander Y35.2Ø2 ☑
        - law enforcement personnel Y35.2Ø1 ☑
        - suspect Y35.2Ø3 ☑
        - unspecified person Y35.2Ø9 ☑

- **Legal** — *continued*
  - intervention — *continued*
    - gas — *continued*
      - specified NEC
        - injuring
          - bystander Y35.292 ☑
          - law enforcement personnel Y35.291 ☑
          - suspect Y35.293 ☑
          - unspecified person Y35.299 ☑
      - tear gas
        - injuring
          - bystander Y35.212 ☑
          - law enforcement personnel Y35.211 ☑
          - suspect Y35.213 ☑
          - unspecified person Y35.219 ☑
    - grenade — *see* Legal, intervention, explosive, grenade
    - injuring
      - bystander Y35.92 ☑
      - law enforcement personnel Y35.91 ☑
      - suspect Y35.93 ☑
      - unspecified person Y35.99 ☑
    - late effect (of) — *see* with 7th character S Y35 ☑
    - manhandling
      - injuring
        - bystander Y35.812 ☑
        - law enforcement personnel Y35.811 ☑
        - suspect Y35.813 ☑
        - unspecified person Y35.819 ☑
    - sequelae (of) — *see* with 7th character S Y35 ☑
    - sharp objects
      - bayonet
        - injuring
          - bystander Y35.412 ☑
          - law enforcement personnel Y35.411 ☑
          - suspect Y35.413 ☑
          - unspecified person Y35.419 ☑
      - injuring
        - bystander Y35.4Ø2 ☑
        - law enforcement personnel Y35.4Ø1 ☑
        - suspect Y35.4Ø3 ☑
        - unspecified person Y35.4Ø9 ☑
      - specified NEC
        - injuring
          - bystander Y35.492 ☑
          - law enforcement personnel Y35.491 ☑
          - suspect Y35.493 ☑
          - unspecified person Y35.499 ☑
    - specified means NEC
      - injuring
        - bystander Y35.892 ☑
        - law enforcement personnel Y35.891 ☑
        - suspect Y35.893 ☑
    - stabbing — *see* Legal, intervention, sharp object
    - stave — *see* Legal, intervention, blunt object, stave
    - stun gun
      - injuring
        - bystander Y35.832 ☑
        - law enforcement personnel Y35.831 ☑
        - suspect Y35.833 ☑
        - unspecified person Y35.839 ☑
    - taser
      - injuring
        - bystander Y35.832 ☑
        - law enforcement personnel Y35.831 ☑
        - suspect Y35.833 ☑
        - unspecified person Y35.839 ☑
    - tear gas — *see* Legal, intervention, gas, tear gas
    - truncheon — *see* Legal, intervention, blunt object, stave
- **Lifting** — *see also* Overexertion
  - heavy objects X5Ø.Ø ☑
  - weights X5Ø.Ø ☑
- **Lightning** (shock) (stroke) (struck by) — *see* subcategory T75.Ø ☑
  - causing fire — *see* Exposure, fire
- **Loss of control** (transport vehicle) NEC — *see* Accident, transport
- **Lost at sea NOS** — *see* Drowning, due to, fall overboard
- **Low**
  - pressure (effects) — *see* Air, pressure, low
  - temperature (effects) — *see* Exposure, cold
- **Lying before train, vehicle or other moving object** X81.8 ☑
  - subway train X81.1 ☑
  - train X81.1 ☑

Place of occurrence — *continued*
  sports area — *continued*
    athletic — *continued*
      court — *continued*
        basketball Y92.31Ø
        specified NEC Y92.318
        squash Y92.311
        tennis Y92.312
      field Y92.328
        baseball Y92.32Ø
        cricket ground Y92.328
        football Y92.321
        hockey Y92.328
        soccer Y92.322
        specified NEC Y92.328
    golf course Y92.39
    gymnasium Y92.39
    riding school Y92.39
    skating rink (roller) Y92.331
      ice Y92.33Ø
    stadium Y92.39
    swimming pool Y92.34
  squash court Y92.311
  stadium Y92.39
  steeplechasing course Y92.39
  store Y92.512
  stream Y92.828
  street and highway Y92.41Ø
    bike path Y92.482
    freeway Y92.411
    highway ramp Y92.415
    interstate highway Y92.411
    local residential or business street Y92.414
    motorway Y92.411
    parking lot Y92.481
    parkway Y92.412
    sidewalk Y92.48Ø
    specified NEC Y92.488
    state road Y92.413
  subway car Y92.816
  supermarket Y92.512
  swamp Y92.828
  swimming pool (public) Y92.34
    private (at) Y92.Ø95
      boarding house Y92.Ø45
      military base Y92.136
      mobile home Y92.Ø26
      nursing home Y92.125
      orphanage Y92.115
      prison Y92.146
      reform school Y92.156
      single family residence Y92.Ø16
  synagogue Y92.22
  television station Y92.59
  tennis court Y92.312
  theater Y92.254
  trade area Y92.59
    bank Y92.51Ø
    cafe Y92.511
    casino Y92.59
    garage Y92.59
    hotel Y92.59
    market Y92.512
    office building Y92.59
    radio station Y92.59
    restaurant Y92.511
    shop Y92.513
    shopping mall Y92.59
    store Y92.512
    supermarket Y92.512
    television station Y92.59
    warehouse Y92.59
  trailer park, residential — *see* Place of occurrence, residence, mobile home
  trailer site NOS Y92.89
  train Y92.815
    station Y92.522
  truck Y92.812
  tunnel under construction Y92.69
  university Y92.214
  urgent (health) care center Y92.532
  vehicle (transport) Y92.818
    airplane Y92.813
    boat Y92.814
    bus Y92.811
    car Y92.81Ø
    specified NEC Y92.818
    subway car Y92.816
    train Y92.815

Place of occurrence — *continued*
  vehicle — *continued*
    truck Y92.812
  warehouse Y92.59
  water reservoir Y92.89
  wilderness area Y92.828
    desert Y92.82Ø
    forest Y92.821
    marsh Y92.828
    mountain Y92.828
    prairie Y92.828
    specified NEC Y92.828
    swamp Y92.828
  workshop Y92.69
  yard, private Y92.Ø96
    boarding house Y92.Ø46
    mobile home Y92.Ø27
    single family house Y92.Ø17
  youth center Y92.29
  zoo (zoological garden) Y92.834
Plumbism — *see* Table of Drugs and Chemicals, lead
Poisoning (accidental) (by) — *see also* Table of Drugs and Chemicals
  by plant, thorns, spines, sharp leaves or other mechanisms NEC X58 ☑
  carbon monoxide
    generated by
      motor vehicle — *see* Accident, transport
      watercraft (in transit) (not in transit) V93.89 ☑
        ferry boat V93.81 ☑
        fishing boat V93.82 ☑
        jet skis V93.83 ☑
        liner V93.81 ☑
        merchant ship V93.8Ø ☑
        passenger ship V93.81 ☑
        powered craft NEC V93.83 ☑
  caused by injection of poisons into skin by plant thorns, spines, sharp leaves X58 ☑
    marine or sea plants (venomous) X58 ☑
  execution — *see* Legal, intervention, gas
    intervention
      by gas — *see* Legal, intervention, gas
      other specified means — *see* Legal, intervention, specified means NEC
  exhaust gas
    generated by
      motor vehicle — *see* Accident, transport
      watercraft (in transit) (not in transit) V93.89 ☑
        ferry boat V93.81 ☑
        fishing boat V93.82 ☑
        jet skis V93.83 ☑
        liner V93.81 ☑
        merchant ship V93.8Ø ☑
        passenger ship V93.81 ☑
        powered craft NEC V93.83 ☑
  fumes or smoke due to
    explosion — *see also* Explosion W4Ø.9 ☑
    fire — *see* Exposure, fire
    ignition — *see* Ignition
  gas
    in legal intervention — *see* Legal, intervention, gas
    legal execution — *see* Legal, intervention, gas
  in war operations — *see* War operations
  legal
Powder burn (by) (from)
  airgun W34.11Ø ☑
  BB gun W34.11Ø ☑
  firearm NEC W34.19 ☑
  gas, air or spring-operated gun NEC W34.118 ☑
  handgun W32.1 ☑
  hunting rifle W33.12 ☑
  larger firearm W33.1Ø ☑
    specified NEC W33.19 ☑
  machine gun W33.13 ☑
  paintball gun W34.111 ☑
  pellet gun W34.11Ø ☑
  shotgun W33.11 ☑
  Very pistol [flare] W34.19 ☑
Premature cessation (of) **surgical and medical care** Y66
Privation (food) (water) X58 ☑
Procedure (operation)
  correct, on wrong side or body part (wrong side) (wrong site) Y65.53
  intended for another patient done on wrong patient Y65.52
  performed on patient not scheduled for surgery Y65.52

Procedure — *continued*
  performed on wrong patient Y65.52
  wrong, performed on correct patient Y65.51
Prolonged
  sitting in transport vehicle — *see* Travel, by type of vehicle
  stay in
    high altitude as cause of anoxia, barodontalgia, barotitis or hypoxia W94.11 ☑
    weightless environment X52 ☑
Pulling, excessive — *see also* Overexertion X5Ø.9- ☑
Puncture, puncturing — *see also* Contact, with, by type of object or machine
  by
    plant thorns, spines, sharp leaves or other mechanisms NEC W6Ø ☑
  during medical or surgical treatment as misadventure — *see* Index to Diseases and Injuries, Complication(s)
Pushed, pushing (accidental) (injury in)
  by other person(s) (accidental) W51 ☑
    as, or caused by, a crowd or human stampede (with fall) W52 ☑
    before moving object NEC YØ2.8 ☑
      motor vehicle YØ2.Ø ☑
      subway train YØ2.1 ☑
      train YØ2.1 ☑
    from
      high place NEC
        in accidental circumstances W17.89 ☑
        stated as
          intentional, homicide (attempt) YØ1 ☑
          undetermined whether accidental or intentional Y3Ø ☑
      transport vehicle NEC — *see also* Accident, transport V89.9 ☑
        stated as
          intentional, homicide (attempt) YØ8.89 ☑
    with fall WØ3 ☑
      due to ice or snow WØØ.Ø ☑
  overexertion X5Ø.9 ☑

R

Radiation (exposure to)
  arc lamps W89.Ø ☑
  atomic power plant (malfunction) NEC W88.1 ☑
  complication of or abnormal reaction to medical radiotherapy Y84.2
  electromagnetic, ionizing W88.Ø ☑
  gamma rays W88.1 ☑
  in
    war operations (from or following nuclear explosion) — *see* War operations
  inadvertent exposure of patient (receiving test or therapy) Y63.3
  infrared (heaters and lamps) W9Ø.1 ☑
    excessive heat from W92 ☑
  ionized, ionizing (particles, artificially accelerated)
    radioisotopes W88.1 ☑
    specified NEC W88.8 ☑
    x-rays W88.Ø ☑
  isotopes, radioactive — *see* Radiation, radioactive isotopes
  laser(s) W9Ø.2 ☑
    in war operations — *see* War operations
    misadventure in medical care Y63.2
  light sources (man-made visible and ultraviolet) W89.9 ☑
    natural X32 ☑
    specified NEC W89.8 ☑
    tanning bed W89.1 ☑
    welding light W89.Ø ☑
  man-made visible light W89.9 ☑
    specified NEC W89.8 ☑
    tanning bed W89.1 ☑
    welding light W89.Ø ☑
  microwave W9Ø.8 ☑
  misadventure in medical or surgical procedure Y63.2
  natural NEC X39.Ø8 ☑
    radon X39.Ø1 ☑
  overdose (in medical or surgical procedure) Y63.2
  radar W9Ø.Ø ☑
  radioactive isotopes (any) W88.1 ☑
    atomic power plant malfunction W88.1 ☑
    misadventure in medical or surgical treatment Y63.2

Radiation — *continued*
- radiofrequency W9Ø.Ø ☑
- radium NEC W88.1 ☑
- sun X32 ☑
- ultraviolet (light) (man-made) W89.9 ☑
  - natural X32 ☑
  - specified NEC W89.8 ☑
  - tanning bed W89.1 ☑
  - welding light W89.Ø ☑
- welding arc, torch, or light W89.Ø ☑
  - excessive heat from W92 ☑
- x-rays (hard) (soft) W88.Ø ☑

Range disease W94.11 ☑

Rape (attempted) T74.2- ☑

Rat bite W53.11 ☑

Reaching (prolonged) (static) X5Ø.1 ☑

Reaction, abnormal to medical procedure — *see also* Complication of or following, by type of procedure Y84.9
- biologicals — *see* Table of Drugs and Chemicals
- drugs — *see* Table of Drugs and Chemicals
- vaccine — *see* Table of Drugs and Chemicals
- with misadventure — *see* Misadventure

Recoil
- airgun W34.11Ø ☑
- BB gun W34.11Ø ☑
- firearn NEC W34.19 ☑
- gas, air or spring-operated gun NEC W34.118 ☑
- handgun W32.1 ☑
- hunting rifle W33.12 ☑
- larger firearm W33.1Ø ☑
  - specified NEC W33.19 ☑
- machine gun W33.13 ☑
- paintball gun W34.111 ☑
- pellet W34.11Ø ☑
- shotgun W33.11 ☑
- Very pistol [flare] W34.19 ☑

Reduction in
- atmospheric pressure — *see* Air, pressure, change

Rock falling on or hitting (accidentally) (person) W2Ø.8 ☑
- in cave-in W2Ø.Ø ☑

Run over (accidentally) (by)
- animal (not being ridden) NEC W55.89 ☑
- machinery — *see* Contact, with, by specified type of machine
- transport vehicle NEC — *see also* Accident, transport VØ9.9 ☑
  - intentional homicide (attempt) YØ3.Ø ☑
  - motor NEC VØ9.2Ø ☑
    - intentional homicide (attempt) YØ3.Ø ☑

Running
- before moving object X81.8 ☑
  - motor vehicle X81.Ø ☑

Running off, away
- animal (being ridden) — *see also* Accident, transport V8Ø.918 ☑
  - not being ridden W55.89 ☑
- animal-drawn vehicle NEC — *see also* Accident, transport V8Ø.928 ☑
- highway, road(way), street
  - transport vehicle NEC — *see also* Accident, transport V89.9 ☑

Rupture pressurized devices — *see* Explosion, by type of device

S

Saturnism — *see* Table of Drugs and Chemicals, lead

Scald, scalding (accidental) (by) (from) (in) X19 ☑
- air (hot) X14.1 ☑
- gases (hot) X14.1 ☑
- homicide (attempt) — *see* Assault, burning, hot object
- inflicted by other person
  - stated as intentional, homicide (attempt) — *see* Assault, burning, hot object
- liquid (boiling) (hot) NEC X12 ☑
  - stated as undetermined whether accidental or intentional Y27.2 ☑
  - suicide (attempt) X77.2 ☑
- local application of externally applied substance in medical or surgical care Y63.5
- metal (molten) (liquid) (hot) NEC X18 ☑
- self-inflicted X77.9 ☑
- stated as undetermined whether accidental or intentional Y27.8 ☑

Scald, scalding — *continued*
- steam X13.1 ☑
  - assault X98.Ø ☑
  - stated as undetermined whether accidental or intentional Y27.Ø ☑
  - suicide (attempt) X77.Ø ☑
- suicide (attempt) X77.9 ☑
- vapor (hot) X13.1 ☑
  - assault X98.Ø ☑
  - stated as undetermined whether accidental or intentional Y27.Ø ☑
  - suicide (attempt) X77.Ø ☑

Scratched by
- cat W55.Ø3 ☑
- person(s) (accidentally) W5Ø.4 ☑
  - with intent to injure or kill YØ4.Ø ☑
  - as, or caused by, a crowd or human stampede (with fall) W52 ☑
  - assault YØ4.Ø ☑
  - homicide (attempt) YØ4.Ø ☑
  - in
    - fight YØ4.Ø ☑
    - legal intervention
      - injuring
        - bystander Y35.892 ☑
        - law enforcement personnel Y35.891 ☑
        - suspect Y35.893 ☑

Seasickness T75.3 ☑

Self-harm NEC — *see also* External cause by type, undetermined whether accidental or intentional
- intentional — *see* Suicide
- poisoning NEC — *see* Table of Drugs and Chemicals, poisoning, accidental

Self-inflicted (injury) **NEC** — *see also* External cause by type, undetermined whether accidental or intentional
- intentional — *see* Suicide
- poisoning NEC — *see* Table of Drugs and Chemicals, poisoning, accidental

Sequelae (of)
- accident NEC — *see* WØØ-X58 with 7th character S
- assault (homicidal) (any means) — *see* X92-YØ8 with 7th character S
- homicide, attempt (any means) — *see* X92-YØ8 with 7th character S
- injury undetermined whether accidentally or purposely inflicted — *see* Y21-Y33 with 7th character S
- intentional self-harm (classifiable to X71-X83) — *see* X71-X83 with 7th character S
- legal intervention — *see* with 7th character S Y35 ☑
- motor vehicle accident — *see* VØØ-V99 with 7th character S
- suicide, attempt (any means) — *see* X71-X83 with 7th character S
- transport accident — *see* VØØ-V99 with 7th character S
- war operations — *see* War operations

Shock
- electric — *see* Exposure, electric current
- from electric appliance (any) (faulty) W86.8 ☑
  - domestic W86.Ø ☑
  - suicide (attempt) X83.1 ☑

Shooting, shot (accidental(ly)) — *see also* Discharge, firearm, by type
- herself or himself — *see* Discharge, firearm by type, self-inflicted
- homicide (attempt) — *see* Discharge, firearm by type, homicide
- in war operations — *see* War operations
- inflicted by other person — *see* Discharge, firearm by type, homicide
  - accidental — *see* Discharge, firearm, by type of firearm
- legal
  - execution — *see* Legal, intervention, firearm
  - intervention — *see* Legal, intervention, firearm
- self-inflicted — *see* Discharge, firearm by type, suicide
  - accidental — *see* Discharge, firearm, by type of firearm
- suicide (attempt) — *see* Discharge, firearm by type, suicide

Shoving (accidentally) **by other person** — *see* Pushed, by other person

Sickness
- alpine W94.11 ☑
- motion — *see* Motion
- mountain W94.11 ☑

Sinking (accidental)
- watercraft (causing drowning, submersion) — *see also* Drowning, due to, accident to, watercraft, sinking
  - causing injury except drowning or submersion — *see* Accident, watercraft, causing, injury NEC

Siriasis X32 ☑

Sitting (prolonged) (static) X5Ø.1 ☑

Slashed wrists — *see* Cut, self-inflicted

Slipping (accidental) (on same level) (with fall) WØ1.Ø ☑
- on
  - ice WØØ.Ø ☑
    - with skates — *see* Accident, transport, pedestrian, conveyance
  - mud WØ1.Ø ☑
  - oil WØ1.Ø ☑
  - snow WØØ.Ø ☑
    - with skis — *see* Accident, transport, pedestrian, conveyance
  - surface (slippery) (wet) NEC WØ1.Ø ☑
- without fall W18.4Ø ☑
  - due to
    - specified NEC W18.49 ☑
    - stepping from one level to another W18.43 ☑
    - stepping into hole or opening W18.42 ☑
    - stepping on object W18.41 ☑

Sliver, wood, contact with W45.8 ☑

Smoldering (due to fire) — *see* Exposure, fire

Sodomy (attempted) **by force** T74.2 ☑

Sound waves (causing injury) W42.9 ☑
- supersonic W42.Ø ☑

Splinter, contact with W45.8 ☑

Stab, stabbing — *see* Cut

Standing (prolonged) (static) X5Ø.1 ☑

Starvation X58 ☑

Status of external cause Y99.9
- child assisting in compensated work for family Y99.8
- civilian activity done for financial or other compensation Y99.Ø
- civilian activity done for income or pay Y99.Ø
- family member assisting in compensated work for other family member Y99.8
- hobby not done for income Y99.8
- leisure activity Y99.8
- military activity Y99.1
- off-duty activity of military personnel Y99.8
- recreation or sport not for income or while a student Y99.8
- specified NEC Y99.8
- student activity Y99.8
- volunteer activity Y99.2

Stepped on
- by
  - animal (not being ridden) NEC W55.89 ☑
  - crowd or human stampede W52 ☑
  - person W5Ø.Ø ☑

Stepping on
- object W22.8 ☑
  - sports equipment W21.9 ☑
  - stationary W22.Ø9 ☑
    - sports equipment W21.89 ☑
  - with fall W18.31 ☑
- person W51 ☑
  - by crowd or human stampede W52 ☑
- sports equipment W21.9 ☑

Sting
- arthropod, nonvenomous W57 ☑
- insect, nonvenomous W57 ☑

Storm (cataclysmic) — *see* Forces of nature, cataclysmic storm

Straining, excessive — *see also* Overexertion X5Ø.9 ☑

Strangling — *see* Strangulation

Strangulation (accidental) T71 ☑

Strenuous movements — *see also* Overexertion X5Ø.9 ☑

Striking against
- airbag (automobile) W22.1Ø ☑
  - driver side W22.11 ☑
  - front passenger side W22.12 ☑
  - specified NEC W22.19 ☑
- bottom when
  - diving or jumping into water (in) W16.822 ☑
    - causing drowning W16.821 ☑
    - from boat W16.722 ☑
      - causing drowning W16.721 ☑
    - natural body W16.622 ☑
      - causing drowning W16.821 ☑

- **Striking against** — *continued*
  - bottom when — *continued*
    - diving or jumping into water — *continued*
      - swimming pool W16.522 ☑
        - causing drowning W16.521 ☑
    - falling into water (in) W16.322 ☑
      - causing drowning W16.321 ☑
      - fountain — *see* Striking against, bottom when, falling into water, specified NEC
      - natural body W16.122 ☑
        - causing drowning W16.121 ☑
      - reservoir — *see* Striking against, bottom when, falling into water, specified NEC
      - specified NEC W16.322 ☑
        - causing drowning W16.321 ☑
      - swimming pool W16.022 ☑
        - causing drowning W16.021 ☑
  - diving board (swimming-pool) W21.4 ☑
  - object W22.8 ☑
    - caused by crowd or human stampede (with fall) W52 ☑
    - furniture W22.03 ☑
    - lamppost W22.02 ☑
    - sports equipment W21.9 ☑
    - stationary W22.09 ☑
      - sports equipment W21.89 ☑
    - wall W22.01 ☑
    - with
      - drowning or submersion — *see* Drowning
      - fall — *see* Fall, due to, bumping against, object
  - person(s) W51 ☑
    - as, or caused by, a crowd or human stampede (with fall) W52 ☑
    - assault Y04.2 ☑
    - homicide (attempt) Y04.2 ☑
    - with fall W03 ☑
      - due to ice or snow W00.0 ☑
  - sports equipment W21.9 ☑
  - wall (when) W22.01 ☑
    - diving or jumping into water (in) W16.832 ☑
      - causing drowning W16.831 ☑
      - swimming pool W16.532 ☑
        - causing drowning W16.531 ☑
    - falling into water (in) W16.332 ☑
      - causing drowning W16.331 ☑
      - fountain — *see* Striking against, wall when, falling into water, specified NEC
      - natural body W16.132 ☑
        - causing drowning W16.131 ☑
      - reservoir — *see* Striking against, wall when, falling into water, specified NEC
      - specified NEC W16.332 ☑
        - causing drowning W16.331 ☑
      - swimming pool W16.032 ☑
        - causing drowning W16.031 ☑
    - swimming pool (when) W22.042 ☑
      - causing drowning W22.041 ☑
      - diving or jumping into water W16.532 ☑
        - causing drowning W16.531 ☑
      - falling into water W16.032 ☑
        - causing drowning W16.031 ☑
- **Struck** (accidentally) **by**
  - airbag (automobile) W22.10 ☑
    - driver side W22.11 ☑
    - front passenger side W22.12 ☑
    - specified NEC W22.19 ☑
  - alligator W58.02 ☑
  - animal (not being ridden) NEC W55.89 ☑
  - avalanche — *see* Landslide
  - ball (hit) (thrown) W21.00 ☑
    - assault Y08.09 ☑
    - baseball W21.03 ☑
    - basketball W21.05 ☑
    - football W21.01 ☑
    - golf ball W21.04 ☑
    - soccer W21.02 ☑
    - softball W21.07 ☑
    - specified NEC W21.09 ☑
    - volleyball W21.06 ☑
  - bat or racquet
    - baseball bat W21.11 ☑
      - assault Y08.02 ☑
    - golf club W21.13 ☑
      - assault Y08.09 ☑
    - specified NEC W21.19 ☑
      - assault Y08.09 ☑
- **Struck** (accidentally) **by** — *continued*
  - bat or racquet — *continued*
    - tennis racquet W21.12 ☑
      - assault Y08.09 ☑
  - bullet — *see also* Discharge, firearm by type
    - in war operations — *see* War operations
  - crocodile W58.12 ☑
  - dog W54.1 ☑
  - flare, Very pistol — *see* Discharge, firearm NEC
  - hailstones X39.8 ☑
  - hockey (ice)
    - field
      - puck W21.221 ☑
      - stick W21.211 ☑
    - puck W21.220 ☑
    - stick W21.210 ☑
      - assault Y08.01 ☑
  - landslide — *see* Landslide
  - law-enforcement agent (on duty) — *see* Legal, intervention, manhandling
    - with blunt object — *see* Legal, intervention, blunt object
  - lightning T75.0 ☑
    - causing fire — *see* Exposure, fire
  - machine — *see* Contact, with, by type of machine
  - mammal NEC W55.89 ☑
    - marine W56.32 ☑
  - marine animal W56.82 ☑
  - missile
    - firearm — *see* Discharge, firearm by type
    - in war operations — *see* War operations, missile
  - object W22.8 ☑
    - blunt W22.8 ☑
      - assault Y00 ☑
      - suicide (attempt) X79 ☑
      - undetermined whether accidental or intentional Y29 ☑
    - falling W20.8 ☑
      - from, in, on
        - building W20.1 ☑
          - burning (uncontrolled fire) X00.4 ☑
        - cataclysmic
          - earth surface movement NEC — *see* Landslide
          - storm — *see* Forces of nature, cataclysmic storm
        - cave-in W20.0 ☑
        - earthquake X34 ☑
        - machine (in operation) — *see* Contact, with, by type of machine
        - structure W20.1 ☑
          - burning X00.4 ☑
        - transport vehicle (in motion) — *see* Accident, transport, by type of vehicle
        - watercraft V93.49 ☑
          - due to
            - accident to craft V91.39 ☑
              - powered craft V91.33 ☑
                - ferry boat V91.31 ☑
                - fishing boat V91.32 ☑
                - jetskis V91.33 ☑
                - liner V91.31 ☑
                - merchant ship V91.30 ☑
                - passenger ship V91.31 ☑
              - unpowered craft V91.38 ☑
                - canoe V91.35 ☑
                - inflatable V91.36 ☑
                - kayak V91.35 ☑
                - sailboat V91.34 ☑
                - surf-board V91.38 ☑
                - windsurfer V91.38 ☑
          - powered craft V93.43 ☑
            - ferry boat V93.41 ☑
            - fishing boat V93.42 ☑
            - jetskis V93.43 ☑
            - liner V93.41 ☑
            - merchant ship V93.40 ☑
            - passenger ship V93.41 ☑
          - unpowered craft V93.48 ☑
            - sailboat V93.44 ☑
            - surf-board V93.48 ☑
            - windsurfer V93.48 ☑
    - moving NEC W20.8 ☑
    - projected W20.8 ☑
      - assault Y00 ☑
      - in sports W21.9 ☑
- **Struck** (accidentally) **by** — *continued*
  - object — *continued*
    - projected — *continued*
      - in sports — *continued*
        - assault Y08.09 ☑
        - ball W21.00 ☑
          - baseball W21.03 ☑
          - basketball W21.05 ☑
          - football W21.01 ☑
          - golf ball W21.04 ☑
          - soccer W21.02 ☑
          - softball W21.07 ☑
          - specified NEC W21.09 ☑
          - volleyball W21.06 ☑
        - bat or racquet
          - baseball bat W21.11 ☑
            - assault Y08.02 ☑
          - golf club W21.13 ☑
            - assault Y08.09 ☑
          - specified NEC W21.19 ☑
            - assault Y08.09 ☑
          - tennis racquet W21.12 ☑
            - assault Y08.09 ☑
        - hockey (ice)
          - field
            - puck W21.221 ☑
            - stick W21.211 ☑
          - puck W21.220 ☑
          - stick W21.210 ☑
            - assault Y08.01 ☑
        - specified NEC W21.89 ☑
    - set in motion by explosion — *see* Explosion
    - thrown W20.8 ☑
      - assault Y00 ☑
      - in sports W21.9 ☑
        - assault Y08.09 ☑
        - ball W21.00 ☑
          - baseball W21.03 ☑
          - basketball W21.05 ☑
          - football W21.01 ☑
          - golf ball W21.04 ☑
          - soccer W21.02 ☑
          - soft ball W21.07 ☑
          - specified NEC W21.09 ☑
          - volleyball W21.06 ☑
        - bat or racquet
          - baseball bat W21.11 ☑
            - assault Y08.02 ☑
          - golf club W21.13 ☑
            - assault Y08.09 ☑
          - specified NEC W21.19 ☑
            - assault Y08.09 ☑
          - tennis racquet W21.12 ☑
            - assault Y08.09 ☑
        - hockey (ice)
          - field
            - puck W21.221 ☑
            - stick W21.211 ☑
          - puck W21.220 ☑
          - stick W21.210 ☑
            - assault Y08.01 ☑
        - specified NEC W21.89 ☑
  - other person(s) W50.0 ☑
    - with
      - blunt object W22.8 ☑
        - intentional, homicide (attempt) Y00 ☑
        - sports equipment W21.9 ☑
        - undetermined whether accidental or intentional Y29 ☑
      - fall W03 ☑
        - due to ice or snow W00.0 ☑
    - as, or caused by, a crowd or human stampede (with fall) W52 ☑
    - assault Y04.2 ☑
    - homicide (attempt) Y04.2 ☑
    - in legal intervention
      - injuring
        - bystander Y35.812 ☑
        - law enforcement personnel Y35.811 ☑
        - suspect Y35.813 ☑
        - unspecified person Y35.819 ☑
    - sports equipment W21.9 ☑
  - police (on duty) — *see* Legal, intervention, manhandling
    - with blunt object — *see* Legal, intervention, blunt object

- **Struck** (accidentally) **by** — *continued*
  - sports equipment W21.9 ☑
    - assault YØ8.Ø9 ☑
    - ball W21.ØØ ☑
      - baseball W21.Ø3 ☑
      - basketball W21.Ø5 ☑
      - football W21.Ø1 ☑
      - golf ball W21.Ø4 ☑
      - soccer W21.Ø2 ☑
      - soft ball W21.Ø7 ☑
      - specified NEC W21.Ø9 ☑
      - volleyball W21.Ø6 ☑
    - bat or racquet
      - baseball bat W21.11 ☑
        - assault YØ8.Ø2 ☑
      - golf club W21.13 ☑
        - assault YØ8.Ø9 ☑
      - specified NEC W21.19 ☑
      - tennis racquet W21.12 ☑
        - assault YØ8.Ø9 ☑
    - cleats (shoe) W21.31 ☑
    - foot wear NEC W21.39 ☑
    - football helmet W21.81 ☑
    - hockey (ice)
      - field
        - puck W21.221 ☑
        - stick W21.211 ☑
      - puck W21.22Ø ☑
      - stick W21.21Ø ☑
        - assault YØ8.Ø1 ☑
    - skate blades W21.32 ☑
    - specified NEC W21.89 ☑
      - assault YØ8.Ø9 ☑
  - thunderbolt — *see* subcategory T75.Ø ☑
    - causing fire — *see* Exposure, fire
  - transport vehicle NEC — *see also* Accident, transport VØ9.9 ☑
    - intentional, homicide (attempt) YØ3.Ø ☑
    - motor NEC — *see also* Accident, transport VØ9.2Ø ☑
      - homicide YØ3.Ø ☑
  - vehicle (transport) NEC — *see* Accident, transport, by type of vehicle
    - stationary (falling from jack, hydraulic lift, ramp) W2Ø.8 ☑
- **Stumbling**
  - over
    - animal NEC WØ1.Ø ☑
      - with fall W18.Ø9 ☑
    - carpet, rug or (small) object W22.8 ☑
      - with fall W18.Ø9 ☑
    - person W51 ☑
      - with fall WØ3 ☑
        - due to ice or snow WØØ.Ø ☑
  - without fall W18.4Ø ☑
    - due to
      - specified NEC W18.49 ☑
      - stepping from one level to another W18.43 ☑
      - stepping into hole or opening W18.42 ☑
      - stepping on object W18.41 ☑
- **Submersion** (accidental) — *see* Drowning
- **Suffocation** (accidental) (by external means) (by pressure) (mechanical) — *see also* category T71 ☑
  - due to, by
    - avalanche — *see* Landslide
    - explosion — *see* Explosion
    - fire — *see* Exposure, fire
    - food, any type (aspiration) (ingestion) (inhalation) — *see* categories T17 and T18 ☑
    - ignition — *see* Ignition
    - landslide — *see* Landslide
    - machine(ry) — *see* Contact, with, by type of machine
    - vomitus (aspiration) (inhalation) T17.81- ☑
  - in
    - burning building XØØ.8 ☑
- **Suicide, suicidal** (attempted) (by) X83.8 ☑
  - blunt object X79 ☑
  - burning, burns X76 ☑
    - hot object X77.9 ☑
      - fluid NEC X77.2 ☑
      - household appliance X77.3 ☑
      - specified NEC X77.8 ☑
      - steam X77.Ø ☑
      - tap water X77.1 ☑
      - vapors X77.Ø ☑
  - caustic substance — *see* Table of Drugs and Chemicals
  - cold, extreme X83.2 ☑
  - collision of motor vehicle with
    - motor vehicle X82.Ø ☑
    - specified NEC X82.8 ☑
    - train X82.1 ☑
    - tree X82.2 ☑
  - crashing of aircraft X83.Ø ☑
  - cut (any part of body) X78.9 ☑
  - cutting or piercing instrument X78.9 ☑
    - dagger X78.2 ☑
    - glass X78.Ø ☑
    - knife X78.1 ☑
    - specified NEC X78.8 ☑
    - sword X78.2 ☑
  - drowning (in) X71.9 ☑
    - bathtub X71.Ø ☑
    - natural water X71.3 ☑
    - specified NEC X71.8 ☑
    - swimming pool X71.1 ☑
      - following fall X71.2 ☑
  - electrocution X83.1 ☑
  - explosive(s) (material) X75 ☑
  - fire, flames X76 ☑
  - firearm X74.9 ☑
    - airgun X74.Ø1 ☑
    - handgun X72 ☑
    - hunting rifle X73.1 ☑
    - larger X73.9 ☑
      - specified NEC X73.8 ☑
    - machine gun X73.2 ☑
    - shotgun X73.Ø ☑
    - specified NEC X74.8 ☑
  - hanging X83.8 ☑
  - hot object — *see* Suicide, burning, hot object
  - jumping
    - before moving object X81.8 ☑
      - motor vehicle X81.Ø ☑
      - subway train X81.1 ☑
      - train X81.1 ☑
    - from high place X8Ø ☑
  - late effect of attempt — *see* X71-X83 with 7th character S
  - lying before moving object, train, vehicle X81.8 ☑
  - poisoning — *see* Table of Drugs and Chemicals
  - puncture (any part of body) — *see* Suicide, cutting or piercing instrument
  - scald — *see* Suicide, burning, hot object
  - sequelae of attempt — *see* X71-X83 with 7th character S
  - sharp object (any) — *see* Suicide, cutting or piercing instrument
  - shooting — *see* Suicide, firearm
  - specified means NEC X83.8 ☑
  - stab (any part of body) — *see* Suicide, cutting or piercing instrument
  - steam, hot vapors X77.Ø ☑
  - strangulation X83.8 ☑
  - submersion — *see* Suicide, drowning
  - suffocation X83.8 ☑
  - wound NEC X83.8 ☑
- **Sunstroke** X32 ☑
- **Supersonic waves** (causing injury) W42.Ø ☑
- **Surgical procedure, complication of** (delayed or as an abnormal reaction without mention of misadventure) — *see also* Complication of or following, by type of procedure
  - due to or as a result of misadventure — *see* Misadventure
- **Swallowed, swallowing**
  - foreign body — *see* Foreign body, alimentary canal
  - poison — *see* Table of Drugs and Chemicals
  - substance
    - caustic or corrosive — *see* Table of Drugs and Chemicals
    - poisonous — *see* Table of Drugs and Chemicals

T

- **Tackle in sport** WØ3 ☑
- **Terrorism** (involving) Y38.8Ø ☑
  - biological weapons Y38.6X- ☑
  - chemical weapons Y38.7X- ☑
  - conflagration Y38.3X- ☑
  - drowning and submersion Y38.89- ☑
  - explosion Y38.2X- ☑
- **Terrorism** — *continued*
  - explosion — *continued*
    - destruction of aircraft Y38.1X- ☑
    - marine weapons Y38.ØX- ☑
  - fire Y38.3X- ☑
  - firearms Y38.4X- ☑
  - hot substances Y38.3X- ☑
  - lasers Y38.89- ☑
  - nuclear weapons Y38.5X- ☑
  - piercing or stabbing instruments Y38.89- ☑
  - secondary effects Y38.9X- ☑
  - specified method NEC Y38.89- ☑
  - suicide bomber Y38.81- ☑
- **Thirst** X58 ☑
- **Threat to breathing**
  - aspiration — *see* Aspiration
  - due to cave-in, falling earth or substance NEC T71 ☑
- **Thrown** (accidentally)
  - against part (any) of or object in transport vehicle (in motion) NEC — *see also* Accident, transport
  - from
    - high place, homicide (attempt) YØ1 ☑
    - machinery — *see* Contact, with, by type of machine
    - transport vehicle NEC — *see also* Accident, transport V89.9 ☑
  - off — *see* Thrown, from
- **Thunderbolt** — *see* subcategory T75.Ø ☑
  - causing fire — *see* Exposure, fire
- **Tidal wave** (any injury) **NEC** — *see* Forces of nature, tidal wave
- **Took**
  - overdose (drug) — *see* Table of Drugs and Chemicals
  - poison — *see* Table of Drugs and Chemicals
- **Tornado** (any injury) X37.1 ☑
- **Torrential rain** (any injury) X37.8 ☑
- **Torture** X58 ☑
- **Trampled by animal NEC** W55.89 ☑
- **Trapped** (accidentally)
  - between objects (moving) (stationary and moving) — *see* Caught
  - by part (any) of
    - motorcycle V29.88 ☑
    - pedal cycle V19.88 ☑
    - transport vehicle NEC — *see also* Accident, transport V89.9 ☑
- **Travel** (effects) (sickness) T75.3 ☑
- **Tree falling on or hitting** (accidentally) (person) W2Ø.8 ☑
- **Tripping**
  - over
    - animal WØ1.Ø ☑
      - with fall WØ1.Ø ☑
    - carpet, rug or (small) object W22.8 ☑
      - with fall W18.Ø9 ☑
    - person W51 ☑
      - with fall WØ3 ☑
        - due to ice or snow WØØ.Ø ☑
  - without fall W18.4Ø ☑
    - due to
      - specified NEC W18.49 ☑
      - stepping from one level to another W18.43 ☑
      - stepping into hole or opening W18.42 ☑
      - stepping on object W18.41 ☑
- **Twisted by person**(s) (accidentally) W5Ø.2 ☑
  - with intent to injure or kill YØ4.Ø ☑
  - as, or caused by, a crowd or human stampede (with fall) W52 ☑
  - assault YØ4.Ø ☑
  - homicide (attempt) YØ4.Ø ☑
  - in
    - fight YØ4.Ø ☑
    - legal intervention — *see* Legal, intervention, manhandling
- **Twisting** (prolonged) (static) X5Ø.1- ☑

U

- **Underdosing of necessary drugs, medicaments or biological substances** Y63.6
- **Undetermined intent** (contact) (exposure)
  - automobile collision Y32 ☑
  - blunt object Y29 ☑
  - drowning (submersion) (in) Y21.9 ☑
    - bathtub Y21.Ø ☑
      - after fall Y21.1 ☑

ICD-10-CM Tabular List of Diseases and Injuries

Chapter 1. Certain Infectious and Parasitic Diseases (AØØ–B99), UØ7.1

Chapter-specific Guidelines with Coding Examples

The chapter-specific guidelines from the ICD-10-CM Official Guidelines for Coding and Reporting have been provided below. Along with these guidelines are coding examples, contained in the shaded boxes, that have been developed to help illustrate the coding and/or sequencing guidance found in these guidelines.

a. Human immunodeficiency virus (HIV) infections

1) Code only confirmed cases

Code only confirmed cases of HIV infection/illness. This is an exception to the hospital inpatient guideline Section II, H.

In this context, "confirmation" does not require documentation of positive serology or culture for HIV; the provider's diagnostic statement that the patient is HIV positive, or has an HIV-related illness is sufficient.

Patient admitted with anemia with possible HIV infection

D64.9	**Anemia, unspecified**

Explanation: Only the anemia is coded in this scenario because it has not been confirmed that an HIV infection is present. This is an exception to the guideline Section II, H for hospital inpatient coding.

2) Selection and sequencing of HIV codes

(a) Patient admitted for HIV-related condition

If a patient is admitted for an HIV-related condition, the principal diagnosis should be B2Ø, Human immunodeficiency virus [HIV] disease followed by additional diagnosis codes for all reported HIV-related conditions.

(b) Patient with HIV disease admitted for unrelated condition

If a patient with HIV disease is admitted for an unrelated condition (such as a traumatic injury), the code for the unrelated condition (e.g., the nature of injury code) should be the principal diagnosis. Other diagnoses would be B2Ø followed by additional diagnosis codes for all reported HIV-related conditions.

Unstable angina, native coronary artery atherosclerosis, HIV

I25.11Ø	**Atherosclerotic heart disease of native coronary artery with unstable angina pectoris**
B2Ø	**Human immunodeficiency virus [HIV] disease**

Explanation: The arteriosclerotic coronary artery disease and the unstable angina are not related to HIV, so those conditions are reported first using a combination code, and HIV is reported secondarily.

(c) Whether the patient is newly diagnosed

Whether the patient is newly diagnosed or has had previous admissions/encounters for HIV conditions is irrelevant to the sequencing decision.

(d) Asymptomatic human immunodeficiency virus

Z21, Asymptomatic human immunodeficiency virus [HIV] infection status, is to be applied when the patient without any documentation of symptoms is listed as being "HIV positive," "known HIV," "HIV test positive," or similar terminology. Do not use this code if the term "AIDS" is used or if the patient is treated for any HIV-related illness or is described as having any condition(s) resulting from his/her HIV positive status; use B2Ø in these cases.

Patient admitted with acute appendicitis. Status positive HIV test on Atripla, with no prior symptoms

K35.8Ø	**Unspecified acute appendicitis**
Z21	**Asymptomatic human immunodeficiency virus [HIV] infection status**

Explanation: Code Z21 is sequenced second since documentation indicates that the patient has had a positive HIV test but has been asymptomatic. Being on medication for HIV is not an indication that code B2Ø is used instead of Z21. Unless there has been documentation that the patient has had current or prior symptoms or HIV-related complications, code B2Ø is not used. The appendicitis is not an AIDS-related complication and is sequenced first.

(e) Patients with inconclusive HIV serology

Patients with inconclusive HIV serology, but no definitive diagnosis or manifestations of the illness, may be assigned code R75, Inconclusive laboratory evidence of human immunodeficiency virus [HIV].

(f) Previously diagnosed HIV-related illness

Patients with any known prior diagnosis of an HIV-related illness should be coded to B2Ø. Once a patient has developed an HIV-related illness, the patient should always be assigned code B2Ø on every subsequent admission/encounter. Patients previously diagnosed with any HIV illness (B2Ø) should never be assigned to R75 or Z21, Asymptomatic human immunodeficiency virus [HIV] infection status.

(g) HIV infection in pregnancy, childbirth and the puerperium

During pregnancy, childbirth or the puerperium, a patient admitted (or presenting for a health care encounter) because of an HIV-related illness should receive a principal diagnosis code of O98.7-, Human immunodeficiency [HIV] disease complicating pregnancy, childbirth and the puerperium, followed by B2Ø and the code(s) for the HIV-related illness(es). Codes from Chapter 15 always take sequencing priority.

Patients with asymptomatic HIV infection status admitted (or presenting for a health care encounter) during pregnancy, childbirth, or the puerperium should receive codes of O98.7- and Z21.

(h) Encounters for testing for HIV

If a patient is being seen to determine his/her HIV status, use code Z11.4, Encounter for screening for human immunodeficiency virus [HIV]. Use additional codes for any associated high-risk behavior.

If a patient with signs or symptoms is being seen for HIV testing, code the signs and symptoms. An additional counseling code Z71.7, Human immunodeficiency virus [HIV] counseling, may be used if counseling is provided during the encounter for the test.

When a patient returns to be informed of his/her HIV test results and the test result is negative, use code Z71.7, Human immunodeficiency virus [HIV] counseling.

If the results are positive, see previous guidelines and assign codes as appropriate.

b. Infectious agents as the cause of diseases classified to other chapters

Certain infections are classified in chapters other than Chapter 1 and no organism is identified as part of the infection code. In these instances, it is necessary to use an additional code from Chapter 1 to identify the organism. A code from category B95, Streptococcus, Staphylococcus, and Enterococcus as the cause of diseases classified to other chapters, B96, Other bacterial agents as the cause of diseases classified to other chapters, or B97, Viral agents as the cause of diseases classified to other chapters, is to be used as an additional code to identify the organism. An instructional note will be found at the infection code advising that an additional organism code is required.

E. coli UTI

N39.Ø	**Urinary tract infection, site not specified**
B96.2Ø	**Unspecified Escherichia coli [E.coli] as the cause of diseases classified elsewhere**

Explanation: An instructional note under the code for the urinary tract infection indicates to code also the specific organism.

c. Infections resistant to antibiotics

Many bacterial infections are resistant to current antibiotics. It is necessary to identify all infections documented as antibiotic resistant. Assign a code from category Z16, Resistance to antimicrobial drugs, following the infection code only if the infection code does not identify drug resistance.

d. Sepsis, severe sepsis, and septic shock

1) Coding of sepsis and severe sepsis

(a) Sepsis

For a diagnosis of sepsis, assign the appropriate code for the underlying systemic infection. If the type of infection or causal organism is not further specified, assign code A41.9, Sepsis, unspecified organism.

A code from subcategory R65.2, Severe sepsis, should not be assigned unless severe sepsis or an associated acute organ dysfunction is documented.

(i) Negative or inconclusive blood cultures and sepsis

Negative or inconclusive blood cultures do not preclude a diagnosis of sepsis in patients with clinical evidence of the condition; however, the provider should be queried.

(ii) Urosepsis

The term urosepsis is a nonspecific term. It is not to be considered synonymous with sepsis. It has no default code in the Alphabetic Index. Should a provider use this term, he/she must be queried for clarification.

(iii)Sepsis with organ dysfunction

If a patient has sepsis and associated acute organ dysfunction or multiple organ dysfunction (MOD), follow the instructions for coding severe sepsis.

(iv) Acute organ dysfunction that is not clearly associated with the sepsis

If a patient has sepsis and an acute organ dysfunction, but the medical record documentation indicates that the acute organ dysfunction is related to a medical condition other than the sepsis, do not assign a code from subcategory R65.2, Severe sepsis. An acute organ dysfunction must be associated with the sepsis in order to assign the severe sepsis code. If the documentation is not clear as to whether an acute organ dysfunction is related to the sepsis or another medical condition, query the provider.

Sepsis and acute respiratory failure due to COPD exacerbation

A41.9	**Sepsis, unspecified organism**
J44.1	**Chronic obstructive pulmonary disease with (acute) exacerbation**
J96.ØØ	**Acute respiratory failure, unspecified whether with hypoxia or hypercapnia**

Explanation: Although acute organ dysfunction is present in the form of acute respiratory failure, severe sepsis (R65.2) is not coded in this example, as the acute respiratory failure is attributed to the COPD exacerbation rather than the sepsis. Sequencing of these codes would be determined by the circumstances of the admission.

(b) Severe sepsis

The coding of severe sepsis requires a minimum of 2 codes: first a code for the underlying systemic infection, followed by a code from subcategory R65.2, Severe sepsis. If the causal organism is not documented, assign code A41.9, Sepsis, unspecified organism, for the infection. Additional code(s) for the associated acute organ dysfunction are also required.

Due to the complex nature of severe sepsis, some cases may require querying the provider prior to assignment of the codes.

2) Septic shock

(a) Septic shock generally refers to circulatory failure associated with severe sepsis, and therefore, it represents a type of acute organ dysfunction.

For cases of septic shock, the code for the systemic infection should be sequenced first, followed by code R65.21, Severe sepsis with septic shock or code T81.12, Postprocedural septic shock. Any additional codes for the other acute organ dysfunctions should also be assigned. As noted in the sequencing instructions in the Tabular List, the code for septic shock cannot be assigned as a principal diagnosis.

Sepsis with septic shock

A41.9	**Sepsis, unspecified organism**
R65.21	**Severe sepsis with septic shock**

Explanation: Documentation of septic shock automatically implies severe sepsis as it is a form of acute organ dysfunction. Septic shock is not coded as the principal diagnosis; it is always preceded by the code for the systemic infection.

3) Sequencing of severe sepsis

If severe sepsis is present on admission, and meets the definition of principal diagnosis, the underlying systemic infection should be assigned as principal diagnosis followed by the appropriate code from subcategory R65.2 as required by the sequencing rules in the Tabular List. A code from subcategory R65.2 can never be assigned as a principal diagnosis.

When severe sepsis develops during an encounter (it was not present on admission), the underlying systemic infection and the appropriate code from subcategory R65.2 should be assigned as secondary diagnoses.

Severe sepsis may be present on admission, but the diagnosis may not be confirmed until sometime after admission. If the documentation is not clear whether severe sepsis was present on admission, the provider should be queried.

4) Sepsis or severe sepsis with a localized infection

If the reason for admission is sepsis or severe sepsis and a localized infection, such as pneumonia or cellulitis, a code(s) for the underlying systemic infection should be assigned first and the code for the localized infection should be assigned as a secondary diagnosis. If the patient has severe sepsis, a code from subcategory R65.2 should also be assigned as a secondary diagnosis. If the patient is admitted with a localized infection, such as pneumonia, and sepsis/severe sepsis doesn't develop until after admission, the localized infection should be assigned first, followed by the appropriate sepsis/severe sepsis codes.

Patient presents with acute renal failure due to severe sepsis from *Pseudomonas* pneumonia

A41.52	**Sepsis due to Pseudomonas**
J15.1	**Pneumonia due to Pseudomonas**
R65.2Ø	**Severe sepsis without septic shock**
N17.9	**Acute kidney failure, unspecified**

Explanation: If all conditions are present on admission, the systemic infection (sepsis) is sequenced first followed by the codes for the localized infection (pneumonia), severe sepsis and any organ dysfunction. If only the pneumonia was present on admission with the sepsis and resulting renal failure developing later in the admission, then the pneumonia would be sequenced first.

5) Sepsis due to a postprocedural infection

(a) Documentation of causal relationship

As with all postprocedural complications, code assignment is based on the provider's documentation of the relationship between the infection and the procedure.

(b) Sepsis due to a postprocedural infection

For infections following a procedure, a code from T81.4Ø, to T81.43 Infection following a procedure, or a code from O86.ØØ to O86.Ø3, Infection of obstetric surgical wound, that identifies the site of the infection should be coded first, if known. Assign an additional code for sepsis following a procedure (T81.44) or sepsis following an obstetrical procedure (O86.Ø4). Use an additional code to identify the infectious agent. If the patient has severe sepsis, the appropriate code from subcategory R65.2 should also be assigned with the additional code(s) for any acute organ dysfunction.

For infections following infusion, transfusion, therapeutic injection, or immunization, a code from subcategory T8Ø.2, Infections following infusion, transfusion, and therapeutic injection, or code T88.Ø-, Infection following immunization, should be coded first, followed by the code for the specific infection. If the patient has severe sepsis, the appropriate code from subcategory R65.2 should also be assigned, with the additional codes(s) for any acute organ dysfunction.

(c) Postprocedural infection and postprocedural septic shock

If a postprocedural infection has resulted in postprocedural septic shock, assign the codes indicated above for sepsis due to a postprocedural infection, followed by code T81.12-, Postprocedural septic shock. Do not assign code R65.21, Severe sepsis with septic shock. Additional code(s) should be assigned for any acute organ dysfunction.

Septic shock following abdominal procedure with intramuscular abscess

T81.42XA	**Infection following a procedure, deep incisional surgical site, initial encounter**
T81.44XA	**Sepsis following a procedure, initial encounter**
A41.9	**Sepsis, unspecified organism**
T81.12XA	**Postprocedural septic shock, initial encounter**

Explanation: The first code reported identifies the site of the postprocedural infection with intramuscular abscess coded to "deep incisional surgical site." If sepsis occurred as a result of the postprocedural infection, code T81.44- should be coded as a secondary diagnosis, followed by a code for the specific type of sepsis. Postprocedural septic shock is captured by code T81.12- and not with code R65.21. If any other acute organ dysfunction was documented as associated with the postprocedural sepsis, additional codes could be assigned to represent those conditions.

6) Sepsis and severe sepsis associated with a noninfectious process (condition)

In some cases, a noninfectious process (condition) such as trauma, may lead to an infection which can result in sepsis or severe sepsis. If sepsis or severe sepsis is documented as associated with a noninfectious condition, such as a burn or serious injury, and this condition meets the definition for principal diagnosis, the code for the noninfectious condition should be sequenced first, followed by the code for the resulting infection. If severe sepsis is present, a code from subcategory R65.2 should also be assigned with any associated organ dysfunction(s) codes. It is not necessary to assign a code from subcategory R65.1, Systemic inflammatory response syndrome (SIRS) of non-infectious origin, for these cases.

If the infection meets the definition of principal diagnosis, it should be sequenced before the non-infectious condition. When both the associated non-infectious condition and the infection meet the definition of principal diagnosis, either may be assigned as principal diagnosis.

Only one code from category R65, Symptoms and signs specifically associated with systemic inflammation and infection, should be assigned. Therefore, when a non-infectious condition leads to an infection resulting in severe sepsis, assign the appropriate code from subcategory R65.2, Severe sepsis. Do not additionally assign a code from subcategory R65.1, Systemic inflammatory response syndrome (SIRS) of non-infectious origin.

See Section I.C.18. SIRS due to non-infectious process

Patient admitted with multiple third-degree burns of right upper arm develops severe MSSA sepsis with septic shock, three days into admission

T22.391A **Burn of third degree of multiple sites of right shoulder and upper arm limb, except wrist and hand, initial encounter**

A41.Ø1 **Sepsis due to Methicillin susceptible Staphylococcus aureus**

R65.21 **Severe sepsis with septic shock**

Explanation: Severe sepsis is coded rather than SIRS from R65 because it is documented as a severe systemic infectious response with septic shock to a noninfectious condition. The code for the systemic infection is not used as the principal diagnosis because it was not present on admission. The patient was admitted for the burn injury.

7) Sepsis and septic shock complicating abortion, pregnancy, childbirth, and the puerperium

See Section I.C.15. Sepsis and septic shock complicating abortion, pregnancy, childbirth and the puerperium

8) Newborn sepsis

See Section I.C.16. f. Bacterial sepsis of Newborn

e. Methicillin resistant Staphylococcus aureus (MRSA) conditions

1) Selection and sequencing of MRSA codes

(a) Combination codes for MRSA infection

When a patient is diagnosed with an infection that is due to methicillin resistant *Staphylococcus aureus* (MRSA), and that infection has a combination code that includes the causal organism (e.g., sepsis, pneumonia) assign the appropriate combination code for the condition (e.g., code A41.Ø2, Sepsis due to Methicillin resistant Staphylococcus aureus or code J15.212, Pneumonia due to Methicillin resistant Staphylococcus aureus). Do not assign code B95.62, Methicillin resistant Staphylococcus aureus infection as the cause of diseases classified elsewhere, as an additional code, because the combination code includes the type of infection and the MRSA organism. Do not assign a code from subcategory Z16.11, Resistance to penicillins, as an additional diagnosis.

See Section C.1. for instructions on coding and sequencing of sepsis and severe sepsis.

(b) Other codes for MRSA infection

When there is documentation of a current infection (e.g., wound infection, stitch abscess, urinary tract infection) due to MRSA, and that infection does not have a combination code that includes the causal organism, assign the appropriate code to identify the condition along with code B95.62, Methicillin resistant Staphylococcus aureus infection as the cause of diseases classified elsewhere for the MRSA infection. Do not assign a code from subcategory Z16.11, Resistance to penicillins.

(c) Methicillin susceptible Staphylococcus aureus (MSSA) and MRSA colonization

The condition or state of being colonized or carrying MSSA or MRSA is called colonization or carriage, while an individual person is described as being colonized or being a carrier. Colonization means that MSSA or MSRA is present on or in the body without necessarily causing illness. A positive MRSA colonization test might be documented by the provider as "MRSA screen positive" or "MRSA nasal swab positive".

Assign code Z22.322, Carrier or suspected carrier of Methicillin resistant Staphylococcus aureus, for patients documented as having MRSA colonization. Assign code Z22.321, Carrier or suspected carrier of Methicillin susceptible Staphylococcus aureus, for patients documented as having MSSA colonization. Colonization is not necessarily indicative of a disease process or as the cause of a specific condition the patient may have unless documented as such by the provider.

(d) MRSA colonization and infection

If a patient is documented as having both MRSA colonization and infection during a hospital admission, code Z22.322, Carrier or suspected carrier of Methicillin resistant Staphylococcus aureus, and a code for the MRSA infection may both be assigned.

f. Zika virus infections

1) Code only confirmed cases

Code only a confirmed diagnosis of Zika virus (A92.5, Zika virus disease) as documented by the provider. This is an exception to the hospital inpatient guideline Section II, H. In this context, "confirmation" does not require documentation of the type of test performed; the provider's diagnostic statement that the condition is confirmed is sufficient. This code should be assigned regardless of the stated mode of transmission.

If the provider documents "suspected", "possible" or "probable" Zika, do not assign code A92.5. Assign a code(s) explaining the reason for encounter (such as fever, rash, or joint pain) or Z2Ø.821, Contact with and (suspected) exposure to Zika virus.

A 45-year-old female recently returned from a Caribbean vacation complaining of fever, headache, joint and muscle aches and is admitted for suspected influenza. Infectious Disease consult diagnoses Zika virus. Patient discharged with Zika virus disease and instructions for hydration, rest, acetaminophen, and follow-up with Infectious Disease.

A92.5 **Zika virus disease**

Explanation: Although only a confirmed diagnosis should be coded, when a provider documents a diagnosis of Zika virus, code A92.5 Zika virus disease, is reported whether or not there is any indication of the type of tests performed. If the patient is pregnant, code first a code from category O98.5- Other viral diseases complicating pregnancy, childbirth and the puerperium, followed by code (A92.5) for the confirmed Zika virus. See also guideline 1.C.15.a.1.

g. Coronavirus infections

1) COVID-19 infection (infection due to SARS-CoV-2)

(a) Code only confirmed cases

Code only a confirmed diagnosis of the 2Ø19 novel coronavirus disease (COVID-19) as documented by the provider or documentation of a positive COVID-19 test result. For a confirmed diagnosis, assign code UØ7.1, COVID-19. This is an exception to the hospital inpatient guideline Section II, H. In this context, "confirmation" does not require documentation of a positive test result for COVID-19; the provider's documentation that the individual has COVID-19 is sufficient.

If the provider documents "suspected," "possible," "probable," or "inconclusive" COVID-19, do not assign code UØ7.1. Instead, code the signs and symptoms reported. See guideline I.C.1.g.1.g.

An elderly patient who is a former smoker is admitted with a productive cough, fatigue, and chest discomfort. CXR and PFTs indicate acute bronchitis. Treatment includes cough suppressants and anti-inflammatory medication, along with isolation precautions. The provider documents acute bronchitis likely due to COVID-19. Laboratory tests were inconclusive.

J2Ø.9 **Acute bronchitis, unspecified**

Z87.891 **History of tobacco dependence**

Explanation: Because the COVID-19 diagnosis was documented as likely by the provider, code UØ7.1 cannot be assigned. Instead a code explaining the reason for the encounter is used, in this case the acute bronchitis. Code J2Ø.9 Acute bronchitis, unspecified, is used because the causative organism, specifically that which causes COVID-19, is not confirmed. Without further documentation of COVID-19 or another causative organism being present, code J2Ø.8 Acute bronchitis due to other specified organisms, does not apply.

A 75-year-old male from a nursing home presents with shortness of breath and fever of 102.7. Patient was diagnosed with pneumonia, confirmed on CXR. Laboratory tests come back positive for COVID-19.

UØ7.1 **COVID-19**

J12.89 **Other viral pneumonia**

Explanation: The provider does not need to explicitly link the test result to the respiratory condition, nor does the provider need to explicitly document a diagnosis of COVID-19; the positive test result alone can be used to assign code UØ7.1. This advice is limited to laboratory tests for COVID-19 only. The significance of all other laboratory test results must be documented by the provider. According to guideline I.C.1.b, code UØ7.1 should be sequenced before the pneumonia code (J12.89).

(b) Sequencing of codes

When COVID-19 meets the definition of principal diagnosis, code UØ7.1, COVID-19, should be sequenced first, followed by the appropriate codes for associated manifestations, except when another guideline requires that certain codes be sequenced first, such as obstetrics, sepsis, or transplant complications.

The patient presents with acute hypoxic respiratory failure due to sepsis from COVID-19 related pneumonia.

A41.89 **Other specified sepsis**

UØ7.1 **COVID-19**

J12.89 **Other viral pneumonia**

J96.Ø1 **Acute respiratory failure with hypoxia**

R65.2Ø **Severe sepsis without septic shock**

Explanation: If all conditions are present on admission, the systemic infection (sepsis) is sequenced first, followed by the code(s) for the localized infection (COVID-19 and pneumonia). The acute respiratory failure (acute organ dysfunction) is clearly documented as being associated with the sepsis, and therefore a severe sepsis code from subcategory R65.2- can also be assigned. If the sepsis had developed later in the admission, with or without any associated respiratory failure, the COVID-19 code would be sequenced first.

For a COVID-19 infection that progresses to sepsis, see Section I.C.1.d. Sepsis, Severe Sepsis, and Septic Shock

See Section I.C.15.s. for COVID-19 infection in pregnancy, childbirth, and the puerperium

See Section I.C.16.h. for COVID-19 infection in newborn

For a COVID-19 infection in a lung transplant patient, see Section I.C.19.g.3.a. Transplant complications other than kidney.

(c) Acute respiratory manifestations of COVID-19

When the reason for the encounter/admission is a respiratory manifestation of COVID-19, assign code UØ7.1, COVID-19, as the principal/first-listed diagnosis and assign code(s) for the respiratory manifestation(s) as additional diagnoses.

The following conditions are examples of common respiratory manifestations of COVID-19.

(i) Pneumonia

For a patient with pneumonia confirmed as due to COVID-19, assign codes UØ7.1, COVID-19, and J12.89, Other viral pneumonia.

(ii) Acute bronchitis

For a patient with acute bronchitis confirmed as due to COVID-19, assign codes UØ7.1, and J2Ø.8, Acute bronchitis due to other specified organisms.

Bronchitis not otherwise specified (NOS) due to COVID-19 should be coded using code UØ7.1 and J4Ø, Bronchitis, not specified as acute or chronic.

(iii) Lower respiratory infection

If the COVID-19 is documented as being associated with a lower respiratory infection, not otherwise specified (NOS), or an acute respiratory infection, NOS, codes UØ7.1 and J22, Unspecified acute lower respiratory infection, should be assigned.

If the COVID-19 is documented as being associated with a respiratory infection, NOS, codes UØ7.1 and J98.8, Other specified respiratory disorders, should be assigned.

(iv) Acute respiratory distress syndrome

For acute respiratory distress syndrome (ARDS) due to COVID-19, assign codes UØ7.1, and J8Ø, Acute respiratory distress syndrome.

(v) Acute respiratory failure

For acute respiratory failure due to COVID-19, assign code UØ7.1, and code J96.Ø-, Acute respiratory failure.

(d) Non-respiratory manifestations of COVID-19

When the reason for the encounter/admission is a non-respiratory manifestation (e.g., viral enteritis) of COVID-19, assign code UØ7.1, COVID-19, as the principal/first-listed diagnosis and assign code(s) for the manifestation(s) as additional diagnoses.

(e) Exposure to COVID-19

For asymptomatic individuals with actual or suspected exposure to COVID-19, assign code Z2Ø.828, Contact with and (suspected) exposure to other viral communicable diseases.

For symptomatic individuals with actual or suspected exposure to COVID-19 and the infection has been ruled out, or test results are inconclusive or unknown, assign code Z2Ø.828, Contact with and (suspected) exposure to other viral communicable diseases. See guideline I.C.21.c.1, Contact/Exposure, for additional guidance regarding the use of category Z2Ø codes.

If COVID-19 is confirmed, see guideline I.C.1.g.1.a.

(f) Screening for COVID-19

During the COVID-19 pandemic, a screening code is generally not appropriate. For encounters for COVID-19 testing, including preoperative testing, code as exposure to COVID-19 (guideline I.C.1.g.1.e).

Coding guidance will be updated as new information concerning any changes in the pandemic status becomes available.

(g) Signs and symptoms without definitive diagnosis of COVID-19

For patients presenting with any signs/symptoms associated with COVID-19 (such as fever, etc.) but a definitive diagnosis has not been established, assign the appropriate code(s) for each of the presenting signs and symptoms such as:

- **RØ5 Cough**
- **RØ6.Ø2 Shortness of breath**
- **R5Ø.9 Fever, unspecified**

If a patient with signs/symptoms associated with COVID-19 also has an actual or suspected contact with or exposure to COVID-19, assign Z2Ø.828, Contact with and (suspected) exposure to other viral communicable diseases, as an additional code.

(h) Asymptomatic individuals who test positive for COVID-19

For asymptomatic individuals who test positive for COVID-19, see guideline I.C.1.g.1.a. Although the individual is asymptomatic, the individual has tested positive and is considered to have the COVID-19 infection.

(i) Personal history of COVID-19

For patients with a history of COVID-19, assign code Z86.19, Personal history of other infectious and parasitic diseases.

(j) Follow-up visits after COVID-19 infection has resolved

For individuals who previously had COVID-19 and are being seen for follow-up evaluation, and COVID-19 test results are negative, assign codes ZØ9, Encounter for follow-up examination after completed treatment for conditions other than malignant neoplasm, and Z86.19, Personal history of other infectious and parasitic diseases.

(k) Encounter for antibody testing

For an encounter for antibody testing that is not being performed to confirm a current COVID-19 infection, nor is a follow-up test after resolution of COVID-19, assign ZØ1.84, Encounter for antibody response examination.

Follow the applicable guidelines above if the individual is being tested to confirm a current COVID-19 infection.

For follow-up testing after a COVID-19 infection, see guideline I.C.1.g.1.j.

Chapter 1. Certain Infectious and Parasitic Diseases (AØØ-B99)

INCLUDES diseases generally recognized as communicable or transmissible

Use additional code to identify resistance to antimicrobial drugs (Z16.-)

EXCLUDES 1 *certain localized infections — see body system-related chapters*

EXCLUDES 2 *carrier or suspected carrier of infectious disease (Z22.-)*
infectious and parasitic diseases complicating pregnancy, childbirth and the puerperium (O98.-)
infectious and parasitic diseases specific to the perinatal period (P35-P39)
influenza and other acute respiratory infections (JØØ-J22)

This chapter contains the following blocks:

AØØ-AØ9 Intestinal infectious diseases
A15-A19 Tuberculosis
A2Ø-A28 Certain zoonotic bacterial diseases
A3Ø-A49 Other bacterial diseases
A5Ø-A64 Infections with a predominantly sexual mode of transmission
A65-A69 Other spirochetal diseases
A7Ø-A74 Other diseases caused by chlamydiae
A75-A79 Rickettsioses
A8Ø-A89 Viral and prion infections of the central nervous system
A9Ø-A99 Arthropod-borne viral fevers and viral hemorrhagic fevers
BØØ-BØ9 Viral infections characterized by skin and mucous membrane lesions
B1Ø Other human herpesviruses
B15-B19 Viral hepatitis
B2Ø Human immunodeficiency virus [HIV] disease
B25-B34 Other viral diseases
B35-B49 Mycoses
B5Ø-B64 Protozoal diseases
B65-B83 Helminthiases
B85-B89 Pediculosis, acariasis and other infestations
B9Ø-B94 Sequelae of infectious and parasitic diseases
B95-B97 Bacterial and viral infectious agents
B99 Other infectious diseases

Intestinal infectious diseases (AØØ-AØ9)

✓4th **AØØ Cholera**

DEF: Acute infection of the bowel due to vibrio cholerae that presents with profuse diarrhea, cramps, and vomiting, resulting in severe dehydration, electrolyte imbalance, and death. It is spread through ingestion of food or water contaminated with feces of infected persons.

AØØ.Ø Cholera due to Vibrio cholerae Ø1, biovar cholerae CC
Classical cholera

AØØ.1 Cholera due to Vibrio cholerae Ø1, biovar eltor CC
Cholera eltor

AØØ.9 Cholera, unspecified CC

✓4th **AØ1 Typhoid and paratyphoid fevers**

DEF: Typhoid fever: Acute generalized illness caused by *Salmonella typhi.* Clinical features include fever, headache, abdominal pain, cough, toxemia, leukopenia, abnormal pulse, rose spots on the skin, bacteremia, hyperplasia of intestinal lymph nodes, mesenteric lymphadenopathy, and Peyer's patches in the intestines.

DEF: Paratyphoid fever: Prolonged febrile illness, caused by *Salmonella* serotypes other than *S. typhi,* especially *S. enterica* serotypes paratyphi A, B, and C.

✓5th **AØ1.Ø Typhoid fever**
Infection due to Salmonella typhi

AØ1.ØØ Typhoid fever, unspecified CC
AØ1.Ø1 Typhoid meningitis CC
AØ1.Ø2 Typhoid fever with heart involvement CC
Typhoid endocarditis
Typhoid myocarditis
AØ1.Ø3 Typhoid pneumonia CC HCC
AØ1.Ø4 Typhoid arthritis CC HCC
AØ1.Ø5 Typhoid osteomyelitis CC HCC
AØ1.Ø9 Typhoid fever with other complications CC

AØ1.1 Paratyphoid fever A CC
AØ1.2 Paratyphoid fever B CC
AØ1.3 Paratyphoid fever C CC
AØ1.4 Paratyphoid fever, unspecified CC
Infection due to Salmonella paratyphi NOS

✓4th **AØ2 Other salmonella infections**

INCLUDES infection or foodborne intoxication due to any Salmonella species other than S. typhi and S. paratyphi

AØ2.Ø Salmonella enteritis CC
Salmonellosis
TIP: Dehydration (E86.0) is a complication of salmonella enteritis and may be reported separately.

AØ2.1 Salmonella sepsis HIV MCC HCC

✓5th **AØ2.2 Localized salmonella infections**

AØ2.2Ø Localized salmonella infection, unspecified HIV
AØ2.21 Salmonella meningitis HIV MCC
AØ2.22 Salmonella pneumonia HIV MCC HCC
AØ2.23 Salmonella arthritis HIV CC HCC
AØ2.24 Salmonella osteomyelitis HIV CC HCC
AØ2.25 Salmonella pyelonephritis HIV CC
Salmonella tubulo-interstitial nephropathy
AØ2.29 Salmonella with other localized infection HIV CC

AØ2.8 Other specified salmonella infections HIV CC
AØ2.9 Salmonella infection, unspecified HIV CC

✓4th **AØ3 Shigellosis**

DEF: Infection caused by the genus *Shigella,* of the family *Enterobacteriaceae* that is known to cause an acute dysenteric infection of the bowel with fever, drowsiness, anorexia, nausea, vomiting, bloody diarrhea, abdominal cramps, and distention.

AØ3.Ø Shigellosis due to Shigella dysenteriae CC
Group A shigellosis [Shiga-Kruse dysentery]
AØ3.1 Shigellosis due to Shigella flexneri
Group B shigellosis
AØ3.2 Shigellosis due to Shigella boydii
Group C shigellosis
AØ3.3 Shigellosis due to Shigella sonnei
Group D shigellosis
AØ3.8 Other shigellosis
AØ3.9 Shigellosis, unspecified
Bacillary dysentery NOS

✓4th **AØ4 Other bacterial intestinal infections**

EXCLUDES 1 *bacterial foodborne intoxications, NEC (AØ5.-)*
tuberculous enteritis (A18.32)

DEF: Escherichia coli: Gram negative, anaerobic of the family *Enterobacteriaceae* found in the large intestine of warm-blooded animals, generally as a nonpathologic entity aiding in digestion. They become pathogenic when an opportunity to grow somewhere outside this relationship presents itself, such as ingestion of fecal contaminated food or water.

AØ4.Ø Enteropathogenic Escherichia coli infection CC
AØ4.1 Enterotoxigenic Escherichia coli infection CC
AØ4.2 Enteroinvasive Escherichia coli infection CC
AØ4.3 Enterohemorrhagic Escherichia coli infection CC
DEF: *E. coli* infection penetrating the intestinal mucosa, producing microscopic ulceration and bleeding.
AØ4.4 Other intestinal Escherichia coli infections CC
Escherichia coli enteritis NOS
AØ4.5 Campylobacter enteritis CC
TIP: For Guillain-Barre syndrome occurring as a sequela of *Campylobacter enteritis*, assign code G61.0 as the first-listed diagnosis followed by B94.8 for the sequelae.
AØ4.6 Enteritis due to Yersinia enterocolitica CC
EXCLUDES 1 *extraintestinal yersiniosis (A28.2)*

✓5th **AØ4.7 Enterocolitis due to Clostridium difficile**
Foodborne intoxication by Clostridium difficile
Pseudomembraneous colitis
AHA: 2017,4Q,4

AØ4.71 Enterocolitis due to Clostridium difficile, recurrent CC
AHA: 2020,1Q,18
AØ4.72 Enterocolitis due to Clostridium difficile, not specified as recurrent CC

AØ4.8 Other specified bacterial intestinal infections CC
AØ4.9 Bacterial intestinal infection, unspecified CC
Bacterial enteritis NOS

A05 Other bacterial foodborne intoxications, not elsewhere classified

EXCLUDES 1 *Clostridium difficile foodborne intoxication and infection (A04.7-)*
Escherichia coli infection (A04.0-A04.4)
listeriosis (A32.-)
salmonella foodborne intoxication and infection (A02.-)
toxic effect of noxious foodstuffs (T61-T62)

A05.0 Foodborne staphylococcal intoxication CC
TIP: Assign code A04.8 to report a staphylococcal infection when it is caused by the ingestion of contaminated food but not caused by *S. aureus* toxins.

A05.1 Botulism food poisoning CC
Botulism NOS
Classical foodborne intoxication due to Clostridium botulinum
EXCLUDES 1 *infant botulism (A48.51)*
wound botulism (A48.52)
DEF: Muscle-paralyzing neurotoxic disease caused by ingesting pre-formed toxin from the bacterium *Clostridium botulinum*. It causes vomiting and diarrhea, vision problems, slurred speech, difficulty swallowing, paralysis, and death.

A05.2 Foodborne Clostridium perfringens [Clostridium welchii] intoxication CC
Enteritis necroticans
Pig-bel

A05.3 Foodborne Vibrio parahaemolyticus intoxication CC

A05.4 Foodborne Bacillus cereus intoxication CC

A05.5 Foodborne Vibrio vulnificus intoxication CC

A05.8 Other specified bacterial foodborne intoxications CC

A05.9 Bacterial foodborne intoxication, unspecified

A06 Amebiasis

INCLUDES infection due to Entamoeba histolytica
EXCLUDES 1 *other protozoal intestinal diseases (A07.-)*
EXCLUDES 2 *acanthamebiasis (B60.1-)*
Naegleriasis (B60.2)

DEF: Infection with a single cell protozoan known as the amoeba. Transmission occurs through ingestion of feces, contaminated food or water, use of human feces as fertilizer, or person-to-person contact.

A06.0 Acute amebic dysentery CC
Acute amebiasis
Intestinal amebiasis NOS

A06.1 Chronic intestinal amebiasis CC

A06.2 Amebic nondysenteric colitis CC

A06.3 Ameboma of intestine CC
Ameboma NOS

A06.4 Amebic liver abscess MCC
Hepatic amebiasis

A06.5 Amebic lung abscess MCC HCC
Amebic abscess of lung (and liver)

A06.6 Amebic brain abscess MCC
Amebic abscess of brain (and liver) (and lung)

A06.7 Cutaneous amebiasis

A06.8 Amebic infection of other sites

A06.81 Amebic cystitis CC

A06.82 Other amebic genitourinary infections CC
Amebic balanitis
Amebic vesiculitis
Amebic vulvovaginitis

A06.89 Other amebic infections CC
Amebic appendicitis
Amebic splenic abscess

A06.9 Amebiasis, unspecified

A07 Other protozoal intestinal diseases

DEF: Protozoa: Group comprised of the simplest, single celled organisms, ranging in size from micro to macroscopic. They can live alone or in colonies, and do not show any differentiation in tissues. Most are motile and can live free in nature, but some are parasitic, causing disease in the variety of hosts they inhabit.

A07.0 Balantidiasis
Balantidial dysentery

A07.1 Giardiasis [lambliasis] CC
DEF: Infection caused by the flagellate protozoan *Giardia lamblia* causing gastrointestinal problems such as vomiting, chronic diarrhea, and weight loss. The most common parasite in the US, this is usually transmitted by ingesting contaminated water while in the cyst state and latches onto the wall of the small intestine.

A07.2 Cryptosporidiosis CC HCC
DEF: Microscopic parasite found in water and one of the most common causes of waterborne gastrointestinal infectious disease in the United States. It is usually transmitted by ingesting contaminated drinking water or recreational water and causes profuse watery diarrhea, flatulence, abdominal pain, and cramping.

A07.3 Isosporiasis HIV CC
Infection due to Isospora belli and Isospora hominis
Intestinal coccidiosis
Isosporosis

A07.4 Cyclosporiasis CC

A07.8 Other specified protozoal intestinal diseases CC
Intestinal microsporidiosis
Intestinal trichomoniasis
Sarcocystosis
Sarcosporidiosis

A07.9 Protozoal intestinal disease, unspecified CC
Flagellate diarrhea
Protozoal colitis
Protozoal diarrhea
Protozoal dysentery

A08 Viral and other specified intestinal infections

EXCLUDES 1 *influenza with involvement of gastrointestinal tract (J09.X3, J10.2, J11.2)*

A08.0 Rotaviral enteritis CC

A08.1 Acute gastroenteropathy due to Norwalk agent and other small round viruses

A08.11 Acute gastroenteropathy due to Norwalk agent CC
Acute gastroenteropathy due to Norovirus
Acute gastroenteropathy due to Norwalk-like agent

A08.19 Acute gastroenteropathy due to other small round viruses CC
Acute gastroenteropathy due to small round virus [SRV] NOS

A08.2 Adenoviral enteritis CC

A08.3 Other viral enteritis

A08.31 Calicivirus enteritis CC

A08.32 Astrovirus enteritis CC

A08.39 Other viral enteritis CC
Coxsackie virus enteritis
Echovirus enteritis
Enterovirus enteritis NEC
Torovirus enteritis

A08.4 Viral intestinal infection, unspecified
Viral enteritis NOS
Viral gastroenteritis NOS
Viral gastroenteropathy NOS
AHA: 2016,3Q,12

A08.8 Other specified intestinal infections

A09 Infectious gastroenteritis and colitis, unspecified CC
Infectious colitis NOS
Infectious enteritis NOS
Infectious gastroenteritis NOS
EXCLUDES 1 *colitis NOS (K52.9)*
diarrhea NOS (R19.7)
enteritis NOS (K52.9)
gastroenteritis NOS (K52.9)
noninfective gastroenteritis and colitis, unspecified (K52.9)

DEF: Colitis: Inflammation of mucous membranes of the colon.
DEF: Enteritis: Inflammation of mucous membranes of the small intestine.
DEF: Gastroenteritis: Inflammation of mucous membranes of the stomach and intestines.

Tuberculosis (A15-A19)

INCLUDES infections due to Mycobacterium tuberculosis and Mycobacterium bovis

EXCLUDES 1 *congenital tuberculosis (P37.Ø)*
nonspecific reaction to test for tuberculosis without active tuberculosis (R76.1-)
pneumoconiosis associated with tuberculosis, any type in A15 (J65)
positive PPD (R76.11)
positive tuberculin skin test without active tuberculosis (R76.11)
sequelae of tuberculosis (B9Ø.-)
silicotuberculosis (J65)

DEF: Bacterial infection that typically spreads by inhalation of an airborne agent that usually attacks the lungs, but may also affect other organs.

✓4th **A15 Respiratory tuberculosis**

A15.Ø Tuberculosis of lung HIV CC
Tuberculous bronchiectasis
Tuberculous fibrosis of lung
Tuberculous pneumonia
Tuberculous pneumothorax

Tuberculosis of Lung

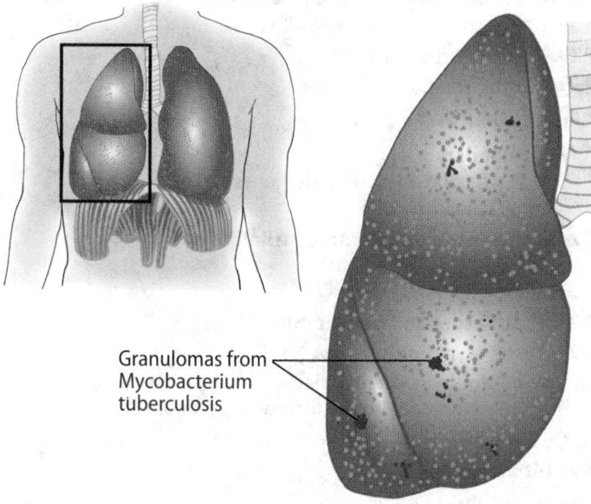

A15.4 Tuberculosis of intrathoracic lymph nodes HIV CC
Tuberculosis of hilar lymph nodes
Tuberculosis of mediastinal lymph nodes
Tuberculosis of tracheobronchial lymph nodes
EXCLUDES 1 *tuberculosis specified as primary (A15.7)*

A15.5 Tuberculosis of larynx, trachea and bronchus HIV CC
Tuberculosis of bronchus
Tuberculosis of glottis
Tuberculosis of larynx
Tuberculosis of trachea

A15.6 Tuberculous pleurisy HIV CC
Tuberculosis of pleura Tuberculous empyema
EXCLUDES 1 *primary respiratory tuberculosis (A15.7)*

A15.7 Primary respiratory tuberculosis HIV CC

A15.8 Other respiratory tuberculosis HIV CC
Mediastinal tuberculosis
Nasopharyngeal tuberculosis
Tuberculosis of nose
Tuberculosis of sinus [any nasal]

A15.9 Respiratory tuberculosis unspecified HIV CC

✓4th **A17 Tuberculosis of nervous system**

A17.Ø Tuberculous meningitis HIV MCC
Tuberculosis of meninges (cerebral)(spinal)
Tuberculous leptomeningitis
EXCLUDES 1 *tuberculous meningoencephalitis (A17.82)*

A17.1 Meningeal tuberculoma HIV MCC
Tuberculoma of meninges (cerebral) (spinal)
EXCLUDES 2 *tuberculoma of brain and spinal cord (A17.81)*

✓5th **A17.8 Other tuberculosis of nervous system**

A17.81 Tuberculoma of brain and spinal cord HIV MCC
Tuberculous abscess of brain and spinal cord

A17.82 Tuberculous meningoencephalitis HIV MCC
Tuberculous myelitis

A17.83 Tuberculous neuritis HIV MCC
Tuberculous mononeuropathy

A17.89 Other tuberculosis of nervous system HIV MCC
Tuberculous polyneuropathy

A17.9 Tuberculosis of nervous system, unspecified HIV CC

✓4th **A18 Tuberculosis of other organs**

✓5th **A18.Ø Tuberculosis of bones and joints**

A18.Ø1 Tuberculosis of spine HIV CC
Pott's disease or curvature of spine
Tuberculous arthritis
Tuberculous osteomyelitis of spine
Tuberculous spondylitis

A18.Ø2 Tuberculous arthritis of other joints HIV CC
Tuberculosis of hip (joint)
Tuberculosis of knee (joint)

A18.Ø3 Tuberculosis of other bones HIV CC
Tuberculous mastoiditis
Tuberculous osteomyelitis

A18.Ø9 Other musculoskeletal tuberculosis HIV CC
Tuberculous myositis
Tuberculous synovitis
Tuberculous tenosynovitis

✓5th **A18.1 Tuberculosis of genitourinary system**

A18.1Ø Tuberculosis of genitourinary system, unspecified HIV CC

A18.11 Tuberculosis of kidney and ureter HIV CC

A18.12 Tuberculosis of bladder HIV CC

A18.13 Tuberculosis of other urinary organs HIV CC
Tuberculous urethritis

A18.14 Tuberculosis of prostate HIV CC A ♂

A18.15 Tuberculosis of other male genital organs HIV CC ♂

A18.16 Tuberculosis of cervix HIV CC ♀

A18.17 Tuberculous female pelvic inflammatory disease HIV CC ♀
Tuberculous endometritis
Tuberculous oophoritis and salpingitis

A18.18 Tuberculosis of other female genital organs HIV CC ♀
Tuberculous ulceration of vulva

A18.2 Tuberculous peripheral lymphadenopathy HIV CC
Tuberculous adenitis
EXCLUDES 2 *tuberculosis of bronchial and mediastinal lymph nodes (A15.4)*
tuberculosis of mesenteric and retroperitoneal lymph nodes (A18.39)
tuberculous tracheobronchial adenopathy (A15.4)

✓5th **A18.3 Tuberculosis of intestines, peritoneum and mesenteric glands**

A18.31 Tuberculous peritonitis HIV MCC
Tuberculous ascites
DEF: Tuberculous inflammation of the membrane lining the abdomen.

A18.32 Tuberculous enteritis HIV CC
Tuberculosis of anus and rectum
Tuberculosis of intestine (large) (small)

A18.39 Retroperitoneal tuberculosis HIV CC
Tuberculosis of mesenteric glands
Tuberculosis of retroperitoneal (lymph glands)

A18.4 Tuberculosis of skin and subcutaneous tissue HIV CC
Erythema induratum, tuberculous
Lupus excedens
Lupus vulgaris NOS
Lupus vulgaris of eyelid
Scrofuloderma
Tuberculosis of external ear
EXCLUDES 2 *lupus erythematosus (L93.-)*
systemic lupus erythematosus (M32.-)

✓5th **A18.5 Tuberculosis of eye**
EXCLUDES 2 *lupus vulgaris of eyelid (A18.4)*

A18.5Ø Tuberculosis of eye, unspecified HIV CC

A18.51 Tuberculous episcleritis HIV CC

A18.52 **Tuberculous keratitis** HIV CC
Tuberculous interstitial keratitis
Tuberculous keratoconjunctivitis (interstitial) (phlyctenular)
A18.53 **Tuberculous chorioretinitis** HIV CC
A18.54 **Tuberculous iridocyclitis** HIV CC
A18.59 **Other tuberculosis of eye** HIV CC
Tuberculous conjunctivitis
A18.6 **Tuberculosis of (inner) (middle) ear** HIV CC
Tuberculous otitis media
EXCLUDES 2 *tuberculosis of external ear (A18.4)*
tuberculous mastoiditis (A18.Ø3)
A18.7 **Tuberculosis of adrenal glands** HIV CC
Tuberculous Addison's disease
✓5th A18.8 **Tuberculosis of other specified organs**
A18.81 **Tuberculosis of thyroid gland** HIV CC
A18.82 **Tuberculosis of other endocrine glands** HIV CC
Tuberculosis of pituitary gland
Tuberculosis of thymus gland
A18.83 **Tuberculosis of digestive tract organs, not elsewhere classified** HIV CC
EXCLUDES 1 *tuberculosis of intestine (A18.32)*
A18.84 **Tuberculosis of heart** HIV CC
Tuberculous cardiomyopathy
Tuberculous endocarditis
Tuberculous myocarditis
Tuberculous pericarditis
A18.85 **Tuberculosis of spleen** HIV CC
A18.89 **Tuberculosis of other sites** HIV CC
Tuberculosis of muscle
Tuberculous cerebral arteritis

✓4th **A19 Miliary tuberculosis**
INCLUDES disseminated tuberculosis
generalized tuberculosis
tuberculous polyserositis
A19.Ø **Acute miliary tuberculosis of a single specified site** HIV MCC
A19.1 **Acute miliary tuberculosis of multiple sites** HIV MCC
A19.2 **Acute miliary tuberculosis, unspecified** HIV MCC
A19.8 **Other miliary tuberculosis** HIV MCC
A19.9 **Miliary tuberculosis, unspecified** HIV MCC

Certain zoonotic bacterial diseases (A2Ø-A28)

✓4th **A2Ø Plague**
INCLUDES infection due to Yersinia pestis
A2Ø.Ø **Bubonic plague** MCC
A2Ø.1 **Cellulocutaneous plague** MCC
A2Ø.2 **Pneumonic plague** MCC HCC
A2Ø.3 **Plague meningitis** MCC
A2Ø.7 **Septicemic plague** MCC HCC
A2Ø.8 **Other forms of plague** MCC
Abortive plague
Asymptomatic plague
Pestis minor
A2Ø.9 **Plague, unspecified** MCC

✓4th **A21 Tularemia**
INCLUDES deer-fly fever
infection due to Francisella tularensis
rabbit fever
DEF: Febrile disease transmitted to humans by the bites of deer flies, fleas, and ticks, by inhaling aerosolized *F. tularensis*, or by ingesting contaminated food or water. Patients quickly develop fever, chills, weakness, headache, backache, and malaise.
A21.Ø **Ulceroglandular tularemia** CC
A21.1 **Oculoglandular tularemia** CC
Ophthalmic tularemia
A21.2 **Pulmonary tularemia** CC HCC
A21.3 **Gastrointestinal tularemia** CC
Abdominal tularemia
A21.7 **Generalized tularemia** CC
A21.8 **Other forms of tularemia** CC
A21.9 **Tularemia, unspecified** CC

✓4th **A22 Anthrax**
INCLUDES infection due to Bacillus anthracis
A22.Ø **Cutaneous anthrax** CC
Malignant carbuncle
Malignant pustule
A22.1 **Pulmonary anthrax** MCC HCC
Inhalation anthrax
Ragpicker's disease
Woolsorter's disease
A22.2 **Gastrointestinal anthrax** CC
A22.7 **Anthrax sepsis** MCC HCC
A22.8 **Other forms of anthrax** CC
Anthrax meningitis
A22.9 **Anthrax, unspecified** CC

✓4th **A23 Brucellosis**
INCLUDES Malta fever
Mediterranean fever
undulant fever
A23.Ø **Brucellosis due to Brucella melitensis**
A23.1 **Brucellosis due to Brucella abortus**
A23.2 **Brucellosis due to Brucella suis**
A23.3 **Brucellosis due to Brucella canis**
A23.8 **Other brucellosis** CC
A23.9 **Brucellosis, unspecified** CC

✓4th **A24 Glanders and melioidosis**
A24.Ø **Glanders** CC
Infection due to Pseudomonas mallei
Malleus
A24.1 **Acute and fulminating melioidosis** CC
Melioidosis pneumonia
Melioidosis sepsis
A24.2 **Subacute and chronic melioidosis** CC
A24.3 **Other melioidosis** CC
A24.9 **Melioidosis, unspecified** CC
Infection due to Pseudomonas pseudomallei NOS
Whitmore's disease

✓4th **A25 Rat-bite fevers**
A25.Ø **Spirillosis** CC
Sodoku
A25.1 **Streptobacillosis** CC
Epidemic arthritic erythema
Haverhill fever
Streptobacillary rat-bite fever
A25.9 **Rat-bite fever, unspecified** CC

✓4th **A26 Erysipeloid**
DEF: Acute cutaneous infection typically caused by trauma to the skin. Presenting as cellulitis, it may become systemic affecting other organs. It is gram positive bacillus and mainly acquired by those who routinely handle meat.
A26.Ø **Cutaneous erysipeloid**
Erythema migrans
A26.7 **Erysipelothrix sepsis** MCC HCC
A26.8 **Other forms of erysipeloid**
A26.9 **Erysipeloid, unspecified**

✓4th **A27 Leptospirosis**
A27.Ø **Leptospirosis icterohemorrhagica** CC
Leptospiral or spirochetal jaundice (hemorrhagic)
Weil's disease
✓5th A27.8 **Other forms of leptospirosis**
A27.81 **Aseptic meningitis in leptospirosis** MCC
A27.89 **Other forms of leptospirosis** CC
A27.9 **Leptospirosis, unspecified** CC

✓4th **A28 Other zoonotic bacterial diseases, not elsewhere classified**
A28.Ø **Pasteurellosis** CC
A28.1 **Cat-scratch disease** CC
Cat-scratch fever
A28.2 **Extraintestinal yersiniosis** CC
EXCLUDES 1 *enteritis due to Yersinia enterocolitica (AØ4.6)*
plague (A2Ø.-)
A28.8 **Other specified zoonotic bacterial diseases, not elsewhere classified** CC
A28.9 **Zoonotic bacterial disease, unspecified** CC

Other bacterial diseases (A30-A49)

AHA: 2016,3Q,8-14

A30 Leprosy [Hansen's disease]
INCLUDES infection due to Mycobacterium leprae
EXCLUDES 1 *sequelae of leprosy (B92)*

A30.0 Indeterminate leprosy CC
I leprosy

A30.1 Tuberculoid leprosy CC
TT leprosy

A30.2 Borderline tuberculoid leprosy CC
BT leprosy

A30.3 Borderline leprosy CC
BB leprosy

A30.4 Borderline lepromatous leprosy CC
BL leprosy

A30.5 Lepromatous leprosy CC
LL leprosy

A30.8 Other forms of leprosy CC

A30.9 Leprosy, unspecified CC

A31 Infection due to other mycobacteria
EXCLUDES 2 *leprosy (A30.-)*
tuberculosis (A15-A19)

A31.0 Pulmonary mycobacterial infection CC HCC
Infection due to Mycobacterium avium
Infection due to Mycobacterium intracellulare [Battey bacillus]
Infection due to Mycobacterium kansasii

A31.1 Cutaneous mycobacterial infection CC
Buruli ulcer
Infection due to Mycobacterium marinum
Infection due to Mycobacterium ulcerans

A31.2 Disseminated mycobacterium avium-intracellulare complex (DMAC) HIV CC HCC
MAC sepsis

A31.8 Other mycobacterial infections HIV CC

A31.9 Mycobacterial infection, unspecified HIV CC
Atypical mycobacterial infection NOS
Mycobacteriosis NOS

A32 Listeriosis
INCLUDES listerial foodborne infection
EXCLUDES 1 *neonatal (disseminated) listeriosis (P37.2)*

A32.0 Cutaneous listeriosis CC

A32.1 Listerial meningitis and meningoencephalitis

A32.11 Listerial meningitis CC

A32.12 Listerial meningoencephalitis CC

A32.7 Listerial sepsis MCC HCC

A32.8 Other forms of listeriosis

A32.81 Oculoglandular listeriosis CC

A32.82 Listerial endocarditis CC

A32.89 Other forms of listeriosis CC
Listerial cerebral arteritis

A32.9 Listeriosis, unspecified CC

A33 Tetanus neonatorum MCC N

A34 Obstetrical tetanus CC M ♀

A35 Other tetanus MCC
Tetanus NOS
EXCLUDES 1 *obstetrical tetanus (A34)*
tetanus neonatorum (A33)

DEF: Tetanus: Acute, often fatal, infectious disease caused by the anaerobic, spore-forming bacillus *Clostridium tetani*. The bacillus enters the body through a contaminated wound, burns, surgical wounds, or cutaneous ulcers. Symptoms include lockjaw, spasms, seizures, and paralysis.

A36 Diphtheria

A36.0 Pharyngeal diphtheria CC
Diphtheritic membranous angina
Tonsillar diphtheria

A36.1 Nasopharyngeal diphtheria CC

A36.2 Laryngeal diphtheria CC
Diphtheritic laryngotracheitis

A36.3 Cutaneous diphtheria CC
EXCLUDES 2 *erythrasma (L08.1)*

A36.8 Other diphtheria

A36.81 Diphtheritic cardiomyopathy CC HCC
Diphtheritic myocarditis

A36.82 Diphtheritic radiculomyelitis CC

A36.83 Diphtheritic polyneuritis CC

A36.84 Diphtheritic tubulo-interstitial nephropathy CC

A36.85 Diphtheritic cystitis CC

A36.86 Diphtheritic conjunctivitis CC

A36.89 Other diphtheritic complications CC
Diphtheritic peritonitis

A36.9 Diphtheria, unspecified CC

A37 Whooping cough
DEF: Acute, highly contagious respiratory tract infection caused by *Bordetella pertussis* and *B. bronchiseptica*. Whooping cough is known by its characteristic paroxysmal cough.

A37.0 Whooping cough due to Bordetella pertussis

A37.00 Whooping cough due to Bordetella pertussis without pneumonia CC

A37.01 Whooping cough due to Bordetella pertussis with pneumonia MCC

A37.1 Whooping cough due to Bordetella parapertussis

A37.10 Whooping cough due to Bordetella parapertussis without pneumonia CC

A37.11 Whooping cough due to Bordetella parapertussis with pneumonia MCC

A37.8 Whooping cough due to other Bordetella species

A37.80 Whooping cough due to other Bordetella species without pneumonia CC

A37.81 Whooping cough due to other Bordetella species with pneumonia MCC

A37.9 Whooping cough, unspecified species

A37.90 Whooping cough, unspecified species without pneumonia CC

A37.91 Whooping cough, unspecified species with pneumonia MCC

A38 Scarlet fever
INCLUDES scarlatina
EXCLUDES 2 *streptococcal sore throat (J02.0)*
DEF: Acute contagious disease caused by Group A bacteria, the same bacterium that causes strep throat. Individuals with strep throat can develop scarlet fever particularly if the infection is not treated with antibiotics. It is characterized by a red blush to the skin of the chest and abdomen and swelling of the nose, throat, and mouth.

A38.0 Scarlet fever with otitis media CC

A38.1 Scarlet fever with myocarditis CC

A38.8 Scarlet fever with other complications CC

A38.9 Scarlet fever, uncomplicated CC
Scarlet fever, NOS

A39 Meningococcal infection
DEF: Condition caused by *Neisseria meningitidis*, a bacteria that may invade the spinal cord, brain, heart, joints, optic nerve, or bloodstream.

A39.0 Meningococcal meningitis MCC

A39.1 Waterhouse-Friderichsen syndrome MCC HCC
Meningococcal hemorrhagic adrenalitis
Meningococcic adrenal syndrome

A39.2 Acute meningococcemia MCC HCC

A39.3 Chronic meningococcemia MCC HCC

A39.4 Meningococcemia, unspecified MCC HCC

A39.5 Meningococcal heart disease

A39.50 Meningococcal carditis, unspecified MCC

A39.51 Meningococcal endocarditis MCC

A39.52 Meningococcal myocarditis MCC

A39.53 Meningococcal pericarditis MCC

A39.8 Other meningococcal infections

A39.81 Meningococcal encephalitis MCC

A39.82 Meningococcal retrobulbar neuritis CC

A39.83 Meningococcal arthritis CC HCC

A39.84 Postmeningococcal arthritis CC HCC

A39.89 Other meningococcal infections CC
Meningococcal conjunctivitis

A39.9 Meningococcal infection, unspecified CC
Meningococcal disease NOS

A40 Streptococcal sepsis
Code first:
postprocedural streptococcal sepsis (T81.4-)
streptococcal sepsis during labor (O75.3)
streptococcal sepsis following abortion or ectopic or molar pregnancy (O03-O07, O08.0)
streptococcal sepsis following immunization (T88.0)
streptococcal sepsis following infusion, transfusion or therapeutic injection (T80.2-)
EXCLUDES 1 *neonatal (P36.0-P36.1)*
puerperal sepsis (O85)
sepsis due to Streptococcus, group D (A41.81)
AHA: 2020,2Q,8,28; 2019,4Q,65; 2018,4Q,89; 2018,1Q,16; 2016,1Q,32

A40.0 Sepsis due to streptococcus, group A MCC HCC
A40.1 Sepsis due to streptococcus, group B MCC HCC
AHA: 2019,1Q,14
A40.3 Sepsis due to Streptococcus pneumoniae MCC HCC
Pneumococcal sepsis
A40.8 Other streptococcal sepsis MCC HCC
A40.9 Streptococcal sepsis, unspecified HIV MCC HCC

A41 Other sepsis
Code first:
postprocedural sepsis (T81.4-)
sepsis during labor (O75.3)
sepsis following abortion, ectopic or molar pregnancy (O03-O07, O08.0)
sepsis following immunization (T88.0)
sepsis following infusion, transfusion or therapeutic injection (T80.2-)
EXCLUDES 1 *bacteremia NOS (R78.81)*
neonatal (P36.-)
puerperal sepsis (O85)
streptococcal sepsis (A40.-)
EXCLUDES 2 *sepsis (due to) (in) actinomycotic (A42.7)*
sepsis (due to) (in) anthrax (A22.7)
sepsis (due to) (in) candidal (B37.7)
sepsis (due to) (in) Erysipelothrix (A26.7)
sepsis (due to) (in) extraintestinal yersiniosis (A28.2)
sepsis (due to) (in) gonococcal (A54.86)
sepsis (due to) (in) herpesviral (B00.7)
sepsis (due to) (in) listerial (A32.7)
sepsis (due to) (in) melioidosis (A24.1)
sepsis (due to) (in) meningococcal (A39.2-A39.4)
sepsis (due to) (in) plague (A20.7)
sepsis (due to) (in) tularemia (A21.7)
toxic shock syndrome (A48.3)
AHA: 2020,2Q,8,28; 2019,4Q,65; 2019,3Q,17; 2018,4Q,18; 2018,1Q,16; 2016,1Q,32; 2014,2Q,13

A41.0 Sepsis due to Staphylococcus aureus
A41.01 Sepsis due to Methicillin susceptible Staphylococcus aureus HIV MCC HCC
MSSA sepsis
Staphylococcus aureus sepsis NOS
AHA: 2020,2Q,17
A41.02 Sepsis due to Methicillin resistant Staphylococcus aureus HIV MCC HCC
A41.1 Sepsis due to other specified staphylococcus HIV MCC HCC
Coagulase negative staphylococcus sepsis
A41.2 Sepsis due to unspecified staphylococcus HIV MCC HCC
A41.3 Sepsis due to Hemophilus influenzae HIV MCC HCC
A41.4 Sepsis due to anaerobes HIV MCC HCC
EXCLUDES 1 *gas gangrene (A48.0)*
A41.5 Sepsis due to other Gram-negative organisms
A41.50 Gram-negative sepsis, unspecified HIV MCC HCC
Gram-negative sepsis NOS
AHA: 2020,2Q,28
A41.51 Sepsis due to Escherichia coli [E. coli] HIV MCC HCC
AHA: 2020,2Q,17
A41.52 Sepsis due to Pseudomonas HIV MCC HCC
Pseudomonas aeroginosa
A41.53 Sepsis due to Serratia HIV MCC HCC
A41.59 Other Gram-negative sepsis HIV MCC HCC
A41.8 Other specified sepsis
A41.81 Sepsis due to Enterococcus HIV MCC HCC
TIP: *E. faecium,* is a species of *Enterococcus* that is highly resistant to multiple antibiotics. Assign a code from category Z16 when resistance to antimicrobial drugs is documented.
A41.89 Other specified sepsis HIV MCC HCC
AHA: 2020,2Q,8; 2017,1Q,51; 2016,3Q,8-14
TIP: Viral sepsis is coded here; assign an additional code to identify the specific viral agent or illness.
A41.9 Sepsis, unspecified organism HIV MCC HCC
Septicemia NOS
AHA: 2020,2Q,28

A42 Actinomycosis
EXCLUDES 1 *actinomycetoma (B47.1)*
A42.0 Pulmonary actinomycosis HIV CC HCC
A42.1 Abdominal actinomycosis HIV CC
A42.2 Cervicofacial actinomycosis HIV CC
A42.7 Actinomycotic sepsis HIV MCC HCC
A42.8 Other forms of actinomycosis
A42.81 Actinomycotic meningitis HIV CC
A42.82 Actinomycotic encephalitis HIV CC
A42.89 Other forms of actinomycosis HIV CC
A42.9 Actinomycosis, unspecified HIV CC

A43 Nocardiosis
DEF: Rare bacterial infection occurring most often in those with weakened immune systems. Can be acquired in soil, decaying plants, or standing water. It typically begins in the lungs and has a tendency to spread to other body systems.
A43.0 Pulmonary nocardiosis HIV CC HCC
A43.1 Cutaneous nocardiosis HIV CC
A43.8 Other forms of nocardiosis HIV CC
A43.9 Nocardiosis, unspecified HIV CC

A44 Bartonellosis
A44.0 Systemic bartonellosis CC
Oroya fever
A44.1 Cutaneous and mucocutaneous bartonellosis CC
Verruga peruana
A44.8 Other forms of bartonellosis CC
A44.9 Bartonellosis, unspecified CC

A46 Erysipelas
EXCLUDES 1 *postpartum or puerperal erysipelas (O86.89)*
DEF: Skin infection affecting the upper dermis and superficial dermal lymphatics. Lesion edges are well-demarcated with distinct raised borders. It is often caused by group A *Streptococci.*

A48 Other bacterial diseases, not elsewhere classified
EXCLUDES 1 *actinomycetoma (B47.1)*
A48.0 Gas gangrene MCC HCC
Clostridial cellulitis
Clostridial myonecrosis
AHA: 2017,4Q,102
A48.1 Legionnaires' disease HIV MCC HCC
DEF: Severe and often fatal infection by *Legionella pneumophila.* Symptoms include high fever, gastrointestinal pain, headache, myalgia, dry cough, and pneumonia and it is usually transmitted through airborne water droplets via air conditioning systems or hot tubs.
A48.2 Nonpneumonic Legionnaires' disease [Pontiac fever]
A48.3 Toxic shock syndrome MCC HCC
Use additional code to identify the organism (B95, B96)
EXCLUDES 1 *endotoxic shock NOS (R57.8)*
sepsis NOS (A41.9)
DEF: Bacteria producing an endotoxin, such as *Staphylococci,* flood the body with the toxins producing a high fever, vomiting and diarrhea, decreasing blood pressure, a skin rash, and shock.
Synonym(s): *TSS.*
A48.4 Brazilian purpuric fever
Systemic Hemophilus aegyptius infection
A48.5 Other specified botulism
Non-foodborne intoxication due to toxins of Clostridium botulinum [C. botulinum]
EXCLUDES 1 *food poisoning due to toxins of Clostridium botulinum (A05.1)*
A48.51 Infant botulism CC P

A48.52 Wound botulism CC
Non-foodborne botulism NOS
Use additional code for associated wound

A48.8 Other specified bacterial diseases

✓4th **A49 Bacterial infection of unspecified site**
EXCLUDES 1 *bacterial agents as the cause of diseases classified elsewhere (B95-B96)*
chlamydial infection NOS (A74.9)
meningococcal infection NOS (A39.9)
rickettsial infection NOS (A79.9)
spirochetal infection NOS (A69.9)

✓5th **A49.Ø Staphylococcal infection, unspecified site**

A49.Ø1 Methicillin susceptible Staphylococcus aureus infection, unspecified site
Methicillin susceptible Staphylococcus aureus (MSSA) infection
Staphylococcus aureus infection NOS

A49.Ø2 Methicillin resistant Staphylococcus aureus infection, unspecified site
Methicillin resistant Staphylococcus aureus (MRSA) infection

A49.1 Streptococcal infection, unspecified site

A49.2 Hemophilus influenzae infection, unspecified site

A49.3 Mycoplasma infection, unspecified site

A49.8 Other bacterial infections of unspecified site

A49.9 Bacterial infection, unspecified
EXCLUDES 1 *bacteremia NOS (R78.81)*

Infections with a predominantly sexual mode of transmission (A5Ø-A64)

EXCLUDES 1 *human immunodeficiency virus [HIV] disease (B2Ø)*
nonspecific and nongonococcal urethritis (N34.1)
Reiter's disease (MØ2.3-)

✓4th **A5Ø Congenital syphilis**

✓5th **A5Ø.Ø Early congenital syphilis, symptomatic**
Any congenital syphilitic condition specified as early or manifest less than two years after birth.

A5Ø.Ø1 Early congenital syphilitic oculopathy CC

A5Ø.Ø2 Early congenital syphilitic osteochondropathy CC

A5Ø.Ø3 Early congenital syphilitic pharyngitis CC
Early congenital syphilitic laryngitis

A5Ø.Ø4 Early congenital syphilitic pneumonia CC

A5Ø.Ø5 Early congenital syphilitic rhinitis CC

A5Ø.Ø6 Early cutaneous congenital syphilis CC

A5Ø.Ø7 Early mucocutaneous congenital syphilis CC

A5Ø.Ø8 Early visceral congenital syphilis CC

A5Ø.Ø9 Other early congenital syphilis, symptomatic CC

A5Ø.1 Early congenital syphilis, latent
Congenital syphilis without clinical manifestations, with positive serological reaction and negative spinal fluid test, less than two years after birth.

A5Ø.2 Early congenital syphilis, unspecified CC
Congenital syphilis NOS less than two years after birth.

✓5th **A5Ø.3 Late congenital syphilitic oculopathy**
EXCLUDES 1 *Hutchinson's triad (A5Ø.53)*

A5Ø.3Ø Late congenital syphilitic oculopathy, unspecified CC

A5Ø.31 Late congenital syphilitic interstitial keratitis CC

A5Ø.32 Late congenital syphilitic chorioretinitis CC

A5Ø.39 Other late congenital syphilitic oculopathy CC

✓5th **A5Ø.4 Late congenital neurosyphilis [juvenile neurosyphilis]**
Use additional code to identify any associated mental disorder
EXCLUDES 1 *Hutchinson's triad (A5Ø.53)*

A5Ø.4Ø Late congenital neurosyphilis, unspecified CC
Juvenile neurosyphilis NOS

A5Ø.41 Late congenital syphilitic meningitis MCC

A5Ø.42 Late congenital syphilitic encephalitis MCC

A5Ø.43 Late congenital syphilitic polyneuropathy CC

A5Ø.44 Late congenital syphilitic optic nerve atrophy CC

A5Ø.45 Juvenile general paresis CC
Dementia paralytica juvenilis
Juvenile tabetoparetic neurosyphilis

A5Ø.49 Other late congenital neurosyphilis CC
Juvenile tabes dorsalis

✓5th **A5Ø.5 Other late congenital syphilis, symptomatic**
Any congenital syphilitic condition specified as late or manifest two years or more after birth.

A5Ø.51 Clutton's joints CC

A5Ø.52 Hutchinson's teeth CC

A5Ø.53 Hutchinson's triad CC

A5Ø.54 Late congenital cardiovascular syphilis CC

A5Ø.55 Late congenital syphilitic arthropathy CC HCC

A5Ø.56 Late congenital syphilitic osteochondropathy CC

A5Ø.57 Syphilitic saddle nose CC

A5Ø.59 Other late congenital syphilis, symptomatic CC

A5Ø.6 Late congenital syphilis, latent
Congenital syphilis without clinical manifestations, with positive serological reaction and negative spinal fluid test, two years or more after birth.

A5Ø.7 Late congenital syphilis, unspecified
Congenital syphilis NOS two years or more after birth.

A5Ø.9 Congenital syphilis, unspecified

✓4th **A51 Early syphilis**
DEF: Syphilis: Sexually transmitted disease caused by the treponema pallidum spirochete. Syphilis usually exhibits cutaneous manifestations and may exist for years without symptoms.

A51.Ø Primary genital syphilis
Syphilitic chancre NOS

A51.1 Primary anal syphilis

A51.2 Primary syphilis of other sites

✓5th **A51.3 Secondary syphilis of skin and mucous membranes**
DEF: Transitory or chronic cutaneous eruptions that present within two to 10 weeks following an initial syphilis infection that may include nontender lymphadenopathy along with alopecia and condylomata lata.

A51.31 Condyloma latum CC

A51.32 Syphilitic alopecia CC

A51.39 Other secondary syphilis of skin CC
Syphilitic leukoderma
Syphilitic mucous patch
EXCLUDES 1 *late syphilitic leukoderma (A52.79)*

✓5th **A51.4 Other secondary syphilis**

A51.41 Secondary syphilitic meningitis MCC

A51.42 Secondary syphilitic female pelvic disease CC ♀

A51.43 Secondary syphilitic oculopathy CC
Secondary syphilitic chorioretinitis
Secondary syphilitic iridocyclitis, iritis
Secondary syphilitic uveitis

A51.44 Secondary syphilitic nephritis CC

A51.45 Secondary syphilitic hepatitis CC

A51.46 Secondary syphilitic osteopathy CC

A51.49 Other secondary syphilitic conditions CC
Secondary syphilitic lymphadenopathy
Secondary syphilitic myositis

A51.5 Early syphilis, latent
Syphilis (acquired) without clinical manifestations, with positive serological reaction and negative spinal fluid test, less than two years after infection.

A51.9 Early syphilis, unspecified

✓4th **A52 Late syphilis**

✓5th **A52.Ø Cardiovascular and cerebrovascular syphilis**

A52.ØØ Cardiovascular syphilis, unspecified CC

A52.Ø1 Syphilitic aneurysm of aorta CC

A52.Ø2 Syphilitic aortitis CC

A52.Ø3 Syphilitic endocarditis CC
Syphilitic aortic valve incompetence or stenosis
Syphilitic mitral valve stenosis
Syphilitic pulmonary valve regurgitation

A52.Ø4 Syphilitic cerebral arteritis CC

A52.Ø5 Other cerebrovascular syphilis CC
Syphilitic cerebral aneurysm (ruptured) (non-ruptured)
Syphilitic cerebral thrombosis

A52.06 Other syphilitic heart involvement CC
Syphilitic coronary artery disease
Syphilitic myocarditis
Syphilitic pericarditis

A52.09 Other cardiovascular syphilis CC

✓5th **A52.1 Symptomatic neurosyphilis**

A52.10 Symptomatic neurosyphilis, unspecified CC

A52.11 Tabes dorsalis CC
Locomotor ataxia (progressive)
Tabetic neurosyphilis

A52.12 Other cerebrospinal syphilis CC

A52.13 Late syphilitic meningitis MCC

A52.14 Late syphilitic encephalitis MCC

A52.15 Late syphilitic neuropathy CC
Late syphilitic acoustic neuritis
Late syphilitic optic (nerve) atrophy
Late syphilitic polyneuropathy
Late syphilitic retrobulbar neuritis

A52.16 Charcôt's arthropathy (tabetic) CC
DEF: Progressive neurologic arthropathy in which chronic degeneration of joints in the weight-bearing areas with peripheral hypertrophy occurs as a complication of a neuropathy disorder. Supporting structures relax from a loss of sensation resulting in chronic joint instability.

A52.17 General paresis CC
Dementia paralytica

A52.19 Other symptomatic neurosyphilis CC
Syphilitic parkinsonism

A52.2 Asymptomatic neurosyphilis CC

A52.3 Neurosyphilis, unspecified CC
Gumma (syphilitic)
Syphilis (late)
Syphiloma

✓5th **A52.7 Other symptomatic late syphilis**

A52.71 Late syphilitic oculopathy CC
Late syphilitic chorioretinitis
Late syphilitic episcleritis

A52.72 Syphilis of lung and bronchus CC

A52.73 Symptomatic late syphilis of other respiratory organs CC

A52.74 Syphilis of liver and other viscera CC
Late syphilitic peritonitis

A52.75 Syphilis of kidney and ureter CC
Syphilitic glomerular disease

A52.76 Other genitourinary symptomatic late syphilis CC
Late syphilitic female pelvic inflammatory disease

A52.77 Syphilis of bone and joint CC

A52.78 Syphilis of other musculoskeletal tissue CC
Late syphilitic bursitis
Syphilis [stage unspecified] of bursa
Syphilis [stage unspecified] of muscle
Syphilis [stage unspecified] of synovium
Syphilis [stage unspecified] of tendon

A52.79 Other symptomatic late syphilis CC
Late syphilitic leukoderma
Syphilis of adrenal gland
Syphilis of pituitary gland
Syphilis of thyroid gland
Syphilitic splenomegaly
EXCLUDES 1 *syphilitic leukoderma (secondary) (A51.39)*

A52.8 Late syphilis, latent
Syphilis (acquired) without clinical manifestations, with positive serological reaction and negative spinal fluid test, two years or more after infection

A52.9 Late syphilis, unspecified

✓4th **A53 Other and unspecified syphilis**

A53.0 Latent syphilis, unspecified as early or late
Latent syphilis NOS
Positive serological reaction for syphilis

A53.9 Syphilis, unspecified
Infection due to Treponema pallidum NOS
Syphilis (acquired) NOS
EXCLUDES 1 *syphilis NOS under two years of age (A50.2)*

✓4th **A54 Gonococcal infection**
DEF: Sexually transmitted bacterial infection caused by *Neisseria gonorrhoeae*. Women are often asymptomatic, while men tend to develop urinary symptoms quickly.

✓5th **A54.0 Gonococcal infection of lower genitourinary tract without periurethral or accessory gland abscess**
EXCLUDES 1 *gonococcal infection with genitourinary gland abscess (A54.1)*
gonococcal infection with periurethral abscess (A54.1)

A54.00 Gonococcal infection of lower genitourinary tract, unspecified CC

A54.01 Gonococcal cystitis and urethritis, unspecified CC

A54.02 Gonococcal vulvovaginitis, unspecified CC ♀

A54.03 Gonococcal cervicitis, unspecified CC ♀

A54.09 Other gonococcal infection of lower genitourinary tract CC

A54.1 Gonococcal infection of lower genitourinary tract with periurethral and accessory gland abscess CC
Gonococcal Bartholin's gland abscess

✓5th **A54.2 Gonococcal pelviperitonitis and other gonococcal genitourinary infection**

A54.21 Gonococcal infection of kidney and ureter CC

A54.22 Gonococcal prostatitis CC ♂

A54.23 Gonococcal infection of other male genital organs CC ♂
Gonococcal epididymitis
Gonococcal orchitis

A54.24 Gonococcal female pelvic inflammatory disease CC ♀
Gonococcal pelviperitonitis
EXCLUDES 1 *gonococcal peritonitis (A54.85)*

A54.29 Other gonococcal genitourinary infections CC

✓5th **A54.3 Gonococcal infection of eye**

A54.30 Gonococcal infection of eye, unspecified CC

A54.31 Gonococcal conjunctivitis CC
Ophthalmia neonatorum due to gonococcus

A54.32 Gonococcal iridocyclitis CC

A54.33 Gonococcal keratitis CC

A54.39 Other gonococcal eye infection CC
Gonococcal endophthalmia

✓5th **A54.4 Gonococcal infection of musculoskeletal system**

A54.40 Gonococcal infection of musculoskeletal system, unspecified CC HCC

A54.41 Gonococcal spondylopathy CC HCC

A54.42 Gonococcal arthritis CC HCC
EXCLUDES 2 *gonococcal infection of spine (A54.41)*

A54.43 Gonococcal osteomyelitis CC HCC
EXCLUDES 2 *gonococcal infection of spine (A54.41)*

A54.49 Gonococcal infection of other musculoskeletal tissue CC HCC
Gonococcal bursitis
Gonococcal myositis
Gonococcal synovitis
Gonococcal tenosynovitis

A54.5 Gonococcal pharyngitis

A54.6 Gonococcal infection of anus and rectum

✓5th **A54.8 Other gonococcal infections**

A54.81 Gonococcal meningitis MCC

A54.82 Gonococcal brain abscess CC

A54.83 Gonococcal heart infection CC
Gonococcal endocarditis
Gonococcal myocarditis
Gonococcal pericarditis

A54.84 Gonococcal pneumonia CC HCC

A54.85 Gonococcal peritonitis CC HCC
EXCLUDES 1 *gonococcal pelviperitonitis (A54.24)*

A54.86 Gonococcal sepsis MCC HCC

A54.89 Other gonococcal infections CC
Gonococcal keratoderma
Gonococcal lymphadenitis

A54.9 Gonococcal infection, unspecified CC

A55 Chlamydial lymphogranuloma (venereum)
Climatic or tropical bubo
Durand-Nicolas-Favre disease
Esthiomene
Lymphogranuloma inguinale

✓4th **A56 Other sexually transmitted chlamydial diseases**
INCLUDES sexually transmitted diseases due to Chlamydia trachomatis
EXCLUDES 1 *neonatal chlamydial conjunctivitis (P39.1)*
neonatal chlamydial pneumonia (P23.1)
EXCLUDES 2 *chlamydial lymphogranuloma (A55)*
conditions classified to A74.-
DEF: Chlamydia trachomatis: Bacterium that causes a common venereal disease. Symptoms of chlamydia are usually mild or absent, however, serious complications may cause irreversible damage, including cystitis, pelvic inflammatory disease, and infertility in women and discharge from the penis, prostatitis, and infertility in men. Genital chlamydial infection can cause arthritis, skin lesions, and inflammation of the eye and urethra.
Synonym(s): *Reiter's syndrome.*

✓5th **A56.0 Chlamydial infection of lower genitourinary tract**
A56.00 Chlamydial infection of lower genitourinary tract, unspecified
A56.01 Chlamydial cystitis and urethritis
A56.02 Chlamydial vulvovaginitis ♀
A56.09 Other chlamydial infection of lower genitourinary tract
Chlamydial cervicitis

✓5th **A56.1 Chlamydial infection of pelviperitoneum and other genitourinary organs**
A56.11 Chlamydial female pelvic inflammatory disease ♀
A56.19 Other chlamydial genitourinary infection
Chlamydial epididymitis
Chlamydial orchitis

A56.2 Chlamydial infection of genitourinary tract, unspecified
A56.3 Chlamydial infection of anus and rectum
A56.4 Chlamydial infection of pharynx
A56.8 Sexually transmitted chlamydial infection of other sites

A57 Chancroid
Ulcus molle
DEF: Localized infection by *Haemophilus ducreyi,* causing genital ulcers and infecting the inguinal lymph nodes.

A58 Granuloma inguinale
Donovanosis

✓4th **A59 Trichomoniasis**
EXCLUDES 2 *intestinal trichomoniasis (A07.8)*
DEF: Infection with the parasitic, flagellated protozoa of the genus *Trichomonas.* This protozoon is found in the intestinal and genitourinary tracts of humans and in the mouth around tartar, cavities, and areas of periodontal disease.

✓5th **A59.0 Urogenital trichomoniasis**
A59.00 Urogenital trichomoniasis, unspecified
Fluor (vaginalis) due to Trichomonas
Leukorrhea (vaginalis) due to Trichomonas
A59.01 Trichomonal vulvovaginitis ♀
A59.02 Trichomonal prostatitis ♂
A59.03 Trichomonal cystitis and urethritis
A59.09 Other urogenital trichomoniasis
Trichomonas cervicitis

A59.8 Trichomoniasis of other sites
A59.9 Trichomoniasis, unspecified

✓4th **A60 Anogenital herpesviral [herpes simplex] infections**
✓5th **A60.0 Herpesviral infection of genitalia and urogenital tract**
A60.00 Herpesviral infection of urogenital system, unspecified HIV
A60.01 Herpesviral infection of penis HIV ♂
A60.02 Herpesviral infection of other male genital organs ♂
A60.03 Herpesviral cervicitis ♀
A60.04 Herpesviral vulvovaginitis HIV ♀
Herpesviral [herpes simplex] ulceration
Herpesviral [herpes simplex] vaginitis
Herpesviral [herpes simplex] vulvitis
A60.09 Herpesviral infection of other urogenital tract HIV
AHA: 2020,1Q,20

A60.1 Herpesviral infection of perianal skin and rectum HIV
A60.9 Anogenital herpesviral infection, unspecified HIV

✓4th **A63 Other predominantly sexually transmitted diseases, not elsewhere classified**
EXCLUDES 2 *molluscum contagiosum (B08.1)*
papilloma of cervix (D26.0)
A63.0 Anogenital (venereal) warts
Anogenital warts due to (human) papillomavirus [HPV]
Condyloma acuminatum
A63.8 Other specified predominantly sexually transmitted diseases

A64 Unspecified sexually transmitted disease

Other spirochetal diseases (A65-A69)

EXCLUDES 2 *leptospirosis (A27.-)*
syphilis (A50-A53)

A65 Nonvenereal syphilis
Bejel
Endemic syphilis
Njovera

✓4th **A66 Yaws**
INCLUDES bouba
frambesia (tropica)
pian
A66.0 Initial lesions of yaws
Chancre of yaws
Frambesia, initial or primary
Initial frambesial ulcer
Mother yaw
A66.1 Multiple papillomata and wet crab yaws
Frambesioma
Pianoma
Plantar or palmar papilloma of yaws
A66.2 Other early skin lesions of yaws
Cutaneous yaws, less than five years after infection
Early yaws (cutaneous) (macular) (maculopapular) (micropapular) (papular)
Frambeside of early yaws
A66.3 Hyperkeratosis of yaws
Ghoul hand
Hyperkeratosis, palmar or plantar (early) (late) due to yaws
Worm-eaten soles
A66.4 Gummata and ulcers of yaws
Gummatous frambeside
Nodular late yaws (ulcerated)
A66.5 Gangosa
Rhinopharyngitis mutilans
A66.6 Bone and joint lesions of yaws HCC
Yaws ganglion
Yaws goundou
Yaws gumma, bone
Yaws gummatous osteitis or periostitis
Yaws hydrarthrosis
Yaws osteitis
Yaws periostitis (hypertrophic)
A66.7 Other manifestations of yaws
Juxta-articular nodules of yaws
Mucosal yaws
A66.8 Latent yaws
Yaws without clinical manifestations, with positive serology
A66.9 Yaws, unspecified

✓4th **A67 Pinta [carate]**
A67.0 Primary lesions of pinta
Chancre (primary) of pinta
Papule (primary) of pinta
A67.1 Intermediate lesions of pinta
Erythematous plaques of pinta
Hyperchromic lesions of pinta
Hyperkeratosis of pinta
Pintids

A67.2 Late **lesions of pinta**
Achromic skin lesions of pinta
Cicatricial skin lesions of pinta
Dyschromic skin lesions of pinta

A67.3 Mixed **lesions of pinta**
Achromic with hyperchromic skin lesions of pinta [carate]

A67.9 **Pinta, unspecified**

✓4th **A68 Relapsing fevers**
INCLUDES recurrent fever
EXCLUDES 2 *Lyme disease (A69.2-)*

A68.Ø Louse-borne **relapsing fever** CC
Relapsing fever due to Borrelia recurrentis

A68.1 Tick-borne **relapsing fever** CC
Relapsing fever due to any Borrelia species other than Borrelia recurrentis

A68.9 **Relapsing fever, unspecified** CC

✓4th **A69 Other spirochetal infections**

A69.Ø **Necrotizing ulcerative stomatitis**
Cancrum oris
Fusospirochetal gangrene
Noma
Stomatitis gangrenosa

A69.1 **Other Vincent's infections** CC
Fusospirochetal pharyngitis
Necrotizing ulcerative (acute) gingivitis
Necrotizing ulcerative (acute) gingivostomatitis
Spirochetal stomatitis
Trench mouth
Vincent's angina
Vincent's gingivitis

✓5th A69.2 **Lyme disease**
Erythema chronicum migrans due to Borrelia burgdorferi
DEF: Recurrent multisystem disorder through tick bites that begins with lesions of erythema chronicum migrans and is followed by arthritis of the large joints, myalgia, malaise, and neurological and cardiac manifestations.

A69.2Ø **Lyme disease, unspecified** CC

A69.21 Meningitis **due to Lyme disease** CC

A69.22 **Other neurologic disorders in Lyme disease** CC
Cranial neuritis
Meningoencephalitis
Polyneuropathy

A69.23 Arthritis **due to Lyme disease** CC HCC

A69.29 **Other conditions associated with Lyme disease** CC
Myopericarditis due to Lyme disease
AHA: 2016,3Q,12

A69.8 **Other specified spirochetal infections**

A69.9 **Spirochetal infection, unspecified**

Other diseases caused by chlamydiae (A7Ø-A74)

EXCLUDES 1 *sexually transmitted chlamydial diseases (A55-A56)*

A7Ø Chlamydia psittaci infections CC
Ornithosis
Parrot fever
Psittacosis

✓4th **A71 Trachoma**
EXCLUDES 1 *sequelae of trachoma (B94.Ø)*

A71.Ø Initial stage **of trachoma**
Trachoma dubium

A71.1 Active stage **of trachoma**
Granular conjunctivitis (trachomatous)
Trachomatous follicular conjunctivitis
Trachomatous pannus

A71.9 **Trachoma, unspecified**

✓4th **A74 Other diseases caused by chlamydiae**
EXCLUDES 1 *neonatal chlamydial conjunctivitis (P39.1)*
neonatal chlamydial pneumonia (P23.1)
Reiter's disease (MØ2.3-)
sexually transmitted chlamydial diseases (A55-A56)
EXCLUDES 2 *chlamydial pneumonia (J16.Ø)*

A74.Ø **Chlamydial** conjunctivitis
Paratrachoma

✓5th A74.8 **Other chlamydial diseases**

A74.81 **Chlamydial** peritonitis

A74.89 **Other chlamydial diseases**

A74.9 **Chlamydial infection, unspecified**
Chlamydiosis NOS

Rickettsioses (A75-A79)

DEF: Rickettsia: Condition caused by bacteria that live in lice/ticks transmitted to humans through bites.

✓4th **A75 Typhus fever**
EXCLUDES 1 *rickettsiosis due to Ehrlichia sennetsu (A79.81)*

A75.Ø **Epidemic louse-borne typhus fever due to** Rickettsia prowazekii CC
Classical typhus (fever)
Epidemic (louse-borne) typhus

A75.1 Recrudescent typhus **[Brill's disease]** CC
Brill-Zinsser disease

A75.2 **Typhus fever due to** Rickettsia typhi CC
Murine (flea-borne) typhus

A75.3 **Typhus fever due to** Rickettsia tsutsugamushi CC
Scrub (mite-borne) typhus
Tsutsugamushi fever
▶Typhus fever due to Orientia Tsutsugamushi (scrub typhus)◀

A75.9 **Typhus fever, unspecified** CC
Typhus (fever) NOS

✓4th **A77 Spotted fever [tick-borne rickettsioses]**

A77.Ø **Spotted fever due to** Rickettsia rickettsii CC
Rocky Mountain spotted fever
Sao Paulo fever

A77.1 **Spotted fever due to** Rickettsia conorii CC
African tick typhus
Boutonneuse fever
India tick typhus
Kenya tick typhus
Marseilles fever
Mediterranean tick fever

A77.2 **Spotted fever due to** Rickettsia siberica CC
North Asian tick fever
Siberian tick typhus

A77.3 **Spotted fever due to** Rickettsia australis CC
Queensland tick typhus

✓5th A77.4 **Ehrlichiosis**
EXCLUDES 1 *Rickettsiosis due to Ehrlichia sennetsu (A79.81)*

A77.4Ø **Ehrlichiosis, unspecified** CC

A77.41 **Ehrlichiosis** chafeensis **[E. chafeensis]** CC

A77.49 **Other ehrlichiosis** CC
▶Ehrlichiosis due to E. ewingii◀
▶Ehrlichiosis due to E. muris euclairensis◀

A77.8 **Other spotted fevers** CC
▶Rickettsia 364D/R. philipii (Pacific Coast tick fever)◀
▶Spotted fever due to Rickettsia africae (African tick bite fever)◀
▶Spotted fever due to Rickettsia parkeri◀

A77.9 **Spotted fever, unspecified** CC
Tick-borne typhus NOS

A78 Q fever CC
Infection due to Coxiella burnetii
Nine Mile fever
Quadrilateral fever

✓4th **A79 Other rickettsioses**

A79.Ø Trench fever CC
Quintan fever
Wolhynian fever

A79.1 **Rickettsialpox due to** Rickettsia akari CC
Kew Garden fever
Vesicular rickettsiosis

✓5th A79.8 **Other specified rickettsioses**

A79.81 **Rickettsiosis due to** Ehrlichia sennetsu CC
▶Rickettsiosis due to Neorickettsia sennetsu◀

A79.89 **Other specified rickettsioses** CC

A79.9 **Rickettsiosis, unspecified** CC
Rickettsial infection NOS

Viral and prion infections of the central nervous system (A8Ø-A89)

EXCLUDES 1 *postpolio syndrome (G14)*
sequelae of poliomyelitis (B91)
sequelae of viral encephalitis (B94.1)

✓4th **A8Ø Acute poliomyelitis**

A8Ø.Ø Acute paralytic poliomyelitis, vaccine-associated MCC
A8Ø.1 Acute paralytic poliomyelitis, wild virus, imported MCC
A8Ø.2 Acute paralytic poliomyelitis, wild virus, indigenous MCC
✓5th **A8Ø.3 Acute paralytic poliomyelitis, other and unspecified**
A8Ø.3Ø Acute paralytic poliomyelitis, unspecified MCC
A8Ø.39 Other acute paralytic poliomyelitis MCC
A8Ø.4 Acute nonparalytic poliomyelitis
A8Ø.9 Acute poliomyelitis, unspecified

✓4th **A81 Atypical virus infections of central nervous system**

INCLUDES diseases of the central nervous system caused by prions
Use additional code to identify:
dementia with behavioral disturbance (FØ2.81)
dementia without behavioral disturbance (FØ2.8Ø)

✓5th **A81.Ø Creutzfeldt-Jakob disease**
DEF: Communicable, rare spongiform encephalopathy occurring later in life with progressive destruction of the pyramidal and extrapyramidal systems eventually leading to death. Progressive dementia, wasting of muscles, tremor, and other symptoms are present.
A81.ØØ Creutzfeldt-Jakob disease, unspecified CC HCC
Jakob-Creutzfeldt disease, unspecified
A81.Ø1 Variant Creutzfeldt-Jakob disease CC HCC
vCJD
A81.Ø9 Other Creutzfeldt-Jakob disease CC HCC
CJD
Familial Creutzfeldt-Jakob disease
Iatrogenic Creutzfeldt-Jakob disease
Sporadic Creutzfeldt-Jakob disease
Subacute spongiform encephalopathy (with dementia)
A81.1 Subacute sclerosing panencephalitis CC HCC
Dawson's inclusion body encephalitis
Van Bogaert's sclerosing leukoencephalopathy
A81.2 Progressive multifocal leukoencephalopathy HIV CC HCC
Multifocal leukoencephalopathy NOS
✓5th **A81.8 Other atypical virus infections of central nervous system**
A81.81 Kuru CC HCC
A81.82 Gerstmann-Sträussler-Scheinker syndrome HIV CC HCC
GSS syndrome
A81.83 Fatal familial insomnia HIV CC HCC
FFI
A81.89 Other atypical virus infections of central nervous system HIV CC HCC
A81.9 Atypical virus infection of central nervous system, unspecified HIV CC HCC
Prion diseases of the central nervous system NOS

✓4th **A82 Rabies**

A82.Ø Sylvatic rabies CC
A82.1 Urban rabies CC
A82.9 Rabies, unspecified CC

✓4th **A83 Mosquito-borne viral encephalitis**

INCLUDES mosquito-borne viral meningoencephalitis
EXCLUDES 2 *Venezuelan equine encephalitis (A92.2)*
West Nile fever (A92.3-)
West Nile virus (A92.3-)

A83.Ø Japanese encephalitis MCC
A83.1 Western equine encephalitis MCC
A83.2 Eastern equine encephalitis MCC
A83.3 St Louis encephalitis MCC
A83.4 Australian encephalitis MCC
Kunjin virus disease
A83.5 California encephalitis MCC
California meningoencephalitis
La Crosse encephalitis
A83.6 Rocio virus disease MCC
A83.8 Other mosquito-borne viral encephalitis MCC
A83.9 Mosquito-borne viral encephalitis, unspecified MCC

✓4th **A84 Tick-borne viral encephalitis**

INCLUDES tick-borne viral meningoencephalitis

A84.Ø Far Eastern tick-borne encephalitis [Russian spring-summer encephalitis] MCC
A84.1 Central European tick-borne encephalitis MCC
▲ ✓5th **A84.8 Other tick-borne viral encephalitis**
~~Louping ill~~
~~Powassan virus disease~~
● **A84.81 Powassan virus disease** MCC
● **A84.89 Other tick-borne viral encephalitis** MCC
Louping ill
Code first, if applicable, transfusion related infection (T8Ø.22-)
A84.9 Tick-borne viral encephalitis, unspecified MCC

✓4th **A85 Other viral encephalitis, not elsewhere classified**

INCLUDES specified viral encephalomyelitis NEC
specified viral meningoencephalitis NEC
EXCLUDES 1 *benign myalgic encephalomyelitis (G93.3)*
encephalitis due to cytomegalovirus (B25.8)
encephalitis due to herpesvirus NEC (B1Ø.Ø-)
encephalitis due to herpesvirus [herpes simplex] (BØØ.4)
encephalitis due to measles virus (BØ5.Ø)
encephalitis due to mumps virus (B26.2)
encephalitis due to poliomyelitis virus (A8Ø.-)
encephalitis due to zoster (BØ2.Ø)
lymphocytic choriomeningitis (A87.2)

A85.Ø Enteroviral encephalitis HIV CC
Enteroviral encephalomyelitis
A85.1 Adenoviral encephalitis HIV CC
Adenoviral meningoencephalitis
A85.2 Arthropod-borne viral encephalitis, unspecified MCC
EXCLUDES 1 *West nile virus with encephalitis (A92.31)*
A85.8 Other specified viral encephalitis HIV CC
Encephalitis lethargica
Von Economo-Cruchet disease

A86 Unspecified viral encephalitis HIV CC
Viral encephalomyelitis NOS
Viral meningoencephalitis NOS

✓4th **A87 Viral meningitis**

EXCLUDES 1 *meningitis due to herpesvirus [herpes simplex] (BØØ.3)*
meningitis due to measles virus (BØ5.1)
meningitis due to mumps virus (B26.1)
meningitis due to poliomyelitis virus (A8Ø.-)
meningitis due to zoster (BØ2.1)
DEF: Meningitis: Inflammation of the meningeal layers of the brain and spine.

A87.Ø Enteroviral meningitis CC
Coxsackievirus meningitis
Echovirus meningitis
A87.1 Adenoviral meningitis CC
A87.2 Lymphocytic choriomeningitis CC
Lymphocytic meningoencephalitis
A87.8 Other viral meningitis CC
A87.9 Viral meningitis, unspecified CC

✓4th **A88 Other viral infections of central nervous system, not elsewhere classified**

EXCLUDES 1 *viral encephalitis NOS (A86)*
viral meningitis NOS (A87.9)

A88.Ø Enteroviral exanthematous fever [Boston exanthem] CC
A88.1 Epidemic vertigo
A88.8 Other specified viral infections of central nervous system HIV CC

A89 Unspecified viral infection of central nervous system HIV CC

Arthropod-borne viral fevers and viral hemorrhagic fevers (A9Ø-A99)

A9Ø Dengue fever [classical dengue] CC
EXCLUDES 1 *dengue hemorrhagic fever (A91)*
AHA: 2016,3Q,13

A91 Dengue hemorrhagic fever CC

A92 Other mosquito-borne viral fevers (4th)
EXCLUDES 1 *Ross River disease (B33.1)*

A92.0 Chikungunya virus disease CC
Chikungunya (hemorrhagic) fever

A92.1 O'nyong-nyong fever CC

A92.2 Venezuelan equine fever CC
Venezuelan equine encephalitis
Venezuelan equine encephalomyelitis virus disease

A92.3 West Nile virus infection (5th)
West Nile fever
AHA: 2016,3Q,12

A92.30 West Nile virus infection, unspecified MCC
West Nile fever NOS
West Nile fever without complications
West Nile virus NOS

A92.31 West Nile virus infection with encephalitis MCC
West Nile encephalitis
West Nile encephalomyelitis

A92.32 West Nile virus infection with other neurologic manifestation MCC
Use additional code to specify the neurologic manifestation

A92.39 West Nile virus infection with other complications MCC
Use additional code to specify the other conditions

A92.4 Rift Valley fever CC

A92.5 Zika virus disease CC
Zika virus fever
Zika virus infection
Zika NOS
EXCLUDES 1 *congenital Zika virus disease (P35.4)*
AHA: 2016,4Q,4-7
DEF: Virus transmitted via a bite from an infected Aedes species mosquito. Common symptoms of the virus include fever, rash, joint pain, and conjunctivitis; they are usually mild in nature and may last from several days to a week. Most people who have the Zika virus do not require medical attention; however, in pregnant women, the Zika virus can cause a serious birth defect called microcephaly, as well as other severe fetal brain defects.
TIP: Code only confirmed diagnoses of Zika virus; documentation by the physician that the disease is confirmed is sufficient.

A92.8 Other specified mosquito-borne viral fevers CC

A92.9 Mosquito-borne viral fever, unspecified CC

A93 Other arthropod-borne viral fevers, not elsewhere classified (4th)

A93.0 Oropouche virus disease CC
Oropouche fever

A93.1 Sandfly fever CC
Pappataci fever
Phlebotomus fever

A93.2 Colorado tick fever CC

A93.8 Other specified arthropod-borne viral fevers CC
Piry virus disease
Vesicular stomatitis virus disease [Indiana fever]

A94 Unspecified arthropod-borne viral fever CC
Arboviral fever NOS
Arbovirus infection NOS

A95 Yellow fever (4th)

A95.0 Sylvatic yellow fever CC
Jungle yellow fever

A95.1 Urban yellow fever CC

A95.9 Yellow fever, unspecified CC

A96 Arenaviral hemorrhagic fever (4th)

A96.0 Junin hemorrhagic fever CC
Argentinian hemorrhagic fever

A96.1 Machupo hemorrhagic fever CC
Bolivian hemorrhagic fever

A96.2 Lassa fever

A96.8 Other arenaviral hemorrhagic fevers CC

A96.9 Arenaviral hemorrhagic fever, unspecified CC

A98 Other viral hemorrhagic fevers, not elsewhere classified (4th)
EXCLUDES 1 *chikungunya hemorrhagic fever (A92.0)*
dengue hemorrhagic fever (A91)

A98.0 Crimean-Congo hemorrhagic fever CC
Central Asian hemorrhagic fever

A98.1 Omsk hemorrhagic fever CC

A98.2 Kyasanur Forest disease CC

A98.3 Marburg virus disease

A98.4 Ebola virus disease

A98.5 Hemorrhagic fever with renal syndrome CC
Epidemic hemorrhagic fever
Korean hemorrhagic fever
Russian hemorrhagic fever
Hantaan virus disease
Hantavirus disease with renal manifestations
Nephropathia epidemica
Songo fever
EXCLUDES 1 *hantavirus (cardio)-pulmonary syndrome (B33.4)*

A98.8 Other specified viral hemorrhagic fevers CC

A99 Unspecified viral hemorrhagic fever CC

Viral infections characterized by skin and mucous membrane lesions (B00-B09)

B00 Herpesviral [herpes simplex] infections (4th)
EXCLUDES 1 *congenital herpesviral infections (P35.2)*
EXCLUDES 2 *anogenital herpesviral infection (A60.-)*
gammaherpesviral mononucleosis (B27.0-)
herpangina (B08.5)

B00.0 Eczema herpeticum HIV
Kaposi's varicelliform eruption

B00.1 Herpesviral vesicular dermatitis HIV
Herpes simplex facialis
Herpes simplex labialis
Herpes simplex otitis externa
Vesicular dermatitis of ear
Vesicular dermatitis of lip

B00.2 Herpesviral gingivostomatitis and pharyngotonsillitis HIV CC
Herpesviral pharyngitis

B00.3 Herpesviral meningitis HIV MCC

B00.4 Herpesviral encephalitis HIV MCC
Herpesviral meningoencephalitis
Simian B disease
EXCLUDES 1 *herpesviral encephalitis due to herpesvirus 6 and 7 (B10.01, B10.09)*
non-simplex herpesviral encephalitis (B10.0-)

B00.5 Herpesviral ocular disease (5th)

B00.50 Herpesviral ocular disease, unspecified HIV CC

B00.51 Herpesviral iridocyclitis HIV CC
Herpesviral iritis
Herpesviral uveitis, anterior

B00.52 Herpesviral keratitis HIV CC
Herpesviral keratoconjunctivitis

B00.53 Herpesviral conjunctivitis HIV CC

B00.59 Other herpesviral disease of eye HIV CC
Herpesviral dermatitis of eyelid

B00.7 Disseminated herpesviral disease HIV MCC HCC
Herpesviral sepsis

B00.8 Other forms of herpesviral infections (5th)

B00.81 Herpesviral hepatitis HIV CC

B00.82 Herpes simplex myelitis MCC HCC

B00.89 Other herpesviral infection HIV CC
Herpesviral whitlow

B00.9 Herpesviral infection, unspecified HIV
Herpes simplex infection NOS

B01 Varicella [chickenpox] (4th)

B01.0 Varicella meningitis CC

B01.1 Varicella encephalitis, myelitis and encephalomyelitis (5th)
Postchickenpox encephalitis, myelitis and encephalomyelitis

B01.11 Varicella encephalitis and encephalomyelitis MCC
Postchickenpox encephalitis and encephalomyelitis

B01.12 Varicella myelitis MCC HCC
Postchickenpox myelitis

B01.2 Varicella pneumonia MCC

✓5th **B01.8 Varicella with other complications**

B01.81 Varicella keratitis CC

B01.89 Other varicella complications CC

B01.9 Varicella without complication CC
Varicella NOS

✓4th **B02 Zoster [herpes zoster]**

INCLUDES shingles
zona

B02.0 Zoster encephalitis HIV CC
Zoster meningoencephalitis

B02.1 Zoster meningitis HIV MCC
AHA: 2019,1Q,18

✓5th **B02.2 Zoster with other nervous system involvement**

B02.21 Postherpetic geniculate ganglionitis HIV CC

B02.22 Postherpetic trigeminal neuralgia HIV CC

B02.23 Postherpetic polyneuropathy HIV CC

B02.24 Postherpetic myelitis MCC HCC
Herpes zoster myelitis

B02.29 Other postherpetic nervous system involvement HIV CC
Postherpetic radiculopathy

✓5th **B02.3 Zoster ocular disease**

B02.30 Zoster ocular disease, unspecified HIV CC

B02.31 Zoster conjunctivitis HIV CC

B02.32 Zoster iridocyclitis HIV CC

B02.33 Zoster keratitis HIV CC
Herpes zoster keratoconjunctivitis

B02.34 Zoster scleritis HIV CC

B02.39 Other herpes zoster eye disease HIV CC
Zoster blepharitis

B02.7 Disseminated zoster HIV CC

B02.8 Zoster with other complications HIV CC
Herpes zoster otitis externa

B02.9 Zoster without complications HIV
Zoster NOS

B03 Smallpox CC

NOTE In 1980 the 33rd World Health Assembly declared that smallpox had been eradicated.
The classification is maintained for surveillance purposes.

B04 Monkeypox CC

✓4th **B05 Measles**

INCLUDES morbilli

EXCLUDES 1 *subacute sclerosing panencephalitis (A81.1)*

B05.0 Measles complicated by encephalitis MCC
Postmeasles encephalitis

B05.1 Measles complicated by meningitis CC
Postmeasles meningitis

B05.2 Measles complicated by pneumonia MCC
Postmeasles pneumonia

B05.3 Measles complicated by otitis media
Postmeasles otitis media

B05.4 Measles with intestinal complications CC

✓5th **B05.8 Measles with other complications**

B05.81 Measles keratitis and keratoconjunctivitis CC

B05.89 Other measles complications CC

B05.9 Measles without complication
Measles NOS

✓4th **B06 Rubella [German measles]**

EXCLUDES 1 *congenital rubella (P35.0)*

DEF: Highly contagious virus in which the symptoms are mild and short-lived in most people. Rubella during pregnancy, however, can result in abortion, stillbirth, or congenital defects.

✓5th **B06.0 Rubella with neurological complications**

B06.00 Rubella with neurological complication, unspecified CC

B06.01 Rubella encephalitis MCC
Rubella meningoencephalitis

B06.02 Rubella meningitis CC

B06.09 Other neurological complications of rubella CC

✓5th **B06.8 Rubella with other complications**

B06.81 Rubella pneumonia CC

B06.82 Rubella arthritis CC HCC

B06.89 Other rubella complications CC

B06.9 Rubella without complication
Rubella NOS

✓4th **B07 Viral warts**

INCLUDES verruca simplex
verruca vulgaris
viral warts due to human papillomavirus

EXCLUDES 2 *anogenital (venereal) warts (A63.0)*
papilloma of bladder (D41.4)
papilloma of cervix (D26.0)
papilloma larynx (D14.1)

B07.0 Plantar wart
Verruca plantaris

B07.8 Other viral warts
Common wart
Flat wart
Verruca plana

B07.9 Viral wart, unspecified

✓4th **B08 Other viral infections characterized by skin and mucous membrane lesions, not elsewhere classified**

EXCLUDES 1 *vesicular stomatitis virus disease (A93.8)*

✓5th **B08.0 Other orthopoxvirus infections**

EXCLUDES 2 *monkeypox (B04)*

✓6th **B08.01 Cowpox and vaccinia not from vaccine**

B08.010 Cowpox
DEF: Disease contracted by milking infected cows. The vesicles usually appear on the fingers, hands, and adjacent areas and usually disappear without scarring. Other symptoms include local edema, lymphangitis, and regional lymphadenitis with or without fever.

B08.011 Vaccinia not from vaccine
EXCLUDES 1 *vaccinia (from vaccination) (generalized) (T88.1)*

B08.02 Orf virus disease
Contagious pustular dermatitis
Ecthyma contagiosum

B08.03 Pseudocowpox [milker's node]

B08.04 Paravaccinia, unspecified

B08.09 Other orthopoxvirus infections
Orthopoxvirus infection NOS

B08.1 Molluscum contagiosum
DEF: Benign poxvirus infection causing small bumps on the skin or conjunctiva and is transmitted by close contact.

✓5th **B08.2 Exanthema subitum [sixth disease]**
Roseola infantum

B08.20 Exanthema subitum [sixth disease], unspecified P
Roseola infantum, unspecified

B08.21 Exanthema subitum [sixth disease] due to human herpesvirus 6 P
Roseola infantum due to human herpesvirus 6

B08.22 Exanthema subitum [sixth disease] due to human herpesvirus 7 P
Roseola infantum due to human herpesvirus 7

B08.3 Erythema infectiosum [fifth disease] CC
DEF: Infection with human parvovirus B19, mainly occurring in children. Symptoms include a low-grade fever, malaise, or a "cold" a few days before the appearance of a mild rash illness that presents as a "slapped-cheek" rash on the face and a lacy red rash on the trunk and limbs.

B08.4 Enteroviral vesicular stomatitis with exanthem
Hand, foot and mouth disease

B08.5 Enteroviral vesicular pharyngitis
Herpangina
DEF: Acute infectious Coxsackie virus infection causing throat lesions, fever, and vomiting that generally affects children in the summer.

✓5th **B08.6 Parapoxvirus infections**

B08.60 Parapoxvirus infection, unspecified

B08.61 Bovine stomatitis

B08.62 Sealpox

B08.69 Other parapoxvirus infections

5th **B08.7 Yatapoxvirus infections**

B08.70 Yatapoxvirus infection, unspecified

B08.71 Tanapox virus disease CC

B08.72 Yaba pox virus disease

Yaba monkey tumor disease

B08.79 Other yatapoxvirus infections

B08.8 Other specified viral infections characterized by skin and mucous membrane lesions

Enteroviral lymphonodular pharyngitis

Foot-and-mouth disease

Poxvirus NEC

B09 Unspecified viral infection characterized by skin and mucous membrane lesions

Viral enanthema NOS

Viral exanthema NOS

Other human herpesviruses (B10)

4th **B10 Other human herpesviruses**

EXCLUDES 2 *cytomegalovirus (B25.9)*
Epstein-Barr virus (B27.0-)
herpes NOS (B00.9)
herpes simplex (B00.-)
herpes zoster (B02.-)
human herpesvirus NOS (B00.-)
human herpesvirus 1 and 2 (B00.-)
human herpesvirus 3 (B01.-, B02.-)
human herpesvirus 4 (B27.0-)
human herpesvirus 5 (B25.-)
varicella (B01.-)
zoster (B02.-)

5th **B10.0 Other human herpesvirus encephalitis**

EXCLUDES 2 *herpes encephalitis NOS (B00.4)*
herpes simplex encephalitis (B00.4)
human herpesvirus encephalitis (B00.4)
simian B herpes virus encephalitis (B00.4)

B10.01 Human herpesvirus 6 encephalitis HIV MCC

B10.09 Other human herpesvirus encephalitis HIV MCC

Human herpesvirus 7 encephalitis

5th **B10.8 Other human herpesvirus infection**

B10.81 Human herpesvirus 6 infection

B10.82 Human herpesvirus 7 infection

B10.89 Other human herpesvirus infection

Human herpesvirus 8 infection

Kaposi's sarcoma-associated herpesvirus infection

Viral hepatitis (B15-B19)

EXCLUDES 1 *sequelae of viral hepatitis (B94.2)*

EXCLUDES 2 *cytomegaloviral hepatitis (B25.1)*
herpesviral [herpes simplex] hepatitis (B00.81)

DEF: Hepatitis A: HAV infection that is self-limiting with flulike symptoms. Transmission is fecal-oral.

DEF: Hepatitis B: HBV infection that can be chronic and systemic. Transmission is bodily fluids.

DEF: Hepatitis C: HCV infection that can be chronic and systemic. Transmission is blood transfusion and unidentified agents.

DEF: Hepatitis D (delta): HDV that occurs only in the presence of hepatitis B virus. Transmission is contaminated blood in contact with mucous membranes.

DEF: Hepatitis E: HEV is an epidemic form. Transmission is fecal-oral, most often from contaminated water.

4th **B15 Acute hepatitis A**

B15.0 Hepatitis A with hepatic coma MCC

B15.9 Hepatitis A without hepatic coma CC

Hepatitis A (acute)(viral) NOS

4th **B16 Acute hepatitis B**

AHA: 2016,3Q,13

B16.0 Acute hepatitis B with delta-agent with hepatic coma MCC

B16.1 Acute hepatitis B with delta-agent without hepatic coma CC

B16.2 Acute hepatitis B without delta-agent with hepatic coma MCC

B16.9 Acute hepatitis B without delta-agent and without hepatic coma CC

Hepatitis B (acute) (viral) NOS

4th **B17 Other acute viral hepatitis**

B17.0 Acute delta-(super) infection of hepatitis B carrier CC

5th **B17.1 Acute hepatitis C**

B17.10 Acute hepatitis C without hepatic coma CC

Acute hepatitis C NOS

B17.11 Acute hepatitis C with hepatic coma MCC

B17.2 Acute hepatitis E CC

B17.8 Other specified acute viral hepatitis CC

Hepatitis non-A non-B (acute) (viral) NEC

B17.9 Acute viral hepatitis, unspecified CC

Acute hepatitis NOS

Acute infectious hepatitis NOS

4th **B18 Chronic viral hepatitis**

INCLUDES carrier of viral hepatitis

AHA: 2017,1Q,41

B18.0 Chronic viral hepatitis B with delta-agent CC HCC

B18.1 Chronic viral hepatitis B without delta-agent CC HCC

Carrier of viral hepatitis B

Chronic (viral) hepatitis B

B18.2 Chronic viral hepatitis C HCC

Carrier of viral hepatitis C

AHA: 2018,1Q,4

B18.8 Other chronic viral hepatitis CC HCC

Carrier of other viral hepatitis

B18.9 Chronic viral hepatitis, unspecified CC HCC

Carrier of unspecified viral hepatitis

4th **B19 Unspecified viral hepatitis**

B19.0 Unspecified viral hepatitis with hepatic coma MCC

5th **B19.1 Unspecified viral hepatitis B**

B19.10 Unspecified viral hepatitis B without hepatic coma CC

Unspecified viral hepatitis B NOS

B19.11 Unspecified viral hepatitis B with hepatic coma MCC

5th **B19.2 Unspecified viral hepatitis C**

B19.20 Unspecified viral hepatitis C without hepatic coma

Viral hepatitis C NOS

B19.21 Unspecified viral hepatitis C with hepatic coma MCC

B19.9 Unspecified viral hepatitis without hepatic coma CC

Viral hepatitis NOS

Human immunodeficiency virus [HIV] disease (B20)

B20 Human immunodeficiency virus [HIV] disease CC HCC

INCLUDES acquired immune deficiency syndrome [AIDS]
AIDS-related complex [ARC]
HIV infection, symptomatic

Code first Human immunodeficiency virus [HIV] disease complicating pregnancy, childbirth and the puerperium, if applicable (O98.7-)

Use additional code(s) to identify all manifestations of HIV infection

EXCLUDES 1 *asymptomatic human immunodeficiency virus [HIV] infection status (Z21)*
exposure to HIV virus (Z20.6)
inconclusive serologic evidence of HIV (R75)

AHA: 2020,2Q,12; 2019,1Q,8-11

Other viral diseases (B25-B34)

4th **B25 Cytomegaloviral disease**

EXCLUDES 1 *congenital cytomegalovirus infection (P35.1)*
cytomegaloviral mononucleosis (B27.1-)

B25.0 Cytomegaloviral pneumonitis MCC HCC

B25.1 Cytomegaloviral hepatitis CC HCC

B25.2 Cytomegaloviral pancreatitis MCC HCC

B25.8 Other cytomegaloviral diseases HIV CC HCC

Cytomegaloviral encephalitis

B25.9 Cytomegaloviral disease, unspecified HIV CC HCC

4th **B26 Mumps**

INCLUDES epidemic parotitis
infectious parotitis

B26.0 Mumps orchitis CC ♂

B26.1 Mumps meningitis MCC

B26.2 Mumps encephalitis MCC

B26.3 Mumps pancreatitis CC

B26.8 Mumps with other complications
B26.81 Mumps hepatitis CC
B26.82 Mumps myocarditis CC
B26.83 Mumps nephritis CC
B26.84 Mumps polyneuropathy CC
B26.85 Mumps arthritis CC HCC
B26.89 Other mumps complications CC
B26.9 Mumps without complication
Mumps NOS
Mumps parotitis NOS

B27 Infectious mononucleosis
INCLUDES glandular fever
monocytic angina
Pfeiffer's disease

B27.Ø Gammaherpesviral mononucleosis
Mononucleosis due to Epstein-Barr virus
B27.ØØ Gammaherpesviral mononucleosis without complication
B27.Ø1 Gammaherpesviral mononucleosis with polyneuropathy
B27.Ø2 Gammaherpesviral mononucleosis with meningitis
B27.Ø9 Gammaherpesviral mononucleosis with other complications
Hepatomegaly in gammaherpesviral mononucleosis

B27.1 Cytomegaloviral mononucleosis
B27.1Ø Cytomegaloviral mononucleosis without complications
B27.11 Cytomegaloviral mononucleosis with polyneuropathy
B27.12 Cytomegaloviral mononucleosis with meningitis
B27.19 Cytomegaloviral mononucleosis with other complication
Hepatomegaly in cytomegaloviral mononucleosis

B27.8 Other infectious mononucleosis
B27.8Ø Other infectious mononucleosis without complication
B27.81 Other infectious mononucleosis with polyneuropathy
B27.82 Other infectious mononucleosis with meningitis
B27.89 Other infectious mononucleosis with other complication
Hepatomegaly in other infectious mononucleosis

B27.9 Infectious mononucleosis, unspecified
B27.9Ø Infectious mononucleosis, unspecified without complication
B27.91 Infectious mononucleosis, unspecified with polyneuropathy
B27.92 Infectious mononucleosis, unspecified with meningitis
B27.99 Infectious mononucleosis, unspecified with other complication
Hepatomegaly in unspecified infectious mononucleosis

B3Ø Viral conjunctivitis
EXCLUDES 1 *herpesviral [herpes simplex] ocular disease (BØØ.5)*
ocular zoster (BØ2.3)

Viral Conjunctivitis

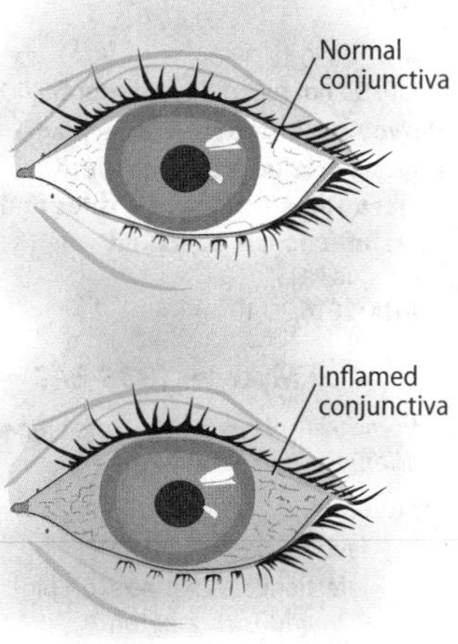

B3Ø.Ø Keratoconjunctivitis due to adenovirus
Epidemic keratoconjunctivitis
Shipyard eye
B3Ø.1 Conjunctivitis due to adenovirus
Acute adenoviral follicular conjunctivitis
Swimming-pool conjunctivitis
B3Ø.2 Viral pharyngoconjunctivitis
B3Ø.3 Acute epidemic hemorrhagic conjunctivitis (enteroviral)
Conjunctivitis due to coxsackievirus 24
Conjunctivitis due to enterovirus 7Ø
Hemorrhagic conjunctivitis (acute)(epidemic)
B3Ø.8 Other viral conjunctivitis
Newcastle conjunctivitis
B3Ø.9 Viral conjunctivitis, unspecified

B33 Other viral diseases, not elsewhere classified
B33.Ø Epidemic myalgia
Bornholm disease
B33.1 Ross River disease CC
Epidemic polyarthritis and exanthema
Ross River fever
B33.2 Viral carditis
Coxsackie (virus) carditis
B33.2Ø Viral carditis, unspecified CC
B33.21 Viral endocarditis CC
B33.22 Viral myocarditis CC
B33.23 Viral pericarditis CC
B33.24 Viral cardiomyopathy HCC
B33.3 Retrovirus infections, not elsewhere classified
Retrovirus infection NOS
B33.4 Hantavirus (cardio)-pulmonary syndrome [HPS] [HCPS] CC
Hantavirus disease with pulmonary manifestations
Sin nombre virus disease
Use additional code to identify any associated acute kidney failure (N17.9)
EXCLUDES 1 *hantavirus disease with renal manifestations (A98.5)*
hemorrhagic fever with renal manifestations (A98.5)
B33.8 Other specified viral diseases
EXCLUDES 1 *anogenital human papillomavirus infection (A63.Ø)*
viral warts due to human papillomavirus infection (BØ7)

B34 Viral infection of unspecified site
EXCLUDES 1 *anogenital human papillomavirus infection (A63.Ø)*
cytomegaloviral disease NOS (B25.9)
herpesvirus [herpes simplex] infection NOS (BØØ.9)
retrovirus infection NOS (B33.3)
viral agents as the cause of diseases classified elsewhere (B97.-)
viral warts due to human papillomavirus infection (BØ7)
B34.Ø Adenovirus infection, unspecified

B34.1 Enterovirus infection, unspecified
Coxsackievirus infection NOS
Echovirus infection NOS

B34.2 Coronavirus infection, unspecified
EXCLUDES 1 ►*COVID-19 (U07.1)*◄
pneumonia due to SARS-associated coronavirus (J12.81)
AHA: 2020,1Q,34-36
TIP: Do not report this code for COVID-19; refer to U07.1.

B34.3 Parvovirus infection, unspecified CC

B34.4 Papovavirus infection, unspecified

B34.8 Other viral infections of unspecified site

B34.9 Viral infection, unspecified
Viremia NOS
AHA: 2016,3Q,10

Mycoses (B35-B49)

EXCLUDES 2 *hypersensitivity pneumonitis due to organic dust (J67.-)*
mycosis fungoides (C84.0-)

✓4th B35 Dermatophytosis

INCLUDES favus
infections due to species of Epidermophyton, Micro-sporum and Trichophyton
tinea, any type except those in B36.-
DEF: Contagious superficial fungal infection of the skin that invades and grows in dead keratin.

B35.0 Tinea barbae and tinea capitis
Beard ringworm
Kerion
Scalp ringworm
Sycosis, mycotic

B35.1 Tinea unguium
Dermatophytic onychia
Dermatophytosis of nail
Onychomycosis
Ringworm of nails

B35.2 Tinea manuum
Dermatophytosis of hand
Hand ringworm

B35.3 Tinea pedis
Athlete's foot
Dermatophytosis of foot
Foot ringworm

B35.4 Tinea corporis
Ringworm of the body

B35.5 Tinea imbricata
Tokelau

B35.6 Tinea cruris
Dhobi itch
Groin ringworm
Jock itch

B35.8 Other dermatophytoses
Disseminated dermatophytosis
Granulomatous dermatophytosis

B35.9 Dermatophytosis, unspecified
Ringworm NOS

✓4th B36 Other superficial mycoses

B36.0 Pityriasis versicolor
Tinea flava
Tinea versicolor

B36.1 Tinea nigra
Keratomycosis nigricans palmaris
Microsporosis nigra
Pityriasis nigra

B36.2 White piedra
Tinea blanca

B36.3 Black piedra

B36.8 Other specified superficial mycoses

B36.9 Superficial mycosis, unspecified

✓4th B37 Candidiasis

INCLUDES candidosis
moniliasis
EXCLUDES 1 *neonatal candidiasis (P37.5)*
DEF: Candida: Genus of yeast-like fungi that are commonly found in the mouth, skin, intestinal tract, and vagina. It may cause a white, cheesy discharge.

B37.0 Candidal stomatitis HIV CC
Oral thrush

B37.1 Pulmonary candidiasis HIV MCC HCC
Candidal bronchitis
Candidal pneumonia

B37.2 Candidiasis of skin and nail HIV
Candidal onychia
Candidal paronychia
EXCLUDES 2 *diaper dermatitis (L22)*

B37.3 Candidiasis of vulva and vagina ♀
Candidal vulvovaginitis
Monilial vulvovaginitis
Vaginal thrush

✓5th **B37.4 Candidiasis of other urogenital sites**

B37.41 Candidal cystitis and urethritis CC H6

B37.42 Candidal balanitis ♂

B37.49 Other urogenital candidiasis CC H6
Candidal pyelonephritis

B37.5 Candidal meningitis HIV MCC

B37.6 Candidal endocarditis HIV MCC

B37.7 Candidal sepsis MCC HCC
Disseminated candidiasis
Systemic candidiasis
AHA: 2014,4Q,46
TIP: This code is assigned when sepsis is documented as due to any *Candida* type. If non-*Candida albicans* is documented, code B48.8 Other specified mycoses, is assigned.

✓5th **B37.8 Candidiasis of other sites**

B37.81 Candidal esophagitis HIV CC HCC

B37.82 Candidal enteritis HIV CC
Candidal proctitis

B37.83 Candidal cheilitis HIV CC

B37.84 Candidal otitis externa HIV CC

B37.89 Other sites of candidiasis HIV CC
Candidal osteomyelitis

B37.9 Candidiasis, unspecified HIV
Thrush NOS

✓4th B38 Coccidioidomycosis

B38.0 Acute pulmonary coccidioidomycosis HIV CC HCC

B38.1 Chronic pulmonary coccidioidomycosis HIV CC HCC

B38.2 Pulmonary coccidioidomycosis, unspecified HIV CC HCC

B38.3 Cutaneous coccidioidomycosis HIV CC

B38.4 Coccidioidomycosis meningitis HIV MCC
DEF: *Coccidioides immitis* infection of the lining of the brain and/or spinal cord.

B38.7 Disseminated coccidioidomycosis HIV CC
Generalized coccidioidomycosis

✓5th **B38.8 Other forms of coccidioidomycosis**

B38.81 Prostatic coccidioidomycosis HIV CC ♂

B38.89 Other forms of coccidioidomycosis HIV CC

B38.9 Coccidioidomycosis, unspecified HIV CC

B39 Histoplasmosis
Code first associated AIDS (B2Ø)
Use additional code for any associated manifestations, such as:
endocarditis (I39)
meningitis (GØ2)
pericarditis (I32)
retinitis (H32)
DEF: Type of lung infection caused by breathing in fungal spores often found in the droppings of bats and birds or soil contaminated by their droppings.

Histoplasmosis

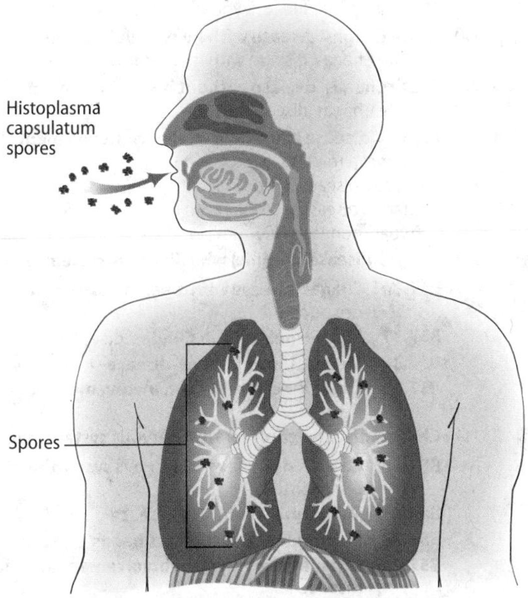

B39.Ø Acute pulmonary histoplasmosis capsulati HIV MCC HCC
B39.1 Chronic pulmonary histoplasmosis capsulati HIV MCC HCC
B39.2 Pulmonary histoplasmosis capsulati, unspecified HIV MCC HCC
B39.3 Disseminated histoplasmosis capsulati HIV CC
Generalized histoplasmosis capsulati
B39.4 Histoplasmosis capsulati, unspecified HIV
American histoplasmosis
B39.5 Histoplasmosis duboisii HIV
African histoplasmosis
B39.9 Histoplasmosis, unspecified HIV

B4Ø Blastomycosis
EXCLUDES 1 *Brazilian blastomycosis (B41.-)*
keloidal blastomycosis (B48.Ø)
B4Ø.Ø Acute pulmonary blastomycosis CC HCC
B4Ø.1 Chronic pulmonary blastomycosis CC HCC
B4Ø.2 Pulmonary blastomycosis, unspecified CC HCC
B4Ø.3 Cutaneous blastomycosis CC
B4Ø.7 Disseminated blastomycosis CC
Generalized blastomycosis
B4Ø.8 Other forms of blastomycosis
B4Ø.81 Blastomycotic meningoencephalitis CC
Meningomyelitis due to blastomycosis
B4Ø.89 Other forms of blastomycosis CC
B4Ø.9 Blastomycosis, unspecified CC

B41 Paracoccidioidomycosis
INCLUDES Brazilian blastomycosis
Lutz' disease
B41.Ø Pulmonary paracoccidioidomycosis CC HCC
B41.7 Disseminated paracoccidioidomycosis CC
Generalized paracoccidioidomycosis
B41.8 Other forms of paracoccidioidomycosis CC
B41.9 Paracoccidioidomycosis, unspecified CC

B42 Sporotrichosis
B42.Ø Pulmonary sporotrichosis
B42.1 Lymphocutaneous sporotrichosis
B42.7 Disseminated sporotrichosis
Generalized sporotrichosis
B42.8 Other forms of sporotrichosis
B42.81 Cerebral sporotrichosis
Meningitis due to sporotrichosis
B42.82 Sporotrichosis arthritis HCC
B42.89 Other forms of sporotrichosis
B42.9 Sporotrichosis, unspecified

B43 Chromomycosis and pheomycotic abscess
B43.Ø Cutaneous chromomycosis
Dermatitis verrucosa
B43.1 Pheomycotic brain abscess
Cerebral chromomycosis
B43.2 Subcutaneous pheomycotic abscess and cyst
B43.8 Other forms of chromomycosis
B43.9 Chromomycosis, unspecified

B44 Aspergillosis
INCLUDES aspergilloma
B44.Ø Invasive pulmonary aspergillosis MCC HCC
B44.1 Other pulmonary aspergillosis CC HCC
B44.2 Tonsillar aspergillosis CC HCC
B44.7 Disseminated aspergillosis CC HCC
Generalized aspergillosis
B44.8 Other forms of aspergillosis
B44.81 Allergic bronchopulmonary aspergillosis CC HCC
B44.89 Other forms of aspergillosis CC HCC
B44.9 Aspergillosis, unspecified CC HCC

B45 Cryptococcosis
B45.Ø Pulmonary cryptococcosis HIV CC HCC
B45.1 Cerebral cryptococcosis MCC HCC
Cryptococcal meningitis
Cryptococcosis meningocerebralis
B45.2 Cutaneous cryptococcosis HIV CC HCC
B45.3 Osseous cryptococcosis HIV CC HCC
B45.7 Disseminated cryptococcosis HIV CC HCC
Generalized cryptococcosis
B45.8 Other forms of cryptococcosis HIV CC HCC
B45.9 Cryptococcosis, unspecified HIV CC HCC

B46 Zygomycosis
B46.Ø Pulmonary mucormycosis MCC HCC
B46.1 Rhinocerebral mucormycosis MCC HCC
B46.2 Gastrointestinal mucormycosis MCC HCC
B46.3 Cutaneous mucormycosis MCC HCC
Subcutaneous mucormycosis
B46.4 Disseminated mucormycosis MCC HCC
Generalized mucormycosis
B46.5 Mucormycosis, unspecified MCC HCC
B46.8 Other zygomycoses MCC HCC
Entomophthoromycosis
B46.9 Zygomycosis, unspecified MCC HCC
Phycomycosis NOS

B47 Mycetoma
B47.Ø Eumycetoma CC
Madura foot, mycotic
Maduromycosis
B47.1 Actinomycetoma HIV CC
B47.9 Mycetoma, unspecified HIV CC
Madura foot NOS

B48 Other mycoses, not elsewhere classified
B48.Ø Lobomycosis
Keloidal blastomycosis
Lobo's disease
B48.1 Rhinosporidiosis
B48.2 Allescheriasis CC
Infection due to Pseudallescheria boydii
EXCLUDES 1 *eumycetoma (B47.Ø)*
B48.3 Geotrichosis CC
Geotrichum stomatitis
B48.4 Penicillosis CC HCC
▶Talaromycosis◀

B48.8 Other specified mycoses HIV CC HCC
Adiaspiromycosis
Infection of tissue and organs by Alternaria
Infection of tissue and organs by Drechslera
Infection of tissue and organs by Fusarium
Infection of tissue and organs by saprophytic fungi NEC
AHA: 2014,4Q,46; 2014,2Q,13
TIP: This code is assigned when sepsis is documented as due to non-*Candida albicans*. If sepsis is due to any *Candida* type, code B37.7 Candidal sepsis, is assigned.

B49 Unspecified mycosis CC
Fungemia NOS

Protozoal diseases (B50-B64)

EXCLUDES 1 *amebiasis (A06.-)*
other protozoal intestinal diseases (A07.-)

✓4th **B50 Plasmodium falciparum malaria**
INCLUDES mixed infections of Plasmodium falciparum with any other Plasmodium species

B50.0 Plasmodium falciparum malaria with cerebral complications CC
Cerebral malaria NOS

B50.8 Other severe and complicated Plasmodium falciparum malaria CC
Severe or complicated Plasmodium falciparum malaria NOS

B50.9 Plasmodium falciparum malaria, unspecified MCC

✓4th **B51 Plasmodium vivax malaria**
INCLUDES mixed infections of Plasmodium vivax with other Plasmodium species, except Plasmodium falciparum
EXCLUDES 1 *Plasmodium vivax with Plasmodium falciparum (B50.-)*

B51.0 Plasmodium vivax malaria with rupture of spleen CC
B51.8 Plasmodium vivax malaria with other complications CC
B51.9 Plasmodium vivax malaria without complication CC
Plasmodium vivax malaria NOS

✓4th **B52 Plasmodium malariae malaria**
INCLUDES mixed infections of Plasmodium malariae with other Plasmodium species, except Plasmodium falciparum and Plasmodium vivax
EXCLUDES 1 *Plasmodium falciparum (B50.-)*
Plasmodium vivax (B51.-)

B52.0 Plasmodium malariae malaria with nephropathy CC
B52.8 Plasmodium malariae malaria with other complications CC
B52.9 Plasmodium malariae malaria without complication CC
Plasmodium malariae malaria NOS

✓4th **B53 Other specified malaria**

B53.0 Plasmodium ovale malaria CC
EXCLUDES 1 *Plasmodium ovale with Plasmodium falciparum (B50.-)*
Plasmodium ovale with Plasmodium malariae (B52.-)
Plasmodium ovale with Plasmodium vivax (B51.-)

B53.1 Malaria due to simian plasmodia CC
EXCLUDES 1 *malaria due to simian plasmodia with Plasmodium falciparum (B50.-)*
malaria due to simian plasmodia with Plasmodium malariae (B52.-)
malaria due to simian plasmodia with Plasmodium ovale (B53.0)
malaria due to simian plasmodia with Plasmodium vivax (B51.-)

B53.8 Other malaria, not elsewhere classified CC

B54 Unspecified malaria CC

✓4th **B55 Leishmaniasis**

B55.0 Visceral leishmaniasis CC
Kala-azar
Post-kala-azar dermal leishmaniasis

B55.1 Cutaneous leishmaniasis CC
B55.2 Mucocutaneous leishmaniasis CC
B55.9 Leishmaniasis, unspecified CC

✓4th **B56 African trypanosomiasis**

B56.0 Gambiense trypanosomiasis CC
Infection due to Trypanosoma brucei gambiense
West African sleeping sickness

B56.1 Rhodesiense trypanosomiasis CC
East African sleeping sickness
Infection due to Trypanosoma brucei rhodesiense

B56.9 African trypanosomiasis, unspecified CC
Sleeping sickness NOS

✓4th **B57 Chagas' disease**
INCLUDES American trypanosomiasis
infection due to Trypanosoma cruzi

B57.0 Acute Chagas' disease with heart involvement CC
Acute Chagas' disease with myocarditis

B57.1 Acute Chagas' disease without heart involvement CC
Acute Chagas' disease NOS

B57.2 Chagas' disease (chronic) with heart involvement CC
American trypanosomiasis NOS
Chagas' disease (chronic) NOS
Chagas' disease (chronic) with myocarditis
Trypanosomiasis NOS

✓5th **B57.3 Chagas' disease (chronic) with digestive system involvement**

B57.30 Chagas' disease with digestive system involvement, unspecified CC
B57.31 Megaesophagus in Chagas' disease CC
B57.32 Megacolon in Chagas' disease CC
B57.39 Other digestive system involvement in Chagas' disease CC

✓5th **B57.4 Chagas' disease (chronic) with nervous system involvement**

B57.40 Chagas' disease with nervous system involvement, unspecified CC
B57.41 Meningitis in Chagas' disease CC
B57.42 Meningoencephalitis in Chagas' disease CC
B57.49 Other nervous system involvement in Chagas' disease CC

B57.5 Chagas' disease (chronic) with other organ involvement CC

✓4th **B58 Toxoplasmosis**
INCLUDES infection due to Toxoplasma gondii
EXCLUDES 1 *congenital toxoplasmosis (P37.1)*

✓5th **B58.0 Toxoplasma oculopathy**

B58.00 Toxoplasma oculopathy, unspecified HIV CC
B58.01 Toxoplasma chorioretinitis HIV CC
B58.09 Other toxoplasma oculopathy HIV CC
Toxoplasma uveitis

B58.1 Toxoplasma hepatitis HIV CC
B58.2 Toxoplasma meningoencephalitis HIV MCC HCC
B58.3 Pulmonary toxoplasmosis HIV MCC HCC

✓5th **B58.8 Toxoplasmosis with other organ involvement**

B58.81 Toxoplasma myocarditis HIV MCC
B58.82 Toxoplasma myositis HIV CC
B58.83 Toxoplasma tubulo-interstitial nephropathy HIV CC
Toxoplasma pyelonephritis
B58.89 Toxoplasmosis with other organ involvement HIV CC

B58.9 Toxoplasmosis, unspecified HIV CC

B59 Pneumocystosis HIV MCC HCC
Pneumonia due to Pneumocystis carinii
Pneumonia due to Pneumocystis jiroveci

✓4th **B60 Other protozoal diseases, not elsewhere classified**
EXCLUDES 1 *cryptosporidiosis (A07.2)*
intestinal microsporidiosis (A07.8)
isosporiasis (A07.3)

▲ ✓5th **B60.0 Babesiosis**
~~Piroplasmosis~~

● **B60.00 Babesiosis, unspecified** CC
Babesiosis due to unspecified Babesia species
Piroplasmosis, unspecified

● **B60.01 Babesiosis due to Babesia microti** CC
Infection due to B. microti

● **B60.02 Babesiosis due to Babesia duncani** CC
Infection due to B. duncani and B. duncani-type species

● **B60.03 Babesiosis due to Babesia divergens** CC
Babesiosis due to Babesia MO-1
Infection due to B. divergens and B. divergens-like strains

● **B60.09 Other babesiosis** CC
Babesiosis due to Babesia KO-1
Babesiosis due to Babesia venatorum
Infection due to other Babesia species
Infection due to other protozoa of the order Piroplasmida
Other piroplasmosis

√5th **B60.1 Acanthamebiasis**
B60.10 Acanthamebiasis, unspecified CC
B60.11 Meningoencephalitis due to Acanthamoeba (culbertsoni)
B60.12 Conjunctivitis due to Acanthamoeba
B60.13 Keratoconjunctivitis due to Acanthamoeba
B60.19 Other acanthamebic disease CC

B60.2 Naegleriasis CC
Primary amebic meningoencephalitis

B60.8 Other specified protozoal diseases HIV
Microsporidiosis

B64 Unspecified protozoal disease

Helminthiases (B65-B83)

√4th **B65 Schistosomiasis [bilharziasis]**
INCLUDES snail fever

B65.0 Schistosomiasis due to Schistosoma haematobium [urinary schistosomiasis] CC

B65.1 Schistosomiasis due to Schistosoma mansoni [intestinal schistosomiasis] CC

B65.2 Schistosomiasis due to Schistosoma japonicum CC
Asiatic schistosomiasis

B65.3 Cercarial dermatitis CC
Swimmer's itch

B65.8 Other schistosomiasis CC
Infection due to Schistosoma intercalatum
Infection due to Schistosoma mattheei
Infection due to Schistosoma mekongi

B65.9 Schistosomiasis, unspecified CC

√4th **B66 Other fluke infections**

B66.0 Opisthorchiasis CC
Infection due to cat liver fluke
Infection due to Opisthorchis (felineus)(viverrini)

B66.1 Clonorchiasis CC
Chinese liver fluke disease
Infection due to Clonorchis sinensis
Oriental liver fluke disease

B66.2 Dicroceliasis CC
Infection due to Dicrocoelium dendriticum
Lancet fluke infection

B66.3 Fascioliasis CC
Infection due to Fasciola gigantica
Infection due to Fasciola hepatica
Infection due to Fasciola indica
Sheep liver fluke disease

B66.4 Paragonimiasis CC HCC
Infection due to Paragonimus species
Lung fluke disease
Pulmonary distomiasis

B66.5 Fasciolopsiasis CC
Infection due to Fasciolopsis buski
Intestinal distomiasis

B66.8 Other specified fluke infections CC
Echinostomiasis
Heterophyiasis
Metagonimiasis
Nanophyetiasis
Watsoniasis

B66.9 Fluke infection, unspecified

√4th **B67 Echinococcosis**
INCLUDES hydatidosis

B67.0 Echinococcus granulosus infection of liver CC
B67.1 Echinococcus granulosus infection of lung CC HCC
B67.2 Echinococcus granulosus infection of bone CC

√5th **B67.3 Echinococcus granulosus infection, other and multiple sites**
B67.31 Echinococcus granulosus infection, thyroid gland CC
B67.32 Echinococcus granulosus infection, multiple sites CC
B67.39 Echinococcus granulosus infection, other sites CC

B67.4 Echinococcus granulosus infection, unspecified CC
Dog tapeworm (infection)

B67.5 Echinococcus multilocularis infection of liver CC

√5th **B67.6 Echinococcus multilocularis infection, other and multiple sites**
B67.61 Echinococcus multilocularis infection, multiple sites CC
B67.69 Echinococcus multilocularis infection, other sites CC

B67.7 Echinococcus multilocularis infection, unspecified CC
B67.8 Echinococcosis, unspecified, of liver CC

√5th **B67.9 Echinococcosis, other and unspecified**
B67.90 Echinococcosis, unspecified CC
Echinococcosis NOS
B67.99 Other echinococcosis CC

√4th **B68 Taeniasis**
EXCLUDES 1 *cysticercosis (B69.-)*

B68.0 Taenia solium taeniasis CC
Pork tapeworm (infection)

B68.1 Taenia saginata taeniasis CC
Beef tapeworm (infection)
Infection due to adult tapeworm Taenia saginata

B68.9 Taeniasis, unspecified CC

√4th **B69 Cysticercosis**
INCLUDES cysticerciasis infection due to larval form of Taenia solium

DEF: Condition that is developed when larvae or eggs of the tapeworm *Taenia solium* are ingested, most commonly in fecally contaminated water or undercooked pork.

B69.0 Cysticercosis of central nervous system CC
B69.1 Cysticercosis of eye CC

√5th **B69.8 Cysticercosis of other sites**
B69.81 Myositis in cysticercosis CC
B69.89 Cysticercosis of other sites CC

B69.9 Cysticercosis, unspecified CC

√4th **B70 Diphyllobothriasis and sparganosis**

B70.0 Diphyllobothriasis CC
Diphyllobothrium (adult) (latum) (pacificum) infection
Fish tapeworm (infection)
EXCLUDES 2 *larval diphyllobothriasis (B70.1)*

B70.1 Sparganosis CC
Infection due to Sparganum (mansoni) (proliferum)
Infection due to Spirometra larva
Larval diphyllobothriasis
Spirometrosis

√4th **B71 Other cestode infections**

B71.0 Hymenolepiasis CC
Dwarf tapeworm infection
Rat tapeworm (infection)

B71.1 Dipylidiasis CC

B71.8 Other specified cestode infections CC
Coenurosis

B71.9 Cestode infection, unspecified
Tapeworm (infection) NOS

B72 Dracunculiasis CC
INCLUDES guinea worm infection
infection due to Dracunculus medinensis

√4th **B73 Onchocerciasis**
INCLUDES onchocerca volvulus infection
onchocercosis
river blindness

√5th **B73.Ø Onchocerciasis with eye disease**
B73.ØØ Onchocerciasis with eye involvement, unspecified CC
B73.Ø1 Onchocerciasis with endophthalmitis CC
B73.Ø2 Onchocerciasis with glaucoma CC
B73.Ø9 Onchocerciasis with other eye involvement CC
Infestation of eyelid due to onchocerciasis

B73.1 Onchocerciasis without eye disease CC

√4th **B74 Filariasis**
EXCLUDES 2 *onchocerciasis (B73)*
tropical (pulmonary) eosinophilia NOS (J82)

B74.Ø Filariasis due to Wuchereria bancrofti CC
Bancroftian elephantiasis
Bancroftian filariasis

B74.1 Filariasis due to Brugia malayi CC
B74.2 Filariasis due to Brugia timori CC
B74.3 Loiasis CC
Calabar swelling
Eyeworm disease of Africa
Loa loa infection

B74.4 Mansonelliasis CC
Infection due to Mansonella ozzardi
Infection due to Mansonella perstans
Infection due to Mansonella streptocerca

B74.8 Other filariases CC
Dirofilariasis

B74.9 Filariasis, unspecified CC

B75 Trichinellosis CC
INCLUDES infection due to Trichinella species
trichiniasis

DEF: Infection by *Trichinella spiralis,* the smallest of the parasitic nematodes, that is transmitted by eating undercooked pork or bear meat. ***Synonym(s):*** *Trichinosis.*

√4th **B76 Hookworm diseases**
INCLUDES uncinariasis

B76.Ø Ancylostomiasis CC
Infection due to Ancylostoma species

B76.1 Necatoriasis CC
Infection due to Necator americanus

B76.8 Other hookworm diseases CC
B76.9 Hookworm disease, unspecified CC
Cutaneous larva migrans NOS

√4th **B77 Ascariasis**
INCLUDES ascaridiasis
roundworm infection

B77.Ø Ascariasis with intestinal complications CC
√5th **B77.8 Ascariasis with other complications**
B77.81 Ascariasis pneumonia MCC
B77.89 Ascariasis with other complications CC

B77.9 Ascariasis, unspecified CC

√4th **B78 Strongyloidiasis**
EXCLUDES 1 *trichostrongyliasis (B81.2)*

B78.Ø Intestinal strongyloidiasis HIV CC
B78.1 Cutaneous strongyloidiasis
B78.7 Disseminated strongyloidiasis HIV CC
B78.9 Strongyloidiasis, unspecified HIV CC

B79 Trichuriasis CC
INCLUDES trichocephaliasis
whipworm (disease)(infection)

B8Ø Enterobiasis CC
INCLUDES oxyuriasis
pinworm infection
threadworm infection

√4th **B81 Other intestinal helminthiases, not elsewhere classified**
EXCLUDES 1 *angiostrongyliasis due to:*
angiostrongylus cantonensis (B83.2)
parastrongylus cantonensis (B83.2)

B81.Ø Anisakiasis CC
Infection due to Anisakis larva

B81.1 Intestinal capillariasis CC
Capillariasis NOS
Infection due to Capillaria philippinensis
EXCLUDES 2 *hepatic capillariasis (B83.8)*

B81.2 Trichostrongyliasis CC
B81.3 Intestinal angiostrongyliasis CC
Angiostrongyliasis due to:
angiostrongylus costaricensis
parastrongylus costaricensis

B81.4 Mixed intestinal helminthiases CC
Infection due to intestinal helminths classified to more than one of the categories B65.Ø-B81.3 and B81.8
Mixed helminthiasis NOS

B81.8 Other specified intestinal helminthiases CC
Infection due to Oesophagostomum species [esophagostomiasis]
Infection due to Ternidens diminutus [ternidensiasis]

√4th **B82 Unspecified intestinal parasitism**
B82.Ø Intestinal helminthiasis, unspecified CC
B82.9 Intestinal parasitism, unspecified

√4th **B83 Other helminthiases**
EXCLUDES 1 *capillariasis NOS (B81.1)*
EXCLUDES 2 *intestinal capillariasis (B81.1)*

B83.Ø Visceral larva migrans
Toxocariasis

B83.1 Gnathostomiasis
Wandering swelling

B83.2 Angiostrongyliasis due to Parastrongylus cantonensis
Eosinophilic meningoencephalitis due to Parastrongylus cantonensis
EXCLUDES 2 *intestinal angiostrongyliasis (B81.3)*

B83.3 Syngamiasis
Syngamosis

B83.4 Internal hirudiniasis
EXCLUDES 2 *external hirudiniasis (B88.3)*

B83.8 Other specified helminthiases
Acanthocephaliasis
Gongylonemiasis
Hepatic capillariasis
Metastrongyliasis
Thelaziasis

B83.9 Helminthiasis, unspecified
Worms NOS
EXCLUDES 1 *intestinal helminthiasis NOS (B82.Ø)*

Pediculosis, acariasis and other infestations (B85-B89)

√4th **B85 Pediculosis and phthiriasis**
B85.Ø Pediculosis due to Pediculus humanus capitis
Head-louse infestation

B85.1 Pediculosis due to Pediculus humanus corporis
Body-louse infestation

B85.2 Pediculosis, unspecified
B85.3 Phthiriasis
Infestation by crab-louse
Infestation by Phthirus pubis

B85.4 Mixed pediculosis and phthiriasis
Infestation classifiable to more than one of the categories B85.Ø-B85.3

B86 Scabies
Sarcoptic itch
DEF: Mite infestation that is caused by *Sarcoptes scabiei.* Scabies causes intense itching and sometimes secondary infection.

√4th **B87 Myiasis**
INCLUDES infestation by larva of flies

B87.Ø Cutaneous myiasis
Creeping myiasis

B87.1 Wound myiasis
Traumatic myiasis
B87.2 Ocular myiasis
B87.3 Nasopharyngeal myiasis
Laryngeal myiasis
B87.4 Aural myiasis
B87.8 Myiasis of other sites
B87.81 Genitourinary myiasis
B87.82 Intestinal myiasis
B87.89 Myiasis of other sites
B87.9 Myiasis, unspecified

B88 Other infestations
B88.Ø Other acariasis
Acarine dermatitis
Dermatitis due to Demodex species
Dermatitis due to Dermanyssus gallinae
Dermatitis due to Liponyssoides sanguineus
Trombiculosis
EXCLUDES 2 *scabies (B86)*
B88.1 Tungiasis [sandflea infestation]
B88.2 Other arthropod infestations
Scarabiasis
B88.3 External hirudiniasis
Leech infestation NOS
EXCLUDES 2 *internal hirudiniasis (B83.4)*
B88.8 Other specified infestations
Ichthyoparasitism due to Vandellia cirrhosa
Linguatulosis
Porocephaliasis
B88.9 Infestation, unspecified
Infestation (skin) NOS
Infestation by mites NOS
Skin parasites NOS

B89 Unspecified parasitic disease

Sequelae of infectious and parasitic diseases (B9Ø-B94)

NOTE Categories B9Ø-B94 are to be used to indicate conditions in categories AØØ-B89 as the cause of sequelae, which are themselves classified elsewhere. The "sequelae" include conditions specified as such; they also include residuals of diseases classifiable to the above categories if there is evidence that the disease itself is no longer present. Codes from these categories are not to be used for chronic infections. Code chronic current infections to active infectious disease as appropriate.

Code first condition resulting from (sequela) the infectious or parasitic disease

B9Ø Sequelae of tuberculosis
B9Ø.Ø Sequelae of central nervous system tuberculosis
B9Ø.1 Sequelae of genitourinary tuberculosis
B9Ø.2 Sequelae of tuberculosis of bones and joints
B9Ø.8 Sequelae of tuberculosis of other organs
EXCLUDES 2 *sequelae of respiratory tuberculosis (B9Ø.9)*
B9Ø.9 Sequelae of respiratory and unspecified tuberculosis
Sequelae of tuberculosis NOS

B91 Sequelae of poliomyelitis
EXCLUDES 1 *postpolio syndrome (G14)*

B92 Sequelae of leprosy

B94 Sequelae of other and unspecified infectious and parasitic diseases
B94.Ø Sequelae of trachoma
B94.1 Sequelae of viral encephalitis
B94.2 Sequelae of viral hepatitis
B94.8 Sequelae of other specified infectious and parasitic diseases
AHA: 2017,4Q,109
B94.9 Sequelae of unspecified infectious and parasitic disease

Bacterial and viral infectious agents (B95-B97)

NOTE These categories are provided for use as supplementary or additional codes to identify the infectious agent(s) in diseases classified elsewhere.

AHA: 2020,2Q,18; 2018,4Q,34; 2018,1Q,16

B95 Streptococcus, Staphylococcus, and Enterococcus as the cause of diseases classified elsewhere
B95.Ø Streptococcus, group A, as the cause of diseases classified elsewhere
B95.1 Streptococcus, group B, as the cause of diseases classified elsewhere
AHA: 2020,1Q,10; 2019,2Q,8-10
B95.2 Enterococcus as the cause of diseases classified elsewhere
B95.3 Streptococcus pneumoniae as the cause of diseases classified elsewhere
B95.4 Other streptococcus as the cause of diseases classified elsewhere
B95.5 Unspecified streptococcus as the cause of diseases classified elsewhere
B95.6 Staphylococcus aureus as the cause of diseases classified elsewhere
B95.61 Methicillin susceptible Staphylococcus aureus infection as the cause of diseases classified elsewhere
Methicillin susceptible Staphylococcus aureus (MSSA) infection as the cause of diseases classified elsewhere
Staphylococcus aureus infection NOS as the cause of diseases classified elsewhere
B95.62 Methicillin resistant Staphylococcus aureus infection as the cause of diseases classified elsewhere
Methicillin resistant staphylococcus aureus (MRSA) infection as the cause of diseases classified elsewhere
AHA: 2016,1Q,12
B95.7 Other staphylococcus as the cause of diseases classified elsewhere
B95.8 Unspecified staphylococcus as the cause of diseases classified elsewhere

B96 Other bacterial agents as the cause of diseases classified elsewhere
B96.Ø Mycoplasma pneumoniae [M. pneumoniae] as the cause of diseases classified elsewhere
Pleuro-pneumonia-like-organism [PPLO]
B96.1 Klebsiella pneumoniae [K. pneumoniae] as the cause of diseases classified elsewhere
B96.2 Escherichia coli [E. coli] as the cause of diseases classified elsewhere
B96.2Ø Unspecified Escherichia coli [E. coli] as the cause of diseases classified elsewhere
Escherichia coli [E. coli] NOS
B96.21 Shiga toxin-producing Escherichia coli [E. coli] [STEC] O157 as the cause of diseases classified elsewhere
E. coli O157:H- (nonmotile) with confirmation of Shiga toxin
E. coli O157 with confirmation of Shiga toxin when H antigen is unknown, or is not H7
O157:H7 Escherichia coli [E.coli] with or without confirmation of Shiga toxin-production
Shiga toxin-producing Escherichia coli [E.coli] O157:H7 with or without confirmation of Shiga toxin-production
STEC O157:H7 with or without confirmation of Shiga toxin-production
B96.22 Other specified Shiga toxin-producing Escherichia coli [E. coli] [STEC] as the cause of diseases classified elsewhere
Non-O157 Shiga toxin-producing Escherichia coli [E.coli]
Non-O157 Shiga toxin-producing Escherichia coli [E.coli] with known O group
B96.23 Unspecified Shiga toxin-producing Escherichia coli [E. coli] [STEC] as the cause of diseases classified elsewhere
Shiga toxin-producing Escherichia coli [E. coli] with unspecified O group
STEC NOS
B96.29 Other Escherichia coli [E. coli] as the cause of diseases classified elsewhere
Non-Shiga toxin-producing E. coli
B96.3 Hemophilus influenzae [H. influenzae] as the cause of diseases classified elsewhere
B96.4 Proteus (mirabilis) (morganii) as the cause of diseases classified elsewhere
B96.5 Pseudomonas (aeruginosa) (mallei) (pseudomallei) as the cause of diseases classified elsewhere
AHA: 2015,1Q,18

B96.6 Bacteroides fragilis [B. fragilis] as the cause of diseases classified elsewhere

B96.7 Clostridium perfringens [C. perfringens] as the cause of diseases classified elsewhere

✓5th **B96.8 Other specified bacterial agents as the cause of diseases classified elsewhere**

B96.81 Helicobacter pylori [H. pylori] as the cause of diseases classified elsewhere

B96.82 Vibrio vulnificus as the cause of diseases classified elsewhere

B96.89 Other specified bacterial agents as the cause of diseases classified elsewhere

✓4th **B97 Viral agents as the cause of diseases classified elsewhere**

AHA: 2016,3Q,8-10,14

B97.Ø Adenovirus as the cause of diseases classified elsewhere

✓5th **B97.1 Enterovirus as the cause of diseases classified elsewhere**

B97.1Ø Unspecified enterovirus as the cause of diseases classified elsewhere

B97.11 Coxsackievirus as the cause of diseases classified elsewhere

B97.12 Echovirus as the cause of diseases classified elsewhere

B97.19 Other enterovirus as the cause of diseases classified elsewhere

✓5th **B97.2 Coronavirus as the cause of diseases classified elsewhere**

TIP: Do not report a code from this subcategory for COVID-19; refer to U07.1.

B97.21 SARS-associated coronavirus as the cause of diseases classified elsewhere CC

EXCLUDES 1 *pneumonia due to SARS-associated coronavirus (J12.81)*

B97.29 Other coronavirus as the cause of diseases classified elsewhere

AHA: 2020,2Q,5; 2020,1Q,34-36

✓5th **B97.3 Retrovirus as the cause of diseases classified elsewhere**

EXCLUDES 1 *human immunodeficiency virus [HIV] disease (B2Ø)*

B97.3Ø Unspecified retrovirus as the cause of diseases classified elsewhere

B97.31 Lentivirus as the cause of diseases classified elsewhere

B97.32 Oncovirus as the cause of diseases classified elsewhere

B97.33 Human T-cell lymphotrophic virus, type I [HTLV-I] as the cause of diseases classified elsewhere CC

B97.34 Human T-cell lymphotrophic virus, type II [HTLV-II] as the cause of diseases classified elsewhere CC

B97.35 Human immunodeficiency virus, type 2 [HIV 2] as the cause of diseases classified elsewhere CC HCC

B97.39 Other retrovirus as the cause of diseases classified elsewhere

B97.4 Respiratory syncytial virus as the cause of diseases classified elsewhere

RSV as the cause of diseases classified elsewhere

Code first related disorders, such as:

otitis media (H65.-)

upper respiratory infection (JØ6.9)

EXCLUDES 2 *acute bronchiolitis due to respiratory syncytial virus (RSV) (J21.Ø)*

acute bronchitis due to respiratory syncytial virus (RSV) (J2Ø.5)

respiratory syncytial virus (RSV) pneumonia (J12.1)

B97.5 Reovirus as the cause of diseases classified elsewhere

B97.6 Parvovirus as the cause of diseases classified elsewhere

B97.7 Papillomavirus as the cause of diseases classified elsewhere

✓5th **B97.8 Other viral agents as the cause of diseases classified elsewhere**

B97.81 Human metapneumovirus as the cause of diseases classified elsewhere

B97.89 Other viral agents as the cause of diseases classified elsewhere

Other infectious diseases (B99)

✓4th **B99 Other and unspecified infectious diseases**

B99.8 Other infectious disease HIV

B99.9 Unspecified infectious disease

Chapter 2. Neoplasms (CØØ–D49)

Chapter-specific Guidelines with Coding Examples

The chapter-specific guidelines from the ICD-10-CM Official Guidelines for Coding and Reporting have been provided below. Along with these guidelines are coding examples, contained in the shaded boxes, that have been developed to help illustrate the coding and/or sequencing guidance found in these guidelines.

General guidelines

Chapter 2 of the ICD-10-CM contains the codes for most benign and all malignant neoplasms. Certain benign neoplasms, such as prostatic adenomas, may be found in the specific body system chapters. To properly code a neoplasm, it is necessary to determine from the record if the neoplasm is benign, in-situ, malignant, or of uncertain histologic behavior. If malignant, any secondary (metastatic) sites should also be determined.

Primary malignant neoplasms overlapping site boundaries

A primary malignant neoplasm that overlaps two or more contiguous (next to each other) sites should be classified to the subcategory/code .8 ('overlapping lesion'), unless the combination is specifically indexed elsewhere. For multiple neoplasms of the same site that are not contiguous such as tumors in different quadrants of the same breast, codes for each site should be assigned.

A 73-year-old white female with a large rapidly growing malignant tumor in the left breast extending from the upper outer quadrant into the axillary tail

C5Ø.812 **Malignant neoplasm of overlapping sites of left female breast**

Explanation: Because this is a single large tumor that overlaps two contiguous sites, a single code for overlapping sites is assigned.

A 52-year old white female with two distinct lesions of the right breast, one (Ø.5 cm) in the upper outer quadrant and a second (1.5 cm) in the lower outer quadrant; path report indicates both lesions are malignant

C5Ø.411 **Malignant neoplasm of upper-outer quadrant of right female breast**

C5Ø.511 **Malignant neoplasm of lower-outer quadrant of right female breast**

Explanation: This patient has two distinct malignant lesions of right breast in adjacent quadrants. Because the lesions are not contiguous, two codes are reported.

Malignant neoplasm of ectopic tissue

Malignant neoplasms of ectopic tissue are to be coded to the site of origin mentioned, e.g., ectopic pancreatic malignant neoplasms involving the stomach are coded to malignant neoplasm of pancreas, unspecified (C25.9).

The neoplasm table in the Alphabetic Index should be referenced first. However, if the histological term is documented, that term should be referenced first, rather than going immediately to the Neoplasm Table, in order to determine which column in the Neoplasm Table is appropriate. For example, if the documentation indicates "adenoma," refer to the term in the Alphabetic Index to review the entries under this term and the instructional note to "see also neoplasm, by site, benign." The table provides the proper code based on the type of neoplasm and the site. It is important to select the proper column in the table that corresponds to the type of neoplasm. The Tabular List should then be referenced to verify that the correct code has been selected from the table and that a more specific site code does not exist.

See Section I.C.21. Factors influencing health status and contact with health services, Status, for information regarding Z15.Ø, codes for genetic susceptibility to cancer.

a. Treatment directed at the malignancy

If the treatment is directed at the malignancy, designate the malignancy as the principal diagnosis.

The only exception to this guideline is if a patient admission/encounter is solely for the administration of chemotherapy, immunotherapy or external beam radiation therapy, assign the appropriate Z51.-- code as the first-listed or principal diagnosis, and the diagnosis or problem for which the service is being performed as a secondary diagnosis.

b. Treatment of secondary site

When a patient is admitted because of a primary neoplasm with metastasis and treatment is directed toward the secondary site only, the secondary neoplasm is designated as the principal diagnosis even though the primary malignancy is still present.

Patient with primary prostate cancer with metastasis to lungs admitted for wedge resection of mass in right lung

C78.Ø1 **Secondary malignant neoplasm of right lung**

C61 **Malignant neoplasm of prostate**

Explanation: Since the admission is for treatment of the lung metastasis, the secondary lung metastasis is sequenced before the primary prostate cancer.

c. Coding and sequencing of complications

Coding and sequencing of complications associated with the malignancies or with the therapy thereof are subject to the following guidelines:

1) Anemia associated with malignancy

When admission/encounter is for management of an anemia associated with the malignancy, and the treatment is only for anemia, the appropriate code for the malignancy is sequenced as the principal or first-listed diagnosis followed by the appropriate code for the anemia (such as code D63.Ø, Anemia in neoplastic disease).

Patient is admitted for treatment of anemia in advanced colon cancer

C18.9 **Malignant neoplasm of colon, unspecified**

D63.Ø **Anemia in neoplastic disease**

Explanation: Even though the admission was solely to treat the anemia, this guideline indicates that the code for the malignancy is sequenced first.

2) Anemia associated with chemotherapy, immunotherapy and radiation therapy

When the admission/encounter is for management of an anemia associated with an adverse effect of the administration of chemotherapy or immunotherapy and the only treatment is for the anemia, the anemia code is sequenced first followed by the appropriate codes for the neoplasm and the adverse effect (T45.1X5, Adverse effect of antineoplastic and immunosuppressive drugs).

A 56-year-old Hispanic male with grade II follicular lymphoma involving multiple lymph node sites referred for blood transfusion to treat anemia due to chemotherapy

D64.81 **Anemia due to antineoplastic chemotherapy**

C82.18 **Follicular lymphoma grade II, lymph nodes of multiple sites**

T45.1X5A **Adverse effect of antineoplastic and immunosuppressive drugs, initial encounter**

Explanation: The code for the anemia is sequenced first followed by the code for the malignant neoplasm and lastly the code for the adverse effect.

When the admission/encounter is for management of an anemia associated with an adverse effect of radiotherapy, the anemia code should be sequenced first, followed by the appropriate neoplasm code and code Y84.2, Radiological procedure and radiotherapy as the cause of abnormal reaction of the patient, or of later complication, without mention of misadventure at the time of the procedure.

A 55-year-old male with a large malignant rectal tumor has been receiving external radiation therapy to shrink the tumor prior to planned surgery. He is admitted today for a blood transfusion to treat anemia related to radiation therapy.

D64.89	**Other specified anemias**
C2Ø	**Malignant neoplasm of rectum**
Y84.2	**Radiological procedure and radiotherapy as the cause of abnormal reaction of the patient, or of later complication, without mention of misadventure at the time of the procedure**

Explanation: The code for the anemia is sequenced first, followed by the code for the malignancy, and lastly the code for the abnormal reaction due to radiotherapy.

3) Management of dehydration due to the malignancy

When the admission/encounter is for management of dehydration due to the malignancy and only the dehydration is being treated (intravenous rehydration), the dehydration is sequenced first, followed by the code(s) for the malignancy.

4) Treatment of a complication resulting from a surgical procedure

When the admission/encounter is for treatment of a complication resulting from a surgical procedure, designate the complication as the principal or first-listed diagnosis if treatment is directed at resolving the complication.

d. Primary malignancy previously excised

When a primary malignancy has been previously excised or eradicated from its site and there is no further treatment directed to that site and there is no evidence of any existing primary malignancy at that site, a code from category Z85, Personal history of malignant neoplasm, should be used to indicate the former site of the malignancy. Any mention of extension, invasion, or metastasis to another site is coded as a secondary malignant neoplasm to that site. The secondary site may be the principal or first-listed diagnosis with the Z85 code used as a secondary code.

History of breast cancer, left radical mastectomy 18 months ago with no current treatment; bronchoscopy with lung biopsy shows metastatic disease in the right lung

C78.Ø1	**Secondary malignant neoplasm of right lung**
Z85.3	**Personal history of malignant neoplasm of breast**

Explanation: The patient has undergone a diagnostic procedure that revealed metastatic breast cancer in the right lung. The code for the secondary (metastatic) site is sequenced first followed by a personal history code to identify the former site of the primary malignancy.

e. Admissions/encounters involving chemotherapy, immunotherapy and radiation therapy

1) Episode of care involves surgical removal of neoplasm

When an episode of care involves the surgical removal of a neoplasm, primary or secondary site, followed by adjunct chemotherapy or radiation treatment during the same episode of care, the code for the neoplasm should be assigned as principal or first-listed diagnosis.

2) Patient admission/encounter solely for administration of chemotherapy, immunotherapy and radiation therapy

If a patient admission/encounter is solely for the administration of chemotherapy, immunotherapy or external beam radiation therapy assign code Z51.Ø, Encounter for antineoplastic radiation therapy, or Z51.11, Encounter for antineoplastic chemotherapy, or Z51.12, Encounter for antineoplastic immunotherapy as the first-listed or principal diagnosis. If a patient receives more than one of these therapies during the same admission more than one of these codes may be assigned, in any sequence.

The malignancy for which the therapy is being administered should be assigned as a secondary diagnosis.

If a patient admission/encounter is for the insertion or implantation of radioactive elements (e.g., brachytherapy) the appropriate code for the malignancy is sequenced as the principal or first-listed diagnosis. Code Z51.Ø should not be assigned.

3) Patient admitted for radiation therapy, chemotherapy or immunotherapy and develops complications

When a patient is admitted for the purpose of external beam radiotherapy, immunotherapy or chemotherapy and develops complications such as uncontrolled nausea and vomiting or dehydration, the principal or first-listed diagnosis is Z51.Ø, Encounter for antineoplastic radiation therapy, or Z51.11, Encounter for antineoplastic chemotherapy, or Z51.12, Encounter for antineoplastic immunotherapy followed by any codes for the complications.

When a patient is admitted for the purpose of insertion or implantation of radioactive elements (e.g., brachytherapy) and develops complications such as uncontrolled nausea and vomiting or dehydration, the principal or first-listed diagnosis is the appropriate code for the malignancy followed by any codes for the complications.

A patient with prostate cancer was admitted for brachytherapy seed implantation and consequently developed urinary retention.

C61	**Malignant neoplasm of prostate**
R33.9	**Retention of urine, unspecified**

Explanation: A code for the malignancy should be listed as the principal diagnosis when insertion of a radioactive element is the reason for admission, even when a complication related to that radioactive element occurs. Codes describing the complications should be listed as secondary codes.

f. Admission/encounter to determine extent of malignancy

When the reason for admission/encounter is to determine the extent of the malignancy, or for a procedure such as paracentesis or thoracentesis, the primary malignancy or appropriate metastatic site is designated as the principal or first-listed diagnosis, even though chemotherapy or radiotherapy is administered.

Patient with left lung cancer with malignant pleural effusion admitted for paracentesis and initiation/administration of chemotherapy

C34.92	**Malignant neoplasm of unspecified part of left bronchus or lung**
J91.Ø	**Malignant pleural effusion**
Z51.11	**Encounter for antineoplastic chemotherapy**

Explanation: The lung cancer is sequenced before the chemotherapy in this instance because the paracentesis for the malignant effusion is also being performed. An instructional note under the malignant effusion instructs that the lung cancer be sequenced first.

g. Symptoms, signs, and abnormal findings listed in Chapter 18 associated with neoplasms

Symptoms, signs, and ill-defined conditions listed in Chapter 18 characteristic of, or associated with, an existing primary or secondary site malignancy cannot be used to replace the malignancy as principal or first-listed diagnosis, regardless of the number of admissions or encounters for treatment and care of the neoplasm.

See Section I.C.21. Factors influencing health status and contact with health services, Encounter for prophylactic organ removal.

h. Admission/encounter for pain control/management

See Section I.C.6. for information on coding admission/encounter for pain control/management.

i. Malignancy in two or more noncontiguous sites

A patient may have more than one malignant tumor in the same organ. These tumors may represent different primaries or metastatic disease, depending on the site. Should the documentation be unclear, the provider should be queried as to the status of each tumor so that the correct codes can be assigned.

j. Disseminated malignant neoplasm, unspecified

Code C8Ø.Ø, Disseminated malignant neoplasm, unspecified, is for use only in those cases where the patient has advanced metastatic disease and no known primary or secondary sites are specified. It should not be used in place of assigning codes for the primary site and all known secondary sites.

Patient who has had no medical care for many years is seen today and diagnosed with carcinomatosis

C8Ø.Ø	**Disseminated malignant neoplasm, unspecified**

Explanation: Carcinomatosis NOS is an "includes" note under this code. Should seldom be used but is available for use in cases such as this.

k. Malignant neoplasm without specification of site

Code C80.1, Malignant (primary) neoplasm, unspecified, equates to Cancer, unspecified. This code should only be used when no determination can be made as to the primary site of a malignancy. This code should rarely be used in the inpatient setting.

l. Sequencing of neoplasm codes

1) Encounter for treatment of primary malignancy

If the reason for the encounter is for treatment of a primary malignancy, assign the malignancy as the principal/first-listed diagnosis. The primary site is to be sequenced first, followed by any metastatic sites.

2) Encounter for treatment of secondary malignancy

When an encounter is for a primary malignancy with metastasis and treatment is directed toward the metastatic (secondary) site(s) only, the metastatic site(s) is designated as the principal/first-listed diagnosis. The primary malignancy is coded as an additional code.

Patient has primary colon cancer with metastasis to rib and is evaluated for possible excision of portion of rib bone

C79.51 **Secondary malignant neoplasm of bone**

C18.9 **Malignant neoplasm of colon, unspecified**

Explanation: The treatment for this encounter is focused on the metastasis to the rib bone rather than the primary colon cancer, thus indicating that the bone metastasis is sequenced as the first-listed code.

3) Malignant neoplasm in a pregnant patient

When a pregnant woman has a malignant neoplasm, a code from subcategory O9A.1-, Malignant neoplasm complicating pregnancy, childbirth, and the puerperium, should be sequenced first, followed by the appropriate code from Chapter 2 to indicate the type of neoplasm.

A 30-year-old pregnant female in second trimester evaluated for thyroid malignancy

O9A.112 **Malignant neoplasm complicating pregnancy, second trimester**

C73 **Malignant neoplasm of thyroid gland**

Explanation: Codes from chapter 15 describing complications of pregnancy are sequenced as first-listed codes, further specified by codes from other chapters such as neoplastic, unless the pregnancy is documented as incidental to the condition. See also guideline 1.C.15.a.1.

4) Encounter for complication associated with a neoplasm

When an encounter is for management of a complication associated with a neoplasm, such as dehydration, and the treatment is only for the complication, the complication is coded first, followed by the appropriate code(s) for the neoplasm.

The exception to this guideline is anemia. When the admission/encounter is for management of an anemia associated with the malignancy, and the treatment is only for anemia, the appropriate code for the malignancy is sequenced as the principal or first-listed diagnosis followed by code D63.0, Anemia in neoplastic disease.

Patient with pancreatic cancer is seen for initiation of TPN for cancer-related moderate protein-calorie malnutrition

E44.0 **Moderate protein-calorie malnutrition**

C25.9 **Malignant neoplasm of pancreas, unspecified**

Explanation: The encounter is to initiate treatment for malnutrition, a common complication of many types of neoplasms, and is sequenced first.

5) Complication from surgical procedure for treatment of a neoplasm

When an encounter is for treatment of a complication resulting from a surgical procedure performed for the treatment of the neoplasm, designate the complication as the principal/first-listed diagnosis. See the guideline regarding the coding of a current malignancy versus personal history to determine if the code for the neoplasm should also be assigned.

6) Pathologic fracture due to a neoplasm

When an encounter is for a pathological fracture due to a neoplasm, and the focus of treatment is the fracture, a code from subcategory M84.5, Pathological fracture in neoplastic disease, should be sequenced first, followed by the code for the neoplasm.

If the focus of treatment is the neoplasm with an associated pathological fracture, the neoplasm code should be sequenced first, followed by a code from M84.5 for the pathological fracture.

m. Current malignancy versus personal history of malignancy

When a primary malignancy has been excised but further treatment, such as an additional surgery for the malignancy, radiation therapy or chemotherapy is directed to that site, the primary malignancy code should be used until treatment is completed.

Female patient with ongoing chemotherapy after right mastectomy for breast cancer

C50.911 **Malignant neoplasm of unspecified site of right female breast**

Z90.11 **Acquired absence of right breast and nipple**

Explanation: Even though the breast has been removed, the breast cancer is still being treated with chemotherapy and therefore is still coded as a current condition rather than personal history.

When a primary malignancy has been previously excised or eradicated from its site, there is no further treatment (of the malignancy) directed to that site, and there is no evidence of any existing primary malignancy at that site, a code from category Z85, Personal history of malignant neoplasm, should be used to indicate the former site of the malignancy.

Codes from subcategories Z85.0–Z85.85 should only be assigned for the former site of a primary malignancy, not the site of a secondary malignancy. **Code Z85.89** may be assigned for the former site(s) of either a primary or secondary malignancy.

See Section I.C.21. Factors influencing health status and contact with health services, History (of)

n. Leukemia, multiple myeloma, and malignant plasma cell neoplasms in remission versus personal history

The categories for leukemia, and category C90, Multiple myeloma and malignant plasma cell neoplasms, have codes indicating whether or not the leukemia has achieved remission. There are also codes Z85.6, Personal history of leukemia, and Z85.79, Personal history of other malignant neoplasms of lymphoid, hematopoietic and related tissues. If the documentation is unclear as to whether the leukemia has achieved remission, the provider should be queried.

See Section I.C.21. Factors influencing health status and contact with health services, History (of)

o. Aftercare following surgery for neoplasm

See Section I.C.21. Factors influencing health status and contact with health services, Aftercare

p. Follow-up care for completed treatment of a malignancy

See Section I.C.21. Factors influencing health status and contact with health services, Follow-up

q. Prophylactic organ removal for prevention of malignancy

See Section I.C. 21, Factors influencing health status and contact with health services, Prophylactic organ removal

r. Malignant neoplasm associated with transplanted organ

A malignant neoplasm of a transplanted organ should be coded as a transplant complication. Assign first the appropriate code from category T86.-, Complications of transplanted organs and tissue, followed by code C80.2, Malignant neoplasm associated with transplanted organ. Use an additional code for the specific malignancy.

Chapter 2. Neoplasms (C00-D49)

NOTE

Functional activity

All neoplasms are classified in this chapter, whether they are functionally active or not. An additional code from Chapter 4 may be used, to identify functional activity associated with any neoplasm.

Morphology [Histology]

Chapter 2 classifies neoplasms primarily by site (topography), with broad groupings for behavior, malignant, in situ, benign, etc. The Table of Neoplasms should be used to identify the correct topography code. In a few cases, such as for malignant melanoma and certain neuroendocrine tumors, the morphology (histologic type) is included in the category and codes.

Primary malignant neoplasms overlapping site boundaries

A primary malignant neoplasm that overlaps two or more contiguous (next to each other) sites should be classified to the subcategory/code .8 ("overlapping lesion"), unless the combination is specifically indexed elsewhere. For multiple neoplasms of the same site that are not contiguous, such as tumors in different quadrants of the same breast, codes for each site should be assigned.

Malignant neoplasm of ectopic tissue

Malignant neoplasms of ectopic tissue are to be coded to the site mentioned, e.g., ectopic pancreatic malignant neoplasms are coded to pancreas, unspecified (C25.9).

AHA: 2017,4Q,103; 2017,1Q,4,5-6,8

This chapter contains the following blocks:

C00-C14	Malignant neoplasms of lip, oral cavity and pharynx
C15-C26	Malignant neoplasms of digestive organs
C30-C39	Malignant neoplasms of respiratory and intrathoracic organs
C40-C41	Malignant neoplasms of bone and articular cartilage
C43-C44	Melanoma and other malignant neoplasms of skin
C45-C49	Malignant neoplasms of mesothelial and soft tissue
C50	Malignant neoplasms of breast
C51-C58	Malignant neoplasms of female genital organs
C60-C63	Malignant neoplasms of male genital organs
C64-C68	Malignant neoplasms of urinary tract
C69-C72	Malignant neoplasms of eye, brain and other parts of central nervous system
C73-C75	Malignant neoplasms of thyroid and other endocrine glands
C7A	Malignant neuroendocrine tumors
C7B	Secondary neuroendocrine tumors
C76-C80	Malignant neoplasms of ill-defined, other secondary and unspecified sites
C81-C96	Malignant neoplasms of lymphoid, hematopoietic and related tissue
D00-D09	In situ neoplasms
D10-D36	Benign neoplasms, except benign neuroendocrine tumors
D3A	Benign neuroendocrine tumors
D37-D48	Neoplasms of uncertain behavior, polycythemia vera and myelodysplastic syndromes
D49	Neoplasms of unspecified behavior

MALIGNANT NEOPLASMS(C00-C96)

Malignant neoplasms, stated or presumed to be primary (of specified sites), and certain specified histologies, except neuroendocrine, and of lymphoid, hematopoietic and related tissue (C00-C75)

Malignant neoplasms of lip, oral cavity and pharynx (C00-C14)

✓4th **C00 Malignant neoplasm of lip**

Use additional code to identify:
- alcohol abuse and dependence (F10.-)
- history of tobacco dependence (Z87.891)
- tobacco dependence (F17.-)
- tobacco use (Z72.0)

EXCLUDES 1 *malignant melanoma of lip (C43.0)*
Merkel cell carcinoma of lip (C4A.0)
other and unspecified malignant neoplasm of skin of lip (C44.0-)

C00.0 Malignant neoplasm of external upper lip
Malignant neoplasm of lipstick area of upper lip
Malignant neoplasm of upper lip NOS
Malignant neoplasm of vermilion border of upper lip

C00.1 Malignant neoplasm of external lower lip
Malignant neoplasm of lower lip NOS
Malignant neoplasm of lipstick area of lower lip
Malignant neoplasm of vermilion border of lower lip

C00.2 Malignant neoplasm of external lip, unspecified
Malignant neoplasm of vermilion border of lip NOS

C00.3 Malignant neoplasm of upper lip, inner aspect
Malignant neoplasm of buccal aspect of upper lip
Malignant neoplasm of frenulum of upper lip
Malignant neoplasm of mucosa of upper lip
Malignant neoplasm of oral aspect of upper lip

C00.4 Malignant neoplasm of lower lip, inner aspect
Malignant neoplasm of buccal aspect of lower lip
Malignant neoplasm of frenulum of lower lip
Malignant neoplasm of mucosa of lower lip
Malignant neoplasm of oral aspect of lower lip

C00.5 Malignant neoplasm of lip, unspecified, inner aspect
Malignant neoplasm of buccal aspect of lip, unspecified
Malignant neoplasm of frenulum of lip, unspecified
Malignant neoplasm of mucosa of lip, unspecified
Malignant neoplasm of oral aspect of lip, unspecified

C00.6 Malignant neoplasm of commissure of lip, unspecified

C00.8 Malignant neoplasm of overlapping sites of lip

C00.9 Malignant neoplasm of lip, unspecified

C01 Malignant neoplasm of base of tongue HCC

Malignant neoplasm of dorsal surface of base of tongue
Malignant neoplasm of fixed part of tongue NOS
Malignant neoplasm of posterior third of tongue

Use additional code to identify:
- alcohol abuse and dependence (F10.-)
- history of tobacco dependence (Z87.891)
- tobacco dependence (F17.-)
- tobacco use (Z72.0)

Malignant Neoplasm of Tongue

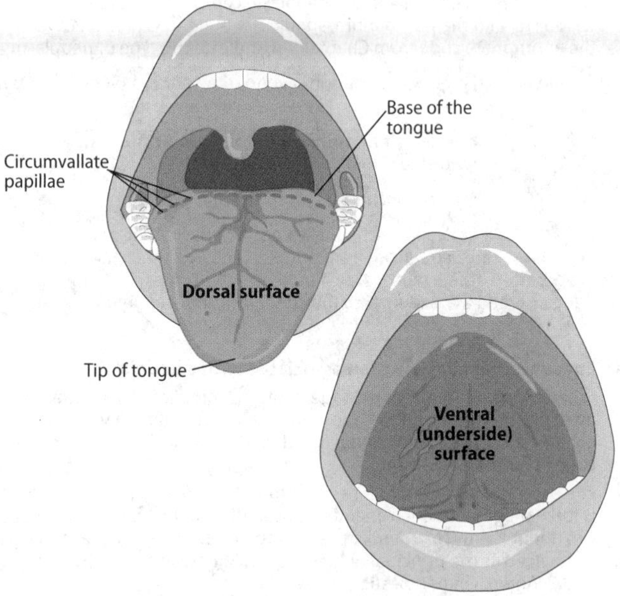

✓4th **C02 Malignant neoplasm of other and unspecified parts of tongue**

Use additional code to identify:
- alcohol abuse and dependence (F10.-)
- history of tobacco dependence (Z87.891)
- tobacco dependence (F17.-)
- tobacco use (Z72.0)

C02.0 Malignant neoplasm of dorsal surface of tongue HCC
Malignant neoplasm of anterior two-thirds of tongue, dorsal surface
EXCLUDES 2 *malignant neoplasm of dorsal surface of base of tongue (C01)*

C02.1 Malignant neoplasm of border of tongue HCC
Malignant neoplasm of tip of tongue

C02.2 Malignant neoplasm of ventral surface of tongue HCC
Malignant neoplasm of anterior two-thirds of tongue, ventral surface
Malignant neoplasm of frenulum linguae

C02.3 Malignant neoplasm of anterior two-thirds of tongue, part unspecified HCC
Malignant neoplasm of middle third of tongue NOS
Malignant neoplasm of mobile part of tongue NOS

CØ2.4 Malignant neoplasm of lingual tonsil HCC
EXCLUDES 2 *malignant neoplasm of tonsil NOS (CØ9.9)*

CØ2.8 Malignant neoplasm of overlapping sites of tongue HCC
Malignant neoplasm of two or more contiguous sites of tongue

CØ2.9 Malignant neoplasm of tongue, unspecified HCC

✓4th **CØ3 Malignant neoplasm of gum**
INCLUDES malignant neoplasm of alveolar (ridge) mucosa
malignant neoplasm of gingiva
Use additional code to identify:
alcohol abuse and dependence (F1Ø.-)
history of tobacco dependence (Z87.891)
tobacco dependence (F17.-)
tobacco use (Z72.Ø)
EXCLUDES 2 *malignant odontogenic neoplasms (C41.Ø-C41.1)*

CØ3.Ø Malignant neoplasm of upper gum HCC

CØ3.1 Malignant neoplasm of lower gum HCC

CØ3.9 Malignant neoplasm of gum, unspecified HCC

✓4th **CØ4 Malignant neoplasm of floor of mouth**
Use additional code to identify:
alcohol abuse and dependence (F1Ø.-)
history of tobacco dependence (Z87.891)
tobacco dependence (F17.-)
tobacco use (Z72.Ø)

CØ4.Ø Malignant neoplasm of anterior floor of mouth HCC
Malignant neoplasm of anterior to the premolar-canine junction

CØ4.1 Malignant neoplasm of lateral floor of mouth HCC

CØ4.8 Malignant neoplasm of overlapping sites of floor of mouth HCC

CØ4.9 Malignant neoplasm of floor of mouth, unspecified HCC

✓4th **CØ5 Malignant neoplasm of palate**
Use additional code to identify:
alcohol abuse and dependence (F1Ø.-)
history of tobacco dependence (Z87.891)
tobacco dependence (F17.-)
tobacco use (Z72.Ø)
EXCLUDES 1 *Kaposi's sarcoma of palate (C46.2)*

CØ5.Ø Malignant neoplasm of hard palate HCC

CØ5.1 Malignant neoplasm of soft palate HCC
EXCLUDES 2 *malignant neoplasm of nasopharyngeal surface of soft palate (C11.3)*

CØ5.2 Malignant neoplasm of uvula HCC

CØ5.8 Malignant neoplasm of overlapping sites of palate HCC

CØ5.9 Malignant neoplasm of palate, unspecified HCC
Malignant neoplasm of roof of mouth

✓4th **CØ6 Malignant neoplasm of other and unspecified parts of mouth**
Use additional code to identify:
alcohol abuse and dependence (F1Ø.-)
history of tobacco dependence (Z87.891)
tobacco dependence (F17.-)
tobacco use (Z72.Ø)

CØ6.Ø Malignant neoplasm of cheek mucosa HCC
Malignant neoplasm of buccal mucosa NOS
Malignant neoplasm of internal cheek

CØ6.1 Malignant neoplasm of vestibule of mouth HCC
Malignant neoplasm of buccal sulcus (upper) (lower)
Malignant neoplasm of labial sulcus (upper) (lower)

CØ6.2 Malignant neoplasm of retromolar area HCC

✓5th **CØ6.8 Malignant neoplasm of overlapping sites of other and unspecified parts of mouth**

CØ6.8Ø Malignant neoplasm of overlapping sites of unspecified parts of mouth HCC

CØ6.89 Malignant neoplasm of overlapping sites of other parts of mouth HCC
"book leaf" neoplasm [ventral surface of tongue and floor of mouth]

CØ6.9 Malignant neoplasm of mouth, unspecified HCC
Malignant neoplasm of minor salivary gland, unspecified site
Malignant neoplasm of oral cavity NOS

CØ7 Malignant neoplasm of parotid gland HCC
Use additional code to identify:
alcohol abuse and dependence (F1Ø.-)
exposure to environmental tobacco smoke (Z77.22)
exposure to tobacco smoke in the perinatal period (P96.81)
history of tobacco dependence (Z87.891)
occupational exposure to environmental tobacco smoke (Z57.31)
tobacco dependence (F17.-)
tobacco use (Z72.Ø)

✓4th **CØ8 Malignant neoplasm of other and unspecified major salivary glands**
INCLUDES malignant neoplasm of salivary ducts
Use additional code to identify:
alcohol abuse and dependence (F1Ø.-)
exposure to environmental tobacco smoke (Z77.22)
exposure to tobacco smoke in the perinatal period (P96.81)
history of tobacco dependence (Z87.891)
occupational exposure to environmental tobacco smoke (Z57.31)
tobacco dependence (F17.-)
tobacco use (Z72.Ø)
EXCLUDES 1 *malignant neoplasms of specified minor salivary glands which are classified according to their anatomical location*
EXCLUDES 2 *malignant neoplasms of minor salivary glands NOS (CØ6.9)*
malignant neoplasm of parotid gland (CØ7)

CØ8.Ø Malignant neoplasm of submandibular gland HCC
Malignant neoplasm of submaxillary gland

CØ8.1 Malignant neoplasm of sublingual gland HCC

CØ8.9 Malignant neoplasm of major salivary gland, unspecified HCC
Malignant neoplasm of salivary gland (major) NOS

✓4th **CØ9 Malignant neoplasm of tonsil**
Use additional code to identify:
alcohol abuse and dependence (F1Ø.-)
exposure to environmental tobacco smoke (Z77.22)
exposure to tobacco smoke in the perinatal period (P96.81)
history of tobacco dependence (Z87.891)
occupational exposure to environmental tobacco smoke (Z57.31)
tobacco dependence (F17.-)
tobacco use (Z72.Ø)
EXCLUDES 2 *malignant neoplasm of lingual tonsil (CØ2.4)*
malignant neoplasm of pharyngeal tonsil (C11.1)

CØ9.Ø Malignant neoplasm of tonsillar fossa HCC

CØ9.1 Malignant neoplasm of tonsillar pillar (anterior) (posterior) HCC

CØ9.8 Malignant neoplasm of overlapping sites of tonsil HCC

CØ9.9 Malignant neoplasm of tonsil, unspecified HCC
Malignant neoplasm of tonsil NOS
Malignant neoplasm of faucial tonsils
Malignant neoplasm of palatine tonsils

✓4th **C1Ø Malignant neoplasm of oropharynx**
Use additional code to identify:
alcohol abuse and dependence (F1Ø.-)
exposure to environmental tobacco smoke (Z77.22)
exposure to tobacco smoke in the perinatal period (P96.81)
history of tobacco dependence (Z87.891)
occupational exposure to environmental tobacco smoke (Z57.31)
tobacco dependence (F17.-)
tobacco use (Z72.Ø)
EXCLUDES 2 *malignant neoplasm of tonsil (CØ9.-)*
DEF: Oropharynx: Middle portion of pharynx (throat); communicates with the oral cavity, nasopharynx and laryngopharynx.

C1Ø.Ø Malignant neoplasm of vallecula HCC

C1Ø.1 Malignant neoplasm of anterior surface of epiglottis HCC
Malignant neoplasm of epiglottis, free border [margin]
Malignant neoplasm of glossoepiglottic fold(s)
EXCLUDES 2 *malignant neoplasm of epiglottis (suprahyoid portion) NOS (C32.1)*

C1Ø.2 Malignant neoplasm of lateral wall of oropharynx HCC

C1Ø.3 Malignant neoplasm of posterior wall of oropharynx HCC

C1Ø.4 Malignant neoplasm of branchial cleft HCC
Malignant neoplasm of branchial cyst [site of neoplasm]

C1Ø.8 Malignant neoplasm of overlapping sites of oropharynx HCC
Malignant neoplasm of junctional region of oropharynx

C1Ø.9 Malignant neoplasm of oropharynx, unspecified HCC

C11 Malignant neoplasm of nasopharynx

Use additional code to identify:
- exposure to environmental tobacco smoke (Z77.22)
- exposure to tobacco smoke in the perinatal period (P96.81)
- history of tobacco dependence (Z87.891)
- occupational exposure to environmental tobacco smoke (Z57.31)
- tobacco dependence (F17.-)
- tobacco use (Z72.Ø)

DEF: Nasopharynx: Upper portion of pharynx (throat); communicates with the nasal cavities, oropharynx and tympanic cavities.

C11.Ø Malignant neoplasm of superior wall of nasopharynx HCC
Malignant neoplasm of roof of nasopharynx

C11.1 Malignant neoplasm of posterior wall of nasopharynx HCC
Malignant neoplasm of adenoid
Malignant neoplasm of pharyngeal tonsil

C11.2 Malignant neoplasm of lateral wall of nasopharynx HCC
Malignant neoplasm of fossa of Rosenmüller
Malignant neoplasm of opening of auditory tube
Malignant neoplasm of pharyngeal recess

C11.3 Malignant neoplasm of anterior wall of nasopharynx HCC
Malignant neoplasm of floor of nasopharynx
Malignant neoplasm of nasopharyngeal (anterior) (posterior) surface of soft palate
Malignant neoplasm of posterior margin of nasal choana
Malignant neoplasm of posterior margin of nasal septum

C11.8 Malignant neoplasm of overlapping sites of nasopharynx HCC

C11.9 Malignant neoplasm of nasopharynx, unspecified HCC
Malignant neoplasm of nasopharyngeal wall NOS

C12 Malignant neoplasm of pyriform sinus HCC

Malignant neoplasm of pyriform fossa

Use additional code to identify:
- exposure to environmental tobacco smoke (Z77.22)
- exposure to tobacco smoke in the perinatal period (P96.81)
- history of tobacco dependence (Z87.891)
- occupational exposure to environmental tobacco smoke (Z57.31)
- tobacco dependence (F17.-)
- tobacco use (Z72.Ø)

C13 Malignant neoplasm of hypopharynx

Use additional code to identify:
- exposure to environmental tobacco smoke (Z77.22)
- exposure to tobacco smoke in the perinatal period (P96.81)
- history of tobacco dependence (Z87.891)
- occupational exposure to environmental tobacco smoke (Z57.31)
- tobacco dependence (F17.-)
- tobacco use (Z72.Ø)

EXCLUDES 2 *malignant neoplasm of pyriform sinus (C12)*

DEF: Hypopharynx: Lower portion of pharynx (throat); communicates with the oropharynx and the esophagus. ***Synonyms:*** *laryngopharynx.*

C13.Ø Malignant neoplasm of postcricoid region HCC

C13.1 Malignant neoplasm of aryepiglottic fold, hypopharyngeal aspect HCC
Malignant neoplasm of aryepiglottic fold, marginal zone
Malignant neoplasm of aryepiglottic fold NOS
Malignant neoplasm of interarytenoid fold, marginal zone
Malignant neoplasm of interarytenoid fold NOS
EXCLUDES 2 *malignant neoplasm of aryepiglottic fold or interarytenoid fold, laryngeal aspect (C32.1)*

C13.2 Malignant neoplasm of posterior wall of hypopharynx HCC

C13.8 Malignant neoplasm of overlapping sites of hypopharynx HCC

C13.9 Malignant neoplasm of hypopharynx, unspecified HCC
Malignant neoplasm of hypopharyngeal wall NOS

C14 Malignant neoplasm of other and ill-defined sites in the lip, oral cavity and pharynx

Use additional code to identify:
- alcohol abuse and dependence (F1Ø.-)
- exposure to environmental tobacco smoke (Z77.22)
- exposure to tobacco smoke in the perinatal period (P96.81)
- history of tobacco dependence (Z87.891)
- occupational exposure to environmental tobacco smoke (Z57.31)
- tobacco dependence (F17.-)
- tobacco use (Z72.Ø)

EXCLUDES 1 *malignant neoplasm of oral cavity NOS (CØ6.9)*

C14.Ø Malignant neoplasm of pharynx, unspecified HCC

C14.2 Malignant neoplasm of Waldeyer's ring HCC
DEF: Waldeyer's ring: Ring of lymphoid tissue that is made up of the two palatine tonsils, the pharyngeal tonsil (adenoid), and the lingual tonsil. It functions as the defense against infection and assists with the development of the immune system.

C14.8 Malignant neoplasm of overlapping sites of lip, oral cavity and pharynx HCC
Primary malignant neoplasm of two or more contiguous sites of lip, oral cavity and pharynx
EXCLUDES 1 *"book leaf" neoplasm [ventral surface of tongue and floor of mouth] (CØ6.89)*

Malignant neoplasms of digestive organs (C15-C26)

EXCLUDES 1 *Kaposi's sarcoma of gastrointestinal sites (C46.4)*
EXCLUDES 2 *gastrointestinal stromal tumors (C49.A-)*

C15 Malignant neoplasm of esophagus

Use additional code to identify:
- alcohol abuse and dependence (F1Ø.-)

C15.3 Malignant neoplasm of upper third of esophagus CC HCC

C15.4 Malignant neoplasm of middle third of esophagus CC HCC

C15.5 Malignant neoplasm of lower third of esophagus CC HCC
EXCLUDES 1 *malignant neoplasm of cardio-esophageal junction (C16.Ø)*

C15.8 Malignant neoplasm of overlapping sites of esophagus CC HCC

C15.9 Malignant neoplasm of esophagus, unspecified CC HCC

C16 Malignant neoplasm of stomach

Use additional code to identify:
- alcohol abuse and dependence (F1Ø.-)

EXCLUDES 2 *malignant carcinoid tumor of the stomach (C7A.Ø92)*

C16.Ø Malignant neoplasm of cardia CC HCC
Malignant neoplasm of cardiac orifice
Malignant neoplasm of cardio-esophageal junction
Malignant neoplasm of esophagus and stomach
Malignant neoplasm of gastro-esophageal junction

C16.1 Malignant neoplasm of fundus of stomach CC HCC

C16.2 Malignant neoplasm of body of stomach CC HCC

C16.3 Malignant neoplasm of pyloric antrum CC HCC
Malignant neoplasm of gastric antrum

C16.4 Malignant neoplasm of pylorus CC HCC
Malignant neoplasm of prepylorus
Malignant neoplasm of pyloric canal

C16.5 Malignant neoplasm of lesser curvature of stomach, unspecified CC HCC
Malignant neoplasm of lesser curvature of stomach, not classifiable to C16.1-C16.4

C16.6 Malignant neoplasm of greater curvature of stomach, unspecified CC HCC
Malignant neoplasm of greater curvature of stomach, not classifiable to C16.Ø-C16.4

C16.8 Malignant neoplasm of overlapping sites of stomach CC HCC

C16.9 Malignant neoplasm of stomach, unspecified CC HCC
Gastric cancer NOS

C17 Malignant neoplasm of small intestine

EXCLUDES 1 *malignant carcinoid tumors of the small intestine (C7A.Ø1)*

AHA: 2016,1Q,19

C17.Ø Malignant neoplasm of duodenum CC HCC

C17.1 Malignant neoplasm of jejunum CC HCC

C17.2 Malignant neoplasm of ileum CC HCC
EXCLUDES 1 *malignant neoplasm of ileocecal valve (C18.Ø)*

C17.3 Meckel's diverticulum, malignant CC HCC
EXCLUDES 1 *Meckel's diverticulum, congenital (Q43.Ø)*
DEF: Congenital, abnormal remnant of embryonic digestive system development that leaves a sacculation or outpouching from the wall of the small intestine near the terminal part of the ileum made of acid-secreting tissue as in the stomach.

C17.8 Malignant neoplasm of overlapping sites of small intestine CC HCC

C17.9 Malignant neoplasm of small intestine, unspecified CC HCC

✓4th C18 Malignant neoplasm of colon

EXCLUDES 1 *malignant carcinoid tumors of the colon (C7A.Ø2-)*

Colon

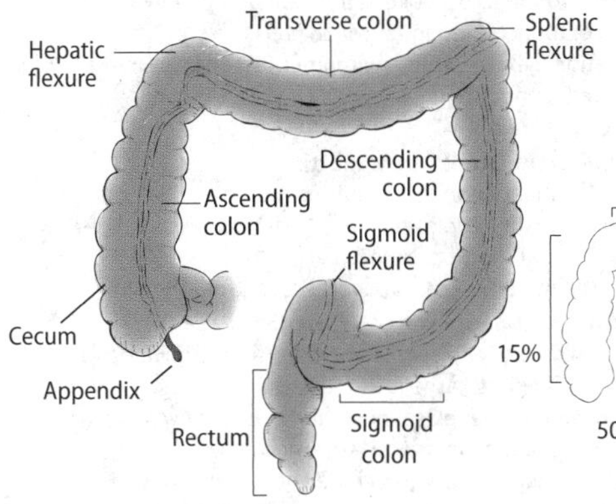

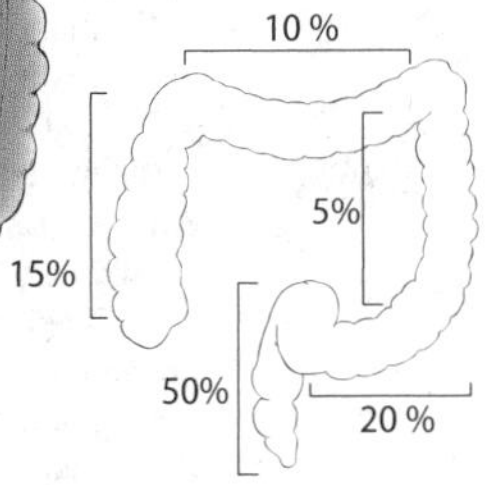

Anatomical distribution of large bowel cancers

C18.Ø Malignant neoplasm of cecum CC HCC
Malignant neoplasm of ileocecal valve

C18.1 Malignant neoplasm of appendix CC HCC

C18.2 Malignant neoplasm of ascending colon CC HCC

C18.3 Malignant neoplasm of hepatic flexure CC HCC

C18.4 Malignant neoplasm of transverse colon CC HCC

C18.5 Malignant neoplasm of splenic flexure CC HCC

C18.6 Malignant neoplasm of descending colon CC HCC

C18.7 Malignant neoplasm of sigmoid colon CC HCC
Malignant neoplasm of sigmoid (flexure)
EXCLUDES 1 *malignant neoplasm of rectosigmoid junction (C19)*

C18.8 Malignant neoplasm of overlapping sites of colon CC HCC

C18.9 Malignant neoplasm of colon, unspecified CC HCC
Malignant neoplasm of large intestine NOS

C19 Malignant neoplasm of rectosigmoid junction CC HCC
Malignant neoplasm of colon with rectum
Malignant neoplasm of rectosigmoid (colon)
EXCLUDES 1 *malignant carcinoid tumors of the colon (C7A.Ø2-)*

C2Ø Malignant neoplasm of rectum CC HCC
Malignant neoplasm of rectal ampulla
EXCLUDES 1 *malignant carcinoid tumor of the rectum (C7A.Ø26)*

✓4th C21 Malignant neoplasm of anus and anal canal

EXCLUDES 2 *malignant carcinoid tumors of the colon (C7A.Ø2-)*
malignant melanoma of anal margin (C43.51)
malignant melanoma of anal skin (C43.51)
malignant melanoma of perianal skin (C43.51)
other and unspecified malignant neoplasm of anal margin (C44.5ØØ, C44.51Ø, C44.52Ø, C44.59Ø)
other and unspecified malignant neoplasm of anal skin (C44.5ØØ, C44.51Ø, C44.52Ø, C44.59Ø)
other and unspecified malignant neoplasm of perianal skin (C44.5ØØ, C44.51Ø, C44.52Ø, C44.59Ø)

C21.Ø Malignant neoplasm of anus, unspecified CC HCC

C21.1 Malignant neoplasm of anal canal CC HCC
Malignant neoplasm of anal sphincter

C21.2 Malignant neoplasm of cloacogenic zone CC HCC

C21.8 Malignant neoplasm of overlapping sites of rectum, anus and anal canal CC HCC
Malignant neoplasm of anorectal junction
Malignant neoplasm of anorectum
Primary malignant neoplasm of two or more contiguous sites of rectum, anus and anal canal

✓4th C22 Malignant neoplasm of liver and intrahepatic bile ducts

EXCLUDES 1 *malignant neoplasm of biliary tract NOS (C24.9)*
secondary malignant neoplasm of liver and intrahepatic bile duct (C78.7)

Use additional code to identify:
alcohol abuse and dependence (F1Ø.-)
hepatitis B (B16.-, B18.Ø-B18.1)
hepatitis C (B17.1-, B18.2)

C22.Ø Liver cell carcinoma CC HCC
Hepatocellular carcinoma
Hepatoma
AHA: 2016,1Q,18

C22.1 Intrahepatic bile duct carcinoma CC HCC
Cholangiocarcinoma
EXCLUDES 1 *malignant neoplasm of hepatic duct (C24.Ø)*

C22.2 Hepatoblastoma CC HCC

C22.3 Angiosarcoma of liver CC HCC
Kupffer cell sarcoma

C22.4 Other sarcomas of liver CC HCC

C22.7 Other specified carcinomas of liver CC HCC

C22.8 Malignant neoplasm of liver, primary, unspecified as to type CC HCC

C22.9 Malignant neoplasm of liver, not specified as primary or secondary CC HCC

C23 Malignant neoplasm of gallbladder CC HCC

✓4th C24 Malignant neoplasm of other and unspecified parts of biliary tract

EXCLUDES 1 *malignant neoplasm of intrahepatic bile duct (C22.1)*

C24.Ø Malignant neoplasm of extrahepatic bile duct CC HCC
Malignant neoplasm of biliary duct or passage NOS
Malignant neoplasm of common bile duct
Malignant neoplasm of cystic duct
Malignant neoplasm of hepatic duct

C24.1 Malignant neoplasm of ampulla of Vater CC HCC
DEF: Malignant neoplasm in the area of dilation at the juncture of the common bile and pancreatic ducts near the opening into the lumen of the duodenum.

C24.8 Malignant neoplasm of overlapping sites of biliary tract CC HCC
Malignant neoplasm involving both intrahepatic and extrahepatic bile ducts
Primary malignant neoplasm of two or more contiguous sites of biliary tract

C24.9 Malignant neoplasm of biliary tract, unspecified CC HCC

✓4th C25 Malignant neoplasm of pancreas

Code also exocrine pancreatic insufficiency (K86.81)
Use additional code to identify:
alcohol abuse and dependence (F1Ø.-)

Pancreas

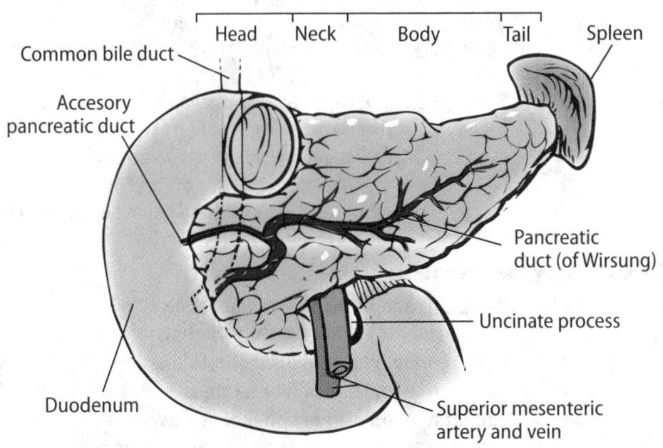

C25.Ø Malignant neoplasm of head of pancreas CC HCC

C25.1 Malignant neoplasm of body of pancreas CC HCC

C25.2 Malignant neoplasm of tail of pancreas CC HCC

C25.3 Malignant neoplasm of pancreatic duct CC HCC

C25.4 Malignant neoplasm of endocrine pancreas CC HCC
Malignant neoplasm of islets of Langerhans
Use additional code to identify any functional activity

C25.7 Malignant neoplasm of other parts of pancreas CC HCC
Malignant neoplasm of neck of pancreas

C25.8 Malignant neoplasm of overlapping sites of pancreas CC HCC

C25.9 Malignant neoplasm of pancreas, unspecified CC HCC

✓4th **C26 Malignant neoplasm of other and ill-defined digestive organs**
EXCLUDES 1 *malignant neoplasm of peritoneum and retroperitoneum (C48.-)*

C26.Ø Malignant neoplasm of intestinal tract, part unspecified HCC
Malignant neoplasm of intestine NOS

C26.1 Malignant neoplasm of spleen HCC
EXCLUDES 1 *Hodgkin lymphoma (C81.-)*
non-Hodgkin lymphoma (C82-C85)

C26.9 Malignant neoplasm of ill-defined sites within the digestive system HCC
Malignant neoplasm of alimentary canal or tract NOS
Malignant neoplasm of gastrointestinal tract NOS
EXCLUDES 1 *malignant neoplasm of abdominal NOS (C76.2)*
malignant neoplasm of intra-abdominal NOS (C76.2)

Malignant neoplasms of respiratory and intrathoracic organs (C3Ø-C39)

INCLUDES malignant neoplasm of middle ear
EXCLUDES 1 *mesothelioma (C45.-)*

✓4th **C3Ø Malignant neoplasm of nasal cavity and middle ear**

C3Ø.Ø Malignant neoplasm of nasal cavity HCC
Malignant neoplasm of cartilage of nose
Malignant neoplasm of nasal concha
Malignant neoplasm of internal nose
Malignant neoplasm of septum of nose
Malignant neoplasm of vestibule of nose
EXCLUDES 1 *malignant neoplasm of nasal bone (C41.Ø)*
malignant neoplasm of nose NOS (C76.Ø)
malignant neoplasm of olfactory bulb (C72.2-)
malignant neoplasm of posterior margin of nasal septum and choana (C11.3)
malignant melanoma of skin of nose (C43.31)
malignant neoplasm of turbinates (C41.Ø)
other and unspecified malignant neoplasm of skin of nose (C44.3Ø1, C44.311, C44.321, C44.391)

C3Ø.1 Malignant neoplasm of middle ear HCC
Malignant neoplasm of antrum tympanicum
Malignant neoplasm of auditory tube
Malignant neoplasm of eustachian tube
Malignant neoplasm of inner ear
Malignant neoplasm of mastoid air cells
Malignant neoplasm of tympanic cavity
EXCLUDES 1 *malignant neoplasm of auricular canal (external) (C43.2-,C44.2-)*
malignant neoplasm of bone of ear (meatus) (C41.Ø)
malignant neoplasm of cartilage of ear (C49.Ø)
malignant melanoma of skin of (external) ear (C43.2-)
other and unspecified malignant neoplasm of skin of (external) ear (C44.2-)

✓4th **C31 Malignant neoplasm of accessory sinuses**

C31.Ø Malignant neoplasm of maxillary sinus HCC
Malignant neoplasm of antrum (Highmore) (maxillary)

C31.1 Malignant neoplasm of ethmoidal sinus HCC

C31.2 Malignant neoplasm of frontal sinus HCC

C31.3 Malignant neoplasm of sphenoid sinus HCC

C31.8 Malignant neoplasm of overlapping sites of accessory sinuses HCC

C31.9 Malignant neoplasm of accessory sinus, unspecified HCC

✓4th **C32 Malignant neoplasm of larynx**
Use additional code to identify:
alcohol abuse and dependence (F1Ø.-)
exposure to environmental tobacco smoke (Z77.22)
exposure to tobacco smoke in the perinatal period (P96.81)
history of tobacco dependence (Z87.891)
occupational exposure to environmental tobacco smoke (Z57.31)
tobacco dependence (F17.-)
tobacco use (Z72.Ø)

C32.Ø Malignant neoplasm of glottis HCC
Malignant neoplasm of intrinsic larynx
Malignant neoplasm of laryngeal commissure (anterior)(posterior)
Malignant neoplasm of vocal cord (true) NOS

C32.1 Malignant neoplasm of supraglottis HCC
Malignant neoplasm of aryepiglottic fold or interarytenoid fold, laryngeal aspect
Malignant neoplasm of epiglottis (suprahyoid portion) NOS
Malignant neoplasm of extrinsic larynx
Malignant neoplasm of false vocal cord
Malignant neoplasm of posterior (laryngeal) surface of epiglottis
Malignant neoplasm of ventricular bands
EXCLUDES 2 *malignant neoplasm of anterior surface of epiglottis (C1Ø.1)*
malignant neoplasm of aryepiglottic fold or interarytenoid fold, hypopharyngeal aspect (C13.1)
malignant neoplasm of aryepiglottic fold or interarytenoid fold, marginal zone (C13.1)
malignant neoplasm of aryepiglottic fold or interarytenoid fold NOS (C13.1)

C32.2 Malignant neoplasm of subglottis HCC

C32.3 Malignant neoplasm of laryngeal cartilage HCC

C32.8 Malignant neoplasm of overlapping sites of larynx HCC

C32.9 Malignant neoplasm of larynx, unspecified HCC

C33 Malignant neoplasm of trachea CC HCC
Use additional code to identify:
exposure to environmental tobacco smoke (Z77.22)
exposure to tobacco smoke in the perinatal period (P96.81)
history of tobacco dependence (Z87.891)
occupational exposure to environmental tobacco smoke (Z57.31)
tobacco dependence (F17.-)
tobacco use (Z72.Ø)

✓4th **C34 Malignant neoplasm of bronchus and lung**
Use additional code to identify:
exposure to environmental tobacco smoke (Z77.22)
exposure to tobacco smoke in the perinatal period (P96.81)
history of tobacco dependence (Z87.891)
occupational exposure to environmental tobacco smoke (Z57.31)
tobacco dependence (F17.-)
tobacco use (Z72.Ø)
EXCLUDES 1 *Kaposi's sarcoma of lung (C46.5-)*
malignant carcinoid tumor of the bronchus and lung (C7A.Ø9Ø)

AHA: 2019,1Q,16

TIP: When documented, assign code I31.3 for associated malignant pericardial effusion. If the sole reason for admission is to treat the effusion with no treatment of the lung malignancy rendered, code I31.3 may be sequenced first.

✓5th **C34.Ø Malignant neoplasm of main bronchus**
Malignant neoplasm of carina
Malignant neoplasm of hilus (of lung)

C34.ØØ Malignant neoplasm of unspecified main bronchus CC HCC

C34.Ø1 Malignant neoplasm of right main bronchus CC HCC

C34.Ø2 Malignant neoplasm of left main bronchus CC HCC

✓5th **C34.1 Malignant neoplasm of upper lobe, bronchus or lung**

C34.1Ø Malignant neoplasm of upper lobe, unspecified bronchus or lung CC HCC

C34.11 Malignant neoplasm of upper lobe, right bronchus or lung CC HCC

C34.12 Malignant neoplasm of upper lobe, left bronchus or lung CC HCC

C34.2 Malignant neoplasm of middle lobe, bronchus or lung CC HCC

✓5th **C34.3 Malignant neoplasm of lower lobe, bronchus or lung**

C34.30 Malignant neoplasm of lower lobe, unspecified bronchus or lung CC HCC

C34.31 Malignant neoplasm of lower lobe, right bronchus or lung CC HCC

C34.32 Malignant neoplasm of lower lobe, left bronchus or lung CC HCC

✓5th **C34.8 Malignant neoplasm of overlapping sites of bronchus and lung**

C34.80 Malignant neoplasm of overlapping sites of unspecified bronchus and lung CC HCC

C34.81 Malignant neoplasm of overlapping sites of right bronchus and lung CC HCC

C34.82 Malignant neoplasm of overlapping sites of left bronchus and lung CC HCC

✓5th **C34.9 Malignant neoplasm of unspecified part of bronchus or lung**

C34.90 Malignant neoplasm of unspecified part of unspecified bronchus or lung CC HCC

Lung cancer NOS

C34.91 Malignant neoplasm of unspecified part of right bronchus or lung CC HCC

C34.92 Malignant neoplasm of unspecified part of left bronchus or lung CC HCC

C37 Malignant neoplasm of thymus CC HCC

EXCLUDES 1 *malignant carcinoid tumor of the thymus (C7A.Ø91)*

✓4th **C38 Malignant neoplasm of heart, mediastinum and pleura**

EXCLUDES 1 *mesothelioma (C45.-)*

C38.Ø Malignant neoplasm of heart CC HCC

Malignant neoplasm of pericardium

EXCLUDES 1 *malignant neoplasm of great vessels (C49.3)*

C38.1 Malignant neoplasm of anterior mediastinum CC HCC

C38.2 Malignant neoplasm of posterior mediastinum CC HCC

C38.3 Malignant neoplasm of mediastinum, part unspecified CC HCC

C38.4 Malignant neoplasm of pleura CC HCC

C38.8 Malignant neoplasm of overlapping sites of heart, mediastinum and pleura CC HCC

✓4th **C39 Malignant neoplasm of other and ill-defined sites in the respiratory system and intrathoracic organs**

Use additional code to identify:
- exposure to environmental tobacco smoke (Z77.22)
- exposure to tobacco smoke in the perinatal period (P96.81)
- history of tobacco dependence (Z87.891)
- occupational exposure to environmental tobacco smoke (Z57.31)
- tobacco dependence (F17.-)
- tobacco use (Z72.Ø)

EXCLUDES 1 *intrathoracic malignant neoplasm NOS (C76.1)*
thoracic malignant neoplasm NOS (C76.1)

C39.Ø Malignant neoplasm of upper respiratory tract, part unspecified HCC

C39.9 Malignant neoplasm of lower respiratory tract, part unspecified HCC

Malignant neoplasm of respiratory tract NOS

Malignant neoplasms of bone and articular cartilage (C4Ø-C41)

INCLUDES malignant neoplasm of cartilage (articular) (joint)
malignant neoplasm of periosteum

EXCLUDES 1 *malignant neoplasm of bone marrow NOS (C96.9)*
malignant neoplasm of synovia (C49.-)

✓4th **C4Ø Malignant neoplasm of bone and articular cartilage of limbs**

Use additional code to identify major osseous defect, if applicable (M89.7-)

✓5th **C4Ø.Ø Malignant neoplasm of scapula and long bones of upper limb**

C4Ø.ØØ Malignant neoplasm of scapula and long bones of unspecified upper limb CC HCC

C4Ø.Ø1 Malignant neoplasm of scapula and long bones of right upper limb CC HCC

C4Ø.Ø2 Malignant neoplasm of scapula and long bones of left upper limb CC HCC

✓5th **C4Ø.1 Malignant neoplasm of short bones of upper limb**

C4Ø.1Ø Malignant neoplasm of short bones of unspecified upper limb CC HCC

C4Ø.11 Malignant neoplasm of short bones of right upper limb CC HCC

C4Ø.12 Malignant neoplasm of short bones of left upper limb CC HCC

✓5th **C4Ø.2 Malignant neoplasm of long bones of lower limb**

C4Ø.2Ø Malignant neoplasm of long bones of unspecified lower limb CC HCC

C4Ø.21 Malignant neoplasm of long bones of right lower limb CC HCC

C4Ø.22 Malignant neoplasm of long bones of left lower limb CC HCC

✓5th **C4Ø.3 Malignant neoplasm of short bones of lower limb**

C4Ø.3Ø Malignant neoplasm of short bones of unspecified lower limb CC HCC

C4Ø.31 Malignant neoplasm of short bones of right lower limb CC HCC

C4Ø.32 Malignant neoplasm of short bones of left lower limb CC HCC

✓5th **C4Ø.8 Malignant neoplasm of overlapping sites of bone and articular cartilage of limb**

C4Ø.8Ø Malignant neoplasm of overlapping sites of bone and articular cartilage of unspecified limb CC HCC

C4Ø.81 Malignant neoplasm of overlapping sites of bone and articular cartilage of right limb CC HCC

C4Ø.82 Malignant neoplasm of overlapping sites of bone and articular cartilage of left limb CC HCC

✓5th **C4Ø.9 Malignant neoplasm of unspecified bones and articular cartilage of limb**

C4Ø.9Ø Malignant neoplasm of unspecified bones and articular cartilage of unspecified limb CC HCC

C4Ø.91 Malignant neoplasm of unspecified bones and articular cartilage of right limb CC HCC

C4Ø.92 Malignant neoplasm of unspecified bones and articular cartilage of left limb CC HCC

✓4th **C41 Malignant neoplasm of bone and articular cartilage of other and unspecified sites**

EXCLUDES 1 *malignant neoplasm of bones of limbs (C4Ø.-)*
malignant neoplasm of cartilage of ear (C49.Ø)
malignant neoplasm of cartilage of eyelid (C49.Ø)
malignant neoplasm of cartilage of larynx (C32.3)
malignant neoplasm of cartilage of limbs (C4Ø.-)
malignant neoplasm of cartilage of nose (C3Ø.Ø)

C41.Ø Malignant neoplasm of bones of skull and face CC HCC

Malignant neoplasm of maxilla (superior)
Malignant neoplasm of orbital bone

EXCLUDES 2 *carcinoma, any type except intraosseous or odontogenic of:*
maxillary sinus (C31.Ø)
upper jaw (CØ3.Ø)
malignant neoplasm of jaw bone (lower) (C41.1)

C41.1 Malignant neoplasm of mandible CC HCC

Malignant neoplasm of inferior maxilla
Malignant neoplasm of lower jaw bone

EXCLUDES 2 *carcinoma, any type except intraosseous or odontogenic of:*
jaw NOS (CØ3.9)
lower (CØ3.1)
malignant neoplasm of upper jaw bone (C41.Ø)

C41.2 Malignant neoplasm of vertebral column CC HCC

EXCLUDES 1 *malignant neoplasm of sacrum and coccyx (C41.4)*

C41.3 Malignant neoplasm of ribs, sternum and clavicle CC HCC

C41.4 Malignant neoplasm of pelvic bones, sacrum and coccyx CC HCC

C41.9 Malignant neoplasm of bone and articular cartilage, unspecified CC HCC

Melanoma and other malignant neoplasms of skin (C43-C44)

✓4th **C43 Malignant melanoma of skin**

EXCLUDES 1 *melanoma in situ (DØ3.-)*

EXCLUDES 2 *malignant melanoma of skin of genital organs (C51-C52, C6Ø.-, C63.-)*
Merkel cell carcinoma (C4A.-)
sites other than skin - code to malignant neoplasm of the site

C43.Ø Malignant melanoma of lip HCC

EXCLUDES 1 *malignant neoplasm of vermilion border of lip (CØØ.Ø-CØØ.2)*

✓5th **C43.1 Malignant melanoma of eyelid, including canthus**
AHA: 2018,4Q,4
C43.10 Malignant melanoma of unspecified eyelid, including canthus HCC
✓6th **C43.11 Malignant melanoma of right eyelid, including canthus**
C43.111 Malignant melanoma of right upper eyelid, including canthus HCC
C43.112 Malignant melanoma of right lower eyelid, including canthus HCC
✓6th **C43.12 Malignant melanoma of left eyelid, including canthus**
C43.121 Malignant melanoma of left upper eyelid, including canthus HCC
C43.122 Malignant melanoma of left lower eyelid, including canthus HCC
✓5th **C43.2 Malignant melanoma of ear and external auricular canal**
C43.20 Malignant melanoma of unspecified ear and external auricular canal HCC
C43.21 Malignant melanoma of right ear and external auricular canal HCC
C43.22 Malignant melanoma of left ear and external auricular canal HCC
✓5th **C43.3 Malignant melanoma of other and unspecified parts of face**
C43.30 Malignant melanoma of unspecified part of face HCC
C43.31 Malignant melanoma of nose HCC
C43.39 Malignant melanoma of other parts of face HCC
C43.4 Malignant melanoma of scalp and neck HCC
✓5th **C43.5 Malignant melanoma of trunk**
EXCLUDES 2 *malignant neoplasm of anus NOS (C21.Ø)*
malignant neoplasm of scrotum (C63.2)
C43.51 Malignant melanoma of anal skin HCC
Malignant melanoma of anal margin
Malignant melanoma of perianal skin
C43.52 Malignant melanoma of skin of breast HCC
C43.59 Malignant melanoma of other part of trunk HCC
✓5th **C43.6 Malignant melanoma of upper limb, including shoulder**
C43.60 Malignant melanoma of unspecified upper limb, including shoulder HCC
C43.61 Malignant melanoma of right upper limb, including shoulder HCC
C43.62 Malignant melanoma of left upper limb, including shoulder HCC
✓5th **C43.7 Malignant melanoma of lower limb, including hip**
C43.70 Malignant melanoma of unspecified lower limb, including hip HCC
C43.71 Malignant melanoma of right lower limb, including hip HCC
C43.72 Malignant melanoma of left lower limb, including hip HCC
C43.8 Malignant melanoma of overlapping sites of skin HCC
C43.9 Malignant melanoma of skin, unspecified HCC
Malignant melanoma of unspecified site of skin
Melanoma (malignant) NOS

✓4th **C4A Merkel cell carcinoma**
DEF: Malignant cutaneous cancer predominantly found in elderly patients with sun exposure that usually presents as a flesh-colored or bluish-red lump typically seen on the neck, head, and face.
C4A.Ø Merkel cell carcinoma of lip HCC
EXCLUDES 1 *malignant neoplasm of vermilion border of lip (CØØ.Ø-CØØ.2)*
✓5th **C4A.1 Merkel cell carcinoma of eyelid, including canthus**
AHA: 2018,4Q,4
C4A.10 Merkel cell carcinoma of unspecified eyelid, including canthus HCC
✓6th **C4A.11 Merkel cell carcinoma of right eyelid, including canthus**
C4A.111 Merkel cell carcinoma of right upper eyelid, including canthus HCC
C4A.112 Merkel cell carcinoma of right lower eyelid, including canthus HCC
✓6th **C4A.12 Merkel cell carcinoma of left eyelid, including canthus**
C4A.121 Merkel cell carcinoma of left upper eyelid, including canthus HCC
C4A.122 Merkel cell carcinoma of left lower eyelid, including canthus HCC
✓5th **C4A.2 Merkel cell carcinoma of ear and external auricular canal**
C4A.20 Merkel cell carcinoma of unspecified ear and external auricular canal HCC
C4A.21 Merkel cell carcinoma of right ear and external auricular canal HCC
C4A.22 Merkel cell carcinoma of left ear and external auricular canal HCC
✓5th **C4A.3 Merkel cell carcinoma of other and unspecified parts of face**
C4A.30 Merkel cell carcinoma of unspecified part of face HCC
C4A.31 Merkel cell carcinoma of nose HCC
C4A.39 Merkel cell carcinoma of other parts of face HCC
C4A.4 Merkel cell carcinoma of scalp and neck HCC
✓5th **C4A.5 Merkel cell carcinoma of trunk**
EXCLUDES 2 *malignant neoplasm of anus NOS (C21.Ø)*
malignant neoplasm of scrotum (C63.2)
C4A.51 Merkel cell carcinoma of anal skin HCC
Merkel cell carcinoma of anal margin
Merkel cell carcinoma of perianal skin
C4A.52 Merkel cell carcinoma of skin of breast HCC
C4A.59 Merkel cell carcinoma of other part of trunk HCC
✓5th **C4A.6 Merkel cell carcinoma of upper limb, including shoulder**
C4A.60 Merkel cell carcinoma of unspecified upper limb, including shoulder HCC
C4A.61 Merkel cell carcinoma of right upper limb, including shoulder HCC
C4A.62 Merkel cell carcinoma of left upper limb, including shoulder HCC
✓5th **C4A.7 Merkel cell carcinoma of lower limb, including hip**
C4A.70 Merkel cell carcinoma of unspecified lower limb, including hip HCC
C4A.71 Merkel cell carcinoma of right lower limb, including hip HCC
C4A.72 Merkel cell carcinoma of left lower limb, including hip HCC
C4A.8 Merkel cell carcinoma of overlapping sites HCC
C4A.9 Merkel cell carcinoma, unspecified HCC
Merkel cell carcinoma of unspecified site
Merkel cell carcinoma NOS

✓4th **C44 Other and unspecified malignant neoplasm of skin**
INCLUDES malignant neoplasm of sebaceous glands
malignant neoplasm of sweat glands
EXCLUDES 1 *Kaposi's sarcoma of skin (C46.Ø)*
malignant melanoma of skin (C43.-)
malignant neoplasm of skin of genital organs (C51-C52, C6Ø.-, C63.2)
Merkel cell carcinoma (C4A.-)
DEF: Basal cell carcinoma: Abnormal growth of skin cells that arises from the deepest layer of the epidermis and may present as an open sore, red patches, pink growth, or scar. Typically caused by sun exposure, it is one of the most common forms of skin cancer.
DEF: Squamous cell carcinoma: Uncontrolled growth of abnormal skin cells that arises from the outer layers of the skin (epidermis) and may present as an open sore. It is characterized by a firm, red nodule, elevated growth with a central depression, or a flat sore with a scaly crust.
✓5th **C44.Ø Other and unspecified malignant neoplasm of skin of lip**
EXCLUDES 1 *malignant neoplasm of lip (CØØ.-)*
C44.ØØ Unspecified malignant neoplasm of skin of lip
C44.Ø1 Basal cell carcinoma of skin of lip
C44.Ø2 Squamous cell carcinoma of skin of lip
C44.Ø9 Other specified malignant neoplasm of skin of lip
✓5th **C44.1 Other and unspecified malignant neoplasm of skin of eyelid, including canthus**
EXCLUDES 1 *connective tissue of eyelid (C49.Ø)*
AHA: 2018,4Q,4
✓6th **C44.10 Unspecified malignant neoplasm of skin of eyelid, including canthus**
C44.101 Unspecified malignant neoplasm of skin of unspecified eyelid, including canthus
✓7th **C44.102 Unspecified malignant neoplasm of skin of right eyelid, including canthus**
C44.1021 Unspecified malignant neoplasm of skin of right upper eyelid, including canthus

C44.1022 Unspecified malignant neoplasm of skin of right lower eyelid, including canthus

C44.109 Unspecified malignant neoplasm of skin of left eyelid, including canthus
C44.1091 Unspecified malignant neoplasm of skin of left upper eyelid, including canthus
C44.1092 Unspecified malignant neoplasm of skin of left lower eyelid, including canthus

C44.11 Basal cell carcinoma of skin of eyelid, including canthus
C44.111 Basal cell carcinoma of skin of unspecified eyelid, including canthus
C44.112 Basal cell carcinoma of skin of right eyelid, including canthus
C44.1121 Basal cell carcinoma of skin of right upper eyelid, including canthus
C44.1122 Basal cell carcinoma of skin of right lower eyelid, including canthus
C44.119 Basal cell carcinoma of skin of left eyelid, including canthus
C44.1191 Basal cell carcinoma of skin of left upper eyelid, including canthus
C44.1192 Basal cell carcinoma of skin of left lower eyelid, including canthus

C44.12 Squamous cell carcinoma of skin of eyelid, including canthus
C44.121 Squamous cell carcinoma of skin of unspecified eyelid, including canthus
C44.122 Squamous cell carcinoma of skin of right eyelid, including canthus
C44.1221 Squamous cell carcinoma of skin of right upper eyelid, including canthus
C44.1222 Squamous cell carcinoma of skin of right lower eyelid, including canthus
C44.129 Squamous cell carcinoma of skin of left eyelid, including canthus
C44.1291 Squamous cell carcinoma of skin of left upper eyelid, including canthus
C44.1292 Squamous cell carcinoma of skin of left lower eyelid, including canthus

C44.13 Sebaceous cell carcinoma of skin of eyelid, including canthus
C44.131 Sebaceous cell carcinoma of skin of unspecified eyelid, including canthus
C44.132 Sebaceous cell carcinoma of skin of right eyelid, including canthus
C44.1321 Sebaceous cell carcinoma of skin of right upper eyelid, including canthus
C44.1322 Sebaceous cell carcinoma of skin of right lower eyelid, including canthus
C44.139 Sebaceous cell carcinoma of skin of left eyelid, including canthus
C44.1391 Sebaceous cell carcinoma of skin of left upper eyelid, including canthus
C44.1392 Sebaceous cell carcinoma of skin of left lower eyelid, including canthus

C44.19 Other specified malignant neoplasm of skin of eyelid, including canthus
C44.191 Other specified malignant neoplasm of skin of unspecified eyelid, including canthus
C44.192 Other specified malignant neoplasm of skin of right eyelid, including canthus
C44.1921 Other specified malignant neoplasm of skin of right upper eyelid, including canthus
C44.1922 Other specified malignant neoplasm of skin of right lower eyelid, including canthus
C44.199 Other specified malignant neoplasm of skin of left eyelid, including canthus
C44.1991 Other specified malignant neoplasm of skin of left upper eyelid, including canthus
C44.1992 Other specified malignant neoplasm of skin of left lower eyelid, including canthus

C44.2 Other and unspecified malignant neoplasm of skin of ear and external auricular canal

EXCLUDES 1 *connective tissue of ear (C49.0)*

C44.20 Unspecified malignant neoplasm of skin of ear and external auricular canal
C44.201 Unspecified malignant neoplasm of skin of unspecified ear and external auricular canal
C44.202 Unspecified malignant neoplasm of skin of right ear and external auricular canal
C44.209 Unspecified malignant neoplasm of skin of left ear and external auricular canal

C44.21 Basal cell carcinoma of skin of ear and external auricular canal
C44.211 Basal cell carcinoma of skin of unspecified ear and external auricular canal
C44.212 Basal cell carcinoma of skin of right ear and external auricular canal
C44.219 Basal cell carcinoma of skin of left ear and external auricular canal

C44.22 Squamous cell carcinoma of skin of ear and external auricular canal
C44.221 Squamous cell carcinoma of skin of unspecified ear and external auricular canal
C44.222 Squamous cell carcinoma of skin of right ear and external auricular canal
C44.229 Squamous cell carcinoma of skin of left ear and external auricular canal

C44.29 Other specified malignant neoplasm of skin of ear and external auricular canal
C44.291 Other specified malignant neoplasm of skin of unspecified ear and external auricular canal
C44.292 Other specified malignant neoplasm of skin of right ear and external auricular canal
C44.299 Other specified malignant neoplasm of skin of left ear and external auricular canal

C44.3 Other and unspecified malignant neoplasm of skin of other and unspecified parts of face

C44.30 Unspecified malignant neoplasm of skin of other and unspecified parts of face
C44.300 Unspecified malignant neoplasm of skin of unspecified part of face
C44.301 Unspecified malignant neoplasm of skin of nose
C44.309 Unspecified malignant neoplasm of skin of other parts of face

C44.31 Basal cell carcinoma of skin of other and unspecified parts of face
C44.310 Basal cell carcinoma of skin of unspecified parts of face
C44.311 Basal cell carcinoma of skin of nose
C44.319 Basal cell carcinoma of skin of other parts of face

C44.32 Squamous cell carcinoma of skin of other and unspecified parts of face
C44.320 Squamous cell carcinoma of skin of unspecified parts of face
C44.321 Squamous cell carcinoma of skin of nose
C44.329 Squamous cell carcinoma of skin of other parts of face

C44.39 Other specified malignant neoplasm of skin of other and unspecified parts of face
C44.390 Other specified malignant neoplasm of skin of unspecified parts of face
C44.391 Other specified malignant neoplasm of skin of nose
C44.399 Other specified malignant neoplasm of skin of other parts of face

5th **C44.4 Other and unspecified malignant neoplasm of skin of scalp and neck**
- **C44.40 Unspecified malignant neoplasm of skin of scalp and neck**
- **C44.41 Basal cell carcinoma of skin of scalp and neck**
- **C44.42 Squamous cell carcinoma of skin of scalp and neck**
- **C44.49 Other specified malignant neoplasm of skin of scalp and neck**

5th **C44.5 Other and unspecified malignant neoplasm of skin of trunk**
EXCLUDES 1 *anus NOS (C21.Ø)*
scrotum (C63.2)
- 6th **C44.5Ø Unspecified malignant neoplasm of skin of trunk**
  - **C44.5ØØ Unspecified malignant neoplasm of anal skin**
    Unspecified malignant neoplasm of anal margin
    Unspecified malignant neoplasm of perianal skin
  - **C44.5Ø1 Unspecified malignant neoplasm of skin of breast**
  - **C44.5Ø9 Unspecified malignant neoplasm of skin of other part of trunk**
- 6th **C44.51 Basal cell carcinoma of skin of trunk**
  - **C44.51Ø Basal cell carcinoma of anal skin**
    Basal cell carcinoma of anal margin
    Basal cell carcinoma of perianal skin
  - **C44.511 Basal cell carcinoma of skin of breast**
  - **C44.519 Basal cell carcinoma of skin of other part of trunk**
- 6th **C44.52 Squamous cell carcinoma of skin of trunk**
  - **C44.52Ø Squamous cell carcinoma of anal skin**
    Squamous cell carcinoma of anal margin
    Squamous cell carcinoma of perianal skin
  - **C44.521 Squamous cell carcinoma of skin of breast**
  - **C44.529 Squamous cell carcinoma of skin of other part of trunk**
- 6th **C44.59 Other specified malignant neoplasm of skin of trunk**
  - **C44.59Ø Other specified malignant neoplasm of anal skin**
    Other specified malignant neoplasm of anal margin
    Other specified malignant neoplasm of perianal skin
  - **C44.591 Other specified malignant neoplasm of skin of breast**
  - **C44.599 Other specified malignant neoplasm of skin of other part of trunk**

5th **C44.6 Other and unspecified malignant neoplasm of skin of upper limb, including shoulder**
- 6th **C44.6Ø Unspecified malignant neoplasm of skin of upper limb, including shoulder**
  - **C44.6Ø1 Unspecified malignant neoplasm of skin of unspecified upper limb, including shoulder**
  - **C44.6Ø2 Unspecified malignant neoplasm of skin of right upper limb, including shoulder**
  - **C44.6Ø9 Unspecified malignant neoplasm of skin of left upper limb, including shoulder**
- 6th **C44.61 Basal cell carcinoma of skin of upper limb, including shoulder**
  - **C44.611 Basal cell carcinoma of skin of unspecified upper limb, including shoulder**
  - **C44.612 Basal cell carcinoma of skin of right upper limb, including shoulder**
  - **C44.619 Basal cell carcinoma of skin of left upper limb, including shoulder**
- 6th **C44.62 Squamous cell carcinoma of skin of upper limb, including shoulder**
  - **C44.621 Squamous cell carcinoma of skin of unspecified upper limb, including shoulder**
  - **C44.622 Squamous cell carcinoma of skin of right upper limb, including shoulder**
  - **C44.629 Squamous cell carcinoma of skin of left upper limb, including shoulder**
- 6th **C44.69 Other specified malignant neoplasm of skin of upper limb, including shoulder**
  - **C44.691 Other specified malignant neoplasm of skin of unspecified upper limb, including shoulder**
  - **C44.692 Other specified malignant neoplasm of skin of right upper limb, including shoulder**
  - **C44.699 Other specified malignant neoplasm of skin of left upper limb, including shoulder**

5th **C44.7 Other and unspecified malignant neoplasm of skin of lower limb, including hip**
- 6th **C44.7Ø Unspecified malignant neoplasm of skin of lower limb, including hip**
  - **C44.7Ø1 Unspecified malignant neoplasm of skin of unspecified lower limb, including hip**
  - **C44.7Ø2 Unspecified malignant neoplasm of skin of right lower limb, including hip**
  - **C44.7Ø9 Unspecified malignant neoplasm of skin of left lower limb, including hip**
- 6th **C44.71 Basal cell carcinoma of skin of lower limb, including hip**
  - **C44.711 Basal cell carcinoma of skin of unspecified lower limb, including hip**
  - **C44.712 Basal cell carcinoma of skin of right lower limb, including hip**
  - **C44.719 Basal cell carcinoma of skin of left lower limb, including hip**
- 6th **C44.72 Squamous cell carcinoma of skin of lower limb, including hip**
  - **C44.721 Squamous cell carcinoma of skin of unspecified lower limb, including hip**
  - **C44.722 Squamous cell carcinoma of skin of right lower limb, including hip**
  - **C44.729 Squamous cell carcinoma of skin of left lower limb, including hip**
- 6th **C44.79 Other specified malignant neoplasm of skin of lower limb, including hip**
  - **C44.791 Other specified malignant neoplasm of skin of unspecified lower limb, including hip**
  - **C44.792 Other specified malignant neoplasm of skin of right lower limb, including hip**
  - **C44.799 Other specified malignant neoplasm of skin of left lower limb, including hip**

5th **C44.8 Other and unspecified malignant neoplasm of overlapping sites of skin**
- **C44.8Ø Unspecified malignant neoplasm of overlapping sites of skin**
- **C44.81 Basal cell carcinoma of overlapping sites of skin**
- **C44.82 Squamous cell carcinoma of overlapping sites of skin**
- **C44.89 Other specified malignant neoplasm of overlapping sites of skin**

5th **C44.9 Other and unspecified malignant neoplasm of skin, unspecified**
- **C44.9Ø Unspecified malignant neoplasm of skin, unspecified**
  Malignant neoplasm of unspecified site of skin
- **C44.91 Basal cell carcinoma of skin, unspecified**
- **C44.92 Squamous cell carcinoma of skin, unspecified**
- **C44.99 Other specified malignant neoplasm of skin, unspecified**

Malignant neoplasms of mesothelial and soft tissue (C45-C49)

4th **C45 Mesothelioma**

DEF: Rare type of cancer that forms in the thin layer of protective tissue that covers the majority of internal organs (mesothelium).

- **C45.Ø Mesothelioma of pleura** CC HCC
  EXCLUDES 1 *other malignant neoplasm of pleura (C38.4)*
  AHA: 2017,2Q,11
  TIP: For pleural mesothelioma that has metastasized to the chest wall, assign this code for the primary site along with C79.89 for metastatic cancer in the chest wall.
- **C45.1 Mesothelioma of peritoneum** CC HCC
  Mesothelioma of cul-de-sac
  Mesothelioma of mesentery
  Mesothelioma of mesocolon
  Mesothelioma of omentum
  Mesothelioma of peritoneum (parietal) (pelvic)
  EXCLUDES 1 *other malignant neoplasm of soft tissue of peritoneum (C48.-)*
- **C45.2 Mesothelioma of pericardium** CC HCC
  EXCLUDES 1 *other malignant neoplasm of pericardium (C38.Ø)*
- **C45.7 Mesothelioma of other sites** HCC

C45.9 Mesothelioma, unspecified HCC

C46 Kaposi's sarcoma

Code first any human immunodeficiency virus [HIV] disease (B20)

DEF: Malignant neoplasm that causes patches of abnormal tissue to grow under the skin, in the lining of the mouth, nose, and throat, in lymph nodes, or in other visceral organs. Kaposi's sarcoma is caused by human herpesvirus8 (HHV8).

C46.0 Kaposi's sarcoma of skin HIV CC HCC

C46.1 Kaposi's sarcoma of soft tissue HIV CC HCC

Kaposi's sarcoma of blood vessel
Kaposi's sarcoma of connective tissue
Kaposi's sarcoma of fascia
Kaposi's sarcoma of ligament
Kaposi's sarcoma of lymphatic(s) NEC
Kaposi's sarcoma of muscle

EXCLUDES 2 *Kaposi's sarcoma of lymph glands and nodes (C46.3)*

C46.2 Kaposi's sarcoma of palate HIV CC HCC

C46.3 Kaposi's sarcoma of lymph nodes HIV CC HCC

C46.4 Kaposi's sarcoma of gastrointestinal sites HIV CC HCC

C46.5 Kaposi's sarcoma of lung

AHA: 2019,1Q,16

TIP: When associated malignant pericardial effusion is documented, assign code I31.3. If the sole reason for admission is to treat the effusion with no treatment of the lung malignancy rendered, code I31.3 may be sequenced first.

C46.50 Kaposi's sarcoma of unspecified lung HIV CC HCC

C46.51 Kaposi's sarcoma of right lung HIV CC HCC

C46.52 Kaposi's sarcoma of left lung HIV CC HCC

C46.7 Kaposi's sarcoma of other sites HIV CC HCC

C46.9 Kaposi's sarcoma, unspecified HIV CC HCC

Kaposi's sarcoma of unspecified site

C47 Malignant neoplasm of peripheral nerves and autonomic nervous system

INCLUDES malignant neoplasm of sympathetic and parasympathetic nerves and ganglia

EXCLUDES 1 *Kaposi's sarcoma of soft tissue (C46.1)*

C47.0 Malignant neoplasm of peripheral nerves of head, face and neck CC HCC

EXCLUDES 1 *malignant neoplasm of peripheral nerves of orbit (C69.6-)*

C47.1 Malignant neoplasm of peripheral nerves of upper limb, including shoulder

C47.10 Malignant neoplasm of peripheral nerves of unspecified upper limb, including shoulder CC HCC

C47.11 Malignant neoplasm of peripheral nerves of right upper limb, including shoulder CC HCC

C47.12 Malignant neoplasm of peripheral nerves of left upper limb, including shoulder CC HCC

C47.2 Malignant neoplasm of peripheral nerves of lower limb, including hip

C47.20 Malignant neoplasm of peripheral nerves of unspecified lower limb, including hip CC HCC

C47.21 Malignant neoplasm of peripheral nerves of right lower limb, including hip CC HCC

C47.22 Malignant neoplasm of peripheral nerves of left lower limb, including hip CC HCC

C47.3 Malignant neoplasm of peripheral nerves of thorax CC HCC

C47.4 Malignant neoplasm of peripheral nerves of abdomen CC HCC

C47.5 Malignant neoplasm of peripheral nerves of pelvis CC HCC

C47.6 Malignant neoplasm of peripheral nerves of trunk, unspecified CC HCC

Malignant neoplasm of peripheral nerves of unspecified part of trunk

C47.8 Malignant neoplasm of overlapping sites of peripheral nerves and autonomic nervous system CC HCC

C47.9 Malignant neoplasm of peripheral nerves and autonomic nervous system, unspecified CC HCC

Malignant neoplasm of unspecified site of peripheral nerves and autonomic nervous system

C48 Malignant neoplasm of retroperitoneum and peritoneum

EXCLUDES 1 *Kaposi's sarcoma of connective tissue (C46.1)*
mesothelioma (C45.-)

C48.0 Malignant neoplasm of retroperitoneum CC HCC

C48.1 Malignant neoplasm of specified parts of peritoneum CC HCC

Malignant neoplasm of cul-de-sac
Malignant neoplasm of mesentery
Malignant neoplasm of mesocolon
Malignant neoplasm of omentum
Malignant neoplasm of parietal peritoneum
Malignant neoplasm of pelvic peritoneum

C48.2 Malignant neoplasm of peritoneum, unspecified CC HCC

C48.8 Malignant neoplasm of overlapping sites of retroperitoneum and peritoneum CC HCC

C49 Malignant neoplasm of other connective and soft tissue

INCLUDES malignant neoplasm of blood vessel
malignant neoplasm of bursa
malignant neoplasm of cartilage
malignant neoplasm of fascia
malignant neoplasm of fat
malignant neoplasm of ligament, except uterine
malignant neoplasm of lymphatic vessel
malignant neoplasm of muscle
malignant neoplasm of synovia
malignant neoplasm of tendon (sheath)

EXCLUDES 1 *malignant neoplasm of cartilage (of):*
articular (C40-C41)
larynx (C32.3)
nose (C30.0)
malignant neoplasm of connective tissue of breast (C50.-)

EXCLUDES 2 *Kaposi's sarcoma of soft tissue (C46.1)*
malignant neoplasm of heart (C38.0)
malignant neoplasm of peripheral nerves and autonomic nervous system (C47.-)
malignant neoplasm of peritoneum (C48.2)
malignant neoplasm of retroperitoneum (C48.0)
malignant neoplasm of uterine ligament (C57.3)
mesothelioma (C45.-)

C49.0 Malignant neoplasm of connective and soft tissue of head, face and neck CC HCC

Malignant neoplasm of connective tissue of ear
Malignant neoplasm of connective tissue of eyelid

EXCLUDES 1 *connective tissue of orbit (C69.6-)*

C49.1 Malignant neoplasm of connective and soft tissue of upper limb, including shoulder

C49.10 Malignant neoplasm of connective and soft tissue of unspecified upper limb, including shoulder CC HCC

C49.11 Malignant neoplasm of connective and soft tissue of right upper limb, including shoulder CC HCC

C49.12 Malignant neoplasm of connective and soft tissue of left upper limb, including shoulder CC HCC

C49.2 Malignant neoplasm of connective and soft tissue of lower limb, including hip

C49.20 Malignant neoplasm of connective and soft tissue of unspecified lower limb, including hip CC HCC

C49.21 Malignant neoplasm of connective and soft tissue of right lower limb, including hip CC HCC

C49.22 Malignant neoplasm of connective and soft tissue of left lower limb, including hip CC HCC

C49.3 Malignant neoplasm of connective and soft tissue of thorax CC HCC

Malignant neoplasm of axilla
Malignant neoplasm of diaphragm
Malignant neoplasm of great vessels

EXCLUDES 1 *malignant neoplasm of breast (C50.-)*
malignant neoplasm of heart (C38.0)
malignant neoplasm of mediastinum (C38.1-C38.3)
malignant neoplasm of thymus (C37)

AHA: 2015,3Q,19

C49.4 Malignant neoplasm of connective and soft tissue of abdomen CC HCC

Malignant neoplasm of abdominal wall
Malignant neoplasm of hypochondrium

C49.5 Malignant neoplasm of connective and soft tissue of pelvis CC HCC

Malignant neoplasm of buttock
Malignant neoplasm of groin
Malignant neoplasm of perineum

C49.6 Malignant neoplasm of connective and soft tissue of trunk, unspecified CC HCC
Malignant neoplasm of back NOS

C49.8 Malignant neoplasm of overlapping sites of connective and soft tissue CC HCC
Primary malignant neoplasm of two or more contiguous sites of connective and soft tissue

C49.9 Malignant neoplasm of connective and soft tissue, unspecified CC HCC

✓5th **C49.A Gastrointestinal stromal tumor**
AHA: 2016,4Q,8
DEF: Uncommon malignant tumor found in the GI tract that originates from interstitial cells of the autonomic nervous system. Most occur in the stomach or small intestine but can originate anywhere in the GI tract.

C49.A0 Gastrointestinal stromal tumor, unspecified site CC HCC
C49.A1 Gastrointestinal stromal tumor of esophagus CC HCC
C49.A2 Gastrointestinal stromal tumor of stomach CC HCC
C49.A3 Gastrointestinal stromal tumor of small intestine CC HCC
C49.A4 Gastrointestinal stromal tumor of large intestine CC HCC
C49.A5 Gastrointestinal stromal tumor of rectum CC HCC
C49.A9 Gastrointestinal stromal tumor of other sites CC HCC

Malignant neoplasms of breast (C50)

✓4th **C50 Malignant neoplasm of breast**
INCLUDES connective tissue of breast
Paget's disease of breast
Paget's disease of nipple
Use additional code to identify estrogen receptor status (Z17.0, Z17.1)
EXCLUDES 1 *skin of breast (C44.501, C44.511, C44.521, C44.591)*
AHA: 2017,4Q,19

Female Breast

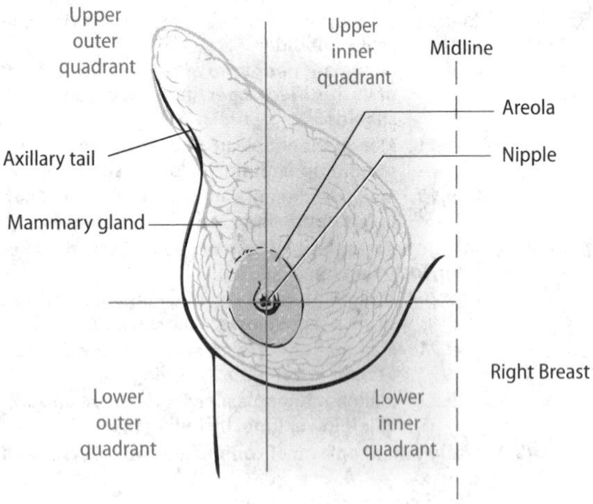

✓5th **C50.0 Malignant neoplasm of nipple and areola**
✓6th **C50.01 Malignant neoplasm of nipple and areola, female**
C50.011 Malignant neoplasm of nipple and areola, right female breast HCC ♀
C50.012 Malignant neoplasm of nipple and areola, left female breast HCC ♀
C50.019 Malignant neoplasm of nipple and areola, unspecified female breast HCC ♀
✓6th **C50.02 Malignant neoplasm of nipple and areola, male**
C50.021 Malignant neoplasm of nipple and areola, right male breast HCC ♂
C50.022 Malignant neoplasm of nipple and areola, left male breast HCC ♂
C50.029 Malignant neoplasm of nipple and areola, unspecified male breast HCC ♂

✓5th **C50.1 Malignant neoplasm of central portion of breast**
✓6th **C50.11 Malignant neoplasm of central portion of breast, female**
C50.111 Malignant neoplasm of central portion of right female breast HCC ♀
C50.112 Malignant neoplasm of central portion of left female breast HCC ♀
C50.119 Malignant neoplasm of central portion of unspecified female breast HCC ♀
✓6th **C50.12 Malignant neoplasm of central portion of breast, male**
C50.121 Malignant neoplasm of central portion of right male breast HCC ♂
C50.122 Malignant neoplasm of central portion of left male breast HCC ♂
C50.129 Malignant neoplasm of central portion of unspecified male breast HCC ♂

✓5th **C50.2 Malignant neoplasm of upper-inner quadrant of breast**
✓6th **C50.21 Malignant neoplasm of upper-inner quadrant of breast, female**
C50.211 Malignant neoplasm of upper-inner quadrant of right female breast HCC ♀
C50.212 Malignant neoplasm of upper-inner quadrant of left female breast HCC ♀
C50.219 Malignant neoplasm of upper-inner quadrant of unspecified female breast HCC ♀
✓6th **C50.22 Malignant neoplasm of upper-inner quadrant of breast, male**
C50.221 Malignant neoplasm of upper-inner quadrant of right male breast HCC ♂
C50.222 Malignant neoplasm of upper-inner quadrant of left male breast HCC ♂
C50.229 Malignant neoplasm of upper-inner quadrant of unspecified male breast HCC ♂

✓5th **C50.3 Malignant neoplasm of lower-inner quadrant of breast**
✓6th **C50.31 Malignant neoplasm of lower-inner quadrant of breast, female**
C50.311 Malignant neoplasm of lower-inner quadrant of right female breast HCC ♀
C50.312 Malignant neoplasm of lower-inner quadrant of left female breast HCC ♀
C50.319 Malignant neoplasm of lower-inner quadrant of unspecified female breast HCC ♀
✓6th **C50.32 Malignant neoplasm of lower-inner quadrant of breast, male**
C50.321 Malignant neoplasm of lower-inner quadrant of right male breast HCC ♂
C50.322 Malignant neoplasm of lower-inner quadrant of left male breast HCC ♂
C50.329 Malignant neoplasm of lower-inner quadrant of unspecified male breast HCC ♂

✓5th **C50.4 Malignant neoplasm of upper-outer quadrant of breast**
✓6th **C50.41 Malignant neoplasm of upper-outer quadrant of breast, female**
C50.411 Malignant neoplasm of upper-outer quadrant of right female breast HCC ♀
C50.412 Malignant neoplasm of upper-outer quadrant of left female breast HCC ♀
C50.419 Malignant neoplasm of upper-outer quadrant of unspecified female breast HCC ♀
✓6th **C50.42 Malignant neoplasm of upper-outer quadrant of breast, male**
C50.421 Malignant neoplasm of upper-outer quadrant of right male breast HCC ♂
C50.422 Malignant neoplasm of upper-outer quadrant of left male breast HCC ♂
C50.429 Malignant neoplasm of upper-outer quadrant of unspecified male breast HCC ♂

✓5th **C50.5 Malignant neoplasm of lower-outer quadrant of breast**
✓6th **C50.51 Malignant neoplasm of lower-outer quadrant of breast, female**
C50.511 Malignant neoplasm of lower-outer quadrant of right female breast HCC ♀
C50.512 Malignant neoplasm of lower-outer quadrant of left female breast HCC ♀

C50.519 Malignant neoplasm of lower-outer quadrant of unspecified female breast HCC ♀

C50.52 Malignant neoplasm of lower-outer quadrant of breast, male

C50.521 Malignant neoplasm of lower-outer quadrant of right male breast HCC ♂

C50.522 Malignant neoplasm of lower-outer quadrant of left male breast HCC ♂

C50.529 Malignant neoplasm of lower-outer quadrant of unspecified male breast HCC ♂

C50.6 Malignant neoplasm of axillary tail of breast

C50.61 Malignant neoplasm of axillary tail of breast, female

C50.611 Malignant neoplasm of axillary tail of right female breast HCC ♀

C50.612 Malignant neoplasm of axillary tail of left female breast HCC ♀

C50.619 Malignant neoplasm of axillary tail of unspecified female breast HCC ♀

C50.62 Malignant neoplasm of axillary tail of breast, male

C50.621 Malignant neoplasm of axillary tail of right male breast HCC ♂

C50.622 Malignant neoplasm of axillary tail of left male breast HCC ♂

C50.629 Malignant neoplasm of axillary tail of unspecified male breast HCC ♂

C50.8 Malignant neoplasm of overlapping sites of breast

C50.81 Malignant neoplasm of overlapping sites of breast, female

C50.811 Malignant neoplasm of overlapping sites of right female breast HCC ♀

C50.812 Malignant neoplasm of overlapping sites of left female breast HCC ♀

C50.819 Malignant neoplasm of overlapping sites of unspecified female breast HCC ♀

C50.82 Malignant neoplasm of overlapping sites of breast, male

C50.821 Malignant neoplasm of overlapping sites of right male breast HCC ♂

C50.822 Malignant neoplasm of overlapping sites of left male breast HCC ♂

C50.829 Malignant neoplasm of overlapping sites of unspecified male breast HCC ♂

C50.9 Malignant neoplasm of breast of unspecified site

C50.91 Malignant neoplasm of breast of unspecified site, female

C50.911 Malignant neoplasm of unspecified site of right female breast HCC ♀

C50.912 Malignant neoplasm of unspecified site of left female breast HCC ♀

C50.919 Malignant neoplasm of unspecified site of unspecified female breast HCC ♀

C50.92 Malignant neoplasm of breast of unspecified site, male

C50.921 Malignant neoplasm of unspecified site of right male breast HCC ♂

C50.922 Malignant neoplasm of unspecified site of left male breast HCC ♂

C50.929 Malignant neoplasm of unspecified site of unspecified male breast HCC ♂

Malignant neoplasms of female genital organs (C51-C58)

INCLUDES malignant neoplasm of skin of female genital organs

C51 Malignant neoplasm of vulva

EXCLUDES 1 *carcinoma in situ of vulva (D07.1)*

C51.0 Malignant neoplasm of labium majus HCC ♀
Malignant neoplasm of Bartholin's [greater vestibular] gland

C51.1 Malignant neoplasm of labium minus HCC ♀

C51.2 Malignant neoplasm of clitoris HCC ♀

C51.8 Malignant neoplasm of overlapping sites of vulva HCC ♀

C51.9 Malignant neoplasm of vulva, unspecified HCC ♀
Malignant neoplasm of external female genitalia NOS
Malignant neoplasm of pudendum

C52 Malignant neoplasm of vagina HCC ♀

EXCLUDES 1 *carcinoma in situ of vagina (D07.2)*

C53 Malignant neoplasm of cervix uteri

EXCLUDES 1 *carcinoma in situ of cervix uteri (D06.-)*

AHA: 2017,4Q,103

C53.0 Malignant neoplasm of endocervix HCC ♀

C53.1 Malignant neoplasm of exocervix HCC ♀

C53.8 Malignant neoplasm of overlapping sites of cervix uteri HCC ♀

C53.9 Malignant neoplasm of cervix uteri, unspecified HCC ♀

C54 Malignant neoplasm of corpus uteri

C54.0 Malignant neoplasm of isthmus uteri HCC ♀
Malignant neoplasm of lower uterine segment

C54.1 Malignant neoplasm of endometrium HCC ♀

C54.2 Malignant neoplasm of myometrium HCC ♀

C54.3 Malignant neoplasm of fundus uteri HCC ♀

C54.8 Malignant neoplasm of overlapping sites of corpus uteri HCC ♀

C54.9 Malignant neoplasm of corpus uteri, unspecified HCC ♀

C55 Malignant neoplasm of uterus, part unspecified HCC ♀

C56 Malignant neoplasm of ovary

Use additional code to identify any functional activity

C56.1 Malignant neoplasm of right ovary CC HCC ♀

C56.2 Malignant neoplasm of left ovary CC HCC ♀

C56.9 Malignant neoplasm of unspecified ovary CC HCC ♀

C57 Malignant neoplasm of other and unspecified female genital organs

C57.0 Malignant neoplasm of fallopian tube
Malignant neoplasm of oviduct
Malignant neoplasm of uterine tube

C57.00 Malignant neoplasm of unspecified fallopian tube HCC ♀

C57.01 Malignant neoplasm of right fallopian tube HCC ♀

C57.02 Malignant neoplasm of left fallopian tube HCC ♀

C57.1 Malignant neoplasm of broad ligament

C57.10 Malignant neoplasm of unspecified broad ligament HCC ♀

C57.11 Malignant neoplasm of right broad ligament HCC ♀

C57.12 Malignant neoplasm of left broad ligament HCC ♀

C57.2 Malignant neoplasm of round ligament

C57.20 Malignant neoplasm of unspecified round ligament HCC ♀

C57.21 Malignant neoplasm of right round ligament HCC ♀

C57.22 Malignant neoplasm of left round ligament HCC ♀

C57.3 Malignant neoplasm of parametrium HCC ♀
Malignant neoplasm of uterine ligament NOS

C57.4 Malignant neoplasm of uterine adnexa, unspecified HCC ♀

C57.7 Malignant neoplasm of other specified female genital organs HCC ♀
Malignant neoplasm of wolffian body or duct

C57.8 Malignant neoplasm of overlapping sites of female genital organs HCC ♀
Primary malignant neoplasm of two or more contiguous sites of the female genital organs whose point of origin cannot be determined
Primary tubo-ovarian malignant neoplasm whose point of origin cannot be determined
Primary utero-ovarian malignant neoplasm whose point of origin cannot be determined

C57.9 Malignant neoplasm of female genital organ, unspecified HCC ♀
Malignant neoplasm of female genitourinary tract NOS

C58 Malignant neoplasm of placenta HCC M ♀

INCLUDES choriocarcinoma NOS
chorionepithelioma NOS

EXCLUDES 1 *chorioadenoma (destruens) (D39.2)*
hydatidiform mole NOS (O01.9)
invasive hydatidiform mole (D39.2)
male choriocarcinoma NOS (C62.9-)
malignant hydatidiform mole (D39.2)

Malignant neoplasms of male genital organs (C60-C63)

INCLUDES malignant neoplasm of skin of male genital organs

✓4th **C60 Malignant neoplasm of penis**

C60.0 Malignant neoplasm of prepuce HCC ♂
Malignant neoplasm of foreskin

C60.1 Malignant neoplasm of glans penis HCC ♂

C60.2 Malignant neoplasm of body of penis HCC ♂
Malignant neoplasm of corpus cavernosum

C60.8 Malignant neoplasm of overlapping sites of penis HCC ♂

C60.9 Malignant neoplasm of penis, unspecified HCC ♂
Malignant neoplasm of skin of penis NOS

C61 Malignant neoplasm of prostate HCC ♂
Use additional code to identify:
hormone sensitivity status (Z19.1-Z19.2)
rising PSA following treatment for malignant neoplasm of prostate (R97.21)

EXCLUDES 1 *malignant neoplasm of seminal vesicle (C63.7)*

AHA: 2017,1Q,17

✓4th **C62 Malignant neoplasm of testis**
Use additional code to identify any functional activity

✓5th **C62.0 Malignant neoplasm of undescended testis**
Malignant neoplasm of ectopic testis
Malignant neoplasm of retained testis

C62.00 Malignant neoplasm of unspecified undescended testis HCC ♂

C62.01 Malignant neoplasm of undescended right testis HCC ♂

C62.02 Malignant neoplasm of undescended left testis HCC ♂

✓5th **C62.1 Malignant neoplasm of descended testis**
Malignant neoplasm of scrotal testis

C62.10 Malignant neoplasm of unspecified descended testis HCC ♂

C62.11 Malignant neoplasm of descended right testis HCC ♂

C62.12 Malignant neoplasm of descended left testis HCC ♂

✓5th **C62.9 Malignant neoplasm of testis, unspecified whether descended or undescended**

C62.90 Malignant neoplasm of unspecified testis, unspecified whether descended or undescended HCC ♂
Malignant neoplasm of testis NOS

C62.91 Malignant neoplasm of right testis, unspecified whether descended or undescended HCC ♂

C62.92 Malignant neoplasm of left testis, unspecified whether descended or undescended HCC ♂

✓4th **C63 Malignant neoplasm of other and unspecified male genital organs**

✓5th **C63.0 Malignant neoplasm of epididymis**

C63.00 Malignant neoplasm of unspecified epididymis HCC ♂

C63.01 Malignant neoplasm of right epididymis HCC ♂

C63.02 Malignant neoplasm of left epididymis HCC ♂

✓5th **C63.1 Malignant neoplasm of spermatic cord**

C63.10 Malignant neoplasm of unspecified spermatic cord HCC ♂

C63.11 Malignant neoplasm of right spermatic cord HCC ♂

C63.12 Malignant neoplasm of left spermatic cord HCC ♂

C63.2 Malignant neoplasm of scrotum HCC ♂
Malignant neoplasm of skin of scrotum

C63.7 Malignant neoplasm of other specified male genital organs HCC ♂
Malignant neoplasm of seminal vesicle
Malignant neoplasm of tunica vaginalis

C63.8 Malignant neoplasm of overlapping sites of male genital organs HCC ♂
Primary malignant neoplasm of two or more contiguous sites of male genital organs whose point of origin cannot be determined

C63.9 Malignant neoplasm of male genital organ, unspecified HCC ♂
Malignant neoplasm of male genitourinary tract NOS

Malignant neoplasms of urinary tract (C64-C68)

✓4th **C64 Malignant neoplasm of kidney, except renal pelvis**

EXCLUDES 1 *malignant carcinoid tumor of the kidney (C7A.093)*
malignant neoplasm of renal calyces (C65.-)
malignant neoplasm of renal pelvis (C65.-)

C64.1 Malignant neoplasm of right kidney, except renal pelvis CC HCC

C64.2 Malignant neoplasm of left kidney, except renal pelvis CC HCC

C64.9 Malignant neoplasm of unspecified kidney, except renal pelvis CC HCC

✓4th **C65 Malignant neoplasm of renal pelvis**

INCLUDES malignant neoplasm of pelviureteric junction
malignant neoplasm of renal calyces

C65.1 Malignant neoplasm of right renal pelvis CC HCC

C65.2 Malignant neoplasm of left renal pelvis CC HCC

C65.9 Malignant neoplasm of unspecified renal pelvis CC HCC

✓4th **C66 Malignant neoplasm of ureter**

EXCLUDES 1 *malignant neoplasm of ureteric orifice of bladder (C67.6)*

C66.1 Malignant neoplasm of right ureter CC HCC

C66.2 Malignant neoplasm of left ureter CC HCC

C66.9 Malignant neoplasm of unspecified ureter CC HCC

✓4th **C67 Malignant neoplasm of bladder**

C67.0 Malignant neoplasm of trigone of bladder HCC

C67.1 Malignant neoplasm of dome of bladder HCC

C67.2 Malignant neoplasm of lateral wall of bladder HCC

C67.3 Malignant neoplasm of anterior wall of bladder HCC

C67.4 Malignant neoplasm of posterior wall of bladder HCC

C67.5 Malignant neoplasm of bladder neck HCC
Malignant neoplasm of internal urethral orifice

C67.6 Malignant neoplasm of ureteric orifice HCC

C67.7 Malignant neoplasm of urachus HCC

C67.8 Malignant neoplasm of overlapping sites of bladder HCC

C67.9 Malignant neoplasm of bladder, unspecified HCC
AHA: 2016,1Q,19

✓4th **C68 Malignant neoplasm of other and unspecified urinary organs**

EXCLUDES 1 *malignant neoplasm of female genitourinary tract NOS (C57.9)*
malignant neoplasm of male genitourinary tract NOS (C63.9)

C68.0 Malignant neoplasm of urethra CC HCC

EXCLUDES 1 *malignant neoplasm of urethral orifice of bladder (C67.5)*

C68.1 Malignant neoplasm of paraurethral glands CC HCC

C68.8 Malignant neoplasm of overlapping sites of urinary organs CC HCC
Primary malignant neoplasm of two or more contiguous sites of urinary organs whose point of origin cannot be determined

C68.9 Malignant neoplasm of urinary organ, unspecified CC HCC
Malignant neoplasm of urinary system NOS

Malignant neoplasms of eye, brain and other parts of central nervous system (C69-C72)

✓4th **C69 Malignant neoplasm of eye and adnexa**

EXCLUDES 1 *malignant neoplasm of connective tissue of eyelid (C49.0)*
malignant neoplasm of eyelid (skin) (C43.1-, C44.1-)
malignant neoplasm of optic nerve (C72.3-)

✓5th **C69.0 Malignant neoplasm of conjunctiva**

C69.00 Malignant neoplasm of unspecified conjunctiva HCC

C69.01 Malignant neoplasm of right conjunctiva HCC

C69.02 Malignant neoplasm of left conjunctiva HCC

✓5th **C69.1 Malignant neoplasm of cornea**

C69.10 Malignant neoplasm of unspecified cornea HCC

C69.11 Malignant neoplasm of right cornea HCC

C69.12 Malignant neoplasm of left cornea HCC

✓5th **C69.2 Malignant neoplasm of retina**

EXCLUDES 1 *dark area on retina (D49.81)*
neoplasm of unspecified behavior of retina and choroid (D49.81)
retinal freckle (D49.81)

C69.20 Malignant neoplasm of unspecified retina HCC
C69.21 Malignant neoplasm of right retina HCC
C69.22 Malignant neoplasm of left retina HCC

✓5th **C69.3 Malignant neoplasm of choroid**

C69.30 Malignant neoplasm of unspecified choroid HCC
C69.31 Malignant neoplasm of right choroid HCC
C69.32 Malignant neoplasm of left choroid HCC

✓5th **C69.4 Malignant neoplasm of ciliary body**

C69.40 Malignant neoplasm of unspecified ciliary body HCC
C69.41 Malignant neoplasm of right ciliary body HCC
C69.42 Malignant neoplasm of left ciliary body HCC

✓5th **C69.5 Malignant neoplasm of lacrimal gland and duct**

Malignant neoplasm of lacrimal sac
Malignant neoplasm of nasolacrimal duct

C69.50 Malignant neoplasm of unspecified lacrimal gland and duct HCC
C69.51 Malignant neoplasm of right lacrimal gland and duct HCC
C69.52 Malignant neoplasm of left lacrimal gland and duct HCC

✓5th **C69.6 Malignant neoplasm of orbit**

Malignant neoplasm of connective tissue of orbit
Malignant neoplasm of extraocular muscle
Malignant neoplasm of peripheral nerves of orbit
Malignant neoplasm of retrobulbar tissue
Malignant neoplasm of retro-ocular tissue

EXCLUDES 1 *malignant neoplasm of orbital bone (C41.Ø)*

C69.6Ø Malignant neoplasm of unspecified orbit HCC
C69.61 Malignant neoplasm of right orbit HCC
C69.62 Malignant neoplasm of left orbit HCC

✓5th **C69.8 Malignant neoplasm of overlapping sites of eye and adnexa**

C69.8Ø Malignant neoplasm of overlapping sites of unspecified eye and adnexa HCC
C69.81 Malignant neoplasm of overlapping sites of right eye and adnexa HCC
C69.82 Malignant neoplasm of overlapping sites of left eye and adnexa HCC

✓5th **C69.9 Malignant neoplasm of unspecified site of eye**

Malignant neoplasm of eyeball

C69.9Ø Malignant neoplasm of unspecified site of unspecified eye HCC
C69.91 Malignant neoplasm of unspecified site of right eye HCC
C69.92 Malignant neoplasm of unspecified site of left eye HCC

✓4th **C7Ø Malignant neoplasm of meninges**

C7Ø.Ø Malignant neoplasm of cerebral meninges CC HCC
C7Ø.1 Malignant neoplasm of spinal meninges CC HCC
C7Ø.9 Malignant neoplasm of meninges, unspecified CC HCC

✓4th **C71 Malignant neoplasm of brain**

EXCLUDES 1 *malignant neoplasm of cranial nerves (C72.2-C72.5)*
retrobulbar malignant neoplasm (C69.6-)

Lobes of the Brain

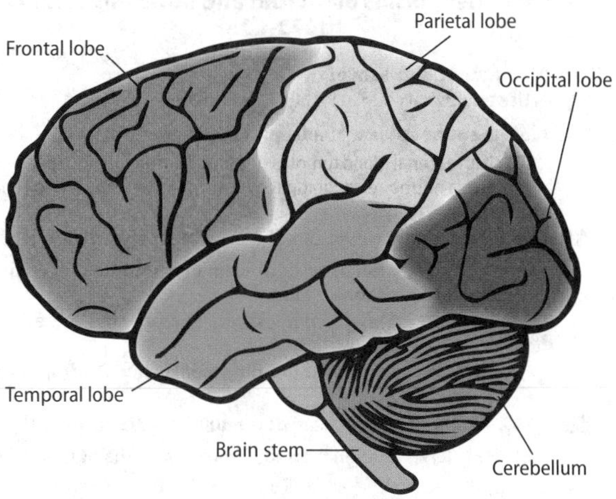

C71.Ø Malignant neoplasm of cerebrum, except lobes and ventricles CC HCC

Malignant neoplasm of supratentorial NOS

C71.1 Malignant neoplasm of frontal lobe CC HCC
C71.2 Malignant neoplasm of temporal lobe CC HCC
C71.3 Malignant neoplasm of parietal lobe CC HCC
C71.4 Malignant neoplasm of occipital lobe CC HCC
C71.5 Malignant neoplasm of cerebral ventricle CC HCC

EXCLUDES 1 *malignant neoplasm of fourth cerebral ventricle (C71.7)*

C71.6 Malignant neoplasm of cerebellum CC HCC
C71.7 Malignant neoplasm of brain stem CC HCC

Malignant neoplasm of fourth cerebral ventricle
Infratentorial malignant neoplasm NOS

C71.8 Malignant neoplasm of overlapping sites of brain CC HCC
C71.9 Malignant neoplasm of brain, unspecified CC HCC

AHA: 2014,3Q,3

✓4th **C72 Malignant neoplasm of spinal cord, cranial nerves and other parts of central nervous system**

EXCLUDES 1 *malignant neoplasm of meninges (C7Ø.-)*
malignant neoplasm of peripheral nerves and autonomic nervous system (C47.-)

C72.Ø Malignant neoplasm of spinal cord CC HCC
C72.1 Malignant neoplasm of cauda equina CC HCC

✓5th **C72.2 Malignant neoplasm of olfactory nerve**

Malignant neoplasm of olfactory bulb

C72.2Ø Malignant neoplasm of unspecified olfactory nerve CC HCC
C72.21 Malignant neoplasm of right olfactory nerve CC HCC
C72.22 Malignant neoplasm of left olfactory nerve CC HCC

✓5th **C72.3 Malignant neoplasm of optic nerve**

C72.3Ø Malignant neoplasm of unspecified optic nerve CC HCC
C72.31 Malignant neoplasm of right optic nerve CC HCC
C72.32 Malignant neoplasm of left optic nerve CC HCC

✓5th **C72.4 Malignant neoplasm of acoustic nerve**

C72.4Ø Malignant neoplasm of unspecified acoustic nerve CC HCC
C72.41 Malignant neoplasm of right acoustic nerve CC HCC
C72.42 Malignant neoplasm of left acoustic nerve CC HCC

✓5th **C72.5 Malignant neoplasm of other and unspecified cranial nerves**

C72.5Ø Malignant neoplasm of unspecified cranial nerve CC HCC

Malignant neoplasm of cranial nerve NOS

C72.59 Malignant neoplasm of other cranial nerves CC HCC

Chapter 2. Neoplasms
C69.2–C72.59

C72.9 Malignant neoplasm of central nervous system, unspecified CC HCC
Malignant neoplasm of unspecified site of central nervous system
Malignant neoplasm of nervous system NOS

Malignant neoplasms of thyroid and other endocrine glands (C73-C75)

C73 Malignant neoplasm of thyroid gland HCC
Use additional code to identify any functional activity

C74 Malignant neoplasm of adrenal gland
TIP: If an adrenal gland tumor is described as functioning (producing too much of a hormone), additional codes should be assigned to report the functional activity.

C74.Ø Malignant neoplasm of cortex of adrenal gland
C74.ØØ Malignant neoplasm of cortex of unspecified adrenal gland CC HCC
C74.Ø1 Malignant neoplasm of cortex of right adrenal gland CC HCC
C74.Ø2 Malignant neoplasm of cortex of left adrenal gland CC HCC

C74.1 Malignant neoplasm of medulla of adrenal gland
C74.1Ø Malignant neoplasm of medulla of unspecified adrenal gland CC HCC
C74.11 Malignant neoplasm of medulla of right adrenal gland CC HCC
C74.12 Malignant neoplasm of medulla of left adrenal gland CC HCC

C74.9 Malignant neoplasm of unspecified part of adrenal gland
C74.9Ø Malignant neoplasm of unspecified part of unspecified adrenal gland CC HCC
C74.91 Malignant neoplasm of unspecified part of right adrenal gland CC HCC
C74.92 Malignant neoplasm of unspecified part of left adrenal gland CC HCC

C75 Malignant neoplasm of other endocrine glands and related structures
EXCLUDES 1 *malignant carcinoid tumors (C7A.Ø-)*
malignant neoplasm of adrenal gland (C74.-)
malignant neoplasm of endocrine pancreas (C25.4)
malignant neoplasm of islets of Langerhans (C25.4)
malignant neoplasm of ovary (C56.-)
malignant neoplasm of testis (C62.-)
malignant neoplasm of thymus (C37)
malignant neoplasm of thyroid gland (C73)
malignant neuroendocrine tumors (C7A.-)

C75.Ø Malignant neoplasm of parathyroid gland CC HCC
C75.1 Malignant neoplasm of pituitary gland CC HCC
C75.2 Malignant neoplasm of craniopharyngeal duct CC HCC
C75.3 Malignant neoplasm of pineal gland CC HCC
C75.4 Malignant neoplasm of carotid body CC HCC
C75.5 Malignant neoplasm of aortic body and other paraganglia CC HCC
C75.8 Malignant neoplasm with pluriglandular involvement, unspecified CC HCC
C75.9 Malignant neoplasm of endocrine gland, unspecified CC HCC

Malignant neuroendocrine tumors (C7A)

C7A Malignant neuroendocrine tumors
Code also any associated multiple endocrine neoplasia [MEN] syndromes (E31.2-)
Use additional code to identify any associated endocrine syndrome, such as:
carcinoid syndrome (E34.Ø)
EXCLUDES 2 *malignant pancreatic islet cell tumors (C25.4)*
Merkel cell carcinoma (C4A.-)
AHA: 2019,3Q,7
DEF: Tumors comprised of cells that are capable of producing hormonal syndromes in which the normal hormonal balance required to support body system functions is adversely affected.

C7A.Ø Malignant carcinoid tumors
AHA: 2019,3Q,7
DEF: Specific type of slow-growing benign or malignant neuroendocrine tumors. Carcinoid tumors occur most commonly in the hormone producing cells of the gastrointestinal tracts and can also occur in the pancreas, testes, ovaries, or lungs.

C7A.ØØ Malignant carcinoid tumor of unspecified site CC HCC

C7A.Ø1 Malignant carcinoid tumors of the small intestine
C7A.Ø1Ø Malignant carcinoid tumor of the duodenum CC HCC
C7A.Ø11 Malignant carcinoid tumor of the jejunum CC HCC
C7A.Ø12 Malignant carcinoid tumor of the ileum CC HCC
C7A.Ø19 Malignant carcinoid tumor of the small intestine, unspecified portion CC HCC

C7A.Ø2 Malignant carcinoid tumors of the appendix, large intestine, and rectum
C7A.Ø2Ø Malignant carcinoid tumor of the appendix CC HCC
C7A.Ø21 Malignant carcinoid tumor of the cecum CC HCC
C7A.Ø22 Malignant carcinoid tumor of the ascending colon CC HCC
C7A.Ø23 Malignant carcinoid tumor of the transverse colon CC HCC
C7A.Ø24 Malignant carcinoid tumor of the descending colon CC HCC
C7A.Ø25 Malignant carcinoid tumor of the sigmoid colon CC HCC
C7A.Ø26 Malignant carcinoid tumor of the rectum CC HCC
C7A.Ø29 Malignant carcinoid tumor of the large intestine, unspecified portion CC HCC
Malignant carcinoid tumor of the colon NOS

C7A.Ø9 Malignant carcinoid tumors of other sites
C7A.Ø9Ø Malignant carcinoid tumor of the bronchus and lung CC HCC
AHA: 2019,1Q,16
TIP: When associated malignant pericardial effusion is documented, assign code I31.3. If the sole reason for admission is to treat the effusion with no treatment of the lung malignancy rendered, code I31.3 may be sequenced first.
C7A.Ø91 Malignant carcinoid tumor of the thymus CC HCC
C7A.Ø92 Malignant carcinoid tumor of the stomach CC HCC
C7A.Ø93 Malignant carcinoid tumor of the kidney CC HCC
C7A.Ø94 Malignant carcinoid tumor of the foregut, unspecified CC HCC
C7A.Ø95 Malignant carcinoid tumor of the midgut, unspecified CC HCC
C7A.Ø96 Malignant carcinoid tumor of the hindgut, unspecified CC HCC
C7A.Ø98 Malignant carcinoid tumors of other sites CC HCC

C7A.1 Malignant poorly differentiated neuroendocrine tumors CC HCC
Malignant poorly differentiated neuroendocrine tumor NOS
Malignant poorly differentiated neuroendocrine carcinoma, any site
High grade neuroendocrine carcinoma, any site

C7A.8 Other malignant neuroendocrine tumors CC HCC
AHA: 2019,3Q,7

Secondary neuroendocrine tumors (C7B)

✓4th **C7B Secondary neuroendocrine tumors**
Use additional code to identify any functional activity

✓5th **C7B.Ø Secondary carcinoid tumors**
AHA: 2019,3Q,7

C7B.ØØ Secondary carcinoid tumors, unspecified site HCC
C7B.Ø1 Secondary carcinoid tumors of distant lymph nodes CC HCC
C7B.Ø2 Secondary carcinoid tumors of liver CC HCC
C7B.Ø3 Secondary carcinoid tumors of bone CC HCC
C7B.Ø4 Secondary carcinoid tumors of peritoneum CC HCC
Mesentary metastasis of carcinoid tumor
C7B.Ø9 Secondary carcinoid tumors of other sites CC HCC

C7B.1 Secondary Merkel cell carcinoma HCC
Merkel cell carcinoma nodal presentation
Merkel cell carcinoma visceral metastatic presentation

C7B.8 Other secondary neuroendocrine tumors CC HCC
AHA: 2019,3Q,7

Malignant neoplasms of ill-defined, other secondary and unspecified sites (C76-C8Ø)

✓4th **C76 Malignant neoplasm of other and ill-defined sites**
EXCLUDES 1 *malignant neoplasm of female genitourinary tract NOS (C57.9)*
malignant neoplasm of male genitourinary tract NOS (C63.9)
malignant neoplasm of lymphoid, hematopoietic and related tissue (C81-C96)
malignant neoplasm of skin (C44.-)
malignant neoplasm of unspecified site NOS (C8Ø.1)

C76.Ø Malignant neoplasm of head, face and neck HCC
Malignant neoplasm of cheek NOS
Malignant neoplasm of nose NOS

C76.1 Malignant neoplasm of thorax HCC
Intrathoracic malignant neoplasm NOS
Malignant neoplasm of axilla NOS
Thoracic malignant neoplasm NOS

C76.2 Malignant neoplasm of abdomen HCC

C76.3 Malignant neoplasm of pelvis HCC
Malignant neoplasm of groin NOS
Malignant neoplasm of sites overlapping systems within the pelvis
Rectovaginal (septum) malignant neoplasm
Rectovesical (septum) malignant neoplasm

✓5th **C76.4 Malignant neoplasm of upper limb**
C76.4Ø Malignant neoplasm of unspecified upper limb HCC
C76.41 Malignant neoplasm of right upper limb HCC
C76.42 Malignant neoplasm of left upper limb HCC

✓5th **C76.5 Malignant neoplasm of lower limb**
C76.5Ø Malignant neoplasm of unspecified lower limb HCC
C76.51 Malignant neoplasm of right lower limb HCC
C76.52 Malignant neoplasm of left lower limb HCC

C76.8 Malignant neoplasm of other specified ill-defined sites HCC
Malignant neoplasm of overlapping ill-defined sites

✓4th **C77 Secondary and unspecified malignant neoplasm of lymph nodes**
EXCLUDES 1 *malignant neoplasm of lymph nodes, specified as primary (C81-C86, C88, C96.-)*
mesentary metastasis of carcinoid tumor (C7B.Ø4)
secondary carcinoid tumors of distant lymph nodes (C7B.Ø1)

C77.Ø Secondary and unspecified malignant neoplasm of lymph nodes of head, face and neck CC HCC
Secondary and unspecified malignant neoplasm of supraclavicular lymph nodes

C77.1 Secondary and unspecified malignant neoplasm of intrathoracic lymph nodes CC HCC

C77.2 Secondary and unspecified malignant neoplasm of intra-abdominal lymph nodes CC HCC

C77.3 Secondary and unspecified malignant neoplasm of axilla and upper limb lymph nodes CC HCC
Secondary and unspecified malignant neoplasm of pectoral lymph nodes

C77.4 Secondary and unspecified malignant neoplasm of inguinal and lower limb lymph nodes CC HCC

C77.5 Secondary and unspecified malignant neoplasm of intrapelvic lymph nodes CC HCC

C77.8 Secondary and unspecified malignant neoplasm of lymph nodes of multiple regions CC HCC

C77.9 Secondary and unspecified malignant neoplasm of lymph node, unspecified CC HCC

✓4th **C78 Secondary malignant neoplasm of respiratory and digestive organs**
EXCLUDES 1 *secondary carcinoid tumors of liver (C7B.Ø2)*
secondary carcinoid tumors of peritoneum (C7B.Ø4)
EXCLUDES 2 *lymph node metastases (C77.Ø)*

✓5th **C78.Ø Secondary malignant neoplasm of lung**
AHA: 2019,1Q,16
C78.ØØ Secondary malignant neoplasm of unspecified lung CC HCC
C78.Ø1 Secondary malignant neoplasm of right lung CC HCC
C78.Ø2 Secondary malignant neoplasm of left lung CC HCC

C78.1 Secondary malignant neoplasm of mediastinum CC HCC
C78.2 Secondary malignant neoplasm of pleura CC HCC

✓5th **C78.3 Secondary malignant neoplasm of other and unspecified respiratory organs**
C78.3Ø Secondary malignant neoplasm of unspecified respiratory organ CC HCC
C78.39 Secondary malignant neoplasm of other respiratory organs CC HCC

C78.4 Secondary malignant neoplasm of small intestine CC HCC
C78.5 Secondary malignant neoplasm of large intestine and rectum CC HCC
C78.6 Secondary malignant neoplasm of retroperitoneum and peritoneum CC HCC
AHA: 2017,2Q,12
C78.7 Secondary malignant neoplasm of liver and intrahepatic bile duct CC HCC

✓5th **C78.8 Secondary malignant neoplasm of other and unspecified digestive organs**
C78.8Ø Secondary malignant neoplasm of unspecified digestive organ CC HCC
C78.89 Secondary malignant neoplasm of other digestive organs CC HCC
Code also exocrine pancreatic insufficiency (K86.81)

✓4th **C79 Secondary malignant neoplasm of other and unspecified sites**
EXCLUDES 1 *secondary carcinoid tumors (C7B.-)*
secondary neuroendocrine tumors (C7B.-)

✓5th **C79.Ø Secondary malignant neoplasm of kidney and renal pelvis**
C79.ØØ Secondary malignant neoplasm of unspecified kidney and renal pelvis CC HCC
C79.Ø1 Secondary malignant neoplasm of right kidney and renal pelvis CC HCC
C79.Ø2 Secondary malignant neoplasm of left kidney and renal pelvis CC HCC

✓5th **C79.1 Secondary malignant neoplasm of bladder and other and unspecified urinary organs**
C79.1Ø Secondary malignant neoplasm of unspecified urinary organs CC HCC

C79.11 **Secondary malignant neoplasm of bladder** CC HCC
EXCLUDES 2 *lymph node metastases (C77.Ø)*

C79.19 **Secondary malignant neoplasm of other urinary organs** CC HCC

C79.2 **Secondary malignant neoplasm of skin** CC HCC
EXCLUDES 1 *secondary Merkel cell carcinoma (C7B.1)*

✓5th C79.3 **Secondary malignant neoplasm of brain and cerebral meninges**

C79.31 **Secondary malignant neoplasm of brain** CC HCC

C79.32 **Secondary malignant neoplasm of cerebral meninges** CC HCC
AHA: 2020,1Q,13

✓5th C79.4 **Secondary malignant neoplasm of other and unspecified parts of nervous system**

C79.4Ø **Secondary malignant neoplasm of unspecified part of nervous system** CC HCC

C79.49 **Secondary malignant neoplasm of other parts of nervous system** CC HCC

✓5th C79.5 **Secondary malignant neoplasm of bone and bone marrow**
EXCLUDES 1 *secondary carcinoid tumors of bone (C7B.Ø3)*

C79.51 **Secondary malignant neoplasm of bone** CC HCC
TIP: Do not assign in addition to a code from subcategory C90.0 when multiple myeloma is described as metastatic to the bone; bone involvement is integral to multiple myeloma.

C79.52 **Secondary malignant neoplasm of bone marrow** CC HCC

✓5th C79.6 **Secondary malignant neoplasm of ovary**

C79.6Ø **Secondary malignant neoplasm of unspecified ovary** CC HCC ♀

C79.61 **Secondary malignant neoplasm of right ovary** CC HCC ♀

C79.62 **Secondary malignant neoplasm of left ovary** CC HCC ♀

✓5th C79.7 **Secondary malignant neoplasm of adrenal gland**

C79.7Ø **Secondary malignant neoplasm of unspecified adrenal gland** CC HCC

C79.71 **Secondary malignant neoplasm of right adrenal gland** CC HCC

C79.72 **Secondary malignant neoplasm of left adrenal gland** CC HCC

✓5th C79.8 **Secondary malignant neoplasm of other specified sites**

C79.81 **Secondary malignant neoplasm of breast** CC HCC

C79.82 **Secondary malignant neoplasm of genital organs** CC HCC

C79.89 **Secondary malignant neoplasm of other specified sites** CC HCC
AHA: 2017,2Q,11

C79.9 **Secondary malignant neoplasm of unspecified site** CC HCC
Metastatic cancer NOS
Metastatic disease NOS
EXCLUDES 1 *carcinomatosis NOS (C8Ø.Ø)*
generalized cancer NOS (C8Ø.Ø)
malignant (primary) neoplasm of unspecified site (C8Ø.1)

✓4th C8Ø **Malignant neoplasm without specification of site**
EXCLUDES 1 *malignant carcinoid tumor of unspecified site (C7A.ØØ)*
malignant neoplasm of specified multiple sites — code to each site

C8Ø.Ø **Disseminated malignant neoplasm, unspecified** CC HCC
Carcinomatosis NOS
Generalized cancer, unspecified site (primary) (secondary)
Generalized malignancy, unspecified site (primary) (secondary)

C8Ø.1 **Malignant (primary) neoplasm, unspecified** HCC
Cancer NOS
Cancer unspecified site (primary)
Carcinoma unspecified site (primary)
Malignancy unspecified site (primary)
EXCLUDES 1 *secondary malignant neoplasm of unspecified site (C79.9)*

C8Ø.2 **Malignant neoplasm associated with transplanted organ** CC HCC
Code first complication of transplanted organ (T86.-)
Use additional code to identify the specific malignancy

Malignant neoplasms of lymphoid, hematopoietic and related tissue (C81-C96)

EXCLUDES 2 *Kaposi's sarcoma of lymph nodes (C46.3)*
secondary and unspecified neoplasm of lymph nodes (C77.-)
secondary neoplasm of bone marrow (C79.52)
secondary neoplasm of spleen (C78.89)

✓4th C81 **Hodgkin lymphoma**
EXCLUDES 1 *personal history of Hodgkin lymphoma (Z85.71)*
DEF: Malignant disorder of lymphoid cells characterized by the presence of progressively swollen lymph nodes and spleen that may also involve the liver. A diagnosis of Hodgkin's lymphoma can be confirmed by the presence of Reed-Sternberg cells. ***Synonym(s):*** *Hodgkin disease.*

✓5th C81.Ø **Nodular lymphocyte predominant Hodgkin lymphoma**

C81.ØØ **Nodular lymphocyte predominant Hodgkin lymphoma, unspecified site** CC HCC

C81.Ø1 **Nodular lymphocyte predominant Hodgkin lymphoma, lymph nodes of head, face, and neck** CC HCC

C81.Ø2 **Nodular lymphocyte predominant Hodgkin lymphoma, intrathoracic lymph nodes** CC HCC

C81.Ø3 **Nodular lymphocyte predominant Hodgkin lymphoma, intra-abdominal lymph nodes** CC HCC

C81.Ø4 **Nodular lymphocyte predominant Hodgkin lymphoma, lymph nodes of axilla and upper limb** CC HCC

C81.Ø5 **Nodular lymphocyte predominant Hodgkin lymphoma, lymph nodes of inguinal region and lower limb** CC HCC

C81.Ø6 **Nodular lymphocyte predominant Hodgkin lymphoma, intrapelvic lymph nodes** CC HCC

C81.Ø7 **Nodular lymphocyte predominant Hodgkin lymphoma, spleen** CC HCC

C81.Ø8 **Nodular lymphocyte predominant Hodgkin lymphoma, lymph nodes of multiple sites** CC HCC

C81.Ø9 **Nodular lymphocyte predominant Hodgkin lymphoma, extranodal and solid organ sites** CC HCC

✓5th C81.1 **Nodular sclerosis Hodgkin lymphoma**
Nodular sclerosis classical Hodgkin lymphoma

C81.1Ø **Nodular sclerosis Hodgkin lymphoma, unspecified site** CC HCC

C81.11 **Nodular sclerosis Hodgkin lymphoma, lymph nodes of head, face, and neck** CC HCC

C81.12 **Nodular sclerosis Hodgkin lymphoma, intrathoracic lymph nodes** CC HCC

C81.13 **Nodular sclerosis Hodgkin lymphoma, intra-abdominal lymph nodes** CC HCC

C81.14 **Nodular sclerosis Hodgkin lymphoma, lymph nodes of axilla and upper limb** CC HCC

C81.15 **Nodular sclerosis Hodgkin lymphoma, lymph nodes of inguinal region and lower limb** CC HCC

C81.16 **Nodular sclerosis Hodgkin lymphoma, intrapelvic lymph nodes** CC HCC

C81.17 **Nodular sclerosis Hodgkin lymphoma, spleen** CC HCC

C81.18 **Nodular sclerosis Hodgkin lymphoma, lymph nodes of multiple sites** CC HCC

C81.19 **Nodular sclerosis Hodgkin lymphoma, extranodal and solid organ sites** CC HCC

✓5th C81.2 **Mixed cellularity Hodgkin lymphoma**
Mixed cellularity classical Hodgkin lymphoma

C81.2Ø **Mixed cellularity Hodgkin lymphoma, unspecified site** CC HCC

C81.21 **Mixed cellularity Hodgkin lymphoma, lymph nodes of head, face, and neck** CC HCC

C81.22 **Mixed cellularity Hodgkin lymphoma, intrathoracic lymph nodes** CC HCC

C81.23 **Mixed cellularity Hodgkin lymphoma, intra-abdominal lymph nodes** CC HCC

C81.24 **Mixed cellularity Hodgkin lymphoma, lymph nodes of axilla and upper limb** CC HCC

C81.25 **Mixed cellularity Hodgkin lymphoma, lymph nodes of inguinal region and lower limb** CC HCC

C81.26 **Mixed cellularity Hodgkin lymphoma, intrapelvic lymph nodes** CC HCC

C81.27 **Mixed cellularity Hodgkin lymphoma, spleen** CC HCC

C81.28 Mixed cellularity Hodgkin lymphoma, lymph nodes of multiple sites CC HCC
C81.29 Mixed cellularity Hodgkin lymphoma, extranodal and solid organ sites CC HCC

√5th C81.3 Lymphocyte depleted Hodgkin lymphoma
Lymphocyte depleted classical Hodgkin lymphoma
C81.30 Lymphocyte depleted Hodgkin lymphoma, unspecified site CC HCC
C81.31 Lymphocyte depleted Hodgkin lymphoma, lymph nodes of head, face, and neck CC HCC
C81.32 Lymphocyte depleted Hodgkin lymphoma, intrathoracic lymph nodes CC HCC
C81.33 Lymphocyte depleted Hodgkin lymphoma, intra-abdominal lymph nodes CC HCC
C81.34 Lymphocyte depleted Hodgkin lymphoma, lymph nodes of axilla and upper limb CC HCC
C81.35 Lymphocyte depleted Hodgkin lymphoma, lymph nodes of inguinal region and lower limb CC HCC
C81.36 Lymphocyte depleted Hodgkin lymphoma, intrapelvic lymph nodes CC HCC
C81.37 Lymphocyte depleted Hodgkin lymphoma, spleen CC HCC
C81.38 Lymphocyte depleted Hodgkin lymphoma, lymph nodes of multiple sites CC HCC
C81.39 Lymphocyte depleted Hodgkin lymphoma, extranodal and solid organ sites CC HCC

√5th C81.4 Lymphocyte-rich Hodgkin lymphoma
Lymphocyte-rich classical Hodgkin lymphoma
EXCLUDES 1 *nodular lymphocyte predominant Hodgkin lymphoma (C81.0-)*
C81.40 Lymphocyte-rich Hodgkin lymphoma, unspecified site CC HCC
C81.41 Lymphocyte-rich Hodgkin lymphoma, lymph nodes of head, face, and neck CC HCC
C81.42 Lymphocyte-rich Hodgkin lymphoma, intrathoracic lymph nodes CC HCC
C81.43 Lymphocyte-rich Hodgkin lymphoma, intra-abdominal lymph nodes CC HCC
C81.44 Lymphocyte-rich Hodgkin lymphoma, lymph nodes of axilla and upper limb CC HCC
C81.45 Lymphocyte-rich Hodgkin lymphoma, lymph nodes of inguinal region and lower limb CC HCC
C81.46 Lymphocyte-rich Hodgkin lymphoma, intrapelvic lymph nodes CC HCC
C81.47 Lymphocyte-rich Hodgkin lymphoma, spleen CC HCC
C81.48 Lymphocyte-rich Hodgkin lymphoma, lymph nodes of multiple sites CC HCC
C81.49 Lymphocyte-rich Hodgkin lymphoma, extranodal and solid organ sites CC HCC

√5th C81.7 Other Hodgkin lymphoma
Classical Hodgkin lymphoma NOS
Other classical Hodgkin lymphoma
C81.70 Other Hodgkin lymphoma, unspecified site CC HCC
C81.71 Other Hodgkin lymphoma, lymph nodes of head, face, and neck CC HCC
C81.72 Other Hodgkin lymphoma, intrathoracic lymph nodes CC HCC
C81.73 Other Hodgkin lymphoma, intra-abdominal lymph nodes CC HCC
C81.74 Other Hodgkin lymphoma, lymph nodes of axilla and upper limb CC HCC
C81.75 Other Hodgkin lymphoma, lymph nodes of inguinal region and lower limb CC HCC
C81.76 Other Hodgkin lymphoma, intrapelvic lymph nodes CC HCC
C81.77 Other Hodgkin lymphoma, spleen CC HCC
C81.78 Other Hodgkin lymphoma, lymph nodes of multiple sites CC HCC
C81.79 Other Hodgkin lymphoma, extranodal and solid organ sites CC HCC

√5th C81.9 Hodgkin lymphoma, unspecified
C81.90 Hodgkin lymphoma, unspecified, unspecified site CC HCC
C81.91 Hodgkin lymphoma, unspecified, lymph nodes of head, face, and neck CC HCC
C81.92 Hodgkin lymphoma, unspecified, intrathoracic lymph nodes CC HCC
C81.93 Hodgkin lymphoma, unspecified, intra-abdominal lymph nodes CC HCC
C81.94 Hodgkin lymphoma, unspecified, lymph nodes of axilla and upper limb CC HCC
C81.95 Hodgkin lymphoma, unspecified, lymph nodes of inguinal region and lower limb CC HCC
C81.96 Hodgkin lymphoma, unspecified, intrapelvic lymph nodes CC HCC
C81.97 Hodgkin lymphoma, unspecified, spleen CC HCC
C81.98 Hodgkin lymphoma, unspecified, lymph nodes of multiple sites CC HCC
C81.99 Hodgkin lymphoma, unspecified, extranodal and solid organ sites CC HCC

√4th C82 Follicular lymphoma
INCLUDES follicular lymphoma with or without diffuse areas
EXCLUDES 1 *mature T/NK-cell lymphomas (C84.-)*
personal history of non-Hodgkin lymphoma (Z85.72)
DEF: Most common subgroup of non-Hodgkin lymphomas (NHL), accounting for 20 to 30 percent of all NHLs. NHL is a B-cell lymphoma that is slow growing and characterized by the circular pattern of malignant cell growth with the cells clustered into identifiable nodules or follicles.

√5th C82.0 Follicular lymphoma grade I
C82.00 Follicular lymphoma grade I, unspecified site CC HCC
C82.01 Follicular lymphoma grade I, lymph nodes of head, face, and neck CC HCC
C82.02 Follicular lymphoma grade I, intrathoracic lymph nodes CC HCC
C82.03 Follicular lymphoma grade I, intra-abdominal lymph nodes CC HCC
C82.04 Follicular lymphoma grade I, lymph nodes of axilla and upper limb CC HCC
C82.05 Follicular lymphoma grade I, lymph nodes of inguinal region and lower limb CC HCC
C82.06 Follicular lymphoma grade I, intrapelvic lymph nodes CC HCC
C82.07 Follicular lymphoma grade I, spleen CC HCC
C82.08 Follicular lymphoma grade I, lymph nodes of multiple sites CC HCC
C82.09 Follicular lymphoma grade I, extranodal and solid organ sites CC HCC

√5th C82.1 Follicular lymphoma grade II
C82.10 Follicular lymphoma grade II, unspecified site CC HCC
C82.11 Follicular lymphoma grade II, lymph nodes of head, face, and neck CC HCC
C82.12 Follicular lymphoma grade II, intrathoracic lymph nodes CC HCC
C82.13 Follicular lymphoma grade II, intra-abdominal lymph nodes CC HCC
C82.14 Follicular lymphoma grade II, lymph nodes of axilla and upper limb CC HCC
C82.15 Follicular lymphoma grade II, lymph nodes of inguinal region and lower limb CC HCC
C82.16 Follicular lymphoma grade II, intrapelvic lymph nodes CC HCC
C82.17 Follicular lymphoma grade II, spleen CC HCC
C82.18 Follicular lymphoma grade II, lymph nodes of multiple sites CC HCC
C82.19 Follicular lymphoma grade II, extranodal and solid organ sites CC HCC

√5th C82.2 Follicular lymphoma grade III, unspecified
C82.20 Follicular lymphoma grade III, unspecified, unspecified site CC HCC
C82.21 Follicular lymphoma grade III, unspecified, lymph nodes of head, face, and neck CC HCC
C82.22 Follicular lymphoma grade III, unspecified, intrathoracic lymph nodes CC HCC
C82.23 Follicular lymphoma grade III, unspecified, intra-abdominal lymph nodes CC HCC
C82.24 Follicular lymphoma grade III, unspecified, lymph nodes of axilla and upper limb CC HCC
C82.25 Follicular lymphoma grade III, unspecified, lymph nodes of inguinal region and lower limb CC HCC
C82.26 Follicular lymphoma grade III, unspecified, intrapelvic lymph nodes CC HCC
C82.27 Follicular lymphoma grade III, unspecified, spleen CC HCC

C82.28 Follicular lymphoma grade III, unspecified, lymph nodes of multiple sites CC HCC
C82.29 Follicular lymphoma grade III, unspecified, extranodal and solid organ sites CC HCC

✓5th C82.3 Follicular lymphoma grade IIIa
C82.3Ø Follicular lymphoma grade IIIa, unspecified site CC HCC
C82.31 Follicular lymphoma grade IIIa, lymph nodes of head, face, and neck CC HCC
C82.32 Follicular lymphoma grade IIIa, intrathoracic lymph nodes CC HCC
C82.33 Follicular lymphoma grade IIIa, intra-abdominal lymph nodes CC HCC
C82.34 Follicular lymphoma grade IIIa, lymph nodes of axilla and upper limb CC HCC
C82.35 Follicular lymphoma grade IIIa, lymph nodes of inguinal region and lower limb CC HCC
C82.36 Follicular lymphoma grade IIIa, intrapelvic lymph nodes CC HCC
C82.37 Follicular lymphoma grade IIIa, spleen CC HCC
C82.38 Follicular lymphoma grade IIIa, lymph nodes of multiple sites CC HCC
C82.39 Follicular lymphoma grade IIIa, extranodal and solid organ sites CC HCC

✓5th C82.4 Follicular lymphoma grade IIIb
C82.4Ø Follicular lymphoma grade IIIb, unspecified site CC HCC
C82.41 Follicular lymphoma grade IIIb, lymph nodes of head, face, and neck CC HCC
C82.42 Follicular lymphoma grade IIIb, intrathoracic lymph nodes CC HCC
C82.43 Follicular lymphoma grade IIIb, intra-abdominal lymph nodes CC HCC
C82.44 Follicular lymphoma grade IIIb, lymph nodes of axilla and upper limb CC HCC
C82.45 Follicular lymphoma grade IIIb, lymph nodes of inguinal region and lower limb CC HCC
C82.46 Follicular lymphoma grade IIIb, intrapelvic lymph nodes CC HCC
C82.47 Follicular lymphoma grade IIIb, spleen CC HCC
C82.48 Follicular lymphoma grade IIIb, lymph nodes of multiple sites CC HCC
C82.49 Follicular lymphoma grade IIIb, extranodal and solid organ sites CC HCC

✓5th C82.5 Diffuse follicle center lymphoma
C82.5Ø Diffuse follicle center lymphoma, unspecified site HIV CC HCC
C82.51 Diffuse follicle center lymphoma, lymph nodes of head, face, and neck HIV CC HCC
C82.52 Diffuse follicle center lymphoma, intrathoracic lymph nodes HIV CC HCC
C82.53 Diffuse follicle center lymphoma, intra-abdominal lymph nodes HIV CC HCC
C82.54 Diffuse follicle center lymphoma, lymph nodes of axilla and upper limb HIV CC HCC
C82.55 Diffuse follicle center lymphoma, lymph nodes of inguinal region and lower limb HIV CC HCC
C82.56 Diffuse follicle center lymphoma, intrapelvic lymph nodes HIV CC HCC
C82.57 Diffuse follicle center lymphoma, spleen HIV CC HCC
C82.58 Diffuse follicle center lymphoma, lymph nodes of multiple sites HIV CC HCC
C82.59 Diffuse follicle center lymphoma, extranodal and solid organ sites HIV CC HCC

✓5th C82.6 Cutaneous follicle center lymphoma
C82.6Ø Cutaneous follicle center lymphoma, unspecified site CC HCC
C82.61 Cutaneous follicle center lymphoma, lymph nodes of head, face, and neck CC HCC
C82.62 Cutaneous follicle center lymphoma, intrathoracic lymph nodes CC HCC
C82.63 Cutaneous follicle center lymphoma, intra-abdominal lymph nodes CC HCC
C82.64 Cutaneous follicle center lymphoma, lymph nodes of axilla and upper limb CC HCC
C82.65 Cutaneous follicle center lymphoma, lymph nodes of inguinal region and lower limb CC HCC
C82.66 Cutaneous follicle center lymphoma, intrapelvic lymph nodes CC HCC
C82.67 Cutaneous follicle center lymphoma, spleen CC HCC
C82.68 Cutaneous follicle center lymphoma, lymph nodes of multiple sites CC HCC
C82.69 Cutaneous follicle center lymphoma, extranodal and solid organ sites CC HCC

✓5th C82.8 Other types of follicular lymphoma
C82.8Ø Other types of follicular lymphoma, unspecified site CC HCC
C82.81 Other types of follicular lymphoma, lymph nodes of head, face, and neck CC HCC
C82.82 Other types of follicular lymphoma, intrathoracic lymph nodes CC HCC
C82.83 Other types of follicular lymphoma, intra-abdominal lymph nodes CC HCC
C82.84 Other types of follicular lymphoma, lymph nodes of axilla and upper limb CC HCC
C82.85 Other types of follicular lymphoma, lymph nodes of inguinal region and lower limb CC HCC
C82.86 Other types of follicular lymphoma, intrapelvic lymph nodes CC HCC
C82.87 Other types of follicular lymphoma, spleen CC HCC
C82.88 Other types of follicular lymphoma, lymph nodes of multiple sites CC HCC
C82.89 Other types of follicular lymphoma, extranodal and solid organ sites CC HCC

✓5th C82.9 Follicular lymphoma, unspecified
C82.9Ø Follicular lymphoma, unspecified, unspecified site CC HCC
C82.91 Follicular lymphoma, unspecified, lymph nodes of head, face, and neck CC HCC
C82.92 Follicular lymphoma, unspecified, intrathoracic lymph nodes CC HCC
C82.93 Follicular lymphoma, unspecified, intra-abdominal lymph nodes CC HCC
C82.94 Follicular lymphoma, unspecified, lymph nodes of axilla and upper limb CC HCC
C82.95 Follicular lymphoma, unspecified, lymph nodes of inguinal region and lower limb CC HCC
C82.96 Follicular lymphoma, unspecified, intrapelvic lymph nodes CC HCC
C82.97 Follicular lymphoma, unspecified, spleen CC HCC
C82.98 Follicular lymphoma, unspecified, lymph nodes of multiple sites CC HCC
C82.99 Follicular lymphoma, unspecified, extranodal and solid organ sites CC HCC

✓4th C83 Non-follicular lymphoma
EXCLUDES 1 *personal history of non-Hodgkin lymphoma (Z85.72)*

✓5th C83.Ø Small cell B-cell lymphoma
Lymphoplasmacytic lymphoma
Nodal marginal zone lymphoma
Non-leukemic variant of B-CLL
Splenic marginal zone lymphoma
EXCLUDES 1 *chronic lymphocytic leukemia (C91.1)*
mature T/NK-cell lymphomas (C84.-)
Waldenström macroglobulinemia (C88.Ø)
DEF: Nonfollicular lymphoma that is rare, slow growing, and usually found in the older population.
C83.ØØ Small cell B-cell lymphoma, unspecified site HIV CC HCC
C83.Ø1 Small cell B-cell lymphoma, lymph nodes of head, face, and neck HIV CC HCC
C83.Ø2 Small cell B-cell lymphoma, intrathoracic lymph nodes HIV CC HCC
C83.Ø3 Small cell B-cell lymphoma, intra-abdominal lymph nodes HIV CC HCC
C83.Ø4 Small cell B-cell lymphoma, lymph nodes of axilla and upper limb HIV CC HCC
C83.Ø5 Small cell B-cell lymphoma, lymph nodes of inguinal region and lower limb HIV CC HCC
C83.Ø6 Small cell B-cell lymphoma, intrapelvic lymph nodes HIV CC HCC
C83.Ø7 Small cell B-cell lymphoma, spleen HIV CC HCC
C83.Ø8 Small cell B-cell lymphoma, lymph nodes of multiple sites HIV CC HCC

C83.Ø9 **Small cell B-cell lymphoma, extranodal and solid organ sites** HIV CC HCC

✓5th **C83.1 Mantle cell lymphoma**

Centrocytic lymphoma
Malignant lymphomatous polyposis
DEF: Rare form of B-cell non-Hodgkin lymphoma named for the location of the tumor cell production, the mantle zone of the lymph nodes.

C83.1Ø **Mantle cell lymphoma, unspecified site** HIV CC HCC
C83.11 **Mantle cell lymphoma, lymph nodes of head, face, and neck** HIV CC HCC
C83.12 **Mantle cell lymphoma, intrathoracic lymph nodes** HIV CC HCC
C83.13 **Mantle cell lymphoma, intra-abdominal lymph nodes** HIV CC HCC
C83.14 **Mantle cell lymphoma, lymph nodes of axilla and upper limb** HIV CC HCC
C83.15 **Mantle cell lymphoma, lymph nodes of inguinal region and lower limb** HIV CC HCC
C83.16 **Mantle cell lymphoma, intrapelvic lymph nodes** HIV CC HCC
C83.17 **Mantle cell lymphoma, spleen** HIV CC HCC
C83.18 **Mantle cell lymphoma, lymph nodes of multiple sites** HIV CC HCC
C83.19 **Mantle cell lymphoma, extranodal and solid organ sites** HIV CC HCC

✓5th **C83.3 Diffuse large B-cell lymphoma**

Anaplastic diffuse large B-cell lymphoma
CD3Ø-positive diffuse large B-cell lymphoma
Centroblastic diffuse large B-cell lymphoma
Diffuse large B-cell lymphoma, subtype not specified
Immunoblastic diffuse large B-cell lymphoma
Plasmablastic diffuse large B-cell lymphoma
T-cell rich diffuse large B-cell lymphoma
EXCLUDES 1 *mediastinal (thymic) large B-cell lymphoma (C85.2-)*
mature T/NK-cell lymphomas (C84.-)
DEF: Nonfollicular lymphoma that is one of the more common types of lymphoma. This cancer is fast growing and affects any age but is found mostly in the older population.

C83.3Ø **Diffuse large B-cell lymphoma, unspecified site** HIV CC HCC
C83.31 **Diffuse large B-cell lymphoma, lymph nodes of head, face, and neck** HIV CC HCC
C83.32 **Diffuse large B-cell lymphoma, intrathoracic lymph nodes** HIV CC HCC
C83.33 **Diffuse large B-cell lymphoma, intra-abdominal lymph nodes** HIV CC HCC
C83.34 **Diffuse large B-cell lymphoma, lymph nodes of axilla and upper limb** HIV CC HCC
C83.35 **Diffuse large B-cell lymphoma, lymph nodes of inguinal region and lower limb** HIV CC HCC
C83.36 **Diffuse large B-cell lymphoma, intrapelvic lymph nodes** HIV CC HCC
C83.37 **Diffuse large B-cell lymphoma, spleen** HIV CC HCC
C83.38 **Diffuse large B-cell lymphoma, lymph nodes of multiple sites** HIV CC HCC
C83.39 **Diffuse large B-cell lymphoma, extranodal and solid organ sites** HIV CC HCC

✓5th **C83.5 Lymphoblastic (diffuse) lymphoma**

B-precursor lymphoma
Lymphoblastic B-cell lymphoma
Lymphoblastic lymphoma NOS
Lymphoblastic T-cell lymphoma
T-precursor lymphoma
DEF: Type of non-Hodgkin lymphoma considered lymphoma or leukemia—the determination is made based on the amount of bone marrow involvement. The cells are small to medium immature T-cells that often originate in the thymus where many of the T-cells are made.

C83.5Ø **Lymphoblastic (diffuse) lymphoma, unspecified site** CC HCC
C83.51 **Lymphoblastic (diffuse) lymphoma, lymph nodes of head, face, and neck** CC HCC
C83.52 **Lymphoblastic (diffuse) lymphoma, intrathoracic lymph nodes** CC HCC
C83.53 **Lymphoblastic (diffuse) lymphoma, intra-abdominal lymph nodes** CC HCC
C83.54 **Lymphoblastic (diffuse) lymphoma, lymph nodes of axilla and upper limb** CC HCC
C83.55 **Lymphoblastic (diffuse) lymphoma, lymph nodes of inguinal region and lower limb** CC HCC
C83.56 **Lymphoblastic (diffuse) lymphoma, intrapelvic lymph nodes** CC HCC
C83.57 **Lymphoblastic (diffuse) lymphoma, spleen** CC HCC
C83.58 **Lymphoblastic (diffuse) lymphoma, lymph nodes of multiple sites** CC HCC
C83.59 **Lymphoblastic (diffuse) lymphoma, extranodal and solid organ sites** CC HCC

✓5th **C83.7 Burkitt lymphoma**

Atypical Burkitt lymphoma
Burkitt-like lymphoma
EXCLUDES 1 *mature B-cell leukemia Burkitt type (C91.A-)*
DEF: Malignancy of the lymphatic system, most often seen as a large bone-deteriorating lesion within the jaw or as an abdominal mass. It is a form of non-Hodgkin's lymphoma and is recognized as the fastest growing human tumor.

C83.7Ø **Burkitt lymphoma, unspecified site** HIV CC HCC
C83.71 **Burkitt lymphoma, lymph nodes of head, face, and neck** HIV CC HCC
C83.72 **Burkitt lymphoma, intrathoracic lymph nodes** HIV CC HCC
C83.73 **Burkitt lymphoma, intra-abdominal lymph nodes** HIV CC HCC
C83.74 **Burkitt lymphoma, lymph nodes of axilla and upper limb** HIV CC HCC
C83.75 **Burkitt lymphoma, lymph nodes of inguinal region and lower limb** HIV CC HCC
C83.76 **Burkitt lymphoma, intrapelvic lymph nodes** HIV CC HCC
C83.77 **Burkitt lymphoma, spleen** HIV CC HCC
C83.78 **Burkitt lymphoma, lymph nodes of multiple sites** HIV CC HCC
C83.79 **Burkitt lymphoma, extranodal and solid organ sites** HIV CC HCC

✓5th **C83.8 Other non-follicular lymphoma**

Intravascular large B-cell lymphoma
Lymphoid granulomatosis
Primary effusion B-cell lymphoma
EXCLUDES 1 *mediastinal (thymic) large B-cell lymphoma (C85.2-)*
T-cell rich B-cell lymphoma (C83.3-)

C83.8Ø **Other non-follicular lymphoma, unspecified site** HIV CC HCC
C83.81 **Other non-follicular lymphoma, lymph nodes of head, face, and neck** HIV CC HCC
C83.82 **Other non-follicular lymphoma, intrathoracic lymph nodes** HIV CC HCC
C83.83 **Other non-follicular lymphoma, intra-abdominal lymph nodes** HIV CC HCC
C83.84 **Other non-follicular lymphoma, lymph nodes of axilla and upper limb** HIV CC HCC
C83.85 **Other non-follicular lymphoma, lymph nodes of inguinal region and lower limb** HIV CC HCC
C83.86 **Other non-follicular lymphoma, intrapelvic lymph nodes** HIV CC HCC
C83.87 **Other non-follicular lymphoma, spleen** HIV CC HCC
C83.88 **Other non-follicular lymphoma, lymph nodes of multiple sites** HIV CC HCC
C83.89 **Other non-follicular lymphoma, extranodal and solid organ sites** HIV CC HCC

✓5th **C83.9 Non-follicular (diffuse) lymphoma, unspecified**

C83.9Ø **Non-follicular (diffuse) lymphoma, unspecified, unspecified site** HIV CC HCC
C83.91 **Non-follicular (diffuse) lymphoma, unspecified, lymph nodes of head, face, and neck** HIV CC HCC
C83.92 **Non-follicular (diffuse) lymphoma, unspecified, intrathoracic lymph nodes** HIV CC HCC
C83.93 **Non-follicular (diffuse) lymphoma, unspecified, intra-abdominal lymph nodes** HIV CC HCC
C83.94 **Non-follicular (diffuse) lymphoma, unspecified, lymph nodes of axilla and upper limb** HIV CC HCC
C83.95 **Non-follicular (diffuse) lymphoma, unspecified, lymph nodes of inguinal region and lower limb** HIV CC HCC

C83.96 **Non-follicular (diffuse) lymphoma, unspecified, intrapelvic lymph nodes** HIV CC HCC

C83.97 **Non-follicular (diffuse) lymphoma, unspecified, spleen** HIV CC HCC

C83.98 **Non-follicular (diffuse) lymphoma, unspecified, lymph nodes of multiple sites** HIV CC HCC

C83.99 **Non-follicular (diffuse) lymphoma, unspecified, extranodal and solid organ sites** HIV CC HCC

✓4th C84 Mature T/NK-cell lymphomas

EXCLUDES 1 *personal history of non-Hodgkin lymphoma (Z85.72)*

✓5th C84.0 Mycosis fungoides

EXCLUDES 1 *peripheral T-cell lymphoma, not classified (C84.4-)*

DEF: Most common form of cutaneous T-cell lymphoma. A type of non-Hodgkin lymphoma in which white blood cells become cancerous and affect the skin and sometimes internal organs.

Synonym(s): *Alibert-Bazin syndrome.*

C84.00 **Mycosis fungoides, unspecified site** CC HCC

C84.01 **Mycosis fungoides, lymph nodes of head, face, and neck** CC HCC

C84.02 **Mycosis fungoides, intrathoracic lymph nodes** CC HCC

C84.03 **Mycosis fungoides, intra-abdominal lymph nodes** CC HCC

C84.04 **Mycosis fungoides, lymph nodes of axilla and upper limb** CC HCC

C84.05 **Mycosis fungoides, lymph nodes of inguinal region and lower limb** CC HCC

C84.06 **Mycosis fungoides, intrapelvic lymph nodes** CC HCC

C84.07 **Mycosis fungoides, spleen** CC HCC

C84.08 **Mycosis fungoides, lymph nodes of multiple sites** CC HCC

C84.09 **Mycosis fungoides, extranodal and solid organ sites** CC HCC

✓5th C84.1 Sézary disease

DEF: Extension of mycosis fungoides that affects the blood and all of the skin, appearing as sunburn, rather than patches. It spreads to the lymph nodes and is often linked to a weakened immune system.

C84.10 **Sézary disease, unspecified site** CC HCC

C84.11 **Sézary disease, lymph nodes of head, face, and neck** CC HCC

C84.12 **Sézary disease, intrathoracic lymph nodes** CC HCC

C84.13 **Sézary disease, intra-abdominal lymph nodes** CC HCC

C84.14 **Sézary disease, lymph nodes of axilla and upper limb** CC HCC

C84.15 **Sézary disease, lymph nodes of inguinal region and lower limb** CC HCC

C84.16 **Sézary disease, intrapelvic lymph nodes** CC HCC

C84.17 **Sézary disease, spleen** CC HCC

C84.18 **Sézary disease, lymph nodes of multiple sites** CC HCC

C84.19 **Sézary disease, extranodal and solid organ sites** CC HCC

✓5th C84.4 Peripheral T-cell lymphoma, not classified

Lennert's lymphoma
Lymphoepithelioid lymphoma
Mature T-cell lymphoma, not elsewhere classified

C84.40 **Peripheral T-cell lymphoma, not classified, unspecified site** HIV CC HCC

C84.41 **Peripheral T-cell lymphoma, not classified, lymph nodes of head, face, and neck** HIV CC HCC

C84.42 **Peripheral T-cell lymphoma, not classified, intrathoracic lymph nodes** HIV CC HCC

C84.43 **Peripheral T-cell lymphoma, not classified, intra-abdominal lymph nodes** HIV CC HCC

C84.44 **Peripheral T-cell lymphoma, not classified, lymph nodes of axilla and upper limb** HIV CC HCC

C84.45 **Peripheral T-cell lymphoma, not classified, lymph nodes of inguinal region and lower limb** HIV CC HCC

C84.46 **Peripheral T-cell lymphoma, not classified, intrapelvic lymph nodes** HIV CC HCC

C84.47 **Peripheral T-cell lymphoma, not classified, spleen** HIV CC HCC

C84.48 **Peripheral T-cell lymphoma, not classified, lymph nodes of multiple sites** HIV CC HCC

C84.49 **Peripheral T-cell lymphoma, not classified, extranodal and solid organ sites** HIV CC HCC

✓5th C84.6 Anaplastic large cell lymphoma, ALK-positive

Anaplastic large cell lymphoma, CD30-positive

C84.60 **Anaplastic large cell lymphoma, ALK-positive, unspecified site** HIV CC HCC

C84.61 **Anaplastic large cell lymphoma, ALK-positive, lymph nodes of head, face, and neck** HIV CC HCC

C84.62 **Anaplastic large cell lymphoma, ALK-positive, intrathoracic lymph nodes** HIV CC HCC

C84.63 **Anaplastic large cell lymphoma, ALK-positive, intra-abdominal lymph nodes** HIV CC HCC

C84.64 **Anaplastic large cell lymphoma, ALK-positive, lymph nodes of axilla and upper limb** HIV CC HCC

C84.65 **Anaplastic large cell lymphoma, ALK-positive, lymph nodes of inguinal region and lower limb** HIV CC HCC

C84.66 **Anaplastic large cell lymphoma, ALK-positive, intrapelvic lymph nodes** HIV CC HCC

C84.67 **Anaplastic large cell lymphoma, ALK-positive, spleen** HIV CC HCC

C84.68 **Anaplastic large cell lymphoma, ALK-positive, lymph nodes of multiple sites** HIV CC HCC

C84.69 **Anaplastic large cell lymphoma, ALK-positive, extranodal and solid organ sites** HIV CC HCC

✓5th C84.7 Anaplastic large cell lymphoma, ALK-negative

EXCLUDES 1 *primary cutaneous CD30-positive T-cell proliferations (C86.6-)*

C84.70 **Anaplastic large cell lymphoma, ALK-negative, unspecified site** HIV CC HCC

C84.71 **Anaplastic large cell lymphoma, ALK-negative, lymph nodes of head, face, and neck** HIV CC HCC

C84.72 **Anaplastic large cell lymphoma, ALK-negative, intrathoracic lymph nodes** HIV CC HCC

C84.73 **Anaplastic large cell lymphoma, ALK-negative, intra-abdominal lymph nodes** HIV CC HCC

C84.74 **Anaplastic large cell lymphoma, ALK-negative, lymph nodes of axilla and upper limb** HIV CC HCC

C84.75 **Anaplastic large cell lymphoma, ALK-negative, lymph nodes of inguinal region and lower limb** HIV CC HCC

C84.76 **Anaplastic large cell lymphoma, ALK-negative, intrapelvic lymph nodes** HIV CC HCC

C84.77 **Anaplastic large cell lymphoma, ALK-negative, spleen** HIV CC HCC

C84.78 **Anaplastic large cell lymphoma, ALK-negative, lymph nodes of multiple sites** HIV CC HCC

C84.79 **Anaplastic large cell lymphoma, ALK-negative, extranodal and solid organ sites** HIV CC HCC

✓5th C84.A Cutaneous T-cell lymphoma, unspecified

C84.A0 **Cutaneous T-cell lymphoma, unspecified, unspecified site** HIV CC HCC

C84.A1 **Cutaneous T-cell lymphoma, unspecified lymph nodes of head, face, and neck** HIV CC HCC

C84.A2 **Cutaneous T-cell lymphoma, unspecified, intrathoracic lymph nodes** HIV CC HCC

C84.A3 **Cutaneous T-cell lymphoma, unspecified, intra-abdominal lymph nodes** HIV CC HCC

C84.A4 **Cutaneous T-cell lymphoma, unspecified, lymph nodes of axilla and upper limb** HIV CC HCC

C84.A5 **Cutaneous T-cell lymphoma, unspecified, lymph nodes of inguinal region and lower limb** HIV CC HCC

C84.A6 **Cutaneous T-cell lymphoma, unspecified, intrapelvic lymph nodes** HIV CC HCC

C84.A7 **Cutaneous T-cell lymphoma, unspecified, spleen** HIV CC HCC

C84.A8 **Cutaneous T-cell lymphoma, unspecified, lymph nodes of multiple sites** HIV CC HCC

C84.A9 **Cutaneous T-cell lymphoma, unspecified, extranodal and solid organ sites** HIV CC HCC

√5th **C84.Z Other mature T/NK-cell lymphomas**

NOTE If T-cell lineage or involvement is mentioned in conjunction with a specific lymphoma, code to the more specific description.

EXCLUDES 1 *angioimmunoblastic T-cell lymphoma (C86.5)*
blastic NK-cell lymphoma (C86.4)
enteropathy-type T-cell lymphoma (C86.2)
extranodal NK-cell lymphoma, nasal type (C86.0)
hepatosplenic T-cell lymphoma (C86.1)
primary cutaneous CD30-positive T-cell proliferations (C86.6)
subcutaneous panniculitis-like T-cell lymphoma (C86.3)
T-cell leukemia (C91.1-)

C84.Z0 Other mature T/NK-cell lymphomas, unspecified site HIV CC HCC
C84.Z1 Other mature T/NK-cell lymphomas, lymph nodes of head, face, and neck HIV CC HCC
C84.Z2 Other mature T/NK-cell lymphomas, intrathoracic lymph nodes HIV CC HCC
C84.Z3 Other mature T/NK-cell lymphomas, intra-abdominal lymph nodes HIV CC HCC
C84.Z4 Other mature T/NK-cell lymphomas, lymph nodes of axilla and upper limb HIV CC HCC
C84.Z5 Other mature T/NK-cell lymphomas, lymph nodes of inguinal region and lower limb HIV CC HCC
C84.Z6 Other mature T/NK-cell lymphomas, intrapelvic lymph nodes HIV CC HCC
C84.Z7 Other mature T/NK-cell lymphomas, spleen HIV CC HCC
C84.Z8 Other mature T/NK-cell lymphomas, lymph nodes of multiple sites HIV CC HCC
C84.Z9 Other mature T/NK-cell lymphomas, extranodal and solid organ sites HIV CC HCC

√5th **C84.9 Mature T/NK-cell lymphomas, unspecified**

NK/T cell lymphoma NOS

EXCLUDES 1 *mature T-cell lymphoma, not elsewhere classified (C84.4-)*

C84.90 Mature T/NK-cell lymphomas, unspecified, unspecified site HIV CC HCC
C84.91 Mature T/NK-cell lymphomas, unspecified, lymph nodes of head, face, and neck HIV CC HCC
C84.92 Mature T/NK-cell lymphomas, unspecified, intrathoracic lymph nodes HIV CC HCC
C84.93 Mature T/NK-cell lymphomas, unspecified, intra-abdominal lymph nodes HIV CC HCC
C84.94 Mature T/NK-cell lymphomas, unspecified, lymph nodes of axilla and upper limb HIV CC HCC
C84.95 Mature T/NK-cell lymphomas, unspecified, lymph nodes of inguinal region and lower limb HIV CC HCC
C84.96 Mature T/NK-cell lymphomas, unspecified, intrapelvic lymph nodes HIV CC HCC
C84.97 Mature T/NK-cell lymphomas, unspecified, spleen HIV CC HCC
C84.98 Mature T/NK-cell lymphomas, unspecified, lymph nodes of multiple sites HIV CC HCC
C84.99 Mature T/NK-cell lymphomas, unspecified, extranodal and solid organ sites HIV CC HCC

√4th **C85 Other specified and unspecified types of non-Hodgkin lymphoma**

EXCLUDES 1 *other specified types of T/NK-cell lymphoma (C86.-)*
personal history of non-Hodgkin lymphoma (Z85.72)

√5th **C85.1 Unspecified B-cell lymphoma**

NOTE If B-cell lineage or involvement is mentioned in conjunction with a specific lymphoma, code to the more specific description.

C85.10 Unspecified B-cell lymphoma, unspecified site HIV CC HCC
C85.11 Unspecified B-cell lymphoma, lymph nodes of head, face, and neck HIV CC HCC
C85.12 Unspecified B-cell lymphoma, intrathoracic lymph nodes HIV CC HCC
C85.13 Unspecified B-cell lymphoma, intra-abdominal lymph nodes HIV CC HCC
C85.14 Unspecified B-cell lymphoma, lymph nodes of axilla and upper limb HIV CC HCC
C85.15 Unspecified B-cell lymphoma, lymph nodes of inguinal region and lower limb HIV CC HCC
C85.16 Unspecified B-cell lymphoma, intrapelvic lymph nodes HIV CC HCC
C85.17 Unspecified B-cell lymphoma, spleen HIV CC HCC
C85.18 Unspecified B-cell lymphoma, lymph nodes of multiple sites HIV CC HCC
C85.19 Unspecified B-cell lymphoma, extranodal and solid organ sites HIV CC HCC

√5th **C85.2 Mediastinal (thymic) large B-cell lymphoma**

C85.20 Mediastinal (thymic) large B-cell lymphoma, unspecified site HIV CC HCC
C85.21 Mediastinal (thymic) large B-cell lymphoma, lymph nodes of head, face, and neck HIV CC HCC
C85.22 Mediastinal (thymic) large B-cell lymphoma, intrathoracic lymph nodes HIV CC HCC
C85.23 Mediastinal (thymic) large B-cell lymphoma, intra-abdominal lymph nodes HIV CC HCC
C85.24 Mediastinal (thymic) large B-cell lymphoma, lymph nodes of axilla and upper limb HIV CC HCC
C85.25 Mediastinal (thymic) large B-cell lymphoma, lymph nodes of inguinal region and lower limb HIV CC HCC
C85.26 Mediastinal (thymic) large B-cell lymphoma, intrapelvic lymph nodes HIV CC HCC
C85.27 Mediastinal (thymic) large B-cell lymphoma, spleen HIV CC HCC
C85.28 Mediastinal (thymic) large B-cell lymphoma, lymph nodes of multiple sites HIV CC HCC
C85.29 Mediastinal (thymic) large B-cell lymphoma, extranodal and solid organ sites HIV CC HCC

√5th **C85.8 Other specified types of non-Hodgkin lymphoma**

C85.80 Other specified types of non-Hodgkin lymphoma, unspecified site HIV CC HCC
C85.81 Other specified types of non-Hodgkin lymphoma, lymph nodes of head, face, and neck HIV CC HCC
C85.82 Other specified types of non-Hodgkin lymphoma, intrathoracic lymph nodes HIV CC HCC
C85.83 Other specified types of non-Hodgkin lymphoma, intra-abdominal lymph nodes HIV CC HCC
C85.84 Other specified types of non-Hodgkin lymphoma, lymph nodes of axilla and upper limb HIV CC HCC
C85.85 Other specified types of non-Hodgkin lymphoma, lymph nodes of inguinal region and lower limb HIV CC HCC
C85.86 Other specified types of non-Hodgkin lymphoma, intrapelvic lymph nodes HIV CC HCC
C85.87 Other specified types of non-Hodgkin lymphoma, spleen HIV CC HCC
C85.88 Other specified types of non-Hodgkin lymphoma, lymph nodes of multiple sites HIV CC HCC
C85.89 Other specified types of non-Hodgkin lymphoma, extranodal and solid organ sites HIV CC HCC

√5th **C85.9 Non-Hodgkin lymphoma, unspecified**

Lymphoma NOS
Malignant lymphoma NOS
Non-Hodgkin lymphoma NOS

C85.90 Non-Hodgkin lymphoma, unspecified, unspecified site HIV CC HCC
C85.91 Non-Hodgkin lymphoma, unspecified, lymph nodes of head, face, and neck HIV CC HCC
C85.92 Non-Hodgkin lymphoma, unspecified, intrathoracic lymph nodes HIV CC HCC
C85.93 Non-Hodgkin lymphoma, unspecified, intra-abdominal lymph nodes HIV CC HCC
C85.94 Non-Hodgkin lymphoma, unspecified, lymph nodes of axilla and upper limb HIV CC HCC
C85.95 Non-Hodgkin lymphoma, unspecified, lymph nodes of inguinal region and lower limb HIV CC HCC
C85.96 Non-Hodgkin lymphoma, unspecified, intrapelvic lymph nodes HIV CC HCC
C85.97 Non-Hodgkin lymphoma, unspecified, spleen HIV CC HCC
C85.98 Non-Hodgkin lymphoma, unspecified, lymph nodes of multiple sites HIV CC HCC
C85.99 Non-Hodgkin lymphoma, unspecified, extranodal and solid organ sites HIV CC HCC

✓4th C86 Other specified types of T/NK-cell lymphoma

EXCLUDES 1 *anaplastic large cell lymphoma, ALK negative (C84.7-)*
anaplastic large cell lymphoma, ALK positive (C84.6-)
mature T/NK-cell lymphomas (C84.-)
other specified types of non-Hodgkin lymphoma (C85.8-)

C86.Ø Extranodal NK/T-cell lymphoma, nasal type HIV CC HCC

C86.1 Hepatosplenic T-cell lymphoma HIV CC HCC
Alpha-beta and gamma delta types

C86.2 Enteropathy-type (intestinal) T-cell lymphoma HIV CC HCC
Enteropathy associated T-cell lymphoma

C86.3 Subcutaneous panniculitis-like T-cell lymphoma HIV CC HCC

C86.4 Blastic NK-cell lymphoma HIV CC HCC
Blastic plasmacytoid dendritic cell neoplasm (BPDCN)

C86.5 Angioimmunoblastic T-cell lymphoma HIV CC HCC
Angioimmunoblastic lymphadenopathy with dysproteinemia (AILD)

C86.6 Primary cutaneous CD3Ø-positive T-cell proliferations HIV CC HCC
Lymphomatoid papulosis
Primary cutaneous anaplastic large cell lymphoma
Primary cutaneous CD3Ø-positive large T-cell lymphoma

✓4th C88 Malignant immunoproliferative diseases and certain other B-cell lymphomas

EXCLUDES 1 *B-cell lymphoma, unspecified (C85.1-)*
personal history of other malignant neoplasms of lymphoid, hematopoietic and related tissues (Z85.79)

C88.Ø Waldenström macroglobulinemia HCC
Lymphoplasmacytic lymphoma with IgM-production
Macroglobulinemia (idiopathic) (primary)
EXCLUDES 1 *small cell B-cell lymphoma (C83.Ø)*

C88.2 Heavy chain disease CC HCC
Franklin disease
Gamma heavy chain disease
Mu heavy chain disease

C88.3 Immunoproliferative small intestinal disease CC HCC
Alpha heavy chain disease
Mediterranean lymphoma

C88.4 Extranodal marginal zone B-cell lymphoma of mucosa-associated lymphoid tissue [MALT-lymphoma] HIV CC HCC
Lymphoma of skin-associated lymphoid tissue [SALT-lymphoma]
Lymphoma of bronchial-associated lymphoid tissue [BALT-lymphoma]
EXCLUDES 1 *high malignant (diffuse large B-cell) lymphoma (C83.3-)*

C88.8 Other malignant immunoproliferative diseases CC HCC

C88.9 Malignant immunoproliferative disease, unspecified CC HCC
Immunoproliferative disease NOS

✓4th C9Ø Multiple myeloma and malignant plasma cell neoplasms

EXCLUDES 1 *personal history of other malignant neoplasms of lymphoid, hematopoietic and related tissues (Z85.79)*

AHA: 2019,2Q,30

✓5th C9Ø.Ø Multiple myeloma
Kahler's disease
Medullary plasmacytoma
Myelomatosis
Plasma cell myeloma
EXCLUDES 1 *solitary myeloma (C9Ø.3-)*
solitary plasmactyoma (C9Ø.3-)

TIP: Do not assign an additional code for bone metastasis (C79.51) when multiple myeloma is described as metastatic to the bone; bone involvement is integral to this disease process.

C9Ø.ØØ Multiple myeloma not having achieved remission CC HCC
Multiple myeloma with failed remission
Multiple myeloma NOS

C9Ø.Ø1 Multiple myeloma in remission CC HCC

C9Ø.Ø2 Multiple myeloma in relapse CC HCC

✓5th C9Ø.1 Plasma cell leukemia
Plasmacytic leukemia
AHA: 2019,2Q,30

C9Ø.1Ø Plasma cell leukemia not having achieved remission CC HCC
Plasma cell leukemia with failed remission
Plasma cell leukemia NOS

C9Ø.11 Plasma cell leukemia in remission CC HCC

C9Ø.12 Plasma cell leukemia in relapse CC HCC

✓5th C9Ø.2 Extramedullary plasmacytoma

C9Ø.2Ø Extramedullary plasmacytoma not having achieved remission CC HCC
Extramedullary plasmacytoma with failed remission
Extramedullary plasmacytoma NOS

C9Ø.21 Extramedullary plasmacytoma in remission CC HCC

C9Ø.22 Extramedullary plasmacytoma in relapse CC HCC

✓5th C9Ø.3 Solitary plasmacytoma
Localized malignant plasma cell tumor NOS
Plasmacytoma NOS
Solitary myeloma

C9Ø.3Ø Solitary plasmacytoma not having achieved remission CC HCC
Solitary plasmacytoma with failed remission
Solitary plasmacytoma NOS

C9Ø.31 Solitary plasmacytoma in remission CC HCC

C9Ø.32 Solitary plasmacytoma in relapse CC HCC

✓4th C91 Lymphoid leukemia

EXCLUDES 1 *personal history of leukemia (Z85.6)*

AHA: 2020,1Q,13

DEF: Malignant proliferation of immature lymphocytes (white blood cells that make up lymphoid tissue), called lymphoblasts, that originate in the bone marrow. Can be acute (ALL) or chronic (CLL).

✓5th C91.Ø Acute lymphoblastic leukemia [ALL]

NOTE Codes in subcategory C91.Ø- should only be used for T-cell and B-cell precursor leukemia

C91.ØØ Acute lymphoblastic leukemia not having achieved remission CC HCC
Acute lymphoblastic leukemia with failed remission
Acute lymphoblastic leukemia NOS

C91.Ø1 Acute lymphoblastic leukemia, in remission CC HCC

C91.Ø2 Acute lymphoblastic leukemia, in relapse CC HCC

✓5th C91.1 Chronic lymphocytic leukemia of B-cell type
Lymphoplasmacytic leukemia
Richter syndrome
EXCLUDES 1 *lymphoplasmacytic lymphoma (C83.Ø-)*

C91.1Ø Chronic lymphocytic leukemia of B-cell type not having achieved remission CC HCC
Chronic lymphocytic leukemia of B-cell type with failed remission
Chronic lymphocytic leukemia of B-cell type NOS

C91.11 Chronic lymphocytic leukemia of B-cell type in remission CC HCC

C91.12 Chronic lymphocytic leukemia of B-cell type in relapse CC HCC

✓5th C91.3 Prolymphocytic leukemia of B-cell type

C91.3Ø Prolymphocytic leukemia of B-cell type not having achieved remission CC HCC
Prolymphocytic leukemia of B-cell type with failed remission
Prolymphocytic leukemia of B-cell type NOS

C91.31 Prolymphocytic leukemia of B-cell type, in remission CC HCC

C91.32 Prolymphocytic leukemia of B-cell type, in relapse CC HCC

C91.4 Hairy cell leukemia
Leukemic reticuloendotheliosis
DEF: Rare type of leukemia that is slow growing and often also considered a type of lymphoma. The small B-cell lymphocytes appear with "hairy" projections under a microscope and are found mostly in the bone marrow, spleen, and blood.
C91.40 Hairy cell leukemia not having achieved remission CC HCC
Hairy cell leukemia with failed remission
Hairy cell leukemia NOS
C91.41 Hairy cell leukemia, in remission CC HCC
C91.42 Hairy cell leukemia, in relapse CC HCC

C91.5 Adult T-cell lymphoma/leukemia (HTLV-1-associated)
Acute variant of adult T-cell lymphoma/leukemia (HTLV-1-associated)
Chronic variant of adult T-cell lymphoma/leukemia (HTLV-1-associated)
Lymphomatoid variant of adult T-cell lymphoma/leukemia (HTLV-1-associated)
Smouldering variant of adult T-cell lymphoma/leukemia (HTLV-1-associated)
C91.50 Adult T-cell lymphoma/leukemia (HTLV-1-associated) not having achieved remission CC HCC A
Adult T-cell lymphoma/leukemia (HTLV-1-associated) with failed remission
Adult T-cell lymphoma/leukemia (HTLV-1-associated) NOS
C91.51 Adult T-cell lymphoma/leukemia (HTLV-1-associated), in remission CC HCC A
C91.52 Adult T-cell lymphoma/leukemia (HTLV-1-associated), in relapse CC HCC A

C91.6 Prolymphocytic leukemia of T-cell type
C91.60 Prolymphocytic leukemia of T-cell type not having achieved remission CC HCC
Prolymphocytic leukemia of T-cell type with failed remission
Prolymphocytic leukemia of T-cell type NOS
C91.61 Prolymphocytic leukemia of T-cell type, in remission CC HCC
C91.62 Prolymphocytic leukemia of T-cell type, in relapse CC HCC

C91.A Mature B-cell leukemia Burkitt-type
EXCLUDES 1 *Burkitt lymphoma (C83.7-)*
C91.A0 Mature B-cell leukemia Burkitt-type not having achieved remission CC HCC
Mature B-cell leukemia Burkitt-type with failed remission
Mature B-cell leukemia Burkitt-type NOS
C91.A1 Mature B-cell leukemia Burkitt-type, in remission CC HCC
C91.A2 Mature B-cell leukemia Burkitt-type, in relapse CC HCC

C91.Z Other lymphoid leukemia
T-cell large granular lymphocytic leukemia (associated with rheumatoid arthritis)
C91.Z0 Other lymphoid leukemia not having achieved remission CC HCC
Other lymphoid leukemia with failed remission
Other lymphoid leukemia NOS
C91.Z1 Other lymphoid leukemia, in remission CC HCC
C91.Z2 Other lymphoid leukemia, in relapse CC HCC

C91.9 Lymphoid leukemia, unspecified
C91.90 Lymphoid leukemia, unspecified not having achieved remission CC HCC
Lymphoid leukemia with failed remission
Lymphoid leukemia NOS
C91.91 Lymphoid leukemia, unspecified, in remission CC HCC
C91.92 Lymphoid leukemia, unspecified, in relapse CC HCC

C92 Myeloid leukemia
INCLUDES granulocytic leukemia
myelogenous leukemia
EXCLUDES 1 *personal history of leukemia (Z85.6)*
AHA: 2020,1Q,13; 2019,1Q,16
DEF: Cancer that develops in immature myelocytes called myeloblasts. These are the cells that become white blood cells (except lymphocytes), red blood cells, or platelet making cells. Can be acute (AML) or chronic (CML).
TIP: Pancytopenia, although common in some types of myeloid leukemias, is not always inherent. When it is documented, code D61.818 can be assigned in addition to a code from this category.

C92.0 Acute myeloblastic leukemia
Acute myeloblastic leukemia, minimal differentiation
Acute myeloblastic leukemia (with maturation)
Acute myeloblastic leukemia 1/ETO
Acute myeloblastic leukemia M0
Acute myeloblastic leukemia M1
Acute myeloblastic leukemia M2
Acute myeloblastic leukemia with t(8;21)
Acute myeloblastic leukemia (without a FAB classification) NOS
Refractory anemia with excess blasts in transformation [RAEBT]
EXCLUDES 1 *acute exacerbation of chronic myeloid leukemia (C92.10)*
refractory anemia with excess of blasts not in transformation (D46.2-)
AHA: 2018,4Q,87
C92.00 Acute myeloblastic leukemia, not having achieved remission CC HCC
Acute myeloblastic leukemia with failed remission
Acute myeloblastic leukemia NOS
C92.01 Acute myeloblastic leukemia, in remission CC HCC
C92.02 Acute myeloblastic leukemia, in relapse CC HCC

C92.1 Chronic myeloid leukemia, BCR/ABL-positive
Chronic myelogenous leukemia, Philadelphia chromosome (Ph1) positive
Chronic myelogenous leukemia, t(9;22) (q34;q11)
Chronic myelogenous leukemia with crisis of blast cells
EXCLUDES 1 *atypical chronic myeloid leukemia BCR/ABL-negative (C92.2-)*
chronic myelomonocytic leukemia (C93.1-)
chronic myeloproliferative disease (D47.1)
C92.10 Chronic myeloid leukemia, BCR/ABL-positive, not having achieved remission CC HCC
Chronic myeloid leukemia, BCR/ABL-positive with failed remission
Chronic myeloid leukemia, BCR/ABL-positive NOS
C92.11 Chronic myeloid leukemia, BCR/ABL-positive, in remission CC HCC
C92.12 Chronic myeloid leukemia, BCR/ABL-positive, in relapse CC HCC

C92.2 Atypical chronic myeloid leukemia, BCR/ABL-negative
C92.20 Atypical chronic myeloid leukemia, BCR/ABL-negative, not having achieved remission CC HCC
Atypical chronic myeloid leukemia, BCR/ABL-negative with failed remission
Atypical chronic myeloid leukemia, BCR/ABL-negative NOS
C92.21 Atypical chronic myeloid leukemia, BCR/ABL-negative, in remission CC HCC
C92.22 Atypical chronic myeloid leukemia, BCR/ABL-negative, in relapse CC HCC

C92.3 Myeloid sarcoma
A malignant tumor of immature myeloid cells
Chloroma
Granulocytic sarcoma
C92.30 Myeloid sarcoma, not having achieved remission CC HCC
Myeloid sarcoma with failed remission
Myeloid sarcoma NOS
C92.31 Myeloid sarcoma, in remission CC HCC
C92.32 Myeloid sarcoma, in relapse CC HCC

✓5th **C92.4 Acute promyelocytic leukemia**
AML M3
AML Me with t(15;17) and variants
C92.40 Acute promyelocytic leukemia, not having achieved remission CC HCC
Acute promyelocytic leukemia with failed remission
Acute promyelocytic leukemia NOS
C92.41 Acute promyelocytic leukemia, in remission CC HCC
C92.42 Acute promyelocytic leukemia, in relapse CC HCC

✓5th **C92.5 Acute myelomonocytic leukemia**
AML M4
AML M4 Eo with inv(16) or t(16;16)
C92.50 Acute myelomonocytic leukemia, not having achieved remission CC HCC
Acute myelomonocytic leukemia with failed remission
Acute myelomonocytic leukemia NOS
C92.51 Acute myelomonocytic leukemia, in remission CC HCC
C92.52 Acute myelomonocytic leukemia, in relapse CC HCC

✓5th **C92.6 Acute myeloid leukemia with 11q23-abnormality**
Acute myeloid leukemia with variation of MLL-gene
C92.60 Acute myeloid leukemia with 11q23-abnormality not having achieved remission CC HCC
Acute myeloid leukemia with 11q23-abnormality with failed remission
Acute myeloid leukemia with 11q23-abnormality NOS
C92.61 Acute myeloid leukemia with 11q23-abnormality in remission CC HCC
C92.62 Acute myeloid leukemia with 11q23-abnormality in relapse CC HCC

✓5th **C92.A Acute myeloid leukemia with multilineage dysplasia**
Acute myeloid leukemia with dysplasia of remaining hematopoesis and/or myelodysplastic disease in its history
C92.A0 Acute myeloid leukemia with multilineage dysplasia, not having achieved remission CC HCC
Acute myeloid leukemia with multilineage dysplasia with failed remission
Acute myeloid leukemia with multilineage dysplasia NOS
C92.A1 Acute myeloid leukemia with multilineage dysplasia, in remission CC HCC
C92.A2 Acute myeloid leukemia with multilineage dysplasia, in relapse CC HCC

✓5th **C92.Z Other myeloid leukemia**
C92.Z0 Other myeloid leukemia not having achieved remission CC HCC
Myeloid leukemia NEC with failed remission
Myeloid leukemia NEC
C92.Z1 Other myeloid leukemia, in remission CC HCC
C92.Z2 Other myeloid leukemia, in relapse CC HCC

✓5th **C92.9 Myeloid leukemia, unspecified**
C92.90 Myeloid leukemia, unspecified, not having achieved remission CC HCC
Myeloid leukemia, unspecified with failed remission
Myeloid leukemia, unspecified NOS
C92.91 Myeloid leukemia, unspecified in remission CC HCC
C92.92 Myeloid leukemia, unspecified in relapse CC HCC

✓4th **C93 Monocytic leukemia**
INCLUDES monocytoid leukemia
EXCLUDES 1 *personal history of leukemia (Z85.6)*
AHA: 2020,1Q,13

✓5th **C93.0 Acute monoblastic/monocytic leukemia**
AML M5
AML M5a
AML M5b
C93.00 Acute monoblastic/monocytic leukemia, not having achieved remission CC HCC
Acute monoblastic/monocytic leukemia with failed remission
Acute monoblastic/monocytic leukemia NOS
C93.01 Acute monoblastic/monocytic leukemia, in remission CC HCC
C93.02 Acute monoblastic/monocytic leukemia, in relapse CC HCC

✓5th **C93.1 Chronic myelomonocytic leukemia**
Chronic monocytic leukemia
CMML-1
CMML-2
CMML with eosinophilia
►Code also, if applicable, eosinophilia (D72.18)◄
C93.10 Chronic myelomonocytic leukemia not having achieved remission CC HCC
Chronic myelomonocytic leukemia with failed remission
Chronic myelomonocytic leukemia NOS
C93.11 Chronic myelomonocytic leukemia, in remission CC HCC
C93.12 Chronic myelomonocytic leukemia, in relapse CC HCC

✓5th **C93.3 Juvenile myelomonocytic leukemia**
C93.30 Juvenile myelomonocytic leukemia, not having achieved remission CC HCC P
Juvenile myelomonocytic leukemia with failed remission
Juvenile myelomonocytic leukemia NOS
C93.31 Juvenile myelomonocytic leukemia, in remission CC HCC P
C93.32 Juvenile myelomonocytic leukemia, in relapse CC HCC P

✓5th **C93.Z Other monocytic leukemia**
C93.Z0 Other monocytic leukemia, not having achieved remission CC HCC
Other monocytic leukemia NOS
C93.Z1 Other monocytic leukemia, in remission CC HCC
C93.Z2 Other monocytic leukemia, in relapse CC HCC

✓5th **C93.9 Monocytic leukemia, unspecified**
C93.90 Monocytic leukemia, unspecified, not having achieved remission CC HCC
Monocytic leukemia, unspecified with failed remission
Monocytic leukemia, unspecified NOS
C93.91 Monocytic leukemia, unspecified in remission CC HCC
C93.92 Monocytic leukemia, unspecified in relapse CC HCC

✓4th **C94 Other leukemias of specified cell type**
EXCLUDES 1 *leukemic reticuloendotheliosis (C91.4-)*
myelodysplastic syndromes (D46.-)
personal history of leukemia (Z85.6)
plasma cell leukemia (C90.1-)
AHA: 2020,1Q,13

✓5th **C94.0 Acute erythroid leukemia**
Acute myeloid leukemia M6(a)(b)
Erythroleukemia
DEF: Erythroleukemia: Malignant blood dyscrasia (a myeloproliferative disorder).
C94.00 Acute erythroid leukemia, not having achieved remission CC HCC
Acute erythroid leukemia with failed remission
Acute erythroid leukemia NOS
C94.01 Acute erythroid leukemia, in remission CC HCC
C94.02 Acute erythroid leukemia, in relapse CC HCC

✓5th **C94.2 Acute megakaryoblastic leukemia**
Acute myeloid leukemia M7
Acute megakaryocytic leukemia
C94.20 Acute megakaryoblastic leukemia not having achieved remission CC HCC
Acute megakaryoblastic leukemia with failed remission
Acute megakaryoblastic leukemia NOS
C94.21 Acute megakaryoblastic leukemia, in remission CC HCC
C94.22 Acute megakaryoblastic leukemia, in relapse CC HCC

✓5th **C94.3 Mast cell leukemia**
AHA: 2017,4Q,5
C94.30 Mast cell leukemia not having achieved remission CC HCC
Mast cell leukemia with failed remission
Mast cell leukemia NOS
C94.31 Mast cell leukemia, in remission CC HCC
C94.32 Mast cell leukemia, in relapse CC HCC

✓5th **C94.4 Acute panmyelosis with myelofibrosis**
Acute myelofibrosis
EXCLUDES 1 *myelofibrosis NOS (D75.81)*
secondary myelofibrosis NOS (D75.81)
C94.40 Acute panmyelosis with myelofibrosis not having achieved remission CC HCC
Acute myelofibrosis NOS
Acute panmyelosis with myelofibrosis with failed remission
Acute panmyelosis NOS
C94.41 Acute panmyelosis with myelofibrosis, in remission CC HCC
C94.42 Acute panmyelosis with myelofibrosis, in relapse CC HCC

C94.6 Myelodysplastic disease, not classified CC HCC
Myeloproliferative disease, not classified

✓5th **C94.8 Other specified leukemias**
Aggressive NK-cell leukemia
Acute basophilic leukemia
C94.80 Other specified leukemias not having achieved remission CC HCC
Other specified leukemia with failed remission
Other specified leukemias NOS
C94.81 Other specified leukemias, in remission CC HCC
C94.82 Other specified leukemias, in relapse CC HCC

✓4th **C95 Leukemia of unspecified cell type**
EXCLUDES 1 *personal history of leukemia (Z85.6)*
AHA: 2020,1Q,13

✓5th **C95.0 Acute leukemia of unspecified cell type**
Acute bilineal leukemia
Acute mixed lineage leukemia
Biphenotypic acute leukemia
Stem cell leukemia of unclear lineage
EXCLUDES 1 *acute exacerbation of unspecified chronic leukemia (C95.10)*
C95.00 Acute leukemia of unspecified cell type not having achieved remission CC HCC
Acute leukemia of unspecified cell type with failed remission
Acute leukemia NOS
C95.01 Acute leukemia of unspecified cell type, in remission CC HCC
C95.02 Acute leukemia of unspecified cell type, in relapse CC HCC

✓5th **C95.1 Chronic leukemia of unspecified cell type**
C95.10 Chronic leukemia of unspecified cell type not having achieved remission CC HCC
Chronic leukemia of unspecified cell type with failed remission
Chronic leukemia NOS
C95.11 Chronic leukemia of unspecified cell type, in remission CC HCC
C95.12 Chronic leukemia of unspecified cell type, in relapse CC HCC

✓5th **C95.9 Leukemia, unspecified**
C95.90 Leukemia, unspecified not having achieved remission CC HCC
Leukemia, unspecified with failed remission
Leukemia NOS
C95.91 Leukemia, unspecified, in remission CC HCC
C95.92 Leukemia, unspecified, in relapse CC HCC

✓4th **C96 Other and unspecified malignant neoplasms of lymphoid, hematopoietic and related tissue**
EXCLUDES 1 *personal history of other malignant neoplasms of lymphoid, hematopoietic and related tissues (Z85.79)*

C96.0 Multifocal and multisystemic (disseminated) Langerhans-cell histiocytosis CC HCC
Histiocytosis X, multisystemic
Letterer-Siwe disease
EXCLUDES 1 *adult pulmonary Langerhans cell histiocytosis (J84.82)*
multifocal and unisystemic Langerhans-cell histiocytosis (C96.5)
unifocal Langerhans-cell histiocytosis (C96.6)

✓5th **C96.2 Malignant mast cell neoplasm**
EXCLUDES 1 *indolent mastocytosis (D47.02)*
mast cell leukemia (C94.30)
mastocytosis (congenital) (cutaneous) (Q82.2)
AHA: 2017,4Q,5
DEF: Mast cell: Type of white blood cell found in the loose connective tissue of blood vessels and bronchioles responsible for acute hypersensitivity reactions, including anaphylactic shock. The IgE receptors on these cells bind with allergens causing cell degranulation and diffuse, widespread histamine release that results in airway constriction and vasodilation with decreased systemic blood pressure.
C96.20 Malignant mast cell neoplasm, unspecified CC HCC
C96.21 Aggressive systemic mastocytosis CC HCC
C96.22 Mast cell sarcoma CC HCC
C96.29 Other malignant mast cell neoplasm CC HCC

C96.4 Sarcoma of dendritic cells (accessory cells) CC HCC
Follicular dendritic cell sarcoma
Interdigitating dendritic cell sarcoma
Langerhans cell sarcoma

C96.5 Multifocal and unisystemic Langerhans-cell histiocytosis CC HCC
Hand-Schüller-Christian disease
Histiocytosis X, multifocal
EXCLUDES 1 *multifocal and multisystemic (disseminated) Langerhans-cell histiocytosis (C96.0)*
unifocal Langerhans-cell histiocytosis (C96.6)

C96.6 Unifocal Langerhans-cell histiocytosis CC HCC
Eosinophilic granuloma
Histiocytosis X, unifocal
Histiocytosis X NOS
Langerhans-cell histiocytosis NOS
EXCLUDES 1 *multifocal and multisysemic (disseminated) Langerhans-cell histiocytosis (C96.0)*
multifocal and unisystemic Langerhans-cell histiocytosis (C96.5)

C96.A Histiocytic sarcoma CC HCC
Malignant histiocytosis

C96.Z Other specified malignant neoplasms of lymphoid, hematopoietic and related tissue CC HCC

C96.9 Malignant neoplasm of lymphoid, hematopoietic and related tissue, unspecified CC HCC

In situ neoplasms (D00-D09)

INCLUDES Bowen's disease
erythroplasia
grade III intraepithelial neoplasia
Queyrat's erythroplasia

✓4th D00 Carcinoma in situ of oral cavity, esophagus and stomach

EXCLUDES 1 *melanoma in situ (D03.-)*

✓5th D00.0 Carcinoma in situ of lip, oral cavity and pharynx

Use additional code to identify:
exposure to environmental tobacco smoke (Z77.22)
exposure to tobacco smoke in the perinatal period (P96.81)
history of tobacco dependence (Z87.891)
occupational exposure to environmental tobacco smoke (Z57.31)
tobacco dependence (F17.-)
tobacco use (Z72.0)

EXCLUDES 1 *carcinoma in situ of aryepiglottic fold or interarytenoid fold, laryngeal aspect (D02.0)*
carcinoma in situ of epiglottis NOS (D02.0)
carcinoma in situ of epiglottis suprahyoid portion (D02.0)
carcinoma in situ of skin of lip (D03.0, D04.0)

D00.00 Carcinoma in situ of oral cavity, unspecified site
D00.01 Carcinoma in situ of labial mucosa and vermilion border
D00.02 Carcinoma in situ of buccal mucosa
D00.03 Carcinoma in situ of gingiva and edentulous alveolar ridge
D00.04 Carcinoma in situ of soft palate
D00.05 Carcinoma in situ of hard palate
D00.06 Carcinoma in situ of floor of mouth
D00.07 Carcinoma in situ of tongue
D00.08 Carcinoma in situ of pharynx

Carcinoma in situ of aryepiglottic fold NOS
Carcinoma in situ of hypopharyngeal aspect of aryepiglottic fold
Carcinoma in situ of marginal zone of aryepiglottic fold

D00.1 Carcinoma in situ of esophagus
D00.2 Carcinoma in situ of stomach

✓4th D01 Carcinoma in situ of other and unspecified digestive organs

EXCLUDES 1 *melanoma in situ (D03.-)*

D01.0 Carcinoma in situ of colon

EXCLUDES 1 *carcinoma in situ of rectosigmoid junction (D01.1)*

D01.1 Carcinoma in situ of rectosigmoid junction
D01.2 Carcinoma in situ of rectum
D01.3 Carcinoma in situ of anus and anal canal

Anal intraepithelial neoplasia III [AIN III]
Severe dysplasia of anus

EXCLUDES 1 *anal intraepithelial neoplasia I and II [AIN I and AIN II] (K62.82)*
carcinoma in situ of anal margin (D04.5)
carcinoma in situ of anal skin (D04.5)
carcinoma in situ of perianal skin (D04.5)

✓5th D01.4 Carcinoma in situ of other and unspecified parts of intestine

EXCLUDES 1 *carcinoma in situ of ampulla of Vater (D01.5)*

D01.40 Carcinoma in situ of unspecified part of intestine
D01.49 Carcinoma in situ of other parts of intestine

D01.5 Carcinoma in situ of liver, gallbladder and bile ducts

Carcinoma in situ of ampulla of Vater

D01.7 Carcinoma in situ of other specified digestive organs

Carcinoma in situ of pancreas

D01.9 Carcinoma in situ of digestive organ, unspecified

✓4th D02 Carcinoma in situ of middle ear and respiratory system

Use additional code to identify:
exposure to environmental tobacco smoke (Z77.22)
exposure to tobacco smoke in the perinatal period (P96.81)
history of tobacco dependence (Z87.891)
occupational exposure to environmental tobacco smoke (Z57.31)
tobacco dependence (F17.-)
tobacco use (Z72.0)

EXCLUDES 1 *melanoma in situ (D03.-)*

D02.0 Carcinoma in situ of larynx

Carcinoma in situ of aryepiglottic fold or interarytenoid fold, laryngeal aspect
Carcinoma in situ of epiglottis (suprahyoid portion)

EXCLUDES 1 *carcinoma in situ of aryepiglottic fold or interarytenoid fold NOS (D00.08)*
carcinoma in situ of hypopharyngeal aspect (D00.08)
carcinoma in situ of marginal zone (D00.08)

D02.1 Carcinoma in situ of trachea

✓5th D02.2 Carcinoma in situ of bronchus and lung

D02.20 Carcinoma in situ of unspecified bronchus and lung
D02.21 Carcinoma in situ of right bronchus and lung
D02.22 Carcinoma in situ of left bronchus and lung

D02.3 Carcinoma in situ of other parts of respiratory system

Carcinoma in situ of accessory sinuses
Carcinoma in situ of middle ear
Carcinoma in situ of nasal cavities

EXCLUDES 1 *carcinoma in situ of ear (external) (skin) (D04.2-)*
carcinoma in situ of nose NOS (D09.8)
carcinoma in situ of skin of nose (D04.3)

D02.4 Carcinoma in situ of respiratory system, unspecified

✓4th D03 Melanoma in situ

D03.0 Melanoma in situ of lip HCC

✓5th D03.1 Melanoma in situ of eyelid, including canthus

AHA: 2018,4Q,4

D03.10 Melanoma in situ of unspecified eyelid, including canthus HCC

✓6th D03.11 Melanoma in situ of right eyelid, including canthus

D03.111 Melanoma in situ of right upper eyelid, including canthus HCC
D03.112 Melanoma in situ of right lower eyelid, including canthus HCC

✓6th D03.12 Melanoma in situ of left eyelid, including canthus

D03.121 Melanoma in situ of left upper eyelid, including canthus HCC
D03.122 Melanoma in situ of left lower eyelid, including canthus HCC

✓5th D03.2 Melanoma in situ of ear and external auricular canal

D03.20 Melanoma in situ of unspecified ear and external auricular canal HCC
D03.21 Melanoma in situ of right ear and external auricular canal HCC
D03.22 Melanoma in situ of left ear and external auricular canal HCC

✓5th D03.3 Melanoma in situ of other and unspecified parts of face

D03.30 Melanoma in situ of unspecified part of face HCC
D03.39 Melanoma in situ of other parts of face HCC

D03.4 Melanoma in situ of scalp and neck HCC

✓5th D03.5 Melanoma in situ of trunk

D03.51 Melanoma in situ of anal skin HCC

Melanoma in situ of anal margin
Melanoma in situ of perianal skin

D03.52 Melanoma in situ of breast (skin) (soft tissue) HCC
D03.59 Melanoma in situ of other part of trunk HCC

✓5th D03.6 Melanoma in situ of upper limb, including shoulder

D03.60 Melanoma in situ of unspecified upper limb, including shoulder HCC
D03.61 Melanoma in situ of right upper limb, including shoulder HCC
D03.62 Melanoma in situ of left upper limb, including shoulder HCC

✓5th D03.7 Melanoma in situ of lower limb, including hip

D03.70 Melanoma in situ of unspecified lower limb, including hip HCC

D03.71 Melanoma in situ of right lower limb, including hip HCC
D03.72 Melanoma in situ of left lower limb, including hip HCC
D03.8 Melanoma in situ of other sites HCC
Melanoma in situ of scrotum
EXCLUDES 1 *carcinoma in situ of scrotum (D07.61)*
D03.9 Melanoma in situ, unspecified HCC

D04 Carcinoma in situ of skin
EXCLUDES 1 *erythroplasia of Queyrat (penis) NOS (D07.4)*
melanoma in situ (D03.-)
D04.0 Carcinoma in situ of skin of lip
EXCLUDES 2 *carcinoma in situ of vermilion border of lip (D00.01)*
D04.1 Carcinoma in situ of skin of eyelid, including canthus
AHA: 2018,4Q,4
D04.10 Carcinoma in situ of skin of unspecified eyelid, including canthus
D04.11 Carcinoma in situ of skin of right eyelid, including canthus
D04.111 Carcinoma in situ of skin of right upper eyelid, including canthus
D04.112 Carcinoma in situ of skin of right lower eyelid, including canthus
D04.12 Carcinoma in situ of skin of left eyelid, including canthus
D04.121 Carcinoma in situ of skin of left upper eyelid, including canthus
D04.122 Carcinoma in situ of skin of left lower eyelid, including canthus
D04.2 Carcinoma in situ of skin of ear and external auricular canal
D04.20 Carcinoma in situ of skin of unspecified ear and external auricular canal
D04.21 Carcinoma in situ of skin of right ear and external auricular canal
D04.22 Carcinoma in situ of skin of left ear and external auricular canal
D04.3 Carcinoma in situ of skin of other and unspecified parts of face
D04.30 Carcinoma in situ of skin of unspecified part of face
D04.39 Carcinoma in situ of skin of other parts of face
D04.4 Carcinoma in situ of skin of scalp and neck
D04.5 Carcinoma in situ of skin of trunk
Carcinoma in situ of anal margin
Carcinoma in situ of anal skin
Carcinoma in situ of perianal skin
Carcinoma in situ of skin of breast
EXCLUDES 1 *carcinoma in situ of anus NOS (D01.3)*
carcinoma in situ of scrotum (D07.61)
carcinoma in situ of skin of genital organs (D07.-)
D04.6 Carcinoma in situ of skin of upper limb, including shoulder
D04.60 Carcinoma in situ of skin of unspecified upper limb, including shoulder
D04.61 Carcinoma in situ of skin of right upper limb, including shoulder
D04.62 Carcinoma in situ of skin of left upper limb, including shoulder
D04.7 Carcinoma in situ of skin of lower limb, including hip
D04.70 Carcinoma in situ of skin of unspecified lower limb, including hip
D04.71 Carcinoma in situ of skin of right lower limb, including hip
D04.72 Carcinoma in situ of skin of left lower limb, including hip
D04.8 Carcinoma in situ of skin of other sites
D04.9 Carcinoma in situ of skin, unspecified

D05 Carcinoma in situ of breast
EXCLUDES 1 *carcinoma in situ of skin of breast (D04.5)*
melanoma in situ of breast (skin) (D03.5)
Paget's disease of breast or nipple (C50.-)
D05.0 Lobular carcinoma in situ of breast
D05.00 Lobular carcinoma in situ of unspecified breast
D05.01 Lobular carcinoma in situ of right breast
D05.02 Lobular carcinoma in situ of left breast
D05.1 Intraductal carcinoma in situ of breast
D05.10 Intraductal carcinoma in situ of unspecified breast
D05.11 Intraductal carcinoma in situ of right breast
D05.12 Intraductal carcinoma in situ of left breast
D05.8 Other specified type of carcinoma in situ of breast
D05.80 Other specified type of carcinoma in situ of unspecified breast
D05.81 Other specified type of carcinoma in situ of right breast
D05.82 Other specified type of carcinoma in situ of left breast
D05.9 Unspecified type of carcinoma in situ of breast
D05.90 Unspecified type of carcinoma in situ of unspecified breast
D05.91 Unspecified type of carcinoma in situ of right breast
D05.92 Unspecified type of carcinoma in situ of left breast

D06 Carcinoma in situ of cervix uteri
INCLUDES cervical adenocarcinoma in situ
cervical intraepithelial glandular neoplasia
cervical intraepithelial neoplasia III [CIN III]
severe dysplasia of cervix uteri
EXCLUDES 1 *cervical intraepithelial neoplasia II [CIN II] (N87.1)*
cytologic evidence of malignancy of cervix without histologic confirmation (R87.614)
high grade squamous intraepithelial lesion (HGSIL) of cervix (R87.613)
melanoma in situ of cervix (D03.5)
moderate cervical dysplasia (N87.1)
D06.0 Carcinoma in situ of endocervix ♀
D06.1 Carcinoma in situ of exocervix ♀
D06.7 Carcinoma in situ of other parts of cervix ♀
D06.9 Carcinoma in situ of cervix, unspecified ♀

D07 Carcinoma in situ of other and unspecified genital organs
EXCLUDES 1 *melanoma in situ of trunk (D03.5)*
D07.0 Carcinoma in situ of endometrium ♀
D07.1 Carcinoma in situ of vulva ♀
Severe dysplasia of vulva
Vulvar intraepithelial neoplasia III [VIN III]
EXCLUDES 1 *moderate dysplasia of vulva (N90.1)*
vulvar intraepithelial neoplasia II [VIN II] (N90.1)
D07.2 Carcinoma in situ of vagina ♀
Severe dysplasia of vagina
Vaginal intraepithelial neoplasia III [VAIN III]
EXCLUDES 1 *moderate dysplasia of vagina (N89.1)*
vaginal intraepithelial neoplasia II [VIN II] (N89.1)
D07.3 Carcinoma in situ of other and unspecified female genital organs
D07.30 Carcinoma in situ of unspecified female genital organs ♀
D07.39 Carcinoma in situ of other female genital organs ♀
D07.4 Carcinoma in situ of penis ♂
Erythroplasia of Queyrat NOS
D07.5 Carcinoma in situ of prostate ♂
Prostatic intraepithelial neoplasia III (PIN III)
Severe dysplasia of prostate
EXCLUDES 1 *dysplasia (mild) (moderate) of prostate (N42.3-)*
prostatic intraepithelial neoplasia II [PIN II] (N42.3-)
D07.6 Carcinoma in situ of other and unspecified male genital organs
D07.60 Carcinoma in situ of unspecified male genital organs ♂
D07.61 Carcinoma in situ of scrotum ♂
D07.69 Carcinoma in situ of other male genital organs ♂

D09 Carcinoma in situ of other and unspecified sites
EXCLUDES 1 *melanoma in situ (D03.-)*
D09.0 Carcinoma in situ of bladder
D09.1 Carcinoma in situ of other and unspecified urinary organs
D09.10 Carcinoma in situ of unspecified urinary organ
D09.19 Carcinoma in situ of other urinary organs
D09.2 Carcinoma in situ of eye
EXCLUDES 1 *carcinoma in situ of skin of eyelid (D04.1-)*
D09.20 Carcinoma in situ of unspecified eye
D09.21 Carcinoma in situ of right eye
D09.22 Carcinoma in situ of left eye

DØ9.3 Carcinoma in situ of thyroid and other endocrine glands
EXCLUDES 1 *carcinoma in situ of endocrine pancreas (DØ1.7)*
carcinoma in situ of ovary (DØ7.39)
carcinoma in situ of testis (DØ7.69)

DØ9.8 Carcinoma in situ of other specified sites

DØ9.9 Carcinoma in situ, unspecified

Benign neoplasms, except benign neuroendocrine tumors (D1Ø-D36)

✓4th D1Ø Benign neoplasm of mouth and pharynx

D1Ø.Ø Benign neoplasm of lip
Benign neoplasm of lip (frenulum) (inner aspect) (mucosa) (vermilion border)
EXCLUDES 1 *benign neoplasm of skin of lip (D22.Ø, D23.Ø)*

D1Ø.1 Benign neoplasm of tongue
Benign neoplasm of lingual tonsil

D1Ø.2 Benign neoplasm of floor of mouth

✓5th D1Ø.3 Benign neoplasm of other and unspecified parts of mouth

D1Ø.3Ø Benign neoplasm of unspecified part of mouth

D1Ø.39 Benign neoplasm of other parts of mouth
Benign neoplasm of minor salivary gland NOS
EXCLUDES 1 *benign odontogenic neoplasms (D16.4-D16.5)*
benign neoplasm of mucosa of lip (D1Ø.Ø)
benign neoplasm of nasopharyngeal surface of soft palate (D1Ø.6)

D1Ø.4 Benign neoplasm of tonsil
Benign neoplasm of tonsil (faucial) (palatine)
EXCLUDES 1 *benign neoplasm of lingual tonsil (D1Ø.1)*
benign neoplasm of pharyngeal tonsil (D1Ø.6)
benign neoplasm of tonsillar fossa (D1Ø.5)
benign neoplasm of tonsillar pillars (D1Ø.5)

D1Ø.5 Benign neoplasm of other parts of oropharynx
Benign neoplasm of epiglottis, anterior aspect
Benign neoplasm of tonsillar fossa
Benign neoplasm of tonsillar pillars
Benign neoplasm of vallecula
EXCLUDES 1 *benign neoplasm of epiglottis NOS (D14.1)*
benign neoplasm of epiglottis, suprahyoid portion (D14.1)
DEF: Oropharynx: Middle portion of pharynx (throat); communicates with the oral cavity, nasopharynx and laryngopharynx.

D1Ø.6 Benign neoplasm of nasopharynx
Benign neoplasm of pharyngeal tonsil
Benign neoplasm of posterior margin of septum and choanae
DEF: Nasopharynx: Upper portion of pharynx (throat); communicates with the nasal cavities, oropharynx and tympanic cavities.

D1Ø.7 Benign neoplasm of hypopharynx
DEF: Hypopharynx: Lower portion of pharynx (throat); communicates with the oropharynx and the esophagus.
Synonyms: *laryngopharynx.*

D1Ø.9 Benign neoplasm of pharynx, unspecified

✓4th D11 Benign neoplasm of major salivary glands
EXCLUDES 1 *benign neoplasms of specified minor salivary glands which are classified according to their anatomical location*
benign neoplasms of minor salivary glands NOS (D1Ø.39)

D11.Ø Benign neoplasm of parotid gland

D11.7 Benign neoplasm of other major salivary glands
Benign neoplasm of sublingual salivary gland
Benign neoplasm of submandibular salivary gland

D11.9 Benign neoplasm of major salivary gland, unspecified

✓4th D12 Benign neoplasm of colon, rectum, anus and anal canal
EXCLUDES 1 *benign carcinoid tumors of the large intestine, and rectum (D3A.Ø2-)*
polyp of colon NOS (K63.5)
AHA: 2018,2Q,14; 2017,1Q,15; 2015,2Q,14
TIP: Code K63.5 Polyp of colon, is assigned when documentation states hyperplastic colon polyps, regardless of the site in the colon. Slow-growing, hyperplastic polyps are not precancerous and are classified differently from benign or adenomatous polyps.

D12.Ø Benign neoplasm of cecum
Benign neoplasm of ileocecal valve

D12.1 Benign neoplasm of appendix
EXCLUDES 1 *benign carcinoid tumor of the appendix (D3A.Ø2Ø)*

D12.2 Benign neoplasm of ascending colon

D12.3 Benign neoplasm of transverse colon
Benign neoplasm of hepatic flexure
Benign neoplasm of splenic flexure
AHA: 2017,1Q,16

D12.4 Benign neoplasm of descending colon

D12.5 Benign neoplasm of sigmoid colon

D12.6 Benign neoplasm of colon, unspecified
Adenomatosis of colon
Benign neoplasm of large intestine NOS
Polyposis (hereditary) of colon
EXCLUDES 1 *inflammatory polyp of colon (K51.4-)*

D12.7 Benign neoplasm of rectosigmoid junction

D12.8 Benign neoplasm of rectum
EXCLUDES 1 *benign carcinoid tumor of the rectum (D3A.Ø26)*
AHA: 2018,1Q,6

D12.9 Benign neoplasm of anus and anal canal
Benign neoplasm of anus NOS
EXCLUDES 1 *benign neoplasm of anal margin (D22.5, D23.5)*
benign neoplasm of anal skin (D22.5, D23.5)
benign neoplasm of perianal skin (D22.5, D23.5)

✓4th D13 Benign neoplasm of other and ill-defined parts of digestive system
EXCLUDES 1 *benign stromal tumors of digestive system (D21.4)*

D13.Ø Benign neoplasm of esophagus

D13.1 Benign neoplasm of stomach
EXCLUDES 1 *benign carcinoid tumor of the stomach (D3A.Ø92)*

D13.2 Benign neoplasm of duodenum
EXCLUDES 1 *benign carcinoid tumor of the duodenum (D3A.Ø1Ø)*

✓5th D13.3 Benign neoplasm of other and unspecified parts of small intestine
EXCLUDES 1 *benign carcinoid tumors of the small intestine (D3A.Ø1-)*
benign neoplasm of ileocecal valve (D12.Ø)

D13.3Ø Benign neoplasm of unspecified part of small intestine

D13.39 Benign neoplasm of other parts of small intestine

D13.4 Benign neoplasm of liver
Benign neoplasm of intrahepatic bile ducts

D13.5 Benign neoplasm of extrahepatic bile ducts

D13.6 Benign neoplasm of pancreas
EXCLUDES 1 *benign neoplasm of endocrine pancreas (D13.7)*

D13.7 Benign neoplasm of endocrine pancreas
Benign neoplasm of islets of Langerhans
Islet cell tumor
Use additional code to identify any functional activity

D13.9 Benign neoplasm of ill-defined sites within the digestive system
Benign neoplasm of digestive system NOS
Benign neoplasm of intestine NOS
Benign neoplasm of spleen

✓4th D14 Benign neoplasm of middle ear and respiratory system

D14.Ø Benign neoplasm of middle ear, nasal cavity and accessory sinuses
Benign neoplasm of cartilage of nose
EXCLUDES 1 *benign neoplasm of auricular canal (external) (D22.2-, D23.2-)*
benign neoplasm of bone of ear (D16.4)
benign neoplasm of bone of nose (D16.4)
benign neoplasm of cartilage of ear (D21.Ø)
benign neoplasm of ear (external)(skin) (D22.2-, D23.2-)
benign neoplasm of nose NOS (D36.7)
benign neoplasm of skin of nose (D22.39, D23.39)
benign neoplasm of olfactory bulb (D33.3)
benign neoplasm of posterior margin of septum and choanae (D1Ø.6)
polyp of accessory sinus (J33.8)
polyp of ear (middle) (H74.4)
polyp of nasal (cavity) (J33.-)

D14.1 **Benign neoplasm of larynx**
Adenomatous polyp of larynx
Benign neoplasm of epiglottis (suprahyoid portion)
EXCLUDES 1 *benign neoplasm of epiglottis, anterior aspect (D1Ø.5)*
polyp (nonadenomatous) of vocal cord or larynx (J38.1)

D14.2 **Benign neoplasm of trachea**

✓5th D14.3 **Benign neoplasm of bronchus and lung**
EXCLUDES 1 *benign carcinoid tumor of the bronchus and lung (D3A.Ø9Ø)*

D14.3Ø **Benign neoplasm of unspecified bronchus and lung**
D14.31 **Benign neoplasm of right bronchus and lung**
D14.32 **Benign neoplasm of left bronchus and lung**

D14.4 **Benign neoplasm of respiratory system, unspecified**

✓4th **D15 Benign neoplasm of other and unspecified intrathoracic organs**
EXCLUDES 1 *benign neoplasm of mesothelial tissue (D19.-)*

D15.Ø **Benign neoplasm of thymus**
EXCLUDES 1 *benign carcinoid tumor of the thymus (D3A.Ø91)*

D15.1 **Benign neoplasm of heart**
EXCLUDES 1 *benign neoplasm of great vessels (D21.3)*

D15.2 **Benign neoplasm of mediastinum**
D15.7 **Benign neoplasm of other specified intrathoracic organs**
D15.9 **Benign neoplasm of intrathoracic organ, unspecified**

✓4th **D16 Benign neoplasm of bone and articular cartilage**
EXCLUDES 1 *benign neoplasm of connective tissue of ear (D21.Ø)*
benign neoplasm of connective tissue of eyelid (D21.Ø)
benign neoplasm of connective tissue of larynx (D14.1)
benign neoplasm of connective tissue of nose (D14.Ø)
benign neoplasm of synovia (D21.-)

✓5th D16.Ø **Benign neoplasm of scapula and long bones of upper limb**
D16.ØØ **Benign neoplasm of scapula and long bones of unspecified upper limb**
D16.Ø1 **Benign neoplasm of scapula and long bones of right upper limb**
D16.Ø2 **Benign neoplasm of scapula and long bones of left upper limb**

✓5th D16.1 **Benign neoplasm of short bones of upper limb**
D16.1Ø **Benign neoplasm of short bones of unspecified upper limb**
D16.11 **Benign neoplasm of short bones of right upper limb**
D16.12 **Benign neoplasm of short bones of left upper limb**

✓5th D16.2 **Benign neoplasm of long bones of lower limb**
D16.2Ø **Benign neoplasm of long bones of unspecified lower limb**
D16.21 **Benign neoplasm of long bones of right lower limb**
D16.22 **Benign neoplasm of long bones of left lower limb**

✓5th D16.3 **Benign neoplasm of short bones of lower limb**
D16.3Ø **Benign neoplasm of short bones of unspecified lower limb**
D16.31 **Benign neoplasm of short bones of right lower limb**
D16.32 **Benign neoplasm of short bones of left lower limb**

D16.4 **Benign neoplasm of bones of skull and face**
Benign neoplasm of maxilla (superior)
Benign neoplasm of orbital bone
Keratocyst of maxilla
Keratocystic odontogenic tumor of maxilla
EXCLUDES 2 *benign neoplasm of lower jaw bone (D16.5)*

D16.5 **Benign neoplasm of lower jaw bone**
Keratocyst of mandible
Keratocystic odontogenic tumor of mandible

D16.6 **Benign neoplasm of vertebral column**
EXCLUDES 1 *benign neoplasm of sacrum and coccyx (D16.8)*

D16.7 **Benign neoplasm of ribs, sternum and clavicle**
D16.8 **Benign neoplasm of pelvic bones, sacrum and coccyx**
D16.9 **Benign neoplasm of bone and articular cartilage, unspecified**

✓4th **D17 Benign lipomatous neoplasm**

D17.Ø **Benign lipomatous neoplasm of skin and subcutaneous tissue of head, face and neck**
D17.1 **Benign lipomatous neoplasm of skin and subcutaneous tissue of trunk**

✓5th D17.2 **Benign lipomatous neoplasm of skin and subcutaneous tissue of limb**
D17.2Ø **Benign lipomatous neoplasm of skin and subcutaneous tissue of unspecified limb**
D17.21 **Benign lipomatous neoplasm of skin and subcutaneous tissue of right arm**
D17.22 **Benign lipomatous neoplasm of skin and subcutaneous tissue of left arm**
D17.23 **Benign lipomatous neoplasm of skin and subcutaneous tissue of right leg**
D17.24 **Benign lipomatous neoplasm of skin and subcutaneous tissue of left leg**

✓5th D17.3 **Benign lipomatous neoplasm of skin and subcutaneous tissue of other and unspecified sites**
D17.3Ø **Benign lipomatous neoplasm of skin and subcutaneous tissue of unspecified sites**
D17.39 **Benign lipomatous neoplasm of skin and subcutaneous tissue of other sites**

D17.4 **Benign lipomatous neoplasm of intrathoracic organs**
D17.5 **Benign lipomatous neoplasm of intra-abdominal organs**
EXCLUDES 1 *benign lipomatous neoplasm of peritoneum and retroperitoneum (D17.79)*

D17.6 **Benign lipomatous neoplasm of spermatic cord** ♂

✓5th D17.7 **Benign lipomatous neoplasm of other sites**
D17.71 **Benign lipomatous neoplasm of kidney**
D17.72 **Benign lipomatous neoplasm of other genitourinary organ**
D17.79 **Benign lipomatous neoplasm of other sites**
Benign lipomatous neoplasm of peritoneum
Benign lipomatous neoplasm of retroperitoneum

D17.9 **Benign lipomatous neoplasm, unspecified**
Lipoma NOS

✓4th **D18 Hemangioma and lymphangioma, any site**
EXCLUDES 1 *benign neoplasm of glomus jugulare (D35.6)*
blue or pigmented nevus (D22.-)
nevus NOS (D22.-)
vascular nevus (Q82.5)

✓5th D18.Ø **Hemangioma**
Angioma NOS
Cavernous nevus
DEF: Common benign tumor usually occurring in infancy that is composed of newly formed blood vessels due to malformation of the angioblastic tissue.

D18.ØØ **Hemangioma unspecified site**
D18.Ø1 **Hemangioma of skin and subcutaneous tissue**
D18.Ø2 **Hemangioma of intracranial structures** HCC
D18.Ø3 **Hemangioma of intra-abdominal structures**
D18.Ø9 **Hemangioma of other sites**

D18.1 **Lymphangioma, any site**
AHA: 2018,3Q,31; 2018,2Q,13

✓4th **D19 Benign neoplasm of mesothelial tissue**

D19.Ø **Benign neoplasm of mesothelial tissue of pleura**
D19.1 **Benign neoplasm of mesothelial tissue of peritoneum**
D19.7 **Benign neoplasm of mesothelial tissue of other sites**
D19.9 **Benign neoplasm of mesothelial tissue, unspecified**
Benign mesothelioma NOS

✓4th **D2Ø Benign neoplasm of soft tissue of retroperitoneum and peritoneum**
EXCLUDES 1 *benign lipomatous neoplasm of peritoneum and retroperitoneum (D17.79)*
benign neoplasm of mesothelial tissue (D19.-)

D2Ø.Ø **Benign neoplasm of soft tissue of retroperitoneum**
D2Ø.1 **Benign neoplasm of soft tissue of peritoneum**

✓4th D21 Other benign neoplasms of connective and other soft tissue

INCLUDES benign neoplasm of blood vessel
benign neoplasm of bursa
benign neoplasm of cartilage
benign neoplasm of fascia
benign neoplasm of fat
benign neoplasm of ligament, except uterine
benign neoplasm of lymphatic channel
benign neoplasm of muscle
benign neoplasm of synovia
benign neoplasm of tendon (sheath)
benign stromal tumors

EXCLUDES 1 *benign neoplasm of articular cartilage (D16.-)*
benign neoplasm of cartilage of larynx (D14.1)
benign neoplasm of cartilage of nose (D14.Ø)
benign neoplasm of connective tissue of breast (D24.-)
benign neoplasm of peripheral nerves and autonomic nervous system (D36.1-)
benign neoplasm of peritoneum (D2Ø.1)
benign neoplasm of retroperitoneum (D2Ø.Ø)
benign neoplasm of uterine ligament, any (D28.2)
benign neoplasm of vascular tissue (D18.-)
hemangioma (D18.Ø-)
lipomatous neoplasm (D17.-)
lymphangioma (D18.1)
uterine leiomyoma (D25.-)

D21.Ø Benign neoplasm of connective and other soft tissue of head, face and neck
Benign neoplasm of connective tissue of ear
Benign neoplasm of connective tissue of eyelid
EXCLUDES 1 *benign neoplasm of connective tissue of orbit (D31.6-)*

✓5th D21.1 Benign neoplasm of connective and other soft tissue of upper limb, including shoulder
D21.1Ø Benign neoplasm of connective and other soft tissue of unspecified upper limb, including shoulder
D21.11 Benign neoplasm of connective and other soft tissue of right upper limb, including shoulder
D21.12 Benign neoplasm of connective and other soft tissue of left upper limb, including shoulder

✓5th D21.2 Benign neoplasm of connective and other soft tissue of lower limb, including hip
D21.2Ø Benign neoplasm of connective and other soft tissue of unspecified lower limb, including hip
D21.21 Benign neoplasm of connective and other soft tissue of right lower limb, including hip
D21.22 Benign neoplasm of connective and other soft tissue of left lower limb, including hip

D21.3 Benign neoplasm of connective and other soft tissue of thorax
Benign neoplasm of axilla
Benign neoplasm of diaphragm
Benign neoplasm of great vessels
EXCLUDES 1 *benign neoplasm of heart (D15.1)*
benign neoplasm of mediastinum (D15.2)
benign neoplasm of thymus (D15.Ø)

D21.4 Benign neoplasm of connective and other soft tissue of abdomen
Benign stromal tumors of abdomen

D21.5 Benign neoplasm of connective and other soft tissue of pelvis
EXCLUDES 1 *benign neoplasm of any uterine ligament (D28.2)*
uterine leiomyoma (D25.-)

D21.6 Benign neoplasm of connective and other soft tissue of trunk, unspecified
▶Benign neoplasm of connective and other soft tissue of back NOS◀

D21.9 Benign neoplasm of connective and other soft tissue, unspecified

✓4th D22 Melanocytic nevi

INCLUDES atypical nevus
blue hairy pigmented nevus
nevus NOS

D22.Ø Melanocytic nevi of lip

✓5th D22.1 Melanocytic nevi of eyelid, including canthus
AHA: 2018,4Q,4
D22.1Ø Melanocytic nevi of unspecified eyelid, including canthus
✓6th D22.11 Melanocytic nevi of right eyelid, including canthus
D22.111 Melanocytic nevi of right upper eyelid, including canthus
D22.112 Melanocytic nevi of right lower eyelid, including canthus
✓6th D22.12 Melanocytic nevi of left eyelid, including canthus
D22.121 Melanocytic nevi of left upper eyelid, including canthus
D22.122 Melanocytic nevi of left lower eyelid, including canthus

✓5th D22.2 Melanocytic nevi of ear and external auricular canal
D22.2Ø Melanocytic nevi of unspecified ear and external auricular canal
D22.21 Melanocytic nevi of right ear and external auricular canal
D22.22 Melanocytic nevi of left ear and external auricular canal

✓5th D22.3 Melanocytic nevi of other and unspecified parts of face
D22.3Ø Melanocytic nevi of unspecified part of face
D22.39 Melanocytic nevi of other parts of face

D22.4 Melanocytic nevi of scalp and neck

D22.5 Melanocytic nevi of trunk
Melanocytic nevi of anal margin
Melanocytic nevi of anal skin
Melanocytic nevi of perianal skin
Melanocytic nevi of skin of breast

✓5th D22.6 Melanocytic nevi of upper limb, including shoulder
D22.6Ø Melanocytic nevi of unspecified upper limb, including shoulder
D22.61 Melanocytic nevi of right upper limb, including shoulder
D22.62 Melanocytic nevi of left upper limb, including shoulder

✓5th D22.7 Melanocytic nevi of lower limb, including hip
D22.7Ø Melanocytic nevi of unspecified lower limb, including hip
D22.71 Melanocytic nevi of right lower limb, including hip
D22.72 Melanocytic nevi of left lower limb, including hip

D22.9 Melanocytic nevi, unspecified

✓4th D23 Other benign neoplasms of skin

INCLUDES benign neoplasm of hair follicles
benign neoplasm of sebaceous glands
benign neoplasm of sweat glands

EXCLUDES 1 *benign lipomatous neoplasms of skin (D17.Ø-D17.3)*
EXCLUDES 2 *melanocytic nevi (D22.-)*

D23.Ø Other benign neoplasm of skin of lip
EXCLUDES 1 *benign neoplasm of vermilion border of lip (D1Ø.Ø)*

✓5th D23.1 Other benign neoplasm of skin of eyelid, including canthus
AHA: 2018,4Q,4
D23.1Ø Other benign neoplasm of skin of unspecified eyelid, including canthus
✓6th D23.11 Other benign neoplasm of skin of right eyelid, including canthus
D23.111 Other benign neoplasm of skin of right upper eyelid, including canthus
D23.112 Other benign neoplasm of skin of right lower eyelid, including canthus
✓6th D23.12 Other benign neoplasm of skin of left eyelid, including canthus
D23.121 Other benign neoplasm of skin of left upper eyelid, including canthus
D23.122 Other benign neoplasm of skin of left lower eyelid, including canthus

✓5th D23.2 Other benign neoplasm of skin of ear and external auricular canal
D23.2Ø Other benign neoplasm of skin of unspecified ear and external auricular canal
D23.21 Other benign neoplasm of skin of right ear and external auricular canal
D23.22 Other benign neoplasm of skin of left ear and external auricular canal

✓5th D23.3 Other benign neoplasm of skin of other and unspecified parts of face
D23.3Ø Other benign neoplasm of skin of unspecified part of face
D23.39 Other benign neoplasm of skin of other parts of face

D23.4 Other benign neoplasm of skin of scalp and neck

D23.5 Other benign neoplasm of skin of trunk
Other benign neoplasm of anal margin
Other benign neoplasm of anal skin
Other benign neoplasm of perianal skin
Other benign neoplasm of skin of breast
EXCLUDES 1 *benign neoplasm of anus NOS (D12.9)*

✓5th **D23.6 Other benign neoplasm of skin of upper limb, including shoulder**
D23.60 Other benign neoplasm of skin of unspecified upper limb, including shoulder
D23.61 Other benign neoplasm of skin of right upper limb, including shoulder
D23.62 Other benign neoplasm of skin of left upper limb, including shoulder

✓5th **D23.7 Other benign neoplasm of skin of lower limb, including hip**
D23.70 Other benign neoplasm of skin of unspecified lower limb, including hip
D23.71 Other benign neoplasm of skin of right lower limb, including hip
D23.72 Other benign neoplasm of skin of left lower limb, including hip

D23.9 Other benign neoplasm of skin, unspecified

✓4th **D24 Benign neoplasm of breast**
INCLUDES benign neoplasm of connective tissue of breast
benign neoplasm of soft parts of breast
fibroadenoma of breast
EXCLUDES 2 *adenofibrosis of breast (N6Ø.2)*
benign cyst of breast (N6Ø.-)
benign mammary dysplasia (N6Ø.-)
benign neoplasm of skin of breast (D22.5, D23.5)
fibrocystic disease of breast (N6Ø.-)

D24.1 Benign neoplasm of right breast
D24.2 Benign neoplasm of left breast
D24.9 Benign neoplasm of unspecified breast

✓4th **D25 Leiomyoma of uterus**
INCLUDES uterine fibroid
uterine fibromyoma
uterine myoma

Uterine Leiomyomas (Fibroids)

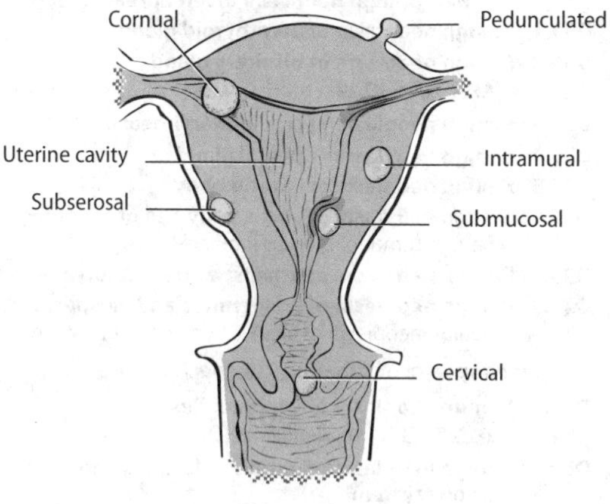

D25.Ø Submucous leiomyoma of uterus ♀
D25.1 Intramural leiomyoma of uterus ♀
Interstitial leiomyoma of uterus
D25.2 Subserosal leiomyoma of uterus ♀
Subperitoneal leiomyoma of uterus
D25.9 Leiomyoma of uterus, unspecified ♀

✓4th **D26 Other benign neoplasms of uterus**
D26.Ø Other benign neoplasm of cervix uteri ♀
D26.1 Other benign neoplasm of corpus uteri ♀
D26.7 Other benign neoplasm of other parts of uterus ♀
D26.9 Other benign neoplasm of uterus, unspecified ♀

✓4th **D27 Benign neoplasm of ovary**
Use additional code to identify any functional activity
EXCLUDES 2 *corpus albicans cyst (N83.2-)*
corpus luteum cyst (N83.1-)
endometrial cyst (N8Ø.1)
follicular (atretic) cyst (N83.Ø-)
graafian follicle cyst (N83.Ø-)
ovarian cyst NEC (N83.2-)
ovarian retention cyst (N83.2-)

D27.Ø Benign neoplasm of right ovary ♀
D27.1 Benign neoplasm of left ovary ♀
D27.9 Benign neoplasm of unspecified ovary ♀

✓4th **D28 Benign neoplasm of other and unspecified female genital organs**
INCLUDES adenomatous polyp
benign neoplasm of skin of female genital organs
benign teratoma
EXCLUDES 1 *epoophoron cyst (Q5Ø.5)*
fimbrial cyst (Q5Ø.4)
Gartner's duct cyst (Q52.4)
parovarian cyst (Q5Ø.5)

D28.Ø Benign neoplasm of vulva ♀
D28.1 Benign neoplasm of vagina ♀
D28.2 Benign neoplasm of uterine tubes and ligaments ♀
Benign neoplasm of fallopian tube
Benign neoplasm of uterine ligament (broad) (round)
D28.7 Benign neoplasm of other specified female genital organs ♀
D28.9 Benign neoplasm of female genital organ, unspecified ♀

✓4th **D29 Benign neoplasm of male genital organs**
INCLUDES benign neoplasm of skin of male genital organs

D29.Ø Benign neoplasm of penis ♂
D29.1 Benign neoplasm of prostate ♂
EXCLUDES 1 *enlarged prostate (N4Ø.-)*

✓5th **D29.2 Benign neoplasm of testis**
Use additional code to identify any functional activity
D29.20 Benign neoplasm of unspecified testis ♂
D29.21 Benign neoplasm of right testis ♂
D29.22 Benign neoplasm of left testis ♂

✓5th **D29.3 Benign neoplasm of epididymis**
D29.30 Benign neoplasm of unspecified epididymis ♂
D29.31 Benign neoplasm of right epididymis ♂
D29.32 Benign neoplasm of left epididymis ♂

D29.4 Benign neoplasm of scrotum ♂
Benign neoplasm of skin of scrotum
D29.8 Benign neoplasm of other specified male genital organs ♂
Benign neoplasm of seminal vesicle
Benign neoplasm of spermatic cord
Benign neoplasm of tunica vaginalis
D29.9 Benign neoplasm of male genital organ, unspecified ♂

✓4th **D3Ø Benign neoplasm of urinary organs**

✓5th **D3Ø.Ø Benign neoplasm of kidney**
EXCLUDES 1 *benign carcinoid tumor of the kidney (D3A.Ø93)*
benign neoplasm of renal calyces (D3Ø.1-)
benign neoplasm of renal pelvis (D3Ø.1-)
D3Ø.ØØ Benign neoplasm of unspecified kidney
D3Ø.Ø1 Benign neoplasm of right kidney
D3Ø.Ø2 Benign neoplasm of left kidney

✓5th **D3Ø.1 Benign neoplasm of renal pelvis**
D3Ø.1Ø Benign neoplasm of unspecified renal pelvis
D3Ø.11 Benign neoplasm of right renal pelvis
D3Ø.12 Benign neoplasm of left renal pelvis

✓5th **D3Ø.2 Benign neoplasm of ureter**
EXCLUDES 1 *benign neoplasm of ureteric orifice of bladder (D3Ø.3)*
D3Ø.2Ø Benign neoplasm of unspecified ureter
D3Ø.21 Benign neoplasm of right ureter
D3Ø.22 Benign neoplasm of left ureter

D3Ø.3 Benign neoplasm of bladder
Benign neoplasm of ureteric orifice of bladder
Benign neoplasm of urethral orifice of bladder

D30.4 Benign neoplasm of urethra
EXCLUDES 1 *benign neoplasm of urethral orifice of bladder (D30.3)*

D30.8 Benign neoplasm of other specified urinary organs
Benign neoplasm of paraurethral glands

D30.9 Benign neoplasm of urinary organ, unspecified
Benign neoplasm of urinary system NOS

✓4th D31 Benign neoplasm of eye and adnexa
EXCLUDES 1 *benign neoplasm of connective tissue of eyelid (D21.0)*
benign neoplasm of optic nerve (D33.3)
benign neoplasm of skin of eyelid (D22.1-, D23.1-)

✓5th D31.0 Benign neoplasm of conjunctiva
D31.00 Benign neoplasm of unspecified conjunctiva
D31.01 Benign neoplasm of right conjunctiva
D31.02 Benign neoplasm of left conjunctiva

✓5th D31.1 Benign neoplasm of cornea
D31.10 Benign neoplasm of unspecified cornea
D31.11 Benign neoplasm of right cornea
D31.12 Benign neoplasm of left cornea

✓5th D31.2 Benign neoplasm of retina
EXCLUDES 1 *dark area on retina (D49.81)*
hemangioma of retina (D49.81)
neoplasm of unspecified behavior of retina and choroid (D49.81)
retinal freckle (D49.81)
D31.20 Benign neoplasm of unspecified retina
D31.21 Benign neoplasm of right retina
D31.22 Benign neoplasm of left retina

✓5th D31.3 Benign neoplasm of choroid
D31.30 Benign neoplasm of unspecified choroid
D31.31 Benign neoplasm of right choroid
D31.32 Benign neoplasm of left choroid

✓5th D31.4 Benign neoplasm of ciliary body
D31.40 Benign neoplasm of unspecified ciliary body
D31.41 Benign neoplasm of right ciliary body
D31.42 Benign neoplasm of left ciliary body

✓5th D31.5 Benign neoplasm of lacrimal gland and duct
Benign neoplasm of lacrimal sac
Benign neoplasm of nasolacrimal duct
D31.50 Benign neoplasm of unspecified lacrimal gland and duct
D31.51 Benign neoplasm of right lacrimal gland and duct
D31.52 Benign neoplasm of left lacrimal gland and duct

✓5th D31.6 Benign neoplasm of unspecified site of orbit
Benign neoplasm of connective tissue of orbit
Benign neoplasm of extraocular muscle
Benign neoplasm of peripheral nerves of orbit
Benign neoplasm of retrobulbar tissue
Benign neoplasm of retro-ocular tissue
EXCLUDES 1 *benign neoplasm of orbital bone (D16.4)*
D31.60 Benign neoplasm of unspecified site of unspecified orbit
D31.61 Benign neoplasm of unspecified site of right orbit
D31.62 Benign neoplasm of unspecified site of left orbit

✓5th D31.9 Benign neoplasm of unspecified part of eye
Benign neoplasm of eyeball
D31.90 Benign neoplasm of unspecified part of unspecified eye
D31.91 Benign neoplasm of unspecified part of right eye
D31.92 Benign neoplasm of unspecified part of left eye

✓4th D32 Benign neoplasm of meninges
D32.0 Benign neoplasm of cerebral meninges HCC
D32.1 Benign neoplasm of spinal meninges HCC
D32.9 Benign neoplasm of meninges, unspecified HCC
Meningioma NOS

✓4th D33 Benign neoplasm of brain and other parts of central nervous system
EXCLUDES 1 *angioma (D18.0-)*
benign neoplasm of meninges (D32.-)
benign neoplasm of peripheral nerves and autonomic nervous system (D36.1-)
hemangioma (D18.0-)
neurofibromatosis (Q85.0-)
retro-ocular benign neoplasm (D31.6-)

D33.0 Benign neoplasm of brain, supratentorial HCC
Benign neoplasm of cerebral ventricle
Benign neoplasm of cerebrum
Benign neoplasm of frontal lobe
Benign neoplasm of occipital lobe
Benign neoplasm of parietal lobe
Benign neoplasm of temporal lobe
EXCLUDES 1 *benign neoplasm of fourth ventricle (D33.1)*

D33.1 Benign neoplasm of brain, infratentorial HCC
Benign neoplasm of brain stem
Benign neoplasm of cerebellum
Benign neoplasm of fourth ventricle

D33.2 Benign neoplasm of brain, unspecified HCC
D33.3 Benign neoplasm of cranial nerves HCC
Benign neoplasm of olfactory bulb
D33.4 Benign neoplasm of spinal cord HCC
D33.7 Benign neoplasm of other specified parts of central nervous system HCC
D33.9 Benign neoplasm of central nervous system, unspecified HCC
Benign neoplasm of nervous system (central) NOS

D34 Benign neoplasm of thyroid gland
Use additional code to identify any functional activity

✓4th D35 Benign neoplasm of other and unspecified endocrine glands
Use additional code to identify any functional activity
EXCLUDES 1 *benign neoplasm of endocrine pancreas (D13.7)*
benign neoplasm of ovary (D27.-)
benign neoplasm of testis (D29.2.-)
benign neoplasm of thymus (D15.0)

✓5th D35.0 Benign neoplasm of adrenal gland
D35.00 Benign neoplasm of unspecified adrenal gland
D35.01 Benign neoplasm of right adrenal gland
D35.02 Benign neoplasm of left adrenal gland

D35.1 Benign neoplasm of parathyroid gland
D35.2 Benign neoplasm of pituitary gland HCC
AHA: 2014,3Q,22
D35.3 Benign neoplasm of craniopharyngeal duct HCC
D35.4 Benign neoplasm of pineal gland HCC
D35.5 Benign neoplasm of carotid body
D35.6 Benign neoplasm of aortic body and other paraganglia
Benign tumor of glomus jugulare
D35.7 Benign neoplasm of other specified endocrine glands
D35.9 Benign neoplasm of endocrine gland, unspecified
Benign neoplasm of unspecified endocrine gland

✓4th D36 Benign neoplasm of other and unspecified sites
D36.0 Benign neoplasm of lymph nodes
EXCLUDES 1 *lymphangioma (D18.1)*

✓5th D36.1 Benign neoplasm of peripheral nerves and autonomic nervous system
EXCLUDES 1 *benign neoplasm of peripheral nerves of orbit (D31.6-)*
neurofibromatosis (Q85.0-)
D36.10 Benign neoplasm of peripheral nerves and autonomic nervous system, unspecified
D36.11 Benign neoplasm of peripheral nerves and autonomic nervous system of face, head, and neck
D36.12 Benign neoplasm of peripheral nerves and autonomic nervous system, upper limb, including shoulder
D36.13 Benign neoplasm of peripheral nerves and autonomic nervous system of lower limb, including hip
D36.14 Benign neoplasm of peripheral nerves and autonomic nervous system of thorax
D36.15 Benign neoplasm of peripheral nerves and autonomic nervous system of abdomen

D36.16 Benign neoplasm of peripheral nerves and autonomic nervous system of pelvis

D36.17 Benign neoplasm of peripheral nerves and autonomic nervous system of trunk, unspecified

D36.7 Benign neoplasm of other specified sites

Benign neoplasm of back NOS

Benign neoplasm of nose NOS

D36.9 Benign neoplasm, unspecified site

Benign neuroendocrine tumors (D3A)

✓4th D3A Benign neuroendocrine tumors

Code also any associated multiple endocrine neoplasia [MEN] syndromes (E31.2-)

Use additional code to identify any associated endocrine syndrome, such as:

carcinoid syndrome (E34.Ø)

EXCLUDES 2 *benign pancreatic islet cell tumors (D13.7)*

✓5th D3A.Ø Benign carcinoid tumors

D3A.ØØ Benign carcinoid tumor of unspecified site

Carcinoid tumor NOS

✓6th D3A.Ø1 Benign carcinoid tumors of the small intestine

D3A.Ø1Ø Benign carcinoid tumor of the duodenum

D3A.Ø11 Benign carcinoid tumor of the jejunum

D3A.Ø12 Benign carcinoid tumor of the ileum

D3A.Ø19 Benign carcinoid tumor of the small intestine, unspecified portion

✓6th D3A.Ø2 Benign carcinoid tumors of the appendix, large intestine, and rectum

D3A.Ø2Ø Benign carcinoid tumor of the appendix

D3A.Ø21 Benign carcinoid tumor of the cecum

D3A.Ø22 Benign carcinoid tumor of the ascending colon

D3A.Ø23 Benign carcinoid tumor of the transverse colon

D3A.Ø24 Benign carcinoid tumor of the descending colon

D3A.Ø25 Benign carcinoid tumor of the sigmoid colon

D3A.Ø26 Benign carcinoid tumor of the rectum

D3A.Ø29 Benign carcinoid tumor of the large intestine, unspecified portion

Benign carcinoid tumor of the colon NOS

✓6th D3A.Ø9 Benign carcinoid tumors of other sites

D3A.Ø9Ø Benign carcinoid tumor of the bronchus and lung

D3A.Ø91 Benign carcinoid tumor of the thymus

D3A.Ø92 Benign carcinoid tumor of the stomach

D3A.Ø93 Benign carcinoid tumor of the kidney

D3A.Ø94 Benign carcinoid tumor of the foregut, unspecified

D3A.Ø95 Benign carcinoid tumor of the midgut, unspecified

D3A.Ø96 Benign carcinoid tumor of the hindgut, unspecified

D3A.Ø98 Benign carcinoid tumors of other sites

D3A.8 Other benign neuroendocrine tumors

Neuroendocrine tumor NOS

Neoplasms of uncertain behavior, polycythemia vera and myelodysplastic syndromes (D37-D48)

NOTE Categories D37-D44, and D48 classify by site neoplasms of uncertain behavior, i.e., histologic confirmation whether the neoplasm is malignant or benign cannot be made.

EXCLUDES 1 *neoplasms of unspecified behavior (D49.-)*

✓4th D37 Neoplasm of uncertain behavior of oral cavity and digestive organs

EXCLUDES 1 *stromal tumors of uncertain behavior of digestive system (D48.1)*

✓5th D37.Ø Neoplasm of uncertain behavior of lip, oral cavity and pharynx

EXCLUDES 1 *neoplasm of uncertain behavior of aryepiglottic fold or interarytenoid fold, laryngeal aspect (D38.Ø)*

neoplasm of uncertain behavior of epiglottis NOS (D38.Ø)

neoplasm of uncertain behavior of skin of lip (D48.5)

neoplasm of uncertain behavior of suprahyoid portion of epiglottis (D38.Ø)

D37.Ø1 Neoplasm of uncertain behavior of lip

Neoplasm of uncertain behavior of vermilion border of lip

D37.Ø2 Neoplasm of uncertain behavior of tongue

✓6th D37.Ø3 Neoplasm of uncertain behavior of the major salivary glands

D37.Ø3Ø Neoplasm of uncertain behavior of the parotid salivary glands

D37.Ø31 Neoplasm of uncertain behavior of the sublingual salivary glands

D37.Ø32 Neoplasm of uncertain behavior of the submandibular salivary glands

D37.Ø39 Neoplasm of uncertain behavior of the major salivary glands, unspecified

D37.Ø4 Neoplasm of uncertain behavior of the minor salivary glands

Neoplasm of uncertain behavior of submucosal salivary glands of lip

Neoplasm of uncertain behavior of submucosal salivary glands of cheek

Neoplasm of uncertain behavior of submucosal salivary glands of hard palate

Neoplasm of uncertain behavior of submucosal salivary glands of soft palate

D37.Ø5 Neoplasm of uncertain behavior of pharynx

Neoplasm of uncertain behavior of aryepiglottic fold of pharynx NOS

Neoplasm of uncertain behavior of hypopharyngeal aspect of aryepiglottic fold of pharynx

Neoplasm of uncertain behavior of marginal zone of aryepiglottic fold of pharynx

D37.Ø9 Neoplasm of uncertain behavior of other specified sites of the oral cavity

D37.1 Neoplasm of uncertain behavior of stomach

D37.2 Neoplasm of uncertain behavior of small intestine

D37.3 Neoplasm of uncertain behavior of appendix

D37.4 Neoplasm of uncertain behavior of colon

D37.5 Neoplasm of uncertain behavior of rectum

Neoplasm of uncertain behavior of rectosigmoid junction

D37.6 Neoplasm of uncertain behavior of liver, gallbladder and bile ducts

Neoplasm of uncertain behavior of ampulla of Vater

D37.8 Neoplasm of uncertain behavior of other specified digestive organs

Neoplasm of uncertain behavior of anal canal

Neoplasm of uncertain behavior of anal sphincter

Neoplasm of uncertain behavior of anus NOS

Neoplasm of uncertain behavior of esophagus

Neoplasm of uncertain behavior of intestine NOS

Neoplasm of uncertain behavior of pancreas

EXCLUDES 1 *neoplasm of uncertain behavior of anal margin (D48.5)*

neoplasm of uncertain behavior of anal skin (D48.5)

neoplasm of uncertain behavior of perianal skin (D48.5)

D37.9 Neoplasm of uncertain behavior of digestive organ, unspecified

4th D38 Neoplasm of uncertain behavior of middle ear and respiratory and intrathoracic organs

EXCLUDES 1 *neoplasm of uncertain behavior of heart (D48.7)*

D38.0 Neoplasm of uncertain behavior of larynx

Neoplasm of uncertain behavior of aryepiglottic fold or interarytenoid fold, laryngeal aspect

Neoplasm of uncertain behavior of epiglottis (suprahyoid portion)

EXCLUDES 1 *neoplasm of uncertain behavior of aryepiglottic fold or interarytenoid fold NOS (D37.05)*
neoplasm of uncertain behavior of hypopharyngeal aspect of aryepiglottic fold (D37.05)
neoplasm of uncertain behavior of marginal zone of aryepiglottic fold (D37.05)

D38.1 Neoplasm of uncertain behavior of trachea, bronchus and lung

D38.2 Neoplasm of uncertain behavior of pleura

D38.3 Neoplasm of uncertain behavior of mediastinum

D38.4 Neoplasm of uncertain behavior of thymus

D38.5 Neoplasm of uncertain behavior of other respiratory organs

Neoplasm of uncertain behavior of accessory sinuses

Neoplasm of uncertain behavior of cartilage of nose

Neoplasm of uncertain behavior of middle ear

Neoplasm of uncertain behavior of nasal cavities

EXCLUDES 1 *neoplasm of uncertain behavior of ear (external) (skin) (D48.5)*
neoplasm of uncertain behavior of nose NOS (D48.7)
neoplasm of uncertain behavior of skin of nose (D48.5)

D38.6 Neoplasm of uncertain behavior of respiratory organ, unspecified

4th D39 Neoplasm of uncertain behavior of female genital organs

D39.0 Neoplasm of uncertain behavior of uterus ♀

5th D39.1 Neoplasm of uncertain behavior of ovary

Use additional code to identify any functional activity

D39.10 Neoplasm of uncertain behavior of unspecified ovary ♀

D39.11 Neoplasm of uncertain behavior of right ovary ♀

D39.12 Neoplasm of uncertain behavior of left ovary ♀

D39.2 Neoplasm of uncertain behavior of placenta M ♀

Chorioadenoma destruens

Invasive hydatidiform mole

Malignant hydatidiform mole

EXCLUDES 1 *hydatidiform mole NOS (O01.9)*

D39.8 Neoplasm of uncertain behavior of other specified female genital organs ♀

Neoplasm of uncertain behavior of skin of female genital organs

D39.9 Neoplasm of uncertain behavior of female genital organ, unspecified ♀

4th D40 Neoplasm of uncertain behavior of male genital organs

D40.0 Neoplasm of uncertain behavior of prostate ♂

5th D40.1 Neoplasm of uncertain behavior of testis

D40.10 Neoplasm of uncertain behavior of unspecified testis ♂

D40.11 Neoplasm of uncertain behavior of right testis ♂

D40.12 Neoplasm of uncertain behavior of left testis ♂

D40.8 Neoplasm of uncertain behavior of other specified male genital organs ♂

Neoplasm of uncertain behavior of skin of male genital organs

D40.9 Neoplasm of uncertain behavior of male genital organ, unspecified ♂

4th D41 Neoplasm of uncertain behavior of urinary organs

5th D41.0 Neoplasm of uncertain behavior of kidney

EXCLUDES 1 *neoplasm of uncertain behavior of renal pelvis (D41.1-)*

D41.00 Neoplasm of uncertain behavior of unspecified kidney

D41.01 Neoplasm of uncertain behavior of right kidney

D41.02 Neoplasm of uncertain behavior of left kidney

5th D41.1 Neoplasm of uncertain behavior of renal pelvis

D41.10 Neoplasm of uncertain behavior of unspecified renal pelvis

D41.11 Neoplasm of uncertain behavior of right renal pelvis

D41.12 Neoplasm of uncertain behavior of left renal pelvis

5th D41.2 Neoplasm of uncertain behavior of ureter

D41.20 Neoplasm of uncertain behavior of unspecified ureter

D41.21 Neoplasm of uncertain behavior of right ureter

D41.22 Neoplasm of uncertain behavior of left ureter

D41.3 Neoplasm of uncertain behavior of urethra

D41.4 Neoplasm of uncertain behavior of bladder

D41.8 Neoplasm of uncertain behavior of other specified urinary organs

D41.9 Neoplasm of uncertain behavior of unspecified urinary organ

4th D42 Neoplasm of uncertain behavior of meninges

D42.0 Neoplasm of uncertain behavior of cerebral meninges HCC

D42.1 Neoplasm of uncertain behavior of spinal meninges HCC

D42.9 Neoplasm of uncertain behavior of meninges, unspecified HCC

4th D43 Neoplasm of uncertain behavior of brain and central nervous system

EXCLUDES 1 *neoplasm of uncertain behavior of peripheral nerves and autonomic nervous system (D48.2)*

D43.0 Neoplasm of uncertain behavior of brain, supratentorial HCC

Neoplasm of uncertain behavior of cerebral ventricle

Neoplasm of uncertain behavior of cerebrum

Neoplasm of uncertain behavior of frontal lobe

Neoplasm of uncertain behavior of occipital lobe

Neoplasm of uncertain behavior of parietal lobe

Neoplasm of uncertain behavior of temporal lobe

EXCLUDES 1 *neoplasm of uncertain behavior of fourth ventricle (D43.1)*

D43.1 Neoplasm of uncertain behavior of brain, infratentorial HCC

Neoplasm of uncertain behavior of brain stem

Neoplasm of uncertain behavior of cerebellum

Neoplasm of uncertain behavior of fourth ventricle

D43.2 Neoplasm of uncertain behavior of brain, unspecified HCC

D43.3 Neoplasm of uncertain behavior of cranial nerves HCC

D43.4 Neoplasm of uncertain behavior of spinal cord HCC

D43.8 Neoplasm of uncertain behavior of other specified parts of central nervous system HCC

D43.9 Neoplasm of uncertain behavior of central nervous system, unspecified HCC

Neoplasm of uncertain behavior of nervous system (central) NOS

4th D44 Neoplasm of uncertain behavior of endocrine glands

EXCLUDES 1 *multiple endocrine adenomatosis (E31.2-)*
multiple endocrine neoplasia (E31.2-)
neoplasm of uncertain behavior of endocrine pancreas (D37.8)
neoplasm of uncertain behavior of ovary (D39.1-)
neoplasm of uncertain behavior of testis (D40.1-)
neoplasm of uncertain behavior of thymus (D38.4)

D44.0 Neoplasm of uncertain behavior of thyroid gland

5th D44.1 Neoplasm of uncertain behavior of adrenal gland

Use additional code to identify any functional activity

D44.10 Neoplasm of uncertain behavior of unspecified adrenal gland

D44.11 Neoplasm of uncertain behavior of right adrenal gland

D44.12 Neoplasm of uncertain behavior of left adrenal gland

D44.2 Neoplasm of uncertain behavior of parathyroid gland

D44.3 Neoplasm of uncertain behavior of pituitary gland HCC

Use additional code to identify any functional activity

D44.4 Neoplasm of uncertain behavior of craniopharyngeal duct HCC

D44.5 Neoplasm of uncertain behavior of pineal gland HCC

D44.6 Neoplasm of uncertain behavior of carotid body HCC

D44.7 Neoplasm of uncertain behavior of aortic body and other paraganglia HCC

AHA: 2016,4Q,26

D44.9 Neoplasm of uncertain behavior of unspecified endocrine gland

D45 Polycythemia vera HCC

EXCLUDES 1 *familial polycythemia (D75.Ø)*
secondary polycythemia (D75.1)

DEF: Abnormal proliferation of all bone marrow elements, increased red cell mass, and total blood volume. The etiology is unknown, but it is frequently associated with splenomegaly, leukocytosis, and thrombocythemia.

✓4th **D46 Myelodysplastic syndromes**

Use additional code for adverse effect, if applicable, to identify drug (T36-T5Ø with fifth or sixth character 5)

EXCLUDES 2 *drug-induced aplastic anemia (D61.1)*

D46.Ø Refractory anemia without ring sideroblasts, so stated HCC
Refractory anemia without sideroblasts, without excess of blasts

D46.1 Refractory anemia with ring sideroblasts HCC
RARS

✓5th **D46.2 Refractory anemia with excess of blasts [RAEB]**

D46.2Ø Refractory anemia with excess of blasts, unspecified HCC
RAEB NOS

D46.21 Refractory anemia with excess of blasts 1 HCC
RAEB 1

D46.22 Refractory anemia with excess of blasts 2 CC HCC
RAEB 2

D46.A Refractory cytopenia with multilineage dysplasia HCC

D46.B Refractory cytopenia with multilineage dysplasia and ring sideroblasts HCC
RCMD RS

D46.C Myelodysplastic syndrome with isolated del(5q) chromosomal abnormality CC HCC
Myelodysplastic syndrome with 5q deletion
5q minus syndrome NOS

D46.4 Refractory anemia, unspecified HCC

D46.Z Other myelodysplastic syndromes HCC
EXCLUDES 1 *chronic myelomonocytic leukemia (C93.1-)*

D46.9 Myelodysplastic syndrome, unspecified HCC
Myelodysplasia NOS

✓4th **D47 Other neoplasms of uncertain behavior of lymphoid, hematopoietic and related tissue**

✓5th **D47.Ø Mast cell neoplasms of uncertain behavior**

EXCLUDES 1 *congenital cutaneous mastocytosis (Q82.2)*
histiocytic neoplasms of uncertain behavior (D47.Z9)
malignant mast cell neoplasm (C96.2-)

AHA: 2017,4Q,5

D47.Ø1 Cutaneous mastocytosis CC
Diffuse cutaneous mastocytosis
Maculopapular cutaneous mastocytosis
Solitary mastocytoma
Telangiectasia macularis eruptiva perstans
Urticaria pigmentosa
EXCLUDES 1 *congenital (diffuse) (maculopapular) cutaneous mastocytosis (Q82.2)*
congenital urticaria pigmentosa (Q82.2)
extracutaneous mastocytoma (D47.Ø9)

D47.Ø2 Systemic mastocytosis CC
Indolent systemic mastocytosis
Isolated bone marrow mastocytosis
Smoldering systemic mastocytosis
Systemic mastocytosis, with an associated hematological non-mast cell lineage disease (SM-AHNMD)
Code also, if applicable, any associated hematological non-mast cell lineage disease, such as:
acute myeloid leukemia (C92.6-, C92.A-)
chronic myelomonocytic leukemia (C93.1-)
essential thrombocytosis (D47.3)
hypereosinophilic syndrome (D72.1)
myelodysplastic syndrome (D46.9)
myeloproliferative syndrome (D47.1)
non-Hodgkin lymphoma (C82-C85)
plasma cell myeloma (C9Ø.Ø-)
polycythemia vera (D45)
EXCLUDES 1 *aggressive systemic mastocytosis (C96.21)*
mast cell leukemia (C94.3-)

D47.Ø9 Other mast cell neoplasms of uncertain behavior CC
Extracutaneous mastocytoma
Mast cell tumor NOS
Mastocytoma NOS
Mastocytosis NOS

D47.1 Chronic myeloproliferative disease CC HCC
Chronic neutrophilic leukemia
Myeloproliferative disease, unspecified
EXCLUDES 1 *atypical chronic myeloid leukemia BCR/ABL-negative (C92.2-)*
chronic myeloid leukemia BCR/ABL-positive (C92.1-)
myelofibrosis NOS (D75.81)
myelophthisic anemia (D61.82)
myelophthisis (D61.82)
secondary myelofibrosis NOS (D75.81)

D47.2 Monoclonal gammopathy
Monoclonal gammopathy of undetermined significance [MGUS]

D47.3 Essential (hemorrhagic) thrombocythemia HCC
Essential thrombocytosis
Idiopathic hemorrhagic thrombocythemia
DEF: Chronic myeloproliferative neoplasm involving production of excess blood platelets that may result in abnormal clotting or hemorrhaging.

D47.4 Osteomyelofibrosis HCC
Chronic idiopathic myelofibrosis
Myelofibrosis (idiopathic) (with myeloid metaplasia)
Myelosclerosis (megakaryocytic) with myeloid metaplasia
Secondary myelofibrosis in myeloproliferative disease
EXCLUDES 1 *acute myelofibrosis (C94.4-)*

✓5th **D47.Z Other specified neoplasms of uncertain behavior of lymphoid, hematopoietic and related tissue**

AHA: 2016,4Q,8

D47.Z1 Post-transplant lymphoproliferative disorder (PTLD) CC HCC
Code first complications of transplanted organs and tissue (T86.-)
DEF: Excessive proliferation of B-cell lymphocytes following Epstein-Barr virus infection in organ transplant patients. It may progress to non-Hodgkin lymphoma.

D47.Z2 Castleman disease CC HCC
Code also if applicable human herpesvirus 8 infection (B1Ø.89)
EXCLUDES 2 *Kaposi's sarcoma ►(C46.-)◄*
DEF: Rare disease of the lymph nodes and lymphoid tissues that closely mimics lymphoma.

D47.Z9 Other specified neoplasms of uncertain behavior of lymphoid, hematopoietic and related tissue CC HCC
Histiocytic tumors of uncertain behavior

D47.9 Neoplasm of uncertain behavior of lymphoid, hematopoietic and related tissue, unspecified CC HCC
Lymphoproliferative disease NOS

✓4th **D48 Neoplasm of uncertain behavior of other and unspecified sites**

EXCLUDES 1 *neurofibromatosis (nonmalignant) (Q85.Ø-)*

D48.Ø Neoplasm of uncertain behavior of bone and articular cartilage
EXCLUDES 1 *neoplasm of uncertain behavior of cartilage of ear (D48.1)*
neoplasm of uncertain behavior of cartilage of larynx (D38.Ø)
neoplasm of uncertain behavior of cartilage of nose (D38.5)
neoplasm of uncertain behavior of connective tissue of eyelid (D48.1)
neoplasm of uncertain behavior of synovia (D48.1)

D48.1 Neoplasm of uncertain behavior of connective and other soft tissue
Neoplasm of uncertain behavior of connective tissue of ear
Neoplasm of uncertain behavior of connective tissue of eyelid
Stromal tumors of uncertain behavior of digestive system
EXCLUDES 1 *neoplasm of uncertain behavior of articular cartilage (D48.Ø)*
neoplasm of uncertain behavior of cartilage of larynx (D38.Ø)
neoplasm of uncertain behavior of cartilage of nose (D38.5)
neoplasm of uncertain behavior of connective tissue of breast (D48.6-)

D48.2 Neoplasm of uncertain behavior of peripheral nerves and autonomic nervous system
EXCLUDES 1 *neoplasm of uncertain behavior of peripheral nerves of orbit (D48.7)*

D48.3 Neoplasm of uncertain behavior of retroperitoneum

D48.4 Neoplasm of uncertain behavior of peritoneum

D48.5 Neoplasm of uncertain behavior of skin
Neoplasm of uncertain behavior of anal margin
Neoplasm of uncertain behavior of anal skin
Neoplasm of uncertain behavior of perianal skin
Neoplasm of uncertain behavior of skin of breast
EXCLUDES 1 *neoplasm of uncertain behavior of anus NOS (D37.8)*
neoplasm of uncertain behavior of skin of genital organs (D39.8, D4Ø.8)
neoplasm of uncertain behavior of vermilion border of lip (D37.Ø)

✓5th **D48.6 Neoplasm of uncertain behavior of breast**
Neoplasm of uncertain behavior of connective tissue of breast
Cystosarcoma phyllodes
EXCLUDES 1 *neoplasm of uncertain behavior of skin of breast (D48.5)*

D48.6Ø Neoplasm of uncertain behavior of unspecified breast

D48.61 Neoplasm of uncertain behavior of right breast

D48.62 Neoplasm of uncertain behavior of left breast

D48.7 Neoplasm of uncertain behavior of other specified sites
Neoplasm of uncertain behavior of eye
Neoplasm of uncertain behavior of heart
Neoplasm of uncertain behavior of peripheral nerves of orbit
EXCLUDES 1 *neoplasm of uncertain behavior of connective tissue (D48.1)*
neoplasm of uncertain behavior of skin of eyelid (D48.5)

D48.9 Neoplasm of uncertain behavior, unspecified

Neoplasms of unspecified behavior (D49)

✓4th **D49 Neoplasms of unspecified behavior**

NOTE Category D49 classifies by site neoplasms of unspecified morphology and behavior. The term "mass", unless otherwise stated, is not to be regarded as a neoplastic growth.

INCLUDES "growth" NOS
neoplasm NOS
new growth NOS
tumor NOS

EXCLUDES 1 *neoplasms of uncertain behavior (D37-D44, D48)*

D49.Ø Neoplasm of unspecified behavior of digestive system
EXCLUDES 1 *neoplasm of unspecified behavior of margin of anus (D49.2)*
neoplasm of unspecified behavior of perianal skin (D49.2)
neoplasm of unspecified behavior of skin of anus (D49.2)

D49.1 Neoplasm of unspecified behavior of respiratory system

D49.2 Neoplasm of unspecified behavior of bone, soft tissue, and skin
EXCLUDES 1 *neoplasm of unspecified behavior of anal canal (D49.Ø)*
neoplasm of unspecified behavior of anus NOS (D49.Ø)
neoplasm of unspecified behavior of bone marrow (D49.89)
neoplasm of unspecified behavior of cartilage of larynx (D49.1)
neoplasm of unspecified behavior of cartilage of nose (D49.1)
neoplasm of unspecified behavior of connective tissue of breast (D49.3)
neoplasm of unspecified behavior of skin of genital organs (D49.59)
neoplasm of unspecified behavior of vermilion border of lip (D49.Ø)

D49.3 Neoplasm of unspecified behavior of breast
EXCLUDES 1 *neoplasm of unspecified behavior of skin of breast (D49.2)*

D49.4 Neoplasm of unspecified behavior of bladder

✓5th **D49.5 Neoplasm of unspecified behavior of other genitourinary organs**
AHA: 2016,4Q,9

✓6th **D49.51 Neoplasm of unspecified behavior of kidney**

D49.511 Neoplasm of unspecified behavior of right kidney

D49.512 Neoplasm of unspecified behavior of left kidney

D49.519 Neoplasm of unspecified behavior of unspecified kidney

D49.59 Neoplasm of unspecified behavior of other genitourinary organ

D49.6 Neoplasm of unspecified behavior of brain HCC
EXCLUDES 1 *neoplasm of unspecified behavior of cerebral meninges (D49.7)*
neoplasm of unspecified behavior of cranial nerves (D49.7)

D49.7 Neoplasm of unspecified behavior of endocrine glands and other parts of nervous system
EXCLUDES 1 *neoplasm of unspecified behavior of peripheral, sympathetic, and parasympathetic nerves and ganglia (D49.2)*

✓5th **D49.8 Neoplasm of unspecified behavior of other specified sites**
EXCLUDES 1 *neoplasm of unspecified behavior of eyelid (skin) (D49.2)*
neoplasm of unspecified behavior of eyelid cartilage (D49.2)
neoplasm of unspecified behavior of great vessels (D49.2)
neoplasm of unspecified behavior of optic nerve (D49.7)

D49.81 Neoplasm of unspecified behavior of retina and choroid
Dark area on retina
Retinal freckle

D49.89 Neoplasm of unspecified behavior of other specified sites

D49.9 Neoplasm of unspecified behavior of unspecified site

Chapter 3. Diseases of the Blood and Blood-forming Organs and Certain Disorders Involving the Immune Mechanism (D5Ø–D89)

Chapter-specific Guidelines with Coding Examples
Reserved for future guideline expansion

Chapter 3. Diseases of the Blood and Blood-forming Organs and Certain Disorders Involving the Immune Mechanism (D5Ø-D89)

EXCLUDES 2 *autoimmune disease (systemic) NOS (M35.9)*
certain conditions originating in the perinatal period (PØØ-P96)
complications of pregnancy, childbirth and the puerperium (OØØ-O9A)
congenital malformations, deformations and chromosomal abnormalities (QØØ-Q99)
endocrine, nutritional and metabolic diseases (EØØ-E88)
human immunodeficiency virus [HIV] disease (B2Ø)
injury, poisoning and certain other consequences of external causes (SØØ-T88)
neoplasms (CØØ-D49)
symptoms, signs and abnormal clinical and laboratory findings, not elsewhere classified (RØØ-R94)

This chapter contains the following blocks:

D5Ø-D53	Nutritional anemias
D55-D59	Hemolytic anemias
D6Ø-D64	Aplastic and other anemias and other bone marrow failure syndromes
D65-D69	Coagulation defects, purpura and other hemorrhagic conditions
D7Ø-D77	Other disorders of blood and blood-forming organs
D78	Intraoperative and postprocedural complications of the spleen
D8Ø-D89	Certain disorders involving the immune mechanism

Nutritional anemias (D5Ø-D53)

DEF: Nutritional anemia: The result of inadequate intake or absorption of a vitamin or mineral that impacts the production of red blood cells or causes them to develop abnormally affecting the size and shape.
TIP: Documentation must identify a link between anemia and the nutritional deficiency; low levels of a particular nutrient may occur concurrently with anemia but not cause the anemia.

✓4th **D5Ø Iron deficiency anemia**
INCLUDES asiderotic anemia
hypochromic anemia

D5Ø.Ø Iron deficiency anemia secondary to blood loss (chronic)
Posthemorrhagic anemia (chronic)
EXCLUDES 1 *acute posthemorrhagic anemia (D62)*
congenital anemia from fetal blood loss (P61.3)
AHA: 2019,3Q,17

D5Ø.1 Sideropenic dysphagia
Kelly-Paterson syndrome
Plummer-Vinson syndrome

D5Ø.8 Other iron deficiency anemias
Iron deficiency anemia due to inadequate dietary iron intake

D5Ø.9 Iron deficiency anemia, unspecified

✓4th **D51 Vitamin B12 deficiency anemia**
EXCLUDES 1 *vitamin B12 deficiency (E53.8)*

D51.Ø Vitamin B12 deficiency anemia due to intrinsic factor deficiency
Addison anemia
Biermer anemia
Pernicious (congenital) anemia
Congenital intrinsic factor deficiency
DEF: Chronic progressive anemia due to vitamin B12 malabsorption, caused by lack of secretion of intrinsic factor, which is produced by the gastric mucosa of the stomach.

D51.1 Vitamin B12 deficiency anemia due to selective vitamin B12 malabsorption with proteinuria
Imerslund (Gräsbeck) syndrome
Megaloblastic hereditary anemia

D51.2 Transcobalamin II deficiency

D51.3 Other dietary vitamin B12 deficiency anemia
Vegan anemia

D51.8 Other vitamin B12 deficiency anemias

D51.9 Vitamin B12 deficiency anemia, unspecified

✓4th **D52 Folate deficiency anemia**
EXCLUDES 1 *folate deficiency without anemia (E53.8)*
DEF: Deficiency in a B complex vitamin needed for the production of healthy red blood cells. Lack of folate, or folic acid, and other absorption conditions can cause anemia resulting in large, misshapen red blood cells called megaloblasts.

D52.Ø Dietary folate deficiency anemia
Nutritional megaloblastic anemia
DEF: Result of a poor diet with inadequate intake of folate, which is needed to produce healthy red blood cells.

D52.1 Drug-induced folate deficiency anemia
Use additional code for adverse effect, if applicable, to identify drug (T36-T5Ø with fifth or sixth character 5)

D52.8 Other folate deficiency anemias

D52.9 Folate deficiency anemia, unspecified
Folic acid deficiency anemia NOS

✓4th **D53 Other nutritional anemias**
INCLUDES megaloblastic anemia unresponsive to vitamin B12 or folate therapy

D53.Ø Protein deficiency anemia
Amino-acid deficiency anemia
Orotaciduric anemia
EXCLUDES 1 *Lesch-Nyhan syndrome (E79.1)*

D53.1 Other megaloblastic anemias, not elsewhere classified
Megaloblastic anemia NOS
EXCLUDES 1 *Di Guglielmo's disease (C94.Ø)*

D53.2 Scorbutic anemia
EXCLUDES 1 *scurvy (E54)*

D53.8 Other specified nutritional anemias
Anemia associated with deficiency of copper
Anemia associated with deficiency of molybdenum
Anemia associated with deficiency of zinc
EXCLUDES 1 *nutritional deficiencies without anemia, such as:*
copper deficiency NOS (E61.Ø)
molybdenum deficiency NOS (E61.5)
zinc deficiency NOS (E6Ø)

D53.9 Nutritional anemia, unspecified
Simple chronic anemia
EXCLUDES 1 *anemia NOS (D64.9)*
AHA: 2018,4Q,88

Hemolytic anemias (D55-D59)

✓4th **D55 Anemia due to enzyme disorders**
EXCLUDES 1 *drug-induced enzyme deficiency anemia (D59.2)*

D55.Ø Anemia due to glucose-6-phosphate dehydrogenase [G6PD] deficiency HCC
Favism
G6PD deficiency anemia
EXCLUDES 1 *glucose-6-phosphate dehydrogenase (G6PD) deficiency without anemia (D75.A)*

D55.1 Anemia due to other disorders of glutathione metabolism HCC
Anemia (due to) enzyme deficiencies, except G6PD, related to the hexose monophosphate [HMP] shunt pathway
Anemia (due to) hemolytic nonspherocytic (hereditary), type I

D55.2 Anemia due to disorders of glycolytic enzymes HCC
Hemolytic nonspherocytic (hereditary) anemia, type II
Hexokinase deficiency anemia
Pyruvate kinase [PK] deficiency anemia
Triose-phosphate isomerase deficiency anemia
EXCLUDES 1 *disorders of glycolysis not associated with anemia ▶(E74.81-)◀*

D55.3 Anemia due to disorders of nucleotide metabolism HCC

D55.8 Other anemias due to enzyme disorders HCC

D55.9 Anemia due to enzyme disorder, unspecified HCC

✓4th D56 Thalassemia

EXCLUDES 1 *sickle-cell thalassemia (D57.4-)*

DEF: Group of inherited disorders of hemoglobin metabolism causing mild to severe anemia. It is usually found in people of Mediterranean, African, Chinese, or Asian descent.

Thalassemia

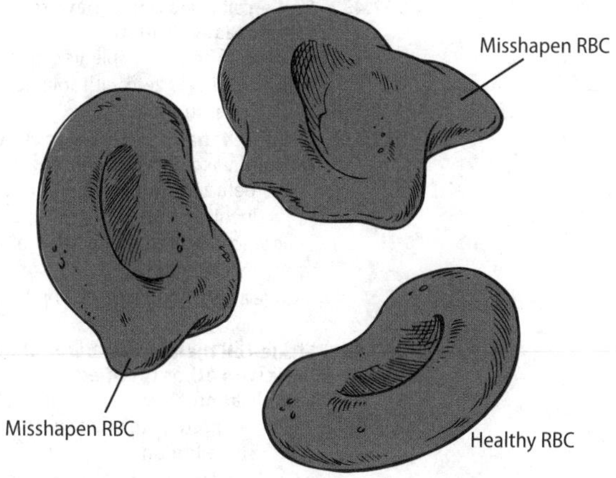

D56.Ø Alpha thalassemia HCC
- Alpha thalassemia major
- Hemoglobin H Constant Spring
- Hemoglobin H disease
- Hydrops fetalis due to alpha thalassemia
- Severe alpha thalassemia
- Triple gene defect alpha thalassemia

Use additional code, if applicable, for hydrops fetalis due to alpha thalassemia (P56.99)

EXCLUDES 1 *alpha thalassemia trait or minor (D56.3)*
asymptomatic alpha thalassemia (D56.3)
hydrops fetalis due to isoimmunization (P56.Ø)
hydrops fetalis not due to immune hemolysis (P83.2)

DEF: HBA1 and HBA2 genetic variant of chromosome 16 prevalent among those of African and Southeast Asian descent. Alpha thalassemia is associated with a wide spectrum of anemic presentation and includes hemoglobin H disease subtypes.

D56.1 Beta thalassemia HCC
- Beta thalassemia major
- Cooley's anemia
- Homozygous beta thalassemia
- Severe beta thalassemia
- Thalassemia intermedia
- Thalassemia major

EXCLUDES 1 *beta thalassemia minor (D56.3)*
beta thalassemia trait (D56.3)
delta-beta thalassemia (D56.2)
hemoglobin E-beta thalassemia (D56.5)
sickle-cell beta thalassemia (D57.4-)

D56.2 Delta-beta thalassemia HCC
- Homozygous delta-beta thalassemia

EXCLUDES 1 *delta-beta thalassemia minor (D56.3)*
delta-beta thalassemia trait (D56.3)

D56.3 Thalassemia minor
- Alpha thalassemia minor
- Alpha thalassemia silent carrier
- Alpha thalassemia trait
- Beta thalassemia minor
- Beta thalassemia trait
- Delta-beta thalassemia minor
- Delta-beta thalassemia trait
- Thalassemia trait NOS

EXCLUDES 1 *alpha thalassemia (D56.Ø)*
beta thalassemia (D56.1)
delta-beta thalassemia (D56.2)
hemoglobin E-beta thalassemia (D56.5)
sickle-cell trait (D57.3)

DEF: Solitary abnormal gene that identifies a carrier of the disease, yet with an absence of symptoms or a clinically mild anemic presentation.

D56.4 Hereditary persistence of fetal hemoglobin [HPFH] HCC

D56.5 Hemoglobin E-beta thalassemia HCC

EXCLUDES 1 *beta thalassemia (D56.1)*
beta thalassemia minor (D56.3)
beta thalassemia trait (D56.3)
delta-beta thalassemia (D56.2)
delta-beta thalassemia trait (D56.3)
hemoglobin E disease (D58.2)
other hemoglobinopathies (D58.2)
sickle-cell beta thalassemia (D57.4-)

D56.8 Other thalassemias HCC
- Dominant thalassemia
- Hemoglobin C thalassemia
- Mixed thalassemia
- Thalassemia with other hemoglobinopathy

EXCLUDES 1 *hemoglobin C disease (D58.2)*
hemoglobin E disease (D58.2)
other hemoglobinopathies (D58.2)
sickle-cell anemia (D57.-)
sickle-cell thalassemia (D57.4)

D56.9 Thalassemia, unspecified
- Mediterranean anemia (with other hemoglobinopathy)

✓4th D57 Sickle-cell disorders

Use additional code for any associated fever (R5Ø.81)

EXCLUDES 1 *other hemoglobinopathies (D58.-)*

DEF: Severe, chronic inherited diseases caused by a genetic variation in hemoglobin protein of the red blood cell. The gene mutation causes the red blood cell to become hard, sticky, and crescent or sickle shaped making it harder for red blood cells to travel through the bloodstream disrupting blood flow and decreasing oxygen transport to tissues.

Sickle cell

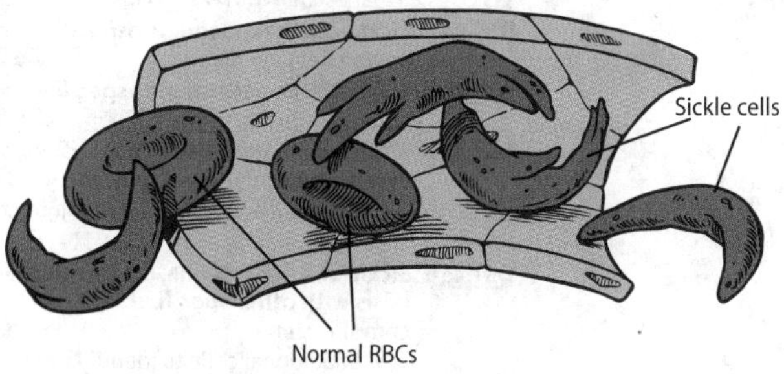

✓5th D57.Ø Hb-SS disease with crisis
- ▶Sickle-cell disease with crisis◀
- Hb-SS disease with vasoocclusive pain

D57.ØØ Hb-SS disease with crisis, unspecified MCC HCC
- ▶Hb-SS disease with (painful) crisis NOS◀
- ▶Hb-SS disease with vasoocclusive pain NOS◀

D57.Ø1 Hb-SS disease with acute chest syndrome MCC HCC

D57.Ø2 Hb-SS disease with splenic sequestration MCC HCC

● **D57.03 Hb-SS disease with cerebral vascular involvement** MCC
Code also, if applicable, cerebral infarction (I63.-)

● **D57.09 Hb-SS disease with crisis with other specified complication** MCC
Use additional code to identify complications, such as:
cholelithiasis (K80.-)
priapism (N48.32)

D57.1 Sickle-cell disease without crisis HCC
Hb-SS disease without crisis
Sickle-cell anemia NOS
Sickle-cell disease NOS
Sickle-cell disorder NOS

✓5th **D57.2 Sickle-cell/Hb-C disease**
Hb-SC disease
Hb-S/Hb-C disease

D57.20 Sickle-cell/Hb-C disease without crisis HCC

✓6th **D57.21 Sickle-cell/Hb-C disease with crisis**

D57.211 Sickle-cell/Hb-C disease with acute chest syndrome MCC HCC

D57.212 Sickle-cell/Hb-C disease with splenic sequestration MCC HCC

● **D57.213 Sickle-cell/Hb-C disease with cerebral vascular involvement** MCC
Code also, if applicable, cerebral infarction (I63.-)

● **D57.218 Sickle-cell/Hb-C disease with crisis with other specified complication** MCC
Use additional code to identify complications, such as:
cholelithiasis (K80.-)
priapism (N48.32)

D57.219 Sickle-cell/Hb-C disease with crisis, unspecified MCC HCC
Sickle-cell/Hb-C disease with crisis NOS
▶Sickle-cell/Hb-C disease with vasoocclusive pain NOS◀

D57.3 Sickle-cell trait HCC
Hb-S trait
Heterozygous hemoglobin S
DEF: Heterozygous genetic makeup characterized by one gene for normal hemoglobin and one for sickle-cell hemoglobin. The clinical disease is rarely present.

✓5th **D57.4 Sickle-cell thalassemia**
Sickle-cell beta thalassemia
Thalassemia Hb-S disease

D57.40 Sickle-cell thalassemia without crisis HCC
Microdrepanocytosis
Sickle-cell thalassemia NOS

▲ ✓6th **D57.41 Sickle-cell thalassemia, unspecified, with crisis**
▶Sickle-cell thalassemia with (painful) crisis NOS◀
▶Sickle-cell thalassemia with vasoocclusive pain NOS◀

▲ **D57.411 Sickle-cell thalassemia, unspecified, with acute chest syndrome** MCC HCC

▲ **D57.412 Sickle-cell thalassemia, unspecified, with splenic sequestration** MCC HCC

● **D57.413 Sickle-cell thalassemia, unspecified, with cerebral vascular involvement** MCC
Code also, if applicable cerebral infarction (I63.-)

● **D57.418 Sickle-cell thalassemia, unspecified, with crisis with other specified complication** MCC
Use additional code to identify complications, such as:
cholelithiasis (K80.-)
priapism (N48.32)

▲ **D57.419 Sickle-cell thalassemia, unspecified, with crisis** MCC HCC
▶Sickle-cell thalassemia with (painful) crisis NOS◀
▶Sickle-cell thalassemia with vasoocclusive pain◀

● **D57.42 Sickle-cell thalassemia beta zero without crisis**
HbS-beta zero without crisis
Sickle-cell beta zero without crisis

● ✓6th **D57.43 Sickle-cell thalassemia beta zero with crisis**
HbS-beta zero with crisis
Sickle-cell beta zero with crisis

● **D57.431 Sickle-cell thalassemia beta zero with acute chest syndrome** MCC
HbS-beta zero with acute chest syndrome
Sickle-cell beta zero with acute chest syndrome

● **D57.432 Sickle-cell thalassemia beta zero with splenic sequestration** MCC
HbS-beta zero with splenic sequestration
Sickle-cell beta zero with splenic sequestration

● **D57.433 Sickle-cell thalassemia beta zero with cerebral vascular involvement** MCC
HbS-beta zero with cerebral vascular involvement
Sickle-cell beta zero with cerebral vascular involvement
Code also, if applicable cerebral infarction (I63.-)

● **D57.438 Sickle-cell thalassemia beta zero with crisis with other specified complication** MCC
HbS-beta zero with other specified complication
Sickle-cell beta zero with other specified complication
Use additional code to identify complications, such as:
cholelithiasis (K80.-)
priapism (N48.32)

● **D57.439 Sickle-cell thalassemia beta zero with crisis, unspecified** MCC
HbS-beta zero with other specified complication
Sickle-cell beta zero with crisis unspecified
Sickle-cell thalassemia beta zero with (painful) crisis NOS
Sickle-cell thalassemia beta zero with vasoocclusive pain

● **D57.44 Sickle-cell thalassemia beta plus without crisis**
HbS-beta plus without crisis
Sickle-cell beta plus without crisis

● ✓6th **D57.45 Sickle-cell thalassemia beta plus with crisis**
HbS-beta plus with crisis
Sickle-cell beta plus with crisis

● **D57.451 Sickle-cell thalassemia beta plus with acute chest syndrome** MCC
HbS-beta plus with acute chest syndrome
Sickle-cell beta plus with acute chest syndrome

● **D57.452 Sickle-cell thalassemia beta plus with splenic sequestration** MCC
HbS-beta plus with splenic sequestration
Sickle-cell beta plus with splenic sequestration

● **D57.453 Sickle-cell thalassemia beta plus with cerebral vascular involvement** MCC
HbS-beta plus with cerebral vascular involvement
Sickle-cell beta plus with cerebral vascular involvement
Code also, if applicable cerebral infarction (I63.-)

● **D57.458 Sickle-cell thalassemia beta plus with crisis with other specified complication** MCC
HbS-beta plus with crisis with other specified complication
Sickle-cell beta plus with crisis with other specified complication
Use additional code to identify complications, such as:
cholelithiasis (K80.-)
priapism (N48.32)

● **D57.459 Sickle-cell thalassemia beta plus with crisis, unspecified** MCC
HbS-beta plus with crisis with unspecified complication
Sickle-cell beta plus with crisis with unspecified complication
Sickle-cell thalassemia beta plus with (painful) crisis NOS
Sickle-cell thalassemia beta plus with vasoocclusive pain

✓5th **D57.8 Other sickle-cell disorders**
Hb-SD disease
Hb-SE disease

D57.80 Other sickle-cell disorders without crisis HCC

✓6th **D57.81 Other sickle-cell disorders with crisis**

D57.811 Other sickle-cell disorders with acute chest syndrome MCC HCC

D57.812 Other sickle-cell disorders with splenic sequestration MCC HCC

● **D57.813 Other sickle-cell disorders with cerebral vascular involvement** MCC
Code also, if applicable: cerebral infarction (I63.-)

● **D57.818 Other sickle-cell disorders with crisis with other specified complication** MCC
Use additional code to identify complications, such as:
cholelithiasis (K80.-)
priapism (N48.32)

D57.819 Other sickle-cell disorders with crisis, unspecified MCC HCC
Other sickle-cell disorders with crisis NOS
▶Other sickle-cell disorders with vasoocclusive pain NOS◀

✓4th **D58 Other hereditary hemolytic anemias**
EXCLUDES 1 *hemolytic anemia of the newborn (P55.-)*

D58.0 Hereditary spherocytosis HCC
Acholuric (familial) jaundice
Congenital (spherocytic) hemolytic icterus
Minkowski-Chauffard syndrome
DEF: Inherited condition caused by mutations to genes responsible for the production of proteins that form the membranes of red blood cells. The shape and flexibility of the red blood cell membrane is altered diminishing the cells ability to traverse the spleen, therefore becoming trapped and destroyed before the red blood cell has reached maturity.

D58.1 Hereditary elliptocytosis HCC
Elliptocytosis (congenital)
Ovalocytosis (congenital) (hereditary)

D58.2 Other hemoglobinopathies HCC
Abnormal hemoglobin NOS
Congenital Heinz body anemia
Hb-C disease
Hb-D disease
Hb-E disease
Hemoglobinopathy NOS
Unstable hemoglobin hemolytic disease
EXCLUDES 1 *familial polycythemia (D75.0)*
Hb-M disease (D74.0)
hemoglobin E-beta thalassemia (D56.5)
hereditary persistence of fetal hemoglobin [HPFH] (D56.4)
high-altitude polycythemia (D75.1)
methemoglobinemia (D74.-)
other hemoglobinopathies with thalassemia (D56.8)

D58.8 Other specified hereditary hemolytic anemias CC HCC
Stomatocytosis

D58.9 Hereditary hemolytic anemia, unspecified CC HCC

✓4th **D59 Acquired hemolytic anemia**
DEF: Non-hereditary anemia characterized by premature destruction of red blood cells caused by infectious organisms, poisons, and physical agents.

D59.0 Drug-induced autoimmune hemolytic anemia CC HCC
Use additional code for adverse effect, if applicable, to identify drug (T36-T50 with fifth or sixth character 5)

▲ ✓5th **D59.1 Other autoimmune hemolytic anemias**
~~Autoimmune hemolytic disease (cold type) (warm type)~~
~~Chronic cold hemagglutinin disease~~
~~Cold agglutinin disease~~
~~Cold agglutinin hemoglobinuria~~
~~Cold type (secondary) (symptomatic) hemolytic anemia~~
~~Warm type (secondary) (symptomatic) hemolytic anemia~~
EXCLUDES 1 ~~*Evans syndrome (D69.41)*~~
~~*hemolytic disease of newborn (P55.-)*~~
~~*paroxysmal cold hemoglobinuria (D59.6)*~~
EXCLUDES 2 ▶*Evans syndrome (D69.41)*◀
▶*hemolytic disease of newborn (P55.-)*◀
▶*paroxysmal cold hemoglobinuria (D59.6)*◀

● **D59.10 Autoimmune hemolytic anemia, unspecified** CC

● **D59.11 Warm autoimmune hemolytic anemia** CC
Warm type (primary) (secondary) (symptomatic) autoimmune hemolytic anemia
Warm type autoimmune hemolytic disease

● **D59.12 Cold autoimmune hemolytic anemia** CC
Chronic cold hemagglutinin disease
Cold agglutinin disease
Cold agglutinin hemoglobinuria
Cold type (primary) (secondary) (symptomatic) autoimmune hemolytic anemia
Cold type autoimmune hemolytic disease

● **D59.13 Mixed type autoimmune hemolytic anemia** CC
Mixed type autoimmune hemolytic disease
Mixed type, cold and warm, (primary) (secondary) (symptomatic) autoimmune hemolytic anemia

● **D59.19 Other autoimmune hemolytic anemia** CC

D59.2 Drug-induced nonautoimmune hemolytic anemia CC HCC
Drug-induced enzyme deficiency anemia
Use additional code for adverse effect, if applicable, to identify drug (T36-T50 with fifth or sixth character 5)

D59.3 Hemolytic-uremic syndrome MCC HCC
Use additional code to identify associated:
E. coli infection (B96.2-)
Pneumococcal pneumonia (J13)
Shigella dysenteriae (A03.9)
DEF: Condition typically precipitated by infection causing low platelets and destruction of red blood cells resulting in hemolytic anemia. This cell damage and blockage of renal capillaries lead to kidney failure. Mainly affects children.

D59.4 Other nonautoimmune hemolytic anemias CC HCC
Mechanical hemolytic anemia
Microangiopathic hemolytic anemia
Toxic hemolytic anemia

D59.5 Paroxysmal nocturnal hemoglobinuria [Marchiafava-Micheli] HCC
EXCLUDES 1 *hemoglobinuria NOS (R82.3)*

D59.6 Hemoglobinuria due to hemolysis from other external causes HCC
Hemoglobinuria from exertion
March hemoglobinuria
Paroxysmal cold hemoglobinuria
Use additional code (Chapter 20) to identify external cause
EXCLUDES 1 *hemoglobinuria NOS (R82.3)*

D59.8 Other acquired hemolytic anemias HCC

D59.9 Acquired hemolytic anemia, unspecified CC HCC
Idiopathic hemolytic anemia, chronic

Aplastic and other anemias and other bone marrow failure syndromes (D60-D64)

✓4th **D60 Acquired pure red cell aplasia [erythroblastopenia]**
INCLUDES red cell aplasia (acquired) (adult) (with thymoma)
EXCLUDES 1 *congenital red cell aplasia (D61.01)*
DEF: Bone marrow failure characterized by underproduction of red blood cells while white blood cell and platelet production remains normal.

D60.0 Chronic acquired pure red cell aplasia MCC HCC

D60.1 Transient acquired pure red cell aplasia MCC HCC

D60.8 Other acquired pure red cell aplasias MCC HCC

D60.9 Acquired pure red cell aplasia, unspecified MCC HCC

√4th D61 Other aplastic anemias and other bone marrow failure syndromes

EXCLUDES 1 ~~*neutropenia (D70.-)*~~

EXCLUDES 2 ►*neutropenia (D70.-)*◄

AHA: 2014,4Q,22

DEF: Aplastic anemia: Bone marrow failure characterized by underproduction of red bloods cells, white blood cells and platelets.

√5th D61.0 Constitutional aplastic anemia

D61.01 Constitutional (pure) red blood cell aplasia CC HCC

Blackfan-Diamond syndrome
Congenital (pure) red cell aplasia
Familial hypoplastic anemia
Primary (pure) red cell aplasia
Red cell (pure) aplasia of infants

EXCLUDES 1 *acquired red cell aplasia (D60.9)*

D61.09 Other constitutional aplastic anemia CC HCC

Fanconi's anemia
Pancytopenia with malformations

D61.1 Drug-induced aplastic anemia MCC HCC

Use additional code for adverse effect, if applicable, to identify drug (T36-T50 with fifth or sixth character 5)

D61.2 Aplastic anemia due to other external agents MCC HCC

Code first, if applicable, toxic effects of substances chiefly nonmedicinal as to source (T51-T65)

D61.3 Idiopathic aplastic anemia MCC HCC

√5th D61.8 Other specified aplastic anemias and other bone marrow failure syndromes

√6th D61.81 Pancytopenia

EXCLUDES 1 *pancytopenia (due to) (with) aplastic anemia (D61.9)*
pancytopenia (due to) (with) bone marrow infiltration (D61.82)
pancytopenia (due to) (with) congenital (pure) red cell aplasia (D61.01)
pancytopenia (due to) (with) hairy cell leukemia (C91.4-)
pancytopenia (due to) (with) human immunodeficiency virus disease (B20)
pancytopenia (due to) (with) leukoerythroblastic anemia (D61.82)
pancytopenia (due to) (with) myeloproliferative disease (D47.1)

EXCLUDES 2 *pancytopenia (due to) (with) myelodysplastic syndromes (D46.-)*

DEF: Shortage of all three blood cells: white, red, and platelets.

D61.810 Antineoplastic chemotherapy induced pancytopenia MCC HCC

EXCLUDES 2 *aplastic anemia due to antineoplastic chemotherapy (D61.1)*

D61.811 Other drug-induced pancytopenia MCC HCC

EXCLUDES 2 *aplastic anemia due to drugs (D61.1)*

D61.818 Other pancytopenia CC HCC

AHA: 2019,1Q,16

TIP: Assign this code in addition to myeloid leukemia codes (C92.-) when pancytopenia is documented. Although common in some types of myeloid leukemia, pancytopenia is not always inherent.

D61.82 Myelophthisis CC HCC

Leukoerythroblastic anemia
Myelophthisic anemia
Panmyelophthisis

Code also the underlying disorder, such as:
malignant neoplasm of breast (C50.-)
tuberculosis (A15.-)

EXCLUDES 1 *idiopathic myelofibrosis (D47.1)*
myelofibrosis NOS (D75.81)
myelofibrosis with myeloid metaplasia (D47.4)
primary myelofibrosis (D47.1)
secondary myelofibrosis (D75.81)

DEF: Condition that occurs when normal hematopoietic tissue in the bone marrow is replaced with abnormal tissue, such as fibrous tissue or tumors. Most commonly seen during the advanced stages of cancer.

D61.89 Other specified aplastic anemias and other bone marrow failure syndromes MCC HCC

D61.9 Aplastic anemia, unspecified CC HCC

Hypoplastic anemia NOS
Medullary hypoplasia

D62 Acute posthemorrhagic anemia CC

EXCLUDES 1 *anemia due to chronic blood loss (D50.0)*
blood loss anemia NOS (D50.0)
congenital anemia from fetal blood loss (P61.3)

AHA: 2019,3Q,11,17

√4th D63 Anemia in chronic diseases classified elsewhere

D63.0 Anemia in neoplastic disease

Code first neoplasm (C00-D49)

EXCLUDES 1 *aplastic anemia due to antineoplastic chemotherapy (D61.1)*

EXCLUDES 2 *anemia due to antineoplastic chemotherapy (D64.81)*

D63.1 Anemia in chronic kidney disease

Erythropoietin resistant anemia (EPO resistant anemia)
Code first underlying chronic kidney disease (CKD) (N18.-)

D63.8 Anemia in other chronic diseases classified elsewhere

Code first underlying disease, such as:
diphyllobothriasis (B70.0)
hookworm disease (B76.0-B76.9)
hypothyroidism (E00.0-E03.9)
malaria (B50.0-B54)
symptomatic late syphilis (A52.79)
tuberculosis (A18.89)

√4th D64 Other anemias

EXCLUDES 1 *refractory anemia (D46.-)*
refractory anemia with excess blasts in transformation [RAEB T] (C92.0-)

DEF: Sideroblastic anemia: Hereditary or secondary disorder in which the red blood cells cannot effectively use iron, a nutrient needed to make hemoglobin. Although the iron can enter the red blood cell it is not assimilated into the hemoglobin molecule and builds up ringed sideroblasts around the cell nucleus.

D64.0 Hereditary sideroblastic anemia HCC

Sex-linked hypochromic sideroblastic anemia

D64.1 Secondary sideroblastic anemia due to disease HCC

Code first underlying disease

D64.2 Secondary sideroblastic anemia due to drugs and toxins HCC

Code first poisoning due to drug or toxin, if applicable (T36-T65 with fifth or sixth character 1-4 or 6)
Use additional code for adverse effect, if applicable, to identify drug (T36-T50 with fifth or sixth character 5)

D64.3 Other sideroblastic anemias HCC

Sideroblastic anemia NOS
Pyridoxine-responsive sideroblastic anemia NEC

D64.4 Congenital dyserythropoietic anemia

Dyshematopoietic anemia (congenital)

EXCLUDES 1 *Blackfan-Diamond syndrome (D61.01)*
Di Guglielmo's disease (C94.0)

√5th **D64.8 Other specified anemias**

D64.81 Anemia due to antineoplastic chemotherapy
Antineoplastic chemotherapy induced anemia
EXCLUDES 1 *aplastic anemia due to antineoplastic chemotherapy (D61.1)*
EXCLUDES 2 *anemia in neoplastic disease (D63.Ø)*
AHA: 2014,4Q,22
DEF: Reversible adverse effect of chemotherapy, causing inhibition of bone marrow production. A decrease in red blood cell production prevents adequate oxygenation of the tissues and organs causing fatigue, shortness of breath (SOB), and exacerbation of other medical conditions.

D64.89 Other specified anemias
Infantile pseudoleukemia

D64.9 Anemia, unspecified
AHA: 2018,4Q,88; 2017,1Q,7

Coagulation defects, purpura and other hemorrhagic conditions (D65-D69)

D65 Disseminated intravascular coagulation [defibrination syndrome] MCC HCC
Afibrinogenemia, acquired
Consumption coagulopathy
Diffuse or disseminated intravascular coagulation [DIC]
Fibrinolytic hemorrhage, acquired
Fibrinolytic purpura
Purpura fulminans
EXCLUDES 1 *disseminated intravascular coagulation (complicating):*
abortion or ectopic or molar pregnancy (OØØ-OØ7, OØ8.1)
in newborn (P6Ø)
pregnancy, childbirth and the puerperium (O45.Ø, O46.Ø, O67.Ø, O72.3)

Coagulation

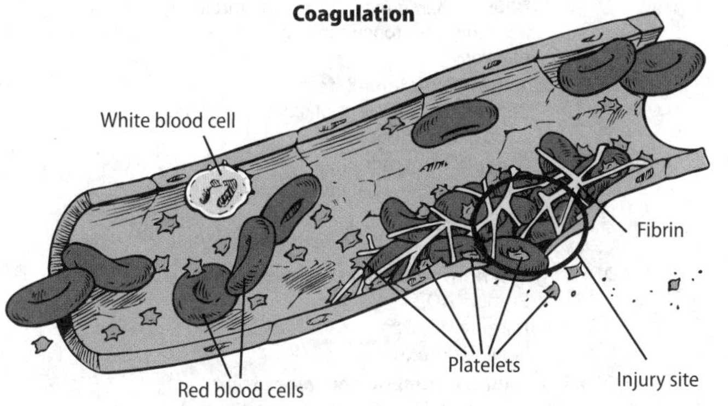

D66 Hereditary factor VIII deficiency MCC HCC
Classical hemophilia
Deficiency factor VIII (with functional defect)
Hemophilia A
Hemophilia NOS
EXCLUDES 1 *factor VIII deficiency with vascular defect (D68.Ø)*
DEF: Hereditary, sex-linked lack of antihemophilic globulin (AHG) (factor VIII) that causes abnormal coagulation characterized by increased bleeding; large bruises of skin; bleeding in the mouth, nose, and gastrointestinal tract; and hemorrhages into joints, resulting in swelling and impaired function.

D67 Hereditary factor IX deficiency MCC HCC
Christmas disease
Factor IX deficiency (with functional defect)
Hemophilia B
Plasma thromboplastin component [PTC] deficiency

√4th **D68 Other coagulation defects**
EXCLUDES 1 *abnormal coagulation profile (R79.1)*
coagulation defects complicating abortion or ectopic or molar pregnancy (OØØ-OØ7, OØ8.1)
coagulation defects complicating pregnancy, childbirth and the puerperium (O45.Ø, O46.Ø, O67.Ø, O72.3)
AHA: 2016,1Q,14

D68.Ø Von Willebrand's disease CC HCC
Angiohemophilia
Factor VIII deficiency with vascular defect
Vascular hemophilia
EXCLUDES 1 *capillary fragility (hereditary) (D69.8)*
factor VIII deficiency NOS (D66)
factor VIII deficiency with functional defect (D66)
DEF: Congenital, abnormal blood coagulation caused by deficient blood factor VII. Symptoms include excess or prolonged bleeding.

D68.1 Hereditary factor XI deficiency CC HCC
Hemophilia C
Plasma thromboplastin antecedent [PTA] deficiency
Rosenthal's disease

D68.2 Hereditary deficiency of other clotting factors CC HCC
AC globulin deficiency
Congenital afibrinogenemia
Deficiency of factor I [fibrinogen]
Deficiency of factor II [prothrombin]
Deficiency of factor V [labile]
Deficiency of factor VII [stable]
Deficiency of factor X [Stuart-Prower]
Deficiency of factor XII [Hageman]
Deficiency of factor XIII [fibrin stabilizing]
Dysfibrinogenemia (congenital)
Hypoproconvertinemia
Owren's disease
Proaccelerin deficiency

√5th **D68.3 Hemorrhagic disorder due to circulating anticoagulants**

√6th **D68.31 Hemorrhagic disorder due to intrinsic circulating anticoagulants, antibodies, or inhibitors**

D68.311 Acquired hemophilia CC HCC
Autoimmune hemophilia
Autoimmune inhibitors to clotting factors
Secondary hemophilia

D68.312 Antiphospholipid antibody with hemorrhagic disorder CC HCC
Lupus anticoagulant (LAC) with hemorrhagic disorder
Systemic lupus erythematosus [SLE] inhibitor with hemorrhagic disorder
EXCLUDES 1 *antiphospholipid antibody, finding without diagnosis (R76.Ø)*
antiphospholipid antibody syndrome (D68.61)
antiphospholipid antibody with hypercoagulable state (D68.61)
lupus anticoagulant (LAC) finding without diagnosis (R76.Ø)
lupus anticoagulant (LAC) with hypercoagulable state (D68.62)
systemic lupus erythematosus [SLE] inhibitor finding without diagnosis (R76.Ø)
systemic lupus erythematosus [SLE] inhibitor with hypercoagulable state (D68.62)

D68.318 Other hemorrhagic disorder due to intrinsic circulating anticoagulants, antibodies, or inhibitors CC HCC
Antithromboplastinemia
Antithromboplastinogenemia
Hemorrhagic disorder due to intrinsic increase in antithrombin
Hemorrhagic disorder due to intrinsic increase in anti-VIIIa
Hemorrhagic disorder due to intrinsic increase in anti-IXa
Hemorrhagic disorder due to intrinsic increase in anti-XIa

D68.32 Hemorrhagic disorder due to extrinsic circulating anticoagulants CC HCC
Drug-induced hemorrhagic disorder
Hemorrhagic disorder due to increase in anti-IIa
Hemorrhagic disorder due to increase in anti-Xa
Hyperheparinemia
Use additional code for adverse effect, if applicable, to identify drug (T45.515, T45.525)
AHA: 2016,1Q,14-15
TIP: Do not assign to identify routine therapeutic anticoagulation effects; assign only for documented adverse effects.

D68.4 Acquired coagulation factor deficiency CC HCC
Deficiency of coagulation factor due to liver disease
Deficiency of coagulation factor due to vitamin K deficiency
EXCLUDES 1 *vitamin K deficiency of newborn (P53)*

√5th **D68.5 Primary thrombophilia**
Primary hypercoagulable states
EXCLUDES 1 *antiphospholipid syndrome (D68.61)*
lupus anticoagulant (D68.62)
secondary activated protein C resistance (D68.69)
secondary antiphospholipid antibody syndrome (D68.69)
secondary lupus anticoagulant with hypercoagulable state (D68.69)
secondary systemic lupus erythematosus [SLE] inhibitor with hypercoagulable state (D68.69)
systemic lupus erythematosus [SLE] inhibitor finding without diagnosis (R76.Ø)
systemic lupus erythematosus [SLE] inhibitor with hemorrhagic disorder (D68.312)
thrombotic thrombocytopenic purpura (M31.1)
DEF: Thrombophilia: Increased tendency of the blood to clot, which can lead to thrombus or embolus formation.

D68.51 Activated protein C resistance CC HCC
Factor V Leiden mutation

D68.52 Prothrombin gene mutation CC HCC

D68.59 Other primary thrombophilia CC HCC
Antithrombin III deficiency
Hypercoagulable state NOS
Primary hypercoagulable state NEC
Primary thrombophilia NEC
Protein C deficiency
Protein S deficiency
Thrombophilia NOS

√5th **D68.6 Other thrombophilia**
Other hypercoagulable states
EXCLUDES 1 *diffuse or disseminated intravascular coagulation [DIC] (D65)*
heparin induced thrombocytopenia (HIT) (D75.82)
hyperhomocysteinemia (E72.11)

D68.61 Antiphospholipid syndrome CC HCC
Anticardiolipin syndrome
Antiphospholipid antibody syndrome
EXCLUDES 1 *anti-phospholipid antibody, finding without diagnosis (R76.Ø)*
anti-phospholipid antibody with hemorrhagic disorder (D68.312)
lupus anticoagulant syndrome (D68.62)

D68.62 Lupus anticoagulant syndrome CC HCC
Lupus anticoagulant
Presence of systemic lupus erythematosus [SLE] inhibitor
EXCLUDES 1 *anticardiolipin syndrome (D68.61)*
antiphospholipid syndrome (D68.61)
lupus anticoagulant (LAC) finding without diagnosis (R76.Ø)
lupus anticoagulant (LAC) with hemorrhagic disorder (D68.312)

D68.69 Other thrombophilia CC HCC
Hypercoagulable states NEC
Secondary hypercoagulable state NOS

D68.8 Other specified coagulation defects CC HCC
EXCLUDES 1 *hemorrhagic disease of newborn (P53)*

D68.9 Coagulation defect, unspecified CC HCC

√4th **D69 Purpura and other hemorrhagic conditions**
EXCLUDES 1 *benign hypergammaglobulinemic purpura (D89.Ø)*
cryoglobulinemic purpura (D89.1)
essential (hemorrhagic) thrombocythemia (D47.3)
hemorrhagic thrombocythemia (D47.3)
purpura fulminans (D65)
thrombotic thrombocytopenic purpura (M31.1)
Waldenström hypergammaglobulinemic purpura (D89.Ø)

D69.Ø Allergic purpura CC HCC
Allergic vasculitis
Nonthrombocytopenic hemorrhagic purpura
Nonthrombocytopenic idiopathic purpura
Purpura anaphylactoid
Purpura Henoch(-Schönlein)
Purpura rheumatica
Vascular purpura
EXCLUDES 1 *thrombocytopenic hemorrhagic purpura (D69.3)*
DEF: Any hemorrhagic condition, thrombocytic or nonthrombocytopenic in origin, caused by a presumed allergic reaction.

D69.1 Qualitative platelet defects HCC
Bernard-Soulier [giant platelet] syndrome
Glanzmann's disease
Grey platelet syndrome
Thromboasthenia (hemorrhagic) (hereditary)
Thrombocytopathy
EXCLUDES 1 *von Willebrand's disease (D68.Ø)*

D69.2 Other nonthrombocytopenic purpura HCC
Purpura NOS
Purpura simplex
Senile purpura

D69.3 Immune thrombocytopenic purpura CC HCC
Hemorrhagic (thrombocytopenic) purpura
Idiopathic thrombocytopenic purpura
Tidal platelet dysgenesis
DEF: Tidal platelet dysgenesis: Fluctuation of platelet counts from normal to very low within periods of 20 to 40 days and may involve autoimmune platelet destruction.

√5th **D69.4 Other primary thrombocytopenia**
EXCLUDES 1 *transient neonatal thrombocytopenia (P61.Ø)*
Wiskott-Aldrich syndrome (D82.Ø)

D69.41 Evans syndrome CC HCC

D69.42 Congenital and hereditary thrombocytopenia purpura CC HCC
Congenital thrombocytopenia
Hereditary thrombocytopenia
Code first congenital or hereditary disorder, such as: thrombocytopenia with absent radius (TAR syndrome) (Q87.2)

D69.49 Other primary thrombocytopenia HCC
Megakaryocytic hypoplasia
Primary thrombocytopenia NOS

√5th **D69.5 Secondary thrombocytopenia**
EXCLUDES 1 *heparin induced thrombocytopenia (HIT) (D75.82)*
transient thrombocytopenia of newborn (P61.Ø)

D69.51 Posttransfusion purpura
Posttransfusion purpura from whole blood (fresh) or blood products
PTP

D69.59 Other secondary thrombocytopenia
AHA: 2014,4Q,22

D69.6 Thrombocytopenia, unspecified HCC

D69.8 Other specified hemorrhagic conditions HCC
Capillary fragility (hereditary)
Vascular pseudohemophilia

D69.9 Hemorrhagic condition, unspecified HCC

Other disorders of blood and blood-forming organs (D70-D77)

√4th **D70 Neutropenia**
INCLUDES agranulocytosis
decreased absolute neurophile count (ANC)
Use additional code for any associated:
fever (R50.81)
mucositis (J34.81, K12.3-, K92.81, N76.81)
EXCLUDES 1 *neutropenic splenomegaly (D73.81)*
transient neonatal neutropenia (P61.5)
DEF: Abnormally low number of neutrophils. Neutrophils are phagocytic, meaning they surround and consume harmful pathogens, primarily bacteria. When neutrophil counts decrease the risk of infection increases.

D70.0 Congenital agranulocytosis HCC
Congenital neutropenia
Infantile genetic agranulocytosis
Kostmann's disease

D70.1 Agranulocytosis secondary to cancer chemotherapy HCC
Code also underlying neoplasm
Use additional code for adverse effect, if applicable, to identify drug (T45.1X5)
AHA: 2014,4Q,22

D70.2 Other drug-induced agranulocytosis HCC
Use additional code for adverse effect, if applicable, to identify drug (T36-T50 with fifth or sixth character 5)

D70.3 Neutropenia due to infection HCC

D70.4 Cyclic neutropenia HCC
Cyclic hematopoiesis
Periodic neutropenia

D70.8 Other neutropenia HCC

D70.9 Neutropenia, unspecified HCC

D71 Functional disorders of polymorphonuclear neutrophils HCC
Cell membrane receptor complex [CR3] defect
Chronic (childhood) granulomatous disease
Congenital dysphagocytosis
Progressive septic granulomatosis

√4th **D72 Other disorders of white blood cells**
EXCLUDES 1 *basophilia (D72.824)*
immunity disorders (D80-D89)
neutropenia (D70)
preleukemia (syndrome) (D46.9)

D72.0 Genetic anomalies of leukocytes HCC
Alder (granulation) (granulocyte) anomaly
Alder syndrome
Hereditary leukocytic hypersegmentation
Hereditary leukocytic hyposegmentation
Hereditary leukomelanopathy
May-Hegglin (granulation) (granulocyte) anomaly
May-Hegglin syndrome
Pelger-Huët (granulation) (granulocyte) anomaly
Pelger-Huët syndrome
EXCLUDES 1 *Chédiak (-Steinbrinck)-Higashi syndrome (E70.330)*

▲ √5th **D72.1 Eosinophilia**
~~Allergic eosinophilia~~
~~Hereditary eosinophilia~~
EXCLUDES 1 ~~*Löffler's syndrome (J82)*~~
~~*pulmonary eosinophilia (J82)*~~
EXCLUDES 2 ►*Löffler's syndrome (J82)*◄
►*pulmonary eosinophilia (J82)*◄

● **D72.10 Eosinophilia, unspecified**

● √6th **D72.11 Hypereosinophilic syndrome [HES]**

● **D72.110 Idiopathic hypereosinophilic syndrome [IHES]**

● **D72.111 Lymphocytic Variant Hypereosinophilic Syndrome [LHES]**
Lymphocyte variant hypereosinophilia
Code also, if applicable, any associated lymphocytic neoplastic disorder

● **D72.118 Other hypereosinophilic syndrome**
Episodic angioedema with eosinophilia
Gleich's syndrome

● **D72.119 Hypereosinophilic syndrome [HES], unspecified**

● **D72.12 Drug rash with eosinophilia and systemic symptoms syndrome**
DRESS syndrome
Use additional code for adverse effect, if applicable, to identify drug (T36-T50 with fifth or sixth character 5)

● ***D72.18 Eosinophilia in diseases classified elsewhere***
Code first underlying disease, such as:
chronic myelomonocytic leukemia (C93.1-)

● **D72.19 Other eosinophilia**
Familial eosinophilia
Hereditary eosinophilia

√5th **D72.8 Other specified disorders of white blood cells**
EXCLUDES 1 *leukemia (C91-C95)*

√6th **D72.81 Decreased white blood cell count**
EXCLUDES 1 *neutropenia (D70.-)*

D72.810 Lymphocytopenia
Decreased lymphocytes

D72.818 Other decreased white blood cell count
Basophilic leukopenia
Eosinophilic leukopenia
Monocytopenia
Other decreased leukocytes
Plasmacytopenia

D72.819 Decreased white blood cell count, unspecified
Decreased leukocytes, unspecified
Leukocytopenia, unspecified
Leukopenia
EXCLUDES 1 *malignant leukopenia (D70.9)*

√6th **D72.82 Elevated white blood cell count**
EXCLUDES 1 *eosinophilia (D72.1)*

D72.820 Lymphocytosis (symptomatic)
Elevated lymphocytes

D72.821 Monocytosis (symptomatic)
EXCLUDES 1 *infectious mononucleosis (B27.-)*

D72.822 Plasmacytosis

D72.823 Leukemoid reaction
Basophilic leukemoid reaction
Leukemoid reaction NOS
Lymphocytic leukemoid reaction
Monocytic leukemoid reaction
Myelocytic leukemoid reaction
Neutrophilic leukemoid reaction

D72.824 Basophilia
DEF: Increase in the basophils of the blood, a type of white blood cell, often seen in conjunction with neoplastic disorders.

D72.825 Bandemia
Bandemia without diagnosis of specific infection
EXCLUDES 1 *confirmed infection — code to infection*
leukemia (C91.-, C92.-, C93.-, C94.-, C95.-)
DEF: Increase in early neutrophil cells, called band cells that may indicate infection.

D72.828 Other elevated white blood cell count

D72.829 Elevated white blood cell count, unspecified
Elevated leukocytes, unspecified
Leukocytosis, unspecified

D72.89 Other specified disorders of white blood cells
Abnormality of white blood cells NEC

D72.9 Disorder of white blood cells, unspecified
Abnormal leukocyte differential NOS

✓4th D73 Diseases of spleen

D73.Ø Hyposplenism
Atrophy of spleen
EXCLUDES 1 *asplenia (congenital) (Q89.Ø1)*
postsurgical absence of spleen (Z9Ø.81)

D73.1 Hypersplenism
EXCLUDES 1 *neutropenic splenomegaly (D73.81)*
primary splenic neutropenia (D73.81)
splenitis, splenomegaly in late syphilis (A52.79)
splenitis, splenomegaly in tuberculosis (A18.85)
splenomegaly NOS (R16.1)
splenomegaly congenital (Q89.Ø)

D73.2 Chronic congestive splenomegaly

D73.3 Abscess of spleen

D73.4 Cyst of spleen

D73.5 Infarction of spleen
Splenic rupture, nontraumatic
Torsion of spleen
EXCLUDES 1 *rupture of spleen due to Plasmodium vivax malaria (B51.Ø)*
traumatic rupture of spleen (S36.Ø3-)

✓5th D73.8 Other diseases of spleen

D73.81 Neutropenic splenomegaly
Werner-Schultz disease

D73.89 Other diseases of spleen
Fibrosis of spleen NOS
Perisplenitis
Splenitis NOS

D73.9 Disease of spleen, unspecified

✓4th D74 Methemoglobinemia

D74.Ø Congenital methemoglobinemia CC
Congenital NADH-methemoglobin reductase deficiency
Hemoglobin-M [Hb-M] disease
Methemoglobinemia, hereditary

D74.8 Other methemoglobinemias CC
Acquired methemoglobinemia (with sulfhemoglobinemia)
Toxic methemoglobinemia

D74.9 Methemoglobinemia, unspecified CC

✓4th D75 Other and unspecified diseases of blood and blood-forming organs
EXCLUDES 2 *acute lymphadenitis (LØ4.-)*
chronic lymphadenitis (I88.1)
enlarged lymph nodes (R59.-)
hypergammaglobulinemia NOS (D89.2)
lymphadenitis NOS (I88.9)
mesenteric lymphadenitis (acute) (chronic) (I88.Ø)

D75.Ø Familial erythrocytosis
Benign polycythemia
Familial polycythemia
EXCLUDES 1 *hereditary ovalocytosis (D58.1)*

D75.1 Secondary polycythemia
Acquired polycythemia
Emotional polycythemia
Erythrocytosis NOS
Hypoxemic polycythemia
Nephrogenous polycythemia
Polycythemia due to erythropoietin
Polycythemia due to fall in plasma volume
Polycythemia due to high altitude
Polycythemia due to stress
Polycythemia NOS
Relative polycythemia
EXCLUDES 1 *polycythemia neonatorum (P61.1)*
polycythemia vera (D45)
DEF: Elevated number of red blood cells in circulating blood as a result of reduced oxygen supply to the tissues.

✓5th D75.8 Other specified diseases of blood and blood-forming organs

D75.81 Myelofibrosis CC HCC
Myelofibrosis NOS
Secondary myelofibrosis NOS
Code first the underlying disorder, such as:
malignant neoplasm of breast (C5Ø.-)
Use additional code, if applicable, for associated therapy-related myelodysplastic syndrome (D46.-)
Use additional code for adverse effect, if applicable, to identify drug (T45.1X5)
EXCLUDES 1 *acute myelofibrosis (C94.4-)*
idiopathic myelofibrosis (D47.1)
leukoerythroblastic anemia (D61.82)
myelofibrosis with myeloid metaplasia (D47.4)
myelophthisic anemia (D61.82)
myelophthisis (D61.82)
primary myelofibrosis (D47.1)

D75.82 Heparin induced thrombocytopenia (HIT) HCC
DEF: Immune-mediated reaction to heparin therapy causing an abrupt fall in platelet count and serious complications such as pulmonary embolism, stroke, AMI, or DVT.

D75.89 Other specified diseases of blood and blood-forming organs

D75.9 Disease of blood and blood-forming organs, unspecified

D75.A Glucose-6-phosphate dehydrogenase (G6PD) deficiency without anemia
EXCLUDES 1 *glucose-6-phosphate dehydrogenase (G6PD) deficiency with anemia (D55.Ø)*
AHA: 2019,4Q,4-5

✓4th D76 Other specified diseases with participation of lymphoreticular and reticulohistiocytic tissue
EXCLUDES 1 *(Abt-) Letterer-Siwe disease (C96.Ø)*
eosinophilic granuloma (C96.6)
Hand-Schüller-Christian disease (C96.5)
histiocytic medullary reticulosis (C96.9)
histiocytic sarcoma (C96.A)
histiocytosis X, multifocal (C96.5)
histiocytosis X, unifocal (C96.6)
Langerhans-cell histiocytosis, multifocal (C96.5)
Langerhans-cell histiocytosis NOS (C96.6)
Langerhans-cell histiocytosis, unifocal (C96.6)
leukemic reticuloendotheliosis (C91.4-)
lipomelanotic reticulosis (I89.8)
malignant histiocytosis (C96.A)
malignant reticulosis (C86.Ø)
nonlipid reticuloendotheliosis (C96.Ø)

D76.1 Hemophagocytic lymphohistiocytosis CC HCC
Familial hemophagocytic reticulosis
Histiocytoses of mononuclear phagocytes

D76.2 Hemophagocytic syndrome, infection-associated CC HCC
Use additional code to identify infectious agent or disease

D76.3 Other histiocytosis syndromes CC HCC
Reticulohistiocytoma (giant-cell)
Sinus histiocytosis with massive lymphadenopathy
Xanthogranuloma

D77 Other disorders of blood and blood-forming organs in diseases classified elsewhere
Code first underlying disease, such as:
amyloidosis (E85.-)
congenital early syphilis (A5Ø.Ø)
echinococcosis (B67.Ø-B67.9)
malaria (B5Ø.Ø-B54)
schistosomiasis [bilharziasis] (B65.Ø-B65.9)
vitamin C deficiency (E54)
EXCLUDES 1 *rupture of spleen due to Plasmodium vivax malaria (B51.Ø)*
splenitis, splenomegaly in late syphilis (A52.79)
splenitis, splenomegaly in tuberculosis (A18.85)

Intraoperative and postprocedural complications of the spleen (D78)

D78 Intraoperative and postprocedural complications of the spleen
AHA: 2016,4Q,9-10

D78.0 Intraoperative hemorrhage and hematoma of the spleen complicating a procedure
EXCLUDES 1 *intraoperative hemorrhage and hematoma of the spleen due to accidental puncture or laceration during a procedure (D78.1-)*

D78.01 Intraoperative hemorrhage and hematoma of the spleen complicating a procedure on the spleen CC
D78.02 Intraoperative hemorrhage and hematoma of the spleen complicating other procedure CC

D78.1 Accidental puncture and laceration of the spleen during a procedure
D78.11 Accidental puncture and laceration of the spleen during a procedure on the spleen CC
D78.12 Accidental puncture and laceration of the spleen during other procedure CC

D78.2 Postprocedural hemorrhage of the spleen following a procedure
D78.21 Postprocedural hemorrhage of the spleen following a procedure on the spleen CC
D78.22 Postprocedural hemorrhage of the spleen following other procedure CC

D78.3 Postprocedural hematoma and seroma of the spleen following a procedure
D78.31 Postprocedural hematoma of the spleen following a procedure on the spleen CC
D78.32 Postprocedural hematoma of the spleen following other procedure CC
D78.33 Postprocedural seroma of the spleen following a procedure on the spleen CC
D78.34 Postprocedural seroma of the spleen following other procedure CC

D78.8 Other intraoperative and postprocedural complications of the spleen
Use additional code, if applicable, to further specify disorder
D78.81 Other intraoperative complications of the spleen CC
D78.89 Other postprocedural complications of the spleen CC

Certain disorders involving the immune mechanism (D8Ø-D89)

INCLUDES defects in the complement system
immunodeficiency disorders, except human immunodeficiency virus [HIV] disease
sarcoidosis

EXCLUDES 1 *autoimmune disease (systemic) NOS (M35.9)*
functional disorders of polymorphonuclear neutrophils (D71)
human immunodeficiency virus [HIV] disease (B2Ø)

D8Ø Immunodeficiency with predominantly antibody defects

D8Ø.Ø Hereditary hypogammaglobulinemia CC HCC
Autosomal recessive agammaglobulinemia (Swiss type)
X-linked agammaglobulinemia [Bruton] (with growth hormone deficiency)

D8Ø.1 Nonfamilial hypogammaglobulinemia CC HCC
Agammaglobulinemia with immunoglobulin-bearing B-lymphocytes
Common variable agammaglobulinemia [CVAgamma]
Hypogammaglobulinemia NOS

D8Ø.2 Selective deficiency of immunoglobulin A [IgA] CC HCC
D8Ø.3 Selective deficiency of immunoglobulin G [IgG] subclasses CC HCC
D8Ø.4 Selective deficiency of immunoglobulin M [IgM] CC HCC
D8Ø.5 Immunodeficiency with increased immunoglobulin M [IgM] CC HCC
D8Ø.6 Antibody deficiency with near-normal immunoglobulins or with hyperimmunoglobulinemia CC HCC
D8Ø.7 Transient hypogammaglobulinemia of infancy CC HCC
D8Ø.8 Other immunodeficiencies with predominantly antibody defects CC HCC
Kappa light chain deficiency
D8Ø.9 Immunodeficiency with predominantly antibody defects, unspecified CC HCC

D81 Combined immunodeficiencies
EXCLUDES 1 *autosomal recessive agammaglobulinemia (Swiss type) (D8Ø.Ø)*

D81.Ø Severe combined immunodeficiency [SCID] with reticular dysgenesis CC HCC
D81.1 Severe combined immunodeficiency [SCID] with low T- and B-cell numbers CC HCC
D81.2 Severe combined immunodeficiency [SCID] with low or normal B-cell numbers CC HCC

D81.3 Adenosine deaminase [ADA] deficiency
AHA: 2019,4Q,5-6

D81.3Ø Adenosine deaminase deficiency, unspecified CC HCC
ADA deficiency NOS

D81.31 Severe combined immunodeficiency due to adenosine deaminase deficiency CC HCC
ADA deficiency with SCID
Adenosine deaminase [ADA] deficiency with severe combined immunodeficiency

D81.32 Adenosine deaminase 2 deficiency CC HCC
ADA2 deficiency
Adenosine deaminase deficiency type 2
Code also, if applicable, any associated manifestations, such as:
polyarteritis nodosa (M3Ø.Ø)
stroke (I63.-)

D81.39 Other adenosine deaminase deficiency CC HCC
Adenosine deaminase [ADA] deficiency type 1, NOS
Adenosine deaminase [ADA] deficiency type 1, without SCID
Adenosine deaminase [ADA] deficiency type 1, without severe combined immunodeficiency
Partial ADA deficiency (type 1)
Partial adenosine deaminase deficiency (type 1)

D81.4 Nezelof's syndrome CC HCC
D81.5 Purine nucleoside phosphorylase [PNP] deficiency CC HCC
D81.6 Major histocompatibility complex class I deficiency CC HCC
Bare lymphocyte syndrome
D81.7 Major histocompatibility complex class II deficiency CC HCC

D81.8 Other combined immunodeficiencies
D81.81 Biotin-dependent carboxylase deficiency
Multiple carboxylase deficiency
EXCLUDES 1 *biotin-dependent carboxylase deficiency due to dietary deficiency of biotin (E53.8)*

D81.81Ø Biotinidase deficiency
D81.818 Other biotin-dependent carboxylase deficiency
Holocarboxylase synthetase deficiency
Other multiple carboxylase deficiency
D81.819 Biotin-dependent carboxylase deficiency, unspecified
Multiple carboxylase deficiency, unspecified

D81.89 Other combined immunodeficiencies CC HCC
D81.9 Combined immunodeficiency, unspecified CC HCC
Severe combined immunodeficiency disorder [SCID] NOS

D82 Immunodeficiency associated with other major defects
EXCLUDES 1 *ataxia telangiectasia [Louis-Bar] (G11.3)*

D82.Ø Wiskott-Aldrich syndrome CC HCC
Immunodeficiency with thrombocytopenia and eczema
D82.1 Di George's syndrome CC HCC
Pharyngeal pouch syndrome
Thymic alymphoplasia
Thymic aplasia or hypoplasia with immunodeficiency
AHA: 2019,3Q,14
D82.2 Immunodeficiency with short-limbed stature HCC
D82.3 Immunodeficiency following hereditary defective response to Epstein-Barr virus HCC
X-linked lymphoproliferative disease
D82.4 Hyperimmunoglobulin E [IgE] syndrome HCC
D82.8 Immunodeficiency associated with other specified major defects HCC
D82.9 Immunodeficiency associated with major defect, unspecified HCC

√4th D83 Common variable immunodeficiency

D83.0 Common variable immunodeficiency with predominant abnormalities of B-cell numbers and function CC HCC

D83.1 Common variable immunodeficiency with predominant immunoregulatory T-cell disorders CC HCC

D83.2 Common variable immunodeficiency with autoantibodies to B- or T-cells CC HCC

D83.8 Other common variable immunodeficiencies CC HCC

D83.9 Common variable immunodeficiency, unspecified CC HCC

√4th D84 Other immunodeficiencies

D84.0 Lymphocyte function antigen-1 [LFA-1] defect HCC

D84.1 Defects in the complement system HCC

C1 esterase inhibitor [C1-INH] deficiency

▲ **√5th D84.8 Other specified immunodeficiencies**

● ***D84.81 Immunodeficiency due to conditions classified elsewhere*** CC

Code first underlying condition, such as:

chromosomal abnormalities (Q90-Q99)

diabetes mellitus (E08-E13)

malignant neoplasms (C00-C96)

EXCLUDES 1 *certain disorders involving the immune mechanism (D80-D83, D84.0, D84.1, D84.9)*

human immunodeficiency virus [HIV] disease (B20)

● **√6th D84.82 Immunodeficiency due to drugs and external causes**

● **D84.821 Immunodeficiency due to drugs** CC

Immunodeficiency due to (current or past) medication

Use additional code for adverse effect if applicable, to identify adverse effect of drug (T36-T50 with fifth or six character 5)

Use additional code, if applicable, for associated long term (current) drug therapy drug or medication such as:

long term (current) drug therapy systemic steroids (Z79.52)

other long term (current) drug therapy (Z79.899)

● **D84.822 Immunodeficiency due to external causes** CC

Code also, if applicable, radiological procedure and radiotherapy (Y84.2)

Use additional code for external cause such as:

exposure to ionizing radiation (W88)

● **D84.89 Other immunodeficiencies** CC

D84.9 Immunodeficiency, unspecified CC HCC

▶Immunocompromised NOS◀

▶Immunodeficient NOS◀

▶Immunosuppressed NOS◀

√4th D86 Sarcoidosis

DEF: Clustering of immune cells resulting in granuloma formation. Often affects the lungs and lymphatic system but can occur in other body sites.

D86.0 Sarcoidosis of lung HCC

D86.1 Sarcoidosis of lymph nodes

D86.2 Sarcoidosis of lung with sarcoidosis of lymph nodes HCC

D86.3 Sarcoidosis of skin

√5th D86.8 Sarcoidosis of other sites

D86.81 Sarcoid meningitis

D86.82 Multiple cranial nerve palsies in sarcoidosis HCC

D86.83 Sarcoid iridocyclitis

D86.84 Sarcoid pyelonephritis

Tubulo-interstitial nephropathy in sarcoidosis

D86.85 Sarcoid myocarditis

D86.86 Sarcoid arthropathy

Polyarthritis in sarcoidosis

D86.87 Sarcoid myositis

D86.89 Sarcoidosis of other sites

Hepatic granuloma

Uveoparotid fever [Heerfordt]

D86.9 Sarcoidosis, unspecified

√4th D89 Other disorders involving the immune mechanism, not elsewhere classified

EXCLUDES 1 *hyperglobulinemia NOS (R77.1)*

monoclonal gammopathy (of undetermined significance) (D47.2)

EXCLUDES 2 *transplant failure and rejection (T86.-)*

D89.0 Polyclonal hypergammaglobulinemia

Benign hypergammaglobulinemic purpura

Polyclonal gammopathy NOS

D89.1 Cryoglobulinemia HCC

Cryoglobulinemic purpura

Cryoglobulinemic vasculitis

Essential cryoglobulinemia

Idiopathic cryoglobulinemia

Mixed cryoglobulinemia

Primary cryoglobulinemia

Secondary cryoglobulinemia

D89.2 Hypergammaglobulinemia, unspecified

D89.3 Immune reconstitution syndrome HCC

Immune reconstitution inflammatory syndrome [IRIS]

Use additional code for adverse effect, if applicable, to identify drug (T36-T50 with fifth or sixth character 5)

√5th D89.4 Mast cell activation syndrome and related disorders

EXCLUDES 1 *aggressive systemic mastocytosis (C96.21)*

congenital cutaneous mastocytosis (Q82.2)

(non-congenital) cutaneous mastocytosis (D47.01)

(indolent) systemic mastocytosis (D47.02)

malignant mast cell neoplasm (C96.2-)

malignant mastocytoma (C96.29)

mast cell leukemia (C94.3-)

mast cell sarcoma (C96.22)

mastocytoma NOS (D47.09)

other mast cell neoplasms of uncertain behavior (D47.09)

systemic mastocytosis associated with a clonal hematologic non-mast cell lineage disease (SM-AHNMD) (D47.02)

AHA: 2016,4Q,11

D89.40 Mast cell activation, unspecified HCC

Mast cell activation disorder, unspecified

Mast cell activation syndrome, NOS

D89.41 Monoclonal mast cell activation syndrome HCC

D89.42 Idiopathic mast cell activation syndrome HCC

D89.43 Secondary mast cell activation HCC

Secondary mast cell activation syndrome

Code also underlying etiology, if known

D89.49 Other mast cell activation disorder HCC

Other mast cell activation syndrome

√5th D89.8 Other specified disorders involving the immune mechanism, not elsewhere classified

√6th D89.81 Graft-versus-host disease

Code first underlying cause, such as:

complications of transplanted organs and tissue (T86.-)

complications of blood transfusion (T80.89)

Use additional code to identify associated manifestations, such as:

desquamative dermatitis (L30.8)

diarrhea (R19.7)

elevated bilirubin (R17)

hair loss (L65.9)

D89.810 Acute graft-versus-host disease CC HCC

D89.811 Chronic graft-versus-host disease CC HCC

D89.812 Acute on chronic graft-versus-host disease CC HCC

D89.813 Graft-versus-host disease, unspecified CC HCC

D89.82 Autoimmune lymphoproliferative syndrome [ALPS] HCC

DEF: Rare genetic alteration of the Fas protein that impairs normal cellular apoptosis (normal cell death), causing abnormal accumulation of lymphocytes in the lymph glands, liver, and spleen. Symptoms include neutropenia, anemia, and thrombocytopenia.

● ✓6th **D89.83 Cytokine release syndrome**

Code first underlying cause, such as:
complications following infusion, transfusion and therapeutic injection (T8Ø.89-)
complications of transplanted organs and tissue (T86.-)

Use additional code to identify associated manifestations

● **D89.831 Cytokine release syndrome, grade 1**

● **D89.832 Cytokine release syndrome, grade 2**

● **D89.833 Cytokine release syndrome, grade 3**

● **D89.834 Cytokine release syndrome, grade 4**

● **D89.835 Cytokine release syndrome, grade 5**

● **D89.839 Cytokine release syndrome, grade unspecified**

D89.89 Other specified disorders involving the immune mechanism, not elsewhere classified HCC

EXCLUDES 1 *human immunodeficiency virus disease (B2Ø)*

AHA: 2017,4Q,109

D89.9 Disorder involving the immune mechanism, unspecified HCC

Immune disease NOS

AHA: 2015,3Q,22

Chapter 4. Endocrine, Nutritional and Metabolic Diseases (E00–E89)

Chapter-specific Guidelines with Coding Examples

The chapter-specific guidelines from the ICD-10-CM Official Guidelines for Coding and Reporting have been provided below. Along with these guidelines are coding examples, contained in the shaded boxes, that have been developed to help illustrate the coding and/or sequencing guidance found in these guidelines.

a. Diabetes mellitus

The diabetes mellitus codes are combination codes that include the type of diabetes mellitus, the body system affected, and the complications affecting that body system. As many codes within a particular category as are necessary to describe all of the complications of the disease may be used. They should be sequenced based on the reason for a particular encounter. Assign as many codes from categories E08–E13 as needed to identify all of the associated conditions that the patient has.

Patient is seen for poorly controlled diabetes, type 2, with diabetic polyneuropathy and diabetic retinopathy with macular edema

E11.65 **Type 2 diabetes mellitus with hyperglycemia**

E11.311 **Type 2 diabetes mellitus with unspecified diabetic retinopathy with macular edema**

E11.42 **Type 2 diabetes mellitus with diabetic polyneuropathy**

Explanation: Use as many codes to describe the diabetic complications as needed. Many are combination codes that describe more than one condition. Code first the reason for the encounter. "Poorly controlled" is described as "with hyperglycemia." Diabetes documented as "uncontrolled" is not assumed to be hyperglycemic but can be classified to either hyperglycemia or hypoglycemia. If documentation is not clear, the provider must be queried so that the appropriate code can be reported.

1) Type of diabetes

The age of a patient is not the sole determining factor, though most type 1 diabetics develop the condition before reaching puberty. For this reason type 1 diabetes mellitus is also referred to as juvenile diabetes.

A 45-year-old patient is diagnosed with type 1 diabetes

E10.9 **Type 1 diabetes mellitus without complications**

Explanation: Although most type 1 diabetics are diagnosed in childhood or adolescence, it can also begin in adults.

2) Type of diabetes mellitus not documented

If the type of diabetes mellitus is not documented in the medical record the default is E11.-, Type 2 diabetes mellitus.

H & P lists diabetes and hypertension on patient problem list

E11.9 **Type 2 diabetes mellitus without complications**

I10 **Essential (primary) hypertension**

Explanation: Since the type of diabetes was not documented and no complications were noted, the default code is E11.9.

3) Diabetes mellitus and the use of insulin, oral hypoglycemics, and injectable non-insulin drugs

If the documentation in a medical record does not indicate the type of diabetes but does indicate that the patient uses insulin, code E11-, Type 2 diabetes mellitus, should be assigned. An additional code should be assigned from category Z79 to identify the long-term (current) use of insulin or oral hypoglycemic drugs. If the patient is treated with both oral medications and insulin, only the code for long-term (current) use of insulin should be assigned. **If the patient is treated with both insulin and an injectable non-insulin antidiabetic drug, assign codes Z79.4, Long-term (current) use of insulin, and Z79.899, Other long term (current) drug therapy. If the patient is treated with both oral hypoglycemic drugs and an injectable non-insulin antidiabetic drug, assign codes Z79.84, Long-term (current) use of oral hypoglycemic drugs, and Z79.899, Other long-term (current) drug therapy.** Code Z79.4 should not be assigned if insulin is given temporarily to bring a type 2 patient's blood sugar under control during an encounter.

Type 2 diabetic patient on daily metformin and Victoza is admitted in ketoacidosis, insulin given to stabilize blood sugars and discontinued at discharge

E11.10 **Type 2 diabetes mellitus with ketoacidosis without coma**

Z79.84 **Long term (current) use of oral hypoglycemic drugs**

Z79.899 **Other long term (current) drug therapy**

Explanation: Documentation indicates the patient is on an oral antidiabetic medication (metformin) and an injectable noninsulin antidiabetic medication (Victoza). Although insulin was given to the patient during the encounter, it was discontinued at discharge, indicating that the patient does not regularly use insulin. A Z code representing long-term use of the oral drug and long-term use of the injectable medication can be applied. Applying code Z79.4 to represent long-term use of insulin would be inappropriate.

4) Diabetes mellitus in pregnancy and gestational diabetes

See Section I.C.15. Diabetes mellitus in pregnancy.

See Section I.C.15. Gestational (pregnancy induced) diabetes

5) Complications due to insulin pump malfunction

(a) Underdose of insulin due to insulin pump failure

An underdose of insulin due to an insulin pump failure should be assigned to a code from subcategory T85.6, Mechanical complication of other specified internal and external prosthetic devices, implants and grafts, that specifies the type of pump malfunction, as the principal or first-listed code, followed by code T38.3X6-, Underdosing of insulin and oral hypoglycemic [antidiabetic] drugs. Additional codes for the type of diabetes mellitus and any associated complications due to the underdosing should also be assigned.

A 24-year-old type 1 diabetic male treated in ED for hyperglycemia; insulin pump found to be malfunctioning and underdosing

T85.614A **Breakdown (mechanical) of insulin pump, initial encounter**

T38.3X6A **Underdosing of insulin and oral hypoglycemic [antidiabetic] drugs, initial encounter**

E10.65 **Type 1 diabetes mellitus with hyperglycemia**

Explanation: The complication code for the mechanical breakdown of the pump is sequenced first, followed by the underdosing code and type of diabetes with complication. Code all other diabetic complication codes necessary to describe the patient's condition.

(b) Overdose of insulin due to insulin pump failure

The principal or first-listed code for an encounter due to an insulin pump malfunction resulting in an overdose of insulin, should also be T85.6-, Mechanical complication of other specified internal and external prosthetic devices, implants and grafts, followed by code T38.3X1-, Poisoning by insulin and oral hypoglycemic [antidiabetic] drugs, accidental (unintentional).

A 24-year-old type 1 diabetic male found down with diabetic coma, brought into ED and treated for hypoglycemia; insulin pump found to be malfunctioning and overdosing

T85.614A **Breakdown (mechanical) of insulin pump, initial encounter**

T38.3X1A **Poisoning by insulin and oral hypoglycemic [antidiabetic] drugs, accidental (unintentional), initial encounter**

E10.641 **Type 1 diabetes mellitus with hypoglycemia with coma**

Explanation: The complication code for the mechanical breakdown of the pump is sequenced first, followed by the poisoning code and type of diabetes with complication. All the characters in the combination code must be used to form a valid code and to fully describe the type of diabetes, the hypoglycemia, and the coma.

6) **Secondary diabetes mellitus**

Codes under categories EØ8, Diabetes mellitus due to underlying condition, EØ9, Drug or chemical induced diabetes mellitus, and E13, Other specified diabetes mellitus, identify complications/manifestations associated with secondary diabetes mellitus. Secondary diabetes is always caused by another condition or event (e.g., cystic fibrosis, malignant neoplasm of pancreas, pancreatectomy, adverse effect of drug, or poisoning).

(a) **Secondary diabetes mellitus and the use of insulin or oral hypoglycemic drugs**

For patients with secondary diabetes mellitus who routinely use insulin or oral hypoglycemic drugs, an additional code from category Z79 should be assigned to identify the long-term (current) use of insulin or oral hypoglycemic drugs. If the patient is treated with both oral medications and insulin, only the code for long-term (current) use of insulin should be assigned. **If the patient is treated with both insulin and an injectable non-insulin antidiabetic drug, assign codes Z79.4, Long-term (current) use of insulin, and Z79.899, Other long term (current) drug therapy. If the patient is treated with both oral hypoglycemic drugs and an injectable non-insulin antidiabetic drug, assign codes Z79.84, Long-term (current) use of oral hypoglycemic drugs, and Z79.899, Other long-term (current) drug therapy.** Code Z79.4 should not be assigned if insulin is given temporarily to bring a secondary diabetic patient's blood sugar under control during an encounter.

The patient, maintained on metformin and insulin, was admitted for treatment of diabetic gangrene. The patient developed diabetes secondary to Nelson's syndrome.

E24.1	**Nelson's syndrome**
EØ8.52	**Diabetes mellitus due to underlying condition with diabetic peripheral angiopathy with gangrene**
Z79.4	**Long term (current) use of insulin**

Explanation: When diabetes is caused by an underlying condition, the underlying condition should always be sequenced before any codes representing the diabetes. Patients with secondary diabetes may be maintained on both insulin and an oral hypoglycemic. Report only the code for the long-term use of insulin when both oral hypoglycemic and insulin are prescribed.

(b) **Assigning and sequencing secondary diabetes codes and its causes**

The sequencing of the secondary diabetes codes in relationship to codes for the cause of the diabetes is based on the Tabular List instructions for categories EØ8, EØ9 and E13.

(i) **Secondary diabetes mellitus due to pancreatectomy**

For postpancreatectomy diabetes mellitus (lack of insulin due to the surgical removal of all or part of the pancreas), assign code E89.1, Postprocedural hypoinsulinemia. Assign a code from category E13 and a code from subcategory Z9Ø.41, Acquired absence of pancreas, as additional codes.

Patient with newly diagnosed diabetes after surgical removal of part of pancreas is discharged with referral for consult to initiate insulin.

E89.1	**Postprocedural hypoinsulinemia**
E13.9	**Other specified diabetes mellitus without complications**
Z9Ø.411	**Acquired partial absence of pancreas**

Explanation: Sequence the postprocedural complication of the hypoinsulinemia due to the partial removal of the pancreas as the first-listed code, followed by the other specified diabetes (NEC) with or without complications and the partial or total acquired absence of the pancreas. Code Z79.4 Long term (current) use of insulin, is not added because the insulin has not yet been started.

(ii) **Secondary diabetes due to drugs**

Secondary diabetes may be caused by an adverse effect of correctly administered medications, poisoning or sequela of poisoning.

See section I.C.19.e for coding of adverse effects and poisoning, and section I.C.20 for external cause code reporting.

Initial encounter for corticosteroid-induced diabetes mellitus

EØ9.9	**Drug or chemical induced diabetes mellitus without complications**
T38.ØX5A	**Adverse effect of glucocorticoids and synthetic analogues, initial encounter**

Explanation: If the diabetes is caused by an adverse effect of a drug, the diabetic condition is coded first. If it occurs from a poisoning or overdose, the poisoning code causing the diabetes is sequenced first.

Chapter 4. Endocrine, Nutritional and Metabolic Diseases (E00-E89)

NOTE All neoplasms, whether functionally active or not, are classified in Chapter 2. Appropriate codes in this chapter (i.e. E05.8, E07.0, E16-E31, E34.-) may be used as additional codes to indicate either functional activity by neoplasms and ectopic endocrine tissue or hyperfunction and hypofunction of endocrine glands associated with neoplasms and other conditions classified elsewhere.

EXCLUDES 1 *transitory endocrine and metabolic disorders specific to newborn (P70-P74)*

AHA: 2018,2Q,6

This chapter contains the following blocks:

E00-E07 Disorders of thyroid gland
E08-E13 Diabetes mellitus
E15-E16 Other disorders of glucose regulation and pancreatic internal secretion
E20-E35 Disorders of other endocrine glands
E36 Intraoperative complications of endocrine system
E40-E46 Malnutrition
E50-E64 Other nutritional deficiencies
E65-E68 Overweight, obesity and other hyperalimentation
E70-E88 Metabolic disorders
E89 Postprocedural endocrine and metabolic complications and disorders, not elsewhere classified

Disorders of thyroid gland (E00-E07)

E00 Congenital iodine-deficiency syndrome (4th)
Use additional code (F70-F79) to identify associated intellectual disabilities
EXCLUDES 1 *subclinical iodine-deficiency hypothyroidism (E02)*

E00.0 Congenital iodine-deficiency syndrome, neurological type
Endemic cretinism, neurological type

E00.1 Congenital iodine-deficiency syndrome, myxedematous type
Endemic hypothyroid cretinism
Endemic cretinism, myxedematous type

E00.2 Congenital iodine-deficiency syndrome, mixed type
Endemic cretinism, mixed type

E00.9 Congenital iodine-deficiency syndrome, unspecified
Congenital iodine-deficiency hypothyroidism NOS
Endemic cretinism NOS

E01 Iodine-deficiency related thyroid disorders and allied conditions (4th)
EXCLUDES 1 *congenital iodine-deficiency syndrome (E00.-)*
subclinical iodine-deficiency hypothyroidism (E02)

E01.0 Iodine-deficiency related diffuse (endemic) goiter

E01.1 Iodine-deficiency related multinodular (endemic) goiter
Iodine-deficiency related nodular goiter

E01.2 Iodine-deficiency related (endemic) goiter, unspecified
Endemic goiter NOS

E01.8 Other iodine-deficiency related thyroid disorders and allied conditions
Acquired iodine-deficiency hypothyroidism NOS

E02 Subclinical iodine-deficiency hypothyroidism

E03 Other hypothyroidism (4th)
EXCLUDES 1 *iodine-deficiency related hypothyroidism (E00-E02)*
postprocedural hypothyroidism (E89.0)
DEF: Hypothyroidism: Underproduction of thyroid hormone.

E03.0 Congenital hypothyroidism with diffuse goiter
Congenital parenchymatous goiter (nontoxic)
Congenital goiter (nontoxic) NOS
EXCLUDES 1 *transitory congenital goiter with normal function (P72.0)*

E03.1 Congenital hypothyroidism without goiter
Aplasia of thyroid (with myxedema)
Congenital atrophy of thyroid
Congenital hypothyroidism NOS

E03.2 Hypothyroidism due to medicaments and other exogenous substances
Code first poisoning due to drug or toxin, if applicable (T36-T65 with fifth or sixth character 1-4 or 6)
Use additional code for adverse effect, if applicable, to identify drug (T36-T50 with fifth or sixth character 5)

E03.3 Postinfectious hypothyroidism

E03.4 Atrophy of thyroid (acquired)
EXCLUDES 1 *congenital atrophy of thyroid (E03.1)*

E03.5 Myxedema coma MCC HCC

E03.8 Other specified hypothyroidism

E03.9 Hypothyroidism, unspecified
Myxedema NOS

E04 Other nontoxic goiter (4th)
EXCLUDES 1 *congenital goiter (NOS) (diffuse) (parenchymatous) (E03.0)*
iodine-deficiency related goiter (E00-E02)

E04.0 Nontoxic diffuse goiter
Diffuse (colloid) nontoxic goiter
Simple nontoxic goiter

E04.1 Nontoxic single thyroid nodule
Colloid nodule (cystic) (thyroid)
Nontoxic uninodular goiter
Thyroid (cystic) nodule NOS
DEF: Enlarged thyroid, commonly due to decreased thyroid production, with a single nodule. No clinical hypothyroidism.

E04.2 Nontoxic multinodular goiter
Cystic goiter NOS
Multinodular (cystic) goiter NOS
DEF: Enlarged thyroid, commonly due to decreased thyroid production with multiple nodules. No clinical hypothyroidism.

E04.8 Other specified nontoxic goiter

E04.9 Nontoxic goiter, unspecified
Goiter NOS
Nodular goiter (nontoxic) NOS

E05 Thyrotoxicosis [hyperthyroidism] (4th)
EXCLUDES 1 *chronic thyroiditis with transient thyrotoxicosis (E06.2)*
neonatal thyrotoxicosis (P72.1)
DEF: Excessive quantities of hormones from the thyroid gland caused by overproduction or loss of storage ability.

E05.0 Thyrotoxicosis with diffuse goiter (5th)
Exophthalmic or toxic goiter NOS
Graves' disease
Toxic diffuse goiter
DEF: Diffuse thyroid enlargement accompanied by hyperthyroidism, bulging eyes, and dermopathy.

E05.00 Thyrotoxicosis with diffuse goiter without thyrotoxic crisis or storm

E05.01 Thyrotoxicosis with diffuse goiter with thyrotoxic crisis or storm MCC

Goiter

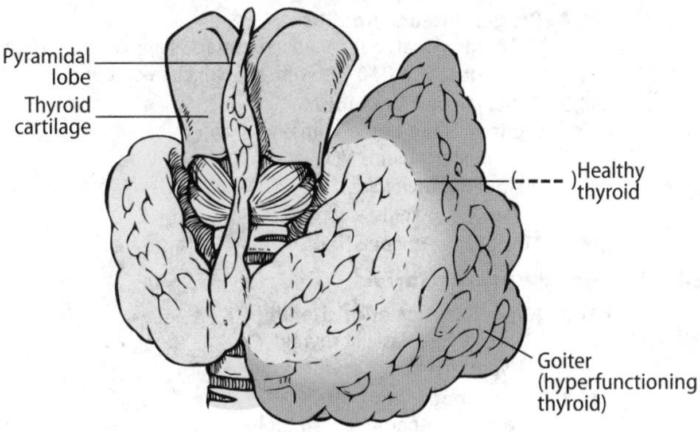

E05.1 Thyrotoxicosis with toxic single thyroid nodule (5th)
Thyrotoxicosis with toxic uninodular goiter
DEF: Symptomatic hyperthyroidism with a single nodule on the enlarged thyroid gland. Onset of symptoms can be abrupt and include extreme nervousness, insomnia, weight loss, tremors, and psychosis or coma.

E05.10 Thyrotoxicosis with toxic single thyroid nodule without thyrotoxic crisis or storm

E05.11 Thyrotoxicosis with toxic single thyroid nodule with thyrotoxic crisis or storm MCC

E05.2 Thyrotoxicosis with toxic multinodular goiter (5th)
Toxic nodular goiter NOS

E05.20 Thyrotoxicosis with toxic multinodular goiter without thyrotoxic crisis or storm

E05.21 Thyrotoxicosis with toxic multinodular goiter with thyrotoxic crisis or storm MCC

E05.3 Thyrotoxicosis from ectopic thyroid tissue (5th)

E05.30 Thyrotoxicosis from ectopic thyroid tissue without thyrotoxic crisis or storm

E05.31 Thyrotoxicosis from ectopic thyroid tissue with thyrotoxic crisis or storm MCC

Chapter 4. Endocrine, Nutritional and Metabolic Diseases

✓5th **EØ5.4 Thyrotoxicosis factitia**

EØ5.4Ø Thyrotoxicosis factitia without thyrotoxic crisis or storm

EØ5.41 Thyrotoxicosis factitia with thyrotoxic crisis or storm MCC

✓5th **EØ5.8 Other thyrotoxicosis**

Overproduction of thyroid-stimulating hormone

EØ5.8Ø Other thyrotoxicosis without thyrotoxic crisis or storm

EØ5.81 Other thyrotoxicosis with thyrotoxic crisis or storm MCC

✓5th **EØ5.9 Thyrotoxicosis, unspecified**

Hyperthyroidism NOS

EØ5.9Ø Thyrotoxicosis, unspecified without thyrotoxic crisis or storm

EØ5.91 Thyrotoxicosis, unspecified with thyrotoxic crisis or storm MCC

✓4th **EØ6 Thyroiditis**

EXCLUDES 1 *postpartum thyroiditis (O9Ø.5)*

DEF: Inflammation of the thyroid gland.

EØ6.Ø Acute thyroiditis CC

Abscess of thyroid
Pyogenic thyroiditis
Suppurative thyroiditis
Use additional code (B95-B97) to identify infectious agent

EØ6.1 Subacute thyroiditis

de Quervain thyroiditis
Giant-cell thyroiditis
Granulomatous thyroiditis
Nonsuppurative thyroiditis
Viral thyroiditis

EXCLUDES 1 *autoimmune thyroiditis (EØ6.3)*

EØ6.2 Chronic thyroiditis with transient thyrotoxicosis

EXCLUDES 1 *autoimmune thyroiditis (EØ6.3)*

EØ6.3 Autoimmune thyroiditis

Hashimoto's thyroiditis
Hashitoxicosis (transient)
Lymphadenoid goiter
Lymphocytic thyroiditis
Struma lymphomatosa

EØ6.4 Drug-induced thyroiditis

Use additional code for adverse effect, if applicable, to identify drug (T36-T5Ø with fifth or sixth character 5)

EØ6.5 Other chronic thyroiditis

Chronic fibrous thyroiditis
Chronic thyroiditis NOS
Ligneous thyroiditis
Riedel thyroiditis

EØ6.9 Thyroiditis, unspecified

✓4th **EØ7 Other disorders of thyroid**

EØ7.Ø Hypersecretion of calcitonin

C-cell hyperplasia of thyroid
Hypersecretion of thyrocalcitonin

EØ7.1 Dyshormogenetic goiter

Familial dyshormogenetic goiter
Pendred's syndrome

EXCLUDES 1 *transitory congenital goiter with normal function (P72.Ø)*

✓5th **EØ7.8 Other specified disorders of thyroid**

EØ7.81 Sick-euthyroid syndrome

Euthyroid sick-syndrome

DEF: Thyroid dysfunction caused by abnormal levels of thyroid hormones T3 and/or T4. This syndrome is often associated with starvation or critical illness.

EØ7.89 Other specified disorders of thyroid

Abnormality of thyroid-binding globulin
Hemorrhage of thyroid
Infarction of thyroid

EØ7.9 Disorder of thyroid, unspecified

Diabetes mellitus (EØ8-E13)

AHA: 2020,1Q,12; 2018,2Q,6; 2017,4Q,100-101; 2016,2Q,36; 2016,1Q,11-13; 2013,4Q,114; 2013,3Q,20

✓4th **EØ8 Diabetes mellitus due to underlying condition**

Code first the underlying condition, such as:
congenital rubella (P35.Ø)
Cushing's syndrome (E24.-)
cystic fibrosis (E84.-)
malignant neoplasm (CØØ-C96)
malnutrition (E4Ø-E46)
pancreatitis and other diseases of the pancreas (K85-K86.-)

Use additional code to identify control using:
insulin (Z79.4)
oral antidiabetic drugs (Z79.84)
oral hypoglycemic drugs (Z79.84)

EXCLUDES 1 *drug or chemical induced diabetes mellitus (EØ9.-)*
gestational diabetes (O24.4-)
neonatal diabetes mellitus (P7Ø.2)
postpancreatectomy diabetes mellitus (E13.-)
postprocedural diabetes mellitus (E13.-)
secondary diabetes mellitus NEC (E13.-)
type 1 diabetes mellitus (E1Ø.-)
type 2 diabetes mellitus (E11.-)

✓5th **EØ8.Ø Diabetes mellitus due to underlying condition with hyperosmolarity**

DEF: Diabetic hyperosmolarity: Extremely high levels of glucose in the blood without ketones.

EØ8.ØØ Diabetes mellitus due to underlying condition with hyperosmolarity without nonketotic hyperglycemic-hyperosmolar coma (NKHHC) MCC H9 HCC

EØ8.Ø1 Diabetes mellitus due to underlying condition with hyperosmolarity with coma MCC H9 HCC

✓5th **EØ8.1 Diabetes mellitus due to underlying condition with ketoacidosis**

DEF: Diabetic ketoacidosis: Potentially life-threatening complication due to a shortage of insulin in which the body switches to burning fatty acids and producing acidic ketone bodies.

EØ8.1Ø Diabetes mellitus due to underlying condition with ketoacidosis without coma MCC H9 HCC

EØ8.11 Diabetes mellitus due to underlying condition with ketoacidosis with coma MCC HCC

✓5th **EØ8.2 Diabetes mellitus due to underlying condition with kidney complications**

AHA: 2019,3Q,3; 2018,4Q,88

EØ8.21 Diabetes mellitus due to underlying condition with diabetic nephropathy HCC

Diabetes mellitus due to underlying condition with intercapillary glomerulosclerosis
Diabetes mellitus due to underlying condition with intracapillary glomerulonephrosis
Diabetes mellitus due to underlying condition with Kimmelstiel-Wilson disease

EØ8.22 Diabetes mellitus due to underlying condition with diabetic chronic kidney disease HCC

Use additional code to identify stage of chronic kidney disease (N18.1-N18.6)

EØ8.29 Diabetes mellitus due to underlying condition with other diabetic kidney complication HCC

Renal tubular degeneration in diabetes mellitus due to underlying condition

EØ8.3 Diabetes mellitus due to underlying condition with ophthalmic complications
AHA: 2016,4Q,11-13

One of the following 7th characters is to be assigned to codes in subcategories EØ8.32, EØ8.33, EØ8.34, EØ8.35, and EØ8.37 to designate laterality of the disease:
1 right eye
2 left eye
3 bilateral
9 unspecified eye

EØ8.31 Diabetes mellitus due to underlying condition with unspecified diabetic retinopathy
DEF: Diabetic retinopathy: Diabetic complication from damage to the retinal vessels resulting in vision problems that can progress to blindness.

EØ8.311 Diabetes mellitus due to underlying condition with unspecified diabetic retinopathy with macular edema HCC

EØ8.319 Diabetes mellitus due to underlying condition with unspecified diabetic retinopathy without macular edema HCC

EØ8.32 Diabetes mellitus due to underlying condition with mild nonproliferative diabetic retinopathy
Diabetes mellitus due to underlying condition with nonproliferative diabetic retinopathy NOS

EØ8.321 Diabetes mellitus due to underlying condition with mild nonproliferative diabetic retinopathy with macular edema HCC

EØ8.329 Diabetes mellitus due to underlying condition with mild nonproliferative diabetic retinopathy without macular edema HCC

EØ8.33 Diabetes mellitus due to underlying condition with moderate nonproliferative diabetic retinopathy

EØ8.331 Diabetes mellitus due to underlying condition with moderate nonproliferative diabetic retinopathy with macular edema HCC

EØ8.339 Diabetes mellitus due to underlying condition with moderate nonproliferative diabetic retinopathy without macular edema HCC

EØ8.34 Diabetes mellitus due to underlying condition with severe nonproliferative diabetic retinopathy

EØ8.341 Diabetes mellitus due to underlying condition with severe nonproliferative diabetic retinopathy with macular edema HCC

EØ8.349 Diabetes mellitus due to underlying condition with severe nonproliferative diabetic retinopathy without macular edema HCC

EØ8.35 Diabetes mellitus due to underlying condition with proliferative diabetic retinopathy

EØ8.351 Diabetes mellitus due to underlying condition with proliferative diabetic retinopathy with macular edema HCC

EØ8.352 Diabetes mellitus due to underlying condition with proliferative diabetic retinopathy with traction retinal detachment involving the macula HCC

EØ8.353 Diabetes mellitus due to underlying condition with proliferative diabetic retinopathy with traction retinal detachment not involving the macula HCC

EØ8.354 Diabetes mellitus due to underlying condition with proliferative diabetic retinopathy with combined traction retinal detachment and rhegmatogenous retinal detachment HCC

EØ8.355 Diabetes mellitus due to underlying condition with stable proliferative diabetic retinopathy HCC

EØ8.359 Diabetes mellitus due to underlying condition with proliferative diabetic retinopathy without macular edema HCC

EØ8.36 Diabetes mellitus due to underlying condition with diabetic cataract HCC
AHA: 2019,2Q,30-31; 2016,4Q,142

EØ8.37 Diabetes mellitus due to underlying condition with diabetic macular edema, resolved following treatment HCC

EØ8.39 Diabetes mellitus due to underlying condition with other diabetic ophthalmic complication HCC
Use additional code to identify manifestation, such as:
diabetic glaucoma (H4Ø-H42)

EØ8.4 Diabetes mellitus due to underlying condition with neurological complications

EØ8.4Ø Diabetes mellitus due to underlying condition with diabetic neuropathy, unspecified HCC

EØ8.41 Diabetes mellitus due to underlying condition with diabetic mononeuropathy HCC

EØ8.42 Diabetes mellitus due to underlying condition with diabetic polyneuropathy HCC
Diabetes mellitus due to underlying condition with diabetic neuralgia

EØ8.43 Diabetes mellitus due to underlying condition with diabetic autonomic (poly)neuropathy HCC
Diabetes mellitus due to underlying condition with diabetic gastroparesis
AHA: 2013,4Q,114

EØ8.44 Diabetes mellitus due to underlying condition with diabetic amyotrophy HCC

EØ8.49 Diabetes mellitus due to underlying condition with other diabetic neurological complication HCC

EØ8.5 Diabetes mellitus due to underlying condition with circulatory complications

EØ8.51 Diabetes mellitus due to underlying condition with diabetic peripheral angiopathy without gangrene HCC
AHA: 2018,3Q,3-4; 2018,2Q,7

EØ8.52 Diabetes mellitus due to underlying condition with diabetic peripheral angiopathy with gangrene CC HCC
Diabetes mellitus due to underlying condition with diabetic gangrene
AHA: 2020,2Q,18; 2018,3Q,3; 2018,2Q,7; 2017,4Q,102

EØ8.59 Diabetes mellitus due to underlying condition with other circulatory complications HCC

EØ8.6 Diabetes mellitus due to underlying condition with other specified complications

EØ8.61 Diabetes mellitus due to underlying condition with diabetic arthropathy

EØ8.61Ø Diabetes mellitus due to underlying condition with diabetic neuropathic arthropathy HCC
Diabetes mellitus due to underlying condition with Charcôt's joints
DEF: Charcot's joint: Progressive neurologic arthropathy in which chronic degeneration of joints in the weight-bearing areas with peripheral hypertrophy occurs as a complication of a neuropathy disorder. Supporting structures relax from a loss of sensation resulting in chronic joint instability.

EØ8.618 Diabetes mellitus due to underlying condition with other diabetic arthropathy HCC
AHA: 2018,2Q,6

EØ8.62 Diabetes mellitus due to underlying condition with skin complications

EØ8.62Ø Diabetes mellitus due to underlying condition with diabetic dermatitis HCC
Diabetes mellitus due to underlying condition with diabetic necrobiosis lipoidica

EØ8.621 Diabetes mellitus due to underlying condition with foot ulcer HCC
Use additional code to identify site of ulcer (L97.4-, L97.5-)
AHA: 2020,2Q,19

E08.622 Diabetes mellitus due to underlying condition with other skin ulcer HCC
Use additional code to identify site of ulcer (L97.1-L97.9, L98.41-L98.49)
AHA: 2017,4Q,17

E08.628 Diabetes mellitus due to underlying condition with other skin complications HCC

✓6th **E08.63 Diabetes mellitus due to underlying condition with oral complications**

E08.630 Diabetes mellitus due to underlying condition with periodontal disease HCC

E08.638 Diabetes mellitus due to underlying condition with other oral complications HCC

✓6th **E08.64 Diabetes mellitus due to underlying condition with hypoglycemia**
AHA: 2017,1Q,42

E08.641 Diabetes mellitus due to underlying condition with hypoglycemia with coma MCC HCC

E08.649 Diabetes mellitus due to underlying condition with hypoglycemia without coma HCC
AHA: 2016,3Q,42; 2015,3Q,21

E08.65 Diabetes mellitus due to underlying condition with hyperglycemia HCC
AHA: 2017,1Q,42; 2013,3Q,20

E08.69 Diabetes mellitus due to underlying condition with other specified complication HCC
Use additional code to identify complication
AHA: 2016,4Q,141; 2016,1Q,13

E08.8 Diabetes mellitus due to underlying condition with unspecified complications HCC

E08.9 Diabetes mellitus due to underlying condition without complications HCC
AHA: 2020,2Q,18

✓4th **E09 Drug or chemical induced diabetes mellitus**

Code first poisoning due to drug or toxin, if applicable (T36-T65 with fifth or sixth character 1-4 or 6)
Use additional code for adverse effect, if applicable, to identify drug (T36-T50 with fifth or sixth character 5)
Use additional code to identify control using:
insulin (Z79.4)
oral antidiabetic drugs (Z79.84)
oral hypoglycemic drugs (Z79.84)

EXCLUDES 1 *diabetes mellitus due to underlying condition (E08.-)*
gestational diabetes (O24.4-)
neonatal diabetes mellitus (P70.2)
postpancreatectomy diabetes mellitus (E13.-)
postprocedural diabetes mellitus (E13.-)
secondary diabetes mellitus NEC (E13.-)
type 1 diabetes mellitus (E10.-)
type 2 diabetes mellitus (E11.-)

✓5th **E09.0 Drug or chemical induced diabetes mellitus with hyperosmolarity**
DEF: Diabetic hyperosmolarity: Extremely high levels of glucose in the blood without ketones.

E09.00 Drug or chemical induced diabetes mellitus with hyperosmolarity without nonketotic hyperglycemic-hyperosmolar coma (NKHHC) MCC H9 HCC

E09.01 Drug or chemical induced diabetes mellitus with hyperosmolarity with coma MCC H9 HCC

✓5th **E09.1 Drug or chemical induced diabetes mellitus with ketoacidosis**
DEF: Diabetic ketoacidosis: Potentially life-threatening complication due to a shortage of insulin in which the body switches to burning fatty acids and producing acidic ketone bodies.

E09.10 Drug or chemical induced diabetes mellitus with ketoacidosis without coma MCC H9 HCC

E09.11 Drug or chemical induced diabetes mellitus with ketoacidosis with coma MCC HCC

✓5th **E09.2 Drug or chemical induced diabetes mellitus with kidney complications**
AHA: 2019,3Q,3; 2018,4Q,88

E09.21 Drug or chemical induced diabetes mellitus with diabetic nephropathy HCC
Drug or chemical induced diabetes mellitus with intercapillary glomerulosclerosis
Drug or chemical induced diabetes mellitus with intracapillary glomerulonephrosis
Drug or chemical induced diabetes mellitus with Kimmelstiel-Wilson disease

E09.22 Drug or chemical induced diabetes mellitus with diabetic chronic kidney disease HCC
Use additional code to identify stage of chronic kidney disease (N18.1-N18.6)

E09.29 Drug or chemical induced diabetes mellitus with other diabetic kidney complication HCC
Drug or chemical induced diabetes mellitus with renal tubular degeneration

✓5th **E09.3 Drug or chemical induced diabetes mellitus with ophthalmic complications**
AHA: 2016,4Q,11-13

One of the following 7th characters is to be assigned to codes in subcategories E09.32, E09.33, E09.34, E09.35, and E09.37 to designate laterality of the disease:
1 right eye
2 left eye
3 bilateral
9 unspecified eye

✓6th **E09.31 Drug or chemical induced diabetes mellitus with unspecified diabetic retinopathy**
DEF: Diabetic retinopathy: Diabetic complication from damage to the retinal vessels resulting in vision problems that can progress to blindness.

E09.311 Drug or chemical induced diabetes mellitus with unspecified diabetic retinopathy with macular edema HCC

E09.319 Drug or chemical induced diabetes mellitus with unspecified diabetic retinopathy without macular edema HCC

✓6th **E09.32 Drug or chemical induced diabetes mellitus with mild nonproliferative diabetic retinopathy**
Drug or chemical induced diabetes mellitus with nonproliferative diabetic retinopathy NOS

✓7th **E09.321 Drug or chemical induced diabetes mellitus with mild nonproliferative diabetic retinopathy with macular edema** HCC

✓7th **E09.329 Drug or chemical induced diabetes mellitus with mild nonproliferative diabetic retinopathy without macular edema** HCC

✓6th **E09.33 Drug or chemical induced diabetes mellitus with moderate nonproliferative diabetic retinopathy**

✓7th **E09.331 Drug or chemical induced diabetes mellitus with moderate nonproliferative diabetic retinopathy with macular edema** HCC

✓7th **E09.339 Drug or chemical induced diabetes mellitus with moderate nonproliferative diabetic retinopathy without macular edema** HCC

✓6th **E09.34 Drug or chemical induced diabetes mellitus with severe nonproliferative diabetic retinopathy**

✓7th **E09.341 Drug or chemical induced diabetes mellitus with severe nonproliferative diabetic retinopathy with macular edema** HCC

✓7th **E09.349 Drug or chemical induced diabetes mellitus with severe nonproliferative diabetic retinopathy without macular edema** HCC

✓6th **E09.35 Drug or chemical induced diabetes mellitus with proliferative diabetic retinopathy**

✓7th **E09.351 Drug or chemical induced diabetes mellitus with proliferative diabetic retinopathy with macular edema** HCC

✓7th **E09.352 Drug or chemical induced diabetes mellitus with proliferative diabetic retinopathy with traction retinal detachment involving the macula** HCC

E09.353 Drug or chemical induced diabetes mellitus with proliferative diabetic retinopathy with traction retinal detachment not involving the macula HCC

E09.354 Drug or chemical induced diabetes mellitus with proliferative diabetic retinopathy with combined traction retinal detachment and rhegmatogenous retinal detachment HCC

E09.355 Drug or chemical induced diabetes mellitus with stable proliferative diabetic retinopathy HCC

E09.359 Drug or chemical induced diabetes mellitus with proliferative diabetic retinopathy without macular edema HCC

E09.36 Drug or chemical induced diabetes mellitus with diabetic cataract HCC

AHA: 2019,2Q,30-31; 2016,4Q,142

E09.37 Drug or chemical induced diabetes mellitus with diabetic macular edema, resolved following treatment HCC

E09.39 Drug or chemical induced diabetes mellitus with other diabetic ophthalmic complication HCC

Use additional code to identify manifestation, such as:

diabetic glaucoma (H40-H42)

E09.4 Drug or chemical induced diabetes mellitus with neurological complications

E09.40 Drug or chemical induced diabetes mellitus with neurological complications with diabetic neuropathy, unspecified HCC

E09.41 Drug or chemical induced diabetes mellitus with neurological complications with diabetic mononeuropathy HCC

E09.42 Drug or chemical induced diabetes mellitus with neurological complications with diabetic polyneuropathy HCC

Drug or chemical induced diabetes mellitus with diabetic neuralgia

E09.43 Drug or chemical induced diabetes mellitus with neurological complications with diabetic autonomic (poly)neuropathy HCC

Drug or chemical induced diabetes mellitus with diabetic gastroparesis

AHA: 2013,4Q,114

E09.44 Drug or chemical induced diabetes mellitus with neurological complications with diabetic amyotrophy HCC

E09.49 Drug or chemical induced diabetes mellitus with neurological complications with other diabetic neurological complication HCC

E09.5 Drug or chemical induced diabetes mellitus with circulatory complications

E09.51 Drug or chemical induced diabetes mellitus with diabetic peripheral angiopathy without gangrene HCC

AHA: 2018,3Q,3-4; 2018,2Q,7

E09.52 Drug or chemical induced diabetes mellitus with diabetic peripheral angiopathy with gangrene CC HCC

Drug or chemical induced diabetes mellitus with diabetic gangrene

AHA: 2020,2Q,18; 2018,3Q,3; 2018,2Q,7; 2017,4Q,102

E09.59 Drug or chemical induced diabetes mellitus with other circulatory complications HCC

E09.6 Drug or chemical induced diabetes mellitus with other specified complications

E09.61 Drug or chemical induced diabetes mellitus with diabetic arthropathy

E09.610 Drug or chemical induced diabetes mellitus with diabetic neuropathic arthropathy HCC

Drug or chemical induced diabetes mellitus with Charcôt's joints

DEF: Charcot's joint: Progressive neurologic arthropathy in which chronic degeneration of joints in the weight-bearing areas with peripheral hypertrophy occurs as a complication of a neuropathy disorder. Supporting structures relax from a loss of sensation resulting in chronic joint instability.

E09.618 Drug or chemical induced diabetes mellitus with other diabetic arthropathy HCC

AHA: 2018,2Q,6

E09.62 Drug or chemical induced diabetes mellitus with skin complications

E09.620 Drug or chemical induced diabetes mellitus with diabetic dermatitis HCC

Drug or chemical induced diabetes mellitus with diabetic necrobiosis lipoidica

E09.621 Drug or chemical induced diabetes mellitus with foot ulcer HCC

Use additional code to identify site of ulcer (L97.4-, L97.5-)

AHA: 2020,2Q,19

E09.622 Drug or chemical induced diabetes mellitus with other skin ulcer HCC

Use additional code to identify site of ulcer (L97.1-L97.9, L98.41-L98.49)

AHA: 2017,4Q,17

E09.628 Drug or chemical induced diabetes mellitus with other skin complications HCC

E09.63 Drug or chemical induced diabetes mellitus with oral complications

E09.630 Drug or chemical induced diabetes mellitus with periodontal disease HCC

E09.638 Drug or chemical induced diabetes mellitus with other oral complications HCC

E09.64 Drug or chemical induced diabetes mellitus with hypoglycemia

AHA: 2017,1Q,42

E09.641 Drug or chemical induced diabetes mellitus with hypoglycemia with coma MCC HCC

E09.649 Drug or chemical induced diabetes mellitus with hypoglycemia without coma HCC

AHA: 2016,3Q,42; 2015,3Q,21

E09.65 Drug or chemical induced diabetes mellitus with hyperglycemia HCC

AHA: 2017,1Q,42; 2013,3Q,20

E09.69 Drug or chemical induced diabetes mellitus with other specified complication HCC

Use additional code to identify complication

AHA: 2016,4Q,141; 2016,1Q,13

E09.8 Drug or chemical induced diabetes mellitus with unspecified complications HCC

E09.9 Drug or chemical induced diabetes mellitus without complications HCC

AHA: 2020,2Q,18

√4th **E10 Type 1 diabetes mellitus**

INCLUDES brittle diabetes (mellitus)
diabetes (mellitus) due to autoimmune process
diabetes (mellitus) due to immune mediated pancreatic islet beta-cell destruction
idiopathic diabetes (mellitus)
juvenile onset diabetes (mellitus)
ketosis-prone diabetes (mellitus)

EXCLUDES 1 *diabetes mellitus due to underlying condition (E08.-)*
drug or chemical induced diabetes mellitus (E09.-)
gestational diabetes (O24.4-)
hyperglycemia NOS (R73.9)
neonatal diabetes mellitus (P70.2)
postpancreatectomy diabetes mellitus (E13.-)
postprocedural diabetes mellitus (E13.-)
secondary diabetes mellitus NEC (E13.-)
type 2 diabetes mellitus (E11.-)

√5th **E10.1 Type 1 diabetes mellitus with ketoacidosis**
AHA: 2013,3Q,20
DEF: Diabetic ketoacidosis: Potentially life-threatening complication due to a shortage of insulin in which the body switches to burning fatty acids and producing acidic ketone bodies.

E10.10 Type 1 diabetes mellitus with ketoacidosis without coma MCC H9 HCC

E10.11 Type 1 diabetes mellitus with ketoacidosis with coma MCC HCC

√5th **E10.2 Type 1 diabetes mellitus with kidney complications**
AHA: 2019,3Q,3; 2018,4Q,88

E10.21 Type 1 diabetes mellitus with diabetic nephropathy HCC
Type 1 diabetes mellitus with intercapillary glomerulosclerosis
Type 1 diabetes mellitus with intracapillary glomerulonephrosis
Type 1 diabetes mellitus with Kimmelstiel-Wilson disease

E10.22 Type 1 diabetes mellitus with diabetic chronic kidney disease HCC
Use additional code to identify stage of chronic kidney disease (N18.1-N18.6)

E10.29 Type 1 diabetes mellitus with other diabetic kidney complication HCC
Type 1 diabetes mellitus with renal tubular degeneration
AHA: 2016,1Q,13

√5th **E10.3 Type 1 diabetes mellitus with ophthalmic complications**
AHA: 2016,4Q,11-13

One of the following 7th characters is to be assigned to codes in subcategories E10.32, E10.33, E10.34, E10.35, and E10.37 to designate laterality of the disease:
1 right eye
2 left eye
3 bilateral
9 unspecified eye

√6th **E10.31 Type 1 diabetes mellitus with unspecified diabetic retinopathy**
DEF: Diabetic retinopathy: Diabetic complication from damage to the retinal vessels resulting in vision problems that can progress to blindness.

E10.311 Type 1 diabetes mellitus with unspecified diabetic retinopathy with macular edema HCC

E10.319 Type 1 diabetes mellitus with unspecified diabetic retinopathy without macular edema HCC

√6th **E10.32 Type 1 diabetes mellitus with mild nonproliferative diabetic retinopathy**
Type 1 diabetes mellitus with nonproliferative diabetic retinopathy NOS

√7th **E10.321 Type 1 diabetes mellitus with mild nonproliferative diabetic retinopathy with macular edema** HCC

√7th **E10.329 Type 1 diabetes mellitus with mild nonproliferative diabetic retinopathy without macular edema** HCC

√6th **E10.33 Type 1 diabetes mellitus with moderate nonproliferative diabetic retinopathy**

√7th **E10.331 Type 1 diabetes mellitus with moderate nonproliferative diabetic retinopathy with macular edema** HCC

√7th **E10.339 Type 1 diabetes mellitus with moderate nonproliferative diabetic retinopathy without macular edema** HCC

√6th **E10.34 Type 1 diabetes mellitus with severe nonproliferative diabetic retinopathy**

√7th **E10.341 Type 1 diabetes mellitus with severe nonproliferative diabetic retinopathy with macular edema** HCC

√7th **E10.349 Type 1 diabetes mellitus with severe nonproliferative diabetic retinopathy without macular edema** HCC

√6th **E10.35 Type 1 diabetes mellitus with proliferative diabetic retinopathy**

√7th **E10.351 Type 1 diabetes mellitus with proliferative diabetic retinopathy with macular edema** HCC

√7th **E10.352 Type 1 diabetes mellitus with proliferative diabetic retinopathy with traction retinal detachment involving the macula** HCC

√7th **E10.353 Type 1 diabetes mellitus with proliferative diabetic retinopathy with traction retinal detachment not involving the macula** HCC

√7th **E10.354 Type 1 diabetes mellitus with proliferative diabetic retinopathy with combined traction retinal detachment and rhegmatogenous retinal detachment** HCC

√7th **E10.355 Type 1 diabetes mellitus with stable proliferative diabetic retinopathy** HCC

√7th **E10.359 Type 1 diabetes mellitus with proliferative diabetic retinopathy without macular edema** HCC

E10.36 Type 1 diabetes mellitus with diabetic cataract HCC
AHA: 2019,2Q,30-31; 2016,4Q,142

√x7th **E10.37 Type 1 diabetes mellitus with diabetic macular edema, resolved following treatment** HCC

E10.39 Type 1 diabetes mellitus with other diabetic ophthalmic complication HCC
Use additional code to identify manifestation, such as:
diabetic glaucoma (H40-H42)

√5th **E10.4 Type 1 diabetes mellitus with neurological complications**

E10.40 Type 1 diabetes mellitus with diabetic neuropathy, unspecified HCC

E10.41 Type 1 diabetes mellitus with diabetic mononeuropathy HCC

E10.42 Type 1 diabetes mellitus with diabetic polyneuropathy HCC
Type 1 diabetes mellitus with diabetic neuralgia

E10.43 Type 1 diabetes mellitus with diabetic autonomic (poly)neuropathy HCC
Type 1 diabetes mellitus with diabetic gastroparesis
AHA: 2013,4Q,114

E10.44 Type 1 diabetes mellitus with diabetic amyotrophy HCC

E10.49 Type 1 diabetes mellitus with other diabetic neurological complication HCC

√5th **E10.5 Type 1 diabetes mellitus with circulatory complications**

E10.51 Type 1 diabetes mellitus with diabetic peripheral angiopathy without gangrene HCC
AHA: 2018,3Q,3-4; 2018,2Q,7

E10.52 Type 1 diabetes mellitus with diabetic peripheral angiopathy with gangrene CC HCC
Type 1 diabetes mellitus with diabetic gangrene
AHA: 2020,2Q,18; 2018,3Q,3; 2018,2Q,7; 2017,4Q,102

E10.59 Type 1 diabetes mellitus with other circulatory complications HCC

E10.6 Type 1 diabetes mellitus with other specified complications

E10.61 Type 1 diabetes mellitus with diabetic arthropathy

E10.610 Type 1 diabetes mellitus with diabetic neuropathic arthropathy HCC

Type 1 diabetes mellitus with Charcôt's joints

DEF: Charcot's joint: Progressive neurologic arthropathy in which chronic degeneration of joints in the weight-bearing areas with peripheral hypertrophy occurs as a complication of a neuropathy disorder. Supporting structures relax from a loss of sensation resulting in chronic joint instability.

E10.618 Type 1 diabetes mellitus with other diabetic arthropathy HCC

AHA: 2018,2Q,6

E10.62 Type 1 diabetes mellitus with skin complications

E10.620 Type 1 diabetes mellitus with diabetic dermatitis HCC

Type 1 diabetes mellitus with diabetic necrobiosis lipoidica

E10.621 Type 1 diabetes mellitus with foot ulcer HCC

Use additional code to identify site of ulcer (L97.4-, L97.5-)

AHA: 2020,2Q,19

E10.622 Type 1 diabetes mellitus with other skin ulcer HCC

Use additional code to identify site of ulcer (L97.1-L97.9, L98.41-L98.49)

AHA: 2017,4Q,17

E10.628 Type 1 diabetes mellitus with other skin complications HCC

E10.63 Type 1 diabetes mellitus with oral complications

E10.630 Type 1 diabetes mellitus with periodontal disease HCC

E10.638 Type 1 diabetes mellitus with other oral complications HCC

E10.64 Type 1 diabetes mellitus with hypoglycemia

AHA: 2017,1Q,42

E10.641 Type 1 diabetes mellitus with hypoglycemia with coma MCC HCC

E10.649 Type 1 diabetes mellitus with hypoglycemia without coma HCC

AHA: 2016,3Q,42; 2016,1Q,13; 2015,3Q,21

E10.65 Type 1 diabetes mellitus with hyperglycemia HCC

AHA: 2017,1Q,42; 2013,3Q,20

E10.69 Type 1 diabetes mellitus with other specified complication HCC

Use additional code to identify complication

AHA: 2016,4Q,141; 2016,1Q,13

E10.8 Type 1 diabetes mellitus with unspecified complications HCC

E10.9 Type 1 diabetes mellitus without complications HCC

AHA: 2020,2Q,18

E11 Type 2 diabetes mellitus

INCLUDES diabetes (mellitus) due to insulin secretory defect
diabetes NOS
insulin resistant diabetes (mellitus)

Use additional code to identify control using:
insulin (Z79.4)
oral antidiabetic drugs (Z79.84)
oral hypoglycemic drugs (Z79.84)

EXCLUDES 1 *diabetes mellitus due to underlying condition (E08.-)*
drug or chemical induced diabetes mellitus (E09.-)
gestational diabetes (O24.4-)
neonatal diabetes mellitus (P70.2)
postpancreatectomy diabetes mellitus (E13.-)
postprocedural diabetes mellitus (E13.-)
secondary diabetes mellitus NEC (E13.-)
type 1 diabetes mellitus (E10.-)

AHA: 2020,1Q,12; 2016,2Q,10; 2013,1Q,26

E11.0 Type 2 diabetes mellitus with hyperosmolarity

DEF: Diabetic hyperosmolarity: Extremely high levels of glucose in the blood without ketones.

E11.00 Type 2 diabetes mellitus with hyperosmolarity without nonketotic hyperglycemic-hyperosmolar coma (NKHHC) MCC H9 HCC

E11.01 Type 2 diabetes mellitus with hyperosmolarity with coma MCC H9 HCC

E11.1 Type 2 diabetes mellitus with ketoacidosis

AHA: 2017,4Q,6

DEF: Diabetic ketoacidosis: Potentially life-threatening complication due to a shortage of insulin in which the body switches to burning fatty acids and producing acidic ketone bodies.

E11.10 Type 2 diabetes mellitus with ketoacidosis without coma MCC HCC

E11.11 Type 2 diabetes mellitus with ketoacidosis with coma MCC HCC

E11.2 Type 2 diabetes mellitus with kidney complications

AHA: 2019,3Q,3; 2018,4Q,88

E11.21 Type 2 diabetes mellitus with diabetic nephropathy HCC

Type 2 diabetes mellitus with intercapillary glomerulosclerosis

Type 2 diabetes mellitus with intracapillary glomerulonephrosis

Type 2 diabetes mellitus with Kimmelstiel-Wilson disease

E11.22 Type 2 diabetes mellitus with diabetic chronic kidney disease HCC

Use additional code to identify stage of chronic kidney disease (N18.1-N18.6)

E11.29 Type 2 diabetes mellitus with other diabetic kidney complication HCC

Type 2 diabetes mellitus with renal tubular degeneration

E11.3 Type 2 diabetes mellitus with ophthalmic complications

AHA: 2016,4Q,11-13

One of the following 7th characters is to be assigned to codes in subcategories E11.32, E11.33, E11.34, E11.35, and E11.37 to designate laterality of the disease:
1 right eye
2 left eye
3 bilateral
9 unspecified eye

E11.31 Type 2 diabetes mellitus with unspecified diabetic retinopathy

DEF: Diabetic retinopathy: Diabetic complication from damage to the retinal vessels resulting in vision problems that can progress to blindness.

E11.311 Type 2 diabetes mellitus with unspecified diabetic retinopathy with macular edema HCC

E11.319 Type 2 diabetes mellitus with unspecified diabetic retinopathy without macular edema HCC

✓6th **E11.32 Type 2 diabetes mellitus with mild nonproliferative diabetic retinopathy**
Type 2 diabetes mellitus with nonproliferative diabetic retinopathy NOS

✓7th **E11.321 Type 2 diabetes mellitus with mild nonproliferative diabetic retinopathy with macular edema** HCC

✓7th **E11.329 Type 2 diabetes mellitus with mild nonproliferative diabetic retinopathy without macular edema** HCC

✓6th **E11.33 Type 2 diabetes mellitus with moderate nonproliferative diabetic retinopathy**

✓7th **E11.331 Type 2 diabetes mellitus with moderate nonproliferative diabetic retinopathy with macular edema** HCC

✓7th **E11.339 Type 2 diabetes mellitus with moderate nonproliferative diabetic retinopathy without macular edema** HCC

✓6th **E11.34 Type 2 diabetes mellitus with severe nonproliferative diabetic retinopathy**

✓7th **E11.341 Type 2 diabetes mellitus with severe nonproliferative diabetic retinopathy with macular edema** HCC

✓7th **E11.349 Type 2 diabetes mellitus with severe nonproliferative diabetic retinopathy without macular edema** HCC

✓6th **E11.35 Type 2 diabetes mellitus with proliferative diabetic retinopathy**

✓7th **E11.351 Type 2 diabetes mellitus with proliferative diabetic retinopathy with macular edema** HCC

✓7th **E11.352 Type 2 diabetes mellitus with proliferative diabetic retinopathy with traction retinal detachment involving the macula** HCC

✓7th **E11.353 Type 2 diabetes mellitus with proliferative diabetic retinopathy with traction retinal detachment not involving the macula** HCC

✓7th **E11.354 Type 2 diabetes mellitus with proliferative diabetic retinopathy with combined traction retinal detachment and rhegmatogenous retinal detachment** HCC

✓7th **E11.355 Type 2 diabetes mellitus with stable proliferative diabetic retinopathy** HCC

✓7th **E11.359 Type 2 diabetes mellitus with proliferative diabetic retinopathy without macular edema** HCC

E11.36 Type 2 diabetes mellitus with diabetic cataract HCC
AHA: 2019,2Q,30-31; 2016,4Q,142

✓x7th **E11.37 Type 2 diabetes mellitus with diabetic macular edema, resolved following treatment** HCC

E11.39 Type 2 diabetes mellitus with other diabetic ophthalmic complication HCC
Use additional code to identify manifestation, such as:
diabetic glaucoma (H4Ø-H42)

✓5th **E11.4 Type 2 diabetes mellitus with neurological complications**

E11.4Ø Type 2 diabetes mellitus with diabetic neuropathy, unspecified HCC
AHA: 2013,4Q,129

E11.41 Type 2 diabetes mellitus with diabetic mononeuropathy HCC

E11.42 Type 2 diabetes mellitus with diabetic polyneuropathy HCC
Type 2 diabetes mellitus with diabetic neuralgia
AHA: 2020,1Q,12

E11.43 Type 2 diabetes mellitus with diabetic autonomic (poly)neuropathy HCC
Type 2 diabetes mellitus with diabetic gastroparesis
AHA: 2013,4Q,114

E11.44 Type 2 diabetes mellitus with diabetic amyotrophy HCC

E11.49 Type 2 diabetes mellitus with other diabetic neurological complication HCC

✓5th **E11.5 Type 2 diabetes mellitus with circulatory complications**

E11.51 Type 2 diabetes mellitus with diabetic peripheral angiopathy without gangrene HCC
AHA: 2018,3Q,3-4; 2018,2Q,7

E11.52 Type 2 diabetes mellitus with diabetic peripheral angiopathy with gangrene CC HCC
Type 2 diabetes mellitus with diabetic gangrene
AHA: 2020,2Q,18; 2018,3Q,3; 2018,2Q,7; 2017,4Q,102

E11.59 Type 2 diabetes mellitus with other circulatory complications HCC

✓5th **E11.6 Type 2 diabetes mellitus with other specified complications**

✓6th **E11.61 Type 2 diabetes mellitus with diabetic arthropathy**

E11.61Ø Type 2 diabetes mellitus with diabetic neuropathic arthropathy HCC
Type 2 diabetes mellitus with Charcôt's joints
DEF: Charcot's joint: Progressive neurologic arthropathy in which chronic degeneration of joints in the weight-bearing areas with peripheral hypertrophy occurs as a complication of a neuropathy disorder. Supporting structures relax from a loss of sensation resulting in chronic joint instability.

E11.618 Type 2 diabetes mellitus with other diabetic arthropathy HCC
AHA: 2018,2Q,6

✓6th **E11.62 Type 2 diabetes mellitus with skin complications**

E11.62Ø Type 2 diabetes mellitus with diabetic dermatitis HCC
Type 2 diabetes mellitus with diabetic necrobiosis lipoidica

E11.621 Type 2 diabetes mellitus with foot ulcer HCC
Use additional code to identify site of ulcer (L97.4-, L97.5-)
AHA: 2020,2Q,19; 2020,1Q,12

E11.622 Type 2 diabetes mellitus with other skin ulcer HCC
Use additional code to identify site of ulcer (L97.1-L97.9, L98.41-L98.49)
AHA: 2017,4Q,17

E11.628 Type 2 diabetes mellitus with other skin complications HCC

✓6th **E11.63 Type 2 diabetes mellitus with oral complications**

E11.63Ø Type 2 diabetes mellitus with periodontal disease HCC

E11.638 Type 2 diabetes mellitus with other oral complications HCC

✓6th **E11.64 Type 2 diabetes mellitus with hypoglycemia**
AHA: 2017,1Q,42

E11.641 Type 2 diabetes mellitus with hypoglycemia with coma MCC HCC

E11.649 Type 2 diabetes mellitus with hypoglycemia without coma HCC
AHA: 2016,3Q,42; 2015,3Q,21

E11.65 Type 2 diabetes mellitus with hyperglycemia HCC
AHA: 2017,1Q,42; 2013,3Q,20

E11.69 Type 2 diabetes mellitus with other specified complication HCC
Use additional code to identify complication
AHA: 2020,1Q,12; 2016,4Q,141; 2016,1Q,13

E11.8 Type 2 diabetes mellitus with unspecified complications HCC

E11.9 Type 2 diabetes mellitus without complications HCC
AHA: 2020,2Q,18

✓4th E13 Other specified diabetes mellitus

INCLUDES diabetes mellitus due to genetic defects of beta-cell function
diabetes mellitus due to genetic defects in insulin action
postpancreatectomy diabetes mellitus
postprocedural diabetes mellitus
secondary diabetes mellitus NEC

Use additional code to identify control using:
insulin (Z79.4)
oral antidiabetic drugs (Z79.84)
oral hypoglycemic drugs (Z79.84)

EXCLUDES 1 *diabetes (mellitus) due to autoimmune process (E1Ø.-)*
diabetes (mellitus) due to immune mediated pancreatic islet beta-cell destruction (E1Ø.-)
diabetes mellitus due to underlying condition (EØ8.-)
drug or chemical induced diabetes mellitus (EØ9.-)
gestational diabetes (O24.4-)
neonatal diabetes mellitus (P7Ø.2)
type 1 diabetes mellitus (E1Ø.-)

AHA: 2018,3Q,4; 2016,1Q,11-13

TIP: Use this category when the diabetes is documented as diabetes type 1.5. Synonymous terms used in the documentation may also include combined diabetes type 1 and type 2, latent autoimmune diabetes of adults (LADA), slow-progressing type 1 diabetes, or double diabetes.

TIP: When postprocedural or postpancreatectomy hypoinsulinemia (E89.1) is documented with postprocedural or postpancreatectomy diabetes mellitus (E13.-), code E89.1 should be sequenced first.

✓5th E13.Ø Other specified diabetes mellitus with hyperosmolarity

DEF: Diabetic hyperosmolarity: Extremely high levels of glucose in the blood without ketones.

E13.ØØ Other specified diabetes mellitus with hyperosmolarity without nonketotic hyperglycemic-hyperosmolar coma (NKHHC) MCC H9 HCC

EXCLUDES 2 *type 2 diabetes mellitus (E11.-)*

E13.Ø1 Other specified diabetes mellitus with hyperosmolarity with coma MCC H9 HCC

✓5th E13.1 Other specified diabetes mellitus with ketoacidosis

AHA: 2016,2Q,10; 2013,1Q,26

DEF: Diabetic ketoacidosis: Potentially life-threatening complication due to a shortage of insulin in which the body switches to burning fatty acids and producing acidic ketone bodies.

E13.1Ø Other specified diabetes mellitus with ketoacidosis without coma MCC H9 HCC

E13.11 Other specified diabetes mellitus with ketoacidosis with coma MCC HCC

✓5th E13.2 Other specified diabetes mellitus with kidney complications

AHA: 2019,3Q,3; 2018,4Q,88

E13.21 Other specified diabetes mellitus with diabetic nephropathy HCC

Other specified diabetes mellitus with intercapillary glomerulosclerosis
Other specified diabetes mellitus with intracapillary glomerulonephrosis
Other specified diabetes mellitus with Kimmelstiel-Wilson disease

E13.22 Other specified diabetes mellitus with diabetic chronic kidney disease HCC

Use additional code to identify stage of chronic kidney disease (N18.1-N18.6)

E13.29 Other specified diabetes mellitus with other diabetic kidney complication HCC

Other specified diabetes mellitus with renal tubular degeneration

✓5th E13.3 Other specified diabetes mellitus with ophthalmic complications

AHA: 2016,4Q,11-13

One of the following 7th characters is to be assigned to codes in subcategories E13.32, E13.33, E13.34, E13.35, and E13.37 to designate laterality of the disease:
1 right eye
2 left eye
3 bilateral
9 unspecified eye

✓6th E13.31 Other specified diabetes mellitus with unspecified diabetic retinopathy

DEF: Diabetic retinopathy: Diabetic complication from damage to the retinal vessels resulting in vision problems that can progress to blindness.

E13.311 Other specified diabetes mellitus with unspecified diabetic retinopathy with macular edema HCC

E13.319 Other specified diabetes mellitus with unspecified diabetic retinopathy without macular edema HCC

✓6th E13.32 Other specified diabetes mellitus with mild nonproliferative diabetic retinopathy

Other specified diabetes mellitus with nonproliferative diabetic retinopathy NOS

✓7th E13.321 Other specified diabetes mellitus with mild nonproliferative diabetic retinopathy with macular edema HCC

✓7th E13.329 Other specified diabetes mellitus with mild nonproliferative diabetic retinopathy without macular edema HCC

✓6th E13.33 Other specified diabetes mellitus with moderate nonproliferative diabetic retinopathy

✓7th E13.331 Other specified diabetes mellitus with moderate nonproliferative diabetic retinopathy with macular edema HCC

✓7th E13.339 Other specified diabetes mellitus with moderate nonproliferative diabetic retinopathy without macular edema HCC

✓6th E13.34 Other specified diabetes mellitus with severe nonproliferative diabetic retinopathy

✓7th E13.341 Other specified diabetes mellitus with severe nonproliferative diabetic retinopathy with macular edema HCC

✓7th E13.349 Other specified diabetes mellitus with severe nonproliferative diabetic retinopathy without macular edema HCC

✓6th E13.35 Other specified diabetes mellitus with proliferative diabetic retinopathy

✓7th E13.351 Other specified diabetes mellitus with proliferative diabetic retinopathy with macular edema HCC

✓7th E13.352 Other specified diabetes mellitus with proliferative diabetic retinopathy with traction retinal detachment involving the macula HCC

✓7th E13.353 Other specified diabetes mellitus with proliferative diabetic retinopathy with traction retinal detachment not involving the macula HCC

✓7th E13.354 Other specified diabetes mellitus with proliferative diabetic retinopathy with combined traction retinal detachment and rhegmatogenous retinal detachment HCC

✓7th E13.355 Other specified diabetes mellitus with stable proliferative diabetic retinopathy HCC

✓7th E13.359 Other specified diabetes mellitus with proliferative diabetic retinopathy without macular edema HCC

E13.36 Other specified diabetes mellitus with diabetic cataract HCC

AHA: 2019,2Q,30-31; 2016,4Q,142

√x7th E13.37 Other specified diabetes mellitus with diabetic macular edema, resolved following treatment HCC

E13.39 Other specified diabetes mellitus with other diabetic ophthalmic complication HCC
Use additional code to identify manifestation, such as:
diabetic glaucoma (H40-H42)

✓5th **E13.4 Other specified diabetes mellitus with neurological complications**

E13.40 Other specified diabetes mellitus with diabetic neuropathy, unspecified HCC

E13.41 Other specified diabetes mellitus with diabetic mononeuropathy HCC

E13.42 Other specified diabetes mellitus with diabetic polyneuropathy HCC
Other specified diabetes mellitus with diabetic neuralgia

E13.43 Other specified diabetes mellitus with diabetic autonomic (poly)neuropathy HCC
Other specified diabetes mellitus with diabetic gastroparesis
AHA: 2013,4Q,114

E13.44 Other specified diabetes mellitus with diabetic amyotrophy HCC

E13.49 Other specified diabetes mellitus with other diabetic neurological complication HCC

✓5th **E13.5 Other specified diabetes mellitus with circulatory complications**

E13.51 Other specified diabetes mellitus with diabetic peripheral angiopathy without gangrene HCC
AHA: 2018,3Q,3-4; 2018,2Q,7

E13.52 Other specified diabetes mellitus with diabetic peripheral angiopathy with gangrene CC HCC
Other specified diabetes mellitus with diabetic gangrene
AHA: 2020,2Q,18; 2018,3Q,3; 2018,2Q,7; 2017,4Q,102

E13.59 Other specified diabetes mellitus with other circulatory complications HCC

✓5th **E13.6 Other specified diabetes mellitus with other specified complications**

✓6th **E13.61 Other specified diabetes mellitus with diabetic arthropathy**

E13.610 Other specified diabetes mellitus with diabetic neuropathic arthropathy HCC
Other specified diabetes mellitus with Charcôt's joints
DEF: Charcot's joint: Progressive neurologic arthropathy in which chronic degeneration of joints in the weight-bearing areas with peripheral hypertrophy occurs as a complication of a neuropathy disorder. Supporting structures relax from a loss of sensation resulting in chronic joint instability.

E13.618 Other specified diabetes mellitus with other diabetic arthropathy HCC
AHA: 2018,2Q,6

✓6th **E13.62 Other specified diabetes mellitus with skin complications**

E13.620 Other specified diabetes mellitus with diabetic dermatitis HCC
Other specified diabetes mellitus with diabetic necrobiosis lipoidica

E13.621 Other specified diabetes mellitus with foot ulcer HCC
Use additional code to identify site of ulcer (L97.4-, L97.5-)
AHA: 2020,2Q,19

E13.622 Other specified diabetes mellitus with other skin ulcer HCC
Use additional code to identify site of ulcer (L97.1-L97.9, L98.41-L98.49)
AHA: 2017,4Q,17

E13.628 Other specified diabetes mellitus with other skin complications HCC

✓6th **E13.63 Other specified diabetes mellitus with oral complications**

E13.630 Other specified diabetes mellitus with periodontal disease HCC

E13.638 Other specified diabetes mellitus with other oral complications HCC

✓6th **E13.64 Other specified diabetes mellitus with hypoglycemia**
AHA: 2017,1Q,42

E13.641 Other specified diabetes mellitus with hypoglycemia with coma MCC HCC

E13.649 Other specified diabetes mellitus with hypoglycemia without coma HCC
AHA: 2016,3Q,42; 2015,3Q,21

E13.65 Other specified diabetes mellitus with hyperglycemia HCC
AHA: 2017,1Q,42; 2013,3Q,20

E13.69 Other specified diabetes mellitus with other specified complication HCC
Use additional code to identify complication
AHA: 2016,4Q,141; 2016,1Q,13

E13.8 Other specified diabetes mellitus with unspecified complications HCC

E13.9 Other specified diabetes mellitus without complications HCC
AHA: 2020,2Q,18

Other disorders of glucose regulation and pancreatic internal secretion (E15-E16)

E15 Nondiabetic hypoglycemic coma CC H9 HCC
INCLUDES drug-induced insulin coma in nondiabetic
hyperinsulinism with hypoglycemic coma
hypoglycemic coma NOS

✓4th **E16 Other disorders of pancreatic internal secretion**

E16.0 Drug-induced hypoglycemia without coma
EXCLUDES 1 *diabetes with hypoglycemia without coma (E09.649)*
Use additional code for adverse effect, if applicable, to identify drug (T36-T50 with fifth or sixth character 5)

E16.1 Other hypoglycemia
Functional hyperinsulinism
Functional nonhyperinsulinemic hypoglycemia
Hyperinsulinism NOS
Hyperplasia of pancreatic islet beta cells NOS
EXCLUDES 1 *diabetes with hypoglycemia (E08.649, E10.649, E11.649, E13.649)*
hypoglycemia in infant of diabetic mother (P70.1)
neonatal hypoglycemia (P70.4)

E16.2 Hypoglycemia, unspecified
EXCLUDES 1 *diabetes with hypoglycemia (E08.649, E10.649, E11.649, E13.649)*
AHA: 2016,3Q,42
TIP: Assign for nondiabetic hypoglycemic encephalopathy not further clarified in the documentation.

E16.3 Increased secretion of glucagon
Hyperplasia of pancreatic endocrine cells with glucagon excess

E16.4 Increased secretion of gastrin
Hypergastrinemia
Hyperplasia of pancreatic endocrine cells with gastrin excess
Zollinger-Ellison syndrome

E16.8 Other specified disorders of pancreatic internal secretion
Increased secretion from endocrine pancreas of growth hormone-releasing hormone
Increased secretion from endocrine pancreas of pancreatic polypeptide
Increased secretion from endocrine pancreas of somatostatin
Increased secretion from endocrine pancreas of vasoactive-intestinal polypeptide

E16.9 Disorder of pancreatic internal secretion, unspecified
Islet-cell hyperplasia NOS
Pancreatic endocrine cell hyperplasia NOS

Disorders of other endocrine glands (E2Ø-E35)

EXCLUDES 1 *galactorrhea (N64.3)*
gynecomastia (N62)

E2Ø Hypoparathyroidism

EXCLUDES 1 *Di George's syndrome (D82.1)*
postprocedural hypoparathyroidism (E89.2)
tetany NOS (R29.Ø)
transitory neonatal hypoparathyroidism (P71.4)

E2Ø.Ø Idiopathic hypoparathyroidism HCC
DEF: Abnormally low secretion of parathyroid hormones, with unknown cause, which causes decreased calcium and increased phosphorus in the blood, resulting in muscle cramps, tetany, tingling, or burning in the lips, fingers, and toes, and cataracts.

E2Ø.1 Pseudohypoparathyroidism

E2Ø.8 Other hypoparathyroidism HCC

E2Ø.9 Hypoparathyroidism, unspecified HCC
Parathyroid tetany

E21 Hyperparathyroidism and other disorders of parathyroid gland

EXCLUDES 1 *adult osteomalacia (M83.-)*
ectopic hyperparathyroidism (E34.2)
familial hypocalciuric hypercalcemia (E83.52)
hungry bone syndrome (E83.81)
infantile and juvenile osteomalacia (E55.Ø)

E21.Ø Primary hyperparathyroidism HCC
Hyperplasia of parathyroid
Osteitis fibrosa cystica generalisata [von Recklinghausen's disease of bone]
DEF: Parathyroid dysfunction commonly caused by hyperplasia of two or more glands. Symptoms include hypercalcemia and increased parathyroid hormone levels.

E21.1 Secondary hyperparathyroidism, not elsewhere classified HCC
EXCLUDES 1 *secondary hyperparathyroidism of renal origin (N25.81)*

E21.2 Other hyperparathyroidism HCC
Tertiary hyperparathyroidism
EXCLUDES 1 *familial hypocalciuric hypercalcemia (E83.52)*

E21.3 Hyperparathyroidism, unspecified HCC

E21.4 Other specified disorders of parathyroid gland HCC

E21.5 Disorder of parathyroid gland, unspecified HCC

E22 Hyperfunction of pituitary gland

EXCLUDES 1 *Cushing's syndrome (E24.-)*
Nelson's syndrome (E24.1)
overproduction of ACTH not associated with Cushing's disease (E27.Ø)
overproduction of pituitary ACTH (E24.Ø)
overproduction of thyroid-stimulating hormone (EØ5.8-)

E22.Ø Acromegaly and pituitary gigantism HCC
Overproduction of growth hormone
EXCLUDES 1 *constitutional gigantism (E34.4)*
constitutional tall stature (E34.4)
increased secretion from endocrine pancreas of growth hormone-releasing hormone (E16.8)
DEF: Acromegaly: Chronic condition caused by overproduction of the pituitary growth hormone resulting in enlarged skeletal parts and facial features.

E22.1 Hyperprolactinemia CC HCC
Use additional code for adverse effect, if applicable, to identify drug (T36-T5Ø with fifth or sixth character 5)

E22.2 Syndrome of inappropriate secretion of antidiuretic hormone CC HCC

E22.8 Other hyperfunction of pituitary gland CC HCC
Central precocious puberty

E22.9 Hyperfunction of pituitary gland, unspecified CC HCC

E23 Hypofunction and other disorders of the pituitary gland

INCLUDES the listed conditions whether the disorder is in the pituitary or the hypothalamus
EXCLUDES 1 *postprocedural hypopituitarism (E89.3)*

E23.Ø Hypopituitarism CC HCC
Fertile eunuch syndrome
Hypogonadotropic hypogonadism
Idiopathic growth hormone deficiency
Isolated deficiency of gonadotropin
Isolated deficiency of growth hormone
Isolated deficiency of pituitary hormone
Kallmann's syndrome
Lorain-Levi short stature
Necrosis of pituitary gland (postpartum)
Panhypopituitarism
Pituitary cachexia
Pituitary insufficiency NOS
Pituitary short stature
Sheehan's syndrome
Simmonds' disease

E23.1 Drug-induced hypopituitarism HCC
Use additional code for adverse effect, if applicable, to identify drug (T36-T5Ø with fifth or sixth character 5)

E23.2 Diabetes insipidus CC HCC
EXCLUDES 1 *nephrogenic diabetes insipidus (N25.1)*

E23.3 Hypothalamic dysfunction, not elsewhere classified HCC
EXCLUDES 1 *Prader-Willi syndrome (Q87.11)*
Russell-Silver syndrome (Q87.19)

E23.6 Other disorders of pituitary gland HCC
Abscess of pituitary
Adiposogenital dystrophy

E23.7 Disorder of pituitary gland, unspecified HCC

E24 Cushing's syndrome

EXCLUDES 1 *congenital adrenal hyperplasia (E25.Ø)*

DEF: Abdominal striae, acne, hypertension, decreased carbohydrate tolerance, moon face, obesity, protein catabolism, and psychiatric disturbances resulting from increased adrenocortical secretion of cortisol caused by ACTH-dependent adrenocortical hyperplasia or tumor, or by steroid effects.

E24.Ø Pituitary-dependent Cushing's disease CC HCC
Overproduction of pituitary ACTH
Pituitary-dependent hypercorticalism

E24.1 Nelson's syndrome HCC

E24.2 Drug-induced Cushing's syndrome CC HCC
Use additional code for adverse effect, if applicable, to identify drug (T36-T5Ø with fifth or sixth character 5)

E24.3 Ectopic ACTH syndrome CC HCC

E24.4 Alcohol-induced pseudo-Cushing's syndrome CC HCC

E24.8 Other Cushing's syndrome CC HCC

E24.9 Cushing's syndrome, unspecified CC HCC

E25 Adrenogenital disorders

INCLUDES adrenogenital syndromes, virilizing or feminizing, whether acquired or due to adrenal hyperplasia
consequent on inborn enzyme defects in hormone synthesis
female adrenal pseudohermaphroditism
female heterosexual precocious pseudopuberty
male isosexual precocious pseudopuberty
male macrogenitosomia praecox
male sexual precocity with adrenal hyperplasia
male virilization (female)
EXCLUDES 1 *indeterminate sex and pseudohermaphroditism (Q56)*
chromosomal abnormalities (Q9Ø-Q99)

E25.Ø Congenital adrenogenital disorders associated with enzyme deficiency HCC
Congenital adrenal hyperplasia
21-Hydroxylase deficiency
Salt-losing congenital adrenal hyperplasia

E25.8 Other adrenogenital disorders HCC
Idiopathic adrenogenital disorder
Use additional code for adverse effect, if applicable, to identify drug (T36-T5Ø with fifth or sixth character 5)

E25.9 Adrenogenital disorder, unspecified HCC
Adrenogenital syndrome NOS

√4th E26 Hyperaldosteronism

√5th E26.Ø Primary hyperaldosteronism

E26.Ø1 Conn's syndrome HCC
Code also adrenal adenoma (D35.Ø-)

E26.Ø2 Glucocorticoid-remediable aldosteronism HCC
Familial aldosteronism type I
DEF: Rare autosomal dominant familial form of primary aldosteronism in which the secretion of aldosterone is under the influence of adrenocorticotrophic hormone (ACTH) rather than the renin-angiotensin mechanism. Moderate hypersecretion of aldosterone and suppressed plasma renin activity that are rapidly reversed by administration of glucosteroids. Symptoms include hypertension and mild hypokalemia.

E26.Ø9 Other primary hyperaldosteronism HCC
Primary aldosteronism due to adrenal hyperplasia (bilateral)

E26.1 Secondary hyperaldosteronism HCC

√5th E26.8 Other hyperaldosteronism

E26.81 Bartter's syndrome HCC

E26.89 Other hyperaldosteronism HCC

E26.9 Hyperaldosteronism, unspecified HCC
Aldosteronism NOS
Hyperaldosteronism NOS

√4th E27 Other disorders of adrenal gland

E27.Ø Other adrenocortical overactivity CC HCC
Overproduction of ACTH, not associated with Cushing's disease
Premature adrenarche
EXCLUDES 1 *Cushing's syndrome (E24.-)*

E27.1 Primary adrenocortical insufficiency CC HCC
Addison's disease
Autoimmune adrenalitis
EXCLUDES 1 *Addison only phenotype adrenoleukodystrophy (E71.528)*
amyloidosis (E85.-)
tuberculous Addison's disease (A18.7)
Waterhouse-Friderichsen syndrome (A39.1)

E27.2 Addisonian crisis CC HCC
Adrenal crisis
Adrenocortical crisis
DEF: Life-threatening condition that occurs when there is not enough cortisol excreted from the adrenal glands. This condition may be due to injury to the adrenal glands or to the pituitary gland, which controls adrenal hormone secretion, or when a patient stops hydrocortisone treatment too quickly or too early.

E27.3 Drug-induced adrenocortical insufficiency CC HCC
Use additional code for adverse effect, if applicable, to identify drug (T36-T5Ø with fifth or sixth character 5)

√5th E27.4 Other and unspecified adrenocortical insufficiency
EXCLUDES 1 *adrenoleukodystrophy [Addison-Schilder] (E71.528)*
Waterhouse-Friderichsen syndrome (A39.1)

E27.4Ø Unspecified adrenocortical insufficiency CC HCC
Adrenocortical insufficiency NOS
Hypoaldosteronism

E27.49 Other adrenocortical insufficiency CC HCC
Adrenal hemorrhage
Adrenal infarction

E27.5 Adrenomedullary hyperfunction CC HCC
Adrenomedullary hyperplasia
Catecholamine hypersecretion

E27.8 Other specified disorders of adrenal gland HCC
Abnormality of cortisol-binding globulin

E27.9 Disorder of adrenal gland, unspecified HCC

√4th E28 Ovarian dysfunction
EXCLUDES 1 *isolated gonadotropin deficiency (E23.Ø)*
postprocedural ovarian failure (E89.4-)

E28.Ø Estrogen excess ♀
Use additional code for adverse effect, if applicable, to identify drug (T36-T5Ø with fifth or sixth character 5)

E28.1 Androgen excess ♀
Hypersecretion of ovarian androgens
Use additional code for adverse effect, if applicable, to identify drug (T36-T5Ø with fifth or sixth character 5)

E28.2 Polycystic ovarian syndrome ♀
Sclerocystic ovary syndrome
Stein-Leventhal syndrome
DEF: Common hormonal disorder among women of reproductive age that involves enlarged ovaries with numerous small cysts located along the outer ovarian edge.

√5th E28.3 Primary ovarian failure
EXCLUDES 1 *pure gonadal dysgenesis (Q99.1)*
Turner's syndrome (Q96.-)

√6th E28.31 Premature menopause

E28.31Ø Symptomatic premature menopause A ♀
Symptoms such as flushing, sleeplessness, headache, lack of concentration, associated with premature menopause

E28.319 Asymptomatic premature menopause A ♀
Premature menopause NOS

E28.39 Other primary ovarian failure ♀
Decreased estrogen
Resistant ovary syndrome

E28.8 Other ovarian dysfunction ♀
Ovarian hyperfunction NOS
EXCLUDES 1 *postprocedural ovarian failure (E89.4-)*

E28.9 Ovarian dysfunction, unspecified ♀

√4th E29 Testicular dysfunction
EXCLUDES 1 *androgen insensitivity syndrome (E34.5-)*
azoospermia or oligospermia NOS (N46.Ø-N46.1)
isolated gonadotropin deficiency (E23.Ø)
Klinefelter's syndrome (Q98.Ø-Q98.1, Q98.4)

E29.Ø Testicular hyperfunction ♂
Hypersecretion of testicular hormones

E29.1 Testicular hypofunction ♂
Defective biosynthesis of testicular androgen NOS
5-delta-Reductase deficiency (with male pseudohermaphroditism)
Testicular hypogonadism NOS
Use additional code for adverse effect, if applicable, to identify drug (T36-T5Ø with fifth or sixth character 5)
EXCLUDES 1 *postprocedural testicular hypofunction (E89.5)*

E29.8 Other testicular dysfunction ♂

E29.9 Testicular dysfunction, unspecified ♂

√4th E3Ø Disorders of puberty, not elsewhere classified

E3Ø.Ø Delayed puberty
Constitutional delay of puberty
Delayed sexual development

E3Ø.1 Precocious puberty P
Precocious menstruation
EXCLUDES 1 *Albright (-McCune) (-Sternberg) syndrome (Q78.1)*
central precocious puberty (E22.8)
congenital adrenal hyperplasia (E25.Ø)
female heterosexual precocious pseudopuberty (E25.-)
male isosexual precocious pseudopuberty (E25.-)

E3Ø.8 Other disorders of puberty P
Premature thelarche

E3Ø.9 Disorder of puberty, unspecified

√4th E31 Polyglandular dysfunction
EXCLUDES 1 *ataxia telangiectasia [Louis-Bar] (G11.3)*
dystrophia myotonica [Steinert] (G71.11)
pseudohypoparathyroidism (E2Ø.1)

E31.Ø Autoimmune polyglandular failure HCC
Schmidt's syndrome

E31.1 Polyglandular hyperfunction HCC
EXCLUDES 1 *multiple endocrine adenomatosis (E31.2-)*
multiple endocrine neoplasia (E31.2-)

✓5th **E31.2 Multiple endocrine neoplasia [MEN] syndromes**
Multiple endocrine adenomatosis
Code also any associated malignancies and other conditions associated with the syndromes
DEF: Group of conditions in which several endocrine glands grow excessively (such as in adenomatous hyperplasia) and/or develop benign or malignant tumors. Tumors and hyperplasia associated with MEN often produce excess hormones, which impede normal physiology. There is no comprehensive cure known for MEN syndrome. Treatment is directed at the hyperplasia or tumors in each individual gland. Tumors are usually surgically removed and oral medications or hormonal injections are used to correct hormone imbalances.

E31.20 Multiple endocrine neoplasia [MEN] syndrome, unspecified HCC
Multiple endocrine adenomatosis NOS
Multiple endocrine neoplasia [MEN] syndrome NOS

E31.21 Multiple endocrine neoplasia [MEN] type I HCC
Wermer's syndrome

E31.22 Multiple endocrine neoplasia [MEN] type IIA HCC
Sipple's syndrome

E31.23 Multiple endocrine neoplasia [MEN] type IIB HCC

E31.8 Other polyglandular dysfunction HCC

E31.9 Polyglandular dysfunction, unspecified HCC

✓4th **E32 Diseases of thymus**
EXCLUDES 1 *aplasia or hypoplasia of thymus with immunodeficiency (D82.1)*
myasthenia gravis (G70.0)

E32.0 Persistent hyperplasia of thymus HCC
Hypertrophy of thymus

E32.1 Abscess of thymus CC HCC

E32.8 Other diseases of thymus HCC
EXCLUDES 1 *aplasia or hypoplasia with immunodeficiency (D82.1)*
thymoma (D15.0)

E32.9 Disease of thymus, unspecified HCC

✓4th **E34 Other endocrine disorders**
EXCLUDES 1 *pseudohypoparathyroidism (E20.1)*

E34.0 Carcinoid syndrome CC HCC
NOTE May be used as an additional code to identify functional activity associated with a carcinoid tumor.

E34.1 Other hypersecretion of intestinal hormones

E34.2 Ectopic hormone secretion, not elsewhere classified
EXCLUDES 1 *ectopic ACTH syndrome (E24.3)*

E34.3 Short stature due to endocrine disorder
Constitutional short stature
Laron-type short stature
EXCLUDES 1 *achondroplastic short stature (Q77.4)*
hypochondroplastic short stature (Q77.4)
nutritional short stature (E45)
pituitary short stature (E23.0)
progeria (E34.8)
renal short stature (N25.0)
Russell-Silver syndrome (Q87.19)
short-limbed stature with immunodeficiency (D82.2)
short stature in specific dysmorphic syndromes — code to syndrome — see Alphabetical Index
short stature NOS (R62.52)

E34.4 Constitutional tall stature HCC
Constitutional gigantism

✓5th **E34.5 Androgen insensitivity syndrome**
DEF: X-linked recessive condition in which individuals that are chromosomally male fail to develop normal male external genitalia due to an abnormality on the X chromosome that prohibits the body, completely or in part, from recognizing the androgens produced. ***Synonym(s):*** *AIS*

E34.50 Androgen insensitivity syndrome, unspecified
Androgen insensitivity NOS

E34.51 Complete androgen insensitivity syndrome
Complete androgen insensitivity
de Quervain syndrome
Goldberg-Maxwell syndrome

E34.52 Partial androgen insensitivity syndrome
Partial androgen insensitivity
Reifenstein syndrome

E34.8 Other specified endocrine disorders
Pineal gland dysfunction
Progeria
EXCLUDES 2 *pseudohypoparathyroidism (E20.1)*

E34.9 Endocrine disorder, unspecified
Endocrine disturbance NOS
Hormone disturbance NOS

E35 Disorders of endocrine glands in diseases classified elsewhere
Code first underlying disease, such as:
late congenital syphilis of thymus gland [Dubois disease] (A50.5)
Use additional code, if applicable, to identify:
sequelae of tuberculosis of other organs (B90.8)
EXCLUDES 1 *Echinococcus granulosus infection of thyroid gland (B67.3)*
meningococcal hemorrhagic adrenalitis (A39.1)
syphilis of endocrine gland (A52.79)
tuberculosis of adrenal gland, except calcification (A18.7)
tuberculosis of endocrine gland NEC (A18.82)
tuberculosis of thyroid gland (A18.81)
Waterhouse-Friderichsen syndrome (A39.1)

Intraoperative complications of endocrine system (E36)

✓4th **E36 Intraoperative complications of endocrine system**
EXCLUDES 2 *postprocedural endocrine and metabolic complications and disorders, not elsewhere classified (E89.-)*

✓5th **E36.0 Intraoperative hemorrhage and hematoma of an endocrine system organ or structure complicating a procedure**
EXCLUDES 1 *intraoperative hemorrhage and hematoma of an endocrine system organ or structure due to accidental puncture or laceration during a procedure (E36.1-)*

E36.01 Intraoperative hemorrhage and hematoma of an endocrine system organ or structure complicating an endocrine system procedure CC
AHA: 2020,1Q,19

E36.02 Intraoperative hemorrhage and hematoma of an endocrine system organ or structure complicating other procedure CC

✓5th **E36.1 Accidental puncture and laceration of an endocrine system organ or structure during a procedure**

E36.11 Accidental puncture and laceration of an endocrine system organ or structure during an endocrine system procedure CC

E36.12 Accidental puncture and laceration of an endocrine system organ or structure during other procedure CC

E36.8 Other intraoperative complications of endocrine system
Use additional code, if applicable, to further specify disorder

Malnutrition (E40-E46)

EXCLUDES 1 *intestinal malabsorption (K90.-)*
sequelae of protein-calorie malnutrition (E64.0)
EXCLUDES 2 *nutritional anemias (D50-D53)*
starvation (T73.0)
AHA: 2020,1Q,4-7; 2017,4Q,108; 2017,3Q,25
TIP: Assign additional code for BMI from category Z68, when documented. BMI can be based on documentation from clinicians who are not the patient's provider.
TIP: Malnutrition is not considered integral to cancer; assign the appropriate code in addition to the code for the specific type of cancer.

E40 Kwashiorkor MCC HCC
Severe malnutrition with nutritional edema with dyspigmentation of skin and hair
EXCLUDES 1 *marasmic kwashiorkor (E42)*

E41 Nutritional marasmus MCC HCC
Severe malnutrition with marasmus
EXCLUDES 1 *marasmic kwashiorkor (E42)*
AHA: 2017,3Q,24
DEF: Protein-calorie malabsorption or malnutrition in children characterized by tissue wasting, dehydration, and subcutaneous fat depletion. It may occur with infectious disease.

E42 Marasmic kwashiorkor MCC HCC
Intermediate form severe protein-calorie malnutrition
Severe protein-calorie malnutrition with signs of both kwashiorkor and marasmus

E43 Unspecified severe protein-calorie malnutrition MCC HCC
Starvation edema
AHA: 2020,1Q,5,6; 2017,4Q,108

E44 Protein-calorie malnutrition of moderate and mild degree
AHA: 2020,1Q,5
E44.Ø Moderate protein-calorie malnutrition CC HCC
E44.1 Mild protein-calorie malnutrition CC HCC

E45 Retarded development following protein-calorie malnutrition CC HCC
Nutritional short stature
Nutritional stunting
Physical retardation due to malnutrition

E46 Unspecified protein-calorie malnutrition CC HCC
Malnutrition NOS
Protein-calorie imbalance NOS
EXCLUDES 1 *nutritional deficiency NOS (E63.9)*
AHA: 2018,4Q,82

Other nutritional deficiencies (E5Ø-E64)

EXCLUDES 2 *nutritional anemias (D5Ø-D53)*

E5Ø Vitamin A deficiency
EXCLUDES 1 *sequelae of vitamin A deficiency (E64.1)*
E5Ø.Ø Vitamin A deficiency with conjunctival xerosis
E5Ø.1 Vitamin A deficiency with Bitot's spot and conjunctival xerosis
Bitot's spot in the young child
DEF: Vitamin A deficiency with conjunctival dryness and superficial spots of keratinized epithelium.
E5Ø.2 Vitamin A deficiency with corneal xerosis
E5Ø.3 Vitamin A deficiency with corneal ulceration and xerosis
E5Ø.4 Vitamin A deficiency with keratomalacia
DEF: Vitamin A deficiency creating corneal dryness that progresses to corneal insensitivity, softness, and necrosis. It is usually bilateral.
E5Ø.5 Vitamin A deficiency with night blindness
E5Ø.6 Vitamin A deficiency with xerophthalmic scars of cornea
E5Ø.7 Other ocular manifestations of vitamin A deficiency
Xerophthalmia NOS
E5Ø.8 Other manifestations of vitamin A deficiency
Follicular keratosis
Xeroderma
E5Ø.9 Vitamin A deficiency, unspecified
Hypovitaminosis A NOS

E51 Thiamine deficiency
EXCLUDES 1 *sequelae of thiamine deficiency (E64.8)*
E51.1 Beriberi
E51.11 Dry beriberi CC
Beriberi NOS
Beriberi with polyneuropathy
E51.12 Wet beriberi CC
Beriberi with cardiovascular manifestations
Cardiovascular beriberi
Shoshin disease
E51.2 Wernicke's encephalopathy CC
DEF: Deficiency of vitamin B1 resulting in a triad of acute mental confusion, ataxia, and ophthalmoplegia. The vast majority of affected patients are alcoholics.
E51.8 Other manifestations of thiamine deficiency CC
E51.9 Thiamine deficiency, unspecified CC

E52 Niacin deficiency [pellagra]
Niacin (-tryptophan) deficiency
Nicotinamide deficiency
Pellagra (alcoholic)
EXCLUDES 1 *sequelae of niacin deficiency (E64.8)*

E53 Deficiency of other B group vitamins
EXCLUDES 1 *sequelae of vitamin B deficiency (E64.8)*
E53.Ø Riboflavin deficiency CC
Ariboflavinosis
Vitamin B2 deficiency
E53.1 Pyridoxine deficiency
Vitamin B6 deficiency
EXCLUDES 1 *pyridoxine-responsive sideroblastic anemia (D64.3)*
E53.8 Deficiency of other specified B group vitamins
Biotin deficiency
Cyanocobalamin deficiency
Folate deficiency
Folic acid deficiency
Pantothenic acid deficiency
Vitamin B12 deficiency
EXCLUDES 1 *folate deficiency anemia (D52.-)*
vitamin B12 deficiency anemia (D51.-)
E53.9 Vitamin B deficiency, unspecified

E54 Ascorbic acid deficiency
Deficiency of vitamin C
Scurvy
EXCLUDES 1 *scorbutic anemia (D53.2)*
sequelae of vitamin C deficiency (E64.2)
DEF: Vitamin C deficiency causing swollen gums, myalgia, weight loss, and weakness.

E55 Vitamin D deficiency
EXCLUDES 1 *adult osteomalacia (M83.-)*
osteoporosis (M8Ø.-)
sequelae of rickets (E64.3)
E55.Ø Rickets, active CC
Infantile osteomalacia
Juvenile osteomalacia
EXCLUDES 1 *celiac rickets (K9Ø.Ø)*
Crohn's rickets (K5Ø.-)
hereditary vitamin D-dependent rickets (E83.32)
inactive rickets (E64.3)
renal rickets (N25.Ø)
sequelae of rickets (E64.3)
vitamin D-resistant rickets (E83.31)
DEF: Rickets: Softening or weakening of the bones due to a lack of vitamin D, calcium, and phosphate.
E55.9 Vitamin D deficiency, unspecified
Avitaminosis D

E56 Other vitamin deficiencies
EXCLUDES 1 *sequelae of other vitamin deficiencies (E64.8)*
E56.Ø Deficiency of vitamin E
E56.1 Deficiency of vitamin K
EXCLUDES 1 *deficiency of coagulation factor due to vitamin K deficiency (D68.4)*
vitamin K deficiency of newborn (P53)
E56.8 Deficiency of other vitamins
E56.9 Vitamin deficiency, unspecified

E58 Dietary calcium deficiency
EXCLUDES 1 *disorders of calcium metabolism (E83.5-)*
sequelae of calcium deficiency (E64.8)

E59 Dietary selenium deficiency
Keshan disease
EXCLUDES 1 *sequelae of selenium deficiency (E64.8)*

E6Ø Dietary zinc deficiency

E61 Deficiency of other nutrient elements
Use additional code for adverse effect, if applicable, to identify drug (T36-T5Ø with fifth or sixth character 5)
EXCLUDES 1 *disorders of mineral metabolism (E83.-)*
iodine deficiency related thyroid disorders (EØØ-EØ2)
sequelae of malnutrition and other nutritional deficiencies (E64.-)
E61.Ø Copper deficiency
E61.1 Iron deficiency
EXCLUDES 1 *iron deficiency anemia (D5Ø.-)*
E61.2 Magnesium deficiency
E61.3 Manganese deficiency
E61.4 Chromium deficiency
E61.5 Molybdenum deficiency
E61.6 Vanadium deficiency
E61.7 Deficiency of multiple nutrient elements
E61.8 Deficiency of other specified nutrient elements
E61.9 Deficiency of nutrient element, unspecified

E63 Other nutritional deficiencies

EXCLUDES 1 *dehydration (E86.Ø)*
failure to thrive, adult (R62.7)
failure to thrive, child (R62.51)
feeding problems in newborn (P92.-)
sequelae of malnutrition and other nutritional deficiencies (E64.-)

E63.Ø Essential fatty acid [EFA] deficiency
E63.1 Imbalance of constituents of food intake
E63.8 Other specified nutritional deficiencies
E63.9 Nutritional deficiency, unspecified

E64 Sequelae of malnutrition and other nutritional deficiencies

NOTE This category is to be used to indicate conditions in categories E43, E44, E46, E5Ø-E63 as the cause of sequelae, which are themselves classified elsewhere. The 'sequelae' include conditions specified as such; they also include the late effects of diseases classifiable to the above categories if the disease itself is no longer present

Code first condition resulting from (sequela) of malnutrition and other nutritional deficiencies

E64.Ø Sequelae of protein-calorie malnutrition CC HCC
EXCLUDES 2 *retarded development following protein-calorie malnutrition (E45)*
E64.1 Sequelae of vitamin A deficiency
E64.2 Sequelae of vitamin C deficiency
E64.3 Sequelae of rickets
E64.8 Sequelae of other nutritional deficiencies
E64.9 Sequelae of unspecified nutritional deficiency

Overweight, obesity and other hyperalimentation (E65-E68)

E65 Localized adiposity
Fat pad

E66 Overweight and obesity
Code first obesity complicating pregnancy, childbirth and the puerperium, if applicable (O99.21-)
Use additional code to identify body mass index (BMI), if known (Z68.-)
EXCLUDES 1 *adiposogenital dystrophy (E23.6)*
lipomatosis NOS (E88.2)
lipomatosis dolorosa [Dercum] (E88.2)
Prader-Willi syndrome (Q87.11)

AHA: 2018,4Q,77,79-80
TIP: Do not assign a BMI code (Z68.-) when a pregnant patient is documented as being overweight or obese. Only a code from subcategory O99.21- and a code from this category should be assigned.

E66.Ø Obesity due to excess calories
E66.Ø1 Morbid (severe) obesity due to excess calories H11 HCC
EXCLUDES 1 *morbid (severe) obesity with alveolar hypoventilation (E66.2)*
E66.Ø9 Other obesity due to excess calories
E66.1 Drug-induced obesity
Use additional code for adverse effect, if applicable, to identify drug (T36-T5Ø with fifth or sixth character 5)
E66.2 Morbid (severe) obesity with alveolar hypoventilation CC HCC
Obesity hypoventilation syndrome (OHS)
Pickwickian syndrome
E66.3 Overweight
AHA: 2018,4Q,78
E66.8 Other obesity
E66.9 Obesity, unspecified
Obesity NOS

E67 Other hyperalimentation
EXCLUDES 1 *hyperalimentation NOS (R63.2)*
sequelae of hyperalimentation (E68)
E67.Ø Hypervitaminosis A
E67.1 Hypercarotenemia
DEF: Elevated blood carotene level as a result of excessive carotenoid ingestion or an inability to convert carotenoids to vitamin A. Characteristics often include yellow discoloration of the skin, which may follow overeating of carotenoid-rich foods such as carrots, sweet potatoes, or squash.
E67.2 Megavitamin-B6 syndrome
E67.3 Hypervitaminosis D
E67.8 Other specified hyperalimentation

E68 Sequelae of hyperalimentation
Code first condition resulting from (sequela) of hyperalimentation

Metabolic disorders (E7Ø-E88)

EXCLUDES 1 *androgen insensitivity syndrome (E34.5-)*
congenital adrenal hyperplasia (E25.Ø)
▶Ehlers-Danlos syndromes◀ (Q79.6-)
hemolytic anemias attributable to enzyme disorders (D55.-)
Marfan's syndrome (Q87.4)
5-alpha-reductase deficiency (E29.1)

AHA: 2018,2Q,6

E7Ø Disorders of aromatic amino-acid metabolism
E7Ø.Ø Classical phenylketonuria CC HCC
E7Ø.1 Other hyperphenylalaninemias CC HCC
E7Ø.2 Disorders of tyrosine metabolism
EXCLUDES 1 *transitory tyrosinemia of newborn (P74.5)*
E7Ø.2Ø Disorder of tyrosine metabolism, unspecified CC HCC
E7Ø.21 Tyrosinemia CC HCC
Hypertyrosinemia
E7Ø.29 Other disorders of tyrosine metabolism CC HCC
Alkaptonuria
Ochronosis
E7Ø.3 Albinism
DEF: Absence of pigment in skin, hair, and eyes. This genetic condition is often accompanied by astigmatism, photophobia, and nystagmus.
E7Ø.3Ø Albinism, unspecified CC HCC
E7Ø.31 Ocular albinism
E7Ø.31Ø X-linked ocular albinism CC HCC
E7Ø.311 Autosomal recessive ocular albinism CC HCC
E7Ø.318 Other ocular albinism CC HCC
E7Ø.319 Ocular albinism, unspecified CC HCC
E7Ø.32 Oculocutaneous albinism
EXCLUDES 1 *Chediak-Higashi syndrome (E7Ø.33Ø)*
Hermansky-Pudlak syndrome (E7Ø.331)
E7Ø.32Ø Tyrosinase negative oculocutaneous albinism CC HCC
Albinism I
Oculocutaneous albinism ty-neg
E7Ø.321 Tyrosinase positive oculocutaneous albinism CC HCC
Albinism II
Oculocutaneous albinism ty-pos
E7Ø.328 Other oculocutaneous albinism CC HCC
Cross syndrome
E7Ø.329 Oculocutaneous albinism, unspecified CC HCC
E7Ø.33 Albinism with hematologic abnormality
E7Ø.33Ø Chediak-Higashi syndrome CC HCC
E7Ø.331 Hermansky-Pudlak syndrome CC HCC
E7Ø.338 Other albinism with hematologic abnormality CC HCC
E7Ø.339 Albinism with hematologic abnormality, unspecified CC HCC
E7Ø.39 Other specified albinism CC HCC
Piebaldism
E7Ø.4 Disorders of histidine metabolism
E7Ø.4Ø Disorders of histidine metabolism, unspecified CC HCC
E7Ø.41 Histidinemia CC HCC
E7Ø.49 Other disorders of histidine metabolism CC HCC
E7Ø.5 Disorders of tryptophan metabolism CC HCC
▲ **E7Ø.8 Other disorders of aromatic amino-acid metabolism**
● **E7Ø.81 Aromatic L-amino acid decarboxylase deficiency** CC
AADC deficiency
● **E7Ø.89 Other disorders of aromatic amino-acid metabolism** CC
E7Ø.9 Disorder of aromatic amino-acid metabolism, unspecified CC HCC

E71 Disorders of branched-chain amino-acid metabolism and fatty-acid metabolism
E71.Ø Maple-syrup-urine disease CC HCC

✓5th **E71.1 Other disorders of branched-chain amino-acid metabolism**
✓6th **E71.11 Branched-chain organic acidurias**
E71.110 Isovaleric acidemia CC HCC
E71.111 3-methylglutaconic aciduria CC HCC
E71.118 Other branched-chain organic acidurias CC HCC
✓6th **E71.12 Disorders of propionate metabolism**
E71.120 Methylmalonic acidemia CC HCC
E71.121 Propionic acidemia CC HCC
E71.128 Other disorders of propionate metabolism CC HCC
E71.19 Other disorders of branched-chain amino-acid metabolism CC HCC
Hyperleucine-isoleucinemia
Hypervalinemia
E71.2 Disorder of branched-chain amino-acid metabolism, unspecified CC HCC
✓5th **E71.3 Disorders of fatty-acid metabolism**
EXCLUDES 1 *peroxisomal disorders (E71.5)*
Refsum's disease (G60.1)
Schilder's disease (G37.0)
EXCLUDES 2 *carnitine deficiency due to inborn error of metabolism (E71.42)*
E71.30 Disorder of fatty-acid metabolism, unspecified
✓6th **E71.31 Disorders of fatty-acid oxidation**
E71.310 Long chain/very long chain acyl CoA dehydrogenase deficiency CC HCC
LCAD
VLCAD
E71.311 Medium chain acyl CoA dehydrogenase deficiency CC HCC
MCAD
E71.312 Short chain acyl CoA dehydrogenase deficiency CC HCC
SCAD
E71.313 Glutaric aciduria type II CC HCC
Glutaric aciduria type II A
Glutaric aciduria type II B
Glutaric aciduria type II C
EXCLUDES 1 *glutaric aciduria (type 1) NOS (E72.3)*
E71.314 Muscle carnitine palmitoyltransferase deficiency CC HCC
E71.318 Other disorders of fatty-acid oxidation CC HCC
E71.32 Disorders of ketone metabolism CC HCC
E71.39 Other disorders of fatty-acid metabolism CC HCC
✓5th **E71.4 Disorders of carnitine metabolism**
EXCLUDES 1 *muscle carnitine palmitoyltransferase deficiency (E71.314)*
E71.40 Disorder of carnitine metabolism, unspecified HCC
E71.41 Primary carnitine deficiency HCC
E71.42 Carnitine deficiency due to inborn errors of metabolism HCC
Code also associated inborn error or metabolism
E71.43 Iatrogenic carnitine deficiency HCC
Carnitine deficiency due to hemodialysis
Carnitine deficiency due to Valproic acid therapy
✓6th **E71.44 Other secondary carnitine deficiency**
E71.440 Ruvalcaba-Myhre-Smith syndrome HCC
E71.448 Other secondary carnitine deficiency HCC
✓5th **E71.5 Peroxisomal disorders**
EXCLUDES 1 *Schilder's disease (G37.0)*
E71.50 Peroxisomal disorder, unspecified CC HCC
✓6th **E71.51 Disorders of peroxisome biogenesis**
Group 1 peroxisomal disorders
EXCLUDES 1 *Refsum's disease (G60.1)*
E71.510 Zellweger syndrome CC HCC
E71.511 Neonatal adrenoleukodystrophy CC HCC
EXCLUDES 1 *X-linked adrenoleukodystrophy (E71.42-)*
E71.518 Other disorders of peroxisome biogenesis CC HCC
✓6th **E71.52 X-linked adrenoleukodystrophy**
E71.520 Childhood cerebral X-linked adrenoleukodystrophy CC HCC
E71.521 Adolescent X-linked adrenoleukodystrophy CC HCC
E71.522 Adrenomyeloneuropathy CC HCC
E71.528 Other X-linked adrenoleukodystrophy CC HCC
Addison only phenotype adrenoleukodystrophy
Addison-Schilder adrenoleukodystrophy
E71.529 X-linked adrenoleukodystrophy, unspecified type CC HCC
E71.53 Other group 2 peroxisomal disorders CC HCC
✓6th **E71.54 Other peroxisomal disorders**
E71.540 Rhizomelic chondrodysplasia punctata CC HCC
EXCLUDES 1 *chondrodysplasia punctata NOS (Q77.3)*
E71.541 Zellweger-like syndrome CC HCC
E71.542 Other group 3 peroxisomal disorders CC HCC
E71.548 Other peroxisomal disorders CC HCC

✓4th **E72 Other disorders of amino-acid metabolism**
EXCLUDES 1 *disorders of:*
aromatic amino-acid metabolism (E70.-)
branched-chain amino-acid metabolism (E71.0-E71.2)
fatty-acid metabolism (E71.3)
purine and pyrimidine metabolism (E79.-)
gout (M1A.-, M10.-)
✓5th **E72.0 Disorders of amino-acid transport**
EXCLUDES 1 *disorders of tryptophan metabolism (E70.5)*
E72.00 Disorders of amino-acid transport, unspecified CC HCC
E72.01 Cystinuria CC HCC
E72.02 Hartnup's disease CC HCC
E72.03 Lowe's syndrome CC HCC
Use additional code for associated glaucoma (H42)
E72.04 Cystinosis CC HCC
Fanconi (-de Toni) (-Debré) syndrome with cystinosis
EXCLUDES 1 *Fanconi (-de Toni) (-Debré) syndrome without cystinosis (E72.09)*
E72.09 Other disorders of amino-acid transport CC HCC
Fanconi (-de Toni) (-Debré) syndrome, unspecified
✓5th **E72.1 Disorders of sulfur-bearing amino-acid metabolism**
EXCLUDES 1 *cystinosis (E72.04)*
cystinuria (E72.01)
transcobalamin II deficiency (D51.2)
E72.10 Disorders of sulfur-bearing amino-acid metabolism, unspecified CC HCC
E72.11 Homocystinuria CC HCC
Cystathionine synthase deficiency
E72.12 Methylenetetrahydrofolate reductase deficiency CC HCC
E72.19 Other disorders of sulfur-bearing amino-acid metabolism CC HCC
Cystathioninuria
Methioninemia
Sulfite oxidase deficiency
✓5th **E72.2 Disorders of urea cycle metabolism**
EXCLUDES 1 *disorders of ornithine metabolism (E72.4)*
E72.20 Disorder of urea cycle metabolism, unspecified CC HCC
Hyperammonemia
EXCLUDES 1 *hyperammonemia- hyperornithinemia-homocitrullinemia syndrome E72.4*
transient hyperammonemia of newborn (P74.6)
E72.21 Argininemia CC HCC
E72.22 Arginosuccinic aciduria CC HCC
E72.23 Citrullinemia CC HCC
E72.29 Other disorders of urea cycle metabolism CC HCC

E72.3 Disorders of lysine and hydroxylysine metabolism CC HCC
Glutaric aciduria NOS
Glutaric aciduria (type I)
Hydroxylysinemia
Hyperlysinemia
EXCLUDES 1 *glutaric aciduria type II (E71.313)*
Refsum's disease (G6Ø.1)
Zellweger syndrome (E71.51Ø)

E72.4 Disorders of ornithine metabolism CC HCC
Hyperammonemia-Hyperornithinemia-Homocitrullinemia syndrome
Ornithinemia (types I, II)
Ornithine transcarbamylase deficiency
EXCLUDES 1 *hereditary choroidal dystrophy (H31.2-)*

✓5th **E72.5 Disorders of glycine metabolism**
E72.5Ø Disorder of glycine metabolism, unspecified CC HCC
E72.51 Non-ketotic hyperglycinemia CC HCC
E72.52 Trimethylaminuria CC HCC
E72.53 Primary hyperoxaluria CC HCC
Oxalosis
Oxaluria
AHA: 2018,4Q,29
E72.59 Other disorders of glycine metabolism CC HCC
D-glycericacidemia
Hyperhydroxyprolinemia
Hyperprolinemia (types I, II)
Sarcosinemia

✓5th **E72.8 Other specified disorders of amino-acid metabolism**
AHA: 2018,4Q,5
E72.81 Disorders of gamma aminobutyric acid metabolism CC HCC
4-hydroxybutyric aciduria
Disorders of GABA metabolism
GABA metabolic defect
GABA transaminase deficiency
GABA-T deficiency
Gamma-hydroxybutyric aciduria
SSADHD
Succinic semialdehyde dehydrogenase deficiency
E72.89 Other specified disorders of amino-acid metabolism CC HCC
Disorders of beta-amino-acid metabolism
Disorders of gamma-glutamyl cycle

E72.9 Disorder of amino-acid metabolism, unspecified CC HCC

✓4th **E73 Lactose intolerance**
DEF: Inability to break down sugar in dairy products due to a deficiency in the enzyme lactase.
E73.Ø Congenital lactase deficiency
E73.1 Secondary lactase deficiency
E73.8 Other lactose intolerance
E73.9 Lactose intolerance, unspecified

✓4th **E74 Other disorders of carbohydrate metabolism**
EXCLUDES 1 *diabetes mellitus (EØ8-E13)*
hypoglycemia NOS (E16.2)
increased secretion of glucagon (E16.3)
mucopolysaccharidosis (E76.Ø-E76.3)

✓5th **E74.Ø Glycogen storage disease**
E74.ØØ Glycogen storage disease, unspecified CC HCC
E74.Ø1 von Gierke disease CC HCC
Type I glycogen storage disease
E74.Ø2 Pompe disease CC HCC
Cardiac glycogenosis
Type II glycogen storage disease
E74.Ø3 Cori disease CC HCC
Forbes disease
Type III glycogen storage disease
E74.Ø4 McArdle disease CC HCC
Type V glycogen storage disease
E74.Ø9 Other glycogen storage disease CC HCC
Andersen disease
Hers disease
Tauri disease
Glycogen storage disease, types Ø, IV, VI-XI
Liver phosphorylase deficiency
Muscle phosphofructokinase deficiency

✓5th **E74.1 Disorders of fructose metabolism**
EXCLUDES 1 *muscle phosphofructokinase deficiency (E74.Ø9)*
E74.1Ø Disorder of fructose metabolism, unspecified
E74.11 Essential fructosuria
Fructokinase deficiency
E74.12 Hereditary fructose intolerance
Fructosemia
E74.19 Other disorders of fructose metabolism
Fructose-1, 6-diphosphatase deficiency

✓5th **E74.2 Disorders of galactose metabolism**
E74.2Ø Disorders of galactose metabolism, unspecified CC HCC
E74.21 Galactosemia CC HCC
DEF: Any of three genetic disorders caused by a defective galactose metabolism. Symptoms include failure to thrive in infancy, jaundice, liver and spleen damage, cataracts, and mental retardation.
E74.29 Other disorders of galactose metabolism CC HCC
Galactokinase deficiency

✓5th **E74.3 Other disorders of intestinal carbohydrate absorption**
EXCLUDES 2 *lactose intolerance (E73.-)*
E74.31 Sucrase-isomaltase deficiency
E74.39 Other disorders of intestinal carbohydrate absorption
Disorder of intestinal carbohydrate absorption NOS
Glucose-galactose malabsorption
Sucrase deficiency

E74.4 Disorders of pyruvate metabolism and gluconeogenesis CC HCC
Deficiency of phosphoenolpyruvate carboxykinase
Deficiency of pyruvate carboxylase
Deficiency of pyruvate dehydrogenase
EXCLUDES 1 *disorders of pyruvate metabolism and gluconeogenesis with anemia (D55.-)*
Leigh's syndrome (G31.82)

▲ ✓5th **E74.8 Other specified disorders of carbohydrate metabolism**
~~Essential pentosuria~~
~~Renal glycosuria~~

● ✓6th **E74.81 Disorders of glucose transport, not elsewhere classified**
● **E74.81Ø Glucose transporter protein type 1 deficiency** CC
De Vivo syndrome
Glucose transport defect, blood-brain barrier
Glut1 deficiency
GLUT1 deficiency syndrome 1, infantile onset
GLUT1 deficiency syndrome 2, childhood onset
● **E74.818 Other disorders of glucose transport** CC
(Familial) renal glycosuria
● **E74.819 Disorders of glucose transport, unspecified** CC
● **E74.89 Other specified disorders of carbohydrate metabolism** CC
Essential pentosuria

E74.9 Disorder of carbohydrate metabolism, unspecified HCC

✓4th **E75 Disorders of sphingolipid metabolism and other lipid storage disorders**
EXCLUDES 1 *mucolipidosis, types I-III (E77.Ø-E77.1)*
Refsum's disease (G6Ø.1)

✓5th **E75.Ø GM2 gangliosidosis**
E75.ØØ GM2 gangliosidosis, unspecified CC HCC
E75.Ø1 Sandhoff disease CC HCC

Chapter 4. Endocrine, Nutritional and Metabolic Diseases
E72.3–E75.Ø1

E75.02 Tay-Sachs disease CC HCC
DEF: Genetic mutation of the HEXA gene that inhibits the breakdown of a toxic substance called ganglioside. The accumulation of ganglioside results in destruction of the neurons in the brain and spinal cord.

Tay-Sachs Disease

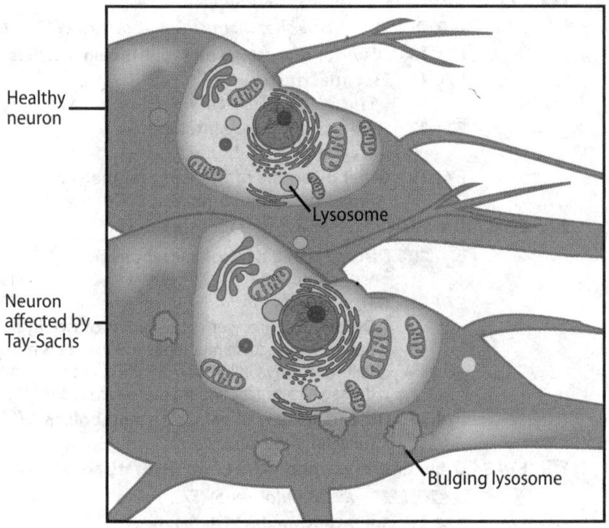

E75.09 Other GM2 gangliosidosis CC HCC
Adult GM2 gangliosidosis
Juvenile GM2 gangliosidosis

√5th **E75.1 Other and unspecified gangliosidosis**

E75.10 Unspecified gangliosidosis CC HCC
Gangliosidosis NOS

E75.11 Mucolipidosis IV CC HCC

E75.19 Other gangliosidosis CC HCC
GM1 gangliosidosis
GM3 gangliosidosis

√5th **E75.2 Other sphingolipidosis**
EXCLUDES 1 *adrenoleukodystrophy [Addison-Schilder] (E71.528)*

E75.21 Fabry (-Anderson) disease HCC

E75.22 Gaucher disease HCC

E75.23 Krabbe disease CC HCC

√6th **E75.24 Niemann-Pick disease**

E75.240 Niemann-Pick disease type A HCC

E75.241 Niemann-Pick disease type B HCC

E75.242 Niemann-Pick disease type C HCC

E75.243 Niemann-Pick disease type D HCC

E75.248 Other Niemann-Pick disease HCC

E75.249 Niemann-Pick disease, unspecified HCC

E75.25 Metachromatic leukodystrophy CC HCC

E75.26 Sulfatase deficiency CC HCC
Multiple sulfatase deficiency (MSD)
AHA: 2018,4Q,5-6

E75.29 Other sphingolipidosis CC HCC
Farber's syndrome
Sulfatide lipidosis

E75.3 Sphingolipidosis, unspecified HCC

E75.4 Neuronal ceroid lipofuscinosis CC HCC
Batten disease
Bielschowsky-Jansky disease
Kufs disease
Spielmeyer-Vogt disease

E75.5 Other lipid storage disorders
Cerebrotendinous cholesterosis [van Bogaert-Scherer-Epstein]
Wolman's disease

E75.6 Lipid storage disorder, unspecified

√4th **E76 Disorders of glycosaminoglycan metabolism**

√5th **E76.0 Mucopolysaccharidosis, type I**

E76.01 Hurler's syndrome CC HCC

E76.02 Hurler-Scheie syndrome CC HCC

E76.03 Scheie's syndrome CC HCC

E76.1 Mucopolysaccharidosis, type II CC HCC
Hunter's syndrome

√5th **E76.2 Other mucopolysaccharidoses**

√6th **E76.21 Morquio mucopolysaccharidoses**

E76.210 Morquio A mucopolysaccharidoses CC HCC
Classic Morquio syndrome
Morquio syndrome A
Mucopolysaccharidosis, type IVA

E76.211 Morquio B mucopolysaccharidoses CC HCC
Morquio-like mucopolysaccharidoses
Morquio-like syndrome
Morquio syndrome B
Mucopolysaccharidosis, type IVB

E76.219 Morquio mucopolysaccharidoses, unspecified CC HCC
Morquio syndrome
Mucopolysaccharidosis, type IV

E76.22 Sanfilippo mucopolysaccharidoses CC HCC
Mucopolysaccharidosis, type III (A) (B) (C) (D)
Sanfilippo A syndrome
Sanfilippo B syndrome
Sanfilippo C syndrome
Sanfilippo D syndrome

E76.29 Other mucopolysaccharidoses CC HCC
beta-Glucuronidase deficiency
Maroteaux-Lamy (mild) (severe) syndrome
Mucopolysaccharidosis, types VI, VII

E76.3 Mucopolysaccharidosis, unspecified CC HCC

E76.8 Other disorders of glucosaminoglycan metabolism CC HCC

E76.9 Glucosaminoglycan metabolism disorder, unspecified CC HCC

√4th **E77 Disorders of glycoprotein metabolism**

E77.0 Defects in post-translational modification of lysosomal enzymes HCC
Mucolipidosis II [I-cell disease]
Mucolipidosis III [pseudo-Hurler polydystrophy]

E77.1 Defects in glycoprotein degradation HCC
Aspartylglucosaminuria
Fucosidosis
Mannosidosis
Sialidosis [mucolipidosis I]

E77.8 Other disorders of glycoprotein metabolism HCC

E77.9 Disorder of glycoprotein metabolism, unspecified HCC

√4th **E78 Disorders of lipoprotein metabolism and other lipidemias**
EXCLUDES 1 *sphingolipidosis (E75.0-E75.3)*

√5th **E78.0 Pure hypercholesterolemia**
AHA: 2016,4Q,13-14

E78.00 Pure hypercholesterolemia, unspecified
Fredrickson's hyperlipoproteinemia, type IIa
Hyperbetalipoproteinemia
Low-density-lipoprotein-type [LDL] hyperlipoproteinemia
(Pure) hypercholesterolemia NOS

E78.01 Familial hypercholesterolemia

E78.1 Pure hyperglyceridemia
Elevated fasting triglycerides
Endogenous hyperglyceridemia
Fredrickson's hyperlipoproteinemia, type IV
Hyperlipidemia, group B
Hyperprebetalipoproteinemia
Very-low-density-lipoprotein-type [VLDL] hyperlipoproteinemia

E78.2 Mixed hyperlipidemia
Broad- or floating-betalipoproteinemia
Combined hyperlipidemia NOS
Elevated cholesterol with elevated triglycerides NEC
Fredrickson's hyperlipoproteinemia, type IIb or III
Hyperbetalipoproteinemia with prebetalipoproteinemia
Hypercholesteremia with endogenous hyperglyceridemia
Hyperlipidemia, group C
Tubo-eruptive xanthoma
Xanthoma tuberosum
EXCLUDES 1 *cerebrotendinous cholesterosis [van Bogaert-Scherer-Epstein] (E75.5)*
familial combined hyperlipidemia (E78.49)

E78.3 Hyperchylomicronemia
Chylomicron retention disease
Fredrickson's hyperlipoproteinemia, type I or V
Hyperlipidemia, group D
Mixed hyperglyceridemia

✓5th **E78.4 Other hyperlipidemia**
AHA: 2018,4Q,6

E78.41 Elevated Lipoprotein(a)
Elevated Lp(a)

E78.49 Other hyperlipidemia
Familial combined hyperlipidemia

E78.5 Hyperlipidemia, unspecified

E78.6 Lipoprotein deficiency
Abetalipoproteinemia
Depressed HDL cholesterol
High-density lipoprotein deficiency
Hypoalphalipoproteinemia
Hypobetalipoproteinemia (familial)
Lecithin cholesterol acyltransferase deficiency
Tangier disease

✓5th **E78.7 Disorders of bile acid and cholesterol metabolism**
EXCLUDES 1 *Niemann-Pick disease type C (E75.242)*

E78.70 Disorder of bile acid and cholesterol metabolism, unspecified

E78.71 Barth syndrome CC

E78.72 Smith-Lemli-Opitz syndrome CC

E78.79 Other disorders of bile acid and cholesterol metabolism

✓5th **E78.8 Other disorders of lipoprotein metabolism**

E78.81 Lipoid dermatoarthritis

E78.89 Other lipoprotein metabolism disorders

E78.9 Disorder of lipoprotein metabolism, unspecified

✓4th **E79 Disorders of purine and pyrimidine metabolism**
EXCLUDES 1 *Ataxia-telangiectasia (Q87.19)*
Bloom's syndrome (Q82.8)
Cockayne's syndrome (Q87.19)
calculus of kidney (N20.0)
combined immunodeficiency disorders (D81.-)
Fanconi's anemia (D61.09)
gout (M1A.-, M10.-)
orotaciduric anemia (D53.0)
progeria (E34.8)
Werner's syndrome (E34.8)
xeroderma pigmentosum (Q82.1)

E79.0 Hyperuricemia without signs of inflammatory arthritis and tophaceous disease
Asymptomatic hyperuricemia

E79.1 Lesch-Nyhan syndrome CC HCC
HGPRT deficiency

E79.2 Myoadenylate deaminase deficiency CC HCC

E79.8 Other disorders of purine and pyrimidine metabolism CC HCC
Hereditary xanthinuria

E79.9 Disorder of purine and pyrimidine metabolism, unspecified CC HCC

✓4th **E80 Disorders of porphyrin and bilirubin metabolism**
INCLUDES defects of catalase and peroxidase

E80.0 Hereditary erythropoietic porphyria CC HCC
Congenital erythropoietic porphyria
Erythropoietic protoporphyria

E80.1 Porphyria cutanea tarda CC HCC

✓5th **E80.2 Other and unspecified porphyria**

E80.20 Unspecified porphyria CC HCC
Porphyria NOS

E80.21 Acute intermittent (hepatic) porphyria CC HCC

E80.29 Other porphyria CC HCC
Hereditary coproporphyria

E80.3 Defects of catalase and peroxidase CC HCC
Acatalasia [Takahara]

E80.4 Gilbert syndrome

E80.5 Crigler-Najjar syndrome

E80.6 Other disorders of bilirubin metabolism
Dubin-Johnson syndrome
Rotor's syndrome

E80.7 Disorder of bilirubin metabolism, unspecified

✓4th **E83 Disorders of mineral metabolism**
EXCLUDES 1 *dietary mineral deficiency (E58-E61)*
parathyroid disorders (E20-E21)
vitamin D deficiency (E55.-)

✓5th **E83.0 Disorders of copper metabolism**

E83.00 Disorder of copper metabolism, unspecified

E83.01 Wilson's disease
Code also associated Kayser Fleischer ring (H18.04-)

E83.09 Other disorders of copper metabolism
Menkes' (kinky hair) (steely hair) disease

✓5th **E83.1 Disorders of iron metabolism**
EXCLUDES 1 *iron deficiency anemia (D50.-)*
sideroblastic anemia (D64.0-D64.3)

E83.10 Disorder of iron metabolism, unspecified

✓6th **E83.11 Hemochromatosis**
EXCLUDES 1 *GALD (P78.84)*
gestational alloimmune liver disease (P78.84)
neonatal hemochromatosis (P78.84)

E83.110 Hereditary hemochromatosis HCC
Bronzed diabetes
Pigmentary cirrhosis (of liver)
Primary (hereditary) hemochromatosis

E83.111 Hemochromatosis due to repeated red blood cell transfusions
Iron overload due to repeated red blood cell transfusions
Transfusion (red blood cell) associated hemochromatosis

E83.118 Other hemochromatosis

E83.119 Hemochromatosis, unspecified

E83.19 Other disorders of iron metabolism
Use additional code, if applicable, for idiopathic pulmonary hemosiderosis (J84.03)

E83.2 Disorders of zinc metabolism
Acrodermatitis enteropathica

✓5th **E83.3 Disorders of phosphorus metabolism and phosphatases**
EXCLUDES 1 *adult osteomalacia (M83.-)*
osteoporosis (M80.-)

E83.30 Disorder of phosphorus metabolism, unspecified

E83.31 Familial hypophosphatemia
Vitamin D-resistant osteomalacia
Vitamin D-resistant rickets
EXCLUDES 1 *vitamin D-deficiency rickets (E55.0)*

E83.32 Hereditary vitamin D-dependent rickets (type 1) (type 2)
25-hydroxyvitamin D 1-alpha-hydroxylase deficiency
Pseudovitamin D deficiency
Vitamin D receptor defect

E83.39 Other disorders of phosphorus metabolism
Acid phosphatase deficiency
Hypophosphatasia

✓5th **E83.4 Disorders of magnesium metabolism**

E83.40 Disorders of magnesium metabolism, unspecified

E83.41 Hypermagnesemia
AHA: 2016,4Q,54

E83.42 Hypomagnesemia

E83.49 Other disorders of magnesium metabolism

✓5th **E83.5 Disorders of calcium metabolism**

EXCLUDES 1 *chondrocalcinosis (M11.1-M11.2)*
hungry bone syndrome (E83.81)
hyperparathyroidism (E21.Ø-E21.3)

E83.5Ø Unspecified disorder of calcium metabolism

E83.51 Hypocalcemia

E83.52 Hypercalcemia
Familial hypocalciuric hypercalcemia

E83.59 Other disorders of calcium metabolism

✓5th **E83.8 Other disorders of mineral metabolism**

E83.81 Hungry bone syndrome

E83.89 Other disorders of mineral metabolism

E83.9 Disorder of mineral metabolism, unspecified

✓4th **E84 Cystic fibrosis**

INCLUDES mucoviscidosis

Code also exocrine pancreatic insufficiency (K86.81)

DEF: Genetic disorder affecting the respiratory, digestive, and reproductive systems in infants to young adults by disturbing exocrine gland function and causing chronic pulmonary disease with excess mucus production and pancreatic deficiency.

E84.Ø Cystic fibrosis with pulmonary manifestations MCC HCC
Use additional code to identify any infectious organism present, such as:
Pseudomonas (B96.5)

✓5th **E84.1 Cystic fibrosis with intestinal manifestations**

E84.11 Meconium ileus in cystic fibrosis MCC HCC N
EXCLUDES 1 *meconium ileus not due to cystic fibrosis (P76.Ø)*

E84.19 Cystic fibrosis with other intestinal manifestations CC HCC
Distal intestinal obstruction syndrome

E84.8 Cystic fibrosis with other manifestations CC HCC

E84.9 Cystic fibrosis, unspecified CC HCC

✓4th **E85 Amyloidosis**

EXCLUDES 2 *Alzheimer's disease (G3Ø.Ø-)*

DEF: Conditions of diverse etiologies characterized by the accumulation of insoluble fibrillar proteins (amyloid) in various organs and tissues of the body, compromising vital functions.

E85.Ø Non-neuropathic heredofamilial amyloidosis CC HCC
Hereditary amyloid nephropathy
Code also associated disorders, such as:
autoinflammatory syndromes (MØ4.-)
EXCLUDES 2 *transthyretin-related (ATTR) familial amyloid cardiomyopathy (E85.4)*

E85.1 Neuropathic heredofamilial amyloidosis CC HCC
Amyloid polyneuropathy (Portuguese)
Transthyretin-related (ATTR) familial amyloid polyneuropathy
AHA: 2012,4Q,99

E85.2 Heredofamilial amyloidosis, unspecified CC HCC

E85.3 Secondary systemic amyloidosis CC HCC
Hemodialysis-associated amyloidosis

E85.4 Organ-limited amyloidosis CC HCC
Localized amyloidosis
Transthyretin-related (ATTR) familial amyloid cardiomyopathy

✓5th **E85.8 Other amyloidosis**
AHA: 2017,4Q,7

E85.81 Light chain (AL) amyloidosis CC HCC

E85.82 Wild-type transthyretin-related (ATTR) amyloidosis CC HCC
Senile systemic amyloidosis (SSA)

E85.89 Other amyloidosis CC HCC

E85.9 Amyloidosis, unspecified CC HCC

✓4th **E86 Volume depletion**

Use additional code(s) for any associated disorders of electrolyte and acid-base balance (E87.-)

EXCLUDES 1 *dehydration of newborn (P74.1)*
~~*hypovolemic shock NOS (R57.1)*~~
postprocedural hypovolemic shock (T81.19)
traumatic hypovolemic shock (T79.4)

EXCLUDES 2 ▶*hypovolemic shock NOS (R57.1)*◀

AHA: 2019,2Q,7; 2018,2Q,6

E86.Ø Dehydration
AHA: 2019,2Q,7; 2019,1Q,12; 2014,1Q,7
TIP: Can be assigned in addition to hypernatremia (E87.0) or hyponatremia (E87.1), when documented.

E86.1 Hypovolemia
Depletion of volume of plasma

E86.9 Volume depletion, unspecified
DEF: Depletion of total body water (dehydration) and/or contraction of total intravascular plasma (hypovolemia).

✓4th **E87 Other disorders of fluid, electrolyte and acid-base balance**

EXCLUDES 1 *diabetes insipidus (E23.2)*
electrolyte imbalance associated with hyperemesis gravidarum (O21.1)
electrolyte imbalance following ectopic or molar pregnancy (OØ8.5)
familial periodic paralysis (G72.3)

AHA: 2018,2Q,6

E87.Ø Hyperosmolality and hypernatremia CC
Sodium [Na] excess
Sodium [Na] overload
AHA: 2014,1Q,7
TIP: Assign an additional code for dehydration (E86.0), when documented.

E87.1 Hypo-osmolality and hyponatremia CC
Sodium [Na] deficiency
EXCLUDES 1 *syndrome of inappropriate secretion of antidiuretic hormone (E22.2)*
AHA: 2014,1Q,7
TIP: Assign an additional code for dehydration (E86.0), when documented.

E87.2 Acidosis CC
Acidosis NOS
Lactic acidosis
Metabolic acidosis
Respiratory acidosis
EXCLUDES 1 *diabetic acidosis — see categories EØ8-E1Ø, E13 with ketoacidosis*
DEF: Reduction of alkaline in the blood and tissues caused by an increase in acid and decrease in bicarbonate.

E87.3 Alkalosis CC
Alkalosis NOS
Metabolic alkalosis
Respiratory alkalosis

E87.4 Mixed disorder of acid-base balance CC

E87.5 Hyperkalemia
Potassium [K] excess
Potassium [K] overload

E87.6 Hypokalemia
Potassium [K] deficiency

✓5th **E87.7 Fluid overload**

EXCLUDES 1 *edema NOS (R6Ø.9)*
fluid retention (R6Ø.9)

E87.7Ø Fluid overload, unspecified

E87.71 Transfusion associated circulatory overload
Fluid overload due to transfusion (blood) (blood components)
TACO

E87.79 Other fluid overload

E87.8 Other disorders of electrolyte and fluid balance, not elsewhere classified
Electrolyte imbalance NOS
Hyperchloremia
Hypochloremia

✓4th E88 Other and unspecified metabolic disorders
Use additional codes for associated conditions
EXCLUDES 1 *histiocytosis X (chronic) (C96.6)*

✓5th E88.Ø Disorders of plasma-protein metabolism, not elsewhere classified
EXCLUDES 1 *~~disorder of lipoprotein metabolism (E78.-)~~*
monoclonal gammopathy (of undetermined significance) (D47.2)
polyclonal hypergammaglobulinemia (D89.Ø)
Waldenström macroglobulinemia (C88.Ø)
EXCLUDES 2 ▶*disorder of lipoprotein metabolism (E78.-)*◀

E88.Ø1 Alpha-1-antitrypsin deficiency HCC
AAT deficiency

E88.Ø2 Plasminogen deficiency CC
Dysplasminogenemia
Hypoplasminogenemia
Type 1 plasminogen deficiency
Type 2 plasminogen deficiency
Code also, if applicable, ligneous conjunctivitis (H1Ø.51)
Use additional code for associated findings, such as:
hydrocephalus (G91.4)
otitis media (H67.-)
respiratory disorder related to plasminogen deficiency (J99)
AHA: 2018,4Q,6-7

E88.Ø9 Other disorders of plasma-protein metabolism, not elsewhere classified
Bisalbuminemia

E88.1 Lipodystrophy, not elsewhere classified
Lipodystrophy NOS
EXCLUDES 1 *Whipple's disease (K9Ø.81)*

E88.2 Lipomatosis, not elsewhere classified
Lipomatosis NOS
Lipomatosis (Check) dolorosa [Dercum]

E88.3 Tumor lysis syndrome MCC
Tumor lysis syndrome (spontaneous)
Tumor lysis syndrome following antineoplastic drug chemotherapy
Use additional code for adverse effect, if applicable, to identify drug (T45.1X5)
AHA: 2020,1Q,37; 2019,2Q,24
DEF: Potentially fatal metabolic complication of tumor necrosis caused by spontaneous or treatment-related accumulation of byproducts from dying cancer cells. Symptoms include hyperkalemia, hyperphosphatemia, hypocalcemia, hyperuricemia, and hyperuricosuria.

✓5th E88.4 Mitochondrial metabolism disorders
EXCLUDES 1 *disorders of pyruvate metabolism (E74.4)*
Kearns-Sayre syndrome (H49.81)
Leber's disease (H47.22)
Leigh's encephalopathy (G31.82)
mitochondrial myopathy, NEC (G71.3)
Reye's syndrome (G93.7)

E88.4Ø Mitochondrial metabolism disorder, unspecified CC HCC

E88.41 MELAS syndrome CC HCC
Mitochondrial myopathy, encephalopathy, lactic acidosis and stroke-like episodes

E88.42 MERRF syndrome CC HCC
Myoclonic epilepsy associated with ragged-red fibers
Code also progressive myoclonic epilepsy (G4Ø.3-)

E88.49 Other mitochondrial metabolism disorders CC HCC

✓5th E88.8 Other specified metabolic disorders

E88.81 Metabolic syndrome
Dysmetabolic syndrome X
Use additional codes for associated manifestations, such as:
obesity (E66.-)
DEF: Group of health risks that increase the likelihood of developing heart disease, stroke, and diabetes. These risks include certain parameters for blood pressure, cholesterol, and glucose levels.

E88.89 Other specified metabolic disorders HCC
Launois-Bensaude adenolipomatosis
EXCLUDES 1 *adult pulmonary Langerhans cell histiocytosis (J84.82)*

E88.9 Metabolic disorder, unspecified

Postprocedural endocrine and metabolic complications and disorders, not elsewhere classified (E89)

✓4th E89 Postprocedural endocrine and metabolic complications and disorders, not elsewhere classified
EXCLUDES 2 *intraoperative complications of endocrine system organ or structure (E36.Ø-, E36.1-, E36.8)*

E89.Ø Postprocedural hypothyroidism
Postirradiation hypothyroidism
Postsurgical hypothyroidism

E89.1 Postprocedural hypoinsulinemia CC
Postpancreatectomy hyperglycemia
Postsurgical hypoinsulinemia
Use additional code, if applicable, to identify:
acquired absence of pancreas (Z9Ø.41-)
diabetes mellitus (postpancreatectomy) (postprocedural) (E13.-)
insulin use (Z79.4)
EXCLUDES 1 *transient postprocedural hyperglycemia (R73.9)*
transient postprocedural hypoglycemia (E16.2)

E89.2 Postprocedural hypoparathyroidism HCC
Parathyroprival tetany

E89.3 Postprocedural hypopituitarism HCC
Postirradiation hypopituitarism

✓5th E89.4 Postprocedural ovarian failure

E89.4Ø Asymptomatic postprocedural ovarian failure ♀
Postprocedural ovarian failure NOS

E89.41 Symptomatic postprocedural ovarian failure ♀
Symptoms such as flushing, sleeplessness, headache, lack of concentration, associated with postprocedural menopause

E89.5 Postprocedural testicular hypofunction ♂

E89.6 Postprocedural adrenocortical (-medullary) hypofunction CC HCC

✓5th E89.8 Other postprocedural endocrine and metabolic complications and disorders
AHA: 2016,4Q,9-10

✓6th E89.81 Postprocedural hemorrhage of an endocrine system organ or structure following a procedure

E89.81Ø Postprocedural hemorrhage of an endocrine system organ or structure following an endocrine system procedure CC

E89.811 Postprocedural hemorrhage of an endocrine system organ or structure following other procedure CC

✓6th E89.82 Postprocedural hematoma and seroma of an endocrine system organ or structure

E89.82Ø Postprocedural hematoma of an endocrine system organ or structure following an endocrine system procedure CC

E89.821 Postprocedural hematoma of an endocrine system organ or structure following other procedure CC

E89.822 Postprocedural seroma of an endocrine system organ or structure following an endocrine system procedure CC

E89.823 Postprocedural seroma of an endocrine system organ or structure following other procedure CC

E89.89 Other postprocedural endocrine and metabolic complications and disorders CC
Use additional code, if applicable, to further specify disorder

Chapter 5. Mental, Behavioral and Neurodevelopmental Disorders (FØ1–F99)

Chapter-specific Guidelines with Coding Examples

The chapter-specific guidelines from the ICD-10-CM Official Guidelines for Coding and Reporting have been provided below. Along with these guidelines are coding examples, contained in the shaded boxes, that have been developed to help illustrate the coding and/or sequencing guidance found in these guidelines.

a. Pain disorders related to psychological factors

Assign code F45.41, for pain that is exclusively related to psychological disorders. As indicated by the Excludes 1 note under category G89, a code from category G89 should not be assigned with code F45.41.

Perceived abdominal pain determined to be persistent somatoform pain disorder

F45.41 Pain disorder exclusively related to psychological factors

Explanation: This pain was diagnosed as being exclusively psychological; therefore, no code from category G89 is added.

Code F45.42, Pain disorders with related psychological factors, should be used with a code from category G89, Pain, not elsewhere classified, if there is documentation of a psychological component for a patient with acute or chronic pain.

See Section I.C.6. Pain

b. Mental and behavioral disorders due to psychoactive substance use

1) In remission

Selection of codes for "in remission" for categories F1Ø-F19, Mental and behavioral disorders due to psychoactive substance use (categories F1Ø-F19 with -11, -.21) requires the provider's clinical judgment. The appropriate codes for "in remission" are assigned only on the basis of provider documentation (as defined in the Official Guidelines for Coding and Reporting), unless otherwise instructed by the classification.

Mild substance use disorders in early or sustained remission are classified to the appropriate codes for substance abuse in remission, and moderate or severe substance use disorders in early or sustained remission are classified to the appropriate codes for substance dependence in remission.

Insomnia in patient with history of methamphetamine abuse; lab results indicate no current drug use

G47.ØØ Insomnia, unspecified

F15.1Ø Other stimulant abuse, uncomplicated

Explanation: Insomnia is a common side-effect of stimulant use, such as methamphetamines. Although lab tests do not indicate that the patient is currently using methamphetamines, there is no specific documentation stating that the stimulant abuse is in remission. "History of" abuse does not equate to "in remission" in this instance.

2) Psychoactive substance use, abuse and dependence

When the provider documentation refers to use, abuse and dependence of the same substance (e.g. alcohol, opioid, cannabis, etc.), only one code should be assigned to identify the pattern of use based on the following hierarchy:

- If both use and abuse are documented, assign only the code for abuse
- If both abuse and dependence are documented, assign only the code for dependence
- If use, abuse and dependence are all documented, assign only the code for dependence
- If both use and dependence are documented, assign only the code for dependence.

History and physical notes cannabis dependence; progress note says cannabis abuse

F12.2Ø Cannabis dependence, uncomplicated

Explanation: In the hierarchy, the dependence code is used if both abuse and dependence are documented.

Discharge summary says cocaine abuse; progress notes list cocaine use

F14.1Ø Cocaine abuse, uncomplicated

Explanation: In the hierarchy, the abuse code is used if both abuse and use are documented.

3) Psychoactive substance use, unspecified

As with all other unspecified diagnoses, the codes for unspecified psychoactive substance use disorders (F1Ø.9-, F11.9-, F12.9-, F13.9-, F14.9-, F15.9-, F16.9-, F18.9-, F19.9-) should only be assigned based on provider documentation and when they meet the definition of a reportable diagnosis (see Section III, Reporting Additional Diagnoses). These codes are to be used only when the psychoactive substance use is associated with a physical **disorder included in chapter 5 (such as sexual dysfunction and sleep disorder), or a** mental or behavioral disorder, and such a relationship is documented by the provider.

c. Factitious disorder

Factitious disorder imposed on self or Munchausen's syndrome is a disorder in which a person falsely reports or causes his or her own physical or psychological signs or symptoms. For patients with documented factitious disorder on self or Munchausen's syndrome, assign the appropriate code from subcategory F68.1-, Factitious disorder imposed on self.

Munchausen's syndrome by proxy (MSBP) is a disorder in which a caregiver (perpetrator) falsely reports or causes an illness or injury in another person (victim) under his or her care, such as a child, an elderly adult, or a person who has a disability. The condition is also referred to as "factitious disorder imposed on another" or "factitious disorder by proxy." The perpetrator, not the victim, receives this diagnosis. Assign code F68.A, Factitious disorder imposed on another, to the perpetrator's record. For the victim of a patient suffering from MSBP, assign the appropriate code from categories T74, Adult and child abuse, neglect and other maltreatment, confirmed, or T76, Adult and child abuse, neglect and other maltreatment, suspected.

See Section I.C.19.f. Adult and child abuse, neglect and other maltreatment

Chapter 5. Mental, Behavioral and Neurodevelopmental Disorders (F01-F99)

INCLUDES disorders of psychological development

EXCLUDES 2 *symptoms, signs and abnormal clinical laboratory findings, not elsewhere classified (R00-R99)*

This chapter contains the following blocks:

F01-F09 Mental disorders due to known physiological conditions
F10-F19 Mental and behavioral disorders due to psychoactive substance use
F20-F29 Schizophrenia, schizotypal, delusional, and other non-mood psychotic disorders
F30-F39 Mood [affective] disorders
F40-F48 Anxiety, dissociative, stress-related, somatoform and other nonpsychotic mental disorders
F50-F59 Behavioral syndromes associated with physiological disturbances and physical factors
F60-F69 Disorders of adult personality and behavior
F70-F79 Intellectual disabilities
F80-F89 Pervasive and specific developmental disorders
F90-F98 Behavioral and emotional disorders with onset usually occurring in childhood and adolescence
F99 Unspecified mental disorder

Mental disorders due to known physiological conditions (F01-F09)

NOTE This block comprises a range of mental disorders grouped together on the basis of their having in common a demonstrable etiology in cerebral disease, brain injury, or other insult leading to cerebral dysfunction. The dysfunction may be primary, as in diseases, injuries, and insults that affect the brain directly and selectively; or secondary, as in systemic diseases and disorders that attack the brain only as one of the multiple organs or systems of the body that are involved.

✓4th F01 Vascular dementia

Vascular dementia as a result of infarction of the brain due to vascular disease, including hypertensive cerebrovascular disease.

INCLUDES arteriosclerotic dementia

Code first the underlying physiological condition or sequelae of cerebrovascular disease.

✓5th F01.5 Vascular dementia

F01.50 Vascular dementia without behavioral disturbance HCC A

Major neurocognitive disorder without behavioral disturbance

F01.51 Vascular dementia with behavioral disturbance CC HCC A

Major neurocognitive disorder due to vascular disease, with behavioral disturbance
Major neurocognitive disorder with aggressive behavior
Major neurocognitive disorder with combative behavior
Major neurocognitive disorder with violent behavior
Vascular dementia with aggressive behavior
Vascular dementia with combative behavior
Vascular dementia with violent behavior
Use additional code, if applicable, to identify wandering in vascular dementia (Z91.83)

✓4th F02 Dementia in other diseases classified elsewhere

INCLUDES major neurocognitive disorder in other diseases classified elsewhere

Code first the underlying physiological condition, such as:
Alzheimer's (G30.-)
cerebral lipidosis (E75.4)
Creutzfeldt-Jakob disease (A81.0-)
dementia with Lewy bodies (G31.83)
dementia with Parkinsonism (G31.83)
epilepsy and recurrent seizures (G40.-)
frontotemporal dementia (G31.09)
hepatolenticular degeneration (E83.0)
human immunodeficiency virus [HIV] disease (B20)
Huntington's disease (G10)
hypercalcemia (E83.52)
hypothyroidism, acquired (E00-E03.-)
intoxications (T36-T65)
Jakob-Creutzfeldt disease (A81.0-)
multiple sclerosis (G35)
neurosyphilis (A52.17)
niacin deficiency [pellagra] (E52)
Parkinson's disease (G20)
Pick's disease (G31.01)
polyarteritis nodosa (M30.0)
prion disease (A81.9)
systemic lupus erythematosus (M32.-)
traumatic brain injury (S06.-)
trypanosomiasis (B56.-, B57.-)
vitamin B deficiency (E53.8)

EXCLUDES 2 *dementia in alcohol and psychoactive substance disorders (F10-F19, with .17, .27, .97)*
vascular dementia (F01.5-)

✓5th F02.8 Dementia in other diseases classified elsewhere

AHA: 2017,2Q,7; 2016,4Q,141; 2016,2Q,6

TIP: A code from this subcategory should always be assigned with a code from category G30 when Alzheimer's disease is documented, even in the absence of documented dementia.

F02.80 Dementia in other diseases classified elsewhere without behavioral disturbance HCC

Dementia in other diseases classified elsewhere NOS
Major neurocognitive disorder in other diseases classified elsewhere

F02.81 Dementia in other diseases classified elsewhere with behavioral disturbance CC HCC

Dementia in other diseases classified elsewhere with aggressive behavior
Dementia in other diseases classified elsewhere with combative behavior
Dementia in other diseases classified elsewhere with violent behavior
Major neurocognitive disorder in other diseases classified elsewhere with aggressive behavior
Major neurocognitive disorder in other diseases classified elsewhere with combative behavior
Major neurocognitive disorder in other diseases classified elsewhere with violent behavior
Use additional code, if applicable, to identify wandering in dementia in conditions classified elsewhere (Z91.83)

✓4th F03 Unspecified dementia

Presenile dementia NOS
Presenile psychosis NOS
Primary degenerative dementia NOS
Senile dementia NOS
Senile dementia depressed or paranoid type
Senile psychosis NOS

EXCLUDES 1 *senility NOS (R41.81)*

EXCLUDES 2 *mild memory disturbance due to known physiological condition (F06.8)*
senile dementia with delirium or acute confusional state (F05)

✓5th F03.9 Unspecified dementia

F03.90 Unspecified dementia without behavioral disturbance HIV HCC A

Dementia NOS
AHA: 2012,4Q,92

F03.91 Unspecified dementia with behavioral disturbance CC HCC A
Unspecified dementia with aggressive behavior
Unspecified dementia with combative behavior
Unspecified dementia with violent behavior
Use additional code, if applicable, to identify wandering in unspecified dementia (Z91.83)

F04 Amnestic disorder due to known physiological condition HCC
Korsakov's psychosis or syndrome, nonalcoholic
Code first the underlying physiological condition
EXCLUDES 1 *amnesia NOS (R41.3)*
anterograde amnesia (R41.1)
dissociative amnesia (F44.0)
retrograde amnesia (R41.2)
EXCLUDES 2 *alcohol-induced or unspecified Korsakov's syndrome (F10.26, F10.96)*
Korsakov's syndrome induced by other psychoactive substances (F13.26, F13.96, F19.16, F19.26, F19.96)

F05 Delirium due to known physiological condition CC
Acute or subacute brain syndrome
Acute or subacute confusional state (nonalcoholic)
Acute or subacute infective psychosis
Acute or subacute organic reaction
Acute or subacute psycho-organic syndrome
Delirium of mixed etiology
Delirium superimposed on dementia
Sundowning
Code first the underlying physiological condition
EXCLUDES 1 *delirium NOS (R41.0)*
EXCLUDES 2 *delirium tremens alcohol-induced or unspecified (F10.231, F10.921)*
AHA: 2019,2Q,34

✓4th **F06 Other mental disorders due to known physiological condition**
INCLUDES mental disorders due to endocrine disorder
mental disorders due to exogenous hormone
mental disorders due to exogenous toxic substance
mental disorders due to primary cerebral disease
mental disorders due to somatic illness
mental disorders due to systemic disease affecting the brain
Code first the underlying physiological condition
EXCLUDES 1 *unspecified dementia (F03)*
EXCLUDES 2 *delirium due to known physiological condition (F05)*
dementia as classified in F01-F02
other mental disorders associated with alcohol and other psychoactive substances (F10-F19)

F06.0 Psychotic disorder with hallucinations due to known physiological condition CC
Organic hallucinatory state (nonalcoholic)
EXCLUDES 2 *hallucinations and perceptual disturbance induced by alcohol and other psychoactive substances (F10-F19 with .151, .251, .951)*
schizophrenia (F20.-)

F06.1 Catatonic disorder due to known physiological condition
Catatonia associated with another mental disorder
Catatonia NOS
EXCLUDES 1 *catatonic stupor (R40.1)*
stupor NOS (R40.1)
EXCLUDES 2 *catatonic schizophrenia (F20.2)*
dissociative stupor (F44.2)
DEF: Catatonic: Abnormal neuropsychiatric state characterized by stupor, immobility or purposeless movements, or unresponsiveness in a person who otherwise appears awake.

F06.2 Psychotic disorder with delusions due to known physiological condition CC
Paranoid and paranoid-hallucinatory organic states
Schizophrenia-like psychosis in epilepsy
EXCLUDES 2 *alcohol and drug-induced psychotic disorder (F10-F19 with .150, .250, .950)*
brief psychotic disorder (F23)
delusional disorder (F22)
schizophrenia (F20.-)

✓5th **F06.3 Mood disorder due to known physiological condition**
EXCLUDES 2 *mood disorders due to alcohol and other psychoactive substances (F10-F19 with .14, .24, .94)*
mood disorders, not due to known physiological condition or unspecified (F30-F39)

F06.30 Mood disorder due to known physiological condition, unspecified

F06.31 Mood disorder due to known physiological condition with depressive features
Depressive disorder due to known physiological condition, with depressive features

F06.32 Mood disorder due to known physiological condition with major depressive-like episode
Depressive disorder due to known physiological condition, with major depressive-like episode

F06.33 Mood disorder due to known physiological condition with manic features
Bipolar and related disorder due to a known physiological condition, with manic features
Bipolar and related disorder due to known physiological condition, with manic- or hypomanic-like episodes

F06.34 Mood disorder due to known physiological condition with mixed features
Bipolar and related disorder due to known physiological condition, with mixed features
Depressive disorder due to known physiological condition, with mixed features

F06.4 Anxiety disorder due to known physiological condition
EXCLUDES 2 *anxiety disorders due to alcohol and other psychoactive substances (F10-F19 with .180, .280, .980)*
anxiety disorders, not due to known physiological condition or unspecified (F40.-, F41.-)

F06.8 Other specified mental disorders due to known physiological condition HIV
Epileptic psychosis NOS
Obsessive-compulsive and related disorder due to a known physiological condition
Organic dissociative disorder
Organic emotionally labile [asthenic] disorder

✓4th **F07 Personality and behavioral disorders due to known physiological condition**
Code first the underlying physiological condition

F07.0 Personality change due to known physiological condition
Frontal lobe syndrome
Limbic epilepsy personality syndrome
Lobotomy syndrome
Organic personality disorder
Organic pseudopsychopathic personality
Organic pseudoretarded personality
Postleucotomy syndrome
Code first underlying physiological condition
EXCLUDES 1 *mild cognitive impairment (G31.84)*
postconcussional syndrome (F07.81)
postencephalitic syndrome (F07.89)
signs and symptoms involving emotional state (R45.-)
EXCLUDES 2 *specific personality disorder (F60.-)*

✓5th **F07.8 Other personality and behavioral disorders due to known physiological condition**

F07.81 Postconcussional syndrome
Postcontusional syndrome (encephalopathy)
Post-traumatic brain syndrome, nonpsychotic
Use additional code to identify associated post-traumatic headache, if applicable (G44.3-)
EXCLUDES 1 *current concussion (brain) (S06.0-)*
postencephalitic syndrome (F07.89)
DEF: Concussion symptoms that persist for weeks or months after a head injury. These symptoms may include headache, giddiness, fatigue, insomnia, mood fluctuation, and a subjective feeling of impaired intellectual function with extreme reaction to normal stressors.

F07.89 Other personality and behavioral disorders due to known physiological condition
Postencephalitic syndrome
Right hemispheric organic affective disorder

FØ7.9 Unspecified personality and behavioral disorder due to known physiological condition HIV
Organic psychosyndrome

FØ9 Unspecified mental disorder due to known physiological condition HIV
Mental disorder NOS due to known physiological condition
Organic brain syndrome NOS
Organic mental disorder NOS
Organic psychosis NOS
Symptomatic psychosis NOS
Code first the underlying physiological condition
EXCLUDES 1 *psychosis NOS (F29)*

Mental and behavioral disorders due to psychoactive substance use (F1Ø-F19)

AHA: 2020,1Q,9; 2018,4Q,69-70; 2017,4Q,8; 2017,2Q,27

✓4th **F1Ø Alcohol related disorders**
Use additional code for blood alcohol level, if applicable (Y9Ø.-)
AHA: 2019,3Q,8

✓5th **F1Ø.1 Alcohol abuse**
EXCLUDES 1 *alcohol dependence (F1Ø.2-)*
alcohol use, unspecified (F1Ø.9-)
AHA: 2018,1Q,16; 2015,2Q,15
TIP: Alcohol withdrawal is classified to dependence only (F10.23-); there is no combination code for alcohol abuse with withdrawal. When alcohol abuse and alcohol withdrawal are documented for the same encounter, query the provider for clarification.
TIP: Assign when documentation indicates alcohol withdrawal without dependence; do not assign an additional code for withdrawal.

F1Ø.1Ø Alcohol abuse, uncomplicated
Alcohol use disorder, mild

F1Ø.11 Alcohol abuse, in remission
Alcohol use disorder, mild, in early remission
Alcohol use disorder, mild, in sustained remission

✓6th **F1Ø.12 Alcohol abuse with intoxication**
F1Ø.12Ø Alcohol abuse with intoxication, uncomplicated HCC
F1Ø.121 Alcohol abuse with intoxication delirium CC HCC
F1Ø.129 Alcohol abuse with intoxication, unspecified HCC

● ✓6th **F1Ø.13 Alcohol abuse, with withdrawal**
● **F1Ø.13Ø Alcohol abuse with withdrawal, uncomplicated** CC
● **F1Ø.131 Alcohol abuse with withdrawal delirium** CC
● **F1Ø.132 Alcohol abuse with withdrawal with perceptual disturbance** CC
● **F1Ø.139 Alcohol abuse with withdrawal, unspecified** CC

F1Ø.14 Alcohol abuse with alcohol-induced mood disorder CC HCC
Alcohol use disorder, mild, with alcohol-induced bipolar or related disorder
Alcohol use disorder, mild, with alcohol-induced depressive disorder

✓6th **F1Ø.15 Alcohol abuse with alcohol-induced psychotic disorder**
F1Ø.15Ø Alcohol abuse with alcohol-induced psychotic disorder with delusions HCC
F1Ø.151 Alcohol abuse with alcohol-induced psychotic disorder with hallucinations CC HCC
DEF: Psychosis lasting less than six months with slight or no clouding of consciousness in which auditory hallucinations predominate.
F1Ø.159 Alcohol abuse with alcohol-induced psychotic disorder, unspecified CC HCC

✓6th **F1Ø.18 Alcohol abuse with other alcohol-induced disorders**
F1Ø.18Ø Alcohol abuse with alcohol-induced anxiety disorder CC HCC
F1Ø.181 Alcohol abuse with alcohol-induced sexual dysfunction CC HCC
F1Ø.182 Alcohol abuse with alcohol-induced sleep disorder HCC
F1Ø.188 Alcohol abuse with other alcohol-induced disorder CC HCC

F1Ø.19 Alcohol abuse with unspecified alcohol-induced disorder CC HCC

✓5th **F1Ø.2 Alcohol dependence**
EXCLUDES 1 *alcohol abuse (F1Ø.1-)*
alcohol use, unspecified (F1Ø.9-)
EXCLUDES 2 *toxic effect of alcohol (T51.Ø-)*

F1Ø.2Ø Alcohol dependence, uncomplicated HCC
Alcohol use disorder, moderate
Alcohol use disorder, severe
AHA: 2020,1Q,9

F1Ø.21 Alcohol dependence, in remission HCC
Alcohol use disorder, moderate, in early remission
Alcohol use disorder, moderate, in sustained remission
Alcohol use disorder, severe, in early remission
Alcohol use disorder, severe, in sustained remission

✓6th **F1Ø.22 Alcohol dependence with intoxication**
Acute drunkenness (in alcoholism)
EXCLUDES 2 *alcohol dependence with withdrawal (F1Ø.23-)*
F1Ø.22Ø Alcohol dependence with intoxication, uncomplicated HCC
F1Ø.221 Alcohol dependence with intoxication delirium CC HCC
F1Ø.229 Alcohol dependence with intoxication, unspecified HCC

✓6th **F1Ø.23 Alcohol dependence with withdrawal**
EXCLUDES 2 *alcohol dependence with intoxication (F1Ø.22-)*
AHA: 2018,1Q,16; 2015,2Q,15
TIP: Do not assign a code from this subcategory when documentation indicates alcohol withdrawal without dependence.
F1Ø.23Ø Alcohol dependence with withdrawal, uncomplicated CC HCC
F1Ø.231 Alcohol dependence with withdrawal delirium CC HCC
F1Ø.232 Alcohol dependence with withdrawal with perceptual disturbance CC HCC
F1Ø.239 Alcohol dependence with withdrawal, unspecified CC HCC

F1Ø.24 Alcohol dependence with alcohol-induced mood disorder CC HCC
Alcohol use disorder, moderate, with alcohol-induced bipolar or related disorder
Alcohol use disorder, moderate, with alcohol-induced depressive disorder
Alcohol use disorder, severe, with alcohol-induced bipolar or related disorder
Alcohol use disorder, severe, with alcohol-induced depressive disorder

✓6th **F1Ø.25 Alcohol dependence with alcohol-induced psychotic disorder**
F1Ø.25Ø Alcohol dependence with alcohol-induced psychotic disorder with delusions HCC
F1Ø.251 Alcohol dependence with alcohol-induced psychotic disorder with hallucinations CC HCC
F1Ø.259 Alcohol dependence with alcohol-induced psychotic disorder, unspecified CC HCC

F1Ø.26 Alcohol dependence with alcohol-induced persisting amnestic disorder HCC
Alcohol use disorder, moderate, with alcohol-induced major neurocognitive disorder, amnestic-confabulatory type
Alcohol use disorder, severe, with alcohol-induced major neurocognitive disorder, amnestic-confabulatory type
DEF: Prominent and lasting reduced memory span and disordered time appreciation and confabulation that occurs in alcoholics as sequel to acute alcoholic psychosis.

F10.27 **Alcohol dependence with alcohol-induced persisting dementia** CC HCC
Alcohol use disorder, moderate, with alcohol-induced major neurocognitive disorder, nonamnestic-confabulatory type
Alcohol use disorder, severe, with alcohol-induced major neurocognitive disorder, nonamnestic-confabulatory type

✓6th F10.28 **Alcohol dependence with other alcohol-induced disorders**
F10.280 **Alcohol dependence with alcohol-induced anxiety disorder** CC HCC
F10.281 **Alcohol dependence with alcohol-induced sexual dysfunction** CC HCC
F10.282 **Alcohol dependence with alcohol-induced sleep disorder** HCC
F10.288 **Alcohol dependence with other alcohol-induced disorder** CC HCC
Alcohol use disorder, moderate, with alcohol-induced mild neurocognitive disorder
Alcohol use disorder, severe, with alcohol-induced mild neurocognitive disorder
AHA: 2020,1Q,9

F10.29 **Alcohol dependence with unspecified alcohol-induced disorder** CC HCC

✓5th F10.9 **Alcohol use, unspecified**
EXCLUDES 1 *alcohol abuse (F10.1-)*
alcohol dependence (F10.2-)
AHA: 2018,2Q,10-11
TIP: Assign a substance use code only when the provider documents a relationship between the use and an associated physical, mental, or behavioral disorder. As with all diagnoses, substance use codes must meet the definition of a reportable diagnosis.

✓6th F10.92 **Alcohol use, unspecified with intoxication**
F10.920 **Alcohol use, unspecified with intoxication, uncomplicated** HCC
AHA: 2018,2Q,10-11
F10.921 **Alcohol use, unspecified with intoxication delirium** CC HCC
F10.929 **Alcohol use, unspecified with intoxication, unspecified** HCC

● ✓6th F10.93 **Alcohol use, unspecified with withdrawal**
● F10.930 **Alcohol use, unspecified with withdrawal, uncomplicated** CC
● F10.931 **Alcohol use, unspecified with withdrawal delirium** CC
● F10.932 **Alcohol use, unspecified with withdrawal with perceptual disturbance** CC
● F10.939 **Alcohol use, unspecified with withdrawal, unspecified** CC

F10.94 **Alcohol use, unspecified with alcohol-induced mood disorder** CC HCC
Alcohol induced bipolar or related disorder, without use disorder
Alcohol induced depressive disorder, without use disorder

✓6th F10.95 **Alcohol use, unspecified with alcohol-induced psychotic disorder**
F10.950 **Alcohol use, unspecified with alcohol-induced psychotic disorder with delusions** HCC
F10.951 **Alcohol use, unspecified with alcohol-induced psychotic disorder with hallucinations** CC HCC
F10.959 **Alcohol use, unspecified with alcohol-induced psychotic disorder, unspecified** CC HCC
Alcohol-induced psychotic disorder without use disorder

F10.96 **Alcohol use, unspecified with alcohol-induced persisting amnestic disorder** HCC
Alcohol-induced major neurocognitive disorder, amnestic-confabulatory type, without use disorder

F10.97 **Alcohol use, unspecified with alcohol-induced persisting dementia** HCC
Alcohol-induced major neurocognitive disorder, nonamnestic-confabulatory type, without use disorder

✓6th F10.98 **Alcohol use, unspecified with other alcohol-induced disorders**
F10.980 **Alcohol use, unspecified with alcohol-induced anxiety disorder** CC HCC
Alcohol induced anxiety disorder, without use disorder
F10.981 **Alcohol use, unspecified with alcohol-induced sexual dysfunction** CC HCC
Alcohol induced sexual dysfunction, without use disorder
F10.982 **Alcohol use, unspecified with alcohol-induced sleep disorder** HCC
Alcohol induced sleep disorder, without use disorder
F10.988 **Alcohol use, unspecified with other alcohol-induced disorder** CC HCC
Alcohol induced mild neurocognitive disorder, without use disorder

F10.99 **Alcohol use, unspecified with unspecified alcohol-induced disorder** CC HCC

✓4th F11 Opioid related disorders

✓5th F11.1 **Opioid abuse**
EXCLUDES 1 *opioid dependence (F11.2-)*
opioid use, unspecified (F11.9-)

F11.10 **Opioid abuse, uncomplicated** HCC
Opioid use disorder, mild
F11.11 **Opioid abuse, in remission** HCC
Opioid use disorder, mild, in early remission
Opioid use disorder, mild, in sustained remission

✓6th F11.12 **Opioid abuse with intoxication**
F11.120 **Opioid abuse with intoxication, uncomplicated** HCC
F11.121 **Opioid abuse with intoxication delirium** CC HCC
F11.122 **Opioid abuse with intoxication with perceptual disturbance** HCC
F11.129 **Opioid abuse with intoxication, unspecified** HCC

● F11.13 **Opioid abuse with withdrawal** CC
F11.14 **Opioid abuse with opioid-induced mood disorder** HCC
Opioid use disorder, mild, with opioid-induced depressive disorder

✓6th F11.15 **Opioid abuse with opioid-induced psychotic disorder**
F11.150 **Opioid abuse with opioid-induced psychotic disorder with delusions** CC HCC
F11.151 **Opioid abuse with opioid-induced psychotic disorder with hallucinations** CC HCC
F11.159 **Opioid abuse with opioid-induced psychotic disorder, unspecified** HCC

✓6th F11.18 **Opioid abuse with other opioid-induced disorder**
F11.181 **Opioid abuse with opioid-induced sexual dysfunction** HCC
F11.182 **Opioid abuse with opioid-induced sleep disorder** HCC
F11.188 **Opioid abuse with other opioid-induced disorder** HCC

F11.19 **Opioid abuse with unspecified opioid-induced disorder** HCC

✓5th F11.2 **Opioid dependence**
EXCLUDES 1 *opioid abuse (F11.1-)*
opioid use, unspecified (F11.9-)
EXCLUDES 2 *opioid poisoning (T40.0-T40.2-)*

F11.20 **Opioid dependence, uncomplicated** CC HCC
Opioid use disorder, moderate
Opioid use disorder, severe

F11.21 **Opioid dependence, in remission** HCC
Opioid use disorder, moderate, in early remission
Opioid use disorder, moderate, in sustained remission
Opioid use disorder, severe, in early remission
Opioid use disorder, severe, in sustained remission

✓6th F11.22 **Opioid dependence with intoxication**
EXCLUDES 1 *opioid dependence with withdrawal (F11.23)*

F11.220 **Opioid dependence with intoxication, uncomplicated** HCC
F11.221 **Opioid dependence with intoxication delirium** CC HCC
F11.222 **Opioid dependence with intoxication with perceptual disturbance** CC HCC
F11.229 **Opioid dependence with intoxication, unspecified** HCC

F11.23 **Opioid dependence with withdrawal** CC HCC
EXCLUDES 1 *opioid dependence with intoxication (F11.22-)*

F11.24 **Opioid dependence with opioid-induced mood disorder** HCC
Opioid use disorder, moderate, with opioid induced depressive disorder

✓6th F11.25 **Opioid dependence with opioid-induced psychotic disorder**
F11.250 **Opioid dependence with opioid-induced psychotic disorder with delusions** CC HCC
F11.251 **Opioid dependence with opioid-induced psychotic disorder with hallucinations** CC HCC
F11.259 **Opioid dependence with opioid-induced psychotic disorder, unspecified** CC HCC

✓6th F11.28 **Opioid dependence with other opioid-induced disorder**
F11.281 **Opioid dependence with opioid-induced sexual dysfunction** CC HCC
F11.282 **Opioid dependence with opioid-induced sleep disorder** CC HCC
F11.288 **Opioid dependence with other opioid-induced disorder** CC HCC

F11.29 **Opioid dependence with unspecified opioid-induced disorder** HCC

✓5th F11.9 **Opioid use, unspecified**
EXCLUDES 1 *opioid abuse (F11.1-)*
opioid dependence (F11.2-)

TIP: Assign a substance use code only when the provider documents a relationship between the use and an associated physical, mental, or behavioral disorder. As with all diagnoses, substance use codes must meet the definition of a reportable diagnosis.

F11.90 **Opioid use, unspecified, uncomplicated**
AHA: 2018,2Q,10-11

✓6th F11.92 **Opioid use, unspecified with intoxication**
EXCLUDES 1 *opioid use, unspecified with withdrawal (F11.93)*

F11.920 **Opioid use, unspecified with intoxication, uncomplicated** HCC
F11.921 **Opioid use, unspecified with intoxication delirium** CC HCC
Opioid-induced delirium
F11.922 **Opioid use, unspecified with intoxication with perceptual disturbance** HCC
F11.929 **Opioid use, unspecified with intoxication, unspecified** HCC

F11.93 **Opioid use, unspecified with withdrawal** CC HCC
EXCLUDES 1 *opioid use, unspecified with intoxication (F11.92-)*

F11.94 **Opioid use, unspecified with opioid-induced mood disorder** HCC
Opioid induced depressive disorder, without use disorder

✓6th F11.95 **Opioid use, unspecified with opioid-induced psychotic disorder**
F11.950 **Opioid use, unspecified with opioid-induced psychotic disorder with delusions** CC HCC
F11.951 **Opioid use, unspecified with opioid-induced psychotic disorder with hallucinations** CC HCC
F11.959 **Opioid use, unspecified with opioid-induced psychotic disorder, unspecified** HCC

✓6th F11.98 **Opioid use, unspecified with other specified opioid-induced disorder**
F11.981 **Opioid use, unspecified with opioid-induced sexual dysfunction** HCC
Opioid induced sexual dysfunction, without use disorder
F11.982 **Opioid use, unspecified with opioid-induced sleep disorder** HCC
Opioid induced sleep disorder, without use disorder
F11.988 **Opioid use, unspecified with other opioid-induced disorder** HCC
Opioid induced anxiety disorder, without use disorder

F11.99 **Opioid use, unspecified with unspecified opioid-induced disorder** HCC

✓4th **F12 Cannabis related disorders**
INCLUDES marijuana
AHA: 2020,1Q,8

✓5th F12.1 **Cannabis abuse**
EXCLUDES 1 *cannabis dependence (F12.2-)*
cannabis use, unspecified (F12.9-)

F12.10 **Cannabis abuse, uncomplicated**
Cannabis use disorder, mild
F12.11 **Cannabis abuse, in remission**
Cannabis use disorder, mild, in early remission
Cannabis use disorder, mild, in sustained remission

✓6th F12.12 **Cannabis abuse with intoxication**
F12.120 **Cannabis abuse with intoxication, uncomplicated** HCC
F12.121 **Cannabis abuse with intoxication delirium** CC HCC
F12.122 **Cannabis abuse with intoxication with perceptual disturbance** HCC
F12.129 **Cannabis abuse with intoxication, unspecified** HCC

● F12.13 **Cannabis abuse with withdrawal**

✓6th F12.15 **Cannabis abuse with psychotic disorder**
F12.150 **Cannabis abuse with psychotic disorder with delusions** CC HCC
F12.151 **Cannabis abuse with psychotic disorder with hallucinations** CC HCC
F12.159 **Cannabis abuse with psychotic disorder, unspecified** HCC

✓6th F12.18 **Cannabis abuse with other cannabis-induced disorder**
F12.180 **Cannabis abuse with cannabis-induced anxiety disorder** HCC
F12.188 **Cannabis abuse with other cannabis-induced disorder** HCC
Cannabis use disorder, mild, with cannabis-induced sleep disorder

F12.19 **Cannabis abuse with unspecified cannabis-induced disorder** HCC

✓5th F12.2 **Cannabis dependence**
EXCLUDES 1 *cannabis abuse (F12.1-)*
cannabis use, unspecified (F12.9-)
EXCLUDES 2 *cannabis poisoning (T40.7-)*

F12.20 **Cannabis dependence, uncomplicated** HCC
Cannabis use disorder, moderate
Cannabis use disorder, severe
F12.21 **Cannabis dependence, in remission** HCC
Cannabis use disorder, moderate, in early remission
Cannabis use disorder, moderate, in sustained remission
Cannabis use disorder, severe, in early remission
Cannabis use disorder, severe, in sustained remission

✓6th F12.22 **Cannabis dependence with intoxication**
F12.220 **Cannabis dependence with intoxication, uncomplicated** HCC
F12.221 **Cannabis dependence with intoxication delirium** CC HCC
F12.222 **Cannabis dependence with intoxication with perceptual disturbance** HCC

F12.229 Cannabis dependence with intoxication, unspecified HCC

F12.23 Cannabis dependence with withdrawal HCC
AHA: 2018,4Q,7

✓6th **F12.25 Cannabis dependence with psychotic disorder**

F12.25Ø Cannabis dependence with psychotic disorder with delusions CC HCC

F12.251 Cannabis dependence with psychotic disorder with hallucinations CC HCC

F12.259 Cannabis dependence with psychotic disorder, unspecified HCC

✓6th **F12.28 Cannabis dependence with other cannabis-induced disorder**

F12.28Ø Cannabis dependence with cannabis-induced anxiety disorder HCC

F12.288 Cannabis dependence with other cannabis-induced disorder HCC
Cannabis use disorder, moderate, with cannabis-induced sleep disorder
Cannabis use disorder, severe, with cannabis-induced sleep disorder

F12.29 Cannabis dependence with unspecified cannabis-induced disorder HCC

✓5th **F12.9 Cannabis use, unspecified**
EXCLUDES 1 *cannabis abuse (F12.1-)*
cannabis dependence (F12.2-)
TIP: Assign a substance use code only when the provider documents a relationship between the use and an associated physical, mental, or behavioral disorder. As with all diagnoses, substance use codes must meet the definition of a reportable diagnosis.

F12.9Ø Cannabis use, unspecified, uncomplicated
AHA: 2018,2Q,10-11

✓6th **F12.92 Cannabis use, unspecified with intoxication**

F12.92Ø Cannabis use, unspecified with intoxication, uncomplicated HCC

F12.921 Cannabis use, unspecified with intoxication delirium CC HCC

F12.922 Cannabis use, unspecified with intoxication with perceptual disturbance HCC

F12.929 Cannabis use, unspecified with intoxication, unspecified HCC

F12.93 Cannabis use, unspecified with withdrawal HCC
AHA: 2018,4Q,7

✓6th **F12.95 Cannabis use, unspecified with psychotic disorder**

F12.95Ø Cannabis use, unspecified with psychotic disorder with delusions CC HCC

F12.951 Cannabis use, unspecified with psychotic disorder with hallucinations CC HCC

F12.959 Cannabis use, unspecified with psychotic disorder, unspecified HCC
Cannabis induced psychotic disorder, without use disorder

✓6th **F12.98 Cannabis use, unspecified with other cannabis-induced disorder**

F12.98Ø Cannabis use, unspecified with anxiety disorder HCC
Cannabis induced anxiety disorder, without use disorder

F12.988 Cannabis use, unspecified with other cannabis-induced disorder HCC
Cannabis induced sleep disorder, without use disorder

F12.99 Cannabis use, unspecified with unspecified cannabis-induced disorder HCC

✓4th **F13 Sedative, hypnotic, or anxiolytic related disorders**

✓5th **F13.1 Sedative, hypnotic or anxiolytic-related abuse**
EXCLUDES 1 *sedative, hypnotic or anxiolytic-related dependence (F13.2-)*
sedative, hypnotic, or anxiolytic use, unspecified (F13.9-)

F13.1Ø Sedative, hypnotic or anxiolytic abuse, uncomplicated HCC
Sedative, hypnotic, or anxiolytic use disorder, mild

F13.11 Sedative, hypnotic or anxiolytic abuse, in remission HCC
Sedative, hypnotic or anxiolytic use disorder, mild, in early remission
Sedative, hypnotic or anxiolytic use disorder, mild, in sustained remission

✓6th **F13.12 Sedative, hypnotic or anxiolytic abuse with intoxication**

F13.12Ø Sedative, hypnotic or anxiolytic abuse with intoxication, uncomplicated HCC

F13.121 Sedative, hypnotic or anxiolytic abuse with intoxication delirium CC HCC

F13.129 Sedative, hypnotic or anxiolytic abuse with intoxication, unspecified HCC

● ✓6th **F13.13 Sedative, hypnotic or anxiolytic abuse with withdrawal**

● **F13.13Ø Sedative, hypnotic or anxiolytic abuse with withdrawal, uncomplicated** CC

● **F13.131 Sedative, hypnotic or anxiolytic abuse with withdrawal delirium** CC

● **F13.132 Sedative, hypnotic or anxiolytic abuse with withdrawal with perceptual disturbance** CC

● **F13.139 Sedative, hypnotic or anxiolytic abuse with withdrawal, unspecified** CC

F13.14 Sedative, hypnotic or anxiolytic abuse with sedative, hypnotic or anxiolytic-induced mood disorder HCC
Sedative, hypnotic, or anxiolytic use disorder, mild, with sedative, hypnotic, or anxiolytic-induced bipolar or related disorder
Sedative, hypnotic, or anxiolytic use disorder, mild, with sedative, hypnotic, or anxiolytic-induced depressive disorder

✓6th **F13.15 Sedative, hypnotic or anxiolytic abuse with sedative, hypnotic or anxiolytic-induced psychotic disorder**

F13.15Ø Sedative, hypnotic or anxiolytic abuse with sedative, hypnotic or anxiolytic-induced psychotic disorder with delusions CC HCC

F13.151 Sedative, hypnotic or anxiolytic abuse with sedative, hypnotic or anxiolytic-induced psychotic disorder with hallucinations CC HCC

F13.159 Sedative, hypnotic or anxiolytic abuse with sedative, hypnotic or anxiolytic-induced psychotic disorder, unspecified HCC

✓6th **F13.18 Sedative, hypnotic or anxiolytic abuse with other sedative, hypnotic or anxiolytic-induced disorders**

F13.18Ø Sedative, hypnotic or anxiolytic abuse with sedative, hypnotic or anxiolytic-induced anxiety disorder HCC

F13.181 Sedative, hypnotic or anxiolytic abuse with sedative, hypnotic or anxiolytic-induced sexual dysfunction HCC

F13.182 Sedative, hypnotic or anxiolytic abuse with sedative, hypnotic or anxiolytic-induced sleep disorder HCC

F13.188 Sedative, hypnotic or anxiolytic abuse with other sedative, hypnotic or anxiolytic-induced disorder HCC

F13.19 Sedative, hypnotic or anxiolytic abuse with unspecified sedative, hypnotic or anxiolytic-induced disorder HCC

✓5th **F13.2 Sedative, hypnotic or anxiolytic-related dependence**
EXCLUDES 1 *sedative, hypnotic or anxiolytic-related abuse (F13.1-)*
sedative, hypnotic, or anxiolytic use, unspecified (F13.9-)
EXCLUDES 2 *sedative, hypnotic, or anxiolytic poisoning (T42.-)*

F13.2Ø Sedative, hypnotic or anxiolytic dependence, uncomplicated CC HCC

F13.21 Sedative, hypnotic or anxiolytic dependence, in remission HCC
Sedative, hypnotic or anxiolytic use disorder, moderate, in early remission
Sedative, hypnotic or anxiolytic use disorder, moderate, in sustained remission
Sedative, hypnotic or anxiolytic use disorder, severe, in early remission
Sedative, hypnotic or anxiolytic use disorder, severe, in sustained remission

√6th **F13.22 Sedative, hypnotic or anxiolytic dependence with intoxication**
EXCLUDES 1 *sedative, hypnotic or anxiolytic dependence with withdrawal (F13.23-)*

F13.220 Sedative, hypnotic or anxiolytic dependence with intoxication, uncomplicated HCC

F13.221 Sedative, hypnotic or anxiolytic dependence with intoxication delirium CC HCC

F13.229 Sedative, hypnotic or anxiolytic dependence with intoxication, unspecified HCC

√6th **F13.23 Sedative, hypnotic or anxiolytic dependence with withdrawal**
Sedative, hypnotic, or anxiolytic use disorder, moderate
Sedative, hypnotic, or anxiolytic use disorder, severe
EXCLUDES 1 *sedative, hypnotic or anxiolytic dependence with intoxication (F13.22-)*

F13.230 Sedative, hypnotic or anxiolytic dependence with withdrawal, uncomplicated CC HCC

F13.231 Sedative, hypnotic or anxiolytic dependence with withdrawal delirium CC HCC

F13.232 Sedative, hypnotic or anxiolytic dependence with withdrawal with perceptual disturbance CC HCC
Sedative, hypnotic, or anxiolytic withdrawal with perceptual disturbances

F13.239 Sedative, hypnotic or anxiolytic dependence with withdrawal, unspecified CC HCC
Sedative, hypnotic, or anxiolytic withdrawal without perceptual disturbances

F13.24 Sedative, hypnotic or anxiolytic dependence with sedative, hypnotic or anxiolytic-induced mood disorder HCC
Sedative, hypnotic, or anxiolytic use disorder, moderate, with sedative, hypnotic, or anxiolytic-induced bipolar or related disorder
Sedative, hypnotic, or anxiolytic use disorder, moderate, with sedative, hypnotic, or anxiolytic-induced depressive disorder
Sedative, hypnotic, or anxiolytic use disorder, severe, with sedative, hypnotic, or anxiolytic-induced bipolar or related disorder
Sedative, hypnotic, or anxiolytic use disorder, severe, with sedative, hypnotic, or anxiolytic-induced depressive disorder

√6th **F13.25 Sedative, hypnotic or anxiolytic dependence with sedative, hypnotic or anxiolytic-induced psychotic disorder**

F13.250 Sedative, hypnotic or anxiolytic dependence with sedative, hypnotic or anxiolytic-induced psychotic disorder with delusions CC HCC

F13.251 Sedative, hypnotic or anxiolytic dependence with sedative, hypnotic or anxiolytic-induced psychotic disorder with hallucinations CC HCC

F13.259 Sedative, hypnotic or anxiolytic dependence with sedative, hypnotic or anxiolytic-induced psychotic disorder, unspecified CC HCC

F13.26 Sedative, hypnotic or anxiolytic dependence with sedative, hypnotic or anxiolytic-induced persisting amnestic disorder CC HCC

F13.27 Sedative, hypnotic or anxiolytic dependence with sedative, hypnotic or anxiolytic-induced persisting dementia CC HCC
Sedative, hypnotic, or anxiolytic use disorder, moderate, with sedative, hypnotic, or anxiolytic induced major neurocognitive disorder
Sedative, hypnotic, or anxiolytic use disorder, severe, with sedative, hypnotic, or anxiolytic-induced major neurocognitive disorder

√6th **F13.28 Sedative, hypnotic or anxiolytic dependence with other sedative, hypnotic or anxiolytic-induced disorders**

F13.280 Sedative, hypnotic or anxiolytic dependence with sedative, hypnotic or anxiolytic-induced anxiety disorder CC HCC

F13.281 Sedative, hypnotic or anxiolytic dependence with sedative, hypnotic or anxiolytic-induced sexual dysfunction CC HCC

F13.282 Sedative, hypnotic or anxiolytic dependence with sedative, hypnotic or anxiolytic-induced sleep disorder CC HCC

F13.288 Sedative, hypnotic or anxiolytic dependence with other sedative, hypnotic or anxiolytic-induced disorder CC HCC
Sedative, hypnotic, or anxiolytic use disorder, moderate, with sedative, hypnotic, or anxiolytic-induced mild neurocognitive disorder
Sedative, hypnotic, or anxiolytic use disorder, severe, with sedative, hypnotic, or anxiolytic-induced mild neurocognitive disorder

F13.29 Sedative, hypnotic or anxiolytic dependence with unspecified sedative, hypnotic or anxiolytic-induced disorder HCC

√5th **F13.9 Sedative, hypnotic or anxiolytic-related use, unspecified**
EXCLUDES 1 *sedative, hypnotic or anxiolytic-related abuse (F13.1-)*
sedative, hypnotic or anxiolytic-related dependence (F13.2-)

TIP: Assign a substance use code only when the provider documents a relationship between the use and an associated physical, mental, or behavioral disorder. As with all diagnoses, substance use codes must meet the definition of a reportable diagnosis.

F13.90 Sedative, hypnotic, or anxiolytic use, unspecified, uncomplicated
AHA: 2018,2Q,10-11

√6th **F13.92 Sedative, hypnotic or anxiolytic use, unspecified with intoxication**
EXCLUDES 1 *sedative, hypnotic or anxiolytic use, unspecified with withdrawal (F13.93-)*

F13.920 Sedative, hypnotic or anxiolytic use, unspecified with intoxication, uncomplicated HCC

F13.921 Sedative, hypnotic or anxiolytic use, unspecified with intoxication delirium CC HCC
Sedative, hypnotic, or anxiolytic-induced delirium

F13.929 Sedative, hypnotic or anxiolytic use, unspecified with intoxication, unspecified HCC

√6th **F13.93 Sedative, hypnotic or anxiolytic use, unspecified with withdrawal**
EXCLUDES 1 *sedative, hypnotic or anxiolytic use, unspecified with intoxication (F13.92-)*

F13.930 Sedative, hypnotic or anxiolytic use, unspecified with withdrawal, uncomplicated CC HCC

F13.931 Sedative, hypnotic or anxiolytic use, unspecified with withdrawal delirium CC HCC

F13.932 **Sedative, hypnotic or anxiolytic use, unspecified with withdrawal with perceptual disturbances** CC HCC

F13.939 **Sedative, hypnotic or anxiolytic use, unspecified with withdrawal, unspecified** CC HCC

F13.94 **Sedative, hypnotic or anxiolytic use, unspecified with sedative, hypnotic or anxiolytic-induced mood disorder** HCC
Sedative, hypnotic, or anxiolytic-induced bipolar or related disorder, without use disorder
Sedative, hypnotic, or anxiolytic-induced depressive disorder, without use disorder

✓6th F13.95 **Sedative, hypnotic or anxiolytic use, unspecified with sedative, hypnotic or anxiolytic-induced psychotic disorder**

F13.95Ø **Sedative, hypnotic or anxiolytic use, unspecified with sedative, hypnotic or anxiolytic-induced psychotic disorder with delusions** CC HCC

F13.951 **Sedative, hypnotic or anxiolytic use, unspecified with sedative, hypnotic or anxiolytic-induced psychotic disorder with hallucinations** CC HCC

F13.959 **Sedative, hypnotic or anxiolytic use, unspecified with sedative, hypnotic or anxiolytic-induced psychotic disorder, unspecified** HCC
Sedative, hypnotic, or anxiolytic-induced psychotic disorder, without use disorder

F13.96 **Sedative, hypnotic or anxiolytic use, unspecified with sedative, hypnotic or anxiolytic-induced persisting amnestic disorder** HCC

F13.97 **Sedative, hypnotic or anxiolytic use, unspecified with sedative, hypnotic or anxiolytic-induced persisting dementia** CC HCC
Sedative, hypnotic, or anxiolytic-induced major neurocognitive disorder, without use disorder

✓6th F13.98 **Sedative, hypnotic or anxiolytic use, unspecified with other sedative, hypnotic or anxiolytic-induced disorders**

F13.98Ø **Sedative, hypnotic or anxiolytic use, unspecified with sedative, hypnotic or anxiolytic-induced anxiety disorder** HCC
Sedative, hypnotic, or anxiolytic-induced anxiety disorder, without use disorder

F13.981 **Sedative, hypnotic or anxiolytic use, unspecified with sedative, hypnotic or anxiolytic-induced sexual dysfunction** HCC
Sedative, hypnotic, or anxiolytic-induced sexual dysfunction disorder, without use disorder

F13.982 **Sedative, hypnotic or anxiolytic use, unspecified with sedative, hypnotic or anxiolytic-induced sleep disorder** HCC
Sedative, hypnotic, or anxiolytic-induced sleep disorder, without use disorder

F13.988 **Sedative, hypnotic or anxiolytic use, unspecified with other sedative, hypnotic or anxiolytic-induced disorder** HCC
Sedative, hypnotic, or anxiolytic-induced mild neurocognitive disorder

F13.99 **Sedative, hypnotic or anxiolytic use, unspecified with unspecified sedative, hypnotic or anxiolytic-induced disorder** HCC

✓4th **F14 Cocaine related disorders**

EXCLUDES 2 *other stimulant-related disorders (F15.-)*

✓5th **F14.1 Cocaine abuse**

EXCLUDES 1 *cocaine dependence (F14.2-)*
cocaine use, unspecified (F14.9-)

F14.1Ø **Cocaine abuse, uncomplicated** HCC
Cocaine use disorder, mild

F14.11 **Cocaine abuse, in remission** HCC
Cocaine use disorder, mild, in early remission
Cocaine use disorder, mild, in sustained remission

✓6th F14.12 **Cocaine abuse with intoxication**

F14.12Ø **Cocaine abuse with intoxication, uncomplicated** HCC

F14.121 **Cocaine abuse with intoxication with delirium** CC HCC

F14.122 **Cocaine abuse with intoxication with perceptual disturbance** HCC

F14.129 **Cocaine abuse with intoxication, unspecified** HCC

● F14.13 **Cocaine abuse, unspecified with withdrawal** CC

F14.14 **Cocaine abuse with cocaine-induced mood disorder** HCC
Cocaine use disorder, mild, with cocaine-induced bipolar or related disorder
Cocaine use disorder, mild, with cocaine-induced depressive disorder

✓6th F14.15 **Cocaine abuse with cocaine-induced psychotic disorder**

F14.15Ø **Cocaine abuse with cocaine-induced psychotic disorder with delusions** CC HCC

F14.151 **Cocaine abuse with cocaine-induced psychotic disorder with hallucinations** CC HCC

F14.159 **Cocaine abuse with cocaine-induced psychotic disorder, unspecified** HCC

✓6th F14.18 **Cocaine abuse with other cocaine-induced disorder**

F14.18Ø **Cocaine abuse with cocaine-induced anxiety disorder** HCC

F14.181 **Cocaine abuse with cocaine-induced sexual dysfunction** HCC

F14.182 **Cocaine abuse with cocaine-induced sleep disorder** HCC

F14.188 **Cocaine abuse with other cocaine-induced disorder** HCC
Cocaine use disorder, mild, with cocaine-induced obsessive compulsive or related disorder

F14.19 **Cocaine abuse with unspecified cocaine-induced disorder** HCC

✓5th **F14.2 Cocaine dependence**

EXCLUDES 1 *cocaine abuse (F14.1-)*
cocaine use, unspecified (F14.9-)

EXCLUDES 2 *cocaine poisoning (T4Ø.5-)*

F14.2Ø **Cocaine dependence, uncomplicated** CC HCC
Cocaine use disorder, moderate
Cocaine use disorder, severe

F14.21 **Cocaine dependence, in remission** HCC
Cocaine use disorder, moderate, in early remission
Cocaine use disorder, moderate, in sustained remission
Cocaine use disorder, severe, in early remission
Cocaine use disorder, severe, in sustained remission

✓6th F14.22 **Cocaine dependence with intoxication**

EXCLUDES 1 *cocaine dependence with withdrawal (F14.23)*

F14.22Ø **Cocaine dependence with intoxication, uncomplicated** HCC

F14.221 **Cocaine dependence with intoxication delirium** CC HCC

F14.222 **Cocaine dependence with intoxication with perceptual disturbance** CC HCC

F14.229 **Cocaine dependence with intoxication, unspecified** CC HCC

F14.23 **Cocaine dependence with withdrawal** CC HCC

EXCLUDES 1 *cocaine dependence with intoxication (F14.22-)*

F14.24 **Cocaine dependence with cocaine-induced mood disorder** HCC
Cocaine use disorder, moderate, with cocaine-induced bipolar or related disorder
Cocaine use disorder, moderate, with cocaine-induced depressive disorder
Cocaine use disorder, severe, with cocaine-induced bipolar or related disorder
Cocaine use disorder, severe, with cocaine-induced depressive disorder

✓6th F14.25 **Cocaine dependence with cocaine-induced psychotic disorder**

F14.25Ø **Cocaine dependence with cocaine-induced psychotic disorder with delusions** CC HCC

F14.251 Cocaine dependence with cocaine-induced psychotic disorder with hallucinations CC HCC

F14.259 Cocaine dependence with cocaine-induced psychotic disorder, unspecified CC HCC

✓6th **F14.28 Cocaine dependence with other cocaine-induced disorder**

F14.280 Cocaine dependence with cocaine-induced anxiety disorder CC HCC

F14.281 Cocaine dependence with cocaine-induced sexual dysfunction CC HCC

F14.282 Cocaine dependence with cocaine-induced sleep disorder CC HCC

F14.288 Cocaine dependence with other cocaine-induced disorder CC HCC

Cocaine use disorder, moderate, with cocaine-induced obsessive compulsive or related disorder

Cocaine use disorder, severe, with cocaine-induced obsessive compulsive or related disorder

F14.29 Cocaine dependence with unspecified cocaine-induced disorder HCC

✓5th **F14.9 Cocaine use, unspecified**

EXCLUDES 1 *cocaine abuse (F14.1-)*
cocaine dependence (F14.2-)

TIP: Assign a substance use code only when the provider documents a relationship between the use and an associated physical, mental, or behavioral disorder. As with all diagnoses, substance use codes must meet the definition of a reportable diagnosis.

F14.90 Cocaine use, unspecified, uncomplicated

AHA: 2018,2Q,10-11

✓6th **F14.92 Cocaine use, unspecified with intoxication**

F14.920 Cocaine use, unspecified with intoxication, uncomplicated HCC

F14.921 Cocaine use, unspecified with intoxication delirium CC HCC

F14.922 Cocaine use, unspecified with intoxication with perceptual disturbance HCC

F14.929 Cocaine use, unspecified with intoxication, unspecified HCC

● **F14.93 Cocaine use, unspecified with withdrawal** CC

F14.94 Cocaine use, unspecified with cocaine-induced mood disorder HCC

Cocaine induced bipolar or related disorder, without use disorder

Cocaine induced depressive disorder, without use disorder

✓6th **F14.95 Cocaine use, unspecified with cocaine-induced psychotic disorder**

F14.950 Cocaine use, unspecified with cocaine-induced psychotic disorder with delusions CC HCC

F14.951 Cocaine use, unspecified with cocaine-induced psychotic disorder with hallucinations CC HCC

F14.959 Cocaine use, unspecified with cocaine-induced psychotic disorder, unspecified HCC

Cocaine induced psychotic disorder, without use disorder

✓6th **F14.98 Cocaine use, unspecified with other specified cocaine-induced disorder**

F14.980 Cocaine use, unspecified with cocaine-induced anxiety disorder HCC

Cocaine induced anxiety disorder, without use disorder

F14.981 Cocaine use, unspecified with cocaine-induced sexual dysfunction HCC

Cocaine induced sexual dysfunction, without use disorder

F14.982 Cocaine use, unspecified with cocaine-induced sleep disorder HCC

Cocaine induced sleep disorder, without use disorder

F14.988 Cocaine use, unspecified with other cocaine-induced disorder HCC

Cocaine induced obsessive compulsive or related disorder

F14.99 Cocaine use, unspecified with unspecified cocaine-induced disorder HCC

✓4th **F15 Other stimulant related disorders**

INCLUDES amphetamine-related disorders
caffeine

EXCLUDES 2 *cocaine-related disorders (F14.-)*

✓5th **F15.1 Other stimulant abuse**

EXCLUDES 1 *other stimulant dependence (F15.2-)*
other stimulant use, unspecified (F15.9-)

F15.10 Other stimulant abuse, uncomplicated HCC

Amphetamine type substance use disorder, mild

Other or unspecified stimulant use disorder, mild

F15.11 Other stimulant abuse, in remission HCC

Amphetamine type substance use disorder, mild, in early remission

Amphetamine type substance use disorder, mild, in sustained remission

Other or unspecified stimulant use disorder, mild, in early remission

Other or unspecified stimulant use disorder, mild, in sustained remission

✓6th **F15.12 Other stimulant abuse with intoxication**

F15.120 Other stimulant abuse with intoxication, uncomplicated HCC

F15.121 Other stimulant abuse with intoxication delirium CC HCC

F15.122 Other stimulant abuse with intoxication with perceptual disturbance HCC

Amphetamine or other stimulant use disorder, mild, with amphetamine or other stimulant intoxication, with perceptual disturbances

F15.129 Other stimulant abuse with intoxication, unspecified HCC

Amphetamine or other stimulant use disorder, mild, with amphetamine or other stimulant intoxication, without perceptual disturbances

● **F15.13 Other stimulant abuse with withdrawal** CC

F15.14 Other stimulant abuse with stimulant-induced mood disorder HCC

Amphetamine or other stimulant use disorder, mild, with amphetamine or other stimulant induced bipolar or related disorder

Amphetamine or other stimulant use disorder, mild, with amphetamine or other stimulant induced depressive disorder

✓6th **F15.15 Other stimulant abuse with stimulant-induced psychotic disorder**

F15.150 Other stimulant abuse with stimulant-induced psychotic disorder with delusions CC HCC

F15.151 Other stimulant abuse with stimulant-induced psychotic disorder with hallucinations CC HCC

F15.159 Other stimulant abuse with stimulant-induced psychotic disorder, unspecified HCC

✓6th **F15.18 Other stimulant abuse with other stimulant-induced disorder**

F15.180 Other stimulant abuse with stimulant-induced anxiety disorder HCC

F15.181 Other stimulant abuse with stimulant-induced sexual dysfunction HCC

F15.182 Other stimulant abuse with stimulant-induced sleep disorder HCC

F15.188 **Other stimulant abuse with other stimulant-induced disorder** HCC
Amphetamine or other stimulant use disorder, mild, with amphetamine or other stimulant induced obsessive-compulsive or related disorder

F15.19 **Other stimulant abuse with unspecified stimulant-induced disorder** HCC

✓5th F15.2 **Other stimulant dependence**
EXCLUDES 1 *other stimulant abuse (F15.1-)*
other stimulant use, unspecified (F15.9-)

F15.20 **Other stimulant dependence, uncomplicated** CC HCC
Amphetamine type substance use disorder, moderate
Amphetamine type substance use disorder, severe
Other or unspecified stimulant use disorder, moderate
Other or unspecified stimulant use disorder, severe

F15.21 **Other stimulant dependence, in remission** HCC
Amphetamine type substance use disorder, moderate, in early remission
Amphetamine type substance use disorder, moderate, in sustained remission
Amphetamine type substance use disorder, severe, in early remission
Amphetamine type substance use disorder, severe, in sustained remission
Other or unspecified stimulant use disorder, moderate, in early remission
Other or unspecified stimulant use disorder, moderate, in sustained remission
Other or unspecified stimulant use disorder, severe, in early remission
Other or unspecified stimulant use disorder, severe, in sustained remission

✓6th F15.22 **Other stimulant dependence with intoxication**
EXCLUDES 1 *other stimulant dependence with withdrawal (F15.23)*

F15.220 **Other stimulant dependence with intoxication, uncomplicated** HCC

F15.221 **Other stimulant dependence with intoxication delirium** CC HCC

F15.222 **Other stimulant dependence with intoxication with perceptual disturbance** CC HCC
Amphetamine or other stimulant use disorder, moderate, with amphetamine or other stimulant intoxication, with perceptual disturbances
Amphetamine or other stimulant use disorder, severe, with amphetamine or other stimulant intoxication, with perceptual disturbances

F15.229 **Other stimulant dependence with intoxication, unspecified** HCC
Amphetamine or other stimulant use disorder, moderate, with amphetamine or other stimulant intoxication, without perceptual disturbances
Amphetamine or other stimulant use disorder, severe, with amphetamine or other stimulant intoxication, without perceptual disturbances

F15.23 **Other stimulant dependence with withdrawal** CC HCC
Amphetamine or other stimulant withdrawal
EXCLUDES 1 *other stimulant dependence with intoxication (F15.22-)*

F15.24 **Other stimulant dependence with stimulant-induced mood disorder** HCC
Amphetamine or other stimulant use disorder, moderate, with amphetamine or other stimulant-induced bipolar or related disorder
Amphetamine or other stimulant use disorder, moderate, with amphetamine or other stimulant induced depressive disorder
Amphetamine or other stimulant use disorder, severe, with amphetamine or other stimulant-induced bipolar or related disorder
Amphetamine or other stimulant use disorder, severe, with amphetamine or other stimulant-induced depressive disorder

✓6th F15.25 **Other stimulant dependence with stimulant-induced psychotic disorder**

F15.250 **Other stimulant dependence with stimulant-induced psychotic disorder with delusions** CC HCC

F15.251 **Other stimulant dependence with stimulant-induced psychotic disorder with hallucinations** CC HCC

F15.259 **Other stimulant dependence with stimulant-induced psychotic disorder, unspecified** CC HCC

✓6th F15.28 **Other stimulant dependence with other stimulant-induced disorder**

F15.280 **Other stimulant dependence with stimulant-induced anxiety disorder** CC HCC

F15.281 **Other stimulant dependence with stimulant-induced sexual dysfunction** CC HCC

F15.282 **Other stimulant dependence with stimulant-induced sleep disorder** CC HCC

F15.288 **Other stimulant dependence with other stimulant-induced disorder** CC HCC
Amphetamine or other stimulant use disorder, moderate, with amphetamine orother stimulant induced obsessive compulsive or related disorder
Amphetamine or other stimulant use disorder, severe, with amphetamine or otherstimulant induced obsessive compulsive or related disorder

F15.29 **Other stimulant dependence with unspecified stimulant-induced disorder** HCC

✓5th F15.9 **Other stimulant use, unspecified**
EXCLUDES 1 *other stimulant abuse (F15.1-)*
other stimulant dependence (F15.2-)

TIP: Assign a substance use code only when the provider documents a relationship between the use and an associated physical, mental, or behavioral disorder. As with all diagnoses, substance use codes must meet the definition of a reportable diagnosis.

F15.90 **Other stimulant use, unspecified, uncomplicated**
AHA: 2018,2Q,10-11

✓6th F15.92 **Other stimulant use, unspecified with intoxication**
EXCLUDES 1 *other stimulant use, unspecified with withdrawal (F15.93)*

F15.920 **Other stimulant use, unspecified with intoxication, uncomplicated** HCC

F15.921 **Other stimulant use, unspecified with intoxication delirium** CC HCC
Amphetamine or other stimulant-induced delirium

F15.922 **Other stimulant use, unspecified with intoxication with perceptual disturbance** HCC

F15.929 **Other stimulant use, unspecified with intoxication, unspecified** HCC
Caffeine intoxication

F15.93 **Other stimulant use, unspecified with withdrawal** CC HCC
Caffeine withdrawal
EXCLUDES 1 *other stimulant use, unspecified with intoxication (F15.92-)*

F15.94 **Other stimulant use, unspecified with stimulant-induced mood disorder** HCC
Amphetamine or other stimulant-induced bipolar or related disorder, without use disorder
Amphetamine or other stimulant-induced depressive disorder, without use disorder

✓6th F15.95 **Other stimulant use, unspecified with stimulant-induced psychotic disorder**

F15.950 **Other stimulant use, unspecified with stimulant-induced psychotic disorder with delusions** CC HCC

F15.951 **Other stimulant use, unspecified with stimulant-induced psychotic disorder with hallucinations** CC HCC

F15.959 **Other stimulant use, unspecified with stimulant-induced psychotic disorder, unspecified** HCC
Amphetamine or other stimulant-induced psychotic disorder, without use disorder

✓6th F15.98 **Other stimulant use, unspecified with other stimulant-induced disorder**

F15.980 **Other stimulant use, unspecified with stimulant-induced anxiety disorder** HCC
Amphetamine or other stimulant-induced anxiety disorder, without use disorder
Caffeine induced anxiety disorder, without use disorder

F15.981 **Other stimulant use, unspecified with stimulant-induced sexual dysfunction** HCC
Amphetamine or other stimulant-induced sexual dysfunction, without use disorder

F15.982 **Other stimulant use, unspecified with stimulant-induced sleep disorder** HCC
Amphetamine or other stimulant-induced sleep disorder, without use disorder
Caffeine induced sleep disorder, without use disorder

F15.988 **Other stimulant use, unspecified with other stimulant-induced disorder** HCC
Amphetamine or other stimulant-induced obsessive compulsive or related disorder, without use disorder

F15.99 **Other stimulant use, unspecified with unspecified stimulant-induced disorder** HCC

✓4th **F16 Hallucinogen related disorders**

INCLUDES ecstasy
PCP
phencyclidine

AHA: 2018,4Q,31

✓5th F16.1 **Hallucinogen abuse**

EXCLUDES 1 *hallucinogen dependence (F16.2-)*
hallucinogen use, unspecified (F16.9-)

F16.10 **Hallucinogen abuse, uncomplicated** HCC
Other hallucinogen use disorder, mild
Phencyclidine use disorder, mild

F16.11 **Hallucinogen abuse, in remission** HCC
Other hallucinogen use disorder, mild, in early remission
Other hallucinogen use disorder, mild, in sustained remission
Phencyclidine use disorder, mild, in early remission
Phencyclidine use disorder, mild, in sustained remission

✓6th F16.12 **Hallucinogen abuse with intoxication**

F16.120 **Hallucinogen abuse with intoxication, uncomplicated** HCC

F16.121 **Hallucinogen abuse with intoxication with delirium** CC HCC

F16.122 **Hallucinogen abuse with intoxication with perceptual disturbance** HCC

F16.129 **Hallucinogen abuse with intoxication, unspecified** HCC

F16.14 **Hallucinogen abuse with hallucinogen-induced mood disorder** HCC
Other hallucinogen use disorder, mild, with other hallucinogen induced bipolar or related disorder
Other hallucinogen use disorder, mild, with other hallucinogen induced depressive disorder
Phencyclidine use disorder, mild, with phencyclidine induced bipolar or related disorder
Phencyclidine use disorder, mild, with phencyclidine induced depressive disorder

✓6th F16.15 **Hallucinogen abuse with hallucinogen-induced psychotic disorder**

F16.150 **Hallucinogen abuse with hallucinogen-induced psychotic disorder with delusions** CC HCC

F16.151 **Hallucinogen abuse with hallucinogen-induced psychotic disorder with hallucinations** CC HCC

F16.159 **Hallucinogen abuse with hallucinogen-induced psychotic disorder, unspecified** HCC

✓6th F16.18 **Hallucinogen abuse with other hallucinogen-induced disorder**

F16.180 **Hallucinogen abuse with hallucinogen-induced anxiety disorder** HCC

F16.183 **Hallucinogen abuse with hallucinogen persisting perception disorder (flashbacks)** HCC

F16.188 **Hallucinogen abuse with other hallucinogen-induced disorder** HCC

F16.19 **Hallucinogen abuse with unspecified hallucinogen-induced disorder** HCC

✓5th F16.2 **Hallucinogen dependence**

EXCLUDES 1 *hallucinogen abuse (F16.1-)*
hallucinogen use, unspecified (F16.9-)

F16.20 **Hallucinogen dependence, uncomplicated** CC HCC
Other hallucinogen use disorder, moderate
Other hallucinogen use disorder, severe
Phencyclidine use disorder, moderate
Phencyclidine use disorder, severe

F16.21 **Hallucinogen dependence, in remission** HCC
Other hallucinogen use disorder, moderate, in early remission
Other hallucinogen use disorder, moderate, in sustained remission
Other hallucinogen use disorder, severe, in early remission
Other hallucinogen use disorder, severe, in sustained remission
Phencyclidine use disorder, moderate, in early remission
Phencyclidine use disorder, moderate, in sustained remission
Phencyclidine use disorder, severe, in early remission
Phencyclidine use disorder, severe, in sustained remission

✓6th F16.22 **Hallucinogen dependence with intoxication**

F16.220 **Hallucinogen dependence with intoxication, uncomplicated** HCC

F16.221 **Hallucinogen dependence with intoxication with delirium** CC HCC

F16.229 **Hallucinogen dependence with intoxication, unspecified** HCC

F16.24 Hallucinogen dependence with hallucinogen-induced mood disorder HCC
- Other hallucinogen use disorder, moderate, with other hallucinogen induced bipolar or related disorder
- Other hallucinogen use disorder, moderate, with other hallucinogen induced depressive disorder
- Other hallucinogen use disorder, severe, with other hallucinogen-induced bipolar or related disorder
- Other hallucinogen use disorder, severe, with other hallucinogen-induced depressive disorder
- Phencyclidine use disorder, moderate, with phencyclidine induced bipolar or related disorder
- Phencyclidine use disorder, moderate, with phencyclidine induced depressive disorder
- Phencyclidine use disorder, severe, with phencyclidine induced bipolar or related disorder
- Phencyclidine use disorder, severe, with phencyclidine-induced depressive disorder

√6th **F16.25 Hallucinogen dependence with hallucinogen-induced psychotic disorder**

F16.250 Hallucinogen dependence with hallucinogen-induced psychotic disorder with delusions CC HCC

F16.251 Hallucinogen dependence with hallucinogen-induced psychotic disorder with hallucinations CC HCC

F16.259 Hallucinogen dependence with hallucinogen-induced psychotic disorder, unspecified CC HCC

√6th **F16.28 Hallucinogen dependence with other hallucinogen-induced disorder**

F16.280 Hallucinogen dependence with hallucinogen-induced anxiety disorder CC HCC

F16.283 Hallucinogen dependence with hallucinogen persisting perception disorder (flashbacks) CC HCC

F16.288 Hallucinogen dependence with other hallucinogen-induced disorder CC HCC

F16.29 Hallucinogen dependence with unspecified hallucinogen-induced disorder HCC

√5th **F16.9 Hallucinogen use, unspecified**

EXCLUDES 1 *hallucinogen abuse (F16.1-)*
hallucinogen dependence (F16.2-)

TIP: Assign a substance use code only when the provider documents a relationship between the use and an associated physical, mental, or behavioral disorder. As with all diagnoses, substance use codes must meet the definition of a reportable diagnosis.

F16.90 Hallucinogen use, unspecified, uncomplicated
AHA: 2018,2Q,10-11

√6th **F16.92 Hallucinogen use, unspecified with intoxication**

F16.920 Hallucinogen use, unspecified with intoxication, uncomplicated HCC

F16.921 Hallucinogen use, unspecified with intoxication with delirium CC HCC
- Other hallucinogen intoxication delirium

F16.929 Hallucinogen use, unspecified with intoxication, unspecified HCC

F16.94 Hallucinogen use, unspecified with hallucinogen-induced mood disorder HCC
- Other hallucinogen induced bipolar or related disorder, without use disorder
- Other hallucinogen induced depressive disorder, without use disorder
- Phencyclidine induced bipolar or related disorder, without use disorder
- Phencyclidine induced depressive disorder, without use disorder

√6th **F16.95 Hallucinogen use, unspecified with hallucinogen-induced psychotic disorder**

F16.950 Hallucinogen use, unspecified with hallucinogen-induced psychotic disorder with delusions CC HCC

F16.951 Hallucinogen use, unspecified with hallucinogen-induced psychotic disorder with hallucinations CC HCC

F16.959 Hallucinogen use, unspecified with hallucinogen-induced psychotic disorder, unspecified HCC
- Other hallucinogen induced psychotic disorder, without use disorder
- Phencyclidine induced psychotic disorder, without use disorder

√6th **F16.98 Hallucinogen use, unspecified with other specified hallucinogen-induced disorder**

F16.980 Hallucinogen use, unspecified with hallucinogen-induced anxiety disorder HCC
- Other hallucinogen-induced anxiety disorder, without use disorder
- Phencyclidine induced anxiety disorder, without use disorder

F16.983 Hallucinogen use, unspecified with hallucinogen persisting perception disorder (flashbacks) HCC

F16.988 Hallucinogen use, unspecified with other hallucinogen-induced disorder HCC

F16.99 Hallucinogen use, unspecified with unspecified hallucinogen-induced disorder HCC

√4th **F17 Nicotine dependence**

EXCLUDES 1 *history of tobacco dependence (Z87.891)*
tobacco use NOS (Z72.0)

EXCLUDES 2 *tobacco use (smoking) during pregnancy, childbirth and the puerperium (O99.33-)*
toxic effect of nicotine (T65.2-)

AHA: 2013,4Q,108-109

√5th **F17.2 Nicotine dependence**

√6th **F17.20 Nicotine dependence, unspecified**

F17.200 Nicotine dependence, unspecified, uncomplicated
- Tobacco use disorder, mild
- Tobacco use disorder, moderate
- Tobacco use disorder, severe

AHA: 2016,1Q,36
TIP: Assign when provider documentation indicates "smoker" without further specification.

F17.201 Nicotine dependence, unspecified, in remission
- Tobacco use disorder, mild, in early remission
- Tobacco use disorder, mild, in sustained remission
- Tobacco use disorder, moderate, in early remission
- Tobacco use disorder, moderate, in sustained remission
- Tobacco use disorder, severe, in early remission
- Tobacco use disorder, severe, in sustained remission

F17.203 Nicotine dependence unspecified, with withdrawal CC
- Tobacco withdrawal

F17.208 Nicotine dependence, unspecified, with other nicotine-induced disorders

F17.209 Nicotine dependence, unspecified, with unspecified nicotine-induced disorders

√6th **F17.21 Nicotine dependence, cigarettes**

F17.210 Nicotine dependence, cigarettes, uncomplicated
AHA: 2017,2Q,28-29

F17.211 **Nicotine dependence, cigarettes, in remission**
Tobacco use disorder, cigarettes, mild, in early remission
Tobacco use disorder, cigarettes, mild, in sustained remission
Tobacco use disorder, cigarettes, moderate, in early remission
Tobacco use disorder, cigarettes, moderate, in sustained remission
Tobacco use disorder, cigarettes, severe, in early remission
Tobacco use disorder, cigarettes, severe, in sustained remission

F17.213 **Nicotine dependence, cigarettes, with withdrawal** CC

F17.218 **Nicotine dependence, cigarettes, with other nicotine-induced disorders**

F17.219 **Nicotine dependence, cigarettes, with unspecified nicotine-induced disorders**

✓6th F17.22 **Nicotine dependence, chewing tobacco**

F17.220 **Nicotine dependence, chewing tobacco, uncomplicated**

F17.221 **Nicotine dependence, chewing tobacco, in remission**
Tobacco use disorder, chewing tobacco, mild, in early remission
Tobacco use disorder, chewing tobacco, mild, in sustained remission
Tobacco use disorder, chewing tobacco, moderate, in early remission
Tobacco use disorder, chewing tobacco, moderate, in sustained remission
Tobacco use disorder, chewing tobacco, severe, in early remission
Tobacco use disorder, chewing tobacco, severe, in sustained remission

F17.223 **Nicotine dependence, chewing tobacco, with withdrawal** CC

F17.228 **Nicotine dependence, chewing tobacco, with other nicotine-induced disorders**

F17.229 **Nicotine dependence, chewing tobacco, with unspecified nicotine-induced disorders**

✓6th F17.29 **Nicotine dependence, other tobacco product**

F17.290 **Nicotine dependence, other tobacco product, uncomplicated**
AHA: 2017,2Q,28-29

F17.291 **Nicotine dependence, other tobacco product, in remission**
Tobacco use disorder, other tobacco product, mild, in early remission
Tobacco use disorder, other tobacco product, mild, in sustained remission
Tobacco use disorder, other tobacco product, moderate, in early remission
Tobacco use disorder, other tobacco product, moderate, in sustained remission
Tobacco use disorder, other tobacco product, severe, in early remission
Tobacco use disorder, other tobacco product, severe, in sustained remission

F17.293 **Nicotine dependence, other tobacco product, with withdrawal** CC

F17.298 **Nicotine dependence, other tobacco product, with other nicotine-induced disorders**

F17.299 **Nicotine dependence, other tobacco product, with unspecified nicotine-induced disorders**

✓4th **F18 Inhalant related disorders**
INCLUDES volatile solvents

✓5th **F18.1 Inhalant abuse**
EXCLUDES 1 *inhalant dependence (F18.2-)*
inhalant use, unspecified (F18.9-)

F18.10 **Inhalant abuse, uncomplicated** HCC
Inhalant use disorder, mild

F18.11 **Inhalant abuse, in remission** HCC
Inhalant use disorder, mild, in early remission
Inhalant use disorder, mild, in sustained remission

✓6th F18.12 **Inhalant abuse with intoxication**

F18.120 **Inhalant abuse with intoxication, uncomplicated** HCC

F18.121 **Inhalant abuse with intoxication delirium** CC HCC

F18.129 **Inhalant abuse with intoxication, unspecified** HCC

F18.14 **Inhalant abuse with inhalant-induced mood disorder** HCC
Inhalant use disorder, mild, with inhalant induced depressive disorder

✓6th F18.15 **Inhalant abuse with inhalant-induced psychotic disorder**

F18.150 **Inhalant abuse with inhalant-induced psychotic disorder with delusions** CC HCC

F18.151 **Inhalant abuse with inhalant-induced psychotic disorder with hallucinations** CC HCC

F18.159 **Inhalant abuse with inhalant-induced psychotic disorder, unspecified** HCC

F18.17 **Inhalant abuse with inhalant-induced dementia** CC HCC
Inhalant use disorder, mild, with inhalant induced major neurocognitive disorder

✓6th F18.18 **Inhalant abuse with other inhalant-induced disorders**

F18.180 **Inhalant abuse with inhalant-induced anxiety disorder** HCC

F18.188 **Inhalant abuse with other inhalant-induced disorder** HCC
Inhalant use disorder, mild, with inhalant induced mild neurocognitive disorder

F18.19 **Inhalant abuse with unspecified inhalant-induced disorder** HCC

✓5th **F18.2 Inhalant dependence**
EXCLUDES 1 *inhalant abuse (F18.1-)*
inhalant use, unspecified (F18.9-)

F18.20 **Inhalant dependence, uncomplicated** CC HCC
Inhalant use disorder, moderate
Inhalant use disorder, severe

F18.21 **Inhalant dependence, in remission** HCC
Inhalant use disorder, moderate, in early remission
Inhalant use disorder, moderate, in sustained remission
Inhalant use disorder, severe, in early remission
Inhalant use disorder, severe, in sustained remission

✓6th F18.22 **Inhalant dependence with intoxication**

F18.220 **Inhalant dependence with intoxication, uncomplicated** HCC

F18.221 **Inhalant dependence with intoxication delirium** CC HCC

F18.229 **Inhalant dependence with intoxication, unspecified** HCC

F18.24 **Inhalant dependence with inhalant-induced mood disorder** HCC
Inhalant use disorder, moderate, with inhalant induced depressive disorder
Inhalant use disorder, severe, with inhalant induced depressive disorder

✓6th F18.25 **Inhalant dependence with inhalant-induced psychotic disorder**

F18.250 **Inhalant dependence with inhalant-induced psychotic disorder with delusions** CC HCC

F18.251 **Inhalant dependence with inhalant-induced psychotic disorder with hallucinations** CC HCC

F18.259 Inhalant dependence with inhalant-induced psychotic disorder, unspecified CC HCC

F18.27 Inhalant dependence with inhalant-induced dementia CC HCC

Inhalant use disorder, moderate, with inhalant induced major neurocognitive disorder

Inhalant use disorder, severe, with inhalant induced major neurocognitive disorder

✓6th **F18.28 Inhalant dependence with other inhalant-induced disorders**

F18.280 Inhalant dependence with inhalant-induced anxiety disorder CC HCC

F18.288 Inhalant dependence with other inhalant-induced disorder CC HCC

Inhalant use disorder, moderate, with inhalant-induced mild neurocognitive disorder

Inhalant use disorder, severe, with inhalant-induced mild neurocognitive disorder

F18.29 Inhalant dependence with unspecified inhalant-induced disorder HCC

✓5th **F18.9 Inhalant use, unspecified**

EXCLUDES 1 *inhalant abuse (F18.1-)*

inhalant dependence (F18.2-)

TIP: Assign a substance use code only when the provider documents a relationship between the use and an associated physical, mental, or behavioral disorder. As with all diagnoses, substance use codes must meet the definition of a reportable diagnosis.

F18.90 Inhalant use, unspecified, uncomplicated

AHA: 2018,2Q,10-11

✓6th **F18.92 Inhalant use, unspecified with intoxication**

F18.920 Inhalant use, unspecified with intoxication, uncomplicated HCC

F18.921 Inhalant use, unspecified with intoxication with delirium CC HCC

F18.929 Inhalant use, unspecified with intoxication, unspecified HCC

F18.94 Inhalant use, unspecified with inhalant-induced mood disorder HCC

Inhalant induced depressive disorder

✓6th **F18.95 Inhalant use, unspecified with inhalant-induced psychotic disorder**

F18.950 Inhalant use, unspecified with inhalant-induced psychotic disorder with delusions CC HCC

F18.951 Inhalant use, unspecified with inhalant-induced psychotic disorder with hallucinations CC HCC

F18.959 Inhalant use, unspecified with inhalant-induced psychotic disorder, unspecified HCC

F18.97 Inhalant use, unspecified with inhalant-induced persisting dementia CC HCC

Inhalant-induced major neurocognitive disorder

✓6th **F18.98 Inhalant use, unspecified with other inhalant-induced disorders**

F18.980 Inhalant use, unspecified with inhalant-induced anxiety disorder HCC

F18.988 Inhalant use, unspecified with other inhalant-induced disorder HCC

Inhalant-induced mild neurocognitive disorder

F18.99 Inhalant use, unspecified with unspecified inhalant-induced disorder HCC

✓4th **F19 Other psychoactive substance related disorders**

INCLUDES polysubstance drug use (indiscriminate drug use)

✓5th **F19.1 Other psychoactive substance abuse**

EXCLUDES 1 *other psychoactive substance dependence (F19.2-)*

other psychoactive substance use, unspecified (F19.9-)

F19.10 Other psychoactive substance abuse, uncomplicated HCC

Other (or unknown) substance use disorder, mild

F19.11 Other psychoactive substance abuse, in remission HCC

Other (or unknown) substance use disorder, mild, in early remission

Other (or unknown) substance use disorder, mild, in sustained remission

✓6th **F19.12 Other psychoactive substance abuse with intoxication**

F19.120 Other psychoactive substance abuse with intoxication, uncomplicated HCC

F19.121 Other psychoactive substance abuse with intoxication delirium CC HCC

F19.122 Other psychoactive substance abuse with intoxication with perceptual disturbances HCC

F19.129 Other psychoactive substance abuse with intoxication, unspecified HCC

● ✓6th **F19.13 Other psychoactive substance abuse with withdrawal**

● **F19.130 Other psychoactive substance abuse with withdrawal, uncomplicated** CC

● **F19.131 Other psychoactive substance abuse with withdrawal delirium** CC

● **F19.132 Other psychoactive substance abuse with withdrawal with perceptual disturbance** CC

● **F19.139 Other psychoactive substance abuse with withdrawal, unspecified** CC

F19.14 Other psychoactive substance abuse with psychoactive substance-induced mood disorder HCC

Other (or unknown) substance use disorder, mild, with other (or unknown) substance-induced bipolar or related disorder

Other (or unknown) substance use disorder, mild, with other (or unknown) substance-induced depressive disorder

✓6th **F19.15 Other psychoactive substance abuse with psychoactive substance-induced psychotic disorder**

F19.150 Other psychoactive substance abuse with psychoactive substance-induced psychotic disorder with delusions CC HCC

F19.151 Other psychoactive substance abuse with psychoactive substance-induced psychotic disorder with hallucinations CC HCC

F19.159 Other psychoactive substance abuse with psychoactive substance-induced psychotic disorder, unspecified HCC

F19.16 Other psychoactive substance abuse with psychoactive substance-induced persisting amnestic disorder HCC

F19.17 Other psychoactive substance abuse with psychoactive substance-induced persisting dementia CC HCC

Other (or unknown) substance use disorder, mild, with other (or unknown) substance-induced major neurocognitive disorder

✓6th **F19.18 Other psychoactive substance abuse with other psychoactive substance-induced disorders**

F19.180 Other psychoactive substance abuse with psychoactive substance-induced anxiety disorder HCC

F19.181 Other psychoactive substance abuse with psychoactive substance-induced sexual dysfunction HCC

F19.182 Other psychoactive substance abuse with psychoactive substance-induced sleep disorder HCC

F19.188 Other psychoactive substance abuse with other psychoactive substance-induced disorder HCC
- Other (or unknown) substance use disorder, mild, with other (or unknown) substance induced mild neurocognitive disorder
- Other (or unknown) substance use disorder, mild, with other (or unknown) substance induced obsessive-compulsive or related disorder

F19.19 Other psychoactive substance abuse with unspecified psychoactive substance-induced disorder HCC

✓5th **F19.2 Other psychoactive substance dependence**

EXCLUDES 1 *other psychoactive substance abuse (F19.1-)*
other psychoactive substance use, unspecified (F19.9-)

F19.20 Other psychoactive substance dependence, uncomplicated CC HCC
- Other (or unknown) substance use disorder, moderate
- Other (or unknown) substance use disorder, severe

F19.21 Other psychoactive substance dependence, in remission HCC
- Other (or unknown) substance use disorder, moderate, in early remission
- Other (or unknown) substance use disorder, moderate, in sustained remission
- Other (or unknown) substance use disorder, severe, in early remission
- Other (or unknown) substance use disorder, severe, in sustained remission

✓6th **F19.22 Other psychoactive substance dependence with intoxication**

EXCLUDES 1 *other psychoactive substance dependence with withdrawal (F19.23-)*

F19.220 Other psychoactive substance dependence with intoxication, uncomplicated HCC

F19.221 Other psychoactive substance dependence with intoxication delirium CC HCC

F19.222 Other psychoactive substance dependence with intoxication with perceptual disturbance CC HCC

F19.229 Other psychoactive substance dependence with intoxication, unspecified HCC

✓6th **F19.23 Other psychoactive substance dependence with withdrawal**

EXCLUDES 1 *other psychoactive substance dependence with intoxication (F19.22-)*

F19.230 Other psychoactive substance dependence with withdrawal, uncomplicated CC HCC

F19.231 Other psychoactive substance dependence with withdrawal delirium CC HCC

F19.232 Other psychoactive substance dependence with withdrawal with perceptual disturbance CC HCC

F19.239 Other psychoactive substance dependence with withdrawal, unspecified CC HCC

F19.24 Other psychoactive substance dependence with psychoactive substance-induced mood disorder HCC
- Other (or unknown) substance use disorder, moderate, with other (or unknown) substance induced bipolar or related disorder
- Other (or unknown) substance use disorder, moderate, with other (or unknown) substance induced depressive disorder
- Other (or unknown) substance use disorder, severe, with other (or unknown) substance induced bipolar or related disorder
- Other (or unknown) substance use disorder, severe, with other (or unknown) substance induced depressive disorder

✓6th **F19.25 Other psychoactive substance dependence with psychoactive substance-induced psychotic disorder**

F19.250 Other psychoactive substance dependence with psychoactive substance-induced psychotic disorder with delusions CC HCC

F19.251 Other psychoactive substance dependence with psychoactive substance-induced psychotic disorder with hallucinations CC HCC

F19.259 Other psychoactive substance dependence with psychoactive substance-induced psychotic disorder, unspecified CC HCC

F19.26 Other psychoactive substance dependence with psychoactive substance-induced persisting amnestic disorder CC HCC

F19.27 Other psychoactive substance dependence with psychoactive substance-induced persisting dementia CC HCC
- Other (or unknown) substance use disorder, moderate, with other (or unknown) substance induced major neurocognitive disorder
- Other (or unknown) substance use disorder, severe, with other (or unknown) substance induced major neurocognitive disorder

✓6th **F19.28 Other psychoactive substance dependence with other psychoactive substance-induced disorders**

F19.280 Other psychoactive substance dependence with psychoactive substance-induced anxiety disorder CC HCC

F19.281 Other psychoactive substance dependence with psychoactive substance-induced sexual dysfunction CC HCC

F19.282 Other psychoactive substance dependence with psychoactive substance-induced sleep disorder CC HCC

F19.288 Other psychoactive substance dependence with other psychoactive substance-induced disorder CC HCC
- Other (or unknown) substance use disorder, moderate, with other (or unknown) substance induced mild neurocognitive disorder
- Other (or unknown) substance use disorder, severe, with other (or unknown) substance induced mild neurocognitive disorder
- Other (or unknown) substance use disorder, moderate, with other (or unknown) substance induced obsessive compulsive or related disorder
- Other (or unknown) substance use disorder, severe, with other (or unknown) substance induced obsessive-compulsive or related disorder

F19.29 Other psychoactive substance dependence with unspecified psychoactive substance-induced disorder HCC

✓5th **F19.9 Other psychoactive substance use, unspecified**

EXCLUDES 1 *other psychoactive substance abuse (F19.1-)*
other psychoactive substance dependence (F19.2-)

TIP: Assign a substance use code only when the provider documents a relationship between the use and an associated physical, mental, or behavioral disorder. As with all diagnoses, substance use codes must meet the definition of a reportable diagnosis.

F19.90 Other psychoactive substance use, unspecified, uncomplicated
AHA: 2018,2Q,10-11

✓6th **F19.92 Other psychoactive substance use, unspecified with intoxication**

EXCLUDES 1 *other psychoactive substance use, unspecified with withdrawal (F19.93)*

F19.920 Other psychoactive substance use, unspecified with intoxication, uncomplicated HCC

F19.921 Other psychoactive substance use, unspecified with intoxication with delirium CC HCC
Other (or unknown) substance-induced delirium

F19.922 Other psychoactive substance use, unspecified with intoxication with perceptual disturbance HCC

F19.929 Other psychoactive substance use, unspecified with intoxication, unspecified HCC

✓6th **F19.93 Other psychoactive substance use, unspecified with withdrawal**

EXCLUDES 1 *other psychoactive substance use, unspecified with intoxication (F19.92-)*

F19.930 Other psychoactive substance use, unspecified with withdrawal, uncomplicated CC HCC

F19.931 Other psychoactive substance use, unspecified with withdrawal delirium CC HCC

F19.932 Other psychoactive substance use, unspecified with withdrawal with perceptual disturbance CC HCC

F19.939 Other psychoactive substance use, unspecified with withdrawal, unspecified CC HCC

F19.94 Other psychoactive substance use, unspecified with psychoactive substance-induced mood disorder HCC
Other (or unknown) substance-induced bipolar or related disorder, without use disorder
Other (or unknown) substance-induced depressive disorder, without use disorder

✓6th **F19.95 Other psychoactive substance use, unspecified with psychoactive substance-induced psychotic disorder**

F19.950 Other psychoactive substance use, unspecified with psychoactive substance-induced psychotic disorder with delusions CC HCC

F19.951 Other psychoactive substance use, unspecified with psychoactive substance-induced psychotic disorder with hallucinations CC HCC

F19.959 Other psychoactive substance use, unspecified with psychoactive substance-induced psychotic disorder, unspecified HCC
Other or unknown substance-induced psychotic disorder, without use disorder

F19.96 Other psychoactive substance use, unspecified with psychoactive substance-induced persisting amnestic disorder HCC

F19.97 Other psychoactive substance use, unspecified with psychoactive substance-induced persisting dementia CC HCC
Other (or unknown) substance-induced major neurocognitive disorder, without use disorder

✓6th **F19.98 Other psychoactive substance use, unspecified with other psychoactive substance-induced disorders**

F19.980 Other psychoactive substance use, unspecified with psychoactive substance-induced anxiety disorder HCC
Other (or unknown) substance-induced anxiety disorder, without use disorder

F19.981 Other psychoactive substance use, unspecified with psychoactive substance-induced sexual dysfunction HCC
Other (or unknown) substance-induced sexual dysfunction, without use disorder

F19.982 Other psychoactive substance use, unspecified with psychoactive substance-induced sleep disorder HCC
Other (or unknown) substance-induced sleep disorder, without use disorder

F19.988 Other psychoactive substance use, unspecified with other psychoactive substance-induced disorder HCC
Other (or unknown) substance-induced mild neurocognitive disorder, without use disorder
Other (or unknown) substance-induced obsessive-compulsive or related disorder, without use disorder

F19.99 Other psychoactive substance use, unspecified with unspecified psychoactive substance-induced disorder HCC

Schizophrenia, schizotypal, delusional, and other non-mood psychotic disorders (F20-F29)

✓4th **F20 Schizophrenia**

EXCLUDES 1 *brief psychotic disorder (F23)*
cyclic schizophrenia (F25.0)
mood [affective] disorders with psychotic symptoms (F30.2, F31.2, F31.5, F31.64, F32.3, F33.3)
schizoaffective disorder (F25.-)
schizophrenic reaction NOS (F23)

EXCLUDES 2 *schizophrenic reaction in:*
alcoholism (F10.15-, F10.25-, F10.95-)
brain disease (F06.2)
epilepsy (F06.2)
psychoactive drug use (F11-F19 with .15, .25, .95)
schizotypal disorder (F21)

DEF: Group of disorders with disturbances in thought (delusions, hallucinations), mood (blunted, flattened, inappropriate affect), and sense of self. Schizophrenia also includes bizarre, purposeless behavior, repetitious activity, or inactivity.

F20.0 Paranoid schizophrenia CC HCC
Paraphrenic schizophrenia

EXCLUDES 1 *involutional paranoid state (F22)*
paranoia (F22)

DEF: Preoccupied with delusional suspicions and auditory hallucinations related to a single theme. This type of schizophrenia is usually hostile, grandiose, threatening, persecutory, and occasionally hypochondriacal.

F20.1 Disorganized schizophrenia CC HCC
Hebephrenic schizophrenia
Hebephrenia

F20.2 Catatonic schizophrenia CC HCC
Schizophrenic catalepsy
Schizophrenic catatonia
Schizophrenic flexibilitas cerea

EXCLUDES 1 *catatonic stupor (R40.1)*

DEF: Extreme changes in motor activity. One extreme is a decreased response or reaction to the environment and the other is spontaneous activity.

F20.3 Undifferentiated schizophrenia HCC
Atypical schizophrenia

EXCLUDES 1 *acute schizophrenia-like psychotic disorder (F23)*

EXCLUDES 2 *post-schizophrenic depression (F32.89)*

F20.5 Residual schizophrenia CC HCC
Restzustand (schizophrenic)
Schizophrenic residual state

✓5th **F20.8 Other schizophrenia**

F20.81 Schizophreniform disorder CC HCC
Schizophreniform psychosis NOS

F20.89 Other schizophrenia CC HCC
Cenesthopathic schizophrenia
Simple schizophrenia

F20.9 Schizophrenia, unspecified HCC
AHA: 2019,2Q,32

F21 Schizotypal disorder HCC
Borderline schizophrenia
Latent schizophrenia
Latent schizophrenic reaction
Prepsychotic schizophrenia
Prodromal schizophrenia
Pseudoneurotic schizophrenia
Pseudopsychopathic schizophrenia
Schizotypal personality disorder
EXCLUDES 2 *Asperger's syndrome (F84.5)*
schizoid personality disorder (F60.1)
DEF: Disorder characterized by various oddities of thinking, perception, communication, and behavior that may be manifested as magical thinking, ideas of reference, paranoid ideation, recurrent illusions and derealization (depersonalization), or social isolation.

F22 Delusional disorders HCC
Delusional dysmorphophobia
Involutional paranoid state
Paranoia
Paranoia querulans
Paranoid psychosis
Paranoid state
Paraphrenia (late)
Sensitiver Beziehungswahn
EXCLUDES 1 *mood [affective] disorders with psychotic symptoms (F30.2, F31.2, F31.5, F31.64, F32.3, F33.3)*
paranoid schizophrenia (F20.0)
EXCLUDES 2 *paranoid personality disorder (F60.0)*
paranoid psychosis, psychogenic (F23)
paranoid reaction (F23)

F23 Brief psychotic disorder CC HCC
Paranoid reaction
Psychogenic paranoid psychosis
EXCLUDES 2 *mood [affective] disorders with psychotic symptoms (F30.2, F31.2, F31.5, F31.64, F32.3, F33.3)*
AHA: 2019,2Q,32

F24 Shared psychotic disorder HCC
Folie à deux
Induced paranoid disorder
Induced psychotic disorder

✓4th **F25 Schizoaffective disorders**
EXCLUDES 1 *mood [affective] disorders with psychotic symptoms (F30.2, F31.2, F31.5, F31.64, F32.3, F33.3)*
schizophrenia (F20.-)

F25.0 Schizoaffective disorder, bipolar type HCC
Cyclic schizophrenia
Schizoaffective disorder, manic type
Schizoaffective disorder, mixed type
Schizoaffective psychosis, bipolar type

F25.1 Schizoaffective disorder, depressive type HCC
Schizoaffective psychosis, depressive type

F25.8 Other schizoaffective disorders HCC

F25.9 Schizoaffective disorder, unspecified HCC
Schizoaffective psychosis NOS

F28 Other psychotic disorder not due to a substance or known physiological condition HIV HCC
Chronic hallucinatory psychosis
Other specified schizophrenia spectrum and other psychotic disorder

F29 Unspecified psychosis not due to a substance or known physiological condition HIV HCC
Psychosis NOS
Unspecified schizophrenia spectrum and other psychotic disorder
EXCLUDES 1 *mental disorder NOS (F99)*
unspecified mental disorder due to known physiological condition (F09)

Mood [affective] disorders (F30-F39)

✓4th **F30 Manic episode**
INCLUDES bipolar disorder, single manic episode
mixed affective episode
EXCLUDES 1 *bipolar disorder (F31.-)*
major depressive disorder, recurrent (F33.-)
major depressive disorder, single episode (F32.-)
DEF: Mania: Characterized by abnormal states of elation or excitement out of keeping with the individual's circumstances and varying from enhanced liveliness (hypomania) to violent, almost uncontrollable, excitement. Aggression and anger, flight of ideas, distractibility, impaired judgment, and grandiose ideas are common.

✓5th **F30.1 Manic episode without psychotic symptoms**

F30.10 Manic episode without psychotic symptoms, unspecified CC HCC

F30.11 Manic episode without psychotic symptoms, mild CC HCC

F30.12 Manic episode without psychotic symptoms, moderate CC HCC

F30.13 Manic episode, severe, without psychotic symptoms CC HCC

F30.2 Manic episode, severe with psychotic symptoms CC HCC
Manic stupor
Mania with mood-congruent psychotic symptoms
Mania with mood-incongruent psychotic symptoms

F30.3 Manic episode in partial remission HCC

F30.4 Manic episode in full remission HCC

F30.8 Other manic episodes HCC
Hypomania

F30.9 Manic episode, unspecified CC HCC
Mania NOS

✓4th **F31 Bipolar disorder**
INCLUDES bipolar I disorder
bipolar type I disorder
manic-depressive illness
manic-depressive psychosis
manic-depressive reaction
EXCLUDES 1 *bipolar disorder, single manic episode (F30.-)*
major depressive disorder, recurrent (F33.-)
major depressive disorder, single episode (F32.-)
EXCLUDES 2 *cyclothymia (F34.0)*
AHA: 2020,1Q,23

F31.0 Bipolar disorder, current episode hypomanic CC HCC

✓5th **F31.1 Bipolar disorder, current episode manic without psychotic features**

F31.10 Bipolar disorder, current episode manic without psychotic features, unspecified CC HCC

F31.11 Bipolar disorder, current episode manic without psychotic features, mild CC HCC

F31.12 Bipolar disorder, current episode manic without psychotic features, moderate CC HCC

F31.13 Bipolar disorder, current episode manic without psychotic features, severe CC HCC

F31.2 Bipolar disorder, current episode manic severe with psychotic features CC HCC
Bipolar disorder, current episode manic with mood-congruent psychotic symptoms
Bipolar disorder, current episode manic with mood-incongruent psychotic symptoms
Bipolar I disorder, current or most recent episode manic with psychotic features

✓5th **F31.3 Bipolar disorder, current episode depressed, mild or moderate severity**

F31.30 Bipolar disorder, current episode depressed, mild or moderate severity, unspecified CC HCC

F31.31 Bipolar disorder, current episode depressed, mild CC HCC

F31.32 Bipolar disorder, current episode depressed, moderate CC HCC

F31.4 Bipolar disorder, current episode depressed, severe, without psychotic features CC HCC

F31.5 Bipolar disorder, current episode depressed, severe, with psychotic features CC HCC
Bipolar disorder, current episode depressed with mood-congruent psychotic symptoms
Bipolar disorder, current episode depressed with mood-incongruent psychotic symptoms
Bipolar I disorder, current or most recent episode depressed, with psychotic features

✓5th **F31.6 Bipolar disorder, current episode mixed**

F31.60 Bipolar disorder, current episode mixed, unspecified CC HCC

F31.61 Bipolar disorder, current episode mixed, mild CC HCC

F31.62 Bipolar disorder, current episode mixed, moderate CC HCC

F31.63 Bipolar disorder, current episode mixed, severe, without psychotic features CC HCC

F31.64 Bipolar disorder, current episode mixed, severe, with psychotic features CC HCC
Bipolar disorder, current episode mixed with mood-congruent psychotic symptoms
Bipolar disorder, current episode mixed with mood-incongruent psychotic symptoms

✓5th **F31.7 Bipolar disorder, currently in remission**

F31.70 Bipolar disorder, currently in remission, most recent episode unspecified HCC

F31.71 Bipolar disorder, in partial remission, most recent episode hypomanic HCC

F31.72 Bipolar disorder, in full remission, most recent episode hypomanic HCC

F31.73 Bipolar disorder, in partial remission, most recent episode manic HCC

F31.74 Bipolar disorder, in full remission, most recent episode manic HCC

F31.75 Bipolar disorder, in partial remission, most recent episode depressed HCC

F31.76 Bipolar disorder, in full remission, most recent episode depressed HCC

F31.77 Bipolar disorder, in partial remission, most recent episode mixed HCC

F31.78 Bipolar disorder, in full remission, most recent episode mixed HCC

✓5th **F31.8 Other bipolar disorders**

F31.81 Bipolar II disorder CC HCC
Bipolar disorder, type 2

F31.89 Other bipolar disorder CC HCC
Recurrent manic episodes NOS

F31.9 Bipolar disorder, unspecified HCC
Manic depression
AHA: 2020,1Q,23

✓4th **F32 Major depressive disorder, single episode**

INCLUDES single episode of agitated depression
single episode of depressive reaction
single episode of major depression
single episode of psychogenic depression
single episode of reactive depression
single episode of vital depression

EXCLUDES 1 *bipolar disorder (F31.-)*
manic episode (F30.-)
recurrent depressive disorder (F33.-)

EXCLUDES 2 *adjustment disorder (F43.2)*

AHA: 2020,1Q,23
DEF: Mood disorder that produces depression that may exhibit as sadness, low self-esteem, or guilt feelings. Other manifestations may be withdrawal from friends and family and interrupted sleep.

F32.0 Major depressive disorder, single episode, mild CC HCC

F32.1 Major depressive disorder, single episode, moderate CC HCC

F32.2 Major depressive disorder, single episode, severe without psychotic features CC HCC

F32.3 Major depressive disorder, single episode, severe with psychotic features CC HCC
Single episode of major depression with mood-congruent psychotic symptoms
Single episode of major depression with mood-incongruent psychotic symptoms
Single episode of major depression with psychotic symptoms
Single episode of psychogenic depressive psychosis
Single episode of psychotic depression
Single episode of reactive depressive psychosis

F32.4 Major depressive disorder, single episode, in partial remission HCC

F32.5 Major depressive disorder, single episode, in full remission HCC

✓5th **F32.8 Other depressive episodes**
AHA: 2016,4Q,14

F32.81 Premenstrual dysphoric disorder ♀
EXCLUDES 1 *premenstrual tension syndrome (N94.3)*
DEF: Severe manifestation of premenstrual syndrome (PMS) that can be disabling and destructive to day-to-day activities. It can exacerbate pre-existing emotional disorders, like depression and anxiety, and cause feelings of loss of control, fatigue, and irritability.

F32.89 Other specified depressive episodes
Atypical depression
Post-schizophrenic depression
Single episode of 'masked' depression NOS

F32.9 Major depressive disorder, single episode, unspecified
Depression NOS
Depressive disorder NOS
Major depression NOS
AHA: 2013,4Q,107

✓4th **F33 Major depressive disorder, recurrent**

INCLUDES recurrent episodes of depressive reaction
recurrent episodes of endogenous depression
recurrent episodes of major depression
recurrent episodes of psychogenic depression
recurrent episodes of reactive depression
recurrent episodes of seasonal depressive disorder
recurrent episodes of vital depression

EXCLUDES 1 *bipolar disorder (F31.-)*
manic episode (F30.-)

AHA: 2020,1Q,23
DEF: Mood disorder that produces depression that may exhibit as sadness, low self-esteem, or guilt feelings. Other manifestations may be withdrawal from friends and family and interrupted sleep.

F33.0 Major depressive disorder, recurrent, mild CC HCC

F33.1 Major depressive disorder, recurrent, moderate CC HCC

F33.2 Major depressive disorder, recurrent, severe without psychotic features CC HCC

F33.3 Major depressive disorder, recurrent, severe with psychotic symptoms CC HCC
Endogenous depression with psychotic symptoms
Major depressive disorder, recurrent, with psychotic features
Recurrent severe episodes of major depression with mood-congruent psychotic symptoms
Recurrent severe episodes of major depression with mood-incongruent psychotic symptoms
Recurrent severe episodes of major depression with psychotic symptoms
Recurrent severe episodes of psychogenic depressive psychosis
Recurrent severe episodes of psychotic depression
Recurrent severe episodes of reactive depressive psychosis

✓5th **F33.4 Major depressive disorder, recurrent, in remission**

F33.40 Major depressive disorder, recurrent, in remission, unspecified CC HCC

F33.41 Major depressive disorder, recurrent, in partial remission HCC

F33.42 Major depressive disorder, recurrent, in full remission HCC

F33.8 Other recurrent depressive disorders CC HCC
Recurrent brief depressive episodes

F33.9 Major depressive disorder, recurrent, unspecified CC HCC
Monopolar depression NOS

✓4th F34 Persistent mood [affective] disorders

F34.0 Cyclothymic disorder
Affective personality disorder
Cycloid personality
Cyclothymia
Cyclothymic personality
DEF: Mood disorder characterized by fast and repeated alterations between hypomanic and depressed moods.

F34.1 Dysthymic disorder
Depressive neurosis
Depressive personality disorder
Dysthymia
Neurotic depression
Persistent anxiety depression
Persistent depressive disorder
EXCLUDES 2 *anxiety depression (mild or not persistent) (F41.8)*
DEF: Depression without psychosis. It is a less severe but persistent depression and is considered a mild to moderate chronic form of depression.

✓5th F34.8 Other persistent mood [affective] disorders
AHA: 2016,4Q,14

F34.81 Disruptive mood dysregulation disorder CC HCC

F34.89 Other specified persistent mood disorders CC HCC

F34.9 Persistent mood [affective] disorder, unspecified CC HCC

F39 Unspecified mood [affective] disorder HCC
Affective psychosis NOS

Anxiety, dissociative, stress-related, somatoform and other nonpsychotic mental disorders (F40-F48)

✓4th F40 Phobic anxiety disorders
DEF: Phobia: Broad-range anxiety with abnormally intense dread of certain objects or specific situations that would not normally have that effect.

✓5th F40.0 Agoraphobia
DEF: Profound anxiety or fear of leaving familiar settings like home, or being in unfamiliar locations or with strangers or crowds. Agoraphobia may or may not be preceded by recurrent panic attacks.

F40.00 Agoraphobia, unspecified

F40.01 Agoraphobia with panic disorder
Panic disorder with agoraphobia
EXCLUDES 1 *panic disorder without agoraphobia (F41.0)*

F40.02 Agoraphobia without panic disorder

✓5th F40.1 Social phobias
Anthropophobia
Social anxiety disorder
Social anxiety disorder of childhood
Social neurosis

F40.10 Social phobia, unspecified

F40.11 Social phobia, generalized

✓5th F40.2 Specific (isolated) phobias
EXCLUDES 2 *dysmorphophobia (nondelusional) (F45.22)*
nosophobia (F45.22)

✓6th F40.21 Animal type phobia

F40.210 Arachnophobia
Fear of spiders

F40.218 Other animal type phobia

✓6th F40.22 Natural environment type phobia

F40.220 Fear of thunderstorms

F40.228 Other natural environment type phobia

✓6th F40.23 Blood, injection, injury type phobia

F40.230 Fear of blood

F40.231 Fear of injections and transfusions

F40.232 Fear of other medical care

F40.233 Fear of injury

✓6th F40.24 Situational type phobia

F40.240 Claustrophobia

F40.241 Acrophobia

F40.242 Fear of bridges

F40.243 Fear of flying

F40.248 Other situational type phobia

✓6th F40.29 Other specified phobia

F40.290 Androphobia
Fear of men

F40.291 Gynephobia
Fear of women

F40.298 Other specified phobia

F40.8 Other phobic anxiety disorders
Phobic anxiety disorder of childhood

F40.9 Phobic anxiety disorder, unspecified
Phobia NOS
Phobic state NOS

✓4th F41 Other anxiety disorders
EXCLUDES 2 *anxiety in:*
acute stress reaction (F43.0)
neurasthenia (F48.8)
psychophysiologic disorders (F45.-)
transient adjustment reaction (F43.2)
separation anxiety (F93.0)

F41.0 Panic disorder [episodic paroxysmal anxiety]
Panic attack
Panic state
EXCLUDES 1 *panic disorder with agoraphobia (F40.01)*
DEF: Neurotic disorder characterized by recurrent panic or anxiety, apprehension, fear, or terror. Symptoms include shortness of breath, palpitations, dizziness, and shakiness; fear of dying may persist.

F41.1 Generalized anxiety disorder
Anxiety neurosis
Anxiety reaction
Anxiety state
Overanxious disorder
EXCLUDES 2 *neurasthenia (F48.8)*

F41.3 Other mixed anxiety disorders

F41.8 Other specified anxiety disorders
Anxiety depression (mild or not persistent)
Anxiety hysteria
Mixed anxiety and depressive disorder

F41.9 Anxiety disorder, unspecified
Anxiety NOS

✓4th F42 Obsessive-compulsive disorder
EXCLUDES 2 *obsessive-compulsive personality (disorder) (F60.5)*
obsessive-compulsive symptoms occurring in depression (F32-F33)
obsessive-compulsive symptoms occurring in schizophrenia (F20.-)
AHA: 2016,4Q,14-15

F42.2 Mixed obsessional thoughts and acts

F42.3 Hoarding disorder

F42.4 Excoriation (skin-picking) disorder
EXCLUDES 1 *factitial dermatitis (L98.1)*
other specified behavioral and emotional disorders with onset usually occurring in early childhood and adolescence (F98.8)

F42.8 Other obsessive-compulsive disorder
Anancastic neurosis
Obsessive-compulsive neurosis

F42.9 Obsessive-compulsive disorder, unspecified

✓4th F43 Reaction to severe stress, and adjustment disorders

F43.0 Acute stress reaction
Acute crisis reaction
Acute reaction to stress
Combat and operational stress reaction
Combat fatigue
Crisis state
Psychic shock

✓5th F43.1 Post-traumatic stress disorder (PTSD)
Traumatic neurosis
DEF: Preoccupation with traumatic events beyond normal experience (i.e., rape, personal assault, etc.) that may also include recurring flashbacks of the trauma. Symptoms include difficulty remembering, sleeping, or concentrating, and guilt feelings for surviving.

F43.10 Post-traumatic stress disorder, unspecified

F43.11 Post-traumatic stress disorder, acute

F43.12 Post-traumatic stress disorder, chronic

F43.2 Adjustment disorders
Culture shock
Grief reaction
Hospitalism in children
EXCLUDES 2 *separation anxiety disorder of childhood (F93.Ø)*

F43.2Ø Adjustment disorder, unspecified
F43.21 Adjustment disorder with depressed mood
AHA: 2014,1Q,25
F43.22 Adjustment disorder with anxiety
F43.23 Adjustment disorder with mixed anxiety and depressed mood
F43.24 Adjustment disorder with disturbance of conduct
F43.25 Adjustment disorder with mixed disturbance of emotions and conduct
F43.29 Adjustment disorder with other symptoms

F43.8 Other reactions to severe stress
Other specified trauma and stressor-related disorder

F43.9 Reaction to severe stress, unspecified
Trauma and stressor-related disorder, NOS

F44 Dissociative and conversion disorders
INCLUDES conversion hysteria
conversion reaction
hysteria
hysterical psychosis
EXCLUDES 2 *malingering [conscious simulation] (Z76.5)*

F44.Ø Dissociative amnesia HCC
EXCLUDES 1 *amnesia NOS (R41.3)*
anterograde amnesia (R41.1)
dissociative amnesia with dissociative fugue (F44.1)
retrograde amnesia (R41.2)
EXCLUDES 2 *alcohol-or other psychoactive substance-induced amnestic disorder (F1Ø, F13, F19 with .26, .96)*
amnestic disorder due to known physiological condition (FØ4)
postictal amnesia in epilepsy (G4Ø.-)

F44.1 Dissociative fugue HCC
Dissociative amnesia with dissociative fugue
EXCLUDES 2 *postictal fugue in epilepsy (G4Ø.-)*
DEF: Dissociative hysteria identified by memory loss and flight from familiar surroundings to a completely separate environment. Episodes may last hours or days. Conscious activity is not associated with perception of surroundings and there is no later memory of the episode.

F44.2 Dissociative stupor
EXCLUDES 1 *catatonic stupor (R4Ø.1)*
stupor NOS (R4Ø.1)
EXCLUDES 2 *catatonic disorder due to known physiological condition (FØ6.1)*
depressive stupor (F32, F33)
manic stupor (F3Ø, F31)

F44.4 Conversion disorder with motor symptom or deficit
Conversion disorder with abnormal movement
Conversion disorder with speech symptoms
Conversion disorder with swallowing symptoms
Conversion disorder with weakness/paralysis
Dissociative motor disorders
Psychogenic aphonia
Psychogenic dysphonia

F44.5 Conversion disorder with seizures or convulsions
Conversion disorder with attacks or seizures
Dissociative convulsions
AHA: 2019,1Q,19

F44.6 Conversion disorder with sensory symptom or deficit
Conversion disorder with anesthesia or sensory loss
Conversion disorder with special sensory symptoms
Dissociative anesthesia and sensory loss
Psychogenic deafness

F44.7 Conversion disorder with mixed symptom presentation

F44.8 Other dissociative and conversion disorders
F44.81 Dissociative identity disorder HCC
Multiple personality disorder
F44.89 Other dissociative and conversion disorders
Ganser's syndrome
Psychogenic confusion
Psychogenic twilight state
Trance and possession disorders

F44.9 Dissociative and conversion disorder, unspecified
Dissociative disorder NOS

F45 Somatoform disorders
EXCLUDES 2 *dissociative and conversion disorders (F44.-)*
factitious disorders (F68.1-, F68.A)
hair-plucking (F63.3)
lalling (F8Ø.Ø)
lisping (F8Ø.Ø)
malingering [conscious simulation] (Z76.5)
nail-biting (F98.8)
psychological or behavioral factors associated with disorders or diseases classified elsewhere (F54)
sexual dysfunction, not due to a substance or known physiological condition (F52.-)
thumb-sucking (F98.8)
tic disorders (in childhood and adolescence) (F95.-)
Tourette's syndrome (F95.2)
trichotillomania (F63.3)
DEF: Types of disorders causing inconsistent physical symptoms that cannot be explained.

F45.Ø Somatization disorder
Briquet's disorder
Multiple psychosomatic disorder

F45.1 Undifferentiated somatoform disorder
Somatic symptom disorder
Undifferentiated psychosomatic disorder

F45.2 Hypochondriacal disorders
EXCLUDES 2 *delusional dysmorphophobia (F22)*
fixed delusions about bodily functions or shape (F22)
F45.2Ø Hypochondriacal disorder, unspecified
F45.21 Hypochondriasis
Hypochondriacal neurosis
Illness anxiety disorder
F45.22 Body dysmorphic disorder
Dysmorphophobia (nondelusional)
Nosophobia
F45.29 Other hypochondriacal disorders

F45.4 Pain disorders related to psychological factors
EXCLUDES 1 *pain NOS (R52)*
F45.41 Pain disorder exclusively related to psychological factors
Somatoform pain disorder (persistent)
F45.42 Pain disorder with related psychological factors
Code also associated acute or chronic pain (G89.-)

F45.8 Other somatoform disorders
Psychogenic dysmenorrhea
Psychogenic dysphagia, including 'globus hystericus'
Psychogenic pruritus
Psychogenic torticollis
Somatoform autonomic dysfunction
Teeth grinding
EXCLUDES 1 *sleep related teeth grinding (G47.63)*

F45.9 Somatoform disorder, unspecified
Psychosomatic disorder NOS

F48 Other nonpsychotic mental disorders

F48.1 Depersonalization-derealization syndrome HCC

F48.2 Pseudobulbar affect
Involuntary emotional expression disorder
Code first underlying cause, if known, such as:
amyotrophic lateral sclerosis (G12.21)
multiple sclerosis (G35)
sequelae of cerebrovascular disease (I69.-)
sequelae of traumatic intracranial injury (SØ6.-)

F48.8 Other specified nonpsychotic mental disorders
Dhat syndrome
Neurasthenia
Occupational neurosis, including writer's cramp
Psychasthenia
Psychasthenic neurosis
Psychogenic syncope

F48.9 Nonpsychotic mental disorder, unspecified
Neurosis NOS

Behavioral syndromes associated with physiological disturbances and physical factors (F5Ø-F59)

✓4th F5Ø Eating disorders

EXCLUDES 1 *anorexia NOS (R63.Ø)*
feeding difficulties (R63.3)
feeding problems of newborn (P92.-)
polyphagia (R63.2)

EXCLUDES 2 *feeding disorder in infancy or childhood (F98.2-)*

AHA: 2018,4Q,82

TIP: Assign additional code for BMI from category Z68, when documented. BMI can be based on documentation from clinicians who are not the patient's provider.

✓5th F5Ø.Ø Anorexia nervosa

EXCLUDES 1 *loss of appetite (R63.Ø)*
psychogenic loss of appetite (F5Ø.89)

DEF: Psychological eating disorder characterized by an intense fear of gaining weight and an unrealistic perception of body image that perpetuates the feeling of being fat or having too much fat. Avoidance of food and restrictive or unhealthy eating are common.

F5Ø.ØØ Anorexia nervosa, unspecified CC
F5Ø.Ø1 Anorexia nervosa, restricting type CC
F5Ø.Ø2 Anorexia nervosa, binge eating/purging type CC
EXCLUDES 1 *bulimia nervosa (F5Ø.2)*

F5Ø.2 Bulimia nervosa CC
Bulimia NOS
Hyperorexia nervosa
EXCLUDES 1 *anorexia nervosa, binge eating/purging type (F5Ø.Ø2)*

DEF: Episodic pattern of overeating (binge eating) followed by purging or extreme exercise accompanied by an awareness of the abnormal eating pattern with a fear of not being able to stop eating.

✓5th F5Ø.8 Other eating disorders

EXCLUDES 2 *pica of infancy and childhood (F98.3)*

AHA: 2017,4Q,9; 2016,4Q,15-16

F5Ø.81 Binge eating disorder
F5Ø.82 Avoidant/restrictive food intake disorder
F5Ø.89 Other specified eating disorder
Pica in adults
Psychogenic loss of appetite

F5Ø.9 Eating disorder, unspecified
Atypical anorexia nervosa
Atypical bulimia nervosa
Feeding or eating disorder, unspecified
Other specified feeding disorder

✓4th F51 Sleep disorders not due to a substance or known physiological condition

EXCLUDES 2 *organic sleep disorders (G47.-)*

✓5th F51.Ø Insomnia not due to a substance or known physiological condition

EXCLUDES 2 *alcohol related insomnia (F1Ø.182, F1Ø.282, F1Ø.982)*
drug-related insomnia (F11.182, F11.282, F11.982, F13.182, F13.282, F13.982, F14.182, F14.282, F14.982, F15.182, F15.282, F15.982, F19.182, F19.282, F19.982)
insomnia NOS (G47.Ø-)
insomnia due to known physiological condition (G47.Ø-)
organic insomnia (G47.Ø-)
sleep deprivation (Z72.82Ø)

F51.Ø1 Primary insomnia
Idiopathic insomnia
F51.Ø2 Adjustment insomnia
F51.Ø3 Paradoxical insomnia
F51.Ø4 Psychophysiologic insomnia
F51.Ø5 Insomnia due to other mental disorder
Code also associated mental disorder
F51.Ø9 Other insomnia not due to a substance or known physiological condition

✓5th F51.1 Hypersomnia not due to a substance or known physiological condition

EXCLUDES 2 *alcohol related hypersomnia (F1Ø.182, F1Ø.282, F1Ø.982)*
drug-related hypersomnia (F11.182, F11.282, F11.982, F13.182, F13.282, F13.982, F14.182, F14.282, F14.982, F15.182, F15.282, F15.982, F19.182, F19.282, F19.982)
hypersomnia NOS (G47.1Ø)
hypersomnia due to known physiological condition (G47.1Ø)
idiopathic hypersomnia (G47.11, G47.12)
narcolepsy (G47.4-)

F51.11 Primary hypersomnia
F51.12 Insufficient sleep syndrome
EXCLUDES 1 *sleep deprivation (Z72.82Ø)*
F51.13 Hypersomnia due to other mental disorder
Code also associated mental disorder
F51.19 Other hypersomnia not due to a substance or known physiological condition

F51.3 Sleepwalking [somnambulism]
Non-rapid eye movement sleep arousal disorders, sleepwalking type

F51.4 Sleep terrors [night terrors]
Non-rapid eye movement sleep arousal disorders, sleep terror type

F51.5 Nightmare disorder
Dream anxiety disorder

F51.8 Other sleep disorders not due to a substance or known physiological condition

F51.9 Sleep disorder not due to a substance or known physiological condition, unspecified
Emotional sleep disorder NOS

✓4th F52 Sexual dysfunction not due to a substance or known physiological condition

EXCLUDES 2 *Dhat syndrome (F48.8)*

F52.Ø Hypoactive sexual desire disorder
Lack or loss of sexual desire
Male hypoactive sexual desire disorder
Sexual anhedonia
EXCLUDES 1 *decreased libido (R68.82)*

F52.1 Sexual aversion disorder
Sexual aversion and lack of sexual enjoyment

✓5th F52.2 Sexual arousal disorders
Failure of genital response

F52.21 Male erectile disorder ♂
Erectile disorder
Psychogenic impotence
EXCLUDES 1 *impotence of organic origin (N52.-)*
impotence NOS (N52.-)

F52.22 Female sexual arousal disorder ♀
Female sexual interest/arousal disorder

✓5th F52.3 Orgasmic disorder
Inhibited orgasm
Psychogenic anorgasmy

F52.31 Female orgasmic disorder ♀
F52.32 Male orgasmic disorder ♂
Delayed ejaculation

F52.4 Premature ejaculation ♂

F52.5 Vaginismus not due to a substance or known physiological condition ♀
Psychogenic vaginismus
EXCLUDES 2 *vaginismus (due to a known physiological condition) (N94.2)*

DEF: Psychogenic response resulting in painful contractions of the vaginal canal muscles. This condition can be severe enough to prevent sexual intercourse.

F52.6 Dyspareunia not due to a substance or known physiological condition
Genito-pelvic pain penetration disorder
Psychogenic dyspareunia
EXCLUDES 2 *dyspareunia (due to a known physiological condition) (N94.1-)*

F52.8 Other sexual dysfunction not due to a substance or known physiological condition
Excessive sexual drive
Nymphomania
Satyriasis

F52.9 Unspecified sexual dysfunction not due to a substance or known physiological condition
Sexual dysfunction NOS

✓4th **F53 Mental and behavioral disorders associated with the puerperium, not elsewhere classified**
EXCLUDES 1 *mood disorders with psychotic features (F30.2, F31.2, F31.5, F31.64, F32.3, F33.3)*
postpartum dysphoria (O90.6)
psychosis in schizophrenia, schizotypal, delusional, and other psychotic disorders (F20-F29)
AHA: 2018,4Q,8

F53.0 Postpartum depression M ♀
Postnatal depression, NOS
Postpartum depression, NOS

F53.1 Puerperal psychosis HCC M ♀
Postpartum psychosis
Puerperal psychosis, NOS

F54 Psychological and behavioral factors associated with disorders or diseases classified elsewhere
Psychological factors affecting physical conditions
Code first the associated physical disorder, such as:
asthma (J45.-)
dermatitis (L23-L25)
gastric ulcer (K25.-)
mucous colitis (K58.-)
ulcerative colitis (K51.-)
urticaria (L50.-)
EXCLUDES 2 *tension-type headache (G44.2)*

✓4th **F55 Abuse of non-psychoactive substances**
EXCLUDES 2 *abuse of psychoactive substances (F10-F19)*

F55.0 Abuse of antacids
F55.1 Abuse of herbal or folk remedies
F55.2 Abuse of laxatives
F55.3 Abuse of steroids or hormones
F55.4 Abuse of vitamins
F55.8 Abuse of other non-psychoactive substances

F59 Unspecified behavioral syndromes associated with physiological disturbances and physical factors
Psychogenic physiological dysfunction NOS

Disorders of adult personality and behavior (F60-F69)

✓4th **F60 Specific personality disorders**

F60.0 Paranoid personality disorder HCC
Expansive paranoid personality (disorder)
Fanatic personality (disorder)
Paranoid personality (disorder)
Querulant personality (disorder)
Sensitive paranoid personality (disorder)
EXCLUDES 2 *paranoia (F22)*
paranoia querulans (F22)
paranoid psychosis (F22)
paranoid schizophrenia (F20.0)
paranoid state (F22)

F60.1 Schizoid personality disorder HCC
EXCLUDES 2 *Asperger's syndrome (F84.5)*
delusional disorder (F22)
schizoid disorder of childhood (F84.5)
schizophrenia (F20.-)
schizotypal disorder (F21)

F60.2 Antisocial personality disorder HCC
Amoral personality (disorder)
Asocial personality (disorder)
Dissocial personality disorder
Psychopathic personality (disorder)
Sociopathic personality (disorder)
EXCLUDES 1 *conduct disorders (F91.-)*
EXCLUDES 2 *borderline personality disorder (F60.3)*

F60.3 Borderline personality disorder HCC
Aggressive personality (disorder)
Emotionally unstable personality disorder
Explosive personality (disorder)
EXCLUDES 2 *antisocial personality disorder (F60.2)*

F60.4 Histrionic personality disorder HCC
Hysterical personality (disorder)
Psychoinfantile personality (disorder)

F60.5 Obsessive-compulsive personality disorder HCC
Anankastic personality (disorder)
Compulsive personality (disorder)
Obsessional personality (disorder)
EXCLUDES 2 *obsessive-compulsive disorder ►(F42.-)◄*

F60.6 Avoidant personality disorder HCC
Anxious personality disorder

F60.7 Dependent personality disorder HCC
Asthenic personality (disorder)
Inadequate personality (disorder)
Passive personality (disorder)
DEF: Lack of self-confidence, fear of abandonment, and an obsessive need to be taken care of.

✓5th **F60.8 Other specific personality disorders**

F60.81 Narcissistic personality disorder HCC

F60.89 Other specific personality disorders HCC
Eccentric personality disorder
"Haltlose" type personality disorder
Immature personality disorder
Passive-aggressive personality disorder
Psychoneurotic personality disorder
Self-defeating personality disorder

F60.9 Personality disorder, unspecified HCC
Character disorder NOS
Character neurosis NOS
Pathological personality NOS

✓4th **F63 Impulse disorders**
EXCLUDES 2 *habitual excessive use of alcohol or psychoactive substances (F10-F19)*
impulse disorders involving sexual behavior (F65.-)

F63.0 Pathological gambling
Compulsive gambling
Gambling disorder
EXCLUDES 1 *gambling and betting NOS (Z72.6)*
EXCLUDES 2 *excessive gambling by manic patients (F30, F31)*
gambling in antisocial personality disorder (F60.2)

F63.1 Pyromania
Pathological fire-setting
EXCLUDES 2 *fire-setting (by) (in):*
adult with antisocial personality disorder (F60.2)
alcohol or psychoactive substance intoxication (F10-F19)
conduct disorders (F91.-)
mental disorders due to known physiological condition (F01-F09)
schizophrenia (F20.-)

F63.2 Kleptomania
Pathological stealing
EXCLUDES 1 *shoplifting as the reason for observation for suspected mental disorder (Z03.8)*
EXCLUDES 2 *depressive disorder with stealing (F31-F33)*
stealing due to underlying mental condition - code to mental condition
stealing in mental disorders due to known physiological condition (F01-F09)

F63.3 Trichotillomania
Hair plucking
EXCLUDES 2 *other stereotyped movement disorder (F98.4)*

✓5th **F63.8 Other impulse disorders**

F63.81 Intermittent explosive disorder
F63.89 Other impulse disorders

F63.9 Impulse disorder, unspecified
Impulse control disorder NOS

✓4th F64 Gender identity disorders
AHA: 2016,4Q,16

F64.0 Transsexualism
Gender identity disorder in adolescence and adulthood
Gender dysphoria in adolescents and adults

F64.1 Dual role transvestism
Use additional code to identify sex reassignment status (Z87.890)
EXCLUDES 1 *gender identity disorder in childhood (F64.2)*
EXCLUDES 2 *fetishistic transvestism (F65.1)*

F64.2 Gender identity disorder of childhood P
Gender dysphoria in children
EXCLUDES 1 *gender identity disorder in adolescence and adulthood (F64.0)*
EXCLUDES 2 *sexual maturation disorder (F66)*

F64.8 Other gender identity disorders
Other specified gender dysphoria

F64.9 Gender identity disorder, unspecified
Gender dysphoria, unspecified
Gender-role disorder NOS

✓4th F65 Paraphilias

F65.0 Fetishism
Fetishistic disorder

F65.1 Transvestic fetishism
Fetishistic transvestism
Transvestic disorder

F65.2 Exhibitionism
Exhibitionistic disorder

F65.3 Voyeurism
Voyeuristic disorder

F65.4 Pedophilia
Pedophilic disorder

✓5th F65.5 Sadomasochism

F65.50 Sadomasochism, unspecified

F65.51 Sexual masochism
Sexual masochism disorder

F65.52 Sexual sadism
Sexual sadism disorder

✓5th F65.8 Other paraphilias

F65.81 Frotteurism
Frotteuristic disorder

F65.89 Other paraphilias
Necrophilia
Other specified paraphilic disorder

F65.9 Paraphilia, unspecified
Paraphilic disorder, unspecified
Sexual deviation NOS

F66 Other sexual disorders
Sexual maturation disorder
Sexual relationship disorder

✓4th F68 Other disorders of adult personality and behavior
AHA: 2018,4Q,9,65

✓5th F68.1 Factitious disorder imposed on self
Compensation neurosis
Elaboration of physical symptoms for psychological reasons
Hospital hopper syndrome
Münchausen's syndrome
Peregrinating patient
EXCLUDES 2 *factitial dermatitis (L98.1)*
person feigning illness (with obvious motivation) (Z76.5)

F68.10 Factitious disorder imposed on self, unspecified CC

F68.11 Factitious disorder imposed on self, with predominantly psychological signs and symptoms

F68.12 Factitious disorder imposed on self, with predominantly physical signs and symptoms CC

F68.13 Factitious disorder imposed on self, with combined psychological and physical signs and symptoms

F68.A Factitious disorder imposed on another CC
Factitious disorder by proxy
Münchausen's by proxy

F68.8 Other specified disorders of adult personality and behavior

F69 Unspecified disorder of adult personality and behavior A

Intellectual disabilities (F70-F79)

Code first any associated physical or developmental disorders
EXCLUDES 1 *borderline intellectual functioning, IQ above 70 to 84 (R41.83)*

F70 Mild intellectual disabilities
IQ level 50-55 to approximately 70
Mild mental subnormality

F71 Moderate intellectual disabilities
IQ level 35-40 to 50-55
Moderate mental subnormality

F72 Severe intellectual disabilities CC
IQ 20-25 to 35-40
Severe mental subnormality

F73 Profound intellectual disabilities CC
IQ level below 20-25
Profound mental subnormality

F78 Other intellectual disabilities

F79 Unspecified intellectual disabilities
Mental deficiency NOS
Mental subnormality NOS

Pervasive and specific developmental disorders (F80-F89)

✓4th F80 Specific developmental disorders of speech and language

F80.0 Phonological disorder
Dyslalia
Functional speech articulation disorder
Lalling
Lisping
Phonological developmental disorder
Speech articulation developmental disorder
Speech-sound disorder
EXCLUDES 1 *speech articulation impairment due to aphasia NOS (R47.01)*
speech articulation impairment due to apraxia (R48.2)
EXCLUDES 2 *speech articulation impairment due to hearing loss (F80.4)*
speech articulation impairment due to intellectual disabilities (F70-F79)
speech articulation impairment with expressive language developmental disorder (F80.1)
speech articulation impairment with mixed receptive expressive language developmental disorder (F80.2)

F80.1 Expressive language disorder
Developmental dysphasia or aphasia, expressive type
EXCLUDES 1 *mixed receptive-expressive language disorder (F80.2)*
dysphasia and aphasia NOS (R47.-)
EXCLUDES 2 *acquired aphasia with epilepsy [Landau-Kleffner] (G40.80-)*
selective mutism (F94.0)
intellectual disabilities (F70-F79)
pervasive developmental disorders (F84.-)

F80.2 Mixed receptive-expressive language disorder
Developmental dysphasia or aphasia, receptive type
Developmental Wernicke's aphasia
EXCLUDES 1 *central auditory processing disorder (H93.25)*
dysphasia or aphasia NOS (R47.-)
expressive language disorder (F80.1)
expressive type dysphasia or aphasia (F80.1)
word deafness (H93.25)
EXCLUDES 2 *acquired aphasia with epilepsy [Landau-Kleffner] (G40.80-)*
pervasive developmental disorders (F84.-)
selective mutism (F94.0)
intellectual disabilities (F70-F79)

F80.4 Speech and language development delay due to hearing loss
Code also type of hearing loss (H90.-, H91.-)

F80.8 Other developmental disorders of speech and language
AHA: 2017,1Q,27

F80.81 Childhood onset fluency disorder
Cluttering NOS
Stuttering NOS
EXCLUDES 1 *adult onset fluency disorder (F98.5)*
fluency disorder in conditions classified elsewhere (R47.82)
fluency disorder (stuttering) following cerebrovascular disease (I69. with final characters -23)

F80.82 Social pragmatic communication disorder
EXCLUDES 1 *Asperger's syndrome (F84.5)*
autistic disorder (F84.0)
AHA: 2016,4Q,16

F80.89 Other developmental disorders of speech and language

F80.9 Developmental disorder of speech and language, unspecified
Communication disorder NOS
Language disorder NOS

F81 Specific developmental disorders of scholastic skills

F81.0 Specific reading disorder
"Backward reading"
Developmental dyslexia
Specific learning disorder, with impairment in reading
Specific reading retardation
EXCLUDES 1 *alexia NOS (R48.0)*
dyslexia NOS (R48.0)
DEF: Serious impairment of reading skills unexplained in relation to general intelligence and teaching processes.

F81.2 Mathematics disorder
Developmental acalculia
Developmental arithmetical disorder
Developmental Gerstmann's syndrome
Specific learning disorder, with impairment in mathematics
EXCLUDES 1 *acalculia NOS (R48.8)*
EXCLUDES 2 *arithmetical difficulties associated with a reading disorder (F81.0)*
arithmetical difficulties associated with a spelling disorder (F81.81)
arithmetical difficulties due to inadequate teaching (Z55.8)

F81.8 Other developmental disorders of scholastic skills

F81.81 Disorder of written expression
Specific learning disorder, with impairment in written expression
Specific spelling disorder

F81.89 Other developmental disorders of scholastic skills

F81.9 Developmental disorder of scholastic skills, unspecified
Knowledge acquisition disability NOS
Learning disability NOS
Learning disorder NOS

F82 Specific developmental disorder of motor function
Clumsy child syndrome
Developmental coordination disorder
Developmental dyspraxia
EXCLUDES 1 *abnormalities of gait and mobility (R26.-)*
lack of coordination (R27.-)
EXCLUDES 2 *lack of coordination secondary to intellectual disabilities (F70-F79)*

F84 Pervasive developmental disorders
Use additional code to identify any associated medical condition and intellectual disabilities.

F84.0 Autistic disorder CC
Autism spectrum disorder
Infantile autism
Infantile psychosis
Kanner's syndrome
EXCLUDES 1 *Asperger's syndrome (F84.5)*
AHA: 2017,1Q,27

F84.2 Rett's syndrome CC
EXCLUDES 1 *Asperger's syndrome (F84.5)*
autistic disorder (F84.0)
other childhood disintegrative disorder (F84.3)

F84.3 Other childhood disintegrative disorder CC P
Dementia infantilis
Disintegrative psychosis
Heller's syndrome
Symbiotic psychosis
Use additional code to identify any associated neurological condition
EXCLUDES 1 *Asperger's syndrome (F84.5)*
autistic disorder (F84.0)
Rett's syndrome (F84.2)

F84.5 Asperger's syndrome CC
Asperger's disorder
Autistic psychopathy
Schizoid disorder of childhood
DEF: High-functioning form of autism. Children with this syndrome usually develop speech on schedule, are generally very intelligent, and communicate well, but have considerable social shortcomings. ***Synonym(s):*** *AS.*

F84.8 Other pervasive developmental disorders CC
Overactive disorder associated with intellectual disabilities and stereotyped movements

F84.9 Pervasive developmental disorder, unspecified CC
Atypical autism

F88 Other disorders of psychological development
Developmental agnosia
Global developmental delay
Other specified neurodevelopmental disorder

F89 Unspecified disorder of psychological development
Developmental disorder NOS
Neurodevelopmental disorder NOS

Behavioral and emotional disorders with onset usually occurring in childhood and adolescence (F90-F98)

NOTE Codes within categories F90-F98 may be used regardless of the age of a patient. These disorders generally have onset within the childhood or adolescent years, but may continue throughout life or not be diagnosed until adulthood

F90 Attention-deficit hyperactivity disorders
INCLUDES attention deficit disorder with hyperactivity
attention deficit syndrome with hyperactivity
EXCLUDES 2 *anxiety disorders (F40.-, F41.-)*
mood [affective] disorders (F30-F39)
pervasive developmental disorders (F84.-)
schizophrenia (F20.-)

F90.0 Attention-deficit hyperactivity disorder, predominantly inattentive type
Attention-deficit/hyperactivity disorder, predominantly inattentive presentation

F90.1 Attention-deficit hyperactivity disorder, predominantly hyperactive type
Attention-deficit/hyperactivity disorder, predominantly hyperactive impulsive presentation

F90.2 Attention-deficit hyperactivity disorder, combined type
Attention-deficit/hyperactivity disorder, combined presentation

F90.8 Attention-deficit hyperactivity disorder, other type

F90.9 Attention-deficit hyperactivity disorder, unspecified type
Attention-deficit hyperactivity disorder of childhood or adolescence NOS
Attention-deficit hyperactivity disorder NOS

F91 Conduct disorders
EXCLUDES 1 *antisocial behavior (Z72.81-)*
antisocial personality disorder (F60.2)
EXCLUDES 2 *conduct problems associated with attention-deficit hyperactivity disorder (F90.-)*
mood [affective] disorders (F30-F39)
pervasive developmental disorders (F84.-)
schizophrenia (F20.-)

F91.0 Conduct disorder confined to family context

F91.1 Conduct disorder, childhood-onset type
Unsocialized conduct disorder
Conduct disorder, solitary aggressive type
Unsocialized aggressive disorder

F91.2 Conduct disorder, adolescent-onset type
Socialized conduct disorder
Conduct disorder, group type

F91.3 Oppositional defiant disorder

F91.8 Other conduct disorders
Other specified conduct disorder
Other specified disruptive disorder

F91.9 Conduct disorder, unspecified
Behavioral disorder NOS
Conduct disorder NOS
Disruptive behavior disorder NOS
Disruptive disorder NOS

✓4th **F93 Emotional disorders with onset specific to childhood**

F93.Ø Separation anxiety disorder of childhood
EXCLUDES 2 *mood [affective] disorders (F3Ø-F39)*
nonpsychotic mental disorders (F4Ø-F48)
phobic anxiety disorder of childhood (F4Ø.8)
social phobia (F4Ø.1)

F93.8 Other childhood emotional disorders
Identity disorder
EXCLUDES 2 *gender identity disorder of childhood (F64.2)*

F93.9 Childhood emotional disorder, unspecified

✓4th **F94 Disorders of social functioning with onset specific to childhood and adolescence**

F94.Ø Selective mutism
Elective mutism
EXCLUDES 2 *pervasive developmental disorders (F84.-)*
schizophrenia (F2Ø.-)
specific developmental disorders of speech and language (F8Ø.-)
transient mutism as part of separation anxiety in young children (F93.Ø)

F94.1 Reactive attachment disorder of childhood
Use additional code to identify any associated failure to thrive or growth retardation
EXCLUDES 1 *disinhibited attachment disorder of childhood (F94.2)*
normal variation in pattern of selective attachment
EXCLUDES 2 *Asperger's syndrome (F84.5)*
maltreatment syndromes (T74.-)
sexual or physical abuse in childhood, resulting in psychosocial problems (Z62.81-)

F94.2 Disinhibited attachment disorder of childhood
Affectionless psychopathy
Institutional syndrome
EXCLUDES 1 *reactive attachment disorder of childhood (F94.1)*
EXCLUDES 2 *Asperger's syndrome (F84.5)*
attention-deficit hyperactivity disorders (F9Ø.-)
hospitalism in children (F43.2-)

F94.8 Other childhood disorders of social functioning

F94.9 Childhood disorder of social functioning, unspecified

✓4th **F95 Tic disorder**

F95.Ø Transient tic disorder
Provisional tic disorder

F95.1 Chronic motor or vocal tic disorder

F95.2 Tourette's disorder
Combined vocal and multiple motor tic disorder [de la Tourette]
Tourette's syndrome

F95.8 Other tic disorders

F95.9 Tic disorder, unspecified
Tic NOS

✓4th **F98 Other behavioral and emotional disorders with onset usually occurring in childhood and adolescence**
EXCLUDES 2 *breath-holding spells (RØ6.89)*
gender identity disorder of childhood (F64.2)
Kleine-Levin syndrome (G47.13)
obsessive-compulsive disorder ►(F42.-)◄
sleep disorders not due to a substance or known physiological condition (F51.-)

F98.Ø Enuresis not due to a substance or known physiological condition
Enuresis (primary) (secondary) of nonorganic origin
Functional enuresis
Psychogenic enuresis
Urinary incontinence of nonorganic origin
EXCLUDES 1 *enuresis NOS (R32)*

F98.1 Encopresis not due to a substance or known physiological condition
Functional encopresis
Incontinence of feces of nonorganic origin
Psychogenic encopresis
Use additional code to identify the cause of any coexisting constipation
EXCLUDES 1 *encopresis NOS (R15.-)*

✓5th **F98.2 Other feeding disorders of infancy and childhood**
EXCLUDES 1 *feeding difficulties (R63.3)*
EXCLUDES 2 *anorexia nervosa and other eating disorders (F5Ø.-)*
feeding problems of newborn (P92.-)
pica of infancy or childhood (F98.3)

F98.21 Rumination disorder of infancy

F98.29 Other feeding disorders of infancy and early childhood

F98.3 Pica of infancy and childhood

F98.4 Stereotyped movement disorders
Stereotype/habit disorder
EXCLUDES 1 *abnormal involuntary movements (R25.-)*
EXCLUDES 2 *compulsions in obsessive-compulsive disorder ►(F42.-)◄*
hair plucking (F63.3)
movement disorders of organic origin (G2Ø-G25)
nail-biting (F98.8)
nose-picking (F98.8)
stereotypies that are part of a broader psychiatric condition (FØ1-F95)
thumb-sucking (F98.8)
tic disorders (F95.-)
trichotillomania (F63.3)

F98.5 Adult onset fluency disorder
EXCLUDES 1 *childhood onset fluency disorder (F8Ø.81)*
dysphasia (R47.Ø2)
fluency disorder in conditions classified elsewhere (R47.82)
fluency disorder (stuttering) following cerebrovascular disease (I69. with final characters -23)
tic disorders (F95.-)

F98.8 Other specified behavioral and emotional disorders with onset usually occurring in childhood and adolescence
Excessive masturbation
Nail-biting
Nose-picking
Thumb-sucking

F98.9 Unspecified behavioral and emotional disorders with onset usually occurring in childhood and adolescence

Unspecified mental disorder (F99)

F99 Mental disorder, not otherwise specified
Mental illness NOS
EXCLUDES 1 *unspecified mental disorder due to known physiological condition (FØ9)*

Chapter 6. Diseases of the Nervous System (GØØ-G99)

Chapter-specific Guidelines with Coding Examples

The chapter-specific guidelines from the ICD-10-CM Official Guidelines for Coding and Reporting have been provided below. Along with these guidelines are coding examples, contained in the shaded boxes, that have been developed to help illustrate the coding and/or sequencing guidance found in these guidelines.

a. Dominant/nondominant side

Codes from category G81, Hemiplegia and hemiparesis, and subcategories G83.1, Monoplegia of lower limb, G83.2, Monoplegia of upper limb, and G83.3, Monoplegia, unspecified, identify whether the dominant or nondominant side is affected. Should the affected side be documented, but not specified as dominant or nondominant, and the classification system does not indicate a default, code selection is as follows:

- For ambidextrous patients, the default should be dominant.
- If the left side is affected, the default is non-dominant.
- If the right side is affected, the default is dominant.

> Hemiplegia affecting left side of ambidextrous patient
>
> **G81.92 Hemiplegia, unspecified affecting left dominant side**
>
> *Explanation*: Documentation states that the left side is affected and dominant is used for ambidextrous persons.

> Right spastic hemiplegia, unknown whether patient is right- or left-handed
>
> **G81.11 Spastic hemiplegia affecting right dominant side**
>
> *Explanation*: Since it is unknown whether the patient is right- or left-handed, if the right side is affected, the default is dominant.

b. Pain—category G89

1) General coding information

Codes in category G89, Pain, not elsewhere classified, may be used in conjunction with codes from other categories and chapters to provide more detail about acute or chronic pain and neoplasm-related pain, unless otherwise indicated below.

If the pain is not specified as acute or chronic, post-thoracotomy, postprocedural, or neoplasm-related, do not assign codes from category G89.

A code from category G89 should not be assigned if the underlying (definitive) diagnosis is known, unless the reason for the encounter is pain control/ management and not management of the underlying condition.

When an admission or encounter is for a procedure aimed at treating the underlying condition (e.g., spinal fusion, kyphoplasty), a code for the underlying condition (e.g., vertebral fracture, spinal stenosis) should be assigned as the principal diagnosis. No code from category G89 should be assigned.

> Elderly patient with back pain is admitted for kyphoplasty for age-related osteopathic compression fracture at vertebra T3
>
> **M8Ø.Ø8XA Age-related osteoporosis with current pathological fracture, vertebra(e), initial encounter for fracture**
>
> *Explanation*: No code is assigned for the pain as it is inherent in the underlying condition being treated.

(a) Category G89 codes as principal or first-listed diagnosis

Category G89 codes are acceptable as principal diagnosis or the first-listed code:

- When pain control or pain management is the reason for the admission/encounter (e.g., a patient with displaced intervertebral disc, nerve impingement and severe back pain presents for injection of steroid into the spinal canal). The underlying cause of the pain should be reported as an additional diagnosis, if known.
- When a patient is admitted for the insertion of a neurostimulator for pain control, assign the appropriate pain code as the principal or first-listed diagnosis. When an admission or encounter is for a procedure aimed at treating the underlying condition and a neurostimulator is inserted for pain control during the same admission/encounter, a code for the underlying condition should be assigned as the principal diagnosis and the appropriate pain code should be assigned as a secondary diagnosis.

> Patient with chronic pain from lumbar spondylosis with radiculopathy not relieved by surgery is admitted for insertion of neurostimulator.
>
> **G89.29 Other chronic pain**
>
> **M47.26 Other spondylosis with radiculopathy, lumbar region**
>
> *Explanation*: Since the patient is admitted specifically for a neurostimulator implantation for pain management and not to treat the underlying spondylosis, the chronic pain code is sequenced first, followed by the underlying condition. Neither code M54.16 nor M54.5 is necessary because M47.26 describes the radiculopathy and the site.

(b) Use of category G89 codes in conjunction with site specific pain codes

(i) Assigning category G89 and site-specific pain codes

Codes from category G89 may be used in conjunction with codes that identify the site of pain (including codes from chapter 18) if the category G89 code provides additional information. For example, if the code describes the site of the pain, but does not fully describe whether the pain is acute or chronic, then both codes should be assigned.

> During hospital stay, patient is seen by orthopaedics to evaluate chronic left shoulder pain.
>
> **M25.512 Pain in left shoulder**
>
> **G89.29 Other chronic pain**
>
> *Explanation*: No underlying condition has been determined yet so the pain would be the reason for the visit. The M25 pain code in this instance does not fully describe the condition as it does not represent that the pain is chronic. The G89 chronic pain code is assigned to provide specificity.

(ii) Sequencing of category G89 codes with site-specific pain codes

The sequencing of category G89 codes with site-specific pain codes (including chapter 18 codes), is dependent on the circumstances of the encounter/admission as follows:

- If the encounter is for pain control or pain management, assign the code from category G89 followed by the code identifying the specific site of pain (e.g., encounter for pain management for acute neck pain from trauma is assigned code G89.11, Acute pain due to trauma, followed by code M54.2, Cervicalgia, to identify the site of pain).

> Management of acute, traumatic right knee pain
>
> **G89.11 Acute pain due to trauma**
>
> **M25.561 Pain in right knee**
>
> *Explanation*: The reason for the encounter is to manage or control the pain, not to treat or evaluate an underlying condition. The G89 pain code is assigned as the principal diagnosis but in this instance does not fully describe the condition as it does not include the site and laterality. The M25 pain code is added to provide this information.

- If the encounter is for any other reason except pain control or pain management, and a related definitive diagnosis has not been established (confirmed) by the provider, assign the code for the specific site of pain first, followed by the appropriate code from category G89.

> Tests are performed to investigate the source of the patient's chronic epigastric abdominal pain
>
> **R1Ø.13 Epigastric pain**
>
> **G89.29 Other chronic pain**
>
> *Explanation*: In this instance the patient's epigastric pain is not being treated; rather the source of the pain is being investigated. A code from chapter 18 for epigastric pain is sequenced before the additional specificity of the G89 code for the chronic pain.

2) Pain due to devices, implants and grafts

See Section I.C.19. Pain due to medical devices

3) Postoperative pain

The provider's documentation should be used to guide the coding of postoperative pain, as well as *Section III. Reporting Additional Diagnoses* and *Section IV. Diagnostic Coding and Reporting in the Outpatient Setting*.

The default for post-thoracotomy and other postoperative pain not specified as acute or chronic is the code for the acute form.

Routine or expected postoperative pain immediately after surgery should not be coded.

> Pain pump dose is increased for the patient's unexpected, extreme pain post-thoracotomy
>
> **G89.12 Acute post-thoracotomy pain**
>
> *Explanation*: When acute or chronic is not documented, default to acute. The use of "unexpected, extreme" and the increase of medication dosage indicate that the pain was more than routine or expected.

(a) Postoperative pain not associated with specific postoperative complication

Postoperative pain not associated with a specific postoperative complication is assigned to the appropriate postoperative pain code in category G89.

(b) Postoperative pain associated with specific postoperative complication

Postoperative pain associated with a specific postoperative complication (such as painful wire sutures) is assigned to the appropriate code(s) found in Chapter 19, Injury, poisoning, and certain other consequences of external causes. If appropriate, use additional code(s) from category G89 to identify acute or chronic pain (G89.18 or G89.28).

4) Chronic pain

Chronic pain is classified to subcategory G89.2. There is no time frame defining when pain becomes chronic pain. The provider's documentation should be used to guide use of these codes.

5) Neoplasm related pain

Code G89.3 is assigned to pain documented as being related, associated or due to cancer, primary or secondary malignancy, or tumor. This code is assigned regardless of whether the pain is acute or chronic.

This code may be assigned as the principal or first-listed code when the stated reason for the admission/encounter is documented as pain control/pain management. The underlying neoplasm should be reported as an additional diagnosis.

> Pain medication adjustment for chronic pain from bone metastasis
>
> **G89.3 Neoplasm related pain (acute)(chronic)**
>
> **C79.51 Secondary malignant neoplasm of bone**
>
> *Explanation*: Since the encounter was for pain medication management, the pain, rather than the neoplasm, was the reason for the encounter and is sequenced first. This "neoplasm-related pain" code includes both acute and chronic pain.

When the reason for the admission/encounter is management of the neoplasm and the pain associated with the neoplasm is also documented, code G89.3 may be assigned as an additional diagnosis. It is not necessary to assign an additional code for the site of the pain.

See Section I.C.2 for instructions on the sequencing of neoplasms for all other stated reasons for the admission/encounter (except for pain control/pain management).

> Patient with lung cancer presents with acute hip pain and is evaluated and found to have iliac bone metastasis
>
> **C79.51 Secondary malignant neoplasm of bone**
>
> **C34.9Ø Malignant neoplasm of unspecified part of unspecified bronchus or lung**
>
> **G89.3 Neoplasm related pain (acute)(chronic)**
>
> *Explanation*: The reason for the encounter was the evaluation and diagnosis of the bone metastasis, whose code would be assigned as first-listed, followed by codes for the primary neoplasm and the pain due to the iliac bone metastasis.

6) Chronic pain syndrome

Central pain syndrome (G89.Ø) and chronic pain syndrome (G89.4) are different than the term "chronic pain," and therefore codes should only be used when the provider has specifically documented this condition.

See Section I.C.5. Pain disorders related to psychological factors

Chapter 6. Diseases of the Nervous System (G00-G99)

EXCLUDES 2 *certain conditions originating in the perinatal period (P04-P96)*
certain infectious and parasitic diseases (A00-B99)
complications of pregnancy, childbirth and the puerperium (O00-O9A)
congenital malformations, deformations, and chromosomal abnormalities (Q00-Q99)
endocrine, nutritional and metabolic diseases (E00-E88)
injury, poisoning and certain other consequences of external causes (S00-T88)
neoplasms (C00-D49)
symptoms, signs and abnormal clinical and laboratory findings, not elsewhere classified (R00-R94)

This chapter contains the following blocks:

- G00-G09 Inflammatory diseases of the central nervous system
- G10-G14 Systemic atrophies primarily affecting the central nervous system
- G20-G26 Extrapyramidal and movement disorders
- G30-G32 Other degenerative diseases of the nervous system
- G35-G37 Demyelinating diseases of the central nervous system
- G40-G47 Episodic and paroxysmal disorders
- G50-G59 Nerve, nerve root and plexus disorders
- G60-G65 Polyneuropathies and other disorders of the peripheral nervous system
- G70-G73 Diseases of myoneural junction and muscle
- G80-G83 Cerebral palsy and other paralytic syndromes
- G89-G99 Other disorders of the nervous system

Inflammatory diseases of the central nervous system (G00-G09)

✓4th G00 Bacterial meningitis, not elsewhere classified

INCLUDES bacterial arachnoiditis
bacterial leptomeningitis
bacterial meningitis
bacterial pachymeningitis

EXCLUDES 1 *bacterial meningoencephalitis (G04.2)*
bacterial meningomyelitis (G04.2)

DEF: Inflammation of meningeal layers of the brain and spinal cord due to a bacterial infection.

G00.0 Hemophilus meningitis MCC
Meningitis due to Hemophilus influenzae

G00.1 Pneumococcal meningitis MCC
Meningtitis due to Streptococcal pneumoniae

G00.2 Streptococcal meningitis MCC
Use additional code to further identify organism (B95.0-B95.5)

G00.3 Staphylococcal meningitis MCC
Use additional code to further identify organism (B95.61-B95.8)

G00.8 Other bacterial meningitis MCC
Meningitis due to Escherichia coli
Meningitis due to Friedländer's bacillus
Meningitis due to Klebsiella
Use additional code to further identify organism (B96.-)

G00.9 Bacterial meningitis, unspecified MCC
Meningitis due to gram-negative bacteria, unspecified
Purulent meningitis NOS
Pyogenic meningitis NOS
Suppurative meningitis NOS

G01 Meningitis in bacterial diseases classified elsewhere MCC
Code first underlying disease

EXCLUDES 1 *meningitis (in):*
gonococcal (A54.81)
leptospirosis (A27.81)
listeriosis (A32.11)
Lyme disease (A69.21)
meningococcal (A39.0)
neurosyphilis (A52.13)
tuberculosis (A17.0)
meningoencephalitis and meningomyelitis in bacterial diseases classified elsewhere (G05)

G02 Meningitis in other infectious and parasitic diseases classified elsewhere MCC
Code first underlying disease, such as:
African trypanosomiasis (B56.-)
poliovirus infection (A80.-)

EXCLUDES 1 *candidal meningitis (B37.5)*
coccidioidomycosis meningitis (B38.4)
cryptococcal meningitis (B45.1)
herpesviral [herpes simplex] meningitis (B00.3)
infectious mononucleosis complicated by meningitis (B27.- with fourth character 2)
measles complicated by meningitis (B05.1)
meningoencephalitis and meningomyelitis in other infectious and parasitic diseases classified elsewhere (G05)
mumps meningitis (B26.1)
rubella meningitis (B06.02)
varicella [chickenpox] meningitis (B01.0)
zoster meningitis (B02.1)

✓4th G03 Meningitis due to other and unspecified causes

INCLUDES arachnoiditis NOS
leptomeningitis NOS
meningitis NOS
pachymeningitis NOS

EXCLUDES 1 *meningoencephalitis (G04.-)*
meningomyelitis (G04.-)

G03.0 Nonpyogenic meningitis MCC
Aseptic meningitis
Nonbacterial meningitis
DEF: Type of meningitis where no bacterial, viral, or other infectious source exists that explains the meningitis symptomology.

G03.1 Chronic meningitis CC

G03.2 Benign recurrent meningitis [Mollaret] CC
DEF: Aseptic or noninfectious inflammation of the meninges with the presence of Mollaret cells in the spinal fluid. The patient experiences recurrent bouts of inflammation, lasting anywhere from two to five days.

G03.8 Meningitis due to other specified causes MCC

G03.9 Meningitis, unspecified MCC
Arachnoiditis (spinal) NOS

✓4th G04 Encephalitis, myelitis and encephalomyelitis

INCLUDES acute ascending myelitis
meningoencephalitis
meningomyelitis

EXCLUDES 1 *encephalopathy NOS (G93.40)*

EXCLUDES 2 *acute transverse myelitis (G37.3-)*
alcoholic encephalopathy (G31.2)
benign myalgic encephalomyelitis (G93.3)
multiple sclerosis (G35)
subacute necrotizing myelitis (G37.4)
toxic encephalitis (G92)
toxic encephalopathy (G92)

DEF: Encephalitis: Inflammation of the brain, often caused by viral or bacterial infection.
DEF: Encephalomyelitis: Inflammatory disease, often viral in nature, that affects the brain and spinal cord.
DEF: Myelitis: Inflammation of the spinal cord.

✓5th G04.0 Acute disseminated encephalitis and encephalomyelitis (ADEM)

EXCLUDES 1 *acute necrotizing hemorrhagic encephalopathy (G04.3-)*
other noninfectious acute disseminated encephalomyelitis (noninfectious ADEM) (G04.81)

G04.00 Acute disseminated encephalitis and encephalomyelitis, unspecified MCC

G04.01 Postinfectious acute disseminated encephalitis and encephalomyelitis (postinfectious ADEM) MCC

EXCLUDES 1 *post chickenpox encephalitis (B01.1)*
post measles encephalitis (B05.0)
post measles myelitis (B05.1)

GØ4.Ø2 Postimmunization acute disseminated encephalitis, myelitis and encephalomyelitis MCC
Encephalitis, post immunization
Encephalomyelitis, post immunization
Use additional code to identify the vaccine (T5Ø.A-, T5Ø.B-, T5Ø.Z-)

GØ4.1 Tropical spastic paraplegia CC HCC

GØ4.2 Bacterial meningoencephalitis and meningomyelitis, not elsewhere classified MCC

✓5th **GØ4.3 Acute necrotizing hemorrhagic encephalopathy**
EXCLUDES 1 *acute disseminated encephalitis and encephalomyelitis (GØ4.Ø-)*

GØ4.3Ø Acute necrotizing hemorrhagic encephalopathy, unspecified MCC

GØ4.31 Postinfectious acute necrotizing hemorrhagic encephalopathy MCC

GØ4.32 Postimmunization acute necrotizing hemorrhagic encephalopathy MCC
Use additional code to identify the vaccine (T5Ø.A-, T5Ø.B-, T5Ø.Z-)

GØ4.39 Other acute necrotizing hemorrhagic encephalopathy MCC
Code also underlying etiology, if applicable

✓5th **GØ4.8 Other encephalitis, myelitis and encephalomyelitis**
Code also any associated seizure (G4Ø.-, R56.9)

GØ4.81 Other encephalitis and encephalomyelitis HIV MCC
Noninfectious acute disseminated encephalomyelitis (noninfectious ADEM)

GØ4.89 Other myelitis HIV MCC HCC
AHA: 2020,1Q,14
TIP: Report for acute flaccid myelitis.

✓5th **GØ4.9 Encephalitis, myelitis and encephalomyelitis, unspecified**

GØ4.9Ø Encephalitis and encephalomyelitis, unspecified HIV MCC
Ventriculitis (cerebral) NOS

GØ4.91 Myelitis, unspecified HIV MCC HCC

✓4th **GØ5 Encephalitis, myelitis and encephalomyelitis in diseases classified elsewhere**
Code first underlying disease, such as:
human immunodeficiency virus [HIV] disease (B2Ø)
poliovirus (A8Ø.-)
suppurative otitis media (H66.Ø1-H66.4)
trichinellosis (B75)
EXCLUDES 1 *adenoviral encephalitis, myelitis and encephalomyelitis (A85.1)*
congenital toxoplasmosis encephalitis, myelitis and encephalomyelitis (P37.1)
cytomegaloviral encephalitis, myelitis and encephalomyelitis (B25.8)
encephalitis, myelitis and encephalomyelitis (in) measles (BØ5.Ø)
encephalitis, myelitis and encephalomyelitis (in) systemic lupus erythematosus (M32.19)
enteroviral encephalitis, myelitis and encephalomyelitis (A85.Ø)
eosinophilic meningoencephalitis (B83.2)
herpesviral [herpes simplex] encephalitis, myelitis and encephalomyelitis (BØØ.4)
listerial encephalitis, myelitis and encephalomyelitis (A32.12)
meningococcal encephalitis, myelitis and encephalomyelitis (A39.81)
mumps encephalitis, myelitis and encephalomyelitis (B26.2)
postchickenpox encephalitis, myelitis and encephalomyelitis (BØ1.1-)
rubella encephalitis, myelitis and encephalomyelitis (BØ6.Ø1)
toxoplasmosis encephalitis, myelitis and encephalomyelitis (B58.2)
zoster encephalitis, myelitis and encephalomyelitis (BØ2.Ø)

GØ5.3 Encephalitis and encephalomyelitis in diseases classified elsewhere MCC
Meningoencephalitis in diseases classified elsewhere

GØ5.4 Myelitis in diseases classified elsewhere MCC HCC
Meningomyelitis in diseases classified elsewhere

✓4th **GØ6 Intracranial and intraspinal abscess and granuloma**
Use additional code (B95-B97) to identify infectious agent
DEF: Abscess: Circumscribed collection of pus resulting from bacteria, frequently associated with swelling and other signs of inflammation.
DEF: Granuloma: Abnormal, dense collections or cells forming a mass or nodule of chronically inflamed tissue with granulations that is usually associated with an infective process.

GØ6.Ø Intracranial abscess and granuloma MCC
Brain [any part] abscess (embolic)
Cerebellar abscess (embolic)
Cerebral abscess (embolic)
Intracranial epidural abscess or granuloma
Intracranial extradural abscess or granuloma
Intracranial subdural abscess or granuloma
Otogenic abscess (embolic)
EXCLUDES 1 *tuberculous intracranial abscess and granuloma (A17.81)*

GØ6.1 Intraspinal abscess and granuloma MCC
Abscess (embolic) of spinal cord [any part]
Intraspinal epidural abscess or granuloma
Intraspinal extradural abscess or granuloma
Intraspinal subdural abscess or granuloma
EXCLUDES 1 *tuberculous intraspinal abscess and granuloma (A17.81)*

GØ6.2 Extradural and subdural abscess, unspecified MCC

GØ7 Intracranial and intraspinal abscess and granuloma in diseases classified elsewhere MCC
Code first underlying disease, such as:
schistosomiasis granuloma of brain (B65.-)
EXCLUDES 1 *abscess of brain:*
amebic (AØ6.6)
chromomycotic (B43.1)
gonococcal (A54.82)
tuberculous (A17.81)
tuberculoma of meninges (A17.1)

GØ8 Intracranial and intraspinal phlebitis and thrombophlebitis MCC
Septic embolism of intracranial or intraspinal venous sinuses and veins
Septic endophlebitis of intracranial or intraspinal venous sinuses and veins
Septic phlebitis of intracranial or intraspinal venous sinuses and veins
Septic thrombophlebitis of intracranial or intraspinal venous sinuses and veins
Septic thrombosis of intracranial or intraspinal venous sinuses and veins
EXCLUDES 1 *intracranial phlebitis and thrombophlebitis complicating:*
abortion, ectopic or molar pregnancy (OØØ-OØ7, OØ8.7)
pregnancy, childbirth and the puerperium (O22.5, O87.3)
nonpyogenic intracranial phlebitis and thrombophlebitis (I67.6)
EXCLUDES 2 *intracranial phlebitis and thrombophlebitis complicating nonpyogenic intraspinal phlebitis and thrombophlebitis (G95.1)*
DEF: Inflammation and formation of a blood clot in a vein within the brain or spine, or their linings.

GØ9 Sequelae of inflammatory diseases of central nervous system
NOTE Category GØ9 is to be used to indicate conditions whose primary classification is to GØØ-GØ8 as the cause of sequelae, themselves classifiable elsewhere. The "sequelae" include conditions specified as residuals.
Code first condition resulting from (sequela) of inflammatory diseases of central nervous system

Systemic atrophies primarily affecting the central nervous system (G1Ø-G14)

G1Ø Huntington's disease CC HCC
Huntington's chorea
Huntington's dementia
Code also dementia in other diseases classified elsewhere without behavioral disturbance (FØ2.8Ø)
DEF: Genetic disease caused by degeneration of nerve cells in the brain, characterized by chronic progressive mental deterioration. Dementia and death occur within 15 to 20 years of onset.

√4th **G11 Hereditary ataxia**

EXCLUDES 2 *cerebral palsy (G8Ø.-)*
hereditary and idiopathic neuropathy (G6Ø.-)
metabolic disorders (E7Ø-E88)

DEF: Ataxia: Defect in muscular control or coordination due to a central nervous system disorder, particularly when voluntary muscular movements are attempted.

G11.Ø Congenital nonprogressive ataxia CC HCC

▲ √5th **G11.1 Early-onset cerebellar ataxia**
~~Early-onset cerebellar ataxia with essential tremor~~
~~Early-onset cerebellar ataxia with myoclonus [Hunt's ataxia]~~
~~Early-onset cerebellar ataxia with retained tendon reflexes~~
~~Friedreich's ataxia (autosomal recessive)~~
~~X-linked recessive spinocerebellar ataxia~~

● **G11.1Ø Early-onset cerebellar ataxia, unspecified** CC

● **G11.11 Friedreich ataxia** CC
Autosomal recessive Friedreich ataxia
Friedreich ataxia with retained reflexes

● **G11.19 Other early-onset cerebellar ataxia** CC
Early-onset cerebellar ataxia with essential tremor
Early-onset cerebellar ataxia with myoclonus [Hunt's ataxia]
Early-onset cerebellar ataxia with retained tendon reflexes
X-linked recessive spinocerebellar ataxia

G11.2 Late-onset cerebellar ataxia CC HCC A

G11.3 Cerebellar ataxia with defective DNA repair CC HCC
Ataxia telangiectasia [Louis-Bar]
EXCLUDES 2 *Cockayne's syndrome (Q87.19)*
other disorders of purine and pyrimidine metabolism (E79.-)
xeroderma pigmentosum (Q82.1)

G11.4 Hereditary spastic paraplegia CC HCC

G11.8 Other hereditary ataxias CC HCC

G11.9 Hereditary ataxia, unspecified CC HCC
Hereditary cerebellar ataxia NOS
Hereditary cerebellar degeneration
Hereditary cerebellar disease
Hereditary cerebellar syndrome

√4th **G12 Spinal muscular atrophy and related syndromes**

G12.Ø Infantile spinal muscular atrophy, type I [Werdnig-Hoffman] CC HCC

G12.1 Other inherited spinal muscular atrophy CC HCC
Adult form spinal muscular atrophy
Childhood form, type II spinal muscular atrophy
Distal spinal muscular atrophy
Juvenile form, type III spinal muscular atrophy [Kugelberg-Welander]
Progressive bulbar palsy of childhood [Fazio-Londe]
Scapuloperoneal form spinal muscular atrophy

√5th **G12.2 Motor neuron disease**
AHA: 2017,4Q,9-10

G12.2Ø Motor neuron disease, unspecified CC HCC

G12.21 Amyotrophic lateral sclerosis CC HCC A

G12.22 Progressive bulbar palsy CC HCC

G12.23 Primary lateral sclerosis CC HCC

G12.24 Familial motor neuron disease CC HCC

G12.25 Progressive spinal muscle atrophy CC HCC

G12.29 Other motor neuron disease CC HCC

G12.8 Other spinal muscular atrophies and related syndromes CC HCC

G12.9 Spinal muscular atrophy, unspecified CC HCC

√4th **G13 Systemic atrophies primarily affecting central nervous system in diseases classified elsewhere**

G13.Ø Paraneoplastic neuromyopathy and neuropathy HCC
Carcinomatous neuromyopathy
Sensorial paraneoplastic neuropathy [Denny Brown]
Code first underlying neoplasm (CØØ-D49)

G13.1 Other systemic atrophy primarily affecting central nervous system in neoplastic disease HCC
Paraneoplastic limbic encephalopathy
Code first underlying neoplasm (CØØ-D49)

G13.2 Systemic atrophy primarily affecting the central nervous system in myxedema HCC
Code first underlying disease, such as:
hypothyroidism (EØ3.-)
myxedematous congenital iodine deficiency (EØØ.1)

G13.8 Systemic atrophy primarily affecting central nervous system in other diseases classified elsewhere HCC
Code first underlying disease

G14 Postpolio syndrome
INCLUDES postpolio myelitic syndrome
EXCLUDES 1 *sequelae of poliomyelitis (B91)*

Extrapyramidal and movement disorders (G2Ø-G26)

G2Ø Parkinson's disease HCC
Hemiparkinsonism
Idiopathic Parkinsonism or Parkinson's disease
Paralysis agitans
Parkinsonism or Parkinson's disease NOS
Primary Parkinsonism or Parkinson's disease
▶Use additional code to identify:◀
▶dementia with behavioral disturbance (FØ2.81)◀
▶dementia without behavioral disturbance (FØ2.8Ø)◀
EXCLUDES 1 *dementia with Parkinsonism (G31.83)*
AHA: 2017,2Q,7; 2016,2Q,6
TIP: Repeated falls (R29.6) are not integral to Parkinson's disease and can be separately coded.

√4th **G21 Secondary parkinsonism**
EXCLUDES 1 *dementia with Parkinsonism (G31.83)*
Huntington's disease (G1Ø)
Shy-Drager syndrome (G9Ø.3)
syphilitic Parkinsonism (A52.19)

G21.Ø Malignant neuroleptic syndrome MCC
Use additional code for adverse effect, if applicable, to identify drug (T43.3X5, T43.4X5, T43.5Ø5, T43.595)
EXCLUDES 1 *neuroleptic induced parkinsonism (G21.11)*

√5th **G21.1 Other drug-induced secondary parkinsonism**

G21.11 Neuroleptic induced parkinsonism CC HCC
Use additional code for adverse effect, if applicable, to identify drug (T43.3X5, T43.4X5, T43.5Ø5, T43.595)
EXCLUDES 1 *malignant neuroleptic syndrome (G21.Ø)*

G21.19 Other drug induced secondary parkinsonism CC HCC
Other medication-induced parkinsonism
Use additional code for adverse effect, if applicable, to identify drug (T36-T5Ø with fifth or sixth character 5)

G21.2 Secondary parkinsonism due to other external agents CC HCC
Code first (T51-T65) to identify external agent

G21.3 Postencephalitic parkinsonism CC HCC

G21.4 Vascular parkinsonism HCC

G21.8 Other secondary parkinsonism CC HCC

G21.9 Secondary parkinsonism, unspecified CC HCC

√4th **G23 Other degenerative diseases of basal ganglia**
EXCLUDES 2 *multi-system degeneration of the autonomic nervous system (G9Ø.3)*

G23.Ø Hallervorden-Spatz disease CC HCC
Pigmentary pallidal degeneration

G23.1 Progressive supranuclear ophthalmoplegia [Steele-Richardson-Olszewski] CC HCC
Progressive supranuclear palsy

G23.2 Striatonigral degeneration CC HCC

G23.8 Other specified degenerative diseases of basal ganglia CC HCC
Calcification of basal ganglia

G23.9 Degenerative disease of basal ganglia, unspecified CC HCC

✓4th G24 Dystonia

INCLUDES dyskinesia

EXCLUDES 2 *athetoid cerebral palsy (G8Ø.3)*

DEF: Disorder of abnormal muscle tone, excessive or inadequate. Involuntary movements and prolonged muscle contractions result in tremors, abnormalities in posture, and twisting body motions that affect an isolated area or the whole body.

✓5th G24.Ø Drug induced dystonia

Use additional code for adverse effect, if applicable, to identify drug (T36-T5Ø with fifth or sixth character 5)

G24.Ø1 Drug induced subacute dyskinesia

Drug induced blepharospasm
Drug induced orofacial dyskinesia
Neuroleptic induced tardive dyskinesia
Tardive dyskinesia

G24.Ø2 Drug induced acute dystonia CC

Acute dystonic reaction to drugs
Neuroleptic induced acute dystonia

G24.Ø9 Other drug induced dystonia CC

G24.1 Genetic torsion dystonia

Dystonia deformans progressiva
Dystonia musculorum deformans
Familial torsion dystonia
Idiopathic familial dystonia
Idiopathic (torsion) dystonia NOS
(Schwalbe-) Ziehen-Oppenheim disease

G24.2 Idiopathic nonfamilial dystonia CC

G24.3 Spasmodic torticollis

EXCLUDES 1 *congenital torticollis (Q68.Ø)*
hysterical torticollis (F44.4)
ocular torticollis (R29.891)
psychogenic torticollis (F45.8)
torticollis NOS (M43.6)
traumatic recurrent torticollis (S13.4)

DEF: Twisted, unnatural position of the neck due to contracted cervical muscles that pull the head to one side or cause involuntary shaking of the head.

G24.4 Idiopathic orofacial dystonia

Orofacial dyskinesia

EXCLUDES 1 *drug induced orofacial dyskinesia (G24.Ø1)*

G24.5 Blepharospasm

EXCLUDES 1 *drug induced blepharospasm (G24.Ø1)*

DEF: Involuntary contraction of the orbicularis oculi muscle, resulting in the eyelids being completely closed.

G24.8 Other dystonia CC

Acquired torsion dystonia NOS

G24.9 Dystonia, unspecified

Dyskinesia NOS

✓4th G25 Other extrapyramidal and movement disorders

EXCLUDES 2 *sleep related movement disorders (G47.6-)*

G25.Ø Essential tremor

Familial tremor

EXCLUDES 1 *tremor NOS (R25.1)*

G25.1 Drug-induced tremor

Use additional code for adverse effect, if applicable, to identify drug (T36-T5Ø with fifth or sixth character 5)

G25.2 Other specified forms of tremor

Intention tremor

G25.3 Myoclonus

Drug-induced myoclonus
Palatal myoclonus
Use additional code for adverse effect, if applicable, to identify drug (T36-T5Ø with fifth or sixth character 5)

EXCLUDES 1 *facial myokymia (G51.4)*
myoclonic epilepsy (G4Ø.-)

DEF: Spasmodic, brief, involuntary muscle contractions that can be due to an undetermined etiology, drug-induced, or caused by a disease process.

G25.4 Drug-induced chorea

Use additional code for adverse effect, if applicable, to identify drug (T36-T5Ø with fifth or sixth character 5)

G25.5 Other chorea

Chorea NOS

EXCLUDES 1 *chorea NOS with heart involvement (IØ2.Ø)*
Huntington's chorea (G1Ø)
rheumatic chorea (IØ2.-)
Sydenham's chorea (IØ2.-)

✓5th G25.6 Drug induced tics and other tics of organic origin

G25.61 Drug induced tics

Use additional code for adverse effect, if applicable, to identify drug (T36-T5Ø with fifth or sixth character 5)

G25.69 Other tics of organic origin

EXCLUDES 1 *habit spasm (F95.9)*
tic NOS (F95.9)
Tourette's syndrome (F95.2)

✓5th G25.7 Other and unspecified drug induced movement disorders

Use additional code for adverse effect, if applicable, to identify drug (T36-T5Ø with fifth or sixth character 5)

G25.7Ø Drug induced movement disorder, unspecified

G25.71 Drug induced akathisia

Drug induced acathisia
Neuroleptic induced acute akathisia
Tardive akathisia

G25.79 Other drug induced movement disorders

✓5th G25.8 Other specified extrapyramidal and movement disorders

G25.81 Restless legs syndrome

DEF: Neurological disorder of unknown etiology creating an irresistible urge to move the legs, which may temporarily relieve the symptoms. This syndrome is accompanied by motor restlessness and sensations of pain, burning, prickling, or tingling.

G25.82 Stiff-man syndrome CC

G25.83 Benign shuddering attacks

G25.89 Other specified extrapyramidal and movement disorders

G25.9 Extrapyramidal and movement disorder, unspecified CC

G26 Extrapyramidal and movement disorders in diseases classified elsewhere

Code first underlying disease

Other degenerative diseases of the nervous system (G3Ø-G32)

✓4th G3Ø Alzheimer's disease

INCLUDES Alzheimer's dementia senile and presenile forms

Use additional code to identify:
delirium, if applicable (FØ5)
dementia with behavioral disturbance (FØ2.81)
dementia without behavioral disturbance (FØ2.8Ø)

EXCLUDES 1 *senile degeneration of brain NEC (G31.1)*
senile dementia NOS (FØ3)
senility NOS (R41.81)

AHA: 2017,1Q,43

TIP: A code from subcategory F02.8 should always be assigned with a code from this category, even in the absence of documented dementia.

TIP: Functional quadriplegia (R53.2) is not integral to Alzheimer's disease and can be coded in addition to codes from category G30.

G3Ø.Ø Alzheimer's disease with early onset HCC

G3Ø.1 Alzheimer's disease with late onset HCC A

G3Ø.8 Other Alzheimer's disease HCC

G3Ø.9 Alzheimer's disease, unspecified HCC

AHA: 2016,2Q,6; 2012,4Q,95

G31 Other degenerative diseases of nervous system, not elsewhere classified
For codes G31.Ø–G31.83, G31.85–G31.9, use additional code to identify:
dementia with behavioral disturbance (FØ2.81)
dementia without behavioral disturbance (FØ2.8Ø)
EXCLUDES 2 *Reye's syndrome (G93.7)*

G31.Ø Frontotemporal dementia

G31.Ø1 Pick's disease HCC
Primary progressive aphasia
Progressive isolated aphasia
DEF: Progressive frontotemporal dementia with asymmetrical atrophy of the frontal and temporal regions of the cerebral cortex and abnormal rounded brain cells called Pick cells with the presence of abnormal staining of protein (called tau). Symptoms include prominent apathy, behavioral changes such as disinhibition and restlessness, echolalia, impairment of language, memory, and intellect, increased carelessness, poor personal hygiene, and decreased attention span.

G31.Ø9 Other frontotemporal dementia HCC
Frontal dementia

G31.1 Senile degeneration of brain, not elsewhere classified HCC
EXCLUDES 1 *Alzheimer's disease (G3Ø.-)*
senility NOS (R41.81)

G31.2 Degeneration of nervous system due to alcohol HCC
Alcoholic cerebellar ataxia
Alcoholic cerebellar degeneration
Alcoholic cerebral degeneration
Alcoholic encephalopathy
Dysfunction of the autonomic nervous system due to alcohol
Code also associated alcoholism (F1Ø.-)

G31.8 Other specified degenerative diseases of nervous system

G31.81 Alpers disease CC HCC
Grey-matter degeneration

G31.82 Leigh's disease CC HCC
Subacute necrotizing encephalopathy

G31.83 Dementia with Lewy bodies HCC
Dementia with Parkinsonism
Lewy body dementia
Lewy body disease
AHA: 2017,2Q,7; 2016,4Q,141
DEF: Cerebral dementia with neurophysiologic changes, increased hippocampal volume, hypoperfusion in the occipital lobes, beta amyloid deposits with neurofibrillary tangles, and atrophy of the cortex and brainstem. Hallmark neuropsychological characteristics include fluctuating cognition with pronounced variation in attention and alertness, recurrent hallucinations, and Parkinsonism.

G31.84 Mild cognitive impairment, so stated
Mild neurocognitive disorder
EXCLUDES 1 *age related cognitive decline (R41.81)*
altered mental status (R41.82)
cerebral degeneration (G31.9)
change in mental status (R41.82)
cognitive deficits following (sequelae of) cerebral hemorrhage or infarction (I69.Ø1-, I69.11-, I69.21-, I69.31-, I69.81-, I69.91-)
cognitive impairment due to intracranial or head injury (SØ6.-)
dementia (FØ1.-, FØ2.-, FØ3)
mild memory disturbance (FØ6.8)
neurologic neglect syndrome (R41.4)
personality change, nonpsychotic (F68.8)

G31.85 Corticobasal degeneration HCC

G31.89 Other specified degenerative diseases of nervous system HCC

G31.9 Degenerative disease of nervous system, unspecified HCC

G32 Other degenerative disorders of nervous system in diseases classified elsewhere

G32.Ø Subacute combined degeneration of spinal cord in diseases classified elsewhere CC HCC
Dana-Putnam syndrome
Sclerosis of spinal cord (combined) (dorsolateral) (posterolateral)
Code first underlying disease, such as:
anemia (D51.9)
dietary (D51.3)
pernicious (D51.Ø)
vitamin B12 deficiency (E53.8)
EXCLUDES 1 *syphilitic combined degeneration of spinal cord (A52.11)*

G32.8 Other specified degenerative disorders of nervous system in diseases classified elsewhere
Code first underlying disease, such as:
amyloidosis cerebral degeneration (E85.-)
cerebral degeneration (due to) hypothyroidism (EØØ.Ø-EØ3.9)
cerebral degeneration (due to) neoplasm (CØØ-D49)
cerebral degeneration (due to) vitamin B deficiency, except thiamine (E52-E53.-)
EXCLUDES 1 *superior hemorrhagic polioencephalitis [Wernicke's encephalopathy] (E51.2)*

G32.81 Cerebellar ataxia in diseases classified elsewhere CC HCC
Code first underlying disease, such as:
celiac disease (with gluten ataxia) (K9Ø.Ø)
cerebellar ataxia (in) neoplastic disease (paraneoplastic cerebellar degeneration) (CØØ-D49)
non-celiac gluten ataxia (M35.9)
EXCLUDES 1 *systemic atrophy primarily affecting the central nervous system in alcoholic cerebellar ataxia (G31.2)*
systemic atrophy primarily affecting the central nervous system in myxedema (G13.2)

G32.89 Other specified degenerative disorders of nervous system in diseases classified elsewhere
Degenerative encephalopathy in diseases classified elsewhere

Demyelinating diseases of the central nervous system (G35-G37)

G35 Multiple sclerosis HCC
Disseminated multiple sclerosis
Generalized multiple sclerosis
Multiple sclerosis NOS
Multiple sclerosis of brain stem
Multiple sclerosis of cord

G36 Other acute disseminated demyelination
EXCLUDES 1 *postinfectious encephalitis and encephalomyelitis NOS (GØ4.Ø1)*
DEF: Demyelination: Abnormal loss of myelin, the protective white matter that insulates nerve endings and facilitates neuroreception and neurotransmission. When this substance is damaged, the nerve is short-circuited, resulting in impaired or loss of function.

G36.Ø Neuromyelitis optica [Devic] CC HCC
Demyelination in optic neuritis
EXCLUDES 1 *optic neuritis NOS (H46)*

G36.1 Acute and subacute hemorrhagic leukoencephalitis [Hurst] CC HCC

G36.8 Other specified acute disseminated demyelination CC HCC

G36.9 Acute disseminated demyelination, unspecified HIV CC HCC

G37 Other demyelinating diseases of central nervous system

G37.Ø Diffuse sclerosis of central nervous system CC HCC
Periaxial encephalitis
Schilder's disease
EXCLUDES 1 *X linked adrenoleukodystrophy (E71.52-)*

G37.1 Central demyelination of corpus callosum CC HCC

G37.2 Central pontine myelinolysis CC HCC

G37.3 Acute transverse myelitis in demyelinating disease of central nervous system CC HCC
Acute transverse myelitis NOS
Acute transverse myelopathy
EXCLUDES 1 *multiple sclerosis (G35)*
neuromyelitis optica [Devic] (G36.0)

G37.4 Subacute necrotizing myelitis of central nervous system HIV MCC HCC

G37.5 Concentric sclerosis [Balo] of central nervous system CC HCC

G37.8 Other specified demyelinating diseases of central nervous system CC HCC

G37.9 Demyelinating disease of central nervous system, unspecified HIV CC HCC

Episodic and paroxysmal disorders (G40-G47)

✓4th G40 Epilepsy and recurrent seizures

NOTE The following terms are to be considered equivalent to intractable: pharmacoresistant (pharmacologically resistant), treatment resistant, refractory (medically) and poorly controlled

EXCLUDES 1 *conversion disorder with seizures (F44.5)*
convulsions NOS (R56.9)
post traumatic seizures (R56.1)
seizure (convulsive) NOS (R56.9)
seizure of newborn (P90)

EXCLUDES 2 *hippocampal sclerosis (G93.81)*
mesial temporal sclerosis (G93.81)
temporal sclerosis (G93.81)
Todd's paralysis (G83.84)

✓5th G40.0 Localization-related (focal) (partial) idiopathic epilepsy and epileptic syndromes with seizures of localized onset
Benign childhood epilepsy with centrotemporal EEG spikes
Childhood epilepsy with occipital EEG paroxysms
EXCLUDES 1 *adult onset localization-related epilepsy (G40.1-, G40.2-)*

✓6th G40.00 Localization-related (focal) (partial) idiopathic epilepsy and epileptic syndromes with seizures of localized onset, not intractable
Localization-related (focal) (partial) idiopathic epilepsy and epileptic syndromes with seizures of localized onset without intractability

G40.001 Localization-related (focal) (partial) idiopathic epilepsy and epileptic syndromes with seizures of localized onset, not intractable, with status epilepticus CC HCC

G40.009 Localization-related (focal) (partial) idiopathic epilepsy and epileptic syndromes with seizures of localized onset, not intractable, without status epilepticus CC HCC
Localization-related (focal) (partial) idiopathic epilepsy and epileptic syndromes with seizures of localized onset NOS

✓6th G40.01 Localization-related (focal) (partial) idiopathic epilepsy and epileptic syndromes with seizures of localized onset, intractable

G40.011 Localization-related (focal) (partial) idiopathic epilepsy and epileptic syndromes with seizures of localized onset, intractable, with status epilepticus CC HCC

G40.019 Localization-related (focal) (partial) idiopathic epilepsy and epileptic syndromes with seizures of localized onset, intractable, without status epilepticus CC HCC

✓5th G40.1 Localization-related (focal) (partial) symptomatic epilepsy and epileptic syndromes with simple partial seizures
Attacks without alteration of consciousness
Epilepsia partialis continua [Kozhevnikof]
Simple partial seizures developing into secondarily generalized seizures

✓6th G40.10 Localization-related (focal) (partial) symptomatic epilepsy and epileptic syndromes with simple partial seizures, not intractable
Localization-related (focal) (partial) symptomatic epilepsy and epileptic syndromes with simple partial seizures without intractability

G40.101 Localization-related (focal) (partial) symptomatic epilepsy and epileptic syndromes with simple partial seizures, not intractable, with status epilepticus CC HCC

G40.109 Localization-related (focal) (partial) symptomatic epilepsy and epileptic syndromes with simple partial seizures, not intractable, without status epilepticus CC HCC
Localization-related (focal) (partial) symptomatic epilepsy and epileptic syndromes with simple partial seizures NOS

✓6th G40.11 Localization-related (focal) (partial) symptomatic epilepsy and epileptic syndromes with simple partial seizures, intractable

G40.111 Localization-related (focal) (partial) symptomatic epilepsy and epileptic syndromes with simple partial seizures, intractable, with status epilepticus CC HCC

G40.119 Localization-related (focal) (partial) symptomatic epilepsy and epileptic syndromes with simple partial seizures, intractable, without status epilepticus CC HCC

✓5th G40.2 Localization-related (focal) (partial) symptomatic epilepsy and epileptic syndromes with complex partial seizures
Attacks with alteration of consciousness, often with automatisms
Complex partial seizures developing into secondarily generalized seizures

✓6th G40.20 Localization-related (focal) (partial) symptomatic epilepsy and epileptic syndromes with complex partial seizures, not intractable
Localization-related (focal) (partial) symptomatic epilepsy and epileptic syndromes with complex partial seizures without intractability

G40.201 Localization-related (focal) (partial) symptomatic epilepsy and epileptic syndromes with complex partial seizures, not intractable, with status epilepticus CC HCC

G40.209 Localization-related (focal) (partial) symptomatic epilepsy and epileptic syndromes with complex partial seizures, not intractable, without status epilepticus CC HCC
Localization-related (focal) (partial) symptomatic epilepsy and epileptic syndromes with complex partial seizures NOS

✓6th G40.21 Localization-related (focal) (partial) symptomatic epilepsy and epileptic syndromes with complex partial seizures, intractable

G40.211 Localization-related (focal) (partial) symptomatic epilepsy and epileptic syndromes with complex partial seizures, intractable, with status epilepticus CC HCC

G40.219 Localization-related (focal) (partial) symptomatic epilepsy and epileptic syndromes with complex partial seizures, intractable, without status epilepticus CC HCC

G40.3 Generalized idiopathic epilepsy and epileptic syndromes
Code also MERRF syndrome, if applicable (E88.42)

G40.30 Generalized idiopathic epilepsy and epileptic syndromes, not intractable
Generalized idiopathic epilepsy and epileptic syndromes without intractability

G40.301 Generalized idiopathic epilepsy and epileptic syndromes, not intractable, with status epilepticus MCC HCC

G40.309 Generalized idiopathic epilepsy and epileptic syndromes, not intractable, without status epilepticus HCC
Generalized idiopathic epilepsy and epileptic syndromes NOS

G40.31 Generalized idiopathic epilepsy and epileptic syndromes, intractable

G40.311 Generalized idiopathic epilepsy and epileptic syndromes, intractable, with status epilepticus MCC HCC

G40.319 Generalized idiopathic epilepsy and epileptic syndromes, intractable, without status epilepticus MCC HCC

G40.A Absence epileptic syndrome
Childhood absence epilepsy [pyknolepsy]
Juvenile absence epilepsy
Absence epileptic syndrome, NOS

G40.A0 Absence epileptic syndrome, not intractable

G40.A01 Absence epileptic syndrome, not intractable, with status epilepticus HCC

G40.A09 Absence epileptic syndrome, not intractable, without status epilepticus HCC

G40.A1 Absence epileptic syndrome, intractable

G40.A11 Absence epileptic syndrome, intractable, with status epilepticus CC HCC

G40.A19 Absence epileptic syndrome, intractable, without status epilepticus CC HCC

G40.B Juvenile myoclonic epilepsy [impulsive petit mal]

G40.B0 Juvenile myoclonic epilepsy, not intractable

G40.B01 Juvenile myoclonic epilepsy, not intractable, with status epilepticus CC HCC

G40.B09 Juvenile myoclonic epilepsy, not intractable, without status epilepticus CC HCC

G40.B1 Juvenile myoclonic epilepsy, intractable

G40.B11 Juvenile myoclonic epilepsy, intractable, with status epilepticus CC HCC

G40.B19 Juvenile myoclonic epilepsy, intractable, without status epilepticus CC HCC

G40.4 Other generalized epilepsy and epileptic syndromes
Epilepsy with grand mal seizures on awakening
Epilepsy with myoclonic absences
Epilepsy with myoclonic-astatic seizures
Grand mal seizure NOS
Nonspecific atonic epileptic seizures
Nonspecific clonic epileptic seizures
Nonspecific myoclonic epileptic seizures
Nonspecific tonic epileptic seizures
Nonspecific tonic-clonic epileptic seizures
Symptomatic early myoclonic encephalopathy

G40.40 Other generalized epilepsy and epileptic syndromes, not intractable
Other generalized epilepsy and epileptic syndromes without intractability
Other generalized epilepsy and epileptic syndromes NOS

G40.401 Other generalized epilepsy and epileptic syndromes, not intractable, with status epilepticus HCC

G40.409 Other generalized epilepsy and epileptic syndromes, not intractable, without status epilepticus HCC

G40.41 Other generalized epilepsy and epileptic syndromes, intractable

G40.411 Other generalized epilepsy and epileptic syndromes, intractable, with status epilepticus CC HCC

G40.419 Other generalized epilepsy and epileptic syndromes, intractable, without status epilepticus CC HCC

● **G40.42 Cyclin-Dependent Kinase-Like 5 Deficiency Disorder**
CDKL5
Use additional code, if known, to identify associated manifestations, such as:
cortical blindness (H47.61-)
global development delay (F88)

G40.5 Epileptic seizures related to external causes
Epileptic seizures related to alcohol
Epileptic seizures related to drugs
Epileptic seizures related to hormonal changes
Epileptic seizures related to sleep deprivation
Epileptic seizures related to stress
Code also, if applicable, associated epilepsy and recurrent seizures (G40.-)
Use additional code for adverse effect, if applicable, to identify drug (T36-T50 with fifth or sixth character 5)

G40.50 Epileptic seizures related to external causes, not intractable

G40.501 Epileptic seizures related to external causes, not intractable, with status epilepticus CC HCC

G40.509 Epileptic seizures related to external causes, not intractable, without status epilepticus CC HCC
Epileptic seizures related to external causes, NOS

G40.8 Other epilepsy and recurrent seizures
Epilepsies and epileptic syndromes undetermined as to whether they are focal or generalized
Landau-Kleffner syndrome

G40.80 Other epilepsy

G40.801 Other epilepsy, not intractable, with status epilepticus CC HCC
Other epilepsy without intractability with status epilepticus

G40.802 Other epilepsy, not intractable, without status epilepticus CC HCC
Other epilepsy NOS
Other epilepsy without intractability without status epilepticus

G40.803 Other epilepsy, intractable, with status epilepticus CC HCC

G40.804 Other epilepsy, intractable, without status epilepticus CC HCC

G40.81 Lennox-Gastaut syndrome
DEF: Severe form of epilepsy with usual onset in early childhood. Seizures are frequent and difficult to treat, causing falls and intellectual impairment.

G40.811 Lennox-Gastaut syndrome, not intractable, with status epilepticus CC HCC

G40.812 Lennox-Gastaut syndrome, not intractable, without status epilepticus CC HCC

G40.813 Lennox-Gastaut syndrome, intractable, with status epilepticus CC HCC

G40.814 Lennox-Gastaut syndrome, intractable, without status epilepticus CC HCC

G40.82 Epileptic spasms
Infantile spasms
Salaam attacks
West's syndrome

G40.821 Epileptic spasms, not intractable, with status epilepticus CC HCC

G40.822 Epileptic spasms, not intractable, without status epilepticus CC HCC

G40.823 Epileptic spasms, intractable, with status epilepticus CC HCC

G40.824 Epileptic spasms, intractable, without status epilepticus CC HCC

● **G40.83 Dravet syndrome**
Polymorphic epilepsy in infancy (PMEI)
Severe myoclonic epilepsy in infancy (SMEI)

● **G40.833 Dravet syndrome, intractable, with status epilepticus** CC

● **G40.834 Dravet syndrome, intractable, without status epilepticus** CC
Dravet syndrome NOS

G40.89 Other seizures CC HCC
EXCLUDES 1 *post traumatic seizures (R56.1)*
recurrent seizures NOS (G40.909)
seizure NOS (R56.9)

✓5th **G40.9 Epilepsy, unspecified**
AHA: 2019,1Q,19

✓6th **G40.90 Epilepsy, unspecified, not intractable**
Epilepsy, unspecified, without intractability

G40.901 Epilepsy, unspecified, not intractable, with status epilepticus HCC

G40.909 Epilepsy, unspecified, not intractable, without status epilepticus HCC
Epilepsy NOS
Epileptic convulsions NOS
Epileptic fits NOS
Epileptic seizures NOS
Recurrent seizures NOS
Seizure disorder NOS

✓6th **G40.91 Epilepsy, unspecified, intractable**
Intractable seizure disorder NOS

G40.911 Epilepsy, unspecified, intractable, with status epilepticus CC HCC

G40.919 Epilepsy, unspecified, intractable, without status epilepticus CC HCC

✓4th **G43 Migraine**

NOTE The following terms are to be considered equivalent to intractable: pharmacoresistant (pharmacologically resistant), treatment resistant, refractory (medically) and poorly controlled

Use additional code for adverse effect, if applicable, to identify drug (T36-T50 with fifth or sixth character 5)

EXCLUDES 1 *headache NOS ▶(R51.9)◀*
lower half migraine (G44.00)

EXCLUDES 2 *headache syndromes (G44.-)*

DEF: Headaches that occur periodically on one or both sides of the head that may be associated with nausea and vomiting, sensitivity to light and sound, dizziness, distorted vision, and cognitive disturbances.

✓5th **G43.0 Migraine without aura**
Common migraine
EXCLUDES 1 *chronic migraine without aura (G43.7-)*

✓6th **G43.00 Migraine without aura, not intractable**
Migraine without aura without mention of refractory migraine

G43.001 Migraine without aura, not intractable, with status migrainosus

G43.009 Migraine without aura, not intractable, without status migrainosus
Migraine without aura NOS

✓6th **G43.01 Migraine without aura, intractable**
Migraine without aura with refractory migraine

G43.011 Migraine without aura, intractable, with status migrainosus

G43.019 Migraine without aura, intractable, without status migrainosus

✓5th **G43.1 Migraine with aura**
Basilar migraine
Classical migraine
Migraine equivalents
Migraine preceded or accompanied by transient focal neurological phenomena
Migraine triggered seizures
Migraine with acute-onset aura
Migraine with aura without headache (migraine equivalents)
Migraine with prolonged aura
Migraine with typical aura
Retinal migraine
Code also any associated seizure (G40.-, R56.9)
EXCLUDES 1 *persistent migraine aura (G43.5-, G43.6-)*

✓6th **G43.10 Migraine with aura, not intractable**
Migraine with aura without mention of refractory migraine

G43.101 Migraine with aura, not intractable, with status migrainosus

G43.109 Migraine with aura, not intractable, without status migrainosus
Migraine with aura NOS

✓6th **G43.11 Migraine with aura, intractable**
Migraine with aura with refractory migraine

G43.111 Migraine with aura, intractable, with status migrainosus

G43.119 Migraine with aura, intractable, without status migrainosus

✓5th **G43.4 Hemiplegic migraine**
Familial migraine
Sporadic migraine

✓6th **G43.40 Hemiplegic migraine, not intractable**
Hemiplegic migraine without refractory migraine

G43.401 Hemiplegic migraine, not intractable, with status migrainosus

G43.409 Hemiplegic migraine, not intractable, without status migrainosus
Hemiplegic migraine NOS

✓6th **G43.41 Hemiplegic migraine, intractable**
Hemiplegic migraine with refractory migraine

G43.411 Hemiplegic migraine, intractable, with status migrainosus

G43.419 Hemiplegic migraine, intractable, without status migrainosus

✓5th **G43.5 Persistent migraine aura without cerebral infarction**

✓6th **G43.50 Persistent migraine aura without cerebral infarction, not intractable**
Persistent migraine aura without cerebral infarction, without refractory migraine

G43.501 Persistent migraine aura without cerebral infarction, not intractable, with status migrainosus

G43.509 Persistent migraine aura without cerebral infarction, not intractable, without status migrainosus
Persistent migraine aura NOS

✓6th **G43.51 Persistent migraine aura without cerebral infarction, intractable**
Persistent migraine aura without cerebral infarction, with refractory migraine

G43.511 Persistent migraine aura without cerebral infarction, intractable, with status migrainosus

G43.519 Persistent migraine aura without cerebral infarction, intractable, without status migrainosus

✓5th **G43.6 Persistent migraine aura with cerebral infarction**
Code also the type of cerebral infarction (I63.-)

✓6th **G43.60 Persistent migraine aura with cerebral infarction, not intractable**
Persistent migraine aura with cerebral infarction, without refractory migraine

G43.601 Persistent migraine aura with cerebral infarction, not intractable, with status migrainosus CC

G43.609 Persistent migraine aura with cerebral infarction, not intractable, without status migrainosus CC

✓6th **G43.61 Persistent migraine aura with cerebral infarction, intractable**
Persistent migraine aura with cerebral infarction, with refractory migraine

G43.611 Persistent migraine aura with cerebral infarction, intractable, with status migrainosus CC

G43.619 Persistent migraine aura with cerebral infarction, intractable, without status migrainosus CC

✓5th **G43.7 Chronic migraine without aura**
Transformed migraine
EXCLUDES 1 *migraine without aura (G43.0-)*

✓6th **G43.70 Chronic migraine without aura, not intractable**
Chronic migraine without aura, without refractory migraine

G43.701 Chronic migraine without aura, not intractable, with status migrainosus

G43.709 **Chronic migraine without aura, not intractable, without status migrainosus**
Chronic migraine without aura NOS

G43.71 **Chronic migraine without aura, intractable**
Chronic migraine without aura, with refractory migraine

G43.711 **Chronic migraine without aura, intractable, with status migrainosus**

G43.719 **Chronic migraine without aura, intractable, without status migrainosus**

G43.A **Cyclical vomiting**
EXCLUDES 1 *cyclical vomiting syndrome unrelated to migraine (R11.15)*
AHA: 2019,4Q,15

G43.A0 **Cyclical vomiting, in migraine, not intractable**
Cyclical vomiting, without refractory migraine

G43.A1 **Cyclical vomiting, in migraine, intractable**
Cyclical vomiting, with refractory migraine

G43.B **Ophthalmoplegic migraine**

G43.B0 **Ophthalmoplegic migraine, not intractable**
Ophthalmoplegic migraine, without refractory migraine

G43.B1 **Ophthalmoplegic migraine, intractable**
Ophthalmoplegic migraine, with refractory migraine

G43.C **Periodic headache syndromes in child or adult**

G43.C0 **Periodic headache syndromes in child or adult, not intractable**
Periodic headache syndromes in child or adult, without refractory migraine

G43.C1 **Periodic headache syndromes in child or adult, intractable**
Periodic headache syndromes in child or adult, with refractory migraine

G43.D **Abdominal migraine**

G43.D0 **Abdominal migraine, not intractable**
Abdominal migraine, without refractory migraine

G43.D1 **Abdominal migraine, intractable**
Abdominal migraine, with refractory migraine

G43.8 **Other migraine**

G43.80 **Other migraine, not intractable**
Other migraine, without refractory migraine

G43.801 **Other migraine, not intractable, with status migrainosus**

G43.809 **Other migraine, not intractable, without status migrainosus**

G43.81 **Other migraine, intractable**
Other migraine, with refractory migraine

G43.811 **Other migraine, intractable, with status migrainosus**

G43.819 **Other migraine, intractable, without status migrainosus**

G43.82 **Menstrual migraine, not intractable**
Menstrual headache, not intractable
Menstrual migraine, without refractory migraine
Menstrually related migraine, not intractable
Pre-menstrual headache, not intractable
Pre-menstrual migraine, not intractable
Pure menstrual migraine, not intractable
Code also associated premenstrual tension syndrome (N94.3)

G43.821 **Menstrual migraine, not intractable, with status migrainosus** ♀

G43.829 **Menstrual migraine, not intractable, without status migrainosus** ♀
Menstrual migraine NOS

G43.83 **Menstrual migraine, intractable**
Menstrual headache, intractable
Menstrual migraine, with refractory migraine
Menstrually related migraine, intractable
Pre-menstrual headache, intractable
Pre-menstrual migraine, intractable
Pure menstrual migraine, intractable
Code also associated premenstrual tension syndrome (N94.3)

G43.831 **Menstrual migraine, intractable, with status migrainosus** ♀

G43.839 **Menstrual migraine, intractable, without status migrainosus** ♀

G43.9 **Migraine, unspecified**

G43.90 **Migraine, unspecified, not intractable**
Migraine, unspecified, without refractory migraine

G43.901 **Migraine, unspecified, not intractable, with status migrainosus**
Status migrainosus NOS

G43.909 **Migraine, unspecified, not intractable, without status migrainosus**
Migraine NOS

G43.91 **Migraine, unspecified, intractable**
Migraine, unspecified, with refractory migraine

G43.911 **Migraine, unspecified, intractable, with status migrainosus**

G43.919 **Migraine, unspecified, intractable, without status migrainosus**

G44 **Other headache syndromes**
EXCLUDES 1 *headache NOS ▶(R51.9)◀*
EXCLUDES 2 *atypical facial pain (G50.1)*
headache due to lumbar puncture (G97.1)
migraines (G43.-)
trigeminal neuralgia (G50.0)

G44.0 **Cluster headaches and other trigeminal autonomic cephalgias (TAC)**
DEF: Cluster headache: Characteristic grouping or clustering of headaches that can last for a number of weeks or months and then completely disappear for months or years. They are typically not associated with gastrointestinal upset or light sensitivity as experienced in migraines.

G44.00 **Cluster headache syndrome, unspecified**
Ciliary neuralgia
Cluster headache NOS
Histamine cephalgia
Lower half migraine
Migrainous neuralgia

G44.001 **Cluster headache syndrome, unspecified, intractable**

G44.009 **Cluster headache syndrome, unspecified, not intractable**
Cluster headache syndrome NOS

G44.01 **Episodic cluster headache**

G44.011 **Episodic cluster headache, intractable**

G44.019 **Episodic cluster headache, not intractable**
Episodic cluster headache NOS

G44.02 **Chronic cluster headache**

G44.021 **Chronic cluster headache, intractable**

G44.029 **Chronic cluster headache, not intractable**
Chronic cluster headache NOS

G44.03 **Episodic paroxysmal hemicrania**
Paroxysmal hemicrania NOS

G44.031 **Episodic paroxysmal hemicrania, intractable**

G44.039 **Episodic paroxysmal hemicrania, not intractable**
Episodic paroxysmal hemicrania NOS

G44.04 **Chronic paroxysmal hemicrania**

G44.041 **Chronic paroxysmal hemicrania, intractable**

G44.049 **Chronic paroxysmal hemicrania, not intractable**
Chronic paroxysmal hemicrania NOS

G44.05 **Short lasting unilateral neuralgiform headache with conjunctival injection and tearing (SUNCT)**

G44.051 **Short lasting unilateral neuralgiform headache with conjunctival injection and tearing (SUNCT), intractable**

G44.059 **Short lasting unilateral neuralgiform headache with conjunctival injection and tearing (SUNCT), not intractable**
Short lasting unilateral neuralgiform headache with conjunctival injection and tearing (SUNCT) NOS

G44.09 **Other trigeminal autonomic cephalgias (TAC)**

G44.091 **Other trigeminal autonomic cephalgias (TAC), intractable**

G44.099 **Other trigeminal autonomic cephalgias (TAC), not intractable**

Chapter 6. Diseases of the Nervous System G43.709–G44.099

G44.1 Vascular headache, not elsewhere classified
EXCLUDES 2 *cluster headache (G44.Ø)*
complicated headache syndromes (G44.5-)
drug-induced headache (G44.4-)
migraine (G43.-)
other specified headache syndromes (G44.8-)
post-traumatic headache (G44.3-)
tension-type headache (G44.2-)

✓5th **G44.2 Tension-type headache**
✓6th **G44.2Ø Tension-type headache, unspecified**
G44.2Ø1 Tension-type headache, unspecified, intractable
G44.2Ø9 Tension-type headache, unspecified, not intractable
Tension headache NOS
✓6th **G44.21 Episodic tension-type headache**
G44.211 Episodic tension-type headache, intractable
G44.219 Episodic tension-type headache, not intractable
Episodic tension-type headache NOS
✓6th **G44.22 Chronic tension-type headache**
G44.221 Chronic tension-type headache, intractable
G44.229 Chronic tension-type headache, not intractable
Chronic tension-type headache NOS

✓5th **G44.3 Post-traumatic headache**
✓6th **G44.3Ø Post-traumatic headache, unspecified**
G44.3Ø1 Post-traumatic headache, unspecified, intractable
G44.3Ø9 Post-traumatic headache, unspecified, not intractable
Post-traumatic headache NOS
✓6th **G44.31 Acute post-traumatic headache**
G44.311 Acute post-traumatic headache, intractable
G44.319 Acute post-traumatic headache, not intractable
Acute post-traumatic headache NOS
✓6th **G44.32 Chronic post-traumatic headache**
G44.321 Chronic post-traumatic headache, intractable
G44.329 Chronic post-traumatic headache, not intractable
Chronic post-traumatic headache NOS

✓5th **G44.4 Drug-induced headache, not elsewhere classified**
Medication overuse headache
Use additional code for adverse effect, if applicable, to identify drug (T36-T5Ø with fifth or sixth character 5)
G44.4Ø Drug-induced headache, not elsewhere classified, not intractable
G44.41 Drug-induced headache, not elsewhere classified, intractable

✓5th **G44.5 Complicated headache syndromes**
G44.51 Hemicrania continua
DEF: Persistent primary headache of unknown causation occurring on one side of the face and head. May last for more than three months, with daily and continuous pain of moderate intensity with severe exacerbations.
G44.52 New daily persistent headache (NDPH)
G44.53 Primary thunderclap headache
G44.59 Other complicated headache syndrome

✓5th **G44.8 Other specified headache syndromes**
EXCLUDES 2 ▶*headache with orthostatic or positional component, not elsewhere classifed (R51.Ø)*◀
G44.81 Hypnic headache
G44.82 Headache associated with sexual activity
Orgasmic headache
Preorgasmic headache
G44.83 Primary cough headache
G44.84 Primary exertional headache
G44.85 Primary stabbing headache
G44.89 Other headache syndrome

✓4th **G45 Transient cerebral ischemic attacks and related syndromes**
EXCLUDES 1 *neonatal cerebral ischemia (P91.Ø)*
transient retinal artery occlusion (H34.Ø-)
AHA: 2018,2Q,9
DEF: Transient cerebral ischemic attack: Intermittent or brief cerebral dysfunction from lack of oxygenation with no persistent neurological deficits associated with occlusive vascular disease. TIA may denote an impending cerebrovascular accident.
G45.Ø Vertebro-basilar artery syndrome CC
G45.1 Carotid artery syndrome (hemispheric) CC
G45.2 Multiple and bilateral precerebral artery syndromes CC
G45.3 Amaurosis fugax CC
G45.4 Transient global amnesia
EXCLUDES 1 *amnesia NOS (R41.3)*
G45.8 Other transient cerebral ischemic attacks and related syndromes CC
G45.9 Transient cerebral ischemic attack, unspecified CC
Spasm of cerebral artery
TIA
Transient cerebral ischemia NOS

✓4th **G46 Vascular syndromes of brain in cerebrovascular diseases**
Code first underlying cerebrovascular disease (I6Ø-I69)
G46.Ø Middle cerebral artery syndrome CC
G46.1 Anterior cerebral artery syndrome CC
G46.2 Posterior cerebral artery syndrome CC
G46.3 Brain stem stroke syndrome
Benedikt syndrome
Claude syndrome
Foville syndrome
Millard-Gubler syndrome
Wallenberg syndrome
Weber syndrome
G46.4 Cerebellar stroke syndrome
G46.5 Pure motor lacunar syndrome
G46.6 Pure sensory lacunar syndrome
G46.7 Other lacunar syndromes
G46.8 Other vascular syndromes of brain in cerebrovascular diseases

✓4th **G47 Sleep disorders**
EXCLUDES 2 *nightmares (F51.5)*
nonorganic sleep disorders (F51.-)
sleep terrors (F51.4)
sleepwalking (F51.3)
✓5th **G47.Ø Insomnia**
EXCLUDES 2 *alcohol related insomnia (F1Ø.182, F1Ø.282, F1Ø.982)*
drug-related insomnia (F11.182, F11.282, F11.982, F13.182, F13.282, F13.982, F14.182, F14.282, F14.982, F15.182, F15.282, F15.982, F19.182, F19.282, F19.982)
idiopathic insomnia (F51.Ø1)
insomnia due to a mental disorder (F51.Ø5)
insomnia not due to a substance or known physiological condition (F51.Ø-)
nonorganic insomnia (F51.Ø-)
primary insomnia (F51.Ø1)
sleep apnea (G47.3-)
G47.ØØ Insomnia, unspecified
Insomnia NOS
G47.Ø1 Insomnia due to medical condition
Code also associated medical condition
G47.Ø9 Other insomnia

✓5th **G47.1 Hypersomnia**

EXCLUDES 2 *alcohol-related hypersomnia (F10.182, F10.282, F10.982)*
drug-related hypersomnia (F11.182, F11.282, F11.982, F13.182, F13.282, F13.982, F14.182, F14.282, F14.982, F15.182, F15.282, F15.982, F19.182, F19.282, F19.982)
hypersomnia due to a mental disorder (F51.13)
hypersomnia not due to a substance or known physiological condition (F51.1-)
primary hypersomnia (F51.11)
sleep apnea (G47.3-)

G47.10 Hypersomnia, unspecified
Hypersomnia NOS

G47.11 Idiopathic hypersomnia with long sleep time
Idiopathic hypersomnia NOS

G47.12 Idiopathic hypersomnia without long sleep time

G47.13 Recurrent hypersomnia
Kleine-Levin syndrome
Menstrual related hypersomnia

G47.14 Hypersomnia due to medical condition
Code also associated medical condition

G47.19 Other hypersomnia

✓5th **G47.2 Circadian rhythm sleep disorders**
Disorders of the sleep wake schedule
Inversion of nyctohemeral rhythm
Inversion of sleep rhythm
DEF: Circadian rhythm: Daily cycle (24-hour period) of physical, mental and behavioral changes. It is largely influenced by environmental ques, such as changes in light or temperature. ***Synonyms:*** *sleep/wake cycle.*

G47.20 Circadian rhythm sleep disorder, unspecified type
Sleep wake schedule disorder NOS

G47.21 Circadian rhythm sleep disorder, delayed sleep phase type
Delayed sleep phase syndrome

G47.22 Circadian rhythm sleep disorder, advanced sleep phase type

G47.23 Circadian rhythm sleep disorder, irregular sleep wake type
Irregular sleep-wake pattern

G47.24 Circadian rhythm sleep disorder, free running type
Circadian rhythm sleep disorder, non-24-hour sleep-wake type

G47.25 Circadian rhythm sleep disorder, jet lag type

G47.26 Circadian rhythm sleep disorder, shift work type

G47.27 Circadian rhythm sleep disorder in conditions classified elsewhere
Code first underlying condition

G47.29 Other circadian rhythm sleep disorder

✓5th **G47.3 Sleep apnea**
Code also any associated underlying condition

EXCLUDES 1 *apnea NOS (R06.81)*
Cheyne-Stokes breathing (R06.3)
pickwickian syndrome (E66.2)
sleep apnea of newborn (P28.3)

G47.30 Sleep apnea, unspecified
Sleep apnea NOS

G47.31 Primary central sleep apnea
Idiopathic central sleep apnea

G47.32 High altitude periodic breathing

G47.33 Obstructive sleep apnea (adult) (pediatric)
Obstructive sleep apnea hypopnea
EXCLUDES 1 *obstructive sleep apnea of newborn (P28.3)*

G47.34 Idiopathic sleep related nonobstructive alveolar hypoventilation
Sleep related hypoxia

G47.35 Congenital central alveolar hypoventilation syndrome

G47.36 Sleep related hypoventilation in conditions classified elsewhere
Sleep related hypoxemia in conditions classified elsewhere
Code first underlying condition

G47.37 Central sleep apnea in conditions classified elsewhere
Code first underlying condition

G47.39 Other sleep apnea

✓5th **G47.4 Narcolepsy and cataplexy**

✓6th **G47.41 Narcolepsy**

G47.411 Narcolepsy with cataplexy

G47.419 Narcolepsy without cataplexy
Narcolepsy NOS

✓6th **G47.42 Narcolepsy in conditions classified elsewhere**
Code first underlying condition

G47.421 Narcolepsy in conditions classified elsewhere with cataplexy

G47.429 Narcolepsy in conditions classified elsewhere without cataplexy

✓5th **G47.5 Parasomnia**

EXCLUDES 1 *alcohol induced parasomnia (F10.182, F10.282, F10.982)*
drug induced parasomnia (F11.182, F11.282, F11.982, F13.182, F13.282, F13.982, F14.182, F14.282, F14.982, F15.182, F15.282, F15.982, F19.182, F19.282, F19.982)
parasomnia not due to a substance or known physiological condition (F51.8)

G47.50 Parasomnia, unspecified
Parasomnia NOS

G47.51 Confusional arousals

G47.52 REM sleep behavior disorder

G47.53 Recurrent isolated sleep paralysis

G47.54 Parasomnia in conditions classified elsewhere
Code first underlying condition

G47.59 Other parasomnia

✓5th **G47.6 Sleep related movement disorders**

EXCLUDES 2 *restless legs syndrome (G25.81)*

G47.61 Periodic limb movement disorder

G47.62 Sleep related leg cramps

G47.63 Sleep related bruxism
EXCLUDES 1 *psychogenic bruxism (F45.8)*

G47.69 Other sleep related movement disorders

G47.8 Other sleep disorders
Other specified sleep-wake disorder

G47.9 Sleep disorder, unspecified
Sleep disorder NOS
Unspecified sleep-wake disorder

Nerve, nerve root and plexus disorders (G50-G59)

EXCLUDES 1 *current traumatic nerve, nerve root and plexus disorders — see Injury, nerve by body region*
neuralgia NOS (M79.2)
neuritis NOS (M79.2)
peripheral neuritis in pregnancy (O26.82-)
radiculitis NOS (M54.1-)

✓4th **G50 Disorders of trigeminal nerve**
INCLUDES disorders of 5th cranial nerve

Trigeminal and Facial Nerve Branches

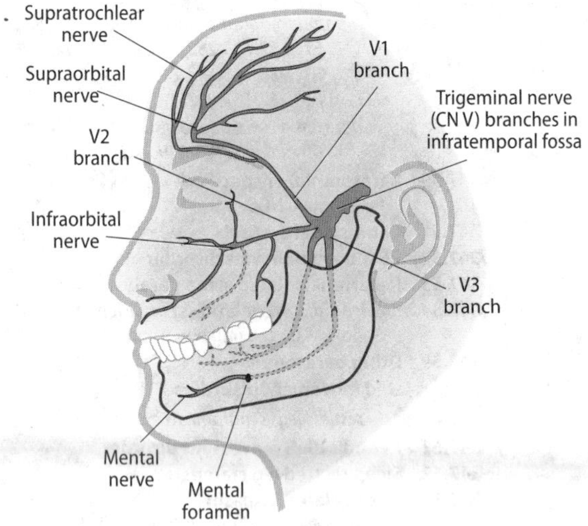

G50.0 Trigeminal neuralgia
Syndrome of paroxysmal facial pain
Tic douloureux

G50.1 Atypical facial pain

G50.8 Other disorders of trigeminal nerve

G50.9 Disorder of trigeminal nerve, unspecified

✓4th **G51 Facial nerve disorders**
INCLUDES disorders of 7th cranial nerve

G51.0 Bell's palsy
Facial palsy

G51.1 Geniculate ganglionitis
EXCLUDES 1 *postherpetic geniculate ganglionitis (B02.21)*

G51.2 Melkersson's syndrome
Melkersson-Rosenthal syndrome

✓5th **G51.3 Clonic hemifacial spasm**
AHA: 2018,4Q,10

G51.31 Clonic hemifacial spasm, right

G51.32 Clonic hemifacial spasm, left

G51.33 Clonic hemifacial spasm, bilateral

G51.39 Clonic hemifacial spasm, unspecified

G51.4 Facial myokymia

G51.8 Other disorders of facial nerve

G51.9 Disorder of facial nerve, unspecified

✓4th **G52 Disorders of other cranial nerves**
EXCLUDES 2 *disorders of acoustic [8th] nerve (H93.3)*
disorders of optic [2nd] nerve (H46, H47.0)
paralytic strabismus due to nerve palsy (H49.0-H49.2)

G52.0 Disorders of olfactory nerve
Disorders of 1st cranial nerve

G52.1 Disorders of glossopharyngeal nerve
Disorder of 9th cranial nerve
Glossopharyngeal neuralgia

G52.2 Disorders of vagus nerve
Disorders of pneumogastric [10th] nerve

G52.3 Disorders of hypoglossal nerve
Disorders of 12th cranial nerve

G52.7 Disorders of multiple cranial nerves
Polyneuritis cranialis

G52.8 Disorders of other specified cranial nerves

G52.9 Cranial nerve disorder, unspecified

G53 Cranial nerve disorders in diseases classified elsewhere
Code first underlying disease, such as:
neoplasm (C00-D49)
EXCLUDES 1 *multiple cranial nerve palsy in sarcoidosis (D86.82)*
multiple cranial nerve palsy in syphilis (A52.15)
postherpetic geniculate ganglionitis (B02.21)
postherpetic trigeminal neuralgia (B02.22)

✓4th **G54 Nerve root and plexus disorders**
EXCLUDES 1 *current traumatic nerve root and plexus disorders — see nerve injury by body region*
intervertebral disc disorders (M50-M51)
neuralgia or neuritis NOS (M79.2)
neuritis or radiculitis brachial NOS (M54.13)
neuritis or radiculitis lumbar NOS (M54.16)
neuritis or radiculitis lumbosacral NOS (M54.17)
neuritis or radiculitis thoracic NOS (M54.14)
radiculitis NOS (M54.10)
radiculopathy NOS (M54.10)
spondylosis (M47.-)

G54.0 Brachial plexus disorders
Thoracic outlet syndrome
DEF: Acquired disorder affecting the spinal nerves that send signals to the shoulder, arm, and hand, causing corresponding motor and sensory dysfunction. This disorder is characterized by regional paresthesia, pain, muscle weakness, and in severe cases paralysis.

G54.1 Lumbosacral plexus disorders

G54.2 Cervical root disorders, not elsewhere classified

G54.3 Thoracic root disorders, not elsewhere classified

G54.4 Lumbosacral root disorders, not elsewhere classified

G54.5 Neuralgic amyotrophy
Parsonage-Aldren-Turner syndrome
Shoulder-girdle neuritis
EXCLUDES 1 *neuralgic amyotrophy in diabetes mellitus (E08-E13 with .44)*

G54.6 Phantom limb syndrome with pain HCC

G54.7 Phantom limb syndrome without pain HCC
Phantom limb syndrome NOS

G54.8 Other nerve root and plexus disorders

G54.9 Nerve root and plexus disorder, unspecified

G55 Nerve root and plexus compressions in diseases classified elsewhere
Code first underlying disease, such as:
neoplasm (C00-D49)
EXCLUDES 1 *nerve root compression (due to) (in) ankylosing spondylitis (M45.-)*
nerve root compression (due to) (in) dorsopathies (M53.-, M54.-)
nerve root compression (due to) (in) intervertebral disc disorders (M50.1.-, M51.1.-)
nerve root compression (due to) (in) spondylopathies (M46.-, M48.-)
nerve root compression (due to) (in) spondylosis (M47.0-M47.2-)

✓4th G56 Mononeuropathies of upper limb

EXCLUDES 1 *current traumatic nerve disorder — see nerve injury by body region*

AHA: 2016,4Q,17-18

Nerves of Upper Limb

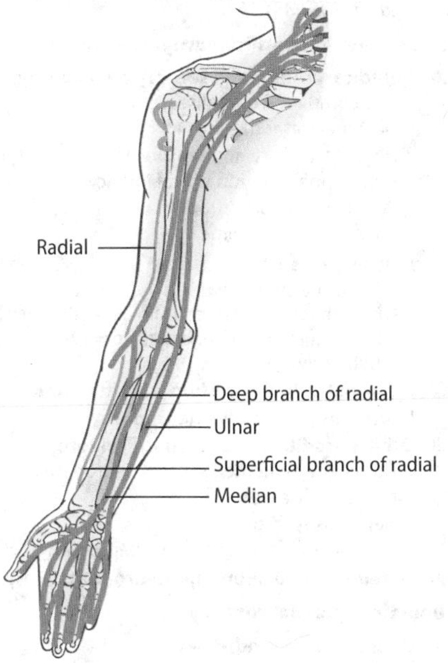

✓5th G56.Ø Carpal tunnel syndrome

DEF: Swelling and inflammation in the tendons or bursa surrounding the median nerve caused by repetitive activity. The resulting compression on the nerve causes pain, numbness, and tingling especially to the palm, index, middle finger, and thumb.

G56.ØØ Carpal tunnel syndrome, unspecified upper limb
G56.Ø1 Carpal tunnel syndrome, right upper limb
G56.Ø2 Carpal tunnel syndrome, left upper limb
G56.Ø3 Carpal tunnel syndrome, bilateral upper limbs

✓5th G56.1 Other lesions of median nerve

G56.1Ø Other lesions of median nerve, unspecified upper limb
G56.11 Other lesions of median nerve, right upper limb
G56.12 Other lesions of median nerve, left upper limb
G56.13 Other lesions of median nerve, bilateral upper limbs

✓5th G56.2 Lesion of ulnar nerve

Tardy ulnar nerve palsy

G56.2Ø Lesion of ulnar nerve, unspecified upper limb
G56.21 Lesion of ulnar nerve, right upper limb
G56.22 Lesion of ulnar nerve, left upper limb
G56.23 Lesion of ulnar nerve, bilateral upper limbs

✓5th G56.3 Lesion of radial nerve

G56.3Ø Lesion of radial nerve, unspecified upper limb
G56.31 Lesion of radial nerve, right upper limb
G56.32 Lesion of radial nerve, left upper limb
G56.33 Lesion of radial nerve, bilateral upper limbs

✓5th G56.4 Causalgia of upper limb

Complex regional pain syndrome II of upper limb

EXCLUDES 1 *complex regional pain syndrome I of lower limb (G9Ø.52-)*
complex regional pain syndrome I of upper limb (G9Ø.51-)
complex regional pain syndrome II of lower limb (G57.7-)
reflex sympathetic dystrophy of lower limb (G9Ø.52-)
reflex sympathetic dystrophy of upper limb (G9Ø.51-)

G56.4Ø Causalgia of unspecified upper limb
G56.41 Causalgia of right upper limb
G56.42 Causalgia of left upper limb
G56.43 Causalgia of bilateral upper limbs

✓5th G56.8 Other specified mononeuropathies of upper limb

Interdigital neuroma of upper limb

G56.8Ø Other specified mononeuropathies of unspecified upper limb
G56.81 Other specified mononeuropathies of right upper limb
G56.82 Other specified mononeuropathies of left upper limb
G56.83 Other specified mononeuropathies of bilateral upper limbs

✓5th G56.9 Unspecified mononeuropathy of upper limb

G56.9Ø Unspecified mononeuropathy of unspecified upper limb
G56.91 Unspecified mononeuropathy of right upper limb
G56.92 Unspecified mononeuropathy of left upper limb
G56.93 Unspecified mononeuropathy of bilateral upper limbs

✓4th G57 Mononeuropathies of lower limb

EXCLUDES 1 *current traumatic nerve disorder — see nerve injury by body region*

AHA: 2016,4Q,17-18

Nerves of Lower Limb

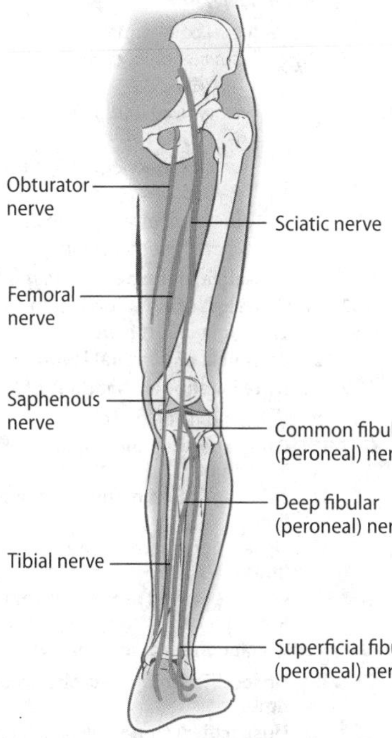

✓5th G57.Ø Lesion of sciatic nerve

EXCLUDES 1 *sciatica NOS (M54.3-)*

EXCLUDES 2 *sciatica attributed to intervertebral disc disorder (M51.1.-)*

G57.ØØ Lesion of sciatic nerve, unspecified lower limb
G57.Ø1 Lesion of sciatic nerve, right lower limb
G57.Ø2 Lesion of sciatic nerve, left lower limb
G57.Ø3 Lesion of sciatic nerve, bilateral lower limbs

✓5th G57.1 Meralgia paresthetica

Lateral cutaneous nerve of thigh syndrome

G57.1Ø Meralgia paresthetica, unspecified lower limb
G57.11 Meralgia paresthetica, right lower limb
G57.12 Meralgia paresthetica, left lower limb
G57.13 Meralgia paresthetica, bilateral lower limbs

✓5th G57.2 Lesion of femoral nerve

G57.2Ø Lesion of femoral nerve, unspecified lower limb
G57.21 Lesion of femoral nerve, right lower limb
G57.22 Lesion of femoral nerve, left lower limb
G57.23 Lesion of femoral nerve, bilateral lower limbs

✓5th G57.3 Lesion of lateral popliteal nerve

Peroneal nerve palsy

G57.3Ø Lesion of lateral popliteal nerve, unspecified lower limb
G57.31 Lesion of lateral popliteal nerve, right lower limb
G57.32 Lesion of lateral popliteal nerve, left lower limb
G57.33 Lesion of lateral popliteal nerve, bilateral lower limbs

✓5th **G57.4 Lesion of medial popliteal nerve**

G57.40 Lesion of medial popliteal nerve, unspecified lower limb

G57.41 Lesion of medial popliteal nerve, right lower limb

G57.42 Lesion of medial popliteal nerve, left lower limb

G57.43 Lesion of medial popliteal nerve, bilateral lower limbs

✓5th **G57.5 Tarsal tunnel syndrome**

G57.50 Tarsal tunnel syndrome, unspecified lower limb

G57.51 Tarsal tunnel syndrome, right lower limb

G57.52 Tarsal tunnel syndrome, left lower limb

G57.53 Tarsal tunnel syndrome, bilateral lower limbs

✓5th **G57.6 Lesion of plantar nerve**

Morton's metatarsalgia

G57.60 Lesion of plantar nerve, unspecified lower limb

G57.61 Lesion of plantar nerve, right lower limb

G57.62 Lesion of plantar nerve, left lower limb

G57.63 Lesion of plantar nerve, bilateral lower limbs

✓5th **G57.7 Causalgia of lower limb**

Complex regional pain syndrome II of lower limb

EXCLUDES 1 *complex regional pain syndrome I of lower limb (G90.52-)*
complex regional pain syndrome I of upper limb (G90.51-)
complex regional pain syndrome II of upper limb (G56.4-)
reflex sympathetic dystrophy of lower limb (G90.52-)
reflex sympathetic dystrophy of upper limb (G90.51-)

G57.70 Causalgia of unspecified lower limb

G57.71 Causalgia of right lower limb

G57.72 Causalgia of left lower limb

G57.73 Causalgia of bilateral lower limbs

✓5th **G57.8 Other specified mononeuropathies of lower limb**

Interdigital neuroma of lower limb

G57.80 Other specified mononeuropathies of unspecified lower limb

G57.81 Other specified mononeuropathies of right lower limb

G57.82 Other specified mononeuropathies of left lower limb

G57.83 Other specified mononeuropathies of bilateral lower limbs

✓5th **G57.9 Unspecified mononeuropathy of lower limb**

G57.90 Unspecified mononeuropathy of unspecified lower limb

G57.91 Unspecified mononeuropathy of right lower limb

G57.92 Unspecified mononeuropathy of left lower limb

G57.93 Unspecified mononeuropathy of bilateral lower limbs

✓4th **G58 Other mononeuropathies**

G58.0 Intercostal neuropathy

G58.7 Mononeuritis multiplex

G58.8 Other specified mononeuropathies

G58.9 Mononeuropathy, unspecified

G59 Mononeuropathy in diseases classified elsewhere

Code first underlying disease

EXCLUDES 1 *diabetic mononeuropathy (E08-E13 with .41)*
syphilitic nerve paralysis (A52.19)
syphilitic neuritis (A52.15)
tuberculous mononeuropathy (A17.83)

Polyneuropathies and other disorders of the peripheral nervous system (G60-G65)

EXCLUDES 1 *neuralgia NOS (M79.2)*
neuritis NOS (M79.2)
peripheral neuritis in pregnancy (O26.82-)
radiculitis NOS (M54.10)

✓4th **G60 Hereditary and idiopathic neuropathy**

G60.0 Hereditary motor and sensory neuropathy

Charcôt-Marie-Tooth disease
Déjérine-Sottas disease
Hereditary motor and sensory neuropathy, types I-IV
Hypertrophic neuropathy of infancy
Peroneal muscular atrophy (axonal type) (hypertrophic type)
Roussy-Levy syndrome

G60.1 Refsum's disease CC

Infantile Refsum disease

DEF: Genetic disorder of the lipid metabolism characterized by retinitis pigmentosa, degenerative nerve disease, ataxia, and dry, rough, scaly skin.

G60.2 Neuropathy in association with hereditary ataxia

G60.3 Idiopathic progressive neuropathy

G60.8 Other hereditary and idiopathic neuropathies

Dominantly inherited sensory neuropathy
Morvan's disease
Nelaton's syndrome
Recessively inherited sensory neuropathy

G60.9 Hereditary and idiopathic neuropathy, unspecified

✓4th **G61 Inflammatory polyneuropathy**

G61.0 Guillain-Barre syndrome CC HCC

Acute (post-)infective polyneuritis
Miller Fisher syndrome

AHA: 2014,2Q,4

DEF: Autoimmune disorder due to an immune response to foreign antigens with paraplegia of limbs, flaccid paralysis, ophthalmoplegia, ataxia, and areflexia. In most cases, this disorder is triggered by a mild viral infection, surgery, or following an immunization.

TIP: Guillain-Barre syndrome can occur as a sequela of *Campylobacter enteritis*. Assign code B94.8 for the sequelae as an additional diagnosis.

G61.1 Serum neuropathy HCC

Use additional code for adverse effect, if applicable, to identify serum (T50.-)

✓5th **G61.8 Other inflammatory polyneuropathies**

G61.81 Chronic inflammatory demyelinating polyneuritis CC HCC

G61.82 Multifocal motor neuropathy HCC

MMN

AHA: 2016,4Q,18

G61.89 Other inflammatory polyneuropathies HCC

G61.9 Inflammatory polyneuropathy, unspecified HCC

✓4th **G62 Other and unspecified polyneuropathies**

G62.0 Drug-induced polyneuropathy HCC

Use additional code for adverse effect, if applicable, to identify drug (T36-T50 with fifth or sixth character 5)

G62.1 Alcoholic polyneuropathy HCC

AHA: 2019,3Q,8

G62.2 Polyneuropathy due to other toxic agents HCC

Code first (T51-T65) to identify toxic agent

✓5th **G62.8 Other specified polyneuropathies**

G62.81 Critical illness polyneuropathy CC HCC

Acute motor neuropathy

G62.82 Radiation-induced polyneuropathy HCC

Use additional external cause code (W88-W90, X39.0-) to identify cause

G62.89 Other specified polyneuropathies

AHA: 2016,2Q,11

G62.9 Polyneuropathy, unspecified

Neuropathy NOS

G63 *Polyneuropathy in diseases classified elsewhere* HCC
Code first underlying disease, such as:
amyloidosis (E85.-)
endocrine disease, except diabetes (E00-E07, E15-E16, E20-E34)
metabolic diseases (E70-E88)
neoplasm (C00-D49)
nutritional deficiency (E40-E64)
EXCLUDES 1 *polyneuropathy (in):*
diabetes mellitus (E08-E13 with .42)
diphtheria (A36.83)
infectious mononucleosis (B27.0-B27.9 with 1)
Lyme disease (A69.22)
mumps (B26.84)
postherpetic (B02.23)
rheumatoid arthritis (M05.5-)
scleroderma (M34.83)
systemic lupus erythematosus (M32.19)
AHA: 2012,4Q,99

G64 Other disorders of peripheral nervous system
Disorder of peripheral nervous system NOS

✓4th **G65 Sequelae of inflammatory and toxic polyneuropathies**
Code first condition resulting from (sequela) of inflammatory and toxic polyneuropathies
G65.0 Sequelae of Guillain-Barré syndrome HCC
G65.1 Sequelae of other inflammatory polyneuropathy HCC
G65.2 Sequelae of toxic polyneuropathy HCC

Diseases of myoneural junction and muscle (G70-G73)

✓4th **G70 Myasthenia gravis and other myoneural disorders**
EXCLUDES 1 *botulism (A05.1, A48.51-A48.52)*
transient neonatal myasthenia gravis (P94.0)

✓5th **G70.0 Myasthenia gravis**
DEF: Autoimmune neuromuscular disorder caused by antibodies to the acetylcholine receptors at the neuromuscular junction, interfering with proper binding of the neurotransmitter from the neuron to the target muscle, causing muscle weakness, fatigue, and exhaustion, without pain or atrophy.
G70.00 Myasthenia gravis without (acute) exacerbation HCC
Myasthenia gravis NOS
G70.01 Myasthenia gravis with (acute) exacerbation MCC HCC
Myasthenia gravis in crisis
G70.1 Toxic myoneural disorders HCC
Code first (T51-T65) to identify toxic agent
G70.2 Congenital and developmental myasthenia HCC
✓5th **G70.8 Other specified myoneural disorders**
● **G70.80 Lambert-Eaton syndrome, unspecified** CC HCC
Lambert-Eaton syndrome NOS
● ***G70.81 Lambert-Eaton syndrome in disease classified elsewhere*** CC HCC
Code first underlying disease
EXCLUDES 1 *Lambert-Eaton syndrome in neoplastic disease (G73.1)*
G70.89 Other specified myoneural disorders HCC
G70.9 Myoneural disorder, unspecified HCC

✓4th **G71 Primary disorders of muscles**
EXCLUDES 2 *arthrogryposis multiplex congenita (Q74.3)*
metabolic disorders (E70-E88)
myositis (M60.-)

✓5th **G71.0 Muscular dystrophy**
AHA: 2018,4Q,11-12
G71.00 Muscular dystrophy, unspecified HCC
G71.01 Duchenne or Becker muscular dystrophy HCC
Autosomal recessive, childhood type, muscular dystrophy resembling Duchenne or Becker muscular dystrophy
Benign [Becker] muscular dystrophy
Severe [Duchenne] muscular dystrophy
G71.02 Facioscapulohumeral muscular dystrophy HCC
Scapulohumeral muscular dystrophy
G71.09 Other specified muscular dystrophies HCC
Benign scapuloperoneal muscular dystrophy with early contractures [Emery-Dreifuss]
Congenital muscular dystrophy NOS
Congenital muscular dystrophy with specific morphological abnormalities of the muscle fiber
Distal muscular dystrophy
Limb-girdle muscular dystrophy
Ocular muscular dystrophy
Oculopharyngeal muscular dystrophy
Scapuloperoneal muscular dystrophy

✓5th **G71.1 Myotonic disorders**
G71.11 Myotonic muscular dystrophy HCC
Dystrophia myotonica [Steinert]
Myotonia atrophica
Myotonic dystrophy
Proximal myotonic myopathy (PROMM)
Steinert disease
G71.12 Myotonia congenita
Acetazolamide responsive myotonia congenita
Dominant myotonia congenita [Thomsen disease]
Myotonia levior
Recessive myotonia congenita [Becker disease]
G71.13 Myotonic chondrodystrophy
Chondrodystrophic myotonia
Congenital myotonic chondrodystrophy
Schwartz-Jampel disease
G71.14 Drug induced myotonia
Use additional code for adverse effect, if applicable, to identify drug (T36-T50 with fifth or sixth character 5)
G71.19 Other specified myotonic disorders
Myotonia fluctuans
Myotonia permanens
Neuromyotonia [Isaacs]
Paramyotonia congenita (of von Eulenburg)
Pseudomyotonia
Symptomatic myotonia

▲ ✓5th **G71.2 Congenital myopathies**
~~Central core disease~~
~~Fiber-type disproportion~~
~~Minicore disease~~
~~Multicore disease~~
~~Myotubular (centronuclear) myopathy~~
~~Nemaline myopathy~~
~~EXCLUDES 1 *arthrogryposis multiplex congenita (Q74.3)*~~
EXCLUDES 2 ▶*arthrogryposis multiplex congenita (Q74.3)*◀
● **G71.20 Congenital myopathy, unspecifed** CC
● **G71.21 Nemaline myopathy** CC
● ✓6th **G71.22 Centronuclear myopathy**
● **G71.220 X-linked myotubular myopathy** CC
Myotubular (centronuclear) myopathy
● **G71.228 Other centronuclear myopathy** CC
Autosomal centronuclear myopathy
Autosomal dominant centronuclear myopathy
Autosomal recessive centronuclear myopathy
Centronuclear myopathy, NOS
● **G71.29 Other congenital myopathy** CC
Central core disease
Minicore disease
Multicore disease
Multiminicore disease
G71.3 Mitochondrial myopathy, not elsewhere classified
EXCLUDES 1 *Kearns-Sayre syndrome (H49.81)*
Leber's disease (H47.21)
Leigh's encephalopathy (G31.82)
mitochondrial metabolism disorders (E88.4.-)
Reye's syndrome (G93.7)
G71.8 Other primary disorders of muscles
G71.9 Primary disorder of muscle, unspecified
Hereditary myopathy NOS

√4th G72 Other and unspecified myopathies

EXCLUDES 1 *arthrogryposis multiplex congenita (Q74.3)*
dermatopolymyositis (M33.-)
ischemic infarction of muscle (M62.2-)
myositis (M6Ø.-)
polymyositis (M33.2.-)

G72.Ø Drug-induced myopathy CC
Use additional code for adverse effect, if applicable, to identify drug (T36-T5Ø with fifth or sixth character 5)

G72.1 Alcoholic myopathy CC
Use additional code to identify alcoholism (F1Ø.-)

G72.2 Myopathy due to other toxic agents CC
Code first (T51-T65) to identify toxic agent

G72.3 Periodic paralysis
Familial periodic paralysis
Hyperkalemic periodic paralysis (familial)
Hypokalemic periodic paralysis (familial)
Myotonic periodic paralysis (familial)
Normokalemic paralysis (familial)
Potassium sensitive periodic paralysis
EXCLUDES 1 *paramyotonia congenita (of von Eulenburg) (G71.19)*

√5th G72.4 Inflammatory and immune myopathies, not elsewhere classified

G72.41 Inclusion body myositis [IBM]

G72.49 Other inflammatory and immune myopathies, not elsewhere classified
Inflammatory myopathy NOS

√5th G72.8 Other specified myopathies

G72.81 Critical illness myopathy CC
Acute necrotizing myopathy
Acute quadriplegic myopathy
Intensive care (ICU) myopathy
Myopathy of critical illness

G72.89 Other specified myopathies

G72.9 Myopathy, unspecified

√4th G73 Disorders of myoneural junction and muscle in diseases classified elsewhere

G73.1 Lambert-Eaton syndrome in neoplastic disease CC HCC
Code first underlying neoplasm (CØØ-D49)
EXCLUDES 1 *Lambert-Eaton syndrome not associated with neoplasm (G7Ø.8Ø-G7Ø.81)*

G73.3 Myasthenic syndromes in other diseases classified elsewhere CC HCC
Code first underlying disease, such as:
neoplasm (CØØ-D49)
thyrotoxicosis (EØ5.-)

G73.7 Myopathy in diseases classified elsewhere
Code first underlying disease, such as:
hyperparathyroidism (E21.Ø, E21.3)
hypoparathyroidism (E2Ø.-)
glycogen storage disease (E74.Ø)
lipid storage disorders (E75.-)
EXCLUDES 1 *myopathy in:*
rheumatoid arthritis (MØ5.32)
sarcoidosis (D86.87)
scleroderma (M34.82)
sicca syndrome [Sjögren] (M35.Ø3)
systemic lupus erythematosus (M32.19)

Cerebral palsy and other paralytic syndromes (G8Ø-G83)

√4th G8Ø Cerebral palsy

EXCLUDES 1 *hereditary spastic paraplegia (G11.4)*

G8Ø.Ø Spastic quadriplegic cerebral palsy MCC HCC
Congenital spastic paralysis (cerebral)

G8Ø.1 Spastic diplegic cerebral palsy CC HCC
Spastic cerebral palsy NOS

G8Ø.2 Spastic hemiplegic cerebral palsy CC HCC

G8Ø.3 Athetoid cerebral palsy CC HCC
Double athetosis (syndrome)
Dyskinetic cerebral palsy
Dystonic cerebral palsy
Vogt disease

G8Ø.4 Ataxic cerebral palsy HCC

G8Ø.8 Other cerebral palsy HCC
Mixed cerebral palsy syndromes

G8Ø.9 Cerebral palsy, unspecified HCC
Cerebral palsy NOS

√4th G81 Hemiplegia and hemiparesis

NOTE This category is to be used only when hemiplegia (complete)(incomplete) is reported without further specification, or is stated to be old or longstanding but of unspecified cause. The category is also for use in multiple coding to identify these types of hemiplegia resulting from any cause.

EXCLUDES 1 *congenital cerebral palsy (G8Ø.-)*
hemiplegia and hemiparesis due to sequela of cerebrovascular disease (I69.Ø5-, I69.15-, I69.25-, I69.35-, I69.85-, I69.95-)

AHA: 2015,1Q,25

TIP: If the documentation specifies the affected side but not whether it is the dominant or nondominant side, the default is as follows: for ambidextrous patients, the default is dominant; when the left side is affected, the default is nondominant; and when the right side is affected, the default is dominant.

√5th G81.Ø Flaccid hemiplegia

G81.ØØ Flaccid hemiplegia affecting unspecified side CC HCC

G81.Ø1 Flaccid hemiplegia affecting right dominant side CC HCC

G81.Ø2 Flaccid hemiplegia affecting left dominant side CC HCC

G81.Ø3 Flaccid hemiplegia affecting right nondominant side CC HCC

G81.Ø4 Flaccid hemiplegia affecting left nondominant side CC HCC

√5th G81.1 Spastic hemiplegia

G81.1Ø Spastic hemiplegia affecting unspecified side CC HCC

G81.11 Spastic hemiplegia affecting right dominant side CC HCC

G81.12 Spastic hemiplegia affecting left dominant side CC HCC

G81.13 Spastic hemiplegia affecting right nondominant side CC HCC

G81.14 Spastic hemiplegia affecting left nondominant side CC HCC

√5th G81.9 Hemiplegia, unspecified
AHA: 2014,1Q,23

G81.9Ø Hemiplegia, unspecified affecting unspecified side CC HCC

G81.91 Hemiplegia, unspecified affecting right dominant side CC HCC

G81.92 Hemiplegia, unspecified affecting left dominant side CC HCC

G81.93 Hemiplegia, unspecified affecting right nondominant side CC HCC

G81.94 Hemiplegia, unspecified affecting left nondominant side CC HCC

√4th G82 Paraplegia (paraparesis) and quadriplegia (quadriparesis)

NOTE This category is to be used only when the listed conditions are reported without further specification, or are stated to be old or longstanding but of unspecified cause. The category is also for use in multiple coding to identify these conditions resulting from any cause

EXCLUDES 1 *congenital cerebral palsy (G8Ø.-)*
functional quadriplegia (R53.2)
hysterical paralysis (F44.4)

√5th G82.2 Paraplegia
Paralysis of both lower limbs NOS
Paraparesis (lower) NOS
Paraplegia (lower) NOS
AHA: 2017,3Q,3

G82.2Ø Paraplegia, unspecified CC HCC

G82.21 Paraplegia, complete CC HCC

G82.22 Paraplegia, incomplete CC HCC

√5th G82.5 Quadriplegia

G82.5Ø Quadriplegia, unspecified MCC HCC

G82.51 Quadriplegia, C1-C4 complete MCC HCC

G82.52 Quadriplegia, C1-C4 incomplete MCC HCC

G82.53 Quadriplegia, C5-C7 complete MCC HCC

G82.54 Quadriplegia, C5-C7 incomplete MCC HCC

G83 Other paralytic syndromes

NOTE This category is to be used only when the listed conditions are reported without further specification, or are stated to be old or longstanding but of unspecified cause. The category is also for use in multiple coding to identify these conditions resulting from any cause.

INCLUDES paralysis (complete) (incomplete), except as in G80-G82

G83.0 Diplegia of upper limbs CC HCC

Diplegia (upper)

Paralysis of both upper limbs

G83.1 Monoplegia of lower limb

Paralysis of lower limb

EXCLUDES 1 *monoplegia of lower limbs due to sequela of cerebrovascular disease (I69.04-, I69.14-, I69.24-, I69.34-, I69.84-, I69.94-)*

TIP: If the documentation specifies the affected side but not whether it is the dominant or nondominant side, the default is as follows: for ambidextrous patients, the default is dominant; when the left side is affected, the default is nondominant; and when the right side is affected, the default is dominant.

G83.10 Monoplegia of lower limb affecting unspecified side HCC

G83.11 Monoplegia of lower limb affecting right dominant side HCC

G83.12 Monoplegia of lower limb affecting left dominant side HCC

G83.13 Monoplegia of lower limb affecting right nondominant side HCC

G83.14 Monoplegia of lower limb affecting left nondominant side HCC

G83.2 Monoplegia of upper limb

Paralysis of upper limb

EXCLUDES 1 *monoplegia of upper limbs due to sequela of cerebrovascular disease (I69.03-, I69.13-, I69.23-, I69.33-, I69.83-, I69.93-)*

TIP: If the documentation specifies the affected side but not whether it is the dominant or nondominant side, the default is as follows: for ambidextrous patients, the default is dominant; when the left side is affected, the default is nondominant; and when the right side is affected, the default is dominant.

G83.20 Monoplegia of upper limb affecting unspecified side HCC

G83.21 Monoplegia of upper limb affecting right dominant side HCC

G83.22 Monoplegia of upper limb affecting left dominant side HCC

G83.23 Monoplegia of upper limb affecting right nondominant side HCC

G83.24 Monoplegia of upper limb affecting left nondominant side HCC

G83.3 Monoplegia, unspecified

TIP: If the documentation specifies the affected side but not whether it is the dominant or nondominant side, the default is as follows: for ambidextrous patients, the default is dominant; when the left side is affected, the default is nondominant; and when the right side is affected, the default is dominant.

G83.30 Monoplegia, unspecified affecting unspecified side HCC

G83.31 Monoplegia, unspecified affecting right dominant side HCC

G83.32 Monoplegia, unspecified affecting left dominant side HCC

G83.33 Monoplegia, unspecified affecting right nondominant side HCC

G83.34 Monoplegia, unspecified affecting left nondominant side HCC

G83.4 Cauda equina syndrome CC HCC

Neurogenic bladder due to cauda equina syndrome

EXCLUDES 1 *cord bladder NOS (G95.89)*

neurogenic bladder NOS (N31.9)

DEF: Compression of the spinal nerve roots presenting with pain and tingling radiating down the buttocks, back of the thigh and calf, and into the foot in a sciatic manner with aching in the bladder, perineum, and sacrum. Loss of bowel and bladder control may also occur.

G83.5 Locked-in state MCC HCC

G83.8 Other specified paralytic syndromes

EXCLUDES 1 *paralytic syndromes due to current spinal cord injury — code to spinal cord injury (S14, S24, S34)*

G83.81 Brown-Séquard syndrome HCC

G83.82 Anterior cord syndrome HCC

G83.83 Posterior cord syndrome HCC

G83.84 Todd's paralysis (postepileptic) HCC

G83.89 Other specified paralytic syndromes HCC

G83.9 Paralytic syndrome, unspecified HCC

Other disorders of the nervous system (G89-G99)

G89 Pain, not elsewhere classified

Code also related psychological factors associated with pain (F45.42)

EXCLUDES 1 *generalized pain NOS (R52)*

pain disorders exclusively related to psychological factors (F45.41)

pain NOS (R52)

EXCLUDES 2 *atypical face pain (G50.1)*

headache syndromes (G44.-)

localized pain, unspecified type — code to pain by site, such as:

- *abdomen pain (R10.-)*
- *back pain (M54.9)*
- *breast pain (N64.4)*
- *chest pain (R07.1-R07.9)*
- *ear pain (H92.0-)*
- *eye pain (H57.1)*
- *headache ►(R51.9)◄*
- *joint pain (M25.5-)*
- *limb pain (M79.6-)*
- *lumbar region pain (M54.5)*
- *painful urination (R30.9)*
- *pelvic and perineal pain (R10.2)*
- *renal colic (N23)*
- *shoulder pain (M25.51-)*
- *spine pain (M54.-)*
- *throat pain (R07.0)*
- *tongue pain (K14.6)*
- *tooth pain (K08.8)*

migraines (G43.-)

myalgia (M79.1-)

pain from prosthetic devices, implants, and grafts (T82.84, T83.84, T84.84, T85.84-)

phantom limb syndrome with pain (G54.6)

vulvar vestibulitis (N94.810)

vulvodynia (N94.81-)

G89.0 Central pain syndrome

Déjérine-Roussy syndrome

Myelopathic pain syndrome

Thalamic pain syndrome (hyperesthetic)

G89.1 Acute pain, not elsewhere classified

G89.11 Acute pain due to trauma

G89.12 Acute post-thoracotomy pain

Post-thoracotomy pain NOS

G89.18 Other acute postprocedural pain

Postoperative pain NOS

Postprocedural pain NOS

G89.2 Chronic pain, not elsewhere classified

EXCLUDES 1 *causalgia, lower limb (G57.7-)*

causalgia, upper limb (G56.4-)

central pain syndrome (G89.0)

chronic pain syndrome (G89.4)

complex regional pain syndrome II, lower limb (G57.7-)

complex regional pain syndrome II, upper limb (G56.4-)

neoplasm related chronic pain (G89.3)

reflex sympathetic dystrophy (G90.5-)

G89.21 Chronic pain due to trauma

G89.22 Chronic post-thoracotomy pain

G89.28 Other chronic postprocedural pain

Other chronic postoperative pain

G89.29 Other chronic pain

G89.3 Neoplasm related pain (acute) (chronic)
Cancer associated pain
Pain due to malignancy (primary) (secondary)
Tumor associated pain

G89.4 Chronic pain syndrome
Chronic pain associated with significant psychosocial dysfunction

✓4th G90 Disorders of autonomic nervous system
EXCLUDES 1 *dysfunction of the autonomic nervous system due to alcohol (G31.2)*

✓5th G90.0 Idiopathic peripheral autonomic neuropathy

G90.01 Carotid sinus syncope
Carotid sinus syndrome
DEF: Vagal activation caused by pressure on the carotid sinus baroreceptors. Sympathetic nerve impulses may cause sinus arrest or AV block.

G90.09 Other idiopathic peripheral autonomic neuropathy
Idiopathic peripheral autonomic neuropathy NOS

G90.1 Familial dysautonomia [Riley-Day] HCC

G90.2 Horner's syndrome
Bernard(-Horner) syndrome
Cervical sympathetic dystrophy or paralysis

G90.3 Multi-system degeneration of the autonomic nervous system CC HCC
Neurogenic orthostatic hypotension [Shy-Drager]
EXCLUDES 1 *orthostatic hypotension NOS (I95.1)*

G90.4 Autonomic dysreflexia
Use additional code to identify the cause, such as:
fecal impaction (K56.41)
pressure ulcer (pressure area) (L89.-)
urinary tract infection (N39.0)

✓5th G90.5 Complex regional pain syndrome I (CRPS I)
Reflex sympathetic dystrophy
EXCLUDES 1 *causalgia of lower limb (G57.7-)*
causalgia of upper limb (G56.4-)
complex regional pain syndrome II of lower limb (G57.7-)
complex regional pain syndrome II of upper limb (G56.4-)

G90.50 Complex regional pain syndrome I, unspecified CC

✓6th G90.51 Complex regional pain syndrome I of upper limb

G90.511 Complex regional pain syndrome I of right upper limb CC

G90.512 Complex regional pain syndrome I of left upper limb CC

G90.513 Complex regional pain syndrome I of upper limb, bilateral CC

G90.519 Complex regional pain syndrome I of unspecified upper limb CC

✓6th G90.52 Complex regional pain syndrome I of lower limb

G90.521 Complex regional pain syndrome I of right lower limb CC

G90.522 Complex regional pain syndrome I of left lower limb CC

G90.523 Complex regional pain syndrome I of lower limb, bilateral CC

G90.529 Complex regional pain syndrome I of unspecified lower limb CC

G90.59 Complex regional pain syndrome I of other specified site CC

G90.8 Other disorders of autonomic nervous system

G90.9 Disorder of the autonomic nervous system, unspecified

✓4th G91 Hydrocephalus
INCLUDES acquired hydrocephalus
EXCLUDES 1 *Arnold-Chiari syndrome with hydrocephalus (Q07.-)*
congenital hydrocephalus (Q03.-)
spina bifida with hydrocephalus (Q05.-)
DEF: Abnormal buildup of cerebrospinal fluid in the brain causing dilation of the ventricles.

Hydrocephalus (Acquired)

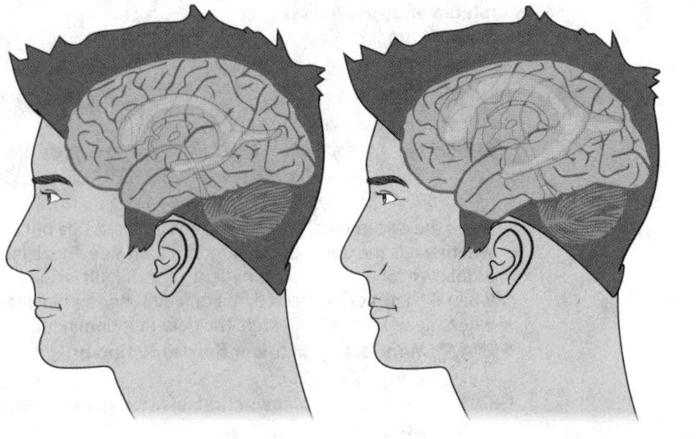

G91.0 Communicating hydrocephalus CC HCC
Secondary normal pressure hydrocephalus

G91.1 Obstructive hydrocephalus CC HCC
DEF: Obstruction of the cerebrospinal fluid passage from the brain into the spinal canal characterized by headaches, drowsiness, poor coordination, urinary incontinence, nausea, vomiting, and papilledema.

G91.2 (Idiopathic) normal pressure hydrocephalus CC HCC
Normal pressure hydrocephalus NOS

G91.3 Post-traumatic hydrocephalus, unspecified CC HCC

G91.4 Hydrocephalus in diseases classified elsewhere HCC
Code first underlying condition, such as:
congenital syphilis (A50.4-)
neoplasm (C00-D49)
plasminogen deficiency (E88.02)
EXCLUDES 1 *hydrocephalus due to congenital toxoplasmosis (P37.1)*
AHA: 2014,3Q,3

G91.8 Other hydrocephalus CC HCC

G91.9 Hydrocephalus, unspecified CC HCC

G92 Toxic encephalopathy MCC
Toxic encephalitis
Toxic metabolic encephalopathy
►Code first, if applicable, drug induced (T36-T50) or use (T51-T65) to identify toxic agent◄
~~Code first (T51-T65) to identify toxic agent~~
AHA: 2017,1Q,39-40
DEF: Brain tissue degeneration due to a toxic substance.

✓4th G93 Other disorders of brain

G93.0 Cerebral cysts
Arachnoid cyst
Porencephalic cyst, acquired
EXCLUDES 1 *acquired periventricular cysts of newborn (P91.1)*
congenital cerebral cysts (Q04.6)

G93.1 Anoxic brain damage, not elsewhere classified CC HCC
EXCLUDES 1 *cerebral anoxia due to anesthesia during labor and delivery (O74.3)*
cerebral anoxia due to anesthesia during the puerperium (O89.2)
neonatal anoxia (P84)
DEF: Brain injury not resulting from birth trauma that is due to lack of oxygen. Brain cells, when deprived of oxygen; begin to expire after 4 minutes.

G93.2 Benign intracranial hypertension
▶Pseudotumor◀
EXCLUDES 1 *hypertensive encephalopathy (I67.4)*
▶obstructive hydrocephalus (G91.1)◀

G93.3 Postviral fatigue syndrome
Benign myalgic encephalomyelitis
EXCLUDES 1 *chronic fatigue syndrome NOS (R53.82)*

✓5th **G93.4 Other and unspecified encephalopathy**
EXCLUDES 1 *alcoholic encephalopathy (G31.2)*
encephalopathy in diseases classified elsewhere (G94)
hypertensive encephalopathy (I67.4)
~~*toxic (metabolic) encephalopathy (G92)*~~
EXCLUDES 2 ▶*toxic (metabolic) encephalopathy (G92)*◀

G93.40 Encephalopathy, unspecified HIV CC
AHA: 2017,2Q,8

G93.41 Metabolic encephalopathy HIV MCC
Septic encephalopathy
AHA: 2017,2Q,8; 2016,3Q,42; 2015,3Q,21
TIP: Assign separately when documented with diabetic hypoglycemia (E08.649, E09.649, E10.649, E11.649, E13.649).

G93.49 Other encephalopathy HIV CC
Encephalopathy NEC
AHA: 2018,4Q,16; 2018,2Q,22,24; 2017,2Q,9

G93.5 Compression of brain MCC HCC
Arnold-Chiari type 1 compression of brain
Compression of brain (stem)
Herniation of brain (stem)
EXCLUDES 1 *diffuse traumatic compression of brain (S06.2-)*
focal traumatic compression of brain (S06.3-)
AHA: 2020,2Q,31

G93.6 Cerebral edema MCC HCC
EXCLUDES 1 *cerebral edema due to birth injury (P11.0)*
traumatic cerebral edema (S06.1-)

G93.7 Reye's syndrome MCC HCC P
Code first poisoning due to salicylates, if applicable (T39.0-, with sixth character 1-4)
Use additional code for adverse effect due to salicylates, if applicable (T39.0-, with sixth character 5)
DEF: Rare childhood illness often developed after a viral upper respiratory infection. Symptoms include vomiting, elevated serum transaminase, brain swelling, disturbances of consciousness, seizures, and changes in liver and other viscera and it can be fatal.

✓5th **G93.8 Other specified disorders of brain**

G93.81 Temporal sclerosis
Hippocampal sclerosis
Mesial temporal sclerosis

G93.82 Brain death MCC

G93.89 Other specified disorders of brain
Postradiation encephalopathy
AHA: 2020,2Q,24; 2019,3Q,8

G93.9 Disorder of brain, unspecified HIV

G94 Other disorders of brain in diseases classified elsewhere
Code first underlying disease
EXCLUDES 1 *encephalopathy in congenital syphilis (A50.49)*
encephalopathy in influenza (J09.X9, J10.81, J11.81)
encephalopathy in syphilis (A52.19)
hydrocephalus in diseases classified elsewhere (G91.4)
AHA: 2018,2Q,22; 2017,2Q,8-9

✓4th **G95 Other and unspecified diseases of spinal cord**
EXCLUDES 2 *myelitis (G04.-)*

G95.0 Syringomyelia and syringobulbia CC HCC

✓5th **G95.1 Vascular myelopathies**
EXCLUDES 2 *intraspinal phlebitis and thrombophlebitis, except non-pyogenic (G08)*

G95.11 Acute infarction of spinal cord (embolic) (nonembolic) MCC HCC
Anoxia of spinal cord
Arterial thrombosis of spinal cord

G95.19 Other vascular myelopathies MCC HCC
Edema of spinal cord
Hematomyelia
Nonpyogenic intraspinal phlebitis and thrombophlebitis
Subacute necrotic myelopathy

✓5th **G95.2 Other and unspecified cord compression**

G95.20 Unspecified cord compression HIV CC HCC

G95.29 Other cord compression HIV CC HCC

✓5th **G95.8 Other specified diseases of spinal cord**
EXCLUDES 1 *neurogenic bladder NOS (N31.9)*
neurogenic bladder due to cauda equina syndrome (G83.4)
neuromuscular dysfunction of bladder without spinal cord lesion (N31.-)

G95.81 Conus medullaris syndrome CC HCC

G95.89 Other specified diseases of spinal cord CC HCC
Cord bladder NOS
Drug-induced myelopathy
Radiation-induced myelopathy
EXCLUDES 1 *myelopathy NOS (G95.9)*

G95.9 Disease of spinal cord, unspecified HIV CC HCC
Myelopathy NOS

✓4th **G96 Other disorders of central nervous system**
▶Code also if applicable:◀
▶intracranial hypotension (G96.81-)◀

▲ ✓5th **G96.0 Cerebrospinal fluid leak**
▶Code also if applicable:◀
▶intracranial hypotension (G96.81-)◀
EXCLUDES 1 *cerebrospinal fluid leak from spinal puncture (G97.0)*
AHA: 2018,2Q,13
DEF: Cerebrospinal fluid discharging from the nose or the ear caused by a fracture of the frontal bone with tearing of dura mater and arachnoid. It is characterized by watery drainage usually from only one side of the nose or one ear, headache, vision changes, and hearing loss.

● **G96.00 Cerebrospinal fluid leak, unspecified** CC
Code also if applicable:
head injury (S00.- to S09.-)

● **G96.01 Cranial cerebrospinal fluid leak, spontaneous** CC
Otorrhea due to spontaneous cerebrospinal fluid CSF leak
Rhinorrhea due to spontaneous cerebrospinal fluid CSF leak
Spontaneous cerebrospinal fluid leak from skull base

● **G96.02 Spinal cerebrospinal fluid leak, spontaneous** CC
Spontaneous cerebrospinal fluid leak from spine

● **G96.08 Other cranial cerebrospinal fluid leak** CC
Postoperative cranial cerebrospinal fluid leak
Traumatic cranial cerebrospinal fluid leak
Code also if applicable:
head injury (S00.- to S09.-)

● **G96.09 Other spinal cerebrospinal fluid leak** CC
Other spinal CSF leak
Postoperative spinal cerebrospinal fluid leak
Traumatic spinal cerebrospinal fluid leak
Code also if applicable:
head injury (S00.- to S09.-)

✓5th **G96.1 Disorders of meninges, not elsewhere classified**

G96.11 Dural tear CC
▶Code also intracranial hypotension, if applicable (G96.81-)◀
EXCLUDES 1 *accidental puncture or laceration of dura during a procedure (G97.41)*
AHA: 2014,4Q,24

G96.12 Meningeal adhesions (cerebral) (spinal)

▲ ✓6th **G96.19 Other disorders of meninges, not elsewhere classified**

● **G96.191 Perineural cyst**
Cervical nerve root cyst
Lumbar nerve root cyst
Sacral nerve root cyst
Tarlov cyst
Thoracic nerve root cyst

● G96.198 **Other disorders of meninges, not elsewhere classified**

▲ ✓5th **G96.8 Other specified disorders of central nervous system**

● ✓6th **G96.81 Intracranial hypotension**

Code also any associated diagnoses, such as:
brachial amyotrophy (G54.5)
cerebrospinal fluid leak from spine (G96.Ø2)
cranial nerve disorders in diseases classified elsewhere (G53)
nerve root and compressions in diseases classified elsewhere (G55)
nonpyogenic thrombosis of intracranial venous system (I67.6)
nontraumatic intracerebral hemorrhage (I61.-)
nontraumatic subdural hemorrhage (I62.Ø-)
other and unspecified cord compression (G95.2-)
other secondary parkinsonism (G21.8)
reversible cerebrovascular vasoconstriction syndrome (I67.841)
spinal cord herniation (G95.89)
stroke (I63.-)
syringomyelia (G95.Ø)

● **G96.81Ø Intracranial hypotension, unspecified**

● **G96.811 Intracranial hypotension, spontaneous**

● **G96.819 Other intracranial hypotension**

● **G96.89 Other specified disorders of central nervous system**

G96.9 Disorder of central nervous system, unspecified HIV

✓4th **G97 Intraoperative and postprocedural complications and disorders of nervous system, not elsewhere classified**

EXCLUDES 2 *intraoperative and postprocedural cerebrovascular infarction (I97.81-, I97.82-)*

AHA: 2016,4Q,9-10

G97.Ø Cerebrospinal fluid leak from spinal puncture CC

▶Code also any associated diagnoses or complications, such as:◀
▶intracranial hypotension following a procedure (G97.83-G97.84)◀

Spinal Puncture

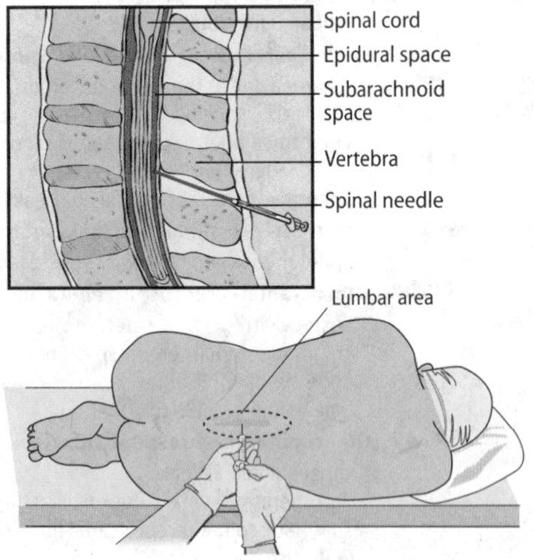

G97.1 Other reaction to spinal and lumbar puncture

Headache due to lumbar puncture
▶Other reaction to spinal dural puncture◀
▶Code also, if applicable, any associated headache with orthostatic component (R51.Ø)◀

G97.2 Intracranial hypotension following ventricular shunting CC

▶Code also any associated diagnoses or complications◀

✓5th **G97.3 Intraoperative hemorrhage and hematoma of a nervous system organ or structure complicating a procedure**

EXCLUDES 1 *intraoperative hemorrhage and hematoma of a nervous system organ or structure due to accidental puncture and laceration during a procedure (G97.4-)*

G97.31 Intraoperative hemorrhage and hematoma of a nervous system organ or structure complicating a nervous system procedure CC

G97.32 Intraoperative hemorrhage and hematoma of a nervous system organ or structure complicating other procedure CC

✓5th **G97.4 Accidental puncture and laceration of a nervous system organ or structure during a procedure**

G97.41 Accidental puncture or laceration of dura during a procedure CC

Incidental (inadvertent) durotomy
▶Code also any associated diagnoses or complications◀
AHA: 2014,4Q,24

G97.48 Accidental puncture and laceration of other nervous system organ or structure during a nervous system procedure CC

G97.49 Accidental puncture and laceration of other nervous system organ or structure during other procedure CC

✓5th **G97.5 Postprocedural hemorrhage of a nervous system organ or structure following a procedure**

G97.51 Postprocedural hemorrhage of a nervous system organ or structure following a nervous system procedure CC

G97.52 Postprocedural hemorrhage of a nervous system organ or structure following other procedure CC

✓5th **G97.6 Postprocedural hematoma and seroma of a nervous system organ or structure following a procedure**

G97.61 Postprocedural hematoma of a nervous system organ or structure following a nervous system procedure CC

G97.62 Postprocedural hematoma of a nervous system organ or structure following other procedure CC

G97.63 Postprocedural seroma of a nervous system organ or structure following a nervous system procedure CC

G97.64 Postprocedural seroma of a nervous system organ or structure following other procedure CC

✓5th **G97.8 Other intraoperative and postprocedural complications and disorders of nervous system**

Use additional code to further specify disorder

G97.81 Other intraoperative complications of nervous system CC

G97.82 Other postprocedural complications and disorders of nervous system CC

● **G97.83 Intracranial hypotension following lumbar cerebrospinal fluid shunting** CC

Code also any associated diagnoses or complications

● **G97.84 Intracranial hypotension following other procedure** CC

Code also, if applicable:
accidental puncture or laceration of dura during a procedure (G97.41)
cerebrospinal fluid leak from spinal puncture (G97.Ø)

✓4th **G98 Other disorders of nervous system not elsewhere classified**

INCLUDES nervous system disorder NOS

G98.Ø Neurogenic arthritis, not elsewhere classified

Nonsyphilitic neurogenic arthropathy NEC
Nonsyphilitic neurogenic spondylopathy NEC

EXCLUDES 1 *spondylopathy (in):*
syringomyelia and syringobulbia (G95.Ø)
tabes dorsalis (A52.11)

G98.8 Other disorders of nervous system HIV

Nervous system disorder NOS

✓4th **G99 Other disorders of nervous system in diseases classified elsewhere**

G99.Ø Autonomic neuropathy in diseases classified elsewhere CC

Code first underlying disease, such as:
amyloidosis (E85.-)
gout (M1A.-, M1Ø.-)
hyperthyroidism (EØ5.-)

EXCLUDES 1 *diabetic autonomic neuropathy (EØ8-E13 with .43)*

G99.2 ***Myelopathy in diseases classified elsewhere*** CC HCC

Code first underlying disease, such as:

neoplasm (CØØ-D49)

EXCLUDES 1 *myelopathy in:*

intervertebral disease (M5Ø.Ø-, M51.Ø-)

spondylosis (M47.Ø-, M47.1-)

AHA: 2018,3Q,18-19

TIP: Use this code in addition to a spondylolisthesis code (M43.1-) or a spinal stenosis code (M48.0-) when either of these disorders is documented as the cause of the myelopathy.

G99.8 ***Other specified disorders of nervous system in diseases classified elsewhere***

Code first underlying disorder, such as:

amyloidosis (E85.-)

avitaminosis (E56.9)

EXCLUDES 1 *nervous system involvement in:*

cysticercosis (B69.Ø)

rubella (BØ6.Ø-)

syphilis (A52.1-)

Chapter 7. Diseases of the Eye and Adnexa (HØØ–H59)

Chapter-specific Guidelines with Coding Examples

The chapter-specific guidelines from the ICD-10-CM Official Guidelines for Coding and Reporting have been provided below. Along with these guidelines are coding examples, contained in the shaded boxes, that have been developed to help illustrate the coding and/or sequencing guidance found in these guidelines.

a. Glaucoma

1) Assigning glaucoma codes

Assign as many codes from category H4Ø, Glaucoma, as needed to identify the type of glaucoma, the affected eye, and the glaucoma stage.

2) Bilateral glaucoma with same type and stage

When a patient has bilateral glaucoma and both eyes are documented as being the same type and stage, and there is a code for bilateral glaucoma, report only the code for the type of glaucoma, bilateral, with the seventh character for the stage.

> Bilateral severe stage pigmentary glaucoma
>
> **H4Ø.1333 Pigmentary glaucoma, bilateral, severe stage**
>
> *Explanation*: In this scenario, the patient has the same type and stage of glaucoma in both eyes. As this type of glaucoma has a code for bilateral, assign only the code for the bilateral glaucoma with the seventh character for the stage.

When a patient has bilateral glaucoma and both eyes are documented as being the same type and stage, and the classification does not provide a code for bilateral glaucoma (i.e. subcategories H4Ø.1Ø and H4Ø.2Ø) report only one code for the type of glaucoma with the appropriate seventh character for the stage.

> Bilateral open-angle glaucoma; not specified as to type and stage indeterminate in both eyes
>
> **H4Ø.1ØX4 Unspecified open-angle glaucoma, indeterminate stage**
>
> *Explanation*: In this scenario, the patient has glaucoma of the same type and stage of both eyes, but there is no code specifically for bilateral glaucoma. Only one code is assigned with the appropriate seventh character for the stage.

3) Bilateral glaucoma stage with different types or stages

When a patient has bilateral glaucoma and each eye is documented as having a different type or stage, and the classification distinguishes laterality, assign the appropriate code for each eye rather than the code for bilateral glaucoma.

When a patient has bilateral glaucoma and each eye is documented as having a different type, and the classification does not distinguish laterality (i.e. subcategories H4Ø.1Ø and H4Ø.2Ø), assign one code for each type of glaucoma with the appropriate seventh character for the stage.

> Documentation relates mild, unspecified primary angle-closure glaucoma of the left eye with mild unspecified open-angle glaucoma of the right eye
>
> **H4Ø.2ØX1 Unspecified primary angle-closure glaucoma, mild stage**
>
> **H4Ø.1ØX1 Unspecified open-angle glaucoma, mild stage**
>
> *Explanation*: In this scenario the patient has a different type of glaucoma in each eye and the classification does not distinguish laterality. A code for each type of glaucoma is assigned, each with the appropriate seventh character for the stage.

When a patient has bilateral glaucoma and each eye is documented as having the same type, but different stage, and the classification does not distinguish laterality (i.e. subcategories H4Ø.1Ø and H4Ø.2Ø), assign a code for the type of glaucoma for each eye with the seventh character for the specific glaucoma stage documented for each eye.

> Bilateral open-angle glaucoma, not specified as to type; the right eye is documented to be in mild stage and the left eye as being in moderate stage
>
> **H4Ø.1ØX1 Unspecified open-angle glaucoma, mild stage**
>
> **H4Ø.1ØX2 Unspecified open-angle glaucoma, moderate stage**
>
> *Explanation*: In this scenario the patient has the same type of glaucoma in each eye but each eye is at a different stage, and the classification does not distinguish laterality at this subcategory level. Two codes are assigned; both codes represent the same type of glaucoma but each has a different seventh character identifying the appropriate stage for each eye.

4) Patient admitted with glaucoma and stage evolves during the admission

If a patient is admitted with glaucoma and the stage progresses during the admission, assign the code for highest stage documented.

> Patient admitted with mild low-tension glaucoma of the right eye, which progresses to moderate stage during the patient's stay
>
> **H4Ø.1212 Low-tension glaucoma, right eye, moderate stage**
>
> *Explanation*: When the glaucoma stage progresses during an admission, assign only the code for the highest stage documented.

5) Indeterminate stage glaucoma

Assignment of the seventh character "4" for "indeterminate stage" should be based on the clinical documentation. The seventh character "4" is used for glaucomas whose stage cannot be clinically determined. This seventh character should not be confused with the seventh character "Ø", unspecified, which should be assigned when there is no documentation regarding the stage of the glaucoma.

b. Blindness

If "blindness" or "low vision" of both eyes is documented but the visual impairment category is not documented, assign code H54.3, Unqualified visual loss, both eyes. If "blindness" or "low vision" in one eye is documented but the visual impairment category is not documented, assign a code from H54.6-, Unqualified visual loss, one eye. If "blindness" or "visual loss" is documented without any information about whether one or both eyes are affected, assign code H54.7, Unspecified visual loss.

> Blindness in 89-year-old male
>
> **H54.7 Unspecified visual loss**
>
> *Explanation*: Blindness is stated, but there is no mention of whether one or both eyes are affected or the severity of this visual impairment.

Chapter 7. Diseases of the Eye and Adnexa (H00-H59)

NOTE Use an external cause code following the code for the eye condition, if applicable, to identify the cause of the eye condition

EXCLUDES 2 *certain conditions originating in the perinatal period (P04-P96)*
certain infectious and parasitic diseases (A00-B99)
complications of pregnancy, childbirth and the puerperium (O00-O9A)
congenital malformations, deformations, and chromosomal abnormalities (Q00-Q99)
diabetes mellitus related eye conditions (E09.3-, E10.3-, E11.3-, E13.3-)
endocrine, nutritional and metabolic diseases (E00-E88)
injury (trauma) of eye and orbit (S05.-)
injury, poisoning and certain other consequences of external causes (S00-T88)
neoplasms (C00-D49)
symptoms, signs and abnormal clinical and laboratory findings, not elsewhere classified (R00-R94)
syphilis related eye disorders (A50.01, A50.3-, A51.43, A52.71)

This chapter contains the following blocks:

H00-H05	Disorders of eyelid, lacrimal system and orbit
H10-H11	Disorders of conjunctiva
H15-H22	Disorders of sclera, cornea, iris and ciliary body
H25-H28	Disorders of lens
H30-H36	Disorders of choroid and retina
H40-H42	Glaucoma
H43-H44	Disorders of vitreous body and globe
H46-H47	Disorders of optic nerve and visual pathways
H49-H52	Disorders of ocular muscles, binocular movement, accommodation and refraction
H53-H54	Visual disturbances and blindness
H55-H57	Other disorders of eye and adnexa
H59	Intraoperative and postprocedural complications and disorders of eye and adnexa, not elsewhere classified

Disorders of eyelid, lacrimal system and orbit (H00-H05)

EXCLUDES 2 *open wound of eyelid (S01.1-)*
superficial injury of eyelid (S00.1-, S00.2-)

✓4th **H00 Hordeolum and chalazion**

✓5th **H00.0 Hordeolum (externum) (internum) of eyelid**

DEF: Acute localized infection of the gland of Zeis (external hordeolum) or Molt or of the meibomian glands (internal hordeolum) of the orbit.

✓6th **H00.01 Hordeolum externum**

Hordeolum NOS
Stye

- **H00.011 Hordeolum externum right upper eyelid**
- **H00.012 Hordeolum externum right lower eyelid**
- **H00.013 Hordeolum externum right eye, unspecified eyelid**
- **H00.014 Hordeolum externum left upper eyelid**
- **H00.015 Hordeolum externum left lower eyelid**
- **H00.016 Hordeolum externum left eye, unspecified eyelid**
- **H00.019 Hordeolum externum unspecified eye, unspecified eyelid**

✓6th **H00.02 Hordeolum internum**

Infection of meibomian gland

- **H00.021 Hordeolum internum right upper eyelid**
- **H00.022 Hordeolum internum right lower eyelid**
- **H00.023 Hordeolum internum right eye, unspecified eyelid**
- **H00.024 Hordeolum internum left upper eyelid**
- **H00.025 Hordeolum internum left lower eyelid**
- **H00.026 Hordeolum internum left eye, unspecified eyelid**
- **H00.029 Hordeolum internum unspecified eye, unspecified eyelid**

✓6th **H00.03 Abscess of eyelid**

Furuncle of eyelid

- **H00.031 Abscess of right upper eyelid**
- **H00.032 Abscess of right lower eyelid**
- **H00.033 Abscess of eyelid right eye, unspecified eyelid**
- **H00.034 Abscess of left upper eyelid**
- **H00.035 Abscess of left lower eyelid**
- **H00.036 Abscess of eyelid left eye, unspecified eyelid**
- **H00.039 Abscess of eyelid unspecified eye, unspecified eyelid**

✓5th **H00.1 Chalazion**

Meibomian (gland) cyst

EXCLUDES 2 *infected meibomian gland (H00.02-)*

DEF: Noninfectious, obstructive mass in the oil gland of the eyelid that results in a small chronic lump or inflammation.

- **H00.11 Chalazion right upper eyelid**
- **H00.12 Chalazion right lower eyelid**
- **H00.13 Chalazion right eye, unspecified eyelid**
- **H00.14 Chalazion left upper eyelid**
- **H00.15 Chalazion left lower eyelid**
- **H00.16 Chalazion left eye, unspecified eyelid**
- **H00.19 Chalazion unspecified eye, unspecified eyelid**

✓4th **H01 Other inflammation of eyelid**

✓5th **H01.0 Blepharitis**

EXCLUDES 1 *blepharoconjunctivitis (H10.5-)*

✓6th **H01.00 Unspecified blepharitis**

AHA: 2018,4Q,13

- **H01.001 Unspecified blepharitis right upper eyelid**
- **H01.002 Unspecified blepharitis right lower eyelid**
- **H01.003 Unspecified blepharitis right eye, unspecified eyelid**
- **H01.004 Unspecified blepharitis left upper eyelid**
- **H01.005 Unspecified blepharitis left lower eyelid**
- **H01.006 Unspecified blepharitis left eye, unspecified eyelid**
- **H01.009 Unspecified blepharitis unspecified eye, unspecified eyelid**
- **H01.00A Unspecified blepharitis right eye, upper and lower eyelids**
- **H01.00B Unspecified blepharitis left eye, upper and lower eyelids**

✓6th **H01.01 Ulcerative blepharitis**

AHA: 2018,4Q,13

- **H01.011 Ulcerative blepharitis right upper eyelid**
- **H01.012 Ulcerative blepharitis right lower eyelid**
- **H01.013 Ulcerative blepharitis right eye, unspecified eyelid**
- **H01.014 Ulcerative blepharitis left upper eyelid**
- **H01.015 Ulcerative blepharitis left lower eyelid**
- **H01.016 Ulcerative blepharitis left eye, unspecified eyelid**
- **H01.019 Ulcerative blepharitis unspecified eye, unspecified eyelid**
- **H01.01A Ulcerative blepharitis right eye, upper and lower eyelids**
- **H01.01B Ulcerative blepharitis left eye, upper and lower eyelids**

✓6th **H01.02 Squamous blepharitis**

AHA: 2018,4Q,13

- **H01.021 Squamous blepharitis right upper eyelid**
- **H01.022 Squamous blepharitis right lower eyelid**
- **H01.023 Squamous blepharitis right eye, unspecified eyelid**
- **H01.024 Squamous blepharitis left upper eyelid**
- **H01.025 Squamous blepharitis left lower eyelid**
- **H01.026 Squamous blepharitis left eye, unspecified eyelid**
- **H01.029 Squamous blepharitis unspecified eye, unspecified eyelid**
- **H01.02A Squamous blepharitis right eye, upper and lower eyelids**
- **H01.02B Squamous blepharitis left eye, upper and lower eyelids**

✓5th **H01.1 Noninfectious dermatoses of eyelid**

✓6th **H01.11 Allergic dermatitis of eyelid**

Contact dermatitis of eyelid

- **H01.111 Allergic dermatitis of right upper eyelid**
- **H01.112 Allergic dermatitis of right lower eyelid**
- **H01.113 Allergic dermatitis of right eye, unspecified eyelid**
- **H01.114 Allergic dermatitis of left upper eyelid**
- **H01.115 Allergic dermatitis of left lower eyelid**
- **H01.116 Allergic dermatitis of left eye, unspecified eyelid**
- **H01.119 Allergic dermatitis of unspecified eye, unspecified eyelid**

√6th **HØ1.12 Discoid lupus erythematosus of eyelid**
- **HØ1.121 Discoid lupus erythematosus of right upper eyelid**
- **HØ1.122 Discoid lupus erythematosus of right lower eyelid**
- **HØ1.123 Discoid lupus erythematosus of right eye, unspecified eyelid**
- **HØ1.124 Discoid lupus erythematosus of left upper eyelid**
- **HØ1.125 Discoid lupus erythematosus of left lower eyelid**
- **HØ1.126 Discoid lupus erythematosus of left eye, unspecified eyelid**
- **HØ1.129 Discoid lupus erythematosus of unspecified eye, unspecified eyelid**

√6th **HØ1.13 Eczematous dermatitis of eyelid**
- **HØ1.131 Eczematous dermatitis of right upper eyelid**
- **HØ1.132 Eczematous dermatitis of right lower eyelid**
- **HØ1.133 Eczematous dermatitis of right eye, unspecified eyelid**
- **HØ1.134 Eczematous dermatitis of left upper eyelid**
- **HØ1.135 Eczematous dermatitis of left lower eyelid**
- **HØ1.136 Eczematous dermatitis of left eye, unspecified eyelid**
- **HØ1.139 Eczematous dermatitis of unspecified eye, unspecified eyelid**

√6th **HØ1.14 Xeroderma of eyelid**
- **HØ1.141 Xeroderma of right upper eyelid**
- **HØ1.142 Xeroderma of right lower eyelid**
- **HØ1.143 Xeroderma of right eye, unspecified eyelid**
- **HØ1.144 Xeroderma of left upper eyelid**
- **HØ1.145 Xeroderma of left lower eyelid**
- **HØ1.146 Xeroderma of left eye, unspecified eyelid**
- **HØ1.149 Xeroderma of unspecified eye, unspecified eyelid**

HØ1.8 Other specified inflammations of eyelid

HØ1.9 Unspecified inflammation of eyelid
Inflammation of eyelid NOS

√4th **HØ2 Other disorders of eyelid**

EXCLUDES 1 *congenital malformations of eyelid (Q1Ø.Ø-Q1Ø.3)*

Entropion and Ectropion

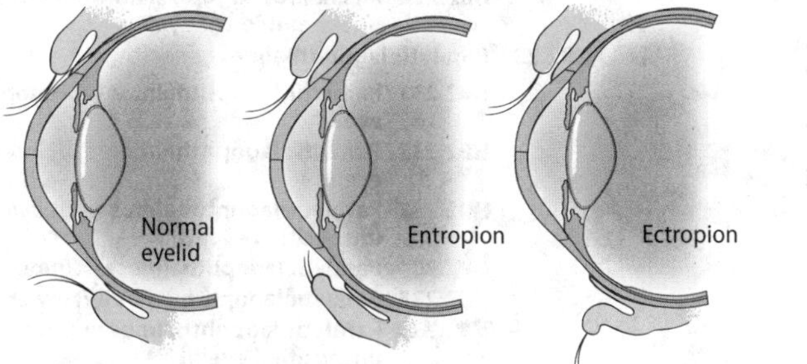

√5th **HØ2.Ø Entropion and trichiasis of eyelid**

DEF: Entropion: Inversion of the eyelid, turning the edge in toward the eyeball and causing irritation from contact of the lashes with the surface of the eye.

DEF: Trichiasis: Condition wherein the eyelid is in a normal position but lashes are ingrown or misdirected in their growth so that they irritate the tissues of the eye.

√6th **HØ2.ØØ Unspecified entropion of eyelid**
- **HØ2.ØØ1 Unspecified entropion of right upper eyelid**
- **HØ2.ØØ2 Unspecified entropion of right lower eyelid**
- **HØ2.ØØ3 Unspecified entropion of right eye, unspecified eyelid**
- **HØ2.ØØ4 Unspecified entropion of left upper eyelid**
- **HØ2.ØØ5 Unspecified entropion of left lower eyelid**
- **HØ2.ØØ6 Unspecified entropion of left eye, unspecified eyelid**
- **HØ2.ØØ9 Unspecified entropion of unspecified eye, unspecified eyelid**

√6th **HØ2.Ø1 Cicatricial entropion of eyelid**
- **HØ2.Ø11 Cicatricial entropion of right upper eyelid**
- **HØ2.Ø12 Cicatricial entropion of right lower eyelid**
- **HØ2.Ø13 Cicatricial entropion of right eye, unspecified eyelid**
- **HØ2.Ø14 Cicatricial entropion of left upper eyelid**
- **HØ2.Ø15 Cicatricial entropion of left lower eyelid**
- **HØ2.Ø16 Cicatricial entropion of left eye, unspecified eyelid**
- **HØ2.Ø19 Cicatricial entropion of unspecified eye, unspecified eyelid**

√6th **HØ2.Ø2 Mechanical entropion of eyelid**
- **HØ2.Ø21 Mechanical entropion of right upper eyelid**
- **HØ2.Ø22 Mechanical entropion of right lower eyelid**
- **HØ2.Ø23 Mechanical entropion of right eye, unspecified eyelid**
- **HØ2.Ø24 Mechanical entropion of left upper eyelid**
- **HØ2.Ø25 Mechanical entropion of left lower eyelid**
- **HØ2.Ø26 Mechanical entropion of left eye, unspecified eyelid**
- **HØ2.Ø29 Mechanical entropion of unspecified eye, unspecified eyelid**

√6th **HØ2.Ø3 Senile entropion of eyelid**
- **HØ2.Ø31 Senile entropion of right upper eyelid** A
- **HØ2.Ø32 Senile entropion of right lower eyelid** A
- **HØ2.Ø33 Senile entropion of right eye, unspecified eyelid** A
- **HØ2.Ø34 Senile entropion of left upper eyelid** A
- **HØ2.Ø35 Senile entropion of left lower eyelid** A
- **HØ2.Ø36 Senile entropion of left eye, unspecified eyelid** A
- **HØ2.Ø39 Senile entropion of unspecified eye, unspecified eyelid** A

√6th **HØ2.Ø4 Spastic entropion of eyelid**
- **HØ2.Ø41 Spastic entropion of right upper eyelid**
- **HØ2.Ø42 Spastic entropion of right lower eyelid**
- **HØ2.Ø43 Spastic entropion of right eye, unspecified eyelid**
- **HØ2.Ø44 Spastic entropion of left upper eyelid**
- **HØ2.Ø45 Spastic entropion of left lower eyelid**
- **HØ2.Ø46 Spastic entropion of left eye, unspecified eyelid**
- **HØ2.Ø49 Spastic entropion of unspecified eye, unspecified eyelid**

√6th **HØ2.Ø5 Trichiasis without entropion**
- **HØ2.Ø51 Trichiasis without entropion right upper eyelid**
- **HØ2.Ø52 Trichiasis without entropion right lower eyelid**
- **HØ2.Ø53 Trichiasis without entropion right eye, unspecified eyelid**
- **HØ2.Ø54 Trichiasis without entropion left upper eyelid**
- **HØ2.Ø55 Trichiasis without entropion left lower eyelid**
- **HØ2.Ø56 Trichiasis without entropion left eye, unspecified eyelid**
- **HØ2.Ø59 Trichiasis without entropion unspecified eye, unspecified eyelid**

√5th **HØ2.1 Ectropion of eyelid**

DEF: Drooping of the lower eyelid away from the eye or outward turning or eversion of the edge of the eyelid, exposing the palpebral conjunctiva and causing irritation.

√6th **HØ2.1Ø Unspecified ectropion of eyelid**
- **HØ2.1Ø1 Unspecified ectropion of right upper eyelid**
- **HØ2.1Ø2 Unspecified ectropion of right lower eyelid**
- **HØ2.1Ø3 Unspecified ectropion of right eye, unspecified eyelid**
- **HØ2.1Ø4 Unspecified ectropion of left upper eyelid**
- **HØ2.1Ø5 Unspecified ectropion of left lower eyelid**

H02.106 Unspecified ectropion of left eye, unspecified eyelid
H02.109 Unspecified ectropion of unspecified eye, unspecified eyelid

√6th **H02.11** Cicatricial ectropion of eyelid
- **H02.111** Cicatricial ectropion of right upper eyelid
- **H02.112** Cicatricial ectropion of right lower eyelid
- **H02.113** Cicatricial ectropion of right eye, unspecified eyelid
- **H02.114** Cicatricial ectropion of left upper eyelid
- **H02.115** Cicatricial ectropion of left lower eyelid
- **H02.116** Cicatricial ectropion of left eye, unspecified eyelid
- **H02.119** Cicatricial ectropion of unspecified eye, unspecified eyelid

√6th **H02.12** Mechanical ectropion of eyelid
- **H02.121** Mechanical ectropion of right upper eyelid
- **H02.122** Mechanical ectropion of right lower eyelid
- **H02.123** Mechanical ectropion of right eye, unspecified eyelid
- **H02.124** Mechanical ectropion of left upper eyelid
- **H02.125** Mechanical ectropion of left lower eyelid
- **H02.126** Mechanical ectropion of left eye, unspecified eyelid
- **H02.129** Mechanical ectropion of unspecified eye, unspecified eyelid

√6th **H02.13** Senile ectropion of eyelid
- **H02.131** Senile ectropion of right upper eyelid A
- **H02.132** Senile ectropion of right lower eyelid A
- **H02.133** Senile ectropion of right eye, unspecified eyelid A
- **H02.134** Senile ectropion of left upper eyelid A
- **H02.135** Senile ectropion of left lower eyelid A
- **H02.136** Senile ectropion of left eye, unspecified eyelid A
- **H02.139** Senile ectropion of unspecified eye, unspecified eyelid A

√6th **H02.14** Spastic ectropion of eyelid
- **H02.141** Spastic ectropion of right upper eyelid
- **H02.142** Spastic ectropion of right lower eyelid
- **H02.143** Spastic ectropion of right eye, unspecified eyelid
- **H02.144** Spastic ectropion of left upper eyelid
- **H02.145** Spastic ectropion of left lower eyelid
- **H02.146** Spastic ectropion of left eye, unspecified eyelid
- **H02.149** Spastic ectropion of unspecified eye, unspecified eyelid

√6th **H02.15** Paralytic ectropion of eyelid

AHA: 2018,4Q,13
- **H02.151** Paralytic ectropion of right upper eyelid
- **H02.152** Paralytic ectropion of right lower eyelid
- **H02.153** Paralytic ectropion of right eye, unspecified eyelid
- **H02.154** Paralytic ectropion of left upper eyelid
- **H02.155** Paralytic ectropion of left lower eyelid
- **H02.156** Paralytic ectropion of left eye, unspecified eyelid
- **H02.159** Paralytic ectropion of unspecified eye, unspecified eyelid

√5th **H02.2 Lagophthalmos**

AHA: 2018,4Q,14

DEF: Condition of the eye that prevents it from closing completely.

√6th **H02.20** Unspecified lagophthalmos
- **H02.201** Unspecified lagophthalmos right upper eyelid
- **H02.202** Unspecified lagophthalmos right lower eyelid
- **H02.203** Unspecified lagophthalmos right eye, unspecified eyelid
- **H02.204** Unspecified lagophthalmos left upper eyelid
- **H02.205** Unspecified lagophthalmos left lower eyelid
- **H02.206** Unspecified lagophthalmos left eye, unspecified eyelid
- **H02.209** Unspecified lagophthalmos unspecified eye, unspecified eyelid
- **H02.20A** Unspecified lagophthalmos right eye, upper and lower eyelids
- **H02.20B** Unspecified lagophthalmos left eye, upper and lower eyelids
- **H02.20C** Unspecified lagophthalmos, bilateral, upper and lower eyelids

√6th **H02.21** Cicatricial lagophthalmos
- **H02.211** Cicatricial lagophthalmos right upper eyelid
- **H02.212** Cicatricial lagophthalmos right lower eyelid
- **H02.213** Cicatricial lagophthalmos right eye, unspecified eyelid
- **H02.214** Cicatricial lagophthalmos left upper eyelid
- **H02.215** Cicatricial lagophthalmos left lower eyelid
- **H02.216** Cicatricial lagophthalmos left eye, unspecified eyelid
- **H02.219** Cicatricial lagophthalmos unspecified eye, unspecified eyelid
- **H02.21A** Cicatricial lagophthalmos right eye, upper and lower eyelids
- **H02.21B** Cicatricial lagophthalmos left eye, upper and lower eyelids
- **H02.21C** Cicatricial lagophthalmos, bilateral, upper and lower eyelids

√6th **H02.22** Mechanical lagophthalmos
- **H02.221** Mechanical lagophthalmos right upper eyelid
- **H02.222** Mechanical lagophthalmos right lower eyelid
- **H02.223** Mechanical lagophthalmos right eye, unspecified eyelid
- **H02.224** Mechanical lagophthalmos left upper eyelid
- **H02.225** Mechanical lagophthalmos left lower eyelid
- **H02.226** Mechanical lagophthalmos left eye, unspecified eyelid
- **H02.229** Mechanical lagophthalmos unspecified eye, unspecified eyelid
- **H02.22A** Mechanical lagophthalmos right eye, upper and lower eyelids
- **H02.22B** Mechanical lagophthalmos left eye, upper and lower eyelids
- **H02.22C** Mechanical lagophthalmos, bilateral, upper and lower eyelids

√6th **H02.23** Paralytic lagophthalmos
- **H02.231** Paralytic lagophthalmos right upper eyelid
- **H02.232** Paralytic lagophthalmos right lower eyelid
- **H02.233** Paralytic lagophthalmos right eye, unspecified eyelid
- **H02.234** Paralytic lagophthalmos left upper eyelid
- **H02.235** Paralytic lagophthalmos left lower eyelid
- **H02.236** Paralytic lagophthalmos left eye, unspecified eyelid
- **H02.239** Paralytic lagophthalmos unspecified eye, unspecified eyelid
- **H02.23A** Paralytic lagophthalmos right eye, upper and lower eyelids
- **H02.23B** Paralytic lagophthalmos left eye, upper and lower eyelids
- **H02.23C** Paralytic lagophthalmos, bilateral, upper and lower eyelids

√5th **H02.3 Blepharochalasis**

Pseudoptosis

DEF: Loss of elasticity and relaxation of skin of the eyelid, thickened or indurated skin on the eyelid associated with recurrent episodes of edema, and intracellular atrophy.
- **H02.30** Blepharochalasis unspecified eye, unspecified eyelid
- **H02.31** Blepharochalasis right upper eyelid
- **H02.32** Blepharochalasis right lower eyelid
- **H02.33** Blepharochalasis right eye, unspecified eyelid
- **H02.34** Blepharochalasis left upper eyelid
- **H02.35** Blepharochalasis left lower eyelid
- **H02.36** Blepharochalasis left eye, unspecified eyelid

✓5th H02.4 Ptosis of eyelid
✓6th H02.40 Unspecified ptosis of eyelid
H02.401 Unspecified ptosis of right eyelid
H02.402 Unspecified ptosis of left eyelid
H02.403 Unspecified ptosis of bilateral eyelids
H02.409 Unspecified ptosis of unspecified eyelid
✓6th H02.41 Mechanical ptosis of eyelid
H02.411 Mechanical ptosis of right eyelid
H02.412 Mechanical ptosis of left eyelid
H02.413 Mechanical ptosis of bilateral eyelids
H02.419 Mechanical ptosis of unspecified eyelid
✓6th H02.42 Myogenic ptosis of eyelid
H02.421 Myogenic ptosis of right eyelid
H02.422 Myogenic ptosis of left eyelid
H02.423 Myogenic ptosis of bilateral eyelids
H02.429 Myogenic ptosis of unspecified eyelid
✓6th H02.43 Paralytic ptosis of eyelid
Neurogenic ptosis of eyelid
H02.431 Paralytic ptosis of right eyelid
H02.432 Paralytic ptosis of left eyelid
H02.433 Paralytic ptosis of bilateral eyelids
H02.439 Paralytic ptosis unspecified eyelid
✓5th H02.5 Other disorders affecting eyelid function
EXCLUDES 2 *blepharospasm (G24.5)*
organic tic (G25.69)
psychogenic tic (F95.-)
✓6th H02.51 Abnormal innervation syndrome
H02.511 Abnormal innervation syndrome right upper eyelid
H02.512 Abnormal innervation syndrome right lower eyelid
H02.513 Abnormal innervation syndrome right eye, unspecified eyelid
H02.514 Abnormal innervation syndrome left upper eyelid
H02.515 Abnormal innervation syndrome left lower eyelid
H02.516 Abnormal innervation syndrome left eye, unspecified eyelid
H02.519 Abnormal innervation syndrome unspecified eye, unspecified eyelid
✓6th H02.52 Blepharophimosis
Ankyloblepharon
H02.521 Blepharophimosis right upper eyelid
H02.522 Blepharophimosis right lower eyelid
H02.523 Blepharophimosis right eye, unspecified eyelid
H02.524 Blepharophimosis left upper eyelid
H02.525 Blepharophimosis left lower eyelid
H02.526 Blepharophimosis left eye, unspecified eyelid
H02.529 Blepharophimosis unspecified eye, unspecified lid
✓6th H02.53 Eyelid retraction
Eyelid lag
H02.531 Eyelid retraction right upper eyelid
H02.532 Eyelid retraction right lower eyelid
H02.533 Eyelid retraction right eye, unspecified eyelid
H02.534 Eyelid retraction left upper eyelid
H02.535 Eyelid retraction left lower eyelid
H02.536 Eyelid retraction left eye, unspecified eyelid
H02.539 Eyelid retraction unspecified eye, unspecified lid
H02.59 Other disorders affecting eyelid function
Deficient blink reflex
Sensory disorders
✓5th H02.6 Xanthelasma of eyelid
DEF: Condition in which there are small yellow tumors that occur on the eyelid, usually appearing near the nose.
H02.60 Xanthelasma of unspecified eye, unspecified eyelid
H02.61 Xanthelasma of right upper eyelid
H02.62 Xanthelasma of right lower eyelid
H02.63 Xanthelasma of right eye, unspecified eyelid
H02.64 Xanthelasma of left upper eyelid
H02.65 Xanthelasma of left lower eyelid
H02.66 Xanthelasma of left eye, unspecified eyelid
✓5th H02.7 Other and unspecified degenerative disorders of eyelid and periocular area
H02.70 Unspecified degenerative disorders of eyelid and periocular area
✓6th H02.71 Chloasma of eyelid and periocular area
Dyspigmentation of eyelid
Hyperpigmentation of eyelid
H02.711 Chloasma of right upper eyelid and periocular area
H02.712 Chloasma of right lower eyelid and periocular area
H02.713 Chloasma of right eye, unspecified eyelid and periocular area
H02.714 Chloasma of left upper eyelid and periocular area
H02.715 Chloasma of left lower eyelid and periocular area
H02.716 Chloasma of left eye, unspecified eyelid and periocular area
H02.719 Chloasma of unspecified eye, unspecified eyelid and periocular area
✓6th H02.72 Madarosis of eyelid and periocular area
Hypotrichosis of eyelid
H02.721 Madarosis of right upper eyelid and periocular area
H02.722 Madarosis of right lower eyelid and periocular area
H02.723 Madarosis of right eye, unspecified eyelid and periocular area
H02.724 Madarosis of left upper eyelid and periocular area
H02.725 Madarosis of left lower eyelid and periocular area
H02.726 Madarosis of left eye, unspecified eyelid and periocular area
H02.729 Madarosis of unspecified eye, unspecified eyelid and periocular area
✓6th H02.73 Vitiligo of eyelid and periocular area
Hypopigmentation of eyelid
H02.731 Vitiligo of right upper eyelid and periocular area
H02.732 Vitiligo of right lower eyelid and periocular area
H02.733 Vitiligo of right eye, unspecified eyelid and periocular area
H02.734 Vitiligo of left upper eyelid and periocular area
H02.735 Vitiligo of left lower eyelid and periocular area
H02.736 Vitiligo of left eye, unspecified eyelid and periocular area
H02.739 Vitiligo of unspecified eye, unspecified eyelid and periocular area
H02.79 Other degenerative disorders of eyelid and periocular area
✓5th H02.8 Other specified disorders of eyelid
✓6th H02.81 Retained foreign body in eyelid
Use additional code to identify the type of retained foreign body (Z18.-)
EXCLUDES 1 *laceration of eyelid with foreign body (S01.12-)*
retained intraocular foreign body (H44.6-, H44.7-)
superficial foreign body of eyelid and periocular area (S00.25-)
H02.811 Retained foreign body in right upper eyelid
H02.812 Retained foreign body in right lower eyelid
H02.813 Retained foreign body in right eye, unspecified eyelid
H02.814 Retained foreign body in left upper eyelid
H02.815 Retained foreign body in left lower eyelid
H02.816 Retained foreign body in left eye, unspecified eyelid
H02.819 Retained foreign body in unspecified eye, unspecified eyelid
✓6th H02.82 Cysts of eyelid
Sebaceous cyst of eyelid
H02.821 Cysts of right upper eyelid
H02.822 Cysts of right lower eyelid

H02.823 Cysts of right eye, unspecified eyelid
H02.824 Cysts of left upper eyelid
H02.825 Cysts of left lower eyelid
H02.826 Cysts of left eye, unspecified eyelid
H02.829 Cysts of unspecified eye, unspecified eyelid

6th H02.83 Dermatochalasis of eyelid
DEF: Acquired form of connective tissue disorder associated with decreased elastic tissue and abnormal elastin formation, resulting in loss of elasticity of the skin of the eyelid. It is generally associated with aging.
H02.831 Dermatochalasis of right upper eyelid
H02.832 Dermatochalasis of right lower eyelid
H02.833 Dermatochalasis of right eye, unspecified eyelid
H02.834 Dermatochalasis of left upper eyelid
H02.835 Dermatochalasis of left lower eyelid
H02.836 Dermatochalasis of left eye, unspecified eyelid
H02.839 Dermatochalasis of unspecified eye, unspecified eyelid

6th H02.84 Edema of eyelid
Hyperemia of eyelid
H02.841 Edema of right upper eyelid
H02.842 Edema of right lower eyelid
H02.843 Edema of right eye, unspecified eyelid
H02.844 Edema of left upper eyelid
H02.845 Edema of left lower eyelid
H02.846 Edema of left eye, unspecified eyelid
H02.849 Edema of unspecified eye, unspecified eyelid

6th H02.85 Elephantiasis of eyelid
H02.851 Elephantiasis of right upper eyelid
H02.852 Elephantiasis of right lower eyelid
H02.853 Elephantiasis of right eye, unspecified eyelid
H02.854 Elephantiasis of left upper eyelid
H02.855 Elephantiasis of left lower eyelid
H02.856 Elephantiasis of left eye, unspecified eyelid
H02.859 Elephantiasis of unspecified eye, unspecified eyelid

6th H02.86 Hypertrichosis of eyelid
H02.861 Hypertrichosis of right upper eyelid
H02.862 Hypertrichosis of right lower eyelid
H02.863 Hypertrichosis of right eye, unspecified eyelid
H02.864 Hypertrichosis of left upper eyelid
H02.865 Hypertrichosis of left lower eyelid
H02.866 Hypertrichosis of left eye, unspecified eyelid
H02.869 Hypertrichosis of unspecified eye, unspecified eyelid

6th H02.87 Vascular anomalies of eyelid
H02.871 Vascular anomalies of right upper eyelid
H02.872 Vascular anomalies of right lower eyelid
H02.873 Vascular anomalies of right eye, unspecified eyelid
H02.874 Vascular anomalies of left upper eyelid
H02.875 Vascular anomalies of left lower eyelid
H02.876 Vascular anomalies of left eye, unspecified eyelid
H02.879 Vascular anomalies of unspecified eye, unspecified eyelid

6th H02.88 Meibomian gland dysfunction of eyelid
AHA: 2018,4Q,14-15
H02.881 Meibomian gland dysfunction right upper eyelid
H02.882 Meibomian gland dysfunction right lower eyelid
H02.883 Meibomian gland dysfunction of right eye, unspecified eyelid
H02.884 Meibomian gland dysfunction left upper eyelid
H02.885 Meibomian gland dysfunction left lower eyelid
H02.886 Meibomian gland dysfunction of left eye, unspecified eyelid
H02.889 Meibomian gland dysfunction of unspecified eye, unspecified eyelid
H02.88A Meibomian gland dysfunction right eye, upper and lower eyelids
H02.88B Meibomian gland dysfunction left eye, upper and lower eyelids

H02.89 Other specified disorders of eyelid
Hemorrhage of eyelid

H02.9 Unspecified disorder of eyelid
Disorder of eyelid NOS

4th H04 Disorders of lacrimal system
EXCLUDES 1 *congenital malformations of lacrimal system (Q10.4-Q10.6)*

5th H04.0 Dacryoadenitis
DEF: Inflammation of the lacrimal gland.

6th H04.00 Unspecified dacryoadenitis
H04.001 Unspecified dacryoadenitis, right lacrimal gland
H04.002 Unspecified dacryoadenitis, left lacrimal gland
H04.003 Unspecified dacryoadenitis, bilateral lacrimal glands
H04.009 Unspecified dacryoadenitis, unspecified lacrimal gland

6th H04.01 Acute dacryoadenitis
H04.011 Acute dacryoadenitis, right lacrimal gland
H04.012 Acute dacryoadenitis, left lacrimal gland
H04.013 Acute dacryoadenitis, bilateral lacrimal glands
H04.019 Acute dacryoadenitis, unspecified lacrimal gland

6th H04.02 Chronic dacryoadenitis
H04.021 Chronic dacryoadenitis, right lacrimal gland
H04.022 Chronic dacryoadenitis, left lacrimal gland
H04.023 Chronic dacryoadenitis, bilateral lacrimal gland
H04.029 Chronic dacryoadenitis, unspecified lacrimal gland

6th H04.03 Chronic enlargement of lacrimal gland
H04.031 Chronic enlargement of right lacrimal gland
H04.032 Chronic enlargement of left lacrimal gland
H04.033 Chronic enlargement of bilateral lacrimal glands
H04.039 Chronic enlargement of unspecified lacrimal gland

5th H04.1 Other disorders of lacrimal gland

6th H04.11 Dacryops
H04.111 Dacryops of right lacrimal gland
H04.112 Dacryops of left lacrimal gland
H04.113 Dacryops of bilateral lacrimal glands
H04.119 Dacryops of unspecified lacrimal gland

6th H04.12 Dry eye syndrome
Tear film insufficiency, NOS
H04.121 Dry eye syndrome of right lacrimal gland
H04.122 Dry eye syndrome of left lacrimal gland
H04.123 Dry eye syndrome of bilateral lacrimal glands
H04.129 Dry eye syndrome of unspecified lacrimal gland

6th H04.13 Lacrimal cyst
Lacrimal cystic degeneration
H04.131 Lacrimal cyst, right lacrimal gland
H04.132 Lacrimal cyst, left lacrimal gland
H04.133 Lacrimal cyst, bilateral lacrimal glands
H04.139 Lacrimal cyst, unspecified lacrimal gland

6th H04.14 Primary lacrimal gland atrophy
H04.141 Primary lacrimal gland atrophy, right lacrimal gland
H04.142 Primary lacrimal gland atrophy, left lacrimal gland
H04.143 Primary lacrimal gland atrophy, bilateral lacrimal glands
H04.149 Primary lacrimal gland atrophy, unspecified lacrimal gland

6th H04.15 Secondary lacrimal gland atrophy
H04.151 Secondary lacrimal gland atrophy, right lacrimal gland

H04.152 Secondary lacrimal gland atrophy, left lacrimal gland
H04.153 Secondary lacrimal gland atrophy, bilateral lacrimal glands
H04.159 Secondary lacrimal gland atrophy, unspecified lacrimal gland

✓6th H04.16 Lacrimal gland dislocation
H04.161 Lacrimal gland dislocation, right lacrimal gland
H04.162 Lacrimal gland dislocation, left lacrimal gland
H04.163 Lacrimal gland dislocation, bilateral lacrimal glands
H04.169 Lacrimal gland dislocation, unspecified lacrimal gland

H04.19 Other specified disorders of lacrimal gland

✓5th H04.2 Epiphora

DEF: Excessive tearing or overflow of tears down the cheeks often due to a stricture in the lacrimal passages but can be caused by other conditions.

✓6th H04.20 Unspecified epiphora
H04.201 Unspecified epiphora, right side
H04.202 Unspecified epiphora, left side
H04.203 Unspecified epiphora, bilateral
H04.209 Unspecified epiphora, unspecified side

✓6th H04.21 Epiphora due to excess lacrimation
H04.211 Epiphora due to excess lacrimation, right lacrimal gland
H04.212 Epiphora due to excess lacrimation, left lacrimal gland
H04.213 Epiphora due to excess lacrimation, bilateral lacrimal glands
H04.219 Epiphora due to excess lacrimation, unspecified lacrimal gland

✓6th H04.22 Epiphora due to insufficient drainage
H04.221 Epiphora due to insufficient drainage, right side
H04.222 Epiphora due to insufficient drainage, left side
H04.223 Epiphora due to insufficient drainage, bilateral
H04.229 Epiphora due to insufficient drainage, unspecified side

✓5th H04.3 Acute and unspecified inflammation of lacrimal passages

EXCLUDES 1 *neonatal dacryocystitis (P39.1)*

✓6th H04.30 Unspecified dacryocystitis
H04.301 Unspecified dacryocystitis of right lacrimal passage
H04.302 Unspecified dacryocystitis of left lacrimal passage
H04.303 Unspecified dacryocystitis of bilateral lacrimal passages
H04.309 Unspecified dacryocystitis of unspecified lacrimal passage

✓6th H04.31 Phlegmonous dacryocystitis
H04.311 Phlegmonous dacryocystitis of right lacrimal passage
H04.312 Phlegmonous dacryocystitis of left lacrimal passage
H04.313 Phlegmonous dacryocystitis of bilateral lacrimal passages
H04.319 Phlegmonous dacryocystitis of unspecified lacrimal passage

✓6th H04.32 Acute dacryocystitis
Acute dacryopericystitis
H04.321 Acute dacryocystitis of right lacrimal passage
H04.322 Acute dacryocystitis of left lacrimal passage
H04.323 Acute dacryocystitis of bilateral lacrimal passages
H04.329 Acute dacryocystitis of unspecified lacrimal passage

✓6th H04.33 Acute lacrimal canaliculitis
H04.331 Acute lacrimal canaliculitis of right lacrimal passage
H04.332 Acute lacrimal canaliculitis of left lacrimal passage
H04.333 Acute lacrimal canaliculitis of bilateral lacrimal passages
H04.339 Acute lacrimal canaliculitis of unspecified lacrimal passage

✓5th H04.4 Chronic inflammation of lacrimal passages

✓6th H04.41 Chronic dacryocystitis
H04.411 Chronic dacryocystitis of right lacrimal passage
H04.412 Chronic dacryocystitis of left lacrimal passage
H04.413 Chronic dacryocystitis of bilateral lacrimal passages
H04.419 Chronic dacryocystitis of unspecified lacrimal passage

✓6th H04.42 Chronic lacrimal canaliculitis
H04.421 Chronic lacrimal canaliculitis of right lacrimal passage
H04.422 Chronic lacrimal canaliculitis of left lacrimal passage
H04.423 Chronic lacrimal canaliculitis of bilateral lacrimal passages
H04.429 Chronic lacrimal canaliculitis of unspecified lacrimal passage

✓6th H04.43 Chronic lacrimal mucocele
H04.431 Chronic lacrimal mucocele of right lacrimal passage
H04.432 Chronic lacrimal mucocele of left lacrimal passage
H04.433 Chronic lacrimal mucocele of bilateral lacrimal passages
H04.439 Chronic lacrimal mucocele of unspecified lacrimal passage

✓5th H04.5 Stenosis and insufficiency of lacrimal passages

✓6th H04.51 Dacryolith
H04.511 Dacryolith of right lacrimal passage
H04.512 Dacryolith of left lacrimal passage
H04.513 Dacryolith of bilateral lacrimal passages
H04.519 Dacryolith of unspecified lacrimal passage

✓6th H04.52 Eversion of lacrimal punctum
H04.521 Eversion of right lacrimal punctum
H04.522 Eversion of left lacrimal punctum
H04.523 Eversion of bilateral lacrimal punctum
H04.529 Eversion of unspecified lacrimal punctum

✓6th H04.53 Neonatal obstruction of nasolacrimal duct

EXCLUDES 1 *congenital stenosis and stricture of lacrimal duct (Q10.5)*

H04.531 Neonatal obstruction of right nasolacrimal duct N
H04.532 Neonatal obstruction of left nasolacrimal duct N
H04.533 Neonatal obstruction of bilateral nasolacrimal duct N
H04.539 Neonatal obstruction of unspecified nasolacrimal duct N

✓6th H04.54 Stenosis of lacrimal canaliculi
H04.541 Stenosis of right lacrimal canaliculi
H04.542 Stenosis of left lacrimal canaliculi
H04.543 Stenosis of bilateral lacrimal canaliculi
H04.549 Stenosis of unspecified lacrimal canaliculi

✓6th H04.55 Acquired stenosis of nasolacrimal duct
H04.551 Acquired stenosis of right nasolacrimal duct
H04.552 Acquired stenosis of left nasolacrimal duct
H04.553 Acquired stenosis of bilateral nasolacrimal duct
H04.559 Acquired stenosis of unspecified nasolacrimal duct

✓6th H04.56 Stenosis of lacrimal punctum
H04.561 Stenosis of right lacrimal punctum
H04.562 Stenosis of left lacrimal punctum
H04.563 Stenosis of bilateral lacrimal punctum
H04.569 Stenosis of unspecified lacrimal punctum

✓6th H04.57 Stenosis of lacrimal sac
H04.571 Stenosis of right lacrimal sac
H04.572 Stenosis of left lacrimal sac
H04.573 Stenosis of bilateral lacrimal sac
H04.579 Stenosis of unspecified lacrimal sac

H04.6 Other changes of lacrimal passages ✓5th
- ✓6th **H04.61 Lacrimal fistula**
  - **H04.611 Lacrimal fistula right lacrimal passage** SW
  - **H04.612 Lacrimal fistula left lacrimal passage** SW
  - **H04.613 Lacrimal fistula bilateral lacrimal passages** SW
  - **H04.619 Lacrimal fistula unspecified lacrimal passage** SW
- **H04.69 Other changes of lacrimal passages**

H04.8 Other disorders of lacrimal system ✓5th
- ✓6th **H04.81 Granuloma of lacrimal passages**
  - **H04.811 Granuloma of right lacrimal passage**
  - **H04.812 Granuloma of left lacrimal passage**
  - **H04.813 Granuloma of bilateral lacrimal passages**
  - **H04.819 Granuloma of unspecified lacrimal passage**
- **H04.89 Other disorders of lacrimal system**

H04.9 Disorder of lacrimal system, unspecified

✓4th H05 Disorders of orbit

EXCLUDES 1 *congenital malformation of orbit (Q10.7)*

H05.0 Acute inflammation of orbit ✓5th
- **H05.00 Unspecified acute inflammation of orbit**
- ✓6th **H05.01 Cellulitis of orbit**
  - Abscess of orbit
  - **H05.011 Cellulitis of right orbit** CC
  - **H05.012 Cellulitis of left orbit** CC
  - **H05.013 Cellulitis of bilateral orbits** CC
  - **H05.019 Cellulitis of unspecified orbit** CC
- ✓6th **H05.02 Osteomyelitis of orbit**
  - **H05.021 Osteomyelitis of right orbit** CC
  - **H05.022 Osteomyelitis of left orbit** CC
  - **H05.023 Osteomyelitis of bilateral orbits** CC
  - **H05.029 Osteomyelitis of unspecified orbit** CC
- ✓6th **H05.03 Periostitis of orbit**
  - **H05.031 Periostitis of right orbit** CC
  - **H05.032 Periostitis of left orbit** CC
  - **H05.033 Periostitis of bilateral orbits** CC
  - **H05.039 Periostitis of unspecified orbit** CC
- ✓6th **H05.04 Tenonitis of orbit**
  - **H05.041 Tenonitis of right orbit**
  - **H05.042 Tenonitis of left orbit**
  - **H05.043 Tenonitis of bilateral orbits**
  - **H05.049 Tenonitis of unspecified orbit**

H05.1 Chronic inflammatory disorders of orbit ✓5th
- **H05.10 Unspecified chronic inflammatory disorders of orbit**
- ✓6th **H05.11 Granuloma of orbit**
  - Pseudotumor (inflammatory) of orbit
  - **H05.111 Granuloma of right orbit**
  - **H05.112 Granuloma of left orbit**
  - **H05.113 Granuloma of bilateral orbits**
  - **H05.119 Granuloma of unspecified orbit**
- ✓6th **H05.12 Orbital myositis**
  - **H05.121 Orbital myositis, right orbit**
  - **H05.122 Orbital myositis, left orbit**
  - **H05.123 Orbital myositis, bilateral**
  - **H05.129 Orbital myositis, unspecified orbit**

H05.2 Exophthalmic conditions ✓5th
- **H05.20 Unspecified exophthalmos**
- ✓6th **H05.21 Displacement (lateral) of globe**
  - **H05.211 Displacement (lateral) of globe, right eye**
  - **H05.212 Displacement (lateral) of globe, left eye**
  - **H05.213 Displacement (lateral) of globe, bilateral**
  - **H05.219 Displacement (lateral) of globe, unspecified eye**
- ✓6th **H05.22 Edema of orbit**
  - Orbital congestion
  - **H05.221 Edema of right orbit**
  - **H05.222 Edema of left orbit**
  - **H05.223 Edema of bilateral orbit**
  - **H05.229 Edema of unspecified orbit**
- ✓6th **H05.23 Hemorrhage of orbit**
  - **H05.231 Hemorrhage of right orbit**
  - **H05.232 Hemorrhage of left orbit**
  - **H05.233 Hemorrhage of bilateral orbit**
  - **H05.239 Hemorrhage of unspecified orbit**
- ✓6th **H05.24 Constant exophthalmos**
  - **H05.241 Constant exophthalmos, right eye**
  - **H05.242 Constant exophthalmos, left eye**
  - **H05.243 Constant exophthalmos, bilateral**
  - **H05.249 Constant exophthalmos, unspecified eye**
- ✓6th **H05.25 Intermittent exophthalmos**
  - **H05.251 Intermittent exophthalmos, right eye**
  - **H05.252 Intermittent exophthalmos, left eye**
  - **H05.253 Intermittent exophthalmos, bilateral**
  - **H05.259 Intermittent exophthalmos, unspecified eye**
- ✓6th **H05.26 Pulsating exophthalmos**
  - **H05.261 Pulsating exophthalmos, right eye**
  - **H05.262 Pulsating exophthalmos, left eye**
  - **H05.263 Pulsating exophthalmos, bilateral**
  - **H05.269 Pulsating exophthalmos, unspecified eye**

H05.3 Deformity of orbit ✓5th

EXCLUDES 1 *congenital deformity of orbit (Q10.7)*
hypertelorism (Q75.2)

- **H05.30 Unspecified deformity of orbit**
- ✓6th **H05.31 Atrophy of orbit**
  - **H05.311 Atrophy of right orbit**
  - **H05.312 Atrophy of left orbit**
  - **H05.313 Atrophy of bilateral orbit**
  - **H05.319 Atrophy of unspecified orbit**
- ✓6th **H05.32 Deformity of orbit due to bone disease**
  - Code also associated bone disease
  - **H05.321 Deformity of right orbit due to bone disease**
  - **H05.322 Deformity of left orbit due to bone disease**
  - **H05.323 Deformity of bilateral orbits due to bone disease**
  - **H05.329 Deformity of unspecified orbit due to bone disease**
- ✓6th **H05.33 Deformity of orbit due to trauma or surgery**
  - **H05.331 Deformity of right orbit due to trauma or surgery**
  - **H05.332 Deformity of left orbit due to trauma or surgery**
  - **H05.333 Deformity of bilateral orbits due to trauma or surgery**
  - **H05.339 Deformity of unspecified orbit due to trauma or surgery**
- ✓6th **H05.34 Enlargement of orbit**
  - **H05.341 Enlargement of right orbit**
  - **H05.342 Enlargement of left orbit**
  - **H05.343 Enlargement of bilateral orbits**
  - **H05.349 Enlargement of unspecified orbit**
- ✓6th **H05.35 Exostosis of orbit**
  - **H05.351 Exostosis of right orbit**
  - **H05.352 Exostosis of left orbit**
  - **H05.353 Exostosis of bilateral orbits**
  - **H05.359 Exostosis of unspecified orbit**

H05.4 Enophthalmos ✓5th
- ✓6th **H05.40 Unspecified enophthalmos**
  - **H05.401 Unspecified enophthalmos, right eye**
  - **H05.402 Unspecified enophthalmos, left eye**
  - **H05.403 Unspecified enophthalmos, bilateral**
  - **H05.409 Unspecified enophthalmos, unspecified eye**
- ✓6th **H05.41 Enophthalmos due to atrophy of orbital tissue**
  - **H05.411 Enophthalmos due to atrophy of orbital tissue, right eye**
  - **H05.412 Enophthalmos due to atrophy of orbital tissue, left eye**
  - **H05.413 Enophthalmos due to atrophy of orbital tissue, bilateral**
  - **H05.419 Enophthalmos due to atrophy of orbital tissue, unspecified eye**
- ✓6th **H05.42 Enophthalmos due to trauma or surgery**
  - **H05.421 Enophthalmos due to trauma or surgery, right eye**
  - **H05.422 Enophthalmos due to trauma or surgery, left eye**

H05.423 Enophthalmos due to trauma or surgery, bilateral
H05.429 Enophthalmos due to trauma or surgery, unspecified eye

H05.5 Retained (old) foreign body following penetrating wound of orbit
Retrobulbar foreign body
Use additional code to identify the type of retained foreign body (Z18.-)
EXCLUDES 1 *current penetrating wound of orbit (S05.4-)*
EXCLUDES 2 *retained foreign body of eyelid (H02.81-)*
retained intraocular foreign body (H44.6-, H44.7-)
H05.50 Retained (old) foreign body following penetrating wound of unspecified orbit
H05.51 Retained (old) foreign body following penetrating wound of right orbit
H05.52 Retained (old) foreign body following penetrating wound of left orbit
H05.53 Retained (old) foreign body following penetrating wound of bilateral orbits

H05.8 Other disorders of orbit
H05.81 Cyst of orbit
Encephalocele of orbit
H05.811 Cyst of right orbit
H05.812 Cyst of left orbit
H05.813 Cyst of bilateral orbits
H05.819 Cyst of unspecified orbit
H05.82 Myopathy of extraocular muscles
H05.821 Myopathy of extraocular muscles, right orbit
H05.822 Myopathy of extraocular muscles, left orbit
H05.823 Myopathy of extraocular muscles, bilateral
H05.829 Myopathy of extraocular muscles, unspecified orbit
H05.89 Other disorders of orbit

H05.9 Unspecified disorder of orbit

Disorders of conjunctiva (H10-H11)

H10 Conjunctivitis
EXCLUDES 1 *keratoconjunctivitis (H16.2-)*

H10.0 Mucopurulent conjunctivitis
H10.01 Acute follicular conjunctivitis
H10.011 Acute follicular conjunctivitis, right eye
H10.012 Acute follicular conjunctivitis, left eye
H10.013 Acute follicular conjunctivitis, bilateral
H10.019 Acute follicular conjunctivitis, unspecified eye
H10.02 Other mucopurulent conjunctivitis
H10.021 Other mucopurulent conjunctivitis, right eye
H10.022 Other mucopurulent conjunctivitis, left eye
H10.023 Other mucopurulent conjunctivitis, bilateral
H10.029 Other mucopurulent conjunctivitis, unspecified eye

H10.1 Acute atopic conjunctivitis
Acute papillary conjunctivitis
H10.10 Acute atopic conjunctivitis, unspecified eye
H10.11 Acute atopic conjunctivitis, right eye
H10.12 Acute atopic conjunctivitis, left eye
H10.13 Acute atopic conjunctivitis, bilateral

H10.2 Other acute conjunctivitis
H10.21 Acute toxic conjunctivitis
Acute chemical conjunctivitis
Code first (T51-T65) to identify chemical and intent
EXCLUDES 1 *burn and corrosion of eye and adnexa (T26.-)*
H10.211 Acute toxic conjunctivitis, right eye
H10.212 Acute toxic conjunctivitis, left eye
H10.213 Acute toxic conjunctivitis, bilateral
H10.219 Acute toxic conjunctivitis, unspecified eye
H10.22 Pseudomembranous conjunctivitis
H10.221 Pseudomembranous conjunctivitis, right eye
H10.222 Pseudomembranous conjunctivitis, left eye
H10.223 Pseudomembranous conjunctivitis, bilateral
H10.229 Pseudomembranous conjunctivitis, unspecified eye
H10.23 Serous conjunctivitis, except viral
EXCLUDES 1 *viral conjunctivitis (B30.-)*
H10.231 Serous conjunctivitis, except viral, right eye
H10.232 Serous conjunctivitis, except viral, left eye
H10.233 Serous conjunctivitis, except viral, bilateral
H10.239 Serous conjunctivitis, except viral, unspecified eye

H10.3 Unspecified acute conjunctivitis
EXCLUDES 1 *ophthalmia neonatorum NOS (P39.1)*
H10.30 Unspecified acute conjunctivitis, unspecified eye
H10.31 Unspecified acute conjunctivitis, right eye
H10.32 Unspecified acute conjunctivitis, left eye
H10.33 Unspecified acute conjunctivitis, bilateral

H10.4 Chronic conjunctivitis
H10.40 Unspecified chronic conjunctivitis
H10.401 Unspecified chronic conjunctivitis, right eye
H10.402 Unspecified chronic conjunctivitis, left eye
H10.403 Unspecified chronic conjunctivitis, bilateral
H10.409 Unspecified chronic conjunctivitis, unspecified eye
H10.41 Chronic giant papillary conjunctivitis
H10.411 Chronic giant papillary conjunctivitis, right eye
H10.412 Chronic giant papillary conjunctivitis, left eye
H10.413 Chronic giant papillary conjunctivitis, bilateral
H10.419 Chronic giant papillary conjunctivitis, unspecified eye
H10.42 Simple chronic conjunctivitis
H10.421 Simple chronic conjunctivitis, right eye
H10.422 Simple chronic conjunctivitis, left eye
H10.423 Simple chronic conjunctivitis, bilateral
H10.429 Simple chronic conjunctivitis, unspecified eye
H10.43 Chronic follicular conjunctivitis
H10.431 Chronic follicular conjunctivitis, right eye
H10.432 Chronic follicular conjunctivitis, left eye
H10.433 Chronic follicular conjunctivitis, bilateral
H10.439 Chronic follicular conjunctivitis, unspecified eye
H10.44 Vernal conjunctivitis
EXCLUDES 1 *vernal keratoconjunctivitis with limbar and corneal involvement (H16.26-)*
H10.45 Other chronic allergic conjunctivitis

H10.5 Blepharoconjunctivitis
H10.50 Unspecified blepharoconjunctivitis
H10.501 Unspecified blepharoconjunctivitis, right eye
H10.502 Unspecified blepharoconjunctivitis, left eye
H10.503 Unspecified blepharoconjunctivitis, bilateral
H10.509 Unspecified blepharoconjunctivitis, unspecified eye
H10.51 Ligneous conjunctivitis
Code also underlying condition if known, such as: plasminogen deficiency (E88.02)
H10.511 Ligneous conjunctivitis, right eye
H10.512 Ligneous conjunctivitis, left eye
H10.513 Ligneous conjunctivitis, bilateral
H10.519 Ligneous conjunctivitis, unspecified eye

- ✓6th **H1Ø.52 Angular blepharoconjunctivitis**
  - **H1Ø.521 Angular blepharoconjunctivitis, right eye**
  - **H1Ø.522 Angular blepharoconjunctivitis, left eye**
  - **H1Ø.523 Angular blepharoconjunctivitis, bilateral**
  - **H1Ø.529 Angular blepharoconjunctivitis, unspecified eye**
- ✓6th **H1Ø.53 Contact blepharoconjunctivitis**
  - **H1Ø.531 Contact blepharoconjunctivitis, right eye**
  - **H1Ø.532 Contact blepharoconjunctivitis, left eye**
  - **H1Ø.533 Contact blepharoconjunctivitis, bilateral**
  - **H1Ø.539 Contact blepharoconjunctivitis, unspecified eye**

✓5th **H1Ø.8 Other conjunctivitis**

- ✓6th **H1Ø.81 Pingueculitis**

  EXCLUDES 1 *pinguecula (H11.15-)*

  - **H1Ø.811 Pingueculitis, right eye**
  - **H1Ø.812 Pingueculitis, left eye**
  - **H1Ø.813 Pingueculitis, bilateral**
  - **H1Ø.819 Pingueculitis, unspecified eye**
- ✓6th **H1Ø.82 Rosacea conjunctivitis**

  Code first underlying rosacea dermatitis (L71.-)

  AHA: 2018,4Q,15

  - **H1Ø.821 Rosacea conjunctivitis, right eye**
  - **H1Ø.822 Rosacea conjunctivitis, left eye**
  - **H1Ø.823 Rosacea conjunctivitis, bilateral**
  - **H1Ø.829 Rosacea conjunctivitis, unspecified eye**
- **H1Ø.89 Other conjunctivitis**

H1Ø.9 Unspecified conjunctivitis

✓4th H11 Other disorders of conjunctiva

EXCLUDES 1 *keratoconjunctivitis (H16.2-)*

✓5th **H11.Ø Pterygium of eye**

EXCLUDES 1 *pseudopterygium (H11.81-)*

DEF: Benign, wedge-shaped, conjunctival thickening that advances from the inner corner of the eye toward the cornea.

Pterygium

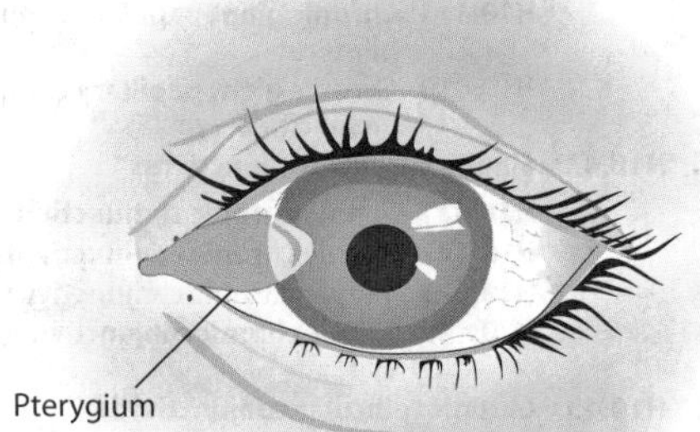

- ✓6th **H11.ØØ Unspecified pterygium of eye**
  - **H11.ØØ1 Unspecified pterygium of right eye**
  - **H11.ØØ2 Unspecified pterygium of left eye**
  - **H11.ØØ3 Unspecified pterygium of eye, bilateral**
  - **H11.ØØ9 Unspecified pterygium of unspecified eye**
- ✓6th **H11.Ø1 Amyloid pterygium**
  - **H11.Ø11 Amyloid pterygium of right eye**
  - **H11.Ø12 Amyloid pterygium of left eye**
  - **H11.Ø13 Amyloid pterygium of eye, bilateral**
  - **H11.Ø19 Amyloid pterygium of unspecified eye**
- ✓6th **H11.Ø2 Central pterygium of eye**
  - **H11.Ø21 Central pterygium of right eye**
  - **H11.Ø22 Central pterygium of left eye**
  - **H11.Ø23 Central pterygium of eye, bilateral**
  - **H11.Ø29 Central pterygium of unspecified eye**
- ✓6th **H11.Ø3 Double pterygium of eye**
  - **H11.Ø31 Double pterygium of right eye**
  - **H11.Ø32 Double pterygium of left eye**
  - **H11.Ø33 Double pterygium of eye, bilateral**
  - **H11.Ø39 Double pterygium of unspecified eye**
- ✓6th **H11.Ø4 Peripheral pterygium of eye, stationary**
  - **H11.Ø41 Peripheral pterygium, stationary, right eye**
  - **H11.Ø42 Peripheral pterygium, stationary, left eye**
  - **H11.Ø43 Peripheral pterygium, stationary, bilateral**
  - **H11.Ø49 Peripheral pterygium, stationary, unspecified eye**
- ✓6th **H11.Ø5 Peripheral pterygium of eye, progressive**
  - **H11.Ø51 Peripheral pterygium, progressive, right eye**
  - **H11.Ø52 Peripheral pterygium, progressive, left eye**
  - **H11.Ø53 Peripheral pterygium, progressive, bilateral**
  - **H11.Ø59 Peripheral pterygium, progressive, unspecified eye**
- ✓6th **H11.Ø6 Recurrent pterygium of eye**
  - **H11.Ø61 Recurrent pterygium of right eye**
  - **H11.Ø62 Recurrent pterygium of left eye**
  - **H11.Ø63 Recurrent pterygium of eye, bilateral**
  - **H11.Ø69 Recurrent pterygium of unspecified eye**

✓5th **H11.1 Conjunctival degenerations and deposits**

EXCLUDES 2 *pseudopterygium (H11.81)*

- **H11.1Ø Unspecified conjunctival degenerations**
- ✓6th **H11.11 Conjunctival deposits**
  - **H11.111 Conjunctival deposits, right eye**
  - **H11.112 Conjunctival deposits, left eye**
  - **H11.113 Conjunctival deposits, bilateral**
  - **H11.119 Conjunctival deposits, unspecified eye**
- ✓6th **H11.12 Conjunctival concretions**
  - **H11.121 Conjunctival concretions, right eye**
  - **H11.122 Conjunctival concretions, left eye**
  - **H11.123 Conjunctival concretions, bilateral**
  - **H11.129 Conjunctival concretions, unspecified eye**
- ✓6th **H11.13 Conjunctival pigmentations**

  Conjunctival argyrosis [argyria]

  - **H11.131 Conjunctival pigmentations, right eye**
  - **H11.132 Conjunctival pigmentations, left eye**
  - **H11.133 Conjunctival pigmentations, bilateral**
  - **H11.139 Conjunctival pigmentations, unspecified eye**
- ✓6th **H11.14 Conjunctival xerosis, unspecified**

  EXCLUDES 1 *xerosis of conjunctiva due to vitamin A deficiency (E5Ø.Ø, E5Ø.1)*

  DEF: Abnormal dryness of the conjunctiva due to lack of insufficient tears or conjunctival secretions.

  - **H11.141 Conjunctival xerosis, unspecified, right eye**
  - **H11.142 Conjunctival xerosis, unspecified, left eye**
  - **H11.143 Conjunctival xerosis, unspecified, bilateral**
  - **H11.149 Conjunctival xerosis, unspecified, unspecified eye**

√6th H11.15 Pinguecula

EXCLUDES 1 *pingueculitis (H10.81-)*

DEF: Proliferation on the conjunctiva near the sclerocorneal junction, usually of the side of the nose and usually in older patients.

Pinguecula

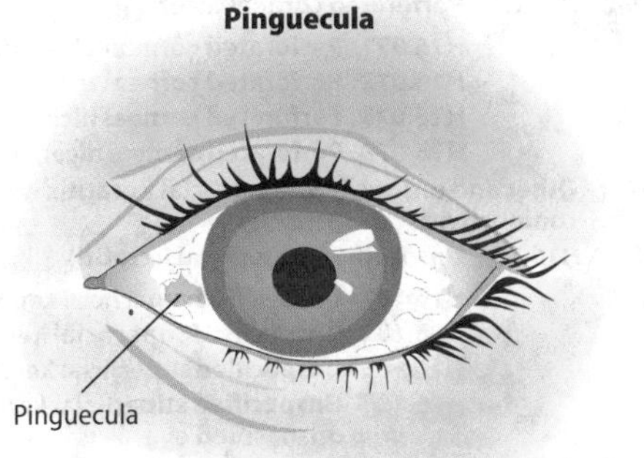

H11.151 Pinguecula, right eye
H11.152 Pinguecula, left eye
H11.153 Pinguecula, bilateral
H11.159 Pinguecula, unspecified eye

√5th H11.2 Conjunctival scars

√6th H11.21 Conjunctival adhesions and strands (localized)
H11.211 Conjunctival adhesions and strands (localized), right eye
H11.212 Conjunctival adhesions and strands (localized), left eye
H11.213 Conjunctival adhesions and strands (localized), bilateral
H11.219 Conjunctival adhesions and strands (localized), unspecified eye

√6th H11.22 Conjunctival granuloma
H11.221 Conjunctival granuloma, right eye
H11.222 Conjunctival granuloma, left eye
H11.223 Conjunctival granuloma, bilateral
H11.229 Conjunctival granuloma, unspecified

√6th H11.23 Symblepharon
H11.231 Symblepharon, right eye
H11.232 Symblepharon, left eye
H11.233 Symblepharon, bilateral
H11.239 Symblepharon, unspecified eye

√6th H11.24 Scarring of conjunctiva
H11.241 Scarring of conjunctiva, right eye
H11.242 Scarring of conjunctiva, left eye
H11.243 Scarring of conjunctiva, bilateral
H11.249 Scarring of conjunctiva, unspecified eye

√5th H11.3 Conjunctival hemorrhage

Subconjunctival hemorrhage

H11.30 Conjunctival hemorrhage, unspecified eye
H11.31 Conjunctival hemorrhage, right eye
H11.32 Conjunctival hemorrhage, left eye
H11.33 Conjunctival hemorrhage, bilateral

√5th H11.4 Other conjunctival vascular disorders and cysts

√6th H11.41 Vascular abnormalities of conjunctiva

Conjunctival aneurysm

H11.411 Vascular abnormalities of conjunctiva, right eye
H11.412 Vascular abnormalities of conjunctiva, left eye
H11.413 Vascular abnormalities of conjunctiva, bilateral
H11.419 Vascular abnormalities of conjunctiva, unspecified eye

√6th H11.42 Conjunctival edema
H11.421 Conjunctival edema, right eye
H11.422 Conjunctival edema, left eye
H11.423 Conjunctival edema, bilateral
H11.429 Conjunctival edema, unspecified eye

√6th H11.43 Conjunctival hyperemia
H11.431 Conjunctival hyperemia, right eye
H11.432 Conjunctival hyperemia, left eye
H11.433 Conjunctival hyperemia, bilateral
H11.439 Conjunctival hyperemia, unspecified eye

√6th H11.44 Conjunctival cysts
H11.441 Conjunctival cysts, right eye
H11.442 Conjunctival cysts, left eye
H11.443 Conjunctival cysts, bilateral
H11.449 Conjunctival cysts, unspecified eye

√5th H11.8 Other specified disorders of conjunctiva

√6th H11.81 Pseudopterygium of conjunctiva
H11.811 Pseudopterygium of conjunctiva, right eye
H11.812 Pseudopterygium of conjunctiva, left eye
H11.813 Pseudopterygium of conjunctiva, bilateral
H11.819 Pseudopterygium of conjunctiva, unspecified eye

√6th H11.82 Conjunctivochalasis
H11.821 Conjunctivochalasis, right eye
H11.822 Conjunctivochalasis, left eye
H11.823 Conjunctivochalasis, bilateral
H11.829 Conjunctivochalasis, unspecified eye

H11.89 Other specified disorders of conjunctiva

H11.9 Unspecified disorder of conjunctiva

Disorders of sclera, cornea, iris and ciliary body (H15-H22)

√4th H15 Disorders of sclera

√5th H15.0 Scleritis

√6th H15.00 Unspecified scleritis
H15.001 Unspecified scleritis, right eye
H15.002 Unspecified scleritis, left eye
H15.003 Unspecified scleritis, bilateral
H15.009 Unspecified scleritis, unspecified eye

√6th H15.01 Anterior scleritis
H15.011 Anterior scleritis, right eye
H15.012 Anterior scleritis, left eye
H15.013 Anterior scleritis, bilateral
H15.019 Anterior scleritis, unspecified eye

√6th H15.02 Brawny scleritis
H15.021 Brawny scleritis, right eye
H15.022 Brawny scleritis, left eye
H15.023 Brawny scleritis, bilateral
H15.029 Brawny scleritis, unspecified eye

√6th H15.03 Posterior scleritis

Sclerotenonitis

H15.031 Posterior scleritis, right eye
H15.032 Posterior scleritis, left eye
H15.033 Posterior scleritis, bilateral
H15.039 Posterior scleritis, unspecified eye

√6th H15.04 Scleritis with corneal involvement
H15.041 Scleritis with corneal involvement, right eye
H15.042 Scleritis with corneal involvement, left eye
H15.043 Scleritis with corneal involvement, bilateral
H15.049 Scleritis with corneal involvement, unspecified eye

√6th H15.05 Scleromalacia perforans
H15.051 Scleromalacia perforans, right eye
H15.052 Scleromalacia perforans, left eye
H15.053 Scleromalacia perforans, bilateral
H15.059 Scleromalacia perforans, unspecified eye

√6th H15.09 Other scleritis

Scleral abscess

H15.091 Other scleritis, right eye
H15.092 Other scleritis, left eye
H15.093 Other scleritis, bilateral
H15.099 Other scleritis, unspecified eye

√5th H15.1 Episcleritis

√6th H15.10 Unspecified episcleritis
H15.101 Unspecified episcleritis, right eye
H15.102 Unspecified episcleritis, left eye
H15.103 Unspecified episcleritis, bilateral
H15.109 Unspecified episcleritis, unspecified eye

✓6th H15.11 Episcleritis periodica fugax
- H15.111 Episcleritis periodica fugax, right eye
- H15.112 Episcleritis periodica fugax, left eye
- H15.113 Episcleritis periodica fugax, bilateral
- H15.119 Episcleritis periodica fugax, unspecified eye

✓6th H15.12 Nodular episcleritis
- H15.121 Nodular episcleritis, right eye
- H15.122 Nodular episcleritis, left eye
- H15.123 Nodular episcleritis, bilateral
- H15.129 Nodular episcleritis, unspecified eye

✓5th H15.8 Other disorders of sclera

EXCLUDES 2 *blue sclera (Q13.5)*
degenerative myopia (H44.2-)

✓6th H15.81 Equatorial staphyloma
- H15.811 Equatorial staphyloma, right eye
- H15.812 Equatorial staphyloma, left eye
- H15.813 Equatorial staphyloma, bilateral
- H15.819 Equatorial staphyloma, unspecified eye

✓6th H15.82 Localized anterior staphyloma
- H15.821 Localized anterior staphyloma, right eye
- H15.822 Localized anterior staphyloma, left eye
- H15.823 Localized anterior staphyloma, bilateral
- H15.829 Localized anterior staphyloma, unspecified eye

✓6th H15.83 Staphyloma posticum
- H15.831 Staphyloma posticum, right eye
- H15.832 Staphyloma posticum, left eye
- H15.833 Staphyloma posticum, bilateral
- H15.839 Staphyloma posticum, unspecified eye

✓6th H15.84 Scleral ectasia
- H15.841 Scleral ectasia, right eye
- H15.842 Scleral ectasia, left eye
- H15.843 Scleral ectasia, bilateral
- H15.849 Scleral ectasia, unspecified eye

✓6th H15.85 Ring staphyloma
- H15.851 Ring staphyloma, right eye
- H15.852 Ring staphyloma, left eye
- H15.853 Ring staphyloma, bilateral
- H15.859 Ring staphyloma, unspecified eye

H15.89 Other disorders of sclera

H15.9 Unspecified disorder of sclera

✓4th H16 Keratitis

DEF: Condition in which the cornea becomes inflamed and irritated.

✓5th H16.Ø Corneal ulcer

✓6th H16.ØØ Unspecified corneal ulcer
- H16.ØØ1 Unspecified corneal ulcer, right eye
- H16.ØØ2 Unspecified corneal ulcer, left eye
- H16.ØØ3 Unspecified corneal ulcer, bilateral
- H16.ØØ9 Unspecified corneal ulcer, unspecified eye

✓6th H16.Ø1 Central corneal ulcer
- H16.Ø11 Central corneal ulcer, right eye
- H16.Ø12 Central corneal ulcer, left eye
- H16.Ø13 Central corneal ulcer, bilateral
- H16.Ø19 Central corneal ulcer, unspecified eye

✓6th H16.Ø2 Ring corneal ulcer
- H16.Ø21 Ring corneal ulcer, right eye
- H16.Ø22 Ring corneal ulcer, left eye
- H16.Ø23 Ring corneal ulcer, bilateral
- H16.Ø29 Ring corneal ulcer, unspecified eye

✓6th H16.Ø3 Corneal ulcer with hypopyon
- H16.Ø31 Corneal ulcer with hypopyon, right eye
- H16.Ø32 Corneal ulcer with hypopyon, left eye
- H16.Ø33 Corneal ulcer with hypopyon, bilateral
- H16.Ø39 Corneal ulcer with hypopyon, unspecified eye

✓6th H16.Ø4 Marginal corneal ulcer
- H16.Ø41 Marginal corneal ulcer, right eye
- H16.Ø42 Marginal corneal ulcer, left eye
- H16.Ø43 Marginal corneal ulcer, bilateral
- H16.Ø49 Marginal corneal ulcer, unspecified eye

✓6th H16.Ø5 Mooren's corneal ulcer
- H16.Ø51 Mooren's corneal ulcer, right eye
- H16.Ø52 Mooren's corneal ulcer, left eye
- H16.Ø53 Mooren's corneal ulcer, bilateral
- H16.Ø59 Mooren's corneal ulcer, unspecified eye

✓6th H16.Ø6 Mycotic corneal ulcer
- H16.Ø61 Mycotic corneal ulcer, right eye
- H16.Ø62 Mycotic corneal ulcer, left eye
- H16.Ø63 Mycotic corneal ulcer, bilateral
- H16.Ø69 Mycotic corneal ulcer, unspecified eye

✓6th H16.Ø7 Perforated corneal ulcer
- H16.Ø71 Perforated corneal ulcer, right eye
- H16.Ø72 Perforated corneal ulcer, left eye
- H16.Ø73 Perforated corneal ulcer, bilateral
- H16.Ø79 Perforated corneal ulcer, unspecified eye

✓5th H16.1 Other and unspecified superficial keratitis without conjunctivitis

✓6th H16.1Ø Unspecified superficial keratitis
- H16.1Ø1 Unspecified superficial keratitis, right eye
- H16.1Ø2 Unspecified superficial keratitis, left eye
- H16.1Ø3 Unspecified superficial keratitis, bilateral
- H16.1Ø9 Unspecified superficial keratitis, unspecified eye

✓6th H16.11 Macular keratitis

Areolar keratitis
Nummular keratitis
Stellate keratitis
Striate keratitis

- H16.111 Macular keratitis, right eye
- H16.112 Macular keratitis, left eye
- H16.113 Macular keratitis, bilateral
- H16.119 Macular keratitis, unspecified eye

✓6th H16.12 Filamentary keratitis
- H16.121 Filamentary keratitis, right eye
- H16.122 Filamentary keratitis, left eye
- H16.123 Filamentary keratitis, bilateral
- H16.129 Filamentary keratitis, unspecified eye

✓6th H16.13 Photokeratitis

Snow blindness
Welders keratitis

- H16.131 Photokeratitis, right eye
- H16.132 Photokeratitis, left eye
- H16.133 Photokeratitis, bilateral
- H16.139 Photokeratitis, unspecified eye

✓6th H16.14 Punctate keratitis
- H16.141 Punctate keratitis, right eye
- H16.142 Punctate keratitis, left eye
- H16.143 Punctate keratitis, bilateral
- H16.149 Punctate keratitis, unspecified eye

✓5th H16.2 Keratoconjunctivitis

✓6th H16.2Ø Unspecified keratoconjunctivitis

Superficial keratitis with conjunctivitis NOS

- H16.2Ø1 Unspecified keratoconjunctivitis, right eye
- H16.2Ø2 Unspecified keratoconjunctivitis, left eye
- H16.2Ø3 Unspecified keratoconjunctivitis, bilateral
- H16.2Ø9 Unspecified keratoconjunctivitis, unspecified eye

✓6th H16.21 Exposure keratoconjunctivitis
- H16.211 Exposure keratoconjunctivitis, right eye
- H16.212 Exposure keratoconjunctivitis, left eye
- H16.213 Exposure keratoconjunctivitis, bilateral
- H16.219 Exposure keratoconjunctivitis, unspecified eye

✓6th H16.22 Keratoconjunctivitis sicca, not specified as Sjögren's

EXCLUDES 1 *Sjögren's syndrome (M35.Ø1)*

- H16.221 Keratoconjunctivitis sicca, not specified as Sjögren's, right eye
- H16.222 Keratoconjunctivitis sicca, not specified as Sjögren's, left eye
- H16.223 Keratoconjunctivitis sicca, not specified as Sjögren's, bilateral
- H16.229 Keratoconjunctivitis sicca, not specified as Sjögren's, unspecified eye

✓6th H16.23 Neurotrophic keratoconjunctivitis
- H16.231 Neurotrophic keratoconjunctivitis, right eye
- H16.232 Neurotrophic keratoconjunctivitis, left eye

H16.233 Neurotrophic keratoconjunctivitis, bilateral
H16.239 Neurotrophic keratoconjunctivitis, unspecified eye

H16.24 Ophthalmia nodosa
H16.241 Ophthalmia nodosa, right eye
H16.242 Ophthalmia nodosa, left eye
H16.243 Ophthalmia nodosa, bilateral
H16.249 Ophthalmia nodosa, unspecified eye

H16.25 Phlyctenular keratoconjunctivitis
H16.251 Phlyctenular keratoconjunctivitis, right eye
H16.252 Phlyctenular keratoconjunctivitis, left eye
H16.253 Phlyctenular keratoconjunctivitis, bilateral
H16.259 Phlyctenular keratoconjunctivitis, unspecified eye

H16.26 Vernal keratoconjunctivitis, with limbar and corneal involvement
EXCLUDES 1 *vernal conjunctivitis without limbar and corneal involvement (H1Ø.44)*
H16.261 Vernal keratoconjunctivitis, with limbar and corneal involvement, right eye
H16.262 Vernal keratoconjunctivitis, with limbar and corneal involvement, left eye
H16.263 Vernal keratoconjunctivitis, with limbar and corneal involvement, bilateral
H16.269 Vernal keratoconjunctivitis, with limbar and corneal involvement, unspecified eye

H16.29 Other keratoconjunctivitis
H16.291 Other keratoconjunctivitis, right eye
H16.292 Other keratoconjunctivitis, left eye
H16.293 Other keratoconjunctivitis, bilateral
H16.299 Other keratoconjunctivitis, unspecified eye

H16.3 Interstitial and deep keratitis

H16.3Ø Unspecified interstitial keratitis
H16.3Ø1 Unspecified interstitial keratitis, right eye
H16.3Ø2 Unspecified interstitial keratitis, left eye
H16.3Ø3 Unspecified interstitial keratitis, bilateral
H16.3Ø9 Unspecified interstitial keratitis, unspecified eye

H16.31 Corneal abscess
H16.311 Corneal abscess, right eye
H16.312 Corneal abscess, left eye
H16.313 Corneal abscess, bilateral
H16.319 Corneal abscess, unspecified eye

H16.32 Diffuse interstitial keratitis
Cogan's syndrome
H16.321 Diffuse interstitial keratitis, right eye
H16.322 Diffuse interstitial keratitis, left eye
H16.323 Diffuse interstitial keratitis, bilateral
H16.329 Diffuse interstitial keratitis, unspecified eye

H16.33 Sclerosing keratitis
H16.331 Sclerosing keratitis, right eye
H16.332 Sclerosing keratitis, left eye
H16.333 Sclerosing keratitis, bilateral
H16.339 Sclerosing keratitis, unspecified eye

H16.39 Other interstitial and deep keratitis
H16.391 Other interstitial and deep keratitis, right eye
H16.392 Other interstitial and deep keratitis, left eye
H16.393 Other interstitial and deep keratitis, bilateral
H16.399 Other interstitial and deep keratitis, unspecified eye

H16.4 Corneal neovascularization

H16.4Ø Unspecified corneal neovascularization
H16.4Ø1 Unspecified corneal neovascularization, right eye
H16.4Ø2 Unspecified corneal neovascularization, left eye
H16.4Ø3 Unspecified corneal neovascularization, bilateral
H16.4Ø9 Unspecified corneal neovascularization, unspecified eye

H16.41 Ghost vessels (corneal)
H16.411 Ghost vessels (corneal), right eye
H16.412 Ghost vessels (corneal), left eye
H16.413 Ghost vessels (corneal), bilateral
H16.419 Ghost vessels (corneal), unspecified eye

H16.42 Pannus (corneal)
H16.421 Pannus (corneal), right eye
H16.422 Pannus (corneal), left eye
H16.423 Pannus (corneal), bilateral
H16.429 Pannus (corneal), unspecified eye

H16.43 Localized vascularization of cornea
H16.431 Localized vascularization of cornea, right eye
H16.432 Localized vascularization of cornea, left eye
H16.433 Localized vascularization of cornea, bilateral
H16.439 Localized vascularization of cornea, unspecified eye

H16.44 Deep vascularization of cornea
H16.441 Deep vascularization of cornea, right eye
H16.442 Deep vascularization of cornea, left eye
H16.443 Deep vascularization of cornea, bilateral
H16.449 Deep vascularization of cornea, unspecified eye

H16.8 Other keratitis
H16.9 Unspecified keratitis

H17 Corneal scars and opacities

H17.Ø Adherent leukoma
H17.ØØ Adherent leukoma, unspecified eye
H17.Ø1 Adherent leukoma, right eye
H17.Ø2 Adherent leukoma, left eye
H17.Ø3 Adherent leukoma, bilateral

H17.1 Central corneal opacity
H17.1Ø Central corneal opacity, unspecified eye
H17.11 Central corneal opacity, right eye
H17.12 Central corneal opacity, left eye
H17.13 Central corneal opacity, bilateral

H17.8 Other corneal scars and opacities

H17.81 Minor opacity of cornea
Corneal nebula
H17.811 Minor opacity of cornea, right eye
H17.812 Minor opacity of cornea, left eye
H17.813 Minor opacity of cornea, bilateral
H17.819 Minor opacity of cornea, unspecified eye

H17.82 Peripheral opacity of cornea
H17.821 Peripheral opacity of cornea, right eye
H17.822 Peripheral opacity of cornea, left eye
H17.823 Peripheral opacity of cornea, bilateral
H17.829 Peripheral opacity of cornea, unspecified eye

H17.89 Other corneal scars and opacities
H17.9 Unspecified corneal scar and opacity

H18 Other disorders of cornea

H18.Ø Corneal pigmentations and deposits

H18.ØØ Unspecified corneal deposit
H18.ØØ1 Unspecified corneal deposit, right eye
H18.ØØ2 Unspecified corneal deposit, left eye
H18.ØØ3 Unspecified corneal deposit, bilateral
H18.ØØ9 Unspecified corneal deposit, unspecified eye

H18.Ø1 Anterior corneal pigmentations
Staehli's line
H18.Ø11 Anterior corneal pigmentations, right eye
H18.Ø12 Anterior corneal pigmentations, left eye
H18.Ø13 Anterior corneal pigmentations, bilateral
H18.Ø19 Anterior corneal pigmentations, unspecified eye

H18.Ø2 Argentous corneal deposits
H18.Ø21 Argentous corneal deposits, right eye
H18.Ø22 Argentous corneal deposits, left eye
H18.Ø23 Argentous corneal deposits, bilateral
H18.Ø29 Argentous corneal deposits, unspecified eye

√6th **H18.03 Corneal deposits in metabolic disorders**

Code also associated metabolic disorder

H18.031 Corneal deposits in metabolic disorders, right eye

H18.032 Corneal deposits in metabolic disorders, left eye

H18.033 Corneal deposits in metabolic disorders, bilateral

H18.039 Corneal deposits in metabolic disorders, unspecified eye

√6th **H18.04 Kayser-Fleischer ring**

Code also associated Wilson's disease (E83.01)

H18.041 Kayser-Fleischer ring, right eye

H18.042 Kayser-Fleischer ring, left eye

H18.043 Kayser-Fleischer ring, bilateral

H18.049 Kayser-Fleischer ring, unspecified eye

√6th **H18.05 Posterior corneal pigmentations**

Krukenberg's spindle

H18.051 Posterior corneal pigmentations, right eye

H18.052 Posterior corneal pigmentations, left eye

H18.053 Posterior corneal pigmentations, bilateral

H18.059 Posterior corneal pigmentations, unspecified eye

√6th **H18.06 Stromal corneal pigmentations**

Hematocornea

H18.061 Stromal corneal pigmentations, right eye

H18.062 Stromal corneal pigmentations, left eye

H18.063 Stromal corneal pigmentations, bilateral

H18.069 Stromal corneal pigmentations, unspecified eye

√5th **H18.1 Bullous keratopathy**

DEF: Corneal swelling due to a damaged corneal endothelium. Bullous keratopathy is characterized by recurring, rupturing epithelial blisters causing glaucoma, iridocyclitis, and Fuchs dystrophy.

H18.10 Bullous keratopathy, unspecified eye

H18.11 Bullous keratopathy, right eye

H18.12 Bullous keratopathy, left eye

H18.13 Bullous keratopathy, bilateral

√5th **H18.2 Other and unspecified corneal edema**

H18.20 Unspecified corneal edema

√6th **H18.21 Corneal edema secondary to contact lens**

EXCLUDES 2 *other corneal disorders due to contact lens (H18.82-)*

H18.211 Corneal edema secondary to contact lens, right eye

H18.212 Corneal edema secondary to contact lens, left eye

H18.213 Corneal edema secondary to contact lens, bilateral

H18.219 Corneal edema secondary to contact lens, unspecified eye

√6th **H18.22 Idiopathic corneal edema**

H18.221 Idiopathic corneal edema, right eye

H18.222 Idiopathic corneal edema, left eye

H18.223 Idiopathic corneal edema, bilateral

H18.229 Idiopathic corneal edema, unspecified eye

√6th **H18.23 Secondary corneal edema**

H18.231 Secondary corneal edema, right eye

H18.232 Secondary corneal edema, left eye

H18.233 Secondary corneal edema, bilateral

H18.239 Secondary corneal edema, unspecified eye

√5th **H18.3 Changes of corneal membranes**

H18.30 Unspecified corneal membrane change

√6th **H18.31 Folds and rupture in Bowman's membrane**

H18.311 Folds and rupture in Bowman's membrane, right eye

H18.312 Folds and rupture in Bowman's membrane, left eye

H18.313 Folds and rupture in Bowman's membrane, bilateral

H18.319 Folds and rupture in Bowman's membrane, unspecified eye

√6th **H18.32 Folds in Descemet's membrane**

H18.321 Folds in Descemet's membrane, right eye

H18.322 Folds in Descemet's membrane, left eye

H18.323 Folds in Descemet's membrane, bilateral

H18.329 Folds in Descemet's membrane, unspecified eye

√6th **H18.33 Rupture in Descemet's membrane**

H18.331 Rupture in Descemet's membrane, right eye

H18.332 Rupture in Descemet's membrane, left eye

H18.333 Rupture in Descemet's membrane, bilateral

H18.339 Rupture in Descemet's membrane, unspecified eye

√5th **H18.4 Corneal degeneration**

EXCLUDES 1 *Mooren's ulcer (H16.0-)*
recurrent erosion of cornea (H18.83-)

H18.40 Unspecified corneal degeneration

√6th **H18.41 Arcus senilis**

Senile corneal changes

H18.411 Arcus senilis, right eye

H18.412 Arcus senilis, left eye

H18.413 Arcus senilis, bilateral

H18.419 Arcus senilis, unspecified eye

√6th **H18.42 Band keratopathy**

H18.421 Band keratopathy, right eye

H18.422 Band keratopathy, left eye

H18.423 Band keratopathy, bilateral

H18.429 Band keratopathy, unspecified eye

H18.43 Other calcerous corneal degeneration

√6th **H18.44 Keratomalacia**

EXCLUDES 1 *keratomalacia due to vitamin A deficiency (E50.4)*

H18.441 Keratomalacia, right eye

H18.442 Keratomalacia, left eye

H18.443 Keratomalacia, bilateral

H18.449 Keratomalacia, unspecified eye

√6th **H18.45 Nodular corneal degeneration**

H18.451 Nodular corneal degeneration, right eye

H18.452 Nodular corneal degeneration, left eye

H18.453 Nodular corneal degeneration, bilateral

H18.459 Nodular corneal degeneration, unspecified eye

√6th **H18.46 Peripheral corneal degeneration**

H18.461 Peripheral corneal degeneration, right eye

H18.462 Peripheral corneal degeneration, left eye

H18.463 Peripheral corneal degeneration, bilateral

H18.469 Peripheral corneal degeneration, unspecified eye

H18.49 Other corneal degeneration

√5th **H18.5 Hereditary corneal dystrophies**

▲ √6th **H18.50 Unspecified hereditary corneal dystrophies**

● **H18.501 Unspecified hereditary corneal dystrophies, right eye**

● **H18.502 Unspecified hereditary corneal dystrophies, left eye**

● **H18.503 Unspecified hereditary corneal dystrophies, bilateral**

● **H18.509 Unspecified hereditary corneal dystrophies, unspecified eye**

▲ √6th **H18.51 Endothelial corneal dystrophy**

Fuchs' dystrophy

● **H18.511 Endothelial corneal dystrophy, right eye**

● **H18.512 Endothelial corneal dystrophy, left eye**

● **H18.513 Endothelial corneal dystrophy, bilateral**

● **H18.519 Endothelial corneal dystrophy, unspecified eye**

▲ √6th **H18.52 Epithelial (juvenile) corneal dystrophy**

● **H18.521 Epithelial (juvenile) corneal dystrophy, right eye**

● **H18.522 Epithelial (juvenile) corneal dystrophy, left eye**

● **H18.523 Epithelial (juvenile) corneal dystrophy, bilateral**

● **H18.529 Epithelial (juvenile) corneal dystrophy, unspecified eye**

▲ ✓6th **H18.53 Granular corneal dystrophy**
● **H18.531 Granular corneal dystrophy, right eye**
● **H18.532 Granular corneal dystrophy, left eye**
● **H18.533 Granular corneal dystrophy, bilateral**
● **H18.539 Granular corneal dystrophy, unspecified eye**
▲ ✓6th **H18.54 Lattice corneal dystrophy**
● **H18.541 Lattice corneal dystrophy, right eye**
● **H18.542 Lattice corneal dystrophy, left eye**
● **H18.543 Lattice corneal dystrophy, bilateral**
● **H18.549 Lattice corneal dystrophy, unspecified eye**
▲ ✓6th **H18.55 Macular corneal dystrophy**
● **H18.551 Macular corneal dystrophy, right eye**
● **H18.552 Macular corneal dystrophy, left eye**
● **H18.553 Macular corneal dystrophy, bilateral**
● **H18.559 Macular corneal dystrophy, unspecified eye**
▲ ✓6th **H18.59 Other hereditary corneal dystrophies**
● **H18.591 Other hereditary corneal dystrophies, right eye**
● **H18.592 Other hereditary corneal dystrophies, left eye**
● **H18.593 Other hereditary corneal dystrophies, bilateral**
● **H18.599 Other hereditary corneal dystrophies, unspecified eye**

✓5th **H18.6 Keratoconus**

✓6th **H18.60 Keratoconus, unspecified**
H18.601 Keratoconus, unspecified, right eye
H18.602 Keratoconus, unspecified, left eye
H18.603 Keratoconus, unspecified, bilateral
H18.609 Keratoconus, unspecified, unspecified eye

✓6th **H18.61 Keratoconus, stable**
H18.611 Keratoconus, stable, right eye
H18.612 Keratoconus, stable, left eye
H18.613 Keratoconus, stable, bilateral
H18.619 Keratoconus, stable, unspecified eye

✓6th **H18.62 Keratoconus, unstable**
Acute hydrops
H18.621 Keratoconus, unstable, right eye
H18.622 Keratoconus, unstable, left eye
H18.623 Keratoconus, unstable, bilateral
H18.629 Keratoconus, unstable, unspecified eye

✓5th **H18.7 Other and unspecified corneal deformities**
EXCLUDES 1 *congenital malformations of cornea (Q13.3-Q13.4)*

H18.70 Unspecified corneal deformity

✓6th **H18.71 Corneal ectasia**
H18.711 Corneal ectasia, right eye
H18.712 Corneal ectasia, left eye
H18.713 Corneal ectasia, bilateral
H18.719 Corneal ectasia, unspecified eye

✓6th **H18.72 Corneal staphyloma**
H18.721 Corneal staphyloma, right eye
H18.722 Corneal staphyloma, left eye
H18.723 Corneal staphyloma, bilateral
H18.729 Corneal staphyloma, unspecified eye

✓6th **H18.73 Descemetocele**
H18.731 Descemetocele, right eye
H18.732 Descemetocele, left eye
H18.733 Descemetocele, bilateral
H18.739 Descemetocele, unspecified eye

✓6th **H18.79 Other corneal deformities**
H18.791 Other corneal deformities, right eye
H18.792 Other corneal deformities, left eye
H18.793 Other corneal deformities, bilateral
H18.799 Other corneal deformities, unspecified eye

✓5th **H18.8 Other specified disorders of cornea**

✓6th **H18.81 Anesthesia and hypoesthesia of cornea**
H18.811 Anesthesia and hypoesthesia of cornea, right eye
H18.812 Anesthesia and hypoesthesia of cornea, left eye
H18.813 Anesthesia and hypoesthesia of cornea, bilateral
H18.819 Anesthesia and hypoesthesia of cornea, unspecified eye

✓6th **H18.82 Corneal disorder due to contact lens**
EXCLUDES 2 *corneal edema due to contact lens (H18.21-)*
H18.821 Corneal disorder due to contact lens, right eye
H18.822 Corneal disorder due to contact lens, left eye
H18.823 Corneal disorder due to contact lens, bilateral
H18.829 Corneal disorder due to contact lens, unspecified eye

✓6th **H18.83 Recurrent erosion of cornea**
H18.831 Recurrent erosion of cornea, right eye
H18.832 Recurrent erosion of cornea, left eye
H18.833 Recurrent erosion of cornea, bilateral
H18.839 Recurrent erosion of cornea, unspecified eye

✓6th **H18.89 Other specified disorders of cornea**
H18.891 Other specified disorders of cornea, right eye
H18.892 Other specified disorders of cornea, left eye
H18.893 Other specified disorders of cornea, bilateral
H18.899 Other specified disorders of cornea, unspecified eye

H18.9 Unspecified disorder of cornea

✓4th **H2Ø Iridocyclitis**

✓5th **H2Ø.Ø Acute and subacute iridocyclitis**
Acute anterior uveitis
Acute cyclitis
Acute iritis
Subacute anterior uveitis
Subacute cyclitis
Subacute iritis
EXCLUDES 1 *iridocyclitis, iritis, uveitis (due to) (in) diabetes mellitus (EØ8-E13 with .39)*
iridocyclitis, iritis, uveitis (due to) (in) diphtheria (A36.89)
iridocyclitis, iritis, uveitis (due to) (in) gonococcal (A54.32)
iridocyclitis, iritis, uveitis (due to) (in) herpes (simplex) (BØØ.51)
iridocyclitis, iritis, uveitis (due to) (in) herpes zoster (BØ2.32)
iridocyclitis, iritis, uveitis (due to) (in) late congenital syphilis (A5Ø.39)
iridocyclitis, iritis, uveitis (due to) (in) late syphilis (A52.71)
iridocyclitis, iritis, uveitis (due to) (in) sarcoidosis (D86.83)
iridocyclitis, iritis, uveitis (due to) (in) syphilis (A51.43)
iridocyclitis, iritis, uveitis (due to) (in) toxoplasmosis (B58.Ø9)
iridocyclitis, iritis, uveitis (due to) (in) tuberculosis (A18.54)

H2Ø.ØØ Unspecified acute and subacute iridocyclitis CC

✓6th **H2Ø.Ø1 Primary iridocyclitis**
H2Ø.Ø11 Primary iridocyclitis, right eye CC
H2Ø.Ø12 Primary iridocyclitis, left eye CC
H2Ø.Ø13 Primary iridocyclitis, bilateral CC
H2Ø.Ø19 Primary iridocyclitis, unspecified eye CC

✓6th **H2Ø.Ø2 Recurrent acute iridocyclitis**
H2Ø.Ø21 Recurrent acute iridocyclitis, right eye CC
H2Ø.Ø22 Recurrent acute iridocyclitis, left eye CC
H2Ø.Ø23 Recurrent acute iridocyclitis, bilateral CC
H2Ø.Ø29 Recurrent acute iridocyclitis, unspecified eye CC

Chapter 7. Diseases of the Eye and Adnexa H18.53–H20.029

√6th **H20.03 Secondary infectious iridocyclitis**
- **H20.031 Secondary infectious iridocyclitis, right eye** CC
- **H20.032 Secondary infectious iridocyclitis, left eye** CC
- **H20.033 Secondary infectious iridocyclitis, bilateral** CC
- **H20.039 Secondary infectious iridocyclitis, unspecified eye** CC

√6th **H20.04 Secondary noninfectious iridocyclitis**
- **H20.041 Secondary noninfectious iridocyclitis, right eye**
- **H20.042 Secondary noninfectious iridocyclitis, left eye**
- **H20.043 Secondary noninfectious iridocyclitis, bilateral**
- **H20.049 Secondary noninfectious iridocyclitis, unspecified eye**

√6th **H20.05 Hypopyon**
- **H20.051 Hypopyon, right eye**
- **H20.052 Hypopyon, left eye**
- **H20.053 Hypopyon, bilateral**
- **H20.059 Hypopyon, unspecified eye**

√5th **H20.1 Chronic iridocyclitis**

Use additional code for any associated cataract (H26.21-)

EXCLUDES 2 *posterior cyclitis (H30.2-)*

- **H20.10 Chronic iridocyclitis, unspecified eye**
- **H20.11 Chronic iridocyclitis, right eye**
- **H20.12 Chronic iridocyclitis, left eye**
- **H20.13 Chronic iridocyclitis, bilateral**

√5th **H20.2 Lens-induced iridocyclitis**
- **H20.20 Lens-induced iridocyclitis, unspecified eye**
- **H20.21 Lens-induced iridocyclitis, right eye**
- **H20.22 Lens-induced iridocyclitis, left eye**
- **H20.23 Lens-induced iridocyclitis, bilateral**

√5th **H20.8 Other iridocyclitis**

EXCLUDES 2 *glaucomatocyclitis crises (H40.4-)*
posterior cyclitis (H30.2-)
sympathetic uveitis (H44.13-)

√6th **H20.81 Fuchs' heterochromic cyclitis**
- **H20.811 Fuchs' heterochromic cyclitis, right eye**
- **H20.812 Fuchs' heterochromic cyclitis, left eye**
- **H20.813 Fuchs' heterochromic cyclitis, bilateral**
- **H20.819 Fuchs' heterochromic cyclitis, unspecified eye**

√6th **H20.82 Vogt-Koyanagi syndrome**
- **H20.821 Vogt-Koyanagi syndrome, right eye**
- **H20.822 Vogt-Koyanagi syndrome, left eye**
- **H20.823 Vogt-Koyanagi syndrome, bilateral**
- **H20.829 Vogt-Koyanagi syndrome, unspecified eye**

H20.9 Unspecified iridocyclitis CC

Uveitis NOS

√4th **H21 Other disorders of iris and ciliary body**

EXCLUDES 2 *sympathetic uveitis (H44.1-)*

√5th **H21.0 Hyphema**

EXCLUDES 1 *traumatic hyphema (S05.1-)*

Hyphema

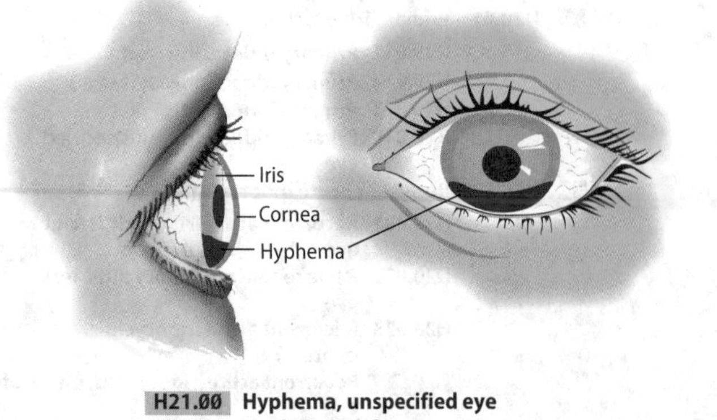

- **H21.00 Hyphema, unspecified eye**
- **H21.01 Hyphema, right eye**
- **H21.02 Hyphema, left eye**
- **H21.03 Hyphema, bilateral**

√5th **H21.1 Other vascular disorders of iris and ciliary body**

Neovascularization of iris or ciliary body
Rubeosis iridis
Rubeosis of iris

√6th **H21.1X Other vascular disorders of iris and ciliary body**
- **H21.1X1 Other vascular disorders of iris and ciliary body, right eye**
- **H21.1X2 Other vascular disorders of iris and ciliary body, left eye**
- **H21.1X3 Other vascular disorders of iris and ciliary body, bilateral**
- **H21.1X9 Other vascular disorders of iris and ciliary body, unspecified eye**

√5th **H21.2 Degeneration of iris and ciliary body**

√6th **H21.21 Degeneration of chamber angle**
- **H21.211 Degeneration of chamber angle, right eye**
- **H21.212 Degeneration of chamber angle, left eye**
- **H21.213 Degeneration of chamber angle, bilateral**
- **H21.219 Degeneration of chamber angle, unspecified eye**

√6th **H21.22 Degeneration of ciliary body**
- **H21.221 Degeneration of ciliary body, right eye**
- **H21.222 Degeneration of ciliary body, left eye**
- **H21.223 Degeneration of ciliary body, bilateral**
- **H21.229 Degeneration of ciliary body, unspecified eye**

√6th **H21.23 Degeneration of iris (pigmentary)**

Translucency of iris

- **H21.231 Degeneration of iris (pigmentary), right eye**
- **H21.232 Degeneration of iris (pigmentary), left eye**
- **H21.233 Degeneration of iris (pigmentary), bilateral**
- **H21.239 Degeneration of iris (pigmentary), unspecified eye**

√6th **H21.24 Degeneration of pupillary margin**
- **H21.241 Degeneration of pupillary margin, right eye**
- **H21.242 Degeneration of pupillary margin, left eye**
- **H21.243 Degeneration of pupillary margin, bilateral**
- **H21.249 Degeneration of pupillary margin, unspecified eye**

√6th **H21.25 Iridoschisis**
- **H21.251 Iridoschisis, right eye**
- **H21.252 Iridoschisis, left eye**
- **H21.253 Iridoschisis, bilateral**
- **H21.259 Iridoschisis, unspecified eye**

√6th **H21.26 Iris atrophy (essential) (progressive)**
- **H21.261 Iris atrophy (essential) (progressive), right eye**
- **H21.262 Iris atrophy (essential) (progressive), left eye**
- **H21.263 Iris atrophy (essential) (progressive), bilateral**
- **H21.269 Iris atrophy (essential) (progressive), unspecified eye**

√6th **H21.27 Miotic pupillary cyst**
- **H21.271 Miotic pupillary cyst, right eye**
- **H21.272 Miotic pupillary cyst, left eye**
- **H21.273 Miotic pupillary cyst, bilateral**
- **H21.279 Miotic pupillary cyst, unspecified eye**

H21.29 Other iris atrophy

√5th **H21.3 Cyst of iris, ciliary body and anterior chamber**

EXCLUDES 2 *miotic pupillary cyst (H21.27-)*

√6th **H21.30 Idiopathic cysts of iris, ciliary body or anterior chamber**

Cyst of iris, ciliary body or anterior chamber NOS

- **H21.301 Idiopathic cysts of iris, ciliary body or anterior chamber, right eye**
- **H21.302 Idiopathic cysts of iris, ciliary body or anterior chamber, left eye**
- **H21.303 Idiopathic cysts of iris, ciliary body or anterior chamber, bilateral**

H21.3Ø9 Idiopathic cysts of iris, ciliary body or anterior chamber, unspecified eye

✓6th **H21.31 Exudative cysts of iris or anterior chamber**

H21.311 Exudative cysts of iris or anterior chamber, right eye

H21.312 Exudative cysts of iris or anterior chamber, left eye

H21.313 Exudative cysts of iris or anterior chamber, bilateral

H21.319 Exudative cysts of iris or anterior chamber, unspecified eye

✓6th **H21.32 Implantation cysts of iris, ciliary body or anterior chamber**

H21.321 Implantation cysts of iris, ciliary body or anterior chamber, right eye

H21.322 Implantation cysts of iris, ciliary body or anterior chamber, left eye

H21.323 Implantation cysts of iris, ciliary body or anterior chamber, bilateral

H21.329 Implantation cysts of iris, ciliary body or anterior chamber, unspecified eye

✓6th **H21.33 Parasitic cyst of iris, ciliary body or anterior chamber**

H21.331 Parasitic cyst of iris, ciliary body or anterior chamber, right eye CC

H21.332 Parasitic cyst of iris, ciliary body or anterior chamber, left eye CC

H21.333 Parasitic cyst of iris, ciliary body or anterior chamber, bilateral CC

H21.339 Parasitic cyst of iris, ciliary body or anterior chamber, unspecified eye CC

✓6th **H21.34 Primary cyst of pars plana**

H21.341 Primary cyst of pars plana, right eye

H21.342 Primary cyst of pars plana, left eye

H21.343 Primary cyst of pars plana, bilateral

H21.349 Primary cyst of pars plana, unspecified eye

✓6th **H21.35 Exudative cyst of pars plana**

DEF: Protein, fatty-filled bullous elevation of the nonpigmented outermost ciliary epithelium of pars plana, due to fluid leak from blood vessels.

H21.351 Exudative cyst of pars plana, right eye

H21.352 Exudative cyst of pars plana, left eye

H21.353 Exudative cyst of pars plana, bilateral

H21.359 Exudative cyst of pars plana, unspecified eye

✓5th **H21.4 Pupillary membranes**

Iris bombé
Pupillary occlusion
Pupillary seclusion

EXCLUDES 1 *congenital pupillary membranes (Q13.8)*

H21.4Ø Pupillary membranes, unspecified eye

H21.41 Pupillary membranes, right eye

H21.42 Pupillary membranes, left eye

H21.43 Pupillary membranes, bilateral

✓5th **H21.5 Other and unspecified adhesions and disruptions of iris and ciliary body**

EXCLUDES 1 *corectopia (Q13.2)*

✓6th **H21.5Ø Unspecified adhesions of iris**

Synechia (iris) NOS

H21.5Ø1 Unspecified adhesions of iris, right eye

H21.5Ø2 Unspecified adhesions of iris, left eye

H21.5Ø3 Unspecified adhesions of iris, bilateral

H21.5Ø9 Unspecified adhesions of iris and ciliary body, unspecified eye

✓6th **H21.51 Anterior synechiae (iris)**

H21.511 Anterior synechiae (iris), right eye

H21.512 Anterior synechiae (iris), left eye

H21.513 Anterior synechiae (iris), bilateral

H21.519 Anterior synechiae (iris), unspecified eye

✓6th **H21.52 Goniosynechiae**

H21.521 Goniosynechiae, right eye

H21.522 Goniosynechiae, left eye

H21.523 Goniosynechiae, bilateral

H21.529 Goniosynechiae, unspecified eye

✓6th **H21.53 Iridodialysis**

H21.531 Iridodialysis, right eye

H21.532 Iridodialysis, left eye

H21.533 Iridodialysis, bilateral

H21.539 Iridodialysis, unspecified eye

✓6th **H21.54 Posterior synechiae (iris)**

H21.541 Posterior synechiae (iris), right eye

H21.542 Posterior synechiae (iris), left eye

H21.543 Posterior synechiae (iris), bilateral

H21.549 Posterior synechiae (iris), unspecified eye

✓6th **H21.55 Recession of chamber angle**

H21.551 Recession of chamber angle, right eye

H21.552 Recession of chamber angle, left eye

H21.553 Recession of chamber angle, bilateral

H21.559 Recession of chamber angle, unspecified eye

✓6th **H21.56 Pupillary abnormalities**

Deformed pupil
Ectopic pupil
Rupture of sphincter, pupil

EXCLUDES 1 *congenital deformity of pupil (Q13.2-)*

H21.561 Pupillary abnormality, right eye

H21.562 Pupillary abnormality, left eye

H21.563 Pupillary abnormality, bilateral

H21.569 Pupillary abnormality, unspecified eye

✓5th **H21.8 Other specified disorders of iris and ciliary body**

H21.81 Floppy iris syndrome

Intraoperative floppy iris syndrome (IFIS)
Use additional code for adverse effect, if applicable, to identify drug (T36-T5Ø with fifth or sixth character 5)

H21.82 Plateau iris syndrome (post-iridectomy) (postprocedural)

H21.89 Other specified disorders of iris and ciliary body

H21.9 Unspecified disorder of iris and ciliary body

H22 Disorders of iris and ciliary body in diseases classified elsewhere

Code first underlying disease, such as:
gout (M1A.-, M1Ø.-)
leprosy (A3Ø.-)
parasitic disease (B89)

Disorders of lens (H25-H28)

✓4th **H25 Age-related cataract**

Senile cataract

EXCLUDES 2 *capsular glaucoma with pseudoexfoliation of lens (H4Ø.1-)*

Cataracts

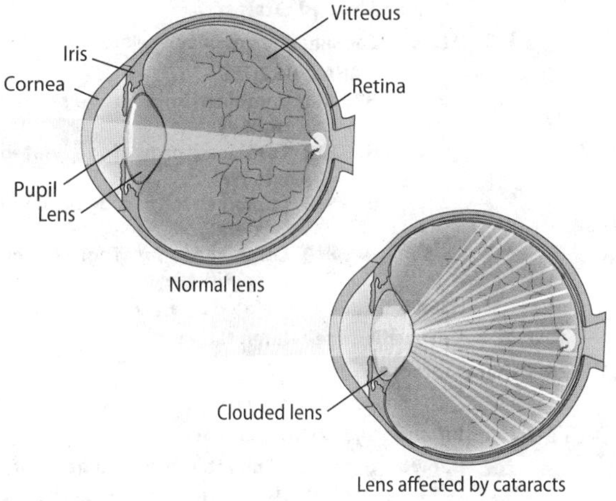

✓5th **H25.Ø Age-related incipient cataract**

✓6th **H25.Ø1 Cortical age-related cataract**

H25.Ø11 Cortical age-related cataract, right eye A

H25.Ø12 Cortical age-related cataract, left eye A

H25.Ø13 Cortical age-related cataract, bilateral A

H25.Ø19 Cortical age-related cataract, unspecified eye A

✓6th **H25.Ø3 Anterior subcapsular polar age-related cataract**

H25.Ø31 Anterior subcapsular polar age-related cataract, right eye A

H25.032 Anterior subcapsular polar age-related cataract, left eye A
H25.033 Anterior subcapsular polar age-related cataract, bilateral A
H25.039 Anterior subcapsular polar age-related cataract, unspecified eye A

√6th H25.04 Posterior subcapsular polar age-related cataract
H25.041 Posterior subcapsular polar age-related cataract, right eye A
H25.042 Posterior subcapsular polar age-related cataract, left eye A
H25.043 Posterior subcapsular polar age-related cataract, bilateral A
H25.049 Posterior subcapsular polar age-related cataract, unspecified eye A

√6th H25.09 Other age-related incipient cataract
Coronary age-related cataract
Punctate age-related cataract
Water clefts
H25.091 Other age-related incipient cataract, right eye A
H25.092 Other age-related incipient cataract, left eye A
H25.093 Other age-related incipient cataract, bilateral A
H25.099 Other age-related incipient cataract, unspecified eye A

√5th H25.1 Age-related nuclear cataract
Cataracta brunescens
Nuclear sclerosis cataract
AHA: 2019,2Q,31; 2016,1Q,32
H25.10 Age-related nuclear cataract, unspecified eye A
H25.11 Age-related nuclear cataract, right eye A
H25.12 Age-related nuclear cataract, left eye A
H25.13 Age-related nuclear cataract, bilateral A

√5th H25.2 Age-related cataract, morgagnian type
Age-related hypermature cataract
H25.20 Age-related cataract, morgagnian type, unspecified eye A
H25.21 Age-related cataract, morgagnian type, right eye A
H25.22 Age-related cataract, morgagnian type, left eye A
H25.23 Age-related cataract, morgagnian type, bilateral A

√5th H25.8 Other age-related cataract
√6th H25.81 Combined forms of age-related cataract
AHA: 2019,2Q,30
H25.811 Combined forms of age-related cataract, right eye A
H25.812 Combined forms of age-related cataract, left eye A
H25.813 Combined forms of age-related cataract, bilateral A
H25.819 Combined forms of age-related cataract, unspecified eye A
H25.89 Other age-related cataract A

H25.9 Unspecified age-related cataract A

√4th H26 Other cataract
EXCLUDES 1 *congenital cataract (Q12.0)*

√5th H26.0 Infantile and juvenile cataract
√6th H26.00 Unspecified infantile and juvenile cataract
H26.001 Unspecified infantile and juvenile cataract, right eye P
H26.002 Unspecified infantile and juvenile cataract, left eye P
H26.003 Unspecified infantile and juvenile cataract, bilateral P
H26.009 Unspecified infantile and juvenile cataract, unspecified eye P

√6th H26.01 Infantile and juvenile cortical, lamellar, or zonular cataract
H26.011 Infantile and juvenile cortical, lamellar, or zonular cataract, right eye P
H26.012 Infantile and juvenile cortical, lamellar, or zonular cataract, left eye P
H26.013 Infantile and juvenile cortical, lamellar, or zonular cataract, bilateral P
H26.019 Infantile and juvenile cortical, lamellar, or zonular cataract, unspecified eye P

√6th H26.03 Infantile and juvenile nuclear cataract
H26.031 Infantile and juvenile nuclear cataract, right eye P
H26.032 Infantile and juvenile nuclear cataract, left eye P
H26.033 Infantile and juvenile nuclear cataract, bilateral P
H26.039 Infantile and juvenile nuclear cataract, unspecified eye P

√6th H26.04 Anterior subcapsular polar infantile and juvenile cataract
H26.041 Anterior subcapsular polar infantile and juvenile cataract, right eye P
H26.042 Anterior subcapsular polar infantile and juvenile cataract, left eye P
H26.043 Anterior subcapsular polar infantile and juvenile cataract, bilateral P
H26.049 Anterior subcapsular polar infantile and juvenile cataract, unspecified eye P

√6th H26.05 Posterior subcapsular polar infantile and juvenile cataract
H26.051 Posterior subcapsular polar infantile and juvenile cataract, right eye P
H26.052 Posterior subcapsular polar infantile and juvenile cataract, left eye P
H26.053 Posterior subcapsular polar infantile and juvenile cataract, bilateral P
H26.059 Posterior subcapsular polar infantile and juvenile cataract, unspecified eye P

√6th H26.06 Combined forms of infantile and juvenile cataract
H26.061 Combined forms of infantile and juvenile cataract, right eye P
H26.062 Combined forms of infantile and juvenile cataract, left eye P
H26.063 Combined forms of infantile and juvenile cataract, bilateral P
H26.069 Combined forms of infantile and juvenile cataract, unspecified eye P
H26.09 Other infantile and juvenile cataract P

√5th H26.1 Traumatic cataract
Use additional code (Chapter 20) to identify external cause
√6th H26.10 Unspecified traumatic cataract
H26.101 Unspecified traumatic cataract, right eye
H26.102 Unspecified traumatic cataract, left eye
H26.103 Unspecified traumatic cataract, bilateral
H26.109 Unspecified traumatic cataract, unspecified eye

√6th H26.11 Localized traumatic opacities
H26.111 Localized traumatic opacities, right eye
H26.112 Localized traumatic opacities, left eye
H26.113 Localized traumatic opacities, bilateral
H26.119 Localized traumatic opacities, unspecified eye

√6th H26.12 Partially resolved traumatic cataract
H26.121 Partially resolved traumatic cataract, right eye
H26.122 Partially resolved traumatic cataract, left eye
H26.123 Partially resolved traumatic cataract, bilateral
H26.129 Partially resolved traumatic cataract, unspecified eye

√6th H26.13 Total traumatic cataract
H26.131 Total traumatic cataract, right eye
H26.132 Total traumatic cataract, left eye
H26.133 Total traumatic cataract, bilateral
H26.139 Total traumatic cataract, unspecified eye

√5th H26.2 Complicated cataract
H26.20 Unspecified complicated cataract
Cataracta complicata NOS
√6th H26.21 Cataract with neovascularization
Code also associated condition, such as:
chronic iridocyclitis (H20.1-)
H26.211 Cataract with neovascularization, right eye

H26.212 Cataract with neovascularization, left eye
H26.213 Cataract with neovascularization, bilateral
H26.219 Cataract with neovascularization, unspecified eye

H26.22 Cataract secondary to ocular disorders (degenerative) (inflammatory)
Code also associated ocular disorder
H26.221 Cataract secondary to ocular disorders (degenerative) (inflammatory), right eye
H26.222 Cataract secondary to ocular disorders (degenerative) (inflammatory), left eye
H26.223 Cataract secondary to ocular disorders (degenerative) (inflammatory), bilateral
H26.229 Cataract secondary to ocular disorders (degenerative) (inflammatory), unspecified eye

H26.23 Glaucomatous flecks (subcapsular)
Code first underlying glaucoma (H40-H42)
H26.231 Glaucomatous flecks (subcapsular), right eye
H26.232 Glaucomatous flecks (subcapsular), left eye
H26.233 Glaucomatous flecks (subcapsular), bilateral
H26.239 Glaucomatous flecks (subcapsular), unspecified eye

H26.3 Drug-induced cataract
Toxic cataract
Use additional code for adverse effect, if applicable, to identify drug (T36-T50 with fifth or sixth character 5)
H26.30 Drug-induced cataract, unspecified eye
H26.31 Drug-induced cataract, right eye
H26.32 Drug-induced cataract, left eye
H26.33 Drug-induced cataract, bilateral

H26.4 Secondary cataract
H26.40 Unspecified secondary cataract
H26.41 Soemmering's ring
H26.411 Soemmering's ring, right eye
H26.412 Soemmering's ring, left eye
H26.413 Soemmering's ring, bilateral
H26.419 Soemmering's ring, unspecified eye
H26.49 Other secondary cataract
AHA: 2018,2Q,14
H26.491 Other secondary cataract, right eye
H26.492 Other secondary cataract, left eye
H26.493 Other secondary cataract, bilateral
H26.499 Other secondary cataract, unspecified eye

H26.8 Other specified cataract
H26.9 Unspecified cataract

H27 Other disorders of lens
EXCLUDES 1 *congenital lens malformations (Q12.-)*
mechanical complications of intraocular lens implant (T85.2)
pseudophakia (Z96.1)

H27.0 Aphakia
Acquired absence of lens
Acquired aphakia
Aphakia due to trauma
EXCLUDES 1 *cataract extraction status (Z98.4-)*
congenital absence of lens (Q12.3)
congenital aphakia (Q12.3)
H27.00 Aphakia, unspecified eye
H27.01 Aphakia, right eye
H27.02 Aphakia, left eye
H27.03 Aphakia, bilateral

H27.1 Dislocation of lens
H27.10 Unspecified dislocation of lens
H27.11 Subluxation of lens
H27.111 Subluxation of lens, right eye
H27.112 Subluxation of lens, left eye
H27.113 Subluxation of lens, bilateral
H27.119 Subluxation of lens, unspecified eye
H27.12 Anterior dislocation of lens
H27.121 Anterior dislocation of lens, right eye
H27.122 Anterior dislocation of lens, left eye
H27.123 Anterior dislocation of lens, bilateral
H27.129 Anterior dislocation of lens, unspecified eye
H27.13 Posterior dislocation of lens
H27.131 Posterior dislocation of lens, right eye
H27.132 Posterior dislocation of lens, left eye
H27.133 Posterior dislocation of lens, bilateral
H27.139 Posterior dislocation of lens, unspecified eye
H27.8 Other specified disorders of lens
H27.9 Unspecified disorder of lens

H28 Cataract in diseases classified elsewhere
Code first underlying disease, such as:
hypoparathyroidism (E20.-)
myotonia (G71.1-)
myxedema (E03.-)
protein-calorie malnutrition (E40-E46)
EXCLUDES 1 *cataract in diabetes mellitus (E08.36, E09.36, E10.36, E11.36, E13.36)*

Disorders of choroid and retina (H30-H36)

H30 Chorioretinal inflammation

H30.0 Focal chorioretinal inflammation
Focal chorioretinitis
Focal choroiditis
Focal retinitis
Focal retinochoroiditis
H30.00 Unspecified focal chorioretinal inflammation
Focal chorioretinitis NOS
Focal choroiditis NOS
Focal retinitis NOS
Focal retinochoroiditis NOS
H30.001 Unspecified focal chorioretinal inflammation, right eye
H30.002 Unspecified focal chorioretinal inflammation, left eye
H30.003 Unspecified focal chorioretinal inflammation, bilateral
H30.009 Unspecified focal chorioretinal inflammation, unspecified eye
H30.01 Focal chorioretinal inflammation, juxtapapillary
H30.011 Focal chorioretinal inflammation, juxtapapillary, right eye
H30.012 Focal chorioretinal inflammation, juxtapapillary, left eye
H30.013 Focal chorioretinal inflammation, juxtapapillary, bilateral
H30.019 Focal chorioretinal inflammation, juxtapapillary, unspecified eye
H30.02 Focal chorioretinal inflammation of posterior pole
H30.021 Focal chorioretinal inflammation of posterior pole, right eye
H30.022 Focal chorioretinal inflammation of posterior pole, left eye
H30.023 Focal chorioretinal inflammation of posterior pole, bilateral
H30.029 Focal chorioretinal inflammation of posterior pole, unspecified eye
H30.03 Focal chorioretinal inflammation, peripheral
H30.031 Focal chorioretinal inflammation, peripheral, right eye
H30.032 Focal chorioretinal inflammation, peripheral, left eye
H30.033 Focal chorioretinal inflammation, peripheral, bilateral
H30.039 Focal chorioretinal inflammation, peripheral, unspecified eye
H30.04 Focal chorioretinal inflammation, macular or paramacular
H30.041 Focal chorioretinal inflammation, macular or paramacular, right eye
H30.042 Focal chorioretinal inflammation, macular or paramacular, left eye
H30.043 Focal chorioretinal inflammation, macular or paramacular, bilateral
H30.049 Focal chorioretinal inflammation, macular or paramacular, unspecified eye

√5th **H30.1 Disseminated chorioretinal inflammation**
Disseminated chorioretinitis
Disseminated choroiditis
Disseminated retinitis
Disseminated retinochoroiditis
EXCLUDES 2 *exudative retinopathy (H35.02-)*

√6th **H30.10 Unspecified disseminated chorioretinal inflammation**
Disseminated chorioretinitis NOS
Disseminated choroiditis NOS
Disseminated retinitis NOS
Disseminated retinochoroiditis NOS
H30.101 Unspecified disseminated chorioretinal inflammation, right eye CC
H30.102 Unspecified disseminated chorioretinal inflammation, left eye CC
H30.103 Unspecified disseminated chorioretinal inflammation, bilateral CC
H30.109 Unspecified disseminated chorioretinal inflammation, unspecified eye CC

√6th **H30.11 Disseminated chorioretinal inflammation of posterior pole**
H30.111 Disseminated chorioretinal inflammation of posterior pole, right eye CC
H30.112 Disseminated chorioretinal inflammation of posterior pole, left eye CC
H30.113 Disseminated chorioretinal inflammation of posterior pole, bilateral CC
H30.119 Disseminated chorioretinal inflammation of posterior pole, unspecified eye CC

√6th **H30.12 Disseminated chorioretinal inflammation, peripheral**
H30.121 Disseminated chorioretinal inflammation, peripheral right eye CC
H30.122 Disseminated chorioretinal inflammation, peripheral, left eye CC
H30.123 Disseminated chorioretinal inflammation, peripheral, bilateral CC
H30.129 Disseminated chorioretinal inflammation, peripheral, unspecified eye CC

√6th **H30.13 Disseminated chorioretinal inflammation, generalized**
H30.131 Disseminated chorioretinal inflammation, generalized, right eye CC
H30.132 Disseminated chorioretinal inflammation, generalized, left eye CC
H30.133 Disseminated chorioretinal inflammation, generalized, bilateral CC
H30.139 Disseminated chorioretinal inflammation, generalized, unspecified eye CC

√6th **H30.14 Acute posterior multifocal placoid pigment epitheliopathy**
H30.141 Acute posterior multifocal placoid pigment epitheliopathy, right eye CC
H30.142 Acute posterior multifocal placoid pigment epitheliopathy, left eye CC
H30.143 Acute posterior multifocal placoid pigment epitheliopathy, bilateral CC
H30.149 Acute posterior multifocal placoid pigment epitheliopathy, unspecified eye CC

√5th **H30.2 Posterior cyclitis**
Pars planitis
H30.20 Posterior cyclitis, unspecified eye
H30.21 Posterior cyclitis, right eye
H30.22 Posterior cyclitis, left eye
H30.23 Posterior cyclitis, bilateral

√5th **H30.8 Other chorioretinal inflammations**

√6th **H30.81 Harada's disease**
H30.811 Harada's disease, right eye
H30.812 Harada's disease, left eye
H30.813 Harada's disease, bilateral
H30.819 Harada's disease, unspecified eye

√6th **H30.89 Other chorioretinal inflammations**
H30.891 Other chorioretinal inflammations, right eye CC
H30.892 Other chorioretinal inflammations, left eye CC
H30.893 Other chorioretinal inflammations, bilateral CC
H30.899 Other chorioretinal inflammations, unspecified eye CC

√5th **H30.9 Unspecified chorioretinal inflammation**
Chorioretinitis NOS
Choroiditis NOS
Neuroretinitis NOS
Retinitis NOS
Retinochoroiditis NOS
H30.90 Unspecified chorioretinal inflammation, unspecified eye CC
H30.91 Unspecified chorioretinal inflammation, right eye CC
H30.92 Unspecified chorioretinal inflammation, left eye CC
H30.93 Unspecified chorioretinal inflammation, bilateral CC

√4th **H31 Other disorders of choroid**

√5th **H31.0 Chorioretinal scars**
EXCLUDES 2 *postsurgical chorioretinal scars (H59.81-)*

√6th **H31.00 Unspecified chorioretinal scars**
H31.001 Unspecified chorioretinal scars, right eye
H31.002 Unspecified chorioretinal scars, left eye
H31.003 Unspecified chorioretinal scars, bilateral
H31.009 Unspecified chorioretinal scars, unspecified eye

√6th **H31.01 Macula scars of posterior pole (postinflammatory) (post-traumatic)**
EXCLUDES 1 *postprocedural chorioretinal scar (H59.81-)*
H31.011 Macula scars of posterior pole (postinflammatory) (post-traumatic), right eye
H31.012 Macula scars of posterior pole (postinflammatory) (post-traumatic), left eye
H31.013 Macula scars of posterior pole (postinflammatory) (post-traumatic), bilateral
H31.019 Macula scars of posterior pole (postinflammatory) (post-traumatic), unspecified eye

√6th **H31.02 Solar retinopathy**
H31.021 Solar retinopathy, right eye
H31.022 Solar retinopathy, left eye
H31.023 Solar retinopathy, bilateral
H31.029 Solar retinopathy, unspecified eye

√6th **H31.09 Other chorioretinal scars**
H31.091 Other chorioretinal scars, right eye
H31.092 Other chorioretinal scars, left eye
H31.093 Other chorioretinal scars, bilateral
H31.099 Other chorioretinal scars, unspecified eye

√5th **H31.1 Choroidal degeneration**
EXCLUDES 2 *angioid streaks of macula (H35.33)*

√6th **H31.10 Unspecified choroidal degeneration**
Choroidal sclerosis NOS
H31.101 Choroidal degeneration, unspecified, right eye
H31.102 Choroidal degeneration, unspecified, left eye
H31.103 Choroidal degeneration, unspecified, bilateral
H31.109 Choroidal degeneration, unspecified, unspecified eye

√6th **H31.11 Age-related choroidal atrophy**
H31.111 Age-related choroidal atrophy, right eye A
H31.112 Age-related choroidal atrophy, left eye A
H31.113 Age-related choroidal atrophy, bilateral A
H31.119 Age-related choroidal atrophy, unspecified eye A

√6th **H31.12 Diffuse secondary atrophy of choroid**
H31.121 Diffuse secondary atrophy of choroid, right eye

H31.122 Diffuse secondary atrophy of choroid, left eye
H31.123 Diffuse secondary atrophy of choroid, bilateral
H31.129 Diffuse secondary atrophy of choroid, unspecified eye

√5th H31.2 Hereditary choroidal dystrophy
EXCLUDES 2 *hyperornithinemia (E72.4)*
ornithinemia (E72.4)
H31.20 Hereditary choroidal dystrophy, unspecified
H31.21 Choroideremia
H31.22 Choroidal dystrophy (central areolar) (generalized) (peripapillary)
H31.23 Gyrate atrophy, choroid
H31.29 Other hereditary choroidal dystrophy

√5th H31.3 Choroidal hemorrhage and rupture
√6th H31.30 Unspecified choroidal hemorrhage
H31.301 Unspecified choroidal hemorrhage, right eye
H31.302 Unspecified choroidal hemorrhage, left eye
H31.303 Unspecified choroidal hemorrhage, bilateral
H31.309 Unspecified choroidal hemorrhage, unspecified eye
√6th H31.31 Expulsive choroidal hemorrhage
H31.311 Expulsive choroidal hemorrhage, right eye
H31.312 Expulsive choroidal hemorrhage, left eye
H31.313 Expulsive choroidal hemorrhage, bilateral
H31.319 Expulsive choroidal hemorrhage, unspecified eye
√6th H31.32 Choroidal rupture
H31.321 Choroidal rupture, right eye CC
H31.322 Choroidal rupture, left eye CC
H31.323 Choroidal rupture, bilateral CC
H31.329 Choroidal rupture, unspecified eye CC

√5th H31.4 Choroidal detachment
√6th H31.40 Unspecified choroidal detachment
H31.401 Unspecified choroidal detachment, right eye CC
H31.402 Unspecified choroidal detachment, left eye CC
H31.403 Unspecified choroidal detachment, bilateral CC
H31.409 Unspecified choroidal detachment, unspecified eye CC
√6th H31.41 Hemorrhagic choroidal detachment
H31.411 Hemorrhagic choroidal detachment, right eye CC
H31.412 Hemorrhagic choroidal detachment, left eye CC
H31.413 Hemorrhagic choroidal detachment, bilateral CC
H31.419 Hemorrhagic choroidal detachment, unspecified eye CC
√6th H31.42 Serous choroidal detachment
H31.421 Serous choroidal detachment, right eye CC
H31.422 Serous choroidal detachment, left eye CC
H31.423 Serous choroidal detachment, bilateral CC
H31.429 Serous choroidal detachment, unspecified eye CC

H31.8 Other specified disorders of choroid
H31.9 Unspecified disorder of choroid

H32 Chorioretinal disorders in diseases classified elsewhere
Code first underlying disease, such as:
congenital toxoplasmosis (P37.1)
histoplasmosis (B39.-)
leprosy (A30.-)
EXCLUDES 1 *chorioretinitis (in):*
toxoplasmosis (acquired) (B58.01)
tuberculosis (A18.53)

√4th **H33 Retinal detachments and breaks**
EXCLUDES 1 *detachment of retinal pigment epithelium (H35.72-, H35.73-)*

Retinal Detachment

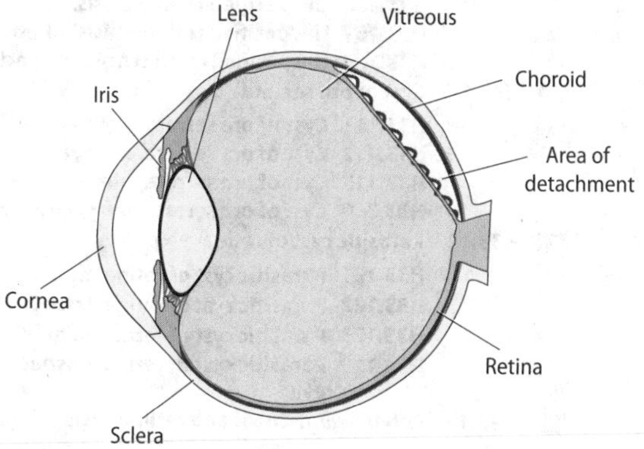

√5th H33.0 Retinal detachment with retinal break
Rhegmatogenous retinal detachment
EXCLUDES 1 *serous retinal detachment (without retinal break) (H33.2-)*
√6th H33.00 Unspecified retinal detachment with retinal break
H33.001 Unspecified retinal detachment with retinal break, right eye
H33.002 Unspecified retinal detachment with retinal break, left eye
H33.003 Unspecified retinal detachment with retinal break, bilateral
H33.009 Unspecified retinal detachment with retinal break, unspecified eye
√6th H33.01 Retinal detachment with single break
H33.011 Retinal detachment with single break, right eye
H33.012 Retinal detachment with single break, left eye
H33.013 Retinal detachment with single break, bilateral
H33.019 Retinal detachment with single break, unspecified eye
√6th H33.02 Retinal detachment with multiple breaks
H33.021 Retinal detachment with multiple breaks, right eye
H33.022 Retinal detachment with multiple breaks, left eye
H33.023 Retinal detachment with multiple breaks, bilateral
H33.029 Retinal detachment with multiple breaks, unspecified eye
√6th H33.03 Retinal detachment with giant retinal tear
H33.031 Retinal detachment with giant retinal tear, right eye
H33.032 Retinal detachment with giant retinal tear, left eye
H33.033 Retinal detachment with giant retinal tear, bilateral
H33.039 Retinal detachment with giant retinal tear, unspecified eye
√6th H33.04 Retinal detachment with retinal dialysis
H33.041 Retinal detachment with retinal dialysis, right eye
H33.042 Retinal detachment with retinal dialysis, left eye
H33.043 Retinal detachment with retinal dialysis, bilateral
H33.049 Retinal detachment with retinal dialysis, unspecified eye
√6th H33.05 Total retinal detachment
H33.051 Total retinal detachment, right eye
H33.052 Total retinal detachment, left eye
H33.053 Total retinal detachment, bilateral
H33.059 Total retinal detachment, unspecified eye

√5th **H33.1 Retinoschisis and retinal cysts**

EXCLUDES 1 *congenital retinoschisis (Q14.1)*
microcystoid degeneration of retina (H35.42-)

√6th **H33.10 Unspecified retinoschisis**

H33.101 Unspecified retinoschisis, right eye
H33.102 Unspecified retinoschisis, left eye
H33.103 Unspecified retinoschisis, bilateral
H33.109 Unspecified retinoschisis, unspecified eye

√6th **H33.11 Cyst of ora serrata**

H33.111 Cyst of ora serrata, right eye
H33.112 Cyst of ora serrata, left eye
H33.113 Cyst of ora serrata, bilateral
H33.119 Cyst of ora serrata, unspecified eye

√6th **H33.12 Parasitic cyst of retina**

H33.121 Parasitic cyst of retina, right eye CC
H33.122 Parasitic cyst of retina, left eye CC
H33.123 Parasitic cyst of retina, bilateral CC
H33.129 Parasitic cyst of retina, unspecified eye CC

√6th **H33.19 Other retinoschisis and retinal cysts**

Pseudocyst of retina

H33.191 Other retinoschisis and retinal cysts, right eye
H33.192 Other retinoschisis and retinal cysts, left eye
H33.193 Other retinoschisis and retinal cysts, bilateral
H33.199 Other retinoschisis and retinal cysts, unspecified eye

√5th **H33.2 Serous retinal detachment**

Retinal detachment NOS
Retinal detachment without retinal break

EXCLUDES 1 *central serous chorioretinopathy (H35.71-)*

H33.20 Serous retinal detachment, unspecified eye CC
H33.21 Serous retinal detachment, right eye CC
H33.22 Serous retinal detachment, left eye CC
H33.23 Serous retinal detachment, bilateral CC

√5th **H33.3 Retinal breaks without detachment**

EXCLUDES 1 *chorioretinal scars after surgery for detachment (H59.81-)*
peripheral retinal degeneration without break (H35.4-)

√6th **H33.30 Unspecified retinal break**

H33.301 Unspecified retinal break, right eye
H33.302 Unspecified retinal break, left eye
H33.303 Unspecified retinal break, bilateral
H33.309 Unspecified retinal break, unspecified eye

√6th **H33.31 Horseshoe tear of retina without detachment**

Operculum of retina without detachment

H33.311 Horseshoe tear of retina without detachment, right eye
H33.312 Horseshoe tear of retina without detachment, left eye
H33.313 Horseshoe tear of retina without detachment, bilateral
H33.319 Horseshoe tear of retina without detachment, unspecified eye

√6th **H33.32 Round hole of retina without detachment**

H33.321 Round hole, right eye
H33.322 Round hole, left eye
H33.323 Round hole, bilateral
H33.329 Round hole, unspecified eye

√6th **H33.33 Multiple defects of retina without detachment**

H33.331 Multiple defects of retina without detachment, right eye
H33.332 Multiple defects of retina without detachment, left eye
H33.333 Multiple defects of retina without detachment, bilateral
H33.339 Multiple defects of retina without detachment, unspecified eye

√5th **H33.4 Traction detachment of retina**

Proliferative vitreo-retinopathy with retinal detachment

H33.40 Traction detachment of retina, unspecified eye CC
H33.41 Traction detachment of retina, right eye CC
H33.42 Traction detachment of retina, left eye CC
H33.43 Traction detachment of retina, bilateral CC

H33.8 Other retinal detachments CC

√4th **H34 Retinal vascular occlusions**

EXCLUDES 1 *amaurosis fugax (G45.3)*

√5th **H34.0 Transient retinal artery occlusion**

H34.00 Transient retinal artery occlusion, unspecified eye CC
H34.01 Transient retinal artery occlusion, right eye CC
H34.02 Transient retinal artery occlusion, left eye CC
H34.03 Transient retinal artery occlusion, bilateral CC

√5th **H34.1 Central retinal artery occlusion**

H34.10 Central retinal artery occlusion, unspecified eye CC
H34.11 Central retinal artery occlusion, right eye CC
H34.12 Central retinal artery occlusion, left eye CC
H34.13 Central retinal artery occlusion, bilateral CC

√5th **H34.2 Other retinal artery occlusions**

√6th **H34.21 Partial retinal artery occlusion**

Hollenhorst's plaque
Retinal microembolism

H34.211 Partial retinal artery occlusion, right eye CC
H34.212 Partial retinal artery occlusion, left eye CC
H34.213 Partial retinal artery occlusion, bilateral CC
H34.219 Partial retinal artery occlusion, unspecified eye CC

√6th **H34.23 Retinal artery branch occlusion**

H34.231 Retinal artery branch occlusion, right eye CC
H34.232 Retinal artery branch occlusion, left eye CC
H34.233 Retinal artery branch occlusion, bilateral CC
H34.239 Retinal artery branch occlusion, unspecified eye CC

√5th **H34.8 Other retinal vascular occlusions**

AHA: 2016,4Q,19

√6th **H34.81 Central retinal vein occlusion**

One of the following 7th characters is to be assigned to codes in subcategory H34.81 to designate the severity of the occlusion:
0 with macular edema
1 with retinal neovascularization
2 stable
old central retinal vein occlusion

√7th **H34.811 Central retinal vein occlusion, right eye** CC
√7th **H34.812 Central retinal vein occlusion, left eye** CC
√7th **H34.813 Central retinal vein occlusion, bilateral** CC
√7th **H34.819 Central retinal vein occlusion, unspecified eye** CC

√6th **H34.82 Venous engorgement**

Incipient retinal vein occlusion
Partial retinal vein occlusion

H34.821 Venous engorgement, right eye
H34.822 Venous engorgement, left eye
H34.823 Venous engorgement, bilateral
H34.829 Venous engorgement, unspecified eye

√6th **H34.83 Tributary (branch) retinal vein occlusion**

One of the following 7th characters is to be assigned to codes in subcategory H34.83 to designate the severity of the occlusion:
0 with macular edema
1 with retinal neovascularization
2 stable
old tributary (branch) retinal vein occlusion

√7th **H34.831 Tributary (branch) retinal vein occlusion, right eye**
√7th **H34.832 Tributary (branch) retinal vein occlusion, left eye**

H34.833 Tributary (branch) retinal vein occlusion, bilateral
H34.839 Tributary (branch) retinal vein occlusion, unspecified eye
H34.9 Unspecified retinal vascular occlusion CC

H35 Other retinal disorders
EXCLUDES 2 *diabetic retinal disorders (EØ8.311-EØ8.359, EØ9.311-EØ9.359, E1Ø.311-E1Ø.359, E11.311-E11.359, E13.311-E13.359)*

H35.Ø Background retinopathy and retinal vascular changes
Code also any associated hypertension (I1Ø.-)
H35.ØØ Unspecified background retinopathy
H35.Ø1 Changes in retinal vascular appearance
Retinal vascular sheathing
H35.Ø11 Changes in retinal vascular appearance, right eye
H35.Ø12 Changes in retinal vascular appearance, left eye
H35.Ø13 Changes in retinal vascular appearance, bilateral
H35.Ø19 Changes in retinal vascular appearance, unspecified eye
H35.Ø2 Exudative retinopathy
Coats retinopathy
H35.Ø21 Exudative retinopathy, right eye
H35.Ø22 Exudative retinopathy, left eye
H35.Ø23 Exudative retinopathy, bilateral
H35.Ø29 Exudative retinopathy, unspecified eye
H35.Ø3 Hypertensive retinopathy
H35.Ø31 Hypertensive retinopathy, right eye
H35.Ø32 Hypertensive retinopathy, left eye
H35.Ø33 Hypertensive retinopathy, bilateral
H35.Ø39 Hypertensive retinopathy, unspecified eye
H35.Ø4 Retinal micro-aneurysms, unspecified
H35.Ø41 Retinal micro-aneurysms, unspecified, right eye
H35.Ø42 Retinal micro-aneurysms, unspecified, left eye
H35.Ø43 Retinal micro-aneurysms, unspecified, bilateral
H35.Ø49 Retinal micro-aneurysms, unspecified, unspecified eye
H35.Ø5 Retinal neovascularization, unspecified
H35.Ø51 Retinal neovascularization, unspecified, right eye
H35.Ø52 Retinal neovascularization, unspecified, left eye
H35.Ø53 Retinal neovascularization, unspecified, bilateral
H35.Ø59 Retinal neovascularization, unspecified, unspecified eye
H35.Ø6 Retinal vasculitis
Eales disease
Retinal perivasculitis
DEF: Sight-threatening intraocular inflammation of the retinal blood vessels that causes minimal, partial, or even complete blindness.
H35.Ø61 Retinal vasculitis, right eye
H35.Ø62 Retinal vasculitis, left eye
H35.Ø63 Retinal vasculitis, bilateral
H35.Ø69 Retinal vasculitis, unspecified eye
H35.Ø7 Retinal telangiectasis
H35.Ø71 Retinal telangiectasis, right eye
H35.Ø72 Retinal telangiectasis, left eye
H35.Ø73 Retinal telangiectasis, bilateral
H35.Ø79 Retinal telangiectasis, unspecified eye
H35.Ø9 Other intraretinal microvascular abnormalities
Retinal varices

H35.1 Retinopathy of prematurity
H35.1Ø Retinopathy of prematurity, unspecified
Retinopathy of prematurity NOS
H35.1Ø1 Retinopathy of prematurity, unspecified, right eye
H35.1Ø2 Retinopathy of prematurity, unspecified, left eye
H35.1Ø3 Retinopathy of prematurity, unspecified, bilateral
H35.1Ø9 Retinopathy of prematurity, unspecified, unspecified eye
H35.11 Retinopathy of prematurity, stage Ø
H35.111 Retinopathy of prematurity, stage Ø, right eye
H35.112 Retinopathy of prematurity, stage Ø, left eye
H35.113 Retinopathy of prematurity, stage Ø, bilateral
H35.119 Retinopathy of prematurity, stage Ø, unspecified eye
H35.12 Retinopathy of prematurity, stage 1
H35.121 Retinopathy of prematurity, stage 1, right eye
H35.122 Retinopathy of prematurity, stage 1, left eye
H35.123 Retinopathy of prematurity, stage 1, bilateral
H35.129 Retinopathy of prematurity, stage 1, unspecified eye
H35.13 Retinopathy of prematurity, stage 2
H35.131 Retinopathy of prematurity, stage 2, right eye
H35.132 Retinopathy of prematurity, stage 2, left eye
H35.133 Retinopathy of prematurity, stage 2, bilateral
H35.139 Retinopathy of prematurity, stage 2, unspecified eye
H35.14 Retinopathy of prematurity, stage 3
H35.141 Retinopathy of prematurity, stage 3, right eye
H35.142 Retinopathy of prematurity, stage 3, left eye
H35.143 Retinopathy of prematurity, stage 3, bilateral
H35.149 Retinopathy of prematurity, stage 3, unspecified eye
H35.15 Retinopathy of prematurity, stage 4
H35.151 Retinopathy of prematurity, stage 4, right eye
H35.152 Retinopathy of prematurity, stage 4, left eye
H35.153 Retinopathy of prematurity, stage 4, bilateral
H35.159 Retinopathy of prematurity, stage 4, unspecified eye
H35.16 Retinopathy of prematurity, stage 5
H35.161 Retinopathy of prematurity, stage 5, right eye
H35.162 Retinopathy of prematurity, stage 5, left eye
H35.163 Retinopathy of prematurity, stage 5, bilateral
H35.169 Retinopathy of prematurity, stage 5, unspecified eye
H35.17 Retrolental fibroplasia
H35.171 Retrolental fibroplasia, right eye
H35.172 Retrolental fibroplasia, left eye
H35.173 Retrolental fibroplasia, bilateral
H35.179 Retrolental fibroplasia, unspecified eye

H35.2 Other non-diabetic proliferative retinopathy
Proliferative vitreo-retinopathy
EXCLUDES 1 *proliferative vitreo-retinopathy with retinal detachment (H33.4-)*
H35.2Ø Other non-diabetic proliferative retinopathy, unspecified eye
H35.21 Other non-diabetic proliferative retinopathy, right eye
H35.22 Other non-diabetic proliferative retinopathy, left eye
H35.23 Other non-diabetic proliferative retinopathy, bilateral

H35.3 Degeneration of macula and posterior pole
H35.3Ø Unspecified macular degeneration A
Age-related macular degeneration

✓6th **H35.31 Nonexudative age-related macular degeneration**

Atrophic age-related macular degeneration
Dry age-related macular degeneration
AHA: 2016,4Q,20-21

One of the following 7th characters is to be assigned to each code in subcategory H35.31 to designate the stage of the disease:
- Ø stage unspecified
- 1 early dry stage
- 2 intermediate dry stage
- 3 advanced atrophic without subfoveal involvement
  advanced dry stage
- 4 advanced atrophic with subfoveal involvement

✓7th **H35.311 Nonexudative age-related macular degeneration, right eye** A
✓7th **H35.312 Nonexudative age-related macular degeneration, left eye** A
✓7th **H35.313 Nonexudative age-related macular degeneration, bilateral** A
✓7th **H35.319 Nonexudative age-related macular degeneration, unspecified eye** A

✓6th **H35.32 Exudative age-related macular degeneration**

Wet age-related macular degeneration
AHA: 2016,4Q,20-21

One of the following 7th characters is to be assigned to each code in subcategory H35.32 to designate the stage of the disease:
- Ø stage unspecified
- 1 with active choroidal neovascularization
- 2 with inactive choroidal neovascularization
  with involuted or regressed neovascularization
- 3 with inactive scar

✓7th **H35.321 Exudative age-related macular degeneration, right eye** HCC A
✓7th **H35.322 Exudative age-related macular degeneration, left eye** HCC A
✓7th **H35.323 Exudative age-related macular degeneration, bilateral** HCC A
✓7th **H35.329 Exudative age-related macular degeneration, unspecified eye** HCC A

H35.33 Angioid streaks of macula

DEF: Degeneration of the choroid; characterized by broad, irregular, dark brown streaks radiating from optic disc; occurs with pseudoxanthoma elasticum or Paget's disease.

✓6th **H35.34 Macular cyst, hole, or pseudohole**

H35.341 Macular cyst, hole, or pseudohole, right eye
H35.342 Macular cyst, hole, or pseudohole, left eye
H35.343 Macular cyst, hole, or pseudohole, bilateral
H35.349 Macular cyst, hole, or pseudohole, unspecified eye

✓6th **H35.35 Cystoid macular degeneration**

EXCLUDES 1 *cystoid macular edema following cataract surgery (H59.Ø3-)*

H35.351 Cystoid macular degeneration, right eye
H35.352 Cystoid macular degeneration, left eye
H35.353 Cystoid macular degeneration, bilateral
H35.359 Cystoid macular degeneration, unspecified eye

✓6th **H35.36 Drusen (degenerative) of macula**

AHA: 2017,1Q,51; 2016,4Q,21

H35.361 Drusen (degenerative) of macula, right eye
H35.362 Drusen (degenerative) of macula, left eye
H35.363 Drusen (degenerative) of macula, bilateral
H35.369 Drusen (degenerative) of macula, unspecified eye

✓6th **H35.37 Puckering of macula**

H35.371 Puckering of macula, right eye
H35.372 Puckering of macula, left eye
H35.373 Puckering of macula, bilateral
H35.379 Puckering of macula, unspecified eye

✓6th **H35.38 Toxic maculopathy**

Code first poisoning due to drug or toxin, if applicable (T36-T65 with fifth or sixth character 1-4 or 6)
Use additional code for adverse effect, if applicable, to identify drug (T36-T5Ø with fifth or sixth character 5)

H35.381 Toxic maculopathy, right eye
H35.382 Toxic maculopathy, left eye
H35.383 Toxic maculopathy, bilateral
H35.389 Toxic maculopathy, unspecified eye

✓5th **H35.4 Peripheral retinal degeneration**

EXCLUDES 1 *hereditary retinal degeneration (dystrophy) (H35.5-)*
peripheral retinal degeneration with retinal break (H33.3-)

H35.4Ø Unspecified peripheral retinal degeneration

✓6th **H35.41 Lattice degeneration of retina**

Palisade degeneration of retina
DEF: Degeneration of the retina, often bilateral, that is usually benign. It is characterized by lines intersecting at irregular intervals in the peripheral retina. Retinal thinning and retinal holes may occur.

H35.411 Lattice degeneration of retina, right eye
H35.412 Lattice degeneration of retina, left eye
H35.413 Lattice degeneration of retina, bilateral
H35.419 Lattice degeneration of retina, unspecified eye

✓6th **H35.42 Microcystoid degeneration of retina**

H35.421 Microcystoid degeneration of retina, right eye
H35.422 Microcystoid degeneration of retina, left eye
H35.423 Microcystoid degeneration of retina, bilateral
H35.429 Microcystoid degeneration of retina, unspecified eye

✓6th **H35.43 Paving stone degeneration of retina**

H35.431 Paving stone degeneration of retina, right eye
H35.432 Paving stone degeneration of retina, left eye
H35.433 Paving stone degeneration of retina, bilateral
H35.439 Paving stone degeneration of retina, unspecified eye

✓6th **H35.44 Age-related reticular degeneration of retina**

H35.441 Age-related reticular degeneration of retina, right eye A
H35.442 Age-related reticular degeneration of retina, left eye A
H35.443 Age-related reticular degeneration of retina, bilateral A
H35.449 Age-related reticular degeneration of retina, unspecified eye A

✓6th **H35.45 Secondary pigmentary degeneration**

H35.451 Secondary pigmentary degeneration, right eye
H35.452 Secondary pigmentary degeneration, left eye
H35.453 Secondary pigmentary degeneration, bilateral
H35.459 Secondary pigmentary degeneration, unspecified eye

✓6th **H35.46 Secondary vitreoretinal degeneration**

H35.461 Secondary vitreoretinal degeneration, right eye
H35.462 Secondary vitreoretinal degeneration, left eye
H35.463 Secondary vitreoretinal degeneration, bilateral
H35.469 Secondary vitreoretinal degeneration, unspecified eye

✓5th **H35.5 Hereditary retinal dystrophy**

EXCLUDES 1 *dystrophies primarily involving Bruch's membrane (H31.1-)*

H35.5Ø Unspecified hereditary retinal dystrophy
H35.51 Vitreoretinal dystrophy

H35.52 Pigmentary retinal dystrophy
Albipunctate retinal dystrophy
Retinitis pigmentosa
Tapetoretinal dystrophy
H35.53 Other dystrophies primarily involving the sensory retina
Stargardt's disease
H35.54 Dystrophies primarily involving the retinal pigment epithelium
Vitelliform retinal dystrophy

✓5th H35.6 Retinal hemorrhage
H35.60 Retinal hemorrhage, unspecified eye
H35.61 Retinal hemorrhage, right eye
H35.62 Retinal hemorrhage, left eye
H35.63 Retinal hemorrhage, bilateral

✓5th H35.7 Separation of retinal layers
EXCLUDES 1 *retinal detachment (serous) (H33.2-)*
rhegmatogenous retinal detachment (H33.Ø-)
H35.70 Unspecified separation of retinal layers CC
✓6th H35.71 Central serous chorioretinopathy
H35.711 Central serous chorioretinopathy, right eye
H35.712 Central serous chorioretinopathy, left eye
H35.713 Central serous chorioretinopathy, bilateral
H35.719 Central serous chorioretinopathy, unspecified eye
✓6th H35.72 Serous detachment of retinal pigment epithelium
H35.721 Serous detachment of retinal pigment epithelium, right eye CC
H35.722 Serous detachment of retinal pigment epithelium, left eye CC
H35.723 Serous detachment of retinal pigment epithelium, bilateral CC
H35.729 Serous detachment of retinal pigment epithelium, unspecified eye CC
✓6th H35.73 Hemorrhagic detachment of retinal pigment epithelium
H35.731 Hemorrhagic detachment of retinal pigment epithelium, right eye CC
H35.732 Hemorrhagic detachment of retinal pigment epithelium, left eye CC
H35.733 Hemorrhagic detachment of retinal pigment epithelium, bilateral CC
H35.739 Hemorrhagic detachment of retinal pigment epithelium, unspecified eye CC

✓5th H35.8 Other specified retinal disorders
EXCLUDES 2 *retinal hemorrhage (H35.6-)*
H35.81 Retinal edema
Retinal cotton wool spots
H35.82 Retinal ischemia CC
H35.89 Other specified retinal disorders
H35.9 Unspecified retinal disorder

H36 Retinal disorders in diseases classified elsewhere
Code first underlying disease, such as:
lipid storage disorders (E75.-)
sickle-cell disorders (D57.-)
EXCLUDES 1 *arteriosclerotic retinopathy (H35.Ø-)*
diabetic retinopathy (EØ8.3-, EØ9.3-, E1Ø.3-, E11.3-, E13.3-)

Glaucoma (H4Ø-H42)

✓4th **H4Ø Glaucoma**
EXCLUDES 1 *absolute glaucoma (H44.51-)*
congenital glaucoma (Q15.Ø)
traumatic glaucoma due to birth injury (P15.3)

Open Angle/Angle Closure Glaucoma

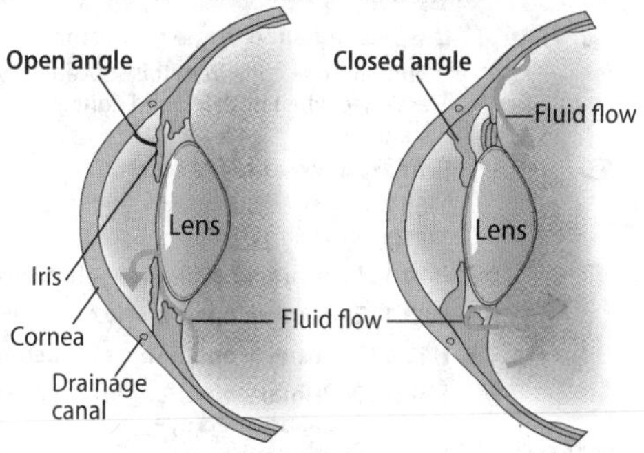

✓5th H4Ø.Ø Glaucoma suspect
✓6th H4Ø.ØØ Preglaucoma, unspecified
H4Ø.ØØ1 Preglaucoma, unspecified, right eye
H4Ø.ØØ2 Preglaucoma, unspecified, left eye
H4Ø.ØØ3 Preglaucoma, unspecified, bilateral
H4Ø.ØØ9 Preglaucoma, unspecified, unspecified eye
✓6th H4Ø.Ø1 Open angle with borderline findings, low risk
Open angle, low risk
H4Ø.Ø11 Open angle with borderline findings, low risk, right eye
H4Ø.Ø12 Open angle with borderline findings, low risk, left eye
H4Ø.Ø13 Open angle with borderline findings, low risk, bilateral
H4Ø.Ø19 Open angle with borderline findings, low risk, unspecified eye
✓6th H4Ø.Ø2 Open angle with borderline findings, high risk
Open angle, high risk
H4Ø.Ø21 Open angle with borderline findings, high risk, right eye
H4Ø.Ø22 Open angle with borderline findings, high risk, left eye
H4Ø.Ø23 Open angle with borderline findings, high risk, bilateral
H4Ø.Ø29 Open angle with borderline findings, high risk, unspecified eye
✓6th H4Ø.Ø3 Anatomical narrow angle
Primary angle closure suspect
H4Ø.Ø31 Anatomical narrow angle, right eye
H4Ø.Ø32 Anatomical narrow angle, left eye
H4Ø.Ø33 Anatomical narrow angle, bilateral
H4Ø.Ø39 Anatomical narrow angle, unspecified eye
✓6th H4Ø.Ø4 Steroid responder
H4Ø.Ø41 Steroid responder, right eye
H4Ø.Ø42 Steroid responder, left eye
H4Ø.Ø43 Steroid responder, bilateral
H4Ø.Ø49 Steroid responder, unspecified eye
✓6th H4Ø.Ø5 Ocular hypertension
H4Ø.Ø51 Ocular hypertension, right eye
H4Ø.Ø52 Ocular hypertension, left eye
H4Ø.Ø53 Ocular hypertension, bilateral
H4Ø.Ø59 Ocular hypertension, unspecified eye
✓6th H4Ø.Ø6 Primary angle closure without glaucoma damage
H4Ø.Ø61 Primary angle closure without glaucoma damage, right eye
H4Ø.Ø62 Primary angle closure without glaucoma damage, left eye
H4Ø.Ø63 Primary angle closure without glaucoma damage, bilateral
H4Ø.Ø69 Primary angle closure without glaucoma damage, unspecified eye

√5th **H40.1 Open-angle glaucoma**

One of the following 7th characters is to be assigned to each code in subcategories H40.10, H40.11, H40.12, H40.13, and H40.14 to designate the stage of glaucoma.
- 0 stage unspecified
- 1 mild stage
- 2 moderate stage
- 3 severe stage
- 4 indeterminate stage

√x7th **H40.10 Unspecified open-angle glaucoma**
TIP: Only one code from this subcategory should be assigned when both left and right eyes are the same stage.

√6th **H40.11 Primary open-angle glaucoma**
Chronic simple glaucoma
AHA: 2016,4Q,22

√7th **H40.111 Primary open-angle glaucoma, right eye**
√7th **H40.112 Primary open-angle glaucoma, left eye**
√7th **H40.113 Primary open-angle glaucoma, bilateral**
√7th **H40.119 Primary open-angle glaucoma, unspecified eye**

√6th **H40.12 Low-tension glaucoma**

√7th **H40.121 Low-tension glaucoma, right eye**
√7th **H40.122 Low-tension glaucoma, left eye**
√7th **H40.123 Low-tension glaucoma, bilateral**
√7th **H40.129 Low-tension glaucoma, unspecified eye**

√6th **H40.13 Pigmentary glaucoma**

√7th **H40.131 Pigmentary glaucoma, right eye**
√7th **H40.132 Pigmentary glaucoma, left eye**
√7th **H40.133 Pigmentary glaucoma, bilateral**
√7th **H40.139 Pigmentary glaucoma, unspecified eye**

√6th **H40.14 Capsular glaucoma with pseudoexfoliation of lens**

√7th **H40.141 Capsular glaucoma with pseudoexfoliation of lens, right eye**
√7th **H40.142 Capsular glaucoma with pseudoexfoliation of lens, left eye**
√7th **H40.143 Capsular glaucoma with pseudoexfoliation of lens, bilateral**
√7th **H40.149 Capsular glaucoma with pseudoexfoliation of lens, unspecified eye**

√6th **H40.15 Residual stage of open-angle glaucoma**

H40.151 Residual stage of open-angle glaucoma, right eye
H40.152 Residual stage of open-angle glaucoma, left eye
H40.153 Residual stage of open-angle glaucoma, bilateral
H40.159 Residual stage of open-angle glaucoma, unspecified eye

√5th **H40.2 Primary angle-closure glaucoma**

EXCLUDES 1 *aqueous misdirection (H40.83-)*
malignant glaucoma (H40.83-)

One of the following 7th characters is to be assigned to code H40.20 and H40.22- to designate the stage of glaucoma.
- 0 stage unspecified
- 1 mild stage
- 2 moderate stage
- 3 severe stage
- 4 indeterminate stage

√x7th **H40.20 Unspecified primary angle-closure glaucoma**
TIP: Only one code from this subcategory should be assigned when both left and right eyes are the same stage.

√6th **H40.21 Acute angle-closure glaucoma**
Acute angle-closure glaucoma attack
Acute angle-closure glaucoma crisis

H40.211 Acute angle-closure glaucoma, right eye CC
H40.212 Acute angle-closure glaucoma, left eye CC
H40.213 Acute angle-closure glaucoma, bilateral CC
H40.219 Acute angle-closure glaucoma, unspecified eye CC

√6th **H40.22 Chronic angle-closure glaucoma**
Chronic primary angle closure glaucoma

√7th **H40.221 Chronic angle-closure glaucoma, right eye**
√7th **H40.222 Chronic angle-closure glaucoma, left eye**
√7th **H40.223 Chronic angle-closure glaucoma, bilateral**
√7th **H40.229 Chronic angle-closure glaucoma, unspecified eye**

√6th **H40.23 Intermittent angle-closure glaucoma**

H40.231 Intermittent angle-closure glaucoma, right eye
H40.232 Intermittent angle-closure glaucoma, left eye
H40.233 Intermittent angle-closure glaucoma, bilateral
H40.239 Intermittent angle-closure glaucoma, unspecified eye

√6th **H40.24 Residual stage of angle-closure glaucoma**

H40.241 Residual stage of angle-closure glaucoma, right eye
H40.242 Residual stage of angle-closure glaucoma, left eye
H40.243 Residual stage of angle-closure glaucoma, bilateral
H40.249 Residual stage of angle-closure glaucoma, unspecified eye

√5th **H40.3 Glaucoma secondary to eye trauma**
Code also underlying condition

One of the following 7th characters is to be assigned to each code in subcategory H40.3- to designate the stage of glaucoma.
- 0 stage unspecified
- 1 mild stage
- 2 moderate stage
- 3 severe stage
- 4 indeterminate stage

√x7th **H40.30 Glaucoma secondary to eye trauma, unspecified eye**
√x7th **H40.31 Glaucoma secondary to eye trauma, right eye**
√x7th **H40.32 Glaucoma secondary to eye trauma, left eye**
√x7th **H40.33 Glaucoma secondary to eye trauma, bilateral**

√5th **H40.4 Glaucoma secondary to eye inflammation**
Code also underlying condition

One of the following 7th characters is to be assigned to each code in subcategory H40.4- to designate the stage of glaucoma.
- 0 stage unspecified
- 1 mild stage
- 2 moderate stage
- 3 severe stage
- 4 indeterminate stage

√x7th **H40.40 Glaucoma secondary to eye inflammation, unspecified eye**
√x7th **H40.41 Glaucoma secondary to eye inflammation, right eye**
√x7th **H40.42 Glaucoma secondary to eye inflammation, left eye**
√x7th **H40.43 Glaucoma secondary to eye inflammation, bilateral**

√5th **H40.5 Glaucoma secondary to other eye disorders**
Code also underlying eye disorder

One of the following 7th characters is to be assigned to each code in subcategory H40.5- to designate the stage of glaucoma.
- 0 stage unspecified
- 1 mild stage
- 2 moderate stage
- 3 severe stage
- 4 indeterminate stage

√x7th **H40.50 Glaucoma secondary to other eye disorders, unspecified eye**
√x7th **H40.51 Glaucoma secondary to other eye disorders, right eye**
√x7th **H40.52 Glaucoma secondary to other eye disorders, left eye**
√x7th **H40.53 Glaucoma secondary to other eye disorders, bilateral**

H40.6 Glaucoma secondary to drugs

Use additional code for adverse effect, if applicable, to identify drug (T36-T50 with fifth or sixth character 5)

One of the following 7th characters is to be assigned to each code in subcategory H40.6- to designate the stage of glaucoma
- 0 stage unspecified
- 1 mild stage
- 2 moderate stage
- 3 severe stage
- 4 indeterminate stage

H40.60 Glaucoma secondary to drugs, unspecified eye
H40.61 Glaucoma secondary to drugs, right eye
H40.62 Glaucoma secondary to drugs, left eye
H40.63 Glaucoma secondary to drugs, bilateral

H40.8 Other glaucoma

H40.81 Glaucoma with increased episcleral venous pressure
H40.811 Glaucoma with increased episcleral venous pressure, right eye
H40.812 Glaucoma with increased episcleral venous pressure, left eye
H40.813 Glaucoma with increased episcleral venous pressure, bilateral
H40.819 Glaucoma with increased episcleral venous pressure, unspecified eye

H40.82 Hypersecretion glaucoma
H40.821 Hypersecretion glaucoma, right eye
H40.822 Hypersecretion glaucoma, left eye
H40.823 Hypersecretion glaucoma, bilateral
H40.829 Hypersecretion glaucoma, unspecified eye

H40.83 Aqueous misdirection
Malignant glaucoma
H40.831 Aqueous misdirection, right eye
H40.832 Aqueous misdirection, left eye
H40.833 Aqueous misdirection, bilateral
H40.839 Aqueous misdirection, unspecified eye

H40.89 Other specified glaucoma

H40.9 Unspecified glaucoma

H42 Glaucoma in diseases classified elsewhere

Code first underlying condition, such as:
amyloidosis (E85.-)
aniridia (Q13.1)
glaucoma (in) diabetes mellitus (E08.39, E09.39, E10.39, E11.39, E13.39)
Lowe's syndrome (E72.03)
Reiger's anomaly (Q13.81)
specified metabolic disorder (E70-E88)

EXCLUDES 1 *glaucoma (in) onchocerciasis (B73.02)*
glaucoma (in) syphilis (A52.71)
glaucoma (in) tuberculous (A18.59)

Disorders of vitreous body and globe (H43-H44)

H43 Disorders of vitreous body

H43.0 Vitreous prolapse

EXCLUDES 1 *traumatic vitreous prolapse (S05.2-)*
vitreous syndrome following cataract surgery (H59.0-)

H43.00 Vitreous prolapse, unspecified eye
H43.01 Vitreous prolapse, right eye
H43.02 Vitreous prolapse, left eye
H43.03 Vitreous prolapse, bilateral

H43.1 Vitreous hemorrhage
H43.10 Vitreous hemorrhage, unspecified eye HCC
H43.11 Vitreous hemorrhage, right eye HCC
H43.12 Vitreous hemorrhage, left eye HCC
H43.13 Vitreous hemorrhage, bilateral HCC

H43.2 Crystalline deposits in vitreous body
H43.20 Crystalline deposits in vitreous body, unspecified eye
H43.21 Crystalline deposits in vitreous body, right eye
H43.22 Crystalline deposits in vitreous body, left eye
H43.23 Crystalline deposits in vitreous body, bilateral

H43.3 Other vitreous opacities

H43.31 Vitreous membranes and strands
H43.311 Vitreous membranes and strands, right eye
H43.312 Vitreous membranes and strands, left eye
H43.313 Vitreous membranes and strands, bilateral
H43.319 Vitreous membranes and strands, unspecified eye

H43.39 Other vitreous opacities
Vitreous floaters
H43.391 Other vitreous opacities, right eye
H43.392 Other vitreous opacities, left eye
H43.393 Other vitreous opacities, bilateral
H43.399 Other vitreous opacities, unspecified eye

H43.8 Other disorders of vitreous body

EXCLUDES 1 *proliferative vitreo-retinopathy with retinal detachment (H33.4-)*
EXCLUDES 2 *vitreous abscess (H44.02-)*

H43.81 Vitreous degeneration
Vitreous detachment
H43.811 Vitreous degeneration, right eye
H43.812 Vitreous degeneration, left eye
H43.813 Vitreous degeneration, bilateral
H43.819 Vitreous degeneration, unspecified eye

H43.82 Vitreomacular adhesion
Vitreomacular traction
H43.821 Vitreomacular adhesion, right eye A
H43.822 Vitreomacular adhesion, left eye A
H43.823 Vitreomacular adhesion, bilateral A
H43.829 Vitreomacular adhesion, unspecified eye A

H43.89 Other disorders of vitreous body

H43.9 Unspecified disorder of vitreous body

H44 Disorders of globe

INCLUDES disorders affecting multiple structures of eye

H44.0 Purulent endophthalmitis

Use additional code to identify organism

EXCLUDES 1 *bleb associated endophthalmitis (H59.4-)*

H44.00 Unspecified purulent endophthalmitis
H44.001 Unspecified purulent endophthalmitis, right eye CC
H44.002 Unspecified purulent endophthalmitis, left eye CC
H44.003 Unspecified purulent endophthalmitis, bilateral CC
H44.009 Unspecified purulent endophthalmitis, unspecified eye CC

H44.01 Panophthalmitis (acute)
H44.011 Panophthalmitis (acute), right eye CC
H44.012 Panophthalmitis (acute), left eye CC
H44.013 Panophthalmitis (acute), bilateral CC
H44.019 Panophthalmitis (acute), unspecified eye CC

H44.02 Vitreous abscess (chronic)
H44.021 Vitreous abscess (chronic), right eye CC
H44.022 Vitreous abscess (chronic), left eye CC
H44.023 Vitreous abscess (chronic), bilateral CC
H44.029 Vitreous abscess (chronic), unspecified eye CC

H44.1 Other endophthalmitis

EXCLUDES 1 *bleb associated endophthalmitis (H59.4-)*
EXCLUDES 2 *ophthalmia nodosa (H16.2-)*

H44.11 Panuveitis

DEF: Inflammation of all layers of the uvea of the eye, including the choroid, iris, and ciliary body. It also typically involves the lens, retina, optic nerve, and vitreous and causes reduced vision or blindness.

H44.111 Panuveitis, right eye CC
H44.112 Panuveitis, left eye CC
H44.113 Panuveitis, bilateral CC
H44.119 Panuveitis, unspecified eye CC

√6th H44.12 Parasitic endophthalmitis, unspecified
- H44.121 Parasitic endophthalmitis, unspecified, right eye CC
- H44.122 Parasitic endophthalmitis, unspecified, left eye CC
- H44.123 Parasitic endophthalmitis, unspecified, bilateral CC
- H44.129 Parasitic endophthalmitis, unspecified, unspecified eye CC

√6th H44.13 Sympathetic uveitis
- H44.131 Sympathetic uveitis, right eye CC
- H44.132 Sympathetic uveitis, left eye CC
- H44.133 Sympathetic uveitis, bilateral CC
- H44.139 Sympathetic uveitis, unspecified eye CC

H44.19 Other endophthalmitis CC

√5th H44.2 Degenerative myopia

Malignant myopia

AHA: 2017,4Q,10-11

- H44.2Ø Degenerative myopia, unspecified eye
- H44.21 Degenerative myopia, right eye
- H44.22 Degenerative myopia, left eye
- H44.23 Degenerative myopia, bilateral

√6th H44.2A Degenerative myopia with choroidal neovascularization

Use additional code for any associated choroid disorders (H31.-)

- H44.2A1 Degenerative myopia with choroidal neovascularization, right eye
- H44.2A2 Degenerative myopia with choroidal neovascularization, left eye
- H44.2A3 Degenerative myopia with choroidal neovascularization, bilateral eye
- H44.2A9 Degenerative myopia with choroidal neovascularization, unspecified eye

√6th H44.2B Degenerative myopia with macular hole
- H44.2B1 Degenerative myopia with macular hole, right eye
- H44.2B2 Degenerative myopia with macular hole, left eye
- H44.2B3 Degenerative myopia with macular hole, bilateral eye
- H44.2B9 Degenerative myopia with macular hole, unspecified eye

√6th H44.2C Degenerative myopia with retinal detachment

Use additional code to identify the retinal detachment (H33.-)

- H44.2C1 Degenerative myopia with retinal detachment, right eye
- H44.2C2 Degenerative myopia with retinal detachment, left eye
- H44.2C3 Degenerative myopia with retinal detachment, bilateral eye
- H44.2C9 Degenerative myopia with retinal detachment, unspecified eye

√6th H44.2D Degenerative myopia with foveoschisis
- H44.2D1 Degenerative myopia with foveoschisis, right eye
- H44.2D2 Degenerative myopia with foveoschisis, left eye
- H44.2D3 Degenerative myopia with foveoschisis, bilateral eye
- H44.2D9 Degenerative myopia with foveoschisis, unspecified eye

√6th H44.2E Degenerative myopia with other maculopathy
- H44.2E1 Degenerative myopia with other maculopathy, right eye
- H44.2E2 Degenerative myopia with other maculopathy, left eye
- H44.2E3 Degenerative myopia with other maculopathy, bilateral eye
- H44.2E9 Degenerative myopia with other maculopathy, unspecified eye

√5th H44.3 Other and unspecified degenerative disorders of globe

H44.3Ø Unspecified degenerative disorder of globe

√6th H44.31 Chalcosis
- H44.311 Chalcosis, right eye
- H44.312 Chalcosis, left eye
- H44.313 Chalcosis, bilateral
- H44.319 Chalcosis, unspecified eye

√6th H44.32 Siderosis of eye

DEF: Iron pigment deposits within tissue of the eyeball caused by high iron content of the blood. Symptoms include cataracts, rust-colored anterior subcapsular deposits, iris heterochromia, pupillary mydriasis, and depressed electroretinogram amplitudes.

- H44.321 Siderosis of eye, right eye
- H44.322 Siderosis of eye, left eye
- H44.323 Siderosis of eye, bilateral
- H44.329 Siderosis of eye, unspecified eye

√6th H44.39 Other degenerative disorders of globe
- H44.391 Other degenerative disorders of globe, right eye
- H44.392 Other degenerative disorders of globe, left eye
- H44.393 Other degenerative disorders of globe, bilateral
- H44.399 Other degenerative disorders of globe, unspecified eye

√5th H44.4 Hypotony of eye

H44.4Ø Unspecified hypotony of eye

√6th H44.41 Flat anterior chamber hypotony of eye
- H44.411 Flat anterior chamber hypotony of right eye
- H44.412 Flat anterior chamber hypotony of left eye
- H44.413 Flat anterior chamber hypotony of eye, bilateral
- H44.419 Flat anterior chamber hypotony of unspecified eye

√6th H44.42 Hypotony of eye due to ocular fistula
- H44.421 Hypotony of right eye due to ocular fistula
- H44.422 Hypotony of left eye due to ocular fistula
- H44.423 Hypotony of eye due to ocular fistula, bilateral
- H44.429 Hypotony of unspecified eye due to ocular fistula

√6th H44.43 Hypotony of eye due to other ocular disorders
- H44.431 Hypotony of eye due to other ocular disorders, right eye
- H44.432 Hypotony of eye due to other ocular disorders, left eye
- H44.433 Hypotony of eye due to other ocular disorders, bilateral
- H44.439 Hypotony of eye due to other ocular disorders, unspecified eye

√6th H44.44 Primary hypotony of eye
- H44.441 Primary hypotony of right eye
- H44.442 Primary hypotony of left eye
- H44.443 Primary hypotony of eye, bilateral
- H44.449 Primary hypotony of unspecified eye

√5th H44.5 Degenerated conditions of globe

H44.5Ø Unspecified degenerated conditions of globe

√6th H44.51 Absolute glaucoma
- H44.511 Absolute glaucoma, right eye
- H44.512 Absolute glaucoma, left eye
- H44.513 Absolute glaucoma, bilateral
- H44.519 Absolute glaucoma, unspecified eye

√6th H44.52 Atrophy of globe

Phthisis bulbi

- H44.521 Atrophy of globe, right eye
- H44.522 Atrophy of globe, left eye
- H44.523 Atrophy of globe, bilateral
- H44.529 Atrophy of globe, unspecified eye

√6th H44.53 Leucocoria
- H44.531 Leucocoria, right eye
- H44.532 Leucocoria, left eye
- H44.533 Leucocoria, bilateral
- H44.539 Leucocoria, unspecified eye

H44.6 Retained (old) intraocular foreign body, magnetic

Use additional code to identify magnetic foreign body (Z18.11)

EXCLUDES 1 *current intraocular foreign body (SØ5.-)*

EXCLUDES 2 *retained foreign body in eyelid (HØ2.81-)*
retained (old) foreign body following penetrating wound of orbit (HØ5.5-)
retained (old) intraocular foreign body, nonmagnetic (H44.7-)

H44.6Ø Unspecified retained (old) intraocular foreign body, magnetic
- **H44.6Ø1 Unspecified retained (old) intraocular foreign body, magnetic, right eye**
- **H44.6Ø2 Unspecified retained (old) intraocular foreign body, magnetic, left eye**
- **H44.6Ø3 Unspecified retained (old) intraocular foreign body, magnetic, bilateral**
- **H44.6Ø9 Unspecified retained (old) intraocular foreign body, magnetic, unspecified eye**

H44.61 Retained (old) magnetic foreign body in anterior chamber
- **H44.611 Retained (old) magnetic foreign body in anterior chamber, right eye**
- **H44.612 Retained (old) magnetic foreign body in anterior chamber, left eye**
- **H44.613 Retained (old) magnetic foreign body in anterior chamber, bilateral**
- **H44.619 Retained (old) magnetic foreign body in anterior chamber, unspecified eye**

H44.62 Retained (old) magnetic foreign body in iris or ciliary body
- **H44.621 Retained (old) magnetic foreign body in iris or ciliary body, right eye**
- **H44.622 Retained (old) magnetic foreign body in iris or ciliary body, left eye**
- **H44.623 Retained (old) magnetic foreign body in iris or ciliary body, bilateral**
- **H44.629 Retained (old) magnetic foreign body in iris or ciliary body, unspecified eye**

H44.63 Retained (old) magnetic foreign body in lens
- **H44.631 Retained (old) magnetic foreign body in lens, right eye**
- **H44.632 Retained (old) magnetic foreign body in lens, left eye**
- **H44.633 Retained (old) magnetic foreign body in lens, bilateral**
- **H44.639 Retained (old) magnetic foreign body in lens, unspecified eye**

H44.64 Retained (old) magnetic foreign body in posterior wall of globe
- **H44.641 Retained (old) magnetic foreign body in posterior wall of globe, right eye**
- **H44.642 Retained (old) magnetic foreign body in posterior wall of globe, left eye**
- **H44.643 Retained (old) magnetic foreign body in posterior wall of globe, bilateral**
- **H44.649 Retained (old) magnetic foreign body in posterior wall of globe, unspecified eye**

H44.65 Retained (old) magnetic foreign body in vitreous body
- **H44.651 Retained (old) magnetic foreign body in vitreous body, right eye**
- **H44.652 Retained (old) magnetic foreign body in vitreous body, left eye**
- **H44.653 Retained (old) magnetic foreign body in vitreous body, bilateral**
- **H44.659 Retained (old) magnetic foreign body in vitreous body, unspecified eye**

H44.69 Retained (old) intraocular foreign body, magnetic, in other or multiple sites
- **H44.691 Retained (old) intraocular foreign body, magnetic, in other or multiple sites, right eye**
- **H44.692 Retained (old) intraocular foreign body, magnetic, in other or multiple sites, left eye**
- **H44.693 Retained (old) intraocular foreign body, magnetic, in other or multiple sites, bilateral**
- **H44.699 Retained (old) intraocular foreign body, magnetic, in other or multiple sites, unspecified eye**

H44.7 Retained (old) intraocular foreign body, nonmagnetic

Use additional code to identify nonmagnetic foreign body (Z18.Ø1-Z18.1Ø, Z18.12, Z18.2-Z18.9)

EXCLUDES 1 *current intraocular foreign body (SØ5.-)*

EXCLUDES 2 *retained foreign body in eyelid (HØ2.81-)*
retained (old) foreign body following penetrating wound of orbit (HØ5.5-)
retained (old) intraocular foreign body, magnetic (H44.6-)

H44.7Ø Unspecified retained (old) intraocular foreign body, nonmagnetic
- **H44.7Ø1 Unspecified retained (old) intraocular foreign body, nonmagnetic, right eye**
- **H44.7Ø2 Unspecified retained (old) intraocular foreign body, nonmagnetic, left eye**
- **H44.7Ø3 Unspecified retained (old) intraocular foreign body, nonmagnetic, bilateral**
- **H44.7Ø9 Unspecified retained (old) intraocular foreign body, nonmagnetic, unspecified eye**
  Retained (old) intraocular foreign body NOS

H44.71 Retained (nonmagnetic) (old) foreign body in anterior chamber
- **H44.711 Retained (nonmagnetic) (old) foreign body in anterior chamber, right eye**
- **H44.712 Retained (nonmagnetic) (old) foreign body in anterior chamber, left eye**
- **H44.713 Retained (nonmagnetic) (old) foreign body in anterior chamber, bilateral**
- **H44.719 Retained (nonmagnetic) (old) foreign body in anterior chamber, unspecified eye**

H44.72 Retained (nonmagnetic) (old) foreign body in iris or ciliary body
- **H44.721 Retained (nonmagnetic) (old) foreign body in iris or ciliary body, right eye**
- **H44.722 Retained (nonmagnetic) (old) foreign body in iris or ciliary body, left eye**
- **H44.723 Retained (nonmagnetic) (old) foreign body in iris or ciliary body, bilateral**
- **H44.729 Retained (nonmagnetic) (old) foreign body in iris or ciliary body, unspecified eye**

H44.73 Retained (nonmagnetic) (old) foreign body in lens
- **H44.731 Retained (nonmagnetic) (old) foreign body in lens, right eye**
- **H44.732 Retained (nonmagnetic) (old) foreign body in lens, left eye**
- **H44.733 Retained (nonmagnetic) (old) foreign body in lens, bilateral**
- **H44.739 Retained (nonmagnetic) (old) foreign body in lens, unspecified eye**

H44.74 Retained (nonmagnetic) (old) foreign body in posterior wall of globe
- **H44.741 Retained (nonmagnetic) (old) foreign body in posterior wall of globe, right eye**
- **H44.742 Retained (nonmagnetic) (old) foreign body in posterior wall of globe, left eye**
- **H44.743 Retained (nonmagnetic) (old) foreign body in posterior wall of globe, bilateral**
- **H44.749 Retained (nonmagnetic) (old) foreign body in posterior wall of globe, unspecified eye**

H44.75 Retained (nonmagnetic) (old) foreign body in vitreous body
- **H44.751 Retained (nonmagnetic) (old) foreign body in vitreous body, right eye**
- **H44.752 Retained (nonmagnetic) (old) foreign body in vitreous body, left eye**
- **H44.753 Retained (nonmagnetic) (old) foreign body in vitreous body, bilateral**
- **H44.759 Retained (nonmagnetic) (old) foreign body in vitreous body, unspecified eye**

H44.79 Retained (old) intraocular foreign body, nonmagnetic, in other or multiple sites
- **H44.791 Retained (old) intraocular foreign body, nonmagnetic, in other or multiple sites, right eye**
- **H44.792 Retained (old) intraocular foreign body, nonmagnetic, in other or multiple sites, left eye**

H44.793 Retained (old) intraocular foreign body, nonmagnetic, in other or multiple sites, bilateral
H44.799 Retained (old) intraocular foreign body, nonmagnetic, in other or multiple sites, unspecified eye

√5th H44.8 Other disorders of globe
√6th H44.81 Hemophthalmos
DEF: Pool of blood within the eyeball, not from a current injury.
H44.811 Hemophthalmos, right eye
H44.812 Hemophthalmos, left eye
H44.813 Hemophthalmos, bilateral
H44.819 Hemophthalmos, unspecified eye
√6th H44.82 Luxation of globe
H44.821 Luxation of globe, right eye
H44.822 Luxation of globe, left eye
H44.823 Luxation of globe, bilateral
H44.829 Luxation of globe, unspecified eye
H44.89 Other disorders of globe
H44.9 Unspecified disorder of globe

Disorders of optic nerve and visual pathways (H46-H47)

√4th **H46 Optic neuritis**
EXCLUDES 2 *ischemic optic neuropathy (H47.Ø1-)*
neuromyelitis optica [Devic] (G36.Ø)
√5th H46.Ø Optic papillitis
H46.ØØ Optic papillitis, unspecified eye CC
H46.Ø1 Optic papillitis, right eye CC
H46.Ø2 Optic papillitis, left eye CC
H46.Ø3 Optic papillitis, bilateral CC
√5th H46.1 Retrobulbar neuritis
Retrobulbar neuritis NOS
EXCLUDES 1 *syphilitic retrobulbar neuritis (A52.15)*
H46.1Ø Retrobulbar neuritis, unspecified eye CC
H46.11 Retrobulbar neuritis, right eye CC
H46.12 Retrobulbar neuritis, left eye CC
H46.13 Retrobulbar neuritis, bilateral CC
H46.2 Nutritional optic neuropathy
H46.3 Toxic optic neuropathy
Code first (T51-T65) to identify cause
H46.8 Other optic neuritis CC
H46.9 Unspecified optic neuritis CC

√4th **H47 Other disorders of optic [2nd] nerve and visual pathways**
√5th H47.Ø Disorders of optic nerve, not elsewhere classified
√6th H47.Ø1 Ischemic optic neuropathy
H47.Ø11 Ischemic optic neuropathy, right eye
H47.Ø12 Ischemic optic neuropathy, left eye
H47.Ø13 Ischemic optic neuropathy, bilateral
H47.Ø19 Ischemic optic neuropathy, unspecified eye
√6th H47.Ø2 Hemorrhage in optic nerve sheath
H47.Ø21 Hemorrhage in optic nerve sheath, right eye
H47.Ø22 Hemorrhage in optic nerve sheath, left eye
H47.Ø23 Hemorrhage in optic nerve sheath, bilateral
H47.Ø29 Hemorrhage in optic nerve sheath, unspecified eye
√6th H47.Ø3 Optic nerve hypoplasia
H47.Ø31 Optic nerve hypoplasia, right eye
H47.Ø32 Optic nerve hypoplasia, left eye
H47.Ø33 Optic nerve hypoplasia, bilateral
H47.Ø39 Optic nerve hypoplasia, unspecified eye
√6th H47.Ø9 Other disorders of optic nerve, not elsewhere classified
Compression of optic nerve
H47.Ø91 Other disorders of optic nerve, not elsewhere classified, right eye
H47.Ø92 Other disorders of optic nerve, not elsewhere classified, left eye
H47.Ø93 Other disorders of optic nerve, not elsewhere classified, bilateral
H47.Ø99 Other disorders of optic nerve, not elsewhere classified, unspecified eye

√5th H47.1 Papilledema
DEF: Swelling of the optic papilla, the raised area connected to the optic disk made up of nerves that enter the eyeball. It may be caused by increased intracranial pressure, decreased ocular pressure, or a retinal disorder.
H47.1Ø Unspecified papilledema CC
H47.11 Papilledema associated with increased intracranial pressure CC
H47.12 Papilledema associated with decreased ocular pressure
H47.13 Papilledema associated with retinal disorder
√6th H47.14 Foster-Kennedy syndrome
H47.141 Foster-Kennedy syndrome, right eye
H47.142 Foster-Kennedy syndrome, left eye
H47.143 Foster-Kennedy syndrome, bilateral
H47.149 Foster-Kennedy syndrome, unspecified eye
√5th H47.2 Optic atrophy
H47.2Ø Unspecified optic atrophy
√6th H47.21 Primary optic atrophy
H47.211 Primary optic atrophy, right eye
H47.212 Primary optic atrophy, left eye
H47.213 Primary optic atrophy, bilateral
H47.219 Primary optic atrophy, unspecified eye
H47.22 Hereditary optic atrophy
Leber's optic atrophy
√6th H47.23 Glaucomatous optic atrophy
H47.231 Glaucomatous optic atrophy, right eye
H47.232 Glaucomatous optic atrophy, left eye
H47.233 Glaucomatous optic atrophy, bilateral
H47.239 Glaucomatous optic atrophy, unspecified eye
√6th H47.29 Other optic atrophy
Temporal pallor of optic disc
H47.291 Other optic atrophy, right eye
H47.292 Other optic atrophy, left eye
H47.293 Other optic atrophy, bilateral
H47.299 Other optic atrophy, unspecified eye
√5th H47.3 Other disorders of optic disc
√6th H47.31 Coloboma of optic disc
H47.311 Coloboma of optic disc, right eye
H47.312 Coloboma of optic disc, left eye
H47.313 Coloboma of optic disc, bilateral
H47.319 Coloboma of optic disc, unspecified eye
√6th H47.32 Drusen of optic disc
H47.321 Drusen of optic disc, right eye
H47.322 Drusen of optic disc, left eye
H47.323 Drusen of optic disc, bilateral
H47.329 Drusen of optic disc, unspecified eye
√6th H47.33 Pseudopapilledema of optic disc
H47.331 Pseudopapilledema of optic disc, right eye
H47.332 Pseudopapilledema of optic disc, left eye
H47.333 Pseudopapilledema of optic disc, bilateral
H47.339 Pseudopapilledema of optic disc, unspecified eye
√6th H47.39 Other disorders of optic disc
H47.391 Other disorders of optic disc, right eye
H47.392 Other disorders of optic disc, left eye
H47.393 Other disorders of optic disc, bilateral
H47.399 Other disorders of optic disc, unspecified eye
√5th H47.4 Disorders of optic chiasm
Code also underlying condition
H47.41 Disorders of optic chiasm in (due to) inflammatory disorders CC
H47.42 Disorders of optic chiasm in (due to) neoplasm CC
H47.43 Disorders of optic chiasm in (due to) vascular disorders CC
H47.49 Disorders of optic chiasm in (due to) other disorders CC

H47.5 Disorders of other visual pathways

Disorders of optic tracts, geniculate nuclei and optic radiations
Code also underlying condition

H47.51 Disorders of visual pathways in (due to) inflammatory disorders

H47.511 Disorders of visual pathways in (due to) inflammatory disorders, right side CC
H47.512 Disorders of visual pathways in (due to) inflammatory disorders, left side CC
H47.519 Disorders of visual pathways in (due to) inflammatory disorders, unspecified side CC

H47.52 Disorders of visual pathways in (due to) neoplasm

H47.521 Disorders of visual pathways in (due to) neoplasm, right side CC
H47.522 Disorders of visual pathways in (due to) neoplasm, left side CC
H47.529 Disorders of visual pathways in (due to) neoplasm, unspecified side CC

H47.53 Disorders of visual pathways in (due to) vascular disorders

H47.531 Disorders of visual pathways in (due to) vascular disorders, right side CC
H47.532 Disorders of visual pathways in (due to) vascular disorders, left side CC
H47.539 Disorders of visual pathways in (due to) vascular disorders, unspecified side CC

H47.6 Disorders of visual cortex

Code also underlying condition
EXCLUDES 1 *injury to visual cortex S04.04-*

H47.61 Cortical blindness

H47.611 Cortical blindness, right side of brain
H47.612 Cortical blindness, left side of brain
H47.619 Cortical blindness, unspecified side of brain

H47.62 Disorders of visual cortex in (due to) inflammatory disorders

H47.621 Disorders of visual cortex in (due to) inflammatory disorders, right side of brain CC
H47.622 Disorders of visual cortex in (due to) inflammatory disorders, left side of brain CC
H47.629 Disorders of visual cortex in (due to) inflammatory disorders, unspecified side of brain CC

H47.63 Disorders of visual cortex in (due to) neoplasm

H47.631 Disorders of visual cortex in (due to) neoplasm, right side of brain CC
H47.632 Disorders of visual cortex in (due to) neoplasm, left side of brain CC
H47.639 Disorders of visual cortex in (due to) neoplasm, unspecified side of brain CC

H47.64 Disorders of visual cortex in (due to) vascular disorders

H47.641 Disorders of visual cortex in (due to) vascular disorders, right side of brain CC
H47.642 Disorders of visual cortex in (due to) vascular disorders, left side of brain CC
H47.649 Disorders of visual cortex in (due to) vascular disorders, unspecified side of brain CC

H47.9 Unspecified disorder of visual pathways

Disorders of ocular muscles, binocular movement, accommodation and refraction (H49-H52)

EXCLUDES 2 *nystagmus and other irregular eye movements (H55)*

H49 Paralytic strabismus

EXCLUDES 2 *internal ophthalmoplegia (H52.51-)*
internuclear ophthalmoplegia (H51.2-)
progressive supranuclear ophthalmoplegia (G23.1)

DEF: Strabismus: Misalignment of the eyes with the inability to move and focus in the same direction due to conditions affecting the muscles controlling them.

H49.0 Third [oculomotor] nerve palsy

H49.00 Third [oculomotor] nerve palsy, unspecified eye
H49.01 Third [oculomotor] nerve palsy, right eye
H49.02 Third [oculomotor] nerve palsy, left eye
H49.03 Third [oculomotor] nerve palsy, bilateral

H49.1 Fourth [trochlear] nerve palsy

H49.10 Fourth [trochlear] nerve palsy, unspecified eye
H49.11 Fourth [trochlear] nerve palsy, right eye
H49.12 Fourth [trochlear] nerve palsy, left eye
H49.13 Fourth [trochlear] nerve palsy, bilateral

H49.2 Sixth [abducent] nerve palsy

H49.20 Sixth [abducent] nerve palsy, unspecified eye
H49.21 Sixth [abducent] nerve palsy, right eye
H49.22 Sixth [abducent] nerve palsy, left eye
H49.23 Sixth [abducent] nerve palsy, bilateral

H49.3 Total (external) ophthalmoplegia

H49.30 Total (external) ophthalmoplegia, unspecified eye
H49.31 Total (external) ophthalmoplegia, right eye
H49.32 Total (external) ophthalmoplegia, left eye
H49.33 Total (external) ophthalmoplegia, bilateral

H49.4 Progressive external ophthalmoplegia

EXCLUDES 1 *Kearns-Sayre syndrome (H49.81-)*

H49.40 Progressive external ophthalmoplegia, unspecified eye
H49.41 Progressive external ophthalmoplegia, right eye
H49.42 Progressive external ophthalmoplegia, left eye
H49.43 Progressive external ophthalmoplegia, bilateral

H49.8 Other paralytic strabismus

H49.81 Kearns-Sayre syndrome

Progressive external ophthalmoplegia with pigmentary retinopathy
Use additional code for other manifestation, such as: heart block (I45.9)

H49.811 Kearns-Sayre syndrome, right eye CC HCC
H49.812 Kearns-Sayre syndrome, left eye CC HCC
H49.813 Kearns-Sayre syndrome, bilateral CC HCC
H49.819 Kearns-Sayre syndrome, unspecified eye CC HCC

H49.88 Other paralytic strabismus

External ophthalmoplegia NOS

H49.881 Other paralytic strabismus, right eye
H49.882 Other paralytic strabismus, left eye
H49.883 Other paralytic strabismus, bilateral
H49.889 Other paralytic strabismus, unspecified eye

H49.9 Unspecified paralytic strabismus

H50 Other strabismus

DEF: Strabismus: Misalignment of the eyes with the inability to move and focus in the same direction due to conditions affecting the muscles controlling them.

H50.0 Esotropia

Convergent concomitant strabismus
EXCLUDES 1 *intermittent esotropia (H50.31-, H50.32)*

H50.00 Unspecified esotropia

H50.01 Monocular esotropia

H50.011 Monocular esotropia, right eye
H50.012 Monocular esotropia, left eye

H50.02 Monocular esotropia with A pattern

H50.021 Monocular esotropia with A pattern, right eye

H50.022 Monocular esotropia with A pattern, left eye

✓6th H50.03 Monocular esotropia with V pattern

H50.031 Monocular esotropia with V pattern, right eye

H50.032 Monocular esotropia with V pattern, left eye

✓6th H50.04 Monocular esotropia with other noncomitancies

H50.041 Monocular esotropia with other noncomitancies, right eye

H50.042 Monocular esotropia with other noncomitancies, left eye

H50.05 Alternating esotropia

H50.06 Alternating esotropia with A pattern

H50.07 Alternating esotropia with V pattern

H50.08 Alternating esotropia with other noncomitancies

Eye Muscle Diseases

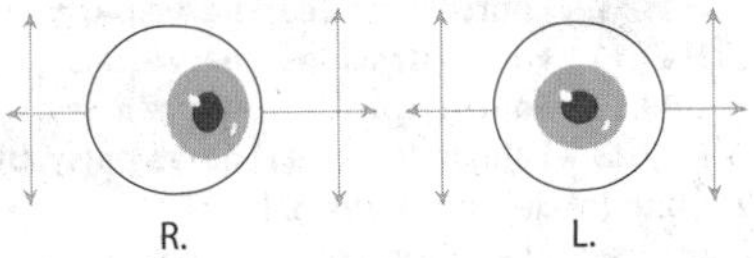

Monocular (one eye only) esotropia (inward)

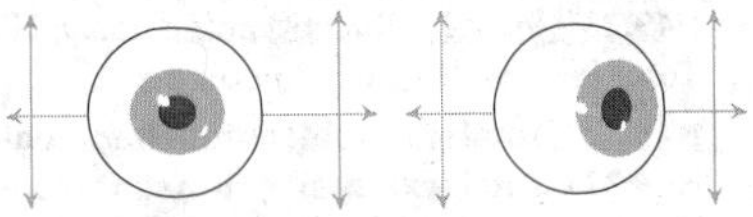

Monocular exotropia (outward)

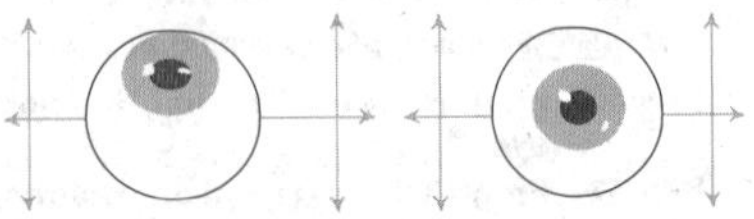

Monocular hypertropia (upward)

✓5th H50.1 Exotropia

Divergent concomitant strabismus

EXCLUDES 1 *intermittent exotropia (H50.33-, H50.34)*

H50.10 Unspecified exotropia

✓6th H50.11 Monocular exotropia

H50.111 Monocular exotropia, right eye

H50.112 Monocular exotropia, left eye

✓6th H50.12 Monocular exotropia with A pattern

H50.121 Monocular exotropia with A pattern, right eye

H50.122 Monocular exotropia with A pattern, left eye

✓6th H50.13 Monocular exotropia with V pattern

H50.131 Monocular exotropia with V pattern, right eye

H50.132 Monocular exotropia with V pattern, left eye

✓6th H50.14 Monocular exotropia with other noncomitancies

H50.141 Monocular exotropia with other noncomitancies, right eye

H50.142 Monocular exotropia with other noncomitancies, left eye

H50.15 Alternating exotropia

H50.16 Alternating exotropia with A pattern

H50.17 Alternating exotropia with V pattern

H50.18 Alternating exotropia with other noncomitancies

✓5th H50.2 Vertical strabismus

Hypertropia

H50.21 Vertical strabismus, right eye

H50.22 Vertical strabismus, left eye

✓5th H50.3 Intermittent heterotropia

H50.30 Unspecified intermittent heterotropia

✓6th H50.31 Intermittent monocular esotropia

H50.311 Intermittent monocular esotropia, right eye

H50.312 Intermittent monocular esotropia, left eye

H50.32 Intermittent alternating esotropia

✓6th H50.33 Intermittent monocular exotropia

H50.331 Intermittent monocular exotropia, right eye

H50.332 Intermittent monocular exotropia, left eye

H50.34 Intermittent alternating exotropia

✓5th H50.4 Other and unspecified heterotropia

H50.40 Unspecified heterotropia

✓6th H50.41 Cyclotropia

H50.411 Cyclotropia, right eye

H50.412 Cyclotropia, left eye

H50.42 Monofixation syndrome

H50.43 Accommodative component in esotropia

✓5th H50.5 Heterophoria

H50.50 Unspecified heterophoria

H50.51 Esophoria

H50.52 Exophoria

H50.53 Vertical heterophoria

H50.54 Cyclophoria

H50.55 Alternating heterophoria

✓5th H50.6 Mechanical strabismus

H50.60 Mechanical strabismus, unspecified

✓6th H50.61 Brown's sheath syndrome

H50.611 Brown's sheath syndrome, right eye

H50.612 Brown's sheath syndrome, left eye

H50.69 Other mechanical strabismus

Strabismus due to adhesions

Traumatic limitation of duction of eye muscle

✓5th H50.8 Other specified strabismus

✓6th H50.81 Duane's syndrome

H50.811 Duane's syndrome, right eye

H50.812 Duane's syndrome, left eye

H50.89 Other specified strabismus

H50.9 Unspecified strabismus

✓4th **H51 Other disorders of binocular movement**

H51.0 Palsy (spasm) of conjugate gaze

✓5th H51.1 Convergence insufficiency and excess

H51.11 Convergence insufficiency

H51.12 Convergence excess

✓5th H51.2 Internuclear ophthalmoplegia

H51.20 Internuclear ophthalmoplegia, unspecified eye

H51.21 Internuclear ophthalmoplegia, right eye

H51.22 Internuclear ophthalmoplegia, left eye

H51.23 Internuclear ophthalmoplegia, bilateral

H51.8 Other specified disorders of binocular movement

H51.9 Unspecified disorder of binocular movement

✓4th **H52 Disorders of refraction and accommodation**

✓5th H52.0 Hypermetropia

H52.00 Hypermetropia, unspecified eye

H52.01 Hypermetropia, right eye

H52.02 Hypermetropia, left eye

H52.03 Hypermetropia, bilateral

✓5th H52.1 Myopia

EXCLUDES 1 *degenerative myopia (H44.2-)*

H52.10 Myopia, unspecified eye

H52.11 Myopia, right eye

H52.12 Myopia, left eye

H52.13 Myopia, bilateral

✓5th H52.2 Astigmatism

✓6th H52.20 Unspecified astigmatism

H52.201 Unspecified astigmatism, right eye

H52.202 Unspecified astigmatism, left eye

H52.203 Unspecified astigmatism, bilateral

H52.209 Unspecified astigmatism, unspecified eye

✓6th H52.21 Irregular astigmatism

H52.211 Irregular astigmatism, right eye

H52.212 Irregular astigmatism, left eye

H52.213 Irregular astigmatism, bilateral

H52.219 Irregular astigmatism, unspecified eye

✓6th **H52.22 Regular astigmatism**
- **H52.221 Regular astigmatism, right eye**
- **H52.222 Regular astigmatism, left eye**
- **H52.223 Regular astigmatism, bilateral**
- **H52.229 Regular astigmatism, unspecified eye**

✓5th **H52.3 Anisometropia and aniseikonia**
- **H52.31 Anisometropia**
- **H52.32 Aniseikonia**

H52.4 Presbyopia

✓5th **H52.5 Disorders of accommodation**

✓6th **H52.51 Internal ophthalmoplegia (complete) (total)**
- **H52.511 Internal ophthalmoplegia (complete) (total), right eye**
- **H52.512 Internal ophthalmoplegia (complete) (total), left eye**
- **H52.513 Internal ophthalmoplegia (complete) (total), bilateral**
- **H52.519 Internal ophthalmoplegia (complete) (total), unspecified eye**

✓6th **H52.52 Paresis of accommodation**
- **H52.521 Paresis of accommodation, right eye**
- **H52.522 Paresis of accommodation, left eye**
- **H52.523 Paresis of accommodation, bilateral**
- **H52.529 Paresis of accommodation, unspecified eye**

✓6th **H52.53 Spasm of accommodation**
- **H52.531 Spasm of accommodation, right eye**
- **H52.532 Spasm of accommodation, left eye**
- **H52.533 Spasm of accommodation, bilateral**
- **H52.539 Spasm of accommodation, unspecified eye**

H52.6 Other disorders of refraction

H52.7 Unspecified disorder of refraction

Visual disturbances and blindness (H53-H54)

✓4th **H53 Visual disturbances**

✓5th **H53.Ø Amblyopia ex anopsia**

EXCLUDES 1 *amblyopia due to vitamin A deficiency (E5Ø.5)*

✓6th **H53.ØØ Unspecified amblyopia**
- **H53.ØØ1 Unspecified amblyopia, right eye**
- **H53.ØØ2 Unspecified amblyopia, left eye**
- **H53.ØØ3 Unspecified amblyopia, bilateral**
- **H53.ØØ9 Unspecified amblyopia, unspecified eye**

✓6th **H53.Ø1 Deprivation amblyopia**
- **H53.Ø11 Deprivation amblyopia, right eye**
- **H53.Ø12 Deprivation amblyopia, left eye**
- **H53.Ø13 Deprivation amblyopia, bilateral**
- **H53.Ø19 Deprivation amblyopia, unspecified eye**

✓6th **H53.Ø2 Refractive amblyopia**
- **H53.Ø21 Refractive amblyopia, right eye**
- **H53.Ø22 Refractive amblyopia, left eye**
- **H53.Ø23 Refractive amblyopia, bilateral**
- **H53.Ø29 Refractive amblyopia, unspecified eye**

✓6th **H53.Ø3 Strabismic amblyopia**

EXCLUDES 1 *strabismus (H5Ø.-)*

- **H53.Ø31 Strabismic amblyopia, right eye**
- **H53.Ø32 Strabismic amblyopia, left eye**
- **H53.Ø33 Strabismic amblyopia, bilateral**
- **H53.Ø39 Strabismic amblyopia, unspecified eye**

✓6th **H53.Ø4 Amblyopia suspect**

AHA: 2016,4Q,22-23

- **H53.Ø41 Amblyopia suspect, right eye**
- **H53.Ø42 Amblyopia suspect, left eye**
- **H53.Ø43 Amblyopia suspect, bilateral**
- **H53.Ø49 Amblyopia suspect, unspecified eye**

✓5th **H53.1 Subjective visual disturbances**

EXCLUDES 1 *subjective visual disturbances due to vitamin A deficiency (E5Ø.5)*
visual hallucinations (R44.1)

H53.1Ø Unspecified subjective visual disturbances

H53.11 Day blindness
Hemeralopia

✓6th **H53.12 Transient visual loss**
Scintillating scotoma

EXCLUDES 1 *amaurosis fugax (G45.3-)*
transient retinal artery occlusion (H34.Ø-)

- **H53.121 Transient visual loss, right eye** CC
- **H53.122 Transient visual loss, left eye** CC
- **H53.123 Transient visual loss, bilateral** CC
- **H53.129 Transient visual loss, unspecified eye** CC

✓6th **H53.13 Sudden visual loss**
- **H53.131 Sudden visual loss, right eye** CC
- **H53.132 Sudden visual loss, left eye** CC
- **H53.133 Sudden visual loss, bilateral** CC
- **H53.139 Sudden visual loss, unspecified eye** CC

✓6th **H53.14 Visual discomfort**
Asthenopia
Photophobia
- **H53.141 Visual discomfort, right eye**
- **H53.142 Visual discomfort, left eye**
- **H53.143 Visual discomfort, bilateral**
- **H53.149 Visual discomfort, unspecified**

H53.15 Visual distortions of shape and size
Metamorphopsia

H53.16 Psychophysical visual disturbances

H53.19 Other subjective visual disturbances
Visual halos

H53.2 Diplopia
Double vision

✓5th **H53.3 Other and unspecified disorders of binocular vision**
- **H53.3Ø Unspecified disorder of binocular vision**
- **H53.31 Abnormal retinal correspondence**
- **H53.32 Fusion with defective stereopsis**
- **H53.33 Simultaneous visual perception without fusion**
- **H53.34 Suppression of binocular vision**

✓5th **H53.4 Visual field defects**

H53.4Ø Unspecified visual field defects

✓6th **H53.41 Scotoma involving central area**
Central scotoma
- **H53.411 Scotoma involving central area, right eye**
- **H53.412 Scotoma involving central area, left eye**
- **H53.413 Scotoma involving central area, bilateral**
- **H53.419 Scotoma involving central area, unspecified eye**

✓6th **H53.42 Scotoma of blind spot area**
Enlarged blind spot
- **H53.421 Scotoma of blind spot area, right eye**
- **H53.422 Scotoma of blind spot area, left eye**
- **H53.423 Scotoma of blind spot area, bilateral**
- **H53.429 Scotoma of blind spot area, unspecified eye**

✓6th **H53.43 Sector or arcuate defects**
Arcuate scotoma
Bjerrum scotoma
- **H53.431 Sector or arcuate defects, right eye**
- **H53.432 Sector or arcuate defects, left eye**
- **H53.433 Sector or arcuate defects, bilateral**
- **H53.439 Sector or arcuate defects, unspecified eye**

✓6th **H53.45 Other localized visual field defect**
Peripheral visual field defect
Ring scotoma NOS
Scotoma NOS
- **H53.451 Other localized visual field defect, right eye**
- **H53.452 Other localized visual field defect, left eye**
- **H53.453 Other localized visual field defect, bilateral**
- **H53.459 Other localized visual field defect, unspecified eye**

✓6th **H53.46 Homonymous bilateral field defects**
Homonymous hemianopia
Homonymous hemianopsia
Quadrant anopia
Quadrant anopsia
- **H53.461 Homonymous bilateral field defects, right side**

H53.462 Homonymous bilateral field defects, left side

H53.469 Homonymous bilateral field defects, unspecified side
Homonymous bilateral field defects NOS

H53.47 Heteronymous bilateral field defects
Heteronymous hemianop(s)ia

✓6th **H53.48 Generalized contraction of visual field**

H53.481 Generalized contraction of visual field, right eye

H53.482 Generalized contraction of visual field, left eye

H53.483 Generalized contraction of visual field, bilateral

H53.489 Generalized contraction of visual field, unspecified eye

✓5th **H53.5 Color vision deficiencies**
Color blindness
EXCLUDES 2 day blindness (H53.11)

H53.50 Unspecified color vision deficiencies
Color blindness NOS

H53.51 Achromatopsia
DEF: Nonprogressive genetic visual disorder characterized by complete color blindness, decreased vision, and light sensitivity.

H53.52 Acquired color vision deficiency

H53.53 Deuteranomaly
Deuteranopia
DEF: Male-only genetic disorder causing difficulty in distinguishing green and red; no shortened spectrum.

H53.54 Protanomaly
Protanopia

H53.55 Tritanomaly
Tritanopia

H53.59 Other color vision deficiencies

✓5th **H53.6 Night blindness**
EXCLUDES 1 night blindness due to vitamin A deficiency (E50.5)

H53.60 Unspecified night blindness

H53.61 Abnormal dark adaptation curve

H53.62 Acquired night blindness

H53.63 Congenital night blindness

H53.69 Other night blindness

✓5th **H53.7 Vision sensitivity deficiencies**

H53.71 Glare sensitivity

H53.72 Impaired contrast sensitivity

H53.8 Other visual disturbances

H53.9 Unspecified visual disturbance

✓4th **H54 Blindness and low vision**

NOTE For definition of visual impairment categories see table below

Code first any associated underlying cause of the blindness
EXCLUDES 1 amaurosis fugax (G45.3)
AHA: 2017,4Q,11-12

✓5th **H54.0 Blindness, both eyes**
Visual impairment categories 3, 4, 5 in both eyes.

✓6th **H54.0X Blindness, both eyes, different category levels**

✓7th **H54.0X3 Blindness right eye, category 3**

H54.0X33 Blindness right eye category 3, blindness left eye category 3

H54.0X34 Blindness right eye category 3, blindness left eye category 4

H54.0X35 Blindness right eye category 3, blindness left eye category 5

✓7th **H54.0X4 Blindness right eye, category 4**

H54.0X43 Blindness right eye category 4, blindness left eye category 3

H54.0X44 Blindness right eye category 4, blindness left eye category 4

H54.0X45 Blindness right eye category 4, blindness left eye category 5

✓7th **H54.0X5 Blindness right eye, category 5**

H54.0X53 Blindness right eye category 5, blindness left eye category 3

H54.0X54 Blindness right eye category 5, blindness left eye category 4

H54.0X55 Blindness right eye category 5, blindness left eye category 5

✓5th **H54.1 Blindness, one eye, low vision other eye**
Visual impairment categories 3, 4, 5 in one eye, with categories 1 or 2 in the other eye.

H54.10 Blindness, one eye, low vision other eye, unspecified eyes

✓6th **H54.11 Blindness, right eye, low vision left eye**

✓7th **H54.113 Blindness right eye category 3, low vision left eye**

H54.1131 Blindness right eye category 3, low vision left eye category 1

H54.1132 Blindness right eye category 3, low vision left eye category 2

✓7th **H54.114 Blindness right eye category 4, low vision left eye**

H54.1141 Blindness right eye category 4, low vision left eye category 1

H54.1142 Blindness right eye category 4, low vision left eye category 2

✓7th **H54.115 Blindness right eye category 5, low vision left eye**

H54.1151 Blindness right eye category 5, low vision left eye category 1

H54.1152 Blindness right eye category 5, low vision left eye category 2

✓6th **H54.12 Blindness, left eye, low vision right eye**

✓7th **H54.121 Low vision right eye category 1, blindness left eye**

H54.1213 Low vision right eye category 1, blindness left eye category 3

H54.1214 Low vision right eye category 1, blindness left eye category 4

H54.1215 Low vision right eye category 1, blindness left eye category 5

✓7th **H54.122 Low vision right eye category 2, blindness left eye**

H54.1223 Low vision right eye category 2, blindness left eye category 3

H54.1224 Low vision right eye category 2, blindness left eye category 4

H54.1225 Low vision right eye category 2, blindness left eye category 5

✓5th **H54.2 Low vision, both eyes**
Visual impairment categories 1 or 2 in both eyes.

✓6th **H54.2X Low vision, both eyes, different category levels**

✓7th **H54.2X1 Low vision, right eye, category 1**

H54.2X11 Low vision right eye category 1, low vision left eye category 1

H54.2X12 Low vision right eye category 1, low vision left eye category 2

✓7th **H54.2X2 Low vision, right eye, category 2**

H54.2X21 Low vision right eye category 2, low vision left eye category 1

H54.2X22 Low vision right eye category 2, low vision left eye category 2

H54.3 Unqualified visual loss, both eyes
Visual impairment category 9 in both eyes.
TIP: Assign only when both eyes are documented as affected by blindness or low vision but the visual impairment category is not documented.

✓5th **H54.4 Blindness, one eye**
Visual impairment categories 3, 4, 5 in one eye [normal vision in other eye]

H54.40 Blindness, one eye, unspecified eye

✓6th **H54.41 Blindness, right eye, normal vision left eye**

✓7th **H54.413 Blindness, right eye, category 3**

H54.413A Blindness right eye category 3, normal vision left eye

✓7th **H54.414 Blindness, right eye, category 4**

H54.414A Blindness right eye category 4, normal vision left eye

H54.415 **Blindness, right eye, category 5**
H54.415A **Blindness right eye category 5, normal vision left eye**

H54.42 **Blindness, left eye, normal vision right eye**
H54.42A **Blindness, left eye, category 3-5**
H54.42A3 **Blindness left eye category 3, normal vision right eye**
H54.42A4 **Blindness left eye category 4, normal vision right eye**
H54.42A5 **Blindness left eye category 5, normal vision right eye**

H54.5 **Low vision, one eye**
Visual impairment categories 1 or 2 in one eye [normal vision in other eye].
H54.5Ø **Low vision, one eye, unspecified eye**
H54.51 **Low vision, right eye, normal vision left eye**
H54.511 **Low vision, right eye, category 1-2**
H54.511A **Low vision right eye category 1, normal vision left eye**
H54.512A **Low vision right eye category 2, normal vision left eye**
H54.52 **Low vision, left eye, normal vision right eye**
H54.52A **Low vision, left eye, category 1-2**
H54.52A1 **Low vision left eye category 1, normal vision right eye**
H54.52A2 **Low vision left eye category 2, normal vision right eye**

H54.6 **Unqualified visual loss, one eye**
Visual impairment category 9 in one eye [normal vision in other eye].
TIP: Assign a code from this category only when one eye is documented as affected by blindness or low vision but the visual impairment category is not documented.
H54.6Ø **Unqualified visual loss, one eye, unspecified**
H54.61 **Unqualified visual loss, right eye, normal vision left eye**
H54.62 **Unqualified visual loss, left eye, normal vision right eye**

H54.7 **Unspecified visual loss**
Visual impairment category 9 NOS
TIP: Assign only when documentation specifies blindness, visual loss, or low vision but not whether one or both eyes are affected or the visual impairment category.

H54.8 **Legal blindness, as defined in USA**
Blindness NOS according to USA definition
EXCLUDES 1 *legal blindness with specification of impairment level (H54.Ø-H54.7)*

NOTE The table below gives a classification of severity of visual impairment recommended by a WHO Study Group on the Prevention of Blindness, Geneva, 6-1Ø November 1972.

The term "low vision" in category H54 comprises categories 1 and 2 of the table, the term "blindness" categories 3, 4 and 5, and the term "unqualified visual loss" category 9.

If the extent of the visual field is taken into account, patients with a field no greater than 1Ø but greater than 5 around central fixation should be placed in category 3 and patients with a field no greater than 5 around central fixation should be placed in category 4, even if the central acuity is not impaired.

Category of visual impairment	Visual acuity with best possible correction	
	Maximum less than:	**Minimum equal to or better than:**
1	6/18 3/1Ø (Ø.3) 2Ø/7Ø	6/6Ø 1/1Ø (Ø.1) 2Ø/2ØØ
2	6/6Ø 1/1Ø (Ø.1) 2Ø/2ØØ	3/6Ø 1/2Ø (Ø.Ø5) 2Ø/4ØØ
3	3/6Ø 1/2ØØ (Ø.Ø5) 2Ø/4ØØ	1/6Ø (finger counting at one meter) 1/5Ø (Ø.Ø2) 5/3ØØ (2Ø/12ØØ)
4	1/6Ø (finger counting at one meter) 1/5Ø (Ø.Ø2) 5/3ØØ	Light perception
5	No light perception	
9	Undetermined or unspecified	

Other disorders of eye and adnexa (H55-H57)

H55 **Nystagmus and other irregular eye movements**
H55.Ø **Nystagmus**
DEF: Rapid, rhythmic, involuntary movements of the eyeball in vertical, horizontal, rotational, or mixed directions.
H55.ØØ **Unspecified nystagmus**
H55.Ø1 **Congenital nystagmus**
H55.Ø2 **Latent nystagmus**
H55.Ø3 **Visual deprivation nystagmus**
H55.Ø4 **Dissociated nystagmus**
H55.Ø9 **Other forms of nystagmus**
H55.8 **Other irregular eye movements**
▲ H55.81 **Deficient saccadic eye movements**
● H55.82 **Deficient smooth pursuit eye movements**
H55.89 **Other irregular eye movements**

H57 **Other disorders of eye and adnexa**
H57.Ø **Anomalies of pupillary function**
H57.ØØ **Unspecified anomaly of pupillary function**
H57.Ø1 **Argyll Robertson pupil, atypical**
EXCLUDES 1 *syphilitic Argyll Robertson pupil (A52.19)*
H57.Ø2 **Anisocoria**
H57.Ø3 **Miosis**
H57.Ø4 **Mydriasis**
H57.Ø5 **Tonic pupil**
H57.Ø51 **Tonic pupil, right eye**
H57.Ø52 **Tonic pupil, left eye**
H57.Ø53 **Tonic pupil, bilateral**
H57.Ø59 **Tonic pupil, unspecified eye**
H57.Ø9 **Other anomalies of pupillary function**
H57.1 **Ocular pain**
H57.1Ø **Ocular pain, unspecified eye**

H57.11 Ocular pain, right eye
H57.12 Ocular pain, left eye
H57.13 Ocular pain, bilateral

✓5th H57.8 Other specified disorders of eye and adnexa
AHA: 2018,4Q,15-16

✓6th H57.81 Brow ptosis
H57.811 Brow ptosis, right
H57.812 Brow ptosis, left
H57.813 Brow ptosis, bilateral
H57.819 Brow ptosis, unspecified

H57.89 Other specified disorders of eye and adnexa

H57.9 Unspecified disorder of eye and adnexa

Intraoperative and postprocedural complications and disorders of eye and adnexa, not elsewhere classified (H59)

✓4th **H59 Intraoperative and postprocedural complications and disorders of eye and adnexa, not elsewhere classified**

EXCLUDES 1 *mechanical complication of intraocular lens (T85.2)*
mechanical complication of other ocular prosthetic devices, implants and grafts (T85.3)
pseudophakia (Z96.1)
secondary cataracts (H26.4-)

✓5th H59.0 Disorders of the eye following cataract surgery

✓6th H59.01 Keratopathy (bullous aphakic) following cataract surgery
Vitreal corneal syndrome
Vitreous (touch) syndrome
H59.011 Keratopathy (bullous aphakic) following cataract surgery, right eye CC
H59.012 Keratopathy (bullous aphakic) following cataract surgery, left eye CC
H59.013 Keratopathy (bullous aphakic) following cataract surgery, bilateral CC
H59.019 Keratopathy (bullous aphakic) following cataract surgery, unspecified eye CC

✓6th H59.02 Cataract (lens) fragments in eye following cataract surgery
H59.021 Cataract (lens) fragments in eye following cataract surgery, right eye
H59.022 Cataract (lens) fragments in eye following cataract surgery, left eye
H59.023 Cataract (lens) fragments in eye following cataract surgery, bilateral
H59.029 Cataract (lens) fragments in eye following cataract surgery, unspecified eye

✓6th H59.03 Cystoid macular edema following cataract surgery
H59.031 Cystoid macular edema following cataract surgery, right eye CC
H59.032 Cystoid macular edema following cataract surgery, left eye CC
H59.033 Cystoid macular edema following cataract surgery, bilateral CC
H59.039 Cystoid macular edema following cataract surgery, unspecified eye CC

✓6th H59.09 Other disorders of the eye following cataract surgery
H59.091 Other disorders of the right eye following cataract surgery CC
H59.092 Other disorders of the left eye following cataract surgery CC
H59.093 Other disorders of the eye following cataract surgery, bilateral CC
H59.099 Other disorders of unspecified eye following cataract surgery CC

✓5th H59.1 Intraoperative hemorrhage and hematoma of eye and adnexa complicating a procedure

EXCLUDES 1 *intraoperative hemorrhage and hematoma of eye and adnexa due to accidental puncture or laceration during a procedure (H59.2-)*

✓6th H59.11 Intraoperative hemorrhage and hematoma of eye and adnexa complicating an ophthalmic procedure
H59.111 Intraoperative hemorrhage and hematoma of right eye and adnexa complicating an ophthalmic procedure CC
H59.112 Intraoperative hemorrhage and hematoma of left eye and adnexa complicating an ophthalmic procedure CC
H59.113 Intraoperative hemorrhage and hematoma of eye and adnexa complicating an ophthalmic procedure, bilateral CC
H59.119 Intraoperative hemorrhage and hematoma of unspecified eye and adnexa complicating an ophthalmic procedure CC

✓6th H59.12 Intraoperative hemorrhage and hematoma of eye and adnexa complicating other procedure
H59.121 Intraoperative hemorrhage and hematoma of right eye and adnexa complicating other procedure CC
H59.122 Intraoperative hemorrhage and hematoma of left eye and adnexa complicating other procedure CC
H59.123 Intraoperative hemorrhage and hematoma of eye and adnexa complicating other procedure, bilateral CC
H59.129 Intraoperative hemorrhage and hematoma of unspecified eye and adnexa complicating other procedure CC

✓5th H59.2 Accidental puncture and laceration of eye and adnexa during a procedure

✓6th H59.21 Accidental puncture and laceration of eye and adnexa during an ophthalmic procedure
H59.211 Accidental puncture and laceration of right eye and adnexa during an ophthalmic procedure CC
H59.212 Accidental puncture and laceration of left eye and adnexa during an ophthalmic procedure CC
H59.213 Accidental puncture and laceration of eye and adnexa during an ophthalmic procedure, bilateral CC
H59.219 Accidental puncture and laceration of unspecified eye and adnexa during an ophthalmic procedure CC

✓6th H59.22 Accidental puncture and laceration of eye and adnexa during other procedure
H59.221 Accidental puncture and laceration of right eye and adnexa during other procedure CC
H59.222 Accidental puncture and laceration of left eye and adnexa during other procedure CC
H59.223 Accidental puncture and laceration of eye and adnexa during other procedure, bilateral CC
H59.229 Accidental puncture and laceration of unspecified eye and adnexa during other procedure CC

✓5th H59.3 Postprocedural hemorrhage, hematoma, and seroma of eye and adnexa following a procedure
AHA: 2016,4Q,9-10

✓6th H59.31 Postprocedural hemorrhage of eye and adnexa following an ophthalmic procedure
H59.311 Postprocedural hemorrhage of right eye and adnexa following an ophthalmic procedure CC
H59.312 Postprocedural hemorrhage of left eye and adnexa following an ophthalmic procedure CC
H59.313 Postprocedural hemorrhage of eye and adnexa following an ophthalmic procedure, bilateral CC
H59.319 Postprocedural hemorrhage of unspecified eye and adnexa following an ophthalmic procedure CC

✓6th H59.32 Postprocedural hemorrhage of eye and adnexa following other procedure
H59.321 Postprocedural hemorrhage of right eye and adnexa following other procedure CC
H59.322 Postprocedural hemorrhage of left eye and adnexa following other procedure CC
H59.323 Postprocedural hemorrhage of eye and adnexa following other procedure, bilateral CC

H59.329 Postprocedural hemorrhage of unspecified eye and adnexa following other procedure CC

H59.33 Postprocedural hematoma of eye and adnexa following an ophthalmic procedure

H59.331 Postprocedural hematoma of right eye and adnexa following an ophthalmic procedure CC

H59.332 Postprocedural hematoma of left eye and adnexa following an ophthalmic procedure CC

H59.333 Postprocedural hematoma of eye and adnexa following an ophthalmic procedure, bilateral CC

H59.339 Postprocedural hematoma of unspecified eye and adnexa following an ophthalmic procedure CC

H59.34 Postprocedural hematoma of eye and adnexa following other procedure

H59.341 Postprocedural hematoma of right eye and adnexa following other procedure CC

H59.342 Postprocedural hematoma of left eye and adnexa following other procedure CC

H59.343 Postprocedural hematoma of eye and adnexa following other procedure, bilateral CC

H59.349 Postprocedural hematoma of unspecified eye and adnexa following other procedure CC

H59.35 Postprocedural seroma of eye and adnexa following an ophthalmic procedure

H59.351 Postprocedural seroma of right eye and adnexa following an ophthalmic procedure CC

H59.352 Postprocedural seroma of left eye and adnexa following an ophthalmic procedure CC

H59.353 Postprocedural seroma of eye and adnexa following an ophthalmic procedure, bilateral CC

H59.359 Postprocedural seroma of unspecified eye and adnexa following an ophthalmic procedure CC

H59.36 Postprocedural seroma of eye and adnexa following other procedure

H59.361 Postprocedural seroma of right eye and adnexa following other procedure CC

H59.362 Postprocedural seroma of left eye and adnexa following other procedure CC

H59.363 Postprocedural seroma of eye and adnexa following other procedure, bilateral CC

H59.369 Postprocedural seroma of unspecified eye and adnexa following other procedure CC

H59.4 Inflammation (infection) of postprocedural bleb

Postprocedural blebitis

EXCLUDES 1 *filtering (vitreous) bleb after glaucoma surgery status (Z98.83)*

H59.40 Inflammation (infection) of postprocedural bleb, unspecified

H59.41 Inflammation (infection) of postprocedural bleb, stage 1

H59.42 Inflammation (infection) of postprocedural bleb, stage 2

H59.43 Inflammation (infection) of postprocedural bleb, stage 3

Bleb endophthalmitis

H59.8 Other intraoperative and postprocedural complications and disorders of eye and adnexa, not elsewhere classified

H59.81 Chorioretinal scars after surgery for detachment

H59.811 Chorioretinal scars after surgery for detachment, right eye CC

H59.812 Chorioretinal scars after surgery for detachment, left eye CC

H59.813 Chorioretinal scars after surgery for detachment, bilateral CC

H59.819 Chorioretinal scars after surgery for detachment, unspecified eye CC

H59.88 Other intraoperative complications of eye and adnexa, not elsewhere classified CC

H59.89 Other postprocedural complications and disorders of eye and adnexa, not elsewhere classified CC

Chapter 8. Diseases of the Ear and Mastoid Process (H6Ø–H95)

Chapter-specific Guidelines with Coding Examples
Reserved for future guideline expansion.

Chapter 8. Diseases of the Ear and Mastoid Process (H60-H95)

NOTE Use an external cause code following the code for the ear condition, if applicable, to identify the cause of the ear condition

EXCLUDES 2 *certain conditions originating in the perinatal period (P04-P96)*
certain infectious and parasitic diseases (A00-B99)
complications of pregnancy, childbirth and the puerperium (O00-O9A)
congenital malformations, deformations and chromosomal abnormalities (Q00-Q99)
endocrine, nutritional and metabolic diseases (E00-E88)
injury, poisoning and certain other consequences of external causes (S00-T88)
neoplasms (C00-D49)
symptoms, signs and abnormal clinical and laboratory findings, not elsewhere classified (R00-R94)

This chapter contains the following blocks:

H60-H62 Diseases of external ear
H65-H75 Diseases of middle ear and mastoid
H80-H83 Diseases of inner ear
H90-H94 Other disorders of ear
H95 Intraoperative and postprocedural complications and disorders of ear and mastoid process, not elsewhere classified

Diseases of external ear (H60-H62)

✓4th **H60 Otitis externa**

TIP: When the specific infectious agent is identified, a code from Chapter 1 is assigned instead of a code from this category.

✓5th **H60.0 Abscess of external ear**

Boil of external ear
Carbuncle of auricle or external auditory canal
Furuncle of external ear

H60.00 Abscess of external ear, unspecified ear
H60.01 Abscess of right external ear
H60.02 Abscess of left external ear
H60.03 Abscess of external ear, bilateral

✓5th **H60.1 Cellulitis of external ear**

Cellulitis of auricle
Cellulitis of external auditory canal

H60.10 Cellulitis of external ear, unspecified ear
H60.11 Cellulitis of right external ear
H60.12 Cellulitis of left external ear
H60.13 Cellulitis of external ear, bilateral

✓5th **H60.2 Malignant otitis externa**

H60.20 Malignant otitis externa, unspecified ear CC
H60.21 Malignant otitis externa, right ear CC
H60.22 Malignant otitis externa, left ear CC
H60.23 Malignant otitis externa, bilateral CC

✓5th **H60.3 Other infective otitis externa**

✓6th **H60.31 Diffuse otitis externa**

H60.311 Diffuse otitis externa, right ear
H60.312 Diffuse otitis externa, left ear
H60.313 Diffuse otitis externa, bilateral
H60.319 Diffuse otitis externa, unspecified ear

✓6th **H60.32 Hemorrhagic otitis externa**

H60.321 Hemorrhagic otitis externa, right ear
H60.322 Hemorrhagic otitis externa, left ear
H60.323 Hemorrhagic otitis externa, bilateral
H60.329 Hemorrhagic otitis externa, unspecified ear

✓6th **H60.33 Swimmer's ear**

DEF: Commonly occurs when water gets trapped in the ear after swimming.

H60.331 Swimmer's ear, right ear
H60.332 Swimmer's ear, left ear
H60.333 Swimmer's ear, bilateral
H60.339 Swimmer's ear, unspecified ear

✓6th **H60.39 Other infective otitis externa**

H60.391 Other infective otitis externa, right ear
H60.392 Other infective otitis externa, left ear
H60.393 Other infective otitis externa, bilateral
H60.399 Other infective otitis externa, unspecified ear

✓5th **H60.4 Cholesteatoma of external ear**

Keratosis obturans of external ear (canal)

EXCLUDES 2 *cholesteatoma of middle ear (H71.-)*
recurrent cholesteatoma of postmastoidectomy cavity (H95.0-)

DEF: Cholesteatoma: Noncancerous cyst-like mass of cell debris, including cholesterol and epithelial cells resulting from trauma, repeated or improperly healed infections, and congenital enclosure of epidermal cells.

H60.40 Cholesteatoma of external ear, unspecified ear
H60.41 Cholesteatoma of right external ear
H60.42 Cholesteatoma of left external ear
H60.43 Cholesteatoma of external ear, bilateral

✓5th **H60.5 Acute noninfective otitis externa**

✓6th **H60.50 Unspecified acute noninfective otitis externa**

Acute otitis externa NOS

H60.501 Unspecified acute noninfective otitis externa, right ear
H60.502 Unspecified acute noninfective otitis externa, left ear
H60.503 Unspecified acute noninfective otitis externa, bilateral
H60.509 Unspecified acute noninfective otitis externa, unspecified ear

✓6th **H60.51 Acute actinic otitis externa**

H60.511 Acute actinic otitis externa, right ear
H60.512 Acute actinic otitis externa, left ear
H60.513 Acute actinic otitis externa, bilateral
H60.519 Acute actinic otitis externa, unspecified ear

✓6th **H60.52 Acute chemical otitis externa**

H60.521 Acute chemical otitis externa, right ear
H60.522 Acute chemical otitis externa, left ear
H60.523 Acute chemical otitis externa, bilateral
H60.529 Acute chemical otitis externa, unspecified ear

✓6th **H60.53 Acute contact otitis externa**

H60.531 Acute contact otitis externa, right ear
H60.532 Acute contact otitis externa, left ear
H60.533 Acute contact otitis externa, bilateral
H60.539 Acute contact otitis externa, unspecified ear

✓6th **H60.54 Acute eczematoid otitis externa**

H60.541 Acute eczematoid otitis externa, right ear
H60.542 Acute eczematoid otitis externa, left ear
H60.543 Acute eczematoid otitis externa, bilateral
H60.549 Acute eczematoid otitis externa, unspecified ear

✓6th **H60.55 Acute reactive otitis externa**

H60.551 Acute reactive otitis externa, right ear
H60.552 Acute reactive otitis externa, left ear
H60.553 Acute reactive otitis externa, bilateral
H60.559 Acute reactive otitis externa, unspecified ear

✓6th **H60.59 Other noninfective acute otitis externa**

H60.591 Other noninfective acute otitis externa, right ear
H60.592 Other noninfective acute otitis externa, left ear
H60.593 Other noninfective acute otitis externa, bilateral
H60.599 Other noninfective acute otitis externa, unspecified ear

✓5th **H60.6 Unspecified chronic otitis externa**

H60.60 Unspecified chronic otitis externa, unspecified ear
H60.61 Unspecified chronic otitis externa, right ear
H60.62 Unspecified chronic otitis externa, left ear
H60.63 Unspecified chronic otitis externa, bilateral

✓5th **H60.8 Other otitis externa**

✓6th **H60.8X Other otitis externa**

H60.8X1 Other otitis externa, right ear
H60.8X2 Other otitis externa, left ear
H60.8X3 Other otitis externa, bilateral
H60.8X9 Other otitis externa, unspecified ear

✓5th **H60.9 Unspecified otitis externa**

H60.90 Unspecified otitis externa, unspecified ear
H60.91 Unspecified otitis externa, right ear

H60.92 Unspecified otitis externa, left ear
H60.93 Unspecified otitis externa, bilateral

H61 Other disorders of external ear

H61.0 Chondritis and perichondritis of external ear
Chondrodermatitis nodularis chronica helicis
Perichondritis of auricle
Perichondritis of pinna

H61.00 Unspecified perichondritis of external ear
H61.001 Unspecified perichondritis of right external ear
H61.002 Unspecified perichondritis of left external ear
H61.003 Unspecified perichondritis of external ear, bilateral
H61.009 Unspecified perichondritis of external ear, unspecified ear

H61.01 Acute perichondritis of external ear
H61.011 Acute perichondritis of right external ear
H61.012 Acute perichondritis of left external ear
H61.013 Acute perichondritis of external ear, bilateral
H61.019 Acute perichondritis of external ear, unspecified ear

H61.02 Chronic perichondritis of external ear
H61.021 Chronic perichondritis of right external ear
H61.022 Chronic perichondritis of left external ear
H61.023 Chronic perichondritis of external ear, bilateral
H61.029 Chronic perichondritis of external ear, unspecified ear

H61.03 Chondritis of external ear
Chondritis of auricle
Chondritis of pinna
AHA: 2015,1Q,18
DEF: Infection that has progressed into the cartilage and presents as indurated and edematous skin over the pinna. Vascular compromise occurs with tissue necrosis and deformity.
H61.031 Chondritis of right external ear
H61.032 Chondritis of left external ear
H61.033 Chondritis of external ear, bilateral
H61.039 Chondritis of external ear, unspecified ear

H61.1 Noninfective disorders of pinna
EXCLUDES 2 *cauliflower ear (M95.1-)*
gouty tophi of ear (M1A.-)

H61.10 Unspecified noninfective disorders of pinna
Disorder of pinna NOS
H61.101 Unspecified noninfective disorders of pinna, right ear
H61.102 Unspecified noninfective disorders of pinna, left ear
H61.103 Unspecified noninfective disorders of pinna, bilateral
H61.109 Unspecified noninfective disorders of pinna, unspecified ear

H61.11 Acquired deformity of pinna
Acquired deformity of auricle
EXCLUDES 2 *cauliflower ear (M95.1-)*
H61.111 Acquired deformity of pinna, right ear
H61.112 Acquired deformity of pinna, left ear
H61.113 Acquired deformity of pinna, bilateral
H61.119 Acquired deformity of pinna, unspecified ear

H61.12 Hematoma of pinna
Hematoma of auricle
H61.121 Hematoma of pinna, right ear
H61.122 Hematoma of pinna, left ear
H61.123 Hematoma of pinna, bilateral
H61.129 Hematoma of pinna, unspecified ear

H61.19 Other noninfective disorders of pinna
H61.191 Noninfective disorders of pinna, right ear
H61.192 Noninfective disorders of pinna, left ear
H61.193 Noninfective disorders of pinna, bilateral
H61.199 Noninfective disorders of pinna, unspecified ear

H61.2 Impacted cerumen
Wax in ear
H61.20 Impacted cerumen, unspecified ear
H61.21 Impacted cerumen, right ear
H61.22 Impacted cerumen, left ear
H61.23 Impacted cerumen, bilateral

H61.3 Acquired stenosis of external ear canal
Collapse of external ear canal
EXCLUDES 1 *postprocedural stenosis of external ear canal (H95.81-)*

H61.30 Acquired stenosis of external ear canal, unspecified
H61.301 Acquired stenosis of right external ear canal, unspecified
H61.302 Acquired stenosis of left external ear canal, unspecified
H61.303 Acquired stenosis of external ear canal, unspecified, bilateral
H61.309 Acquired stenosis of external ear canal, unspecified, unspecified ear

H61.31 Acquired stenosis of external ear canal secondary to trauma
H61.311 Acquired stenosis of right external ear canal secondary to trauma
H61.312 Acquired stenosis of left external ear canal secondary to trauma
H61.313 Acquired stenosis of external ear canal secondary to trauma, bilateral
H61.319 Acquired stenosis of external ear canal secondary to trauma, unspecified ear

H61.32 Acquired stenosis of external ear canal secondary to inflammation and infection
DEF: Narrowing of the external ear canal due to chronic inflammation or infection.
H61.321 Acquired stenosis of right external ear canal secondary to inflammation and infection
H61.322 Acquired stenosis of left external ear canal secondary to inflammation and infection
H61.323 Acquired stenosis of external ear canal secondary to inflammation and infection, bilateral
H61.329 Acquired stenosis of external ear canal secondary to inflammation and infection, unspecified ear

H61.39 Other acquired stenosis of external ear canal
H61.391 Other acquired stenosis of right external ear canal
H61.392 Other acquired stenosis of left external ear canal
H61.393 Other acquired stenosis of external ear canal, bilateral
H61.399 Other acquired stenosis of external ear canal, unspecified ear

H61.8 Other specified disorders of external ear

H61.81 Exostosis of external canal
H61.811 Exostosis of right external canal
H61.812 Exostosis of left external canal
H61.813 Exostosis of external canal, bilateral
H61.819 Exostosis of external canal, unspecified ear

H61.89 Other specified disorders of external ear
H61.891 Other specified disorders of right external ear
H61.892 Other specified disorders of left external ear
H61.893 Other specified disorders of external ear, bilateral
H61.899 Other specified disorders of external ear, unspecified ear

H61.9 Disorder of external ear, unspecified
H61.90 Disorder of external ear, unspecified, unspecified ear
H61.91 Disorder of right external ear, unspecified
H61.92 Disorder of left external ear, unspecified
H61.93 Disorder of external ear, unspecified, bilateral

✓4th **H62 Disorders of external ear in diseases classified elsewhere**

✓5th **H62.4 Otitis externa in other diseases classified elsewhere**

Code first underlying disease, such as:
erysipelas (A46)
impetigo (LØ1.Ø)

EXCLUDES 1 *otitis externa (in):*
candidiasis (B37.84)
herpes viral [herpes simplex] (BØØ.1)
herpes zoster (BØ2.8)

H62.4Ø Otitis externa in other diseases classified elsewhere, unspecified ear
H62.41 Otitis externa in other diseases classified elsewhere, right ear
H62.42 Otitis externa in other diseases classified elsewhere, left ear
H62.43 Otitis externa in other diseases classified elsewhere, bilateral

✓5th **H62.8 Other disorders of external ear in diseases classified elsewhere**

Code first underlying disease, such as:
gout (M1A.-, M1Ø.-)

✓6th **H62.8X Other disorders of external ear in diseases classified elsewhere**

H62.8X1 Other disorders of right external ear in diseases classified elsewhere
H62.8X2 Other disorders of left external ear in diseases classified elsewhere
H62.8X3 Other disorders of external ear in diseases classified elsewhere, bilateral
H62.8X9 Other disorders of external ear in diseases classified elsewhere, unspecified ear

Diseases of middle ear and mastoid (H65-H75)

✓4th **H65 Nonsuppurative otitis media**

INCLUDES nonsuppurative otitis media with myringitis

Use additional code for any associated perforated tympanic membrane (H72.-)

Use additional code, if applicable, to identify:
exposure to environmental tobacco smoke (Z77.22)
exposure to tobacco smoke in the perinatal period (P96.81)
history of tobacco dependence (Z87.891)
infectious agent (B95-B97)
occupational exposure to environmental tobacco smoke (Z57.31)
tobacco dependence (F17.-)
tobacco use (Z72.Ø)

✓5th **H65.Ø Acute serous otitis media**

Acute and subacute secretory otitis

H65.ØØ Acute serous otitis media, unspecified ear
H65.Ø1 Acute serous otitis media, right ear
H65.Ø2 Acute serous otitis media, left ear
H65.Ø3 Acute serous otitis media, bilateral
H65.Ø4 Acute serous otitis media, recurrent, right ear
H65.Ø5 Acute serous otitis media, recurrent, left ear
H65.Ø6 Acute serous otitis media, recurrent, bilateral
H65.Ø7 Acute serous otitis media, recurrent, unspecified ear

✓5th **H65.1 Other acute nonsuppurative otitis media**

EXCLUDES 1 *otitic barotrauma (T7Ø.Ø)*
otitis media (acute) NOS (H66.9)

✓6th **H65.11 Acute and subacute allergic otitis media (mucoid) (sanguinous) (serous)**

H65.111 Acute and subacute allergic otitis media (mucoid) (sanguinous) (serous), right ear
H65.112 Acute and subacute allergic otitis media (mucoid) (sanguinous) (serous), left ear
H65.113 Acute and subacute allergic otitis media (mucoid) (sanguinous) (serous), bilateral
H65.114 Acute and subacute allergic otitis media (mucoid) (sanguinous) (serous), recurrent, right ear
H65.115 Acute and subacute allergic otitis media (mucoid) (sanguinous) (serous), recurrent, left ear
H65.116 Acute and subacute allergic otitis media (mucoid) (sanguinous) (serous), recurrent, bilateral
H65.117 Acute and subacute allergic otitis media (mucoid) (sanguinous) (serous), recurrent, unspecified ear
H65.119 Acute and subacute allergic otitis media (mucoid) (sanguinous) (serous), unspecified ear

✓6th **H65.19 Other acute nonsuppurative otitis media**

Acute and subacute mucoid otitis media
Acute and subacute nonsuppurative otitis media NOS
Acute and subacute sanguinous otitis media
Acute and subacute seromucinous otitis media

H65.191 Other acute nonsuppurative otitis media, right ear
H65.192 Other acute nonsuppurative otitis media, left ear
H65.193 Other acute nonsuppurative otitis media, bilateral
H65.194 Other acute nonsuppurative otitis media, recurrent, right ear
H65.195 Other acute nonsuppurative otitis media, recurrent, left ear
H65.196 Other acute nonsuppurative otitis media, recurrent, bilateral
H65.197 Other acute nonsuppurative otitis media recurrent, unspecified ear
H65.199 Other acute nonsuppurative otitis media, unspecified ear

✓5th **H65.2 Chronic serous otitis media**

Chronic tubotympanal catarrh

H65.2Ø Chronic serous otitis media, unspecified ear
H65.21 Chronic serous otitis media, right ear
H65.22 Chronic serous otitis media, left ear
H65.23 Chronic serous otitis media, bilateral

✓5th **H65.3 Chronic mucoid otitis media**

Chronic mucinous otitis media
Chronic secretory otitis media
Chronic transudative otitis media
Glue ear

EXCLUDES 1 *adhesive middle ear disease (H74.1)*

H65.3Ø Chronic mucoid otitis media, unspecified ear
H65.31 Chronic mucoid otitis media, right ear
H65.32 Chronic mucoid otitis media, left ear
H65.33 Chronic mucoid otitis media, bilateral

✓5th **H65.4 Other chronic nonsuppurative otitis media**

✓6th **H65.41 Chronic allergic otitis media**

H65.411 Chronic allergic otitis media, right ear
H65.412 Chronic allergic otitis media, left ear
H65.413 Chronic allergic otitis media, bilateral
H65.419 Chronic allergic otitis media, unspecified ear

✓6th **H65.49 Other chronic nonsuppurative otitis media**

Chronic exudative otitis media
Chronic nonsuppurative otitis media NOS
Chronic otitis media with effusion (nonpurulent)
Chronic seromucinous otitis media

H65.491 Other chronic nonsuppurative otitis media, right ear
H65.492 Other chronic nonsuppurative otitis media, left ear
H65.493 Other chronic nonsuppurative otitis media, bilateral
H65.499 Other chronic nonsuppurative otitis media, unspecified ear

✓5th **H65.9 Unspecified nonsuppurative otitis media**

Allergic otitis media NOS
Catarrhal otitis media NOS
Exudative otitis media NOS
Mucoid otitis media NOS
Otitis media with effusion (nonpurulent) NOS
Secretory otitis media NOS
Seromucinous otitis media NOS
Serous otitis media NOS
Transudative otitis media NOS

H65.9Ø Unspecified nonsuppurative otitis media, unspecified ear
H65.91 Unspecified nonsuppurative otitis media, right ear
H65.92 Unspecified nonsuppurative otitis media, left ear
H65.93 Unspecified nonsuppurative otitis media, bilateral

✓4th H66 Suppurative and unspecified otitis media

INCLUDES suppurative and unspecified otitis media with myringitis

Use additional code to identify:
- exposure to environmental tobacco smoke (Z77.22)
- exposure to tobacco smoke in the perinatal period (P96.81)
- history of tobacco dependence (Z87.891)
- occupational exposure to environmental tobacco smoke (Z57.31)
- tobacco dependence (F17.-)
- tobacco use (Z72.Ø)

AHA: 2016,1Q,34

✓5th H66.Ø Acute suppurative otitis media

✓6th H66.ØØ Acute suppurative otitis media without spontaneous rupture of ear drum

H66.ØØ1 Acute suppurative otitis media without spontaneous rupture of ear drum, right ear

H66.ØØ2 Acute suppurative otitis media without spontaneous rupture of ear drum, left ear

H66.ØØ3 Acute suppurative otitis media without spontaneous rupture of ear drum, bilateral

H66.ØØ4 Acute suppurative otitis media without spontaneous rupture of ear drum, recurrent, right ear

H66.ØØ5 Acute suppurative otitis media without spontaneous rupture of ear drum, recurrent, left ear

H66.ØØ6 Acute suppurative otitis media without spontaneous rupture of ear drum, recurrent, bilateral

H66.ØØ7 Acute suppurative otitis media without spontaneous rupture of ear drum, recurrent, unspecified ear

H66.ØØ9 Acute suppurative otitis media without spontaneous rupture of ear drum, unspecified ear

✓6th H66.Ø1 Acute suppurative otitis media with spontaneous rupture of ear drum

DEF: Sudden, severe inflammation of the middle ear, causing pressure that perforates the ear drum tissue.

H66.Ø11 Acute suppurative otitis media with spontaneous rupture of ear drum, right ear

H66.Ø12 Acute suppurative otitis media with spontaneous rupture of ear drum, left ear

H66.Ø13 Acute suppurative otitis media with spontaneous rupture of ear drum, bilateral

H66.Ø14 Acute suppurative otitis media with spontaneous rupture of ear drum, recurrent, right ear

H66.Ø15 Acute suppurative otitis media with spontaneous rupture of ear drum, recurrent, left ear

H66.Ø16 Acute suppurative otitis media with spontaneous rupture of ear drum, recurrent, bilateral

H66.Ø17 Acute suppurative otitis media with spontaneous rupture of ear drum, recurrent, unspecified ear

H66.Ø19 Acute suppurative otitis media with spontaneous rupture of ear drum, unspecified ear

✓5th H66.1 Chronic tubotympanic suppurative otitis media

Benign chronic suppurative otitis media
Chronic tubotympanic disease
Use additional code for any associated perforated tympanic membrane (H72.-)

H66.1Ø Chronic tubotympanic suppurative otitis media, unspecified

H66.11 Chronic tubotympanic suppurative otitis media, right ear

H66.12 Chronic tubotympanic suppurative otitis media, left ear

H66.13 Chronic tubotympanic suppurative otitis media, bilateral

✓5th H66.2 Chronic atticoantral suppurative otitis media

Chronic atticoantral disease
Use additional code for any associated perforated tympanic membrane (H72.-)

H66.2Ø Chronic atticoantral suppurative otitis media, unspecified ear

H66.21 Chronic atticoantral suppurative otitis media, right ear

H66.22 Chronic atticoantral suppurative otitis media, left ear

H66.23 Chronic atticoantral suppurative otitis media, bilateral

✓5th H66.3 Other chronic suppurative otitis media

Chronic suppurative otitis media NOS
Use additional code for any associated perforated tympanic membrane (H72.-)

EXCLUDES 1 *tuberculous otitis media (A18.6)*

✓6th H66.3X Other chronic suppurative otitis media

H66.3X1 Other chronic suppurative otitis media, right ear

H66.3X2 Other chronic suppurative otitis media, left ear

H66.3X3 Other chronic suppurative otitis media, bilateral

H66.3X9 Other chronic suppurative otitis media, unspecified ear

✓5th H66.4 Suppurative otitis media, unspecified

Purulent otitis media NOS
Use additional code for any associated perforated tympanic membrane (H72.-)

H66.4Ø Suppurative otitis media, unspecified, unspecified ear

H66.41 Suppurative otitis media, unspecified, right ear

H66.42 Suppurative otitis media, unspecified, left ear

H66.43 Suppurative otitis media, unspecified, bilateral

✓5th H66.9 Otitis media, unspecified

Otitis media NOS
Acute otitis media NOS
Chronic otitis media NOS
Use additional code for any associated perforated tympanic membrane (H72.-)

H66.9Ø Otitis media, unspecified, unspecified ear

H66.91 Otitis media, unspecified, right ear

H66.92 Otitis media, unspecified, left ear

H66.93 Otitis media, unspecified, bilateral

✓4th H67 Otitis media in diseases classified elsewhere

Code first underlying disease, such as:
- plasminogen deficiency (E88.Ø2)
- viral disease NEC (BØØ-B34)

Use additional code for any associated perforated tympanic membrane (H72.-)

EXCLUDES 1 *otitis media in:*
- *influenza (JØ9.X9, J1Ø.83, J11.83)*
- *measles (BØ5.3)*
- *scarlet fever (A38.Ø)*
- *tuberculosis (A18.6)*

H67.1 Otitis media in diseases classified elsewhere, right ear

H67.2 Otitis media in diseases classified elsewhere, left ear

H67.3 Otitis media in diseases classified elsewhere, bilateral

H67.9 Otitis media in diseases classified elsewhere, unspecified ear

✓4th H68 Eustachian salpingitis and obstruction

DEF: Eustachian tube: Internal channel between the tympanic cavity and the nasopharynx that equalizes internal pressure to the outside pressure and drains mucous production from the middle ear.

✓5th H68.Ø Eustachian salpingitis

✓6th H68.ØØ Unspecified Eustachian salpingitis

H68.ØØ1 Unspecified Eustachian salpingitis, right ear

H68.ØØ2 Unspecified Eustachian salpingitis, left ear

H68.ØØ3 Unspecified Eustachian salpingitis, bilateral

H68.ØØ9 Unspecified Eustachian salpingitis, unspecified ear

✓6th H68.Ø1 Acute Eustachian salpingitis

H68.Ø11 Acute Eustachian salpingitis, right ear

H68.Ø12 Acute Eustachian salpingitis, left ear

H68.Ø13 Acute Eustachian salpingitis, bilateral

H68.Ø19 Acute Eustachian salpingitis, unspecified ear

✓6th H68.Ø2 Chronic Eustachian salpingitis

H68.Ø21 Chronic Eustachian salpingitis, right ear

H68.Ø22 Chronic Eustachian salpingitis, left ear

H68.023 Chronic Eustachian salpingitis, bilateral
H68.029 Chronic Eustachian salpingitis, unspecified ear

H68.1 Obstruction of Eustachian tube
Stenosis of Eustachian tube
Stricture of Eustachian tube

H68.10 Unspecified obstruction of Eustachian tube
H68.101 Unspecified obstruction of Eustachian tube, right ear
H68.102 Unspecified obstruction of Eustachian tube, left ear
H68.103 Unspecified obstruction of Eustachian tube, bilateral
H68.109 Unspecified obstruction of Eustachian tube, unspecified ear

H68.11 Osseous obstruction of Eustachian tube
H68.111 Osseous obstruction of Eustachian tube, right ear
H68.112 Osseous obstruction of Eustachian tube, left ear
H68.113 Osseous obstruction of Eustachian tube, bilateral
H68.119 Osseous obstruction of Eustachian tube, unspecified ear

H68.12 Intrinsic cartilagenous obstruction of Eustachian tube
H68.121 Intrinsic cartilagenous obstruction of Eustachian tube, right ear
H68.122 Intrinsic cartilagenous obstruction of Eustachian tube, left ear
H68.123 Intrinsic cartilagenous obstruction of Eustachian tube, bilateral
H68.129 Intrinsic cartilagenous obstruction of Eustachian tube, unspecified ear

H68.13 Extrinsic cartilagenous obstruction of Eustachian tube
Compression of Eustachian tube
H68.131 Extrinsic cartilagenous obstruction of Eustachian tube, right ear
H68.132 Extrinsic cartilagenous obstruction of Eustachian tube, left ear
H68.133 Extrinsic cartilagenous obstruction of Eustachian tube, bilateral
H68.139 Extrinsic cartilagenous obstruction of Eustachian tube, unspecified ear

H69 Other and unspecified disorders of Eustachian tube
DEF: Eustachian tube: Internal channel between the tympanic cavity and the nasopharynx that equalizes internal pressure to the outside pressure and drains mucous production from the middle ear.

H69.0 Patulous Eustachian tube
H69.00 Patulous Eustachian tube, unspecified ear
H69.01 Patulous Eustachian tube, right ear
H69.02 Patulous Eustachian tube, left ear
H69.03 Patulous Eustachian tube, bilateral

H69.8 Other specified disorders of Eustachian tube
H69.80 Other specified disorders of Eustachian tube, unspecified ear
H69.81 Other specified disorders of Eustachian tube, right ear
H69.82 Other specified disorders of Eustachian tube, left ear
H69.83 Other specified disorders of Eustachian tube, bilateral

H69.9 Unspecified Eustachian tube disorder
H69.90 Unspecified Eustachian tube disorder, unspecified ear
H69.91 Unspecified Eustachian tube disorder, right ear
H69.92 Unspecified Eustachian tube disorder, left ear
H69.93 Unspecified Eustachian tube disorder, bilateral

H70 Mastoiditis and related conditions

H70.0 Acute mastoiditis
Abscess of mastoid
Empyema of mastoid

H70.00 Acute mastoiditis without complications
H70.001 Acute mastoiditis without complications, right ear CC
H70.002 Acute mastoiditis without complications, left ear CC
H70.003 Acute mastoiditis without complications, bilateral CC
H70.009 Acute mastoiditis without complications, unspecified ear CC

H70.01 Subperiosteal abscess of mastoid
H70.011 Subperiosteal abscess of mastoid, right ear CC
H70.012 Subperiosteal abscess of mastoid, left ear CC
H70.013 Subperiosteal abscess of mastoid, bilateral CC
H70.019 Subperiosteal abscess of mastoid, unspecified ear CC

H70.09 Acute mastoiditis with other complications
H70.091 Acute mastoiditis with other complications, right ear CC
H70.092 Acute mastoiditis with other complications, left ear CC
H70.093 Acute mastoiditis with other complications, bilateral CC
H70.099 Acute mastoiditis with other complications, unspecified ear CC

H70.1 Chronic mastoiditis
Caries of mastoid
Fistula of mastoid
EXCLUDES 1 *tuberculous mastoiditis (A18.03)*
H70.10 Chronic mastoiditis, unspecified ear
H70.11 Chronic mastoiditis, right ear
H70.12 Chronic mastoiditis, left ear
H70.13 Chronic mastoiditis, bilateral

H70.2 Petrositis
Inflammation of petrous bone

H70.20 Unspecified petrositis
H70.201 Unspecified petrositis, right ear
H70.202 Unspecified petrositis, left ear
H70.203 Unspecified petrositis, bilateral
H70.209 Unspecified petrositis, unspecified ear

H70.21 Acute petrositis
DEF: Sudden, severe inflammation of the petrous temporal bone behind the ear, associated with a middle ear infection.
H70.211 Acute petrositis, right ear
H70.212 Acute petrositis, left ear
H70.213 Acute petrositis, bilateral
H70.219 Acute petrositis, unspecified ear

H70.22 Chronic petrositis
H70.221 Chronic petrositis, right ear
H70.222 Chronic petrositis, left ear
H70.223 Chronic petrositis, bilateral
H70.229 Chronic petrositis, unspecified ear

H70.8 Other mastoiditis and related conditions
EXCLUDES 1 *preauricular sinus and cyst (Q18.1)*
sinus, fistula, and cyst of branchial cleft (Q18.0)

H70.81 Postauricular fistula
H70.811 Postauricular fistula, right ear SW
H70.812 Postauricular fistula, left ear SW
H70.813 Postauricular fistula, bilateral SW
H70.819 Postauricular fistula, unspecified ear SW

H70.89 Other mastoiditis and related conditions
H70.891 Other mastoiditis and related conditions, right ear
H70.892 Other mastoiditis and related conditions, left ear
H70.893 Other mastoiditis and related conditions, bilateral
H70.899 Other mastoiditis and related conditions, unspecified ear

H70.9 Unspecified mastoiditis
H70.90 Unspecified mastoiditis, unspecified ear
H70.91 Unspecified mastoiditis, right ear
H70.92 Unspecified mastoiditis, left ear
H70.93 Unspecified mastoiditis, bilateral

H71 Cholesteatoma of middle ear

EXCLUDES 2 *cholesteatoma of external ear (H60.4-)*
recurrent cholesteatoma of postmastoidectomy cavity (H95.0-)

DEF: Cholesteatoma: Noncancerous cyst-like mass of cell debris, including cholesterol and epithelial cells resulting from trauma, repeated or improperly healed infections, and congenital enclosure of epidermal cells.

Cholesteatoma of Middle Ear

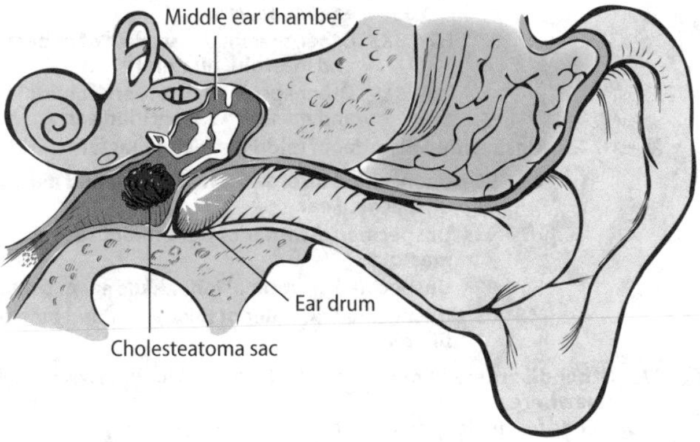

H71.0 Cholesteatoma of attic
- **H71.00 Cholesteatoma of attic, unspecified ear**
- **H71.01 Cholesteatoma of attic, right ear**
- **H71.02 Cholesteatoma of attic, left ear**
- **H71.03 Cholesteatoma of attic, bilateral**

H71.1 Cholesteatoma of tympanum
- **H71.10 Cholesteatoma of tympanum, unspecified ear**
- **H71.11 Cholesteatoma of tympanum, right ear**
- **H71.12 Cholesteatoma of tympanum, left ear**
- **H71.13 Cholesteatoma of tympanum, bilateral**

H71.2 Cholesteatoma of mastoid
- **H71.20 Cholesteatoma of mastoid, unspecified ear**
- **H71.21 Cholesteatoma of mastoid, right ear**
- **H71.22 Cholesteatoma of mastoid, left ear**
- **H71.23 Cholesteatoma of mastoid, bilateral**

H71.3 Diffuse cholesteatosis
- **H71.30 Diffuse cholesteatosis, unspecified ear**
- **H71.31 Diffuse cholesteatosis, right ear**
- **H71.32 Diffuse cholesteatosis, left ear**
- **H71.33 Diffuse cholesteatosis, bilateral**

H71.9 Unspecified cholesteatoma
- **H71.90 Unspecified cholesteatoma, unspecified ear**
- **H71.91 Unspecified cholesteatoma, right ear**
- **H71.92 Unspecified cholesteatoma, left ear**
- **H71.93 Unspecified cholesteatoma, bilateral**

H72 Perforation of tympanic membrane

INCLUDES persistent post-traumatic perforation of ear drum
postinflammatory perforation of ear drum

Code first any associated otitis media (H65.-, H66.1-, H66.2-, H66.3-, H66.4-, H66.9-, H67.-)

EXCLUDES 1 *acute suppurative otitis media with rupture of the tympanic membrane (H66.01-)*
traumatic rupture of ear drum (S09.2-)

H72.0 Central perforation of tympanic membrane
- **H72.00 Central perforation of tympanic membrane, unspecified ear**
- **H72.01 Central perforation of tympanic membrane, right ear**
- **H72.02 Central perforation of tympanic membrane, left ear**
- **H72.03 Central perforation of tympanic membrane, bilateral**

H72.1 Attic perforation of tympanic membrane

Perforation of pars flaccida
- **H72.10 Attic perforation of tympanic membrane, unspecified ear**
- **H72.11 Attic perforation of tympanic membrane, right ear**
- **H72.12 Attic perforation of tympanic membrane, left ear**
- **H72.13 Attic perforation of tympanic membrane, bilateral**

H72.2 Other marginal perforations of tympanic membrane

H72.2X Other marginal perforations of tympanic membrane
- **H72.2X1 Other marginal perforations of tympanic membrane, right ear**
- **H72.2X2 Other marginal perforations of tympanic membrane, left ear**
- **H72.2X3 Other marginal perforations of tympanic membrane, bilateral**
- **H72.2X9 Other marginal perforations of tympanic membrane, unspecified ear**

H72.8 Other perforations of tympanic membrane

H72.81 Multiple perforations of tympanic membrane
- **H72.811 Multiple perforations of tympanic membrane, right ear**
- **H72.812 Multiple perforations of tympanic membrane, left ear**
- **H72.813 Multiple perforations of tympanic membrane, bilateral**
- **H72.819 Multiple perforations of tympanic membrane, unspecified ear**

H72.82 Total perforations of tympanic membrane
- **H72.821 Total perforations of tympanic membrane, right ear**
- **H72.822 Total perforations of tympanic membrane, left ear**
- **H72.823 Total perforations of tympanic membrane, bilateral**
- **H72.829 Total perforations of tympanic membrane, unspecified ear**

H72.9 Unspecified perforation of tympanic membrane
- **H72.90 Unspecified perforation of tympanic membrane, unspecified ear**
- **H72.91 Unspecified perforation of tympanic membrane, right ear**
- **H72.92 Unspecified perforation of tympanic membrane, left ear**
- **H72.93 Unspecified perforation of tympanic membrane, bilateral**

H73 Other disorders of tympanic membrane

H73.0 Acute myringitis

EXCLUDES 1 *acute myringitis with otitis media (H65, H66)*

H73.00 Unspecified acute myringitis

Acute tympanitis NOS
- **H73.001 Acute myringitis, right ear**
- **H73.002 Acute myringitis, left ear**
- **H73.003 Acute myringitis, bilateral**
- **H73.009 Acute myringitis, unspecified ear**

H73.01 Bullous myringitis

DEF: Bacterial or viral otitis media that is characterized by the appearance of serous or hemorrhagic blebs on the ear drum and sudden onset of severe pain in ear.
- **H73.011 Bullous myringitis, right ear**
- **H73.012 Bullous myringitis, left ear**
- **H73.013 Bullous myringitis, bilateral**
- **H73.019 Bullous myringitis, unspecified ear**

H73.09 Other acute myringitis
- **H73.091 Other acute myringitis, right ear**
- **H73.092 Other acute myringitis, left ear**
- **H73.093 Other acute myringitis, bilateral**
- **H73.099 Other acute myringitis, unspecified ear**

H73.1 Chronic myringitis

Chronic tympanitis

EXCLUDES 1 *chronic myringitis with otitis media (H65, H66)*
- **H73.10 Chronic myringitis, unspecified ear**
- **H73.11 Chronic myringitis, right ear**
- **H73.12 Chronic myringitis, left ear**
- **H73.13 Chronic myringitis, bilateral**

H73.2 Unspecified myringitis
- **H73.20 Unspecified myringitis, unspecified ear**
- **H73.21 Unspecified myringitis, right ear**
- **H73.22 Unspecified myringitis, left ear**
- **H73.23 Unspecified myringitis, bilateral**

H73.8 Other specified disorders of tympanic membrane

H73.81 Atrophic flaccid tympanic membrane
- **H73.811 Atrophic flaccid tympanic membrane, right ear**

H73.812 Atrophic flaccid tympanic membrane, left ear
H73.813 Atrophic flaccid tympanic membrane, bilateral
H73.819 Atrophic flaccid tympanic membrane, unspecified ear

6th H73.82 Atrophic nonflaccid tympanic membrane
H73.821 Atrophic nonflaccid tympanic membrane, right ear
H73.822 Atrophic nonflaccid tympanic membrane, left ear
H73.823 Atrophic nonflaccid tympanic membrane, bilateral
H73.829 Atrophic nonflaccid tympanic membrane, unspecified ear

6th H73.89 Other specified disorders of tympanic membrane
H73.891 Other specified disorders of tympanic membrane, right ear
H73.892 Other specified disorders of tympanic membrane, left ear
H73.893 Other specified disorders of tympanic membrane, bilateral
H73.899 Other specified disorders of tympanic membrane, unspecified ear

5th H73.9 Unspecified disorder of tympanic membrane
H73.90 Unspecified disorder of tympanic membrane, unspecified ear
H73.91 Unspecified disorder of tympanic membrane, right ear
H73.92 Unspecified disorder of tympanic membrane, left ear
H73.93 Unspecified disorder of tympanic membrane, bilateral

4th **H74 Other disorders of middle ear mastoid**
EXCLUDES 2 *mastoiditis (H70.-)*

5th H74.0 Tympanosclerosis
DEF: Calcification of tissue in the ear drum, middle ear bones, and middle ear canal.
H74.01 Tympanosclerosis, right ear
H74.02 Tympanosclerosis, left ear
H74.03 Tympanosclerosis, bilateral
H74.09 Tympanosclerosis, unspecified ear

5th H74.1 Adhesive middle ear disease
Adhesive otitis
EXCLUDES 1 *glue ear (H65.3-)*
H74.11 Adhesive right middle ear disease
H74.12 Adhesive left middle ear disease
H74.13 Adhesive middle ear disease, bilateral
H74.19 Adhesive middle ear disease, unspecified ear

5th H74.2 Discontinuity and dislocation of ear ossicles
H74.20 Discontinuity and dislocation of ear ossicles, unspecified ear
H74.21 Discontinuity and dislocation of right ear ossicles
H74.22 Discontinuity and dislocation of left ear ossicles
H74.23 Discontinuity and dislocation of ear ossicles, bilateral

5th H74.3 Other acquired abnormalities of ear ossicles
6th H74.31 Ankylosis of ear ossicles
H74.311 Ankylosis of ear ossicles, right ear
H74.312 Ankylosis of ear ossicles, left ear
H74.313 Ankylosis of ear ossicles, bilateral
H74.319 Ankylosis of ear ossicles, unspecified ear

6th H74.32 Partial loss of ear ossicles
H74.321 Partial loss of ear ossicles, right ear
H74.322 Partial loss of ear ossicles, left ear
H74.323 Partial loss of ear ossicles, bilateral
H74.329 Partial loss of ear ossicles, unspecified ear

6th H74.39 Other acquired abnormalities of ear ossicles
H74.391 Other acquired abnormalities of right ear ossicles
H74.392 Other acquired abnormalities of left ear ossicles
H74.393 Other acquired abnormalities of ear ossicles, bilateral
H74.399 Other acquired abnormalities of ear ossicles, unspecified ear

5th H74.4 Polyp of middle ear
H74.40 Polyp of middle ear, unspecified ear
H74.41 Polyp of right middle ear
H74.42 Polyp of left middle ear
H74.43 Polyp of middle ear, bilateral

5th H74.8 Other specified disorders of middle ear and mastoid
6th H74.8X Other specified disorders of middle ear and mastoid
H74.8X1 Other specified disorders of right middle ear and mastoid
H74.8X2 Other specified disorders of left middle ear and mastoid
H74.8X3 Other specified disorders of middle ear and mastoid, bilateral
H74.8X9 Other specified disorders of middle ear and mastoid, unspecified ear

5th H74.9 Unspecified disorder of middle ear and mastoid
H74.90 Unspecified disorder of middle ear and mastoid, unspecified ear
H74.91 Unspecified disorder of right middle ear and mastoid
H74.92 Unspecified disorder of left middle ear and mastoid
H74.93 Unspecified disorder of middle ear and mastoid, bilateral

4th **H75 Other disorders of middle ear and mastoid in diseases classified elsewhere**
Code first underlying disease

5th H75.0 Mastoiditis in infectious and parasitic diseases classified elsewhere
EXCLUDES 1 *mastoiditis (in):*
syphilis (A52.77)
tuberculosis (A18.03)
H75.00 Mastoiditis in infectious and parasitic diseases classified elsewhere, unspecified ear
H75.01 Mastoiditis in infectious and parasitic diseases classified elsewhere, right ear
H75.02 Mastoiditis in infectious and parasitic diseases classified elsewhere, left ear
H75.03 Mastoiditis in infectious and parasitic diseases classified elsewhere, bilateral

5th H75.8 Other specified disorders of middle ear and mastoid in diseases classified elsewhere
H75.80 Other specified disorders of middle ear and mastoid in diseases classified elsewhere, unspecified ear
H75.81 Other specified disorders of right middle ear and mastoid in diseases classified elsewhere
H75.82 Other specified disorders of left middle ear and mastoid in diseases classified elsewhere
H75.83 Other specified disorders of middle ear and mastoid in diseases classified elsewhere, bilateral

Diseases of inner ear (H80-H83)

4th **H80 Otosclerosis**
INCLUDES otospongiosis

5th H80.0 Otosclerosis involving oval window, nonobliterative
H80.00 Otosclerosis involving oval window, nonobliterative, unspecified ear
H80.01 Otosclerosis involving oval window, nonobliterative, right ear
H80.02 Otosclerosis involving oval window, nonobliterative, left ear
H80.03 Otosclerosis involving oval window, nonobliterative, bilateral

5th H80.1 Otosclerosis involving oval window, obliterative
H80.10 Otosclerosis involving oval window, obliterative, unspecified ear
H80.11 Otosclerosis involving oval window, obliterative, right ear
H80.12 Otosclerosis involving oval window, obliterative, left ear
H80.13 Otosclerosis involving oval window, obliterative, bilateral

5th H80.2 Cochlear otosclerosis
Otosclerosis involving otic capsule
Otosclerosis involving round window
H80.20 Cochlear otosclerosis, unspecified ear
H80.21 Cochlear otosclerosis, right ear
H80.22 Cochlear otosclerosis, left ear
H80.23 Cochlear otosclerosis, bilateral

H80.8 Other otosclerosis
- H80.80 Other otosclerosis, unspecified ear
- H80.81 Other otosclerosis, right ear
- H80.82 Other otosclerosis, left ear
- H80.83 Other otosclerosis, bilateral

H80.9 Unspecified otosclerosis
- H80.90 Unspecified otosclerosis, unspecified ear
- H80.91 Unspecified otosclerosis, right ear
- H80.92 Unspecified otosclerosis, left ear
- H80.93 Unspecified otosclerosis, bilateral

H81 Disorders of vestibular function

EXCLUDES 1 *epidemic vertigo (A88.1)*
vertigo NOS (R42)

H81.0 Ménière's disease
Labyrinthine hydrops
Ménière's syndrome or vertigo
DEF: Distended membranous labyrinth of the middle ear from fluctuating pressure of fluid (hydrops) that causes vertigo, tinnitus, pressure, and hearing loss that may last on and off for several hours. Episodes may occur in clusters or may subside for weeks, months, or even years.
- H81.01 Ménière's disease, right ear
- H81.02 Ménière's disease, left ear
- H81.03 Ménière's disease, bilateral
- H81.09 Ménière's disease, unspecified ear

H81.1 Benign paroxysmal vertigo
- H81.10 Benign paroxysmal vertigo, unspecified ear
- H81.11 Benign paroxysmal vertigo, right ear
- H81.12 Benign paroxysmal vertigo, left ear
- H81.13 Benign paroxysmal vertigo, bilateral

H81.2 Vestibular neuronitis
DEF: Transient benign vertigo caused by inflammation of the vestibular nerve. It is characterized by response to caloric stimulation on one side and nystagmus with rhythmic movement of the eyes. Normal auditory function is present.
- H81.20 Vestibular neuronitis, unspecified ear
- H81.21 Vestibular neuronitis, right ear
- H81.22 Vestibular neuronitis, left ear
- H81.23 Vestibular neuronitis, bilateral

H81.3 Other peripheral vertigo

H81.31 Aural vertigo
- H81.311 Aural vertigo, right ear
- H81.312 Aural vertigo, left ear
- H81.313 Aural vertigo, bilateral
- H81.319 Aural vertigo, unspecified ear

H81.39 Other peripheral vertigo
Lermoyez' syndrome
Otogenic vertigo
Peripheral vertigo NOS
- H81.391 Other peripheral vertigo, right ear
- H81.392 Other peripheral vertigo, left ear
- H81.393 Other peripheral vertigo, bilateral
- H81.399 Other peripheral vertigo, unspecified ear

H81.4 Vertigo of central origin
Central positional nystagmus
- H81.41 Vertigo of central origin, right ear
- H81.42 Vertigo of central origin, left ear
- H81.43 Vertigo of central origin, bilateral
- H81.49 Vertigo of central origin, unspecified ear

H81.8 Other disorders of vestibular function

H81.8X Other disorders of vestibular function
- H81.8X1 Other disorders of vestibular function, right ear
- H81.8X2 Other disorders of vestibular function, left ear
- H81.8X3 Other disorders of vestibular function, bilateral
- H81.8X9 Other disorders of vestibular function, unspecified ear

H81.9 Unspecified disorder of vestibular function
Vertiginous syndrome NOS
- H81.90 Unspecified disorder of vestibular function, unspecified ear
- H81.91 Unspecified disorder of vestibular function, right ear
- H81.92 Unspecified disorder of vestibular function, left ear
- H81.93 Unspecified disorder of vestibular function, bilateral

H82 Vertiginous syndromes in diseases classified elsewhere

Code first underlying disease

EXCLUDES 1 *epidemic vertigo (A88.1)*
- *H82.1* ***Vertiginous syndromes in diseases classified elsewhere, right ear***
- *H82.2* ***Vertiginous syndromes in diseases classified elsewhere, left ear***
- *H82.3* ***Vertiginous syndromes in diseases classified elsewhere, bilateral***
- *H82.9* ***Vertiginous syndromes in diseases classified elsewhere, unspecified ear***

H83 Other diseases of inner ear

H83.0 Labyrinthitis
DEF: Inflammation of the inner ear, or labyrinth, characterized by pus, vertigo, dizziness, nausea, and hearing loss.
- H83.01 Labyrinthitis, right ear
- H83.02 Labyrinthitis, left ear
- H83.03 Labyrinthitis, bilateral
- H83.09 Labyrinthitis, unspecified ear

H83.1 Labyrinthine fistula
- H83.11 Labyrinthine fistula, right ear
- H83.12 Labyrinthine fistula, left ear SW
- H83.13 Labyrinthine fistula, bilateral SW
- H83.19 Labyrinthine fistula, unspecified ear SW

H83.2 Labyrinthine dysfunction
Labyrinthine hypersensitivity
Labyrinthine hypofunction
Labyrinthine loss of function
DEF: Decreased function of the labyrinth sensors.

H83.2X Labyrinthine dysfunction
- H83.2X1 Labyrinthine dysfunction, right ear
- H83.2X2 Labyrinthine dysfunction, left ear
- H83.2X3 Labyrinthine dysfunction, bilateral
- H83.2X9 Labyrinthine dysfunction, unspecified ear

H83.3 Noise effects on inner ear
Acoustic trauma of inner ear
Noise-induced hearing loss of inner ear

H83.3X Noise effects on inner ear
- H83.3X1 Noise effects on right inner ear
- H83.3X2 Noise effects on left inner ear
- H83.3X3 Noise effects on inner ear, bilateral
- H83.3X9 Noise effects on inner ear, unspecified ear

H83.8 Other specified diseases of inner ear

H83.8X Other specified diseases of inner ear
- H83.8X1 Other specified diseases of right inner ear
- H83.8X2 Other specified diseases of left inner ear
- H83.8X3 Other specified diseases of inner ear, bilateral
- H83.8X9 Other specified diseases of inner ear, unspecified ear

H83.9 Unspecified disease of inner ear
- H83.90 Unspecified disease of inner ear, unspecified ear
- H83.91 Unspecified disease of right inner ear
- H83.92 Unspecified disease of left inner ear
- H83.93 Unspecified disease of inner ear, bilateral

Other disorders of ear (H90-H94)

H90 Conductive and sensorineural hearing loss

EXCLUDES 1 *deaf nonspeaking NEC (H91.3)*
deafness NOS (H91.9-)
hearing loss NOS (H91.9-)
noise-induced hearing loss (H83.3-)
ototoxic hearing loss (H91.0-)
sudden (idiopathic) hearing loss (H91.2-)

AHA: 2015,2Q,7

DEF: Conductive hearing loss: Hearing Loss due to the inability of sound waves to move from the outer (external ear) to the inner ear.

DEF: Sensorineural hearing loss: Hearing loss that occurs from damage to the hair cells of the inner ear or problems with the nerve pathways from the inner ear to the brain.

- H90.0 Conductive hearing loss, bilateral

✓5th **H90.1 Conductive hearing loss, unilateral with unrestricted hearing on the contralateral side**
- **H90.11 Conductive hearing loss, unilateral, right ear, with unrestricted hearing on the contralateral side**
- **H90.12 Conductive hearing loss, unilateral, left ear, with unrestricted hearing on the contralateral side**

H90.2 Conductive hearing loss, unspecified
Conductive deafness NOS

H90.3 Sensorineural hearing loss, bilateral

✓5th **H90.4 Sensorineural hearing loss, unilateral with unrestricted hearing on the contralateral side**
- **H90.41 Sensorineural hearing loss, unilateral, right ear, with unrestricted hearing on the contralateral side**
- **H90.42 Sensorineural hearing loss, unilateral, left ear, with unrestricted hearing on the contralateral side**

H90.5 Unspecified sensorineural hearing loss
Central hearing loss NOS
Congenital deafness NOS
Neural hearing loss NOS
Perceptive hearing loss NOS
Sensorineural deafness NOS
Sensory hearing loss NOS
EXCLUDES 1 *abnormal auditory perception (H93.2-)*
psychogenic deafness (F44.6)

H90.6 Mixed conductive and sensorineural hearing loss, bilateral
AHA: 2015,2Q,7

✓5th **H90.7 Mixed conductive and sensorineural hearing loss, unilateral with unrestricted hearing on the contralateral side**
- **H90.71 Mixed conductive and sensorineural hearing loss, unilateral, right ear, with unrestricted hearing on the contralateral side**
- **H90.72 Mixed conductive and sensorineural hearing loss, unilateral, left ear, with unrestricted hearing on the contralateral side**

H90.8 Mixed conductive and sensorineural hearing loss, unspecified

✓5th **H90.A Conductive and sensorineural hearing loss with restricted hearing on the contralateral side**
AHA: 2016,4Q,23-25

✓6th **H90.A1 Conductive hearing loss, unilateral, with restricted hearing on the contralateral side**
- **H90.A11 Conductive hearing loss, unilateral, right ear with restricted hearing on the contralateral side**
- **H90.A12 Conductive hearing loss, unilateral, left ear with restricted hearing on the contralateral side**

✓6th **H90.A2 Sensorineural hearing loss, unilateral, with restricted hearing on the contralateral side**
- **H90.A21 Sensorineural hearing loss, unilateral, right ear, with restricted hearing on the contralateral side**
- **H90.A22 Sensorineural hearing loss, unilateral, left ear, with restricted hearing on the contralateral side**

✓6th **H90.A3 Mixed conductive and sensorineural hearing loss, unilateral with restricted hearing on the contralateral side**
- **H90.A31 Mixed conductive and sensorineural hearing loss, unilateral, right ear with restricted hearing on the contralateral side**
- **H90.A32 Mixed conductive and sensorineural hearing, unilateral, left ear with restricted hearing on the contralateral side**

✓4th **H91 Other and unspecified hearing loss**
EXCLUDES 1 *abnormal auditory perception (H93.2-)*
hearing loss as classified in H90.-
impacted cerumen (H61.2-)
noise-induced hearing loss (H83.3-)
psychogenic deafness (F44.6)
transient ischemic deafness (H93.01-)

✓5th **H91.0 Ototoxic hearing loss**
Code first poisoning due to drug or toxin, if applicable (T36-T65 with fifth or sixth character 1-4 or 6)
Use additional code for adverse effect, if applicable, to identify drug (T36-T50 with fifth or sixth character 5)
- **H91.01 Ototoxic hearing loss, right ear**
- **H91.02 Ototoxic hearing loss, left ear**
- **H91.03 Ototoxic hearing loss, bilateral**
- **H91.09 Ototoxic hearing loss, unspecified ear**

✓5th **H91.1 Presbycusis**
Presbyacusia
- **H91.10 Presbycusis, unspecified ear**
- **H91.11 Presbycusis, right ear**
- **H91.12 Presbycusis, left ear**
- **H91.13 Presbycusis, bilateral**

✓5th **H91.2 Sudden idiopathic hearing loss**
Sudden hearing loss NOS
- **H91.20 Sudden idiopathic hearing loss, unspecified ear**
- **H91.21 Sudden idiopathic hearing loss, right ear**
- **H91.22 Sudden idiopathic hearing loss, left ear**
- **H91.23 Sudden idiopathic hearing loss, bilateral**

H91.3 Deaf nonspeaking, not elsewhere classified

✓5th **H91.8 Other specified hearing loss**

✓6th **H91.8X Other specified hearing loss**
- **H91.8X1 Other specified hearing loss, right ear**
- **H91.8X2 Other specified hearing loss, left ear**
- **H91.8X3 Other specified hearing loss, bilateral**
- **H91.8X9 Other specified hearing loss, unspecified ear**

✓5th **H91.9 Unspecified hearing loss**
Deafness NOS
High frequency deafness
Low frequency deafness
- **H91.90 Unspecified hearing loss, unspecified ear**
- **H91.91 Unspecified hearing loss, right ear**
- **H91.92 Unspecified hearing loss, left ear**
- **H91.93 Unspecified hearing loss, bilateral**

✓4th **H92 Otalgia and effusion of ear**

✓5th **H92.0 Otalgia**
- **H92.01 Otalgia, right ear**
- **H92.02 Otalgia, left ear**
- **H92.03 Otalgia, bilateral**
- **H92.09 Otalgia, unspecified ear**

✓5th **H92.1 Otorrhea**
EXCLUDES 1 *leakage of cerebrospinal fluid through ear (G96.0)*
- **H92.10 Otorrhea, unspecified ear**
- **H92.11 Otorrhea, right ear**
- **H92.12 Otorrhea, left ear**
- **H92.13 Otorrhea, bilateral**

✓5th **H92.2 Otorrhagia**
EXCLUDES 1 *traumatic otorrhagia — code to injury*
- **H92.20 Otorrhagia, unspecified ear**
- **H92.21 Otorrhagia, right ear**
- **H92.22 Otorrhagia, left ear**
- **H92.23 Otorrhagia, bilateral**

✓4th **H93 Other disorders of ear, not elsewhere classified**

✓5th **H93.0 Degenerative and vascular disorders of ear**
EXCLUDES 1 *presbycusis (H91.1)*

✓6th **H93.01 Transient ischemic deafness**
- **H93.011 Transient ischemic deafness, right ear**
- **H93.012 Transient ischemic deafness, left ear**
- **H93.013 Transient ischemic deafness, bilateral**
- **H93.019 Transient ischemic deafness, unspecified ear**

✓6th **H93.09 Unspecified degenerative and vascular disorders of ear**
- **H93.091 Unspecified degenerative and vascular disorders of right ear**
- **H93.092 Unspecified degenerative and vascular disorders of left ear**
- **H93.093 Unspecified degenerative and vascular disorders of ear, bilateral**
- **H93.099 Unspecified degenerative and vascular disorders of unspecified ear**

✓5th **H93.1 Tinnitus**
- **H93.11 Tinnitus, right ear**
- **H93.12 Tinnitus, left ear**
- **H93.13 Tinnitus, bilateral**
- **H93.19 Tinnitus, unspecified ear**

✓5th **H93.A Pulsatile tinnitus**
AHA: 2016,4Q,25-26
- **H93.A1 Pulsatile tinnitus, right ear**
- **H93.A2 Pulsatile tinnitus, left ear**
- **H93.A3 Pulsatile tinnitus, bilateral**

H93.A9 Pulsatile tinnitus, unspecified ear

H93.2 Other abnormal auditory perceptions

EXCLUDES 2 *auditory hallucinations (R44.Ø)*

H93.21 Auditory recruitment

H93.211 Auditory recruitment, right ear

H93.212 Auditory recruitment, left ear

H93.213 Auditory recruitment, bilateral

H93.219 Auditory recruitment, unspecified ear

H93.22 Diplacusis

H93.221 Diplacusis, right ear

H93.222 Diplacusis, left ear

H93.223 Diplacusis, bilateral

H93.229 Diplacusis, unspecified ear

H93.23 Hyperacusis

DEF: Exceptionally acute sense of hearing caused by such conditions as Bell's palsy. This term may also refer to painful sensitivity to sounds.

H93.231 Hyperacusis, right ear

H93.232 Hyperacusis, left ear

H93.233 Hyperacusis, bilateral

H93.239 Hyperacusis, unspecified ear

H93.24 Temporary auditory threshold shift

H93.241 Temporary auditory threshold shift, right ear

H93.242 Temporary auditory threshold shift, left ear

H93.243 Temporary auditory threshold shift, bilateral

H93.249 Temporary auditory threshold shift, unspecified ear

H93.25 Central auditory processing disorder

Congenital auditory imperception

Word deafness

EXCLUDES 1 *mixed receptive-expressive language disorder (F8Ø.2)*

H93.29 Other abnormal auditory perceptions

H93.291 Other abnormal auditory perceptions, right ear

H93.292 Other abnormal auditory perceptions, left ear

H93.293 Other abnormal auditory perceptions, bilateral

H93.299 Other abnormal auditory perceptions, unspecified ear

H93.3 Disorders of acoustic nerve

Disorder of 8th cranial nerve

EXCLUDES 1 *acoustic neuroma (D33.3)*

syphilitic acoustic neuritis (A52.15)

H93.3X Disorders of acoustic nerve

H93.3X1 Disorders of right acoustic nerve

H93.3X2 Disorders of left acoustic nerve

H93.3X3 Disorders of bilateral acoustic nerves

H93.3X9 Disorders of unspecified acoustic nerve

H93.8 Other specified disorders of ear

H93.8X Other specified disorders of ear

H93.8X1 Other specified disorders of right ear

H93.8X2 Other specified disorders of left ear

H93.8X3 Other specified disorders of ear, bilateral

H93.8X9 Other specified disorders of ear, unspecified ear

H93.9 Unspecified disorder of ear

H93.9Ø Unspecified disorder of ear, unspecified ear

H93.91 Unspecified disorder of right ear

H93.92 Unspecified disorder of left ear

H93.93 Unspecified disorder of ear, bilateral

H94 Other disorders of ear in diseases classified elsewhere

H94.Ø Acoustic neuritis in infectious and parasitic diseases classified elsewhere

Code first underlying disease, such as:

parasitic disease (B65-B89)

EXCLUDES 1 *acoustic neuritis (in):*

herpes zoster (BØ2.29)

syphilis (A52.15)

H94.ØØ Acoustic neuritis in infectious and parasitic diseases classified elsewhere, unspecified ear

H94.Ø1 Acoustic neuritis in infectious and parasitic diseases classified elsewhere, right ear

H94.Ø2 Acoustic neuritis in infectious and parasitic diseases classified elsewhere, left ear

H94.Ø3 Acoustic neuritis in infectious and parasitic diseases classified elsewhere, bilateral

H94.8 Other specified disorders of ear in diseases classified elsewhere

Code first underlying disease, such as:

congenital syphilis (A5Ø.Ø)

EXCLUDES 1 *aural myiasis (B87.4)*

syphilitic labyrinthitis (A52.79)

H94.8Ø Other specified disorders of ear in diseases classified elsewhere, unspecified ear

H94.81 Other specified disorders of right ear in diseases classified elsewhere

H94.82 Other specified disorders of left ear in diseases classified elsewhere

H94.83 Other specified disorders of ear in diseases classified elsewhere, bilateral

Intraoperative and postprocedural complications and disorders of ear and mastoid process, not elsewhere classified (H95)

H95 Intraoperative and postprocedural complications and disorders of ear and mastoid process, not elsewhere classified

AHA: 2016,4Q,9-10

H95.Ø Recurrent cholesteatoma of postmastoidectomy cavity

H95.ØØ Recurrent cholesteatoma of postmastoidectomy cavity, unspecified ear

H95.Ø1 Recurrent cholesteatoma of postmastoidectomy cavity, right ear

H95.Ø2 Recurrent cholesteatoma of postmastoidectomy cavity, left ear

H95.Ø3 Recurrent cholesteatoma of postmastoidectomy cavity, bilateral ears

H95.1 Other disorders of ear and mastoid process following mastoidectomy

H95.11 Chronic inflammation of postmastoidectomy cavity

H95.111 Chronic inflammation of postmastoidectomy cavity, right ear

H95.112 Chronic inflammation of postmastoidectomy cavity, left ear

H95.113 Chronic inflammation of postmastoidectomy cavity, bilateral ears

H95.119 Chronic inflammation of postmastoidectomy cavity, unspecified ear

H95.12 Granulation of postmastoidectomy cavity

H95.121 Granulation of postmastoidectomy cavity, right ear

H95.122 Granulation of postmastoidectomy cavity, left ear

H95.123 Granulation of postmastoidectomy cavity, bilateral ears

H95.129 Granulation of postmastoidectomy cavity, unspecified ear

H95.13 Mucosal cyst of postmastoidectomy cavity

H95.131 Mucosal cyst of postmastoidectomy cavity, right ear

H95.132 Mucosal cyst of postmastoidectomy cavity, left ear

H95.133 Mucosal cyst of postmastoidectomy cavity, bilateral ears

H95.139 Mucosal cyst of postmastoidectomy cavity, unspecified ear

H95.19 Other disorders following mastoidectomy

H95.191 Other disorders following mastoidectomy, right ear

H95.192 Other disorders following mastoidectomy, left ear

H95.193 Other disorders following mastoidectomy, bilateral ears

H95.199 Other disorders following mastoidectomy, unspecified ear

√5th **H95.2 Intraoperative hemorrhage and hematoma of ear and mastoid process complicating a procedure**

EXCLUDES 1 *intraoperative hemorrhage and hematoma of ear and mastoid process due to accidental puncture or laceration during a procedure (H95.3-)*

H95.21 Intraoperative hemorrhage and hematoma of ear and mastoid process complicating a procedure on the ear and mastoid process CC

H95.22 Intraoperative hemorrhage and hematoma of ear and mastoid process complicating other procedure CC

√5th **H95.3 Accidental puncture and laceration of ear and mastoid process during a procedure**

H95.31 Accidental puncture and laceration of the ear and mastoid process during a procedure on the ear and mastoid process CC

H95.32 Accidental puncture and laceration of the ear and mastoid process during other procedure CC

√5th **H95.4 Postprocedural hemorrhage of ear and mastoid process following a procedure**

H95.41 Postprocedural hemorrhage of ear and mastoid process following a procedure on the ear and mastoid process CC

H95.42 Postprocedural hemorrhage of ear and mastoid process following other procedure CC

√5th **H95.5 Postprocedural hematoma and seroma of ear and mastoid process following a procedure**

H95.51 Postprocedural hematoma of ear and mastoid process following a procedure on the ear and mastoid process CC

H95.52 Postprocedural hematoma of ear and mastoid process following other procedure CC

H95.53 Postprocedural seroma of ear and mastoid process following a procedure on the ear and mastoid process CC

H95.54 Postprocedural seroma of ear and mastoid process following other procedure CC

√5th **H95.8 Other intraoperative and postprocedural complications and disorders of the ear and mastoid process, not elsewhere classified**

EXCLUDES 2 *postprocedural complications and disorders following mastoidectomy (H95.Ø-, H95.1-)*

√6th **H95.81 Postprocedural stenosis of external ear canal**

H95.811 Postprocedural stenosis of right external ear canal CC

H95.812 Postprocedural stenosis of left external ear canal CC

H95.813 Postprocedural stenosis of external ear canal, bilateral CC

H95.819 Postprocedural stenosis of unspecified external ear canal CC

H95.88 Other intraoperative complications and disorders of the ear and mastoid process, not elsewhere classified CC

Use additional code, if applicable, to further specify disorder

H95.89 Other postprocedural complications and disorders of the ear and mastoid process, not elsewhere classified CC

Use additional code, if applicable, to further specify disorder

Chapter 9. Diseases of the Circulatory System (I00–I99)

Chapter-specific Guidelines with Coding Examples

The chapter-specific guidelines from the ICD-10-CM Official Guidelines for Coding and Reporting have been provided below. Along with these guidelines are coding examples, contained in the shaded boxes, that have been developed to help illustrate the coding and/or sequencing guidance found in these guidelines.

a. Hypertension

The classification presumes a causal relationship between hypertension and heart involvement and between hypertension and kidney involvement, as the two conditions are linked by the term "with" in the Alphabetic Index. These conditions should be coded as related even in the absence of provider documentation explicitly linking them, unless the documentation clearly states the conditions are unrelated.

For hypertension and conditions not specifically linked by relational terms such as "with," "associated with" or "due to" in the classification, provider documentation must link the conditions in order to code them as related.

1) Hypertension with heart disease

Hypertension with heart conditions classified to I50.- or I51.4-I51.7, I51.89, I51.9, are assigned to a code from category I11, Hypertensive heart disease. Use additional code(s) from category I50, Heart failure, to identify the type(s) of heart failure in those patients with heart failure.

The same heart conditions (I50.-, I51.4-I51.7, I51.89, I51.9) with hypertension are coded separately if the provider has documented they are unrelated to the hypertension. Sequence according to the circumstances of the admission/encounter.

Patient is admitted in left heart failure. Patient also has a history of hypertension managed by medication.

I11.0	**Hypertensive heart disease with heart failure**
I50.1	**Left ventricular failure, unspecified**

Explanation: Without a diagnostic statement to the contrary, hypertension and heart failure have an assumed causal relationship, and a combination code should be used. An additional code to identify the type of heart failure (I50.-) should also be provided.

2) Hypertensive chronic kidney disease

Assign codes from category I12, Hypertensive chronic kidney disease, when both hypertension and a condition classifiable to category N18, Chronic kidney disease (CKD), are present. CKD should not be coded as hypertensive if the provider indicates the CKD is not related to the hypertension.

The appropriate code from category N18 should be used as a secondary code with a code from category I12 to identify the stage of chronic kidney disease.

See Section I.C.14. Chronic kidney disease.

If a patient has hypertensive chronic kidney disease and acute renal failure, **the acute renal failure should also be coded. Sequence according to the circumstances of the admission/encounter.**

Patient is admitted with stage IV chronic kidney disease (CKD) due to polycystic kidney disease. Patient also is on lisinopril for hypertension.

N18.4	**Chronic kidney disease, stage 4 (severe)**
Q61.3	**Polycystic kidney, unspecified**
I10	**Essential (primary) hypertension**

Explanation: A combination code describing a relationship between hypertension and CKD is not used because the physician documentation identifies the polycystic kidney disease as the cause for the CKD.

3) Hypertensive heart and chronic kidney disease

Assign codes from combination category I13, Hypertensive heart and chronic kidney disease, when there is hypertension with both heart and kidney involvement. If heart failure is present, assign an additional code from category I50 to identify the type of heart failure.

The appropriate code from category N18, Chronic kidney disease, should be used as a secondary code with a code from category I13 to identify the stage of chronic kidney disease.

See Section I.C.14. Chronic kidney disease.

The codes in category I13, Hypertensive heart and chronic kidney disease, are combination codes that include hypertension, heart disease and chronic kidney disease. The Includes note at I13 specifies that the conditions included at I11 and I12 are included together in I13. If a patient has hypertension, heart disease and chronic kidney disease, then a code from I13 should be used, not individual codes for hypertension, heart disease and chronic kidney disease, or codes from I11 or I12.

For patients with both acute renal failure and chronic kidney disease, **the** acute renal failure **should also be coded. Sequence according to the circumstances of the admission/encounter.**

Patient admitted with acute tubular necrosis, history of hypertensive heart and kidney disease with congestive heart failure and stage 3a chronic kidney disease

N17.0	**Acute kidney failure with tubular necrosis**
I13.0	**Hypertensive heart and chronic kidney disease with heart failure and stage 1 through stage 4 chronic kidney disease, or unspecified chronic kidney disease**
I50.9	**Heart failure, unspecified**
N18.31	**Chronic kidney disease, stage 3a**

Explanation: It is appropriate to report an acute kidney failure code and a chronic kidney failure code when both conditions are treated during an encounter. In this instance, the acute renal failure was the focus of treatment and therefore sequenced as principal diagnosis. Combination codes in category I13 are used to report conditions classifiable to *both* categories I11 and I12. Do not report conditions classifiable to I11 and I12 separately. Use additional codes to report the type of heart failure and stage of CKD.

4) Hypertensive cerebrovascular disease

For hypertensive cerebrovascular disease, first assign the appropriate code from categories I60-I69, followed by the appropriate hypertension code.

Rupture of cerebral aneurysm caused by malignant hypertension

I60.7	**Nontraumatic subarachnoid hemorrhage from unspecified intracranial artery**
I10	**Essential (primary) hypertension**

Explanation: Hypertensive cerebrovascular disease requires two codes: the appropriate I60–I69 code followed by the appropriate hypertension code.

5) Hypertensive retinopathy

Subcategory H35.0, Background retinopathy and retinal vascular changes, should be used with a code from category I10 – I15, Hypertensive disease to include the systemic hypertension. The sequencing is based on the reason for the encounter.

6) Hypertension, secondary

Secondary hypertension is due to an underlying condition. Two codes are required: one to identify the underlying etiology and one from category I15 to identify the hypertension. Sequencing of codes is determined by the reason for admission/encounter.

Renovascular hypertension due to renal artery atherosclerosis

I15.0	**Renovascular hypertension**
I70.1	**Atherosclerosis of renal artery**

Explanation: Secondary hypertension requires two codes: a code to identify the etiology and the appropriate I15 code.

7) Hypertension, transient

Assign code R03.0, Elevated blood pressure reading without diagnosis of hypertension, unless patient has an established diagnosis of hypertension. Assign code O13.-, Gestational [pregnancy-induced] hypertension without significant proteinuria, or O14.-, Pre-eclampsia, for transient hypertension of pregnancy.

8) Hypertension, controlled

This diagnostic statement usually refers to an existing state of hypertension under control by therapy. Assign the appropriate code from categories I10-I15, Hypertensive diseases.

9) Hypertension, uncontrolled

Uncontrolled hypertension may refer to untreated hypertension or hypertension not responding to current therapeutic regimen. In either case, assign the appropriate code from categories I10-I15, Hypertensive diseases.

10) Hypertensive crisis

Assign a code from category I16, Hypertensive crisis, for documented hypertensive urgency, hypertensive emergency or unspecified hypertensive crisis. Code also any identified hypertensive disease (I10-I15). The sequencing is based on the reason for the encounter.

11) Pulmonary hypertension

Pulmonary hypertension is classified to category I27, Other pulmonary heart diseases. For secondary pulmonary hypertension (I27.1, I27.2-), code also any associated conditions or adverse effects of drugs or toxins. The sequencing is based on the reason for the encounter, except for adverse effects of drugs (See Section I.C.19.e.).

b. Atherosclerotic coronary artery disease and angina

ICD-10-CM has combination codes for atherosclerotic heart disease with angina pectoris. The subcategories for these codes are I25.11, Atherosclerotic heart disease of native coronary artery with angina pectoris and I25.7, Atherosclerosis of coronary artery bypass graft(s) and coronary artery of transplanted heart with angina pectoris.

When using one of these combination codes it is not necessary to use an additional code for angina pectoris. A causal relationship can be assumed in a patient with both atherosclerosis and angina pectoris, unless the documentation indicates the angina is due to something other than the atherosclerosis.

If a patient with coronary artery disease is admitted due to an acute myocardial infarction (AMI), the AMI should be sequenced before the coronary artery disease.

See Section I.C.9. Acute myocardial infarction (AMI)

c. Intraoperative and postprocedural cerebrovascular accident

Medical record documentation should clearly specify the cause- and- effect relationship between the medical intervention and the cerebrovascular accident in order to assign a code for intraoperative or postprocedural cerebrovascular accident.

Proper code assignment depends on whether it was an infarction or hemorrhage and whether it occurred intraoperatively or postoperatively. If it was a cerebral hemorrhage, code assignment depends on the type of procedure performed.

> Embolic cerebral infarction of the right middle cerebral artery that occurred during hip replacement surgery. The surgeon documented as due to the surgery.
>
> **I97.811 Intraoperative cerebrovascular infarction during other surgery**
>
> **I63.411 Cerebral infarction due to embolism of right middle cerebral artery**
>
> *Explanation*: Code assignment for intraoperative or postprocedural cerebrovascular accident is based on the provider's documentation of a cause-and-effect relationship between the condition and the procedure. Proper code assignment also depends on whether the cerebrovascular accident was an infarction or hemorrhage, occurred intraoperatively or postoperatively, and the type of procedure performed.

d. Sequelae of cerebrovascular disease

1) Category I69, Sequelae of cerebrovascular disease

Category I69 is used to indicate conditions classifiable to categories I60-I67 as the causes of sequela (neurologic deficits), themselves classified elsewhere. These "late effects" include neurologic deficits that persist after initial onset of conditions classifiable to categories I60-I67. The neurologic deficits caused by cerebrovascular disease may be present from the onset or may arise at any time after the onset of the condition classifiable to categories I60-I67.

Codes from category I69, Sequelae of cerebrovascular disease, that specify hemiplegia, hemiparesis and monoplegia identify whether the dominant or nondominant side is affected. Should the affected side be documented, but not specified as dominant or nondominant, and the classification system does not indicate a default, code selection is as follows:

- For ambidextrous patients, the default should be dominant.
- If the left side is affected, the default is non-dominant.
- If the right side is affected, the default is dominant.

2) Codes from category I69 with codes from I60–I67

Codes from category I69 may be assigned on a health care record with codes from I60-I67, if the patient has a current cerebrovascular disease and deficits from an old cerebrovascular disease.

3) Codes from category I69 and personal history of transient ischemic attack (TIA) and cerebral infarction (Z86.73)

Codes from category I69 should not be assigned if the patient does not have neurologic deficits.

See Section I.C.21. 4. History (of) for use of personal history codes

e. Acute myocardial infarction (AMI)

1) Type 1 ST elevation myocardial infarction (STEMI) and non ST elevation myocardial infarction (NSTEMI)

The ICD-10-CM codes for type 1 acute myocardial infarction (AMI) identify the site, such as anterolateral wall or true posterior wall. Subcategories I21.0-I21.2 and code I21.3 are used for type 1 ST elevation myocardial infarction (STEMI). Code I21.4, Non-ST elevation (NSTEMI) myocardial infarction, is used for type 1 non-ST elevation myocardial infarction (NSTEMI) and nontransmural MIs.

If a type 1 NSTEMI evolves to STEMI, assign the STEMI code. If a type 1 STEMI converts to NSTEMI due to thrombolytic therapy, it is still coded as STEMI.

For encounters occurring while the myocardial infarction is equal to, or less than, four weeks old, including transfers to another acute setting or a postacute setting, and the myocardial infarction meets the definition for "other diagnoses" (see Section III, Reporting Additional Diagnoses), codes from category I21 may continue to be reported. For encounters after the 4 week time frame and the patient is still receiving care related to the myocardial infarction, the appropriate aftercare code should be assigned, rather than a code from category I21. For old or healed myocardial infarctions not requiring further care, code I25.2, Old myocardial infarction, may be assigned.

2) Acute myocardial infarction, unspecified

Code I21.9, Acute myocardial infarction, unspecified, is the default for unspecified acute myocardial infarction or unspecified type. If only type 1 STEMI or transmural MI without the site is documented, assign code I21.3, ST elevation (STEMI) myocardial infarction of unspecified site.

3) AMI documented as nontransmural or subendocardial but site provided

If an AMI is documented as nontransmural or subendocardial, but the site is provided, it is still coded as a subendocardial AMI.

See Section I.C.21.3 for information on coding status post administration of tPA in a different facility within the last 24 hours.

4) Subsequent acute myocardial infarction

A code from category I22, Subsequent ST elevation (STEMI) and non-ST elevation (NSTEMI) myocardial infarction, is to be used when a patient who has suffered a type 1 or unspecified AMI has a new AMI within the 4 week time frame of the initial AMI. A code from category I22 must be used in conjunction with a code from category I21. The sequencing of the I22 and I21 codes depends on the circumstances of the encounter.

Do not assign code I22 for subsequent myocardial infarctions other than type 1 or unspecified. For subsequent type 2 AMI assign only code I21.A1. For subsequent type 4 or type 5 AMI, assign only code I21.A9.

If a subsequent myocardial infarction of one type occurs within 4 weeks of a myocardial infarction of a different type, assign the appropriate codes from category I21 to identify each type. Do not assign a code from I22. Codes from category I22 should only be assigned if both the initial and subsequent myocardial infarctions are type 1 or unspecified.

5) Other types of myocardial infarction

The ICD-10-CM provides codes for different types of myocardial infarction. Type 1 myocardial infarctions are assigned to codes I21.0-I21.4.

Type 2 myocardial infarction (myocardial infarction due to demand ischemia or secondary to ischemic imbalance) is assigned to code I21.A1, Myocardial infarction type 2 with the underlying cause coded first. Do not assign code I24.8, Other forms of acute ischemic heart disease, for the demand ischemia. If a type 2 AMI is described as NSTEMI or STEMI, only assign code I21.A1. Codes I21.01-I21.4 should only be assigned for type 1 AMIs.

Acute myocardial infarctions type 3, 4a, 4b, 4c and 5 are assigned to code I21.A9, Other myocardial infarction type.

The "Code also" and "Code first" notes should be followed related to complications, and for coding of postprocedural myocardial infarctions during or following cardiac surgery.

> Myocardial infarction involving the left circumflex artery occurring during PTCA with stent insertion to treat coronary artery disease
>
> **I25.10 Atherosclerotic heart disease of native coronary artery without angina pectoris**
>
> **I97.790 Other intraoperative cardiac functional disturbances during cardiac surgery**
>
> **I21.A9 Other myocardial infarction type**
>
> *Explanation*: A myocardial infarction occurring during a revascularization procedure is not considered a type 1 myocardial infarction (MI) and should not be coded to a type 1 MI code (I21.0-, I21.1-, I21.2-, I21.3) even when the specific site of the MI is documented. According to the code first instruction at I21.A9, the complication code (I97.790) should be sequenced before code I21.A9.

Chapter 9. Diseases of the Circulatory System (I00-I99)

EXCLUDES 2 *certain conditions originating in the perinatal period (P04-P96)*
certain infectious and parasitic diseases (A00-B99)
complications of pregnancy, childbirth and the puerperium (O00-O9A)
congenital malformations, deformations, and chromosomal abnormalities (Q00-Q99)
endocrine, nutritional and metabolic diseases (E00-E88)
injury, poisoning and certain other consequences of external causes (S00-T88)
neoplasms (C00-D49)
symptoms, signs and abnormal clinical and laboratory findings, not elsewhere classified (R00-R94)
systemic connective tissue disorders (M30-M36)
transient cerebral ischemic attacks and related syndromes (G45.-)

This chapter contains the following blocks:

I00-I02	Acute rheumatic fever
I05-I09	Chronic rheumatic heart diseases
I10-I16	Hypertensive diseases
I20-I25	Ischemic heart diseases
I26-I28	Pulmonary heart disease and diseases of pulmonary circulation
I30-I52	Other forms of heart disease
I60-I69	Cerebrovascular diseases
I70-I79	Diseases of arteries, arterioles and capillaries
I80-I89	Diseases of veins, lymphatic vessels and lymph nodes, not elsewhere classified
I95-I99	Other and unspecified disorders of the circulatory system

Acute rheumatic fever (I00-I02)

DEF: Inflammatory disease that can follow a throat infection by group A streptococci. Complications can involve the joints (arthritis), subcutaneous tissue (nodules), skin (erythema marginatum), heart (carditis), or brain (chorea).

I00 Rheumatic fever without heart involvement
INCLUDES arthritis, rheumatic, acute or subacute
EXCLUDES 1 *rheumatic fever with heart involvement (I01.0-I01.9)*

✓4th **I01 Rheumatic fever with heart involvement**
EXCLUDES 1 *chronic diseases of rheumatic origin (I05-I09) unless rheumatic fever is also present or there is evidence of reactivation or activity of the rheumatic process*

I01.0 Acute rheumatic pericarditis CC
Any condition in I00 with pericarditis
Rheumatic pericarditis (acute)
EXCLUDES 1 *acute pericarditis not specified as rheumatic (I30.-)*

I01.1 Acute rheumatic endocarditis CC
Any condition in I00 with endocarditis or valvulitis
Acute rheumatic valvulitis

I01.2 Acute rheumatic myocarditis CC
Any condition in I00 with myocarditis

I01.8 Other acute rheumatic heart disease CC
Any condition in I00 with other or multiple types of heart involvement
Acute rheumatic pancarditis

I01.9 Acute rheumatic heart disease, unspecified CC
Any condition in I00 with unspecified type of heart involvement
Rheumatic carditis, acute
Rheumatic heart disease, active or acute

✓4th **I02 Rheumatic chorea**
INCLUDES Sydenham's chorea
EXCLUDES 1 *chorea NOS (G25.5)*
Huntington's chorea (G10)

I02.0 Rheumatic chorea with heart involvement CC
Chorea NOS with heart involvement
Rheumatic chorea with heart involvement of any type classifiable under I01.-

I02.9 Rheumatic chorea without heart involvement CC
Rheumatic chorea NOS

Chronic rheumatic heart diseases (I05-I09)

✓4th **I05 Rheumatic mitral valve diseases**
INCLUDES conditions classifiable to both I05.0 and I05.2-I05.9, whether specified as rheumatic or not
EXCLUDES 1 *mitral valve disease specified as nonrheumatic (I34.-)*
mitral valve disease with aortic and/or tricuspid valve involvement (I08.-)

I05.0 Rheumatic mitral stenosis
Mitral (valve) obstruction (rheumatic)
DEF: Narrowing of the mitral valve between the left atrium and left ventricle due to rheumatic fever. Symptoms include shortness of breath during or after exercise, fatigue, palpitations, chest discomfort, and swelling of feet or legs.

I05.1 Rheumatic mitral insufficiency
Rheumatic mitral incompetence
Rheumatic mitral regurgitation
EXCLUDES 1 *mitral insufficiency not specified as rheumatic (I34.0)*

I05.2 Rheumatic mitral stenosis with insufficiency
Rheumatic mitral stenosis with incompetence or regurgitation

I05.8 Other rheumatic mitral valve diseases
Rheumatic mitral (valve) failure

I05.9 Rheumatic mitral valve disease, unspecified
Rheumatic mitral (valve) disorder (chronic) NOS

✓4th **I06 Rheumatic aortic valve diseases**
EXCLUDES 1 *aortic valve disease not specified as rheumatic (I35.-)*
aortic valve disease with mitral and/or tricuspid valve involvement (I08.-)

I06.0 Rheumatic aortic stenosis
Rheumatic aortic (valve) obstruction

I06.1 Rheumatic aortic insufficiency
Rheumatic aortic incompetence
Rheumatic aortic regurgitation

I06.2 Rheumatic aortic stenosis with insufficiency
Rheumatic aortic stenosis with incompetence or regurgitation

I06.8 Other rheumatic aortic valve diseases

I06.9 Rheumatic aortic valve disease, unspecified
Rheumatic aortic (valve) disease NOS

✓4th **I07 Rheumatic tricuspid valve diseases**
INCLUDES rheumatic tricuspid valve diseases specified as rheumatic or unspecified
EXCLUDES 1 *tricuspid valve disease specified as nonrheumatic (I36.-)*
tricuspid valve disease with aortic and/or mitral valve involvement (I08.-)

I07.0 Rheumatic tricuspid stenosis
Tricuspid (valve) stenosis (rheumatic)

I07.1 Rheumatic tricuspid insufficiency
Tricuspid (valve) insufficiency (rheumatic)

I07.2 Rheumatic tricuspid stenosis and insufficiency

I07.8 Other rheumatic tricuspid valve diseases

I07.9 Rheumatic tricuspid valve disease, unspecified
Rheumatic tricuspid valve disorder NOS

✓4th **I08 Multiple valve diseases**
INCLUDES multiple valve diseases specified as rheumatic or unspecified
EXCLUDES 1 *endocarditis, valve unspecified (I38)*
multiple valve disease specified a nonrheumatic (I34.-, I35.-, I36.-, I37.-, I38.-, Q22.-, Q23.-, Q24.8-)
rheumatic valve disease NOS (I09.1)

I08.0 Rheumatic disorders of both mitral and aortic valves
Involvement of both mitral and aortic valves specified as rheumatic or unspecified
AHA: 2019,2Q,5

I08.1 Rheumatic disorders of both mitral and tricuspid valves

I08.2 Rheumatic disorders of both aortic and tricuspid valves

I08.3 Combined rheumatic disorders of mitral, aortic and tricuspid valves

I08.8 Other rheumatic multiple valve diseases

I08.9 Rheumatic multiple valve disease, unspecified

✓4th **I09 Other rheumatic heart diseases**

I09.0 Rheumatic myocarditis CC
EXCLUDES 1 *myocarditis not specified as rheumatic (I51.4)*

I09.1 Rheumatic diseases of endocardium, valve unspecified
Rheumatic endocarditis (chronic)
Rheumatic valvulitis (chronic)
EXCLUDES 1 *endocarditis, valve unspecified (I38)*

I09.2 Chronic rheumatic pericarditis CC
Adherent pericardium, rheumatic
Chronic rheumatic mediastinopericarditis
Chronic rheumatic myopericarditis
EXCLUDES 1 *chronic pericarditis not specified as rheumatic (I31.-)*

✓5th **I09.8 Other specified rheumatic heart diseases**

I09.81 Rheumatic heart failure CC HCC
Use additional code to identify type of heart failure (I50.-)
DEF: Decreased cardiac output, edema, and hypertension due to rheumatic heart disease.

I09.89 Other specified rheumatic heart diseases
Rheumatic disease of pulmonary valve

I09.9 Rheumatic heart disease, unspecified
Rheumatic carditis
EXCLUDES 1 *rheumatoid carditis (M05.31)*

Hypertensive diseases (I10-I16)

Use additional code to identify:
exposure to environmental tobacco smoke (Z77.22)
history of tobacco dependence (Z87.891)
occupational exposure to environmental tobacco smoke (Z57.31)
tobacco dependence (F17.-)
tobacco use (Z72.0)

EXCLUDES 1 *neonatal hypertension (P29.2)*
primary pulmonary hypertension (I27.0)
EXCLUDES 2 *hypertensive disease complicating pregnancy, childbirth and the puerperium (O10-O11, O13-O16)*

I10 Essential (primary) hypertension
INCLUDES high blood pressure
hypertension (arterial) (benign) (essential) (malignant) (primary) (systemic)
EXCLUDES 1 *hypertensive disease complicating pregnancy, childbirth and the puerperium (O10-O11, O13-O16)*
EXCLUDES 2 *essential (primary) hypertension involving vessels of brain (I60-I69)*
essential (primary) hypertension involving vessels of eye (H35.0-)
AHA: 2020,1Q,12; 2018,2Q,9; 2016,4Q,27

✓4th **I11 Hypertensive heart disease**
INCLUDES ▶any condition in I50.- or I51.4-I51.7, I51.89, I51.9 due to hypertension◀
AHA: 2018,2Q,9
TIP: Do not assign a code from this category when provider documentation indicates the heart disease is attributable to another cause.

I11.0 Hypertensive heart disease with heart failure HCC
Hypertensive heart failure
Use additional code to identify type of heart failure (I50.-)
AHA: 2017,1Q,47

I11.9 Hypertensive heart disease without heart failure
Hypertensive heart disease NOS

✓4th **I12 Hypertensive chronic kidney disease**
INCLUDES any condition in N18 and N26 — due to hypertension
arteriosclerosis of kidney
arteriosclerotic nephritis (chronic) (interstitial)
hypertensive nephropathy
nephrosclerosis
EXCLUDES 1 *hypertension due to kidney disease (I15.0, I15.1)*
renovascular hypertension (I15.0)
secondary hypertension (I15.-)
EXCLUDES 2 *acute kidney failure (N17.-)*
AHA: 2019,3Q,3; 2018,4Q,88; 2016,3Q,22
TIP: Do not assign a code from this category when provider documentation indicates the chronic kidney disease (CKD) is attributable to another cause.

I12.0 Hypertensive chronic kidney disease with stage 5 chronic kidney disease or end stage renal disease CC HCC
Use additional code to identify the stage of chronic kidney disease (N18.5, N18.6)

I12.9 Hypertensive chronic kidney disease with stage 1 through stage 4 chronic kidney disease, or unspecified chronic kidney disease
Hypertensive chronic kidney disease NOS
Hypertensive renal disease NOS
Use additional code to identify the stage of chronic kidney disease (N18.1-N18.4, N18.9)

✓4th **I13 Hypertensive heart and chronic kidney disease**
INCLUDES any condition in I11.- with any condition in I12.-
cardiorenal disease
cardiovascular renal disease
TIP: Do not assign a code from this category when provider documentation indicates the heart and/or chronic kidney disease is attributable to another cause.

I13.0 Hypertensive heart and chronic kidney disease with heart failure and stage 1 through stage 4 chronic kidney disease, or unspecified chronic kidney disease CC HCC
Use additional code to identify type of heart failure (I50.-)
Use additional code to identify stage of chronic kidney disease (N18.1-N18.4, N18.9)

✓5th **I13.1 Hypertensive heart and chronic kidney disease without heart failure**

I13.10 Hypertensive heart and chronic kidney disease without heart failure, with stage 1 through stage 4 chronic kidney disease, or unspecified chronic kidney disease
Hypertensive heart disease and hypertensive chronic kidney disease NOS
Use additional code to identify the stage of chronic kidney disease (N18.1-N18.4, N18.9)

I13.11 Hypertensive heart and chronic kidney disease without heart failure, with stage 5 chronic kidney disease, or end stage renal disease CC HCC
Use additional code to identify the stage of chronic kidney disease (N18.5, N18.6)

I13.2 Hypertensive heart and chronic kidney disease with heart failure and with stage 5 chronic kidney disease, or end stage renal disease CC HCC
Use additional code to identify type of heart failure (I50.-)
Use additional code to identify the stage of chronic kidney disease (N18.5, N18.6)

✓4th **I15 Secondary hypertension**
Code also underlying condition
EXCLUDES 1 *postprocedural hypertension (I97.3)*
EXCLUDES 2 *secondary hypertension involving vessels of brain (I60-I69)*
secondary hypertension involving vessels of eye (H35.0-)

I15.0 Renovascular hypertension
I15.1 Hypertension secondary to other renal disorders
AHA: 2016,3Q,22
I15.2 Hypertension secondary to endocrine disorders
I15.8 Other secondary hypertension
I15.9 Secondary hypertension, unspecified

✓4th **I16 Hypertensive crisis**
Code also any identified hypertensive disease (I10-I15)
AHA: 2016,4Q,26-28

I16.0 Hypertensive urgency
I16.1 Hypertensive emergency CC
I16.9 Hypertensive crisis, unspecified CC

Ischemic heart diseases (I2Ø-I25)

Use additional code to identify presence of hypertension (I1Ø-I16)

I2Ø Angina pectoris

Use additional code to identify:
exposure to environmental tobacco smoke (Z77.22)
history of tobacco dependence (Z87.891)
occupational exposure to environmental tobacco smoke (Z57.31)
tobacco dependence (F17.-)
tobacco use (Z72.Ø)

EXCLUDES 1 *angina pectoris with atherosclerotic heart disease of native coronary arteries (I25.1-)*
atherosclerosis of coronary artery bypass graft(s) and coronary artery of transplanted heart with angina pectoris (I25.7-)
postinfarction angina (I23.7)

DEF: Chest pain due to reduced blood flow resulting in a lack of oxygen to the heart muscles.

I2Ø.Ø Unstable angina CC HCC
Accelerated angina
Crescendo angina
De novo effort angina
Intermediate coronary syndrome
Preinfarction syndrome
Worsening effort angina
DEF: Condition representing an intermediate stage between angina of effort and acute myocardial infarction.

I2Ø.1 Angina pectoris with documented spasm CC HCC
Angiospastic angina
Prinzmetal angina
Spasm-induced angina
Variant angina

I2Ø.8 Other forms of angina pectoris HCC
Angina equivalent
Angina of effort
Coronary slow flow syndrome
Stable angina
Stenocardia
Use additional code(s) for symptoms associated with angina equivalent

I2Ø.9 Angina pectoris, unspecified HCC
Angina NOS
Anginal syndrome
Cardiac angina
Ischemic chest pain

I21 Acute myocardial infarction

INCLUDES cardiac infarction
coronary (artery) embolism
coronary (artery) occlusion
coronary (artery) rupture
coronary (artery) thrombosis
infarction of heart, myocardium, or ventricle
myocardial infarction specified as acute or with a stated duration of 4 weeks (28 days) or less from onset

Use additional code, if applicable, to identify:
exposure to environmental tobacco smoke (Z77.22)
history of tobacco dependence (Z87.891)
occupational exposure to environmental tobacco smoke (Z57.31)
status post administration of tPA (rtPA) in a different facility within the last 24 hours prior to admission to current facility (Z92.82)
tobacco dependence (F17.-)
tobacco use (Z72.Ø)

EXCLUDES 2 *old myocardial infarction (I25.2)*
postmyocardial infarction syndrome (I24.1)
subsequent type 1 myocardial infarction (I22.-)

AHA: 2019,2Q,5; 2018,4Q,68; 2018,3Q,5; 2017,4Q,12-14; 2017,1Q,44-45; 2016,4Q,140; 2015,2Q,16; 2013,1Q,25; 2012,4Q,96,102-103

TIP: When chronic total occlusion and myocardial infarction are documented as being in different vessels, assign code I25.82 Chronic total occlusion of coronary artery, in addition to the myocardial infarction code.

I21.Ø ST elevation (STEMI) myocardial infarction of anterior wall
Type 1 ST elevation myocardial infarction of anterior wall
DEF: ST elevation myocardial infarction: Complete obstruction of one or more coronary arteries causing decreased blood flow (ischemia) and necrosis of myocardial muscle cells.

I21.Ø1 ST elevation (STEMI) myocardial infarction involving left main coronary artery MCC HCC

I21.Ø2 ST elevation (STEMI) myocardial infarction involving left anterior descending coronary artery MCC HCC
ST elevation (STEMI) myocardial infarction involving diagonal coronary artery
AHA: 2013,1Q,25

I21.Ø9 ST elevation (STEMI) myocardial infarction involving other coronary artery of anterior wall MCC HCC
Acute transmural myocardial infarction of anterior wall
Anteroapical transmural (Q wave) infarction (acute)
Anterolateral transmural (Q wave) infarction (acute)
Anteroseptal transmural (Q wave) infarction (acute)
Transmural (Q wave) infarction (acute) (of) anterior (wall) NOS
AHA: 2012,4Q,102-103

I21.1 ST elevation (STEMI) myocardial infarction of inferior wall
Type 1 ST elevation myocardial infarction of inferior wall
DEF: ST elevation myocardial infarction: Complete obstruction of one or more coronary arteries causing decreased blood flow (ischemia) and necrosis of myocardial muscle cells.

I21.11 ST elevation (STEMI) myocardial infarction involving right coronary artery MCC HCC
Inferoposterior transmural (Q wave) infarction (acute)

I21.19 ST elevation (STEMI) myocardial infarction involving other coronary artery of inferior wall MCC HCC
Acute transmural myocardial infarction of inferior wall
Inferolateral transmural (Q wave) infarction (acute)
Transmural (Q wave) infarction (acute) (of) diaphragmatic wall
Transmural (Q wave) infarction (acute) (of) inferior (wall) NOS
EXCLUDES 2 *ST elevation (STEMI) myocardial infarction involving left circumflex coronary artery (I21.21)*
AHA: 2012,4Q,96

I21.2 ST elevation (STEMI) myocardial infarction of other sites
Type 1 ST elevation myocardial infarction of other sites
DEF: ST elevation myocardial infarction: Complete obstruction of one or more coronary arteries causing decreased blood flow (ischemia) and necrosis of myocardial muscle cells.

I21.21 ST elevation (STEMI) myocardial infarction involving left circumflex coronary artery MCC HCC
ST elevation (STEMI) myocardial infarction involving oblique marginal coronary artery

I21.29 ST elevation (STEMI) myocardial infarction involving other sites MCC HCC
Acute transmural myocardial infarction of other sites
Apical-lateral transmural (Q wave) infarction (acute)
Basal-lateral transmural (Q wave) infarction (acute)
High lateral transmural (Q wave) infarction (acute)
Lateral (wall) NOS transmural (Q wave) infarction (acute)
Posterior (true) transmural (Q wave) infarction (acute)
Posterobasal transmural (Q wave) infarction (acute)
Posterolateral transmural (Q wave) infarction (acute)
Posteroseptal transmural (Q wave) infarction (acute)
Septal transmural (Q wave) infarction (acute) NOS

I21.3 ST elevation (STEMI) myocardial infarction of unspecified site MCC HCC
Acute transmural myocardial infarction of unspecified site
Transmural (Q wave) myocardial infarction NOS
Type 1 ST elevation myocardial infarction of unspecified site
DEF: ST elevation myocardial infarction: Complete obstruction of one or more coronary arteries causing decreased blood flow (ischemia) and necrosis of myocardial muscle cells.

I21.4 Non-ST elevation (NSTEMI) myocardial infarction MCC HCC
Acute subendocardial myocardial infarction
Non-Q wave myocardial infarction NOS
Nontransmural myocardial infarction NOS
Type 1 non-ST elevation myocardial infarction
AHA: 2019,2Q,33; 2017,1Q,44-45
DEF: Partial obstruction of one or more coronary arteries that causes decreased blood flow (ischemia) and may cause partial thickness necrosis of myocardial muscle cells.

I21.9 Acute myocardial infarction, unspecified MCC HCC
Myocardial infarction (acute) NOS

✓5th **I21.A Other type of myocardial infarction**
AHA: 2019,2Q,5

I21.A1 Myocardial infarction type 2 MCC HCC
Myocardial infarction due to demand ischemia
Myocardial infarction secondary to ischemic imbalance
Code first the underlying cause, such as:
anemia (D5Ø.Ø-D64.9)
chronic obstructive pulmonary disease (J44.-)
paroxysmal tachycardia (I47.Ø-I47.9)
shock (R57.Ø-R57.9)
AHA: 2019,4Q,53; 2017,4Q,13-14
DEF: Often referred to as due to demand ischemia, myocardial infarction (MI) type 2 refers to an MI due to ischemia and necrosis resulting from an oxygen imbalance to the heart. This mismatch between oxygen decreased supply and increased demand is caused by conditions other than coronary artery disease such as vasospasm, embolism, anemia, hypertension, hypotension, or arrhythmias.

I21.A9 Other myocardial infarction type MCC HCC
Myocardial infarction associated with revascularization procedure
Myocardial infarction type 3
Myocardial infarction type 4a
Myocardial infarction type 4b
Myocardial infarction type 4c
Myocardial infarction type 5
Code first, if applicable, postprocedural myocardial infarction following cardiac surgery (I97.19Ø), or postprocedural myocardial infarction during cardiac surgery (I97.79Ø)
Code also complication, if known and applicable, such as:
(acute) stent occlusion (T82.897-)
(acute) stent stenosis (T82.855-)
(acute) stent thrombosis (T82.867-)
cardiac arrest due to underlying cardiac condition (I46.2)
complication of percutaneous coronary intervention (PCI) (I97.89)
occlusion of coronary artery bypass graft (T82.218-)
AHA: 2019,2Q,33

✓4th **I22 Subsequent ST elevation (STEMI) and non-ST elevation (NSTEMI) myocardial infarction**
INCLUDES acute myocardial infarction occurring within four weeks (28 days) of a previous acute myocardial infarction, regardless of site
cardiac infarction
coronary (artery) embolism
coronary (artery) occlusion
coronary (artery) rupture
coronary (artery) thrombosis
infarction of heart, myocardium, or ventricle
recurrent myocardial infarction
reinfarction of myocardium
rupture of heart, myocardium, or ventricle
subsequent type 1 myocardial infarction
Use additional code, if applicable, to identify:
exposure to environmental tobacco smoke (Z77.22)
history of tobacco dependence (Z87.891)
occupational exposure to environmental tobacco smoke (Z57.31)
status post administration of tPA (rtPA) in a different facility within the last 24 hours prior to admission to current facility (Z92.82)
tobacco dependence (F17.-)
tobacco use (Z72.Ø)
EXCLUDES 1 *subsequent myocardial infarction, type 2 (I21.A1)*
subsequent myocardial infarction of other type (type 3) (type 4) (type 5) (I21.A9)
AHA: 2018,4Q,68; 2018,3Q,5; 2017,4Q,12-13; 2017,2Q,11; 2013,1Q,25; 2012,4Q,97,102-103
DEF: Non-ST elevation myocardial infarction: Partial obstruction of one or more coronary arteries that causes decreased blood flow (ischemia) and may cause partial thickness necrosis of myocardial muscle cells.
DEF: ST elevation myocardial infarction: Complete obstruction of one or more coronary arteries causing decreased blood flow (ischemia) and necrosis of myocardial muscle cells.
TIP: When chronic total occlusion and myocardial infarction are documented as being in different vessels, assign code I25.82 Chronic total occlusion of coronary artery, in addition to the myocardial infarction code.

I22.Ø Subsequent ST elevation (STEMI) myocardial infarction of anterior wall MCC HCC
Subsequent acute transmural myocardial infarction of anterior wall
Subsequent transmural (Q wave) infarction (acute)(of) anterior (wall) NOS
Subsequent anteroapical transmural (Q wave) infarction (acute)
Subsequent anterolateral transmural (Q wave) infarction (acute)
Subsequent anteroseptal transmural (Q wave) infarction (acute)

I22.1 Subsequent ST elevation (STEMI) myocardial infarction of inferior wall MCC HCC
Subsequent acute transmural myocardial infarction of inferior wall
Subsequent transmural (Q wave) infarction (acute)(of) diaphragmatic wall
Subsequent transmural (Q wave) infarction (acute)(of) inferior (wall) NOS
Subsequent inferolateral transmural (Q wave) infarction (acute)
Subsequent inferoposterior transmural (Q wave) infarction (acute)
AHA: 2012,4Q,102

I22.2 Subsequent non-ST elevation (NSTEMI) myocardial infarction MCC HCC
Subsequent acute subendocardial myocardial infarction
Subsequent non-Q wave myocardial infarction NOS
Subsequent nontransmural myocardial infarction NOS

I22.8 Subsequent ST elevation (STEMI) myocardial infarction of other sites MCC HCC
Subsequent acute transmural myocardial infarction of other sites
Subsequent apical-lateral transmural (Q wave) myocardial infarction (acute)
Subsequent basal-lateral transmural (Q wave) myocardial infarction (acute)
Subsequent high lateral transmural (Q wave) myocardial infarction (acute)
Subsequent transmural (Q wave) myocardial infarction (acute)(of) lateral (wall) NOS
Subsequent posterior (true) transmural (Q wave) myocardial infarction (acute)
Subsequent posterobasal transmural (Q wave) myocardial infarction (acute)
Subsequent posterolateral transmural (Q wave) myocardial infarction (acute)
Subsequent posteroseptal transmural (Q wave) myocardial infarction (acute)
Subsequent septal NOS transmural (Q wave) myocardial infarction (acute)

I22.9 Subsequent ST elevation (STEMI) myocardial infarction of unspecified site MCC HCC
Subsequent acute myocardial infarction of unspecified site
Subsequent myocardial infarction (acute) NOS

✓4th **I23 Certain current complications following ST elevation (STEMI) and non-ST elevation (NSTEMI) myocardial infarction (within the 28 day period)**
AHA: 2017,2Q,11
DEF: ST elevation myocardial infarction: Complete obstruction of one or more coronary arteries causing decreased blood flow (ischemia) and necrosis of myocardial muscle cells.
DEF: Non-ST elevation myocardial infarction: Partial obstruction of one or more coronary arteries that causes decreased blood flow (ischemia) and may cause partial thickness necrosis of myocardial muscle cells.

I23.Ø Hemopericardium as current complication following acute myocardial infarction CC HCC A
EXCLUDES 1 *hemopericardium not specified as current complication following acute myocardial infarction (I31.2)*

I23.1 Atrial septal defect as current complication following acute myocardial infarction CC HCC A
EXCLUDES 1 *acquired atrial septal defect not specified as current complication following acute myocardial infarction (I51.Ø)*

I23.2 Ventricular septal defect as current complication following acute myocardial infarction CC HCC A
EXCLUDES 1 *acquired ventricular septal defect not specified as current complication following acute myocardial infarction (I51.Ø)*

I23.3 Rupture of cardiac wall without hemopericardium as current complication following acute myocardial infarction CC HCC A

I23.4 Rupture of chordae tendineae as current complication following acute myocardial infarction MCC HCC
EXCLUDES 1 *rupture of chordae tendineae not specified as current complication following acute myocardial infarction (I51.1)*

I23.5 Rupture of papillary muscle as current complication following acute myocardial infarction MCC HCC
EXCLUDES 1 *rupture of papillary muscle not specified as current complication following acute myocardial infarction (I51.2)*

I23.6 Thrombosis of atrium, auricular appendage, and ventricle as current complications following acute myocardial infarction CC HCC A
EXCLUDES 1 *thrombosis of atrium, auricular appendage, and ventricle not specified as current complication following acute myocardial infarction (I51.3)*

I23.7 Postinfarction angina CC HCC A
AHA: 2015,2Q,16
TIP: When postinfarction angina occurs with atherosclerotic coronary artery disease, code both I23.7 and I25.118 for atherosclerotic disease with other forms of angina pectoris.

I23.8 Other current complications following acute myocardial infarction CC HCC A

✓4th **I24 Other acute ischemic heart diseases**
EXCLUDES 1 *angina pectoris (I2Ø.-)*
transient myocardial ischemia in newborn (P29.4)

I24.Ø Acute coronary thrombosis not resulting in myocardial infarction CC HCC
Acute coronary (artery) (vein) embolism not resulting in myocardial infarction
Acute coronary (artery) (vein) occlusion not resulting in myocardial infarction
Acute coronary (artery) (vein) thromboembolism not resulting in myocardial infarction
EXCLUDES 1 *atherosclerotic heart disease (I25.1-)*
AHA: 2013,1Q,24

I24.1 Dressler's syndrome CC HCC
Postmyocardial infarction syndrome
EXCLUDES 1 *postinfarction angina (I23.7)*
DEF: Fever, leukocytosis, chest pain, evidence of pericarditis, pleurisy, and pneumonia occurring days or weeks after a myocardial infarction.

I24.8 Other forms of acute ischemic heart disease CC HCC
EXCLUDES 1 *myocardial infarction due to demand ischemia (I21.A1)*
AHA: 2019,4Q,53; 2017,4Q,13

I24.9 Acute ischemic heart disease, unspecified CC HCC
EXCLUDES 1 *ischemic heart disease (chronic) NOS (I25.9)*

✓4th **I25 Chronic ischemic heart disease**
Use additional code to identify:
chronic total occlusion of coronary artery (I25.82)
exposure to environmental tobacco smoke (Z77.22)
history of tobacco dependence (Z87.891)
occupational exposure to environmental tobacco smoke (Z57.31)
tobacco dependence (F17.-)
tobacco use (Z72.Ø)

✓5th **I25.1 Atherosclerotic heart disease of native coronary artery**
Atherosclerotic cardiovascular disease
Coronary (artery) atheroma
Coronary (artery) atherosclerosis
Coronary (artery) disease
Coronary (artery) sclerosis
Use additional code, if applicable, to identify:
coronary atherosclerosis due to calcified coronary lesion (I25.84)
coronary atherosclerosis due to lipid rich plaque (I25.83)
EXCLUDES 2 *atheroembolism (I75.-)*
atherosclerosis of coronary artery bypass graft(s) and transplanted heart (I25.7-)

Atheromas

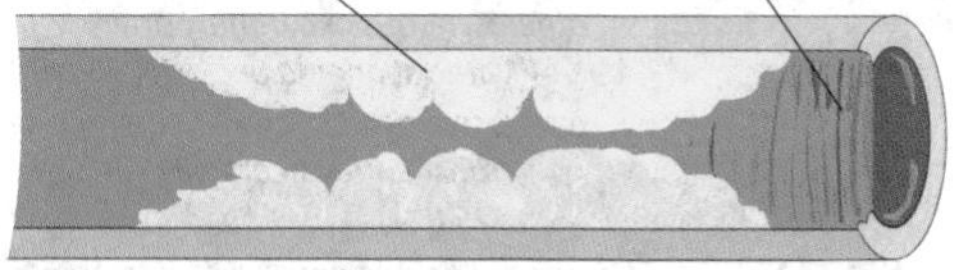

I25.1Ø Atherosclerotic heart disease of native coronary artery without angina pectoris A
Atherosclerotic heart disease NOS
AHA: 2015,2Q,16; 2012,4Q,92

✓6th **I25.11 Atherosclerotic heart disease of native coronary artery with angina pectoris**

I25.11Ø Atherosclerotic heart disease of native coronary artery with unstable angina pectoris CC HCC A
EXCLUDES 1 *unstable angina without atherosclerotic heart disease (I2Ø.Ø)*

Chapter 9. Diseases of the Circulatory System

I22.8–I25.11Ø

I25.111 Atherosclerotic heart disease of native coronary artery with angina pectoris with documented spasm HCC A
EXCLUDES 1 *angina pectoris with documented spasm without atherosclerotic heart disease (I2Ø.1)*

I25.118 Atherosclerotic heart disease of native coronary artery with other forms of angina pectoris HCC A
EXCLUDES 1 *other forms of angina pectoris without atherosclerotic heart disease (I2Ø.8)*
AHA: 2015,2Q,16
TIP: When postinfarction angina occurs with atherosclerotic coronary artery disease, code both I23.7 and I25.118 for atherosclerotic disease with other forms of angina pectoris.

I25.119 Atherosclerotic heart disease of native coronary artery with unspecified angina pectoris HCC A
Atherosclerotic heart disease with angina NOS
Atherosclerotic heart disease with ischemic chest pain
EXCLUDES 1 *unspecified angina pectoris without atherosclerotic heart disease (I2Ø.9)*

I25.2 Old myocardial infarction
Healed myocardial infarction
Past myocardial infarction diagnosed by ECG or other investigation, but currently presenting no symptoms

I25.3 Aneurysm of heart CC
Mural aneurysm
Ventricular aneurysm

✓5th **I25.4 Coronary artery aneurysm and dissection**

I25.41 Coronary artery aneurysm
Coronary arteriovenous fistula, acquired
EXCLUDES 1 *congenital coronary (artery) aneurysm (Q24.5)*

I25.42 Coronary artery dissection MCC
DEF: Tear in the intimal arterial wall of a coronary artery resulting in the sudden intrusion of blood within the layers of the wall.

I25.5 Ischemic cardiomyopathy
EXCLUDES 2 *coronary atherosclerosis (I25.1-, I25.7-)*

I25.6 Silent myocardial ischemia

✓5th **I25.7 Atherosclerosis of coronary artery bypass graft(s) and coronary artery of transplanted heart with angina pectoris**
Use additional code, if applicable, to identify:
coronary atherosclerosis due to calcified coronary lesion (I25.84)
coronary atherosclerosis due to lipid rich plaque (I25.83)
EXCLUDES 1 *atherosclerosis of bypass graft(s) of transplanted heart without angina pectoris (I25.812)*
atherosclerosis of coronary artery bypass graft(s) without angina pectoris (I25.81Ø)
atherosclerosis of native coronary artery of transplanted heart without angina pectoris (I25.811)

✓6th **I25.7Ø Atherosclerosis of coronary artery bypass graft(s), unspecified, with angina pectoris**

I25.7ØØ Atherosclerosis of coronary artery bypass graft(s), unspecified, with unstable angina pectoris CC HCC A
EXCLUDES 1 *unstable angina pectoris without atherosclerosis of coronary artery bypass graft (I2Ø.Ø)*

I25.7Ø1 Atherosclerosis of coronary artery bypass graft(s), unspecified, with angina pectoris with documented spasm HCC A
EXCLUDES 1 *angina pectoris with documented spasm without atherosclerosis of coronary artery bypass graft (I2Ø.1)*

I25.7Ø8 Atherosclerosis of coronary artery bypass graft(s), unspecified, with other forms of angina pectoris HCC A
EXCLUDES 1 *other forms of angina pectoris without atherosclerosis of coronary artery bypass graft (I2Ø.8)*

I25.7Ø9 Atherosclerosis of coronary artery bypass graft(s), unspecified, with unspecified angina pectoris HCC A
EXCLUDES 1 *unspecified angina pectoris without atherosclerosis of coronary artery bypass graft (I2Ø.9)*

✓6th **I25.71 Atherosclerosis of autologous vein coronary artery bypass graft(s) with angina pectoris**

I25.71Ø Atherosclerosis of autologous vein coronary artery bypass graft(s) with unstable angina pectoris CC HCC A
EXCLUDES 1 *unstable angina without atherosclerosis of autologous vein coronary artery bypass graft(s) (I2Ø.Ø)*
EXCLUDES 2 *embolism or thrombus of coronary artery bypass graft(s) (T82.8-)*

I25.711 Atherosclerosis of autologous vein coronary artery bypass graft(s) with angina pectoris with documented spasm CC HCC A
EXCLUDES 1 *angina pectoris with documented spasm without atherosclerosis of autologous vein coronary artery bypass graft(s) (I2Ø.1)*

I25.718 Atherosclerosis of autologous vein coronary artery bypass graft(s) with other forms of angina pectoris CC HCC A
EXCLUDES 1 *other forms of angina pectoris without atherosclerosis of autologous vein coronary artery bypass graft(s) (I2Ø.8)*

I25.719 Atherosclerosis of autologous vein coronary artery bypass graft(s) with unspecified angina pectoris CC HCC A
EXCLUDES 1 *unspecified angina pectoris without atherosclerosis of autologous vein coronary artery bypass graft(s) (I2Ø.9)*

✓6th **I25.72 Atherosclerosis of autologous artery coronary artery bypass graft(s) with angina pectoris**
Atherosclerosis of internal mammary artery graft with angina pectoris

I25.72Ø Atherosclerosis of autologous artery coronary artery bypass graft(s) with unstable angina pectoris CC HCC A
EXCLUDES 1 *unstable angina without atherosclerosis of autologous artery coronary artery bypass graft(s) (I2Ø.Ø)*

I25.721 Atherosclerosis of autologous artery coronary artery bypass graft(s) with angina pectoris with documented spasm CC HCC A
EXCLUDES 1 *angina pectoris with documented spasm without atherosclerosis of autologous artery coronary artery bypass graft(s) (I2Ø.1)*

I25.728 Atherosclerosis of autologous artery coronary artery bypass graft(s) with other forms of angina pectoris CC HCC A
EXCLUDES 1 *other forms of angina pectoris without atherosclerosis of autologous artery coronary artery bypass graft(s) (I20.8)*

I25.729 Atherosclerosis of autologous artery coronary artery bypass graft(s) with unspecified angina pectoris CC HCC A
EXCLUDES 1 *unspecified angina pectoris without atherosclerosis of autologous artery coronary artery bypass graft(s) (I20.9)*

✓6th **I25.73 Atherosclerosis of nonautologous biological coronary artery bypass graft(s) with angina pectoris**

I25.730 Atherosclerosis of nonautologous biological coronary artery bypass graft(s) with unstable angina pectoris CC HCC A
EXCLUDES 1 *unstable angina without atherosclerosis of nonautologous biological coronary artery bypass graft(s) (I20.0)*

I25.731 Atherosclerosis of nonautologous biological coronary artery bypass graft(s) with angina pectoris with documented spasm CC HCC A
EXCLUDES 1 *angina pectoris with documented spasm without atherosclerosis of nonautologous biological coronary artery bypass graft(s) (I20.1)*

I25.738 Atherosclerosis of nonautologous biological coronary artery bypass graft(s) with other forms of angina pectoris CC HCC A
EXCLUDES 1 *other forms of angina pectoris without atherosclerosis of nonautologous biological coronary artery bypass graft(s) (I20.8)*

I25.739 Atherosclerosis of nonautologous biological coronary artery bypass graft(s) with unspecified angina pectoris CC HCC A
EXCLUDES 1 *unspecified angina pectoris without atherosclerosis of nonautologous biological coronary artery bypass graft(s) (I20.9)*

✓6th **I25.75 Atherosclerosis of native coronary artery of transplanted heart with angina pectoris**
EXCLUDES 1 *atherosclerosis of native coronary artery of transplanted heart without angina pectoris (I25.811)*

I25.750 Atherosclerosis of native coronary artery of transplanted heart with unstable angina CC HCC

I25.751 Atherosclerosis of native coronary artery of transplanted heart with angina pectoris with documented spasm CC HCC

I25.758 Atherosclerosis of native coronary artery of transplanted heart with other forms of angina pectoris CC HCC

I25.759 Atherosclerosis of native coronary artery of transplanted heart with unspecified angina pectoris CC HCC

✓6th **I25.76 Atherosclerosis of bypass graft of coronary artery of transplanted heart with angina pectoris**
EXCLUDES 1 *atherosclerosis of bypass graft of coronary artery of transplanted heart without angina pectoris (I25.812)*

I25.760 Atherosclerosis of bypass graft of coronary artery of transplanted heart with unstable angina CC HCC A

I25.761 Atherosclerosis of bypass graft of coronary artery of transplanted heart with angina pectoris with documented spasm CC HCC A

I25.768 Atherosclerosis of bypass graft of coronary artery of transplanted heart with other forms of angina pectoris CC HCC A

I25.769 Atherosclerosis of bypass graft of coronary artery of transplanted heart with unspecified angina pectoris CC HCC A

✓6th **I25.79 Atherosclerosis of other coronary artery bypass graft(s) with angina pectoris**

I25.790 Atherosclerosis of other coronary artery bypass graft(s) with unstable angina pectoris CC HCC A
EXCLUDES 1 *unstable angina without atherosclerosis of other coronary artery bypass graft(s) (I20.0)*

I25.791 Atherosclerosis of other coronary artery bypass graft(s) with angina pectoris with documented spasm CC HCC A
EXCLUDES 1 *angina pectoris with documented spasm without atherosclerosis of other coronary artery bypass graft(s) (I20.1)*

I25.798 Atherosclerosis of other coronary artery bypass graft(s) with other forms of angina pectoris CC HCC A
EXCLUDES 1 *other forms of angina pectoris without atherosclerosis of other coronary artery bypass graft(s) (I20.8)*

I25.799 Atherosclerosis of other coronary artery bypass graft(s) with unspecified angina pectoris CC HCC A
EXCLUDES 1 *unspecified angina pectoris without atherosclerosis of other coronary artery bypass graft(s) (I20.9)*

✓5th **I25.8 Other forms of chronic ischemic heart disease**

✓6th **I25.81 Atherosclerosis of other coronary vessels without angina pectoris**
Use additional code, if applicable, to identify:
coronary atherosclerosis due to calcified coronary lesion (I25.84)
coronary atherosclerosis due to lipid rich plaque (I25.83)
EXCLUDES 2 *atherosclerotic heart disease of native coronary artery without angina pectoris (I25.10)*

I25.810 Atherosclerosis of coronary artery bypass graft(s) without angina pectoris CC A
Atherosclerosis of coronary artery bypass graft NOS
EXCLUDES 1 *atherosclerosis of coronary bypass graft(s) with angina pectoris (I25.70-I25.73-, I25.79-)*

I25.811 Atherosclerosis of native coronary artery of transplanted heart without angina pectoris CC
Atherosclerosis of native coronary artery of transplanted heart NOS
EXCLUDES 1 *atherosclerosis of native coronary artery of transplanted heart with angina pectoris (I25.75-)*

I25.812 Atherosclerosis of bypass graft of coronary artery of transplanted heart without angina pectoris CC A
Atherosclerosis of bypass graft of transplanted heart NOS
EXCLUDES 1 *atherosclerosis of bypass graft of transplanted heart with angina pectoris (I25.76)*

I25.82 Chronic total occlusion of coronary artery
Complete occlusion of coronary artery
Total occlusion of coronary artery
Code first coronary atherosclerosis (I25.1-, I25.7-, I25.81-)
EXCLUDES 1 *acute coronary occulsion with myocardial infarction (I21.Ø-I21.9, I22.-)*
acute coronary occlusion without myocardial infarction (I24.Ø)
AHA: 2018,3Q,5
DEF: Complete blockage of the coronary artery due to plaque accumulation over an extended period of time, resulting in substantial reduction of blood flow. Symptoms include angina or chest pain.
TIP: Report this code in addition to a code from category I21 or I22 when the chronic total occlusion and the myocardial infarction are documented as being in different vessels.

I25.83 Coronary atherosclerosis due to lipid rich plaque A
Code first coronary atherosclerosis (I25.1-, I25.7-, I25.81-)

I25.84 Coronary atherosclerosis due to calcified coronary lesion
Coronary atherosclerosis due to severely calcified coronary lesion
Code first coronary atherosclerosis (I25.1-, I25.7-, I25.81-)

I25.89 Other forms of chronic ischemic heart disease

I25.9 Chronic ischemic heart disease, unspecified
Ischemic heart disease (chronic) NOS

Pulmonary heart disease and diseases of pulmonary circulation (I26-I28)

✓4th **I26 Pulmonary embolism**
INCLUDES pulmonary (acute)(artery)(vein) infarction
pulmonary (acute) (artery)(vein) thromboembolism
pulmonary (acute)(artery)(vein) thrombosis
EXCLUDES 2 *chronic pulmonary embolism (I27.82)*
personal history of pulmonary embolism (Z86.711)
pulmonary embolism complicating abortion, ectopic or molar pregnancy (OØØ-OØ7, OØ8.2)
pulmonary embolism complicating pregnancy, childbirth and the puerperium (O88.-)
pulmonary embolism due to trauma (T79.Ø, T79.1)
pulmonary embolism due to complications of surgical and medical care (T8Ø.Ø, T81.7-, T82.8-)
septic (non-pulmonary) arterial embolism (I76)

✓5th **I26.Ø Pulmonary embolism with acute cor pulmonale**
DEF: Cor pulmonale: Heart-lung disease appearing in identifiable forms as chronic or acute. The chronic form of this heart-lung disease is marked by dilation, hypertrophy and failure of the right ventricle due to a disease that has affected the function of the lungs, excluding congenital or left heart diseases and is also called chronic cardiopulmonary disease. The acute form is an overload of the right ventricle from a rapid onset of pulmonary hypertension, usually arising from a pulmonary embolism.

I26.Ø1 Septic pulmonary embolism with acute cor pulmonale MCC HCC
Code first underlying infection

I26.Ø2 Saddle embolus of pulmonary artery with acute cor pulmonale MCC H10 HCC

I26.Ø9 Other pulmonary embolism with acute cor pulmonale MCC H10 HCC
Acute cor pulmonale NOS
AHA: 2014,4Q,21

✓5th **I26.9 Pulmonary embolism without acute cor pulmonale**

I26.9Ø Septic pulmonary embolism without acute cor pulmonale MCC HCC
Code first underlying infection

I26.92 Saddle embolus of pulmonary artery without acute cor pulmonale MCC H10 HCC

I26.93 Single subsegmental pulmonary embolism without acute cor pulmonale MCC H10 HCC
Subsegmental pulmonary embolism NOS
AHA: 2019,4Q,6-7

I26.94 Multiple subsegmental pulmonary emboli without acute cor pulmonale MCC H10 HCC
AHA: 2019,4Q,6-7

I26.99 Other pulmonary embolism without acute cor pulmonale MCC H10 HCC
Acute pulmonary embolism NOS
Pulmonary embolism NOS
AHA: 2019,2Q,22

✓4th **I27 Other pulmonary heart diseases**

I27.Ø Primary pulmonary hypertension CC HCC
Heritable pulmonary arterial hypertension
Idiopathic pulmonary arterial hypertension
Primary group 1 pulmonary hypertension
Primary pulmonary arterial hypertension
EXCLUDES 1 *persistent pulmonary hypertension of newborn (P29.3Ø)*
pulmonary hypertension NOS (I27.2Ø)
secondary pulmonary arterial hypertension (I27.21)
secondary pulmonary hypertension (I27.29)
DEF: Condition that occurs when pressure within the pulmonary artery is elevated and vascular resistance is observed in the lungs.

I27.1 Kyphoscoliotic heart disease CC HCC

✓5th **I27.2 Other secondary pulmonary hypertension**
Code also associated underlying condition
EXCLUDES 1 *Eisenmenger's syndrome (I27.83)*
AHA: 2017,4Q,14-15; 2014,4Q,21
DEF: Condition that occurs when pressure within the pulmonary artery is elevated and vascular resistance is observed in the lungs.

I27.2Ø Pulmonary hypertension, unspecified HCC
Pulmonary hypertension NOS

I27.21 Secondary pulmonary arterial hypertension HCC
(Associated) (drug-induced) (toxin-induced) pulmonary arterial hypertension NOS
(Associated) (drug-induced) (toxin-induced) (secondary) group 1 pulmonary hypertension
Code also associated conditions if applicable, or adverse effects of drugs or toxins, such as:
adverse effect of appetite depressants (T5Ø.5X5)
congenital heart disease (Q2Ø-Q28)
human immunodeficiency virus [HIV] disease (B2Ø)
polymyositis (M33.2-)
portal hypertension (K76.6)
rheumatoid arthritis (MØ5.-)
schistosomiasis (B65.-)
Sjögren syndrome (M35.Ø-)
systemic sclerosis (M34.-)

I27.22 Pulmonary hypertension due to left heart disease HCC
Group 2 pulmonary hypertension
Code also associated left heart disease, if known, such as:
multiple valve disease (IØ8.-)
rheumatic aortic valve diseases (IØ6.-)
rheumatic mitral valve diseases (IØ5.-)

I27.23 Pulmonary hypertension due to lung diseases and hypoxia HCC
Group 3 pulmonary hypertension
Code also associated lung disease, if known, such as:
bronchiectasis (J47.-)
cystic fibrosis with pulmonary manifestations (E84.Ø)
interstitial lung disease (J84.-)
pleural effusion (J9Ø)
sleep apnea (G47.3-)

I27.24 Chronic thromboembolic pulmonary hypertension HCC
Group 4 pulmonary hypertension
Code also associated pulmonary embolism, if applicable (I26.-, I27.82)

I27.29 Other secondary pulmonary hypertension HCC
Group 5 pulmonary hypertension
Pulmonary hypertension with unclear multifactorial mechanisms
Pulmonary hypertension due to hematologic disorders
Pulmonary hypertension due to metabolic disorders
Pulmonary hypertension due to other systemic disorders
Code also other associated disorders, if known, such as:
chronic myeloid leukemia ►(C92.1Ø-C92.22)◄
essential thrombocythemia (D47.3)
Gaucher disease (E75.22)
hypertensive chronic kidney disease with end stage renal disease (I12.Ø, I13.11, I13.2)
hyperthyroidism (EØ5.-)
hypothyroidism (EØØ-EØ3)
polycythemia vera (D45)
sarcoidosis (D86.-)
AHA: 2016,2Q,8

✓5th **I27.8 Other specified pulmonary heart diseases**

I27.81 Cor pulmonale (chronic) HCC
Cor pulmonale NOS
EXCLUDES 1 *acute cor pulmonale (I26.Ø-)*
AHA: 2014,4Q,21
DEF: Heart-lung disease appearing in identifiable forms as chronic or acute. The chronic form of this heart-lung disease is marked by dilation, hypertrophy and failure of the right ventricle due to a disease that has affected the function of the lungs, excluding congenital or left heart diseases and is also called chronic cardiopulmonary disease. The acute form is an overload of the right ventricle from a rapid onset of pulmonary hypertension, usually arising from a pulmonary embolism.

I27.82 Chronic pulmonary embolism CC HCC
Use additional code, if applicable, for associated long-term (current) use of anticoagulants (Z79.Ø1)
EXCLUDES 1 *personal history of pulmonary embolism (Z86.711)*
DEF: Long-standing condition commonly associated with pulmonary hypertension in which small blood clots travel to the lungs repeatedly over many weeks, months, or years, requiring continuation of established anticoagulant or thrombolytic therapy.

I27.83 Eisenmenger's syndrome HCC
Eisenmenger's complex
(Irreversible) Eisenmenger's disease
Pulmonary hypertension with right to left shunt related to congenital heart disease
Code also underlying heart defect, if known, such as:
atrial septal defect (Q21.1)
Eisenmenger's defect (Q21.8)
patent ductus arteriosus (Q25.Ø)
ventricular septal defect (Q21.Ø)
DEF: Pulmonary hypertension with congenital communication between two circulations resulting in a right to left shunt. This causes reduced oxygen saturation in the arterial blood, leading to cyanosis and organ damage. Once it develops, this life-threating condition is irreversible.

I27.89 Other specified pulmonary heart diseases HCC

I27.9 Pulmonary heart disease, unspecified HCC
Chronic cardiopulmonary disease

✓4th **I28 Other diseases of pulmonary vessels**

I28.Ø Arteriovenous fistula of pulmonary vessels CC HCC
EXCLUDES 1 *congenital arteriovenous fistula (Q25.72)*

I28.1 Aneurysm of pulmonary artery CC HCC
EXCLUDES 1 *congenital aneurysm (Q25.79)*
congenital arteriovenous aneurysm (Q25.72)

I28.8 Other diseases of pulmonary vessels HCC
Pulmonary arteritis
Pulmonary endarteritis
Rupture of pulmonary vessels
Stenosis of pulmonary vessels
Stricture of pulmonary vessels

I28.9 Disease of pulmonary vessels, unspecified HCC

Other forms of heart disease (I3Ø-I52)

✓4th **I3Ø Acute pericarditis**
INCLUDES acute mediastinopericarditis
acute myopericarditis
acute pericardial effusion
acute pleuropericarditis
acute pneumopericarditis
EXCLUDES 1 *Dressler's syndrome (I24.1)*
rheumatic pericarditis (acute) (IØ1.Ø)
viral pericarditis due to Coxsakie virus (B33.23)
DEF: Pericarditis: Inflammation affecting the pericardium, the fibroserous membrane that surrounds the heart.

I3Ø.Ø Acute nonspecific idiopathic pericarditis CC

I3Ø.1 Infective pericarditis CC
Pneumococcal pericarditis
Pneumopyopericardium
Purulent pericarditis
Pyopericarditis
Pyopericardium
Pyopneumopericardium
Staphylococcal pericarditis
Streptococcal pericarditis
Suppurative pericarditis
Viral pericarditis
Use additional code (B95-B97) to identify infectious agent

I3Ø.8 Other forms of acute pericarditis CC

I3Ø.9 Acute pericarditis, unspecified CC

✓4th **I31 Other diseases of pericardium**
EXCLUDES 1 *diseases of pericardium specified as rheumatic (IØ9.2)*
postcardiotomy syndrome (I97.Ø)
traumatic injury to pericardium (S26.-)

I31.Ø Chronic adhesive pericarditis CC
Accretio cordis
Adherent pericardium
Adhesive mediastinopericarditis

I31.1 Chronic constrictive pericarditis CC
Concretio cordis
Pericardial calcification

I31.2 Hemopericardium, not elsewhere classified CC
EXCLUDES 1 *hemopericardium as current complication following acute myocardial infarction (I23.Ø)*
DEF: Presence of blood in the pericardial sac (pericardium). It can lead to potentially fatal cardiac tamponade if enough blood enters the pericardial cavity.

I31.3 Pericardial effusion (noninflammatory) CC
Chyloperircardium
EXCLUDES 1 *acute pericardial effusion (I3Ø.9)*
AHA: 2019,1Q,16
TIP: Assign this code for documented malignant pericardial effusion. If the sole reason for admission is to treat the effusion with no treatment rendered for the associated malignancy, this code may be sequenced first.

I31.4 Cardiac tamponade CC
Code first underlying cause
DEF: Life-threatening condition in which fluid or blood accumulates in the space between the muscle of the heart (myocardium) and the outer sac that covers the heart (pericardium), resulting in compression of the heart.

Cardiac Tamponade

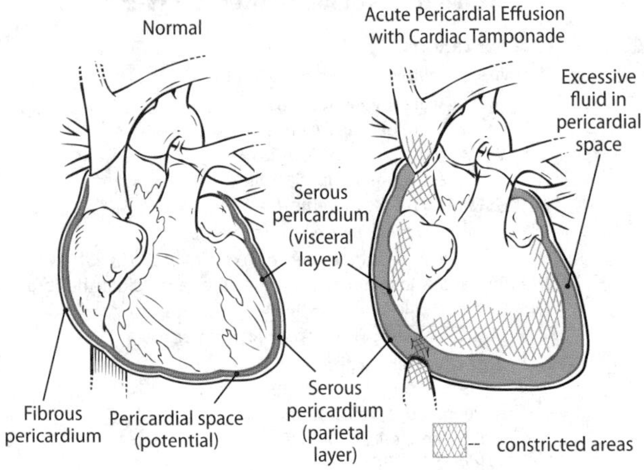

I31.8 Other specified diseases of pericardium CC
Epicardial plaques
Focal pericardial adhesions

I31.9 Disease of pericardium, unspecified CC
Pericarditis (chronic) NOS

I32 Pericarditis in diseases classified elsewhere CC
Code first underlying disease
EXCLUDES 1 *pericarditis (in):*
coxsackie (virus) (B33.23)
gonococcal (A54.83)
meningococcal (A39.53)
rheumatoid (arthritis) (MØ5.31)
syphilitic (A52.Ø6)
systemic lupus erythematosus (M32.12)
tuberculosis (A18.84)
DEF: Pericarditis: Inflammation affecting the pericardium, the fibroserous membrane that surrounds the heart.

✓4th **I33 Acute and subacute endocarditis**
EXCLUDES 1 *acute rheumatic endocarditis (IØ1.1)*
endocarditis NOS (I38)
DEF: Endocarditis: Inflammatory disease of the interior lining of the heart chamber and heart valves.

I33.Ø Acute and subacute infective endocarditis HIV MCC
Bacterial endocarditis (acute) (subacute)
Infective endocarditis (acute) (subacute) NOS
Endocarditis lenta (acute) (subacute)
Malignant endocarditis (acute) (subacute)
Purulent endocarditis (acute) (subacute)
Septic endocarditis (acute) (subacute)
Ulcerative endocarditis (acute) (subacute)
Vegetative endocarditis (acute) (subacute)
Use additional code (B95-B97) to identify infectious agent

I33.9 Acute and subacute endocarditis, unspecified HIV MCC
Acute endocarditis NOS
Acute myoendocarditis NOS
Acute periendocarditis NOS
Subacute endocarditis NOS
Subacute myoendocarditis NOS
Subacute periendocarditis NOS

✓4th **I34 Nonrheumatic mitral valve disorders**
EXCLUDES 1 *mitral valve disease (IØ5.9)*
mitral valve failure (IØ5.8)
mitral valve stenosis (IØ5.Ø)
mitral valve disorder of unspecified cause with diseases of aortic and/or tricuspid valve(s) (IØ8.-)
mitral valve disorder of unspecified cause with mitral stenosis or obstruction (IØ5.Ø)
mitral valve disorder specified as congenital (Q23.2, Q23.9)
mitral valve disorder specified as rheumatic (IØ5.-)

I34.Ø Nonrheumatic mitral (valve) insufficiency
Nonrheumatic mitral (valve) incompetence NOS
Nonrheumatic mitral (valve) regurgitation NOS

I34.1 Nonrheumatic mitral (valve) prolapse
Floppy nonrheumatic mitral valve syndrome
EXCLUDES 1 *Marfan's syndrome (Q87.4-)*

I34.2 Nonrheumatic mitral (valve) stenosis

I34.8 Other nonrheumatic mitral valve disorders

I34.9 Nonrheumatic mitral valve disorder, unspecified

✓4th **I35 Nonrheumatic aortic valve disorders**
EXCLUDES 1 *aortic valve disorder of unspecified cause but with diseases of mitral and/or tricuspid valve(s) (IØ8.-)*
aortic valve disorder specified as congenital (Q23.Ø, Q23.1)
aortic valve disorder specified as rheumatic (IØ6.-)
hypertrophic subaortic stenosis (I42.1)

I35.Ø Nonrheumatic aortic (valve) stenosis

I35.1 Nonrheumatic aortic (valve) insufficiency
Nonrheumatic aortic (valve) incompetence NOS
Nonrheumatic aortic (valve) regurgitation NOS

I35.2 Nonrheumatic aortic (valve) stenosis with insufficiency

I35.8 Other nonrheumatic aortic valve disorders

I35.9 Nonrheumatic aortic valve disorder, unspecified

✓4th **I36 Nonrheumatic tricuspid valve disorders**
EXCLUDES 1 *tricuspid valve disorders of unspecified cause (IØ7.-)*
tricuspid valve disorders specified as congenital (Q22.4, Q22.8, Q22.9)
tricuspid valve disorders specified as rheumatic (IØ7.-)
tricuspid valve disorders with aortic and/or mitral valve involvement (IØ8.-)

I36.Ø Nonrheumatic tricuspid (valve) stenosis

I36.1 Nonrheumatic tricuspid (valve) insufficiency
Nonrheumatic tricuspid (valve) incompetence
Nonrheumatic tricuspid (valve) regurgitation

I36.2 Nonrheumatic tricuspid (valve) stenosis with insufficiency

I36.8 Other nonrheumatic tricuspid valve disorders

I36.9 Nonrheumatic tricuspid valve disorder, unspecified

✓4th **I37 Nonrheumatic pulmonary valve disorders**
EXCLUDES 1 *pulmonary valve disorder specified as congenital (Q22.1, Q22.2, Q22.3)*
pulmonary valve disorder specified as rheumatic (IØ9.89)

I37.Ø Nonrheumatic pulmonary valve stenosis

I37.1 Nonrheumatic pulmonary valve insufficiency
Nonrheumatic pulmonary valve incompetence
Nonrheumatic pulmonary valve regurgitation

I37.2 Nonrheumatic pulmonary valve stenosis with insufficiency

I37.8 Other nonrheumatic pulmonary valve disorders

I37.9 Nonrheumatic pulmonary valve disorder, unspecified

I38 Endocarditis, valve unspecified CC
INCLUDES endocarditis (chronic) NOS
valvular incompetence NOS
valvular insufficiency NOS
valvular regurgitation NOS
valvular stenosis NOS
valvulitis (chronic) NOS
EXCLUDES 1 *congenital insufficiency of cardiac valve NOS (Q24.8)*
congenital stenosis of cardiac valve NOS (Q24.8)
endocardial fibroelastosis (I42.4)
endocarditis specified as rheumatic (IØ9.1)
DEF: Endocarditis: Inflammatory disease of the interior lining of the heart chamber and heart valves.

I39 Endocarditis and heart valve disorders in diseases classified elsewhere CC

Code first underlying disease, such as:
Q fever (A78)

EXCLUDES 1 *endocardial involvement in:*
candidiasis (B37.6)
gonococcal infection (A54.83)
Libman-Sacks disease (M32.11)
listerosis (A32.82)
meningococcal infection (A39.51)
rheumatoid arthritis (MØ5.31)
syphilis (A52.Ø3)
tuberculosis (A18.84)
typhoid fever (AØ1.Ø2)

DEF: Endocarditis: Inflammatory disease of the interior lining of the heart chamber and heart valves.

✓4th **I4Ø Acute myocarditis**

INCLUDES subacute myocarditis

EXCLUDES 1 *acute rheumatic myocarditis (IØ1.2)*

DEF: Myocarditis: Inflammation of the middle layer of the heart, which is composed of muscle tissue.

I4Ø.Ø Infective myocarditis HIV MCC
Septic myocarditis
Use additional code (B95-B97) to identify infectious agent

I4Ø.1 Isolated myocarditis HIV MCC
Fiedler's myocarditis
Giant cell myocarditis
Idiopathic myocarditis

I4Ø.8 Other acute myocarditis HIV MCC

I4Ø.9 Acute myocarditis, unspecified HIV MCC

I41 Myocarditis in diseases classified elsewhere MCC

Code first underlying disease, such as:
typhus (A75.Ø-A75.9)

EXCLUDES 1 *myocarditis (in):*
Chagas' disease (chronic) (B57.2)
acute (B57.Ø)
coxsackie (virus) infection (B33.22)
diphtheritic (A36.81)
gonococcal (A54.83)
influenzal (JØ9.X9, J1Ø.82, J11.82)
meningococcal (A39.52)
mumps (B26.82)
rheumatoid arthritis (MØ5.31)
sarcoid (D86.85)
syphilis (A52.Ø6)
toxoplasmosis (B58.81)
tuberculous (A18.84)

DEF: Myocarditis: Inflammation of the middle layer of the heart, which is composed of muscle tissue.

✓4th **I42 Cardiomyopathy**

INCLUDES myocardiopathy

Code first pre-existing cardiomyopathy complicating pregnancy and puerperium (O99.4)

EXCLUDES 2 *ischemic cardiomyopathy (I25.5)*
peripartum cardiomyopathy (O9Ø.3)
ventricular hypertrophy (I51.7)

I42.Ø Dilated cardiomyopathy CC HCC
Congestive cardiomyopathy

I42.1 Obstructive hypertrophic cardiomyopathy CC HCC
Hypertrophic subaortic stenosis (idiopathic)
DEF: Cardiomyopathy marked by left ventricle hypertrophy and an enlarged septum that result in obstructed blood flow, arrhythmias, mitral regurgitation, and sudden cardiac death.
TIP: When this condition is described as inherited, assign code Q24.8.

I42.2 Other hypertrophic cardiomyopathy CC HCC
Nonobstructive hypertrophic cardiomyopathy

I42.3 Endomyocardial (eosinophilic) disease CC HCC
Endomyocardial (tropical) fibrosis
Löffler's endocarditis

I42.4 Endocardial fibroelastosis CC HCC
Congenital cardiomyopathy
Elastomyofibrosis

I42.5 Other restrictive cardiomyopathy CC HCC
Constrictive cardiomyopathy NOS

I42.6 Alcoholic cardiomyopathy CC HCC
Code also presence of alcoholism (F1Ø.-)

I42.7 Cardiomyopathy due to drug and external agent CC HCC
Code first poisoning due to drug or toxin, if applicable (T36-T65 with fifth or sixth character 1-4 or 6)
Use additional code for adverse effect, if applicable, to identify drug (T36-T5Ø with fifth or sixth character 5)

I42.8 Other cardiomyopathies CC HCC

I42.9 Cardiomyopathy, unspecified CC HCC
Cardiomyopathy (primary) (secondary) NOS

I43 Cardiomyopathy in diseases classified elsewhere CC HCC

Code first underlying disease, such as:
amyloidosis (E85.-)
glycogen storage disease (E74.Ø)
gout (M1Ø.Ø-)
thyrotoxicosis (EØ5.Ø-EØ5.9-)

EXCLUDES 1 *cardiomyopathy (in):*
coxsackie (virus) (B33.24)
diphtheria (A36.81)
sarcoidosis (D86.85)
tuberculosis (A18.84)

✓4th **I44 Atrioventricular and left bundle-branch block**

I44.Ø Atrioventricular block, first degree

I44.1 Atrioventricular block, second degree
Atrioventricular block, type I and II
Möbitz block, type I and II
Second degree block, type I and II
Wenckebach's block

I44.2 Atrioventricular block, complete CC HCC
Complete heart block NOS
Third degree block
AHA: 2019,2Q,4

✓5th **I44.3 Other and unspecified atrioventricular block**
Atrioventricular block NOS

I44.3Ø Unspecified atrioventricular block

I44.39 Other atrioventricular block

I44.4 Left anterior fascicular block

I44.5 Left posterior fascicular block

✓5th **I44.6 Other and unspecified fascicular block**

I44.6Ø Unspecified fascicular block
Left bundle-branch hemiblock NOS

I44.69 Other fascicular block

I44.7 Left bundle-branch block, unspecified

Conduction Disorders

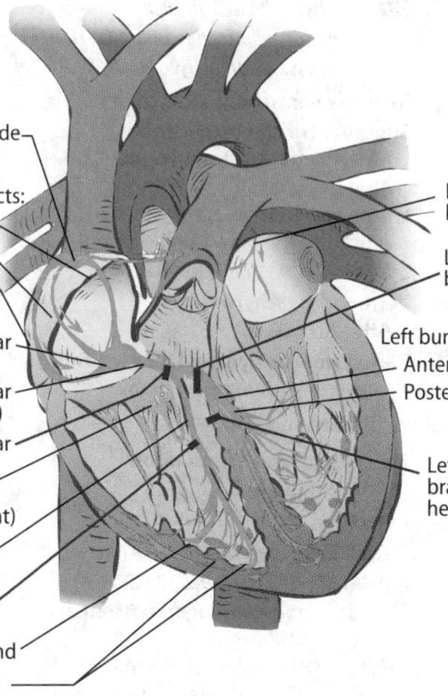

✓4th **I45 Other conduction disorders**

I45.Ø Right fascicular block

√5th **I45.1 Other and unspecified right bundle-branch block**

I45.10 Unspecified right bundle-branch block
Right bundle-branch block NOS

I45.19 Other right bundle-branch block

I45.2 Bifascicular block CC

I45.3 Trifascicular block CC

I45.4 Nonspecific intraventricular block
Bundle-branch block NOS

I45.5 Other specified heart block
Sinoatrial block
Sinoauricular block
EXCLUDES 1 *heart block NOS (I45.9)*

I45.6 Pre-excitation syndrome
Accelerated atrioventricular conduction
Accessory atrioventricular conduction
Anomalous atrioventricular excitation
Lown-Ganong-Levine syndrome
Pre-excitation atrioventricular conduction
Wolff-Parkinson-White syndrome

√5th **I45.8 Other specified conduction disorders**

I45.81 Long QT syndrome
DEF: Condition characterized by recurrent syncope, malignant arrhythmias, and sudden death. This syndrome has a characteristic prolonged Q-T interval on an electrocardiogram.

I45.89 Other specified conduction disorders CC
Atrioventricular [AV] dissociation
Interference dissociation
Isorhythmic dissociation
Nonparoxysmal AV nodal tachycardia
AHA: 2013,2Q,31

I45.9 Conduction disorder, unspecified
Heart block NOS
Stokes-Adams syndrome

√4th **I46 Cardiac arrest**
EXCLUDES 1 ~~*cardiogenic shock (R57.Ø)*~~
EXCLUDES 2 ►*cardiogenic shock (R57.Ø)*◄
AHA: 2019,2Q,4-5

I46.2 Cardiac arrest due to underlying cardiac condition MCC HCC
Code first underlying cardiac condition

I46.8 Cardiac arrest due to other underlying condition MCC HCC
Code first underlying condition

I46.9 Cardiac arrest, cause unspecified MCC HCC

√4th **I47 Paroxysmal tachycardia**
Code first tachycardia complicating:
abortion or ectopic or molar pregnancy (OØØ-OØ7, OØ8.8)
obstetric surgery and procedures (O75.4)
EXCLUDES 1 *tachycardia NOS (RØØ.Ø)*
sinoauricular tachycardia NOS (RØØ.Ø)
sinus [sinusal] tachycardia NOS (RØØ.Ø)

I47.Ø Re-entry ventricular arrhythmia CC HCC

I47.1 Supraventricular tachycardia CC HCC
Atrial (paroxysmal) tachycardia
Atrioventricular [AV] (paroxysmal) tachycardia
Atrioventricular re-entrant (nodal) tachycardia [AVNRT] [AVRT]
Junctional (paroxysmal) tachycardia
Nodal (paroxysmal) tachycardia

I47.2 Ventricular tachycardia CC HCC
AHA: 2013,3Q,23

I47.9 Paroxysmal tachycardia, unspecified HCC
Bouveret (-Hoffman) syndrome

√4th **I48 Atrial fibrillation and flutter**

I48.Ø Paroxysmal atrial fibrillation HCC
AHA: 2018,3Q,6

√5th **I48.1 Persistent atrial fibrillation**
EXCLUDES 1 *permanent atrial fibrillation (I48.21)*
AHA: 2019,4Q,7; 2019,2Q,3; 2018,3Q,6

I48.11 Longstanding persistent atrial fibrillation CC HCC

I48.19 Other persistent atrial fibrillation CC HCC
Chronic persistent atrial fibrillation
Persistent atrial fibrillation, NOS
AHA: 2019,4Q,7

√5th **I48.2 Chronic atrial fibrillation**
AHA: 2019,4Q,7; 2019,2Q,3; 2018,3Q,6

I48.20 Chronic atrial fibrillation, unspecified CC HCC
EXCLUDES 1 *chronic persistent atrial fibrillation (I48.19)*

I48.21 Permanent atrial fibrillation CC HCC

I48.3 Typical atrial flutter CC HCC
Type I atrial flutter

I48.4 Atypical atrial flutter CC HCC
Type II atrial flutter

√5th **I48.9 Unspecified atrial fibrillation and atrial flutter**

I48.91 Unspecified atrial fibrillation HCC

I48.92 Unspecified atrial flutter CC HCC

√4th **I49 Other cardiac arrhythmias**
Code first cardiac arrhythmia complicating:
abortion or ectopic or molar pregnancy (OØØ-OØ7, OØ8.8)
obstetric surgery and procedures (O75.4)
EXCLUDES 1 *neonatal dysrhythmia (P29.1-)*
sinoatrial bradycardia (RØØ.1)
sinus bradycardia (RØØ.1)
vagal bradycardia (RØØ.1)
EXCLUDES 2 *bradycardia NOS (RØØ.1)*

√5th **I49.Ø Ventricular fibrillation and flutter**

I49.Ø1 Ventricular fibrillation MCC HCC

I49.Ø2 Ventricular flutter MCC HCC

I49.1 Atrial premature depolarization
Atrial premature beats

I49.2 Junctional premature depolarization CC HCC

I49.3 Ventricular premature depolarization
AHA: 2020,2Q,23

√5th **I49.4 Other and unspecified premature depolarization**

I49.40 Unspecified premature depolarization
Premature beats NOS

I49.49 Other premature depolarization
Ectopic beats
Extrasystoles
Extrasystolic arrhythmias
Premature contractions

I49.5 Sick sinus syndrome HCC
Tachycardia-bradycardia syndrome
AHA: 2019,1Q,33
TIP: The presence of a pacemaker controls but does not cure sick sinus syndrome and therefore is considered a reportable chronic condition. When a pacemaker is evaluated by a provider, this code and code Z95.0 Presence of cardiac pacemaker, should be reported, even in the absence of any notable changes or management.

I49.8 Other specified cardiac arrhythmias
Brugada syndrome
Coronary sinus rhythm disorder
Ectopic rhythm disorder
Nodal rhythm disorder

I49.9 Cardiac arrhythmia, unspecified
Arrhythmia (cardiac) NOS

I50 Heart failure

Code first:
heart failure complicating abortion or ectopic or molar pregnancy (O00-O07, O08.8)
heart failure due to hypertension (I11.0)
heart failure due to hypertension with chronic kidney disease (I13.-)
heart failure following surgery (I97.13-)
obstetric surgery and procedures (O75.4)
rheumatic heart failure (I09.81)

EXCLUDES 1 *neonatal cardiac failure (P29.0)*

EXCLUDES 2 *cardiac arrest (I46.-)*

AHA: 2018,4Q,67; 2018,2Q,9; 2017,1Q,47; 2014,1Q,25; 2013,2Q,33

I50.1 Left ventricular failure, unspecified CC HCC
Cardiac asthma
Edema of lung with heart disease NOS
Edema of lung with heart failure
Left heart failure
Pulmonary edema with heart disease NOS
Pulmonary edema with heart failure
EXCLUDES 1 *edema of lung without heart disease or heart failure (J81.-)*
pulmonary edema without heart disease or failure (J81.-)

I50.2 Systolic (congestive) heart failure
Heart failure with reduced ejection fraction [HFrEF]
Systolic left ventricular heart failure
Code also end stage heart failure, if applicable (I50.84)
EXCLUDES 1 *combined systolic (congestive) and diastolic (congestive) heart failure (I50.4-)*
AHA: 2017,1Q,46; 2016,1Q,10

I50.20 Unspecified systolic (congestive) heart failure CC HCC
I50.21 Acute systolic (congestive) heart failure MCC HCC
I50.22 Chronic systolic (congestive) heart failure CC HCC
I50.23 Acute on chronic systolic (congestive) heart failure MCC HCC

I50.3 Diastolic (congestive) heart failure
Diastolic left ventricular heart failure
Heart failure with normal ejection fraction
Heart failure with preserved ejection fraction [HFpEF]
Code also end stage heart failure, if applicable (I50.84)
EXCLUDES 1 *combined systolic (congestive) and diastolic (congestive) heart failure (I50.4-)*
AHA: 2017,1Q,46; 2016,1Q,10

I50.30 Unspecified diastolic (congestive) heart failure CC HCC
I50.31 Acute diastolic (congestive) heart failure MCC HCC
I50.32 Chronic diastolic (congestive) heart failure CC HCC
I50.33 Acute on chronic diastolic (congestive) heart failure MCC HCC

I50.4 Combined systolic (congestive) and diastolic (congestive) heart failure
Combined systolic and diastolic left ventricular heart failure
Heart failure with reduced ejection fraction and diastolic dysfunction
Code also end stage heart failure, if applicable (I50.84)
AHA: 2017,1Q,46; 2016,1Q,10

I50.40 Unspecified combined systolic (congestive) and diastolic (congestive) heart failure CC HCC
I50.41 Acute combined systolic (congestive) and diastolic (congestive) heart failure MCC HCC
I50.42 Chronic combined systolic (congestive) and diastolic (congestive) heart failure CC HCC
I50.43 Acute on chronic combined systolic (congestive) and diastolic (congestive) heart failure MCC HCC

I50.8 Other heart failure
AHA: 2017,4Q,15-16

I50.81 Right heart failure
Right ventricular failure

I50.810 Right heart failure, unspecified HCC
Right heart failure without mention of left heart failure
Right ventricular failure NOS

I50.811 Acute right heart failure HCC
Acute isolated right heart failure
Acute (isolated) right ventricular failure

I50.812 Chronic right heart failure HCC
Chronic isolated right heart failure
Chronic (isolated) right ventricular failure

I50.813 Acute on chronic right heart failure HCC
Acute on chronic isolated right heart failure
Acute on chronic (isolated) right ventricular failure
Acute decompensation of chronic (isolated) right ventricular failure
Acute exacerbation of chronic (isolated) right ventricular failure

I50.814 Right heart failure due to left heart failure HCC
Right ventricular failure secondary to left ventricular failure
Code also the type of left ventricular failure, if known (I50.2-I50.43)
EXCLUDES 1 *right heart failure with but not due to left heart failure (I50.82)*

I50.82 Biventricular heart failure HCC
Code also the type of left ventricular failure as systolic, diastolic, or combined, if known (I50.2-I50.43)

I50.83 High output heart failure HCC
DEF: Occurs when the high demand for blood exceeds the capacity of a normally functioning heart to meet the demand.

I50.84 End stage heart failure HCC
Stage D heart failure
Code also the type of heart failure as systolic, diastolic, or combined, if known (I50.2-I50.43)

I50.89 Other heart failure HCC

I50.9 Heart failure, unspecified HCC
Cardiac, heart or myocardial failure NOS
Congestive heart disease
Congestive heart failure NOS
EXCLUDES 2 *fluid overload unrelated to congestive heart failure (E87.70)*
AHA: 2017,4Q,15-16; 2017,1Q,45-46; 2014,4Q,21; 2012,4Q,92

I51 Complications and ill-defined descriptions of heart disease

EXCLUDES 1 *any condition in I51.4-I51.9 due to hypertension (I11.-)*
any condition in I51.4-I51.9 due to hypertension and chronic kidney disease (I13.-)
heart disease specified as rheumatic (I00-I09)

I51.0 Cardiac septal defect, acquired CC A
Acquired septal atrial defect (old)
Acquired septal auricular defect (old)
Acquired septal ventricular defect (old)
EXCLUDES 1 *cardiac septal defect as current complication following acute myocardial infarction (I23.1, I23.2)*
DEF: Abnormal communication between opposite heart chambers due to a defect of the septum. It is not present at birth.

I51.1 Rupture of chordae tendineae, not elsewhere classified MCC HCC
EXCLUDES 1 *rupture of chordae tendineae as current complication following acute myocardial infarction (I23.4)*

I51.2 Rupture of papillary muscle, not elsewhere classified MCC HCC
EXCLUDES 1 *rupture of papillary muscle as current complication following acute myocardial infarction (I23.5)*

I51.3 Intracardiac thrombosis, not elsewhere classified
Apical thrombosis (old)
Atrial thrombosis (old)
Auricular thrombosis (old)
Mural thrombosis (old)
Ventricular thrombosis (old)
EXCLUDES 1 *intracardiac thrombosis as current complication following acute myocardial infarction (I23.6)*
AHA: 2013,1Q,24

I51.4 Myocarditis, unspecified HCC
Chronic (interstitial) myocarditis
Myocardial fibrosis
Myocarditis NOS
EXCLUDES 1 *acute or subacute myocarditis (I40.-)*
AHA: 2018,4Q,67; 2018,2Q,9

I51.5 Myocardial degeneration HCC
Fatty degeneration of heart or myocardium
Myocardial disease
Senile degeneration of heart or myocardium
AHA: 2018,4Q,67; 2018,2Q,9

I51.7 Cardiomegaly
Cardiac dilatation
Cardiac hypertrophy
Ventricular dilatation
AHA: 2018,4Q,67; 2018,2Q,9

✓5th **I51.8 Other ill-defined heart diseases**
AHA: 2018,2Q,9

I51.81 Takotsubo syndrome CC
Reversible left ventricular dysfunction following sudden emotional stress
Stress induced cardiomyopathy
Takotsubo cardiomyopathy
Transient left ventricular apical ballooning syndrome
DEF: Complex of symptoms mimicking myocardial infarct in absence of heart disease, with the majority of cases occurring in postmenopausal women. Heart muscles are temporarily weakened, and a sudden, massive surge of adrenalin stuns the heart, greatly reducing the ability to pump blood.

I51.89 Other ill-defined heart diseases
Carditis (acute)(chronic)
Pancarditis (acute)(chronic)
AHA: 2019,2Q,5; 2018,4Q,67

I51.9 Heart disease, unspecified
AHA: 2018,4Q,67; 2018,2Q,9

I52 Other heart disorders in diseases classified elsewhere
Code first underlying disease, such as:
congenital syphilis (A50.5)
mucopolysaccharidosis (E76.3)
schistosomiasis (B65.0-B65.9)
EXCLUDES 1 *heart disease (in):*
gonococcal infection (A54.83)
meningococcal infection (A39.50)
rheumatoid arthritis (M05.31)
syphilis (A52.06)

Cerebrovascular diseases (I60-I69)

Use additional code to identify presence of:
alcohol abuse and dependence (F10.-)
exposure to environmental tobacco smoke (Z77.22)
history of tobacco dependence (Z87.891)
hypertension (I10-I16)
occupational exposure to environmental tobacco smoke (Z57.31)
tobacco dependence (F17.-)
tobacco use (Z72.0)
EXCLUDES 1 *traumatic intracranial hemorrhage (S06.-)*
AHA: 2014,3Q,5; 2012,4Q,91-92

✓4th **I60 Nontraumatic subarachnoid hemorrhage**
EXCLUDES 1 *syphilitic ruptured cerebral aneurysm (A52.05)*
EXCLUDES 2 *sequelae of subarachnoid hemorrhage (I69.0-)*

✓5th **I60.0 Nontraumatic subarachnoid hemorrhage from carotid siphon and bifurcation**
I60.00 Nontraumatic subarachnoid hemorrhage from unspecified carotid siphon and bifurcation MCC HCC
I60.01 Nontraumatic subarachnoid hemorrhage from right carotid siphon and bifurcation MCC HCC
I60.02 Nontraumatic subarachnoid hemorrhage from left carotid siphon and bifurcation MCC HCC

✓5th **I60.1 Nontraumatic subarachnoid hemorrhage from middle cerebral artery**
I60.10 Nontraumatic subarachnoid hemorrhage from unspecified middle cerebral artery MCC HCC
I60.11 Nontraumatic subarachnoid hemorrhage from right middle cerebral artery MCC HCC
I60.12 Nontraumatic subarachnoid hemorrhage from left middle cerebral artery MCC HCC

I60.2 Nontraumatic subarachnoid hemorrhage from anterior communicating artery MCC HCC

✓5th **I60.3 Nontraumatic subarachnoid hemorrhage from posterior communicating artery**
I60.30 Nontraumatic subarachnoid hemorrhage from unspecified posterior communicating artery MCC HCC
I60.31 Nontraumatic subarachnoid hemorrhage from right posterior communicating artery MCC HCC
I60.32 Nontraumatic subarachnoid hemorrhage from left posterior communicating artery MCC HCC

I60.4 Nontraumatic subarachnoid hemorrhage from basilar artery MCC HCC

✓5th **I60.5 Nontraumatic subarachnoid hemorrhage from vertebral artery**
I60.50 Nontraumatic subarachnoid hemorrhage from unspecified vertebral artery MCC HCC
I60.51 Nontraumatic subarachnoid hemorrhage from right vertebral artery MCC HCC
I60.52 Nontraumatic subarachnoid hemorrhage from left vertebral artery MCC HCC

I60.6 Nontraumatic subarachnoid hemorrhage from other intracranial arteries MCC HCC

I60.7 Nontraumatic subarachnoid hemorrhage from unspecified intracranial artery MCC HCC
Ruptured (congenital) berry aneurysm
Ruptured (congenital) cerebral aneurysm
Subarachnoid hemorrhage (nontraumatic) from cerebral artery NOS
Subarachnoid hemorrhage (nontraumatic) from communicating artery NOS
EXCLUDES 1 *berry aneurysm, nonruptured (I67.1)*

I60.8 Other nontraumatic subarachnoid hemorrhage MCC HCC
Meningeal hemorrhage
Rupture of cerebral arteriovenous malformation

I60.9 Nontraumatic subarachnoid hemorrhage, unspecified MCC HCC

✓4th **I61 Nontraumatic intracerebral hemorrhage**
EXCLUDES 2 *sequelae of intracerebral hemorrhage (I69.1-)*
AHA: 2017,2Q,9-10

I61.0 Nontraumatic intracerebral hemorrhage in hemisphere, subcortical MCC HCC
Deep intracerebral hemorrhage (nontraumatic)
AHA: 2016,4Q,27

I61.1 Nontraumatic intracerebral hemorrhage in hemisphere, cortical MCC HCC
Cerebral lobe hemorrhage (nontraumatic)
Superficial intracerebral hemorrhage (nontraumatic)

I61.2 Nontraumatic intracerebral hemorrhage in hemisphere, unspecified MCC HCC
I61.3 Nontraumatic intracerebral hemorrhage in brain stem MCC HCC
I61.4 Nontraumatic intracerebral hemorrhage in cerebellum MCC HCC
I61.5 Nontraumatic intracerebral hemorrhage, intraventricular MCC HCC
I61.6 Nontraumatic intracerebral hemorrhage, multiple localized MCC HCC
I61.8 Other nontraumatic intracerebral hemorrhage MCC HCC
I61.9 Nontraumatic intracerebral hemorrhage, unspecified MCC HCC

✓4th **I62 Other and unspecified nontraumatic intracranial hemorrhage**
EXCLUDES 2 *sequelae of intracranial hemorrhage (I69.2)*

✓5th **I62.0 Nontraumatic subdural hemorrhage**
I62.00 Nontraumatic subdural hemorrhage, unspecified MCC HCC
I62.01 Nontraumatic acute subdural hemorrhage MCC HCC
I62.02 Nontraumatic subacute subdural hemorrhage MCC HCC
I62.03 Nontraumatic chronic subdural hemorrhage MCC HCC

I62.1 Nontraumatic extradural hemorrhage MCC HCC
Nontraumatic epidural hemorrhage

I62.9 Nontraumatic intracranial hemorrhage, unspecified CC HCC

I63 Cerebral infarction (4th)

INCLUDES occlusion and stenosis of cerebral and precerebral arteries, resulting in cerebral infarction

Use additional code, if applicable, to identify status post administration of tPA (rtPA) in a different facility within the last 24 hours prior to admission to current facility (Z92.82)

Use additional code, if known, to indicate National Institutes of Health Stroke Scale (NIHSS) score (R29.7-)

EXCLUDES 1 ▶*neonatal cerebral infarction (P91.82-)*◀

EXCLUDES 2 *sequelae of cerebral infarction (I69.3-)*

AHA: 2017,2Q,9-10; 2016,4Q,28,61-62; 2014,1Q,23

TIP: Weakness on one side of the body documented as secondary to stroke is synonymous with hemiparesis/hemiplegia (G81.-). Weakness of one limb documented as secondary to stroke is synonymous with monoplegia (G83.1-, G83.2-, G83.3-).

- (5th) **I63.0 Cerebral infarction due to thrombosis of precerebral arteries**
  - **I63.00 Cerebral infarction due to thrombosis of unspecified precerebral artery** MCC HCC
  - (6th) **I63.01 Cerebral infarction due to thrombosis of vertebral artery**
    - **I63.011 Cerebral infarction due to thrombosis of right vertebral artery** MCC HCC
    - **I63.012 Cerebral infarction due to thrombosis of left vertebral artery** MCC HCC
    - **I63.013 Cerebral infarction due to thrombosis of bilateral vertebral arteries** MCC HCC
    - **I63.019 Cerebral infarction due to thrombosis of unspecified vertebral artery** MCC HCC
  - **I63.02 Cerebral infarction due to thrombosis of basilar artery** MCC HCC
  - (6th) **I63.03 Cerebral infarction due to thrombosis of carotid artery**
    - **I63.031 Cerebral infarction due to thrombosis of right carotid artery** MCC HCC
    - **I63.032 Cerebral infarction due to thrombosis of left carotid artery** MCC HCC
    - **I63.033 Cerebral infarction due to thrombosis of bilateral carotid arteries** MCC HCC
    - **I63.039 Cerebral infarction due to thrombosis of unspecified carotid artery** MCC HCC
  - **I63.09 Cerebral infarction due to thrombosis of other precerebral artery** MCC HCC
- (5th) **I63.1 Cerebral infarction due to embolism of precerebral arteries**
  - **I63.10 Cerebral infarction due to embolism of unspecified precerebral artery** MCC HCC
  - (6th) **I63.11 Cerebral infarction due to embolism of vertebral artery**
    - **I63.111 Cerebral infarction due to embolism of right vertebral artery** MCC HCC
    - **I63.112 Cerebral infarction due to embolism of left vertebral artery** MCC HCC
    - **I63.113 Cerebral infarction due to embolism of bilateral vertebral arteries** MCC HCC
    - **I63.119 Cerebral infarction due to embolism of unspecified vertebral artery** MCC HCC
  - **I63.12 Cerebral infarction due to embolism of basilar artery** MCC HCC
  - (6th) **I63.13 Cerebral infarction due to embolism of carotid artery**
    - **I63.131 Cerebral infarction due to embolism of right carotid artery** MCC HCC
    - **I63.132 Cerebral infarction due to embolism of left carotid artery** MCC HCC
    - **I63.133 Cerebral infarction due to embolism of bilateral carotid arteries** MCC HCC
    - **I63.139 Cerebral infarction due to embolism of unspecified carotid artery** MCC HCC
  - **I63.19 Cerebral infarction due to embolism of other precerebral artery** MCC HCC
- (5th) **I63.2 Cerebral infarction due to unspecified occlusion or stenosis of precerebral arteries**
  - **I63.20 Cerebral infarction due to unspecified occlusion or stenosis of unspecified precerebral arteries** MCC HCC
  - (6th) **I63.21 Cerebral infarction due to unspecified occlusion or stenosis of vertebral arteries**
    - **I63.211 Cerebral infarction due to unspecified occlusion or stenosis of right vertebral artery** MCC HCC
    - **I63.212 Cerebral infarction due to unspecified occlusion or stenosis of left vertebral artery** MCC HCC
    - **I63.213 Cerebral infarction due to unspecified occlusion or stenosis of bilateral vertebral arteries** MCC HCC
    - **I63.219 Cerebral infarction due to unspecified occlusion or stenosis of unspecified vertebral artery** MCC HCC
  - **I63.22 Cerebral infarction due to unspecified occlusion or stenosis of basilar artery** MCC HCC
  - (6th) **I63.23 Cerebral infarction due to unspecified occlusion or stenosis of carotid arteries**
    - **I63.231 Cerebral infarction due to unspecified occlusion or stenosis of right carotid arteries** MCC HCC
    - **I63.232 Cerebral infarction due to unspecified occlusion or stenosis of left carotid arteries** MCC HCC
    - **I63.233 Cerebral infarction due to unspecified occlusion or stenosis of bilateral carotid arteries** MCC HCC
    - **I63.239 Cerebral infarction due to unspecified occlusion or stenosis of unspecified carotid artery** MCC HCC
  - **I63.29 Cerebral infarction due to unspecified occlusion or stenosis of other precerebral arteries** MCC HCC
- (5th) **I63.3 Cerebral infarction due to thrombosis of cerebral arteries**
  - **I63.30 Cerebral infarction due to thrombosis of unspecified cerebral artery** MCC HCC
  - (6th) **I63.31 Cerebral infarction due to thrombosis of middle cerebral artery**
    - **I63.311 Cerebral infarction due to thrombosis of right middle cerebral artery** MCC HCC
    - **I63.312 Cerebral infarction due to thrombosis of left middle cerebral artery** MCC HCC
    - **I63.313 Cerebral infarction due to thrombosis of bilateral middle cerebral arteries** MCC HCC
    - **I63.319 Cerebral infarction due to thrombosis of unspecified middle cerebral artery** MCC HCC
  - (6th) **I63.32 Cerebral infarction due to thrombosis of anterior cerebral artery**
    - **I63.321 Cerebral infarction due to thrombosis of right anterior cerebral artery** MCC HCC
    - **I63.322 Cerebral infarction due to thrombosis of left anterior cerebral artery** MCC HCC
    - **I63.323 Cerebral infarction due to thrombosis of bilateral anterior cerebral arteries** MCC HCC
    - **I63.329 Cerebral infarction due to thrombosis of unspecified anterior cerebral artery** MCC HCC
  - (6th) **I63.33 Cerebral infarction due to thrombosis of posterior cerebral artery**
    - **I63.331 Cerebral infarction due to thrombosis of right posterior cerebral artery** MCC HCC
    - **I63.332 Cerebral infarction due to thrombosis of left posterior cerebral artery** MCC HCC
    - **I63.333 Cerebral infarction due to thrombosis of bilateral posterior cerebral arteries** MCC HCC
    - **I63.339 Cerebral infarction due to thrombosis of unspecified posterior cerebral artery** MCC HCC
  - (6th) **I63.34 Cerebral infarction due to thrombosis of cerebellar artery**
    - **I63.341 Cerebral infarction due to thrombosis of right cerebellar artery** MCC HCC
    - **I63.342 Cerebral infarction due to thrombosis of left cerebellar artery** MCC HCC
    - **I63.343 Cerebral infarction due to thrombosis of bilateral cerebellar arteries** MCC HCC
    - **I63.349 Cerebral infarction due to thrombosis of unspecified cerebellar artery** MCC HCC
  - **I63.39 Cerebral infarction due to thrombosis of other cerebral artery** MCC HCC
- (5th) **I63.4 Cerebral infarction due to embolism of cerebral arteries**
  - **I63.40 Cerebral infarction due to embolism of unspecified cerebral artery** MCC HCC

√6th **I63.41 Cerebral infarction due to embolism of middle cerebral artery**
- **I63.411 Cerebral infarction due to embolism of right middle cerebral artery** MCC HCC
- **I63.412 Cerebral infarction due to embolism of left middle cerebral artery** MCC HCC
- **I63.413 Cerebral infarction due to embolism of bilateral middle cerebral arteries** MCC HCC
- **I63.419 Cerebral infarction due to embolism of unspecified middle cerebral artery** MCC HCC

√6th **I63.42 Cerebral infarction due to embolism of anterior cerebral artery**
- **I63.421 Cerebral infarction due to embolism of right anterior cerebral artery** MCC HCC
- **I63.422 Cerebral infarction due to embolism of left anterior cerebral artery** MCC HCC
- **I63.423 Cerebral infarction due to embolism of bilateral anterior cerebral arteries** MCC HCC
- **I63.429 Cerebral infarction due to embolism of unspecified anterior cerebral artery** MCC HCC

√6th **I63.43 Cerebral infarction due to embolism of posterior cerebral artery**
- **I63.431 Cerebral infarction due to embolism of right posterior cerebral artery** MCC HCC
- **I63.432 Cerebral infarction due to embolism of left posterior cerebral artery** MCC HCC
- **I63.433 Cerebral infarction due to embolism of bilateral posterior cerebral arteries** MCC HCC
- **I63.439 Cerebral infarction due to embolism of unspecified posterior cerebral artery** MCC HCC

√6th **I63.44 Cerebral infarction due to embolism of cerebellar artery**
- **I63.441 Cerebral infarction due to embolism of right cerebellar artery** MCC HCC
- **I63.442 Cerebral infarction due to embolism of left cerebellar artery** MCC HCC
- **I63.443 Cerebral infarction due to embolism of bilateral cerebellar arteries** MCC HCC
- **I63.449 Cerebral infarction due to embolism of unspecified cerebellar artery** MCC HCC

I63.49 Cerebral infarction due to embolism of other cerebral artery MCC HCC

√5th **I63.5 Cerebral infarction due to unspecified occlusion or stenosis of cerebral arteries**

I63.50 Cerebral infarction due to unspecified occlusion or stenosis of unspecified cerebral artery MCC HCC

√6th **I63.51 Cerebral infarction due to unspecified occlusion or stenosis of middle cerebral artery**
- **I63.511 Cerebral infarction due to unspecified occlusion or stenosis of right middle cerebral artery** MCC HCC
- **I63.512 Cerebral infarction due to unspecified occlusion or stenosis of left middle cerebral artery** MCC HCC
- **I63.513 Cerebral infarction due to unspecified occlusion or stenosis of bilateral middle cerebral arteries** MCC HCC
- **I63.519 Cerebral infarction due to unspecified occlusion or stenosis of unspecified middle cerebral artery** MCC HCC

√6th **I63.52 Cerebral infarction due to unspecified occlusion or stenosis of anterior cerebral artery**
- **I63.521 Cerebral infarction due to unspecified occlusion or stenosis of right anterior cerebral artery** MCC HCC
- **I63.522 Cerebral infarction due to unspecified occlusion or stenosis of left anterior cerebral artery** MCC HCC
- **I63.523 Cerebral infarction due to unspecified occlusion or stenosis of bilateral anterior cerebral arteries** MCC HCC
- **I63.529 Cerebral infarction due to unspecified occlusion or stenosis of unspecified anterior cerebral artery** MCC HCC

√6th **I63.53 Cerebral infarction due to unspecified occlusion or stenosis of posterior cerebral artery**
- **I63.531 Cerebral infarction due to unspecified occlusion or stenosis of right posterior cerebral artery** MCC HCC
- **I63.532 Cerebral infarction due to unspecified occlusion or stenosis of left posterior cerebral artery** MCC HCC
- **I63.533 Cerebral infarction due to unspecified occlusion or stenosis of bilateral posterior cerebral arteries** MCC HCC
- **I63.539 Cerebral infarction due to unspecified occlusion or stenosis of unspecified posterior cerebral artery** MCC HCC

√6th **I63.54 Cerebral infarction due to unspecified occlusion or stenosis of cerebellar artery**
- **I63.541 Cerebral infarction due to unspecified occlusion or stenosis of right cerebellar artery** MCC HCC
- **I63.542 Cerebral infarction due to unspecified occlusion or stenosis of left cerebellar artery** MCC HCC
- **I63.543 Cerebral infarction due to unspecified occlusion or stenosis of bilateral cerebellar arteries** MCC HCC
- **I63.549 Cerebral infarction due to unspecified occlusion or stenosis of unspecified cerebellar artery** MCC HCC

I63.59 Cerebral infarction due to unspecified occlusion or stenosis of other cerebral artery MCC HCC

I63.6 Cerebral infarction due to cerebral venous thrombosis, nonpyogenic MCC HCC

√5th **I63.8 Other cerebral infarction**

AHA: 2018,4Q,16

- **I63.81 Other cerebral infarction due to occlusion or stenosis of small artery** MCC HCC
  Lacunar infarction
- **I63.89 Other cerebral infarction** MCC HCC

I63.9 Cerebral infarction, unspecified MCC HCC

Stroke NOS

EXCLUDES 2 *transient cerebral ischemic attacks and related syndromes (G45.-)*

AHA: 2020,2Q,29; 2015,1Q,25

TIP: When provider documentation does not identify the location of an infarction, imaging reports can be used to pinpoint the location and lead to a more specific infarction code.

√4th **I65 Occlusion and stenosis of precerebral arteries, not resulting in cerebral infarction**

INCLUDES embolism of precerebral artery
narrowing of precerebral artery
obstruction (complete) (partial) of precerebral artery
thrombosis of precerebral artery

EXCLUDES 1 *insufficiency, NOS, of precerebral artery (G45.-)*
insufficiency of precerebral arteries causing cerebral infarction (I63.0-I63.2)

AHA: 2018,2Q,9

√5th **I65.0 Occlusion and stenosis of vertebral artery**
- **I65.01 Occlusion and stenosis of right vertebral artery**
- **I65.02 Occlusion and stenosis of left vertebral artery**
- **I65.03 Occlusion and stenosis of bilateral vertebral arteries**
- **I65.09 Occlusion and stenosis of unspecified vertebral artery**

I65.1 Occlusion and stenosis of basilar artery

√5th **I65.2 Occlusion and stenosis of carotid artery**
- **I65.21 Occlusion and stenosis of right carotid artery**
- **I65.22 Occlusion and stenosis of left carotid artery**
- **I65.23 Occlusion and stenosis of bilateral carotid arteries**
- **I65.29 Occlusion and stenosis of unspecified carotid artery**

I65.8 Occlusion and stenosis of other precerebral arteries

I65.9 Occlusion and stenosis of unspecified precerebral artery

Occlusion and stenosis of precerebral artery NOS

✓4th **I66 Occlusion and stenosis of cerebral arteries, not resulting in cerebral infarction**

INCLUDES embolism of cerebral artery
narrowing of cerebral artery
obstruction (complete) (partial) of cerebral artery
thrombosis of cerebral artery

EXCLUDES 1 *occlusion and stenosis of cerebral artery causing cerebral infarction (I63.3-I63.5)*

✓5th **I66.Ø Occlusion and stenosis of middle cerebral artery**

I66.Ø1 Occlusion and stenosis of right middle cerebral artery

I66.Ø2 Occlusion and stenosis of left middle cerebral artery

I66.Ø3 Occlusion and stenosis of bilateral middle cerebral arteries

I66.Ø9 Occlusion and stenosis of unspecified middle cerebral artery

✓5th **I66.1 Occlusion and stenosis of anterior cerebral artery**

I66.11 Occlusion and stenosis of right anterior cerebral artery

I66.12 Occlusion and stenosis of left anterior cerebral artery

I66.13 Occlusion and stenosis of bilateral anterior cerebral arteries

I66.19 Occlusion and stenosis of unspecified anterior cerebral artery

✓5th **I66.2 Occlusion and stenosis of posterior cerebral artery**

I66.21 Occlusion and stenosis of right posterior cerebral artery

I66.22 Occlusion and stenosis of left posterior cerebral artery

I66.23 Occlusion and stenosis of bilateral posterior cerebral arteries

I66.29 Occlusion and stenosis of unspecified posterior cerebral artery

I66.3 Occlusion and stenosis of cerebellar arteries

I66.8 Occlusion and stenosis of other cerebral arteries
Occlusion and stenosis of perforating arteries

I66.9 Occlusion and stenosis of unspecified cerebral artery

✓4th **I67 Other cerebrovascular diseases**

EXCLUDES 2 *sequelae of the listed conditions (I69.8)*

I67.Ø Dissection of cerebral arteries, nonruptured MCC HCC

EXCLUDES 1 *ruptured cerebral arteries (I6Ø.7)*

I67.1 Cerebral aneurysm, nonruptured
Cerebral aneurysm NOS
Cerebral arteriovenous fistula, acquired
Internal carotid artery aneurysm, intracranial portion
Internal carotid artery aneurysm, NOS

EXCLUDES 1 *congenital cerebral aneurysm, nonruptured (Q28.-)*
ruptured cerebral aneurysm (I6Ø.7)

Berry Aneurysm

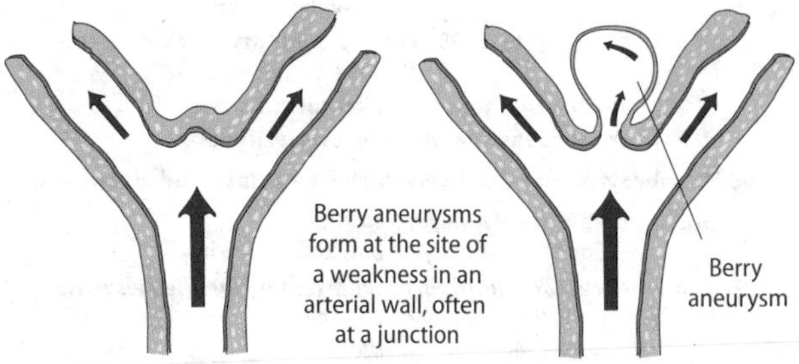

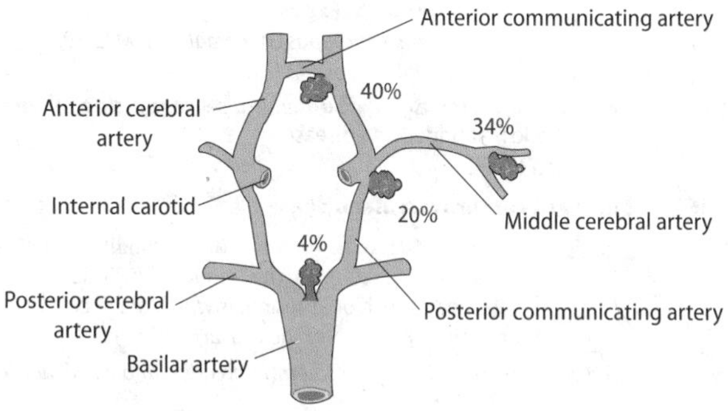

Common sites of berry aneurysms in the circle of Willis arteries

I67.2 Cerebral atherosclerosis A
Atheroma of cerebral and precerebral arteries

I67.3 Progressive vascular leukoencephalopathy HIV CC HCC
Binswanger's disease

I67.4 Hypertensive encephalopathy CC

EXCLUDES 2 *insufficiency, NOS, of precerebral arteries (G45.2)*

I67.5 Moyamoya disease CC
DEF: Cerebrovascular ischemia. Vessels occlude and rupture, causing tiny hemorrhages at the base of brain. It affects predominantly Japanese people.

I67.6 Nonpyogenic thrombosis of intracranial venous system CC
Nonpyogenic thrombosis of cerebral vein
Nonpyogenic thrombosis of intracranial venous sinus

EXCLUDES 1 *nonpyogenic thrombosis of intracranial venous system causing infarction (I63.6)*

I67.7 Cerebral arteritis, not elsewhere classified CC
Granulomatous angiitis of the nervous system

EXCLUDES 1 *allergic granulomatous angiitis (M3Ø.1)*

✓5th **I67.8 Other specified cerebrovascular diseases**

I67.81 Acute cerebrovascular insufficiency CC
Acute cerebrovascular insufficiency unspecified as to location or reversibility

I67.82 Cerebral ischemia CC
Chronic cerebral ischemia

I67.83 Posterior reversible encephalopathy syndrome HIV MCC
PRES

✓6th **I67.84 Cerebral vasospasm and vasoconstriction**

I67.841 Reversible cerebrovascular vasoconstriction syndrome CC
Call-Fleming syndrome
Code first underlying condition, if applicable, such as eclampsia (O15.ØØ-O15.9)

I67.848 Other cerebrovascular vasospasm and vasoconstriction CC

✓6th **I67.85 Hereditary cerebrovascular diseases**
AHA: 2018,4Q,17

I67.850 Cerebral autosomal dominant arteriopathy with subcortical infarcts and leukoencephalopathy CC
CADASIL
Code also any associated diagnoses, such as:
epilepsy (G40.-)
stroke (I63.-)
vascular dementia (F01.-)

I67.858 Other hereditary cerebrovascular disease CC

I67.89 Other cerebrovascular disease CC

I67.9 Cerebrovascular disease, unspecified

✓4th **I68 Cerebrovascular disorders in diseases classified elsewhere**

I68.0 Cerebral amyloid angiopathy
Code first underlying amyloidosis (E85.-)

I68.2 Cerebral arteritis in other diseases classified elsewhere CC
Code first underlying disease
EXCLUDES 1 *cerebral arteritis (in):*
listerosis (A32.89)
syphilis (A52.04)
systemic lupus erythematosus (M32.19)
tuberculosis (A18.89)

I68.8 Other cerebrovascular disorders in diseases classified elsewhere
Code first underlying disease
EXCLUDES 1 *syphilitic cerebral aneurysm (A52.05)*

✓4th **I69 Sequelae of cerebrovascular disease**

NOTE Category I69 is to be used to indicate conditions in I60-I67 as the cause of sequelae. The "sequelae" include conditions specified as such or as residuals which may occur at any time after the onset of the causal condition

EXCLUDES 1 *personal history of cerebral infarction without residual deficit (Z86.73)*
personal history of prolonged reversible ischemic neurologic deficit (PRIND) (Z86.73)
personal history of reversible ischemic neurologcial deficit (RIND) (Z86.73)
sequelae of traumatic intracranial injury (S06.-)

AHA: 2020,2Q,29; 2017,1Q,47; 2016,4Q,28; 2015,1Q,25; 2012,4Q,106

TIP: Weakness on one side of the body (unilateral weakness) documented as secondary to old cerebrovascular disease is synonymous with hemiparesis/hemiplegia. Weakness of one limb documented as secondary to old cerebrovascular disease is synonymous with monoplegia.

TIP: For codes describing hemiplegia, hemiparesis, and monoplegia; if the documentation identifies the affected side but not whether it is the dominant or nondominant side, the default is as follows: for ambidextrous patients, the default is dominant; when the left side is affected, the default is nondominant; and when the right side is affected, the default is dominant.

✓5th **I69.0 Sequelae of nontraumatic subarachnoid hemorrhage**

I69.00 Unspecified sequelae of nontraumatic subarachnoid hemorrhage

✓6th **I69.01 Cognitive deficits following nontraumatic subarachnoid hemorrhage**

I69.010 Attention and concentration deficit following nontraumatic subarachnoid hemorrhage

I69.011 Memory deficit following nontraumatic subarachnoid hemorrhage

I69.012 Visuospatial deficit and spatial neglect following nontraumatic subarachnoid hemorrhage

I69.013 Psychomotor deficit following nontraumatic subarachnoid hemorrhage

I69.014 Frontal lobe and executive function deficit following nontraumatic subarachnoid hemorrhage

I69.015 Cognitive social or emotional deficit following nontraumatic subarachnoid hemorrhage

I69.018 Other symptoms and signs involving cognitive functions following nontraumatic subarachnoid hemorrhage

I69.019 Unspecified symptoms and signs involving cognitive functions following nontraumatic subarachnoid hemorrhage

✓6th **I69.02 Speech and language deficits following nontraumatic subarachnoid hemorrhage**

I69.020 Aphasia following nontraumatic subarachnoid hemorrhage

I69.021 Dysphasia following nontraumatic subarachnoid hemorrhage

I69.022 Dysarthria following nontraumatic subarachnoid hemorrhage

I69.023 Fluency disorder following nontraumatic subarachnoid hemorrhage
Stuttering following nontraumatic subarachnoid hemorrhage

I69.028 Other speech and language deficits following nontraumatic subarachnoid hemorrhage

✓6th **I69.03 Monoplegia of upper limb following nontraumatic subarachnoid hemorrhage**
AHA: 2017,1Q,47

I69.031 Monoplegia of upper limb following nontraumatic subarachnoid hemorrhage affecting right dominant side HCC

I69.032 Monoplegia of upper limb following nontraumatic subarachnoid hemorrhage affecting left dominant side HCC

I69.033 Monoplegia of upper limb following nontraumatic subarachnoid hemorrhage affecting right non-dominant side HCC

I69.034 Monoplegia of upper limb following nontraumatic subarachnoid hemorrhage affecting left non-dominant side HCC

I69.039 Monoplegia of upper limb following nontraumatic subarachnoid hemorrhage affecting unspecified side HCC

✓6th **I69.04 Monoplegia of lower limb following nontraumatic subarachnoid hemorrhage**
AHA: 2017,1Q,47

I69.041 Monoplegia of lower limb following nontraumatic subarachnoid hemorrhage affecting right dominant side HCC

I69.042 Monoplegia of lower limb following nontraumatic subarachnoid hemorrhage affecting left dominant side HCC

I69.043 Monoplegia of lower limb following nontraumatic subarachnoid hemorrhage affecting right non-dominant side HCC

I69.044 Monoplegia of lower limb following nontraumatic subarachnoid hemorrhage affecting left non-dominant side HCC

I69.049 Monoplegia of lower limb following nontraumatic subarachnoid hemorrhage affecting unspecified side HCC

✓6th **I69.05 Hemiplegia and hemiparesis following nontraumatic subarachnoid hemorrhage**
AHA: 2015,1Q,25

I69.051 Hemiplegia and hemiparesis following nontraumatic subarachnoid hemorrhage affecting right dominant side CC HCC

I69.052 Hemiplegia and hemiparesis following nontraumatic subarachnoid hemorrhage affecting left dominant side CC HCC

I69.053 Hemiplegia and hemiparesis following nontraumatic subarachnoid hemorrhage affecting right non-dominant side CC HCC

I69.054 Hemiplegia and hemiparesis following nontraumatic subarachnoid hemorrhage affecting left non-dominant side CC HCC

I69.059 Hemiplegia and hemiparesis following nontraumatic subarachnoid hemorrhage affecting unspecified side CC HCC

I69.06 Other paralytic syndrome following nontraumatic subarachnoid hemorrhage
Use additional code to identify type of paralytic syndrome, such as:
locked-in state (G83.5)
quadriplegia (G82.5-)
EXCLUDES 1 *hemiplegia/hemiparesis following nontraumatic subarachnoid hemorrhage (I69.05-)*
monoplegia of lower limb following nontraumatic subarachnoid hemorrhage (I69.04-)
monoplegia of upper limb following nontraumatic subarachnoid hemorrhage (I69.03-)

I69.061 Other paralytic syndrome following nontraumatic subarachnoid hemorrhage affecting right dominant side HCC
I69.062 Other paralytic syndrome following nontraumatic subarachnoid hemorrhage affecting left dominant side HCC
I69.063 Other paralytic syndrome following nontraumatic subarachnoid hemorrhage affecting right non-dominant side HCC
I69.064 Other paralytic syndrome following nontraumatic subarachnoid hemorrhage affecting left non-dominant side HCC
I69.065 Other paralytic syndrome following nontraumatic subarachnoid hemorrhage, bilateral HCC
I69.069 Other paralytic syndrome following nontraumatic subarachnoid hemorrhage affecting unspecified side HCC

I69.09 Other sequelae of nontraumatic subarachnoid hemorrhage

I69.090 Apraxia following nontraumatic subarachnoid hemorrhage
I69.091 Dysphagia following nontraumatic subarachnoid hemorrhage
Use additional code to identify the type of dysphagia, if known (R13.1-)
I69.092 Facial weakness following nontraumatic subarachnoid hemorrhage
Facial droop following nontraumatic subarachnoid hemorrhage
I69.093 Ataxia following nontraumatic subarachnoid hemorrhage
I69.098 Other sequelae following nontraumatic subarachnoid hemorrhage
Alterations of sensation following nontraumatic subarachnoid hemorrhage
Disturbance of vision following nontraumatic subarachnoid hemorrhage
Use additional code to identify the sequelae

I69.1 Sequelae of nontraumatic intracerebral hemorrhage

I69.10 Unspecified sequelae of nontraumatic intracerebral hemorrhage

I69.11 Cognitive deficits following nontraumatic intracerebral hemorrhage

I69.110 Attention and concentration deficit following nontraumatic intracerebral hemorrhage
I69.111 Memory deficit following nontraumatic intracerebral hemorrhage
I69.112 Visuospatial deficit and spatial neglect following nontraumatic intracerebral hemorrhage
I69.113 Psychomotor deficit following nontraumatic intracerebral hemorrhage
I69.114 Frontal lobe and executive function deficit following nontraumatic intracerebral hemorrhage
I69.115 Cognitive social or emotional deficit following nontraumatic intracerebral hemorrhage
I69.118 Other symptoms and signs involving cognitive functions following nontraumatic intracerebral hemorrhage
I69.119 Unspecified symptoms and signs involving cognitive functions following nontraumatic intracerebral hemorrhage

I69.12 Speech and language deficits following nontraumatic intracerebral hemorrhage

I69.120 Aphasia following nontraumatic intracerebral hemorrhage
I69.121 Dysphasia following nontraumatic intracerebral hemorrhage
I69.122 Dysarthria following nontraumatic intracerebral hemorrhage
I69.123 Fluency disorder following nontraumatic intracerebral hemorrhage
Stuttering following nontraumatic intracerebral hemorrhage
I69.128 Other speech and language deficits following nontraumatic intracerebral hemorrhage

I69.13 Monoplegia of upper limb following nontraumatic intracerebral hemorrhage
AHA: 2017,1Q,47

I69.131 Monoplegia of upper limb following nontraumatic intracerebral hemorrhage affecting right dominant side HCC
I69.132 Monoplegia of upper limb following nontraumatic intracerebral hemorrhage affecting left dominant side HCC
I69.133 Monoplegia of upper limb following nontraumatic intracerebral hemorrhage affecting right non-dominant side HCC
I69.134 Monoplegia of upper limb following nontraumatic intracerebral hemorrhage affecting left non-dominant side HCC
I69.139 Monoplegia of upper limb following nontraumatic intracerebral hemorrhage affecting unspecified side HCC

I69.14 Monoplegia of lower limb following nontraumatic intracerebral hemorrhage
AHA: 2017,1Q,47

I69.141 Monoplegia of lower limb following nontraumatic intracerebral hemorrhage affecting right dominant side HCC
I69.142 Monoplegia of lower limb following nontraumatic intracerebral hemorrhage affecting left dominant side HCC
I69.143 Monoplegia of lower limb following nontraumatic intracerebral hemorrhage affecting right non-dominant side HCC
I69.144 Monoplegia of lower limb following nontraumatic intracerebral hemorrhage affecting left non-dominant side HCC
I69.149 Monoplegia of lower limb following nontraumatic intracerebral hemorrhage affecting unspecified side HCC

I69.15 Hemiplegia and hemiparesis following nontraumatic intracerebral hemorrhage
AHA: 2015,1Q,25

I69.151 Hemiplegia and hemiparesis following nontraumatic intracerebral hemorrhage affecting right dominant side CC HCC
I69.152 Hemiplegia and hemiparesis following nontraumatic intracerebral hemorrhage affecting left dominant side CC HCC
I69.153 Hemiplegia and hemiparesis following nontraumatic intracerebral hemorrhage affecting right non-dominant side CC HCC
I69.154 Hemiplegia and hemiparesis following nontraumatic intracerebral hemorrhage affecting left non-dominant side CC HCC
I69.159 Hemiplegia and hemiparesis following nontraumatic intracerebral hemorrhage affecting unspecified side CC HCC

√6th **I69.16 Other paralytic syndrome following nontraumatic intracerebral hemorrhage**
Use additional code to identify type of paralytic syndrome, such as:
locked-in state (G83.5)
quadriplegia (G82.5-)
EXCLUDES 1 *hemiplegia/hemiparesis following nontraumatic intracerebral hemorrhage (I69.15-)*
monoplegia of lower limb following nontraumatic intracerebral hemorrhage (I69.14-)
monoplegia of upper limb following nontraumatic intracerebral hemorrhage (I69.13-)

I69.161 Other paralytic syndrome following nontraumatic intracerebral hemorrhage affecting right dominant side HCC

I69.162 Other paralytic syndrome following nontraumatic intracerebral hemorrhage affecting left dominant side HCC

I69.163 Other paralytic syndrome following nontraumatic intracerebral hemorrhage affecting right non-dominant side HCC

I69.164 Other paralytic syndrome following nontraumatic intracerebral hemorrhage affecting left non-dominant side HCC

I69.165 Other paralytic syndrome following nontraumatic intracerebral hemorrhage, bilateral HCC

I69.169 Other paralytic syndrome following nontraumatic intracerebral hemorrhage affecting unspecified side HCC

√6th **I69.19 Other sequelae of nontraumatic intracerebral hemorrhage**

I69.190 Apraxia following nontraumatic intracerebral hemorrhage

I69.191 Dysphagia following nontraumatic intracerebral hemorrhage
Use additional code to identify the type of dysphagia, if known (R13.1-)

I69.192 Facial weakness following nontraumatic intracerebral hemorrhage
Facial droop following nontraumatic intracerebral hemorrhage

I69.193 Ataxia following nontraumatic intracerebral hemorrhage

I69.198 Other sequelae of nontraumatic intracerebral hemorrhage
Alteration of sensations following nontraumatic intracerebral hemorrhage
Disturbance of vision following nontraumatic intracerebral hemorrhage
Use additional code to identify the sequelae

√5th **I69.2 Sequelae of other nontraumatic intracranial hemorrhage**

I69.20 Unspecified sequelae of other nontraumatic intracranial hemorrhage

√6th **I69.21 Cognitive deficits following other nontraumatic intracranial hemorrhage**

I69.210 Attention and concentration deficit following other nontraumatic intracranial hemorrhage

I69.211 Memory deficit following other nontraumatic intracranial hemorrhage

I69.212 Visuospatial deficit and spatial neglect following other nontraumatic intracranial hemorrhage

I69.213 Psychomotor deficit following other nontraumatic intracranial hemorrhage

I69.214 Frontal lobe and executive function deficit following other nontraumatic intracranial hemorrhage

I69.215 Cognitive social or emotional deficit following other nontraumatic intracranial hemorrhage

I69.218 Other symptoms and signs involving cognitive functions following other nontraumatic intracranial hemorrhage

I69.219 Unspecified symptoms and signs involving cognitive functions following other nontraumatic intracranial hemorrhage

√6th **I69.22 Speech and language deficits following other nontraumatic intracranial hemorrhage**

I69.220 Aphasia following other nontraumatic intracranial hemorrhage

I69.221 Dysphasia following other nontraumatic intracranial hemorrhage

I69.222 Dysarthria following other nontraumatic intracranial hemorrhage

I69.223 Fluency disorder following other nontraumatic intracranial hemorrhage
Stuttering following other nontraumatic intracranial hemorrhage

I69.228 Other speech and language deficits following other nontraumatic intracranial hemorrhage

√6th **I69.23 Monoplegia of upper limb following other nontraumatic intracranial hemorrhage**
AHA: 2017,1Q,47

I69.231 Monoplegia of upper limb following other nontraumatic intracranial hemorrhage affecting right dominant side HCC

I69.232 Monoplegia of upper limb following other nontraumatic intracranial hemorrhage affecting left dominant side HCC

I69.233 Monoplegia of upper limb following other nontraumatic intracranial hemorrhage affecting right non-dominant side HCC

I69.234 Monoplegia of upper limb following other nontraumatic intracranial hemorrhage affecting left non-dominant side HCC

I69.239 Monoplegia of upper limb following other nontraumatic intracranial hemorrhage affecting unspecified side HCC

√6th **I69.24 Monoplegia of lower limb following other nontraumatic intracranial hemorrhage**
AHA: 2017,1Q,47

I69.241 Monoplegia of lower limb following other nontraumatic intracranial hemorrhage affecting right dominant side HCC

I69.242 Monoplegia of lower limb following other nontraumatic intracranial hemorrhage affecting left dominant side HCC

I69.243 Monoplegia of lower limb following other nontraumatic intracranial hemorrhage affecting right non-dominant side HCC

I69.244 Monoplegia of lower limb following other nontraumatic intracranial hemorrhage affecting left non-dominant side HCC

I69.249 Monoplegia of lower limb following other nontraumatic intracranial hemorrhage affecting unspecified side HCC

√6th **I69.25 Hemiplegia and hemiparesis following other nontraumatic intracranial hemorrhage**
AHA: 2015,1Q,25

I69.251 Hemiplegia and hemiparesis following other nontraumatic intracranial hemorrhage affecting right dominant side CC HCC

I69.252 Hemiplegia and hemiparesis following other nontraumatic intracranial hemorrhage affecting left dominant side CC HCC

I69.253 Hemiplegia and hemiparesis following other nontraumatic intracranial hemorrhage affecting right non-dominant side CC HCC

I69.254 Hemiplegia and hemiparesis following other nontraumatic intracranial hemorrhage affecting left non-dominant side CC HCC

I69.259 Hemiplegia and hemiparesis following other nontraumatic intracranial hemorrhage affecting unspecified side CC HCC

I69.26 Other paralytic syndrome following other nontraumatic intracranial hemorrhage
Use additional code to identify type of paralytic syndrome, such as:
locked-in state (G83.5)
quadriplegia (G82.5-)
EXCLUDES 1 *hemiplegia/hemiparesis following other nontraumatic intracranial hemorrhage (I69.25-)*
monoplegia of lower limb following other nontraumatic intracranial hemorrhage (I69.24-)
monoplegia of upper limb following other nontraumatic intracranial hemorrhage (I69.23-)

I69.261 Other paralytic syndrome following other nontraumatic intracranial hemorrhage affecting right dominant side HCC
I69.262 Other paralytic syndrome following other nontraumatic intracranial hemorrhage affecting left dominant side HCC
I69.263 Other paralytic syndrome following other nontraumatic intracranial hemorrhage affecting right non-dominant side HCC
I69.264 Other paralytic syndrome following other nontraumatic intracranial hemorrhage affecting left non-dominant side HCC
I69.265 Other paralytic syndrome following other nontraumatic intracranial hemorrhage, bilateral HCC
I69.269 Other paralytic syndrome following other nontraumatic intracranial hemorrhage affecting unspecified side HCC

I69.29 Other sequelae of other nontraumatic intracranial hemorrhage
I69.290 Apraxia following other nontraumatic intracranial hemorrhage
I69.291 Dysphagia following other nontraumatic intracranial hemorrhage
Use additional code to identify the type of dysphagia, if known (R13.1-)
I69.292 Facial weakness following other nontraumatic intracranial hemorrhage
Facial droop following other nontraumatic intracranial hemorrhage
I69.293 Ataxia following other nontraumatic intracranial hemorrhage
I69.298 Other sequelae of other nontraumatic intracranial hemorrhage
Alteration of sensation following other nontraumatic intracranial hemorrhage
Disturbance of vision following other nontraumatic intracranial hemorrhage
Use additional code to identify the sequelae

I69.3 Sequelae of cerebral infarction
Sequelae of stroke NOS
AHA: 2013,4Q,127-128; 2012,4Q,92,94

I69.30 Unspecified sequelae of cerebral infarction

I69.31 Cognitive deficits following cerebral infarction
I69.310 Attention and concentration deficit following cerebral infarction
I69.311 Memory deficit following cerebral infarction
I69.312 Visuospatial deficit and spatial neglect following cerebral infarction
I69.313 Psychomotor deficit following cerebral infarction
I69.314 Frontal lobe and executive function deficit following cerebral infarction
I69.315 Cognitive social or emotional deficit following cerebral infarction
I69.318 Other symptoms and signs involving cognitive functions following cerebral infarction
I69.319 Unspecified symptoms and signs involving cognitive functions following cerebral infarction

I69.32 Speech and language deficits following cerebral infarction
I69.320 Aphasia following cerebral infarction
I69.321 Dysphasia following cerebral infarction
AHA: 2012,4Q,91
I69.322 Dysarthria following cerebral infarction
EXCLUDES 2 *transient ischemic attack (TIA) (G45.9)*
I69.323 Fluency disorder following cerebral infarction
Stuttering following cerebral infarction
I69.328 Other speech and language deficits following cerebral infarction

I69.33 Monoplegia of upper limb following cerebral infarction
AHA: 2017,1Q,47
I69.331 Monoplegia of upper limb following cerebral infarction affecting right dominant side HCC
I69.332 Monoplegia of upper limb following cerebral infarction affecting left dominant side HCC
I69.333 Monoplegia of upper limb following cerebral infarction affecting right non-dominant side HCC
I69.334 Monoplegia of upper limb following cerebral infarction affecting left non-dominant side HCC
I69.339 Monoplegia of upper limb following cerebral infarction affecting unspecified side HCC

I69.34 Monoplegia of lower limb following cerebral infarction
AHA: 2017,1Q,47
I69.341 Monoplegia of lower limb following cerebral infarction affecting right dominant side HCC
I69.342 Monoplegia of lower limb following cerebral infarction affecting left dominant side HCC
I69.343 Monoplegia of lower limb following cerebral infarction affecting right non-dominant side HCC
I69.344 Monoplegia of lower limb following cerebral infarction affecting left non-dominant side HCC
I69.349 Monoplegia of lower limb following cerebral infarction affecting unspecified side HCC

I69.35 Hemiplegia and hemiparesis following cerebral infarction
AHA: 2015,1Q,25
I69.351 Hemiplegia and hemiparesis following cerebral infarction affecting right dominant side CC HCC
EXCLUDES 2 *transient ischemic attack (TIA) (G45.9)*
I69.352 Hemiplegia and hemiparesis following cerebral infarction affecting left dominant side CC HCC
I69.353 Hemiplegia and hemiparesis following cerebral infarction affecting right non-dominant side CC HCC
I69.354 Hemiplegia and hemiparesis following cerebral infarction affecting left non-dominant side CC HCC
AHA: 2012,4Q,91
I69.359 Hemiplegia and hemiparesis following cerebral infarction affecting unspecified side CC HCC

✓6th **I69.36 Other paralytic syndrome following cerebral infarction**
Use additional code to identify type of paralytic syndrome, such as:
locked-in state (G83.5)
quadriplegia (G82.5-)
EXCLUDES 1 *hemiplegia/hemiparesis following cerebral infarction (I69.35-)*
monoplegia of lower limb following cerebral infarction (I69.34-)
monoplegia of upper limb following cerebral infarction (I69.33-)

I69.361 Other paralytic syndrome following cerebral infarction affecting right dominant side HCC
I69.362 Other paralytic syndrome following cerebral infarction affecting left dominant side HCC
I69.363 Other paralytic syndrome following cerebral infarction affecting right non-dominant side HCC
I69.364 Other paralytic syndrome following cerebral infarction affecting left non-dominant side HCC
I69.365 Other paralytic syndrome following cerebral infarction, bilateral HCC
I69.369 Other paralytic syndrome following cerebral infarction affecting unspecified side HCC

✓6th **I69.39 Other sequelae of cerebral infarction**
I69.390 Apraxia following cerebral infarction
I69.391 Dysphagia following cerebral infarction
Use additional code to identify the type of dysphagia, if known (R13.1-)
I69.392 Facial weakness following cerebral infarction
Facial droop following cerebral infarction
I69.393 Ataxia following cerebral infarction
I69.398 Other sequelae of cerebral infarction
Alteration of sensation following cerebral infarction
Disturbance of vision following cerebral infarction
Use additional code to identify the sequelae
AHA: 2020,2Q,29

✓5th **I69.8 Sequelae of other cerebrovascular diseases**
EXCLUDES 1 *sequelae of traumatic intracranial injury (S06.-)*
I69.80 Unspecified sequelae of other cerebrovascular disease

✓6th **I69.81 Cognitive deficits following other cerebrovascular disease**
I69.810 Attention and concentration deficit following other cerebrovascular disease
I69.811 Memory deficit following other cerebrovascular disease
I69.812 Visuospatial deficit and spatial neglect following other cerebrovascular disease
I69.813 Psychomotor deficit following other cerebrovascular disease
I69.814 Frontal lobe and executive function deficit following other cerebrovascular disease
I69.815 Cognitive social or emotional deficit following other cerebrovascular disease
I69.818 Other symptoms and signs involving cognitive functions following other cerebrovascular disease
I69.819 Unspecified symptoms and signs involving cognitive functions following other cerebrovascular disease

✓6th **I69.82 Speech and language deficits following other cerebrovascular disease**
I69.820 Aphasia following other cerebrovascular disease
I69.821 Dysphasia following other cerebrovascular disease
I69.822 Dysarthria following other cerebrovascular disease
I69.823 Fluency disorder following other cerebrovascular disease
Stuttering following other cerebrovascular disease
I69.828 Other speech and language deficits following other cerebrovascular disease
AHA: 2019,3Q,8

✓6th **I69.83 Monoplegia of upper limb following other cerebrovascular disease**
AHA: 2017,1Q,47
I69.831 Monoplegia of upper limb following other cerebrovascular disease affecting right dominant side HCC
I69.832 Monoplegia of upper limb following other cerebrovascular disease affecting left dominant side HCC
I69.833 Monoplegia of upper limb following other cerebrovascular disease affecting right non-dominant side HCC
I69.834 Monoplegia of upper limb following other cerebrovascular disease affecting left non-dominant side HCC
I69.839 Monoplegia of upper limb following other cerebrovascular disease affecting unspecified side HCC

✓6th **I69.84 Monoplegia of lower limb following other cerebrovascular disease**
AHA: 2017,1Q,47
I69.841 Monoplegia of lower limb following other cerebrovascular disease affecting right dominant side HCC
I69.842 Monoplegia of lower limb following other cerebrovascular disease affecting left dominant side HCC
I69.843 Monoplegia of lower limb following other cerebrovascular disease affecting right non-dominant side HCC
I69.844 Monoplegia of lower limb following other cerebrovascular disease affecting left non-dominant side HCC
I69.849 Monoplegia of lower limb following other cerebrovascular disease affecting unspecified side HCC

✓6th **I69.85 Hemiplegia and hemiparesis following other cerebrovascular disease**
AHA: 2015,1Q,25
I69.851 Hemiplegia and hemiparesis following other cerebrovascular disease affecting right dominant side CC HCC
I69.852 Hemiplegia and hemiparesis following other cerebrovascular disease affecting left dominant side CC HCC
I69.853 Hemiplegia and hemiparesis following other cerebrovascular disease affecting right non-dominant side CC HCC
I69.854 Hemiplegia and hemiparesis following other cerebrovascular disease affecting left non-dominant side CC HCC
I69.859 Hemiplegia and hemiparesis following other cerebrovascular disease affecting unspecified side CC HCC

✓6th **I69.86 Other paralytic syndrome following other cerebrovascular disease**
Use additional code to identify type of paralytic syndrome, such as:
locked-in state (G83.5)
quadriplegia (G82.5-)
EXCLUDES 1 *hemiplegia/hemiparesis following other cerebrovascular disease (I69.85-)*
monoplegia of lower limb following other cerebrovascular disease (I69.84-)
monoplegia of upper limb following other cerebrovascular disease (I69.83-)

I69.861 Other paralytic syndrome following other cerebrovascular disease affecting right dominant side HCC
I69.862 Other paralytic syndrome following other cerebrovascular disease affecting left dominant side HCC
I69.863 Other paralytic syndrome following other cerebrovascular disease affecting right non-dominant side HCC

I69.864 **Other paralytic syndrome following other cerebrovascular disease affecting left non-dominant side** HCC

I69.865 **Other paralytic syndrome following other cerebrovascular disease, bilateral** HCC

I69.869 **Other paralytic syndrome following other cerebrovascular disease affecting unspecified side** HCC

✓6th I69.89 **Other sequelae of other cerebrovascular disease**

I69.890 **Apraxia following other cerebrovascular disease**

I69.891 **Dysphagia following other cerebrovascular disease**

Use additional code to identify the type of dysphagia, if known (R13.1-)

I69.892 **Facial weakness following other cerebrovascular disease**

Facial droop following other cerebrovascular disease

I69.893 **Ataxia following other cerebrovascular disease**

I69.898 **Other sequelae of other cerebrovascular disease**

Alteration of sensation following other cerebrovascular disease

Disturbance of vision following other cerebrovascular disease

Use additional code to identify the sequelae

✓5th I69.9 **Sequelae of unspecified cerebrovascular diseases**

EXCLUDES 1 *sequelae of stroke (I69.3)*

sequelae of traumatic intracranial injury (S06.-)

I69.90 **Unspecified sequelae of unspecified cerebrovascular disease**

✓6th I69.91 **Cognitive deficits following unspecified cerebrovascular disease**

I69.910 **Attention and concentration deficit following unspecified cerebrovascular disease**

I69.911 **Memory deficit following unspecified cerebrovascular disease**

I69.912 **Visuospatial deficit and spatial neglect following unspecified cerebrovascular disease**

I69.913 **Psychomotor deficit following unspecified cerebrovascular disease**

I69.914 **Frontal lobe and executive function deficit following unspecified cerebrovascular disease**

I69.915 **Cognitive social or emotional deficit following unspecified cerebrovascular disease**

I69.918 **Other symptoms and signs involving cognitive functions following unspecified cerebrovascular disease**

I69.919 **Unspecified symptoms and signs involving cognitive functions following unspecified cerebrovascular disease**

✓6th I69.92 **Speech and language deficits following unspecified cerebrovascular disease**

I69.920 **Aphasia following unspecified cerebrovascular disease**

I69.921 **Dysphasia following unspecified cerebrovascular disease**

I69.922 **Dysarthria following unspecified cerebrovascular disease**

I69.923 **Fluency disorder following unspecified cerebrovascular disease**

Stuttering following unspecified cerebrovascular disease

I69.928 **Other speech and language deficits following unspecified cerebrovascular disease**

✓6th I69.93 **Monoplegia of upper limb following unspecified cerebrovascular disease**

AHA: 2017,1Q,47

I69.931 **Monoplegia of upper limb following unspecified cerebrovascular disease affecting right dominant side** HCC

I69.932 **Monoplegia of upper limb following unspecified cerebrovascular disease affecting left dominant side** HCC

I69.933 **Monoplegia of upper limb following unspecified cerebrovascular disease affecting right non-dominant side** HCC

I69.934 **Monoplegia of upper limb following unspecified cerebrovascular disease affecting left non-dominant side** HCC

I69.939 **Monoplegia of upper limb following unspecified cerebrovascular disease affecting unspecified side** HCC

✓6th I69.94 **Monoplegia of lower limb following unspecified cerebrovascular disease**

AHA: 2017,1Q,47

I69.941 **Monoplegia of lower limb following unspecified cerebrovascular disease affecting right dominant side** HCC

I69.942 **Monoplegia of lower limb following unspecified cerebrovascular disease affecting left dominant side** HCC

I69.943 **Monoplegia of lower limb following unspecified cerebrovascular disease affecting right non-dominant side** HCC

I69.944 **Monoplegia of lower limb following unspecified cerebrovascular disease affecting left non-dominant side** HCC

I69.949 **Monoplegia of lower limb following unspecified cerebrovascular disease affecting unspecified side** HCC

✓6th I69.95 **Hemiplegia and hemiparesis following unspecified cerebrovascular disease**

AHA: 2015,1Q,25

I69.951 **Hemiplegia and hemiparesis following unspecified cerebrovascular disease affecting right dominant side** CC HCC

I69.952 **Hemiplegia and hemiparesis following unspecified cerebrovascular disease affecting left dominant side** CC HCC

I69.953 **Hemiplegia and hemiparesis following unspecified cerebrovascular disease affecting right non-dominant side** CC HCC

I69.954 **Hemiplegia and hemiparesis following unspecified cerebrovascular disease affecting left non-dominant side** CC HCC

I69.959 **Hemiplegia and hemiparesis following unspecified cerebrovascular disease affecting unspecified side** CC HCC

✓6th I69.96 **Other paralytic syndrome following unspecified cerebrovascular disease**

Use additional code to identify type of paralytic syndrome, such as:

locked-in state (G83.5)

quadriplegia (G82.5-)

EXCLUDES 1 *hemiplegia/hemiparesis following unspecified cerebrovascular disease (I69.95-)*

monoplegia of lower limb following unspecified cerebrovascular disease (I69.94-)

monoplegia of upper limb following unspecified cerebrovascular disease (I69.93-)

I69.961 **Other paralytic syndrome following unspecified cerebrovascular disease affecting right dominant side** HCC

I69.962 **Other paralytic syndrome following unspecified cerebrovascular disease affecting left dominant side** HCC

I69.963 **Other paralytic syndrome following unspecified cerebrovascular disease affecting right non-dominant side** HCC

I69.964 **Other paralytic syndrome following unspecified cerebrovascular disease affecting left non-dominant side** HCC

I69.965 **Other paralytic syndrome following unspecified cerebrovascular disease, bilateral** HCC

I69.969 **Other paralytic syndrome following unspecified cerebrovascular disease affecting unspecified side** HCC

√6th **I69.99 Other sequelae of unspecified cerebrovascular disease**

I69.990 Apraxia following unspecified cerebrovascular disease

I69.991 Dysphagia following unspecified cerebrovascular disease

Use additional code to identify the type of dysphagia, if known (R13.1-)

I69.992 Facial weakness following unspecified cerebrovascular disease

Facial droop following unspecified cerebrovascular disease

I69.993 Ataxia following unspecified cerebrovascular disease

I69.998 Other sequelae following unspecified cerebrovascular disease

Alteration in sensation following unspecified cerebrovascular disease

Disturbance of vision following unspecified cerebrovascular disease

Use additional code to identify the sequelae

Diseases of arteries, arterioles and capillaries (I70-I79)

√4th **I70 Atherosclerosis**

INCLUDES arterial degeneration
arteriolosclerosis
arteriosclerosis
arteriosclerotic vascular disease
arteriovascular degeneration
atheroma
endarteritis deformans or obliterans
senile arteritis
senile endarteritis
vascular degeneration

Use additional code to identify:
exposure to environmental tobacco smoke (Z77.22)
history of tobacco dependence (Z87.891)
occupational exposure to environmental tobacco smoke (Z57.31)
tobacco dependence (F17.-)
tobacco use (Z72.0)

EXCLUDES 2 *arteriosclerotic cardiovascular disease (I25.1-)*
arteriosclerotic heart disease (I25.1-)
atheroembolism (I75.-)
cerebral atherosclerosis (I67.2)
coronary atherosclerosis (I25.1-)
mesenteric atherosclerosis (K55.1)
precerebral atherosclerosis (I67.2)
primary pulmonary atherosclerosis (I27.0)

I70.0 Atherosclerosis of aorta HCC A

I70.1 Atherosclerosis of renal artery HCC A

Goldblatt's kidney

EXCLUDES 2 *atherosclerosis of renal arterioles (I12.-)*

√5th **I70.2 Atherosclerosis of native arteries of the extremities**

Mönckeberg's (medial) sclerosis

Use additional code, if applicable, to identify chronic total occlusion of artery of extremity (I70.92)

EXCLUDES 2 *atherosclerosis of bypass graft of extremities (I70.30-I70.79)*

AHA: 2018,3Q,4; 2018,2Q,7

√6th **I70.20 Unspecified atherosclerosis of native arteries of extremities**

I70.201 Unspecified atherosclerosis of native arteries of extremities, right leg HCC A

I70.202 Unspecified atherosclerosis of native arteries of extremities, left leg HCC A

I70.203 Unspecified atherosclerosis of native arteries of extremities, bilateral legs HCC A

I70.208 Unspecified atherosclerosis of native arteries of extremities, other extremity HCC A

I70.209 Unspecified atherosclerosis of native arteries of extremities, unspecified extremity HCC A

√6th **I70.21 Atherosclerosis of native arteries of extremities with intermittent claudication**

I70.211 Atherosclerosis of native arteries of extremities with intermittent claudication, right leg HCC A

I70.212 Atherosclerosis of native arteries of extremities with intermittent claudication, left leg HCC A

I70.213 Atherosclerosis of native arteries of extremities with intermittent claudication, bilateral legs HCC A

I70.218 Atherosclerosis of native arteries of extremities with intermittent claudication, other extremity HCC A

I70.219 Atherosclerosis of native arteries of extremities with intermittent claudication, unspecified extremity HCC A

√6th **I70.22 Atherosclerosis of native arteries of extremities with rest pain**

INCLUDES any condition classifiable to I70.21-
▶chronic limb-threatening ischemia NOS of native arteries of extremities◀
▶chronic limb-threatening ischemia of native arteries of extremities with rest pain◀
▶critical limb ischemia NOS of native arteries of extremities◀
▶critical limb ischemia of native arteries of extremities with rest pain◀

I70.221 Atherosclerosis of native arteries of extremities with rest pain, right leg HCC A

I70.222 Atherosclerosis of native arteries of extremities with rest pain, left leg HCC A

I70.223 Atherosclerosis of native arteries of extremities with rest pain, bilateral legs HCC A

I70.228 Atherosclerosis of native arteries of extremities with rest pain, other extremity HCC A

I70.229 Atherosclerosis of native arteries of extremities with rest pain, unspecified extremity HCC A

√6th **I70.23 Atherosclerosis of native arteries of right leg with ulceration**

INCLUDES any condition classifiable to I70.211 and I70.221
▶chronic limb-threatening ischemia of native arteries of right leg with ulceration◀
▶critical limb ischemia of native arteries of right leg with ulceration◀

Use additional code to identify severity of ulcer (L97.-)

I70.231 Atherosclerosis of native arteries of right leg with ulceration of thigh HCC A

I70.232 Atherosclerosis of native arteries of right leg with ulceration of calf HCC A

I70.233 Atherosclerosis of native arteries of right leg with ulceration of ankle HCC A

I70.234 Atherosclerosis of native arteries of right leg with ulceration of heel and midfoot HCC A

Atherosclerosis of native arteries of right leg with ulceration of plantar surface of midfoot

I70.235 Atherosclerosis of native arteries of right leg with ulceration of other part of foot HCC A

Atherosclerosis of native arteries of right leg extremities with ulceration of toe

I70.238 Atherosclerosis of native arteries of right leg with ulceration of other part of lower leg HCC A

I70.239 Atherosclerosis of native arteries of right leg with ulceration of unspecified site HCC A

✓6th **I70.24 Atherosclerosis of native arteries of left leg with ulceration**
INCLUDES any condition classifiable to I70.212 and I70.222
▶chronic limb-threatening ischemia of native arteries of left leg with ulceration◀
▶critical limb ischemia of native arteries of left leg with ulceration◀
Use additional code to identify severity of ulcer (L97.-)

I70.241 Atherosclerosis of native arteries of left leg with ulceration of thigh HCC A

I70.242 Atherosclerosis of native arteries of left leg with ulceration of calf HCC A

I70.243 Atherosclerosis of native arteries of left leg with ulceration of ankle HCC A

I70.244 Atherosclerosis of native arteries of left leg with ulceration of heel and midfoot HCC A
Atherosclerosis of native arteries of left leg with ulceration of plantar surface of midfoot

I70.245 Atherosclerosis of native arteries of left leg with ulceration of other part of foot HCC A
Atherosclerosis of native arteries of left leg extremities with ulceration of toe

I70.248 Atherosclerosis of native arteries of left leg with ulceration of other part of lower leg HCC A

I70.249 Atherosclerosis of native arteries of left leg with ulceration of unspecified site HCC A

I70.25 Atherosclerosis of native arteries of other extremities with ulceration HCC A
INCLUDES any condition classifiable to I70.218 and I70.228
Use additional code to identify the severity of the ulcer (L98.49-)

✓6th **I70.26 Atherosclerosis of native arteries of extremities with gangrene**
INCLUDES any condition classifiable to I70.21-, I70.22-, I70.23-, I70.24-, and I70.25-
▶chronic limb-threatening ischemia of native arteries of extremities with gangrene◀
▶critical limb ischemia of native arteries of extremities with gangrene◀
Use additional code to identify the severity of any ulcer (L97.-, L98.49-), if applicable

I70.261 Atherosclerosis of native arteries of extremities with gangrene, right leg CC HCC A

I70.262 Atherosclerosis of native arteries of extremities with gangrene, left leg CC HCC A

I70.263 Atherosclerosis of native arteries of extremities with gangrene, bilateral legs CC HCC A

I70.268 Atherosclerosis of native arteries of extremities with gangrene, other extremity CC HCC A

I70.269 Atherosclerosis of native arteries of extremities with gangrene, unspecified extremity CC HCC A

✓6th **I70.29 Other atherosclerosis of native arteries of extremities**

I70.291 Other atherosclerosis of native arteries of extremities, right leg HCC A

I70.292 Other atherosclerosis of native arteries of extremities, left leg HCC A

I70.293 Other atherosclerosis of native arteries of extremities, bilateral legs HCC A

I70.298 Other atherosclerosis of native arteries of extremities, other extremity HCC A

I70.299 Other atherosclerosis of native arteries of extremities, unspecified extremity HCC A

✓5th **I70.3 Atherosclerosis of unspecified type of bypass graft(s) of the extremities**
Use additional code, if applicable, to identify chronic total occlusion of artery of extremity (I70.92)
EXCLUDES 1 *embolism or thrombus of bypass graft(s) of extremities (T82.8-)*

✓6th **I70.30 Unspecified atherosclerosis of unspecified type of bypass graft(s) of the extremities**

I70.301 Unspecified atherosclerosis of unspecified type of bypass graft(s) of the extremities, right leg HCC A

I70.302 Unspecified atherosclerosis of unspecified type of bypass graft(s) of the extremities, left leg HCC A

I70.303 Unspecified atherosclerosis of unspecified type of bypass graft(s) of the extremities, bilateral legs HCC A

I70.308 Unspecified atherosclerosis of unspecified type of bypass graft(s) of the extremities, other extremity HCC A

I70.309 Unspecified atherosclerosis of unspecified type of bypass graft(s) of the extremities, unspecified extremity HCC A

✓6th **I70.31 Atherosclerosis of unspecified type of bypass graft(s) of the extremities with intermittent claudication**

I70.311 Atherosclerosis of unspecified type of bypass graft(s) of the extremities with intermittent claudication, right leg HCC A

I70.312 Atherosclerosis of unspecified type of bypass graft(s) of the extremities with intermittent claudication, left leg HCC A

I70.313 Atherosclerosis of unspecified type of bypass graft(s) of the extremities with intermittent claudication, bilateral legs HCC A

I70.318 Atherosclerosis of unspecified type of bypass graft(s) of the extremities with intermittent claudication, other extremity HCC A

I70.319 Atherosclerosis of unspecified type of bypass graft(s) of the extremities with intermittent claudication, unspecified extremity HCC A

✓6th **I70.32 Atherosclerosis of unspecified type of bypass graft(s) of the extremities with rest pain**
INCLUDES any condition classifiable to I70.31-
▶chronic limb-threatening ischemia NOS of unspecified type of bypass graft(s) of the extremities◀
▶chronic limb-threatening ischemia of unspecified type of bypass graft(s) of the extremities with rest pain, right leg◀
▶critical limb ischemia NOS of unspecified type of bypass graft(s) of the extremities◀
▶critical limb ischemia of unspecified type of bypass graft(s) of the extremities with rest pain◀

I70.321 Atherosclerosis of unspecified type of bypass graft(s) of the extremities with rest pain, right leg HCC A

I70.322 Atherosclerosis of unspecified type of bypass graft(s) of the extremities with rest pain, left leg HCC A

I70.323 Atherosclerosis of unspecified type of bypass graft(s) of the extremities with rest pain, bilateral legs HCC A

I70.328 Atherosclerosis of unspecified type of bypass graft(s) of the extremities with rest pain, other extremity HCC A

I70.329 Atherosclerosis of unspecified type of bypass graft(s) of the extremities with rest pain, unspecified extremity HCC A

✓6th **I70.33 Atherosclerosis of unspecified type of bypass graft(s) of the right leg with ulceration**
INCLUDES any condition classifiable to I70.311 and I70.321
▶chronic limb-threatening ischemia of unspecified type of bypass graft(s) of the right leg with ulceration◀
▶critical limb ischemia of unspecified type of bypass graft(s) of the right leg with ulceration◀
Use additional code to identify severity of ulcer (L97.-)

I70.331 Atherosclerosis of unspecified type of bypass graft(s) of the right leg with ulceration of thigh CC HCC A

I70.332 Atherosclerosis of unspecified type of bypass graft(s) of the right leg with ulceration of calf CC HCC A

I70.333 Atherosclerosis of unspecified type of bypass graft(s) of the right leg with ulceration of ankle CC HCC A

I70.334 Atherosclerosis of unspecified type of bypass graft(s) of the right leg with ulceration of heel and midfoot CC HCC A
Atherosclerosis of unspecified type of bypass graft(s) of right leg with ulceration of plantar surface of midfoot

I70.335 Atherosclerosis of unspecified type of bypass graft(s) of the right leg with ulceration of other part of foot HCC A
Atherosclerosis of unspecified type of bypass graft(s) of the right leg with ulceration of toe

I70.338 Atherosclerosis of unspecified type of bypass graft(s) of the right leg with ulceration of other part of lower leg CC HCC A

I70.339 Atherosclerosis of unspecified type of bypass graft(s) of the right leg with ulceration of unspecified site CC HCC A

✓6th **I70.34 Atherosclerosis of unspecified type of bypass graft(s) of the left leg with ulceration**
INCLUDES any condition classifiable to I70.312 and I70.322
▶chronic limb-threatening ischemia of unspecified type of bypass graft(s) of the left leg with ulceration◀
▶critical limb ischemia of unspecified type of bypass graft(s) of the left leg with ulceration◀
Use additional code to identify severity of ulcer (L97.-)

I70.341 Atherosclerosis of unspecified type of bypass graft(s) of the left leg with ulceration of thigh CC HCC A

I70.342 Atherosclerosis of unspecified type of bypass graft(s) of the left leg with ulceration of calf CC HCC A

I70.343 Atherosclerosis of unspecified type of bypass graft(s) of the left leg with ulceration of ankle CC HCC A

I70.344 Atherosclerosis of unspecified type of bypass graft(s) of the left leg with ulceration of heel and midfoot CC HCC A
Atherosclerosis of unspecified type of bypass graft(s) of left leg with ulceration of plantar surface of midfoot

I70.345 Atherosclerosis of unspecified type of bypass graft(s) of the left leg with ulceration of other part of foot HCC A
Atherosclerosis of unspecified type of bypass graft(s) of the left leg with ulceration of toe

I70.348 Atherosclerosis of unspecified type of bypass graft(s) of the left leg with ulceration of other part of lower leg CC HCC A

I70.349 Atherosclerosis of unspecified type of bypass graft(s) of the left leg with ulceration of unspecified site CC HCC A

I70.35 Atherosclerosis of unspecified type of bypass graft(s) of other extremity with ulceration HCC A
INCLUDES any condition classifiable to I70.318 and I70.328
Use additional code to identify severity of ulcer (L98.49-)

✓6th **I70.36 Atherosclerosis of unspecified type of bypass graft(s) of the extremities with gangrene**
INCLUDES any condition classifiable to I70.31-, I70.32-, I70.33-, I70.34-, I70.35
▶chronic limb-threatening ischemia of unspecified type of bypass graft(s) of the extremities with gangrene◀
▶critical limb ischemia of unspecified type of bypass graft(s) of the extremities with gangrene◀
Use additional code to identify the severity of any ulcer (L97.-, L98.49-), if applicable

I70.361 Atherosclerosis of unspecified type of bypass graft(s) of the extremities with gangrene, right leg CC HCC A

I70.362 Atherosclerosis of unspecified type of bypass graft(s) of the extremities with gangrene, left leg CC HCC A

I70.363 Atherosclerosis of unspecified type of bypass graft(s) of the extremities with gangrene, bilateral legs CC HCC A

I70.368 Atherosclerosis of unspecified type of bypass graft(s) of the extremities with gangrene, other extremity CC HCC A

I70.369 Atherosclerosis of unspecified type of bypass graft(s) of the extremities with gangrene, unspecified extremity CC HCC A

✓6th **I70.39 Other atherosclerosis of unspecified type of bypass graft(s) of the extremities**

I70.391 Other atherosclerosis of unspecified type of bypass graft(s) of the extremities, right leg HCC A

I70.392 Other atherosclerosis of unspecified type of bypass graft(s) of the extremities, left leg HCC A

I70.393 Other atherosclerosis of unspecified type of bypass graft(s) of the extremities, bilateral legs HCC A

I70.398 Other atherosclerosis of unspecified type of bypass graft(s) of the extremities, other extremity HCC A

I70.399 Other atherosclerosis of unspecified type of bypass graft(s) of the extremities, unspecified extremity HCC A

✓5th **I70.4 Atherosclerosis of autologous vein bypass graft(s) of the extremities**
Use additional code, if applicable, to identify chronic total occlusion of artery of extremity (I70.92)

✓6th **I70.40 Unspecified atherosclerosis of autologous vein bypass graft(s) of the extremities**

I70.401 Unspecified atherosclerosis of autologous vein bypass graft(s) of the extremities, right leg HCC A

I70.402 Unspecified atherosclerosis of autologous vein bypass graft(s) of the extremities, left leg HCC A

I70.403 Unspecified atherosclerosis of autologous vein bypass graft(s) of the extremities, bilateral legs HCC A

I70.408 Unspecified atherosclerosis of autologous vein bypass graft(s) of the extremities, other extremity HCC A

I70.409 Unspecified atherosclerosis of autologous vein bypass graft(s) of the extremities, unspecified extremity HCC A

✓6th **I70.41 Atherosclerosis of autologous vein bypass graft(s) of the extremities with intermittent claudication**

I70.411 Atherosclerosis of autologous vein bypass graft(s) of the extremities with intermittent claudication, right leg HCC A

I70.412 Atherosclerosis of autologous vein bypass graft(s) of the extremities with intermittent claudication, left leg HCC A

I70.413 Atherosclerosis of autologous vein bypass graft(s) of the extremities with intermittent claudication, bilateral legs HCC A

I70.418 Atherosclerosis of autologous vein bypass graft(s) of the extremities with intermittent claudication, other extremity HCC A

I70.419 Atherosclerosis of autologous vein bypass graft(s) of the extremities with intermittent claudication, unspecified extremity HCC A

✓6th **I70.42 Atherosclerosis of autologous vein bypass graft(s) of the extremities with rest pain**

INCLUDES any condition classifiable to I70.41-
▶chronic limb-threatening ischemia NOS of autologous vein bypass graft(s) of the extremities◀
▶chronic limb-threatening ischemia of autologous vein bypass graft(s) of the extremities with rest pain◀
▶critical limb ischemia NOS of autologous vein bypass graft(s) of the extremities◀
▶critical limb ischemia of autologous vein bypass graft(s) of the extremities with rest pain◀

I70.421 Atherosclerosis of autologous vein bypass graft(s) of the extremities with rest pain, right leg HCC A

I70.422 Atherosclerosis of autologous vein bypass graft(s) of the extremities with rest pain, left leg HCC A

I70.423 Atherosclerosis of autologous vein bypass graft(s) of the extremities with rest pain, bilateral legs HCC A

I70.428 Atherosclerosis of autologous vein bypass graft(s) of the extremities with rest pain, other extremity HCC A

I70.429 Atherosclerosis of autologous vein bypass graft(s) of the extremities with rest pain, unspecified extremity HCC A

✓6th **I70.43 Atherosclerosis of autologous vein bypass graft(s) of the right leg with ulceration**

INCLUDES any condition classifiable to I70.411 and I70.421
▶chronic limb-threatening ischemia of autologous vein bypass graft(s) of the right leg with ulceration◀
▶critical limb ischemia of autologous vein bypass graft(s) of the right leg with ulceration◀

Use additional code to identify severity of ulcer (L97.-)

I70.431 Atherosclerosis of autologous vein bypass graft(s) of the right leg with ulceration of thigh CC HCC A

I70.432 Atherosclerosis of autologous vein bypass graft(s) of the right leg with ulceration of calf CC HCC A

I70.433 Atherosclerosis of autologous vein bypass graft(s) of the right leg with ulceration of ankle CC HCC A

I70.434 Atherosclerosis of autologous vein bypass graft(s) of the right leg with ulceration of heel and midfoot CC HCC A

Atherosclerosis of autologous vein bypass graft(s) of right leg with ulceration of plantar surface of midfoot

I70.435 Atherosclerosis of autologous vein bypass graft(s) of the right leg with ulceration of other part of foot HCC A

Atherosclerosis of autologous vein bypass graft(s) of right leg with ulceration of toe

I70.438 Atherosclerosis of autologous vein bypass graft(s) of the right leg with ulceration of other part of lower leg CC HCC A

I70.439 Atherosclerosis of autologous vein bypass graft(s) of the right leg with ulceration of unspecified site CC HCC A

✓6th **I70.44 Atherosclerosis of autologous vein bypass graft(s) of the left leg with ulceration**

INCLUDES any condition classifiable to I70.412 and I70.422
▶chronic limb-threatening ischemia of autologous vein bypass graft(s) of the left leg with ulceration◀
▶critical limb ischemia of autologous vein bypass graft(s) of the left leg with ulceration◀

Use additional code to identify severity of ulcer (L97.-)

I70.441 Atherosclerosis of autologous vein bypass graft(s) of the left leg with ulceration of thigh CC HCC A

I70.442 Atherosclerosis of autologous vein bypass graft(s) of the left leg with ulceration of calf CC HCC A

I70.443 Atherosclerosis of autologous vein bypass graft(s) of the left leg with ulceration of ankle CC HCC A

I70.444 Atherosclerosis of autologous vein bypass graft(s) of the left leg with ulceration of heel and midfoot CC HCC A

Atherosclerosis of autologous vein bypass graft(s) of left leg with ulceration of plantar surface of midfoot

I70.445 Atherosclerosis of autologous vein bypass graft(s) of the left leg with ulceration of other part of foot HCC A

Atherosclerosis of autologous vein bypass graft(s) of left leg with ulceration of toe

I70.448 Atherosclerosis of autologous vein bypass graft(s) of the left leg with ulceration of other part of lower leg CC HCC A

I70.449 Atherosclerosis of autologous vein bypass graft(s) of the left leg with ulceration of unspecified site CC HCC A

I70.45 Atherosclerosis of autologous vein bypass graft(s) of other extremity with ulceration HCC A

INCLUDES any condition classifiable to I70.418, I70.428, and I70.438

Use additional code to identify severity of ulcer (L98.49)

✓6th **I70.46 Atherosclerosis of autologous vein bypass graft(s) of the extremities with gangrene**

INCLUDES any condition classifiable to I70.41-, I70.42-, and I70.43-, I70.44-, I70.45
▶chronic limb-threatening ischemia of autologous vein bypass graft(s) of the extremities with gangrene◀
▶critical limb ischemia of autologous vein bypass graft(s) of the extremities with gangrene◀

Use additional code to identify the severity of any ulcer (L97.-, L98.49-), if applicable

I70.461 Atherosclerosis of autologous vein bypass graft(s) of the extremities with gangrene, right leg CC HCC A

I70.462 Atherosclerosis of autologous vein bypass graft(s) of the extremities with gangrene, left leg CC HCC A

I70.463 Atherosclerosis of autologous vein bypass graft(s) of the extremities with gangrene, bilateral legs CC HCC A

I70.468 Atherosclerosis of autologous vein bypass graft(s) of the extremities with gangrene, other extremity CC HCC A

I70.469 Atherosclerosis of autologous vein bypass graft(s) of the extremities with gangrene, unspecified extremity CC HCC A

✓6th **I70.49 Other atherosclerosis of autologous vein bypass graft(s) of the extremities**

I70.491 Other atherosclerosis of autologous vein bypass graft(s) of the extremities, right leg HCC A

I70.492 Other atherosclerosis of autologous vein bypass graft(s) of the extremities, left leg HCC A

I7Ø.493 Other atherosclerosis of autologous vein bypass graft(s) of the extremities, bilateral legs HCC A

I7Ø.498 Other atherosclerosis of autologous vein bypass graft(s) of the extremities, other extremity HCC A

I7Ø.499 Other atherosclerosis of autologous vein bypass graft(s) of the extremities, unspecified extremity HCC A

√5th **I7Ø.5 Atherosclerosis of nonautologous biological bypass graft(s) of the extremities**

Use additional code, if applicable, to identify chronic total occlusion of artery of extremity (I7Ø.92)

√6th **I7Ø.5Ø Unspecified atherosclerosis of nonautologous biological bypass graft(s) of the extremities**

I7Ø.5Ø1 Unspecified atherosclerosis of nonautologous biological bypass graft(s) of the extremities, right leg HCC A

I7Ø.5Ø2 Unspecified atherosclerosis of nonautologous biological bypass graft(s) of the extremities, left leg HCC A

I7Ø.5Ø3 Unspecified atherosclerosis of nonautologous biological bypass graft(s) of the extremities, bilateral legs HCC A

I7Ø.5Ø8 Unspecified atherosclerosis of nonautologous biological bypass graft(s) of the extremities, other extremity HCC A

I7Ø.5Ø9 Unspecified atherosclerosis of nonautologous biological bypass graft(s) of the extremities, unspecified extremity HCC A

√6th **I7Ø.51 Atherosclerosis of nonautologous biological bypass graft(s) of the extremities intermittent claudication**

I7Ø.511 Atherosclerosis of nonautologous biological bypass graft(s) of the extremities with intermittent claudication, right leg HCC A

I7Ø.512 Atherosclerosis of nonautologous biological bypass graft(s) of the extremities with intermittent claudication, left leg HCC A

I7Ø.513 Atherosclerosis of nonautologous biological bypass graft(s) of the extremities with intermittent claudication, bilateral legs HCC A

I7Ø.518 Atherosclerosis of nonautologous biological bypass graft(s) of the extremities with intermittent claudication, other extremity HCC A

I7Ø.519 Atherosclerosis of nonautologous biological bypass graft(s) of the extremities with intermittent claudication, unspecified extremity HCC A

√6th **I7Ø.52 Atherosclerosis of nonautologous biological bypass graft(s) of the extremities with rest pain**

INCLUDES any condition classifiable to I7Ø.51-
▶chronic limb-threatening ischemia NOS of nonautologous biological bypass graft(s) of the extremities◀
▶chronic limb-threatening ischemia of nonautologous biological bypass graft(s) of the extremities with rest pain◀
▶critical limb ischemia NOS of nonautologous biological bypass graft(s) of the extremities◀
▶critical limb ischemia of nonautologous biological bypass graft(s) of the extremities with rest pain◀

I7Ø.521 Atherosclerosis of nonautologous biological bypass graft(s) of the extremities with rest pain, right leg HCC A

I7Ø.522 Atherosclerosis of nonautologous biological bypass graft(s) of the extremities with rest pain, left leg HCC A

I7Ø.523 Atherosclerosis of nonautologous biological bypass graft(s) of the extremities with rest pain, bilateral legs HCC A

I7Ø.528 Atherosclerosis of nonautologous biological bypass graft(s) of the extremities with rest pain, other extremity HCC A

I7Ø.529 Atherosclerosis of nonautologous biological bypass graft(s) of the extremities with rest pain, unspecified extremity HCC A

√6th **I7Ø.53 Atherosclerosis of nonautologous biological bypass graft(s) of the right leg with ulceration**

INCLUDES any condition classifiable to I7Ø.511 and I7Ø.521
▶chronic limb-threatening ischemia of nonautologous biological bypass graft(s) of the right leg with ulceration◀
▶critical limb ischemia of nonautologous biological bypass graft(s) of the right leg with ulceration◀

Use additional code to identify severity of ulcer (L97.-)

I7Ø.531 Atherosclerosis of nonautologous biological bypass graft(s) of the right leg with ulceration of thigh CC HCC A

I7Ø.532 Atherosclerosis of nonautologous biological bypass graft(s) of the right leg with ulceration of calf CC HCC A

I7Ø.533 Atherosclerosis of nonautologous biological bypass graft(s) of the right leg with ulceration of ankle CC HCC A

I7Ø.534 Atherosclerosis of nonautologous biological bypass graft(s) of the right leg with ulceration of heel and midfoot CC HCC A

Atherosclerosis of nonautologous biological bypass graft(s) of right leg with ulceration of plantar surface of midfoot

I7Ø.535 Atherosclerosis of nonautologous biological bypass graft(s) of the right leg with ulceration of other part of foot HCC A

Atherosclerosis of nonautologous biological bypass graft(s) of the right leg with ulceration of toe

I7Ø.538 Atherosclerosis of nonautologous biological bypass graft(s) of the right leg with ulceration of other part of lower leg CC HCC A

I7Ø.539 Atherosclerosis of nonautologous biological bypass graft(s) of the right leg with ulceration of unspecified site CC HCC A

√6th **I7Ø.54 Atherosclerosis of nonautologous biological bypass graft(s) of the left leg with ulceration**

INCLUDES any condition classifiable to I7Ø.512 and I7Ø.522
▶chronic limb-threatening ischemia of nonautologous biological bypass graft(s) of the left leg with ulceration◀
▶critical limb ischemia of nonautologous biological bypass graft(s) of the left leg with ulceration◀

Use additional code to identify severity of ulcer (L97.-)

I7Ø.541 Atherosclerosis of nonautologous biological bypass graft(s) of the left leg with ulceration of thigh CC HCC A

I7Ø.542 Atherosclerosis of nonautologous biological bypass graft(s) of the left leg with ulceration of calf CC HCC A

I7Ø.543 Atherosclerosis of nonautologous biological bypass graft(s) of the left leg with ulceration of ankle CC HCC A

I7Ø.544 Atherosclerosis of nonautologous biological bypass graft(s) of the left leg with ulceration of heel and midfoot CC HCC A

Atherosclerosis of nonautologous biological bypass graft(s) of left leg with ulceration of plantar surface of midfoot

I70.545 **Atherosclerosis of nonautologous biological bypass graft(s) of the left leg with ulceration of other part of foot** HCC A

Atherosclerosis of nonautologous biological bypass graft(s) of the left leg with ulceration of toe

I70.548 **Atherosclerosis of nonautologous biological bypass graft(s) of the left leg with ulceration of other part of lower leg** CC HCC A

I70.549 **Atherosclerosis of nonautologous biological bypass graft(s) of the left leg with ulceration of unspecified site** CC HCC A

I70.55 **Atherosclerosis of nonautologous biological bypass graft(s) of other extremity with ulceration** HCC A

INCLUDES any condition classifiable to I70.518, I70.528, and I70.538

Use additional code to identify severity of ulcer (L98.49)

✓6th I70.56 **Atherosclerosis of nonautologous biological bypass graft(s) of the extremities with gangrene**

INCLUDES any condition classifiable to I70.51-, I70.52-, and I70.53-, I70.54-, I70.55

▶chronic limb-threatening ischemia of nonautologous biological bypass graft(s) of the extremities with gangrene◀

▶critical limb ischemia of nonautologous biological bypass graft(s) of the extremities with gangrene◀

Use additional code to identify the severity of any ulcer (L97.-, L98.49-), if applicable

I70.561 **Atherosclerosis of nonautologous biological bypass graft(s) of the extremities with gangrene, right leg** CC HCC A

I70.562 **Atherosclerosis of nonautologous biological bypass graft(s) of the extremities with gangrene, left leg** CC HCC A

I70.563 **Atherosclerosis of nonautologous biological bypass graft(s) of the extremities with gangrene, bilateral legs** CC HCC A

I70.568 **Atherosclerosis of nonautologous biological bypass graft(s) of the extremities with gangrene, other extremity** CC HCC A

I70.569 **Atherosclerosis of nonautologous biological bypass graft(s) of the extremities with gangrene, unspecified extremity** CC HCC A

✓6th I70.59 **Other atherosclerosis of nonautologous biological bypass graft(s) of the extremities**

I70.591 **Other atherosclerosis of nonautologous biological bypass graft(s) of the extremities, right leg** HCC A

I70.592 **Other atherosclerosis of nonautologous biological bypass graft(s) of the extremities, left leg** HCC A

I70.593 **Other atherosclerosis of nonautologous biological bypass graft(s) of the extremities, bilateral legs** HCC A

I70.598 **Other atherosclerosis of nonautologous biological bypass graft(s) of the extremities, other extremity** HCC A

I70.599 **Other atherosclerosis of nonautologous biological bypass graft(s) of the extremities, unspecified extremity** HCC A

✓5th I70.6 **Atherosclerosis of nonbiological bypass graft(s) of the extremities**

Use additional code, if applicable, to identify chronic total occlusion of artery of extremity (I70.92)

✓6th I70.60 **Unspecified atherosclerosis of nonbiological bypass graft(s) of the extremities**

I70.601 **Unspecified atherosclerosis of nonbiological bypass graft(s) of the extremities, right leg** HCC A

I70.602 **Unspecified atherosclerosis of nonbiological bypass graft(s) of the extremities, left leg** HCC A

I70.603 **Unspecified atherosclerosis of nonbiological bypass graft(s) of the extremities, bilateral legs** HCC A

I70.608 **Unspecified atherosclerosis of nonbiological bypass graft(s) of the extremities, other extremity** HCC A

I70.609 **Unspecified atherosclerosis of nonbiological bypass graft(s) of the extremities, unspecified extremity** HCC A

✓6th I70.61 **Atherosclerosis of nonbiological bypass graft(s) of the extremities with intermittent claudication**

I70.611 **Atherosclerosis of nonbiological bypass graft(s) of the extremities with intermittent claudication, right leg** HCC A

I70.612 **Atherosclerosis of nonbiological bypass graft(s) of the extremities with intermittent claudication, left leg** HCC A

I70.613 **Atherosclerosis of nonbiological bypass graft(s) of the extremities with intermittent claudication, bilateral legs** HCC A

I70.618 **Atherosclerosis of nonbiological bypass graft(s) of the extremities with intermittent claudication, other extremity** HCC A

I70.619 **Atherosclerosis of nonbiological bypass graft(s) of the extremities with intermittent claudication, unspecified extremity** HCC A

✓6th I70.62 **Atherosclerosis of nonbiological bypass graft(s) of the extremities with rest pain**

INCLUDES any condition classifiable to I70.61-

▶chronic limb-threatening ischemia NOS of nonbiological bypass graft(s) of the extremities◀

▶chronic limb-threatening ischemia of nonbiological bypass graft(s) of the extremities with rest pain◀

▶critical limb ischemia NOS of nonbiological bypass graft(s) of the extremities◀

▶critical limb ischemia of nonbiological bypass graft(s) of the extremities with rest pain◀

I70.621 **Atherosclerosis of nonbiological bypass graft(s) of the extremities with rest pain, right leg** HCC A

I70.622 **Atherosclerosis of nonbiological bypass graft(s) of the extremities with rest pain, left leg** HCC A

I70.623 **Atherosclerosis of nonbiological bypass graft(s) of the extremities with rest pain, bilateral legs** HCC A

I70.628 **Atherosclerosis of nonbiological bypass graft(s) of the extremities with rest pain, other extremity** HCC A

I70.629 **Atherosclerosis of nonbiological bypass graft(s) of the extremities with rest pain, unspecified extremity** HCC A

✓6th I70.63 **Atherosclerosis of nonbiological bypass graft(s) of the right leg with ulceration**

INCLUDES any condition classifiable to I70.611 and I70.621

▶chronic limb-threatening ischemia of nonbiological bypass graft(s) of the right leg with ulceration◀

▶critical limb ischemia of nonbiological bypass graft(s) of the right leg with ulceration◀

Use additional code to identify severity of ulcer (L97.-)

I70.631 **Atherosclerosis of nonbiological bypass graft(s) of the right leg with ulceration of thigh** CC HCC A

I70.632 **Atherosclerosis of nonbiological bypass graft(s) of the right leg with ulceration of calf** CC HCC A

Chapter 9. Diseases of the Circulatory System

I70.545–I70.632

I70.633 Atherosclerosis of nonbiological bypass graft(s) of the right leg with ulceration of ankle CC HCC A

I70.634 Atherosclerosis of nonbiological bypass graft(s) of the right leg with ulceration of heel and midfoot CC HCC A

Atherosclerosis of nonbiological bypass graft(s) of right leg with ulceration of plantar surface of midfoot

I70.635 Atherosclerosis of nonbiological bypass graft(s) of the right leg with ulceration of other part of foot HCC A

Atherosclerosis of nonbiological bypass graft(s) of the right leg with ulceration of toe

I70.638 Atherosclerosis of nonbiological bypass graft(s) of the right leg with ulceration of other part of lower leg CC HCC A

I70.639 Atherosclerosis of nonbiological bypass graft(s) of the right leg with ulceration of unspecified site CC HCC A

✓6th **I70.64 Atherosclerosis of nonbiological bypass graft(s) of the left leg with ulceration**

INCLUDES any condition classifiable to I70.612 and I70.622

▶chronic limb-threatening ischemia of nonbiological bypass graft(s) of the left leg with ulceration◀

▶critical limb ischemia of nonbiological bypass graft(s) of the left leg with ulceration◀

Use additional code to identify severity of ulcer (L97.-)

I70.641 Atherosclerosis of nonbiological bypass graft(s) of the left leg with ulceration of thigh CC HCC A

I70.642 Atherosclerosis of nonbiological bypass graft(s) of the left leg with ulceration of calf CC HCC A

I70.643 Atherosclerosis of nonbiological bypass graft(s) of the left leg with ulceration of ankle CC HCC A

I70.644 Atherosclerosis of nonbiological bypass graft(s) of the left leg with ulceration of heel and midfoot CC HCC A

Atherosclerosis of nonbiological bypass graft(s) of left leg with ulceration of plantar surface of midfoot

I70.645 Atherosclerosis of nonbiological bypass graft(s) of the left leg with ulceration of other part of foot HCC A

Atherosclerosis of nonbiological bypass graft(s) of the left leg with ulceration of toe

I70.648 Atherosclerosis of nonbiological bypass graft(s) of the left leg with ulceration of other part of lower leg CC HCC A

I70.649 Atherosclerosis of nonbiological bypass graft(s) of the left leg with ulceration of unspecified site CC HCC A

I70.65 Atherosclerosis of nonbiological bypass graft(s) of other extremity with ulceration HCC A

INCLUDES any condition classifiable to I70.618 and I70.628

Use additional code to identify severity of ulcer (L98.49)

✓6th **I70.66 Atherosclerosis of nonbiological bypass graft(s) of the extremities with gangrene**

INCLUDES any condition classifiable to I70.61-, I70.62-, I70.63-, I70.64-, I70.65

▶chronic limb-threatening ischemia of nonbiological bypass graft(s) of the extremities with gangrene◀

▶critical limb ischemia of nonbiological bypass graft(s) of the extremities with gangrene◀

Use additional code to identify the severity of any ulcer (L97.-, L98.49-), if applicable

I70.661 Atherosclerosis of nonbiological bypass graft(s) of the extremities with gangrene, right leg CC HCC A

I70.662 Atherosclerosis of nonbiological bypass graft(s) of the extremities with gangrene, left leg CC HCC A

I70.663 Atherosclerosis of nonbiological bypass graft(s) of the extremities with gangrene, bilateral legs CC HCC A

I70.668 Atherosclerosis of nonbiological bypass graft(s) of the extremities with gangrene, other extremity CC HCC A

I70.669 Atherosclerosis of nonbiological bypass graft(s) of the extremities with gangrene, unspecified extremity CC HCC A

✓6th **I70.69 Other atherosclerosis of nonbiological bypass graft(s) of the extremities**

I70.691 Other atherosclerosis of nonbiological bypass graft(s) of the extremities, right leg HCC A

I70.692 Other atherosclerosis of nonbiological bypass graft(s) of the extremities, left leg HCC A

I70.693 Other atherosclerosis of nonbiological bypass graft(s) of the extremities, bilateral legs HCC A

I70.698 Other atherosclerosis of nonbiological bypass graft(s) of the extremities, other extremity HCC A

I70.699 Other atherosclerosis of nonbiological bypass graft(s) of the extremities, unspecified extremity HCC A

✓5th **I70.7 Atherosclerosis of other type of bypass graft(s) of the extremities**

Use additional code, if applicable, to identify chronic total occlusion of artery of extremity (I70.92)

✓6th **I70.70 Unspecified atherosclerosis of other type of bypass graft(s) of the extremities**

I70.701 Unspecified atherosclerosis of other type of bypass graft(s) of the extremities, right leg HCC A

I70.702 Unspecified atherosclerosis of other type of bypass graft(s) of the extremities, left leg HCC A

I70.703 Unspecified atherosclerosis of other type of bypass graft(s) of the extremities, bilateral legs HCC A

I70.708 Unspecified atherosclerosis of other type of bypass graft(s) of the extremities, other extremity HCC A

I70.709 Unspecified atherosclerosis of other type of bypass graft(s) of the extremities, unspecified extremity HCC A

✓6th **I70.71 Atherosclerosis of other type of bypass graft(s) of the extremities with intermittent claudication**

I70.711 Atherosclerosis of other type of bypass graft(s) of the extremities with intermittent claudication, right leg HCC A

I70.712 Atherosclerosis of other type of bypass graft(s) of the extremities with intermittent claudication, left leg HCC A

I70.713 Atherosclerosis of other type of bypass graft(s) of the extremities with intermittent claudication, bilateral legs HCC A

I70.718 Atherosclerosis of other type of bypass graft(s) of the extremities with intermittent claudication, other extremity HCC A

I70.719 Atherosclerosis of other type of bypass graft(s) of the extremities with intermittent claudication, unspecified extremity HCC A

I70.72 **Atherosclerosis of other type of bypass graft(s) of the extremities with rest pain**
INCLUDES any condition classifiable to I70.71-
▶chronic limb-threatening ischemia NOS of other type of bypass graft(s) of the extremities◀
▶chronic limb-threatening ischemia of other type of bypass graft(s) of the extremities with rest pain◀
▶critical limb ischemia NOS of other type of bypass graft(s) of the extremities◀
▶critical limb ischemia of other type of bypass graft(s) of the extremities with rest pain◀

I70.721 **Atherosclerosis of other type of bypass graft(s) of the extremities with rest pain, right leg** HCC A
I70.722 **Atherosclerosis of other type of bypass graft(s) of the extremities with rest pain, left leg** HCC A
I70.723 **Atherosclerosis of other type of bypass graft(s) of the extremities with rest pain, bilateral legs** HCC A
I70.728 **Atherosclerosis of other type of bypass graft(s) of the extremities with rest pain, other extremity** HCC A
I70.729 **Atherosclerosis of other type of bypass graft(s) of the extremities with rest pain, unspecified extremity** HCC A

I70.73 **Atherosclerosis of other type of bypass graft(s) of the right leg with ulceration**
INCLUDES any condition classifiable to I70.711 and I70.721
▶chronic limb-threatening ischemia of other type of bypass graft(s) of the right leg with ulceration◀
▶critical limb ischemia of other type of bypass graft(s) of the right leg with ulceration◀
Use additional code to identify severity of ulcer (L97.-)

I70.731 **Atherosclerosis of other type of bypass graft(s) of the right leg with ulceration of thigh** CC HCC A
I70.732 **Atherosclerosis of other type of bypass graft(s) of the right leg with ulceration of calf** CC HCC A
I70.733 **Atherosclerosis of other type of bypass graft(s) of the right leg with ulceration of ankle** CC HCC A
I70.734 **Atherosclerosis of other type of bypass graft(s) of the right leg with ulceration of heel and midfoot** CC HCC A
Atherosclerosis of other type of bypass graft(s) of right leg with ulceration of plantar surface of midfoot
I70.735 **Atherosclerosis of other type of bypass graft(s) of the right leg with ulceration of other part of foot** HCC A
Atherosclerosis of other type of bypass graft(s) of right leg with ulceration of toe
I70.738 **Atherosclerosis of other type of bypass graft(s) of the right leg with ulceration of other part of lower leg** CC HCC A
I70.739 **Atherosclerosis of other type of bypass graft(s) of the right leg with ulceration of unspecified site** CC HCC A

I70.74 **Atherosclerosis of other type of bypass graft(s) of the left leg with ulceration**
INCLUDES any condition classifiable to I70.712 and I70.722
▶chronic limb-threatening ischemia of other type of bypass graft(s) of the left leg with ulceration◀
▶critical limb ischemia of other type of bypass graft(s) of the left leg with ulceration◀
Use additional code to identify severity of ulcer (L97.-)

I70.741 **Atherosclerosis of other type of bypass graft(s) of the left leg with ulceration of thigh** CC HCC A
I70.742 **Atherosclerosis of other type of bypass graft(s) of the left leg with ulceration of calf** CC HCC A
I70.743 **Atherosclerosis of other type of bypass graft(s) of the left leg with ulceration of ankle** CC HCC A
I70.744 **Atherosclerosis of other type of bypass graft(s) of the left leg with ulceration of heel and midfoot** CC HCC A
Atherosclerosis of other type of bypass graft(s) of left leg with ulceration of plantar surface of midfoot
I70.745 **Atherosclerosis of other type of bypass graft(s) of the left leg with ulceration of other part of foot** HCC A
Atherosclerosis of other type of bypass graft(s) of left leg with ulceration of toe
I70.748 **Atherosclerosis of other type of bypass graft(s) of the left leg with ulceration of other part of lower leg** CC HCC A
I70.749 **Atherosclerosis of other type of bypass graft(s) of the left leg with ulceration of unspecified site** CC HCC A

I70.75 **Atherosclerosis of other type of bypass graft(s) of other extremity with ulceration** HCC A
INCLUDES any condition classifiable to I70.718 and I70.728
Use additional code to identify severity of ulcer (L98.49)

I70.76 **Atherosclerosis of other type of bypass graft(s) of the extremities with gangrene**
INCLUDES any condition classifiable to I70.71-, I70.72-, I70.73-, I70.74-, I70.75
▶chronic limb-threatening ischemia of other type of bypass graft(s) of the extremities with gangrene◀
▶critical limb ischemia of other type of bypass graft(s) of the extremities with gangrene◀
Use additional code to identify the severity of any ulcer (L97.-, L98.49-), if applicable

I70.761 **Atherosclerosis of other type of bypass graft(s) of the extremities with gangrene, right leg** CC HCC A
I70.762 **Atherosclerosis of other type of bypass graft(s) of the extremities with gangrene, left leg** CC HCC A
I70.763 **Atherosclerosis of other type of bypass graft(s) of the extremities with gangrene, bilateral legs** CC HCC A
I70.768 **Atherosclerosis of other type of bypass graft(s) of the extremities with gangrene, other extremity** CC HCC A
I70.769 **Atherosclerosis of other type of bypass graft(s) of the extremities with gangrene, unspecified extremity** CC HCC A

I70.79 **Other atherosclerosis of other type of bypass graft(s) of the extremities**
I70.791 **Other atherosclerosis of other type of bypass graft(s) of the extremities, right leg** HCC A
I70.792 **Other atherosclerosis of other type of bypass graft(s) of the extremities, left leg** HCC A
I70.793 **Other atherosclerosis of other type of bypass graft(s) of the extremities, bilateral legs** HCC A
I70.798 **Other atherosclerosis of other type of bypass graft(s) of the extremities, other extremity** HCC A
I70.799 **Other atherosclerosis of other type of bypass graft(s) of the extremities, unspecified extremity** HCC A

I70.8 **Atherosclerosis of other arteries** A
TIP: Arteriosclerosis of the iliac arteries is coded here.

I70.9 **Other and unspecified atherosclerosis**
I70.90 **Unspecified atherosclerosis** A
I70.91 **Generalized atherosclerosis** A

I7Ø.92 Chronic total occlusion of artery of the extremities CC HCC A
Complete occlusion of artery of the extremities
Total occlusion of artery of the extremities
Code first atherosclerosis of arteries of the extremities (I7Ø.2-, I7Ø.3-, I7Ø.4-, I7Ø.5-, I7Ø.6-, I7Ø.7-)

✓4th I71 Aortic aneurysm and dissection

EXCLUDES 1 *aortic ectasia (I77.81-)*
syphilitic aortic aneurysm (A52.Ø1)
traumatic aortic aneurysm (S25.Ø9, S35.Ø9)

✓5th I71.Ø Dissection of aorta

I71.ØØ Dissection of unspecified site of aorta MCC HCC
I71.Ø1 Dissection of thoracic aorta MCC HCC
I71.Ø2 Dissection of abdominal aorta MCC HCC
I71.Ø3 Dissection of thoracoabdominal aorta MCC HCC

I71.1 Thoracic aortic aneurysm, ruptured MCC HCC
I71.2 Thoracic aortic aneurysm, without rupture HCC
I71.3 Abdominal aortic aneurysm, ruptured MCC HCC
I71.4 Abdominal aortic aneurysm, without rupture HCC
I71.5 Thoracoabdominal aortic aneurysm, ruptured MCC HCC
I71.6 Thoracoabdominal aortic aneurysm, without rupture HCC
I71.8 Aortic aneurysm of unspecified site, ruptured MCC HCC
Rupture of aorta NOS
I71.9 Aortic aneurysm of unspecified site, without rupture HCC
Aneurysm of aorta
Dilatation of aorta
Hyaline necrosis of aorta

✓4th I72 Other aneurysm

INCLUDES aneurysm (cirsoid) (false) (ruptured)
EXCLUDES 2 *acquired aneurysm (I77.Ø)*
aneurysm (of) aorta (I71.-)
aneurysm (of) arteriovenous NOS (Q27.3-)
carotid artery dissection (I77.71)
cerebral (nonruptured) aneurysm (I67.1)
coronary aneurysm (I25.4)
coronary artery dissection (I25.42)
dissection of artery NEC (I77.79)
dissection of precerebral artery, congenital (nonruptured) (Q28.1)
heart aneurysm (I25.3)
iliac artery dissection (I77.72)
precerebral artery, congential (nonruptured) (Q28.1)
pulmonary artery aneurysm (I28.1)
renal artery dissection (I77.73)
retinal aneurysm (H35.Ø)
ruptured cerebral aneurysm (I6Ø.7)
varicose aneurysm (I77.Ø)
vertebral artery dissection (I77.74)

AHA: 2016,4Q,28-29

I72.Ø Aneurysm of carotid artery HCC
Aneurysm of common carotid artery
Aneurysm of external carotid artery
Aneurysm of internal carotid artery, extracranial portion
EXCLUDES 1 *aneurysm of internal carotid artery, intracranial portion (I67.1)*
aneurysm of internal carotid artery NOS (I67.1)

I72.1 Aneurysm of artery of upper extremity HCC
I72.2 Aneurysm of renal artery HCC
I72.3 Aneurysm of iliac artery HCC
I72.4 Aneurysm of artery of lower extremity HCC
AHA: 2019,2Q,21
I72.5 Aneurysm of other precerebral arteries HCC
Aneurysm of basilar artery (trunk)
EXCLUDES 2 *aneurysm of carotid artery (I72.Ø)*
aneurysm of vertebral artery (I72.6)
dissection of carotid artery (I77.71)
dissection of other precerebral arteries (I77.75)
dissection of vertebral artery (I77.74)
I72.6 Aneurysm of vertebral artery HCC
EXCLUDES 2 *dissection of vertebral artery (I77.74)*
I72.8 Aneurysm of other specified arteries HCC
I72.9 Aneurysm of unspecified site HCC

Aneurysm

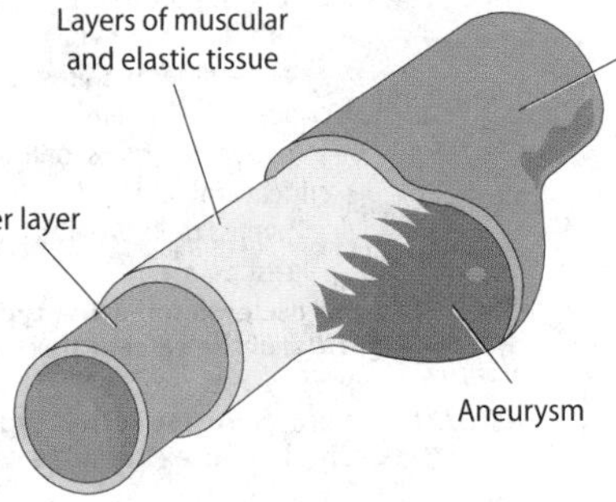

✓4th I73 Other peripheral vascular diseases

EXCLUDES 2 *chilblains (T69.1)*
frostbite (T33-T34)
immersion hand or foot (T69.Ø-)
spasm of cerebral artery (G45.9)

AHA: 2018,4Q,87

✓5th I73.Ø Raynaud's syndrome
Raynaud's disease
Raynaud's phenomenon (secondary)
DEF: Constriction of the arteries of the digits caused by cold or by nerve or arterial damage and can be prompted by stress or emotion. Blood cannot reach the skin and soft tissues and the skin turns white with blue mottling.

I73.ØØ Raynaud's syndrome without gangrene
I73.Ø1 Raynaud's syndrome with gangrene CC HCC

I73.1 Thromboangiitis obliterans [Buerger's disease] HCC
DEF: Inflammatory disease of the extremity blood vessels, mainly the lower blood vessels. This disease is associated with heavy tobacco use. The arteries are more affected than veins. It occurs primarily in young men and leads to tissue ischemia and gangrene.

✓5th I73.8 Other specified peripheral vascular diseases
EXCLUDES 1 *diabetic (peripheral) angiopathy (EØ8-E13 with .51-.52)*

I73.81 Erythromelalgia HCC
I73.89 Other specified peripheral vascular diseases HCC
Acrocyanosis
Erythrocyanosis
Simple acroparesthesia [Schultze's type]
Vasomotor acroparesthesia [Nothnagel's type]

I73.9 Peripheral vascular disease, unspecified HCC
Intermittent claudication
Peripheral angiopathy NOS
Spasm of artery
EXCLUDES 1 *atherosclerosis of the extremities (I7Ø.2-I7Ø.7-)*
AHA: 2018,2Q,7

I74 Arterial embolism and thrombosis

INCLUDES embolic infarction
embolic occlusion
thrombotic infarction
thrombotic occlusion

Code first:
embolism and thrombosis complicating abortion or ectopic or molar pregnancy (O00-O07, O08.2)
embolism and thrombosis complicating pregnancy, childbirth and the puerperium (O88.-)

EXCLUDES 2 *atheroembolism (I75.-)*
basilar embolism and thrombosis (I63.0-I63.2, I65.1)
carotid embolism and thrombosis (I63.0-I63.2, I65.2)
cerebral embolism and thrombosis (I63.3-I63.5, I66.-)
coronary embolism and thrombosis (I21-I25)
mesenteric embolism and thrombosis (K55.0-)
ophthalmic embolism and thrombosis (H34.-)
precerebral embolism and thrombosis NOS (I63.0-I63.2, I65.9)
pulmonary embolism and thrombosis (I26.-)
renal embolism and thrombosis (N28.0)
retinal embolism and thrombosis (H34.-)
septic embolism and thrombosis (I76)
vertebral embolism and thrombosis (I63.0-I63.2, I65.0)

I74.0 Embolism and thrombosis of abdominal aorta

I74.01 Saddle embolus of abdominal aorta MCC HCC

I74.09 Other arterial embolism and thrombosis of abdominal aorta CC HCC
Aortic bifurcation syndrome
Aortoiliac obstruction
Leriche's syndrome

I74.1 Embolism and thrombosis of other and unspecified parts of aorta

I74.10 Embolism and thrombosis of unspecified parts of aorta CC HCC

I74.11 Embolism and thrombosis of thoracic aorta CC HCC

I74.19 Embolism and thrombosis of other parts of aorta CC HCC

I74.2 Embolism and thrombosis of arteries of the upper extremities CC HCC

I74.3 Embolism and thrombosis of arteries of the lower extremities CC HCC

I74.4 Embolism and thrombosis of arteries of extremities, unspecified CC HCC
Peripheral arterial embolism NOS

I74.5 Embolism and thrombosis of iliac artery CC HCC

I74.8 Embolism and thrombosis of other arteries CC HCC

I74.9 Embolism and thrombosis of unspecified artery CC HCC

I75 Atheroembolism

INCLUDES atherothrombotic microembolism
cholesterol embolism

I75.0 Atheroembolism of extremities

I75.01 Atheroembolism of upper extremity

I75.011 Atheroembolism of right upper extremity CC HCC

I75.012 Atheroembolism of left upper extremity CC HCC

I75.013 Atheroembolism of bilateral upper extremities CC HCC

I75.019 Atheroembolism of unspecified upper extremity CC HCC

I75.02 Atheroembolism of lower extremity

I75.021 Atheroembolism of right lower extremity CC HCC

I75.022 Atheroembolism of left lower extremity CC HCC

I75.023 Atheroembolism of bilateral lower extremities CC HCC

I75.029 Atheroembolism of unspecified lower extremity CC HCC

I75.8 Atheroembolism of other sites

I75.81 Atheroembolism of kidney CC HCC
Use additional code for any associated acute kidney failure and chronic kidney disease (N17.-, N18.-)

I75.89 Atheroembolism of other site CC HCC

I76 Septic arterial embolism CC HCC
Code first underlying infection, such as:
infective endocarditis (I33.0)
lung abscess (J85.-)
Use additional code to identify the site of the embolism (I74.-)
EXCLUDES 2 *septic pulmonary embolism (I26.01, I26.90)*

I77 Other disorders of arteries and arterioles

EXCLUDES 2 *collagen (vascular) diseases (M30-M36)*
hypersensitivity angiitis (M31.0)
pulmonary artery (I28.-)

I77.0 Arteriovenous fistula, acquired HCC
Aneurysmal varix
Arteriovenous aneurysm, acquired
EXCLUDES 1 *arteriovenous aneurysm NOS (Q27.3-)*
presence of arteriovenous shunt (fistula) for dialysis (Z99.2)
traumatic — see injury of blood vessel by body region
EXCLUDES 2 *cerebral (I67.1)*
coronary (I25.4)
DEF: Communication between an artery and vein caused by trauma or invasive procedures.

I77.1 Stricture of artery HCC
Narrowing of artery

I77.2 Rupture of artery CC HCC
Erosion of artery
Fistula of artery
Ulcer of artery
EXCLUDES 1 *traumatic rupture of artery — see injury of blood vessel by body region*

I77.3 Arterial fibromuscular dysplasia HCC
Fibromuscular hyperplasia (of) carotid artery
Fibromuscular hyperplasia (of) renal artery

I77.4 Celiac artery compression syndrome CC HCC

I77.5 Necrosis of artery CC HCC

I77.6 Arteritis, unspecified HCC
Aortitis NOS
Endarteritis NOS
EXCLUDES 1 *arteritis or endarteritis:*
aortic arch (M31.4)
cerebral NEC (I67.7)
coronary (I25.89)
deformans (I70.-)
giant cell (M31.5, M31.6)
obliterans (I70.-)
senile (I70.-)

I77.7 Other arterial dissection
EXCLUDES 2 *dissection of aorta (I71.0-)*
dissection of coronary artery (I25.42)
AHA: 2016,4Q,28-29

I77.70 Dissection of unspecified artery MCC HCC

I77.71 Dissection of carotid artery MCC HCC

I77.72 Dissection of iliac artery MCC HCC

I77.73 Dissection of renal artery MCC HCC

I77.74 Dissection of vertebral artery MCC HCC
EXCLUDES 2 *aneurysm of vertebral artery (I72.6)*

I77.75 Dissection of other precerebral arteries MCC HCC
Dissection of basilar artery (trunk)
EXCLUDES 2 *aneurysm of carotid artery (I72.0)*
aneurysm of other precerebral arteries (I72.5)
aneurysm of vertebral artery (I72.6)
dissection of carotid artery (I77.71)
dissection of vertebral artery (I77.74)

I77.76 Dissection of artery of upper extremity MCC HCC

I77.77 Dissection of artery of lower extremity MCC HCC

I77.79 Dissection of other specified artery MCC HCC

I77.8 Other specified disorders of arteries and arterioles

I77.81 Aortic ectasia
Ectasis aorta
EXCLUDES 1 *aortic aneurysm and dissection (I71.0-)*

I77.810 Thoracic aortic ectasia HCC

I77.811 Abdominal aortic ectasia HCC

I77.812 Thoracoabdominal aortic ectasia HCC

I77.819 Aortic ectasia, unspecified site HCC

Chapter 9. Diseases of the Circulatory System

I74–I77.819

I77.89 Other specified disorders of arteries and arterioles HCC

I77.9 Disorder of arteries and arterioles, unspecified HCC
AHA: 2018,2Q,7

✓4th **I78 Diseases of capillaries**

I78.Ø Hereditary hemorrhagic telangiectasia HCC
Rendu-Osler-Weber disease

I78.1 Nevus, non-neoplastic
Araneus nevus
Senile nevus
Spider nevus
Stellar nevus
EXCLUDES 1 *nevus NOS (D22.-)*
vascular NOS (Q82.5)
EXCLUDES 2 *blue nevus (D22.-)*
flammeus nevus (Q82.5)
hairy nevus (D22.-)
melanocytic nevus (D22.-)
pigmented nevus (D22.-)
portwine nevus (Q82.5)
sanguineous nevus (Q82.5)
strawberry nevus (Q82.5)
verrucous nevus (Q82.5)
AHA: 2019,1Q,21

I78.8 Other diseases of capillaries

I78.9 Disease of capillaries, unspecified

✓4th **I79 Disorders of arteries, arterioles and capillaries in diseases classified elsewhere**

I79.Ø ***Aneurysm of aorta in diseases classified elsewhere*** HCC
Code first underlying disease
EXCLUDES 1 *syphilitic aneurysm (A52.Ø1)*

I79.1 ***Aortitis in diseases classified elsewhere*** HCC
Code first underlying disease
EXCLUDES 1 *syphilitic aortitis (A52.Ø2)*

I79.8 ***Other disorders of arteries, arterioles and capillaries in diseases classified elsewhere*** HCC
Code first underlying disease, such as:
amyloidosis (E85.-)
EXCLUDES 1 *diabetic (peripheral) angiopathy (EØ8-E13 with .51-.52)*
syphilitic endarteritis (A52.Ø9)
tuberculous endarteritis (A18.89)

Diseases of veins, lymphatic vessels and lymph nodes, not elsewhere classified (I8Ø-I89)

✓4th **I8Ø Phlebitis and thrombophlebitis**
INCLUDES endophlebitis
inflammation, vein
periphlebitis
suppurative phlebitis
Code first:
phlebitis and thrombophlebitis complicating abortion, ectopic or molar pregnancy (OØØ-OØ7, OØ8.7)
phlebitis and thrombophlebitis complicating pregnancy, childbirth and the puerperium (O22.-, O87.-)
EXCLUDES 1 *venous embolism and thrombosis of lower extremities (I82.4-, I82.5-, I82.81-)*

✓5th **I8Ø.Ø Phlebitis and thrombophlebitis of superficial vessels of lower extremities**
Phlebitis and thrombophlebitis of femoropopliteal vein

I8Ø.ØØ Phlebitis and thrombophlebitis of superficial vessels of unspecified lower extremity

I8Ø.Ø1 Phlebitis and thrombophlebitis of superficial vessels of right lower extremity

I8Ø.Ø2 Phlebitis and thrombophlebitis of superficial vessels of left lower extremity

I8Ø.Ø3 Phlebitis and thrombophlebitis of superficial vessels of lower extremities, bilateral

✓5th **I8Ø.1 Phlebitis and thrombophlebitis of femoral vein**
Phlebitis and thrombophlebitis of common femoral vein
Phlebitis and thrombophlebitis of deep femoral vein

I8Ø.1Ø Phlebitis and thrombophlebitis of unspecified femoral vein CC HCC

I8Ø.11 Phlebitis and thrombophlebitis of right femoral vein CC HCC

I8Ø.12 Phlebitis and thrombophlebitis of left femoral vein CC HCC

I8Ø.13 Phlebitis and thrombophlebitis of femoral vein, bilateral CC HCC

✓5th **I8Ø.2 Phlebitis and thrombophlebitis of other and unspecified deep vessels of lower extremities**

✓6th **I8Ø.2Ø Phlebitis and thrombophlebitis of unspecified deep vessels of lower extremities**

I8Ø.2Ø1 Phlebitis and thrombophlebitis of unspecified deep vessels of right lower extremity CC HCC

I8Ø.2Ø2 Phlebitis and thrombophlebitis of unspecified deep vessels of left lower extremity CC HCC

I8Ø.2Ø3 Phlebitis and thrombophlebitis of unspecified deep vessels of lower extremities, bilateral CC HCC

I8Ø.2Ø9 Phlebitis and thrombophlebitis of unspecified deep vessels of unspecified lower extremity CC HCC

✓6th **I8Ø.21 Phlebitis and thrombophlebitis of iliac vein**
Phlebitis and thrombophlebitis of common iliac vein
Phlebitis and thrombophlebitis of external iliac vein
Phlebitis and thrombophlebitis of internal iliac vein

I8Ø.211 Phlebitis and thrombophlebitis of right iliac vein CC HCC

I8Ø.212 Phlebitis and thrombophlebitis of left iliac vein CC HCC

I8Ø.213 Phlebitis and thrombophlebitis of iliac vein, bilateral CC HCC

I8Ø.219 Phlebitis and thrombophlebitis of unspecified iliac vein CC HCC

✓6th **I8Ø.22 Phlebitis and thrombophlebitis of popliteal vein**

I8Ø.221 Phlebitis and thrombophlebitis of right popliteal vein CC HCC

I8Ø.222 Phlebitis and thrombophlebitis of left popliteal vein CC HCC

I8Ø.223 Phlebitis and thrombophlebitis of popliteal vein, bilateral CC HCC

I8Ø.229 Phlebitis and thrombophlebitis of unspecified popliteal vein CC HCC

✓6th **I8Ø.23 Phlebitis and thrombophlebitis of tibial vein**
Phlebitis and thrombophlebitis of anterior tibial vein
Phlebitis and thrombophlebitis of posterior tibial vein

I8Ø.231 Phlebitis and thrombophlebitis of right tibial vein CC HCC

I8Ø.232 Phlebitis and thrombophlebitis of left tibial vein CC HCC

I8Ø.233 Phlebitis and thrombophlebitis of tibial vein, bilateral CC HCC

I8Ø.239 Phlebitis and thrombophlebitis of unspecified tibial vein CC HCC

✓6th **I8Ø.24 Phlebitis and thrombophlebitis of peroneal vein**
AHA: 2019,4Q,8

I8Ø.241 Phlebitis and thrombophlebitis of right peroneal vein CC HCC

I8Ø.242 Phlebitis and thrombophlebitis of left peroneal vein CC HCC

I8Ø.243 Phlebitis and thrombophlebitis of peroneal vein, bilateral CC HCC

I8Ø.249 Phlebitis and thrombophlebitis of unspecified peroneal vein CC HCC

✓6th **I8Ø.25 Phlebitis and thrombophlebitis of calf muscular vein**
Phlebitis and thrombophlebitis of calf muscular vein, NOS
Phlebitis and thrombophlebitis of gastrocnemial vein
Phlebitis and thrombophlebitis of soleal vein
AHA: 2019,4Q,8

I8Ø.251 Phlebitis and thrombophlebitis of right calf muscular vein HCC

I8Ø.252 Phlebitis and thrombophlebitis of left calf muscular vein HCC

I8Ø.253 Phlebitis and thrombophlebitis of calf muscular vein, bilateral HCC

I8Ø.259 Phlebitis and thrombophlebitis of unspecified calf muscular vein HCC

√6th **I80.29 Phlebitis and thrombophlebitis of other deep vessels of lower extremities**

I80.291 Phlebitis and thrombophlebitis of other deep vessels of right lower extremity CC HCC

I80.292 Phlebitis and thrombophlebitis of other deep vessels of left lower extremity CC HCC

I80.293 Phlebitis and thrombophlebitis of other deep vessels of lower extremity, bilateral CC HCC

I80.299 Phlebitis and thrombophlebitis of other deep vessels of unspecified lower extremity CC HCC

I80.3 Phlebitis and thrombophlebitis of lower extremities, unspecified

I80.8 Phlebitis and thrombophlebitis of other sites

I80.9 Phlebitis and thrombophlebitis of unspecified site

I81 Portal vein thrombosis MCC

Portal (vein) obstruction

EXCLUDES 2 *hepatic vein thrombosis (I82.0)*

phlebitis of portal vein (K75.1)

AHA: 2019,4Q,68

√4th **I82 Other venous embolism and thrombosis**

Code first venous embolism and thrombosis complicating:

abortion, ectopic or molar pregnancy (O00-O07, O08.7)

pregnancy, childbirth and the puerperium (O22.-, O87.-)

EXCLUDES 2 *venous embolism and thrombosis (of):*

cerebral (I63.6, I67.6)

coronary (I21-I25)

intracranial and intraspinal, septic or NOS (G08)

intracranial, nonpyogenic (I67.6)

intraspinal, nonpyogenic (G95.1)

mesenteric (K55.0-)

portal (I81)

pulmonary (I26.-)

I82.0 Budd-Chiari syndrome MCC HCC

Hepatic vein thrombosis

DEF: Thrombosis or other obstruction of the hepatic veins. Symptoms include an enlarged liver, extensive collateral vessels, intractable ascites, and severe portal hypertension.

I82.1 Thrombophlebitis migrans CC

√5th **I82.2 Embolism and thrombosis of vena cava and other thoracic veins**

√6th **I82.21 Embolism and thrombosis of superior vena cava**

I82.210 Acute embolism and thrombosis of superior vena cava CC HCC

Embolism and thrombosis of superior vena cava NOS

I82.211 Chronic embolism and thrombosis of superior vena cava CC HCC

√6th **I82.22 Embolism and thrombosis of inferior vena cava**

I82.220 Acute embolism and thrombosis of inferior vena cava MCC HCC

Embolism and thrombosis of inferior vena cava NOS

I82.221 Chronic embolism and thrombosis of inferior vena cava MCC HCC

√6th **I82.29 Embolism and thrombosis of other thoracic veins**

Embolism and thrombosis of brachiocephalic (innominate) vein

I82.290 Acute embolism and thrombosis of other thoracic veins CC HCC

I82.291 Chronic embolism and thrombosis of other thoracic veins CC HCC

I82.3 Embolism and thrombosis of renal vein CC HCC

√5th **I82.4 Acute embolism and thrombosis of deep veins of lower extremity**

√6th **I82.40 Acute embolism and thrombosis of unspecified deep veins of lower extremity**

Deep vein thrombosis NOS

DVT NOS

EXCLUDES 1 *acute embolism and thrombosis of unspecified deep veins of distal lower extremity (I82.4Z-)*

acute embolism and thrombosis of unspecified deep veins of proximal lower extremity (I82.4Y-)

I82.401 Acute embolism and thrombosis of unspecified deep veins of right lower extremity CC H10 HCC

I82.402 Acute embolism and thrombosis of unspecified deep veins of left lower extremity CC H10 HCC

I82.403 Acute embolism and thrombosis of unspecified deep veins of lower extremity, bilateral CC H10 HCC

I82.409 Acute embolism and thrombosis of unspecified deep veins of unspecified lower extremity CC H10 HCC

√6th **I82.41 Acute embolism and thrombosis of femoral vein**

Acute embolism and thrombosis of common femoral vein

Acute embolism and thrombosis of deep femoral vein

I82.411 Acute embolism and thrombosis of right femoral vein CC H10 HCC

I82.412 Acute embolism and thrombosis of left femoral vein CC H10 HCC

I82.413 Acute embolism and thrombosis of femoral vein, bilateral CC H10 HCC

I82.419 Acute embolism and thrombosis of unspecified femoral vein CC H10 HCC

√6th **I82.42 Acute embolism and thrombosis of iliac vein**

Acute embolism and thrombosis of common iliac vein

Acute embolism and thrombosis of external iliac vein

Acute embolism and thrombosis of internal iliac vein

I82.421 Acute embolism and thrombosis of right iliac vein CC H10 HCC

I82.422 Acute embolism and thrombosis of left iliac vein CC H10 HCC

I82.423 Acute embolism and thrombosis of iliac vein, bilateral CC H10 HCC

I82.429 Acute embolism and thrombosis of unspecified iliac vein CC H10 HCC

√6th **I82.43 Acute embolism and thrombosis of popliteal vein**

I82.431 Acute embolism and thrombosis of right popliteal vein CC H10 HCC

I82.432 Acute embolism and thrombosis of left popliteal vein CC H10 HCC

I82.433 Acute embolism and thrombosis of popliteal vein, bilateral CC H10 HCC

I82.439 Acute embolism and thrombosis of unspecified popliteal vein CC H10 HCC

√6th **I82.44 Acute embolism and thrombosis of tibial vein**

Acute embolism and thrombosis of anterior tibial vein

Acute embolism and thrombosis of posterior tibial vein

I82.441 Acute embolism and thrombosis of right tibial vein CC H10 HCC

I82.442 Acute embolism and thrombosis of left tibial vein CC H10 HCC

I82.443 Acute embolism and thrombosis of tibial vein, bilateral CC H10 HCC

I82.449 Acute embolism and thrombosis of unspecified tibial vein CC H10 HCC

√6th **I82.45 Acute embolism and thrombosis of peroneal vein**

AHA: 2019,4Q,8-10

I82.451 Acute embolism and thrombosis of right peroneal vein CC H10 HCC

I82.452 Acute embolism and thrombosis of left peroneal vein CC H10 HCC

I82.453 Acute embolism and thrombosis of peroneal vein, bilateral CC H10 HCC

I82.459 Acute embolism and thrombosis of unspecified peroneal vein CC H10 HCC

√6th **I82.46 Acute embolism and thrombosis of calf muscular vein**

Acute embolism and thrombosis of calf muscular vein, NOS

Acute embolism and thrombosis of gastrocnemial vein

Acute embolism and thrombosis of soleal vein

AHA: 2019,4Q,8-10

I82.461 Acute embolism and thrombosis of right calf muscular vein HCC

I82.462 Acute embolism and thrombosis of left calf muscular vein HCC

I82.463 Acute embolism and thrombosis of calf muscular vein, bilateral HCC

I82.469 Acute embolism and thrombosis of unspecified calf muscular vein HCC

√6th **I82.49 Acute embolism and thrombosis of other specified deep vein of lower extremity**

I82.491 Acute embolism and thrombosis of other specified deep vein of right lower extremity CC H10 HCC

I82.492 Acute embolism and thrombosis of other specified deep vein of left lower extremity CC H10 HCC

I82.493 Acute embolism and thrombosis of other specified deep vein of lower extremity, bilateral CC H10 HCC

I82.499 Acute embolism and thrombosis of other specified deep vein of unspecified lower extremity CC H10 HCC

√6th **I82.4Y Acute embolism and thrombosis of unspecified deep veins of proximal lower extremity**

Acute embolism and thrombosis of deep vein of thigh NOS

Acute embolism and thrombosis of deep vein of upper leg NOS

I82.4Y1 Acute embolism and thrombosis of unspecified deep veins of right proximal lower extremity CC H10 HCC

I82.4Y2 Acute embolism and thrombosis of unspecified deep veins of left proximal lower extremity CC H10 HCC

I82.4Y3 Acute embolism and thrombosis of unspecified deep veins of proximal lower extremity, bilateral CC H10 HCC

I82.4Y9 Acute embolism and thrombosis of unspecified deep veins of unspecified proximal lower extremity CC H10 HCC

√6th **I82.4Z Acute embolism and thrombosis of unspecified deep veins of distal lower extremity**

Acute embolism and thrombosis of deep vein of calf NOS

Acute embolism and thrombosis of deep vein of lower leg NOS

I82.4Z1 Acute embolism and thrombosis of unspecified deep veins of right distal lower extremity CC H10 HCC

I82.4Z2 Acute embolism and thrombosis of unspecified deep veins of left distal lower extremity CC H10 HCC

I82.4Z3 Acute embolism and thrombosis of unspecified deep veins of distal lower extremity, bilateral CC H10 HCC

I82.4Z9 Acute embolism and thrombosis of unspecified deep veins of unspecified distal lower extremity CC H10 HCC

√5th **I82.5 Chronic embolism and thrombosis of deep veins of lower extremity**

Use additional code, if applicable, for associated long-term (current) use of anticoagulants (Z79.01)

EXCLUDES 1 *personal history of venous embolism and thrombosis (Z86.718)*

AHA: 2020,2Q,20

√6th **I82.50 Chronic embolism and thrombosis of unspecified deep veins of lower extremity**

EXCLUDES 1 *chronic embolism and thrombosis of unspecified deep veins of distal lower extremity (I82.5Z-)*

chronic embolism and thrombosis of unspecified deep veins of proximal lower extremity (I82.5Y-)

I82.501 Chronic embolism and thrombosis of unspecified deep veins of right lower extremity CC HCC

I82.502 Chronic embolism and thrombosis of unspecified deep veins of left lower extremity CC HCC

I82.503 Chronic embolism and thrombosis of unspecified deep veins of lower extremity, bilateral CC HCC

I82.509 Chronic embolism and thrombosis of unspecified deep veins of unspecified lower extremity CC HCC

√6th **I82.51 Chronic embolism and thrombosis of femoral vein**

Chronic embolism and thrombosis of common femoral vein

Chronic embolism and thrombosis of deep femoral vein

I82.511 Chronic embolism and thrombosis of right femoral vein CC HCC

I82.512 Chronic embolism and thrombosis of left femoral vein CC HCC

I82.513 Chronic embolism and thrombosis of femoral vein, bilateral CC HCC

I82.519 Chronic embolism and thrombosis of unspecified femoral vein CC HCC

√6th **I82.52 Chronic embolism and thrombosis of iliac vein**

Chronic embolism and thrombosis of common iliac vein

Chronic embolism and thrombosis of external iliac vein

Chronic embolism and thrombosis of internal iliac vein

I82.521 Chronic embolism and thrombosis of right iliac vein CC HCC

I82.522 Chronic embolism and thrombosis of left iliac vein CC HCC

I82.523 Chronic embolism and thrombosis of iliac vein, bilateral CC HCC

I82.529 Chronic embolism and thrombosis of unspecified iliac vein CC HCC

√6th **I82.53 Chronic embolism and thrombosis of popliteal vein**

I82.531 Chronic embolism and thrombosis of right popliteal vein CC HCC

I82.532 Chronic embolism and thrombosis of left popliteal vein CC HCC

I82.533 Chronic embolism and thrombosis of popliteal vein, bilateral CC HCC

I82.539 Chronic embolism and thrombosis of unspecified popliteal vein CC HCC

√6th **I82.54 Chronic embolism and thrombosis of tibial vein**

Chronic embolism and thrombosis of anterior tibial vein

Chronic embolism and thrombosis of posterior tibial vein

I82.541 Chronic embolism and thrombosis of right tibial vein CC HCC

I82.542 Chronic embolism and thrombosis of left tibial vein CC HCC

I82.543 Chronic embolism and thrombosis of tibial vein, bilateral CC HCC

I82.549 Chronic embolism and thrombosis of unspecified tibial vein CC HCC

I82.55 Chronic embolism and thrombosis of peroneal vein
AHA: 2019,4Q,8-10
- **I82.551 Chronic embolism and thrombosis of right peroneal vein** CC HCC
- **I82.552 Chronic embolism and thrombosis of left peroneal vein** CC HCC
- **I82.553 Chronic embolism and thrombosis of peroneal vein, bilateral** CC HCC
- **I82.559 Chronic embolism and thrombosis of unspecified peroneal vein** CC HCC

I82.56 Chronic embolism and thrombosis of calf muscular vein
Chronic embolism and thrombosis of calf muscular vein NOS
Chronic embolism and thrombosis of gastrocnemial vein
Chronic embolism and thrombosis of soleal vein
AHA: 2019,4Q,8-10
- **I82.561 Chronic embolism and thrombosis of right calf muscular vein** HCC
- **I82.562 Chronic embolism and thrombosis of left calf muscular vein** HCC
- **I82.563 Chronic embolism and thrombosis of calf muscular vein, bilateral** HCC
- **I82.569 Chronic embolism and thrombosis of unspecified calf muscular vein** HCC

I82.59 Chronic embolism and thrombosis of other specified deep vein of lower extremity
- **I82.591 Chronic embolism and thrombosis of other specified deep vein of right lower extremity** CC HCC
- **I82.592 Chronic embolism and thrombosis of other specified deep vein of left lower extremity** CC HCC
- **I82.593 Chronic embolism and thrombosis of other specified deep vein of lower extremity, bilateral** CC HCC
- **I82.599 Chronic embolism and thrombosis of other specified deep vein of unspecified lower extremity** CC HCC

I82.5Y Chronic embolism and thrombosis of unspecified deep veins of proximal lower extremity
Chronic embolism and thrombosis of deep veins of thigh NOS
Chronic embolism and thrombosis of deep veins of upper leg NOS
- **I82.5Y1 Chronic embolism and thrombosis of unspecified deep veins of right proximal lower extremity** CC HCC
- **I82.5Y2 Chronic embolism and thrombosis of unspecified deep veins of left proximal lower extremity** CC HCC
- **I82.5Y3 Chronic embolism and thrombosis of unspecified deep veins of proximal lower extremity, bilateral** CC HCC
- **I82.5Y9 Chronic embolism and thrombosis of unspecified deep veins of unspecified proximal lower extremity** CC HCC

I82.5Z Chronic embolism and thrombosis of unspecified deep veins of distal lower extremity
Chronic embolism and thrombosis of deep veins of calf NOS
Chronic embolism and thrombosis of deep veins of lower leg NOS
- **I82.5Z1 Chronic embolism and thrombosis of unspecified deep veins of right distal lower extremity** CC HCC
- **I82.5Z2 Chronic embolism and thrombosis of unspecified deep veins of left distal lower extremity** CC HCC
- **I82.5Z3 Chronic embolism and thrombosis of unspecified deep veins of distal lower extremity, bilateral** CC HCC
- **I82.5Z9 Chronic embolism and thrombosis of unspecified deep veins of unspecified distal lower extremity** CC HCC

I82.6 Acute embolism and thrombosis of veins of upper extremity

I82.60 Acute embolism and thrombosis of unspecified veins of upper extremity
- **I82.601 Acute embolism and thrombosis of unspecified veins of right upper extremity** CC
- **I82.602 Acute embolism and thrombosis of unspecified veins of left upper extremity** CC
- **I82.603 Acute embolism and thrombosis of unspecified veins of upper extremity, bilateral** CC
- **I82.609 Acute embolism and thrombosis of unspecified veins of unspecified upper extremity** CC

I82.61 Acute embolism and thrombosis of superficial veins of upper extremity
Acute embolism and thrombosis of antecubital vein
Acute embolism and thrombosis of basilic vein
Acute embolism and thrombosis of cephalic vein
- **I82.611 Acute embolism and thrombosis of superficial veins of right upper extremity** CC
- **I82.612 Acute embolism and thrombosis of superficial veins of left upper extremity** CC
- **I82.613 Acute embolism and thrombosis of superficial veins of upper extremity, bilateral** CC
- **I82.619 Acute embolism and thrombosis of superficial veins of unspecified upper extremity** CC

I82.62 Acute embolism and thrombosis of deep veins of upper extremity
Acute embolism and thrombosis of brachial vein
Acute embolism and thrombosis of radial vein
Acute embolism and thrombosis of ulnar vein
- **I82.621 Acute embolism and thrombosis of deep veins of right upper extremity** CC HCC
- **I82.622 Acute embolism and thrombosis of deep veins of left upper extremity** CC HCC
- **I82.623 Acute embolism and thrombosis of deep veins of upper extremity, bilateral** CC HCC
- **I82.629 Acute embolism and thrombosis of deep veins of unspecified upper extremity** CC HCC

I82.7 Chronic embolism and thrombosis of veins of upper extremity
Use additional code, if applicable, for associated long-term (current) use of anticoagulants (Z79.01)
EXCLUDES 1 *personal history of venous embolism and thrombosis (Z86.718)*

I82.70 Chronic embolism and thrombosis of unspecified veins of upper extremity
- **I82.701 Chronic embolism and thrombosis of unspecified veins of right upper extremity** CC
- **I82.702 Chronic embolism and thrombosis of unspecified veins of left upper extremity** CC
- **I82.703 Chronic embolism and thrombosis of unspecified veins of upper extremity, bilateral** CC
- **I82.709 Chronic embolism and thrombosis of unspecified veins of unspecified upper extremity** CC

I82.71 Chronic embolism and thrombosis of superficial veins of upper extremity
Chronic embolism and thrombosis of antecubital vein
Chronic embolism and thrombosis of basilic vein
Chronic embolism and thrombosis of cephalic vein
- **I82.711 Chronic embolism and thrombosis of superficial veins of right upper extremity** CC
- **I82.712 Chronic embolism and thrombosis of superficial veins of left upper extremity** CC
- **I82.713 Chronic embolism and thrombosis of superficial veins of upper extremity, bilateral** CC

I82.719 Chronic embolism and thrombosis of superficial veins of unspecified upper extremity CC

I82.72 Chronic embolism and thrombosis of deep veins of upper extremity
Chronic embolism and thrombosis of brachial vein
Chronic embolism and thrombosis of radial vein
Chronic embolism and thrombosis of ulnar vein

I82.721 Chronic embolism and thrombosis of deep veins of right upper extremity CC HCC
I82.722 Chronic embolism and thrombosis of deep veins of left upper extremity CC HCC
I82.723 Chronic embolism and thrombosis of deep veins of upper extremity, bilateral CC HCC
I82.729 Chronic embolism and thrombosis of deep veins of unspecified upper extremity CC HCC

I82.A Embolism and thrombosis of axillary vein

I82.A1 Acute embolism and thrombosis of axillary vein
I82.A11 Acute embolism and thrombosis of right axillary vein CC HCC
I82.A12 Acute embolism and thrombosis of left axillary vein CC HCC
I82.A13 Acute embolism and thrombosis of axillary vein, bilateral CC HCC
I82.A19 Acute embolism and thrombosis of unspecified axillary vein CC HCC

I82.A2 Chronic embolism and thrombosis of axillary vein
I82.A21 Chronic embolism and thrombosis of right axillary vein CC HCC
I82.A22 Chronic embolism and thrombosis of left axillary vein CC HCC
I82.A23 Chronic embolism and thrombosis of axillary vein, bilateral CC HCC
I82.A29 Chronic embolism and thrombosis of unspecified axillary vein CC HCC

I82.B Embolism and thrombosis of subclavian vein

I82.B1 Acute embolism and thrombosis of subclavian vein
I82.B11 Acute embolism and thrombosis of right subclavian vein CC HCC
I82.B12 Acute embolism and thrombosis of left subclavian vein CC HCC
I82.B13 Acute embolism and thrombosis of subclavian vein, bilateral CC HCC
I82.B19 Acute embolism and thrombosis of unspecified subclavian vein CC HCC

I82.B2 Chronic embolism and thrombosis of subclavian vein
I82.B21 Chronic embolism and thrombosis of right subclavian vein CC HCC
I82.B22 Chronic embolism and thrombosis of left subclavian vein CC HCC
I82.B23 Chronic embolism and thrombosis of subclavian vein, bilateral CC HCC
I82.B29 Chronic embolism and thrombosis of unspecified subclavian vein CC HCC

I82.C Embolism and thrombosis of internal jugular vein

I82.C1 Acute embolism and thrombosis of internal jugular vein
I82.C11 Acute embolism and thrombosis of right internal jugular vein CC HCC
I82.C12 Acute embolism and thrombosis of left internal jugular vein CC HCC
I82.C13 Acute embolism and thrombosis of internal jugular vein, bilateral CC HCC
I82.C19 Acute embolism and thrombosis of unspecified internal jugular vein CC HCC

I82.C2 Chronic embolism and thrombosis of internal jugular vein
I82.C21 Chronic embolism and thrombosis of right internal jugular vein CC HCC
I82.C22 Chronic embolism and thrombosis of left internal jugular vein CC HCC
I82.C23 Chronic embolism and thrombosis of internal jugular vein, bilateral CC HCC
I82.C29 Chronic embolism and thrombosis of unspecified internal jugular vein CC HCC

I82.8 Embolism and thrombosis of other specified veins
Use additional code, if applicable, for associated long-term (current) use of anticoagulants (Z79.Ø1)

I82.81 Embolism and thrombosis of superficial veins of lower extremities
Embolism and thrombosis of saphenous vein (greater) (lesser)
I82.811 Embolism and thrombosis of superficial veins of right lower extremity CC
I82.812 Embolism and thrombosis of superficial veins of left lower extremity CC
I82.813 Embolism and thrombosis of superficial veins of lower extremities, bilateral CC
I82.819 Embolism and thrombosis of superficial veins of unspecified lower extremity CC

I82.89 Embolism and thrombosis of other specified veins
I82.89Ø Acute embolism and thrombosis of other specified veins CC
I82.891 Chronic embolism and thrombosis of other specified veins CC

I82.9 Embolism and thrombosis of unspecified vein
I82.9Ø Acute embolism and thrombosis of unspecified vein CC
Embolism of vein NOS
Thrombosis (vein) NOS
I82.91 Chronic embolism and thrombosis of unspecified vein CC

I83 Varicose veins of lower extremities

EXCLUDES 1 *varicose veins complicating pregnancy (O22.Ø-)*
varicose veins complicating the puerperium (O87.4)

I83.Ø Varicose veins of lower extremities with ulcer
Use additional code to identify severity of ulcer (L97.-)

I83.ØØ Varicose veins of unspecified lower extremity with ulcer
I83.ØØ1 Varicose veins of unspecified lower extremity with ulcer of thigh HCC A
I83.ØØ2 Varicose veins of unspecified lower extremity with ulcer of calf HCC A
I83.ØØ3 Varicose veins of unspecified lower extremity with ulcer of ankle HCC A
I83.ØØ4 Varicose veins of unspecified lower extremity with ulcer of heel and midfoot HCC A
Varicose veins of unspecified lower extremity with ulcer of plantar surface of midfoot
I83.ØØ5 Varicose veins of unspecified lower extremity with ulcer other part of foot HCC A
Varicose veins of unspecified lower extremity with ulcer of toe
I83.ØØ8 Varicose veins of unspecified lower extremity with ulcer other part of lower leg HCC A
I83.ØØ9 Varicose veins of unspecified lower extremity with ulcer of unspecified site HCC A

I83.Ø1 Varicose veins of right lower extremity with ulcer
I83.Ø11 Varicose veins of right lower extremity with ulcer of thigh HCC A
I83.Ø12 Varicose veins of right lower extremity with ulcer of calf HCC A
I83.Ø13 Varicose veins of right lower extremity with ulcer of ankle HCC A
I83.Ø14 Varicose veins of right lower extremity with ulcer of heel and midfoot HCC A
Varicose veins of right lower extremity with ulcer of plantar surface of midfoot
I83.Ø15 Varicose veins of right lower extremity with ulcer other part of foot HCC A
Varicose veins of right lower extremity with ulcer of toe

I83.018 Varicose veins of right lower extremity with ulcer other part of lower leg HCC A

I83.019 Varicose veins of right lower extremity with ulcer of unspecified site HCC A

✓6th I83.02 Varicose veins of left lower extremity with ulcer

I83.021 Varicose veins of left lower extremity with ulcer of thigh HCC A

I83.022 Varicose veins of left lower extremity with ulcer of calf HCC A

I83.023 Varicose veins of left lower extremity with ulcer of ankle HCC A

I83.024 Varicose veins of left lower extremity with ulcer of heel and midfoot HCC A
Varicose veins of left lower extremity with ulcer of plantar surface of midfoot

I83.025 Varicose veins of left lower extremity with ulcer other part of foot HCC A
Varicose veins of left lower extremity with ulcer of toe

I83.028 Varicose veins of left lower extremity with ulcer other part of lower leg HCC A

I83.029 Varicose veins of left lower extremity with ulcer of unspecified site HCC A

✓5th I83.1 Varicose veins of lower extremities with inflammation

I83.10 Varicose veins of unspecified lower extremity with inflammation A

I83.11 Varicose veins of right lower extremity with inflammation A

I83.12 Varicose veins of left lower extremity with inflammation A

✓5th I83.2 Varicose veins of lower extremities with both ulcer and inflammation
Use additional code to identify severity of ulcer (L97.-)

✓6th I83.20 Varicose veins of unspecified lower extremity with both ulcer and inflammation

I83.201 Varicose veins of unspecified lower extremity with both ulcer of thigh and inflammation CC HCC A

I83.202 Varicose veins of unspecified lower extremity with both ulcer of calf and inflammation CC HCC A

I83.203 Varicose veins of unspecified lower extremity with both ulcer of ankle and inflammation CC HCC A

I83.204 Varicose veins of unspecified lower extremity with both ulcer of heel and midfoot and inflammation CC HCC A
Varicose veins of unspecified lower extremity with both ulcer of plantar surface of midfoot and inflammation

I83.205 Varicose veins of unspecified lower extremity with both ulcer of other part of foot and inflammation CC HCC A
Varicose veins of unspecified lower extremity with both ulcer of toe and inflammation

I83.208 Varicose veins of unspecified lower extremity with both ulcer of other part of lower extremity and inflammation CC HCC A

I83.209 Varicose veins of unspecified lower extremity with both ulcer of unspecified site and inflammation CC HCC A

✓6th I83.21 Varicose veins of right lower extremity with both ulcer and inflammation

I83.211 Varicose veins of right lower extremity with both ulcer of thigh and inflammation CC HCC A

I83.212 Varicose veins of right lower extremity with both ulcer of calf and inflammation CC HCC A

I83.213 Varicose veins of right lower extremity with both ulcer of ankle and inflammation CC HCC A

I83.214 Varicose veins of right lower extremity with both ulcer of heel and midfoot and inflammation CC HCC A
Varicose veins of right lower extremity with both ulcer of plantar surface of midfoot and inflammation

I83.215 Varicose veins of right lower extremity with both ulcer other part of foot and inflammation CC HCC A
Varicose veins of right lower extremity with both ulcer of toe and inflammation

I83.218 Varicose veins of right lower extremity with both ulcer of other part of lower extremity and inflammation CC HCC A

I83.219 Varicose veins of right lower extremity with both ulcer of unspecified site and inflammation CC HCC A

✓6th I83.22 Varicose veins of left lower extremity with both ulcer and inflammation

I83.221 Varicose veins of left lower extremity with both ulcer of thigh and inflammation CC HCC A

I83.222 Varicose veins of left lower extremity with both ulcer of calf and inflammation CC HCC A

I83.223 Varicose veins of left lower extremity with both ulcer of ankle and inflammation CC HCC A

I83.224 Varicose veins of left lower extremity with both ulcer of heel and midfoot and inflammation CC HCC A
Varicose veins of left lower extremity with both ulcer of plantar surface of midfoot and inflammation

I83.225 Varicose veins of left lower extremity with both ulcer other part of foot and inflammation CC HCC A
Varicose veins of left lower extremity with both ulcer of toe and inflammation

I83.228 Varicose veins of left lower extremity with both ulcer of other part of lower extremity and inflammation CC HCC A

I83.229 Varicose veins of left lower extremity with both ulcer of unspecified site and inflammation CC HCC A

✓5th I83.8 Varicose veins of lower extremities with other complications

✓6th I83.81 Varicose veins of lower extremities with pain

I83.811 Varicose veins of right lower extremity with pain A

I83.812 Varicose veins of left lower extremity with pain A

I83.813 Varicose veins of bilateral lower extremities with pain A

I83.819 Varicose veins of unspecified lower extremity with pain A

✓6th I83.89 Varicose veins of lower extremities with other complications
Varicose veins of lower extremities with edema
Varicose veins of lower extremities with swelling

I83.891 Varicose veins of right lower extremity with other complications A

I83.892 Varicose veins of left lower extremity with other complications A

I83.893 Varicose veins of bilateral lower extremities with other complications A

I83.899 Varicose veins of unspecified lower extremity with other complications A

✓5th I83.9 Asymptomatic varicose veins of lower extremities
Phlebectasia of lower extremities
Varicose veins of lower extremities
Varix of lower extremities

I83.90 Asymptomatic varicose veins of unspecified lower extremity A
Varicose veins NOS

I83.91 Asymptomatic varicose veins of right lower extremity A

I83.92 Asymptomatic varicose veins of left lower extremity A

I83.93 Asymptomatic varicose veins of bilateral lower extremities A

√4th **I85 Esophageal varices**
Use additional code to identify:
alcohol abuse and dependence (F1Ø.-)

√5th **I85.Ø Esophageal varices**
Idiopathic esophageal varices
Primary esophageal varices

I85.ØØ Esophageal varices without bleeding CC HCC
Esophageal varices NOS

I85.Ø1 Esophageal varices with bleeding MCC HCC

√5th **I85.1 Secondary esophageal varices**
Esophageal varices secondary to alcoholic liver disease
Esophageal varices secondary to cirrhosis of liver
Esophageal varices secondary to schistosomiasis
Esophageal varices secondary to toxic liver disease
Code first underlying disease

I85.1Ø Secondary esophageal varices without bleeding CC HCC

I85.11 Secondary esophageal varices with bleeding MCC HCC

√4th **I86 Varicose veins of other sites**
EXCLUDES 1 *varicose veins of unspecified site (I83.9-)*
EXCLUDES 2 *retinal varices (H35.Ø-)*

I86.Ø Sublingual varices
DEF: Distended, tortuous veins beneath the tongue.

I86.1 Scrotal varices ♂
Varicocele

I86.2 Pelvic varices

I86.3 Vulval varices ♀
EXCLUDES 1 *vulval varices complicating childbirth and the puerperium (O87.8)*
vulval varices complicating pregnancy (O22.1-)

I86.4 Gastric varices

I86.8 Varicose veins of other specified sites A
Varicose ulcer of nasal septum

√4th **I87 Other disorders of veins**

√5th **I87.Ø Postthrombotic syndrome**
Chronic venous hypertension due to deep vein thrombosis
Postphlebitic syndrome
EXCLUDES 1 *chronic venous hypertension without deep vein thrombosis (I87.3-)*

√6th **I87.ØØ Postthrombotic syndrome without complications**
Asymptomatic postthrombotic syndrome

I87.ØØ1 Postthrombotic syndrome without complications of right lower extremity

I87.ØØ2 Postthrombotic syndrome without complications of left lower extremity

I87.ØØ3 Postthrombotic syndrome without complications of bilateral lower extremity

I87.ØØ9 Postthrombotic syndrome without complications of unspecified extremity
Postthrombotic syndrome NOS

√6th **I87.Ø1 Postthrombotic syndrome with ulcer**
Use additional code to specify site and severity of ulcer (L97.-)

I87.Ø11 Postthrombotic syndrome with ulcer of right lower extremity CC HCC

I87.Ø12 Postthrombotic syndrome with ulcer of left lower extremity CC HCC

I87.Ø13 Postthrombotic syndrome with ulcer of bilateral lower extremity CC HCC

I87.Ø19 Postthrombotic syndrome with ulcer of unspecified lower extremity CC HCC

√6th **I87.Ø2 Postthrombotic syndrome with inflammation**

I87.Ø21 Postthrombotic syndrome with inflammation of right lower extremity

I87.Ø22 Postthrombotic syndrome with inflammation of left lower extremity

I87.Ø23 Postthrombotic syndrome with inflammation of bilateral lower extremity

I87.Ø29 Postthrombotic syndrome with inflammation of unspecified lower extremity

√6th **I87.Ø3 Postthrombotic syndrome with ulcer and inflammation**
Use additional code to specify site and severity of ulcer (L97.-)

I87.Ø31 Postthrombotic syndrome with ulcer and inflammation of right lower extremity CC HCC

I87.Ø32 Postthrombotic syndrome with ulcer and inflammation of left lower extremity CC HCC

I87.Ø33 Postthrombotic syndrome with ulcer and inflammation of bilateral lower extremity CC HCC

I87.Ø39 Postthrombotic syndrome with ulcer and inflammation of unspecified lower extremity CC HCC

√6th **I87.Ø9 Postthrombotic syndrome with other complications**

I87.Ø91 Postthrombotic syndrome with other complications of right lower extremity

I87.Ø92 Postthrombotic syndrome with other complications of left lower extremity

I87.Ø93 Postthrombotic syndrome with other complications of bilateral lower extremity

I87.Ø99 Postthrombotic syndrome with other complications of unspecified lower extremity

I87.1 Compression of vein CC
Stricture of vein
Vena cava syndrome (inferior) (superior)
EXCLUDES 2 *compression of pulmonary vein (I28.8)*

I87.2 Venous insufficiency (chronic) (peripheral)
Stasis dermatitis
EXCLUDES 1 *stasis dermatitis with varicose veins of lower extremities (I83.1-, I83.2-)*
DEF: Insufficient drainage of venous blood in any part of the body that results in edema or dermatosis.

√5th **I87.3 Chronic venous hypertension (idiopathic)**
Stasis edema
EXCLUDES 1 *chronic venous hypertension due to deep vein thrombosis (I87.Ø-)*
varicose veins of lower extremities (I83.-)

√6th **I87.3Ø Chronic venous hypertension (idiopathic) without complications**
Asymptomatic chronic venous hypertension (idiopathic)

I87.3Ø1 Chronic venous hypertension (idiopathic) without complications of right lower extremity

I87.3Ø2 Chronic venous hypertension (idiopathic) without complications of left lower extremity

I87.3Ø3 Chronic venous hypertension (idiopathic) without complications of bilateral lower extremity

I87.3Ø9 Chronic venous hypertension (idiopathic) without complications of unspecified lower extremity
Chronic venous hypertension NOS

√6th **I87.31 Chronic venous hypertension (idiopathic) with ulcer**
Use additional code to specify site and severity of ulcer (L97.-)

I87.311 Chronic venous hypertension (idiopathic) with ulcer of right lower extremity CC HCC

I87.312 Chronic venous hypertension (idiopathic) with ulcer of left lower extremity CC HCC

I87.313 Chronic venous hypertension (idiopathic) with ulcer of bilateral lower extremity CC HCC

I87.319 Chronic venous hypertension (idiopathic) with ulcer of unspecified lower extremity CC HCC

√6th **I87.32 Chronic venous hypertension (idiopathic) with inflammation**

I87.321 Chronic venous hypertension (idiopathic) with inflammation of right lower extremity

I87.322 Chronic venous hypertension (idiopathic) with inflammation of left lower extremity

I87.323 **Chronic venous hypertension (idiopathic) with inflammation of bilateral lower extremity**

I87.329 **Chronic venous hypertension (idiopathic) with inflammation of unspecified lower extremity**

✓6th I87.33 **Chronic venous hypertension (idiopathic) with ulcer and inflammation**

Use additional code to specify site and severity of ulcer (L97.-)

I87.331 **Chronic venous hypertension (idiopathic) with ulcer and inflammation of right lower extremity** CC HCC

I87.332 **Chronic venous hypertension (idiopathic) with ulcer and inflammation of left lower extremity** CC HCC

I87.333 **Chronic venous hypertension (idiopathic) with ulcer and inflammation of bilateral lower extremity** CC HCC

I87.339 **Chronic venous hypertension (idiopathic) with ulcer and inflammation of unspecified lower extremity** CC HCC

✓6th I87.39 **Chronic venous hypertension (idiopathic) with other complications**

I87.391 **Chronic venous hypertension (idiopathic) with other complications of right lower extremity**

I87.392 **Chronic venous hypertension (idiopathic) with other complications of left lower extremity**

I87.393 **Chronic venous hypertension (idiopathic) with other complications of bilateral lower extremity**

I87.399 **Chronic venous hypertension (idiopathic) with other complications of unspecified lower extremity**

I87.8 **Other specified disorders of veins**

Phlebosclerosis
Venofibrosis

I87.9 **Disorder of vein, unspecified**

✓4th **I88 Nonspecific lymphadenitis**

EXCLUDES 1 *acute lymphadenitis, except mesenteric (LØ4.-)*
enlarged lymph nodes NOS (R59.-)
human immunodeficiency virus [HIV] disease resulting in generalized lymphadenopathy (B2Ø)

I88.Ø **Nonspecific mesenteric lymphadenitis**

Mesenteric lymphadenitis (acute)(chronic)

I88.1 **Chronic lymphadenitis, except mesenteric**

Adenitis
Lymphadenitis

I88.8 **Other nonspecific lymphadenitis**

I88.9 **Nonspecific lymphadenitis, unspecified**

Lymphadenitis NOS

✓4th **I89 Other noninfective disorders of lymphatic vessels and lymph nodes**

EXCLUDES 1 *chylocele, tunica vaginalis (nonfilarial) NOS (N5Ø.89)*
enlarged lymph nodes NOS (R59.-)
filarial chylocele (B74.-)
hereditary lymphedema (Q82.Ø)

I89.Ø **Lymphedema, not elsewhere classified**

Elephantiasis (nonfilarial) NOS
Lymphangiectasis
Obliteration, lymphatic vessel
Praecox lymphedema
Secondary lymphedema

EXCLUDES 1 *postmastectomy lymphedema (I97.2)*

I89.1 **Lymphangitis**

Chronic lymphangitis
Lymphangitis NOS
Subacute lymphangitis

EXCLUDES 1 *acute lymphangitis (LØ3.-)*

I89.8 **Other specified noninfective disorders of lymphatic vessels and lymph nodes**

Chylocele (nonfilarial)
Chylous ascites
Chylous cyst
Lipomelanotic reticulosis
Lymph node or vessel fistula
Lymph node or vessel infarction
Lymph node or vessel rupture

I89.9 **Noninfective disorder of lymphatic vessels and lymph nodes, unspecified**

Disease of lymphatic vessels NOS

Other and unspecified disorders of the circulatory system (I95-I99)

✓4th **I95 Hypotension**

EXCLUDES 1 *cardiovascular collapse (R57.9) (~R57.9)*
maternal hypotension syndrome (O26.5-)
nonspecific low blood pressure reading NOS (RØ3.1)

I95.Ø **Idiopathic hypotension**

I95.1 **Orthostatic hypotension**

Hypotension, postural

EXCLUDES 1 *neurogenic orthostatic hypotension [Shy-Drager] (G9Ø.3)*
orthostatic hypotension due to drugs (I95.2)

I95.2 **Hypotension due to drugs**

Orthostatic hypotension due to drugs

Use additional code for adverse effect, if applicable, to identify drug (T36-T5Ø with fifth or sixth character 5)

I95.3 **Hypotension of hemodialysis**

Intra-dialytic hypotension

✓5th I95.8 **Other hypotension**

I95.81 **Postprocedural hypotension**

I95.89 **Other hypotension**

Chronic hypotension

I95.9 **Hypotension, unspecified**

I96 Gangrene, not elsewhere classified CC HCC

Gangrenous cellulitis

EXCLUDES 1 *gangrene in atherosclerosis of native arteries of the extremities (I7Ø.26)*
gangrene in hernia (K4Ø.1, K4Ø.4, K41.1, K41.4, K42.1, K43.1-, K44.1, K45.1, K46.1)
gangrene in other peripheral vascular diseases (I73.-)
gangrene of certain specified sites — see Alphabetical Index
gas gangrene (A48.Ø)
pyoderma gangrenosum (L88)

EXCLUDES 2 *gangrene in diabetes mellitus (EØ8-E13 with .52)*

AHA: 2018,4Q,87; 2018,3Q,3; 2017,3Q,6; 2013,2Q,34

✓4th **I97 Intraoperative and postprocedural complications and disorders of circulatory system, not elsewhere classified**

EXCLUDES 2 *postprocedural shock (T81.1-)*

AHA: 2019,2Q,21

I97.Ø **Postcardiotomy syndrome**

✓5th I97.1 **Other postprocedural cardiac functional disturbances**

EXCLUDES 2 *acute pulmonary insufficiency following thoracic surgery (J95.1)*
intraoperative cardiac functional disturbances (I97.7-)

✓6th I97.11 **Postprocedural cardiac insufficiency**

I97.11Ø **Postprocedural cardiac insufficiency following cardiac surgery** CC

I97.111 **Postprocedural cardiac insufficiency following other surgery** CC

✓6th I97.12 **Postprocedural cardiac arrest**

I97.12Ø **Postprocedural cardiac arrest following cardiac surgery** CC

I97.121 **Postprocedural cardiac arrest following other surgery** CC

✓6th I97.13 **Postprocedural heart failure**

Use additional code to identify the heart failure (I5Ø.-)

I97.13Ø **Postprocedural heart failure following cardiac surgery** CC

I97.131 **Postprocedural heart failure following other surgery** CC

✓6th **I97.19 Other postprocedural cardiac functional disturbances**
Use additional code, if applicable, to further specify disorder

I97.190 Other postprocedural cardiac functional disturbances following cardiac surgery CC
Use additional code, if applicable, for type 4 or type 5 myocardial infarction, to further specify disorder
AHA: 2019,2Q,33

I97.191 Other postprocedural cardiac functional disturbances following other surgery CC

I97.2 Postmastectomy lymphedema syndrome A
Elephantiasis due to mastectomy
Obliteration of lymphatic vessels

I97.3 Postprocedural hypertension

✓5th **I97.4 Intraoperative hemorrhage and hematoma of a circulatory system organ or structure complicating a procedure**
EXCLUDES 1 *intraoperative hemorrhage and hematoma of a circulatory system organ or structure due to accidental puncture and laceration during a procedure (I97.5-)*
EXCLUDES 2 *intraoperative cerebrovascular hemorrhage complicating a procedure (G97.3-)*

✓6th **I97.41 Intraoperative hemorrhage and hematoma of a circulatory system organ or structure complicating a circulatory system procedure**

I97.410 Intraoperative hemorrhage and hematoma of a circulatory system organ or structure complicating a cardiac catheterization CC

I97.411 Intraoperative hemorrhage and hematoma of a circulatory system organ or structure complicating a cardiac bypass CC

I97.418 Intraoperative hemorrhage and hematoma of a circulatory system organ or structure complicating other circulatory system procedure CC

I97.42 Intraoperative hemorrhage and hematoma of a circulatory system organ or structure complicating other procedure CC
AHA: 2020,1Q,19

✓5th **I97.5 Accidental puncture and laceration of a circulatory system organ or structure during a procedure**
EXCLUDES 2 *accidental puncture and laceration of brain during a procedure (G97.4-)*

I97.51 Accidental puncture and laceration of a circulatory system organ or structure during a circulatory system procedure CC
AHA: 2019,2Q,24

I97.52 Accidental puncture and laceration of a circulatory system organ or structure during other procedure CC

✓5th **I97.6 Postprocedural hemorrhage, hematoma and seroma of a circulatory system organ or structure following a procedure**
EXCLUDES 2 *postprocedural cerebrovascular hemorrhage complicating a procedure (G97.5-)*
AHA: 2016,4Q,9-10

✓6th **I97.61 Postprocedural hemorrhage of a circulatory system organ or structure following a circulatory system procedure**

I97.610 Postprocedural hemorrhage of a circulatory system organ or structure following a cardiac catheterization CC

I97.611 Postprocedural hemorrhage of a circulatory system organ or structure following cardiac bypass CC

I97.618 Postprocedural hemorrhage of a circulatory system organ or structure following other circulatory system procedure CC

✓6th **I97.62 Postprocedural hemorrhage, hematoma and seroma of a circulatory system organ or structure following other procedure**

I97.620 Postprocedural hemorrhage of a circulatory system organ or structure following other procedure CC

I97.621 Postprocedural hematoma of a circulatory system organ or structure following other procedure CC

I97.622 Postprocedural seroma of a circulatory system organ or structure following other procedure CC

✓6th **I97.63 Postprocedural hematoma of a circulatory system organ or structure following a circulatory system procedure**

I97.630 Postprocedural hematoma of a circulatory system organ or structure following a cardiac catheterization CC

I97.631 Postprocedural hematoma of a circulatory system organ or structure following cardiac bypass CC

I97.638 Postprocedural hematoma of a circulatory system organ or structure following other circulatory system procedure CC

✓6th **I97.64 Postprocedural seroma of a circulatory system organ or structure following a circulatory system procedure**

I97.640 Postprocedural seroma of a circulatory system organ or structure following a cardiac catheterization CC

I97.641 Postprocedural seroma of a circulatory system organ or structure following cardiac bypass CC

I97.648 Postprocedural seroma of a circulatory system organ or structure following other circulatory system procedure CC

✓5th **I97.7 Intraoperative cardiac functional disturbances**
EXCLUDES 2 *acute pulmonary insufficiency following thoracic surgery (J95.1)*
postprocedural cardiac functional disturbances (I97.1-)

✓6th **I97.71 Intraoperative cardiac arrest**

I97.710 Intraoperative cardiac arrest during cardiac surgery CC

I97.711 Intraoperative cardiac arrest during other surgery CC

✓6th **I97.79 Other intraoperative cardiac functional disturbances**
Use additional code, if applicable, to further specify disorder

I97.790 Other intraoperative cardiac functional disturbances during cardiac surgery CC

I97.791 Other intraoperative cardiac functional disturbances during other surgery CC

✓5th **I97.8 Other intraoperative and postprocedural complications and disorders of the circulatory system, not elsewhere classified**
Use additional code, if applicable, to further specify disorder

✓6th **I97.81 Intraoperative cerebrovascular infarction**

I97.810 Intraoperative cerebrovascular infarction during cardiac surgery CC HCC

I97.811 Intraoperative cerebrovascular infarction during other surgery CC HCC

✓6th **I97.82 Postprocedural cerebrovascular infarction**

I97.820 Postprocedural cerebrovascular infarction following cardiac surgery CC HCC

I97.821 Postprocedural cerebrovascular infarction following other surgery CC HCC

I97.88 Other intraoperative complications of the circulatory system, not elsewhere classified CC

I97.89 Other postprocedural complications and disorders of the circulatory system, not elsewhere classified CC
AHA: 2019,2Q,33

✓4th **I99 Other and unspecified disorders of circulatory system**

I99.8 Other disorder of circulatory system

I99.9 Unspecified disorder of circulatory system

Chapter 10. Diseases of the Respiratory System (J00–J99), U07.0

Chapter-specific Guidelines with Coding Examples

The chapter-specific guidelines from the ICD-10-CM Official Guidelines for Coding and Reporting have been provided below. Along with these guidelines are coding examples, contained in the shaded boxes, that have been developed to help illustrate the coding and/or sequencing guidance found in these guidelines.

a. Chronic obstructive pulmonary disease [COPD] and asthma

1) Acute exacerbation of chronic obstructive bronchitis and asthma

The codes in categories J44 and J45 distinguish between uncomplicated cases and those in acute exacerbation. An acute exacerbation is a worsening or a decompensation of a chronic condition. An acute exacerbation is not equivalent to an infection superimposed on a chronic condition, though an exacerbation may be triggered by an infection.

Vancomycin IV was started to treat a patient with acute pneumonia due to *Streptococcus pneumoniae*. Patient also with acute exacerbation of COPD continued on home meds.

J13 **Pneumonia due to Streptococcus pneumoniae**

J44.0 **Chronic obstructive pulmonary disease with (acute) lower respiratory infection**

J44.1 **Chronic obstructive pulmonary disease with (acute) exacerbation**

Explanation: ICD-10-CM uses combination codes to create organism-specific classifications for acute pneumonia. Category J44 codes include combination codes with severity components, which differentiate between COPD with acute lower respiratory infection (acute pneumonia), COPD with acute exacerbation, and COPD without mention of a complication (unspecified).

An acute exacerbation is a worsening or a decompensation of a chronic condition. An acute exacerbation is not equivalent to an infection superimposed on a chronic condition, though an exacerbation may be triggered by an infection, as in this example. Treatment of the pneumonia necessitated the inpatient admission. Instructional notes at J44.0 say to "code also to identify the infection," which informs the coder that another code must be assigned if applicable. Sequencing of the pneumonia and COPD exacerbation are governed by the Section II, "Selection of Principal Diagnosis," guidelines. In this case it was the pneumonia that was "chiefly responsible for occasioning the admission" with the IV vancomycin treatment.

Exacerbation of moderate persistent asthma with status asthmaticus

J45.42 **Moderate persistent asthma with status asthmaticus**

Explanation: Category J45 Asthma includes severity-specific subcategories and fifth-character codes to distinguish between uncomplicated cases, those in acute exacerbation, and those with status asthmaticus.

b. Acute respiratory failure

1) Acute respiratory failure as principal diagnosis

A code from subcategory J96.0, Acute respiratory failure, or subcategory J96.2, Acute and chronic respiratory failure, may be assigned as a principal diagnosis when it is the condition established after study to be chiefly responsible for occasioning the admission to the hospital, and the selection is supported by the Alphabetic Index and Tabular List. However, chapter-specific coding guidelines (such as obstetrics, poisoning, HIV, newborn) that provide sequencing direction take precedence.

Acute hypoxic respiratory failure due to COPD exacerbation

J96.01 **Acute respiratory failure with hypoxia**

J44.1 **Chronic obstructive pulmonary disease with (acute) exacerbation**

Explanation: Category J96 classifies respiratory failure with combination codes that designate the severity and the presence of hypoxia and hypercapnia. Code J96.01 is sequenced as the first-listed diagnosis, as the reason for the admission. Respiratory failure may be assigned as a principal diagnosis when it is the condition established after study to be chiefly responsible for occasioning the admission to the hospital and the selection is supported by the Alphabetic Index and Tabular List.

2) Acute respiratory failure as secondary diagnosis

Respiratory failure may be listed as a secondary diagnosis if it occurs after admission, or if it is present on admission, but does not meet the definition of principal diagnosis.

Acute respiratory failure due to accidental oxycodone overdose

T40.2X1A **Poisoning by other opioids, accidental (unintentional), initial encounter**

J96.00 **Acute respiratory failure, unspecified whether with hypoxia or hypercapnia**

Explanation: Respiratory failure may be assigned as a principal diagnosis when it is the condition established after study to be chiefly responsible for occasioning the admission to the hospital, and the selection is supported by the Alphabetic Index and Tabular List. However, chapter-specific coding guidelines, such as poisoning, that provide sequencing direction take precedence. When coding a poisoning or reaction to the improper use of a medication (e.g. overdose, wrong substance given or taken in error, wrong route of administration), first assign the appropriate code from categories T36–T50. Use additional code(s) for all manifestations of the poisoning. In this instance, the respiratory failure is a manifestation of the poisoning and is sequenced as a secondary diagnosis.

Acute pneumococcal pneumonia with subsequent development of acute respiratory failure

J13 **Pneumonia due to Streptococcus pneumoniae**

J96.00 **Acute respiratory failure, unspecified whether with hypoxia or hypercapnia**

Explanation: Acute respiratory failure may be listed as a secondary diagnosis if it occurs after admission, or if it is present on admission but does not meet the definition of principal diagnosis.

3) Sequencing of acute respiratory failure and another acute condition

When a patient is admitted with respiratory failure and another acute condition, (e.g., myocardial infarction, cerebrovascular accident, aspiration pneumonia), the principal diagnosis will not be the same in every situation. This applies whether the other acute condition is a respiratory or nonrespiratory condition. Selection of the principal diagnosis will be dependent on the circumstances of admission. If both the respiratory failure and the other acute condition are equally responsible for occasioning the admission to the hospital, and there are no chapter-specific sequencing rules, the guideline regarding two or more diagnoses that equally meet the definition for principal diagnosis (*Section II, C.*) may be applied in these situations.

If the documentation is not clear as to whether acute respiratory failure and another condition are equally responsible for occasioning the admission, query the provider for clarification.

Acute pneumococcal pneumonia and acute respiratory failure, both present on admission

J96.00 **Acute respiratory failure, unspecified whether with hypoxia or hypercapnia**

J13 **Pneumonia due to Streptococcus pneumoniae**

Explanation: When a patient is admitted with respiratory failure and another acute condition, such as a bacterial pneumonia, the principal diagnosis is not the same in every situation. This applies whether the other acute condition is a respiratory or nonrespiratory condition. The principal diagnosis depends on the circumstances of admission.

c. Influenza due to certain identified influenza viruses

Code only confirmed cases of influenza due to certain identified influenza viruses (category J09), and due to other identified influenza virus (category J10). This is an exception to the hospital inpatient guideline Section II, H. (Uncertain Diagnosis).

In this context, "confirmation" does not require documentation of positive laboratory testing specific for avian or other novel influenza A or other identified influenza virus. However, coding should be based on the provider's diagnostic statement that the patient has avian influenza, or other novel influenza A, for category J09, or has another particular identified strain of influenza, such as H1N1 or H3N2, but not identified as novel or variant, for category J10.

If the provider records "suspected" or "possible" or "probable" avian influenza, or novel influenza, or other identified influenza, then the appropriate influenza code from category J11, Influenza due to unidentified influenza virus, should be assigned. A code from category JØ9, Influenza due to certain identified influenza viruses, should not be assigned nor should a code from category J1Ø, Influenza due to other identified influenza virus.

Influenza due to avian influenza virus with pneumonia

JØ9.X1	**Influenza due to identified novel influenza A virus with pneumonia**

Explanation: Codes in category JØ9 Influenza due to certain identified influenza viruses should be assigned only for confirmed cases. "Confirmation" does not require positive laboratory testing of a specific influenza virus but does need to be based on the provider's diagnostic statement, which should not include terms such as "possible,""probable," or "suspected."

d. Ventilator associated pneumonia

1) Documentation of ventilator associated pneumonia

As with all procedural or postprocedural complications, code assignment is based on the provider's documentation of the relationship between the condition and the procedure.

Code J95.851, Ventilator associated pneumonia, should be assigned only when the provider has documented ventilator associated pneumonia (VAP). An additional code to identify the organism (e.g., Pseudomonas aeruginosa, code B96.5) should also be assigned. Do not assign an additional code from categories J12-J18 to identify the type of pneumonia.

Code J95.851 should not be assigned for cases where the patient has pneumonia and is on a mechanical ventilator and the provider has not specifically stated that the pneumonia is ventilator-associated pneumonia. If the documentation is unclear as to whether the patient has a pneumonia that is a complication attributable to the mechanical ventilator, query the provider.

2) Ventilator associated pneumonia develops after admission

A patient may be admitted with one type of pneumonia (e.g., code J13, Pneumonia due to Streptococcus pneumonia) and subsequently develop VAP. In this instance, the principal diagnosis would be the appropriate code from categories J12-J18 for the pneumonia diagnosed at the time of admission. Code J95.851, Ventilator associated pneumonia, would be assigned as an additional diagnosis when the provider has also documented the presence of ventilator associated pneumonia.

Patient with pneumonia due to *Klebsiella pneumoniae* develops superimposed MRSA ventilator-associated pneumonia

J15.Ø	**Pneumonia due to Klebsiella pneumoniae**
J95.851	**Ventilator associated pneumonia**
B95.62	**Methicillin resistant Staphylococcus aureus infection as the cause of diseases classified elsewhere**

Explanation: Code assignment for ventilator-associated pneumonia is based on the provider's documentation of the relationship between the condition and the procedure and is reported only when the provider has documented ventilator-associated pneumonia (VAP).

A patient may be admitted with one type of pneumonia and subsequently develop VAP. In this example, the principal diagnosis code describes the pneumonia diagnosed at the time of admission, with code J95.851 Ventilator associated pneumonia, assigned as secondary.

e. Vaping-related disorders

For patients presenting with condition(s) related to vaping, assign code UØ7.Ø, Vaping-related disorder, as the principal diagnosis. For lung injury due to vaping, assign only code UØ7.Ø. Assign additional codes for other manifestations, such as acute respiratory failure (subcategory J96.Ø-) or pneumonitis (code J68.Ø).

Associated respiratory signs and symptoms due to vaping, such as cough, shortness of breath, etc., are not coded separately, when a definitive diagnosis has been established. However, it would be appropriate to code separately any gastrointestinal symptoms, such as diarrhea and abdominal pain.

23-year-old patient with history of anxiety disorder admitted with fever, dyspnea and nonproductive cough. Patient's respiratory function continued to clinically worsen, requiring intubation for suspected ARDS and required OGT suction for coffee ground hematemesis. Following extubating, patient confirmed the use of THC vaping cartridge preceding development of symptoms. Discharge diagnosis is ARDS due to EVALI and anxiety disorder.

UØ7.Ø	**Vaping related disorder**
J8Ø	**Acute respiratory distress syndrome**
K92.Ø	**Hematemesis**
F41.9	**Anxiety disorder, unspecified**

Explanation: Codes UØ7.Ø and J8Ø represent the vaping-related disorder and its associated manifestation, the acute respiratory distress syndrome (ARDS). The symptoms that brought the patient in are not coded separately because these are integral to the vaping disorder and the ARDS, unlike the hematemesis (vomiting blood) a gastrointestinal symptom that is not integral to either of these conditions.

Chapter 10. Diseases of the Respiratory System (J00-J99)

NOTE When a respiratory condition is described as occurring in more than one site and is not specifically indexed, it should be classified to the lower anatomic site (e.g., tracheobronchitis to bronchitis in J40).

Use additional code, where applicable, to identify:
exposure to environmental tobacco smoke (Z77.22)
exposure to tobacco smoke in the perinatal period (P96.81)
history of tobacco dependence (Z87.891)
occupational exposure to environmental tobacco smoke (Z57.31)
tobacco dependence (F17.-)
tobacco use (Z72.0)

EXCLUDES 2 *certain conditions originating in the perinatal period (P04-P96)*
certain infectious and parasitic diseases (A00-B99)
complications of pregnancy, childbirth and the puerperium (O00-O9A)
congenital malformations, deformations and chromosomal abnormalities (Q00-Q99)
endocrine, nutritional and metabolic diseases (E00-E88)
injury, poisoning and certain other consequences of external causes (S00-T88)
neoplasms (C00-D49)
smoke inhalation (T59.81-)
symptoms, signs and abnormal clinical and laboratory findings, not elsewhere classified (R00-R94)

This chapter contains the following blocks:

J00-J06	Acute upper respiratory infections
J09-J18	Influenza and pneumonia
J20-J22	Other acute lower respiratory infections
J30-J39	Other diseases of upper respiratory tract
J40-J47	Chronic lower respiratory diseases
J60-J70	Lung diseases due to external agents
J80-J84	Other respiratory diseases principally affecting the interstitium
J85-J86	Suppurative and necrotic conditions of the lower respiratory tract
J90-J94	Other diseases of the pleura
J95	Intraoperative and postprocedural complications and disorders of respiratory system, not elsewhere classified
J96-J99	Other diseases of the respiratory system

Acute upper respiratory infections (J00-J06)

EXCLUDES 1 *chronic obstructive pulmonary disease with acute lower respiratory infection (J44.0)*
~~*influenza virus with other respiratory manifestations (J09.X2, J10.1, J11.1)*~~

J00 Acute nasopharyngitis [common cold]
Acute rhinitis
Coryza (acute)
Infective nasopharyngitis NOS
Infective rhinitis
Nasal catarrh, acute
Nasopharyngitis NOS
EXCLUDES 1 *acute pharyngitis (J02.-)*
acute sore throat NOS (J02.9)
▶*influenza virus with other respiratory manifestations (J09.X2, J10.1, J11.1)*◀
pharyngitis NOS (J02.9)
rhinitis NOS (J31.0)
sore throat NOS (J02.9)
EXCLUDES 2 *allergic rhinitis (J30.1-J30.9)*
chronic pharyngitis (J31.2)
chronic rhinitis (J31.0)
chronic sore throat (J31.2)
nasopharyngitis, chronic (J31.1)
vasomotor rhinitis (J30.0)
DEF: Acute inflammation of the mucous membranes that extends from the nares to the pharynx. It is characterized by nasal obstruction, sneezing, runny nose, and sore throat.

✓4th **J01 Acute sinusitis**
INCLUDES acute abscess of sinus
acute empyema of sinus
acute infection of sinus
acute inflammation of sinus
acute suppuration of sinus
Use additional code (B95-B97) to identify infectious agent
EXCLUDES 1 *sinusitis NOS (J32.9)*
EXCLUDES 2 *chronic sinusitis (J32.0-J32.8)*

✓5th **J01.0 Acute maxillary sinusitis**
Acute antritis
J01.00 Acute maxillary sinusitis, unspecified
J01.01 Acute recurrent maxillary sinusitis

✓5th **J01.1 Acute frontal sinusitis**
J01.10 Acute frontal sinusitis, unspecified
J01.11 Acute recurrent frontal sinusitis

✓5th **J01.2 Acute ethmoidal sinusitis**
J01.20 Acute ethmoidal sinusitis, unspecified
J01.21 Acute recurrent ethmoidal sinusitis

✓5th **J01.3 Acute sphenoidal sinusitis**
J01.30 Acute sphenoidal sinusitis, unspecified
J01.31 Acute recurrent sphenoidal sinusitis

✓5th **J01.4 Acute pansinusitis**
J01.40 Acute pansinusitis, unspecified
J01.41 Acute recurrent pansinusitis

✓5th **J01.8 Other acute sinusitis**
J01.80 Other acute sinusitis
Acute sinusitis involving more than one sinus but not pansinusitis
J01.81 Other acute recurrent sinusitis
Acute recurrent sinusitis involving more than one sinus but not pansinusitis

✓5th **J01.9 Acute sinusitis, unspecified**
J01.90 Acute sinusitis, unspecified
J01.91 Acute recurrent sinusitis, unspecified

✓4th **J02 Acute pharyngitis**
INCLUDES acute sore throat
EXCLUDES 1 *acute laryngopharyngitis (J06.0)*
peritonsillar abscess (J36)
pharyngeal abscess (J39.1)
retropharyngeal abscess (J39.0)
EXCLUDES 2 *chronic pharyngitis (J31.2)*

J02.0 Streptococcal pharyngitis
Septic pharyngitis
Streptococcal sore throat
EXCLUDES 2 *scarlet fever (A38.-)*

J02.8 Acute pharyngitis due to other specified organisms
Use additional code (B95-B97) to identify infectious agent
EXCLUDES 1 *acute pharyngitis due to coxsackie virus (B08.5)*
acute pharyngitis due to gonococcus (A54.5)
acute pharyngitis due to herpes [simplex] virus (B00.2)
acute pharyngitis due to infectious mononucleosis (B27.-)
enteroviral vesicular pharyngitis (B08.5)

J02.9 Acute pharyngitis, unspecified
Gangrenous pharyngitis (acute)
Infective pharyngitis (acute) NOS
Pharyngitis (acute) NOS
Sore throat (acute) NOS
Suppurative pharyngitis (acute)
Ulcerative pharyngitis (acute)
EXCLUDES 1 ▶*influenza virus with other respiratory manifestations (J09.X2, J10.1, J11.1)*◀

✓4th **J03 Acute tonsillitis**
EXCLUDES 1 *acute sore throat (J02.-)*
hypertrophy of tonsils (J35.1)
peritonsillar abscess (J36)
sore throat NOS (J02.9)
streptococcal sore throat (J02.0)
EXCLUDES 2 *chronic tonsillitis (J35.0)*

✓5th **J03.0 Streptococcal tonsillitis**
J03.00 Acute streptococcal tonsillitis, unspecified
J03.01 Acute recurrent streptococcal tonsillitis

✓5th **J03.8 Acute tonsillitis due to other specified organisms**
Use additional code (B95-B97) to identify infectious agent
EXCLUDES 1 *diphtheritic tonsillitis (A36.0)*
herpesviral pharyngotonsillitis (B00.2)
streptococcal tonsillitis (J03.0)
tuberculous tonsillitis (A15.8)
Vincent's tonsillitis (A69.1)
J03.80 Acute tonsillitis due to other specified organisms
J03.81 Acute recurrent tonsillitis due to other specified organisms

√5th **J03.9 Acute tonsillitis, unspecified**
Follicular tonsillitis (acute)
Gangrenous tonsillitis (acute)
Infective tonsillitis (acute)
Tonsillitis (acute) NOS
Ulcerative tonsillitis (acute)
EXCLUDES 1 ▶*influenza virus with other respiratory manifestations (J09.X2, J10.1, J11.1)*◀

J03.90 Acute tonsillitis, unspecified
J03.91 Acute recurrent tonsillitis, unspecified

√4th **J04 Acute laryngitis and tracheitis**
▶Code also influenza, if present, such as:◀
▶influenza due to identified novel influenza A virus with other respiratory manifestations (J09.X2)◀
▶influenza due to other identified influenza virus with other respiratory manifestations (J10.1)◀
▶influenza due to unidentified influenza virus with other respiratory manifestations (J11.1)◀
Use additional code (B95-B97) to identify infectious agent
EXCLUDES 1 *acute obstructive laryngitis [croup] and epiglottitis (J05.-)*
EXCLUDES 2 *laryngismus (stridulus) (J38.5)*

J04.0 Acute laryngitis
Edematous laryngitis (acute)
Laryngitis (acute) NOS
Subglottic laryngitis (acute)
Suppurative laryngitis (acute)
Ulcerative laryngitis (acute)
EXCLUDES 1 *acute obstructive laryngitis (J05.0)*
EXCLUDES 2 *chronic laryngitis (J37.0)*

√5th **J04.1 Acute tracheitis**
Acute viral tracheitis
Catarrhal tracheitis (acute)
Tracheitis (acute) NOS
EXCLUDES 2 *chronic tracheitis (J42)*

J04.10 Acute tracheitis without obstruction
J04.11 Acute tracheitis with obstruction MCC

J04.2 Acute laryngotracheitis
Laryngotracheitis NOS
Tracheitis (acute) with laryngitis (acute)
EXCLUDES 1 *acute obstructive laryngotracheitis (J05.0)*
EXCLUDES 2 *chronic laryngotracheitis (J37.1)*

√5th **J04.3 Supraglottitis, unspecified**

J04.30 Supraglottitis, unspecified, without obstruction
J04.31 Supraglottitis, unspecified, with obstruction MCC

√4th **J05 Acute obstructive laryngitis [croup] and epiglottitis**
▶Code also, if present, such as:◀
▶influenza due to identified novel influenza A virus with other respiratory manifestations (J09.X2)◀
▶influenza due to other identified influenza virus with other respiratory manifestations (J10.1)◀
▶influenza due to unidentified influenza virus with other respiratory manifestations (J11.1)◀
Use additional code (B95-B97) to identify infectious agent

J05.0 Acute obstructive laryngitis [croup]
Obstructive laryngitis (acute) NOS
Obstructive laryngotracheitis NOS
DEF: Acute laryngeal obstruction due to allergies, foreign bodies, or in the majority of cases a viral infection. Symptoms include a harsh, barking cough, hoarseness, and a persistent, high-pitched respiratory sound (stridor).

√5th **J05.1 Acute epiglottitis**
EXCLUDES 2 *epiglottitis, chronic (J37.0)*

J05.10 Acute epiglottitis without obstruction CC
Epiglottitis NOS
J05.11 Acute epiglottitis with obstruction MCC

√4th **J06 Acute upper respiratory infections of multiple and unspecified sites**
EXCLUDES 1 *acute respiratory infection NOS (J22)*
▶*influenza virus with other respiratory manifestations (J09.X2, J10.1, J11.1)*◀
streptococcal pharyngitis (J02.0)

J06.0 Acute laryngopharyngitis

J06.9 Acute upper respiratory infection, unspecified
Upper respiratory disease, acute
Upper respiratory infection NOS
Use additional code (B95-B97) to identify infectious agent, if known, such as:
respiratory syncytial virus (RSV) (B97.4)
AHA: 2020,1Q,22

Influenza and pneumonia (J09-J18)

EXCLUDES 2 *allergic or eosinophilic pneumonia (J82)*
aspiration pneumonia NOS (J69.0)
meconium pneumonia (P24.01)
neonatal aspiration pneumonia (P24.-)
pneumonia due to solids and liquids (J69.-)
congenital pneumonia (P23.9)
lipid pneumonia (J69.1)
rheumatic pneumonia (I00)
ventilator associated pneumonia (J95.851)

AHA: 2017,4Q,96
TIP: Assign J18.1 only when the provider specifically documents "lobar pneumonia" without specifying a causal organism. Lobar pneumonia may not be assumed based on an imaging report that identifies pneumonia in a specific lobe.
TIP: Documentation of lobar pneumonia or multilobar pneumonia should be coded to J18.1 when the specific organism causing the pneumonia is not identified. When the organism is documented, lobar pneumonia or multilobar pneumonia should be coded using categories J12-J16, depending on the organism that is present.
TIP: Hemoptysis (R04.2) is not customarily associated with pneumonia and may be reported separately.

√4th **J09 Influenza due to certain identified influenza viruses**
EXCLUDES 1 *influenza A/H1N1 (J10.-)*
influenza due to other identified influenza virus (J10.-)
influenza due to unidentified influenza virus (J11.-)
seasonal influenza due to other identified influenza virus (J10.-)
seasonal influenza due to unidentified influenza virus (J11.-)

√5th **J09.X Influenza due to identified novel influenza A virus**
Avian influenza
Bird influenza
Influenza A/H5N1
Influenza of other animal origin, not bird or swine
Swine influenza virus (viruses that normally cause infections in pigs)
AHA: 2016,3Q,10

J09.X1 Influenza due to identified novel influenza A virus with pneumonia HIV MCC
Code also, if applicable, associated:
lung abscess (J85.1)
other specified type of pneumonia

J09.X2 Influenza due to identified novel influenza A virus with other respiratory manifestations
Influenza due to identified novel influenza A virus NOS
Influenza due to identified novel influenza A virus with laryngitis
Influenza due to identified novel influenza A virus with pharyngitis
Influenza due to identified novel influenza A virus with upper respiratory symptoms
Use additional code, if applicable, for associated:
pleural effusion (J91.8)
sinusitis (J01.-)

J09.X3 Influenza due to identified novel influenza A virus with gastrointestinal manifestations
Influenza due to identified novel influenza A virus gastroenteritis
EXCLUDES 1 *'intestinal flu' [viral gastroenteritis] (A08.-)*

J09.X9 Influenza due to identified novel influenza A virus with other manifestations
Influenza due to identified novel influenza A virus with encephalopathy
Influenza due to identified novel influenza A virus with myocarditis
Influenza due to identified novel influenza A virus with otitis media
Use additional code to identify manifestation

J10 Influenza due to other identified influenza virus

INCLUDES ▶influenza A (non-novel)◀
▶influenza B◀
▶influenza C◀

EXCLUDES 1 *influenza due to avian influenza virus (J09.X-)*
influenza due to swine flu (J09.X-)
influenza due to unidentifed influenza virus (J11.-)

J10.0 Influenza due to other identified influenza virus with pneumonia
Code also associated lung abscess, if applicable (J85.1)

J10.00 Influenza due to other identified influenza virus with unspecified type of pneumonia MCC

J10.01 Influenza due to other identified influenza virus with the same other identified influenza virus pneumonia MCC

J10.08 Influenza due to other identified influenza virus with other specified pneumonia HIV MCC
Code also other specified type of pneumonia

J10.1 Influenza due to other identified influenza virus with other respiratory manifestations
Influenza due to other identified influenza virus NOS
Influenza due to other identified influenza virus with laryngitis
Influenza due to other identified influenza virus with pharyngitis
Influenza due to other identified influenza virus with upper respiratory symptoms
Use additional code for associated pleural effusion, if applicable (J91.8)
Use additional code for associated sinusitis, if applicable (J01.-)
AHA: 2016,3Q,10-11

J10.2 Influenza due to other identified influenza virus with gastrointestinal manifestations
Influenza due to other identified influenza virus gastroenteritis
EXCLUDES 1 *"intestinal flu" [viral gastroenteritis] (A08.-)*

J10.8 Influenza due to other identified influenza virus with other manifestations

J10.81 Influenza due to other identified influenza virus with encephalopathy

J10.82 Influenza due to other identified influenza virus with myocarditis

J10.83 Influenza due to other identified influenza virus with otitis media
Use additional code for any associated perforated tympanic membrane (H72.-)

J10.89 Influenza due to other identified influenza virus with other manifestations
Use additional codes to identify the manifestations

J11 Influenza due to unidentified influenza virus

J11.0 Influenza due to unidentified influenza virus with pneumonia
Code also associated lung abscess, if applicable (J85.1)
AHA: 2016,3Q,11

J11.00 Influenza due to unidentified influenza virus with unspecified type of pneumonia MCC
Influenza with pneumonia NOS

J11.08 Influenza due to unidentified influenza virus with specified pneumonia MCC
Code also other specified type of pneumonia

J11.1 Influenza due to unidentified influenza virus with other respiratory manifestations
Influenza NOS
Influenzal laryngitis NOS
Influenzal pharyngitis NOS
Influenza with upper respiratory symptoms NOS
Use additional code for associated pleural effusion, if applicable (J91.8)
Use additional code for associated sinusitis, if applicable (J01.-)

J11.2 Influenza due to unidentified influenza virus with gastrointestinal manifestations
Influenza gastroenteritis NOS
EXCLUDES 1 *"intestinal flu" [viral gastroenteritis] (A08.-)*

J11.8 Influenza due to unidentified influenza virus with other manifestations

J11.81 Influenza due to unidentified influenza virus with encephalopathy
Influenzal encephalopathy NOS

J11.82 Influenza due to unidentified influenza virus with myocarditis
Influenzal myocarditis NOS

J11.83 Influenza due to unidentified influenza virus with otitis media
Influenzal otitis media NOS
Use additional code for any associated perforated tympanic membrane (H72.-)

J11.89 Influenza due to unidentified influenza virus with other manifestations
Use additional codes to identify the manifestations

J12 Viral pneumonia, not elsewhere classified

INCLUDES bronchopneumonia due to viruses other than influenza viruses

Code first associated influenza, if applicable (J09.X1, J10.0-, J11.0-)
Code also associated abscess, if applicable (J85.1)

EXCLUDES 1 *aspiration pneumonia due to anesthesia during labor and delivery (O74.0)*
aspiration pneumonia due to anesthesia during pregnancy (O29)
aspiration pneumonia due to anesthesia during puerperium (O89.0)
aspiration pneumonia due to solids and liquids (J69.-)
aspiration pneumonia NOS (J69.0)
congenital pneumonia (P23.0)
congenital rubella pneumonitis (P35.0)
interstitial pneumonia NOS (J84.9)
lipid pneumonia (J69.1)
neonatal aspiration pneumonia (P24.-)

AHA: 2020,2Q,28; 2019,1Q,35; 2018,3Q,24; 2016,3Q,15; 2013,4Q,118

J12.0 Adenoviral pneumonia MCC

J12.1 Respiratory syncytial virus pneumonia MCC
RSV pneumonia

J12.2 Parainfluenza virus pneumonia MCC

J12.3 Human metapneumovirus pneumonia HIV MCC

J12.8 Other viral pneumonia

J12.81 Pneumonia due to SARS-associated coronavirus HIV MCC
Severe acute respiratory syndrome NOS
DEF: Severe adult respiratory syndrome caused by the coronavirus, specified as inflammation of the lungs with consolidation.

J12.89 Other viral pneumonia HIV MCC
AHA: 2020,2Q,8,11; 2020,1Q,34-36
TIP: For pneumonia confirmed as due to COVID-19, assign code U07.1 as the primary or first-listed diagnosis and J12.89 as a secondary diagnosis.

J12.9 Viral pneumonia, unspecified HIV MCC

J13 Pneumonia due to Streptococcus pneumoniae HIV MCC HCC
Bronchopneumonia due to S. pneumoniae
Code first associated influenza, if applicable (J09.X1, J10.0-, J11.0-)
Code also associated abscess, if applicable (J85.1)

EXCLUDES 1 *congenital pneumonia due to S. pneumoniae (P23.6)*
lobar pneumonia, unspecified organism (J18.1)
pneumonia due to other streptococci (J15.3-J15.4)

AHA: 2020,2Q,28; 2019,1Q,35; 2018,3Q,24; 2016,3Q,15; 2013,4Q,118

J14 Pneumonia due to Hemophilus influenzae HIV MCC HCC
Bronchopneumonia due to H. influenzae
Code first associated influenza, if applicable (J09.X1, J10.0-, J11.0-)
Code also associated abscess, if applicable (J85.1)
EXCLUDES 1 *congenital pneumonia due to H. influenzae (P23.6)*
AHA: 2020,2Q,28; 2019,1Q,35; 2018,3Q,24; 2016,3Q,15; 2013,4Q,118

J15 Bacterial pneumonia, not elsewhere classified

INCLUDES Bronchopneumonia due to bacteria other than S. pneumoniae and H. influenzae

Code first associated influenza, if applicable (J09.X1, J10.0-, -J11.0-)
Code also associated abscess, if applicable (J85.1)

EXCLUDES 1 *chlamydial pneumonia (J16.0)*
congenital pneumonia (P23.-)
Legionnaires' disease (A48.1)
spirochetal pneumonia (A69.8)

AHA: 2020,2Q,28; 2019,1Q,35; 2018,3Q,24; 2016,3Q,15; 2013,4Q,118

J15.0 Pneumonia due to Klebsiella pneumoniae HIV MCC HCC

J15.1 Pneumonia due to Pseudomonas HIV MCC HCC

J15.2 Pneumonia due to staphylococcus

J15.20 Pneumonia due to staphylococcus, unspecified HIV MCC HCC

✓6th **J15.21 Pneumonia due to Staphylococcus aureus**

J15.211 Pneumonia due to methicillin susceptible Staphylococcus aureus HIV MCC HCC
MSSA pneumonia
Pneumonia due to Staphylococcus aureus NOS

J15.212 Pneumonia due to methicillin resistant Staphylococcus aureus HIV MCC HCC

J15.29 Pneumonia due to other staphylococcus HIV MCC HCC

J15.3 Pneumonia due to streptococcus, group B HIV MCC HCC

J15.4 Pneumonia due to other streptococci HIV MCC HCC
EXCLUDES 1 *pneumonia due to streptococcus, group B (J15.3)*
pneumonia due to Streptococcus pneumoniae (J13)

J15.5 Pneumonia due to Escherichia coli HIV MCC HCC

J15.6 Pneumonia due to other Gram-negative bacteria HIV MCC HCC
Pneumonia due to other aerobic Gram-negative bacteria
Pneumonia due to Serratia marcescens
AHA: 2020,2Q,28

J15.7 Pneumonia due to Mycoplasma pneumoniae MCC

J15.8 Pneumonia due to other specified bacteria HIV MCC HCC

J15.9 Unspecified bacterial pneumonia HIV MCC
Pneumonia due to gram-positive bacteria

✓4th **J16 Pneumonia due to other infectious organisms, not elsewhere classified**
Code first associated influenza, if applicable (J09.X1, J10.0-, J11.0-)
Code also associated abscess, if applicable (J85.1)
EXCLUDES 1 *congenital pneumonia (P23.-)*
ornithosis (A70)
pneumocystosis (B59)
pneumonia NOS (J18.9)
AHA: 2020,2Q,28; 2019,1Q,35; 2018,3Q,24; 2016,3Q,15; 2013,4Q,118

J16.0 Chlamydial pneumonia MCC

J16.8 Pneumonia due to other specified infectious organisms MCC

J17 Pneumonia in diseases classified elsewhere MCC
Code first underlying disease, such as:
Q fever (A78)
rheumatic fever (I00)
schistosomiasis (B65.0-B65.9)
EXCLUDES 1 *candidial pneumonia (B37.1)*
chlamydial pneumonia (J16.0)
gonorrheal pneumonia (A54.84)
histoplasmosis pneumonia (B39.0-B39.2)
measles pneumonia (B05.2)
nocardiosis pneumonia (A43.0)
pneumocystosis (B59)
pneumonia due to Pneumocystis carinii (B59)
pneumonia due to Pneumocystis jiroveci (B59)
pneumonia in actinomycosis (A42.0)
pneumonia in anthrax (A22.1)
pneumonia in ascariasis (B77.81)
pneumonia in aspergillosis (B44.0-B44.1)
pneumonia in coccidioidomycosis (B38.0-B38.2)
pneumonia in cytomegalovirus disease (B25.0)
pneumonia in toxoplasmosis (B58.3)
rubella pneumonia (B06.81)
salmonella pneumonia (A02.22)
spirochetal infection NEC with pneumonia (A69.8)
tularemia pneumonia (A21.2)
typhoid fever with pneumonia (A01.03)
varicella pneumonia (B01.2)
whooping cough with pneumonia (A37 with fifth character 1)
AHA: 2020,2Q,28; 2019,1Q,35; 2016,3Q,15; 2013,4Q,118

✓4th **J18 Pneumonia, unspecified organism**
Code first associated influenza, if applicable (J09.X1, J10.0-, J11.0-)
EXCLUDES 1 *abscess of lung with pneumonia (J85.1)*
aspiration pneumonia due to anesthesia during labor and delivery (O74.0)
aspiration pneumonia due to anesthesia during pregnancy (O29)
aspiration pneumonia due to anesthesia during puerperium (O89.0)
aspiration pneumonia due to solids and liquids (J69.-)
aspiration pneumonia NOS (J69.0)
congenital pneumonia (P23.0)
drug-induced interstitial lung disorder (J70.2-J70.4)
interstitial pneumonia NOS (J84.9)
lipid pneumonia (J69.1)
neonatal aspiration pneumonia (P24.-)
pneumonitis due to external agents (J67-J70)
pneumonitis due to fumes and vapors (J68.0)
usual interstitial pneumonia ►(J84.178)◄
AHA: 2020,2Q,28; 2019,1Q,35; 2016,3Q,15; 2013,4Q,118

J18.0 Bronchopneumonia, unspecified organism MCC
EXCLUDES 1 *hypostatic bronchopneumonia (J18.2)*
lipid pneumonia (J69.1)
EXCLUDES 2 *acute bronchiolitis (J21.-)*
chronic bronchiolitis (J44.9)

J18.1 Lobar pneumonia, unspecified organism HIV MCC HCC
AHA: 2019,3Q,37; 2018,3Q,24
TIP: Assign J18.1 only when the provider specifically documents "lobar pneumonia" without specifying a causal organism. Lobar pneumonia may not be assumed based on an imaging report that identifies pneumonia in a specific lobe.
TIP: Use this code for documented lobar pneumonia or multilobar pneumonia when the causal organism is not identified. If the causal organism is identified, codes from categories J12-J16 should be used, depending on the organism that is present.

J18.2 Hypostatic pneumonia, unspecified organism CC
Hypostatic bronchopneumonia
Passive pneumonia

J18.8 Other pneumonia, unspecified organism HIV MCC

J18.9 Pneumonia, unspecified organism HIV MCC
AHA: 2020,2Q,28; 2019,3Q,15; 2019,2Q,28; 2014,3Q,4; 2013,4Q,119; 2012,4Q,94

Other acute lower respiratory infections (J20-J22)

EXCLUDES 2 *chronic obstructive pulmonary disease with acute lower respiratory infection (J44.0)*

✓4th **J20 Acute bronchitis**
INCLUDES acute and subacute bronchitis (with) bronchospasm
acute and subacute bronchitis (with) tracheitis
acute and subacute bronchitis (with) tracheobronchitis, acute
acute and subacute fibrinous bronchitis
acute and subacute membranous bronchitis
acute and subacute purulent bronchitis
acute and subacute septic bronchitis
EXCLUDES 1 *bronchitis NOS (J40)*
tracheobronchitis NOS (J40)
EXCLUDES 2 *acute bronchitis with bronchiectasis (J47.0)*
acute bronchitis with chronic obstructive asthma (J44.0)
acute bronchitis with chronic obstructive pulmonary disease (J44.0)
allergic bronchitis NOS (J45.909-)
bronchitis due to chemicals, fumes and vapors (J68.0)
chronic bronchitis NOS (J42)
chronic mucopurulent bronchitis (J41.1)
chronic obstructive bronchitis (J44.-)
chronic obstructive tracheobronchitis (J44.-)
chronic simple bronchitis (J41.0)
chronic tracheobronchitis (J42)
AHA: 2019,1Q,35; 2016,3Q,10,16
DEF: Acute inflammation of the main branches of the bronchial tree due to infectious or irritant agents. Symptoms include cough with a varied production of sputum, fever, substernal soreness, and lung rales. Bronchitis usually lasts three to 10 days.

J20.0 Acute bronchitis due to Mycoplasma pneumoniae

J20.1 Acute bronchitis due to Hemophilus influenzae

J2Ø.2 Acute bronchitis due to streptococcus

J2Ø.3 Acute bronchitis due to coxsackievirus

J2Ø.4 Acute bronchitis due to parainfluenza virus

J2Ø.5 Acute bronchitis due to respiratory syncytial virus
Acute bronchitis due to RSV

J2Ø.6 Acute bronchitis due to rhinovirus

J2Ø.7 Acute bronchitis due to echovirus

J2Ø.8 Acute bronchitis due to other specified organisms
AHA: 2020,1Q,34-36
TIP: Assign as a secondary code for a patient with acute bronchitis confirmed as due to COVID-19; assign U07.1 as the principal or first-listed code.

J2Ø.9 Acute bronchitis, unspecified

✓4th J21 Acute bronchiolitis
INCLUDES acute bronchiolitis with bronchospasm
EXCLUDES 2 *respiratory bronchiolitis interstitial lung disease (J84.115)*

J21.Ø Acute bronchiolitis due to respiratory syncytial virus CC
Acute bronchiolitis due to RSV

J21.1 Acute bronchiolitis due to human metapneumovirus CC

J21.8 Acute bronchiolitis due to other specified organisms CC

J21.9 Acute bronchiolitis, unspecified CC
Bronchiolitis (acute)
EXCLUDES 1 *chronic bronchiolitis (J44.-)*

J22 Unspecified acute lower respiratory infection
Acute (lower) respiratory (tract) infection NOS
EXCLUDES 1 *upper respiratory infection (acute) (JØ6.9)*
AHA: 2020,1Q,22,34-36
TIP: Assign as a secondary code for a patient with a respiratory infection specified as acute or lower that is documented as being associated with COVID-19; assign U07.1 as the principal or first-listed code. If the respiratory infection documentation does not specify acute or lower, assign J98.8.

Other diseases of upper respiratory tract (J3Ø-J39)

✓4th J3Ø Vasomotor and allergic rhinitis
INCLUDES spasmodic rhinorrhea
EXCLUDES 1 *allergic rhinitis with asthma (bronchial) (J45.9Ø9)*
rhinitis NOS (J31.Ø)

J3Ø.Ø Vasomotor rhinitis
DEF: Noninfectious and nonallergic type of rhinitis for which the cause is often unknown. Symptoms often mimic those of allergic rhinitis with a diagnosis of vasomotor rhinitis typically made after ruling out allergens as the cause.

J3Ø.1 Allergic rhinitis due to pollen
Allergy NOS due to pollen
Hay fever
Pollinosis

J3Ø.2 Other seasonal allergic rhinitis

J3Ø.5 Allergic rhinitis due to food

✓5th J3Ø.8 Other allergic rhinitis

J3Ø.81 Allergic rhinitis due to animal (cat) (dog) hair and dander

J3Ø.89 Other allergic rhinitis
Perennial allergic rhinitis

J3Ø.9 Allergic rhinitis, unspecified

✓4th J31 Chronic rhinitis, nasopharyngitis and pharyngitis
Use additional code to identify:
exposure to environmental tobacco smoke (Z77.22)
exposure to tobacco smoke in the perinatal period (P96.81)
history of tobacco dependence (Z87.891)
occupational exposure to environmental tobacco smoke (Z57.31)
tobacco dependence (F17.-)
tobacco use (Z72.Ø)

J31.Ø Chronic rhinitis
Atrophic rhinitis (chronic)
Granulomatous rhinitis (chronic)
Hypertrophic rhinitis (chronic)
Obstructive rhinitis (chronic)
Ozena
Purulent rhinitis (chronic)
Rhinitis (chronic) NOS
Ulcerative rhinitis (chronic)
EXCLUDES 1 *allergic rhinitis (J3Ø.1-J3Ø.9)*
vasomotor rhinitis (J3Ø.Ø)
DEF: Persistent inflammation of the mucous membranes of the nose, characterized by a postnasal drip.

J31.1 Chronic nasopharyngitis
EXCLUDES 2 *acute nasopharyngitis (JØØ)*
DEF: Persistent inflammation of the mucous membranes extending from the nares to the pharynx. It is characterized by constant irritation in the nasopharynx and postnasal drip.

J31.2 Chronic pharyngitis
Atrophic pharyngitis (chronic)
Chronic sore throat
Granular pharyngitis (chronic)
Hypertrophic pharyngitis (chronic)
EXCLUDES 2 *acute pharyngitis (JØ2.9)*

✓4th J32 Chronic sinusitis
INCLUDES sinus abscess
sinus empyema
sinus infection
sinus suppuration
Use additional code to identify:
exposure to environmental tobacco smoke (Z77.22)
exposure to tobacco smoke in the perinatal period (P96.81)
history of tobacco dependence (Z87.891)
infectious agent (B95-B97)
occupational exposure to environmental tobacco smoke (Z57.31)
tobacco dependence (F17.-)
tobacco use (Z72.Ø)
EXCLUDES 2 *acute sinusitis (JØ1.-)*

J32.Ø Chronic maxillary sinusitis
Antritis (chronic)
Maxillary sinusitis NOS

J32.1 Chronic frontal sinusitis
Frontal sinusitis NOS

J32.2 Chronic ethmoidal sinusitis
Ethmoidal sinusitis NOS
EXCLUDES 1 *Woakes' ethmoiditis (J33.1)*

J32.3 Chronic sphenoidal sinusitis
Sphenoidal sinusitis NOS

J32.4 Chronic pansinusitis
Pansinusitis NOS

J32.8 Other chronic sinusitis
Sinusitis (chronic) involving more than one sinus but not pansinusitis

J32.9 Chronic sinusitis, unspecified
Sinusitis (chronic) NOS

✓4th J33 Nasal polyp
Use additional code to identify:
exposure to environmental tobacco smoke (Z77.22)
exposure to tobacco smoke in the perinatal period (P96.81)
history of tobacco dependence (Z87.891)
occupational exposure to environmental tobacco smoke (Z57.31)
tobacco dependence (F17.-)
tobacco use (Z72.Ø)
EXCLUDES 1 *adenomatous polyps (D14.Ø)*

J33.Ø Polyp of nasal cavity
Choanal polyp
Nasopharyngeal polyp

J33.1 Polypoid sinus degeneration
Woakes' syndrome or ethmoiditis

J33.8 Other polyp of sinus
Accessory polyp of sinus
Ethmoidal polyp of sinus
Maxillary polyp of sinus
Sphenoidal polyp of sinus

J33.9 Nasal polyp, unspecified

✓4th J34 Other and unspecified disorders of nose and nasal sinuses
EXCLUDES 2 *varicose ulcer of nasal septum (I86.8)*

J34.Ø Abscess, furuncle and carbuncle of nose
Cellulitis of nose
Necrosis of nose
Ulceration of nose

J34.1 Cyst and mucocele of nose and nasal sinus

J34.2 Deviated nasal septum
Deflection or deviation of septum (nasal) (acquired)
EXCLUDES 1 *congenital deviated nasal septum (Q67.4)*
DEF: Condition in which the nasal septum, a thin wall composed of cartilage and bone that separates the two nostrils, is crooked or displaced from the midline.

J34.3 Hypertrophy of nasal turbinates
DEF: Overgrowth of bones within the nasal turbinate, which are ridges of bone and soft tissue that project from the sidewalls of the nasal passages. Hypertrophy can cause obstruction of the nasal passages.

✓5th **J34.8 Other specified disorders of nose and nasal sinuses**

J34.81 Nasal mucositis (ulcerative)
Code also type of associated therapy, such as:
antineoplastic and immunosuppressive drugs (T45.1X-)
radiological procedure and radiotherapy (Y84.2)
EXCLUDES 2 *gastrointestinal mucositis (ulcerative) (K92.81)*
mucositis (ulcerative) of vagina and vulva (N76.81)
oral mucositis (ulcerative) (K12.3-)

J34.89 Other specified disorders of nose and nasal sinuses
Perforation of nasal septum NOS
Rhinolith

J34.9 Unspecified disorder of nose and nasal sinuses

✓4th **J35 Chronic diseases of tonsils and adenoids**
Use additional code to identify:
exposure to environmental tobacco smoke (Z77.22)
exposure to tobacco smoke in the perinatal period (P96.81)
history of tobacco dependence (Z87.891)
occupational exposure to environmental tobacco smoke (Z57.31)
tobacco dependence (F17.-)
tobacco use (Z72.Ø)

✓5th **J35.Ø Chronic tonsillitis and adenoiditis**
EXCLUDES 2 *acute tonsillitis (JØ3.-)*

J35.Ø1 Chronic tonsillitis
J35.Ø2 Chronic adenoiditis
J35.Ø3 Chronic tonsillitis and adenoiditis

J35.1 Hypertrophy of tonsils
Enlargement of tonsils
EXCLUDES 1 *hypertrophy of tonsils with tonsillitis (J35.Ø-)*

J35.2 Hypertrophy of adenoids
Enlargement of adenoids
EXCLUDES 1 *hypertrophy of adenoids with adenoiditis (J35.Ø-)*

J35.3 Hypertrophy of tonsils with hypertrophy of adenoids
EXCLUDES 1 *hypertrophy of tonsils and adenoids with tonsillitis and adenoiditis (J35.Ø3)*

J35.8 Other chronic diseases of tonsils and adenoids
Adenoid vegetations
Amygdalolith
Calculus, tonsil
Cicatrix of tonsil (and adenoid)
Tonsillar tag
Ulcer of tonsil

J35.9 Chronic disease of tonsils and adenoids, unspecified
Disease (chronic) of tonsils and adenoids NOS

J36 Peritonsillar abscess CC
INCLUDES abscess of tonsil
peritonsillar cellulitis
quinsy
Use additional code (B95-B97) to identify infectious agent
EXCLUDES 1 *acute tonsillitis (JØ3.-)*
chronic tonsillitis (J35.Ø)
retropharyngeal abscess (J39.Ø)
tonsillitis NOS (JØ3.9-)

✓4th **J37 Chronic laryngitis and laryngotracheitis**
Use additional code to identify:
exposure to environmental tobacco smoke (Z77.22)
exposure to tobacco smoke in the perinatal period (P96.81)
history of tobacco dependence (Z87.891)
infectious agent (B95-B97)
occupational exposure to environmental tobacco smoke (Z57.31)
tobacco dependence (F17.-)
tobacco use (Z72.Ø)

J37.Ø Chronic laryngitis
Catarrhal laryngitis
Hypertrophic laryngitis
Sicca laryngitis
EXCLUDES 2 *acute laryngitis (JØ4.Ø)*
obstructive (acute) laryngitis (JØ5.Ø)

J37.1 Chronic laryngotracheitis
Laryngitis, chronic, with tracheitis (chronic)
Tracheitis, chronic, with laryngitis
EXCLUDES 1 *chronic tracheitis (J42)*
EXCLUDES 2 *acute laryngotracheitis (JØ4.2)*
acute tracheitis (JØ4.1)

✓4th **J38 Diseases of vocal cords and larynx, not elsewhere classified**
Use additional code to identify:
exposure to environmental tobacco smoke (Z77.22)
exposure to tobacco smoke in the perinatal period (P96.81)
history of tobacco dependence (Z87.891)
occupational exposure to environmental tobacco smoke (Z57.31)
tobacco dependence (F17.-)
tobacco use (Z72.Ø)
EXCLUDES 1 *congenital laryngeal stridor (P28.89)*
obstructive laryngitis (acute) (JØ5.Ø)
postprocedural subglottic stenosis (J95.5)
stridor (RØ6.1)
ulcerative laryngitis (JØ4.Ø)

✓5th **J38.Ø Paralysis of vocal cords and larynx**
Laryngoplegia
Paralysis of glottis

J38.ØØ Paralysis of vocal cords and larynx, unspecified
J38.Ø1 Paralysis of vocal cords and larynx, unilateral
J38.Ø2 Paralysis of vocal cords and larynx, bilateral

J38.1 Polyp of vocal cord and larynx
EXCLUDES 1 *adenomatous polyps (D14.1)*

J38.2 Nodules of vocal cords
Chorditis (fibrinous)(nodosa)(tuberosa)
Singer's nodes
Teacher's nodes

J38.3 Other diseases of vocal cords
Abscess of vocal cords
Cellulitis of vocal cords
Granuloma of vocal cords
Leukokeratosis of vocal cords
Leukoplakia of vocal cords

J38.4 Edema of larynx
Edema (of) glottis
Subglottic edema
Supraglottic edema
EXCLUDES 1 *acute obstructive laryngitis [croup] (JØ5.Ø)*
edematous laryngitis (JØ4.Ø)

J38.5 Laryngeal spasm
Laryngismus (stridulus)

J38.6 Stenosis of larynx

J38.7 Other diseases of larynx
Abscess of larynx
Cellulitis of larynx
Disease of larynx NOS
Necrosis of larynx
Pachyderma of larynx
Perichondritis of larynx
Ulcer of larynx

✓4th **J39 Other diseases of upper respiratory tract**
EXCLUDES 1 *acute respiratory infection NOS (J22)*
acute upper respiratory infection (JØ6.9)
upper respiratory inflammation due to chemicals, gases, fumes or vapors (J68.2)

J39.Ø Retropharyngeal and parapharyngeal abscess CC
Peripharyngeal abscess
EXCLUDES 1 *peritonsillar abscess (J36)*
DEF: Purulent infection behind the pharynx and the front of the precerebral fascia, characterized by neck stiffness, cervical lymphadenopathy, sore throat, fever, and stridor.

J39.1 Other abscess of pharynx CC
Cellulitis of pharynx
Nasopharyngeal abscess

J39.2 Other diseases of pharynx
Cyst of pharynx
Edema of pharynx
EXCLUDES 2 *chronic pharyngitis (J31.2)*
ulcerative pharyngitis (JØ2.9)

J39.3 Upper respiratory tract hypersensitivity reaction, site unspecified

EXCLUDES 1 *hypersensitivity reaction of upper respiratory tract, such as:*
extrinsic allergic alveolitis (J67.9)
pneumoconiosis (J6Ø-J67.9)

J39.8 Other specified diseases of upper respiratory tract

J39.9 Disease of upper respiratory tract, unspecified

Chronic lower respiratory diseases (J4Ø-J47)

EXCLUDES 1 *bronchitis due to chemicals, gases, fumes and vapors (J68.Ø)*
EXCLUDES 2 *cystic fibrosis (E84.-)*

J4Ø Bronchitis, not specified as acute or chronic
Bronchitis NOS
Bronchitis with tracheitis NOS
Catarrhal bronchitis
Tracheobronchitis NOS
Use additional code to identify:
exposure to environmental tobacco smoke (Z77.22)
exposure to tobacco smoke in the perinatal period (P96.81)
history of tobacco dependence (Z87.891)
occupational exposure to environmental tobacco smoke (Z57.31)
tobacco dependence (F17.-)
tobacco use (Z72.Ø)

EXCLUDES 1 *acute bronchitis (J2Ø.-)*
allergic bronchitis NOS (J45.9Ø9-)
asthmatic bronchitis NOS (J45.9-)
bronchitis due to chemicals, gases, fumes and vapors (J68.Ø)

AHA: 2020,1Q,34-36
TIP: Assign as a secondary code for a patient with bronchitis of unspecified acuity due to COVID-19; assign U07.1 as the principal or first-listed code.

✓4th **J41 Simple and mucopurulent chronic bronchitis**
Use additional code to identify:
exposure to environmental tobacco smoke (Z77.22)
exposure to tobacco smoke in the perinatal period (P96.81)
history of tobacco dependence (Z87.891)
occupational exposure to environmental tobacco smoke (Z57.31)
tobacco dependence (F17.-)
tobacco use (Z72.Ø)

EXCLUDES 1 *chronic bronchitis NOS (J42)*
chronic obstructive bronchitis (J44.-)

J41.Ø Simple chronic bronchitis HCC
J41.1 Mucopurulent chronic bronchitis HCC
J41.8 Mixed simple and mucopurulent chronic bronchitis HCC

J42 Unspecified chronic bronchitis HCC
Chronic bronchitis NOS
Chronic tracheitis
Chronic tracheobronchitis
Use additional code to identify:
exposure to environmental tobacco smoke (Z77.22)
exposure to tobacco smoke in the perinatal period (P96.81)
history of tobacco dependence (Z87.891)
occupational exposure to environmental tobacco smoke (Z57.31)
tobacco dependence (F17.-)
tobacco use (Z72.Ø)

EXCLUDES 1 *chronic asthmatic bronchitis (J44.-)*
chronic bronchitis with airways obstruction (J44.-)
chronic emphysematous bronchitis (J44.-)
chronic obstructive pulmonary disease NOS (J44.9)
simple and mucopurulent chronic bronchitis (J41.-)

✓4th **J43 Emphysema**
Use additional code to identify:
exposure to environmental tobacco smoke (Z77.22)
history of tobacco dependence (Z87.891)
occupational exposure to environmental tobacco smoke (Z57.31)
tobacco dependence (F17.-)
tobacco use (Z72.Ø)

EXCLUDES 1 *compensatory emphysema (J98.3)*
emphysema due to inhalation of chemicals, gases, fumes or vapors (J68.4)
emphysema with chronic (obstructive) bronchitis (J44.-)
emphysematous (obstructive) bronchitis (J44.-)
interstitial emphysema (J98.2)
mediastinal emphysema (J98.2)
neonatal interstitial emphysema (P25.Ø)
surgical (subcutaneous) emphysema (T81.82)
~~*traumatic subcutaneous emphysema (T79.7)*~~

EXCLUDES 2 ▶*traumatic subcutaneous emphysema (T79.7)*◀

DEF: Pathological condition in which there is destructive enlargement of the air sacs in the lungs resulting in damage and lack of elasticity to the alveolar walls, commonly seen in long-term smokers.

Emphysema

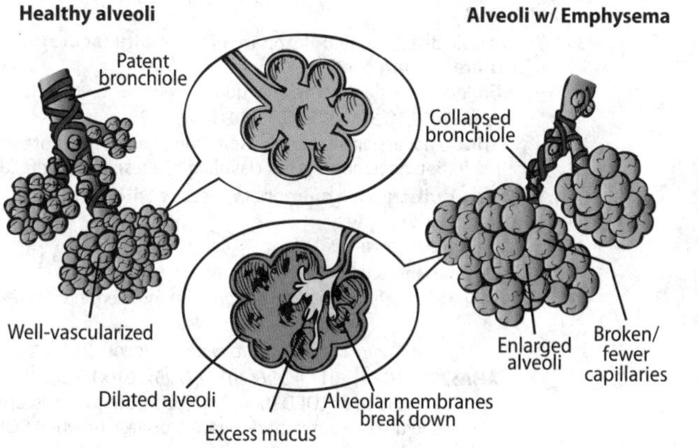

J43.Ø Unilateral pulmonary emphysema [MacLeod's syndrome] HCC
Swyer-James syndrome
Unilateral emphysema
Unilateral hyperlucent lung
Unilateral pulmonary artery functional hypoplasia
Unilateral transparency of lung

J43.1 Panlobular emphysema HCC
Panacinar emphysema

J43.2 Centrilobular emphysema HCC

J43.8 Other emphysema HCC

J43.9 Emphysema, unspecified HCC
Bullous emphysema (lung)(pulmonary)
Emphysema (lung)(pulmonary) NOS
Emphysematous bleb
Vesicular emphysema (lung)(pulmonary)
AHA: 2019,1Q,34-36; 2017,4Q,97-98

√4th J44 Other chronic obstructive pulmonary disease

INCLUDES asthma with chronic obstructive pulmonary disease
chronic asthmatic (obstructive) bronchitis
chronic bronchitis with airways obstruction
chronic bronchitis with emphysema
chronic emphysematous bronchitis
chronic obstructive asthma
chronic obstructive bronchitis
chronic obstructive tracheobronchitis

Code also type of asthma, if applicable (J45.-)

Use additional code to identify:
exposure to environmental tobacco smoke (Z77.22)
history of tobacco dependence (Z87.891)
occupational exposure to environmental tobacco smoke (Z57.31)
tobacco dependence (F17.-)
tobacco use (Z72.Ø)

EXCLUDES 1 *bronchiectasis (J47.-)*
chronic bronchitis NOS (J42)
chronic simple and mucopurulent bronchitis (J41.-)
chronic tracheitis (J42)
chronic tracheobronchitis (J42)
emphysema without chronic bronchitis (J43.-)

AHA: 2019,1Q,34-36; 2017,4Q,97-98; 2017,1Q,25-26; 2016,3Q,15-16; 2013,4Q,109

J44.Ø Chronic obstructive pulmonary disease with (acute) lower respiratory infection CC HCC
Code also to identify the infection
AHA: 2019,1Q,35; 2017,4Q,96; 2017,1Q,24-25
TIP: Do not assign when only aspiration pneumonia is present. Aspiration pneumonia is not classified as a respiratory infection.

J44.1 Chronic obstructive pulmonary disease with (acute) exacerbation CC HCC
Decompensated COPD
Decompensated COPD with (acute) exacerbation
EXCLUDES 2 *chronic obstructive pulmonary disease [COPD] with acute bronchitis (J44.Ø)*
lung diseases due to external agents (J6Ø-J7Ø)
AHA: 2019,1Q,34; 2017,4Q,96; 2017,1Q,26; 2016,1Q,36
TIP: Exacerbation of COPD should not be assumed based upon worsening of a concomitant respiratory disease or when COPD is described as end-stage.

J44.9 Chronic obstructive pulmonary disease, unspecified HCC
Chronic obstructive airway disease NOS
Chronic obstructive lung disease NOS
EXCLUDES 2 *lung diseases due to external agents (J6Ø-J7Ø)*
AHA: 2019,1Q,36; 2017,4Q,96-97; 2016,1Q,36; 2014,4Q,21; 2013,4Q,109

√4th J45 Asthma

INCLUDES allergic (predominantly) asthma
allergic bronchitis NOS
allergic rhinitis with asthma
atopic asthma
extrinsic allergic asthma
hay fever with asthma
idiosyncratic asthma
intrinsic nonallergic asthma
nonallergic asthma

Use additional code to identify:
▶eosinophilic asthma (J82.83) ◀
exposure to environmental tobacco smoke (Z77.22)
exposure to tobacco smoke in the perinatal period (P96.81)
history of tobacco dependence (Z87.891)
occupational exposure to environmental tobacco smoke (Z57.31)
tobacco dependence (F17.-)
tobacco use (Z72.Ø)

EXCLUDES 1 *detergent asthma (J69.8)*
eosinophilic asthma (J82)
miner's asthma (J6Ø)
wheezing NOS (RØ6.2)
wood asthma (J67.8)

EXCLUDES 2 *asthma with chronic obstructive pulmonary disease (J44.9)*
chronic asthmatic (obstructive) bronchitis (J44.9)
chronic obstructive asthma (J44.9)

AHA: 2019,1Q,36; 2017,1Q,25-26; 2012,4Q,99
DEF: Status asthmaticus: Severe, intractable episode of asthma that is unresponsive to normal therapeutic measures.

Asthma

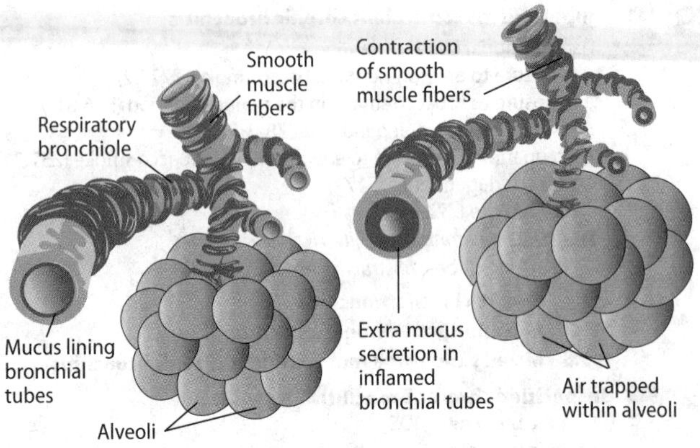

√5th J45.2 Mild intermittent asthma

J45.2Ø Mild intermittent asthma, uncomplicated
Mild intermittent asthma NOS

J45.21 Mild intermittent asthma with (acute) exacerbation CC

J45.22 Mild intermittent asthma with status asthmaticus CC

√5th J45.3 Mild persistent asthma

J45.3Ø Mild persistent asthma, uncomplicated
Mild persistent asthma NOS

J45.31 Mild persistent asthma with (acute) exacerbation CC
AHA: 2016,1Q,35

J45.32 Mild persistent asthma with status asthmaticus CC

√5th J45.4 Moderate persistent asthma

J45.4Ø Moderate persistent asthma, uncomplicated
Moderate persistent asthma NOS

J45.41 Moderate persistent asthma with (acute) exacerbation CC
AHA: 2017,1Q,26

J45.42 Moderate persistent asthma with status asthmaticus CC

✓5th **J45.5 Severe persistent asthma**

J45.50 Severe persistent asthma, uncomplicated
Severe persistent asthma NOS

J45.51 Severe persistent asthma with (acute) exacerbation CC

J45.52 Severe persistent asthma with status asthmaticus CC

✓5th **J45.9 Other and unspecified asthma**

✓6th **J45.90 Unspecified asthma**
Asthmatic bronchitis NOS
Childhood asthma NOS
Late onset asthma
AHA: 2017,4Q,96; 2017,1Q,25

J45.901 Unspecified asthma with (acute) exacerbation CC

J45.902 Unspecified asthma with status asthmaticus CC

J45.909 Unspecified asthma, uncomplicated
Asthma NOS
EXCLUDES 2 *lung diseases due to external agents (J60-J70)*
AHA: 2017,1Q,25

✓6th **J45.99 Other asthma**

J45.990 Exercise induced bronchospasm

J45.991 Cough variant asthma

J45.998 Other asthma

✓4th **J47 Bronchiectasis**

INCLUDES bronchiolectasis

Use additional code to identify:
exposure to environmental tobacco smoke (Z77.22)
exposure to tobacco smoke in the perinatal period (P96.81)
history of tobacco dependence (Z87.891)
occupational exposure to environmental tobacco smoke (Z57.31)
tobacco dependence (F17.-)
tobacco use (Z72.0)

EXCLUDES 1 *congenital bronchiectasis (Q33.4)*
tuberculous bronchiectasis (current disease) (A15.0)

DEF: Dilation of the bronchi with mucus production and persistent cough due to infection or chronic conditions that causes diminished lung capacity and frequent infections of the lung.

J47.0 Bronchiectasis with acute lower respiratory infection CC HCC
Bronchiectasis with acute bronchitis
Use additional code to identify the infection

J47.1 Bronchiectasis with (acute) exacerbation CC HCC

J47.9 Bronchiectasis, uncomplicated HCC
Bronchiectasis NOS

Lung diseases due to external agents (J60-J70)

EXCLUDES 2 *asthma (J45.-)*
malignant neoplasm of bronchus and lung (C34.-)

DEF: Pneumoconiosis: Condition caused by inhaling inorganic dust particles, typically associated with occupations that require regular exposure to mineral dusts. A form of interstitial lung disease that contributes to the inflammation of the air sacs, causing the lung tissue to harden.

J60 Coalworker's pneumoconiosis HCC A
Anthracosilicosis
Anthracosis
Black lung disease
Coalworker's lung
EXCLUDES 1 *coalworker pneumoconiosis with tuberculosis, any type in A15 (J65)*

J61 Pneumoconiosis due to asbestos and other mineral fibers HCC A
Asbestosis
EXCLUDES 1 *pleural plaque with asbestosis (J92.0)*
pneumoconiosis with tuberculosis, any type in A15 (J65)

✓4th **J62 Pneumoconiosis due to dust containing silica**

INCLUDES silicotic fibrosis (massive) of lung
EXCLUDES 1 *pneumoconiosis with tuberculosis, any type in A15 (J65)*

J62.0 Pneumoconiosis due to talc dust HCC

J62.8 Pneumoconiosis due to other dust containing silica HCC
Silicosis NOS

✓4th **J63 Pneumoconiosis due to other inorganic dusts**

EXCLUDES 1 *pneumoconiosis with tuberculosis, any type in A15 (J65)*

J63.0 Aluminosis (of lung) HCC

J63.1 Bauxite fibrosis (of lung) HCC

J63.2 Berylliosis HCC

J63.3 Graphite fibrosis (of lung) HCC

J63.4 Siderosis HCC
AHA: 2019,3Q,8

J63.5 Stannosis HCC

J63.6 Pneumoconiosis due to other specified inorganic dusts HCC

J64 Unspecified pneumoconiosis HCC
EXCLUDES 1 *pneumonoconiosis with tuberculosis, any type in A15 (J65)*

J65 Pneumoconiosis associated with tuberculosis HCC
Any condition in J60-J64 with tuberculosis, any type in A15
Silicotuberculosis

✓4th **J66 Airway disease due to specific organic dust**

EXCLUDES 2 *allergic alveolitis (J67.-)*
asbestosis (J61)
bagassosis (J67.1)
farmer's lung (J67.0)
hypersensitivity pneumonitis due to organic dust (J67.-)
reactive airways dysfunction syndrome (J68.3)

J66.0 Byssinosis HCC
Airway disease due to cotton dust

J66.1 Flax-dressers' disease HCC

J66.2 Cannabinosis HCC

J66.8 Airway disease due to other specific organic dusts HCC

✓4th **J67 Hypersensitivity pneumonitis due to organic dust**

INCLUDES allergic alveolitis and pneumonitis due to inhaled organic dust and particles of fungal, actinomycetic or other origin
EXCLUDES 1 *pneumonitis due to inhalation of chemicals, gases, fumes or vapors (J68.0)*

J67.0 Farmer's lung HCC
Harvester's lung
Haymaker's lung
Moldy hay disease

J67.1 Bagassosis HCC
Bagasse disease
Bagasse pneumonitis

J67.2 Bird fancier's lung HCC
Budgerigar fancier's disease or lung
Pigeon fancier's disease or lung

J67.3 Suberosis HCC
Corkhandler's disease or lung
Corkworker's disease or lung

J67.4 Maltworker's lung HCC
Alveolitis due to Aspergillus clavatus

J67.5 Mushroom-worker's lung HCC

J67.6 Maple-bark-stripper's lung HCC
Alveolitis due to Cryptostroma corticale
Cryptostromosis

J67.7 Air conditioner and humidifier lung CC HCC
Allergic alveolitis due to fungal, thermophilic actinomycetes and other organisms growing in ventilation [air conditioning] systems

J67.8 Hypersensitivity pneumonitis due to other organic dusts CC HCC
Cheese-washer's lung
Coffee-worker's lung
Fish-meal worker's lung
Furrier's lung
Sequoiosis

J67.9 Hypersensitivity pneumonitis due to unspecified organic dust CC HCC
Allergic alveolitis (extrinsic) NOS
Hypersensitivity pneumonitis NOS

Chapter 10. Diseases of the Respiratory System

J45.5–J67.9

J68 Respiratory conditions due to inhalation of chemicals, gases, fumes and vapors
Code first (T51-T65) to identify cause
Use additional code to identify associated respiratory conditions, such as:
acute respiratory failure (J96.Ø-)

J68.Ø Bronchitis and pneumonitis due to chemicals, gases, fumes and vapors CC HCC
Chemical bronchitis (acute)
AHA: 2019,2Q,31

J68.1 Pulmonary edema due to chemicals, gases, fumes and vapors MCC HCC
Chemical pulmonary edema (acute) (chronic)
EXCLUDES 1 *pulmonary edema (acute) (chronic) NOS (J81.-)*

J68.2 Upper respiratory inflammation due to chemicals, gases, fumes and vapors, not elsewhere classified HCC

J68.3 Other acute and subacute respiratory conditions due to chemicals, gases, fumes and vapors HCC
Reactive airways dysfunction syndrome

J68.4 Chronic respiratory conditions due to chemicals, gases, fumes and vapors HCC
Emphysema (diffuse) (chronic) due to inhalation of chemicals, gases, fumes and vapors
Obliterative bronchiolitis (chronic) (subacute) due to inhalation of chemicals, gases, fumes and vapors
Pulmonary fibrosis (chronic) due to inhalation of chemicals, gases, fumes and vapors
EXCLUDES 1 *chronic pulmonary edema due to chemicals, gases, fumes and vapors (J68.1)*

J68.8 Other respiratory conditions due to chemicals, gases, fumes and vapors HCC

J68.9 Unspecified respiratory condition due to chemicals, gases, fumes and vapors HCC

J69 Pneumonitis due to solids and liquids
EXCLUDES 1 *neonatal aspiration syndromes (P24.-)*
postprocedural pneumonitis (J95.4)
AHA: 2017,1Q,24
DEF: Pneumonitis: Noninfectious inflammation of the walls of the alveoli in the lung tissue due to inhalation of food, vomit, oils, essences, or other solids or liquids.

J69.Ø Pneumonitis due to inhalation of food and vomit MCC HCC
Aspiration pneumonia NOS
Aspiration pneumonia (due to) food (regurgitated)
Aspiration pneumonia (due to) gastric secretions
Aspiration pneumonia (due to) milk
Aspiration pneumonia (due to) vomit
Code also any associated foreign body in respiratory tract (T17.-)
EXCLUDES 1 *chemical pneumonitis due to anesthesia (J95.4)*
obstetric aspiration pneumonitis (O74.Ø)
AHA: 2020,2Q,11,28; 2019,3Q,17; 2019,2Q,6,31

J69.1 Pneumonitis due to inhalation of oils and essences MCC HCC
Exogenous lipoid pneumonia
Lipid pneumonia NOS
Code first (T51-T65) to identify substance
EXCLUDES 1 *endogenous lipoid pneumonia (J84.89)*

J69.8 Pneumonitis due to inhalation of other solids and liquids MCC HCC
Pneumonitis due to aspiration of blood
Pneumonitis due to aspiration of detergent
Code first (T51-T65) to identify substance

J7Ø Respiratory conditions due to other external agents

J7Ø.Ø Acute pulmonary manifestations due to radiation CC HCC
Radiation pneumonitis
Use additional code (W88-W9Ø, X39.Ø-) to identify the external cause

J7Ø.1 Chronic and other pulmonary manifestations due to radiation CC HCC
Fibrosis of lung following radiation
Use additional code (W88-W9Ø, X39.Ø-) to identify the external cause

J7Ø.2 Acute drug-induced interstitial lung disorders HCC
Use additional code for adverse effect, if applicable, to identify drug (T36-T5Ø with fifth or sixth character 5)
EXCLUDES 1 *interstitial pneumonia NOS (J84.9)*
lymphoid interstitial pneumonia (J84.2)
AHA: 2019,2Q,28

J7Ø.3 Chronic drug-induced interstitial lung disorders HCC
Use additional code for adverse effect, if applicable, to identify drug (T36-T5Ø with fifth or sixth character 5)
EXCLUDES 1 *interstitial pneumonia NOS (J84.9)*
lymphoid interstitial pneumonia (J84.2)

J7Ø.4 Drug-induced interstitial lung disorders, unspecified HCC
Use additional code for adverse effect, if applicable, to identify drug (T36-T5Ø with fifth or sixth character 5)
EXCLUDES 1 *interstitial pneumonia NOS (J84.9)*
lymphoid interstitial pneumonia (J84.2)
AHA: 2019,2Q,28

J7Ø.5 Respiratory conditions due to smoke inhalation HCC
~~Smoke inhalation NOS~~
▶Code first smoke inhalation (T59.81-)◀
EXCLUDES 1 ~~*smoke inhalation due to chemicals, gases, fumes and vapors (J68.9)*~~
EXCLUDES 2 ▶*smoke inhalation due to chemicals, gases, fumes and vapors (J68.9)*◀
AHA: 2013,4Q,121

J7Ø.8 Respiratory conditions due to other specified external agents HCC
Code first (T51-T65) to identify the external agent

J7Ø.9 Respiratory conditions due to unspecified external agent HCC
Code first (T51-T65) to identify the external agent

Other respiratory diseases principally affecting the interstitium (J8Ø-J84)

J8Ø Acute respiratory distress syndrome MCC HCC
Acute respiratory distress syndrome in adult or child
Adult hyaline membrane disease
EXCLUDES 1 *respiratory distress syndrome in newborn (perinatal) (P22.Ø)*
AHA: 2020,1Q,34-36; 2017,1Q,26
DEF: Lung inflammation or injury resulting in a build-up of fluid in the air sacs, preventing the passage of oxygen from the air into the bloodstream.
TIP: Assign as a secondary code for a patient with acute respiratory distress syndrome (ARDS) due to COVID-19; assign code U07.1 as the principal or first-listed code.

J81 Pulmonary edema
Use additional code to identify:
exposure to environmental tobacco smoke (Z77.22)
history of tobacco dependence (Z87.891)
occupational exposure to environmental tobacco smoke (Z57.31)
tobacco dependence (F17.-)
tobacco use (Z72.Ø)
EXCLUDES 1 *chemical (acute) pulmonary edema (J68.1)*
hypostatic pneumonia (J18.2)
passive pneumonia (J18.2)
pulmonary edema due to external agents (J6Ø-J7Ø)
pulmonary edema with heart disease NOS (I5Ø.1)
pulmonary edema with heart failure (I5Ø.1)
DEF: Accumulation of fluid in the air sacs of the lungs, making it difficult to breathe.

J81.Ø Acute pulmonary edema MCC HCC
Acute edema of lung

J81.1 Chronic pulmonary edema CC
Pulmonary congestion (chronic) (passive)
Pulmonary edema NOS

▲✓4th **J82 Pulmonary eosinophilia, not elsewhere classified**

~~Allergic pneumonia~~
~~Eosinophilic asthma~~
~~Eosinophilic pneumonia~~
~~Löffler's pneumonia~~
~~Tropical (pulmonary) eosinophilia NOS~~

EXCLUDES 1 ~~*pulmonary eosinophilia due to aspergillosis (B44.-)*~~
~~*pulmonary eosinophilia due to drugs (J70.2-J70.4)*~~
~~*pulmonary eosinophilia due to specified parasitic infection (B50-B83)*~~
~~*pulmonary eosinophilia due to systemic connective tissue disorders (M30-M36)*~~
~~*pulmonary infiltrate NOS (R91.8)*~~

EXCLUDES 2 ▶*pulmonary eosinophilia due to aspergillosis (B44.-)*◀
▶*pulmonary eosinophilia due to drugs (J70.2-J70.4)*◀
▶*pulmonary eosinophilia due to specified parasitic infection (B50-B83)*◀
▶*pulmonary eosinophilia due to systemic connective tissue disorders (M30-M36)*◀
▶*pulmonary infiltrate NOS (R91.8)*◀

DEF: Infiltration of eosinophils (white blood cells of the immune system) into the parenchyma of the lungs, resulting in cough, fever, and dyspnea.

● ✓5th **J82.8 Pulmonary eosinophilia, not elsewhere classified**

● **J82.81 Chronic eosinophilic pneumonia** CC
Eosinophilic pneumonia, NOS

● **J82.82 Acute eosinophilic pneumonia** CC

● **J82.83 Eosinophilic asthma** CC
Code first asthma, by type, such as:
mild intermittent asthma (J45.2-)
mild persistent asthma (J45.3-)
moderate persistent asthma (J45.4-)
severe persistent asthma (J45.5-)

● **J82.89 Other pulmonary eosinophilia, not elsewhere classified** CC
Allergic pneumonia
Löffler's pneumonia
Tropical (pulmonary) eosinophilia NOS

✓4th **J84 Other interstitial pulmonary diseases**

EXCLUDES 1 *drug-induced interstitial lung disorders (J70.2-J70.4)*
interstitial emphysema (J98.2)

EXCLUDES 2 *lung diseases due to external agents (J60-J70)*

DEF: Interstitial: Within the small spaces or gaps occurring in tissue or organs.

✓5th **J84.0 Alveolar and parieto-alveolar conditions**

J84.01 Alveolar proteinosis CC HCC
DEF: Reduced ventilation due to proteinaceous deposits on alveoli. Symptoms include dyspnea, cough, chest pain, weakness, weight loss, and hemoptysis.

J84.02 Pulmonary alveolar microlithiasis CC HCC

J84.03 Idiopathic pulmonary hemosiderosis CC HCC
Essential brown induration of lung
Code first underlying disease, such as:
disorders of iron metabolism (E83.1-)
EXCLUDES 1 *acute idiopathic pulmonary hemorrhage in infants [AIPHI] (R04.81)*
DEF: Fibrosis of the alveolar walls marked by abnormal accumulation of iron as hemosiderin in the lungs. It primarily affects children and symptoms include anemia, fluid in the lungs, and blood in the sputum. Etiology is unknown.

J84.09 Other alveolar and parieto-alveolar conditions CC HCC

✓5th **J84.1 Other interstitial pulmonary diseases with fibrosis**

EXCLUDES 1 *pulmonary fibrosis (chronic) due to inhalation of chemicals, gases, fumes or vapors (J68.4)*
pulmonary fibrosis (chronic) following radiation (J70.1)

J84.10 Pulmonary fibrosis, unspecified HCC
Capillary fibrosis of lung
Cirrhosis of lung (chronic) NOS
Fibrosis of lung (atrophic) (chronic) (confluent) (massive) (perialveolar) (peribronchial) NOS
Induration of lung (chronic) NOS
Postinflammatory pulmonary fibrosis

✓6th **J84.11 Idiopathic interstitial pneumonia**

EXCLUDES 1 *lymphoid interstitial pneumonia (J84.2)*
pneumocystis pneumonia (B59)

J84.111 Idiopathic interstitial pneumonia, not otherwise specified HCC

J84.112 Idiopathic pulmonary fibrosis HCC
Cryptogenic fibrosing alveolitis
Idiopathic fibrosing alveolitis

J84.113 Idiopathic non-specific interstitial pneumonitis HCC
EXCLUDES 1 *non-specific interstitial pneumonia NOS, or due to known underlying cause (J84.89)*

J84.114 Acute interstitial pneumonitis CC HCC
Hamman-Rich syndrome
EXCLUDES 1 *pneumocystis pneumonia (B59)*

J84.115 Respiratory bronchiolitis interstitial lung disease HCC

J84.116 Cryptogenic organizing pneumonia CC HCC
EXCLUDES 1 *organizing pneumonia NOS, or due to known underlying cause (J84.89)*

J84.117 Desquamative interstitial pneumonia CC HCC

▲ ✓6th **J84.17 Other interstitial pulmonary diseases with fibrosis in diseases classified elsewhere**

~~Interstitial pneumonia (nonspecific) (usual) due to collagen vascular disease~~
~~Interstitial pneumonia (nonspecific) (usual) in diseases classified elsewhere~~
~~Organizing pneumonia due to collagen vascular disease~~
~~Organizing pneumonia in diseases classified elsewhere~~
~~Code first underlying disease, such as:~~
~~progressive systemic sclerosis (M34.0)~~
~~rheumatoid arthritis (M05.00-M06.9)~~
~~systemic lupus erythematosis (M32.0-M32.9)~~

● ***J84.170 Interstitial lung disease with progressive fibrotic phenotype in diseases classified elsewhere***
Progressive fibrotic interstitial lung disease
Code first underlying disease, such as:
lung diseases due to external agents (J60-J70)
rheumatoid arthritis (M05.00-M06.9)
sarcoidosis (D86)
systemic connective tissue disorders (M30-M36)

● ***J84.178 Other interstitial pulmonary diseases with fibrosis in diseases classified elsewhere***
Interstitial pneumonia (nonspecific) (usual) due to collagen vascular disease
Interstitial pneumonia (nonspecific) (usual) in diseases classified elsewhere
Organizing pneumonia due to collagen vascular disease
Organizing pneumonia in diseases classified elsewhere
Code first underlying disease, such as:
progressive systemic sclerosis (M34.0)
rheumatoid arthritis (M05.00-M06.9)
systemic lupus erythematosis (M32.0-M32.9)

J84.2 Lymphoid interstitial pneumonia CC HCC
Lymphoid interstitial pneumonitis

✓5th **J84.8 Other specified interstitial pulmonary diseases**

EXCLUDES 1 *exogenous lipoid pneumonia (J69.1)*
unspecified lipoid pneumonia (J69.1)

J84.81 Lymphangioleiomyomatosis MCC HCC
Lymphangiomyomatosis

J84.82 Adult pulmonary Langerhans cell histiocytosis CC HCC A
Adult PLCH

J84.83 Surfactant mutations of the lung MCC HCC
DEF: Genetic disorder resulting in insufficient secretion of a complex mixture of phospholipids and proteins that reduce surface tension in the alveoli following the onset of breathing to facilitate lung expansion in the newborn. It is the leading indication for pediatric lung transplantation.

✓6th **J84.84 Other interstitial lung diseases of childhood**

J84.841 Neuroendocrine cell hyperplasia of infancy MCC HCC

J84.842 Pulmonary interstitial glycogenosis MCC HCC

J84.843 Alveolar capillary dysplasia with vein misalignment MCC HCC

J84.848 Other interstitial lung diseases of childhood MCC HCC

J84.89 Other specified interstitial pulmonary diseases HCC
Endogenous lipoid pneumonia
Interstitial pneumonitis
Non-specific interstitial pneumonitis NOS
Organizing pneumonia NOS
Code first, if applicable:
poisoning due to drug or toxin (T51-T65 with fifth or sixth character to indicate intent), for toxic pneumonopathy
underlying cause of pneumonopathy, if known
Use additional code, for adverse effect, to identify drug (T36-T5Ø with fifth or sixth character 5), if drug-induced
EXCLUDES 1 *cryptogenic organizing pneumonia (J84.116)*
idiopathic non-specific interstitial pneumonitis (J84.113)
lymphoid interstitial pneumonia (J84.2)
lipoid pneumonia, exogenous or unspecified (J69.1)
AHA: 2019,2Q,28

J84.9 Interstitial pulmonary disease, unspecified CC HCC
Interstitial pneumonia NOS

Suppurative and necrotic conditions of the lower respiratory tract (J85-J86)

✓4th **J85 Abscess of lung and mediastinum**
Use additional code (B95-B97) to identify infectious agent

J85.Ø Gangrene and necrosis of lung MCC HCC

J85.1 Abscess of lung with pneumonia MCC HCC
Code also the type of pneumonia

J85.2 Abscess of lung without pneumonia MCC HCC
Abscess of lung NOS

J85.3 Abscess of mediastinum MCC HCC

✓4th **J86 Pyothorax**
Use additional code (B95-B97) to identify infectious agent
EXCLUDES 1 *abscess of lung (J85.-)*
pyothorax due to tuberculosis (A15.6)
DEF: Collection of pus in the pleural space that is commonly caused by an infection that spreads from the lung, such as bacterial pneumonia or a lung abscess.

J86.Ø Pyothorax with fistula MCC HCC SW
Bronchocutaneous fistula
Bronchopleural fistula
Hepatopleural fistula
Mediastinal fistula
Pleural fistula
Thoracic fistula
Any condition classifiable to J86.9 with fistula
DEF: Purulent infection of the respiratory cavity, with communication from a cavity to another structure.

J86.9 Pyothorax without fistula MCC HCC
Abscess of pleura
Abscess of thorax
Empyema (chest) (lung) (pleura)
Fibrinopurulent pleurisy
Purulent pleurisy
Pyopneumothorax
Septic pleurisy
Seropurulent pleurisy
Suppurative pleurisy

Other diseases of the pleura (J9Ø-J94)

J9Ø Pleural effusion, not elsewhere classified CC
Encysted pleurisy
Pleural effusion NOS
Pleurisy with effusion (exudative) (serous)
EXCLUDES 1 *chylous (pleural) effusion (J94.Ø)*
malignant pleural effusion (J91.Ø))
pleurisy NOS (RØ9.1)
tuberculous pleural effusion (A15.6)
DEF: Collection of lymph and other fluid within the pleural space.

✓4th **J91 Pleural effusion in conditions classified elsewhere**
EXCLUDES 2 *pleural effusion in heart failure (I5Ø.-)*
pleural effusion in systemic lupus erythematosus (M32.13)
DEF: Collection of lymph and other fluid within the pleural space.

J91.Ø Malignant pleural effusion CC
Code first underlying neoplasm

J91.8 Pleural effusion in other conditions classified elsewhere CC
Code first underlying disease, such as:
filariasis (B74.Ø-B74.9)
influenza (JØ9.X2, J1Ø.1, J11.1)
AHA: 2015,2Q,15
TIP: Assign this code as a secondary diagnosis to congestive heart failure (I50.-) only if pleural effusion is specifically evaluated or treated.

Pleural Effusion

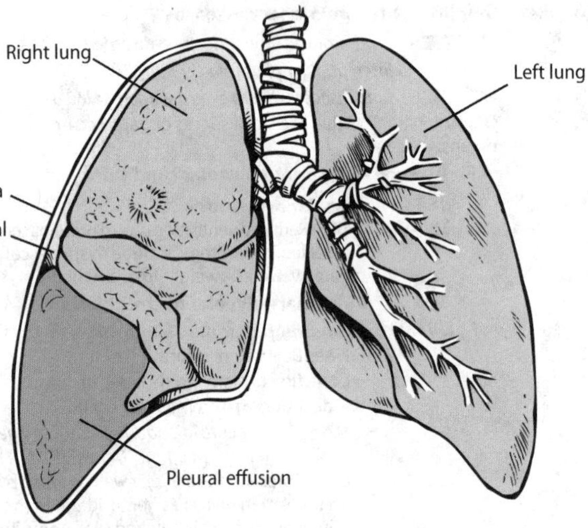

✓4th **J92 Pleural plaque**
INCLUDES pleural thickening
DEF: Areas of fibrous thickening that form on the parietal or visceral pleura, the membranes that line the ribs and lungs.

J92.Ø Pleural plaque with presence of asbestos

J92.9 Pleural plaque without asbestos
Pleural plaque NOS

J93 Pneumothorax and air leak

EXCLUDES 1 *congenital or perinatal pneumothorax (P25.1)*
postprocedural air leak (J95.812)
postprocedural pneumothorax (J95.811)
pyopneumothorax (J86.-)
traumatic pneumothorax (S27.Ø)
tuberculous (current disease) pneumothorax (A15.-)

DEF: Pneumothorax: Lung displacement due to abnormal leakage of air or gas that is trapped in the pleural space formed by the membrane that encloses the lungs and lines the thoracic cavity.

J93.Ø Spontaneous tension pneumothorax MCC
DEF: Leaking air from the lung into the lining, causing collapse.

J93.1 Other spontaneous pneumothorax

J93.11 Primary spontaneous pneumothorax CC

J93.12 Secondary spontaneous pneumothorax CC
Code first underlying condition, such as:
catamenial pneumothorax due to endometriosis (N8Ø.8)
cystic fibrosis (E84.-)
eosinophilic pneumonia (J82)
lymphangioleiomyomatosis (J84.81)
malignant neoplasm of bronchus and lung (C34.-)
Marfan's syndrome (Q87.4)
pneumonia due to Pneumocystis carinii (B59)
secondary malignant neoplasm of lung (C78.Ø-)
spontaneous rupture of the esophagus (K22.3)

J93.8 Other pneumothorax and air leak

J93.81 Chronic pneumothorax CC

J93.82 Other air leak CC
Persistent air leak

J93.83 Other pneumothorax CC
Acute pneumothorax
Spontaneous pneumothorax NOS

J93.9 Pneumothorax, unspecified CC
Pneumothorax NOS

J94 Other pleural conditions

EXCLUDES 1 *pleurisy NOS (RØ9.1)*
traumatic hemopneumothorax (S27.2)
traumatic hemothorax (S27.1)
tuberculous pleural conditions (current disease) (A15.-)

J94.Ø Chylous effusion CC
Chyliform effusion
DEF: Fluid within the pleural space due to the leaking of lymph contents into the space, usually as a result of thoracic duct damage or injury or mediastinal lymphoma.

J94.1 Fibrothorax
DEF: Fibrosis within the pleural lining of the lungs commonly seen as a stiff layer surrounding the lung typically attributed to traumatic hemothorax or pleural effusion.

J94.2 Hemothorax CC
Hemopneumothorax

J94.8 Other specified pleural conditions CC
Hydropneumothorax
Hydrothorax

J94.9 Pleural condition, unspecified

Intraoperative and postprocedural complications and disorders of respiratory system, not elsewhere classified (J95)

J95 Intraoperative and postprocedural complications and disorders of respiratory system, not elsewhere classified

EXCLUDES 2 *aspiration pneumonia (J69.-)*
emphysema (subcutaneous) resulting from a procedure (T81.82)
hypostatic pneumonia (J18.2)
pulmonary manifestations due to radiation (J7Ø.Ø-J7Ø.1)

J95.Ø Tracheostomy complications
DEF: Tracheostomy: Formation of a tracheal opening on the neck surface with tube insertion to allow for respiration in cases of obstruction or decreased patency. A tracheostomy may be planned or performed on an emergency basis for temporary or long-term use.

Tracheostomy

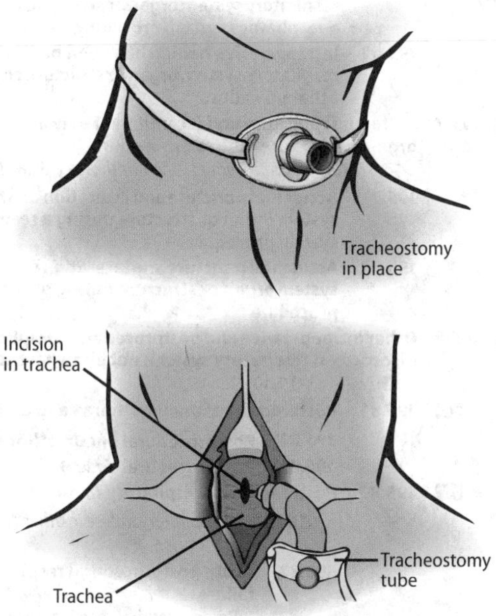

J95.ØØ Unspecified tracheostomy complication CC HCC

J95.Ø1 Hemorrhage from tracheostomy stoma CC HCC

J95.Ø2 Infection of tracheostomy stoma CC HCC
Use additional code to identify type of infection, such as:
cellulitis of neck (LØ3.221)
sepsis (A4Ø, A41.-)

J95.Ø3 Malfunction of tracheostomy stoma CC HCC
Mechanical complication of tracheostomy stoma
Obstruction of tracheostomy airway
Tracheal stenosis due to tracheostomy

J95.Ø4 Tracheo-esophageal fistula following tracheostomy CC HCC

J95.Ø9 Other tracheostomy complication CC HCC

J95.1 Acute pulmonary insufficiency following thoracic surgery MCC HCC
EXCLUDES 2 *functional disturbances following cardiac surgery (I97.Ø, I97.1-)*

J95.2 Acute pulmonary insufficiency following nonthoracic surgery MCC HCC
EXCLUDES 2 *functional disturbances following cardiac surgery (I97.Ø, I97.1-)*

J95.3 Chronic pulmonary insufficiency following surgery MCC HCC
EXCLUDES 2 *functional disturbances following cardiac surgery (I97.Ø, I97.1-)*

J95.4 Chemical pneumonitis due to anesthesia CC
Mendelson's syndrome
Postprocedural aspiration pneumonia
Use additional code for adverse effect, if applicable, to identify drug (T41.- with fifth or sixth character 5)
EXCLUDES 1 *aspiration pneumonitis due to anesthesia complicating labor and delivery (O74.Ø)*
aspiration pneumonitis due to anesthesia complicating pregnancy (O29)
aspiration pneumonitis due to anesthesia complicating the puerperium (O89.Ø1)

J95.5 Postprocedural subglottic stenosis CC

√5th **J95.6 Intraoperative hemorrhage and hematoma of a respiratory system organ or structure complicating a procedure**
EXCLUDES 1 *intraoperative hemorrhage and hematoma of a respiratory system organ or structure due to accidental puncture and laceration during procedure (J95.7-)*

J95.61 Intraoperative hemorrhage and hematoma of a respiratory system organ or structure complicating a respiratory system procedure CC

J95.62 Intraoperative hemorrhage and hematoma of a respiratory system organ or structure complicating other procedure CC

√5th **J95.7 Accidental puncture and laceration of a respiratory system organ or structure during a procedure**
EXCLUDES 2 *postprocedural pneumothorax (J95.811)*

J95.71 Accidental puncture and laceration of a respiratory system organ or structure during a respiratory system procedure CC

J95.72 Accidental puncture and laceration of a respiratory system organ or structure during other procedure CC

√5th **J95.8 Other intraoperative and postprocedural complications and disorders of respiratory system, not elsewhere classified**
AHA: 2016,4Q,9-10

√6th **J95.81 Postprocedural pneumothorax and air leak**

J95.811 Postprocedural pneumothorax CC H14

J95.812 Postprocedural air leak CC

√6th **J95.82 Postprocedural respiratory failure**
EXCLUDES 1 *respiratory failure in other conditions (J96.-)*

J95.821 Acute postprocedural respiratory failure MCC HCC
Postprocedural respiratory failure NOS

J95.822 Acute and chronic postprocedural respiratory failure MCC HCC

√6th **J95.83 Postprocedural hemorrhage of a respiratory system organ or structure following a procedure**

J95.830 Postprocedural hemorrhage of a respiratory system organ or structure following a respiratory system procedure CC

J95.831 Postprocedural hemorrhage of a respiratory system organ or structure following other procedure CC

J95.84 Transfusion-related acute lung injury (TRALI) CC
DEF: Relatively rare, but serious, pulmonary complication of blood transfusion, with acute respiratory distress, noncardiogenic pulmonary edema, cyanosis, hypoxemia, hypotension, fever, and chills.

√6th **J95.85 Complication of respirator [ventilator]**

J95.850 Mechanical complication of respirator CC HCC
EXCLUDES 1 *encounter for respirator [ventilator] dependence during power failure (Z99.12)*

J95.851 Ventilator associated pneumonia CC HCC
Ventilator associated pneumonitis
Use additional code to identify the organism, if known (B95.-, B96.-, B97.-)
EXCLUDES 1 *ventilator lung in newborn (P27.8)*
AHA: 2020,2Q,17; 2017,1Q,25

J95.859 Other complication of respirator [ventilator] CC HCC

√6th **J95.86 Postprocedural hematoma and seroma of a respiratory system organ or structure following a procedure**

J95.86Ø Postprocedural hematoma of a respiratory system organ or structure following a respiratory system procedure CC

J95.861 Postprocedural hematoma of a respiratory system organ or structure following other procedure CC

J95.862 Postprocedural seroma of a respiratory system organ or structure following a respiratory system procedure CC

J95.863 Postprocedural seroma of a respiratory system organ or structure following other procedure CC

J95.88 Other intraoperative complications of respiratory system, not elsewhere classified CC

J95.89 Other postprocedural complications and disorders of respiratory system, not elsewhere classified CC
Use additional code to identify disorder, such as:
aspiration pneumonia (J69.-)
bacterial or viral pneumonia (J12-J18)
EXCLUDES 2 *acute pulmonary insufficiency following thoracic surgery (J95.1)*
postprocedural subglottic stenosis (J95.5)

Other diseases of the respiratory system (J96-J99)

√4th **J96 Respiratory failure, not elsewhere classified**
EXCLUDES 1 *acute respiratory distress syndrome (J8Ø)*
cardiorespiratory failure (RØ9.2)
newborn respiratory distress syndrome (P22.Ø)
postprocedural respiratory failure (J95.82-)
respiratory arrest (RØ9.2)
respiratory arrest of newborn (P28.81)
respiratory failure of newborn (P28.5)

√5th **J96.Ø Acute respiratory failure**

J96.ØØ Acute respiratory failure, unspecified whether with hypoxia or hypercapnia MCC HCC
AHA: 2016,3Q,14; 2013,4Q,121

J96.Ø1 Acute respiratory failure with hypoxia MCC HCC

J96.Ø2 Acute respiratory failure with hypercapnia MCC HCC

√5th **J96.1 Chronic respiratory failure**

J96.1Ø Chronic respiratory failure, unspecified whether with hypoxia or hypercapnia CC HCC
AHA: 2016,1Q,38; 2015,1Q,21

J96.11 Chronic respiratory failure with hypoxia CC HCC
AHA: 2013,4Q,129

J96.12 Chronic respiratory failure with hypercapnia CC HCC

√5th **J96.2 Acute and chronic respiratory failure**
Acute on chronic respiratory failure

J96.2Ø Acute and chronic respiratory failure, unspecified whether with hypoxia or hypercapnia MCC HCC

J96.21 Acute and chronic respiratory failure with hypoxia MCC HCC

J96.22 Acute and chronic respiratory failure with hypercapnia MCC HCC

√5th **J96.9 Respiratory failure, unspecified**

J96.9Ø Respiratory failure, unspecified, unspecified whether with hypoxia or hypercapnia MCC HCC

J96.91 Respiratory failure, unspecified with hypoxia MCC HCC

J96.92 Respiratory failure, unspecified with hypercapnia MCC HCC

✓4th J98 Other respiratory disorders

Use additional code to identify:
- exposure to environmental tobacco smoke (Z77.22)
- exposure to tobacco smoke in the perinatal period (P96.81)
- history of tobacco dependence (Z87.891)
- occupational exposure to environmental tobacco smoke (Z57.31)
- tobacco dependence (F17.-)
- tobacco use (Z72.Ø)

EXCLUDES 1 *newborn apnea (P28.4)*
newborn sleep apnea (P28.3)

EXCLUDES 2 *apnea NOS (RØ6.81)*
sleep apnea (G47.3-)

✓5th J98.Ø Diseases of bronchus, not elsewhere classified

J98.Ø1 Acute bronchospasm

EXCLUDES 1 *acute bronchiolitis with bronchospasm (J21.-)*
acute bronchitis with bronchospasm (J2Ø.-)
asthma (J45.-)
exercise induced bronchospasm (J45.99Ø)

J98.Ø9 Other diseases of bronchus, not elsewhere classified

Broncholithiasis
Calcification of bronchus
Stenosis of bronchus
Tracheobronchial collapse
Tracheobronchial dyskinesia
Ulcer of bronchus

✓5th J98.1 Pulmonary collapse

EXCLUDES 1 *therapeutic collapse of lung status (Z98.3)*

J98.11 Atelectasis CC

EXCLUDES 1 *newborn atelectasis*
tuberculous atelectasis (current disease) (A15)

DEF: Collapse of lung tissue affecting part or all of one lung, preventing normal oxygen absorption to healthy tissues.

J98.19 Other pulmonary collapse CC

J98.2 Interstitial emphysema HCC

Mediastinal emphysema

EXCLUDES 1 *emphysema NOS (J43.9)*
emphysema in newborn (P25.Ø)
surgical emphysema (subcutaneous) (T81.82)
traumatic subcutaneous emphysema (T79.7)

J98.3 Compensatory emphysema HCC

DEF: Distention of all or part of the lung caused by disease processes or surgical intervention that decreased volume in another part of the lung, causing an overcompensation reaction. Compensatory emphysema occurs in association with pneumonias, pleural effusions, atelectasis, empyema, and pneumothorax.

J98.4 Other disorders of lung

Calcification of lung
Cystic lung disease (acquired)
Lung disease NOS
Pulmolithiasis

EXCLUDES 1 *acute interstitial pneumonitis (J84.114)*
pulmonary insufficiency following surgery (J95.1-J95.2)

✓5th J98.5 Diseases of mediastinum, not elsewhere classified

EXCLUDES 2 *abscess of mediastinum (J85.3)*

AHA: 2016,4Q,29

J98.51 Mediastinitis MCC H8

Code first underlying condition, if applicable, such as postoperative mediastinitis (T81.-)

J98.59 Other diseases of mediastinum, not elsewhere classified MCC H8

Fibrosis of mediastinum
Hernia of mediastinum
Retraction of mediastinum

J98.6 Disorders of diaphragm

Diaphragmatitis
Paralysis of diaphragm
Relaxation of diaphragm

EXCLUDES 1 *congenital malformation of diaphragm NEC (Q79.1)*
congenital diaphragmatic hernia (Q79.Ø)

EXCLUDES 2 *diaphragmatic hernia (K44.-)*

J98.8 Other specified respiratory disorders

AHA: 2020,1Q,34-36

TIP: Assign as a secondary code for a patient with a respiratory infection that is not further specified but is documented as being associated with COVID-19; assign U07.1 as the principal or first-listed code. If the respiratory infection documentation specifies acute or lower respiratory infection (NOS), assign J22 instead.

J98.9 Respiratory disorder, unspecified

Respiratory disease (chronic) NOS

J99 Respiratory disorders in diseases classified elsewhere HCC

Code first underlying disease, such as:
- amyloidosis (E85.-)
- ankylosing spondylitis (M45)
- congenital syphilis (A5Ø.5)
- cryoglobulinemia (D89.1)
- early congenital syphilis (A5Ø.Ø)
- plasminogen deficiency (E88.Ø2)
- schistosomiasis (B65.Ø-B65.9)

EXCLUDES 1 *respiratory disorders in:*
amebiasis (AØ6.5)
blastomycosis (B4Ø.Ø-B4Ø.2)
candidiasis (B37.1)
coccidioidomycosis (B38.Ø-B38.2)
cystic fibrosis with pulmonary manifestations (E84.Ø)
dermatomyositis (M33.Ø1, M33.11)
histoplasmosis (B39.Ø-B39.2)
late syphilis (A52.72, A52.73)
polymyositis (M33.21)
sicca syndrome (M35.Ø2)
systemic lupus erythematosus (M32.13)
systemic sclerosis (M34.81)
Wegener's granulomatosis (M31.3Ø-M31.31)

Chapter 11. Diseases of the Digestive System (KØØ–K95)

Chapter-specific Guidelines with Coding Examples
Reserved for future guideline expansion.

Chapter 11. Diseases of the Digestive System (KØØ-K95)

EXCLUDES 2 *certain conditions originating in the perinatal period (PØ4-P96)*
certain infectious and parasitic diseases (AØØ-B99)
complications of pregnancy, childbirth and the puerperium (OØØ-O9A)
congenital malformations, deformations and chromosomal abnormalities (QØØ-Q99)
endocrine, nutritional and metabolic diseases (EØØ-E88)
injury, poisoning and certain other consequences of external causes (SØØ-T88)
neoplasms (CØØ-D49)
symptoms, signs and abnormal clinical and laboratory findings, not elsewhere classified (RØØ-R94)

This chapter contains the following blocks:

KØØ-K14 Diseases of oral cavity and salivary glands
K2Ø-K31 Diseases of esophagus, stomach and duodenum
K35-K38 Diseases of appendix
K4Ø-K46 Hernia
K5Ø-K52 Noninfective enteritis and colitis
K55-K64 Other diseases of intestines
K65-K68 Diseases of peritoneum and retroperitoneum
K7Ø-K77 Diseases of liver
K8Ø-K87 Disorders of gallbladder, biliary tract and pancreas
K9Ø-K95 Other diseases of the digestive system

Diseases of oral cavity and salivary glands (KØØ-K14)

✓4th **KØØ Disorders of tooth development and eruption**
EXCLUDES 2 *embedded and impacted teeth (KØ1.-)*

KØØ.Ø Anodontia
Hypodontia
Oligodontia
EXCLUDES 1 *acquired absence of teeth (KØ8.1-)*
DEF: Partial or complete absence of teeth due to a congenital defect involving the tooth bud.

KØØ.1 Supernumerary teeth
Distomolar
Fourth molar
Mesiodens
Paramolar
Supplementary teeth
EXCLUDES 2 *supernumerary roots (KØØ.2)*

KØØ.2 Abnormalities of size and form of teeth
Concrescence of teeth
Fusion of teeth
Gemination of teeth
Dens evaginatus
Dens in dente
Dens invaginatus
Enamel pearls
Macrodontia
Microdontia
Peg-shaped [conical] teeth
Supernumerary roots
Taurodontism
Tuberculum paramolare
EXCLUDES 1 *abnormalities of teeth due to congenital syphilis (A5Ø.5)*
tuberculum Carabelli, which is regarded as a normal variation and should not be coded

KØØ.3 Mottled teeth
Dental fluorosis
Mottling of enamel
Nonfluoride enamel opacities
EXCLUDES 2 *deposits [accretions] on teeth (KØ3.6)*

KØØ.4 Disturbances in tooth formation
Aplasia and hypoplasia of cementum
Dilaceration of tooth
Enamel hypoplasia (neonatal) (postnatal) (prenatal)
Regional odontodysplasia
Turner's tooth
EXCLUDES 1 *Hutchinson's teeth and mulberry molars in congenital syphilis (A5Ø.5)*
EXCLUDES 2 *mottled teeth (KØØ.3)*

KØØ.5 Hereditary disturbances in tooth structure, not elsewhere classified
Amelogenesis imperfecta
Dentinogenesis imperfecta
Odontogenesis imperfecta
Dentinal dysplasia
Shell teeth

KØØ.6 Disturbances in tooth eruption
Dentia praecox
Natal tooth
Neonatal tooth
Premature eruption of tooth
Premature shedding of primary [deciduous] tooth
Prenatal teeth
Retained [persistent] primary tooth
EXCLUDES 2 *embedded and impacted teeth (KØ1.-)*

KØØ.7 Teething syndrome

KØØ.8 Other disorders of tooth development
Color changes during tooth formation
Intrinsic staining of teeth NOS
EXCLUDES 2 *posteruptive color changes (KØ3.7)*

KØØ.9 Disorder of tooth development, unspecified
Disorder of odontogenesis NOS

✓4th **KØ1 Embedded and impacted teeth**
EXCLUDES 1 *abnormal position of fully erupted teeth (M26.3-)*

KØ1.Ø Embedded teeth

KØ1.1 Impacted teeth

✓4th **KØ2 Dental caries**
INCLUDES caries of dentine
dental cavities
early childhood caries
pre-eruptive caries
recurrent caries (dentino enamel junction) (enamel) (to the pulp)
tooth decay

DEF: Localized section of tooth decay that begins on the tooth surface with destruction of the calcified enamel, allowing bacterial destruction to continue and form cavities and may extend to the dentin and pulp.

Tooth Anatomy

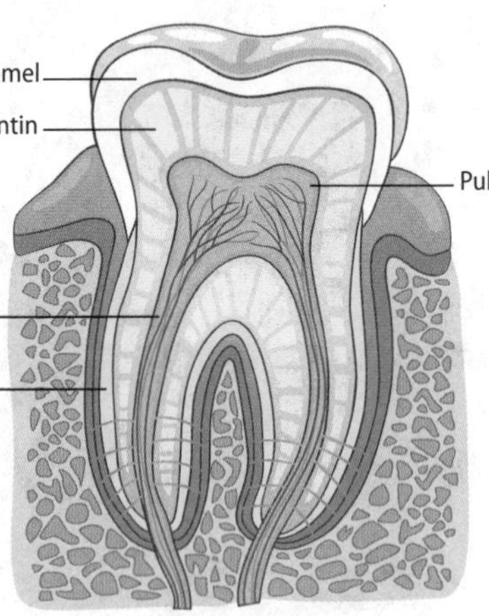

KØ2.3 Arrested dental caries
Arrested coronal and root caries

✓5th **KØ2.5 Dental caries on pit and fissure surface**
Dental caries on chewing surface of tooth

KØ2.51 Dental caries on pit and fissure surface limited to enamel
White spot lesions [initial caries] on pit and fissure surface of tooth

KØ2.52 Dental caries on pit and fissure surface penetrating into dentin
Primary dental caries, cervical origin

KØ2.53 Dental caries on pit and fissure surface penetrating into pulp

5th **KØ2.6 Dental caries on smooth surface**

KØ2.61 Dental caries on smooth surface limited to enamel
White spot lesions [initial caries] on smooth surface of tooth

KØ2.62 Dental caries on smooth surface penetrating into dentin

KØ2.63 Dental caries on smooth surface penetrating into pulp

KØ2.7 Dental root caries

KØ2.9 Dental caries, unspecified

4th **KØ3 Other diseases of hard tissues of teeth**

EXCLUDES 2 *bruxism (F45.8)*
dental caries (KØ2.-)
teeth-grinding NOS (F45.8)

KØ3.Ø Excessive attrition of teeth
Approximal wear of teeth
Occlusal wear of teeth
DEF: Attrition: In dentistry, wearing away or erosion of tooth surface from abrasive food or grinding teeth.

KØ3.1 Abrasion of teeth
Dentifrice abrasion of teeth
Habitual abrasion of teeth
Occupational abrasion of teeth
Ritual abrasion of teeth
Traditional abrasion of teeth
Wedge defect NOS

KØ3.2 Erosion of teeth
Erosion of teeth due to diet
Erosion of teeth due to drugs and medicaments
Erosion of teeth due to persistent vomiting
Erosion of teeth NOS
Idiopathic erosion of teeth
Occupational erosion of teeth

KØ3.3 Pathological resorption of teeth
Internal granuloma of pulp
Resorption of teeth (external)

KØ3.4 Hypercementosis
Cementation hyperplasia

KØ3.5 Ankylosis of teeth

KØ3.6 Deposits [accretions] on teeth
Betel deposits [accretions] on teeth
Black deposits [accretions] on teeth
Extrinsic staining of teeth NOS
Green deposits [accretions] on teeth
Materia alba deposits [accretions] on teeth
Orange deposits [accretions] on teeth
Staining of teeth NOS
Subgingival dental calculus
Supragingival dental calculus
Tobacco deposits [accretions] on teeth

KØ3.7 Posteruptive color changes of dental hard tissues
EXCLUDES 2 *deposits [accretions] on teeth (KØ3.6)*

5th **KØ3.8 Other specified diseases of hard tissues of teeth**

KØ3.81 Cracked tooth
EXCLUDES 1 *asymptomatic craze lines in enamel - omit code*
broken or fractured tooth due to trauma (SØ2.5)

KØ3.89 Other specified diseases of hard tissues of teeth

KØ3.9 Disease of hard tissues of teeth, unspecified

4th **KØ4 Diseases of pulp and periapical tissues**
AHA: 2016,4Q,29-30

5th **KØ4.Ø Pulpitis**
Acute pulpitis
Chronic (hyperplastic) (ulcerative) pulpitis

KØ4.Ø1 Reversible pulpitis CC

KØ4.Ø2 Irreversible pulpitis CC

KØ4.1 Necrosis of pulp
Pulpal gangrene

KØ4.2 Pulp degeneration
Denticles
Pulpal calcifications
Pulpal stones

KØ4.3 Abnormal hard tissue formation in pulp
Secondary or irregular dentine

KØ4.4 Acute apical periodontitis of pulpal origin CC
Acute apical periodontitis NOS
EXCLUDES 1 *acute periodontitis (KØ5.2-)*
DEF: Severe inflammation of the area surrounding the tip of a tooth's root that is often secondary to infection or trauma.

KØ4.5 Chronic apical periodontitis
Apical or periapical granuloma
Apical periodontitis NOS
EXCLUDES 1 *chronic periodontitis (KØ5.3-)*

KØ4.6 Periapical abscess with sinus SW
Dental abscess with sinus
Dentoalveolar abscess with sinus

KØ4.7 Periapical abscess without sinus
Dental abscess without sinus
Dentoalveolar abscess without sinus

KØ4.8 Radicular cyst
Apical (periodontal) cyst
Periapical cyst
Residual radicular cyst
EXCLUDES 2 *lateral periodontal cyst (KØ9.Ø)*
DEF: Most common odontogenic cyst in tissue around the tooth apex due to chronic inflammation of dental pulp.

5th **KØ4.9 Other and unspecified diseases of pulp and periapical tissues**

KØ4.9Ø Unspecified diseases of pulp and periapical tissues

KØ4.99 Other diseases of pulp and periapical tissues

4th **KØ5 Gingivitis and periodontal diseases**
Use additional code to identify:
alcohol abuse and dependence (F1Ø.-)
exposure to environmental tobacco smoke (Z77.22)
exposure to tobacco smoke in the perinatal period (P96.81)
history of tobacco dependence (Z87.891)
occupational exposure to environmental tobacco smoke (Z57.31)
tobacco dependence (F17.-)
tobacco use (Z72.Ø)
AHA: 2016,4Q,29-30

5th **KØ5.Ø Acute gingivitis**
EXCLUDES 1 *acute necrotizing ulcerative gingivitis (A69.1)*
herpesviral [herpes simplex] gingivostomatitis (BØØ.2)

KØ5.ØØ Acute gingivitis, plaque induced
Acute gingivitis NOS
Plaque induced gingival disease

KØ5.Ø1 Acute gingivitis, non-plaque induced

5th **KØ5.1 Chronic gingivitis**
Desquamative gingivitis (chronic)
Gingivitis (chronic) NOS
Hyperplastic gingivitis (chronic)
Pregnancy associated gingivitis
Simple marginal gingivitis (chronic)
Ulcerative gingivitis (chronic)
Code first, if applicable, diseases of the digestive system complicating pregnacy (O99.61-)

KØ5.1Ø Chronic gingivitis, plaque induced
Chronic gingivitis NOS
Gingivitis NOS

KØ5.11 Chronic gingivitis, non-plaque induced

5th **KØ5.2 Aggressive periodontitis**
Acute pericoronitis
EXCLUDES 1 *acute apical periodontitis (KØ4.4)*
periapical abscess (KØ4.7)
periapical abscess with sinus (KØ4.6)

KØ5.2Ø Aggressive periodontitis, unspecified

6th **KØ5.21 Aggressive periodontitis, localized**
Periodontal abscess

KØ5.211 Aggressive periodontitis, localized, slight

KØ5.212 Aggressive periodontitis, localized, moderate

KØ5.213 Aggressive periodontitis, localized, severe

KØ5.219 Aggressive periodontitis, localized, unspecified severity

6th **KØ5.22 Aggressive periodontitis, generalized**

KØ5.221 Aggressive periodontitis, generalized, slight

KØ5.222 Aggressive periodontitis, generalized, moderate

KØ5.223 Aggressive periodontitis, generalized, severe

KØ5.229 Aggressive periodontitis, generalized, unspecified severity

KØ5.3 Chronic periodontitis
Chronic pericoronitis
Complex periodontitis
Periodontitis NOS
Simplex periodontitis
EXCLUDES 1 *chronic apical periodontitis (KØ4.5)*

KØ5.30 Chronic periodontitis, unspecified

KØ5.31 Chronic periodontitis, localized
KØ5.311 Chronic periodontitis, localized, slight
KØ5.312 Chronic periodontitis, localized, moderate
KØ5.313 Chronic periodontitis, localized, severe
KØ5.319 Chronic periodontitis, localized, unspecified severity

KØ5.32 Chronic periodontitis, generalized
KØ5.321 Chronic periodontitis, generalized, slight
KØ5.322 Chronic periodontitis, generalized, moderate
KØ5.323 Chronic periodontitis, generalized, severe
KØ5.329 Chronic periodontitis, generalized, unspecified

KØ5.4 Periodontosis
Juvenile periodontosis

KØ5.5 Other periodontal diseases
Combined periodontic-endodontic lesion
Narrow gingival width (of periodontal soft tissue)
EXCLUDES 2 *leukoplakia of gingiva (K13.21)*

KØ5.6 Periodontal disease, unspecified

KØ6 Other disorders of gingiva and edentulous alveolar ridge
EXCLUDES 2 *acute gingivitis (KØ5.Ø)*
atrophy of edentulous alveolar ridge (KØ8.2)
chronic gingivitis (KØ5.1)
gingivitis NOS (KØ5.1)
AHA: 2016,4Q,29-30

KØ6.Ø Gingival recession
Gingival recession (postinfective) (postprocedural)
AHA: 2017,4Q,16

KØ6.Ø1 Gingival recession, localized
KØ6.Ø1Ø Localized gingival recession, unspecified
Localized gingival recession, NOS
KØ6.Ø11 Localized gingival recession, minimal
KØ6.Ø12 Localized gingival recession, moderate
KØ6.Ø13 Localized gingival recession, severe

KØ6.Ø2 Gingival recession, generalized
KØ6.Ø2Ø Generalized gingival recession, unspecified
Generalized gingival recession, NOS
KØ6.Ø21 Generalized gingival recession, minimal
KØ6.Ø22 Generalized gingival recession, moderate
KØ6.Ø23 Generalized gingival recession, severe

KØ6.1 Gingival enlargement
Gingival fibromatosis

KØ6.2 Gingival and edentulous alveolar ridge lesions associated with trauma
Irritative hyperplasia of edentulous ridge [denture hyperplasia]
Use additional code (Chapter 2Ø) to identify external cause or denture status (Z97.2)

KØ6.3 Horizontal alveolar bone loss

KØ6.8 Other specified disorders of gingiva and edentulous alveolar ridge
Fibrous epulis
Flabby alveolar ridge
Giant cell epulis
Peripheral giant cell granuloma of gingiva
Pyogenic granuloma of gingiva
Vertical ridge deficiency
EXCLUDES 2 *gingival cyst (KØ9.Ø)*

KØ6.9 Disorder of gingiva and edentulous alveolar ridge, unspecified

KØ8 Other disorders of teeth and supporting structures
EXCLUDES 2 *dentofacial anomalies [including malocclusion] (M26.-)*
disorders of jaw (M27.-)
AHA: 2016,4Q,29-30

KØ8.Ø Exfoliation of teeth due to systemic causes
Code also underlying systemic condition

KØ8.1 Complete loss of teeth
Acquired loss of teeth, complete
EXCLUDES 1 *congenital absence of teeth (KØØ.Ø)*
exfoliation of teeth due to systemic causes (KØ8.Ø)
partial loss of teeth (KØ8.4-)
DEF: Loss of all teeth as a result of caries, trauma, extraction, periodontal disease, or other specified or unspecified causes.
Synonym(s): *complete edentulism*

KØ8.1Ø Complete loss of teeth, unspecified cause
KØ8.1Ø1 Complete loss of teeth, unspecified cause, class I
KØ8.1Ø2 Complete loss of teeth, unspecified cause, class II
KØ8.1Ø3 Complete loss of teeth, unspecified cause, class III
KØ8.1Ø4 Complete loss of teeth, unspecified cause, class IV
KØ8.1Ø9 Complete loss of teeth, unspecified cause, unspecified class
Edentulism NOS

KØ8.11 Complete loss of teeth due to trauma
KØ8.111 Complete loss of teeth due to trauma, class I
KØ8.112 Complete loss of teeth due to trauma, class II
KØ8.113 Complete loss of teeth due to trauma, class III
KØ8.114 Complete loss of teeth due to trauma, class IV
KØ8.119 Complete loss of teeth due to trauma, unspecified class

KØ8.12 Complete loss of teeth due to periodontal diseases
KØ8.121 Complete loss of teeth due to periodontal diseases, class I
KØ8.122 Complete loss of teeth due to periodontal diseases, class II
KØ8.123 Complete loss of teeth due to periodontal diseases, class III
KØ8.124 Complete loss of teeth due to periodontal diseases, class IV
KØ8.129 Complete loss of teeth due to periodontal diseases, unspecified class

KØ8.13 Complete loss of teeth due to caries
KØ8.131 Complete loss of teeth due to caries, class I
KØ8.132 Complete loss of teeth due to caries, class II
KØ8.133 Complete loss of teeth due to caries, class III
KØ8.134 Complete loss of teeth due to caries, class IV
KØ8.139 Complete loss of teeth due to caries, unspecified class

KØ8.19 Complete loss of teeth due to other specified cause
KØ8.191 Complete loss of teeth due to other specified cause, class I
KØ8.192 Complete loss of teeth due to other specified cause, class II
KØ8.193 Complete loss of teeth due to other specified cause, class III
KØ8.194 Complete loss of teeth due to other specified cause, class IV
KØ8.199 Complete loss of teeth due to other specified cause, unspecified class

KØ8.2 Atrophy of edentulous alveolar ridge
KØ8.2Ø Unspecified atrophy of edentulous alveolar ridge
Atrophy of the mandible NOS
Atrophy of the maxilla NOS
KØ8.21 Minimal atrophy of the mandible
Minimal atrophy of the edentulous mandible
KØ8.22 Moderate atrophy of the mandible
Moderate atrophy of the edentulous mandible

K08.23 Severe atrophy of the mandible
Severe atrophy of the edentulous mandible

K08.24 Minimal atrophy of maxilla
Minimal atrophy of the edentulous maxilla

K08.25 Moderate atrophy of the maxilla
Moderate atrophy of the edentulous maxilla

K08.26 Severe atrophy of the maxilla
Severe atrophy of the edentulous maxilla

K08.3 Retained dental root

✓5th **K08.4 Partial loss of teeth**
Acquired loss of teeth, partial
EXCLUDES 1 *complete loss of teeth (K08.1-)*
congenital absence of teeth (K00.0)
EXCLUDES 2 *exfoliation of teeth due to systemic causes (K08.0)*

✓6th **K08.40 Partial loss of teeth, unspecified cause**
K08.401 Partial loss of teeth, unspecified cause, class I
K08.402 Partial loss of teeth, unspecified cause, class II
K08.403 Partial loss of teeth, unspecified cause, class III
K08.404 Partial loss of teeth, unspecified cause, class IV
K08.409 Partial loss of teeth, unspecified cause, unspecified class
Tooth extraction status NOS

✓6th **K08.41 Partial loss of teeth due to trauma**
K08.411 Partial loss of teeth due to trauma, class I
K08.412 Partial loss of teeth due to trauma, class II
K08.413 Partial loss of teeth due to trauma, class III
K08.414 Partial loss of teeth due to trauma, class IV
K08.419 Partial loss of teeth due to trauma, unspecified class

✓6th **K08.42 Partial loss of teeth due to periodontal diseases**
K08.421 Partial loss of teeth due to periodontal diseases, class I
K08.422 Partial loss of teeth due to periodontal diseases, class II
K08.423 Partial loss of teeth due to periodontal diseases, class III
K08.424 Partial loss of teeth due to periodontal diseases, class IV
K08.429 Partial loss of teeth due to periodontal diseases, unspecified class

✓6th **K08.43 Partial loss of teeth due to caries**
K08.431 Partial loss of teeth due to caries, class I
K08.432 Partial loss of teeth due to caries, class II
K08.433 Partial loss of teeth due to caries, class III
K08.434 Partial loss of teeth due to caries, class IV
K08.439 Partial loss of teeth due to caries, unspecified class

✓6th **K08.49 Partial loss of teeth due to other specified cause**
K08.491 Partial loss of teeth due to other specified cause, class I
K08.492 Partial loss of teeth due to other specified cause, class II
K08.493 Partial loss of teeth due to other specified cause, class III
K08.494 Partial loss of teeth due to other specified cause, class IV
K08.499 Partial loss of teeth due to other specified cause, unspecified class

✓5th **K08.5 Unsatisfactory restoration of tooth**
Defective bridge, crown, filling
Defective dental restoration
EXCLUDES 1 *dental restoration status (Z98.811)*
EXCLUDES 2 *endosseous dental implant failure (M27.6-)*
unsatisfactory endodontic treatment (M27.5-)

K08.50 Unsatisfactory restoration of tooth, unspecified
Defective dental restoration NOS

K08.51 Open restoration margins of tooth
Dental restoration failure of marginal integrity
Open margin on tooth restoration
Poor gingival margin to tooth restoration

K08.52 Unrepairable overhanging of dental restorative materials
Overhanging of tooth restoration

✓6th **K08.53 Fractured dental restorative material**
EXCLUDES 1 *cracked tooth (K03.81)*
traumatic fracture of tooth (S02.5)
K08.530 Fractured dental restorative material without loss of material
K08.531 Fractured dental restorative material with loss of material
K08.539 Fractured dental restorative material, unspecified

K08.54 Contour of existing restoration of tooth biologically incompatible with oral health
Dental restoration failure of periodontal anatomical integrity
Unacceptable contours of existing restoration of tooth
Unacceptable morphology of existing restoration of tooth

K08.55 Allergy to existing dental restorative material
Use additional code to identify the specific type of allergy

K08.56 Poor aesthetic of existing restoration of tooth
Dental restoration aesthetically inadequate or displeasing

K08.59 Other unsatisfactory restoration of tooth
Other defective dental restoration

✓5th **K08.8 Other specified disorders of teeth and supporting structures**
K08.81 Primary occlusal trauma
K08.82 Secondary occlusal trauma
K08.89 Other specified disorders of teeth and supporting structures
Enlargement of alveolar ridge NOS
Insufficient anatomic crown height
Insufficient clinical crown length
Irregular alveolar process
Toothache NOS

K08.9 Disorder of teeth and supporting structures, unspecified

✓4th **K09 Cysts of oral region, not elsewhere classified**
INCLUDES lesions showing histological features both of aneurysmal cyst and of another fibro-osseous lesion
EXCLUDES 2 *cysts of jaw (M27.0-, M27.4-)*
radicular cyst (K04.8)

K09.0 Developmental odontogenic cysts
Dentigerous cyst
Eruption cyst
Follicular cyst
Gingival cyst
Lateral periodontal cyst
Primordial cyst
EXCLUDES 2 *keratocysts (D16.4, D16.5)*
odontogenic keratocystic tumors (D16.4, D16.5)

K09.1 Developmental (nonodontogenic) cysts of oral region
Cyst (of) incisive canal
Cyst (of) palatine of papilla
Globulomaxillary cyst
Median palatal cyst
Nasoalveolar cyst
Nasolabial cyst
Nasopalatine duct cyst

K09.8 Other cysts of oral region, not elsewhere classified
Dermoid cyst
Epidermoid cyst
Lymphoepithelial cyst
Epstein's pearl

K09.9 Cyst of oral region, unspecified

✓4th **K11 Diseases of salivary glands**
Use additional code to identify:
alcohol abuse and dependence (F10.-)
exposure to environmental tobacco smoke (Z77.22)
exposure to tobacco smoke in the perinatal period (P96.81)
history of tobacco dependence (Z87.891)
occupational exposure to environmental tobacco smoke (Z57.31)
tobacco dependence (F17.-)
tobacco use (Z72.0)

K11.0 Atrophy of salivary gland

K11.1 Hypertrophy of salivary gland
DEF: Overgrowth of or enlarged salivary gland tissue caused by infection, salivary duct blockage, autoimmune diseases, and benign and malignant tumors.

✓5th **K11.2 Sialoadenitis**
Parotitis
EXCLUDES 1 *epidemic parotitis (B26.-)*
mumps (B26.-)
uveoparotid fever [Heerfordt] (D86.89)
DEF: Inflammation of the salivary gland.

K11.20 Sialoadenitis, unspecified
K11.21 Acute sialoadenitis
EXCLUDES 1 *acute recurrent sialoadenitis (K11.22)*
K11.22 Acute recurrent sialoadenitis
K11.23 Chronic sialoadenitis

K11.3 Abscess of salivary gland CC
K11.4 Fistula of salivary gland CC SW
EXCLUDES 1 *congenital fistula of salivary gland (Q38.4)*

K11.5 Sialolithiasis
Calculus of salivary gland or duct
Stone of salivary gland or duct

K11.6 Mucocele of salivary gland
Mucous extravasation cyst of salivary gland
Mucous retention cyst of salivary gland
Ranula

K11.7 Disturbances of salivary secretion
Hypoptyalism
Ptyalism
Xerostomia
EXCLUDES 2 *dry mouth NOS (R68.2)*

K11.8 Other diseases of salivary glands
Benign lymphoepithelial lesion of salivary gland
Mikulicz' disease
Necrotizing sialometaplasia
Sialectasia
Stenosis of salivary duct
Stricture of salivary duct
EXCLUDES 1 *sicca syndrome [Sjögren] (M35.0-)*

K11.9 Disease of salivary gland, unspecified
Sialoadenopathy NOS

✓4th **K12 Stomatitis and related lesions**
Use additional code to identify:
alcohol abuse and dependence (F10.-)
exposure to environmental tobacco smoke (Z77.22)
exposure to tobacco smoke in the perinatal period (P96.81)
history of tobacco dependence (Z87.891)
occupational exposure to environmental tobacco smoke (Z57.31)
tobacco dependence (F17.-)
tobacco use (Z72.0)
EXCLUDES 1 *cancrum oris (A69.0)*
cheilitis (K13.0)
gangrenous stomatitis (A69.0)
herpesviral [herpes simplex] gingivostomatitis (B00.2)
noma (A69.0)

K12.0 Recurrent oral aphthae
Aphthous stomatitis (major) (minor)
Bednar's aphthae
Periadenitis mucosa necrotica recurrens
Recurrent aphthous ulcer
Stomatitis herpetiformis
DEF: Disorder of unknown etiology with small oval or round painful ulcers of the mouth marked by a grayish exudate and a red halo effect.

K12.1 Other forms of stomatitis
Stomatitis NOS
Denture stomatitis
Ulcerative stomatitis
Vesicular stomatitis
EXCLUDES 1 *acute necrotizing ulcerative stomatitis (A69.1)*
Vincent's stomatitis (A69.1)

K12.2 Cellulitis and abscess of mouth CC
Cellulitis of mouth (floor)
Submandibular abscess
EXCLUDES 2 *abscess of salivary gland (K11.3)*
abscess of tongue (K14.0)
periapical abscess (K04.6-K04.7)
periodontal abscess (K05.21)
peritonsillar abscess (J36)

✓5th **K12.3 Oral mucositis (ulcerative)**
Mucositis (oral) (oropharyneal)
EXCLUDES 2 *gastrointestinal mucositis (ulcerative) (K92.81)*
mucositis (ulcerative) of vagina and vulva (N76.81)
nasal mucositis (ulcerative) (J34.81)

K12.30 Oral mucositis (ulcerative), unspecified
K12.31 Oral mucositis (ulcerative) due to antineoplastic therapy
Use additional code for adverse effect, if applicable, to identify antineoplastic and immunosuppressive drugs (T45.1X5)
Use additional code for other antineoplastic therapy, such as:
radiological procedure and radiotherapy (Y84.2)
K12.32 Oral mucositis (ulcerative) due to other drugs
Use additional code for adverse effect, if applicable, to identify drug (T36-T50 with fifth or sixth character 5)
K12.33 Oral mucositis (ulcerative) due to radiation
Use additional external cause code (W88-W90, X39.0-) to identify cause
K12.39 Other oral mucositis (ulcerative)
Viral oral mucositis (ulcerative)

✓4th **K13 Other diseases of lip and oral mucosa**
INCLUDES epithelial disturbances of tongue
Use additional code to identify:
alcohol abuse and dependence (F10.-)
exposure to environmental tobacco smoke (Z77.22)
exposure to tobacco smoke in the perinatal period (P96.81)
history of tobacco dependence (Z87.891)
occupational exposure to environmental tobacco smoke (Z57.31)
tobacco dependence (F17.-)
tobacco use (Z72.0)
EXCLUDES 2 *certain disorders of gingiva and edentulous alveolar ridge (K05-K06)*
cysts of oral region (K09.-)
diseases of tongue (K14.-)
stomatitis and related lesions (K12.-)

K13.0 Diseases of lips
Abscess of lips
Angular cheilitis
Cellulitis of lips
Cheilitis NOS
Cheilodynia
Cheilosis
Exfoliative cheilitis
Fistula of lips
Glandular cheilitis
Hypertrophy of lips
Perlèche NEC
EXCLUDES 1 *ariboflavinosis (E53.0)*
cheilitis due to radiation-related disorders (L55-L59)
congenital fistula of lips (Q38.0)
congenital hypertrophy of lips (Q18.6)
perlèche due to candidiasis (B37.83)
perlèche due to riboflavin deficiency (E53.0)

K13.1 Cheek and lip biting

K13.2 Leukoplakia and other disturbances of oral epithelium, including tongue
EXCLUDES 1 *carcinoma in situ of oral epithelium (DØØ.Ø-)*
hairy leukoplakia (K13.3)
DEF: Leukoplakia: Thickened white patches or lesions appearing on a mucous membrane, such as oral mucosa or tongue.

K13.21 Leukoplakia of oral mucosa, including tongue
Leukokeratosis of oral mucosa
Leukoplakia of gingiva, lips, tongue
EXCLUDES 1 *hairy leukoplakia (K13.3)*
leukokeratosis nicotina palati (K13.24)

K13.22 Minimal keratinized residual ridge mucosa
Minimal keratinization of alveolar ridge mucosa

K13.23 Excessive keratinized residual ridge mucosa
Excessive keratinization of alveolar ridge mucosa

K13.24 Leukokeratosis nicotina palati
Smoker's palate

K13.29 Other disturbances of oral epithelium, including tongue
Erythroplakia of mouth or tongue
Focal epithelial hyperplasia of mouth or tongue
Leukoedema of mouth or tongue
Other oral epithelium disturbances

K13.3 Hairy leukoplakia

K13.4 Granuloma and granuloma-like lesions of oral mucosa
Eosinophilic granuloma
Granuloma pyogenicum
Verrucous xanthoma

K13.5 Oral submucous fibrosis
Submucous fibrosis of tongue

K13.6 Irritative hyperplasia of oral mucosa
EXCLUDES 2 *irritative hyperplasia of edentulous ridge [denture hyperplasia] (KØ6.2)*

K13.7 Other and unspecified lesions of oral mucosa

K13.7Ø Unspecified lesions of oral mucosa

K13.79 Other lesions of oral mucosa
Focal oral mucinosis

K14 Diseases of tongue
Use additional code to identify:
alcohol abuse and dependence (F1Ø.-)
exposure to environmental tobacco smoke (Z77.22)
history of tobacco dependence (Z87.891)
occupational exposure to environmental tobacco smoke (Z57.31)
tobacco dependence (F17.-)
tobacco use (Z72.Ø)
EXCLUDES 2 *erythroplakia (K13.29)*
focal epithelial hyperplasia (K13.29)
leukedema of tongue (K13.29)
leukoplakia of tongue (K13.21)
hairy leukoplakia (K13.3)
macroglossia (congenital) (Q38.2)
submucous fibrosis of tongue (K13.5)

K14.Ø Glossitis
Abscess of tongue
Ulceration (traumatic) of tongue
EXCLUDES 1 *atrophic glossitis (K14.4)*
DEF: Inflammation and swelling of the tongue that may be associated with infection, adverse drug reactions, smoking, or injury.

K14.1 Geographic tongue
Benign migratory glossitis
Glossitis areata exfoliativa

K14.2 Median rhomboid glossitis

K14.3 Hypertrophy of tongue papillae
Black hairy tongue
Coated tongue
Hypertrophy of foliate papillae
Lingua villosa nigra

K14.4 Atrophy of tongue papillae
Atrophic glossitis

K14.5 Plicated tongue
Fissured tongue
Furrowed tongue
Scrotal tongue
EXCLUDES 1 *fissured tongue, congenital (Q38.3)*

K14.6 Glossodynia
Glossopyrosis
Painful tongue

K14.8 Other diseases of tongue
Atrophy of tongue
Crenated tongue
Enlargement of tongue
Glossocele
Glossoptosis
Hypertrophy of tongue

K14.9 Disease of tongue, unspecified
Glossopathy NOS

Diseases of esophagus, stomach and duodenum (K2Ø-K31)

EXCLUDES 2 *hiatus hernia (K44.-)*

K2Ø Esophagitis
Use additional code to identify:
alcohol abuse and dependence (F1Ø.-)
EXCLUDES 1 *erosion of esophagus (K22.1-)*
esophagitis with gastro-esophageal reflux disease ►(K21.Ø-)◄
reflux esophagitis ►(K21.Ø-)◄
ulcerative esophagitis (K22.1-)
EXCLUDES 2 *eosinophilic gastritis or gastroenteritis (K52.81)*

K2Ø.Ø Eosinophilic esophagitis

▲ **K2Ø.8 Other esophagitis**
~~Abscess of esophagus~~

● **K2Ø.8Ø Other esophagitis without bleeding**
Abscess of esophagus
Other esophagitis NOS

● **K2Ø.81 Other esophagitis with bleeding** MCC

▲ **K2Ø.9 Esophagitis, unspecified**
~~Esophagitis NOS~~

● **K2Ø.9Ø Esophagitis, unspecified without bleeding**
Esophagitis NOS

● **K2Ø.91 Esophagitis, unspecified with bleeding** MCC

K21 Gastro-esophageal reflux disease
EXCLUDES 1 *newborn esophageal reflux (P78.83)*

▲ **K21.Ø Gastro-esophageal reflux disease with esophagitis**
~~Reflux esophagitis~~

● **K21.ØØ Gastro-esophageal reflux disease with esophagitis, without bleeding**
Reflux esophagitis

● **K21.Ø1 Gastro-esophageal reflux disease with esophagitis, with bleeding** MCC

K21.9 Gastro-esophageal reflux disease without esophagitis
Esophageal reflux NOS
AHA: 2016,1Q,18

K22 Other diseases of esophagus
EXCLUDES 2 *esophageal varices (I85.-)*

K22.Ø Achalasia of cardia
Achalasia NOS
Cardiospasm
EXCLUDES 1 *congenital cardiospasm (Q39.5)*
DEF: Esophageal motility disorder that is caused by absence of the esophageal peristalsis and impaired relaxation of the lower esophageal sphincter. It is characterized by dysphagia, regurgitation, and heartburn.

✓5th **K22.1 Ulcer of esophagus**
Barrett's ulcer
Erosion of esophagus
Fungal ulcer of esophagus
Peptic ulcer of esophagus
Ulcer of esophagus due to ingestion of chemicals
Ulcer of esophagus due to ingestion of drugs and medicaments
Ulcerative esophagitis
Code first poisoning due to drug or toxin, if applicable (T36-T65 with fifth or sixth character 1-4 or 6)
Use additional code for adverse effect, if applicable, to identify drug (T36-T5Ø with fifth or sixth character 5)
EXCLUDES 1 *Barrett's esophagus (K22.7-)*
AHA: 2018,3Q,22; 2017,3Q,27
TIP: Assign a code for "with bleeding" when an esophageal ulcer and bleeding (hematemesis) are documented. The ICD-10-CM classification assumes the two are related without the provider linking the two conditions. Evidence of bleeding during a procedure is not required.
TIP: For bleeding ulcers resulting from anticoagulant therapy, code D68.32 Hemorrhagic disorder due to extrinsic circulating anticoagulant, and an adverse-effect code from subcategory T45.5- should also be assigned. Either the bleeding ulcer code or code D68.32 may be sequenced first, depending on the circumstances of admission.

K22.1Ø Ulcer of esophagus without bleeding CC
Ulcer of esophagus NOS

K22.11 Ulcer of esophagus with bleeding MCC
EXCLUDES 2 *bleeding esophageal varices (I85.Ø1, I85.11)*

K22.2 Esophageal obstruction
Compression of esophagus
Constriction of esophagus
Stenosis of esophagus
Stricture of esophagus
EXCLUDES 1 *congenital stenosis or stricture of esophagus (Q39.3)*

K22.3 Perforation of esophagus MCC
Rupture of esophagus
EXCLUDES 1 *traumatic perforation of (thoracic) esophagus (S27.8-)*

K22.4 Dyskinesia of esophagus
Corkscrew esophagus
Diffuse esophageal spasm
Spasm of esophagus
EXCLUDES 1 *cardiospasm (K22.Ø)*

K22.5 Diverticulum of esophagus, acquired
Esophageal pouch, acquired
EXCLUDES 1 *diverticulum of esophagus (congenital) (Q39.6)*

K22.6 Gastro-esophageal laceration-hemorrhage syndrome MCC
Mallory-Weiss syndrome

✓5th **K22.7 Barrett's esophagus**
Barrett's disease
Barrett's syndrome
EXCLUDES 1 *Barrett's ulcer (K22.1)*
malignant neoplasm of esophagus (C15.-)
DEF: Metaplastic disorder in which specialized columnar epithelial cells replace the normal squamous epithelial cells. Secondary to chronic gastroesophageal reflux damage to the mucosa, this disorder increases the risk of developing adenocarcinoma.

K22.7Ø Barrett's esophagus without dysplasia
Barrett's esophagus NOS

✓6th **K22.71 Barrett's esophagus with dysplasia**
K22.71Ø Barrett's esophagus with low grade dysplasia
K22.711 Barrett's esophagus with high grade dysplasia
K22.719 Barrett's esophagus with dysplasia, unspecified

K22.8 Other specified diseases of esophagus
Hemorrhage of esophagus NOS
EXCLUDES 2 *esophageal varices (I85.-)*
Paterson-Kelly syndrome (D5Ø.1)
AHA: 2020,1Q,16

K22.9 Disease of esophagus, unspecified

K23 Disorders of esophagus in diseases classified elsewhere
Code first underlying disease, such as:
congenital syphilis (A5Ø.5)
EXCLUDES 1 *late syphilis (A52.79)*
megaesophagus due to Chagas' disease (B57.31)
tuberculosis (A18.83)

✓4th **K25 Gastric ulcer**
INCLUDES erosion (acute) of stomach
pylorus ulcer (peptic)
stomach ulcer (peptic)
Use additional code to identify:
alcohol abuse and dependence (F1Ø.-)
EXCLUDES 1 *acute gastritis (K29.Ø-)*
peptic ulcer NOS (K27.-)
AHA: 2017,3Q,27
TIP: Assign a code for "with hemorrhage" when a gastric ulcer and GI bleeding are documented. The ICD-10-CM classification assumes the two are related without the provider linking the two conditions. Evidence of bleeding during a procedure is not required.
TIP: For bleeding ulcers resulting from anticoagulant therapy, code D68.32 Hemorrhagic disorder due to extrinsic circulating anticoagulant, and an adverse-effect code from subcategory T45.5- should also be assigned. Either the bleeding ulcer code or code D68.32 may be sequenced first, depending on the circumstances of admission.

K25.Ø Acute gastric ulcer with hemorrhage MCC
K25.1 Acute gastric ulcer with perforation MCC HCC
K25.2 Acute gastric ulcer with both hemorrhage and perforation MCC HCC
K25.3 Acute gastric ulcer without hemorrhage or perforation CC
K25.4 Chronic or unspecified gastric ulcer with hemorrhage MCC
K25.5 Chronic or unspecified gastric ulcer with perforation MCC HCC
K25.6 Chronic or unspecified gastric ulcer with both hemorrhage and perforation MCC HCC
K25.7 Chronic gastric ulcer without hemorrhage or perforation
K25.9 Gastric ulcer, unspecified as acute or chronic, without hemorrhage or perforation

Gastrointestinal Ulcers

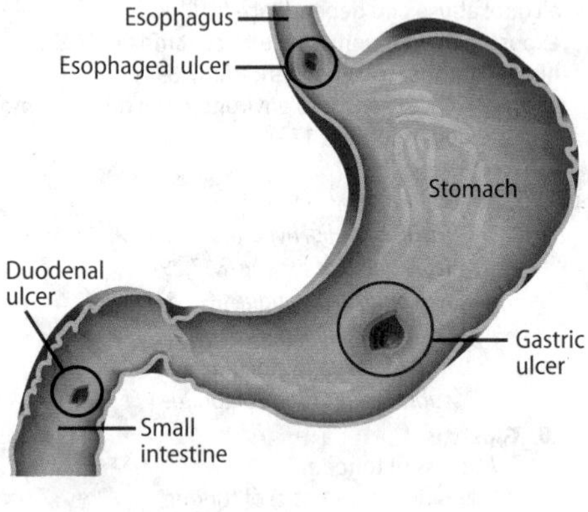

✓4th **K26 Duodenal ulcer**
INCLUDES erosion (acute) of duodenum
duodenum ulcer (peptic)
postpyloric ulcer (peptic)
Use additional code to identify:
alcohol abuse and dependence (F1Ø.-)
EXCLUDES 1 *peptic ulcer NOS (K27.-)*
AHA: 2017,3Q,27
TIP: Assign a code for "with hemorrhage" when a duodenal ulcer and GI bleeding are documented. The ICD-10-CM classification assumes the two are related without the provider linking the two conditions. Evidence of bleeding during a procedure is not required.
TIP: For bleeding ulcers resulting from anticoagulant therapy, code D68.32 Hemorrhagic disorder due to extrinsic circulating anticoagulant, and an adverse-effect code from subcategory T45.5- should also be assigned. Either the bleeding ulcer code or code D68.32 may be sequenced first, depending on the circumstances of admission.

K26.Ø Acute duodenal ulcer with hemorrhage MCC
K26.1 Acute duodenal ulcer with perforation MCC HCC
K26.2 Acute duodenal ulcer with both hemorrhage and perforation MCC HCC

K26.3 Acute duodenal ulcer without hemorrhage or perforation CC

K26.4 Chronic or unspecified duodenal ulcer with hemorrhage MCC
AHA: 2016,1Q,14

K26.5 Chronic or unspecified duodenal ulcer with perforation MCC HCC

K26.6 Chronic or unspecified duodenal ulcer with both hemorrhage and perforation MCC HCC

K26.7 Chronic duodenal ulcer without hemorrhage or perforation

K26.9 Duodenal ulcer, unspecified as acute or chronic, without hemorrhage or perforation

✓4th **K27 Peptic ulcer, site unspecified**

INCLUDES gastroduodenal ulcer NOS
peptic ulcer NOS

Use additional code to identify:
alcohol abuse and dependence (F1Ø.-)

EXCLUDES 1 *peptic ulcer of newborn (P78.82)*

AHA: 2017,3Q,27

TIP: Assign a code for "with hemorrhage" when a peptic ulcer and GI bleeding are documented. The ICD-10-CM classification assumes the two are related without the provider linking the two conditions. Evidence of bleeding during a procedure is not required.

TIP: For bleeding ulcers resulting from anticoagulant therapy, code D68.32 Hemorrhagic disorder due to extrinsic circulating anticoagulant, and an adverse-effect code from subcategory T45.5- should also be assigned. Either the bleeding ulcer code or code D68.32 may be sequenced first, depending on the circumstances of admission.

K27.Ø Acute peptic ulcer, site unspecified, with hemorrhage MCC

K27.1 Acute peptic ulcer, site unspecified, with perforation MCC HCC

K27.2 Acute peptic ulcer, site unspecified, with both hemorrhage and perforation MCC HCC

K27.3 Acute peptic ulcer, site unspecified, without hemorrhage or perforation CC

K27.4 Chronic or unspecified peptic ulcer, site unspecified, with hemorrhage MCC

K27.5 Chronic or unspecified peptic ulcer, site unspecified, with perforation MCC HCC

K27.6 Chronic or unspecified peptic ulcer, site unspecified, with both hemorrhage and perforation MCC HCC

K27.7 Chronic peptic ulcer, site unspecified, without hemorrhage or perforation

K27.9 Peptic ulcer, site unspecified, unspecified as acute or chronic, without hemorrhage or perforation

✓4th **K28 Gastrojejunal ulcer**

INCLUDES anastomotic ulcer (peptic) or erosion
gastrocolic ulcer (peptic) or erosion
gastrointestinal ulcer (peptic) or erosion
gastrojejunal ulcer (peptic) or erosion
jejunal ulcer (peptic) or erosion
marginal ulcer (peptic) or erosion
stomal ulcer (peptic) or erosion

Use additional code to identify:
alcohol abuse and dependence (F1Ø.-)

EXCLUDES 1 *primary ulcer of small intestine (K63.3)*

AHA: 2017,3Q,27

TIP: Assign a code for "with hemorrhage" when a gastrojejunal ulcer and GI bleeding are documented. The ICD-10-CM classification assumes the two are related without the provider linking the two conditions. Evidence of bleeding during a procedure is not required.

TIP: For bleeding ulcers resulting from anticoagulant therapy, code D68.32 Hemorrhagic disorder due to extrinsic circulating anticoagulant, and an adverse-effect code from subcategory T45.5- should also be assigned. Either the bleeding ulcer code or code D68.32 may be sequenced first, depending on the circumstances of admission.

K28.Ø Acute gastrojejunal ulcer with hemorrhage MCC

K28.1 Acute gastrojejunal ulcer with perforation MCC HCC

K28.2 Acute gastrojejunal ulcer with both hemorrhage and perforation MCC HCC

K28.3 Acute gastrojejunal ulcer without hemorrhage or perforation CC

K28.4 Chronic or unspecified gastrojejunal ulcer with hemorrhage MCC

K28.5 Chronic or unspecified gastrojejunal ulcer with perforation MCC HCC

K28.6 Chronic or unspecified gastrojejunal ulcer with both hemorrhage and perforation MCC HCC

K28.7 Chronic gastrojejunal ulcer without hemorrhage or perforation

K28.9 Gastrojejunal ulcer, unspecified as acute or chronic, without hemorrhage or perforation

✓4th **K29 Gastritis and duodenitis**

EXCLUDES 1 *eosinophilic gastritis or gastroenteritis (K52.81)*
Zollinger-Ellison syndrome (E16.4)

AHA: 2018,3Q,22

TIP: Assign a code for "with bleeding" when gastritis or duodenitis and GI bleeding are documented. The ICD-10-CM classification assumes the two are related without the provider linking the two conditions. Evidence of bleeding during a procedure is not required.

TIP: For bleeding resulting from anticoagulant therapy, code D68.32 Hemorrhagic disorder due to extrinsic circulating anticoagulant, and an adverse-effect code from subcategory T45.5- should also be assigned. Either code K29 or code D68.32 may be sequenced first, depending on the circumstances of admission.

✓5th K29.Ø Acute gastritis
Use additional code to identify:
alcohol abuse and dependence (F1Ø.-)
EXCLUDES 1 *erosion (acute) of stomach (K25.-)*

K29.ØØ Acute gastritis without bleeding
K29.Ø1 Acute gastritis with bleeding MCC

✓5th K29.2 Alcoholic gastritis
Use additional code to identify:
alcohol abuse and dependence (F1Ø.-)

K29.2Ø Alcoholic gastritis without bleeding
K29.21 Alcoholic gastritis with bleeding MCC

✓5th K29.3 Chronic superficial gastritis

K29.3Ø Chronic superficial gastritis without bleeding
K29.31 Chronic superficial gastritis with bleeding MCC

✓5th K29.4 Chronic atrophic gastritis
Gastric atrophy

K29.4Ø Chronic atrophic gastritis without bleeding
K29.41 Chronic atrophic gastritis with bleeding MCC

✓5th K29.5 Unspecified chronic gastritis
Chronic antral gastritis
Chronic fundal gastritis

K29.5Ø Unspecified chronic gastritis without bleeding
K29.51 Unspecified chronic gastritis with bleeding MCC

✓5th K29.6 Other gastritis
Giant hypertrophic gastritis
Granulomatous gastritis
Ménétrier's disease

K29.6Ø Other gastritis without bleeding
K29.61 Other gastritis with bleeding MCC

✓5th K29.7 Gastritis, unspecified

K29.7Ø Gastritis, unspecified, without bleeding
K29.71 Gastritis, unspecified, with bleeding MCC

✓5th K29.8 Duodenitis

K29.8Ø Duodenitis without bleeding
K29.81 Duodenitis with bleeding MCC

✓5th K29.9 Gastroduodenitis, unspecified

K29.9Ø Gastroduodenitis, unspecified, without bleeding
K29.91 Gastroduodenitis, unspecified, with bleeding MCC

K3Ø Functional dyspepsia
Indigestion

EXCLUDES 1 *dyspepsia NOS (R1Ø.13)*
heartburn (R12)
nervous dyspepsia (F45.8)
neurotic dyspepsia (F45.8)
psychogenic dyspepsia (F45.8)

✓4th **K31 Other diseases of stomach and duodenum**

INCLUDES functional disorders of stomach

EXCLUDES 2 *diabetic gastroparesis (EØ8.43, EØ9.43, E1Ø.43, E11.43, E13.43)*
diverticulum of duodenum (K57.ØØ-K57.13)

K31.Ø Acute dilatation of stomach CC
Acute distention of stomach

K31.1 Adult hypertrophic pyloric stenosis CC A
Pyloric stenosis NOS
EXCLUDES 1 *congenital or infantile pyloric stenosis (Q4Ø.Ø)*

K31.2 Hourglass stricture and stenosis of stomach
EXCLUDES 1 *congenital hourglass stomach (Q40.2)*
hourglass contraction of stomach (K31.89)

K31.3 Pylorospasm, not elsewhere classified
EXCLUDES 1 *congenital or infantile pylorospasm (Q40.0)*
neurotic pylorospasm (F45.8)
psychogenic pylorospasm (F45.8)

K31.4 Gastric diverticulum
EXCLUDES 1 *congenital diverticulum of stomach (Q40.2)*

K31.5 Obstruction of duodenum CC
Constriction of duodenum
Duodenal ileus (chronic)
Stenosis of duodenum
Stricture of duodenum
Volvulus of duodenum
EXCLUDES 1 *congenital stenosis of duodenum (Q41.0)*

K31.6 Fistula of stomach and duodenum CC SW
Gastrocolic fistula
Gastrojejunocolic fistula

K31.7 Polyp of stomach and duodenum
EXCLUDES 1 *adenomatous polyp of stomach (D13.1)*
AHA: 2020,1Q,16

✓5th **K31.8 Other specified diseases of stomach and duodenum**

✓6th **K31.81 Angiodysplasia of stomach and duodenum**
TIP: Assign a code for "with bleeding" when angiodysplasia of the stomach or the duodenum and GI bleeding are documented. The ICD-10-CM classification assumes the two are related without the provider linking the two conditions. Evidence of bleeding during a procedure is not required.

K31.811 Angiodysplasia of stomach and duodenum with bleeding MCC

K31.819 Angiodysplasia of stomach and duodenum without bleeding
Angiodysplasia of stomach and duodenum NOS

K31.82 Dieulafoy lesion (hemorrhagic) of stomach and duodenum MCC
EXCLUDES 2 *Dieulafoy lesion of intestine (K63.81)*
DEF: Abnormally large submucosal artery protruding through a defect in the stomach mucosa or intestines that can cause massive and life-threatening hemorrhaging.

K31.83 Achlorhydria
DEF: Absence of hydrochloric acid in gastric secretions due to gastric mucosa atrophy. Achlorhydria is unresponsive to histamines.

K31.84 Gastroparesis
Gastroparalysis
Code first underlying disease, if known, such as:
anorexia nervosa (F50.0-)
diabetes mellitus (E08.43, E09.43, E10.43, E11.43, E13.43)
scleroderma (M34.-)
AHA: 2013,4Q,114

K31.89 Other diseases of stomach and duodenum
AHA: 2020,1Q,15; 2017,1Q,28

K31.9 Disease of stomach and duodenum, unspecified

Diseases of appendix (K35-K38)

✓4th **K35 Acute appendicitis**
AHA: 2018,4Q,17-18

✓5th **K35.2 Acute appendicitis with generalized peritonitis**
Appendicitis (acute) with generalized (diffuse) peritonitis following rupture or perforation of appendix

K35.20 Acute appendicitis with generalized peritonitis, without abscess CC
(Acute) appendicitis with generalized peritonitis NOS

K35.21 Acute appendicitis with generalized peritonitis, with abscess MCC

✓5th **K35.3 Acute appendicitis with localized peritonitis**

K35.30 Acute appendicitis with localized peritonitis, without perforation or gangrene CC
Acute appendicitis with localized peritonitis NOS

K35.31 Acute appendicitis with localized peritonitis and gangrene, without perforation CC

K35.32 Acute appendicitis with perforation and localized peritonitis, without abscess MCC
(Acute) appendicitis with perforation NOS
Perforated appendix NOS
Ruptured appendix (with localized peritonitis) NOS
AHA: 2020,1Q,16

K35.33 Acute appendicitis with perforation and localized peritonitis, with abscess MCC
(Acute) appendicitis with (peritoneal) abscess NOS
Ruptured appendix with localized peritonitis and abscess

✓5th **K35.8 Other and unspecified acute appendicitis**

K35.80 Unspecified acute appendicitis CC
Acute appendicitis NOS
Acute appendicitis without (localized) (generalized) peritonitis

✓6th **K35.89 Other acute appendicitis**
AHA: 2020,1Q,16

K35.890 Other acute appendicitis without perforation or gangrene CC

K35.891 Other acute appendicitis without perforation, with gangrene CC
(Acute) appendicitis with gangrene NOS

K36 Other appendicitis
Chronic appendicitis
Recurrent appendicitis

K37 Unspecified appendicitis
EXCLUDES 1 *unspecified appendicitis with peritonitis (K35.2-, K35.3-)*

✓4th **K38 Other diseases of appendix**

K38.0 Hyperplasia of appendix

K38.1 Appendicular concretions
Fecalith of appendix
Stercolith of appendix

K38.2 Diverticulum of appendix

K38.3 Fistula of appendix

K38.8 Other specified diseases of appendix
Intussusception of appendix

K38.9 Disease of appendix, unspecified

Hernia (K40-K46)

NOTE Hernia with both gangrene and obstruction is classified to hernia with gangrene.

INCLUDES acquired hernia
congenital [except diaphragmatic or hiatus] hernia
recurrent hernia

✓4th **K40 Inguinal hernia**
INCLUDES bubonocele
direct inguinal hernia
double inguinal hernia
indirect inguinal hernia
inguinal hernia NOS
oblique inguinal hernia
scrotal hernia
DEF: Within the groin region.

✓5th **K40.0 Bilateral inguinal hernia, with obstruction, without gangrene**
Inguinal hernia (bilateral) causing obstruction without gangrene
Incarcerated inguinal hernia (bilateral) without gangrene
Irreducible inguinal hernia (bilateral) without gangrene
Strangulated inguinal hernia (bilateral) without gangrene

K40.00 Bilateral inguinal hernia, with obstruction, without gangrene, not specified as recurrent CC
Bilateral inguinal hernia, with obstruction, without gangrene NOS

K40.01 Bilateral inguinal hernia, with obstruction, without gangrene, recurrent CC

✓5th **K40.1 Bilateral inguinal hernia, with gangrene**

K40.10 Bilateral inguinal hernia, with gangrene, not specified as recurrent MCC
Bilateral inguinal hernia, with gangrene NOS

K40.11 Bilateral inguinal hernia, with gangrene, recurrent MCC

K40.2 Bilateral inguinal hernia, without obstruction or gangrene

K40.20 Bilateral inguinal hernia, without obstruction or gangrene, not specified as recurrent
Bilateral inguinal hernia NOS

K40.21 Bilateral inguinal hernia, without obstruction or gangrene, recurrent

K40.3 Unilateral inguinal hernia, with obstruction, without gangrene
Inguinal hernia (unilateral) causing obstruction without gangrene
Incarcerated inguinal hernia (unilateral) without gangrene
Irreducible inguinal hernia (unilateral) without gangrene
Strangulated inguinal hernia (unilateral) without gangrene

K40.30 Unilateral inguinal hernia, with obstruction, without gangrene, not specified as recurrent CC
Inguinal hernia, with obstruction NOS
Unilateral inguinal hernia, with obstruction, without gangrene NOS

K40.31 Unilateral inguinal hernia, with obstruction, without gangrene, recurrent CC

K40.4 Unilateral inguinal hernia, with gangrene

K40.40 Unilateral inguinal hernia, with gangrene, not specified as recurrent MCC
Inguinal hernia with gangrene NOS
Unilateral inguinal hernia with gangrene NOS

K40.41 Unilateral inguinal hernia, with gangrene, recurrent MCC

K40.9 Unilateral inguinal hernia, without obstruction or gangrene

K40.90 Unilateral inguinal hernia, without obstruction or gangrene, not specified as recurrent
Inguinal hernia NOS
Unilateral inguinal hernia NOS

K40.91 Unilateral inguinal hernia, without obstruction or gangrene, recurrent

Hernia Sites

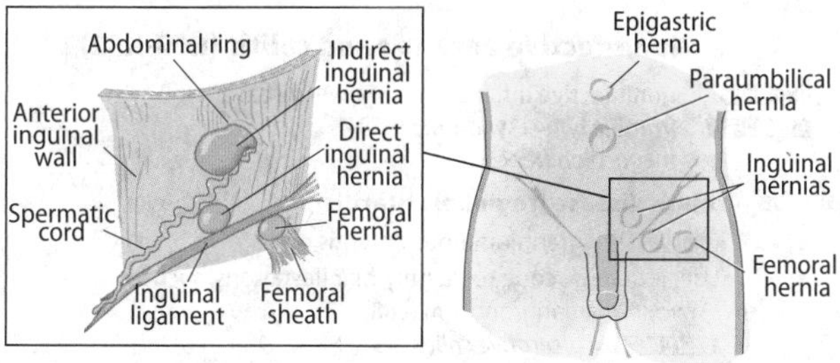

K41 Femoral hernia

K41.0 Bilateral femoral hernia, with obstruction, without gangrene
Femoral hernia (bilateral) causing obstruction, without gangrene
Incarcerated femoral hernia (bilateral), without gangrene
Irreducible femoral hernia (bilateral), without gangrene
Strangulated femoral hernia (bilateral), without gangrene

K41.00 Bilateral femoral hernia, with obstruction, without gangrene, not specified as recurrent CC
Bilateral femoral hernia, with obstruction, without gangrene NOS

K41.01 Bilateral femoral hernia, with obstruction, without gangrene, recurrent CC

K41.1 Bilateral femoral hernia, with gangrene

K41.10 Bilateral femoral hernia, with gangrene, not specified as recurrent MCC
Bilateral femoral hernia, with gangrene NOS

K41.11 Bilateral femoral hernia, with gangrene, recurrent MCC

K41.2 Bilateral femoral hernia, without obstruction or gangrene

K41.20 Bilateral femoral hernia, without obstruction or gangrene, not specified as recurrent
Bilateral femoral hernia NOS

K41.21 Bilateral femoral hernia, without obstruction or gangrene, recurrent

K41.3 Unilateral femoral hernia, with obstruction, without gangrene
Femoral hernia (unilateral) causing obstruction, without gangrene
Incarcerated femoral hernia (unilateral), without gangrene
Irreducible femoral hernia (unilateral), without gangrene
Strangulated femoral hernia (unilateral), without gangrene

K41.30 Unilateral femoral hernia, with obstruction, without gangrene, not specified as recurrent CC
Femoral hernia, with obstruction NOS
Unilateral femoral hernia, with obstruction NOS

K41.31 Unilateral femoral hernia, with obstruction, without gangrene, recurrent CC

K41.4 Unilateral femoral hernia, with gangrene

K41.40 Unilateral femoral hernia, with gangrene, not specified as recurrent MCC
Femoral hernia, with gangrene NOS
Unilateral femoral hernia, with gangrene NOS

K41.41 Unilateral femoral hernia, with gangrene, recurrent MCC

K41.9 Unilateral femoral hernia, without obstruction or gangrene

K41.90 Unilateral femoral hernia, without obstruction or gangrene, not specified as recurrent
Femoral hernia NOS
Unilateral femoral hernia NOS

K41.91 Unilateral femoral hernia, without obstruction or gangrene, recurrent

K42 Umbilical hernia

INCLUDES paraumbilical hernia
EXCLUDES 1 *omphalocele (Q79.2)*

K42.0 Umbilical hernia with obstruction, without gangrene CC
Umbilical hernia causing obstruction, without gangrene
Incarcerated umbilical hernia, without gangrene
Irreducible umbilical hernia, without gangrene
Strangulated umbilical hernia, without gangrene

K42.1 Umbilical hernia with gangrene MCC
Gangrenous umbilical hernia

K42.9 Umbilical hernia without obstruction or gangrene
Umbilical hernia NOS

K43 Ventral hernia

DEF: Condition in which a loop of bowel protrudes through a weakness in the abdominal wall muscles that may occur as a birth defect, past surgical site (incisional), or form at a stomal site (parastomal).

K43.0 Incisional hernia with obstruction, without gangrene CC
Incisional hernia causing obstruction, without gangrene
Incarcerated incisional hernia, without gangrene
Irreducible incisional hernia, without gangrene
Strangulated incisional hernia, without gangrene

K43.1 Incisional hernia with gangrene MCC
Gangrenous incisional hernia
AHA: 2020,2Q,22

K43.2 Incisional hernia without obstruction or gangrene
Incisional hernia NOS

K43.3 Parastomal hernia with obstruction, without gangrene CC
Incarcerated parastomal hernia, without gangrene
Irreducible parastomal hernia, without gangrene
Parastomal hernia causing obstruction, without gangrene
Strangulated parastomal hernia, without gangrene

K43.4 Parastomal hernia with gangrene MCC
Gangrenous parastomal hernia

K43.5 Parastomal hernia without obstruction or gangrene
Parastomal hernia NOS

K43.6 Other and unspecified ventral hernia with obstruction, without gangrene CC
Epigastric hernia causing obstruction, without gangrene
Hypogastric hernia causing obstruction, without gangrene
Incarcerated epigastric hernia without gangrene
Incarcerated hypogastric hernia without gangrene
Incarcerated midline hernia without gangrene
Incarcerated spigelian hernia without gangrene
Incarcerated subxiphoid hernia without gangrene
Irreducible epigastric hernia without gangrene
Irreducible hypogastric hernia without gangrene
Irreducible midline hernia without gangrene
Irreducible spigelian hernia without gangrene
Irreducible subxiphoid hernia without gangrene
Midline hernia causing obstruction, without gangrene
Spigelian hernia causing obstruction, without gangrene
Strangulated epigastric hernia without gangrene
Strangulated hypogastric hernia without gangrene
Strangulated midline hernia without gangrene
Strangulated spigelian hernia without gangrene
Strangulated subxiphoid hernia without gangrene
Subxiphoid hernia causing obstruction, without gangrene

K43.7 Other and unspecified ventral hernia with gangrene MCC
Any condition listed under K43.6 specified as gangrenous

K43.9 Ventral hernia without obstruction or gangrene
Epigastric hernia
Ventral hernia NOS

✓4th K44 Diaphragmatic hernia
INCLUDES hiatus hernia (esophageal) (sliding)
paraesophageal hernia
EXCLUDES 1 *congenital diaphragmatic hernia (Q79.0)*
congenital hiatus hernia (Q40.1)
DEF: Protrusion of an abdominal organ, usually the stomach, through the esophageal opening within the diaphragm and occurring in two types: the sliding hiatal hernia and the paraesophageal hernia.

Hiatal Hernia

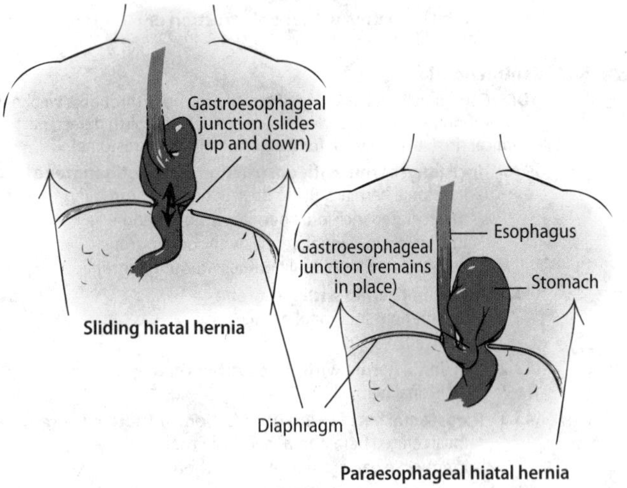

K44.0 Diaphragmatic hernia with obstruction, without gangrene CC
Diaphragmatic hernia causing obstruction
Incarcerated diaphragmatic hernia
Irreducible diaphragmatic hernia
Strangulated diaphragmatic hernia

K44.1 Diaphragmatic hernia with gangrene MCC
Gangrenous diaphragmatic hernia

K44.9 Diaphragmatic hernia without obstruction or gangrene
Diaphragmatic hernia NOS

✓4th K45 Other abdominal hernia
INCLUDES abdominal hernia, specified site NEC
lumbar hernia
obturator hernia
pudendal hernia
retroperitoneal hernia
sciatic hernia

K45.0 Other specified abdominal hernia with obstruction, without gangrene CC
Other specified abdominal hernia causing obstruction
Other specified incarcerated abdominal hernia
Other specified irreducible abdominal hernia
Other specified strangulated abdominal hernia

K45.1 Other specified abdominal hernia with gangrene MCC
Any condition listed under K45 specified as gangrenous

K45.8 Other specified abdominal hernia without obstruction or gangrene

✓4th K46 Unspecified abdominal hernia
INCLUDES enterocele
epiplocele
hernia NOS
interstitial hernia
intestinal hernia
intra-abdominal hernia
EXCLUDES 1 *vaginal enterocele (N81.5)*

K46.0 Unspecified abdominal hernia with obstruction, without gangrene CC
Unspecified abdominal hernia causing obstruction
Unspecified incarcerated abdominal hernia
Unspecified irreducible abdominal hernia
Unspecified strangulated abdominal hernia

K46.1 Unspecified abdominal hernia with gangrene MCC
Any condition listed under K46 specified as gangrenous

K46.9 Unspecified abdominal hernia without obstruction or gangrene
Abdominal hernia NOS

Noninfective enteritis and colitis (K50-K52)

INCLUDES noninfective inflammatory bowel disease
EXCLUDES 1 *irritable bowel syndrome (K58.-)*
megacolon (K59.3-)

✓4th K50 Crohn's disease [regional enteritis]
INCLUDES granulomatous enteritis
Use additional code to identify manifestations, such as:
pyoderma gangrenosum (L88)
EXCLUDES 1 *ulcerative colitis (K51.-)*
AHA: 2019,3Q,5; 2012,4Q,104
DEF: Chronic inflammation of the gastrointestinal tract characterized by chronic granulomatous disease, most commonly affecting the intestines and the terminal ileum.

✓5th K50.0 Crohn's disease of small intestine
Crohn's disease [regional enteritis] of duodenum
Crohn's disease [regional enteritis] of ileum
Crohn's disease [regional enteritis] of jejunum
Regional ileitis
Terminal ileitis
EXCLUDES 1 *Crohn's disease of both small and large intestine (K50.8-)*

K50.00 Crohn's disease of small intestine without complications CC HCC

✓6th K50.01 Crohn's disease of small intestine with complications

K50.011 Crohn's disease of small intestine with rectal bleeding CC HCC

K50.012 Crohn's disease of small intestine with intestinal obstruction CC HCC

K50.013 Crohn's disease of small intestine with fistula CC HCC SW

K50.014 Crohn's disease of small intestine with abscess CC HCC
AHA: 2012,4Q,104

K50.018 Crohn's disease of small intestine with other complication CC HCC

K50.019 Crohn's disease of small intestine with unspecified complications CC HCC

✓5th **K5Ø.1 Crohn's disease of large intestine**
Crohn's disease [regional enteritis] of colon
Crohn's disease [regional enteritis] of large bowel
Crohn's disease [regional enteritis] of rectum
Granulomatous colitis
Regional colitis
EXCLUDES 1 *Crohn's disease of both small and large intestine (K5Ø.8)*

K5Ø.1Ø Crohn's disease of large intestine without complications CC HCC

✓6th **K5Ø.11 Crohn's disease of large intestine with complications**

K5Ø.111 Crohn's disease of large intestine with rectal bleeding CC HCC
K5Ø.112 Crohn's disease of large intestine with intestinal obstruction CC HCC
K5Ø.113 Crohn's disease of large intestine with fistula CC HCC SW
K5Ø.114 Crohn's disease of large intestine with abscess CC HCC
K5Ø.118 Crohn's disease of large intestine with other complication CC HCC
K5Ø.119 Crohn's disease of large intestine with unspecified complications CC HCC

✓5th **K5Ø.8 Crohn's disease of both small and large intestine**

K5Ø.8Ø Crohn's disease of both small and large intestine without complications CC HCC

✓6th **K5Ø.81 Crohn's disease of both small and large intestine with complications**

K5Ø.811 Crohn's disease of both small and large intestine with rectal bleeding CC HCC
K5Ø.812 Crohn's disease of both small and large intestine with intestinal obstruction CC HCC
K5Ø.813 Crohn's disease of both small and large intestine with fistula CC HCC SW
K5Ø.814 Crohn's disease of both small and large intestine with abscess CC HCC
K5Ø.818 Crohn's disease of both small and large intestine with other complication CC HCC
K5Ø.819 Crohn's disease of both small and large intestine with unspecified complications CC HCC

✓5th **K5Ø.9 Crohn's disease, unspecified**

K5Ø.9Ø Crohn's disease, unspecified, without complications CC HCC
Crohn's disease NOS
Regional enteritis NOS

✓6th **K5Ø.91 Crohn's disease, unspecified, with complications**

K5Ø.911 Crohn's disease, unspecified, with rectal bleeding CC HCC
K5Ø.912 Crohn's disease, unspecified, with intestinal obstruction CC HCC
K5Ø.913 Crohn's disease, unspecified, with fistula CC HCC SW
K5Ø.914 Crohn's disease, unspecified, with abscess CC HCC
K5Ø.918 Crohn's disease, unspecified, with other complication CC HCC
K5Ø.919 Crohn's disease, unspecified, with unspecified complications CC HCC

✓4th **K51 Ulcerative colitis**

Use additional code to identify manifestations, such as:
pyoderma gangrenosum (L88)
EXCLUDES 1 *Crohn's disease [regional enteritis] (K5Ø.-)*

✓5th **K51.Ø Ulcerative (chronic) pancolitis**
Backwash ileitis

K51.ØØ Ulcerative (chronic) pancolitis without complications CC HCC
Ulcerative (chronic) pancolitis NOS

✓6th **K51.Ø1 Ulcerative (chronic) pancolitis with complications**

K51.Ø11 Ulcerative (chronic) pancolitis with rectal bleeding CC HCC
K51.Ø12 Ulcerative (chronic) pancolitis with intestinal obstruction CC HCC
K51.Ø13 Ulcerative (chronic) pancolitis with fistula CC HCC SW
K51.Ø14 Ulcerative (chronic) pancolitis with abscess CC HCC
K51.Ø18 Ulcerative (chronic) pancolitis with other complication CC HCC
K51.Ø19 Ulcerative (chronic) pancolitis with unspecified complications CC HCC

✓5th **K51.2 Ulcerative (chronic) proctitis**

K51.2Ø Ulcerative (chronic) proctitis without complications CC HCC
Ulcerative (chronic) proctitis NOS

✓6th **K51.21 Ulcerative (chronic) proctitis with complications**

K51.211 Ulcerative (chronic) proctitis with rectal bleeding CC HCC
K51.212 Ulcerative (chronic) proctitis with intestinal obstruction CC HCC
K51.213 Ulcerative (chronic) proctitis with fistula CC HCC SW
K51.214 Ulcerative (chronic) proctitis with abscess CC HCC
K51.218 Ulcerative (chronic) proctitis with other complication CC HCC
K51.219 Ulcerative (chronic) proctitis with unspecified complications CC HCC

✓5th **K51.3 Ulcerative (chronic) rectosigmoiditis**

K51.3Ø Ulcerative (chronic) rectosigmoiditis without complications CC HCC
Ulcerative (chronic) rectosigmoiditis NOS

✓6th **K51.31 Ulcerative (chronic) rectosigmoiditis with complications**

K51.311 Ulcerative (chronic) rectosigmoiditis with rectal bleeding CC HCC
K51.312 Ulcerative (chronic) rectosigmoiditis with intestinal obstruction CC HCC
K51.313 Ulcerative (chronic) rectosigmoiditis with fistula CC HCC SW
K51.314 Ulcerative (chronic) rectosigmoiditis with abscess CC HCC
K51.318 Ulcerative (chronic) rectosigmoiditis with other complication CC HCC
K51.319 Ulcerative (chronic) rectosigmoiditis with unspecified complications CC HCC

✓5th **K51.4 Inflammatory polyps of colon**
EXCLUDES 1 *adenomatous polyp of colon (D12.6)*
polyposis of colon (D12.6)
polyps of colon NOS (K63.5)

K51.4Ø Inflammatory polyps of colon without complications CC HCC
Inflammatory polyps of colon NOS

✓6th **K51.41 Inflammatory polyps of colon with complications**

K51.411 Inflammatory polyps of colon with rectal bleeding CC HCC
K51.412 Inflammatory polyps of colon with intestinal obstruction CC HCC
K51.413 Inflammatory polyps of colon with fistula CC HCC SW
K51.414 Inflammatory polyps of colon with abscess CC HCC
K51.418 Inflammatory polyps of colon with other complication CC HCC
K51.419 Inflammatory polyps of colon with unspecified complications CC HCC

✓5th **K51.5 Left sided colitis**
Left hemicolitis

K51.5Ø Left sided colitis without complications CC HCC
Left sided colitis NOS

✓6th **K51.51 Left sided colitis with complications**

K51.511 Left sided colitis with rectal bleeding CC HCC
K51.512 Left sided colitis with intestinal obstruction CC HCC
K51.513 Left sided colitis with fistula CC HCC SW
K51.514 Left sided colitis with abscess CC HCC
K51.518 Left sided colitis with other complication CC HCC
K51.519 Left sided colitis with unspecified complications CC HCC

Chapter 11. Diseases of the Digestive System

✓5th **K51.8 Other ulcerative colitis**

K51.80 Other ulcerative colitis without complications CC HCC

✓6th **K51.81 Other ulcerative colitis with complications**

K51.811 Other ulcerative colitis with rectal bleeding CC HCC

K51.812 Other ulcerative colitis with intestinal obstruction CC HCC

K51.813 Other ulcerative colitis with fistula CC HCC SW

K51.814 Other ulcerative colitis with abscess CC HCC

K51.818 Other ulcerative colitis with other complication CC HCC

K51.819 Other ulcerative colitis with unspecified complications CC HCC

✓5th **K51.9 Ulcerative colitis, unspecified**

K51.90 Ulcerative colitis, unspecified, without complications CC HCC

✓6th **K51.91 Ulcerative colitis, unspecified, with complications**

K51.911 Ulcerative colitis, unspecified with rectal bleeding CC HCC

K51.912 Ulcerative colitis, unspecified with intestinal obstruction CC HCC

K51.913 Ulcerative colitis, unspecified with fistula CC HCC SW

K51.914 Ulcerative colitis, unspecified with abscess CC HCC

K51.918 Ulcerative colitis, unspecified with other complication CC HCC

K51.919 Ulcerative colitis, unspecified with unspecified complications CC HCC

✓4th **K52 Other and unspecified noninfective gastroenteritis and colitis**

AHA: 2016,4Q,30-31

K52.0 Gastroenteritis and colitis due to radiation CC

K52.1 Toxic gastroenteritis and colitis CC

Drug-induced gastroenteritis and colitis

Code first (T51-T65) to identify toxic agent

Use additional code for adverse effect, if applicable, to identify drug (T36-T50 with fifth or sixth character 5)

AHA: 2019,1Q,17

✓5th **K52.2 Allergic and dietetic gastroenteritis and colitis**

Food hypersensitivity gastroenteritis or colitis

Use additional code to identify type of food allergy (Z91.01-, Z91.02-)

EXCLUDES 2 *allergic eosinophilic colitis (K52.82)*
allergic eosinophilic esophagitis (K20.0)
allergic eosinophilic gastritis (K52.81)
allergic eosinophilic gastroenteritis (K52.81)
food protein-induced proctocolitis (K52.82)

DEF: True immunoglobulin E (IgE)-mediated allergic reaction of the lining of the stomach, intestines, or colon to food proteins. It causes nausea, vomiting, diarrhea, and abdominal cramping.

TIP: Assign a code for "with hemorrhage" when angiodysplasia and GI bleeding are documented. The ICD-10-CM classification assumes the two are related without the provider linking the two conditions. Evidence of bleeding during a procedure is not required.

K52.21 Food protein-induced enterocolitis syndrome

FPIES

Use additional code for hypovolemic shock, if present (R57.1)

K52.22 Food protein-induced enteropathy

K52.29 Other allergic and dietetic gastroenteritis and colitis

Food hypersensitivity gastroenteritis or colitis

Immediate gastrointestinal hypersensitivity

K52.3 Indeterminate colitis

Colonic inflammatory bowel disease unclassified (IBDU)

EXCLUDES 1 *unspecified colitis (K52.9)*

✓5th **K52.8 Other specified noninfective gastroenteritis and colitis**

K52.81 Eosinophilic gastritis or gastroenteritis

Eosinophilic enteritis

EXCLUDES 2 *eosinophilic esophagitis (K20.0)*

DEF: Disorder involving the accumulation of eosinophil in the lining of the stomach or multiple levels of the gastrointestinal tract, but without a known cause such as connective tissue disease, drug reaction, malignancy, or parasitic infection.

K52.82 Eosinophilic colitis

Allergic proctocolitis

Food-induced eosinophilic proctocolitis

Food protein-induced proctocolitis

Milk protein-induced proctocolitis

DEF: Disorder involving the accumulation of eosinophil in the tissues lining the colon, but without a known cause such as connective tissue disease, drug reaction, malignancy, or parasitic infection. The resultant inflammation may cause extreme abdominal pain, diarrhea, or bloody stool.

✓6th **K52.83 Microscopic colitis**

K52.831 Collagenous colitis

K52.832 Lymphocytic colitis

K52.838 Other microscopic colitis

K52.839 Microscopic colitis, unspecified

K52.89 Other specified noninfective gastroenteritis and colitis

AHA: 2019,1Q,20

K52.9 Noninfective gastroenteritis and colitis, unspecified

Colitis NOS

Enteritis NOS

Gastroenteritis NOS

Ileitis NOS

Jejunitis NOS

Sigmoiditis NOS

EXCLUDES 1 *diarrhea NOS (R19.7)*
functional diarrhea (K59.1)
infectious gastroenteritis and colitis NOS (A09)
neonatal diarrhea (noninfective) (P78.3)
psychogenic diarrhea (F45.8)

Other diseases of intestines (K55-K64)

✓4th **K55 Vascular disorders of intestine**

EXCLUDES 1 *necrotizing enterocolitis of newborn (P77.-)*

AHA: 2016,4Q,32

✓5th **K55.0 Acute vascular disorders of intestine**

Infarction of appendices epiploicae

Mesenteric (artery) (vein) embolism

Mesenteric (artery) (vein) infarction

Mesenteric (artery) (vein) thrombosis

AHA: 2019,4Q,68

✓6th **K55.01 Acute (reversible) ischemia of small intestine**

K55.011 Focal (segmental) acute (reversible) ischemia of small intestine MCC HCC

K55.012 Diffuse acute (reversible) ischemia of small intestine MCC HCC

K55.019 Acute (reversible) ischemia of small intestine, extent unspecified MCC HCC

✓6th **K55.02 Acute infarction of small intestine**

Gangrene of small intestine

Necrosis of small intestine

K55.021 Focal (segmental) acute infarction of small intestine MCC HCC

K55.022 Diffuse acute infarction of small intestine MCC HCC

K55.029 Acute infarction of small intestine, extent unspecified MCC HCC

✓6th **K55.03 Acute (reversible) ischemia of large intestine**

Acute fulminant ischemic colitis

Subacute ischemic colitis

K55.031 Focal (segmental) acute (reversible) ischemia of large intestine MCC HCC

K55.032 Diffuse acute (reversible) ischemia of large intestine MCC HCC

K55.Ø39 Acute (reversible) ischemia of large intestine, extent unspecified MCC HCC
AHA: 2019,4Q,68

K55.Ø4 Acute infarction of large intestine
Gangrene of large intestine
Necrosis of large intestine

K55.Ø41 Focal (segmental) acute infarction of large intestine MCC HCC

K55.Ø42 Diffuse acute infarction of large intestine MCC HCC

K55.Ø49 Acute infarction of large intestine, extent unspecified MCC HCC

K55.Ø5 Acute (reversible) ischemia of intestine, part unspecified

K55.Ø51 Focal (segmental) acute (reversible) ischemia of intestine, part unspecified MCC HCC

K55.Ø52 Diffuse acute (reversible) ischemia of intestine, part unspecified MCC HCC

K55.Ø59 Acute (reversible) ischemia of intestine, part and extent unspecified MCC HCC

K55.Ø6 Acute infarction of intestine, part unspecified
Acute intestinal infarction
Gangrene of intestine
Necrosis of intestine

K55.Ø61 Focal (segmental) acute infarction of intestine, part unspecified MCC HCC

K55.Ø62 Diffuse acute infarction of intestine, part unspecified MCC HCC

K55.Ø69 Acute infarction of intestine, part and extent unspecified MCC HCC

K55.1 Chronic vascular disorders of intestine CC HCC
Chronic ischemic colitis
Chronic ischemic enteritis
Chronic ischemic enterocolitis
Ischemic stricture of intestine
Mesenteric atherosclerosis
Mesenteric vascular insufficiency

K55.2 Angiodysplasia of colon
AHA: 2018,3Q,21
TIP: Assign a code for "with hemorrhage" when angiodysplasia and GI bleeding are documented. The ICD-10-CM classification assumes the two are related without the provider linking the two conditions. Evidence of bleeding during a procedure is not required.

K55.2Ø Angiodysplasia of colon without hemorrhage

K55.21 Angiodysplasia of colon with hemorrhage MCC
DEF: Small vascular abnormalities due to fragile blood vessels in the colon, resulting in blood loss from the gastrointestinal (GI) tract.

K55.3 Necrotizing enterocolitis
EXCLUDES 1 *necrotizing enterocolitis of newborn (P77.-)*
EXCLUDES 2 *necrotizing enterocolitis due to Clostridium difficile (AØ4.7-)*

K55.3Ø Necrotizing enterocolitis, unspecified MCC HCC
Necrotizing enterocolitis, NOS

K55.31 Stage 1 necrotizing enterocolitis MCC HCC
Necrotizing enterocolitis without pneumatosis, without perforation

K55.32 Stage 2 necrotizing enterocolitis MCC HCC
Necrotizing enterocolitis with pneumatosis, without perforation

K55.33 Stage 3 necrotizing enterocolitis MCC HCC
Necrotizing enterocolitis with perforation
Necrotizing enterocolitis with pneumatosis and perforation

K55.8 Other vascular disorders of intestine CC HCC

K55.9 Vascular disorder of intestine, unspecified CC HCC
Ischemic colitis
Ischemic enteritis
Ischemic enterocolitis

K56 Paralytic ileus and intestinal obstruction without hernia
EXCLUDES 1 *congenital stricture or stenosis of intestine (Q41-Q42)*
cystic fibrosis with meconium ileus (E84.11)
ischemic stricture of intestine (K55.1)
meconium ileus NOS (P76.Ø)
neonatal intestinal obstructions classifiable to P76.-
obstruction of duodenum (K31.5)
postprocedural intestinal obstruction (K91.3-)
~~*stenosis of anus or rectum (K62.4)*~~
EXCLUDES 2 ►*stenosis of anus or rectum (K62.4)*◄

K56.Ø Paralytic ileus CC HCC
Paralysis of bowel
Paralysis of colon
Paralysis of intestine
EXCLUDES 1 *gallstone ileus (K56.3)*
ileus NOS (K56.7)
obstructive ileus NOS (K56.69-)
DEF: Intestinal obstruction due to paralysis of bowel motility or peristalsis.

K56.1 Intussusception CC HCC
Intussusception or invagination of bowel
Intussusception or invagination of colon
Intussusception or invagination of intestine
Intussusception or invagination of rectum
EXCLUDES 2 *intussusception of appendix (K38.8)*
DEF: Intestinal obstruction due to prolapse of a bowel section into an adjacent section. It occurs primarily in children and symptoms include acute abdominal pain, vomiting, and passage of blood and mucus from the rectum.

K56.2 Volvulus MCC HCC
Strangulation of colon or intestine
Torsion of colon or intestine
Twist of colon or intestine
EXCLUDES 2 *volvulus of duodenum (K31.5)*
DEF: Twisting, knotting, or entanglement of the bowel on itself that may quickly compromise oxygen supply to the intestinal tissues. A volvulus usually occurs at the sigmoid and ileocecal areas of the intestines.

Volvulus

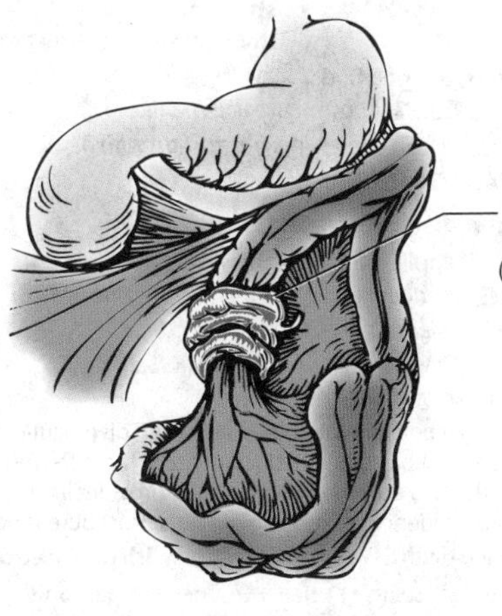

K56.3 Gallstone ileus CC HCC
Obstruction of intestine by gallstone

K56.4 Other impaction of intestine

K56.41 Fecal impaction HCC
EXCLUDES 1 *constipation (K59.Ø-)*
incomplete defecation (R15.Ø)

K56.49 Other impaction of intestine CC HCC

✓5th **K56.5 Intestinal adhesions [bands] with obstruction (postinfection)**
Abdominal hernia due to adhesions with obstruction
Peritoneal adhesions [bands] with intestinal obstruction (postinfection)
AHA: 2017,4Q,16-17

K56.50 Intestinal adhesions [bands], unspecified as to partial versus complete obstruction CC HCC
Intestinal adhesions with obstruction NOS

K56.51 Intestinal adhesions [bands], with partial obstruction CC HCC
Intestinal adhesions with incomplete obstruction

K56.52 Intestinal adhesions [bands] with complete obstruction CC HCC

✓5th **K56.6 Other and unspecified intestinal obstruction**
AHA: 2017,4Q,16-17; 2017,2Q,12

✓6th **K56.60 Unspecified intestinal obstruction**
EXCLUDES 1 ~~*intestinal obstruction due to specified condition - code to condition*~~

K56.600 Partial intestinal obstruction, unspecified as to cause CC HCC
Incomplete intestinal obstruction, NOS

K56.601 Complete intestinal obstruction, unspecified as to cause CC HCC

K56.609 Unspecified intestinal obstruction, unspecified as to partial versus complete obstruction CC HCC
Intestinal obstruction NOS

✓6th **K56.69 Other intestinal obstruction**
Enterostenosis NOS
Obstructive ileus NOS
Occlusion of colon or intestine NOS
Stenosis of colon or intestine NOS
Stricture of colon or intestine NOS
EXCLUDES 1 *intestinal obstruction due to specified condition - code to condition*

K56.690 Other partial intestinal obstruction CC HCC
Other incomplete intestinal obstruction

K56.691 Other complete intestinal obstruction CC HCC

K56.699 Other intestinal obstruction unspecified as to partial versus complete obstruction CC HCC
Other intestinal obstruction, NEC

K56.7 Ileus, unspecified CC HCC
EXCLUDES 1 *obstructive ileus (K56.69-)*
EXCLUDES 2 *intestinal obstruction with hernia (K40-K46)*
AHA: 2017,1Q,40

✓4th **K57 Diverticular disease of intestine**
Code also if applicable peritonitis K65.-
EXCLUDES 1 *congenital diverticulum of intestine (Q43.8)*
Meckel's diverticulum (Q43.0)
EXCLUDES 2 *diverticulum of appendix (K38.2)*
AHA: 2018,3Q,21
TIP: Assign a code for "with bleeding" when diverticular disease of the intestine and GI bleeding are documented. The ICD-10-CM classification assumes the two are related without the provider linking the two conditions. Evidence of bleeding during a procedure is not required.

✓5th **K57.0 Diverticulitis of small intestine with perforation and abscess**
~~Diverticulitis of small intestine with peritonitis~~
EXCLUDES 1 *diverticulitis of both small and large intestine with perforation and abscess (K57.4-)*

K57.00 Diverticulitis of small intestine with perforation and abscess without bleeding CC

K57.01 Diverticulitis of small intestine with perforation and abscess with bleeding MCC

✓5th **K57.1 Diverticular disease of small intestine without perforation or abscess**
EXCLUDES 1 *diverticular disease of both small and large intestine without perforation or abscess (K57.5-)*

K57.10 Diverticulosis of small intestine without perforation or abscess without bleeding
Diverticular disease of small intestine NOS

K57.11 Diverticulosis of small intestine without perforation or abscess with bleeding MCC

K57.12 Diverticulitis of small intestine without perforation or abscess without bleeding CC

K57.13 Diverticulitis of small intestine without perforation or abscess with bleeding MCC

✓5th **K57.2 Diverticulitis of large intestine with perforation and abscess**
~~Diverticulitis of colon with peritonitis~~
EXCLUDES 1 *diverticulitis of both small and large intestine with perforation and abscess (K57.4-)*

K57.20 Diverticulitis of large intestine with perforation and abscess without bleeding CC

K57.21 Diverticulitis of large intestine with perforation and abscess with bleeding MCC

✓5th **K57.3 Diverticular disease of large intestine without perforation or abscess**
EXCLUDES 1 *diverticular disease of both small and large intestine without perforation or abscess (K57.5-)*

K57.30 Diverticulosis of large intestine without perforation or abscess without bleeding
Diverticular disease of colon NOS

K57.31 Diverticulosis of large intestine without perforation or abscess with bleeding MCC

K57.32 Diverticulitis of large intestine without perforation or abscess without bleeding CC

K57.33 Diverticulitis of large intestine without perforation or abscess with bleeding MCC

✓5th **K57.4 Diverticulitis of both small and large intestine with perforation and abscess**
~~Diverticulitis of both small and large intestine with peritonitis~~

K57.40 Diverticulitis of both small and large intestine with perforation and abscess without bleeding CC

K57.41 Diverticulitis of both small and large intestine with perforation and abscess with bleeding MCC

✓5th **K57.5 Diverticular disease of both small and large intestine without perforation or abscess**

K57.50 Diverticulosis of both small and large intestine without perforation or abscess without bleeding
Diverticular disease of both small and large intestine NOS

K57.51 Diverticulosis of both small and large intestine without perforation or abscess with bleeding MCC

K57.52 Diverticulitis of both small and large intestine without perforation or abscess without bleeding CC

K57.53 Diverticulitis of both small and large intestine without perforation or abscess with bleeding MCC

✓5th **K57.8 Diverticulitis of intestine, part unspecified, with perforation and abscess**
~~Diverticulitis of intestine NOS with peritonitis~~

K57.80 Diverticulitis of intestine, part unspecified, with perforation and abscess without bleeding CC

K57.81 Diverticulitis of intestine, part unspecified, with perforation and abscess with bleeding MCC

✓5th **K57.9 Diverticular disease of intestine, part unspecified, without perforation or abscess**

K57.90 Diverticulosis of intestine, part unspecified, without perforation or abscess without bleeding
Diverticular disease of intestine NOS

K57.91 Diverticulosis of intestine, part unspecified, without perforation or abscess with bleeding MCC

K57.92 Diverticulitis of intestine, part unspecified, without perforation or abscess without bleeding CC

K57.93 Diverticulitis of intestine, part unspecified, without perforation or abscess with bleeding MCC

✓4th **K58 Irritable bowel syndrome**
INCLUDES irritable colon
spastic colon
AHA: 2016,4Q,32-33

K58.0 Irritable bowel syndrome with diarrhea
K58.1 Irritable bowel syndrome with constipation
K58.2 Mixed irritable bowel syndrome
K58.8 Other irritable bowel syndrome
K58.9 Irritable bowel syndrome without diarrhea
Irritable bowel syndrome NOS

K59 Other functional intestinal disorders

EXCLUDES 1 *change in bowel habit NOS (R19.4)*
intestinal malabsorption (K90.-)
psychogenic intestinal disorders (F45.8)

EXCLUDES 2 *functional disorders of stomach (K31.-)*

K59.0 Constipation

EXCLUDES 1 *fecal impaction (K56.41)*
incomplete defecation (R15.0)

AHA: 2016,4Q,33

K59.00 Constipation, unspecified

K59.01 Slow transit constipation

DEF: Delay in the transit of fecal material through the colon secondary to smooth muscle dysfunction or decreased peristaltic contractions along the colon.

K59.02 Outlet dysfunction constipation

K59.03 Drug induced constipation

Use additional code for adverse effect, if applicable, to identify drug (T36-T50 with fifth or sixth character 5)

K59.04 Chronic idiopathic constipation

Functional constipation

K59.09 Other constipation

Chronic constipation

K59.1 Functional diarrhea

EXCLUDES 1 *diarrhea NOS (R19.7)*
irritable bowel syndrome with diarrhea (K58.0)

K59.2 Neurogenic bowel, not elsewhere classified CC

DEF: Disorder of bowel due to a spinal cord lesion due to injury or as a complication of conditions such as multiple sclerosis (MS) or spina bifida. Loss of bowel control is the primary symptom, manifested as constipation or bowel incontinence.

K59.3 Megacolon, not elsewhere classified

Dilatation of colon

Code first, if applicable (T51-T65) to identify toxic agent

EXCLUDES 1 *congenital megacolon (aganglionic) (Q43.1)*
megacolon (due to) (in) Chagas' disease (B57.32)
megacolon (due to) (in) Clostridium difficile (A04.7-)
megacolon (due to) (in) Hirschsprung's disease (Q43.1)

AHA: 2016,4Q,33-34

K59.31 Toxic megacolon CC HCC

K59.39 Other megacolon CC

Megacolon NOS

K59.4 Anal spasm

Proctalgia fugax

▲ **K59.8 Other specified functional intestinal disorders**

~~Atony of colon~~

~~Pseudo-obstruction (acute) (chronic) of intestine~~

● **K59.81 Ogilvie syndrome**

Acute colonic pseudo-obstruction (ACPO)

● **K59.89 Other specified functional intestinal disorders**

Atony of colon

Pseudo-obstruction (acute) (chronic) of intestine

K59.9 Functional intestinal disorder, unspecified

K60 Fissure and fistula of anal and rectal regions

EXCLUDES 1 *fissure and fistula of anal and rectal regions with abscess or cellulitis (K61.-)*

EXCLUDES 2 *anal sphincter tear (healed) (nontraumatic) (old) (K62.81)*

K60.0 Acute anal fissure

K60.1 Chronic anal fissure

K60.2 Anal fissure, unspecified

K60.3 Anal fistula SW

K60.4 Rectal fistula SW

Fistula of rectum to skin

EXCLUDES 1 *rectovaginal fistula (N82.3)*
vesicorectal fistual (N32.1)

K60.5 Anorectal fistula SW

K61 Abscess of anal and rectal regions

INCLUDES abscess of anal and rectal regions
cellulitis of anal and rectal regions

K61.0 Anal abscess CC

Perianal abscess

EXCLUDES 2 *intrasphincteric abscess (K61.4)*

K61.1 Rectal abscess CC

Perirectal abscess

EXCLUDES 1 *ischiorectal abscess (K61.39)*

AHA: 2012,4Q,104

K61.2 Anorectal abscess CC

K61.3 Ischiorectal abscess

AHA: 2018,4Q,19

K61.31 Horseshoe abscess

K61.39 Other ischiorectal abscess

Abscess of ischiorectal fossa

Ischiorectal abscess, NOS

K61.4 Intrasphincteric abscess CC

Intersphincteric abscess

K61.5 Supralevator abscess

AHA: 2018,4Q,19

K62 Other diseases of anus and rectum

INCLUDES anal canal

EXCLUDES 2 *colostomy and enterostomy malfunction (K94.0-, K94.1-)*
fecal incontinence (R15.-)
hemorrhoids (K64.-)

K62.0 Anal polyp

K62.1 Rectal polyp

EXCLUDES 1 *adenomatous polyp (D12.8)*

AHA: 2018,1Q,6

K62.2 Anal prolapse

Prolapse of anal canal

K62.3 Rectal prolapse

Prolapse of rectal mucosa

K62.4 Stenosis of anus and rectum

Stricture of anus (sphincter)

AHA: 2019,2Q,13

K62.5 Hemorrhage of anus and rectum CC

EXCLUDES 1 *gastrointestinal bleeding NOS (K92.2)*
melena (K92.1)
neonatal rectal hemorrhage (P54.2)

AHA: 2019,1Q,21

K62.6 Ulcer of anus and rectum CC

Solitary ulcer of anus and rectum

Stercoral ulcer of anus and rectum

EXCLUDES 1 *fissure and fistula of anus and rectum (K60.-)*
ulcerative colitis (K51.-)

K62.7 Radiation proctitis

▶Use additional code to identify the type of radiation (W88.-) or radiation therapy (Y84.2)◀

AHA: 2019,1Q,21

K62.8 Other specified diseases of anus and rectum

EXCLUDES 2 *ulcerative proctitis (K51.2)*

K62.81 Anal sphincter tear (healed) (nontraumatic) (old)

Tear of anus, nontraumatic

Use additional code for any associated fecal incontinence (R15.-)

EXCLUDES 2 *anal fissure (K60.-)*
anal sphincter tear (healed) (old) complicating delivery (O34.7-)
traumatic tear of anal sphincter (S31.831)

K62.82 Dysplasia of anus

Anal intraepithelial neoplasia I and II (AIN I and II) (histologically confirmed)

Dysplasia of anus NOS

Mild and moderate dysplasia of anus (histologically confirmed)

EXCLUDES 1 *abnormal results from anal cytologic examination without histologic confirmation (R85.61-)*
anal intraepithelial neoplasia III (D01.3)
carcinoma in situ of anus (D01.3)
HGSIL of anus (R85.613)
severe dysplasia of anus (D01.3)

K62.89 Other specified diseases of anus and rectum

Proctitis NOS

Use additional code for any associated fecal incontinence (R15.-)

K62.9 Disease of anus and rectum, unspecified

✓4th K63 Other diseases of intestine

K63.Ø Abscess of intestine CC

EXCLUDES 1 *abscess of intestine with Crohn's disease (K5Ø.Ø14, K5Ø.114, K5Ø.814, K5Ø.914)*
abscess of intestine with diverticular disease (K57.Ø, K57.2, K57.4, K57.8)
abscess of intestine with ulcerative colitis (K51.Ø14, K51.214, K51.314, K51.414, K51.514, K51.814, K51.914)

EXCLUDES 2 *abscess of anal and rectal regions (K61.-)*
abscess of appendix (K35.3-)

K63.1 Perforation of intestine (nontraumatic) MCC HCC

Perforation (nontraumatic) of rectum

EXCLUDES 1 *perforation (nontraumatic) of duodenum (K26.-)*
perforation (nontraumatic) of intestine with diverticular disease (K57.Ø, K57.2, K57.4, K57.8)

EXCLUDES 2 *perforation (nontraumatic) of appendix (K35.2-, K35.3-)*

AHA: 2020,2Q,22

K63.2 Fistula of intestine CC SW

EXCLUDES 1 *fistula of duodenum (K31.6)*
fistula of intestine with Crohn's disease (K5Ø.Ø13, K5Ø.113, K5Ø.813, K5Ø.913)
fistula of intestine with ulcerative colitis (K51.Ø13, K51.213, K51.313, K51.413, K51.513, K51.813, K51.913)

EXCLUDES 2 *fistula of anal and rectal regions (K6Ø.-)*
fistula of appendix (K38.3)
intestinal-genital fistula, female (N82.2-N82.4)
vesicointestinal fistula (N32.1)

AHA: 2017,3Q,4

K63.3 Ulcer of intestine CC

Primary ulcer of small intestine

EXCLUDES 1 *duodenal ulcer (K26.-)*
gastrointestinal ulcer (K28.-)
gastrojejunal ulcer (K28.-)
jejunal ulcer (K28.-)
peptic ulcer, site unspecified (K27.-)
ulcer of intestine with perforation (K63.1)
ulcer of anus or rectum (K62.6)
ulcerative colitis (K51.-)

K63.4 Enteroptosis

K63.5 Polyp of colon

EXCLUDES 1 *adenomatous polyp of colon (D12.-)*
inflammatory polyp of colon (K51.4-)
polyposis of colon (D12.6)

AHA: 2019,1Q,33; 2018,2Q,14; 2017,1Q,15; 2015,2Q,14

TIP: Assign this code when documentation states hyperplastic colon polyp regardless of the site in the colon. Slow-growing, hyperplastic polyps are not precancerous and are classified differently from benign or adenomatous polyps.

✓5th K63.8 Other specified diseases of intestine

K63.81 Dieulafoy lesion of intestine MCC

EXCLUDES 2 *Dieulafoy lesion of stomach and duodenum (K31.82)*

DEF: Abnormally large submucosal artery protruding through a defect in the stomach mucosa or intestines that can cause massive and life-threatening hemorrhaging.

K63.89 Other specified diseases of intestine

AHA: 2013,2Q,31

K63.9 Disease of intestine, unspecified

✓4th K64 Hemorrhoids and perianal venous thrombosis

INCLUDES piles

EXCLUDES 1 *hemorrhoids complicating childbirth and the puerperium (O87.2)*
hemorrhoids complicating pregnancy (O22.4)

Hemorrhoids

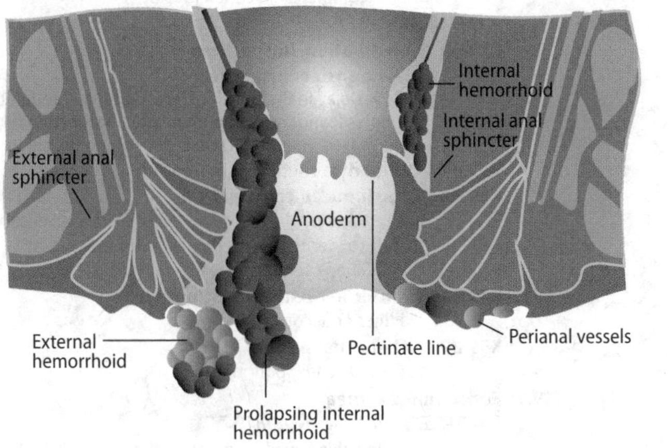

K64.Ø First degree hemorrhoids

Grade/stage I hemorrhoids
Hemorrhoids (bleeding) without prolapse outside of anal canal

K64.1 Second degree hemorrhoids

Grade/stage II hemorrhoids
Hemorrhoids (bleeding) that prolapse with straining, but retract spontaneously

K64.2 Third degree hemorrhoids

Grade/stage III hemorrhoids
Hemorrhoids (bleeding) that prolapse with straining and require manual replacement back inside anal canal

K64.3 Fourth degree hemorrhoids

Grade/stage IV hemorrhoids
Hemorrhoids (bleeding) with prolapsed tissue that cannot be manually replaced

K64.4 Residual hemorrhoidal skin tags

External hemorrhoids, NOS
Skin tags of anus

K64.5 Perianal venous thrombosis

External hemorrhoids with thrombosis
Perianal hematoma
Thrombosed hemorrhoids NOS

K64.8 Other hemorrhoids

Internal hemorrhoids, without mention of degree
Prolapsed hemorrhoids, degree not specified

K64.9 Unspecified hemorrhoids

Hemorrhoids (bleeding) NOS
Hemorrhoids (bleeding) without mention of degree

Diseases of peritoneum and retroperitoneum (K65-K68)

K65 Peritonitis
Use additional code (B95-B97), to identify infectious agent, if known
Code also if applicable diverticular disease of intestine (K57.-)
EXCLUDES 1 *acute appendicitis with generalized peritonitis (K35.2-)*
aseptic peritonitis (T81.6)
benign paroxysmal peritonitis (E85.Ø)
chemical peritonitis (T81.6)
gonococcal peritonitis (A54.85)
neonatal peritonitis (P78.Ø-P78.1)
pelvic peritonitis, female (N73.3-N73.5)
periodic familial peritonitis (E85.Ø)
peritonitis due to talc or other foreign substance (T81.6)
peritonitis in chlamydia (A74.81)
peritonitis in diphtheria (A36.89)
peritonitis in syphilis (late) (A52.74)
peritonitis in tuberculosis (A18.31)
peritonitis with or following abortion or ectopic or molar pregnancy (OØØ-OØ7, OØ8.Ø)
peritonitis with or following appendicitis (K35.-)
puerperal peritonitis (O85)
retroperitoneal infections (K68.-)

K65.Ø Generalized (acute) peritonitis MCC HCC
Pelvic peritonitis (acute), male
Subphrenic peritonitis (acute)
Suppurative peritonitis (acute)

K65.1 Peritoneal abscess MCC HCC
Abdominopelvic abscess
Abscess (of) omentum
Abscess (of) peritoneum
Mesenteric abscess
Retrocecal abscess
Subdiaphragmatic abscess
Subhepatic abscess
Subphrenic abscess
AHA: 2019,1Q,15

K65.2 Spontaneous bacterial peritonitis MCC HCC
EXCLUDES 1 *bacterial peritonitis NOS (K65.9)*

K65.3 Choleperitonitis MCC HCC
Peritonitis due to bile
DEF: Inflammation of the peritoneum due to leakage of bile into the peritoneal cavity resulting from rupture of the bile passages or gallbladder.

K65.4 Sclerosing mesenteritis CC HCC
Fat necrosis of peritoneum
(Idiopathic) sclerosing mesenteric fibrosis
Mesenteric lipodystrophy
Mesenteric panniculitis
Retractile mesenteritis

K65.8 Other peritonitis MCC HCC
Chronic proliferative peritonitis
Peritonitis due to urine

K65.9 Peritonitis, unspecified MCC HCC
Bacterial peritonitis NOS
AHA: 2013,2Q,31

K66 Other disorders of peritoneum
EXCLUDES 2 *ascites (R18.-)*
peritoneal effusion (chronic) (R18.8)

K66.Ø Peritoneal adhesions (postprocedural) (postinfection)
Adhesions (of) abdominal (wall)
Adhesions (of) diaphragm
Adhesions (of) intestine
Adhesions (of) male pelvis
Adhesions (of) omentum
Adhesions (of) stomach
Adhesive bands
Mesenteric adhesions
EXCLUDES 1 *female pelvic adhesions [bands] (N73.6)*
peritoneal adhesions with intestinal obstruction (K56.5-)

K66.1 Hemoperitoneum MCC
EXCLUDES 1 *traumatic hemoperitoneum (S36.8-)*

K66.8 Other specified disorders of peritoneum

K66.9 Disorder of peritoneum, unspecified

K67 Disorders of peritoneum in infectious diseases classified elsewhere MCC HCC
Code first underlying disease, such as:
congenital syphilis (A5Ø.Ø)
helminthiasis (B65.Ø-B83.9)
EXCLUDES 1 *peritonitis in chlamydia (A74.81)*
peritonitis in diphtheria (A36.89)
peritonitis in gonococcal (A54.85)
peritonitis in syphilis (late) (A52.74)
peritonitis in tuberculosis (A18.31)

K68 Disorders of retroperitoneum

K68.1 Retroperitoneal abscess

K68.11 Postprocedural retroperitoneal abscess CC H11 H12 H13
EXCLUDES 2 *infection following procedure (T81.4-)*

K68.12 Psoas muscle abscess MCC HCC

K68.19 Other retroperitoneal abscess MCC HCC
AHA: 2019,1Q,15
TIP: This code should be used for a diagnosis of internal presacral abscess. If an intra-abdominal abscess is also present, code K65.1 can also be assigned; sequencing depends on the circumstances of admission.

K68.9 Other disorders of retroperitoneum MCC

Diseases of liver (K7Ø-K77)

EXCLUDES 1 *jaundice NOS (R17)*
EXCLUDES 2 *hemochromatosis (E83.11-)*
Reye's syndrome (G93.7)
viral hepatitis (B15-B19)
Wilson's disease (E83.Ø)

K7Ø Alcoholic liver disease
Use additional code to identify:
alcohol abuse and dependence (F1Ø.-)

K7Ø.Ø Alcoholic fatty liver A

K7Ø.1 Alcoholic hepatitis

K7Ø.1Ø Alcoholic hepatitis without ascites A

K7Ø.11 Alcoholic hepatitis with ascites A

K7Ø.2 Alcoholic fibrosis and sclerosis of liver A

K7Ø.3 Alcoholic cirrhosis of liver
Alcoholic cirrhosis NOS

K7Ø.3Ø Alcoholic cirrhosis of liver without ascites HCC A

K7Ø.31 Alcoholic cirrhosis of liver with ascites HCC A
AHA: 2018,1Q,4

K7Ø.4 Alcoholic hepatic failure
Acute alcoholic hepatic failure
Alcoholic hepatic failure NOS
Chronic alcoholic hepatic failure
Subacute alcoholic hepatic failure

K7Ø.4Ø Alcoholic hepatic failure without coma HCC A

K7Ø.41 Alcoholic hepatic failure with coma MCC HCC A

K7Ø.9 Alcoholic liver disease, unspecified HCC A

K71 Toxic liver disease
INCLUDES drug-induced idiosyncratic (unpredictable) liver disease
drug-induced toxic (predictable) liver disease
Code first poisoning due to drug or toxin, if applicable (T36-T65 with fifth or sixth character 1-4 or 6)
Use additional code for adverse effect, if applicable, to identify drug (T36-T5Ø with fifth or sixth character 5)
EXCLUDES 2 *alcoholic liver disease (K7Ø.-)*
Budd-Chiari syndrome (I82.Ø)

K71.Ø Toxic liver disease with cholestasis
Cholestasis with hepatocyte injury
"Pure" cholestasis

K71.1 Toxic liver disease with hepatic necrosis
Hepatic failure (acute) (chronic) due to drugs

K71.1Ø Toxic liver disease with hepatic necrosis, without coma

K71.11 Toxic liver disease with hepatic necrosis, with coma MCC HCC

K71.2 Toxic liver disease with acute hepatitis

K71.3 Toxic liver disease with chronic persistent hepatitis

K71.4 Toxic liver disease with chronic lobular hepatitis

K71.5 **Toxic liver disease with chronic active hepatitis**
Toxic liver disease with lupoid hepatitis
K71.50 **Toxic liver disease with chronic active hepatitis without ascites**
K71.51 **Toxic liver disease with chronic active hepatitis with ascites**
AHA: 2018,1Q,4
K71.6 **Toxic liver disease with hepatitis, not elsewhere classified**
K71.7 **Toxic liver disease with fibrosis and cirrhosis of liver**
K71.8 **Toxic liver disease with other disorders of liver**
Toxic liver disease with focal nodular hyperplasia
Toxic liver disease with hepatic granulomas
Toxic liver disease with peliosis hepatis
Toxic liver disease with veno-occlusive disease of liver
K71.9 **Toxic liver disease, unspecified**

K72 Hepatic failure, not elsewhere classified

INCLUDES fulminant hepatitis NEC, with hepatic failure
hepatic encephalopathy NOS
liver (cell) necrosis with hepatic failure
malignant hepatitis NEC, with hepatic failure
yellow liver atrophy or dystrophy
EXCLUDES 1 *alcoholic hepatic failure (K70.4)*
hepatic failure with toxic liver disease (K71.1-)
icterus of newborn (P55-P59)
postprocedural hepatic failure (K91.82)
EXCLUDES 2 *hepatic failure complicating abortion or ectopic or molar pregnancy (O00-O07, O08.8)*
hepatic failure complicating pregnancy, childbirth and the puerperium (O26.6-)
viral hepatitis with hepatic coma (B15-B19)
AHA: 2017,1Q,41

K72.0 **Acute and subacute hepatic failure**
Acute non-viral hepatitis NOS
AHA: 2015,2Q,17; 2014,2Q,13
K72.00 **Acute and subacute hepatic failure without coma** MCC
K72.01 **Acute and subacute hepatic failure with coma** MCC HCC
K72.1 **Chronic hepatic failure**
K72.10 **Chronic hepatic failure without coma** HCC
K72.11 **Chronic hepatic failure with coma** MCC HCC
K72.9 **Hepatic failure, unspecified**
K72.90 **Hepatic failure, unspecified without coma** HCC
AHA: 2018,4Q,20; 2016,2Q,35
K72.91 **Hepatic failure, unspecified with coma** MCC HCC
Hepatic coma NOS

K73 Chronic hepatitis, not elsewhere classified

EXCLUDES 1 *alcoholic hepatitis (chronic) (K70.1-)*
drug-induced hepatitis (chronic) (K71.-)
granulomatous hepatitis (chronic) NEC (K75.3)
reactive, nonspecific hepatitis (chronic) (K75.2)
viral hepatitis (chronic) (B15-B19)

K73.0 **Chronic persistent hepatitis, not elsewhere classified** HCC
K73.1 **Chronic lobular hepatitis, not elsewhere classified** HCC
K73.2 **Chronic active hepatitis, not elsewhere classified** HCC
K73.8 **Other chronic hepatitis, not elsewhere classified** HCC
K73.9 **Chronic hepatitis, unspecified** HCC

K74 Fibrosis and cirrhosis of liver

Code also, if applicable, viral hepatitis (acute) (chronic) (B15-B19)
EXCLUDES 1 *alcoholic cirrhosis (of liver) (K70.3)*
alcoholic fibrosis of liver (K70.2)
cardiac sclerosis of liver (K76.1)
cirrhosis (of liver) with toxic liver disease (K71.7)
congenital cirrhosis (of liver) (P78.81)
pigmentary cirrhosis (of liver) (E83.110)

▲ K74.0 **Hepatic fibrosis**
▶Code first underlying liver disease, such as:◀
▶nonalcoholic steatohepatitis (NASH) (K75.81)◀
● K74.00 **Hepatic fibrosis, unspecified**
● K74.01 **Hepatic fibrosis, early fibrosis**
Hepatic fibrosis, stage F1 or stage F2
● K74.02 **Hepatic fibrosis, advanced fibrosis**
Hepatic fibrosis, stage F3
EXCLUDES 1 *cirrhosis of liver (K74.6-)*
hepatic fibrosis, stage F4 (K74.6-)
K74.1 **Hepatic sclerosis**
K74.2 **Hepatic fibrosis with hepatic sclerosis**
K74.3 **Primary biliary cirrhosis** HCC
Chronic nonsuppurative destructive cholangitis
Primary biliary cholangitis
EXCLUDES 2 *primary sclerosing cholangitis (K83.01)*
K74.4 **Secondary biliary cirrhosis** HCC
K74.5 **Biliary cirrhosis, unspecified** HCC
K74.6 **Other and unspecified cirrhosis of liver**
K74.60 **Unspecified cirrhosis of liver** HCC
Cirrhosis (of liver) NOS
AHA: 2018,1Q,4
K74.69 **Other cirrhosis of liver** HCC
Cryptogenic cirrhosis (of liver)
Macronodular cirrhosis (of liver)
Micronodular cirrhosis (of liver)
Mixed type cirrhosis (of liver)
Portal cirrhosis (of liver)
Postnecrotic cirrhosis (of liver)

K75 Other inflammatory liver diseases

EXCLUDES 2 *toxic liver disease (K71.-)*

K75.0 **Abscess of liver** MCC
Cholangitic hepatic abscess
Hematogenic hepatic abscess
Hepatic abscess NOS
Lymphogenic hepatic abscess
Pylephlebitic hepatic abscess
EXCLUDES 1 *amebic liver abscess (A06.4)*
cholangitis without liver abscess (K83.09)
pylephlebitis without liver abscess (K75.1)
EXCLUDES 2 *acute or subacute hepatitis NOS (B17.9)*
acute or subacute non-viral hepatitis (K72.0)
chronic hepatitis NEC (K73.8)
K75.1 **Phlebitis of portal vein** MCC
Pylephlebitis
EXCLUDES 1 *pylephlebitic liver abscess (K75.0)*
DEF: Inflammation of the portal vein or branches due to diverticulitis, perforated appendicitis, or peritonitis. Symptoms include fever, chills, jaundice, sweating, and abscess in various body parts.
K75.2 **Nonspecific reactive hepatitis**
EXCLUDES 1 *acute or subacute hepatitis (K72.0-)*
chronic hepatitis NEC (K73.-)
viral hepatitis (B15-B19)
K75.3 **Granulomatous hepatitis, not elsewhere classified**
EXCLUDES 1 *acute or subacute hepatitis (K72.0-)*
chronic hepatitis NEC (K73.-)
viral hepatitis (B15-B19)
K75.4 **Autoimmune hepatitis** HCC
Lupoid hepatitis NEC
K75.8 **Other specified inflammatory liver diseases**
K75.81 **Nonalcoholic steatohepatitis (NASH)**
▶Use additional code, if applicable, hepatic fibrosis (K74.0-)◀
K75.89 **Other specified inflammatory liver diseases**
K75.9 **Inflammatory liver disease, unspecified**
Hepatitis NOS
EXCLUDES 1 *acute or subacute hepatitis (K72.0-)*
chronic hepatitis NEC (K73.-)
viral hepatitis (B15-B19)
AHA: 2015,2Q,17

K76 Other diseases of liver

EXCLUDES 2 *alcoholic liver disease (K70.-)*
amyloid degeneration of liver (E85.-)
cystic disease of liver (congenital) (Q44.6)
hepatic vein thrombosis (I82.0)
hepatomegaly NOS (R16.0)
pigmentary cirrhosis (of liver) (E83.110)
portal vein thrombosis (I81)
toxic liver disease (K71.-)

K76.0 Fatty (change of) liver, not elsewhere classified
Nonalcoholic fatty liver disease (NAFLD)
EXCLUDES 1 *nonalcoholic steatohepatitis (NASH) (K75.81)*

K76.1 Chronic passive congestion of liver
Cardiac cirrhosis
Cardiac sclerosis

K76.2 Central hemorrhagic necrosis of liver MCC
EXCLUDES 1 *liver necrosis with hepatic failure (K72.-)*

K76.3 Infarction of liver MCC

K76.4 Peliosis hepatis
Hepatic angiomatosis

K76.5 Hepatic veno-occlusive disease
EXCLUDES 1 *Budd-Chiari syndrome (I82.0)*

K76.6 Portal hypertension CC HCC
Use additional code for any associated complications, such as:
portal hypertensive gastropathy (K31.89)
AHA: 2020,1Q,15

K76.7 Hepatorenal syndrome MCC HCC
EXCLUDES 1 *hepatorenal syndrome following labor and delivery (O90.4)*
postprocedural hepatorenal syndrome (K91.83)

K76.8 Other specified diseases of liver

K76.81 Hepatopulmonary syndrome HCC
Code first underlying liver disease, such as:
alcoholic cirrhosis of liver (K70.3-)
cirrhosis of liver without mention of alcohol (K74.6-)

K76.89 Other specified diseases of liver
Cyst (simple) of liver
Focal nodular hyperplasia of liver
Hepatoptosis

K76.9 Liver disease, unspecified

K77 Liver disorders in diseases classified elsewhere CC
Code first underlying disease, such as:
amyloidosis (E85.-)
congenital syphilis (A50.0, A50.5)
congenital toxoplasmosis (P37.1)
schistosomiasis (B65.0-B65.9)

EXCLUDES 1 *alcoholic hepatitis (K70.1-)*
alcoholic liver disease (K70.-)
cytomegaloviral hepatitis (B25.1)
herpesviral [herpes simplex] hepatitis (B00.81)
infectious mononucleosis with liver disease (B27.0-B27.9 with .9)
mumps hepatitis (B26.81)
sarcoidosis with liver disease (D86.89)
secondary syphilis with liver disease (A51.45)
syphilis (late) with liver disease (A52.74)
toxoplasmosis (acquired) hepatitis (B58.1)
tuberculosis with liver disease (A18.83)

Disorders of gallbladder, biliary tract and pancreas (K80-K87)

K80 Cholelithiasis
EXCLUDES 1 *retained cholelithiasis following cholecystectomy (K91.86)*
AHA: 2018,4Q,20
DEF: Presence or formation of concretions (calculi or "gallstones") in the gallbladder. The stones contain cholesterol, calcium carbonate, or calcium bilirubinate in pure forms or in various combinations.

Cholelithiasis

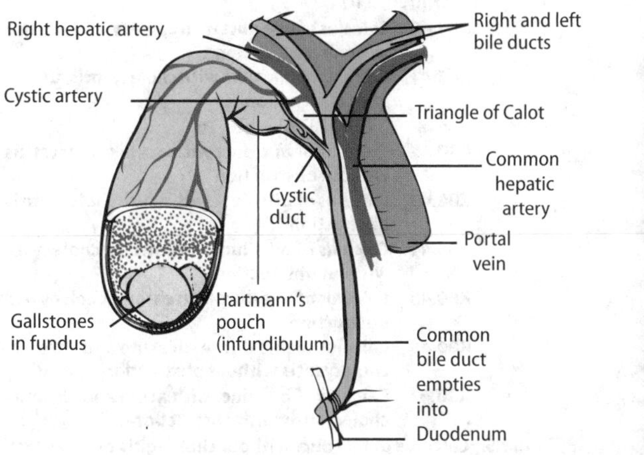

K80.0 Calculus of gallbladder with acute cholecystitis
Any condition listed in K80.2 with acute cholecystitis
Use additional code if applicable for associated gangrene of gallbladder (K82.A1), or perforation of gallbladder (K82.A2)

K80.00 Calculus of gallbladder with acute cholecystitis without obstruction CC

K80.01 Calculus of gallbladder with acute cholecystitis with obstruction CC

K80.1 Calculus of gallbladder with other cholecystitis
Use additional code if applicable for associated gangrene of gallbladder (K82.A1), or perforation of gallbladder (K82.A2)

K80.10 Calculus of gallbladder with chronic cholecystitis without obstruction CC
Cholelithiasis with cholecystitis NOS

K80.11 Calculus of gallbladder with chronic cholecystitis with obstruction CC

K80.12 Calculus of gallbladder with acute and chronic cholecystitis without obstruction CC

K80.13 Calculus of gallbladder with acute and chronic cholecystitis with obstruction CC

K80.18 Calculus of gallbladder with other cholecystitis without obstruction CC

K80.19 Calculus of gallbladder with other cholecystitis with obstruction CC

K80.2 Calculus of gallbladder without cholecystitis
Cholecystolithiasis without cholecystitis
Cholelithiasis (without cholecystitis)
Colic (recurrent) of gallbladder (without cholecystitis)
Gallstone (impacted) of cystic duct (without cholecystitis)
Gallstone (impacted) of gallbladder (without cholecystitis)

K80.20 Calculus of gallbladder without cholecystitis without obstruction

K80.21 Calculus of gallbladder without cholecystitis with obstruction CC

K80.3 Calculus of bile duct with cholangitis
Any condition listed in K80.5 with cholangitis
DEF: Cholangitis: Inflammation of the bile ducts.

K80.30 Calculus of bile duct with cholangitis, unspecified, without obstruction CC

K80.31 Calculus of bile duct with cholangitis, unspecified, with obstruction CC

K80.32 Calculus of bile duct with acute cholangitis without obstruction CC

K80.33 Calculus of bile duct with acute cholangitis with obstruction CC

K80.34 Calculus of bile duct with chronic cholangitis without obstruction CC

K80.35 **Calculus of bile duct with chronic cholangitis with obstruction** CC

K80.36 **Calculus of bile duct with acute and chronic cholangitis without obstruction** CC

K80.37 **Calculus of bile duct with acute and chronic cholangitis with obstruction** CC

✓5th K80.4 **Calculus of bile duct with cholecystitis**

Any condition listed in K80.5 with cholecystitis (with cholangitis)

▶Codes also fistula of bile duct (K83.3)◀

Use additional code if applicable for associated gangrene of gallbladder (K82.A1), or perforation of gallbladder (K82.A2)

AHA: 2019,1Q,17

K80.40 **Calculus of bile duct with cholecystitis, unspecified, without obstruction** CC

K80.41 **Calculus of bile duct with cholecystitis, unspecified, with obstruction** CC

AHA: 2019,1Q,17

K80.42 **Calculus of bile duct with acute cholecystitis without obstruction** CC

K80.43 **Calculus of bile duct with acute cholecystitis with obstruction** CC

K80.44 **Calculus of bile duct with chronic cholecystitis without obstruction** CC

K80.45 **Calculus of bile duct with chronic cholecystitis with obstruction** CC

K80.46 **Calculus of bile duct with acute and chronic cholecystitis without obstruction** CC

K80.47 **Calculus of bile duct with acute and chronic cholecystitis with obstruction** CC

✓5th K80.5 **Calculus of bile duct without cholangitis or cholecystitis**

Choledocholithiasis (without cholangitis or cholecystitis)

Gallstone (impacted) of bile duct NOS (without cholangitis or cholecystitis)

Gallstone (impacted) of common duct (without cholangitis or cholecystitis)

Gallstone (impacted) of hepatic duct (without cholangitis or cholecystitis)

Hepatic cholelithiasis (without cholangitis or cholecystitis)

Hepatic colic (recurrent) (without cholangitis or cholecystitis)

DEF: Cholangitis: Inflammation of the bile ducts.

K80.50 **Calculus of bile duct without cholangitis or cholecystitis without obstruction**

K80.51 **Calculus of bile duct without cholangitis or cholecystitis with obstruction** CC

✓5th K80.6 **Calculus of gallbladder and bile duct with cholecystitis**

Use additional code if applicable for associated gangrene of gallbladder (K82.A1), or perforation of gallbladder (K82.A2)

K80.60 **Calculus of gallbladder and bile duct with cholecystitis, unspecified, without obstruction** CC

K80.61 **Calculus of gallbladder and bile duct with cholecystitis, unspecified, with obstruction** CC

K80.62 **Calculus of gallbladder and bile duct with acute cholecystitis without obstruction** CC

K80.63 **Calculus of gallbladder and bile duct with acute cholecystitis with obstruction** CC

K80.64 **Calculus of gallbladder and bile duct with chronic cholecystitis without obstruction** CC

K80.65 **Calculus of gallbladder and bile duct with chronic cholecystitis with obstruction** CC

K80.66 **Calculus of gallbladder and bile duct with acute and chronic cholecystitis without obstruction** CC

K80.67 **Calculus of gallbladder and bile duct with acute and chronic cholecystitis with obstruction** MCC

✓5th K80.7 **Calculus of gallbladder and bile duct without cholecystitis**

K80.70 **Calculus of gallbladder and bile duct without cholecystitis without obstruction**

K80.71 **Calculus of gallbladder and bile duct without cholecystitis with obstruction** CC

✓5th K80.8 **Other cholelithiasis**

K80.80 **Other cholelithiasis without obstruction**

K80.81 **Other cholelithiasis with obstruction** CC

✓4th K81 **Cholecystitis**

Use additional code if applicable for associated gangrene of gallbladder (K82.A1), or perforation of gallbladder (K82.A2)

EXCLUDES 1 *cholecystitis with cholelithiasis (K80.-)*

AHA: 2018,4Q,20

K81.0 **Acute cholecystitis** CC

Abscess of gallbladder
Angiocholecystitis
Emphysematous (acute) cholecystitis
Empyema of gallbladder
Gangrene of gallbladder
Gangrenous cholecystitis
Suppurative cholecystitis

K81.1 **Chronic cholecystitis**

K81.2 **Acute cholecystitis with chronic cholecystitis** CC

K81.9 **Cholecystitis, unspecified**

✓4th K82 **Other diseases of gallbladder**

EXCLUDES 1 *nonvisualization of gallbladder (R93.2)*
postcholecystectomy syndrome (K91.5)

K82.0 **Obstruction of gallbladder** CC

Occlusion of cystic duct or gallbladder without cholelithiasis
Stenosis of cystic duct or gallbladder without cholelithiasis
Stricture of cystic duct or gallbladder without cholelithiasis

EXCLUDES 1 *obstruction of gallbladder with cholelithiasis (K80.-)*

K82.1 **Hydrops of gallbladder** CC

Mucocele of gallbladder

K82.2 **Perforation of gallbladder** MCC

Rupture of cystic duct or gallbladder

EXCLUDES 1 *perforation of gallbladder in cholecystitis (K82.A2)*

K82.3 **Fistula of gallbladder** CC

Cholecystocolic fistula
Cholecystoduodenal fistula

K82.4 **Cholesterolosis of gallbladder**

Strawberry gallbladder

EXCLUDES 1 *cholesterolosis of gallbladder with cholecystitis (K81.-)*
cholesterolosis of gallbladder with cholelithiasis (K80.-)

K82.8 **Other specified diseases of gallbladder**

Adhesions of cystic duct or gallbladder
Atrophy of cystic duct or gallbladder
Cyst of cystic duct or gallbladder
Dyskinesia of cystic duct or gallbladder
Hypertrophy of cystic duct or gallbladder
Nonfunctioning of cystic duct or gallbladder
Ulcer of cystic duct or gallbladder

K82.9 **Disease of gallbladder, unspecified**

✓5th K82.A **Disorders of gallbladder in diseases classified elsewhere**

Code first the type of cholecystitis (K81.-), or cholelithiasis with cholecystitis (K80.00-K80.19, K80.40-K80.47, K80.60-K80.67)

AHA: 2018,4Q,19-20

K82.A1 ***Gangrene of gallbladder in cholecystitis***

K82.A2 ***Perforation of gallbladder in cholecystitis*** CC

✓4th K83 **Other diseases of biliary tract**

EXCLUDES 1 *postcholecystectomy syndrome (K91.5)*

EXCLUDES 2 *conditions involving the gallbladder (K81-K82)*
conditions involving the cystic duct (K81-K82)

✓5th K83.0 **Cholangitis**

EXCLUDES 1 *cholangitic liver abscess (K75.0)*
cholangitis with choledocholithiasis (K80.3-, K80.4-)

EXCLUDES 2 *chronic nonsuppurative destructive cholangitis (K74.3)*
primary biliary cholangitis (K74.3)
primary biliary cirrhosis (K74.3)

AHA: 2018,4Q,20

K83.01 **Primary sclerosing cholangitis** CC

K83.09 **Other cholangitis** CC
Ascending cholangitis
Cholangitis NOS
Primary cholangitis
Recurrent cholangitis
Sclerosing cholangitis
Secondary cholangitis
Stenosing cholangitis
Suppurative cholangitis

K83.1 **Obstruction of bile duct** MCC
Occlusion of bile duct without cholelithiasis
Stenosis of bile duct without cholelithiasis
Stricture of bile duct without cholelithiasis
EXCLUDES 1 *congenital obstruction of bile duct (Q44.3)*
obstruction of bile duct with cholelithiasis (K80.-)
AHA: 2016,1Q,18

K83.2 **Perforation of bile duct** MCC
Rupture of bile duct

K83.3 **Fistula of bile duct** CC
Choledochoduodenal fistula
AHA: 2019,1Q,17

K83.4 **Spasm of sphincter of Oddi**

K83.5 **Biliary cyst**

K83.8 **Other specified diseases of biliary tract**
Adhesions of biliary tract
Atrophy of biliary tract
Hypertrophy of biliary tract
Ulcer of biliary tract

K83.9 **Disease of biliary tract, unspecified**

K85 **Acute pancreatitis**
INCLUDES acute (recurrent) pancreatitis
subacute pancreatitis
AHA: 2016,4Q,34

K85.0 **Idiopathic acute pancreatitis**
K85.00 **Idiopathic acute pancreatitis without necrosis or infection** MCC
K85.01 **Idiopathic acute pancreatitis with uninfected necrosis** MCC
K85.02 **Idiopathic acute pancreatitis with infected necrosis** MCC

K85.1 **Biliary acute pancreatitis**
Gallstone pancreatitis
K85.10 **Biliary acute pancreatitis without necrosis or infection** MCC
K85.11 **Biliary acute pancreatitis with uninfected necrosis** MCC
K85.12 **Biliary acute pancreatitis with infected necrosis** MCC

K85.2 **Alcohol induced acute pancreatitis**
EXCLUDES 2 *alcohol induced chronic pancreatitis (K86.0)*
K85.20 **Alcohol induced acute pancreatitis without necrosis or infection** MCC
AHA: 2020,1Q,9
K85.21 **Alcohol induced acute pancreatitis with uninfected necrosis** MCC
K85.22 **Alcohol induced acute pancreatitis with infected necrosis** MCC

K85.3 **Drug induced acute pancreatitis**
Use additional code for adverse effect, if applicable, to identify drug (T36-T50 with fifth or sixth character 5)
Use additional code to identify drug abuse and dependence (F11.- F17.-)
K85.30 **Drug induced acute pancreatitis without necrosis or infection** MCC
K85.31 **Drug induced acute pancreatitis with uninfected necrosis** MCC
K85.32 **Drug induced acute pancreatitis with infected necrosis** MCC

K85.8 **Other acute pancreatitis**
K85.80 **Other acute pancreatitis without necrosis or infection** MCC
K85.81 **Other acute pancreatitis with uninfected necrosis** MCC
K85.82 **Other acute pancreatitis with infected necrosis** MCC

K85.9 **Acute pancreatitis, unspecified**
Pancreatitis NOS
K85.90 **Acute pancreatitis without necrosis or infection, unspecified** MCC
K85.91 **Acute pancreatitis with uninfected necrosis, unspecified** MCC
K85.92 **Acute pancreatitis with infected necrosis, unspecified** MCC

K86 **Other diseases of pancreas**
EXCLUDES 2 *fibrocystic disease of pancreas (E84.-)*
islet cell tumor (of pancreas) (D13.7)
pancreatic steatorrhea (K90.3)

K86.0 **Alcohol-induced chronic pancreatitis** CC HCC
Use additional code to identify:
alcohol abuse and dependence (F10.-)
Code also exocrine pancreatic insufficiency (K86.81)
EXCLUDES 2 *alcohol induced acute pancreatitis (K85.2-)*

K86.1 **Other chronic pancreatitis** CC HCC
Chronic pancreatitis NOS
Infectious chronic pancreatitis
Recurrent chronic pancreatitis
Relapsing chronic pancreatitis
Code also exocrine pancreatic insufficiency (K86.81)

K86.2 **Cyst of pancreas** CC

K86.3 **Pseudocyst of pancreas** CC

K86.8 **Other specified diseases of pancreas**
AHA: 2016,4Q,34-35
K86.81 **Exocrine pancreatic insufficiency**
K86.89 **Other specified diseases of pancreas**
Aseptic pancreatic necrosis, unrelated to acute pancreatitis
Atrophy of pancreas
Calculus of pancreas
Cirrhosis of pancreas
Fibrosis of pancreas
Pancreatic fat necrosis, unrelated to acute pancreatitis
Pancreatic infantilism
Pancreatic necrosis NOS, unrelated to acute pancreatitis

K86.9 **Disease of pancreas, unspecified**

K87 ***Disorders of gallbladder, biliary tract and pancreas in diseases classified elsewhere***
Code first underlying disease
EXCLUDES 1 *cytomegaloviral pancreatitis (B25.2)*
mumps pancreatitis (B26.3)
syphilitic gallbladder (A52.74)
syphilitic pancreas (A52.74)
tuberculosis of gallbladder (A18.83)
tuberculosis of pancreas (A18.83)

Other diseases of the digestive system (K90-K95)

K90 **Intestinal malabsorption**
EXCLUDES 1 *intestinal malabsorption following gastrointestinal surgery (K91.2)*
AHA: 2017,4Q,108

K90.0 **Celiac disease**
Celiac disease with steatorrhea
Celiac gluten-sensitive enteropathy
Nontropical sprue
Use additional code for associated disorders including:
dermatitis herpetiformis (L13.0)
gluten ataxia (G32.81)
Code also exocrine pancreatic insufficiency (K86.81)
DEF: Malabsorption syndrome due to gluten consumption. Symptoms include fetid, bulky, frothy, oily stools; a distended abdomen; gas; asthenia; electrolyte depletion; and vitamin B, D, and K deficiency.

K90.1 **Tropical sprue** CC
Sprue NOS
Tropical steatorrhea

K90.2 **Blind loop syndrome, not elsewhere classified** CC
Blind loop syndrome NOS
EXCLUDES 1 *congenital blind loop syndrome (Q43.8)*
postsurgical blind loop syndrome (K91.2)

K90.3 **Pancreatic steatorrhea** CC

✓5th **K90.4 Other malabsorption due to intolerance**
EXCLUDES 2 *celiac gluten-sensitive enteropathy (K90.0)*
lactose intolerance (E73.-)
AHA: 2016,4Q,35-36
K90.41 Non-celiac gluten sensitivity CC
Gluten sensitivity NOS
Non-celiac gluten sensitive enteropathy
K90.49 Malabsorption due to intolerance, not elsewhere classified CC
Malabsorption due to intolerance to carbohydrate
Malabsorption due to intolerance to fat
Malabsorption due to intolerance to protein
Malabsorption due to intolerance to starch
✓5th **K90.8 Other intestinal malabsorption**
K90.81 Whipple's disease CC
K90.89 Other intestinal malabsorption CC
K90.9 Intestinal malabsorption, unspecified CC

✓4th **K91 Intraoperative and postprocedural complications and disorders of digestive system, not elsewhere classified**
EXCLUDES 2 *complications of artificial opening of digestive system (K94.-)*
complications of bariatric procedures (K95.-)
gastrojejunal ulcer (K28.-)
postprocedural (radiation) retroperitoneal abscess (K68.11)
radiation colitis (K52.0)
radiation gastroenteritis (K52.0)
radiation proctitis (K62.7)
AHA: 2016,4Q,9-10
K91.0 Vomiting following gastrointestinal surgery
K91.1 Postgastric surgery syndromes
Dumping syndrome
Postgastrectomy syndrome
Postvagotomy syndrome
K91.2 Postsurgical malabsorption, not elsewhere classified CC
Postsurgical blind loop syndrome
EXCLUDES 1 *malabsorption osteomalacia in adults (M83.2)*
malabsorption osteoporosis, postsurgical (M80.8-, M81.8)
✓5th **K91.3 Postprocedural intestinal obstruction**
AHA: 2017,4Q,16-17; 2017,1Q,40
K91.30 Postprocedural intestinal obstruction, unspecified as to partial versus complete CC
Postprocedural intestinal obstruction NOS
K91.31 Postprocedural partial intestinal obstruction CC
Postprocedural incomplete intestinal obstruction
K91.32 Postprocedural complete intestinal obstruction CC
K91.5 Postcholecystectomy syndrome
✓5th **K91.6 Intraoperative hemorrhage and hematoma of a digestive system organ or structure complicating a procedure**
EXCLUDES 1 *intraoperative hemorrhage and hematoma of a digestive system organ or structure due to accidental puncture and laceration during a procedure (K91.7-)*
K91.61 Intraoperative hemorrhage and hematoma of a digestive system organ or structure complicating a digestive system procedure CC
AHA: 2020,1Q,19
K91.62 Intraoperative hemorrhage and hematoma of a digestive system organ or structure complicating other procedure CC
✓5th **K91.7 Accidental puncture and laceration of a digestive system organ or structure during a procedure**
K91.71 Accidental puncture and laceration of a digestive system organ or structure during a digestive system procedure CC
K91.72 Accidental puncture and laceration of a digestive system organ or structure during other procedure CC
AHA: 2019,2Q,23
✓5th **K91.8 Other intraoperative and postprocedural complications and disorders of digestive system**
K91.81 Other intraoperative complications of digestive system CC
K91.82 Postprocedural hepatic failure CC
K91.83 Postprocedural hepatorenal syndrome CC
✓6th **K91.84 Postprocedural hemorrhage of a digestive system organ or structure following a procedure**
K91.840 Postprocedural hemorrhage of a digestive system organ or structure following a digestive system procedure CC
AHA: 2016,1Q,15
K91.841 Postprocedural hemorrhage of a digestive system organ or structure following other procedure CC
✓6th **K91.85 Complications of intestinal pouch**
K91.850 Pouchitis CC HCC
Inflammation of internal ileoanal pouch
DEF: Inflammatory complication of an existing surgically created ileoanal pouch, resulting in multiple GI complaints, including diarrhea, abdominal pain, rectal bleeding, fecal urgency, or incontinence.
K91.858 Other complications of intestinal pouch CC HCC
AHA: 2019,2Q,13
K91.86 Retained cholelithiasis following cholecystectomy CC
✓6th **K91.87 Postprocedural hematoma and seroma of a digestive system organ or structure following a procedure**
K91.870 Postprocedural hematoma of a digestive system organ or structure following a digestive system procedure CC
K91.871 Postprocedural hematoma of a digestive system organ or structure following other procedure CC
K91.872 Postprocedural seroma of a digestive system organ or structure following a digestive system procedure CC
K91.873 Postprocedural seroma of a digestive system organ or structure following other procedure CC
K91.89 Other postprocedural complications and disorders of digestive system CC
Use additional code, if applicable, to further specify disorder
EXCLUDES 2 *postprocedural retroperitoneal abscess (K68.11)*
AHA: 2020,2Q,22; 2017,1Q,40

✓4th **K92 Other diseases of digestive system**
EXCLUDES 1 *neonatal gastrointestinal hemorrhage (P54.0-P54.3)*
K92.0 Hematemesis CC
K92.1 Melena CC
EXCLUDES 1 *occult blood in feces (R19.5)*
K92.2 Gastrointestinal hemorrhage, unspecified CC
Gastric hemorrhage NOS
Intestinal hemorrhage NOS
EXCLUDES 1 *acute hemorrhagic gastritis (K29.01)*
hemorrhage of anus and rectum (K62.5)
angiodysplasia of stomach with hemorrhage (K31.811)
diverticular disease with hemorrhage (K57.-)
gastritis and duodenitis with hemorrhage (K29.-)
peptic ulcer with hemorrhage (K25-K28)
✓5th **K92.8 Other specified diseases of the digestive system**
K92.81 Gastrointestinal mucositis (ulcerative) CC
Code also type of associated therapy, such as:
antineoplastic and immunosuppressive drugs (T45.1X-)
radiological procedure and radiotherapy (Y84.2)
EXCLUDES 2 *mucositis (ulcerative) of vagina and vulva (N76.81)*
nasal mucositis (ulcerative) (J34.81)
oral mucositis (ulcerative) (K12.3-)
K92.89 Other specified diseases of the digestive system
K92.9 Disease of digestive system, unspecified

✓4th **K94 Complications of artificial openings of the digestive system**
✓5th **K94.0 Colostomy complications**
K94.00 Colostomy complication, unspecified HCC
K94.01 Colostomy hemorrhage CC HCC

K94.Ø2 Colostomy infection CC HCC
Use additional code to specify type of infection, such as:
cellulitis of abdominal wall (LØ3.311)
sepsis (A4Ø.-, A41.-)

K94.Ø3 Colostomy malfunction CC HCC
Mechanical complication of colostomy

K94.Ø9 Other complications of colostomy CC HCC

K94.1 Enterostomy complications

K94.1Ø Enterostomy complication, unspecified HCC

K94.11 Enterostomy hemorrhage CC HCC

K94.12 Enterostomy infection CC HCC
Use additional code to specify type of infection, such as:
cellulitis of abdominal wall (LØ3.311)
sepsis (A4Ø.-, A41.-)

K94.13 Enterostomy malfunction CC HCC
Mechanical complication of enterostomy

K94.19 Other complications of enterostomy CC HCC

K94.2 Gastrostomy complications

K94.2Ø Gastrostomy complication, unspecified HCC

K94.21 Gastrostomy hemorrhage HCC

K94.22 Gastrostomy infection CC HCC
Use additional code to specify type of infection, such as:
cellulitis of abdominal wall (LØ3.311)
sepsis (A4Ø.-, A41.-)

K94.23 Gastrostomy malfunction CC HCC
Mechanical complication of gastrostomy
AHA: 2019,1Q,26

K94.29 Other complications of gastrostomy HCC

K94.3 Esophagostomy complications

K94.3Ø Esophagostomy complications, unspecified CC HCC

K94.31 Esophagostomy hemorrhage CC HCC

K94.32 Esophagostomy infection CC HCC
Use additional code to identify the infection

K94.33 Esophagostomy malfunction CC HCC
Mechanical complication of esophagostomy

K94.39 Other complications of esophagostomy CC HCC

K95 Complications of bariatric procedures

K95.Ø Complications of gastric band procedure

K95.Ø1 Infection due to gastric band procedure CC H11
Use additional code to specify type of infection or organism, such as:
bacterial and viral infectious agents (B95.-, B96.-)
cellulitis of abdominal wall (LØ3.311)
sepsis (A4Ø.-, A41.-)

K95.Ø9 Other complications of gastric band procedure CC
Use additional code, if applicable, to further specify complication

K95.8 Complications of other bariatric procedure
EXCLUDES 1 *complications of gastric band surgery (K95.Ø-)*

K95.81 Infection due to other bariatric procedure CC H11
Use additional code to specify type of infection or organism, such as:
bacterial and viral infectious agents (B95.-, B96.-)
cellulitis of abdominal wall (LØ3.311)
sepsis (A4Ø.-, A41.-)

K95.89 Other complications of other bariatric procedure CC
Use additional code, if applicable, to further specify complication

Chapter 12. Diseases of the Skin and Subcutaneous Tissue (LØØ–L99)

Chapter-specific Guidelines with Coding Examples

The chapter-specific guidelines from the ICD-10-CM Official Guidelines for Coding and Reporting have been provided below. Along with these guidelines are coding examples, contained in the shaded boxes, that have been developed to help illustrate the coding and/or sequencing guidance found in these guidelines.

a. Pressure ulcer stage codes

1) Pressure ulcer stages

Codes in category L89, Pressure ulcer, identify the site and stage of the pressure ulcer.

The ICD-10-CM classifies pressure ulcer stages based on severity, which is designated by stages 1-4, deep tissue pressure injury, unspecified stage, and unstageable.

Assign as many codes from category L89 as needed to identify all the pressure ulcers the patient has, if applicable.

See Section I.B.14 for pressure ulcer stage documentation by clinicians other than patient's provider

> Nursing notes: Dressings changed daily on stage 4 ulcer on heel and stage 2 ulcer on elbow
>
> Discharge summary: Pressure ulcers on right heel and left elbow
>
> **L89.614 Pressure ulcer of right heel, stage 4**
>
> **L89.Ø22 Pressure ulcer of left elbow, stage 2**
>
> *Explanation:* Right heel and left elbow pressure ulcers were documented by the patient's provider in the discharge summary. Although the stage of these ulcers was not included in the provider's diagnostic statement, it is appropriate to code the stage from documentation from other clinicians involved in the patient's care, such as the nurse's notes, according to section I.B.14. Combination codes from category L89 Pressure ulcer, identify the site of the pressure ulcer as well as the stage. Assign as many codes from category L89 as needed to identify all the pressure ulcers the patient has.

2) Unstageable pressure ulcers

Assignment of the code for unstageable pressure ulcer (L89.--Ø) should be based on the clinical documentation. These codes are used for pressure ulcers whose stage cannot be clinically determined (e.g., the ulcer is covered by eschar or has been treated with a skin or muscle graft). This code should not be confused with the codes for unspecified stage (L89.--9). When there is no documentation regarding the stage of the pressure ulcer, assign the appropriate code for unspecified stage (L89.--9).

> Pressure ulcer of the right lower back documented as unstageable due to the presence of thick eschar covering the ulcer
>
> **L89.13Ø Pressure ulcer of right lower back, unstageable**
>
> *Explanation:* Codes for unstageable pressure ulcers are assigned when the stage cannot be clinically determined (e.g., the ulcer is covered by eschar or has been treated with a skin or muscle graft).

3) Documented pressure ulcer stage

Assignment of the pressure ulcer stage code should be guided by clinical documentation of the stage or documentation of the terms found in the Alphabetic Index. For clinical terms describing the stage that are not found in the Alphabetic Index, and there is no documentation of the stage, the provider should be queried.

> Left heel pressure ulcer with partial thickness skin loss involving the dermis
>
> **L89.622 Pressure ulcer of left heel, stage 2**
>
> *Explanation:* Code assignment for the pressure ulcer stage should be guided by either the clinical documentation of the stage or the documentation of terms found in the Alphabetic Index. The clinical documentation describing the left heel pressure ulcer "partial thickness skin loss involving the dermis" matches the ICD-10-CM index parenthetical description for stage 2 "(abrasion, blister, partial thickness skin loss involving epidermis and/or dermis)."

4) Patients admitted with pressure ulcers documented as healed

No code is assigned if the documentation states that the pressure ulcer is completely healed at the time of admission.

5) Pressure ulcers documented as healing

Pressure ulcers described as healing should be assigned the appropriate pressure ulcer stage code based on the documentation in the medical record. If the documentation does not provide information about the stage of the healing pressure ulcer, assign the appropriate code for unspecified stage.

If the documentation is unclear as to whether the patient has a current (new) pressure ulcer or if the patient is being treated for a healing pressure ulcer, query the provider.

For ulcers that were present on admission but healed at the time of discharge, assign the code for the site and stage of the pressure ulcer at the time of admission.

> H & P noted healing stage 2 sacral pressure ulcer. Resolved at time of discharge summary.
>
> **L89.152 Pressure ulcer of sacral region, stage 2**
>
> *Explanation:* Although completely healed upon discharge, the pressure ulcer required observation and/or treatment and should be coded based on the site and stage upon admission.

6) Patient admitted with pressure ulcer evolving into another stage during the admission

If a patient is admitted to an inpatient hospital with a pressure ulcer at one stage and it progresses to a higher stage, two separate codes should be assigned: one code for the site and stage of the ulcer on admission and a second code for the same ulcer site and the highest stage reported during the stay.

> Stage 3 right hip pressure ulcer worsened during admission to a stage 4
>
> **L89.213 Pressure ulcer of right hip, stage 3**
>
> **L89.214 Pressure ulcer of right hip, stage 4**
>
> *Explanation:* A pressure ulcer that progresses from a lower stage to a higher stage is assigned two codes, one for the documented stage upon admission and one for the documented stage at discharge.

7) Pressure-induced deep tissue damage

For pressure-induced deep tissue damage or deep tissue pressure injury, assign only the appropriate code for pressure-induced deep tissue damage (L89.--6).

b. Non-pressure chronic ulcers

1) Patients admitted with non-pressure ulcers documented as healed

No code is assigned if the documentation states that the non-pressure ulcer is completely healed at the time of admission.

2) Non-pressure ulcers documented as healing

Non-pressure ulcers described as healing should be assigned the appropriate non-pressure ulcer code based on the documentation in the medical record. If the documentation does not provide information about the severity of the healing non-pressure ulcer, assign the appropriate code for unspecified severity.

If the documentation is unclear as to whether the patient has a current (new) non-pressure ulcer or if the patient is being treated for a healing non-pressure ulcer, query the provider.

For ulcers that were present on admission but healed at the time of discharge, assign the code for the site and severity of the non-pressure ulcer at the time of admission.

> Admission diagnosis: Chronic ulcer, fat layer exposed, on left ankle
>
> Discharge diagnosis: Resolution of ulcer on the left ankle
>
> **L97.322 Non-pressure chronic ulcer of left ankle with fat layer exposed**
>
> *Explanation:* Although the ulcer was documented as resolved (healed) at discharge, a code representing the site and severity of the ulcer upon admission should be appended.

3) Patient admitted with non-pressure ulcer that progresses to another severity level during the admission

If a patient is admitted to an inpatient hospital with a non-pressure ulcer at one severity level and it progresses to a higher severity level, two separate codes should be assigned: one code for the site and severity level of the ulcer on admission and a second code for the same ulcer site and the highest severity level reported during the stay.

See Section I.B.14 for pressure ulcer stage documentation by clinicians other than patient's provider

Chapter 12. Diseases of the Skin and Subcutaneous Tissue (LØØ-L99)

EXCLUDES 2 *certain conditions originating in the perinatal period (PØ4-P96)*
certain infectious and parasitic diseases (AØØ-B99)
complications of pregnancy, childbirth and the puerperium (OØØ-O9A)
congenital malformations, deformations, and chromosomal abnormalities (QØØ-Q99)
endocrine, nutritional and metabolic diseases (EØØ-E88)
lipomelanotic reticulosis (I89.8)
neoplasms (CØØ-D49)
symptoms, signs and abnormal clinical and laboratory findings, not elsewhere classified (RØØ-R94)
systemic connective tissue disorders (M3Ø-M36)
viral warts (BØ7.-)

This chapter contains the following blocks:

LØØ-LØ8	Infections of the skin and subcutaneous tissue
L1Ø-L14	Bullous disorders
L2Ø-L3Ø	Dermatitis and eczema
L4Ø-L45	Papulosquamous disorders
L49-L54	Urticaria and erythema
L55-L59	Radiation-related disorders of the skin and subcutaneous tissue
L6Ø-L75	Disorders of skin appendages
L76	Intraoperative and postprocedural complications of skin and subcutaneous tissue
L8Ø-L99	Other disorders of the skin and subcutaneous tissue

Infections of the skin and subcutaneous tissue (LØØ-LØ8)

Use additional code (B95-B97) to identify infectious agent

EXCLUDES 2 *hordeolum (HØØ.Ø)*
infective dermatitis (L3Ø.3)
local infections of skin classified in Chapter 1
lupus panniculitis (L93.2)
panniculitis NOS (M79.3)
panniculitis of neck and back (M54.Ø-)
perlèche NOS (K13.Ø)
perlèche due to candidiasis (B37.Ø)
perlèche due to riboflavin deficiency (E53.Ø)
pyogenic granuloma (L98.Ø)
relapsing panniculitis [Weber-Christian] (M35.6)
viral warts (BØ7.-)
zoster (BØ2.-)

LØØ Staphylococcal scalded skin syndrome
Ritter's disease
Use additional code to identify percentage of skin exfoliation (L49.-)
EXCLUDES 1 *bullous impetigo (LØ1.Ø3)*
pemphigus neonatorum (LØ1.Ø3)
toxic epidermal necrolysis [Lyell] (L51.2)
DEF: Infectious skin disease of children younger than 5 years marked by eruptions ranging from a few localized blisters to widespread, easily ruptured, fine vesicles and bullae affecting almost the entire body. It results in exfoliation of large planes of skin and leaves raw areas.

✓4th **LØ1 Impetigo**
EXCLUDES 1 *impetigo herpetiformis (L4Ø.1)*
DEF: Acute, superficial, highly contagious skin infection commonly occurring in children. Skin lesions usually appear on the face and consist of vesicles and bullae that burst and form yellow crusts.

✓5th **LØ1.Ø Impetigo**
Impetigo contagiosa
Impetigo vulgaris

LØ1.ØØ Impetigo, unspecified
Impetigo NOS

LØ1.Ø1 Non-bullous impetigo

LØ1.Ø2 Bockhart's impetigo
Impetigo follicularis
Perifolliculitis NOS
Superficial pustular perifolliculitis
DEF: Superficial inflammation of the hair follicles most commonly caused by staph aureus that manifests as rounded, sphere-shaped, pustular eruptions in the areas of the scalp, beard, underarms, extremities, and buttocks.

LØ1.Ø3 Bullous impetigo
Impetigo neonatorum
Pemphigus neonatorum

LØ1.Ø9 Other impetigo
Ulcerative impetigo

LØ1.1 Impetiginization of other dermatoses

✓4th **LØ2 Cutaneous abscess, furuncle and carbuncle**
Use additional code to identify organism (B95-B96)
EXCLUDES 2 *abscess of anus and rectal regions (K61.-)*
abscess of female genital organs (external) (N76.4)
abscess of male genital organs (external) (N48.2, N49.-)
DEF: Carbuncle: Infection of the skin that arises from a collection of interconnected infected boils or furuncles, usually from hair follicles infected by *Staphylococcus*. This condition can produce pus and form drainage cavities.
DEF: Furuncle: Inflamed, painful abscess, cyst, or nodule on the skin caused by bacteria, often *Staphylococcus*, entering along the hair follicle.

✓5th **LØ2.Ø Cutaneous abscess, furuncle and carbuncle of face**
EXCLUDES 2 *abscess of ear, external (H6Ø.Ø)*
abscess of eyelid (HØØ.Ø)
abscess of head [any part, except face] (LØ2.8)
abscess of lacrimal gland (HØ4.Ø)
abscess of lacrimal passages (HØ4.3)
abscess of mouth (K12.2)
abscess of nose (J34.Ø)
abscess of orbit (HØ5.Ø)
submandibular abscess (K12.2)

LØ2.Ø1 Cutaneous abscess of face CC

LØ2.Ø2 Furuncle of face
Boil of face
Folliculitis of face

LØ2.Ø3 Carbuncle of face

✓5th **LØ2.1 Cutaneous abscess, furuncle and carbuncle of neck**

LØ2.11 Cutaneous abscess of neck CC

LØ2.12 Furuncle of neck
Boil of neck
Folliculitis of neck

LØ2.13 Carbuncle of neck

✓5th **LØ2.2 Cutaneous abscess, furuncle and carbuncle of trunk**
EXCLUDES 1 *non-newborn omphalitis (LØ8.82)*
omphalitis of newborn (P38.-)
EXCLUDES 2 *abscess of breast (N61.1)*
abscess of buttocks (LØ2.3)
abscess of female external genital organs (N76.4)
abscess of hip (LØ2.4)
abscess of male external genital organs (N48.2, N49.-)

✓6th **LØ2.21 Cutaneous abscess of trunk**
LØ2.211 Cutaneous abscess of abdominal wall CC
LØ2.212 Cutaneous abscess of back [any part, except buttock] CC
LØ2.213 Cutaneous abscess of chest wall CC
LØ2.214 Cutaneous abscess of groin CC
LØ2.215 Cutaneous abscess of perineum CC
LØ2.216 Cutaneous abscess of umbilicus CC
LØ2.219 Cutaneous abscess of trunk, unspecified CC

✓6th **LØ2.22 Furuncle of trunk**
Boil of trunk
Folliculitis of trunk
LØ2.221 Furuncle of abdominal wall
LØ2.222 Furuncle of back [any part, except buttock]
LØ2.223 Furuncle of chest wall
LØ2.224 Furuncle of groin
LØ2.225 Furuncle of perineum
LØ2.226 Furuncle of umbilicus
LØ2.229 Furuncle of trunk, unspecified

✓6th **LØ2.23 Carbuncle of trunk**
LØ2.231 Carbuncle of abdominal wall
LØ2.232 Carbuncle of back [any part, except buttock]
LØ2.233 Carbuncle of chest wall
LØ2.234 Carbuncle of groin
LØ2.235 Carbuncle of perineum
LØ2.236 Carbuncle of umbilicus
LØ2.239 Carbuncle of trunk, unspecified

✓5th **LØ2.3 Cutaneous abscess, furuncle and carbuncle of buttock**
EXCLUDES 1 *pilonidal cyst with abscess (LØ5.Ø1)*

LØ2.31 Cutaneous abscess of buttock CC
Cutaneous abscess of gluteal region

LØ2.32 Furuncle of buttock
Boil of buttock
Folliculitis of buttock
Furuncle of gluteal region
LØ2.33 Carbuncle of buttock
Carbuncle of gluteal region

✓5th LØ2.4 Cutaneous abscess, furuncle and carbuncle of limb
EXCLUDES 2 *cutaneous abscess, furuncle and carbuncle of groin (LØ2.214, LØ2.224, LØ2.234)*
cutaneous abscess, furuncle and carbuncle of hand (LØ2.5-)
cutaneous abscess, furuncle and carbuncle of foot (LØ2.6-)

✓6th LØ2.41 Cutaneous abscess of limb
LØ2.411 Cutaneous abscess of right axilla CC
LØ2.412 Cutaneous abscess of left axilla CC
LØ2.413 Cutaneous abscess of right upper limb CC
LØ2.414 Cutaneous abscess of left upper limb CC
LØ2.415 Cutaneous abscess of right lower limb CC
LØ2.416 Cutaneous abscess of left lower limb CC
LØ2.419 Cutaneous abscess of limb, unspecified CC

✓6th LØ2.42 Furuncle of limb
Boil of limb
Folliculitis of limb
LØ2.421 Furuncle of right axilla
LØ2.422 Furuncle of left axilla
LØ2.423 Furuncle of right upper limb
LØ2.424 Furuncle of left upper limb
LØ2.425 Furuncle of right lower limb
LØ2.426 Furuncle of left lower limb
LØ2.429 Furuncle of limb, unspecified

✓6th LØ2.43 Carbuncle of limb
LØ2.431 Carbuncle of right axilla
LØ2.432 Carbuncle of left axilla
LØ2.433 Carbuncle of right upper limb
LØ2.434 Carbuncle of left upper limb
LØ2.435 Carbuncle of right lower limb
LØ2.436 Carbuncle of left lower limb
LØ2.439 Carbuncle of limb, unspecified

✓5th LØ2.5 Cutaneous abscess, furuncle and carbuncle of hand

✓6th LØ2.51 Cutaneous abscess of hand
LØ2.511 Cutaneous abscess of right hand CC
LØ2.512 Cutaneous abscess of left hand CC
LØ2.519 Cutaneous abscess of unspecified hand CC

✓6th LØ2.52 Furuncle hand
Boil of hand
Folliculitis of hand
LØ2.521 Furuncle right hand
LØ2.522 Furuncle left hand
LØ2.529 Furuncle unspecified hand

✓6th LØ2.53 Carbuncle of hand
LØ2.531 Carbuncle of right hand
LØ2.532 Carbuncle of left hand
LØ2.539 Carbuncle of unspecified hand

✓5th LØ2.6 Cutaneous abscess, furuncle and carbuncle of foot

✓6th LØ2.61 Cutaneous abscess of foot
LØ2.611 Cutaneous abscess of right foot CC
LØ2.612 Cutaneous abscess of left foot CC
LØ2.619 Cutaneous abscess of unspecified foot CC

✓6th LØ2.62 Furuncle of foot
Boil of foot
Folliculitis of foot
LØ2.621 Furuncle of right foot
LØ2.622 Furuncle of left foot
LØ2.629 Furuncle of unspecified foot

✓6th LØ2.63 Carbuncle of foot
LØ2.631 Carbuncle of right foot
LØ2.632 Carbuncle of left foot
LØ2.639 Carbuncle of unspecified foot

✓5th LØ2.8 Cutaneous abscess, furuncle and carbuncle of other sites

✓6th LØ2.81 Cutaneous abscess of other sites
LØ2.811 Cutaneous abscess of head [any part, except face] CC
LØ2.818 Cutaneous abscess of other sites CC

✓6th LØ2.82 Furuncle of other sites
Boil of other sites
Folliculitis of other sites
LØ2.821 Furuncle of head [any part, except face]
LØ2.828 Furuncle of other sites

✓6th LØ2.83 Carbuncle of other sites
LØ2.831 Carbuncle of head [any part, except face]
LØ2.838 Carbuncle of other sites

✓5th LØ2.9 Cutaneous abscess, furuncle and carbuncle, unspecified
LØ2.91 Cutaneous abscess, unspecified CC
LØ2.92 Furuncle, unspecified
Boil NOS
Furunculosis NOS
LØ2.93 Carbuncle, unspecified

✓4th LØ3 Cellulitis and acute lymphangitis

EXCLUDES 2 *cellulitis of anal and rectal region (K61.-)*
cellulitis of external auditory canal (H6Ø.1)
cellulitis of eyelid (HØØ.Ø)
cellulitis of female external genital organs (N76.4)
cellulitis of lacrimal apparatus (HØ4.3)
cellulitis of male external genital organs (N48.2, N49.-)
cellulitis of mouth (K12.2)
cellulitis of nose (J34.Ø)
eosinophilic cellulitis [Wells] (L98.3)
febrile neutrophilic dermatosis [Sweet] (L98.2)
lymphangitis (chronic) (subacute) (I89.1)

AHA: 2017,4Q,100
DEF: Cellulitis: Infection of the skin and subcutaneous tissues, most often caused by *Staphylococcus* or *Streptococcus* bacteria secondary to a cutaneous lesion. Progression of the inflammation may lead to abscess and tissue death, or even systemic infection-like bacteremia.
DEF: Lymphangitis: Inflammation of the lymph channels most often caused by *Streptococcus*.

✓5th LØ3.Ø Cellulitis and acute lymphangitis of finger and toe
Infection of nail
Onychia
Paronychia
Perionychia

✓6th LØ3.Ø1 Cellulitis of finger
Felon
Whitlow
EXCLUDES 1 *herpetic whitlow (BØØ.89)*
DEF: Felon: Superficial bacterial skin infection at the tip of the finger.
LØ3.Ø11 Cellulitis of right finger
LØ3.Ø12 Cellulitis of left finger
LØ3.Ø19 Cellulitis of unspecified finger

✓6th LØ3.Ø2 Acute lymphangitis of finger
Hangnail with lymphangitis of finger
LØ3.Ø21 Acute lymphangitis of right finger
LØ3.Ø22 Acute lymphangitis of left finger
LØ3.Ø29 Acute lymphangitis of unspecified finger

✓6th LØ3.Ø3 Cellulitis of toe
LØ3.Ø31 Cellulitis of right toe
LØ3.Ø32 Cellulitis of left toe
LØ3.Ø39 Cellulitis of unspecified toe

✓6th LØ3.Ø4 Acute lymphangitis of toe
Hangnail with lymphangitis of toe
LØ3.Ø41 Acute lymphangitis of right toe
LØ3.Ø42 Acute lymphangitis of left toe
LØ3.Ø49 Acute lymphangitis of unspecified toe

✓5th LØ3.1 Cellulitis and acute lymphangitis of other parts of limb

✓6th LØ3.11 Cellulitis of other parts of limb
EXCLUDES 2 *cellulitis of fingers (LØ3.Ø1-)*
cellulitis of toes (LØ3.Ø3-)
groin (LØ3.314)
LØ3.111 Cellulitis of right axilla CC
LØ3.112 Cellulitis of left axilla CC
LØ3.113 Cellulitis of right upper limb CC
LØ3.114 Cellulitis of left upper limb CC

LØ3.115 Cellulitis of right lower limb CC
LØ3.116 Cellulitis of left lower limb CC
LØ3.119 Cellulitis of unspecified part of limb CC

√6th **LØ3.12 Acute lymphangitis of other parts of limb**
EXCLUDES 2 *acute lymphangitis of fingers (LØ3.2-)*
acute lymphangitis of groin (LØ3.324)
acute lymphangitis of toes (LØ3.Ø4-)

LØ3.121 Acute lymphangitis of right axilla CC
LØ3.122 Acute lymphangitis of left axilla CC
LØ3.123 Acute lymphangitis of right upper limb CC
LØ3.124 Acute lymphangitis of left upper limb CC
LØ3.125 Acute lymphangitis of right lower limb CC
LØ3.126 Acute lymphangitis of left lower limb CC
LØ3.129 Acute lymphangitis of unspecified part of limb CC

√5th **LØ3.2 Cellulitis and acute lymphangitis of face and neck**

√6th **LØ3.21 Cellulitis and acute lymphangitis of face**

LØ3.211 Cellulitis of face CC
EXCLUDES 2 *abscess of orbit (HØ5.Ø1-)*
cellulitis of ear (H6Ø.1-)
cellulitis of eyelid (HØØ.Ø-)
cellulitis of head (LØ3.81)
cellulitis of lacrimal apparatus (HØ4.3)
cellulitis of lip (K13.Ø)
cellulitis of mouth (K12.2)
cellulitis of nose (internal) (J34.Ø)
cellulitis of orbit (HØ5.Ø1-)
cellulitis of scalp (LØ3.81)
AHA: 2013,4Q,123

LØ3.212 Acute lymphangitis of face CC
LØ3.213 Periorbital cellulitis CC
Preseptal cellulitis
AHA: 2016,4Q,36

√6th **LØ3.22 Cellulitis and acute lymphangitis of neck**

LØ3.221 Cellulitis of neck CC
LØ3.222 Acute lymphangitis of neck CC

√5th **LØ3.3 Cellulitis and acute lymphangitis of trunk**

√6th **LØ3.31 Cellulitis of trunk**
EXCLUDES 2 *cellulitis of anal and rectal regions (K61.-)*
cellulitis of breast NOS (N61.Ø)
cellulitis of female external genital organs (N76.4)
cellulitis of male external genital organs (N48.2, N49.-)
omphalitis of newborn (P38.-)
puerperal cellulitis of breast (O91.2)

LØ3.311 Cellulitis of abdominal wall CC
EXCLUDES 2 *cellulitis of umbilicus (LØ3.316)*
cellulitis of groin (LØ3.314)

LØ3.312 Cellulitis of back [any part except buttock] CC
LØ3.313 Cellulitis of chest wall CC
LØ3.314 Cellulitis of groin CC
LØ3.315 Cellulitis of perineum CC
LØ3.316 Cellulitis of umbilicus CC
LØ3.317 Cellulitis of buttock CC
LØ3.319 Cellulitis of trunk, unspecified CC

√6th **LØ3.32 Acute lymphangitis of trunk**

LØ3.321 Acute lymphangitis of abdominal wall CC
LØ3.322 Acute lymphangitis of back [any part except buttock] CC
LØ3.323 Acute lymphangitis of chest wall CC
LØ3.324 Acute lymphangitis of groin CC
LØ3.325 Acute lymphangitis of perineum CC
LØ3.326 Acute lymphangitis of umbilicus CC
LØ3.327 Acute lymphangitis of buttock CC
LØ3.329 Acute lymphangitis of trunk, unspecified CC

√5th **LØ3.8 Cellulitis and acute lymphangitis of other sites**

√6th **LØ3.81 Cellulitis of other sites**

LØ3.811 Cellulitis of head [any part, except face] CC
Cellulitis of scalp
EXCLUDES 2 *cellulitis of face (LØ3.211)*

LØ3.818 Cellulitis of other sites CC

√6th **LØ3.89 Acute lymphangitis of other sites**

LØ3.891 Acute lymphangitis of head [any part, except face] CC
LØ3.898 Acute lymphangitis of other sites CC

√5th **LØ3.9 Cellulitis and acute lymphangitis, unspecified**

LØ3.9Ø Cellulitis, unspecified CC
LØ3.91 Acute lymphangitis, unspecified CC
EXCLUDES 1 *lymphangitis NOS (I89.1)*

√4th **LØ4 Acute lymphadenitis**
INCLUDES abscess (acute) of lymph nodes, except mesenteric
acute lymphadenitis, except mesenteric
EXCLUDES 1 *chronic or subacute lymphadenitis, except mesenteric (I88.1)*
enlarged lymph nodes (R59.-)
human immunodeficiency virus [HIV] disease resulting in generalized lymphadenopathy (B2Ø)
lymphadenitis NOS (I88.9)
nonspecific mesenteric lymphadenitis (I88.Ø)
DEF: Inflammation or enlargement of the lymph nodes.

LØ4.Ø Acute lymphadenitis of face, head and neck
LØ4.1 Acute lymphadenitis of trunk
LØ4.2 Acute lymphadenitis of upper limb
Acute lymphadenitis of axilla
Acute lymphadenitis of shoulder
LØ4.3 Acute lymphadenitis of lower limb
Acute lymphadenitis of hip
EXCLUDES 2 *acute lymphadenitis of groin (LØ4.1)*
LØ4.8 Acute lymphadenitis of other sites
LØ4.9 Acute lymphadenitis, unspecified

√4th **LØ5 Pilonidal cyst and sinus**
DEF: Pilonidal cyst: Sac or sinus cavity of trapped epithelial tissues in the sacrococcygeal region, usually associated with ingrown hair.
DEF: Pilonidal sinus: Fistula, tract, or channel that extends from an infected area of ingrown hair to another site within the skin or out to the skin surface.

Pilonidal Cyst

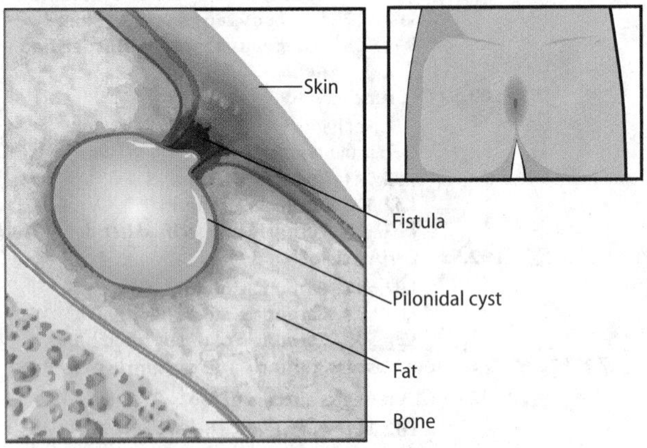

√5th **LØ5.Ø Pilonidal cyst and sinus with abscess**

LØ5.Ø1 Pilonidal cyst with abscess CC SW
Pilonidal abscess
Pilonidal dimple with abscess
Postanal dimple with abscess
EXCLUDES 2 *congenital sacral dimple (Q82.6)*
parasacral dimple (Q82.6)

LØ5.Ø2 Pilonidal sinus with abscess CC SW
Coccygeal fistula with abscess
Coccygeal sinus with abscess
Pilonidal fistula with abscess

✓5th **LØ5.9 Pilonidal cyst and sinus without abscess**

LØ5.91 Pilonidal cyst without abscess
Pilonidal dimple
Postanal dimple
Pilonidal cyst NOS
EXCLUDES 2 *congenital sacral dimple (Q82.6)*
parasacral dimple (Q82.6)

LØ5.92 Pilonidal sinus without abscess SW
Coccygeal fistula
Coccygeal sinus without abscess
Pilonidal fistula

✓4th **LØ8 Other local infections of skin and subcutaneous tissue**

LØ8.Ø Pyoderma
Dermatitis gangrenosa
Purulent dermatitis
Septic dermatitis
Suppurative dermatitis
EXCLUDES 1 *pyoderma gangrenosum (L88)*
pyoderma vegetans (LØ8.81)
DEF: Any superficial skin disease commonly characterized by the discharging of pus not attributed to another condition.

LØ8.1 Erythrasma HIV CC
DEF: Chronic, superficial skin infection of brown scaly patches, commonly found in skin folds most prevalent in the overweight or diabetic population.

✓5th **LØ8.8 Other specified local infections of the skin and subcutaneous tissue**

LØ8.81 Pyoderma vegetans
EXCLUDES 1 *pyoderma gangrenosum (L88)*
pyoderma NOS (LØ8.Ø)

LØ8.82 Omphalitis not of newborn
EXCLUDES 1 *omphalitis of newborn (P38.-)*

LØ8.89 Other specified local infections of the skin and subcutaneous tissue

LØ8.9 Local infection of the skin and subcutaneous tissue, unspecified

Bullous disorders (L1Ø-L14)

EXCLUDES 1 *benign familial pemphigus [Hailey-Hailey] (Q82.8)*
staphylococcal scalded skin syndrome (LØØ)
toxic epidermal necrolysis [Lyell] (L51.2)

✓4th **L1Ø Pemphigus**
EXCLUDES 1 *pemphigus neonatorum (LØ1.Ø3)*

L1Ø.Ø Pemphigus vulgaris CC
L1Ø.1 Pemphigus vegetans CC
L1Ø.2 Pemphigus foliaceous CC
L1Ø.3 Brazilian pemphigus [fogo selvagem] CC
L1Ø.4 Pemphigus erythematosus CC
Senear-Usher syndrome
L1Ø.5 Drug-induced pemphigus CC
Use additional code for adverse effect, if applicable, to identify drug (T36-T5Ø with fifth or sixth character 5)

✓5th **L1Ø.8 Other pemphigus**
L1Ø.81 Paraneoplastic pemphigus CC
L1Ø.89 Other pemphigus CC

L1Ø.9 Pemphigus, unspecified CC

✓4th **L11 Other acantholytic disorders**

L11.Ø Acquired keratosis follicularis
EXCLUDES 1 *keratosis follicularis (congenital) [Darier-White] (Q82.8)*
L11.1 Transient acantholytic dermatosis [Grover]
L11.8 Other specified acantholytic disorders
L11.9 Acantholytic disorder, unspecified

✓4th **L12 Pemphigoid**
EXCLUDES 1 *herpes gestationis (O26.4-)*
impetigo herpetiformis (L4Ø.1)

L12.Ø Bullous pemphigoid CC

L12.1 Cicatricial pemphigoid
Benign mucous membrane pemphigoid
DEF: Chronic autoimmune disease characterized by subepidermal blistering lesions of the mucosa, including the conjunctiva. It is seen predominantly in the elderly and produces adhesions and scarring.

L12.2 Chronic bullous disease of childhood P
Juvenile dermatitis herpetiformis

✓5th **L12.3 Acquired epidermolysis bullosa**
EXCLUDES 1 *epidermolysis bullosa (congenital) (Q81.-)*

L12.3Ø Acquired epidermolysis bullosa, unspecified CC HCC
L12.31 Epidermolysis bullosa due to drug CC HCC
Use additional code for adverse effect, if applicable, to identify drug (T36-T5Ø with fifth or sixth character 5)
L12.35 Other acquired epidermolysis bullosa CC HCC

L12.8 Other pemphigoid CC
L12.9 Pemphigoid, unspecified CC

✓4th **L13 Other bullous disorders**

L13.Ø Dermatitis herpetiformis
Duhring's disease
Hydroa herpetiformis
EXCLUDES 1 *juvenile dermatitis herpetiformis (L12.2)*
senile dermatitis herpetiformis (L12.Ø)
DEF: Skin disease to which people are genetically predisposed resulting from an immunological response to gluten. Dermatitis herpetiformis is an extremely pruritic eruption of various lesions that frequently heal, leaving hyperpigmentation or hypopigmentation and occasionally scarring. It is usually associated with asymptomatic gluten-sensitive enteropathy.

L13.1 Subcorneal pustular dermatitis
Sneddon-Wilkinson disease
L13.8 Other specified bullous disorders
L13.9 Bullous disorder, unspecified

L14 Bullous disorders in diseases classified elsewhere
Code first underlying disease

Dermatitis and eczema (L2Ø-L3Ø)

NOTE In this block the terms dermatitis and eczema are used synonymously and interchangeably.

EXCLUDES 2 *chronic (childhood) granulomatous disease (D71)*
dermatitis gangrenosa (LØ8.Ø)
dermatitis herpetiformis (L13.Ø)
dry skin dermatitis (L85.3)
factitial dermatitis (L98.1)
perioral dermatitis (L71.Ø)
radiation-related disorders of the skin and subcutaneous tissue (L55-L59)
stasis dermatitis (I87.2)

✓4th **L2Ø Atopic dermatitis**

L2Ø.Ø Besnier's prurigo

✓5th **L2Ø.8 Other atopic dermatitis**
EXCLUDES 2 *circumscribed neurodermatitis (L28.Ø)*

L2Ø.81 Atopic neurodermatitis
Diffuse neurodermatitis
L2Ø.82 Flexural eczema
L2Ø.83 Infantile (acute) (chronic) eczema P
L2Ø.84 Intrinsic (allergic) eczema
L2Ø.89 Other atopic dermatitis

L2Ø.9 Atopic dermatitis, unspecified

✓4th **L21 Seborrheic dermatitis**
EXCLUDES 2 *infective dermatitis (L3Ø.3)*
seborrheic keratosis (L82.-)

L21.Ø Seborrhea capitis
Cradle cap
AHA: 2018,1Q,6
TIP: Assign for dandruff in an adult patient.
L21.1 Seborrheic infantile dermatitis P
L21.8 Other seborrheic dermatitis
L21.9 Seborrheic dermatitis, unspecified
Seborrhea NOS

L22 Diaper dermatitis
Diaper erythema
Diaper rash
Psoriasiform diaper rash

√4th **L23 Allergic contact dermatitis**
EXCLUDES 1 *allergy NOS (T78.4Ø)*
contact dermatitis NOS (L25.9)
dermatitis NOS (L3Ø.9)
EXCLUDES 2 *dermatitis due to substances taken internally (L27.-)*
dermatitis of eyelid (HØ1.1-)
diaper dermatitis (L22)
eczema of external ear (H6Ø.5-)
irritant contact dermatitis (L24.-)
perioral dermatitis (L71.Ø)
radiation-related disorders of the skin and subcutaneous tissue (L55-L59)

L23.Ø Allergic contact dermatitis due to metals
Allergic contact dermatitis due to chromium
Allergic contact dermatitis due to nickel

L23.1 Allergic contact dermatitis due to adhesives

L23.2 Allergic contact dermatitis due to cosmetics

L23.3 Allergic contact dermatitis due to drugs in contact with skin
Use additional code for adverse effect, if applicable, to identify drug (T36-T5Ø with fifth or sixth character 5)
EXCLUDES 2 *dermatitis due to ingested drugs and medicaments (L27.Ø-L27.1)*

L23.4 Allergic contact dermatitis due to dyes

L23.5 Allergic contact dermatitis due to other chemical products
Allergic contact dermatitis due to cement
Allergic contact dermatitis due to insecticide
Allergic contact dermatitis due to plastic
Allergic contact dermatitis due to rubber

L23.6 Allergic contact dermatitis due to food in contact with the skin
EXCLUDES 2 *dermatitis due to ingested food (L27.2)*

L23.7 Allergic contact dermatitis due to plants, except food
EXCLUDES 2 *allergy NOS due to pollen (J3Ø.1)*

√5th **L23.8 Allergic contact dermatitis due to other agents**

L23.81 Allergic contact dermatitis due to animal (cat) (dog) dander
Allergic contact dermatitis due to animal (cat) (dog) hair

L23.89 Allergic contact dermatitis due to other agents

L23.9 Allergic contact dermatitis, unspecified cause
Allergic contact eczema NOS

√4th **L24 Irritant contact dermatitis**
EXCLUDES 1 *allergy NOS (T78.4Ø)*
contact dermatitis NOS (L25.9)
dermatitis NOS (L3Ø.9)
EXCLUDES 2 *allergic contact dermatitis (L23.-)*
dermatitis due to substances taken internally (L27.-)
dermatitis of eyelid (HØ1.1-)
diaper dermatitis (L22)
eczema of external ear (H6Ø.5-)
perioral dermatitis (L71.Ø)
radiation-related disorders of the skin and subcutaneous tissue (L55-L59)

L24.Ø Irritant contact dermatitis due to detergents

L24.1 Irritant contact dermatitis due to oils and greases

L24.2 Irritant contact dermatitis due to solvents
Irritant contact dermatitis due to chlorocompound
Irritant contact dermatitis due to cyclohexane
Irritant contact dermatitis due to ester
Irritant contact dermatitis due to glycol
Irritant contact dermatitis due to hydrocarbon
Irritant contact dermatitis due to ketone

L24.3 Irritant contact dermatitis due to cosmetics

L24.4 Irritant contact dermatitis due to drugs in contact with skin
Use additional code for adverse effect, if applicable, to identify drug (T36-T5Ø with fifth or sixth character 5)

L24.5 Irritant contact dermatitis due to other chemical products
Irritant contact dermatitis due to cement
Irritant contact dermatitis due to insecticide
Irritant contact dermatitis due to plastic
Irritant contact dermatitis due to rubber

L24.6 Irritant contact dermatitis due to food in contact with skin
EXCLUDES 2 *dermatitis due to ingested food (L27.2)*

L24.7 Irritant contact dermatitis due to plants, except food
EXCLUDES 2 *allergy NOS to pollen (J3Ø.1)*

√5th **L24.8 Irritant contact dermatitis due to other agents**

L24.81 Irritant contact dermatitis due to metals
Irritant contact dermatitis due to chromium
Irritant contact dermatitis due to nickel

L24.89 Irritant contact dermatitis due to other agents
Irritant contact dermatitis due to dyes

L24.9 Irritant contact dermatitis, unspecified cause
Irritant contact eczema NOS

√4th **L25 Unspecified contact dermatitis**
EXCLUDES 1 *allergic contact dermatitis (L23.-)*
allergy NOS (T78.4Ø)
dermatitis NOS (L3Ø.9)
irritant contact dermatitis (L24.-)
EXCLUDES 2 *dermatitis due to ingested substances (L27.-)*
dermatitis of eyelid (HØ1.1-)
eczema of external ear (H6Ø.5-)
perioral dermatitis (L71.Ø)
radiation-related disorders of the skin and subcutaneous tissue (L55-L59)

L25.Ø Unspecified contact dermatitis due to cosmetics

L25.1 Unspecified contact dermatitis due to drugs in contact with skin
Use additional code for adverse effect, if applicable, to identify drug (T36-T5Ø with fifth or sixth character 5)
EXCLUDES 2 *dermatitis due to ingested drugs and medicaments (L27.Ø-L27.1)*

L25.2 Unspecified contact dermatitis due to dyes

L25.3 Unspecified contact dermatitis due to other chemical products
Unspecified contact dermatitis due to cement
Unspecified contact dermatitis due to insecticide

L25.4 Unspecified contact dermatitis due to food in contact with skin
EXCLUDES 2 *dermatitis due to ingested food (L27.2)*

L25.5 Unspecified contact dermatitis due to plants, except food
EXCLUDES 1 *nettle rash (L5Ø.9)*
EXCLUDES 2 *allergy NOS due to pollen (J3Ø.1)*

L25.8 Unspecified contact dermatitis due to other agents

L25.9 Unspecified contact dermatitis, unspecified cause
Contact dermatitis (occupational) NOS
Contact eczema (occupational) NOS

L26 Exfoliative dermatitis
Hebra's pityriasis
EXCLUDES 1 *Ritter's disease (LØØ)*

√4th **L27 Dermatitis due to substances taken internally**
EXCLUDES 1 *allergy NOS (T78.4Ø)*
EXCLUDES 2 *adverse food reaction, except dermatitis (T78.Ø-T78.1)*
contact dermatitis (L23-L25)
drug photoallergic response (L56.1)
drug phototoxic response (L56.Ø)
urticaria (L5Ø.-)

L27.Ø Generalized skin eruption due to drugs and medicaments taken internally
Use additional code for adverse effect, if applicable, to identify drug (T36-T5Ø with fifth or sixth character 5)

L27.1 Localized skin eruption due to drugs and medicaments taken internally
Use additional code for adverse effect, if applicable, to identify drug (T36-T5Ø with fifth or sixth character 5)

L27.2 Dermatitis due to ingested food
EXCLUDES 2 *dermatitis due to food in contact with skin (L23.6, L24.6, L25.4)*

L27.8 Dermatitis due to other substances taken internally

L27.9 Dermatitis due to unspecified substance taken internally

L28 Lichen simplex chronicus and prurigo

L28.0 Lichen simplex chronicus
Circumscribed neurodermatitis
Lichen NOS

L28.1 Prurigo nodularis

L28.2 Other prurigo
Prurigo NOS
Prurigo Hebra
Prurigo mitis
Urticaria papulosa

L29 Pruritus

EXCLUDES 1 *neurotic excoriation (L98.1)*
psychogenic pruritus (F45.8)

L29.0 Pruritus ani

L29.1 Pruritus scroti ♂

L29.2 Pruritus vulvae ♀

L29.3 Anogenital pruritus, unspecified

L29.8 Other pruritus

L29.9 Pruritus, unspecified
Itch NOS

L30 Other and unspecified dermatitis

EXCLUDES 2 *contact dermatitis (L23-L25)*
dry skin dermatitis (L85.3)
small plaque parapsoriasis (L41.3)
stasis dermatitis (I87.2)

L30.0 Nummular dermatitis

L30.1 Dyshidrosis [pompholyx]

L30.2 Cutaneous autosensitization
Candidid [levurid]
Dermatophytid
Eczematid

L30.3 Infective dermatitis
Infectious eczematoid dermatitis

L30.4 Erythema intertrigo

L30.5 Pityriasis alba
AHA: 2018,1Q,6

L30.8 Other specified dermatitis

L30.9 Dermatitis, unspecified
Eczema NOS

Papulosquamous disorders (L40-L45)

L40 Psoriasis

DEF: Chronic autoimmune condition that speeds up skin cell growth, causing excessive immature skin cells to form raised, rounded erythematous lesions covered by dry, silvery scaling patches. Most commonly found on the scalp, elbows, knees, hands, feet, and genitals, it can also affect the joints with stiffness and swelling.

L40.0 Psoriasis vulgaris
Nummular psoriasis
Plaque psoriasis

L40.1 Generalized pustular psoriasis
Impetigo herpetiformis
Von Zumbusch's disease

L40.2 Acrodermatitis continua

L40.3 Pustulosis palmaris et plantaris

L40.4 Guttate psoriasis

L40.5 Arthropathic psoriasis

L40.50 Arthropathic psoriasis, unspecified HCC

L40.51 Distal interphalangeal psoriatic arthropathy HCC

L40.52 Psoriatic arthritis mutilans HCC

L40.53 Psoriatic spondylitis HCC

L40.54 Psoriatic juvenile arthropathy HCC

L40.59 Other psoriatic arthropathy HCC

L40.8 Other psoriasis
Flexural psoriasis

L40.9 Psoriasis, unspecified

L41 Parapsoriasis

EXCLUDES 1 *poikiloderma vasculare atrophicans (L94.5)*

L41.0 Pityriasis lichenoides et varioliformis acuta
Mucha-Habermann disease

L41.1 Pityriasis lichenoides chronica

L41.3 Small plaque parapsoriasis

L41.4 Large plaque parapsoriasis

L41.5 Retiform parapsoriasis

L41.8 Other parapsoriasis

L41.9 Parapsoriasis, unspecified

L42 Pityriasis rosea

L43 Lichen planus

EXCLUDES 1 *lichen planopilaris (L66.1)*

L43.0 Hypertrophic lichen planus

L43.1 Bullous lichen planus

L43.2 Lichenoid drug reaction
Use additional code for adverse effect, if applicable, to identify drug (T36-T50 with fifth or sixth character 5)

L43.3 Subacute (active) lichen planus
Lichen planus tropicus

L43.8 Other lichen planus

L43.9 Lichen planus, unspecified

L44 Other papulosquamous disorders

L44.0 Pityriasis rubra pilaris

L44.1 Lichen nitidus
DEF: Chronic, inflammatory, asymptomatic skin disorder, characterized by numerous glistening, flat-topped, discrete, skin-colored micropapules, most often on the penis, lower abdomen, inner thighs, wrists, forearms, breasts, and buttocks.

L44.2 Lichen striatus

L44.3 Lichen ruber moniliformis

L44.4 Infantile papular acrodermatitis [Gianotti-Crosti] P

L44.8 Other specified papulosquamous disorders

L44.9 Papulosquamous disorder, unspecified

L45 Papulosquamous disorders in diseases classified elsewhere
Code first underlying disease

Urticaria and erythema (L49-L54)

EXCLUDES 1 *Lyme disease (A69.2-)*
rosacea (L71.-)

L49 Exfoliation due to erythematous conditions according to extent of body surface involved
Code first erythematous condition causing exfoliation, such as:
Ritter's disease (L00)
(Staphylococcal) scalded skin syndrome (L00)
Stevens-Johnson syndrome (L51.1)
Stevens-Johnson syndrome-toxic epidermal necrolysis overlap syndrome (L51.3)
toxic epidermal necrolysis (L51.2)
DEF: Exfoliation: Falling or sloughing off skin in layers.

L49.0 Exfoliation due to erythematous condition involving less than 10 percent of body surface
Exfoliation due to erythematous condition NOS

L49.1 Exfoliation due to erythematous condition involving 10-19 percent of body surface

L49.2 Exfoliation due to erythematous condition involving 20-29 percent of body surface

L49.3 Exfoliation due to erythematous condition involving 30-39 percent of body surface CC

L49.4 Exfoliation due to erythematous condition involving 40-49 percent of body surface CC

L49.5 Exfoliation due to erythematous condition involving 50-59 percent of body surface CC

L49.6 Exfoliation due to erythematous condition involving 60-69 percent of body surface CC

L49.7 Exfoliation due to erythematous condition involving 70-79 percent of body surface CC

L49.8 Exfoliation due to erythematous condition involving 80-89 percent of body surface CC

L49.9 Exfoliation due to erythematous condition involving 90 or more percent of body surface CC

✓4th L50 Urticaria

EXCLUDES 1 *allergic contact dermatitis (L23.-)*
angioneurotic edema (T78.3)
giant urticaria (T78.3)
hereditary angio-edema (D84.1)
Quincke's edema (T78.3)
serum urticaria (T80.6-)
solar urticaria (L56.3)
urticaria neonatorum (P83.8)
urticaria papulosa (L28.2)
urticaria pigmentosa (D47.01)

DEF: Eruption of itching edema of the skin. ***Synonym(s):*** *hives.*

L50.0 Allergic urticaria
L50.1 Idiopathic urticaria
L50.2 Urticaria due to cold and heat
EXCLUDES 2 *familial cold urticaria (M04.2)*
L50.3 Dermatographic urticaria
L50.4 Vibratory urticaria
L50.5 Cholinergic urticaria
L50.6 Contact urticaria
L50.8 Other urticaria
Chronic urticaria
Recurrent periodic urticaria
L50.9 Urticaria, unspecified

✓4th L51 Erythema multiforme

Use additional code for adverse effect, if applicable, to identify drug (T36-T50 with fifth or sixth character 5)
Use additional code to identify associated manifestations, such as:
arthropathy associated with dermatological disorders (M14.8-)
conjunctival edema (H11.42)
conjunctivitis (H10.22-)
corneal scars and opacities (H17.-)
corneal ulcer (H16.0-)
edema of eyelid (H02.84-)
inflammation of eyelid (H01.8)
keratoconjunctivitis sicca (H16.22-)
mechanical lagophthalmos (H02.22-)
stomatitis (K12.-)
symblepharon (H11.23-)
Use additional code to identify percentage of skin exfoliation (L49.-)

EXCLUDES 1 *staphylococcal scalded skin syndrome (L00)*
Ritter's disease (L00)

DEF: Acute complex of symptoms with a varied pattern of skin eruptions, such as macular, bullous, popular, nodose, or vesicular lesions on the neck, face, and legs. Erythema (redness of skin and mucous membranes) multiforme (multiple forms) is a hypersensitivity (allergic) reaction that can occur at any age but primarily affects children or young adults.

L51.0 Nonbullous erythema multiforme
L51.1 Stevens-Johnson syndrome CC HCC
L51.2 Toxic epidermal necrolysis [Lyell] CC HCC
L51.3 Stevens-Johnson syndrome-toxic epidermal necrolysis overlap syndrome CC HCC
SJS-TEN overlap syndrome
L51.8 Other erythema multiforme
L51.9 Erythema multiforme, unspecified
Erythema iris
Erythema multiforme major NOS
Erythema multiforme minor NOS
Herpes iris

L52 Erythema nodosum

EXCLUDES 1 *tuberculous erythema nodosum (A18.4)*

DEF: Form of panniculitis (inflammation of the fat layer beneath the skin) most often occurring in women. Commonly seen as a hypersensitivity reaction to infections, drugs, sarcoidosis, and specific enteropathies. The acute stage is associated with fever, malaise, and arthralgia. The lesions are pink to blue in color as tender nodules and are found on the front of the legs below the knees.

✓4th L53 Other erythematous conditions

EXCLUDES 1 *erythema ab igne (L59.0)*
erythema due to external agents in contact with skin (L23-L25)
erythema intertrigo (L30.4)

L53.0 Toxic erythema CC
Code first poisoning due to drug or toxin, if applicable (T36-T65 with fifth or sixth character 1-4 or 6)
Use additional code for adverse effect, if applicable, to identify drug (T36-T50 with fifth or sixth character 5)
EXCLUDES 1 *neonatal erythema toxicum (P83.1)*
L53.1 Erythema annulare centrifugum CC
L53.2 Erythema marginatum CC
L53.3 Other chronic figurate erythema CC
L53.8 Other specified erythematous conditions
L53.9 Erythematous condition, unspecified
Erythema NOS
Erythroderma NOS

L54 Erythema in diseases classified elsewhere

Code first underlying disease

Radiation-related disorders of the skin and subcutaneous tissue (L55-L59)

✓4th L55 Sunburn

L55.0 Sunburn of first degree
L55.1 Sunburn of second degree
L55.2 Sunburn of third degree
L55.9 Sunburn, unspecified

✓4th L56 Other acute skin changes due to ultraviolet radiation

Use additional code to identify the source of the ultraviolet radiation (W89, X32)

L56.0 Drug phototoxic response
Use additional code for adverse effect, if applicable, to identify drug (T36-T50 with fifth or sixth character 5)
L56.1 Drug photoallergic response
Use additional code for adverse effect, if applicable, to identify drug (T36-T50 with fifth or sixth character 5)
L56.2 Photocontact dermatitis [berloque dermatitis]
L56.3 Solar urticaria
L56.4 Polymorphous light eruption
L56.5 Disseminated superficial actinic porokeratosis (DSAP)
DEF: Autosomal dominant skin condition occurring in sun-exposed areas of the skin (particularly the arms and legs), characterized by superficial annular, keratotic, brownish-red spots or thickenings with depressed centers and sharp, ridged borders. It may evolve into squamous cell carcinoma.
L56.8 Other specified acute skin changes due to ultraviolet radiation
L56.9 Acute skin change due to ultraviolet radiation, unspecified

✓4th L57 Skin changes due to chronic exposure to nonionizing radiation

▶Use additional code to identify the source of the ultraviolet radiation (W89), or other nonionizing radiation (W90)◀

L57.0 Actinic keratosis
Keratosis NOS
Senile keratosis
Solar keratosis
L57.1 Actinic reticuloid
L57.2 Cutis rhomboidalis nuchae
L57.3 Poikiloderma of Civatte
L57.4 Cutis laxa senilis
Elastosis senilis
L57.5 Actinic granuloma
L57.8 Other skin changes due to chronic exposure to nonionizing radiation
Farmer's skin
Sailor's skin
Solar dermatitis
L57.9 Skin changes due to chronic exposure to nonionizing radiation, unspecified

✓4th L58 Radiodermatitis

Use additional code to identify the source of the radiation (W88, W90)

L58.0 Acute radiodermatitis
L58.1 Chronic radiodermatitis
L58.9 Radiodermatitis, unspecified

✓4th L59 Other disorders of skin and subcutaneous tissue related to radiation

L59.Ø Erythema ab igne [dermatitis ab igne]

L59.8 Other specified disorders of the skin and subcutaneous tissue related to radiation
AHA: 2017,1Q,33

L59.9 Disorder of the skin and subcutaneous tissue related to radiation, unspecified

Disorders of skin appendages (L6Ø-L75)

EXCLUDES 1 *congenital malformations of integument (Q84.-)*

✓4th L6Ø Nail disorders

EXCLUDES 2 *clubbing of nails (R68.3)*
onychia and paronychia (LØ3.Ø-)

Nail Disorders

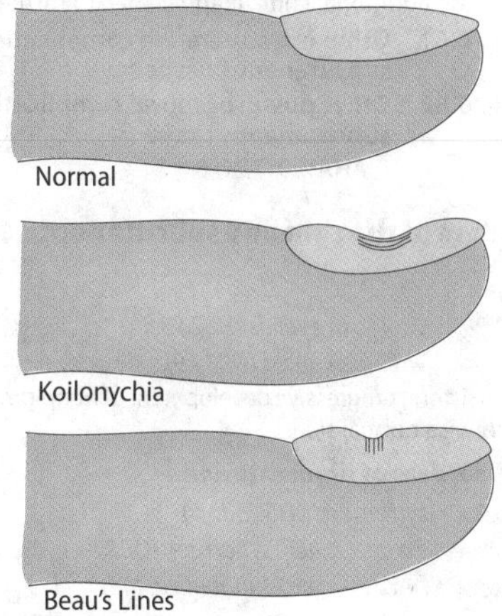

L6Ø.Ø Ingrowing nail

L6Ø.1 Onycholysis

L6Ø.2 Onychogryphosis

L6Ø.3 Nail dystrophy

L6Ø.4 Beau's lines

L6Ø.5 Yellow nail syndrome

L6Ø.8 Other nail disorders

L6Ø.9 Nail disorder, unspecified

L62 Nail disorders in diseases classified elsewhere
Code first underlying disease, such as:
pachydermoperiostosis (M89.4-)

✓4th L63 Alopecia areata

L63.Ø Alopecia (capitis) totalis

L63.1 Alopecia universalis

L63.2 Ophiasis

L63.8 Other alopecia areata

L63.9 Alopecia areata, unspecified

✓4th L64 Androgenic alopecia

INCLUDES male-pattern baldness

L64.Ø Drug-induced androgenic alopecia
Use additional code for adverse effect, if applicable, to identify drug (T36-T5Ø with fifth or sixth character 5)

L64.8 Other androgenic alopecia

L64.9 Androgenic alopecia, unspecified

✓4th L65 Other nonscarring hair loss

Use additional code for adverse effect, if applicable, to identify drug (T36-T5Ø with fifth or sixth character 5)

EXCLUDES 1 *trichotillomania (F63.3)*

L65.Ø Telogen effluvium
DEF: Form of nonscarring alopecia characterized by shedding of hair from premature telogen development in follicles due to stress, including shock, childbirth, surgery, drugs, or weight loss.

L65.1 Anagen effluvium

L65.2 Alopecia mucinosa

L65.8 Other specified nonscarring hair loss

L65.9 Nonscarring hair loss, unspecified
Alopecia NOS

✓4th L66 Cicatricial alopecia [scarring hair loss]

L66.Ø Pseudopelade

L66.1 Lichen planopilaris
Follicular lichen planus

L66.2 Folliculitis decalvans

L66.3 Perifolliculitis capitis abscedens

L66.4 Folliculitis ulerythematosa reticulata

L66.8 Other cicatricial alopecia
AHA: 2015,1Q,19

L66.9 Cicatricial alopecia, unspecified

✓4th L67 Hair color and hair shaft abnormalities

EXCLUDES 1 *monilethrix (Q84.1)*
pili annulati (Q84.1)
telogen effluvium (L65.Ø)

L67.Ø Trichorrhexis nodosa

L67.1 Variations in hair color
Canities
Greyness, hair (premature)
Heterochromia of hair
Poliosis circumscripta, acquired
Poliosis NOS

L67.8 Other hair color and hair shaft abnormalities
Fragilitas crinium

L67.9 Hair color and hair shaft abnormality, unspecified

✓4th L68 Hypertrichosis

INCLUDES excess hair

EXCLUDES 1 *congenital hypertrichosis (Q84.2)*
persistent lanugo (Q84.2)

L68.Ø Hirsutism

L68.1 Acquired hypertrichosis lanuginosa

L68.2 Localized hypertrichosis

L68.3 Polytrichia

L68.8 Other hypertrichosis

L68.9 Hypertrichosis, unspecified

✓4th L7Ø Acne

EXCLUDES 2 *acne keloid (L73.Ø)*

L7Ø.Ø Acne vulgaris

L7Ø.1 Acne conglobata

L7Ø.2 Acne varioliformis
Acne necrotica miliaris
DEF: Rare form of acne characterized by development of persistent brown papulopustules followed by scar formation. This type of acne usually presents on the brow and temporoparietal part of the scalp.

L7Ø.3 Acne tropica

L7Ø.4 Infantile acne P

L7Ø.5 Acné excoriée
Acné excoriée des jeunes filles
Picker's acne

L7Ø.8 Other acne

L7Ø.9 Acne, unspecified

✓4th L71 Rosacea

Use additional code for adverse effect, if applicable, to identify drug (T36-T5Ø with fifth or sixth character 5)

L71.Ø Perioral dermatitis

L71.1 Rhinophyma

L71.8 Other rosacea
AHA: 2018,4Q,15

L71.9 Rosacea, unspecified

✓4th L72 Follicular cysts of skin and subcutaneous tissue

L72.Ø Epidermal cyst

✓5th L72.1 Pilar and trichodermal cyst

L72.11 Pilar cyst

L72.12 Trichodermal cyst
Trichilemmal (proliferating) cyst

L72.2 Steatocystoma multiplex

L72.3 Sebaceous cyst
EXCLUDES 2 *pilar cyst (L72.11)*
trichilemmal (proliferating) cyst (L72.12)

L72.8 Other follicular cysts of the skin and subcutaneous tissue

L72.9 Follicular cyst of the skin and subcutaneous tissue, unspecified

✓4th L73 Other follicular disorders

L73.Ø Acne keloid

L73.1 Pseudofolliculitis barbae

L73.2 **Hidradenitis suppurativa**

L73.8 **Other specified follicular disorders**
Sycosis barbae

L73.9 **Follicular disorder, unspecified**

✓4th **L74 Eccrine sweat disorders**

EXCLUDES 2 *generalized hyperhidrosis (R61)*

DEF: Eccrine sweat glands: Glands found in the dermal and hypodermal layer of the skin throughout the body, particularly on the forehead, scalp, axillae, palms, and soles. These glands produce watery and neutral or slightly acidic sweat.

L74.0 **Miliaria rubra**

L74.1 **Miliaria crystallina**

L74.2 **Miliaria profunda**
Miliaria tropicalis

L74.3 **Miliaria, unspecified**

L74.4 **Anhidrosis**
Hypohidrosis
DEF: Inability to sweat normally. When the body can't cool itself through perspiration it can lead to heatstroke, a life-threatening condition.

✓5th L74.5 **Focal hyperhidrosis**

✓6th L74.51 **Primary focal hyperhidrosis**

L74.510 **Primary focal hyperhidrosis, axilla**

L74.511 **Primary focal hyperhidrosis, face**

L74.512 **Primary focal hyperhidrosis, palms**

L74.513 **Primary focal hyperhidrosis, soles**

L74.519 **Primary focal hyperhidrosis, unspecified**

L74.52 **Secondary focal hyperhidrosis**
Frey's syndrome

L74.8 **Other eccrine sweat disorders**

L74.9 **Eccrine sweat disorder, unspecified**
Sweat gland disorder NOS

✓4th **L75 Apocrine sweat disorders**

EXCLUDES 1 *dyshidrosis (L30.1)*
hidradenitis suppurativa (L73.2)

DEF: Apocrine sweat glands: Found in the axilla, areola, and circumanal region, these glands begin to function in puberty and produce viscid milky secretions in response to external stimuli.

L75.0 **Bromhidrosis**

L75.1 **Chromhidrosis**

L75.2 **Apocrine miliaria**
Fox-Fordyce disease
DEF: Chronic, usually pruritic disease evidenced by small follicular papular eruptions, especially in the axillary and pubic areas. Apocrine miliaria develops from the closure and rupture of the affected apocrine glands' intraepidermal portion of the ducts.

L75.8 **Other apocrine sweat disorders**

L75.9 **Apocrine sweat disorder, unspecified**

Intraoperative and postprocedural complications of skin and subcutaneous tissue (L76)

✓4th **L76 Intraoperative and postprocedural complications of skin and subcutaneous tissue**

AHA: 2016,4Q,9-10

✓5th L76.0 **Intraoperative hemorrhage and hematoma of skin and subcutaneous tissue complicating a procedure**

EXCLUDES 1 *intraoperative hemorrhage and hematoma of skin and subcutaneous tissue due to accidental puncture and laceration during a procedure (L76.1-)*

L76.01 **Intraoperative hemorrhage and hematoma of skin and subcutaneous tissue complicating a dermatologic procedure** CC

L76.02 **Intraoperative hemorrhage and hematoma of skin and subcutaneous tissue complicating other procedure** CC

✓5th L76.1 **Accidental puncture and laceration of skin and subcutaneous tissue during a procedure**

L76.11 **Accidental puncture and laceration of skin and subcutaneous tissue during a dermatologic procedure** CC

L76.12 **Accidental puncture and laceration of skin and subcutaneous tissue during other procedure** CC

✓5th L76.2 **Postprocedural hemorrhage of skin and subcutaneous tissue following a procedure**

L76.21 **Postprocedural hemorrhage of skin and subcutaneous tissue following a dermatologic procedure** CC

L76.22 **Postprocedural hemorrhage of skin and subcutaneous tissue following other procedure** CC

✓5th L76.3 **Postprocedural hematoma and seroma of skin and subcutaneous tissue following a procedure**

L76.31 **Postprocedural hematoma of skin and subcutaneous tissue following a dermatologic procedure** CC

L76.32 **Postprocedural hematoma of skin and subcutaneous tissue following other procedure** CC

L76.33 **Postprocedural seroma of skin and subcutaneous tissue following a dermatologic procedure** CC

L76.34 **Postprocedural seroma of skin and subcutaneous tissue following other procedure** CC

✓5th L76.8 **Other intraoperative and postprocedural complications of skin and subcutaneous tissue**
Use additional code, if applicable, to further specify disorder

L76.81 **Other intraoperative complications of skin and subcutaneous tissue**

L76.82 **Other postprocedural complications of skin and subcutaneous tissue**
AHA: 2017,3Q,6

Other disorders of the skin and subcutaneous tissue (L80-L99)

L80 Vitiligo

EXCLUDES 2 *vitiligo of eyelids (H02.73-)*
vitiligo of vulva (N90.89)

DEF: Persistent, progressive development of nonpigmented white patches on otherwise normal skin.

✓4th **L81 Other disorders of pigmentation**

EXCLUDES 1 *birthmark NOS (Q82.5)*
Peutz-Jeghers syndrome (Q85.8)

EXCLUDES 2 *nevus — see Alphabetical Index*

L81.0 **Postinflammatory hyperpigmentation**

L81.1 **Chloasma**

L81.2 **Freckles**

L81.3 **Café au lait spots**

L81.4 **Other melanin hyperpigmentation**
Lentigo

L81.5 **Leukoderma, not elsewhere classified**

L81.6 **Other disorders of diminished melanin formation**

L81.7 **Pigmented purpuric dermatosis**
Angioma serpiginosum

L81.8 **Other specified disorders of pigmentation**
Iron pigmentation
Tattoo pigmentation

L81.9 **Disorder of pigmentation, unspecified**

✓4th **L82 Seborrheic keratosis**

INCLUDES basal cell papilloma
dermatosis papulosa nigra
Leser-Trélat disease

EXCLUDES 2 *seborrheic dermatitis (L21.-)*

DEF: Common, benign, noninvasive, lightly pigmented, warty growth composed of basaloid cells that usually appear at middle age as soft, easily crumbling plaques on the face, trunk, and extremities.

L82.0 **Inflamed seborrheic keratosis**

L82.1 **Other seborrheic keratosis**
Seborrheic keratosis NOS

L83 Acanthosis nigricans
Confluent and reticulated papillomatosis
DEF: Diffuse, velvety hyperplasia of the spinous skin layer of the axilla and other body folds marked by gray, brown, or black pigmentation. In adult form, it is often associated with malignant acanthosis nigricans in a benign, nevoid form relatively generalized.

L84 Corns and callosities
Callus
Clavus

✓4th **L85 Other epidermal thickening**

EXCLUDES 2 *hypertrophic disorders of the skin (L91.-)*

L85.0 **Acquired ichthyosis**
EXCLUDES 1 *congenital ichthyosis (Q80.-)*

L85.1 **Acquired keratosis [keratoderma] palmaris et plantaris**
EXCLUDES 1 *inherited keratosis palmaris et plantaris (Q82.8)*

L85.2 **Keratosis punctata (palmaris et plantaris)**

L85.3 Xerosis cutis
Dry skin dermatitis

L85.8 Other specified epidermal thickening
Cutaneous horn

L85.9 Epidermal thickening, unspecified

L86 Keratoderma in diseases classified elsewhere
Code first underlying disease, such as:
Reiter's disease (MØ2.3-)
EXCLUDES 1 *gonococcal keratoderma (A54.89)*
gonococcal keratosis (A54.89)
keratoderma due to vitamin A deficiency (E5Ø.8)
keratosis due to vitamin A deficiency (E5Ø.8)
xeroderma due to vitamin A deficiency (E5Ø.8)

✓4th **L87 Transepidermal elimination disorders**
EXCLUDES 1 *granuloma annulare (perforating) (L92.Ø)*

L87.Ø Keratosis follicularis et parafollicularis in cutem penetrans
Hyperkeratosis follicularis penetrans
Kyrle disease

L87.1 Reactive perforating collagenosis

L87.2 Elastosis perforans serpiginosa

L87.8 Other transepidermal elimination disorders

L87.9 Transepidermal elimination disorder, unspecified

L88 Pyoderma gangrenosum CC
Phagedenic pyoderma
EXCLUDES 1 *dermatitis gangrenosa (LØ8.Ø)*
DEF: Persistent debilitating skin disease characterized by irregular, boggy, blue-red ulcerations, with central healing and undermined edges.

✓4th **L89 Pressure ulcer**
INCLUDES bed sore
decubitus ulcer
plaster ulcer
pressure area
pressure sore
Code first any associated gangrene (I96)
EXCLUDES 2 *decubitus (trophic) ulcer of cervix (uteri) (N86)*
diabetic ulcers (EØ8.621, EØ8.622, EØ9.621, EØ9.622, E1Ø.621, E1Ø.622, E11.621, E11.622, E13.621, E13.622)
non-pressure chronic ulcer of skin (L97.-)
skin infections (LØØ-LØ8)
varicose ulcer (I83.Ø, I83.2)
AHA: 2019,4Q,10-11,54; 2018,4Q,69; 2018,3Q,3; 2018,2Q,21; 2017,4Q,109; 2017,1Q,49; 2016,4Q,143
TIP: The stage of a diagnosed pressure ulcer can be based on documentation from clinicians who are not the patient's provider.

Four Stages of Pressure Ulcer

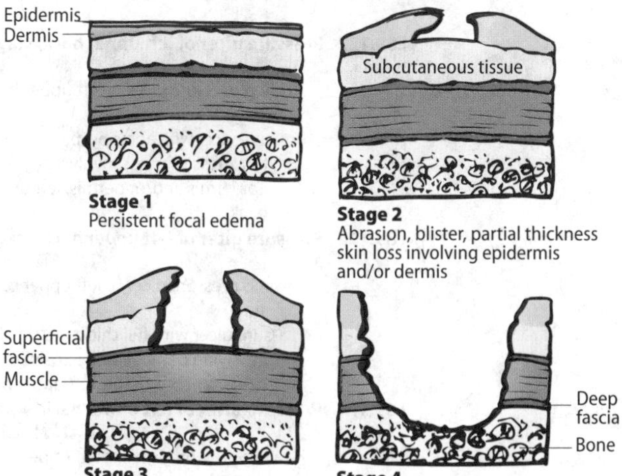

Stage 1 Persistent focal edema

Stage 2 Abrasion, blister, partial thickness skin loss involving epidermis and/or dermis

Stage 3 Full thickness skin loss involving damage or necrosis of subcutaneous tissue

Stage 4 Necrosis of soft tissues through to underlying muscle, tendon, or bone

✓5th **L89.Ø Pressure ulcer of elbow**

✓6th **L89.ØØ Pressure ulcer of unspecified elbow**

L89.ØØØ Pressure ulcer of unspecified elbow, unstageable HCC SW

L89.ØØ1 Pressure ulcer of unspecified elbow, stage 1
Healing pressure ulcer of unspecified elbow, stage 1
Pressure pre-ulcer skin changes limited to persistent focal edema, unspecified elbow

L89.ØØ2 Pressure ulcer of unspecified elbow, stage 2 HCC
Healing pressure ulcer of unspecified elbow, stage 2
Pressure ulcer with abrasion, blister, partial thickness skin loss involving epidermis and/or dermis, unspecified elbow

L89.ØØ3 Pressure ulcer of unspecified elbow, stage 3 MCC H4 HCC SW
Healing pressure ulcer of unspecified elbow, stage 3
Pressure ulcer with full thickness skin loss involving damage or necrosis of subcutaneous tissue, unspecified elbow

L89.ØØ4 Pressure ulcer of unspecified elbow, stage 4 MCC H4 HCC SW
Healing pressure ulcer of unspecified elbow, stage 4
Pressure ulcer with necrosis of soft tissues through to underlying muscle, tendon, or bone, unspecified elbow

L89.ØØ6 Pressure-induced deep tissue damage of unspecified elbow

L89.ØØ9 Pressure ulcer of unspecified elbow, unspecified stage
Healing pressure ulcer of elbow NOS
Healing pressure ulcer of unspecified elbow, unspecified stage

✓6th **L89.Ø1 Pressure ulcer of right elbow**

L89.Ø1Ø Pressure ulcer of right elbow, unstageable HCC SW

L89.Ø11 Pressure ulcer of right elbow, stage 1
Healing pressure ulcer of right elbow, stage 1
Pressure pre-ulcer skin changes limited to persistent focal edema, right elbow

L89.Ø12 Pressure ulcer of right elbow, stage 2 HCC
Healing pressure ulcer of right elbow, stage 2
Pressure ulcer with abrasion, blister, partial thickness skin loss involving epidermis and/or dermis, right elbow

L89.Ø13 Pressure ulcer of right elbow, stage 3 MCC H4 HCC SW
Healing pressure ulcer of right elbow, stage 3
Pressure ulcer with full thickness skin loss involving damage or necrosis of subcutaneous tissue, right elbow

L89.Ø14 Pressure ulcer of right elbow, stage 4 MCC H4 HCC SW
Healing pressure ulcer of right elbow, stage 4
Pressure ulcer with necrosis of soft tissues through to underlying muscle, tendon, or bone, right elbow

L89.Ø16 Pressure-induced deep tissue damage of right elbow

L89.Ø19 Pressure ulcer of right elbow, unspecified stage
Healing pressure right of elbow NOS
Healing pressure ulcer of right elbow, unspecified stage

✓6th **L89.Ø2 Pressure ulcer of left elbow**

L89.Ø2Ø Pressure ulcer of left elbow, unstageable HCC SW

L89.021 Pressure ulcer of left elbow, stage 1
Healing pressure ulcer of left elbow, stage 1
Pressure pre-ulcer skin changes limited to persistent focal edema, left elbow

L89.022 Pressure ulcer of left elbow, stage 2 HCC
Healing pressure ulcer of left elbow, stage 2
Pressure ulcer with abrasion, blister, partial thickness skin loss involving epidermis and/or dermis, left elbow

L89.023 Pressure ulcer of left elbow, stage 3 MCC H4 HCC SW
Healing pressure ulcer of left elbow, stage 3
Pressure ulcer with full thickness skin loss involving damage or necrosis of subcutaneous tissue, left elbow

L89.024 Pressure ulcer of left elbow, stage 4 MCC H4 HCC SW
Healing pressure ulcer of left elbow, stage 4
Pressure ulcer with necrosis of soft tissues through to underlying muscle, tendon, or bone, left elbow

L89.026 Pressure-induced deep tissue damage of left elbow

L89.029 Pressure ulcer of left elbow, unspecified stage
Healing pressure ulcer of left of elbow NOS
Healing pressure ulcer of left elbow, unspecified stage

✓5th **L89.1 Pressure ulcer of back**

✓6th **L89.10 Pressure ulcer of unspecified part of back**

L89.100 Pressure ulcer of unspecified part of back, unstageable HCC SW

L89.101 Pressure ulcer of unspecified part of back, stage 1
Healing pressure ulcer of unspecified part of back, stage 1
Pressure pre-ulcer skin changes limited to persistent focal edema, unspecified part of back

L89.102 Pressure ulcer of unspecified part of back, stage 2 HCC
Healing pressure ulcer of unspecified part of back, stage 2
Pressure ulcer with abrasion, blister, partial thickness skin loss involving epidermis and/or dermis, unspecified part of back

L89.103 Pressure ulcer of unspecified part of back, stage 3 MCC H4 HCC SW
Healing pressure ulcer of unspecified part of back, stage 3
Pressure ulcer with full thickness skin loss involving damage or necrosis of subcutaneous tissue, unspecified part of back

L89.104 Pressure ulcer of unspecified part of back, stage 4 MCC H4 HCC SW
Healing pressure ulcer of unspecified part of back, stage 4
Pressure ulcer with necrosis of soft tissues through to underlying muscle, tendon, or bone, unspecified part of back

L89.106 Pressure-induced deep tissue damage of unspecified part of back

L89.109 Pressure ulcer of unspecified part of back, unspecified stage
Healing pressure ulcer of unspecified part of back NOS
Healing pressure ulcer of unspecified part of back, unspecified stage

✓6th **L89.11 Pressure ulcer of right upper back**
Pressure ulcer of right shoulder blade

L89.110 Pressure ulcer of right upper back, unstageable HCC SW

L89.111 Pressure ulcer of right upper back, stage 1
Healing pressure ulcer of right upper back, stage 1
Pressure pre-ulcer skin changes limited to persistent focal edema, right upper back

L89.112 Pressure ulcer of right upper back, stage 2 HCC
Healing pressure ulcer of right upper back, stage 2
Pressure ulcer with abrasion, blister, partial thickness skin loss involving epidermis and/or dermis, right upper back

L89.113 Pressure ulcer of right upper back, stage 3 MCC H4 HCC SW
Healing pressure ulcer of right upper back, stage 3
Pressure ulcer with full thickness skin loss involving damage or necrosis of subcutaneous tissue, right upper back

L89.114 Pressure ulcer of right upper back, stage 4 MCC H4 HCC SW
Healing pressure ulcer of right upper back, stage 4
Pressure ulcer with necrosis of soft tissues through to underlying muscle, tendon, or bone, right upper back

L89.116 Pressure-induced deep tissue damage of right upper back

L89.119 Pressure ulcer of right upper back, unspecified stage
Healing pressure ulcer of right upper back NOS
Healing pressure ulcer of right upper back, unspecified stage

✓6th **L89.12 Pressure ulcer of left upper back**
Pressure ulcer of left shoulder blade

L89.120 Pressure ulcer of left upper back, unstageable HCC SW

L89.121 Pressure ulcer of left upper back, stage 1
Healing pressure ulcer of left upper back, stage 1
Pressure pre-ulcer skin changes limited to persistent focal edema, left upper back

L89.122 Pressure ulcer of left upper back, stage 2 HCC
Healing pressure ulcer of left upper back, stage 2
Pressure ulcer with abrasion, blister, partial thickness skin loss involving epidermis and/or dermis, left upper back

L89.123 Pressure ulcer of left upper back, stage 3 MCC H4 HCC SW
Healing pressure ulcer of left upper back, stage 3
Pressure ulcer with full thickness skin loss involving damage or necrosis of subcutaneous tissue, left upper back

L89.124 Pressure ulcer of left upper back, stage 4 MCC H4 HCC SW
Healing pressure ulcer of left upper back, stage 4
Pressure ulcer with necrosis of soft tissues through to underlying muscle, tendon, or bone, left upper back

L89.126 Pressure-induced deep tissue damage of left upper back

L89.129 Pressure ulcer of left upper back, unspecified stage
Healing pressure ulcer of left upper back NOS
Healing pressure ulcer of left upper back, unspecified stage

✓6th **L89.13 Pressure ulcer of right lower back**

L89.130 Pressure ulcer of right lower back, unstageable HCC SW

L89.131 Pressure ulcer of right lower back, stage 1
Healing pressure ulcer of right lower back, stage 1
Pressure pre-ulcer skin changes limited to persistent focal edema, right lower back

L89.132 Pressure ulcer of right lower back, stage 2 HCC
Healing pressure ulcer of right lower back, stage 2
Pressure ulcer with abrasion, blister, partial thickness skin loss involving epidermis and/or dermis, right lower back

L89.133 Pressure ulcer of right lower back, stage 3 MCC H4 HCC SW
Healing pressure ulcer of right lower back, stage 3
Pressure ulcer with full thickness skin loss involving damage or necrosis of subcutaneous tissue, right lower back

L89.134 Pressure ulcer of right lower back, stage 4 MCC H4 HCC SW
Healing pressure ulcer of right lower back, stage 4
Pressure ulcer with necrosis of soft tissues through to underlying muscle, tendon, or bone, right lower back

L89.136 Pressure-induced deep tissue damage of right lower back

L89.139 Pressure ulcer of right lower back, unspecified stage
Healing pressure ulcer of right lower back NOS
Healing pressure ulcer of right lower back, unspecified stage

✓6th **L89.14 Pressure ulcer of left lower back**

L89.140 Pressure ulcer of left lower back, unstageable HCC SW

L89.141 Pressure ulcer of left lower back, stage 1
Healing pressure ulcer of left lower back, stage 1
Pressure pre-ulcer skin changes limited to persistent focal edema, left lower back

L89.142 Pressure ulcer of left lower back, stage 2 HCC
Healing pressure ulcer of left lower back, stage 2
Pressure ulcer with abrasion, blister, partial thickness skin loss involving epidermis and/or dermis, left lower back

L89.143 Pressure ulcer of left lower back, stage 3 MCC H4 HCC SW
Healing pressure ulcer of left lower back, stage 3
Pressure ulcer with full thickness skin loss involving damage or necrosis of subcutaneous tissue, left lower back

L89.144 Pressure ulcer of left lower back, stage 4 MCC H4 HCC SW
Healing pressure ulcer of left lower back, stage 4
Pressure ulcer with necrosis of soft tissues through to underlying muscle, tendon, or bone, left lower back

L89.146 Pressure-induced deep tissue damage of left lower back

L89.149 Pressure ulcer of left lower back, unspecified stage
Healing pressure ulcer of left lower back NOS
Healing pressure ulcer of left lower back, unspecified stage

✓6th **L89.15 Pressure ulcer of sacral region**
Pressure ulcer of coccyx
Pressure ulcer of tailbone

L89.150 Pressure ulcer of sacral region, unstageable HCC SW

L89.151 Pressure ulcer of sacral region, stage 1
Healing pressure ulcer of sacral region, stage 1
Pressure pre-ulcer skin changes limited to persistent focal edema, sacral region

L89.152 Pressure ulcer of sacral region, stage 2 HCC
Healing pressure ulcer of sacral region, stage 2
Pressure ulcer with abrasion, blister, partial thickness skin loss involving epidermis and/or dermis, sacral region

L89.153 Pressure ulcer of sacral region, stage 3 MCC H4 HCC SW
Healing pressure ulcer of sacral region, stage 3
Pressure ulcer with full thickness skin loss involving damage or necrosis of subcutaneous tissue, sacral region

L89.154 Pressure ulcer of sacral region, stage 4 MCC H4 HCC SW
Healing pressure ulcer of sacral region, stage 4
Pressure ulcer with necrosis of soft tissues through to underlying muscle, tendon, or bone, sacral region

L89.156 Pressure-induced deep tissue damage of sacral region

L89.159 Pressure ulcer of sacral region, unspecified stage
Healing pressure ulcer of sacral region NOS
Healing pressure ulcer of sacral region, unspecified stage

✓5th **L89.2 Pressure ulcer of hip**

✓6th **L89.20 Pressure ulcer of unspecified hip**

L89.200 Pressure ulcer of unspecified hip, unstageable HCC SW

L89.201 Pressure ulcer of unspecified hip, stage 1
Healing pressure ulcer of unspecified hip back, stage 1
Pressure pre-ulcer skin changes limited to persistent focal edema, unspecified hip

L89.202 Pressure ulcer of unspecified hip, stage 2 HCC
Healing pressure ulcer of unspecified hip, stage 2
Pressure ulcer with abrasion, blister, partial thickness skin loss involving epidermis and/or dermis, unspecified hip

L89.203 Pressure ulcer of unspecified hip, stage 3 MCC H4 HCC SW
Healing pressure ulcer of unspecified hip, stage 3
Pressure ulcer with full thickness skin loss involving damage or necrosis of subcutaneous tissue, unspecified hip

L89.204 Pressure ulcer of unspecified hip, stage 4 MCC H4 HCC SW
Healing pressure ulcer of unspecified hip, stage 4
Pressure ulcer with necrosis of soft tissues through to underlying muscle, tendon, or bone, unspecified hip

L89.206 **Pressure-induced deep tissue damage of unspecified hip**

L89.209 **Pressure ulcer of unspecified hip, unspecified stage**
Healing pressure ulcer of unspecified hip NOS
Healing pressure ulcer of unspecified hip, unspecified stage

✓6th L89.21 **Pressure ulcer of right hip**

L89.210 **Pressure ulcer of right hip, unstageable** HCC SW

L89.211 **Pressure ulcer of right hip, stage 1**
Healing pressure ulcer of right hip back, stage 1
Pressure pre-ulcer skin changes limited to persistent focal edema, right hip

L89.212 **Pressure ulcer of right hip, stage 2** HCC
Healing pressure ulcer of right hip, stage 2
Pressure ulcer with abrasion, blister, partial thickness skin loss involving epidermis and/or dermis, right hip

L89.213 **Pressure ulcer of right hip, stage 3** MCC H4 HCC SW
Healing pressure ulcer of right hip, stage 3
Pressure ulcer with full thickness skin loss involving damage or necrosis of subcutaneous tissue, right hip

L89.214 **Pressure ulcer of right hip, stage 4** MCC H4 HCC SW
Healing pressure ulcer of right hip, stage 4
Pressure ulcer with necrosis of soft tissues through to underlying muscle, tendon, or bone, right hip

L89.216 **Pressure-induced deep tissue damage of right hip**

L89.219 **Pressure ulcer of right hip, unspecified stage**
Healing pressure ulcer of right hip NOS
Healing pressure ulcer of right hip, unspecified stage

✓6th L89.22 **Pressure ulcer of left hip**

L89.220 **Pressure ulcer of left hip, unstageable** HCC SW

L89.221 **Pressure ulcer of left hip, stage 1**
Healing pressure ulcer of left hip back, stage 1
Pressure pre-ulcer skin changes limited to persistent focal edema, left hip

L89.222 **Pressure ulcer of left hip, stage 2** HCC
Healing pressure ulcer of left hip, stage 2
Pressure ulcer with abrasion, blister, partial thickness skin loss involving epidermis and/or dermis, left hip

L89.223 **Pressure ulcer of left hip, stage 3** MCC H4 HCC SW
Healing pressure ulcer of left hip, stage 3
Pressure ulcer with full thickness skin loss involving damage or necrosis of subcutaneous tissue, left hip

L89.224 **Pressure ulcer of left hip, stage 4** MCC H4 HCC SW
Healing pressure ulcer of left hip, stage 4
Pressure ulcer with necrosis of soft tissues through to underlying muscle, tendon, or bone, left hip

L89.226 **Pressure-induced deep tissue damage of left hip**

L89.229 **Pressure ulcer of left hip, unspecified stage**
Healing pressure ulcer of left hip NOS
Healing pressure ulcer of left hip, unspecified stage

✓5th L89.3 **Pressure ulcer of buttock**

✓6th L89.30 **Pressure ulcer of unspecified buttock**

L89.300 **Pressure ulcer of unspecified buttock, unstageable** HCC SW

L89.301 **Pressure ulcer of unspecified buttock, stage 1**
Healing pressure ulcer of unspecified buttock, stage 1
Pressure pre-ulcer skin changes limited to persistent focal edema, unspecified buttock

L89.302 **Pressure ulcer of unspecified buttock, stage 2** HCC
Healing pressure ulcer of unspecified buttock, stage 2
Pressure ulcer with abrasion, blister, partial thickness skin loss involving epidermis and/or dermis, unspecified buttock

L89.303 **Pressure ulcer of unspecified buttock, stage 3** MCC H4 HCC SW
Healing pressure ulcer of unspecified buttock, stage 3
Pressure ulcer with full thickness skin loss involving damage or necrosis of subcutaneous tissue, unspecified buttock

L89.304 **Pressure ulcer of unspecified buttock, stage 4** MCC H4 HCC SW
Healing pressure ulcer of unspecified buttock, stage 4
Pressure ulcer with necrosis of soft tissues through to underlying muscle, tendon, or bone, unspecified buttock

L89.306 **Pressure-induced deep tissue damage of unspecified buttock**

L89.309 **Pressure ulcer of unspecified buttock, unspecified stage**
Healing pressure ulcer of unspecified buttock NOS
Healing pressure ulcer of unspecified buttock, unspecified stage

✓6th L89.31 **Pressure ulcer of right buttock**

L89.310 **Pressure ulcer of right buttock, unstageable** HCC SW

L89.311 **Pressure ulcer of right buttock, stage 1**
Healing pressure ulcer of right buttock, stage 1
Pressure pre-ulcer skin changes limited to persistent focal edema, right buttock

L89.312 **Pressure ulcer of right buttock, stage 2** HCC
Healing pressure ulcer of right buttock, stage 2
Pressure ulcer with abrasion, blister, partial thickness skin loss involving epidermis and/or dermis, right buttock

L89.313 **Pressure ulcer of right buttock, stage 3** MCC H4 HCC SW
Healing pressure ulcer of right buttock, stage 3
Pressure ulcer with full thickness skin loss involving damage or necrosis of subcutaneous tissue, right buttock

L89.314 **Pressure ulcer of right buttock, stage 4** MCC H4 HCC SW
Healing pressure ulcer of right buttock, stage 4
Pressure ulcer with necrosis of soft tissues through to underlying muscle, tendon, or bone, right buttock

L89.316 **Pressure-induced deep tissue damage of right buttock**

L89.319 **Pressure ulcer of right buttock, unspecified stage**
Healing pressure ulcer of right buttock NOS
Healing pressure ulcer of right buttock, unspecified stage

✓6th L89.32 **Pressure ulcer of left buttock**

L89.320 **Pressure ulcer of left buttock, unstageable** HCC SW

L89.321 Pressure ulcer of left buttock, stage 1
Healing pressure ulcer of left buttock, stage 1
Pressure pre-ulcer skin changes limited to persistent focal edema, left buttock

L89.322 Pressure ulcer of left buttock, stage 2 HCC
Healing pressure ulcer of left buttock, stage 2
Pressure ulcer with abrasion, blister, partial thickness skin loss involving epidermis and/or dermis, left buttock

L89.323 Pressure ulcer of left buttock, stage 3 MCC H4 HCC SW
Healing pressure ulcer of left buttock, stage 3
Pressure ulcer with full thickness skin loss involving damage or necrosis of subcutaneous tissue, left buttock

L89.324 Pressure ulcer of left buttock, stage 4 MCC H4 HCC SW
Healing pressure ulcer of left buttock, stage 4
Pressure ulcer with necrosis of soft tissues through to underlying muscle, tendon, or bone, left buttock

L89.326 Pressure-induced deep tissue damage of left buttock

L89.329 Pressure ulcer of left buttock, unspecified stage
Healing pressure ulcer of left buttock NOS
Healing pressure ulcer of left buttock, unspecified stage

✓5th **L89.4 Pressure ulcer of contiguous site of back, buttock and hip**

L89.4Ø Pressure ulcer of contiguous site of back, buttock and hip, unspecified stage
Healing pressure ulcer of contiguous site of back, buttock and hip NOS
Healing pressure ulcer of contiguous site of back, buttock and hip, unspecified stage

L89.41 Pressure ulcer of contiguous site of back, buttock and hip, stage 1
Healing pressure ulcer of contiguous site of back, buttock and hip, stage 1
Pressure pre-ulcer skin changes limited to persistent focal edema, contiguous site of back, buttock and hip

L89.42 Pressure ulcer of contiguous site of back, buttock and hip, stage 2 HCC
Healing pressure ulcer of contiguous site of back, buttock and hip, stage 2
Pressure ulcer with abrasion, blister, partial thickness skin loss involving epidermis and/or dermis, contiguous site of back, buttock and hip

L89.43 Pressure ulcer of contiguous site of back, buttock and hip, stage 3 MCC H4 HCC SW
Healing pressure ulcer of contiguous site of back, buttock and hip, stage 3
Pressure ulcer with full thickness skin loss involving damage or necrosis of subcutaneous tissue, contiguous site of back, buttock and hip

L89.44 Pressure ulcer of contiguous site of back, buttock and hip, stage 4 MCC H4 HCC SW
Healing pressure ulcer of contiguous site of back, buttock and hip, stage 4
Pressure ulcer with necrosis of soft tissues through to underlying muscle, tendon, or bone, contiguous site of back, buttock and hip

L89.45 Pressure ulcer of contiguous site of back, buttock and hip, unstageable HCC SW

L89.46 Pressure-induced deep tissue damage of contiguous site of back, buttock and hip

✓5th **L89.5 Pressure ulcer of ankle**

✓6th **L89.5Ø Pressure ulcer of unspecified ankle**

L89.5ØØ Pressure ulcer of unspecified ankle, unstageable HCC SW

L89.5Ø1 Pressure ulcer of unspecified ankle, stage 1
Healing pressure ulcer of unspecified ankle, stage 1
Pressure pre-ulcer skin changes limited to persistent focal edema, unspecified ankle

L89.5Ø2 Pressure ulcer of unspecified ankle, stage 2 HCC
Healing pressure ulcer of unspecified ankle, stage 2
Pressure ulcer with abrasion, blister, partial thickness skin loss involving epidermis and/or dermis, unspecified ankle

L89.5Ø3 Pressure ulcer of unspecified ankle, stage 3 MCC H4 HCC SW
Healing pressure ulcer of unspecified ankle, stage 3
Pressure ulcer with full thickness skin loss involving damage or necrosis of subcutaneous tissue, unspecified ankle

L89.5Ø4 Pressure ulcer of unspecified ankle, stage 4 MCC H4 HCC SW
Healing pressure ulcer of unspecified ankle, stage 4
Pressure ulcer with necrosis of soft tissues through to underlying muscle, tendon, or bone, unspecified ankle

L89.5Ø6 Pressure-induced deep tissue damage of unspecified ankle

L89.5Ø9 Pressure ulcer of unspecified ankle, unspecified stage
Healing pressure ulcer of unspecified ankle NOS
Healing pressure ulcer of unspecified ankle, unspecified stage

✓6th **L89.51 Pressure ulcer of right ankle**

L89.51Ø Pressure ulcer of right ankle, unstageable HCC SW

L89.511 Pressure ulcer of right ankle, stage 1
Healing pressure ulcer of right ankle, stage 1
Pressure pre-ulcer skin changes limited to persistent focal edema, right ankle

L89.512 Pressure ulcer of right ankle, stage 2 HCC
Healing pressure ulcer of right ankle, stage 2
Pressure ulcer with abrasion, blister, partial thickness skin loss involving epidermis and/or dermis, right ankle

L89.513 Pressure ulcer of right ankle, stage 3 MCC H4 HCC SW
Healing pressure ulcer of right ankle, stage 3
Pressure ulcer with full thickness skin loss involving damage or necrosis of subcutaneous tissue, right ankle

L89.514 Pressure ulcer of right ankle, stage 4 MCC H4 HCC SW
Healing pressure ulcer of right ankle, stage 4
Pressure ulcer with necrosis of soft tissues through to underlying muscle, tendon, or bone, right ankle

L89.516 Pressure-induced deep tissue damage of right ankle

L89.519 Pressure ulcer of right ankle, unspecified stage
Healing pressure ulcer of right ankle NOS
Healing pressure ulcer of right ankle, unspecified stage

✓6th **L89.52 Pressure ulcer of left ankle**

L89.52Ø Pressure ulcer of left ankle, unstageable HCC SW

L89.521 Pressure ulcer of left ankle, stage 1
Healing pressure ulcer of left ankle, stage 1
Pressure pre-ulcer skin changes limited to persistent focal edema, left ankle

L89.522 Pressure ulcer of left ankle, stage 2 HCC
Healing pressure ulcer of left ankle, stage 2
Pressure ulcer with abrasion, blister, partial thickness skin loss involving epidermis and/or dermis, left ankle

L89.523 Pressure ulcer of left ankle, stage 3 MCC H4 HCC SW
Healing pressure ulcer of left ankle, stage 3
Pressure ulcer with full thickness skin loss involving damage or necrosis of subcutaneous tissue, left ankle

L89.524 Pressure ulcer of left ankle, stage 4 MCC H4 HCC SW
Healing pressure ulcer of left ankle, stage 4
Pressure ulcer with necrosis of soft tissues through to underlying muscle, tendon, or bone, left ankle

L89.526 Pressure-induced deep tissue damage of left ankle

L89.529 Pressure ulcer of left ankle, unspecified stage
Healing pressure ulcer of left ankle NOS
Healing pressure ulcer of left ankle, unspecified stage

✓5th **L89.6 Pressure ulcer of heel**

✓6th **L89.60 Pressure ulcer of unspecified heel**

L89.600 Pressure ulcer of unspecified heel, unstageable HCC SW

L89.601 Pressure ulcer of unspecified heel, stage 1
Healing pressure ulcer of unspecified heel, stage 1
Pressure pre-ulcer skin changes limited to persistent focal edema, unspecified heel

L89.602 Pressure ulcer of unspecified heel, stage 2 HCC
Healing pressure ulcer of unspecified heel, stage 2
Pressure ulcer with abrasion, blister, partial thickness skin loss involving epidermis and/or dermis, unspecified heel

L89.603 Pressure ulcer of unspecified heel, stage 3 MCC H4 HCC SW
Healing pressure ulcer of unspecified heel, stage 3
Pressure ulcer with full thickness skin loss involving damage or necrosis of subcutaneous tissue, unspecified heel

L89.604 Pressure ulcer of unspecified heel, stage 4 MCC H4 HCC SW
Healing pressure ulcer of unspecified heel, stage 4
Pressure ulcer with necrosis of soft tissues through to underlying muscle, tendon, or bone, unspecified heel

L89.606 Pressure-induced deep tissue damage of unspecified heel

L89.609 Pressure ulcer of unspecified heel, unspecified stage
Healing pressure ulcer of unspecified heel NOS
Healing pressure ulcer of unspecified heel, unspecified stage

✓6th **L89.61 Pressure ulcer of right heel**

L89.610 Pressure ulcer of right heel, unstageable HCC SW

L89.611 Pressure ulcer of right heel, stage 1
Healing pressure ulcer of right heel, stage 1
Pressure pre-ulcer skin changes limited to persistent focal edema, right heel

L89.612 Pressure ulcer of right heel, stage 2 HCC
Healing pressure ulcer of right heel, stage 2
Pressure ulcer with abrasion, blister, partial thickness skin loss involving epidermis and/or dermis, right heel

L89.613 Pressure ulcer of right heel, stage 3 MCC H4 HCC SW
Healing pressure ulcer of right heel, stage 3
Pressure ulcer with full thickness skin loss involving damage or necrosis of subcutaneous tissue, right heel

L89.614 Pressure ulcer of right heel, stage 4 MCC H4 HCC SW
Healing pressure ulcer of right heel, stage 4
Pressure ulcer with necrosis of soft tissues through to underlying muscle, tendon, or bone, right heel

L89.616 Pressure-induced deep tissue damage of right heel

L89.619 Pressure ulcer of right heel, unspecified stage
Healing pressure ulcer of right heel NOS
Healing pressure ulcer of right heel, unspecified stage

✓6th **L89.62 Pressure ulcer of left heel**

L89.620 Pressure ulcer of left heel, unstageable HCC SW

L89.621 Pressure ulcer of left heel, stage 1
Healing pressure ulcer of left heel, stage 1
Pressure pre-ulcer skin changes limited to persistent focal edema, left heel

L89.622 Pressure ulcer of left heel, stage 2 HCC
Healing pressure ulcer of left heel, stage 2
Pressure ulcer with abrasion, blister, partial thickness skin loss involving epidermis and/or dermis, left heel

L89.623 Pressure ulcer of left heel, stage 3 MCC H4 HCC SW
Healing pressure ulcer of left heel, stage 3
Pressure ulcer with full thickness skin loss involving damage or necrosis of subcutaneous tissue, left heel

L89.624 Pressure ulcer of left heel, stage 4 MCC H4 HCC SW
Healing pressure ulcer of left heel, stage 4
Pressure ulcer with necrosis of soft tissues through to underlying muscle, tendon, or bone, left heel

L89.626 Pressure-induced deep tissue damage of left heel

L89.629 Pressure ulcer of left heel, unspecified stage
Healing pressure ulcer of left heel NOS
Healing pressure ulcer of left heel, unspecified stage

✓5th **L89.8 Pressure ulcer of other site**

✓6th **L89.81 Pressure ulcer of head**
Pressure ulcer of face

L89.810 Pressure ulcer of head, unstageable HCC SW

L89.811 Pressure ulcer of head, stage 1
Healing pressure ulcer of head, stage 1
Pressure pre-ulcer skin changes limited to persistent focal edema, head

L89.812 Pressure ulcer of head, stage 2 HCC
Healing pressure ulcer of head, stage 2
Pressure ulcer with abrasion, blister, partial thickness skin loss involving epidermis and/or dermis, head

L89.813 Pressure ulcer of head, stage 3 MCC H4 HCC SW
Healing pressure ulcer of head, stage 3
Pressure ulcer with full thickness skin loss involving damage or necrosis of subcutaneous tissue, head

L89.814 **Pressure ulcer of head, stage 4** MCC H4 HCC SW
Healing pressure ulcer of head, stage 4
Pressure ulcer with necrosis of soft tissues through to underlying muscle, tendon, or bone, head

L89.816 **Pressure-induced deep tissue damage of head**

L89.819 **Pressure ulcer of head, unspecified stage**
Healing pressure ulcer of head NOS
Healing pressure ulcer of head, unspecified stage

6th L89.89 **Pressure ulcer of other site**

L89.890 **Pressure ulcer of other site, unstageable** HCC SW

L89.891 **Pressure ulcer of other site, stage 1**
Healing pressure ulcer of other site, stage 1
Pressure pre-ulcer skin changes limited to persistent focal edema, other site

L89.892 **Pressure ulcer of other site, stage 2** HCC
Healing pressure ulcer of other site, stage 2
Pressure ulcer with abrasion, blister, partial thickness skin loss involving epidermis and/or dermis, other site

L89.893 **Pressure ulcer of other site, stage 3** MCC H4 HCC SW
Healing pressure ulcer of other site, stage 3
Pressure ulcer with full thickness skin loss involving damage or necrosis of subcutaneous tissue, other site

L89.894 **Pressure ulcer of other site, stage 4** MCC H4 HCC SW
Healing pressure ulcer of other site, stage 4
Pressure ulcer with necrosis of soft tissues through to underlying muscle, tendon, or bone, other site

L89.896 **Pressure-induced deep tissue damage of other site**

L89.899 **Pressure ulcer of other site, unspecified stage**
Healing pressure ulcer of other site NOS
Healing pressure ulcer of other site, unspecified stage

5th L89.9 **Pressure ulcer of unspecified site**

L89.90 **Pressure ulcer of unspecified site, unspecified stage**
Healing pressure ulcer of unspecified site NOS
Healing pressure ulcer of unspecified site, unspecified stage

L89.91 **Pressure ulcer of unspecified site, stage 1**
Healing pressure ulcer of unspecified site, stage 1
Pressure pre-ulcer skin changes limited to persistent focal edema, unspecified site

L89.92 **Pressure ulcer of unspecified site, stage 2** HCC
Healing pressure ulcer of unspecified site, stage 2
Pressure ulcer with abrasion, blister, partial thickness skin loss involving epidermis and/or dermis, unspecified site

L89.93 **Pressure ulcer of unspecified site, stage 3** MCC H4 HCC SW
Healing pressure ulcer of unspecified site, stage 3
Pressure ulcer with full thickness skin loss involving damage or necrosis of subcutaneous tissue, unspecified site

L89.94 **Pressure ulcer of unspecified site, stage 4** MCC H4 HCC SW
Healing pressure ulcer of unspecified site, stage 4
Pressure ulcer with necrosis of soft tissues through to underlying muscle, tendon, or bone, unspecified site

L89.95 **Pressure ulcer of unspecified site, unstageable** HCC SW

L89.96 **Pressure-induced deep tissue damage of unspecified site**

4th L90 **Atrophic disorders of skin**

L90.0 **Lichen sclerosus et atrophicus**
EXCLUDES 2 *lichen sclerosus of external female genital organs (N90.4)*
lichen sclerosus of external male genital organs (N48.0)

L90.1 **Anetoderma of Schweninger-Buzzi**

L90.2 **Anetoderma of Jadassohn-Pellizzari**

L90.3 **Atrophoderma of Pasini and Pierini**

L90.4 **Acrodermatitis chronica atrophicans**

L90.5 **Scar conditions and fibrosis of skin**
Adherent scar (skin)
Cicatrix
Disfigurement of skin due to scar
Fibrosis of skin NOS
Scar NOS
EXCLUDES 2 *hypertrophic scar (L91.0)*
keloid scar (L91.0)
AHA: 2016,2Q,5; 2015,1Q,19

L90.6 **Striae atrophicae**

L90.8 **Other atrophic disorders of skin**

L90.9 **Atrophic disorder of skin, unspecified**

4th L91 **Hypertrophic disorders of skin**

L91.0 **Hypertrophic scar**
Keloid
Keloid scar
EXCLUDES 2 *acne keloid (L73.0)*
scar NOS (L90.5)
DEF: Overgrowth of scar tissue due to excess amounts of collagen during connective tissue repair, occurring mainly on the upper trunk and face.

L91.8 **Other hypertrophic disorders of the skin**

L91.9 **Hypertrophic disorder of the skin, unspecified**

4th L92 **Granulomatous disorders of skin and subcutaneous tissue**
EXCLUDES 2 *actinic granuloma (L57.5)*

L92.0 **Granuloma annulare**
Perforating granuloma annulare

L92.1 **Necrobiosis lipoidica, not elsewhere classified**
EXCLUDES 1 *necrobiosis lipoidica associated with diabetes mellitus (E08-E13 with .620)*

L92.2 **Granuloma faciale [eosinophilic granuloma of skin]**

L92.3 **Foreign body granuloma of the skin and subcutaneous tissue**
Use additional code to identify the type of retained foreign body (Z18.-)

L92.8 **Other granulomatous disorders of the skin and subcutaneous tissue**

L92.9 **Granulomatous disorder of the skin and subcutaneous tissue, unspecified**
EXCLUDES 2 *umbilical granuloma (P83.81)*
AHA: 2017,4Q,21-22

4th L93 **Lupus erythematosus**
Use additional code for adverse effect, if applicable, to identify drug (T36-T50 with fifth or sixth character 5)
EXCLUDES 1 *lupus exedens (A18.4)*
lupus vulgaris (A18.4)
scleroderma (M34.-)
systemic lupus erythematosus (M32.-)
DEF: Inflammatory, autoimmune skin condition in which the body's autoimmune system attacks healthy tissue of the integumentary system.

L93.0 **Discoid lupus erythematosus**
Lupus erythematosus NOS

L93.1 **Subacute cutaneous lupus erythematosus**

L93.2 **Other local lupus erythematosus**
Lupus erythematosus profundus
Lupus panniculitis

4th L94 **Other localized connective tissue disorders**
EXCLUDES 1 *systemic connective tissue disorders (M30-M36)*

L94.0 **Localized scleroderma [morphea]**
Circumscribed scleroderma

L94.1 **Linear scleroderma**
En coup de sabre lesion

L94.2 **Calcinosis cutis**

L94.3 **Sclerodactyly**

L94.4 **Gottron's papules**

L94.5 **Poikiloderma vasculare atrophicans**

L94.6 Ainhum

L94.8 Other specified localized connective tissue disorders

L94.9 Localized connective tissue disorder, unspecified

✓4th L95 Vasculitis limited to skin, not elsewhere classified

EXCLUDES 1 *angioma serpiginosum (L81.7)*
Henoch(-Schönlein) purpura (D69.Ø)
hypersensitivity angiitis (M31.Ø)
lupus panniculitis (L93.2)
panniculitis NOS (M79.3)
panniculitis of neck and back (M54.Ø-)
polyarteritis nodosa (M3Ø.Ø)
relapsing panniculitis (M35.6)
rheumatoid vasculitis (MØ5.2)
serum sickness (T8Ø.6-)
urticaria (L5Ø.-)
Wegener's granulomatosis (M31.3-)

L95.Ø Livedoid vasculitis

Atrophie blanche (en plaque)

L95.1 Erythema elevatum diutinum

L95.8 Other vasculitis limited to the skin

L95.9 Vasculitis limited to the skin, unspecified

✓4th L97 Non-pressure chronic ulcer of lower limb, not elsewhere classified

INCLUDES chronic ulcer of skin of lower limb NOS
non-healing ulcer of skin
non-infected sinus of skin
trophic ulcer NOS
tropical ulcer NOS
ulcer of skin of lower limb NOS

Code first any associated underlying condition, such as:
any associated gangrene (I96)
atherosclerosis of the lower extremities (I7Ø.23-, I7Ø.24-, I7Ø.33-, I7Ø.34-, I7Ø.43-, I7Ø.44-, I7Ø.53-, I7Ø.54-, I7Ø.63-, I7Ø.64-, I7Ø.73-, I7Ø.74-)
chronic venous hypertension (I87.31-, I87.33-)
diabetic ulcers (EØ8.621, EØ8.622, EØ9.621, EØ9.622, E1Ø.621, E1Ø.622, E11.621, E11.622, E13.621, E13.622)
postphlebitic syndrome (I87.Ø1-, I87.Ø3-)
postthrombotic syndrome (I87.Ø1-, I87.Ø3-)
varicose ulcer (I83.Ø-, I83.2-)

EXCLUDES 2 *pressure ulcer (pressure area) (L89.-)*
skin infections (LØØ-LØ8)
specific infections classified to AØØ-B99

AHA: 2020,2Q,19; 2018,4Q,69; 2017,4Q,17

TIP: The depth and/or severity of a diagnosed nonpressure ulcer can be determined based on medical record documentation from clinicians who are not the patient's provider.

TIP: Assign a code from this category/subcategory for nonpressure ulcers documented as acute.

✓5th L97.1 Non-pressure chronic ulcer of thigh

✓6th L97.1Ø Non-pressure chronic ulcer of unspecified thigh

L97.1Ø1 Non-pressure chronic ulcer of unspecified thigh limited to breakdown of skin CC HCC

L97.1Ø2 Non-pressure chronic ulcer of unspecified thigh with fat layer exposed CC HCC SW

L97.1Ø3 Non-pressure chronic ulcer of unspecified thigh with necrosis of muscle CC HCC SW

L97.1Ø4 Non-pressure chronic ulcer of unspecified thigh with necrosis of bone CC HCC SW

L97.1Ø5 Non-pressure chronic ulcer of unspecified thigh with muscle involvement without evidence of necrosis CC HCC

L97.1Ø6 Non-pressure chronic ulcer of unspecified thigh with bone involvement without evidence of necrosis CC HCC

L97.1Ø8 Non-pressure chronic ulcer of unspecified thigh with other specified severity CC HCC

L97.1Ø9 Non-pressure chronic ulcer of unspecified thigh with unspecified severity CC HCC

✓6th L97.11 Non-pressure chronic ulcer of right thigh

L97.111 Non-pressure chronic ulcer of right thigh limited to breakdown of skin CC HCC

L97.112 Non-pressure chronic ulcer of right thigh with fat layer exposed CC HCC SW

L97.113 Non-pressure chronic ulcer of right thigh with necrosis of muscle CC HCC SW

L97.114 Non-pressure chronic ulcer of right thigh with necrosis of bone CC HCC SW

L97.115 Non-pressure chronic ulcer of right thigh with muscle involvement without evidence of necrosis CC HCC

L97.116 Non-pressure chronic ulcer of right thigh with bone involvement without evidence of necrosis CC HCC

L97.118 Non-pressure chronic ulcer of right thigh with other specified severity CC HCC

L97.119 Non-pressure chronic ulcer of right thigh with unspecified severity CC HCC

✓6th L97.12 Non-pressure chronic ulcer of left thigh

L97.121 Non-pressure chronic ulcer of left thigh limited to breakdown of skin CC HCC

L97.122 Non-pressure chronic ulcer of left thigh with fat layer exposed CC HCC SW

L97.123 Non-pressure chronic ulcer of left thigh with necrosis of muscle CC HCC SW

L97.124 Non-pressure chronic ulcer of left thigh with necrosis of bone CC HCC SW

L97.125 Non-pressure chronic ulcer of left thigh with muscle involvement without evidence of necrosis CC HCC

L97.126 Non-pressure chronic ulcer of left thigh with bone involvement without evidence of necrosis CC HCC

L97.128 Non-pressure chronic ulcer of left thigh with other specified severity CC HCC

L97.129 Non-pressure chronic ulcer of left thigh with unspecified severity CC HCC

✓5th L97.2 Non-pressure chronic ulcer of calf

✓6th L97.2Ø Non-pressure chronic ulcer of unspecified calf

L97.2Ø1 Non-pressure chronic ulcer of unspecified calf limited to breakdown of skin CC HCC

L97.2Ø2 Non-pressure chronic ulcer of unspecified calf with fat layer exposed CC HCC SW

L97.2Ø3 Non-pressure chronic ulcer of unspecified calf with necrosis of muscle CC HCC SW

L97.2Ø4 Non-pressure chronic ulcer of unspecified calf with necrosis of bone CC HCC SW

L97.2Ø5 Non-pressure chronic ulcer of unspecified calf with muscle involvement without evidence of necrosis CC HCC

L97.2Ø6 Non-pressure chronic ulcer of unspecified calf with bone involvement without evidence of necrosis CC HCC

L97.2Ø8 Non-pressure chronic ulcer of unspecified calf with other specified severity CC HCC

L97.2Ø9 Non-pressure chronic ulcer of unspecified calf with unspecified severity CC HCC

✓6th L97.21 Non-pressure chronic ulcer of right calf

L97.211 Non-pressure chronic ulcer of right calf limited to breakdown of skin CC HCC

L97.212 Non-pressure chronic ulcer of right calf with fat layer exposed CC HCC SW

L97.213 Non-pressure chronic ulcer of right calf with necrosis of muscle CC HCC SW

L97.214 Non-pressure chronic ulcer of right calf with necrosis of bone CC HCC SW

L97.215 Non-pressure chronic ulcer of right calf with muscle involvement without evidence of necrosis CC HCC

L97.216 Non-pressure chronic ulcer of right calf with bone involvement without evidence of necrosis CC HCC

L97.218 Non-pressure chronic ulcer of right calf with other specified severity CC HCC

L97.219 Non-pressure chronic ulcer of right calf with unspecified severity CC HCC

✓6th L97.22 Non-pressure chronic ulcer of left calf

L97.221 Non-pressure chronic ulcer of left calf limited to breakdown of skin CC HCC

L97.222 Non-pressure chronic ulcer of left calf with fat layer exposed CC HCC SW

L97.223 Non-pressure chronic ulcer of left calf with necrosis of muscle CC HCC SW
L97.224 Non-pressure chronic ulcer of left calf with necrosis of bone CC HCC SW
L97.225 Non-pressure chronic ulcer of left calf with muscle involvement without evidence of necrosis CC HCC
L97.226 Non-pressure chronic ulcer of left calf with bone involvement without evidence of necrosis CC HCC
L97.228 Non-pressure chronic ulcer of left calf with other specified severity CC HCC
L97.229 Non-pressure chronic ulcer of left calf with unspecified severity CC HCC

5th L97.3 Non-pressure chronic ulcer of ankle

6th L97.30 Non-pressure chronic ulcer of unspecified ankle
L97.301 Non-pressure chronic ulcer of unspecified ankle limited to breakdown of skin CC HCC
L97.302 Non-pressure chronic ulcer of unspecified ankle with fat layer exposed CC HCC SW
L97.303 Non-pressure chronic ulcer of unspecified ankle with necrosis of muscle CC HCC SW
L97.304 Non-pressure chronic ulcer of unspecified ankle with necrosis of bone CC HCC SW
L97.305 Non-pressure chronic ulcer of unspecified ankle with muscle involvement without evidence of necrosis CC HCC
L97.306 Non-pressure chronic ulcer of unspecified ankle with bone involvement without evidence of necrosis CC HCC
L97.308 Non-pressure chronic ulcer of unspecified ankle with other specified severity CC HCC
L97.309 Non-pressure chronic ulcer of unspecified ankle with unspecified severity CC HCC

6th L97.31 Non-pressure chronic ulcer of right ankle
L97.311 Non-pressure chronic ulcer of right ankle limited to breakdown of skin CC HCC
L97.312 Non-pressure chronic ulcer of right ankle with fat layer exposed CC HCC SW
L97.313 Non-pressure chronic ulcer of right ankle with necrosis of muscle CC HCC SW
L97.314 Non-pressure chronic ulcer of right ankle with necrosis of bone CC HCC SW
L97.315 Non-pressure chronic ulcer of right ankle with muscle involvement without evidence of necrosis CC HCC
L97.316 Non-pressure chronic ulcer of right ankle with bone involvement without evidence of necrosis CC HCC
L97.318 Non-pressure chronic ulcer of right ankle with other specified severity CC HCC
L97.319 Non-pressure chronic ulcer of right ankle with unspecified severity CC HCC

6th L97.32 Non-pressure chronic ulcer of left ankle
L97.321 Non-pressure chronic ulcer of left ankle limited to breakdown of skin CC HCC
L97.322 Non-pressure chronic ulcer of left ankle with fat layer exposed CC HCC SW
L97.323 Non-pressure chronic ulcer of left ankle with necrosis of muscle CC HCC SW
L97.324 Non-pressure chronic ulcer of left ankle with necrosis of bone CC HCC SW
L97.325 Non-pressure chronic ulcer of left ankle with muscle involvement without evidence of necrosis CC HCC
L97.326 Non-pressure chronic ulcer of left ankle with bone involvement without evidence of necrosis CC HCC
L97.328 Non-pressure chronic ulcer of left ankle with other specified severity CC HCC
L97.329 Non-pressure chronic ulcer of left ankle with unspecified severity CC HCC

5th L97.4 Non-pressure chronic ulcer of heel and midfoot
Non-pressure chronic ulcer of plantar surface of midfoot

6th L97.40 Non-pressure chronic ulcer of unspecified heel and midfoot
L97.401 Non-pressure chronic ulcer of unspecified heel and midfoot limited to breakdown of skin CC HCC
L97.402 Non-pressure chronic ulcer of unspecified heel and midfoot with fat layer exposed CC HCC SW
L97.403 Non-pressure chronic ulcer of unspecified heel and midfoot with necrosis of muscle CC HCC SW
L97.404 Non-pressure chronic ulcer of unspecified heel and midfoot with necrosis of bone CC HCC SW
L97.405 Non-pressure chronic ulcer of unspecified heel and midfoot with muscle involvement without evidence of necrosis CC HCC
L97.406 Non-pressure chronic ulcer of unspecified heel and midfoot with bone involvement without evidence of necrosis CC HCC
L97.408 Non-pressure chronic ulcer of unspecified heel and midfoot with other specified severity CC HCC
L97.409 Non-pressure chronic ulcer of unspecified heel and midfoot with unspecified severity CC HCC

6th L97.41 Non-pressure chronic ulcer of right heel and midfoot
L97.411 Non-pressure chronic ulcer of right heel and midfoot limited to breakdown of skin CC HCC
L97.412 Non-pressure chronic ulcer of right heel and midfoot with fat layer exposed CC HCC SW
AHA: 2020,2Q,19
L97.413 Non-pressure chronic ulcer of right heel and midfoot with necrosis of muscle CC HCC SW
L97.414 Non-pressure chronic ulcer of right heel and midfoot with necrosis of bone CC HCC SW
L97.415 Non-pressure chronic ulcer of right heel and midfoot with muscle involvement without evidence of necrosis CC HCC
L97.416 Non-pressure chronic ulcer of right heel and midfoot with bone involvement without evidence of necrosis CC HCC
L97.418 Non-pressure chronic ulcer of right heel and midfoot with other specified severity CC HCC
L97.419 Non-pressure chronic ulcer of right heel and midfoot with unspecified severity CC HCC

6th L97.42 Non-pressure chronic ulcer of left heel and midfoot
L97.421 Non-pressure chronic ulcer of left heel and midfoot limited to breakdown of skin CC HCC
AHA: 2016,1Q,12
L97.422 Non-pressure chronic ulcer of left heel and midfoot with fat layer exposed CC HCC SW
AHA: 2020,2Q,19
L97.423 Non-pressure chronic ulcer of left heel and midfoot with necrosis of muscle CC HCC SW
L97.424 Non-pressure chronic ulcer of left heel and midfoot with necrosis of bone CC HCC SW
L97.425 Non-pressure chronic ulcer of left heel and midfoot with muscle involvement without evidence of necrosis CC HCC
L97.426 Non-pressure chronic ulcer of left heel and midfoot with bone involvement without evidence of necrosis CC HCC
L97.428 Non-pressure chronic ulcer of left heel and midfoot with other specified severity CC HCC

L97.429 Non-pressure chronic ulcer of left heel and midfoot with unspecified severity CC HCC

✓5th L97.5 Non-pressure chronic ulcer of other part of foot
Non-pressure chronic ulcer of toe

✓6th L97.50 Non-pressure chronic ulcer of other part of unspecified foot

L97.501 Non-pressure chronic ulcer of other part of unspecified foot limited to breakdown of skin HCC

L97.502 Non-pressure chronic ulcer of other part of unspecified foot with fat layer exposed HCC SW

L97.503 Non-pressure chronic ulcer of other part of unspecified foot with necrosis of muscle HCC SW

L97.504 Non-pressure chronic ulcer of other part of unspecified foot with necrosis of bone HCC SW

L97.505 Non-pressure chronic ulcer of other part of unspecified foot with muscle involvement without evidence of necrosis CC HCC

L97.506 Non-pressure chronic ulcer of other part of unspecified foot with bone involvement without evidence of necrosis CC HCC

L97.508 Non-pressure chronic ulcer of other part of unspecified foot with other specified severity CC HCC

L97.509 Non-pressure chronic ulcer of other part of unspecified foot with unspecified severity HCC

✓6th L97.51 Non-pressure chronic ulcer of other part of right foot
AHA: 2020,1Q,12

L97.511 Non-pressure chronic ulcer of other part of right foot limited to breakdown of skin HCC

L97.512 Non-pressure chronic ulcer of other part of right foot with fat layer exposed HCC SW
AHA: 2020,2Q,19

L97.513 Non-pressure chronic ulcer of other part of right foot with necrosis of muscle HCC SW

L97.514 Non-pressure chronic ulcer of other part of right foot with necrosis of bone HCC SW

L97.515 Non-pressure chronic ulcer of other part of right foot with muscle involvement without evidence of necrosis CC HCC

L97.516 Non-pressure chronic ulcer of other part of right foot with bone involvement without evidence of necrosis CC HCC

L97.518 Non-pressure chronic ulcer of other part of right foot with other specified severity CC HCC

L97.519 Non-pressure chronic ulcer of other part of right foot with unspecified severity HCC

✓6th L97.52 Non-pressure chronic ulcer of other part of left foot
AHA: 2020,1Q,12

L97.521 Non-pressure chronic ulcer of other part of left foot limited to breakdown of skin HCC

L97.522 Non-pressure chronic ulcer of other part of left foot with fat layer exposed HCC SW
AHA: 2020,2Q,19

L97.523 Non-pressure chronic ulcer of other part of left foot with necrosis of muscle HCC SW

L97.524 Non-pressure chronic ulcer of other part of left foot with necrosis of bone HCC SW

L97.525 Non-pressure chronic ulcer of other part of left foot with muscle involvement without evidence of necrosis CC HCC

L97.526 Non-pressure chronic ulcer of other part of left foot with bone involvement without evidence of necrosis CC HCC

L97.528 Non-pressure chronic ulcer of other part of left foot with other specified severity CC HCC

L97.529 Non-pressure chronic ulcer of other part of left foot with unspecified severity HCC

✓5th L97.8 Non-pressure chronic ulcer of other part of lower leg

✓6th L97.80 Non-pressure chronic ulcer of other part of unspecified lower leg

L97.801 Non-pressure chronic ulcer of other part of unspecified lower leg limited to breakdown of skin CC HCC

L97.802 Non-pressure chronic ulcer of other part of unspecified lower leg with fat layer exposed CC HCC SW

L97.803 Non-pressure chronic ulcer of other part of unspecified lower leg with necrosis of muscle CC HCC SW

L97.804 Non-pressure chronic ulcer of other part of unspecified lower leg with necrosis of bone CC HCC SW

L97.805 Non-pressure chronic ulcer of other part of unspecified lower leg with muscle involvement without evidence of necrosis CC HCC

L97.806 Non-pressure chronic ulcer of other part of unspecified lower leg with bone involvement without evidence of necrosis CC HCC

L97.808 Non-pressure chronic ulcer of other part of unspecified lower leg with other specified severity CC HCC

L97.809 Non-pressure chronic ulcer of other part of unspecified lower leg with unspecified severity CC HCC

✓6th L97.81 Non-pressure chronic ulcer of other part of right lower leg

L97.811 Non-pressure chronic ulcer of other part of right lower leg limited to breakdown of skin CC HCC

L97.812 Non-pressure chronic ulcer of other part of right lower leg with fat layer exposed CC HCC SW

L97.813 Non-pressure chronic ulcer of other part of right lower leg with necrosis of muscle CC HCC SW

L97.814 Non-pressure chronic ulcer of other part of right lower leg with necrosis of bone CC HCC SW

L97.815 Non-pressure chronic ulcer of other part of right lower leg with muscle involvement without evidence of necrosis CC HCC

L97.816 Non-pressure chronic ulcer of other part of right lower leg with bone involvement without evidence of necrosis CC HCC

L97.818 Non-pressure chronic ulcer of other part of right lower leg with other specified severity CC HCC

L97.819 Non-pressure chronic ulcer of other part of right lower leg with unspecified severity CC HCC

✓6th L97.82 Non-pressure chronic ulcer of other part of left lower leg

L97.821 Non-pressure chronic ulcer of other part of left lower leg limited to breakdown of skin CC HCC

L97.822 Non-pressure chronic ulcer of other part of left lower leg with fat layer exposed CC HCC SW

L97.823 Non-pressure chronic ulcer of other part of left lower leg with necrosis of muscle CC HCC SW

L97.824 Non-pressure chronic ulcer of other part of left lower leg with necrosis of bone CC HCC SW

L97.825 Non-pressure chronic ulcer of other part of left lower leg with muscle involvement without evidence of necrosis CC HCC

L97.826 Non-pressure chronic ulcer of other part of left lower leg with bone involvement without evidence of necrosis CC HCC

L97.828 Non-pressure chronic ulcer of other part of left lower leg with other specified severity CC HCC

L97.829 Non-pressure chronic ulcer of other part of left lower leg with unspecified severity CC HCC

✓5th L97.9 Non-pressure chronic ulcer of unspecified part of lower leg

✓6th L97.90 Non-pressure chronic ulcer of unspecified part of unspecified lower leg

L97.901 Non-pressure chronic ulcer of unspecified part of unspecified lower leg limited to breakdown of skin CC HCC

L97.902 Non-pressure chronic ulcer of unspecified part of unspecified lower leg with fat layer exposed CC HCC SW

L97.903 Non-pressure chronic ulcer of unspecified part of unspecified lower leg with necrosis of muscle CC HCC SW

L97.904 Non-pressure chronic ulcer of unspecified part of unspecified lower leg with necrosis of bone CC HCC SW

L97.905 Non-pressure chronic ulcer of unspecified part of unspecified lower leg with muscle involvement without evidence of necrosis CC HCC

L97.906 Non-pressure chronic ulcer of unspecified part of unspecified lower leg with bone involvement without evidence of necrosis CC HCC

L97.908 Non-pressure chronic ulcer of unspecified part of unspecified lower leg with other specified severity CC HCC

L97.909 Non-pressure chronic ulcer of unspecified part of unspecified lower leg with unspecified severity CC HCC

✓6th L97.91 Non-pressure chronic ulcer of unspecified part of right lower leg

L97.911 Non-pressure chronic ulcer of unspecified part of right lower leg limited to breakdown of skin CC HCC

L97.912 Non-pressure chronic ulcer of unspecified part of right lower leg with fat layer exposed CC HCC SW

L97.913 Non-pressure chronic ulcer of unspecified part of right lower leg with necrosis of muscle CC HCC SW

L97.914 Non-pressure chronic ulcer of unspecified part of right lower leg with necrosis of bone CC HCC SW

L97.915 Non-pressure chronic ulcer of unspecified part of right lower leg with muscle involvement without evidence of necrosis CC HCC

L97.916 Non-pressure chronic ulcer of unspecified part of right lower leg with bone involvement without evidence of necrosis CC HCC

L97.918 Non-pressure chronic ulcer of unspecified part of right lower leg with other specified severity CC HCC

L97.919 Non-pressure chronic ulcer of unspecified part of right lower leg with unspecified severity CC HCC

✓6th L97.92 Non-pressure chronic ulcer of unspecified part of left lower leg

L97.921 Non-pressure chronic ulcer of unspecified part of left lower leg limited to breakdown of skin CC HCC SW

L97.922 Non-pressure chronic ulcer of unspecified part of left lower leg with fat layer exposed CC HCC SW

L97.923 Non-pressure chronic ulcer of unspecified part of left lower leg with necrosis of muscle CC HCC SW

L97.924 Non-pressure chronic ulcer of unspecified part of left lower leg with necrosis of bone CC HCC SW

L97.925 Non-pressure chronic ulcer of unspecified part of left lower leg with muscle involvement without evidence of necrosis CC HCC

L97.926 Non-pressure chronic ulcer of unspecified part of left lower leg with bone involvement without evidence of necrosis CC HCC

L97.928 Non-pressure chronic ulcer of unspecified part of left lower leg with other specified severity CC HCC

L97.929 Non-pressure chronic ulcer of unspecified part of left lower leg with unspecified severity CC HCC

✓4th **L98 Other disorders of skin and subcutaneous tissue, not elsewhere classified**

L98.Ø Pyogenic granuloma

EXCLUDES 2 *pyogenic granuloma of gingiva (KØ6.8)*
pyogenic granuloma of maxillary alveolar ridge (KØ4.5)
pyogenic granuloma of oral mucosa (K13.4)

DEF: Solitary polypoid capillary hemangioma often associated with local irritation, trauma, and superimposed inflammation. Located on the skin and gingival or oral mucosa, they bleed easily and may ulcerate and form crusted sores.

L98.1 Factitial dermatitis

Neurotic excoriation

EXCLUDES 1 *excoriation (skin-picking) disorder (F42.4)*

AHA: 2016,4Q,15

DEF: Self-inflicted skin lesions to satisfy an unconscious psychological or emotional need. Methods used to injure the skin include deep excoriations with a sharp instrument, scarification with a knife, or the application of caustic chemicals and burning, sometimes with a cigarette.

L98.2 Febrile neutrophilic dermatosis [Sweet]

L98.3 Eosinophilic cellulitis [Wells] CC

✓5th **L98.4 Non-pressure chronic ulcer of skin, not elsewhere classified**

Chronic ulcer of skin NOS
Tropical ulcer NOS
Ulcer of skin NOS

EXCLUDES 2 *gangrene (I96)*
pressure ulcer (pressure area) (L89.-)
skin infections (LØØ-LØ8)
specific infections classified to AØØ-B99
ulcer of lower limb NEC (L97.-)
varicose ulcer ►(I83.Ø-I83.93)◄

AHA: 2017,4Q,17

TIP: The depth and/or severity of a diagnosed nonpressure ulcer can be determined based on medical record documentation from clinicians who are not the patient's provider.

TIP: Assign a code from this category/subcategory for nonpressure ulcers documented as acute.

✓6th L98.41 Non-pressure chronic ulcer of buttock

L98.411 Non-pressure chronic ulcer of buttock limited to breakdown of skin HCC

L98.412 Non-pressure chronic ulcer of buttock with fat layer exposed HCC SW

L98.413 Non-pressure chronic ulcer of buttock with necrosis of muscle HCC SW

L98.414 Non-pressure chronic ulcer of buttock with necrosis of bone HCC SW

L98.415 Non-pressure chronic ulcer of buttock with muscle involvement without evidence of necrosis CC HCC

L98.416 Non-pressure chronic ulcer of buttock with bone involvement without evidence of necrosis CC HCC

L98.418 Non-pressure chronic ulcer of buttock with other specified severity CC HCC

L98.419 Non-pressure chronic ulcer of buttock with unspecified severity HCC

✓6th L98.42 Non-pressure chronic ulcer of back

L98.421 Non-pressure chronic ulcer of back limited to breakdown of skin HCC

L98.422 Non-pressure chronic ulcer of back with fat layer exposed HCC SW

L98.423 Non-pressure chronic ulcer of back with necrosis of muscle HCC SW

L98.424 Non-pressure chronic ulcer of back with necrosis of bone HCC SW

L98.425 Non-pressure chronic ulcer of back with muscle involvement without evidence of necrosis CC HCC

L98.426 Non-pressure chronic ulcer of back with bone involvement without evidence of necrosis CC HCC

L98.428 Non-pressure chronic ulcer of back with other specified severity CC HCC

L98.429 Non-pressure chronic ulcer of back with unspecified severity HCC

✓6th **L98.49 Non-pressure chronic ulcer of skin of other sites**

Non-pressure chronic ulcer of skin NOS

L98.491 Non-pressure chronic ulcer of skin of other sites limited to breakdown of skin HCC

L98.492 Non-pressure chronic ulcer of skin of other sites with fat layer exposed HCC SW

L98.493 Non-pressure chronic ulcer of skin of other sites with necrosis of muscle HCC SW

L98.494 Non-pressure chronic ulcer of skin of other sites with necrosis of bone HCC SW

L98.495 Non-pressure chronic ulcer of skin of other sites with muscle involvement without evidence of necrosis CC HCC

L98.496 Non-pressure chronic ulcer of skin of other sites with bone involvement without evidence of necrosis CC HCC

L98.498 Non-pressure chronic ulcer of skin of other sites with other specified severity CC HCC

L98.499 Non-pressure chronic ulcer of skin of other sites with unspecified severity HCC

L98.5 Mucinosis of the skin

Focal mucinosis

Lichen myxedematosus

Reticular erythematous mucinosis

EXCLUDES 1 *focal oral mucinosis (K13.79)*

myxedema (EØ3.9)

L98.6 Other infiltrative disorders of the skin and subcutaneous tissue

EXCLUDES 1 *hyalinosis cutis et mucosae (E78.89)*

L98.7 Excessive and redundant skin and subcutaneous tissue

Loose or sagging skin, following bariatric surgery weight loss

Loose or sagging skin following dietary weight loss

Loose or sagging skin, NOS

EXCLUDES 2 *acquired excess or redundant skin of eyelid (HØ2.3-)*

congenital excess or redundant skin of eyelid (Q1Ø.3)

skin changes due to chronic exposure to nonionizing radiation (L57.-)

AHA: 2016,4Q,36

L98.8 Other specified disorders of the skin and subcutaneous tissue

AHA: 2013,2Q,32

L98.9 Disorder of the skin and subcutaneous tissue, unspecified

L99 Other disorders of skin and subcutaneous tissue in diseases classified elsewhere

Code first underlying disease, such as:

amyloidosis (E85.-)

EXCLUDES 1 *skin disorders in diabetes (EØ8-E13 with .62)*

skin disorders in gonorrhea (A54.89)

skin disorders in syphilis (A51.31, A52.79)

Chapter 13. Diseases of the Musculoskeletal System and Connective Tissue (MØØ–M99)

Chapter-specific Guidelines with Coding Examples

The chapter-specific guidelines from the ICD-10-CM Official Guidelines for Coding and Reporting have been provided below. Along with these guidelines are coding examples, contained in the shaded boxes, that have been developed to help illustrate the coding and/or sequencing guidance found in these guidelines.

a. Site and laterality

Most of the codes within Chapter 13 have site and laterality designations. The site represents the bone, joint or the muscle involved. For some conditions where more than one bone, joint or muscle is usually involved, such as osteoarthritis, there is a "multiple sites" code available. For categories where no multiple site code is provided and more than one bone, joint or muscle is involved, multiple codes should be used to indicate the different sites involved.

Rheumatoid arthritis of multiple sites without rheumatoid factor

MØ6.Ø9 Rheumatoid arthritis without rheumatoid factor, multiple sites

Explanation: For some conditions where more than one bone, joint or muscle is usually involved, such as rheumatoid arthritis, there is a "multiple sites" code available.

Osteomyelitis of the fourth thoracic and second lumbar vertebrae

M46.24 Osteomyelitis of vertebra, thoracic region

M46.26 Osteomyelitis of vertebra, lumbar region

Explanation: For categories without a multiple site code and more than one bone, joint, or muscle is involved, multiple codes should be used to indicate the different sites involved.

1) Bone versus joint

For certain conditions, the bone may be affected at the upper or lower end, (e.g., avascular necrosis of bone, M87, Osteoporosis, M8Ø, M81). Though the portion of the bone affected may be at the joint, the site designation will be the bone, not the joint.

Idiopathic avascular necrosis of the femoral head of the left hip joint

M87.Ø52 Idiopathic aseptic necrosis of left femur

Explanation: For certain conditions such as avascular necrosis, the bone may be affected at the joint, but the site designation is the bone, not the joint.

b. Acute traumatic versus chronic or recurrent musculoskeletal conditions

Many musculoskeletal conditions are a result of previous injury or trauma to a site, or are recurrent conditions. Bone, joint or muscle conditions that are the result of a healed injury are usually found in chapter 13. Recurrent bone, joint or muscle conditions are also usually found in chapter 13. Any current, acute injury should be coded to the appropriate injury code from chapter 19. Chronic or recurrent conditions should generally be coded with a code from chapter 13. If it is difficult to determine from the documentation in the record which code is best to describe a condition, query the provider.

Acute traumatic bucket-handle tear of right medial meniscus

S83.211A Bucket-handle tear of medial meniscus, current injury, right knee, initial encounter

Explanation: Any current, acute injury is not coded in chapter 13. It should instead be coded to the appropriate injury code from chapter 19.

Old bucket-handle tear of right medial meniscus

M23.2Ø3 Derangement of unspecified medial meniscus due to old tear or injury, right knee

Explanation: Chronic or recurrent conditions should generally be coded with a code from chapter 13.

c. Coding of pathologic fractures

7th character A is for use as long as the patient is receiving active treatment for the fracture. Examples of active treatment are: surgical treatment, emergency department encounter, evaluation and continuing treatment by the same or a different physician. While the patient may be seen by a new or different provider over the course of treatment for a pathological fracture, assignment of the 7th character is based on whether the patient is undergoing active treatment and not whether the provider is seeing the patient for the first time.

Patient admitted for repair of pathologic fracture of left foot, unknown cause. The surgery will be performed by his orthopedic specialist who he has been seeing for this fracture for the past month.

M84.475A Pathological fracture, left foot, initial encounter for fracture

Explanation: Seventh character A is for use as long as the patient is receiving active treatment for a pathologic fracture. Examples of active treatment are surgical treatment, emergency department encounter, evaluation, and continuing treatment by the same or a different physician.

The seventh character is based on whether the patient is undergoing active treatment such as surgery, and not whether the provider is seeing the patient for the first time.

7th character D is to be used for encounters after the patient has completed active treatment for the fracture and is receiving routine care for the fracture during the healing or recovery phase. The other 7th characters, listed under each subcategory in the Tabular List, are to be used for subsequent encounters for treatment of problems associated with the healing, such as malunions, nonunions, and sequelae.

Care for complications of surgical treatment for fracture repairs during the healing or recovery phase should be coded with the appropriate complication codes.

See Section I.C.19. Coding of traumatic fractures.

d. Osteoporosis

Osteoporosis is a systemic condition, meaning that all bones of the musculoskeletal system are affected. Therefore, site is not a component of the codes under category M81, Osteoporosis without current pathological fracture. The site codes under category M8Ø, Osteoporosis with current pathological fracture, identify the site of the fracture, not the osteoporosis.

1) Osteoporosis without pathological fracture

Category M81, Osteoporosis without current pathological fracture, is for use for patients with osteoporosis who do not currently have a pathologic fracture due to the osteoporosis, even if they have had a fracture in the past. For patients with a history of osteoporosis fractures, status code Z87.31Ø, Personal history of (healed) osteoporosis fracture, should follow the code from M81.

Age-related osteoporosis with healed osteoporotic fracture of the lumbar vertebra

M81.Ø Age-related osteoporosis without current pathological fracture

Z87.31Ø Personal history of (healed) osteoporosis fracture

Explanation: Category M81 is used for patients with osteoporosis who do not currently have a pathologic fracture due to the osteoporosis. To report a previous (healed) fracture, status code Z87.31Ø Personal history of (healed) osteoporosis fracture, should follow the code from M81.

2) Osteoporosis with current pathological fracture

Category M8Ø, Osteoporosis with current pathological fracture, is for patients who have a current pathologic fracture at the time of an encounter. The codes under M8Ø identify the site of the fracture. A code from category M8Ø, not a traumatic fracture code, should be used for any patient with known osteoporosis who suffers a fracture, even if the patient had a minor fall or trauma, if that fall or trauma would not usually break a normal, healthy bone.

Disuse osteoporosis with current fracture of right shoulder sustained lifting a grocery bag, initial encounter

M8Ø.811A Other osteoporosis with current pathological fracture, right shoulder, initial encounter for fracture

Explanation: A code from category M8Ø, not a traumatic fracture code, should be used for any patient with known osteoporosis who suffers a fracture, even if the patient had a minor fall or trauma, if that fall or trauma would not usually break a normal, healthy bone.

Muscle/Tendon Table

ICD-10-CM categorizes certain muscles and tendons in the upper and lower extremities by their action (e.g., extension, flexion), their anatomical location (e.g., posterior, anterior), and/or whether they are intrinsic or extrinsic to a certain anatomical area. The Muscle/Tendon Table is provided at the beginning of chapters 13 and 19 as a resource to help users when code selection depends on one or more of these characteristics. Please note that this table is not all-inclusive, and proper code assignment should be based on the provider's documentation.

Body Region	Muscle	Extensor Tendon	Flexor Tendon	Other Tendon
Shoulder				
	Deltoid	Posterior deltoid	Anterior deltoid	
	Rotator cuff			
	Infraspinatus			Infraspinatus
	Subscapularis			Subscapularis
	Supraspinatus			Supraspinatus
	Teres minor			Teres minor
	Teres major	Teres major		
Upper arm				
	Anterior muscles			
	Biceps brachii — long head		Biceps brachii — long head	
	Biceps brachii — short head		Biceps brachii — short head	
	Brachialis		Brachialis	
	Coracobrachialis		Coracobrachialis	
	Posterior muscles			
	Triceps brachii	Triceps brachii		
Forearm				
	Anterior muscles			
	Flexors			
	Deep			
	Flexor digitorum profundus		Flexor digitorum profundus	
	Flexor pollicis longus		Flexor pollicis longus	
	Intermediate			
	Flexor digitorum superficialis		Flexor digitorum superficialis	
	Superficial			
	Flexor carpi radialis		Flexor carpi radialis	
	Flexor carpi ulnaris		Flexor carpi ulnaris	
	Palmaris longus		Palmaris longus	
	Pronators			
	Pronator quadratus			Pronator quadratus
	Pronator teres			Pronator teres
	Posterior muscles			
	Extensors			
	Deep			
	Abductor pollicis longus			Abductor pollicis longus
	Extensor indicis	Extensor indicis		
	Extensor pollicis brevis	Extensor pollicis brevis		
	Extensor pollicis longus	Extensor pollicis longus		
	Superficial			
	Brachioradialis			Brachioradialis
	Extensor carpi radialis brevis	Extensor carpi radialis brevis		
	Extensor carpi radialis longus	Extensor carpi radialis longus		
	Extensor carpi ulnaris	Extensor carpi ulnaris		
	Extensor digiti minimi	Extensor digiti minimi		
	Extensor digitorum	Extensor digitorum		
	Anconeus	Anconeus		
	Supinator			Supinator

Body Region	Muscle	Extensor Tendon	Flexor Tendon	Other Tendon
Hand				
Extrinsic — attach to a site in the forearm as well as a site in the hand with action related to hand movement at the wrist				
	Extensor carpi radialis brevis	Extensor carpi radialis brevis		
	Extensor carpi radialis longus	Extensor carpi radialis longus		
	Extensor carpi ulnaris	Extensor carpi ulnaris		
	Flexor carpi radialis		Flexor carpi radialis	
	Flexor carpi ulnaris		Flexor carpi ulnaris	
	Flexor digitorum superficialis		Flexor digitorum superficialis	
	Palmaris longus		Palmaris longus	
Extrinsic — attach to a site in the forearm as well as a site in the hand with action in the hand related to finger movement				
	Adductor pollicis longus			Adductor pollicis longus
	Extensor digiti minimi	Extensor digiti minimi		
	Extensor digitorum	Extensor digitorum		
	Extensor indicis	Extensor indicis		
	Flexor digitorum profundus		Flexor digitorum profundus	
	Flexor digitorum superficialis		Flexor digitorum superficialis	
Extrinsic — attach to a site in the forearm as well as a site in the hand with action in the hand related to thumb movement				
	Extensor pollicis brevis	Extensor pollicis brevis		
	Extensor pollicis longus	Extensor pollicis longus		
	Flexor pollicis longus		Flexor pollicis longus	
Intrinsic — found within the hand only				
	Adductor pollicis			Adductor pollicis
	Dorsal interossei	Dorsal interossei	Dorsal interossei	
	Lumbricals	Lumbricals	Lumbricals	
	Palmaris brevis			Palmaris brevis
	Palmar interossei	Palmar interossei	Palmar interossei	
	Hypothenar muscles			
	Abductor digiti minimi			Abductor digiti minimi
	Flexor digiti minimi brevis		Flexor digiti minimi brevis	
	Opponens digiti minimi		Opponens digiti minimi	
	Thenar muscles			
	Abductor pollicis brevis			Abductor pollicis brevis
	Flexor pollicis brevis		Flexor pollicis brevis	
	Opponens pollicis		Opponens pollicis	
Thigh				
	Anterior muscles			
	Iliopsoas		Iliopsoas	
	Pectineus		Pectineus	
	Quadriceps	Quadriceps		
	Rectus femoris	Rectus femoris — Extends knee	Rectus femoris — Flexes hip	
	Vastus intermedius	Vastus intermedius		
	Vastus lateralis	Vastus lateralis		
	Vastus medialis	Vastus medialis		
	Sartorius		Sartorius	
	Medial muscles			
	Adductor brevis			Adductor brevis
	Adductor longus			Adductor longus
	Adductor magnus			Adductor magnus
	Gracilis			Gracilis
	Obturator externus			Obturator externus
	Posterior muscles			
	Hamstring	Hamstring — Extends hip	Hamstring — Flexes knee	
	Biceps femoris	Biceps femoris	Biceps femoris	
	Semimembranosus	Semimembranosus	Semimembranosus	
	Semitendinosus	Semitendinosus	Semitendinosus	

Body Region	Muscle	Extensor Tendon	Flexor Tendon	Other Tendon
Lower leg				
	Anterior muscles			
	Extensor digitorum longus	Extensor digitorum longus		
	Extensor hallucis longus	Extensor hallucis longus		
	Fibularis (peroneus) tertius	Fibularis (peroneus) tertius		
	Tibialis anterior	Tibialis anterior		Tibialis anterior
	Lateral muscles			
	Fibularis (peroneus) brevis		Fibularis (peroneus) brevis	
	Fibularis (peroneus) longus		Fibularis (peroneus) longus	
	Posterior muscles			
	Deep			
	Flexor digitorum longus		Flexor digitorum longus	
	Flexor hallucis longus		Flexor hallucis longus	
	Popliteus		Popliteus	
	Tibialis posterior		Tibialis posterior	
	Superficial			
	Gastrocnemius		Gastrocnemius	
	Plantaris		Plantaris	
	Soleus		Soleus	
				Calcaneal (Achilles)
Ankle/Foot				
Extrinsic — attach to a site in the lower leg as well as a site in the foot with action related to foot movement at the ankle				
	Plantaris		Plantaris	
	Soleus		Soleus	
	Tibialis anterior	Tibialis anterior		
	Tibialis posterior		Tibialis posterior	
Extrinsic — attach to a site in the lower leg as well as a site in the foot with action in the foot related to toe movement				
	Extensor digitorum longus	Extensor digitorum longus		
	Extensor hallucis longus	Extensor hallucis longus		
	Flexor digitorum longus		Flexor digitorum longus	
	Flexor hallucis longus		Flexor hallucis longus	
Intrinsic — found within the ankle/foot only				
	Dorsal muscles			
	Extensor digitorum brevis	Extensor digitorum brevis		
	Extensor hallucis brevis	Extensor hallucis brevis		
	Plantar muscles			
	Abductor digiti minimi		Abductor digiti minimi	
	Abductor hallucis		Abductor hallucis	
	Dorsal interossei	Dorsal interossei	Dorsal interossei	
	Flexor digiti minimi brevis		Flexor digiti minimi brevis	
	Flexor digitorum brevis		Flexor digitorum brevis	
	Flexor hallucis brevis		Flexor hallucis brevis	
	Lumbricals	Lumbricals	Lumbricals	
	Quadratus plantae		Quadratus plantae	
	Plantar interossei	Plantar interossei	Plantar interossei	

Chapter 13. Diseases of the Musculoskeletal System and Connective Tissue (M00-M99)

NOTE Use an external cause code following the code for the musculoskeletal condition, if applicable, to identify the cause of the musculoskeletal condition

EXCLUDES 2 *arthropathic psoriasis (L40.5-)*
certain conditions originating in the perinatal period (P04-P96)
certain infectious and parasitic diseases (A00-B99)
compartment syndrome (traumatic) (T79.A-)
complications of pregnancy, childbirth and the puerperium (O00-O9A)
congenital malformations, deformations, and chromosomal abnormalities (Q00-Q99)
endocrine, nutritional and metabolic diseases (E00-E88)
injury, poisoning and certain other consequences of external causes (S00-T88)
neoplasms (C00-D49)
symptoms, signs and abnormal clinical and laboratory findings, not elsewhere classified (R00-R94)

This chapter contains the following blocks:

M00-M02	Infectious arthropathies
M04	Autoinflammatory syndromes
M05-M14	Inflammatory polyarthropathies
M15-M19	Osteoarthritis
M20-M25	Other joint disorders
M26-M27	Dentofacial anomalies [including malocclusion] and other disorders of jaw
M30-M36	Systemic connective tissue disorders
M40-M43	Deforming dorsopathies
M45-M49	Spondylopathies
M50-M54	Other dorsopathies
M60-M63	Disorders of muscles
M65-M67	Disorders of synovium and tendon
M70-M79	Other soft tissue disorders
M80-M85	Disorders of bone density and structure
M86-M90	Other osteopathies
M91-M94	Chondropathies
M95	Other disorders of the musculoskeletal system and connective tissue
M96	Intraoperative and postprocedural complications and disorders of musculoskeletal system, not elsewhere classified
M97	Periprosthetic fracture around internal prosthetic joint
M99	Biomechanical lesions, not elsewhere classified

ARTHROPATHIES (M00-M25)

INCLUDES disorders affecting predominantly peripheral (limb) joints

Infectious arthropathies (M00-M02)

NOTE This block comprises arthropathies due to microbiological agents. Distinction is made between the following types of etiological relationship:

a) direct infection of joint, where organisms invade synovial tissue and microbial antigen is present in the joint;

b) indirect infection, which may be of two types: a reactive arthropathy, where microbial infection of the body is established but neither organisms nor antigens can be identified in the joint, and a postinfective arthropathy, where microbial antigen is present but recovery of an organism is inconstant and evidence of local multiplication is lacking.

AHA: 2019,3Q,16

✓4th M00 Pyogenic arthritis

EXCLUDES 2 ▶*infection and inflammatory reaction due to internal joint prosthesis (T84.5-)*◀

DEF: Pyogenic: Relating to or involving pus production, often referred to as suppurative or purulent.

✓5th M00.0 Staphylococcal arthritis and polyarthritis

Use additional code (B95.61-B95.8) to identify bacterial agent

EXCLUDES 2 ~~*infection and inflammatory reaction due to internal joint prosthesis (T84.5-)*~~

M00.00 Staphylococcal arthritis, unspecified joint CC HCC

✓6th M00.01 Staphylococcal arthritis, shoulder

M00.011 Staphylococcal arthritis, right shoulder CC HCC

M00.012 Staphylococcal arthritis, left shoulder CC HCC

M00.019 Staphylococcal arthritis, unspecified shoulder CC HCC

✓6th M00.02 Staphylococcal arthritis, elbow

M00.021 Staphylococcal arthritis, right elbow CC HCC

M00.022 Staphylococcal arthritis, left elbow CC HCC

M00.029 Staphylococcal arthritis, unspecified elbow CC HCC

✓6th M00.03 Staphylococcal arthritis, wrist

Staphylococcal arthritis of carpal bones

M00.031 Staphylococcal arthritis, right wrist CC HCC

M00.032 Staphylococcal arthritis, left wrist CC HCC

M00.039 Staphylococcal arthritis, unspecified wrist CC HCC

✓6th M00.04 Staphylococcal arthritis, hand

Staphylococcal arthritis of metacarpus and phalanges

M00.041 Staphylococcal arthritis, right hand CC HCC

M00.042 Staphylococcal arthritis, left hand CC HCC

M00.049 Staphylococcal arthritis, unspecified hand CC HCC

✓6th M00.05 Staphylococcal arthritis, hip

M00.051 Staphylococcal arthritis, right hip CC HCC

M00.052 Staphylococcal arthritis, left hip CC HCC

M00.059 Staphylococcal arthritis, unspecified hip CC HCC

✓6th M00.06 Staphylococcal arthritis, knee

M00.061 Staphylococcal arthritis, right knee CC HCC

M00.062 Staphylococcal arthritis, left knee CC HCC

M00.069 Staphylococcal arthritis, unspecified knee CC HCC

✓6th M00.07 Staphylococcal arthritis, ankle and foot

Staphylococcal arthritis, tarsus, metatarsus and phalanges

M00.071 Staphylococcal arthritis, right ankle and foot CC HCC

M00.072 Staphylococcal arthritis, left ankle and foot CC HCC

M00.079 Staphylococcal arthritis, unspecified ankle and foot CC HCC

M00.08 Staphylococcal arthritis, vertebrae CC HCC

M00.09 Staphylococcal polyarthritis CC HCC

✓5th M00.1 Pneumococcal arthritis and polyarthritis

M00.10 Pneumococcal arthritis, unspecified joint CC HCC

✓6th M00.11 Pneumococcal arthritis, shoulder

M00.111 Pneumococcal arthritis, right shoulder CC HCC

M00.112 Pneumococcal arthritis, left shoulder CC HCC

M00.119 Pneumococcal arthritis, unspecified shoulder CC HCC

✓6th M00.12 Pneumococcal arthritis, elbow

M00.121 Pneumococcal arthritis, right elbow CC HCC

M00.122 Pneumococcal arthritis, left elbow CC HCC

M00.129 Pneumococcal arthritis, unspecified elbow CC HCC

✓6th M00.13 Pneumococcal arthritis, wrist

Pneumococcal arthritis of carpal bones

M00.131 Pneumococcal arthritis, right wrist CC HCC

M00.132 Pneumococcal arthritis, left wrist CC HCC

M00.139 Pneumococcal arthritis, unspecified wrist CC HCC

✓6th M00.14 Pneumococcal arthritis, hand

Pneumococcal arthritis of metacarpus and phalanges

M00.141 Pneumococcal arthritis, right hand CC HCC

M00.142 Pneumococcal arthritis, left hand CC HCC

M00.149 Pneumococcal arthritis, unspecified hand CC HCC

✓6th **MØØ.15 Pneumococcal arthritis, hip**
- **MØØ.151 Pneumococcal arthritis, right hip** CC HCC
- **MØØ.152 Pneumococcal arthritis, left hip** CC HCC
- **MØØ.159 Pneumococcal arthritis, unspecified hip** CC HCC

✓6th **MØØ.16 Pneumococcal arthritis, knee**
- **MØØ.161 Pneumococcal arthritis, right knee** CC HCC
- **MØØ.162 Pneumococcal arthritis, left knee** CC HCC
- **MØØ.169 Pneumococcal arthritis, unspecified knee** CC HCC

✓6th **MØØ.17 Pneumococcal arthritis, ankle and foot**

Pneumococcal arthritis, tarsus, metatarsus and phalanges
- **MØØ.171 Pneumococcal arthritis, right ankle and foot** CC HCC
- **MØØ.172 Pneumococcal arthritis, left ankle and foot** CC HCC
- **MØØ.179 Pneumococcal arthritis, unspecified ankle and foot** CC HCC

MØØ.18 Pneumococcal arthritis, vertebrae CC HCC

MØØ.19 Pneumococcal polyarthritis CC HCC

✓5th **MØØ.2 Other streptococcal arthritis and polyarthritis**

Use additional code (B95.Ø-B95.2, B95.4-B95.5) to identify bacterial agent

MØØ.2Ø Other streptococcal arthritis, unspecified joint CC HCC

✓6th **MØØ.21 Other streptococcal arthritis, shoulder**
- **MØØ.211 Other streptococcal arthritis, right shoulder** CC HCC
- **MØØ.212 Other streptococcal arthritis, left shoulder** CC HCC
- **MØØ.219 Other streptococcal arthritis, unspecified shoulder** CC HCC

✓6th **MØØ.22 Other streptococcal arthritis, elbow**
- **MØØ.221 Other streptococcal arthritis, right elbow** CC HCC
- **MØØ.222 Other streptococcal arthritis, left elbow** CC HCC
- **MØØ.229 Other streptococcal arthritis, unspecified elbow** CC HCC

✓6th **MØØ.23 Other streptococcal arthritis, wrist**

Other streptococcal arthritis of carpal bones
- **MØØ.231 Other streptococcal arthritis, right wrist** CC HCC
- **MØØ.232 Other streptococcal arthritis, left wrist** CC HCC
- **MØØ.239 Other streptococcal arthritis, unspecified wrist** CC HCC

✓6th **MØØ.24 Other streptococcal arthritis, hand**

Other streptococcal arthritis metacarpus and phalanges
- **MØØ.241 Other streptococcal arthritis, right hand** CC HCC
- **MØØ.242 Other streptococcal arthritis, left hand** CC HCC
- **MØØ.249 Other streptococcal arthritis, unspecified hand** CC HCC

✓6th **MØØ.25 Other streptococcal arthritis, hip**
- **MØØ.251 Other streptococcal arthritis, right hip** CC HCC
- **MØØ.252 Other streptococcal arthritis, left hip** CC HCC
- **MØØ.259 Other streptococcal arthritis, unspecified hip** CC HCC

✓6th **MØØ.26 Other streptococcal arthritis, knee**
- **MØØ.261 Other streptococcal arthritis, right knee** CC HCC
- **MØØ.262 Other streptococcal arthritis, left knee** CC HCC
- **MØØ.269 Other streptococcal arthritis, unspecified knee** CC HCC

✓6th **MØØ.27 Other streptococcal arthritis, ankle and foot**

Other streptococcal arthritis, tarsus, metatarsus and phalanges
- **MØØ.271 Other streptococcal arthritis, right ankle and foot** CC HCC
- **MØØ.272 Other streptococcal arthritis, left ankle and foot** CC HCC
- **MØØ.279 Other streptococcal arthritis, unspecified ankle and foot** CC HCC

MØØ.28 Other streptococcal arthritis, vertebrae CC HCC

MØØ.29 Other streptococcal polyarthritis CC HCC

✓5th **MØØ.8 Arthritis and polyarthritis due to other bacteria**

Use additional code (B96) to identify bacteria

MØØ.8Ø Arthritis due to other bacteria, unspecified joint CC HCC

✓6th **MØØ.81 Arthritis due to other bacteria, shoulder**
- **MØØ.811 Arthritis due to other bacteria, right shoulder** CC HCC
- **MØØ.812 Arthritis due to other bacteria, left shoulder** CC HCC
- **MØØ.819 Arthritis due to other bacteria, unspecified shoulder** CC HCC

✓6th **MØØ.82 Arthritis due to other bacteria, elbow**
- **MØØ.821 Arthritis due to other bacteria, right elbow** CC HCC
- **MØØ.822 Arthritis due to other bacteria, left elbow** CC HCC
- **MØØ.829 Arthritis due to other bacteria, unspecified elbow** CC HCC

✓6th **MØØ.83 Arthritis due to other bacteria, wrist**

Arthritis due to other bacteria, carpal bones
- **MØØ.831 Arthritis due to other bacteria, right wrist** CC HCC
- **MØØ.832 Arthritis due to other bacteria, left wrist** CC HCC
- **MØØ.839 Arthritis due to other bacteria, unspecified wrist** CC HCC

✓6th **MØØ.84 Arthritis due to other bacteria, hand**

Arthritis due to other bacteria, metacarpus and phalanges
- **MØØ.841 Arthritis due to other bacteria, right hand** CC HCC
- **MØØ.842 Arthritis due to other bacteria, left hand** CC HCC
- **MØØ.849 Arthritis due to other bacteria, unspecified hand** CC HCC

✓6th **MØØ.85 Arthritis due to other bacteria, hip**
- **MØØ.851 Arthritis due to other bacteria, right hip** CC HCC
- **MØØ.852 Arthritis due to other bacteria, left hip** CC HCC
- **MØØ.859 Arthritis due to other bacteria, unspecified hip** CC HCC

✓6th **MØØ.86 Arthritis due to other bacteria, knee**

AHA: 2019,3Q,16
- **MØØ.861 Arthritis due to other bacteria, right knee** CC HCC
- **MØØ.862 Arthritis due to other bacteria, left knee** CC HCC
- **MØØ.869 Arthritis due to other bacteria, unspecified knee** CC HCC

✓6th **MØØ.87 Arthritis due to other bacteria, ankle and foot**

Arthritis due to other bacteria, tarsus, metatarsus, and phalanges
- **MØØ.871 Arthritis due to other bacteria, right ankle and foot** CC HCC
- **MØØ.872 Arthritis due to other bacteria, left ankle and foot** CC HCC
- **MØØ.879 Arthritis due to other bacteria, unspecified ankle and foot** CC HCC

MØØ.88 Arthritis due to other bacteria, vertebrae CC HCC

MØØ.89 Polyarthritis due to other bacteria CC HCC

MØØ.9 Pyogenic arthritis, unspecified CC HCC

Infective arthritis NOS

M01 Direct infections of joint in infectious and parasitic diseases classified elsewhere

Code first underlying disease, such as:
- leprosy [Hansen's disease] (A30.-)
- mycoses (B35-B49)
- O'nyong-nyong fever (A92.1)
- paratyphoid fever (A01.1-A01.4)

EXCLUDES 1
- *arthropathy in Lyme disease (A69.23)*
- *gonococcal arthritis (A54.42)*
- *meningococcal arthritis (A39.83)*
- *mumps arthritis (B26.85)*
- *postinfective arthropathy (M02.-)*
- *postmeningococcal arthritis (A39.84)*
- *reactive arthritis (M02.3)*
- *rubella arthritis (B06.82)*
- *sarcoidosis arthritis (D86.86)*
- *typhoid fever arthritis (A01.04)*
- *tuberculosis arthritis (A18.01-A18.02)*

M01.X Direct infection of joint in infectious and parasitic diseases classified elsewhere

M01.X0 Direct infection of unspecified joint in infectious and parasitic diseases classified elsewhere CC HCC

M01.X1 Direct infection of shoulder joint in infectious and parasitic diseases classified elsewhere

M01.X11 Direct infection of right shoulder in infectious and parasitic diseases classified elsewhere CC HCC

M01.X12 Direct infection of left shoulder in infectious and parasitic diseases classified elsewhere CC HCC

M01.X19 Direct infection of unspecified shoulder in infectious and parasitic diseases classified elsewhere CC HCC

M01.X2 Direct infection of elbow in infectious and parasitic diseases classified elsewhere

M01.X21 Direct infection of right elbow in infectious and parasitic diseases classified elsewhere CC HCC

M01.X22 Direct infection of left elbow in infectious and parasitic diseases classified elsewhere CC HCC

M01.X29 Direct infection of unspecified elbow in infectious and parasitic diseases classified elsewhere CC HCC

M01.X3 Direct infection of wrist in infectious and parasitic diseases classified elsewhere

Direct infection of carpal bones in infectious and parasitic diseases classified elsewhere

M01.X31 Direct infection of right wrist in infectious and parasitic diseases classified elsewhere CC HCC

M01.X32 Direct infection of left wrist in infectious and parasitic diseases classified elsewhere CC HCC

M01.X39 Direct infection of unspecified wrist in infectious and parasitic diseases classified elsewhere CC HCC

M01.X4 Direct infection of hand in infectious and parasitic diseases classified elsewhere

Direct infection of metacarpus and phalanges in infectious and parasitic diseases classified elsewhere

M01.X41 Direct infection of right hand in infectious and parasitic diseases classified elsewhere CC HCC

M01.X42 Direct infection of left hand in infectious and parasitic diseases classified elsewhere CC HCC

M01.X49 Direct infection of unspecified hand in infectious and parasitic diseases classified elsewhere CC HCC

M01.X5 Direct infection of hip in infectious and parasitic diseases classified elsewhere

M01.X51 Direct infection of right hip in infectious and parasitic diseases classified elsewhere CC HCC

M01.X52 Direct infection of left hip in infectious and parasitic diseases classified elsewhere CC HCC

M01.X59 Direct infection of unspecified hip in infectious and parasitic diseases classified elsewhere CC HCC

M01.X6 Direct infection of knee in infectious and parasitic diseases classified elsewhere

M01.X61 Direct infection of right knee in infectious and parasitic diseases classified elsewhere CC HCC

M01.X62 Direct infection of left knee in infectious and parasitic diseases classified elsewhere CC HCC

M01.X69 Direct infection of unspecified knee in infectious and parasitic diseases classified elsewhere CC HCC

M01.X7 Direct infection of ankle and foot in infectious and parasitic diseases classified elsewhere

Direct infection of tarsus, metatarsus and phalanges in infectious and parasitic diseases classified elsewhere

M01.X71 Direct infection of right ankle and foot in infectious and parasitic diseases classified elsewhere CC HCC

M01.X72 Direct infection of left ankle and foot in infectious and parasitic diseases classified elsewhere CC HCC

M01.X79 Direct infection of unspecified ankle and foot in infectious and parasitic diseases classified elsewhere CC HCC

M01.X8 Direct infection of vertebrae in infectious and parasitic diseases classified elsewhere CC HCC

M01.X9 Direct infection of multiple joints in infectious and parasitic diseases classified elsewhere CC HCC

M02 Postinfective and reactive arthropathies

Code first underlying disease, such as:
- congenital syphilis [Clutton's joints] (A50.5)
- enteritis due to Yersinia enterocolitica (A04.6)
- infective endocarditis (I33.0)
- viral hepatitis (B15-B19)

EXCLUDES 1
- *Behçet's disease (M35.2)*
- *direct infections of joint in infectious and parasitic diseases classified elsewhere (M01.-)*
- *mumps arthritis (B26.85)*
- *postmeningococcal arthritis (A39.84)*
- *rheumatic fever (I00)*
- *rubella arthritis (B06.82)*
- *syphilis arthritis (late) (A52.77)*
- *tabetic arthropathy [Charcôt's] (A52.16)*

M02.0 Arthropathy following intestinal bypass

M02.00 Arthropathy following intestinal bypass, unspecified site

M02.01 Arthropathy following intestinal bypass, shoulder

M02.011 Arthropathy following intestinal bypass, right shoulder

M02.012 Arthropathy following intestinal bypass, left shoulder

M02.019 Arthropathy following intestinal bypass, unspecified shoulder

M02.02 Arthropathy following intestinal bypass, elbow

M02.021 Arthropathy following intestinal bypass, right elbow

M02.022 Arthropathy following intestinal bypass, left elbow

M02.029 Arthropathy following intestinal bypass, unspecified elbow

M02.03 Arthropathy following intestinal bypass, wrist

Arthropathy following intestinal bypass, carpal bones

M02.031 Arthropathy following intestinal bypass, right wrist

M02.032 Arthropathy following intestinal bypass, left wrist

M02.039 Arthropathy following intestinal bypass, unspecified wrist

M02.04 Arthropathy following intestinal bypass, hand

Arthropathy following intestinal bypass, metacarpals and phalanges

M02.041 Arthropathy following intestinal bypass, right hand

M02.042 Arthropathy following intestinal bypass, left hand

MØ2.Ø49 Arthropathy following intestinal bypass, unspecified hand

✓6th MØ2.Ø5 Arthropathy following intestinal bypass, hip

MØ2.Ø51 Arthropathy following intestinal bypass, right hip

MØ2.Ø52 Arthropathy following intestinal bypass, left hip

MØ2.Ø59 Arthropathy following intestinal bypass, unspecified hip

✓6th MØ2.Ø6 Arthropathy following intestinal bypass, knee

MØ2.Ø61 Arthropathy following intestinal bypass, right knee

MØ2.Ø62 Arthropathy following intestinal bypass, left knee

MØ2.Ø69 Arthropathy following intestinal bypass, unspecified knee

✓6th MØ2.Ø7 Arthropathy following intestinal bypass, ankle and foot

Arthropathy following intestinal bypass, tarsus, metatarsus and phalanges

MØ2.Ø71 Arthropathy following intestinal bypass, right ankle and foot

MØ2.Ø72 Arthropathy following intestinal bypass, left ankle and foot

MØ2.Ø79 Arthropathy following intestinal bypass, unspecified ankle and foot

MØ2.Ø8 Arthropathy following intestinal bypass, vertebrae

MØ2.Ø9 Arthropathy following intestinal bypass, multiple sites

✓5th MØ2.1 Postdysenteric arthropathy

MØ2.1Ø Postdysenteric arthropathy, unspecified site CC HCC

✓6th MØ2.11 Postdysenteric arthropathy, shoulder

MØ2.111 Postdysenteric arthropathy, right shoulder CC HCC

MØ2.112 Postdysenteric arthropathy, left shoulder CC HCC

MØ2.119 Postdysenteric arthropathy, unspecified shoulder CC HCC

✓6th MØ2.12 Postdysenteric arthropathy, elbow

MØ2.121 Postdysenteric arthropathy, right elbow CC HCC

MØ2.122 Postdysenteric arthropathy, left elbow CC HCC

MØ2.129 Postdysenteric arthropathy, unspecified elbow CC HCC

✓6th MØ2.13 Postdysenteric arthropathy, wrist

Postdysenteric arthropathy, carpal bones

MØ2.131 Postdysenteric arthropathy, right wrist CC HCC

MØ2.132 Postdysenteric arthropathy, left wrist CC HCC

MØ2.139 Postdysenteric arthropathy, unspecified wrist CC HCC

✓6th MØ2.14 Postdysenteric arthropathy, hand

Postdysenteric arthropathy, metacarpus and phalanges

MØ2.141 Postdysenteric arthropathy, right hand CC HCC

MØ2.142 Postdysenteric arthropathy, left hand CC HCC

MØ2.149 Postdysenteric arthropathy, unspecified hand CC HCC

✓6th MØ2.15 Postdysenteric arthropathy, hip

MØ2.151 Postdysenteric arthropathy, right hip CC HCC

MØ2.152 Postdysenteric arthropathy, left hip CC HCC

MØ2.159 Postdysenteric arthropathy, unspecified hip CC HCC

✓6th MØ2.16 Postdysenteric arthropathy, knee

MØ2.161 Postdysenteric arthropathy, right knee CC HCC

MØ2.162 Postdysenteric arthropathy, left knee CC HCC

MØ2.169 Postdysenteric arthropathy, unspecified knee CC HCC

✓6th MØ2.17 Postdysenteric arthropathy, ankle and foot

Postdysenteric arthropathy, tarsus, metatarsus and phalanges

MØ2.171 Postdysenteric arthropathy, right ankle and foot CC HCC

MØ2.172 Postdysenteric arthropathy, left ankle and foot CC HCC

MØ2.179 Postdysenteric arthropathy, unspecified ankle and foot CC HCC

MØ2.18 Postdysenteric arthropathy, vertebrae CC HCC

MØ2.19 Postdysenteric arthropathy, multiple sites CC HCC

✓5th MØ2.2 Postimmunization arthropathy

MØ2.2Ø Postimmunization arthropathy, unspecified site

✓6th MØ2.21 Postimmunization arthropathy, shoulder

MØ2.211 Postimmunization arthropathy, right shoulder

MØ2.212 Postimmunization arthropathy, left shoulder

MØ2.219 Postimmunization arthropathy, unspecified shoulder

✓6th MØ2.22 Postimmunization arthropathy, elbow

MØ2.221 Postimmunization arthropathy, right elbow

MØ2.222 Postimmunization arthropathy, left elbow

MØ2.229 Postimmunization arthropathy, unspecified elbow

✓6th MØ2.23 Postimmunization arthropathy, wrist

Postimmunization arthropathy, carpal bones

MØ2.231 Postimmunization arthropathy, right wrist

MØ2.232 Postimmunization arthropathy, left wrist

MØ2.239 Postimmunization arthropathy, unspecified wrist

✓6th MØ2.24 Postimmunization arthropathy, hand

Postimmunization arthropathy, metacarpus and phalanges

MØ2.241 Postimmunization arthropathy, right hand

MØ2.242 Postimmunization arthropathy, left hand

MØ2.249 Postimmunization arthropathy, unspecified hand

✓6th MØ2.25 Postimmunization arthropathy, hip

MØ2.251 Postimmunization arthropathy, right hip

MØ2.252 Postimmunization arthropathy, left hip

MØ2.259 Postimmunization arthropathy, unspecified hip

✓6th MØ2.26 Postimmunization arthropathy, knee

MØ2.261 Postimmunization arthropathy, right knee

MØ2.262 Postimmunization arthropathy, left knee

MØ2.269 Postimmunization arthropathy, unspecified knee

✓6th MØ2.27 Postimmunization arthropathy, ankle and foot

Postimmunization arthropathy, tarsus, metatarsus and phalanges

MØ2.271 Postimmunization arthropathy, right ankle and foot

MØ2.272 Postimmunization arthropathy, left ankle and foot

MØ2.279 Postimmunization arthropathy, unspecified ankle and foot

MØ2.28 Postimmunization arthropathy, vertebrae

MØ2.29 Postimmunization arthropathy, multiple sites

✓5th MØ2.3 Reiter's disease

Reactive arthritis

DEF: Arthritis, iridocyclitis, and urethritis, sometimes with diarrhea. While symptoms may recur, arthritis is constant.

MØ2.3Ø Reiter's disease, unspecified site CC HCC

✓6th MØ2.31 Reiter's disease, shoulder

MØ2.311 Reiter's disease, right shoulder CC HCC

MØ2.312 Reiter's disease, left shoulder CC HCC

MØ2.319 Reiter's disease, unspecified shoulder CC HCC

✓6th MØ2.32 Reiter's disease, elbow

MØ2.321 Reiter's disease, right elbow CC HCC

MØ2.322 Reiter's disease, left elbow CC HCC

M02.329 Reiter's disease, unspecified elbow CC HCC

✓6th M02.33 Reiter's disease, wrist

Reiter's disease, carpal bones

M02.331 Reiter's disease, right wrist CC HCC

M02.332 Reiter's disease, left wrist CC HCC

M02.339 Reiter's disease, unspecified wrist CC HCC

✓6th M02.34 Reiter's disease, hand

Reiter's disease, metacarpus and phalanges

M02.341 Reiter's disease, right hand CC HCC

M02.342 Reiter's disease, left hand CC HCC

M02.349 Reiter's disease, unspecified hand CC HCC

✓6th M02.35 Reiter's disease, hip

M02.351 Reiter's disease, right hip CC HCC

M02.352 Reiter's disease, left hip CC HCC

M02.359 Reiter's disease, unspecified hip CC HCC

✓6th M02.36 Reiter's disease, knee

M02.361 Reiter's disease, right knee CC HCC

M02.362 Reiter's disease, left knee CC HCC

M02.369 Reiter's disease, unspecified knee CC HCC

✓6th M02.37 Reiter's disease, ankle and foot

Reiter's disease, tarsus, metatarsus and phalanges

M02.371 Reiter's disease, right ankle and foot CC HCC

M02.372 Reiter's disease, left ankle and foot CC HCC

M02.379 Reiter's disease, unspecified ankle and foot CC HCC

M02.38 Reiter's disease, vertebrae CC HCC

M02.39 Reiter's disease, multiple sites CC HCC

✓5th M02.8 Other reactive arthropathies

M02.80 Other reactive arthropathies, unspecified site CC HCC

✓6th M02.81 Other reactive arthropathies, shoulder

M02.811 Other reactive arthropathies, right shoulder CC HCC

M02.812 Other reactive arthropathies, left shoulder CC HCC

M02.819 Other reactive arthropathies, unspecified shoulder CC HCC

✓6th M02.82 Other reactive arthropathies, elbow

M02.821 Other reactive arthropathies, right elbow CC HCC

M02.822 Other reactive arthropathies, left elbow CC HCC

M02.829 Other reactive arthropathies, unspecified elbow CC HCC

✓6th M02.83 Other reactive arthropathies, wrist

Other reactive arthropathies, carpal bones

M02.831 Other reactive arthropathies, right wrist CC HCC

M02.832 Other reactive arthropathies, left wrist CC HCC

M02.839 Other reactive arthropathies, unspecified wrist CC HCC

✓6th M02.84 Other reactive arthropathies, hand

Other reactive arthropathies, metacarpus and phalanges

M02.841 Other reactive arthropathies, right hand CC HCC

M02.842 Other reactive arthropathies, left hand CC HCC

M02.849 Other reactive arthropathies, unspecified hand CC HCC

✓6th M02.85 Other reactive arthropathies, hip

M02.851 Other reactive arthropathies, right hip CC HCC

M02.852 Other reactive arthropathies, left hip CC HCC

M02.859 Other reactive arthropathies, unspecified hip CC HCC

✓6th M02.86 Other reactive arthropathies, knee

M02.861 Other reactive arthropathies, right knee CC HCC

M02.862 Other reactive arthropathies, left knee CC HCC

M02.869 Other reactive arthropathies, unspecified knee CC HCC

✓6th M02.87 Other reactive arthropathies, ankle and foot

Other reactive arthropathies, tarsus, metatarsus and phalanges

M02.871 Other reactive arthropathies, right ankle and foot CC HCC

M02.872 Other reactive arthropathies, left ankle and foot CC HCC

M02.879 Other reactive arthropathies, unspecified ankle and foot CC HCC

M02.88 Other reactive arthropathies, vertebrae CC HCC

M02.89 Other reactive arthropathies, multiple sites CC HCC

M02.9 Reactive arthropathy, unspecified HCC

Autoinflammatory syndromes (M04)

✓4th M04 Autoinflammatory syndromes

EXCLUDES 2 *Crohn's disease (K50.-)*

AHA: 2016,4Q,37

M04.1 Periodic fever syndromes HCC

Familial Mediterranean fever

Hyperimmunoglobin D syndrome

Mevalonate kinase deficiency

Tumor necrosis factor receptor associated periodic syndrome [TRAPS]

M04.2 Cryopyrin-associated periodic syndromes HCC

Chronic infantile neurological, cutaneous and articular syndrome [CINCA]

Familial cold autoinflammatory syndrome

Familial cold urticaria

Muckle-Wells syndrome

Neonatal onset multisystemic inflammatory disorder [NOMID]

M04.8 Other autoinflammatory syndromes HCC

Blau syndrome

Deficiency of interleukin 1 receptor antagonist [DIRA]

Majeed syndrome

Periodic fever, aphthous stomatitis, pharyngitis, and adenopathy syndrome [PFAPA]

Pyogenic arthritis, pyoderma gangrenosum, and acne syndrome [PAPA]

M04.9 Autoinflammatory syndrome, unspecified HCC

Inflammatory polyarthropathies (M05-M14)

✓4th M05 Rheumatoid arthritis with rheumatoid factor

EXCLUDES 1 *rheumatic fever (I00)*

juvenile rheumatoid arthritis (M08.-)

rheumatoid arthritis of spine (M45.-)

DEF: Rheumatoid arthritis: Autoimmune systemic disease that causes chronic inflammation of the joints and other areas of the body, manifested by inflammatory changes in articular structures and synovial membranes, atrophy, and loss in bone density.

✓5th M05.0 Felty's syndrome

Rheumatoid arthritis with splenoadenomegaly and leukopenia

M05.00 Felty's syndrome, unspecified site HCC

✓6th M05.01 Felty's syndrome, shoulder

M05.011 Felty's syndrome, right shoulder HCC

M05.012 Felty's syndrome, left shoulder HCC

M05.019 Felty's syndrome, unspecified shoulder HCC

✓6th M05.02 Felty's syndrome, elbow

M05.021 Felty's syndrome, right elbow HCC

M05.022 Felty's syndrome, left elbow HCC

M05.029 Felty's syndrome, unspecified elbow HCC

✓6th M05.03 Felty's syndrome, wrist

Felty's syndrome, carpal bones

M05.031 Felty's syndrome, right wrist HCC

M05.032 Felty's syndrome, left wrist HCC

MØ5.Ø39 Felty's syndrome, unspecified wrist HCC

✓6th MØ5.Ø4 Felty's syndrome, hand

Felty's syndrome, metacarpus and phalanges

MØ5.Ø41 Felty's syndrome, right hand HCC

MØ5.Ø42 Felty's syndrome, left hand HCC

MØ5.Ø49 Felty's syndrome, unspecified hand HCC

✓6th MØ5.Ø5 Felty's syndrome, hip

MØ5.Ø51 Felty's syndrome, right hip HCC

MØ5.Ø52 Felty's syndrome, left hip HCC

MØ5.Ø59 Felty's syndrome, unspecified hip HCC

✓6th MØ5.Ø6 Felty's syndrome, knee

MØ5.Ø61 Felty's syndrome, right knee HCC

MØ5.Ø62 Felty's syndrome, left knee HCC

MØ5.Ø69 Felty's syndrome, unspecified knee HCC

✓6th MØ5.Ø7 Felty's syndrome, ankle and foot

Felty's syndrome, tarsus, metatarsus and phalanges

MØ5.Ø71 Felty's syndrome, right ankle and foot HCC

MØ5.Ø72 Felty's syndrome, left ankle and foot HCC

MØ5.Ø79 Felty's syndrome, unspecified ankle and foot HCC

MØ5.Ø9 Felty's syndrome, multiple sites HCC

✓5th MØ5.1 Rheumatoid lung disease with rheumatoid arthritis

DEF: Lung disorders associated with rheumatoid arthritis.

MØ5.1Ø Rheumatoid lung disease with rheumatoid arthritis of unspecified site HCC

✓6th MØ5.11 Rheumatoid lung disease with rheumatoid arthritis of shoulder

MØ5.111 Rheumatoid lung disease with rheumatoid arthritis of right shoulder HCC

MØ5.112 Rheumatoid lung disease with rheumatoid arthritis of left shoulder HCC

MØ5.119 Rheumatoid lung disease with rheumatoid arthritis of unspecified shoulder HCC

✓6th MØ5.12 Rheumatoid lung disease with rheumatoid arthritis of elbow

MØ5.121 Rheumatoid lung disease with rheumatoid arthritis of right elbow HCC

MØ5.122 Rheumatoid lung disease with rheumatoid arthritis of left elbow HCC

MØ5.129 Rheumatoid lung disease with rheumatoid arthritis of unspecified elbow HCC

✓6th MØ5.13 Rheumatoid lung disease with rheumatoid arthritis of wrist

Rheumatoid lung disease with rheumatoid arthritis, carpal bones

MØ5.131 Rheumatoid lung disease with rheumatoid arthritis of right wrist HCC

MØ5.132 Rheumatoid lung disease with rheumatoid arthritis of left wrist HCC

MØ5.139 Rheumatoid lung disease with rheumatoid arthritis of unspecified wrist HCC

✓6th MØ5.14 Rheumatoid lung disease with rheumatoid arthritis of hand

Rheumatoid lung disease with rheumatoid arthritis, metacarpus and phalanges

MØ5.141 Rheumatoid lung disease with rheumatoid arthritis of right hand HCC

MØ5.142 Rheumatoid lung disease with rheumatoid arthritis of left hand HCC

MØ5.149 Rheumatoid lung disease with rheumatoid arthritis of unspecified hand HCC

✓6th MØ5.15 Rheumatoid lung disease with rheumatoid arthritis of hip

MØ5.151 Rheumatoid lung disease with rheumatoid arthritis of right hip HCC

MØ5.152 Rheumatoid lung disease with rheumatoid arthritis of left hip HCC

MØ5.159 Rheumatoid lung disease with rheumatoid arthritis of unspecified hip HCC

✓6th MØ5.16 Rheumatoid lung disease with rheumatoid arthritis of knee

MØ5.161 Rheumatoid lung disease with rheumatoid arthritis of right knee HCC

MØ5.162 Rheumatoid lung disease with rheumatoid arthritis of left knee HCC

MØ5.169 Rheumatoid lung disease with rheumatoid arthritis of unspecified knee HCC

✓6th MØ5.17 Rheumatoid lung disease with rheumatoid arthritis of ankle and foot

Rheumatoid lung disease with rheumatoid arthritis, tarsus, metatarsus and phalanges

MØ5.171 Rheumatoid lung disease with rheumatoid arthritis of right ankle and foot HCC

MØ5.172 Rheumatoid lung disease with rheumatoid arthritis of left ankle and foot HCC

MØ5.179 Rheumatoid lung disease with rheumatoid arthritis of unspecified ankle and foot HCC

MØ5.19 Rheumatoid lung disease with rheumatoid arthritis of multiple sites HCC

✓5th MØ5.2 Rheumatoid vasculitis with rheumatoid arthritis

MØ5.2Ø Rheumatoid vasculitis with rheumatoid arthritis of unspecified site HCC

✓6th MØ5.21 Rheumatoid vasculitis with rheumatoid arthritis of shoulder

MØ5.211 Rheumatoid vasculitis with rheumatoid arthritis of right shoulder HCC

MØ5.212 Rheumatoid vasculitis with rheumatoid arthritis of left shoulder HCC

MØ5.219 Rheumatoid vasculitis with rheumatoid arthritis of unspecified shoulder HCC

✓6th MØ5.22 Rheumatoid vasculitis with rheumatoid arthritis of elbow

MØ5.221 Rheumatoid vasculitis with rheumatoid arthritis of right elbow HCC

MØ5.222 Rheumatoid vasculitis with rheumatoid arthritis of left elbow HCC

MØ5.229 Rheumatoid vasculitis with rheumatoid arthritis of unspecified elbow HCC

✓6th MØ5.23 Rheumatoid vasculitis with rheumatoid arthritis of wrist

Rheumatoid vasculitis with rheumatoid arthritis, carpal bones

MØ5.231 Rheumatoid vasculitis with rheumatoid arthritis of right wrist HCC

MØ5.232 Rheumatoid vasculitis with rheumatoid arthritis of left wrist HCC

MØ5.239 Rheumatoid vasculitis with rheumatoid arthritis of unspecified wrist HCC

✓6th MØ5.24 Rheumatoid vasculitis with rheumatoid arthritis of hand

Rheumatoid vasculitis with rheumatoid arthritis, metacarpus and phalanges

MØ5.241 Rheumatoid vasculitis with rheumatoid arthritis of right hand HCC

MØ5.242 Rheumatoid vasculitis with rheumatoid arthritis of left hand HCC

MØ5.249 Rheumatoid vasculitis with rheumatoid arthritis of unspecified hand HCC

✓6th MØ5.25 Rheumatoid vasculitis with rheumatoid arthritis of hip

MØ5.251 Rheumatoid vasculitis with rheumatoid arthritis of right hip HCC

MØ5.252 Rheumatoid vasculitis with rheumatoid arthritis of left hip HCC

MØ5.259 Rheumatoid vasculitis with rheumatoid arthritis of unspecified hip HCC

✓6th MØ5.26 Rheumatoid vasculitis with rheumatoid arthritis of knee

MØ5.261 Rheumatoid vasculitis with rheumatoid arthritis of right knee HCC

MØ5.262 Rheumatoid vasculitis with rheumatoid arthritis of left knee HCC

M05.269 **Rheumatoid vasculitis with rheumatoid arthritis of unspecified knee** HCC

✓6th **M05.27 Rheumatoid vasculitis with rheumatoid arthritis of ankle and foot**

Rheumatoid vasculitis with rheumatoid arthritis, tarsus, metatarsus and phalanges

M05.271 **Rheumatoid vasculitis with rheumatoid arthritis of right ankle and foot** HCC

M05.272 **Rheumatoid vasculitis with rheumatoid arthritis of left ankle and foot** HCC

M05.279 **Rheumatoid vasculitis with rheumatoid arthritis of unspecified ankle and foot** HCC

M05.29 Rheumatoid vasculitis with rheumatoid arthritis of multiple sites HCC

✓5th **M05.3 Rheumatoid heart disease with rheumatoid arthritis**

Rheumatoid carditis
Rheumatoid endocarditis
Rheumatoid myocarditis
Rheumatoid pericarditis

M05.30 **Rheumatoid heart disease with rheumatoid arthritis of unspecified site** HCC

✓6th **M05.31 Rheumatoid heart disease with rheumatoid arthritis of shoulder**

M05.311 **Rheumatoid heart disease with rheumatoid arthritis of right shoulder** HCC

M05.312 **Rheumatoid heart disease with rheumatoid arthritis of left shoulder** HCC

M05.319 **Rheumatoid heart disease with rheumatoid arthritis of unspecified shoulder** HCC

✓6th **M05.32 Rheumatoid heart disease with rheumatoid arthritis of elbow**

M05.321 **Rheumatoid heart disease with rheumatoid arthritis of right elbow** HCC

M05.322 **Rheumatoid heart disease with rheumatoid arthritis of left elbow** HCC

M05.329 **Rheumatoid heart disease with rheumatoid arthritis of unspecified elbow** HCC

✓6th **M05.33 Rheumatoid heart disease with rheumatoid arthritis of wrist**

Rheumatoid heart disease with rheumatoid arthritis, carpal bones

M05.331 **Rheumatoid heart disease with rheumatoid arthritis of right wrist** HCC

M05.332 **Rheumatoid heart disease with rheumatoid arthritis of left wrist** HCC

M05.339 **Rheumatoid heart disease with rheumatoid arthritis of unspecified wrist** HCC

✓6th **M05.34 Rheumatoid heart disease with rheumatoid arthritis of hand**

Rheumatoid heart disease with rheumatoid arthritis, metacarpus and phalanges

M05.341 **Rheumatoid heart disease with rheumatoid arthritis of right hand** HCC

M05.342 **Rheumatoid heart disease with rheumatoid arthritis of left hand** HCC

M05.349 **Rheumatoid heart disease with rheumatoid arthritis of unspecified hand** HCC

✓6th **M05.35 Rheumatoid heart disease with rheumatoid arthritis of hip**

M05.351 **Rheumatoid heart disease with rheumatoid arthritis of right hip** HCC

M05.352 **Rheumatoid heart disease with rheumatoid arthritis of left hip** HCC

M05.359 **Rheumatoid heart disease with rheumatoid arthritis of unspecified hip** HCC

✓6th **M05.36 Rheumatoid heart disease with rheumatoid arthritis of knee**

M05.361 **Rheumatoid heart disease with rheumatoid arthritis of right knee** HCC

M05.362 **Rheumatoid heart disease with rheumatoid arthritis of left knee** HCC

M05.369 **Rheumatoid heart disease with rheumatoid arthritis of unspecified knee** HCC

✓6th **M05.37 Rheumatoid heart disease with rheumatoid arthritis of ankle and foot**

Rheumatoid heart disease with rheumatoid arthritis, tarsus, metatarsus and phalanges

M05.371 **Rheumatoid heart disease with rheumatoid arthritis of right ankle and foot** HCC

M05.372 **Rheumatoid heart disease with rheumatoid arthritis of left ankle and foot** HCC

M05.379 **Rheumatoid heart disease with rheumatoid arthritis of unspecified ankle and foot** HCC

M05.39 Rheumatoid heart disease with rheumatoid arthritis of multiple sites HCC

✓5th **M05.4 Rheumatoid myopathy with rheumatoid arthritis**

M05.40 **Rheumatoid myopathy with rheumatoid arthritis of unspecified site** CC HCC

✓6th **M05.41 Rheumatoid myopathy with rheumatoid arthritis of shoulder**

M05.411 **Rheumatoid myopathy with rheumatoid arthritis of right shoulder** CC HCC

M05.412 **Rheumatoid myopathy with rheumatoid arthritis of left shoulder** CC HCC

M05.419 **Rheumatoid myopathy with rheumatoid arthritis of unspecified shoulder** CC HCC

✓6th **M05.42 Rheumatoid myopathy with rheumatoid arthritis of elbow**

M05.421 **Rheumatoid myopathy with rheumatoid arthritis of right elbow** CC HCC

M05.422 **Rheumatoid myopathy with rheumatoid arthritis of left elbow** CC HCC

M05.429 **Rheumatoid myopathy with rheumatoid arthritis of unspecified elbow** CC HCC

✓6th **M05.43 Rheumatoid myopathy with rheumatoid arthritis of wrist**

Rheumatoid myopathy with rheumatoid arthritis, carpal bones

M05.431 **Rheumatoid myopathy with rheumatoid arthritis of right wrist** CC HCC

M05.432 **Rheumatoid myopathy with rheumatoid arthritis of left wrist** CC HCC

M05.439 **Rheumatoid myopathy with rheumatoid arthritis of unspecified wrist** CC HCC

✓6th **M05.44 Rheumatoid myopathy with rheumatoid arthritis of hand**

Rheumatoid myopathy with rheumatoid arthritis, metacarpus and phalanges

M05.441 **Rheumatoid myopathy with rheumatoid arthritis of right hand** CC HCC

M05.442 **Rheumatoid myopathy with rheumatoid arthritis of left hand** CC HCC

M05.449 **Rheumatoid myopathy with rheumatoid arthritis of unspecified hand** CC HCC

✓6th **M05.45 Rheumatoid myopathy with rheumatoid arthritis of hip**

M05.451 **Rheumatoid myopathy with rheumatoid arthritis of right hip** CC HCC

M05.452 **Rheumatoid myopathy with rheumatoid arthritis of left hip** CC HCC

M05.459 **Rheumatoid myopathy with rheumatoid arthritis of unspecified hip** CC HCC

✓6th **M05.46 Rheumatoid myopathy with rheumatoid arthritis of knee**

M05.461 **Rheumatoid myopathy with rheumatoid arthritis of right knee** CC HCC

M05.462 **Rheumatoid myopathy with rheumatoid arthritis of left knee** CC HCC

M05.469 **Rheumatoid myopathy with rheumatoid arthritis of unspecified knee** CC HCC

✓6th **M05.47 Rheumatoid myopathy with rheumatoid arthritis of ankle and foot**

Rheumatoid myopathy with rheumatoid arthritis, tarsus, metatarsus and phalanges

M05.471 **Rheumatoid myopathy with rheumatoid arthritis of right ankle and foot** CC HCC

MØ5.472 Rheumatoid myopathy with rheumatoid arthritis of left ankle and foot CC HCC
MØ5.479 Rheumatoid myopathy with rheumatoid arthritis of unspecified ankle and foot CC HCC
MØ5.49 Rheumatoid myopathy with rheumatoid arthritis of multiple sites CC HCC
✓5th MØ5.5 Rheumatoid polyneuropathy with rheumatoid arthritis
MØ5.5Ø Rheumatoid polyneuropathy with rheumatoid arthritis of unspecified site HCC
✓6th MØ5.51 Rheumatoid polyneuropathy with rheumatoid arthritis of shoulder
MØ5.511 Rheumatoid polyneuropathy with rheumatoid arthritis of right shoulder HCC
MØ5.512 Rheumatoid polyneuropathy with rheumatoid arthritis of left shoulder HCC
MØ5.519 Rheumatoid polyneuropathy with rheumatoid arthritis of unspecified shoulder HCC
✓6th MØ5.52 Rheumatoid polyneuropathy with rheumatoid arthritis of elbow
MØ5.521 Rheumatoid polyneuropathy with rheumatoid arthritis of right elbow HCC
MØ5.522 Rheumatoid polyneuropathy with rheumatoid arthritis of left elbow HCC
MØ5.529 Rheumatoid polyneuropathy with rheumatoid arthritis of unspecified elbow HCC
✓6th MØ5.53 Rheumatoid polyneuropathy with rheumatoid arthritis of wrist
Rheumatoid polyneuropathy with rheumatoid arthritis, carpal bones
MØ5.531 Rheumatoid polyneuropathy with rheumatoid arthritis of right wrist HCC
MØ5.532 Rheumatoid polyneuropathy with rheumatoid arthritis of left wrist HCC
MØ5.539 Rheumatoid polyneuropathy with rheumatoid arthritis of unspecified wrist HCC
✓6th MØ5.54 Rheumatoid polyneuropathy with rheumatoid arthritis of hand
Rheumatoid polyneuropathy with rheumatoid arthritis, metacarpus and phalanges
MØ5.541 Rheumatoid polyneuropathy with rheumatoid arthritis of right hand HCC
MØ5.542 Rheumatoid polyneuropathy with rheumatoid arthritis of left hand HCC
MØ5.549 Rheumatoid polyneuropathy with rheumatoid arthritis of unspecified hand HCC
✓6th MØ5.55 Rheumatoid polyneuropathy with rheumatoid arthritis of hip
MØ5.551 Rheumatoid polyneuropathy with rheumatoid arthritis of right hip HCC
MØ5.552 Rheumatoid polyneuropathy with rheumatoid arthritis of left hip HCC
MØ5.559 Rheumatoid polyneuropathy with rheumatoid arthritis of unspecified hip HCC
✓6th MØ5.56 Rheumatoid polyneuropathy with rheumatoid arthritis of knee
MØ5.561 Rheumatoid polyneuropathy with rheumatoid arthritis of right knee HCC
MØ5.562 Rheumatoid polyneuropathy with rheumatoid arthritis of left knee HCC
MØ5.569 Rheumatoid polyneuropathy with rheumatoid arthritis of unspecified knee HCC
✓6th MØ5.57 Rheumatoid polyneuropathy with rheumatoid arthritis of ankle and foot
Rheumatoid polyneuropathy with rheumatoid arthritis, tarsus, metatarsus and phalanges
MØ5.571 Rheumatoid polyneuropathy with rheumatoid arthritis of right ankle and foot HCC
MØ5.572 Rheumatoid polyneuropathy with rheumatoid arthritis of left ankle and foot HCC
MØ5.579 Rheumatoid polyneuropathy with rheumatoid arthritis of unspecified ankle and foot HCC
MØ5.59 Rheumatoid polyneuropathy with rheumatoid arthritis of multiple sites HCC
✓5th MØ5.6 Rheumatoid arthritis with involvement of other organs and systems
MØ5.6Ø Rheumatoid arthritis of unspecified site with involvement of other organs and systems HCC
✓6th MØ5.61 Rheumatoid arthritis of shoulder with involvement of other organs and systems
MØ5.611 Rheumatoid arthritis of right shoulder with involvement of other organs and systems HCC
MØ5.612 Rheumatoid arthritis of left shoulder with involvement of other organs and systems HCC
MØ5.619 Rheumatoid arthritis of unspecified shoulder with involvement of other organs and systems HCC
✓6th MØ5.62 Rheumatoid arthritis of elbow with involvement of other organs and systems
MØ5.621 Rheumatoid arthritis of right elbow with involvement of other organs and systems HCC
MØ5.622 Rheumatoid arthritis of left elbow with involvement of other organs and systems HCC
MØ5.629 Rheumatoid arthritis of unspecified elbow with involvement of other organs and systems HCC
✓6th MØ5.63 Rheumatoid arthritis of wrist with involvement of other organs and systems
Rheumatoid arthritis of carpal bones with involvement of other organs and systems
MØ5.631 Rheumatoid arthritis of right wrist with involvement of other organs and systems HCC
MØ5.632 Rheumatoid arthritis of left wrist with involvement of other organs and systems HCC
MØ5.639 Rheumatoid arthritis of unspecified wrist with involvement of other organs and systems HCC
✓6th MØ5.64 Rheumatoid arthritis of hand with involvement of other organs and systems
Rheumatoid arthritis of metacarpus and phalanges with involvement of other organs and systems
MØ5.641 Rheumatoid arthritis of right hand with involvement of other organs and systems HCC
MØ5.642 Rheumatoid arthritis of left hand with involvement of other organs and systems HCC
MØ5.649 Rheumatoid arthritis of unspecified hand with involvement of other organs and systems HCC
✓6th MØ5.65 Rheumatoid arthritis of hip with involvement of other organs and systems
MØ5.651 Rheumatoid arthritis of right hip with involvement of other organs and systems HCC
MØ5.652 Rheumatoid arthritis of left hip with involvement of other organs and systems HCC
MØ5.659 Rheumatoid arthritis of unspecified hip with involvement of other organs and systems HCC
✓6th MØ5.66 Rheumatoid arthritis of knee with involvement of other organs and systems
MØ5.661 Rheumatoid arthritis of right knee with involvement of other organs and systems HCC
MØ5.662 Rheumatoid arthritis of left knee with involvement of other organs and systems HCC
MØ5.669 Rheumatoid arthritis of unspecified knee with involvement of other organs and systems HCC

✓6th **MØ5.67 Rheumatoid arthritis of ankle and foot with involvement of other organs and systems**
Rheumatoid arthritis of tarsus, metatarsus and phalanges with involvement of other organs and systems

MØ5.671 Rheumatoid arthritis of right ankle and foot with involvement of other organs and systems HCC

MØ5.672 Rheumatoid arthritis of left ankle and foot with involvement of other organs and systems HCC

MØ5.679 Rheumatoid arthritis of unspecified ankle and foot with involvement of other organs and systems HCC

MØ5.69 Rheumatoid arthritis of multiple sites with involvement of other organs and systems HCC

✓5th **MØ5.7 Rheumatoid arthritis with rheumatoid factor without organ or systems involvement**

MØ5.7Ø Rheumatoid arthritis with rheumatoid factor of unspecified site without organ or systems involvement HCC

✓6th **MØ5.71 Rheumatoid arthritis with rheumatoid factor of shoulder without organ or systems involvement**

MØ5.711 Rheumatoid arthritis with rheumatoid factor of right shoulder without organ or systems involvement HCC

MØ5.712 Rheumatoid arthritis with rheumatoid factor of left shoulder without organ or systems involvement HCC

MØ5.719 Rheumatoid arthritis with rheumatoid factor of unspecified shoulder without organ or systems involvement HCC

✓6th **MØ5.72 Rheumatoid arthritis with rheumatoid factor of elbow without organ or systems involvement**

MØ5.721 Rheumatoid arthritis with rheumatoid factor of right elbow without organ or systems involvement HCC

MØ5.722 Rheumatoid arthritis with rheumatoid factor of left elbow without organ or systems involvement HCC

MØ5.729 Rheumatoid arthritis with rheumatoid factor of unspecified elbow without organ or systems involvement HCC

✓6th **MØ5.73 Rheumatoid arthritis with rheumatoid factor of wrist without organ or systems involvement**

MØ5.731 Rheumatoid arthritis with rheumatoid factor of right wrist without organ or systems involvement HCC

MØ5.732 Rheumatoid arthritis with rheumatoid factor of left wrist without organ or systems involvement HCC

MØ5.739 Rheumatoid arthritis with rheumatoid factor of unspecified wrist without organ or systems involvement HCC

✓6th **MØ5.74 Rheumatoid arthritis with rheumatoid factor of hand without organ or systems involvement**

MØ5.741 Rheumatoid arthritis with rheumatoid factor of right hand without organ or systems involvement HCC

MØ5.742 Rheumatoid arthritis with rheumatoid factor of left hand without organ or systems involvement HCC

MØ5.749 Rheumatoid arthritis with rheumatoid factor of unspecified hand without organ or systems involvement HCC

✓6th **MØ5.75 Rheumatoid arthritis with rheumatoid factor of hip without organ or systems involvement**

MØ5.751 Rheumatoid arthritis with rheumatoid factor of right hip without organ or systems involvement HCC

MØ5.752 Rheumatoid arthritis with rheumatoid factor of left hip without organ or systems involvement HCC

MØ5.759 Rheumatoid arthritis with rheumatoid factor of unspecified hip without organ or systems involvement HCC

✓6th **MØ5.76 Rheumatoid arthritis with rheumatoid factor of knee without organ or systems involvement**

MØ5.761 Rheumatoid arthritis with rheumatoid factor of right knee without organ or systems involvement HCC

MØ5.762 Rheumatoid arthritis with rheumatoid factor of left knee without organ or systems involvement HCC

MØ5.769 Rheumatoid arthritis with rheumatoid factor of unspecified knee without organ or systems involvement HCC

✓6th **MØ5.77 Rheumatoid arthritis with rheumatoid factor of ankle and foot without organ or systems involvement**

MØ5.771 Rheumatoid arthritis with rheumatoid factor of right ankle and foot without organ or systems involvement HCC

MØ5.772 Rheumatoid arthritis with rheumatoid factor of left ankle and foot without organ or systems involvement HCC

MØ5.779 Rheumatoid arthritis with rheumatoid factor of unspecified ankle and foot without organ or systems involvement HCC

MØ5.79 Rheumatoid arthritis with rheumatoid factor of multiple sites without organ or systems involvement HCC

● **MØ5.7A Rheumatoid arthritis with rheumatoid factor of other specified site without organ or systems involvement**

✓5th **MØ5.8 Other rheumatoid arthritis with rheumatoid factor**

MØ5.8Ø Other rheumatoid arthritis with rheumatoid factor of unspecified site HCC

✓6th **MØ5.81 Other rheumatoid arthritis with rheumatoid factor of shoulder**

MØ5.811 Other rheumatoid arthritis with rheumatoid factor of right shoulder HCC

MØ5.812 Other rheumatoid arthritis with rheumatoid factor of left shoulder HCC

MØ5.819 Other rheumatoid arthritis with rheumatoid factor of unspecified shoulder HCC

✓6th **MØ5.82 Other rheumatoid arthritis with rheumatoid factor of elbow**

MØ5.821 Other rheumatoid arthritis with rheumatoid factor of right elbow HCC

MØ5.822 Other rheumatoid arthritis with rheumatoid factor of left elbow HCC

MØ5.829 Other rheumatoid arthritis with rheumatoid factor of unspecified elbow HCC

✓6th **MØ5.83 Other rheumatoid arthritis with rheumatoid factor of wrist**

MØ5.831 Other rheumatoid arthritis with rheumatoid factor of right wrist HCC

MØ5.832 Other rheumatoid arthritis with rheumatoid factor of left wrist HCC

MØ5.839 Other rheumatoid arthritis with rheumatoid factor of unspecified wrist HCC

✓6th **MØ5.84 Other rheumatoid arthritis with rheumatoid factor of hand**

MØ5.841 Other rheumatoid arthritis with rheumatoid factor of right hand HCC

MØ5.842 Other rheumatoid arthritis with rheumatoid factor of left hand HCC

MØ5.849 Other rheumatoid arthritis with rheumatoid factor of unspecified hand HCC

✓6th **MØ5.85 Other rheumatoid arthritis with rheumatoid factor of hip**

MØ5.851 Other rheumatoid arthritis with rheumatoid factor of right hip HCC

MØ5.852 Other rheumatoid arthritis with rheumatoid factor of left hip HCC

MØ5.859 Other rheumatoid arthritis with rheumatoid factor of unspecified hip HCC

✓6th **MØ5.86 Other rheumatoid arthritis with rheumatoid factor of knee**

MØ5.861 Other rheumatoid arthritis with rheumatoid factor of right knee HCC

MØ5.862 Other rheumatoid arthritis with rheumatoid factor of left knee HCC

M05.869 Other rheumatoid arthritis with rheumatoid factor of unspecified knee HCC

6th M05.87 Other rheumatoid arthritis with rheumatoid factor of ankle and foot

M05.871 Other rheumatoid arthritis with rheumatoid factor of right ankle and foot HCC

M05.872 Other rheumatoid arthritis with rheumatoid factor of left ankle and foot HCC

M05.879 Other rheumatoid arthritis with rheumatoid factor of unspecified ankle and foot HCC

M05.89 Other rheumatoid arthritis with rheumatoid factor of multiple sites HCC

● M05.8A Other rheumatoid arthritis with rheumatoid factor of other specified site

M05.9 Rheumatoid arthritis with rheumatoid factor, unspecified HCC

4th M06 Other rheumatoid arthritis

DEF: Rheumatoid arthritis: Autoimmune systemic disease that causes chronic inflammation of the joints and other areas of the body, manifested by inflammatory changes in articular structures and synovial membranes, atrophy, and loss in bone density.

5th M06.0 Rheumatoid arthritis without rheumatoid factor

M06.00 Rheumatoid arthritis without rheumatoid factor, unspecified site HCC

6th M06.01 Rheumatoid arthritis without rheumatoid factor, shoulder

M06.011 Rheumatoid arthritis without rheumatoid factor, right shoulder HCC

M06.012 Rheumatoid arthritis without rheumatoid factor, left shoulder HCC

M06.019 Rheumatoid arthritis without rheumatoid factor, unspecified shoulder HCC

6th M06.02 Rheumatoid arthritis without rheumatoid factor, elbow

M06.021 Rheumatoid arthritis without rheumatoid factor, right elbow HCC

M06.022 Rheumatoid arthritis without rheumatoid factor, left elbow HCC

M06.029 Rheumatoid arthritis without rheumatoid factor, unspecified elbow HCC

6th M06.03 Rheumatoid arthritis without rheumatoid factor, wrist

M06.031 Rheumatoid arthritis without rheumatoid factor, right wrist HCC

M06.032 Rheumatoid arthritis without rheumatoid factor, left wrist HCC

M06.039 Rheumatoid arthritis without rheumatoid factor, unspecified wrist HCC

6th M06.04 Rheumatoid arthritis without rheumatoid factor, hand

M06.041 Rheumatoid arthritis without rheumatoid factor, right hand HCC

M06.042 Rheumatoid arthritis without rheumatoid factor, left hand HCC

M06.049 Rheumatoid arthritis without rheumatoid factor, unspecified hand HCC

6th M06.05 Rheumatoid arthritis without rheumatoid factor, hip

M06.051 Rheumatoid arthritis without rheumatoid factor, right hip HCC

M06.052 Rheumatoid arthritis without rheumatoid factor, left hip HCC

M06.059 Rheumatoid arthritis without rheumatoid factor, unspecified hip HCC

6th M06.06 Rheumatoid arthritis without rheumatoid factor, knee

M06.061 Rheumatoid arthritis without rheumatoid factor, right knee HCC

M06.062 Rheumatoid arthritis without rheumatoid factor, left knee HCC

M06.069 Rheumatoid arthritis without rheumatoid factor, unspecified knee HCC

6th M06.07 Rheumatoid arthritis without rheumatoid factor, ankle and foot

M06.071 Rheumatoid arthritis without rheumatoid factor, right ankle and foot HCC

M06.072 Rheumatoid arthritis without rheumatoid factor, left ankle and foot HCC

M06.079 Rheumatoid arthritis without rheumatoid factor, unspecified ankle and foot HCC

M06.08 Rheumatoid arthritis without rheumatoid factor, vertebrae HCC

M06.09 Rheumatoid arthritis without rheumatoid factor, multiple sites HCC

● M06.0A Rheumatoid arthritis without rheumatoid factor, other specified site

M06.1 Adult-onset Still's disease HCC A

EXCLUDES 1 *Still's disease NOS (M08.2-)*

DEF: Type of systemic arthritis characterized by a transient rash and spiking fevers. This condition may resolve or develop into a chronic condition and may affect internal organs, as well as joints.

Synonym(s): *AOSD*

5th M06.2 Rheumatoid bursitis

M06.20 Rheumatoid bursitis, unspecified site HCC

6th M06.21 Rheumatoid bursitis, shoulder

M06.211 Rheumatoid bursitis, right shoulder HCC

M06.212 Rheumatoid bursitis, left shoulder HCC

M06.219 Rheumatoid bursitis, unspecified shoulder HCC

6th M06.22 Rheumatoid bursitis, elbow

M06.221 Rheumatoid bursitis, right elbow HCC

M06.222 Rheumatoid bursitis, left elbow HCC

M06.229 Rheumatoid bursitis, unspecified elbow HCC

6th M06.23 Rheumatoid bursitis, wrist

M06.231 Rheumatoid bursitis, right wrist HCC

M06.232 Rheumatoid bursitis, left wrist HCC

M06.239 Rheumatoid bursitis, unspecified wrist HCC

6th M06.24 Rheumatoid bursitis, hand

M06.241 Rheumatoid bursitis, right hand HCC

M06.242 Rheumatoid bursitis, left hand HCC

M06.249 Rheumatoid bursitis, unspecified hand HCC

6th M06.25 Rheumatoid bursitis, hip

M06.251 Rheumatoid bursitis, right hip HCC

M06.252 Rheumatoid bursitis, left hip HCC

M06.259 Rheumatoid bursitis, unspecified hip HCC

6th M06.26 Rheumatoid bursitis, knee

M06.261 Rheumatoid bursitis, right knee HCC

M06.262 Rheumatoid bursitis, left knee HCC

M06.269 Rheumatoid bursitis, unspecified knee HCC

6th M06.27 Rheumatoid bursitis, ankle and foot

M06.271 Rheumatoid bursitis, right ankle and foot HCC

M06.272 Rheumatoid bursitis, left ankle and foot HCC

M06.279 Rheumatoid bursitis, unspecified ankle and foot HCC

M06.28 Rheumatoid bursitis, vertebrae HCC

M06.29 Rheumatoid bursitis, multiple sites HCC

5th M06.3 Rheumatoid nodule

M06.30 Rheumatoid nodule, unspecified site HCC

6th M06.31 Rheumatoid nodule, shoulder

M06.311 Rheumatoid nodule, right shoulder HCC

M06.312 Rheumatoid nodule, left shoulder HCC

M06.319 Rheumatoid nodule, unspecified shoulder HCC

6th M06.32 Rheumatoid nodule, elbow

M06.321 Rheumatoid nodule, right elbow HCC

M06.322 Rheumatoid nodule, left elbow HCC

M06.329 Rheumatoid nodule, unspecified elbow HCC

6th M06.33 Rheumatoid nodule, wrist

M06.331 Rheumatoid nodule, right wrist HCC

M06.332 Rheumatoid nodule, left wrist HCC

M06.339 Rheumatoid nodule, unspecified wrist HCC

M06.34 Rheumatoid nodule, hand
M06.341 Rheumatoid nodule, right hand HCC
M06.342 Rheumatoid nodule, left hand HCC
M06.349 Rheumatoid nodule, unspecified hand HCC
M06.35 Rheumatoid nodule, hip
M06.351 Rheumatoid nodule, right hip HCC
M06.352 Rheumatoid nodule, left hip HCC
M06.359 Rheumatoid nodule, unspecified hip HCC
M06.36 Rheumatoid nodule, knee
M06.361 Rheumatoid nodule, right knee HCC
M06.362 Rheumatoid nodule, left knee HCC
M06.369 Rheumatoid nodule, unspecified knee HCC
M06.37 Rheumatoid nodule, ankle and foot
M06.371 Rheumatoid nodule, right ankle and foot HCC
M06.372 Rheumatoid nodule, left ankle and foot HCC
M06.379 Rheumatoid nodule, unspecified ankle and foot HCC
M06.38 Rheumatoid nodule, vertebrae HCC
M06.39 Rheumatoid nodule, multiple sites HCC
M06.4 Inflammatory polyarthropathy HCC
EXCLUDES 1 *polyarthritis NOS (M13.0)*
M06.8 Other specified rheumatoid arthritis
M06.80 Other specified rheumatoid arthritis, unspecified site HCC
M06.81 Other specified rheumatoid arthritis, shoulder
M06.811 Other specified rheumatoid arthritis, right shoulder HCC
M06.812 Other specified rheumatoid arthritis, left shoulder HCC
M06.819 Other specified rheumatoid arthritis, unspecified shoulder HCC
M06.82 Other specified rheumatoid arthritis, elbow
M06.821 Other specified rheumatoid arthritis, right elbow HCC
M06.822 Other specified rheumatoid arthritis, left elbow HCC
M06.829 Other specified rheumatoid arthritis, unspecified elbow HCC
M06.83 Other specified rheumatoid arthritis, wrist
M06.831 Other specified rheumatoid arthritis, right wrist HCC
M06.832 Other specified rheumatoid arthritis, left wrist HCC
M06.839 Other specified rheumatoid arthritis, unspecified wrist HCC
M06.84 Other specified rheumatoid arthritis, hand
M06.841 Other specified rheumatoid arthritis, right hand HCC
M06.842 Other specified rheumatoid arthritis, left hand HCC
M06.849 Other specified rheumatoid arthritis, unspecified hand HCC
M06.85 Other specified rheumatoid arthritis, hip
M06.851 Other specified rheumatoid arthritis, right hip HCC
M06.852 Other specified rheumatoid arthritis, left hip HCC
M06.859 Other specified rheumatoid arthritis, unspecified hip HCC
M06.86 Other specified rheumatoid arthritis, knee
M06.861 Other specified rheumatoid arthritis, right knee HCC
M06.862 Other specified rheumatoid arthritis, left knee HCC
M06.869 Other specified rheumatoid arthritis, unspecified knee HCC
M06.87 Other specified rheumatoid arthritis, ankle and foot
M06.871 Other specified rheumatoid arthritis, right ankle and foot HCC
M06.872 Other specified rheumatoid arthritis, left ankle and foot HCC
M06.879 Other specified rheumatoid arthritis, unspecified ankle and foot HCC
M06.88 Other specified rheumatoid arthritis, vertebrae HCC
M06.89 Other specified rheumatoid arthritis, multiple sites HCC
● M06.8A Other specified rheumatoid arthritis, other specified site
M06.9 Rheumatoid arthritis, unspecified HCC

M07 Enteropathic arthropathies

Code also associated enteropathy, such as:
regional enteritis [Crohn's disease] (K50.-)
ulcerative colitis (K51.-)
EXCLUDES 1 *psoriatic arthropathies (L40.5-)*

M07.6 Enteropathic arthropathies
M07.60 Enteropathic arthropathies, unspecified site
M07.61 Enteropathic arthropathies, shoulder
M07.611 Enteropathic arthropathies, right shoulder
M07.612 Enteropathic arthropathies, left shoulder
M07.619 Enteropathic arthropathies, unspecified shoulder
M07.62 Enteropathic arthropathies, elbow
M07.621 Enteropathic arthropathies, right elbow
M07.622 Enteropathic arthropathies, left elbow
M07.629 Enteropathic arthropathies, unspecified elbow
M07.63 Enteropathic arthropathies, wrist
M07.631 Enteropathic arthropathies, right wrist
M07.632 Enteropathic arthropathies, left wrist
M07.639 Enteropathic arthropathies, unspecified wrist
M07.64 Enteropathic arthropathies, hand
M07.641 Enteropathic arthropathies, right hand
M07.642 Enteropathic arthropathies, left hand
M07.649 Enteropathic arthropathies, unspecified hand
M07.65 Enteropathic arthropathies, hip
M07.651 Enteropathic arthropathies, right hip
M07.652 Enteropathic arthropathies, left hip
M07.659 Enteropathic arthropathies, unspecified hip
M07.66 Enteropathic arthropathies, knee
M07.661 Enteropathic arthropathies, right knee
M07.662 Enteropathic arthropathies, left knee
M07.669 Enteropathic arthropathies, unspecified knee
M07.67 Enteropathic arthropathies, ankle and foot
M07.671 Enteropathic arthropathies, right ankle and foot
M07.672 Enteropathic arthropathies, left ankle and foot
M07.679 Enteropathic arthropathies, unspecified ankle and foot
M07.68 Enteropathic arthropathies, vertebrae
M07.69 Enteropathic arthropathies, multiple sites

M08 Juvenile arthritis

Code also any associated underlying condition, such as:
regional enteritis [Crohn's disease] (K50.-)
ulcerative colitis (K51.-)
EXCLUDES 1 *arthropathy in Whipple's disease (M14.8)*
Felty's syndrome (M05.0)
juvenile dermatomyositis (M33.0-)
psoriatic juvenile arthropathy (L40.54)

M08.0 Unspecified juvenile rheumatoid arthritis
Juvenile rheumatoid arthritis with or without rheumatoid factor
M08.00 Unspecified juvenile rheumatoid arthritis of unspecified site HCC
M08.01 Unspecified juvenile rheumatoid arthritis, shoulder
M08.011 Unspecified juvenile rheumatoid arthritis, right shoulder HCC
M08.012 Unspecified juvenile rheumatoid arthritis, left shoulder HCC
M08.019 Unspecified juvenile rheumatoid arthritis, unspecified shoulder HCC

√6th **MØ8.Ø2 Unspecified juvenile rheumatoid arthritis of elbow**
- **MØ8.Ø21 Unspecified juvenile rheumatoid arthritis, right elbow** HCC
- **MØ8.Ø22 Unspecified juvenile rheumatoid arthritis, left elbow** HCC
- **MØ8.Ø29 Unspecified juvenile rheumatoid arthritis, unspecified elbow** HCC

√6th **MØ8.Ø3 Unspecified juvenile rheumatoid arthritis, wrist**
- **MØ8.Ø31 Unspecified juvenile rheumatoid arthritis, right wrist** HCC
- **MØ8.Ø32 Unspecified juvenile rheumatoid arthritis, left wrist** HCC
- **MØ8.Ø39 Unspecified juvenile rheumatoid arthritis, unspecified wrist** HCC

√6th **MØ8.Ø4 Unspecified juvenile rheumatoid arthritis, hand**
- **MØ8.Ø41 Unspecified juvenile rheumatoid arthritis, right hand** HCC
- **MØ8.Ø42 Unspecified juvenile rheumatoid arthritis, left hand** HCC
- **MØ8.Ø49 Unspecified juvenile rheumatoid arthritis, unspecified hand** HCC

√6th **MØ8.Ø5 Unspecified juvenile rheumatoid arthritis, hip**
- **MØ8.Ø51 Unspecified juvenile rheumatoid arthritis, right hip** HCC
- **MØ8.Ø52 Unspecified juvenile rheumatoid arthritis, left hip** HCC
- **MØ8.Ø59 Unspecified juvenile rheumatoid arthritis, unspecified hip** HCC

√6th **MØ8.Ø6 Unspecified juvenile rheumatoid arthritis, knee**
- **MØ8.Ø61 Unspecified juvenile rheumatoid arthritis, right knee** HCC
- **MØ8.Ø62 Unspecified juvenile rheumatoid arthritis, left knee** HCC
- **MØ8.Ø69 Unspecified juvenile rheumatoid arthritis, unspecified knee** HCC

√6th **MØ8.Ø7 Unspecified juvenile rheumatoid arthritis, ankle and foot**
- **MØ8.Ø71 Unspecified juvenile rheumatoid arthritis, right ankle and foot** HCC
- **MØ8.Ø72 Unspecified juvenile rheumatoid arthritis, left ankle and foot** HCC
- **MØ8.Ø79 Unspecified juvenile rheumatoid arthritis, unspecified ankle and foot** HCC

MØ8.Ø8 Unspecified juvenile rheumatoid arthritis, vertebrae HCC

MØ8.Ø9 Unspecified juvenile rheumatoid arthritis, multiple sites HCC

● **MØ8.ØA Unspecified juvenile rheumatoid arthritis, other specified site**

MØ8.1 Juvenile ankylosing spondylitis HCC

EXCLUDES 1 *ankylosing spondylitis in adults (M45.Ø-)*

√5th **MØ8.2 Juvenile rheumatoid arthritis with systemic onset**

Still's disease NOS

EXCLUDES 1 *adult-onset Still's disease (MØ6.1-)*

DEF: Systemic juvenile rheumatoid arthritis characterized by a transient rash and spiking fevers that may affect internal organs, as well as joints.

MØ8.2Ø Juvenile rheumatoid arthritis with systemic onset, unspecified site HCC

√6th **MØ8.21 Juvenile rheumatoid arthritis with systemic onset, shoulder**
- **MØ8.211 Juvenile rheumatoid arthritis with systemic onset, right shoulder** HCC
- **MØ8.212 Juvenile rheumatoid arthritis with systemic onset, left shoulder** HCC
- **MØ8.219 Juvenile rheumatoid arthritis with systemic onset, unspecified shoulder** HCC

√6th **MØ8.22 Juvenile rheumatoid arthritis with systemic onset, elbow**
- **MØ8.221 Juvenile rheumatoid arthritis with systemic onset, right elbow** HCC
- **MØ8.222 Juvenile rheumatoid arthritis with systemic onset, left elbow** HCC
- **MØ8.229 Juvenile rheumatoid arthritis with systemic onset, unspecified elbow** HCC

√6th **MØ8.23 Juvenile rheumatoid arthritis with systemic onset, wrist**
- **MØ8.231 Juvenile rheumatoid arthritis with systemic onset, right wrist** HCC
- **MØ8.232 Juvenile rheumatoid arthritis with systemic onset, left wrist** HCC
- **MØ8.239 Juvenile rheumatoid arthritis with systemic onset, unspecified wrist** HCC

√6th **MØ8.24 Juvenile rheumatoid arthritis with systemic onset, hand**
- **MØ8.241 Juvenile rheumatoid arthritis with systemic onset, right hand** HCC
- **MØ8.242 Juvenile rheumatoid arthritis with systemic onset, left hand** HCC
- **MØ8.249 Juvenile rheumatoid arthritis with systemic onset, unspecified hand** HCC

√6th **MØ8.25 Juvenile rheumatoid arthritis with systemic onset, hip**
- **MØ8.251 Juvenile rheumatoid arthritis with systemic onset, right hip** HCC
- **MØ8.252 Juvenile rheumatoid arthritis with systemic onset, left hip** HCC
- **MØ8.259 Juvenile rheumatoid arthritis with systemic onset, unspecified hip** HCC

√6th **MØ8.26 Juvenile rheumatoid arthritis with systemic onset, knee**
- **MØ8.261 Juvenile rheumatoid arthritis with systemic onset, right knee** HCC
- **MØ8.262 Juvenile rheumatoid arthritis with systemic onset, left knee** HCC
- **MØ8.269 Juvenile rheumatoid arthritis with systemic onset, unspecified knee** HCC

√6th **MØ8.27 Juvenile rheumatoid arthritis with systemic onset, ankle and foot**
- **MØ8.271 Juvenile rheumatoid arthritis with systemic onset, right ankle and foot** HCC
- **MØ8.272 Juvenile rheumatoid arthritis with systemic onset, left ankle and foot** HCC
- **MØ8.279 Juvenile rheumatoid arthritis with systemic onset, unspecified ankle and foot** HCC

MØ8.28 Juvenile rheumatoid arthritis with systemic onset, vertebrae HCC

MØ8.29 Juvenile rheumatoid arthritis with systemic onset, multiple sites HCC

● **MØ8.2A Juvenile rheumatoid arthritis with systemic onset, other specified site**

MØ8.3 Juvenile rheumatoid polyarthritis (seronegative) HCC

√5th **MØ8.4 Pauciarticular juvenile rheumatoid arthritis**

MØ8.4Ø Pauciarticular juvenile rheumatoid arthritis, unspecified site HCC

√6th **MØ8.41 Pauciarticular juvenile rheumatoid arthritis, shoulder**
- **MØ8.411 Pauciarticular juvenile rheumatoid arthritis, right shoulder** HCC
- **MØ8.412 Pauciarticular juvenile rheumatoid arthritis, left shoulder** HCC
- **MØ8.419 Pauciarticular juvenile rheumatoid arthritis, unspecified shoulder** HCC

√6th **MØ8.42 Pauciarticular juvenile rheumatoid arthritis, elbow**
- **MØ8.421 Pauciarticular juvenile rheumatoid arthritis, right elbow** HCC
- **MØ8.422 Pauciarticular juvenile rheumatoid arthritis, left elbow** HCC
- **MØ8.429 Pauciarticular juvenile rheumatoid arthritis, unspecified elbow** HCC

√6th **MØ8.43 Pauciarticular juvenile rheumatoid arthritis, wrist**
- **MØ8.431 Pauciarticular juvenile rheumatoid arthritis, right wrist** HCC
- **MØ8.432 Pauciarticular juvenile rheumatoid arthritis, left wrist** HCC
- **MØ8.439 Pauciarticular juvenile rheumatoid arthritis, unspecified wrist** HCC

√6th **MØ8.44 Pauciarticular juvenile rheumatoid arthritis, hand**
- **MØ8.441 Pauciarticular juvenile rheumatoid arthritis, right hand** HCC
- **MØ8.442 Pauciarticular juvenile rheumatoid arthritis, left hand** HCC
- **MØ8.449 Pauciarticular juvenile rheumatoid arthritis, unspecified hand** HCC

√6th **MØ8.45 Pauciarticular juvenile rheumatoid arthritis, hip**
- **MØ8.451 Pauciarticular juvenile rheumatoid arthritis, right hip** HCC

M08.452 Pauciarticular juvenile rheumatoid arthritis, left hip HCC
M08.459 Pauciarticular juvenile rheumatoid arthritis, unspecified hip HCC
M08.46 Pauciarticular juvenile rheumatoid arthritis, knee
M08.461 Pauciarticular juvenile rheumatoid arthritis, right knee HCC
M08.462 Pauciarticular juvenile rheumatoid arthritis, left knee HCC
M08.469 Pauciarticular juvenile rheumatoid arthritis, unspecified knee HCC
M08.47 Pauciarticular juvenile rheumatoid arthritis, ankle and foot
M08.471 Pauciarticular juvenile rheumatoid arthritis, right ankle and foot HCC
M08.472 Pauciarticular juvenile rheumatoid arthritis, left ankle and foot HCC
M08.479 Pauciarticular juvenile rheumatoid arthritis, unspecified ankle and foot HCC
M08.48 Pauciarticular juvenile rheumatoid arthritis, vertebrae HCC
● M08.4A Pauciarticular juvenile rheumatoid arthritis, other specified site

M08.8 Other juvenile arthritis
M08.80 Other juvenile arthritis, unspecified site HCC
M08.81 Other juvenile arthritis, shoulder
M08.811 Other juvenile arthritis, right shoulder HCC
M08.812 Other juvenile arthritis, left shoulder HCC
M08.819 Other juvenile arthritis, unspecified shoulder HCC
M08.82 Other juvenile arthritis, elbow
M08.821 Other juvenile arthritis, right elbow HCC
M08.822 Other juvenile arthritis, left elbow HCC
M08.829 Other juvenile arthritis, unspecified elbow HCC
M08.83 Other juvenile arthritis, wrist
M08.831 Other juvenile arthritis, right wrist HCC
M08.832 Other juvenile arthritis, left wrist HCC
M08.839 Other juvenile arthritis, unspecified wrist HCC
M08.84 Other juvenile arthritis, hand
M08.841 Other juvenile arthritis, right hand HCC
M08.842 Other juvenile arthritis, left hand HCC
M08.849 Other juvenile arthritis, unspecified hand HCC
M08.85 Other juvenile arthritis, hip
M08.851 Other juvenile arthritis, right hip HCC
M08.852 Other juvenile arthritis, left hip HCC
M08.859 Other juvenile arthritis, unspecified hip HCC
M08.86 Other juvenile arthritis, knee
M08.861 Other juvenile arthritis, right knee HCC
M08.862 Other juvenile arthritis, left knee HCC
M08.869 Other juvenile arthritis, unspecified knee HCC
M08.87 Other juvenile arthritis, ankle and foot
M08.871 Other juvenile arthritis, right ankle and foot HCC
M08.872 Other juvenile arthritis, left ankle and foot HCC
M08.879 Other juvenile arthritis, unspecified ankle and foot HCC
M08.88 Other juvenile arthritis, other specified site HCC
Other juvenile arthritis, vertebrae
M08.89 Other juvenile arthritis, multiple sites HCC

M08.9 Juvenile arthritis, unspecified
EXCLUDES 1 *juvenile rheumatoid arthritis, unspecified (M08.0-)*
M08.90 Juvenile arthritis, unspecified, unspecified site HCC
M08.91 Juvenile arthritis, unspecified, shoulder
M08.911 Juvenile arthritis, unspecified, right shoulder HCC
M08.912 Juvenile arthritis, unspecified, left shoulder HCC
M08.919 Juvenile arthritis, unspecified, unspecified shoulder HCC
M08.92 Juvenile arthritis, unspecified, elbow
M08.921 Juvenile arthritis, unspecified, right elbow HCC
M08.922 Juvenile arthritis, unspecified, left elbow HCC
M08.929 Juvenile arthritis, unspecified, unspecified elbow HCC
M08.93 Juvenile arthritis, unspecified, wrist
M08.931 Juvenile arthritis, unspecified, right wrist HCC
M08.932 Juvenile arthritis, unspecified, left wrist HCC
M08.939 Juvenile arthritis, unspecified, unspecified wrist HCC
M08.94 Juvenile arthritis, unspecified, hand
M08.941 Juvenile arthritis, unspecified, right hand HCC
M08.942 Juvenile arthritis, unspecified, left hand HCC
M08.949 Juvenile arthritis, unspecified, unspecified hand HCC
M08.95 Juvenile arthritis, unspecified, hip
M08.951 Juvenile arthritis, unspecified, right hip HCC
M08.952 Juvenile arthritis, unspecified, left hip HCC
M08.959 Juvenile arthritis, unspecified, unspecified hip HCC
M08.96 Juvenile arthritis, unspecified, knee
M08.961 Juvenile arthritis, unspecified, right knee HCC
M08.962 Juvenile arthritis, unspecified, left knee HCC
M08.969 Juvenile arthritis, unspecified, unspecified knee HCC
M08.97 Juvenile arthritis, unspecified, ankle and foot
M08.971 Juvenile arthritis, unspecified, right ankle and foot HCC
M08.972 Juvenile arthritis, unspecified, left ankle and foot HCC
M08.979 Juvenile arthritis, unspecified, unspecified ankle and foot HCC
M08.98 Juvenile arthritis, unspecified, vertebrae HCC
M08.99 Juvenile arthritis, unspecified, multiple sites HCC
● M08.9A Juvenile arthritis, unspecified, other specified site

M1A Chronic gout

Use additional code to identify:
autonomic neuropathy in diseases classified elsewhere (G99.0)
calculus of urinary tract in diseases classified elsewhere (N22)
cardiomyopathy in diseases classified elsewhere (I43)
disorders of external ear in diseases classified elsewhere (H61.1-, H62.8-)
disorders of iris and ciliary body in diseases classified elsewhere (H22)
glomerular disorders in diseases classified elsewhere (N08)

EXCLUDES 1 *gout NOS (M10.-)*
EXCLUDES 2 *acute gout (M10.-)*

The appropriate 7th character is to be added to each code from category M1A.
0 without tophus (tophi)
1 with tophus (tophi)

M1A.0 Idiopathic chronic gout
Chronic gouty bursitis
Primary chronic gout
M1A.00 Idiopathic chronic gout, unspecified site
M1A.01 Idiopathic chronic gout, shoulder
M1A.011 Idiopathic chronic gout, right shoulder
M1A.012 Idiopathic chronic gout, left shoulder
M1A.019 Idiopathic chronic gout, unspecified shoulder
M1A.02 Idiopathic chronic gout, elbow
M1A.021 Idiopathic chronic gout, right elbow

√7th M1A.022 Idiopathic chronic gout, left elbow
√7th M1A.029 Idiopathic chronic gout, unspecified elbow
√6th M1A.03 Idiopathic chronic gout, wrist
√7th M1A.031 Idiopathic chronic gout, right wrist
√7th M1A.032 Idiopathic chronic gout, left wrist
√7th M1A.039 Idiopathic chronic gout, unspecified wrist
√6th M1A.04 Idiopathic chronic gout, hand
√7th M1A.041 Idiopathic chronic gout, right hand
√7th M1A.042 Idiopathic chronic gout, left hand
√7th M1A.049 Idiopathic chronic gout, unspecified hand
√6th M1A.05 Idiopathic chronic gout, hip
√7th M1A.051 Idiopathic chronic gout, right hip
√7th M1A.052 Idiopathic chronic gout, left hip
√7th M1A.059 Idiopathic chronic gout, unspecified hip
√6th M1A.06 Idiopathic chronic gout, knee
√7th M1A.061 Idiopathic chronic gout, right knee
√7th M1A.062 Idiopathic chronic gout, left knee
√7th M1A.069 Idiopathic chronic gout, unspecified knee
√6th M1A.07 Idiopathic chronic gout, ankle and foot
√7th M1A.071 Idiopathic chronic gout, right ankle and foot
√7th M1A.072 Idiopathic chronic gout, left ankle and foot
√7th M1A.079 Idiopathic chronic gout, unspecified ankle and foot
√x7th M1A.08 Idiopathic chronic gout, vertebrae
√x7th M1A.09 Idiopathic chronic gout, multiple sites

√5th M1A.1 Lead-induced chronic gout

Code first toxic effects of lead and its compounds (T56.Ø-)

√x7th M1A.1Ø Lead-induced chronic gout, unspecified site
√6th M1A.11 Lead-induced chronic gout, shoulder
√7th M1A.111 Lead-induced chronic gout, right shoulder
√7th M1A.112 Lead-induced chronic gout, left shoulder
√7th M1A.119 Lead-induced chronic gout, unspecified shoulder
√6th M1A.12 Lead-induced chronic gout, elbow
√7th M1A.121 Lead-induced chronic gout, right elbow
√7th M1A.122 Lead-induced chronic gout, left elbow
√7th M1A.129 Lead-induced chronic gout, unspecified elbow
√6th M1A.13 Lead-induced chronic gout, wrist
√7th M1A.131 Lead-induced chronic gout, right wrist
√7th M1A.132 Lead-induced chronic gout, left wrist
√7th M1A.139 Lead-induced chronic gout, unspecified wrist
√6th M1A.14 Lead-induced chronic gout, hand
√7th M1A.141 Lead-induced chronic gout, right hand
√7th M1A.142 Lead-induced chronic gout, left hand
√7th M1A.149 Lead-induced chronic gout, unspecified hand
√6th M1A.15 Lead-induced chronic gout, hip
√7th M1A.151 Lead-induced chronic gout, right hip
√7th M1A.152 Lead-induced chronic gout, left hip
√7th M1A.159 Lead-induced chronic gout, unspecified hip
√6th M1A.16 Lead-induced chronic gout, knee
√7th M1A.161 Lead-induced chronic gout, right knee
√7th M1A.162 Lead-induced chronic gout, left knee
√7th M1A.169 Lead-induced chronic gout, unspecified knee
√6th M1A.17 Lead-induced chronic gout, ankle and foot
√7th M1A.171 Lead-induced chronic gout, right ankle and foot
√7th M1A.172 Lead-induced chronic gout, left ankle and foot
√7th M1A.179 Lead-induced chronic gout, unspecified ankle and foot
√x7th M1A.18 Lead-induced chronic gout, vertebrae
√x7th M1A.19 Lead-induced chronic gout, multiple sites

√5th M1A.2 Drug-induced chronic gout

Use additional code for adverse effect, if applicable, to identify drug (T36-T5Ø with fifth or sixth character 5)

√x7th M1A.2Ø Drug-induced chronic gout, unspecified site
√6th M1A.21 Drug-induced chronic gout, shoulder
√7th M1A.211 Drug-induced chronic gout, right shoulder
√7th M1A.212 Drug-induced chronic gout, left shoulder
√7th M1A.219 Drug-induced chronic gout, unspecified shoulder
√6th M1A.22 Drug-induced chronic gout, elbow
√7th M1A.221 Drug-induced chronic gout, right elbow
√7th M1A.222 Drug-induced chronic gout, left elbow
√7th M1A.229 Drug-induced chronic gout, unspecified elbow
√6th M1A.23 Drug-induced chronic gout, wrist
√7th M1A.231 Drug-induced chronic gout, right wrist
√7th M1A.232 Drug-induced chronic gout, left wrist
√7th M1A.239 Drug-induced chronic gout, unspecified wrist
√6th M1A.24 Drug-induced chronic gout, hand
√7th M1A.241 Drug-induced chronic gout, right hand
√7th M1A.242 Drug-induced chronic gout, left hand
√7th M1A.249 Drug-induced chronic gout, unspecified hand
√6th M1A.25 Drug-induced chronic gout, hip
√7th M1A.251 Drug-induced chronic gout, right hip
√7th M1A.252 Drug-induced chronic gout, left hip
√7th M1A.259 Drug-induced chronic gout, unspecified hip
√6th M1A.26 Drug-induced chronic gout, knee
√7th M1A.261 Drug-induced chronic gout, right knee
√7th M1A.262 Drug-induced chronic gout, left knee
√7th M1A.269 Drug-induced chronic gout, unspecified knee
√6th M1A.27 Drug-induced chronic gout, ankle and foot
√7th M1A.271 Drug-induced chronic gout, right ankle and foot
√7th M1A.272 Drug-induced chronic gout, left ankle and foot
√7th M1A.279 Drug-induced chronic gout, unspecified ankle and foot
√x7th M1A.28 Drug-induced chronic gout, vertebrae
√x7th M1A.29 Drug-induced chronic gout, multiple sites

√5th M1A.3 Chronic gout due to renal impairment

Code first associated renal disease

√x7th M1A.3Ø Chronic gout due to renal impairment, unspecified site
√6th M1A.31 Chronic gout due to renal impairment, shoulder
√7th M1A.311 Chronic gout due to renal impairment, right shoulder
√7th M1A.312 Chronic gout due to renal impairment, left shoulder
√7th M1A.319 Chronic gout due to renal impairment, unspecified shoulder
√6th M1A.32 Chronic gout due to renal impairment, elbow
√7th M1A.321 Chronic gout due to renal impairment, right elbow
√7th M1A.322 Chronic gout due to renal impairment, left elbow
√7th M1A.329 Chronic gout due to renal impairment, unspecified elbow
√6th M1A.33 Chronic gout due to renal impairment, wrist
√7th M1A.331 Chronic gout due to renal impairment, right wrist
√7th M1A.332 Chronic gout due to renal impairment, left wrist
√7th M1A.339 Chronic gout due to renal impairment, unspecified wrist
√6th M1A.34 Chronic gout due to renal impairment, hand
√7th M1A.341 Chronic gout due to renal impairment, right hand
√7th M1A.342 Chronic gout due to renal impairment, left hand
√7th M1A.349 Chronic gout due to renal impairment, unspecified hand

6th **M1A.35 Chronic gout due to renal impairment, hip**
- 7th **M1A.351 Chronic gout due to renal impairment, right hip**
- 7th **M1A.352 Chronic gout due to renal impairment, left hip**
- 7th **M1A.359 Chronic gout due to renal impairment, unspecified hip**

6th **M1A.36 Chronic gout due to renal impairment, knee**
- 7th **M1A.361 Chronic gout due to renal impairment, right knee**
- 7th **M1A.362 Chronic gout due to renal impairment, left knee**
- 7th **M1A.369 Chronic gout due to renal impairment, unspecified knee**

6th **M1A.37 Chronic gout due to renal impairment, ankle and foot**
- 7th **M1A.371 Chronic gout due to renal impairment, right ankle and foot**
- 7th **M1A.372 Chronic gout due to renal impairment, left ankle and foot**
- 7th **M1A.379 Chronic gout due to renal impairment, unspecified ankle and foot**

x7th **M1A.38 Chronic gout due to renal impairment, vertebrae**

x7th **M1A.39 Chronic gout due to renal impairment, multiple sites**

5th **M1A.4 Other secondary chronic gout**

Code first associated condition

x7th **M1A.40 Other secondary chronic gout, unspecified site**

6th **M1A.41 Other secondary chronic gout, shoulder**
- 7th **M1A.411 Other secondary chronic gout, right shoulder**
- 7th **M1A.412 Other secondary chronic gout, left shoulder**
- 7th **M1A.419 Other secondary chronic gout, unspecified shoulder**

6th **M1A.42 Other secondary chronic gout, elbow**
- 7th **M1A.421 Other secondary chronic gout, right elbow**
- 7th **M1A.422 Other secondary chronic gout, left elbow**
- 7th **M1A.429 Other secondary chronic gout, unspecified elbow**

6th **M1A.43 Other secondary chronic gout, wrist**
- 7th **M1A.431 Other secondary chronic gout, right wrist**
- 7th **M1A.432 Other secondary chronic gout, left wrist**
- 7th **M1A.439 Other secondary chronic gout, unspecified wrist**

6th **M1A.44 Other secondary chronic gout, hand**
- 7th **M1A.441 Other secondary chronic gout, right hand**
- 7th **M1A.442 Other secondary chronic gout, left hand**
- 7th **M1A.449 Other secondary chronic gout, unspecified hand**

6th **M1A.45 Other secondary chronic gout, hip**
- 7th **M1A.451 Other secondary chronic gout, right hip**
- 7th **M1A.452 Other secondary chronic gout, left hip**
- 7th **M1A.459 Other secondary chronic gout, unspecified hip**

6th **M1A.46 Other secondary chronic gout, knee**
- 7th **M1A.461 Other secondary chronic gout, right knee**
- 7th **M1A.462 Other secondary chronic gout, left knee**
- 7th **M1A.469 Other secondary chronic gout, unspecified knee**

6th **M1A.47 Other secondary chronic gout, ankle and foot**
- 7th **M1A.471 Other secondary chronic gout, right ankle and foot**
- 7th **M1A.472 Other secondary chronic gout, left ankle and foot**
- 7th **M1A.479 Other secondary chronic gout, unspecified ankle and foot**

x7th **M1A.48 Other secondary chronic gout, vertebrae**

x7th **M1A.49 Other secondary chronic gout, multiple sites**

x7th **M1A.9 Chronic gout, unspecified**

4th **M10 Gout**

Acute gout
Gout attack
Gout flare
Podagra
Use additional code to identify:
- autonomic neuropathy in diseases classified elsewhere (G99.0)
- calculus of urinary tract in diseases classified elsewhere (N22)
- cardiomyopathy in diseases classified elsewhere (I43)
- disorders of external ear in diseases classified elsewhere (H61.1-, H62.8-)
- disorders of iris and ciliary body in diseases classified elsewhere (H22)
- glomerular disorders in diseases classified elsewhere (N08)

EXCLUDES 2 *chronic gout (M1A.-)*

DEF: Purine and pyrimidine metabolic disorders, manifested by hyperuricemia and recurrent acute inflammatory arthritis. Monosodium urate or monohydrate crystals may be deposited in and around the joints, leading to joint destruction and severe crippling.

5th **M10.0 Idiopathic gout**

Gouty bursitis
Primary gout

M10.00 Idiopathic gout, unspecified site

6th **M10.01 Idiopathic gout, shoulder**
- **M10.011 Idiopathic gout, right shoulder**
- **M10.012 Idiopathic gout, left shoulder**
- **M10.019 Idiopathic gout, unspecified shoulder**

6th **M10.02 Idiopathic gout, elbow**
- **M10.021 Idiopathic gout, right elbow**
- **M10.022 Idiopathic gout, left elbow**
- **M10.029 Idiopathic gout, unspecified elbow**

6th **M10.03 Idiopathic gout, wrist**
- **M10.031 Idiopathic gout, right wrist**
- **M10.032 Idiopathic gout, left wrist**
- **M10.039 Idiopathic gout, unspecified wrist**

6th **M10.04 Idiopathic gout, hand**
- **M10.041 Idiopathic gout, right hand**
- **M10.042 Idiopathic gout, left hand**
- **M10.049 Idiopathic gout, unspecified hand**

6th **M10.05 Idiopathic gout, hip**
- **M10.051 Idiopathic gout, right hip**
- **M10.052 Idiopathic gout, left hip**
- **M10.059 Idiopathic gout, unspecified hip**

6th **M10.06 Idiopathic gout, knee**
- **M10.061 Idiopathic gout, right knee**
- **M10.062 Idiopathic gout, left knee**
- **M10.069 Idiopathic gout, unspecified knee**

6th **M10.07 Idiopathic gout, ankle and foot**
- **M10.071 Idiopathic gout, right ankle and foot**
- **M10.072 Idiopathic gout, left ankle and foot**
- **M10.079 Idiopathic gout, unspecified ankle and foot**

M10.08 Idiopathic gout, vertebrae

M10.09 Idiopathic gout, multiple sites

5th **M10.1 Lead-induced gout**

Code first toxic effects of lead and its compounds (T56.0-)

M10.10 Lead-induced gout, unspecified site

6th **M10.11 Lead-induced gout, shoulder**
- **M10.111 Lead-induced gout, right shoulder**
- **M10.112 Lead-induced gout, left shoulder**
- **M10.119 Lead-induced gout, unspecified shoulder**

6th **M10.12 Lead-induced gout, elbow**
- **M10.121 Lead-induced gout, right elbow**
- **M10.122 Lead-induced gout, left elbow**
- **M10.129 Lead-induced gout, unspecified elbow**

6th **M10.13 Lead-induced gout, wrist**
- **M10.131 Lead-induced gout, right wrist**
- **M10.132 Lead-induced gout, left wrist**
- **M10.139 Lead-induced gout, unspecified wrist**

6th **M10.14 Lead-induced gout, hand**
- **M10.141 Lead-induced gout, right hand**
- **M10.142 Lead-induced gout, left hand**
- **M10.149 Lead-induced gout, unspecified hand**

6th **M10.15 Lead-induced gout, hip**
- **M10.151 Lead-induced gout, right hip**
- **M10.152 Lead-induced gout, left hip**
- **M10.159 Lead-induced gout, unspecified hip**

√6th M10.16 Lead-induced gout, knee
M10.161 Lead-induced gout, right knee
M10.162 Lead-induced gout, left knee
M10.169 Lead-induced gout, unspecified knee
√6th M10.17 Lead-induced gout, ankle and foot
M10.171 Lead-induced gout, right ankle and foot
M10.172 Lead-induced gout, left ankle and foot
M10.179 Lead-induced gout, unspecified ankle and foot
M10.18 Lead-induced gout, vertebrae
M10.19 Lead-induced gout, multiple sites
√5th M10.2 Drug-induced gout
Use additional code for adverse effect, if applicable, to identify drug (T36-T50 with fifth or sixth character 5)
M10.20 Drug-induced gout, unspecified site
√6th M10.21 Drug-induced gout, shoulder
M10.211 Drug-induced gout, right shoulder
M10.212 Drug-induced gout, left shoulder
M10.219 Drug-induced gout, unspecified shoulder
√6th M10.22 Drug-induced gout, elbow
M10.221 Drug-induced gout, right elbow
M10.222 Drug-induced gout, left elbow
M10.229 Drug-induced gout, unspecified elbow
√6th M10.23 Drug-induced gout, wrist
M10.231 Drug-induced gout, right wrist
M10.232 Drug-induced gout, left wrist
M10.239 Drug-induced gout, unspecified wrist
√6th M10.24 Drug-induced gout, hand
M10.241 Drug-induced gout, right hand
M10.242 Drug-induced gout, left hand
M10.249 Drug-induced gout, unspecified hand
√6th M10.25 Drug-induced gout, hip
M10.251 Drug-induced gout, right hip
M10.252 Drug-induced gout, left hip
M10.259 Drug-induced gout, unspecified hip
√6th M10.26 Drug-induced gout, knee
M10.261 Drug-induced gout, right knee
M10.262 Drug-induced gout, left knee
M10.269 Drug-induced gout, unspecified knee
√6th M10.27 Drug-induced gout, ankle and foot
M10.271 Drug-induced gout, right ankle and foot
M10.272 Drug-induced gout, left ankle and foot
M10.279 Drug-induced gout, unspecified ankle and foot
M10.28 Drug-induced gout, vertebrae
M10.29 Drug-induced gout, multiple sites
√5th M10.3 Gout due to renal impairment
Code first associated renal disease
M10.30 Gout due to renal impairment, unspecified site
√6th M10.31 Gout due to renal impairment, shoulder
M10.311 Gout due to renal impairment, right shoulder
M10.312 Gout due to renal impairment, left shoulder
M10.319 Gout due to renal impairment, unspecified shoulder
√6th M10.32 Gout due to renal impairment, elbow
M10.321 Gout due to renal impairment, right elbow
M10.322 Gout due to renal impairment, left elbow
M10.329 Gout due to renal impairment, unspecified elbow
√6th M10.33 Gout due to renal impairment, wrist
M10.331 Gout due to renal impairment, right wrist
M10.332 Gout due to renal impairment, left wrist
M10.339 Gout due to renal impairment, unspecified wrist
√6th M10.34 Gout due to renal impairment, hand
M10.341 Gout due to renal impairment, right hand
M10.342 Gout due to renal impairment, left hand
M10.349 Gout due to renal impairment, unspecified hand
√6th M10.35 Gout due to renal impairment, hip
M10.351 Gout due to renal impairment, right hip
M10.352 Gout due to renal impairment, left hip
M10.359 Gout due to renal impairment, unspecified hip
√6th M10.36 Gout due to renal impairment, knee
M10.361 Gout due to renal impairment, right knee
M10.362 Gout due to renal impairment, left knee
M10.369 Gout due to renal impairment, unspecified knee
√6th M10.37 Gout due to renal impairment, ankle and foot
M10.371 Gout due to renal impairment, right ankle and foot
M10.372 Gout due to renal impairment, left ankle and foot
M10.379 Gout due to renal impairment, unspecified ankle and foot
M10.38 Gout due to renal impairment, vertebrae
M10.39 Gout due to renal impairment, multiple sites
√5th M10.4 Other secondary gout
Code first associated condition
M10.40 Other secondary gout, unspecified site
√6th M10.41 Other secondary gout, shoulder
M10.411 Other secondary gout, right shoulder
M10.412 Other secondary gout, left shoulder
M10.419 Other secondary gout, unspecified shoulder
√6th M10.42 Other secondary gout, elbow
M10.421 Other secondary gout, right elbow
M10.422 Other secondary gout, left elbow
M10.429 Other secondary gout, unspecified elbow
√6th M10.43 Other secondary gout, wrist
M10.431 Other secondary gout, right wrist
M10.432 Other secondary gout, left wrist
M10.439 Other secondary gout, unspecified wrist
√6th M10.44 Other secondary gout, hand
M10.441 Other secondary gout, right hand
M10.442 Other secondary gout, left hand
M10.449 Other secondary gout, unspecified hand
√6th M10.45 Other secondary gout, hip
M10.451 Other secondary gout, right hip
M10.452 Other secondary gout, left hip
M10.459 Other secondary gout, unspecified hip
√6th M10.46 Other secondary gout, knee
M10.461 Other secondary gout, right knee
M10.462 Other secondary gout, left knee
M10.469 Other secondary gout, unspecified knee
√6th M10.47 Other secondary gout, ankle and foot
M10.471 Other secondary gout, right ankle and foot
M10.472 Other secondary gout, left ankle and foot
M10.479 Other secondary gout, unspecified ankle and foot
M10.48 Other secondary gout, vertebrae
M10.49 Other secondary gout, multiple sites
M10.9 Gout, unspecified
Gout NOS

√4th **M11 Other crystal arthropathies**
√5th M11.0 Hydroxyapatite deposition disease
DEF: Disease caused by deposits of calcium phosphate crystals in the soft tissues close to the joint (especially tendons) or in the joints. These calcifications can be mono or polyarticular and can cause destruction of the joint involved.
M11.00 Hydroxyapatite deposition disease, unspecified site
√6th M11.01 Hydroxyapatite deposition disease, shoulder
M11.011 Hydroxyapatite deposition disease, right shoulder
M11.012 Hydroxyapatite deposition disease, left shoulder
M11.019 Hydroxyapatite deposition disease, unspecified shoulder
√6th M11.02 Hydroxyapatite deposition disease, elbow
M11.021 Hydroxyapatite deposition disease, right elbow
M11.022 Hydroxyapatite deposition disease, left elbow
M11.029 Hydroxyapatite deposition disease, unspecified elbow

✓6th M11.Ø3 Hydroxyapatite deposition disease, wrist
M11.Ø31 Hydroxyapatite deposition disease, right wrist
M11.Ø32 Hydroxyapatite deposition disease, left wrist
M11.Ø39 Hydroxyapatite deposition disease, unspecified wrist
✓6th M11.Ø4 Hydroxyapatite deposition disease, hand
M11.Ø41 Hydroxyapatite deposition disease, right hand
M11.Ø42 Hydroxyapatite deposition disease, left hand
M11.Ø49 Hydroxyapatite deposition disease, unspecified hand
✓6th M11.Ø5 Hydroxyapatite deposition disease, hip
M11.Ø51 Hydroxyapatite deposition disease, right hip
M11.Ø52 Hydroxyapatite deposition disease, left hip
M11.Ø59 Hydroxyapatite deposition disease, unspecified hip
✓6th M11.Ø6 Hydroxyapatite deposition disease, knee
M11.Ø61 Hydroxyapatite deposition disease, right knee
M11.Ø62 Hydroxyapatite deposition disease, left knee
M11.Ø69 Hydroxyapatite deposition disease, unspecified knee
✓6th M11.Ø7 Hydroxyapatite deposition disease, ankle and foot
M11.Ø71 Hydroxyapatite deposition disease, right ankle and foot
M11.Ø72 Hydroxyapatite deposition disease, left ankle and foot
M11.Ø79 Hydroxyapatite deposition disease, unspecified ankle and foot
M11.Ø8 Hydroxyapatite deposition disease, vertebrae
M11.Ø9 Hydroxyapatite deposition disease, multiple sites

✓5th M11.1 Familial chondrocalcinosis
M11.1Ø Familial chondrocalcinosis, unspecified site
✓6th M11.11 Familial chondrocalcinosis, shoulder
M11.111 Familial chondrocalcinosis, right shoulder
M11.112 Familial chondrocalcinosis, left shoulder
M11.119 Familial chondrocalcinosis, unspecified shoulder
✓6th M11.12 Familial chondrocalcinosis, elbow
M11.121 Familial chondrocalcinosis, right elbow
M11.122 Familial chondrocalcinosis, left elbow
M11.129 Familial chondrocalcinosis, unspecified elbow
✓6th M11.13 Familial chondrocalcinosis, wrist
M11.131 Familial chondrocalcinosis, right wrist
M11.132 Familial chondrocalcinosis, left wrist
M11.139 Familial chondrocalcinosis, unspecified wrist
✓6th M11.14 Familial chondrocalcinosis, hand
M11.141 Familial chondrocalcinosis, right hand
M11.142 Familial chondrocalcinosis, left hand
M11.149 Familial chondrocalcinosis, unspecified hand
✓6th M11.15 Familial chondrocalcinosis, hip
M11.151 Familial chondrocalcinosis, right hip
M11.152 Familial chondrocalcinosis, left hip
M11.159 Familial chondrocalcinosis, unspecified hip
✓6th M11.16 Familial chondrocalcinosis, knee
M11.161 Familial chondrocalcinosis, right knee
M11.162 Familial chondrocalcinosis, left knee
M11.169 Familial chondrocalcinosis, unspecified knee
✓6th M11.17 Familial chondrocalcinosis, ankle and foot
M11.171 Familial chondrocalcinosis, right ankle and foot
M11.172 Familial chondrocalcinosis, left ankle and foot
M11.179 Familial chondrocalcinosis, unspecified ankle and foot
M11.18 Familial chondrocalcinosis, vertebrae
M11.19 Familial chondrocalcinosis, multiple sites

✓5th M11.2 Other chondrocalcinosis
Chondrocalcinosis NOS
AHA: 2018,3Q,20
TIP: Pseudogout is captured with codes in this subcategory.
M11.2Ø Other chondrocalcinosis, unspecified site
✓6th M11.21 Other chondrocalcinosis, shoulder
M11.211 Other chondrocalcinosis, right shoulder
M11.212 Other chondrocalcinosis, left shoulder
M11.219 Other chondrocalcinosis, unspecified shoulder
✓6th M11.22 Other chondrocalcinosis, elbow
M11.221 Other chondrocalcinosis, right elbow
M11.222 Other chondrocalcinosis, left elbow
M11.229 Other chondrocalcinosis, unspecified elbow
✓6th M11.23 Other chondrocalcinosis, wrist
M11.231 Other chondrocalcinosis, right wrist
M11.232 Other chondrocalcinosis, left wrist
M11.239 Other chondrocalcinosis, unspecified wrist
✓6th M11.24 Other chondrocalcinosis, hand
M11.241 Other chondrocalcinosis, right hand
M11.242 Other chondrocalcinosis, left hand
M11.249 Other chondrocalcinosis, unspecified hand
✓6th M11.25 Other chondrocalcinosis, hip
M11.251 Other chondrocalcinosis, right hip
M11.252 Other chondrocalcinosis, left hip
M11.259 Other chondrocalcinosis, unspecified hip
✓6th M11.26 Other chondrocalcinosis, knee
M11.261 Other chondrocalcinosis, right knee
M11.262 Other chondrocalcinosis, left knee
M11.269 Other chondrocalcinosis, unspecified knee
✓6th M11.27 Other chondrocalcinosis, ankle and foot
M11.271 Other chondrocalcinosis, right ankle and foot
M11.272 Other chondrocalcinosis, left ankle and foot
M11.279 Other chondrocalcinosis, unspecified ankle and foot
M11.28 Other chondrocalcinosis, vertebrae
M11.29 Other chondrocalcinosis, multiple sites

✓5th M11.8 Other specified crystal arthropathies
M11.8Ø Other specified crystal arthropathies, unspecified site
✓6th M11.81 Other specified crystal arthropathies, shoulder
M11.811 Other specified crystal arthropathies, right shoulder
M11.812 Other specified crystal arthropathies, left shoulder
M11.819 Other specified crystal arthropathies, unspecified shoulder
✓6th M11.82 Other specified crystal arthropathies, elbow
M11.821 Other specified crystal arthropathies, right elbow
M11.822 Other specified crystal arthropathies, left elbow
M11.829 Other specified crystal arthropathies, unspecified elbow
✓6th M11.83 Other specified crystal arthropathies, wrist
M11.831 Other specified crystal arthropathies, right wrist
M11.832 Other specified crystal arthropathies, left wrist
M11.839 Other specified crystal arthropathies, unspecified wrist
✓6th M11.84 Other specified crystal arthropathies, hand
M11.841 Other specified crystal arthropathies, right hand
M11.842 Other specified crystal arthropathies, left hand
M11.849 Other specified crystal arthropathies, unspecified hand
✓6th M11.85 Other specified crystal arthropathies, hip
M11.851 Other specified crystal arthropathies, right hip

M11.852 Other specified crystal arthropathies, left hip
M11.859 Other specified crystal arthropathies, unspecified hip
✓6th M11.86 Other specified crystal arthropathies, knee
M11.861 Other specified crystal arthropathies, right knee
M11.862 Other specified crystal arthropathies, left knee
M11.869 Other specified crystal arthropathies, unspecified knee
✓6th M11.87 Other specified crystal arthropathies, ankle and foot
M11.871 Other specified crystal arthropathies, right ankle and foot
M11.872 Other specified crystal arthropathies, left ankle and foot
M11.879 Other specified crystal arthropathies, unspecified ankle and foot
M11.88 Other specified crystal arthropathies, vertebrae
M11.89 Other specified crystal arthropathies, multiple sites
M11.9 Crystal arthropathy, unspecified

✓4th **M12 Other and unspecified arthropathy**

EXCLUDES 1 *arthrosis (M15-M19)*
cricoarytenoid arthropathy (J38.7)

✓5th M12.Ø Chronic postrheumatic arthropathy [Jaccoud]
M12.ØØ Chronic postrheumatic arthropathy [Jaccoud], unspecified site HCC
✓6th M12.Ø1 Chronic postrheumatic arthropathy [Jaccoud], shoulder
M12.Ø11 Chronic postrheumatic arthropathy [Jaccoud], right shoulder HCC
M12.Ø12 Chronic postrheumatic arthropathy [Jaccoud], left shoulder HCC
M12.Ø19 Chronic postrheumatic arthropathy [Jaccoud], unspecified shoulder HCC
✓6th M12.Ø2 Chronic postrheumatic arthropathy [Jaccoud], elbow
M12.Ø21 Chronic postrheumatic arthropathy [Jaccoud], right elbow HCC
M12.Ø22 Chronic postrheumatic arthropathy [Jaccoud], left elbow HCC
M12.Ø29 Chronic postrheumatic arthropathy [Jaccoud], unspecified elbow HCC
✓6th M12.Ø3 Chronic postrheumatic arthropathy [Jaccoud], wrist
M12.Ø31 Chronic postrheumatic arthropathy [Jaccoud], right wrist HCC
M12.Ø32 Chronic postrheumatic arthropathy [Jaccoud], left wrist HCC
M12.Ø39 Chronic postrheumatic arthropathy [Jaccoud], unspecified wrist HCC
✓6th M12.Ø4 Chronic postrheumatic arthropathy [Jaccoud], hand
M12.Ø41 Chronic postrheumatic arthropathy [Jaccoud], right hand HCC
M12.Ø42 Chronic postrheumatic arthropathy [Jaccoud], left hand HCC
M12.Ø49 Chronic postrheumatic arthropathy [Jaccoud], unspecified hand HCC
✓6th M12.Ø5 Chronic postrheumatic arthropathy [Jaccoud], hip
M12.Ø51 Chronic postrheumatic arthropathy [Jaccoud], right hip HCC
M12.Ø52 Chronic postrheumatic arthropathy [Jaccoud], left hip HCC
M12.Ø59 Chronic postrheumatic arthropathy [Jaccoud], unspecified hip HCC
✓6th M12.Ø6 Chronic postrheumatic arthropathy [Jaccoud], knee
M12.Ø61 Chronic postrheumatic arthropathy [Jaccoud], right knee HCC
M12.Ø62 Chronic postrheumatic arthropathy [Jaccoud], left knee HCC
M12.Ø69 Chronic postrheumatic arthropathy [Jaccoud], unspecified knee HCC
✓6th M12.Ø7 Chronic postrheumatic arthropathy [Jaccoud], ankle and foot
M12.Ø71 Chronic postrheumatic arthropathy [Jaccoud], right ankle and foot HCC
M12.Ø72 Chronic postrheumatic arthropathy [Jaccoud], left ankle and foot HCC
M12.Ø79 Chronic postrheumatic arthropathy [Jaccoud], unspecified ankle and foot HCC
M12.Ø8 Chronic postrheumatic arthropathy [Jaccoud], other specified site HCC
Chronic postrheumatic arthropathy [Jaccoud], vertebrae
M12.Ø9 Chronic postrheumatic arthropathy [Jaccoud], multiple sites HCC

✓5th M12.1 Kaschin-Beck disease
Osteochondroarthrosis deformans endemica
M12.1Ø Kaschin-Beck disease, unspecified site
✓6th M12.11 Kaschin-Beck disease, shoulder
M12.111 Kaschin-Beck disease, right shoulder
M12.112 Kaschin-Beck disease, left shoulder
M12.119 Kaschin-Beck disease, unspecified shoulder
✓6th M12.12 Kaschin-Beck disease, elbow
M12.121 Kaschin-Beck disease, right elbow
M12.122 Kaschin-Beck disease, left elbow
M12.129 Kaschin-Beck disease, unspecified elbow
✓6th M12.13 Kaschin-Beck disease, wrist
M12.131 Kaschin-Beck disease, right wrist
M12.132 Kaschin-Beck disease, left wrist
M12.139 Kaschin-Beck disease, unspecified wrist
✓6th M12.14 Kaschin-Beck disease, hand
M12.141 Kaschin-Beck disease, right hand
M12.142 Kaschin-Beck disease, left hand
M12.149 Kaschin-Beck disease, unspecified hand
✓6th M12.15 Kaschin-Beck disease, hip
M12.151 Kaschin-Beck disease, right hip
M12.152 Kaschin-Beck disease, left hip
M12.159 Kaschin-Beck disease, unspecified hip
✓6th M12.16 Kaschin-Beck disease, knee
M12.161 Kaschin-Beck disease, right knee
M12.162 Kaschin-Beck disease, left knee
M12.169 Kaschin-Beck disease, unspecified knee
✓6th M12.17 Kaschin-Beck disease, ankle and foot
M12.171 Kaschin-Beck disease, right ankle and foot
M12.172 Kaschin-Beck disease, left ankle and foot
M12.179 Kaschin-Beck disease, unspecified ankle and foot
M12.18 Kaschin-Beck disease, vertebrae
M12.19 Kaschin-Beck disease, multiple sites

✓5th M12.2 Villonodular synovitis (pigmented)
M12.2Ø Villonodular synovitis (pigmented), unspecified site
✓6th M12.21 Villonodular synovitis (pigmented), shoulder
M12.211 Villonodular synovitis (pigmented), right shoulder
M12.212 Villonodular synovitis (pigmented), left shoulder
M12.219 Villonodular synovitis (pigmented), unspecified shoulder
✓6th M12.22 Villonodular synovitis (pigmented), elbow
M12.221 Villonodular synovitis (pigmented), right elbow
M12.222 Villonodular synovitis (pigmented), left elbow
M12.229 Villonodular synovitis (pigmented), unspecified elbow
✓6th M12.23 Villonodular synovitis (pigmented), wrist
M12.231 Villonodular synovitis (pigmented), right wrist
M12.232 Villonodular synovitis (pigmented), left wrist
M12.239 Villonodular synovitis (pigmented), unspecified wrist
✓6th M12.24 Villonodular synovitis (pigmented), hand
M12.241 Villonodular synovitis (pigmented), right hand
M12.242 Villonodular synovitis (pigmented), left hand
M12.249 Villonodular synovitis (pigmented), unspecified hand

✓6th M12.25 **Villonodular synovitis (pigmented), hip**
- M12.251 Villonodular synovitis (pigmented), right hip
- M12.252 Villonodular synovitis (pigmented), left hip
- M12.259 Villonodular synovitis (pigmented), unspecified hip

✓6th M12.26 **Villonodular synovitis (pigmented), knee**
- M12.261 Villonodular synovitis (pigmented), right knee
- M12.262 Villonodular synovitis (pigmented), left knee
- M12.269 Villonodular synovitis (pigmented), unspecified knee

✓6th M12.27 **Villonodular synovitis (pigmented), ankle and foot**
- M12.271 Villonodular synovitis (pigmented), right ankle and foot
- M12.272 Villonodular synovitis (pigmented), left ankle and foot
- M12.279 Villonodular synovitis (pigmented), unspecified ankle and foot

M12.28 **Villonodular synovitis (pigmented), other specified site**
Villonodular synovitis (pigmented), vertebrae

M12.29 **Villonodular synovitis (pigmented), multiple sites**

✓5th **M12.3 Palindromic rheumatism**

DEF: Sudden and recurring attacks of moderate to severe joint pain and swelling generally occurring in the hands or feet of unknown etiology. After the attack subsides, the joints appear normal again.

M12.30 **Palindromic rheumatism, unspecified site**

✓6th M12.31 **Palindromic rheumatism, shoulder**
- M12.311 Palindromic rheumatism, right shoulder
- M12.312 Palindromic rheumatism, left shoulder
- M12.319 Palindromic rheumatism, unspecified shoulder

✓6th M12.32 **Palindromic rheumatism, elbow**
- M12.321 Palindromic rheumatism, right elbow
- M12.322 Palindromic rheumatism, left elbow
- M12.329 Palindromic rheumatism, unspecified elbow

✓6th M12.33 **Palindromic rheumatism, wrist**
- M12.331 Palindromic rheumatism, right wrist
- M12.332 Palindromic rheumatism, left wrist
- M12.339 Palindromic rheumatism, unspecified wrist

✓6th M12.34 **Palindromic rheumatism, hand**
- M12.341 Palindromic rheumatism, right hand
- M12.342 Palindromic rheumatism, left hand
- M12.349 Palindromic rheumatism, unspecified hand

✓6th M12.35 **Palindromic rheumatism, hip**
- M12.351 Palindromic rheumatism, right hip
- M12.352 Palindromic rheumatism, left hip
- M12.359 Palindromic rheumatism, unspecified hip

✓6th M12.36 **Palindromic rheumatism, knee**
- M12.361 Palindromic rheumatism, right knee
- M12.362 Palindromic rheumatism, left knee
- M12.369 Palindromic rheumatism, unspecified knee

✓6th M12.37 **Palindromic rheumatism, ankle and foot**
- M12.371 Palindromic rheumatism, right ankle and foot
- M12.372 Palindromic rheumatism, left ankle and foot
- M12.379 Palindromic rheumatism, unspecified ankle and foot

M12.38 **Palindromic rheumatism, other specified site**
Palindromic rheumatism, vertebrae

M12.39 **Palindromic rheumatism, multiple sites**

✓5th **M12.4 Intermittent hydrarthrosis**

M12.40 **Intermittent hydrarthrosis, unspecified site**

✓6th M12.41 **Intermittent hydrarthrosis, shoulder**
- M12.411 Intermittent hydrarthrosis, right shoulder
- M12.412 Intermittent hydrarthrosis, left shoulder
- M12.419 Intermittent hydrarthrosis, unspecified shoulder

✓6th M12.42 **Intermittent hydrarthrosis, elbow**
- M12.421 Intermittent hydrarthrosis, right elbow
- M12.422 Intermittent hydrarthrosis, left elbow
- M12.429 Intermittent hydrarthrosis, unspecified elbow

✓6th M12.43 **Intermittent hydrarthrosis, wrist**
- M12.431 Intermittent hydrarthrosis, right wrist
- M12.432 Intermittent hydrarthrosis, left wrist
- M12.439 Intermittent hydrarthrosis, unspecified wrist

✓6th M12.44 **Intermittent hydrarthrosis, hand**
- M12.441 Intermittent hydrarthrosis, right hand
- M12.442 Intermittent hydrarthrosis, left hand
- M12.449 Intermittent hydrarthrosis, unspecified hand

✓6th M12.45 **Intermittent hydrarthrosis, hip**
- M12.451 Intermittent hydrarthrosis, right hip
- M12.452 Intermittent hydrarthrosis, left hip
- M12.459 Intermittent hydrarthrosis, unspecified hip

✓6th M12.46 **Intermittent hydrarthrosis, knee**
- M12.461 Intermittent hydrarthrosis, right knee
- M12.462 Intermittent hydrarthrosis, left knee
- M12.469 Intermittent hydrarthrosis, unspecified knee

✓6th M12.47 **Intermittent hydrarthrosis, ankle and foot**
- M12.471 Intermittent hydrarthrosis, right ankle and foot
- M12.472 Intermittent hydrarthrosis, left ankle and foot
- M12.479 Intermittent hydrarthrosis, unspecified ankle and foot

M12.48 **Intermittent hydrarthrosis, other site**

M12.49 **Intermittent hydrarthrosis, multiple sites**

✓5th **M12.5 Traumatic arthropathy**

EXCLUDES 1
current injury-see Alphabetic Index
post-traumatic osteoarthritis of first carpometacarpal joint (M18.2-M18.3)
post-traumatic osteoarthritis of hip (M16.4-M16.5)
post-traumatic osteoarthritis of knee (M17.2-M17.3)
post-traumatic osteoarthritis NOS (M19.1-)
post-traumatic osteoarthritis of other single joints (M19.1-)

AHA: 2015,1Q,17

M12.50 **Traumatic arthropathy, unspecified site**

✓6th M12.51 **Traumatic arthropathy, shoulder**
- M12.511 Traumatic arthropathy, right shoulder
- M12.512 Traumatic arthropathy, left shoulder
- M12.519 Traumatic arthropathy, unspecified shoulder

✓6th M12.52 **Traumatic arthropathy, elbow**
- M12.521 Traumatic arthropathy, right elbow
- M12.522 Traumatic arthropathy, left elbow
- M12.529 Traumatic arthropathy, unspecified elbow

✓6th M12.53 **Traumatic arthropathy, wrist**
- M12.531 Traumatic arthropathy, right wrist
- M12.532 Traumatic arthropathy, left wrist
- M12.539 Traumatic arthropathy, unspecified wrist

✓6th M12.54 **Traumatic arthropathy, hand**
- M12.541 Traumatic arthropathy, right hand
- M12.542 Traumatic arthropathy, left hand
- M12.549 Traumatic arthropathy, unspecified hand

✓6th M12.55 **Traumatic arthropathy, hip**
- M12.551 Traumatic arthropathy, right hip
- M12.552 Traumatic arthropathy, left hip
- M12.559 Traumatic arthropathy, unspecified hip

✓6th M12.56 **Traumatic arthropathy, knee**
- M12.561 Traumatic arthropathy, right knee
- M12.562 Traumatic arthropathy, left knee
- M12.569 Traumatic arthropathy, unspecified knee

✓6th M12.57 **Traumatic arthropathy, ankle and foot**
- M12.571 Traumatic arthropathy, right ankle and foot
- M12.572 Traumatic arthropathy, left ankle and foot

M12.579 **Traumatic arthropathy, unspecified ankle and foot**

M12.58 **Traumatic arthropathy, other specified site**
Traumatic arthropathy, vertebrae

M12.59 **Traumatic arthropathy, multiple sites**

✓5th **M12.8** **Other specific arthropathies, not elsewhere classified**
Transient arthropathy

M12.80 **Other specific arthropathies, not elsewhere classified, unspecified site**

✓6th **M12.81** **Other specific arthropathies, not elsewhere classified, shoulder**

M12.811 **Other specific arthropathies, not elsewhere classified, right shoulder**

M12.812 **Other specific arthropathies, not elsewhere classified, left shoulder**

M12.819 **Other specific arthropathies, not elsewhere classified, unspecified shoulder**

✓6th **M12.82** **Other specific arthropathies, not elsewhere classified, elbow**

M12.821 **Other specific arthropathies, not elsewhere classified, right elbow**

M12.822 **Other specific arthropathies, not elsewhere classified, left elbow**

M12.829 **Other specific arthropathies, not elsewhere classified, unspecified elbow**

✓6th **M12.83** **Other specific arthropathies, not elsewhere classified, wrist**

M12.831 **Other specific arthropathies, not elsewhere classified, right wrist**

M12.832 **Other specific arthropathies, not elsewhere classified, left wrist**

M12.839 **Other specific arthropathies, not elsewhere classified, unspecified wrist**

✓6th **M12.84** **Other specific arthropathies, not elsewhere classified, hand**

M12.841 **Other specific arthropathies, not elsewhere classified, right hand**

M12.842 **Other specific arthropathies, not elsewhere classified, left hand**

M12.849 **Other specific arthropathies, not elsewhere classified, unspecified hand**

✓6th **M12.85** **Other specific arthropathies, not elsewhere classified, hip**

M12.851 **Other specific arthropathies, not elsewhere classified, right hip**

M12.852 **Other specific arthropathies, not elsewhere classified, left hip**

M12.859 **Other specific arthropathies, not elsewhere classified, unspecified hip**

✓6th **M12.86** **Other specific arthropathies, not elsewhere classified, knee**

M12.861 **Other specific arthropathies, not elsewhere classified, right knee**

M12.862 **Other specific arthropathies, not elsewhere classified, left knee**

M12.869 **Other specific arthropathies, not elsewhere classified, unspecified knee**

✓6th **M12.87** **Other specific arthropathies, not elsewhere classified, ankle and foot**

M12.871 **Other specific arthropathies, not elsewhere classified, right ankle and foot**

M12.872 **Other specific arthropathies, not elsewhere classified, left ankle and foot**

M12.879 **Other specific arthropathies, not elsewhere classified, unspecified ankle and foot**

M12.88 **Other specific arthropathies, not elsewhere classified, other specified site**
Other specific arthropathies, not elsewhere classified, vertebrae

M12.89 **Other specific arthropathies, not elsewhere classified, multiple sites**

M12.9 **Arthropathy, unspecified**

✓4th **M13** **Other arthritis**

EXCLUDES 1 *arthrosis (M15-M19)*
osteoarthritis (M15-M19)

M13.0 **Polyarthritis, unspecified**

✓5th **M13.1** **Monoarthritis, not elsewhere classified**

M13.10 **Monoarthritis, not elsewhere classified, unspecified site**

✓6th **M13.11** **Monoarthritis, not elsewhere classified, shoulder**

M13.111 **Monoarthritis, not elsewhere classified, right shoulder**

M13.112 **Monoarthritis, not elsewhere classified, left shoulder**

M13.119 **Monoarthritis, not elsewhere classified, unspecified shoulder**

✓6th **M13.12** **Monoarthritis, not elsewhere classified, elbow**

M13.121 **Monoarthritis, not elsewhere classified, right elbow**

M13.122 **Monoarthritis, not elsewhere classified, left elbow**

M13.129 **Monoarthritis, not elsewhere classified, unspecified elbow**

✓6th **M13.13** **Monoarthritis, not elsewhere classified, wrist**

M13.131 **Monoarthritis, not elsewhere classified, right wrist**

M13.132 **Monoarthritis, not elsewhere classified, left wrist**

M13.139 **Monoarthritis, not elsewhere classified, unspecified wrist**

✓6th **M13.14** **Monoarthritis, not elsewhere classified, hand**

M13.141 **Monoarthritis, not elsewhere classified, right hand**

M13.142 **Monoarthritis, not elsewhere classified, left hand**

M13.149 **Monoarthritis, not elsewhere classified, unspecified hand**

✓6th **M13.15** **Monoarthritis, not elsewhere classified, hip**

M13.151 **Monoarthritis, not elsewhere classified, right hip**

M13.152 **Monoarthritis, not elsewhere classified, left hip**

M13.159 **Monoarthritis, not elsewhere classified, unspecified hip**

✓6th **M13.16** **Monoarthritis, not elsewhere classified, knee**

M13.161 **Monoarthritis, not elsewhere classified, right knee**

M13.162 **Monoarthritis, not elsewhere classified, left knee**

M13.169 **Monoarthritis, not elsewhere classified, unspecified knee**

✓6th **M13.17** **Monoarthritis, not elsewhere classified, ankle and foot**

M13.171 **Monoarthritis, not elsewhere classified, right ankle and foot**

M13.172 **Monoarthritis, not elsewhere classified, left ankle and foot**

M13.179 **Monoarthritis, not elsewhere classified, unspecified ankle and foot**

✓5th **M13.8** **Other specified arthritis**
Allergic arthritis

EXCLUDES 1 *osteoarthritis (M15-M19)*

M13.80 **Other specified arthritis, unspecified site**

✓6th **M13.81** **Other specified arthritis, shoulder**

M13.811 **Other specified arthritis, right shoulder**

M13.812 **Other specified arthritis, left shoulder**

M13.819 **Other specified arthritis, unspecified shoulder**

✓6th **M13.82** **Other specified arthritis, elbow**

M13.821 **Other specified arthritis, right elbow**

M13.822 **Other specified arthritis, left elbow**

M13.829 **Other specified arthritis, unspecified elbow**

✓6th **M13.83** **Other specified arthritis, wrist**

M13.831 **Other specified arthritis, right wrist**

M13.832 **Other specified arthritis, left wrist**

M13.839 **Other specified arthritis, unspecified wrist**

✓6th **M13.84** **Other specified arthritis, hand**

M13.841 **Other specified arthritis, right hand**

M13.842 **Other specified arthritis, left hand**

M13.849 **Other specified arthritis, unspecified hand**

✓6th **M13.85** **Other specified arthritis, hip**

M13.851 **Other specified arthritis, right hip**

M13.852 **Other specified arthritis, left hip**

M13.859 **Other specified arthritis, unspecified hip**

√6th M13.86 Other specified arthritis, knee
M13.861 Other specified arthritis, right knee
M13.862 Other specified arthritis, left knee
M13.869 Other specified arthritis, unspecified knee
√6th M13.87 Other specified arthritis, ankle and foot
M13.871 Other specified arthritis, right ankle and foot
M13.872 Other specified arthritis, left ankle and foot
M13.879 Other specified arthritis, unspecified ankle and foot
M13.88 Other specified arthritis, other site
M13.89 Other specified arthritis, multiple sites

√4th M14 Arthropathies in other diseases classified elsewhere

EXCLUDES 1 *arthropathy in:*
diabetes mellitus (EØ8-E13 with .61-)
hematological disorders (M36.2-M36.3)
hypersensitivity reactions (M36.4)
neoplastic disease (M36.1)
neurosyphillis (A52.16)
sarcoidosis (D86.86)
enteropathic arthropathies (MØ7.-)
juvenile psoriatic arthropathy (L4Ø.54)
lipoid dermatoarthritis (E78.81)

√5th M14.6 Charcôt's joint
Neuropathic arthropathy
EXCLUDES 1 *Charcôt's joint in diabetes mellitus (EØ8-E13 with .61Ø)*
Charcôt's joint in tabes dorsalis (A52.16)
DEF: Progressive neurologic arthropathy in which chronic degeneration of joints in the weight-bearing areas with peripheral hypertrophy occurs as a complication of a neuropathy disorder. Supporting structures relax from a loss of sensation resulting in chronic joint instability.
M14.6Ø Charcôt's joint, unspecified site
√6th M14.61 Charcôt's joint, shoulder
M14.611 Charcôt's joint, right shoulder
M14.612 Charcôt's joint, left shoulder
M14.619 Charcôt's joint, unspecified shoulder
√6th M14.62 Charcôt's joint, elbow
M14.621 Charcôt's joint, right elbow
M14.622 Charcôt's joint, left elbow
M14.629 Charcôt's joint, unspecified elbow
√6th M14.63 Charcôt's joint, wrist
M14.631 Charcôt's joint, right wrist
M14.632 Charcôt's joint, left wrist
M14.639 Charcôt's joint, unspecified wrist
√6th M14.64 Charcôt's joint, hand
M14.641 Charcôt's joint, right hand
M14.642 Charcôt's joint, left hand
M14.649 Charcôt's joint, unspecified hand
√6th M14.65 Charcôt's joint, hip
M14.651 Charcôt's joint, right hip
M14.652 Charcôt's joint, left hip
M14.659 Charcôt's joint, unspecified hip
√6th M14.66 Charcôt's joint, knee
M14.661 Charcôt's joint, right knee
M14.662 Charcôt's joint, left knee
M14.669 Charcôt's joint, unspecified knee
√6th M14.67 Charcôt's joint, ankle and foot
M14.671 Charcôt's joint, right ankle and foot
M14.672 Charcôt's joint, left ankle and foot
M14.679 Charcôt's joint, unspecified ankle and foot
M14.68 Charcôt's joint, vertebrae
M14.69 Charcôt's joint, multiple sites

√5th M14.8 Arthropathies in other specified diseases classified elsewhere
Code first underlying disease, such as:
amyloidosis (E85.-)
erythema multiforme (L51.-)
erythema nodosum (L52)
hemochromatosis (E83.11-)
hyperparathyroidism (E21.-)
hypothyroidism (EØØ-EØ3)
sickle-cell disorders (D57.-)
thyrotoxicosis [hyperthyroidism] (EØ5.-)
Whipple's disease (K9Ø.81)
M14.8Ø Arthropathies in other specified diseases classified elsewhere, unspecified site
√6th M14.81 Arthropathies in other specified diseases classified elsewhere, shoulder
M14.811 Arthropathies in other specified diseases classified elsewhere, right shoulder
M14.812 Arthropathies in other specified diseases classified elsewhere, left shoulder
M14.819 Arthropathies in other specified diseases classified elsewhere, unspecified shoulder
√6th M14.82 Arthropathies in other specified diseases classified elsewhere, elbow
M14.821 Arthropathies in other specified diseases classified elsewhere, right elbow
M14.822 Arthropathies in other specified diseases classified elsewhere, left elbow
M14.829 Arthropathies in other specified diseases classified elsewhere, unspecified elbow
√6th M14.83 Arthropathies in other specified diseases classified elsewhere, wrist
M14.831 Arthropathies in other specified diseases classified elsewhere, right wrist
M14.832 Arthropathies in other specified diseases classified elsewhere, left wrist
M14.839 Arthropathies in other specified diseases classified elsewhere, unspecified wrist
√6th M14.84 Arthropathies in other specified diseases classified elsewhere, hand
M14.841 Arthropathies in other specified diseases classified elsewhere, right hand
M14.842 Arthropathies in other specified diseases classified elsewhere, left hand
M14.849 Arthropathies in other specified diseases classified elsewhere, unspecified hand
√6th M14.85 Arthropathies in other specified diseases classified elsewhere, hip
M14.851 Arthropathies in other specified diseases classified elsewhere, right hip
M14.852 Arthropathies in other specified diseases classified elsewhere, left hip
M14.859 Arthropathies in other specified diseases classified elsewhere, unspecified hip
√6th M14.86 Arthropathies in other specified diseases classified elsewhere, knee
M14.861 Arthropathies in other specified diseases classified elsewhere, right knee
M14.862 Arthropathies in other specified diseases classified elsewhere, left knee
M14.869 Arthropathies in other specified diseases classified elsewhere, unspecified knee
√6th M14.87 Arthropathies in other specified diseases classified elsewhere, ankle and foot
M14.871 Arthropathies in other specified diseases classified elsewhere, right ankle and foot
M14.872 Arthropathies in other specified diseases classified elsewhere, left ankle and foot
M14.879 Arthropathies in other specified diseases classified elsewhere, unspecified ankle and foot
M14.88 Arthropathies in other specified diseases classified elsewhere, vertebrae
M14.89 Arthropathies in other specified diseases classified elsewhere, multiple sites

Osteoarthritis (M15-M19)

EXCLUDES 2 *osteoarthritis of spine (M47.-)*

AHA: 2020,2Q,14; 2016,4Q,147

TIP: Assign a primary osteoarthritis code when the site of the osteoarthritis is documented but the type of osteoarthritis — primary, secondary, generalized, or post-traumatic — is not documented. Primary is considered the default.

✓4th **M15 Polyosteoarthritis**

INCLUDES arthritis of multiple sites

EXCLUDES 1 *bilateral involvement of single joint (M16-M19)*

M15.Ø Primary generalized (osteo)arthritis

M15.1 Heberden's nodes (with arthropathy)

Interphalangeal distal osteoarthritis

M15.2 Bouchard's nodes (with arthropathy)

Juxtaphalangeal distal osteoarthritis

M15.3 Secondary multiple arthritis

Post-traumatic polyosteoarthritis

M15.4 Erosive (osteo)arthritis

M15.8 Other polyosteoarthritis

M15.9 Polyosteoarthritis, unspecified

Generalized osteoarthritis NOS

✓4th **M16 Osteoarthritis of hip**

AHA: 2016,4Q,146

M16.Ø Bilateral primary osteoarthritis of hip

AHA: 2018,2Q,15

✓5th **M16.1 Unilateral primary osteoarthritis of hip**

Primary osteoarthritis of hip NOS

AHA: 2018,2Q,15

M16.1Ø Unilateral primary osteoarthritis, unspecified hip

M16.11 Unilateral primary osteoarthritis, right hip

M16.12 Unilateral primary osteoarthritis, left hip

M16.2 Bilateral osteoarthritis resulting from hip dysplasia

✓5th **M16.3 Unilateral osteoarthritis resulting from hip dysplasia**

Dysplastic osteoarthritis of hip NOS

M16.3Ø Unilateral osteoarthritis resulting from hip dysplasia, unspecified hip

M16.31 Unilateral osteoarthritis resulting from hip dysplasia, right hip

M16.32 Unilateral osteoarthritis resulting from hip dysplasia, left hip

M16.4 Bilateral post-traumatic osteoarthritis of hip

✓5th **M16.5 Unilateral post-traumatic osteoarthritis of hip**

Post-traumatic osteoarthritis of hip NOS

M16.5Ø Unilateral post-traumatic osteoarthritis, unspecified hip

M16.51 Unilateral post-traumatic osteoarthritis, right hip

M16.52 Unilateral post-traumatic osteoarthritis, left hip

M16.6 Other bilateral secondary osteoarthritis of hip

M16.7 Other unilateral secondary osteoarthritis of hip

Secondary osteoarthritis of hip NOS

M16.9 Osteoarthritis of hip, unspecified

✓4th **M17 Osteoarthritis of knee**

AHA: 2016,4Q,146-147

M17.Ø Bilateral primary osteoarthritis of knee

AHA: 2018,2Q,15

✓5th **M17.1 Unilateral primary osteoarthritis of knee**

Primary osteoarthritis of knee NOS

AHA: 2018,2Q,15

M17.1Ø Unilateral primary osteoarthritis, unspecified knee

M17.11 Unilateral primary osteoarthritis, right knee

M17.12 Unilateral primary osteoarthritis, left knee

M17.2 Bilateral post-traumatic osteoarthritis of knee

✓5th **M17.3 Unilateral post-traumatic osteoarthritis of knee**

Post-traumatic osteoarthritis of knee NOS

M17.3Ø Unilateral post-traumatic osteoarthritis, unspecified knee

M17.31 Unilateral post-traumatic osteoarthritis, right knee

M17.32 Unilateral post-traumatic osteoarthritis, left knee

M17.4 Other bilateral secondary osteoarthritis of knee

M17.5 Other unilateral secondary osteoarthritis of knee

Secondary osteoarthritis of knee NOS

M17.9 Osteoarthritis of knee, unspecified

✓4th **M18 Osteoarthritis of first carpometacarpal joint**

M18.Ø Bilateral primary osteoarthritis of first carpometacarpal joints

✓5th **M18.1 Unilateral primary osteoarthritis of first carpometacarpal joint**

Primary osteoarthritis of first carpometacarpal joint NOS

M18.1Ø Unilateral primary osteoarthritis of first carpometacarpal joint, unspecified hand

M18.11 Unilateral primary osteoarthritis of first carpometacarpal joint, right hand

M18.12 Unilateral primary osteoarthritis of first carpometacarpal joint, left hand

M18.2 Bilateral post-traumatic osteoarthritis of first carpometacarpal joints

✓5th **M18.3 Unilateral post-traumatic osteoarthritis of first carpometacarpal joint**

Post-traumatic osteoarthritis of first carpometacarpal joint NOS

M18.3Ø Unilateral post-traumatic osteoarthritis of first carpometacarpal joint, unspecified hand

M18.31 Unilateral post-traumatic osteoarthritis of first carpometacarpal joint, right hand

M18.32 Unilateral post-traumatic osteoarthritis of first carpometacarpal joint, left hand

M18.4 Other bilateral secondary osteoarthritis of first carpometacarpal joints

✓5th **M18.5 Other unilateral secondary osteoarthritis of first carpometacarpal joint**

Secondary osteoarthritis of first carpometacarpal joint NOS

M18.5Ø Other unilateral secondary osteoarthritis of first carpometacarpal joint, unspecified hand

M18.51 Other unilateral secondary osteoarthritis of first carpometacarpal joint, right hand

M18.52 Other unilateral secondary osteoarthritis of first carpometacarpal joint, left hand

M18.9 Osteoarthritis of first carpometacarpal joint, unspecified

✓4th **M19 Other and unspecified osteoarthritis**

EXCLUDES 1 *polyarthritis (M15.-)*

EXCLUDES 2 *arthrosis of spine (M47.-)*
hallux rigidus (M2Ø.2)
osteoarthritis of spine (M47.-)

✓5th **M19.Ø Primary osteoarthritis of other joints**

AHA: 2018,2Q,15; 2016,4Q,145

✓6th **M19.Ø1 Primary osteoarthritis, shoulder**

M19.Ø11 Primary osteoarthritis, right shoulder

M19.Ø12 Primary osteoarthritis, left shoulder

M19.Ø19 Primary osteoarthritis, unspecified shoulder

✓6th **M19.Ø2 Primary osteoarthritis, elbow**

M19.Ø21 Primary osteoarthritis, right elbow

M19.Ø22 Primary osteoarthritis, left elbow

M19.Ø29 Primary osteoarthritis, unspecified elbow

✓6th **M19.Ø3 Primary osteoarthritis, wrist**

M19.Ø31 Primary osteoarthritis, right wrist

M19.Ø32 Primary osteoarthritis, left wrist

M19.Ø39 Primary osteoarthritis, unspecified wrist

✓6th **M19.Ø4 Primary osteoarthritis, hand**

EXCLUDES 2 *primary osteoarthritis of first carpometacarpal joint (M18.Ø-, M18.1-)*

M19.Ø41 Primary osteoarthritis, right hand

M19.Ø42 Primary osteoarthritis, left hand

M19.Ø49 Primary osteoarthritis, unspecified hand

✓6th **M19.Ø7 Primary osteoarthritis ankle and foot**

M19.Ø71 Primary osteoarthritis, right ankle and foot

M19.Ø72 Primary osteoarthritis, left ankle and foot

M19.Ø79 Primary osteoarthritis, unspecified ankle and foot

● **M19.Ø9 Primary osteoarthritis, other specified site**

✓5th **M19.1 Post-traumatic osteoarthritis of other joints**

✓6th **M19.11 Post-traumatic osteoarthritis, shoulder**

M19.111 Post-traumatic osteoarthritis, right shoulder

M19.112 Post-traumatic osteoarthritis, left shoulder

M19.119 Post-traumatic osteoarthritis, unspecified shoulder

✓6th **M19.12 Post-traumatic osteoarthritis, elbow**

M19.121 Post-traumatic osteoarthritis, right elbow

M19.122 Post-traumatic osteoarthritis, left elbow

M19.129 Post-traumatic osteoarthritis, unspecified elbow

M19.13 Post-traumatic osteoarthritis, wrist

M19.131 Post-traumatic osteoarthritis, right wrist

M19.132 Post-traumatic osteoarthritis, left wrist

M19.139 Post-traumatic osteoarthritis, unspecified wrist

M19.14 Post-traumatic osteoarthritis, hand

EXCLUDES 2 *post-traumatic osteoarthritis of first carpometacarpal joint (M18.2-, M18.3-)*

M19.141 Post-traumatic osteoarthritis, right hand

M19.142 Post-traumatic osteoarthritis, left hand

M19.149 Post-traumatic osteoarthritis, unspecified hand

M19.17 Post-traumatic osteoarthritis, ankle and foot

M19.171 Post-traumatic osteoarthritis, right ankle and foot

M19.172 Post-traumatic osteoarthritis, left ankle and foot

M19.179 Post-traumatic osteoarthritis, unspecified ankle and foot

● M19.19 Post-traumatic osteoarthritis, other specified site

M19.2 Secondary osteoarthritis of other joints

M19.21 Secondary osteoarthritis, shoulder

M19.211 Secondary osteoarthritis, right shoulder

M19.212 Secondary osteoarthritis, left shoulder

M19.219 Secondary osteoarthritis, unspecified shoulder

M19.22 Secondary osteoarthritis, elbow

M19.221 Secondary osteoarthritis, right elbow

M19.222 Secondary osteoarthritis, left elbow

M19.229 Secondary osteoarthritis, unspecified elbow

M19.23 Secondary osteoarthritis, wrist

M19.231 Secondary osteoarthritis, right wrist

M19.232 Secondary osteoarthritis, left wrist

M19.239 Secondary osteoarthritis, unspecified wrist

M19.24 Secondary osteoarthritis, hand

M19.241 Secondary osteoarthritis, right hand

M19.242 Secondary osteoarthritis, left hand

M19.249 Secondary osteoarthritis, unspecified hand

M19.27 Secondary osteoarthritis, ankle and foot

M19.271 Secondary osteoarthritis, right ankle and foot

M19.272 Secondary osteoarthritis, left ankle and foot

M19.279 Secondary osteoarthritis, unspecified ankle and foot

● M19.29 Secondary osteoarthritis, other specified site

M19.9 Osteoarthritis, unspecified site

TIP: Assign M19.90 when neither the site nor the type of osteoarthritis — primary, secondary, or post-traumatic — is documented.

M19.90 Unspecified osteoarthritis, unspecified site
Arthrosis NOS
Arthritis NOS
Osteoarthritis NOS
AHA: 2016,4Q,145-147

M19.91 Primary osteoarthritis, unspecified site
Primary osteoarthritis NOS

M19.92 Post-traumatic osteoarthritis, unspecified site
Post-traumatic osteoarthritis NOS

M19.93 Secondary osteoarthritis, unspecified site
Secondary osteoarthritis NOS

Other joint disorders (M20-M25)

EXCLUDES 2 *joints of the spine (M40-M54)*

M20 Acquired deformities of fingers and toes

EXCLUDES 1 *acquired absence of fingers and toes (Z89.-)*
congenital absence of fingers and toes (Q71.3-, Q72.3-)
congenital deformities and malformations of fingers and toes (Q66.-, Q68-Q70, Q74.-)

M20.0 Deformity of finger(s)

EXCLUDES 1 *clubbing of fingers (R68.3)*
palmar fascial fibromatosis [Dupuytren] (M72.0)
trigger finger (M65.3)

M20.00 Unspecified deformity of finger(s)

M20.001 Unspecified deformity of right finger(s)

M20.002 Unspecified deformity of left finger(s)

M20.009 Unspecified deformity of unspecified finger(s)

M20.01 Mallet finger

M20.011 Mallet finger of right finger(s)

M20.012 Mallet finger of left finger(s)

M20.019 Mallet finger of unspecified finger(s)

M20.02 Boutonnière deformity

DEF: Deformity of the finger caused by flexion of the proximal interphalangeal joint and hyperextension of the distal joint. The deformity results from rheumatoid arthritis, osteoarthritis, or injury.

M20.021 Boutonnière deformity of right finger(s)

M20.022 Boutonnière deformity of left finger(s)

M20.029 Boutonnière deformity of unspecified finger(s)

M20.03 Swan-neck deformity

DEF: Flexed distal and hyperextended proximal interphalangeal joint most commonly caused by rheumatoid arthritis.

M20.031 Swan-neck deformity of right finger(s)

M20.032 Swan-neck deformity of left finger(s)

M20.039 Swan-neck deformity of unspecified finger(s)

M20.09 Other deformity of finger(s)

M20.091 Other deformity of right finger(s)

M20.092 Other deformity of left finger(s)

M20.099 Other deformity of finger(s), unspecified finger(s)

M20.1 Hallux valgus (acquired)

EXCLUDES 2 *bunion (M21.6-)*

AHA: 2016,4Q,38

DEF: Deformity in which the great toe deviates toward the other toes and may even be positioned over or under the second toe.

Hallux Valgus

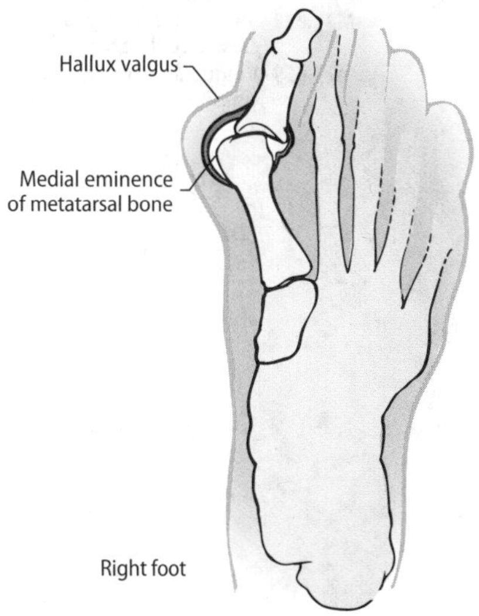

M20.10 Hallux valgus (acquired), unspecified foot

M20.11 Hallux valgus (acquired), right foot

M20.12 Hallux valgus (acquired), left foot

✓5th **M20.2 Hallux rigidus**

- **M20.20 Hallux rigidus, unspecified foot**
- **M20.21 Hallux rigidus, right foot**
- **M20.22 Hallux rigidus, left foot**

✓5th **M20.3 Hallux varus (acquired)**

DEF: Deformity in which the great toe deviates away from the other toes.

- **M20.30 Hallux varus (acquired), unspecified foot**
- **M20.31 Hallux varus (acquired), right foot**
- **M20.32 Hallux varus (acquired), left foot**

✓5th **M20.4 Other hammer toe(s) (acquired)**

- **M20.40 Other hammer toe(s) (acquired), unspecified foot**
- **M20.41 Other hammer toe(s) (acquired), right foot**
- **M20.42 Other hammer toe(s) (acquired), left foot**

✓5th **M20.5 Other deformities of toe(s) (acquired)**

✓6th **M20.5X Other deformities of toe(s) (acquired)**

- **M20.5X1 Other deformities of toe(s) (acquired), right foot**
- **M20.5X2 Other deformities of toe(s) (acquired), left foot**
- **M20.5X9 Other deformities of toe(s) (acquired), unspecified foot**

✓5th **M20.6 Acquired deformities of toe(s), unspecified**

- **M20.60 Acquired deformities of toe(s), unspecified, unspecified foot**
- **M20.61 Acquired deformities of toe(s), unspecified, right foot**
- **M20.62 Acquired deformities of toe(s), unspecified, left foot**

✓4th **M21 Other acquired deformities of limbs**

EXCLUDES 1 *acquired absence of limb (Z89.-)*
congenital absence of limbs (Q71-Q73)
congenital deformities and malformations of limbs (Q65-Q66, Q68-Q74)

EXCLUDES 2 *acquired deformities of fingers or toes (M20.-)*
coxa plana (M91.2)

✓5th **M21.0 Valgus deformity, not elsewhere classified**

EXCLUDES 1 *metatarsus valgus (Q66.6)*
talipes calcaneovalgus (Q66.4-)

- **M21.00 Valgus deformity, not elsewhere classified, unspecified site**

✓6th **M21.02 Valgus deformity, not elsewhere classified, elbow**

Cubitus valgus

- **M21.021 Valgus deformity, not elsewhere classified, right elbow**
- **M21.022 Valgus deformity, not elsewhere classified, left elbow**
- **M21.029 Valgus deformity, not elsewhere classified, unspecified elbow**

✓6th **M21.05 Valgus deformity, not elsewhere classified, hip**

- **M21.051 Valgus deformity, not elsewhere classified, right hip**
- **M21.052 Valgus deformity, not elsewhere classified, left hip**
- **M21.059 Valgus deformity, not elsewhere classified, unspecified hip**

✓6th **M21.06 Valgus deformity, not elsewhere classified, knee**

Genu valgum
Knock knee

DEF: Genu valga/valgum: Condition in which the thighs slant inward, causing the knees to be angled abnormally close together, leaving the space between the ankles wider than normal.

Genu Valga (knock-knee)

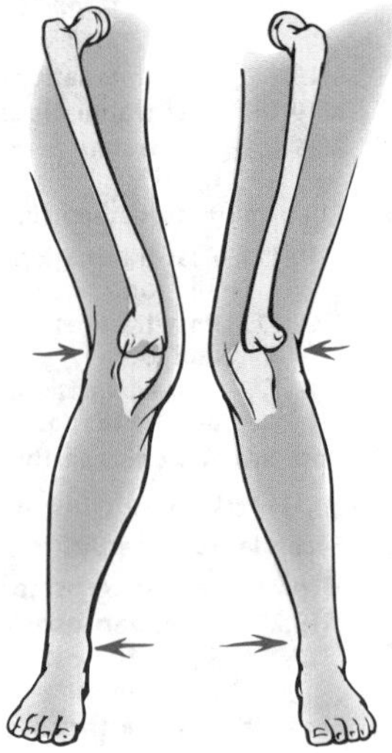

- **M21.061 Valgus deformity, not elsewhere classified, right knee**
- **M21.062 Valgus deformity, not elsewhere classified, left knee**
- **M21.069 Valgus deformity, not elsewhere classified, unspecified knee**

✓6th **M21.07 Valgus deformity, not elsewhere classified, ankle**

- **M21.071 Valgus deformity, not elsewhere classified, right ankle**
- **M21.072 Valgus deformity, not elsewhere classified, left ankle**
- **M21.079 Valgus deformity, not elsewhere classified, unspecified ankle**

✓5th **M21.1 Varus deformity, not elsewhere classified**

EXCLUDES 1 *metatarsus varus (Q66.22-)*
tibia vara ▶(M92.51-)◀

- **M21.10 Varus deformity, not elsewhere classified, unspecified site**

✓6th **M21.12 Varus deformity, not elsewhere classified, elbow**

Cubitus varus, elbow

- **M21.121 Varus deformity, not elsewhere classified, right elbow**
- **M21.122 Varus deformity, not elsewhere classified, left elbow**
- **M21.129 Varus deformity, not elsewhere classified, unspecified elbow**

✓6th **M21.15 Varus deformity, not elsewhere classified, hip**

- **M21.151 Varus deformity, not elsewhere classified, right hip**
- **M21.152 Varus deformity, not elsewhere classified, left hip**
- **M21.159 Varus deformity, not elsewhere classified, unspecified**

M21.16 Varus deformity, not elsewhere classified, knee

Bow leg

Genu varum

DEF: Genu varus/varum: Condition in which the thighs and/or legs are bowed in an outward curve with an abnormally increased space between the knees.

Genu Varus (bowleg)

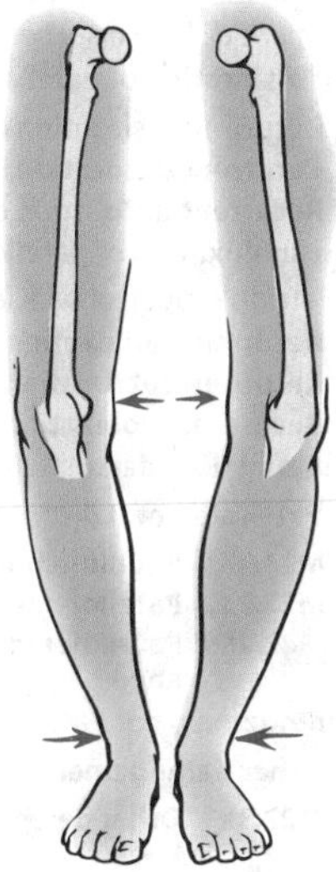

M21.161 Varus deformity, not elsewhere classified, right knee

M21.162 Varus deformity, not elsewhere classified, left knee

M21.169 Varus deformity, not elsewhere classified, unspecified knee

M21.17 Varus deformity, not elsewhere classified, ankle

M21.171 Varus deformity, not elsewhere classified, right ankle

M21.172 Varus deformity, not elsewhere classified, left ankle

M21.179 Varus deformity, not elsewhere classified, unspecified ankle

M21.2 Flexion deformity

M21.20 Flexion deformity, unspecified site

M21.21 Flexion deformity, shoulder

M21.211 Flexion deformity, right shoulder

M21.212 Flexion deformity, left shoulder

M21.219 Flexion deformity, unspecified shoulder

M21.22 Flexion deformity, elbow

M21.221 Flexion deformity, right elbow

M21.222 Flexion deformity, left elbow

M21.229 Flexion deformity, unspecified elbow

M21.23 Flexion deformity, wrist

M21.231 Flexion deformity, right wrist

M21.232 Flexion deformity, left wrist

M21.239 Flexion deformity, unspecified wrist

M21.24 Flexion deformity, finger joints

M21.241 Flexion deformity, right finger joints

M21.242 Flexion deformity, left finger joints

M21.249 Flexion deformity, unspecified finger joints

M21.25 Flexion deformity, hip

M21.251 Flexion deformity, right hip

M21.252 Flexion deformity, left hip

M21.259 Flexion deformity, unspecified hip

M21.26 Flexion deformity, knee

M21.261 Flexion deformity, right knee

M21.262 Flexion deformity, left knee

M21.269 Flexion deformity, unspecified knee

M21.27 Flexion deformity, ankle and toes

M21.271 Flexion deformity, right ankle and toes

M21.272 Flexion deformity, left ankle and toes

M21.279 Flexion deformity, unspecified ankle and toes

M21.3 Wrist or foot drop (acquired)

M21.33 Wrist drop (acquired)

M21.331 Wrist drop, right wrist

M21.332 Wrist drop, left wrist

M21.339 Wrist drop, unspecified wrist

M21.37 Foot drop (acquired)

M21.371 Foot drop, right foot

M21.372 Foot drop, left foot

M21.379 Foot drop, unspecified foot

M21.4 Flat foot [pes planus] (acquired)

EXCLUDES 1 *congenital pes planus (Q66.5-)*

M21.40 Flat foot [pes planus] (acquired), unspecified foot

M21.41 Flat foot [pes planus] (acquired), right foot

M21.42 Flat foot [pes planus] (acquired), left foot

M21.5 Acquired clawhand, clubhand, clawfoot and clubfoot

EXCLUDES 1 *clubfoot, not specified as acquired (Q66.89)*

M21.51 Acquired clawhand

M21.511 Acquired clawhand, right hand

M21.512 Acquired clawhand, left hand

M21.519 Acquired clawhand, unspecified hand

M21.52 Acquired clubhand

M21.521 Acquired clubhand, right hand

M21.522 Acquired clubhand, left hand

M21.529 Acquired clubhand, unspecified hand

M21.53 Acquired clawfoot

DEF: High foot arch with hyperextended toes at the metatarsophalangeal joint and flexed toes at the distal joints.

M21.531 Acquired clawfoot, right foot

M21.532 Acquired clawfoot, left foot

M21.539 Acquired clawfoot, unspecified foot

M21.54 Acquired clubfoot

DEF: Acquired anomaly of the foot with the heel elevated and rotated outward and the toes pointing inward.

M21.541 Acquired clubfoot, right foot

M21.542 Acquired clubfoot, left foot

M21.549 Acquired clubfoot, unspecified foot

M21.6 Other acquired deformities of foot

EXCLUDES 2 *deformities of toe (acquired) (M20.1-M20.6-)*

AHA: 2016,4Q,38

M21.61 Bunion

M21.611 Bunion of right foot

M21.612 Bunion of left foot

M21.619 Bunion of unspecified foot

M21.62 Bunionette

M21.621 Bunionette of right foot

M21.622 Bunionette of left foot

M21.629 Bunionette of unspecified foot

M21.6X Other acquired deformities of foot

M21.6X1 Other acquired deformities of right foot

M21.6X2 Other acquired deformities of left foot

M21.6X9 Other acquired deformities of unspecified foot

M21.7 Unequal limb length (acquired)

NOTE The site used should correspond to the shorter limb

M21.70 Unequal limb length (acquired), unspecified site

M21.72 Unequal limb length (acquired), humerus

M21.721 Unequal limb length (acquired), right humerus

M21.722 Unequal limb length (acquired), left humerus

M21.729 Unequal limb length (acquired), unspecified humerus

M21.73 Unequal limb length (acquired), ulna and radius

M21.731 Unequal limb length (acquired), right ulna

M21.732 Unequal limb length (acquired), left ulna

M21.733 Unequal limb length (acquired), right radius

M21.734 Unequal limb length (acquired), left radius

M21.739 Unequal limb length (acquired), unspecified ulna and radius

6th M21.75 Unequal limb length (acquired), femur
- M21.751 Unequal limb length (acquired), right femur
- M21.752 Unequal limb length (acquired), left femur
- M21.759 Unequal limb length (acquired), unspecified femur

6th M21.76 Unequal limb length (acquired), tibia and fibula
- M21.761 Unequal limb length (acquired), right tibia
- M21.762 Unequal limb length (acquired), left tibia
- M21.763 Unequal limb length (acquired), right fibula
- M21.764 Unequal limb length (acquired), left fibula
- M21.769 Unequal limb length (acquired), unspecified tibia and fibula

5th M21.8 Other specified acquired deformities of limbs

EXCLUDES 2 *coxa plana (M91.2)*

- M21.80 Other specified acquired deformities of unspecified limb

6th M21.82 Other specified acquired deformities of upper arm
- M21.821 Other specified acquired deformities of right upper arm
- M21.822 Other specified acquired deformities of left upper arm
- M21.829 Other specified acquired deformities of unspecified upper arm

6th M21.83 Other specified acquired deformities of forearm
- M21.831 Other specified acquired deformities of right forearm
- M21.832 Other specified acquired deformities of left forearm
- M21.839 Other specified acquired deformities of unspecified forearm

6th M21.85 Other specified acquired deformities of thigh
- M21.851 Other specified acquired deformities of right thigh
- M21.852 Other specified acquired deformities of left thigh
- M21.859 Other specified acquired deformities of unspecified thigh

6th M21.86 Other specified acquired deformities of lower leg
- M21.861 Other specified acquired deformities of right lower leg
- M21.862 Other specified acquired deformities of left lower leg
- M21.869 Other specified acquired deformities of unspecified lower leg

5th M21.9 Unspecified acquired deformity of limb and hand
- M21.90 Unspecified acquired deformity of unspecified limb

6th M21.92 Unspecified acquired deformity of upper arm
- M21.921 Unspecified acquired deformity of right upper arm
- M21.922 Unspecified acquired deformity of left upper arm
- M21.929 Unspecified acquired deformity of unspecified upper arm

6th M21.93 Unspecified acquired deformity of forearm
- M21.931 Unspecified acquired deformity of right forearm
- M21.932 Unspecified acquired deformity of left forearm
- M21.939 Unspecified acquired deformity of unspecified forearm

6th M21.94 Unspecified acquired deformity of hand
- M21.941 Unspecified acquired deformity of hand, right hand
- M21.942 Unspecified acquired deformity of hand, left hand
- M21.949 Unspecified acquired deformity of hand, unspecified hand

6th M21.95 Unspecified acquired deformity of thigh
- M21.951 Unspecified acquired deformity of right thigh
- M21.952 Unspecified acquired deformity of left thigh
- M21.959 Unspecified acquired deformity of unspecified thigh

6th M21.96 Unspecified acquired deformity of lower leg
- M21.961 Unspecified acquired deformity of right lower leg
- M21.962 Unspecified acquired deformity of left lower leg
- M21.969 Unspecified acquired deformity of unspecified lower leg

4th M22 Disorder of patella

EXCLUDES 1 ~~*traumatic dislocation of patella (S83.0-)*~~

EXCLUDES 2 ▶*traumatic dislocation of patella (S83.0-)*◀

5th M22.0 Recurrent dislocation of patella
- M22.00 Recurrent dislocation of patella, unspecified knee
- M22.01 Recurrent dislocation of patella, right knee
- M22.02 Recurrent dislocation of patella, left knee

5th M22.1 Recurrent subluxation of patella

Incomplete dislocation of patella
- M22.10 Recurrent subluxation of patella, unspecified knee
- M22.11 Recurrent subluxation of patella, right knee
- M22.12 Recurrent subluxation of patella, left knee

5th M22.2 Patellofemoral disorders

6th M22.2X Patellofemoral disorders
- M22.2X1 Patellofemoral disorders, right knee
- M22.2X2 Patellofemoral disorders, left knee
- M22.2X9 Patellofemoral disorders, unspecified knee

5th M22.3 Other derangements of patella

6th M22.3X Other derangements of patella
- M22.3X1 Other derangements of patella, right knee
- M22.3X2 Other derangements of patella, left knee
- M22.3X9 Other derangements of patella, unspecified knee

5th M22.4 Chondromalacia patellae
- M22.40 Chondromalacia patellae, unspecified knee
- M22.41 Chondromalacia patellae, right knee
- M22.42 Chondromalacia patellae, left knee

5th M22.8 Other disorders of patella

6th M22.8X Other disorders of patella
- M22.8X1 Other disorders of patella, right knee
- M22.8X2 Other disorders of patella, left knee
- M22.8X9 Other disorders of patella, unspecified knee

5th M22.9 Unspecified disorder of patella
- M22.90 Unspecified disorder of patella, unspecified knee
- M22.91 Unspecified disorder of patella, right knee
- M22.92 Unspecified disorder of patella, left knee

4th M23 Internal derangement of knee

EXCLUDES 1 *ankylosis (M24.66)*
~~*current injury — see injury of knee and lower leg (S80-S89)*~~
deformity of knee (M21.-)
osteochondritis dissecans (M93.2)
~~*recurrent dislocation or subluxation of joints (M24.4)*~~
~~*recurrent dislocation or subluxation of patella (M22.0-M22.1)*~~

EXCLUDES 2 ▶*current injury — see injury of knee and lower leg (S80-S89)*◀
▶*recurrent dislocation or subluxation of joints (M24.4)*◀
▶*recurrent dislocation or subluxation of patella (M22.0-M22.1)*◀

5th M23.0 Cystic meniscus

6th M23.00 Cystic meniscus, unspecified meniscus

Cystic meniscus, unspecified lateral meniscus
Cystic meniscus, unspecified medial meniscus
- M23.000 Cystic meniscus, unspecified lateral meniscus, right knee
- M23.001 Cystic meniscus, unspecified lateral meniscus, left knee
- M23.002 Cystic meniscus, unspecified lateral meniscus, unspecified knee
- M23.003 Cystic meniscus, unspecified medial meniscus, right knee
- M23.004 Cystic meniscus, unspecified medial meniscus, left knee
- M23.005 Cystic meniscus, unspecified medial meniscus, unspecified knee
- M23.006 Cystic meniscus, unspecified meniscus, right knee

M23.007 Cystic meniscus, unspecified meniscus, left knee
M23.009 Cystic meniscus, unspecified meniscus, unspecified knee

✓6th M23.01 Cystic meniscus, anterior horn of medial meniscus
M23.011 Cystic meniscus, anterior horn of medial meniscus, right knee
M23.012 Cystic meniscus, anterior horn of medial meniscus, left knee
M23.019 Cystic meniscus, anterior horn of medial meniscus, unspecified knee

✓6th M23.02 Cystic meniscus, posterior horn of medial meniscus
M23.021 Cystic meniscus, posterior horn of medial meniscus, right knee
M23.022 Cystic meniscus, posterior horn of medial meniscus, left knee
M23.029 Cystic meniscus, posterior horn of medial meniscus, unspecified knee

✓6th M23.03 Cystic meniscus, other medial meniscus
M23.031 Cystic meniscus, other medial meniscus, right knee
M23.032 Cystic meniscus, other medial meniscus, left knee
M23.039 Cystic meniscus, other medial meniscus, unspecified knee

✓6th M23.04 Cystic meniscus, anterior horn of lateral meniscus
M23.041 Cystic meniscus, anterior horn of lateral meniscus, right knee
M23.042 Cystic meniscus, anterior horn of lateral meniscus, left knee
M23.049 Cystic meniscus, anterior horn of lateral meniscus, unspecified knee

✓6th M23.05 Cystic meniscus, posterior horn of lateral meniscus
M23.051 Cystic meniscus, posterior horn of lateral meniscus, right knee
M23.052 Cystic meniscus, posterior horn of lateral meniscus, left knee
M23.059 Cystic meniscus, posterior horn of lateral meniscus, unspecified knee

✓6th M23.06 Cystic meniscus, other lateral meniscus
M23.061 Cystic meniscus, other lateral meniscus, right knee
M23.062 Cystic meniscus, other lateral meniscus, left knee
M23.069 Cystic meniscus, other lateral meniscus, unspecified knee

✓5th M23.2 Derangement of meniscus due to old tear or injury
Old bucket-handle tear
AHA: 2019,2Q,26

Derangement of Meniscus

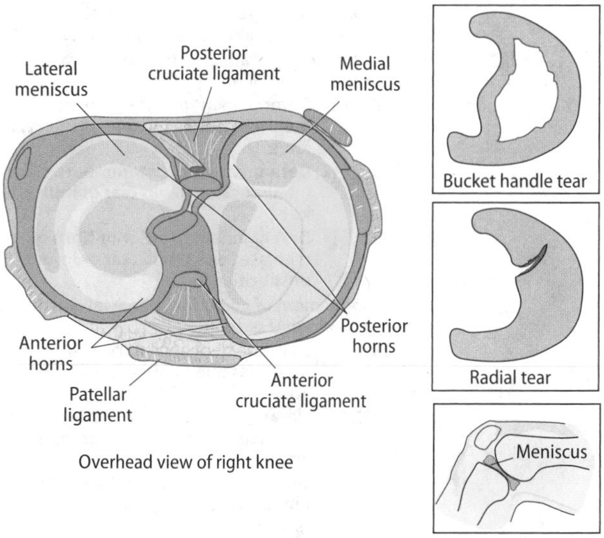

Overhead view of right knee

✓6th M23.20 Derangement of unspecified meniscus due to old tear or injury
Derangement of unspecified lateral meniscus due to old tear or injury
Derangement of unspecified medial meniscus due to old tear or injury
M23.200 Derangement of unspecified lateral meniscus due to old tear or injury, right knee
M23.201 Derangement of unspecified lateral meniscus due to old tear or injury, left knee
M23.202 Derangement of unspecified lateral meniscus due to old tear or injury, unspecified knee
M23.203 Derangement of unspecified medial meniscus due to old tear or injury, right knee
M23.204 Derangement of unspecified medial meniscus due to old tear or injury, left knee
M23.205 Derangement of unspecified medial meniscus due to old tear or injury, unspecified knee
M23.206 Derangement of unspecified meniscus due to old tear or injury, right knee
M23.207 Derangement of unspecified meniscus due to old tear or injury, left knee
M23.209 Derangement of unspecified meniscus due to old tear or injury, unspecified knee

✓6th M23.21 Derangement of anterior horn of medial meniscus due to old tear or injury
M23.211 Derangement of anterior horn of medial meniscus due to old tear or injury, right knee
M23.212 Derangement of anterior horn of medial meniscus due to old tear or injury, left knee
M23.219 Derangement of anterior horn of medial meniscus due to old tear or injury, unspecified knee

✓6th M23.22 Derangement of posterior horn of medial meniscus due to old tear or injury
M23.221 Derangement of posterior horn of medial meniscus due to old tear or injury, right knee
M23.222 Derangement of posterior horn of medial meniscus due to old tear or injury, left knee
M23.229 Derangement of posterior horn of medial meniscus due to old tear or injury, unspecified knee

√6th **M23.23 Derangement of other medial meniscus due to old tear or injury**
- **M23.231 Derangement of other medial meniscus due to old tear or injury, right knee**
- **M23.232 Derangement of other medial meniscus due to old tear or injury, left knee**
- **M23.239 Derangement of other medial meniscus due to old tear or injury, unspecified knee**

√6th **M23.24 Derangement of anterior horn of lateral meniscus due to old tear or injury**
- **M23.241 Derangement of anterior horn of lateral meniscus due to old tear or injury, right knee**
- **M23.242 Derangement of anterior horn of lateral meniscus due to old tear or injury, left knee**
- **M23.249 Derangement of anterior horn of lateral meniscus due to old tear or injury, unspecified knee**

√6th **M23.25 Derangement of posterior horn of lateral meniscus due to old tear or injury**
- **M23.251 Derangement of posterior horn of lateral meniscus due to old tear or injury, right knee**
- **M23.252 Derangement of posterior horn of lateral meniscus due to old tear or injury, left knee**
- **M23.259 Derangement of posterior horn of lateral meniscus due to old tear or injury, unspecified knee**

√6th **M23.26 Derangement of other lateral meniscus due to old tear or injury**
- **M23.261 Derangement of other lateral meniscus due to old tear or injury, right knee**
- **M23.262 Derangement of other lateral meniscus due to old tear or injury, left knee**
- **M23.269 Derangement of other lateral meniscus due to old tear or injury, unspecified knee**

√5th **M23.3 Other meniscus derangements**

Degenerate meniscus
Detached meniscus
Retained meniscus

√6th **M23.30 Other meniscus derangements, unspecified meniscus**

Other meniscus derangements, unspecified lateral meniscus
Other meniscus derangements, unspecified medial meniscus

- **M23.300 Other meniscus derangements, unspecified lateral meniscus, right knee**
- **M23.301 Other meniscus derangements, unspecified lateral meniscus, left knee**
- **M23.302 Other meniscus derangements, unspecified lateral meniscus, unspecified knee**
- **M23.303 Other meniscus derangements, unspecified medial meniscus, right knee**
- **M23.304 Other meniscus derangements, unspecified medial meniscus, left knee**
- **M23.305 Other meniscus derangements, unspecified medial meniscus, unspecified knee**
- **M23.306 Other meniscus derangements, unspecified meniscus, right knee**
- **M23.307 Other meniscus derangements, unspecified meniscus, left knee**
- **M23.309 Other meniscus derangements, unspecified meniscus, unspecified knee**

√6th **M23.31 Other meniscus derangements, anterior horn of medial meniscus**
- **M23.311 Other meniscus derangements, anterior horn of medial meniscus, right knee**
- **M23.312 Other meniscus derangements, anterior horn of medial meniscus, left knee**
- **M23.319 Other meniscus derangements, anterior horn of medial meniscus, unspecified knee**

√6th **M23.32 Other meniscus derangements, posterior horn of medial meniscus**
- **M23.321 Other meniscus derangements, posterior horn of medial meniscus, right knee**
- **M23.322 Other meniscus derangements, posterior horn of medial meniscus, left knee**
- **M23.329 Other meniscus derangements, posterior horn of medial meniscus, unspecified knee**

√6th **M23.33 Other meniscus derangements, other medial meniscus**
- **M23.331 Other meniscus derangements, other medial meniscus, right knee**
- **M23.332 Other meniscus derangements, other medial meniscus, left knee**
- **M23.339 Other meniscus derangements, other medial meniscus, unspecified knee**

√6th **M23.34 Other meniscus derangements, anterior horn of lateral meniscus**
- **M23.341 Other meniscus derangements, anterior horn of lateral meniscus, right knee**
- **M23.342 Other meniscus derangements, anterior horn of lateral meniscus, left knee**
- **M23.349 Other meniscus derangements, anterior horn of lateral meniscus, unspecified knee**

√6th **M23.35 Other meniscus derangements, posterior horn of lateral meniscus**
- **M23.351 Other meniscus derangements, posterior horn of lateral meniscus, right knee**
- **M23.352 Other meniscus derangements, posterior horn of lateral meniscus, left knee**
- **M23.359 Other meniscus derangements, posterior horn of lateral meniscus, unspecified knee**

√6th **M23.36 Other meniscus derangements, other lateral meniscus**
- **M23.361 Other meniscus derangements, other lateral meniscus, right knee**
- **M23.362 Other meniscus derangements, other lateral meniscus, left knee**
- **M23.369 Other meniscus derangements, other lateral meniscus, unspecified knee**

√5th **M23.4 Loose body in knee**
- **M23.40 Loose body in knee, unspecified knee**
- **M23.41 Loose body in knee, right knee**
- **M23.42 Loose body in knee, left knee**

√5th **M23.5 Chronic instability of knee**
- **M23.50 Chronic instability of knee, unspecified knee**
- **M23.51 Chronic instability of knee, right knee**
- **M23.52 Chronic instability of knee, left knee**

√5th **M23.6 Other spontaneous disruption of ligament(s) of knee**

√6th **M23.60 Other spontaneous disruption of unspecified ligament of knee**
- **M23.601 Other spontaneous disruption of unspecified ligament of right knee**
- **M23.602 Other spontaneous disruption of unspecified ligament of left knee**
- **M23.609 Other spontaneous disruption of unspecified ligament of unspecified knee**

√6th **M23.61 Other spontaneous disruption of anterior cruciate ligament of knee**
- **M23.611 Other spontaneous disruption of anterior cruciate ligament of right knee**
- **M23.612 Other spontaneous disruption of anterior cruciate ligament of left knee**
- **M23.619 Other spontaneous disruption of anterior cruciate ligament of unspecified knee**

√6th **M23.62 Other spontaneous disruption of posterior cruciate ligament of knee**
- **M23.621 Other spontaneous disruption of posterior cruciate ligament of right knee**
- **M23.622 Other spontaneous disruption of posterior cruciate ligament of left knee**
- **M23.629 Other spontaneous disruption of posterior cruciate ligament of unspecified knee**

√6th **M23.63 Other spontaneous disruption of medial collateral ligament of knee**
- **M23.631 Other spontaneous disruption of medial collateral ligament of right knee**
- **M23.632 Other spontaneous disruption of medial collateral ligament of left knee**
- **M23.639 Other spontaneous disruption of medial collateral ligament of unspecified knee**

√6th M23.64 Other spontaneous disruption of lateral collateral ligament of knee
M23.641 Other spontaneous disruption of lateral collateral ligament of right knee
M23.642 Other spontaneous disruption of lateral collateral ligament of left knee
M23.649 Other spontaneous disruption of lateral collateral ligament of unspecified knee
√6th M23.67 Other spontaneous disruption of capsular ligament of knee
M23.671 Other spontaneous disruption of capsular ligament of right knee
M23.672 Other spontaneous disruption of capsular ligament of left knee
M23.679 Other spontaneous disruption of capsular ligament of unspecified knee
√5th M23.8 Other internal derangements of knee
Laxity of ligament of knee
Snapping knee
√6th M23.8X Other internal derangements of knee
M23.8X1 Other internal derangements of right knee
M23.8X2 Other internal derangements of left knee
M23.8X9 Other internal derangements of unspecified knee
√5th M23.9 Unspecified internal derangement of knee
M23.90 Unspecified internal derangement of unspecified knee
M23.91 Unspecified internal derangement of right knee
M23.92 Unspecified internal derangement of left knee

√4th **M24 Other specific joint derangements**
EXCLUDES 1 *current injury — see injury of joint by body region*
EXCLUDES 2 *ganglion (M67.4)*
snapping knee (M23.8-)
temporomandibular joint disorders (M26.6-)
√5th M24.0 Loose body in joint
EXCLUDES 2 *loose body in knee (M23.4)*
M24.00 Loose body in unspecified joint
√6th M24.01 Loose body in shoulder
M24.011 Loose body in right shoulder
M24.012 Loose body in left shoulder
M24.019 Loose body in unspecified shoulder
√6th M24.02 Loose body in elbow
M24.021 Loose body in right elbow
M24.022 Loose body in left elbow
M24.029 Loose body in unspecified elbow
√6th M24.03 Loose body in wrist
M24.031 Loose body in right wrist
M24.032 Loose body in left wrist
M24.039 Loose body in unspecified wrist
√6th M24.04 Loose body in finger joints
M24.041 Loose body in right finger joint(s)
M24.042 Loose body in left finger joint(s)
M24.049 Loose body in unspecified finger joint(s)
√6th M24.05 Loose body in hip
M24.051 Loose body in right hip
M24.052 Loose body in left hip
M24.059 Loose body in unspecified hip
√6th M24.07 Loose body in ankle and toe joints
M24.071 Loose body in right ankle
M24.072 Loose body in left ankle
M24.073 Loose body in unspecified ankle
M24.074 Loose body in right toe joint(s)
M24.075 Loose body in left toe joint(s)
M24.076 Loose body in unspecified toe joints
M24.08 Loose body, other site
√5th M24.1 Other articular cartilage disorders
EXCLUDES 2 *chondrocalcinosis (M11.1, M11.2-)*
internal derangement of knee (M23.-)
metastatic calcification (E83.5)
ochronosis (E70.2)
M24.10 Other articular cartilage disorders, unspecified site
√6th M24.11 Other articular cartilage disorders, shoulder
M24.111 Other articular cartilage disorders, right shoulder
M24.112 Other articular cartilage disorders, left shoulder
M24.119 Other articular cartilage disorders, unspecified shoulder
√6th M24.12 Other articular cartilage disorders, elbow
M24.121 Other articular cartilage disorders, right elbow
M24.122 Other articular cartilage disorders, left elbow
M24.129 Other articular cartilage disorders, unspecified elbow
√6th M24.13 Other articular cartilage disorders, wrist
M24.131 Other articular cartilage disorders, right wrist
M24.132 Other articular cartilage disorders, left wrist
M24.139 Other articular cartilage disorders, unspecified wrist
√6th M24.14 Other articular cartilage disorders, hand
M24.141 Other articular cartilage disorders, right hand
M24.142 Other articular cartilage disorders, left hand
M24.149 Other articular cartilage disorders, unspecified hand
√6th M24.15 Other articular cartilage disorders, hip
M24.151 Other articular cartilage disorders, right hip
M24.152 Other articular cartilage disorders, left hip
M24.159 Other articular cartilage disorders, unspecified hip
√6th M24.17 Other articular cartilage disorders, ankle and foot
M24.171 Other articular cartilage disorders, right ankle
M24.172 Other articular cartilage disorders, left ankle
M24.173 Other articular cartilage disorders, unspecified ankle
M24.174 Other articular cartilage disorders, right foot
M24.175 Other articular cartilage disorders, left foot
M24.176 Other articular cartilage disorders, unspecified foot
● M24.19 Other articular cartilage disorders, other specified site
√5th M24.2 Disorder of ligament
Instability secondary to old ligament injury
Ligamentous laxity NOS
EXCLUDES 1 *familial ligamentous laxity (M35.7)*
EXCLUDES 2 *internal derangement of knee (M23.5-M23.8X9)*
M24.20 Disorder of ligament, unspecified site
√6th M24.21 Disorder of ligament, shoulder
M24.211 Disorder of ligament, right shoulder
M24.212 Disorder of ligament, left shoulder
M24.219 Disorder of ligament, unspecified shoulder
√6th M24.22 Disorder of ligament, elbow
M24.221 Disorder of ligament, right elbow
M24.222 Disorder of ligament, left elbow
M24.229 Disorder of ligament, unspecified elbow
√6th M24.23 Disorder of ligament, wrist
M24.231 Disorder of ligament, right wrist
M24.232 Disorder of ligament, left wrist
M24.239 Disorder of ligament, unspecified wrist
√6th M24.24 Disorder of ligament, hand
M24.241 Disorder of ligament, right hand
M24.242 Disorder of ligament, left hand
M24.249 Disorder of ligament, unspecified hand
√6th M24.25 Disorder of ligament, hip
M24.251 Disorder of ligament, right hip
M24.252 Disorder of ligament, left hip
M24.259 Disorder of ligament, unspecified hip
√6th M24.27 Disorder of ligament, ankle and foot
M24.271 Disorder of ligament, right ankle
M24.272 Disorder of ligament, left ankle
M24.273 Disorder of ligament, unspecified ankle

M24.274 Disorder of ligament, right foot
M24.275 Disorder of ligament, left foot
M24.276 Disorder of ligament, unspecified foot
M24.28 Disorder of ligament, vertebrae
● M24.29 Disorder of ligament, other specified site

✓5th M24.3 Pathological dislocation of joint, not elsewhere classified
EXCLUDES 1 *congenital dislocation or displacement of joint — see congenital malformations and deformations of the musculoskeletal system (Q65-Q79)*
current injury — see injury of joints and ligaments by body region
recurrent dislocation of joint (M24.4-)

M24.3Ø Pathological dislocation of unspecified joint, not elsewhere classified
✓6th M24.31 Pathological dislocation of shoulder, not elsewhere classified
M24.311 Pathological dislocation of right shoulder, not elsewhere classified
M24.312 Pathological dislocation of left shoulder, not elsewhere classified
M24.319 Pathological dislocation of unspecified shoulder, not elsewhere classified
✓6th M24.32 Pathological dislocation of elbow, not elsewhere classified
M24.321 Pathological dislocation of right elbow, not elsewhere classified
M24.322 Pathological dislocation of left elbow, not elsewhere classified
M24.329 Pathological dislocation of unspecified elbow, not elsewhere classified
✓6th M24.33 Pathological dislocation of wrist, not elsewhere classified
M24.331 Pathological dislocation of right wrist, not elsewhere classified
M24.332 Pathological dislocation of left wrist, not elsewhere classified
M24.339 Pathological dislocation of unspecified wrist, not elsewhere classified
✓6th M24.34 Pathological dislocation of hand, not elsewhere classified
M24.341 Pathological dislocation of right hand, not elsewhere classified
M24.342 Pathological dislocation of left hand, not elsewhere classified
M24.349 Pathological dislocation of unspecified hand, not elsewhere classified
✓6th M24.35 Pathological dislocation of hip, not elsewhere classified
M24.351 Pathological dislocation of right hip, not elsewhere classified
M24.352 Pathological dislocation of left hip, not elsewhere classified
M24.359 Pathological dislocation of unspecified hip, not elsewhere classified
✓6th M24.36 Pathological dislocation of knee, not elsewhere classified
M24.361 Pathological dislocation of right knee, not elsewhere classified
M24.362 Pathological dislocation of left knee, not elsewhere classified
M24.369 Pathological dislocation of unspecified knee, not elsewhere classified
✓6th M24.37 Pathological dislocation of ankle and foot, not elsewhere classified
M24.371 Pathological dislocation of right ankle, not elsewhere classified
M24.372 Pathological dislocation of left ankle, not elsewhere classified
M24.373 Pathological dislocation of unspecified ankle, not elsewhere classified
M24.374 Pathological dislocation of right foot, not elsewhere classified
M24.375 Pathological dislocation of left foot, not elsewhere classified
M24.376 Pathological dislocation of unspecified foot, not elsewhere classified
● M24.39 Pathological dislocation of other specified joint, not elsewhere classified

✓5th M24.4 Recurrent dislocation of joint
Recurrent subluxation of joint
EXCLUDES 2 *recurrent dislocation of patella (M22.Ø-M22.1)*
recurrent vertebral dislocation (M43.3-, M43.4, M43.5-)

M24.4Ø Recurrent dislocation, unspecified joint
✓6th M24.41 Recurrent dislocation, shoulder
M24.411 Recurrent dislocation, right shoulder
M24.412 Recurrent dislocation, left shoulder
M24.419 Recurrent dislocation, unspecified shoulder
✓6th M24.42 Recurrent dislocation, elbow
M24.421 Recurrent dislocation, right elbow
M24.422 Recurrent dislocation, left elbow
M24.429 Recurrent dislocation, unspecified elbow
✓6th M24.43 Recurrent dislocation, wrist
M24.431 Recurrent dislocation, right wrist
M24.432 Recurrent dislocation, left wrist
M24.439 Recurrent dislocation, unspecified wrist
✓6th M24.44 Recurrent dislocation, hand and finger(s)
M24.441 Recurrent dislocation, right hand
M24.442 Recurrent dislocation, left hand
M24.443 Recurrent dislocation, unspecified hand
M24.444 Recurrent dislocation, right finger
M24.445 Recurrent dislocation, left finger
M24.446 Recurrent dislocation, unspecified finger
✓6th M24.45 Recurrent dislocation, hip
M24.451 Recurrent dislocation, right hip
M24.452 Recurrent dislocation, left hip
M24.459 Recurrent dislocation, unspecified hip
✓6th M24.46 Recurrent dislocation, knee
M24.461 Recurrent dislocation, right knee
M24.462 Recurrent dislocation, left knee
M24.469 Recurrent dislocation, unspecified knee
✓6th M24.47 Recurrent dislocation, ankle, foot and toes
M24.471 Recurrent dislocation, right ankle
M24.472 Recurrent dislocation, left ankle
M24.473 Recurrent dislocation, unspecified ankle
M24.474 Recurrent dislocation, right foot
M24.475 Recurrent dislocation, left foot
M24.476 Recurrent dislocation, unspecified foot
M24.477 Recurrent dislocation, right toe(s)
M24.478 Recurrent dislocation, left toe(s)
M24.479 Recurrent dislocation, unspecified toe(s)
● M24.49 Recurrent dislocation, other specified joint

✓5th M24.5 Contracture of joint
EXCLUDES 1 *contracture of muscle without contracture of joint (M62.4-)*
contracture of tendon (sheath) without contracture of joint (M62.4-)
Dupuytren's contracture (M72.Ø)
EXCLUDES 2 *acquired deformities of limbs (M2Ø-M21)*
AHA: 2016,2Q,6

M24.5Ø Contracture, unspecified joint
✓6th M24.51 Contracture, shoulder
M24.511 Contracture, right shoulder
M24.512 Contracture, left shoulder
M24.519 Contracture, unspecified shoulder
✓6th M24.52 Contracture, elbow
M24.521 Contracture, right elbow
M24.522 Contracture, left elbow
M24.529 Contracture, unspecified elbow
✓6th M24.53 Contracture, wrist
M24.531 Contracture, right wrist
M24.532 Contracture, left wrist
M24.539 Contracture, unspecified wrist
✓6th M24.54 Contracture, hand
M24.541 Contracture, right hand
M24.542 Contracture, left hand
M24.549 Contracture, unspecified hand
✓6th M24.55 Contracture, hip
M24.551 Contracture, right hip
M24.552 Contracture, left hip
M24.559 Contracture, unspecified hip

M24.56 Contracture, knee
M24.561 Contracture, right knee
M24.562 Contracture, left knee
M24.569 Contracture, unspecified knee
M24.57 Contracture, ankle and foot
M24.571 Contracture, right ankle
M24.572 Contracture, left ankle
M24.573 Contracture, unspecified ankle
M24.574 Contracture, right foot
M24.575 Contracture, left foot
M24.576 Contracture, unspecified foot
● M24.59 Contracture, other specified joint

M24.6 Ankylosis of joint
EXCLUDES 1 *stiffness of joint without ankylosis (M25.6-)*
EXCLUDES 2 *spine (M43.2-)*
DEF: Ankylosis: Abnormal union or fusion of bones in a joint, which is normally moveable.
M24.60 Ankylosis, unspecified joint
M24.61 Ankylosis, shoulder
M24.611 Ankylosis, right shoulder
M24.612 Ankylosis, left shoulder
M24.619 Ankylosis, unspecified shoulder
M24.62 Ankylosis, elbow
M24.621 Ankylosis, right elbow
M24.622 Ankylosis, left elbow
M24.629 Ankylosis, unspecified elbow
M24.63 Ankylosis, wrist
M24.631 Ankylosis, right wrist
M24.632 Ankylosis, left wrist
M24.639 Ankylosis, unspecified wrist
M24.64 Ankylosis, hand
M24.641 Ankylosis, right hand
M24.642 Ankylosis, left hand
M24.649 Ankylosis, unspecified hand
M24.65 Ankylosis, hip
M24.651 Ankylosis, right hip
M24.652 Ankylosis, left hip
M24.659 Ankylosis, unspecified hip
M24.66 Ankylosis, knee
M24.661 Ankylosis, right knee
M24.662 Ankylosis, left knee
M24.669 Ankylosis, unspecified knee
M24.67 Ankylosis, ankle and foot
M24.671 Ankylosis, right ankle
M24.672 Ankylosis, left ankle
M24.673 Ankylosis, unspecified ankle
M24.674 Ankylosis, right foot
M24.675 Ankylosis, left foot
M24.676 Ankylosis, unspecified foot
● M24.69 Ankylosis, other specified joint

M24.7 Protrusio acetabuli
DEF: Intrapelvic protrusion of the acetabulum characterized by the sinking of the floor of the acetabulum, causing the femoral head to protrude. It limits hip movement and is of unknown etiology. ***Synonym(s):*** *Otto's pelvis.*

M24.8 Other specific joint derangements, not elsewhere classified
EXCLUDES 2 *iliotibial band syndrome (M76.3)*
M24.80 Other specific joint derangements of unspecified joint, not elsewhere classified
M24.81 Other specific joint derangements of shoulder, not elsewhere classified
M24.811 Other specific joint derangements of right shoulder, not elsewhere classified
M24.812 Other specific joint derangements of left shoulder, not elsewhere classified
M24.819 Other specific joint derangements of unspecified shoulder, not elsewhere classified
M24.82 Other specific joint derangements of elbow, not elsewhere classified
M24.821 Other specific joint derangements of right elbow, not elsewhere classified
M24.822 Other specific joint derangements of left elbow, not elsewhere classified
M24.829 Other specific joint derangements of unspecified elbow, not elsewhere classified
M24.83 Other specific joint derangements of wrist, not elsewhere classified
M24.831 Other specific joint derangements of right wrist, not elsewhere classified
M24.832 Other specific joint derangements of left wrist, not elsewhere classified
M24.839 Other specific joint derangements of unspecified wrist, not elsewhere classified
M24.84 Other specific joint derangements of hand, not elsewhere classified
M24.841 Other specific joint derangements of right hand, not elsewhere classified
M24.842 Other specific joint derangements of left hand, not elsewhere classified
M24.849 Other specific joint derangements of unspecified hand, not elsewhere classified
M24.85 Other specific joint derangements of hip, not elsewhere classified
Irritable hip
M24.851 Other specific joint derangements of right hip, not elsewhere classified
M24.852 Other specific joint derangements of left hip, not elsewhere classified
M24.859 Other specific joint derangements of unspecified hip, not elsewhere classified
M24.87 Other specific joint derangements of ankle and foot, not elsewhere classified
M24.871 Other specific joint derangements of right ankle, not elsewhere classified
M24.872 Other specific joint derangements of left ankle, not elsewhere classified
M24.873 Other specific joint derangements of unspecified ankle, not elsewhere classified
M24.874 Other specific joint derangements of right foot, not elsewhere classified
M24.875 Other specific joint derangements left foot, not elsewhere classified
M24.876 Other specific joint derangements of unspecified foot, not elsewhere classified
● M24.89 Other specific joint derangement of other specified joint, not elsewhere classified
M24.9 Joint derangement, unspecified

M25 Other joint disorder, not elsewhere classified
EXCLUDES 2 *abnormality of gait and mobility (R26.-)*
acquired deformities of limb (M20-M21)
calcification of bursa (M71.4-)
calcification of shoulder (joint) (M75.3)
calcification of tendon (M65.2-)
difficulty in walking (R26.2)
temporomandibular joint disorder (M26.6-)

M25.0 Hemarthrosis
EXCLUDES 1 *current injury — see injury of joint by body region*
hemophilic arthropathy (M36.2)
M25.00 Hemarthrosis, unspecified joint CC
M25.01 Hemarthrosis, shoulder
M25.011 Hemarthrosis, right shoulder CC
M25.012 Hemarthrosis, left shoulder CC
M25.019 Hemarthrosis, unspecified shoulder CC
M25.02 Hemarthrosis, elbow
M25.021 Hemarthrosis, right elbow CC
M25.022 Hemarthrosis, left elbow CC
M25.029 Hemarthrosis, unspecified elbow CC
M25.03 Hemarthrosis, wrist
M25.031 Hemarthrosis, right wrist CC
M25.032 Hemarthrosis, left wrist CC
M25.039 Hemarthrosis, unspecified wrist CC
M25.04 Hemarthrosis, hand
M25.041 Hemarthrosis, right hand CC
M25.042 Hemarthrosis, left hand CC
M25.049 Hemarthrosis, unspecified hand CC
M25.05 Hemarthrosis, hip
M25.051 Hemarthrosis, right hip CC
M25.052 Hemarthrosis, left hip CC
M25.059 Hemarthrosis, unspecified hip CC

✓6th M25.06 Hemarthrosis, knee
M25.061 Hemarthrosis, right knee CC
M25.062 Hemarthrosis, left knee CC
M25.069 Hemarthrosis, unspecified knee CC
✓6th M25.07 Hemarthrosis, ankle and foot
M25.071 Hemarthrosis, right ankle CC
M25.072 Hemarthrosis, left ankle CC
M25.073 Hemarthrosis, unspecified ankle CC
M25.074 Hemarthrosis, right foot CC
M25.075 Hemarthrosis, left foot CC
M25.076 Hemarthrosis, unspecified foot CC
M25.08 Hemarthrosis, other specified site CC
Hemarthrosis, vertebrae

✓5th M25.1 Fistula of joint
M25.10 Fistula, unspecified joint SW
✓6th M25.11 Fistula, shoulder
M25.111 Fistula, right shoulder SW
M25.112 Fistula, left shoulder SW
M25.119 Fistula, unspecified shoulder SW
✓6th M25.12 Fistula, elbow
M25.121 Fistula, right elbow SW
M25.122 Fistula, left elbow SW
M25.129 Fistula, unspecified elbow SW
✓6th M25.13 Fistula, wrist
M25.131 Fistula, right wrist SW
M25.132 Fistula, left wrist SW
M25.139 Fistula, unspecified wrist SW
✓6th M25.14 Fistula, hand
M25.141 Fistula, right hand SW
M25.142 Fistula, left hand SW
M25.149 Fistula, unspecified hand SW
✓6th M25.15 Fistula, hip
M25.151 Fistula, right hip SW
M25.152 Fistula, left hip SW
M25.159 Fistula, unspecified hip SW
✓6th M25.16 Fistula, knee
M25.161 Fistula, right knee SW
M25.162 Fistula, left knee SW
M25.169 Fistula, unspecified knee SW
✓6th M25.17 Fistula, ankle and foot
M25.171 Fistula, right ankle SW
M25.172 Fistula, left ankle SW
M25.173 Fistula, unspecified ankle SW
M25.174 Fistula, right foot SW
M25.175 Fistula, left foot SW
M25.176 Fistula, unspecified foot SW
M25.18 Fistula, other specified site SW
Fistula, vertebrae

✓5th M25.2 Flail joint
DEF: Hinged joint that exhibits an abnormal or excessive degree of range and mobility.
M25.20 Flail joint, unspecified joint
✓6th M25.21 Flail joint, shoulder
M25.211 Flail joint, right shoulder
M25.212 Flail joint, left shoulder
M25.219 Flail joint, unspecified shoulder
✓6th M25.22 Flail joint, elbow
M25.221 Flail joint, right elbow
M25.222 Flail joint, left elbow
M25.229 Flail joint, unspecified elbow
✓6th M25.23 Flail joint, wrist
M25.231 Flail joint, right wrist
M25.232 Flail joint, left wrist
M25.239 Flail joint, unspecified wrist
✓6th M25.24 Flail joint, hand
M25.241 Flail joint, right hand
M25.242 Flail joint, left hand
M25.249 Flail joint, unspecified hand
✓6th M25.25 Flail joint, hip
M25.251 Flail joint, right hip
M25.252 Flail joint, left hip
M25.259 Flail joint, unspecified hip
✓6th M25.26 Flail joint, knee
M25.261 Flail joint, right knee
M25.262 Flail joint, left knee
M25.269 Flail joint, unspecified knee
✓6th M25.27 Flail joint, ankle and foot
M25.271 Flail joint, right ankle and foot
M25.272 Flail joint, left ankle and foot
M25.279 Flail joint, unspecified ankle and foot
M25.28 Flail joint, other site

✓5th M25.3 Other instability of joint
EXCLUDES 1 *instability of joint secondary to old ligament injury (M24.2-)*
instability of joint secondary to removal of joint prosthesis (M96.8-)
EXCLUDES 2 *spinal instabilities (M53.2-)*
M25.30 Other instability, unspecified joint
✓6th M25.31 Other instability, shoulder
M25.311 Other instability, right shoulder
M25.312 Other instability, left shoulder
M25.319 Other instability, unspecified shoulder
✓6th M25.32 Other instability, elbow
M25.321 Other instability, right elbow
M25.322 Other instability, left elbow
M25.329 Other instability, unspecified elbow
✓6th M25.33 Other instability, wrist
M25.331 Other instability, right wrist
M25.332 Other instability, left wrist
M25.339 Other instability, unspecified wrist
✓6th M25.34 Other instability, hand
M25.341 Other instability, right hand
M25.342 Other instability, left hand
M25.349 Other instability, unspecified hand
✓6th M25.35 Other instability, hip
M25.351 Other instability, right hip
M25.352 Other instability, left hip
M25.359 Other instability, unspecified hip
✓6th M25.36 Other instability, knee
M25.361 Other instability, right knee
M25.362 Other instability, left knee
M25.369 Other instability, unspecified knee
✓6th M25.37 Other instability, ankle and foot
M25.371 Other instability, right ankle
M25.372 Other instability, left ankle
M25.373 Other instability, unspecified ankle
M25.374 Other instability, right foot
M25.375 Other instability, left foot
M25.376 Other instability, unspecified foot
● M25.39 Other instability, other specified joint

✓5th M25.4 Effusion of joint
EXCLUDES 1 *hydrarthrosis in yaws (A66.6)*
intermittent hydrarthrosis (M12.4-)
other infective (teno)synovitis (M65.1-)
M25.40 Effusion, unspecified joint
✓6th M25.41 Effusion, shoulder
M25.411 Effusion, right shoulder
M25.412 Effusion, left shoulder
M25.419 Effusion, unspecified shoulder
✓6th M25.42 Effusion, elbow
M25.421 Effusion, right elbow
M25.422 Effusion, left elbow
M25.429 Effusion, unspecified elbow
✓6th M25.43 Effusion, wrist
M25.431 Effusion, right wrist
M25.432 Effusion, left wrist
M25.439 Effusion, unspecified wrist
✓6th M25.44 Effusion, hand
M25.441 Effusion, right hand
M25.442 Effusion, left hand
M25.449 Effusion, unspecified hand
✓6th M25.45 Effusion, hip
M25.451 Effusion, right hip
M25.452 Effusion, left hip
M25.459 Effusion, unspecified hip

√6th M25.46 Effusion, knee
M25.461 Effusion, right knee
M25.462 Effusion, left knee
M25.469 Effusion, unspecified knee
√6th M25.47 Effusion, ankle and foot
M25.471 Effusion, right ankle
M25.472 Effusion, left ankle
M25.473 Effusion, unspecified ankle
M25.474 Effusion, right foot
M25.475 Effusion, left foot
M25.476 Effusion, unspecified foot
M25.48 Effusion, other site
√5th M25.5 Pain in joint
EXCLUDES 2 *pain in hand (M79.64-)*
pain in fingers (M79.64-)
pain in foot (M79.67-)
pain in limb (M79.6-)
pain in toes (M79.67-)
M25.50 Pain in unspecified joint
√6th M25.51 Pain in shoulder
M25.511 Pain in right shoulder
M25.512 Pain in left shoulder
M25.519 Pain in unspecified shoulder
√6th M25.52 Pain in elbow
M25.521 Pain in right elbow
M25.522 Pain in left elbow
M25.529 Pain in unspecified elbow
√6th M25.53 Pain in wrist
M25.531 Pain in right wrist
M25.532 Pain in left wrist
M25.539 Pain in unspecified wrist
√6th M25.54 Pain in joints of hand
AHA: 2016,4Q,38
M25.541 Pain in joints of right hand
M25.542 Pain in joints of left hand
M25.549 Pain in joints of unspecified hand
Pain in joints of hand NOS
√6th M25.55 Pain in hip
M25.551 Pain in right hip
M25.552 Pain in left hip
M25.559 Pain in unspecified hip
√6th M25.56 Pain in knee
M25.561 Pain in right knee
M25.562 Pain in left knee
M25.569 Pain in unspecified knee
√6th M25.57 Pain in ankle and joints of foot
M25.571 Pain in right ankle and joints of right foot
M25.572 Pain in left ankle and joints of left foot
M25.579 Pain in unspecified ankle and joints of unspecified foot
● M25.59 Pain in other specified joint
√5th M25.6 Stiffness of joint, not elsewhere classified
EXCLUDES 1 *ankylosis of joint (M24.6-)*
contracture of joint (M24.5-)
M25.60 Stiffness of unspecified joint, not elsewhere classified
√6th M25.61 Stiffness of shoulder, not elsewhere classified
M25.611 Stiffness of right shoulder, not elsewhere classified
M25.612 Stiffness of left shoulder, not elsewhere classified
M25.619 Stiffness of unspecified shoulder, not elsewhere classified
√6th M25.62 Stiffness of elbow, not elsewhere classified
M25.621 Stiffness of right elbow, not elsewhere classified
M25.622 Stiffness of left elbow, not elsewhere classified
M25.629 Stiffness of unspecified elbow, not elsewhere classified
√6th M25.63 Stiffness of wrist, not elsewhere classified
M25.631 Stiffness of right wrist, not elsewhere classified
M25.632 Stiffness of left wrist, not elsewhere classified
M25.639 Stiffness of unspecified wrist, not elsewhere classified
√6th M25.64 Stiffness of hand, not elsewhere classified
M25.641 Stiffness of right hand, not elsewhere classified
M25.642 Stiffness of left hand, not elsewhere classified
M25.649 Stiffness of unspecified hand, not elsewhere classified
√6th M25.65 Stiffness of hip, not elsewhere classified
M25.651 Stiffness of right hip, not elsewhere classified
M25.652 Stiffness of left hip, not elsewhere classified
M25.659 Stiffness of unspecified hip, not elsewhere classified
√6th M25.66 Stiffness of knee, not elsewhere classified
M25.661 Stiffness of right knee, not elsewhere classified
M25.662 Stiffness of left knee, not elsewhere classified
M25.669 Stiffness of unspecified knee, not elsewhere classified
√6th M25.67 Stiffness of ankle and foot, not elsewhere classified
M25.671 Stiffness of right ankle, not elsewhere classified
M25.672 Stiffness of left ankle, not elsewhere classified
M25.673 Stiffness of unspecified ankle, not elsewhere classified
M25.674 Stiffness of right foot, not elsewhere classified
M25.675 Stiffness of left foot, not elsewhere classified
M25.676 Stiffness of unspecified foot, not elsewhere classified
● M25.69 Stiffness of other specified joint, not elsewhere classified
√5th M25.7 Osteophyte
M25.70 Osteophyte, unspecified joint
√6th M25.71 Osteophyte, shoulder
M25.711 Osteophyte, right shoulder
M25.712 Osteophyte, left shoulder
M25.719 Osteophyte, unspecified shoulder
√6th M25.72 Osteophyte, elbow
M25.721 Osteophyte, right elbow
M25.722 Osteophyte, left elbow
M25.729 Osteophyte, unspecified elbow
√6th M25.73 Osteophyte, wrist
M25.731 Osteophyte, right wrist
M25.732 Osteophyte, left wrist
M25.739 Osteophyte, unspecified wrist
√6th M25.74 Osteophyte, hand
M25.741 Osteophyte, right hand
M25.742 Osteophyte, left hand
M25.749 Osteophyte, unspecified hand
√6th M25.75 Osteophyte, hip
M25.751 Osteophyte, right hip
M25.752 Osteophyte, left hip
M25.759 Osteophyte, unspecified hip
√6th M25.76 Osteophyte, knee
M25.761 Osteophyte, right knee
M25.762 Osteophyte, left knee
M25.769 Osteophyte, unspecified knee
√6th M25.77 Osteophyte, ankle and foot
M25.771 Osteophyte, right ankle
M25.772 Osteophyte, left ankle
M25.773 Osteophyte, unspecified ankle
M25.774 Osteophyte, right foot
M25.775 Osteophyte, left foot
M25.776 Osteophyte, unspecified foot
M25.78 Osteophyte, vertebrae
√5th M25.8 Other specified joint disorders
M25.80 Other specified joint disorders, unspecified joint
√6th M25.81 Other specified joint disorders, shoulder
M25.811 Other specified joint disorders, right shoulder

M25.812 **Other specified joint disorders, left shoulder**
M25.819 **Other specified joint disorders, unspecified shoulder**

√6th M25.82 **Other specified joint disorders, elbow**
M25.821 **Other specified joint disorders, right elbow**
M25.822 **Other specified joint disorders, left elbow**
M25.829 **Other specified joint disorders, unspecified elbow**

√6th M25.83 **Other specified joint disorders, wrist**
M25.831 **Other specified joint disorders, right wrist**
M25.832 **Other specified joint disorders, left wrist**
M25.839 **Other specified joint disorders, unspecified wrist**

√6th M25.84 **Other specified joint disorders, hand**
M25.841 **Other specified joint disorders, right hand**
M25.842 **Other specified joint disorders, left hand**
M25.849 **Other specified joint disorders, unspecified hand**

√6th M25.85 **Other specified joint disorders, hip**
AHA: 2014,4Q,25
M25.851 **Other specified joint disorders, right hip**
M25.852 **Other specified joint disorders, left hip**
M25.859 **Other specified joint disorders, unspecified hip**

√6th M25.86 **Other specified joint disorders, knee**
M25.861 **Other specified joint disorders, right knee**
M25.862 **Other specified joint disorders, left knee**
M25.869 **Other specified joint disorders, unspecified knee**

√6th M25.87 **Other specified joint disorders, ankle and foot**
M25.871 **Other specified joint disorders, right ankle and foot**
M25.872 **Other specified joint disorders, left ankle and foot**
M25.879 **Other specified joint disorders, unspecified ankle and foot**

M25.9 **Joint disorder, unspecified**

Dentofacial anomalies [including malocclusion] and other disorders of jaw (M26-M27)

EXCLUDES 1 *hemifacial atrophy or hypertrophy (Q67.4)*
unilateral condylar hyperplasia or hypoplasia (M27.8)

√4th **M26 Dentofacial anomalies [including malocclusion]**

√5th M26.0 **Major anomalies of jaw size**
EXCLUDES 1 *acromegaly (E22.0)*
Robin's syndrome (Q87.0)
M26.00 **Unspecified anomaly of jaw size**
M26.01 **Maxillary hyperplasia**
M26.02 **Maxillary hypoplasia**
AHA: 2014,3Q,23
M26.03 **Mandibular hyperplasia**
M26.04 **Mandibular hypoplasia**
M26.05 **Macrogenia**
M26.06 **Microgenia**
M26.07 **Excessive tuberosity of jaw**
Entire maxillary tuberosity
M26.09 **Other specified anomalies of jaw size**

√5th M26.1 **Anomalies of jaw-cranial base relationship**
M26.10 **Unspecified anomaly of jaw-cranial base relationship**
M26.11 **Maxillary asymmetry**
M26.12 **Other jaw asymmetry**
M26.19 **Other specified anomalies of jaw-cranial base relationship**
AHA: 2020,1Q,21

√5th M26.2 **Anomalies of dental arch relationship**
M26.20 **Unspecified anomaly of dental arch relationship**
√6th M26.21 **Malocclusion, Angle's class**
M26.211 **Malocclusion, Angle's class I**
Neutro-occlusion
M26.212 **Malocclusion, Angle's class II**
Disto-occlusion Division I
Disto-occlusion Division II
M26.213 **Malocclusion, Angle's class III**
Mesio-occlusion
M26.219 **Malocclusion, Angle's class, unspecified**
√6th M26.22 **Open occlusal relationship**
M26.220 **Open anterior occlusal relationship**
Anterior open bite
M26.221 **Open posterior occlusal relationship**
Posterior open bite
M26.23 **Excessive horizontal overlap**
Excessive horizontal overjet
M26.24 **Reverse articulation**
Crossbite (anterior) (posterior)
M26.25 **Anomalies of interarch distance**
M26.29 **Other anomalies of dental arch relationship**
Midline deviation of dental arch
Overbite (excessive) deep
Overbite (excessive) horizontal
Overbite (excessive) vertical
Posterior lingual occlusion of mandibular teeth

√5th M26.3 **Anomalies of tooth position of fully erupted tooth or teeth**
EXCLUDES 2 *embedded and impacted teeth (K01.-)*
M26.30 **Unspecified anomaly of tooth position of fully erupted tooth or teeth**
Abnormal spacing of fully erupted tooth or teeth NOS
Displacement of fully erupted tooth or teeth NOS
Transposition of fully erupted tooth or teeth NOS
M26.31 **Crowding of fully erupted teeth**
M26.32 **Excessive spacing of fully erupted teeth**
Diastema of fully erupted tooth or teeth NOS
M26.33 **Horizontal displacement of fully erupted tooth or teeth**
Tipped tooth or teeth
Tipping of fully erupted tooth
M26.34 **Vertical displacement of fully erupted tooth or teeth**
Extruded tooth
Infraeruption of tooth or teeth
Supraeruption of tooth or teeth
M26.35 **Rotation of fully erupted tooth or teeth**
M26.36 **Insufficient interocclusal distance of fully erupted teeth (ridge)**
Lack of adequate intermaxillary vertical dimension of fully erupted teeth
M26.37 **Excessive interocclusal distance of fully erupted teeth**
Excessive intermaxillary vertical dimension of fully erupted teeth
Loss of occlusal vertical dimension of fully erupted teeth
M26.39 **Other anomalies of tooth position of fully erupted tooth or teeth**

M26.4 **Malocclusion, unspecified**

√5th M26.5 **Dentofacial functional abnormalities**
EXCLUDES 1 *bruxism (F45.8)*
teeth-grinding NOS (F45.8)
M26.50 **Dentofacial functional abnormalities, unspecified**
M26.51 **Abnormal jaw closure**
M26.52 **Limited mandibular range of motion**
M26.53 **Deviation in opening and closing of the mandible**
M26.54 **Insufficient anterior guidance**
Insufficient anterior occlusal guidance
M26.55 **Centric occlusion maximum intercuspation discrepancy**
EXCLUDES 1 *centric occlusion NOS (M26.59)*
M26.56 **Non-working side interference**
Balancing side interference
M26.57 **Lack of posterior occlusal support**
M26.59 **Other dentofacial functional abnormalities**
Centric occlusion (of teeth) NOS
Malocclusion due to abnormal swallowing
Malocclusion due to mouth breathing
Malocclusion due to tongue, lip or finger habits

M26.6 Temporomandibular joint disorders
EXCLUDES 2 *current temporomandibular joint dislocation (SØ3.Ø)*
current temporomandibular joint sprain (SØ3.4)
AHA: 2016,4Q,38-39

Temporomandibular Joint

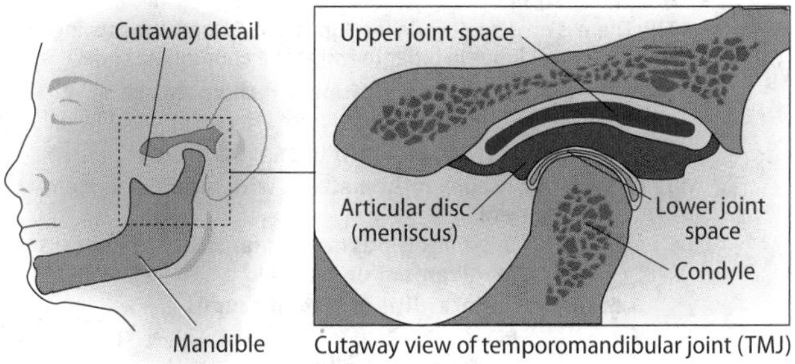

Cutaway view of temporomandibular joint (TMJ)

M26.60 Temporomandibular joint disorder, unspecified
M26.601 Right temporomandibular joint disorder, unspecified
M26.602 Left temporomandibular joint disorder, unspecified
M26.603 Bilateral temporomandibular joint disorder, unspecified
M26.609 Unspecified temporomandibular joint disorder, unspecified side
Temporomandibular joint disorder NOS
M26.61 Adhesions and ankylosis of temporomandibular joint
M26.611 Adhesions and ankylosis of right temporomandibular joint
M26.612 Adhesions and ankylosis of left temporomandibular joint
M26.613 Adhesions and ankylosis of bilateral temporomandibular joint
M26.619 Adhesions and ankylosis of temporomandibular joint, unspecified side
M26.62 Arthralgia of temporomandibular joint
M26.621 Arthralgia of right temporomandibular joint
M26.622 Arthralgia of left temporomandibular joint
M26.623 Arthralgia of bilateral temporomandibular joint
M26.629 Arthralgia of temporomandibular joint, unspecified side
M26.63 Articular disc disorder of temporomandibular joint
M26.631 Articular disc disorder of right temporomandibular joint
M26.632 Articular disc disorder of left temporomandibular joint
M26.633 Articular disc disorder of bilateral temporomandibular joint
M26.639 Articular disc disorder of temporomandibular joint, unspecified side
● **M26.64 Arthritis of temporomandibular joint**
● **M26.641 Arthritis of right temporomandibular joint**
● **M26.642 Arthritis of left temporomandibular joint**
● **M26.643 Arthritis of bilateral temporomandibular joint**
● **M26.649 Arthritis of unspecified temporomandibular joint**
● **M26.65 Arthropathy of temporomandibular joint**
● **M26.651 Arthropathy of right temporomandibular joint**
● **M26.652 Arthropathy of left temporomandibular joint**
● **M26.653 Arthropathy of bilateral temporomandibular joint**
● **M26.659 Arthropathy of unspecified temporomandibular joint**
M26.69 Other specified disorders of temporomandibular joint

M26.7 Dental alveolar anomalies
M26.70 Unspecified alveolar anomaly
M26.71 Alveolar maxillary hyperplasia
M26.72 Alveolar mandibular hyperplasia
M26.73 Alveolar maxillary hypoplasia
M26.74 Alveolar mandibular hypoplasia
M26.79 Other specified alveolar anomalies
M26.8 Other dentofacial anomalies
M26.81 Anterior soft tissue impingement
Anterior soft tissue impingement on teeth
M26.82 Posterior soft tissue impingement
Posterior soft tissue impingement on teeth
M26.89 Other dentofacial anomalies
M26.9 Dentofacial anomaly, unspecified

M27 Other diseases of jaws
M27.Ø Developmental disorders of jaws
Latent bone cyst of jaw
Stafne's cyst
Torus mandibularis
Torus palatinus
M27.1 Giant cell granuloma, central
Giant cell granuloma NOS
EXCLUDES 1 *peripheral giant cell granuloma (KØ6.8)*
M27.2 Inflammatory conditions of jaws
Osteitis of jaw(s)
Osteomyelitis (neonatal) jaw(s)
Osteoradionecrosis jaw(s)
Periostitis jaw(s)
Sequestrum of jaw bone
Use additional code (W88-W9Ø, X39.Ø) to identify radiation, if radiation-induced
EXCLUDES 2 *osteonecrosis of jaw due to drug (M87.18Ø)*
M27.3 Alveolitis of jaws
Alveolar osteitis
Dry socket
M27.4 Other and unspecified cysts of jaw
EXCLUDES 1 *cysts of oral region (KØ9.-)*
latent bone cyst of jaw (M27.Ø)
Stafne's cyst (M27.Ø)
M27.4Ø Unspecified cyst of jaw
Cyst of jaw NOS
M27.49 Other cysts of jaw
Aneurysmal cyst of jaw
Hemorrhagic cyst of jaw
Traumatic cyst of jaw
M27.5 Periradicular pathology associated with previous endodontic treatment
M27.51 Perforation of root canal space due to endodontic treatment
M27.52 Endodontic overfill
M27.53 Endodontic underfill
M27.59 Other periradicular pathology associated with previous endodontic treatment
M27.6 Endosseous dental implant failure
M27.61 Osseointegration failure of dental implant
Hemorrhagic complications of dental implant placement
Iatrogenic osseointegration failure of dental implant
Osseointegration failure of dental implant due to complications of systemic disease
Osseointegration failure of dental implant due to poor bone quality
Pre-integration failure of dental implant NOS
Pre-osseointegration failure of dental implant

Chapter 13. Diseases of the Musculoskeletal System and Connective Tissue

M26.6–M27.61

M27.62 Post-osseointegration biological failure of dental implant
Failure of dental implant due to lack of attached gingiva
Failure of dental implant due to occlusal trauma (caused by poor prosthetic design)
Failure of dental implant due to parafunctional habits
Failure of dental implant due to periodontal infection (peri-implantitis)
Failure of dental implant due to poor oral hygiene
Iatrogenic post-osseointegration failure of dental implant
Post-osseointegration failure of dental implant due to complications of systemic disease

M27.63 Post-osseointegration mechanical failure of dental implant
Failure of dental prosthesis causing loss of dental implant
Fracture of dental implant
EXCLUDES 2 *cracked tooth (KØ3.81)*
fractured dental restorative material with loss of material (KØ8.531)
fractured dental restorative material without loss of material (KØ8.53Ø)
fractured tooth (SØ2.5)

M27.69 Other endosseous dental implant failure
Dental implant failure NOS

M27.8 Other specified diseases of jaws
Cherubism
Exostosis
Fibrous dysplasia
Unilateral condylar hyperplasia
Unilateral condylar hypoplasia
EXCLUDES 1 *jaw pain (R68.84)*

M27.9 Disease of jaws, unspecified

Systemic connective tissue disorders (M3Ø-M36)

INCLUDES autoimmune disease NOS
collagen (vascular) disease NOS
systemic autoimmune disease
systemic collagen (vascular) disease
EXCLUDES 1 *autoimmune disease, single organ or single cell-type-code to relevant condition category*

4th M3Ø Polyarteritis nodosa and related conditions
EXCLUDES 1 *microscopic polyarteritis (M31.7)*

M3Ø.Ø Polyarteritis nodosa CC HCC

M3Ø.1 Polyarteritis with lung involvement [Churg-Strauss] CC HCC
Allergic granulomatous angiitis
►Eosinophilic granulomatosis with polyangiitis [EGPA]◄

M3Ø.2 Juvenile polyarteritis CC HCC

M3Ø.3 Mucocutaneous lymph node syndrome [Kawasaki] CC HCC

M3Ø.8 Other conditions related to polyarteritis nodosa CC HCC
Polyangiitis overlap syndrome

4th M31 Other necrotizing vasculopathies

M31.Ø Hypersensitivity angiitis CC HCC
Goodpasture's syndrome

M31.1 Thrombotic microangiopathy MCC HCC
Thrombotic thrombocytopenic purpura

M31.2 Lethal midline granuloma CC HCC

5th M31.3 Wegener's granulomatosis
►Granulomatosis with polyangiitis◄
Necrotizing respiratory granulomatosis

M31.3Ø Wegener's granulomatosis without renal involvement CC HCC
Wegener's granulomatosis NOS

M31.31 Wegener's granulomatosis with renal involvement CC HCC

M31.4 Aortic arch syndrome [Takayasu] CC HCC

M31.5 Giant cell arteritis with polymyalgia rheumatica HCC

M31.6 Other giant cell arteritis HCC

M31.7 Microscopic polyangiitis CC HCC
Microscopic polyarteritis
EXCLUDES 1 *polyarteritis nodosa (M3Ø.Ø)*

M31.8 Other specified necrotizing vasculopathies CC HCC
Hypocomplementemic vasculitis
Septic vasculitis

M31.9 Necrotizing vasculopathy, unspecified CC HCC

4th M32 Systemic lupus erythematosus (SLE)
EXCLUDES 1 *lupus erythematosus (discoid) (NOS) (L93.Ø)*
AHA: 2018,3Q,14
TIP: There is no default code for "lupus NOS." Query the provider for the specific type of lupus in order to assign the appropriate code.

M32.Ø Drug-induced systemic lupus erythematosus HCC
Use additional code for adverse effect, if applicable, to identify drug (T36-T5Ø with fifth or sixth character 5)

5th M32.1 Systemic lupus erythematosus with organ or system involvement

M32.1Ø Systemic lupus erythematosus, organ or system involvement unspecified HCC

M32.11 Endocarditis in systemic lupus erythematosus CC HCC
Libman-Sacks disease

M32.12 Pericarditis in systemic lupus erythematosus CC HCC
Lupus pericarditis

M32.13 Lung involvement in systemic lupus erythematosus HCC
Pleural effusion due to systemic lupus erythematosus

M32.14 Glomerular disease in systemic lupus erythematosus HCC
Lupus renal disease NOS
AHA: 2013,4Q,125

M32.15 Tubulo-interstitial nephropathy in systemic lupus erythematosus HCC

M32.19 Other organ or system involvement in systemic lupus erythematosus HCC

M32.8 Other forms of systemic lupus erythematosus HCC

M32.9 Systemic lupus erythematosus, unspecified HCC
SLE NOS
Systemic lupus erythematosus NOS
Systemic lupus erythematosus without organ involvement

4th M33 Dermatopolymyositis
AHA: 2017,4Q,18

5th M33.Ø Juvenile dermatomyositis

M33.ØØ Juvenile dermatomyositis, organ involvement unspecified CC HCC

M33.Ø1 Juvenile dermatomyositis with respiratory involvement CC HCC

M33.Ø2 Juvenile dermatomyositis with myopathy CC HCC

M33.Ø3 Juvenile dermatomyositis without myopathy CC HCC

M33.Ø9 Juvenile dermatomyositis with other organ involvement CC HCC

5th M33.1 Other dermatomyositis
Adult dermatomyositis

M33.1Ø Other dermatomyositis, organ involvement unspecified CC HCC

M33.11 Other dermatomyositis with respiratory involvement CC HCC

M33.12 Other dermatomyositis with myopathy CC HCC

M33.13 Other dermatomyositis without myopathy CC HCC
Dermatomyositis NOS

M33.19 Other dermatomyositis with other organ involvement CC HCC

5th M33.2 Polymyositis

M33.2Ø Polymyositis, organ involvement unspecified CC HCC

M33.21 Polymyositis with respiratory involvement CC HCC

M33.22 Polymyositis with myopathy CC HCC

M33.29 Polymyositis with other organ involvement CC HCC

5th M33.9 Dermatopolymyositis, unspecified

M33.9Ø Dermatopolymyositis, unspecified, organ involvement unspecified CC HCC

M33.91 Dermatopolymyositis, unspecified with respiratory involvement CC HCC

M33.92 **Dermatopolymyositis, unspecified with myopathy** CC HCC
M33.93 **Dermatopolymyositis, unspecified without myopathy** CC HCC
M33.99 **Dermatopolymyositis, unspecified with other organ involvement** CC HCC

M34 Systemic sclerosis [scleroderma]
EXCLUDES 1 *circumscribed scleroderma (L94.Ø)*
neonatal scleroderma (P83.88)

M34.Ø **Progressive systemic sclerosis** HCC
M34.1 **CR(E)ST syndrome** HCC
Combination of calcinosis, Raynaud's phenomenon, esophageal dysfunction, sclerodactyly, telangiectasia
M34.2 **Systemic sclerosis induced by drug and chemical** HCC
Code first poisoning due to drug or toxin, if applicable (T36-T65 with fifth or sixth character 1-4 or 6)
Use additional code for adverse effect, if applicable, to identify drug (T36-T5Ø with fifth or sixth character 5)
M34.8 **Other forms of systemic sclerosis**
M34.81 **Systemic sclerosis with lung involvement** CC HCC
M34.82 **Systemic sclerosis with myopathy** CC HCC
M34.83 **Systemic sclerosis with polyneuropathy** HCC
M34.89 **Other systemic sclerosis** HCC
M34.9 **Systemic sclerosis, unspecified** HCC

M35 Other systemic involvement of connective tissue
EXCLUDES 1 *reactive perforating collagenosis (L87.1)*

M35.Ø **Sicca syndrome [Sjögren]**
DEF: Autoimmune disease associated with keratoconjunctivitis, laryngopharyngitis, rhinitis, dry mouth, enlarged parotid gland, and chronic polyarthritis.
M35.ØØ **Sicca syndrome, unspecified** HCC
M35.Ø1 **Sicca syndrome with keratoconjunctivitis** HCC
M35.Ø2 **Sicca syndrome with lung involvement** HCC
M35.Ø3 **Sicca syndrome with myopathy** CC HCC
M35.Ø4 **Sicca syndrome with tubulo-interstitial nephropathy** HCC
Renal tubular acidosis in sicca syndrome
M35.Ø9 **Sicca syndrome with other organ involvement** HCC
M35.1 **Other overlap syndromes** CC HCC
Mixed connective tissue disease
EXCLUDES 1 *polyangiitis overlap syndrome (M3Ø.8)*
M35.2 **Behçet's disease** CC HCC
M35.3 **Polymyalgia rheumatica** HCC
EXCLUDES 1 *polymyalgia rheumatica with giant cell arteritis (M31.5)*
M35.4 **Diffuse (eosinophilic) fasciitis**
M35.5 **Multifocal fibrosclerosis** CC HCC
M35.6 **Relapsing panniculitis [Weber-Christian]**
EXCLUDES 1 *lupus panniculitis (L93.2)*
panniculitis NOS (M79.3-)
M35.7 **Hypermobility syndrome**
Familial ligamentous laxity
EXCLUDES 1 *►Ehlers-Danlos syndromes◄ (Q79.6-)*
ligamentous laxity, NOS (M24.2-)
M35.8 **Other specified systemic involvement of connective tissue** CC HCC
M35.9 **Systemic involvement of connective tissue, unspecified** HCC
Autoimmune disease (systemic) NOS
Collagen (vascular) disease NOS

M36 Systemic disorders of connective tissue in diseases classified elsewhere
EXCLUDES 2 *arthropathies in diseases classified elsewhere (M14.-)*

M36.Ø ***Dermato(poly)myositis in neoplastic disease*** CC HCC
Code first underlying neoplasm (CØØ-D49)
M36.1 ***Arthropathy in neoplastic disease***
Code first underlying neoplasm, such as:
leukemia (C91-C95)
malignant histiocytosis (C96.A)
multiple myeloma (C9Ø.Ø)
M36.2 ***Hemophilic arthropathy***
Hemarthrosis in hemophilic arthropathy
Code first underlying disease, such as:
factor VIII deficiency (D66)
with vascular defect (D68.Ø)
factor IX deficiency (D67)
hemophilia (classical) (D66)
hemophilia B (D67)
hemophilia C (D68.1)
M36.3 ***Arthropathy in other blood disorders***
M36.4 ***Arthropathy in hypersensitivity reactions classified elsewhere***
Code first underlying disease, such as:
Henoch (-Schönlein) purpura (D69.Ø)
serum sickness (T8Ø.6-)
M36.8 ***Systemic disorders of connective tissue in other diseases classified elsewhere*** HCC
Code first underlying disease, such as:
alkaptonuria (E7Ø.2)
hypogammaglobulinemia (D8Ø.-)
ochronosis (E7Ø.2)

DORSOPATHIES (M4Ø-M54)

Deforming dorsopathies (M4Ø-M43)

M4Ø Kyphosis and lordosis
EXCLUDES 1 *congenital kyphosis and lordosis (Q76.4)*
kyphoscoliosis (M41.-)
postprocedural kyphosis and lordosis (M96.-)

Kyphosis and Lordosis

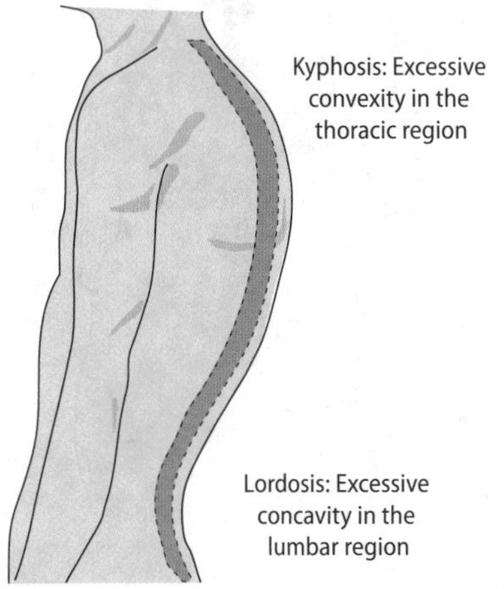

M4Ø.Ø **Postural kyphosis**
EXCLUDES 1 *osteochondrosis of spine (M42.-)*
M4Ø.ØØ **Postural kyphosis, site unspecified**
M4Ø.Ø3 **Postural kyphosis, cervicothoracic region**
M4Ø.Ø4 **Postural kyphosis, thoracic region**
M4Ø.Ø5 **Postural kyphosis, thoracolumbar region**
M4Ø.1 **Other secondary kyphosis**
M4Ø.1Ø **Other secondary kyphosis, site unspecified**
M4Ø.12 **Other secondary kyphosis, cervical region**
M4Ø.13 **Other secondary kyphosis, cervicothoracic region**
M4Ø.14 **Other secondary kyphosis, thoracic region**
M4Ø.15 **Other secondary kyphosis, thoracolumbar region**
M4Ø.2 **Other and unspecified kyphosis**
M4Ø.2Ø **Unspecified kyphosis**
M4Ø.2Ø2 **Unspecified kyphosis, cervical region**
M4Ø.2Ø3 **Unspecified kyphosis, cervicothoracic region**
M4Ø.2Ø4 **Unspecified kyphosis, thoracic region**
M4Ø.2Ø5 **Unspecified kyphosis, thoracolumbar region**
M4Ø.2Ø9 **Unspecified kyphosis, site unspecified**
M4Ø.29 **Other kyphosis**
M4Ø.292 **Other kyphosis, cervical region**
M4Ø.293 **Other kyphosis, cervicothoracic region**
M4Ø.294 **Other kyphosis, thoracic region**
M4Ø.295 **Other kyphosis, thoracolumbar region**

M40.299 Other kyphosis, site unspecified

√5th M40.3 Flatback syndrome

M40.30 Flatback syndrome, site unspecified
M40.35 Flatback syndrome, thoracolumbar region
M40.36 Flatback syndrome, lumbar region
M40.37 Flatback syndrome, lumbosacral region

√5th M40.4 Postural lordosis

Acquired lordosis

M40.40 Postural lordosis, site unspecified
M40.45 Postural lordosis, thoracolumbar region
M40.46 Postural lordosis, lumbar region
M40.47 Postural lordosis, lumbosacral region

√5th M40.5 Lordosis, unspecified

M40.50 Lordosis, unspecified, site unspecified
M40.55 Lordosis, unspecified, thoracolumbar region
M40.56 Lordosis, unspecified, lumbar region
M40.57 Lordosis, unspecified, lumbosacral region

√4th M41 Scoliosis

INCLUDES kyphoscoliosis

EXCLUDES 1 *congenital scoliosis due to bony malformation (Q76.3)*
congenital scoliosis NOS (Q67.5)
kyphoscoliotic heart disease (I27.1)
postprocedural scoliosis (M96.-)
postural congenital scoliosis (Q67.5)

Scoliosis

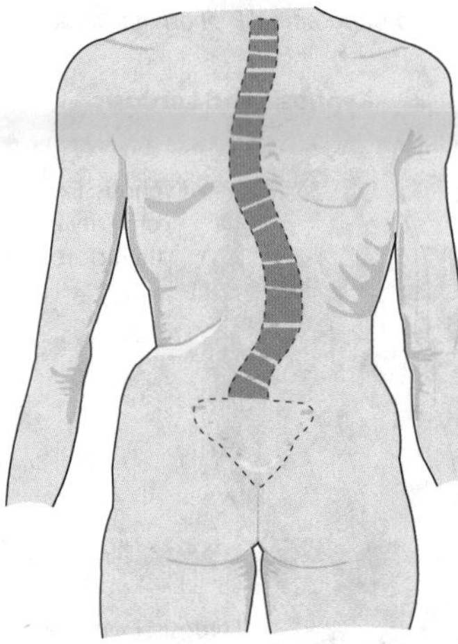

Lateral curvature of spine

√5th M41.0 Infantile idiopathic scoliosis

AHA: 2014,4Q,26

M41.00 Infantile idiopathic scoliosis, site unspecified
M41.02 Infantile idiopathic scoliosis, cervical region
M41.03 Infantile idiopathic scoliosis, cervicothoracic region
M41.04 Infantile idiopathic scoliosis, thoracic region
M41.05 Infantile idiopathic scoliosis, thoracolumbar region
M41.06 Infantile idiopathic scoliosis, lumbar region
M41.07 Infantile idiopathic scoliosis, lumbosacral region
M41.08 Infantile idiopathic scoliosis, sacral and sacrococcygeal region

√5th M41.1 Juvenile and adolescent idiopathic scoliosis

√6th M41.11 Juvenile idiopathic scoliosis

AHA: 2014,4Q,28

M41.112 Juvenile idiopathic scoliosis, cervical region
M41.113 Juvenile idiopathic scoliosis, cervicothoracic region
M41.114 Juvenile idiopathic scoliosis, thoracic region
M41.115 Juvenile idiopathic scoliosis, thoracolumbar region
M41.116 Juvenile idiopathic scoliosis, lumbar region
M41.117 Juvenile idiopathic scoliosis, lumbosacral region
M41.119 Juvenile idiopathic scoliosis, site unspecified

√6th M41.12 Adolescent scoliosis

M41.122 Adolescent idiopathic scoliosis, cervical region
M41.123 Adolescent idiopathic scoliosis, cervicothoracic region
M41.124 Adolescent idiopathic scoliosis, thoracic region
M41.125 Adolescent idiopathic scoliosis, thoracolumbar region
M41.126 Adolescent idiopathic scoliosis, lumbar region
M41.127 Adolescent idiopathic scoliosis, lumbosacral region
M41.129 Adolescent idiopathic scoliosis, site unspecified

√5th M41.2 Other idiopathic scoliosis

M41.20 Other idiopathic scoliosis, site unspecified
M41.22 Other idiopathic scoliosis, cervical region
M41.23 Other idiopathic scoliosis, cervicothoracic region
M41.24 Other idiopathic scoliosis, thoracic region
M41.25 Other idiopathic scoliosis, thoracolumbar region
M41.26 Other idiopathic scoliosis, lumbar region
M41.27 Other idiopathic scoliosis, lumbosacral region

√5th M41.3 Thoracogenic scoliosis

M41.30 Thoracogenic scoliosis, site unspecified
M41.34 Thoracogenic scoliosis, thoracic region
M41.35 Thoracogenic scoliosis, thoracolumbar region

√5th M41.4 Neuromuscular scoliosis

Scoliosis secondary to cerebral palsy, Friedreich's ataxia, poliomyelitis and other neuromuscular disorders
Code also underlying condition
AHA: 2014,4Q,27

M41.40 Neuromuscular scoliosis, site unspecified
M41.41 Neuromuscular scoliosis, occipito-atlanto-axial region
M41.42 Neuromuscular scoliosis, cervical region
M41.43 Neuromuscular scoliosis, cervicothoracic region
M41.44 Neuromuscular scoliosis, thoracic region
M41.45 Neuromuscular scoliosis, thoracolumbar region
M41.46 Neuromuscular scoliosis, lumbar region
M41.47 Neuromuscular scoliosis, lumbosacral region

√5th M41.5 Other secondary scoliosis

AHA: 2019,1Q,19

M41.50 Other secondary scoliosis, site unspecified
M41.52 Other secondary scoliosis, cervical region
M41.53 Other secondary scoliosis, cervicothoracic region
M41.54 Other secondary scoliosis, thoracic region
M41.55 Other secondary scoliosis, thoracolumbar region
M41.56 Other secondary scoliosis, lumbar region
M41.57 Other secondary scoliosis, lumbosacral region

√5th M41.8 Other forms of scoliosis

M41.80 Other forms of scoliosis, site unspecified
M41.82 Other forms of scoliosis, cervical region
M41.83 Other forms of scoliosis, cervicothoracic region
M41.84 Other forms of scoliosis, thoracic region
M41.85 Other forms of scoliosis, thoracolumbar region
M41.86 Other forms of scoliosis, lumbar region
M41.87 Other forms of scoliosis, lumbosacral region

M41.9 Scoliosis, unspecified

√4th M42 Spinal osteochondrosis

√5th M42.0 Juvenile osteochondrosis of spine

Calvé's disease
Scheuermann's disease

EXCLUDES 1 *postural kyphosis (M40.0)*

M42.00 Juvenile osteochondrosis of spine, site unspecified
M42.01 Juvenile osteochondrosis of spine, occipito-atlanto-axial region
M42.02 Juvenile osteochondrosis of spine, cervical region
M42.03 Juvenile osteochondrosis of spine, cervicothoracic region
M42.04 Juvenile osteochondrosis of spine, thoracic region
M42.05 Juvenile osteochondrosis of spine, thoracolumbar region
M42.06 Juvenile osteochondrosis of spine, lumbar region
M42.07 Juvenile osteochondrosis of spine, lumbosacral region

M42.Ø8 Juvenile osteochondrosis of spine, sacral and sacrococcygeal region
M42.Ø9 Juvenile osteochondrosis of spine, multiple sites in spine

M42.1 Adult osteochondrosis of spine
M42.1Ø Adult osteochondrosis of spine, site unspecified A
M42.11 Adult osteochondrosis of spine, occipito-atlanto-axial region A
M42.12 Adult osteochondrosis of spine, cervical region A
M42.13 Adult osteochondrosis of spine, cervicothoracic region A
M42.14 Adult osteochondrosis of spine, thoracic region A
M42.15 Adult osteochondrosis of spine, thoracolumbar region A
M42.16 Adult osteochondrosis of spine, lumbar region A
M42.17 Adult osteochondrosis of spine, lumbosacral region A
M42.18 Adult osteochondrosis of spine, sacral and sacrococcygeal region A
M42.19 Adult osteochondrosis of spine, multiple sites in spine A

M42.9 Spinal osteochondrosis, unspecified

M43 Other deforming dorsopathies

EXCLUDES 1 *congenital spondylolysis and spondylolisthesis (Q76.2)*
hemivertebra (Q76.3-Q76.4)
Klippel-Feil syndrome (Q76.1)
lumbarization and sacralization (Q76.4)
platyspondylisis (Q76.4)
spina bifida occulta (Q76.Ø)
spinal curvature in osteoporosis (M8Ø.-)
spinal curvature in Paget's disease of bone [osteitis deformans] (M88.-)

M43.Ø Spondylolysis
EXCLUDES 1 *congenital spondylolysis (Q76.2)*
spondylolisthesis (M43.1)
M43.ØØ Spondylolysis, site unspecified
M43.Ø1 Spondylolysis, occipito-atlanto-axial region
M43.Ø2 Spondylolysis, cervical region
M43.Ø3 Spondylolysis, cervicothoracic region
M43.Ø4 Spondylolysis, thoracic region
M43.Ø5 Spondylolysis, thoracolumbar region
M43.Ø6 Spondylolysis, lumbar region
M43.Ø7 Spondylolysis, lumbosacral region
M43.Ø8 Spondylolysis, sacral and sacrococcygeal region
M43.Ø9 Spondylolysis, multiple sites in spine

M43.1 Spondylolisthesis
EXCLUDES 1 *acute traumatic of lumbosacral region (S33.1)*
acute traumatic of sites other than lumbosacral — code to Fracture, vertebra, by region
congenital spondylolisthesis (Q76.2)
AHA: 2020,2Q,21; 2018,3Q,18
TIP: Code also any associated radiculopathy (M54.1-) and/or myelopathy (G99.2).
M43.1Ø Spondylolisthesis, site unspecified
M43.11 Spondylolisthesis, occipito-atlanto-axial region
M43.12 Spondylolisthesis, cervical region
M43.13 Spondylolisthesis, cervicothoracic region
M43.14 Spondylolisthesis, thoracic region
M43.15 Spondylolisthesis, thoracolumbar region
M43.16 Spondylolisthesis, lumbar region
M43.17 Spondylolisthesis, lumbosacral region
M43.18 Spondylolisthesis, sacral and sacrococcygeal region
M43.19 Spondylolisthesis, multiple sites in spine

M43.2 Fusion of spine
Ankylosis of spinal joint
EXCLUDES 1 *ankylosing spondylitis (M45.Ø-)*
congenital fusion of spine (Q76.4)
EXCLUDES 2 *arthrodesis status (Z98.1)*
pseudoarthrosis after fusion or arthrodesis (M96.Ø)
M43.2Ø Fusion of spine, site unspecified
M43.21 Fusion of spine, occipito-atlanto-axial region
M43.22 Fusion of spine, cervical region
M43.23 Fusion of spine, cervicothoracic region
M43.24 Fusion of spine, thoracic region
M43.25 Fusion of spine, thoracolumbar region
M43.26 Fusion of spine, lumbar region
M43.27 Fusion of spine, lumbosacral region
M43.28 Fusion of spine, sacral and sacrococcygeal region

M43.3 Recurrent atlantoaxial dislocation with myelopathy

M43.4 Other recurrent atlantoaxial dislocation

M43.5 Other recurrent vertebral dislocation
EXCLUDES 1 *biomechanical lesions NEC (M99.-)*

M43.5X Other recurrent vertebral dislocation
M43.5X2 Other recurrent vertebral dislocation, cervical region
M43.5X3 Other recurrent vertebral dislocation, cervicothoracic region
M43.5X4 Other recurrent vertebral dislocation, thoracic region
M43.5X5 Other recurrent vertebral dislocation, thoracolumbar region
M43.5X6 Other recurrent vertebral dislocation, lumbar region
M43.5X7 Other recurrent vertebral dislocation, lumbosacral region
M43.5X8 Other recurrent vertebral dislocation, sacral and sacrococcygeal region
M43.5X9 Other recurrent vertebral dislocation, site unspecified

M43.6 Torticollis
EXCLUDES 1 *congenital (sternomastoid) torticollis (Q68.Ø)*
current injury — see Injury, of spine, by body region
ocular torticollis (R29.891)
psychogenic torticollis (F45.8)
spasmodic torticollis (G24.3)
torticollis due to birth injury (P15.2)
DEF: Twisted, unnatural position of the neck due to contracted cervical muscles that pull the head to one side.

M43.8 Other specified deforming dorsopathies
EXCLUDES 2 *kyphosis and lordosis (M4Ø.-)*
scoliosis (M41.-)

M43.8X Other specified deforming dorsopathies
M43.8X1 Other specified deforming dorsopathies, occipito-atlanto-axial region
M43.8X2 Other specified deforming dorsopathies, cervical region
M43.8X3 Other specified deforming dorsopathies, cervicothoracic region
M43.8X4 Other specified deforming dorsopathies, thoracic region
M43.8X5 Other specified deforming dorsopathies, thoracolumbar region
M43.8X6 Other specified deforming dorsopathies, lumbar region
M43.8X7 Other specified deforming dorsopathies, lumbosacral region
M43.8X8 Other specified deforming dorsopathies, sacral and sacrococcygeal region
M43.8X9 Other specified deforming dorsopathies, site unspecified

M43.9 Deforming dorsopathy, unspecified
Curvature of spine NOS

Spondylopathies (M45-M49)

M45 Ankylosing spondylitis

Rheumatoid arthritis of spine
EXCLUDES 1 *arthropathy in Reiter's disease (MØ2.3-)*
juvenile (ankylosing) spondylitis (MØ8.1)
EXCLUDES 2 *Behçet's disease (M35.2)*

M45.Ø Ankylosing spondylitis of multiple sites in spine HCC
M45.1 Ankylosing spondylitis of occipito-atlanto-axial region HCC
M45.2 Ankylosing spondylitis of cervical region HCC
M45.3 Ankylosing spondylitis of cervicothoracic region HCC
M45.4 Ankylosing spondylitis of thoracic region HCC
M45.5 Ankylosing spondylitis of thoracolumbar region HCC
M45.6 Ankylosing spondylitis lumbar region HCC
M45.7 Ankylosing spondylitis of lumbosacral region HCC

M45.8 Ankylosing spondylitis sacral and sacrococcygeal region HCC

M45.9 Ankylosing spondylitis of unspecified sites in spine HCC

M46 Other inflammatory spondylopathies

M46.Ø Spinal enthesopathy

Disorder of ligamentous or muscular attachments of spine

M46.ØØ Spinal enthesopathy, site unspecified HCC

M46.Ø1 Spinal enthesopathy, occipito-atlanto-axial region HCC

M46.Ø2 Spinal enthesopathy, cervical region HCC

M46.Ø3 Spinal enthesopathy, cervicothoracic region HCC

M46.Ø4 Spinal enthesopathy, thoracic region HCC

M46.Ø5 Spinal enthesopathy, thoracolumbar region HCC

M46.Ø6 Spinal enthesopathy, lumbar region HCC

M46.Ø7 Spinal enthesopathy, lumbosacral region HCC

M46.Ø8 Spinal enthesopathy, sacral and sacrococcygeal region HCC

M46.Ø9 Spinal enthesopathy, multiple sites in spine HCC

M46.1 Sacroiliitis, not elsewhere classified HCC

AHA: 2020,2Q,14

DEF: Inflammation of the sacroiliac joint (situated at the juncture of the sacrum and hip). Symptoms include pain in the buttocks or lower back that can extend down one or both legs.

M46.2 Osteomyelitis of vertebra

M46.2Ø Osteomyelitis of vertebra, site unspecified CC HCC

M46.21 Osteomyelitis of vertebra, occipito-atlanto-axial region CC HCC

M46.22 Osteomyelitis of vertebra, cervical region CC HCC

M46.23 Osteomyelitis of vertebra, cervicothoracic region CC HCC

M46.24 Osteomyelitis of vertebra, thoracic region CC HCC

M46.25 Osteomyelitis of vertebra, thoracolumbar region CC HCC

M46.26 Osteomyelitis of vertebra, lumbar region CC HCC

M46.27 Osteomyelitis of vertebra, lumbosacral region CC HCC

M46.28 Osteomyelitis of vertebra, sacral and sacrococcygeal region CC HCC

M46.3 Infection of intervertebral disc (pyogenic)

Use additional code (B95-B97) to identify infectious agent

M46.3Ø Infection of intervertebral disc (pyogenic), site unspecified CC HCC

M46.31 Infection of intervertebral disc (pyogenic), occipito-atlanto-axial region CC HCC

M46.32 Infection of intervertebral disc (pyogenic), cervical region CC HCC

M46.33 Infection of intervertebral disc (pyogenic), cervicothoracic region CC HCC

M46.34 Infection of intervertebral disc (pyogenic), thoracic region CC HCC

M46.35 Infection of intervertebral disc (pyogenic), thoracolumbar region CC HCC

M46.36 Infection of intervertebral disc (pyogenic), lumbar region CC HCC

M46.37 Infection of intervertebral disc (pyogenic), lumbosacral region CC HCC

M46.38 Infection of intervertebral disc (pyogenic), sacral and sacrococcygeal region CC HCC

M46.39 Infection of intervertebral disc (pyogenic), multiple sites in spine CC HCC

M46.4 Discitis, unspecified

M46.4Ø Discitis, unspecified, site unspecified

M46.41 Discitis, unspecified, occipito-atlanto-axial region

M46.42 Discitis, unspecified, cervical region

M46.43 Discitis, unspecified, cervicothoracic region

M46.44 Discitis, unspecified, thoracic region

M46.45 Discitis, unspecified, thoracolumbar region

M46.46 Discitis, unspecified, lumbar region

M46.47 Discitis, unspecified, lumbosacral region

M46.48 Discitis, unspecified, sacral and sacrococcygeal region

M46.49 Discitis, unspecified, multiple sites in spine

M46.5 Other infective spondylopathies

M46.5Ø Other infective spondylopathies, site unspecified HCC

M46.51 Other infective spondylopathies, occipito-atlanto-axial region HCC

M46.52 Other infective spondylopathies, cervical region HCC

M46.53 Other infective spondylopathies, cervicothoracic region HCC

M46.54 Other infective spondylopathies, thoracic region HCC

M46.55 Other infective spondylopathies, thoracolumbar region HCC

M46.56 Other infective spondylopathies, lumbar region HCC

M46.57 Other infective spondylopathies, lumbosacral region HCC

M46.58 Other infective spondylopathies, sacral and sacrococcygeal region HCC

M46.59 Other infective spondylopathies, multiple sites in spine HCC

M46.8 Other specified inflammatory spondylopathies

M46.8Ø Other specified inflammatory spondylopathies, site unspecified HCC

M46.81 Other specified inflammatory spondylopathies, occipito-atlanto-axial region HCC

M46.82 Other specified inflammatory spondylopathies, cervical region HCC

M46.83 Other specified inflammatory spondylopathies, cervicothoracic region HCC

M46.84 Other specified inflammatory spondylopathies, thoracic region HCC

M46.85 Other specified inflammatory spondylopathies, thoracolumbar region HCC

M46.86 Other specified inflammatory spondylopathies, lumbar region HCC

M46.87 Other specified inflammatory spondylopathies, lumbosacral region HCC

M46.88 Other specified inflammatory spondylopathies, sacral and sacrococcygeal region HCC

M46.89 Other specified inflammatory spondylopathies, multiple sites in spine HCC

M46.9 Unspecified inflammatory spondylopathy

M46.9Ø Unspecified inflammatory spondylopathy, site unspecified HCC

M46.91 Unspecified inflammatory spondylopathy, occipito-atlanto-axial region HCC

M46.92 Unspecified inflammatory spondylopathy, cervical region HCC

AHA: 2019,3Q,10

M46.93 Unspecified inflammatory spondylopathy, cervicothoracic region HCC

M46.94 Unspecified inflammatory spondylopathy, thoracic region HCC

M46.95 Unspecified inflammatory spondylopathy, thoracolumbar region HCC

M46.96 Unspecified inflammatory spondylopathy, lumbar region HCC

M46.97 Unspecified inflammatory spondylopathy, lumbosacral region HCC

M46.98 Unspecified inflammatory spondylopathy, sacral and sacrococcygeal region HCC

M46.99 Unspecified inflammatory spondylopathy, multiple sites in spine HCC

M47 Spondylosis

INCLUDES arthrosis or osteoarthritis of spine
degeneration of facet joints

AHA: 2020,1Q,17; 2019,3Q,10-11; 2016,4Q,147

M47.Ø Anterior spinal and vertebral artery compression syndromes

M47.Ø1 Anterior spinal artery compression syndromes

M47.Ø11 Anterior spinal artery compression syndromes, occipito-atlanto-axial region CC

M47.Ø12 Anterior spinal artery compression syndromes, cervical region CC

M47.Ø13 Anterior spinal artery compression syndromes, cervicothoracic region CC

M47.Ø14 Anterior spinal artery compression syndromes, thoracic region CC

M47.Ø15 Anterior spinal artery compression syndromes, thoracolumbar region CC

M47.Ø16 Anterior spinal artery compression syndromes, lumbar region CC

M47.Ø19 Anterior spinal artery compression syndromes, site unspecified CC

√6th M47.Ø2 Vertebral artery compression syndromes

M47.Ø21 Vertebral artery compression syndromes, occipito-atlanto-axial region CC

M47.Ø22 Vertebral artery compression syndromes, cervical region CC

M47.Ø29 Vertebral artery compression syndromes, site unspecified CC

√5th M47.1 Other spondylosis with myelopathy

Spondylogenic compression of spinal cord

EXCLUDES 1 *vertebral subluxation (M43.3-M43.5X9)*

AHA: 2020,1Q,17

M47.1Ø Other spondylosis with myelopathy, site unspecified CC

M47.11 Other spondylosis with myelopathy, occipito-atlanto-axial region CC

M47.12 Other spondylosis with myelopathy, cervical region CC

M47.13 Other spondylosis with myelopathy, cervicothoracic region CC

M47.14 Other spondylosis with myelopathy, thoracic region CC

M47.15 Other spondylosis with myelopathy, thoracolumbar region CC

M47.16 Other spondylosis with myelopathy, lumbar region CC

√5th M47.2 Other spondylosis with radiculopathy

AHA: 2020,1Q,17

M47.2Ø Other spondylosis with radiculopathy, site unspecified

M47.21 Other spondylosis with radiculopathy, occipito-atlanto-axial region

M47.22 Other spondylosis with radiculopathy, cervical region

M47.23 Other spondylosis with radiculopathy, cervicothoracic region

M47.24 Other spondylosis with radiculopathy, thoracic region

M47.25 Other spondylosis with radiculopathy, thoracolumbar region

M47.26 Other spondylosis with radiculopathy, lumbar region

M47.27 Other spondylosis with radiculopathy, lumbosacral region

M47.28 Other spondylosis with radiculopathy, sacral and sacrococcygeal region

√5th M47.8 Other spondylosis

√6th M47.81 Spondylosis without myelopathy or radiculopathy

AHA: 2019,3Q,10-11; 2018,2Q,14

M47.811 Spondylosis without myelopathy or radiculopathy, occipito-atlanto-axial region

M47.812 Spondylosis without myelopathy or radiculopathy, cervical region

M47.813 Spondylosis without myelopathy or radiculopathy, cervicothoracic region

M47.814 Spondylosis without myelopathy or radiculopathy, thoracic region

M47.815 Spondylosis without myelopathy or radiculopathy, thoracolumbar region

M47.816 Spondylosis without myelopathy or radiculopathy, lumbar region

M47.817 Spondylosis without myelopathy or radiculopathy, lumbosacral region

M47.818 Spondylosis without myelopathy or radiculopathy, sacral and sacrococcygeal region

M47.819 Spondylosis without myelopathy or radiculopathy, site unspecified

√6th M47.89 Other spondylosis

M47.891 Other spondylosis, occipito-atlanto-axial region

M47.892 Other spondylosis, cervical region

M47.893 Other spondylosis, cervicothoracic region

M47.894 Other spondylosis, thoracic region

M47.895 Other spondylosis, thoracolumbar region

M47.896 Other spondylosis, lumbar region

M47.897 Other spondylosis, lumbosacral region

M47.898 Other spondylosis, sacral and sacrococcygeal region

M47.899 Other spondylosis, site unspecified

M47.9 Spondylosis, unspecified

√4th M48 Other spondylopathies

√5th M48.Ø Spinal stenosis

Caudal stenosis

AHA: 2020,1Q,17; 2018,3Q,18-19

TIP: Code also any associated radiculopathy (M54.1-) and/or myelopathy (G99.2).

M48.ØØ Spinal stenosis, site unspecified

M48.Ø1 Spinal stenosis, occipito-atlanto-axial region

M48.Ø2 Spinal stenosis, cervical region

M48.Ø3 Spinal stenosis, cervicothoracic region

M48.Ø4 Spinal stenosis, thoracic region

M48.Ø5 Spinal stenosis, thoracolumbar region

√6th M48.Ø6 Spinal stenosis, lumbar region

AHA: 2018,3Q,19; 2017,4Q,18-19

DEF: Spinal canal narrowing in the lumbar area with nerve root compression, causing muscle pain, fatigue, and weakness during extension of the lumbar spine. Pain is relieved by sitting or bending.

M48.Ø61 Spinal stenosis, lumbar region without neurogenic claudication

Spinal stenosis, lumbar region NOS

M48.Ø62 Spinal stenosis, lumbar region with neurogenic claudication

M48.Ø7 Spinal stenosis, lumbosacral region

M48.Ø8 Spinal stenosis, sacral and sacrococcygeal region

√5th M48.1 Ankylosing hyperostosis [Forestier]

Diffuse idiopathic skeletal hyperostosis [DISH]

M48.1Ø Ankylosing hyperostosis [Forestier], site unspecified

M48.11 Ankylosing hyperostosis [Forestier], occipito-atlanto-axial region

M48.12 Ankylosing hyperostosis [Forestier], cervical region

M48.13 Ankylosing hyperostosis [Forestier], cervicothoracic region

M48.14 Ankylosing hyperostosis [Forestier], thoracic region

M48.15 Ankylosing hyperostosis [Forestier], thoracolumbar region

M48.16 Ankylosing hyperostosis [Forestier], lumbar region

M48.17 Ankylosing hyperostosis [Forestier], lumbosacral region

M48.18 Ankylosing hyperostosis [Forestier], sacral and sacrococcygeal region

M48.19 Ankylosing hyperostosis [Forestier], multiple sites in spine

√5th M48.2 Kissing spine

M48.2Ø Kissing spine, site unspecified

M48.21 Kissing spine, occipito-atlanto-axial region

M48.22 Kissing spine, cervical region

M48.23 Kissing spine, cervicothoracic region

M48.24 Kissing spine, thoracic region

M48.25 Kissing spine, thoracolumbar region

M48.26 Kissing spine, lumbar region

M48.27 Kissing spine, lumbosacral region

√5th M48.3 Traumatic spondylopathy

M48.3Ø Traumatic spondylopathy, site unspecified CC

M48.31 Traumatic spondylopathy, occipito-atlanto-axial region CC

M48.32 Traumatic spondylopathy, cervical region CC

M48.33 Traumatic spondylopathy, cervicothoracic region CC

M48.34 Traumatic spondylopathy, thoracic region CC

M48.35 Traumatic spondylopathy, thoracolumbar region CC

M48.36 Traumatic spondylopathy, lumbar region CC

M48.37 Traumatic spondylopathy, lumbosacral region CC

M48.38 Traumatic spondylopathy, sacral and sacrococcygeal region CC

√5th **M48.4 Fatigue fracture of vertebra**

Stress fracture of vertebra

EXCLUDES 1 *pathological fracture NOS (M84.4-)*
pathological fracture of vertebra due to neoplasm (M84.58)
pathological fracture of vertebra due to osteoporosis (M80.-)
pathological fracture of vertebra due to other diagnosis (M84.68)
traumatic fracture of vertebrae (S12.0-S12.3-, S22.0-, S32.0-)

The appropriate 7th character is to be added to each code from subcategory M48.4.
A initial encounter for fracture
D subsequent encounter for fracture with routine healing
G subsequent encounter for fracture with delayed healing
S sequela of fracture

√x7th **M48.40 Fatigue fracture of vertebra, site unspecified**
√x7th **M48.41 Fatigue fracture of vertebra, occipito-atlanto-axial region**
√x7th **M48.42 Fatigue fracture of vertebra, cervical region**
√x7th **M48.43 Fatigue fracture of vertebra, cervicothoracic region**
√x7th **M48.44 Fatigue fracture of vertebra, thoracic region**
√x7th **M48.45 Fatigue fracture of vertebra, thoracolumbar region**
√x7th **M48.46 Fatigue fracture of vertebra, lumbar region**
√x7th **M48.47 Fatigue fracture of vertebra, lumbosacral region**
√x7th **M48.48 Fatigue fracture of vertebra, sacral and sacrococcygeal region**

√5th **M48.5 Collapsed vertebra, not elsewhere classified**

Collapsed vertebra NOS
Compression fracture of vertebra NOS
Wedging of vertebra NOS

EXCLUDES 1 *current injury — see Injury of spine, by body region*
fatigue fracture of vertebra (M48.4)
pathological fracture NOS (M84.4-)
pathological fracture of vertebra due to neoplasm (M84.58)
pathological fracture of vertebra due to osteoporosis (M80.-)
pathological fracture of vertebra due to other diagnosis (M84.68)
stress fracture of vertebra (M48.4-)
traumatic fracture of vertebra (S12.-, S22.-, S32.-)

The appropriate 7th character is to be added to each code from subcategory M48.5.
A initial encounter for fracture
D subsequent encounter for fracture with routine healing
G subsequent encounter for fracture with delayed healing
S sequela of fracture

6 √x7th **M48.50 Collapsed vertebra, not elsewhere classified, site unspecified** CC HCC
6 √x7th **M48.51 Collapsed vertebra, not elsewhere classified, occipito-atlanto-axial region** CC HCC
6 √x7th **M48.52 Collapsed vertebra, not elsewhere classified, cervical region** CC HCC
6 √x7th **M48.53 Collapsed vertebra, not elsewhere classified, cervicothoracic region** CC HCC
6 √x7th **M48.54 Collapsed vertebra, not elsewhere classified, thoracic region** CC HCC
6 √x7th **M48.55 Collapsed vertebra, not elsewhere classified, thoracolumbar region** CC HCC
6 √x7th **M48.56 Collapsed vertebra, not elsewhere classified, lumbar region** CC HCC
6 √x7th **M48.57 Collapsed vertebra, not elsewhere classified, lumbosacral region** CC HCC
6 √x7th **M48.58 Collapsed vertebra, not elsewhere classified, sacral and sacrococcygeal region** CC HCC

√5th **M48.8 Other specified spondylopathies**

Ossification of posterior longitudinal ligament

√6th **M48.8X Other specified spondylopathies**

M48.8X1 Other specified spondylopathies, occipito-atlanto-axial region HCC
M48.8X2 Other specified spondylopathies, cervical region HCC
M48.8X3 Other specified spondylopathies, cervicothoracic region HCC
M48.8X4 Other specified spondylopathies, thoracic region HCC
M48.8X5 Other specified spondylopathies, thoracolumbar region HCC
M48.8X6 Other specified spondylopathies, lumbar region HCC
M48.8X7 Other specified spondylopathies, lumbosacral region HCC
M48.8X8 Other specified spondylopathies, sacral and sacrococcygeal region HCC
M48.8X9 Other specified spondylopathies, site unspecified HCC

M48.9 Spondylopathy, unspecified

√4th **M49 Spondylopathies in diseases classified elsewhere**

INCLUDES curvature of spine in diseases classified elsewhere
deformity of spine in diseases classified elsewhere
kyphosis in diseases classified elsewhere
scoliosis in diseases classified elsewhere
spondylopathy in diseases classified elsewhere

Code first underlying disease, such as:
brucellosis (A23.-)
Charcôt-Marie-Tooth disease (G60.0)
enterobacterial infections (A01-A04)
osteitis fibrosa cystica (E21.0)

EXCLUDES 1 *curvature of spine in tuberculosis [Pott's] (A18.01)*
enteropathic arthropathies (M07.-)
gonococcal spondylitis (A54.41)
neuropathic spondylopathy in syringomyelia (G95.0)
neuropathic spondylopathy in tabes dorsalis (A52.11)
neuropathic [tabes dorsalis] spondylitis (A52.11)
nonsyphilitic neuropathic spondylopathy NEC (G98.0)
spondylitis in syphilis (acquired) (A52.77)
tuberculous spondylitis (A18.01)
typhoid fever spondylitis (A01.05)

√5th **M49.8 Spondylopathy in diseases classified elsewhere**

M49.80 Spondylopathy in diseases classified elsewhere, site unspecified HCC
M49.81 Spondylopathy in diseases classified elsewhere, occipito-atlanto-axial region HCC
M49.82 Spondylopathy in diseases classified elsewhere, cervical region HCC
M49.83 Spondylopathy in diseases classified elsewhere, cervicothoracic region HCC
M49.84 Spondylopathy in diseases classified elsewhere, thoracic region HCC
M49.85 Spondylopathy in diseases classified elsewhere, thoracolumbar region HCC
M49.86 Spondylopathy in diseases classified elsewhere, lumbar region HCC
M49.87 Spondylopathy in diseases classified elsewhere, lumbosacral region HCC
M49.88 Spondylopathy in diseases classified elsewhere, sacral and sacrococcygeal region HCC
M49.89 Spondylopathy in diseases classified elsewhere, multiple sites in spine HCC

Other dorsopathies (M50-M54)

EXCLUDES 1 *current injury — see injury of spine by body region*
discitis NOS (M46.4-)

√4th **M50 Cervical disc disorders**

NOTE Code to the most superior level of disorder

INCLUDES cervicothoracic disc disorders
cervicothoracic disc disorders with cervicalgia

AHA: 2016,4Q,39-40; 2016,1Q,17

√5th **M50.0 Cervical disc disorder with myelopathy**

AHA: 2018,3Q,19

M50.00 Cervical disc disorder with myelopathy, unspecified cervical region CC
M50.01 Cervical disc disorder with myelopathy, high cervical region CC

C2-C3 disc disorder with myelopathy
C3-C4 disc disorder with myelopathy

M50.02 Cervical disc disorder with myelopathy, mid-cervical region

M50.020 Cervical disc disorder with myelopathy, mid-cervical region, unspecified level CC

M50.021 Cervical disc disorder at C4-C5 level with myelopathy CC

C4-C5 disc disorder with myelopathy

M50.022 Cervical disc disorder at C5-C6 level with myelopathy CC

C5-C6 disc disorder with myelopathy

M50.023 Cervical disc disorder at C6-C7 level with myelopathy CC

C6-C7 disc disorder with myelopathy

M50.03 Cervical disc disorder with myelopathy, cervicothoracic region CC

C7-T1 disc disorder with myelopathy

M50.1 Cervical disc disorder with radiculopathy

EXCLUDES 2 *brachial radiculitis NOS (M54.13)*

AHA: 2018,3Q,19

M50.10 Cervical disc disorder with radiculopathy, unspecified cervical region

M50.11 Cervical disc disorder with radiculopathy, high cervical region

C2-C3 disc disorder with radiculopathy

C3 radiculopathy due to disc disorder

C3-C4 disc disorder with radiculopathy

C4 radiculopathy due to disc disorder

M50.12 Cervical disc disorder with radiculopathy, mid-cervical region

M50.120 Mid-cervical disc disorder, unspecified level

M50.121 Cervical disc disorder at C4-C5 level with radiculopathy

C4-C5 disc disorder with radiculopathy

C5 radiculopathy due to disc disorder

M50.122 Cervical disc disorder at C5-C6 level with radiculopathy

C5-C6 disc disorder with radiculopathy

C6 radiculopathy due to disc disorder

M50.123 Cervical disc disorder at C6-C7 level with radiculopathy

C6-C7 disc disorder with radiculopathy

C7 radiculopathy due to disc disorder

M50.13 Cervical disc disorder with radiculopathy, cervicothoracic region

C7-T1 disc disorder with radiculopathy

C8 radiculopathy due to disc disorder

M50.2 Other cervical disc displacement

M50.20 Other cervical disc displacement, unspecified cervical region

M50.21 Other cervical disc displacement, high cervical region

Other C2-C3 cervical disc displacement

Other C3-C4 cervical disc displacement

M50.22 Other cervical disc displacement, mid-cervical region

M50.220 Other cervical disc displacement, mid-cervical region, unspecified level

M50.221 Other cervical disc displacement at C4-C5 level

Other C4-C5 cervical disc displacement

M50.222 Other cervical disc displacement at C5-C6 level

Other C5-C6 cervical disc displacement

M50.223 Other cervical disc displacement at C6-C7 level

Other C6-C7 cervical disc displacement

M50.23 Other cervical disc displacement, cervicothoracic region

Other C7-T1 cervical disc displacement

M50.3 Other cervical disc degeneration

M50.30 Other cervical disc degeneration, unspecified cervical region

M50.31 Other cervical disc degeneration, high cervical region

Other C2-C3 cervical disc degeneration

Other C3-C4 cervical disc degeneration

M50.32 Other cervical disc degeneration, mid-cervical region

M50.320 Other cervical disc degeneration, mid-cervical region, unspecified level

M50.321 Other cervical disc degeneration at C4-C5 level

Other C4-C5 cervical disc degeneration

M50.322 Other cervical disc degeneration at C5-C6 level

Other C5-C6 cervical disc degeneration

M50.323 Other cervical disc degeneration at C6-C7 level

Other C6-C7 cervical disc degeneration

M50.33 Other cervical disc degeneration, cervicothoracic region

Other C7-T1 cervical disc degeneration

M50.8 Other cervical disc disorders

M50.80 Other cervical disc disorders, unspecified cervical region

M50.81 Other cervical disc disorders, high cervical region

Other C2-C3 cervical disc disorders

Other C3-C4 cervical disc disorders

M50.82 Other cervical disc disorders, mid-cervical region

M50.820 Other cervical disc disorders, mid-cervical region, unspecified level

M50.821 Other cervical disc disorders at C4-C5 level

Other C4-C5 cervical disc disorders

M50.822 Other cervical disc disorders at C5-C6 level

Other C5-C6 cervical disc disorders

M50.823 Other cervical disc disorders at C6-C7 level

Other C6-C7 cervical disc disorders

M50.83 Other cervical disc disorders, cervicothoracic region

Other C7-T1 cervical disc disorders

M50.9 Cervical disc disorder, unspecified

M50.90 Cervical disc disorder, unspecified, unspecified cervical region

M50.91 Cervical disc disorder, unspecified, high cervical region

C2-C3 cervical disc disorder, unspecified

C3-C4 cervical disc disorder, unspecified

M50.92 Cervical disc disorder, unspecified, mid-cervical region

M50.920 Unspecified cervical disc disorder, mid-cervical region, unspecified level

M50.921 Unspecified cervical disc disorder at C4-C5 level

Unspecified C4-C5 cervical disc disorder

M50.922 Unspecified cervical disc disorder at C5-C6 level

Unspecified C5-C6 cervical disc disorder

M50.923 Unspecified cervical disc disorder at C6-C7 level

Unspecified C6-C7 cervical disc disorder

M50.93 Cervical disc disorder, unspecified, cervicothoracic region

C7-T1 cervical disc disorder, unspecified

M51 Thoracic, thoracolumbar, and lumbosacral intervertebral disc disorders

EXCLUDES 2 *cervical and cervicothoracic disc disorders (M50.-)*

sacral and sacrococcygeal disorders (M53.3)

M51.0 Thoracic, thoracolumbar and lumbosacral intervertebral disc disorders with myelopathy

M51.04 Intervertebral disc disorders with myelopathy, thoracic region CC

M51.05 Intervertebral disc disorders with myelopathy, thoracolumbar region CC

M51.06 Intervertebral disc disorders with myelopathy, lumbar region CC

M51.1 Thoracic, thoracolumbar and lumbosacral intervertebral disc disorders with radiculopathy

Sciatica due to intervertebral disc disorder

EXCLUDES 1 *lumbar radiculitis NOS (M54.16)*

sciatica NOS (M54.3)

AHA: 2018,3Q,18

M51.14 Intervertebral disc disorders with radiculopathy, thoracic region

M51.15 **Intervertebral disc disorders with radiculopathy, thoracolumbar region**

M51.16 **Intervertebral disc disorders with radiculopathy, lumbar region**

M51.17 **Intervertebral disc disorders with radiculopathy, lumbosacral region**

✓5th **M51.2** **Other thoracic, thoracolumbar and lumbosacral intervertebral disc displacement**

Lumbago due to displacement of intervertebral disc

Displacement Intervertebral Disc

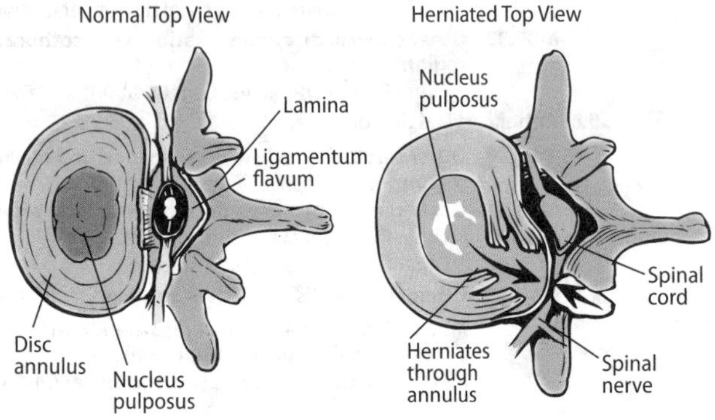

M51.24 **Other intervertebral disc displacement, thoracic region**

M51.25 **Other intervertebral disc displacement, thoracolumbar region**

M51.26 **Other intervertebral disc displacement, lumbar region**

M51.27 **Other intervertebral disc displacement, lumbosacral region**

✓5th **M51.3** **Other thoracic, thoracolumbar and lumbosacral intervertebral disc degeneration**

AHA: 2018,2Q,15; 2013,3Q,22

M51.34 **Other intervertebral disc degeneration, thoracic region**

M51.35 **Other intervertebral disc degeneration, thoracolumbar region**

M51.36 **Other intervertebral disc degeneration, lumbar region**

M51.37 **Other intervertebral disc degeneration, lumbosacral region**

✓5th **M51.4** **Schmorl's nodes**

DEF: Irregular bone defect in the margin of the vertebral body that causes herniation into the end plate of the vertebral body.

M51.44 **Schmorl's nodes, thoracic region**

M51.45 **Schmorl's nodes, thoracolumbar region**

M51.46 **Schmorl's nodes, lumbar region**

M51.47 **Schmorl's nodes, lumbosacral region**

✓5th **M51.8** **Other thoracic, thoracolumbar and lumbosacral intervertebral disc disorders**

M51.84 **Other intervertebral disc disorders, thoracic region**

M51.85 **Other intervertebral disc disorders, thoracolumbar region**

M51.86 **Other intervertebral disc disorders, lumbar region**

M51.87 **Other intervertebral disc disorders, lumbosacral region**

M51.9 **Unspecified thoracic, thoracolumbar and lumbosacral intervertebral disc disorder**

✓4th **M53** **Other and unspecified dorsopathies, not elsewhere classified**

M53.Ø **Cervicocranial syndrome**

Posterior cervical sympathetic syndrome

M53.1 **Cervicobrachial syndrome**

EXCLUDES 2 *cervical disc disorder (M5Ø.-)*
thoracic outlet syndrome (G54.Ø)

✓5th **M53.2** **Spinal instabilities**

✓6th **M53.2X** **Spinal instabilities**

M53.2X1 **Spinal instabilities, occipito-atlanto-axial region**

M53.2X2 **Spinal instabilities, cervical region**

M53.2X3 **Spinal instabilities, cervicothoracic region**

M53.2X4 **Spinal instabilities, thoracic region**

M53.2X5 **Spinal instabilities, thoracolumbar region**

M53.2X6 **Spinal instabilities, lumbar region**

M53.2X7 **Spinal instabilities, lumbosacral region**

M53.2X8 **Spinal instabilities, sacral and sacrococcygeal region**

M53.2X9 **Spinal instabilities, site unspecified**

M53.3 **Sacrococcygeal disorders, not elsewhere classified**

Coccygodynia

✓5th **M53.8** **Other specified dorsopathies**

M53.8Ø **Other specified dorsopathies, site unspecified**

M53.81 **Other specified dorsopathies, occipito-atlanto-axial region**

M53.82 **Other specified dorsopathies, cervical region**

M53.83 **Other specified dorsopathies, cervicothoracic region**

M53.84 **Other specified dorsopathies, thoracic region**

M53.85 **Other specified dorsopathies, thoracolumbar region**

M53.86 **Other specified dorsopathies, lumbar region**

M53.87 **Other specified dorsopathies, lumbosacral region**

M53.88 **Other specified dorsopathies, sacral and sacrococcygeal region**

M53.9 **Dorsopathy, unspecified**

✓4th **M54** **Dorsalgia**

EXCLUDES 1 *psychogenic dorsalgia (F45.41)*

✓5th **M54.Ø** **Panniculitis affecting regions of neck and back**

EXCLUDES 1 *lupus panniculitis (L93.2)*
panniculitis NOS (M79.3)
relapsing [Weber-Christian] panniculitis (M35.6)

M54.ØØ **Panniculitis affecting regions of neck and back, site unspecified**

M54.Ø1 **Panniculitis affecting regions of neck and back, occipito-atlanto-axial region**

M54.Ø2 **Panniculitis affecting regions of neck and back, cervical region**

M54.Ø3 **Panniculitis affecting regions of neck and back, cervicothoracic region**

M54.Ø4 **Panniculitis affecting regions of neck and back, thoracic region**

M54.Ø5 **Panniculitis affecting regions of neck and back, thoracolumbar region**

M54.Ø6 **Panniculitis affecting regions of neck and back, lumbar region**

M54.Ø7 **Panniculitis affecting regions of neck and back, lumbosacral region**

M54.Ø8 **Panniculitis affecting regions of neck and back, sacral and sacrococcygeal region**

M54.Ø9 **Panniculitis affecting regions, neck and back, multiple sites in spine**

✓5th **M54.1** **Radiculopathy**

Brachial neuritis or radiculitis NOS
Lumbar neuritis or radiculitis NOS
Lumbosacral neuritis or radiculitis NOS
Thoracic neuritis or radiculitis NOS
Radiculitis NOS

EXCLUDES 1 *neuralgia and neuritis NOS (M79.2)*
radiculopathy with cervical disc disorder (M5Ø.1)
radiculopathy with lumbar and other intervertebral disc disorder (M51.1-)
radiculopathy with spondylosis (M47.2-)

AHA: 2018,3Q,18

TIP: A code from this subcategory can be used in addition to a spondylolisthesis code (M43.1-) or a spinal stenosis code (M48.0-) when either condition is documented as the cause of the radiculopathy.

M54.1Ø **Radiculopathy, site unspecified**

M54.11 **Radiculopathy, occipito-atlanto-axial region**

M54.12 **Radiculopathy, cervical region**

M54.13 **Radiculopathy, cervicothoracic region**

M54.14 **Radiculopathy, thoracic region**

M54.15 **Radiculopathy, thoracolumbar region**

M54.16 **Radiculopathy, lumbar region**

M54.17 **Radiculopathy, lumbosacral region**

M54.18 **Radiculopathy, sacral and sacrococcygeal region**

M54.2 **Cervicalgia**

EXCLUDES 1 *cervicalgia due to intervertebral cervical disc disorder (M5Ø.-)*

M54.3 Sciatica

EXCLUDES 1 *lesion of sciatic nerve (G57.0)*
sciatica due to intervertebral disc disorder (M51.1-)
sciatica with lumbago (M54.4-)

M54.30 Sciatica, unspecified side
M54.31 Sciatica, right side
M54.32 Sciatica, left side

M54.4 Lumbago with sciatica

EXCLUDES 1 *lumbago with sciatica due to intervertebral disc disorder (M51.1-)*

AHA: 2016,2Q,7

M54.40 Lumbago with sciatica, unspecified side
M54.41 Lumbago with sciatica, right side
M54.42 Lumbago with sciatica, left side

M54.5 Low back pain
Loin pain
Lumbago NOS

EXCLUDES 1 *low back strain (S39.012)*
lumbago due to intervertebral disc displacement (M51.2-)
lumbago with sciatica (M54.4-)

M54.6 Pain in thoracic spine

EXCLUDES 1 *pain in thoracic spine due to intervertebral disc disorder (M51.-)*

M54.8 Other dorsalgia

EXCLUDES 1 *dorsalgia in thoracic region (M54.6)*
low back pain (M54.5)

M54.81 Occipital neuralgia
M54.89 Other dorsalgia

M54.9 Dorsalgia, unspecified
Backache NOS
Back pain NOS

SOFT TISSUE DISORDERS (M60-M79)

Disorders of muscles (M60-M63)

EXCLUDES 1 *dermatopolymyositis (M33.-)*
muscular dystrophies and myopathies (G71-G72)
myopathy in amyloidosis (E85.-)
myopathy in polyarteritis nodosa (M30.0)
myopathy in rheumatoid arthritis (M05.32)
myopathy in scleroderma (M34.-)
myopathy in Sjögren's syndrome (M35.03)
myopathy in systemic lupus erythematosus (M32.-)

M60 Myositis

EXCLUDES 2 *inclusion body myositis [IBM] (G72.41)*

M60.0 Infective myositis
Tropical pyomyositis
Use additional code (B95-B97) to identify infectious agent

M60.00 Infective myositis, unspecified site

M60.000 Infective myositis, unspecified right arm CC
Infective myositis, right upper limb NOS
M60.001 Infective myositis, unspecified left arm CC
Infective myositis, left upper limb NOS
M60.002 Infective myositis, unspecified arm CC
Infective myositis, upper limb NOS
M60.003 Infective myositis, unspecified right leg CC
Infective myositis, right lower limb NOS
M60.004 Infective myositis, unspecified left leg CC
Infective myositis, left lower limb NOS
M60.005 Infective myositis, unspecified leg CC
Infective myositis, lower limb NOS
M60.009 Infective myositis, unspecified site CC

M60.01 Infective myositis, shoulder

M60.011 Infective myositis, right shoulder CC
M60.012 Infective myositis, left shoulder CC
M60.019 Infective myositis, unspecified shoulder CC

M60.02 Infective myositis, upper arm

M60.021 Infective myositis, right upper arm CC
M60.022 Infective myositis, left upper arm CC
M60.029 Infective myositis, unspecified upper arm CC

M60.03 Infective myositis, forearm

M60.031 Infective myositis, right forearm CC
M60.032 Infective myositis, left forearm CC
M60.039 Infective myositis, unspecified forearm CC

M60.04 Infective myositis, hand and fingers

M60.041 Infective myositis, right hand CC
M60.042 Infective myositis, left hand CC
M60.043 Infective myositis, unspecified hand CC
M60.044 Infective myositis, right finger(s) CC
M60.045 Infective myositis, left finger(s) CC
M60.046 Infective myositis, unspecified finger(s) CC

M60.05 Infective myositis, thigh

M60.051 Infective myositis, right thigh CC
M60.052 Infective myositis, left thigh CC
M60.059 Infective myositis, unspecified thigh CC

M60.06 Infective myositis, lower leg

M60.061 Infective myositis, right lower leg CC
M60.062 Infective myositis, left lower leg CC
M60.069 Infective myositis, unspecified lower leg CC

M60.07 Infective myositis, ankle, foot and toes

M60.070 Infective myositis, right ankle CC
M60.071 Infective myositis, left ankle CC
M60.072 Infective myositis, unspecified ankle CC
M60.073 Infective myositis, right foot CC
M60.074 Infective myositis, left foot CC
M60.075 Infective myositis, unspecified foot CC
M60.076 Infective myositis, right toe(s) CC
M60.077 Infective myositis, left toe(s) CC
M60.078 Infective myositis, unspecified toe(s) CC

M60.08 Infective myositis, other site CC
M60.09 Infective myositis, multiple sites CC

M60.1 Interstitial myositis

M60.10 Interstitial myositis of unspecified site

M60.11 Interstitial myositis, shoulder

M60.111 Interstitial myositis, right shoulder
M60.112 Interstitial myositis, left shoulder
M60.119 Interstitial myositis, unspecified shoulder

M60.12 Interstitial myositis, upper arm

M60.121 Interstitial myositis, right upper arm
M60.122 Interstitial myositis, left upper arm
M60.129 Interstitial myositis, unspecified upper arm

M60.13 Interstitial myositis, forearm

M60.131 Interstitial myositis, right forearm
M60.132 Interstitial myositis, left forearm
M60.139 Interstitial myositis, unspecified forearm

M60.14 Interstitial myositis, hand

M60.141 Interstitial myositis, right hand
M60.142 Interstitial myositis, left hand
M60.149 Interstitial myositis, unspecified hand

M60.15 Interstitial myositis, thigh

M60.151 Interstitial myositis, right thigh
M60.152 Interstitial myositis, left thigh
M60.159 Interstitial myositis, unspecified thigh

M60.16 Interstitial myositis, lower leg

M60.161 Interstitial myositis, right lower leg
M60.162 Interstitial myositis, left lower leg
M60.169 Interstitial myositis, unspecified lower leg

M60.17 Interstitial myositis, ankle and foot

M60.171 Interstitial myositis, right ankle and foot
M60.172 Interstitial myositis, left ankle and foot
M60.179 Interstitial myositis, unspecified ankle and foot

M60.18 Interstitial myositis, other site
M60.19 Interstitial myositis, multiple sites

✓5th **M60.2 Foreign body granuloma of soft tissue, not elsewhere classified**

Use additional code to identify the type of retained foreign body (Z18.-)

EXCLUDES 1 *foreign body granuloma of skin and subcutaneous tissue (L92.3)*

M60.20 Foreign body granuloma of soft tissue, not elsewhere classified, unspecified site

✓6th **M60.21 Foreign body granuloma of soft tissue, not elsewhere classified, shoulder**

M60.211 Foreign body granuloma of soft tissue, not elsewhere classified, right shoulder

M60.212 Foreign body granuloma of soft tissue, not elsewhere classified, left shoulder

M60.219 Foreign body granuloma of soft tissue, not elsewhere classified, unspecified shoulder

✓6th **M60.22 Foreign body granuloma of soft tissue, not elsewhere classified, upper arm**

M60.221 Foreign body granuloma of soft tissue, not elsewhere classified, right upper arm

M60.222 Foreign body granuloma of soft tissue, not elsewhere classified, left upper arm

M60.229 Foreign body granuloma of soft tissue, not elsewhere classified, unspecified upper arm

✓6th **M60.23 Foreign body granuloma of soft tissue, not elsewhere classified, forearm**

M60.231 Foreign body granuloma of soft tissue, not elsewhere classified, right forearm

M60.232 Foreign body granuloma of soft tissue, not elsewhere classified, left forearm

M60.239 Foreign body granuloma of soft tissue, not elsewhere classified, unspecified forearm

✓6th **M60.24 Foreign body granuloma of soft tissue, not elsewhere classified, hand**

M60.241 Foreign body granuloma of soft tissue, not elsewhere classified, right hand

M60.242 Foreign body granuloma of soft tissue, not elsewhere classified, left hand

M60.249 Foreign body granuloma of soft tissue, not elsewhere classified, unspecified hand

✓6th **M60.25 Foreign body granuloma of soft tissue, not elsewhere classified, thigh**

M60.251 Foreign body granuloma of soft tissue, not elsewhere classified, right thigh

M60.252 Foreign body granuloma of soft tissue, not elsewhere classified, left thigh

M60.259 Foreign body granuloma of soft tissue, not elsewhere classified, unspecified thigh

✓6th **M60.26 Foreign body granuloma of soft tissue, not elsewhere classified, lower leg**

M60.261 Foreign body granuloma of soft tissue, not elsewhere classified, right lower leg

M60.262 Foreign body granuloma of soft tissue, not elsewhere classified, left lower leg

M60.269 Foreign body granuloma of soft tissue, not elsewhere classified, unspecified lower leg

✓6th **M60.27 Foreign body granuloma of soft tissue, not elsewhere classified, ankle and foot**

M60.271 Foreign body granuloma of soft tissue, not elsewhere classified, right ankle and foot

M60.272 Foreign body granuloma of soft tissue, not elsewhere classified, left ankle and foot

M60.279 Foreign body granuloma of soft tissue, not elsewhere classified, unspecified ankle and foot

M60.28 Foreign body granuloma of soft tissue, not elsewhere classified, other site

✓5th **M60.8 Other myositis**

M60.80 Other myositis, unspecified site

✓6th **M60.81 Other myositis shoulder**

M60.811 Other myositis, right shoulder

M60.812 Other myositis, left shoulder

M60.819 Other myositis, unspecified shoulder

✓6th **M60.82 Other myositis, upper arm**

M60.821 Other myositis, right upper arm

M60.822 Other myositis, left upper arm

M60.829 Other myositis, unspecified upper arm

✓6th **M60.83 Other myositis, forearm**

M60.831 Other myositis, right forearm

M60.832 Other myositis, left forearm

M60.839 Other myositis, unspecified forearm

✓6th **M60.84 Other myositis, hand**

M60.841 Other myositis, right hand

M60.842 Other myositis, left hand

M60.849 Other myositis, unspecified hand

✓6th **M60.85 Other myositis, thigh**

M60.851 Other myositis, right thigh

M60.852 Other myositis, left thigh

M60.859 Other myositis, unspecified thigh

✓6th **M60.86 Other myositis, lower leg**

M60.861 Other myositis, right lower leg

M60.862 Other myositis, left lower leg

M60.869 Other myositis, unspecified lower leg

✓6th **M60.87 Other myositis, ankle and foot**

M60.871 Other myositis, right ankle and foot

M60.872 Other myositis, left ankle and foot

M60.879 Other myositis, unspecified ankle and foot

M60.88 Other myositis, other site

M60.89 Other myositis, multiple sites

M60.9 Myositis, unspecified

✓4th **M61 Calcification and ossification of muscle**

✓5th **M61.0 Myositis ossificans traumatica**

M61.00 Myositis ossificans traumatica, unspecified site

✓6th **M61.01 Myositis ossificans traumatica, shoulder**

M61.011 Myositis ossificans traumatica, right shoulder

M61.012 Myositis ossificans traumatica, left shoulder

M61.019 Myositis ossificans traumatica, unspecified shoulder

✓6th **M61.02 Myositis ossificans traumatica, upper arm**

M61.021 Myositis ossificans traumatica, right upper arm

M61.022 Myositis ossificans traumatica, left upper arm

M61.029 Myositis ossificans traumatica, unspecified upper arm

✓6th **M61.03 Myositis ossificans traumatica, forearm**

M61.031 Myositis ossificans traumatica, right forearm

M61.032 Myositis ossificans traumatica, left forearm

M61.039 Myositis ossificans traumatica, unspecified forearm

✓6th **M61.04 Myositis ossificans traumatica, hand**

M61.041 Myositis ossificans traumatica, right hand

M61.042 Myositis ossificans traumatica, left hand

M61.049 Myositis ossificans traumatica, unspecified hand

✓6th **M61.05 Myositis ossificans traumatica, thigh**

M61.051 Myositis ossificans traumatica, right thigh

M61.052 Myositis ossificans traumatica, left thigh

M61.059 Myositis ossificans traumatica, unspecified thigh

✓6th **M61.06 Myositis ossificans traumatica, lower leg**

M61.061 Myositis ossificans traumatica, right lower leg

M61.062 Myositis ossificans traumatica, left lower leg

M61.069 Myositis ossificans traumatica, unspecified lower leg

✓6th **M61.07 Myositis ossificans traumatica, ankle and foot**

M61.071 Myositis ossificans traumatica, right ankle and foot

M61.072 Myositis ossificans traumatica, left ankle and foot

M61.079 Myositis ossificans traumatica, unspecified ankle and foot

M61.08 Myositis ossificans traumatica, other site

M60.2–M61.08

M61.09 Myositis ossificans traumatica, multiple sites

M61.1 Myositis ossificans progressiva
Fibrodysplasia ossificans progressiva
- M61.10 Myositis ossificans progressiva, unspecified site
- M61.11 Myositis ossificans progressiva, shoulder
  - M61.111 Myositis ossificans progressiva, right shoulder
  - M61.112 Myositis ossificans progressiva, left shoulder
  - M61.119 Myositis ossificans progressiva, unspecified shoulder
- M61.12 Myositis ossificans progressiva, upper arm
  - M61.121 Myositis ossificans progressiva, right upper arm
  - M61.122 Myositis ossificans progressiva, left upper arm
  - M61.129 Myositis ossificans progressiva, unspecified arm
- M61.13 Myositis ossificans progressiva, forearm
  - M61.131 Myositis ossificans progressiva, right forearm
  - M61.132 Myositis ossificans progressiva, left forearm
  - M61.139 Myositis ossificans progressiva, unspecified forearm
- M61.14 Myositis ossificans progressiva, hand and finger(s)
  - M61.141 Myositis ossificans progressiva, right hand
  - M61.142 Myositis ossificans progressiva, left hand
  - M61.143 Myositis ossificans progressiva, unspecified hand
  - M61.144 Myositis ossificans progressiva, right finger(s)
  - M61.145 Myositis ossificans progressiva, left finger(s)
  - M61.146 Myositis ossificans progressiva, unspecified finger(s)
- M61.15 Myositis ossificans progressiva, thigh
  - M61.151 Myositis ossificans progressiva, right thigh
  - M61.152 Myositis ossificans progressiva, left thigh
  - M61.159 Myositis ossificans progressiva, unspecified thigh
- M61.16 Myositis ossificans progressiva, lower leg
  - M61.161 Myositis ossificans progressiva, right lower leg
  - M61.162 Myositis ossificans progressiva, left lower leg
  - M61.169 Myositis ossificans progressiva, unspecified lower leg
- M61.17 Myositis ossificans progressiva, ankle, foot and toe(s)
  - M61.171 Myositis ossificans progressiva, right ankle
  - M61.172 Myositis ossificans progressiva, left ankle
  - M61.173 Myositis ossificans progressiva, unspecified ankle
  - M61.174 Myositis ossificans progressiva, right foot
  - M61.175 Myositis ossificans progressiva, left foot
  - M61.176 Myositis ossificans progressiva, unspecified foot
  - M61.177 Myositis ossificans progressiva, right toe(s)
  - M61.178 Myositis ossificans progressiva, left toe(s)
  - M61.179 Myositis ossificans progressiva, unspecified toe(s)
- M61.18 Myositis ossificans progressiva, other site
- M61.19 Myositis ossificans progressiva, multiple sites

M61.2 Paralytic calcification and ossification of muscle
Myositis ossificans associated with quadriplegia or paraplegia
- M61.20 Paralytic calcification and ossification of muscle, unspecified site
- M61.21 Paralytic calcification and ossification of muscle, shoulder
  - M61.211 Paralytic calcification and ossification of muscle, right shoulder
  - M61.212 Paralytic calcification and ossification of muscle, left shoulder
  - M61.219 Paralytic calcification and ossification of muscle, unspecified shoulder
- M61.22 Paralytic calcification and ossification of muscle, upper arm
  - M61.221 Paralytic calcification and ossification of muscle, right upper arm
  - M61.222 Paralytic calcification and ossification of muscle, left upper arm
  - M61.229 Paralytic calcification and ossification of muscle, unspecified upper arm
- M61.23 Paralytic calcification and ossification of muscle, forearm
  - M61.231 Paralytic calcification and ossification of muscle, right forearm
  - M61.232 Paralytic calcification and ossification of muscle, left forearm
  - M61.239 Paralytic calcification and ossification of muscle, unspecified forearm
- M61.24 Paralytic calcification and ossification of muscle, hand
  - M61.241 Paralytic calcification and ossification of muscle, right hand
  - M61.242 Paralytic calcification and ossification of muscle, left hand
  - M61.249 Paralytic calcification and ossification of muscle, unspecified hand
- M61.25 Paralytic calcification and ossification of muscle, thigh
  - M61.251 Paralytic calcification and ossification of muscle, right thigh
  - M61.252 Paralytic calcification and ossification of muscle, left thigh
  - M61.259 Paralytic calcification and ossification of muscle, unspecified thigh
- M61.26 Paralytic calcification and ossification of muscle, lower leg
  - M61.261 Paralytic calcification and ossification of muscle, right lower leg
  - M61.262 Paralytic calcification and ossification of muscle, left lower leg
  - M61.269 Paralytic calcification and ossification of muscle, unspecified lower leg
- M61.27 Paralytic calcification and ossification of muscle, ankle and foot
  - M61.271 Paralytic calcification and ossification of muscle, right ankle and foot
  - M61.272 Paralytic calcification and ossification of muscle, left ankle and foot
  - M61.279 Paralytic calcification and ossification of muscle, unspecified ankle and foot
- M61.28 Paralytic calcification and ossification of muscle, other site
- M61.29 Paralytic calcification and ossification of muscle, multiple sites

M61.3 Calcification and ossification of muscles associated with burns
Myositis ossificans associated with burns
- M61.30 Calcification and ossification of muscles associated with burns, unspecified site
- M61.31 Calcification and ossification of muscles associated with burns, shoulder
  - M61.311 Calcification and ossification of muscles associated with burns, right shoulder
  - M61.312 Calcification and ossification of muscles associated with burns, left shoulder
  - M61.319 Calcification and ossification of muscles associated with burns, unspecified shoulder
- M61.32 Calcification and ossification of muscles associated with burns, upper arm
  - M61.321 Calcification and ossification of muscles associated with burns, right upper arm
  - M61.322 Calcification and ossification of muscles associated with burns, left upper arm
  - M61.329 Calcification and ossification of muscles associated with burns, unspecified upper arm
- M61.33 Calcification and ossification of muscles associated with burns, forearm
  - M61.331 Calcification and ossification of muscles associated with burns, right forearm
  - M61.332 Calcification and ossification of muscles associated with burns, left forearm

M61.339 Calcification and ossification of muscles associated with burns, unspecified forearm

✓6th M61.34 Calcification and ossification of muscles associated with burns, hand

M61.341 Calcification and ossification of muscles associated with burns, right hand

M61.342 Calcification and ossification of muscles associated with burns, left hand

M61.349 Calcification and ossification of muscles associated with burns, unspecified hand

✓6th M61.35 Calcification and ossification of muscles associated with burns, thigh

M61.351 Calcification and ossification of muscles associated with burns, right thigh

M61.352 Calcification and ossification of muscles associated with burns, left thigh

M61.359 Calcification and ossification of muscles associated with burns, unspecified thigh

✓6th M61.36 Calcification and ossification of muscles associated with burns, lower leg

M61.361 Calcification and ossification of muscles associated with burns, right lower leg

M61.362 Calcification and ossification of muscles associated with burns, left lower leg

M61.369 Calcification and ossification of muscles associated with burns, unspecified lower leg

✓6th M61.37 Calcification and ossification of muscles associated with burns, ankle and foot

M61.371 Calcification and ossification of muscles associated with burns, right ankle and foot

M61.372 Calcification and ossification of muscles associated with burns, left ankle and foot

M61.379 Calcification and ossification of muscles associated with burns, unspecified ankle and foot

M61.38 Calcification and ossification of muscles associated with burns, other site

M61.39 Calcification and ossification of muscles associated with burns, multiple sites

✓5th M61.4 Other calcification of muscle

EXCLUDES 1 *calcific tendinitis NOS (M65.2-)*
calcific tendinitis of shoulder (M75.3)

M61.4Ø Other calcification of muscle, unspecified site

✓6th M61.41 Other calcification of muscle, shoulder

M61.411 Other calcification of muscle, right shoulder

M61.412 Other calcification of muscle, left shoulder

M61.419 Other calcification of muscle, unspecified shoulder

✓6th M61.42 Other calcification of muscle, upper arm

M61.421 Other calcification of muscle, right upper arm

M61.422 Other calcification of muscle, left upper arm

M61.429 Other calcification of muscle, unspecified upper arm

✓6th M61.43 Other calcification of muscle, forearm

M61.431 Other calcification of muscle, right forearm

M61.432 Other calcification of muscle, left forearm

M61.439 Other calcification of muscle, unspecified forearm

✓6th M61.44 Other calcification of muscle, hand

M61.441 Other calcification of muscle, right hand

M61.442 Other calcification of muscle, left hand

M61.449 Other calcification of muscle, unspecified hand

✓6th M61.45 Other calcification of muscle, thigh

M61.451 Other calcification of muscle, right thigh

M61.452 Other calcification of muscle, left thigh

M61.459 Other calcification of muscle, unspecified thigh

✓6th M61.46 Other calcification of muscle, lower leg

M61.461 Other calcification of muscle, right lower leg

M61.462 Other calcification of muscle, left lower leg

M61.469 Other calcification of muscle, unspecified lower leg

✓6th M61.47 Other calcification of muscle, ankle and foot

M61.471 Other calcification of muscle, right ankle and foot

M61.472 Other calcification of muscle, left ankle and foot

M61.479 Other calcification of muscle, unspecified ankle and foot

M61.48 Other calcification of muscle, other site

M61.49 Other calcification of muscle, multiple sites

✓5th M61.5 Other ossification of muscle

M61.5Ø Other ossification of muscle, unspecified site

✓6th M61.51 Other ossification of muscle, shoulder

M61.511 Other ossification of muscle, right shoulder

M61.512 Other ossification of muscle, left shoulder

M61.519 Other ossification of muscle, unspecified shoulder

✓6th M61.52 Other ossification of muscle, upper arm

M61.521 Other ossification of muscle, right upper arm

M61.522 Other ossification of muscle, left upper arm

M61.529 Other ossification of muscle, unspecified upper arm

✓6th M61.53 Other ossification of muscle, forearm

M61.531 Other ossification of muscle, right forearm

M61.532 Other ossification of muscle, left forearm

M61.539 Other ossification of muscle, unspecified forearm

✓6th M61.54 Other ossification of muscle, hand

M61.541 Other ossification of muscle, right hand

M61.542 Other ossification of muscle, left hand

M61.549 Other ossification of muscle, unspecified hand

✓6th M61.55 Other ossification of muscle, thigh

M61.551 Other ossification of muscle, right thigh

M61.552 Other ossification of muscle, left thigh

M61.559 Other ossification of muscle, unspecified thigh

✓6th M61.56 Other ossification of muscle, lower leg

M61.561 Other ossification of muscle, right lower leg

M61.562 Other ossification of muscle, left lower leg

M61.569 Other ossification of muscle, unspecified lower leg

✓6th M61.57 Other ossification of muscle, ankle and foot

M61.571 Other ossification of muscle, right ankle and foot

M61.572 Other ossification of muscle, left ankle and foot

M61.579 Other ossification of muscle, unspecified ankle and foot

M61.58 Other ossification of muscle, other site

M61.59 Other ossification of muscle, multiple sites

M61.9 Calcification and ossification of muscle, unspecified

✓4th M62 Other disorders of muscle

EXCLUDES 1 *alcoholic myopathy (G72.1)*
cramp and spasm (R25.2)
drug-induced myopathy (G72.Ø)
myalgia (M79.1-)
stiff-man syndrome (G25.82)

EXCLUDES 2 *nontraumatic hematoma of muscle (M79.81)*

✓5th M62.Ø Separation of muscle (nontraumatic)

Diastasis of muscle

EXCLUDES 1 *diastasis recti complicating pregnancy, labor and delivery (O71.8)*
traumatic separation of muscle — see strain of muscle by body region

M62.ØØ Separation of muscle (nontraumatic), unspecified site

✓6th M62.Ø1 Separation of muscle (nontraumatic), shoulder

M62.Ø11 Separation of muscle (nontraumatic), right shoulder

M62.Ø12 Separation of muscle (nontraumatic), left shoulder
M62.Ø19 Separation of muscle (nontraumatic), unspecified shoulder

✓6th M62.Ø2 Separation of muscle (nontraumatic), upper arm
M62.Ø21 Separation of muscle (nontraumatic), right upper arm
M62.Ø22 Separation of muscle (nontraumatic), left upper arm
M62.Ø29 Separation of muscle (nontraumatic), unspecified upper arm

✓6th M62.Ø3 Separation of muscle (nontraumatic), forearm
M62.Ø31 Separation of muscle (nontraumatic), right forearm
M62.Ø32 Separation of muscle (nontraumatic), left forearm
M62.Ø39 Separation of muscle (nontraumatic), unspecified forearm

✓6th M62.Ø4 Separation of muscle (nontraumatic), hand
M62.Ø41 Separation of muscle (nontraumatic), right hand
M62.Ø42 Separation of muscle (nontraumatic), left hand
M62.Ø49 Separation of muscle (nontraumatic), unspecified hand

✓6th M62.Ø5 Separation of muscle (nontraumatic), thigh
M62.Ø51 Separation of muscle (nontraumatic), right thigh
M62.Ø52 Separation of muscle (nontraumatic), left thigh
M62.Ø59 Separation of muscle (nontraumatic), unspecified thigh

✓6th M62.Ø6 Separation of muscle (nontraumatic), lower leg
M62.Ø61 Separation of muscle (nontraumatic), right lower leg
M62.Ø62 Separation of muscle (nontraumatic), left lower leg
M62.Ø69 Separation of muscle (nontraumatic), unspecified lower leg

✓6th M62.Ø7 Separation of muscle (nontraumatic), ankle and foot
M62.Ø71 Separation of muscle (nontraumatic), right ankle and foot
M62.Ø72 Separation of muscle (nontraumatic), left ankle and foot
M62.Ø79 Separation of muscle (nontraumatic), unspecified ankle and foot

M62.Ø8 Separation of muscle (nontraumatic), other site

✓5th M62.1 Other rupture of muscle (nontraumatic)

EXCLUDES 1 *traumatic rupture of muscle — see strain of muscle by body region*
EXCLUDES 2 *rupture of tendon (M66.-)*

M62.1Ø Other rupture of muscle (nontraumatic), unspecified site

✓6th M62.11 Other rupture of muscle (nontraumatic), shoulder
M62.111 Other rupture of muscle (nontraumatic), right shoulder
M62.112 Other rupture of muscle (nontraumatic), left shoulder
M62.119 Other rupture of muscle (nontraumatic), unspecified shoulder

✓6th M62.12 Other rupture of muscle (nontraumatic), upper arm
M62.121 Other rupture of muscle (nontraumatic), right upper arm
M62.122 Other rupture of muscle (nontraumatic), left upper arm
M62.129 Other rupture of muscle (nontraumatic), unspecified upper arm

✓6th M62.13 Other rupture of muscle (nontraumatic), forearm
M62.131 Other rupture of muscle (nontraumatic), right forearm
M62.132 Other rupture of muscle (nontraumatic), left forearm
M62.139 Other rupture of muscle (nontraumatic), unspecified forearm

✓6th M62.14 Other rupture of muscle (nontraumatic), hand
M62.141 Other rupture of muscle (nontraumatic), right hand
M62.142 Other rupture of muscle (nontraumatic), left hand
M62.149 Other rupture of muscle (nontraumatic), unspecified hand

✓6th M62.15 Other rupture of muscle (nontraumatic), thigh
M62.151 Other rupture of muscle (nontraumatic), right thigh
M62.152 Other rupture of muscle (nontraumatic), left thigh
M62.159 Other rupture of muscle (nontraumatic), unspecified thigh

✓6th M62.16 Other rupture of muscle (nontraumatic), lower leg
M62.161 Other rupture of muscle (nontraumatic), right lower leg
M62.162 Other rupture of muscle (nontraumatic), left lower leg
M62.169 Other rupture of muscle (nontraumatic), unspecified lower leg

✓6th M62.17 Other rupture of muscle (nontraumatic), ankle and foot
M62.171 Other rupture of muscle (nontraumatic), right ankle and foot
M62.172 Other rupture of muscle (nontraumatic), left ankle and foot
M62.179 Other rupture of muscle (nontraumatic), unspecified ankle and foot

M62.18 Other rupture of muscle (nontraumatic), other site

✓5th M62.2 Nontraumatic ischemic infarction of muscle

EXCLUDES 1 *compartment syndrome (traumatic) (T79.A-)*
nontraumatic compartment syndrome (M79.A-)
rhabdomyolysis (M62.82)
traumatic ischemia of muscle (T79.6)
Volkmann's ischemic contracture (T79.6)

M62.2Ø Nontraumatic ischemic infarction of muscle, unspecified site

✓6th M62.21 Nontraumatic ischemic infarction of muscle, shoulder
M62.211 Nontraumatic ischemic infarction of muscle, right shoulder
M62.212 Nontraumatic ischemic infarction of muscle, left shoulder
M62.219 Nontraumatic ischemic infarction of muscle, unspecified shoulder

✓6th M62.22 Nontraumatic ischemic infarction of muscle, upper arm
M62.221 Nontraumatic ischemic infarction of muscle, right upper arm
M62.222 Nontraumatic ischemic infarction of muscle, left upper arm
M62.229 Nontraumatic ischemic infarction of muscle, unspecified upper arm

✓6th M62.23 Nontraumatic ischemic infarction of muscle, forearm
M62.231 Nontraumatic ischemic infarction of muscle, right forearm
M62.232 Nontraumatic ischemic infarction of muscle, left forearm
M62.239 Nontraumatic ischemic infarction of muscle, unspecified forearm

✓6th M62.24 Nontraumatic ischemic infarction of muscle, hand
M62.241 Nontraumatic ischemic infarction of muscle, right hand
M62.242 Nontraumatic ischemic infarction of muscle, left hand
M62.249 Nontraumatic ischemic infarction of muscle, unspecified hand

✓6th M62.25 Nontraumatic ischemic infarction of muscle, thigh
M62.251 Nontraumatic ischemic infarction of muscle, right thigh
M62.252 Nontraumatic ischemic infarction of muscle, left thigh
M62.259 Nontraumatic ischemic infarction of muscle, unspecified thigh

✓6th M62.26 Nontraumatic ischemic infarction of muscle, lower leg
M62.261 Nontraumatic ischemic infarction of muscle, right lower leg
M62.262 Nontraumatic ischemic infarction of muscle, left lower leg
M62.269 Nontraumatic ischemic infarction of muscle, unspecified lower leg

√6th **M62.27 Nontraumatic ischemic infarction of muscle, ankle and foot**
- **M62.271 Nontraumatic ischemic infarction of muscle, right ankle and foot**
- **M62.272 Nontraumatic ischemic infarction of muscle, left ankle and foot**
- **M62.279 Nontraumatic ischemic infarction of muscle, unspecified ankle and foot**

M62.28 Nontraumatic ischemic infarction of muscle, other site

M62.3 Immobility syndrome (paraplegic)

√5th **M62.4 Contracture of muscle**

Contracture of tendon (sheath)

EXCLUDES 1 *contracture of joint (M24.5-)*

M62.40 Contracture of muscle, unspecified site

√6th **M62.41 Contracture of muscle, shoulder**
- **M62.411 Contracture of muscle, right shoulder**
- **M62.412 Contracture of muscle, left shoulder**
- **M62.419 Contracture of muscle, unspecified shoulder**

√6th **M62.42 Contracture of muscle, upper arm**
- **M62.421 Contracture of muscle, right upper arm**
- **M62.422 Contracture of muscle, left upper arm**
- **M62.429 Contracture of muscle, unspecified upper arm**

√6th **M62.43 Contracture of muscle, forearm**
- **M62.431 Contracture of muscle, right forearm**
- **M62.432 Contracture of muscle, left forearm**
- **M62.439 Contracture of muscle, unspecified forearm**

√6th **M62.44 Contracture of muscle, hand**
- **M62.441 Contracture of muscle, right hand**
- **M62.442 Contracture of muscle, left hand**
- **M62.449 Contracture of muscle, unspecified hand**

√6th **M62.45 Contracture of muscle, thigh**
- **M62.451 Contracture of muscle, right thigh**
- **M62.452 Contracture of muscle, left thigh**
- **M62.459 Contracture of muscle, unspecified thigh**

√6th **M62.46 Contracture of muscle, lower leg**
- **M62.461 Contracture of muscle, right lower leg**
- **M62.462 Contracture of muscle, left lower leg**
- **M62.469 Contracture of muscle, unspecified lower leg**

√6th **M62.47 Contracture of muscle, ankle and foot**
- **M62.471 Contracture of muscle, right ankle and foot**
- **M62.472 Contracture of muscle, left ankle and foot**
- **M62.479 Contracture of muscle, unspecified ankle and foot**

M62.48 Contracture of muscle, other site

M62.49 Contracture of muscle, multiple sites

√5th **M62.5 Muscle wasting and atrophy, not elsewhere classified**

Disuse atrophy NEC

EXCLUDES 1 *neuralgic amyotrophy (G54.5)*
progressive muscular atrophy (G12.21)
sarcopenia (M62.84)

EXCLUDES 2 *pelvic muscle wasting (N81.84)*

M62.50 Muscle wasting and atrophy, not elsewhere classified, unspecified site

√6th **M62.51 Muscle wasting and atrophy, not elsewhere classified, shoulder**
- **M62.511 Muscle wasting and atrophy, not elsewhere classified, right shoulder**
- **M62.512 Muscle wasting and atrophy, not elsewhere classified, left shoulder**
- **M62.519 Muscle wasting and atrophy, not elsewhere classified, unspecified shoulder**

√6th **M62.52 Muscle wasting and atrophy, not elsewhere classified, upper arm**
- **M62.521 Muscle wasting and atrophy, not elsewhere classified, right upper arm**
- **M62.522 Muscle wasting and atrophy, not elsewhere classified, left upper arm**
- **M62.529 Muscle wasting and atrophy, not elsewhere classified, unspecified upper arm**

√6th **M62.53 Muscle wasting and atrophy, not elsewhere classified, forearm**
- **M62.531 Muscle wasting and atrophy, not elsewhere classified, right forearm**
- **M62.532 Muscle wasting and atrophy, not elsewhere classified, left forearm**
- **M62.539 Muscle wasting and atrophy, not elsewhere classified, unspecified forearm**

√6th **M62.54 Muscle wasting and atrophy, not elsewhere classified, hand**
- **M62.541 Muscle wasting and atrophy, not elsewhere classified, right hand**
- **M62.542 Muscle wasting and atrophy, not elsewhere classified, left hand**
- **M62.549 Muscle wasting and atrophy, not elsewhere classified, unspecified hand**

√6th **M62.55 Muscle wasting and atrophy, not elsewhere classified, thigh**
- **M62.551 Muscle wasting and atrophy, not elsewhere classified, right thigh**
- **M62.552 Muscle wasting and atrophy, not elsewhere classified, left thigh**
- **M62.559 Muscle wasting and atrophy, not elsewhere classified, unspecified thigh**

√6th **M62.56 Muscle wasting and atrophy, not elsewhere classified, lower leg**
- **M62.561 Muscle wasting and atrophy, not elsewhere classified, right lower leg**
- **M62.562 Muscle wasting and atrophy, not elsewhere classified, left lower leg**
- **M62.569 Muscle wasting and atrophy, not elsewhere classified, unspecified lower leg**

√6th **M62.57 Muscle wasting and atrophy, not elsewhere classified, ankle and foot**
- **M62.571 Muscle wasting and atrophy, not elsewhere classified, right ankle and foot**
- **M62.572 Muscle wasting and atrophy, not elsewhere classified, left ankle and foot**
- **M62.579 Muscle wasting and atrophy, not elsewhere classified, unspecified ankle and foot**

M62.58 Muscle wasting and atrophy, not elsewhere classified, other site

M62.59 Muscle wasting and atrophy, not elsewhere classified, multiple sites

√5th **M62.8 Other specified disorders of muscle**

EXCLUDES 2 *nontraumatic hematoma of muscle (M79.81)*

M62.81 Muscle weakness (generalized)

EXCLUDES 1 *muscle weakness in sarcopenia (M62.84)*

M62.82 Rhabdomyolysis CC

EXCLUDES 1 *traumatic rhabdomyolysis (T79.6)*

AHA: 2019,2Q,12

DEF: Rapid disintegration or destruction of skeletal muscle caused by direct or indirect injury, resulting in the excretion of muscle protein myoglobin into the urine.

√6th **M62.83 Muscle spasm**
- **M62.830 Muscle spasm of back**
- **M62.831 Muscle spasm of calf**
  Charley-horse
- **M62.838 Other muscle spasm**

M62.84 Sarcopenia

Age-related sarcopenia

Code first underlying disease, if applicable, such as:
- disorders of myoneural junction and muscle disease in diseases classified elsewhere (G73.-)
- other and unspecified myopathies (G72.-)
- primary disorders of muscles (G71.-)

AHA: 2016,4Q,41

M62.89 Other specified disorders of muscle

Muscle (sheath) hernia

M62.9 Disorder of muscle, unspecified

M63 Disorders of muscle in diseases classified elsewhere

Code first underlying disease, such as:
leprosy (A3Ø.-)
neoplasm (C49.-, C79.89, D21.-, D48.1)
schistosomiasis (B65.-)
trichinellosis (B75)

EXCLUDES 1 *myopathy in cysticercosis (B69.81)*
myopathy in endocrine diseases (G73.7)
myopathy in metabolic diseases (G73.7)
myopathy in sarcoidosis (D86.87)
myopathy in secondary syphilis (A51.49)
myopathy in syphilis (late) (A52.78)
myopathy in toxoplasmosis (B58.82)
myopathy in tuberculosis (A18.Ø9)

M63.8 Disorders of muscle in diseases classified elsewhere

M63.8Ø Disorders of muscle in diseases classified elsewhere, unspecified site

M63.81 Disorders of muscle in diseases classified elsewhere, shoulder

M63.811 Disorders of muscle in diseases classified elsewhere, right shoulder
M63.812 Disorders of muscle in diseases classified elsewhere, left shoulder
M63.819 Disorders of muscle in diseases classified elsewhere, unspecified shoulder

M63.82 Disorders of muscle in diseases classified elsewhere, upper arm

M63.821 Disorders of muscle in diseases classified elsewhere, right upper arm
M63.822 Disorders of muscle in diseases classified elsewhere, left upper arm
M63.829 Disorders of muscle in diseases classified elsewhere, unspecified upper arm

M63.83 Disorders of muscle in diseases classified elsewhere, forearm

M63.831 Disorders of muscle in diseases classified elsewhere, right forearm
M63.832 Disorders of muscle in diseases classified elsewhere, left forearm
M63.839 Disorders of muscle in diseases classified elsewhere, unspecified forearm

M63.84 Disorders of muscle in diseases classified elsewhere, hand

M63.841 Disorders of muscle in diseases classified elsewhere, right hand
M63.842 Disorders of muscle in diseases classified elsewhere, left hand
M63.849 Disorders of muscle in diseases classified elsewhere, unspecified hand

M63.85 Disorders of muscle in diseases classified elsewhere, thigh

M63.851 Disorders of muscle in diseases classified elsewhere, right thigh
M63.852 Disorders of muscle in diseases classified elsewhere, left thigh
M63.859 Disorders of muscle in diseases classified elsewhere, unspecified thigh

M63.86 Disorders of muscle in diseases classified elsewhere, lower leg

M63.861 Disorders of muscle in diseases classified elsewhere, right lower leg
M63.862 Disorders of muscle in diseases classified elsewhere, left lower leg
M63.869 Disorders of muscle in diseases classified elsewhere, unspecified lower leg

M63.87 Disorders of muscle in diseases classified elsewhere, ankle and foot

M63.871 Disorders of muscle in diseases classified elsewhere, right ankle and foot
M63.872 Disorders of muscle in diseases classified elsewhere, left ankle and foot
M63.879 Disorders of muscle in diseases classified elsewhere, unspecified ankle and foot

M63.88 Disorders of muscle in diseases classified elsewhere, other site
M63.89 Disorders of muscle in diseases classified elsewhere, multiple sites

Disorders of synovium and tendon (M65-M67)

M65 Synovitis and tenosynovitis

EXCLUDES 1 *chronic crepitant synovitis of hand and wrist (M7Ø.Ø-)*
current injury — see injury of ligament or tendon by body region
soft tissue disorders related to use, overuse and pressure (M7Ø.-)

M65.Ø Abscess of tendon sheath

Use additional code (B95-B96) to identify bacterial agent.

M65.ØØ Abscess of tendon sheath, unspecified site

M65.Ø1 Abscess of tendon sheath, shoulder

M65.Ø11 Abscess of tendon sheath, right shoulder
M65.Ø12 Abscess of tendon sheath, left shoulder
M65.Ø19 Abscess of tendon sheath, unspecified shoulder

M65.Ø2 Abscess of tendon sheath, upper arm

M65.Ø21 Abscess of tendon sheath, right upper arm
M65.Ø22 Abscess of tendon sheath, left upper arm
M65.Ø29 Abscess of tendon sheath, unspecified upper arm

M65.Ø3 Abscess of tendon sheath, forearm

M65.Ø31 Abscess of tendon sheath, right forearm
M65.Ø32 Abscess of tendon sheath, left forearm
M65.Ø39 Abscess of tendon sheath, unspecified forearm

M65.Ø4 Abscess of tendon sheath, hand

M65.Ø41 Abscess of tendon sheath, right hand
M65.Ø42 Abscess of tendon sheath, left hand
M65.Ø49 Abscess of tendon sheath, unspecified hand

M65.Ø5 Abscess of tendon sheath, thigh

M65.Ø51 Abscess of tendon sheath, right thigh
M65.Ø52 Abscess of tendon sheath, left thigh
M65.Ø59 Abscess of tendon sheath, unspecified thigh

M65.Ø6 Abscess of tendon sheath, lower leg

M65.Ø61 Abscess of tendon sheath, right lower leg
M65.Ø62 Abscess of tendon sheath, left lower leg
M65.Ø69 Abscess of tendon sheath, unspecified lower leg

M65.Ø7 Abscess of tendon sheath, ankle and foot

M65.Ø71 Abscess of tendon sheath, right ankle and foot
M65.Ø72 Abscess of tendon sheath, left ankle and foot
M65.Ø79 Abscess of tendon sheath, unspecified ankle and foot

M65.Ø8 Abscess of tendon sheath, other site

M65.1 Other infective (teno)synovitis

M65.1Ø Other infective (teno)synovitis, unspecified site

M65.11 Other infective (teno)synovitis, shoulder

M65.111 Other infective (teno)synovitis, right shoulder
M65.112 Other infective (teno)synovitis, left shoulder
M65.119 Other infective (teno)synovitis, unspecified shoulder

M65.12 Other infective (teno)synovitis, elbow

M65.121 Other infective (teno)synovitis, right elbow
M65.122 Other infective (teno)synovitis, left elbow
M65.129 Other infective (teno)synovitis, unspecified elbow

M65.13 Other infective (teno)synovitis, wrist

M65.131 Other infective (teno)synovitis, right wrist
M65.132 Other infective (teno)synovitis, left wrist
M65.139 Other infective (teno)synovitis, unspecified wrist

M65.14 Other infective (teno)synovitis, hand

M65.141 Other infective (teno)synovitis, right hand
M65.142 Other infective (teno)synovitis, left hand
M65.149 Other infective (teno)synovitis, unspecified hand

✓6th **M65.15 Other infective (teno)synovitis, hip**
- **M65.151 Other infective (teno)synovitis, right hip**
- **M65.152 Other infective (teno)synovitis, left hip**
- **M65.159 Other infective (teno)synovitis, unspecified hip**

✓6th **M65.16 Other infective (teno)synovitis, knee**
- **M65.161 Other infective (teno)synovitis, right knee**
- **M65.162 Other infective (teno)synovitis, left knee**
- **M65.169 Other infective (teno)synovitis, unspecified knee**

✓6th **M65.17 Other infective (teno)synovitis, ankle and foot**
- **M65.171 Other infective (teno)synovitis, right ankle and foot**
- **M65.172 Other infective (teno)synovitis, left ankle and foot**
- **M65.179 Other infective (teno)synovitis, unspecified ankle and foot**

M65.18 Other infective (teno)synovitis, other site

M65.19 Other infective (teno)synovitis, multiple sites

✓5th **M65.2 Calcific tendinitis**

EXCLUDES 1 *tendinitis as classified in M75-M77*
calcified tendinitis of shoulder (M75.3)

M65.20 Calcific tendinitis, unspecified site

✓6th **M65.22 Calcific tendinitis, upper arm**
- **M65.221 Calcific tendinitis, right upper arm**
- **M65.222 Calcific tendinitis, left upper arm**
- **M65.229 Calcific tendinitis, unspecified upper arm**

✓6th **M65.23 Calcific tendinitis, forearm**
- **M65.231 Calcific tendinitis, right forearm**
- **M65.232 Calcific tendinitis, left forearm**
- **M65.239 Calcific tendinitis, unspecified forearm**

✓6th **M65.24 Calcific tendinitis, hand**
- **M65.241 Calcific tendinitis, right hand**
- **M65.242 Calcific tendinitis, left hand**
- **M65.249 Calcific tendinitis, unspecified hand**

✓6th **M65.25 Calcific tendinitis, thigh**
- **M65.251 Calcific tendinitis, right thigh**
- **M65.252 Calcific tendinitis, left thigh**
- **M65.259 Calcific tendinitis, unspecified thigh**

✓6th **M65.26 Calcific tendinitis, lower leg**
- **M65.261 Calcific tendinitis, right lower leg**
- **M65.262 Calcific tendinitis, left lower leg**
- **M65.269 Calcific tendinitis, unspecified lower leg**

✓6th **M65.27 Calcific tendinitis, ankle and foot**
- **M65.271 Calcific tendinitis, right ankle and foot**
- **M65.272 Calcific tendinitis, left ankle and foot**
- **M65.279 Calcific tendinitis, unspecified ankle and foot**

M65.28 Calcific tendinitis, other site

M65.29 Calcific tendinitis, multiple sites

✓5th **M65.3 Trigger finger**

Nodular tendinous disease

M65.30 Trigger finger, unspecified finger

✓6th **M65.31 Trigger thumb**
- **M65.311 Trigger thumb, right thumb**
- **M65.312 Trigger thumb, left thumb**
- **M65.319 Trigger thumb, unspecified thumb**

✓6th **M65.32 Trigger finger, index finger**
- **M65.321 Trigger finger, right index finger**
- **M65.322 Trigger finger, left index finger**
- **M65.329 Trigger finger, unspecified index finger**

✓6th **M65.33 Trigger finger, middle finger**
- **M65.331 Trigger finger, right middle finger**
- **M65.332 Trigger finger, left middle finger**
- **M65.339 Trigger finger, unspecified middle finger**

✓6th **M65.34 Trigger finger, ring finger**
- **M65.341 Trigger finger, right ring finger**
- **M65.342 Trigger finger, left ring finger**
- **M65.349 Trigger finger, unspecified ring finger**

✓6th **M65.35 Trigger finger, little finger**
- **M65.351 Trigger finger, right little finger**
- **M65.352 Trigger finger, left little finger**
- **M65.359 Trigger finger, unspecified little finger**

M65.4 Radial styloid tenosynovitis [de Quervain]

✓5th **M65.8 Other synovitis and tenosynovitis**

M65.80 Other synovitis and tenosynovitis, unspecified site

✓6th **M65.81 Other synovitis and tenosynovitis, shoulder**
- **M65.811 Other synovitis and tenosynovitis, right shoulder**
- **M65.812 Other synovitis and tenosynovitis, left shoulder**
- **M65.819 Other synovitis and tenosynovitis, unspecified shoulder**

✓6th **M65.82 Other synovitis and tenosynovitis, upper arm**
- **M65.821 Other synovitis and tenosynovitis, right upper arm**
- **M65.822 Other synovitis and tenosynovitis, left upper arm**
- **M65.829 Other synovitis and tenosynovitis, unspecified upper arm**

✓6th **M65.83 Other synovitis and tenosynovitis, forearm**
- **M65.831 Other synovitis and tenosynovitis, right forearm**
- **M65.832 Other synovitis and tenosynovitis, left forearm**
- **M65.839 Other synovitis and tenosynovitis, unspecified forearm**

✓6th **M65.84 Other synovitis and tenosynovitis, hand**
- **M65.841 Other synovitis and tenosynovitis, right hand**
- **M65.842 Other synovitis and tenosynovitis, left hand**
- **M65.849 Other synovitis and tenosynovitis, unspecified hand**

✓6th **M65.85 Other synovitis and tenosynovitis, thigh**
- **M65.851 Other synovitis and tenosynovitis, right thigh**
- **M65.852 Other synovitis and tenosynovitis, left thigh**
- **M65.859 Other synovitis and tenosynovitis, unspecified thigh**

✓6th **M65.86 Other synovitis and tenosynovitis, lower leg**
- **M65.861 Other synovitis and tenosynovitis, right lower leg**
- **M65.862 Other synovitis and tenosynovitis, left lower leg**
- **M65.869 Other synovitis and tenosynovitis, unspecified lower leg**

✓6th **M65.87 Other synovitis and tenosynovitis, ankle and foot**
- **M65.871 Other synovitis and tenosynovitis, right ankle and foot**
- **M65.872 Other synovitis and tenosynovitis, left ankle and foot**
- **M65.879 Other synovitis and tenosynovitis, unspecified ankle and foot**

M65.88 Other synovitis and tenosynovitis, other site

M65.89 Other synovitis and tenosynovitis, multiple sites

M65.9 Synovitis and tenosynovitis, unspecified

✓4th **M66 Spontaneous rupture of synovium and tendon**

INCLUDES rupture that occurs when a normal force is applied to tissues that are inferred to have less than normal strength

EXCLUDES 2 *rotator cuff syndrome (M75.1-)*
rupture where an abnormal force is applied to normal tissue — see injury of tendon by body region

M66.0 Rupture of popliteal cyst

✓5th **M66.1 Rupture of synovium**

Rupture of synovial cyst

EXCLUDES 2 *rupture of popliteal cyst (M66.0)*

M66.10 Rupture of synovium, unspecified joint

✓6th **M66.11 Rupture of synovium, shoulder**
- **M66.111 Rupture of synovium, right shoulder**
- **M66.112 Rupture of synovium, left shoulder**
- **M66.119 Rupture of synovium, unspecified shoulder**

✓6th **M66.12 Rupture of synovium, elbow**
- **M66.121 Rupture of synovium, right elbow**
- **M66.122 Rupture of synovium, left elbow**
- **M66.129 Rupture of synovium, unspecified elbow**

✓6th **M66.13 Rupture of synovium, wrist**
- **M66.131 Rupture of synovium, right wrist**
- **M66.132 Rupture of synovium, left wrist**

M66.139 Rupture of synovium, unspecified wrist

M66.14 Rupture of synovium, hand and fingers
- M66.141 Rupture of synovium, right hand
- M66.142 Rupture of synovium, left hand
- M66.143 Rupture of synovium, unspecified hand
- M66.144 Rupture of synovium, right finger(s)
- M66.145 Rupture of synovium, left finger(s)
- M66.146 Rupture of synovium, unspecified finger(s)

M66.15 Rupture of synovium, hip
- M66.151 Rupture of synovium, right hip
- M66.152 Rupture of synovium, left hip
- M66.159 Rupture of synovium, unspecified hip

M66.17 Rupture of synovium, ankle, foot and toes
- M66.171 Rupture of synovium, right ankle
- M66.172 Rupture of synovium, left ankle
- M66.173 Rupture of synovium, unspecified ankle
- M66.174 Rupture of synovium, right foot
- M66.175 Rupture of synovium, left foot
- M66.176 Rupture of synovium, unspecified foot
- M66.177 Rupture of synovium, right toe(s)
- M66.178 Rupture of synovium, left toe(s)
- M66.179 Rupture of synovium, unspecified toe(s)

M66.18 Rupture of synovium, other site

M66.2 Spontaneous rupture of extensor tendons

TIP: Refer to the Muscle/Tendon table at the beginning of this chapter.

M66.20 Spontaneous rupture of extensor tendons, unspecified site

M66.21 Spontaneous rupture of extensor tendons, shoulder
- M66.211 Spontaneous rupture of extensor tendons, right shoulder
- M66.212 Spontaneous rupture of extensor tendons, left shoulder
- M66.219 Spontaneous rupture of extensor tendons, unspecified shoulder

M66.22 Spontaneous rupture of extensor tendons, upper arm
- M66.221 Spontaneous rupture of extensor tendons, right upper arm
- M66.222 Spontaneous rupture of extensor tendons, left upper arm
- M66.229 Spontaneous rupture of extensor tendons, unspecified upper arm

M66.23 Spontaneous rupture of extensor tendons, forearm
- M66.231 Spontaneous rupture of extensor tendons, right forearm
- M66.232 Spontaneous rupture of extensor tendons, left forearm
- M66.239 Spontaneous rupture of extensor tendons, unspecified forearm

M66.24 Spontaneous rupture of extensor tendons, hand
- M66.241 Spontaneous rupture of extensor tendons, right hand
- M66.242 Spontaneous rupture of extensor tendons, left hand
- M66.249 Spontaneous rupture of extensor tendons, unspecified hand

M66.25 Spontaneous rupture of extensor tendons, thigh
- M66.251 Spontaneous rupture of extensor tendons, right thigh
- M66.252 Spontaneous rupture of extensor tendons, left thigh
- M66.259 Spontaneous rupture of extensor tendons, unspecified thigh

M66.26 Spontaneous rupture of extensor tendons, lower leg
- M66.261 Spontaneous rupture of extensor tendons, right lower leg
- M66.262 Spontaneous rupture of extensor tendons, left lower leg
- M66.269 Spontaneous rupture of extensor tendons, unspecified lower leg

M66.27 Spontaneous rupture of extensor tendons, ankle and foot
- M66.271 Spontaneous rupture of extensor tendons, right ankle and foot
- M66.272 Spontaneous rupture of extensor tendons, left ankle and foot
- M66.279 Spontaneous rupture of extensor tendons, unspecified ankle and foot

M66.28 Spontaneous rupture of extensor tendons, other site

M66.29 Spontaneous rupture of extensor tendons, multiple sites

M66.3 Spontaneous rupture of flexor tendons

TIP: Refer to the Muscle/Tendon table at the beginning of this chapter.

M66.30 Spontaneous rupture of flexor tendons, unspecified site

M66.31 Spontaneous rupture of flexor tendons, shoulder
- M66.311 Spontaneous rupture of flexor tendons, right shoulder
- M66.312 Spontaneous rupture of flexor tendons, left shoulder
- M66.319 Spontaneous rupture of flexor tendons, unspecified shoulder

M66.32 Spontaneous rupture of flexor tendons, upper arm
- M66.321 Spontaneous rupture of flexor tendons, right upper arm
- M66.322 Spontaneous rupture of flexor tendons, left upper arm
- M66.329 Spontaneous rupture of flexor tendons, unspecified upper arm

M66.33 Spontaneous rupture of flexor tendons, forearm
- M66.331 Spontaneous rupture of flexor tendons, right forearm
- M66.332 Spontaneous rupture of flexor tendons, left forearm
- M66.339 Spontaneous rupture of flexor tendons, unspecified forearm

M66.34 Spontaneous rupture of flexor tendons, hand
- M66.341 Spontaneous rupture of flexor tendons, right hand
- M66.342 Spontaneous rupture of flexor tendons, left hand
- M66.349 Spontaneous rupture of flexor tendons, unspecified hand

M66.35 Spontaneous rupture of flexor tendons, thigh
- M66.351 Spontaneous rupture of flexor tendons, right thigh
- M66.352 Spontaneous rupture of flexor tendons, left thigh
- M66.359 Spontaneous rupture of flexor tendons, unspecified thigh

M66.36 Spontaneous rupture of flexor tendons, lower leg
- M66.361 Spontaneous rupture of flexor tendons, right lower leg
- M66.362 Spontaneous rupture of flexor tendons, left lower leg
- M66.369 Spontaneous rupture of flexor tendons, unspecified lower leg

M66.37 Spontaneous rupture of flexor tendons, ankle and foot
- M66.371 Spontaneous rupture of flexor tendons, right ankle and foot
- M66.372 Spontaneous rupture of flexor tendons, left ankle and foot
- M66.379 Spontaneous rupture of flexor tendons, unspecified ankle and foot

M66.38 Spontaneous rupture of flexor tendons, other site

M66.39 Spontaneous rupture of flexor tendons, multiple sites

M66.8 Spontaneous rupture of other tendons

TIP: Refer to the Muscle/Tendon table at the beginning of this chapter.

M66.80 Spontaneous rupture of other tendons, unspecified site

M66.81 Spontaneous rupture of other tendons, shoulder
- M66.811 Spontaneous rupture of other tendons, right shoulder
- M66.812 Spontaneous rupture of other tendons, left shoulder
- M66.819 Spontaneous rupture of other tendons, unspecified shoulder

M66.82 Spontaneous rupture of other tendons, upper arm
- M66.821 Spontaneous rupture of other tendons, right upper arm

M66.822 Spontaneous rupture of other tendons, left upper arm
M66.829 Spontaneous rupture of other tendons, unspecified upper arm
√6th **M66.83** Spontaneous rupture of other tendons, forearm
M66.831 Spontaneous rupture of other tendons, right forearm
M66.832 Spontaneous rupture of other tendons, left forearm
M66.839 Spontaneous rupture of other tendons, unspecified forearm
√6th **M66.84** Spontaneous rupture of other tendons, hand
M66.841 Spontaneous rupture of other tendons, right hand
M66.842 Spontaneous rupture of other tendons, left hand
M66.849 Spontaneous rupture of other tendons, unspecified hand
√6th **M66.85** Spontaneous rupture of other tendons, thigh
M66.851 Spontaneous rupture of other tendons, right thigh
M66.852 Spontaneous rupture of other tendons, left thigh
M66.859 Spontaneous rupture of other tendons, unspecified thigh
√6th **M66.86** Spontaneous rupture of other tendons, lower leg
M66.861 Spontaneous rupture of other tendons, right lower leg
M66.862 Spontaneous rupture of other tendons, left lower leg
M66.869 Spontaneous rupture of other tendons, unspecified lower leg
√6th **M66.87** Spontaneous rupture of other tendons, ankle and foot
M66.871 Spontaneous rupture of other tendons, right ankle and foot
M66.872 Spontaneous rupture of other tendons, left ankle and foot
M66.879 Spontaneous rupture of other tendons, unspecified ankle and foot
M66.88 Spontaneous rupture of other tendons, other sites
M66.89 Spontaneous rupture of other tendons, multiple sites
M66.9 Spontaneous rupture of unspecified tendon
Rupture at musculotendinous junction, nontraumatic

√4th **M67 Other disorders of synovium and tendon**
EXCLUDES 1 *palmar fascial fibromatosis [Dupuytren] (M72.Ø)*
tendinitis NOS (M77.9-)
xanthomatosis localized to tendons (E78.2)

√5th **M67.Ø** Short Achilles tendon (acquired)
M67.ØØ Short Achilles tendon (acquired), unspecified ankle
M67.Ø1 Short Achilles tendon (acquired), right ankle
M67.Ø2 Short Achilles tendon (acquired), left ankle
√5th **M67.2** Synovial hypertrophy, not elsewhere classified
EXCLUDES 1 *villonodular synovitis (pigmented) (M12.2-)*
M67.2Ø Synovial hypertrophy, not elsewhere classified, unspecified site
√6th **M67.21** Synovial hypertrophy, not elsewhere classified, shoulder
M67.211 Synovial hypertrophy, not elsewhere classified, right shoulder
M67.212 Synovial hypertrophy, not elsewhere classified, left shoulder
M67.219 Synovial hypertrophy, not elsewhere classified, unspecified shoulder
√6th **M67.22** Synovial hypertrophy, not elsewhere classified, upper arm
M67.221 Synovial hypertrophy, not elsewhere classified, right upper arm
M67.222 Synovial hypertrophy, not elsewhere classified, left upper arm
M67.229 Synovial hypertrophy, not elsewhere classified, unspecified upper arm
√6th **M67.23** Synovial hypertrophy, not elsewhere classified, forearm
M67.231 Synovial hypertrophy, not elsewhere classified, right forearm
M67.232 Synovial hypertrophy, not elsewhere classified, left forearm
M67.239 Synovial hypertrophy, not elsewhere classified, unspecified forearm
√6th **M67.24** Synovial hypertrophy, not elsewhere classified, hand
M67.241 Synovial hypertrophy, not elsewhere classified, right hand
M67.242 Synovial hypertrophy, not elsewhere classified, left hand
M67.249 Synovial hypertrophy, not elsewhere classified, unspecified hand
√6th **M67.25** Synovial hypertrophy, not elsewhere classified, thigh
M67.251 Synovial hypertrophy, not elsewhere classified, right thigh
M67.252 Synovial hypertrophy, not elsewhere classified, left thigh
M67.259 Synovial hypertrophy, not elsewhere classified, unspecified thigh
√6th **M67.26** Synovial hypertrophy, not elsewhere classified, lower leg
M67.261 Synovial hypertrophy, not elsewhere classified, right lower leg
M67.262 Synovial hypertrophy, not elsewhere classified, left lower leg
M67.269 Synovial hypertrophy, not elsewhere classified, unspecified lower leg
√6th **M67.27** Synovial hypertrophy, not elsewhere classified, ankle and foot
M67.271 Synovial hypertrophy, not elsewhere classified, right ankle and foot
M67.272 Synovial hypertrophy, not elsewhere classified, left ankle and foot
M67.279 Synovial hypertrophy, not elsewhere classified, unspecified ankle and foot
M67.28 Synovial hypertrophy, not elsewhere classified, other site
M67.29 Synovial hypertrophy, not elsewhere classified, multiple sites
√5th **M67.3** Transient synovitis
Toxic synovitis
EXCLUDES 1 *palindromic rheumatism (M12.3-)*
M67.3Ø Transient synovitis, unspecified site
√6th **M67.31** Transient synovitis, shoulder
M67.311 Transient synovitis, right shoulder
M67.312 Transient synovitis, left shoulder
M67.319 Transient synovitis, unspecified shoulder
√6th **M67.32** Transient synovitis, elbow
M67.321 Transient synovitis, right elbow
M67.322 Transient synovitis, left elbow
M67.329 Transient synovitis, unspecified elbow
√6th **M67.33** Transient synovitis, wrist
M67.331 Transient synovitis, right wrist
M67.332 Transient synovitis, left wrist
M67.339 Transient synovitis, unspecified wrist
√6th **M67.34** Transient synovitis, hand
M67.341 Transient synovitis, right hand
M67.342 Transient synovitis, left hand
M67.349 Transient synovitis, unspecified hand
√6th **M67.35** Transient synovitis, hip
M67.351 Transient synovitis, right hip
M67.352 Transient synovitis, left hip
M67.359 Transient synovitis, unspecified hip
√6th **M67.36** Transient synovitis, knee
M67.361 Transient synovitis, right knee
M67.362 Transient synovitis, left knee
M67.369 Transient synovitis, unspecified knee
√6th **M67.37** Transient synovitis, ankle and foot
M67.371 Transient synovitis, right ankle and foot
M67.372 Transient synovitis, left ankle and foot
M67.379 Transient synovitis, unspecified ankle and foot
M67.38 Transient synovitis, other site
M67.39 Transient synovitis, multiple sites

✓5th M67.4 **Ganglion**

Ganglion of joint or tendon (sheath)

EXCLUDES 1 *ganglion in yaws (A66.6)*

EXCLUDES 2 *cyst of bursa (M71.2-M71.3)*

cyst of synovium (M71.2-M71.3)

DEF: Fluid-filled, benign cyst appearing on a tendon sheath or aponeurosis, frequently connecting to an underlying joint.

M67.40 Ganglion, unspecified site

✓6th **M67.41 Ganglion, shoulder**

M67.411 Ganglion, right shoulder

M67.412 Ganglion, left shoulder

M67.419 Ganglion, unspecified shoulder

✓6th **M67.42 Ganglion, elbow**

M67.421 Ganglion, right elbow

M67.422 Ganglion, left elbow

M67.429 Ganglion, unspecified elbow

✓6th **M67.43 Ganglion, wrist**

Ganglion of Wrist

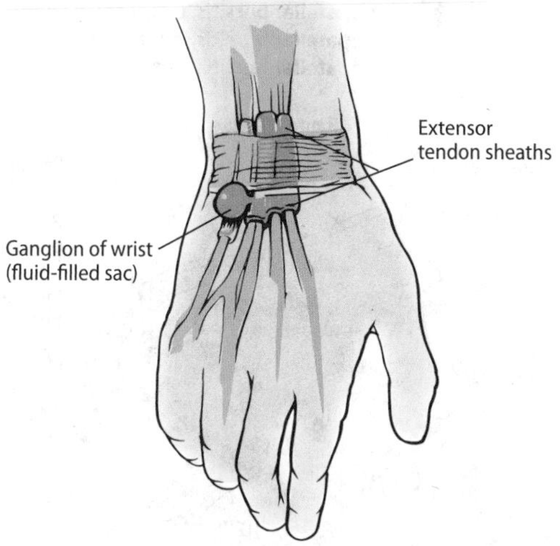

M67.431 Ganglion, right wrist

M67.432 Ganglion, left wrist

M67.439 Ganglion, unspecified wrist

✓6th **M67.44 Ganglion, hand**

M67.441 Ganglion, right hand

M67.442 Ganglion, left hand

M67.449 Ganglion, unspecified hand

✓6th **M67.45 Ganglion, hip**

M67.451 Ganglion, right hip

M67.452 Ganglion, left hip

M67.459 Ganglion, unspecified hip

✓6th **M67.46 Ganglion, knee**

M67.461 Ganglion, right knee

M67.462 Ganglion, left knee

M67.469 Ganglion, unspecified knee

✓6th **M67.47 Ganglion, ankle and foot**

M67.471 Ganglion, right ankle and foot

M67.472 Ganglion, left ankle and foot

M67.479 Ganglion, unspecified ankle and foot

M67.48 Ganglion, other site

M67.49 Ganglion, multiple sites

✓5th **M67.5 Plica syndrome**

Plica knee

M67.50 Plica syndrome, unspecified knee

M67.51 Plica syndrome, right knee

M67.52 Plica syndrome, left knee

✓5th **M67.8 Other specified disorders of synovium and tendon**

M67.80 Other specified disorders of synovium and tendon, unspecified site

✓6th **M67.81 Other specified disorders of synovium and tendon, shoulder**

M67.811 Other specified disorders of synovium, right shoulder

M67.812 Other specified disorders of synovium, left shoulder

M67.813 Other specified disorders of tendon, right shoulder

M67.814 Other specified disorders of tendon, left shoulder

M67.819 Other specified disorders of synovium and tendon, unspecified shoulder

✓6th **M67.82 Other specified disorders of synovium and tendon, elbow**

M67.821 Other specified disorders of synovium, right elbow

M67.822 Other specified disorders of synovium, left elbow

M67.823 Other specified disorders of tendon, right elbow

M67.824 Other specified disorders of tendon, left elbow

M67.829 Other specified disorders of synovium and tendon, unspecified elbow

✓6th **M67.83 Other specified disorders of synovium and tendon, wrist**

M67.831 Other specified disorders of synovium, right wrist

M67.832 Other specified disorders of synovium, left wrist

M67.833 Other specified disorders of tendon, right wrist

M67.834 Other specified disorders of tendon, left wrist

M67.839 Other specified disorders of synovium and tendon, unspecified wrist

✓6th **M67.84 Other specified disorders of synovium and tendon, hand**

M67.841 Other specified disorders of synovium, right hand

M67.842 Other specified disorders of synovium, left hand

M67.843 Other specified disorders of tendon, right hand

M67.844 Other specified disorders of tendon, left hand

M67.849 Other specified disorders of synovium and tendon, unspecified hand

✓6th **M67.85 Other specified disorders of synovium and tendon, hip**

M67.851 Other specified disorders of synovium, right hip

M67.852 Other specified disorders of synovium, left hip

M67.853 Other specified disorders of tendon, right hip

M67.854 Other specified disorders of tendon, left hip

M67.859 Other specified disorders of synovium and tendon, unspecified hip

✓6th **M67.86 Other specified disorders of synovium and tendon, knee**

M67.861 Other specified disorders of synovium, right knee

M67.862 Other specified disorders of synovium, left knee

M67.863 Other specified disorders of tendon, right knee

M67.864 Other specified disorders of tendon, left knee

M67.869 Other specified disorders of synovium and tendon, unspecified knee

✓6th **M67.87 Other specified disorders of synovium and tendon, ankle and foot**

M67.871 Other specified disorders of synovium, right ankle and foot

M67.872 Other specified disorders of synovium, left ankle and foot

M67.873 Other specified disorders of tendon, right ankle and foot

M67.874 Other specified disorders of tendon, left ankle and foot

M67.879 Other specified disorders of synovium and tendon, unspecified ankle and foot

M67.88 Other specified disorders of synovium and tendon, other site

M67.89 Other specified disorders of synovium and tendon, multiple sites

✓5th M67.9 Unspecified disorder of synovium and tendon

M67.90 Unspecified disorder of synovium and tendon, unspecified site

✓6th M67.91 Unspecified disorder of synovium and tendon, shoulder

M67.911 Unspecified disorder of synovium and tendon, right shoulder

M67.912 Unspecified disorder of synovium and tendon, left shoulder

M67.919 Unspecified disorder of synovium and tendon, unspecified shoulder

✓6th M67.92 Unspecified disorder of synovium and tendon, upper arm

M67.921 Unspecified disorder of synovium and tendon, right upper arm

M67.922 Unspecified disorder of synovium and tendon, left upper arm

M67.929 Unspecified disorder of synovium and tendon, unspecified upper arm

✓6th M67.93 Unspecified disorder of synovium and tendon, forearm

M67.931 Unspecified disorder of synovium and tendon, right forearm

M67.932 Unspecified disorder of synovium and tendon, left forearm

M67.939 Unspecified disorder of synovium and tendon, unspecified forearm

✓6th M67.94 Unspecified disorder of synovium and tendon, hand

M67.941 Unspecified disorder of synovium and tendon, right hand

M67.942 Unspecified disorder of synovium and tendon, left hand

M67.949 Unspecified disorder of synovium and tendon, unspecified hand

✓6th M67.95 Unspecified disorder of synovium and tendon, thigh

M67.951 Unspecified disorder of synovium and tendon, right thigh

M67.952 Unspecified disorder of synovium and tendon, left thigh

M67.959 Unspecified disorder of synovium and tendon, unspecified thigh

✓6th M67.96 Unspecified disorder of synovium and tendon, lower leg

M67.961 Unspecified disorder of synovium and tendon, right lower leg

M67.962 Unspecified disorder of synovium and tendon, left lower leg

M67.969 Unspecified disorder of synovium and tendon, unspecified lower leg

✓6th M67.97 Unspecified disorder of synovium and tendon, ankle and foot

M67.971 Unspecified disorder of synovium and tendon, right ankle and foot

M67.972 Unspecified disorder of synovium and tendon, left ankle and foot

M67.979 Unspecified disorder of synovium and tendon, unspecified ankle and foot

M67.98 Unspecified disorder of synovium and tendon, other site

M67.99 Unspecified disorder of synovium and tendon, multiple sites

Other soft tissue disorders (M70-M79)

✓4th M70 Soft tissue disorders related to use, overuse and pressure

INCLUDES soft tissue disorders of occupational origin

Use additional external cause code to identify activity causing disorder (Y93.-)

EXCLUDES 1 *bursitis NOS (M71.9-)*

EXCLUDES 2 *bursitis of shoulder (M75.5)*

enthesopathies (M76-M77)

pressure ulcer (pressure area) (L89.-)

✓5th M70.0 Crepitant synovitis (acute) (chronic) of hand and wrist

✓6th M70.03 Crepitant synovitis (acute) (chronic), wrist

M70.031 Crepitant synovitis (acute) (chronic), right wrist

M70.032 Crepitant synovitis (acute) (chronic), left wrist

M70.039 Crepitant synovitis (acute) (chronic), unspecified wrist

✓6th M70.04 Crepitant synovitis (acute) (chronic), hand

M70.041 Crepitant synovitis (acute) (chronic), right hand

M70.042 Crepitant synovitis (acute) (chronic), left hand

M70.049 Crepitant synovitis (acute) (chronic), unspecified hand

✓5th M70.1 Bursitis of hand

M70.10 Bursitis, unspecified hand

M70.11 Bursitis, right hand

M70.12 Bursitis, left hand

✓5th M70.2 Olecranon bursitis

M70.20 Olecranon bursitis, unspecified elbow

M70.21 Olecranon bursitis, right elbow

M70.22 Olecranon bursitis, left elbow

✓5th M70.3 Other bursitis of elbow

M70.30 Other bursitis of elbow, unspecified elbow

M70.31 Other bursitis of elbow, right elbow

M70.32 Other bursitis of elbow, left elbow

✓5th M70.4 Prepatellar bursitis

M70.40 Prepatellar bursitis, unspecified knee

M70.41 Prepatellar bursitis, right knee

M70.42 Prepatellar bursitis, left knee

Knee Bursae

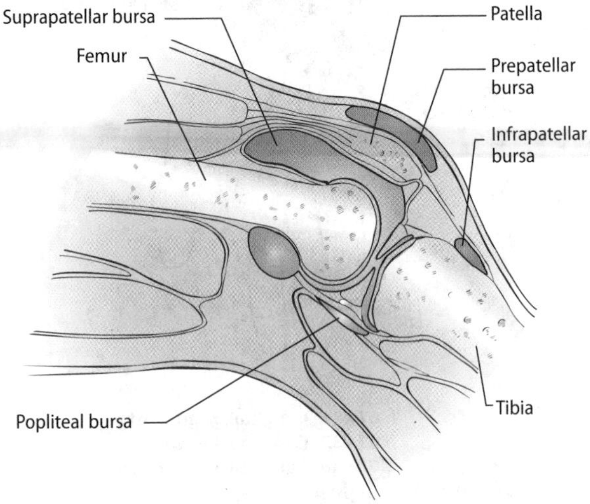

✓5th M70.5 Other bursitis of knee

M70.50 Other bursitis of knee, unspecified knee

M70.51 Other bursitis of knee, right knee

M70.52 Other bursitis of knee, left knee

✓5th M70.6 Trochanteric bursitis

Trochanteric tendinitis

M70.60 Trochanteric bursitis, unspecified hip

M70.61 Trochanteric bursitis, right hip

M70.62 Trochanteric bursitis, left hip

✓5th M70.7 Other bursitis of hip

Ischial bursitis

M70.70 Other bursitis of hip, unspecified hip

M70.71 Other bursitis of hip, right hip

M70.72 Other bursitis of hip, left hip

✓5th M70.8 Other soft tissue disorders related to use, overuse and pressure

M70.80 Other soft tissue disorders related to use, overuse and pressure of unspecified site

✓6th M70.81 Other soft tissue disorders related to use, overuse and pressure of shoulder

M70.811 Other soft tissue disorders related to use, overuse and pressure, right shoulder

M70.812 Other soft tissue disorders related to use, overuse and pressure, left shoulder

M70.819 Other soft tissue disorders related to use, overuse and pressure, unspecified shoulder

✓6th M70.82 Other soft tissue disorders related to use, overuse and pressure of upper arm

M70.821 Other soft tissue disorders related to use, overuse and pressure, right upper arm

M7Ø.822 Other soft tissue disorders related to use, overuse and pressure, left upper arm
M7Ø.829 Other soft tissue disorders related to use, overuse and pressure, unspecified upper arms

✓6th M7Ø.83 Other soft tissue disorders related to use, overuse and pressure of forearm
M7Ø.831 Other soft tissue disorders related to use, overuse and pressure, right forearm
M7Ø.832 Other soft tissue disorders related to use, overuse and pressure, left forearm
M7Ø.839 Other soft tissue disorders related to use, overuse and pressure, unspecified forearm

✓6th M7Ø.84 Other soft tissue disorders related to use, overuse and pressure of hand
M7Ø.841 Other soft tissue disorders related to use, overuse and pressure, right hand
M7Ø.842 Other soft tissue disorders related to use, overuse and pressure, left hand
M7Ø.849 Other soft tissue disorders related to use, overuse and pressure, unspecified hand

✓6th M7Ø.85 Other soft tissue disorders related to use, overuse and pressure of thigh
M7Ø.851 Other soft tissue disorders related to use, overuse and pressure, right thigh
M7Ø.852 Other soft tissue disorders related to use, overuse and pressure, left thigh
M7Ø.859 Other soft tissue disorders related to use, overuse and pressure, unspecified thigh

✓6th M7Ø.86 Other soft tissue disorders related to use, overuse and pressure lower leg
M7Ø.861 Other soft tissue disorders related to use, overuse and pressure, right lower leg
M7Ø.862 Other soft tissue disorders related to use, overuse and pressure, left lower leg
M7Ø.869 Other soft tissue disorders related to use, overuse and pressure, unspecified leg

✓6th M7Ø.87 Other soft tissue disorders related to use, overuse and pressure of ankle and foot
M7Ø.871 Other soft tissue disorders related to use, overuse and pressure, right ankle and foot
M7Ø.872 Other soft tissue disorders related to use, overuse and pressure, left ankle and foot
M7Ø.879 Other soft tissue disorders related to use, overuse and pressure, unspecified ankle and foot

M7Ø.88 Other soft tissue disorders related to use, overuse and pressure other site

M7Ø.89 Other soft tissue disorders related to use, overuse and pressure multiple sites

✓5th M7Ø.9 Unspecified soft tissue disorder related to use, overuse and pressure

M7Ø.9Ø Unspecified soft tissue disorder related to use, overuse and pressure of unspecified site

✓6th M7Ø.91 Unspecified soft tissue disorder related to use, overuse and pressure of shoulder
M7Ø.911 Unspecified soft tissue disorder related to use, overuse and pressure, right shoulder
M7Ø.912 Unspecified soft tissue disorder related to use, overuse and pressure, left shoulder
M7Ø.919 Unspecified soft tissue disorder related to use, overuse and pressure, unspecified shoulder

✓6th M7Ø.92 Unspecified soft tissue disorder related to use, overuse and pressure of upper arm
M7Ø.921 Unspecified soft tissue disorder related to use, overuse and pressure, right upper arm
M7Ø.922 Unspecified soft tissue disorder related to use, overuse and pressure, left upper arm
M7Ø.929 Unspecified soft tissue disorder related to use, overuse and pressure, unspecified upper arm

✓6th M7Ø.93 Unspecified soft tissue disorder related to use, overuse and pressure of forearm
M7Ø.931 Unspecified soft tissue disorder related to use, overuse and pressure, right forearm
M7Ø.932 Unspecified soft tissue disorder related to use, overuse and pressure, left forearm
M7Ø.939 Unspecified soft tissue disorder related to use, overuse and pressure, unspecified forearm

✓6th M7Ø.94 Unspecified soft tissue disorder related to use, overuse and pressure of hand
M7Ø.941 Unspecified soft tissue disorder related to use, overuse and pressure, right hand
M7Ø.942 Unspecified soft tissue disorder related to use, overuse and pressure, left hand
M7Ø.949 Unspecified soft tissue disorder related to use, overuse and pressure, unspecified hand

✓6th M7Ø.95 Unspecified soft tissue disorder related to use, overuse and pressure of thigh
M7Ø.951 Unspecified soft tissue disorder related to use, overuse and pressure, right thigh
M7Ø.952 Unspecified soft tissue disorder related to use, overuse and pressure, left thigh
M7Ø.959 Unspecified soft tissue disorder related to use, overuse and pressure, unspecified thigh

✓6th M7Ø.96 Unspecified soft tissue disorder related to use, overuse and pressure lower leg
M7Ø.961 Unspecified soft tissue disorder related to use, overuse and pressure, right lower leg
M7Ø.962 Unspecified soft tissue disorder related to use, overuse and pressure, left lower leg
M7Ø.969 Unspecified soft tissue disorder related to use, overuse and pressure, unspecified lower leg

✓6th M7Ø.97 Unspecified soft tissue disorder related to use, overuse and pressure of ankle and foot
M7Ø.971 Unspecified soft tissue disorder related to use, overuse and pressure, right ankle and foot
M7Ø.972 Unspecified soft tissue disorder related to use, overuse and pressure, left ankle and foot
M7Ø.979 Unspecified soft tissue disorder related to use, overuse and pressure, unspecified ankle and foot

M7Ø.98 Unspecified soft tissue disorder related to use, overuse and pressure other

M7Ø.99 Unspecified soft tissue disorder related to use, overuse and pressure multiple sites

✓4th M71 Other bursopathies

EXCLUDES 1 *bunion (M2Ø.1)*
bursitis related to use, overuse or pressure (M7Ø.-)
enthesopathies (M76-M77)

✓5th M71.Ø Abscess of bursa

Use additional code (B95.-, B96.-) to identify causative organism

M71.ØØ Abscess of bursa, unspecified site

✓6th M71.Ø1 Abscess of bursa, shoulder
M71.Ø11 Abscess of bursa, right shoulder
M71.Ø12 Abscess of bursa, left shoulder
M71.Ø19 Abscess of bursa, unspecified shoulder

✓6th M71.Ø2 Abscess of bursa, elbow
M71.Ø21 Abscess of bursa, right elbow
M71.Ø22 Abscess of bursa, left elbow
M71.Ø29 Abscess of bursa, unspecified elbow

✓6th M71.Ø3 Abscess of bursa, wrist
M71.Ø31 Abscess of bursa, right wrist
M71.Ø32 Abscess of bursa, left wrist
M71.Ø39 Abscess of bursa, unspecified wrist

✓6th M71.Ø4 Abscess of bursa, hand
M71.Ø41 Abscess of bursa, right hand
M71.Ø42 Abscess of bursa, left hand
M71.Ø49 Abscess of bursa, unspecified hand

✓6th M71.Ø5 Abscess of bursa, hip
M71.Ø51 Abscess of bursa, right hip
M71.Ø52 Abscess of bursa, left hip
M71.Ø59 Abscess of bursa, unspecified hip

✓6th M71.Ø6 Abscess of bursa, knee
M71.Ø61 Abscess of bursa, right knee
M71.Ø62 Abscess of bursa, left knee
M71.Ø69 Abscess of bursa, unspecified knee

✓6th **M71.07 Abscess of bursa, ankle and foot**

M71.071 Abscess of bursa, right ankle and foot

M71.072 Abscess of bursa, left ankle and foot

M71.079 Abscess of bursa, unspecified ankle and foot

M71.08 Abscess of bursa, other site

M71.09 Abscess of bursa, multiple sites

✓5th **M71.1 Other infective bursitis**

Use additional code (B95.-, B96.-) to identify causative organism

M71.10 Other infective bursitis, unspecified site

✓6th **M71.11 Other infective bursitis, shoulder**

M71.111 Other infective bursitis, right shoulder

M71.112 Other infective bursitis, left shoulder

M71.119 Other infective bursitis, unspecified shoulder

✓6th **M71.12 Other infective bursitis, elbow**

M71.121 Other infective bursitis, right elbow

M71.122 Other infective bursitis, left elbow

M71.129 Other infective bursitis, unspecified elbow

✓6th **M71.13 Other infective bursitis, wrist**

M71.131 Other infective bursitis, right wrist

M71.132 Other infective bursitis, left wrist

M71.139 Other infective bursitis, unspecified wrist

✓6th **M71.14 Other infective bursitis, hand**

M71.141 Other infective bursitis, right hand

M71.142 Other infective bursitis, left hand

M71.149 Other infective bursitis, unspecified hand

✓6th **M71.15 Other infective bursitis, hip**

M71.151 Other infective bursitis, right hip

M71.152 Other infective bursitis, left hip

M71.159 Other infective bursitis, unspecified hip

✓6th **M71.16 Other infective bursitis, knee**

M71.161 Other infective bursitis, right knee

M71.162 Other infective bursitis, left knee

M71.169 Other infective bursitis, unspecified knee

✓6th **M71.17 Other infective bursitis, ankle and foot**

M71.171 Other infective bursitis, right ankle and foot

M71.172 Other infective bursitis, left ankle and foot

M71.179 Other infective bursitis, unspecified ankle and foot

M71.18 Other infective bursitis, other site

M71.19 Other infective bursitis, multiple sites

✓5th **M71.2 Synovial cyst of popliteal space [Baker]**

EXCLUDES 1 *synovial cyst of popliteal space with rupture (M66.0)*

DEF: Sac filled with clear synovial fluid in adults, usually secondary to disease inside the joint, located on the back of the knee in the popliteal fossa area. In children, the cyst usually represents a ganglion of one of the tendons in the knee.

Baker's Cyst

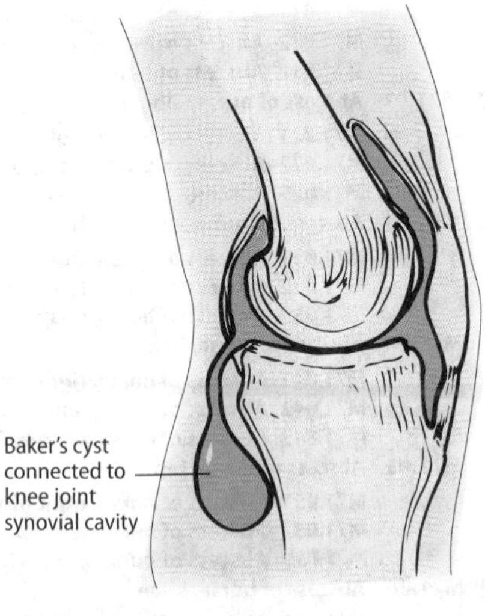

M71.20 Synovial cyst of popliteal space [Baker], unspecified knee

M71.21 Synovial cyst of popliteal space [Baker], right knee

M71.22 Synovial cyst of popliteal space [Baker], left knee

✓5th **M71.3 Other bursal cyst**

Synovial cyst NOS

EXCLUDES 1 *synovial cyst with rupture (M66.1-)*

M71.30 Other bursal cyst, unspecified site

✓6th **M71.31 Other bursal cyst, shoulder**

M71.311 Other bursal cyst, right shoulder

M71.312 Other bursal cyst, left shoulder

M71.319 Other bursal cyst, unspecified shoulder

✓6th **M71.32 Other bursal cyst, elbow**

M71.321 Other bursal cyst, right elbow

M71.322 Other bursal cyst, left elbow

M71.329 Other bursal cyst, unspecified elbow

✓6th **M71.33 Other bursal cyst, wrist**

M71.331 Other bursal cyst, right wrist

M71.332 Other bursal cyst, left wrist

M71.339 Other bursal cyst, unspecified wrist

✓6th **M71.34 Other bursal cyst, hand**

M71.341 Other bursal cyst, right hand

M71.342 Other bursal cyst, left hand

M71.349 Other bursal cyst, unspecified hand

✓6th **M71.35 Other bursal cyst, hip**

M71.351 Other bursal cyst, right hip

M71.352 Other bursal cyst, left hip

M71.359 Other bursal cyst, unspecified hip

✓6th **M71.37 Other bursal cyst, ankle and foot**

M71.371 Other bursal cyst, right ankle and foot

M71.372 Other bursal cyst, left ankle and foot

M71.379 Other bursal cyst, unspecified ankle and foot

M71.38 Other bursal cyst, other site

M71.39 Other bursal cyst, multiple sites

✓5th **M71.4 Calcium deposit in bursa**

EXCLUDES 2 *calcium deposit in bursa of shoulder (M75.3)*

M71.40 Calcium deposit in bursa, unspecified site

✓6th **M71.42 Calcium deposit in bursa, elbow**

M71.421 Calcium deposit in bursa, right elbow

M71.422 Calcium deposit in bursa, left elbow

M71.429 Calcium deposit in bursa, unspecified elbow

✓6th **M71.43 Calcium deposit in bursa, wrist**

M71.431 Calcium deposit in bursa, right wrist

M71.432 Calcium deposit in bursa, left wrist

M71.439 Calcium deposit in bursa, unspecified wrist

✓6th **M71.44 Calcium deposit in bursa, hand**

M71.441 Calcium deposit in bursa, right hand

M71.442 Calcium deposit in bursa, left hand

M71.449 Calcium deposit in bursa, unspecified hand

✓6th **M71.45 Calcium deposit in bursa, hip**

M71.451 Calcium deposit in bursa, right hip

M71.452 Calcium deposit in bursa, left hip

M71.459 Calcium deposit in bursa, unspecified hip

✓6th **M71.46 Calcium deposit in bursa, knee**

M71.461 Calcium deposit in bursa, right knee

M71.462 Calcium deposit in bursa, left knee

M71.469 Calcium deposit in bursa, unspecified knee

✓6th **M71.47 Calcium deposit in bursa, ankle and foot**

M71.471 Calcium deposit in bursa, right ankle and foot

M71.472 Calcium deposit in bursa, left ankle and foot

M71.479 Calcium deposit in bursa, unspecified ankle and foot

M71.48 Calcium deposit in bursa, other site

M71.49 Calcium deposit in bursa, multiple sites

✓5th **M71.5 Other bursitis, not elsewhere classified**

EXCLUDES 1 *bursitis NOS (M71.9-)*

EXCLUDES 2 *bursitis of shoulder (M75.5)*

bursitis of tibial collateral [Pellegrini-Stieda] (M76.4-)

M71.50 Other bursitis, not elsewhere classified, unspecified site

✓6th M71.52 **Other bursitis, not elsewhere classified, elbow**
- M71.521 **Other bursitis, not elsewhere classified, right elbow**
- M71.522 **Other bursitis, not elsewhere classified, left elbow**
- M71.529 **Other bursitis, not elsewhere classified, unspecified elbow**

✓6th M71.53 **Other bursitis, not elsewhere classified, wrist**
- M71.531 **Other bursitis, not elsewhere classified, right wrist**
- M71.532 **Other bursitis, not elsewhere classified, left wrist**
- M71.539 **Other bursitis, not elsewhere classified, unspecified wrist**

✓6th M71.54 **Other bursitis, not elsewhere classified, hand**
- M71.541 **Other bursitis, not elsewhere classified, right hand**
- M71.542 **Other bursitis, not elsewhere classified, left hand**
- M71.549 **Other bursitis, not elsewhere classified, unspecified hand**

✓6th M71.55 **Other bursitis, not elsewhere classified, hip**
- M71.551 **Other bursitis, not elsewhere classified, right hip**
- M71.552 **Other bursitis, not elsewhere classified, left hip**
- M71.559 **Other bursitis, not elsewhere classified, unspecified hip**

✓6th M71.56 **Other bursitis, not elsewhere classified, knee**
- M71.561 **Other bursitis, not elsewhere classified, right knee**
- M71.562 **Other bursitis, not elsewhere classified, left knee**
- M71.569 **Other bursitis, not elsewhere classified, unspecified knee**

✓6th M71.57 **Other bursitis, not elsewhere classified, ankle and foot**
- M71.571 **Other bursitis, not elsewhere classified, right ankle and foot**
- M71.572 **Other bursitis, not elsewhere classified, left ankle and foot**
- M71.579 **Other bursitis, not elsewhere classified, unspecified ankle and foot**

M71.58 **Other bursitis, not elsewhere classified, other site**

✓5th M71.8 **Other specified bursopathies**

M71.8Ø **Other specified bursopathies, unspecified site**

✓6th M71.81 **Other specified bursopathies, shoulder**
- M71.811 **Other specified bursopathies, right shoulder**
- M71.812 **Other specified bursopathies, left shoulder**
- M71.819 **Other specified bursopathies, unspecified shoulder**

✓6th M71.82 **Other specified bursopathies, elbow**
- M71.821 **Other specified bursopathies, right elbow**
- M71.822 **Other specified bursopathies, left elbow**
- M71.829 **Other specified bursopathies, unspecified elbow**

✓6th M71.83 **Other specified bursopathies, wrist**
- M71.831 **Other specified bursopathies, right wrist**
- M71.832 **Other specified bursopathies, left wrist**
- M71.839 **Other specified bursopathies, unspecified wrist**

✓6th M71.84 **Other specified bursopathies, hand**
- M71.841 **Other specified bursopathies, right hand**
- M71.842 **Other specified bursopathies, left hand**
- M71.849 **Other specified bursopathies, unspecified hand**

✓6th M71.85 **Other specified bursopathies, hip**
- M71.851 **Other specified bursopathies, right hip**
- M71.852 **Other specified bursopathies, left hip**
- M71.859 **Other specified bursopathies, unspecified hip**

✓6th M71.86 **Other specified bursopathies, knee**
- M71.861 **Other specified bursopathies, right knee**
- M71.862 **Other specified bursopathies, left knee**
- M71.869 **Other specified bursopathies, unspecified knee**

✓6th M71.87 **Other specified bursopathies, ankle and foot**
- M71.871 **Other specified bursopathies, right ankle and foot**
- M71.872 **Other specified bursopathies, left ankle and foot**
- M71.879 **Other specified bursopathies, unspecified ankle and foot**

M71.88 **Other specified bursopathies, other site**

M71.89 **Other specified bursopathies, multiple sites**

M71.9 **Bursopathy, unspecified**
Bursitis NOS

✓4th M72 Fibroblastic disorders

EXCLUDES 2 *retroperitoneal fibromatosis (D48.3)*

M72.Ø **Palmar fascial fibromatosis [Dupuytren]** A
DEF: Dupuytren's contracture: Flexion deformity of a finger, due to shortened, thickened fibrosing of palmar fascia. The cause is unknown, but it is associated with long-standing epilepsy.

M72.1 **Knuckle pads**

M72.2 **Plantar fascial fibromatosis**
Plantar fasciitis
DEF: Rapid-growing and multiplanar nodular swellings and pain in the foot that is not associated with contractures.

M72.4 **Pseudosarcomatous fibromatosis**
Nodular fasciitis

M72.6 **Necrotizing fasciitis** MCC HCC
Use additional code (B95.-, B96.-) to identify causative organism

M72.8 **Other fibroblastic disorders**
Abscess of fascia
Fasciitis NEC
Other infective fasciitis
Use additional code to (B95.-, B96.-) identify causative organism
EXCLUDES 1 *diffuse (eosinophilic) fasciitis (M35.4)*
necrotizing fasciitis (M72.6)
nodular fasciitis (M72.4)
perirenal fasciitis NOS (N13.5)
perirenal fasciitis with infection (N13.6)
plantar fasciitis (M72.2)

M72.9 **Fibroblastic disorder, unspecified**
Fasciitis NOS
Fibromatosis NOS

✓4th M75 Shoulder lesions

EXCLUDES 2 *shoulder-hand syndrome (M89.Ø-)*

✓5th M75.Ø **Adhesive capsulitis of shoulder**
Frozen shoulder
Periarthritis of shoulder
AHA: 2015,2Q,23
- M75.ØØ **Adhesive capsulitis of unspecified shoulder**
- M75.Ø1 **Adhesive capsulitis of right shoulder**
- M75.Ø2 **Adhesive capsulitis of left shoulder**

✓5th M75.1 **Rotator cuff tear or rupture, not specified as traumatic**
Rotator cuff syndrome
Supraspinatus syndrome
Supraspinatus tear or rupture, not specified as traumatic
EXCLUDES 1 *tear of rotator cuff, traumatic (S46.Ø1-)*

✓6th M75.1Ø **Unspecified rotator cuff tear or rupture, not specified as traumatic**
- M75.1ØØ **Unspecified rotator cuff tear or rupture of unspecified shoulder, not specified as traumatic**
- M75.1Ø1 **Unspecified rotator cuff tear or rupture of right shoulder, not specified as traumatic**
- M75.1Ø2 **Unspecified rotator cuff tear or rupture of left shoulder, not specified as traumatic**

✓6th M75.11 **Incomplete rotator cuff tear or rupture not specified as traumatic**
- M75.11Ø **Incomplete rotator cuff tear or rupture of unspecified shoulder, not specified as traumatic**
- M75.111 **Incomplete rotator cuff tear or rupture of right shoulder, not specified as traumatic**
- M75.112 **Incomplete rotator cuff tear or rupture of left shoulder, not specified as traumatic**

M75.12 Complete rotator cuff tear or rupture not specified as traumatic
- **M75.120 Complete rotator cuff tear or rupture of unspecified shoulder, not specified as traumatic**
- **M75.121 Complete rotator cuff tear or rupture of right shoulder, not specified as traumatic**
- **M75.122 Complete rotator cuff tear or rupture of left shoulder, not specified as traumatic**

M75.2 Bicipital tendinitis
- **M75.20 Bicipital tendinitis, unspecified shoulder**
- **M75.21 Bicipital tendinitis, right shoulder**
- **M75.22 Bicipital tendinitis, left shoulder**

M75.3 Calcific tendinitis of shoulder

Calcified bursa of shoulder
- **M75.30 Calcific tendinitis of unspecified shoulder**
- **M75.31 Calcific tendinitis of right shoulder**
- **M75.32 Calcific tendinitis of left shoulder**

M75.4 Impingement syndrome of shoulder
- **M75.40 Impingement syndrome of unspecified shoulder**
- **M75.41 Impingement syndrome of right shoulder**
- **M75.42 Impingement syndrome of left shoulder**

M75.5 Bursitis of shoulder
- **M75.50 Bursitis of unspecified shoulder**
- **M75.51 Bursitis of right shoulder**
- **M75.52 Bursitis of left shoulder**

M75.8 Other shoulder lesions
- **M75.80 Other shoulder lesions, unspecified shoulder**
- **M75.81 Other shoulder lesions, right shoulder**
- **M75.82 Other shoulder lesions, left shoulder**

M75.9 Shoulder lesion, unspecified
- **M75.90 Shoulder lesion, unspecified, unspecified shoulder**
- **M75.91 Shoulder lesion, unspecified, right shoulder**
- **M75.92 Shoulder lesion, unspecified, left shoulder**

M76 Enthesopathies, lower limb, excluding foot

EXCLUDES 2 *bursitis due to use, overuse and pressure (M70.-)*
enthesopathies of ankle and foot (M77.5-)

M76.0 Gluteal tendinitis
- **M76.00 Gluteal tendinitis, unspecified hip**
- **M76.01 Gluteal tendinitis, right hip**
- **M76.02 Gluteal tendinitis, left hip**

M76.1 Psoas tendinitis
- **M76.10 Psoas tendinitis, unspecified hip**
- **M76.11 Psoas tendinitis, right hip**
- **M76.12 Psoas tendinitis, left hip**

M76.2 Iliac crest spur
- **M76.20 Iliac crest spur, unspecified hip**
- **M76.21 Iliac crest spur, right hip**
- **M76.22 Iliac crest spur, left hip**

M76.3 Iliotibial band syndrome
- **M76.30 Iliotibial band syndrome, unspecified leg**
- **M76.31 Iliotibial band syndrome, right leg**
- **M76.32 Iliotibial band syndrome, left leg**

M76.4 Tibial collateral bursitis [Pellegrini-Stieda]
- **M76.40 Tibial collateral bursitis [Pellegrini-Stieda], unspecified leg**
- **M76.41 Tibial collateral bursitis [Pellegrini-Stieda], right leg**
- **M76.42 Tibial collateral bursitis [Pellegrini-Stieda], left leg**

M76.5 Patellar tendinitis
- **M76.50 Patellar tendinitis, unspecified knee**
- **M76.51 Patellar tendinitis, right knee**
- **M76.52 Patellar tendinitis, left knee**

M76.6 Achilles tendinitis

Achilles bursitis
- **M76.60 Achilles tendinitis, unspecified leg**
- **M76.61 Achilles tendinitis, right leg**
- **M76.62 Achilles tendinitis, left leg**

M76.7 Peroneal tendinitis
- **M76.70 Peroneal tendinitis, unspecified leg**
- **M76.71 Peroneal tendinitis, right leg**
- **M76.72 Peroneal tendinitis, left leg**

M76.8 Other specified enthesopathies of lower limb, excluding foot

M76.81 Anterior tibial syndrome
- **M76.811 Anterior tibial syndrome, right leg**
- **M76.812 Anterior tibial syndrome, left leg**
- **M76.819 Anterior tibial syndrome, unspecified leg**

M76.82 Posterior tibial tendinitis
- **M76.821 Posterior tibial tendinitis, right leg**
- **M76.822 Posterior tibial tendinitis, left leg**
- **M76.829 Posterior tibial tendinitis, unspecified leg**

M76.89 Other specified enthesopathies of lower limb, excluding foot
- **M76.891 Other specified enthesopathies of right lower limb, excluding foot**
- **M76.892 Other specified enthesopathies of left lower limb, excluding foot**
- **M76.899 Other specified enthesopathies of unspecified lower limb, excluding foot**

M76.9 Unspecified enthesopathy, lower limb, excluding foot

M77 Other enthesopathies

EXCLUDES 1 *bursitis NOS (M71.9-)*

EXCLUDES 2 *bursitis due to use, overuse and pressure (M70.-)*
osteophyte (M25.7)
spinal enthesopathy (M46.0-)

M77.0 Medial epicondylitis
- **M77.00 Medial epicondylitis, unspecified elbow**
- **M77.01 Medial epicondylitis, right elbow**
- **M77.02 Medial epicondylitis, left elbow**

M77.1 Lateral epicondylitis

Tennis elbow
- **M77.10 Lateral epicondylitis, unspecified elbow**
- **M77.11 Lateral epicondylitis, right elbow**
- **M77.12 Lateral epicondylitis, left elbow**

M77.2 Periarthritis of wrist
- **M77.20 Periarthritis, unspecified wrist**
- **M77.21 Periarthritis, right wrist**
- **M77.22 Periarthritis, left wrist**

M77.3 Calcaneal spur

DEF: Overgrowth of calcaneus bone on the underside of the heel that causes pain on walking. Calcaneal spur is due to a chronic avulsion injury of the plantar fascia from the calcaneus.
- **M77.30 Calcaneal spur, unspecified foot**
- **M77.31 Calcaneal spur, right foot**
- **M77.32 Calcaneal spur, left foot**

M77.4 Metatarsalgia

EXCLUDES 1 *Morton's metatarsalgia (G57.6)*
- **M77.40 Metatarsalgia, unspecified foot**
- **M77.41 Metatarsalgia, right foot**
- **M77.42 Metatarsalgia, left foot**

M77.5 Other enthesopathy of foot and ankle
- **M77.50 Other enthesopathy of unspecified foot and ankle**
- **M77.51 Other enthesopathy of right foot and ankle**
- **M77.52 Other enthesopathy of left foot and ankle**

M77.8 Other enthesopathies, not elsewhere classified

M77.9 Enthesopathy, unspecified

Bone spur NOS
Capsulitis NOS
Periarthritis NOS
Tendinitis NOS

M79 Other and unspecified soft tissue disorders, not elsewhere classified

EXCLUDES 1 *psychogenic rheumatism (F45.8)*
soft tissue pain, psychogenic (F45.41)

M79.0 Rheumatism, unspecified

EXCLUDES 1 *fibromyalgia (M79.7)*
palindromic rheumatism (M12.3-)

M79.1 Myalgia

Myofascial pain syndrome

EXCLUDES 1 *fibromyalgia (M79.7)*
myositis (M60.-)

AHA: 2018,4Q,21
- **M79.10 Myalgia, unspecified site**
- **M79.11 Myalgia of mastication muscle**
- **M79.12 Myalgia of auxiliary muscles, head and neck**
- **M79.18 Myalgia, other site**

M79.2 Neuralgia and neuritis, unspecified
EXCLUDES 1 *brachial radiculitis NOS (M54.1)*
lumbosacral radiculitis NOS (M54.1)
mononeuropathies (G56-G58)
radiculitis NOS (M54.1)
sciatica (M54.3-M54.4)
TIP: Assign for documented neuropathic pain.

M79.3 Panniculitis, unspecified
EXCLUDES 1 *lupus panniculitis (L93.2)*
neck and back panniculitis (M54.0-)
relapsing [Weber-Christian] panniculitis (M35.6)

M79.4 Hypertrophy of (infrapatellar) fat pad

M79.5 Residual foreign body in soft tissue
EXCLUDES 1 *foreign body granuloma of skin and subcutaneous tissue (L92.3)*
foreign body granuloma of soft tissue (M60.2-)

✓5th **M79.6 Pain in limb, hand, foot, fingers and toes**
EXCLUDES 2 *pain in joint (M25.5-)*

✓6th **M79.60 Pain in limb, unspecified**
M79.601 Pain in right arm
Pain in right upper limb NOS
M79.602 Pain in left arm
Pain in left upper limb NOS
M79.603 Pain in arm, unspecified
Pain in upper limb NOS
M79.604 Pain in right leg
Pain in right lower limb NOS
M79.605 Pain in left leg
Pain in left lower limb NOS
M79.606 Pain in leg, unspecified
Pain in lower limb NOS
M79.609 Pain in unspecified limb
Pain in limb NOS

✓6th **M79.62 Pain in upper arm**
Pain in axillary region
M79.621 Pain in right upper arm
M79.622 Pain in left upper arm
M79.629 Pain in unspecified upper arm

✓6th **M79.63 Pain in forearm**
M79.631 Pain in right forearm
M79.632 Pain in left forearm
M79.639 Pain in unspecified forearm

✓6th **M79.64 Pain in hand and fingers**
M79.641 Pain in right hand
M79.642 Pain in left hand
M79.643 Pain in unspecified hand
M79.644 Pain in right finger(s)
M79.645 Pain in left finger(s)
M79.646 Pain in unspecified finger(s)

✓6th **M79.65 Pain in thigh**
M79.651 Pain in right thigh
M79.652 Pain in left thigh
M79.659 Pain in unspecified thigh

✓6th **M79.66 Pain in lower leg**
M79.661 Pain in right lower leg
M79.662 Pain in left lower leg
M79.669 Pain in unspecified lower leg

✓6th **M79.67 Pain in foot and toes**
M79.671 Pain in right foot
M79.672 Pain in left foot
M79.673 Pain in unspecified foot
M79.674 Pain in right toe(s)
M79.675 Pain in left toe(s)
M79.676 Pain in unspecified toe(s)

M79.7 Fibromyalgia
Fibromyositis
Fibrositis
Myofibrositis

✓5th **M79.A Nontraumatic compartment syndrome**
Code first, if applicable, associated postprocedural complication
EXCLUDES 1 *compartment syndrome NOS (T79.A-)*
fibromyalgia (M79.7)
nontraumatic ischemic infarction of muscle (M62.2-)
traumatic compartment syndrome (T79.A-)

✓6th **M79.A1 Nontraumatic compartment syndrome of upper extremity**
Nontraumatic compartment syndrome of shoulder, arm, forearm, wrist, hand, and fingers
M79.A11 Nontraumatic compartment syndrome of right upper extremity CC
M79.A12 Nontraumatic compartment syndrome of left upper extremity CC
M79.A19 Nontraumatic compartment syndrome of unspecified upper extremity CC

✓6th **M79.A2 Nontraumatic compartment syndrome of lower extremity**
Nontraumatic compartment syndrome of hip, buttock, thigh, leg, foot, and toes
M79.A21 Nontraumatic compartment syndrome of right lower extremity CC
M79.A22 Nontraumatic compartment syndrome of left lower extremity CC
M79.A29 Nontraumatic compartment syndrome of unspecified lower extremity CC

M79.A3 Nontraumatic compartment syndrome of abdomen CC
M79.A9 Nontraumatic compartment syndrome of other sites CC

✓5th **M79.8 Other specified soft tissue disorders**
M79.81 Nontraumatic hematoma of soft tissue
Nontraumatic hematoma of muscle
Nontraumatic seroma of muscle and soft tissue
M79.89 Other specified soft tissue disorders
Polyalgia

M79.9 Soft tissue disorder, unspecified

OSTEOPATHIES AND CHONDROPATHIES (M80-M94)

Disorders of bone density and structure (M80-M85)

✓4th **M80 Osteoporosis with current pathological fracture**
INCLUDES osteoporosis with current fragility fracture
Use additional code to identify major osseous defect, if applicable (M89.7-)
EXCLUDES 1 *collapsed vertebra NOS (M48.5)*
pathological fracture NOS (M84.4)
wedging of vertebra NOS (M48.5)
EXCLUDES 2 *personal history of (healed) osteoporosis fracture (Z87.310)*
AHA: 2018,2Q,12
TIP: The site codes in this category identify the site of the fracture, not the site of the osteoporosis.

The appropriate 7th character is to be added to each code from category M80:
- A initial encounter for fracture
- D subsequent encounter for fracture with routine healing
- G subsequent encounter for fracture with delayed healing
- K subsequent encounter for fracture with nonunion
- P subsequent encounter for fracture with malunion
- S sequela

✓5th **M80.0 Age-related osteoporosis with current pathological fracture**
Involutional osteoporosis with current pathological fracture
Osteoporosis NOS with current pathological fracture
Postmenopausal osteoporosis with current pathological fracture
Senile osteoporosis with current pathological fracture

3 √x7th **M80.00 Age-related osteoporosis with current pathological fracture, unspecified site** CC A

✓6th **M80.01 Age-related osteoporosis with current pathological fracture, shoulder**
3 ✓7th **M80.011 Age-related osteoporosis with current pathological fracture, right shoulder** CC A
3 ✓7th **M80.012 Age-related osteoporosis with current pathological fracture, left shoulder** CC A

3 ✓7th **M80.019 Age-related osteoporosis with current pathological fracture, unspecified shoulder** CC A

✓6th **M80.02 Age-related osteoporosis with current pathological fracture, humerus**

3 ✓7th **M80.021 Age-related osteoporosis with current pathological fracture, right humerus** CC A

3 ✓7th **M80.022 Age-related osteoporosis with current pathological fracture, left humerus** CC A

3 ✓7th **M80.029 Age-related osteoporosis with current pathological fracture, unspecified humerus** CC A

✓6th **M80.03 Age-related osteoporosis with current pathological fracture, forearm**

Age-related osteoporosis with current pathological fracture of wrist

3 ✓7th **M80.031 Age-related osteoporosis with current pathological fracture, right forearm** CC A

3 ✓7th **M80.032 Age-related osteoporosis with current pathological fracture, left forearm** CC A

3 ✓7th **M80.039 Age-related osteoporosis with current pathological fracture, unspecified forearm** CC A

✓6th **M80.04 Age-related osteoporosis with current pathological fracture, hand**

3 ✓7th **M80.041 Age-related osteoporosis with current pathological fracture, right hand** CC A

3 ✓7th **M80.042 Age-related osteoporosis with current pathological fracture, left hand** CC A

3 ✓7th **M80.049 Age-related osteoporosis with current pathological fracture, unspecified hand** CC A

✓6th **M80.05 Age-related osteoporosis with current pathological fracture, femur**

Age-related osteoporosis with current pathological fracture of hip

3,6 ✓7th **M80.051 Age-related osteoporosis with current pathological fracture, right femur** CC HCC A

3,6 ✓7th **M80.052 Age-related osteoporosis with current pathological fracture, left femur** CC HCC A

3,6 ✓7th **M80.059 Age-related osteoporosis with current pathological fracture, unspecified femur** CC HCC A

✓6th **M80.06 Age-related osteoporosis with current pathological fracture, lower leg**

3 ✓7th **M80.061 Age-related osteoporosis with current pathological fracture, right lower leg** CC A

3 ✓7th **M80.062 Age-related osteoporosis with current pathological fracture, left lower leg** CC A

3 ✓7th **M80.069 Age-related osteoporosis with current pathological fracture, unspecified lower leg** CC A

✓6th **M80.07 Age-related osteoporosis with current pathological fracture, ankle and foot**

3 ✓7th **M80.071 Age-related osteoporosis with current pathological fracture, right ankle and foot** CC A

3 ✓7th **M80.072 Age-related osteoporosis with current pathological fracture, left ankle and foot** CC A

3 ✓7th **M80.079 Age-related osteoporosis with current pathological fracture, unspecified ankle and foot** CC A

3,6 ✓x7th **M80.08 Age-related osteoporosis with current pathological fracture, vertebra(e)** CC HCC A

● 3 ✓x7th **M80.0A Age-related osteoporosis with current pathological fracture, other site** CC A

✓5th **M80.8 Other osteoporosis with current pathological fracture**

Drug-induced osteoporosis with current pathological fracture
Idiopathic osteoporosis with current pathological fracture
Osteoporosis of disuse with current pathological fracture
Postoophorectomy osteoporosis with current pathological fracture
Postsurgical malabsorption osteoporosis with current pathological fracture
Post-traumatic osteoporosis with current pathological fracture
Use additional code for adverse effect, if applicable, to identify drug (T36-T50 with fifth or sixth character 5)

3 ✓x7th **M80.80 Other osteoporosis with current pathological fracture, unspecified site** CC

✓6th **M80.81 Other osteoporosis with pathological fracture, shoulder**

3 ✓7th **M80.811 Other osteoporosis with current pathological fracture, right shoulder** CC

3 ✓7th **M80.812 Other osteoporosis with current pathological fracture, left shoulder** CC

3 ✓7th **M80.819 Other osteoporosis with current pathological fracture, unspecified shoulder** CC

✓6th **M80.82 Other osteoporosis with current pathological fracture, humerus**

3 ✓7th **M80.821 Other osteoporosis with current pathological fracture, right humerus** CC

3 ✓7th **M80.822 Other osteoporosis with current pathological fracture, left humerus** CC

3 ✓7th **M80.829 Other osteoporosis with current pathological fracture, unspecified humerus** CC

✓6th **M80.83 Other osteoporosis with current pathological fracture, forearm**

Other osteoporosis with current pathological fracture of wrist

3 ✓7th **M80.831 Other osteoporosis with current pathological fracture, right forearm** CC

3 ✓7th **M80.832 Other osteoporosis with current pathological fracture, left forearm** CC

3 ✓7th **M80.839 Other osteoporosis with current pathological fracture, unspecified forearm** CC

✓6th **M80.84 Other osteoporosis with current pathological fracture, hand**

3 ✓7th **M80.841 Other osteoporosis with current pathological fracture, right hand** CC

3 ✓7th **M80.842 Other osteoporosis with current pathological fracture, left hand** CC

3 ✓7th **M80.849 Other osteoporosis with current pathological fracture, unspecified hand** CC

✓6th **M80.85 Other osteoporosis with current pathological fracture, femur**

Other osteoporosis with current pathological fracture of hip

3,6 ✓7th **M80.851 Other osteoporosis with current pathological fracture, right femur** CC HCC

3,6 ✓7th **M80.852 Other osteoporosis with current pathological fracture, left femur** CC HCC

3,6 ✓7th **M80.859 Other osteoporosis with current pathological fracture, unspecified femur** CC HCC

✓6th **M80.86 Other osteoporosis with current pathological fracture, lower leg**

3 ✓7th **M80.861 Other osteoporosis with current pathological fracture, right lower leg** CC

3 ✓7th **M80.862 Other osteoporosis with current pathological fracture, left lower leg** CC

3 ✓7th **M80.869 Other osteoporosis with current pathological fracture, unspecified lower leg** CC

√6th **M8Ø.87 Other osteoporosis with current pathological fracture, ankle and foot**

3 √7th **M8Ø.871 Other osteoporosis with current pathological fracture, right ankle and foot** CC

3 √7th **M8Ø.872 Other osteoporosis with current pathological fracture, left ankle and foot** CC

3 √7th **M8Ø.879 Other osteoporosis with current pathological fracture, unspecified ankle and foot** CC

3,6 √x7th **M8Ø.88 Other osteoporosis with current pathological fracture, vertebra(e)** CC HCC

● 3 √x7th **M8Ø.8A Other osteoporosis with current pathological fracture, other site** CC

√4th **M81 Osteoporosis without current pathological fracture**

Use additional code to identify:
major osseous defect, if applicable (M89.7-)
personal history of (healed) osteoporosis fracture, if applicable (Z87.31Ø)

EXCLUDES 1 *osteoporosis with current pathological fracture (M8Ø.-)*
Sudeck's atrophy (M89.Ø)

M81.Ø Age-related osteoporosis without current pathological fracture A

Involutional osteoporosis without current pathological fracture
Osteoporosis NOS
Postmenopausal osteoporosis without current pathological fracture
Senile osteoporosis without current pathological fracture

M81.6 Localized osteoporosis [Lequesne]

EXCLUDES 1 *Sudeck's atrophy (M89.Ø)*

M81.8 Other osteoporosis without current pathological fracture

Drug-induced osteoporosis without current pathological fracture
Idiopathic osteoporosis without current pathological fracture
Osteoporosis of disuse without current pathological fracture
Postoophorectomy osteoporosis without current pathological fracture
Postsurgical malabsorption osteoporosis without current pathological fracture
Post-traumatic osteoporosis without current pathological fracture
Use additional code for adverse effect, if applicable, to identify drug (T36-T5Ø with fifth or sixth character 5)

√4th **M83 Adult osteomalacia**

EXCLUDES 1 *infantile and juvenile osteomalacia (E55.Ø)*
renal osteodystrophy (N25.Ø)
rickets (active) (E55.Ø)
rickets (active) sequelae (E64.3)
vitamin D-resistant osteomalacia (E83.3)
vitamin D-resistant rickets (active) (E83.3)

M83.Ø Puerperal osteomalacia M ♀

M83.1 Senile osteomalacia A

M83.2 Adult osteomalacia due to malabsorption A

Postsurgical malabsorption osteomalacia in adults

M83.3 Adult osteomalacia due to malnutrition A

M83.4 Aluminum bone disease

M83.5 Other drug-induced osteomalacia in adults A

Use additional code for adverse effect, if applicable, to identify drug (T36-T5Ø with fifth or sixth character 5)

M83.8 Other adult osteomalacia A

M83.9 Adult osteomalacia, unspecified A

√4th **M84 Disorder of continuity of bone**

EXCLUDES 2 *traumatic fracture of bone-see fracture, by site*

√5th **M84.3 Stress fracture**

Fatigue fracture
March fracture
Stress fracture NOS
Stress reaction
Use additional external cause code(s) to identify the cause of the stress fracture

EXCLUDES 1 *pathological fracture due to osteoporosis (M8Ø.-)*
pathological fracture NOS (M84.4.-)
traumatic fracture (S12.-, S22.-, S32.-, S42.-, S52.-, S62.-, S72.-, S82.-, S92.-)

EXCLUDES 2 *personal history of (healed) stress (fatigue) fracture (Z87.312)*
stress fracture of vertebra (M48.4-)

The appropriate 7th character is to be added to each code from subcategory M84.3.
A initial encounter for fracture
D subsequent encounter for fracture with routine healing
G subsequent encounter for fracture with delayed healing
K subsequent encounter for fracture with nonunion
P subsequent encounter for fracture with malunion
S sequela

4 √x7th **M84.3Ø Stress fracture, unspecified site** CC

√6th **M84.31 Stress fracture, shoulder**

4 √7th **M84.311 Stress fracture, right shoulder** CC

4 √7th **M84.312 Stress fracture, left shoulder** CC

4 √7th **M84.319 Stress fracture, unspecified shoulder** CC

√6th **M84.32 Stress fracture, humerus**

4 √7th **M84.321 Stress fracture, right humerus** CC

4 √7th **M84.322 Stress fracture, left humerus** CC

4 √7th **M84.329 Stress fracture, unspecified humerus** CC

√6th **M84.33 Stress fracture, ulna and radius**

4 √7th **M84.331 Stress fracture, right ulna** CC

4 √7th **M84.332 Stress fracture, left ulna** CC

4 √7th **M84.333 Stress fracture, right radius** CC

4 √7th **M84.334 Stress fracture, left radius** CC

4 √7th **M84.339 Stress fracture, unspecified ulna and radius** CC

√6th **M84.34 Stress fracture, hand and fingers**

4 √7th **M84.341 Stress fracture, right hand** CC

4 √7th **M84.342 Stress fracture, left hand** CC

4 √7th **M84.343 Stress fracture, unspecified hand** CC

4 √7th **M84.344 Stress fracture, right finger(s)** CC

4 √7th **M84.345 Stress fracture, left finger(s)** CC

4 √7th **M84.346 Stress fracture, unspecified finger(s)** CC

√6th **M84.35 Stress fracture, pelvis and femur**

Stress fracture, hip

4 √7th **M84.35Ø Stress fracture, pelvis** CC

4 √7th **M84.351 Stress fracture, right femur** CC

4 √7th **M84.352 Stress fracture, left femur** CC

4 √7th **M84.353 Stress fracture, unspecified femur** CC

4 √7th **M84.359 Stress fracture, hip, unspecified** CC

√6th **M84.36 Stress fracture, tibia and fibula**

4 √7th **M84.361 Stress fracture, right tibia** CC

4 √7th **M84.362 Stress fracture, left tibia** CC

4 √7th **M84.363 Stress fracture, right fibula** CC

4 √7th **M84.364 Stress fracture, left fibula** CC

4 √7th **M84.369 Stress fracture, unspecified tibia and fibula** CC

√6th **M84.37 Stress fracture, ankle, foot and toes**

4 √7th **M84.371 Stress fracture, right ankle** CC

4 √7th **M84.372 Stress fracture, left ankle** CC

4 √7th **M84.373 Stress fracture, unspecified ankle** CC

4 √7th **M84.374 Stress fracture, right foot** CC

4 √7th **M84.375 Stress fracture, left foot** CC

4 ✓7th **M84.376 Stress fracture, unspecified foot** CC
4 ✓7th **M84.377 Stress fracture, right toe(s)** CC
4 ✓7th **M84.378 Stress fracture, left toe(s)** CC
4 ✓7th **M84.379 Stress fracture, unspecified toe(s)** CC
4 ✓x7th **M84.38 Stress fracture, other site** CC
EXCLUDES 2 *stress fracture of vertebra (M48.4-)*

✓5th **M84.4 Pathological fracture, not elsewhere classified**
Chronic fracture
Pathological fracture NOS
EXCLUDES 1 *collapsed vertebra NEC (M48.5)*
pathological fracture in neoplastic disease (M84.5-)
pathological fracture in osteoporosis (M80.-)
pathological fracture in other disease (M84.6-)
stress fracture (M84.3-)
traumatic fracture (S12.-, S22.-, S32.-, S42.-, S52.-, S62.-, S72.-, S82.-, S92.-)
EXCLUDES 2 *personal history of (healed) pathological fracture (Z87.311)*

The appropriate 7th character is to be added to each code from subcategory M84.4.
A initial encounter for fracture
D subsequent encounter for fracture with routine healing
G subsequent encounter for fracture with delayed healing
K subsequent encounter for fracture with nonunion
P subsequent encounter for fracture with malunion
S sequela

3 ✓x7th **M84.40 Pathological fracture, unspecified site** CC
✓6th **M84.41 Pathological fracture, shoulder**
3 ✓7th **M84.411 Pathological fracture, right shoulder** CC
3 ✓7th **M84.412 Pathological fracture, left shoulder** CC
3 ✓7th **M84.419 Pathological fracture, unspecified shoulder** CC
✓6th **M84.42 Pathological fracture, humerus**
3 ✓7th **M84.421 Pathological fracture, right humerus** CC
3 ✓7th **M84.422 Pathological fracture, left humerus** CC
3 ✓7th **M84.429 Pathological fracture, unspecified humerus** CC
✓6th **M84.43 Pathological fracture, ulna and radius**
3 ✓7th **M84.431 Pathological fracture, right ulna** CC
3 ✓7th **M84.432 Pathological fracture, left ulna** CC
3 ✓7th **M84.433 Pathological fracture, right radius** CC
3 ✓7th **M84.434 Pathological fracture, left radius** CC
3 ✓7th **M84.439 Pathological fracture, unspecified ulna and radius** CC
✓6th **M84.44 Pathological fracture, hand and fingers**
3 ✓7th **M84.441 Pathological fracture, right hand** CC
3 ✓7th **M84.442 Pathological fracture, left hand** CC
3 ✓7th **M84.443 Pathological fracture, unspecified hand** CC
3 ✓7th **M84.444 Pathological fracture, right finger(s)** CC
3 ✓7th **M84.445 Pathological fracture, left finger(s)** CC
3 ✓7th **M84.446 Pathological fracture, unspecified finger(s)** CC
✓6th **M84.45 Pathological fracture, femur and pelvis**
AHA: 2016,4Q,43
3,6 ✓7th **M84.451 Pathological fracture, right femur** CC HCC
3,6 ✓7th **M84.452 Pathological fracture, left femur** CC HCC
3,6 ✓7th **M84.453 Pathological fracture, unspecified femur** CC HCC
3 ✓7th **M84.454 Pathological fracture, pelvis** CC
3,6 ✓7th **M84.459 Pathological fracture, hip, unspecified** CC HCC
✓6th **M84.46 Pathological fracture, tibia and fibula**
3 ✓7th **M84.461 Pathological fracture, right tibia** CC
3 ✓7th **M84.462 Pathological fracture, left tibia** CC
3 ✓7th **M84.463 Pathological fracture, right fibula** CC
3 ✓7th **M84.464 Pathological fracture, left fibula** CC
3 ✓7th **M84.469 Pathological fracture, unspecified tibia and fibula** CC
✓6th **M84.47 Pathological fracture, ankle, foot and toes**
3 ✓7th **M84.471 Pathological fracture, right ankle** CC
3 ✓7th **M84.472 Pathological fracture, left ankle** CC
3 ✓7th **M84.473 Pathological fracture, unspecified ankle** CC
3 ✓7th **M84.474 Pathological fracture, right foot** CC
3 ✓7th **M84.475 Pathological fracture, left foot** CC
3 ✓7th **M84.476 Pathological fracture, unspecified foot** CC
3 ✓7th **M84.477 Pathological fracture, right toe(s)** CC
3 ✓7th **M84.478 Pathological fracture, left toe(s)** CC
3 ✓7th **M84.479 Pathological fracture, unspecified toe(s)** CC
3 ✓x7th **M84.48 Pathological fracture, other site** CC

✓5th **M84.5 Pathological fracture in neoplastic disease**
Code also underlying neoplasm

The appropriate 7th character is to be added to each code from subcategory M84.5.
A initial encounter for fracture
D subsequent encounter for fracture with routine healing
G subsequent encounter for fracture with delayed healing
K subsequent encounter for fracture with nonunion
P subsequent encounter for fracture with malunion
S sequela

3 ✓x7th **M84.50 Pathological fracture in neoplastic disease, unspecified site** CC
✓6th **M84.51 Pathological fracture in neoplastic disease, shoulder**
3 ✓7th **M84.511 Pathological fracture in neoplastic disease, right shoulder** CC
3 ✓7th **M84.512 Pathological fracture in neoplastic disease, left shoulder** CC
3 ✓7th **M84.519 Pathological fracture in neoplastic disease, unspecified shoulder** CC
✓6th **M84.52 Pathological fracture in neoplastic disease, humerus**
3 ✓7th **M84.521 Pathological fracture in neoplastic disease, right humerus** CC
3 ✓7th **M84.522 Pathological fracture in neoplastic disease, left humerus** CC
3 ✓7th **M84.529 Pathological fracture in neoplastic disease, unspecified humerus** CC
✓6th **M84.53 Pathological fracture in neoplastic disease, ulna and radius**
3 ✓7th **M84.531 Pathological fracture in neoplastic disease, right ulna** CC
3 ✓7th **M84.532 Pathological fracture in neoplastic disease, left ulna** CC
3 ✓7th **M84.533 Pathological fracture in neoplastic disease, right radius** CC
3 ✓7th **M84.534 Pathological fracture in neoplastic disease, left radius** CC
3 ✓7th **M84.539 Pathological fracture in neoplastic disease, unspecified ulna and radius** CC
✓6th **M84.54 Pathological fracture in neoplastic disease, hand**
3 ✓7th **M84.541 Pathological fracture in neoplastic disease, right hand** CC
3 ✓7th **M84.542 Pathological fracture in neoplastic disease, left hand** CC
3 ✓7th **M84.549 Pathological fracture in neoplastic disease, unspecified hand** CC
✓6th **M84.55 Pathological fracture in neoplastic disease, pelvis and femur**
3 ✓7th **M84.550 Pathological fracture in neoplastic disease, pelvis** CC
3,6 ✓7th **M84.551 Pathological fracture in neoplastic disease, right femur** CC HCC
3,6 ✓7th **M84.552 Pathological fracture in neoplastic disease, left femur** CC HCC
3,6 ✓7th **M84.553 Pathological fracture in neoplastic disease, unspecified femur** CC HCC
3,6 ✓7th **M84.559 Pathological fracture in neoplastic disease, hip, unspecified** CC HCC

√6th **M84.56 Pathological fracture in neoplastic disease, tibia and fibula**
- 3 √7th **M84.561 Pathological fracture in neoplastic disease, right tibia** CC
- 3 √7th **M84.562 Pathological fracture in neoplastic disease, left tibia** CC
- 3 √7th **M84.563 Pathological fracture in neoplastic disease, right fibula** CC
- 3 √7th **M84.564 Pathological fracture in neoplastic disease, left fibula** CC
- 3 √7th **M84.569 Pathological fracture in neoplastic disease, unspecified tibia and fibula** CC

√6th **M84.57 Pathological fracture in neoplastic disease, ankle and foot**
- 3 √7th **M84.571 Pathological fracture in neoplastic disease, right ankle** CC
- 3 √7th **M84.572 Pathological fracture in neoplastic disease, left ankle** CC
- 3 √7th **M84.573 Pathological fracture in neoplastic disease, unspecified ankle** CC
- 3 √7th **M84.574 Pathological fracture in neoplastic disease, right foot** CC
- 3 √7th **M84.575 Pathological fracture in neoplastic disease, left foot** CC
- 3 √7th **M84.576 Pathological fracture in neoplastic disease, unspecified foot** CC

3 √x7th **M84.58 Pathological fracture in neoplastic disease, other specified site** CC

Pathological fracture in neoplastic disease, vertebrae

√5th **M84.6 Pathological fracture in other disease**

Code also underlying condition

EXCLUDES 1 *pathological fracture in osteoporosis (M80.-)*

The appropriate 7th character is to be added to each code from subcategory M84.6.
- A initial encounter for fracture
- D subsequent encounter for fracture with routine healing
- G subsequent encounter for fracture with delayed healing
- K subsequent encounter for fracture with nonunion
- P subsequent encounter for fracture with malunion
- S sequela

3 √x7th **M84.60 Pathological fracture in other disease, unspecified site** CC

√6th **M84.61 Pathological fracture in other disease, shoulder**
- 3 √7th **M84.611 Pathological fracture in other disease, right shoulder** CC
- 3 √7th **M84.612 Pathological fracture in other disease, left shoulder** CC
- 3 √7th **M84.619 Pathological fracture in other disease, unspecified shoulder** CC

√6th **M84.62 Pathological fracture in other disease, humerus**
- 3 √7th **M84.621 Pathological fracture in other disease, right humerus** CC
- 3 √7th **M84.622 Pathological fracture in other disease, left humerus** CC
- 3 √7th **M84.629 Pathological fracture in other disease, unspecified humerus** CC

√6th **M84.63 Pathological fracture in other disease, ulna and radius**
- 3 √7th **M84.631 Pathological fracture in other disease, right ulna** CC
- 3 √7th **M84.632 Pathological fracture in other disease, left ulna** CC
- 3 √7th **M84.633 Pathological fracture in other disease, right radius** CC
- 3 √7th **M84.634 Pathological fracture in other disease, left radius** CC
- 3 √7th **M84.639 Pathological fracture in other disease, unspecified ulna and radius** CC

√6th **M84.64 Pathological fracture in other disease, hand**
- 3 √7th **M84.641 Pathological fracture in other disease, right hand** CC
- 3 √7th **M84.642 Pathological fracture in other disease, left hand** CC
- 3 √7th **M84.649 Pathological fracture in other disease, unspecified hand** CC

√6th **M84.65 Pathological fracture in other disease, pelvis and femur**
- 3 √7th **M84.650 Pathological fracture in other disease, pelvis** CC
- 3,6 √7th **M84.651 Pathological fracture in other disease, right femur** CC HCC
- 3,6 √7th **M84.652 Pathological fracture in other disease, left femur** CC HCC
- 3,6 √7th **M84.653 Pathological fracture in other disease, unspecified femur** CC HCC
- 3,6 √7th **M84.659 Pathological fracture in other disease, hip, unspecified** CC HCC

√6th **M84.66 Pathological fracture in other disease, tibia and fibula**
- 3 √7th **M84.661 Pathological fracture in other disease, right tibia** CC
- 3 √7th **M84.662 Pathological fracture in other disease, left tibia** CC
- 3 √7th **M84.663 Pathological fracture in other disease, right fibula** CC
- 3 √7th **M84.664 Pathological fracture in other disease, left fibula** CC
- 3 √7th **M84.669 Pathological fracture in other disease, unspecified tibia and fibula** CC

√6th **M84.67 Pathological fracture in other disease, ankle and foot**
- 3 √7th **M84.671 Pathological fracture in other disease, right ankle** CC
- 3 √7th **M84.672 Pathological fracture in other disease, left ankle** CC
- 3 √7th **M84.673 Pathological fracture in other disease, unspecified ankle** CC
- 3 √7th **M84.674 Pathological fracture in other disease, right foot** CC
- 3 √7th **M84.675 Pathological fracture in other disease, left foot** CC
- 3 √7th **M84.676 Pathological fracture in other disease, unspecified foot** CC

3 √x7th **M84.68 Pathological fracture in other disease, other site** CC

√5th **M84.7 Nontraumatic fracture, not elsewhere classified**

√6th **M84.75 Atypical femoral fracture**

AHA: 2016,4Q,41-42

The appropriate 7th character is to be added to each code from M84.75.
- A initial encounter for fracture
- D subsequent encounter for fracture with routine healing
- G subsequent encounter for fracture with delayed healing
- K subsequent encounter for fracture with nonunion
- P subsequent encounter for fracture with malunion
- S sequela

- 3 √7th **M84.750 Atypical femoral fracture, unspecified** CC
- 3 √7th **M84.751 Incomplete atypical femoral fracture, right leg** CC
- 3 √7th **M84.752 Incomplete atypical femoral fracture, left leg** CC
- 3 √7th **M84.753 Incomplete atypical femoral fracture, unspecified leg** CC
- 3,6 √7th **M84.754 Complete transverse atypical femoral fracture, right leg** CC HCC
- 3,6 √7th **M84.755 Complete transverse atypical femoral fracture, left leg** CC HCC
- 3,6 √7th **M84.756 Complete transverse atypical femoral fracture, unspecified leg** CC HCC
- 3,6 √7th **M84.757 Complete oblique atypical femoral fracture, right leg** CC HCC
- 3,6 √7th **M84.758 Complete oblique atypical femoral fracture, left leg** CC HCC
- 3,6 √7th **M84.759 Complete oblique atypical femoral fracture, unspecified leg** CC HCC

√5th **M84.8 Other disorders of continuity of bone**

M84.80 Other disorders of continuity of bone, unspecified site

√6th **M84.81 Other disorders of continuity of bone, shoulder**
- **M84.811 Other disorders of continuity of bone, right shoulder**
- **M84.812 Other disorders of continuity of bone, left shoulder**
- **M84.819 Other disorders of continuity of bone, unspecified shoulder**

√6th **M84.82 Other disorders of continuity of bone, humerus**
- **M84.821 Other disorders of continuity of bone, right humerus**
- **M84.822 Other disorders of continuity of bone, left humerus**
- **M84.829 Other disorders of continuity of bone, unspecified humerus**

√6th **M84.83 Other disorders of continuity of bone, ulna and radius**
- **M84.831 Other disorders of continuity of bone, right ulna**
- **M84.832 Other disorders of continuity of bone, left ulna**
- **M84.833 Other disorders of continuity of bone, right radius**
- **M84.834 Other disorders of continuity of bone, left radius**
- **M84.839 Other disorders of continuity of bone, unspecified ulna and radius**

√6th **M84.84 Other disorders of continuity of bone, hand**
- **M84.841 Other disorders of continuity of bone, right hand**
- **M84.842 Other disorders of continuity of bone, left hand**
- **M84.849 Other disorders of continuity of bone, unspecified hand**

√6th **M84.85 Other disorders of continuity of bone, pelvic region and thigh**
- **M84.851 Other disorders of continuity of bone, right pelvic region and thigh**
- **M84.852 Other disorders of continuity of bone, left pelvic region and thigh**
- **M84.859 Other disorders of continuity of bone, unspecified pelvic region and thigh**

√6th **M84.86 Other disorders of continuity of bone, tibia and fibula**
- **M84.861 Other disorders of continuity of bone, right tibia**
- **M84.862 Other disorders of continuity of bone, left tibia**
- **M84.863 Other disorders of continuity of bone, right fibula**
- **M84.864 Other disorders of continuity of bone, left fibula**
- **M84.869 Other disorders of continuity of bone, unspecified tibia and fibula**

√6th **M84.87 Other disorders of continuity of bone, ankle and foot**
- **M84.871 Other disorders of continuity of bone, right ankle and foot**
- **M84.872 Other disorders of continuity of bone, left ankle and foot**
- **M84.879 Other disorders of continuity of bone, unspecified ankle and foot**

M84.88 Other disorders of continuity of bone, other site

M84.9 Disorder of continuity of bone, unspecified

√4th M85 Other disorders of bone density and structure

EXCLUDES 1 *osteogenesis imperfecta (Q78.Ø)*
osteopetrosis (Q78.2)
osteopoikilosis (Q78.8)
polyostotic fibrous dysplasia (Q78.1)

√5th **M85.Ø Fibrous dysplasia (monostotic)**

EXCLUDES 2 *fibrous dysplasia of jaw (M27.8)*

M85.ØØ Fibrous dysplasia (monostotic), unspecified site

√6th **M85.Ø1 Fibrous dysplasia (monostotic), shoulder**
- **M85.Ø11 Fibrous dysplasia (monostotic), right shoulder**
- **M85.Ø12 Fibrous dysplasia (monostotic), left shoulder**
- **M85.Ø19 Fibrous dysplasia (monostotic), unspecified shoulder**

√6th **M85.Ø2 Fibrous dysplasia (monostotic), upper arm**
- **M85.Ø21 Fibrous dysplasia (monostotic), right upper arm**
- **M85.Ø22 Fibrous dysplasia (monostotic), left upper arm**
- **M85.Ø29 Fibrous dysplasia (monostotic), unspecified upper arm**

√6th **M85.Ø3 Fibrous dysplasia (monostotic), forearm**
- **M85.Ø31 Fibrous dysplasia (monostotic), right forearm**
- **M85.Ø32 Fibrous dysplasia (monostotic), left forearm**
- **M85.Ø39 Fibrous dysplasia (monostotic), unspecified forearm**

√6th **M85.Ø4 Fibrous dysplasia (monostotic), hand**
- **M85.Ø41 Fibrous dysplasia (monostotic), right hand**
- **M85.Ø42 Fibrous dysplasia (monostotic), left hand**
- **M85.Ø49 Fibrous dysplasia (monostotic), unspecified hand**

√6th **M85.Ø5 Fibrous dysplasia (monostotic), thigh**
- **M85.Ø51 Fibrous dysplasia (monostotic), right thigh**
- **M85.Ø52 Fibrous dysplasia (monostotic), left thigh**
- **M85.Ø59 Fibrous dysplasia (monostotic), unspecified thigh**

√6th **M85.Ø6 Fibrous dysplasia (monostotic), lower leg**
- **M85.Ø61 Fibrous dysplasia (monostotic), right lower leg**
- **M85.Ø62 Fibrous dysplasia (monostotic), left lower leg**
- **M85.Ø69 Fibrous dysplasia (monostotic), unspecified lower leg**

√6th **M85.Ø7 Fibrous dysplasia (monostotic), ankle and foot**
- **M85.Ø71 Fibrous dysplasia (monostotic), right ankle and foot**
- **M85.Ø72 Fibrous dysplasia (monostotic), left ankle and foot**
- **M85.Ø79 Fibrous dysplasia (monostotic), unspecified ankle and foot**

M85.Ø8 Fibrous dysplasia (monostotic), other site

M85.Ø9 Fibrous dysplasia (monostotic), multiple sites

√5th **M85.1 Skeletal fluorosis**

M85.1Ø Skeletal fluorosis, unspecified site

√6th **M85.11 Skeletal fluorosis, shoulder**
- **M85.111 Skeletal fluorosis, right shoulder**
- **M85.112 Skeletal fluorosis, left shoulder**
- **M85.119 Skeletal fluorosis, unspecified shoulder**

√6th **M85.12 Skeletal fluorosis, upper arm**
- **M85.121 Skeletal fluorosis, right upper arm**
- **M85.122 Skeletal fluorosis, left upper arm**
- **M85.129 Skeletal fluorosis, unspecified upper arm**

√6th **M85.13 Skeletal fluorosis, forearm**
- **M85.131 Skeletal fluorosis, right forearm**
- **M85.132 Skeletal fluorosis, left forearm**
- **M85.139 Skeletal fluorosis, unspecified forearm**

√6th **M85.14 Skeletal fluorosis, hand**
- **M85.141 Skeletal fluorosis, right hand**
- **M85.142 Skeletal fluorosis, left hand**
- **M85.149 Skeletal fluorosis, unspecified hand**

√6th **M85.15 Skeletal fluorosis, thigh**
- **M85.151 Skeletal fluorosis, right thigh**
- **M85.152 Skeletal fluorosis, left thigh**
- **M85.159 Skeletal fluorosis, unspecified thigh**

√6th **M85.16 Skeletal fluorosis, lower leg**
- **M85.161 Skeletal fluorosis, right lower leg**
- **M85.162 Skeletal fluorosis, left lower leg**
- **M85.169 Skeletal fluorosis, unspecified lower leg**

√6th **M85.17 Skeletal fluorosis, ankle and foot**
- **M85.171 Skeletal fluorosis, right ankle and foot**
- **M85.172 Skeletal fluorosis, left ankle and foot**
- **M85.179 Skeletal fluorosis, unspecified ankle and foot**

M85.18 Skeletal fluorosis, other site

M85.19 Skeletal fluorosis, multiple sites

M85.2 Hyperostosis of skull
DEF: Abnormal bone growth on the inner aspect of the cranial bones.

✓5th **M85.3 Osteitis condensans**
M85.30 Osteitis condensans, unspecified site
✓6th **M85.31 Osteitis condensans, shoulder**
M85.311 Osteitis condensans, right shoulder
M85.312 Osteitis condensans, left shoulder
M85.319 Osteitis condensans, unspecified shoulder
✓6th **M85.32 Osteitis condensans, upper arm**
M85.321 Osteitis condensans, right upper arm
M85.322 Osteitis condensans, left upper arm
M85.329 Osteitis condensans, unspecified upper arm
✓6th **M85.33 Osteitis condensans, forearm**
M85.331 Osteitis condensans, right forearm
M85.332 Osteitis condensans, left forearm
M85.339 Osteitis condensans, unspecified forearm
✓6th **M85.34 Osteitis condensans, hand**
M85.341 Osteitis condensans, right hand
M85.342 Osteitis condensans, left hand
M85.349 Osteitis condensans, unspecified hand
✓6th **M85.35 Osteitis condensans, thigh**
M85.351 Osteitis condensans, right thigh
M85.352 Osteitis condensans, left thigh
M85.359 Osteitis condensans, unspecified thigh
✓6th **M85.36 Osteitis condensans, lower leg**
M85.361 Osteitis condensans, right lower leg
M85.362 Osteitis condensans, left lower leg
M85.369 Osteitis condensans, unspecified lower leg
✓6th **M85.37 Osteitis condensans, ankle and foot**
M85.371 Osteitis condensans, right ankle and foot
M85.372 Osteitis condensans, left ankle and foot
M85.379 Osteitis condensans, unspecified ankle and foot
M85.38 Osteitis condensans, other site
M85.39 Osteitis condensans, multiple sites

✓5th **M85.4 Solitary bone cyst**
EXCLUDES 2 *solitary cyst of jaw (M27.4)*
M85.40 Solitary bone cyst, unspecified site
✓6th **M85.41 Solitary bone cyst, shoulder**
M85.411 Solitary bone cyst, right shoulder
M85.412 Solitary bone cyst, left shoulder
M85.419 Solitary bone cyst, unspecified shoulder
✓6th **M85.42 Solitary bone cyst, humerus**
M85.421 Solitary bone cyst, right humerus
M85.422 Solitary bone cyst, left humerus
M85.429 Solitary bone cyst, unspecified humerus
✓6th **M85.43 Solitary bone cyst, ulna and radius**
M85.431 Solitary bone cyst, right ulna and radius
M85.432 Solitary bone cyst, left ulna and radius
M85.439 Solitary bone cyst, unspecified ulna and radius
✓6th **M85.44 Solitary bone cyst, hand**
M85.441 Solitary bone cyst, right hand
M85.442 Solitary bone cyst, left hand
M85.449 Solitary bone cyst, unspecified hand
✓6th **M85.45 Solitary bone cyst, pelvis**
M85.451 Solitary bone cyst, right pelvis
M85.452 Solitary bone cyst, left pelvis
M85.459 Solitary bone cyst, unspecified pelvis
✓6th **M85.46 Solitary bone cyst, tibia and fibula**
M85.461 Solitary bone cyst, right tibia and fibula
M85.462 Solitary bone cyst, left tibia and fibula
M85.469 Solitary bone cyst, unspecified tibia and fibula
✓6th **M85.47 Solitary bone cyst, ankle and foot**
M85.471 Solitary bone cyst, right ankle and foot
M85.472 Solitary bone cyst, left ankle and foot
M85.479 Solitary bone cyst, unspecified ankle and foot
M85.48 Solitary bone cyst, other site

✓5th **M85.5 Aneurysmal bone cyst**
EXCLUDES 2 *aneurysmal cyst of jaw (M27.4)*
DEF: Solitary bone lesion that bulges into the periosteum and is marked by a calcified rim.
M85.50 Aneurysmal bone cyst, unspecified site
✓6th **M85.51 Aneurysmal bone cyst, shoulder**
M85.511 Aneurysmal bone cyst, right shoulder
M85.512 Aneurysmal bone cyst, left shoulder
M85.519 Aneurysmal bone cyst, unspecified shoulder
✓6th **M85.52 Aneurysmal bone cyst, upper arm**
M85.521 Aneurysmal bone cyst, right upper arm
M85.522 Aneurysmal bone cyst, left upper arm
M85.529 Aneurysmal bone cyst, unspecified upper arm
✓6th **M85.53 Aneurysmal bone cyst, forearm**
M85.531 Aneurysmal bone cyst, right forearm
M85.532 Aneurysmal bone cyst, left forearm
M85.539 Aneurysmal bone cyst, unspecified forearm
✓6th **M85.54 Aneurysmal bone cyst, hand**
M85.541 Aneurysmal bone cyst, right hand
M85.542 Aneurysmal bone cyst, left hand
M85.549 Aneurysmal bone cyst, unspecified hand
✓6th **M85.55 Aneurysmal bone cyst, thigh**
M85.551 Aneurysmal bone cyst, right thigh
M85.552 Aneurysmal bone cyst, left thigh
M85.559 Aneurysmal bone cyst, unspecified thigh
✓6th **M85.56 Aneurysmal bone cyst, lower leg**
M85.561 Aneurysmal bone cyst, right lower leg
M85.562 Aneurysmal bone cyst, left lower leg
M85.569 Aneurysmal bone cyst, unspecified lower leg
✓6th **M85.57 Aneurysmal bone cyst, ankle and foot**
M85.571 Aneurysmal bone cyst, right ankle and foot
M85.572 Aneurysmal bone cyst, left ankle and foot
M85.579 Aneurysmal bone cyst, unspecified ankle and foot
M85.58 Aneurysmal bone cyst, other site
M85.59 Aneurysmal bone cyst, multiple sites

✓5th **M85.6 Other cyst of bone**
EXCLUDES 1 *cyst of jaw NEC (M27.4)*
osteitis fibrosa cystica generalisata [von Recklinghausen's disease of bone] (E21.0)
M85.60 Other cyst of bone, unspecified site
✓6th **M85.61 Other cyst of bone, shoulder**
M85.611 Other cyst of bone, right shoulder
M85.612 Other cyst of bone, left shoulder
M85.619 Other cyst of bone, unspecified shoulder
✓6th **M85.62 Other cyst of bone, upper arm**
M85.621 Other cyst of bone, right upper arm
M85.622 Other cyst of bone, left upper arm
M85.629 Other cyst of bone, unspecified upper arm
✓6th **M85.63 Other cyst of bone, forearm**
M85.631 Other cyst of bone, right forearm
M85.632 Other cyst of bone, left forearm
M85.639 Other cyst of bone, unspecified forearm
✓6th **M85.64 Other cyst of bone, hand**
M85.641 Other cyst of bone, right hand
M85.642 Other cyst of bone, left hand
M85.649 Other cyst of bone, unspecified hand
✓6th **M85.65 Other cyst of bone, thigh**
M85.651 Other cyst of bone, right thigh
M85.652 Other cyst of bone, left thigh
M85.659 Other cyst of bone, unspecified thigh
✓6th **M85.66 Other cyst of bone, lower leg**
M85.661 Other cyst of bone, right lower leg
M85.662 Other cyst of bone, left lower leg
M85.669 Other cyst of bone, unspecified lower leg
✓6th **M85.67 Other cyst of bone, ankle and foot**
M85.671 Other cyst of bone, right ankle and foot
M85.672 Other cyst of bone, left ankle and foot
M85.679 Other cyst of bone, unspecified ankle and foot
M85.68 Other cyst of bone, other site

M85.69 **Other cyst of bone, multiple sites**

✓5th **M85.8** **Other specified disorders of bone density and structure**

Hyperostosis of bones, except skull
Osteosclerosis, acquired

EXCLUDES 1 *diffuse idiopathic skeletal hyperostosis [DISH] (M48.1)*
osteosclerosis congenita (Q77.4)
osteosclerosis fragilitas (generalista) (Q78.2)
osteosclerosis myelofibrosis (D75.81)

M85.80 **Other specified disorders of bone density and structure, unspecified site**

✓6th **M85.81** **Other specified disorders of bone density and structure, shoulder**

M85.811 **Other specified disorders of bone density and structure, right shoulder**

M85.812 **Other specified disorders of bone density and structure, left shoulder**

M85.819 **Other specified disorders of bone density and structure, unspecified shoulder**

✓6th **M85.82** **Other specified disorders of bone density and structure, upper arm**

M85.821 **Other specified disorders of bone density and structure, right upper arm**

M85.822 **Other specified disorders of bone density and structure, left upper arm**

M85.829 **Other specified disorders of bone density and structure, unspecified upper arm**

✓6th **M85.83** **Other specified disorders of bone density and structure, forearm**

M85.831 **Other specified disorders of bone density and structure, right forearm**

M85.832 **Other specified disorders of bone density and structure, left forearm**

M85.839 **Other specified disorders of bone density and structure, unspecified forearm**

✓6th **M85.84** **Other specified disorders of bone density and structure, hand**

M85.841 **Other specified disorders of bone density and structure, right hand**

M85.842 **Other specified disorders of bone density and structure, left hand**

M85.849 **Other specified disorders of bone density and structure, unspecified hand**

✓6th **M85.85** **Other specified disorders of bone density and structure, thigh**

M85.851 **Other specified disorders of bone density and structure, right thigh**

M85.852 **Other specified disorders of bone density and structure, left thigh**

M85.859 **Other specified disorders of bone density and structure, unspecified thigh**

✓6th **M85.86** **Other specified disorders of bone density and structure, lower leg**

M85.861 **Other specified disorders of bone density and structure, right lower leg**

M85.862 **Other specified disorders of bone density and structure, left lower leg**

M85.869 **Other specified disorders of bone density and structure, unspecified lower leg**

✓6th **M85.87** **Other specified disorders of bone density and structure, ankle and foot**

M85.871 **Other specified disorders of bone density and structure, right ankle and foot**

M85.872 **Other specified disorders of bone density and structure, left ankle and foot**

M85.879 **Other specified disorders of bone density and structure, unspecified ankle and foot**

M85.88 **Other specified disorders of bone density and structure, other site**

M85.89 **Other specified disorders of bone density and structure, multiple sites**

M85.9 **Disorder of bone density and structure, unspecified**

Other osteopathies (M86-M90)

EXCLUDES 1 *postprocedural osteopathies (M96.-)*

✓4th **M86** **Osteomyelitis**

Use additional code (B95-B97) to identify infectious agent
Use additional code to identify major osseous defect, if applicable (M89.7-)

EXCLUDES 1 *osteomyelitis due to:*
echinococcus (B67.2)
gonococcus (A54.43)
salmonella (A02.24)

EXCLUDES 2 *ostemyelitis of:*
orbit (H05.0-)
petrous bone (H70.2-)
vertebra (M46.2-)

✓5th **M86.0** **Acute hematogenous osteomyelitis**

M86.00 **Acute hematogenous osteomyelitis, unspecified site** CC HCC

✓6th **M86.01** **Acute hematogenous osteomyelitis, shoulder**

M86.011 **Acute hematogenous osteomyelitis, right shoulder** CC HCC

M86.012 **Acute hematogenous osteomyelitis, left shoulder** CC HCC

M86.019 **Acute hematogenous osteomyelitis, unspecified shoulder** CC HCC

✓6th **M86.02** **Acute hematogenous osteomyelitis, humerus**

M86.021 **Acute hematogenous osteomyelitis, right humerus** CC HCC

M86.022 **Acute hematogenous osteomyelitis, left humerus** CC HCC

M86.029 **Acute hematogenous osteomyelitis, unspecified humerus** CC HCC

✓6th **M86.03** **Acute hematogenous osteomyelitis, radius and ulna**

M86.031 **Acute hematogenous osteomyelitis, right radius and ulna** CC HCC

M86.032 **Acute hematogenous osteomyelitis, left radius and ulna** CC HCC

M86.039 **Acute hematogenous osteomyelitis, unspecified radius and ulna** CC HCC

✓6th **M86.04** **Acute hematogenous osteomyelitis, hand**

M86.041 **Acute hematogenous osteomyelitis, right hand** CC HCC

M86.042 **Acute hematogenous osteomyelitis, left hand** CC HCC

M86.049 **Acute hematogenous osteomyelitis, unspecified hand** CC HCC

✓6th **M86.05** **Acute hematogenous osteomyelitis, femur**

M86.051 **Acute hematogenous osteomyelitis, right femur** CC HCC

M86.052 **Acute hematogenous osteomyelitis, left femur** CC HCC

M86.059 **Acute hematogenous osteomyelitis, unspecified femur** CC HCC

✓6th **M86.06** **Acute hematogenous osteomyelitis, tibia and fibula**

M86.061 **Acute hematogenous osteomyelitis, right tibia and fibula** CC HCC

M86.062 **Acute hematogenous osteomyelitis, left tibia and fibula** CC HCC

M86.069 **Acute hematogenous osteomyelitis, unspecified tibia and fibula** CC HCC

✓6th **M86.07** **Acute hematogenous osteomyelitis, ankle and foot**

M86.071 **Acute hematogenous osteomyelitis, right ankle and foot** CC HCC

M86.072 **Acute hematogenous osteomyelitis, left ankle and foot** CC HCC

M86.079 **Acute hematogenous osteomyelitis, unspecified ankle and foot** CC HCC

M86.08 **Acute hematogenous osteomyelitis, other sites** CC HCC

M86.09 **Acute hematogenous osteomyelitis, multiple sites** CC HCC

✓5th **M86.1** **Other acute osteomyelitis**

M86.10 **Other acute osteomyelitis, unspecified site** CC HCC

M86.11 Other acute osteomyelitis, shoulder
M86.111 Other acute osteomyelitis, right shoulder CC HCC
M86.112 Other acute osteomyelitis, left shoulder CC HCC
M86.119 Other acute osteomyelitis, unspecified shoulder CC HCC
M86.12 Other acute osteomyelitis, humerus
M86.121 Other acute osteomyelitis, right humerus CC HCC
M86.122 Other acute osteomyelitis, left humerus CC HCC
M86.129 Other acute osteomyelitis, unspecified humerus CC HCC
M86.13 Other acute osteomyelitis, radius and ulna
M86.131 Other acute osteomyelitis, right radius and ulna CC HCC
M86.132 Other acute osteomyelitis, left radius and ulna CC HCC
M86.139 Other acute osteomyelitis, unspecified radius and ulna CC HCC
M86.14 Other acute osteomyelitis, hand
M86.141 Other acute osteomyelitis, right hand CC HCC
M86.142 Other acute osteomyelitis, left hand CC HCC
M86.149 Other acute osteomyelitis, unspecified hand CC HCC
M86.15 Other acute osteomyelitis, femur
M86.151 Other acute osteomyelitis, right femur CC HCC
M86.152 Other acute osteomyelitis, left femur CC HCC
M86.159 Other acute osteomyelitis, unspecified femur CC HCC
M86.16 Other acute osteomyelitis, tibia and fibula
M86.161 Other acute osteomyelitis, right tibia and fibula CC HCC
M86.162 Other acute osteomyelitis, left tibia and fibula CC HCC
M86.169 Other acute osteomyelitis, unspecified tibia and fibula CC HCC
M86.17 Other acute osteomyelitis, ankle and foot
AHA: 2020,1Q,12
M86.171 Other acute osteomyelitis, right ankle and foot CC HCC
M86.172 Other acute osteomyelitis, left ankle and foot CC HCC
M86.179 Other acute osteomyelitis, unspecified ankle and foot CC HCC
M86.18 Other acute osteomyelitis, other site CC HCC
M86.19 Other acute osteomyelitis, multiple sites CC HCC
M86.2 Subacute osteomyelitis
M86.2Ø Subacute osteomyelitis, unspecified site CC HCC
M86.21 Subacute osteomyelitis, shoulder
M86.211 Subacute osteomyelitis, right shoulder CC HCC
M86.212 Subacute osteomyelitis, left shoulder CC HCC
M86.219 Subacute osteomyelitis, unspecified shoulder CC HCC
M86.22 Subacute osteomyelitis, humerus
M86.221 Subacute osteomyelitis, right humerus CC HCC
M86.222 Subacute osteomyelitis, left humerus CC HCC
M86.229 Subacute osteomyelitis, unspecified humerus CC HCC
M86.23 Subacute osteomyelitis, radius and ulna
M86.231 Subacute osteomyelitis, right radius and ulna CC HCC
M86.232 Subacute osteomyelitis, left radius and ulna CC HCC
M86.239 Subacute osteomyelitis, unspecified radius and ulna CC HCC
M86.24 Subacute osteomyelitis, hand
M86.241 Subacute osteomyelitis, right hand CC HCC
M86.242 Subacute osteomyelitis, left hand CC HCC
M86.249 Subacute osteomyelitis, unspecified hand CC HCC
M86.25 Subacute osteomyelitis, femur
M86.251 Subacute osteomyelitis, right femur CC HCC
M86.252 Subacute osteomyelitis, left femur CC HCC
M86.259 Subacute osteomyelitis, unspecified femur CC HCC
M86.26 Subacute osteomyelitis, tibia and fibula
M86.261 Subacute osteomyelitis, right tibia and fibula CC HCC
M86.262 Subacute osteomyelitis, left tibia and fibula CC HCC
M86.269 Subacute osteomyelitis, unspecified tibia and fibula CC HCC
M86.27 Subacute osteomyelitis, ankle and foot
M86.271 Subacute osteomyelitis, right ankle and foot CC HCC
M86.272 Subacute osteomyelitis, left ankle and foot CC HCC
M86.279 Subacute osteomyelitis, unspecified ankle and foot CC HCC
M86.28 Subacute osteomyelitis, other site CC HCC
M86.29 Subacute osteomyelitis, multiple sites CC HCC
M86.3 Chronic multifocal osteomyelitis
M86.3Ø Chronic multifocal osteomyelitis, unspecified site CC HCC
M86.31 Chronic multifocal osteomyelitis, shoulder
M86.311 Chronic multifocal osteomyelitis, right shoulder CC HCC
M86.312 Chronic multifocal osteomyelitis, left shoulder CC HCC
M86.319 Chronic multifocal osteomyelitis, unspecified shoulder CC HCC
M86.32 Chronic multifocal osteomyelitis, humerus
M86.321 Chronic multifocal osteomyelitis, right humerus CC HCC
M86.322 Chronic multifocal osteomyelitis, left humerus CC HCC
M86.329 Chronic multifocal osteomyelitis, unspecified humerus CC HCC
M86.33 Chronic multifocal osteomyelitis, radius and ulna
M86.331 Chronic multifocal osteomyelitis, right radius and ulna CC HCC
M86.332 Chronic multifocal osteomyelitis, left radius and ulna CC HCC
M86.339 Chronic multifocal osteomyelitis, unspecified radius and ulna CC HCC
M86.34 Chronic multifocal osteomyelitis, hand
M86.341 Chronic multifocal osteomyelitis, right hand CC HCC
M86.342 Chronic multifocal osteomyelitis, left hand CC HCC
M86.349 Chronic multifocal osteomyelitis, unspecified hand CC HCC
M86.35 Chronic multifocal osteomyelitis, femur
M86.351 Chronic multifocal osteomyelitis, right femur CC HCC
M86.352 Chronic multifocal osteomyelitis, left femur CC HCC
M86.359 Chronic multifocal osteomyelitis, unspecified femur CC HCC
M86.36 Chronic multifocal osteomyelitis, tibia and fibula
M86.361 Chronic multifocal osteomyelitis, right tibia and fibula CC HCC
M86.362 Chronic multifocal osteomyelitis, left tibia and fibula CC HCC
M86.369 Chronic multifocal osteomyelitis, unspecified tibia and fibula CC HCC
M86.37 Chronic multifocal osteomyelitis, ankle and foot
M86.371 Chronic multifocal osteomyelitis, right ankle and foot CC HCC
M86.372 Chronic multifocal osteomyelitis, left ankle and foot CC HCC

M86.379 Chronic multifocal osteomyelitis, unspecified ankle and foot CC HCC
M86.38 Chronic multifocal osteomyelitis, other site CC HCC
M86.39 Chronic multifocal osteomyelitis, multiple sites CC HCC

5th M86.4 Chronic osteomyelitis with draining sinus
M86.40 Chronic osteomyelitis with draining sinus, unspecified site CC HCC
6th M86.41 Chronic osteomyelitis with draining sinus, shoulder
M86.411 Chronic osteomyelitis with draining sinus, right shoulder CC HCC
M86.412 Chronic osteomyelitis with draining sinus, left shoulder CC HCC
M86.419 Chronic osteomyelitis with draining sinus, unspecified shoulder CC HCC
6th M86.42 Chronic osteomyelitis with draining sinus, humerus
M86.421 Chronic osteomyelitis with draining sinus, right humerus CC HCC
M86.422 Chronic osteomyelitis with draining sinus, left humerus CC HCC
M86.429 Chronic osteomyelitis with draining sinus, unspecified humerus CC HCC
6th M86.43 Chronic osteomyelitis with draining sinus, radius and ulna
M86.431 Chronic osteomyelitis with draining sinus, right radius and ulna CC HCC
M86.432 Chronic osteomyelitis with draining sinus, left radius and ulna CC HCC
M86.439 Chronic osteomyelitis with draining sinus, unspecified radius and ulna CC HCC
6th M86.44 Chronic osteomyelitis with draining sinus, hand
M86.441 Chronic osteomyelitis with draining sinus, right hand CC HCC
M86.442 Chronic osteomyelitis with draining sinus, left hand CC HCC
M86.449 Chronic osteomyelitis with draining sinus, unspecified hand CC HCC
6th M86.45 Chronic osteomyelitis with draining sinus, femur
M86.451 Chronic osteomyelitis with draining sinus, right femur CC HCC
M86.452 Chronic osteomyelitis with draining sinus, left femur CC HCC
M86.459 Chronic osteomyelitis with draining sinus, unspecified femur CC HCC
6th M86.46 Chronic osteomyelitis with draining sinus, tibia and fibula
M86.461 Chronic osteomyelitis with draining sinus, right tibia and fibula CC HCC
M86.462 Chronic osteomyelitis with draining sinus, left tibia and fibula CC HCC
M86.469 Chronic osteomyelitis with draining sinus, unspecified tibia and fibula CC HCC
6th M86.47 Chronic osteomyelitis with draining sinus, ankle and foot
M86.471 Chronic osteomyelitis with draining sinus, right ankle and foot CC HCC
M86.472 Chronic osteomyelitis with draining sinus, left ankle and foot CC HCC
M86.479 Chronic osteomyelitis with draining sinus, unspecified ankle and foot CC HCC
M86.48 Chronic osteomyelitis with draining sinus, other site CC HCC
M86.49 Chronic osteomyelitis with draining sinus, multiple sites CC HCC

5th M86.5 Other chronic hematogenous osteomyelitis
M86.50 Other chronic hematogenous osteomyelitis, unspecified site CC HCC
6th M86.51 Other chronic hematogenous osteomyelitis, shoulder
M86.511 Other chronic hematogenous osteomyelitis, right shoulder CC HCC
M86.512 Other chronic hematogenous osteomyelitis, left shoulder CC HCC
M86.519 Other chronic hematogenous osteomyelitis, unspecified shoulder CC HCC
6th M86.52 Other chronic hematogenous osteomyelitis, humerus
M86.521 Other chronic hematogenous osteomyelitis, right humerus CC HCC
M86.522 Other chronic hematogenous osteomyelitis, left humerus CC HCC
M86.529 Other chronic hematogenous osteomyelitis, unspecified humerus CC HCC
6th M86.53 Other chronic hematogenous osteomyelitis, radius and ulna
M86.531 Other chronic hematogenous osteomyelitis, right radius and ulna CC HCC
M86.532 Other chronic hematogenous osteomyelitis, left radius and ulna CC HCC
M86.539 Other chronic hematogenous osteomyelitis, unspecified radius and ulna CC HCC
6th M86.54 Other chronic hematogenous osteomyelitis, hand
M86.541 Other chronic hematogenous osteomyelitis, right hand CC HCC
M86.542 Other chronic hematogenous osteomyelitis, left hand CC HCC
M86.549 Other chronic hematogenous osteomyelitis, unspecified hand CC HCC
6th M86.55 Other chronic hematogenous osteomyelitis, femur
M86.551 Other chronic hematogenous osteomyelitis, right femur CC HCC
M86.552 Other chronic hematogenous osteomyelitis, left femur CC HCC
M86.559 Other chronic hematogenous osteomyelitis, unspecified femur CC HCC
6th M86.56 Other chronic hematogenous osteomyelitis, tibia and fibula
M86.561 Other chronic hematogenous osteomyelitis, right tibia and fibula CC HCC
M86.562 Other chronic hematogenous osteomyelitis, left tibia and fibula CC HCC
M86.569 Other chronic hematogenous osteomyelitis, unspecified tibia and fibula CC HCC
6th M86.57 Other chronic hematogenous osteomyelitis, ankle and foot
M86.571 Other chronic hematogenous osteomyelitis, right ankle and foot CC HCC
M86.572 Other chronic hematogenous osteomyelitis, left ankle and foot CC HCC
M86.579 Other chronic hematogenous osteomyelitis, unspecified ankle and foot CC HCC
M86.58 Other chronic hematogenous osteomyelitis, other site CC HCC
M86.59 Other chronic hematogenous osteomyelitis, multiple sites CC HCC

5th M86.6 Other chronic osteomyelitis
M86.60 Other chronic osteomyelitis, unspecified site CC HCC
6th M86.61 Other chronic osteomyelitis, shoulder
M86.611 Other chronic osteomyelitis, right shoulder CC HCC
M86.612 Other chronic osteomyelitis, left shoulder CC HCC
M86.619 Other chronic osteomyelitis, unspecified shoulder CC HCC
6th M86.62 Other chronic osteomyelitis, humerus
M86.621 Other chronic osteomyelitis, right humerus CC HCC
M86.622 Other chronic osteomyelitis, left humerus CC HCC
M86.629 Other chronic osteomyelitis, unspecified humerus CC HCC

✓6th **M86.63 Other chronic osteomyelitis, radius and ulna**
- **M86.631 Other chronic osteomyelitis, right radius and ulna** CC HCC
- **M86.632 Other chronic osteomyelitis, left radius and ulna** CC HCC
- **M86.639 Other chronic osteomyelitis, unspecified radius and ulna** CC HCC

✓6th **M86.64 Other chronic osteomyelitis, hand**
- **M86.641 Other chronic osteomyelitis, right hand** CC HCC
- **M86.642 Other chronic osteomyelitis, left hand** CC HCC
- **M86.649 Other chronic osteomyelitis, unspecified hand** CC HCC

✓6th **M86.65 Other chronic osteomyelitis, thigh**
- **M86.651 Other chronic osteomyelitis, right thigh** CC HCC
- **M86.652 Other chronic osteomyelitis, left thigh** CC HCC
- **M86.659 Other chronic osteomyelitis, unspecified thigh** CC HCC

✓6th **M86.66 Other chronic osteomyelitis, tibia and fibula**
- **M86.661 Other chronic osteomyelitis, right tibia and fibula** CC HCC
- **M86.662 Other chronic osteomyelitis, left tibia and fibula** CC HCC
- **M86.669 Other chronic osteomyelitis, unspecified tibia and fibula** CC HCC

✓6th **M86.67 Other chronic osteomyelitis, ankle and foot**
- **M86.671 Other chronic osteomyelitis, right ankle and foot** CC HCC
  AHA: 2016,1Q,13
- **M86.672 Other chronic osteomyelitis, left ankle and foot** CC HCC
- **M86.679 Other chronic osteomyelitis, unspecified ankle and foot** CC HCC

M86.68 Other chronic osteomyelitis, other site CC HCC

M86.69 Other chronic osteomyelitis, multiple sites CC HCC

✓5th **M86.8 Other osteomyelitis**

Brodie's abscess

✓6th **M86.8X Other osteomyelitis**
- **M86.8X0 Other osteomyelitis, multiple sites** CC HCC
- **M86.8X1 Other osteomyelitis, shoulder** CC HCC
- **M86.8X2 Other osteomyelitis, upper arm** CC HCC
- **M86.8X3 Other osteomyelitis, forearm** CC HCC
- **M86.8X4 Other osteomyelitis, hand** CC HCC
- **M86.8X5 Other osteomyelitis, thigh** CC HCC
- **M86.8X6 Other osteomyelitis, lower leg** CC HCC
- **M86.8X7 Other osteomyelitis, ankle and foot** CC HCC
- **M86.8X8 Other osteomyelitis, other site** CC HCC
- **M86.8X9 Other osteomyelitis, unspecified sites** CC HCC

M86.9 Osteomyelitis, unspecified CC HCC

Infection of bone NOS

Periostitis without osteomyelitis

✓4th **M87 Osteonecrosis**

INCLUDES avascular necrosis of bone

Use additional code to identify major osseous defect, if applicable (M89.7-)

EXCLUDES 1 *juvenile osteonecrosis (M91-M92)*
osteochondropathies (M90-M93)

✓5th **M87.0 Idiopathic aseptic necrosis of bone**

M87.00 Idiopathic aseptic necrosis of unspecified bone CC HCC

✓6th **M87.01 Idiopathic aseptic necrosis of shoulder**

Idiopathic aseptic necrosis of clavicle and scapula
- **M87.011 Idiopathic aseptic necrosis of right shoulder** CC HCC
- **M87.012 Idiopathic aseptic necrosis of left shoulder** CC HCC
- **M87.019 Idiopathic aseptic necrosis of unspecified shoulder** CC HCC

✓6th **M87.02 Idiopathic aseptic necrosis of humerus**
- **M87.021 Idiopathic aseptic necrosis of right humerus** CC HCC
- **M87.022 Idiopathic aseptic necrosis of left humerus** CC HCC
- **M87.029 Idiopathic aseptic necrosis of unspecified humerus** CC HCC

✓6th **M87.03 Idiopathic aseptic necrosis of radius, ulna and carpus**
- **M87.031 Idiopathic aseptic necrosis of right radius** CC HCC
- **M87.032 Idiopathic aseptic necrosis of left radius** CC HCC
- **M87.033 Idiopathic aseptic necrosis of unspecified radius** CC HCC
- **M87.034 Idiopathic aseptic necrosis of right ulna** CC HCC
- **M87.035 Idiopathic aseptic necrosis of left ulna** CC HCC
- **M87.036 Idiopathic aseptic necrosis of unspecified ulna** CC HCC
- **M87.037 Idiopathic aseptic necrosis of right carpus** CC HCC
- **M87.038 Idiopathic aseptic necrosis of left carpus** CC HCC
- **M87.039 Idiopathic aseptic necrosis of unspecified carpus** CC HCC

✓6th **M87.04 Idiopathic aseptic necrosis of hand and fingers**

Idiopathic aseptic necrosis of metacarpals and phalanges of hands
- **M87.041 Idiopathic aseptic necrosis of right hand** CC HCC
- **M87.042 Idiopathic aseptic necrosis of left hand** CC HCC
- **M87.043 Idiopathic aseptic necrosis of unspecified hand** CC HCC
- **M87.044 Idiopathic aseptic necrosis of right finger(s)** CC HCC
- **M87.045 Idiopathic aseptic necrosis of left finger(s)** CC HCC
- **M87.046 Idiopathic aseptic necrosis of unspecified finger(s)** CC HCC

✓6th **M87.05 Idiopathic aseptic necrosis of pelvis and femur**
- **M87.050 Idiopathic aseptic necrosis of pelvis** CC HCC
- **M87.051 Idiopathic aseptic necrosis of right femur** CC HCC
- **M87.052 Idiopathic aseptic necrosis of left femur** CC HCC
- **M87.059 Idiopathic aseptic necrosis of unspecified femur** CC HCC

✓6th **M87.06 Idiopathic aseptic necrosis of tibia and fibula**
- **M87.061 Idiopathic aseptic necrosis of right tibia** CC HCC
- **M87.062 Idiopathic aseptic necrosis of left tibia** CC HCC
- **M87.063 Idiopathic aseptic necrosis of unspecified tibia** CC HCC
- **M87.064 Idiopathic aseptic necrosis of right fibula** CC HCC
- **M87.065 Idiopathic aseptic necrosis of left fibula** CC HCC
- **M87.066 Idiopathic aseptic necrosis of unspecified fibula** CC HCC

✓6th **M87.07 Idiopathic aseptic necrosis of ankle, foot and toes**

Idiopathic aseptic necrosis of metatarsus, tarsus, and phalanges of toes
- **M87.071 Idiopathic aseptic necrosis of right ankle** CC HCC
- **M87.072 Idiopathic aseptic necrosis of left ankle** CC HCC
- **M87.073 Idiopathic aseptic necrosis of unspecified ankle** CC HCC
- **M87.074 Idiopathic aseptic necrosis of right foot** CC HCC
- **M87.075 Idiopathic aseptic necrosis of left foot** CC HCC
- **M87.076 Idiopathic aseptic necrosis of unspecified foot** CC HCC

M87.077 Idiopathic aseptic necrosis of right toe(s) CC HCC
M87.078 Idiopathic aseptic necrosis of left toe(s) CC HCC
M87.079 Idiopathic aseptic necrosis of unspecified toe(s) CC HCC
M87.08 Idiopathic aseptic necrosis of bone, other site CC HCC
M87.09 Idiopathic aseptic necrosis of bone, multiple sites CC HCC

✓5th M87.1 Osteonecrosis due to drugs
Use additional code for adverse effect, if applicable, to identify drug (T36-T5Ø with fifth or sixth character 5)
M87.1Ø Osteonecrosis due to drugs, unspecified bone CC HCC
✓6th M87.11 Osteonecrosis due to drugs, shoulder
M87.111 Osteonecrosis due to drugs, right shoulder CC HCC
M87.112 Osteonecrosis due to drugs, left shoulder CC HCC
M87.119 Osteonecrosis due to drugs, unspecified shoulder CC HCC
✓6th M87.12 Osteonecrosis due to drugs, humerus
M87.121 Osteonecrosis due to drugs, right humerus CC HCC
M87.122 Osteonecrosis due to drugs, left humerus CC HCC
M87.129 Osteonecrosis due to drugs, unspecified humerus CC HCC
✓6th M87.13 Osteonecrosis due to drugs of radius, ulna and carpus
M87.131 Osteonecrosis due to drugs of right radius CC HCC
M87.132 Osteonecrosis due to drugs of left radius CC HCC
M87.133 Osteonecrosis due to drugs of unspecified radius CC HCC
M87.134 Osteonecrosis due to drugs of right ulna CC HCC
M87.135 Osteonecrosis due to drugs of left ulna CC HCC
M87.136 Osteonecrosis due to drugs of unspecified ulna CC HCC
M87.137 Osteonecrosis due to drugs of right carpus CC HCC
M87.138 Osteonecrosis due to drugs of left carpus CC HCC
M87.139 Osteonecrosis due to drugs of unspecified carpus CC HCC
✓6th M87.14 Osteonecrosis due to drugs, hand and fingers
M87.141 Osteonecrosis due to drugs, right hand CC HCC
M87.142 Osteonecrosis due to drugs, left hand CC HCC
M87.143 Osteonecrosis due to drugs, unspecified hand CC HCC
M87.144 Osteonecrosis due to drugs, right finger(s) CC HCC
M87.145 Osteonecrosis due to drugs, left finger(s) CC HCC
M87.146 Osteonecrosis due to drugs, unspecified finger(s) CC HCC
✓6th M87.15 Osteonecrosis due to drugs, pelvis and femur
M87.15Ø Osteonecrosis due to drugs, pelvis CC HCC
M87.151 Osteonecrosis due to drugs, right femur CC HCC
M87.152 Osteonecrosis due to drugs, left femur CC HCC
M87.159 Osteonecrosis due to drugs, unspecified femur CC HCC
✓6th M87.16 Osteonecrosis due to drugs, tibia and fibula
M87.161 Osteonecrosis due to drugs, right tibia CC HCC
M87.162 Osteonecrosis due to drugs, left tibia CC HCC
M87.163 Osteonecrosis due to drugs, unspecified tibia CC HCC
M87.164 Osteonecrosis due to drugs, right fibula CC HCC
M87.165 Osteonecrosis due to drugs, left fibula CC HCC
M87.166 Osteonecrosis due to drugs, unspecified fibula CC HCC
✓6th M87.17 Osteonecrosis due to drugs, ankle, foot and toes
M87.171 Osteonecrosis due to drugs, right ankle CC HCC
M87.172 Osteonecrosis due to drugs, left ankle CC HCC
M87.173 Osteonecrosis due to drugs, unspecified ankle CC HCC
M87.174 Osteonecrosis due to drugs, right foot CC HCC
M87.175 Osteonecrosis due to drugs, left foot CC HCC
M87.176 Osteonecrosis due to drugs, unspecified foot CC HCC
M87.177 Osteonecrosis due to drugs, right toe(s) CC HCC
M87.178 Osteonecrosis due to drugs, left toe(s) CC HCC
M87.179 Osteonecrosis due to drugs, unspecified toe(s) CC HCC
✓6th M87.18 Osteonecrosis due to drugs, other site
M87.18Ø Osteonecrosis due to drugs, jaw CC HCC
M87.188 Osteonecrosis due to drugs, other site CC HCC
M87.19 Osteonecrosis due to drugs, multiple sites CC HCC

✓5th M87.2 Osteonecrosis due to previous trauma
M87.2Ø Osteonecrosis due to previous trauma, unspecified bone CC HCC
✓6th M87.21 Osteonecrosis due to previous trauma, shoulder
M87.211 Osteonecrosis due to previous trauma, right shoulder CC HCC
M87.212 Osteonecrosis due to previous trauma, left shoulder CC HCC
M87.219 Osteonecrosis due to previous trauma, unspecified shoulder CC HCC
✓6th M87.22 Osteonecrosis due to previous trauma, humerus
M87.221 Osteonecrosis due to previous trauma, right humerus CC HCC
M87.222 Osteonecrosis due to previous trauma, left humerus CC HCC
M87.229 Osteonecrosis due to previous trauma, unspecified humerus CC HCC
✓6th M87.23 Osteonecrosis due to previous trauma of radius, ulna and carpus
M87.231 Osteonecrosis due to previous trauma of right radius CC HCC
M87.232 Osteonecrosis due to previous trauma of left radius CC HCC
M87.233 Osteonecrosis due to previous trauma of unspecified radius CC HCC
M87.234 Osteonecrosis due to previous trauma of right ulna CC HCC
M87.235 Osteonecrosis due to previous trauma of left ulna CC HCC
M87.236 Osteonecrosis due to previous trauma of unspecified ulna CC HCC
M87.237 Osteonecrosis due to previous trauma of right carpus CC HCC
M87.238 Osteonecrosis due to previous trauma of left carpus CC HCC
M87.239 Osteonecrosis due to previous trauma of unspecified carpus CC HCC
✓6th M87.24 Osteonecrosis due to previous trauma, hand and fingers
M87.241 Osteonecrosis due to previous trauma, right hand CC HCC
M87.242 Osteonecrosis due to previous trauma, left hand CC HCC
M87.243 Osteonecrosis due to previous trauma, unspecified hand CC HCC
M87.244 Osteonecrosis due to previous trauma, right finger(s) CC HCC

M87.245 Osteonecrosis due to previous trauma, left finger(s) CC HCC
M87.246 Osteonecrosis due to previous trauma, unspecified finger(s) CC HCC
✓6th M87.25 Osteonecrosis due to previous trauma, pelvis and femur
M87.250 Osteonecrosis due to previous trauma, pelvis CC HCC
M87.251 Osteonecrosis due to previous trauma, right femur CC HCC
M87.252 Osteonecrosis due to previous trauma, left femur CC HCC
M87.256 Osteonecrosis due to previous trauma, unspecified femur CC HCC
✓6th M87.26 Osteonecrosis due to previous trauma, tibia and fibula
M87.261 Osteonecrosis due to previous trauma, right tibia CC HCC
M87.262 Osteonecrosis due to previous trauma, left tibia CC HCC
M87.263 Osteonecrosis due to previous trauma, unspecified tibia CC HCC
M87.264 Osteonecrosis due to previous trauma, right fibula CC HCC
M87.265 Osteonecrosis due to previous trauma, left fibula CC HCC
M87.266 Osteonecrosis due to previous trauma, unspecified fibula CC HCC
✓6th M87.27 Osteonecrosis due to previous trauma, ankle, foot and toes
M87.271 Osteonecrosis due to previous trauma, right ankle CC HCC
M87.272 Osteonecrosis due to previous trauma, left ankle CC HCC
M87.273 Osteonecrosis due to previous trauma, unspecified ankle CC HCC
M87.274 Osteonecrosis due to previous trauma, right foot CC HCC
M87.275 Osteonecrosis due to previous trauma, left foot CC HCC
M87.276 Osteonecrosis due to previous trauma, unspecified foot CC HCC
M87.277 Osteonecrosis due to previous trauma, right toe(s) CC HCC
M87.278 Osteonecrosis due to previous trauma, left toe(s) CC HCC
M87.279 Osteonecrosis due to previous trauma, unspecified toe(s) CC HCC
M87.28 Osteonecrosis due to previous trauma, other site CC HCC
M87.29 Osteonecrosis due to previous trauma, multiple sites CC HCC
✓5th M87.3 Other secondary osteonecrosis
M87.30 Other secondary osteonecrosis, unspecified bone CC HCC
✓6th M87.31 Other secondary osteonecrosis, shoulder
M87.311 Other secondary osteonecrosis, right shoulder CC HCC
M87.312 Other secondary osteonecrosis, left shoulder CC HCC
M87.319 Other secondary osteonecrosis, unspecified shoulder CC HCC
✓6th M87.32 Other secondary osteonecrosis, humerus
M87.321 Other secondary osteonecrosis, right humerus CC HCC
M87.322 Other secondary osteonecrosis, left humerus CC HCC
M87.329 Other secondary osteonecrosis, unspecified humerus CC HCC
✓6th M87.33 Other secondary osteonecrosis of radius, ulna and carpus
M87.331 Other secondary osteonecrosis of right radius CC HCC
M87.332 Other secondary osteonecrosis of left radius CC HCC
M87.333 Other secondary osteonecrosis of unspecified radius CC HCC
M87.334 Other secondary osteonecrosis of right ulna CC HCC
M87.335 Other secondary osteonecrosis of left ulna CC HCC
M87.336 Other secondary osteonecrosis of unspecified ulna CC HCC
M87.337 Other secondary osteonecrosis of right carpus CC HCC
M87.338 Other secondary osteonecrosis of left carpus CC HCC
M87.339 Other secondary osteonecrosis of unspecified carpus CC HCC
✓6th M87.34 Other secondary osteonecrosis, hand and fingers
M87.341 Other secondary osteonecrosis, right hand CC HCC
M87.342 Other secondary osteonecrosis, left hand CC HCC
M87.343 Other secondary osteonecrosis, unspecified hand CC HCC
M87.344 Other secondary osteonecrosis, right finger(s) CC HCC
M87.345 Other secondary osteonecrosis, left finger(s) CC HCC
M87.346 Other secondary osteonecrosis, unspecified finger(s) CC HCC
✓6th M87.35 Other secondary osteonecrosis, pelvis and femur
M87.350 Other secondary osteonecrosis, pelvis CC HCC
M87.351 Other secondary osteonecrosis, right femur CC HCC
M87.352 Other secondary osteonecrosis, left femur CC HCC
M87.353 Other secondary osteonecrosis, unspecified femur CC HCC
✓6th M87.36 Other secondary osteonecrosis, tibia and fibula
M87.361 Other secondary osteonecrosis, right tibia CC HCC
M87.362 Other secondary osteonecrosis, left tibia CC HCC
M87.363 Other secondary osteonecrosis, unspecified tibia CC HCC
M87.364 Other secondary osteonecrosis, right fibula CC HCC
M87.365 Other secondary osteonecrosis, left fibula CC HCC
M87.366 Other secondary osteonecrosis, unspecified fibula CC HCC
✓6th M87.37 Other secondary osteonecrosis, ankle and foot
M87.371 Other secondary osteonecrosis, right ankle CC HCC
M87.372 Other secondary osteonecrosis, left ankle CC HCC
M87.373 Other secondary osteonecrosis, unspecified ankle CC HCC
M87.374 Other secondary osteonecrosis, right foot CC HCC
M87.375 Other secondary osteonecrosis, left foot CC HCC
M87.376 Other secondary osteonecrosis, unspecified foot CC HCC
M87.377 Other secondary osteonecrosis, right toe(s) CC HCC
M87.378 Other secondary osteonecrosis, left toe(s) CC HCC
M87.379 Other secondary osteonecrosis, unspecified toe(s) CC HCC
M87.38 Other secondary osteonecrosis, other site CC HCC
M87.39 Other secondary osteonecrosis, multiple sites CC HCC
✓5th M87.8 Other osteonecrosis
M87.80 Other osteonecrosis, unspecified bone CC HCC
✓6th M87.81 Other osteonecrosis, shoulder
M87.811 Other osteonecrosis, right shoulder CC HCC
M87.812 Other osteonecrosis, left shoulder CC HCC
M87.819 Other osteonecrosis, unspecified shoulder CC HCC
✓6th M87.82 Other osteonecrosis, humerus
M87.821 Other osteonecrosis, right humerus CC HCC

M87.822 Other osteonecrosis, left humerus CC HCC
M87.829 Other osteonecrosis, unspecified humerus CC HCC

✓6th M87.83 Other osteonecrosis of radius, ulna and carpus
M87.831 Other osteonecrosis of right radius CC HCC
M87.832 Other osteonecrosis of left radius CC HCC
M87.833 Other osteonecrosis of unspecified radius CC HCC
M87.834 Other osteonecrosis of right ulna CC HCC
M87.835 Other osteonecrosis of left ulna CC HCC
M87.836 Other osteonecrosis of unspecified ulna CC HCC
M87.837 Other osteonecrosis of right carpus CC HCC
M87.838 Other osteonecrosis of left carpus CC HCC
M87.839 Other osteonecrosis of unspecified carpus CC HCC

✓6th M87.84 Other osteonecrosis, hand and fingers
M87.841 Other osteonecrosis, right hand CC HCC
M87.842 Other osteonecrosis, left hand CC HCC
M87.843 Other osteonecrosis, unspecified hand CC HCC
M87.844 Other osteonecrosis, right finger(s) CC HCC
M87.845 Other osteonecrosis, left finger(s) CC HCC
M87.849 Other osteonecrosis, unspecified finger(s) CC HCC

✓6th M87.85 Other osteonecrosis, pelvis and femur
M87.85Ø Other osteonecrosis, pelvis CC HCC
M87.851 Other osteonecrosis, right femur CC HCC
M87.852 Other osteonecrosis, left femur CC HCC
M87.859 Other osteonecrosis, unspecified femur CC HCC

✓6th M87.86 Other osteonecrosis, tibia and fibula
M87.861 Other osteonecrosis, right tibia CC HCC
M87.862 Other osteonecrosis, left tibia CC HCC
M87.863 Other osteonecrosis, unspecified tibia CC HCC
M87.864 Other osteonecrosis, right fibula CC HCC
M87.865 Other osteonecrosis, left fibula CC HCC
M87.869 Other osteonecrosis, unspecified fibula CC HCC

✓6th M87.87 Other osteonecrosis, ankle, foot and toes
M87.871 Other osteonecrosis, right ankle CC HCC
M87.872 Other osteonecrosis, left ankle CC HCC
M87.873 Other osteonecrosis, unspecified ankle CC HCC
M87.874 Other osteonecrosis, right foot CC HCC
M87.875 Other osteonecrosis, left foot CC HCC
M87.876 Other osteonecrosis, unspecified foot CC HCC
M87.877 Other osteonecrosis, right toe(s) CC HCC
M87.878 Other osteonecrosis, left toe(s) CC HCC
M87.879 Other osteonecrosis, unspecified toe(s) CC HCC

M87.88 Other osteonecrosis, other site CC HCC
M87.89 Other osteonecrosis, multiple sites CC HCC

M87.9 Osteonecrosis, unspecified CC HCC
Necrosis of bone NOS

✓4th **M88 Osteitis deformans [Paget's disease of bone]**

EXCLUDES 1 *osteitis deformans in neoplastic disease (M9Ø.6)*

DEF: Bone disease characterized by numerous cycles of bone resorption by the body. Resorption is followed by accelerated repair attempts, causing bone deformities and bowing, with associated fractures and pain.

M88.Ø Osteitis deformans of skull
M88.1 Osteitis deformans of vertebrae

✓5th M88.8 Osteitis deformans of other bones

✓6th M88.81 Osteitis deformans of shoulder
M88.811 Osteitis deformans of right shoulder
M88.812 Osteitis deformans of left shoulder
M88.819 Osteitis deformans of unspecified shoulder

✓6th M88.82 Osteitis deformans of upper arm
M88.821 Osteitis deformans of right upper arm
M88.822 Osteitis deformans of left upper arm
M88.829 Osteitis deformans of unspecified upper arm

✓6th M88.83 Osteitis deformans of forearm
M88.831 Osteitis deformans of right forearm
M88.832 Osteitis deformans of left forearm
M88.839 Osteitis deformans of unspecified forearm

✓6th M88.84 Osteitis deformans of hand
M88.841 Osteitis deformans of right hand
M88.842 Osteitis deformans of left hand
M88.849 Osteitis deformans of unspecified hand

✓6th M88.85 Osteitis deformans of thigh
M88.851 Osteitis deformans of right thigh
M88.852 Osteitis deformans of left thigh
M88.859 Osteitis deformans of unspecified thigh

✓6th M88.86 Osteitis deformans of lower leg
M88.861 Osteitis deformans of right lower leg
M88.862 Osteitis deformans of left lower leg
M88.869 Osteitis deformans of unspecified lower leg

✓6th M88.87 Osteitis deformans of ankle and foot
M88.871 Osteitis deformans of right ankle and foot
M88.872 Osteitis deformans of left ankle and foot
M88.879 Osteitis deformans of unspecified ankle and foot

M88.88 Osteitis deformans of other bones
EXCLUDES 2 *osteitis deformans of skull (M88.Ø)*
osteitis deformans of vertebrae (M88.1)

M88.89 Osteitis deformans of multiple sites

M88.9 Osteitis deformans of unspecified bone

✓4th **M89 Other disorders of bone**

✓5th M89.Ø Algoneurodystrophy
Shoulder-hand syndrome
Sudeck's atrophy
EXCLUDES 1 *causalgia, lower limb (G57.7-)*
causalgia, upper limb (G56.4-)
complex regional pain syndrome II, lower limb (G57.7-)
complex regional pain syndrome II, upper limb (G56.4-)
reflex sympathetic dystrophy (G9Ø.5-)

M89.ØØ Algoneurodystrophy, unspecified site

✓6th M89.Ø1 Algoneurodystrophy, shoulder
M89.Ø11 Algoneurodystrophy, right shoulder
M89.Ø12 Algoneurodystrophy, left shoulder
M89.Ø19 Algoneurodystrophy, unspecified shoulder

✓6th M89.Ø2 Algoneurodystrophy, upper arm
M89.Ø21 Algoneurodystrophy, right upper arm
M89.Ø22 Algoneurodystrophy, left upper arm
M89.Ø29 Algoneurodystrophy, unspecified upper arm

✓6th M89.Ø3 Algoneurodystrophy, forearm
M89.Ø31 Algoneurodystrophy, right forearm
M89.Ø32 Algoneurodystrophy, left forearm
M89.Ø39 Algoneurodystrophy, unspecified forearm

✓6th M89.Ø4 Algoneurodystrophy, hand
M89.Ø41 Algoneurodystrophy, right hand
M89.Ø42 Algoneurodystrophy, left hand
M89.Ø49 Algoneurodystrophy, unspecified hand

✓6th M89.Ø5 Algoneurodystrophy, thigh
M89.Ø51 Algoneurodystrophy, right thigh
M89.Ø52 Algoneurodystrophy, left thigh
M89.Ø59 Algoneurodystrophy, unspecified thigh

M89.Ø6 Algoneurodystrophy, lower leg
M89.Ø61 Algoneurodystrophy, right lower leg
M89.Ø62 Algoneurodystrophy, left lower leg
M89.Ø69 Algoneurodystrophy, unspecified lower leg
M89.Ø7 Algoneurodystrophy, ankle and foot
M89.Ø71 Algoneurodystrophy, right ankle and foot
M89.Ø72 Algoneurodystrophy, left ankle and foot
M89.Ø79 Algoneurodystrophy, unspecified ankle and foot
M89.Ø8 Algoneurodystrophy, other site
M89.Ø9 Algoneurodystrophy, multiple sites

M89.1 Physeal arrest
Arrest of growth plate
Epiphyseal arrest
Growth plate arrest

M89.12 Physeal arrest, humerus
M89.121 Complete physeal arrest, right proximal humerus
M89.122 Complete physeal arrest, left proximal humerus
M89.123 Partial physeal arrest, right proximal humerus
M89.124 Partial physeal arrest, left proximal humerus
M89.125 Complete physeal arrest, right distal humerus
M89.126 Complete physeal arrest, left distal humerus
M89.127 Partial physeal arrest, right distal humerus
M89.128 Partial physeal arrest, left distal humerus
M89.129 Physeal arrest, humerus, unspecified
M89.13 Physeal arrest, forearm
M89.131 Complete physeal arrest, right distal radius
M89.132 Complete physeal arrest, left distal radius
M89.133 Partial physeal arrest, right distal radius
M89.134 Partial physeal arrest, left distal radius
M89.138 Other physeal arrest of forearm
M89.139 Physeal arrest, forearm, unspecified
M89.15 Physeal arrest, femur
M89.151 Complete physeal arrest, right proximal femur
M89.152 Complete physeal arrest, left proximal femur
M89.153 Partial physeal arrest, right proximal femur
M89.154 Partial physeal arrest, left proximal femur
M89.155 Complete physeal arrest, right distal femur
M89.156 Complete physeal arrest, left distal femur
M89.157 Partial physeal arrest, right distal femur
M89.158 Partial physeal arrest, left distal femur
M89.159 Physeal arrest, femur, unspecified
M89.16 Physeal arrest, lower leg
M89.16Ø Complete physeal arrest, right proximal tibia
M89.161 Complete physeal arrest, left proximal tibia
M89.162 Partial physeal arrest, right proximal tibia
M89.163 Partial physeal arrest, left proximal tibia
M89.164 Complete physeal arrest, right distal tibia
M89.165 Complete physeal arrest, left distal tibia
M89.166 Partial physeal arrest, right distal tibia
M89.167 Partial physeal arrest, left distal tibia
M89.168 Other physeal arrest of lower leg
M89.169 Physeal arrest, lower leg, unspecified
M89.18 Physeal arrest, other site

M89.2 Other disorders of bone development and growth
M89.2Ø Other disorders of bone development and growth, unspecified site
M89.21 Other disorders of bone development and growth, shoulder
M89.211 Other disorders of bone development and growth, right shoulder
M89.212 Other disorders of bone development and growth, left shoulder
M89.219 Other disorders of bone development and growth, unspecified shoulder
M89.22 Other disorders of bone development and growth, humerus
M89.221 Other disorders of bone development and growth, right humerus
M89.222 Other disorders of bone development and growth, left humerus
M89.229 Other disorders of bone development and growth, unspecified humerus
M89.23 Other disorders of bone development and growth, ulna and radius
M89.231 Other disorders of bone development and growth, right ulna
M89.232 Other disorders of bone development and growth, left ulna
M89.233 Other disorders of bone development and growth, right radius
M89.234 Other disorders of bone development and growth, left radius
M89.239 Other disorders of bone development and growth, unspecified ulna and radius
M89.24 Other disorders of bone development and growth, hand
M89.241 Other disorders of bone development and growth, right hand
M89.242 Other disorders of bone development and growth, left hand
M89.249 Other disorders of bone development and growth, unspecified hand
M89.25 Other disorders of bone development and growth, femur
M89.251 Other disorders of bone development and growth, right femur
M89.252 Other disorders of bone development and growth, left femur
M89.259 Other disorders of bone development and growth, unspecified femur
M89.26 Other disorders of bone development and growth, tibia and fibula
M89.261 Other disorders of bone development and growth, right tibia
M89.262 Other disorders of bone development and growth, left tibia
M89.263 Other disorders of bone development and growth, right fibula
M89.264 Other disorders of bone development and growth, left fibula
M89.269 Other disorders of bone development and growth, unspecified lower leg
M89.27 Other disorders of bone development and growth, ankle and foot
M89.271 Other disorders of bone development and growth, right ankle and foot
M89.272 Other disorders of bone development and growth, left ankle and foot
M89.279 Other disorders of bone development and growth, unspecified ankle and foot
M89.28 Other disorders of bone development and growth, other site
M89.29 Other disorders of bone development and growth, multiple sites

M89.3 Hypertrophy of bone
M89.3Ø Hypertrophy of bone, unspecified site
M89.31 Hypertrophy of bone, shoulder
M89.311 Hypertrophy of bone, right shoulder
M89.312 Hypertrophy of bone, left shoulder
M89.319 Hypertrophy of bone, unspecified shoulder
M89.32 Hypertrophy of bone, humerus
M89.321 Hypertrophy of bone, right humerus
M89.322 Hypertrophy of bone, left humerus
M89.329 Hypertrophy of bone, unspecified humerus
M89.33 Hypertrophy of bone, ulna and radius
M89.331 Hypertrophy of bone, right ulna
M89.332 Hypertrophy of bone, left ulna
M89.333 Hypertrophy of bone, right radius
M89.334 Hypertrophy of bone, left radius
M89.339 Hypertrophy of bone, unspecified ulna and radius

✓6th **M89.34 Hypertrophy of bone, hand**
- **M89.341 Hypertrophy of bone, right hand**
- **M89.342 Hypertrophy of bone, left hand**
- **M89.349 Hypertrophy of bone, unspecified hand**

✓6th **M89.35 Hypertrophy of bone, femur**
- **M89.351 Hypertrophy of bone, right femur**
- **M89.352 Hypertrophy of bone, left femur**
- **M89.359 Hypertrophy of bone, unspecified femur**

✓6th **M89.36 Hypertrophy of bone, tibia and fibula**
- **M89.361 Hypertrophy of bone, right tibia**
- **M89.362 Hypertrophy of bone, left tibia**
- **M89.363 Hypertrophy of bone, right fibula**
- **M89.364 Hypertrophy of bone, left fibula**
- **M89.369 Hypertrophy of bone, unspecified tibia and fibula**

✓6th **M89.37 Hypertrophy of bone, ankle and foot**
- **M89.371 Hypertrophy of bone, right ankle and foot**
- **M89.372 Hypertrophy of bone, left ankle and foot**
- **M89.379 Hypertrophy of bone, unspecified ankle and foot**

M89.38 Hypertrophy of bone, other site

M89.39 Hypertrophy of bone, multiple sites

✓5th **M89.4 Other hypertrophic osteoarthropathy**

Marie-Bamberger disease
Pachydermoperiostosis

M89.40 Other hypertrophic osteoarthropathy, unspecified site

✓6th **M89.41 Other hypertrophic osteoarthropathy, shoulder**
- **M89.411 Other hypertrophic osteoarthropathy, right shoulder**
- **M89.412 Other hypertrophic osteoarthropathy, left shoulder**
- **M89.419 Other hypertrophic osteoarthropathy, unspecified shoulder**

✓6th **M89.42 Other hypertrophic osteoarthropathy, upper arm**
- **M89.421 Other hypertrophic osteoarthropathy, right upper arm**
- **M89.422 Other hypertrophic osteoarthropathy, left upper arm**
- **M89.429 Other hypertrophic osteoarthropathy, unspecified upper arm**

✓6th **M89.43 Other hypertrophic osteoarthropathy, forearm**
- **M89.431 Other hypertrophic osteoarthropathy, right forearm**
- **M89.432 Other hypertrophic osteoarthropathy, left forearm**
- **M89.439 Other hypertrophic osteoarthropathy, unspecified forearm**

✓6th **M89.44 Other hypertrophic osteoarthropathy, hand**
- **M89.441 Other hypertrophic osteoarthropathy, right hand**
- **M89.442 Other hypertrophic osteoarthropathy, left hand**
- **M89.449 Other hypertrophic osteoarthropathy, unspecified hand**

✓6th **M89.45 Other hypertrophic osteoarthropathy, thigh**
- **M89.451 Other hypertrophic osteoarthropathy, right thigh**
- **M89.452 Other hypertrophic osteoarthropathy, left thigh**
- **M89.459 Other hypertrophic osteoarthropathy, unspecified thigh**

✓6th **M89.46 Other hypertrophic osteoarthropathy, lower leg**
- **M89.461 Other hypertrophic osteoarthropathy, right lower leg**
- **M89.462 Other hypertrophic osteoarthropathy, left lower leg**
- **M89.469 Other hypertrophic osteoarthropathy, unspecified lower leg**

✓6th **M89.47 Other hypertrophic osteoarthropathy, ankle and foot**
- **M89.471 Other hypertrophic osteoarthropathy, right ankle and foot**
- **M89.472 Other hypertrophic osteoarthropathy, left ankle and foot**
- **M89.479 Other hypertrophic osteoarthropathy, unspecified ankle and foot**

M89.48 Other hypertrophic osteoarthropathy, other site

M89.49 Other hypertrophic osteoarthropathy, multiple sites

✓5th **M89.5 Osteolysis**

Use additional code to identify major osseous defect, if applicable (M89.7-)

EXCLUDES 2 *periprosthetic osteolysis of internal prosthetic joint (T84.05-)*

M89.50 Osteolysis, unspecified site

✓6th **M89.51 Osteolysis, shoulder**
- **M89.511 Osteolysis, right shoulder**
- **M89.512 Osteolysis, left shoulder**
- **M89.519 Osteolysis, unspecified shoulder**

✓6th **M89.52 Osteolysis, upper arm**
- **M89.521 Osteolysis, right upper arm**
- **M89.522 Osteolysis, left upper arm**
- **M89.529 Osteolysis, unspecified upper arm**

✓6th **M89.53 Osteolysis, forearm**
- **M89.531 Osteolysis, right forearm**
- **M89.532 Osteolysis, left forearm**
- **M89.539 Osteolysis, unspecified forearm**

✓6th **M89.54 Osteolysis, hand**
- **M89.541 Osteolysis, right hand**
- **M89.542 Osteolysis, left hand**
- **M89.549 Osteolysis, unspecified hand**

✓6th **M89.55 Osteolysis, thigh**
- **M89.551 Osteolysis, right thigh**
- **M89.552 Osteolysis, left thigh**
- **M89.559 Osteolysis, unspecified thigh**

✓6th **M89.56 Osteolysis, lower leg**
- **M89.561 Osteolysis, right lower leg**
- **M89.562 Osteolysis, left lower leg**
- **M89.569 Osteolysis, unspecified lower leg**

✓6th **M89.57 Osteolysis, ankle and foot**
- **M89.571 Osteolysis, right ankle and foot**
- **M89.572 Osteolysis, left ankle and foot**
- **M89.579 Osteolysis, unspecified ankle and foot**

M89.58 Osteolysis, other site

M89.59 Osteolysis, multiple sites

✓5th **M89.6 Osteopathy after poliomyelitis**

Use additional code (B91) to identify previous poliomyelitis

EXCLUDES 1 *postpolio syndrome (G14)*

M89.60 Osteopathy after poliomyelitis, unspecified site HCC

✓6th **M89.61 Osteopathy after poliomyelitis, shoulder**
- **M89.611 Osteopathy after poliomyelitis, right shoulder** HCC
- **M89.612 Osteopathy after poliomyelitis, left shoulder** HCC
- **M89.619 Osteopathy after poliomyelitis, unspecified shoulder** HCC

✓6th **M89.62 Osteopathy after poliomyelitis, upper arm**
- **M89.621 Osteopathy after poliomyelitis, right upper arm** HCC
- **M89.622 Osteopathy after poliomyelitis, left upper arm** HCC
- **M89.629 Osteopathy after poliomyelitis, unspecified upper arm** HCC

✓6th **M89.63 Osteopathy after poliomyelitis, forearm**
- **M89.631 Osteopathy after poliomyelitis, right forearm** HCC
- **M89.632 Osteopathy after poliomyelitis, left forearm** HCC
- **M89.639 Osteopathy after poliomyelitis, unspecified forearm** HCC

✓6th **M89.64 Osteopathy after poliomyelitis, hand**
- **M89.641 Osteopathy after poliomyelitis, right hand** HCC
- **M89.642 Osteopathy after poliomyelitis, left hand** HCC
- **M89.649 Osteopathy after poliomyelitis, unspecified hand** HCC

✓6th **M89.65 Osteopathy after poliomyelitis, thigh**
- **M89.651 Osteopathy after poliomyelitis, right thigh** HCC
- **M89.652 Osteopathy after poliomyelitis, left thigh** HCC

M89.659 Osteopathy after poliomyelitis, unspecified thigh HCC

✓6th M89.66 Osteopathy after poliomyelitis, lower leg

M89.661 Osteopathy after poliomyelitis, right lower leg HCC

M89.662 Osteopathy after poliomyelitis, left lower leg HCC

M89.669 Osteopathy after poliomyelitis, unspecified lower leg HCC

✓6th M89.67 Osteopathy after poliomyelitis, ankle and foot

M89.671 Osteopathy after poliomyelitis, right ankle and foot HCC

M89.672 Osteopathy after poliomyelitis, left ankle and foot HCC

M89.679 Osteopathy after poliomyelitis, unspecified ankle and foot HCC

M89.68 Osteopathy after poliomyelitis, other site HCC

M89.69 Osteopathy after poliomyelitis, multiple sites HCC

✓5th M89.7 Major osseous defect

Code first underlying disease, if known, such as:
- aseptic necrosis of bone (M87.-)
- malignant neoplasm of bone (C4Ø.-)
- osteolysis (M89.5)
- osteomyelitis (M86.-)
- osteonecrosis (M87.-)
- osteoporosis (M8Ø.-, M81.-)
- periprosthetic osteolysis (T84.Ø5-)

M89.7Ø Major osseous defect, unspecified site

✓6th M89.71 Major osseous defect, shoulder region

Major osseous defect clavicle or scapula

M89.711 Major osseous defect, right shoulder region

M89.712 Major osseous defect, left shoulder region

M89.719 Major osseous defect, unspecified shoulder region

✓6th M89.72 Major osseous defect, humerus

M89.721 Major osseous defect, right humerus

M89.722 Major osseous defect, left humerus

M89.729 Major osseous defect, unspecified humerus

✓6th M89.73 Major osseous defect, forearm

Major osseous defect of radius and ulna

M89.731 Major osseous defect, right forearm

M89.732 Major osseous defect, left forearm

M89.739 Major osseous defect, unspecified forearm

✓6th M89.74 Major osseous defect, hand

Major osseous defect of carpus, fingers, metacarpus

M89.741 Major osseous defect, right hand

M89.742 Major osseous defect, left hand

M89.749 Major osseous defect, unspecified hand

✓6th M89.75 Major osseous defect, pelvic region and thigh

Major osseous defect of femur and pelvis

M89.751 Major osseous defect, right pelvic region and thigh

M89.752 Major osseous defect, left pelvic region and thigh

M89.759 Major osseous defect, unspecified pelvic region and thigh

✓6th M89.76 Major osseous defect, lower leg

Major osseous defect of fibula and tibia

M89.761 Major osseous defect, right lower leg

M89.762 Major osseous defect, left lower leg

M89.769 Major osseous defect, unspecified lower leg

✓6th M89.77 Major osseous defect, ankle and foot

Major osseous defect of metatarsus, tarsus, toes

M89.771 Major osseous defect, right ankle and foot

M89.772 Major osseous defect, left ankle and foot

M89.779 Major osseous defect, unspecified ankle and foot

M89.78 Major osseous defect, other site

M89.79 Major osseous defect, multiple sites

✓5th M89.8 Other specified disorders of bone

Infantile cortical hyperostoses
Post-traumatic subperiosteal ossification

✓6th M89.8X Other specified disorders of bone

M89.8XØ Other specified disorders of bone, multiple sites

M89.8X1 Other specified disorders of bone, shoulder

M89.8X2 Other specified disorders of bone, upper arm

M89.8X3 Other specified disorders of bone, forearm

AHA: 2019,3Q,9

M89.8X4 Other specified disorders of bone, hand

M89.8X5 Other specified disorders of bone, thigh

M89.8X6 Other specified disorders of bone, lower leg

M89.8X7 Other specified disorders of bone, ankle and foot

M89.8X8 Other specified disorders of bone, other site

M89.8X9 Other specified disorders of bone, unspecified site

M89.9 Disorder of bone, unspecified

✓4th M9Ø Osteopathies in diseases classified elsewhere

EXCLUDES 1 *osteochondritis, osteomyelitis, and osteopathy (in):*
- *cryptococcosis (B45.3)*
- *diabetes mellitus (EØ8-E13 with .69-)*
- *gonococcal (A54.43)*
- *neurogenic syphilis (A52.11)*
- *renal osteodystrophy (N25.Ø)*
- *salmonellosis (AØ2.24)*
- *secondary syphilis (A51.46)*
- *syphilis (late) (A52.77)*

✓5th M9Ø.5 Osteonecrosis in diseases classified elsewhere

Code first underlying disease, such as:
- caisson disease (T7Ø.3)
- hemoglobinopathy (D5Ø-D64)

M9Ø.5Ø Osteonecrosis in diseases classified elsewhere, unspecified site CC HCC

✓6th M9Ø.51 Osteonecrosis in diseases classified elsewhere, shoulder

M9Ø.511 Osteonecrosis in diseases classified elsewhere, right shoulder CC HCC

M9Ø.512 Osteonecrosis in diseases classified elsewhere, left shoulder CC HCC

M9Ø.519 Osteonecrosis in diseases classified elsewhere, unspecified shoulder CC HCC

✓6th M9Ø.52 Osteonecrosis in diseases classified elsewhere, upper arm

M9Ø.521 Osteonecrosis in diseases classified elsewhere, right upper arm CC HCC

M9Ø.522 Osteonecrosis in diseases classified elsewhere, left upper arm CC HCC

M9Ø.529 Osteonecrosis in diseases classified elsewhere, unspecified upper arm CC HCC

✓6th M9Ø.53 Osteonecrosis in diseases classified elsewhere, forearm

M9Ø.531 Osteonecrosis in diseases classified elsewhere, right forearm CC HCC

M9Ø.532 Osteonecrosis in diseases classified elsewhere, left forearm CC HCC

M9Ø.539 Osteonecrosis in diseases classified elsewhere, unspecified forearm CC HCC

✓6th M9Ø.54 Osteonecrosis in diseases classified elsewhere, hand

M9Ø.541 Osteonecrosis in diseases classified elsewhere, right hand CC HCC

M9Ø.542 Osteonecrosis in diseases classified elsewhere, left hand CC HCC

M9Ø.549 Osteonecrosis in diseases classified elsewhere, unspecified hand CC HCC

✓6th M9Ø.55 Osteonecrosis in diseases classified elsewhere, thigh

M9Ø.551 Osteonecrosis in diseases classified elsewhere, right thigh CC HCC

M9Ø.552 Osteonecrosis in diseases classified elsewhere, left thigh CC HCC

M90.559 *Osteonecrosis in diseases classified elsewhere, unspecified thigh* CC HCC

✓6th M90.56 **Osteonecrosis in diseases classified elsewhere, lower leg**

M90.561 *Osteonecrosis in diseases classified elsewhere, right lower leg* CC HCC

M90.562 *Osteonecrosis in diseases classified elsewhere, left lower leg* CC HCC

M90.569 *Osteonecrosis in diseases classified elsewhere, unspecified lower leg* CC HCC

✓6th M90.57 **Osteonecrosis in diseases classified elsewhere, ankle and foot**

M90.571 *Osteonecrosis in diseases classified elsewhere, right ankle and foot* CC HCC

M90.572 *Osteonecrosis in diseases classified elsewhere, left ankle and foot* CC HCC

M90.579 *Osteonecrosis in diseases classified elsewhere, unspecified ankle and foot* CC HCC

M90.58 *Osteonecrosis in diseases classified elsewhere, other site* CC HCC

M90.59 *Osteonecrosis in diseases classified elsewhere, multiple sites* CC HCC

✓5th M90.6 **Osteitis deformans in neoplastic diseases**

Osteitis deformans in malignant neoplasm of bone

Code first the neoplasm (C40.-, C41.-)

EXCLUDES 1 *osteitis deformans [Paget's disease of bone] (M88.-)*

M90.60 *Osteitis deformans in neoplastic diseases, unspecified site*

✓6th M90.61 **Osteitis deformans in neoplastic diseases, shoulder**

M90.611 *Osteitis deformans in neoplastic diseases, right shoulder*

M90.612 *Osteitis deformans in neoplastic diseases, left shoulder*

M90.619 *Osteitis deformans in neoplastic diseases, unspecified shoulder*

✓6th M90.62 **Osteitis deformans in neoplastic diseases, upper arm**

M90.621 *Osteitis deformans in neoplastic diseases, right upper arm*

M90.622 *Osteitis deformans in neoplastic diseases, left upper arm*

M90.629 *Osteitis deformans in neoplastic diseases, unspecified upper arm*

✓6th M90.63 **Osteitis deformans in neoplastic diseases, forearm**

M90.631 *Osteitis deformans in neoplastic diseases, right forearm*

M90.632 *Osteitis deformans in neoplastic diseases, left forearm*

M90.639 *Osteitis deformans in neoplastic diseases, unspecified forearm*

✓6th M90.64 **Osteitis deformans in neoplastic diseases, hand**

M90.641 *Osteitis deformans in neoplastic diseases, right hand*

M90.642 *Osteitis deformans in neoplastic diseases, left hand*

M90.649 *Osteitis deformans in neoplastic diseases, unspecified hand*

✓6th M90.65 **Osteitis deformans in neoplastic diseases, thigh**

M90.651 *Osteitis deformans in neoplastic diseases, right thigh*

M90.652 *Osteitis deformans in neoplastic diseases, left thigh*

M90.659 *Osteitis deformans in neoplastic diseases, unspecified thigh*

✓6th M90.66 **Osteitis deformans in neoplastic diseases, lower leg**

M90.661 *Osteitis deformans in neoplastic diseases, right lower leg*

M90.662 *Osteitis deformans in neoplastic diseases, left lower leg*

M90.669 *Osteitis deformans in neoplastic diseases, unspecified lower leg*

✓6th M90.67 **Osteitis deformans in neoplastic diseases, ankle and foot**

M90.671 *Osteitis deformans in neoplastic diseases, right ankle and foot*

M90.672 *Osteitis deformans in neoplastic diseases, left ankle and foot*

M90.679 *Osteitis deformans in neoplastic diseases, unspecified ankle and foot*

M90.68 *Osteitis deformans in neoplastic diseases, other site*

M90.69 *Osteitis deformans in neoplastic diseases, multiple sites*

✓5th M90.8 **Osteopathy in diseases classified elsewhere**

Code first underlying disease, such as:

rickets (E55.0)

vitamin-D-resistant rickets (E83.3)

M90.80 *Osteopathy in diseases classified elsewhere, unspecified site*

✓6th M90.81 **Osteopathy in diseases classified elsewhere, shoulder**

M90.811 *Osteopathy in diseases classified elsewhere, right shoulder*

M90.812 *Osteopathy in diseases classified elsewhere, left shoulder*

M90.819 *Osteopathy in diseases classified elsewhere, unspecified shoulder*

✓6th M90.82 **Osteopathy in diseases classified elsewhere, upper arm**

M90.821 *Osteopathy in diseases classified elsewhere, right upper arm*

M90.822 *Osteopathy in diseases classified elsewhere, left upper arm*

M90.829 *Osteopathy in diseases classified elsewhere, unspecified upper arm*

✓6th M90.83 **Osteopathy in diseases classified elsewhere, forearm**

M90.831 *Osteopathy in diseases classified elsewhere, right forearm*

M90.832 *Osteopathy in diseases classified elsewhere, left forearm*

M90.839 *Osteopathy in diseases classified elsewhere, unspecified forearm*

✓6th M90.84 **Osteopathy in diseases classified elsewhere, hand**

M90.841 *Osteopathy in diseases classified elsewhere, right hand*

M90.842 *Osteopathy in diseases classified elsewhere, left hand*

M90.849 *Osteopathy in diseases classified elsewhere, unspecified hand*

✓6th M90.85 **Osteopathy in diseases classified elsewhere, thigh**

M90.851 *Osteopathy in diseases classified elsewhere, right thigh*

M90.852 *Osteopathy in diseases classified elsewhere, left thigh*

M90.859 *Osteopathy in diseases classified elsewhere, unspecified thigh*

✓6th M90.86 **Osteopathy in diseases classified elsewhere, lower leg**

M90.861 *Osteopathy in diseases classified elsewhere, right lower leg*

M90.862 *Osteopathy in diseases classified elsewhere, left lower leg*

M90.869 *Osteopathy in diseases classified elsewhere, unspecified lower leg*

✓6th M90.87 **Osteopathy in diseases classified elsewhere, ankle and foot**

M90.871 *Osteopathy in diseases classified elsewhere, right ankle and foot*

M90.872 *Osteopathy in diseases classified elsewhere, left ankle and foot*

M90.879 *Osteopathy in diseases classified elsewhere, unspecified ankle and foot*

M90.88 *Osteopathy in diseases classified elsewhere, other site*

M90.89 *Osteopathy in diseases classified elsewhere, multiple sites*

Chondropathies (M91-M94)

EXCLUDES 1 *postprocedural chondropathies (M96.-)*

✓4th M91 **Juvenile osteochondrosis of hip and pelvis**

EXCLUDES 1 *slipped upper femoral epiphysis (nontraumatic) (M93.0)*

M91.0 **Juvenile osteochondrosis of pelvis**

Osteochondrosis (juvenile) of acetabulum

Osteochondrosis (juvenile) of iliac crest [Buchanan]

Osteochondrosis (juvenile) of ischiopubic synchondrosis [van Neck]

Osteochondrosis (juvenile) of symphysis pubis [Pierson]

✓5th **M91.1 Juvenile osteochondrosis of head of femur [Legg-Calvé-Perthes]**
- **M91.10 Juvenile osteochondrosis of head of femur [Legg-Calvé-Perthes], unspecified leg**
- **M91.11 Juvenile osteochondrosis of head of femur [Legg-Calvé-Perthes], right leg**
- **M91.12 Juvenile osteochondrosis of head of femur [Legg-Calvé-Perthes], left leg**

✓5th **M91.2 Coxa plana**

Hip deformity due to previous juvenile osteochondrosis
- **M91.20 Coxa plana, unspecified hip**
- **M91.21 Coxa plana, right hip**
- **M91.22 Coxa plana, left hip**

✓5th **M91.3 Pseudocoxalgia**
- **M91.30 Pseudocoxalgia, unspecified hip**
- **M91.31 Pseudocoxalgia, right hip**
- **M91.32 Pseudocoxalgia, left hip**

✓5th **M91.4 Coxa magna**
- **M91.40 Coxa magna, unspecified hip**
- **M91.41 Coxa magna, right hip**
- **M91.42 Coxa magna, left hip**

✓5th **M91.8 Other juvenile osteochondrosis of hip and pelvis**

Juvenile osteochondrosis after reduction of congenital dislocation of hip
- **M91.80 Other juvenile osteochondrosis of hip and pelvis, unspecified leg**
- **M91.81 Other juvenile osteochondrosis of hip and pelvis, right leg**
- **M91.82 Other juvenile osteochondrosis of hip and pelvis, left leg**

✓5th **M91.9 Juvenile osteochondrosis of hip and pelvis, unspecified**
- **M91.90 Juvenile osteochondrosis of hip and pelvis, unspecified, unspecified leg**
- **M91.91 Juvenile osteochondrosis of hip and pelvis, unspecified, right leg**
- **M91.92 Juvenile osteochondrosis of hip and pelvis, unspecified, left leg**

✓4th **M92 Other juvenile osteochondrosis**

✓5th **M92.0 Juvenile osteochondrosis of humerus**

Osteochondrosis (juvenile) of capitulum of humerus [Panner]
Osteochondrosis (juvenile) of head of humerus [Haas]
- **M92.00 Juvenile osteochondrosis of humerus, unspecified arm**
- **M92.01 Juvenile osteochondrosis of humerus, right arm**
- **M92.02 Juvenile osteochondrosis of humerus, left arm**

✓5th **M92.1 Juvenile osteochondrosis of radius and ulna**

Osteochondrosis (juvenile) of lower ulna [Burns]
Osteochondrosis (juvenile) of radial head [Brailsford]
- **M92.10 Juvenile osteochondrosis of radius and ulna, unspecified arm**
- **M92.11 Juvenile osteochondrosis of radius and ulna, right arm**
- **M92.12 Juvenile osteochondrosis of radius and ulna, left arm**

✓5th **M92.2 Juvenile osteochondrosis, hand**

✓6th **M92.20 Unspecified juvenile osteochondrosis, hand**
- **M92.201 Unspecified juvenile osteochondrosis, right hand**
- **M92.202 Unspecified juvenile osteochondrosis, left hand**
- **M92.209 Unspecified juvenile osteochondrosis, unspecified hand**

✓6th **M92.21 Osteochondrosis (juvenile) of carpal lunate [Kienböck]**
- **M92.211 Osteochondrosis (juvenile) of carpal lunate [Kienböck], right hand**
- **M92.212 Osteochondrosis (juvenile) of carpal lunate [Kienböck], left hand**
- **M92.219 Osteochondrosis (juvenile) of carpal lunate [Kienböck], unspecified hand**

✓6th **M92.22 Osteochondrosis (juvenile) of metacarpal heads [Mauclaire]**
- **M92.221 Osteochondrosis (juvenile) of metacarpal heads [Mauclaire], right hand**
- **M92.222 Osteochondrosis (juvenile) of metacarpal heads [Mauclaire], left hand**
- **M92.229 Osteochondrosis (juvenile) of metacarpal heads [Mauclaire], unspecified hand**

✓6th **M92.29 Other juvenile osteochondrosis, hand**
- **M92.291 Other juvenile osteochondrosis, right hand**
- **M92.292 Other juvenile osteochondrosis, left hand**
- **M92.299 Other juvenile osteochondrosis, unspecified hand**

✓5th **M92.3 Other juvenile osteochondrosis, upper limb**
- **M92.30 Other juvenile osteochondrosis, unspecified upper limb**
- **M92.31 Other juvenile osteochondrosis, right upper limb**
- **M92.32 Other juvenile osteochondrosis, left upper limb**

✓5th **M92.4 Juvenile osteochondrosis of patella**

Osteochondrosis (juvenile) of primary patellar center [Köhler]
Osteochondrosis (juvenile) of secondary patellar centre [Sinding Larsen]
- **M92.40 Juvenile osteochondrosis of patella, unspecified knee**
- **M92.41 Juvenile osteochondrosis of patella, right knee**
- **M92.42 Juvenile osteochondrosis of patella, left knee**

✓5th **M92.5 Juvenile osteochondrosis of tibia and fibula**

~~Osteochondrosis (juvenile) of proximal tibia [Blount]~~
~~Osteochondrosis (juvenile) of tibial tubercle [Osgood-Schlatter]~~
~~Tibia vara~~

▲ ✓6th **M92.50 Unspecified juvenile osteochondrosis of tibia and fibula**
- ● **M92.501 Unspecified juvenile osteochondrosis, right leg**
- ● **M92.502 Unspecified juvenile osteochondrosis, left leg**
- ● **M92.503 Unspecified juvenile osteochondrosis, bilateral leg**
- ● **M92.509 Unspecified juvenile osteochondrosis, unspecified leg**

▲ ✓6th **M92.51 Juvenile osteochondrosis of proximal tibia**

▶Blount disease◀
▶Tibia vara◀
- ● **M92.511 Juvenile osteochondrosis of proximal tibia, right leg**
- ● **M92.512 Juvenile osteochondrosis of proximal tibia,left leg**
- ● **M92.513 Juvenile osteochondrosis of proximal tibia, bilateral**
- ● **M92.519 Juvenile osteochondrosis of proximal tibia, unspecified leg**

▲ ✓6th **M92.52 Juvenile osteochondrosis of tibia tubercle**

▶Osgood-Schlatter disease◀
- ● **M92.521 Juvenile osteochondrosis of tibia tubercle, right leg**
- ● **M92.522 Juvenile osteochondrosis of tibia tubercle, left leg**
- ● **M92.523 Juvenile osteochondrosis of tibia tubercle, bilateral**
- ● **M92.529 Juvenile osteochondrosis of tibia tubercle, unspecified leg**

● ✓6th **M92.59 Other juvenile osteochondrosis of tibia and fibula**
- ● **M92.591 Other juvenile osteochondrosis of tibia and fibula, right leg**
- ● **M92.592 Other juvenile osteochondrosis of tibia and fibula, left leg**
- ● **M92.593 Other juvenile osteochondrosis of tibia and fibula, bilateral**
- ● **M92.599 Other juvenile osteochondrosis of tibia and fibula, unspecified leg**

✓5th **M92.6 Juvenile osteochondrosis of tarsus**

Osteochondrosis (juvenile) of calcaneum [Sever]
Osteochondrosis (juvenile) of os tibiale externum [Haglund]
Osteochondrosis (juvenile) of talus [Diaz]
Osteochondrosis (juvenile) of tarsal navicular [Köhler]
- **M92.60 Juvenile osteochondrosis of tarsus, unspecified ankle**
- **M92.61 Juvenile osteochondrosis of tarsus, right ankle**
- **M92.62 Juvenile osteochondrosis of tarsus, left ankle**

✓5th **M92.7 Juvenile osteochondrosis of metatarsus**

Osteochondrosis (juvenile) of fifth metatarsus [Iselin]
Osteochondrosis (juvenile) of second metatarsus [Freiberg]
- **M92.70 Juvenile osteochondrosis of metatarsus, unspecified foot**
- **M92.71 Juvenile osteochondrosis of metatarsus, right foot**
- **M92.72 Juvenile osteochondrosis of metatarsus, left foot**

M92.8 Other specified juvenile osteochondrosis
Calcaneal apophysitis
DEF: Calcaneal apophysitis: Inflammation of the calcaneus at the point of Achilles tendon insertion usually occurring in boys ages 8 to 14. Pain, tenderness, and localized swelling are present.

M92.9 Juvenile osteochondrosis, unspecified
Juvenile apophysitis NOS
Juvenile epiphysitis NOS
Juvenile osteochondritis NOS
Juvenile osteochondrosis NOS

✓4th M93 Other osteochondropathies
EXCLUDES 2 *osteochondrosis of spine (M42.-)*

✓5th M93.Ø Slipped upper femoral epiphysis (nontraumatic)
Use additional code for associated chondrolysis (M94.3)

✓6th M93.ØØ Unspecified slipped upper femoral epiphysis (nontraumatic)
M93.ØØ1 Unspecified slipped upper femoral epiphysis (nontraumatic), right hip
M93.ØØ2 Unspecified slipped upper femoral epiphysis (nontraumatic), left hip
M93.ØØ3 Unspecified slipped upper femoral epiphysis (nontraumatic), unspecified hip

✓6th M93.Ø1 Acute slipped upper femoral epiphysis (nontraumatic)
M93.Ø11 Acute slipped upper femoral epiphysis (nontraumatic), right hip
M93.Ø12 Acute slipped upper femoral epiphysis (nontraumatic), left hip
M93.Ø13 Acute slipped upper femoral epiphysis (nontraumatic), unspecified hip

✓6th M93.Ø2 Chronic slipped upper femoral epiphysis (nontraumatic)
M93.Ø21 Chronic slipped upper femoral epiphysis (nontraumatic), right hip
M93.Ø22 Chronic slipped upper femoral epiphysis (nontraumatic), left hip
M93.Ø23 Chronic slipped upper femoral epiphysis (nontraumatic), unspecified hip

✓6th M93.Ø3 Acute on chronic slipped upper femoral epiphysis (nontraumatic)
M93.Ø31 Acute on chronic slipped upper femoral epiphysis (nontraumatic), right hip
M93.Ø32 Acute on chronic slipped upper femoral epiphysis (nontraumatic), left hip
M93.Ø33 Acute on chronic slipped upper femoral epiphysis (nontraumatic), unspecified hip

M93.1 Kienböck's disease of adults A
Adult osteochondrosis of carpal lunates

✓5th M93.2 Osteochondritis dissecans
DEF: Avascular necrosis caused by lack of blood flow to the bone and cartilage of a joint causing the bone to die. This can result in splinters or pieces of cartilage breaking off in the joint.

M93.2Ø Osteochondritis dissecans of unspecified site

✓6th M93.21 Osteochondritis dissecans of shoulder
M93.211 Osteochondritis dissecans, right shoulder
M93.212 Osteochondritis dissecans, left shoulder
M93.219 Osteochondritis dissecans, unspecified shoulder

✓6th M93.22 Osteochondritis dissecans of elbow
M93.221 Osteochondritis dissecans, right elbow
M93.222 Osteochondritis dissecans, left elbow
M93.229 Osteochondritis dissecans, unspecified elbow

✓6th M93.23 Osteochondritis dissecans of wrist
M93.231 Osteochondritis dissecans, right wrist
M93.232 Osteochondritis dissecans, left wrist
M93.239 Osteochondritis dissecans, unspecified wrist

✓6th M93.24 Osteochondritis dissecans of joints of hand
M93.241 Osteochondritis dissecans, joints of right hand
M93.242 Osteochondritis dissecans, joints of left hand
M93.249 Osteochondritis dissecans, joints of unspecified hand

✓6th M93.25 Osteochondritis dissecans of hip
M93.251 Osteochondritis dissecans, right hip
M93.252 Osteochondritis dissecans, left hip
M93.259 Osteochondritis dissecans, unspecified hip

✓6th M93.26 Osteochondritis dissecans knee
M93.261 Osteochondritis dissecans, right knee
M93.262 Osteochondritis dissecans, left knee
M93.269 Osteochondritis dissecans, unspecified knee

✓6th M93.27 Osteochondritis dissecans of ankle and joints of foot
M93.271 Osteochondritis dissecans, right ankle and joints of right foot
M93.272 Osteochondritis dissecans, left ankle and joints of left foot
M93.279 Osteochondritis dissecans, unspecified ankle and joints of foot

M93.28 Osteochondritis dissecans other site
M93.29 Osteochondritis dissecans multiple sites

✓5th M93.8 Other specified osteochondropathies

M93.8Ø Other specified osteochondropathies of unspecified site

✓6th M93.81 Other specified osteochondropathies of shoulder
M93.811 Other specified osteochondropathies, right shoulder
M93.812 Other specified osteochondropathies, left shoulder
M93.819 Other specified osteochondropathies, unspecified shoulder

✓6th M93.82 Other specified osteochondropathies of upper arm
M93.821 Other specified osteochondropathies, right upper arm
M93.822 Other specified osteochondropathies, left upper arm
M93.829 Other specified osteochondropathies, unspecified upper arm

✓6th M93.83 Other specified osteochondropathies of forearm
M93.831 Other specified osteochondropathies, right forearm
M93.832 Other specified osteochondropathies, left forearm
M93.839 Other specified osteochondropathies, unspecified forearm

✓6th M93.84 Other specified osteochondropathies of hand
M93.841 Other specified osteochondropathies, right hand
M93.842 Other specified osteochondropathies, left hand
M93.849 Other specified osteochondropathies, unspecified hand

✓6th M93.85 Other specified osteochondropathies of thigh
M93.851 Other specified osteochondropathies, right thigh
M93.852 Other specified osteochondropathies, left thigh
M93.859 Other specified osteochondropathies, unspecified thigh

✓6th M93.86 Other specified osteochondropathies lower leg
M93.861 Other specified osteochondropathies, right lower leg
M93.862 Other specified osteochondropathies, left lower leg
M93.869 Other specified osteochondropathies, unspecified lower leg

✓6th M93.87 Other specified osteochondropathies of ankle and foot
M93.871 Other specified osteochondropathies, right ankle and foot
M93.872 Other specified osteochondropathies, left ankle and foot
M93.879 Other specified osteochondropathies, unspecified ankle and foot

M93.88 Other specified osteochondropathies other site
M93.89 Other specified osteochondropathies multiple sites

✓5th M93.9 Osteochondropathy, unspecified
Apophysitis NOS
Epiphysitis NOS
Osteochondritis NOS
Osteochondrosis NOS

M93.9Ø Osteochondropathy, unspecified of unspecified site

√6th M93.91 Osteochondropathy, unspecified of shoulder
M93.911 Osteochondropathy, unspecified, right shoulder
M93.912 Osteochondropathy, unspecified, left shoulder
M93.919 Osteochondropathy, unspecified, unspecified shoulder
√6th M93.92 Osteochondropathy, unspecified of upper arm
M93.921 Osteochondropathy, unspecified, right upper arm
M93.922 Osteochondropathy, unspecified, left upper arm
M93.929 Osteochondropathy, unspecified, unspecified upper arm
√6th M93.93 Osteochondropathy, unspecified of forearm
M93.931 Osteochondropathy, unspecified, right forearm
M93.932 Osteochondropathy, unspecified, left forearm
M93.939 Osteochondropathy, unspecified, unspecified forearm
√6th M93.94 Osteochondropathy, unspecified of hand
M93.941 Osteochondropathy, unspecified, right hand
M93.942 Osteochondropathy, unspecified, left hand
M93.949 Osteochondropathy, unspecified, unspecified hand
√6th M93.95 Osteochondropathy, unspecified of thigh
M93.951 Osteochondropathy, unspecified, right thigh
M93.952 Osteochondropathy, unspecified, left thigh
M93.959 Osteochondropathy, unspecified, unspecified thigh
√6th M93.96 Osteochondropathy, unspecified lower leg
M93.961 Osteochondropathy, unspecified, right lower leg
M93.962 Osteochondropathy, unspecified, left lower leg
M93.969 Osteochondropathy, unspecified, unspecified lower leg
√6th M93.97 Osteochondropathy, unspecified of ankle and foot
M93.971 Osteochondropathy, unspecified, right ankle and foot
M93.972 Osteochondropathy, unspecified, left ankle and foot
M93.979 Osteochondropathy, unspecified, unspecified ankle and foot
M93.98 Osteochondropathy, unspecified other site
M93.99 Osteochondropathy, unspecified multiple sites

√4th M94 Other disorders of cartilage

M94.Ø Chondrocostal junction syndrome [Tietze]
Costochondritis
M94.1 Relapsing polychondritis
√5th M94.2 Chondromalacia
EXCLUDES 1 *chondromalacia patellae (M22.4)*
M94.2Ø Chondromalacia, unspecified site
√6th M94.21 Chondromalacia, shoulder
M94.211 Chondromalacia, right shoulder
M94.212 Chondromalacia, left shoulder
M94.219 Chondromalacia, unspecified shoulder
√6th M94.22 Chondromalacia, elbow
M94.221 Chondromalacia, right elbow
M94.222 Chondromalacia, left elbow
M94.229 Chondromalacia, unspecified elbow
√6th M94.23 Chondromalacia, wrist
M94.231 Chondromalacia, right wrist
M94.232 Chondromalacia, left wrist
M94.239 Chondromalacia, unspecified wrist
√6th M94.24 Chondromalacia, joints of hand
M94.241 Chondromalacia, joints of right hand
M94.242 Chondromalacia, joints of left hand
M94.249 Chondromalacia, joints of unspecified hand
√6th M94.25 Chondromalacia, hip
M94.251 Chondromalacia, right hip
M94.252 Chondromalacia, left hip
M94.259 Chondromalacia, unspecified hip
√6th M94.26 Chondromalacia, knee
M94.261 Chondromalacia, right knee
M94.262 Chondromalacia, left knee
M94.269 Chondromalacia, unspecified knee
√6th M94.27 Chondromalacia, ankle and joints of foot
M94.271 Chondromalacia, right ankle and joints of right foot
M94.272 Chondromalacia, left ankle and joints of left foot
M94.279 Chondromalacia, unspecified ankle and joints of foot
M94.28 Chondromalacia, other site
M94.29 Chondromalacia, multiple sites
√5th M94.3 Chondrolysis
Code first any associated slipped upper femoral epiphysis (nontraumatic) (M93.Ø-)
√6th M94.35 Chondrolysis, hip
M94.351 Chondrolysis, right hip
M94.352 Chondrolysis, left hip
M94.359 Chondrolysis, unspecified hip
√5th M94.8 Other specified disorders of cartilage
√6th M94.8X Other specified disorders of cartilage
M94.8XØ Other specified disorders of cartilage, multiple sites
M94.8X1 Other specified disorders of cartilage, shoulder
M94.8X2 Other specified disorders of cartilage, upper arm
M94.8X3 Other specified disorders of cartilage, forearm
M94.8X4 Other specified disorders of cartilage, hand
M94.8X5 Other specified disorders of cartilage, thigh
M94.8X6 Other specified disorders of cartilage, lower leg
M94.8X7 Other specified disorders of cartilage, ankle and foot
M94.8X8 Other specified disorders of cartilage, other site
M94.8X9 Other specified disorders of cartilage, unspecified sites
M94.9 Disorder of cartilage, unspecified

Other disorders of the musculoskeletal system and connective tissue (M95)

√4th M95 Other acquired deformities of musculoskeletal system and connective tissue
EXCLUDES 2 *acquired absence of limbs and organs (Z89-Z9Ø)*
acquired deformities of limbs (M2Ø-M21)
congenital malformations and deformations of the musculoskeletal system (Q65-Q79)
deforming dorsopathies (M4Ø-M43)
dentofacial anomalies [including malocclusion] (M26.-)
postprocedural musculoskeletal disorders (M96.-)
M95.Ø Acquired deformity of nose
EXCLUDES 2 *deviated nasal septum (J34.2)*
√5th M95.1 Cauliflower ear
EXCLUDES 2 *other acquired deformities of ear (H61.1)*
DEF: Acquired deformity of the external ear due to injury or subsequent perichondritis.
M95.1Ø Cauliflower ear, unspecified ear
M95.11 Cauliflower ear, right ear
M95.12 Cauliflower ear, left ear
M95.2 Other acquired deformity of head
M95.3 Acquired deformity of neck
M95.4 Acquired deformity of chest and rib
AHA: 2014,4Q,26-27
M95.5 Acquired deformity of pelvis
EXCLUDES 1 *maternal care for known or suspected disproportion (O33.-)*
M95.8 Other specified acquired deformities of musculoskeletal system
M95.9 Acquired deformity of musculoskeletal system, unspecified

Intraoperative and postprocedural complications and disorders of musculoskeletal system, not elsewhere classified (M96)

√4th **M96 Intraoperative and postprocedural complications and disorders of musculoskeletal system, not elsewhere classified**

EXCLUDES 2 *arthropathy following intestinal bypass (MØ2.Ø-)*
complications of internal orthopedic prosthetic devices, implants and grafts (T84.-)
disorders associated with osteoporosis (M8Ø)
periprosthetic fracture around internal prosthetic joint (M97.-)
presence of functional implants and other devices (Z96-Z97)

M96.Ø Pseudarthrosis after fusion or arthrodesis CC

M96.1 Postlaminectomy syndrome, not elsewhere classified

M96.2 Postradiation kyphosis

M96.3 Postlaminectomy kyphosis

M96.4 Postsurgical lordosis

M96.5 Postradiation scoliosis

√5th **M96.6 Fracture of bone following insertion of orthopedic implant, joint prosthesis, or bone plate**

Intraoperative fracture of bone during insertion of orthopedic implant, joint prosthesis, or bone plate

EXCLUDES 2 *complication of internal orthopedic devices, implants or grafts (T84.-)*

√6th **M96.62 Fracture of humerus following insertion of orthopedic implant, joint prosthesis, or bone plate**

M96.621 Fracture of humerus following insertion of orthopedic implant, joint prosthesis, or bone plate, right arm CC HCC

M96.622 Fracture of humerus following insertion of orthopedic implant, joint prosthesis, or bone plate, left arm CC HCC

M96.629 Fracture of humerus following insertion of orthopedic implant, joint prosthesis, or bone plate, unspecified arm CC HCC

√6th **M96.63 Fracture of radius or ulna following insertion of orthopedic implant, joint prosthesis, or bone plate**

M96.631 Fracture of radius or ulna following insertion of orthopedic implant, joint prosthesis, or bone plate, right arm CC HCC

M96.632 Fracture of radius or ulna following insertion of orthopedic implant, joint prosthesis, or bone plate, left arm CC HCC

M96.639 Fracture of radius or ulna following insertion of orthopedic implant, joint prosthesis, or bone plate, unspecified arm CC HCC

M96.65 Fracture of pelvis following insertion of orthopedic implant, joint prosthesis, or bone plate CC HCC

√6th **M96.66 Fracture of femur following insertion of orthopedic implant, joint prosthesis, or bone plate**

M96.661 Fracture of femur following insertion of orthopedic implant, joint prosthesis, or bone plate, right leg CC HCC

M96.662 Fracture of femur following insertion of orthopedic implant, joint prosthesis, or bone plate, left leg CC HCC

M96.669 Fracture of femur following insertion of orthopedic implant, joint prosthesis, or bone plate, unspecified leg CC HCC

√6th **M96.67 Fracture of tibia or fibula following insertion of orthopedic implant, joint prosthesis, or bone plate**

M96.671 Fracture of tibia or fibula following insertion of orthopedic implant, joint prosthesis, or bone plate, right leg CC HCC

M96.672 Fracture of tibia or fibula following insertion of orthopedic implant, joint prosthesis, or bone plate, left leg CC HCC

M96.679 Fracture of tibia or fibula following insertion of orthopedic implant, joint prosthesis, or bone plate, unspecified leg CC HCC

M96.69 Fracture of other bone following insertion of orthopedic implant, joint prosthesis, or bone plate CC HCC

√5th **M96.8 Other intraoperative and postprocedural complications and disorders of musculoskeletal system, not elsewhere classified**

AHA: 2016,4Q,9-10

√6th **M96.81 Intraoperative hemorrhage and hematoma of a musculoskeletal structure complicating a procedure**

EXCLUDES 1 *intraoperative hemorrhage and hematoma of a musculoskeletal structure due to accidental puncture and laceration during a procedure (M96.82-)*

M96.81Ø Intraoperative hemorrhage and hematoma of a musculoskeletal structure complicating a musculoskeletal system procedure CC

M96.811 Intraoperative hemorrhage and hematoma of a musculoskeletal structure complicating other procedure CC

√6th **M96.82 Accidental puncture and laceration of a musculoskeletal structure during a procedure**

M96.82Ø Accidental puncture and laceration of a musculoskeletal structure during a musculoskeletal system procedure CC

M96.821 Accidental puncture and laceration of a musculoskeletal structure during other procedure CC

√6th **M96.83 Postprocedural hemorrhage of a musculoskeletal structure following a procedure**

M96.83Ø Postprocedural hemorrhage of a musculoskeletal structure following a musculoskeletal system procedure CC

M96.831 Postprocedural hemorrhage of a musculoskeletal structure following other procedure CC

√6th **M96.84 Postprocedural hematoma and seroma of a musculoskeletal structure following a procedure**

M96.84Ø Postprocedural hematoma of a musculoskeletal structure following a musculoskeletal system procedure CC

M96.841 Postprocedural hematoma of a musculoskeletal structure following other procedure CC

AHA: 2016,4Q,10

M96.842 Postprocedural seroma of a musculoskeletal structure following a musculoskeletal system procedure CC

M96.843 Postprocedural seroma of a musculoskeletal structure following other procedure CC

AHA: 2018,3Q,6

M96.89 Other intraoperative and postprocedural complications and disorders of the musculoskeletal system CC

Instability of joint secondary to removal of joint prosthesis

Use additional code, if applicable, to further specify disorder

Periprosthetic fractures around internal prosthetic joint (M97)

√4th **M97 Periprosthetic fracture around internal prosthetic joint**

EXCLUDES 2 *breakage (fracture) of prosthetic joint (T84.Ø1-)*
fracture of bone following insertion of orthopedic implant, joint prosthesis or bone plate (M96.6-)

AHA: 2016,4Q,42-43

The appropriate 7th character is to be added to each code from category M97.
A initial encounter
D subsequent encounter
S sequela

√5th **M97.Ø Periprosthetic fracture around internal prosthetic hip joint**

AHA: 2018,1Q,21; 2016,4Q,42

√x7th **M97.Ø1 Periprosthetic fracture around internal prosthetic right hip joint** CC HCC

√x7th **M97.Ø2 Periprosthetic fracture around internal prosthetic left hip joint** CC HCC

√5th **M97.1 Periprosthetic fracture around internal prosthetic knee joint**

√x7th **M97.11 Periprosthetic fracture around internal prosthetic right knee joint** CC

√x7th **M97.12 Periprosthetic fracture around internal prosthetic left knee joint** CC

M97.2 Periprosthetic fracture around internal prosthetic ankle joint
- M97.21 Periprosthetic fracture around internal prosthetic right ankle joint CC
- M97.22 Periprosthetic fracture around internal prosthetic left ankle joint CC

M97.3 Periprosthetic fracture around internal prosthetic shoulder joint
- M97.31 Periprosthetic fracture around internal prosthetic right shoulder joint CC
- M97.32 Periprosthetic fracture around internal prosthetic left shoulder joint CC

M97.4 Periprosthetic fracture around internal prosthetic elbow joint
- M97.41 Periprosthetic fracture around internal prosthetic right elbow joint CC
- M97.42 Periprosthetic fracture around internal prosthetic left elbow joint CC

M97.8 Periprosthetic fracture around other internal prosthetic joint CC

Periprosthetic fracture around internal prosthetic finger joint
Periprosthetic fracture around internal prosthetic spinal joint
Periprosthetic fracture around internal prosthetic toe joint
Periprosthetic fracture around internal prosthetic wrist joint
Use additional code to identify the joint (Z96.6-)

M97.9 Periprosthetic fracture around unspecified internal prosthetic joint CC

Biomechanical lesions, not elsewhere classified (M99)

M99 Biomechanical lesions, not elsewhere classified

NOTE This category should not be used if the condition can be classified elsewhere.

DEF: Biomechanical lesion: Term used by osteopathic and chiropractic physicians to describe musculoskeletal conditions treated that are not more appropriately classified elsewhere.

M99.0 Segmental and somatic dysfunction
- M99.00 Segmental and somatic dysfunction of head region
- M99.01 Segmental and somatic dysfunction of cervical region
- M99.02 Segmental and somatic dysfunction of thoracic region
- M99.03 Segmental and somatic dysfunction of lumbar region
- M99.04 Segmental and somatic dysfunction of sacral region
- M99.05 Segmental and somatic dysfunction of pelvic region
- M99.06 Segmental and somatic dysfunction of lower extremity
- M99.07 Segmental and somatic dysfunction of upper extremity
- M99.08 Segmental and somatic dysfunction of rib cage
- M99.09 Segmental and somatic dysfunction of abdomen and other regions

M99.1 Subluxation complex (vertebral)
- M99.10 Subluxation complex (vertebral) of head region CC H5
- M99.11 Subluxation complex (vertebral) of cervical region CC H5
- M99.12 Subluxation complex (vertebral) of thoracic region
- M99.13 Subluxation complex (vertebral) of lumbar region
- M99.14 Subluxation complex (vertebral) of sacral region
- M99.15 Subluxation complex (vertebral) of pelvic region
- M99.16 Subluxation complex (vertebral) of lower extremity
- M99.17 Subluxation complex (vertebral) of upper extremity
- M99.18 Subluxation complex (vertebral) of rib cage CC H5
- M99.19 Subluxation complex (vertebral) of abdomen and other regions

M99.2 Subluxation stenosis of neural canal
- M99.20 Subluxation stenosis of neural canal of head region
- M99.21 Subluxation stenosis of neural canal of cervical region
- M99.22 Subluxation stenosis of neural canal of thoracic region
- M99.23 Subluxation stenosis of neural canal of lumbar region
- M99.24 Subluxation stenosis of neural canal of sacral region
- M99.25 Subluxation stenosis of neural canal of pelvic region
- M99.26 Subluxation stenosis of neural canal of lower extremity
- M99.27 Subluxation stenosis of neural canal of upper extremity
- M99.28 Subluxation stenosis of neural canal of rib cage
- M99.29 Subluxation stenosis of neural canal of abdomen and other regions

M99.3 Osseous stenosis of neural canal
- M99.30 Osseous stenosis of neural canal of head region
- M99.31 Osseous stenosis of neural canal of cervical region
- M99.32 Osseous stenosis of neural canal of thoracic region
- M99.33 Osseous stenosis of neural canal of lumbar region
- M99.34 Osseous stenosis of neural canal of sacral region
- M99.35 Osseous stenosis of neural canal of pelvic region
- M99.36 Osseous stenosis of neural canal of lower extremity
- M99.37 Osseous stenosis of neural canal of upper extremity
- M99.38 Osseous stenosis of neural canal of rib cage
- M99.39 Osseous stenosis of neural canal of abdomen and other regions

M99.4 Connective tissue stenosis of neural canal
- M99.40 Connective tissue stenosis of neural canal of head region
- M99.41 Connective tissue stenosis of neural canal of cervical region
- M99.42 Connective tissue stenosis of neural canal of thoracic region
- M99.43 Connective tissue stenosis of neural canal of lumbar region
- M99.44 Connective tissue stenosis of neural canal of sacral region
- M99.45 Connective tissue stenosis of neural canal of pelvic region
- M99.46 Connective tissue stenosis of neural canal of lower extremity
- M99.47 Connective tissue stenosis of neural canal of upper extremity
- M99.48 Connective tissue stenosis of neural canal of rib cage
- M99.49 Connective tissue stenosis of neural canal of abdomen and other regions

M99.5 Intervertebral disc stenosis of neural canal
- M99.50 Intervertebral disc stenosis of neural canal of head region
- M99.51 Intervertebral disc stenosis of neural canal of cervical region
- M99.52 Intervertebral disc stenosis of neural canal of thoracic region
- M99.53 Intervertebral disc stenosis of neural canal of lumbar region
- M99.54 Intervertebral disc stenosis of neural canal of sacral region
- M99.55 Intervertebral disc stenosis of neural canal of pelvic region
- M99.56 Intervertebral disc stenosis of neural canal of lower extremity
- M99.57 Intervertebral disc stenosis of neural canal of upper extremity
- M99.58 Intervertebral disc stenosis of neural canal of rib cage
- M99.59 Intervertebral disc stenosis of neural canal of abdomen and other regions

M99.6 Osseous and subluxation stenosis of intervertebral foramina
- M99.60 Osseous and subluxation stenosis of intervertebral foramina of head region
- M99.61 Osseous and subluxation stenosis of intervertebral foramina of cervical region
- M99.62 Osseous and subluxation stenosis of intervertebral foramina of thoracic region
- M99.63 Osseous and subluxation stenosis of intervertebral foramina of lumbar region
- M99.64 Osseous and subluxation stenosis of intervertebral foramina of sacral region
- M99.65 Osseous and subluxation stenosis of intervertebral foramina of pelvic region
- M99.66 Osseous and subluxation stenosis of intervertebral foramina of lower extremity
- M99.67 Osseous and subluxation stenosis of intervertebral foramina of upper extremity
- M99.68 Osseous and subluxation stenosis of intervertebral foramina of rib cage
- M99.69 Osseous and subluxation stenosis of intervertebral foramina of abdomen and other regions

✓5th **M99.7 Connective tissue and disc stenosis of intervertebral foramina**

- **M99.70** Connective tissue and disc stenosis of intervertebral foramina of head region
- **M99.71** Connective tissue and disc stenosis of intervertebral foramina of cervical region
- **M99.72** Connective tissue and disc stenosis of intervertebral foramina of thoracic region
- **M99.73** Connective tissue and disc stenosis of intervertebral foramina of lumbar region
- **M99.74** Connective tissue and disc stenosis of intervertebral foramina of sacral region
- **M99.75** Connective tissue and disc stenosis of intervertebral foramina of pelvic region
- **M99.76** Connective tissue and disc stenosis of intervertebral foramina of lower extremity
- **M99.77** Connective tissue and disc stenosis of intervertebral foramina of upper extremity
- **M99.78** Connective tissue and disc stenosis of intervertebral foramina of rib cage
- **M99.79** Connective tissue and disc stenosis of intervertebral foramina of abdomen and other regions

✓5th **M99.8 Other biomechanical lesions**

- **M99.80** Other biomechanical lesions of head region
- **M99.81** Other biomechanical lesions of cervical region
- **M99.82** Other biomechanical lesions of thoracic region
- **M99.83** Other biomechanical lesions of lumbar region
- **M99.84** Other biomechanical lesions of sacral region
- **M99.85** Other biomechanical lesions of pelvic region
- **M99.86** Other biomechanical lesions of lower extremity
- **M99.87** Other biomechanical lesions of upper extremity
- **M99.88** Other biomechanical lesions of rib cage
- **M99.89** Other biomechanical lesions of abdomen and other regions

M99.9 Biomechanical lesion, unspecified

Chapter 14. Diseases of Genitourinary System (NØØ–N99)

Chapter-specific Guidelines with Coding Examples

The chapter-specific guidelines from the ICD-10-CM Official Guidelines for Coding and Reporting have been provided below. Along with these guidelines are coding examples, contained in the shaded boxes, that have been developed to help illustrate the coding and/or sequencing guidance found in these guidelines.

a. Chronic kidney disease

1) Stages of chronic kidney disease (CKD)

The ICD-10-CM classifies CKD based on severity. The severity of CKD is designated by stages 1-5. Stage 2, code N18.2, equates to mild CKD; stage 3, **codes N18.3Ø-N18.32,** equate to moderate CKD; and stage 4, code N18.4, equates to severe CKD. Code N18.6, End stage renal disease (ESRD), is assigned when the provider has documented end-stage renal disease (ESRD).

If both a stage of CKD and ESRD are documented, assign code N18.6 only.

Stage 5 chronic kidney disease with ESRD requiring chronic dialysis

N18.6	**End stage renal disease**
Z99.2	**Dependence on renal dialysis**

Explanation: The diagnostic statement indicates the patient has chronic kidney disease, documented both as stage 5 and as ESRD requiring chronic dialysis. Code N18.6 End stage renal disease (ESRD), is assigned when the provider has documented end-stage-renal disease (ESRD). If both a stage of CKD and ESRD are documented, assign code N18.6 only.

2) Chronic kidney disease and kidney transplant status

Patients who have undergone kidney transplant may still have some form of chronic kidney disease (CKD) because the kidney transplant may not fully restore kidney function. Therefore, the presence of CKD alone does not constitute a transplant complication. Assign the appropriate N18 code for the patient's stage of CKD and code Z94.Ø, Kidney transplant status. If a transplant complication such as failure or rejection or other transplant complication is documented, see section I.C.19.g for information on coding complications of a kidney transplant. If the documentation is unclear as to whether the patient has a complication of the transplant, query the provider.

Patient with residual chronic kidney disease stage 1 after kidney transplant

N18.1	**Chronic kidney disease, stage 1**
Z94.Ø	**Kidney transplant status**

Explanation: Patients who have undergone kidney transplant may still have some form of chronic kidney disease (CKD) because the kidney transplant may not fully restore kidney function. The presence of CKD alone does not constitute a transplant complication. Assign the appropriate N18 code for the patient's stage of CKD and code Z94.Ø Kidney transplant status.

3) Chronic kidney disease with other conditions

Patients with CKD may also suffer from other serious conditions, most commonly diabetes mellitus and hypertension. The sequencing of the CKD code in relationship to codes for other contributing conditions is based on the conventions in the Tabular List.

See I.C.9. Hypertensive chronic kidney disease.

See I.C.19. Chronic kidney disease and kidney transplant complications.

Type 1 diabetic chronic kidney disease, stage 2

E1Ø.22	**Type 1 diabetes mellitus with diabetic chronic kidney disease**
N18.2	**Chronic kidney disease, stage 2 (mild)**

Explanation: Patients with CKD may also suffer from other serious conditions such as diabetes mellitus. The sequencing of the CKD code in relationship to codes for other contributing conditions is based on the conventions in the Tabular List. Diabetic CKD code E1Ø.22 includes an instructional note to "Use additional code to identify stage of chronic kidney disease (N18.1–N18.6)," thus providing sequencing direction.

Chapter 14. Diseases of the Genitourinary System (NØØ-N99)

EXCLUDES 2 *certain conditions originating in the perinatal period (PØ4-P96)*
certain infectious and parasitic diseases (AØØ-B99)
complications of pregnancy, childbirth and the puerperium (OØØ-O9A)
congenital malformations, deformations and chromosomal abnormalities (QØØ-Q99)
endocrine, nutritional and metabolic diseases (EØØ-E88)
injury, poisoning and certain other consequences of external causes (SØØ-T88)
neoplasms (CØØ-D49)
symptoms, signs and abnormal clinical and laboratory findings, not elsewhere classified (RØØ-R94)

This chapter contains the following blocks:

NØØ-NØ8 Glomerular diseases
N1Ø-N16 Renal tubulo-interstitial diseases
N17-N19 Acute kidney failure and chronic kidney disease
N2Ø-N23 Urolithiasis
N25-N29 Other disorders of kidney and ureter
N3Ø-N39 Other diseases of the urinary system
N4Ø-N53 Diseases of male genital organs
N6Ø-N65 Disorders of breast
N7Ø-N77 Inflammatory diseases of female pelvic organs
N8Ø-N98 Noninflammatory disorders of female genital tract
N99 Intraoperative and postprocedural complications and disorders of genitourinary system, not elsewhere classified

Glomerular diseases (NØØ-NØ8)

Code also any associated kidney failure (N17-N19).

EXCLUDES 1 *hypertensive chronic kidney disease (I12.-)*

DEF: Glomeruli: Clusters of microscopic blood vessels located within the kidneys containing small pores through which waste products are filtered from the blood and urine is formed.

DEF: Glomerulonephritis: Disease of the kidney with diffuse inflammation of the capillary loops of the glomeruli.

✓4th **NØØ Acute nephritic syndrome**

INCLUDES acute glomerular disease
acute glomerulonephritis
acute nephritis

EXCLUDES 1 *acute tubulo-interstitial nephritis (N1Ø)*
nephritic syndrome NOS (NØ5.-)

NØØ.Ø Acute nephritic syndrome with minor glomerular abnormality MCC
Acute nephritic syndrome with minimal change lesion

NØØ.1 Acute nephritic syndrome with focal and segmental glomerular lesions MCC
Acute nephritic syndrome with focal and segmental hyalinosis
Acute nephritic syndrome with focal and segmental sclerosis
Acute nephritic syndrome with focal glomerulonephritis

NØØ.2 Acute nephritic syndrome with diffuse membranous glomerulonephritis MCC

NØØ.3 Acute nephritic syndrome with diffuse mesangial proliferative glomerulonephritis MCC

NØØ.4 Acute nephritic syndrome with diffuse endocapillary proliferative glomerulonephritis MCC

NØØ.5 Acute nephritic syndrome with diffuse mesangiocapillary glomerulonephritis MCC
Acute nephritic syndrome with membranoproliferative glomerulonephritis, types 1 and 3, or NOS

EXCLUDES 1 ▶*acute nephritic syndrome with C3 glomerulonephritis (NØØ.A)*◀
▶*acute nephritic syndrome with C3 glomerulopathy (NØØ.A)*◀

NØØ.6 Acute nephritic syndrome with dense deposit disease MCC
▶Acute nephritic syndrome with C3 glomerulopathy with dense deposit disease◀
Acute nephritic syndrome with membranoproliferative glomerulonephritis, type 2

NØØ.7 Acute nephritic syndrome with diffuse crescentic glomerulonephritis MCC
Acute nephritic syndrome with extracapillary glomerulonephritis

NØØ.8 Acute nephritic syndrome with other morphologic changes MCC
Acute nephritic syndrome with proliferative glomerulonephritis NOS

NØØ.9 Acute nephritic syndrome with unspecified morphologic changes MCC

● **NØØ.A Acute nephritic syndrome with C3 glomerulonephritis** MCC
Acute nephritic syndrome with C3 glomerulopathy, NOS

EXCLUDES 1 *acute nephritic syndrome (with C3 glomerulopathy) with dense deposit disease (NØØ.6)*

✓4th **NØ1 Rapidly progressive nephritic syndrome**

INCLUDES rapidly progressive glomerular disease
rapidly progressive glomerulonephritis
rapidly progressive nephritis

EXCLUDES 1 *nephritic syndrome NOS (NØ5.-)*

NØ1.Ø Rapidly progressive nephritic syndrome with minor glomerular abnormality MCC
Rapidly progressive nephritic syndrome with minimal change lesion

NØ1.1 Rapidly progressive nephritic syndrome with focal and segmental glomerular lesions MCC
Rapidly progressive nephritic syndrome with focal and segmental hyalinosis
Rapidly progressive nephritic syndrome with focal and segmental sclerosis
Rapidly progressive nephritic syndrome with focal glomerulonephritis

NØ1.2 Rapidly progressive nephritic syndrome with diffuse membranous glomerulonephritis MCC

NØ1.3 Rapidly progressive nephritic syndrome with diffuse mesangial proliferative glomerulonephritis MCC

NØ1.4 Rapidly progressive nephritic syndrome with diffuse endocapillary proliferative glomerulonephritis MCC

NØ1.5 Rapidly progressive nephritic syndrome with diffuse mesangiocapillary glomerulonephritis MCC
Rapidly progressive nephritic syndrome with membranoproliferative glomerulonephritis, types 1 and 3, or NOS

EXCLUDES 1 ▶*rapidly progressive nephritic syndrome with C3 glomerulonephritis (NØ1.A)*◀
▶*rapidly progressive nephritic syndrome with C3 glomerulopathy (NØ1.A)*◀

NØ1.6 Rapidly progressive nephritic syndrome with dense deposit disease MCC
▶Rapidly progressive nephritic syndrome with C3 glomerulopathy with dense deposit disease◀
Rapidly progressive nephritic syndrome with membranoproliferative glomerulonephritis, type 2

NØ1.7 Rapidly progressive nephritic syndrome with diffuse crescentic glomerulonephritis MCC
Rapidly progressive nephritic syndrome with extracapillary glomerulonephritis

NØ1.8 Rapidly progressive nephritic syndrome with other morphologic changes MCC
Rapidly progressive nephritic syndrome with proliferative glomerulonephritis NOS

NØ1.9 Rapidly progressive nephritic syndrome with unspecified morphologic changes MCC

● **NØ1.A Rapidly progressive nephritic syndrome with C3 glomerulonephritis** MCC
Rapidly progressive nephritic syndrome with C3 glomerulopathy, NOS

EXCLUDES 1 *rapidly progressive nephritic syndrome (with C3 glomerulopathy) with dense deposit disease (NØ1.6)*

✓4th **NØ2 Recurrent and persistent hematuria**

EXCLUDES 1 *acute cystitis with hematuria (N3Ø.Ø1)*
hematuria NOS (R31.9)
hematuria not associated with specified morphologic lesions (R31.-)

NØ2.Ø Recurrent and persistent hematuria with minor glomerular abnormality CC
Recurrent and persistent hematuria with minimal change lesion

NØ2.1 Recurrent and persistent hematuria with focal and segmental glomerular lesions CC
Recurrent and persistent hematuria with focal and segmental hyalinosis
Recurrent and persistent hematuria with focal and segmental sclerosis
Recurrent and persistent hematuria with focal glomerulonephritis

NØ2.2 Recurrent and persistent hematuria with diffuse membranous glomerulonephritis CC

NØ2.3 Recurrent and persistent hematuria with diffuse mesangial proliferative glomerulonephritis CC

NØ2.4 Recurrent and persistent hematuria with diffuse endocapillary proliferative glomerulonephritis CC

NØ2.5 Recurrent and persistent hematuria with diffuse mesangiocapillary glomerulonephritis CC

Recurrent and persistent hematuria with membranoproliferative glomerulonephritis, types 1 and 3, or NOS

EXCLUDES 1 ▶*recurrent and persistent hematuria with C3 glomerulonephritis (NØ2.A)*◀

▶*recurrent and persistent hematuria with C3 glomerulopathy (NØ2.A)*◀

NØ2.6 Recurrent and persistent hematuria with dense deposit disease CC

▶Recurrent and persistent hematuria with C3 glomerulopathy with dense deposit disease◀

Recurrent and persistent hematuria with membranoproliferative glomerulonephritis, type 2

NØ2.7 Recurrent and persistent hematuria with diffuse crescentic glomerulonephritis CC

Recurrent and persistent hematuria with extracapillary glomerulonephritis

NØ2.8 Recurrent and persistent hematuria with other morphologic changes CC

Recurrent and persistent hematuria with proliferative glomerulonephritis NOS

NØ2.9 Recurrent and persistent hematuria with unspecified morphologic changes CC

AHA: 2017,2Q,5

● **NØ2.A Recurrent and persistent hematuria with C3 glomerulonephritis** CC

Recurrent and persistent hematuria with C3 glomerulopathy

EXCLUDES 1 *recurrent and persistent hematuria (with C3 glomerulopathy) with dense deposit disease (NØ2.6)*

✓4th NØ3 Chronic nephritic syndrome

INCLUDES chronic glomerular disease
chronic glomerulonephritis
chronic nephritis

EXCLUDES 1 *chronic tubulo-interstitial nephritis (N11.-)*
diffuse sclerosing glomerulonephritis (NØ5.8-)
nephritic syndrome NOS (NØ5.-)

DEF: Slow, progressive type of nephritis characterized by inflammation of the capillary loops in the glomeruli of the kidney, which leads to renal failure.

NØ3.Ø Chronic nephritic syndrome with minor glomerular abnormality CC

Chronic nephritic syndrome with minimal change lesion

NØ3.1 Chronic nephritic syndrome with focal and segmental glomerular lesions CC

Chronic nephritic syndrome with focal and segmental hyalinosis
Chronic nephritic syndrome with focal and segmental sclerosis
Chronic nephritic syndrome with focal glomerulonephritis

NØ3.2 Chronic nephritic syndrome with diffuse membranous glomerulonephritis CC

NØ3.3 Chronic nephritic syndrome with diffuse mesangial proliferative glomerulonephritis CC

NØ3.4 Chronic nephritic syndrome with diffuse endocapillary proliferative glomerulonephritis CC

NØ3.5 Chronic nephritic syndrome with diffuse mesangiocapillary glomerulonephritis CC

Chronic nephritic syndrome with membranoproliferative glomerulonephritis, types 1 and 3, or NOS

EXCLUDES 1 ▶*chronic nephritic syndrome with C3 glomerulonephritis (NØ3.A)*◀

▶*chronic nephritic syndrome with C3 glomerulopathy (NØ3.A)*◀

NØ3.6 Chronic nephritic syndrome with dense deposit disease CC

▶Chronic nephritic syndrome with C3 glomerulopathy with dense deposit disease◀

Chronic nephritic syndrome with membranoproliferative glomerulonephritis, type 2

NØ3.7 Chronic nephritic syndrome with diffuse crescentic glomerulonephritis CC

Chronic nephritic syndrome with extracapillary glomerulonephritis

NØ3.8 Chronic nephritic syndrome with other morphologic changes CC

Chronic nephritic syndrome with proliferative glomerulonephritis NOS

NØ3.9 Chronic nephritic syndrome with unspecified morphologic changes CC

● **NØ3.A Chronic nephritic syndrome with C3 glomerulonephritis** CC

Chronic nephritic syndrome with C3 glomerulopathy

EXCLUDES 1 *chronic nephritic syndrome (with C3 glomerulopathy) with dense deposit disease (NØ3.6)*

✓4th NØ4 Nephrotic syndrome

INCLUDES congenital nephrotic syndrome
lipoid nephrosis

NØ4.Ø Nephrotic syndrome with minor glomerular abnormality CC

Nephrotic syndrome with minimal change lesion

NØ4.1 Nephrotic syndrome with focal and segmental glomerular lesions CC

Nephrotic syndrome with focal and segmental hyalinosis
Nephrotic syndrome with focal and segmental sclerosis
Nephrotic syndrome with focal glomerulonephritis

NØ4.2 Nephrotic syndrome with diffuse membranous glomerulonephritis CC

NØ4.3 Nephrotic syndrome with diffuse mesangial proliferative glomerulonephritis CC

NØ4.4 Nephrotic syndrome with diffuse endocapillary proliferative glomerulonephritis CC

NØ4.5 Nephrotic syndrome with diffuse mesangiocapillary glomerulonephritis CC

Nephrotic syndrome with membranoproliferative glomerulonephritis, types 1 and 3, or NOS

EXCLUDES 1 ▶*nephrotic syndrome with C3 glomerulonephritis (NØ4.A)*◀

▶*nephrotic syndrome with C3 glomerulopathy (NØ4.A)*◀

NØ4.6 Nephrotic syndrome with dense deposit disease CC

▶Nephrotic syndrome with C3 glomerulopathy with dense deposit disease◀

Nephrotic syndrome with membranoproliferative glomerulonephritis, type 2

NØ4.7 Nephrotic syndrome with diffuse crescentic glomerulonephritis CC

Nephrotic syndrome with extracapillary glomerulonephritis

NØ4.8 Nephrotic syndrome with other morphologic changes CC

Nephrotic syndrome with proliferative glomerulonephritis NOS

NØ4.9 Nephrotic syndrome with unspecified morphologic changes CC

● **NØ4.A Nephrotic syndrome with C3 glomerulonephritis** CC

Nephrotic syndrome with C3 glomerulopathy

EXCLUDES 1 *nephrotic syndrome (with C3 glomerulopathy) with dense deposit disease (NØ4.6)*

✓4th NØ5 Unspecified nephritic syndrome

INCLUDES glomerular disease NOS
glomerulonephritis NOS
nephritis NOS
nephropathy NOS and renal disease NOS with morphological lesion specified in .Ø-.8

EXCLUDES 1 *nephropathy NOS with no stated morphological lesion (N28.9)*
renal disease NOS with no stated morphological lesion (N28.9)
tubulo-interstitial nephritis NOS (N12)

NØ5.Ø Unspecified nephritic syndrome with minor glomerular abnormality

Unspecified nephritic syndrome with minimal change lesion

NØ5.1 Unspecified nephritic syndrome with focal and segmental glomerular lesions

Unspecified nephritic syndrome with focal and segmental hyalinosis
Unspecified nephritic syndrome with focal and segmental sclerosis
Unspecified nephritic syndrome with focal glomerulonephritis

NØ5.2 Unspecified nephritic syndrome with diffuse membranous glomerulonephritis CC

NØ5.3 Unspecified nephritic syndrome with diffuse mesangial proliferative glomerulonephritis CC

NØ5.4 Unspecified nephritic syndrome with diffuse endocapillary proliferative glomerulonephritis CC

NØ5.5 Unspecified nephritic syndrome with diffuse mesangiocapillary glomerulonephritis CC
Unspecified nephritic syndrome with membranoproliferative glomerulonephritis, types 1 and 3, or NOS
EXCLUDES 1 ▶*unspecified nephritic syndrome with C3 glomerulonephritis (NØ5.A)*◀
▶*unspecified nephritic syndrome with C3 glomerulopathy (NØ5.A)*◀

NØ5.6 Unspecified nephritic syndrome with dense deposit disease
▶Unspecified nephritic syndrome with C3 glomerulopathy with dense deposit disease◀
Unspecified nephritic syndrome with membranoproliferative glomerulonephritis, type 2

NØ5.7 Unspecified nephritic syndrome with diffuse crescentic glomerulonephritis
Unspecified nephritic syndrome with extracapillary glomerulonephritis

NØ5.8 Unspecified nephritic syndrome with other morphologic changes
Unspecified nephritic syndrome with proliferative glomerulonephritis NOS

NØ5.9 Unspecified nephritic syndrome with unspecified morphologic changes

● **NØ5.A Unspecified nephritic syndrome with C3 glomerulonephritis** CC
Unspecified nephritic syndrome with C3 glomerulopathy
EXCLUDES 1 *unspecified nephritic syndrome (with C3 glomerulopathy) with dense deposit disease (NØ5.6)*

✓4th NØ6 Isolated proteinuria with specified morphological lesion
EXCLUDES 1 *proteinuria not associated with specific morphologic lesions (R8Ø.Ø)*

NØ6.Ø Isolated proteinuria with minor glomerular abnormality
Isolated proteinuria with minimal change lesion

NØ6.1 Isolated proteinuria with focal and segmental glomerular lesions
Isolated proteinuria with focal and segmental hyalinosis
Isolated proteinuria with focal and segmental sclerosis
Isolated proteinuria with focal glomerulonephritis

NØ6.2 Isolated proteinuria with diffuse membranous glomerulonephritis CC

NØ6.3 Isolated proteinuria with diffuse mesangial proliferative glomerulonephritis CC

NØ6.4 Isolated proteinuria with diffuse endocapillary proliferative glomerulonephritis CC

NØ6.5 Isolated proteinuria with diffuse mesangiocapillary glomerulonephritis CC
Isolated proteinuria with membranoproliferative glomerulonephritis, types 1 and 3, or NOS
EXCLUDES 1 ▶*isolated proteinuria with C3 glomerulonephritis (NØ6.A)*◀
▶*isolated proteinuria with C3 glomerulopathy (NØ6.A)*◀

NØ6.6 Isolated proteinuria with dense deposit disease
▶Isolated proteinuria with C3 glomerulopathy with dense deposit disease◀
Isolated proteinuria with membranoproliferative glomerulonephritis, type 2

NØ6.7 Isolated proteinuria with diffuse crescentic glomerulonephritis
Isolated proteinuria with extracapillary glomerulonephritis

NØ6.8 Isolated proteinuria with other morphologic lesion
Isolated proteinuria with proliferative glomerulonephritis NOS

NØ6.9 Isolated proteinuria with unspecified morphologic lesion

● **NØ6.A Isolated proteinuria with C3 glomerulonephritis** CC
Isolated proteinuria with C3 glomerulopathy
EXCLUDES 1 *isolated proteinuria (with C3 glomerulopathy) with dense deposit disease (NØ6.6)*

✓4th NØ7 Hereditary nephropathy, not elsewhere classified
EXCLUDES 2 *Alport's syndrome (Q87.81-)*
hereditary amyloid nephropathy (E85.-)
nail patella syndrome (Q87.2)
non-neuropathic heredofamilial amyloidosis (E85.-)

NØ7.Ø Hereditary nephropathy, not elsewhere classified with minor glomerular abnormality
Hereditary nephropathy, not elsewhere classified with minimal change lesion

NØ7.1 Hereditary nephropathy, not elsewhere classified with focal and segmental glomerular lesions
Hereditary nephropathy, not elsewhere classified with focal and segmental hyalinosis
Hereditary nephropathy, not elsewhere classified with focal and segmental sclerosis
Hereditary nephropathy, not elsewhere classified with focal glomerulonephritis

NØ7.2 Hereditary nephropathy, not elsewhere classified with diffuse membranous glomerulonephritis CC

NØ7.3 Hereditary nephropathy, not elsewhere classified with diffuse mesangial proliferative glomerulonephritis CC

NØ7.4 Hereditary nephropathy, not elsewhere classified with diffuse endocapillary proliferative glomerulonephritis CC

NØ7.5 Hereditary nephropathy, not elsewhere classified with diffuse mesangiocapillary glomerulonephritis CC
Hereditary nephropathy, not elsewhere classified with membranoproliferative glomerulonephritis, types 1 and 3, or NOS
EXCLUDES 1 ▶*hereditary nephropathy, not elsewhere classified with C3 glomerulonephritis (NØ7.A)*◀
▶*hereditary nephropathy, not elsewhere classified with C3 glomerulopathy (NØ7.A)*◀

NØ7.6 Hereditary nephropathy, not elsewhere classified with dense deposit disease
▶Hereditary nephropathy, not elsewhere classified with C3 glomerulopathy with dense deposit disease◀
Hereditary nephropathy, not elsewhere classified with membranoproliferative glomerulonephritis, type 2

NØ7.7 Hereditary nephropathy, not elsewhere classified with diffuse crescentic glomerulonephritis
Hereditary nephropathy, not elsewhere classified with extracapillary glomerulonephritis

NØ7.8 Hereditary nephropathy, not elsewhere classified with other morphologic lesions
Hereditary nephropathy, not elsewhere classified with proliferative glomerulonephritis NOS

NØ7.9 Hereditary nephropathy, not elsewhere classified with unspecified morphologic lesions

● **NØ7.A Hereditary nephropathy, not elsewhere classified with C3 glomerulonephritis** CC
Hereditary nephropathy, not elsewhere classified with C3 glomerulopathy
EXCLUDES 1 *hereditary nephropathy, not elsewhere classified (with C3 glomerulopathy) with dense deposit disease (NØ7.6)*

N08 Glomerular disorders in diseases classified elsewhere
Glomerulonephritis
Nephritis
Nephropathy
Code first underlying disease, such as:
amyloidosis (E85.-)
congenital syphilis (A50.5)
cryoglobulinemia (D89.1)
disseminated intravascular coagulation (D65)
gout (M1A.-, M10.-)
microscopic polyangiitis (M31.7)
multiple myeloma (C90.0-)
sepsis (A40.0-A41.9)
sickle-cell disease (D57.0-D57.8)
EXCLUDES 1 *glomerulonephritis, nephritis and nephropathy (in):*
antiglomerular basement membrane disease (M31.0)
diabetes (E08-E13 with .21)
gonococcal (A54.21)
Goodpasture's syndrome (M31.0)
hemolytic-uremic syndrome (D59.3)
lupus (M32.14)
mumps (B26.83)
syphilis (A52.75)
systemic lupus erythematosus (M32.14)
Wegener's granulomatosis (M31.31)
pyelonephritis in diseases classified elsewhere (N16)
renal tubulo-interstitial disorders classified elsewhere (N16)

Renal tubulo-interstitial diseases (N10-N16)

INCLUDES pyelonephritis
EXCLUDES 1 *pyeloureteritis cystica (N28.85)*

N10 Acute pyelonephritis CC H6
Acute infectious interstitial nephritis
Acute pyelitis
Acute tubulo-interstitial nephritis
Hemoglobin nephrosis
Myoglobin nephrosis
Use additional code (B95-B97), to identify infectious agent
AHA: 2019,3Q,13

✓4th **N11 Chronic tubulo-interstitial nephritis**
INCLUDES chronic infectious interstitial nephritis
chronic pyelitis
chronic pyelonephritis
Use additional code (B95-B97), to identify infectious agent

N11.0 Nonobstructive reflux-associated chronic pyelonephritis
Pyelonephritis (chronic) associated with (vesicoureteral) reflux
EXCLUDES 1 *vesicoureteral reflux NOS (N13.70)*

N11.1 Chronic obstructive pyelonephritis CC
Pyelonephritis (chronic) associated with anomaly of pelviureteric junction
Pyelonephritis (chronic) associated with anomaly of pyeloureteric junction
Pyelonephritis (chronic) associated with crossing of vessel
Pyelonephritis (chronic) associated with kinking of ureter
Pyelonephritis (chronic) associated with obstruction of ureter
Pyelonephritis (chronic) associated with stricture of pelviureteric junction
Pyelonephritis (chronic) associated with stricture of ureter
EXCLUDES 1 *calculous pyelonephritis (N20.9)*
obstructive uropathy (N13.-)

N11.8 Other chronic tubulo-interstitial nephritis CC
Nonobstructive chronic pyelonephritis NOS

N11.9 Chronic tubulo-interstitial nephritis, unspecified CC H6
Chronic interstitial nephritis NOS
Chronic pyelitis NOS
Chronic pyelonephritis NOS

N12 Tubulo-interstitial nephritis, not specified as acute or chronic CC H6
Interstitial nephritis NOS
Pyelitis NOS
Pyelonephritis NOS
EXCLUDES 1 *calculous pyelonephritis (N20.9)*

✓4th **N13 Obstructive and reflux uropathy**
EXCLUDES 2 *calculus of kidney and ureter without hydronephrosis (N20.-)*
congenital obstructive defects of renal pelvis and ureter (Q62.0-Q62.3)
hydronephrosis with ureteropelvic junction obstruction (Q62.11)
obstructive pyelonephritis (N11.1)
DEF: Hydronephrosis: Distension of the kidney caused by an accumulation of urine that cannot flow out due to an obstruction that may be caused by conditions such as kidney stones or vesicoureteral reflux.

N13.0 Hydronephrosis with ureteropelvic junction obstruction CC
Hydronephrosis due to acquired occlusion of ureteropelvic junction
EXCLUDES 2 *hydronephrosis with ureteropelvic junction obstruction due to calculus (N13.2)*
AHA: 2016,4Q,43

Hydronephrosis/UPJ Obstruction

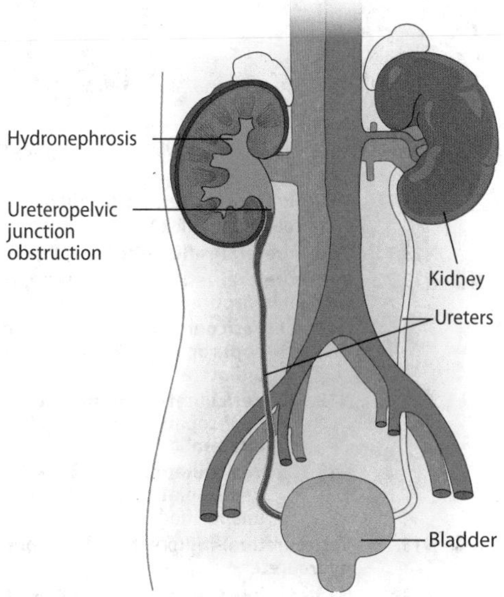

N13.1 Hydronephrosis with ureteral stricture, not elsewhere classified CC
EXCLUDES 1 *hydronephrosis with ureteral stricture with infection (N13.6)*

N13.2 Hydronephrosis with renal and ureteral calculous obstruction CC
EXCLUDES 1 *hydronephrosis with renal and ureteral calculous obstruction with infection (N13.6)*

✓5th **N13.3 Other and unspecified hydronephrosis**
EXCLUDES 1 *hydronephrosis with infection (N13.6)*

N13.30 Unspecified hydronephrosis CC
N13.39 Other hydronephrosis CC

N13.4 Hydroureter CC
EXCLUDES 1 *congenital hydroureter (Q62.3-)*
hydroureter with infection (N13.6)
vesicoureteral-reflux with hydroureter (N13.73-)
DEF: Abnormal enlargement or distension of the ureter with water or urine caused by an obstruction.

N13.5 Crossing vessel and stricture of ureter without hydronephrosis
Kinking and stricture of ureter without hydronephrosis
EXCLUDES 1 *crossing vessel and stricture of ureter without hydronephrosis with infection (N13.6)*

N13.6 Pyonephrosis CC H6
Conditions in N13.0-N13.5 with infection
Obstructive uropathy with infection
Use additional code (B95-B97), to identify infectious agent
AHA: 2018,2Q,21

✓5th **N13.7 Vesicoureteral-reflux**

EXCLUDES 1 *reflux-associated pyelonephritis (N11.Ø)*

DEF: Urine passage from the bladder flows backward up into the ureter and kidneys that can lead to bacterial infection and an increase in hydrostatic pressure, causing kidney damage.

Vesicoureteral Reflux

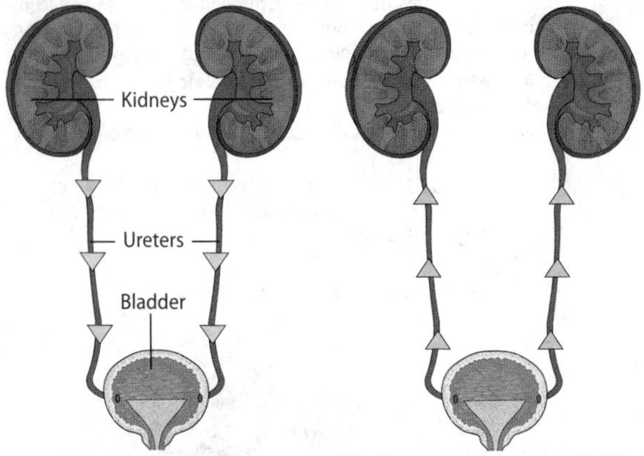

Normal flow of urine — Urine flowing the wrong way (VUR)

N13.70 Vesicoureteral-reflux, unspecified
Vesicoureteral-reflux NOS

N13.71 Vesicoureteral-reflux without reflux nephropathy

✓6th **N13.72 Vesicoureteral-reflux with reflux nephropathy without hydroureter**

N13.721 Vesicoureteral-reflux with reflux nephropathy without hydroureter, unilateral

N13.722 Vesicoureteral-reflux with reflux nephropathy without hydroureter, bilateral

N13.729 Vesicoureteral-reflux with reflux nephropathy without hydroureter, unspecified

✓6th **N13.73 Vesicoureteral-reflux with reflux nephropathy with hydroureter**

N13.731 Vesicoureteral-reflux with reflux nephropathy with hydroureter, unilateral

N13.732 Vesicoureteral-reflux with reflux nephropathy with hydroureter, bilateral

N13.739 Vesicoureteral-reflux with reflux nephropathy with hydroureter, unspecified

N13.8 Other obstructive and reflux uropathy CC
Urinary tract obstruction due to specified cause
Code first, if applicable, any causal condition, such as:
enlarged prostate (N4Ø.1)

N13.9 Obstructive and reflux uropathy, unspecified
Urinary tract obstruction NOS

✓4th **N14 Drug- and heavy-metal-induced tubulo-interstitial and tubular conditions**

Code first poisoning due to drug or toxin, if applicable (T36-T65 with fifth or sixth character 1-4 or 6)

Use additional code for adverse effect, if applicable, to identify drug (T36-T5Ø with fifth or sixth character 5)

N14.Ø Analgesic nephropathy

N14.1 Nephropathy induced by other drugs, medicaments and biological substances

N14.2 Nephropathy induced by unspecified drug, medicament or biological substance

N14.3 Nephropathy induced by heavy metals

N14.4 Toxic nephropathy, not elsewhere classified

✓4th **N15 Other renal tubulo-interstitial diseases**

N15.Ø Balkan nephropathy
Balkan endemic nephropathy

N15.1 Renal and perinephric abscess MCC H6

N15.8 Other specified renal tubulo-interstitial diseases

N15.9 Renal tubulo-interstitial disease, unspecified
Infection of kidney NOS
EXCLUDES 1 *urinary tract infection NOS (N39.Ø)*

N16 Renal tubulo-interstitial disorders in diseases classified elsewhere

Pyelonephritis
Tubulo-interstitial nephritis
Code first underlying disease, such as:
brucellosis (A23.Ø-A23.9)
cryoglobulinemia (D89.1)
glycogen storage disease (E74.Ø)
leukemia (C91-C95)
lymphoma (C81.Ø-C85.9, C96.Ø-C96.9)
multiple myeloma (C9Ø.Ø-)
sepsis (A4Ø.Ø-A41.9)
Wilson's disease (E83.Ø)

EXCLUDES 1 *diphtheritic pyelonephritis and tubulo-interstitial nephritis (A36.84)*
pyelonephritis and tubulo-interstitial nephritis in candidiasis (B37.49)
pyelonephritis and tubulo-interstitial nephritis in cystinosis (E72.Ø4)
pyelonephritis and tubulo-interstitial nephritis in salmonella infection (AØ2.25)
pyelonephritis and tubulo-interstitial nephritis in sarcoidosis (D86.84)
pyelonephritis and tubulo-interstitial nephritis in sicca syndrome [Sjogren's] (M35.Ø4)
pyelonephritis and tubulo-interstitial nephritis in systemic lupus erythematosus (M32.15)
pyelonephritis and tubulo-interstitial nephritis in toxoplasmosis (B58.83)
renal tubular degeneration in diabetes (EØ8-E13 with .29)
syphilitic pyelonephritis and tubulo-interstitial nephritis (A52.75)

Acute kidney failure and chronic kidney disease (N17-N19)

EXCLUDES 2 *congenital renal failure (P96.Ø)*
drug- and heavy-metal-induced tubulo-interstitial and tubular conditions (N14.-)
extrarenal uremia (R39.2)
hemolytic-uremic syndrome (D59.3)
hepatorenal syndrome (K76.7)
postpartum hepatorenal syndrome (O9Ø.4)
posttraumatic renal failure (T79.5)
prerenal uremia (R39.2)
renal failure complicating abortion or ectopic or molar pregnancy (OØØ-OØ7, OØ8.4)
renal failure following labor and delivery (O9Ø.4)
renal failure postprocedural (N99.Ø)

✓4th **N17 Acute kidney failure**

Code also associated underlying condition
EXCLUDES 1 *posttraumatic renal failure (T79.5)*
AHA: 2019,2Q,7; 2019,1Q,12; 2013,4Q,124

N17.Ø Acute kidney failure with tubular necrosis MCC HCC
Acute tubular necrosis
Renal tubular necrosis
Tubular necrosis NOS

N17.1 Acute kidney failure with acute cortical necrosis MCC HCC
Acute cortical necrosis
Cortical necrosis NOS
Renal cortical necrosis

N17.2 Acute kidney failure with medullary necrosis MCC HCC
Medullary [papillary] necrosis NOS
Acute medullary [papillary] necrosis
Renal medullary [papillary] necrosis

N17.8 Other acute kidney failure CC HCC

N17.9 Acute kidney failure, unspecified CC HCC
Acute kidney injury (nontraumatic)
EXCLUDES 2 *traumatic kidney injury (S37.Ø-)*

✓4th **N18 Chronic kidney disease (CKD)**

Code first any associated:
diabetic chronic kidney disease (EØ8.22, EØ9.22, E1Ø.22, E11.22, E13.22)
hypertensive chronic kidney disease (I12.-, I13.-)
Use additional code to identify kidney transplant status, if applicable, (Z94.Ø)
AHA: 2019,3Q,3; 2018,4Q,88; 2013,1Q,24

N18.1 Chronic kidney disease, stage 1

N18.2 Chronic kidney disease, stage 2 (mild)

▲ √5th **N18.3 Chronic kidney disease, stage 3 (moderate)**

● **N18.30 Chronic kidney disease, stage 3 unspecified**

● **N18.31 Chronic kidney disease, stage 3a**

● **N18.32 Chronic kidney disease, stage 3b**

N18.4 Chronic kidney disease, stage 4 (severe) CC HCC

N18.5 Chronic kidney disease, stage 5 CC HCC

EXCLUDES 1 *chronic kidney disease, stage 5 requiring chronic dialysis (N18.6)*

DEF: End-stage renal disease (ESRD) with a GFR value of 15 ml/min or less not yet requiring chronic dialysis.

TIP: When both ESRD and CKD 5 are documented, code only for ESRD.

N18.6 End stage renal disease MCC HCC

Chronic kidney disease requiring chronic dialysis

Use additional code to identify dialysis status (Z99.2)

AHA: 2016,3Q,22; 2016,1Q,12; 2013,4Q,124-125

TIP: When both ESRD and CKD 5 are documented, code only for ESRD.

N18.9 Chronic kidney disease, unspecified

Chronic renal disease
Chronic renal failure NOS
Chronic renal insufficiency
Chronic uremia NOS
Diffuse sclerosing glomerulonephritis NOS

N19 Unspecified kidney failure

Uremia NOS

EXCLUDES 1 *acute kidney failure (N17.-)*
chronic kidney disease (N18.-)
chronic uremia (N18.9)
extrarenal uremia (R39.2)
prerenal uremia (R39.2)
renal insufficiency (acute) (N28.9)
uremia of newborn (P96.0)

Urolithiasis (N20-N23)

AHA: 2017,1Q,5; 2015,2Q,8

TIP: Codes from this code block can be assigned based on the diagnosis listed in a radiology report when authenticated by a radiologist and available at the time of code assignment.

√4th **N20 Calculus of kidney and ureter**

Calculous pyelonephritis

EXCLUDES 1 *nephrocalcinosis (E83.5)*
that with hydronephrosis (N13.2)

AHA: 2019,3Q,13

N20.0 Calculus of kidney

Nephrolithiasis NOS
Renal calculus
Renal stone
Staghorn calculus
Stone in kidney

AHA: 2019,3Q,13

N20.1 Calculus of ureter CC

▶Calculus of the ureteropelvic junction◀
Ureteric stone

AHA: 2016,3Q,22

N20.2 Calculus of kidney with calculus of ureter CC

N20.9 Urinary calculus, unspecified

√4th **N21 Calculus of lower urinary tract**

INCLUDES calculus of lower urinary tract with cystitis and urethritis

N21.0 Calculus in bladder

Calculus in diverticulum of bladder
Urinary bladder stone

EXCLUDES 2 *staghorn calculus (N20.0)*

N21.1 Calculus in urethra

EXCLUDES 2 *calculus of prostate (N42.0)*

N21.8 Other lower urinary tract calculus

N21.9 Calculus of lower urinary tract, unspecified

EXCLUDES 1 *calculus of urinary tract NOS (N20.9)*

N22 Calculus of urinary tract in diseases classified elsewhere

Code first underlying disease, such as:
gout (M1A.-, M10.-)
schistosomiasis (B65.0-B65.9)

N23 Unspecified renal colic

Other disorders of kidney and ureter (N25-N29)

EXCLUDES 2 *disorders of kidney and ureter with urolithiasis (N20-N23)*

√4th **N25 Disorders resulting from impaired renal tubular function**

N25.0 Renal osteodystrophy

Azotemic osteodystrophy
Phosphate-losing tubular disorders
Renal rickets
Renal short stature

EXCLUDES 2 *metabolic disorders classifiable to E70-E88*

DEF: Various bone diseases occurring when kidney function is impaired or fails. Abnormal levels of phosphorous and calcium can lead to osteomalacia, osteoporosis, or osteosclerosis.

N25.1 Nephrogenic diabetes insipidus CC HCC

EXCLUDES 1 *diabetes insipidus NOS (E23.2)*

DEF: Type of diabetes due to the inability of renal tubules to reabsorb water back into the body. It is not responsive to vasopressin (antidiuretic hormone) and it is characterized by excessive thirst and excessive urine production. It may develop into chronic renal insufficiency.

√5th **N25.8 Other disorders resulting from impaired renal tubular function**

N25.81 Secondary hyperparathyroidism of renal origin CC HCC

EXCLUDES 1 *secondary hyperparathyroidism, non-renal (E21.1)*

EXCLUDES 2 *metabolic disorders classifiable to E70-E88*

DEF: Parathyroid dysfunction caused by chronic renal failure. Phosphate clearance and vitamin D production is impaired resulting in lowered calcium blood levels and an excessive production of parathyroid hormone.

N25.89 Other disorders resulting from impaired renal tubular function

Hypokalemic nephropathy
Lightwood-Albright syndrome
Renal tubular acidosis NOS

N25.9 Disorder resulting from impaired renal tubular function, unspecified

√4th **N26 Unspecified contracted kidney**

EXCLUDES 1 *contracted kidney due to hypertension (I12.-)*
diffuse sclerosing glomerulonephritis (N05.8.-)
hypertensive nephrosclerosis (arteriolar) (arteriosclerotic) (I12.-)
small kidney of unknown cause (N27.-)

N26.1 Atrophy of kidney (terminal)

N26.2 Page kidney

N26.9 Renal sclerosis, unspecified

√4th **N27 Small kidney of unknown cause**

INCLUDES oligonephronia

N27.0 Small kidney, unilateral

N27.1 Small kidney, bilateral

N27.9 Small kidney, unspecified

√4th **N28 Other disorders of kidney and ureter, not elsewhere classified**

N28.0 Ischemia and infarction of kidney CC HCC

Renal artery embolism
Renal artery obstruction
Renal artery occlusion
Renal artery thrombosis
Renal infarct

EXCLUDES 1 *atherosclerosis of renal artery (extrarenal part) (I70.1)*
congenital stenosis of renal artery (Q27.1)
Goldblatt's kidney (I70.1)

N28.1 Cyst of kidney, acquired

Cyst (multiple) (solitary) of kidney (acquired)

EXCLUDES 1 *cystic kidney disease (congenital) (Q61.-)*

√5th **N28.8 Other specified disorders of kidney and ureter**

EXCLUDES 1 *hydroureter (N13.4)*
ureteric stricture with hydronephrosis (N13.1)
ureteric stricture without hydronephrosis (N13.5)

N28.81 Hypertrophy of kidney

N28.82 Megaloureter

N28.83 Nephroptosis

N28.84 Pyelitis cystica CC H6

N28.85 Pyeloureteritis cystica CC H6

N28.86 Ureteritis cystica CC H6

N28.89 Other specified disorders of kidney and ureter

N28.9 Disorder of kidney and ureter, unspecified
Nephropathy NOS
Renal disease (acute) NOS
Renal insufficiency (acute)
EXCLUDES 1 *chronic renal insufficiency (N18.9)*
unspecified nephritic syndrome (NØ5.-)
AHA: 2016,1Q,13

N29 Other disorders of kidney and ureter in diseases classified elsewhere
Code first underlying disease, such as:
amyloidosis (E85.-)
nephrocalcinosis (E83.5)
schistosomiasis (B65.Ø-B65.9)
EXCLUDES 1 *disorders of kidney and ureter in:*
cystinosis (E72.Ø)
gonorrhea (A54.21)
syphilis (A52.75)
tuberculosis (A18.11)

Other diseases of the urinary system (N3Ø-N39)

EXCLUDES 1 *urinary infection (complicating):*
abortion or ectopic or molar pregnancy (OØØ-OØ7, OØ8.8)
pregnancy, childbirth and the puerperium (O23.-, O75.3, O86.2-)

√4th **N3Ø Cystitis**
Use additional code to identify infectious agent (B95-B97)
EXCLUDES 1 *prostatocystitis (N41.3)*
AHA: 2017,1Q,6
DEF: Inflammation of the urinary bladder. Symptoms include dysuria, frequency of urination, urgency, and hematuria.

√5th **N3Ø.Ø Acute cystitis**
EXCLUDES 1 *irradiation cystitis (N3Ø.4-)*
trigonitis (N3Ø.3-)
N3Ø.ØØ Acute cystitis without hematuria CC H6
N3Ø.Ø1 Acute cystitis with hematuria CC H6

√5th **N3Ø.1 Interstitial cystitis (chronic)**
N3Ø.1Ø Interstitial cystitis (chronic) without hematuria
N3Ø.11 Interstitial cystitis (chronic) with hematuria

√5th **N3Ø.2 Other chronic cystitis**
N3Ø.2Ø Other chronic cystitis without hematuria
N3Ø.21 Other chronic cystitis with hematuria

√5th **N3Ø.3 Trigonitis**
Urethrotrigonitis
N3Ø.3Ø Trigonitis without hematuria
N3Ø.31 Trigonitis with hematuria

√5th **N3Ø.4 Irradiation cystitis**
N3Ø.4Ø Irradiation cystitis without hematuria CC
N3Ø.41 Irradiation cystitis with hematuria CC

√5th **N3Ø.8 Other cystitis**
Abscess of bladder
N3Ø.8Ø Other cystitis without hematuria
N3Ø.81 Other cystitis with hematuria

√5th **N3Ø.9 Cystitis, unspecified**
N3Ø.9Ø Cystitis, unspecified without hematuria
N3Ø.91 Cystitis, unspecified with hematuria

√4th **N31 Neuromuscular dysfunction of bladder, not elsewhere classified**
Use additional code to identify any associated urinary incontinence (N39.3-N39.4-)
EXCLUDES 1 *cord bladder NOS (G95.89)*
neurogenic bladder due to cauda equina syndrome (G83.4)
neuromuscular dysfunction due to spinal cord lesion (G95.89)

N31.Ø Uninhibited neuropathic bladder, not elsewhere classified

N31.1 Reflex neuropathic bladder, not elsewhere classified

N31.2 Flaccid neuropathic bladder, not elsewhere classified
Atonic (motor) (sensory) neuropathic bladder
Autonomous neuropathic bladder
Nonreflex neuropathic bladder

N31.8 Other neuromuscular dysfunction of bladder

N31.9 Neuromuscular dysfunction of bladder, unspecified
Neurogenic bladder dysfunction NOS

√4th **N32 Other disorders of bladder**
EXCLUDES 2 *calculus of bladder (N21.Ø)*
cystocele (N81.1-)
hernia or prolapse of bladder, female (N81.1-)

N32.Ø Bladder-neck obstruction
Bladder-neck stenosis (acquired)
EXCLUDES 1 *congenital bladder-neck obstruction (Q64.3-)*
DEF: Bladder outlet and vesicourethral obstruction that occurs as a consequence of benign prostatic hypertrophy or prostatic cancer. It may also occur in either sex due to strictures, radiation, cystoscopy, catheterization, injury, infection, blood clots, bladder cancer, impaction, or other disease that compresses the bladder neck.

N32.1 Vesicointestinal fistula CC
Vesicorectal fistula

N32.2 Vesical fistula, not elsewhere classified CC
EXCLUDES 1 *fistula between bladder and female genital tract (N82.Ø-N82.1)*

N32.3 Diverticulum of bladder
EXCLUDES 1 *congenital diverticulum of bladder (Q64.6)*
diverticulitis of bladder (N3Ø.8-)

√5th **N32.8 Other specified disorders of bladder**
N32.81 Overactive bladder
Detrusor muscle hyperactivity
EXCLUDES 1 *frequent urination due to specified bladder condition — code to condition*
DEF: Sudden involuntary contractions of the muscular wall of the bladder that results in a sudden, strong urge to urinate.
N32.89 Other specified disorders of bladder
Bladder hemorrhage
Bladder hypertrophy
Calcified bladder
Contracted bladder

N32.9 Bladder disorder, unspecified

N33 Bladder disorders in diseases classified elsewhere
Code first underlying disease, such as:
schistosomiasis (B65.Ø-B65.9)
EXCLUDES 1 *bladder disorder in syphilis (A52.76)*
bladder disorder in tuberculosis (A18.12)
candidal cystitis (B37.41)
chlamydial cystitis (A56.Ø1)
cystitis in gonorrhea (A54.Ø1)
cystitis in neurogenic bladder (N31.-)
diphtheritic cystitis (A36.85)
neurogenic bladder (N31.-)
syphilitic cystitis (A52.76)
trichomonal cystitis (A59.Ø3)

√4th **N34 Urethritis and urethral syndrome**
Use additional code (B95-B97), to identify infectious agent
EXCLUDES 2 *Reiter's disease (MØ2.3-)*
urethritis in diseases with a predominantly sexual mode of transmission (A5Ø-A64)
urethrotrigonitis (N3Ø.3-)
AHA: 2017,1Q,6

N34.Ø Urethral abscess CC H6
Abscess (of) Cowper's gland
Abscess (of) Littré's gland
Abscess (of) urethral (gland)
Periurethral abscess
EXCLUDES 1 *urethral caruncle (N36.2)*

N34.1 Nonspecific urethritis
Nongonococcal urethritis
Nonvenereal urethritis

N34.2 Other urethritis
Meatitis, urethral
Postmenopausal urethritis
Ulcer of urethra (meatus)
Urethritis NOS

N34.3 Urethral syndrome, unspecified

N35 Urethral stricture
EXCLUDES 1 *congenital urethral stricture (Q64.3-)*
postprocedural urethral stricture (N99.1-)
AHA: 2018,4Q,21-22

N35.0 Post-traumatic urethral stricture
Urethral stricture due to injury
EXCLUDES 1 *postprocedural urethral stricture (N99.1-)*

N35.01 Post-traumatic urethral stricture, male
N35.010 Post-traumatic urethral stricture, male, meatal ♂
N35.011 Post-traumatic bulbous urethral stricture ♂
N35.012 Post-traumatic membranous urethral stricture ♂
N35.013 Post-traumatic anterior urethral stricture ♂
N35.014 Post-traumatic urethral stricture, male, unspecified ♂
N35.016 Post-traumatic urethral stricture, male, overlapping sites ♂

N35.02 Post-traumatic urethral stricture, female
N35.021 Urethral stricture due to childbirth ♀
N35.028 Other post-traumatic urethral stricture, female ♀

N35.1 Postinfective urethral stricture, not elsewhere classified
EXCLUDES 1 *gonococcal urethral stricture (A54.01)*
syphilitic urethral stricture (A52.76)
urethral stricture associated with schistosomiasis (B65.-, N29)

N35.11 Postinfective urethral stricture, not elsewhere classified, male
N35.111 Postinfective urethral stricture, not elsewhere classified, male, meatal ♂
N35.112 Postinfective bulbous urethral stricture, not elsewhere classified, male ♂
N35.113 Postinfective membranous urethral stricture, not elsewhere classified, male ♂
N35.114 Postinfective anterior urethral stricture, not elsewhere classified, male ♂
N35.116 Postinfective urethral stricture, not elsewhere classified, male, overlapping sites ♂
N35.119 Postinfective urethral stricture, not elsewhere classified, male, unspecified ♂
N35.12 Postinfective urethral stricture, not elsewhere classified, female ♀

N35.8 Other urethral stricture
EXCLUDES 1 *postprocedural urethral stricture (N99.1-)*

N35.81 Other urethral stricture, male
N35.811 Other urethral stricture, male, meatal ♂
N35.812 Other urethral bulbous stricture, male ♂
N35.813 Other membranous urethral stricture, male ♂
N35.814 Other anterior urethral stricture, male ♂
N35.816 Other urethral stricture, male, overlapping sites ♂
N35.819 Other urethral stricture, male, unspecified site ♂
N35.82 Other urethral stricture, female ♀

N35.9 Urethral stricture, unspecified
N35.91 Urethral stricture, unspecified, male
N35.911 Unspecified urethral stricture, male, meatal ♂
N35.912 Unspecified bulbous urethral stricture, male ♂
N35.913 Unspecified membranous urethral stricture, male ♂
N35.914 Unspecified anterior urethral stricture, male ♂
N35.916 Unspecified urethral stricture, male, overlapping sites ♂
N35.919 Unspecified urethral stricture, male, unspecified site ♂
Pinhole meatus NOS
Urethral stricture NOS
N35.92 Unspecified urethral stricture, female ♀

N36 Other disorders of urethra
N36.0 Urethral fistula CC
Urethroperineal fistula
Urethrorectal fistula
Urinary fistula NOS
EXCLUDES 1 *urethroscrotal fistula (N50.89)*
urethrovaginal fistula (N82.1)
urethrovesicovaginal fistula (N82.1)
N36.1 Urethral diverticulum
N36.2 Urethral caruncle
N36.4 Urethral functional and muscular disorders
Use additional code to identify associated urinary stress incontinence (N39.3)
N36.41 Hypermobility of urethra
N36.42 Intrinsic sphincter deficiency (ISD)
N36.43 Combined hypermobility of urethra and intrinsic sphincter deficiency
N36.44 Muscular disorders of urethra
Bladder sphincter dyssynergy
N36.5 Urethral false passage
N36.8 Other specified disorders of urethra
EXCLUDES 1 *congenital urethrocele (Q64.7)*
female urethrocele (N81.0)
N36.9 Urethral disorder, unspecified

N37 Urethral disorders in diseases classified elsewhere
Code first underlying disease
EXCLUDES 1 *urethritis (in):*
candidal infection (B37.41)
chlamydial (A56.01)
gonorrhea (A54.01)
syphilis (A52.76)
trichomonal infection (A59.03)
tuberculosis (A18.13)

N39 Other disorders of urinary system
EXCLUDES 2 *hematuria NOS (R31.-)*
recurrent or persistent hematuria (N02.-)
recurrent or persistent hematuria with specified morphological lesion (N02.-)
proteinuria NOS (R80.-)

N39.0 Urinary tract infection, site not specified CC H6
Use additional code (B95-B97), to identify infectious agent
EXCLUDES 1 *candidiasis of urinary tract (B37.4-)*
neonatal urinary tract infection (P39.3)
pyuria (R82.81)
urinary tract infection of specified site, such as:
cystitis (N30.-)
urethritis (N34.-)
AHA: 2019,3Q,17; 2018,2Q,21,22; 2018,1Q,16; 2017,1Q,6; 2012,4Q,94
N39.3 Stress incontinence (female) (male)
Code also any associated overactive bladder (N32.81)
EXCLUDES 1 *mixed incontinence (N39.46)*
N39.4 Other specified urinary incontinence
Code also any associated overactive bladder (N32.81)
EXCLUDES 1 *enuresis NOS (R32)*
functional urinary incontinence (R39.81)
urinary incontinence associated with cognitive impairment (R39.81)
urinary incontinence NOS (R32)
urinary incontinence of nonorganic origin (F98.0)
N39.41 Urge incontinence
EXCLUDES 1 *mixed incontinence (N39.46)*
N39.42 Incontinence without sensory awareness
Insensible (urinary) incontinence
N39.43 Post-void dribbling
N39.44 Nocturnal enuresis
N39.45 Continuous leakage

N39.46 Mixed incontinence
Urge and stress incontinence

✓6th **N39.49 Other specified urinary incontinence**
AHA: 2016,4Q,44

N39.49Ø Overflow incontinence
N39.491 Coital incontinence
N39.492 Postural (urinary) incontinence
N39.498 Other specified urinary incontinence
Reflex incontinence
Total incontinence

N39.8 Other specified disorders of urinary system
N39.9 Disorder of urinary system, unspecified

Diseases of male genital organs (N4Ø-N53)

✓4th **N4Ø Benign prostatic hyperplasia**

INCLUDES adenofibromatous hypertrophy of prostate
benign hypertrophy of the prostate
benign prostatic hypertrophy
BPH
enlarged prostate
nodular prostate
polyp of prostate

EXCLUDES 1 *benign neoplasms of prostate (adenoma, benign) (fibroadenoma) (fibroma) (myoma) (D29.1)*

EXCLUDES 2 *malignant neoplasm of prostate (C61)*

DEF: Enlargement of the prostate gland due to an abnormal proliferation of fibrostromal tissue in the paraurethral glands. This condition causes impingement of the urethra resulting in obstructed urinary flow.

N4Ø.Ø Benign prostatic hyperplasia without lower urinary tract symptoms A ♂
Enlarged prostate NOS
Enlarged prostate without LUTS

N4Ø.1 Benign prostatic hyperplasia with lower urinary tract symptoms A ♂
Enlarged prostate with LUTS
Use additional code for associated symptoms, when specified:
incomplete bladder emptying (R39.14)
nocturia (R35.1)
straining on urination (R39.16)
urinary frequency (R35.Ø)
urinary hesitancy (R39.11)
urinary incontinence (N39.4-)
urinary obstruction (N13.8)
urinary retention (R33.8)
urinary urgency (R39.15)
weak urinary stream (R39.12)
AHA: 2018,4Q,55

N4Ø.2 Nodular prostate without lower urinary tract symptoms A ♂
Nodular prostate without LUTS

N4Ø.3 Nodular prostate with lower urinary tract symptoms A ♂
Use additional code for associated symptoms, when specified:
incomplete bladder emptying (R39.14)
nocturia (R35.1)
straining on urination (R39.16)
urinary frequency (R35.Ø)
urinary hesitancy (R39.11)
urinary incontinence (N39.4-)
urinary obstruction (N13.8)
urinary retention (R33.8)
urinary urgency (R39.15)
weak urinary stream (R39.12)

✓4th **N41 Inflammatory diseases of prostate**
Use additional code (B95-B97), to identify infectious agent

N41.Ø Acute prostatitis CC A ♂
N41.1 Chronic prostatitis A ♂
N41.2 Abscess of prostate CC A ♂
N41.3 Prostatocystitis A ♂
N41.4 Granulomatous prostatitis A ♂
N41.8 Other inflammatory diseases of prostate A ♂
N41.9 Inflammatory disease of prostate, unspecified A ♂
Prostatitis NOS

✓4th **N42 Other and unspecified disorders of prostate**

N42.Ø Calculus of prostate A ♂
Prostatic stone
DEF: Formation of a small, solid stone often composed of calcium carbonate or calcium phosphate in the prostate gland.

N42.1 Congestion and hemorrhage of prostate A ♂
EXCLUDES 1 *enlarged prostate (N4Ø.-)*
hematuria (R31.-)
hyperplasia of prostate (N4Ø.-)
inflammatory diseases of prostate (N41.-)

✓5th **N42.3 Dysplasia of prostate**
AHA: 2016,4Q,44

N42.3Ø Unspecified dysplasia of prostate ♂
N42.31 Prostatic intraepithelial neoplasia ♂
PIN
Prostatic intraepithelial neoplasia I (PIN I)
Prostatic intraepithelial neoplasia II (PIN II)
EXCLUDES 1 *prostatic intraepithelial neoplasia III (PIN III) (DØ7.5)*
DEF: Abnormality of shape and size of the intraepithelial tissues of the prostate. It is a premalignant condition characterized by stalks and absence of a basilar cell layer.
N42.32 Atypical small acinar proliferation of prostate ♂
N42.39 Other dysplasia of prostate ♂

✓5th **N42.8 Other specified disorders of prostate**

N42.81 Prostatodynia syndrome A ♂
Painful prostate syndrome
N42.82 Prostatosis syndrome A ♂
N42.83 Cyst of prostate A ♂
N42.89 Other specified disorders of prostate A ♂

N42.9 Disorder of prostate, unspecified A ♂

✓4th **N43 Hydrocele and spermatocele**

INCLUDES hydrocele of spermatic cord, testis or tunica vaginalis

EXCLUDES 1 *congenital hydrocele (P83.5)*

DEF: Hydrocele: Serous fluid that collects in the tunica vaginalis of the scrotum along the spermatic cord in males.

N43.Ø Encysted hydrocele ♂
N43.1 Infected hydrocele CC ♂
Use additional code (B95-B97), to identify infectious agent
N43.2 Other hydrocele ♂

Hydrocele

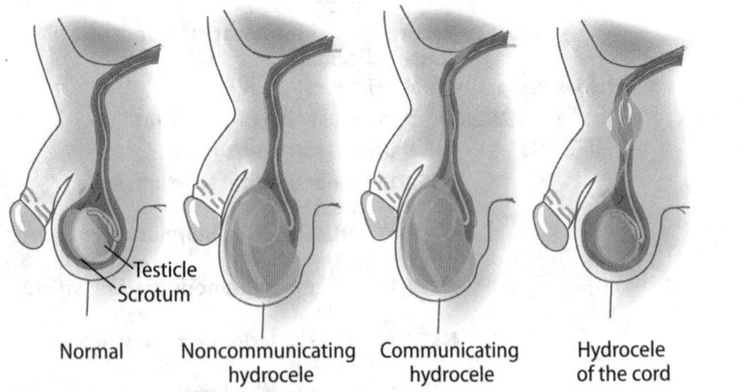

N43.3 Hydrocele, unspecified ♂

✓5th **N43.4 Spermatocele of epididymis**
Spermatic cyst
DEF: Spermatocele: Noncancerous accumulation of fluid and dead sperm cells normally located at the head of the epididymis that exhibits itself as a hard, smooth scrotal mass and do not normally require treatment unless they become enlarged or cause pain.

N43.4Ø Spermatocele of epididymis, unspecified ♂
N43.41 Spermatocele of epididymis, single ♂
N43.42 Spermatocele of epididymis, multiple ♂

✓4th **N44 Noninflammatory disorders of testis**

✓5th **N44.Ø Torsion of testis**

N44.ØØ Torsion of testis, unspecified CC ♂

N44.01 Extravaginal torsion of spermatic cord CC ♂
DEF: Torsion of the spermatic cord just below the tunica vaginalis attachments.

N44.02 Intravaginal torsion of spermatic cord CC ♂
Torsion of spermatic cord NOS

N44.03 Torsion of appendix testis CC ♂

N44.04 Torsion of appendix epididymis CC ♂

N44.1 Cyst of tunica albuginea testis ♂

N44.2 Benign cyst of testis ♂

N44.8 Other noninflammatory disorders of the testis ♂

✓4th N45 Orchitis and epididymitis
Use additional code (B95-B97), to identify infectious agent

N45.1 Epididymitis ♂

N45.2 Orchitis ♂

N45.3 Epididymo-orchitis ♂

N45.4 Abscess of epididymis or testis CC ♂

✓4th N46 Male infertility
EXCLUDES 1 *vasectomy status (Z98.52)*

✓5th N46.0 Azoospermia
Absolute male infertility
Male infertility due to germinal (cell) aplasia
Male infertility due to spermatogenic arrest (complete)
DEF: Failure of the development of sperm or the absence of sperm in semen.

N46.01 Organic azoospermia A ♂
Azoospermia NOS

✓6th N46.02 Azoospermia due to extratesticular causes
Code also associated cause

N46.021 Azoospermia due to drug therapy A ♂

N46.022 Azoospermia due to infection A ♂

N46.023 Azoospermia due to obstruction of efferent ducts A ♂

N46.024 Azoospermia due to radiation A ♂

N46.025 Azoospermia due to systemic disease A ♂

N46.029 Azoospermia due to other extratesticular causes A ♂

✓5th N46.1 Oligospermia
Male infertility due to germinal cell desquamation
Male infertility due to hypospermatogenesis
Male infertility due to incomplete spermatogenic arrest
DEF: Insufficient production of sperm in semen.

N46.11 Organic oligospermia A ♂
Oligospermia NOS

✓6th N46.12 Oligospermia due to extratesticular causes
Code also associated cause

N46.121 Oligospermia due to drug therapy A ♂

N46.122 Oligospermia due to infection A ♂

N46.123 Oligospermia due to obstruction of efferent ducts A ♂

N46.124 Oligospermia due to radiation A ♂

N46.125 Oligospermia due to systemic disease A ♂

N46.129 Oligospermia due to other extratesticular causes A ♂

N46.8 Other male infertility A ♂

N46.9 Male infertility, unspecified A ♂

✓4th N47 Disorders of prepuce

N47.0 Adherent prepuce, newborn N ♂

N47.1 Phimosis ♂
DEF: Condition in which the foreskin is contracted and cannot be drawn back behind the glans penis.

N47.2 Paraphimosis ♂

N47.3 Deficient foreskin ♂

N47.4 Benign cyst of prepuce ♂

N47.5 Adhesions of prepuce and glans penis ♂

N47.6 Balanoposthitis ♂
Use additional code (B95-B97), to identify infectious agent
EXCLUDES 1 *balanitis (N48.1)*

N47.7 Other inflammatory diseases of prepuce ♂
Use additional code (B95-B97), to identify infectious agent

N47.8 Other disorders of prepuce ♂

✓4th N48 Other disorders of penis

N48.0 Leukoplakia of penis ♂
Balanitis xerotica obliterans
Kraurosis of penis
Lichen sclerosus of external male genital organs
EXCLUDES 1 *carcinoma in situ of penis (D07.4)*

N48.1 Balanitis ♂
Use additional code (B95-B97), to identify infectious agent
EXCLUDES 1 *amebic balanitis (A06.8)*
balanitis xerotica obliterans (N48.0)
candidal balanitis (B37.42)
gonococcal balanitis (A54.23)
herpesviral [herpes simplex] balanitis (A60.01)
DEF: Inflammation of the glans penis, most often affecting uncircumcised males.

✓5th N48.2 Other inflammatory disorders of penis
Use additional code (B95-B97), to identify infectious agent
EXCLUDES 1 *balanitis (N48.1)*
balanitis xerotica obliterans (N48.0)
balanoposthitis (N47.6)

N48.21 Abscess of corpus cavernosum and penis ♂

N48.22 Cellulitis of corpus cavernosum and penis ♂

N48.29 Other inflammatory disorders of penis ♂

✓5th N48.3 Priapism
Painful erection
Code first underlying cause

N48.30 Priapism, unspecified CC ♂

N48.31 Priapism due to trauma CC ♂

N48.32 Priapism due to disease classified elsewhere CC ♂

N48.33 Priapism, drug-induced CC ♂

N48.39 Other priapism CC ♂

N48.5 Ulcer of penis ♂

N48.6 Induration penis plastica ♂
Peyronie's disease
Plastic induration of penis

✓5th N48.8 Other specified disorders of penis

N48.81 Thrombosis of superficial vein of penis ♂

N48.82 Acquired torsion of penis ♂
Acquired torsion of penis NOS
EXCLUDES 1 *congenital torsion of penis (Q55.63)*

N48.83 Acquired buried penis ♂
EXCLUDES 1 *congenital hidden penis (Q55.64)*

N48.89 Other specified disorders of penis ♂

N48.9 Disorder of penis, unspecified ♂

✓4th N49 Inflammatory disorders of male genital organs, not elsewhere classified
Use additional code (B95-B97), to identify infectious agent
EXCLUDES 1 *inflammation of penis (N48.1, N48.2-)*
orchitis and epididymitis (N45.-)

N49.0 Inflammatory disorders of seminal vesicle ♂
Vesiculitis NOS

N49.1 Inflammatory disorders of spermatic cord, tunica vaginalis and vas deferens ♂
Vasitis

N49.2 Inflammatory disorders of scrotum ♂

N49.3 Fournier gangrene ♂
AHA: 2020,2Q,18

N49.8 Inflammatory disorders of other specified male genital organs ♂
Inflammation of multiple sites in male genital organs

N49.9 Inflammatory disorder of unspecified male genital organ ♂
Abscess of unspecified male genital organ
Boil of unspecified male genital organ
Carbuncle of unspecified male genital organ
Cellulitis of unspecified male genital organ

✓4th N50 Other and unspecified disorders of male genital organs
EXCLUDES 2 *torsion of testis (N44.0-)*

N50.0 Atrophy of testis ♂

N50.1 Vascular disorders of male genital organs ♂
Hematocele, NOS, of male genital organs
Hemorrhage of male genital organs
Thrombosis of male genital organs

N50.3 Cyst of epididymis ♂

N50.8 Other specified disorders of male genital organs

AHA: 2016,4Q,45

N50.81 Testicular pain

N50.811 Right testicular pain ♂

N50.812 Left testicular pain ♂

N50.819 Testicular pain, unspecified ♂

N50.82 Scrotal pain ♂

N50.89 Other specified disorders of the male genital organs ♂

Atrophy of scrotum, seminal vesicle, spermatic cord, tunica vaginalis and vas deferens

Chylocele, tunica vaginalis (nonfilarial) NOS

Edema of scrotum, seminal vesicle, spermatic cord, tunica vaginalis and vas deferens

Hypertrophy of scrotum, seminal vesicle, spermatic cord, tunica vaginalis and vas deferens

Stricture of spermatic cord, tunica vaginalis, and vas deferens

Ulcer of scrotum, seminal vesicle, spermatic cord, testis, tunica vaginalis and vas deferens

Urethroscrotal fistula

N50.9 Disorder of male genital organs, unspecified ♂

N51 Disorders of male genital organs in diseases classified elsewhere ♂

Code first underlying disease, such as:

filariasis (B74.0-B74.9)

EXCLUDES 1 *amebic balanitis (A06.8)*

candidal balanitis (B37.42)

gonococcal balanitis (A54.23)

gonococcal prostatitis (A54.22)

herpesviral [herpes simplex] balanitis (A60.01)

trichomonal prostatitis (A59.02)

tuberculous prostatitis (A18.14)

N52 Male erectile dysfunction

EXCLUDES 1 *psychogenic impotence (F52.21)*

N52.0 Vasculogenic erectile dysfunction

N52.01 Erectile dysfunction due to arterial insufficiency A ♂

N52.02 Corporo-venous occlusive erectile dysfunction A ♂

N52.03 Combined arterial insufficiency and corporo-venous occlusive erectile dysfunction A ♂

N52.1 Erectile dysfunction due to diseases classified elsewhere A ♂

Code first underlying disease

N52.2 Drug-induced erectile dysfunction A ♂

N52.3 Postprocedural erectile dysfunction

AHA: 2016,4Q,45

N52.31 Erectile dysfunction following radical prostatectomy A ♂

N52.32 Erectile dysfunction following radical cystectomy A ♂

N52.33 Erectile dysfunction following urethral surgery A ♂

N52.34 Erectile dysfunction following simple prostatectomy A ♂

N52.35 Erectile dysfunction following radiation therapy A ♂

N52.36 Erectile dysfunction following interstitial seed therapy A ♂

N52.37 Erectile dysfunction following prostate ablative therapy A ♂

Erectile dysfunction following cryotherapy

Erectile dysfunction following other prostate ablative therapies

Erectile dysfunction following ultrasound ablative therapies

N52.39 Other and unspecified postprocedural erectile dysfunction A ♂

N52.8 Other male erectile dysfunction A ♂

N52.9 Male erectile dysfunction, unspecified A ♂

Impotence NOS

N53 Other male sexual dysfunction

EXCLUDES 1 *psychogenic sexual dysfunction (F52.-)*

N53.1 Ejaculatory dysfunction

EXCLUDES 1 *premature ejaculation (F52.4)*

N53.11 Retarded ejaculation ♂

N53.12 Painful ejaculation ♂

N53.13 Anejaculatory orgasm ♂

N53.14 Retrograde ejaculation ♂

DEF: Form of male sexual dysfunction in which the semen enters the bladder instead of going out through the urethra during ejaculation.

N53.19 Other ejaculatory dysfunction ♂

Ejaculatory dysfunction NOS

N53.8 Other male sexual dysfunction ♂

N53.9 Unspecified male sexual dysfunction ♂

Disorders of breast (N60-N65)

EXCLUDES 1 *disorders of breast associated with childbirth (O91-O92)*

N60 Benign mammary dysplasia

INCLUDES fibrocystic mastopathy

N60.0 Solitary cyst of breast

Cyst of breast

N60.01 Solitary cyst of right breast

N60.02 Solitary cyst of left breast

N60.09 Solitary cyst of unspecified breast

N60.1 Diffuse cystic mastopathy

Cystic breast

Fibrocystic disease of breast

EXCLUDES 1 *diffuse cystic mastopathy with epithelial proliferation (N60.3-)*

N60.11 Diffuse cystic mastopathy of right breast A

N60.12 Diffuse cystic mastopathy of left breast A

N60.19 Diffuse cystic mastopathy of unspecified breast A

N60.2 Fibroadenosis of breast

Adenofibrosis of breast

EXCLUDES 2 *fibroadenoma of breast (D24.-)*

N60.21 Fibroadenosis of right breast

N60.22 Fibroadenosis of left breast

N60.29 Fibroadenosis of unspecified breast

N60.3 Fibrosclerosis of breast

Cystic mastopathy with epithelial proliferation

N60.31 Fibrosclerosis of right breast

N60.32 Fibrosclerosis of left breast

N60.39 Fibrosclerosis of unspecified breast

N60.4 Mammary duct ectasia

N60.41 Mammary duct ectasia of right breast

N60.42 Mammary duct ectasia of left breast

N60.49 Mammary duct ectasia of unspecified breast

N60.8 Other benign mammary dysplasias

N60.81 Other benign mammary dysplasias of right breast

N60.82 Other benign mammary dysplasias of left breast

N60.89 Other benign mammary dysplasias of unspecified breast

N60.9 Unspecified benign mammary dysplasia

N60.91 Unspecified benign mammary dysplasia of right breast

N60.92 Unspecified benign mammary dysplasia of left breast

N60.99 Unspecified benign mammary dysplasia of unspecified breast

N61 Inflammatory disorders of breast

EXCLUDES 1 *inflammatory carcinoma of breast (C50.9)*

inflammatory disorder of breast associated with childbirth (O91.-)

neonatal infective mastitis (P39.0)

thrombophlebitis of breast [Mondor's disease] (I80.8)

N61.0 Mastitis without abscess

Infective mastitis (acute) (nonpuerperal) (subacute)

Mastitis (acute) (nonpuerperal) (subacute) NOS

Cellulitis (acute) (nonpuerperal) (subacute) of breast NOS

Cellulitis (acute) (nonpuerperal) (subacute) of nipple NOS

N61.1 Abscess of the breast and nipple
Abscess (acute) (chronic) (nonpuerperal) of areola
Abscess (acute) (chronic) (nonpuerperal) of breast
Carbuncle of breast
Mastitis with abscess

● **N61.2 Granulomatous mastitis**
● **N61.20 Granulomatous mastitis, unspecified breast**
● **N61.21 Granulomatous mastitis, right breast**
● **N61.22 Granulomatous mastitis, left breast**
● **N61.23 Granulomatous mastitis, bilateral breast**

N62 Hypertrophy of breast
Gynecomastia
Hypertrophy of breast NOS
Massive pubertal hypertrophy of breast
EXCLUDES 1 *breast engorgement of newborn (P83.4)*
disproportion of reconstructed breast (N65.1)

N63 Unspecified lump in breast
Nodule(s) NOS in breast
AHA: 2019,4Q,12; 2017,4Q,19
N63.0 Unspecified lump in unspecified breast
N63.1 Unspecified lump in the right breast
N63.10 Unspecified lump in the right breast, unspecified quadrant
N63.11 Unspecified lump in the right breast, upper outer quadrant
N63.12 Unspecified lump in the right breast, upper inner quadrant
N63.13 Unspecified lump in the right breast, lower outer quadrant
N63.14 Unspecified lump in the right breast, lower inner quadrant
N63.15 Unspecified lump in the right breast, overlapping quadrants
N63.2 Unspecified lump in the left breast
N63.20 Unspecified lump in the left breast, unspecified quadrant
N63.21 Unspecified lump in the left breast, upper outer quadrant
N63.22 Unspecified lump in the left breast, upper inner quadrant
N63.23 Unspecified lump in the left breast, lower outer quadrant
N63.24 Unspecified lump in the left breast, lower inner quadrant
N63.25 Unspecified lump in the left breast, overlapping quadrants
N63.3 Unspecified lump in axillary tail
N63.31 Unspecified lump in axillary tail of the right breast
N63.32 Unspecified lump in axillary tail of the left breast
N63.4 Unspecified lump in breast, subareolar
N63.41 Unspecified lump in right breast, subareolar
N63.42 Unspecified lump in left breast, subareolar

N64 Other disorders of breast
EXCLUDES 2 *mechanical complication of breast prosthesis and implant (T85.4-)*
N64.0 Fissure and fistula of nipple
N64.1 Fat necrosis of breast
Fat necrosis (segmental) of breast
Code first breast necrosis due to breast graft (T85.898)
N64.2 Atrophy of breast
N64.3 Galactorrhea not associated with childbirth
N64.4 Mastodynia
N64.5 Other signs and symptoms in breast
EXCLUDES 2 *abnormal findings on diagnostic imaging of breast (R92.-)*
N64.51 Induration of breast
N64.52 Nipple discharge
EXCLUDES 1 *abnormal findings in nipple discharge (R89.-)*
N64.53 Retraction of nipple
N64.59 Other signs and symptoms in breast
N64.8 Other specified disorders of breast
N64.81 Ptosis of breast A
EXCLUDES 1 *ptosis of native breast in relation to reconstructed breast (N65.1)*
N64.82 Hypoplasia of breast A
Micromastia
EXCLUDES 1 *congenital absence of breast (Q83.0)*
hypoplasia of native breast in relation to reconstructed breast (N65.1)
N64.89 Other specified disorders of breast
Galactocele
Subinvolution of breast (postlactational)
AHA: 2019,1Q,32; 2018,1Q,3
N64.9 Disorder of breast, unspecified

N65 Deformity and disproportion of reconstructed breast
N65.0 Deformity of reconstructed breast A
Contour irregularity in reconstructed breast
Excess tissue in reconstructed breast
Misshapen reconstructed breast
N65.1 Disproportion of reconstructed breast A
Breast asymmetry between native breast and reconstructed breast
Disproportion between native breast and reconstructed breast

Inflammatory diseases of female pelvic organs (N70-N77)

EXCLUDES 1 *inflammatory diseases of female pelvic organs complicating:*
abortion or ectopic or molar pregnancy (O00-O07, O08.0)
pregnancy, childbirth and the puerperium (O23.-, O75.3, O85, O86.-)

N70 Salpingitis and oophoritis
INCLUDES abscess (of) fallopian tube
abscess (of) ovary
pyosalpinx
salpingo-oophoritis
tubo-ovarian abscess
tubo-ovarian inflammatory disease
Use additional code (B95-B97), to identify infectious agent
EXCLUDES 1 *gonococcal infection (A54.24)*
tuberculous infection (A18.17)
N70.0 Acute salpingitis and oophoritis
N70.01 Acute salpingitis CC ♀
N70.02 Acute oophoritis CC ♀
N70.03 Acute salpingitis and oophoritis CC ♀
N70.1 Chronic salpingitis and oophoritis
Hydrosalpinx
N70.11 Chronic salpingitis ♀
N70.12 Chronic oophoritis ♀
N70.13 Chronic salpingitis and oophoritis ♀
N70.9 Salpingitis and oophoritis, unspecified
N70.91 Salpingitis, unspecified ♀
N70.92 Oophoritis, unspecified ♀
N70.93 Salpingitis and oophoritis, unspecified ♀

N71 Inflammatory disease of uterus, except cervix
INCLUDES endo (myo) metritis
metritis
myometritis
pyometra
uterine abscess
Use additional code (B95-B97), to identify infectious agent
EXCLUDES 1 *hyperplastic endometritis (N85.0-)*
infection of uterus following delivery (O85, O86.-)
N71.0 Acute inflammatory disease of uterus CC ♀
N71.1 Chronic inflammatory disease of uterus ♀
N71.9 Inflammatory disease of uterus, unspecified ♀

N72 Inflammatory disease of cervix uteri ♀
INCLUDES cervicitis (with or without erosion or ectropion)
endocervicitis (with or without erosion or ectropion)
exocervicitis (with or without erosion or ectropion)
Use additional code (B95-B97), to identify infectious agent
EXCLUDES 1 *erosion and ectropion of cervix without cervicitis (N86)*

✓4th N73 Other female pelvic inflammatory diseases

Use additional code (B95-B97), to identify infectious agent

N73.0 Acute parametritis and pelvic cellulitis CC ♀
- Abscess of broad ligament
- Abscess of parametrium
- Pelvic cellulitis, female
- **DEF:** Parametritis: Inflammation of the parametrium.

N73.1 Chronic parametritis and pelvic cellulitis ♀
- Any condition in N73.0 specified as chronic
- EXCLUDES 1 *tuberculous parametritis and pelvic cellutis (A18.17)*

N73.2 Unspecified parametritis and pelvic cellulitis ♀
- Any condition in N73.0 unspecified whether acute or chronic

N73.3 Female acute pelvic peritonitis MCC ♀

N73.4 Female chronic pelvic peritonitis CC ♀
- EXCLUDES 1 *tuberculous pelvic (female) peritonitis (A18.17)*

N73.5 Female pelvic peritonitis, unspecified ♀

N73.6 Female pelvic peritoneal adhesions (postinfective) ♀
- EXCLUDES 2 *postprocedural pelvic peritoneal adhesions (N99.4)*
- **AHA:** 2014,1Q,6

N73.8 Other specified female pelvic inflammatory diseases ♀

N73.9 Female pelvic inflammatory disease, unspecified ♀
- Female pelvic infection or inflammation NOS

N74 Female pelvic inflammatory disorders in diseases classified elsewhere ♀

Code first underlying disease

EXCLUDES 1
- *chlamydial cervicitis (A56.02)*
- *chlamydial pelvic inflammatory disease (A56.11)*
- *gonococcal cervicitis (A54.03)*
- *gonococcal pelvic inflammatory disease (A54.24)*
- *herpesviral [herpes simplex] cervicitis (A60.03)*
- *herpesviral [herpes simplex] pelvic inflammatory disease (A60.09)*
- *syphilitic cervicitis (A52.76)*
- *syphilitic pelvic inflammatory disease (A52.76)*
- *trichomonal cervicitis (A59.09)*
- *tuberculous cervicitis (A18.16)*
- *tuberculous pelvic inflammatory disease (A18.17)*

✓4th N75 Diseases of Bartholin's gland

DEF: Bartholin's gland: Mucous-producing gland found in the vestibular bulbs on either side of the vaginal orifice and connected to the mucosal membrane at the opening by a duct.

N75.0 Cyst of Bartholin's gland ♀

N75.1 Abscess of Bartholin's gland CC ♀

N75.8 Other diseases of Bartholin's gland ♀
- Bartholinitis

N75.9 Disease of Bartholin's gland, unspecified ♀

✓4th N76 Other inflammation of vagina and vulva

Use additional code (B95-B97), to identify infectious agent

EXCLUDES 2
- *senile (atrophic) vaginitis (N95.2)*
- *vulvar vestibulitis (N94.810)*

N76.0 Acute vaginitis ♀
- Acute vulvovaginitis
- Vaginitis NOS
- Vulvovaginitis NOS

N76.1 Subacute and chronic vaginitis ♀
- Chronic vulvovaginitis
- Subacute vulvovaginitis

N76.2 Acute vulvitis ♀
- Vulvitis NOS

N76.3 Subacute and chronic vulvitis ♀

N76.4 Abscess of vulva CC ♀
- Furuncle of vulva

N76.5 Ulceration of vagina ♀

N76.6 Ulceration of vulva ♀

✓5th N76.8 Other specified inflammation of vagina and vulva

N76.81 Mucositis (ulcerative) of vagina and vulva CC ♀
- Code also type of associated therapy, such as:
  - antineoplastic and immunosuppressive drugs (T45.1X-)
  - radiological procedure and radiotherapy (Y84.2)
- EXCLUDES 2
  - *gastrointestinal mucositis (ulcerative) (K92.81)*
  - *nasal mucositis (ulcerative) (J34.81)*
  - *oral mucositis (ulcerative) (K12.3-)*

N76.89 Other specified inflammation of vagina and vulva ♀

✓4th N77 Vulvovaginal ulceration and inflammation in diseases classified elsewhere

N77.0 Ulceration of vulva in diseases classified elsewhere ♀
- Code first underlying disease, such as:
  - Behçet's disease (M35.2)
- EXCLUDES 1
  - *ulceration of vulva in gonococcal infection (A54.02)*
  - *ulceration of vulva in herpesviral [herpes simplex] infection (A60.04)*
  - *ulceration of vulva in syphilis (A51.0)*
  - *ulceration of vulva in tuberculosis (A18.18)*

N77.1 Vaginitis, vulvitis and vulvovaginitis in diseases classified elsewhere ♀
- Code first underlying disease, such as:
  - pinworm (B80)
- EXCLUDES 1
  - *candidal vulvovaginitis (B37.3)*
  - *chlamydial vulvovaginitis (A56.02)*
  - *gonococcal vulvovaginitis (A54.02)*
  - *herpesviral [herpes simplex] vulvovaginitis (A60.04)*
  - *trichomonal vulvovaginitis (A59.01)*
  - *tuberculous vulvovaginitis (A18.18)*
  - *vulvovaginitis in early syphilis (A51.0)*
  - *vulvovaginitis in late syphilis (A52.76)*

Noninflammatory disorders of female genital tract (N80-N98)

✓4th N80 Endometriosis

DEF: Aberrant uterine mucosal tissue appearing in areas of the pelvic cavity outside of its normal location, lining the uterus, and inflaming surrounding tissues often resulting in infertility or spontaneous abortion.

N80.0 Endometriosis of uterus ♀
- Adenomyosis
- EXCLUDES 1 *stromal endometriosis (D39.0)*

N80.1 Endometriosis of ovary ♀

N80.2 Endometriosis of fallopian tube ♀

N80.3 Endometriosis of pelvic peritoneum ♀

N80.4 Endometriosis of rectovaginal septum and vagina ♀

N80.5 Endometriosis of intestine ♀

N80.6 Endometriosis in cutaneous scar ♀

N80.8 Other endometriosis ♀
- Endometriosis of thorax

N80.9 Endometriosis, unspecified ♀

✓4th N81 Female genital prolapse

EXCLUDES 1 *genital prolapse complicating pregnancy, labor or delivery (O34.5-)*
prolapse and hernia of ovary and fallopian tube (N83.4-)
prolapse of vaginal vault after hysterectomy (N99.3)

Types of Pelvic Organ Prolapse

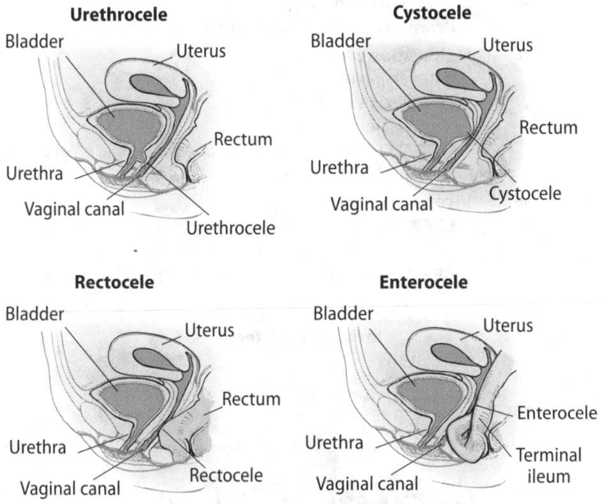

N81.Ø Urethrocele ♀
EXCLUDES 1 *urethrocele with cystocele (N81.1-)*
urethrocele with prolapse of uterus (N81.2-N81.4)

✓5th **N81.1 Cystocele**
Cystocele with urethrocele
Cystourethrocele
EXCLUDES 1 *cystocele with prolapse of uterus (N81.2-N81.4)*

N81.1Ø Cystocele, unspecified ♀
Prolapse of (anterior) vaginal wall NOS

N81.11 Cystocele, midline ♀

N81.12 Cystocele, lateral ♀
Paravaginal cystocele
DEF: Detachment of the lateral support connections of the vagina at the arcus tendineus fasciae pelvis (ATFP) that results in bladder drop. The bladder herniates into the vagina laterally.

N81.2 Incomplete uterovaginal prolapse ♀
First degree uterine prolapse
Prolapse of cervix NOS
Second degree uterine prolapse
EXCLUDES 1 *cervical stump prolapse (N81.85)*

N81.3 Complete uterovaginal prolapse ♀
Procidentia (uteri) NOS
Third degree uterine prolapse

N81.4 Uterovaginal prolapse, unspecified ♀
Prolapse of uterus NOS

N81.5 Vaginal enterocele ♀
EXCLUDES 1 *enterocele with prolapse of uterus (N81.2-N81.4)*

N81.6 Rectocele ♀
Prolapse of posterior vaginal wall
Use additional code for any associated fecal incontinence, if applicable (R15.-)
EXCLUDES 2 *perineocele (N81.81)*
rectal prolapse (K62.3)
rectocele with prolapse of uterus (N81.2-N81.4)

✓5th **N81.8 Other female genital prolapse**

N81.81 Perineocele ♀

N81.82 Incompetence or weakening of pubocervical tissue ♀

N81.83 Incompetence or weakening of rectovaginal tissue ♀

N81.84 Pelvic muscle wasting ♀
Disuse atrophy of pelvic muscles and anal sphincter

N81.85 Cervical stump prolapse ♀

N81.89 Other female genital prolapse ♀
Deficient perineum
Old laceration of muscles of pelvic floor

N81.9 Female genital prolapse, unspecified ♀

✓4th N82 Fistulae involving female genital tract

EXCLUDES 1 *vesicointestinal fistulae (N32.1)*

N82.Ø Vesicovaginal fistula CC SW ♀

N82.1 Other female urinary-genital tract fistulae CC ♀
Cervicovesical fistula
Ureterovaginal fistula
Urethrovaginal fistula
Uteroureteric fistula
Uterovesical fistula
AHA: 2017,3Q,3

N82.2 Fistula of vagina to small intestine CC SW ♀

N82.3 Fistula of vagina to large intestine CC SW ♀
Rectovaginal fistula

N82.4 Other female intestinal-genital tract fistulae CC SW ♀
Intestinouterine fistula

N82.5 Female genital tract-skin fistulae CC SW ♀
Uterus to abdominal wall fistula
Vaginoperineal fistula

N82.8 Other female genital tract fistulae CC ♀

N82.9 Female genital tract fistula, unspecified CC ♀

✓4th N83 Noninflammatory disorders of ovary, fallopian tube and broad ligament

EXCLUDES 2 *hydrosalpinx (N7Ø.1-)*
AHA: 2016,4Q,46

✓5th **N83.Ø Follicular cyst of ovary**
Cyst of graafian follicle
Hemorrhagic follicular cyst (of ovary)

N83.ØØ Follicular cyst of ovary, unspecified side ♀

N83.Ø1 Follicular cyst of right ovary ♀

N83.Ø2 Follicular cyst of left ovary ♀

✓5th **N83.1 Corpus luteum cyst**
Hemorrhagic corpus luteum cyst

N83.1Ø Corpus luteum cyst of ovary, unspecified side ♀

N83.11 Corpus luteum cyst of right ovary ♀

N83.12 Corpus luteum cyst of left ovary ♀

✓5th **N83.2 Other and unspecified ovarian cysts**
EXCLUDES 1 *developmental ovarian cyst (Q5Ø.1)*
neoplastic ovarian cyst (D27.-)
polycystic ovarian syndrome (E28.2)
Stein-Leventhal syndrome (E28.2)

✓6th **N83.2Ø Unspecified ovarian cysts**

N83.2Ø1 Unspecified ovarian cyst, right side ♀

N83.2Ø2 Unspecified ovarian cyst, left side ♀

N83.2Ø9 Unspecified ovarian cyst, unspecified side ♀
Ovarian cyst, NOS

✓6th **N83.29 Other ovarian cysts**
Retention cyst of ovary
Simple cyst of ovary

N83.291 Other ovarian cyst, right side ♀

N83.292 Other ovarian cyst, left side ♀

N83.299 Other ovarian cyst, unspecified side ♀

✓5th **N83.3 Acquired atrophy of ovary and fallopian tube**

✓6th **N83.31 Acquired atrophy of ovary**

N83.311 Acquired atrophy of right ovary ♀

N83.312 Acquired atrophy of left ovary ♀

N83.319 Acquired atrophy of ovary, unspecified side ♀
Acquired atrophy of ovary, NOS

✓6th **N83.32 Acquired atrophy of fallopian tube**

N83.321 Acquired atrophy of right fallopian tube ♀

N83.322 Acquired atrophy of left fallopian tube ♀

N83.329 Acquired atrophy of fallopian tube, unspecified side ♀
Acquired atrophy of fallopian tube, NOS

✓6th **N83.33 Acquired atrophy of ovary and fallopian tube**

N83.331 Acquired atrophy of right ovary and fallopian tube ♀

N83.332 **Acquired atrophy of left ovary and fallopian tube** ♀

N83.339 **Acquired atrophy of ovary and fallopian tube, unspecified side** ♀
Acquired atrophy of ovary and fallopian tube, NOS

✓5th N83.4 **Prolapse and hernia of ovary and fallopian tube**

N83.40 **Prolapse and hernia of ovary and fallopian tube, unspecified side** ♀
Prolapse and hernia of ovary and fallopian tube, NOS

N83.41 **Prolapse and hernia of right ovary and fallopian tube** ♀

N83.42 **Prolapse and hernia of left ovary and fallopian tube** ♀

✓5th N83.5 **Torsion of ovary, ovarian pedicle and fallopian tube**
Torsion of accessory tube

✓6th N83.51 **Torsion of ovary and ovarian pedicle**

N83.511 **Torsion of right ovary and ovarian pedicle** CC ♀

N83.512 **Torsion of left ovary and ovarian pedicle** CC ♀

N83.519 **Torsion of ovary and ovarian pedicle, unspecified side** CC ♀
Torsion of ovary and ovarian pedicle, NOS

✓6th N83.52 **Torsion of fallopian tube**
Torsion of hydatid of Morgagni

N83.521 **Torsion of right fallopian tube** CC ♀

N83.522 **Torsion of left fallopian tube** CC ♀

N83.529 **Torsion of fallopian tube, unspecified side** CC ♀
Torsion of fallopian tube, NOS

N83.53 **Torsion of ovary, ovarian pedicle and fallopian tube** CC ♀

N83.6 **Hematosalpinx** ♀
EXCLUDES 1 *hematosalpinx (with) (in):*
hematocolpos (N89.7)
hematometra (N85.7)
tubal pregnancy (OØØ.1-)

N83.7 **Hematoma of broad ligament** ♀

N83.8 **Other noninflammatory disorders of ovary, fallopian tube and broad ligament** ♀
Broad ligament laceration syndrome [Allen-Masters]

N83.9 **Noninflammatory disorder of ovary, fallopian tube and broad ligament, unspecified** ♀

✓4th N84 **Polyp of female genital tract**
EXCLUDES 1 *adenomatous polyp (D28.-)*
placental polyp (O9Ø.89)

N84.Ø **Polyp of corpus uteri** ♀
Polyp of endometrium
Polyp of uterus NOS
EXCLUDES 1 *polypoid endometrial hyperplasia (N85.Ø-)*

N84.1 **Polyp of cervix uteri** ♀
Mucous polyp of cervix

N84.2 **Polyp of vagina** ♀

N84.3 **Polyp of vulva** ♀
Polyp of labia

N84.8 **Polyp of other parts of female genital tract** ♀

N84.9 **Polyp of female genital tract, unspecified** ♀

✓4th N85 **Other noninflammatory disorders of uterus, except cervix**
EXCLUDES 1 *endometriosis (N8Ø.-)*
inflammatory diseases of uterus (N71.-)
noninflammatory disorders of cervix, except malposition (N86-N88)
polyp of corpus uteri (N84.Ø)
uterine prolapse (N81.-)

✓5th N85.Ø **Endometrial hyperplasia**

N85.ØØ **Endometrial hyperplasia, unspecified** ♀
Hyperplasia (adenomatous) (cystic) (glandular) of endometrium
Hyperplastic endometritis

N85.Ø1 **Benign endometrial hyperplasia** ♀
Endometrial hyperplasia (complex) (simple) without atypia

N85.Ø2 **Endometrial intraepithelial neoplasia [EIN]** ♀
Endometrial hyperplasia with atypia
EXCLUDES 1 *malignant neoplasm of endometrium (with endometrial intraepithelial neoplasia [EIN]) (C54.1)*

N85.2 **Hypertrophy of uterus** ♀
Bulky or enlarged uterus
EXCLUDES 1 *puerperal hypertrophy of uterus (O9Ø.89)*

N85.3 **Subinvolution of uterus** ♀
EXCLUDES 1 *puerperal subinvolution of uterus (O9Ø.89)*

N85.4 **Malposition of uterus** ♀
Anteversion of uterus
Retroflexion of uterus
Retroversion of uterus
EXCLUDES 1 *malposition of uterus complicating pregnancy, labor or delivery (O34.5-, O65.5)*

N85.5 **Inversion of uterus** ♀
EXCLUDES 1 *current obstetric trauma (O71.2)*
postpartum inversion of uterus (O71.2)
DEF: Abnormality in which the uterus turns inside out.

Inversion of Uterus

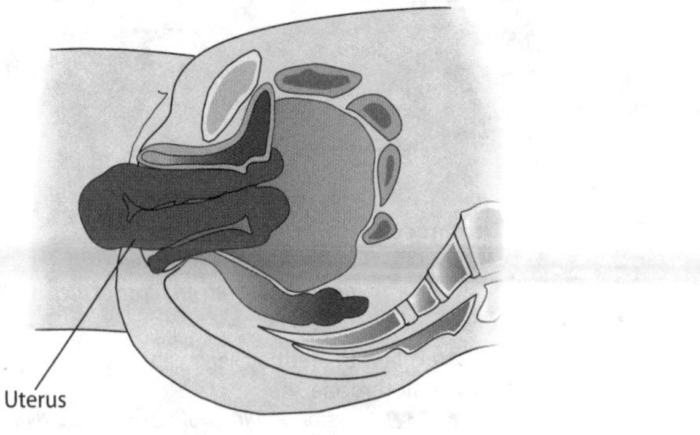

N85.6 **Intrauterine synechiae** ♀

N85.7 **Hematometra** ♀
Hematosalpinx with hematometra
EXCLUDES 1 *hematometra with hematocolpos (N89.7)*
DEF: Accumulation of blood within the uterus.

N85.8 **Other specified noninflammatory disorders of uterus** ♀
Atrophy of uterus, acquired
Fibrosis of uterus NOS

N85.9 **Noninflammatory disorder of uterus, unspecified** ♀
Disorder of uterus NOS

N86 **Erosion and ectropion of cervix uteri** ♀
Decubitus (trophic) ulcer of cervix
Eversion of cervix
EXCLUDES 1 *erosion and ectropion of cervix with cervicitis (N72)*

✓4th N87 **Dysplasia of cervix uteri**
EXCLUDES 1 *abnormal results from cervical cytologic examination without histologic confirmation (R87.61-)*
carcinoma in situ of cervix uteri (DØ6.-)
cervical intraepithelial neoplasia III [CIN III] (DØ6.-)
HGSIL of cervix (R87.613)
severe dysplasia of cervix uteri (DØ6.-)

N87.Ø **Mild cervical dysplasia** ♀
Cervical intraepithelial neoplasia I [CIN I]

N87.1 **Moderate cervical dysplasia** ♀
Cervical intraepithelial neoplasia II [CIN II]

N87.9 **Dysplasia of cervix uteri, unspecified** ♀
Anaplasia of cervix
Cervical atypism
Cervical dysplasia NOS

✓4th N88 **Other noninflammatory disorders of cervix uteri**
EXCLUDES 2 *inflammatory disease of cervix (N72)*
polyp of cervix (N84.1)

N88.Ø **Leukoplakia of cervix uteri** ♀

N88.1 Old laceration of cervix uteri ♀
Adhesions of cervix
EXCLUDES 1 *current obstetric trauma (O71.3)*

N88.2 Stricture and stenosis of cervix uteri ♀
EXCLUDES 1 *stricture and stenosis of cervix uteri complicating labor (O65.5)*

N88.3 Incompetence of cervix uteri ♀
Investigation and management of (suspected) cervical incompetence in a nonpregnant woman
EXCLUDES 1 *cervical incompetence complicating pregnancy (O34.3-)*
DEF: Inadequate functioning of the cervix marked by abnormal widening during pregnancy and causing premature birth or miscarriage.

N88.4 Hypertrophic elongation of cervix uteri ♀

N88.8 Other specified noninflammatory disorders of cervix uteri ♀
EXCLUDES 1 *current obstetric trauma (O71.3)*

N88.9 Noninflammatory disorder of cervix uteri, unspecified ♀

✓4th N89 Other noninflammatory disorders of vagina
EXCLUDES 1 *abnormal results from vaginal cytologic examination without histologic confirmation (R87.62-)*
carcinoma in situ of vagina (DØ7.2)
HGSIL of vagina (R87.623)
inflammation of vagina (N76.-)
senile (atrophic) vaginitis (N95.2)
severe dysplasia of vagina (DØ7.2)
trichomonal leukorrhea (A59.ØØ)
vaginal intraepithelial neoplasia [VAIN], grade III (DØ7.2)

N89.Ø Mild vaginal dysplasia ♀
Vaginal intraepithelial neoplasia [VAIN], grade I

N89.1 Moderate vaginal dysplasia ♀
Vaginal intraepithelial neoplasia [VAIN], grade II

N89.3 Dysplasia of vagina, unspecified ♀

N89.4 Leukoplakia of vagina ♀

N89.5 Stricture and atresia of vagina ♀
Vaginal adhesions
Vaginal stenosis
EXCLUDES 1 *congenital atresia or stricture (Q52.4)*
postprocedural adhesions of vagina (N99.2)

N89.6 Tight hymenal ring ♀
Rigid hymen
Tight introitus
EXCLUDES 1 *imperforate hymen (Q52.3)*

N89.7 Hematocolpos ♀
Hematocolpos with hematometra or hematosalpinx
AHA: 2016,4Q,58

N89.8 Other specified noninflammatory disorders of vagina ♀
Leukorrhea NOS
Old vaginal laceration
Pessary ulcer of vagina
EXCLUDES 1 *current obstetric trauma (O7Ø.-, O71.4, O71.7-O71.8)*
old laceration involving muscles of pelvic floor (N81.8)

N89.9 Noninflammatory disorder of vagina, unspecified ♀

✓4th N9Ø Other noninflammatory disorders of vulva and perineum
EXCLUDES 1 *anogenital (venereal) warts (A63.Ø)*
carcinoma in situ of vulva (DØ7.1)
condyloma acuminatum (A63.Ø)
current obstetric trauma (O7Ø.-, O71.7-O71.8)
inflammation of vulva (N76.-)
severe dysplasia of vulva (DØ7.1)
vulvar intraepithelial neoplasm III [VIN III] (DØ7.1)

N9Ø.Ø Mild vulvar dysplasia ♀
Vulvar intraepithelial neoplasia [VIN], grade I

N9Ø.1 Moderate vulvar dysplasia ♀
Vulvar intraepithelial neoplasia [VIN], grade II

N9Ø.3 Dysplasia of vulva, unspecified ♀

N9Ø.4 Leukoplakia of vulva ♀
Dystrophy of vulva
Kraurosis of vulva
Lichen sclerosus of external female genital organs

N9Ø.5 Atrophy of vulva ♀
Stenosis of vulva

✓5th **N9Ø.6 Hypertrophy of vulva**
AHA: 2016,4Q,46

N9Ø.6Ø Unspecified hypertrophy of vulva ♀
Unspecified hypertrophy of labia

N9Ø.61 Childhood asymmetric labium majus enlargement ♀
CALME

N9Ø.69 Other specified hypertrophy of vulva ♀
Other specified hypertrophy of labia

N9Ø.7 Vulvar cyst ♀

✓5th **N9Ø.8 Other specified noninflammatory disorders of vulva and perineum**

✓6th **N9Ø.81 Female genital mutilation status**
Female genital cutting status

N9Ø.81Ø Female genital mutilation status, unspecified ♀
Female genital cutting status, unspecified
Female genital mutilation status NOS

N9Ø.811 Female genital mutilation Type I status ♀
Clitorectomy status
Female genital cutting Type I status

N9Ø.812 Female genital mutilation Type II status ♀
Clitorectomy with excision of labia minora status
Female genital cutting Type II status

N9Ø.813 Female genital mutilation Type III status ♀
Female genital cutting Type III status
Infibulation status

N9Ø.818 Other female genital mutilation status ♀
Female genital cutting Type IV status
Female genital mutilation Type IV status
Other female genital cutting status

N9Ø.89 Other specified noninflammatory disorders of vulva and perineum ♀
Adhesions of vulva
Hypertrophy of clitoris

N9Ø.9 Noninflammatory disorder of vulva and perineum, unspecified ♀

✓4th N91 Absent, scanty and rare menstruation
EXCLUDES 1 *ovarian dysfunction (E28.-)*

N91.Ø Primary amenorrhea ♀

N91.1 Secondary amenorrhea ♀

N91.2 Amenorrhea, unspecified ♀

N91.3 Primary oligomenorrhea ♀

N91.4 Secondary oligomenorrhea ♀

N91.5 Oligomenorrhea, unspecified ♀
Hypomenorrhea NOS

✓4th N92 Excessive, frequent and irregular menstruation
EXCLUDES 1 *postmenopausal bleeding (N95.Ø)*
precocious puberty (menstruation) (E3Ø.1)

N92.Ø Excessive and frequent menstruation with regular cycle ♀
Heavy periods NOS
Menorrhagia NOS
Polymenorrhea

N92.1 Excessive and frequent menstruation with irregular cycle ♀
Irregular intermenstrual bleeding
Irregular, shortened intervals between menstrual bleeding
Menometrorrhagia
Metrorrhagia

N92.2 Excessive menstruation at puberty P ♀
Excessive bleeding associated with onset of menstrual periods
Pubertal menorrhagia
Puberty bleeding

N92.3 Ovulation bleeding ♀
Regular intermenstrual bleeding

N92.4 Excessive bleeding in the premenopausal period ♀
Climacteric menorrhagia or metrorrhagia
Menopausal menorrhagia or metrorrhagia
Perimenopausal bleeding
Perimenopausal menorrhagia or metrorrhagia
Preclimacteric menorrhagia or metrorrhagia
Premenopausal menorrhagia or metrorrhagia

N92.5 Other specified irregular menstruation ♀

N92.6 Irregular menstruation, unspecified ♀
Irregular bleeding NOS
Irregular periods NOS
EXCLUDES 1 *irregular menstruation with:*
lengthened intervals or scanty bleeding (N91.3-N91.5)
shortened intervals or excessive bleeding (N92.1)

✓4th **N93 Other abnormal uterine and vaginal bleeding**
EXCLUDES 1 *neonatal vaginal hemorrhage (P54.6)*
precocious puberty (menstruation) (E3Ø.1)
pseudomenses (P54.6)

N93.Ø Postcoital and contact bleeding ♀

N93.1 Pre-pubertal vaginal bleeding ♀
AHA: 2016,4Q,47

N93.8 Other specified abnormal uterine and vaginal bleeding ♀
Dysfunctional or functional uterine or vaginal bleeding NOS

N93.9 Abnormal uterine and vaginal bleeding, unspecified ♀

✓4th **N94 Pain and other conditions associated with female genital organs and menstrual cycle**

N94.Ø Mittelschmerz ♀
DEF: One-sided, lower abdominal pain occurring between menstrual periods that is associated with ovulation.

✓5th **N94.1 Dyspareunia**
EXCLUDES 1 *psychogenic dyspareunia (F52.6)*
AHA: 2016,4Q,47

N94.1Ø Unspecified dyspareunia ♀
N94.11 Superficial (introital) dyspareunia ♀
N94.12 Deep dyspareunia ♀
N94.19 Other specified dyspareunia ♀

N94.2 Vaginismus ♀
EXCLUDES 1 *psychogenic vaginismus (F52.5)*
DEF: Spontaneous contractions of the muscles surrounding the vagina, causing it to constrict or close.

N94.3 Premenstrual tension syndrome ♀
Code also associated menstrual migraine (G43.82-, G43.83-)
EXCLUDES 1 *premenstrual dysphoric disorder (F32.81)*

N94.4 Primary dysmenorrhea ♀

N94.5 Secondary dysmenorrhea ♀

N94.6 Dysmenorrhea, unspecified ♀
EXCLUDES 1 *psychogenic dysmenorrhea (F45.8)*

✓5th **N94.8 Other specified conditions associated with female genital organs and menstrual cycle**

✓6th **N94.81 Vulvodynia**
N94.81Ø Vulvar vestibulitis ♀
N94.818 Other vulvodynia ♀
N94.819 Vulvodynia, unspecified ♀
Vulvodynia NOS

N94.89 Other specified conditions associated with female genital organs and menstrual cycle ♀
DEF: Hydrocele: Serous fluid that collects in the canal of Nuck in females.

N94.9 Unspecified condition associated with female genital organs and menstrual cycle ♀

✓4th **N95 Menopausal and other perimenopausal disorders**
Menopausal and other perimenopausal disorders due to naturally occurring (age-related) menopause and perimenopause
EXCLUDES 1 *excessive bleeding in the premenopausal period (N92.4)*
menopausal and perimenopausal disorders due to artificial or premature menopause (E89.4-, E28.31-)
premature menopause (E28.31-)
EXCLUDES 2 *postmenopausal osteoporosis (M81.Ø-)*
postmenopausal osteoporosis with current pathological fracture (M8Ø.Ø-)
postmenopausal urethritis (N34.2)

N95.Ø Postmenopausal bleeding ♀

N95.1 Menopausal and female climacteric states ♀
Symptoms such as flushing, sleeplessness, headache, lack of concentration, associated with natural (age-related) menopause
Use additional code for associated symptoms
EXCLUDES 1 *asymptomatic menopausal state (Z78.Ø)*
symptoms associated with artificial menopause (E89.41)
symptoms associated with premature menopause (E28.31Ø)

N95.2 Postmenopausal atrophic vaginitis ♀
Senile (atrophic) vaginitis

N95.8 Other specified menopausal and perimenopausal disorders ♀

N95.9 Unspecified menopausal and perimenopausal disorder ♀

N96 Recurrent pregnancy loss ♀
Investigation or care in a nonpregnant woman with history of recurrent pregnancy loss
EXCLUDES 1 *recurrent pregnancy loss with current pregnancy (O26.2-)*

✓4th **N97 Female infertility**
INCLUDES inability to achieve a pregnancy
sterility, female NOS
EXCLUDES 1 *female infertility associated with:*
hypopituitarism (E23.Ø)
Stein-Leventhal syndrome (E28.2)
EXCLUDES 2 *incompetence of cervix uteri (N88.3)*
DEF: Infertility: Inability to conceive for at least one year with regular intercourse.
DEF: Primary infertility: Infertility occurring in patients who have never conceived.
DEF: Secondary infertility: Infertility occurring in patients who have previously conceived.

N97.Ø Female infertility associated with anovulation ♀

N97.1 Female infertility of tubal origin ♀
Female infertility associated with congenital anomaly of tube
Female infertility due to tubal block
Female infertility due to tubal occlusion
Female infertility due to tubal stenosis

N97.2 Female infertility of uterine origin ♀
Female infertility associated with congenital anomaly of uterus
Female infertility due to nonimplantation of ovum

N97.8 Female infertility of other origin ♀

N97.9 Female infertility, unspecified ♀

✓4th **N98 Complications associated with artificial fertilization**

N98.Ø Infection associated with artificial insemination CC ♀

N98.1 Hyperstimulation of ovaries CC ♀
Hyperstimulation of ovaries NOS
Hyperstimulation of ovaries associated with induced ovulation

N98.2 Complications of attempted introduction of fertilized ovum following in vitro fertilization CC ♀

N98.3 Complications of attempted introduction of embryo in embryo transfer CC ♀

N98.8 Other complications associated with artificial fertilization CC ♀

N98.9 Complication associated with artificial fertilization, unspecified CC ♀

Intraoperative and postprocedural complications and disorders of genitourinary system, not elsewhere classified (N99)

✓4th **N99 Intraoperative and postprocedural complications and disorders of genitourinary system, not elsewhere classified**
EXCLUDES 2 *irradiation cystitis (N3Ø.4-)*
postoophorectomy osteoporosis with current pathological fracture (M8Ø.8-)
postoophorectomy osteoporosis without current pathological fracture (M81.8)

N99.Ø Postprocedural (acute) (chronic) kidney failure
Use additional code to type of kidney disease

✓5th **N99.1 Postprocedural urethral stricture**
Postcatheterization urethral stricture

✓6th **N99.11 Postprocedural urethral stricture, male**
AHA: 2016,4Q,47-48

N99.11Ø Postprocedural urethral stricture, male, meatal ♂

N99.111 Postprocedural bulbous urethral stricture, male ♂
N99.112 Postprocedural membranous urethral stricture, male ♂
N99.113 Postprocedural anterior bulbous urethral stricture, male ♂
N99.114 Postprocedural urethral stricture, male, unspecified ♂
N99.115 Postprocedural fossa navicularis urethral stricture ♂
N99.116 Postprocedural urethral stricture, male, overlapping sites ♂

N99.12 Postprocedural urethral stricture, female ♀

N99.2 Postprocedural adhesions of vagina ♀

N99.3 Prolapse of vaginal vault after hysterectomy ♀

N99.4 Postprocedural pelvic peritoneal adhesions

EXCLUDES 2 *pelvic peritoneal adhesions NOS (N73.6)*
postinfective pelvic peritoneal adhesions (N73.6)

✓5th N99.5 Complications of stoma of urinary tract

EXCLUDES 2 *mechanical complication of urinary catheter (T83.Ø-)*

AHA: 2016,4Q,48

✓6th N99.51 Complication of cystostomy

N99.51Ø Cystostomy hemorrhage CC HCC
N99.511 Cystostomy infection CC HCC
N99.512 Cystostomy malfunction CC HCC
N99.518 Other cystostomy complication CC HCC

✓6th N99.52 Complication of incontinent external stoma of urinary tract

N99.52Ø Hemorrhage of incontinent external stoma of urinary tract HCC
N99.521 Infection of incontinent external stoma of urinary tract HCC
N99.522 Malfunction of incontinent external stoma of urinary tract HCC
N99.523 Herniation of incontinent stoma of urinary tract HCC
N99.524 Stenosis of incontinent stoma of urinary tract HCC
N99.528 Other complication of incontinent external stoma of urinary tract HCC

✓6th N99.53 Complication of continent stoma of urinary tract

N99.53Ø Hemorrhage of continent stoma of urinary tract HCC
N99.531 Infection of continent stoma of urinary tract HCC
N99.532 Malfunction of continent stoma of urinary tract HCC
N99.533 Herniation of continent stoma of urinary tract HCC
N99.534 Stenosis of continent stoma of urinary tract HCC
N99.538 Other complication of continent stoma of urinary tract HCC

✓5th N99.6 Intraoperative hemorrhage and hematoma of a genitourinary system organ or structure complicating a procedure

EXCLUDES 1 *intraoperative hemorrhage and hematoma of a genitourinary system organ or structure due to accidental puncture or laceration during a procedure (N99.7-)*

N99.61 Intraoperative hemorrhage and hematoma of a genitourinary system organ or structure complicating a genitourinary system procedure CC

N99.62 Intraoperative hemorrhage and hematoma of a genitourinary system organ or structure complicating other procedure CC

✓5th N99.7 Accidental puncture and laceration of a genitourinary system organ or structure during a procedure

N99.71 Accidental puncture and laceration of a genitourinary system organ or structure during a genitourinary system procedure CC

N99.72 Accidental puncture and laceration of a genitourinary system organ or structure during other procedure CC

✓5th N99.8 Other intraoperative and postprocedural complications and disorders of genitourinary system

AHA: 2016,4Q,9-10

N99.81 Other intraoperative complications of genitourinary system

✓6th N99.82 Postprocedural hemorrhage of a genitourinary system organ or structure following a procedure

N99.82Ø Postprocedural hemorrhage of a genitourinary system organ or structure following a genitourinary system procedure CC
N99.821 Postprocedural hemorrhage of a genitourinary system organ or structure following other procedure CC

N99.83 Residual ovary syndrome ♀

✓6th N99.84 Postprocedural hematoma and seroma of a genitourinary system organ or structure following a procedure

N99.84Ø Postprocedural hematoma of a genitourinary system organ or structure following a genitourinary system procedure CC
N99.841 Postprocedural hematoma of a genitourinary system organ or structure following other procedure CC
N99.842 Postprocedural seroma of a genitourinary system organ or structure following a genitourinary system procedure CC
N99.843 Postprocedural seroma of a genitourinary system organ or structure following other procedure CC

N99.85 Post endometrial ablation syndrome ♀

AHA: 2019,4Q,12

N99.89 Other postprocedural complications and disorders of genitourinary system

Chapter 15. Pregnancy, Childbirth and the Puerperium (O00–O9A)

Chapter-specific Guidelines with Coding Examples

The chapter-specific guidelines from the ICD-10-CM Official Guidelines for Coding and Reporting have been provided below. Along with these guidelines are coding examples, contained in the shaded boxes, that have been developed to help illustrate the coding and/or sequencing guidance found in these guidelines.

a. General rules for obstetric cases

1) Codes from Chapter 15 and sequencing priority

Obstetric cases require codes from chapter 15, codes in the range O00-O9A, Pregnancy, Childbirth, and the Puerperium. Chapter 15 codes have sequencing priority over codes from other chapters. Additional codes from other chapters may be used in conjunction with chapter 15 codes to further specify conditions. Should the provider document that the pregnancy is incidental to the encounter, then code Z33.1, Pregnant state, incidental, should be used in place of any chapter 15 codes. It is the provider's responsibility to state that the condition being treated is not affecting the pregnancy.

Pregnant patient at 25 weeks' gestation admitted for bladder abscess

O23.12 Infections of bladder in pregnancy, second trimester

N30.80 Other cystitis without hematuria

Z3A.25 25 weeks gestation of pregnancy

Explanation: The documentation does not indicate that the pregnancy is incidental or in any way unaffected by the bladder abscess; therefore, an obstetrics code should be sequenced first. An additional code was provided to identify the specific bladder condition as this information is not called out specifically in the obstetrics code.

2) Chapter 15 codes used only on the maternal record

Chapter 15 codes are to be used only on the maternal record, never on the record of the newborn.

3) Final character for trimester

The majority of codes in Chapter 15 have a final character indicating the trimester of pregnancy. The timeframes for the trimesters are indicated at the beginning of the chapter. If trimester is not a component of a code, it is because the condition always occurs in a specific trimester, or the concept of trimester of pregnancy is not applicable. Certain codes have characters for only certain trimesters because the condition does not occur in all trimesters, but it may occur in more than just one.

Assignment of the final character for trimester should be based on the provider's documentation of the trimester (or number of weeks) for the current admission/encounter. This applies to the assignment of trimester for pre-existing conditions as well as those that develop during or are due to the pregnancy. The provider's documentation of the number of weeks may be used to assign the appropriate code identifying the trimester.

Whenever delivery occurs during the current admission, and there is an "in childbirth" option for the obstetric complication being coded, the "in childbirth" code should be assigned.

Pregnant patient at 21 weeks' gestation admitted with excessive vomiting

O21.2 Late vomiting of pregnancy

Z3A.21 21 weeks gestation of pregnancy

Explanation: Category O21 classifies vomiting in pregnancy. Although code selection is based on whether the vomiting is before or after 20 completed weeks, these codes are not further classified by trimester. If vomiting only in the second trimester was documented, the provider should be queried for the specific week of gestation, as this will affect code selection.

4) Selection of trimester for inpatient admissions that encompass more than one trimester

In instances when a patient is admitted to a hospital for complications of pregnancy during one trimester and remains in the hospital into a subsequent trimester, the trimester character for the antepartum complication code should be assigned on the basis of the trimester when the complication developed, not the trimester of the discharge. If the condition developed prior to the current admission/encounter or represents a pre-existing condition, the trimester character for the trimester at the time of the admission/encounter should be assigned.

Patient admitted at 27 6/7 weeks' gestation for hemorrhaging from partial placenta previa; three days after admission at 28 1/7 weeks' gestation, she developed gestational hypertension

O44.32 Partial placenta previa with hemorrhage, second trimester

O13.3 Gestational [pregnancy-induced] hypertension without significant proteinuria, third trimester

Z3A.27 27 weeks gestation of pregnancy

Explanation: The patient presented with hemorrhaging from partial placenta previa while still in her 27th week, which falls within the second trimester. The gestational hypertension did not occur until three days after admission, putting the patient in her 28th week of pregnancy or what is considered to be the third trimester. The weeks of gestation captured by a code from category Z3A should represent only the gestational weeks upon admission.

5) Unspecified trimester

Each category that includes codes for trimester has a code for "unspecified trimester." The "unspecified trimester" code should rarely be used, such as when the documentation in the record is insufficient to determine the trimester and it is not possible to obtain clarification.

6) 7th character for fetus identification

Where applicable, a 7th character is to be assigned for certain categories (O31, O32, O33.3 - O33.6, O35, O36, O40, O41, O60.1, O60.2, O64, and O69) to identify the fetus for which the complication code applies.

Assign 7th character "0":

- For single gestations
- When the documentation in the record is insufficient to determine the fetus affected and it is not possible to obtain clarification.
- When it is not possible to clinically determine which fetus is affected.

Maternal patient with twin gestations is seen after ultrasound identifies fetus B to be in breech presentation

O32.1XX2 Maternal care for breech presentation, fetus 2

Explanation: The documentation indicates that although there are two fetuses, only one fetus is determined to be in breech presentation. Whether fetus 2 or fetus B is used, the coder can assign the seventh character of 2 to identify the second fetus as the one in breech.

b. Selection of OB principal or first-listed diagnosis

1) Routine outpatient prenatal visits

For routine outpatient prenatal visits when no complications are present, a code from category Z34, Encounter for supervision of normal pregnancy, should be used as the first-listed diagnosis. These codes should not be used in conjunction with chapter 15 codes.

2) Supervision of high-risk pregnancy

Codes from category O09, Supervision of high-risk pregnancy, are intended for use only during the prenatal period. For complications during the labor or delivery episode as a result of a high-risk pregnancy, assign the applicable complication codes from Chapter 15. If there are no complications during the labor or delivery episode, assign code O80, Encounter for full-term uncomplicated delivery.

For routine prenatal outpatient visits for patients with high-risk pregnancies, a code from category O09, Supervision of high-risk pregnancy, should be used as the first-listed diagnosis. Secondary chapter 15 codes may be used in conjunction with these codes if appropriate.

36-year-old with history of preterm labor admitted in labor with second child at 39 weeks' gestation, delivered healthy baby without complications

O80 Encounter for full-term uncomplicated delivery

Z3A.39 39 weeks gestation of pregnancy

Z37.0 Single live birth

Explanation: Although this patient is over 35 and having her second child (elderly multigravida) and has a history of preterm labor with her first child, no codes from category O09.- should be appended. In the absence of any other complications noted during the encounter, code O80 is the most appropriate code to describe the principal diagnosis.

3) Episodes when no delivery occurs

In episodes when no delivery occurs, the principal diagnosis should correspond to the principal complication of the pregnancy which necessitated the encounter. Should more than one complication exist, all of which are treated or monitored, any of the complication codes may be sequenced first.

4) When a delivery occurs

When an obstetric patient is admitted and delivers during that admission, the condition that prompted the admission should be sequenced as the principal diagnosis. If multiple conditions prompted the admission, sequence the one most related to the delivery as the principal diagnosis. A code for any complication of the delivery should be assigned as an additional diagnosis. In cases of cesarean delivery, if the patient was admitted with a condition that resulted in the performance of a cesarean procedure, that condition should be selected as the principal diagnosis. If the reason for the admission was unrelated to the condition resulting in the cesarean delivery, the condition related to the reason for the admission should be selected as the principal diagnosis.

Maternal patient with diet-controlled gestational diabetes was admitted at 38 weeks' gestation in obstructed labor due to footling presentation; cesarean performed for the malpresentation

O64.8XXØ	**Obstructed labor due to other malposition and malpresentation, not applicable or unspecified**
O24.42Ø	**Gestational diabetes mellitus in childbirth, diet controlled**
Z3A.38	**38 weeks gestation of pregnancy**
Z37.Ø	**Single live birth**

Explanation: The obstructed labor necessitated the cesarean procedure.

At 39 weeks' gestation, a maternal patient presents with hemorrhage with coagulation defect; the next day the patient goes into labor and eventually delivers via cesarean section due to arrested active phase of labor

O46.ØØ3	**Antepartum hemorrhage with coagulation defect, unspecified, third trimester**
O62.1	**Secondary uterine inertia**
Z3A.39	**39 weeks gestation of pregnancy**
Z37.Ø	**Single live birth**

Explanation: The patient was admitted because of the antepartum hemorrhage with coagulation defect. The arrested active phase, although the reason for the cesarean delivery, did not develop until later into the stay.

5) Outcome of delivery

A code from category Z37, Outcome of delivery, should be included on every maternal record when a delivery has occurred. These codes are not to be used on subsequent records or on the newborn record.

c. Pre-existing conditions versus conditions due to the pregnancy

Certain categories in Chapter 15 distinguish between conditions of the mother that existed prior to pregnancy (pre-existing) and those that are a direct result of pregnancy. When assigning codes from Chapter 15, it is important to assess if a condition was pre-existing prior to pregnancy or developed during or due to the pregnancy in order to assign the correct code.

Categories that do not distinguish between pre-existing and pregnancy-related conditions may be used for either. It is acceptable to use codes specifically for the puerperium with codes complicating pregnancy and childbirth if a condition arises postpartum during the delivery encounter.

d. Pre-existing hypertension in pregnancy

Category O1Ø, Pre-existing hypertension complicating pregnancy, childbirth and the puerperium, includes codes for hypertensive heart and hypertensive chronic kidney disease. When assigning one of the O1Ø codes that includes hypertensive heart disease or hypertensive chronic kidney disease, it is necessary to add a secondary code from the appropriate hypertension category to specify the type of heart failure or chronic kidney disease.

See Section I.C.9. Hypertension.

e. Fetal conditions affecting the management of the mother

1) Codes from categories O35 and O36

Codes from categories O35, Maternal care for known or suspected fetal abnormality and damage, and O36, Maternal care for other fetal problems, are assigned only when the fetal condition is actually responsible for modifying the management of the mother, i.e., by requiring diagnostic studies, additional observation, special care, or termination of pregnancy. The fact that the fetal condition exists does not justify assigning a code from this series to the mother's record.

A patient is seen in ED for spotting 15 weeks into her pregnancy; the doctors also suspect fetal hydrocephalus.

O26.852	**Spotting complicating pregnancy, second trimester**
Z3A.15	**15 weeks gestation of pregnancy**

Explanation: Whether the fetal hydrocephalus was suspected or confirmed, an additional code is not warranted for this condition as the documentation does not indicate that this fetal condition is in any way altering the management of the mother or complicating her pregnancy.

2) In utero surgery

In cases when surgery is performed on the fetus, a diagnosis code from category O35, Maternal care for known or suspected fetal abnormality and damage, should be assigned identifying the fetal condition. Assign the appropriate procedure code for the procedure performed.

No code from Chapter 16, the perinatal codes, should be used on the mother's record to identify fetal conditions. Surgery performed in utero on a fetus is still to be coded as an obstetric encounter.

f. HIV infection in pregnancy, childbirth and the puerperium

During pregnancy, childbirth or the puerperium, a patient admitted because of an HIV-related illness should receive a principal diagnosis from subcategory O98.7-, Human immunodeficiency [HIV] disease complicating pregnancy, childbirth and the puerperium, followed by the code(s) for the HIV-related illness(es).

Patients with asymptomatic HIV infection status admitted during pregnancy, childbirth, or the puerperium should receive codes of O98.7- and Z21, Asymptomatic human immunodeficiency virus [HIV] infection status.

A previously asymptomatic HIV patient who is 13 weeks pregnant is admitted with oral thrush.

O98.711	**Human immunodeficiency virus [HIV] disease complicating pregnancy, first trimester**
B2Ø	**Human immunodeficiency virus [HIV] disease**
B37.Ø	**Candidal stomatitis**
Z3A.13	**13 weeks gestation of pregnancy**

Explanation: Because oral thrush is an HIV-related condition, this patient is now considered to have HIV disease. An obstetrics code indicating that HIV is complicating the pregnancy is coded first, followed by B2Ø for HIV disease as well as a code for the oral thrush.

g. Diabetes mellitus in pregnancy

Diabetes mellitus is a significant complicating factor in pregnancy. Pregnant women who are diabetic should be assigned a code from category O24, Diabetes mellitus in pregnancy, childbirth, and the puerperium, first, followed by the appropriate diabetes code(s) (EØ8-E13) from Chapter 4.

h. Long term use of insulin and oral hypoglycemics

See section I.C.4.a.3 for information on the long-term use of insulin and oral hypoglycemics.

i. Gestational (pregnancy induced) diabetes

Gestational (pregnancy induced) diabetes can occur during the second and third trimester of pregnancy in women who were not diabetic prior to pregnancy. Gestational diabetes can cause complications in the pregnancy similar to those of pre-existing diabetes mellitus. It also puts the woman at greater risk of developing diabetes after the pregnancy. Codes for gestational diabetes are in subcategory O24.4, Gestational diabetes mellitus. No other code from category O24, Diabetes mellitus in pregnancy, childbirth, and the puerperium, should be used with a code from O24.4.

The codes under subcategory O24.4 include diet controlled, insulin controlled, and controlled by oral hypoglycemic drugs. If a patient with gestational diabetes is treated with both diet and insulin, only the code for insulin-controlled is required. If a patient with gestational diabetes is treated with both diet and oral hypoglycemic medications, only the code for "controlled by oral hypoglycemic drugs" is required. Code Z79.4, Long-term (current) use of insulin or code Z79.84, Long-term (current) use of oral hypoglycemic drugs, should not be assigned with codes from subcategory O24.4.

An abnormal glucose tolerance in pregnancy is assigned a code from subcategory O99.81, Abnormal glucose complicating pregnancy, childbirth, and the puerperium.

Patient at 39 weeks term pregnancy with gestational diabetes was admitted in labor and delivered a healthy newborn. Patient is on a diabetic diet with daily metformin.

O24.425	**Gestational diabetes mellitus in childbirth, controlled by oral hypoglycemic drugs**
Z3A.39	**39 weeks gestation of pregnancy**
Z37.Ø	**Single live birth**

Explanation: When the patient is admitted for delivery and the patient's gestational diabetes is controlled by both diet and oral hypoglycemic medications, only the combination code in subcategory O24.4- Gestational diabetes mellitus, is reported. No code is added for diet controlled diabetes, and no Z code for long-term use of oral hypoglycemics is reported with the O24.4 combination codes.

j. Sepsis and septic shock complicating abortion, pregnancy, childbirth and the puerperium

When assigning a chapter 15 code for sepsis complicating abortion, pregnancy, childbirth, and the puerperium, a code for the specific type of infection should be assigned as an additional diagnosis. If severe sepsis is present, a code from subcategory R65.2, Severe sepsis, and code(s) for associated organ dysfunction(s) should also be assigned as additional diagnoses.

Patient is seen several days after a miscarriage with sepsis; cultures return MSSA

OØ3.87	**Sepsis following complete or unspecified spontaneous abortion**
B95.61	**Methicillin susceptible Staphylococcus aureus infection as the cause of diseases classified elsewhere**

Explanation: The type of infection that caused this patient to become septic was methicillin susceptible *Staphylococcus aureus* (MSSA), which as a secondary code helps capture all aspects related to this patient's septic condition.

k. Puerperal sepsis

Code O85, Puerperal sepsis, should be assigned with a secondary code to identify the causal organism (e.g., for a bacterial infection, assign a code from category B95-B96, Bacterial infections in conditions classified elsewhere). A code from category A4Ø, Streptococcal sepsis, or A41, Other sepsis, should not be used for puerperal sepsis. If applicable, use additional codes to identify severe sepsis (R65.2-) and any associated acute organ dysfunction.

Code O85 should not be assigned for sepsis following an obstetrical procedure (See Section I.C.1.d.5.b., Sepsis due to a postprocedural infection).

l. Alcohol, tobacco and drug use during pregnancy, childbirth and the puerperium

1) Alcohol use during pregnancy, childbirth and the puerperium

Codes under subcategory O99.31, Alcohol use complicating pregnancy, childbirth, and the puerperium, should be assigned for any pregnancy case when a mother uses alcohol during the pregnancy or postpartum. A secondary code from category F1Ø, Alcohol related disorders, should also be assigned to identify manifestations of the alcohol use.

2) Tobacco use during pregnancy, childbirth and the puerperium

Codes under subcategory O99.33, Smoking (tobacco) complicating pregnancy, childbirth, and the puerperium, should be assigned for any pregnancy case when a mother uses any type of tobacco product during the pregnancy or postpartum. A secondary code from category F17, Nicotine dependence, should also be assigned to identify the type of nicotine dependence.

3) Drug use during pregnancy, childbirth and the puerperium

Codes under subcategory O99.32, Drug use complicating pregnancy, childbirth, and the puerperium, should be assigned for any pregnancy case when a mother uses drugs during the pregnancy or postpartum. This can involve illegal drugs, or inappropriate use or abuse of prescription drugs. Secondary code(s) from categories F11-F16 and F18-F19 should also be assigned to identify manifestations of the drug use.

m. Poisoning, toxic effects, adverse effects and underdosing in a pregnant patient

A code from subcategory O9A.2, Injury, poisoning and certain other consequences of external causes complicating pregnancy, childbirth, and the puerperium, should be sequenced first, followed by the appropriate injury, poisoning, toxic effect, adverse effect or underdosing code, and then the additional code(s) that specifies the condition caused by the poisoning, toxic effect, adverse effect or underdosing.

See Section I.C.19. Adverse effects, poisoning, underdosing and toxic effects.

Patient admitted with accidental carbon monoxide poisoning from a gas heating implement; the patient is 18 weeks' pregnant

O9A.212	**Injury, poisoning and certain other consequences of external causes complicating pregnancy, second trimester**
T58.11XA	**Toxic effect of carbon monoxide from utility gas, accidental (unintentional), initial encounter**
Z3A.18	**18 weeks gestation of pregnancy**

Explanation: Although the carbon monoxide poisoning is the reason the patient was admitted, a code from the obstetrics chapter must be sequenced first. Chapter 15 codes have sequencing priority over codes from other chapters.

n. Normal delivery, code O8Ø

1) Encounter for full term uncomplicated delivery

Code O8Ø should be assigned when a woman is admitted for a full-term normal delivery and delivers a single, healthy infant without any complications antepartum, during the delivery, or postpartum during the delivery episode. Code O8Ø is always a principal diagnosis. It is not to be used if any other code from chapter 15 is needed to describe a current complication of the antenatal, delivery, or postnatal period. Additional codes from other chapters may be used with code O8Ø if they are not related to or are in any way complicating the pregnancy.

2) Uncomplicated delivery with resolved antepartum complication

Code O8Ø may be used if the patient had a complication at some point during the pregnancy, but the complication is not present at the time of the admission for delivery.

Patient presents in labor at 39 weeks' gestation and delivers a healthy newborn; patient had abnormal glucose levels in her first trimester, which have since resolved

O8Ø	**Encounter for full-term uncomplicated delivery**
Z37.Ø	**Single live birth**

Explanation: The abnormal glucose levels during the first trimester cannot be coded if they are not affecting the patient's current trimester. Without additional complications associated with the pregnancy, fetus, or mother, code O8Ø is appropriate.

3) Outcome of delivery for O8Ø

Z37.Ø, Single live birth, is the only outcome of delivery code appropriate for use with O8Ø.

o. The peripartum and postpartum periods

1) Peripartum and postpartum periods

The postpartum period begins immediately after delivery and continues for six weeks following delivery. The peripartum period is defined as the last month of pregnancy to five months postpartum.

2) Peripartum and postpartum complication

A postpartum complication is any complication occurring within the six-week period.

3) Pregnancy-related complications after 6-week period

Chapter 15 codes may also be used to describe pregnancy-related complications after the peripartum or postpartum period if the provider documents that a condition is pregnancy related.

> Patient admitted for varicose veins. She had a baby boy three months ago; the varicose veins started to appear one month ago. The doctor attributes the patient's pregnancy as the cause of the varicose veins, which continue to be painful and bother the patient. She is seeking surgical relief.
>
> **O87.4 Varicose veins of the lower extremity in the puerperium**
>
> *Explanation:* Although the varicose veins occurred several months after the delivery of the newborn, the doctor attributed the varicose veins to pregnancy and therefore a code from chapter 15 is appropriate.

4) Admission for routine postpartum care following delivery outside hospital

When the mother delivers outside the hospital prior to admission and is admitted for routine postpartum care and no complications are noted, code Z39.Ø, Encounter for care and examination of mother immediately after delivery, should be assigned as the principal diagnosis.

5) Pregnancy associated cardiomyopathy

Pregnancy associated cardiomyopathy, code O9Ø.3, is unique in that it may be diagnosed in the third trimester of pregnancy but may continue to progress months after delivery. For this reason, it is referred to as peripartum cardiomyopathy. Code O9Ø.3 is only for use when the cardiomyopathy develops as a result of pregnancy in a woman who did not have pre-existing heart disease.

p. Code O94, Sequelae of complication of pregnancy, childbirth, and the puerperium

1) Code O94

Code O94, Sequelae of complication of pregnancy, childbirth, and the puerperium, is for use in those cases when an initial complication of a pregnancy develops a sequelae requiring care or treatment at a future date.

2) After the initial postpartum period

This code may be used at any time after the initial postpartum period.

3) Sequencing of code O94

This code, like all sequela codes, is to be sequenced following the code describing the sequelae of the complication.

q. Termination of pregnancy and spontaneous abortions

1) Abortion with liveborn fetus

When an attempted termination of pregnancy results in a liveborn fetus, assign code Z33.2, Encounter for elective termination of pregnancy and a code from category Z37, Outcome of Delivery.

2) Retained products of conception following an abortion

Subsequent encounters for retained products of conception following a spontaneous abortion or elective termination of pregnancy, without complications are assigned OØ3.4, Incomplete spontaneous, abortion without complication, or code OØ7.4, Failed attempted termination of pregnancy without complication. This advice is appropriate even when the patient was discharged previously with a discharge diagnosis of complete abortion. If the patient has a specific complication associated with the spontaneous abortion or elective termination of pregnancy in addition to retained products of conception, assign the appropriate complication code (e.g., OØ3.-, OØ4.-, OØ7.-) instead of code OØ3.4 or OØ7.4.

> Patient was seen two days ago for complete spontaneous abortion but returns today for urinary tract infection (UTI) with ultrasound showing retained products of conception
>
> **OØ3.38 Urinary tract infection following incomplete spontaneous abortion**
>
> *Explanation:* Although the diagnosis from the patient's previous stay indicated that the patient had a complete abortion, it is now determined that there were actually retained products of conception (POC). An abortion with retained POC is considered incomplete and in this case resulted in the patient developing a UTI.

3) Complications leading to abortion

Codes from Chapter 15 may be used as additional codes to identify any documented complications of the pregnancy in conjunction with codes in categories in OØ4, OØ7 and OØ8.

r. Abuse in a pregnant patient

For suspected or confirmed cases of abuse of a pregnant patient, a code(s) from subcategories O9A.3, Physical abuse complicating pregnancy, childbirth, and the puerperium, O9A.4, Sexual abuse complicating pregnancy, childbirth, and the puerperium, and O9A.5, Psychological abuse complicating pregnancy, childbirth, and the puerperium, should be sequenced first, followed by the appropriate codes (if applicable) to identify any associated current injury due to physical abuse, sexual abuse, and the perpetrator of abuse.

See Section I.C.19. Adult and child abuse, neglect and other maltreatment.

s. COVID-19 infection in pregnancy, childbirth, and the puerperium

During pregnancy, childbirth or the puerperium, when COVID-19 is the reason for admission/encounter , code O98.5-, Other viral diseases complicating pregnancy, childbirth and the puerperium, should be sequenced as the principal/first-listed diagnosis, and code UØ7.1, COVID-19, and the appropriate codes for associated manifestation(s) should be assigned as additional diagnoses. Codes from Chapter 15 always take sequencing priority.

If the reason for admission/encounter is unrelated to COVID-19 but the patient tests positive for COVID-19 during the admission/encounter, the appropriate code for the reason for admission/encounter should be sequenced as the principal/first-listed diagnosis, and codes O98.5- and UØ7.1, as well as the appropriate codes for associated COVID-19 manifestations, should be assigned as additional diagnoses.

> Patient admitted in labor at 39 weeks' gestation and delivered a healthy newborn. Prenatal care consisted of some hyperemesis early in the pregnancy that has since resolved. No complications encountered during or following delivery. As per hospital protocol, during the pandemic, all patients are to be screened for COVID-19, and the patient tested positive. She remains asymptomatic, will be sent home to quarantine for 14 days.
>
> **O98.52 Other viral diseases complicating childbirth**
>
> **UØ7.1 COVID-19**
>
> **Z3A.39 39 weeks gestation of pregnancy**
>
> **Z37.Ø Single live birth**
>
> *Explanation:* No code is assigned for the hyperemesis as it resolved prior to this admission. Per guideline I.C.1.g.1.f, a screening code is generally not appropriate during the pandemic phase of COVID-19. Most hospitals screen their patients upon admission to the hospital to ensure proper protocols are in place for monitoring and treating those patients who do test positive for the disease. A positive test result alone is confirmation of the disease, according to guideline I.C.1.g.1.a, and code UØ7.1 should be assigned. A claim for any patient admitted during pregnancy, childbirth, or the puerperium and who tests positive or is treated for COVID-19 should have a code from subcategory O98.5- sequenced first, followed by code UØ7.1. As the patient was asymptomatic, no additional codes are assigned to represent any manifestation of the COVID-19 infection.

Chapter 15. Pregnancy, Childbirth and the Puerperium (O00-O9A)

NOTE CODES FROM THIS CHAPTER ARE FOR USE ONLY ON MATERNAL RECORDS, NEVER ON NEWBORN RECORDS

Codes from this chapter are for use for conditions related to or aggravated by the pregnancy, childbirth, or by the puerperium (maternal causes or obstetric causes)

NOTE Trimesters are counted from the first day of the last menstrual period. They are defined as follows:

1st trimester- less than 14 weeks 0 days

2nd trimester- 14 weeks 0 days to less than 28 weeks 0 days

3rd trimester- 28 weeks 0 days until delivery

Use additional code from category Z3A, Weeks of gestation, to identify the specific week of the pregnancy, if known.

EXCLUDES 1 *supervision of normal pregnancy (Z34.-)*

EXCLUDES 2 *mental and behavioral disorders associated with the puerperium (F53.-)*
obstetrical tetanus (A34)
postpartum necrosis of pituitary gland (E23.0)
puerperal osteomalacia (M83.0)

AHA: 2016,1Q,3-5; 2014,3Q,17

This chapter contains the following blocks:

O00-O08 Pregnancy with abortive outcome
O09 Supervision of high risk pregnancy
O10-O16 Edema, proteinuria and hypertensive disorders in pregnancy, childbirth and the puerperium
O20-O29 Other maternal disorders predominantly related to pregnancy
O30-O48 Maternal care related to the fetus and amniotic cavity and possible delivery problems
O60-O77 Complications of labor and delivery
O80-O82 Encounter for delivery
O85-O92 Complications predominantly related to the puerperium
O94-O9A Other obstetric conditions, not elsewhere classified

Pregnancy with abortive outcome (O00-O08)

EXCLUDES 1 *continuing pregnancy in multiple gestation after abortion of one fetus or more (O31.1-, O31.3-)*

TIP: Do not assign a code from category Z3A with codes in this code block.

✓4th **O00 Ectopic pregnancy**

INCLUDES ruptured ectopic pregnancy

Use additional code from category O08 to identify any associated complication

AHA: 2016,4Q,48-50; 2014,3Q,17

DEF: Implantation of a fertilized egg outside the uterus, usually in the fallopian tube or abdomen that requires emergency treatment.

Ectopic Pregnancy

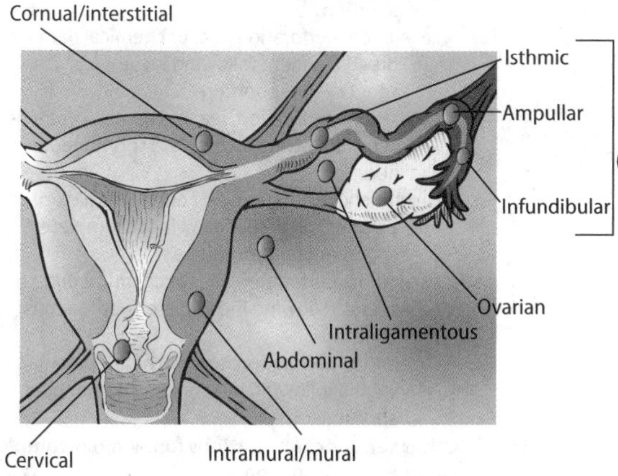

✓5th **O00.0 Abdominal pregnancy**

EXCLUDES 1 *maternal care for viable fetus in abdominal pregnancy (O36.7-)*

O00.00 Abdominal pregnancy without intrauterine pregnancy CC M ♀
Abdominal pregnancy NOS

O00.01 Abdominal pregnancy with intrauterine pregnancy CC M ♀

✓5th **O00.1 Tubal pregnancy**
Fallopian pregnancy
Rupture of (fallopian) tube due to pregnancy
Tubal abortion
AHA: 2017,4Q,20

✓6th **O00.10 Tubal pregnancy without intrauterine pregnancy**
Tubal pregnancy NOS

O00.101 Right tubal pregnancy without intrauterine pregnancy CC M ♀
O00.102 Left tubal pregnancy without intrauterine pregnancy CC M ♀
O00.109 Unspecified tubal pregnancy without intrauterine pregnancy CC M ♀

✓6th **O00.11 Tubal pregnancy with intrauterine pregnancy**

O00.111 Right tubal pregnancy with intrauterine pregnancy CC M ♀
O00.112 Left tubal pregnancy with intrauterine pregnancy CC M ♀
O00.119 Unspecified tubal pregnancy with intrauterine pregnancy CC M ♀

✓5th **O00.2 Ovarian pregnancy**
AHA: 2017,4Q,20

✓6th **O00.20 Ovarian pregnancy without intrauterine pregnancy**
Ovarian pregnancy NOS

O00.201 Right ovarian pregnancy without intrauterine pregnancy CC M ♀
O00.202 Left ovarian pregnancy without intrauterine pregnancy CC M ♀
O00.209 Unspecified ovarian pregnancy without intrauterine pregnancy CC M ♀

✓6th **O00.21 Ovarian pregnancy with intrauterine pregnancy**

O00.211 Right ovarian pregnancy with intrauterine pregnancy CC M ♀
O00.212 Left ovarian pregnancy with intrauterine pregnancy CC M ♀
O00.219 Unspecified ovarian pregnancy with intrauterine pregnancy CC M ♀

✓5th **O00.8 Other ectopic pregnancy**
Cervical pregnancy
Cornual pregnancy
Intraligamentous pregnancy
Mural pregnancy

O00.80 Other ectopic pregnancy without intrauterine pregnancy CC M ♀
Other ectopic pregnancy NOS

O00.81 Other ectopic pregnancy with intrauterine pregnancy CC M ♀

✓5th **O00.9 Ectopic pregnancy, unspecified**

O00.90 Unspecified ectopic pregnancy without intrauterine pregnancy CC M ♀
Ectopic pregnancy NOS

O00.91 Unspecified ectopic pregnancy with intrauterine pregnancy CC M ♀

✓4th **O01 Hydatidiform mole**

Use additional code from category O08 to identify any associated complication

EXCLUDES 1 *chorioadenoma (destruens) (D39.2)*
malignant hydatidiform mole (D39.2)

AHA: 2014,3Q,17

DEF: Abnormal product of pregnancy, marked by a mass of cysts resembling a bunch of grapes due to chorionic villi proliferation and dissolution. It must be surgically removed.

O01.0 Classical hydatidiform mole M ♀
Complete hydatidiform mole

O01.1 Incomplete and partial hydatidiform mole M ♀

O01.9 Hydatidiform mole, unspecified M ♀
Trophoblastic disease NOS
Vesicular mole NOS

√4th O02 Other abnormal products of conception

Use additional code from category O08 to identify any associated complication

EXCLUDES 1 *papyraceous fetus (O31.0-)*

AHA: 2014,3Q,17

O02.0 Blighted ovum and nonhydatidiform mole M ♀

Carneous mole
Fleshy mole
Intrauterine mole NOS
Molar pregnancy NEC
Pathological ovum

O02.1 Missed abortion M ♀

Early fetal death, before completion of 20 weeks of gestation, with retention of dead fetus

EXCLUDES 1 *failed induced abortion (O07.-)*
fetal death (intrauterine) (late) (O36.4)
missed abortion with blighted ovum (O02.0)
missed abortion with hydatidiform mole (O01.-)
missed abortion with nonhydatidiform (O02.0)
missed abortion with other abnormal products of conception (O02.8-)
missed delivery (O36.4)
stillbirth (P95)

AHA: 2019,3Q,11

√5th O02.8 Other specified abnormal products of conception

EXCLUDES 1 *abnormal products of conception with blighted ovum (O02.0)*
abnormal products of conception with hydatidiform mole (O01.-)
abnormal products of conception with nonhydatidiform mole (O02.0)

O02.81 Inappropriate change in quantitative human chorionic gonadotropin (hCG) in early pregnancy M ♀

Biochemical pregnancy
Chemical pregnancy
Inappropriate level of quantitative human chorionic gonadotropin (hCG) for gestational age in early pregnancy

O02.89 Other abnormal products of conception M ♀

O02.9 Abnormal product of conception, unspecified M ♀

√4th O03 Spontaneous abortion

NOTE Incomplete abortion includes retained products of conception following spontaneous abortion

INCLUDES miscarriage

O03.0 Genital tract and pelvic infection following incomplete spontaneous abortion CC M ♀

Endometritis following incomplete spontaneous abortion
Oophoritis following incomplete spontaneous abortion
Parametritis following incomplete spontaneous abortion
Pelvic peritonitis following incomplete spontaneous abortion
Salpingitis following incomplete spontaneous abortion
Salpingo-oophoritis following incomplete spontaneous abortion

EXCLUDES 1 *sepsis following incomplete spontaneous abortion (O03.37)*
urinary tract infection following incomplete spontaneous abortion (O03.38)

O03.1 Delayed or excessive hemorrhage following incomplete spontaneous abortion M ♀

Afibrinogenemia following incomplete spontaneous abortion
Defibrination syndrome following incomplete spontaneous abortion
Hemolysis following incomplete spontaneous abortion
Intravascular coagulation following incomplete spontaneous abortion

O03.2 Embolism following incomplete spontaneous abortion MCC M ♀

Air embolism following incomplete spontaneous abortion
Amniotic fluid embolism following incomplete spontaneous abortion
Blood-clot embolism following incomplete spontaneous abortion
Embolism NOS following incomplete spontaneous abortion
Fat embolism following incomplete spontaneous abortion
Pulmonary embolism following incomplete spontaneous abortion
Pyemic embolism following incomplete spontaneous abortion
Septic or septicopyemic embolism following incomplete spontaneous abortion
Soap embolism following incomplete spontaneous abortion

√5th O03.3 Other and unspecified complications following incomplete spontaneous abortion

O03.30 Unspecified complication following incomplete spontaneous abortion CC M ♀

O03.31 Shock following incomplete spontaneous abortion MCC M ♀

Circulatory collapse following incomplete spontaneous abortion
Shock (postprocedural) following incomplete spontaneous abortion

EXCLUDES 1 *shock due to infection following incomplete spontaneous abortion (O03.37)*

O03.32 Renal failure following incomplete spontaneous abortion MCC M ♀

Kidney failure (acute) following incomplete spontaneous abortion
Oliguria following incomplete spontaneous abortion
Renal shutdown following incomplete spontaneous abortion
Renal tubular necrosis following incomplete spontaneous abortion
Uremia following incomplete spontaneous abortion

O03.33 Metabolic disorder following incomplete spontaneous abortion CC M ♀

O03.34 Damage to pelvic organs following incomplete spontaneous abortion CC M ♀

Laceration, perforation, tear or chemical damage of bladder following incomplete spontaneous abortion
Laceration, perforation, tear or chemical damage of bowel following incomplete spontaneous abortion
Laceration, perforation, tear or chemical damage of broad ligament following incomplete spontaneous abortion
Laceration, perforation, tear or chemical damage of cervix following incomplete spontaneous abortion
Laceration, perforation, tear or chemical damage of periurethral tissue following incomplete spontaneous abortion
Laceration, perforation, tear or chemical damage of uterus following incomplete spontaneous abortion
Laceration, perforation, tear or chemical damage of vagina following incomplete spontaneous abortion

O03.35 Other venous complications following incomplete spontaneous abortion CC M ♀

O03.36 Cardiac arrest following incomplete spontaneous abortion CC M ♀

O03.37 Sepsis following incomplete spontaneous abortion CC M ♀

Use additional code to identify infectious agent (B95-B97)
Use additional code to identify severe sepsis, if applicable (R65.2-)

EXCLUDES 1 *septic or septicopyemic embolism following incomplete spontaneous abortion (O03.2)*

O03.38 Urinary tract infection **following** incomplete **spontaneous abortion** CC M ♀
Cystitis following incomplete spontaneous abortion

O03.39 **Incomplete spontaneous abortion with other complications** CC M ♀

O03.4 Incomplete **spontaneous abortion** without complication M ♀

O03.5 Genital tract and pelvic infection **following** complete or unspecified **spontaneous abortion** CC M ♀
Endometritis following complete or unspecified spontaneous abortion
Oophoritis following complete or unspecified spontaneous abortion
Parametritis following complete or unspecified spontaneous abortion
Pelvic peritonitis following complete or unspecified spontaneous abortion
Salpingitis following complete or unspecified spontaneous abortion
Salpingo-oophoritis following complete or unspecified spontaneous abortion
EXCLUDES 1 *sepsis following complete or unspecified spontaneous abortion (O03.87)*
urinary tract infection following complete or unspecified spontaneous abortion (O03.88)

O03.6 Delayed or excessive hemorrhage **following** complete or unspecified **spontaneous abortion** M ♀
Afibrinogenemia following complete or unspecified spontaneous abortion
Defibrination syndrome following complete or unspecified spontaneous abortion
Hemolysis following complete or unspecified spontaneous abortion
Intravascular coagulation following complete or unspecified spontaneous abortion

O03.7 Embolism **following** complete or unspecified **spontaneous abortion** CC M ♀
Air embolism following complete or unspecified spontaneous abortion
Amniotic fluid embolism following complete or unspecified spontaneous abortion
Blood-clot embolism following complete or unspecified spontaneous abortion
Embolism NOS following complete or unspecified spontaneous abortion
Fat embolism following complete or unspecified spontaneous abortion
Pulmonary embolism following complete or unspecified spontaneous abortion
Pyemic embolism following complete or unspecified spontaneous abortion
Septic or septicopyemic embolism following complete or unspecified spontaneous abortion
Soap embolism following complete or unspecified spontaneous abortion

✓5th **O03.8** **Other and unspecified complications following complete or unspecified spontaneous abortion**

O03.80 **Unspecified complication following** complete or unspecified **spontaneous abortion** CC M ♀

O03.81 Shock **following** complete or unspecified **spontaneous abortion** MCC M ♀
Circulatory collapse following complete or unspecified spontaneous abortion
Shock (postprocedural) following complete or unspecified spontaneous abortion
EXCLUDES 1 *shock due to infection following complete or unspecified spontaneous abortion (O03.87)*

O03.82 Renal failure **following** complete or unspecified **spontaneous abortion** MCC M ♀
Kidney failure (acute) following complete or unspecified spontaneous abortion
Oliguria following complete or unspecified spontaneous abortion
Renal shutdown following complete or unspecified spontaneous abortion
Renal tubular necrosis following complete or unspecified spontaneous abortion
Uremia following complete or unspecified spontaneous abortion

O03.83 Metabolic **disorder following** complete or unspecified **spontaneous abortion** CC M ♀

O03.84 Damage to pelvic organs **following** complete or unspecified **spontaneous abortion** CC M ♀
Laceration, perforation, tear or chemical damage of bladder following complete or unspecified spontaneous abortion
Laceration, perforation, tear or chemical damage of bowel following complete or unspecified spontaneous abortion
Laceration, perforation, tear or chemical damage of broad ligament following complete or unspecified spontaneous abortion
Laceration, perforation, tear or chemical damage of cervix following complete or unspecified spontaneous abortion
Laceration, perforation, tear or chemical damage of periurethral tissue following complete or unspecified spontaneous abortion
Laceration, perforation, tear or chemical damage of uterus following complete or unspecified spontaneous abortion
Laceration, perforation, tear or chemical damage of vagina following complete or unspecified spontaneous abortion

O03.85 **Other** venous **complications following** complete or unspecified **spontaneous abortion** CC M ♀

O03.86 Cardiac arrest **following** complete or unspecified **spontaneous abortion** CC M ♀

O03.87 Sepsis **following** complete or unspecified **spontaneous abortion** CC M ♀
Use additional code to identify infectious agent (B95-B97)
Use additional code to identify severe sepsis, if applicable (R65.2-)
EXCLUDES 1 *septic or septicopyemic embolism following complete or unspecified spontaneous abortion (O03.7)*

O03.88 Urinary tract infection **following** complete or unspecified **spontaneous abortion** CC M ♀
Cystitis following complete or unspecified spontaneous abortion

O03.89 Complete or unspecified **spontaneous abortion with other complications** CC M ♀

O03.9 Complete or unspecified **spontaneous abortion** without complication M ♀
Miscarriage NOS
Spontaneous abortion NOS

Chapter 15. Pregnancy, Childbirth and the Puerperium

O03.38–O03.9

√4th **O04 Complications following (induced) termination of pregnancy**

INCLUDES complications following (induced) termination of pregnancy

EXCLUDES 1 *encounter for elective termination of pregnancy, uncomplicated (Z33.2)*
failed attempted termination of pregnancy (O07.-)

O04.5 Genital tract and pelvic infection following (induced) termination of pregnancy CC M ♀
Endometritis following (induced) termination of pregnancy
Oophoritis following (induced) termination of pregnancy
Parametritis following (induced) termination of pregnancy
Pelvic peritonitis following (induced) termination of pregnancy
Salpingitis following (induced) termination of pregnancy
Salpingo-oophoritis following (induced) termination of pregnancy

EXCLUDES 1 *sepsis following (induced) termination of pregnancy (O04.87)*
urinary tract infection following (induced) termination of pregnancy (O04.88)

O04.6 Delayed or excessive hemorrhage following (induced) termination of pregnancy M ♀
Afibrinogenemia following (induced) termination of pregnancy
Defibrination syndrome following (induced) termination of pregnancy
Hemolysis following (induced) termination of pregnancy
Intravascular coagulation following (induced) termination of pregnancy
AHA: 2019,3Q,11

O04.7 Embolism following (induced) termination of pregnancy MCC M ♀
Air embolism following (induced) termination of pregnancy
Amniotic fluid embolism following (induced) termination of pregnancy
Blood-clot embolism following (induced) termination of pregnancy
Embolism NOS following (induced) termination of pregnancy
Fat embolism following (induced) termination of pregnancy
Pulmonary embolism following (induced) termination of pregnancy
Pyemic embolism following (induced) termination of pregnancy
Septic or septicopyemic embolism following (induced) termination of pregnancy
Soap embolism following (induced) termination of pregnancy

√5th **O04.8 (Induced) termination of pregnancy with other and unspecified complications**

O04.80 (Induced) termination of pregnancy with unspecified complications CC M ♀

O04.81 Shock following (induced) termination of pregnancy MCC M ♀
Circulatory collapse following (induced) termination of pregnancy
Shock (postprocedural) following (induced) termination of pregnancy

EXCLUDES 1 *shock due to infection following (induced) termination of pregnancy (O04.87)*

O04.82 Renal failure following (induced) termination of pregnancy MCC ♀
Kidney failure (acute) following (induced) termination of pregnancy
Oliguria following (induced) termination of pregnancy
Renal shutdown following (induced) termination of pregnancy
Renal tubular necrosis following (induced) termination of pregnancy
Uremia following (induced) termination of pregnancy

O04.83 Metabolic disorder following (induced) termination of pregnancy CC M ♀

O04.84 Damage to pelvic organs following (induced) termination of pregnancy CC M ♀
Laceration, perforation, tear or chemical damage of bladder following (induced) termination of pregnancy
Laceration, perforation, tear or chemical damage of bowel following (induced) termination of pregnancy
Laceration, perforation, tear or chemical damage of broad ligament following (induced) termination of pregnancy
Laceration, perforation, tear or chemical damage of cervix following (induced) termination of pregnancy
Laceration, perforation, tear or chemical damage of periurethral tissue following (induced) termination of pregnancy
Laceration, perforation, tear or chemical damage of uterus following (induced) termination of pregnancy
Laceration, perforation, tear or chemical damage of vagina following (induced) termination of pregnancy

O04.85 Other venous complications following (induced) termination of pregnancy CC M ♀

O04.86 Cardiac arrest following (induced) termination of pregnancy CC M ♀

O04.87 Sepsis following (induced) termination of pregnancy CC M ♀
Use additional code to identify infectious agent (B95-B97)
Use additional code to identify severe sepsis, if applicable (R65.2-)

EXCLUDES 1 *septic or septicopyemic embolism following (induced) termination of pregnancy (O04.7)*

O04.88 Urinary tract infection following (induced) termination of pregnancy CC M ♀
Cystitis following (induced) termination of pregnancy

O04.89 (Induced) termination of pregnancy with other complications CC M ♀

√4th **O07 Failed attempted termination of pregnancy**

INCLUDES failure of attempted induction of termination of pregnancy
incomplete elective abortion

EXCLUDES 1 *incomplete spontaneous abortion (O03.0-)*

O07.0 Genital tract and pelvic infection following failed attempted termination of pregnancy CC M ♀
Endometritis following failed attempted termination of pregnancy
Oophoritis following failed attempted termination of pregnancy
Parametritis following failed attempted termination of pregnancy
Pelvic peritonitis following failed attempted termination of pregnancy
Salpingitis following failed attempted termination of pregnancy
Salpingo-oophoritis following failed attempted termination of pregnancy

EXCLUDES 1 *sepsis following failed attempted termination of pregnancy (O07.37)*
urinary tract infection following failed attempted termination of pregnancy (O07.38)

O07.1 Delayed or excessive hemorrhage following failed attempted termination of pregnancy CC M ♀
Afibrinogenemia following failed attempted termination of pregnancy
Defibrination syndrome following failed attempted termination of pregnancy
Hemolysis following failed attempted termination of pregnancy
Intravascular coagulation following failed attempted termination of pregnancy

O07.2 Embolism following failed attempted termination of pregnancy MCC M ♀
- Air embolism following failed attempted termination of pregnancy
- Amniotic fluid embolism following failed attempted termination of pregnancy
- Blood-clot embolism following failed attempted termination of pregnancy
- Embolism NOS following failed attempted termination of pregnancy
- Fat embolism following failed attempted termination of pregnancy
- Pulmonary embolism following failed attempted termination of pregnancy
- Pyemic embolism following failed attempted termination of pregnancy
- Septic or septicopyemic embolism following failed attempted termination of pregnancy
- Soap embolism following failed attempted termination of pregnancy

✓5th **O07.3 Failed attempted termination of pregnancy with other and unspecified complications**

O07.30 Failed attempted termination of pregnancy with unspecified complications CC M ♀

O07.31 Shock following failed attempted termination of pregnancy MCC M ♀
- Circulatory collapse following failed attempted termination of pregnancy
- Shock (postprocedural) following failed attempted termination of pregnancy

EXCLUDES 1 *shock due to infection following failed attempted termination of pregnancy (O07.37)*

O07.32 Renal failure following failed attempted termination of pregnancy MCC M ♀
- Kidney failure (acute) following failed attempted termination of pregnancy
- Oliguria following failed attempted termination of pregnancy
- Renal shutdown following failed attempted termination of pregnancy
- Renal tubular necrosis following failed attempted termination of pregnancy
- Uremia following failed attempted termination of pregnancy

O07.33 Metabolic disorder following failed attempted termination of pregnancy CC M ♀

O07.34 Damage to pelvic organs following failed attempted termination of pregnancy CC M ♀
- Laceration, perforation, tear or chemical damage of bladder following failed attempted termination of pregnancy
- Laceration, perforation, tear or chemical damage of bowel following failed attempted termination of pregnancy
- Laceration, perforation, tear or chemical damage of broad ligament following failed attempted termination of pregnancy
- Laceration, perforation, tear or chemical damage of cervix following failed attempted termination of pregnancy
- Laceration, perforation, tear or chemical damage of periurethral tissue following failed attempted termination of pregnancy
- Laceration, perforation, tear or chemical damage of uterus following failed attempted termination of pregnancy
- Laceration, perforation, tear or chemical damage of vagina following failed attempted termination of pregnancy

O07.35 Other venous complications following failed attempted termination of pregnancy CC M ♀

O07.36 Cardiac arrest following failed attempted termination of pregnancy CC M ♀

O07.37 Sepsis following failed attempted termination of pregnancy CC M ♀

Use additional code (B95-B97), to identify infectious agent

Use additional code (R65.2-) to identify severe sepsis, if applicable

EXCLUDES 1 *septic or septicopyemic embolism following failed attempted termination of pregnancy (O07.2)*

O07.38 Urinary tract infection following failed attempted termination of pregnancy CC M ♀
- Cystitis following failed attempted termination of pregnancy

O07.39 Failed attempted termination of pregnancy with other complications CC M ♀

O07.4 Failed attempted termination of pregnancy without complication M ♀

✓4th **O08 Complications following ectopic and molar pregnancy**

This category is for use with categories O00-O02 to identify any associated complications

O08.0 Genital tract and pelvic infection following ectopic and molar pregnancy CC M ♀
- Endometritis following ectopic and molar pregnancy
- Oophoritis following ectopic and molar pregnancy
- Parametritis following ectopic and molar pregnancy
- Pelvic peritonitis following ectopic and molar pregnancy
- Salpingitis following ectopic and molar pregnancy
- Salpingo-oophoritis following ectopic and molar pregnancy

EXCLUDES 1 *sepsis following ectopic and molar pregnancy (O08.82)*
urinary tract infection (O08.83)

O08.1 Delayed or excessive hemorrhage following ectopic and molar pregnancy CC M ♀
- Afibrinogenemia following ectopic and molar pregnancy
- Defibrination syndrome following ectopic and molar pregnancy
- Hemolysis following ectopic and molar pregnancy
- Intravascular coagulation following ectopic and molar pregnancy

EXCLUDES 1 *delayed or excessive hemorrhage due to incomplete abortion (O03.1)*

O08.2 Embolism following ectopic and molar pregnancy MCC M ♀
- Air embolism following ectopic and molar pregnancy
- Amniotic fluid embolism following ectopic and molar pregnancy
- Blood-clot embolism following ectopic and molar pregnancy
- Embolism NOS following ectopic and molar pregnancy
- Fat embolism following ectopic and molar pregnancy
- Pulmonary embolism following ectopic and molar pregnancy
- Pyemic embolism following ectopic and molar pregnancy
- Septic or septicopyemic embolism following ectopic and molar pregnancy
- Soap embolism following ectopic and molar pregnancy

O08.3 Shock following ectopic and molar pregnancy MCC M ♀
- Circulatory collapse following ectopic and molar pregnancy
- Shock (postprocedural) following ectopic and molar pregnancy

EXCLUDES 1 *shock due to infection following ectopic and molar pregnancy (O08.82)*

O08.4 Renal failure following ectopic and molar pregnancy MCC M ♀
- Kidney failure (acute) following ectopic and molar pregnancy
- Oliguria following ectopic and molar pregnancy
- Renal shutdown following ectopic and molar pregnancy
- Renal tubular necrosis following ectopic and molar pregnancy
- Uremia following ectopic and molar pregnancy

O08.5 Metabolic disorders following an ectopic and molar pregnancy CC M ♀

O08.6 Damage to pelvic organs and tissues following an ectopic and molar pregnancy CC M ♀

Laceration, perforation, tear or chemical damage of bladder following an ectopic and molar pregnancy

Laceration, perforation, tear or chemical damage of bowel following an ectopic and molar pregnancy

Laceration, perforation, tear or chemical damage of broad ligament following an ectopic and molar pregnancy

Laceration, perforation, tear or chemical damage of cervix following an ectopic and molar pregnancy

Laceration, perforation, tear or chemical damage of periurethral tissue following an ectopic and molar pregnancy

Laceration, perforation, tear or chemical damage of uterus following an ectopic and molar pregnancy

Laceration, perforation, tear or chemical damage of vagina following an ectopic and molar pregnancy

O08.7 Other venous complications following an ectopic and molar pregnancy CC M ♀

✓5th **O08.8 Other complications following an ectopic and molar pregnancy**

O08.81 Cardiac arrest following an ectopic and molar pregnancy CC M ♀

O08.82 Sepsis following ectopic and molar pregnancy CC M ♀

Use additional code (B95-B97), to identify infectious agent

Use additional code (R65.2-) to identify severe sepsis, if applicable

EXCLUDES 1 *septic or septicopyemic embolism following ectopic and molar pregnancy (O08.2)*

O08.83 Urinary tract infection following an ectopic and molar pregnancy CC M ♀

Cystitis following an ectopic and molar pregnancy

O08.89 Other complications following an ectopic and molar pregnancy CC M ♀

O08.9 Unspecified complication following an ectopic and molar pregnancy CC M ♀

Supervision of high risk pregnancy (O09)

✓4th **O09 Supervision of high risk pregnancy**

AHA: 2019,3Q,5; 2016,4Q,48-50,150

✓5th **O09.0 Supervision of pregnancy with history of infertility**

DEF: Infertility: Inability to conceive for at least one year with regular intercourse.

O09.00 Supervision of pregnancy with history of infertility, unspecified trimester M ♀

O09.01 Supervision of pregnancy with history of infertility, first trimester M ♀

O09.02 Supervision of pregnancy with history of infertility, second trimester M ♀

O09.03 Supervision of pregnancy with history of infertility, third trimester M ♀

✓5th **O09.1 Supervision of pregnancy with history of ectopic pregnancy**

DEF: Ectopic pregnancy: Implantation of a fertilized egg outside the uterus, usually in the fallopian tube or abdomen that requires emergency treatment.

O09.10 Supervision of pregnancy with history of ectopic pregnancy, unspecified trimester M ♀

O09.11 Supervision of pregnancy with history of ectopic pregnancy, first trimester M ♀

O09.12 Supervision of pregnancy with history of ectopic pregnancy, second trimester M ♀

O09.13 Supervision of pregnancy with history of ectopic pregnancy, third trimester M ♀

✓5th **O09.A Supervision of pregnancy with history of molar pregnancy**

DEF: Molar pregnancy: Trophoblastic neoplasm that mimics pregnancy by proliferating from a pathologic ovum and resulting only in a mass of cysts resembling grapes, 80 percent of which are benign, but require surgical removal.

O09.A0 Supervision of pregnancy with history of molar pregnancy, unspecified trimester M ♀

O09.A1 Supervision of pregnancy with history of molar pregnancy, first trimester M ♀

O09.A2 Supervision of pregnancy with history of molar pregnancy, second trimester M ♀

O09.A3 Supervision of pregnancy with history of molar pregnancy, third trimester M ♀

✓5th **O09.2 Supervision of pregnancy with other poor reproductive or obstetric history**

EXCLUDES 2 *pregnancy care for patient with history of recurrent pregnancy loss (O26.2-)*

✓6th **O09.21 Supervision of pregnancy with history of pre-term labor**

O09.211 Supervision of pregnancy with history of pre-term labor, first trimester M ♀

O09.212 Supervision of pregnancy with history of pre-term labor, second trimester M ♀

O09.213 Supervision of pregnancy with history of pre-term labor, third trimester M ♀

O09.219 Supervision of pregnancy with history of pre-term labor, unspecified trimester M ♀

✓6th **O09.29 Supervision of pregnancy with other poor reproductive or obstetric history**

Supervision of pregnancy with history of neonatal death

Supervision of pregnancy with history of stillbirth

O09.291 Supervision of pregnancy with other poor reproductive or obstetric history, first trimester M ♀

O09.292 Supervision of pregnancy with other poor reproductive or obstetric history, second trimester M ♀

O09.293 Supervision of pregnancy with other poor reproductive or obstetric history, third trimester M ♀

O09.299 Supervision of pregnancy with other poor reproductive or obstetric history, unspecified trimester M ♀

✓5th **O09.3 Supervision of pregnancy with insufficient antenatal care**

Supervision of concealed pregnancy

Supervision of hidden pregnancy

O09.30 Supervision of pregnancy with insufficient antenatal care, unspecified trimester M ♀

O09.31 Supervision of pregnancy with insufficient antenatal care, first trimester M ♀

O09.32 Supervision of pregnancy with insufficient antenatal care, second trimester M ♀

O09.33 Supervision of pregnancy with insufficient antenatal care, third trimester M ♀

✓5th **O09.4 Supervision of pregnancy with grand multiparity**

O09.40 Supervision of pregnancy with grand multiparity, unspecified trimester M ♀

O09.41 Supervision of pregnancy with grand multiparity, first trimester M ♀

O09.42 Supervision of pregnancy with grand multiparity, second trimester M ♀

O09.43 Supervision of pregnancy with grand multiparity, third trimester M ♀

✓5th **O09.5 Supervision of elderly primigravida and multigravida**

Pregnancy for a female 35 years and older at expected date of delivery

✓6th **O09.51 Supervision of elderly primigravida**

O09.511 Supervision of elderly primigravida, first trimester M ♀

O09.512 Supervision of elderly primigravida, second trimester M ♀

O09.513 Supervision of elderly primigravida, third trimester M ♀

O09.519 Supervision of elderly primigravida, unspecified trimester M ♀

✓6th **O09.52 Supervision of elderly multigravida**

O09.521 Supervision of elderly multigravida, first trimester M ♀

O09.522 Supervision of elderly multigravida, second trimester M ♀

O09.523 Supervision of elderly multigravida, third trimester M ♀

O09.529 Supervision of elderly multigravida, unspecified trimester M ♀

✓5th **O09.6 Supervision of young primigravida and multigravida**

Supervision of pregnancy for a female less than 16 years old at expected date of delivery

✓6th **O09.61 Supervision of young primigravida**

O09.611 Supervision of young primigravida, first trimester M ♀

O09.612 Supervision of young primigravida, second trimester M ♀
O09.613 Supervision of young primigravida, third trimester M ♀
O09.619 Supervision of young primigravida, unspecified trimester M ♀
✓6th O09.62 Supervision of young multigravida
O09.621 Supervision of young multigravida, first trimester M ♀
O09.622 Supervision of young multigravida, second trimester M ♀
O09.623 Supervision of young multigravida, third trimester M ♀
O09.629 Supervision of young multigravida, unspecified trimester M ♀
✓5th O09.7 Supervision of high risk pregnancy due to social problems
O09.70 Supervision of high risk pregnancy due to social problems, unspecified trimester M ♀
O09.71 Supervision of high risk pregnancy due to social problems, first trimester M ♀
O09.72 Supervision of high risk pregnancy due to social problems, second trimester M ♀
O09.73 Supervision of high risk pregnancy due to social problems, third trimester M ♀
✓5th O09.8 Supervision of other high risk pregnancies
✓6th O09.81 Supervision of pregnancy resulting from assisted reproductive technology
Supervision of pregnancy resulting from in-vitro fertilization
EXCLUDES 2 *gestational carrier status (Z33.3)*
O09.811 Supervision of pregnancy resulting from assisted reproductive technology, first trimester M ♀
O09.812 Supervision of pregnancy resulting from assisted reproductive technology, second trimester M ♀
O09.813 Supervision of pregnancy resulting from assisted reproductive technology, third trimester M ♀
O09.819 Supervision of pregnancy resulting from assisted reproductive technology, unspecified trimester M ♀
✓6th O09.82 Supervision of pregnancy with history of in utero procedure during previous pregnancy
O09.821 Supervision of pregnancy with history of in utero procedure during previous pregnancy, first trimester M ♀
O09.822 Supervision of pregnancy with history of in utero procedure during previous pregnancy, second trimester M ♀
O09.823 Supervision of pregnancy with history of in utero procedure during previous pregnancy, third trimester M ♀
O09.829 Supervision of pregnancy with history of in utero procedure during previous pregnancy, unspecified trimester M ♀
EXCLUDES 1 *supervision of pregnancy affected by in utero procedure during current pregnancy (O35.7)*
✓6th O09.89 Supervision of other high risk pregnancies
O09.891 Supervision of other high risk pregnancies, first trimester M ♀
O09.892 Supervision of other high risk pregnancies, second trimester M ♀
O09.893 Supervision of other high risk pregnancies, third trimester M ♀
O09.899 Supervision of other high risk pregnancies, unspecified trimester M ♀
✓5th O09.9 Supervision of high risk pregnancy, unspecified
O09.90 Supervision of high risk pregnancy, unspecified, unspecified trimester M ♀
O09.91 Supervision of high risk pregnancy, unspecified, first trimester M ♀
O09.92 Supervision of high risk pregnancy, unspecified, second trimester M ♀
O09.93 Supervision of high risk pregnancy, unspecified, third trimester M ♀

Edema, proteinuria and hypertensive disorders in pregnancy, childbirth and the puerperium (O10-O16)

AHA: 2016,4Q,50

✓4th **O10 Pre-existing hypertension complicating pregnancy, childbirth and the puerperium**
INCLUDES pre-existing hypertension with pre-existing proteinuria complicating pregnancy, childbirth and the puerperium
EXCLUDES 2 *pre-existing hypertension with superimposed pre-eclampsia complicating pregnancy, childbirth and the puerperium (O11.-)*
✓5th O10.0 Pre-existing essential hypertension complicating pregnancy, childbirth and the puerperium
Any condition in I10 specified as a reason for obstetric care during pregnancy, childbirth or the puerperium
✓6th O10.01 Pre-existing essential hypertension complicating pregnancy
O10.011 Pre-existing essential hypertension complicating pregnancy, first trimester CC M ♀
O10.012 Pre-existing essential hypertension complicating pregnancy, second trimester CC M ♀
O10.013 Pre-existing essential hypertension complicating pregnancy, third trimester CC M ♀
O10.019 Pre-existing essential hypertension complicating pregnancy, unspecified trimester M ♀
O10.02 Pre-existing essential hypertension complicating childbirth CC M ♀
O10.03 Pre-existing essential hypertension complicating the puerperium M ♀
✓5th O10.1 Pre-existing hypertensive heart disease complicating pregnancy, childbirth and the puerperium
Any condition in I11 specified as a reason for obstetric care during pregnancy, childbirth or the puerperium
Use additional code from I11 to identify the type of hypertensive heart disease
✓6th O10.11 Pre-existing hypertensive heart disease complicating pregnancy
O10.111 Pre-existing hypertensive heart disease complicating pregnancy, first trimester M ♀
O10.112 Pre-existing hypertensive heart disease complicating pregnancy, second trimester M ♀
O10.113 Pre-existing hypertensive heart disease complicating pregnancy, third trimester M ♀
O10.119 Pre-existing hypertensive heart disease complicating pregnancy, unspecified trimester M ♀
O10.12 Pre-existing hypertensive heart disease complicating childbirth M ♀
O10.13 Pre-existing hypertensive heart disease complicating the puerperium M ♀
✓5th O10.2 Pre-existing hypertensive chronic kidney disease complicating pregnancy, childbirth and the puerperium
Any condition in I12 specified as a reason for obstetric care during pregnancy, childbirth or the puerperium
Use additional code from I12 to identify the type of hypertensive chronic kidney disease
✓6th O10.21 Pre-existing hypertensive chronic kidney disease complicating pregnancy
O10.211 Pre-existing hypertensive chronic kidney disease complicating pregnancy, first trimester M ♀
O10.212 Pre-existing hypertensive chronic kidney disease complicating pregnancy, second trimester M ♀
O10.213 Pre-existing hypertensive chronic kidney disease complicating pregnancy, third trimester M ♀
O10.219 Pre-existing hypertensive chronic kidney disease complicating pregnancy, unspecified trimester M ♀
O10.22 Pre-existing hypertensive chronic kidney disease complicating childbirth M ♀

O10.23 Pre-existing hypertensive chronic kidney disease complicating the puerperium M ♀

✓5th **O10.3 Pre-existing hypertensive heart and chronic kidney disease complicating pregnancy, childbirth and the puerperium**
Any condition in I13 specified as a reason for obstetric care during pregnancy, childbirth or the puerperium
Use additional code from I13 to identify the type of hypertensive heart and chronic kidney disease

✓6th **O10.31 Pre-existing hypertensive heart and chronic kidney disease complicating pregnancy**

O10.311 Pre-existing hypertensive heart and chronic kidney disease complicating pregnancy, first trimester M ♀

O10.312 Pre-existing hypertensive heart and chronic kidney disease complicating pregnancy, second trimester M ♀

O10.313 Pre-existing hypertensive heart and chronic kidney disease complicating pregnancy, third trimester M ♀

O10.319 Pre-existing hypertensive heart and chronic kidney disease complicating pregnancy, unspecified trimester M ♀

O10.32 Pre-existing hypertensive heart and chronic kidney disease complicating childbirth M ♀

O10.33 Pre-existing hypertensive heart and chronic kidney disease complicating the puerperium M ♀

✓5th **O10.4 Pre-existing secondary hypertension complicating pregnancy, childbirth and the puerperium**
Any condition in I15 specified as a reason for obstetric care during pregnancy, childbirth or the puerperium
Use additional code from I15 to identify the type of secondary hypertension

✓6th **O10.41 Pre-existing secondary hypertension complicating pregnancy**

O10.411 Pre-existing secondary hypertension complicating pregnancy, first trimester CC M ♀

O10.412 Pre-existing secondary hypertension complicating pregnancy, second trimester CC M ♀

O10.413 Pre-existing secondary hypertension complicating pregnancy, third trimester CC M ♀

O10.419 Pre-existing secondary hypertension complicating pregnancy, unspecified trimester M ♀

O10.42 Pre-existing secondary hypertension complicating childbirth MCC M ♀

O10.43 Pre-existing secondary hypertension complicating the puerperium CC M ♀

✓5th **O10.9 Unspecified pre-existing hypertension complicating pregnancy, childbirth and the puerperium**

✓6th **O10.91 Unspecified pre-existing hypertension complicating pregnancy**

O10.911 Unspecified pre-existing hypertension complicating pregnancy, first trimester CC M ♀

O10.912 Unspecified pre-existing hypertension complicating pregnancy, second trimester CC M ♀

O10.913 Unspecified pre-existing hypertension complicating pregnancy, third trimester CC M ♀

O10.919 Unspecified pre-existing hypertension complicating pregnancy, unspecified trimester M ♀

O10.92 Unspecified pre-existing hypertension complicating childbirth CC M ♀

O10.93 Unspecified pre-existing hypertension complicating the puerperium M ♀

✓4th **O11 Pre-existing hypertension with pre-eclampsia**
INCLUDES conditions in O10 complicated by pre-eclampsia
pre-eclampsia superimposed pre-existing in hypertension
Use additional code from O10 to identify the type of hypertension
DEF: Complication of pregnancy manifesting in the development of borderline hypertension, protein in the urine, and unresponsive swelling between the 20th week of pregnancy and the end of the first week following birth in mild to moderate cases. Severe preeclampsia presents with hypertension, associated with marked swelling, proteinuria, abdominal pain, and/or visual changes.

O11.1 Pre-existing hypertension with pre-eclampsia, first trimester MCC M ♀

O11.2 Pre-existing hypertension with pre-eclampsia, second trimester MCC M ♀

O11.3 Pre-existing hypertension with pre-eclampsia, third trimester MCC M ♀

O11.4 Pre-existing hypertension with pre-eclampsia, complicating childbirth M ♀

O11.5 Pre-existing hypertension with pre-eclampsia, complicating the puerperium M ♀

O11.9 Pre-existing hypertension with pre-eclampsia, unspecified trimester M ♀

✓4th **O12 Gestational [pregnancy-induced] edema and proteinuria without hypertension**

✓5th **O12.0 Gestational edema**

O12.00 Gestational edema, unspecified trimester M ♀

O12.01 Gestational edema, first trimester M ♀

O12.02 Gestational edema, second trimester M ♀

O12.03 Gestational edema, third trimester M ♀

O12.04 Gestational edema, complicating childbirth M ♀

O12.05 Gestational edema, complicating the puerperium M ♀

✓5th **O12.1 Gestational proteinuria**

O12.10 Gestational proteinuria, unspecified trimester M ♀

O12.11 Gestational proteinuria, first trimester CC M ♀

O12.12 Gestational proteinuria, second trimester CC M ♀

O12.13 Gestational proteinuria, third trimester CC M ♀

O12.14 Gestational proteinuria, complicating childbirth M ♀

O12.15 Gestational proteinuria, complicating the puerperium M ♀

✓5th **O12.2 Gestational edema with proteinuria**

O12.20 Gestational edema with proteinuria, unspecified trimester M ♀

O12.21 Gestational edema with proteinuria, first trimester CC M ♀

O12.22 Gestational edema with proteinuria, second trimester CC M ♀

O12.23 Gestational edema with proteinuria, third trimester CC M ♀

O12.24 Gestational edema with proteinuria, complicating childbirth M ♀

O12.25 Gestational edema with proteinuria, complicating the puerperium M ♀

✓4th **O13 Gestational [pregnancy-induced] hypertension without significant proteinuria**
INCLUDES gestational hypertension NOS
transient hypertension of pregnancy
AHA: 2016,1Q,5

O13.1 Gestational [pregnancy-induced] hypertension without significant proteinuria, first trimester M ♀

O13.2 Gestational [pregnancy-induced] hypertension without significant proteinuria, second trimester M ♀

O13.3 Gestational [pregnancy-induced] hypertension without significant proteinuria, third trimester M ♀

O13.4 Gestational [pregnancy-induced] hypertension without significant proteinuria, complicating childbirth M ♀

O13.5 Gestational [pregnancy-induced] hypertension without significant proteinuria, complicating the puerperium M ♀

O13.9 Gestational [pregnancy-induced] hypertension without significant proteinuria, unspecified trimester M ♀

O14 Pre-eclampsia

EXCLUDES 1 *pre-existing hypertension with pre-eclampsia (O11)*

DEF: Complication of pregnancy manifesting in the development of borderline hypertension, protein in the urine, and unresponsive swelling between the 20th week of pregnancy and the end of the first week following birth in mild to moderate cases. Severe preeclampsia presents with hypertension, associated with marked swelling, proteinuria, abdominal pain, and/or visual changes.

O14.Ø Mild to moderate pre-eclampsia

AHA: 2019,3Q,12; 2019,2Q,8

O14.ØØ Mild to moderate pre-eclampsia, unspecified trimester M ♀

O14.Ø2 Mild to moderate pre-eclampsia, second trimester CC M ♀

O14.Ø3 Mild to moderate pre-eclampsia, third trimester CC M ♀

O14.Ø4 Mild to moderate pre-eclampsia, complicating childbirth M ♀

AHA: 2019,2Q,8

O14.Ø5 Mild to moderate pre-eclampsia, complicating the puerperium M ♀

O14.1 Severe pre-eclampsia

EXCLUDES 1 *HELLP syndrome (O14.2-)*

AHA: 2019,3Q,12

O14.1Ø Severe pre-eclampsia, unspecified trimester M ♀

O14.12 Severe pre-eclampsia, second trimester MCC M ♀

O14.13 Severe pre-eclampsia, third trimester MCC M ♀

O14.14 Severe pre-eclampsia complicating childbirth M ♀

O14.15 Severe pre-eclampsia, complicating the puerperium M ♀

O14.2 HELLP syndrome

Severe pre-eclampsia with hemolysis, elevated liver enzymes and low platelet count (HELLP)

AHA: 2019,3Q,12

O14.2Ø HELLP syndrome (HELLP), unspecified trimester M ♀

O14.22 HELLP syndrome (HELLP), second trimester MCC M ♀

O14.23 HELLP syndrome (HELLP), third trimester MCC M ♀

O14.24 HELLP syndrome, complicating childbirth M ♀

O14.25 HELLP syndrome, complicating the puerperium M ♀

O14.9 Unspecified pre-eclampsia

O14.9Ø Unspecified pre-eclampsia, unspecified trimester M ♀

O14.92 Unspecified pre-eclampsia, second trimester CC M ♀

O14.93 Unspecified pre-eclampsia, third trimester CC M ♀

O14.94 Unspecified pre-eclampsia, complicating childbirth M ♀

O14.95 Unspecified pre-eclampsia, complicating the puerperium M ♀

O15 Eclampsia

INCLUDES convulsions following conditions in O1Ø-O14 and O16

DEF: Tetany and toxemia producing seizure activity or coma in a pregnant patient who most often has presented with prior preeclampsia (i.e., hypertension, albuminuria, and edema).

O15.Ø Eclampsia complicating pregnancy

O15.ØØ Eclampsia complicating pregnancy, unspecified trimester M ♀

O15.Ø2 Eclampsia complicating pregnancy, second trimester MCC M ♀

O15.Ø3 Eclampsia complicating pregnancy, third trimester MCC M ♀

O15.1 Eclampsia complicating labor MCC M ♀

O15.2 Eclampsia complicating the puerperium MCC M ♀

O15.9 Eclampsia, unspecified as to time period M ♀

Eclampsia NOS

O16 Unspecified maternal hypertension

O16.1 Unspecified maternal hypertension, first trimester CC M ♀

O16.2 Unspecified maternal hypertension, second trimester CC M ♀

O16.3 Unspecified maternal hypertension, third trimester CC M ♀

O16.4 Unspecified maternal hypertension, complicating childbirth M ♀

O16.5 Unspecified maternal hypertension, complicating the puerperium M ♀

O16.9 Unspecified maternal hypertension, unspecified trimester M ♀

Other maternal disorders predominantly related to pregnancy (O2Ø-O29)

EXCLUDES 2 *maternal care related to the fetus and amniotic cavity and possible delivery problems (O3Ø-O48)*
maternal diseases classifiable elsewhere but complicating pregnancy, labor and delivery, and the puerperium (O98-O99)

O2Ø Hemorrhage in early pregnancy

INCLUDES hemorrhage before completion of 2Ø weeks gestation

EXCLUDES 1 *pregnancy with abortive outcome (OØØ-OØ8)*

O2Ø.Ø Threatened abortion CC M ♀

Hemorrhage specified as due to threatened abortion

DEF: Bloody discharge during pregnancy. The cervix may be dilated and pregnancy threatened, but the pregnancy is not terminated.

O2Ø.8 Other hemorrhage in early pregnancy M ♀

O2Ø.9 Hemorrhage in early pregnancy, unspecified CC M ♀

O21 Excessive vomiting in pregnancy

O21.Ø Mild hyperemesis gravidarum M ♀

Hyperemesis gravidarum, mild or unspecified, starting before the end of the 2Øth week of gestation

O21.1 Hyperemesis gravidarum with metabolic disturbance M ♀

Hyperemesis gravidarum, starting before the end of the 2Øth week of gestation, with metabolic disturbance such as carbohydrate depletion

Hyperemesis gravidarum, starting before the end of the 2Øth week of gestation, with metabolic disturbance such as dehydration

Hyperemesis gravidarum, starting before the end of the 2Øth week of gestation, with metabolic disturbance such as electrolyte imbalance

O21.2 Late vomiting of pregnancy M ♀

Excessive vomiting starting after 2Ø completed weeks of gestation

O21.8 Other vomiting complicating pregnancy M ♀

Vomiting due to diseases classified elsewhere, complicating pregnancy

Use additional code, to identify cause

O21.9 Vomiting of pregnancy, unspecified M ♀

O22 Venous complications and hemorrhoids in pregnancy

EXCLUDES 1 *venous complications of:*
abortion NOS (OØ3.9)
ectopic or molar pregnancy (OØ8.7)
failed attempted abortion (OØ7.35)
induced abortion (OØ4.85)
spontaneous abortion (OØ3.89)

EXCLUDES 2 *obstetric pulmonary embolism (O88.-)*
venous complications and hemorrhoids of childbirth and the puerperium (O87.-)

O22.Ø Varicose veins of lower extremity in pregnancy

Varicose veins NOS in pregnancy

DEF: Distended, tortuous veins of the lower extremities associated with pregnancy.

O22.ØØ Varicose veins of lower extremity in pregnancy, unspecified trimester M ♀

O22.Ø1 Varicose veins of lower extremity in pregnancy, first trimester M ♀

O22.Ø2 Varicose veins of lower extremity in pregnancy, second trimester M ♀

O22.Ø3 Varicose veins of lower extremity in pregnancy, third trimester M ♀

O22.1 Genital varices in pregnancy

Perineal varices in pregnancy
Vaginal varices in pregnancy
Vulval varices in pregnancy

O22.1Ø Genital varices in pregnancy, unspecified trimester M ♀

O22.11 Genital varices in pregnancy, first trimester M ♀

O22.12 Genital varices in pregnancy, second trimester M ♀

O22.13 **Genital varices in pregnancy, third trimester** M♀

✓5th **O22.2 Superficial thrombophlebitis in pregnancy**
Phlebitis in pregnancy NOS
Thrombophlebitis of legs in pregnancy
Thrombosis in pregnancy NOS
Use additional code to identify the superficial thrombophlebitis (I80.0-)

O22.20 **Superficial thrombophlebitis in pregnancy, unspecified trimester** CC M♀
O22.21 **Superficial thrombophlebitis in pregnancy, first trimester** CC M♀
O22.22 **Superficial thrombophlebitis in pregnancy, second trimester** CC M♀
O22.23 **Superficial thrombophlebitis in pregnancy, third trimester** CC M♀

✓5th **O22.3 Deep phlebothrombosis in pregnancy**
Deep vein thrombosis, antepartum
Use additional code to identify the deep vein thrombosis (I82.4-, I82.5-, I82.62-. I82.72-)
Use additional code, if applicable, for associated long-term (current) use of anticoagulants (Z79.01)

O22.30 **Deep phlebothrombosis in pregnancy, unspecified trimester** CC M♀
O22.31 **Deep phlebothrombosis in pregnancy, first trimester** MCC M♀
O22.32 **Deep phlebothrombosis in pregnancy, second trimester** MCC M♀
O22.33 **Deep phlebothrombosis in pregnancy, third trimester** MCC M♀

✓5th **O22.4 Hemorrhoids in pregnancy**
O22.40 **Hemorrhoids in pregnancy, unspecified trimester** CC M♀
O22.41 **Hemorrhoids in pregnancy, first trimester** CC M♀
O22.42 **Hemorrhoids in pregnancy, second trimester** CC M♀
O22.43 **Hemorrhoids in pregnancy, third trimester** CC M♀

✓5th **O22.5 Cerebral venous thrombosis in pregnancy**
Cerebrovenous sinus thrombosis in pregnancy

O22.50 **Cerebral venous thrombosis in pregnancy, unspecified trimester** CC M♀
O22.51 **Cerebral venous thrombosis in pregnancy, first trimester** CC M♀
O22.52 **Cerebral venous thrombosis in pregnancy, second trimester** CC M♀
O22.53 **Cerebral venous thrombosis in pregnancy, third trimester** CC M♀

✓5th **O22.8 Other venous complications in pregnancy**
✓6th **O22.8X Other venous complications in pregnancy**
O22.8X1 **Other venous complications in pregnancy, first trimester** CC M♀
O22.8X2 **Other venous complications in pregnancy, second trimester** CC M♀
O22.8X3 **Other venous complications in pregnancy, third trimester** CC M♀
O22.8X9 **Other venous complications in pregnancy, unspecified trimester** CC M♀

✓5th **O22.9 Venous complication in pregnancy, unspecified**
Gestational phlebitis NOS
Gestational phlebopathy NOS
Gestational thrombosis NOS

O22.90 **Venous complication in pregnancy, unspecified, unspecified trimester** CC M♀
O22.91 **Venous complication in pregnancy, unspecified, first trimester** M♀
O22.92 **Venous complication in pregnancy, unspecified, second trimester** M♀
O22.93 **Venous complication in pregnancy, unspecified, third trimester** M♀

✓4th **O23 Infections of genitourinary tract in pregnancy**
Use additional code to identify organism (B95.-, B96.-)
EXCLUDES 2 *gonococcal infections complicating pregnancy, childbirth and the puerperium (O98.2)*
infections with a predominantly sexual mode of transmission NOS complicating pregnancy, childbirth and the puerperium (O98.3)
syphilis complicating pregnancy, childbirth and the puerperium (O98.1)
tuberculosis of genitourinary system complicating pregnancy, childbirth and the puerperium (O98.0)
venereal disease NOS complicating pregnancy, childbirth and the puerperium (O98.3)

AHA: 2018,2Q,20

✓5th **O23.0 Infections of kidney in pregnancy**
Pyelonephritis in pregnancy

O23.00 **Infections of kidney in pregnancy, unspecified trimester** M♀
O23.01 **Infections of kidney in pregnancy, first trimester** CC M♀
O23.02 **Infections of kidney in pregnancy, second trimester** CC M♀
O23.03 **Infections of kidney in pregnancy, third trimester** CC M♀

✓5th **O23.1 Infections of bladder in pregnancy**
O23.10 **Infections of bladder in pregnancy, unspecified trimester** M♀
O23.11 **Infections of bladder in pregnancy, first trimester** CC M♀
O23.12 **Infections of bladder in pregnancy, second trimester** CC M♀
O23.13 **Infections of bladder in pregnancy, third trimester** CC M♀

✓5th **O23.2 Infections of urethra in pregnancy**
O23.20 **Infections of urethra in pregnancy, unspecified trimester** M♀
O23.21 **Infections of urethra in pregnancy, first trimester** CC M♀
O23.22 **Infections of urethra in pregnancy, second trimester** CC M♀
O23.23 **Infections of urethra in pregnancy, third trimester** CC M♀

✓5th **O23.3 Infections of other parts of urinary tract in pregnancy**
O23.30 **Infections of other parts of urinary tract in pregnancy, unspecified trimester** M♀
O23.31 **Infections of other parts of urinary tract in pregnancy, first trimester** CC M♀
O23.32 **Infections of other parts of urinary tract in pregnancy, second trimester** CC M♀
O23.33 **Infections of other parts of urinary tract in pregnancy, third trimester** CC M♀

✓5th **O23.4 Unspecified infection of urinary tract in pregnancy**
O23.40 **Unspecified infection of urinary tract in pregnancy, unspecified trimester** M♀
O23.41 **Unspecified infection of urinary tract in pregnancy, first trimester** CC M♀
O23.42 **Unspecified infection of urinary tract in pregnancy, second trimester** CC M♀
O23.43 **Unspecified infection of urinary tract in pregnancy, third trimester** CC M♀

✓5th **O23.5 Infections of the genital tract in pregnancy**
✓6th **O23.51 Infection of cervix in pregnancy**
O23.511 **Infections of cervix in pregnancy, first trimester** CC M♀
O23.512 **Infections of cervix in pregnancy, second trimester** CC M♀
O23.513 **Infections of cervix in pregnancy, third trimester** CC M♀
O23.519 **Infections of cervix in pregnancy, unspecified trimester** M♀

✓6th **O23.52 Salpingo-oophoritis in pregnancy**
Oophoritis in pregnancy
Salpingitis in pregnancy

O23.521 **Salpingo-oophoritis in pregnancy, first trimester** CC M♀
O23.522 **Salpingo-oophoritis in pregnancy, second trimester** CC M♀

O23.523 **Salpingo-oophoritis in pregnancy, third trimester** CC M ♀

O23.529 **Salpingo-oophoritis in pregnancy, unspecified trimester** M ♀

√6th O23.59 **Infection of other part of genital tract in pregnancy**

O23.591 **Infection of other part of genital tract in pregnancy, first trimester** CC M ♀

O23.592 **Infection of other part of genital tract in pregnancy, second trimester** CC M ♀

O23.593 **Infection of other part of genital tract in pregnancy, third trimester** CC M ♀

O23.599 **Infection of other part of genital tract in pregnancy, unspecified trimester** M ♀

√5th O23.9 **Unspecified genitourinary tract infection in pregnancy**

Genitourinary tract infection in pregnancy NOS

O23.90 **Unspecified genitourinary tract infection in pregnancy, unspecified trimester** M ♀

O23.91 **Unspecified genitourinary tract infection in pregnancy, first trimester** CC M ♀

O23.92 **Unspecified genitourinary tract infection in pregnancy, second trimester** CC M ♀

O23.93 **Unspecified genitourinary tract infection in pregnancy, third trimester** CC M ♀

√4th **O24 Diabetes mellitus in pregnancy, childbirth and the puerperium**

√5th O24.0 **Pre-existing type 1 diabetes mellitus, in pregnancy, childbirth and the puerperium**

Juvenile onset diabetes mellitus, in pregnancy, childbirth and the puerperium

Ketosis-prone diabetes mellitus in pregnancy, childbirth and the puerperium

Use additional code from category E10 to further identify any manifestations

√6th O24.01 **Pre-existing type 1 diabetes mellitus, in pregnancy**

O24.011 **Pre-existing type 1 diabetes mellitus, in pregnancy, first trimester** CC M ♀

O24.012 **Pre-existing type 1 diabetes mellitus, in pregnancy, second trimester** CC M ♀

O24.013 **Pre-existing type 1 diabetes mellitus, in pregnancy, third trimester** CC M ♀

O24.019 **Pre-existing type 1 diabetes mellitus, in pregnancy, unspecified trimester** CC M ♀

O24.02 **Pre-existing type 1 diabetes mellitus, in childbirth** MCC M ♀

O24.03 **Pre-existing type 1 diabetes mellitus, in the puerperium** CC M ♀

√5th O24.1 **Pre-existing type 2 diabetes mellitus, in pregnancy, childbirth and the puerperium**

Insulin-resistant diabetes mellitus in pregnancy, childbirth and the puerperium

Use additional code (for):

from category E11 to further identify any manifestations

long-term (current) use of insulin (Z79.4)

√6th O24.11 **Pre-existing type 2 diabetes mellitus, in pregnancy**

O24.111 **Pre-existing type 2 diabetes mellitus, in pregnancy, first trimester** CC M ♀

O24.112 **Pre-existing type 2 diabetes mellitus, in pregnancy, second trimester** CC M ♀

O24.113 **Pre-existing type 2 diabetes mellitus, in pregnancy, third trimester** CC M ♀

O24.119 **Pre-existing type 2 diabetes mellitus, in pregnancy, unspecified trimester** CC M ♀

O24.12 **Pre-existing type 2 diabetes mellitus, in childbirth** MCC M ♀

O24.13 **Pre-existing type 2 diabetes mellitus, in the puerperium** CC M ♀

√5th O24.3 **Unspecified pre-existing diabetes mellitus in pregnancy, childbirth and the puerperium**

Use additional code (for):

from category E11 to further identify any manifestation

long-term (current) use of insulin (Z79.4)

√6th O24.31 **Unspecified pre-existing diabetes mellitus in pregnancy**

O24.311 **Unspecified pre-existing diabetes mellitus in pregnancy, first trimester** CC M ♀

O24.312 **Unspecified pre-existing diabetes mellitus in pregnancy, second trimester** CC M ♀

O24.313 **Unspecified pre-existing diabetes mellitus in pregnancy, third trimester** CC M ♀

O24.319 **Unspecified pre-existing diabetes mellitus in pregnancy, unspecified trimester** CC M ♀

O24.32 **Unspecified pre-existing diabetes mellitus in childbirth** MCC M ♀

O24.33 **Unspecified pre-existing diabetes mellitus in the puerperium** CC M ♀

√5th O24.4 **Gestational diabetes mellitus**

Diabetes mellitus arising in pregnancy

Gestational diabetes mellitus NOS

AHA: 2016,4Q,50; 2015,4Q,34

√6th O24.41 **Gestational diabetes mellitus in pregnancy**

O24.410 **Gestational diabetes mellitus in pregnancy, diet controlled** M ♀

O24.414 **Gestational diabetes mellitus in pregnancy, insulin controlled** M ♀

O24.415 **Gestational diabetes mellitus in pregnancy, controlled by oral hypoglycemic drugs** M ♀

Gestational diabetes mellitus in pregnancy, controlled by oral antidiabetic drugs

O24.419 **Gestational diabetes mellitus in pregnancy, unspecified control** M ♀

√6th O24.42 **Gestational diabetes mellitus in childbirth**

AHA: 2016,1Q,5

O24.420 **Gestational diabetes mellitus in childbirth, diet controlled** M ♀

O24.424 **Gestational diabetes mellitus in childbirth, insulin controlled** M ♀

O24.425 **Gestational diabetes mellitus in childbirth, controlled by oral hypoglycemic drugs** M ♀

Gestational diabetes mellitus in childbirth, controlled by oral antidiabetic drugs

O24.429 **Gestational diabetes mellitus in childbirth, unspecified control** M ♀

√6th O24.43 **Gestational diabetes mellitus in the puerperium**

O24.430 **Gestational diabetes mellitus in the puerperium, diet controlled** M ♀

O24.434 **Gestational diabetes mellitus in the puerperium, insulin controlled** M ♀

O24.435 **Gestational diabetes mellitus in puerperium, controlled by oral hypoglycemic drugs** M ♀

Gestational diabetes mellitus in puerperium, controlled by oral antidiabetic drugs

O24.439 **Gestational diabetes mellitus in the puerperium, unspecified control** M ♀

√5th O24.8 **Other pre-existing diabetes mellitus in pregnancy, childbirth, and the puerperium**

Use additional code (for):

from categories E08, E09 and E13 to further identify any manifestation

long-term (current) use of insulin (Z79.4)

√6th O24.81 **Other pre-existing diabetes mellitus in pregnancy**

O24.811 **Other pre-existing diabetes mellitus in pregnancy, first trimester** CC M ♀

O24.812 **Other pre-existing diabetes mellitus in pregnancy, second trimester** CC M ♀

O24.813 **Other pre-existing diabetes mellitus in pregnancy, third trimester** CC M ♀

O24.819 **Other pre-existing diabetes mellitus in pregnancy, unspecified trimester** CC M ♀

O24.82 **Other pre-existing diabetes mellitus in childbirth** MCC M ♀

O24.83 **Other pre-existing diabetes mellitus in the puerperium** CC M ♀

✓5th **O24.9 Unspecified diabetes mellitus in pregnancy, childbirth and the puerperium**
Use additional code for long-term (current) use of insulin (Z79.4)

✓6th **O24.91 Unspecified diabetes mellitus in pregnancy**
- **O24.911 Unspecified diabetes mellitus in pregnancy, first trimester** CC M ♀
- **O24.912 Unspecified diabetes mellitus in pregnancy, second trimester** CC M ♀
- **O24.913 Unspecified diabetes mellitus in pregnancy, third trimester** CC M ♀
- **O24.919 Unspecified diabetes mellitus in pregnancy, unspecified trimester** CC M ♀

O24.92 Unspecified diabetes mellitus in childbirth M ♀
O24.93 Unspecified diabetes mellitus in the puerperium CC M ♀

✓4th **O25 Malnutrition in pregnancy, childbirth and the puerperium**

✓5th **O25.1 Malnutrition in pregnancy**
- **O25.10 Malnutrition in pregnancy, unspecified trimester** M ♀
- **O25.11 Malnutrition in pregnancy, first trimester** M ♀
- **O25.12 Malnutrition in pregnancy, second trimester** M ♀
- **O25.13 Malnutrition in pregnancy, third trimester** M ♀

O25.2 Malnutrition in childbirth M ♀
O25.3 Malnutrition in the puerperium M ♀

✓4th **O26 Maternal care for other conditions predominantly related to pregnancy**

✓5th **O26.0 Excessive weight gain in pregnancy**
EXCLUDES 2 *gestational edema (O12.0, O12.2)*
- **O26.00 Excessive weight gain in pregnancy, unspecified trimester** M ♀
- **O26.01 Excessive weight gain in pregnancy, first trimester** M ♀
- **O26.02 Excessive weight gain in pregnancy, second trimester** M ♀
- **O26.03 Excessive weight gain in pregnancy, third trimester** M ♀

✓5th **O26.1 Low weight gain in pregnancy**
- **O26.10 Low weight gain in pregnancy, unspecified trimester** M ♀
- **O26.11 Low weight gain in pregnancy, first trimester** M ♀
- **O26.12 Low weight gain in pregnancy, second trimester** M ♀
- **O26.13 Low weight gain in pregnancy, third trimester** M ♀

✓5th **O26.2 Pregnancy care for patient with recurrent pregnancy loss**
- **O26.20 Pregnancy care for patient with recurrent pregnancy loss, unspecified trimester** M ♀
- **O26.21 Pregnancy care for patient with recurrent pregnancy loss, first trimester** M ♀
- **O26.22 Pregnancy care for patient with recurrent pregnancy loss, second trimester** M ♀
- **O26.23 Pregnancy care for patient with recurrent pregnancy loss, third trimester** M ♀

✓5th **O26.3 Retained intrauterine contraceptive device in pregnancy**
- **O26.30 Retained intrauterine contraceptive device in pregnancy, unspecified trimester** M ♀
- **O26.31 Retained intrauterine contraceptive device in pregnancy, first trimester** M ♀
- **O26.32 Retained intrauterine contraceptive device in pregnancy, second trimester** M ♀
- **O26.33 Retained intrauterine contraceptive device in pregnancy, third trimester** M ♀

✓5th **O26.4 Herpes gestationis**
DEF: Rare skin disorder of unknown origin that appears on the abdomen in the second and third trimester as intensely itchy blisters that spread to other sites.
- **O26.40 Herpes gestationis, unspecified trimester** M ♀
- **O26.41 Herpes gestationis, first trimester** M ♀
- **O26.42 Herpes gestationis, second trimester** M ♀
- **O26.43 Herpes gestationis, third trimester** M ♀

✓5th **O26.5 Maternal hypotension syndrome**
Supine hypotensive syndrome
- **O26.50 Maternal hypotension syndrome, unspecified trimester** M ♀
- **O26.51 Maternal hypotension syndrome, first trimester** M ♀
- **O26.52 Maternal hypotension syndrome, second trimester** M ♀
- **O26.53 Maternal hypotension syndrome, third trimester** M ♀

✓5th **O26.6 Liver and biliary tract disorders in pregnancy, childbirth and the puerperium**
Use additional code to identify the specific disorder
EXCLUDES 2 *hepatorenal syndrome following labor and delivery (O90.4)*

✓6th **O26.61 Liver and biliary tract disorders in pregnancy**
- **O26.611 Liver and biliary tract disorders in pregnancy, first trimester** CC M ♀
- **O26.612 Liver and biliary tract disorders in pregnancy, second trimester** CC M ♀
- **O26.613 Liver and biliary tract disorders in pregnancy, third trimester** CC M ♀
- **O26.619 Liver and biliary tract disorders in pregnancy, unspecified trimester** M ♀

O26.62 Liver and biliary tract disorders in childbirth CC M ♀
O26.63 Liver and biliary tract disorders in the puerperium M ♀

✓5th **O26.7 Subluxation of symphysis (pubis) in pregnancy, childbirth and the puerperium**
EXCLUDES 1 *traumatic separation of symphysis (pubis) during childbirth (O71.6)*

✓6th **O26.71 Subluxation of symphysis (pubis) in pregnancy**
- **O26.711 Subluxation of symphysis (pubis) in pregnancy, first trimester** M ♀
- **O26.712 Subluxation of symphysis (pubis) in pregnancy, second trimester** M ♀
- **O26.713 Subluxation of symphysis (pubis) in pregnancy, third trimester** M ♀
- **O26.719 Subluxation of symphysis (pubis) in pregnancy, unspecified trimester** M ♀

O26.72 Subluxation of symphysis (pubis) in childbirth M ♀
O26.73 Subluxation of symphysis (pubis) in the puerperium M ♀

✓5th **O26.8 Other specified pregnancy related conditions**

✓6th **O26.81 Pregnancy related exhaustion and fatigue**
- **O26.811 Pregnancy related exhaustion and fatigue, first trimester** M ♀
- **O26.812 Pregnancy related exhaustion and fatigue, second trimester** M ♀
- **O26.813 Pregnancy related exhaustion and fatigue, third trimester** M ♀
- **O26.819 Pregnancy related exhaustion and fatigue, unspecified trimester** M ♀

✓6th **O26.82 Pregnancy related peripheral neuritis**
- **O26.821 Pregnancy related peripheral neuritis, first trimester** M ♀
- **O26.822 Pregnancy related peripheral neuritis, second trimester** M ♀
- **O26.823 Pregnancy related peripheral neuritis, third trimester** M ♀
- **O26.829 Pregnancy related peripheral neuritis, unspecified trimester** M ♀

✓6th **O26.83 Pregnancy related renal disease**
Use additional code to identify the specific disorder
- **O26.831 Pregnancy related renal disease, first trimester** CC M ♀
- **O26.832 Pregnancy related renal disease, second trimester** CC M ♀
- **O26.833 Pregnancy related renal disease, third trimester** CC M ♀
- **O26.839 Pregnancy related renal disease, unspecified trimester** M ♀

✓6th **O26.84 Uterine size-date discrepancy complicating pregnancy**
EXCLUDES 1 *encounter for suspected problem with fetal growth ruled out (Z03.74)*
- **O26.841 Uterine size-date discrepancy, first trimester** M ♀
- **O26.842 Uterine size-date discrepancy, second trimester** M ♀

O26.843 Uterine size-date discrepancy, third trimester M ♀

O26.849 Uterine size-date discrepancy, unspecified trimester M ♀

O26.85 Spotting complicating pregnancy

O26.851 Spotting complicating pregnancy, first trimester M ♀

O26.852 Spotting complicating pregnancy, second trimester M ♀

O26.853 Spotting complicating pregnancy, third trimester M ♀

O26.859 Spotting complicating pregnancy, unspecified trimester M ♀

O26.86 Pruritic urticarial papules and plaques of pregnancy (PUPPP) M ♀

Polymorphic eruption of pregnancy

O26.87 Cervical shortening

EXCLUDES 1 *encounter for suspected cervical shortening ruled out (Z03.75)*

DEF: Cervix that has shortened to less than 25 mm before the 24th week of pregnancy. A shortened cervix is a warning sign for impending premature delivery and is treated by cervical cerclage placement or progesterone.

O26.872 Cervical shortening, second trimester CC M ♀

O26.873 Cervical shortening, third trimester CC M ♀

O26.879 Cervical shortening, unspecified trimester CC M ♀

O26.89 Other specified pregnancy related conditions

AHA: 2015,3Q,40

O26.891 Other specified pregnancy related conditions, first trimester M ♀

O26.892 Other specified pregnancy related conditions, second trimester M ♀

O26.893 Other specified pregnancy related conditions, third trimester M ♀

O26.899 Other specified pregnancy related conditions, unspecified trimester M ♀

O26.9 Pregnancy related conditions, unspecified

O26.90 Pregnancy related conditions, unspecified, unspecified trimester M ♀

O26.91 Pregnancy related conditions, unspecified, first trimester M ♀

O26.92 Pregnancy related conditions, unspecified, second trimester M ♀

O26.93 Pregnancy related conditions, unspecified, third trimester M ♀

O28 Abnormal findings on antenatal screening of mother

EXCLUDES 1 *diagnostic findings classified elsewhere — see Alphabetical Index*

O28.0 Abnormal hematological finding on antenatal screening of mother M ♀

O28.1 Abnormal biochemical finding on antenatal screening of mother M ♀

O28.2 Abnormal cytological finding on antenatal screening of mother M ♀

O28.3 Abnormal ultrasonic finding on antenatal screening of mother M ♀

O28.4 Abnormal radiological finding on antenatal screening of mother M ♀

O28.5 Abnormal chromosomal and genetic finding on antenatal screening of mother M ♀

O28.8 Other abnormal findings on antenatal screening of mother M ♀

O28.9 Unspecified abnormal findings on antenatal screening of mother M ♀

O29 Complications of anesthesia during pregnancy

INCLUDES maternal complications arising from the administration of a general, regional or local anesthetic, analgesic or other sedation during pregnancy

Use additional code, if necessary, to identify the complication

EXCLUDES 2 *complications of anesthesia during labor and delivery (O74.-)*
complications of anesthesia during the puerperium (O89.-)

O29.0 Pulmonary complications of anesthesia during pregnancy

O29.01 Aspiration pneumonitis due to anesthesia during pregnancy

Inhalation of stomach contents or secretions NOS due to anesthesia during pregnancy

Mendelson's syndrome due to anesthesia during pregnancy

O29.011 Aspiration pneumonitis due to anesthesia during pregnancy, first trimester M ♀

O29.012 Aspiration pneumonitis due to anesthesia during pregnancy, second trimester M ♀

O29.013 Aspiration pneumonitis due to anesthesia during pregnancy, third trimester M ♀

O29.019 Aspiration pneumonitis due to anesthesia during pregnancy, unspecified trimester M ♀

O29.02 Pressure collapse of lung due to anesthesia during pregnancy

O29.021 Pressure collapse of lung due to anesthesia during pregnancy, first trimester M ♀

O29.022 Pressure collapse of lung due to anesthesia during pregnancy, second trimester M ♀

O29.023 Pressure collapse of lung due to anesthesia during pregnancy, third trimester M ♀

O29.029 Pressure collapse of lung due to anesthesia during pregnancy, unspecified trimester M ♀

O29.09 Other pulmonary complications of anesthesia during pregnancy

O29.091 Other pulmonary complications of anesthesia during pregnancy, first trimester M ♀

O29.092 Other pulmonary complications of anesthesia during pregnancy, second trimester M ♀

O29.093 Other pulmonary complications of anesthesia during pregnancy, third trimester M ♀

O29.099 Other pulmonary complications of anesthesia during pregnancy, unspecified trimester M ♀

O29.1 Cardiac complications of anesthesia during pregnancy

O29.11 Cardiac arrest due to anesthesia during pregnancy

O29.111 Cardiac arrest due to anesthesia during pregnancy, first trimester M ♀

O29.112 Cardiac arrest due to anesthesia during pregnancy, second trimester M ♀

O29.113 Cardiac arrest due to anesthesia during pregnancy, third trimester M ♀

O29.119 Cardiac arrest due to anesthesia during pregnancy, unspecified trimester M ♀

O29.12 Cardiac failure due to anesthesia during pregnancy

O29.121 Cardiac failure due to anesthesia during pregnancy, first trimester M ♀

O29.122 Cardiac failure due to anesthesia during pregnancy, second trimester M ♀

O29.123 Cardiac failure due to anesthesia during pregnancy, third trimester M ♀

O29.129 Cardiac failure due to anesthesia during pregnancy, unspecified trimester M ♀

O29.19 Other cardiac complications of anesthesia during pregnancy

O29.191 Other cardiac complications of anesthesia during pregnancy, first trimester M ♀

O29.192 Other cardiac complications of anesthesia during pregnancy, second trimester M ♀

O29.193 Other cardiac complications of anesthesia during pregnancy, third trimester M ♀

O29.199 Other cardiac complications of anesthesia during pregnancy, unspecified trimester M ♀

✓5th O29.2 Central nervous system complications of anesthesia during pregnancy

✓6th O29.21 Cerebral anoxia due to anesthesia during pregnancy

O29.211 Cerebral anoxia due to anesthesia during pregnancy, first trimester M ♀

O29.212 Cerebral anoxia due to anesthesia during pregnancy, second trimester M ♀

O29.213 Cerebral anoxia due to anesthesia during pregnancy, third trimester M ♀

O29.219 Cerebral anoxia due to anesthesia during pregnancy, unspecified trimester M ♀

✓6th O29.29 Other central nervous system complications of anesthesia during pregnancy

O29.291 Other central nervous system complications of anesthesia during pregnancy, first trimester M ♀

O29.292 Other central nervous system complications of anesthesia during pregnancy, second trimester M ♀

O29.293 Other central nervous system complications of anesthesia during pregnancy, third trimester M ♀

O29.299 Other central nervous system complications of anesthesia during pregnancy, unspecified trimester M ♀

✓5th O29.3 Toxic reaction to local anesthesia during pregnancy

✓6th O29.3X Toxic reaction to local anesthesia during pregnancy

O29.3X1 Toxic reaction to local anesthesia during pregnancy, first trimester M ♀

O29.3X2 Toxic reaction to local anesthesia during pregnancy, second trimester M ♀

O29.3X3 Toxic reaction to local anesthesia during pregnancy, third trimester M ♀

O29.3X9 Toxic reaction to local anesthesia during pregnancy, unspecified trimester M ♀

✓5th O29.4 Spinal and epidural anesthesia induced headache during pregnancy

O29.40 Spinal and epidural anesthesia induced headache during pregnancy, unspecified trimester M ♀

O29.41 Spinal and epidural anesthesia induced headache during pregnancy, first trimester M ♀

O29.42 Spinal and epidural anesthesia induced headache during pregnancy, second trimester M ♀

O29.43 Spinal and epidural anesthesia induced headache during pregnancy, third trimester M ♀

✓5th O29.5 Other complications of spinal and epidural anesthesia during pregnancy

✓6th O29.5X Other complications of spinal and epidural anesthesia during pregnancy

O29.5X1 Other complications of spinal and epidural anesthesia during pregnancy, first trimester M ♀

O29.5X2 Other complications of spinal and epidural anesthesia during pregnancy, second trimester M ♀

O29.5X3 Other complications of spinal and epidural anesthesia during pregnancy, third trimester M ♀

O29.5X9 Other complications of spinal and epidural anesthesia during pregnancy, unspecified trimester M ♀

✓5th O29.6 Failed or difficult intubation for anesthesia during pregnancy

O29.60 Failed or difficult intubation for anesthesia during pregnancy, unspecified trimester M ♀

O29.61 Failed or difficult intubation for anesthesia during pregnancy, first trimester M ♀

O29.62 Failed or difficult intubation for anesthesia during pregnancy, second trimester M ♀

O29.63 Failed or difficult intubation for anesthesia during pregnancy, third trimester M ♀

✓5th O29.8 Other complications of anesthesia during pregnancy

✓6th O29.8X Other complications of anesthesia during pregnancy

O29.8X1 Other complications of anesthesia during pregnancy, first trimester M ♀

O29.8X2 Other complications of anesthesia during pregnancy, second trimester M ♀

O29.8X3 Other complications of anesthesia during pregnancy, third trimester M ♀

O29.8X9 Other complications of anesthesia during pregnancy, unspecified trimester M ♀

✓5th O29.9 Unspecified complication of anesthesia during pregnancy

O29.90 Unspecified complication of anesthesia during pregnancy, unspecified trimester M ♀

O29.91 Unspecified complication of anesthesia during pregnancy, first trimester M ♀

O29.92 Unspecified complication of anesthesia during pregnancy, second trimester M ♀

O29.93 Unspecified complication of anesthesia during pregnancy, third trimester M ♀

Maternal care related to the fetus and amniotic cavity and possible delivery problems (O30-O48)

✓4th **O30 Multiple gestation**

Code also any complications specific to multiple gestation

AHA: 2016,4Q,51

✓5th O30.0 Twin pregnancy

✓6th O30.00 Twin pregnancy, unspecified number of placenta and unspecified number of amniotic sacs

O30.001 Twin pregnancy, unspecified number of placenta and unspecified number of amniotic sacs, first trimester M ♀

O30.002 Twin pregnancy, unspecified number of placenta and unspecified number of amniotic sacs, second trimester M ♀

O30.003 Twin pregnancy, unspecified number of placenta and unspecified number of amniotic sacs, third trimester M ♀

O30.009 Twin pregnancy, unspecified number of placenta and unspecified number of amniotic sacs, unspecified trimester M ♀

✓6th O30.01 Twin pregnancy, monochorionic/monoamniotic

Twin pregnancy, one placenta, one amniotic sac

EXCLUDES 1 *conjoined twins (O30.02-)*

Twin Gestation – Monochorionic/Monoamniotic

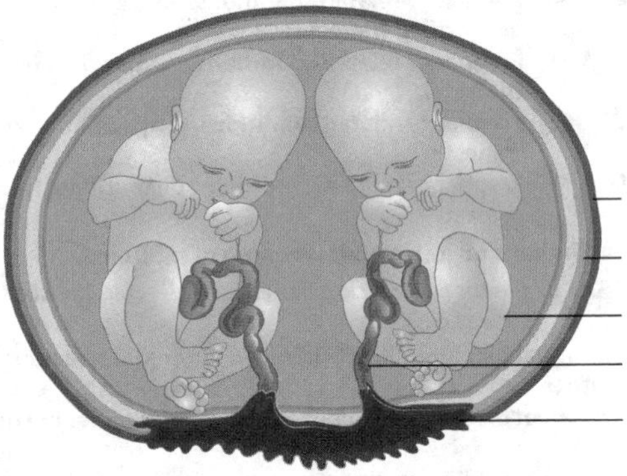

O30.011 Twin pregnancy, monochorionic/monoamniotic, first trimester M ♀

O30.012 Twin pregnancy, monochorionic/monoamniotic, second trimester M ♀

O30.013 Twin pregnancy, monochorionic/monoamniotic, third trimester M ♀

O30.019 Twin pregnancy, monochorionic/monoamniotic, unspecified trimester M ♀

✓6th O30.02 Conjoined twin pregnancy

O30.021 Conjoined twin pregnancy, first trimester M ♀

O30.022 Conjoined twin pregnancy, second trimester M ♀

O30.023 Conjoined twin pregnancy, third trimester M ♀

O30.029 Conjoined twin pregnancy, unspecified trimester M ♀

✓6th **O30.03 Twin pregnancy, monochorionic/diamniotic**
Twin pregnancy, one placenta, two amniotic sacs

Twin Gestation – Monochorionic/Diamniotic

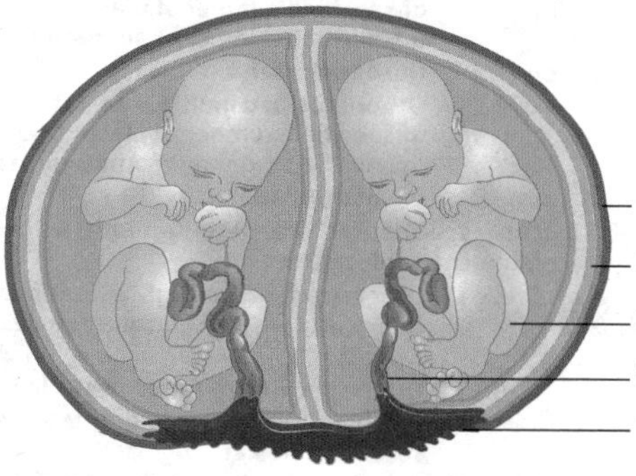

O30.031 Twin pregnancy, monochorionic/diamniotic, first trimester M ♀
O30.032 Twin pregnancy, monochorionic/diamniotic, second trimester M ♀
O30.033 Twin pregnancy, monochorionic/diamniotic, third trimester M ♀
O30.039 Twin pregnancy, monochorionic/diamniotic, unspecified trimester M ♀

✓6th **O30.04 Twin pregnancy, dichorionic/diamniotic**
Twin pregnancy, two placentae, two amniotic sacs

Twin Gestation – Dichorionic/Diamniotic

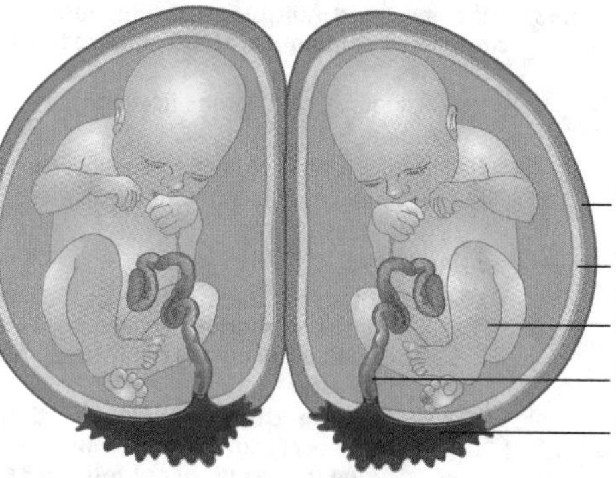

O30.041 Twin pregnancy, dichorionic/diamniotic, first trimester M ♀
O30.042 Twin pregnancy, dichorionic/diamniotic, second trimester M ♀
O30.043 Twin pregnancy, dichorionic/diamniotic, third trimester M ♀
O30.049 Twin pregnancy, dichorionic/diamniotic, unspecified trimester M ♀

✓6th **O30.09 Twin pregnancy, unable to determine number of placenta and number of amniotic sacs**
O30.091 Twin pregnancy, unable to determine number of placenta and number of amniotic sacs, first trimester M ♀
O30.092 Twin pregnancy, unable to determine number of placenta and number of amniotic sacs, second trimester M ♀
O30.093 Twin pregnancy, unable to determine number of placenta and number of amniotic sacs, third trimester M ♀
O30.099 Twin pregnancy, unable to determine number of placenta and number of amniotic sacs, unspecified trimester M ♀

✓5th **O30.1 Triplet pregnancy**
✓6th **O30.10 Triplet pregnancy, unspecified number of placenta and unspecified number of amniotic sacs**
AHA: 2016,2Q,8
O30.101 Triplet pregnancy, unspecified number of placenta and unspecified number of amniotic sacs, first trimester CC M ♀
O30.102 Triplet pregnancy, unspecified number of placenta and unspecified number of amniotic sacs, second trimester CC M ♀
O30.103 Triplet pregnancy, unspecified number of placenta and unspecified number of amniotic sacs, third trimester CC M ♀
O30.109 Triplet pregnancy, unspecified number of placenta and unspecified number of amniotic sacs, unspecified trimester M ♀

✓6th **O30.11 Triplet pregnancy with two or more monochorionic fetuses**
O30.111 Triplet pregnancy with two or more monochorionic fetuses, first trimester CC M ♀
O30.112 Triplet pregnancy with two or more monochorionic fetuses, second trimester CC M ♀
O30.113 Triplet pregnancy with two or more monochorionic fetuses, third trimester CC M ♀
O30.119 Triplet pregnancy with two or more monochorionic fetuses, unspecified trimester M ♀

✓6th **O30.12 Triplet pregnancy with two or more monoamniotic fetuses**
O30.121 Triplet pregnancy with two or more monoamniotic fetuses, first trimester CC M ♀
O30.122 Triplet pregnancy with two or more monoamniotic fetuses, second trimester CC M ♀
O30.123 Triplet pregnancy with two or more monoamniotic fetuses, third trimester CC M ♀
O30.129 Triplet pregnancy with two or more monoamniotic fetuses, unspecified trimester M ♀

✓6th **O30.13 Triplet pregnancy, trichorionic/triamniotic**
AHA: 2018,4Q,22
O30.131 Triplet pregnancy, trichorionic/triamniotic, first trimester CC M ♀
O30.132 Triplet pregnancy, trichorionic/triamniotic, second trimester CC M ♀
O30.133 Triplet pregnancy, trichorionic/triamniotic, third trimester CC M ♀
O30.139 Triplet pregnancy, trichorionic/triamniotic, unspecified trimester M ♀

✓6th **O30.19 Triplet pregnancy, unable to determine number of placenta and number of amniotic sacs**
O30.191 Triplet pregnancy, unable to determine number of placenta and number of amniotic sacs, first trimester CC M ♀
O30.192 Triplet pregnancy, unable to determine number of placenta and number of amniotic sacs, second trimester CC M ♀
O30.193 Triplet pregnancy, unable to determine number of placenta and number of amniotic sacs, third trimester CC M ♀
O30.199 Triplet pregnancy, unable to determine number of placenta and number of amniotic sacs, unspecified trimester M ♀

✓5th **O30.2 Quadruplet pregnancy**
✓6th **O30.20 Quadruplet pregnancy, unspecified number of placenta and unspecified number of amniotic sacs**
O30.201 Quadruplet pregnancy, unspecified number of placenta and unspecified number of amniotic sacs, first trimester CC M ♀

O30.202 Quadruplet pregnancy, unspecified number of placenta and unspecified number of amniotic sacs, second trimester CC M ♀

O30.203 Quadruplet pregnancy, unspecified number of placenta and unspecified number of amniotic sacs, third trimester CC M ♀

O30.209 Quadruplet pregnancy, unspecified number of placenta and unspecified number of amniotic sacs, unspecified trimester M ♀

✓6th **O30.21 Quadruplet pregnancy with two or more monochorionic fetuses**

O30.211 Quadruplet pregnancy with two or more monochorionic fetuses, first trimester CC M ♀

O30.212 Quadruplet pregnancy with two or more monochorionic fetuses, second trimester CC M ♀

O30.213 Quadruplet pregnancy with two or more monochorionic fetuses, third trimester CC M ♀

O30.219 Quadruplet pregnancy with two or more monochorionic fetuses, unspecified trimester M ♀

✓6th **O30.22 Quadruplet pregnancy with two or more monoamniotic fetuses**

O30.221 Quadruplet pregnancy with two or more monoamniotic fetuses, first trimester CC M ♀

O30.222 Quadruplet pregnancy with two or more monoamniotic fetuses, second trimester CC M ♀

O30.223 Quadruplet pregnancy with two or more monoamniotic fetuses, third trimester CC M ♀

O30.229 Quadruplet pregnancy with two or more monoamniotic fetuses, unspecified trimester M ♀

✓6th **O30.23 Quadruplet pregnancy, quadrachorionic/quadra-amniotic**

AHA: 2018,4Q,22

O30.231 Quadruplet pregnancy, quadrachorionic/quadra-amniotic, first trimester CC M ♀

O30.232 Quadruplet pregnancy, quadrachorionic/quadra-amniotic, second trimester CC M ♀

O30.233 Quadruplet pregnancy, quadrachorionic/quadra-amniotic, third trimester CC M ♀

O30.239 Quadruplet pregnancy, quadrachorionic/quadra-amniotic, unspecified trimester M ♀

✓6th **O30.29 Quadruplet pregnancy, unable to determine number of placenta and number of amniotic sacs**

O30.291 Quadruplet pregnancy, unable to determine number of placenta and number of amniotic sacs, first trimester CC M ♀

O30.292 Quadruplet pregnancy, unable to determine number of placenta and number of amniotic sacs, second trimester CC M ♀

O30.293 Quadruplet pregnancy, unable to determine number of placenta and number of amniotic sacs, third trimester CC M ♀

O30.299 Quadruplet pregnancy, unable to determine number of placenta and number of amniotic sacs, unspecified trimester M ♀

✓5th **O30.8 Other specified multiple gestation**

Multiple gestation pregnancy greater then quadruplets

✓6th **O30.80 Other specified multiple gestation, unspecified number of placenta and unspecified number of amniotic sacs**

O30.801 Other specified multiple gestation, unspecified number of placenta and unspecified number of amniotic sacs, first trimester CC M ♀

O30.802 Other specified multiple gestation, unspecified number of placenta and unspecified number of amniotic sacs, second trimester CC M ♀

O30.803 Other specified multiple gestation, unspecified number of placenta and unspecified number of amniotic sacs, third trimester CC M ♀

O30.809 Other specified multiple gestation, unspecified number of placenta and unspecified number of amniotic sacs, unspecified trimester M ♀

✓6th **O30.81 Other specified multiple gestation with two or more monochorionic fetuses**

O30.811 Other specified multiple gestation with two or more monochorionic fetuses, first trimester CC M ♀

O30.812 Other specified multiple gestation with two or more monochorionic fetuses, second trimester CC M ♀

O30.813 Other specified multiple gestation with two or more monochorionic fetuses, third trimester CC M ♀

O30.819 Other specified multiple gestation with two or more monochorionic fetuses, unspecified trimester M ♀

✓6th **O30.82 Other specified multiple gestation with two or more monoamniotic fetuses**

O30.821 Other specified multiple gestation with two or more monoamniotic fetuses, first trimester CC M ♀

O30.822 Other specified multiple gestation with two or more monoamniotic fetuses, second trimester CC M ♀

O30.823 Other specified multiple gestation with two or more monoamniotic fetuses, third trimester CC M ♀

O30.829 Other specified multiple gestation with two or more monoamniotic fetuses, unspecified trimester M ♀

✓6th **O30.83 Other specified multiple gestation, number of chorions and amnions are both equal to the number of fetuses**

Pentachorionic, penta-amniotic pregnancy (quintuplets)

Hexachorionic, hexa-amniotic pregnancy (sextuplets)

Heptachorionic, hepta-amniotic pregnancy (septuplets)

AHA: 2018,4Q,22

O30.831 Other specified multiple gestation, number of chorions and amnions are both equal to the number of fetuses, first trimester CC M ♀

O30.832 Other specified multiple gestation, number of chorions and amnions are both equal to the number of fetuses, second trimester CC M ♀

O30.833 Other specified multiple gestation, number of chorions and amnions are both equal to the number of fetuses, third trimester CC M ♀

O30.839 Other specified multiple gestation, number of chorions and amnions are both equal to the number of fetuses, unspecified trimester M ♀

✓6th **O30.89 Other specified multiple gestation, unable to determine number of placenta and number of amniotic sacs**

O30.891 Other specified multiple gestation, unable to determine number of placenta and number of amniotic sacs, first trimester CC M ♀

O30.892 Other specified multiple gestation, unable to determine number of placenta and number of amniotic sacs, second trimester CC M ♀

O30.893 Other specified multiple gestation, unable to determine number of placenta and number of amniotic sacs, third trimester CC M ♀

O30.899 Other specified multiple gestation, unable to determine number of placenta and number of amniotic sacs, unspecified trimester M ♀

√5th **O30.9 Multiple gestation, unspecified**

Multiple pregnancy NOS

O30.90 Multiple gestation, unspecified, unspecified trimester M ♀

O30.91 Multiple gestation, unspecified, first trimester M ♀

O30.92 Multiple gestation, unspecified, second trimester M ♀

O30.93 Multiple gestation, unspecified, third trimester M ♀

√4th **O31 Complications specific to multiple gestation**

EXCLUDES 2 *delayed delivery of second twin, triplet, etc. (O63.2)*
malpresentation of one fetus or more (O32.9)
placental transfusion syndromes (O43.0-)

AHA: 2012,4Q,107

One of the following 7th characters is to be assigned to each code under category O31. 7th character 0 is for single gestations and multiple gestations where the fetus is unspecified. 7th characters 1 through 9 are for cases of multiple gestations to identify the fetus for which the code applies. The appropriate code from category O30, Multiple gestation, must also be assigned when assigning a code from category O31 that has a 7th character of 1 through 9.

0 not applicable or unspecified
1 fetus 1
2 fetus 2
3 fetus 3
4 fetus 4
5 fetus 5
9 other fetus

√5th **O31.0 Papyraceous fetus**

Fetus compressus

DEF: Fetus that has died, but remains in utero for weeks before delivery, becoming compacted and mummified in appearance, with skin resembling parchment. Occurs most commonly in multigestational pregnancies. ***Synonym(s):*** *paper doll fetus.*

√x7th **O31.00 Papyraceous fetus, unspecified trimester** M ♀

√x7th **O31.01 Papyraceous fetus, first trimester** M ♀

√x7th **O31.02 Papyraceous fetus, second trimester** M ♀

√x7th **O31.03 Papyraceous fetus, third trimester** M ♀

√5th **O31.1 Continuing pregnancy after spontaneous abortion of one fetus or more**

√x7th **O31.10 Continuing pregnancy after spontaneous abortion of one fetus or more, unspecified trimester** M ♀

√x7th **O31.11 Continuing pregnancy after spontaneous abortion of one fetus or more, first trimester** M ♀

√x7th **O31.12 Continuing pregnancy after spontaneous abortion of one fetus or more, second trimester** M ♀

√x7th **O31.13 Continuing pregnancy after spontaneous abortion of one fetus or more, third trimester** M ♀

√5th **O31.2 Continuing pregnancy after intrauterine death of one fetus or more**

√x7th **O31.20 Continuing pregnancy after intrauterine death of one fetus or more, unspecified trimester** M ♀

√x7th **O31.21 Continuing pregnancy after intrauterine death of one fetus or more, first trimester** M ♀

√x7th **O31.22 Continuing pregnancy after intrauterine death of one fetus or more, second trimester** M ♀

√x7th **O31.23 Continuing pregnancy after intrauterine death of one fetus or more, third trimester** M ♀

√5th **O31.3 Continuing pregnancy after elective fetal reduction of one fetus or more**

Continuing pregnancy after selective termination of one fetus or more

√x7th **O31.30 Continuing pregnancy after elective fetal reduction of one fetus or more, unspecified trimester** M ♀

√x7th **O31.31 Continuing pregnancy after elective fetal reduction of one fetus or more, first trimester** M ♀

√x7th **O31.32 Continuing pregnancy after elective fetal reduction of one fetus or more, second trimester** M ♀

√x7th **O31.33 Continuing pregnancy after elective fetal reduction of one fetus or more, third trimester** M ♀

√5th **O31.8 Other complications specific to multiple gestation**

√6th **O31.8X Other complications specific to multiple gestation**

√7th **O31.8X1 Other complications specific to multiple gestation, first trimester** CC M ♀

√7th **O31.8X2 Other complications specific to multiple gestation, second trimester** CC M ♀

√7th **O31.8X3 Other complications specific to multiple gestation, third trimester** CC M ♀

√7th **O31.8X9 Other complications specific to multiple gestation, unspecified trimester** CC M ♀

√4th **O32 Maternal care for malpresentation of fetus**

INCLUDES the listed conditions as a reason for observation, hospitalization or other obstetric care of the mother, or for cesarean delivery before onset of labor

EXCLUDES 1 *malpresentation of fetus with obstructed labor (O64.-)*

AHA: 2012,4Q,107

One of the following 7th characters is to be assigned to each code under category O32. 7th character 0 is for single gestations and multiple gestations where the fetus is unspecified. 7th characters 1 through 9 are for cases of multiple gestations to identify the fetus for which the code applies. The appropriate code from category O30, Multiple gestation, must also be assigned when assigning a code from category O32 that has a 7th character of 1 through 9.

0 not applicable or unspecified
1 fetus 1
2 fetus 2
3 fetus 3
4 fetus 4
5 fetus 5
9 other fetus

√x7th **O32.0 Maternal care for unstable lie** M ♀

√x7th **O32.1 Maternal care for breech presentation** M ♀

Maternal care for buttocks presentation
Maternal care for complete breech
Maternal care for frank breech

EXCLUDES 1 *footling presentation (O32.8)*
incomplete breech (O32.8)

DEF: Fetus presentation in a longitudinal lie with the buttocks or feet closest to birth canal that may require external cephalic version or cesarean delivery.

√x7th **O32.2 Maternal care for transverse and oblique lie** M ♀

Maternal care for oblique presentation
Maternal care for transverse presentation

√x7th **O32.3 Maternal care for face, brow and chin presentation** M ♀

√x7th **O32.4 Maternal care for high head at term** M ♀

Maternal care for failure of head to enter pelvic brim

√x7th **O32.6 Maternal care for compound presentation** M ♀

√x7th **O32.8 Maternal care for other malpresentation of fetus** M ♀

Maternal care for footling presentation
Maternal care for incomplete breech

√x7th **O32.9 Maternal care for malpresentation of fetus, unspecified** M ♀

Fetal Malpresentation

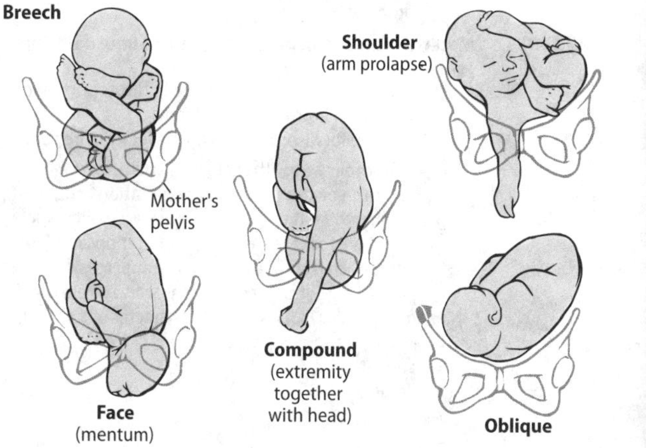

Chapter 15. Pregnancy, Childbirth and the Puerperium
O30.9–O32.9

4th O33 Maternal care for disproportion

INCLUDES the listed conditions as a reason for observation, hospitalization or other obstetric care of the mother, or for cesarean delivery before onset of labor

EXCLUDES 1 *disproportion with obstructed labor (O65-O66)*

O33.Ø Maternal care for disproportion due to deformity of maternal pelvic bones CC M ♀

Maternal care for disproportion due to pelvic deformity causing disproportion NOS

O33.1 Maternal care for disproportion due to generally contracted pelvis M ♀

Maternal care for disproportion due to contracted pelvis NOS causing disproportion

O33.2 Maternal care for disproportion due to inlet contraction of pelvis M ♀

Maternal care for disproportion due to inlet contraction (pelvis) causing disproportion

x7th O33.3 Maternal care for disproportion due to outlet contraction of pelvis M ♀

Maternal care for disproportion due to mid-cavity contraction (pelvis)

Maternal care for disproportion due to outlet contraction (pelvis)

One of the following 7th characters is to be assigned to code O33.3. 7th character Ø is for single gestations and multiple gestations where the fetus is unspecified. 7th characters 1 through 9 are for cases of multiple gestations to identify the fetus for which the code applies. The appropriate code from category O3Ø, Multiple gestation, must also be assigned when assigning code O33.3 with a 7th character of 1 through 9.

Ø not applicable or unspecified
1 fetus 1
2 fetus 2
3 fetus 3
4 fetus 4
5 fetus 5
9 other fetus

x7th O33.4 Maternal care for disproportion of mixed maternal and fetal origin M ♀

One of the following 7th characters is to be assigned to code O33.4. 7th character Ø is for single gestations and multiple gestations where the fetus is unspecified. 7th characters 1 through 9 are for cases of multiple gestations to identify the fetus for which the code applies. The appropriate code from category O3Ø, Multiple gestation, must also be assigned when assigning code O33.4 with a 7th character of 1 through 9.

Ø not applicable or unspecified
1 fetus 1
2 fetus 2
3 fetus 3
4 fetus 4
5 fetus 5
9 other fetus

x7th O33.5 Maternal care for disproportion due to unusually large fetus M ♀

Maternal care for disproportion due to disproportion of fetal origin with normally formed fetus

Maternal care for disproportion due to fetal disproportion NOS

One of the following 7th characters is to be assigned to code O33.5. 7th character Ø is for single gestations and multiple gestations where the fetus is unspecified. 7th characters 1 through 9 are for cases of multiple gestations to identify the fetus for which the code applies. The appropriate code from category O3Ø, Multiple gestation, must also be assigned when assigning code O33.5 with a 7th character of 1 through 9.

Ø not applicable or unspecified
1 fetus 1
2 fetus 2
3 fetus 3
4 fetus 4
5 fetus 5
9 other fetus

x7th O33.6 Maternal care for disproportion due to hydrocephalic fetus M ♀

One of the following 7th characters is to be assigned to code O33.6. 7th character Ø is for single gestations and multiple gestations where the fetus is unspecified. 7th characters 1 through 9 are for cases of multiple gestations to identify the fetus for which the code applies. The appropriate code from category O3Ø, Multiple gestation, must also be assigned when assigning code O33.6 with a 7th character of 1 through 9.

Ø not applicable or unspecified
1 fetus 1
2 fetus 2
3 fetus 3
4 fetus 4
5 fetus 5
9 other fetus

x7th O33.7 Maternal care for disproportion due to other fetal deformities M ♀

Maternal care for disproportion due to fetal ascites
Maternal care for disproportion due to fetal hydrops
Maternal care for disproportion due to fetal meningomyelocele
Maternal care for disproportion due to fetal sacral teratoma
Maternal care for disproportion due to fetal tumor

EXCLUDES 1 *obstructed labor due to other fetal deformities (O66.3)*

AHA: 2016,4Q,51

One of the following 7th characters is to be assigned to code O33.7. 7th character Ø is for single gestations and multiple gestations where the fetus is unspecified. 7th characters 1 through 9 are for cases of multiple gestations to identify the fetus for which the code applies. The appropriate code from category O3Ø, Multiple gestation, must also be assigned when assigning code O33.7 with a 7th character of 1 through 9.

Ø not applicable or unspecified
1 fetus 1
2 fetus 2
3 fetus 3
4 fetus 4
5 fetus 5
9 other fetus

O33.8 Maternal care for disproportion of other origin M ♀

O33.9 Maternal care for disproportion, unspecified M ♀

Maternal care for disproportion due to cephalopelvic disproportion NOS

Maternal care for disproportion due to fetopelvic disproportion NOS

4th O34 Maternal care for abnormality of pelvic organs

INCLUDES the listed conditions as a reason for hospitalization or other obstetric care of the mother, or for cesarean delivery before onset of labor

Code first any associated obstructed labor (O65.5)

Use additional code for specific condition

5th O34.Ø Maternal care for congenital malformation of uterus

Maternal care for double uterus
Maternal care for uterus bicornis

O34.ØØ Maternal care for unspecified congenital malformation of uterus, unspecified trimester M ♀

O34.Ø1 Maternal care for unspecified congenital malformation of uterus, first trimester M ♀

O34.Ø2 Maternal care for unspecified congenital malformation of uterus, second trimester M ♀

O34.Ø3 Maternal care for unspecified congenital malformation of uterus, third trimester M ♀

5th O34.1 Maternal care for benign tumor of corpus uteri

EXCLUDES 2 *maternal care for benign tumor of cervix (O34.4-)*
maternal care for malignant neoplasm of uterus (O9A.1-)

O34.1Ø Maternal care for benign tumor of corpus uteri, unspecified trimester M ♀

O34.11 Maternal care for benign tumor of corpus uteri, first trimester M ♀

O34.12 Maternal care for benign tumor of corpus uteri, second trimester M ♀

O34.13 Maternal care for benign tumor of corpus uteri, third trimester M ♀

✓5th O34.2 **Maternal care due to uterine scar from previous surgery**
AHA: 2016,4Q,76

✓6th O34.21 **Maternal care for scar from previous cesarean delivery**
AHA: 2018,3Q,23; 2016,4Q,51-52

O34.211 **Maternal care for low transverse scar from previous cesarean delivery** M ♀

O34.212 **Maternal care for vertical scar from previous cesarean delivery** M ♀
Maternal care for classical scar from previous cesarean delivery

● O34.218 **Maternal care for other type scar from previous cesarean delivery** M ♀
Mid-transverse T incision

O34.219 **Maternal care for unspecified type scar from previous cesarean delivery** M ♀

● O34.22 **Maternal care for cesarean scar defect (isthmocele)** M ♀

O34.29 **Maternal care due to uterine scar from other previous surgery** M ♀
Maternal care due to uterine scar from other transmural uterine incision

✓5th O34.3 **Maternal care for cervical incompetence**
Maternal care for cerclage with or without cervical incompetence
Maternal care for Shirodkar suture with or without cervical incompetence
DEF: Inadequate functioning of the cervix marked by abnormal widening during pregnancy and causing premature birth or miscarriage.

O34.30 **Maternal care for cervical incompetence, unspecified trimester** M ♀

O34.31 **Maternal care for cervical incompetence, first trimester** MCC M ♀

O34.32 **Maternal care for cervical incompetence, second trimester** MCC M ♀

O34.33 **Maternal care for cervical incompetence, third trimester** MCC M ♀

✓5th O34.4 **Maternal care for other abnormalities of cervix**

O34.40 **Maternal care for other abnormalities of cervix, unspecified trimester** M ♀

O34.41 **Maternal care for other abnormalities of cervix, first trimester** M ♀

O34.42 **Maternal care for other abnormalities of cervix, second trimester** M ♀

O34.43 **Maternal care for other abnormalities of cervix, third trimester** M ♀

✓5th O34.5 **Maternal care for other abnormalities of gravid uterus**

✓6th O34.51 **Maternal care for incarceration of gravid uterus**

O34.511 **Maternal care for incarceration of gravid uterus, first trimester** M ♀

O34.512 **Maternal care for incarceration of gravid uterus, second trimester** M ♀

O34.513 **Maternal care for incarceration of gravid uterus, third trimester** M ♀

O34.519 **Maternal care for incarceration of gravid uterus, unspecified trimester** M ♀

✓6th O34.52 **Maternal care for prolapse of gravid uterus**

O34.521 **Maternal care for prolapse of gravid uterus, first trimester** M ♀

O34.522 **Maternal care for prolapse of gravid uterus, second trimester** M ♀

O34.523 **Maternal care for prolapse of gravid uterus, third trimester** M ♀

O34.529 **Maternal care for prolapse of gravid uterus, unspecified trimester** M ♀

✓6th O34.53 **Maternal care for retroversion of gravid uterus**

O34.531 **Maternal care for retroversion of gravid uterus, first trimester** M ♀

O34.532 **Maternal care for retroversion of gravid uterus, second trimester** M ♀

O34.533 **Maternal care for retroversion of gravid uterus, third trimester** M ♀

O34.539 **Maternal care for retroversion of gravid uterus, unspecified trimester** M ♀

✓6th O34.59 **Maternal care for other abnormalities of gravid uterus**

O34.591 **Maternal care for other abnormalities of gravid uterus, first trimester** M ♀

O34.592 **Maternal care for other abnormalities of gravid uterus, second trimester** M ♀

O34.593 **Maternal care for other abnormalities of gravid uterus, third trimester** M ♀

O34.599 **Maternal care for other abnormalities of gravid uterus, unspecified trimester** M ♀

✓5th O34.6 **Maternal care for abnormality of vagina**
EXCLUDES 2 *maternal care for vaginal varices in pregnancy (O22.1-)*

O34.60 **Maternal care for abnormality of vagina, unspecified trimester** M ♀

O34.61 **Maternal care for abnormality of vagina, first trimester** M ♀

O34.62 **Maternal care for abnormality of vagina, second trimester** M ♀

O34.63 **Maternal care for abnormality of vagina, third trimester** M ♀

✓5th O34.7 **Maternal care for abnormality of vulva and perineum**
EXCLUDES 2 *maternal care for perineal and vulval varices in pregnancy (O22.1-)*

O34.70 **Maternal care for abnormality of vulva and perineum, unspecified trimester** M ♀

O34.71 **Maternal care for abnormality of vulva and perineum, first trimester** M ♀

O34.72 **Maternal care for abnormality of vulva and perineum, second trimester** M ♀

O34.73 **Maternal care for abnormality of vulva and perineum, third trimester** M ♀

✓5th O34.8 **Maternal care for other abnormalities of pelvic organs**

O34.80 **Maternal care for other abnormalities of pelvic organs, unspecified trimester** M ♀

O34.81 **Maternal care for other abnormalities of pelvic organs, first trimester** M ♀

O34.82 **Maternal care for other abnormalities of pelvic organs, second trimester** M ♀

O34.83 **Maternal care for other abnormalities of pelvic organs, third trimester** M ♀

✓5th O34.9 **Maternal care for abnormality of pelvic organ, unspecified**

O34.90 **Maternal care for abnormality of pelvic organ, unspecified, unspecified trimester** M ♀

O34.91 **Maternal care for abnormality of pelvic organ, unspecified, first trimester** M ♀

O34.92 **Maternal care for abnormality of pelvic organ, unspecified, second trimester** M ♀

O34.93 **Maternal care for abnormality of pelvic organ, unspecified, third trimester** M ♀

✓4th **O35 Maternal care for known or suspected fetal abnormality and damage**
INCLUDES the listed conditions in the fetus as a reason for hospitalization or other obstetric care to the mother, or for termination of pregnancy
Code also any associated maternal condition
EXCLUDES 1 *encounter for suspected maternal and fetal conditions ruled out (Z03.7-)*

One of the following 7th characters is to be assigned to each code under category O35. 7th character 0 is for single gestations and multiple gestations where the fetus is unspecified. 7th characters 1 through 9 are for cases of multiple gestations to identify the fetus for which the code applies. The appropriate code from category O30, Multiple gestation, must also be assigned when assigning a code from category O35 that has a 7th character of 1 through 9.
0 not applicable or unspecified
1 fetus 1
2 fetus 2
3 fetus 3
4 fetus 4
5 fetus 5
9 other fetus

✓x7th O35.0 **Maternal care for (suspected) central nervous system malformation in fetus** M ♀
Maternal care for fetal anencephaly
Maternal care for fetal hydrocephalus
Maternal care for fetal spina bifida
EXCLUDES 2 *chromosomal abnormality in fetus (O35.1)*

✓x7th O35.1 **Maternal care for (suspected) chromosomal abnormality in fetus** M ♀

√x7th **O35.2 Maternal care for (suspected) hereditary disease in fetus** M ♀
EXCLUDES 2 *chromosomal abnormality in fetus (O35.1)*

√x7th **O35.3 Maternal care for (suspected) damage to fetus from viral disease in mother** M ♀
Maternal care for damage to fetus from maternal cytomegalovirus infection
Maternal care for damage to fetus from maternal rubella

√x7th **O35.4 Maternal care for (suspected) damage to fetus from alcohol** M ♀

√x7th **O35.5 Maternal care for (suspected) damage to fetus by drugs** M ♀
Maternal care for damage to fetus from drug addiction

√x7th **O35.6 Maternal care for (suspected) damage to fetus by radiation** M ♀

√x7th **O35.7 Maternal care for (suspected) damage to fetus by other medical procedures** M ♀
Maternal care for damage to fetus by amniocentesis
Maternal care for damage to fetus by biopsy procedures
Maternal care for damage to fetus by hematological investigation
Maternal care for damage to fetus by intrauterine contraceptive device
Maternal care for damage to fetus by intrauterine surgery

√x7th **O35.8 Maternal care for other (suspected) fetal abnormality and damage** M ♀
Maternal care for damage to fetus from maternal listeriosis
Maternal care for damage to fetus from maternal toxoplasmosis

√x7th **O35.9 Maternal care for (suspected) fetal abnormality and damage, unspecified** M ♀

√4th **O36 Maternal care for other fetal problems**

INCLUDES the listed conditions in the fetus as a reason for hospitalization or other obstetric care of the mother, or for termination of pregnancy

EXCLUDES 1 *encounter for suspected maternal and fetal conditions ruled out (Z03.7-)*
placental transfusion syndromes (O43.0-)

EXCLUDES 2 *labor and delivery complicated by fetal stress (O77.-)*

AHA: 2015,3Q,40

One of the following 7th characters is to be assigned to each code under category O36. 7th character 0 is for single gestations and multiple gestations where the fetus is unspecified. 7th characters 1 through 9 are for cases of multiple gestations to identify the fetus for which the code applies. The appropriate code from category O30, Multiple gestation, must also be assigned when assigning a code from category O36 that has a 7th character of 1 through 9.

0 not applicable or unspecified
1 fetus 1
2 fetus 2
3 fetus 3
4 fetus 4
5 fetus 5
9 other fetus

√5th **O36.0 Maternal care for rhesus isoimmunization**
Maternal care for Rh incompatibility (with hydrops fetalis)

√6th **O36.01 Maternal care for anti-D [Rh] antibodies**
AHA: 2014,4Q,17

√7th **O36.011 Maternal care for anti-D [Rh] antibodies, first trimester** CC M ♀

√7th **O36.012 Maternal care for anti-D [Rh] antibodies, second trimester** CC M ♀

√7th **O36.013 Maternal care for anti-D [Rh] antibodies, third trimester** CC M ♀

√7th **O36.019 Maternal care for anti-D [Rh] antibodies, unspecified trimester** M ♀

√6th **O36.09 Maternal care for other rhesus isoimmunization**

√7th **O36.091 Maternal care for other rhesus isoimmunization, first trimester** CC M ♀

√7th **O36.092 Maternal care for other rhesus isoimmunization, second trimester** CC M ♀

√7th **O36.093 Maternal care for other rhesus isoimmunization, third trimester** CC M ♀

√7th **O36.099 Maternal care for other rhesus isoimmunization, unspecified trimester** M ♀

√5th **O36.1 Maternal care for other isoimmunization**
Maternal care for ABO isoimmunization

√6th **O36.11 Maternal care for Anti-A sensitization**
Maternal care for isoimmunization NOS (with hydrops fetalis)

√7th **O36.111 Maternal care for Anti-A sensitization, first trimester** M ♀

√7th **O36.112 Maternal care for Anti-A sensitization, second trimester** M ♀

√7th **O36.113 Maternal care for Anti-A sensitization, third trimester** M ♀

√7th **O36.119 Maternal care for Anti-A sensitization, unspecified trimester** M ♀

√6th **O36.19 Maternal care for other isoimmunization**
Maternal care for Anti-B sensitization

√7th **O36.191 Maternal care for other isoimmunization, first trimester** M ♀

√7th **O36.192 Maternal care for other isoimmunization, second trimester** M ♀

√7th **O36.193 Maternal care for other isoimmunization, third trimester** M ♀

√7th **O36.199 Maternal care for other isoimmunization, unspecified trimester** M ♀

√5th **O36.2 Maternal care for hydrops fetalis**
Maternal care for hydrops fetalis NOS
Maternal care for hydrops fetalis not associated with isoimmunization

EXCLUDES 1 *hydrops fetalis associated with ABO isoimmunization (O36.1-)*
hydrops fetalis associated with rhesus isoimmunization (O36.0-)

DEF: Hydrops fetalis: Abnormal fluid buildup in at least two of the following fetal organ spaces: the skin (edema), abdomen (ascites), around the heart (pericardia effusion), and around the lung (pleural effusion). Fluid accumulation may also occur in the mother as polyhydramnios and edema of the placenta.

√x7th **O36.20 Maternal care for hydrops fetalis, unspecified trimester** M ♀

√x7th **O36.21 Maternal care for hydrops fetalis, first trimester** M ♀

√x7th **O36.22 Maternal care for hydrops fetalis, second trimester** M ♀

√x7th **O36.23 Maternal care for hydrops fetalis, third trimester** M ♀

√x7th **O36.4 Maternal care for intrauterine death** CC M ♀
Maternal care for intrauterine fetal death NOS
Maternal care for intrauterine fetal death after completion of 20 weeks of gestation
Maternal care for late fetal death
Maternal care for missed delivery

EXCLUDES 1 *missed abortion (O02.1)*
stillbirth (P95)

√5th **O36.5 Maternal care for known or suspected poor fetal growth**

√6th **O36.51 Maternal care for known or suspected placental insufficiency**

√7th **O36.511 Maternal care for known or suspected placental insufficiency, first trimester** M ♀

√7th **O36.512 Maternal care for known or suspected placental insufficiency, second trimester** M ♀

√7th **O36.513 Maternal care for known or suspected placental insufficiency, third trimester** M ♀

√7th **O36.519 Maternal care for known or suspected placental insufficiency, unspecified trimester** M ♀

√6th **O36.59 Maternal care for other known or suspected poor fetal growth**
Maternal care for known or suspected light-for-dates NOS
Maternal care for known or suspected small-for-dates NOS

√7th **O36.591 Maternal care for other known or suspected poor fetal growth, first trimester** M ♀

√7th **O36.592 Maternal care for other known or suspected poor fetal growth, second trimester** M ♀

O36.593 Maternal care for other known or suspected poor fetal growth, third trimester

O36.599 Maternal care for other known or suspected poor fetal growth, unspecified trimester

O36.6 Maternal care for excessive fetal growth

Maternal care for known or suspected large-for-dates

O36.60 Maternal care for excessive fetal growth, unspecified trimester

O36.61 Maternal care for excessive fetal growth, first trimester

O36.62 Maternal care for excessive fetal growth, second trimester

O36.63 Maternal care for excessive fetal growth, third trimester

O36.7 Maternal care for viable fetus in abdominal pregnancy

O36.70 Maternal care for viable fetus in abdominal pregnancy, unspecified trimester

O36.71 Maternal care for viable fetus in abdominal pregnancy, first trimester

O36.72 Maternal care for viable fetus in abdominal pregnancy, second trimester

O36.73 Maternal care for viable fetus in abdominal pregnancy, third trimester

O36.8 Maternal care for other specified fetal problems

O36.80 Pregnancy with inconclusive fetal viability

Encounter to determine fetal viability of pregnancy

AHA: 2019,2Q,29

O36.81 Decreased fetal movements

O36.812 Decreased fetal movements, second trimester

O36.813 Decreased fetal movements, third trimester

O36.819 Decreased fetal movements, unspecified trimester

O36.82 Fetal anemia and thrombocytopenia

O36.821 Fetal anemia and thrombocytopenia, first trimester

O36.822 Fetal anemia and thrombocytopenia, second trimester

O36.823 Fetal anemia and thrombocytopenia, third trimester

O36.829 Fetal anemia and thrombocytopenia, unspecified trimester

O36.83 Maternal care for abnormalities of the fetal heart rate or rhythm

Maternal care for depressed fetal heart rate tones
Maternal care for fetal bradycardia
Maternal care for fetal heart rate abnormal variability
Maternal care for fetal heart rate decelerations
Maternal care for fetal heart rate irregularity
Maternal care for fetal tachycardia
Maternal care for non-reassuring fetal heart rate or rhythm

AHA: 2017,4Q,20

TIP: Assign for documented fetal tachycardia, bradycardia, decelerations, or loss of variability detected during antenatal testing.

O36.831 Maternal care for abnormalities of the fetal heart rate or rhythm, first trimester

O36.832 Maternal care for abnormalities of the fetal heart rate or rhythm, second trimester

O36.833 Maternal care for abnormalities of the fetal heart rate or rhythm, third trimester

O36.839 Maternal care for abnormalities of the fetal heart rate or rhythm, unspecified trimester

O36.89 Maternal care for other specified fetal problems

O36.891 Maternal care for other specified fetal problems, first trimester

O36.892 Maternal care for other specified fetal problems, second trimester

O36.893 Maternal care for other specified fetal problems, third trimester

O36.899 Maternal care for other specified fetal problems, unspecified trimester

O36.9 Maternal care for fetal problem, unspecified

O36.90 Maternal care for fetal problem, unspecified, unspecified trimester

O36.91 Maternal care for fetal problem, unspecified, first trimester

O36.92 Maternal care for fetal problem, unspecified, second trimester

O36.93 Maternal care for fetal problem, unspecified, third trimester

O40 Polyhydramnios

INCLUDES hydramnios

EXCLUDES 1 *encounter for suspected maternal and fetal conditions ruled out (Z03.7-)*

AHA: 2016,1Q,4

DEF: Excess amniotic fluid surrounding the fetus, typically defined as a total fluid volume of greater than 24.0 cc.

One of the following 7th characters is to be assigned to each code under category O40. 7th character 0 is for single gestations and multiple gestations where the fetus is unspecified. 7th characters 1 through 9 are for cases of multiple gestations to identify the fetus for which the code applies. The appropriate code from category O30, Multiple gestation, must also be assigned when assigning a code from category O40 that has a 7th character of 1 through 9.
0 not applicable or unspecified
1 fetus 1
2 fetus 2
3 fetus 3
4 fetus 4
5 fetus 5
9 other fetus

O40.1 Polyhydramnios, first trimester

O40.2 Polyhydramnios, second trimester

O40.3 Polyhydramnios, third trimester

O40.9 Polyhydramnios, unspecified trimester

O41 Other disorders of amniotic fluid and membranes

EXCLUDES 1 *encounter for suspected maternal and fetal conditions ruled out (Z03.7-)*

One of the following 7th characters is to be assigned to each code under category O41. 7th character 0 is for single gestations and multiple gestations where the fetus is unspecified. 7th characters 1 through 9 are for cases of multiple gestations to identify the fetus for which the code applies. The appropriate code from category O30, Multiple gestation, must also be assigned when assigning a code from category O41 that has a 7th character of 1 through 9.
0 not applicable or unspecified
1 fetus 1
2 fetus 2
3 fetus 3
4 fetus 4
5 fetus 5
9 other fetus

O41.0 Oligohydramnios

Oligohydramnios without rupture of membranes

DEF: Low amniotic fluid, occurring most frequently in the last trimester.

O41.00 Oligohydramnios, unspecified trimester

O41.01 Oligohydramnios, first trimester CC

O41.02 Oligohydramnios, second trimester CC

O41.03 Oligohydramnios, third trimester CC

O41.1 Infection of amniotic sac and membranes

O41.10 Infection of amniotic sac and membranes, unspecified

O41.101 Infection of amniotic sac and membranes, unspecified, first trimester MCC

O41.102 Infection of amniotic sac and membranes, unspecified, second trimester MCC

O41.103 Infection of amniotic sac and membranes, unspecified, third trimester MCC

O41.109 Infection of amniotic sac and membranes, unspecified, unspecified trimester

✓6th **O41.12 Chorioamnionitis**
AHA: 2019,2Q,34

✓7th **O41.121 Chorioamnionitis, first trimester** MCC M ♀

✓7th **O41.122 Chorioamnionitis, second trimester** MCC M ♀

✓7th **O41.123 Chorioamnionitis, third trimester** MCC M ♀

✓7th **O41.129 Chorioamnionitis, unspecified trimester** M ♀

✓6th **O41.14 Placentitis**

✓7th **O41.141 Placentitis, first trimester** MCC M ♀

✓7th **O41.142 Placentitis, second trimester** MCC M ♀

✓7th **O41.143 Placentitis, third trimester** MCC M ♀

✓7th **O41.149 Placentitis, unspecified trimester** M ♀

✓5th **O41.8 Other specified disorders of amniotic fluid and membranes**

✓6th **O41.8X Other specified disorders of amniotic fluid and membranes**

✓7th **O41.8X1 Other specified disorders of amniotic fluid and membranes, first trimester** M ♀

✓7th **O41.8X2 Other specified disorders of amniotic fluid and membranes, second trimester** M ♀

✓7th **O41.8X3 Other specified disorders of amniotic fluid and membranes, third trimester** M ♀

✓7th **O41.8X9 Other specified disorders of amniotic fluid and membranes, unspecified trimester** M ♀

✓5th **O41.9 Disorder of amniotic fluid and membranes, unspecified**

✓x7th **O41.9Ø Disorder of amniotic fluid and membranes, unspecified, unspecified trimester** M ♀

✓x7th **O41.91 Disorder of amniotic fluid and membranes, unspecified, first trimester** M ♀

✓x7th **O41.92 Disorder of amniotic fluid and membranes, unspecified, second trimester** M ♀

✓x7th **O41.93 Disorder of amniotic fluid and membranes, unspecified, third trimester** M ♀

✓4th **O42 Premature rupture of membranes**
AHA: 2016,1Q,3

✓5th **O42.Ø Premature rupture of membranes, onset of labor within 24 hours of rupture**

O42.ØØ Premature rupture of membranes, onset of labor within 24 hours of rupture, unspecified weeks of gestation M ♀

✓6th **O42.Ø1 Preterm premature rupture of membranes, onset of labor within 24 hours of rupture**
Premature rupture of membranes before 37 completed weeks of gestation

O42.Ø11 Preterm premature rupture of membranes, onset of labor within 24 hours of rupture, first trimester M ♀

O42.Ø12 Preterm premature rupture of membranes, onset of labor within 24 hours of rupture, second trimester M ♀

O42.Ø13 Preterm premature rupture of membranes, onset of labor within 24 hours of rupture, third trimester M ♀

O42.Ø19 Preterm premature rupture of membranes, onset of labor within 24 hours of rupture, unspecified trimester M ♀

O42.Ø2 Full-term premature rupture of membranes, onset of labor within 24 hours of rupture M ♀
Premature rupture of membranes at or after 37 completed weeks of gestation, onset of labor within 24 hours of rupture

✓5th **O42.1 Premature rupture of membranes, onset of labor more than 24 hours following rupture**
AHA: 2016,1Q,5

O42.1Ø Premature rupture of membranes, onset of labor more than 24 hours following rupture, unspecified weeks of gestation M ♀

✓6th **O42.11 Preterm premature rupture of membranes, onset of labor more than 24 hours following rupture**
Premature rupture of membranes before 37 completed weeks of gestation

O42.111 Preterm premature rupture of membranes, onset of labor more than 24 hours following rupture, first trimester M ♀

O42.112 Preterm premature rupture of membranes, onset of labor more than 24 hours following rupture, second trimester M ♀

O42.113 Preterm premature rupture of membranes, onset of labor more than 24 hours following rupture, third trimester M ♀

O42.119 Preterm premature rupture of membranes, onset of labor more than 24 hours following rupture, unspecified trimester M ♀

O42.12 Full-term premature rupture of membranes, onset of labor more than 24 hours following rupture M ♀
Premature rupture of membranes at or after 37 completed weeks of gestation, onset of labor more than 24 hours following rupture

✓5th **O42.9 Premature rupture of membranes, unspecified as to length of time between rupture and onset of labor**

O42.9Ø Premature rupture of membranes, unspecified as to length of time between rupture and onset of labor, unspecified weeks of gestation M ♀

✓6th **O42.91 Preterm premature rupture of membranes, unspecified as to length of time between rupture and onset of labor**
Premature rupture of membranes before 37 completed weeks of gestation

O42.911 Preterm premature rupture of membranes, unspecified as to length of time between rupture and onset of labor, first trimester M ♀

O42.912 Preterm premature rupture of membranes, unspecified as to length of time between rupture and onset of labor, second trimester M ♀

O42.913 Preterm premature rupture of membranes, unspecified as to length of time between rupture and onset of labor, third trimester M ♀

O42.919 Preterm premature rupture of membranes, unspecified as to length of time between rupture and onset of labor, unspecified trimester M ♀

O42.92 Full-term premature rupture of membranes, unspecified as to length of time between rupture and onset of labor M ♀
Premature rupture of membranes at or after 37 completed weeks of gestation, unspecified as to length of time between rupture and onset of labor

✓4th **O43 Placental disorders**

EXCLUDES 2 *maternal care for poor fetal growth due to placental insufficiency (O36.5-)*
placenta previa (O44.-)
placental polyp (O9Ø.89)
placentitis (O41.14-)
premature separation of placenta [abruptio placentae] (O45.-)

✓5th **O43.Ø Placental transfusion syndromes**

✓6th **O43.Ø1 Fetomaternal placental transfusion syndrome**
Maternofetal placental transfusion syndrome

O43.Ø11 Fetomaternal placental transfusion syndrome, first trimester M ♀

O43.Ø12 Fetomaternal placental transfusion syndrome, second trimester M ♀

O43.Ø13 Fetomaternal placental transfusion syndrome, third trimester M ♀

O43.Ø19 Fetomaternal placental transfusion syndrome, unspecified trimester M ♀

✓6th **O43.Ø2 Fetus-to-fetus placental transfusion syndrome**

DEF: Condition in which an imbalance in amniotic fluid occurs due to uneven blood flow between twins sharing a placenta.

Twin to Twin Transfusion Syndrome (TTTS)

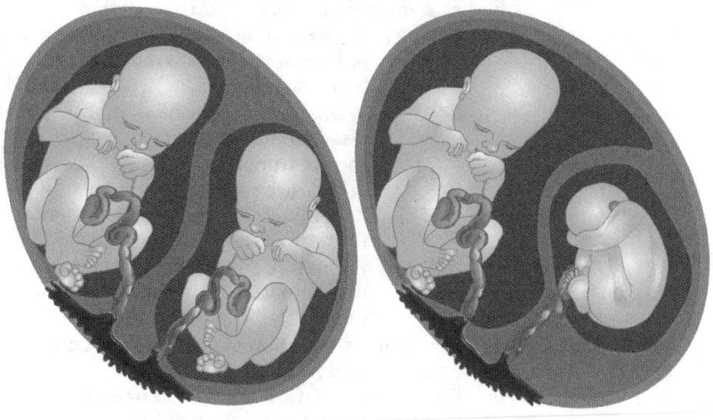

Healthy twins — Twins with TTTS

- **O43.Ø21 Fetus-to-fetus placental transfusion syndrome, first trimester** M ♀
- **O43.Ø22 Fetus-to-fetus placental transfusion syndrome, second trimester** M ♀
- **O43.Ø23 Fetus-to-fetus placental transfusion syndrome, third trimester** M ♀
- **O43.Ø29 Fetus-to-fetus placental transfusion syndrome, unspecified trimester** M ♀

✓5th **O43.1 Malformation of placenta**

✓6th **O43.1Ø Malformation of placenta, unspecified**

Abnormal placenta NOS

- **O43.1Ø1 Malformation of placenta, unspecified, first trimester** M ♀
- **O43.1Ø2 Malformation of placenta, unspecified, second trimester** M ♀
- **O43.1Ø3 Malformation of placenta, unspecified, third trimester** M ♀
- **O43.1Ø9 Malformation of placenta, unspecified, unspecified trimester** M ♀

✓6th **O43.11 Circumvallate placenta**

- **O43.111 Circumvallate placenta, first trimester** M ♀
- **O43.112 Circumvallate placenta, second trimester** M ♀
- **O43.113 Circumvallate placenta, third trimester** M ♀
- **O43.119 Circumvallate placenta, unspecified trimester** M ♀

✓6th **O43.12 Velamentous insertion of umbilical cord**

- **O43.121 Velamentous insertion of umbilical cord, first trimester** M ♀
- **O43.122 Velamentous insertion of umbilical cord, second trimester** M ♀
- **O43.123 Velamentous insertion of umbilical cord, third trimester** M ♀
- **O43.129 Velamentous insertion of umbilical cord, unspecified trimester** M ♀

✓6th **O43.19 Other malformation of placenta**

- **O43.191 Other malformation of placenta, first trimester** M ♀
- **O43.192 Other malformation of placenta, second trimester** M ♀
- **O43.193 Other malformation of placenta, third trimester** M ♀
- **O43.199 Other malformation of placenta, unspecified trimester** M ♀

✓5th **O43.2 Morbidly adherent placenta**

Code also associated third stage postpartum hemorrhage, if applicable (O72.Ø)

EXCLUDES 1 *retained placenta (O73.-)*

✓6th **O43.21 Placenta accreta**

DEF: Condition where the placenta adheres too deeply to the uterine wall; often associated with placenta previa.

- **O43.211 Placenta accreta, first trimester** M ♀
- **O43.212 Placenta accreta, second trimester** M ♀
- **O43.213 Placenta accreta, third trimester** M ♀
- **O43.219 Placenta accreta, unspecified trimester** M ♀

✓6th **O43.22 Placenta increta**

DEF: Condition where the placenta adheres too deeply to the uterine wall and penetrates the muscle; often associated with placenta previa.

- **O43.221 Placenta increta, first trimester** M ♀
- **O43.222 Placenta increta, second trimester** M ♀
- **O43.223 Placenta increta, third trimester** M ♀
- **O43.229 Placenta increta, unspecified trimester** M ♀

✓6th **O43.23 Placenta percreta**

DEF: Condition where the placenta attaches through the uterine muscle and may invade other organs, resulting in antenatal complications, premature delivery, retention of all or a portion of the placenta, or postpartum bleeding.

- **O43.231 Placenta percreta, first trimester** M ♀
- **O43.232 Placenta percreta, second trimester** M ♀
- **O43.233 Placenta percreta, third trimester** M ♀
- **O43.239 Placenta percreta, unspecified trimester** M ♀

✓5th **O43.8 Other placental disorders**

✓6th **O43.81 Placental infarction**

- **O43.811 Placental infarction, first trimester** M ♀
- **O43.812 Placental infarction, second trimester** M ♀
- **O43.813 Placental infarction, third trimester** M ♀
- **O43.819 Placental infarction, unspecified trimester** M ♀

✓6th **O43.89 Other placental disorders**

Placental dysfunction

- **O43.891 Other placental disorders, first trimester** M ♀
- **O43.892 Other placental disorders, second trimester** M ♀
- **O43.893 Other placental disorders, third trimester** M ♀
- **O43.899 Other placental disorders, unspecified trimester** M ♀

✓5th **O43.9 Unspecified placental disorder**

- **O43.9Ø Unspecified placental disorder, unspecified trimester** M ♀
- **O43.91 Unspecified placental disorder, first trimester** M ♀
- **O43.92 Unspecified placental disorder, second trimester** M ♀
- **O43.93 Unspecified placental disorder, third trimester** M ♀

✓4th **O44 Placenta previa**

AHA: 2016,4Q,52-53

DEF: Placenta implanted in the lower segment of the uterus, which commonly causes hemorrhage in the last trimester of pregnancy.

✓5th **O44.Ø Complete placenta previa NOS or without hemorrhage**

Placenta previa NOS

- **O44.ØØ Complete placenta previa NOS or without hemorrhage, unspecified trimester** M ♀
- **O44.Ø1 Complete placenta previa NOS or without hemorrhage, first trimester** CC M ♀
- **O44.Ø2 Complete placenta previa NOS or without hemorrhage, second trimester** CC M ♀

O44.03 **Complete placenta previa NOS or without hemorrhage, third trimester** CC M ♀

✓5th O44.1 **Complete placenta previa with hemorrhage**

EXCLUDES 1 *labor and delivery complicated by hemorrhage from vasa previa (O69.4)*

O44.10 **Complete placenta previa with hemorrhage, unspecified trimester** M ♀

O44.11 **Complete placenta previa with hemorrhage, first trimester** MCC M ♀

O44.12 **Complete placenta previa with hemorrhage, second trimester** MCC M ♀

O44.13 **Complete placenta previa with hemorrhage, third trimester** MCC M ♀

✓5th O44.2 **Partial placenta previa without hemorrhage**

Marginal placenta previa, NOS or without hemorrhage

O44.20 **Partial placenta previa NOS or without hemorrhage, unspecified trimester** M ♀

O44.21 **Partial placenta previa NOS or without hemorrhage, first trimester** CC M ♀

O44.22 **Partial placenta previa NOS or without hemorrhage, second trimester** CC M ♀

O44.23 **Partial placenta previa NOS or without hemorrhage, third trimester** CC M ♀

✓5th O44.3 **Partial placenta previa with hemorrhage**

Marginal placenta previa with hemorrhage

O44.30 **Partial placenta previa with hemorrhage, unspecified trimester** M ♀

O44.31 **Partial placenta previa with hemorrhage, first trimester** MCC M ♀

O44.32 **Partial placenta previa with hemorrhage, second trimester** MCC M ♀

O44.33 **Partial placenta previa with hemorrhage, third trimester** MCC M ♀

✓5th O44.4 **Low lying placenta NOS or without hemorrhage**

Low implantation of placenta NOS or without hemorrhage

O44.40 **Low lying placenta NOS or without hemorrhage, unspecified trimester** M ♀

O44.41 **Low lying placenta NOS or without hemorrhage, first trimester** CC M ♀

O44.42 **Low lying placenta NOS or without hemorrhage, second trimester** CC M ♀

O44.43 **Low lying placenta NOS or without hemorrhage, third trimester** CC M ♀

✓5th O44.5 **Low lying placenta with hemorrhage**

Low implantation of placenta with hemorrhage

O44.50 **Low lying placenta with hemorrhage, unspecified trimester** M ♀

O44.51 **Low lying placenta with hemorrhage, first trimester** MCC M ♀

O44.52 **Low lying placenta with hemorrhage, second trimester** MCC M ♀

O44.53 **Low lying placenta with hemorrhage, third trimester** MCC M ♀

✓4th O45 **Premature separation of placenta [abruptio placentae]**

✓5th O45.0 **Premature separation of placenta with coagulation defect**

✓6th O45.00 **Premature separation of placenta with coagulation defect, unspecified**

O45.001 **Premature separation of placenta with coagulation defect, unspecified, first trimester** MCC M ♀

O45.002 **Premature separation of placenta with coagulation defect, unspecified, second trimester** MCC M ♀

O45.003 **Premature separation of placenta with coagulation defect, unspecified, third trimester** MCC M ♀

O45.009 **Premature separation of placenta with coagulation defect, unspecified, unspecified trimester** M ♀

✓6th O45.01 **Premature separation of placenta with afibrinogenemia**

Premature separation of placenta with hypofibrinogenemia

O45.011 **Premature separation of placenta with afibrinogenemia, first trimester** MCC M ♀

O45.012 **Premature separation of placenta with afibrinogenemia, second trimester** MCC M ♀

O45.013 **Premature separation of placenta with afibrinogenemia, third trimester** MCC M ♀

O45.019 **Premature separation of placenta with afibrinogenemia, unspecified trimester** M ♀

✓6th O45.02 **Premature separation of placenta with disseminated intravascular coagulation**

O45.021 **Premature separation of placenta with disseminated intravascular coagulation, first trimester** MCC M ♀

O45.022 **Premature separation of placenta with disseminated intravascular coagulation, second trimester** MCC M ♀

O45.023 **Premature separation of placenta with disseminated intravascular coagulation, third trimester** MCC M ♀

O45.029 **Premature separation of placenta with disseminated intravascular coagulation, unspecified trimester** M ♀

✓6th O45.09 **Premature separation of placenta with other coagulation defect**

O45.091 **Premature separation of placenta with other coagulation defect, first trimester** MCC M ♀

O45.092 **Premature separation of placenta with other coagulation defect, second trimester** MCC M ♀

O45.093 **Premature separation of placenta with other coagulation defect, third trimester** MCC M ♀

O45.099 **Premature separation of placenta with other coagulation defect, unspecified trimester** M ♀

✓5th O45.8 **Other premature separation of placenta**

✓6th O45.8X **Other premature separation of placenta**

O45.8X1 **Other premature separation of placenta, first trimester** MCC M ♀

O45.8X2 **Other premature separation of placenta, second trimester** MCC M ♀

O45.8X3 **Other premature separation of placenta, third trimester** MCC M ♀

O45.8X9 **Other premature separation of placenta, unspecified trimester** M ♀

✓5th O45.9 **Premature separation of placenta, unspecified**

Abruptio placentae NOS

O45.90 **Premature separation of placenta, unspecified, unspecified trimester** M ♀

O45.91 **Premature separation of placenta, unspecified, first trimester** MCC M ♀

O45.92 **Premature separation of placenta, unspecified, second trimester** MCC M ♀

O45.93 **Premature separation of placenta, unspecified, third trimester** MCC M ♀

✓4th O46 **Antepartum hemorrhage, not elsewhere classified**

EXCLUDES 1 *hemorrhage in early pregnancy (O20.-)*
intrapartum hemorrhage NEC (O67.-)
placenta previa (O44.-)
premature separation of placenta [abruptio placentae] (O45.-)

DEF: Uterine hemorrhage prior to delivery that is not related to placenta previa or abruptio placentae.

✓5th O46.0 **Antepartum hemorrhage with coagulation defect**

✓6th O46.00 **Antepartum hemorrhage with coagulation defect, unspecified**

O46.001 **Antepartum hemorrhage with coagulation defect, unspecified, first trimester** MCC M ♀

O46.002 **Antepartum hemorrhage with coagulation defect, unspecified, second trimester** MCC M ♀

O46.003 **Antepartum hemorrhage with coagulation defect, unspecified, third trimester** MCC M ♀

O46.009 **Antepartum hemorrhage with coagulation defect, unspecified, unspecified trimester** M ♀

√6th **O46.Ø1 Antepartum hemorrhage with afibrinogenemia**
Antepartum hemorrhage with hypofibrinogenemia
O46.Ø11 Antepartum hemorrhage with afibrinogenemia, first trimester MCC M ♀
O46.Ø12 Antepartum hemorrhage with afibrinogenemia, second trimester MCC M ♀
O46.Ø13 Antepartum hemorrhage with afibrinogenemia, third trimester MCC M ♀
O46.Ø19 Antepartum hemorrhage with afibrinogenemia, unspecified trimester M ♀

√6th **O46.Ø2 Antepartum hemorrhage with disseminated intravascular coagulation**
O46.Ø21 Antepartum hemorrhage with disseminated intravascular coagulation, first trimester MCC M ♀
O46.Ø22 Antepartum hemorrhage with disseminated intravascular coagulation, second trimester MCC M ♀
O46.Ø23 Antepartum hemorrhage with disseminated intravascular coagulation, third trimester MCC M ♀
O46.Ø29 Antepartum hemorrhage with disseminated intravascular coagulation, unspecified trimester M ♀

√6th **O46.Ø9 Antepartum hemorrhage with other coagulation defect**
O46.Ø91 Antepartum hemorrhage with other coagulation defect, first trimester MCC M ♀
O46.Ø92 Antepartum hemorrhage with other coagulation defect, second trimester MCC M ♀
O46.Ø93 Antepartum hemorrhage with other coagulation defect, third trimester MCC M ♀
O46.Ø99 Antepartum hemorrhage with other coagulation defect, unspecified trimester M ♀

√5th **O46.8 Other antepartum hemorrhage**
√6th **O46.8X Other antepartum hemorrhage**
O46.8X1 Other antepartum hemorrhage, first trimester M ♀
O46.8X2 Other antepartum hemorrhage, second trimester M ♀
O46.8X3 Other antepartum hemorrhage, third trimester M ♀
O46.8X9 Other antepartum hemorrhage, unspecified trimester M ♀

√5th **O46.9 Antepartum hemorrhage, unspecified**
O46.9Ø Antepartum hemorrhage, unspecified, unspecified trimester M ♀
O46.91 Antepartum hemorrhage, unspecified, first trimester M ♀
O46.92 Antepartum hemorrhage, unspecified, second trimester M ♀
O46.93 Antepartum hemorrhage, unspecified, third trimester M ♀

√4th **O47 False labor**
INCLUDES Braxton Hicks contractions
threatened labor
EXCLUDES 1 *preterm labor (O6Ø.-)*

√5th **O47.Ø False labor before 37 completed weeks of gestation**
O47.ØØ False labor before 37 completed weeks of gestation, unspecified trimester M ♀
O47.Ø2 False labor before 37 completed weeks of gestation, second trimester CC M ♀
O47.Ø3 False labor before 37 completed weeks of gestation, third trimester CC M ♀

O47.1 False labor at or after 37 completed weeks of gestation CC M ♀
O47.9 False labor, unspecified M ♀

√4th **O48 Late pregnancy**
O48.Ø Post-term pregnancy M ♀
Pregnancy over 4Ø completed weeks to 42 completed weeks gestation
O48.1 Prolonged pregnancy M ♀
Pregnancy which has advanced beyond 42 completed weeks gestation
AHA: 2016,1Q,5

Complications of labor and delivery (O6Ø-O77)

√4th **O6Ø Preterm labor**
INCLUDES onset (spontaneous) of labor before 37 completed weeks of gestation
EXCLUDES 1 *false labor (O47.Ø-)*
threatened labor NOS (O47.Ø-)

√5th **O6Ø.Ø Preterm labor without delivery**
O6Ø.ØØ Preterm labor without delivery, unspecified trimester M ♀
O6Ø.Ø2 Preterm labor without delivery, second trimester MCC M ♀
O6Ø.Ø3 Preterm labor without delivery, third trimester MCC M ♀

√5th **O6Ø.1 Preterm labor with preterm delivery**
AHA: 2016,2Q,10

One of the following 7th characters is to be assigned to each code under subcategory O6Ø.1. 7th character Ø is for single gestations and multiple gestations where the fetus is unspecified. 7th characters 1 through 9 are for cases of multiple gestations to identify the fetus for which the code applies. The appropriate code from category O3Ø, Multiple gestation, must also be assigned when assigning a code from subcategory O6Ø.1 that has a 7th character of 1 through 9.
Ø not applicable or unspecified
1 fetus 1
2 fetus 2
3 fetus 3
4 fetus 4
5 fetus 5
9 other fetus

√x7th **O6Ø.1Ø Preterm labor with preterm delivery, unspecified trimester** CC M ♀
Preterm labor with delivery NOS
√x7th **O6Ø.12 Preterm labor second trimester with preterm delivery second trimester** MCC M ♀
√x7th **O6Ø.13 Preterm labor second trimester with preterm delivery third trimester** MCC M ♀
√x7th **O6Ø.14 Preterm labor third trimester with preterm delivery third trimester** MCC M ♀

√5th **O6Ø.2 Term delivery with preterm labor**

One of the following 7th characters is to be assigned to each code under subcategory O6Ø.2. 7th character Ø is for single gestations and multiple gestations where the fetus is unspecified. 7th characters 1 through 9 are for cases of multiple gestations to identify the fetus for which the code applies. The appropriate code from category O3Ø, Multiple gestation, must also be assigned when assigning a code from subcategory O6Ø.2 that has a 7th character of 1 through 9.
Ø not applicable or unspecified
1 fetus 1
2 fetus 2
3 fetus 3
4 fetus 4
5 fetus 5
9 other fetus

√x7th **O6Ø.2Ø Term delivery with preterm labor, unspecified trimester** CC M ♀
√x7th **O6Ø.22 Term delivery with preterm labor, second trimester** MCC M ♀
√x7th **O6Ø.23 Term delivery with preterm labor, third trimester** MCC M ♀

√4th **O61 Failed induction of labor**
O61.Ø Failed medical induction of labor M ♀
Failed induction (of labor) by oxytocin
Failed induction (of labor) by prostaglandins

O61.1 Failed instrumental induction of labor M ♀
Failed mechanical induction (of labor)
Failed surgical induction (of labor)

O61.8 Other failed induction of labor M ♀

O61.9 Failed induction of labor, unspecified M ♀

✓4th O62 Abnormalities of forces of labor

DEF: Uterine inertia: Weak or poorly coordinated contractions of the uterus during labor.

O62.Ø Primary inadequate contractions M ♀
Failure of cervical dilatation
Primary hypotonic uterine dysfunction
Uterine inertia during latent phase of labor

O62.1 Secondary uterine inertia M ♀
Arrested active phase of labor
Secondary hypotonic uterine dysfunction

O62.2 Other uterine inertia M ♀
Atony of uterus without hemorrhage
Atony of uterus NOS
Desultory labor
Hypotonic uterine dysfunction NOS
Irregular labor
Poor contractions
Slow slope active phase of labor
Uterine inertia NOS

EXCLUDES 1 *atony of uterus with hemorrhage (postpartum) (O72.1)*
postpartum atony of uterus without hemorrhage (O75.89)

DEF: Uterine atony: Failure of the uterine muscles to contract after the fetus and placenta are delivered.

O62.3 Precipitate labor M ♀
DEF: Rapid labor with delivery occurring in three hours or less from the onset of contractions.

O62.4 Hypertonic, incoordinate, and prolonged uterine contractions M ♀
Cervical spasm
Contraction ring dystocia
Dyscoordinate labor
Hour-glass contraction of uterus
Hypertonic uterine dysfunction
Incoordinate uterine action
Tetanic contractions
Uterine dystocia NOS
Uterine spasm

EXCLUDES 1 *dystocia (fetal) (maternal) NOS (O66.9)*

O62.8 Other abnormalities of forces of labor M ♀

O62.9 Abnormality of forces of labor, unspecified M ♀

✓4th O63 Long labor

O63.Ø Prolonged first stage (of labor) M ♀

O63.1 Prolonged second stage (of labor) M ♀

O63.2 Delayed delivery of second twin, triplet, etc. M ♀

O63.9 Long labor, unspecified CC M ♀
Prolonged labor NOS

✓4th O64 Obstructed labor due to malposition and malpresentation of fetus

One of the following 7th characters is to be assigned to each code under category O64. 7th character Ø is for single gestations and multiple gestations where the fetus is unspecified. 7th characters 1 through 9 are for cases of multiple gestations to identify the fetus for which the code applies. The appropriate code from category O3Ø, Multiple gestation, must also be assigned when assigning a code from category O64 that has a 7th character of 1 through 9.
Ø not applicable or unspecified
1 fetus 1
2 fetus 2
3 fetus 3
4 fetus 4
5 fetus 5
9 other fetus

Fetal Malposition

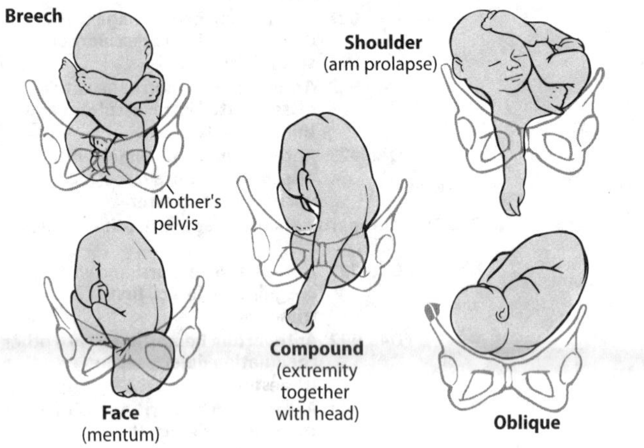

✓x7th O64.Ø Obstructed labor due to incomplete rotation of fetal head M ♀
Deep transverse arrest
Obstructed labor due to persistent occipitoiliac (position)
Obstructed labor due to persistent occipitoposterior (position)
Obstructed labor due to persistent occipitosacral (position)
Obstructed labor due to persistent occipitotransverse (position)

✓x7th O64.1 Obstructed labor due to breech presentation M ♀
Obstructed labor due to buttocks presentation
Obstructed labor due to complete breech presentation
Obstructed labor due to frank breech presentation

✓x7th O64.2 Obstructed labor due to face presentation M ♀
Obstructed labor due to chin presentation

✓x7th O64.3 Obstructed labor due to brow presentation M ♀

✓x7th O64.4 Obstructed labor due to shoulder presentation M ♀
Prolapsed arm

EXCLUDES 1 *impacted shoulders (O66.Ø)*
shoulder dystocia (O66.Ø)

✓x7th O64.5 Obstructed labor due to compound presentation M ♀

✓x7th O64.8 Obstructed labor due to other malposition and malpresentation M ♀
Obstructed labor due to footling presentation
Obstructed labor due to incomplete breech presentation

✓x7th O64.9 Obstructed labor due to malposition and malpresentation, unspecified M ♀

✓4th O65 Obstructed labor due to maternal pelvic abnormality

O65.Ø Obstructed labor due to deformed pelvis M ♀

O65.1 Obstructed labor due to generally contracted pelvis M ♀

O65.2 Obstructed labor due to pelvic inlet contraction M ♀

O65.3 Obstructed labor due to pelvic outlet and mid-cavity contraction M ♀

O65.4 Obstructed labor due to fetopelvic disproportion, unspecified M ♀

EXCLUDES 1 *dystocia due to abnormality of fetus (O66.2-O66.3)*

O65.5 Obstructed labor due to abnormality of maternal pelvic organs M ♀
Obstructed labor due to conditions listed in O34.-
Use additional code to identify abnormality of pelvic organs O34.-

O65.8 Obstructed labor due to other maternal pelvic abnormalities M ♀

O65.9 Obstructed labor due to maternal pelvic abnormality, unspecified M ♀

✓4th **O66 Other obstructed labor**

O66.Ø Obstructed labor due to shoulder dystocia M ♀
Impacted shoulders
DEF: Obstructed labor due to impacted fetal shoulders. It is an emergency condition that may require cesarean section, forceps delivery, vacuum extraction, or symphysiotomy.

O66.1 Obstructed labor due to locked twins M ♀

O66.2 Obstructed labor due to unusually large fetus M ♀

O66.3 Obstructed labor due to other abnormalities of fetus M ♀
Dystocia due to fetal ascites
Dystocia due to fetal hydrops
Dystocia due to fetal meningomyelocele
Dystocia due to fetal sacral teratoma
Dystocia due to fetal tumor
Dystocia due to hydrocephalic fetus
Use additional code to identify cause of obstruction

✓5th **O66.4 Failed trial of labor**

O66.4Ø Failed trial of labor, unspecified M ♀

O66.41 Failed attempted vaginal birth after previous cesarean delivery M ♀
Code first rupture of uterus, if applicable (O71.Ø-, O71.1)

O66.5 Attempted application of vacuum extractor and forceps M ♀
Attempted application of vacuum or forceps, with subsequent delivery by forceps or cesarean delivery

O66.6 Obstructed labor due to other multiple fetuses M ♀

O66.8 Other specified obstructed labor M ♀
Use additional code to identify cause of obstruction

O66.9 Obstructed labor, unspecified M ♀
Dystocia NOS
Fetal dystocia NOS
Maternal dystocia NOS

✓4th **O67 Labor and delivery complicated by intrapartum hemorrhage, not elsewhere classified**

EXCLUDES 1 *antepartum hemorrhage NEC (O46.-)*
placenta previa (O44.-)
premature separation of placenta [abruptio placentae] (O45.-)
EXCLUDES 2 *postpartum hemorrhage (O72.-)*

O67.Ø Intrapartum hemorrhage with coagulation defect MCC M ♀
Intrapartum hemorrhage (excessive) associated with afibrinogenemia
Intrapartum hemorrhage (excessive) associated with disseminated intravascular coagulation
Intrapartum hemorrhage (excessive) associated with hyperfibrinolysis
Intrapartum hemorrhage (excessive) associated with hypofibrinogenemia

O67.8 Other intrapartum hemorrhage M ♀
Excessive intrapartum hemorrhage

O67.9 Intrapartum hemorrhage, unspecified M ♀

O68 Labor and delivery complicated by abnormality of fetal acid-base balance CC M ♀
Fetal acidemia complicating labor and delivery
Fetal acidosis complicating labor and delivery
Fetal alkalosis complicating labor and delivery
Fetal metabolic acidemia complicating labor and delivery
EXCLUDES 1 *fetal stress NOS (O77.9)*
labor and delivery complicated by electrocardiographic evidence of fetal stress (O77.8)
labor and delivery complicated by ultrasonic evidence of fetal stress (O77.8)
EXCLUDES 2 *abnormality in fetal heart rate or rhythm (O76)*
labor and delivery complicated by meconium in amniotic fluid (O77.Ø)

✓4th **O69 Labor and delivery complicated by umbilical cord complications**
AHA: 2016,1Q,5

One of the following 7th characters is to be assigned to each code under category O69. 7th character Ø is for single gestations and multiple gestations where the fetus is unspecified. 7th characters 1 through 9 are for cases of multiple gestations to identify the fetus for which the code applies. The appropriate code from category O3Ø, Multiple gestation, must also be assigned when assigning a code from category O69 that has a 7th character of 1 through 9.
Ø not applicable or unspecified
1 fetus 1
2 fetus 2
3 fetus 3
4 fetus 4
5 fetus 5
9 other fetus

✓x7th **O69.Ø Labor and delivery complicated by prolapse of cord** M ♀
DEF: Abnormal presentation of the fetus marked by a protruding umbilical cord during labor. It can cause fetal death.

✓x7th **O69.1 Labor and delivery complicated by cord around neck, with compression** M ♀
EXCLUDES 1 *labor and delivery complicated by cord around neck, without compression (O69.81)*

✓x7th **O69.2 Labor and delivery complicated by other cord entanglement, with compression** M ♀
Labor and delivery complicated by compression of cord NOS
Labor and delivery complicated by entanglement of cords of twins in monoamniotic sac
Labor and delivery complicated by knot in cord
EXCLUDES 1 *labor and delivery complicated by other cord entanglement, without compression (O69.82)*

✓x7th **O69.3 Labor and delivery complicated by short cord** M ♀

✓x7th **O69.4 Labor and delivery complicated by vasa previa** M ♀
Labor and delivery complicated by hemorrhage from vasa previa

✓x7th **O69.5 Labor and delivery complicated by vascular lesion of cord** M ♀
Labor and delivery complicated by cord bruising
Labor and delivery complicated by cord hematoma
Labor and delivery complicated by thrombosis of umbilical vessels

✓5th **O69.8 Labor and delivery complicated by other cord complications**

✓x7th **O69.81 Labor and delivery complicated by cord around neck, without compression** M ♀
AHA: 2016,1Q,5

✓x7th **O69.82 Labor and delivery complicated by other cord entanglement, without compression** M ♀

✓x7th **O69.89 Labor and delivery complicated by other cord complications** M ♀

✓x7th **O69.9 Labor and delivery complicated by cord complication, unspecified** M ♀

✓4th **O7Ø Perineal laceration during delivery**
INCLUDES episiotomy extended by laceration
EXCLUDES 1 *obstetric high vaginal laceration alone (O71.4)*
AHA: 2016,2Q,34; 2016,1Q,3-4,5

O7Ø.Ø First degree perineal laceration during delivery M ♀
Perineal laceration, rupture or tear involving fourchette during delivery
Perineal laceration, rupture or tear involving labia during delivery
Perineal laceration, rupture or tear involving skin during delivery
Perineal laceration, rupture or tear involving vagina during delivery
Perineal laceration, rupture or tear involving vulva during delivery
Slight perineal laceration, rupture or tear during delivery

O7Ø.1 Second degree perineal laceration during delivery M ♀
Perineal laceration, rupture or tear during delivery as in O7Ø.Ø, also involving pelvic floor
Perineal laceration, rupture or tear during delivery as in O7Ø.Ø, also involving perineal muscles
Perineal laceration, rupture or tear during delivery as in O7Ø.Ø, also involving vaginal muscles
EXCLUDES 1 *perineal laceration involving anal sphincter (O7Ø.2)*

O7Ø.2 Third degree perineal laceration during delivery
Perineal laceration, rupture or tear during delivery as in O7Ø.1, also involving anal sphincter
Perineal laceration, rupture or tear during delivery as in O7Ø.1, also involving rectovaginal septum
Perineal laceration, rupture or tear during delivery as in O7Ø.1, also involving sphincter NOS
EXCLUDES 1 *anal sphincter tear during delivery without third degree perineal laceration (O7Ø.4)*
perineal laceration involving anal or rectal mucosa (O7Ø.3)
AHA: 2016,4Q,53-54

O7Ø.2Ø Third degree perineal laceration during delivery, unspecified CC M ♀

O7Ø.21 Third degree perineal laceration during delivery, IIIa CC M ♀
Third degree perineal laceration during delivery with less than 5Ø% of external anal sphincter (EAS) thickness torn

O7Ø.22 Third degree perineal laceration during delivery, IIIb CC M ♀
Third degree perineal laceration during delivery with more than 5Ø% external anal sphincter (EAS) thickness torn

O7Ø.23 Third degree perineal laceration during delivery, IIIc CC M ♀
Third degree perineal laceration during delivery with both external anal sphincter (EAS) and internal anal sphincter (IAS) torn

O7Ø.3 Fourth degree perineal laceration during delivery CC M ♀
Perineal laceration, rupture or tear during delivery as in O7Ø.2, also involving anal mucosa
Perineal laceration, rupture or tear during delivery as in O7Ø.2, also involving rectal mucosa

O7Ø.4 Anal sphincter tear complicating delivery, not associated with third degree laceration CC M ♀
EXCLUDES 1 *anal sphincter tear with third degree perineal laceration (O7Ø.2)*

O7Ø.9 Perineal laceration during delivery, unspecified M ♀

O71 Other obstetric trauma
INCLUDES obstetric damage from instruments

O71.Ø Rupture of uterus (spontaneous) before onset of labor
EXCLUDES 1 *disruption of (current) cesarean delivery wound (O9Ø.Ø)*
laceration of uterus, NEC (O71.81)

O71.ØØ Rupture of uterus before onset of labor, unspecified trimester M ♀

O71.Ø2 Rupture of uterus before onset of labor, second trimester MCC M ♀

O71.Ø3 Rupture of uterus before onset of labor, third trimester MCC M ♀

O71.1 Rupture of uterus during labor MCC M ♀
Rupture of uterus not stated as occurring before onset of labor
EXCLUDES 1 *disruption of cesarean delivery wound (O9Ø.Ø)*
laceration of uterus, NEC (O71.81)

O71.2 Postpartum inversion of uterus CC M ♀

O71.3 Obstetric laceration of cervix CC M ♀
Annular detachment of cervix

O71.4 Obstetric high vaginal laceration alone CC M ♀
Laceration of vaginal wall without perineal laceration
EXCLUDES 1 *obstetric high vaginal laceration with perineal laceration (O7Ø.-)*
AHA: 2016,1Q,5

O71.5 Other obstetric injury to pelvic organs CC M ♀
Obstetric injury to bladder
Obstetric injury to urethra
EXCLUDES 2 *obstetric periurethral trauma (O71.82)*
AHA: 2014,4Q,18

O71.6 Obstetric damage to pelvic joints and ligaments CC M ♀
Obstetric avulsion of inner symphyseal cartilage
Obstetric damage to coccyx
Obstetric traumatic separation of symphysis (pubis)

O71.7 Obstetric hematoma of pelvis CC M ♀
Obstetric hematoma of perineum
Obstetric hematoma of vagina
Obstetric hematoma of vulva

O71.8 Other specified obstetric trauma

O71.81 Laceration of uterus, not elsewhere classified M ♀

O71.82 Other specified trauma to perineum and vulva M ♀
Obstetric periurethral trauma
AHA: 2016,1Q,4; 2014,4Q,18

O71.89 Other specified obstetric trauma M ♀

O71.9 Obstetric trauma, unspecified M ♀

O72 Postpartum hemorrhage
INCLUDES hemorrhage after delivery of fetus or infant

O72.Ø Third-stage hemorrhage CC M ♀
Hemorrhage associated with retained, trapped or adherent placenta
Retained placenta NOS
Code also type of adherent placenta (O43.2-)
AHA: 2019,3Q,11

O72.1 Other immediate postpartum hemorrhage CC M ♀
Hemorrhage following delivery of placenta
Postpartum hemorrhage (atonic) NOS
Uterine atony with hemorrhage
EXCLUDES 1 *uterine atony NOS (O62.2)*
uterine atony without hemorrhage (O62.2)
postpartum atony of uterus without hemorrhage (O75.89)
AHA: 2016,1Q,4
DEF: Uterine atony: Failure of the uterine muscles to contract after the fetus and placenta are delivered.

O72.2 Delayed and secondary postpartum hemorrhage CC M ♀
Hemorrhage associated with retained portions of placenta or membranes after the first 24 hours following delivery of placenta
Retained products of conception NOS, following delivery

O72.3 Postpartum coagulation defects M ♀
Postpartum afibrinogenemia
Postpartum fibrinolysis

O73 Retained placenta and membranes, without hemorrhage
EXCLUDES 1 *placenta accreta (O43.21-)*
placenta increta (O43.22-)
placenta percreta (O43.23-)
DEF: Postpartum condition resulting from failure to expel placental membrane tissues due to failed contractions of the uterine wall.

O73.Ø Retained placenta without hemorrhage M ♀
Adherent placenta, without hemorrhage
Trapped placenta without hemorrhage

O73.1 Retained portions of placenta and membranes, without hemorrhage M ♀
Retained products of conception following delivery, without hemorrhage

O74 Complications of anesthesia during labor and delivery
INCLUDES maternal complications arising from the administration of a general, regional or local anesthetic, analgesic or other sedation during labor and delivery
Use additional code, if applicable, to identify specific complication

O74.Ø Aspiration pneumonitis due to anesthesia during labor and delivery M ♀
Inhalation of stomach contents or secretions NOS due to anesthesia during labor and delivery
Mendelson's syndrome due to anesthesia during labor and delivery

O74.1 Other pulmonary complications of anesthesia during labor and delivery M ♀

O74.2 Cardiac complications of anesthesia during labor and delivery M ♀

O74.3 Central nervous system complications of anesthesia during labor and delivery M ♀

O74.4 Toxic reaction to local anesthesia during labor and delivery M ♀

O74.5 Spinal and epidural anesthesia-induced headache during labor and delivery M ♀

O74.6 Other complications of spinal and epidural anesthesia during labor and delivery M ♀

O74.7 Failed or difficult intubation for anesthesia during labor and delivery M ♀

O74.8 Other complications of anesthesia during labor and delivery M ♀

O74.9 Complication of anesthesia during labor and delivery, unspecified M ♀

✓4th O75 Other complications of labor and delivery, not elsewhere classified

EXCLUDES 2 *puerperal (postpartum) infection (O86.-)*
puerperal (postpartum) sepsis (O85)

O75.0 Maternal distress during labor and delivery M ♀

O75.1 Shock during or following labor and delivery MCC M ♀
Obstetric shock following labor and delivery

O75.2 Pyrexia during labor, not elsewhere classified CC M ♀

O75.3 Other infection during labor MCC M ♀
Sepsis during labor
Use additional code (B95-B97), to identify infectious agent

O75.4 Other complications of obstetric surgery and procedures M ♀
Cardiac arrest following obstetric surgery or procedures
Cardiac failure following obstetric surgery or procedures
Cerebral anoxia following obstetric surgery or procedures
Pulmonary edema following obstetric surgery or procedures
Use additional code to identify specific complication
EXCLUDES 2 *complications of anesthesia during labor and delivery (O74.-)*
disruption of obstetrical (surgical) wound (O90.0-O90.1)
hematoma of obstetrical (surgical) wound (O90.2)
infection of obstetrical (surgical) wound (O86.0-)

O75.5 Delayed delivery after artificial rupture of membranes M ♀

✓5th O75.8 Other specified complications of labor and delivery

O75.81 Maternal exhaustion complicating labor and delivery M ♀

O75.82 Onset (spontaneous) of labor after 37 completed weeks of gestation but before 39 completed weeks gestation, with delivery by (planned) cesarean section M ♀
Delivery by (planned) cesarean section occurring after 37 completed weeks of gestation but before 39 completed weeks gestation due to (spontaneous) onset of labor
Code first to specify reason for planned cesarean section such as:
cephalopelvic disproportion (normally formed fetus) (O33.9)
previous cesarean delivery (O34.21)

O75.89 Other specified complications of labor and delivery M ♀

O75.9 Complication of labor and delivery, unspecified M ♀

O76 Abnormality in fetal heart rate and rhythm complicating labor and delivery M ♀
Depressed fetal heart rate tones complicating labor and delivery
Fetal bradycardia complicating labor and delivery
Fetal heart rate decelerations complicating labor and delivery
Fetal heart rate irregularity complicating labor and delivery
Fetal heart rate abnormal variability complicating labor and delivery
Fetal tachycardia complicating labor and delivery
Non-reassuring fetal heart rate or rhythm complicating labor and delivery
EXCLUDES 1 *fetal stress NOS (O77.9)*
labor and delivery complicated by electrocardiographic evidence of fetal stress (O77.8)
labor and delivery complicated by ultrasonic evidence of fetal stress (O77.8)
EXCLUDES 2 *fetal metabolic acidemia (O68)*
other fetal stress (O77.0-O77.1)
AHA: 2013,4Q,118

✓4th O77 Other fetal stress complicating labor and delivery

O77.0 Labor and delivery complicated by meconium in amniotic fluid M ♀
AHA: 2013,4Q,117-118

O77.1 Fetal stress in labor or delivery due to drug administration M ♀

O77.8 Labor and delivery complicated by other evidence of fetal stress M ♀
Labor and delivery complicated by electrocardiographic evidence of fetal stress
Labor and delivery complicated by ultrasonic evidence of fetal stress
EXCLUDES 1 *abnormality of fetal acid-base balance (O68)*
abnormality in fetal heart rate or rhythm (O76)
fetal metabolic acidemia (O68)

O77.9 Labor and delivery complicated by fetal stress, unspecified M ♀
EXCLUDES 1 *abnormality of fetal acid-base balance (O68)*
abnormality in fetal heart rate or rhythm (O76)
fetal metabolic acidemia (O68)

Encounter for delivery (O80-O82)

O80 Encounter for full-term uncomplicated delivery M ♀
NOTE Delivery requiring minimal or no assistance, with or without episiotomy, without fetal manipulation [e.g., rotation version] or instrumentation [forceps] of a spontaneous, cephalic, vaginal, full-term, single, live-born infant. This code is for use as a single diagnosis code and is not to be used with any other code from chapter 15.
Use additional code to indicate outcome of delivery (Z37.0)
AHA: 2016,4Q,150; 2014,2Q,9

O82 Encounter for cesarean delivery without indication M ♀
Use additional code to indicate outcome of delivery (Z37.0)

Complications predominantly related to the puerperium (O85-O92)

EXCLUDES 2 *mental and behavioral disorders associated with the puerperium (F53.-)*
obstetrical tetanus (A34)
puerperal osteomalacia (M83.0)

O85 Puerperal sepsis MCC M ♀
Postpartum sepsis
Puerperal peritonitis
Puerperal pyemia
Use additional code (B95-B97), to identify infectious agent
Use additional code (R65.2-) to identify severe sepsis, if applicable
EXCLUDES 1 *fever of unknown origin following delivery (O86.4)*
genital tract infection following delivery (O86.1-)
obstetric pyemic and septic embolism (O88.3-)
puerperal septic thrombophlebitis (O86.81)
urinary tract infection following delivery (O86.2-)
EXCLUDES 2 *sepsis during labor (O75.3)*
AHA: 2020,2Q,32; 2019,2Q,39; 2018,4Q,23

✓4th O86 Other puerperal infections
Use additional code (B95-B97), to identify infectious agent
EXCLUDES 2 *infection during labor (O75.3)*
obstetrical tetanus (A34)

✓5th O86.0 Infection of obstetric surgical wound
Infected cesarean delivery wound following delivery
Infected perineal repair following delivery
EXCLUDES 1 *complications of procedures, not elsewhere classified (T81.4-)*
postprocedural fever NOS (R50.82)
postprocedural retroperitoneal abscess (K68.11)
AHA: 2020,2Q,32; 2018,4Q,22-23,62

O86.00 Infection of obstetric surgical wound, unspecified M ♀

O86.01 Infection of obstetric surgical wound, superficial incisional site M ♀
Subcutaneous abscess following an obstetrical procedure
Stitch abscess following an obstetrical procedure

O86.02 Infection of obstetric surgical wound, deep incisional site M ♀
Intramuscular abscess following an obstetrical procedure
Sub-fascial abscess following an obstetrical procedure
AHA: 2020,2Q,32

O86.03 Infection of obstetric surgical wound, organ and space site M ♀
Intraabdominal abscess following an obstetrical procedure
Subphrenic abscess following an obstetrical procedure

O86.04 Sepsis following an obstetrical procedure MCC M ♀
Use additional code to identify the sepsis
AHA: 2020,2Q,32; 2019,2Q,39

O86.09 Infection of obstetric surgical wound, other surgical site M ♀

√5th **O86.1 Other infection of genital tract following delivery**

O86.11 Cervicitis following delivery CC M ♀
O86.12 Endometritis following delivery CC M ♀
O86.13 Vaginitis following delivery CC M ♀
O86.19 Other infection of genital tract following delivery CC M ♀

√5th **O86.2 Urinary tract infection following delivery**

O86.20 Urinary tract infection following delivery, unspecified CC M ♀
Puerperal urinary tract infection NOS

O86.21 Infection of kidney following delivery CC M ♀
O86.22 Infection of bladder following delivery CC M ♀
Infection of urethra following delivery

O86.29 Other urinary tract infection following delivery CC M ♀

O86.4 Pyrexia of unknown origin following delivery CC M ♀
Puerperal infection NOS following delivery
Puerperal pyrexia NOS following delivery
EXCLUDES 2 *pyrexia during labor (O75.2)*
DEF: Fever of unknown origin experienced by the mother after childbirth.

√5th **O86.8 Other specified puerperal infections**

O86.81 Puerperal septic thrombophlebitis MCC M ♀
O86.89 Other specified puerperal infections MCC M ♀

√4th **O87 Venous complications and hemorrhoids in the puerperium**

INCLUDES venous complications in labor, delivery and the puerperium
EXCLUDES 2 *obstetric embolism (O88.-)*
puerperal septic thrombophlebitis (O86.81)
venous complications in pregnancy (O22.-)

O87.0 Superficial thrombophlebitis in the puerperium CC M ♀
Puerperal phlebitis NOS
Puerperal thrombosis NOS

O87.1 Deep phlebothrombosis in the puerperium MCC M ♀
Deep vein thrombosis, postpartum
Pelvic thrombophlebitis, postpartum
Use additional code to identify the deep vein thrombosis (I82.4-, I82.5-, I82.62-. I82.72-)
Use additional code, if applicable, for associated long-term (current) use of anticoagulants (Z79.01)

O87.2 Hemorrhoids in the puerperium CC M ♀
O87.3 Cerebral venous thrombosis in the puerperium CC M ♀
Cerebrovenous sinus thrombosis in the puerperium

O87.4 Varicose veins of lower extremity in the puerperium M ♀
O87.8 Other venous complications in the puerperium CC M ♀
Genital varices in the puerperium

O87.9 Venous complication in the puerperium, unspecified M ♀
Puerperal phlebopathy NOS

√4th **O88 Obstetric embolism**

EXCLUDES 1 *embolism complicating abortion NOS (O03.2)*
embolism complicating ectopic or molar pregnancy (O08.2)
embolism complicating failed attempted abortion (O07.2)
embolism complicating induced abortion (O04.7)
embolism complicating spontaneous abortion (O03.2, O03.7)

√5th **O88.0 Obstetric air embolism**
DEF: Sudden blocking of the pulmonary artery or right ventricle with air or nitrogen bubbles.

√6th **O88.01 Obstetric air embolism in pregnancy**

O88.011 Air embolism in pregnancy, first trimester MCC M ♀
O88.012 Air embolism in pregnancy, second trimester MCC M ♀
O88.013 Air embolism in pregnancy, third trimester MCC M ♀
O88.019 Air embolism in pregnancy, unspecified trimester M ♀

O88.02 Air embolism in childbirth MCC M ♀
O88.03 Air embolism in the puerperium MCC M ♀

√5th **O88.1 Amniotic fluid embolism**
Anaphylactoid syndrome in pregnancy

√6th **O88.11 Amniotic fluid embolism in pregnancy**

O88.111 Amniotic fluid embolism in pregnancy, first trimester MCC M ♀
O88.112 Amniotic fluid embolism in pregnancy, second trimester MCC M ♀
O88.113 Amniotic fluid embolism in pregnancy, third trimester MCC M ♀
O88.119 Amniotic fluid embolism in pregnancy, unspecified trimester M ♀

O88.12 Amniotic fluid embolism in childbirth MCC M ♀
O88.13 Amniotic fluid embolism in the puerperium MCC M ♀

√5th **O88.2 Obstetric thromboembolism**

√6th **O88.21 Thromboembolism in pregnancy**
Obstetric (pulmonary) embolism NOS

O88.211 Thromboembolism in pregnancy, first trimester MCC M ♀
O88.212 Thromboembolism in pregnancy, second trimester MCC M ♀
O88.213 Thromboembolism in pregnancy, third trimester MCC M ♀
O88.219 Thromboembolism in pregnancy, unspecified trimester M ♀

O88.22 Thromboembolism in childbirth MCC M ♀
O88.23 Thromboembolism in the puerperium MCC M ♀
Puerperal (pulmonary) embolism NOS

√5th **O88.3 Obstetric pyemic and septic embolism**

√6th **O88.31 Pyemic and septic embolism in pregnancy**

O88.311 Pyemic and septic embolism in pregnancy, first trimester MCC M ♀
O88.312 Pyemic and septic embolism in pregnancy, second trimester MCC M ♀
O88.313 Pyemic and septic embolism in pregnancy, third trimester MCC M ♀
O88.319 Pyemic and septic embolism in pregnancy, unspecified trimester CC M ♀

O88.32 Pyemic and septic embolism in childbirth MCC M ♀
O88.33 Pyemic and septic embolism in the puerperium MCC M ♀

√5th **O88.8 Other obstetric embolism**
Obstetric fat embolism

√6th **O88.81 Other embolism in pregnancy**

O88.811 Other embolism in pregnancy, first trimester MCC M ♀
O88.812 Other embolism in pregnancy, second trimester MCC M ♀
O88.813 Other embolism in pregnancy, third trimester MCC M ♀
O88.819 Other embolism in pregnancy, unspecified trimester M ♀

O88.82 Other embolism in childbirth MCC M ♀
O88.83 Other embolism in the puerperium MCC M ♀

√4th **O89 Complications of anesthesia during the puerperium**

INCLUDES maternal complications arising from the administration of a general, regional or local anesthetic, analgesic or other sedation during the puerperium

Use additional code, if applicable, to identify specific complication

√5th **O89.0 Pulmonary complications of anesthesia during the puerperium**

O89.01 Aspiration pneumonitis due to anesthesia during the puerperium M ♀
Inhalation of stomach contents or secretions NOS due to anesthesia during the puerperium
Mendelson's syndrome due to anesthesia during the puerperium

O89.09 Other pulmonary complications of anesthesia during the puerperium M ♀

O89.1 Cardiac complications of anesthesia during the puerperium M ♀

O89.2 Central nervous system complications of anesthesia during the puerperium M ♀

O89.3 Toxic reaction to local anesthesia during the puerperium M ♀

O89.4 Spinal and epidural anesthesia-induced headache during the puerperium M ♀

O89.5 Other complications of spinal and epidural anesthesia during the puerperium M ♀

O89.6 Failed or difficult intubation for anesthesia during the puerperium M ♀

O89.8 Other complications of anesthesia during the puerperium M ♀

O89.9 Complication of anesthesia during the puerperium, unspecified M ♀

✓4th O90 Complications of the puerperium, not elsewhere classified

O90.0 Disruption of cesarean delivery wound M ♀
Dehiscence of cesarean delivery wound
EXCLUDES 1 *rupture of uterus (spontaneous) before onset of labor (O71.0-)*
rupture of uterus during labor (O71.1)

O90.1 Disruption of perineal obstetric wound M ♀
Disruption of wound of episiotomy
Disruption of wound of perineal laceration
Secondary perineal tear

O90.2 Hematoma of obstetric wound M ♀

O90.3 Peripartum cardiomyopathy MCC M ♀
Conditions in I42- arising during pregnancy and the puerperium
EXCLUDES 1 *pre-existing heart disease complicating pregnancy and the puerperium (O99.4-)*
DEF: Any structural or functional abnormality of the ventricular myocardium. It is a noninflammatory disease of obscure or unknown etiology with onset during the postpartum period.

O90.4 Postpartum acute kidney failure MCC M ♀
Hepatorenal syndrome following labor and delivery

O90.5 Postpartum thyroiditis M ♀

O90.6 Postpartum mood disturbance M ♀
Postpartum blues
Postpartum dysphoria
Postpartum sadness
EXCLUDES 1 *postpartum depression (F53.0)*
puerperal psychosis (F53.1)

✓5th O90.8 Other complications of the puerperium, not elsewhere classified

O90.81 Anemia of the puerperium M ♀
Postpartum anemia NOS
EXCLUDES 1 *pre-existing anemia complicating the puerperium (O99.03)*
AHA: 2019,3Q,11

O90.89 Other complications of the puerperium, not elsewhere classified M ♀
Placental polyp

O90.9 Complication of the puerperium, unspecified M ♀

✓4th O91 Infections of breast associated with pregnancy, the puerperium and lactation
Use additional code to identify infection

✓5th O91.0 Infection of nipple associated with pregnancy, the puerperium and lactation

✓6th O91.01 Infection of nipple associated with pregnancy
Gestational abscess of nipple

O91.011 Infection of nipple associated with pregnancy, first trimester M ♀

O91.012 Infection of nipple associated with pregnancy, second trimester M ♀

O91.013 Infection of nipple associated with pregnancy, third trimester M ♀

O91.019 Infection of nipple associated with pregnancy, unspecified trimester M ♀

O91.02 Infection of nipple associated with the puerperium M ♀
Puerperal abscess of nipple

O91.03 Infection of nipple associated with lactation M ♀
Abscess of nipple associated with lactation

✓5th O91.1 Abscess of breast associated with pregnancy, the puerperium and lactation

✓6th O91.11 Abscess of breast associated with pregnancy
Gestational mammary abscess
Gestational purulent mastitis
Gestational subareolar abscess

O91.111 Abscess of breast associated with pregnancy, first trimester M ♀

O91.112 Abscess of breast associated with pregnancy, second trimester M ♀

O91.113 Abscess of breast associated with pregnancy, third trimester M ♀

O91.119 Abscess of breast associated with pregnancy, unspecified trimester M ♀

O91.12 Abscess of breast associated with the puerperium M ♀
Puerperal mammary abscess
Puerperal purulent mastitis
Puerperal subareolar abscess

O91.13 Abscess of breast associated with lactation M ♀
Mammary abscess associated with lactation
Purulent mastitis associated with lactation
Subareolar abscess associated with lactation

✓5th O91.2 Nonpurulent mastitis associated with pregnancy, the puerperium and lactation

✓6th O91.21 Nonpurulent mastitis associated with pregnancy
Gestational interstitial mastitis
Gestational lymphangitis of breast
Gestational mastitis NOS
Gestational parenchymatous mastitis

O91.211 Nonpurulent mastitis associated with pregnancy, first trimester M ♀

O91.212 Nonpurulent mastitis associated with pregnancy, second trimester M ♀

O91.213 Nonpurulent mastitis associated with pregnancy, third trimester M ♀

O91.219 Nonpurulent mastitis associated with pregnancy, unspecified trimester M ♀

O91.22 Nonpurulent mastitis associated with the puerperium M ♀
Puerperal interstitial mastitis
Puerperal lymphangitis of breast
Puerperal mastitis NOS
Puerperal parenchymatous mastitis

O91.23 Nonpurulent mastitis associated with lactation M ♀
Interstitial mastitis associated with lactation
Lymphangitis of breast associated with lactation
Mastitis NOS associated with lactation
Parenchymatous mastitis associated with lactation

✓4th O92 Other disorders of breast and disorders of lactation associated with pregnancy and the puerperium

✓5th O92.0 Retracted nipple associated with pregnancy, the puerperium, and lactation

✓6th O92.01 Retracted nipple associated with pregnancy

O92.011 Retracted nipple associated with pregnancy, first trimester M ♀

O92.012 Retracted nipple associated with pregnancy, second trimester M ♀

O92.013 Retracted nipple associated with pregnancy, third trimester M ♀

O92.019 Retracted nipple associated with pregnancy, unspecified trimester M ♀

O92.02 Retracted nipple associated with the puerperium M ♀

O92.03 Retracted nipple associated with lactation M ♀

✓5th O92.1 Cracked nipple associated with pregnancy, the puerperium, and lactation
Fissure of nipple, gestational or puerperal

✓6th O92.11 Cracked nipple associated with pregnancy

O92.111 Cracked nipple associated with pregnancy, first trimester M ♀

O92.112 Cracked nipple associated with pregnancy, second trimester M ♀

O92.113 Cracked nipple associated with pregnancy, third trimester M ♀

O92.119 Cracked nipple associated with pregnancy, unspecified trimester M ♀

O92.12 **Cracked nipple associated with the puerperium** M ♀

O92.13 **Cracked nipple associated with lactation** M ♀

✓5th O92.2 **Other and unspecified disorders of breast associated with pregnancy and the puerperium**

O92.20 **Unspecified disorder of breast associated with pregnancy and the puerperium** M ♀

O92.29 **Other disorders of breast associated with pregnancy and the puerperium** M ♀

O92.3 **Agalactia** M ♀

Primary agalactia

EXCLUDES 1 *elective agalactia (O92.5)*
secondary agalactia (O92.5)
therapeutic agalactia (O92.5)

DEF: Absence of milk secretion in a female after delivery.

O92.4 **Hypogalactia** M ♀

O92.5 **Suppressed lactation** M ♀

Elective agalactia
Secondary agalactia
Therapeutic agalactia

EXCLUDES 1 *primary agalactia (O92.3)*

O92.6 **Galactorrhea** M ♀

DEF: Excessive or persistent milk secretion by the breast that may occur in the absence of nursing.

✓5th O92.7 **Other and unspecified disorders of lactation**

O92.70 **Unspecified disorders of lactation** M ♀

O92.79 **Other disorders of lactation** M ♀

Puerperal galactocele

Other obstetric conditions, not elsewhere classified (O94-O9A)

O94 **Sequelae of complication of pregnancy, childbirth, and the puerperium** M ♀

NOTE This category is to be used to indicate conditions in O00-O77.-, O85-O94 and O98-O9A.- as the cause of late effects. The sequelae include conditions specified as such, or as late effects, which may occur at any time after the puerperium

Code first condition resulting from (sequela) of complication of pregnancy, childbirth, and the puerperium

✓4th O98 **Maternal infectious and parasitic diseases classifiable elsewhere but complicating pregnancy, childbirth and the puerperium**

INCLUDES the listed conditions when complicating the pregnant state, when aggravated by the pregnancy, or as a reason for obstetric care

Use additional code (Chapter 1), to identify specific infectious or parasitic disease

EXCLUDES 2 *herpes gestationis (O26.4-)*
infectious carrier state (O99.82-, O99.83-)
obstetrical tetanus (A34)
puerperal infection (O86.-)
puerperal sepsis (O85)
when the reason for maternal care is that the disease is known or suspected to have affected the fetus (O35-O36)

✓5th O98.0 **Tuberculosis complicating pregnancy, childbirth and the puerperium**

Conditions in A15-A19

✓6th O98.01 **Tuberculosis complicating pregnancy**

O98.011 **Tuberculosis complicating pregnancy, first trimester** CC M ♀

O98.012 **Tuberculosis complicating pregnancy, second trimester** CC M ♀

O98.013 **Tuberculosis complicating pregnancy, third trimester** CC M ♀

O98.019 **Tuberculosis complicating pregnancy, unspecified trimester** M ♀

O98.02 **Tuberculosis complicating childbirth** CC M ♀

O98.03 **Tuberculosis complicating the puerperium** CC M ♀

✓5th O98.1 **Syphilis complicating pregnancy, childbirth and the puerperium**

Conditions in A50-A53

✓6th O98.11 **Syphilis complicating pregnancy**

O98.111 **Syphilis complicating pregnancy, first trimester** CC M ♀

O98.112 **Syphilis complicating pregnancy, second trimester** CC M ♀

O98.113 **Syphilis complicating pregnancy, third trimester** CC M ♀

O98.119 **Syphilis complicating pregnancy, unspecified trimester** M ♀

O98.12 **Syphilis complicating childbirth** CC M ♀

O98.13 **Syphilis complicating the puerperium** CC M ♀

✓5th O98.2 **Gonorrhea complicating pregnancy, childbirth and the puerperium**

Conditions in A54.-

✓6th O98.21 **Gonorrhea complicating pregnancy**

O98.211 **Gonorrhea complicating pregnancy, first trimester** CC M ♀

O98.212 **Gonorrhea complicating pregnancy, second trimester** CC M ♀

O98.213 **Gonorrhea complicating pregnancy, third trimester** CC M ♀

O98.219 **Gonorrhea complicating pregnancy, unspecified trimester** M ♀

O98.22 **Gonorrhea complicating childbirth** CC M ♀

O98.23 **Gonorrhea complicating the puerperium** CC M ♀

✓5th O98.3 **Other infections with a predominantly sexual mode of transmission complicating pregnancy, childbirth and the puerperium**

Conditions in A55-A64

AHA: 2020,1Q,20

✓6th O98.31 **Other infections with a predominantly sexual mode of transmission complicating pregnancy**

O98.311 **Other infections with a predominantly sexual mode of transmission complicating pregnancy, first trimester** CC M ♀

O98.312 **Other infections with a predominantly sexual mode of transmission complicating pregnancy, second trimester** CC M ♀

O98.313 **Other infections with a predominantly sexual mode of transmission complicating pregnancy, third trimester** CC M ♀

O98.319 **Other infections with a predominantly sexual mode of transmission complicating pregnancy, unspecified trimester** M ♀

O98.32 **Other infections with a predominantly sexual mode of transmission complicating childbirth** CC M ♀

O98.33 **Other infections with a predominantly sexual mode of transmission complicating the puerperium** CC M ♀

✓5th O98.4 **Viral hepatitis complicating pregnancy, childbirth and the puerperium**

Conditions in B15-B19

✓6th O98.41 **Viral hepatitis complicating pregnancy**

O98.411 **Viral hepatitis complicating pregnancy, first trimester** CC M ♀

O98.412 **Viral hepatitis complicating pregnancy, second trimester** CC M ♀

O98.413 **Viral hepatitis complicating pregnancy, third trimester** CC M ♀

O98.419 **Viral hepatitis complicating pregnancy, unspecified trimester** M ♀

O98.42 **Viral hepatitis complicating childbirth** CC M ♀

O98.43 **Viral hepatitis complicating the puerperium** CC M ♀

✓5th O98.5 **Other viral diseases complicating pregnancy, childbirth and the puerperium**

Conditions in A80-B09, B25-B34, R87.81-, R87.82-

EXCLUDES 1 *human immunodeficiency virus [HIV] disease complicating pregnancy, childbirth and the puerperium (O98.7-)*

TIP: Assign a code from this subcategory as the principal or first-listed diagnosis for a patient admitted/presenting during pregnancy, childbirth, or the puerperium because of COVID-19; assign U07.1 and codes for associated manifestations as secondary codes.

✓6th O98.51 **Other viral diseases complicating pregnancy**

O98.511 **Other viral diseases complicating pregnancy, first trimester** CC M ♀

O98.512 **Other viral diseases complicating pregnancy, second trimester** CC M ♀

O98.513 **Other viral diseases complicating pregnancy, third trimester** CC M ♀

O98.519 Other viral diseases complicating pregnancy, unspecified trimester M ♀

O98.52 Other viral diseases complicating childbirth CC M ♀

O98.53 Other viral diseases complicating the puerperium CC M ♀

√5th O98.6 Protozoal diseases complicating pregnancy, childbirth and the puerperium
Conditions in B5Ø-B64

√6th O98.61 Protozoal diseases complicating pregnancy

O98.611 Protozoal diseases complicating pregnancy, first trimester CC M ♀

O98.612 Protozoal diseases complicating pregnancy, second trimester CC M ♀

O98.613 Protozoal diseases complicating pregnancy, third trimester CC M ♀

O98.619 Protozoal diseases complicating pregnancy, unspecified trimester M ♀

O98.62 Protozoal diseases complicating childbirth CC M ♀

O98.63 Protozoal diseases complicating the puerperium CC M ♀

√5th O98.7 Human immunodeficiency virus [HIV] disease complicating pregnancy, childbirth and the puerperium
Use additional code to identify the type of HIV disease:
acquired immune deficiency syndrome (AIDS) (B2Ø)
asymptomatic HIV status (Z21)
HIV positive NOS (Z21)
symptomatic HIV disease (B2Ø)

√6th O98.71 Human immunodeficiency virus [HIV] disease complicating pregnancy

O98.711 Human immunodeficiency virus [HIV] disease complicating pregnancy, first trimester CC M ♀

O98.712 Human immunodeficiency virus [HIV] disease complicating pregnancy, second trimester CC M ♀

O98.713 Human immunodeficiency virus [HIV] disease complicating pregnancy, third trimester CC M ♀

O98.719 Human immunodeficiency virus [HIV] disease complicating pregnancy, unspecified trimester M ♀

O98.72 Human immunodeficiency virus [HIV] disease complicating childbirth CC M ♀

O98.73 Human immunodeficiency virus [HIV] disease complicating the puerperium CC M ♀

√5th O98.8 Other maternal infectious and parasitic diseases complicating pregnancy, childbirth and the puerperium
AHA: 2020,1Q,10

√6th O98.81 Other maternal infectious and parasitic diseases complicating pregnancy

O98.811 Other maternal infectious and parasitic diseases complicating pregnancy, first trimester CC M ♀

O98.812 Other maternal infectious and parasitic diseases complicating pregnancy, second trimester CC M ♀

O98.813 Other maternal infectious and parasitic diseases complicating pregnancy, third trimester CC M ♀

O98.819 Other maternal infectious and parasitic diseases complicating pregnancy, unspecified trimester M ♀

O98.82 Other maternal infectious and parasitic diseases complicating childbirth CC M ♀

O98.83 Other maternal infectious and parasitic diseases complicating the puerperium CC M ♀

√5th O98.9 Unspecified maternal infectious and parasitic disease complicating pregnancy, childbirth and the puerperium

√6th O98.91 Unspecified maternal infectious and parasitic disease complicating pregnancy

O98.911 Unspecified maternal infectious and parasitic disease complicating pregnancy, first trimester CC M ♀

O98.912 Unspecified maternal infectious and parasitic disease complicating pregnancy, second trimester CC M ♀

O98.913 Unspecified maternal infectious and parasitic disease complicating pregnancy, third trimester CC M ♀

O98.919 Unspecified maternal infectious and parasitic disease complicating pregnancy, unspecified trimester M ♀

O98.92 Unspecified maternal infectious and parasitic disease complicating childbirth CC M ♀

O98.93 Unspecified maternal infectious and parasitic disease complicating the puerperium CC M ♀

√4th **O99 Other maternal diseases classifiable elsewhere but complicating pregnancy, childbirth and the puerperium**

INCLUDES conditions which complicate the pregnant state, are aggravated by the pregnancy or are a main reason for obstetric care

Use additional code to identify specific condition

EXCLUDES 2 *when the reason for maternal care is that the condition is known or suspected to have affected the fetus (O35-O36)*

√5th O99.Ø Anemia complicating pregnancy, childbirth and the puerperium
Conditions in D5Ø-D64

EXCLUDES 1 *anemia arising in the puerperium (O9Ø.81)*
postpartum anemia NOS (O9Ø.81)

AHA: 2019,3Q,11

√6th O99.Ø1 Anemia complicating pregnancy
AHA: 2016,1Q,4

O99.Ø11 Anemia complicating pregnancy, first trimester M ♀

O99.Ø12 Anemia complicating pregnancy, second trimester M ♀

O99.Ø13 Anemia complicating pregnancy, third trimester M ♀

O99.Ø19 Anemia complicating pregnancy, unspecified trimester M ♀

O99.Ø2 Anemia complicating childbirth M ♀

O99.Ø3 Anemia complicating the puerperium M ♀

EXCLUDES 1 *postpartum anemia not pre-existing prior to delivery (O9Ø.81)*

√5th O99.1 Other diseases of the blood and blood-forming organs and certain disorders involving the immune mechanism complicating pregnancy, childbirth and the puerperium
Conditions in D65-D89

EXCLUDES 1 *hemorrhage with coagulation defects (O45.-, O46.Ø-, O67.Ø, O72.3)*

√6th O99.11 Other diseases of the blood and blood-forming organs and certain disorders involving the immune mechanism complicating pregnancy

O99.111 Other diseases of the blood and blood-forming organs and certain disorders involving the immune mechanism complicating pregnancy, first trimester CC M ♀

O99.112 Other diseases of the blood and blood-forming organs and certain disorders involving the immune mechanism complicating pregnancy, second trimester CC M ♀

O99.113 Other diseases of the blood and blood-forming organs and certain disorders involving the immune mechanism complicating pregnancy, third trimester CC M ♀

O99.119 Other diseases of the blood and blood-forming organs and certain disorders involving the immune mechanism complicating pregnancy, unspecified trimester CC M ♀

O99.12 Other diseases of the blood and blood-forming organs and certain disorders involving the immune mechanism complicating childbirth CC M ♀

O99.13 Other diseases of the blood and blood-forming organs and certain disorders involving the immune mechanism complicating the puerperium CC M ♀

✓5th **O99.2 Endocrine, nutritional and metabolic diseases complicating pregnancy, childbirth and the puerperium**
▶Conditions in EØØ-E89◀
EXCLUDES 2 *diabetes mellitus (O24.-)*
malnutrition (O25.-)
postpartum thyroiditis (O9Ø.5)

✓6th **O99.21 Obesity complicating pregnancy, childbirth, and the puerperium**
Use additional code to identify the type of obesity (E66.-)
AHA: 2018,4Q,80
TIP: Do not assign a BMI code (Z68.-) for obese or overweight patients who are pregnant.

O99.21Ø Obesity complicating pregnancy, unspecified trimester M ♀
O99.211 Obesity complicating pregnancy, first trimester M ♀
O99.212 Obesity complicating pregnancy, second trimester M ♀
O99.213 Obesity complicating pregnancy, third trimester M ♀
O99.214 Obesity complicating childbirth M ♀
O99.215 Obesity complicating the puerperium M ♀

✓6th **O99.28 Other endocrine, nutritional and metabolic diseases complicating pregnancy, childbirth and the puerperium**

O99.28Ø Endocrine, nutritional and metabolic diseases complicating pregnancy, unspecified trimester M ♀
O99.281 Endocrine, nutritional and metabolic diseases complicating pregnancy, first trimester M ♀
O99.282 Endocrine, nutritional and metabolic diseases complicating pregnancy, second trimester M ♀
O99.283 Endocrine, nutritional and metabolic diseases complicating pregnancy, third trimester M ♀
O99.284 Endocrine, nutritional and metabolic diseases complicating childbirth M ♀
O99.285 Endocrine, nutritional and metabolic diseases complicating the puerperium M ♀

✓5th **O99.3 Mental disorders and diseases of the nervous system complicating pregnancy, childbirth and the puerperium**

✓6th **O99.31 Alcohol use complicating pregnancy, childbirth, and the puerperium**
Use additional code(s) from F1Ø to identify manifestations of the alcohol use

O99.31Ø Alcohol use complicating pregnancy, unspecified trimester M ♀
O99.311 Alcohol use complicating pregnancy, first trimester M ♀
O99.312 Alcohol use complicating pregnancy, second trimester M ♀
O99.313 Alcohol use complicating pregnancy, third trimester M ♀
O99.314 Alcohol use complicating childbirth M ♀
O99.315 Alcohol use complicating the puerperium M ♀

✓6th **O99.32 Drug use complicating pregnancy, childbirth, and the puerperium**
Use additional code(s) from F11-F16 and F18-F19 to identify manifestations of the drug use
AHA: 2018,4Q,69-70; 2018,2Q,10
TIP: When drug use is documented during pregnancy, assign first a code from this subcategory followed by an additional code from F11-F16 and F18-F19 identifying the specific drug use even if not documented as associated with a physical, mental, or behavioral disorder. According to chapter 15 guidelines, it is the provider's responsibility to state that the condition being treated is *not* affecting the pregnancy.

O99.32Ø Drug use complicating pregnancy, unspecified trimester M ♀
O99.321 Drug use complicating pregnancy, first trimester CC M ♀
O99.322 Drug use complicating pregnancy, second trimester CC M ♀
O99.323 Drug use complicating pregnancy, third trimester CC M ♀
O99.324 Drug use complicating childbirth CC M ♀
O99.325 Drug use complicating the puerperium CC M ♀

✓6th **O99.33 Tobacco use disorder complicating pregnancy, childbirth, and the puerperium**
Smoking complicating pregnancy, childbirth, and the puerperium
Use additional code from category F17 to identify type of tobacco nicotine dependence

O99.33Ø Smoking (tobacco) complicating pregnancy, unspecified trimester M ♀
O99.331 Smoking (tobacco) complicating pregnancy, first trimester M ♀
O99.332 Smoking (tobacco) complicating pregnancy, second trimester M ♀
O99.333 Smoking (tobacco) complicating pregnancy, third trimester M ♀
O99.334 Smoking (tobacco) complicating childbirth M ♀
O99.335 Smoking (tobacco) complicating the puerperium M ♀

✓6th **O99.34 Other mental disorders complicating pregnancy, childbirth, and the puerperium**
▶Conditions in FØ1-FØ9, F2Ø-F52 and F54-F99◀
EXCLUDES 2 *postpartum mood disturbance (O9Ø.6)*
postnatal psychosis (F53.1)
puerperal psychosis (F53.1)

O99.34Ø Other mental disorders complicating pregnancy, unspecified trimester M ♀
O99.341 Other mental disorders complicating pregnancy, first trimester M ♀
O99.342 Other mental disorders complicating pregnancy, second trimester M ♀
O99.343 Other mental disorders complicating pregnancy, third trimester M ♀
O99.344 Other mental disorders complicating childbirth M ♀
O99.345 Other mental disorders complicating the puerperium M ♀
AHA: 2018,4Q,8

✓6th **O99.35 Diseases of the nervous system complicating pregnancy, childbirth, and the puerperium**
Conditions in GØØ-G99
EXCLUDES 2 *pregnancy related peripheral neuritis (O26.8-)*

O99.35Ø Diseases of the nervous system complicating pregnancy, unspecified trimester M ♀
O99.351 Diseases of the nervous system complicating pregnancy, first trimester M ♀
O99.352 Diseases of the nervous system complicating pregnancy, second trimester M ♀
O99.353 Diseases of the nervous system complicating pregnancy, third trimester M ♀
O99.354 Diseases of the nervous system complicating childbirth CC M ♀
O99.355 Diseases of the nervous system complicating the puerperium CC M ♀

O99.4 Diseases of the circulatory system complicating pregnancy, childbirth and the puerperium
Conditions in I00-I99
EXCLUDES 1 *peripartum cardiomyopathy (O90.3)*
EXCLUDES 2 *hypertensive disorders (O10-O16)*
obstetric embolism (O88.-)
venous complications and cerebrovenous sinus thrombosis in labor, childbirth and the puerperium (O87.-)
venous complications and cerebrovenous sinus thrombosis in pregnancy (O22.-)
AHA: 2016,2Q,8

O99.41 Diseases of the circulatory system complicating pregnancy
O99.411 Diseases of the circulatory system complicating pregnancy, first trimester CC M ♀
O99.412 Diseases of the circulatory system complicating pregnancy, second trimester CC M ♀
O99.413 Diseases of the circulatory system complicating pregnancy, third trimester CC M ♀
O99.419 Diseases of the circulatory system complicating pregnancy, unspecified trimester M ♀
O99.42 Diseases of the circulatory system complicating childbirth MCC M ♀
O99.43 Diseases of the circulatory system complicating the puerperium CC M ♀

O99.5 Diseases of the respiratory system complicating pregnancy, childbirth and the puerperium
Conditions in J00-J99

O99.51 Diseases of the respiratory system complicating pregnancy
O99.511 Diseases of the respiratory system complicating pregnancy, first trimester M ♀
O99.512 Diseases of the respiratory system complicating pregnancy, second trimester M ♀
O99.513 Diseases of the respiratory system complicating pregnancy, third trimester M ♀
O99.519 Diseases of the respiratory system complicating pregnancy, unspecified trimester M ♀
O99.52 Diseases of the respiratory system complicating childbirth M ♀
O99.53 Diseases of the respiratory system complicating the puerperium M ♀

O99.6 Diseases of the digestive system complicating pregnancy, childbirth and the puerperium
Conditions in K00-K93
EXCLUDES 2 *hemorrhoids in pregnancy (O22.4-)*
liver and biliary tract disorders in pregnancy, childbirth and the puerperium (O26.6-)

O99.61 Diseases of the digestive system complicating pregnancy
AHA: 2016,1Q,4
O99.611 Diseases of the digestive system complicating pregnancy, first trimester M ♀
O99.612 Diseases of the digestive system complicating pregnancy, second trimester M ♀
O99.613 Diseases of the digestive system complicating pregnancy, third trimester M ♀
O99.619 Diseases of the digestive system complicating pregnancy, unspecified trimester M ♀
O99.62 Diseases of the digestive system complicating childbirth M ♀
O99.63 Diseases of the digestive system complicating the puerperium M ♀

O99.7 Diseases of the skin and subcutaneous tissue complicating pregnancy, childbirth and the puerperium
Conditions in L00-L99
EXCLUDES 2 *herpes gestationis (O26.4)*
pruritic urticarial papules and plaques of pregnancy (PUPPP) (O26.86)

O99.71 Diseases of the skin and subcutaneous tissue complicating pregnancy
O99.711 Diseases of the skin and subcutaneous tissue complicating pregnancy, first trimester M ♀
O99.712 Diseases of the skin and subcutaneous tissue complicating pregnancy, second trimester M ♀
O99.713 Diseases of the skin and subcutaneous tissue complicating pregnancy, third trimester M ♀
O99.719 Diseases of the skin and subcutaneous tissue complicating pregnancy, unspecified trimester M ♀
O99.72 Diseases of the skin and subcutaneous tissue complicating childbirth M ♀
O99.73 Diseases of the skin and subcutaneous tissue complicating the puerperium M ♀

O99.8 Other specified diseases and conditions complicating pregnancy, childbirth and the puerperium
Conditions in D00-D48, H00-H95, M00-N99, and Q00-Q99
Use additional code to identify condition
EXCLUDES 2 *genitourinary infections in pregnancy (O23.-)*
infection of genitourinary tract following delivery (O86.1-O86.4)
malignant neoplasm complicating pregnancy, childbirth and the puerperium (O9A.1-)
maternal care for known or suspected abnormality of maternal pelvic organs (O34.-)
postpartum acute kidney failure (O90.4)
traumatic injuries in pregnancy (O9A.2-)

O99.81 Abnormal glucose complicating pregnancy, childbirth and the puerperium
EXCLUDES 1 *gestational diabetes (O24.4-)*
O99.810 Abnormal glucose complicating pregnancy M ♀
O99.814 Abnormal glucose complicating childbirth M ♀
O99.815 Abnormal glucose complicating the puerperium M ♀

O99.82 Streptococcus B carrier state complicating pregnancy, childbirth and the puerperium
EXCLUDES 1 *carrier of streptococcus group B (GBS) in a nonpregnant woman (Z22.330)*
DEF: *Streptococcus* group B colonization: Bacteria normally found in the vagina or lower intestine of many healthy adult women that may infect the fetus during childbirth, causing mental or physical handicaps or death. Women who test positive for *streptococcus* Group B during pregnancy are considered a "colonized" status and are treated with IV antibiotics at the time of delivery and may also be treated with oral antibiotics during the pregnancy.
O99.820 Streptococcus B carrier state complicating pregnancy M ♀
O99.824 Streptococcus B carrier state complicating childbirth M ♀
AHA: 2019,2Q,8
O99.825 Streptococcus B carrier state complicating the puerperium M ♀

O99.83 Other infection carrier state complicating pregnancy, childbirth and the puerperium
Use additional code to identify the carrier state (Z22.-)
O99.830 Other infection carrier state complicating pregnancy CC M ♀
O99.834 Other infection carrier state complicating childbirth CC M ♀
O99.835 Other infection carrier state complicating the puerperium CC M ♀

√6th **O99.84 Bariatric surgery status complicating pregnancy, childbirth and the puerperium**
Gastric banding status complicating pregnancy, childbirth and the puerperium
Gastric bypass status for obesity complicating pregnancy, childbirth and the puerperium
Obesity surgery status complicating pregnancy, childbirth and the puerperium

O99.840 Bariatric surgery status complicating pregnancy, unspecified trimester M ♀
O99.841 Bariatric surgery status complicating pregnancy, first trimester M ♀
O99.842 Bariatric surgery status complicating pregnancy, second trimester M ♀
O99.843 Bariatric surgery status complicating pregnancy, third trimester M ♀
O99.844 Bariatric surgery status complicating childbirth M ♀
O99.845 Bariatric surgery status complicating the puerperium M ♀

▲ √6th **O99.89 Other specified diseases and conditions complicating pregnancy, childbirth and the puerperium**

● **O99.891 Other specified diseases and conditions complicating pregnancy** M ♀
● **O99.892 Other specified diseases and conditions complicating childbirth** M ♀
● **O99.893 Other specified diseases and conditions complicating puerperium** M ♀

√4th **O9A Maternal malignant neoplasms, traumatic injuries and abuse classifiable elsewhere but complicating pregnancy, childbirth and the puerperium**

√5th **O9A.1 Malignant neoplasm complicating pregnancy, childbirth and the puerperium**
Conditions in C00-C96
Use additional code to identify neoplasm
EXCLUDES 2 *maternal care for benign tumor of corpus uteri (O34.1-)*
maternal care for benign tumor of cervix (O34.4-)
AHA: 2015,3Q,19

√6th **O9A.11 Malignant neoplasm complicating pregnancy**

O9A.111 Malignant neoplasm complicating pregnancy, first trimester M ♀
O9A.112 Malignant neoplasm complicating pregnancy, second trimester M ♀
O9A.113 Malignant neoplasm complicating pregnancy, third trimester M ♀
O9A.119 Malignant neoplasm complicating pregnancy, unspecified trimester M ♀

O9A.12 Malignant neoplasm complicating childbirth M ♀
O9A.13 Malignant neoplasm complicating the puerperium M ♀

√5th **O9A.2 Injury, poisoning and certain other consequences of external causes complicating pregnancy, childbirth and the puerperium**
Conditions in S00-T88, except T74 and T76
Use additional code(s) to identify the injury or poisoning
EXCLUDES 2 *physical, sexual and psychological abuse complicating pregnancy, childbirth and the puerperium (O9A.3-, O9A.4-, O9A.5-)*

√6th **O9A.21 Injury, poisoning and certain other consequences of external causes complicating pregnancy**

O9A.211 Injury, poisoning and certain other consequences of external causes complicating pregnancy, first trimester M ♀
O9A.212 Injury, poisoning and certain other consequences of external causes complicating pregnancy, second trimester M ♀
O9A.213 Injury, poisoning and certain other consequences of external causes complicating pregnancy, third trimester M ♀
O9A.219 Injury, poisoning and certain other consequences of external causes complicating pregnancy, unspecified trimester M ♀

O9A.22 Injury, poisoning and certain other consequences of external causes complicating childbirth M ♀
O9A.23 Injury, poisoning and certain other consequences of external causes complicating the puerperium M ♀

√5th **O9A.3 Physical abuse complicating pregnancy, childbirth and the puerperium**
Conditions in T74.11 or T76.11
Use additional code (if applicable):
to identify any associated current injury due to physical abuse
to identify the perpetrator of abuse (Y07.-)
EXCLUDES 2 *sexual abuse complicating pregnancy, childbirth and the puerperium (O9A.4)*

√6th **O9A.31 Physical abuse complicating pregnancy**

O9A.311 Physical abuse complicating pregnancy, first trimester M ♀
O9A.312 Physical abuse complicating pregnancy, second trimester M ♀
O9A.313 Physical abuse complicating pregnancy, third trimester M ♀
O9A.319 Physical abuse complicating pregnancy, unspecified trimester M ♀

O9A.32 Physical abuse complicating childbirth M ♀
O9A.33 Physical abuse complicating the puerperium M ♀

√5th **O9A.4 Sexual abuse complicating pregnancy, childbirth and the puerperium**
Conditions in T74.21 or T76.21
Use additional code (if applicable):
to identify any associated current injury due to sexual abuse
to identify the perpetrator of abuse (Y07.-)

√6th **O9A.41 Sexual abuse complicating pregnancy**

O9A.411 Sexual abuse complicating pregnancy, first trimester M ♀
O9A.412 Sexual abuse complicating pregnancy, second trimester M ♀
O9A.413 Sexual abuse complicating pregnancy, third trimester M ♀
O9A.419 Sexual abuse complicating pregnancy, unspecified trimester M ♀

O9A.42 Sexual abuse complicating childbirth M ♀
O9A.43 Sexual abuse complicating the puerperium M ♀

√5th **O9A.5 Psychological abuse complicating pregnancy, childbirth and the puerperium**
Conditions in T74.31 or T76.31
Use additional code to identify the perpetrator of abuse (Y07.-)

√6th **O9A.51 Psychological abuse complicating pregnancy**

O9A.511 Psychological abuse complicating pregnancy, first trimester M ♀
O9A.512 Psychological abuse complicating pregnancy, second trimester M ♀
O9A.513 Psychological abuse complicating pregnancy, third trimester M ♀
O9A.519 Psychological abuse complicating pregnancy, unspecified trimester M ♀

O9A.52 Psychological abuse complicating childbirth M ♀
O9A.53 Psychological abuse complicating the puerperium M ♀

Chapter 16. Certain Conditions Originating in the Perinatal Period (PØØ–P96)

Chapter-specific Guidelines with Coding Examples

The chapter-specific guidelines from the ICD-10-CM Official Guidelines for Coding and Reporting have been provided below. Along with these guidelines are coding examples, contained in the shaded boxes, that have been developed to help illustrate the coding and/or sequencing guidance found in these guidelines.

For coding and reporting purposes the perinatal period is defined as before birth through the 28th day following birth. The following guidelines are provided for reporting purposes

a. General perinatal rules

1) Use of Chapter 16 codes

Codes in this chapter are never for use on the maternal record. Codes from Chapter 15, the obstetric chapter, are never permitted on the newborn record. Chapter 16 codes may be used throughout the life of the patient if the condition is still present.

2) Principal diagnosis for birth record

When coding the birth episode in a newborn record, assign a code from category Z38, Liveborn infants according to place of birth and type of delivery, as the principal diagnosis. A code from category Z38 is assigned only once, to a newborn at the time of birth. If a newborn is transferred to another institution, a code from category Z38 should not be used at the receiving hospital.

A code from category Z38 is used only on the newborn record, not on the mother's record.

> Newborn delivered via vaginal delivery in Rural Hospital A, experienced meconium aspiration resulting in pneumonia. Rural Hospital A is not equipped to handle the extensive respiratory therapy this baby needs and transfers the patient to Metropolis Hospital B, where the pneumonia resolves and the newborn is eventually discharged.
>
> *Rural Hospital A*
>
> **Z38.ØØ Single liveborn infant, delivered vaginally**
>
> **P24.Ø1 Meconium aspiration with respiratory symptoms**
>
> *Metropolis Hospital B*
>
> **P24.Ø1 Meconium aspiration with respiratory symptoms**
>
> *Explanation:* A code from category Z38 is a one-time use only code. The hospital that actually delivered the newborn, in this case Rural Hospital A, can append a code from category Z38 but for the delivery admission only. Once the patient is transferred or discharged, the Z38 category no longer applies for that patient.
>
> The reason for the transfer to Metropolis Hospital B was for the respiratory symptoms (pneumonia) the newborn was exhibiting secondary to aspirating meconium.

3) Use of codes from other chapters with codes from Chapter 16

Codes from other chapters may be used with codes from chapter 16 if the codes from the other chapters provide more specific detail. Codes for signs and symptoms may be assigned when a definitive diagnosis has not been established. If the reason for the encounter is a perinatal condition, the code from chapter 16 should be sequenced first.

4) Use of Chapter 16 codes after the perinatal period

Should a condition originate in the perinatal period, and continue throughout the life of the patient, the perinatal code should continue to be used regardless of the patient's age.

> A 7-year-old patient with history of birth injury that resulted in Erb's palsy is seen for subscapularis release
>
> **P14.Ø Erb's paralysis due to birth injury**
>
> *Explanation:* Although in this instance Erb's palsy is specifically related to a birth injury, it has not resolved and continues to be a health concern. A perinatal code is appropriate even though this patient is beyond the perinatal period.

5) Birth process or community acquired conditions

If a newborn has a condition that may be either due to the birth process or community acquired and the documentation does not indicate which it is, the default is due to the birth process and the code from Chapter 16 should be used. If the condition is community-acquired, a code from Chapter 16 should not be assigned.

For COVID-19 infection in a newborn, see guideline I.C.16.h.

6) Code all clinically significant conditions

All clinically significant conditions noted on routine newborn examination should be coded. A condition is clinically significant if it requires:

clinical evaluation; or

therapeutic treatment; or

diagnostic procedures; or

extended length of hospital stay; or

increased nursing care and/or monitoring; or

has implications for future health care needs

Note: The perinatal guidelines listed above are the same as the general coding guidelines for "additional diagnoses", except for the final point regarding implications for future health care needs. Codes should be assigned for conditions that have been specified by the provider as having implications for future health care needs.

b. Observation and evaluation of newborns for suspected conditions not found

1) Use of ZØ5 codes

Assign a code from category ZØ5, Observation and evaluation of newborns and infants for suspected conditions ruled out, to identify those instances when a healthy newborn is evaluated for a suspected condition that is determined after study not to be present. Do not use a code from category ZØ5 when the patient has identified signs or symptoms of a suspected problem; in such cases code the sign or symptom.

2) ZØ5 on Other than the birth record

A code from category ZØ5 may also be assigned as a principal or first-listed code for readmissions or encounters when the code from category Z38 code no longer applies. Codes from category ZØ5 are for use only for healthy newborns and infants for which no condition after study is found to be present.

3) ZØ5 on a birth record

A code from category ZØ5 is to be used as a secondary code after the code from category Z38, Liveborn infants according to place of birth and type of delivery.

> Newborn delivered via vaginal delivery; previous ultrasounds showed what appeared to be an abnormality of the right kidney. Kidney function tests were performed and ultrasounds taken and any genitourinary conditions ruled out.
>
> **Z38.ØØ Single liveborn infant, delivered vaginally**
>
> **ZØ5.6 Observation and evaluation of newborn for suspected genitourinary condition ruled out**
>
> Explanation: The newborn had no signs or symptoms of kidney or other genitourinary condition but was evaluated after delivery due to the abnormal prenatal ultrasound findings. A Z code describing the type and place of birth should be coded first, followed by a Z05 category code for the work performed to rule out a suspected genitourinary condition.

c. Coding additional perinatal diagnoses

1) Assigning codes for conditions that require treatment

Assign codes for conditions that require treatment or further investigation, prolong the length of stay, or require resource utilization.

2) **Codes for conditions specified as having implications for future health care needs**

Assign codes for conditions that have been specified by the provider as having implications for future health care needs.

Note: This guideline should not be used for adult patients.

> An abnormal noise was heard in the left hip of a post-term newborn during a physical examination. The pediatrician would like to follow the patient after discharge as a hip click can be an early sign of hip dysplasia. The newborn was delivered via cesarean at 41 weeks.
>
> **Z38.Ø1** **Single liveborn infant, delivered by cesarean**
>
> **PØ8.21** **Post-term newborn**
>
> **R29.4** **Clicking hip**
>
> *Explanation:* The abnormal hip noise or click is appended as a secondary diagnosis not only because it is an abnormal finding upon examination, but also due to its potential to be part of a bigger health issue. The hip dysplasia has not yet been diagnosed and does not warrant a code at this time.

d. Prematurity and fetal growth retardation

Providers utilize different criteria in determining prematurity. A code for prematurity should not be assigned unless it is documented. Assignment of codes in categories PØ5, Disorders of newborn related to slow fetal growth and fetal malnutrition, and PØ7, Disorders of newborn related to short gestation and low birth weight, not elsewhere classified, should be based on the recorded birth weight and estimated gestational age.

When both birth weight and gestational age are available, two codes from category PØ7 should be assigned, with the code for birth weight sequenced before the code for gestational age.

e. Low birth weight and immaturity status

Codes from category PØ7, Disorders of newborn related to short gestation and low birth weight, not elsewhere classified, are for use for a child or adult who was premature or had a low birth weight as a newborn and this is affecting the patient's current health status.

See Section I.C.21. Factors influencing health status and contact with health services, Status.

> A 35-year-old patient, who weighed 659 grams at birth, is seen for heart disease documented as being a consequence of the low birth weight
>
> **I51.9** **Heart disease, unspecified**
>
> **PØ7.Ø2** **Extremely low birth weight newborn, 5ØØ–749 grams**
>
> *Explanation:* A code from subcategories PØ7.Ø- and PØ7.1- is appropriate, regardless of the age of the patient, as long as the documentation provides a clear link between the patient's current illness and the low birth weight.

f. Bacterial sepsis of newborn

Category P36, Bacterial sepsis of newborn, includes congenital sepsis. If a perinate is documented as having sepsis without documentation of congenital or community acquired, the default is congenital and a code from category P36 should be assigned. If the P36 code includes the causal organism, an additional code from category B95, Streptococcus, Staphylococcus, and Enterococcus as the cause of diseases classified elsewhere, or B96, Other bacterial agents as the cause of diseases classified elsewhere, should not be assigned. If the P36 code does not include the causal organism, assign an additional code from category B96. If applicable, use additional codes to identify severe sepsis (R65.2-) and any associated acute organ dysfunction.

> A full-term infant develops severe sepsis 24 hours after discharge from the hospital and is readmitted; cultures identified *E. coli* as the infective agent
>
> **P36.4** **Sepsis of newborn due to Escherichia coli**
>
> **R65.2Ø** **Severe sepsis without septic shock**
>
> *Explanation:* Even though this newborn was discharged and could have acquired *E. coli* from his/her external environment, due to the lack of documentation specifying specifically how this pathogen was acquired, the default is to code the *E. coli* sepsis as congenital. A code from chapter 1, "Certain Infectious and Parasitic Diseases," is not required because the perinatal sepsis code identifies both the sepsis and the bacteria causing the sepsis.

g. Stillbirth

Code P95, Stillbirth, is only for use in institutions that maintain separate records for stillbirths. No other code should be used with P95. Code P95 should not be used on the mother's record.

h. COVID-19 Infection in Newborn

For a newborn that tests positive for COVID-19, assign code UØ7.1, COVID-19, and the appropriate codes for associated manifestation(s) in neonates/newborns in the absence of documentation indicating a specific type of transmission. For a newborn that tests positive for COVID-19 and the provider documents the condition was contracted in utero or during the birth process, assign codes P35.8, Other congenital viral diseases, and UØ7.1, COVID-19. When coding the birth episode in a newborn record, the appropriate code from category Z38, Liveborn infants according to place of birth and type of delivery, should be assigned as the principal diagnosis.

Chapter 16. Certain Conditions Originating in the Perinatal Period (PØØ-P96)

NOTE Codes from this chapter are for use on newborn records only, never on maternal records

INCLUDES conditions that have their origin in the fetal or perinatal period (before birth through the first 28 days after birth) even if morbidity occurs later

EXCLUDES 2 *congenital malformations, deformations and chromosomal abnormalities (QØØ-Q99)*
endocrine, nutritional and metabolic diseases (EØØ-E88)
injury, poisoning and certain other consequences of external causes (SØØ-T88)
neoplasms (CØØ-D49)
tetanus neonatorum (A33)

This chapter contains the following blocks:

PØØ-PØ4 Newborn affected by maternal factors and by complications of pregnancy, labor, and delivery
PØ5-PØ8 Disorders of newborn related to length of gestation and fetal growth
PØ9 Abnormal findings on neonatal screening
P1Ø-P15 Birth trauma
P19-P29 Respiratory and cardiovascular disorders specific to the perinatal period
P35-P39 Infections specific to the perinatal period
P5Ø-P61 Hemorrhagic and hematological disorders of newborn
P7Ø-P74 Transitory endocrine and metabolic disorders specific to newborn
P76-P78 Digestive system disorders of newborn
P8Ø-P83 Conditions involving the integument and temperature regulation of newborn
P84 Other problems with newborn
P9Ø-P96 Other disorders originating in the perinatal period

Newborn affected by maternal factors and by complications of pregnancy, labor, and delivery (PØØ-PØ4)

NOTE These codes are for use when the listed maternal conditions are specified as the cause of confirmed morbidity or potential morbidity which have their origin in the perinatal period (before birth through the first 28 days after birth).

AHA: 2016,4Q,54-55

✓4th **PØØ Newborn affected by maternal conditions that may be unrelated to present pregnancy**
Code first any current condition in newborn
EXCLUDES 2 *encounter for observation of newborn for suspected diseases and conditions ruled out (ZØ5.-)*
newborn affected by maternal complications of pregnancy (PØ1.-)
newborn affected by maternal endocrine and metabolic disorders (P7Ø-P74)
newborn affected by noxious substances transmitted via placenta or breast milk (PØ4.-)

PØØ.Ø Newborn affected by maternal hypertensive disorders
Newborn affected by maternal conditions classifiable to O1Ø-O11, O13-O16

PØØ.1 Newborn affected by maternal renal and urinary tract diseases
Newborn affected by maternal conditions classifiable to NØØ-N39

PØØ.2 Newborn affected by maternal infectious and parasitic diseases
Newborn affected by maternal infectious disease classifiable to AØØ-B99, JØ9 and J1Ø
EXCLUDES 1 *maternal genital tract or other localized infections (PØØ.8)*
EXCLUDES 2 *infections specific to the perinatal period (P35-P39)*
AHA: 2019,2Q,10; 2015,3Q,20

PØØ.3 Newborn affected by other maternal circulatory and respiratory diseases
Newborn affected by maternal conditions classifiable to IØØ-I99, JØØ-J99, Q2Ø-Q34 and not included in PØØ.Ø, PØØ.2

PØØ.4 Newborn affected by maternal nutritional disorders
Newborn affected by maternal disorders classifiable to E4Ø-E64
Maternal malnutrition NOS

PØØ.5 Newborn affected by maternal injury
Newborn affected by maternal conditions classifiable to O9A.2-

PØØ.6 Newborn affected by surgical procedure on mother
Newborn affected by amniocentesis
EXCLUDES 1 *Cesarean delivery for present delivery (PØ3.4)*
damage to placenta from amniocentesis, Cesarean delivery or surgical induction (PØ2.1)
previous surgery to uterus or pelvic organs (PØ3.89)
EXCLUDES 2 *newborn affected by complication of (fetal) intrauterine procedure (P96.5)*

PØØ.7 Newborn affected by other medical procedures on mother, not elsewhere classified
Newborn affected by radiation to mother
EXCLUDES 1 *damage to placenta from amniocentesis, cesarean delivery or surgical induction (PØ2.1)*
newborn affected by other complications of labor and delivery (PØ3.-)

✓5th **PØØ.8 Newborn affected by other maternal conditions**

PØØ.81 Newborn affected by periodontal disease in mother

PØØ.89 Newborn affected by other maternal conditions
Newborn affected by conditions classifiable to T8Ø-T88
Newborn affected by maternal genital tract or other localized infections
Newborn affected by maternal systemic lupus erythematosus
►Use additional code to identify infectious agent, if known◄
AHA: 2019,2Q,9

PØØ.9 Newborn affected by unspecified maternal condition

✓4th **PØ1 Newborn affected by maternal complications of pregnancy**
Code first any current condition in newborn
EXCLUDES 2 *encounter for observation of newborn for suspected diseases and conditions ruled out (ZØ5.-)*

PØ1.Ø Newborn affected by incompetent cervix

PØ1.1 Newborn affected by premature rupture of membranes

PØ1.2 Newborn affected by oligohydramnios
EXCLUDES 1 *oligohydramnios due to premature rupture of membranes (PØ1.1)*
DEF: Oligohydramnios: Low amniotic fluid level, resulting in underdeveloped organs in the fetus.

PØ1.3 Newborn affected by polyhydramnios
Newborn affected by hydramnios
DEF: Polyhydramnios: Excess amniotic fluid surrounding the fetus, typically defined as a total fluid volume of greater than 24.0 cc.

PØ1.4 Newborn affected by ectopic pregnancy
Newborn affected by abdominal pregnancy

PØ1.5 Newborn affected by multiple pregnancy
Newborn affected by triplet (pregnancy)
Newborn affected by twin (pregnancy)

PØ1.6 Newborn affected by maternal death

PØ1.7 Newborn affected by malpresentation before labor
Newborn affected by breech presentation before labor
Newborn affected by external version before labor
Newborn affected by face presentation before labor
Newborn affected by transverse lie before labor
Newborn affected by unstable lie before labor

PØ1.8 Newborn affected by other maternal complications of pregnancy

PØ1.9 Newborn affected by maternal complication of pregnancy, unspecified

✓4th **PØ2 Newborn affected by complications of placenta, cord and membranes**
Code first any current condition in newborn
EXCLUDES 2 *encounter for observation of newborn for suspected diseases and conditions ruled out (ZØ5.-)*

PØ2.Ø Newborn affected by placenta previa
DEF: Placenta developed in the lower segment of the uterus that can cause hemorrhaging leading to preterm delivery.

PØ2.1 Newborn affected by other forms of placental separation and hemorrhage
Newborn affected by abruptio placenta
Newborn affected by accidental hemorrhage
Newborn affected by antepartum hemorrhage
Newborn affected by damage to placenta from amniocentesis, cesarean delivery or surgical induction
Newborn affected by maternal blood loss
Newborn affected by premature separation of placenta

✓5th **P02.2 Newborn affected by other and unspecified morphological and functional abnormalities of placenta**

P02.20 Newborn affected by unspecified morphological and functional abnormalities of placenta

P02.29 Newborn affected by other morphological and functional abnormalities of placenta
Newborn affected by placental dysfunction
Newborn affected by placental infarction
Newborn affected by placental insufficiency

P02.3 Newborn affected by placental transfusion syndromes
Newborn affected by placental and cord abnormalities resulting in twin-to-twin or other transplacental transfusion

P02.4 Newborn affected by prolapsed cord

P02.5 Newborn affected by other compression of umbilical cord
Newborn affected by umbilical cord (tightly) around neck
Newborn affected by entanglement of umbilical cord
Newborn affected by knot in umbilical cord

✓5th **P02.6 Newborn affected by other and unspecified conditions of umbilical cord**

P02.60 Newborn affected by unspecified conditions of umbilical cord

P02.69 Newborn affected by other conditions of umbilical cord
Newborn affected by short umbilical cord
Newborn affected by vasa previa
EXCLUDES 1 *newborn affected by single umbilical artery (Q27.0)*

✓5th **P02.7 Newborn affected by chorioamnionitis**
AHA: 2018,4Q,23-24
DEF: Inflammation of the fetal membranes due to maternal infection characterized by fetal tachycardia, respiratory distress, apnea, weak cries, and poor sucking.

P02.70 Newborn affected by fetal inflammatory response syndrome HCC
Newborn affected by FIRS

P02.78 Newborn affected by other conditions from chorioamnionitis
Newborn affected by amnionitis
Newborn affected by membranitis
Newborn affected by placentitis

P02.8 Newborn affected by other abnormalities of membranes

P02.9 Newborn affected by abnormality of membranes, unspecified

✓4th **P03 Newborn affected by other complications of labor and delivery**
Code first any current condition in newborn
EXCLUDES 2 *encounter for observation of newborn for suspected diseases and conditions ruled out (Z05.-)*

P03.0 Newborn affected by breech delivery and extraction

P03.1 Newborn affected by other malpresentation, malposition and disproportion during labor and delivery
Newborn affected by contracted pelvis
Newborn affected by conditions classifiable to O64-O66
Newborn affected by persistent occipitoposterior
Newborn affected by transverse lie

P03.2 Newborn affected by forceps delivery

Forceps Assisted Birth

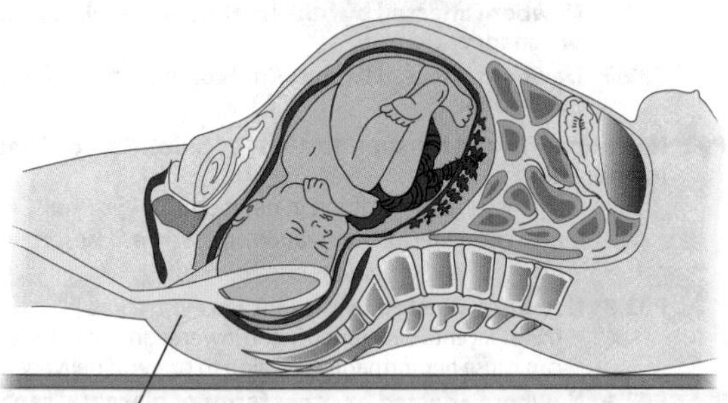

P03.3 Newborn affected by delivery by vacuum extractor [ventouse]

Vacuum Assisted Birth

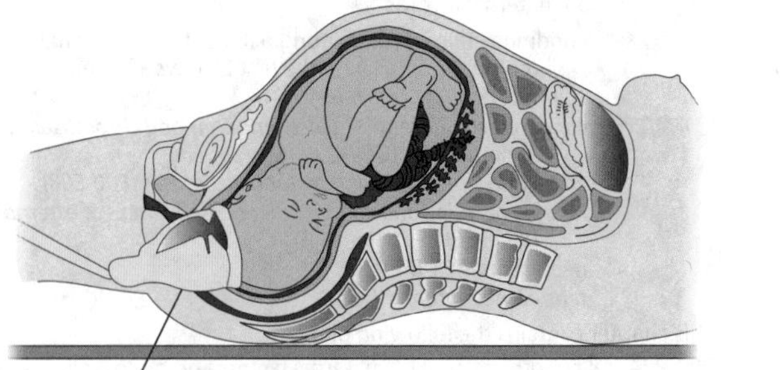

P03.4 Newborn affected by Cesarean delivery

P03.5 Newborn affected by precipitate delivery
Newborn affected by rapid second stage

P03.6 Newborn affected by abnormal uterine contractions
Newborn affected by conditions classifiable to O62.-, except O62.3
Newborn affected by hypertonic labor
Newborn affected by uterine inertia

✓5th **P03.8 Newborn affected by other specified complications of labor and delivery**

✓6th **P03.81 Newborn affected by abnormality in fetal (intrauterine) heart rate or rhythm**
EXCLUDES 1 *neonatal cardiac dysrhythmia (P29.1-)*

P03.810 Newborn affected by abnormality in fetal (intrauterine) heart rate or rhythm before the onset of labor

P03.811 Newborn affected by abnormality in fetal (intrauterine) heart rate or rhythm during labor

P03.819 Newborn affected by abnormality in fetal (intrauterine) heart rate or rhythm, unspecified as to time of onset

P03.82 Meconium passage during delivery
EXCLUDES 1 *meconium aspiration (P24.00, P24.01)*
meconium staining (P96.83)
DEF: Fetal intestinal activity that increases in response to a fetomaternal distressed state during delivery. The anal sphincter relaxes and meconium is passed into the amniotic fluid.

P03.89 Newborn affected by other specified complications of labor and delivery
Newborn affected by abnormality of maternal soft tissues
Newborn affected by conditions classifiable to O60-O75 and by procedures used in labor and delivery not included in P02.- and P03.0-P03.6
Newborn affected by induction of labor

P03.9 Newborn affected by complication of labor and delivery, unspecified

✓4th **P04 Newborn affected by noxious substances transmitted via placenta or breast milk**
INCLUDES nonteratogenic effects of substances transmitted via placenta
EXCLUDES 2 *congenital malformations (Q00-Q99)*
encounter for observation of newborn for suspected diseases and conditions ruled out (Z05.-)
neonatal jaundice from excessive hemolysis due to drugs or toxins transmitted from mother (P58.4)
newborn in contact with and (suspected) exposures hazardous to health not transmitted via placenta or breast milk (Z77.-)

P04.0 Newborn affected by maternal anesthesia and analgesia in pregnancy, labor and delivery
Newborn affected by reactions and intoxications from maternal opiates and tranquilizers administered for procedures during pregnancy or labor and delivery
EXCLUDES 2 *newborn affected by other maternal medication (P04.1-)*

✓5th **P04.1 Newborn affected by other maternal medication**

Code first withdrawal symptoms from maternal use of drugs of addiction, if applicable (P96.1)

EXCLUDES 1 *dysmorphism due to warfarin (Q86.2)*
fetal hydantoin syndrome (Q86.1)

EXCLUDES 2 *maternal anesthesia and analgesia in pregnancy, labor and delivery (P04.0)*
maternal use of drugs of addiction (P04.4-)

AHA: 2018,4Q,24-25

P04.11 Newborn affected by maternal antineoplastic chemotherapy
P04.12 Newborn affected by maternal cytotoxic drugs
P04.13 Newborn affected by maternal use of anticonvulsants
P04.14 Newborn affected by maternal use of opiates
P04.15 Newborn affected by maternal use of antidepressants
P04.16 Newborn affected by maternal use of amphetamines
P04.17 Newborn affected by maternal use of sedative-hypnotics
P04.1A Newborn affected by maternal use of anxiolytics
P04.18 Newborn affected by other maternal medication
P04.19 Newborn affected by maternal use of unspecified medication

P04.2 Newborn affected by maternal use of tobacco

Newborn affected by exposure in utero to tobacco smoke

EXCLUDES 2 *newborn exposure to environmental tobacco smoke (P96.81)*

P04.3 Newborn affected by maternal use of alcohol

EXCLUDES 1 *fetal alcohol syndrome (Q86.0)*

✓5th **P04.4 Newborn affected by maternal use of drugs of addiction**

AHA: 2018,4Q,25

P04.40 Newborn affected by maternal use of unspecified drugs of addiction
P04.41 Newborn affected by maternal use of cocaine
P04.42 Newborn affected by maternal use of hallucinogens

EXCLUDES 2 *newborn affected by other maternal medication (P04.1-)*

P04.49 Newborn affected by maternal use of other drugs of addiction

EXCLUDES 2 *newborn affected by maternal anesthesia and analgesia (P04.0)*
withdrawal symptoms from maternal use of drugs of addiction (P96.1)

P04.5 Newborn affected by maternal use of nutritional chemical substances

P04.6 Newborn affected by maternal exposure to environmental chemical substances

✓5th **P04.8 Newborn affected by other maternal noxious substances**

AHA: 2018,4Q,25

P04.81 Newborn affected by maternal use of cannabis
P04.89 Newborn affected by other maternal noxious substances

P04.9 Newborn affected by maternal noxious substance, unspecified

Disorders of newborn related to length of gestation and fetal growth (P05-P08)

✓4th **P05 Disorders of newborn related to slow fetal growth and fetal malnutrition**

AHA: 2016,4Q,55-56

✓5th **P05.0 Newborn light for gestational age**

Newborn light-for-dates
Weight below but length above 10th percentile for gestational age

P05.00 Newborn light for gestational age, unspecified weight
P05.01 Newborn light for gestational age, less than 500 grams
P05.02 Newborn light for gestational age, 500-749 grams
P05.03 Newborn light for gestational age, 750-999 grams
P05.04 Newborn light for gestational age, 1000-1249 grams
P05.05 Newborn light for gestational age, 1250-1499 grams
P05.06 Newborn light for gestational age, 1500-1749 grams
P05.07 Newborn light for gestational age, 1750-1999 grams
P05.08 Newborn light for gestational age, 2000-2499 grams
P05.09 Newborn light for gestational age, 2500 grams and over

Newborn light for gestational age, other

✓5th **P05.1 Newborn small for gestational age**

Newborn small-and-light-for-dates
Newborn small-for-dates
Weight and length below 10th percentile for gestational age

P05.10 Newborn small for gestational age, unspecified weight
P05.11 Newborn small for gestational age, less than 500 grams
P05.12 Newborn small for gestational age, 500-749 grams
P05.13 Newborn small for gestational age, 750-999 grams
P05.14 Newborn small for gestational age, 1000-1249 grams
P05.15 Newborn small for gestational age, 1250-1499 grams
P05.16 Newborn small for gestational age, 1500-1749 grams
P05.17 Newborn small for gestational age, 1750-1999 grams
P05.18 Newborn small for gestational age, 2000-2499 grams
P05.19 Newborn small for gestational age, other

Newborn small for gestational age, 2500 grams and over

P05.2 Newborn affected by fetal (intrauterine) malnutrition not light or small for gestational age

Infant, not light or small for gestational age, showing signs of fetal malnutrition, such as dry, peeling skin and loss of subcutaneous tissue

EXCLUDES 1 *newborn affected by fetal malnutrition with light for gestational age (P05.0-)*
newborn affected by fetal malnutrition with small for gestational age (P05.1-)

P05.9 Newborn affected by slow intrauterine growth, unspecified

Newborn affected by fetal growth retardation NOS

✓4th **P07 Disorders of newborn related to short gestation and low birth weight, not elsewhere classified**

NOTE When both birth weight and gestational age of the newborn are available, both should be coded with birth weight sequenced before gestational age

INCLUDES the listed conditions, without further specification, as the cause of morbidity or additional care, in newborn

✓5th **P07.0 Extremely low birth weight newborn**

Newborn birth weight 999 g. or less

EXCLUDES 1 *low birth weight due to slow fetal growth and fetal malnutrition (P05.-)*

P07.00 Extremely low birth weight newborn, unspecified weight
P07.01 Extremely low birth weight newborn, less than 500 grams
P07.02 Extremely low birth weight newborn, 500-749 grams
P07.03 Extremely low birth weight newborn, 750-999 grams

✓5th **P07.1 Other low birth weight newborn**

Newborn birth weight 1000-2499 g.

EXCLUDES 1 *low birth weight due to slow fetal growth and fetal malnutrition (P05.-)*

P07.10 Other low birth weight newborn, unspecified weight
P07.14 Other low birth weight newborn, 1000-1249 grams
P07.15 Other low birth weight newborn, 1250-1499 grams
P07.16 Other low birth weight newborn, 1500-1749 grams
P07.17 Other low birth weight newborn, 1750-1999 grams
P07.18 Other low birth weight newborn, 2000-2499 grams

✓5th **P07.2 Extreme immaturity of newborn**

Less than 28 completed weeks (less than 196 completed days) of gestation.

P07.20 Extreme immaturity of newborn, unspecified weeks of gestation

Gestational age less than 28 completed weeks NOS

P07.21 Extreme immaturity of newborn, gestational age less than 23 completed weeks
Extreme immaturity of newborn, gestational age less than 23 weeks, 0 days

P07.22 Extreme immaturity of newborn, gestational age 23 completed weeks
Extreme immaturity of newborn, gestational age 23 weeks, 0 days through 23 weeks, 6 days

P07.23 Extreme immaturity of newborn, gestational age 24 completed weeks
Extreme immaturity of newborn, gestational age 24 weeks, 0 days through 24 weeks, 6 days

P07.24 Extreme immaturity of newborn, gestational age 25 completed weeks
Extreme immaturity of newborn, gestational age 25 weeks, 0 days through 25 weeks, 6 days

P07.25 Extreme immaturity of newborn, gestational age 26 completed weeks
Extreme immaturity of newborn, gestational age 26 weeks, 0 days through 26 weeks, 6 days

P07.26 Extreme immaturity of newborn, gestational age 27 completed weeks
Extreme immaturity of newborn, gestational age 27 weeks, 0 days through 27 weeks, 6 days

✓5th **P07.3 Preterm [premature] newborn [other]**
28 completed weeks or more but less than 37 completed weeks (196 completed days but less than 259 completed days) of gestation
Prematurity NOS
AHA: 2017,3Q,26

P07.30 Preterm newborn, unspecified weeks of gestation

P07.31 Preterm newborn, gestational age 28 completed weeks
Preterm newborn, gestational age 28 weeks, 0 days through 28 weeks, 6 days

P07.32 Preterm newborn, gestational age 29 completed weeks
Preterm newborn, gestational age 29 weeks, 0 days through 29 weeks, 6 days

P07.33 Preterm newborn, gestational age 30 completed weeks
Preterm newborn, gestational age 30 weeks, 0 days through 30 weeks, 6 days

P07.34 Preterm newborn, gestational age 31 completed weeks
Preterm newborn, gestational age 31 weeks, 0 days through 31 weeks, 6 days

P07.35 Preterm newborn, gestational age 32 completed weeks
Preterm newborn, gestational age 32 weeks, 0 days through 32 weeks, 6 days

P07.36 Preterm newborn, gestational age 33 completed weeks
Preterm newborn, gestational age 33 weeks, 0 days through 33 weeks, 6 days

P07.37 Preterm newborn, gestational age 34 completed weeks
Preterm newborn, gestational age 34 weeks, 0 days through 34 weeks, 6 days

P07.38 Preterm newborn, gestational age 35 completed weeks
Preterm newborn, gestational age 35 weeks, 0 days through 35 weeks, 6 days

P07.39 Preterm newborn, gestational age 36 completed weeks
Preterm newborn, gestational age 36 weeks, 0 days through 36 weeks, 6 days

✓4th **P08 Disorders of newborn related to long gestation and high birth weight**

NOTE When both birth weight and gestational age of the newborn are available, priority of assignment should be given to birth weight

INCLUDES the listed conditions, without further specification, as causes of morbidity or additional care, in newborn

P08.0 Exceptionally large newborn baby
Usually implies a birth weight of 4500 g. or more
EXCLUDES 1 *syndrome of infant of diabetic mother (P70.1)*
syndrome of infant of mother with gestational diabetes (P70.0)

P08.1 Other heavy for gestational age newborn
Other newborn heavy- or large-for-dates regardless of period of gestation
Usually implies a birth weight of 4000 g. to 4499 g.
EXCLUDES 1 *newborn with a birth weight of 4500 or more (P08.0)*
syndrome of infant of diabetic mother (P70.1)
syndrome of infant of mother with gestational diabetes (P70.0).

✓5th **P08.2 Late newborn, not heavy for gestational age**
AHA: 2014,1Q,14

P08.21 Post-term newborn
Newborn with gestation period over 40 completed weeks to 42 completed weeks

P08.22 Prolonged gestation of newborn
Newborn with gestation period over 42 completed weeks (294 days or more), not heavy- or large-for-dates.
Postmaturity NOS

Abnormal findings on neonatal screening (P09)

P09 Abnormal findings on neonatal screening
Use additional code to identify signs, symptoms and conditions associated with the screening
EXCLUDES 2 *nonspecific serologic evidence of human immunodeficiency virus [HIV] (R75)*

Birth trauma (P10-P15)

✓4th **P10 Intracranial laceration and hemorrhage due to birth injury**
EXCLUDES 1 *intracranial hemorrhage of newborn NOS (P52.9)*
intracranial hemorrhage of newborn due to anoxia or hypoxia (P52.-)
nontraumatic intracranial hemorrhage of newborn (P52.-)

P10.0 Subdural hemorrhage due to birth injury MCC
Subdural hematoma (localized) due to birth injury
EXCLUDES 1 *subdural hemorrhage accompanying tentorial tear (P10.4)*

P10.1 Cerebral hemorrhage due to birth injury MCC

P10.2 Intraventricular hemorrhage due to birth injury CC

P10.3 Subarachnoid hemorrhage due to birth injury MCC

P10.4 Tentorial tear due to birth injury MCC

P10.8 Other intracranial lacerations and hemorrhages due to birth injury MCC

P10.9 Unspecified intracranial laceration and hemorrhage due to birth injury MCC

✓4th **P11 Other birth injuries to central nervous system**

P11.0 Cerebral edema due to birth injury MCC

P11.1 Other specified brain damage due to birth injury

P11.2 Unspecified brain damage due to birth injury MCC

P11.3 Birth injury to facial nerve
Facial palsy due to birth injury

P11.4 Birth injury to other cranial nerves

P11.5 Birth injury to spine and spinal cord
Fracture of spine due to birth injury

P11.9 Birth injury to central nervous system, unspecified MCC

P12 Birth injury to scalp

Birth Injuries to Scalp

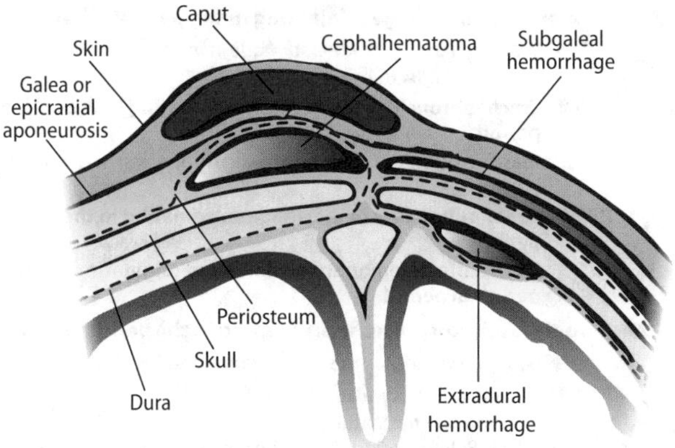

P12.Ø Cephalhematoma due to birth injury
DEF: Condition that occurs in a neonate when blood vessels between the skull and periosteum rupture and blood collects in the subperiosteal space (below the periosteum). It is typically caused by prolonged labor or trauma due to instrument-assisted delivery (e.g., forceps, vacuum extraction), although in rare circumstances, it may indicate a linear skull fracture with intracranial hemorrhage.

P12.1 Chignon (from vacuum extraction) due to birth injury
DEF: Artificial swelling of the scalp that occurs when a collection of interstitial fluid and blood forms in the area of the scalp where the suction cup was applied during a vacuum-assisted delivery.

P12.2 Epicranial subaponeurotic hemorrhage due to birth injury CC
Subgaleal hemorrhage

P12.3 Bruising of scalp due to birth injury

P12.4 Injury of scalp of newborn due to monitoring equipment
Sampling incision of scalp of newborn
Scalp clip (electrode) injury of newborn

P12.8 Other birth injuries to scalp

P12.81 Caput succedaneum
DEF: Swelling of the scalp as a result of pressure being exerted on the head from the vaginal walls, uterus, or instrumentation used in assisting a delivery (e.g., vacuum).

P12.89 Other birth injuries to scalp

P12.9 Birth injury to scalp, unspecified

P13 Birth injury to skeleton
EXCLUDES 2 *birth injury to spine (P11.5)*

P13.Ø Fracture of skull due to birth injury

P13.1 Other birth injuries to skull
EXCLUDES 1 *cephalhematoma (P12.Ø)*

P13.2 Birth injury to femur

P13.3 Birth injury to other long bones

P13.4 Fracture of clavicle due to birth injury

P13.8 Birth injuries to other parts of skeleton

P13.9 Birth injury to skeleton, unspecified

P14 Birth injury to peripheral nervous system

P14.Ø Erb's paralysis due to birth injury
DEF: Erb's paralysis: Most common type of brachial plexus (peripheral nerve) injury in a neonate that involves nerve damage at the level of C5-C6. ***Synonym(s):*** *Erb's palsy*

P14.1 Klumpke's paralysis due to birth injury

P14.2 Phrenic nerve paralysis due to birth injury

P14.3 Other brachial plexus birth injuries

P14.8 Birth injuries to other parts of peripheral nervous system

P14.9 Birth injury to peripheral nervous system, unspecified

P15 Other birth injuries

P15.Ø Birth injury to liver
Rupture of liver due to birth injury

P15.1 Birth injury to spleen
Rupture of spleen due to birth injury

P15.2 Sternomastoid injury due to birth injury

P15.3 Birth injury to eye
Subconjunctival hemorrhage due to birth injury
Traumatic glaucoma due to birth injury

P15.4 Birth injury to face
Facial congestion due to birth injury

P15.5 Birth injury to external genitalia

P15.6 Subcutaneous fat necrosis due to birth injury

P15.8 Other specified birth injuries

P15.9 Birth injury, unspecified

Respiratory and cardiovascular disorders specific to the perinatal period (P19-P29)

P19 Metabolic acidemia in newborn
INCLUDES metabolic acidemia in newborn

P19.Ø Metabolic acidemia in newborn first noted before onset of labor

P19.1 Metabolic acidemia in newborn first noted during labor

P19.2 Metabolic acidemia noted at birth

P19.9 Metabolic acidemia, unspecified

P22 Respiratory distress of newborn
AHA: 2019,2Q,29

P22.Ø Respiratory distress syndrome of newborn MCC
Cardiorespiratory distress syndrome of newborn
Hyaline membrane disease
Idiopathic respiratory distress syndrome [IRDS or RDS] of newborn
Pulmonary hypoperfusion syndrome
Respiratory distress syndrome, type I
EXCLUDES 2 *respiratory arrest of newborn (P28.81)*
respiratory failure of newborn NOS (P28.5)
AHA: 2019,2Q,29
DEF: Severe chest contractions upon air intake and expiratory grunting. The infant appears blue due to oxygen deficiency and has a rapid respiratory rate, formerly called hyaline membrane disease.

P22.1 Transient tachypnea of newborn
Idiopathic tachypnea of newborn
Respiratory distress syndrome, type II
Wet lung syndrome
DEF: Rapid, labored breathing of a newborn. It is a short-term problem that begins after birth and lasts about three days.

P22.8 Other respiratory distress of newborn
EXCLUDES 1 *respiratory arrest of newborn (P28.81)*
respiratory failure of newborn NOS (P28.5)

P22.9 Respiratory distress of newborn, unspecified
EXCLUDES 1 *respiratory arrest of newborn (P28.81)*
respiratory failure of newborn NOS (P28.5)

P23 Congenital pneumonia
INCLUDES infective pneumonia acquired in utero or during birth
EXCLUDES 1 *neonatal pneumonia resulting from aspiration (P24.-)*

P23.Ø Congenital pneumonia due to viral agent MCC
Use additional code (B97) to identify organism
EXCLUDES 1 *congenital rubella pneumonitis (P35.Ø)*

P23.1 Congenital pneumonia due to Chlamydia MCC

P23.2 Congenital pneumonia due to staphylococcus MCC

P23.3 Congenital pneumonia due to streptococcus, group B MCC

P23.4 Congenital pneumonia due to Escherichia coli MCC

P23.5 Congenital pneumonia due to Pseudomonas MCC

P23.6 Congenital pneumonia due to other bacterial agents MCC
Congenital pneumonia due to Hemophilus influenzae
Congenital pneumonia due to Klebsiella pneumoniae
Congenital pneumonia due to Mycoplasma
Congenital pneumonia due to Streptococcus, except group B
Use additional code (B95-B96) to identify organism

P23.8 Congenital pneumonia due to other organisms MCC

P23.9 Congenital pneumonia, unspecified MCC

P24 Neonatal aspiration

INCLUDES aspiration in utero and during delivery

P24.0 Meconium aspiration

EXCLUDES 1 *meconium passage (without aspiration) during delivery (P03.82)*
meconium staining (P96.83)

DEF: Meconium in the trachea or seen on chest x-ray after birth.

P24.00 Meconium aspiration without respiratory symptoms
Meconium aspiration NOS

P24.01 Meconium aspiration with respiratory symptoms MCC
Meconium aspiration pneumonia
Meconium aspiration pneumonitis
Meconium aspiration syndrome NOS
Use additional code to identify any secondary pulmonary hypertension, if applicable (I27.2-)
DEF: Aspiration of fetal intestinal material during or prior to delivery. If is usually a complication of placental insufficiency, causing pneumonitis and bronchial obstruction (inflammatory reaction of lungs).

P24.1 Neonatal aspiration of (clear) amniotic fluid and mucus
Neonatal aspiration of liquor (amnii)

P24.10 Neonatal aspiration of (clear) amniotic fluid and mucus without respiratory symptoms
Neonatal aspiration of amniotic fluid and mucus NOS

P24.11 Neonatal aspiration of (clear) amniotic fluid and mucus with respiratory symptoms MCC
Neonatal aspiration of amniotic fluid and mucus with pneumonia
Neonatal aspiration of amniotic fluid and mucus with pneumonitis
Use additional code to identify any secondary pulmonary hypertension, if applicable (I27.2-)

P24.2 Neonatal aspiration of blood

P24.20 Neonatal aspiration of blood without respiratory symptoms
Neonatal aspiration of blood NOS

P24.21 Neonatal aspiration of blood with respiratory symptoms MCC
Neonatal aspiration of blood with pneumonia
Neonatal aspiration of blood with pneumonitis
Use additional code to identify any secondary pulmonary hypertension, if applicable (I27.2-)

P24.3 Neonatal aspiration of milk and regurgitated food
Neonatal aspiration of stomach contents

P24.30 Neonatal aspiration of milk and regurgitated food without respiratory symptoms
Neonatal aspiration of milk and regurgitated food NOS

P24.31 Neonatal aspiration of milk and regurgitated food with respiratory symptoms MCC
Neonatal aspiration of milk and regurgitated food with pneumonia
Neonatal aspiration of milk and regurgitated food with pneumonitis
Use additional code to identify any secondary pulmonary hypertension, if applicable (I27.2-)

P24.8 Other neonatal aspiration

P24.80 Other neonatal aspiration without respiratory symptoms
Neonatal aspiration NEC

P24.81 Other neonatal aspiration with respiratory symptoms MCC
Neonatal aspiration pneumonia NEC
Neonatal aspiration with pneumonitis NEC
Neonatal aspiration with pneumonia NOS
Neonatal aspiration with pneumonitis NOS
Use additional code to identify any secondary pulmonary hypertension, if applicable (I27.2-)

P24.9 Neonatal aspiration, unspecified

P25 Interstitial emphysema and related conditions originating in the perinatal period

P25.0 Interstitial emphysema originating in the perinatal period MCC

P25.1 Pneumothorax originating in the perinatal period MCC

P25.2 Pneumomediastinum originating in the perinatal period MCC

P25.3 Pneumopericardium originating in the perinatal period MCC

P25.8 Other conditions related to interstitial emphysema originating in the perinatal period MCC

P26 Pulmonary hemorrhage originating in the perinatal period

EXCLUDES 1 *acute idiopathic hemorrhage in infants over 28 days old (R04.81)*

P26.0 Tracheobronchial hemorrhage originating in the perinatal period MCC

P26.1 Massive pulmonary hemorrhage originating in the perinatal period MCC

P26.8 Other pulmonary hemorrhages originating in the perinatal period MCC

P26.9 Unspecified pulmonary hemorrhage originating in the perinatal period MCC

P27 Chronic respiratory disease originating in the perinatal period

EXCLUDES 2 *respiratory distress of newborn (P22.0-P22.9)*

P27.0 Wilson-Mikity syndrome MCC
Pulmonary dysmaturity
DEF: Pulmonary insufficiency in newborn babies, especially those with low birth weight. Rapid onset of hypercapnia and cyanosis occur during the first month of life frequently resulting in death.

P27.1 Bronchopulmonary dysplasia originating in the perinatal period MCC

P27.8 Other chronic respiratory diseases originating in the perinatal period MCC
Congenital pulmonary fibrosis
Ventilator lung in newborn

P27.9 Unspecified chronic respiratory disease originating in the perinatal period MCC

P28 Other respiratory conditions originating in the perinatal period

EXCLUDES 1 *congenital malformations of the respiratory system (Q30-Q34)*

P28.0 Primary atelectasis of newborn CC
Primary failure to expand terminal respiratory units
Pulmonary hypoplasia associated with short gestation
Pulmonary immaturity NOS

P28.1 Other and unspecified atelectasis of newborn

P28.10 Unspecified atelectasis of newborn CC
Atelectasis of newborn NOS

P28.11 Resorption atelectasis without respiratory distress syndrome CC
EXCLUDES 1 *resorption atelectasis with respiratory distress syndrome (P22.0)*

P28.19 Other atelectasis of newborn CC
Partial atelectasis of newborn
Secondary atelectasis of newborn

P28.2 Cyanotic attacks of newborn CC
EXCLUDES 1 *apnea of newborn (P28.3-P28.4)*

P28.3 Primary sleep apnea of newborn CC
Central sleep apnea of newborn
Obstructive sleep apnea of newborn
Sleep apnea of newborn NOS
DEF: Unexplained cessation of breathing when a neonate makes no respiratory effort for 20 seconds or longer or when a neonate's breathing cessation is accompanied by cyanosis, bradycardia, or hypotonia.

P28.4 Other apnea of newborn CC
Apnea of prematurity
Obstructive apnea of newborn
EXCLUDES 1 *obstructive sleep apnea of newborn (P28.3)*

P28.5 Respiratory failure of newborn MCC
EXCLUDES 1 *respiratory arrest of newborn (P28.81)*
respiratory distress of newborn (P22.0-)
AHA: 2019,2Q,29

P28.8 Other specified respiratory conditions of newborn

P28.81 Respiratory arrest of newborn MCC

P28.89 Other specified respiratory conditions of newborn
Congenital laryngeal stridor
Sniffles in newborn
Snuffles in newborn
EXCLUDES 1 *early congenital syphilitic rhinitis (A50.05)*

P28.9 Respiratory condition of newborn, unspecified
Respiratory depression in newborn

P29 Cardiovascular disorders originating in the perinatal period

EXCLUDES 1 *congenital malformations of the circulatory system (Q2Ø-Q28)*

P29.Ø Neonatal cardiac failure

P29.1 Neonatal cardiac dysrhythmia

P29.11 Neonatal tachycardia

P29.12 Neonatal bradycardia

P29.2 Neonatal hypertension

P29.3 Persistent fetal circulation

AHA: 2017,4Q,20-21

P29.3Ø Pulmonary hypertension of newborn MCC

Persistent pulmonary hypertension of newborn

DEF: Condition that occurs when pressure within the pulmonary artery is elevated and vascular resistance is observed in the lungs.

P29.38 Other persistent fetal circulation MCC

Delayed closure of ductus arteriosus

P29.4 Transient myocardial ischemia in newborn

P29.8 Other cardiovascular disorders originating in the perinatal period

P29.81 Cardiac arrest of newborn MCC

P29.89 Other cardiovascular disorders originating in the perinatal period

AHA: 2014,4Q,23

P29.9 Cardiovascular disorder originating in the perinatal period, unspecified

Infections specific to the perinatal period (P35-P39)

Infections acquired in utero, during birth via the umbilicus, or during the first 28 days after birth

EXCLUDES 2 *asymptomatic human immunodeficiency virus [HIV] infection status (Z21)*
congenital gonococcal infection (A54.-)
congenital pneumonia (P23.-)
congenital syphilis (A5Ø.-)
human immunodeficiency virus [HIV] disease (B2Ø)
infant botulism (A48.51)
infectious diseases not specific to the perinatal period (AØØ-B99, JØ9, J1Ø.-)
intestinal infectious disease (AØØ-AØ9)
laboratory evidence of human immunodeficiency virus [HIV] (R75)
tetanus neonatorum (A33)

P35 Congenital viral diseases

INCLUDES infections acquired in utero or during birth

P35.Ø Congenital rubella syndrome CC

Congenital rubella pneumonitis

P35.1 Congenital cytomegalovirus infection MCC

P35.2 Congenital herpesviral [herpes simplex] infection MCC

P35.3 Congenital viral hepatitis MCC

P35.4 Congenital Zika virus disease MCC

Use additional code to identify manifestations of congenital Zika virus disease

AHA: 2018,4Q,25-26

P35.8 Other congenital viral diseases MCC

Congenital varicella [chickenpox]

AHA: 2020,2Q,13

P35.9 Congenital viral disease, unspecified MCC

P36 Bacterial sepsis of newborn

INCLUDES congenital sepsis

Use additional code(s), if applicable, to identify severe sepsis (R65.2-) and associated acute organ dysfunction(s)

P36.Ø Sepsis of newborn due to streptococcus, group B MCC HCC

P36.1 Sepsis of newborn due to other and unspecified streptococci

P36.1Ø Sepsis of newborn due to unspecified streptococci MCC HCC

P36.19 Sepsis of newborn due to other streptococci MCC HCC

P36.2 Sepsis of newborn due to Staphylococcus aureus MCC HCC

P36.3 Sepsis of newborn due to other and unspecified staphylococci

P36.3Ø Sepsis of newborn due to unspecified staphylococci MCC HCC

P36.39 Sepsis of newborn due to other staphylococci MCC HCC

P36.4 Sepsis of newborn due to Escherichia coli MCC HCC

P36.5 Sepsis of newborn due to anaerobes MCC HCC

P36.8 Other bacterial sepsis of newborn MCC HCC

Use additional code from category B96 to identify organism

P36.9 Bacterial sepsis of newborn, unspecified MCC HCC

P37 Other congenital infectious and parasitic diseases

EXCLUDES 2 *congenital syphilis (A5Ø.-)*
infectious neonatal diarrhea (AØØ-AØ9)
necrotizing enterocolitis in newborn (P77.-)
noninfectious neonatal diarrhea (P78.3)
ophthalmia neonatorum due to gonococcus (A54.31)
tetanus neonatorum (A33)

P37.Ø Congenital tuberculosis MCC

P37.1 Congenital toxoplasmosis MCC

Hydrocephalus due to congenital toxoplasmosis

P37.2 Neonatal (disseminated) listeriosis MCC

P37.3 Congenital falciparum malaria MCC

P37.4 Other congenital malaria MCC

P37.5 Neonatal candidiasis

P37.8 Other specified congenital infectious and parasitic diseases MCC

P37.9 Congenital infectious or parasitic disease, unspecified MCC

P38 Omphalitis of newborn

EXCLUDES 1 *omphalitis not of newborn (LØ8.82)*
tetanus omphalitis (A33)
umbilical hemorrhage of newborn (P51.-)

DEF: Omphalitis: Infection and inflammation of the umbilical stump, often due to bacteria that can spread beyond the umbilical stump to the fascia, muscle, or even the umbilical vessels.

P38.1 Omphalitis with mild hemorrhage CC

P38.9 Omphalitis without hemorrhage CC

Omphalitis of newborn NOS

P39 Other infections specific to the perinatal period

Use additional code to identify organism or specific infection

P39.Ø Neonatal infective mastitis CC

EXCLUDES 1 *breast engorgement of newborn (P83.4)*
noninfective mastitis of newborn (P83.4)

P39.1 Neonatal conjunctivitis and dacryocystitis

Neonatal chlamydial conjunctivitis

Ophthalmia neonatorum NOS

EXCLUDES 1 *gonococcal conjunctivitis (A54.31)*

P39.2 Intra-amniotic infection affecting newborn, not elsewhere classified CC

P39.3 Neonatal urinary tract infection CC

P39.4 Neonatal skin infection CC

Neonatal pyoderma

EXCLUDES 1 *pemphigus neonatorum (LØØ)*
staphylococcal scalded skin syndrome (LØØ)

P39.8 Other specified infections specific to the perinatal period CC

P39.9 Infection specific to the perinatal period, unspecified CC

Hemorrhagic and hematological disorders of newborn (P5Ø-P61)

EXCLUDES 1 *congenital stenosis and stricture of bile ducts (Q44.3)*
Crigler-Najjar syndrome (E8Ø.5)
Dubin-Johnson syndrome (E8Ø.6)
Gilbert syndrome (E8Ø.4)
hereditary hemolytic anemias (D55-D58)

P5Ø Newborn affected by intrauterine (fetal) blood loss

EXCLUDES 1 *congenital anemia from intrauterine (fetal) blood loss (P61.3)*

P5Ø.Ø Newborn affected by intrauterine (fetal) blood loss from vasa previa

P5Ø.1 Newborn affected by intrauterine (fetal) blood loss from ruptured cord

P5Ø.2 Newborn affected by intrauterine (fetal) blood loss from placenta

P5Ø.3 Newborn affected by hemorrhage into co-twin

P5Ø.4 Newborn affected by hemorrhage into maternal circulation

P5Ø.5 Newborn affected by intrauterine (fetal) blood loss from cut end of co-twin's cord

P5Ø.8 Newborn affected by other intrauterine (fetal) blood loss

P5Ø.9 Newborn affected by intrauterine (fetal) blood loss, unspecified

Newborn affected by fetal hemorrhage NOS

√4th **P51 Umbilical hemorrhage of newborn**
EXCLUDES 1 *omphalitis with mild hemorrhage (P38.1)*
umbilical hemorrhage from cut end of co-twins cord (P50.5)
P51.0 Massive umbilical hemorrhage of newborn
P51.8 Other umbilical hemorrhages of newborn
Slipped umbilical ligature NOS
P51.9 Umbilical hemorrhage of newborn, unspecified

√4th **P52 Intracranial nontraumatic hemorrhage of newborn**
INCLUDES intracranial hemorrhage due to anoxia or hypoxia
EXCLUDES 1 *intracranial hemorrhage due to birth injury (P10.-)*
intracranial hemorrhage due to other injury (S06.-)
P52.0 Intraventricular (nontraumatic) hemorrhage, grade 1, of newborn CC
Subependymal hemorrhage (without intraventricular extension)
Bleeding into germinal matrix
P52.1 Intraventricular (nontraumatic) hemorrhage, grade 2, of newborn CC
Subependymal hemorrhage with intraventricular extension
Bleeding into ventricle
√5th **P52.2 Intraventricular (nontraumatic) hemorrhage, grade 3 and grade 4, of newborn**
P52.21 Intraventricular (nontraumatic) hemorrhage, grade 3, of newborn MCC
Subependymal hemorrhage with intraventricular extension with enlargement of ventricle
P52.22 Intraventricular (nontraumatic) hemorrhage, grade 4, of newborn MCC
Bleeding into cerebral cortex
Subependymal hemorrhage with intracerebral extension
P52.3 Unspecified intraventricular (nontraumatic) hemorrhage of newborn CC
P52.4 Intracerebral (nontraumatic) hemorrhage of newborn MCC
P52.5 Subarachnoid (nontraumatic) hemorrhage of newborn MCC
P52.6 Cerebellar (nontraumatic) and posterior fossa hemorrhage of newborn MCC
P52.8 Other intracranial (nontraumatic) hemorrhages of newborn MCC
P52.9 Intracranial (nontraumatic) hemorrhage of newborn, unspecified MCC

P53 Hemorrhagic disease of newborn CC
Vitamin K deficiency of newborn

√4th **P54 Other neonatal hemorrhages**
EXCLUDES 1 *newborn affected by (intrauterine) blood loss (P50.-)*
pulmonary hemorrhage originating in the perinatal period (P26.-)
P54.0 Neonatal hematemesis
EXCLUDES 1 *neonatal hematemesis due to swallowed maternal blood (P78.2)*
P54.1 Neonatal melena MCC
EXCLUDES 1 *neonatal melena due to swallowed maternal blood (P78.2)*
P54.2 Neonatal rectal hemorrhage MCC
P54.3 Other neonatal gastrointestinal hemorrhage MCC
P54.4 Neonatal adrenal hemorrhage CC
P54.5 Neonatal cutaneous hemorrhage
Neonatal bruising
Neonatal ecchymoses
Neonatal petechiae
Neonatal superficial hematomata
EXCLUDES 2 *bruising of scalp due to birth injury (P12.3)*
cephalhematoma due to birth injury (P12.0)
P54.6 Neonatal vaginal hemorrhage ♀
Neonatal pseudomenses
P54.8 Other specified neonatal hemorrhages
P54.9 Neonatal hemorrhage, unspecified

√4th **P55 Hemolytic disease of newborn**
P55.0 Rh isoimmunization of newborn
DEF: Incompatible Rh fetal-maternal blood grouping that prematurely destroys red blood cells. Symptoms include jaundice, asphyxia, pulmonary hypertension, edema, respiratory distress, kernicterus, and coagulopathies. It is detected by a Coombs test.
TIP: A positive Coombs test without documentation of associated Rh isoimmunization should be coded to R79.89 Other specified abnormal findings of blood chemistry.
P55.1 ABO isoimmunization of newborn
AHA: 2015,3Q,20
P55.8 Other hemolytic diseases of newborn
AHA: 2018,3Q,24
P55.9 Hemolytic disease of newborn, unspecified

√4th **P56 Hydrops fetalis due to hemolytic disease**
EXCLUDES 1 *hydrops fetalis NOS (P83.2)*
P56.0 Hydrops fetalis due to isoimmunization MCC
√5th **P56.9 Hydrops fetalis due to other and unspecified hemolytic disease**
P56.90 Hydrops fetalis due to unspecified hemolytic disease MCC
P56.99 Hydrops fetalis due to other hemolytic disease MCC

√4th **P57 Kernicterus**
P57.0 Kernicterus due to isoimmunization MCC
DEF: Complication of erythroblastosis fetalis associated with severe neural symptoms, high blood bilirubin levels, and nerve cell destruction. It results in bilirubin-pigmented gray matter of the central nervous system.
P57.8 Other specified kernicterus MCC
EXCLUDES 1 *Crigler-Najjar syndrome (E80.5)*
P57.9 Kernicterus, unspecified MCC

√4th **P58 Neonatal jaundice due to other excessive hemolysis**
EXCLUDES 1 *jaundice due to isoimmunization (P55-P57)*
P58.0 Neonatal jaundice due to bruising
P58.1 Neonatal jaundice due to bleeding
P58.2 Neonatal jaundice due to infection
P58.3 Neonatal jaundice due to polycythemia
√5th **P58.4 Neonatal jaundice due to drugs or toxins transmitted from mother or given to newborn**
Code first poisoning due to drug or toxin, if applicable (T36-T65 with fifth or sixth character 1-4 or 6)
Use additional code for adverse effect, if applicable, to identify drug (T36-T50 with fifth or sixth character 5)
P58.41 Neonatal jaundice due to drugs or toxins transmitted from mother
P58.42 Neonatal jaundice due to drugs or toxins given to newborn
P58.5 Neonatal jaundice due to swallowed maternal blood
P58.8 Neonatal jaundice due to other specified excessive hemolysis
P58.9 Neonatal jaundice due to excessive hemolysis, unspecified

√4th **P59 Neonatal jaundice from other and unspecified causes**
EXCLUDES 1 *jaundice due to inborn errors of metabolism (E70-E88)*
kernicterus (P57.-)
P59.0 Neonatal jaundice associated with preterm delivery
Hyperbilirubinemia of prematurity
Jaundice due to delayed conjugation associated with preterm delivery
P59.1 Inspissated bile syndrome MCC
DEF: Biliary obstruction in newborn resulting from obstruction of outflow tract.
√5th **P59.2 Neonatal jaundice from other and unspecified hepatocellular damage**
EXCLUDES 1 *congenital viral hepatitis (P35.3)*
P59.20 Neonatal jaundice from unspecified hepatocellular damage MCC
P59.29 Neonatal jaundice from other hepatocellular damage MCC
Neonatal giant cell hepatitis
Neonatal (idiopathic) hepatitis
P59.3 Neonatal jaundice from breast milk inhibitor
P59.8 Neonatal jaundice from other specified causes
P59.9 Neonatal jaundice, unspecified
Neonatal physiological jaundice (intense)(prolonged) NOS
AHA: 2015,3Q,20

P60 Disseminated intravascular coagulation of newborn MCC
Defibrination syndrome of newborn

P61 Other perinatal hematological disorders
EXCLUDES 1 *transient hypogammaglobulinemia of infancy (D80.7)*

P61.0 Transient neonatal thrombocytopenia MCC
Neonatal thrombocytopenia due to exchange transfusion
Neonatal thrombocytopenia due to idiopathic maternal thrombocytopenia
Neonatal thrombocytopenia due to isoimmunization
DEF: Temporary decrease in blood platelets of a newborn that is secondary to placental insufficiency.

P61.1 Polycythemia neonatorum
DEF: Abnormal increase of total red blood cells of a newborn that results in hyperviscosity, which slows the flow of blood through small blood vessels.

P61.2 Anemia of prematurity CC

P61.3 Congenital anemia from fetal blood loss CC

P61.4 Other congenital anemias, not elsewhere classified CC
Congenital anemia NOS

P61.5 Transient neonatal neutropenia MCC
EXCLUDES 1 *congenital neutropenia (nontransient) (D70.0)*
DEF: Low blood neutrophil counts of newborn that occurs due to maternal hypertension, sepsis, twin-twin transfusion, alloimmunization, and hemolytic disease.

P61.6 Other transient neonatal disorders of coagulation CC

P61.8 Other specified perinatal hematological disorders

P61.9 Perinatal hematological disorder, unspecified

Transitory endocrine and metabolic disorders specific to newborn (P70-P74)

INCLUDES transitory endocrine and metabolic disturbances caused by the infant's response to maternal endocrine and metabolic factors, or its adjustment to extrauterine environment

AHA: 2018,2Q,6

P70 Transitory disorders of carbohydrate metabolism specific to newborn

P70.0 Syndrome of infant of mother with gestational diabetes
Newborn (with hypoglycemia) affected by maternal gestational diabetes
EXCLUDES 1 *newborn (with hypoglycemia) affected by maternal (pre-existing) diabetes mellitus (P70.1)*
syndrome of infant of a diabetic mother (P70.1)

P70.1 Syndrome of infant of a diabetic mother
Newborn (with hypoglycemia) affected by maternal (pre-existing) diabetes mellitus
EXCLUDES 1 *newborn (with hypoglycemia) affected by maternal gestational diabetes (P70.0)*
syndrome of infant of mother with gestational diabetes (P70.0)

P70.2 Neonatal diabetes mellitus CC

P70.3 Iatrogenic neonatal hypoglycemia

P70.4 Other neonatal hypoglycemia
Transitory neonatal hypoglycemia

P70.8 Other transitory disorders of carbohydrate metabolism of newborn CC

P70.9 Transitory disorder of carbohydrate metabolism of newborn, unspecified

P71 Transitory neonatal disorders of calcium and magnesium metabolism

P71.0 Cow's milk hypocalcemia in newborn CC

P71.1 Other neonatal hypocalcemia CC
EXCLUDES 1 *neonatal hypoparathyroidism (P71.4)*

P71.2 Neonatal hypomagnesemia CC

P71.3 Neonatal tetany without calcium or magnesium deficiency CC
Neonatal tetany NOS

P71.4 Transitory neonatal hypoparathyroidism CC

P71.8 Other transitory neonatal disorders of calcium and magnesium metabolism CC
AHA: 2016,4Q,54

P71.9 Transitory neonatal disorder of calcium and magnesium metabolism, unspecified CC

P72 Other transitory neonatal endocrine disorders
EXCLUDES 1 *congenital hypothyroidism with or without goiter (E03.0-E03.1)*
dyshormogenetic goiter (E07.1)
Pendred's syndrome (E07.1)

P72.0 Neonatal goiter, not elsewhere classified CC
Transitory congenital goiter with normal functioning

P72.1 Transitory neonatal hyperthyroidism CC
Neonatal thyrotoxicosis

P72.2 Other transitory neonatal disorders of thyroid function, not elsewhere classified CC
Transitory neonatal hypothyroidism

P72.8 Other specified transitory neonatal endocrine disorders CC

P72.9 Transitory neonatal endocrine disorder, unspecified

P74 Other transitory neonatal electrolyte and metabolic disturbances
AHA: 2018,4Q,26-27

P74.0 Late metabolic acidosis of newborn MCC
EXCLUDES 1 *(fetal) metabolic acidosis of newborn (P19)*

P74.1 Dehydration of newborn

P74.2 Disturbances of sodium balance of newborn

P74.21 Hypernatremia of newborn

P74.22 Hyponatremia of newborn

P74.3 Disturbances of potassium balance of newborn

P74.31 Hyperkalemia of newborn

P74.32 Hypokalemia of newborn

P74.4 Other transitory electrolyte disturbances of newborn

P74.41 Alkalosis of newborn CC
Hyperbicarbonatemia

P74.42 Disturbances of chlorine balance of newborn

P74.421 Hyperchloremia of newborn
Hyperchloremic metabolic acidosis
EXCLUDES 2 *late metabolic acidosis of the newborn (P74.0)*

P74.422 Hypochloremia of newborn

P74.49 Other transitory electrolyte disturbance of newborn

P74.5 Transitory tyrosinemia of newborn CC

P74.6 Transitory hyperammonemia of newborn CC

P74.8 Other transitory metabolic disturbances of newborn CC
Amino-acid metabolic disorders described as transitory

P74.9 Transitory metabolic disturbance of newborn, unspecified

Digestive system disorders of newborn (P76-P78)

P76 Other intestinal obstruction of newborn

P76.0 Meconium plug syndrome
Meconium ileus NOS
EXCLUDES 1 *meconium ileus in cystic fibrosis (E84.11)*
DEF: Meconium obstruction of a newborn's intestines, resulting from unusually thick or hard meconium.

P76.1 Transitory ileus of newborn CC
EXCLUDES 1 *Hirschsprung's disease (Q43.1)*

P76.2 Intestinal obstruction due to inspissated milk

P76.8 Other specified intestinal obstruction of newborn
EXCLUDES 1 *intestinal obstruction classifiable to K56.-*

P76.9 Intestinal obstruction of newborn, unspecified

P77 Necrotizing enterocolitis of newborn
DEF: Serious intestinal infection and inflammation in preterm infants. Severity is measured by stages and may progress to life-threatening perforation or peritonitis. Resection surgical treatment may be necessary.

P77.1 Stage 1 necrotizing enterocolitis in newborn MCC
Necrotizing enterocolitis without pneumatosis, without perforation
DEF: Broad-spectrum symptoms with nonspecific signs, including feeding intolerance, abdominal distention, bradycardia, and metabolic abnormalities.

P77.2 Stage 2 necrotizing enterocolitis in newborn MCC
Necrotizing enterocolitis with pneumatosis, without perforation
DEF: Radiographic confirmation of necrotizing enterocolitis showing intestinal dilatation, fixed loops of bowels, pneumatosis intestinalis, metabolic acidosis, and thrombocytopenia.

P77.3 Stage 3 necrotizing enterocolitis in newborn MCC
Necrotizing enterocolitis with perforation
Necrotizing enterocolitis with pneumatosis and perforation
DEF: Advanced stage in which an infant demonstrates signs of bowel perforation, septic shock, metabolic acidosis, ascites, disseminated intravascular coagulopathy, and neutropenia.

P77.9 Necrotizing enterocolitis in newborn, unspecified MCC
Necrotizing enterocolitis in newborn, NOS

✓4th **P78 Other perinatal digestive system disorders**
EXCLUDES 1 *cystic fibrosis (E84.Ø-E84.9)*
neonatal gastrointestinal hemorrhages (P54.Ø-P54.3)

P78.Ø Perinatal intestinal perforation MCC
Meconium peritonitis

P78.1 Other neonatal peritonitis
Neonatal peritonitis NOS

P78.2 Neonatal hematemesis and melena due to swallowed maternal blood

P78.3 Noninfective neonatal diarrhea
Neonatal diarrhea NOS

✓5th **P78.8 Other specified perinatal digestive system disorders**

P78.81 Congenital cirrhosis (of liver)

P78.82 Peptic ulcer of newborn

P78.83 Newborn esophageal reflux
Neonatal esophageal reflux

P78.84 Gestational alloimmune liver disease
GALD
Neonatal hemochromatosis
EXCLUDES 1 *hemochromatosis (E83.11-)*
AHA: 2017,4Q,21
DEF: Severe hepatic injury with onset during fetal development with manifestations beginning during fetal life. It is due to maternal antibodies to fetal hepatic cells (hepatocytes) that cross the placenta into the fetal circulation, causing hepatic cell necrosis.

P78.89 Other specified perinatal digestive system disorders

P78.9 Perinatal digestive system disorder, unspecified

Conditions involving the integument and temperature regulation of newborn (P8Ø-P83)

✓4th **P8Ø Hypothermia of newborn**
DEF: Decrease in newborn body temperature due to their larger ratio of surface area to body weight, thin skin with blood vessels close to the surface, and a limited amount of subcutaneous fat.

P8Ø.Ø Cold injury syndrome
Severe and usually chronic hypothermia associated with a pink flushed appearance, edema and neurological and biochemical abnormalities.
EXCLUDES 1 *mild hypothermia of newborn (P8Ø.8)*

P8Ø.8 Other hypothermia of newborn
Mild hypothermia of newborn

P8Ø.9 Hypothermia of newborn, unspecified

✓4th **P81 Other disturbances of temperature regulation of newborn**

P81.Ø Environmental hyperthermia of newborn

P81.8 Other specified disturbances of temperature regulation of newborn

P81.9 Disturbance of temperature regulation of newborn, unspecified
Fever of newborn NOS

✓4th **P83 Other conditions of integument specific to newborn**
EXCLUDES 1 *congenital malformations of skin and integument (Q8Ø-Q84)*
hydrops fetalis due to hemolytic disease (P56.-)
neonatal skin infection (P39.4)
staphylococcal scalded skin syndrome (LØØ)
EXCLUDES 2 *cradle cap (L21.Ø)*
diaper [napkin] dermatitis (L22)

P83.Ø Sclerema neonatorum CC
DEF: Diffuse, rapidly progressing white, waxy, nonpitting hardening of tissue, usually of legs and feet that is life-threatening. It is found in preterm or debilitated infants. Etiology is unknown.

P83.1 Neonatal erythema toxicum

P83.2 Hydrops fetalis not due to hemolytic disease MCC
Hydrops fetalis NOS
DEF: Severe, life-threatening problem of a newborn characterized by severe edema of the entire body. It is unrelated to immune response.

✓5th **P83.3 Other and unspecified edema specific to newborn**

P83.3Ø Unspecified edema specific to newborn CC

P83.39 Other edema specific to newborn CC

P83.4 Breast engorgement of newborn
Noninfective mastitis of newborn

P83.5 Congenital hydrocele ♂
DEF: Hydrocele: Serous fluid that collects in the tunica vaginalis of the scrotum along the spermatic cord in males.

P83.6 Umbilical polyp of newborn

✓5th **P83.8 Other specified conditions of integument specific to newborn**
AHA: 2017,4Q,21-22

P83.81 Umbilical granuloma
EXCLUDES 2 *granulomatous disorder of the skin and subcutaneous tissue, unspecified (L92.9)*

P83.88 Other specified conditions of integument specific to newborn
Bronze baby syndrome
Neonatal scleroderma
Urticaria neonatorum

P83.9 Condition of the integument specific to newborn, unspecified

Other problems with newborn (P84)

P84 Other problems with newborn
Acidemia of newborn
Acidosis of newborn
Anoxia of newborn NOS
Asphyxia of newborn NOS
Hypercapnia of newborn
Hypoxemia of newborn
Hypoxia of newborn NOS
Mixed metabolic and respiratory acidosis of newborn
EXCLUDES 1 *intracranial hemorrhage due to anoxia or hypoxia (P52.-)*
hypoxic ischemic encephalopathy [HIE] (P91.6-)
late metabolic acidosis of newborn (P74.Ø)

Other disorders originating in the perinatal period (P9Ø-P96)

P9Ø Convulsions of newborn MCC
EXCLUDES 1 *benign myoclonic epilepsy in infancy (G4Ø.3-)*
benign neonatal convulsions (familial) (G4Ø.3-)

✓4th **P91 Other disturbances of cerebral status of newborn**

P91.Ø Neonatal cerebral ischemia MCC
EXCLUDES 1 ►*neonatal cerebral infarction (P91.82-)*◄

P91.1 Acquired periventricular cysts of newborn MCC

P91.2 Neonatal cerebral leukomalacia MCC
Periventricular leukomalacia

P91.3 Neonatal cerebral irritability MCC

P91.4 Neonatal cerebral depression MCC

P91.5 Neonatal coma MCC

✓5th **P91.6 Hypoxic ischemic encephalopathy [HIE]**
EXCLUDES 1 *neonatal cerebral depression (P91.4)*
neonatal cerebral irritability (P91.3)
neonatal coma (P91.5)
AHA: 2017,4Q,22

P91.6Ø Hypoxic ischemic encephalopathy [HIE], unspecified CC

P91.61 Mild hypoxic ischemic encephalopathy [HIE] CC

P91.62 Moderate hypoxic ischemic encephalopathy [HIE] CC

P91.63 Severe hypoxic ischemic encephalopathy [HIE] MCC

✓5th **P91.8 Other specified disturbances of cerebral status of newborn**
AHA: 2017,4Q,22

✓6th **P91.81 Neonatal encephalopathy**

P91.811 Neonatal encephalopathy in diseases classified elsewhere
Code first underlying condition, if known, such as:
congenital cirrhosis (of liver) (P78.81)
intracranial nontraumatic hemorrhage of newborn (P52.-)
kernicterus (P57.-)

P91.819 Neonatal encephalopathy, unspecified

● ✓6th **P91.82 Neonatal cerebral infarction**
Neonatal stroke
Perinatal arterial ischemic stroke
Perinatal cerebral infarction
EXCLUDES 1 *cerebral infarction (I63.-)*
EXCLUDES 2 *intracranial hemorrhage of newborn (P52.-)*

● **P91.821 Neonatal cerebral infarction, right side of brain** MCC

● **P91.822 Neonatal cerebral infarction, left side of brain** MCC

● **P91.823 Neonatal cerebral infarction, bilateral** MCC

● **P91.829 Neonatal cerebral infarction, unspecified side** MCC

P91.88 Other specified disturbances of cerebral status of newborn

P91.9 Disturbance of cerebral status of newborn, unspecified

✓4th **P92 Feeding problems of newborn**
EXCLUDES 1 *eating disorders (F50.-)*
feeding problems in child over 28 days old (R63.3)
AHA: 2016,3Q,19
TIP: Continue to assign a code from this category for feeding problems in a patient greater than 28 days old when that feeding problem was initially diagnosed between day 0 and day 28. Do not assign code R63.3.

✓5th **P92.0 Vomiting of newborn**
EXCLUDES 1 *vomiting of child over 28 days old (R11.-)*

P92.01 Bilious vomiting of newborn MCC
EXCLUDES 1 *bilious vomiting in child over 28 days old (R11.14)*

P92.09 Other vomiting of newborn
EXCLUDES 1 *regurgitation of food in newborn (P92.1)*

P92.1 Regurgitation and rumination of newborn

P92.2 Slow feeding of newborn

P92.3 Underfeeding of newborn

P92.4 Overfeeding of newborn

P92.5 Neonatal difficulty in feeding at breast
AHA: 2017,1Q,28

P92.6 Failure to thrive in newborn
EXCLUDES 1 *failure to thrive in child over 28 days old (R62.51)*

P92.8 Other feeding problems of newborn

P92.9 Feeding problem of newborn, unspecified

✓4th **P93 Reactions and intoxications due to drugs administered to newborn**
INCLUDES reactions and intoxications due to drugs administered to fetus affecting newborn
EXCLUDES 1 *jaundice due to drugs or toxins transmitted from mother or given to newborn (P58.4-)*
reactions and intoxications from maternal opiates, tranquilizers and other medication (P04.0-P04.1, P04.4-)
withdrawal symptoms from maternal use of drugs of addiction (P96.1)
withdrawal symptoms from therapeutic use of drugs in newborn (P96.2)

P93.0 Grey baby syndrome CC
Grey syndrome from chloramphenicol administration in newborn

P93.8 Other reactions and intoxications due to drugs administered to newborn CC
Use additional code for adverse effect, if applicable, to identify drug (T36-T50 with fifth or sixth character 5)

✓4th **P94 Disorders of muscle tone of newborn**

P94.0 Transient neonatal myasthenia gravis CC
EXCLUDES 1 *myasthenia gravis (G70.0)*

P94.1 Congenital hypertonia

P94.2 Congenital hypotonia
Floppy baby syndrome, unspecified

P94.8 Other disorders of muscle tone of newborn

P94.9 Disorder of muscle tone of newborn, unspecified

P95 Stillbirth
Deadborn fetus NOS
Fetal death of unspecified cause
Stillbirth NOS
EXCLUDES 1 *maternal care for intrauterine death (O36.4)*
missed abortion (O02.1)
outcome of delivery, stillbirth (Z37.1, Z37.3, Z37.4, Z37.7)

✓4th **P96 Other conditions originating in the perinatal period**

P96.0 Congenital renal failure
Uremia of newborn

P96.1 Neonatal withdrawal symptoms from maternal use of drugs of addiction CC
Drug withdrawal syndrome in infant of dependent mother
Neonatal abstinence syndrome
EXCLUDES 1 *reactions and intoxications from maternal opiates and tranquilizers administered during labor and delivery (P04.0)*
AHA: 2018,4Q,24-25

P96.2 Withdrawal symptoms from therapeutic use of drugs in newborn CC

P96.3 Wide cranial sutures of newborn
Neonatal craniotabes

P96.5 Complication to newborn due to (fetal) intrauterine procedure
EXCLUDES 2 *newborn affected by amniocentesis (P00.6)*

✓5th **P96.8 Other specified conditions originating in the perinatal period**

P96.81 Exposure to (parental) (environmental) tobacco smoke in the perinatal period
EXCLUDES 2 *newborn affected by in utero exposure to tobacco (P04.2)*
exposure to environmental tobacco smoke after the perinatal period (Z77.22)

P96.82 Delayed separation of umbilical cord

P96.83 Meconium staining
EXCLUDES 1 *meconium aspiration (P24.00, P24.01)*
meconium passage during delivery (P03.82)
DEF: Meconium passed in utero causing discoloration on the fetal skin and nails or on the umbilicus. This staining may be incidental or may be an indicator of significant fetal stress that could affect outcomes.

P96.89 Other specified conditions originating in the perinatal period
Use additional code to specify condition

P96.9 Condition originating in the perinatal period, unspecified
Congenital debility NOS

Chapter 17. Congenital Malformations, Deformations and Chromosomal Abnormalities (QØØ–Q99)

Chapter-specific Guidelines with Coding Examples

The chapter-specific guidelines from the ICD-10-CM Official Guidelines for Coding and Reporting have been provided below. Along with these guidelines are coding examples, contained in the shaded boxes, that have been developed to help illustrate the coding and/or sequencing guidance found in these guidelines.

Assign an appropriate code(s) from categories QØØ-Q99, Congenital malformations, deformations, and chromosomal abnormalities when a malformation/deformation or chromosomal abnormality is documented. A malformation/deformation/or chromosomal abnormality may be the principal/first-listed diagnosis on a record or a secondary diagnosis.

When a malformation/deformation/or chromosomal abnormality does not have a unique code assignment, assign additional code(s) for any manifestations that may be present.

When the code assignment specifically identifies the malformation/deformation/or chromosomal abnormality, manifestations that are an inherent component of the anomaly should not be coded separately. Additional codes should be assigned for manifestations that are not an inherent component.

8-day-old infant with tetralogy of Fallot and pulmonary stenosis

Q21.3 **Tetralogy of Fallot**

Explanation: Pulmonary stenosis is inherent in the disease process of tetralogy of Fallot. When the code assignment specifically identifies the malformation/deformation/or chromosomal abnormality, manifestations that are inherent components of the anomaly should not be coded separately.

7-month-old infant with Down syndrome and common atrioventricular canal

Q9Ø.9 **Down syndrome, unspecified**

Q21.2 **Atrioventricular septal defect**

Explanation: While a common atrioventricular canal is often associated with patients with Down syndrome, this manifestation is not an inherent component and may be reported separately. When the code assignment specifically identifies the anomaly, manifestations that are inherent components of the condition should not be coded separately. Additional codes should be assigned for manifestations that are not inherent components.

Codes from Chapter 17 may be used throughout the life of the patient. If a congenital malformation or deformity has been corrected, a personal history code should be used to identify the history of the malformation or deformity. Although present at birth, a malformation/deformation/or chromosomal abnormality may not be identified until later in life. Whenever the condition is diagnosed by the provider, it is appropriate to assign a code from codes QØØ-Q99. For the birth admission, the appropriate code from category Z38, Liveborn infants, according to place of birth and type of delivery, should be sequenced as the principal diagnosis, followed by any congenital anomaly codes, QØØ- Q99.

Three-year-old with history of corrected ventricular septal defect

Z87.74 **Personal history of (corrected) congenital malformations of heart and circulatory system**

Explanation: If a congenital malformation or deformity has been corrected, a personal history code should be used to identify the history of the malformation or deformity.

Forty-year-old man with headaches diagnosed with congenital arteriovenous malformation of cerebral vessels by brain scan

Q28.2 **Arteriovenous malformation of cerebral vessels**

Explanation: Although present at birth, malformations may not be identified until later in life. Whenever a congenital condition is diagnosed by the physician, it is appropriate to assign a code from the range QØØ–Q99.

Newborn with anencephaly delivered vaginally in hospital

Z38.ØØ **Single liveborn infant, delivered vaginally**

QØØ.Ø **Anencephaly**

Explanation: For the birth admission, the appropriate code from category Z38 Liveborn infants, according to place of birth and type of delivery, should be sequenced as the principal diagnosis, followed by any congenital anomaly codes, QØØ–Q99.

Chapter 17. Congenital Malformations, Deformations and Chromosomal Abnormalities (Q00-Q99)

NOTE Codes from this chapter are not for use on maternal records

EXCLUDES 2 *inborn errors of metabolism (E70-E88)*

This chapter contains the following blocks:

Q00-Q07 Congenital malformations of the nervous system
Q10-Q18 Congenital malformations of eye, ear, face and neck
Q20-Q28 Congenital malformations of the circulatory system
Q30-Q34 Congenital malformations of the respiratory system
Q35-Q37 Cleft lip and cleft palate
Q38-Q45 Other congenital malformations of the digestive system
Q50-Q56 Congenital malformations of genital organs
Q60-Q64 Congenital malformations of the urinary system
Q65-Q79 Congenital malformations and deformations of the musculoskeletal system
Q80-Q89 Other congenital malformations
Q90-Q99 Chromosomal abnormalities, not elsewhere classified

Congenital malformations of the nervous system (Q00-Q07)

✓4th **Q00 Anencephaly and similar malformations**

Q00.0 Anencephaly MCC HCC
- Acephaly
- Acrania
- Amyelencephaly
- Hemianencephaly
- Hemicephaly

Q00.1 Craniorachischisis MCC HCC

Q00.2 Iniencephaly MCC HCC

✓4th **Q01 Encephalocele**

INCLUDES Arnold-Chiari syndrome, type III
encephalocystocele
encephalomyelocele
hydroencephalocele
hydromeningocele, cranial
meningocele, cerebral
meningoencephalocele

EXCLUDES 1 *Meckel-Gruber syndrome (Q61.9)*

DEF: Congenital protrusion of brain tissue through a defect in the skull.

Q01.0 Frontal encephalocele CC HCC

Q01.1 Nasofrontal encephalocele CC HCC

Q01.2 Occipital encephalocele CC HCC

Q01.8 Encephalocele of other sites CC HCC

Q01.9 Encephalocele, unspecified CC HCC

Q02 Microcephaly HCC

INCLUDES hydromicrocephaly
micrencephalon

Code first, if applicable, congenital Zika virus disease

EXCLUDES 1 *Meckel-Gruber syndrome (Q61.9)*

AHA: 2018,4Q,26

DEF: Congenital disorder in which the head circumference is more than two standard deviations below the mean for age, sex, race, and gestation and associated with a decreased life expectancy.

✓4th **Q03 Congenital hydrocephalus**

INCLUDES hydrocephalus in newborn

EXCLUDES 1 *Arnold-Chiari syndrome, type II (Q07.0-)*
acquired hydrocephalus (G91.-)
hydrocephalus due to congenital toxoplasmosis (P37.1)
hydrocephalus with spina bifida (Q05.0-Q05.4)

DEF: Hydrocephalus: Abnormal buildup of cerebrospinal fluid in the brain causing dilation of the ventricles.

Congenital Hydrocephalus

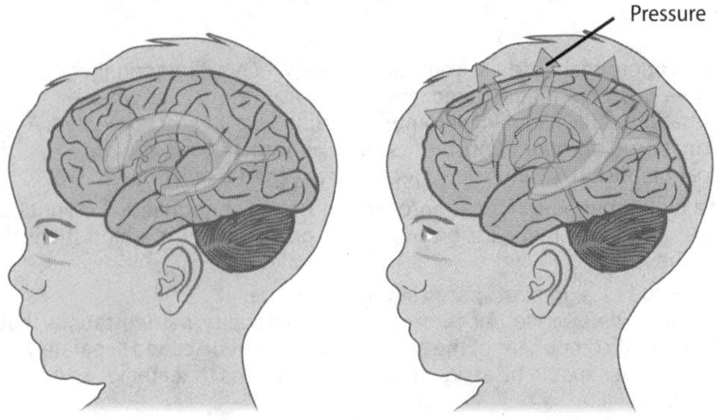

Q03.0 Malformations of aqueduct of Sylvius HCC
- Anomaly of aqueduct of Sylvius
- Obstruction of aqueduct of Sylvius, congenital
- Stenosis of aqueduct of Sylvius

Q03.1 Atresia of foramina of Magendie and Luschka HCC
- Dandy-Walker syndrome

Q03.8 Other congenital hydrocephalus HCC

Q03.9 Congenital hydrocephalus, unspecified HCC

✓4th **Q04 Other congenital malformations of brain**

EXCLUDES 1 *cyclopia (Q87.0)*
macrocephaly (Q75.3)

Q04.0 Congenital malformations of corpus callosum MCC HCC
- Agenesis of corpus callosum

Q04.1 Arhinencephaly MCC HCC

Q04.2 Holoprosencephaly MCC HCC

Q04.3 Other reduction deformities of brain MCC HCC
- Absence of part of brain
- Agenesis of part of brain
- Agyria
- Aplasia of part of brain
- Hydranencephaly
- Hypoplasia of part of brain
- Lissencephaly
- Microgyria
- Pachygyria

EXCLUDES 1 *congenital malformations of corpus callosum (Q04.0)*

Q04.4 Septo-optic dysplasia of brain CC HCC

Q04.5 Megalencephaly CC HCC

Q04.6 Congenital cerebral cysts CC HCC
- Porencephaly
- Schizencephaly

EXCLUDES 1 *acquired porencephalic cyst (G93.0)*

Q04.8 Other specified congenital malformations of brain CC HCC
- Arnold-Chiari syndrome, type IV
- Macrogyria

Q04.9 Congenital malformation of brain, unspecified HCC
- Congenital anomaly NOS of brain
- Congenital deformity NOS of brain
- Congenital disease or lesion NOS of brain
- Multiple anomalies NOS of brain, congenital

Q05 Spina bifida

INCLUDES hydromeningocele (spinal)
meningocele (spinal)
meningomyelocele
myelocele
myelomeningocele
rachischisis
spina bifida (aperta)(cystica)
syringomyelocele

Use additional code for any associated paraplegia (paraparesis) (G82.2-)

EXCLUDES 1 *Arnold-Chiari syndrome, type II (Q07.0-)*
spina bifida occulta (Q76.0)

DEF: Lack of closure in the vertebral column with protrusion of the spinal cord through the defect, often in the lumbosacral area. This condition can be recognized by the presence of alpha-fetoproteins in the amniotic fluid.

Spina Bifida

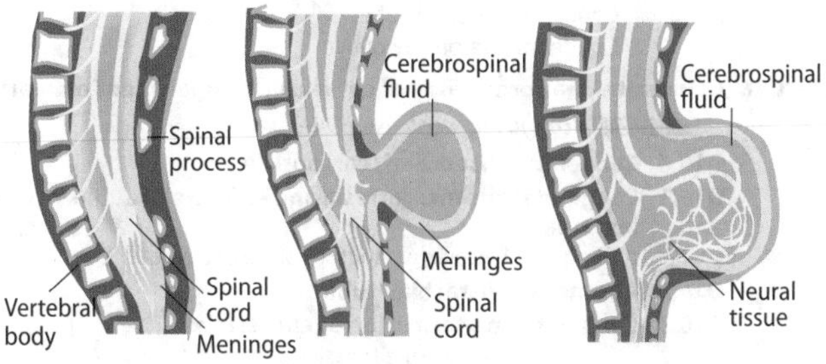

- **Q05.0 Cervical spina bifida with hydrocephalus** CC HCC
- **Q05.1 Thoracic spina bifida with hydrocephalus** CC HCC
  - Dorsal spina bifida with hydrocephalus
  - Thoracolumbar spina bifida with hydrocephalus
- **Q05.2 Lumbar spina bifida with hydrocephalus** CC HCC
  - Lumbosacral spina bifida with hydrocephalus
- **Q05.3 Sacral spina bifida with hydrocephalus** CC HCC
- **Q05.4 Unspecified spina bifida with hydrocephalus** CC HCC
- **Q05.5 Cervical spina bifida without hydrocephalus** HCC
- **Q05.6 Thoracic spina bifida without hydrocephalus** HCC
  - Dorsal spina bifida NOS
  - Thoracolumbar spina bifida NOS
- **Q05.7 Lumbar spina bifida without hydrocephalus** HCC
  - Lumbosacral spina bifida NOS
- **Q05.8 Sacral spina bifida without hydrocephalus** HCC
- **Q05.9 Spina bifida, unspecified** HCC

Q06 Other congenital malformations of spinal cord

- **Q06.0 Amyelia** HCC
- **Q06.1 Hypoplasia and dysplasia of spinal cord** HCC
  - Atelomyelia
  - Myelatelia
  - Myelodysplasia of spinal cord
- **Q06.2 Diastematomyelia** HCC
  - **DEF:** Rare congenital anomaly often associated with spina bifida. The spinal cord is separated into longitudinal halves by a bony, cartilaginous or fibrous septum, each half surrounded by a dural sac.
- **Q06.3 Other congenital cauda equina malformations** HCC
- **Q06.4 Hydromyelia** HCC
  - Hydrorachis
- **Q06.8 Other specified congenital malformations of spinal cord** HCC
- **Q06.9 Congenital malformation of spinal cord, unspecified** HCC
  - Congenital anomaly NOS of spinal cord
  - Congenital deformity NOS of spinal cord
  - Congenital disease or lesion NOS of spinal cord

Q07 Other congenital malformations of nervous system

EXCLUDES 2 *congenital central alveolar hypoventilation syndrome (G47.35)*
familial dysautonomia [Riley-Day] (G90.1)
neurofibromatosis (nonmalignant) (Q85.0-)

Q07.0 Arnold-Chiari syndrome

Arnold-Chiari syndrome, type II

EXCLUDES 1 *Arnold-Chiari syndrome, type III (Q01.-)*
Arnold-Chiari syndrome, type IV (Q04.8)

DEF: Congenital malformation of the brain in which the cerebellum protrudes through the foramen magnum into the spinal canal.

- **Q07.00 Arnold-Chiari syndrome without spina bifida or hydrocephalus** HCC
- **Q07.01 Arnold-Chiari syndrome with spina bifida** HCC
- **Q07.02 Arnold-Chiari syndrome with hydrocephalus** CC HCC
- **Q07.03 Arnold-Chiari syndrome with spina bifida and hydrocephalus** CC HCC

- **Q07.8 Other specified congenital malformations of nervous system** HCC
  - Agenesis of nerve
  - Displacement of brachial plexus
  - Jaw-winking syndrome
  - Marcus Gunn's syndrome
- **Q07.9 Congenital malformation of nervous system, unspecified** HCC
  - Congenital anomaly NOS of nervous system
  - Congenital deformity NOS of nervous system
  - Congenital disease or lesion NOS of nervous system

Congenital malformations of eye, ear, face and neck (Q10-Q18)

EXCLUDES 2 *cleft lip and cleft palate (Q35-Q37)*
congenital malformation of cervical spine (Q05.0, Q05.5, Q67.5, Q76.0-Q76.4)
congenital malformation of larynx (Q31.-)
congenital malformation of lip NEC (Q38.0)
congenital malformation of nose (Q30.-)
congenital malformation of parathyroid gland (Q89.2)
congenital malformation of thyroid gland (Q89.2)

Q10 Congenital malformations of eyelid, lacrimal apparatus and orbit

EXCLUDES 1 *cryptophthalmos NOS (Q11.2)*
cryptophthalmos syndrome (Q87.0)

- **Q10.0 Congenital ptosis**
  - **DEF:** Congenital drooping of the eyelid. Ptosis is mostly idiopathic, but may occur genetically.
- **Q10.1 Congenital ectropion**
- **Q10.2 Congenital entropion**
- **Q10.3 Other congenital malformations of eyelid**
  - Ablepharon
  - Blepharophimosis, congenital
  - Coloboma of eyelid
  - Congenital absence or agenesis of cilia
  - Congenital absence or agenesis of eyelid
  - Congenital accessory eyelid
  - Congenital accessory eye muscle
  - Congenital malformation of eyelid NOS
- **Q10.4 Absence and agenesis of lacrimal apparatus**
  - Congenital absence of punctum lacrimale
- **Q10.5 Congenital stenosis and stricture of lacrimal duct**
- **Q10.6 Other congenital malformations of lacrimal apparatus**
  - Congenital malformation of lacrimal apparatus NOS
- **Q10.7 Congenital malformation of orbit**

Q11 Anophthalmos, microphthalmos and macrophthalmos

- **Q11.0 Cystic eyeball**
- **Q11.1 Other anophthalmos**
  - Anophthalmos NOS
  - Agenesis of eye
  - Aplasia of eye
- **Q11.2 Microphthalmos**
  - Cryptophthalmos NOS
  - Dysplasia of eye
  - Hypoplasia of eye
  - Rudimentary eye
  - EXCLUDES 1 *cryptophthalmos syndrome (Q87.0)*

Q11.3 Macrophthalmos
EXCLUDES 1 *macrophthalmos in congenital glaucoma (Q15.Ø)*

✓4th **Q12 Congenital lens malformations**

Q12.Ø Congenital cataract
Q12.1 Congenital displaced lens
Q12.2 Coloboma of lens

Coloboma of Lens

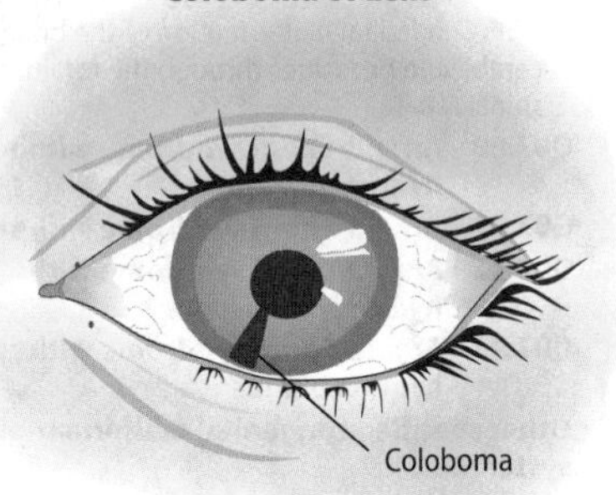

Q12.3 Congenital aphakia
Q12.4 Spherophakia
Q12.8 Other congenital lens malformations
Microphakia
Q12.9 Congenital lens malformation, unspecified

✓4th **Q13 Congenital malformations of anterior segment of eye**

Q13.Ø Coloboma of iris
Coloboma NOS
DEF: Defective or absent section of ocular tissue that may present as mild cupping or a small pit in the ocular disc due to extensive defects in the iris, ciliary body, choroids, and retina.
Q13.1 Absence of iris
Aniridia
Use additional code for associated glaucoma (H42)
DEF: Incompletely formed or absent iris. It affects both eyes and is a dominant trait.
Q13.2 Other congenital malformations of iris
Anisocoria, congenital
Atresia of pupil
Congenital malformation of iris NOS
Corectopia
Q13.3 Congenital corneal opacity
Q13.4 Other congenital corneal malformations
Congenital malformation of cornea NOS
Microcornea
Peter's anomaly
Q13.5 Blue sclera
✓5th **Q13.8 Other congenital malformations of anterior segment of eye**
Q13.81 Rieger's anomaly
Use additional code for associated glaucoma (H42)
Q13.89 Other congenital malformations of anterior segment of eye
Q13.9 Congenital malformation of anterior segment of eye, unspecified

✓4th **Q14 Congenital malformations of posterior segment of eye**
EXCLUDES 2 *optic nerve hypoplasia (H47.Ø3-)*

Q14.Ø Congenital malformation of vitreous humor
Congenital vitreous opacity
Q14.1 Congenital malformation of retina
Congenital retinal aneurysm
Q14.2 Congenital malformation of optic disc
Coloboma of optic disc
Q14.3 Congenital malformation of choroid
Q14.8 Other congenital malformations of posterior segment of eye
Coloboma of the fundus
Q14.9 Congenital malformation of posterior segment of eye, unspecified

✓4th **Q15 Other congenital malformations of eye**
EXCLUDES 1 *congenital nystagmus (H55.Ø1)*
ocular albinism (E7Ø.31-)
optic nerve hypoplasia (H47.Ø3-)
retinitis pigmentosa (H35.52)

Q15.Ø Congenital glaucoma
Axenfeld's anomaly
Buphthalmos
Glaucoma of childhood
Glaucoma of newborn
Hydrophthalmos
Keratoglobus, congenital, with glaucoma
Macrocornea with glaucoma
Macrophthalmos in congenital glaucoma
Megalocornea with glaucoma
Q15.8 Other specified congenital malformations of eye
Q15.9 Congenital malformation of eye, unspecified
Congenital anomaly of eye
Congenital deformity of eye

✓4th **Q16 Congenital malformations of ear causing impairment of hearing**
EXCLUDES 1 *congenital deafness (H9Ø.-)*

Q16.Ø Congenital absence of (ear) auricle
Q16.1 Congenital absence, atresia and stricture of auditory canal (external)
Congenital atresia or stricture of osseous meatus
Q16.2 Absence of eustachian tube
Q16.3 Congenital malformation of ear ossicles
Congenital fusion of ear ossicles
Q16.4 Other congenital malformations of middle ear
Congenital malformation of middle ear NOS
Q16.5 Congenital malformation of inner ear
Congenital anomaly of membranous labyrinth
Congenital anomaly of organ of Corti
Q16.9 Congenital malformation of ear causing impairment of hearing, unspecified
Congenital absence of ear NOS

✓4th **Q17 Other congenital malformations of ear**
EXCLUDES 1 *congenital malformations of ear with impairment of hearing (Q16.Ø-Q16.9)*
preauricular sinus (Q18.1)

Q17.Ø Accessory auricle
Accessory tragus
Polyotia
Preauricular appendage or tag
Supernumerary ear
Supernumerary lobule
Q17.1 Macrotia
DEF: Birth defect characterized by abnormal enlargement of the pinna of the ear.
Q17.2 Microtia
Q17.3 Other misshapen ear
Pointed ear
Q17.4 Misplaced ear
Low-set ears
EXCLUDES 1 *cervical auricle (Q18.2)*
Q17.5 Prominent ear
Bat ear
Q17.8 Other specified congenital malformations of ear
Congenital absence of lobe of ear
Q17.9 Congenital malformation of ear, unspecified
Congenital anomaly of ear NOS

✓4th **Q18 Other congenital malformations of face and neck**
EXCLUDES 1 *cleft lip and cleft palate (Q35-Q37)*
conditions classified to Q67.Ø-Q67.4
congenital malformations of skull and face bones (Q75.-)
cyclopia (Q87.Ø)
dentofacial anomalies [including malocclusion] (M26.-)
malformation syndromes affecting facial appearance (Q87.Ø)
persistent thyroglossal duct (Q89.2)

Q18.Ø Sinus, fistula and cyst of branchial cleft
Branchial vestige
Q18.1 Preauricular sinus and cyst SW
Fistula of auricle, congenital
Cervicoaural fistula

Q18.2 Other branchial cleft malformations
Branchial cleft malformation NOS
Cervical auricle
Otocephaly

Q18.3 Webbing of neck
Pterygium colli
DEF: Congenital malformation characterized by a thick, triangular skinfold that stretches from the lateral side of the neck across the shoulder. It is associated with genetic conditions such as Turner's and Noonan's syndromes.

Q18.4 Macrostomia
DEF: Rare congenital craniofacial bilateral or unilateral anomaly of the mouth due to malformed maxillary and mandibular processes. It results in an abnormally large mouth extending toward the ear.

Q18.5 Microstomia

Q18.6 Macrocheilia
Hypertrophy of lip, congenital

Q18.7 Microcheilia

Q18.8 Other specified congenital malformations of face and neck
Medial cyst of face and neck
Medial fistula of face and neck
Medial sinus of face and neck

Q18.9 Congenital malformation of face and neck, unspecified
Congenital anomaly NOS of face and neck

Congenital malformations of the circulatory system (Q2Ø-Q28)

✓4th Q2Ø Congenital malformations of cardiac chambers and connections
EXCLUDES 1 *dextrocardia with situs inversus (Q89.3)*
mirror-image atrial arrangement with situs inversus (Q89.3)

Q2Ø.Ø Common arterial trunk MCC
Persistent truncus arteriosus
EXCLUDES 1 *aortic septal defect (Q21.4)*

Q2Ø.1 Double outlet right ventricle MCC
Taussig-Bing syndrome

Q2Ø.2 Double outlet left ventricle MCC

Q2Ø.3 Discordant ventriculoarterial connection MCC
Dextrotransposition of aorta
Transposition of great vessels (complete)

Q2Ø.4 Double inlet ventricle MCC
Common ventricle
Cor triloculare biatriatum
Single ventricle

Q2Ø.5 Discordant atrioventricular connection CC
Corrected transposition
Levotransposition
Ventricular inversion

Q2Ø.6 Isomerism of atrial appendages
Isomerism of atrial appendages with asplenia or polysplenia

Q2Ø.8 Other congenital malformations of cardiac chambers and connections
Cor binoculare

Q2Ø.9 Congenital malformation of cardiac chambers and connections, unspecified

✓4th Q21 Congenital malformations of cardiac septa
EXCLUDES 1 *acquired cardiac septal defect (I51.Ø)*

Q21.Ø Ventricular septal defect CC
Roger's disease

Ventricular Septal Defect

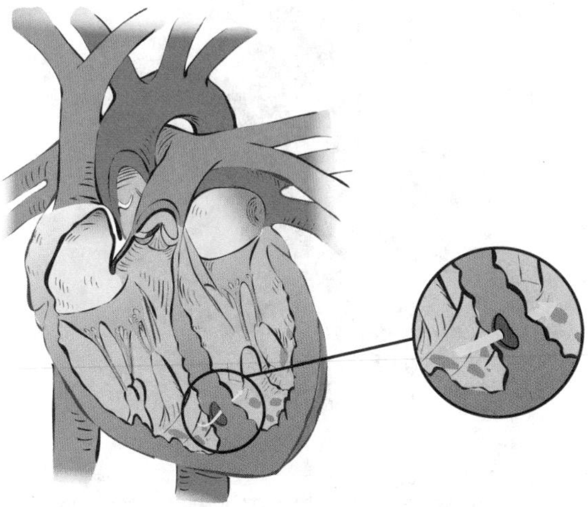

Q21.1 Atrial septal defect CC
Coronary sinus defect
Patent or persistent foramen ovale
Patent or persistent ostium secundum defect (type II)
Patent or persistent sinus venosus defect

Atrial Septal Defect

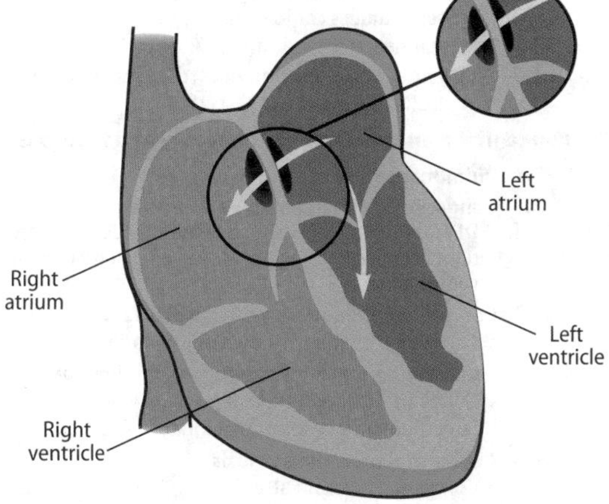

Q21.2 Atrioventricular septal defect CC
Common atrioventricular canal
Endocardial cushion defect
Ostium primum atrial septal defect (type I)

Atrioventricular Septal Defect

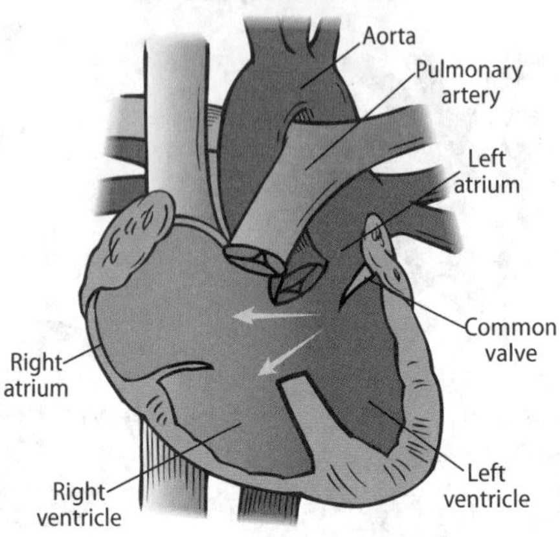

Q21.3 Tetralogy of Fallot MCC
Ventricular septal defect with pulmonary stenosis or atresia, dextroposition of aorta and hypertrophy of right ventricle.
AHA: 2014,3Q,16

Q21.4 Aortopulmonary septal defect
Aortic septal defect
Aortopulmonary window

Q21.8 Other congenital malformations of cardiac septa
Eisenmenger's defect
Pentalogy of Fallot
Code also if applicable:
Eisenmenger's complex (I27.83)
Eisenmenger's syndrome (I27.83)

Q21.9 Congenital malformation of cardiac septum, unspecified
Septal (heart) defect NOS

✓4th Q22 Congenital malformations of pulmonary and tricuspid valves

Q22.Ø Pulmonary valve atresia MCC

Q22.1 Congenital pulmonary valve stenosis CC
DEF: Stenosis of the opening between the pulmonary artery and right ventricle, causing obstructed blood outflow from the right ventricle.

Q22.2 Congenital pulmonary valve insufficiency CC
Congenital pulmonary valve regurgitation

Q22.3 Other congenital malformations of pulmonary valve CC
Congenital malformation of pulmonary valve NOS
Supernumerary cusps of pulmonary valve

Q22.4 Congenital tricuspid stenosis MCC
Congenital tricuspid atresia

Q22.5 Ebstein's anomaly MCC
DEF: Malformation of the tricuspid valve characterized by septal and posterior leaflets attaching to the wall of the right ventricle. Ebstein's anomaly causes the right ventricle to fuse with the atrium into a large right atrium and a small ventricle and leads to heart failure and abnormal cardiac rhythm.

Q22.6 Hypoplastic right heart syndrome MCC

Q22.8 Other congenital malformations of tricuspid valve MCC

Q22.9 Congenital malformation of tricuspid valve, unspecified MCC

✓4th Q23 Congenital malformations of aortic and mitral valves

Q23.Ø Congenital stenosis of aortic valve CC
Congenital aortic atresia
Congenital aortic stenosis NOS
EXCLUDES 1 *congenital stenosis of aortic valve in hypoplastic left heart syndrome (Q23.4)*
congenital subaortic stenosis (Q24.4)
supravalvular aortic stenosis (congenital) (Q25.3)

Q23.1 Congenital insufficiency of aortic valve CC
Bicuspid aortic valve
Congenital aortic insufficiency

Q23.2 Congenital mitral stenosis CC
Congenital mitral atresia
DEF: Congenital stenosis of the mitral valve orifice between the left atrium and ventricle, at the supravalvular, valvular, or subvalvular levels, causing obstruction to left ventricular filling.

Q23.3 Congenital mitral insufficiency CC

Q23.4 Hypoplastic left heart syndrome MCC

Q23.8 Other congenital malformations of aortic and mitral valves

Q23.9 Congenital malformation of aortic and mitral valves, unspecified

✓4th Q24 Other congenital malformations of heart
EXCLUDES 1 *endocardial fibroelastosis (I42.4)*

Q24.Ø Dextrocardia CC
EXCLUDES 1 *dextrocardia with situs inversus (Q89.3)*
isomerism of atrial appendages (with asplenia or polysplenia) (Q2Ø.6)
mirror-image atrial arrangement with situs inversus (Q89.3)
DEF: Congenital condition in which the heart is located on the right side of the chest rather than in its normal position on the left.

Q24.1 Levocardia CC

Q24.2 Cor triatriatum MCC

Q24.3 Pulmonary infundibular stenosis CC
Subvalvular pulmonic stenosis

Q24.4 Congenital subaortic stenosis MCC
DEF: Congenital heart defect characterized by stenosis of the left ventricular outflow tract due to a fibrous tissue ring or septal hypertrophy below the aortic valve.

Q24.5 Malformation of coronary vessels CC
Congenital coronary (artery) aneurysm

Q24.6 Congenital heart block MCC

Q24.8 Other specified congenital malformations of heart
Congenital diverticulum of left ventricle
Congenital malformation of myocardium
Congenital malformation of pericardium
Malposition of heart
Uhl's disease

Q24.9 Congenital malformation of heart, unspecified
Congenital anomaly of heart
Congenital disease of heart

✓4th Q25 Congenital malformations of great arteries

Q25.Ø Patent ductus arteriosus CC
Patent ductus Botallo
Persistent ductus arteriosus
DEF: Condition in which the normal channel between the pulmonary artery and the aorta fails to close at birth, causing arterial blood to recirculate in the lungs and inhibiting the blood supply to the aorta. ***Synonym(s):*** *PDA.*

Patent Ductus Arteriosus

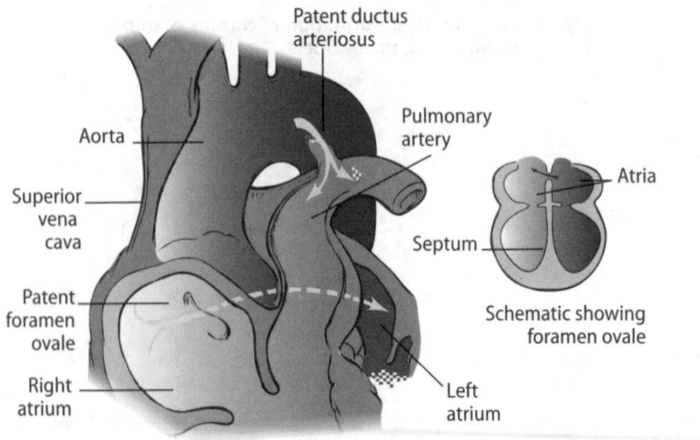

Q25.1 Coarctation of aorta CC
Coarctation of aorta (preductal) (postductal)
Stenosis of aorta
AHA: 2016,4Q,56-57

✓5th **Q25.2 Atresia of aorta**
AHA: 2016,4Q,56-57
Q25.21 Interruption of aortic arch CC
Atresia of aortic arch
Q25.29 Other atresia of aorta CC
Atresia of aorta
Q25.3 Supravalvular aortic stenosis CC
EXCLUDES 1 *congenital aortic stenosis NOS (Q23.Ø)*
congenital stenosis of aortic valve (Q23.Ø)
✓5th **Q25.4 Other congenital malformations of aorta**
EXCLUDES 1 *hypoplasia of aorta in hypoplastic left heart syndrome (Q23.4)*
AHA: 2016,4Q,57
Q25.4Ø Congenital malformation of aorta unspecified CC
Q25.41 Absence and aplasia of aorta CC
Q25.42 Hypoplasia of aorta CC
Q25.43 Congenital aneurysm of aorta CC
Congenital aneurysm of aortic root
Congenital aneurysm of aortic sinus
Q25.44 Congenital dilation of aorta CC
Q25.45 Double aortic arch CC
Vascular ring of aorta

Aortic Arch Anomalies

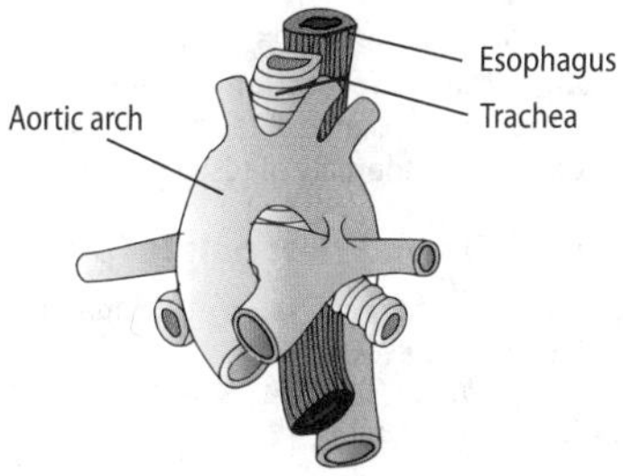

Normal aortic arch

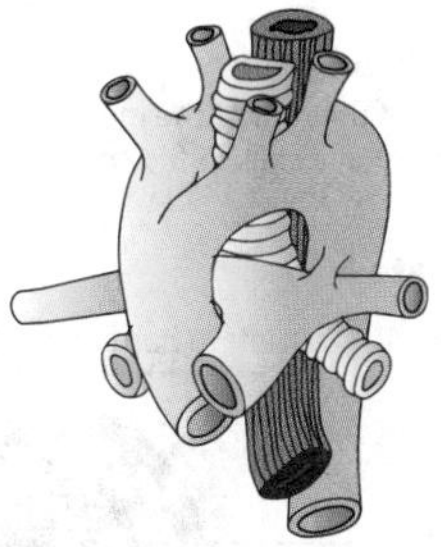
Double aortic arch

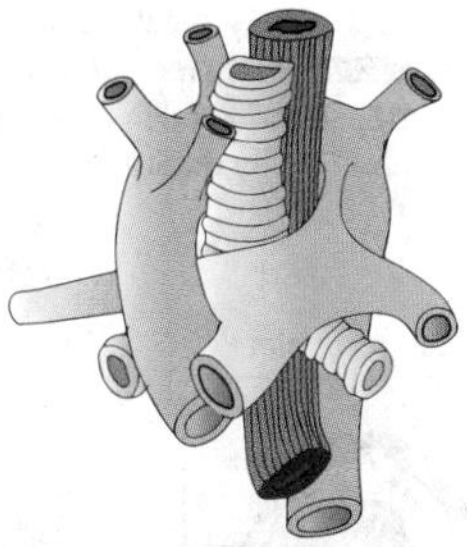
Right aortic arch

Q25.46 Tortuous aortic arch CC
Persistent convolutions of aortic arch
Q25.47 Right aortic arch CC
Persistent right aortic arch
Q25.48 Anomalous origin of subclavian artery CC
Q25.49 Other congenital malformations of aorta CC
Aortic arch
Bovine arch
Q25.5 Atresia of pulmonary artery MCC
Q25.6 Stenosis of pulmonary artery MCC
Supravalvular pulmonary stenosis
✓5th **Q25.7 Other congenital malformations of pulmonary artery**
Q25.71 Coarctation of pulmonary artery MCC
Q25.72 Congenital pulmonary arteriovenous malformation MCC
Congenital pulmonary arteriovenous aneurysm
Q25.79 Other congenital malformations of pulmonary artery MCC
Aberrant pulmonary artery
Agenesis of pulmonary artery
Congenital aneurysm of pulmonary artery
Congenital anomaly of pulmonary artery
Hypoplasia of pulmonary artery
Q25.8 Other congenital malformations of other great arteries CC
Q25.9 Congenital malformation of great arteries, unspecified CC

✓4th **Q26 Congenital malformations of great veins**
Q26.Ø Congenital stenosis of vena cava CC
Congenital stenosis of vena cava (inferior)(superior)
Q26.1 Persistent left superior vena cava CC
Q26.2 Total anomalous pulmonary venous connection CC
Total anomalous pulmonary venous return [TAPVR], subdiaphragmatic
Total anomalous pulmonary venous return [TAPVR], supradiaphragmatic
Q26.3 Partial anomalous pulmonary venous connection CC
Partial anomalous pulmonary venous return
Q26.4 Anomalous pulmonary venous connection, unspecified CC
Q26.5 Anomalous portal venous connection
Q26.6 Portal vein-hepatic artery fistula
Q26.8 Other congenital malformations of great veins CC
Absence of vena cava (inferior) (superior)
Azygos continuation of inferior vena cava
Persistent left posterior cardinal vein
Scimitar syndrome
Q26.9 Congenital malformation of great vein, unspecified CC
Congenital anomaly of vena cava (inferior) (superior) NOS
✓4th **Q27 Other congenital malformations of peripheral vascular system**
EXCLUDES 2 *anomalies of cerebral and precerebral vessels (Q28.Ø-Q28.3)*
anomalies of coronary vessels (Q24.5)
anomalies of pulmonary artery (Q25.5-Q25.7)
congenital retinal aneurysm (Q14.1)
hemangioma and lymphangioma (D18.-)
Q27.Ø Congenital absence and hypoplasia of umbilical artery
Single umbilical artery
Q27.1 Congenital renal artery stenosis
Q27.2 Other congenital malformations of renal artery
Congenital malformation of renal artery NOS
Multiple renal arteries
✓5th **Q27.3 Arteriovenous malformation (peripheral)**
Arteriovenous aneurysm
EXCLUDES 1 *acquired arteriovenous aneurysm (I77.Ø)*
EXCLUDES 2 *arteriovenous malformation of cerebral vessels (Q28.2)*
arteriovenous malformation of precerebral vessels (Q28.Ø)
DEF: Arteriovenous malformation: Connecting passage between an artery and a vein.
Q27.3Ø Arteriovenous malformation, site unspecified CC
Q27.31 Arteriovenous malformation of vessel of upper limb
Q27.32 Arteriovenous malformation of vessel of lower limb
Q27.33 Arteriovenous malformation of digestive system vessel
AHA: 2018,3Q,21
Q27.34 Arteriovenous malformation of renal vessel
Q27.39 Arteriovenous malformation, other site
Q27.4 Congenital phlebectasia CC
Q27.8 Other specified congenital malformations of peripheral vascular system
Absence of peripheral vascular system
Atresia of peripheral vascular system
Congenital aneurysm (peripheral)
Congenital stricture, artery
Congenital varix
EXCLUDES 1 *arteriovenous malformation (Q27.3-)*
Q27.9 Congenital malformation of peripheral vascular system, unspecified
Anomaly of artery or vein NOS
✓4th **Q28 Other congenital malformations of circulatory system**
EXCLUDES 1 *congenital aneurysm NOS (Q27.8)*
congenital coronary aneurysm (Q24.5)
ruptured cerebral arteriovenous malformation (I6Ø.8)
ruptured malformation of precerebral vessels (I72.Ø)
EXCLUDES 2 *congenital peripheral aneurysm (Q27.8)*
congenital pulmonary aneurysm (Q25.79)
congenital retinal aneurysm (Q14.1)
Q28.Ø Arteriovenous malformation of precerebral vessels CC
Congenital arteriovenous precerebral aneurysm (nonruptured)

Q28.1 Other malformations of precerebral vessels CC
Congenital malformation of precerebral vessels NOS
Congenital precerebral aneurysm (nonruptured)

Q28.2 Arteriovenous malformation of cerebral vessels MCC
Arteriovenous malformation of brain NOS
Congenital arteriovenous cerebral aneurysm (nonruptured)

Q28.3 Other malformations of cerebral vessels MCC
Congenital cerebral aneurysm (nonruptured)
Congenital malformation of cerebral vessels NOS
Developmental venous anomaly

Q28.8 Other specified congenital malformations of circulatory system CC
Congenital aneurysm, specified site NEC
Spinal vessel anomaly

Q28.9 Congenital malformation of circulatory system, unspecified CC

Congenital malformations of the respiratory system (Q3Ø-Q34)

✓4th Q3Ø Congenital malformations of nose
EXCLUDES 1 *congenital deviation of nasal septum (Q67.4)*

Q3Ø.Ø Choanal atresia
Atresia of nares (anterior) (posterior)
Congenital stenosis of nares (anterior) (posterior)

Q3Ø.1 Agenesis and underdevelopment of nose
Congenital absent of nose

Q3Ø.2 Fissured, notched and cleft nose

Q3Ø.3 Congenital perforated nasal septum

Q3Ø.8 Other congenital malformations of nose
Accessory nose
Congenital anomaly of nasal sinus wall

Q3Ø.9 Congenital malformation of nose, unspecified

✓4th Q31 Congenital malformations of larynx
EXCLUDES 1 *congenital laryngeal stridor NOS (P28.89)*

Q31.Ø Web of larynx
Glottic web of larynx
Subglottic web of larynx
Web of larynx NOS
DEF: Congenital malformation of the larynx marked by thin, translucent, or thick fibrotic membrane-like structure between the vocal folds. It is characterized by shortness of breath and stridor.

Q31.1 Congenital subglottic stenosis CC

Q31.2 Laryngeal hypoplasia CC

Q31.3 Laryngocele CC

Q31.5 Congenital laryngomalacia CC

Q31.8 Other congenital malformations of larynx CC
Absence of larynx
Agenesis of larynx
Atresia of larynx
Congenital cleft thyroid cartilage
Congenital fissure of epiglottis
Congenital stenosis of larynx NEC
Posterior cleft of cricoid cartilage

Q31.9 Congenital malformation of larynx, unspecified CC

✓4th Q32 Congenital malformations of trachea and bronchus
EXCLUDES 1 *congenital bronchiectasis (Q33.4)*

Q32.Ø Congenital tracheomalacia CC

Q32.1 Other congenital malformations of trachea CC
Atresia of trachea
Congenital anomaly of tracheal cartilage
Congenital dilatation of trachea
Congenital malformation of trachea
Congenital stenosis of trachea
Congenital tracheocele

Q32.2 Congenital bronchomalacia CC

Q32.3 Congenital stenosis of bronchus CC

Q32.4 Other congenital malformations of bronchus CC
Absence of bronchus
Agenesis of bronchus
Atresia of bronchus
Congenital diverticulum of bronchus
Congenital malformation of bronchus NOS

✓4th Q33 Congenital malformations of lung

Q33.Ø Congenital cystic lung CC
Congenital cystic lung disease
Congenital honeycomb lung
Congenital polycystic lung disease
EXCLUDES 1 *cystic fibrosis (E84.Ø)*
cystic lung disease, acquired or unspecified (J98.4)

Q33.1 Accessory lobe of lung
Azygos lobe (fissured), lung

Q33.2 Sequestration of lung MCC

Q33.3 Agenesis of lung MCC
Congenital absence of lung (lobe)

Q33.4 Congenital bronchiectasis CC

Q33.5 Ectopic tissue in lung

Q33.6 Congenital hypoplasia and dysplasia of lung MCC
EXCLUDES 1 *pulmonary hypoplasia associated with short gestation (P28.Ø)*

Q33.8 Other congenital malformations of lung

Q33.9 Congenital malformation of lung, unspecified

✓4th Q34 Other congenital malformations of respiratory system
EXCLUDES 2 *congenital central alveolar hypoventilation syndrome (G47.35)*

Q34.Ø Anomaly of pleura

Q34.1 Congenital cyst of mediastinum

Q34.8 Other specified congenital malformations of respiratory system
Atresia of nasopharynx

Q34.9 Congenital malformation of respiratory system, unspecified
Congenital absence of respiratory system
Congenital anomaly of respiratory system NOS

Cleft lip and cleft palate (Q35-Q37)

Use additional code to identify associated malformation of the nose (Q3Ø.2)
EXCLUDES 1 ~~*Robin's syndrome (Q87.Ø)*~~
EXCLUDES 2 ▶*Robin's syndrome (Q87.Ø)*◀

✓4th Q35 Cleft palate
INCLUDES fissure of palate
palatoschisis
EXCLUDES 1 *cleft palate with cleft lip (Q37.-)*
DEF: Congenital fissure or defect of the roof of the mouth opening to the nasal cavity due to failure of embryonic cells to fuse completely.

Cleft Palate

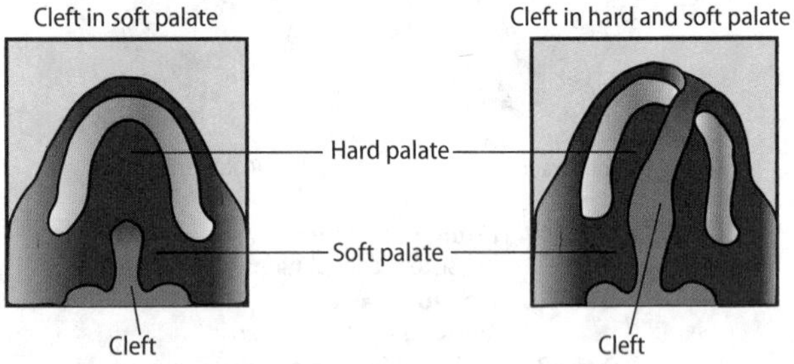

Q35.1 Cleft hard palate

Q35.3 Cleft soft palate

Q35.5 Cleft hard palate with cleft soft palate

Q35.7 Cleft uvula

Q35.9 Cleft palate, unspecified
Cleft palate NOS

Q36 Cleft lip

INCLUDES cheiloschisis
congenital fissure of lip
harelip
labium leporinum

EXCLUDES 1 *cleft lip with cleft palate (Q37.-)*

DEF: Congenital fissure or opening in the upper lip due to failure of embryonic cells to fuse completely.

Cleft Lip

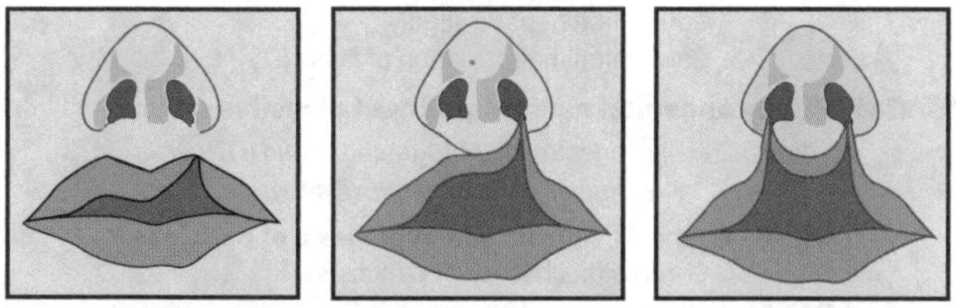

Unilateral incomplete | Unilateral complete | Bilateral complete

Q36.Ø Cleft lip, bilateral

Q36.1 Cleft lip, median

Q36.9 Cleft lip, unilateral
Cleft lip NOS

Q37 Cleft palate with cleft lip

INCLUDES cheilopalatoschisis

Q37.Ø Cleft hard palate with bilateral cleft lip

Q37.1 Cleft hard palate with unilateral cleft lip
Cleft hard palate with cleft lip NOS

Q37.2 Cleft soft palate with bilateral cleft lip

Q37.3 Cleft soft palate with unilateral cleft lip
Cleft soft palate with cleft lip NOS

Q37.4 Cleft hard and soft palate with bilateral cleft lip

Q37.5 Cleft hard and soft palate with unilateral cleft lip
Cleft hard and soft palate with cleft lip NOS

Q37.8 Unspecified cleft palate with bilateral cleft lip

Q37.9 Unspecified cleft palate with unilateral cleft lip
Cleft palate with cleft lip NOS

Other congenital malformations of the digestive system (Q38-Q45)

Q38 Other congenital malformations of tongue, mouth and pharynx

EXCLUDES 1 *dentofacial anomalies (M26.-)*
macrostomia (Q18.4)
microstomia (Q18.5)

Q38.Ø Congenital malformations of lips, not elsewhere classified
Congenital fistula of lip
Congenital malformation of lip NOS
Van der Woude's syndrome

EXCLUDES 1 *cleft lip (Q36.-)*
cleft lip with cleft palate (Q37.-)
macrocheilia (Q18.6)
microcheilia (Q18.7)

Q38.1 Ankyloglossia
Tongue tie

Q38.2 Macroglossia
Congenital hypertrophy of tongue

Q38.3 Other congenital malformations of tongue
Aglossia
Bifid tongue
Congenital adhesion of tongue
Congenital fissure of tongue
Congenital malformation of tongue NOS
Double tongue
Hypoglossia
Hypoplasia of tongue
Microglossia

Q38.4 Congenital malformations of salivary glands and ducts
Atresia of salivary glands and ducts
Congenital absence of salivary glands and ducts
Congenital accessory salivary glands and ducts
Congenital fistula of salivary gland

Q38.5 Congenital malformations of palate, not elsewhere classified
Congenital absence of uvula
Congenital malformation of palate NOS
Congenital high arched palate

EXCLUDES 1 *cleft palate (Q35.-)*
cleft palate with cleft lip (Q37.-)

Q38.6 Other congenital malformations of mouth
Congenital malformation of mouth NOS

Q38.7 Congenital pharyngeal pouch
Congenital diverticulum of pharynx

EXCLUDES 1 *pharyngeal pouch syndrome (D82.1)*

Q38.8 Other congenital malformations of pharynx
Congenital malformation of pharynx NOS
Imperforate pharynx

Q39 Congenital malformations of esophagus

Q39.Ø Atresia of esophagus without fistula MCC
Atresia of esophagus NOS

Q39.1 Atresia of esophagus with tracheo-esophageal fistula MCC
Atresia of esophagus with broncho-esophageal fistula

Q39.2 Congenital tracheo-esophageal fistula without atresia MCC
Congenital tracheo-esophageal fistula NOS

Q39.3 Congenital stenosis and stricture of esophagus MCC

Q39.4 Esophageal web MCC

Q39.5 Congenital dilatation of esophagus CC
Congenital cardiospasm

Q39.6 Congenital diverticulum of esophagus CC
Congenital esophageal pouch

Q39.8 Other congenital malformations of esophagus CC
Congenital absence of esophagus
Congenital displacement of esophagus
Congenital duplication of esophagus

Q39.9 Congenital malformation of esophagus, unspecified CC

Q4Ø Other congenital malformations of upper alimentary tract

Q4Ø.Ø Congenital hypertrophic pyloric stenosis
Congenital or infantile constriction
Congenital or infantile hypertrophy
Congenital or infantile spasm
Congenital or infantile stenosis
Congenital or infantile stricture

Q4Ø.1 Congenital hiatus hernia
Congenital displacement of cardia through esophageal hiatus

EXCLUDES 1 *congenital diaphragmatic hernia (Q79.Ø)*

Q4Ø.2 Other specified congenital malformations of stomach
Congenital displacement of stomach
Congenital diverticulum of stomach
Congenital hourglass stomach
Congenital duplication of stomach
Megalogastria
Microgastria

Q4Ø.3 Congenital malformation of stomach, unspecified

Q4Ø.8 Other specified congenital malformations of upper alimentary tract

Q4Ø.9 Congenital malformation of upper alimentary tract, unspecified
Congenital anomaly of upper alimentary tract
Congenital deformity of upper alimentary tract

Q41 Congenital absence, atresia and stenosis of small intestine

INCLUDES congenital obstruction, occlusion or stricture of small intestine or intestine NOS

EXCLUDES 1 *cystic fibrosis with intestinal manifestation (E84.11)*
meconium ileus NOS (without cystic fibrosis) (P76.Ø)

Q41.Ø Congenital absence, atresia and stenosis of duodenum CC

Q41.1 Congenital absence, atresia and stenosis of jejunum CC
Apple peel syndrome
Imperforate jejunum

Q41.2 Congenital absence, atresia and stenosis of ileum CC

Q41.8 Congenital absence, atresia and stenosis of other specified parts of small intestine CC

Q41.9 Congenital absence, atresia and stenosis of small intestine, part unspecified CC
Congenital absence, atresia and stenosis of intestine NOS

✓4th Q42 Congenital absence, atresia and stenosis of large intestine
INCLUDES congenital obstruction, occlusion and stricture of large intestine

Q42.Ø Congenital absence, atresia and stenosis of rectum with fistula CC

Q42.1 Congenital absence, atresia and stenosis of rectum without fistula CC
Imperforate rectum

Q42.2 Congenital absence, atresia and stenosis of anus with fistula CC

Q42.3 Congenital absence, atresia and stenosis of anus without fistula CC
Imperforate anus

Q42.8 Congenital absence, atresia and stenosis of other parts of large intestine CC

Q42.9 Congenital absence, atresia and stenosis of large intestine, part unspecified CC

✓4th Q43 Other congenital malformations of intestine

Q43.Ø Meckel's diverticulum (displaced) (hypertrophic)
Persistent omphalomesenteric duct
Persistent vitelline duct
DEF: Congenital, abnormal remnant of embryonic digestive system development that leaves a sacculation or outpouching from the wall of the small intestine near the terminal part of the ileum made of acid-secreting tissue as in the stomach.

Q43.1 Hirschsprung's disease CC
Aganglionosis
Congenital (aganglionic) megacolon
DEF: Congenital enlargement or dilation of the colon, with the absence of nerve cells in a segment of colon distally that causes the inability to defecate.

Q43.2 Other congenital functional disorders of colon CC
Congenital dilatation of colon

Q43.3 Congenital malformations of intestinal fixation CC
Congenital omental, anomalous adhesions [bands]
Congenital peritoneal adhesions [bands]
Incomplete rotation of cecum and colon
Insufficient rotation of cecum and colon
Jackson's membrane
Malrotation of colon
Rotation failure of cecum and colon
Universal mesentery

Q43.4 Duplication of intestine CC

Q43.5 Ectopic anus CC

Q43.6 Congenital fistula of rectum and anus CC
EXCLUDES 1 *congenital fistula of anus with absence, atresia and stenosis (Q42.2)*
congenital fistula of rectum with absence, atresia and stenosis (Q42.Ø)
congenital rectovaginal fistula (Q52.2)
congenital urethrorectal fistula (Q64.73)
pilonidal fistula or sinus (LØ5.-)

Q43.7 Persistent cloaca CC
Cloaca NOS

Q43.8 Other specified congenital malformations of intestine CC
Congenital blind loop syndrome
Congenital diverticulitis, colon
Congenital diverticulum, intestine
Dolichocolon
Megaloappendix
Megaloduodenum
Microcolon
Transposition of appendix
Transposition of colon
Transposition of intestine
AHA: 2013,2Q,31

Q43.9 Congenital malformation of intestine, unspecified CC

✓4th Q44 Congenital malformations of gallbladder, bile ducts and liver

Q44.Ø Agenesis, aplasia and hypoplasia of gallbladder CC
Congenital absence of gallbladder

Q44.1 Other congenital malformations of gallbladder CC
Congenital malformation of gallbladder NOS
Intrahepatic gallbladder

Q44.2 Atresia of bile ducts MCC

Q44.3 Congenital stenosis and stricture of bile ducts MCC

Q44.4 Choledochal cyst CC

Q44.5 Other congenital malformations of bile ducts CC
Accessory hepatic duct
Biliary duct duplication
Congenital malformation of bile duct NOS
Cystic duct duplication

Q44.6 Cystic disease of liver CC
Fibrocystic disease of liver

Q44.7 Other congenital malformations of liver CC
Accessory liver
Alagille's syndrome
Congenital absence of liver
Congenital hepatomegaly
Congenital malformation of liver NOS

✓4th Q45 Other congenital malformations of digestive system
EXCLUDES 2 *congenital diaphragmatic hernia (Q79.Ø)*
congenital hiatus hernia (Q4Ø.1)

Q45.Ø Agenesis, aplasia and hypoplasia of pancreas CC
Congenital absence of pancreas

Q45.1 Annular pancreas CC

Q45.2 Congenital pancreatic cyst CC

Q45.3 Other congenital malformations of pancreas and pancreatic duct CC
Accessory pancreas
Congenital malformation of pancreas or pancreatic duct NOS
EXCLUDES 1 *congenital diabetes mellitus (E1Ø.-)*
cystic fibrosis (E84.Ø-E84.9)
fibrocystic disease of pancreas (E84.-)
neonatal diabetes mellitus (P7Ø.2)

Q45.8 Other specified congenital malformations of digestive system
Absence (complete) (partial) of alimentary tract NOS
Duplication of digestive system
Malposition, congenital of digestive system

Q45.9 Congenital malformation of digestive system, unspecified
Congenital anomaly of digestive system
Congenital deformity of digestive system

Congenital malformations of genital organs (Q5Ø-Q56)

EXCLUDES 1 *androgen insensitivity syndrome (E34.5-)*
syndromes associated with anomalies in the number and form of chromosomes (Q9Ø-Q99)

✓4th Q5Ø Congenital malformations of ovaries, fallopian tubes and broad ligaments

✓5th Q5Ø.Ø Congenital absence of ovary
EXCLUDES 1 *Turner's syndrome (Q96.-)*

Q5Ø.Ø1 Congenital absence of ovary, unilateral ♀

Q5Ø.Ø2 Congenital absence of ovary, bilateral ♀

Q5Ø.1 Developmental ovarian cyst ♀

Q5Ø.2 Congenital torsion of ovary ♀

✓5th Q5Ø.3 Other congenital malformations of ovary

Q5Ø.31 Accessory ovary ♀

Q5Ø.32 Ovarian streak ♀
46, XX with streak gonads

Q5Ø.39 Other congenital malformation of ovary ♀
Congenital malformation of ovary NOS

Q5Ø.4 Embryonic cyst of fallopian tube ♀
Fimbrial cyst

Q5Ø.5 Embryonic cyst of broad ligament ♀
Epoophoron cyst
Parovarian cyst

Q5Ø.6 Other congenital malformations of fallopian tube and broad ligament ♀
Absence of fallopian tube and broad ligament
Accessory fallopian tube and broad ligament
Atresia of fallopian tube and broad ligament
Congenital malformation of fallopian tube or broad ligament NOS

✓4th Q51 Congenital malformations of uterus and cervix

Q51.Ø Agenesis and aplasia of uterus ♀
Congenital absence of uterus

✓5th **Q51.1 Doubling of uterus with doubling of cervix and vagina**

Q51.1Ø Doubling of uterus with doubling of cervix and vagina without obstruction ♀
Doubling of uterus with doubling of cervix and vagina NOS

Q51.11 Doubling of uterus with doubling of cervix and vagina with obstruction ♀

✓5th **Q51.2 Other doubling of uterus**
Doubling of uterus NOS
Septate uterus
AHA: 2018,4Q,27

~~**Q51.2Ø Other doubling of uterus, unspecified**~~

▲ **Q51.21 Complete doubling of uterus** ♀
Complete septate uterus

▲ **Q51.22 Partial doubling of uterus** ♀
Partial septate uterus

▲ **Q51.28 Other and unspecified doubling of uterus** ♀
▶Septate uterus NOS◀

Q51.3 Bicornate uterus ♀
Bicornate uterus, complete or partial

Q51.4 Unicornate uterus ♀
Unicornate uterus with or without a separate uterine horn
Uterus with only one functioning horn

Q51.5 Agenesis and aplasia of cervix ♀
Congenital absence of cervix

Q51.6 Embryonic cyst of cervix ♀

Q51.7 Congenital fistulae between uterus and digestive and urinary tracts ♀

✓5th **Q51.8 Other congenital malformations of uterus and cervix**

✓6th **Q51.81 Other congenital malformations of uterus**

Q51.81Ø Arcuate uterus ♀
Arcuatus uterus

Q51.811 Hypoplasia of uterus ♀

Q51.818 Other congenital malformations of uterus ♀
Müllerian anomaly of uterus NEC

✓6th **Q51.82 Other congenital malformations of cervix**

Q51.82Ø Cervical duplication ♀

Q51.821 Hypoplasia of cervix ♀

Q51.828 Other congenital malformations of cervix ♀

Q51.9 Congenital malformation of uterus and cervix, unspecified ♀

✓4th **Q52 Other congenital malformations of female genitalia**

Q52.Ø Congenital absence of vagina ♀
Vaginal agenesis, total or partial

✓5th **Q52.1 Doubling of vagina**
EXCLUDES 1 *doubling of vagina with doubling of uterus and cervix (Q51.1-)*

Q52.1Ø Doubling of vagina, unspecified ♀
Septate vagina NOS

Q52.11 Transverse vaginal septum ♀

✓6th **Q52.12 Longitudinal vaginal septum**
AHA: 2016,4Q,58-59

Q52.12Ø Longitudinal vaginal septum, nonobstructing ♀

Q52.121 Longitudinal vaginal septum, obstructing, right side ♀

Q52.122 Longitudinal vaginal septum, obstructing, left side ♀

Q52.123 Longitudinal vaginal septum, microperforate, right side ♀

Q52.124 Longitudinal vaginal septum, microperforate, left side ♀

Q52.129 Other and unspecified longitudinal vaginal septum ♀

Q52.2 Congenital rectovaginal fistula ♀
EXCLUDES 1 *cloaca (Q43.7)*

Q52.3 Imperforate hymen ♀
DEF: Obstructive anomaly of vagina, characterized by complete closure of the membranous fold around the external opening of the vagina, obstructing the vaginal introitus.

Q52.4 Other congenital malformations of vagina ♀
Canal of Nuck cyst, congenital
Congenital malformation of vagina NOS
Embryonic vaginal cyst
Gartner's duct cyst

Q52.5 Fusion of labia ♀

Q52.6 Congenital malformation of clitoris ♀

✓5th **Q52.7 Other and unspecified congenital malformations of vulva**

Q52.7Ø Unspecified congenital malformations of vulva ♀
Congenital malformation of vulva NOS

Q52.71 Congenital absence of vulva ♀

Q52.79 Other congenital malformations of vulva ♀
Congenital cyst of vulva

Q52.8 Other specified congenital malformations of female genitalia ♀

Q52.9 Congenital malformation of female genitalia, unspecified ♀

✓4th **Q53 Undescended and ectopic testicle**

✓5th **Q53.Ø Ectopic testis**

Q53.ØØ Ectopic testis, unspecified ♂

Q53.Ø1 Ectopic testis, unilateral ♂

Q53.Ø2 Ectopic testes, bilateral ♂

✓5th **Q53.1 Undescended testicle, unilateral**
AHA: 2017,4Q,22-23

Q53.1Ø Unspecified undescended testicle, unilateral ♂

✓6th **Q53.11 Abdominal testis, unilateral**

Q53.111 Unilateral intraabdominal testis ♂

Q53.112 Unilateral inguinal testis ♂

Q53.12 Ectopic perineal testis, unilateral ♂

Q53.13 Unilateral high scrotal testis ♂

✓5th **Q53.2 Undescended testicle, bilateral**
AHA: 2017,4Q,22-23

Q53.2Ø Undescended testicle, unspecified, bilateral ♂

✓6th **Q53.21 Abdominal testis, bilateral**

Q53.211 Bilateral intraabdominal testes ♂

Q53.212 Bilateral inguinal testes ♂

Q53.22 Ectopic perineal testis, bilateral ♂

Q53.23 Bilateral high scrotal testes ♂

Q53.9 Undescended testicle, unspecified ♂
Cryptorchism NOS

✓4th **Q54 Hypospadias**
EXCLUDES 1 *epispadias (Q64.Ø)*
DEF: Abnormal opening of the urethra on the ventral (underside) surface of the penis.

Hypospadias

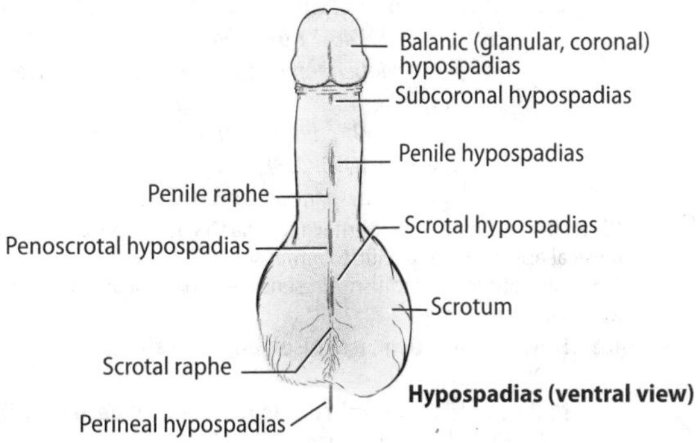

Q54.Ø Hypospadias, balanic ♂
Hypospadias, coronal
Hypospadias, glandular

Q54.1 Hypospadias, penile ♂

Q54.2 Hypospadias, penoscrotal ♂

Q54.3 Hypospadias, perineal ♂

Q54.4 Congenital chordee ♂
Chordee without hypospadias

Q54.8 Other hypospadias ♂
Hypospadias with intersex state

Q54.9 Hypospadias, unspecified ♂

√4th **Q55 Other congenital malformations of male genital organs**

EXCLUDES 1 *congenital hydrocele (P83.5)*
hypospadias (Q54.-)

Q55.Ø Absence and aplasia of testis ♂
Monorchism

Q55.1 Hypoplasia of testis and scrotum ♂
Fusion of testes

√5th **Q55.2 Other and unspecified congenital malformations of testis and scrotum**

Q55.2Ø Unspecified congenital malformations of testis and scrotum ♂
Congenital malformation of testis or scrotum NOS

Q55.21 Polyorchism ♂
DEF: Congenital anomaly in which there are more than two testes.

Q55.22 Retractile testis ♂

Q55.23 Scrotal transposition ♂

Q55.29 Other congenital malformations of testis and scrotum ♂

Q55.3 Atresia of vas deferens ♂
Code first any associated cystic fibrosis (E84.-)

Q55.4 Other congenital malformations of vas deferens, epididymis, seminal vesicles and prostate ♂
Absence or aplasia of prostate
Absence or aplasia of spermatic cord
Congenital malformation of vas deferens, epididymis, seminal vesicles or prostate NOS

Q55.5 Congenital absence and aplasia of penis ♂

√5th **Q55.6 Other congenital malformations of penis**

Q55.61 Curvature of penis (lateral) ♂

Q55.62 Hypoplasia of penis ♂
Micropenis

Q55.63 Congenital torsion of penis ♂
EXCLUDES 1 *acquired torsion of penis (N48.82)*

Q55.64 Hidden penis ♂
Buried penis
Concealed penis
EXCLUDES 1 *acquired buried penis (N48.83)*

Q55.69 Other congenital malformation of penis ♂
Congenital malformation of penis NOS

Q55.7 Congenital vasocutaneous fistula ♂

Q55.8 Other specified congenital malformations of male genital organs ♂

Q55.9 Congenital malformation of male genital organ, unspecified ♂
Congenital anomaly of male genital organ
Congenital deformity of male genital organ

√4th **Q56 Indeterminate sex and pseudohermaphroditism**

EXCLUDES 1 *46, XX true hermaphrodite (Q99.1)*
androgen insensitivity syndrome (E34.5-)
chimera 46, XX/46, XY true hermaphrodite (Q99.Ø)
female pseudohermaphroditism with adrenocortical disorder (E25.-)
pseudohermaphroditism with specified chromosomal anomaly (Q96-Q99)
pure gonadal dysgenesis (Q99.1)

DEF: Indeterminate sex: External genitalia that is nondescript, lacking the physical appearance specific to either sex.
DEF: Pseudohermaphroditism: Presence of gonads of one sex and external genitalia of another sex.

Q56.Ø Hermaphroditism, not elsewhere classified
Ovotestis

Q56.1 Male pseudohermaphroditism, not elsewhere classified ♂
46, XY with streak gonads
Male pseudohermaphroditism NOS

Q56.2 Female pseudohermaphroditism, not elsewhere classified ♀
Female pseudohermaphroditism NOS

Q56.3 Pseudohermaphroditism, unspecified

Q56.4 Indeterminate sex, unspecified
Ambiguous genitalia

Congenital malformations of the urinary system (Q6Ø-Q64)

√4th **Q6Ø Renal agenesis and other reduction defects of kidney**

INCLUDES congenital absence of kidney
congenital atrophy of kidney
infantile atrophy of kidney

Q6Ø.Ø Renal agenesis, unilateral CC

Q6Ø.1 Renal agenesis, bilateral CC

Q6Ø.2 Renal agenesis, unspecified CC

Q6Ø.3 Renal hypoplasia, unilateral CC

Q6Ø.4 Renal hypoplasia, bilateral CC

Q6Ø.5 Renal hypoplasia, unspecified CC

Q6Ø.6 Potter's syndrome CC

√4th **Q61 Cystic kidney disease**

EXCLUDES 1 *acquired cyst of kidney (N28.1)*
Potter's syndrome (Q6Ø.6)

√5th **Q61.Ø Congenital renal cyst**

Q61.ØØ Congenital renal cyst, unspecified CC
Cyst of kidney NOS (congenital)

Q61.Ø1 Congenital single renal cyst CC

Q61.Ø2 Congenital multiple renal cysts CC

√5th **Q61.1 Polycystic kidney, infantile type**
Polycystic kidney, autosomal recessive

Q61.11 Cystic dilatation of collecting ducts CC

Q61.19 Other polycystic kidney, infantile type CC

Q61.2 Polycystic kidney, adult type CC
Polycystic kidney, autosomal dominant

Q61.3 Polycystic kidney, unspecified CC
AHA: 2016,3Q,22

Q61.4 Renal dysplasia CC
Multicystic dysplastic kidney
Multicystic kidney (development)
Multicystic kidney disease
Multicystic renal dysplasia
EXCLUDES 1 *polycystic kidney disease (Q61.11-Q61.3)*

Q61.5 Medullary cystic kidney CC
Nephronopthisis
Sponge kidney NOS
DEF: Sponge kidney: Dilated collecting tubules that are usually asymptomatic. Calcinosis in tubules may cause renal insufficiency.

Q61.8 Other cystic kidney diseases CC
Fibrocystic kidney
Fibrocystic renal degeneration or disease

Q61.9 Cystic kidney disease, unspecified CC
Meckel-Gruber syndrome

√4th **Q62 Congenital obstructive defects of renal pelvis and congenital malformations of ureter**

Q62.Ø Congenital hydronephrosis CC

√5th **Q62.1 Congenital occlusion of ureter**
Atresia and stenosis of ureter

Q62.1Ø Congenital occlusion of ureter, unspecified CC

Q62.11 Congenital occlusion of ureteropelvic junction CC

Q62.12 Congenital occlusion of ureterovesical orifice CC

Q62.2 Congenital megaureter CC
Congenital dilatation of ureter

√5th **Q62.3 Other obstructive defects of renal pelvis and ureter**

Q62.31 Congenital ureterocele, orthotopic CC

Q62.32 Cecoureterocele CC
Ectopic ureterocele

Q62.39 Other obstructive defects of renal pelvis and ureter CC
Ureteropelvic junction obstruction NOS

Q62.4 Agenesis of ureter
Congenital absence ureter

Q62.5 Duplication of ureter
Accessory ureter
Double ureter

√5th **Q62.6 Malposition of ureter**

Q62.6Ø Malposition of ureter, unspecified

Q62.61 Deviation of ureter

Q62.62 Displacement of ureter

Q62.63 Anomalous implantation of ureter
Ectopia of ureter
Ectopic ureter
Q62.69 Other malposition of ureter
Q62.7 Congenital vesico-uretero-renal reflux
Q62.8 Other congenital malformations of ureter
Anomaly of ureter NOS

Q63 Other congenital malformations of kidney
EXCLUDES 1 *congenital nephrotic syndrome (NØ4.-)*
Q63.Ø Accessory kidney
Q63.1 Lobulated, fused and horseshoe kidney
Q63.2 Ectopic kidney
Congenital displaced kidney
Malrotation of kidney
Q63.3 Hyperplastic and giant kidney
Compensatory hypertrophy of kidney
Q63.8 Other specified congenital malformations of kidney
Congenital renal calculi
Q63.9 Congenital malformation of kidney, unspecified

Q64 Other congenital malformations of urinary system
Q64.Ø Epispadias
EXCLUDES 1 *hypospadias (Q54.-)*

Epispadias

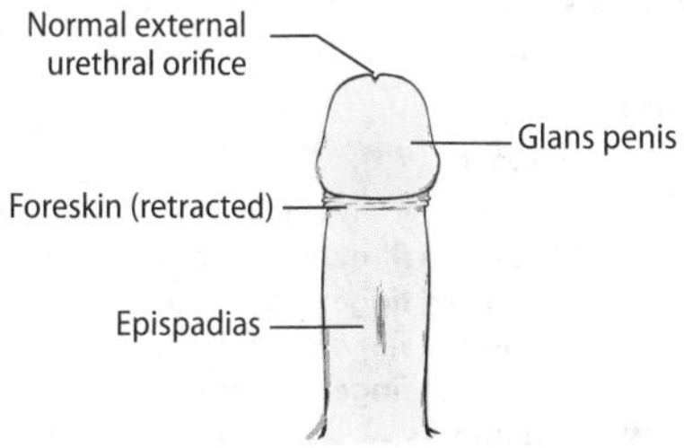

Epispadias (dorsal view)

Q64.1 Exstrophy of urinary bladder
Q64.1Ø Exstrophy of urinary bladder, unspecified CC
Ectopia vesicae
Q64.11 Supravesical fissure of urinary bladder CC
Q64.12 Cloacal exstrophy of urinary bladder CC
Q64.19 Other exstrophy of urinary bladder CC
Extroversion of bladder
Q64.2 Congenital posterior urethral valves CC
Q64.3 Other atresia and stenosis of urethra and bladder neck
Q64.31 Congenital bladder neck obstruction CC
Congenital obstruction of vesicourethral orifice
Q64.32 Congenital stricture of urethra CC
Q64.33 Congenital stricture of urinary meatus CC
Q64.39 Other atresia and stenosis of urethra and bladder neck CC
Atresia and stenosis of urethra and bladder neck NOS
Q64.4 Malformation of urachus
Cyst of urachus
Patent urachus
Prolapse of urachus
Q64.5 Congenital absence of bladder and urethra
Q64.6 Congenital diverticulum of bladder
Q64.7 Other and unspecified congenital malformations of bladder and urethra
EXCLUDES 1 *congenital prolapse of bladder (mucosa) (Q79.4)*
Q64.7Ø Unspecified congenital malformation of bladder and urethra
Malformation of bladder or urethra NOS
Q64.71 Congenital prolapse of urethra
Q64.72 Congenital prolapse of urinary meatus
Q64.73 Congenital urethrorectal fistula
Q64.74 Double urethra
Q64.75 Double urinary meatus
Q64.79 Other congenital malformations of bladder and urethra
Q64.8 Other specified congenital malformations of urinary system
Q64.9 Congenital malformation of urinary system, unspecified
Congenital anomaly NOS of urinary system
Congenital deformity NOS of urinary system

Congenital malformations and deformations of the musculoskeletal system (Q65-Q79)

Q65 Congenital deformities of hip
EXCLUDES 1 *clicking hip (R29.4)*
Q65.Ø Congenital dislocation of hip, unilateral
Q65.ØØ Congenital dislocation of unspecified hip, unilateral
Q65.Ø1 Congenital dislocation of right hip, unilateral
Q65.Ø2 Congenital dislocation of left hip, unilateral
Q65.1 Congenital dislocation of hip, bilateral
Q65.2 Congenital dislocation of hip, unspecified
Q65.3 Congenital partial dislocation of hip, unilateral
Q65.3Ø Congenital partial dislocation of unspecified hip, unilateral
Q65.31 Congenital partial dislocation of right hip, unilateral
Q65.32 Congenital partial dislocation of left hip, unilateral
Q65.4 Congenital partial dislocation of hip, bilateral
Q65.5 Congenital partial dislocation of hip, unspecified
Q65.6 Congenital unstable hip
Congenital dislocatable hip
Q65.8 Other congenital deformities of hip
Q65.81 Congenital coxa valga
Q65.82 Congenital coxa vara
Q65.89 Other specified congenital deformities of hip
Anteversion of femoral neck
Congenital acetabular dysplasia
Q65.9 Congenital deformity of hip, unspecified

Q66 Congenital deformities of feet
EXCLUDES 1 *reduction defects of feet (Q72.-)*
valgus deformities (acquired) (M21.Ø-)
varus deformities (acquired) (M21.1-)
AHA: 2019,4Q,13
Q66.Ø Congenital talipes equinovarus
Q66.ØØ Congenital talipes equinovarus, unspecified foot
Q66.Ø1 Congenital talipes equinovarus, right foot
Q66.Ø2 Congenital talipes equinovarus, left foot
Q66.1 Congenital talipes calcaneovarus
Q66.1Ø Congenital talipes calcaneovarus, unspecified foot
Q66.11 Congenital talipes calcaneovarus, right foot
Q66.12 Congenital talipes calcaneovarus, left foot
Q66.2 Congenital metatarsus (primus) varus
AHA: 2016,4Q,59
Q66.21 Congenital metatarsus primus varus
Q66.211 Congenital metatarsus primus varus, right foot
Q66.212 Congenital metatarsus primus varus, left foot
Q66.219 Congenital metatarsus primus varus, unspecified foot
Q66.22 Congenital metatarsus adductus
Congenital metatarsus varus
Q66.221 Congenital metatarsus adductus, right foot
Q66.222 Congenital metatarsus adductus, left foot
Q66.229 Congenital metatarsus adductus, unspecified foot
Q66.3 Other congenital varus deformities of feet
Hallux varus, congenital
Q66.3Ø Other congenital varus deformities of feet, unspecified foot
Q66.31 Other congenital varus deformities of feet, right foot
Q66.32 Other congenital varus deformities of feet, left foot
Q66.4 Congenital talipes calcaneovalgus
Q66.4Ø Congenital talipes calcaneovalgus, unspecified foot
Q66.41 Congenital talipes calcaneovalgus, right foot
Q66.42 Congenital talipes calcaneovalgus, left foot

√5th **Q66.5 Congenital pes planus**
Congenital flat foot
Congenital rigid flat foot
Congenital spastic (everted) flat foot
EXCLUDES 1 *pes planus, acquired (M21.4)*
Q66.50 Congenital pes planus, unspecified foot
Q66.51 Congenital pes planus, right foot
Q66.52 Congenital pes planus, left foot

Q66.6 Other congenital valgus deformities of feet
Congenital metatarsus valgus

√5th **Q66.7 Congenital pes cavus**
Q66.70 Congenital pes cavus, unspecified foot
Q66.71 Congenital pes cavus, right foot
Q66.72 Congenital pes cavus, left foot

√5th **Q66.8 Other congenital deformities of feet**
Q66.80 Congenital vertical talus deformity, unspecified foot
Q66.81 Congenital vertical talus deformity, right foot
Q66.82 Congenital vertical talus deformity, left foot
Q66.89 Other specified congenital deformities of feet
Congenital asymmetric talipes
Congenital clubfoot NOS
Congenital talipes NOS
Congenital tarsal coalition
Hammer toe, congenital
DEF: Clubfoot: Congenital anomaly of the foot with the heel elevated and rotated outward and the toes pointing inward.

√5th **Q66.9 Congenital deformity of feet, unspecified**
Q66.90 Congenital deformity of feet, unspecified, unspecified foot
Q66.91 Congenital deformity of feet, unspecified, right foot
Q66.92 Congenital deformity of feet, unspecified, left foot

√4th **Q67 Congenital musculoskeletal deformities of head, face, spine and chest**
EXCLUDES 1 *congenital malformation syndromes classified to Q87.-*
Potter's syndrome (Q60.6)

Q67.0 Congenital facial asymmetry
Q67.1 Congenital compression facies
Q67.2 Dolichocephaly
Q67.3 Plagiocephaly
Q67.4 Other congenital deformities of skull, face and jaw
Congenital depressions in skull
Congenital hemifacial atrophy or hypertrophy
Deviation of nasal septum, congenital
Squashed or bent nose, congenital
EXCLUDES 1 *dentofacial anomalies [including malocclusion] (M26.-)*
syphilitic saddle nose (A50.5)
DEF: Deviated septum: Condition in which the nasal septum, a thin wall composed of cartilage and bone that separates the two nostrils, is crooked or displaced from the midline.

Q67.5 Congenital deformity of spine CC
Congenital postural scoliosis
Congenital scoliosis NOS
EXCLUDES 1 *infantile idiopathic scoliosis (M41.0)*
scoliosis due to congenital bony malformation (Q76.3)
AHA: 2014,4Q,26

Q67.6 Pectus excavatum
Congenital funnel chest
Q67.7 Pectus carinatum
Congenital pigeon chest
Q67.8 Other congenital deformities of chest CC
Congenital deformity of chest wall NOS

√4th **Q68 Other congenital musculoskeletal deformities**
EXCLUDES 1 *reduction defects of limb(s) (Q71-Q73)*
EXCLUDES 2 *congenital myotonic chondrodystrophy (G71.13)*

Q68.0 Congenital deformity of sternocleidomastoid muscle
Congenital contracture of sternocleidomastoid (muscle)
Congenital (sternomastoid) torticollis
Sternomastoid tumor (congenital)

Q68.1 Congenital deformity of finger(s) and hand CC
Congenital clubfinger
Spade-like hand (congenital)
Q68.2 Congenital deformity of knee
Congenital dislocation of knee
Congenital genu recurvatum
Q68.3 Congenital bowing of femur
EXCLUDES 1 *anteversion of femur (neck) (Q65.89)*
Q68.4 Congenital bowing of tibia and fibula
Q68.5 Congenital bowing of long bones of leg, unspecified
Q68.6 Discoid meniscus
Q68.8 Other specified congenital musculoskeletal deformities
Congenital deformity of clavicle
Congenital deformity of elbow
Congenital deformity of forearm
Congenital deformity of scapula
Congenital deformity of wrist
Congenital dislocation of elbow
Congenital dislocation of shoulder
Congenital dislocation of wrist

√4th **Q69 Polydactyly**
Q69.0 Accessory finger(s)
Q69.1 Accessory thumb(s)
Q69.2 Accessory toe(s)
Accessory hallux
Q69.9 Polydactyly, unspecified
Supernumerary digit(s) NOS

√4th **Q70 Syndactyly**
√5th **Q70.0 Fused fingers**
Complex syndactyly of fingers with synostosis
Q70.00 Fused fingers, unspecified hand
Q70.01 Fused fingers, right hand
Q70.02 Fused fingers, left hand
Q70.03 Fused fingers, bilateral
√5th **Q70.1 Webbed fingers**
Simple syndactyly of fingers without synostosis
Q70.10 Webbed fingers, unspecified hand
Q70.11 Webbed fingers, right hand
Q70.12 Webbed fingers, left hand
Q70.13 Webbed fingers, bilateral
√5th **Q70.2 Fused toes**
Complex syndactyly of toes with synostosis
Q70.20 Fused toes, unspecified foot
Q70.21 Fused toes, right foot
Q70.22 Fused toes, left foot
Q70.23 Fused toes, bilateral
√5th **Q70.3 Webbed toes**
Simple syndactyly of toes without synostosis
Q70.30 Webbed toes, unspecified foot
Q70.31 Webbed toes, right foot
Q70.32 Webbed toes, left foot
Q70.33 Webbed toes, bilateral
Q70.4 Polysyndactyly, unspecified
EXCLUDES 1 *specified syndactyly of hand and feet — code to specified conditions (Q70.0-Q70.3-)*
Q70.9 Syndactyly, unspecified
Symphalangy NOS

√4th **Q71 Reduction defects of upper limb**
√5th **Q71.0 Congenital complete absence of upper limb**
Q71.00 Congenital complete absence of unspecified upper limb
Q71.01 Congenital complete absence of right upper limb
Q71.02 Congenital complete absence of left upper limb
Q71.03 Congenital complete absence of upper limb, bilateral
√5th **Q71.1 Congenital absence of upper arm and forearm with hand present**
Q71.10 Congenital absence of unspecified upper arm and forearm with hand present
Q71.11 Congenital absence of right upper arm and forearm with hand present
Q71.12 Congenital absence of left upper arm and forearm with hand present
Q71.13 Congenital absence of upper arm and forearm with hand present, bilateral

✓5th Q71.2 Congenital absence of both forearm and hand
- Q71.20 Congenital absence of both forearm and hand, unspecified upper limb
- Q71.21 Congenital absence of both forearm and hand, right upper limb
- Q71.22 Congenital absence of both forearm and hand, left upper limb
- Q71.23 Congenital absence of both forearm and hand, bilateral

✓5th Q71.3 Congenital absence of hand and finger
- Q71.30 Congenital absence of unspecified hand and finger
- Q71.31 Congenital absence of right hand and finger
- Q71.32 Congenital absence of left hand and finger
- Q71.33 Congenital absence of hand and finger, bilateral

✓5th Q71.4 Longitudinal reduction defect of radius
Clubhand (congenital)
Radial clubhand
- Q71.40 Longitudinal reduction defect of unspecified radius
- Q71.41 Longitudinal reduction defect of right radius
- Q71.42 Longitudinal reduction defect of left radius
- Q71.43 Longitudinal reduction defect of radius, bilateral

✓5th Q71.5 Longitudinal reduction defect of ulna
- Q71.50 Longitudinal reduction defect of unspecified ulna
- Q71.51 Longitudinal reduction defect of right ulna
- Q71.52 Longitudinal reduction defect of left ulna
- Q71.53 Longitudinal reduction defect of ulna, bilateral

✓5th Q71.6 Lobster-claw hand
- Q71.60 Lobster-claw hand, unspecified hand
- Q71.61 Lobster-claw right hand
- Q71.62 Lobster-claw left hand
- Q71.63 Lobster-claw hand, bilateral

✓5th Q71.8 Other reduction defects of upper limb

✓6th Q71.81 Congenital shortening of upper limb
- Q71.811 Congenital shortening of right upper limb
- Q71.812 Congenital shortening of left upper limb
- Q71.813 Congenital shortening of upper limb, bilateral
- Q71.819 Congenital shortening of unspecified upper limb

✓6th Q71.89 Other reduction defects of upper limb
- Q71.891 Other reduction defects of right upper limb
- Q71.892 Other reduction defects of left upper limb
- Q71.893 Other reduction defects of upper limb, bilateral
- Q71.899 Other reduction defects of unspecified upper limb

✓5th Q71.9 Unspecified reduction defect of upper limb
- Q71.90 Unspecified reduction defect of unspecified upper limb
- Q71.91 Unspecified reduction defect of right upper limb
- Q71.92 Unspecified reduction defect of left upper limb
- Q71.93 Unspecified reduction defect of upper limb, bilateral

✓4th Q72 Reduction defects of lower limb

✓5th Q72.0 Congenital complete absence of lower limb
- Q72.00 Congenital complete absence of unspecified lower limb
- Q72.01 Congenital complete absence of right lower limb
- Q72.02 Congenital complete absence of left lower limb
- Q72.03 Congenital complete absence of lower limb, bilateral

✓5th Q72.1 Congenital absence of thigh and lower leg with foot present
- Q72.10 Congenital absence of unspecified thigh and lower leg with foot present
- Q72.11 Congenital absence of right thigh and lower leg with foot present
- Q72.12 Congenital absence of left thigh and lower leg with foot present
- Q72.13 Congenital absence of thigh and lower leg with foot present, bilateral

✓5th Q72.2 Congenital absence of both lower leg and foot
- Q72.20 Congenital absence of both lower leg and foot, unspecified lower limb
- Q72.21 Congenital absence of both lower leg and foot, right lower limb
- Q72.22 Congenital absence of both lower leg and foot, left lower limb
- Q72.23 Congenital absence of both lower leg and foot, bilateral

✓5th Q72.3 Congenital absence of foot and toe(s)
- Q72.30 Congenital absence of unspecified foot and toe(s)
- Q72.31 Congenital absence of right foot and toe(s)
- Q72.32 Congenital absence of left foot and toe(s)
- Q72.33 Congenital absence of foot and toe(s), bilateral

✓5th Q72.4 Longitudinal reduction defect of femur
Proximal femoral focal deficiency
- Q72.40 Longitudinal reduction defect of unspecified femur
- Q72.41 Longitudinal reduction defect of right femur
- Q72.42 Longitudinal reduction defect of left femur
- Q72.43 Longitudinal reduction defect of femur, bilateral

✓5th Q72.5 Longitudinal reduction defect of tibia
- Q72.50 Longitudinal reduction defect of unspecified tibia
- Q72.51 Longitudinal reduction defect of right tibia
- Q72.52 Longitudinal reduction defect of left tibia
- Q72.53 Longitudinal reduction defect of tibia, bilateral

✓5th Q72.6 Longitudinal reduction defect of fibula
- Q72.60 Longitudinal reduction defect of unspecified fibula
- Q72.61 Longitudinal reduction defect of right fibula
- Q72.62 Longitudinal reduction defect of left fibula
- Q72.63 Longitudinal reduction defect of fibula, bilateral

✓5th Q72.7 Split foot
- Q72.70 Split foot, unspecified lower limb
- Q72.71 Split foot, right lower limb
- Q72.72 Split foot, left lower limb
- Q72.73 Split foot, bilateral

✓5th Q72.8 Other reduction defects of lower limb

✓6th Q72.81 Congenital shortening of lower limb
- Q72.811 Congenital shortening of right lower limb
- Q72.812 Congenital shortening of left lower limb
- Q72.813 Congenital shortening of lower limb, bilateral
- Q72.819 Congenital shortening of unspecified lower limb

✓6th Q72.89 Other reduction defects of lower limb
- Q72.891 Other reduction defects of right lower limb
- Q72.892 Other reduction defects of left lower limb
- Q72.893 Other reduction defects of lower limb, bilateral
- Q72.899 Other reduction defects of unspecified lower limb

✓5th Q72.9 Unspecified reduction defect of lower limb
- Q72.90 Unspecified reduction defect of unspecified lower limb
- Q72.91 Unspecified reduction defect of right lower limb
- Q72.92 Unspecified reduction defect of left lower limb
- Q72.93 Unspecified reduction defect of lower limb, bilateral

✓4th Q73 Reduction defects of unspecified limb

Q73.0 Congenital absence of unspecified limb(s)
Amelia NOS

Q73.1 Phocomelia, unspecified limb(s)
Phocomelia NOS

Q73.8 Other reduction defects of unspecified limb(s)
Longitudinal reduction deformity of unspecified limb(s)
Ectromelia of limb NOS
Hemimelia of limb NOS
Reduction defect of limb NOS

Q74 Other congenital malformations of limb(s)
EXCLUDES 1 *polydactyly (Q69.-)*
reduction defect of limb (Q71-Q73)
syndactyly (Q70.-)

Q74.0 Other congenital malformations of upper limb(s), including shoulder girdle
Accessory carpal bones
Cleidocranial dysostosis
Congenital pseudarthrosis of clavicle
Macrodactylia (fingers)
Madelung's deformity
Radioulnar synostosis
Sprengel's deformity
Triphalangeal thumb

Q74.1 Congenital malformation of knee
Congenital absence of patella
Congenital dislocation of patella
Congenital genu valgum
Congenital genu varum
Rudimentary patella
EXCLUDES 1 *congenital dislocation of knee (Q68.2)*
congenital genu recurvatum (Q68.2)
nail patella syndrome (Q87.2)

Q74.2 Other congenital malformations of lower limb(s), including pelvic girdle
Congenital fusion of sacroiliac joint
Congenital malformation of ankle joint
Congenital malformation of sacroiliac joint
EXCLUDES 1 *anteversion of femur (neck) (Q65.89)*

Q74.3 Arthrogryposis multiplex congenita CC

Q74.8 Other specified congenital malformations of limb(s)

Q74.9 Unspecified congenital malformation of limb(s)
Congenital anomaly of limb(s) NOS

Q75 Other congenital malformations of skull and face bones
EXCLUDES 1 *congenital malformation of face NOS (Q18.-)*
congenital malformation syndromes classified to Q87.-
dentofacial anomalies [including malocclusion] (M26.-)
musculoskeletal deformities of head and face (Q67.0-Q67.4)
skull defects associated with congenital anomalies of brain such as:
anencephaly (Q00.0)
encephalocele (Q01.-)
hydrocephalus (Q03.-)
microcephaly (Q02)

Q75.0 Craniosynostosis
Acrocephaly
Imperfect fusion of skull
Oxycephaly
Trigonocephaly
DEF: Congenital condition in which one or more of the cranial sutures fuse prematurely, creating a deformed or aberrant head shape.

Q75.1 Craniofacial dysostosis
Crouzon's disease

Q75.2 Hypertelorism

Q75.3 Macrocephaly

Q75.4 Mandibulofacial dysostosis
Franceschetti syndrome
Treacher Collins syndrome

Q75.5 Oculomandibular dysostosis

Q75.8 Other specified congenital malformations of skull and face bones
Absence of skull bone, congenital
Congenital deformity of forehead
Platybasia

Q75.9 Congenital malformation of skull and face bones, unspecified
Congenital anomaly of face bones NOS
Congenital anomaly of skull NOS

Q76 Congenital malformations of spine and bony thorax
EXCLUDES 1 *congenital musculoskeletal deformities of spine and chest (Q67.5-Q67.8)*

Q76.0 Spina bifida occulta
EXCLUDES 1 *meningocele (spinal) (Q05.-)*
spina bifida (aperta) (cystica) (Q05.-)

Q76.1 Klippel-Feil syndrome
Cervical fusion syndrome

Q76.2 Congenital spondylolisthesis
Congenital spondylolysis
EXCLUDES 1 *spondylolisthesis (acquired) (M43.1-)*
spondylolysis (acquired) (M43.0-)

Q76.3 Congenital scoliosis due to congenital bony malformation CC
Hemivertebra fusion or failure of segmentation with scoliosis

Q76.4 Other congenital malformations of spine, not associated with scoliosis

Q76.41 Congenital kyphosis

Q76.411 Congenital kyphosis, occipito-atlanto-axial region

Q76.412 Congenital kyphosis, cervical region

Q76.413 Congenital kyphosis, cervicothoracic region

Q76.414 Congenital kyphosis, thoracic region

Q76.415 Congenital kyphosis, thoracolumbar region

Q76.419 Congenital kyphosis, unspecified region

Q76.42 Congenital lordosis

Q76.425 Congenital lordosis, thoracolumbar region CC

Q76.426 Congenital lordosis, lumbar region CC

Q76.427 Congenital lordosis, lumbosacral region CC

Q76.428 Congenital lordosis, sacral and sacrococcygeal region CC

Q76.429 Congenital lordosis, unspecified region CC

Q76.49 Other congenital malformations of spine, not associated with scoliosis
Congenital absence of vertebra NOS
Congenital fusion of spine NOS
Congenital malformation of lumbosacral (joint) (region) NOS
Congenital malformation of spine NOS
Hemivertebra NOS
Malformation of spine NOS
Platyspondylisis NOS
Supernumerary vertebra NOS

Q76.5 Cervical rib
Supernumerary rib in cervical region

Q76.6 Other congenital malformations of ribs CC
Accessory rib
Congenital absence of rib
Congenital fusion of ribs
Congenital malformation of ribs NOS
EXCLUDES 1 *short rib syndrome (Q77.2)*

Q76.7 Congenital malformation of sternum CC
Congenital absence of sternum
Sternum bifidum

Q76.8 Other congenital malformations of bony thorax CC

Q76.9 Congenital malformation of bony thorax, unspecified CC

Q77 Osteochondrodysplasia with defects of growth of tubular bones and spine
EXCLUDES 1 *mucopolysaccharidosis (E76.0-E76.3)*
EXCLUDES 2 *congenital myotonic chondrodystrophy (G71.13)*

Q77.0 Achondrogenesis
Hypochondrogenesis

Q77.1 Thanatophoric short stature

Q77.2 Short rib syndrome CC
Asphyxiating thoracic dysplasia [Jeune]

Q77.3 Chondrodysplasia punctata
EXCLUDES 1 *Rhizomelic chondrodysplasia punctata (E71.43)*

Q77.4 Achondroplasia
Hypochondroplasia
Osteosclerosis congenita

Q77.5 Diastrophic dysplasia

Q77.6 Chondroectodermal dysplasia
Ellis-van Creveld syndrome

Q77.7 Spondyloepiphyseal dysplasia

Q77.8 Other osteochondrodysplasia with defects of growth of tubular bones and spine

Q77.9 Osteochondrodysplasia with defects of growth of tubular bones and spine, unspecified

Q78 Other osteochondrodysplasias
EXCLUDES 2 *congenital myotonic chondrodystrophy (G71.13)*

Q78.0 Osteogenesis imperfecta CC
Fragilitas ossium
Osteopsathyrosis

Q78.1 Polyostotic fibrous dysplasia
Albright(-McCune)(-Sternberg) syndrome

Q78.2 Osteopetrosis CC
Albers-Schönberg syndrome
Osteosclerosis NOS
DEF: Rare congenital condition in which the bones are excessively dense, resulting from a discrepancy in the formation and breakdown of bone.

Q78.3 Progressive diaphyseal dysplasia
Camurati-Engelmann syndrome

Q78.4 Enchondromatosis
Maffucci's syndrome
Ollier's disease

Q78.5 Metaphyseal dysplasia
Pyle's syndrome

Q78.6 Multiple congenital exostoses
Diaphyseal aclasis

Q78.8 Other specified osteochondrodysplasias
Osteopoikilosis

Q78.9 Osteochondrodysplasia, unspecified
Chondrodystrophy NOS
Osteodystrophy NOS

Q79 Congenital malformations of musculoskeletal system, not elsewhere classified
EXCLUDES 2 *congenital (sternomastoid) torticollis (Q68.0)*

Q79.0 Congenital diaphragmatic hernia MCC
EXCLUDES 1 *congenital hiatus hernia (Q40.1)*

Q79.1 Other congenital malformations of diaphragm MCC
Absence of diaphragm
Congenital malformation of diaphragm NOS
Eventration of diaphragm

Q79.2 Exomphalos MCC
Omphalocele
EXCLUDES 1 *umbilical hernia (K42.-)*

Q79.3 Gastroschisis MCC

Gastroschisis

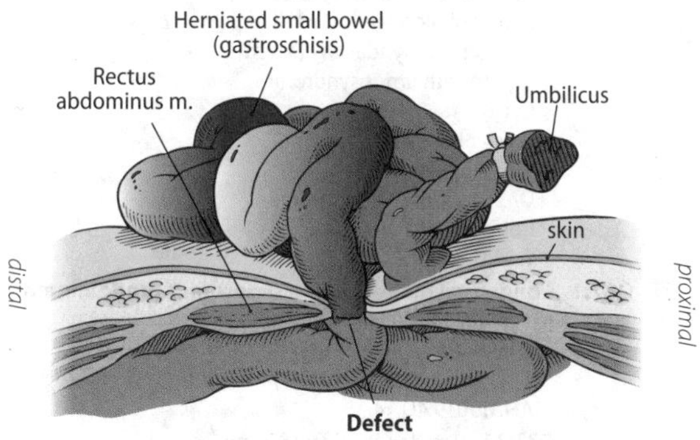

Q79.4 Prune belly syndrome MCC
Congenital prolapse of bladder mucosa
Eagle-Barrett syndrome

Q79.5 Other congenital malformations of abdominal wall
EXCLUDES 1 *umbilical hernia (K42.-)*

Q79.51 Congenital hernia of bladder MCC

Q79.59 Other congenital malformations of abdominal wall MCC

Q79.6 Ehlers-Danlos syndromes
AHA: 2019,4Q,13-14
DEF: Connective tissue disorder that causes hyperextended skin and joints and results in fragile blood vessels with bleeding, poor wound healing, and subcutaneous pseudotumors.

Q79.60 Ehlers-Danlos syndrome, unspecified CC

Q79.61 Classical Ehlers-Danlos syndrome CC
Classical EDS (cEDS)

Q79.62 Hypermobile Ehlers-Danlos syndrome CC
Hypermobile EDS (hEDS)

Q79.63 Vascular Ehlers-Danlos syndrome CC
Vascular EDS (vEDS)

Q79.69 Other Ehlers-Danlos syndromes CC

Q79.8 Other congenital malformations of musculoskeletal system
Absence of muscle
Absence of tendon
Accessory muscle
Amyotrophia congenita
Congenital constricting bands
Congenital shortening of tendon
Poland syndrome

Q79.9 Congenital malformation of musculoskeletal system, unspecified
Congenital anomaly of musculoskeletal system NOS
Congenital deformity of musculoskeletal system NOS

Other congenital malformations (Q80-Q89)

Q80 Congenital ichthyosis
EXCLUDES 1 *Refsum's disease (G60.1)*
DEF: Excessive production of skin cells resulting in red, dry, scaly skin.

Q80.0 Ichthyosis vulgaris

Q80.1 X-linked ichthyosis

Q80.2 Lamellar ichthyosis
Collodion baby

Q80.3 Congenital bullous ichthyosiform erythroderma

Q80.4 Harlequin fetus

Q80.8 Other congenital ichthyosis

Q80.9 Congenital ichthyosis, unspecified

Q81 Epidermolysis bullosa

Q81.0 Epidermolysis bullosa simplex
EXCLUDES 1 *Cockayne's syndrome (Q87.19)*

Q81.1 Epidermolysis bullosa letalis
Herlitz' syndrome

Q81.2 Epidermolysis bullosa dystrophica

Q81.8 Other epidermolysis bullosa

Q81.9 Epidermolysis bullosa, unspecified

Q82 Other congenital malformations of skin
EXCLUDES 1 *acrodermatitis enteropathica (E83.2)*
congenital erythropoietic porphyria (E80.0)
pilonidal cyst or sinus (L05.-)
Sturge-Weber (-Dimitri) syndrome (Q85.8)

Q82.0 Hereditary lymphedema

Q82.1 Xeroderma pigmentosum

Q82.2 Congenital cutaneous mastocytosis
Congenital diffuse cutaneous mastocytosis
Congenital maculopapular cutaneous mastocytosis
Congenital urticaria pigmentosa
EXCLUDES 1 *cutaneous mastocytosis NOS (D47.01)*
diffuse cutaneous mastocytosis (with onset after newborn period) (D47.01)
malignant mastocytosis (C96.2-)
systemic mastocytosis (D47.02)
urticaria pigmentosa (non-congenital) (with onset after newborn period) (D47.01)
AHA: 2017,4Q,5

Q82.3 Incontinentia pigmenti

Q82.4 Ectodermal dysplasia (anhidrotic)
EXCLUDES 1 *Ellis-van Creveld syndrome (Q77.6)*

Q82.5 Congenital non-neoplastic nevus
Birthmark NOS
Flammeus Nevus
Portwine Nevus
Sanguineous Nevus
Strawberry Nevus
Vascular Nevus NOS
Verrucous Nevus
EXCLUDES 2 *araneus nevus (I78.1)*
Café au lait spots (L81.3)
lentigo (L81.4)
melanocytic nevus (D22.-)
nevus NOS (D22.-)
pigmented nevus (D22.-)
spider nevus (I78.1)
stellar nevus (I78.1)

Q82.6 Congenital sacral dimple
Parasacral dimple
EXCLUDES 2 *pilonidal cyst with abscess (LØ5.Ø1)*
pilonidal cyst without abscess (LØ5.91)
AHA: 2016,4Q,60

Q82.8 Other specified congenital malformations of skin
Abnormal palmar creases
Accessory skin tags
Benign familial pemphigus [Hailey-Hailey]
Congenital poikiloderma
Cutis laxa (hyperelastica)
Dermatoglyphic anomalies
Inherited keratosis palmaris et plantaris
Keratosis follicularis [Darier-White]
EXCLUDES 1 *►Ehlers-Danlos syndromes◄ (Q79.6-)*
AHA: 2016,1Q,17

Q82.9 Congenital malformation of skin, unspecified

✓4th **Q83 Congenital malformations of breast**
EXCLUDES 2 *absence of pectoral muscle (Q79.8)*
hypoplasia of breast (N64.82)
micromastia (N64.82)

Q83.Ø Congenital absence of breast with absent nipple
Q83.1 Accessory breast
Supernumerary breast
Q83.2 Absent nipple
Q83.3 Accessory nipple
Supernumerary nipple
Q83.8 Other congenital malformations of breast
Q83.9 Congenital malformation of breast, unspecified

✓4th **Q84 Other congenital malformations of integument**

Q84.Ø Congenital alopecia
Congenital atrichosis
Q84.1 Congenital morphological disturbances of hair, not elsewhere classified
Beaded hair
Monilethrix
Pili annulati
EXCLUDES 1 *Menkes' kinky hair syndrome (E83.Ø)*
Q84.2 Other congenital malformations of hair
Congenital hypertrichosis
Congenital malformation of hair NOS
Persistent lanugo
Q84.3 Anonychia
EXCLUDES 1 *nail patella syndrome (Q87.2)*
Q84.4 Congenital leukonychia
Q84.5 Enlarged and hypertrophic nails
Congenital onychauxis
Pachyonychia
Q84.6 Other congenital malformations of nails
Congenital clubnail
Congenital koilonychia
Congenital malformation of nail NOS
Q84.8 Other specified congenital malformations of integument
Aplasia cutis congenita
Q84.9 Congenital malformation of integument, unspecified
Congenital anomaly of integument NOS
Congenital deformity of integument NOS

✓4th **Q85 Phakomatoses, not elsewhere classified**
EXCLUDES 1 *ataxia telangiectasia [Louis-Bar] (G11.3)*
familial dysautonomia [Riley-Day] (G9Ø.1)

✓5th **Q85.Ø Neurofibromatosis (nonmalignant)**
Q85.ØØ Neurofibromatosis, unspecified HCC
Q85.Ø1 Neurofibromatosis, type 1 HCC
Von Recklinghausen disease
Q85.Ø2 Neurofibromatosis, type 2 HCC
Acoustic neurofibromatosis
DEF: Inherited condition with cutaneous lesions, benign tumors of peripheral nerves, and bilateral 8th nerve masses.
Q85.Ø3 Schwannomatosis HCC
DEF: Genetic mutation (SMARCB1/INI1) causing multiple benign tumors along the nerve pathways, except on the 8th cranial (vestibular) nerve.
Q85.Ø9 Other neurofibromatosis HCC
Q85.1 Tuberous sclerosis CC HCC
Bourneville's disease
Epiloia
Q85.8 Other phakomatoses, not elsewhere classified CC HCC
Peutz-Jeghers Syndrome
Sturge-Weber(-Dimitri) syndrome
von Hippel-Lindau syndrome
EXCLUDES 1 *Meckel-Gruber syndrome (Q61.9)*
Q85.9 Phakomatosis, unspecified CC HCC
Hamartosis NOS

✓4th **Q86 Congenital malformation syndromes due to known exogenous causes, not elsewhere classified**
EXCLUDES 2 *iodine-deficiency-related hypothyroidism (EØØ-EØ2)*
nonteratogenic effects of substances transmitted via placenta or breast milk (PØ4.-)

Q86.Ø Fetal alcohol syndrome (dysmorphic)
Q86.1 Fetal hydantoin syndrome
Meadow's syndrome
Q86.2 Dysmorphism due to warfarin
Q86.8 Other congenital malformation syndromes due to known exogenous causes

✓4th **Q87 Other specified congenital malformation syndromes affecting multiple systems**
Use additional code(s) to identify all associated manifestations

Q87.Ø Congenital malformation syndromes predominantly affecting facial appearance
Acrocephalopolysyndactyly
Acrocephalosyndactyly [Apert]
Cryptophthalmos syndrome
Cyclopia
Goldenhar syndrome
Moebius syndrome
Oro-facial-digital syndrome
Robin syndrome
Whistling face

✓5th **Q87.1 Congenital malformation syndromes predominantly associated with short stature**
EXCLUDES 1 *Ellis-van Creveld syndrome (Q77.6)*
Smith-Lemli-Opitz syndrome (E78.72)
AHA: 2019,4Q,14-15
Q87.11 Prader-Willi syndrome CC
Q87.19 Other congenital malformation syndromes predominantly associated with short stature CC
Aarskog syndrome
Cockayne syndrome
De Lange syndrome
Dubowitz syndrome
Noonan syndrome
Robinow-Silverman-Smith syndrome
Russell-Silver syndrome
Seckel syndrome

Q87.2 Congenital malformation syndromes predominantly involving limbs CC
Holt-Oram syndrome
Klippel-Trenaunay-Weber syndrome
Nail patella syndrome
Rubinstein-Taybi syndrome
Sirenomelia syndrome
Thrombocytopenia with absent radius [TAR] syndrome
VATER syndrome

Q87.3 Congenital malformation syndromes involving early overgrowth CC
Beckwith-Wiedemann syndrome
Sotos syndrome
Weaver syndrome

✓5th **Q87.4 Marfan's syndrome**
DEF: Disorder that affects the connective tissue of multiple systems, including disproportionally long or abnormal bone structure and eye and cardiovascular complications.

Q87.40 Marfan's syndrome, unspecified CC

✓6th **Q87.41 Marfan's syndrome with cardiovascular manifestations**

Q87.410 Marfan's syndrome with aortic dilation CC

Q87.418 Marfan's syndrome with other cardiovascular manifestations CC

Q87.42 Marfan's syndrome with ocular manifestations CC

Q87.43 Marfan's syndrome with skeletal manifestation CC

Q87.5 Other congenital malformation syndromes with other skeletal changes CC

✓5th **Q87.8 Other specified congenital malformation syndromes, not elsewhere classified**
EXCLUDES 1 *Zellweger syndrome (E71.510)*

Q87.81 Alport syndrome CC
Use additional code to identify stage of chronic kidney disease (N18.1-N18.6)

Q87.82 Arterial tortuosity syndrome CC
AHA: 2016,4Q,60-61

Q87.89 Other specified congenital malformation syndromes, not elsewhere classified CC
Laurence-Moon (-Bardet)-Biedl syndrome

✓4th **Q89 Other congenital malformations, not elsewhere classified**

✓5th **Q89.0 Congenital absence and malformations of spleen**
EXCLUDES 1 *isomerism of atrial appendages (with asplenia or polysplenia) (Q20.6)*

Q89.01 Asplenia (congenital) CC

Q89.09 Congenital malformations of spleen CC
Congenital splenomegaly

Q89.1 Congenital malformations of adrenal gland
EXCLUDES 1 *adrenogenital disorders (E25.-)*
congenital adrenal hyperplasia (E25.0)

Q89.2 Congenital malformations of other endocrine glands
Congenital malformation of parathyroid or thyroid gland
Persistent thyroglossal duct
Thyroglossal cyst
EXCLUDES 1 *congenital goiter (E03.0)*
congenital hypothyroidism (E03.1)

Q89.3 Situs inversus CC
Dextrocardia with situs inversus
Mirror-image atrial arrangement with situs inversus
Situs inversus or transversus abdominalis
Situs inversus or transversus thoracis
Transposition of abdominal viscera
Transposition of thoracic viscera
EXCLUDES 1 *dextrocardia NOS (Q24.0)*
DEF: Congenital anomaly in which the internal thoracic and abdominal organs are transposed laterally and found on the opposite side from the normal position.

Q89.4 Conjoined twins MCC
Craniopagus
Dicephaly
Pygopagus
Thoracopagus

Q89.7 Multiple congenital malformations, not elsewhere classified CC
Multiple congenital anomalies NOS
Multiple congenital deformities NOS
EXCLUDES 1 *congenital malformation syndromes affecting multiple systems (Q87.-)*

Q89.8 Other specified congenital malformations CC
Use additional code(s) to identify all associated manifestations

Q89.9 Congenital malformation, unspecified
Congenital anomaly NOS
Congenital deformity NOS

Chromosomal abnormalities, not elsewhere classified (Q90-Q99)

EXCLUDES 2 *mitochondrial metabolic disorders (E88.4-)*

✓4th **Q90 Down syndrome**
Use additional code(s) to identify any associated physical conditions and degree of intellectual disabilities (F70-F79)

Q90.0 Trisomy 21, nonmosaicism (meiotic nondisjunction)

Q90.1 Trisomy 21, mosaicism (mitotic nondisjunction)

Q90.2 Trisomy 21, translocation

Q90.9 Down syndrome, unspecified
Trisomy 21 NOS

✓4th **Q91 Trisomy 18 and Trisomy 13**

Q91.0 Trisomy 18, nonmosaicism (meiotic nondisjunction) CC

Q91.1 Trisomy 18, mosaicism (mitotic nondisjunction) CC

Q91.2 Trisomy 18, translocation CC

Q91.3 Trisomy 18, unspecified CC

Q91.4 Trisomy 13, nonmosaicism (meiotic nondisjunction) CC

Q91.5 Trisomy 13, mosaicism (mitotic nondisjunction) CC

Q91.6 Trisomy 13, translocation CC

Q91.7 Trisomy 13, unspecified CC

✓4th **Q92 Other trisomies and partial trisomies of the autosomes, not elsewhere classified**
INCLUDES unbalanced translocations and insertions
EXCLUDES 1 *trisomies of chromosomes 13, 18, 21 (Q90-Q91)*

Q92.0 Whole chromosome trisomy, nonmosaicism (meiotic nondisjunction)

Q92.1 Whole chromosome trisomy, mosaicism (mitotic nondisjunction)

Q92.2 Partial trisomy
Less than whole arm duplicated
Whole arm or more duplicated
EXCLUDES 1 *partial trisomy due to unbalanced translocation (Q92.5)*

Q92.5 Duplications with other complex rearrangements
Partial trisomy due to unbalanced translocations
Code also any associated deletions due to unbalanced translocations, inversions and insertions (Q93.7)

✓5th **Q92.6 Marker chromosomes**
Trisomies due to dicentrics
Trisomies due to extra rings
Trisomies due to isochromosomes
Individual with marker heterochromatin

Q92.61 Marker chromosomes in normal individual

Q92.62 Marker chromosomes in abnormal individual

Q92.7 Triploidy and polyploidy

Q92.8 Other specified trisomies and partial trisomies of autosomes
Duplications identified by fluorescence in situ hybridization (FISH)
Duplications identified by in situ hybridization (ISH)
Duplications seen only at prometaphase

Q92.9 Trisomy and partial trisomy of autosomes, unspecified

✓4th **Q93 Monosomies and deletions from the autosomes, not elsewhere classified**

Q93.0 Whole chromosome monosomy, nonmosaicism (meiotic nondisjunction)

Q93.1 Whole chromosome monosomy, mosaicism (mitotic nondisjunction)

Q93.2 Chromosome replaced with ring, dicentric or isochromosome

Q93.3 Deletion of short arm of chromosome 4 CC
Wolff-Hirschorn syndrome

Q93.4 Deletion of short arm of chromosome 5 CC
Cri-du-chat syndrome

✓5th **Q93.5 Other deletions of part of a chromosome**
AHA: 2018,4Q,28
Q93.51 Angelman syndrome CC
Q93.59 Other deletions of part of a chromosome CC
Q93.7 Deletions with other complex rearrangements CC
Deletions due to unbalanced translocations, inversions and insertions
Code also any associated duplications due to unbalanced translocations, inversions and insertions (Q92.5)

✓5th **Q93.8 Other deletions from the autosomes**
Q93.81 Velo-cardio-facial syndrome MCC
Deletion 22q11.2
AHA: 2019,3Q,14
DEF: Microdeletion syndrome affecting multiple organs characterized by a cleft palate, heart defects, an elongated face with almond-shaped eyes, wide nose, small ears, weak immune system, weak musculature, hypothyroidism, short stature, and scoliosis. The deletion occurs at q11.2 on the long arm of the chromosome 22.
Q93.82 Williams syndrome CC
AHA: 2018,4Q,28-29
Q93.88 Other microdeletions CC
Miller-Dieker syndrome
Smith-Magenis syndrome
Q93.89 Other deletions from the autosomes CC
Deletions identified by fluorescence in situ hybridization (FISH)
Deletions identified by in situ hybridization (ISH)
Deletions seen only at prometaphase
Q93.9 Deletion from autosomes, unspecified CC

✓4th **Q95 Balanced rearrangements and structural markers, not elsewhere classified**
INCLUDES Robertsonian and balanced reciprocal translocations and insertions
Q95.0 Balanced translocation and insertion in normal individual
Q95.1 Chromosome inversion in normal individual
Q95.2 Balanced autosomal rearrangement in abnormal individual
Q95.3 Balanced sex/autosomal rearrangement in abnormal individual
Q95.5 Individual with autosomal fragile site
Q95.8 Other balanced rearrangements and structural markers
Q95.9 Balanced rearrangement and structural marker, unspecified

✓4th **Q96 Turner's syndrome**
EXCLUDES 1 *Noonan syndrome (Q87.19)*
Q96.0 Karyotype 45, X ♀
Q96.1 Karyotype 46, X iso (Xq) ♀
Karyotype 46, isochromosome Xq
Q96.2 Karyotype 46, X with abnormal sex chromosome, except iso (Xq) ♀
Karyotype 46, X with abnormal sex chromosome, except isochromosome Xq
Q96.3 Mosaicism, 45, X/46, XX or XY ♀
Q96.4 Mosaicism, 45, X/other cell line(s) with abnormal sex chromosome ♀
Q96.8 Other variants of Turner's syndrome ♀
Q96.9 Turner's syndrome, unspecified ♀

✓4th **Q97 Other sex chromosome abnormalities, female phenotype, not elsewhere classified**
EXCLUDES 1 *Turner's syndrome (Q96.-)*
Q97.0 Karyotype 47, XXX ♀
Q97.1 Female with more than three X chromosomes ♀
Q97.2 Mosaicism, lines with various numbers of X chromosomes ♀
Q97.3 Female with 46, XY karyotype ♀
Q97.8 Other specified sex chromosome abnormalities, female phenotype ♀
Q97.9 Sex chromosome abnormality, female phenotype, unspecified ♀

✓4th **Q98 Other sex chromosome abnormalities, male phenotype, not elsewhere classified**
Q98.0 Klinefelter syndrome karyotype 47, XXY ♂
Q98.1 Klinefelter syndrome, male with more than two X chromosomes ♂
Q98.3 Other male with 46, XX karyotype ♂
Q98.4 Klinefelter syndrome, unspecified ♂
Q98.5 Karyotype 47, XYY
Q98.6 Male with structurally abnormal sex chromosome ♂
Q98.7 Male with sex chromosome mosaicism ♂
Q98.8 Other specified sex chromosome abnormalities, male phenotype ♂
Q98.9 Sex chromosome abnormality, male phenotype, unspecified ♂

✓4th **Q99 Other chromosome abnormalities, not elsewhere classified**
Q99.0 Chimera 46, XX/46, XY
Chimera 46, XX/46, XY true hermaphrodite
Q99.1 46, XX true hermaphrodite
46, XX with streak gonads
46, XY with streak gonads
Pure gonadal dysgenesis
Q99.2 Fragile X chromosome
Fragile X syndrome
Q99.8 Other specified chromosome abnormalities
Q99.9 Chromosomal abnormality, unspecified

Chapter 18. Symptoms, Signs and Abnormal Clinical and Laboratory Findings (RØØ–R99)

Chapter-specific Guidelines with Coding Examples

The chapter-specific guidelines from the ICD-10-CM Official Guidelines for Coding and Reporting have been provided below. Along with these guidelines are coding examples, contained in the shaded boxes, that have been developed to help illustrate the coding and/or sequencing guidance found in these guidelines.

Chapter 18 includes symptoms, signs, abnormal results of clinical or other investigative procedures, and ill-defined conditions regarding which no diagnosis classifiable elsewhere is recorded. Signs and symptoms that point to a specific diagnosis have been assigned to a category in other chapters of the classification.

a. Use of symptom codes

Codes that describe symptoms and signs are acceptable for reporting purposes when a related definitive diagnosis has not been established (confirmed) by the provider.

Chest pain of unknown origin

RØ7.9 Chest pain, unspecified

Explanation: Codes that describe symptoms such as chest pain are acceptable for reporting purposes when the provider has not established (confirmed) a related definitive diagnosis.

b. Use of a symptom code with a definitive diagnosis code

Codes for signs and symptoms may be reported in addition to a related definitive diagnosis when the sign or symptom is not routinely associated with that diagnosis, such as the various signs and symptoms associated with complex syndromes. The definitive diagnosis code should be sequenced before the symptom code.

Signs or symptoms that are associated routinely with a disease process should not be assigned as additional codes, unless otherwise instructed by the classification.

Pneumonia with hemoptysis

J18.9 Pneumonia, unspecified organism

RØ4.2 Hemoptysis

Explanation: Codes for signs and symptoms may be reported in addition to a related definitive diagnosis when the sign or symptom is not routinely associated with that diagnosis.

Abdominal pain due to acute appendicitis

K35.8Ø Unspecified acute appendicitis

Explanation: Codes for signs or symptoms routinely associated with a disease process should not be assigned unless the classification instructs otherwise.

c. Combination codes that include symptoms

ICD-10-CM contains a number of combination codes that identify both the definitive diagnosis and common symptoms of that diagnosis. When using one of these combination codes, an additional code should not be assigned for the symptom.

Acute gastritis with hemorrhage

K29.Ø1 Acute gastritis with bleeding

Explanation: When a combination code identifies both the definitive diagnosis and the symptom, an additional code should not be assigned for the symptom.

d. Repeated falls

Code R29.6, Repeated falls, is for use for encounters when a patient has recently fallen and the reason for the fall is being investigated.

Code Z91.81, History of falling, is for use when a patient has fallen in the past and is at risk for future falls. When appropriate, both codes R29.6 and Z91.81 may be assigned together.

e. Coma scale

The coma scale codes (R4Ø.2-) can be used in conjunction with traumatic brain injury codes. These codes are primarily for use by trauma registries, but they may be used in any setting where this information is collected. The coma scale codes should be sequenced after the diagnosis code(s).

These codes, one from each subcategory, are needed to complete the scale. The 7th character indicates when the scale was recorded. The 7th character should match for all three codes.

At a minimum, report the initial score documented on presentation at your facility. This may be a score from the emergency medicine technician (EMT) or in the emergency department. If desired, a facility may choose to capture multiple coma scale scores.

Assign code R4Ø.24, Glasgow coma scale, total score, when only the total score is documented in the medical record and not the individual score(s).

Do not report codes for individual or total Glasgow coma scale scores for a patient with a medically induced coma or a sedated patient.

See Section I.B.14 for coma scale documentation by clinicians other than patient's provider

23-year-old man found down after unknown injury with skull fracture and with concussion and loss of consciousness of unknown duration. EMS evaluated the patient in the field and reported the individual Glasgow coma scores:

Eye opening response—3: eyes open to speech

Verbal response—4: confused but coherent speech

Motor response—6: obeys commands fully

SØ2.ØXXA Fracture of vault of skull, initial encounter for closed fracture

SØ6.ØX9A Concussion with loss of consciousness of unspecified duration, initial encounter

R4Ø.2131 Coma scale, eyes open, to sound, in the field [EMT or ambulance]

R4Ø.2241 Coma scale, best verbal response, confused conversation, in the field [EMT or ambulance]

R4Ø.2361 Coma scale, best motor response, obeys commands, in the field [EMT or ambulance]

Explanation: When individual scores for the Glasgow coma scale are documented, one code from each category is needed to complete the scale. The seventh character indicates when the scale was recorded and should match for all three codes. Assign a code from subcategory R4Ø.24- Glasgow coma scale, total score, when only the total and not the individual score(s) is documented.

Patient with intractable epilepsy with status epilepticus arrives to ED with alteration of consciousness. Coma scale performed en route by EMT documented total coma score as 11. Another coma score was performed upon hospital admission that was documented as 14.

G4Ø.911 Epilepsy, unspecified, intractable, with status epilepticus

R4Ø.2421 Glasgow coma scale score 9-12, in the field [EMT or ambulance]

R4Ø.2413 Glasgow coma scale score 13-15, at hospital admission

Explanation: Coma scores may be used to assess mental status in non-trauma conditions. Use only code R4Ø.24- Glasgow coma scale, total scores when individual scores are unavailable. Multiple scores may be reported with the seventh character representing where or when the assessment was made.

f. Functional quadriplegia

GUIDELINE HAS BEEN DELETED EFFECTIVE OCTOBER 1, 2Ø17

g. SIRS due to non-infectious process

The systemic inflammatory response syndrome (SIRS) can develop as a result of certain non-infectious disease processes, such as trauma, malignant neoplasm, or pancreatitis. When SIRS is documented with a noninfectious condition, and no subsequent infection is documented, the code for the underlying condition, such as an injury, should be assigned, followed by code R65.10, Systemic inflammatory response syndrome (SIRS) of non-infectious origin without acute organ dysfunction, or code R65.11, Systemic inflammatory response syndrome (SIRS) of non-infectious origin with acute organ dysfunction. If an associated acute organ dysfunction is documented, the appropriate code(s) for the specific type of organ dysfunction(s) should be assigned in addition to code R65.11. If acute organ dysfunction is documented, but it cannot be determined if the acute organ dysfunction is associated with SIRS or due to another condition (e.g., directly due to the trauma), the provider should be queried.

Systemic inflammatory response syndrome (SIRS) due to acute gallstone pancreatitis

K85.10	**Biliary acute pancreatitis without necrosis or infection**
R65.10	**Systemic inflammatory response syndrome [SIRS] of non-infectious origin without acute organ dysfunction**

Explanation: When SIRS is documented with a non-infectious condition without subsequent infection documented, the code for the underlying condition such as pancreatitis should be assigned followed by the appropriate code for SIRS of noninfectious origin, either with or without associated organ dysfunction.

h. Death NOS

Code R99, Ill-defined and unknown cause of mortality, is only for use in the very limited circumstance when a patient who has already died is brought into an emergency department or other healthcare facility and is pronounced dead upon arrival. It does not represent the discharge disposition of death.

i. NIHSS stroke scale

The NIH stroke scale (NIHSS) codes (R29.7- -) can be used in conjunction with acute stroke codes (I63) to identify the patient's neurological status and the severity of the stroke. The stroke scale codes should be sequenced after the acute stroke diagnosis code(s).

At a minimum, report the initial score documented. If desired, a facility may choose to capture multiple stroke scale scores.

See Section I.B.14 for NIHSS stroke scale documentation by clinicians other than patient's provider

Patient admitted with CVA seen by neurology consult who documents moderate to severe stroke, 17 on NIHSS stroke scale.

I63.9	**Cerebral infarction, unspecified**
R29.717	**NIHSS score 17**

Explanation: Unspecified cerebral vascular accident (CVA) is sequenced before the NIHSS stroke scale score code. The stroke scale is an assessment tool to help measure stroke-related neurological deficits. Fifteen items are evaluated by trained observers and include such conditions as levels of consciousness, language, dysarthria, ataxia, and sensory loss. A facility may report multiple stroke scale scores if it wants to.

Chapter 18. Symptoms, Signs and Abnormal Clinical and Laboratory Findings, Not Elsewhere Classified (R00-R99)

NOTE This chapter includes symptoms, signs, abnormal results of clinical or other investigative procedures, and ill-defined conditions regarding which no diagnosis classifiable elsewhere is recorded.

Signs and symptoms that point rather definitely to a given diagnosis have been assigned to a category in other chapters of the classification. In general, categories in this chapter include the less well-defined conditions and symptoms that, without the necessary study of the case to establish a final diagnosis, point perhaps equally to two or more diseases or to two or more systems of the body. Practically all categories in the chapter could be designated 'not otherwise specified', 'unknown etiology' or 'transient'. The Alphabetical Index should be consulted to determine which symptoms and signs are to be allocated here and which to other chapters. The residual subcategories, numbered .8, are generally provided for other relevant symptoms that cannot be allocated elsewhere in the classification.

The conditions and signs or symptoms included in categories R00-R94 consist of:

(a) cases for which no more specific diagnosis can be made even after all the facts bearing on the case have been investigated;
(b) signs or symptoms existing at the time of initial encounter that proved to be transient and whose causes could not be determined;
(c) provisional diagnosis in a patient who failed to return for further investigation or care;
(d) cases referred elsewhere for investigation or treatment before the diagnosis was made;
(e) cases in which a more precise diagnosis was not available for any other reason;
(f) certain symptoms, for which supplementary information is provided, that represent important problems in medical care in their own right.

EXCLUDES 2 *abnormal findings on antenatal screening of mother (O28.-)*
certain conditions originating in the perinatal period (P04-P96)
signs and symptoms classified in the body system chapters
signs and symptoms of breast (N63, N64.5)

AHA: 2017,1Q,6,7

This chapter contains the following blocks:

R00-R09 Symptoms and signs involving the circulatory and respiratory systems
R10-R19 Symptoms and signs involving the digestive system and abdomen
R20-R23 Symptoms and signs involving the skin and subcutaneous tissue
R25-R29 Symptoms and signs involving the nervous and musculoskeletal systems
R30-R39 Symptoms and signs involving the genitourinary system
R40-R46 Symptoms and signs involving cognition, perception, emotional state and behavior
R47-R49 Symptoms and signs involving speech and voice
R50-R69 General symptoms and signs
R70-R79 Abnormal findings on examination of blood, without diagnosis
R80-R82 Abnormal findings on examination of urine, without diagnosis
R83-R89 Abnormal findings on examination of other body fluids, substances and tissues, without diagnosis
R90-R94 Abnormal findings on diagnostic imaging and in function studies, without diagnosis
R97 Abnormal tumor markers
R99 Ill-defined and unknown cause of mortality

Symptoms and signs involving the circulatory and respiratory systems (R00-R09)

✓4th **R00 Abnormalities of heart beat**

EXCLUDES 1 *abnormalities originating in the perinatal period (P29.1-)*
EXCLUDES 2 *specified arrhythmias (I47-I49)*

R00.0 Tachycardia, unspecified
Rapid heart beat
Sinoauricular tachycardia NOS
Sinus [sinusal] tachycardia NOS
EXCLUDES 1 *neonatal tachycardia (P29.11)*
paroxysmal tachycardia (I47.-)
DEF: Excessively rapid heart rate of more than 100 beats per minute.

R00.1 Bradycardia, unspecified
Sinoatrial bradycardia
Sinus bradycardia
Slow heart beat
Vagal bradycardia
Use additional code for adverse effect, if applicable, to identify drug (T36-T50 with fifth or sixth character 5)
EXCLUDES 1 *neonatal bradycardia (P29.12)*
AHA: 2020,2Q,23
DEF: Slowed heartbeat, usually defined as a rate fewer than 60 beats per minute. Heart rhythm may be slow as a result of a congenital defect or an acquired problem.

R00.2 Palpitations
Awareness of heart beat

R00.8 Other abnormalities of heart beat

R00.9 Unspecified abnormalities of heart beat

✓4th **R01 Cardiac murmurs and other cardiac sounds**

EXCLUDES 1 *cardiac murmurs and sounds originating in the perinatal period (P29.8)*

R01.0 Benign and innocent cardiac murmurs
Functional cardiac murmur

R01.1 Cardiac murmur, unspecified
Cardiac bruit NOS
Heart murmur NOS
Systolic murmur NOS

R01.2 Other cardiac sounds
Cardiac dullness, increased or decreased
Precordial friction

✓4th **R03 Abnormal blood-pressure reading, without diagnosis**

R03.0 Elevated blood-pressure reading, without diagnosis of hypertension
NOTE This category is to be used to record an episode of elevated blood pressure in a patient in whom no formal diagnosis of hypertension has been made, or as an isolated incidental finding.

R03.1 Nonspecific low blood-pressure reading
EXCLUDES 1 *hypotension (I95.-)*
maternal hypotension syndrome (O26.5-)
neurogenic orthostatic hypotension (G90.3)

✓4th **R04 Hemorrhage from respiratory passages**

R04.0 Epistaxis
Hemorrhage from nose
Nosebleed

R04.1 Hemorrhage from throat
EXCLUDES 2 *hemoptysis (R04.2)*

R04.2 Hemoptysis CC
Blood-stained sputum
Cough with hemorrhage
AHA: 2013,4Q,118

✓5th **R04.8 Hemorrhage from other sites in respiratory passages**

R04.81 Acute idiopathic pulmonary hemorrhage in infants CC P
AIPHI
Acute idiopathic hemorrhage in infants over 28 days old
EXCLUDES 1 *perinatal pulmonary hemorrhage (P26.-)*
von Willebrand's disease (D68.0)

R04.89 Hemorrhage from other sites in respiratory passages CC
Pulmonary hemorrhage NOS

R04.9 Hemorrhage from respiratory passages, unspecified CC

R05 Cough
EXCLUDES 1 *cough with hemorrhage (R04.2)*
smoker's cough (J41.0)
AHA: 2016,2Q,33

✓4th RØ6 Abnormalities of breathing

EXCLUDES 1 *acute respiratory distress syndrome (J8Ø)*
respiratory arrest (RØ9.2)
respiratory arrest of newborn (P28.81)
respiratory distress syndrome of newborn (P22.-)
respiratory failure (J96.-)
respiratory failure of newborn (P28.5)

✓5th RØ6.Ø Dyspnea

EXCLUDES 1 *tachypnea NOS (RØ6.82)*
transient tachypnea of newborn (P22.1)

RØ6.ØØ Dyspnea, unspecified
AHA: 2017,1Q,26

RØ6.Ø1 Orthopnea

RØ6.Ø2 Shortness of breath

RØ6.Ø3 Acute respiratory distress
AHA: 2017,4Q,23

RØ6.Ø9 Other forms of dyspnea

RØ6.1 Stridor

EXCLUDES 1 *congenital laryngeal stridor (P28.89)*
laryngismus (stridulus) (J38.5)

DEF: Certain type of wheezing described as a loud, constant, musical sound produced when breathing with an obstructed airway, like the inspiratory sound heard when laryngeal or esophageal obstruction is present.

RØ6.2 Wheezing

EXCLUDES 1 *asthma (J45.-)*

AHA: 2016,2Q,33

DEF: High-pitched whistling sound during breathing due to stenosis of the respiratory passageway. Wheezing is associated with asthma, sleep apnea, bronchiectasis, bronchiolitis, COPD, and pleural effusion.

RØ6.3 Periodic breathing CC
Cheyne-Stokes breathing

RØ6.4 Hyperventilation

EXCLUDES 1 *psychogenic hyperventilation (F45.8)*

RØ6.5 Mouth breathing

EXCLUDES 2 *dry mouth NOS (R68.2)*

RØ6.6 Hiccough

EXCLUDES 1 *psychogenic hiccough (F45.8)*

RØ6.7 Sneezing

✓5th RØ6.8 Other abnormalities of breathing

RØ6.81 Apnea, not elsewhere classified
Apnea NOS

EXCLUDES 1 *apnea (of) newborn (P28.4)*
sleep apnea (G47.3-)
sleep apnea of newborn (primary) (P28.3)

RØ6.82 Tachypnea, not elsewhere classified
Tachypnea NOS

EXCLUDES 1 *transitory tachypnea of newborn (P22.1)*

RØ6.83 Snoring

RØ6.89 Other abnormalities of breathing
Breath-holding (spells)
Sighing

RØ6.9 Unspecified abnormalities of breathing

✓4th RØ7 Pain in throat and chest

EXCLUDES 1 *epidemic myalgia (B33.Ø)*
EXCLUDES 2 *jaw pain R68.84*
pain in breast (N64.4)

RØ7.Ø Pain in throat

EXCLUDES 1 *chronic sore throat (J31.2)*
sore throat (acute) NOS (JØ2.9)
EXCLUDES 2 *dysphagia (R13.1-)*
pain in neck (M54.2)

RØ7.1 Chest pain on breathing
Painful respiration

RØ7.2 Precordial pain

DEF: Pain felt in the anterior (front) chest wall over the region of the heart. This type of pain is generally felt slightly to the left of the sternum, but may also extend into the surrounding chest wall region.

✓5th RØ7.8 Other chest pain

RØ7.81 Pleurodynia
Pleurodynia NOS

EXCLUDES 1 *epidemic pleurodynia (B33.Ø)*

RØ7.82 Intercostal pain

RØ7.89 Other chest pain
Anterior chest-wall pain NOS

RØ7.9 Chest pain, unspecified

✓4th RØ9 Other symptoms and signs involving the circulatory and respiratory system

EXCLUDES 1 *acute respiratory distress syndrome (J8Ø)*
respiratory arrest of newborn (P28.81)
respiratory distress syndrome of newborn (P22.Ø)
respiratory failure (J96.-)
respiratory failure of newborn (P28.5)

✓5th RØ9.Ø Asphyxia and hypoxemia

EXCLUDES 1 *asphyxia due to carbon monoxide (T58.-)*
asphyxia due to foreign body in respiratory tract (T17.-)
birth (intrauterine) asphyxia (P84)
hyperventilation (RØ6.4)
traumatic asphyxia (T71.-)
EXCLUDES 2 *hypercapnia (RØ6.89)*

RØ9.Ø1 Asphyxia CC

DEF: Interference of oxygen intake due to obstruction or injury of airways resulting in a lack of oxygen perfusion to the tissues or excessive carbon dioxide in the blood. Can cause unconsciousness or death.

RØ9.Ø2 Hypoxemia
AHA: 2019,3Q,15

DEF: Insufficient oxygen in the arterial blood resulting in inadequate delivery of oxygen to the body tissues.

RØ9.1 Pleurisy

EXCLUDES 1 *pleurisy with effusion (J9Ø)*

1 **RØ9.2 Respiratory arrest** MCC HCC
Cardiorespiratory failure

EXCLUDES 1 *cardiac arrest (I46.-)*
respiratory arrest of newborn (P28.81)
respiratory distress of newborn (P22.Ø)
respiratory failure (J96.-)
respiratory failure of newborn (P28.5)
respiratory insufficiency (RØ6.89)
respiratory insufficiency of newborn (P28.5)

RØ9.3 Abnormal sputum
Abnormal amount of sputum
Abnormal color of sputum
Abnormal odor of sputum
Excessive sputum

EXCLUDES 1 *blood-stained sputum (RØ4.2)*

✓5th RØ9.8 Other specified symptoms and signs involving the circulatory and respiratory systems

RØ9.81 Nasal congestion

RØ9.82 Postnasal drip

RØ9.89 Other specified symptoms and signs involving the circulatory and respiratory systems
Abnormal chest percussion
Bruit (arterial)
Chest tympany
Choking sensation
Feeling of foreign body in throat
Friction sounds in chest
Rales
Weak pulse

EXCLUDES 2 *foreign body in throat (T17.2-)*
wheezing (RØ6.2)

Symptoms and signs involving the digestive system and abdomen (R10-R19)

EXCLUDES 2 *congenital or infantile pylorospasm (Q40.0)*
gastrointestinal hemorrhage (K92.0-K92.2)
intestinal obstruction (K56.-)
newborn gastrointestinal hemorrhage (P54.0-P54.3)
newborn intestinal obstruction (P76.-)
pylorospasm (K31.3)
signs and symptoms involving the urinary system (R30-R39)
symptoms referable to female genital organs (N94.-)
symptoms referable to male genital organs (N48-N50)

R10 Abdominal and pelvic pain
EXCLUDES 1 *renal colic (N23)*
EXCLUDES 2 *dorsalgia (M54.-)*
flatulence and related conditions (R14.-)

R10.0 Acute abdomen
Severe abdominal pain (generalized) (with abdominal rigidity)
EXCLUDES 1 *abdominal rigidity NOS (R19.3)*
generalized abdominal pain NOS (R10.84)
localized abdominal pain (R10.1-R10.3-)

R10.1 Pain localized to upper abdomen
R10.10 Upper abdominal pain, unspecified
R10.11 Right upper quadrant pain
R10.12 Left upper quadrant pain
R10.13 Epigastric pain
Dyspepsia
EXCLUDES 1 *functional dyspepsia (K30)*

Abdominal Pain

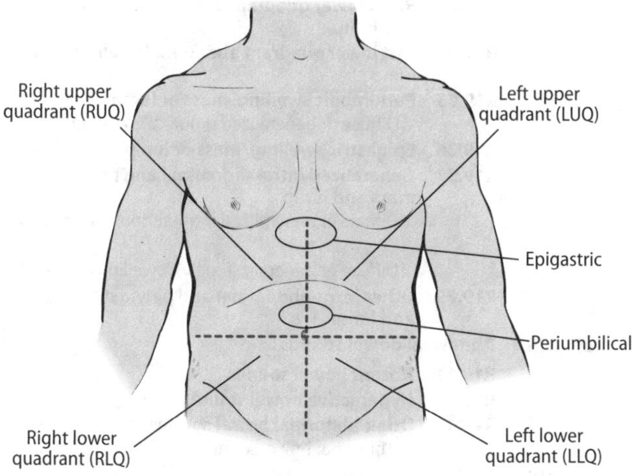

R10.2 Pelvic and perineal pain
EXCLUDES 1 *vulvodynia (N94.81)*

R10.3 Pain localized to other parts of lower abdomen
R10.30 Lower abdominal pain, unspecified
R10.31 Right lower quadrant pain
R10.32 Left lower quadrant pain
R10.33 Periumbilical pain

R10.8 Other abdominal pain
R10.81 Abdominal tenderness
Abdominal tenderness NOS
R10.811 Right upper quadrant abdominal tenderness
R10.812 Left upper quadrant abdominal tenderness
R10.813 Right lower quadrant abdominal tenderness
R10.814 Left lower quadrant abdominal tenderness
R10.815 Periumbilic abdominal tenderness
R10.816 Epigastric abdominal tenderness
R10.817 Generalized abdominal tenderness
R10.819 Abdominal tenderness, unspecified site
R10.82 Rebound abdominal tenderness
R10.821 Right upper quadrant rebound abdominal tenderness
R10.822 Left upper quadrant rebound abdominal tenderness
R10.823 Right lower quadrant rebound abdominal tenderness
R10.824 Left lower quadrant rebound abdominal tenderness
R10.825 Periumbilic rebound abdominal tenderness
R10.826 Epigastric rebound abdominal tenderness
R10.827 Generalized rebound abdominal tenderness
R10.829 Rebound abdominal tenderness, unspecified site
R10.83 Colic P
Colic NOS
Infantile colic
EXCLUDES 1 *colic in adult and child over 12 months old (R10.84)*
DEF: Inconsolable crying in an otherwise well-fed and healthy infant for more than three hours a day, three days a week, for more than three weeks.
R10.84 Generalized abdominal pain
EXCLUDES 1 *generalized abdominal pain associated with acute abdomen (R10.0)*

R10.9 Unspecified abdominal pain

R11 Nausea and vomiting
EXCLUDES 1 *cyclical vomiting associated with migraine (G43.A-)*
excessive vomiting in pregnancy (O21.-)
hematemesis (K92.0)
neonatal hematemesis (P54.0)
newborn vomiting (P92.0-)
psychogenic vomiting (F50.89)
vomiting associated with bulimia nervosa (F50.2)
vomiting following gastrointestinal surgery (K91.0)
AHA: 2017,1Q,28
TIP: Assign a code from this category along with K31.89 Other diseases of stomach and duodenum, to describe cyclical vomiting not due to migraine.

R11.0 Nausea
Nausea NOS
Nausea without vomiting

R11.1 Vomiting
R11.10 Vomiting, unspecified
Vomiting NOS
R11.11 Vomiting without nausea
R11.12 Projectile vomiting
R11.13 Vomiting of fecal matter
R11.14 Bilious vomiting
Bilious emesis
R11.15 Cyclical vomiting syndrome unrelated to migraine
Cyclic vomiting syndrome NOS
Persistent vomiting
EXCLUDES 1 *cyclical vomiting in migraine (G43.A-)*
EXCLUDES 2 *bulimia nervosa (F50.2)*
diabetes mellitus due to underlying condition (E08.-)
AHA: 2019,4Q,15

R11.2 Nausea with vomiting, unspecified
Persistent nausea with vomiting NOS
AHA: 2020,1Q,8

R12 Heartburn
EXCLUDES 1 *dyspepsia NOS (R10.13)*
functional dyspepsia (K30)

R13 Aphagia and dysphagia
R13.0 Aphagia
Inability to swallow
EXCLUDES 1 *psychogenic aphagia (F50.9)*

√5th **R13.1 Dysphagia**

Code first, if applicable, dysphagia following cerebrovascular disease (I69. with final characters -91)

EXCLUDES 1 *psychogenic dysphagia (F45.8)*

Swallowing Function

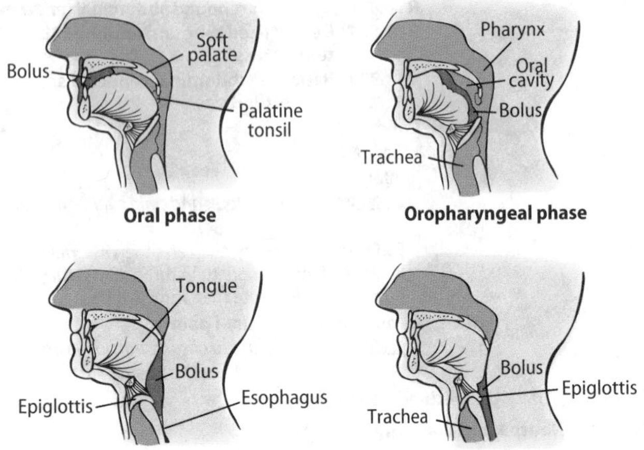

Oral phase **Oropharyngeal phase**

Pharyngeal phase **Pharyngoesophageal phase**

R13.1Ø Dysphagia, unspecified
Difficulty in swallowing NOS

R13.11 Dysphagia, oral phase

R13.12 Dysphagia, oropharyngeal phase

R13.13 Dysphagia, pharyngeal phase

R13.14 Dysphagia, pharyngoesophageal phase

R13.19 Other dysphagia
Cervical dysphagia
Neurogenic dysphagia

√4th **R14 Flatulence and related conditions**

EXCLUDES 1 *psychogenic aerophagy (F45.8)*

R14.Ø Abdominal distension (gaseous)
Bloating
Tympanites (abdominal) (intestinal)

R14.1 Gas pain

R14.2 Eructation

R14.3 Flatulence

√4th **R15 Fecal incontinence**

INCLUDES encopresis NOS

EXCLUDES 1 *fecal incontinence of nonorganic origin (F98.1)*

R15.Ø Incomplete defecation

EXCLUDES 1 *constipation (K59.Ø-)*
fecal impaction (K56.41)

R15.1 Fecal smearing
Fecal soiling

R15.2 Fecal urgency

R15.9 Full incontinence of feces
Fecal incontinence NOS

√4th **R16 Hepatomegaly and splenomegaly, not elsewhere classified**

R16.Ø Hepatomegaly, not elsewhere classified
Hepatomegaly NOS

R16.1 Splenomegaly, not elsewhere classified
Splenomegaly NOS

R16.2 Hepatomegaly with splenomegaly, not elsewhere classified
Hepatosplenomegaly NOS

R17 Unspecified jaundice CC

EXCLUDES 1 *neonatal jaundice (P55, P57-P59)*

√4th **R18 Ascites**

INCLUDES fluid in peritoneal cavity

EXCLUDES 1 *ascites in alcoholic cirrhosis (K7Ø.31)*
ascites in alcoholic hepatitis (K7Ø.11)
ascites in toxic liver disease with chronic active hepatitis (K71.51)

DEF: Abnormal accumulation of free fluid in the abdominal cavity, causing distention and tightness in addition to shortness of breath as the fluid accumulates. Ascites is usually an underlying disorder and can be a manifestation of any number of diseases.

R18.Ø Malignant ascites CC
Code first malignancy, such as:
malignant neoplasm of ovary (C56.-)
secondary malignant neoplasm of retroperitoneum and peritoneum (C78.6)

R18.8 Other ascites CC
Ascites NOS
Peritoneal effusion (chronic)
AHA: 2018,1Q,4

√4th **R19 Other symptoms and signs involving the digestive system and abdomen**

EXCLUDES 1 *acute abdomen (R1Ø.Ø)*

√5th **R19.Ø Intra-abdominal and pelvic swelling, mass and lump**

EXCLUDES 1 *abdominal distension (gaseous) (R14.-)*
ascites (R18.-)

R19.ØØ Intra-abdominal and pelvic swelling, mass and lump, unspecified site

R19.Ø1 Right upper quadrant abdominal swelling, mass and lump

R19.Ø2 Left upper quadrant abdominal swelling, mass and lump

R19.Ø3 Right lower quadrant abdominal swelling, mass and lump

R19.Ø4 Left lower quadrant abdominal swelling, mass and lump

R19.Ø5 Periumbilic swelling, mass or lump
Diffuse or generalized umbilical swelling or mass

R19.Ø6 Epigastric swelling, mass or lump

R19.Ø7 Generalized intra-abdominal and pelvic swelling, mass and lump
Diffuse or generalized intra-abdominal swelling or mass NOS
Diffuse or generalized pelvic swelling or mass NOS

R19.Ø9 Other intra-abdominal and pelvic swelling, mass and lump

√5th **R19.1 Abnormal bowel sounds**

R19.11 Absent bowel sounds

R19.12 Hyperactive bowel sounds

R19.15 Other abnormal bowel sounds
Abnormal bowel sounds NOS

R19.2 Visible peristalsis
Hyperperistalsis
DEF: Visible movements of muscular attempts to move food through the digestive tract due to pyloric obstruction, stomach obstruction, or intestinal obstruction.

√5th **R19.3 Abdominal rigidity**

EXCLUDES 1 *abdominal rigidity with severe abdominal pain (R1Ø.Ø)*

R19.3Ø Abdominal rigidity, unspecified site

R19.31 Right upper quadrant abdominal rigidity

R19.32 Left upper quadrant abdominal rigidity

R19.33 Right lower quadrant abdominal rigidity

R19.34 Left lower quadrant abdominal rigidity

R19.35 Periumbilic abdominal rigidity

R19.36 Epigastric abdominal rigidity

R19.37 Generalized abdominal rigidity

R19.4 Change in bowel habit

EXCLUDES 1 *constipation (K59.Ø-)*
functional diarrhea (K59.1)

R19.5 Other fecal abnormalities
Abnormal stool color
Bulky stools
Mucus in stools
Occult blood in feces
Occult blood in stools
EXCLUDES 1 *melena (K92.1)*
neonatal melena (P54.1)
AHA: 2019,1Q,32

R19.6 Halitosis

R19.7 Diarrhea, unspecified
Diarrhea NOS
EXCLUDES 1 *functional diarrhea (K59.1)*
neonatal diarrhea (P78.3)
psychogenic diarrhea (F45.8)

R19.8 Other specified symptoms and signs involving the digestive system and abdomen

Symptoms and signs involving the skin and subcutaneous tissue (R2Ø-R23)

EXCLUDES 2 *symptoms relating to breast (N64.4-N64.5)*

✓4th **R2Ø Disturbances of skin sensation**
EXCLUDES 1 *dissociative anesthesia and sensory loss (F44.6)*
psychogenic disturbances (F45.8)

R2Ø.Ø Anesthesia of skin
R2Ø.1 Hypoesthesia of skin
R2Ø.2 Paresthesia of skin
Formication
Pins and needles
Tingling skin
EXCLUDES 1 *acroparesthesia (I73.8)*
R2Ø.3 Hyperesthesia
R2Ø.8 Other disturbances of skin sensation
R2Ø.9 Unspecified disturbances of skin sensation

R21 Rash and other nonspecific skin eruption
INCLUDES rash NOS
EXCLUDES 1 *specified type of rash — code to condition*
vesicular eruption (R23.8)

✓4th **R22 Localized swelling, mass and lump of skin and subcutaneous tissue**
INCLUDES subcutaneous nodules (localized)(superficial)
EXCLUDES 1 *abnormal findings on diagnostic imaging (R9Ø-R93)*
edema (R6Ø.-)
enlarged lymph nodes (R59.-)
localized adiposity (E65)
swelling of joint (M25.4-)

R22.Ø Localized swelling, mass and lump, head
R22.1 Localized swelling, mass and lump, neck
R22.2 Localized swelling, mass and lump, trunk
EXCLUDES 1 *intra-abdominal or pelvic mass and lump (R19.Ø-)*
intra-abdominal or pelvic swelling (R19.Ø-)
EXCLUDES 2 *breast mass and lump (N63)*

✓5th **R22.3 Localized swelling, mass and lump, upper limb**
R22.3Ø Localized swelling, mass and lump, unspecified upper limb
R22.31 Localized swelling, mass and lump, right upper limb
R22.32 Localized swelling, mass and lump, left upper limb
R22.33 Localized swelling, mass and lump, upper limb, bilateral

✓5th **R22.4 Localized swelling, mass and lump, lower limb**
R22.4Ø Localized swelling, mass and lump, unspecified lower limb
R22.41 Localized swelling, mass and lump, right lower limb
R22.42 Localized swelling, mass and lump, left lower limb
R22.43 Localized swelling, mass and lump, lower limb, bilateral

R22.9 Localized swelling, mass and lump, unspecified

✓4th **R23 Other skin changes**
R23.Ø Cyanosis
EXCLUDES 1 *acrocyanosis (I73.8)*
cyanotic attacks of newborn (P28.2)
DEF: Bluish or purplish discoloration of the skin due to an inadequate oxygen blood level.

R23.1 Pallor
Clammy skin

R23.2 Flushing
Excessive blushing
Code first, if applicable, menopausal and female climacteric states (N95.1)

R23.3 Spontaneous ecchymoses
Petechiae
EXCLUDES 1 *ecchymoses of newborn (P54.5)*
purpura (D69.-)

R23.4 Changes in skin texture
Desquamation of skin
Induration of skin
Scaling of skin
EXCLUDES 1 *epidermal thickening NOS (L85.9)*

R23.8 Other skin changes
R23.9 Unspecified skin changes

Symptoms and signs involving the nervous and musculoskeletal systems (R25-R29)

✓4th **R25 Abnormal involuntary movements**
EXCLUDES 1 *specific movement disorders (G2Ø-G26)*
stereotyped movement disorders (F98.4)
tic disorders (F95.-)

R25.Ø Abnormal head movements
R25.1 Tremor, unspecified
EXCLUDES 1 *chorea NOS (G25.5)*
essential tremor (G25.Ø)
hysterical tremor (F44.4)
intention tremor (G25.2)

R25.2 Cramp and spasm
EXCLUDES 2 *carpopedal spasm (R29.Ø)*
charley-horse (M62.831)
infantile spasms (G4Ø.4-)
muscle spasm of back (M62.83Ø)
muscle spasm of calf (M62.831)

R25.3 Fasciculation
Twitching NOS
R25.8 Other abnormal involuntary movements
R25.9 Unspecified abnormal involuntary movements

✓4th **R26 Abnormalities of gait and mobility**
EXCLUDES 1 *ataxia NOS (R27.Ø)*
hereditary ataxia (G11.-)
locomotor (syphilitic) ataxia (A52.11)
immobility syndrome (paraplegic) (M62.3)

R26.Ø Ataxic gait
Staggering gait
R26.1 Paralytic gait
Spastic gait
R26.2 Difficulty in walking, not elsewhere classified
EXCLUDES 1 *falling (R29.6)*
unsteadiness on feet (R26.81)
AHA: 2016,2Q,7

✓5th **R26.8 Other abnormalities of gait and mobility**
R26.81 Unsteadiness on feet
R26.89 Other abnormalities of gait and mobility
AHA: 2020,2Q,29

R26.9 Unspecified abnormalities of gait and mobility

✓4th **R27 Other lack of coordination**
EXCLUDES 1 *ataxic gait (R26.Ø)*
hereditary ataxia (G11.-)
vertigo NOS (R42)

R27.Ø Ataxia, unspecified
EXCLUDES 1 *ataxia following cerebrovascular disease (I69. with final characters -93)*
R27.8 Other lack of coordination
R27.9 Unspecified lack of coordination

✓4th R29 Other symptoms and signs involving the nervous and musculoskeletal systems

R29.Ø Tetany CC
Carpopedal spasm
EXCLUDES 1 *hysterical tetany (F44.5)*
neonatal tetany (P71.3)
parathyroid tetany (E2Ø.9)
post-thyroidectomy tetany (E89.2)
DEF: Calcium or other mineral imbalance causing voluntary muscles such as hands, feet, or larynx to spasm rhythmically.

R29.1 Meningismus CC

R29.2 Abnormal reflex
EXCLUDES 2 *abnormal pupillary reflex (H57.Ø)*
hyperactive gag reflex (J39.2)
vasovagal reaction or syncope (R55)

R29.3 Abnormal posture

R29.4 Clicking hip
EXCLUDES 1 *congenital deformities of hip (Q65.-)*

R29.5 Transient paralysis CC
Code first any associated spinal cord injury (S14.Ø, S14.1-, S24.Ø, S24.1-, S34.Ø-, S34.1-)
EXCLUDES 1 *transient ischemic attack (G45.9)*

R29.6 Repeated falls
Falling
Tendency to fall
EXCLUDES 2 *at risk for falling (Z91.81)*
history of falling (Z91.81)
AHA: 2016,2Q,6
TIP: Code in addition to Parkinson's disease (G20), when documented.

✓5th R29.7 National Institutes of Health Stroke Scale (NIHSS) score
Code first the type of cerebral infarction ▶(I63.-)◀
AHA: 2016,4Q,61-62
TIP: Codes from this subcategory may be assigned based on medical record documentation from clinicians who are not the patient's provider.

✓6th R29.7Ø NIHSS score Ø-9
R29.7ØØ NIHSS score Ø
R29.7Ø1 NIHSS score 1
R29.7Ø2 NIHSS score 2
R29.7Ø3 NIHSS score 3
R29.7Ø4 NIHSS score 4
R29.7Ø5 NIHSS score 5
R29.7Ø6 NIHSS score 6
R29.7Ø7 NIHSS score 7
R29.7Ø8 NIHSS score 8
R29.7Ø9 NIHSS score 9

✓6th R29.71 NIHSS score 1Ø-19
R29.71Ø NIHSS score 1Ø
R29.711 NIHSS score 11
R29.712 NIHSS score 12
R29.713 NIHSS score 13
R29.714 NIHSS score 14
R29.715 NIHSS score 15
R29.716 NIHSS score 16
R29.717 NIHSS score 17
R29.718 NIHSS score 18
R29.719 NIHSS score 19

✓6th R29.72 NIHSS score 2Ø-29
R29.72Ø NIHSS score 2Ø
R29.721 NIHSS score 21
R29.722 NIHSS score 22
R29.723 NIHSS score 23
R29.724 NIHSS score 24
R29.725 NIHSS score 25
R29.726 NIHSS score 26
R29.727 NIHSS score 27
R29.728 NIHSS score 28
R29.729 NIHSS score 29

✓6th R29.73 NIHSS score 3Ø-39
R29.73Ø NIHSS score 3Ø
R29.731 NIHSS score 31
R29.732 NIHSS score 32
R29.733 NIHSS score 33
R29.734 NIHSS score 34
R29.735 NIHSS score 35
R29.736 NIHSS score 36
R29.737 NIHSS score 37
R29.738 NIHSS score 38
R29.739 NIHSS score 39

✓6th R29.74 NIHSS score 4Ø-42
R29.74Ø NIHSS score 4Ø
R29.741 NIHSS score 41
R29.742 NIHSS score 42

✓5th R29.8 Other symptoms and signs involving the nervous and musculoskeletal systems

✓6th R29.81 Other symptoms and signs involving the nervous system
R29.81Ø Facial weakness
Facial droop
EXCLUDES 1 *Bell's palsy (G51.Ø)*
facial weakness following cerebrovascular disease (I69. with final characters -92)
R29.818 Other symptoms and signs involving the nervous system

✓6th R29.89 Other symptoms and signs involving the musculoskeletal system
EXCLUDES 2 *pain in limb (M79.6-)*
R29.89Ø Loss of height
EXCLUDES 1 *osteoporosis (M8Ø-M81)*
R29.891 Ocular torticollis
EXCLUDES 1 *congenital (sternomastoid) torticollis Q68.Ø*
psychogenic torticollis (F45.8)
spasmodic torticollis (G24.3)
torticollis due to birth injury (P15.8)
torticollis NOS M43.6
DEF: Abnormal head posture as a result of a contracted state of cervical muscles to correct a visual disturbance, either double vision or a visual field defect.
R29.898 Other symptoms and signs involving the musculoskeletal system

✓5th R29.9 Unspecified symptoms and signs involving the nervous and musculoskeletal systems
R29.9Ø Unspecified symptoms and signs involving the nervous system
R29.91 Unspecified symptoms and signs involving the musculoskeletal system

Symptoms and signs involving the genitourinary system (R3Ø-R39)

✓4th R3Ø Pain associated with micturition
EXCLUDES 1 *psychogenic pain associated with micturition (F45.8)*

R3Ø.Ø Dysuria
Strangury

R3Ø.1 Vesical tenesmus
DEF: Feeling of a full bladder even when there is little or no urine in the bladder.

R3Ø.9 Painful micturition, unspecified
Painful urination NOS

✓4th R31 Hematuria
EXCLUDES 1 *hematuria included with underlying conditions, such as:*
acute cystitis with hematuria (N3Ø.Ø1)
recurrent and persistent hematuria in glomerular diseases (NØ2.-)
AHA: 2017,1Q,17

R31.Ø Gross hematuria

R31.1 Benign essential microscopic hematuria

✓5th R31.2 Other microscopic hematuria
AHA: 2016,4Q,62
R31.21 Asymptomatic microscopic hematuria
AMH
R31.29 Other microscopic hematuria

R31.9 Hematuria, unspecified

R32 Unspecified urinary incontinence
Enuresis NOS
EXCLUDES 1 *functional urinary incontinence (R39.81)*
nonorganic enuresis (F98.0)
stress incontinence and other specified urinary incontinence (N39.3-N39.4-)
urinary incontinence associated with cognitive impairment (R39.81)

R33 Retention of urine
EXCLUDES 1 *psychogenic retention of urine (F45.8)*
R33.0 Drug induced retention of urine
Use additional code for adverse effect, if applicable, to identify drug (T36-T50 with fifth or sixth character 5)
R33.8 Other retention of urine
Code first, if applicable, any causal condition, such as:
enlarged prostate (N40.1)
AHA: 2018,4Q,55
R33.9 Retention of urine, unspecified

R34 Anuria and oliguria
EXCLUDES 1 *anuria and oliguria complicating abortion or ectopic or molar pregnancy (O00-O07, O08.4)*
anuria and oliguria complicating pregnancy (O26.83-)
anuria and oliguria complicating the puerperium (O90.4)

R35 Polyuria
Code first, if applicable, any causal condition, such as:
enlarged prostate (N40.1)
EXCLUDES 1 *psychogenic polyuria (F45.8)*
R35.0 Frequency of micturition
R35.1 Nocturia
R35.8 Other polyuria
Polyuria NOS

R36 Urethral discharge
R36.0 Urethral discharge without blood
R36.1 Hematospermia ♂
R36.9 Urethral discharge, unspecified
Penile discharge NOS
Urethrorrhea

R37 Sexual dysfunction, unspecified

R39 Other and unspecified symptoms and signs involving the genitourinary system
R39.0 Extravasation of urine CC
R39.1 Other difficulties with micturition
Code first, if applicable, any causal condition, such as:
enlarged prostate (N40.1)
R39.11 Hesitancy of micturition
R39.12 Poor urinary stream
Weak urinary steam
R39.13 Splitting of urinary stream
R39.14 Feeling of incomplete bladder emptying
R39.15 Urgency of urination
EXCLUDES 1 *urge incontinence (N39.41, N39.46)*
R39.16 Straining to void
R39.19 Other difficulties with micturition
AHA: 2016,4Q,63
R39.191 Need to immediately re-void
R39.192 Position dependent micturition
R39.198 Other difficulties with micturition
R39.2 Extrarenal uremia
Prerenal uremia
EXCLUDES 1 *uremia NOS (N19)*
R39.8 Other symptoms and signs involving the genitourinary system
AHA: 2017,4Q,22-23
R39.81 Functional urinary incontinence
Urinary incontinence due to cognitive impairment, or severe physical disability or immobility
EXCLUDES 1 *stress incontinence and other specified urinary incontinence (N39.3-N39.4-)*
urinary incontinence NOS (R32)
R39.82 Chronic bladder pain
AHA: 2016,4Q,64
R39.83 Unilateral non-palpable testicle ♂
R39.84 Bilateral non-palpable testicles ♂
R39.89 Other symptoms and signs involving the genitourinary system
R39.9 Unspecified symptoms and signs involving the genitourinary system

Symptoms and signs involving cognition, perception, emotional state and behavior (R40-R46)

EXCLUDES 2 *symptoms and signs constituting part of a pattern of mental disorder (F01-F99)*

R40 Somnolence, stupor and coma
EXCLUDES 1 *neonatal coma (P91.5)*
somnolence, stupor and coma in diabetes (E08-E13)
somnolence, stupor and coma in hepatic failure (K72.-)
somnolence, stupor and coma in hypoglycemia (nondiabetic) (E15)
R40.0 Somnolence
Drowsiness
EXCLUDES 1 *coma (R40.2-)*
R40.1 Stupor
Catatonic stupor
Semicoma
EXCLUDES 1 *catatonic schizophrenia (F20.2)*
coma (R40.2-)
depressive stupor (F31-F33)
dissociative stupor (F44.2)
manic stupor (F30.2)
R40.2 Coma
Code first any associated:
fracture of skull (S02.-)
intracranial injury (S06.-)
NOTE One code from each subcategory, R40.21-R40.23, is required to complete the coma scale
AHA: 2019,2Q,12; 2018,4Q,70; 2017,4Q,23-25,95; 2015,2Q,17; 2014,1Q,19
TIP: Codes for individual (R40.21-, R40.22, R40.23-) or total (R40.24-) coma scale scores may be assigned based on medical record documentation from clinicians who are not the patient's provider.
TIP: It is not appropriate to assign individual (R40.21- , R40.22-, R40.23-) or total (R40.24-) coma scale score codes for patients who are sedated or in medically induced comas.
R40.20 Unspecified coma MCC HCC
Coma NOS
Unconsciousness NOS
R40.21 Coma scale, eyes open

The following appropriate 7th character is to be added to subcategory R40.21-, R40.22-, R40.23-, and R40.24-.
0 unspecified time
1 in the field [EMT or ambulance]
2 at arrival to emergency department
3 at hospital admission
4 24 hours or more after hospital admission

R40.211 Coma scale, eyes open, never MCC HCC
Coma scale eye opening score of 1
R40.212 Coma scale, eyes open, to pain MCC HCC
Coma scale eye opening score of 2
R40.213 Coma scale, eyes open, to sound
Coma scale eye opening score of 3
R40.214 Coma scale, eyes open, spontaneous
Coma scale eye opening score of 4
R40.22 Coma scale, best verbal response
R40.221 Coma scale, best verbal response, none MCC HCC
Coma scale verbal score of 1
R40.222 Coma scale, best verbal response, incomprehensible words MCC HCC
Coma scale verbal score of 2
Incomprehensible sounds (2-5 years of age)
Moans/grunts to pain; restless (< 2 years old)

√7th **R4Ø.223 Coma scale, best verbal response, inappropriate words**
Coma scale verbal score of 3
Inappropriate crying or screaming (< 2 years of age)
Screaming (2-5 years of age)

√7th **R4Ø.224 Coma scale, best verbal response, confused conversation**
Coma scale verbal score of 4
Inappropriate words (2-5 years of age)
Irritable cries (< 2 years of age)

√7th **R4Ø.225 Coma scale, best verbal response, oriented**
Coma scale verbal score of 5
Cooing or babbling or crying appropriately (< 2 years of age)
Uses appropriate words (2-5 years of age)

√6th **R4Ø.23 Coma scale, best motor response**

√7th **R4Ø.231 Coma scale, best motor response, none** MCC HCC
Coma scale motor score of 1

√7th **R4Ø.232 Coma scale, best motor response, extension** MCC HCC
Abnormal extensor posturing to pain or noxious stimuli (< 2 years of age)
Coma scale motor score of 2
Extensor posturing to pain or noxious stimuli (2-5 years of age)

√7th **R4Ø.233 Coma scale, best motor response, abnormal flexion**
Abnormal flexure posturing to pain or noxious stimuli (2-5 years of age)
Coma scale motor score of 3
Flexion/decorticate posturing (< 2 years of age)

√7th **R4Ø.234 Coma scale, best motor response, flexion withdrawal** MCC HCC
Coma scale motor score of 4
Withdraws from pain or noxious stimuli (2-5 years of age)

√7th **R4Ø.235 Coma scale, best motor response, localizes pain**
Coma scale motor score of 5
Localizes pain (2-5 years of age)
Withdraws to touch (< 2 years of age)

√7th **R4Ø.236 Coma scale, best motor response, obeys commands**
Coma scale motor score of 6
Normal or spontaneous movement (< 2 years of age)
Obeys commands (2-5 years of age)

√6th **R4Ø.24 Glasgow coma scale, total score**

NOTE Assign a code from subcategory R4Ø.24, when only the total coma score is documented

AHA: 2016,4Q,64-65

√7th **R4Ø.241 Glasgow coma scale score 13-15**

√7th **R4Ø.242 Glasgow coma scale score 9-12**

√7th **R4Ø.243 Glasgow coma scale score 3-8** HCC

√7th **R4Ø.244 Other coma, without documented Glasgow coma scale score, or with partial score reported** HCC

R4Ø.3 Persistent vegetative state CC HCC
DEF: Persistent wakefulness without consciousness due to a nonfunctioning cerebral cortex.

R4Ø.4 Transient alteration of awareness
AHA: 2020,2Q,24

√4th **R41 Other symptoms and signs involving cognitive functions and awareness**
EXCLUDES 1 *dissociative [conversion] disorders (F44.-)*
mild cognitive impairment, so stated (G31.84)

R41.Ø Disorientation, unspecified
Confusion NOS
Delirium NOS
AHA: 2019,2Q,34

R41.1 Anterograde amnesia

R41.2 Retrograde amnesia

R41.3 Other amnesia
Amnesia NOS
Memory loss NOS
EXCLUDES 1 *amnestic disorder due to known physiologic condition (FØ4)*
amnestic syndrome due to psychoactive substance use (F1Ø-F19 with 5th character .6)
mild memory disturbance due to known physiological condition (FØ6.8)
transient global amnesia (G45.4)

R41.4 Neurologic neglect syndrome CC
Asomatognosia
Hemi-akinesia
Hemi-inattention
Hemispatial neglect
Left-sided neglect
Sensory neglect
Visuospatial neglect
EXCLUDES 1 *visuospatial deficit (R41.842)*

√5th **R41.8 Other symptoms and signs involving cognitive functions and awareness**

R41.81 Age-related cognitive decline A
Senility NOS

R41.82 Altered mental status, unspecified
Change in mental status NOS
EXCLUDES 1 *altered level of consciousness (R4Ø.-)*
altered mental status due to known condition — code to condition
delirium NOS (R41.Ø)
AHA: 2012,4Q,97

R41.83 Borderline intellectual functioning
IQ level 71 to 84
EXCLUDES 1 *intellectual disabilities (F7Ø-F79)*

√6th **R41.84 Other specified cognitive deficit**
EXCLUDES 1 *cognitive deficits as sequelae of cerebrovascular disease (I69.Ø1-, I69.11-, I69.21-, I69.31-, I69.81-, I69.91-)*

R41.84Ø Attention and concentration deficit
EXCLUDES 1 *attention-deficit hyperactivity disorders (F9Ø.-)*

R41.841 Cognitive communication deficit

R41.842 Visuospatial deficit

R41.843 Psychomotor deficit

R41.844 Frontal lobe and executive function deficit

R41.89 Other symptoms and signs involving cognitive functions and awareness
Anosognosia

R41.9 Unspecified symptoms and signs involving cognitive functions and awareness
Unspecified neurocognitive disorder

R42 Dizziness and giddiness
Light-headedness
Vertigo NOS
EXCLUDES 1 *vertiginous syndromes (H81.-)*
vertigo from infrasound (T75.23)

√4th **R43 Disturbances of smell and taste**

R43.Ø Anosmia
DEF: Permanent or transient absence of smell that may be congenital or acquired.

R43.1 Parosmia
DEF: Abnormal perception of smell usually triggered by environmental odors.

R43.2 Parageusia
DEF: Abnormal perception of taste.

R43.8 Other disturbances of smell and taste
Mixed disturbance of smell and taste

R43.9 Unspecified disturbances of smell and taste

R44 Other symptoms and signs involving general sensations and perceptions

EXCLUDES 1 *alcoholic hallucinations ▶(F10.151, F10.251, F10.951)◀*
hallucinations in drug psychosis ▶(F11-F19 with fifth to sixth characters 51)◀
hallucinations in mood disorders with psychotic symptoms (F30.2, F31.5, F32.3, F33.3)
hallucinations in schizophrenia, schizotypal and delusional disorders (F20-F29)

EXCLUDES 2 *disturbances of skin sensation (R20.-)*

R44.0 Auditory hallucinations CC
R44.1 Visual hallucinations
R44.2 Other hallucinations CC
R44.3 Hallucinations, unspecified CC
R44.8 Other symptoms and signs involving general sensations and perceptions
R44.9 Unspecified symptoms and signs involving general sensations and perceptions

R45 Symptoms and signs involving emotional state

R45.0 Nervousness
Nervous tension
R45.1 Restlessness and agitation
R45.2 Unhappiness
R45.3 Demoralization and apathy
EXCLUDES 1 *anhedonia (R45.84)*
R45.4 Irritability and anger
R45.5 Hostility
R45.6 Violent behavior
R45.7 State of emotional shock and stress, unspecified
R45.8 Other symptoms and signs involving emotional state
R45.81 Low self-esteem
R45.82 Worries
R45.83 Excessive crying of child, adolescent or adult
EXCLUDES 1 *excessive crying of infant (baby) R68.11*
R45.84 Anhedonia
R45.85 Homicidal and suicidal ideations
EXCLUDES 1 *suicide attempt (T14.91)*
R45.850 Homicidal ideations
R45.851 Suicidal ideations CC
DEF: Thoughts of committing suicide but no actual attempt of suicide has been made.
R45.86 Emotional lability
R45.87 Impulsiveness
R45.89 Other symptoms and signs involving emotional state

R46 Symptoms and signs involving appearance and behavior

EXCLUDES 1 *appearance and behavior in schizophrenia, schizotypal and delusional disorders (F20-F29)*
mental and behavioral disorders (F01-F99)

R46.0 Very low level of personal hygiene
R46.1 Bizarre personal appearance
R46.2 Strange and inexplicable behavior
R46.3 Overactivity
R46.4 Slowness and poor responsiveness
EXCLUDES 1 *stupor (R40.1)*
R46.5 Suspiciousness and marked evasiveness
R46.6 Undue concern and preoccupation with stressful events
R46.7 Verbosity and circumstantial detail obscuring reason for contact
R46.8 Other symptoms and signs involving appearance and behavior
R46.81 Obsessive-compulsive behavior
EXCLUDES 1 *obsessive-compulsive disorder ▶(F42.-)◀*
R46.89 Other symptoms and signs involving appearance and behavior

Symptoms and signs involving speech and voice (R47-R49)

R47 Speech disturbances, not elsewhere classified

EXCLUDES 1 *autism (F84.0)*
cluttering (F80.81)
specific developmental disorders of speech and language (F80.-)
stuttering (F80.81)

R47.0 Dysphasia and aphasia
R47.01 Aphasia CC
EXCLUDES 1 *aphasia following cerebrovascular disease (I69. with final characters -20)*
progressive isolated aphasia (G31.01)
R47.02 Dysphasia
EXCLUDES 1 *dysphasia following cerebrovascular disease (I69. with final characters -21)*
R47.1 Dysarthria and anarthria
EXCLUDES 1 *dysarthria following cerebrovascular disease (I69. with final characters -22)*
R47.8 Other speech disturbances
EXCLUDES 1 *dysarthria following cerebrovascular disease (I69. with final characters -28)*
R47.81 Slurred speech
R47.82 Fluency disorder in conditions classified elsewhere
Stuttering in conditions classified elsewhere
Code first underlying disease or condition, such as:
Parkinson's disease (G20)
EXCLUDES 1 *adult onset fluency disorder (F98.5)*
childhood onset fluency disorder (F80.81)
fluency disorder (stuttering) following cerebrovascular disease (I69. with final characters -23)
R47.89 Other speech disturbances
R47.9 Unspecified speech disturbances

R48 Dyslexia and other symbolic dysfunctions, not elsewhere classified

EXCLUDES 1 *specific developmental disorders of scholastic skills (F81.-)*

R48.0 Dyslexia and alexia
R48.1 Agnosia
Astereognosia (astereognosis)
Autotopagnosia
EXCLUDES 1 *visual object agnosia (R48.3)*
DEF: Inability to recognize common things such as faces, objects, smells, or voices.
R48.2 Apraxia
EXCLUDES 1 *apraxia following cerebrovascular disease (I69. with final characters -90)*
R48.3 Visual agnosia
Prosopagnosia
Simultanagnosia (asimultagnosia)
R48.8 Other symbolic dysfunctions
Acalculia
Agraphia
AHA: 2017,1Q,27
R48.9 Unspecified symbolic dysfunctions

R49 Voice and resonance disorders

EXCLUDES 1 *psychogenic voice and resonance disorders (F44.4)*

R49.0 Dysphonia
Hoarseness
R49.1 Aphonia
Loss of voice
R49.2 Hypernasality and hyponasality
R49.21 Hypernasality
R49.22 Hyponasality
R49.8 Other voice and resonance disorders
R49.9 Unspecified voice and resonance disorder
Change in voice NOS
Resonance disorder NOS

General symptoms and signs (R50-R69)

✓4th R50 Fever of other and unknown origin

EXCLUDES 1 *chills without fever (R68.83)*
febrile convulsions (R56.0-)
fever of unknown origin during labor (O75.2)
fever of unknown origin in newborn (P81.9)
hypothermia due to illness (R68.0)
malignant hyperthermia due to anesthesia (T88.3)
puerperal pyrexia NOS (O86.4)

R50.2 Drug induced fever
Use additional code for adverse effect, if applicable, to identify drug (T36-T50 with fifth or sixth character 5)
EXCLUDES 1 *postvaccination (postimmunization) fever (R50.83)*

✓5th R50.8 Other specified fever

R50.81 Fever presenting with conditions classified elsewhere
Code first underlying condition when associated fever is present, such as with:
leukemia (C91-C95)
neutropenia (D70.-)
sickle-cell disease (D57.-)
AHA: 2014,4Q,22

R50.82 Postprocedural fever
EXCLUDES 1 *postprocedural infection (T81.4-)*
posttransfusion fever (R50.84)
postvaccination (postimmunization) fever (R50.83)

R50.83 Postvaccination fever
Postimmunization fever

R50.84 Febrile nonhemolytic transfusion reaction
FNHTR
Posttransfusion fever

R50.9 Fever, unspecified
Fever NOS
Fever of unknown origin [FUO]
Fever with chills
Fever with rigors
Hyperpyrexia NOS
Persistent fever
Pyrexia NOS

▲✓4th R51 Headache
~~Facial pain NOS~~
EXCLUDES 1 ~~*atypical face pain (G50.1)*~~
~~*migraine and other headache syndromes (G43-G44)*~~
~~*trigeminal neuralgia (G50.0)*~~
EXCLUDES 2 ▶*atypical face pain (G50.1)*◀
▶*migraine and other headache syndromes (G43-G44)*◀
▶*trigeminal neuralgia (G50.0)*◀

● **R51.0 Headache with orthostatic component, not elsewhere classified**
Headache with positional component, not elsewhere classified

● **R51.9 Headache, unspecified**
Facial pain NOS

R52 Pain, unspecified
Acute pain NOS
Generalized pain NOS
Pain NOS
EXCLUDES 1 *acute and chronic pain, not elsewhere classified (G89.-)*
localized pain, unspecified type — code to pain by site, such as:
abdomen pain (R10.-)
back pain (M54.9)
breast pain (N64.4)
chest pain (R07.1-R07.9)
ear pain (H92.0-)
eye pain (H57.1)
headache ▶(R51.9)◀
joint pain (M25.5-)
limb pain (M79.6-)
lumbar region pain (M54.5)
pelvic and perineal pain (R10.2)
renal colic (N23)
shoulder pain (M25.51-)
spine pain (M54.-)
throat pain (R07.0)
tongue pain (K14.6)
tooth pain (K08.8)
pain disorders exclusively related to psychological factors (F45.41)

✓4th R53 Malaise and fatigue

R53.0 Neoplastic (malignant) related fatigue
Code first associated neoplasm

R53.1 Weakness
Asthenia NOS
EXCLUDES 1 *age-related weakness (R54)*
▶*muscle weakness (generalized) (M62.81)*◀
sarcopenia (M62.84)
senile asthenia (R54)
AHA: 2017,1Q,7; 2015,1Q,25

R53.2 Functional quadriplegia MCC HCC
Complete immobility due to severe physical disability or frailty
EXCLUDES 1 *frailty NOS (R54)*
hysterical paralysis (F44.4)
immobility syndrome (M62.3)
neurologic quadriplegia (G82.5-)
quadriplegia (G82.50)
AHA: 2016,2Q,6
DEF: Inability to move due to a nonphysiological condition, such as dementia. The patient has no mental ability to move independently.

✓5th R53.8 Other malaise and fatigue
EXCLUDES 1 *combat exhaustion and fatigue (F43.0)*
congenital debility (P96.9)
exhaustion and fatigue due to excessive exertion (T73.3)
exhaustion and fatigue due to exposure (T73.2)
exhaustion and fatigue due to heat (T67.-)
exhaustion and fatigue due to pregnancy (O26.8-)
exhaustion and fatigue due to recurrent depressive episode (F33)
exhaustion and fatigue due to senile debility (R54)

R53.81 Other malaise
Chronic debility
Debility NOS
General physical deterioration
Malaise NOS
Nervous debility
EXCLUDES 1 *age-related physical debility (R54)*

R53.82 Chronic fatigue, unspecified
Chronic fatigue syndrome NOS
EXCLUDES 1 *postviral fatigue syndrome (G93.3)*

R53.83 Other fatigue
Fatigue NOS
Lack of energy
Lethargy
Tiredness
EXCLUDES 2 *exhaustion and fatigue due to depressive episode (F32.-)*

R54 Age-related physical debility A
Frailty
Old age
Senescence
Senile asthenia
Senile debility
EXCLUDES 1 *age-related cognitive decline (R41.81)*
sarcopenia (M62.84)
senile psychosis (FØ3)
senility NOS (R41.81)

R55 Syncope and collapse
Blackout
Fainting
Vasovagal attack
EXCLUDES 1 *cardiogenic shock (R57.Ø)*
carotid sinus syncope (G9Ø.Ø1)
heat syncope (T67.1)
neurocirculatory asthenia (F45.8)
neurogenic orthostatic hypotension (G9Ø.3)
orthostatic hypotension (I95.1)
postprocedural shock (T81.1-)
psychogenic syncope (F48.8)
shock NOS (R57.9)
shock complicating or following abortion or ectopic or molar pregnancy (OØØ-OØ7, OØ8.3)
shock complicating or following labor and delivery (O75.1)
Stokes-Adams attack (I45.9)
unconsciousness NOS (R4Ø.2-)

✓4th **R56 Convulsions, not elsewhere classified**
EXCLUDES 1 *dissociative convulsions and seizures (F44.5)*
epileptic convulsions and seizures (G4Ø.-)
newborn convulsions and seizures (P9Ø)

✓5th **R56.Ø Febrile convulsions**

R56.ØØ Simple febrile convulsions CC HCC
Febrile convulsion NOS
Febrile seizure NOS

R56.Ø1 Complex febrile convulsions CC HCC
Atypical febrile seizure
Complex febrile seizure
Complicated febrile seizure
EXCLUDES 1 *status epilepticus (G4Ø.9Ø1)*

R56.1 Post traumatic seizures CC HCC
EXCLUDES 1 *post traumatic epilepsy (G4Ø.-)*

R56.9 Unspecified convulsions HCC
Convulsion disorder
Fit NOS
Recurrent convulsions
Seizure(s) (convulsive) NOS
AHA: 2019,1Q,19

✓4th **R57 Shock, not elsewhere classified**
EXCLUDES 1 *anaphylactic shock NOS (T78.2)*
anaphylactic reaction or shock due to adverse food reaction (T78.Ø-)
anaphylactic shock due to adverse effect of correct drug or medicament properly administered (T88.6)
anaphylactic shock due to serum (T8Ø.5-)
anesthetic shock (T88.3)
electric shock (T75.4)
obstetric shock (O75.1)
postprocedural shock (T81.1-)
psychic shock (F43.Ø)
shock complicating or following ectopic or molar pregnancy (OØØ-OØ7, OØ8.3)
shock due to lightning (T75.Ø1)
traumatic shock (T79.4)
toxic shock syndrome (A48.3)

1 **R57.Ø Cardiogenic shock** MCC HCC
EXCLUDES 2 *septic shock (R65.21)*
DEF: Associated with myocardial infarction, cardiac tamponade, and massive pulmonary embolism. Symptoms include mental confusion, reduced blood pressure, tachycardia, pallor, and cold, clammy skin.

1 **R57.1 Hypovolemic shock** MCC HCC
AHA: 2019,2Q,7

1 **R57.8 Other shock** MCC HCC

R57.9 Shock, unspecified CC HCC
Failure of peripheral circulation NOS

R58 Hemorrhage, not elsewhere classified
Hemorrhage NOS
EXCLUDES 1 *hemorrhage included with underlying conditions, such as:*
acute duodenal ulcer with hemorrhage (K26.Ø)
acute gastritis with bleeding (K29.Ø1)
ulcerative enterocolitis with rectal bleeding (K51.Ø1)

✓4th **R59 Enlarged lymph nodes**
INCLUDES swollen glands
EXCLUDES 1 *acute lymphadenitis (LØ4.-)*
chronic lymphadenitis (I88.1)
lymphadenitis NOS (I88.9)
mesenteric (acute) (chronic) lymphadenitis (I88.Ø)

R59.Ø Localized enlarged lymph nodes

R59.1 Generalized enlarged lymph nodes
Lymphadenopathy NOS

R59.9 Enlarged lymph nodes, unspecified

✓4th **R6Ø Edema, not elsewhere classified**
EXCLUDES 1 *angioneurotic edema (T78.3)*
ascites (R18.-)
cerebral edema (G93.6)
cerebral edema due to birth injury (P11.Ø)
edema of larynx (J38.4)
edema of nasopharynx (J39.2)
edema of pharynx (J39.2)
gestational edema (O12.Ø-)
hereditary edema (Q82.Ø)
hydrops fetalis NOS (P83.2)
hydrothorax (J94.8)
hydrops fetalis NOS (P83.2)
newborn edema (P83.3)
pulmonary edema (J81.-)

R6Ø.Ø Localized edema

R6Ø.1 Generalized edema
EXCLUDES 2 *nutritional edema (E4Ø-E46)*

R6Ø.9 Edema, unspecified
Fluid retention NOS

R61 Generalized hyperhidrosis
Excessive sweating
Night sweats
Secondary hyperhidrosis
Code first, if applicable, menopausal and female climacteric states (N95.1)
EXCLUDES 1 *focal (primary) (secondary) hyperhidrosis (L74.5-)*
Frey's syndrome (L74.52)
localized (primary) (secondary) hyperhidrosis (L74.5-)

√4th **R62 Lack of expected normal physiological development in childhood and adults**
EXCLUDES 1 *delayed puberty (E30.0)*
gonadal dysgenesis (Q99.1)
hypopituitarism (E23.0)

R62.0 Delayed milestone in childhood P
Delayed attainment of expected physiological developmental stage
Late talker
Late walker

√5th **R62.5 Other and unspecified lack of expected normal physiological development in childhood**
EXCLUDES 1 *HIV disease resulting in failure to thrive (B20)*
physical retardation due to malnutrition (E45)

R62.50 Unspecified lack of expected normal physiological development in childhood
Infantilism NOS

R62.51 Failure to thrive (child) P
Failure to gain weight
EXCLUDES 1 *failure to thrive in child under 28 days old (P92.6)*
AHA: 2018,4Q,82
DEF: Organic failure to thrive (FTT): Acute or chronic illness that interferes with nutritional intake, absorption, metabolism excretion, and energy requirements.
DEF: Nonorganic failure to thrive (FTT): Symptom of neglect or abuse.

R62.52 Short stature (child)
Lack of growth
Physical retardation
Short stature NOS
EXCLUDES 1 *short stature due to endocrine disorder (E34.3)*

R62.59 Other lack of expected normal physiological development in childhood

R62.7 Adult failure to thrive A

√4th **R63 Symptoms and signs concerning food and fluid intake**
EXCLUDES 1 *bulimia NOS (F50.2)*

R63.0 Anorexia
Loss of appetite
EXCLUDES 1 *anorexia nervosa (F50.0-)*
loss of appetite of nonorganic origin (F50.89)
AHA: 2018,4Q,82
TIP: Assign an additional code from category Z68 when BMI is documented. BMI can be based on documentation from clinicians who are not the patient's provider.

R63.1 Polydipsia
Excessive thirst

R63.2 Polyphagia
Excessive eating
Hyperalimentation NOS

R63.3 Feeding difficulties
Feeding problem (elderly) (infant) NOS
Picky eater
EXCLUDES 1 *eating disorders (F50.-)*
feeding problems of newborn (P92.-)
infant feeding disorder of nonorganic origin (F98.2-)
AHA: 2017,1Q,28; 2016,3Q,19
TIP: Do not assign for feeding problems in a patient greater than 28 days old if the feeding problem was initially diagnosed between day 0 and day 28; use a code from category P92 instead.

R63.4 Abnormal weight loss
AHA: 2018,4Q,82
TIP: Assign an additional code from category Z68 when BMI is documented. BMI can be based on documentation from clinicians who are not the patient's provider.

R63.5 Abnormal weight gain
EXCLUDES 1 *excessive weight gain in pregnancy (O26.0-)*
obesity (E66.-)
AHA: 2018,4Q,82
TIP: Assign an additional code from category Z68 when BMI is documented. BMI can be based on documentation from clinicians who are not the patient's provider.

R63.6 Underweight
Use additional code to identify body mass index (BMI), if known (Z68.-)
EXCLUDES 1 *abnormal weight loss (R63.4)*
anorexia nervosa (F50.0-)
malnutrition (E40-E46)
AHA: 2018,4Q,82

R63.8 Other symptoms and signs concerning food and fluid intake

R64 Cachexia CC HCC
Wasting syndrome
Code first underlying condition, if known
EXCLUDES 1 *abnormal weight loss (R63.4)*
nutritional marasmus (E41)
AHA: 2018,4Q,82; 2017,3Q,24

√4th **R65 Symptoms and signs specifically associated with systemic inflammation and infection**
AHA: 2019,2Q,38
TIP: When documentation states SIRS with an infection, assign only a code for the infection. ICD-10-CM does not offer a code for SIRS due to infectious process. If sepsis is suspected, query the provider.

√5th **R65.1 Systemic inflammatory response syndrome [SIRS] of non-infectious origin**
Code first underlying condition, such as:
heatstroke (T67.0-)
injury and trauma (S00-T88)
EXCLUDES 1 *sepsis — code to infection*
severe sepsis (R65.2)

R65.10 Systemic inflammatory response syndrome [SIRS] of non-infectious origin without acute organ dysfunction CC HCC
Systemic inflammatory response syndrome (SIRS) NOS
AHA: 2019,2Q,24

R65.11 Systemic inflammatory response syndrome [SIRS] of non-infectious origin with acute organ dysfunction MCC HCC
Use additional code to identify specific acute organ dysfunction, such as:
acute kidney failure (N17.-)
acute respiratory failure (J96.0-)
critical illness myopathy (G72.81)
critical illness polyneuropathy (G62.81)
disseminated intravascular coagulopathy [DIC] (D65)
encephalopathy (metabolic) (septic) (G93.41)
hepatic failure (K72.0-)

√5th **R65.2 Severe sepsis**
Infection with associated acute organ dysfunction
Sepsis with acute organ dysfunction
Sepsis with multiple organ dysfunction
Systemic inflammatory response syndrome due to infectious process with acute organ dysfunction
Code first underlying infection, such as:
infection following a procedure (T81.4-)
infections following infusion, transfusion and therapeutic injection (T80.2-)
puerperal sepsis (O85)
sepsis following complete or unspecified spontaneous abortion (O03.87)
sepsis following ectopic and molar pregnancy (O08.82)
sepsis following incomplete spontaneous abortion (O03.37)
sepsis following (induced) termination of pregnancy (O04.87)
sepsis NOS (A41.9)
Use additional code to identify specific acute organ dysfunction, such as:
acute kidney failure (N17.-)
acute respiratory failure (J96.0-)
critical illness myopathy (G72.81)
critical illness polyneuropathy (G62.81)
disseminated intravascular coagulopathy [DIC] (D65)
encephalopathy (metabolic) (septic) (G93.41)
hepatic failure (K72.0-)
AHA: 2020,2Q,17; 2018,4Q,62-63; 2017,4Q,98-99; 2016,3Q,8

R65.20 Severe sepsis without septic shock MCC HCC
Severe sepsis NOS
AHA: 2020,2Q,17; 2016,3Q,14; 2013,4Q,119

R65.21 Severe sepsis with septic shock MCC HCC
AHA: 2018,4Q,63

R68 Other general symptoms and signs

R68.Ø Hypothermia, not associated with low environmental temperature
EXCLUDES 1 *hypothermia NOS (accidental) (T68)*
hypothermia due to anesthesia (T88.51)
hypothermia due to low environmental temperature (T68)
newborn hypothermia (P8Ø.-)

R68.1 Nonspecific symptoms peculiar to infancy
EXCLUDES 1 *colic, infantile (R1Ø.83)*
neonatal cerebral irritability (P91.3)
teething syndrome (KØØ.7)

R68.11 Excessive crying of infant (baby) P
EXCLUDES 1 *excessive crying of child, adolescent, or adult (R45.83)*

R68.12 Fussy infant (baby) P
Irritable infant

R68.13 Apparent life threatening event in infant (ALTE) P
Apparent life threatening event in newborn
Brief resolved unexplained event (BRUE)
Code first confirmed diagnosis, if known
Use additional code(s) for associated signs and symptoms if no confirmed diagnosis established, or if signs and symptoms are not associated routinely with confirmed diagnosis, or provide additional information for cause of ALTE

R68.19 Other nonspecific symptoms peculiar to infancy P

R68.2 Dry mouth, unspecified
EXCLUDES 1 *dry mouth due to dehydration (E86.Ø)*
dry mouth due to sicca syndrome [Sjögren] (M35.Ø-)
salivary gland hyposecretion (K11.7)

R68.3 Clubbing of fingers
Clubbing of nails
EXCLUDES 1 *congenital clubfinger (Q68.1)*
DEF: Enlarged soft tissue of the distal fingers that usually occurs in heart and lung diseases.

R68.8 Other general symptoms and signs

R68.81 Early satiety
DEF: Premature feeling of being full after eating only a small amount of food. The mechanism of satiety is multifactorial.

R68.82 Decreased libido A
Decreased sexual desire

R68.83 Chills (without fever)
Chills NOS
EXCLUDES 1 *chills with fever (R5Ø.9)*

R68.84 Jaw pain
Mandibular pain
Maxilla pain
EXCLUDES 1 *temporomandibular joint arthralgia (M26.62-)*

R68.89 Other general symptoms and signs

R69 Illness, unspecified
Unknown and unspecified cases of morbidity

Abnormal findings on examination of blood, without diagnosis (R7Ø-R79)

EXCLUDES 2 *abnormal findings on antenatal screening of mother (O28.-)*
abnormalities of lipids (E78.-)
abnormalities of platelets and thrombocytes (D69.-)
abnormalities of white blood cells classified elsewhere (D7Ø-D72)
coagulation hemorrhagic disorders (D65-D68)
diagnostic abnormal findings classified elsewhere — see Alphabetical Index
hemorrhagic and hematological disorders of newborn (P5Ø-P61)

R7Ø Elevated erythrocyte sedimentation rate and abnormality of plasma viscosity

R7Ø.Ø Elevated erythrocyte sedimentation rate

R7Ø.1 Abnormal plasma viscosity

R71 Abnormality of red blood cells
EXCLUDES 1 *anemias (D5Ø-D64)*
anemia of premature infant (P61.2)
benign (familial) polycythemia (D75.Ø)
congenital anemias (P61.2-P61.4)
newborn anemia due to isoimmunization (P55.-)
polycythemia neonatorum (P61.1)
polycythemia NOS (D75.1)
polycythemia vera (D45)
secondary polycythemia (D75.1)

R71.Ø Precipitous drop in hematocrit CC
Drop (precipitous) in hemoglobin
Drop in hematocrit

R71.8 Other abnormality of red blood cells
Abnormal red-cell morphology NOS
Abnormal red-cell volume NOS
Anisocytosis
Poikilocytosis

R73 Elevated blood glucose level
EXCLUDES 1 *diabetes mellitus (EØ8-E13)*
diabetes mellitus in pregnancy, childbirth and the puerperium (O24.-)
neonatal disorders (P7Ø.Ø-P7Ø.2)
postsurgical hypoinsulinemia (E89.1)

R73.Ø Abnormal glucose
EXCLUDES 1 *abnormal glucose in pregnancy (O99.81-)*
diabetes mellitus (EØ8-E13)
dysmetabolic syndrome X (E88.81)
gestational diabetes (O24.4-)
glycosuria (R81)
hypoglycemia (E16.2)

R73.Ø1 Impaired fasting glucose
Elevated fasting glucose

R73.Ø2 Impaired glucose tolerance (oral)
Elevated glucose tolerance

R73.Ø3 Prediabetes
Latent diabetes
AHA: 2016,4Q,65

R73.Ø9 Other abnormal glucose
Abnormal glucose NOS
Abnormal non-fasting glucose tolerance

R73.9 Hyperglycemia, unspecified

R74 Abnormal serum enzyme levels

▲ **R74.Ø Nonspecific elevation of levels of transaminase and lactic acid dehydrogenase [LDH]**

● **R74.01 Elevation of levels of liver transaminase levels**
Elevation of levels of alanine transaminase (ALT)
Elevation of levels of aspartate transaminase (AST)

● **R74.02 Elevation of levels of lactic acid dehydrogenase [LDH]**

R74.8 Abnormal levels of other serum enzymes
Abnormal level of acid phosphatase
Abnormal level of alkaline phosphatase
Abnormal level of amylase
Abnormal level of lipase [triacylglycerol lipase]
AHA: 2019,2Q,6

R74.9 Abnormal serum enzyme level, unspecified

R75 Inconclusive laboratory evidence of human immunodeficiency virus [HIV]
Nonconclusive HIV-test finding in infants
EXCLUDES 1 *asymptomatic human immunodeficiency virus [HIV] infection status (Z21)*
human immunodeficiency virus [HIV] disease (B2Ø)
TIP: Do not assign for patients previously diagnosed with an HIV-related illness; assign code B20 instead.

R76 Other abnormal immunological findings in serum

R76.Ø Raised antibody titer
EXCLUDES 1 *isoimmunization in pregnancy (O36.Ø-O36.1)*
isoimmunization affecting newborn (P55.-)

√5th **R76.1 Nonspecific reaction to test for tuberculosis**

R76.11 Nonspecific reaction to tuberculin skin test without active tuberculosis
Abnormal result of Mantoux test
PPD positive
Tuberculin (skin test) positive
Tuberculin (skin test) reactor
EXCLUDES 1 *nonspecific reaction to cell mediated immunity measurement of gamma interferon antigen response without active tuberculosis (R76.12)*

R76.12 Nonspecific reaction to cell mediated immunity measurement of gamma interferon antigen response without active tuberculosis
Nonspecific reaction to QuantiFERON-TB test (QFT) without active tuberculosis
EXCLUDES 1 *nonspecific reaction to tuberculin skin test without active tuberculosis (R76.11)*
positive tuberculin skin test (R76.11)

R76.8 Other specified abnormal immunological findings in serum
Raised level of immunoglobulins NOS

R76.9 Abnormal immunological finding in serum, unspecified

√4th **R77 Other abnormalities of plasma proteins**
EXCLUDES 1 *disorders of plasma-protein metabolism (E88.Ø-)*

R77.Ø Abnormality of albumin
R77.1 Abnormality of globulin
Hyperglobulinemia NOS
R77.2 Abnormality of alphafetoprotein
R77.8 Other specified abnormalities of plasma proteins
R77.9 Abnormality of plasma protein, unspecified
AHA: 2019,2Q,6

√4th **R78 Findings of drugs and other substances, not normally found in blood**
Use additional code to identify the any retained foreign body, if applicable (Z18.-)
EXCLUDES 1 *mental or behavioral disorders due to psychoactive substance use (F1Ø-F19)*

R78.Ø Finding of alcohol in blood
Use additional external cause code (Y9Ø.-), for detail regarding alcohol level
R78.1 Finding of opiate drug in blood
R78.2 Finding of cocaine in blood
R78.3 Finding of hallucinogen in blood
R78.4 Finding of other drugs of addictive potential in blood
R78.5 Finding of other psychotropic drug in blood
R78.6 Finding of steroid agent in blood

√5th **R78.7 Finding of abnormal level of heavy metals in blood**

R78.71 Abnormal lead level in blood
EXCLUDES 1 *lead poisoning (T56.Ø-)*
R78.79 Finding of abnormal level of heavy metals in blood

√5th **R78.8 Finding of other specified substances, not normally found in blood**

R78.81 Bacteremia CC
EXCLUDES 1 *sepsis — code to specified infection*
DEF: Laboratory finding of bacteria in the blood in the absence of two or more signs of sepsis. Transient in nature, it can progress to septicemia with a severe infectious process.
R78.89 Finding of other specified substances, not normally found in blood
Finding of abnormal level of lithium in blood

R78.9 Finding of unspecified substance, not normally found in blood

√4th **R79 Other abnormal findings of blood chemistry**
Use additional code to identify any retained foreign body, if applicable (Z18.-)
EXCLUDES 1 *asymptomatic hyperuricemia (E79.Ø)*
hyperglycemia NOS (R73.9)
hypoglycemia NOS (E16.2)
neonatal hypoglycemia (P7Ø.3-P7Ø.4)
specific findings indicating disorder of amino-acid metabolism (E7Ø-E72)
specific findings indicating disorder of carbohydrate metabolism (E73-E74)
specific findings indicating disorder of lipid metabolism (E75.-)

R79.Ø Abnormal level of blood mineral
Abnormal blood level of cobalt
Abnormal blood level of copper
Abnormal blood level of iron
Abnormal blood level of magnesium
Abnormal blood level of mineral NEC
Abnormal blood level of zinc
EXCLUDES 1 *abnormal level of lithium (R78.89)*
disorders of mineral metabolism (E83.-)
neonatal hypomagnesemia (P71.2)
nutritional mineral deficiency (E58-E61)

R79.1 Abnormal coagulation profile
Abnormal or prolonged bleeding time
Abnormal or prolonged coagulation time
Abnormal or prolonged partial thromboplastin time [PTT]
Abnormal or prolonged prothrombin time [PT]
EXCLUDES 1 *coagulation defects (D68.-)*
EXCLUDES 2 *abnormality of fluid, electrolyte or acid-base balance (E86-E87)*

√5th **R79.8 Other specified abnormal findings of blood chemistry**

R79.81 Abnormal blood-gas level
R79.82 Elevated C-reactive protein [CRP]
R79.89 Other specified abnormal findings of blood chemistry
AHA: 2019,2Q,6
TIP: Assign for documented abnormal or elevated troponin level when a definitive diagnosis has not been established.
TIP: Assign for positive Coombs test when not further clarified in the documentation.

R79.9 Abnormal finding of blood chemistry, unspecified

Abnormal findings on examination of urine, without diagnosis (R8Ø-R82)

EXCLUDES 1 *abnormal findings on antenatal screening of mother (O28.-)*
diagnostic abnormal findings classified elsewhere — see Alphabetical Index
specific findings indicating disorder of amino-acid metabolism (E7Ø-E72)
specific findings indicating disorder of carbohydrate metabolism (E73-E74)

√4th **R8Ø Proteinuria**
EXCLUDES 1 *gestational proteinuria (O12.1-)*

R8Ø.Ø Isolated proteinuria
Idiopathic proteinuria
EXCLUDES 1 *isolated proteinuria with specific morphological lesion (NØ6.-)*
R8Ø.1 Persistent proteinuria, unspecified
R8Ø.2 Orthostatic proteinuria, unspecified
Postural proteinuria
R8Ø.3 Bence Jones proteinuria
R8Ø.8 Other proteinuria
R8Ø.9 Proteinuria, unspecified
Albuminuria NOS

R81 Glycosuria
EXCLUDES 1 *renal glycosuria ►(E74.818)◄*

√4th **R82 Other and unspecified abnormal findings in urine**
INCLUDES chromoabnormalities in urine
Use additional code to identify any retained foreign body, if applicable (Z18.-)
EXCLUDES 2 *hematuria (R31.-)*

R82.Ø Chyluria CC
EXCLUDES 1 *filarial chyluria (B74.-)*
R82.1 Myoglobinuria CC

R82.2 Biliuria

R82.3 Hemoglobinuria

EXCLUDES 1 *hemoglobinuria due to hemolysis from external causes NEC (D59.6)*
hemoglobinuria due to paroxysmal nocturnal [Marchiafava-Micheli] (D59.5)

DEF: Free hemoglobin in blood due to rapid hemolysis of red blood cells. Causes include burns, crushed injury, sickle cell anemia, thalassemia, parasitic infections, or kidney infections.

R82.4 Acetonuria

Ketonuria

DEF: Excessive excretion of acetone in urine that commonly occurs in diabetic acidosis.

R82.5 Elevated urine levels of drugs, medicaments and biological substances

Elevated urine levels of catecholamines
Elevated urine levels of indoleacetic acid
Elevated urine levels of 17-ketosteroids
Elevated urine levels of steroids

R82.6 Abnormal urine levels of substances chiefly nonmedicinal as to source

Abnormal urine level of heavy metals

✓5th **R82.7 Abnormal findings on microbiological examination of urine**

EXCLUDES 1 *colonization status (Z22.-)*

AHA: 2016,4Q,65

R82.71 Bacteriuria

R82.79 Other abnormal findings on microbiological examination of urine

Positive culture findings of urine

✓5th **R82.8 Abnormal findings on cytological and histological examination of urine**

AHA: 2019,4Q,16

R82.81 Pyuria

Sterile pyuria

R82.89 Other abnormal findings on cytological and histological examination of urine

✓5th **R82.9 Other and unspecified abnormal findings in urine**

R82.90 Unspecified abnormal findings in urine

R82.91 Other chromoabnormalities of urine

Chromoconversion (dipstick)
Idiopathic dipstick converts positive for blood with no cellular forms in sediment

EXCLUDES 1 *hemoglobinuria (R82.3)*
myoglobinuria (R82.1)

✓6th **R82.99 Other abnormal findings in urine**

AHA: 2018,4Q,29-30

R82.991 Hypocitraturia

R82.992 Hyperoxaluria

EXCLUDES 1 *primary hyperoxaluria (E72.53)*

R82.993 Hyperuricosuria

R82.994 Hypercalciuria

Idiopathic hypercalciuria

R82.998 Other abnormal findings in urine

Cells and casts in urine
Crystalluria
Melanuria

Abnormal findings on examination of other body fluids, substances and tissues, without diagnosis (R83-R89)

EXCLUDES 1 *abnormal findings on antenatal screening of mother (O28.-)*
diagnostic abnormal findings classified elsewhere — see Alphabetical Index

EXCLUDES 2 *abnormal findings on examination of blood, without diagnosis (R70-R79)*
abnormal findings on examination of urine, without diagnosis (R80-R82)
abnormal tumor markers (R97.-)

✓4th **R83 Abnormal findings in cerebrospinal fluid**

Cerebrospinal Fluid

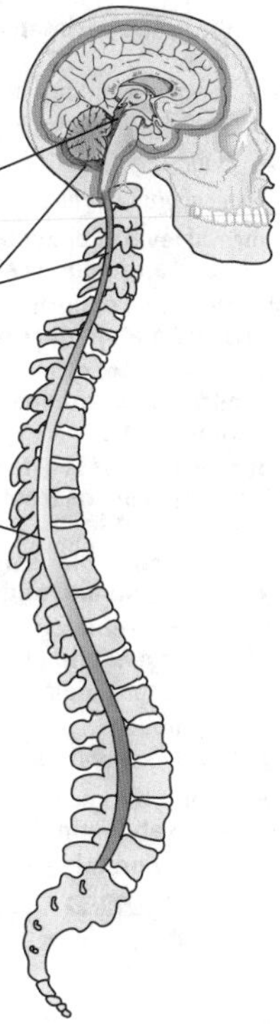

R83.0 Abnormal level of enzymes in cerebrospinal fluid

R83.1 Abnormal level of hormones in cerebrospinal fluid

R83.2 Abnormal level of other drugs, medicaments and biological substances in cerebrospinal fluid

R83.3 Abnormal level of substances chiefly nonmedicinal as to source in cerebrospinal fluid

R83.4 Abnormal immunological findings in cerebrospinal fluid

R83.5 Abnormal microbiological findings in cerebrospinal fluid

Positive culture findings in cerebrospinal fluid

EXCLUDES 1 *colonization status (Z22.-)*

R83.6 Abnormal cytological findings in cerebrospinal fluid

R83.8 Other abnormal findings in cerebrospinal fluid

Abnormal chromosomal findings in cerebrospinal fluid

R83.9 Unspecified abnormal finding in cerebrospinal fluid

✓4th **R84 Abnormal findings in specimens from respiratory organs and thorax**

INCLUDES abnormal findings in bronchial washings
abnormal findings in nasal secretions
abnormal findings in pleural fluid
abnormal findings in sputum
abnormal findings in throat scrapings

EXCLUDES 1 *blood-stained sputum (R04.2)*

R84.0 Abnormal level of enzymes in specimens from respiratory organs and thorax

R84.1 Abnormal level of hormones in specimens from respiratory organs and thorax

R84.2 Abnormal level of other drugs, medicaments and biological substances in specimens from respiratory organs and thorax

R84.3 Abnormal level of substances chiefly nonmedicinal as to source in specimens from respiratory organs and thorax

R84.4 Abnormal immunological findings in specimens from respiratory organs and thorax

R84.5 Abnormal microbiological findings in specimens from respiratory organs and thorax
Positive culture findings in specimens from respiratory organs and thorax
EXCLUDES 1 *colonization status (Z22.-)*

R84.6 Abnormal cytological findings in specimens from respiratory organs and thorax

R84.7 Abnormal histological findings in specimens from respiratory organs and thorax

R84.8 Other abnormal findings in specimens from respiratory organs and thorax
Abnormal chromosomal findings in specimens from respiratory organs and thorax

R84.9 Unspecified abnormal finding in specimens from respiratory organs and thorax

✓4th **R85 Abnormal findings in specimens from digestive organs and abdominal cavity**
INCLUDES abnormal findings in peritoneal fluid
abnormal findings in saliva
EXCLUDES 1 *cloudy peritoneal dialysis effluent (R88.Ø)*
fecal abnormalities (R19.5)

R85.Ø Abnormal level of enzymes in specimens from digestive organs and abdominal cavity

R85.1 Abnormal level of hormones in specimens from digestive organs and abdominal cavity

R85.2 Abnormal level of other drugs, medicaments and biological substances in specimens from digestive organs and abdominal cavity

R85.3 Abnormal level of substances chiefly nonmedicinal as to source in specimens from digestive organs and abdominal cavity

R85.4 Abnormal immunological findings in specimens from digestive organs and abdominal cavity

R85.5 Abnormal microbiological findings in specimens from digestive organs and abdominal cavity
Positive culture findings in specimens from digestive organs and abdominal cavity
EXCLUDES 1 *colonization status (Z22.-)*

✓5th **R85.6 Abnormal cytological findings in specimens from digestive organs and abdominal cavity**

✓6th **R85.61 Abnormal cytologic smear of anus**
EXCLUDES 1 *abnormal cytological findings in specimens from other digestive organs and abdominal cavity (R85.69)*
anal intraepithelial neoplasia I [AIN I] (K62.82)
anal intraepithelial neoplasia II [AIN II] (K62.82)
anal intraepithelial neoplasia III [AIN III] (DØ1.3)
carcinoma in situ of anus (histologically confirmed) (DØ1.3)
dysplasia (mild) (moderate) of anus (histologically confirmed) (K62.82)
severe dysplasia of anus (histologically confirmed) (DØ1.3)
EXCLUDES 2 *anal high risk human papillomavirus (HPV) DNA test positive (R85.81)*
anal low risk human papillomavirus (HPV) DNA test positive (R85.82)

R85.61Ø Atypical squamous cells of undetermined significance on cytologic smear of anus [ASC-US]

R85.611 Atypical squamous cells cannot exclude high grade squamous intraepithelial lesion on cytologic smear of anus [ASC-H]

R85.612 Low grade squamous intraepithelial lesion on cytologic smear of anus [LGSIL]

R85.613 High grade squamous intraepithelial lesion on cytologic smear of anus [HGSIL]

R85.614 Cytologic evidence of malignancy on smear of anus

R85.615 Unsatisfactory cytologic smear of anus
Inadequate sample of cytologic smear of anus

R85.616 Satisfactory anal smear but lacking transformation zone

R85.618 Other abnormal cytological findings on specimens from anus

R85.619 Unspecified abnormal cytological findings in specimens from anus
Abnormal anal cytology NOS
Atypical glandular cells of anus NOS

R85.69 Abnormal cytological findings in specimens from other digestive organs and abdominal cavity

R85.7 Abnormal histological findings in specimens from digestive organs and abdominal cavity

✓5th **R85.8 Other abnormal findings in specimens from digestive organs and abdominal cavity**

R85.81 Anal high risk human papillomavirus [HPV] DNA test positive
EXCLUDES 1 *anogenital warts due to human papillomavirus (HPV) (A63.Ø)*
condyloma acuminatum (A63.Ø)

R85.82 Anal low risk human papillomavirus [HPV] DNA test positive
Use additional code for associated human papillomavirus (B97.7)

R85.89 Other abnormal findings in specimens from digestive organs and abdominal cavity
Abnormal chromosomal findings in specimens from digestive organs and abdominal cavity

R85.9 Unspecified abnormal finding in specimens from digestive organs and abdominal cavity

✓4th **R86 Abnormal findings in specimens from male genital organs**
INCLUDES abnormal findings in prostatic secretions
abnormal findings in semen, seminal fluid
abnormal spermatozoa
EXCLUDES 1 *azoospermia (N46.Ø-)*
oligospermia (N46.1-)

R86.Ø Abnormal level of enzymes in specimens from male genital organs ♂

R86.1 Abnormal level of hormones in specimens from male genital organs ♂

R86.2 Abnormal level of other drugs, medicaments and biological substances in specimens from male genital organs ♂

R86.3 Abnormal level of substances chiefly nonmedicinal as to source in specimens from male genital organs ♂

R86.4 Abnormal immunological findings in specimens from male genital organs ♂

R86.5 Abnormal microbiological findings in specimens from male genital organs ♂
Positive culture findings in specimens from male genital organs
EXCLUDES 1 *colonization status (Z22.-)*

R86.6 Abnormal cytological findings in specimens from male genital organs ♂

R86.7 Abnormal histological findings in specimens from male genital organs ♂

R86.8 Other abnormal findings in specimens from male genital organs ♂
Abnormal chromosomal findings in specimens from male genital organs

R86.9 Unspecified abnormal finding in specimens from male genital organs ♂

✓4th **R87 Abnormal findings in specimens from female genital organs**
INCLUDES abnormal findings in secretion and smears from cervix uteri
abnormal findings in secretion and smears from vagina
abnormal findings in secretion and smears from vulva

R87.Ø Abnormal level of enzymes in specimens from female genital organs ♀

R87.1 Abnormal level of hormones in specimens from female genital organs ♀

R87.2 Abnormal level of other drugs, medicaments and biological substances in specimens from female genital organs ♀

R87.3 Abnormal level of substances chiefly nonmedicinal as to source in specimens from female genital organs ♀

R87.4 Abnormal immunological findings in specimens from female genital organs ♀

R87.5 Abnormal microbiological findings in specimens from female genital organs ♀
Positive culture findings in specimens from female genital organs
EXCLUDES 1 *colonization status (Z22.-)*

√5th **R87.6 Abnormal cytological findings in specimens from female genital organs**

√6th **R87.61 Abnormal cytological findings in specimens from cervix uteri**

EXCLUDES 1 *abnormal cytological findings in specimens from other female genital organs (R87.69)*
abnormal cytological findings in specimens from vagina (R87.62-)
carcinoma in situ of cervix uteri (histologically confirmed) (DØ6.-)
cervical intraepithelial neoplasia I [CIN I] (N87.Ø)
cervical intraepithelial neoplasia II [CIN II] (N87.1)
cervical intraepithelial neoplasia III [CIN III] (DØ6.-)
dysplasia (mild) (moderate) of cervix uteri (histologically confirmed) (N87.-)
severe dysplasia of cervix uteri (histologically confirmed) (DØ6.-)

EXCLUDES 2 *cervical high risk human papillomavirus (HPV) DNA test positive (R87.81Ø)*
cervical low risk human papillomavirus (HPV) DNA test positive (R87.82Ø)

R87.61Ø Atypical squamous cells of undetermined significance on cytologic smear of cervix [ASC-US] ♀

R87.611 Atypical squamous cells cannot exclude high grade squamous intraepithelial lesion on cytologic smear of cervix [ASC-H] ♀

R87.612 Low grade squamous intraepithelial lesion on cytologic smear of cervix [LGSIL] ♀

R87.613 High grade squamous intraepithelial lesion on cytologic smear of cervix [HGSIL] ♀

R87.614 Cytologic evidence of malignancy on smear of cervix ♀

R87.615 Unsatisfactory cytologic smear of cervix ♀
Inadequate sample of cytologic smear of cervix

R87.616 Satisfactory cervical smear but lacking transformation zone ♀

R87.618 Other abnormal cytological findings on specimens from cervix uteri ♀

R87.619 Unspecified abnormal cytological findings in specimens from cervix uteri ♀
Abnormal cervical cytology NOS
Abnormal Papanicolaou smear of cervix NOS
Abnormal thin preparation smear of cervix NOS
Atypical endocervial cells of cervix NOS
Atypical endometrial cells of cervix NOS
Atypical glandular cells of cervix NOS

√6th **R87.62 Abnormal cytological findings in specimens from vagina**
Use additional code to identify acquired absence of uterus and cervix, if applicable (Z9Ø.71-)

EXCLUDES 1 *abnormal cytological findings in specimens from cervix uteri (R87.61-)*
abnormal cytological findings in specimens from other female genital organs (R87.69)
carcinoma in situ of vagina (histologically confirmed) (DØ7.2)
dysplasia (mild) (moderate) of vagina (histologically confirmed) (N89.-)
severe dysplasia of vagina (histologically confirmed) (DØ7.2)
vaginal intraepithelial neoplasia I [VAIN I] (N89.Ø)
vaginal intraepithelial neoplasia II [VAIN II] (N89.1)
vaginal intraepithelial neoplasia III [VAIN III] (DØ7.2)

EXCLUDES 2 *vaginal high risk human papillomavirus (HPV) DNA test positive (R87.811)*
vaginal low risk human papillomavirus (HPV) DNA test positive (R87.821)

R87.62Ø Atypical squamous cells of undetermined significance on cytologic smear of vagina [ASC-US] ♀

R87.621 Atypical squamous cells cannot exclude high grade squamous intraepithelial lesion on cytologic smear of vagina [ASC-H] ♀

R87.622 Low grade squamous intraepithelial lesion on cytologic smear of vagina [LGSIL] ♀

R87.623 High grade squamous intraepithelial lesion on cytologic smear of vagina [HGSIL] ♀

R87.624 Cytologic evidence of malignancy on smear of vagina ♀

R87.625 Unsatisfactory cytologic smear of vagina ♀
Inadequate sample of cytologic smear of vagina

R87.628 Other abnormal cytological findings on specimens from vagina ♀

R87.629 Unspecified abnormal cytological findings in specimens from vagina ♀
Abnormal Papanicolaou smear of vagina NOS
Abnormal thin preparation smear of vagina NOS
Abnormal vaginal cytology NOS
Atypical endocervical cells of vagina NOS
Atypical endometrial cells of vagina NOS
Atypical glandular cells of vagina NOS

R87.69 Abnormal cytological findings in specimens from other female genital organs ♀
Abnormal cytological findings in specimens from female genital organs NOS

EXCLUDES 1 *dysplasia of vulva (histologically confirmed) (N9Ø.Ø-N9Ø.3)*

R87.7 Abnormal histological findings in specimens from female genital organs ♀

EXCLUDES 1 *carcinoma in situ (histologically confirmed) of female genital organs (DØ6-DØ7.3)*
cervical intraepithelial neoplasia I [CIN I] (N87.Ø)
cervical intraepithelial neoplasia II [CIN II] (N87.1)
cervical intraepithelial neoplasia III [CIN III] (DØ6.-)
dysplasia (mild) (moderate) of cervix uteri (histologically confirmed) (N87.-)
dysplasia (mild) (moderate) of vagina (histologically confirmed) (N89.-)
severe dysplasia of cervix uteri (histologically confirmed) (DØ6.-)
severe dysplasia of vagina (histologically confirmed) (DØ7.2)
vaginal intraepithelial neoplasia I [VAIN I] (N89.Ø)
vaginal intraepithelial neoplasia II [VAIN II] (N89.1)
vaginal intraepithelial neoplasia III [VAIN III] (DØ7.2)

✓5th **R87.8 Other abnormal findings in specimens from female genital organs**

✓6th **R87.81 High risk human papillomavirus [HPV] DNA test positive from female genital organs**

EXCLUDES 1 *anogenital warts due to human papillomavirus (HPV) (A63.Ø)*
condyloma acuminatum (A63.Ø)

R87.81Ø Cervical high risk human papillomavirus [HPV] DNA test positive ♀

R87.811 Vaginal high risk human papillomavirus [HPV] DNA test positive ♀

✓6th **R87.82 Low risk human papillomavirus [HPV] DNA test positive from female genital organs**

Use additional code for associated human papillomavirus (B97.7)

R87.82Ø Cervical low risk human papillomavirus [HPV] DNA test positive ♀

R87.821 Vaginal low risk human papillomavirus [HPV] DNA test positive ♀

R87.89 Other abnormal findings in specimens from female genital organs ♀

Abnormal chromosomal findings in specimens from female genital organs

R87.9 Unspecified abnormal finding in specimens from female genital organs ♀

✓4th **R88 Abnormal findings in other body fluids and substances**

R88.Ø Cloudy (hemodialysis) (peritoneal) dialysis effluent

R88.8 Abnormal findings in other body fluids and substances

✓4th **R89 Abnormal findings in specimens from other organs, systems and tissues**

INCLUDES abnormal findings in nipple discharge
abnormal findings in synovial fluid
abnormal findings in wound secretions

R89.Ø Abnormal level of enzymes in specimens from other organs, systems and tissues

R89.1 Abnormal level of hormones in specimens from other organs, systems and tissues

R89.2 Abnormal level of other drugs, medicaments and biological substances in specimens from other organs, systems and tissues

R89.3 Abnormal level of substances chiefly nonmedicinal as to source in specimens from other organs, systems and tissues

R89.4 Abnormal immunological findings in specimens from other organs, systems and tissues

R89.5 Abnormal microbiological findings in specimens from other organs, systems and tissues

Positive culture findings in specimens from other organs, systems and tissues

EXCLUDES 1 *colonization status (Z22.-)*

R89.6 Abnormal cytological findings in specimens from other organs, systems and tissues

R89.7 Abnormal histological findings in specimens from other organs, systems and tissues

R89.8 Other abnormal findings in specimens from other organs, systems and tissues

Abnormal chromosomal findings in specimens from other organs, systems and tissues

R89.9 Unspecified abnormal finding in specimens from other organs, systems and tissues

Abnormal findings on diagnostic imaging and in function studies, without diagnosis (R9Ø-R94)

INCLUDES nonspecific abnormal findings on diagnostic imaging by computerized axial tomography [CAT scan]
nonspecific abnormal findings on diagnostic imaging by magnetic resonance imaging [MRI][NMR]
nonspecific abnormal findings on diagnostic imaging by positron emission tomography [PET scan]
nonspecific abnormal findings on diagnostic imaging by thermography
nonspecific abnormal findings on diagnostic imaging by ultrasound [echogram]
nonspecific abnormal findings on diagnostic imaging by X-ray examination

EXCLUDES 1 *abnormal findings on antenatal screening of mother (O28.-)*
diagnostic abnormal findings classified elsewhere — see Alphabetical Index

✓4th **R9Ø Abnormal findings on diagnostic imaging of central nervous system**

R9Ø.Ø Intracranial space-occupying lesion found on diagnostic imaging of central nervous system

✓5th **R9Ø.8 Other abnormal findings on diagnostic imaging of central nervous system**

R9Ø.81 Abnormal echoencephalogram

R9Ø.82 White matter disease, unspecified

R9Ø.89 Other abnormal findings on diagnostic imaging of central nervous system

Other cerebrovascular abnormality found on diagnostic imaging of central nervous system

✓4th **R91 Abnormal findings on diagnostic imaging of lung**

R91.1 Solitary pulmonary nodule

Coin lesion lung
Solitary pulmonary nodule, subsegmental branch of the bronchial tree

R91.8 Other nonspecific abnormal finding of lung field

Lung mass NOS found on diagnostic imaging of lung
Pulmonary infiltrate NOS
Shadow, lung

✓4th **R92 Abnormal and inconclusive findings on diagnostic imaging of breast**

R92.Ø Mammographic microcalcification found on diagnostic imaging of breast

EXCLUDES 2 *mammographic calcification (calculus) found on diagnostic imaging of breast (R92.1)*

DEF: Calcium and cellular debris deposits in the breast that cannot be felt but can be detected on a mammogram. The deposits can be a sign of cancer, benign conditions, or changes in the breast tissue as a result of inflammation, injury, or an obstructed duct.

R92.1 Mammographic calcification found on diagnostic imaging of breast

Mammographic calculus found on diagnostic imaging of breast

R92.2 Inconclusive mammogram

Dense breasts NOS
Inconclusive mammogram NEC
Inconclusive mammography due to dense breasts
Inconclusive mammography NEC
AHA: 2015,1Q,24

R92.8 Other abnormal and inconclusive findings on diagnostic imaging of breast

✓4th **R93 Abnormal findings on diagnostic imaging of other body structures**

R93.Ø Abnormal findings on diagnostic imaging of skull and head, not elsewhere classified

EXCLUDES 1 *intracranial space-occupying lesion found on diagnostic imaging (R9Ø.Ø)*

R93.1 Abnormal findings on diagnostic imaging of heart and coronary circulation

Abnormal echocardiogram NOS
Abnormal heart shadow

R93.2 Abnormal findings on diagnostic imaging of liver and biliary tract

Nonvisualization of gallbladder

R93.3 Abnormal findings on diagnostic imaging of other parts of digestive tract

✓5th **R93.4 Abnormal findings on diagnostic imaging of urinary organs**
EXCLUDES 2 *hypertrophy of kidney (N28.81)*
AHA: 2016,4Q,66

R93.41 Abnormal radiologic findings on diagnostic imaging of renal pelvis, ureter, or bladder
Filling defect of bladder found on diagnostic imaging
Filling defect of renal pelvis found on diagnostic imaging
Filling defect of ureter found on diagnostic imaging

✓6th **R93.42 Abnormal radiologic findings on diagnostic imaging of kidney**
R93.421 Abnormal radiologic findings on diagnostic imaging of right kidney
R93.422 Abnormal radiologic findings on diagnostic imaging of left kidney
R93.429 Abnormal radiologic findings on diagnostic imaging of unspecified kidney

R93.49 Abnormal radiologic findings on diagnostic imaging of other urinary organs

R93.5 Abnormal findings on diagnostic imaging of other abdominal regions, including retroperitoneum

R93.6 Abnormal findings on diagnostic imaging of limbs
EXCLUDES 2 *abnormal finding in skin and subcutaneous tissue (R93.8-)*
AHA: 2020,1Q,14

R93.7 Abnormal findings on diagnostic imaging of other parts of musculoskeletal system
EXCLUDES 2 *abnormal findings on diagnostic imaging of skull (R93.Ø)*

✓5th **R93.8 Abnormal findings on diagnostic imaging of other specified body structures**
AHA: 2018,4Q,30

✓6th **R93.81 Abnormal radiologic findings on diagnostic imaging of testis**
R93.811 Abnormal radiologic findings on diagnostic imaging of right testicle ♂
R93.812 Abnormal radiologic findings on diagnostic imaging of left testicle ♂
R93.813 Abnormal radiologic findings on diagnostic imaging of testicles, bilateral ♂
R93.819 Abnormal radiologic findings on diagnostic imaging of unspecified testicle ♂

R93.89 Abnormal findings on diagnostic imaging of other specified body structures
Abnormal finding by radioisotope localization of placenta
Abnormal radiological finding in skin and subcutaneous tissue
Mediastinal shift

R93.9 Diagnostic imaging inconclusive due to excess body fat of patient

✓4th **R94 Abnormal results of function studies**
INCLUDES abnormal results of radionuclide [radioisotope] uptake studies
abnormal results of scintigraphy

✓5th **R94.Ø Abnormal results of function studies of central nervous system**
R94.Ø1 Abnormal electroencephalogram [EEG]
R94.Ø2 Abnormal brain scan
R94.Ø9 Abnormal results of other function studies of central nervous system

✓5th **R94.1 Abnormal results of function studies of peripheral nervous system and special senses**

✓6th **R94.11 Abnormal results of function studies of eye**
R94.11Ø Abnormal electro-oculogram [EOG]
R94.111 Abnormal electroretinogram [ERG]
Abnormal retinal function study
R94.112 Abnormal visually evoked potential [VEP]
R94.113 Abnormal oculomotor study
R94.118 Abnormal results of other function studies of eye

✓6th **R94.12 Abnormal results of function studies of ear and other special senses**
AHA: 2016,3Q,17
R94.12Ø Abnormal auditory function study
R94.121 Abnormal vestibular function study
R94.128 Abnormal results of other function studies of ear and other special senses

✓6th **R94.13 Abnormal results of function studies of peripheral nervous system**
R94.13Ø Abnormal response to nerve stimulation, unspecified
R94.131 Abnormal electromyogram [EMG]
EXCLUDES 1 *electromyogram of eye (R94.113)*
R94.138 Abnormal results of other function studies of peripheral nervous system

R94.2 Abnormal results of pulmonary function studies
Reduced ventilatory capacity
Reduced vital capacity

✓5th **R94.3 Abnormal results of cardiovascular function studies**
R94.3Ø Abnormal result of cardiovascular function study, unspecified
R94.31 Abnormal electrocardiogram [ECG] [EKG]
EXCLUDES 1 *long QT syndrome (I45.81)*
R94.39 Abnormal result of other cardiovascular function study
Abnormal electrophysiological intracardiac studies
Abnormal phonocardiogram
Abnormal vectorcardiogram

R94.4 Abnormal results of kidney function studies
Abnormal renal function test

R94.5 Abnormal results of liver function studies

R94.6 Abnormal results of thyroid function studies

R94.7 Abnormal results of other endocrine function studies
EXCLUDES 2 *abnormal glucose (R73.Ø-)*

R94.8 Abnormal results of function studies of other organs and systems
Abnormal basal metabolic rate [BMR]
Abnormal bladder function test
Abnormal splenic function test

Abnormal tumor markers (R97)

✓4th **R97 Abnormal tumor markers**
Elevated tumor associated antigens [TAA]
Elevated tumor specific antigens [TSA]

R97.Ø Elevated carcinoembryonic antigen [CEA]

R97.1 Elevated cancer antigen 125 [CA 125]

✓5th **R97.2 Elevated prostate specific antigen [PSA]**
AHA: 2016,4Q,66
R97.2Ø Elevated prostate specific antigen [PSA] A ♂
R97.21 Rising PSA following treatment for malignant neoplasm of prostate A ♂

R97.8 Other abnormal tumor markers

Ill-defined and unknown cause of mortality (R99)

R99 Ill-defined and unknown cause of mortality
Death (unexplained) NOS
Unspecified cause of mortality

Chapter 19. Injury, Poisoning and Certain Other Consequences of External Causes (SØØ–T88)

Chapter-specific Guidelines with Coding Examples

The chapter-specific guidelines from the ICD-10-CM Official Guidelines for Coding and Reporting have been provided below. Along with these guidelines are coding examples, contained in the shaded boxes, that have been developed to help illustrate the coding and/or sequencing guidance found in these guidelines.

a. Application of 7th characters in Chapter 19

Most categories in chapter 19 have a 7th character requirement for each applicable code. Most categories in this chapter have three 7th character values (with the exception of fractures): A, initial encounter, D, subsequent encounter and S, sequela. Categories for traumatic fractures have additional 7th character values. While the patient may be seen by a new or different provider over the course of treatment for an injury, assignment of the 7th character is based on whether the patient is undergoing active treatment and not whether the provider is seeing the patient for the first time.

For complication codes, active treatment refers to treatment for the condition described by the code, even though it may be related to an earlier precipitating problem. For example, code T84.50XA, Infection and inflammatory reaction due to unspecified internal joint prosthesis, initial encounter, is used when active treatment is provided for the infection, even though the condition relates to the prosthetic device, implant or graft that was placed at a previous encounter.

7th character "A", initial encounter is used for each encounter where the patient is receiving active treatment for the condition.

Patient admitted after fall from a skateboard onto the sidewalk, x-rays identify a nondisplaced fracture to the distal pole of the right scaphoid bone. The patient is placed in a cast.

S62.Ø14A	**Nondisplaced fracture of distal pole of navicular [scaphoid] bone of right wrist, initial encounter for closed fracture**
VØØ.131A	**Fall from skateboard, initial encounter**
Y92.48Ø	**Sidewalk as the place of occurrence of the external cause**
Y93.51	**Activity, roller skating (inline) and skateboarding**
Y99.8	**Other external cause status**

Explanation: This fracture would be coded with a seventh character A for initial encounter because the patient received x-rays to identify the site of the fracture and treatment was rendered; this would be considered active treatment.

7th character "D" subsequent encounter is used for encounters after the patient has completed active treatment of the condition and is receiving routine care for the condition during the healing or recovery phase.

Patient admitted after fall from a skateboard onto the sidewalk resulted in casting of the right arm. X-rays are taken to evaluate how well the nondisplaced fracture to the distal pole of the right scaphoid bone is healing. The physician feels the fracture is healing appropriately; no adjustments to the cast are made.

S62.Ø14D	**Nondisplaced fracture of distal pole of navicular [scaphoid] bone of right wrist, subsequent encounter for fracture with routine healing**
VØØ.131D	**Fall from skateboard, subsequent encounter**

Explanation: This fracture would be coded with a seventh character D for subsequent encounter, whether the same physician who provided the initial cast application or a different physician is now seeing the patient. Although the patient received x-rays, the intent of the x-rays was to assess how the fracture was healing. There was no active treatment rendered and the visit is therefore considered a subsequent encounter.

The aftercare Z codes should not be used for aftercare for conditions such as injuries or poisonings, where 7th characters are provided to identify subsequent care. For example, for aftercare of an injury, assign the acute injury code with the 7th character "D" (subsequent encounter).

7th character "S", sequela, is for use for complications or conditions that arise as a direct result of a condition, such as scar formation after a burn. The scars are sequelae of the burn. When using 7th character "S", it is necessary to use both the injury code that precipitated the sequela and the code for the sequela itself. The "S" is added only to the injury code, not the sequela code. The 7th character "S" identifies the injury responsible for the sequela. The specific type of sequela (e.g. scar) is sequenced first, followed by the injury code.

See Section I.B.1Ø Sequelae, (Late Effects)

Patient with a history of a nondisplaced fracture to the distal pole of the right scaphoid bone due to a fall from a skateboard is admitted for evaluation of arthritis to the right wrist that has developed as a consequence of the traumatic fracture.

M12.531	**Traumatic arthropathy, right wrist**
S62.Ø14S	**Nondisplaced fracture of distal pole of navicular [scaphoid] bone of right wrist, sequela**
VØØ.131S	**Fall from skateboard, sequela**

Explanation: The code identifying the specific sequela condition (traumatic arthritis) should be coded first followed by the injury that instigated the development of the sequela (fracture). The scaphoid fracture injury code is given a 7th character S for sequela to represent its role as the inciting injury. The fracture has healed and is not being managed or treated on this admit and therefore is not applicable as a first listed or principal diagnosis. However, it is directly related to the development of the arthritis and should be appended as a secondary code to signify this cause and effect relationship.

b. Coding of injuries

When coding injuries, assign separate codes for each injury unless a combination code is provided, in which case the combination code is assigned. Codes from category TØ7, Unspecified multiple injuries should not be assigned in the inpatient setting unless information for a more specific code is not available. Traumatic injury codes (SØØ-T14.9) are not to be used for normal, healing surgical wounds or to identify complications of surgical wounds.

The code for the most serious injury, as determined by the provider and the focus of treatment, is sequenced first.

1) Superficial injuries

Superficial injuries such as abrasions or contusions are not coded when associated with more severe injuries of the same site.

2) Primary injury with damage to nerves/blood vessels

When a primary injury results in minor damage to peripheral nerves or blood vessels, the primary injury is sequenced first with additional code(s) for injuries to nerves and spinal cord (such as category SØ4), and/or injury to blood vessels (such as category S15). When the primary injury is to the blood vessels or nerves, that injury should be sequenced first.

3) Iatrogenic injuries

Injury codes from Chapter 19 should not be assigned for injuries that occur during, or as a result of, a medical intervention. Assign the appropriate complication code(s).

c. Coding of traumatic fractures

The principles of multiple coding of injuries should be followed in coding fractures. Fractures of specified sites are coded individually by site in accordance with both the provisions within categories SØ2, S12, S22, S32, S42, S49, S52, S59, S62, S72, S79, S82, S89, S92 and the level of detail furnished by medical record content.

A fracture not indicated as open or closed should be coded to closed. A fracture not indicated whether displaced or not displaced should be coded to displaced.

More specific guidelines are as follows:

1) Initial vs. subsequent encounter for fractures

Traumatic fractures are coded using the appropriate 7th character for initial encounter (A, B, C) for each encounter where the patient is receiving active treatment for the fracture. The appropriate 7th character for initial encounter should also be assigned for a patient who delayed seeking treatment for the fracture or nonunion.

Fractures are coded using the appropriate 7th character for subsequent care for encounters after the patient has completed active treatment of the fracture and is receiving routine care for the fracture during the healing or recovery phase.

Care for complications of surgical treatment for fracture repairs during the healing or recovery phase should be coded with the appropriate complication codes.

Care of complications of fractures, such as malunion and nonunion, should be reported with the appropriate 7th character for subsequent care with nonunion (K, M, N,) or subsequent care with malunion (P, Q, R).

Malunion/nonunion: The appropriate 7th character for initial encounter should also be assigned for a patient who delayed seeking treatment for the fracture or nonunion.

Female patient fell during a forest hiking excursion almost six months ago and until recently did not feel she needed to seek medical attention for her left ankle pain; x-rays show nonunion of lateral malleolus and surgery has been scheduled

S82.62XA	**Displaced fracture of lateral malleolus of left fibula, initial encounter for closed fracture**
WØ1.ØXXA	**Fall on same level from slipping, tripping and stumbling without subsequent striking against object, initial encounter**
Y92.821	**Forest as place of occurrence of the external cause**
Y93.Ø1	**Activity, walking, marching and hiking**
Y99.8	**Other external cause status**

Explanation: A seventh character of A is used for the lateral malleolus nonunion fracture to signify that the fracture is receiving active treatment. The delayed care for the fracture has resulted in a nonunion, but capturing the nonunion in the seventh character is trumped by the provision of active care.

The open fracture designations in the assignment of the 7th character for fractures of the forearm, femur and lower leg, including ankle are based on the Gustilo open fracture classification. When the Gustilo classification type is not specified for an open fracture, the 7th character for open fracture type I or II should be assigned (B, E, H, M, Q).

A 17-year-old arrives at the trauma center with open, displaced right forearm fracture with extensive soft tissue damage. He fell while being tackled playing football for his high school team. On-call orthopaedic specialist documents segmental type IIIA fracture of radial shaft with no need for plastic consult.

S52.361C	**Displaced segmental fracture of shaft of radius, right arm, initial encounter for open fracture type IIIA, IIIB, or IIIC**
WØ3.XXXA	**Other fall on same level due to collision with another person, initial encounter**
Y92.321	**Football field as the place of occurrence of the external cause**
Y93.61	**Activity, American tackle football**

Explanation: The seventh character for forearm fractures capture the type of encounter and whether the fracture is open or closed; open fractures are broken down further by the type of fracture based on the Gustilo classification. The Gustilo classification describes the severity of open fracture and soft tissue injury. Type IIIA describes an open fracture with extensive soft tissue injury but adequate soft tissue remaining for wound coverage. A segmental fracture means that the bone is broken in two places, leaving at least one segment unattached to the bone. There is no need to report an additional code for the soft tissue injury as it is captured in the fracture code.

A code from category M8Ø, not a traumatic fracture code, should be used for any patient with known osteoporosis who suffers a fracture, even if the patient had a minor fall or trauma, if that fall or trauma would not usually break a normal, healthy bone.

See Section I.C.13. Osteoporosis.

The aftercare Z codes should not be used for aftercare for traumatic fractures. For aftercare of a traumatic fracture, assign the acute fracture code with the appropriate 7th character.

2) Multiple fractures sequencing

Multiple fractures are sequenced in accordance with the severity of the fracture.

3) Physeal fractures

For physeal fractures, assign only the code identifying the type of physeal fracture. Do not assign a separate code to identify the specific bone that is fractured.

d. Coding of burns and corrosions

The ICD-10-CM makes a distinction between burns and corrosions. The burn codes are for thermal burns, except sunburns, that come from a heat source, such as a fire or hot appliance. The burn codes are also for burns resulting from electricity and radiation. Corrosions are burns due to chemicals. The guidelines are the same for burns and corrosions.

Current burns (T2Ø-T25) are classified by depth, extent and by agent (X code). Burns are classified by depth as first degree (erythema), second degree (blistering), and third degree (full-thickness involvement). Burns of the eye and internal organs (T26-T28) are classified by site, but not by degree.

1) Sequencing of burn and related condition codes

Sequence first the code that reflects the highest degree of burn when more than one burn is present.

a. When the reason for the admission or encounter is for treatment of external multiple burns, sequence first the code that reflects the burn of the highest degree.

b. When a patient has both internal and external burns, the circumstances of admission govern the selection of the principal diagnosis or first-listed diagnosis.

c. When a patient is admitted for burn injuries and other related conditions such as smoke inhalation and/or respiratory failure, the circumstances of admission govern the selection of the principal or first-listed diagnosis.

Patient admitted with minor first-degree burns to multiple sites of her right and left hands as well as severe smoke inhalation. While she was sleeping at home, a candle on her dresser lit the bedroom curtains on fire.

T59.811A	**Toxic effect of smoke, accidental (unintentional), initial encounter**
J7Ø.5	**Respiratory conditions due to smoke inhalation**
T23.191A	**Burn of first degree of multiple sites of right wrist and hand, initial encounter**
T23.192A	**Burn of first degree of multiple sites of left wrist and hand, initial encounter**
XØ8.8XXA	**Exposure to other specified smoke, fire and flames, initial encounter**
Y92.ØØ3	**Bedroom of unspecified non-institutional (private) residence as the place of occurrence of the external cause**
Y93.84	**Activity, sleeping**

Explanation: Based on the documentation, the inhalation injury is more severe than the first-degree burns and is sequenced first. The burns to the hands are appended as secondary diagnoses.

2) Burns of the same anatomic site

Classify burns of the same anatomic site and on the same side but of different degrees to the subcategory identifying the highest degree recorded in the diagnosis (e.g., for second and third degree burns of right thigh, assign only code T24.311-).

3) Non-healing burns

Non-healing burns are coded as acute burns.

Necrosis of burned skin should be coded as a non-healed burn.

4) Infected burn

For any documented infected burn site, use an additional code for the infection.

5) Assign separate codes for each burn site

When coding burns, assign separate codes for each burn site. Category T3Ø, Burn and corrosion, body region unspecified is extremely vague and should rarely be used.

Codes for burns of "multiple sites" should only be assigned when the medical record documentation does not specify the individual sites.

> Patient is admitted with third-degree burns of the scalp as well as second-degree burns to the back of the right hand
>
> **T2Ø.35XA Burn of third degree of scalp [any part], initial encounter**
>
> **T23.261A Burn of second degree of back of right hand, initial encounter**
>
> *Explanation:* Two codes may be reported as the hand and face represent distinct burn sites.

6) Burns and corrosions classified according to extent of body surface involved

Assign codes from category T31, Burns classified according to extent of body surface involved, or T32, Corrosions classified according to extent of body surface involved, when the site of the burn is not specified or when there is a need for additional data. It is advisable to use category T31 as additional coding when needed to provide data for evaluating burn mortality, such as that needed by burn units. It is also advisable to use category T31 as an additional code for reporting purposes when there is mention of a third-degree burn involving 20 percent or more of the body surface.

Categories T31 and T32 are based on the classic "rule of nines" in estimating body surface involved: head and neck are assigned nine percent, each arm nine percent, each leg 18 percent, the anterior trunk 18 percent, posterior trunk 18 percent, and genitalia one percent. Providers may change these percentage assignments where necessary to accommodate infants and children who have proportionately larger heads than adults, and patients who have large buttocks, thighs, or abdomen that involve burns.

> Patient seen in burn unit for dressing change after he accidentally spilled acetic acid on himself two days ago. The second-degree burns to his right thigh, covering about 3 percent of his body surface, are healing appropriately.
>
> **T54.2X1D Toxic effect of corrosive acids and acid-like substances, accidental (unintentional), subsequent encounter**
>
> **T24.611D Corrosion of second degree of right thigh, subsequent encounter**
>
> **T32.Ø Corrosions involving less than 1Ø% of body surface**
>
> *Explanation:* Code T32.Ø provides additional information as to how much of the patient's body was affected by the corrosive substance.

7) Encounters for treatment of sequela of burns

Encounters for the treatment of the late effects of burns or corrosions (i.e., scars or joint contractures) should be coded with a burn or corrosion code with the 7th character "S" for sequela.

8) Sequelae with a late effect code and current burn

When appropriate, both a code for a current burn or corrosion with 7th character "A" or "D" and a burn or corrosion code with 7th character "S" may be assigned on the same record (when both a current burn and sequelae of an old burn exist). Burns and corrosions do not heal at the same rate and a current healing wound may still exist with sequela of a healed burn or corrosion.

See Section I.B.1Ø Sequela (Late Effects)

> Female patient seen in ED for second-degree burn to the left ear; she also has significant scarring on her left elbow from a third-degree burn from childhood
>
> **T2Ø.212A Burn of second degree of left ear [any part, except ear drum], initial encounter**
>
> **L9Ø.5 Scar conditions and fibrosis of skin**
>
> **T22.322S Burn of third degree of left elbow, sequela**
>
> *Explanation:* The patient is being seen for management of a current second-degree burn, which is reflected in the code by appending the seventh character of A, indicating active treatment or management of this burn. The elbow scarring is a sequela of a previous third-degree burn. The sequela condition precedes the original burn injury, which is appended with a seventh character of S.

9) Use of an external cause code with burns and corrosions

An external cause code should be used with burns and corrosions to identify the source and intent of the burn, as well as the place where it occurred.

e. Adverse effects, poisoning, underdosing and toxic effects

Codes in categories T36-T65 are combination codes that include the substance that was taken as well as the intent. No additional external cause code is required for poisonings, toxic effects, adverse effects and underdosing codes.

1) Do not code directly from the Table of Drugs

Do not code directly from the Table of Drugs and Chemicals. Always refer back to the Tabular List.

2) Use as many codes as necessary to describe

Use as many codes as necessary to describe completely all drugs, medicinal or biological substances.

3) If the same code would describe the causative agent

If the same code would describe the causative agent for more than one adverse reaction, poisoning, toxic effect or underdosing, assign the code only once.

4) If two or more drugs, medicinal or biological substances

If two or more drugs, medicinal or biological substances are taken, code each individually unless a combination code is listed in the Table of Drugs and Chemicals.

If multiple unspecified drugs, medicinal or biological substances were taken, assign the appropriate code from subcategory T5Ø.91, Poisoning by, adverse effect of and underdosing of multiple unspecified drugs, medicaments and biological substances.

5) The occurrence of drug toxicity is classified in ICD-10-CM as follows:

(a) Adverse effect

When coding an adverse effect of a drug that has been correctly prescribed and properly administered, assign the appropriate code for the nature of the adverse effect followed by the appropriate code for the adverse effect of the drug (T36-T5Ø). The code for the drug should have a 5th or 6th character "5" (for example T36.ØX5-) Examples of the nature of an adverse effect are tachycardia, delirium, gastrointestinal hemorrhaging, vomiting, hypokalemia, hepatitis, renal failure, or respiratory failure.

> Patient admitted for stomach pain and jaundice, indicated by physician as possible side-effects of Inderal, recently started for hypertension. Inderal was discontinued and the patient switched to Atenolol instead.
>
> **R1Ø.9 Unspecified abdominal pain**
>
> **R17 Unspecified jaundice**
>
> **T44.7X5A Adverse effect of beta-adrenoreceptor antagonists, initial encounter**
>
> **I1Ø Essential (primary) hypertension**
>
> *Explanation:* The side-effects caused by the drug are listed first, followed by the code for the adverse effect of the drug to capture the specific drug that was used.

(b) Poisoning

When coding a poisoning or reaction to the improper use of a medication (e.g., overdose, wrong substance given or taken in error, wrong route of administration), first assign the appropriate code from categories T36-T5Ø. The poisoning codes have an associated intent as their 5th or 6th character (accidental, intentional self-harm, assault and undetermined. If the intent of the poisoning is unknown or unspecified, code the intent as accidental intent. The undetermined intent is only for use if the documentation in the record specifies that the intent cannot be determined. Use additional code(s) for all manifestations of poisonings.

A 55-year-old female status post recent left knee replacement is admitted due to confusion, dizziness, and nausea. Her spouse brought in her prescribed Xanax, Ambien, and Percocet bottles but has no idea how many she took. It is suspected that her symptoms are due to an overdose of these medications.

T42.4X1A	**Poisoning by benzodiazepines, accidental (unintentional), initial encounter**
T42.6X1A	**Poisoning by other antiepileptic and sedative-hypnotic drugs, accidental (unintentional), initial encounter**
T40.2X1A	**Poisoning by other opioids, accidental (unintentional), initial encounter**
R41.0	**Disorientation, unspecified**
R42	**Dizziness and giddiness**
R11.0	**Nausea**

Explanation: It was not documented whether the overdose of the drugs was accidental or intentional; therefore the correct reporting of the poisoning codes is accidental intent. The poisoning codes are sequenced first, followed by manifestations of the poisoning.

If there is also a diagnosis of abuse or dependence of the substance, the abuse or dependence is assigned as an additional code.

Examples of poisoning include:

(i) Error was made in drug prescription

Errors made in drug prescription or in the administration of the drug by provider, nurse, patient, or other person.

(ii Overdose of a drug intentionally taken

If an overdose of a drug was intentionally taken or administered and resulted in drug toxicity, it would be coded as a poisoning.

(iii) Nonprescribed drug taken with correctly prescribed and properly administered drug

If a nonprescribed drug or medicinal agent was taken in combination with a correctly prescribed and properly administered drug, any drug toxicity or other reaction resulting from the interaction of the two drugs would be classified as a poisoning.

(iv) Interaction of drug(s) and alcohol

When a reaction results from the interaction of a drug(s) and alcohol, this would be classified as poisoning.

See Section I.C.4. if poisoning is the result of insulin pump malfunctions.

(c) Underdosing

Underdosing refers to taking less of a medication than is prescribed by a provider or a manufacturer's instruction. Discontinuing the use of a prescribed medication on the patient's own initiative (not directed by the patient's provider) is also classified as an underdosing. For underdosing, assign the code from categories T36-T50 (fifth or sixth character "6").

Codes for underdosing should never be assigned as principal or first-listed codes. If a patient has a relapse or exacerbation of the medical condition for which the drug is prescribed because of the reduction in dose, then the medical condition itself should be coded.

Noncompliance (Z91.12-, Z91.13- and Z91.14-) or complication of care (Y63.6-Y63.9) codes are to be used with an underdosing code to indicate intent, if known.

Patient admitted for atrial fibrillation with history of chronic atrial fibrillation for which she is prescribed amiodarone. Financial concerns have left the patient unable to pay for her prescriptions and she has been skipping her amiodarone dose every other day to offset the cost.

I48.20	**Chronic atrial fibrillation, unspecified**
T46.2X6A	**Underdosing of other antidysrhythmic drugs, initial encounter**
Z91.120	**Patient's intentional underdosing of medication regimen due to financial hardship**

Explanation: By skipping her amiodarone pill every other day, the patient's atrial fibrillation returned. The condition for which the drug was being taken is reported first, followed by an underdosing code to show that the patient was not adhering to her prescription regimen. The Z code helps elaborate on the patient's social and/or economic circumstances that led to the patient taking less then what she was prescribed.

(d) Toxic effects

When a harmful substance is ingested or comes in contact with a person, this is classified as a toxic effect. The toxic effect codes are in categories T51-T65.

Toxic effect codes have an associated intent: accidental, intentional self-harm, assault and undetermined.

f. Adult and child abuse, neglect and other maltreatment

Sequence first the appropriate code from categories T74.- (Adult and child abuse, neglect and other maltreatment, confirmed) or T76.- (Adult and child abuse, neglect and other maltreatment, suspected) for abuse, neglect and other maltreatment, followed by any accompanying mental health or injury code(s).

If the documentation in the medical record states abuse or neglect it is coded as confirmed (T74.-). It is coded as suspected if it is documented as suspected (T76.-).

For cases of confirmed abuse or neglect an external cause code from the assault section (X92-Y09) should be added to identify the cause of any physical injuries. A perpetrator code (Y07) should be added when the perpetrator of the abuse is known. For suspected cases of abuse or neglect, do not report external cause or perpetrator code.

If a suspected case of abuse, neglect or mistreatment is ruled out during an encounter code Z04.71, Encounter for examination and observation following alleged physical adult abuse, ruled out, or code Z04.72, Encounter for examination and observation following alleged child physical abuse, ruled out, should be used, not a code from T76.

If a suspected case of alleged rape or sexual abuse is ruled out during an encounter code Z04.41, Encounter for examination and observation following alleged adult rape or code Z04.42, Encounter for examination and observation following alleged child rape, should be used, not a code from T76.

If a suspected case of forced sexual exploitation or forced labor exploitation is ruled out during an encounter, code Z04.81, Encounter for examination and observation of victim following forced sexual exploitation, or code Z04.82, Encounter for examination and observation of victim following forced labor exploitation, should be used, not a code from T76.

See Section I.C.15. Abuse in a pregnant patient.

g. Complications of care

1) General guidelines for complications of care

(a) Documentation of complications of care

See Section I.B.16. for information on documentation of complications of care.

2) Pain due to medical devices

Pain associated with devices, implants or grafts left in a surgical site (for example painful hip prosthesis) is assigned to the appropriate code(s) found in Chapter 19, Injury, poisoning, and certain other consequences of external causes. Specific codes for pain due to medical devices are found in the T code section of the ICD-10-CM. Use additional code(s) from category G89 to identify acute or chronic pain due to presence of the device, implant or graft (G89.18 or G89.28).

Chronic left breast pain secondary to breast implant

T85.848A Pain due to other internal prosthetic devices, implants and grafts, initial encounter

N64.4 Mastodynia

G89.28 Other chronic postprocedural pain

Explanation: As the pain is a complication related to the breast implant, the complication code is sequenced first. The T code does not describe the site or type of pain, so additional codes may be appended to indicate that the patient is experiencing chronic pain in the breast.

3) Transplant complications

(a) Transplant complications other than kidney

Codes under category T86, Complications of transplanted organs and tissues, are for use for both complications and rejection of transplanted organs. A transplant complication code is only assigned if the complication affects the function of the transplanted organ. Two codes are required to fully describe a transplant complication: the appropriate code from category T86 and a secondary code that identifies the complication.

Pre-existing conditions or conditions that develop after the transplant are not coded as complications unless they affect the function of the transplanted organs.

See I.C.21. for transplant organ removal status

See I.C.2. for malignant neoplasm associated with transplanted organ.

(b) Kidney transplant complications

Patients who have undergone kidney transplant may still have some form of chronic kidney disease (CKD) because the kidney transplant may not fully restore kidney function. Code T86.1- should be assigned for documented complications of a kidney transplant, such as transplant failure or rejection or other transplant complication. Code T86.1- should not be assigned for post kidney transplant patients who have chronic kidney (CKD) unless a transplant complication such as transplant failure or rejection is documented. If the documentation is unclear as to whether the patient has a complication of the transplant, query the provider.

Conditions that affect the function of the transplanted kidney, other than CKD, should be assigned a code from subcategory T86.1, Complications of transplanted organ, Kidney, and a secondary code that identifies the complication.

For patients with CKD following a kidney transplant, but who do not have a complication such as failure or rejection, *see section I.C.14. Chronic kidney disease and kidney transplant status*.

Patient with chronic kidney disease stage 2; history of successful kidney transplant with no complications identified

N18.2 Chronic kidney disease, stage 2 (mild)

Z94.Ø Kidney transplant status

Explanation: This patient's stage 2 CKD is not indicated as being due to the transplanted kidney but instead is just the residual disease the patient had prior to the transplant.

4) Complication codes that include the external cause

As with certain other T codes, some of the complications of care codes have the external cause included in the code. The code includes the nature of the complication as well as the type of procedure that caused the complication. No external cause code indicating the type of procedure is necessary for these codes.

5) Complications of care codes within the body system chapters

Intraoperative and postprocedural complication codes are found within the body system chapters with codes specific to the organs and structures of that body system. These codes should be sequenced first, followed by a code(s) for the specific complication, if applicable.

Complication codes from the body system chapters should be assigned for intraoperative and postprocedural complications (e.g., the appropriate complication code from chapter 9 would be assigned for a vascular intraoperative or postprocedural complication) unless the complication is specifically indexed to a
T code in chapter 19.

During a spinal fusion procedure, the surgeon inadvertently punctured the dura. The midline durotomy was repaired, and the fusion procedure was completed.

G97.41 Accidental puncture or laceration of dura during a procedure

Explanation: The accidental durotomy is not coded to an injury code in chapter 19 but instead is categorized to the nervous system chapter.

Muscle/Tendon Table

ICD-10-CM categorizes certain muscles and tendons in the upper and lower extremities by their action (e.g., extension, flexion), their anatomical location (e.g., posterior, anterior), and/or whether they are intrinsic or extrinsic to a certain anatomical area. The Muscle/Tendon Table is provided at the beginning of chapters 13 and 19 as a resource to help users when code selection depends on one or more of these characteristics. Please note that this table is not all-inclusive, and proper code assignment should be based on the provider's documentation.

Body Region	Muscle	Extensor Tendon	Flexor Tendon	Other Tendon
Shoulder				
	Deltoid	Posterior deltoid	Anterior deltoid	
	Rotator cuff			
	Infraspinatus			Infraspinatus
	Subscapularis			Subscapularis
	Supraspinatus			Supraspinatus
	Teres minor			Teres minor
	Teres major	Teres major		
Upper arm				
	Anterior muscles			
	Biceps brachii — long head		Biceps brachii — long head	
	Biceps brachii — short head		Biceps brachii — short head	
	Brachialis		Brachialis	
	Coracobrachialis		Coracobrachialis	
	Posterior muscles			
	Triceps brachii	Triceps brachii		
Forearm				
	Anterior muscles			
	Flexors			
	Deep			
	Flexor digitorum profundus		Flexor digitorum profundus	
	Flexor pollicis longus		Flexor pollicis longus	
	Intermediate			
	Flexor digitorum superficialis		Flexor digitorum superficialis	
	Superficial			
	Flexor carpi radialis		Flexor carpi radialis	
	Flexor carpi ulnaris		Flexor carpi ulnaris	
	Palmaris longus		Palmaris longus	
	Pronators			
	Pronator quadratus			Pronator quadratus
	Pronator teres			Pronator teres
	Posterior muscles			
	Extensors			
	Deep			
	Abductor pollicis longus			Abductor pollicis longus
	Extensor indicis	Extensor indicis		
	Extensor pollicis brevis	Extensor pollicis brevis		
	Extensor pollicis longus	Extensor pollicis longus		
	Superficial			
	Brachioradialis			Brachioradialis
	Extensor carpi radialis brevis	Extensor carpi radialis brevis		
	Extensor carpi radialis longus	Extensor carpi radialis longus		
	Extensor carpi ulnaris	Extensor carpi ulnaris		
	Extensor digiti minimi	Extensor digiti minimi		
	Extensor digitorum	Extensor digitorum		
	Anconeus	Anconeus		
	Supinator			Supinator

Body Region	Muscle	Extensor Tendon	Flexor Tendon	Other Tendon
Hand				
Extrinsic — attach to a site in the forearm as well as a site in the hand with action related to hand movement at the wrist				
	Extensor carpi radialis brevis	Extensor carpi radialis brevis		
	Extensor carpi radialis longus	Extensor carpi radialis longus		
	Extensor carpi ulnaris	Extensor carpi ulnaris		
	Flexor carpi radialis		Flexor carpi radialis	
	Flexor carpi ulnaris		Flexor carpi ulnaris	
	Flexor digitorum superficialis		Flexor digitorum superficialis	
	Palmaris longus		Palmaris longus	
Extrinsic — attach to a site in the forearm as well as a site in the hand with action in the hand related to finger movement				
	Adductor pollicis longus			Adductor pollicis longus
	Extensor digiti minimi	Extensor digiti minimi		
	Extensor digitorum	Extensor digitorum		
	Extensor indicis	Extensor indicis		
	Flexor digitorum profundus		Flexor digitorum profundus	
	Flexor digitorum superficialis		Flexor digitorum superficialis	
Extrinsic — attach to a site in the forearm as well as a site in the hand with action in the hand related to thumb movement				
	Extensor pollicis brevis	Extensor pollicis brevis		
	Extensor pollicis longus	Extensor pollicis longus		
	Flexor pollicis longus		Flexor pollicis longus	
Intrinsic — found within the hand only				
	Adductor pollicis			Adductor pollicis
	Dorsal interossei	Dorsal interossei	Dorsal interossei	
	Lumbricals	Lumbricals	Lumbricals	
	Palmaris brevis			Palmaris brevis
	Palmar interossei	Palmar interossei	Palmar interossei	
	Hypothenar muscles			
	Abductor digiti minimi			Abductor digiti minimi
	Flexor digiti minimi brevis		Flexor digiti minimi brevis	
	Opponens digiti minimi		Opponens digiti minimi	
	Thenar muscles			
	Abductor pollicis brevis			Abductor pollicis brevis
	Flexor pollicis brevis		Flexor pollicis brevis	
	Opponens pollicis		Opponens pollicis	
Thigh				
	Anterior muscles			
	Iliopsoas		Iliopsoas	
	Pectineus		Pectineus	
	Quadriceps	Quadriceps		
	Rectus femoris	Rectus femoris — Extends knee	Rectus femoris — Flexes hip	
	Vastus intermedius	Vastus intermedius		
	Vastus lateralis	Vastus lateralis		
	Vastus medialis	Vastus medialis		
	Sartorius		Sartorius	
	Medial muscles			
	Adductor brevis			Adductor brevis
	Adductor longus			Adductor longus
	Adductor magnus			Adductor magnus
	Gracilis			Gracilis
	Obturator externus			Obturator externus
	Posterior muscles			
	Hamstring	Hamstring — Extends hip	Hamstring — Flexes knee	
	Biceps femoris	Biceps femoris	Biceps femoris	
	Semimembranosus	Semimembranosus	Semimembranosus	
	Semitendinosus	Semitendinosus	Semitendinosus	

Body Region	Muscle	Extensor Tendon	Flexor Tendon	Other Tendon
Lower leg				
	Anterior muscles			
	Extensor digitorum longus	Extensor digitorum longus		
	Extensor hallucis longus	Extensor hallucis longus		
	Fibularis (peroneus) tertius	Fibularis (peroneus) tertius		
	Tibialis anterior	Tibialis anterior		Tibialis anterior
	Lateral muscles			
	Fibularis (peroneus) brevis		Fibularis (peroneus) brevis	
	Fibularis (peroneus) longus		Fibularis (peroneus) longus	
	Posterior muscles			
	Deep			
	Flexor digitorum longus		Flexor digitorum longus	
	Flexor hallucis longus		Flexor hallucis longus	
	Popliteus		Popliteus	
	Tibialis posterior		Tibialis posterior	
	Superficial			
	Gastrocnemius		Gastrocnemius	
	Plantaris		Plantaris	
	Soleus		Soleus	
				Calcaneal (Achilles)
Ankle/Foot				
Extrinsic — attach to a site in the lower leg as well as a site in the foot with action related to foot movement at the ankle				
	Plantaris		Plantaris	
	Soleus		Soleus	
	Tibialis anterior	Tibialis anterior		
	Tibialis posterior		Tibialis posterior	
Extrinsic — attach to a site in the lower leg as well as a site in the foot with action in the foot related to toe movement				
	Extensor digitorum longus	Extensor digitorum longus		
	Extensor hallucis longus	Extensor hallucis longus		
	Flexor digitorum longus		Flexor digitorum longus	
	Flexor hallucis longus		Flexor hallucis longus	
Intrinsic — found within the ankle/foot only				
	Dorsal muscles			
	Extensor digitorum brevis	Extensor digitorum brevis		
	Extensor hallucis brevis	Extensor hallucis brevis		
	Plantar muscles			
	Abductor digiti minimi		Abductor digiti minimi	
	Abductor hallucis		Abductor hallucis	
	Dorsal interossei	Dorsal interossei	Dorsal interossei	
	Flexor digiti minimi brevis		Flexor digiti minimi brevis	
	Flexor digitorum brevis		Flexor digitorum brevis	
	Flexor hallucis brevis		Flexor hallucis brevis	
	Lumbricals	Lumbricals	Lumbricals	
	Quadratus plantae		Quadratus plantae	
	Plantar interossei	Plantar interossei	Plantar interossei	

Chapter 19. Injury, Poisoning and Certain Other Consequences of External Causes (S00-T88)

NOTE Use secondary code(s) from Chapter 20, External causes of morbidity, to indicate cause of injury. Codes within the T section that include the external cause do not require an additional external cause code.

Use additional code to identify any retained foreign body, if applicable (Z18.-)

EXCLUDES 1 *birth trauma (P10-P15)*
obstetric trauma (O70-O71)

NOTE The chapter uses the S-section for coding different types of injuries related to single body regions and the T-section to cover injuries to unspecified body regions as well as poisoning and certain other consequences of external causes.

AHA: 2016,2Q,3-7; 2015,4Q,35-38; 2015,3Q,37-39,40; 2015,2Q,6; 2015,1Q,3-21

TIP: The specific site of an injury can be determined from the radiology report when authenticated by a radiologist and available at the time of code assignment.

This chapter contains the following blocks:

S00-S09 Injuries to the head
S10-S19 Injuries to the neck
S20-S29 Injuries to the thorax
S30-S39 Injuries to the abdomen, lower back, lumbar spine, pelvis and external genitals
S40-S49 Injuries to the shoulder and upper arm
S50-S59 Injuries to the elbow and forearm
S60-S69 Injuries to the wrist, hand and fingers
S70-S79 Injuries to the hip and thigh
S80-S89 Injuries to the knee and lower leg
S90-S99 Injuries to the ankle and foot
T07 Injuries involving multiple body regions
T14 Injury of unspecified body region
T15-T19 Effects of foreign body entering through natural orifice
T20-T25 Burns and corrosions of external body surface, specified by site
T26-T28 Burns and corrosions confined to eye and internal organs
T30-T32 Burns and corrosions of multiple and unspecified body regions
T33-T34 Frostbite
T36-T50 Poisoning by, adverse effect of and underdosing of drugs, medicaments and biological substances
T51-T65 Toxic effects of substances chiefly nonmedicinal as to source
T66-T78 Other and unspecified effects of external causes
T79 Certain early complications of trauma
T80-T88 Complications of surgical and medical care, not elsewhere classified

Injuries to the head (S00-S09)

INCLUDES injuries of ear
injuries of eye
injuries of face [any part]
injuries of gum
injuries of jaw
injuries of oral cavity
injuries of palate
injuries of periocular area
injuries of scalp
injuries of temporomandibular joint area
injuries of tongue
injuries of tooth

Code also for any associated infection

EXCLUDES 2 *burns and corrosions (T20-T32)*
effects of foreign body in ear (T16)
effects of foreign body in larynx (T17.3)
effects of foreign body in mouth NOS (T18.0)
effects of foreign body in nose (T17.0-T17.1)
effects of foreign body in pharynx (T17.2)
effects of foreign body on external eye (T15.-)
frostbite (T33-T34)
insect bite or sting, venomous (T63.4)

✓4th **S00 Superficial injury of head**

EXCLUDES 1 *diffuse cerebral contusion (S06.2-)*
focal cerebral contusion (S06.3-)
injury of eye and orbit (S05.-)
open wound of head (S01.-)

The appropriate 7th character is to be added to each code from category S00.
A initial encounter
D subsequent encounter
S sequela

✓5th **S00.0 Superficial injury of scalp**
✓x7th **S00.00 Unspecified superficial injury of scalp**
✓x7th **S00.01 Abrasion of scalp**
✓x7th **S00.02 Blister (nonthermal) of scalp**
✓x7th **S00.03 Contusion of scalp**
Bruise of scalp
Hematoma of scalp
✓x7th **S00.04 External constriction of part of scalp**
✓x7th **S00.05 Superficial foreign body of scalp**
Splinter in the scalp
✓x7th **S00.06 Insect bite (nonvenomous) of scalp**
✓x7th **S00.07 Other superficial bite of scalp**
EXCLUDES 1 *open bite of scalp (S01.05)*

✓5th **S00.1 Contusion of eyelid and periocular area**
Black eye
EXCLUDES 2 *contusion of eyeball and orbital tissues (S05.1)*
✓x7th **S00.10 Contusion of unspecified eyelid and periocular area**
✓x7th **S00.11 Contusion of right eyelid and periocular area**
✓x7th **S00.12 Contusion of left eyelid and periocular area**

✓5th **S00.2 Other and unspecified superficial injuries of eyelid and periocular area**
EXCLUDES 2 *superficial injury of conjunctiva and cornea (S05.0-)*
✓6th **S00.20 Unspecified superficial injury of eyelid and periocular area**
✓7th **S00.201 Unspecified superficial injury of right eyelid and periocular area**
✓7th **S00.202 Unspecified superficial injury of left eyelid and periocular area**
✓7th **S00.209 Unspecified superficial injury of unspecified eyelid and periocular area**
✓6th **S00.21 Abrasion of eyelid and periocular area**
✓7th **S00.211 Abrasion of right eyelid and periocular area**
✓7th **S00.212 Abrasion of left eyelid and periocular area**
✓7th **S00.219 Abrasion of unspecified eyelid and periocular area**
✓6th **S00.22 Blister (nonthermal) of eyelid and periocular area**
✓7th **S00.221 Blister (nonthermal) of right eyelid and periocular area**
✓7th **S00.222 Blister (nonthermal) of left eyelid and periocular area**
✓7th **S00.229 Blister (nonthermal) of unspecified eyelid and periocular area**
✓6th **S00.24 External constriction of eyelid and periocular area**
✓7th **S00.241 External constriction of right eyelid and periocular area**
✓7th **S00.242 External constriction of left eyelid and periocular area**
✓7th **S00.249 External constriction of unspecified eyelid and periocular area**
✓6th **S00.25 Superficial foreign body of eyelid and periocular area**
Splinter of eyelid and periocular area
EXCLUDES 2 *retained foreign body in eyelid (H02.81-)*
✓7th **S00.251 Superficial foreign body of right eyelid and periocular area**
✓7th **S00.252 Superficial foreign body of left eyelid and periocular area**
✓7th **S00.259 Superficial foreign body of unspecified eyelid and periocular area**
✓6th **S00.26 Insect bite (nonvenomous) of eyelid and periocular area**
✓7th **S00.261 Insect bite (nonvenomous) of right eyelid and periocular area**
✓7th **S00.262 Insect bite (nonvenomous) of left eyelid and periocular area**
✓7th **S00.269 Insect bite (nonvenomous) of unspecified eyelid and periocular area**
✓6th **S00.27 Other superficial bite of eyelid and periocular area**
EXCLUDES 1 *open bite of eyelid and periocular area (S01.15)*
✓7th **S00.271 Other superficial bite of right eyelid and periocular area**
✓7th **S00.272 Other superficial bite of left eyelid and periocular area**
✓7th **S00.279 Other superficial bite of unspecified eyelid and periocular area**

✓5th **S00.3 Superficial injury of nose**
✓x7th **S00.30 Unspecified superficial injury of nose**
✓x7th **S00.31 Abrasion of nose**
✓x7th **S00.32 Blister (nonthermal) of nose**

√x7th **S00.33 Contusion of nose**
Bruise of nose
Hematoma of nose
√x7th **S00.34 External constriction of nose**
√x7th **S00.35 Superficial foreign body of nose**
Splinter in the nose
√x7th **S00.36 Insect bite (nonvenomous) of nose**
√x7th **S00.37 Other superficial bite of nose**
EXCLUDES 1 *open bite of nose (S01.25)*

√5th **S00.4 Superficial injury of ear**
√6th **S00.40 Unspecified superficial injury of ear**
√7th **S00.401 Unspecified superficial injury of right ear**
√7th **S00.402 Unspecified superficial injury of left ear**
√7th **S00.409 Unspecified superficial injury of unspecified ear**
√6th **S00.41 Abrasion of ear**
√7th **S00.411 Abrasion of right ear**
√7th **S00.412 Abrasion of left ear**
√7th **S00.419 Abrasion of unspecified ear**
√6th **S00.42 Blister (nonthermal) of ear**
√7th **S00.421 Blister (nonthermal) of right ear**
√7th **S00.422 Blister (nonthermal) of left ear**
√7th **S00.429 Blister (nonthermal) of unspecified ear**
√6th **S00.43 Contusion of ear**
Bruise of ear
Hematoma of ear
√7th **S00.431 Contusion of right ear**
√7th **S00.432 Contusion of left ear**
√7th **S00.439 Contusion of unspecified ear**
√6th **S00.44 External constriction of ear**
√7th **S00.441 External constriction of right ear**
√7th **S00.442 External constriction of left ear**
√7th **S00.449 External constriction of unspecified ear**
√6th **S00.45 Superficial foreign body of ear**
Splinter in the ear
√7th **S00.451 Superficial foreign body of right ear**
√7th **S00.452 Superficial foreign body of left ear**
√7th **S00.459 Superficial foreign body of unspecified ear**
√6th **S00.46 Insect bite (nonvenomous) of ear**
√7th **S00.461 Insect bite (nonvenomous) of right ear**
√7th **S00.462 Insect bite (nonvenomous) of left ear**
√7th **S00.469 Insect bite (nonvenomous) of unspecified ear**
√6th **S00.47 Other superficial bite of ear**
EXCLUDES 1 *open bite of ear (S01.35)*
√7th **S00.471 Other superficial bite of right ear**
√7th **S00.472 Other superficial bite of left ear**
√7th **S00.479 Other superficial bite of unspecified ear**

√5th **S00.5 Superficial injury of lip and oral cavity**
√6th **S00.50 Unspecified superficial injury of lip and oral cavity**
√7th **S00.501 Unspecified superficial injury of lip**
√7th **S00.502 Unspecified superficial injury of oral cavity**
√6th **S00.51 Abrasion of lip and oral cavity**
√7th **S00.511 Abrasion of lip**
√7th **S00.512 Abrasion of oral cavity**
√6th **S00.52 Blister (nonthermal) of lip and oral cavity**
√7th **S00.521 Blister (nonthermal) of lip**
√7th **S00.522 Blister (nonthermal) of oral cavity**
√6th **S00.53 Contusion of lip and oral cavity**
√7th **S00.531 Contusion of lip**
Bruise of lip
Hematoma of lip
√7th **S00.532 Contusion of oral cavity**
Bruise of oral cavity
Hematoma of oral cavity
√6th **S00.54 External constriction of lip and oral cavity**
√7th **S00.541 External constriction of lip**
√7th **S00.542 External constriction of oral cavity**
√6th **S00.55 Superficial foreign body of lip and oral cavity**
√7th **S00.551 Superficial foreign body of lip**
Splinter of lip and oral cavity
√7th **S00.552 Superficial foreign body of oral cavity**
Splinter of lip and oral cavity
√6th **S00.56 Insect bite (nonvenomous) of lip and oral cavity**
√7th **S00.561 Insect bite (nonvenomous) of lip**
√7th **S00.562 Insect bite (nonvenomous) of oral cavity**
√6th **S00.57 Other superficial bite of lip and oral cavity**
√7th **S00.571 Other superficial bite of lip**
EXCLUDES 1 *open bite of lip (S01.551)*
√7th **S00.572 Other superficial bite of oral cavity**
EXCLUDES 1 *open bite of oral cavity (S01.552)*

√5th **S00.8 Superficial injury of other parts of head**
Superficial injuries of face [any part]
√x7th **S00.80 Unspecified superficial injury of other part of head**
√x7th **S00.81 Abrasion of other part of head**
√x7th **S00.82 Blister (nonthermal) of other part of head**
√x7th **S00.83 Contusion of other part of head**
Bruise of other part of head
Hematoma of other part of head
√x7th **S00.84 External constriction of other part of head**
√x7th **S00.85 Superficial foreign body of other part of head**
Splinter in other part of head
√x7th **S00.86 Insect bite (nonvenomous) of other part of head**
√x7th **S00.87 Other superficial bite of other part of head**
EXCLUDES 1 *open bite of other part of head (S01.85)*

√5th **S00.9 Superficial injury of unspecified part of head**
√x7th **S00.90 Unspecified superficial injury of unspecified part of head**
√x7th **S00.91 Abrasion of unspecified part of head**
√x7th **S00.92 Blister (nonthermal) of unspecified part of head**
√x7th **S00.93 Contusion of unspecified part of head**
Bruise of head
Hematoma of head
√x7th **S00.94 External constriction of unspecified part of head**
√x7th **S00.95 Superficial foreign body of unspecified part of head**
Splinter of head
√x7th **S00.96 Insect bite (nonvenomous) of unspecified part of head**
√x7th **S00.97 Other superficial bite of unspecified part of head**
EXCLUDES 1 *open bite of head (S01.95)*

√4th **S01 Open wound of head**
Code also any associated:
injury of cranial nerve (S04.-)
injury of muscle and tendon of head (S09.1-)
intracranial injury (S06.-)
wound infection
EXCLUDES 1 *open skull fracture (S02.- with 7th character B)*
EXCLUDES 2 *injury of eye and orbit (S05.-)*
traumatic amputation of part of head (S08.-)

The appropriate 7th character is to be added to each code from category S01.
A initial encounter
D subsequent encounter
S sequela

√5th **S01.0 Open wound of scalp**
EXCLUDES 1 *avulsion of scalp (S08.0)*
√x7th **S01.00 Unspecified open wound of scalp**
√x7th **S01.01 Laceration without foreign body of scalp**
√x7th **S01.02 Laceration with foreign body of scalp**
√x7th **S01.03 Puncture wound without foreign body of scalp**
√x7th **S01.04 Puncture wound with foreign body of scalp**
√x7th **S01.05 Open bite of scalp**
Bite of scalp NOS
EXCLUDES 1 *superficial bite of scalp (S00.06, S00.07-)*

- S01.1 Open wound of eyelid and periocular area
  - Open wound of eyelid and periocular area with or without involvement of lacrimal passages
  - S01.10 Unspecified open wound of eyelid and periocular area
    - S01.101 Unspecified open wound of right eyelid and periocular area CC
    - S01.102 Unspecified open wound of left eyelid and periocular area CC
    - S01.109 Unspecified open wound of unspecified eyelid and periocular area CC
  - S01.11 Laceration without foreign body of eyelid and periocular area
    - S01.111 Laceration without foreign body of right eyelid and periocular area
    - S01.112 Laceration without foreign body of left eyelid and periocular area
    - S01.119 Laceration without foreign body of unspecified eyelid and periocular area
  - S01.12 Laceration with foreign body of eyelid and periocular area
    - S01.121 Laceration with foreign body of right eyelid and periocular area
    - S01.122 Laceration with foreign body of left eyelid and periocular area
    - S01.129 Laceration with foreign body of unspecified eyelid and periocular area
  - S01.13 Puncture wound without foreign body of eyelid and periocular area
    - S01.131 Puncture wound without foreign body of right eyelid and periocular area
    - S01.132 Puncture wound without foreign body of left eyelid and periocular area
    - S01.139 Puncture wound without foreign body of unspecified eyelid and periocular area
  - S01.14 Puncture wound with foreign body of eyelid and periocular area
    - S01.141 Puncture wound with foreign body of right eyelid and periocular area
    - S01.142 Puncture wound with foreign body of left eyelid and periocular area
    - S01.149 Puncture wound with foreign body of unspecified eyelid and periocular area
  - S01.15 Open bite of eyelid and periocular area
    - Bite of eyelid and periocular area NOS
    - EXCLUDES 1 *superficial bite of eyelid and periocular area (S00.26, S00.27)*
    - S01.151 Open bite of right eyelid and periocular area
    - S01.152 Open bite of left eyelid and periocular area
    - S01.159 Open bite of unspecified eyelid and periocular area
- S01.2 Open wound of nose
  - S01.20 Unspecified open wound of nose
  - S01.21 Laceration without foreign body of nose
  - S01.22 Laceration with foreign body of nose
  - S01.23 Puncture wound without foreign body of nose
  - S01.24 Puncture wound with foreign body of nose
  - S01.25 Open bite of nose
    - Bite of nose NOS
    - EXCLUDES 1 *superficial bite of nose (S00.36, S00.37)*
- S01.3 Open wound of ear
  - S01.30 Unspecified open wound of ear
    - S01.301 Unspecified open wound of right ear
    - S01.302 Unspecified open wound of left ear
    - S01.309 Unspecified open wound of unspecified ear
  - S01.31 Laceration without foreign body of ear
    - S01.311 Laceration without foreign body of right ear
    - S01.312 Laceration without foreign body of left ear
    - S01.319 Laceration without foreign body of unspecified ear
  - S01.32 Laceration with foreign body of ear
    - S01.321 Laceration with foreign body of right ear
    - S01.322 Laceration with foreign body of left ear
    - S01.329 Laceration with foreign body of unspecified ear
  - S01.33 Puncture wound without foreign body of ear
    - S01.331 Puncture wound without foreign body of right ear
    - S01.332 Puncture wound without foreign body of left ear
    - S01.339 Puncture wound without foreign body of unspecified ear
  - S01.34 Puncture wound with foreign body of ear
    - S01.341 Puncture wound with foreign body of right ear
    - S01.342 Puncture wound with foreign body of left ear
    - S01.349 Puncture wound with foreign body of unspecified ear
  - S01.35 Open bite of ear
    - Bite of ear NOS
    - EXCLUDES 1 *superficial bite of ear (S00.46, S00.47)*
    - S01.351 Open bite of right ear
    - S01.352 Open bite of left ear
    - S01.359 Open bite of unspecified ear
- S01.4 Open wound of cheek and temporomandibular area
  - S01.40 Unspecified open wound of cheek and temporomandibular area
    - S01.401 Unspecified open wound of right cheek and temporomandibular area
    - S01.402 Unspecified open wound of left cheek and temporomandibular area
    - S01.409 Unspecified open wound of unspecified cheek and temporomandibular area
  - S01.41 Laceration without foreign body of cheek and temporomandibular area
    - S01.411 Laceration without foreign body of right cheek and temporomandibular area
    - S01.412 Laceration without foreign body of left cheek and temporomandibular area
    - S01.419 Laceration without foreign body of unspecified cheek and temporomandibular area
  - S01.42 Laceration with foreign body of cheek and temporomandibular area
    - S01.421 Laceration with foreign body of right cheek and temporomandibular area
    - S01.422 Laceration with foreign body of left cheek and temporomandibular area
    - S01.429 Laceration with foreign body of unspecified cheek and temporomandibular area
  - S01.43 Puncture wound without foreign body of cheek and temporomandibular area
    - S01.431 Puncture wound without foreign body of right cheek and temporomandibular area
    - S01.432 Puncture wound without foreign body of left cheek and temporomandibular area
    - S01.439 Puncture wound without foreign body of unspecified cheek and temporomandibular area
  - S01.44 Puncture wound with foreign body of cheek and temporomandibular area
    - S01.441 Puncture wound with foreign body of right cheek and temporomandibular area
    - S01.442 Puncture wound with foreign body of left cheek and temporomandibular area
    - S01.449 Puncture wound with foreign body of unspecified cheek and temporomandibular area
  - S01.45 Open bite of cheek and temporomandibular area
    - Bite of cheek and temporomandibular area NOS
    - EXCLUDES 2 *superficial bite of cheek and temporomandibular area (S00.86, S00.87)*
    - S01.451 Open bite of right cheek and temporomandibular area
    - S01.452 Open bite of left cheek and temporomandibular area
    - S01.459 Open bite of unspecified cheek and temporomandibular area

√5th **S01.5 Open wound of lip and oral cavity**
EXCLUDES 2 *tooth dislocation (S03.2)*
tooth fracture (S02.5)

√6th **S01.50 Unspecified open wound of lip and oral cavity**
√7th **S01.501 Unspecified open wound of lip**
√7th **S01.502 Unspecified open wound of oral cavity**

√6th **S01.51 Laceration of lip and oral cavity without foreign body**
√7th **S01.511 Laceration without foreign body of lip**
√7th **S01.512 Laceration without foreign body of oral cavity**

√6th **S01.52 Laceration of lip and oral cavity with foreign body**
√7th **S01.521 Laceration with foreign body of lip**
√7th **S01.522 Laceration with foreign body of oral cavity**

√6th **S01.53 Puncture wound of lip and oral cavity without foreign body**
√7th **S01.531 Puncture wound without foreign body of lip**
√7th **S01.532 Puncture wound without foreign body of oral cavity**

√6th **S01.54 Puncture wound of lip and oral cavity with foreign body**
√7th **S01.541 Puncture wound with foreign body of lip**
√7th **S01.542 Puncture wound with foreign body of oral cavity**

√6th **S01.55 Open bite of lip and oral cavity**
√7th **S01.551 Open bite of lip**
Bite of lip NOS
EXCLUDES 1 *superficial bite of lip (S00.571)*
√7th **S01.552 Open bite of oral cavity**
Bite of oral cavity NOS
EXCLUDES 1 *superficial bite of oral cavity (S00.572)*

√5th **S01.8 Open wound of other parts of head**
√x7th **S01.80 Unspecified open wound of other part of head**
√x7th **S01.81 Laceration without foreign body of other part of head**
√x7th **S01.82 Laceration with foreign body of other part of head**
√x7th **S01.83 Puncture wound without foreign body of other part of head**
√x7th **S01.84 Puncture wound with foreign body of other part of head**
√x7th **S01.85 Open bite of other part of head**
Bite of other part of head NOS
EXCLUDES 1 *superficial bite of other part of head (S00.87)*

√5th **S01.9 Open wound of unspecified part of head**
√x7th **S01.90 Unspecified open wound of unspecified part of head**
√x7th **S01.91 Laceration without foreign body of unspecified part of head**
√x7th **S01.92 Laceration with foreign body of unspecified part of head**
√x7th **S01.93 Puncture wound without foreign body of unspecified part of head**
√x7th **S01.94 Puncture wound with foreign body of unspecified part of head**
√x7th **S01.95 Open bite of unspecified part of head**
Bite of head NOS
EXCLUDES 1 *superficial bite of head NOS (S00.97)*

√4th **S02 Fracture of skull and facial bones**
NOTE A fracture not indicated as open or closed should be coded to closed.

Code also any associated intracranial injury (S06.-)
AHA: 2017,1Q,42; 2016,4Q,66-67

The appropriate 7th character is to be added to each code from category S02.
A initial encounter for closed fracture
B initial encounter for open fracture
D subsequent encounter for fracture with routine healing
G subsequent encounter for fracture with delayed healing
K subsequent encounter for fracture with nonunion
S sequela

2,3,7 √x7th **S02.0 Fracture of vault of skull** MCC CC H5 HCC
Fracture of frontal bone
Fracture of parietal bone

√5th **S02.1 Fracture of base of skull**
EXCLUDES 2 *lateral orbital wall (S02.84-)*
medial orbital wall (S02.83-)
orbital floor (S02.3-)
AHA: 2019,4Q,16-17

√6th **S02.10 Unspecified fracture of base of skull**
2,3,7 √7th **S02.101 Fracture of base of skull, right side** MCC CC H5 HCC
2,3,7 √7th **S02.102 Fracture of base of skull, left side** MCC CC H5 HCC
2,3,7 √7th **S02.109 Fracture of base of skull, unspecified side** MCC CC H5 HCC

√6th **S02.11 Fracture of occiput**
2,3,7 √7th **S02.110 Type I occipital condyle fracture, unspecified side** MCC CC H5 HCC
2,3,7 √7th **S02.111 Type II occipital condyle fracture, unspecified side** MCC CC H5 HCC
2,3,7 √7th **S02.112 Type III occipital condyle fracture, unspecified side** MCC CC H5 HCC
2,3,7 √7th **S02.113 Unspecified occipital condyle fracture** MCC CC H5 HCC
2,3,7 √7th **S02.118 Other fracture of occiput, unspecified side** MCC CC H5 HCC
2,3,7 √7th **S02.119 Unspecified fracture of occiput** MCC CC H5 HCC
2,3,7 √7th **S02.11A Type I occipital condyle fracture, right side** MCC CC H5 HCC
2,3,7 √7th **S02.11B Type I occipital condyle fracture, left side** MCC CC H5 HCC
2,3,7 √7th **S02.11C Type II occipital condyle fracture, right side** MCC CC H5 HCC
2,3,7 √7th **S02.11D Type II occipital condyle fracture, left side** MCC CC H5 HCC
2,3,7 √7th **S02.11E Type III occipital condyle fracture, right side** MCC CC H5 HCC
2,3,7 √7th **S02.11F Type III occipital condyle fracture, left side** MCC CC H5 HCC
2,3,7 √7th **S02.11G Other fracture of occiput, right side** MCC CC H5 HCC
2,3,7 √7th **S02.11H Other fracture of occiput, left side** MCC CC H5 HCC

√6th **S02.12 Fracture of orbital roof**
AHA: 2019,4Q,16-17
2,3,7 √7th **S02.121 Fracture of orbital roof, right side** MCC CC H5 HCC
2,3,7 √7th **S02.122 Fracture of orbital roof, left side** MCC CC H5 HCC
2,3,7 √7th **S02.129 Fracture of orbital roof, unspecified side** MCC CC H5 HCC

2,3,7 √x7th **S02.19 Other fracture of base of skull** MCC CC H5 HCC
Fracture of anterior fossa of base of skull
Fracture of ethmoid sinus
Fracture of frontal sinus
Fracture of middle fossa of base of skull
Fracture of posterior fossa of base of skull
Fracture of sphenoid
Fracture of temporal bone

3 √x7th **S02.2 Fracture of nasal bones** CC H5

S02.3 Fracture of orbital floor
Fracture of inferior orbital wall
EXCLUDES 1 *orbit NOS (S02.85)*
EXCLUDES 2 *lateral orbital wall (S02.84-)*
medial orbital wall (S02.83-)
orbital roof (S02.1-)

3,7 S02.30 Fracture of orbital floor, unspecified side CC H5 HCC
3,7 S02.31 Fracture of orbital floor, right side CC H5 HCC
3,7 S02.32 Fracture of orbital floor, left side CC H5 HCC

S02.4 Fracture of malar, maxillary and zygoma bones
Fracture of superior maxilla
Fracture of upper jaw (bone)
Fracture of zygomatic process of temporal bone

S02.40 Fracture of malar, maxillary and zygoma bones, unspecified
3,7 S02.400 Malar fracture, unspecified side CC H5 HCC
3,7 S02.401 Maxillary fracture, unspecified side CC H5 HCC
3,7 S02.402 Zygomatic fracture, unspecified side CC H5 HCC
3,7 S02.40A Malar fracture, right side CC H5 HCC
3,7 S02.40B Malar fracture, left side CC H5 HCC
3,7 S02.40C Maxillary fracture, right side CC H5 HCC
3,7 S02.40D Maxillary fracture, left side CC H5 HCC
3,7 S02.40E Zygomatic fracture, right side CC H5 HCC
3,7 S02.40F Zygomatic fracture, left side CC H5 HCC

S02.41 LeFort fracture
DEF: Named for Rene Le Fort, these fractures describe different combinations of multiple fractures that occur from significant force to the midface. A common denominator in all three types of LeFort fractures is fracture of the pterygoid processes, which are two bony plates resembling wings that extend downward from the sphenoid bone.

LeFort Fracture Types

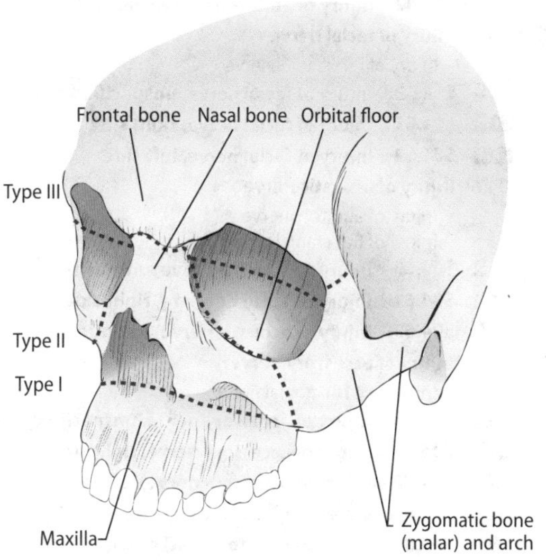

3,7 S02.411 LeFort I fracture CC H5 HCC
3,7 S02.412 LeFort II fracture CC H5 HCC
3,7 S02.413 LeFort III fracture CC H5 HCC

3,7 S02.42 Fracture of alveolus of maxilla CC H5 HCC

4 S02.5 Fracture of tooth (traumatic) CC
Broken tooth
EXCLUDES 1 *cracked tooth (nontraumatic) (K03.81)*

S02.6 Fracture of mandible
Fracture of lower jaw (bone)

S02.60 Fracture of mandible, unspecified
3,7 S02.600 Fracture of unspecified part of body of mandible, unspecified side CC H5 HCC
3,7 S02.601 Fracture of unspecified part of body of right mandible CC H5 HCC
3,7 S02.602 Fracture of unspecified part of body of left mandible CC H5 HCC
3,7 S02.609 Fracture of mandible, unspecified CC H5 HCC

S02.61 Fracture of condylar process of mandible
3,7 S02.610 Fracture of condylar process of mandible, unspecified side CC H5 HCC
3,7 S02.611 Fracture of condylar process of right mandible CC H5 HCC
3,7 S02.612 Fracture of condylar process of left mandible CC H5 HCC

S02.62 Fracture of subcondylar process of mandible
3,7 S02.620 Fracture of subcondylar process of mandible, unspecified side CC H5 HCC
3,7 S02.621 Fracture of subcondylar process of right mandible CC H5 HCC
3,7 S02.622 Fracture of subcondylar process of left mandible CC H5 HCC

S02.63 Fracture of coronoid process of mandible
3,7 S02.630 Fracture of coronoid process of mandible, unspecified side CC H5 HCC
3,7 S02.631 Fracture of coronoid process of right mandible CC H5 HCC
3,7 S02.632 Fracture of coronoid process of left mandible CC H5 HCC

S02.64 Fracture of ramus of mandible
3,7 S02.640 Fracture of ramus of mandible, unspecified side CC H5 HCC
3,7 S02.641 Fracture of ramus of right mandible CC H5 HCC
3,7 S02.642 Fracture of ramus of left mandible CC H5 HCC

S02.65 Fracture of angle of mandible
3,7 S02.650 Fracture of angle of mandible, unspecified side CC H5 HCC
3,7 S02.651 Fracture of angle of right mandible CC H5 HCC
3,7 S02.652 Fracture of angle of left mandible CC H5 HCC

3,7 S02.66 Fracture of symphysis of mandible CC H5 HCC

S02.67 Fracture of alveolus of mandible
3,7 S02.670 Fracture of alveolus of mandible, unspecified side CC H5 HCC
3,7 S02.671 Fracture of alveolus of right mandible CC H5 HCC
3,7 S02.672 Fracture of alveolus of left mandible CC H5 HCC

3,7 S02.69 Fracture of mandible of other specified site CC H5 HCC

S02.8 Fractures of other specified skull and facial bones
Fracture of palate
EXCLUDES 2 *fracture of orbital floor (S02.3-)*
fracture of orbital roof (S02.12-)

3,7 S02.80 Fracture of other specified skull and facial bones, unspecified side CC H5 HCC
3,7 S02.81 Fracture of other specified skull and facial bones, right side CC H5 HCC
3,7 S02.82 Fracture of other specified skull and facial bones, left side CC H5 HCC

S02.83 Fracture of medial orbital wall
EXCLUDES 2 *orbital floor (S02.3-)*
orbital roof (S02.12-)
AHA: 2019,4Q,16-17
3,7 S02.831 Fracture of medial orbital wall, right side CC H5 HCC
3,7 S02.832 Fracture of medial orbital wall, left side CC H5 HCC
3,7 S02.839 Fracture of medial orbital wall, unspecified side CC H5 HCC

S02.84 Fracture of lateral orbital wall
EXCLUDES 2 *orbital floor (S02.3-)*
orbital roof (S02.12-)
AHA: 2019,4Q,16-17
3,7 S02.841 Fracture of lateral orbital wall, right side CC H5 HCC

3,7 √7th **S02.842 Fracture of lateral orbital wall, left side** CC H5 HCC

3,7 √7th **S02.849 Fracture of lateral orbital wall, unspecified side** CC H5 HCC

3,7 √x7th **S02.85 Fracture of orbit, unspecified** CC H5 HCC

Fracture of orbit NOS
Fracture of orbit wall NOS

EXCLUDES 1 *lateral orbital wall (S02.84-)*
medial orbital wall (S02.83-)
orbital floor (S02.3-)
orbital roof (S02.12-)

√5th **S02.9 Fracture of unspecified skull and facial bones**

2,3,7 √x7th **S02.91 Unspecified fracture of skull** MCC CC H5 HCC

AHA: 2020,2Q,24

3,7 √x7th **S02.92 Unspecified fracture of facial bones** CC H5 HCC

√4th **S03 Dislocation and sprain of joints and ligaments of head**

INCLUDES avulsion of joint (capsule) or ligament of head
laceration of cartilage, joint (capsule) or ligament of head
sprain of cartilage, joint (capsule) or ligament of head
traumatic hemarthrosis of joint or ligament of head
traumatic rupture of joint or ligament of head
traumatic subluxation of joint or ligament of head
traumatic tear of joint or ligament of head

Code also any associated open wound

EXCLUDES 2 *strain of muscle or tendon of head (S09.1)*

The appropriate 7th character is to be added to each code from category S03.
A initial encounter
D subsequent encounter
S sequela

√5th **S03.0 Dislocation of jaw**

Dislocation of jaw (cartilage) (meniscus)
Dislocation of mandible
Dislocation of temporomandibular (joint)
AHA: 2016,4Q,67

√x7th **S03.00 Dislocation of jaw, unspecified side**

√x7th **S03.01 Dislocation of jaw, right side**

√x7th **S03.02 Dislocation of jaw, left side**

√x7th **S03.03 Dislocation of jaw, bilateral**

√x7th **S03.1 Dislocation of septal cartilage of nose**

√x7th **S03.2 Dislocation of tooth**

√5th **S03.4 Sprain of jaw**

Sprain of temporomandibular (joint) (ligament)
AHA: 2016,4Q,67

√x7th **S03.40 Sprain of jaw, unspecified side**

√x7th **S03.41 Sprain of jaw, right side**

√x7th **S03.42 Sprain of jaw, left side**

√x7th **S03.43 Sprain of jaw, bilateral**

√x7th **S03.8 Sprain of joints and ligaments of other parts of head**

√x7th **S03.9 Sprain of joints and ligaments of unspecified parts of head**

√4th **S04 Injury of cranial nerve**

The selection of side should be based on the side of the body being affected
Code first any associated intracranial injury (S06.-)
Code also any associated:
open wound of head (S01.-)
skull fracture (S02.-)

The appropriate 7th character is to be added to each code from category S04.
A initial encounter
D subsequent encounter
S sequela

√5th **S04.0 Injury of optic nerve and pathways**

Use additional code to identify any visual field defect or blindness (H53.4-, H54.-)

√6th **S04.01 Injury of optic nerve**

Injury of 2nd cranial nerve

√7th **S04.011 Injury of optic nerve, right eye** CC

√7th **S04.012 Injury of optic nerve, left eye** CC

√7th **S04.019 Injury of optic nerve, unspecified eye** CC

Injury of optic nerve NOS

√x7th **S04.02 Injury of optic chiasm** CC

√6th **S04.03 Injury of optic tract and pathways**

Injury of optic radiation

√7th **S04.031 Injury of optic tract and pathways, right side** CC

√7th **S04.032 Injury of optic tract and pathways, left side** CC

√7th **S04.039 Injury of optic tract and pathways, unspecified side** CC

Injury of optic tract and pathways NOS

√6th **S04.04 Injury of visual cortex**

√7th **S04.041 Injury of visual cortex, right side** CC

√7th **S04.042 Injury of visual cortex, left side** CC

√7th **S04.049 Injury of visual cortex, unspecified side** CC

Injury of visual cortex NOS

√5th **S04.1 Injury of oculomotor nerve**

Injury of 3rd cranial nerve

√x7th **S04.10 Injury of oculomotor nerve, unspecified side** CC

√x7th **S04.11 Injury of oculomotor nerve, right side** CC

√x7th **S04.12 Injury of oculomotor nerve, left side** CC

√5th **S04.2 Injury of trochlear nerve**

Injury of 4th cranial nerve

√x7th **S04.20 Injury of trochlear nerve, unspecified side** CC

√x7th **S04.21 Injury of trochlear nerve, right side** CC

√x7th **S04.22 Injury of trochlear nerve, left side** CC

√5th **S04.3 Injury of trigeminal nerve**

Injury of 5th cranial nerve

√x7th **S04.30 Injury of trigeminal nerve, unspecified side** CC

√x7th **S04.31 Injury of trigeminal nerve, right side** CC

√x7th **S04.32 Injury of trigeminal nerve, left side** CC

√5th **S04.4 Injury of abducent nerve**

Injury of 6th cranial nerve

√x7th **S04.40 Injury of abducent nerve, unspecified side** CC

√x7th **S04.41 Injury of abducent nerve, right side** CC

√x7th **S04.42 Injury of abducent nerve, left side** CC

√5th **S04.5 Injury of facial nerve**

Injury of 7th cranial nerve

√x7th **S04.50 Injury of facial nerve, unspecified side** CC

√x7th **S04.51 Injury of facial nerve, right side** CC

√x7th **S04.52 Injury of facial nerve, left side** CC

√5th **S04.6 Injury of acoustic nerve**

Injury of auditory nerve
Injury of 8th cranial nerve

√x7th **S04.60 Injury of acoustic nerve, unspecified side** CC

√x7th **S04.61 Injury of acoustic nerve, right side** CC

√x7th **S04.62 Injury of acoustic nerve, left side** CC

√5th **S04.7 Injury of accessory nerve**

Injury of 11th cranial nerve

√x7th **S04.70 Injury of accessory nerve, unspecified side** CC

√x7th **S04.71 Injury of accessory nerve, right side** CC

√x7th **S04.72 Injury of accessory nerve, left side** CC

√5th **S04.8 Injury of other cranial nerves**

√6th **S04.81 Injury of olfactory [1st] nerve**

√7th **S04.811 Injury of olfactory [1st] nerve, right side** CC

√7th **S04.812 Injury of olfactory [1st] nerve, left side** CC

√7th **S04.819 Injury of olfactory [1st] nerve, unspecified side** CC

√6th **S04.89 Injury of other cranial nerves**

Injury of vagus [10th] nerve

√7th **S04.891 Injury of other cranial nerves, right side** CC

√7th **S04.892 Injury of other cranial nerves, left side** CC

√7th **S04.899 Injury of other cranial nerves, unspecified side** CC

S04.9 Injury of unspecified cranial nerve CC

S05 Injury of eye and orbit

INCLUDES open wound of eye and orbit

EXCLUDES 2 *2nd cranial [optic] nerve injury (S04.0-)*
3rd cranial [oculomotor] nerve injury (S04.1-)
open wound of eyelid and periocular area (S01.1-)
orbital bone fracture (S02.1-, S02.3-, S02.8-)
superficial injury of eyelid (S00.1-S00.2)

The appropriate 7th character is to be added to each code from category S05.
A initial encounter
D subsequent encounter
S sequela

S05.0 Injury of conjunctiva and corneal abrasion without foreign body

EXCLUDES 1 *foreign body in conjunctival sac (T15.1)*
foreign body in cornea (T15.0)

S05.00 Injury of conjunctiva and corneal abrasion without foreign body, unspecified eye
S05.01 Injury of conjunctiva and corneal abrasion without foreign body, right eye
S05.02 Injury of conjunctiva and corneal abrasion without foreign body, left eye

S05.1 Contusion of eyeball and orbital tissues

Traumatic hyphema

EXCLUDES 2 *black eye NOS (S00.1)*
contusion of eyelid and periocular area (S00.1)

S05.10 Contusion of eyeball and orbital tissues, unspecified eye
S05.11 Contusion of eyeball and orbital tissues, right eye
S05.12 Contusion of eyeball and orbital tissues, left eye

S05.2 Ocular laceration and rupture with prolapse or loss of intraocular tissue

S05.20 Ocular laceration and rupture with prolapse or loss of intraocular tissue, unspecified eye CC
S05.21 Ocular laceration and rupture with prolapse or loss of intraocular tissue, right eye CC
S05.22 Ocular laceration and rupture with prolapse or loss of intraocular tissue, left eye CC

S05.3 Ocular laceration without prolapse or loss of intraocular tissue

Laceration of eye NOS

DEF: Tear in ocular tissue without displacing structures that is due to blunt trauma. It is characterized by pain, redness, and decreased vision.

S05.30 Ocular laceration without prolapse or loss of intraocular tissue, unspecified eye CC
S05.31 Ocular laceration without prolapse or loss of intraocular tissue, right eye CC
S05.32 Ocular laceration without prolapse or loss of intraocular tissue, left eye CC

S05.4 Penetrating wound of orbit with or without foreign body

EXCLUDES 2 *retained (old) foreign body following penetrating wound in orbit (H05.5-)*

S05.40 Penetrating wound of orbit with or without foreign body, unspecified eye CC
S05.41 Penetrating wound of orbit with or without foreign body, right eye CC
S05.42 Penetrating wound of orbit with or without foreign body, left eye CC

S05.5 Penetrating wound with foreign body of eyeball

EXCLUDES 2 *retained (old) intraocular foreign body (H44.6-, H44.7)*

S05.50 Penetrating wound with foreign body of unspecified eyeball CC
S05.51 Penetrating wound with foreign body of right eyeball CC
S05.52 Penetrating wound with foreign body of left eyeball CC

S05.6 Penetrating wound without foreign body of eyeball

Ocular penetration NOS

S05.60 Penetrating wound without foreign body of unspecified eyeball
S05.61 Penetrating wound without foreign body of right eyeball
S05.62 Penetrating wound without foreign body of left eyeball

S05.7 Avulsion of eye

Traumatic enucleation

S05.70 Avulsion of unspecified eye CC
S05.71 Avulsion of right eye CC
S05.72 Avulsion of left eye CC

S05.8 Other injuries of eye and orbit

Lacrimal duct injury

S05.8X Other injuries of eye and orbit

S05.8X1 Other injuries of right eye and orbit CC
S05.8X2 Other injuries of left eye and orbit CC
S05.8X9 Other injuries of unspecified eye and orbit CC

S05.9 Unspecified injury of eye and orbit

Injury of eye NOS

S05.90 Unspecified injury of unspecified eye and orbit
S05.91 Unspecified injury of right eye and orbit CC
S05.92 Unspecified injury of left eye and orbit CC

S06 Intracranial injury

NOTE 7th characters D and S do not apply to codes in category S06 with 6th character 7 – death due to brain injury prior to regaining consciousness, or 8 – death due to other cause prior to regaining consciousness.

INCLUDES traumatic brain injury

Code also any associated:
open wound of head (S01.-)
skull fracture (S02.-)

EXCLUDES 1 *head injury NOS (S09.90)*

AHA: 2017,4Q,25; 2017,1Q,42; 2015,3Q,37

TIP: Do not assign Z87.820 Personal history of traumatic brain injury, when residual conditions persist after an intracranial injury. The codes for the residual conditions should be first listed, followed by a code from category S06 using seventh character S to identify sequelae.

The appropriate 7th character is to be added to each code from category S06.
A initial encounter
D subsequent encounter
S sequela

S06.0 Concussion

Commotio cerebri

EXCLUDES 1 *concussion with other intracranial injuries classified in subcategories S06.1- to S06.6-, S06.81- and S06.82- — code to specified intracranial injury*

AHA: 2016,4Q,67-68

S06.0X Concussion

8 S06.0X0 Concussion without loss of consciousness CC HCC
8 S06.0X1 Concussion with loss of consciousness of 30 minutes or less CC H5 HCC
8 S06.0X9 Concussion with loss of consciousness of unspecified duration CC H5 HCC
Concussion NOS

S06.1 Traumatic cerebral edema

Diffuse traumatic cerebral edema
Focal traumatic cerebral edema

AHA: 2019,3Q,35; 2015,1Q,12-13

S06.1X Traumatic cerebral edema

7 S06.1X0 Traumatic cerebral edema without loss of consciousness MCC HCC
7 S06.1X1 Traumatic cerebral edema with loss of consciousness of 30 minutes or less MCC H5 HCC
7 S06.1X2 Traumatic cerebral edema with loss of consciousness of 31 minutes to 59 minutes MCC H5 HCC
7 S06.1X3 Traumatic cerebral edema with loss of consciousness of 1 hour to 5 hours 59 minutes MCC H5 HCC
7 S06.1X4 Traumatic cerebral edema with loss of consciousness of 6 hours to 24 hours MCC H5 HCC
7 S06.1X5 Traumatic cerebral edema with loss of consciousness greater than 24 hours with return to pre-existing conscious level MCC H5 HCC

7 √7th **S06.1X6 Traumatic cerebral edema with loss of consciousness greater than 24 hours without return to pre-existing conscious level with patient surviving** MCC H5 HCC

√7th **S06.1X7 Traumatic cerebral edema with loss of consciousness of any duration with death due to brain injury prior to regaining consciousness** MCC H5

√7th **S06.1X8 Traumatic cerebral edema with loss of consciousness of any duration with death due to other cause prior to regaining consciousness** MCC H5

7 √7th **S06.1X9 Traumatic cerebral edema with loss of consciousness of unspecified duration** MCC H5 HCC
Traumatic cerebral edema NOS

√5th **S06.2 Diffuse traumatic brain injury**
Diffuse axonal brain injury
EXCLUDES 1 *traumatic diffuse cerebral edema (S06.1X-)*

√6th **S06.2X Diffuse traumatic brain injury**

7 √7th **S06.2X0 Diffuse traumatic brain injury without loss of consciousness** HCC

7 √7th **S06.2X1 Diffuse traumatic brain injury with loss of consciousness of 30 minutes or less** CC H5 HCC

7 √7th **S06.2X2 Diffuse traumatic brain injury with loss of consciousness of 31 minutes to 59 minutes** CC H5 HCC

7 √7th **S06.2X3 Diffuse traumatic brain injury with loss of consciousness of 1 hour to 5 hours 59 minutes** CC H5 HCC

7 √7th **S06.2X4 Diffuse traumatic brain injury with loss of consciousness of 6 hours to 24 hours** CC H5 HCC

7 √7th **S06.2X5 Diffuse traumatic brain injury with loss of consciousness greater than 24 hours with return to pre-existing conscious levels** CC H5 HCC

7 √7th **S06.2X6 Diffuse traumatic brain injury with loss of consciousness greater than 24 hours without return to pre-existing conscious level with patient surviving** MCC H5 HCC

√7th **S06.2X7 Diffuse traumatic brain injury with loss of consciousness of any duration with death due to brain injury prior to regaining consciousness** MCC H5

√7th **S06.2X8 Diffuse traumatic brain injury with loss of consciousness of any duration with death due to other cause prior to regaining consciousness** MCC H5

7 √7th **S06.2X9 Diffuse traumatic brain injury with loss of consciousness of unspecified duration** CC H5 HCC
Diffuse traumatic brain injury NOS

√5th **S06.3 Focal traumatic brain injury**
EXCLUDES 1 *any condition classifiable to S06.4-S06.6*
~~focal cerebral edema (S06.1)~~
EXCLUDES 2 ▶*focal cerebral edema (S06.1)*◀
AHA: 2019,3Q,35; 2015,1Q,12-13

√6th **S06.30 Unspecified focal traumatic brain injury**

7 √7th **S06.300 Unspecified focal traumatic brain injury without loss of consciousness** HCC

7 √7th **S06.301 Unspecified focal traumatic brain injury with loss of consciousness of 30 minutes or less** CC H5 HCC

7 √7th **S06.302 Unspecified focal traumatic brain injury with loss of consciousness of 31 minutes to 59 minutes** CC H5 HCC

7 √7th **S06.303 Unspecified focal traumatic brain injury with loss of consciousness of 1 hour to 5 hours 59 minutes** CC H5 HCC

7 √7th **S06.304 Unspecified focal traumatic brain injury with loss of consciousness of 6 hours to 24 hours** CC H5 HCC

7 √7th **S06.305 Unspecified focal traumatic brain injury with loss of consciousness greater than 24 hours with return to pre-existing conscious level** CC H5 HCC

7 √7th **S06.306 Unspecified focal traumatic brain injury with loss of consciousness greater than 24 hours without return to pre-existing conscious level with patient surviving** MCC H5 HCC

√7th **S06.307 Unspecified focal traumatic brain injury with loss of consciousness of any duration with death due to brain injury prior to regaining consciousness** MCC H5

√7th **S06.308 Unspecified focal traumatic brain injury with loss of consciousness of any duration with death due to other cause prior to regaining consciousness** MCC H5

7 √7th **S06.309 Unspecified focal traumatic brain injury with loss of consciousness of unspecified duration** CC H5 HCC
Unspecified focal traumatic brain injury NOS

√6th **S06.31 Contusion and laceration of right cerebrum**

7 √7th **S06.310 Contusion and laceration of right cerebrum without loss of consciousness** MCC H5 HCC

7 √7th **S06.311 Contusion and laceration of right cerebrum with loss of consciousness of 30 minutes or less** MCC H5 HCC

7 √7th **S06.312 Contusion and laceration of right cerebrum with loss of consciousness of 31 minutes to 59 minutes** MCC H5 HCC

7 √7th **S06.313 Contusion and laceration of right cerebrum with loss of consciousness of 1 hour to 5 hours 59 minutes** MCC H5 HCC

7 √7th **S06.314 Contusion and laceration of right cerebrum with loss of consciousness of 6 hours to 24 hours** MCC H5 HCC

7 √7th **S06.315 Contusion and laceration of right cerebrum with loss of consciousness greater than 24 hours with return to pre-existing conscious level** MCC H5 HCC

7 √7th **S06.316 Contusion and laceration of right cerebrum with loss of consciousness greater than 24 hours without return to pre-existing conscious level with patient surviving** MCC H5 HCC

√7th **S06.317 Contusion and laceration of right cerebrum with loss of consciousness of any duration with death due to brain injury prior to regaining consciousness** MCC H5

√7th **S06.318 Contusion and laceration of right cerebrum with loss of consciousness of any duration with death due to other cause prior to regaining consciousness** MCC H5

7 √7th **S06.319 Contusion and laceration of right cerebrum with loss of consciousness of unspecified duration** MCC H5 HCC
Contusion and laceration of right cerebrum NOS

√6th **S06.32 Contusion and laceration of left cerebrum**

7 √7th **S06.320 Contusion and laceration of left cerebrum without loss of consciousness** MCC H5 HCC

7 √7th **S06.321 Contusion and laceration of left cerebrum with loss of consciousness of 30 minutes or less** MCC H5 HCC

7 √7th **S06.322 Contusion and laceration of left cerebrum with loss of consciousness of 31 minutes to 59 minutes** MCC H5 HCC

7 √7th **S06.323 Contusion and laceration of left cerebrum with loss of consciousness of 1 hour to 5 hours 59 minutes** MCC H5 HCC

7 √7th **S06.324 Contusion and laceration of left cerebrum with loss of consciousness of 6 hours to 24 hours** MCC H5 HCC

7 √7th **S06.325 Contusion and laceration of left cerebrum with loss of consciousness greater than 24 hours with return to pre-existing conscious level** MCC H5 HCC

7 S06.326 **Contusion and laceration of left cerebrum with loss of consciousness greater than 24 hours without return to pre-existing conscious level with patient surviving** MCC H5 HCC

S06.327 **Contusion and laceration of left cerebrum with loss of consciousness of any duration with death due to brain injury prior to regaining consciousness** MCC H5

S06.328 **Contusion and laceration of left cerebrum with loss of consciousness of any duration with death due to other cause prior to regaining consciousness** MCC H5

7 S06.329 **Contusion and laceration of left cerebrum with loss of consciousness of unspecified duration** MCC H5 HCC
Contusion and laceration of left cerebrum NOS

S06.33 **Contusion and laceration of cerebrum, unspecified**

7 S06.330 **Contusion and laceration of cerebrum, unspecified, without loss of consciousness** MCC H5 HCC

7 S06.331 **Contusion and laceration of cerebrum, unspecified, with loss of consciousness of 30 minutes or less** MCC H5 HCC

7 S06.332 **Contusion and laceration of cerebrum, unspecified, with loss of consciousness of 31 minutes to 59 minutes** MCC H5 HCC

7 S06.333 **Contusion and laceration of cerebrum, unspecified, with loss of consciousness of 1 hour to 5 hours 59 minutes** MCC H5 HCC

7 S06.334 **Contusion and laceration of cerebrum, unspecified, with loss of consciousness of 6 hours to 24 hours** MCC H5 HCC

7 S06.335 **Contusion and laceration of cerebrum, unspecified, with loss of consciousness greater than 24 hours with return to pre-existing conscious level** MCC H5 HCC

7 S06.336 **Contusion and laceration of cerebrum, unspecified, with loss of consciousness greater than 24 hours without return to pre-existing conscious level with patient surviving** MCC H5 HCC

S06.337 **Contusion and laceration of cerebrum, unspecified, with loss of consciousness of any duration with death due to brain injury prior to regaining consciousness** MCC H5

S06.338 **Contusion and laceration of cerebrum, unspecified, with loss of consciousness of any duration with death due to other cause prior to regaining consciousness** MCC H5

7 S06.339 **Contusion and laceration of cerebrum, unspecified, with loss of consciousness of unspecified duration** MCC H5 HCC
Contusion and laceration of cerebrum NOS

S06.34 **Traumatic hemorrhage of right cerebrum**
Traumatic intracerebral hemorrhage and hematoma of right cerebrum

7 S06.340 **Traumatic hemorrhage of right cerebrum without loss of consciousness** MCC H5 HCC

7 S06.341 **Traumatic hemorrhage of right cerebrum with loss of consciousness of 30 minutes or less** MCC H5 HCC

7 S06.342 **Traumatic hemorrhage of right cerebrum with loss of consciousness of 31 minutes to 59 minutes** MCC H5 HCC

7 S06.343 **Traumatic hemorrhage of right cerebrum with loss of consciousness of 1 hours to 5 hours 59 minutes** MCC H5 HCC

7 S06.344 **Traumatic hemorrhage of right cerebrum with loss of consciousness of 6 hours to 24 hours** MCC H5 HCC

7 S06.345 **Traumatic hemorrhage of right cerebrum with loss of consciousness greater than 24 hours with return to pre-existing conscious level** MCC H5 HCC

7 S06.346 **Traumatic hemorrhage of right cerebrum with loss of consciousness greater than 24 hours without return to pre-existing conscious level with patient surviving** MCC H5 HCC

S06.347 **Traumatic hemorrhage of right cerebrum with loss of consciousness of any duration with death due to brain injury prior to regaining consciousness** MCC H5

S06.348 **Traumatic hemorrhage of right cerebrum with loss of consciousness of any duration with death due to other cause prior to regaining consciousness** MCC H5

7 S06.349 **Traumatic hemorrhage of right cerebrum with loss of consciousness of unspecified duration** MCC H5 HCC
Traumatic hemorrhage of right cerebrum NOS

S06.35 **Traumatic hemorrhage of left cerebrum**
Traumatic intracerebral hemorrhage and hematoma of left cerebrum

7 S06.350 **Traumatic hemorrhage of left cerebrum without loss of consciousness** MCC H5 HCC

7 S06.351 **Traumatic hemorrhage of left cerebrum with loss of consciousness of 30 minutes or less** MCC H5 HCC

7 S06.352 **Traumatic hemorrhage of left cerebrum with loss of consciousness of 31 minutes to 59 minutes** MCC H5 HCC

7 S06.353 **Traumatic hemorrhage of left cerebrum with loss of consciousness of 1 hours to 5 hours 59 minutes** MCC H5 HCC

7 S06.354 **Traumatic hemorrhage of left cerebrum with loss of consciousness of 6 hours to 24 hours** MCC H5 HCC

7 S06.355 **Traumatic hemorrhage of left cerebrum with loss of consciousness greater than 24 hours with return to pre-existing conscious level** MCC H5 HCC

7 S06.356 **Traumatic hemorrhage of left cerebrum with loss of consciousness greater than 24 hours without return to pre-existing conscious level with patient surviving** MCC H5 HCC

S06.357 **Traumatic hemorrhage of left cerebrum with loss of consciousness of any duration with death due to brain injury prior to regaining consciousness** MCC H5

S06.358 **Traumatic hemorrhage of left cerebrum with loss of consciousness of any duration with death due to other cause prior to regaining consciousness** MCC H5

7 S06.359 **Traumatic hemorrhage of left cerebrum with loss of consciousness of unspecified duration** MCC H5 HCC
Traumatic hemorrhage of left cerebrum NOS

S06.36 **Traumatic hemorrhage of cerebrum, unspecified**
Traumatic intracerebral hemorrhage and hematoma, unspecified

7 S06.360 **Traumatic hemorrhage of cerebrum, unspecified, without loss of consciousness** MCC H5 HCC

7 S06.361 **Traumatic hemorrhage of cerebrum, unspecified, with loss of consciousness of 30 minutes or less** MCC H5 HCC

7 S06.362 **Traumatic hemorrhage of cerebrum, unspecified, with loss of consciousness of 31 minutes to 59 minutes** MCC H5 HCC

7 S06.363 **Traumatic hemorrhage of cerebrum, unspecified, with loss of consciousness of 1 hours to 5 hours 59 minutes** MCC H5 HCC

7 S06.364 **Traumatic hemorrhage of cerebrum, unspecified, with loss of consciousness of 6 hours to 24 hours** MCC H5 HCC

7 S06.365 **Traumatic hemorrhage of cerebrum, unspecified, with loss of consciousness greater than 24 hours with return to pre-existing conscious level** MCC H5 HCC

7 √7th **S06.366 Traumatic hemorrhage of cerebrum, unspecified, with loss of consciousness greater than 24 hours without return to pre-existing conscious level with patient surviving** MCC H5 HCC

√7th **S06.367 Traumatic hemorrhage of cerebrum, unspecified, with loss of consciousness of any duration with death due to brain injury prior to regaining consciousness** MCC H5

√7th **S06.368 Traumatic hemorrhage of cerebrum, unspecified, with loss of consciousness of any duration with death due to other cause prior to regaining consciousness** MCC H5

7 √7th **S06.369 Traumatic hemorrhage of cerebrum, unspecified, with loss of consciousness of unspecified duration** MCC H5 HCC
Traumatic hemorrhage of cerebrum NOS

√6th **S06.37 Contusion, laceration, and hemorrhage of cerebellum**

7 √7th **S06.370 Contusion, laceration, and hemorrhage of cerebellum without loss of consciousness** MCC H5 HCC

7 √7th **S06.371 Contusion, laceration, and hemorrhage of cerebellum with loss of consciousness of 30 minutes or less** CC H5 HCC

7 √7th **S06.372 Contusion, laceration, and hemorrhage of cerebellum with loss of consciousness of 31 minutes to 59 minutes** CC H5 HCC

7 √7th **S06.373 Contusion, laceration, and hemorrhage of cerebellum with loss of consciousness of 1 hour to 5 hours 59 minutes** CC H5 HCC

7 √7th **S06.374 Contusion, laceration, and hemorrhage of cerebellum with loss of consciousness of 6 hours to 24 hours** CC H5 HCC

7 √7th **S06.375 Contusion, laceration, and hemorrhage of cerebellum with loss of consciousness greater than 24 hours with return to pre-existing conscious level** CC H5 HCC

7 √7th **S06.376 Contusion, laceration, and hemorrhage of cerebellum with loss of consciousness greater than 24 hours without return to pre-existing conscious level with patient surviving** MCC H5 HCC

√7th **S06.377 Contusion, laceration, and hemorrhage of cerebellum with loss of consciousness of any duration with death due to brain injury prior to regaining consciousness** MCC H5

√7th **S06.378 Contusion, laceration, and hemorrhage of cerebellum with loss of consciousness of any duration with death due to other cause prior to regaining consciousness** MCC H5

7 √7th **S06.379 Contusion, laceration, and hemorrhage of cerebellum with loss of consciousness of unspecified duration** CC H5 HCC
Contusion, laceration, and hemorrhage of cerebellum NOS

√6th **S06.38 Contusion, laceration, and hemorrhage of brainstem**

7 √7th **S06.380 Contusion, laceration, and hemorrhage of brainstem without loss of consciousness** MCC H5 HCC

7 √7th **S06.381 Contusion, laceration, and hemorrhage of brainstem with loss of consciousness of 30 minutes or less** CC H5 HCC

7 √7th **S06.382 Contusion, laceration, and hemorrhage of brainstem with loss of consciousness of 31 minutes to 59 minutes** CC H5 HCC

7 √7th **S06.383 Contusion, laceration, and hemorrhage of brainstem with loss of consciousness of 1 hour to 5 hours 59 minutes** CC H5 HCC

7 √7th **S06.384 Contusion, laceration, and hemorrhage of brainstem with loss of consciousness of 6 hours to 24 hours** CC H5 HCC

7 √7th **S06.385 Contusion, laceration, and hemorrhage of brainstem with loss of consciousness greater than 24 hours with return to pre-existing conscious level** CC H5 HCC

7 √7th **S06.386 Contusion, laceration, and hemorrhage of brainstem with loss of consciousness greater than 24 hours without return to pre-existing conscious level with patient surviving** MCC H5 HCC

√7th **S06.387 Contusion, laceration, and hemorrhage of brainstem with loss of consciousness of any duration with death due to brain injury prior to regaining consciousness** MCC H5

√7th **S06.388 Contusion, laceration, and hemorrhage of brainstem with loss of consciousness of any duration with death due to other cause prior to regaining consciousness** MCC H5

7 √7th **S06.389 Contusion, laceration, and hemorrhage of brainstem with loss of consciousness of unspecified duration** CC H5 HCC
Contusion, laceration, and hemorrhage of brainstem NOS

√5th **S06.4 Epidural hemorrhage**
Extradural hemorrhage NOS
Extradural hemorrhage (traumatic)
DEF: Epidural space: Space between the endosteum of the cranium (skull) and the dura mater, the outermost layer of a three-layer membrane that covers the brain.

√6th **S06.4X Epidural hemorrhage**

7 √7th **S06.4X0 Epidural hemorrhage without loss of consciousness** MCC H5 HCC

7 √7th **S06.4X1 Epidural hemorrhage with loss of consciousness of 30 minutes or less** MCC H5 HCC

7 √7th **S06.4X2 Epidural hemorrhage with loss of consciousness of 31 minutes to 59 minutes** MCC H5 HCC

7 √7th **S06.4X3 Epidural hemorrhage with loss of consciousness of 1 hour to 5 hours 59 minutes** MCC H5 HCC

7 √7th **S06.4X4 Epidural hemorrhage with loss of consciousness of 6 hours to 24 hours** MCC H5 HCC

7 √7th **S06.4X5 Epidural hemorrhage with loss of consciousness greater than 24 hours with return to pre-existing conscious level** MCC H5 HCC

7 √7th **S06.4X6 Epidural hemorrhage with loss of consciousness greater than 24 hours without return to pre-existing conscious level with patient surviving** MCC H5 HCC

√7th **S06.4X7 Epidural hemorrhage with loss of consciousness of any duration with death due to brain injury prior to regaining consciousness** MCC H5

√7th **S06.4X8 Epidural hemorrhage with loss of consciousness of any duration with death due to other causes prior to regaining consciousness** MCC H5

7 √7th **S06.4X9 Epidural hemorrhage with loss of consciousness of unspecified duration** MCC H5 HCC
Epidural hemorrhage NOS

√5th **S06.5 Traumatic subdural hemorrhage**
DEF: Subdural: Potential space between the dura mater and arachnoid membrane around the brain.

√6th **S06.5X Traumatic subdural hemorrhage**

7 √7th **S06.5X0 Traumatic subdural hemorrhage without loss of consciousness** MCC H5 HCC

7 √7th **S06.5X1 Traumatic subdural hemorrhage with loss of consciousness of 30 minutes or less** MCC H5 HCC

7 √7th **S06.5X2 Traumatic subdural hemorrhage with loss of consciousness of 31 minutes to 59 minutes** MCC H5 HCC

7 √7th **S06.5X3 Traumatic subdural hemorrhage with loss of consciousness of 1 hour to 5 hours 59 minutes** MCC H5 HCC

7 √7th **S06.5X4 Traumatic subdural hemorrhage with loss of consciousness of 6 hours to 24 hours** MCC H5 HCC

7 ✓7th **S06.5X5 Traumatic subdural hemorrhage with loss of consciousness greater than 24 hours with return to pre-existing conscious level** MCC H5 HCC

7 ✓7th **S06.5X6 Traumatic subdural hemorrhage with loss of consciousness greater than 24 hours without return to pre-existing conscious level with patient surviving** MCC H5 HCC

✓7th **S06.5X7 Traumatic subdural hemorrhage with loss of consciousness of any duration with death due to brain injury before regaining consciousness** MCC H5

✓7th **S06.5X8 Traumatic subdural hemorrhage with loss of consciousness of any duration with death due to other cause before regaining consciousness** MCC H5

7 ✓7th **S06.5X9 Traumatic subdural hemorrhage with loss of consciousness of unspecified duration** MCC H5 HCC
Traumatic subdural hemorrhage NOS

✓5th **S06.6 Traumatic subarachnoid hemorrhage**
DEF: Subarachnoid: Space located between the arachnoid membrane and the pia mater that contains cerebrospinal fluid.

✓6th **S06.6X Traumatic subarachnoid hemorrhage**

7 ✓7th **S06.6X0 Traumatic subarachnoid hemorrhage without loss of consciousness** MCC H5 HCC

7 ✓7th **S06.6X1 Traumatic subarachnoid hemorrhage with loss of consciousness of 30 minutes or less** MCC H5 HCC

7 ✓7th **S06.6X2 Traumatic subarachnoid hemorrhage with loss of consciousness of 31 minutes to 59 minutes** MCC H5 HCC

7 ✓7th **S06.6X3 Traumatic subarachnoid hemorrhage with loss of consciousness of 1 hour to 5 hours 59 minutes** MCC H5 HCC

7 ✓7th **S06.6X4 Traumatic subarachnoid hemorrhage with loss of consciousness of 6 hours to 24 hours** MCC H5 HCC

7 ✓7th **S06.6X5 Traumatic subarachnoid hemorrhage with loss of consciousness greater than 24 hours with return to pre-existing conscious level** MCC H5 HCC

7 ✓7th **S06.6X6 Traumatic subarachnoid hemorrhage with loss of consciousness greater than 24 hours without return to pre-existing conscious level with patient surviving** MCC H5 HCC

✓7th **S06.6X7 Traumatic subarachnoid hemorrhage with loss of consciousness of any duration with death due to brain injury prior to regaining consciousness** MCC H5

✓7th **S06.6X8 Traumatic subarachnoid hemorrhage with loss of consciousness of any duration with death due to other cause prior to regaining consciousness** MCC H5

7 ✓7th **S06.6X9 Traumatic subarachnoid hemorrhage with loss of consciousness of unspecified duration** MCC H5 HCC
Traumatic subarachnoid hemorrhage NOS

✓5th **S06.8 Other specified intracranial injuries**

✓6th **S06.81 Injury of right internal carotid artery, intracranial portion, not elsewhere classified**

7 ✓7th **S06.810 Injury of right internal carotid artery, intracranial portion, not elsewhere classified without loss of consciousness** HCC

7 ✓7th **S06.811 Injury of right internal carotid artery, intracranial portion, not elsewhere classified with loss of consciousness of 30 minutes or less** CC H5 HCC

7 ✓7th **S06.812 Injury of right internal carotid artery, intracranial portion, not elsewhere classified with loss of consciousness of 31 minutes to 59 minutes** CC H5 HCC

7 ✓7th **S06.813 Injury of right internal carotid artery, intracranial portion, not elsewhere classified with loss of consciousness of 1 hour to 5 hours 59 minutes** CC H5 HCC

7 ✓7th **S06.814 Injury of right internal carotid artery, intracranial portion, not elsewhere classified with loss of consciousness of 6 hours to 24 hours** CC H5 HCC

7 ✓7th **S06.815 Injury of right internal carotid artery, intracranial portion, not elsewhere classified with loss of consciousness greater than 24 hours with return to pre-existing conscious level** CC H5 HCC

7 ✓7th **S06.816 Injury of right internal carotid artery, intracranial portion, not elsewhere classified with loss of consciousness greater than 24 hours without return to pre-existing conscious level with patient surviving** MCC H5 HCC

✓7th **S06.817 Injury of right internal carotid artery, intracranial portion, not elsewhere classified with loss of consciousness of any duration with death due to brain injury prior to regaining consciousness** MCC H5

✓7th **S06.818 Injury of right internal carotid artery, intracranial portion, not elsewhere classified with loss of consciousness of any duration with death due to other cause prior to regaining consciousness** MCC H5

7 ✓7th **S06.819 Injury of right internal carotid artery, intracranial portion, not elsewhere classified with loss of consciousness of unspecified duration** CC H5 HCC
Injury of right internal carotid artery, intracranial portion, not elsewhere classified NOS

✓6th **S06.82 Injury of left internal carotid artery, intracranial portion, not elsewhere classified**

7 ✓7th **S06.820 Injury of left internal carotid artery, intracranial portion, not elsewhere classified without loss of consciousness** HCC

7 ✓7th **S06.821 Injury of left internal carotid artery, intracranial portion, not elsewhere classified with loss of consciousness of 30 minutes or less** CC H5 HCC

7 ✓7th **S06.822 Injury of left internal carotid artery, intracranial portion, not elsewhere classified with loss of consciousness of 31 minutes to 59 minutes** CC H5 HCC

7 ✓7th **S06.823 Injury of left internal carotid artery, intracranial portion, not elsewhere classified with loss of consciousness of 1 hour to 5 hours 59 minutes** CC H5 HCC

7 ✓7th **S06.824 Injury of left internal carotid artery, intracranial portion, not elsewhere classified with loss of consciousness of 6 hours to 24 hours** CC H5 HCC

7 ✓7th **S06.825 Injury of left internal carotid artery, intracranial portion, not elsewhere classified with loss of consciousness greater than 24 hours with return to pre-existing conscious level** CC H5 HCC

7 ✓7th **S06.826 Injury of left internal carotid artery, intracranial portion, not elsewhere classified with loss of consciousness greater than 24 hours without return to pre-existing conscious level with patient surviving** MCC H5 HCC

✓7th **S06.827 Injury of left internal carotid artery, intracranial portion, not elsewhere classified with loss of consciousness of any duration with death due to brain injury prior to regaining consciousness** MCC H5

✓7th **S06.828 Injury of left internal carotid artery, intracranial portion, not elsewhere classified with loss of consciousness of any duration with death due to other cause prior to regaining consciousness** MCC H5

7 √7th **S06.829 Injury of left internal carotid artery, intracranial portion, not elsewhere classified with loss of consciousness of unspecified duration** CC H5 HCC
Injury of left internal carotid artery, intracranial portion, not elsewhere classified NOS

√6th **S06.89 Other specified intracranial injury**
EXCLUDES 1 *concussion (S06.0X-)*

7 √7th **S06.890 Other specified intracranial injury without loss of consciousness** HCC
7 √7th **S06.891 Other specified intracranial injury with loss of consciousness of 30 minutes or less** CC H5 HCC
7 √7th **S06.892 Other specified intracranial injury with loss of consciousness of 31 minutes to 59 minutes** CC H5 HCC
7 √7th **S06.893 Other specified intracranial injury with loss of consciousness of 1 hour to 5 hours 59 minutes** CC H5 HCC
7 √7th **S06.894 Other specified intracranial injury with loss of consciousness of 6 hours to 24 hours** CC H5 HCC
7 √7th **S06.895 Other specified intracranial injury with loss of consciousness greater than 24 hours with return to pre-existing conscious level** CC H5 HCC
7 √7th **S06.896 Other specified intracranial injury with loss of consciousness greater than 24 hours without return to pre-existing conscious level with patient surviving** MCC H5 HCC
√7th **S06.897 Other specified intracranial injury with loss of consciousness of any duration with death due to brain injury prior to regaining consciousness** MCC H5
√7th **S06.898 Other specified intracranial injury with loss of consciousness of any duration with death due to other cause prior to regaining consciousness** MCC H5
7 √7th **S06.899 Other specified intracranial injury with loss of consciousness of unspecified duration** CC H5 HCC

√5th **S06.9 Unspecified intracranial injury**
Brain injury NOS
Head injury NOS with loss of consciousness
Traumatic brain injury NOS
EXCLUDES 1 *conditions classifiable to S06.0- to S06.8- code to specified intracranial injury*
head injury NOS (S09.90)
AHA: 2020,2Q,31

√6th **S06.9X Unspecified intracranial injury**

7 √7th **S06.9X0 Unspecified intracranial injury without loss of consciousness** HCC
7 √7th **S06.9X1 Unspecified intracranial injury with loss of consciousness of 30 minutes or less** CC H5 HCC
7 √7th **S06.9X2 Unspecified intracranial injury with loss of consciousness of 31 minutes to 59 minutes** CC H5 HCC
7 √7th **S06.9X3 Unspecified intracranial injury with loss of consciousness of 1 hour to 5 hours 59 minutes** CC H5 HCC
7 √7th **S06.9X4 Unspecified intracranial injury with loss of consciousness of 6 hours to 24 hours** CC H5 HCC
7 √7th **S06.9X5 Unspecified intracranial injury with loss of consciousness greater than 24 hours with return to pre-existing conscious level** CC H5 HCC
7 √7th **S06.9X6 Unspecified intracranial injury with loss of consciousness greater than 24 hours without return to pre-existing conscious level with patient surviving** MCC H5 HCC
√7th **S06.9X7 Unspecified intracranial injury with loss of consciousness of any duration with death due to brain injury prior to regaining consciousness** MCC H5
√7th **S06.9X8 Unspecified intracranial injury with loss of consciousness of any duration with death due to other cause prior to regaining consciousness** MCC H5
7 √7th **S06.9X9 Unspecified intracranial injury with loss of consciousness of unspecified duration** CC H5 HCC

√4th **S07 Crushing injury of head**
Use additional code for all associated injuries, such as:
intracranial injuries (S06.-)
skull fractures (S02.-)

The appropriate 7th character is to be added to each code from category S07.
A initial encounter
D subsequent encounter
S sequela

√x7th **S07.0 Crushing injury of face** CC H5
√x7th **S07.1 Crushing injury of skull** CC H5
√x7th **S07.8 Crushing injury of other parts of head** CC H5
√x7th **S07.9 Crushing injury of head, part unspecified** CC H5

√4th **S08 Avulsion and traumatic amputation of part of head**
An amputation not identified as partial or complete should be coded to complete

The appropriate 7th character is to be added to each code from category S08.
A initial encounter
D subsequent encounter
S sequela

√x7th **S08.0 Avulsion of scalp**
√5th **S08.1 Traumatic amputation of ear**
√6th **S08.11 Complete traumatic amputation of ear**
√7th **S08.111 Complete traumatic amputation of right ear**
√7th **S08.112 Complete traumatic amputation of left ear**
√7th **S08.119 Complete traumatic amputation of unspecified ear**
√6th **S08.12 Partial traumatic amputation of ear**
√7th **S08.121 Partial traumatic amputation of right ear**
√7th **S08.122 Partial traumatic amputation of left ear**
√7th **S08.129 Partial traumatic amputation of unspecified ear**
√5th **S08.8 Traumatic amputation of other parts of head**
√6th **S08.81 Traumatic amputation of nose**
√7th **S08.811 Complete traumatic amputation of nose**
√7th **S08.812 Partial traumatic amputation of nose**
√x7th **S08.89 Traumatic amputation of other parts of head**

√4th **S09 Other and unspecified injuries of head**

The appropriate 7th character is to be added to each code from category S09.
A initial encounter
D subsequent encounter
S sequela

√x7th **S09.0 Injury of blood vessels of head, not elsewhere classified** CC
EXCLUDES 1 *injury of cerebral blood vessels (S06.-)*
injury of precerebral blood vessels (S15.-)
√5th **S09.1 Injury of muscle and tendon of head**
Code also any associated open wound (S01.-)
EXCLUDES 2 *sprain to joints and ligament of head (S03.9)*
√x7th **S09.10 Unspecified injury of muscle and tendon of head**
Injury of muscle and tendon of head NOS
√x7th **S09.11 Strain of muscle and tendon of head**
√x7th **S09.12 Laceration of muscle and tendon of head**
√x7th **S09.19 Other specified injury of muscle and tendon of head**
√5th **S09.2 Traumatic rupture of ear drum**
EXCLUDES 1 *traumatic rupture of ear drum due to blast injury (S09.31-)*
√x7th **S09.20 Traumatic rupture of unspecified ear drum** CC
√x7th **S09.21 Traumatic rupture of right ear drum** CC
√x7th **S09.22 Traumatic rupture of left ear drum** CC

S09.3 Other specified and unspecified injury of middle and inner ear
EXCLUDES 1 *injury to ear NOS (S09.91-)*
EXCLUDES 2 *injury to external ear (S00.4-, S01.3-, S08.1-)*

S09.30 Unspecified injury of middle and inner ear
- **S09.301 Unspecified injury of right middle and inner ear** CC
- **S09.302 Unspecified injury of left middle and inner ear** CC
- **S09.309 Unspecified injury of unspecified middle and inner ear** CC

S09.31 Primary blast injury of ear
Blast injury of ear NOS
- **S09.311 Primary blast injury of right ear** CC
- **S09.312 Primary blast injury of left ear** CC
- **S09.313 Primary blast injury of ear, bilateral** CC
- **S09.319 Primary blast injury of unspecified ear** CC

S09.39 Other specified injury of middle and inner ear
Secondary blast injury to ear
- **S09.391 Other specified injury of right middle and inner ear** CC
- **S09.392 Other specified injury of left middle and inner ear** CC
- **S09.399 Other specified injury of unspecified middle and inner ear** CC

S09.8 Other specified injuries of head

S09.9 Unspecified injury of face and head

S09.90 Unspecified injury of head
Head injury NOS
EXCLUDES 1 *brain injury NOS (S06.9-)*
head injury NOS with loss of consciousness (S06.9-)
intracranial injury NOS (S06.9-)

S09.91 Unspecified injury of ear
Injury of ear NOS

S09.92 Unspecified injury of nose
Injury of nose NOS

S09.93 Unspecified injury of face
Injury of face NOS
AHA: 2019,2Q,23

Injuries to the neck (S10-S19)

INCLUDES injuries of nape
injuries of supraclavicular region
injuries of throat

EXCLUDES 2 *burns and corrosions (T20-T32)*
effects of foreign body in esophagus (T18.1)
effects of foreign body in larynx (T17.3)
effects of foreign body in pharynx (T17.2)
effects of foreign body in trachea (T17.4)
frostbite (T33-T34)
insect bite or sting, venomous (T63.4)

S10 Superficial injury of neck

The appropriate 7th character is to be added to each code from category S10.
A initial encounter
D subsequent encounter
S sequela

S10.0 Contusion of throat
Contusion of cervical esophagus
Contusion of larynx
Contusion of pharynx
Contusion of trachea

S10.1 Other and unspecified superficial injuries of throat
- **S10.10 Unspecified superficial injuries of throat**
- **S10.11 Abrasion of throat**
- **S10.12 Blister (nonthermal) of throat**
- **S10.14 External constriction of part of throat**
- **S10.15 Superficial foreign body of throat**
  Splinter in the throat
- **S10.16 Insect bite (nonvenomous) of throat**
- **S10.17 Other superficial bite of throat**
  EXCLUDES 1 *open bite of throat (S11.85)*

S10.8 Superficial injury of other specified parts of neck
- **S10.80 Unspecified superficial injury of other specified part of neck**
- **S10.81 Abrasion of other specified part of neck**
- **S10.82 Blister (nonthermal) of other specified part of neck**
- **S10.83 Contusion of other specified part of neck**
- **S10.84 External constriction of other specified part of neck**
- **S10.85 Superficial foreign body of other specified part of neck**
  Splinter in other specified part of neck
- **S10.86 Insect bite of other specified part of neck**
- **S10.87 Other superficial bite of other specified part of neck**
  EXCLUDES 1 *open bite of other specified parts of neck (S11.85)*

S10.9 Superficial injury of unspecified part of neck
- **S10.90 Unspecified superficial injury of unspecified part of neck**
- **S10.91 Abrasion of unspecified part of neck**
- **S10.92 Blister (nonthermal) of unspecified part of neck**
- **S10.93 Contusion of unspecified part of neck**
- **S10.94 External constriction of unspecified part of neck**
- **S10.95 Superficial foreign body of unspecified part of neck**
- **S10.96 Insect bite of unspecified part of neck**
- **S10.97 Other superficial bite of unspecified part of neck**

S11 Open wound of neck

Code also any associated:
spinal cord injury (S14.0, S14.1-)
wound infection
EXCLUDES 2 *open fracture of vertebra (S12.- with 7th character B)*

The appropriate 7th character is to be added to each code from category S11.
A initial encounter
D subsequent encounter
S sequela

S11.0 Open wound of larynx and trachea

S11.01 Open wound of larynx
EXCLUDES 2 *open wound of vocal cord (S11.03)*
- **S11.011 Laceration without foreign body of larynx** MCC
- **S11.012 Laceration with foreign body of larynx** MCC
- **S11.013 Puncture wound without foreign body of larynx** MCC
- **S11.014 Puncture wound with foreign body of larynx** MCC
- **S11.015 Open bite of larynx** MCC
  Bite of larynx NOS
- **S11.019 Unspecified open wound of larynx** MCC

S11.02 Open wound of trachea
Open wound of cervical trachea
Open wound of trachea NOS
EXCLUDES 2 *open wound of thoracic trachea (S27.5-)*
- **S11.021 Laceration without foreign body of trachea** MCC
- **S11.022 Laceration with foreign body of trachea** MCC
- **S11.023 Puncture wound without foreign body of trachea** MCC
- **S11.024 Puncture wound with foreign body of trachea** MCC
- **S11.025 Open bite of trachea** MCC
  Bite of trachea NOS
- **S11.029 Unspecified open wound of trachea** MCC

S11.03 Open wound of vocal cord
- **S11.031 Laceration without foreign body of vocal cord** MCC
- **S11.032 Laceration with foreign body of vocal cord** MCC
- **S11.033 Puncture wound without foreign body of vocal cord** MCC

√7th S11.034 Puncture wound with foreign body of vocal cord MCC

√7th S11.035 Open bite of vocal cord MCC

Bite of vocal cord NOS

√7th S11.039 Unspecified open wound of vocal cord MCC

√5th S11.1 Open wound of thyroid gland

√x7th S11.10 Unspecified open wound of thyroid gland CC

√x7th S11.11 Laceration without foreign body of thyroid gland CC

√x7th S11.12 Laceration with foreign body of thyroid gland CC

√x7th S11.13 Puncture wound without foreign body of thyroid gland CC

√x7th S11.14 Puncture wound with foreign body of thyroid gland CC

√x7th S11.15 Open bite of thyroid gland CC

Bite of thyroid gland NOS

√5th S11.2 Open wound of pharynx and cervical esophagus

EXCLUDES 1 *open wound of esophagus NOS (S27.8-)*

√x7th S11.20 Unspecified open wound of pharynx and cervical esophagus CC

√x7th S11.21 Laceration without foreign body of pharynx and cervical esophagus CC

√x7th S11.22 Laceration with foreign body of pharynx and cervical esophagus CC

√x7th S11.23 Puncture wound without foreign body of pharynx and cervical esophagus CC

√x7th S11.24 Puncture wound with foreign body of pharynx and cervical esophagus CC

√x7th S11.25 Open bite of pharynx and cervical esophagus CC

Bite of pharynx and cervical esophagus NOS

√5th S11.8 Open wound of other specified parts of neck

√x7th S11.80 Unspecified open wound of other specified part of neck

√x7th S11.81 Laceration without foreign body of other specified part of neck

√x7th S11.82 Laceration with foreign body of other specified part of neck

√x7th S11.83 Puncture wound without foreign body of other specified part of neck

√x7th S11.84 Puncture wound with foreign body of other specified part of neck

√x7th S11.85 Open bite of other specified part of neck

Bite of other specified part of neck NOS

EXCLUDES 1 *superficial bite of other specified part of neck (S10.87)*

√x7th S11.89 Other open wound of other specified part of neck

√5th S11.9 Open wound of unspecified part of neck

√x7th S11.90 Unspecified open wound of unspecified part of neck

√x7th S11.91 Laceration without foreign body of unspecified part of neck

√x7th S11.92 Laceration with foreign body of unspecified part of neck

√x7th S11.93 Puncture wound without foreign body of unspecified part of neck

√x7th S11.94 Puncture wound with foreign body of unspecified part of neck

√x7th S11.95 Open bite of unspecified part of neck

Bite of neck NOS

EXCLUDES 1 *superficial bite of neck (S10.97)*

√4th S12 Fracture of cervical vertebra and other parts of neck

NOTE A fracture not indicated as displaced or nondisplaced should be coded to displaced.

A fracture not indicated as open or closed should be coded to closed.

INCLUDES fracture of cervical neural arch
fracture of cervical spine
fracture of cervical spinous process
fracture of cervical transverse process
fracture of cervical vertebral arch
fracture of neck

Code first any associated cervical spinal cord injury (S14.0, S14.1-)

AHA: 2018,2Q,12; 2015,3Q,37-39

The appropriate 7th character is to be added to all codes from subcategories S12.0-S12.6.

A initial encounter for closed fracture
B initial encounter for open fracture
D subsequent encounter for fracture with routine healing
G subsequent encounter for fracture with delayed healing
K subsequent encounter for fracture with nonunion
S sequela

√5th S12.0 Fracture of first cervical vertebra

Atlas

√6th S12.00 Unspecified fracture of first cervical vertebra

2,3,6 √7th S12.000 Unspecified displaced fracture of first cervical vertebra MCC CC H5 HCC

2,3,6 √7th S12.001 Unspecified nondisplaced fracture of first cervical vertebra MCC CC H5 HCC

2,3,6 √x7th S12.01 Stable burst fracture of first cervical vertebra MCC CC H5 HCC

2,3,6 √x7th S12.02 Unstable burst fracture of first cervical vertebra MCC CC H5 HCC

√6th S12.03 Posterior arch fracture of first cervical vertebra

2,3,6 √7th S12.030 Displaced posterior arch fracture of first cervical vertebra MCC CC H5 HCC

2,3,6 √7th S12.031 Nondisplaced posterior arch fracture of first cervical vertebra MCC CC H5 HCC

√6th S12.04 Lateral mass fracture of first cervical vertebra

2,3,6 √7th S12.040 Displaced lateral mass fracture of first cervical vertebra MCC CC H5 HCC

2,3,6 √7th S12.041 Nondisplaced lateral mass fracture of first cervical vertebra MCC CC H5 HCC

√6th S12.09 Other fracture of first cervical vertebra

2,3,6 √7th S12.090 Other displaced fracture of first cervical vertebra MCC CC H5 HCC

2,3,6 √7th S12.091 Other nondisplaced fracture of first cervical vertebra MCC CC H5 HCC

√5th S12.1 Fracture of second cervical vertebra

Axis

√6th S12.10 Unspecified fracture of second cervical vertebra

2,3,6 √7th S12.100 Unspecified displaced fracture of second cervical vertebra MCC CC H5 HCC

2,3,6 √7th S12.101 Unspecified nondisplaced fracture of second cervical vertebra MCC CC H5 HCC

√6th S12.11 Type II dens fracture

2,3,6 √7th S12.110 Anterior displaced Type II dens fracture MCC CC H5 HCC

2,3,6 √7th S12.111 Posterior displaced Type II dens fracture MCC CC H5 HCC

2,3,6 √7th S12.112 Nondisplaced Type II dens fracture MCC CC H5 HCC

√6th S12.12 Other dens fracture

2,3,6 √7th S12.120 Other displaced dens fracture MCC CC H5 HCC

2,3,6 √7th S12.121 Other nondisplaced dens fracture MCC CC H5 HCC

√6th S12.13 Unspecified traumatic spondylolisthesis of second cervical vertebra

2,3,6 √7th S12.130 Unspecified traumatic displaced spondylolisthesis of second cervical vertebra MCC CC H5 HCC

2,3,6 √7th S12.131 Unspecified traumatic nondisplaced spondylolisthesis of second cervical vertebra MCC CC H5 HCC

2,3,6 √x7th S12.14 Type III traumatic spondylolisthesis of second cervical vertebra MCC CC H5 HCC
√6th S12.15 Other traumatic spondylolisthesis of second cervical vertebra
2,3,6 √7th S12.150 Other traumatic displaced spondylolisthesis of second cervical vertebra MCC CC H5 HCC
2,3,6 √7th S12.151 Other traumatic nondisplaced spondylolisthesis of second cervical vertebra MCC CC H5 HCC
√6th S12.19 Other fracture of second cervical vertebra
2,3,6 √7th S12.190 Other displaced fracture of second cervical vertebra MCC CC H5 HCC
2,3,6 √7th S12.191 Other nondisplaced fracture of second cervical vertebra MCC CC H5 HCC
√5th S12.2 Fracture of third cervical vertebra
√6th S12.20 Unspecified fracture of third cervical vertebra
2,3,6 √7th S12.200 Unspecified displaced fracture of third cervical vertebra MCC CC H5 HCC
2,3,6 √7th S12.201 Unspecified nondisplaced fracture of third cervical vertebra MCC CC H5 HCC
√6th S12.23 Unspecified traumatic spondylolisthesis of third cervical vertebra
2,3,6 √7th S12.230 Unspecified traumatic displaced spondylolisthesis of third cervical vertebra MCC CC H5 HCC
2,3,6 √7th S12.231 Unspecified traumatic nondisplaced spondylolisthesis of third cervical vertebra MCC CC H5 HCC
2,3,6 √x7th S12.24 Type III traumatic spondylolisthesis of third cervical vertebra MCC CC H5 HCC
√6th S12.25 Other traumatic spondylolisthesis of third cervical vertebra
2,3,6 √7th S12.250 Other traumatic displaced spondylolisthesis of third cervical vertebra MCC CC H5 HCC
2,3,6 √7th S12.251 Other traumatic nondisplaced spondylolisthesis of third cervical vertebra MCC CC H5 HCC
√6th S12.29 Other fracture of third cervical vertebra
2,3,6 √7th S12.290 Other displaced fracture of third cervical vertebra MCC CC H5 HCC
2,3,6 √7th S12.291 Other nondisplaced fracture of third cervical vertebra MCC CC H5 HCC
√5th S12.3 Fracture of fourth cervical vertebra
√6th S12.30 Unspecified fracture of fourth cervical vertebra
2,3,6 √7th S12.300 Unspecified displaced fracture of fourth cervical vertebra MCC CC H5 HCC
2,3,6 √7th S12.301 Unspecified nondisplaced fracture of fourth cervical vertebra MCC CC H5 HCC
√6th S12.33 Unspecified traumatic spondylolisthesis of fourth cervical vertebra
2,3,6 √7th S12.330 Unspecified traumatic displaced spondylolisthesis of fourth cervical vertebra MCC CC H5 HCC
2,3,6 √7th S12.331 Unspecified traumatic nondisplaced spondylolisthesis of fourth cervical vertebra MCC CC H5 HCC
2,3,6 √x7th S12.34 Type III traumatic spondylolisthesis of fourth cervical vertebra MCC CC H5 HCC
√6th S12.35 Other traumatic spondylolisthesis of fourth cervical vertebra
2,3,6 √7th S12.350 Other traumatic displaced spondylolisthesis of fourth cervical vertebra MCC CC H5 HCC
2,3,6 √7th S12.351 Other traumatic nondisplaced spondylolisthesis of fourth cervical vertebra MCC CC H5 HCC
√6th S12.39 Other fracture of fourth cervical vertebra
2,3,6 √7th S12.390 Other displaced fracture of fourth cervical vertebra MCC CC H5 HCC
2,3,6 √7th S12.391 Other nondisplaced fracture of fourth cervical vertebra MCC CC H5 HCC
√5th S12.4 Fracture of fifth cervical vertebra
√6th S12.40 Unspecified fracture of fifth cervical vertebra
2,3,6 √7th S12.400 Unspecified displaced fracture of fifth cervical vertebra MCC CC H5 HCC
2,3,6 √7th S12.401 Unspecified nondisplaced fracture of fifth cervical vertebra MCC CC H5 HCC
√6th S12.43 Unspecified traumatic spondylolisthesis of fifth cervical vertebra
2,3,6 √7th S12.430 Unspecified traumatic displaced spondylolisthesis of fifth cervical vertebra MCC CC H5 HCC
2,3,6 √7th S12.431 Unspecified traumatic nondisplaced spondylolisthesis of fifth cervical vertebra MCC CC H5 HCC
2,3,6 √x7th S12.44 Type III traumatic spondylolisthesis of fifth cervical vertebra MCC CC H5 HCC
√6th S12.45 Other traumatic spondylolisthesis of fifth cervical vertebra
2,3,6 √7th S12.450 Other traumatic displaced spondylolisthesis of fifth cervical vertebra MCC CC H5 HCC
2,3,6 √7th S12.451 Other traumatic nondisplaced spondylolisthesis of fifth cervical vertebra MCC CC H5 HCC
√6th S12.49 Other fracture of fifth cervical vertebra
2,3,6 √7th S12.490 Other displaced fracture of fifth cervical vertebra MCC CC H5 HCC
2,3,6 √7th S12.491 Other nondisplaced fracture of fifth cervical vertebra MCC CC H5 HCC
√5th S12.5 Fracture of sixth cervical vertebra
√6th S12.50 Unspecified fracture of sixth cervical vertebra
2,3,6 √7th S12.500 Unspecified displaced fracture of sixth cervical vertebra MCC CC H5 HCC
2,3,6 √7th S12.501 Unspecified nondisplaced fracture of sixth cervical vertebra MCC CC H5 HCC
√6th S12.53 Unspecified traumatic spondylolisthesis of sixth cervical vertebra
2,3,6 √7th S12.530 Unspecified traumatic displaced spondylolisthesis of sixth cervical vertebra MCC CC H5 HCC
2,3,6 √7th S12.531 Unspecified traumatic nondisplaced spondylolisthesis of sixth cervical vertebra MCC CC H5 HCC
2,3,6 √x7th S12.54 Type III traumatic spondylolisthesis of sixth cervical vertebra MCC CC H5 HCC
√6th S12.55 Other traumatic spondylolisthesis of sixth cervical vertebra
2,3,6 √7th S12.550 Other traumatic displaced spondylolisthesis of sixth cervical vertebra MCC CC H5 HCC
2,3,6 √7th S12.551 Other traumatic nondisplaced spondylolisthesis of sixth cervical vertebra MCC CC H5 HCC
√6th S12.59 Other fracture of sixth cervical vertebra
2,3,6 √7th S12.590 Other displaced fracture of sixth cervical vertebra MCC CC H5 HCC
2,3,6 √7th S12.591 Other nondisplaced fracture of sixth cervical vertebra MCC CC H5 HCC
√5th S12.6 Fracture of seventh cervical vertebra
√6th S12.60 Unspecified fracture of seventh cervical vertebra
2,3,6 √7th S12.600 Unspecified displaced fracture of seventh cervical vertebra MCC CC H5 HCC
2,3,6 √7th S12.601 Unspecified nondisplaced fracture of seventh cervical vertebra MCC CC H5 HCC
√6th S12.63 Unspecified traumatic spondylolisthesis of seventh cervical vertebra
2,3,6 √7th S12.630 Unspecified traumatic displaced spondylolisthesis of seventh cervical vertebra MCC CC H5 HCC
2,3,6 √7th S12.631 Unspecified traumatic nondisplaced spondylolisthesis of seventh cervical vertebra MCC CC H5 HCC
2,3,6 √x7th S12.64 Type III traumatic spondylolisthesis of seventh cervical vertebra MCC CC H5 HCC
√6th S12.65 Other traumatic spondylolisthesis of seventh cervical vertebra
2,3,6 √7th S12.650 Other traumatic displaced spondylolisthesis of seventh cervical vertebra MCC CC H5 HCC
2,3,6 √7th S12.651 Other traumatic nondisplaced spondylolisthesis of seventh cervical vertebra MCC CC H5 HCC
√6th S12.69 Other fracture of seventh cervical vertebra
2,3,6 √7th S12.690 Other displaced fracture of seventh cervical vertebra MCC CC H5 HCC

2,3,6 √7th **S12.691 Other nondisplaced fracture of seventh cervical vertebra** MCC CC H5 HCC

6 √x7th **S12.8 Fracture of other parts of neck** MCC H5 HCC
Hyoid bone
Larynx
Thyroid cartilage
Trachea

The appropriate 7th character is to be added to code S12.8.
A initial encounter
D subsequent encounter
S sequela

6 √x7th **S12.9 Fracture of neck, unspecified** CC H5 HCC
Fracture of neck NOS
Fracture of cervical spine NOS
Fracture of cervical vertebra NOS

The appropriate 7th character is to be added to code S12.9.
A initial encounter
D subsequent encounter
S sequela

√4th **S13 Dislocation and sprain of joints and ligaments at neck level**
INCLUDES avulsion of joint or ligament at neck level
laceration of cartilage, joint or ligament at neck level
sprain of cartilage, joint or ligament at neck level
traumatic hemarthrosis of joint or ligament at neck level
traumatic rupture of joint or ligament at neck level
traumatic subluxation of joint or ligament at neck level
traumatic tear of joint or ligament at neck level
Code also any associated open wound
EXCLUDES 2 *strain of muscle or tendon at neck level (S16.1)*

The appropriate 7th character is to be added to each code from category S13.
A initial encounter
D subsequent encounter
S sequela

√x7th **S13.Ø Traumatic rupture of cervical intervertebral disc** CC H5
EXCLUDES 1 *rupture or displacement (nontraumatic) of cervical intervertebral disc NOS (M5Ø.-)*

√5th **S13.1 Subluxation and dislocation of cervical vertebrae**
Code also any associated:
open wound of neck (S11.-)
spinal cord injury (S14.1-)
EXCLUDES 2 *fracture of cervical vertebrae (S12.Ø-S12.3-)*

√6th **S13.1Ø Subluxation and dislocation of unspecified cervical vertebrae**
√7th **S13.1ØØ Subluxation of unspecified cervical vertebrae** CC H5
√7th **S13.1Ø1 Dislocation of unspecified cervical vertebrae** CC H5

√6th **S13.11 Subluxation and dislocation of CØ/C1 cervical vertebrae**
Subluxation and dislocation of atlantooccipital joint
Subluxation and dislocation of atloidooccipital joint
Subluxation and dislocation of occipitoatloid joint
√7th **S13.11Ø Subluxation of CØ/C1 cervical vertebrae** CC H5
√7th **S13.111 Dislocation of CØ/C1 cervical vertebrae** CC H5

√6th **S13.12 Subluxation and dislocation of C1/C2 cervical vertebrae**
Subluxation and dislocation of atlantoaxial joint
√7th **S13.12Ø Subluxation of C1/C2 cervical vertebrae** CC H5
√7th **S13.121 Dislocation of C1/C2 cervical vertebrae** CC H5

√6th **S13.13 Subluxation and dislocation of C2/C3 cervical vertebrae**
√7th **S13.13Ø Subluxation of C2/C3 cervical vertebrae** CC H5
√7th **S13.131 Dislocation of C2/C3 cervical vertebrae** CC H5

√6th **S13.14 Subluxation and dislocation of C3/C4 cervical vertebrae**
√7th **S13.14Ø Subluxation of C3/C4 cervical vertebrae** CC H5
√7th **S13.141 Dislocation of C3/C4 cervical vertebrae** CC H5

√6th **S13.15 Subluxation and dislocation of C4/C5 cervical vertebrae**
√7th **S13.15Ø Subluxation of C4/C5 cervical vertebrae** CC H5
√7th **S13.151 Dislocation of C4/C5 cervical vertebrae** CC H5

√6th **S13.16 Subluxation and dislocation of C5/C6 cervical vertebrae**
√7th **S13.16Ø Subluxation of C5/C6 cervical vertebrae** CC H5
√7th **S13.161 Dislocation of C5/C6 cervical vertebrae** CC H5

√6th **S13.17 Subluxation and dislocation of C6/C7 cervical vertebrae**
√7th **S13.17Ø Subluxation of C6/C7 cervical vertebrae** CC H5
√7th **S13.171 Dislocation of C6/C7 cervical vertebrae** CC H5

√6th **S13.18 Subluxation and dislocation of C7/T1 cervical vertebrae**
√7th **S13.18Ø Subluxation of C7/T1 cervical vertebrae** CC H5
√7th **S13.181 Dislocation of C7/T1 cervical vertebrae** CC H5

√5th **S13.2 Dislocation of other and unspecified parts of neck**
√x7th **S13.2Ø Dislocation of unspecified parts of neck** CC H5
√x7th **S13.29 Dislocation of other parts of neck** CC H5

√x7th **S13.4 Sprain of ligaments of cervical spine**
Sprain of anterior longitudinal (ligament), cervical
Sprain of atlanto-axial (joints)
Sprain of atlanto-occipital (joints)
Whiplash injury of cervical spine

√x7th **S13.5 Sprain of thyroid region**
Sprain of cricoarytenoid (joint) (ligament)
Sprain of cricothyroid (joint) (ligament)
Sprain of thyroid cartilage

√x7th **S13.8 Sprain of joints and ligaments of other parts of neck**
√x7th **S13.9 Sprain of joints and ligaments of unspecified parts of neck**

√4th **S14 Injury of nerves and spinal cord at neck level**
NOTE Code to highest level of cervical cord injury
Code also any associated:
fracture of cervical vertebra (S12.Ø- — S12.6.-)
open wound of neck (S11.-)
transient paralysis (R29.5)

The appropriate 7th character is to be added to each code from category S14.
A initial encounter
D subsequent encounter
S sequela

√x7th **S14.Ø Concussion and edema of cervical spinal cord** MCC HCC

√5th **S14.1 Other and unspecified injuries of cervical spinal cord**
√6th **S14.1Ø Unspecified injury of cervical spinal cord**
√7th **S14.1Ø1 Unspecified injury at C1 level of cervical spinal cord** MCC H5 HCC
√7th **S14.1Ø2 Unspecified injury at C2 level of cervical spinal cord** MCC H5 HCC
√7th **S14.1Ø3 Unspecified injury at C3 level of cervical spinal cord** MCC H5 HCC
√7th **S14.1Ø4 Unspecified injury at C4 level of cervical spinal cord** MCC H5 HCC
√7th **S14.1Ø5 Unspecified injury at C5 level of cervical spinal cord** MCC H5 HCC
√7th **S14.1Ø6 Unspecified injury at C6 level of cervical spinal cord** MCC H5 HCC
√7th **S14.1Ø7 Unspecified injury at C7 level of cervical spinal cord** MCC H5 HCC
√7th **S14.1Ø8 Unspecified injury at C8 level of cervical spinal cord** MCC HCC
√7th **S14.1Ø9 Unspecified injury at unspecified level of cervical spinal cord** HCC
Injury of cervical spinal cord NOS

√6th **S14.11 Complete lesion of cervical spinal cord**
√7th **S14.111 Complete lesion at C1 level of cervical spinal cord** MCC H5 HCC
√7th **S14.112 Complete lesion at C2 level of cervical spinal cord** MCC H5 HCC

7th S14.113 Complete lesion at C3 level of cervical spinal cord MCC H5 HCC
7th S14.114 Complete lesion at C4 level of cervical spinal cord MCC H5 HCC
7th S14.115 Complete lesion at C5 level of cervical spinal cord MCC H5 HCC
7th S14.116 Complete lesion at C6 level of cervical spinal cord MCC H5 HCC
7th S14.117 Complete lesion at C7 level of cervical spinal cord MCC H5 HCC
7th S14.118 Complete lesion at C8 level of cervical spinal cord MCC HCC
7th S14.119 Complete lesion at unspecified level of cervical spinal cord HCC

6th S14.12 Central cord syndrome of cervical spinal cord
7th S14.121 Central cord syndrome at C1 level of cervical spinal cord MCC H5 HCC
7th S14.122 Central cord syndrome at C2 level of cervical spinal cord MCC H5 HCC
7th S14.123 Central cord syndrome at C3 level of cervical spinal cord MCC H5 HCC
7th S14.124 Central cord syndrome at C4 level of cervical spinal cord MCC H5 HCC
7th S14.125 Central cord syndrome at C5 level of cervical spinal cord MCC H5 HCC
7th S14.126 Central cord syndrome at C6 level of cervical spinal cord MCC H5 HCC
7th S14.127 Central cord syndrome at C7 level of cervical spinal cord MCC H5 HCC
7th S14.128 Central cord syndrome at C8 level of cervical spinal cord MCC HCC
7th S14.129 Central cord syndrome at unspecified level of cervical spinal cord HCC

6th S14.13 Anterior cord syndrome of cervical spinal cord
7th S14.131 Anterior cord syndrome at C1 level of cervical spinal cord MCC H5 HCC
7th S14.132 Anterior cord syndrome at C2 level of cervical spinal cord MCC H5 HCC
7th S14.133 Anterior cord syndrome at C3 level of cervical spinal cord MCC H5 HCC
7th S14.134 Anterior cord syndrome at C4 level of cervical spinal cord MCC H5 HCC
7th S14.135 Anterior cord syndrome at C5 level of cervical spinal cord MCC H5 HCC
7th S14.136 Anterior cord syndrome at C6 level of cervical spinal cord MCC H5 HCC
7th S14.137 Anterior cord syndrome at C7 level of cervical spinal cord MCC H5 HCC
7th S14.138 Anterior cord syndrome at C8 level of cervical spinal cord MCC HCC
7th S14.139 Anterior cord syndrome at unspecified level of cervical spinal cord HCC

6th S14.14 Brown-Séquard syndrome of cervical spinal cord
7th S14.141 Brown-Séquard syndrome at C1 level of cervical spinal cord MCC HCC
7th S14.142 Brown-Séquard syndrome at C2 level of cervical spinal cord MCC HCC
7th S14.143 Brown-Séquard syndrome at C3 level of cervical spinal cord MCC HCC
7th S14.144 Brown-Séquard syndrome at C4 level of cervical spinal cord MCC HCC
7th S14.145 Brown-Séquard syndrome at C5 level of cervical spinal cord MCC HCC
7th S14.146 Brown-Séquard syndrome at C6 level of cervical spinal cord MCC HCC
7th S14.147 Brown-Séquard syndrome at C7 level of cervical spinal cord MCC HCC
7th S14.148 Brown-Séquard syndrome at C8 level of cervical spinal cord MCC HCC
7th S14.149 Brown-Séquard syndrome at unspecified level of cervical spinal cord HCC

6th S14.15 Other incomplete lesions of cervical spinal cord
Incomplete lesion of cervical spinal cord NOS
Posterior cord syndrome of cervical spinal cord
7th S14.151 Other incomplete lesion at C1 level of cervical spinal cord MCC H5 HCC
7th S14.152 Other incomplete lesion at C2 level of cervical spinal cord MCC H5 HCC
7th S14.153 Other incomplete lesion at C3 level of cervical spinal cord MCC H5 HCC
7th S14.154 Other incomplete lesion at C4 level of cervical spinal cord MCC H5 HCC
7th S14.155 Other incomplete lesion at C5 level of cervical spinal cord MCC H5 HCC
7th S14.156 Other incomplete lesion at C6 level of cervical spinal cord MCC H5 HCC
7th S14.157 Other incomplete lesion at C7 level of cervical spinal cord MCC H5 HCC
7th S14.158 Other incomplete lesion at C8 level of cervical spinal cord MCC HCC
7th S14.159 Other incomplete lesion at unspecified level of cervical spinal cord HCC

x7th S14.2 Injury of nerve root of cervical spine
x7th S14.3 Injury of brachial plexus
x7th S14.4 Injury of peripheral nerves of neck
x7th S14.5 Injury of cervical sympathetic nerves
x7th S14.8 Injury of other specified nerves of neck
x7th S14.9 Injury of unspecified nerves of neck

4th S15 Injury of blood vessels at neck level

Code also any associated open wound (S11.-)

The appropriate 7th character is to be added to each code from category S15.
A initial encounter
D subsequent encounter
S sequela

5th S15.0 Injury of carotid artery of neck
Injury of carotid artery (common) (external) (internal, extracranial portion)
Injury of carotid artery NOS
EXCLUDES 1 *injury of internal carotid artery, intracranial portion (S06.8)*

6th S15.00 Unspecified injury of carotid artery
7th S15.001 Unspecified injury of right carotid artery CC
7th S15.002 Unspecified injury of left carotid artery CC
7th S15.009 Unspecified injury of unspecified carotid artery CC

6th S15.01 Minor laceration of carotid artery
Incomplete transection of carotid artery
Laceration of carotid artery NOS
Superficial laceration of carotid artery
7th S15.011 Minor laceration of right carotid artery CC
7th S15.012 Minor laceration of left carotid artery CC
7th S15.019 Minor laceration of unspecified carotid artery CC

6th S15.02 Major laceration of carotid artery
Complete transection of carotid artery
Traumatic rupture of carotid artery
7th S15.021 Major laceration of right carotid artery CC
7th S15.022 Major laceration of left carotid artery CC
7th S15.029 Major laceration of unspecified carotid artery CC

6th S15.09 Other specified injury of carotid artery
7th S15.091 Other specified injury of right carotid artery CC
7th S15.092 Other specified injury of left carotid artery CC
7th S15.099 Other specified injury of unspecified carotid artery CC

5th S15.1 Injury of vertebral artery
6th S15.10 Unspecified injury of vertebral artery
7th S15.101 Unspecified injury of right vertebral artery CC
7th S15.102 Unspecified injury of left vertebral artery CC
7th S15.109 Unspecified injury of unspecified vertebral artery CC

√6th S15.11 Minor laceration of vertebral artery
Incomplete transection of vertebral artery
Laceration of vertebral artery NOS
Superficial laceration of vertebral artery
√7th S15.111 Minor laceration of right vertebral artery CC
√7th S15.112 Minor laceration of left vertebral artery CC
√7th S15.119 Minor laceration of unspecified vertebral artery CC
√6th S15.12 Major laceration of vertebral artery
Complete transection of vertebral artery
Traumatic rupture of vertebral artery
√7th S15.121 Major laceration of right vertebral artery CC
√7th S15.122 Major laceration of left vertebral artery CC
√7th S15.129 Major laceration of unspecified vertebral artery CC
√6th S15.19 Other specified injury of vertebral artery
√7th S15.191 Other specified injury of right vertebral artery CC
√7th S15.192 Other specified injury of left vertebral artery CC
√7th S15.199 Other specified injury of unspecified vertebral artery CC
√5th S15.2 Injury of external jugular vein
√6th S15.20 Unspecified injury of external jugular vein
√7th S15.201 Unspecified injury of right external jugular vein CC
√7th S15.202 Unspecified injury of left external jugular vein CC
√7th S15.209 Unspecified injury of unspecified external jugular vein CC
√6th S15.21 Minor laceration of external jugular vein
Incomplete transection of external jugular vein
Laceration of external jugular vein NOS
Superficial laceration of external jugular vein
√7th S15.211 Minor laceration of right external jugular vein CC
√7th S15.212 Minor laceration of left external jugular vein CC
√7th S15.219 Minor laceration of unspecified external jugular vein CC
√6th S15.22 Major laceration of external jugular vein
Complete transection of external jugular vein
Traumatic rupture of external jugular vein
√7th S15.221 Major laceration of right external jugular vein CC
√7th S15.222 Major laceration of left external jugular vein CC
√7th S15.229 Major laceration of unspecified external jugular vein CC
√6th S15.29 Other specified injury of external jugular vein
√7th S15.291 Other specified injury of right external jugular vein CC
√7th S15.292 Other specified injury of left external jugular vein CC
√7th S15.299 Other specified injury of unspecified external jugular vein CC
√5th S15.3 Injury of internal jugular vein
√6th S15.30 Unspecified injury of internal jugular vein
√7th S15.301 Unspecified injury of right internal jugular vein CC
√7th S15.302 Unspecified injury of left internal jugular vein CC
√7th S15.309 Unspecified injury of unspecified internal jugular vein CC
√6th S15.31 Minor laceration of internal jugular vein
Incomplete transection of internal jugular vein
Laceration of internal jugular vein NOS
Superficial laceration of internal jugular vein
√7th S15.311 Minor laceration of right internal jugular vein CC
√7th S15.312 Minor laceration of left internal jugular vein CC
√7th S15.319 Minor laceration of unspecified internal jugular vein CC
√6th S15.32 Major laceration of internal jugular vein
Complete transection of internal jugular vein
Traumatic rupture of internal jugular vein
√7th S15.321 Major laceration of right internal jugular vein CC
√7th S15.322 Major laceration of left internal jugular vein CC
√7th S15.329 Major laceration of unspecified internal jugular vein CC
√6th S15.39 Other specified injury of internal jugular vein
√7th S15.391 Other specified injury of right internal jugular vein CC
√7th S15.392 Other specified injury of left internal jugular vein CC
√7th S15.399 Other specified injury of unspecified internal jugular vein CC
√x7th S15.8 Injury of other specified blood vessels at neck level CC
√x7th S15.9 Injury of unspecified blood vessel at neck level CC

√4th **S16 Injury of muscle, fascia and tendon at neck level**
Code also any associated open wound (S11.-)
EXCLUDES 2 *sprain of joint or ligament at neck level (S13.9)*

The appropriate 7th character is to be added to each code from category S16.
A initial encounter
D subsequent encounter
S sequela

√x7th S16.1 Strain of muscle, fascia and tendon at neck level
√x7th S16.2 Laceration of muscle, fascia and tendon at neck level
√x7th S16.8 Other specified injury of muscle, fascia and tendon at neck level
√x7th S16.9 Unspecified injury of muscle, fascia and tendon at neck level

√4th **S17 Crushing injury of neck**
Use additional code for all associated injuries, such as:
injury of blood vessels (S15.-)
open wound of neck (S11.-)
spinal cord injury (S14.0, S14.1-)
vertebral fracture (S12.0- — S12.3-)

The appropriate 7th character is to be added to each code from category S17.
A initial encounter
D subsequent encounter
S sequela

√x7th S17.0 Crushing injury of larynx and trachea CC H5
√x7th S17.8 Crushing injury of other specified parts of neck CC H5
√x7th S17.9 Crushing injury of neck, part unspecified CC H5

√4th **S19 Other specified and unspecified injuries of neck**

The appropriate 7th character is to be added to each code from category S19.
A initial encounter
D subsequent encounter
S sequela

√5th S19.8 Other specified injuries of neck
√x7th S19.80 Other specified injuries of unspecified part of neck
√x7th S19.81 Other specified injuries of larynx
√x7th S19.82 Other specified injuries of cervical trachea
EXCLUDES 2 *other specified injury of thoracic trachea (S27.5-)*
√x7th S19.83 Other specified injuries of vocal cord
√x7th S19.84 Other specified injuries of thyroid gland
√x7th S19.85 Other specified injuries of pharynx and cervical esophagus
√x7th S19.89 Other specified injuries of other specified part of neck
√x7th S19.9 Unspecified injury of neck

Injuries to the thorax (S2Ø-S29)

INCLUDES injuries of breast
injuries of chest (wall)
injuries of interscapular area

EXCLUDES 2 *burns and corrosions (T2Ø-T32)*
effects of foreign body in bronchus (T17.5)
effects of foreign body in esophagus (T18.1)
effects of foreign body in lung (T17.8)
effects of foreign body in trachea (T17.4)
frostbite (T33-T34)
injuries of axilla
injuries of clavicle
injuries of scapular region
injuries of shoulder
insect bite or sting, venomous (T63.4)

S2Ø Superficial injury of thorax

The appropriate 7th character is to be added to each code from category S2Ø.
A initial encounter
D subsequent encounter
S sequela

S2Ø.Ø Contusion of breast
- **S2Ø.ØØ Contusion of breast, unspecified breast**
- **S2Ø.Ø1 Contusion of right breast**
- **S2Ø.Ø2 Contusion of left breast**

S2Ø.1 Other and unspecified superficial injuries of breast
- **S2Ø.1Ø Unspecified superficial injuries of breast**
  - **S2Ø.1Ø1 Unspecified superficial injuries of breast, right breast**
  - **S2Ø.1Ø2 Unspecified superficial injuries of breast, left breast**
  - **S2Ø.1Ø9 Unspecified superficial injuries of breast, unspecified breast**
- **S2Ø.11 Abrasion of breast**
  - **S2Ø.111 Abrasion of breast, right breast**
  - **S2Ø.112 Abrasion of breast, left breast**
  - **S2Ø.119 Abrasion of breast, unspecified breast**
- **S2Ø.12 Blister (nonthermal) of breast**
  - **S2Ø.121 Blister (nonthermal) of breast, right breast**
  - **S2Ø.122 Blister (nonthermal) of breast, left breast**
  - **S2Ø.129 Blister (nonthermal) of breast, unspecified breast**
- **S2Ø.14 External constriction of part of breast**
  - **S2Ø.141 External constriction of part of breast, right breast**
  - **S2Ø.142 External constriction of part of breast, left breast**
  - **S2Ø.149 External constriction of part of breast, unspecified breast**
- **S2Ø.15 Superficial foreign body of breast**
  Splinter in the breast
  - **S2Ø.151 Superficial foreign body of breast, right breast**
  - **S2Ø.152 Superficial foreign body of breast, left breast**
  - **S2Ø.159 Superficial foreign body of breast, unspecified breast**
- **S2Ø.16 Insect bite (nonvenomous) of breast**
  - **S2Ø.161 Insect bite (nonvenomous) of breast, right breast**
  - **S2Ø.162 Insect bite (nonvenomous) of breast, left breast**
  - **S2Ø.169 Insect bite (nonvenomous) of breast, unspecified breast**
- **S2Ø.17 Other superficial bite of breast**
  EXCLUDES 1 *open bite of breast (S21.Ø5-)*
  - **S2Ø.171 Other superficial bite of breast, right breast**
  - **S2Ø.172 Other superficial bite of breast, left breast**
  - **S2Ø.179 Other superficial bite of breast, unspecified breast**

S2Ø.2 Contusion of thorax
- **S2Ø.2Ø Contusion of thorax, unspecified**
- **S2Ø.21 Contusion of front wall of thorax**
  - **S2Ø.211 Contusion of right front wall of thorax**
  - **S2Ø.212 Contusion of left front wall of thorax**
  - ● **S2Ø.213 Contusion of bilateral front wall of thorax**
  - ● **S2Ø.214 Contusion of middle front wall of thorax**
  - **S2Ø.219 Contusion of unspecified front wall of thorax**
- **S2Ø.22 Contusion of back wall of thorax**
  - **S2Ø.221 Contusion of right back wall of thorax**
  - **S2Ø.222 Contusion of left back wall of thorax**
  - ● **S2Ø.223 Contusion of bilateral back wall of thorax**
  - ● **S2Ø.224 Contusion of middle back wall of thorax**
  - **S2Ø.229 Contusion of unspecified back wall of thorax**

S2Ø.3 Other and unspecified superficial injuries of front wall of thorax
- **S2Ø.3Ø Unspecified superficial injuries of front wall of thorax**
  - **S2Ø.3Ø1 Unspecified superficial injuries of right front wall of thorax**
  - **S2Ø.3Ø2 Unspecified superficial injuries of left front wall of thorax**
  - ● **S2Ø.3Ø3 Unspecified superficial injuries of bilateral front wall of thorax**
  - ● **S2Ø.3Ø4 Unspecified superficial injuries of middle front wall of thorax**
  - **S2Ø.3Ø9 Unspecified superficial injuries of unspecified front wall of thorax**
- **S2Ø.31 Abrasion of front wall of thorax**
  - **S2Ø.311 Abrasion of right front wall of thorax**
  - **S2Ø.312 Abrasion of left front wall of thorax**
  - ● **S2Ø.313 Abrasion of bilateral front wall of thorax**
  - ● **S2Ø.314 Abrasion of middle front wall of thorax**
  - **S2Ø.319 Abrasion of unspecified front wall of thorax**
- **S2Ø.32 Blister (nonthermal) of front wall of thorax**
  - **S2Ø.321 Blister (nonthermal) of right front wall of thorax**
  - **S2Ø.322 Blister (nonthermal) of left front wall of thorax**
  - ● **S2Ø.323 Blister (nonthermal) of bilateral front wall of thorax**
  - ● **S2Ø.324 Blister (nonthermal) of middle front wall of thorax**
  - **S2Ø.329 Blister (nonthermal) of unspecified front wall of thorax**
- **S2Ø.34 External constriction of front wall of thorax**
  - **S2Ø.341 External constriction of right front wall of thorax**
  - **S2Ø.342 External constriction of left front wall of thorax**
  - ● **S2Ø.343 External constriction of bilateral front wall of thorax**
  - ● **S2Ø.344 External constriction of middle front wall of thorax**
  - **S2Ø.349 External constriction of unspecified front wall of thorax**
- **S2Ø.35 Superficial foreign body of front wall of thorax**
  Splinter in front wall of thorax
  - **S2Ø.351 Superficial foreign body of right front wall of thorax**
  - **S2Ø.352 Superficial foreign body of left front wall of thorax**
  - ● **S2Ø.353 Superficial foreign body of bilateral front wall of thorax**
  - ● **S2Ø.354 Superficial foreign body of middle front wall of thorax**
  - **S2Ø.359 Superficial foreign body of unspecified front wall of thorax**
- **S2Ø.36 Insect bite (nonvenomous) of front wall of thorax**
  - **S2Ø.361 Insect bite (nonvenomous) of right front wall of thorax**
  - **S2Ø.362 Insect bite (nonvenomous) of left front wall of thorax**
  - ● **S2Ø.363 Insect bite (nonvenomous) of bilateral front wall of thorax**
  - ● **S2Ø.364 Insect bite (nonvenomous) of middle front wall of thorax**

- √7th **S20.369 Insect bite (nonvenomous) of unspecified front wall of thorax**
- √6th **S20.37 Other superficial bite of front wall of thorax**
  - EXCLUDES 1 *open bite of front wall of thorax (S21.15)*
  - √7th **S20.371 Other superficial bite of right front wall of thorax**
  - √7th **S20.372 Other superficial bite of left front wall of thorax**
  - • √7th **S20.373 Other superficial bite of bilateral front wall of thorax**
  - • √7th **S20.374 Other superficial bite of middle front wall of thorax**
  - √7th **S20.379 Other superficial bite of unspecified front wall of thorax**
- √5th **S20.4 Other and unspecified superficial injuries of back wall of thorax**
  - √6th **S20.40 Unspecified superficial injuries of back wall of thorax**
    - √7th **S20.401 Unspecified superficial injuries of right back wall of thorax**
    - √7th **S20.402 Unspecified superficial injuries of left back wall of thorax**
    - √7th **S20.409 Unspecified superficial injuries of unspecified back wall of thorax**
  - √6th **S20.41 Abrasion of back wall of thorax**
    - √7th **S20.411 Abrasion of right back wall of thorax**
    - √7th **S20.412 Abrasion of left back wall of thorax**
    - √7th **S20.419 Abrasion of unspecified back wall of thorax**
  - √6th **S20.42 Blister (nonthermal) of back wall of thorax**
    - √7th **S20.421 Blister (nonthermal) of right back wall of thorax**
    - √7th **S20.422 Blister (nonthermal) of left back wall of thorax**
    - √7th **S20.429 Blister (nonthermal) of unspecified back wall of thorax**
  - √6th **S20.44 External constriction of back wall of thorax**
    - √7th **S20.441 External constriction of right back wall of thorax**
    - √7th **S20.442 External constriction of left back wall of thorax**
    - √7th **S20.449 External constriction of unspecified back wall of thorax**
  - √6th **S20.45 Superficial foreign body of back wall of thorax**
    - Splinter of back wall of thorax
    - √7th **S20.451 Superficial foreign body of right back wall of thorax**
    - √7th **S20.452 Superficial foreign body of left back wall of thorax**
    - √7th **S20.459 Superficial foreign body of unspecified back wall of thorax**
  - √6th **S20.46 Insect bite (nonvenomous) of back wall of thorax**
    - √7th **S20.461 Insect bite (nonvenomous) of right back wall of thorax**
    - √7th **S20.462 Insect bite (nonvenomous) of left back wall of thorax**
    - √7th **S20.469 Insect bite (nonvenomous) of unspecified back wall of thorax**
  - √6th **S20.47 Other superficial bite of back wall of thorax**
    - EXCLUDES 1 *open bite of back wall of thorax (S21.25)*
    - √7th **S20.471 Other superficial bite of right back wall of thorax**
    - √7th **S20.472 Other superficial bite of left back wall of thorax**
    - √7th **S20.479 Other superficial bite of unspecified back wall of thorax**
- √5th **S20.9 Superficial injury of unspecified parts of thorax**
  - EXCLUDES 1 *contusion of thorax NOS (S20.20)*
  - √x7th **S20.90 Unspecified superficial injury of unspecified parts of thorax**
    - Superficial injury of thoracic wall NOS
  - √x7th **S20.91 Abrasion of unspecified parts of thorax**
  - √x7th **S20.92 Blister (nonthermal) of unspecified parts of thorax**
  - √x7th **S20.94 External constriction of unspecified parts of thorax**
  - √x7th **S20.95 Superficial foreign body of unspecified parts of thorax**
    - Splinter in thorax NOS
  - √x7th **S20.96 Insect bite (nonvenomous) of unspecified parts of thorax**
  - √x7th **S20.97 Other superficial bite of unspecified parts of thorax**
    - EXCLUDES 1 *open bite of thorax NOS (S21.95)*

√4th **S21 Open wound of thorax**

Code also any associated injury, such as:
- injury of heart (S26.-)
- injury of intrathoracic organs (S27.-)
- rib fracture (S22.3-, S22.4-)
- spinal cord injury (S24.0-, S24.1-)
- traumatic hemopneumothorax (S27.3)
- traumatic hemothorax (S27.1)
- traumatic pneumothorax (S27.0)
- wound infection

EXCLUDES 1 *traumatic amputation (partial) of thorax (S28.1)*

> The appropriate 7th character is to be added to each code from category S21.
> A initial encounter
> D subsequent encounter
> S sequela

- √5th **S21.0 Open wound of breast**
  - √6th **S21.00 Unspecified open wound of breast**
    - √7th **S21.001 Unspecified open wound of right breast**
    - √7th **S21.002 Unspecified open wound of left breast**
    - √7th **S21.009 Unspecified open wound of unspecified breast**
  - √6th **S21.01 Laceration without foreign body of breast**
    - √7th **S21.011 Laceration without foreign body of right breast**
    - √7th **S21.012 Laceration without foreign body of left breast**
    - √7th **S21.019 Laceration without foreign body of unspecified breast**
  - √6th **S21.02 Laceration with foreign body of breast**
    - √7th **S21.021 Laceration with foreign body of right breast**
    - √7th **S21.022 Laceration with foreign body of left breast**
    - √7th **S21.029 Laceration with foreign body of unspecified breast**
  - √6th **S21.03 Puncture wound without foreign body of breast**
    - √7th **S21.031 Puncture wound without foreign body of right breast**
    - √7th **S21.032 Puncture wound without foreign body of left breast**
    - √7th **S21.039 Puncture wound without foreign body of unspecified breast**
  - √6th **S21.04 Puncture wound with foreign body of breast**
    - √7th **S21.041 Puncture wound with foreign body of right breast**
    - √7th **S21.042 Puncture wound with foreign body of left breast**
    - √7th **S21.049 Puncture wound with foreign body of unspecified breast**
  - √6th **S21.05 Open bite of breast**
    - Bite of breast NOS
    - EXCLUDES 1 *superficial bite of breast (S20.17)*
    - √7th **S21.051 Open bite of right breast**
    - √7th **S21.052 Open bite of left breast**
    - √7th **S21.059 Open bite of unspecified breast**
- √5th **S21.1 Open wound of front wall of thorax without penetration into thoracic cavity**
  - Open wound of chest without penetration into thoracic cavity
  - √6th **S21.10 Unspecified open wound of front wall of thorax without penetration into thoracic cavity**
    - √7th **S21.101 Unspecified open wound of right front wall of thorax without penetration into thoracic cavity** CC
    - √7th **S21.102 Unspecified open wound of left front wall of thorax without penetration into thoracic cavity** CC
    - √7th **S21.109 Unspecified open wound of unspecified front wall of thorax without penetration into thoracic cavity** CC
  - √6th **S21.11 Laceration without foreign body of front wall of thorax without penetration into thoracic cavity**
    - √7th **S21.111 Laceration without foreign body of right front wall of thorax without penetration into thoracic cavity** CC

S21.112 Laceration without foreign body of left front wall of thorax without penetration into thoracic cavity CC

S21.119 Laceration without foreign body of unspecified front wall of thorax without penetration into thoracic cavity CC

S21.12 Laceration with foreign body of front wall of thorax without penetration into thoracic cavity

S21.121 Laceration with foreign body of right front wall of thorax without penetration into thoracic cavity CC

S21.122 Laceration with foreign body of left front wall of thorax without penetration into thoracic cavity CC

S21.129 Laceration with foreign body of unspecified front wall of thorax without penetration into thoracic cavity CC

S21.13 Puncture wound without foreign body of front wall of thorax without penetration into thoracic cavity

S21.131 Puncture wound without foreign body of right front wall of thorax without penetration into thoracic cavity CC

S21.132 Puncture wound without foreign body of left front wall of thorax without penetration into thoracic cavity CC

S21.139 Puncture wound without foreign body of unspecified front wall of thorax without penetration into thoracic cavity CC

S21.14 Puncture wound with foreign body of front wall of thorax without penetration into thoracic cavity

S21.141 Puncture wound with foreign body of right front wall of thorax without penetration into thoracic cavity CC

S21.142 Puncture wound with foreign body of left front wall of thorax without penetration into thoracic cavity CC

S21.149 Puncture wound with foreign body of unspecified front wall of thorax without penetration into thoracic cavity CC

S21.15 Open bite of front wall of thorax without penetration into thoracic cavity

Bite of front wall of thorax NOS

EXCLUDES 1 *superficial bite of front wall of thorax (S20.37)*

S21.151 Open bite of right front wall of thorax without penetration into thoracic cavity CC

S21.152 Open bite of left front wall of thorax without penetration into thoracic cavity CC

S21.159 Open bite of unspecified front wall of thorax without penetration into thoracic cavity CC

S21.2 Open wound of back wall of thorax without penetration into thoracic cavity

S21.20 Unspecified open wound of back wall of thorax without penetration into thoracic cavity

S21.201 Unspecified open wound of right back wall of thorax without penetration into thoracic cavity

S21.202 Unspecified open wound of left back wall of thorax without penetration into thoracic cavity

S21.209 Unspecified open wound of unspecified back wall of thorax without penetration into thoracic cavity

S21.21 Laceration without foreign body of back wall of thorax without penetration into thoracic cavity

S21.211 Laceration without foreign body of right back wall of thorax without penetration into thoracic cavity

S21.212 Laceration without foreign body of left back wall of thorax without penetration into thoracic cavity

S21.219 Laceration without foreign body of unspecified back wall of thorax without penetration into thoracic cavity

S21.22 Laceration with foreign body of back wall of thorax without penetration into thoracic cavity

S21.221 Laceration with foreign body of right back wall of thorax without penetration into thoracic cavity

S21.222 Laceration with foreign body of left back wall of thorax without penetration into thoracic cavity

S21.229 Laceration with foreign body of unspecified back wall of thorax without penetration into thoracic cavity

S21.23 Puncture wound without foreign body of back wall of thorax without penetration into thoracic cavity

S21.231 Puncture wound without foreign body of right back wall of thorax without penetration into thoracic cavity

S21.232 Puncture wound without foreign body of left back wall of thorax without penetration into thoracic cavity

S21.239 Puncture wound without foreign body of unspecified back wall of thorax without penetration into thoracic cavity

S21.24 Puncture wound with foreign body of back wall of thorax without penetration into thoracic cavity

S21.241 Puncture wound with foreign body of right back wall of thorax without penetration into thoracic cavity

S21.242 Puncture wound with foreign body of left back wall of thorax without penetration into thoracic cavity

S21.249 Puncture wound with foreign body of unspecified back wall of thorax without penetration into thoracic cavity

S21.25 Open bite of back wall of thorax without penetration into thoracic cavity

Bite of back wall of thorax NOS

EXCLUDES 1 *superficial bite of back wall of thorax (S20.47)*

S21.251 Open bite of right back wall of thorax without penetration into thoracic cavity

S21.252 Open bite of left back wall of thorax without penetration into thoracic cavity

S21.259 Open bite of unspecified back wall of thorax without penetration into thoracic cavity

S21.3 Open wound of front wall of thorax with penetration into thoracic cavity

Open wound of chest with penetration into thoracic cavity

S21.30 Unspecified open wound of front wall of thorax with penetration into thoracic cavity

S21.301 Unspecified open wound of right front wall of thorax with penetration into thoracic cavity MCC

S21.302 Unspecified open wound of left front wall of thorax with penetration into thoracic cavity MCC

S21.309 Unspecified open wound of unspecified front wall of thorax with penetration into thoracic cavity MCC

S21.31 Laceration without foreign body of front wall of thorax with penetration into thoracic cavity

S21.311 Laceration without foreign body of right front wall of thorax with penetration into thoracic cavity MCC

S21.312 Laceration without foreign body of left front wall of thorax with penetration into thoracic cavity MCC

S21.319 Laceration without foreign body of unspecified front wall of thorax with penetration into thoracic cavity MCC

S21.32 Laceration with foreign body of front wall of thorax with penetration into thoracic cavity

S21.321 Laceration with foreign body of right front wall of thorax with penetration into thoracic cavity MCC

S21.322 Laceration with foreign body of left front wall of thorax with penetration into thoracic cavity MCC

S21.329 Laceration with foreign body of unspecified front wall of thorax with penetration into thoracic cavity MCC

S21.33 Puncture wound without foreign body of front wall of thorax with penetration into thoracic cavity

S21.331 Puncture wound without foreign body of right front wall of thorax with penetration into thoracic cavity MCC

S21.332 Puncture wound without foreign body of left front wall of thorax with penetration into thoracic cavity MCC

√7th **S21.339 Puncture wound without foreign body of unspecified front wall of thorax with penetration into thoracic cavity** MCC

√6th **S21.34 Puncture wound with foreign body of front wall of thorax with penetration into thoracic cavity**

√7th **S21.341 Puncture wound with foreign body of right front wall of thorax with penetration into thoracic cavity** MCC

√7th **S21.342 Puncture wound with foreign body of left front wall of thorax with penetration into thoracic cavity** MCC

√7th **S21.349 Puncture wound with foreign body of unspecified front wall of thorax with penetration into thoracic cavity** MCC

√6th **S21.35 Open bite of front wall of thorax with penetration into thoracic cavity**

EXCLUDES 1 *superficial bite of front wall of thorax (S20.37)*

√7th **S21.351 Open bite of right front wall of thorax with penetration into thoracic cavity** MCC

√7th **S21.352 Open bite of left front wall of thorax with penetration into thoracic cavity** MCC

√7th **S21.359 Open bite of unspecified front wall of thorax with penetration into thoracic cavity** MCC

√5th **S21.4 Open wound of back wall of thorax with penetration into thoracic cavity**

√6th **S21.40 Unspecified open wound of back wall of thorax with penetration into thoracic cavity**

√7th **S21.401 Unspecified open wound of right back wall of thorax with penetration into thoracic cavity** MCC

√7th **S21.402 Unspecified open wound of left back wall of thorax with penetration into thoracic cavity** MCC

√7th **S21.409 Unspecified open wound of unspecified back wall of thorax with penetration into thoracic cavity** MCC

√6th **S21.41 Laceration without foreign body of back wall of thorax with penetration into thoracic cavity**

√7th **S21.411 Laceration without foreign body of right back wall of thorax with penetration into thoracic cavity** MCC

√7th **S21.412 Laceration without foreign body of left back wall of thorax with penetration into thoracic cavity** MCC

√7th **S21.419 Laceration without foreign body of unspecified back wall of thorax with penetration into thoracic cavity** MCC

√6th **S21.42 Laceration with foreign body of back wall of thorax with penetration into thoracic cavity**

√7th **S21.421 Laceration with foreign body of right back wall of thorax with penetration into thoracic cavity** MCC

√7th **S21.422 Laceration with foreign body of left back wall of thorax with penetration into thoracic cavity** MCC

√7th **S21.429 Laceration with foreign body of unspecified back wall of thorax with penetration into thoracic cavity** MCC

√6th **S21.43 Puncture wound without foreign body of back wall of thorax with penetration into thoracic cavity**

√7th **S21.431 Puncture wound without foreign body of right back wall of thorax with penetration into thoracic cavity** MCC

√7th **S21.432 Puncture wound without foreign body of left back wall of thorax with penetration into thoracic cavity** MCC

√7th **S21.439 Puncture wound without foreign body of unspecified back wall of thorax with penetration into thoracic cavity** MCC

√6th **S21.44 Puncture wound with foreign body of back wall of thorax with penetration into thoracic cavity**

√7th **S21.441 Puncture wound with foreign body of right back wall of thorax with penetration into thoracic cavity** MCC

√7th **S21.442 Puncture wound with foreign body of left back wall of thorax with penetration into thoracic cavity** MCC

√7th **S21.449 Puncture wound with foreign body of unspecified back wall of thorax with penetration into thoracic cavity** MCC

√6th **S21.45 Open bite of back wall of thorax with penetration into thoracic cavity**

Bite of back wall of thorax NOS

EXCLUDES 1 *superficial bite of back wall of thorax (S20.47)*

√7th **S21.451 Open bite of right back wall of thorax with penetration into thoracic cavity** MCC

√7th **S21.452 Open bite of left back wall of thorax with penetration into thoracic cavity** MCC

√7th **S21.459 Open bite of unspecified back wall of thorax with penetration into thoracic cavity** MCC

√5th **S21.9 Open wound of unspecified part of thorax**

Open wound of thoracic wall NOS

√x7th **S21.90 Unspecified open wound of unspecified part of thorax** CC

√x7th **S21.91 Laceration without foreign body of unspecified part of thorax** CC

√x7th **S21.92 Laceration with foreign body of unspecified part of thorax** CC

√x7th **S21.93 Puncture wound without foreign body of unspecified part of thorax** CC

√x7th **S21.94 Puncture wound with foreign body of unspecified part of thorax** CC

√x7th **S21.95 Open bite of unspecified part of thorax** CC

EXCLUDES 1 *superficial bite of thorax (S20.97)*

√4th **S22 Fracture of rib(s), sternum and thoracic spine**

NOTE A fracture not indicated as displaced or nondisplaced should be coded to displaced

A fracture not indicated as open or closed should be coded to closed

INCLUDES fracture of thoracic neural arch
fracture of thoracic spinous process
fracture of thoracic transverse process
fracture of thoracic vertebra
fracture of thoracic vertebral arch

Code first any associated:
injury of intrathoracic organ (S27.-)
spinal cord injury (S24.0-, S24.1-)

EXCLUDES 1 *transection of thorax (S28.1)*

EXCLUDES 2 *fracture of clavicle (S42.0-)*
fracture of scapula (S42.1-)

AHA: 2018,2Q,12; 2015,3Q,37-39

The appropriate 7th character is to be added to each code from category S22.

A initial encounter for closed fracture
B initial encounter for open fracture
D subsequent encounter for fracture with routine healing
G subsequent encounter for fracture with delayed healing
K subsequent encounter for fracture with nonunion
S sequela

√5th **S22.0 Fracture of thoracic vertebra**

√6th **S22.00 Fracture of unspecified thoracic vertebra**

2,3,6 √7th **S22.000 Wedge compression fracture of unspecified thoracic vertebra** MCC CC HS HCC

2,3,6 √7th **S22.001 Stable burst fracture of unspecified thoracic vertebra** MCC CC HS HCC

2,3,6 √7th **S22.002 Unstable burst fracture of unspecified thoracic vertebra** MCC CC HS HCC

2,3,6 √7th **S22.008 Other fracture of unspecified thoracic vertebra** MCC CC HS HCC

2,3,6 √7th **S22.009 Unspecified fracture of unspecified thoracic vertebra** MCC CC HS HCC

√6th **S22.01 Fracture of first thoracic vertebra**

2,3,6 √7th **S22.010 Wedge compression fracture of first thoracic vertebra** MCC CC HS HCC

2,3,6 √7th **S22.011 Stable burst fracture of first thoracic vertebra** MCC CC HS HCC

2,3,6 √7th **S22.012 Unstable burst fracture of first thoracic vertebra** MCC CC HS HCC

2,3,6 √7th **S22.018 Other fracture of first thoracic vertebra** MCC CC HS HCC

2,3,6 √7th **S22.019 Unspecified fracture of first thoracic vertebra** MCC CC HS HCC

✓6th S22.02 Fracture of second thoracic vertebra
- 2,3,6 ✓7th S22.020 Wedge compression fracture of second thoracic vertebra MCC CC H5 HCC
- 2,3,6 ✓7th S22.021 Stable burst fracture of second thoracic vertebra MCC CC H5 HCC
- 2,3,6 ✓7th S22.022 Unstable burst fracture of second thoracic vertebra MCC CC H5 HCC
- 2,3,6 ✓7th S22.028 Other fracture of second thoracic vertebra MCC CC H5 HCC
- 2,3,6 ✓7th S22.029 Unspecified fracture of second thoracic vertebra MCC CC H5 HCC

✓6th S22.03 Fracture of third thoracic vertebra
- 2,3,6 ✓7th S22.030 Wedge compression fracture of third thoracic vertebra MCC CC H5 HCC
- 2,3,6 ✓7th S22.031 Stable burst fracture of third thoracic vertebra MCC CC H5 HCC
- 2,3,6 ✓7th S22.032 Unstable burst fracture of third thoracic vertebra MCC CC H5 HCC
- 2,3,6 ✓7th S22.038 Other fracture of third thoracic vertebra MCC CC H5 HCC
- 2,3,6 ✓7th S22.039 Unspecified fracture of third thoracic vertebra MCC CC H5 HCC

✓6th S22.04 Fracture of fourth thoracic vertebra
- 2,3,6 ✓7th S22.040 Wedge compression fracture of fourth thoracic vertebra MCC CC H5 HCC
- 2,3,6 ✓7th S22.041 Stable burst fracture of fourth thoracic vertebra MCC CC H5 HCC
- 2,3,6 ✓7th S22.042 Unstable burst fracture of fourth thoracic vertebra MCC CC H5 HCC
- 2,3,6 ✓7th S22.048 Other fracture of fourth thoracic vertebra MCC CC H5 HCC
- 2,3,6 ✓7th S22.049 Unspecified fracture of fourth thoracic vertebra MCC CC H5 HCC

✓6th S22.05 Fracture of T5-T6 vertebra
- 2,3,6 ✓7th S22.050 Wedge compression fracture of T5-T6 vertebra MCC CC H5 HCC
- 2,3,6 ✓7th S22.051 Stable burst fracture of T5-T6 vertebra MCC CC H5 HCC
- 2,3,6 ✓7th S22.052 Unstable burst fracture of T5-T6 vertebra MCC CC H5 HCC
- 2,3,6 ✓7th S22.058 Other fracture of T5-T6 vertebra MCC CC H5 HCC
- 2,3,6 ✓7th S22.059 Unspecified fracture of T5-T6 vertebra MCC CC H5 HCC

✓6th S22.06 Fracture of T7-T8 vertebra
- 2,3,6 ✓7th S22.060 Wedge compression fracture of T7-T8 vertebra MCC CC H5 HCC
- 2,3,6 ✓7th S22.061 Stable burst fracture of T7-T8 vertebra MCC CC H5 HCC
- 2,3,6 ✓7th S22.062 Unstable burst fracture of T7-T8 vertebra MCC CC H5 HCC
- 2,3,6 ✓7th S22.068 Other fracture of T7-T8 thoracic vertebra MCC CC H5 HCC
- 2,3,6 ✓7th S22.069 Unspecified fracture of T7-T8 vertebra MCC CC H5 HCC

✓6th S22.07 Fracture of T9-T10 vertebra
- 2,3,6 ✓7th S22.070 Wedge compression fracture of T9-T10 vertebra MCC CC H5 HCC
- 2,3,6 ✓7th S22.071 Stable burst fracture of T9-T10 vertebra MCC CC H5 HCC
- 2,3,6 ✓7th S22.072 Unstable burst fracture of T9-T10 vertebra MCC CC H5 HCC
- 2,3,6 ✓7th S22.078 Other fracture of T9-T10 vertebra MCC CC H5 HCC
- 2,3,6 ✓7th S22.079 Unspecified fracture of T9-T10 vertebra MCC CC H5 HCC

✓6th S22.08 Fracture of T11-T12 vertebra
- 2,3,6 ✓7th S22.080 Wedge compression fracture of T11-T12 vertebra MCC CC H5 HCC
- 2,3,6 ✓7th S22.081 Stable burst fracture of T11-T12 vertebra MCC CC H5 HCC
- 2,3,6 ✓7th S22.082 Unstable burst fracture of T11-T12 vertebra MCC CC H5 HCC
- 2,3,6 ✓7th S22.088 Other fracture of T11-T12 vertebra MCC CC H5 HCC
- 2,3,6 ✓7th S22.089 Unspecified fracture of T11-T12 vertebra MCC CC H5 HCC

✓5th S22.2 Fracture of sternum

DEF: Break in flat bone (breast bone) in the anterior thorax caused by blunt trauma to the anterior chest.

- 2,3 ✓x7th S22.20 Unspecified fracture of sternum MCC CC H5
- 2,3 ✓x7th S22.21 Fracture of manubrium MCC CC H5
- 2,3 ✓x7th S22.22 Fracture of body of sternum MCC CC H5
- 2,3 ✓x7th S22.23 Sternal manubrial dissociation MCC CC H5
- 2,3 ✓x7th S22.24 Fracture of xiphoid process MCC CC H5

✓5th S22.3 Fracture of one rib
- 2,3 ✓x7th S22.31 Fracture of one rib, right side MCC CC H5
- 2,3 ✓x7th S22.32 Fracture of one rib, left side MCC CC H5
- 2,3 ✓x7th S22.39 Fracture of one rib, unspecified side MCC CC H5

✓5th S22.4 Multiple fractures of ribs

Fractures of two or more ribs

EXCLUDES 1 *flail chest (S22.5-)*

- 2,3 ✓x7th S22.41 Multiple fractures of ribs, right side MCC CC H5
- 2,3 ✓x7th S22.42 Multiple fractures of ribs, left side MCC CC H5
- 2,3 ✓x7th S22.43 Multiple fractures of ribs, bilateral MCC CC H5
- 2,3 ✓x7th S22.49 Multiple fractures of ribs, unspecified side MCC CC H5

4 ✓x7th S22.5 Flail chest MCC CC H5

2,3 ✓x7th S22.9 Fracture of bony thorax, part unspecified MCC CC H5

✓4th S23 Dislocation and sprain of joints and ligaments of thorax

INCLUDES
- avulsion of joint or ligament of thorax
- laceration of cartilage, joint or ligament of thorax
- sprain of cartilage, joint or ligament of thorax
- traumatic hemarthrosis of joint or ligament of thorax
- traumatic rupture of joint or ligament of thorax
- traumatic subluxation of joint or ligament of thorax
- traumatic tear of joint or ligament of thorax

Code also any associated open wound

EXCLUDES 2 *dislocation, sprain of sternoclavicular joint (S43.2, S43.6)*
strain of muscle or tendon of thorax (S29.01-)

The appropriate 7th character is to be added to each code from category S23.
- A initial encounter
- D subsequent encounter
- S sequela

✓x7th S23.0 Traumatic rupture of thoracic intervertebral disc

EXCLUDES 1 *rupture or displacement (nontraumatic) of thoracic intervertebral disc NOS (M51.- with fifth character 4)*

✓5th S23.1 Subluxation and dislocation of thoracic vertebra

Code also any associated:
- open wound of thorax (S21.-)
- spinal cord injury (S24.0-, S24.1-)

EXCLUDES 2 *fracture of thoracic vertebrae (S22.0-)*

✓6th S23.10 Subluxation and dislocation of unspecified thoracic vertebra
- ✓7th S23.100 Subluxation of unspecified thoracic vertebra
- ✓7th S23.101 Dislocation of unspecified thoracic vertebra

✓6th S23.11 Subluxation and dislocation of T1/T2 thoracic vertebra
- ✓7th S23.110 Subluxation of T1/T2 thoracic vertebra
- ✓7th S23.111 Dislocation of T1/T2 thoracic vertebra

✓6th S23.12 Subluxation and dislocation of T2/T3-T3/T4 thoracic vertebra
- ✓7th S23.120 Subluxation of T2/T3 thoracic vertebra
- ✓7th S23.121 Dislocation of T2/T3 thoracic vertebra
- ✓7th S23.122 Subluxation of T3/T4 thoracic vertebra
- ✓7th S23.123 Dislocation of T3/T4 thoracic vertebra

✓6th S23.13 Subluxation and dislocation of T4/T5-T5/T6 thoracic vertebra
- ✓7th S23.130 Subluxation of T4/T5 thoracic vertebra
- ✓7th S23.131 Dislocation of T4/T5 thoracic vertebra
- ✓7th S23.132 Subluxation of T5/T6 thoracic vertebra
- ✓7th S23.133 Dislocation of T5/T6 thoracic vertebra

✓6th S23.14 Subluxation and dislocation of T6/T7-T7/T8 thoracic vertebra
- ✓7th S23.140 Subluxation of T6/T7 thoracic vertebra

✓7th **S23.141** Dislocation of T6/T7 thoracic vertebra
✓7th **S23.142** Subluxation of T7/T8 thoracic vertebra
✓7th **S23.143** Dislocation of T7/T8 thoracic vertebra
✓6th **S23.15** Subluxation and dislocation of T8/T9-T9/T1Ø thoracic vertebra
✓7th **S23.15Ø** Subluxation of T8/T9 thoracic vertebra
✓7th **S23.151** Dislocation of T8/T9 thoracic vertebra
✓7th **S23.152** Subluxation of T9/T1Ø thoracic vertebra
✓7th **S23.153** Dislocation of T9/T1Ø thoracic vertebra
✓6th **S23.16** Subluxation and dislocation of T1Ø/T11-T11/T12 thoracic vertebra
✓7th **S23.16Ø** Subluxation of T1Ø/T11 thoracic vertebra
✓7th **S23.161** Dislocation of T1Ø/T11 thoracic vertebra
✓7th **S23.162** Subluxation of T11/T12 thoracic vertebra
✓7th **S23.163** Dislocation of T11/T12 thoracic vertebra
✓6th **S23.17** Subluxation and dislocation of T12/L1 thoracic vertebra
✓7th **S23.17Ø** Subluxation of T12/L1 thoracic vertebra
✓7th **S23.171** Dislocation of T12/L1 thoracic vertebra
✓5th **S23.2** Dislocation of other and unspecified parts of thorax
✓x7th **S23.2Ø** Dislocation of unspecified part of thorax
✓x7th **S23.29** Dislocation of other parts of thorax
✓x7th **S23.3** Sprain of ligaments of thoracic spine
✓5th **S23.4** Sprain of ribs and sternum
✓x7th **S23.41** Sprain of ribs
✓6th **S23.42** Sprain of sternum
✓7th **S23.42Ø** Sprain of sternoclavicular (joint) (ligament)
✓7th **S23.421** Sprain of chondrosternal joint
✓7th **S23.428** Other sprain of sternum
✓7th **S23.429** Unspecified sprain of sternum
✓x7th **S23.8** Sprain of other specified parts of thorax
✓x7th **S23.9** Sprain of unspecified parts of thorax

✓4th **S24 Injury of nerves and spinal cord at thorax level**

NOTE Code to highest level of thoracic spinal cord injury.
Injuries to the spinal cord (S24.Ø and S24.1) refer to the cord level and not bone level injury, and can affect nerve roots at and below the level given.

Code also any associated:
fracture of thoracic vertebra (S22.Ø-)
open wound of thorax (S21.-)
transient paralysis (R29.5)

EXCLUDES 2 *injury of brachial plexus (S14.3)*

The appropriate 7th character is to be added to each code from category S24.
A initial encounter
D subsequent encounter
S sequela

✓x7th **S24.Ø** Concussion and edema of thoracic spinal cord MCC HCC
✓5th **S24.1** Other and unspecified injuries of thoracic spinal cord
✓6th **S24.1Ø** Unspecified injury of thoracic spinal cord
✓7th **S24.1Ø1** Unspecified injury at T1 level of thoracic spinal cord MCC H5 HCC
✓7th **S24.1Ø2** Unspecified injury at T2-T6 level of thoracic spinal cord MCC H5 HCC
✓7th **S24.1Ø3** Unspecified injury at T7-T1Ø level of thoracic spinal cord MCC H5 HCC
✓7th **S24.1Ø4** Unspecified injury at T11-T12 level of thoracic spinal cord MCC H5 HCC
✓7th **S24.1Ø9** Unspecified injury at unspecified level of thoracic spinal cord HCC
Injury of thoracic spinal cord NOS
✓6th **S24.11** Complete lesion of thoracic spinal cord
✓7th **S24.111** Complete lesion at T1 level of thoracic spinal cord MCC H5 HCC
✓7th **S24.112** Complete lesion at T2-T6 level of thoracic spinal cord MCC H5 HCC
✓7th **S24.113** Complete lesion at T7-T1Ø level of thoracic spinal cord MCC H5 HCC
✓7th **S24.114** Complete lesion at T11-T12 level of thoracic spinal cord MCC H5 HCC
✓7th **S24.119** Complete lesion at unspecified level of thoracic spinal cord HCC
✓6th **S24.13** Anterior cord syndrome of thoracic spinal cord
✓7th **S24.131** Anterior cord syndrome at T1 level of thoracic spinal cord MCC H5 HCC
✓7th **S24.132** Anterior cord syndrome at T2-T6 level of thoracic spinal cord MCC H5 HCC
✓7th **S24.133** Anterior cord syndrome at T7-T1Ø level of thoracic spinal cord MCC H5 HCC
✓7th **S24.134** Anterior cord syndrome at T11-T12 level of thoracic spinal cord MCC H5 HCC
✓7th **S24.139** Anterior cord syndrome at unspecified level of thoracic spinal cord HCC
✓6th **S24.14** Brown-Séquard syndrome of thoracic spinal cord
✓7th **S24.141** Brown-Séquard syndrome at T1 level of thoracic spinal cord MCC HCC
✓7th **S24.142** Brown-Séquard syndrome at T2-T6 level of thoracic spinal cord MCC HCC
✓7th **S24.143** Brown-Séquard syndrome at T7-T1Ø level of thoracic spinal cord MCC HCC
✓7th **S24.144** Brown-Séquard syndrome at T11-T12 level of thoracic spinal cord MCC HCC
✓7th **S24.149** Brown-Séquard syndrome at unspecified level of thoracic spinal cord HCC
✓6th **S24.15** Other incomplete lesions of thoracic spinal cord
Incomplete lesion of thoracic spinal cord NOS
Posterior cord syndrome of thoracic spinal cord
✓7th **S24.151** Other incomplete lesion at T1 level of thoracic spinal cord MCC H5 HCC
✓7th **S24.152** Other incomplete lesion at T2-T6 level of thoracic spinal cord MCC H5 HCC
✓7th **S24.153** Other incomplete lesion at T7-T1Ø level of thoracic spinal cord MCC H5 HCC
✓7th **S24.154** Other incomplete lesion at T11-T12 level of thoracic spinal cord MCC H5 HCC
✓7th **S24.159** Other incomplete lesion at unspecified level of thoracic spinal cord HCC
✓x7th **S24.2** Injury of nerve root of thoracic spine
✓x7th **S24.3** Injury of peripheral nerves of thorax
✓x7th **S24.4** Injury of thoracic sympathetic nervous system
Injury of cardiac plexus
Injury of esophageal plexus
Injury of pulmonary plexus
Injury of stellate ganglion
Injury of thoracic sympathetic ganglion
✓x7th **S24.8** Injury of other specified nerves of thorax
✓x7th **S24.9** Injury of unspecified nerve of thorax

✓4th **S25 Injury of blood vessels of thorax**

Code also any associated open wound (S21.-)

The appropriate 7th character is to be added to each code from category S25.
A initial encounter
D subsequent encounter
S sequela

✓5th **S25.Ø** Injury of thoracic aorta
Injury of aorta NOS
✓x7th **S25.ØØ** Unspecified injury of thoracic aorta MCC
✓x7th **S25.Ø1** Minor laceration of thoracic aorta MCC
Incomplete transection of thoracic aorta
Laceration of thoracic aorta NOS
Superficial laceration of thoracic aorta
✓x7th **S25.Ø2** Major laceration of thoracic aorta MCC
Complete transection of thoracic aorta
Traumatic rupture of thoracic aorta
✓x7th **S25.Ø9** Other specified injury of thoracic aorta MCC
✓5th **S25.1** Injury of innominate or subclavian artery
✓6th **S25.1Ø** Unspecified injury of innominate or subclavian artery
✓7th **S25.1Ø1** Unspecified injury of right innominate or subclavian artery MCC
✓7th **S25.1Ø2** Unspecified injury of left innominate or subclavian artery MCC
✓7th **S25.1Ø9** Unspecified injury of unspecified innominate or subclavian artery MCC

✓6th S25.11 Minor laceration of innominate or subclavian artery
Incomplete transection of innominate or subclavian artery
Laceration of innominate or subclavian artery NOS
Superficial laceration of innominate or subclavian artery
✓7th S25.111 Minor laceration of right innominate or subclavian artery MCC
✓7th S25.112 Minor laceration of left innominate or subclavian artery MCC
✓7th S25.119 Minor laceration of unspecified innominate or subclavian artery MCC
✓6th S25.12 Major laceration of innominate or subclavian artery
Complete transection of innominate or subclavian artery
Traumatic rupture of innominate or subclavian artery
✓7th S25.121 Major laceration of right innominate or subclavian artery MCC
✓7th S25.122 Major laceration of left innominate or subclavian artery MCC
✓7th S25.129 Major laceration of unspecified innominate or subclavian artery MCC
✓6th S25.19 Other specified injury of innominate or subclavian artery
✓7th S25.191 Other specified injury of right innominate or subclavian artery MCC
✓7th S25.192 Other specified injury of left innominate or subclavian artery MCC
✓7th S25.199 Other specified injury of unspecified innominate or subclavian artery MCC
✓5th S25.2 Injury of superior vena cava
Injury of vena cava NOS
✓x7th S25.20 Unspecified injury of superior vena cava MCC
✓x7th S25.21 Minor laceration of superior vena cava MCC
Incomplete transection of superior vena cava
Laceration of superior vena cava NOS
Superficial laceration of superior vena cava
✓x7th S25.22 Major laceration of superior vena cava MCC
Complete transection of superior vena cava
Traumatic rupture of superior vena cava
✓x7th S25.29 Other specified injury of superior vena cava MCC
✓5th S25.3 Injury of innominate or subclavian vein
✓6th S25.30 Unspecified injury of innominate or subclavian vein
✓7th S25.301 Unspecified injury of right innominate or subclavian vein MCC
✓7th S25.302 Unspecified injury of left innominate or subclavian vein MCC
✓7th S25.309 Unspecified injury of unspecified innominate or subclavian vein MCC
✓6th S25.31 Minor laceration of innominate or subclavian vein
Incomplete transection of innominate or subclavian vein
Laceration of innominate or subclavian vein NOS
Superficial laceration of innominate or subclavian vein
✓7th S25.311 Minor laceration of right innominate or subclavian vein MCC
✓7th S25.312 Minor laceration of left innominate or subclavian vein MCC
✓7th S25.319 Minor laceration of unspecified innominate or subclavian vein MCC
✓6th S25.32 Major laceration of innominate or subclavian vein
Complete transection of innominate or subclavian vein
Traumatic rupture of innominate or subclavian vein
✓7th S25.321 Major laceration of right innominate or subclavian vein MCC
✓7th S25.322 Major laceration of left innominate or subclavian vein MCC
✓7th S25.329 Major laceration of unspecified innominate or subclavian vein MCC
✓6th S25.39 Other specified injury of innominate or subclavian vein
✓7th S25.391 Other specified injury of right innominate or subclavian vein MCC
✓7th S25.392 Other specified injury of left innominate or subclavian vein MCC
✓7th S25.399 Other specified injury of unspecified innominate or subclavian vein MCC
✓5th S25.4 Injury of pulmonary blood vessels
✓6th S25.40 Unspecified injury of pulmonary blood vessels
✓7th S25.401 Unspecified injury of right pulmonary blood vessels MCC
✓7th S25.402 Unspecified injury of left pulmonary blood vessels MCC
✓7th S25.409 Unspecified injury of unspecified pulmonary blood vessels MCC
✓6th S25.41 Minor laceration of pulmonary blood vessels
Incomplete transection of pulmonary blood vessels
Laceration of pulmonary blood vessels NOS
Superficial laceration of pulmonary blood vessels
✓7th S25.411 Minor laceration of right pulmonary blood vessels MCC
✓7th S25.412 Minor laceration of left pulmonary blood vessels MCC
✓7th S25.419 Minor laceration of unspecified pulmonary blood vessels MCC
✓6th S25.42 Major laceration of pulmonary blood vessels
Complete transection of pulmonary blood vessels
Traumatic rupture of pulmonary blood vessels
✓7th S25.421 Major laceration of right pulmonary blood vessels MCC
✓7th S25.422 Major laceration of left pulmonary blood vessels MCC
✓7th S25.429 Major laceration of unspecified pulmonary blood vessels MCC
✓6th S25.49 Other specified injury of pulmonary blood vessels
✓7th S25.491 Other specified injury of right pulmonary blood vessels MCC
✓7th S25.492 Other specified injury of left pulmonary blood vessels MCC
✓7th S25.499 Other specified injury of unspecified pulmonary blood vessels MCC
✓5th S25.5 Injury of intercostal blood vessels
✓6th S25.50 Unspecified injury of intercostal blood vessels
✓7th S25.501 Unspecified injury of intercostal blood vessels, right side CC
✓7th S25.502 Unspecified injury of intercostal blood vessels, left side CC
✓7th S25.509 Unspecified injury of intercostal blood vessels, unspecified side CC
✓6th S25.51 Laceration of intercostal blood vessels
✓7th S25.511 Laceration of intercostal blood vessels, right side CC
✓7th S25.512 Laceration of intercostal blood vessels, left side CC
✓7th S25.519 Laceration of intercostal blood vessels, unspecified side CC
✓6th S25.59 Other specified injury of intercostal blood vessels
✓7th S25.591 Other specified injury of intercostal blood vessels, right side CC
✓7th S25.592 Other specified injury of intercostal blood vessels, left side CC
✓7th S25.599 Other specified injury of intercostal blood vessels, unspecified side CC
✓5th S25.8 Injury of other blood vessels of thorax
Injury of azygos vein
Injury of mammary artery or vein
✓6th S25.80 Unspecified injury of other blood vessels of thorax
✓7th S25.801 Unspecified injury of other blood vessels of thorax, right side CC
✓7th S25.802 Unspecified injury of other blood vessels of thorax, left side CC
✓7th S25.809 Unspecified injury of other blood vessels of thorax, unspecified side CC
✓6th S25.81 Laceration of other blood vessels of thorax
✓7th S25.811 Laceration of other blood vessels of thorax, right side CC
✓7th S25.812 Laceration of other blood vessels of thorax, left side CC
✓7th S25.819 Laceration of other blood vessels of thorax, unspecified side CC

√6th **S25.89 Other specified injury of other blood vessels of thorax**

√7th **S25.891 Other specified injury of other blood vessels of thorax, right side** CC

√7th **S25.892 Other specified injury of other blood vessels of thorax, left side** CC

√7th **S25.899 Other specified injury of other blood vessels of thorax, unspecified side** CC

√5th **S25.9 Injury of unspecified blood vessel of thorax**

√x7th **S25.90 Unspecified injury of unspecified blood vessel of thorax** CC

√x7th **S25.91 Laceration of unspecified blood vessel of thorax** CC

√x7th **S25.99 Other specified injury of unspecified blood vessel of thorax** CC

√4th **S26 Injury of heart**

Code also any associated:
open wound of thorax (S21.-)
traumatic hemopneumothorax (S27.2)
traumatic hemothorax (S27.1)
traumatic pneumothorax (S27.Ø)

The appropriate 7th character is to be added to each code from category S26.
A initial encounter
D subsequent encounter
S sequela

√5th **S26.Ø Injury of heart with hemopericardium**

√x7th **S26.ØØ Unspecified injury of heart with hemopericardium** CC

√x7th **S26.Ø1 Contusion of heart with hemopericardium** CC

√6th **S26.Ø2 Laceration of heart with hemopericardium**

√7th **S26.Ø2Ø Mild laceration of heart with hemopericardium** MCC

Laceration of heart without penetration of heart chamber

√7th **S26.Ø21 Moderate laceration of heart with hemopericardium** MCC

Laceration of heart with penetration of heart chamber

√7th **S26.Ø22 Major laceration of heart with hemopericardium** MCC

Laceration of heart with penetration of multiple heart chambers

√x7th **S26.Ø9 Other injury of heart with hemopericardium** CC

√5th **S26.1 Injury of heart without hemopericardium**

√x7th **S26.1Ø Unspecified injury of heart without hemopericardium** CC

√x7th **S26.11 Contusion of heart without hemopericardium** CC

√x7th **S26.12 Laceration of heart without hemopericardium** MCC

√x7th **S26.19 Other injury of heart without hemopericardium** CC

√5th **S26.9 Injury of heart, unspecified with or without hemopericardium**

√x7th **S26.9Ø Unspecified injury of heart, unspecified with or without hemopericardium** CC

√x7th **S26.91 Contusion of heart, unspecified with or without hemopericardium** CC

DEF: Bruising within the heart muscle, with no mention of an open wound, usually caused by blunt chest trauma in motor vehicle accidents, falling from great heights, or receiving CPR.

√x7th **S26.92 Laceration of heart, unspecified with or without hemopericardium** MCC

Laceration of heart NOS

AHA: 2019,2Q,24

√x7th **S26.99 Other injury of heart, unspecified with or without hemopericardium** CC

√4th **S27 Injury of other and unspecified intrathoracic organs**

Code also any associated open wound of thorax (S21.-)

EXCLUDES 2 *injury of cervical esophagus (S1Ø-S19)*
injury of trachea (cervical) (S1Ø-S19)

The appropriate 7th character is to be added to each code from category S27.
A initial encounter
D subsequent encounter
S sequela

√x7th **S27.Ø Traumatic pneumothorax** CC

EXCLUDES 1 *spontaneous pneumothorax (J93.-)*

√x7th **S27.1 Traumatic hemothorax** MCC

√x7th **S27.2 Traumatic hemopneumothorax** MCC

√5th **S27.3 Other and unspecified injuries of lung**

√6th **S27.3Ø Unspecified injury of lung**

√7th **S27.3Ø1 Unspecified injury of lung, unilateral** CC

√7th **S27.3Ø2 Unspecified injury of lung, bilateral** CC

√7th **S27.3Ø9 Unspecified injury of lung, unspecified** CC

√6th **S27.31 Primary blast injury of lung**

Blast injury of lung NOS

√7th **S27.311 Primary blast injury of lung, unilateral** CC

√7th **S27.312 Primary blast injury of lung, bilateral** CC

√7th **S27.319 Primary blast injury of lung, unspecified** CC

√6th **S27.32 Contusion of lung**

DEF: Bruising of the lung without mention of an open wound.

√7th **S27.321 Contusion of lung, unilateral** CC

√7th **S27.322 Contusion of lung, bilateral** CC

√7th **S27.329 Contusion of lung, unspecified** CC

√6th **S27.33 Laceration of lung**

√7th **S27.331 Laceration of lung, unilateral** MCC

√7th **S27.332 Laceration of lung, bilateral** MCC

√7th **S27.339 Laceration of lung, unspecified** MCC

√6th **S27.39 Other injuries of lung**

Secondary blast injury of lung

√7th **S27.391 Other injuries of lung, unilateral** CC

√7th **S27.392 Other injuries of lung, bilateral** CC

√7th **S27.399 Other injuries of lung, unspecified** CC

√5th **S27.4 Injury of bronchus**

√6th **S27.4Ø Unspecified injury of bronchus**

√7th **S27.4Ø1 Unspecified injury of bronchus, unilateral** MCC

√7th **S27.4Ø2 Unspecified injury of bronchus, bilateral** MCC

√7th **S27.4Ø9 Unspecified injury of bronchus, unspecified** MCC

√6th **S27.41 Primary blast injury of bronchus**

Blast injury of bronchus NOS

√7th **S27.411 Primary blast injury of bronchus, unilateral** MCC

√7th **S27.412 Primary blast injury of bronchus, bilateral** MCC

√7th **S27.419 Primary blast injury of bronchus, unspecified** MCC

√6th **S27.42 Contusion of bronchus**

√7th **S27.421 Contusion of bronchus, unilateral** MCC

√7th **S27.422 Contusion of bronchus, bilateral** MCC

√7th **S27.429 Contusion of bronchus, unspecified** MCC

√6th **S27.43 Laceration of bronchus**

√7th **S27.431 Laceration of bronchus, unilateral** MCC

√7th **S27.432 Laceration of bronchus, bilateral** MCC

√7th **S27.439 Laceration of bronchus, unspecified** MCC

S27.49 Other injury of bronchus
Secondary blast injury of bronchus
S27.491 Other injury of bronchus, unilateral MCC
S27.492 Other injury of bronchus, bilateral MCC
S27.499 Other injury of bronchus, unspecified MCC

S27.5 Injury of thoracic trachea
S27.50 Unspecified injury of thoracic trachea CC
S27.51 Primary blast injury of thoracic trachea CC
Blast injury of thoracic trachea NOS
S27.52 Contusion of thoracic trachea CC
S27.53 Laceration of thoracic trachea CC
S27.59 Other injury of thoracic trachea CC
Secondary blast injury of thoracic trachea

S27.6 Injury of pleura
S27.60 Unspecified injury of pleura CC
S27.63 Laceration of pleura CC
S27.69 Other injury of pleura CC

S27.8 Injury of other specified intrathoracic organs
S27.80 Injury of diaphragm
S27.802 Contusion of diaphragm CC
S27.803 Laceration of diaphragm CC
S27.808 Other injury of diaphragm CC
S27.809 Unspecified injury of diaphragm CC
S27.81 Injury of esophagus (thoracic part)
S27.812 Contusion of esophagus (thoracic part) MCC
S27.813 Laceration of esophagus (thoracic part) MCC
S27.818 Other injury of esophagus (thoracic part) MCC
S27.819 Unspecified injury of esophagus (thoracic part) MCC
S27.89 Injury of other specified intrathoracic organs
Injury of lymphatic thoracic duct
Injury of thymus gland
S27.892 Contusion of other specified intrathoracic organs CC
S27.893 Laceration of other specified intrathoracic organs CC
S27.898 Other injury of other specified intrathoracic organs CC
S27.899 Unspecified injury of other specified intrathoracic organs CC
S27.9 Injury of unspecified intrathoracic organ CC

S28 Crushing injury of thorax, and traumatic amputation of part of thorax

The appropriate 7th character is to be added to each code from category S28.
A initial encounter
D subsequent encounter
S sequela

S28.0 Crushed chest
Use additional code for all associated injuries
EXCLUDES 1 *flail chest (S22.5)*
S28.1 Traumatic amputation (partial) of part of thorax, except breast CC
S28.2 Traumatic amputation of breast
S28.21 Complete traumatic amputation of breast
Traumatic amputation of breast NOS
S28.211 Complete traumatic amputation of right breast
S28.212 Complete traumatic amputation of left breast
S28.219 Complete traumatic amputation of unspecified breast
S28.22 Partial traumatic amputation of breast
S28.221 Partial traumatic amputation of right breast
S28.222 Partial traumatic amputation of left breast
S28.229 Partial traumatic amputation of unspecified breast

S29 Other and unspecified injuries of thorax

Code also any associated open wound (S21.-)

The appropriate 7th character is to be added to each code from category S29.
A initial encounter
D subsequent encounter
S sequela

S29.0 Injury of muscle and tendon at thorax level
S29.00 Unspecified injury of muscle and tendon of thorax
S29.001 Unspecified injury of muscle and tendon of front wall of thorax
S29.002 Unspecified injury of muscle and tendon of back wall of thorax
S29.009 Unspecified injury of muscle and tendon of unspecified wall of thorax
S29.01 Strain of muscle and tendon of thorax
S29.011 Strain of muscle and tendon of front wall of thorax
S29.012 Strain of muscle and tendon of back wall of thorax
S29.019 Strain of muscle and tendon of unspecified wall of thorax
S29.02 Laceration of muscle and tendon of thorax
S29.021 Laceration of muscle and tendon of front wall of thorax CC
S29.022 Laceration of muscle and tendon of back wall of thorax
S29.029 Laceration of muscle and tendon of unspecified wall of thorax CC
S29.09 Other injury of muscle and tendon of thorax
S29.091 Other injury of muscle and tendon of front wall of thorax
S29.092 Other injury of muscle and tendon of back wall of thorax
S29.099 Other injury of muscle and tendon of unspecified wall of thorax
S29.8 Other specified injuries of thorax
S29.9 Unspecified injury of thorax

Injuries to the abdomen, lower back, lumbar spine, pelvis and external genitals (S30-S39)

INCLUDES injuries to the abdominal wall
injuries to the anus
injuries to the buttock
injuries to the external genitalia
injuries to the flank
injuries to the groin

EXCLUDES 2 *burns and corrosions (T20-T32)*
effects of foreign body in anus and rectum (T18.5)
effects of foreign body in genitourinary tract (T19.-)
effects of foreign body in stomach, small intestine and colon (T18.2-T18.4)
frostbite (T33-T34)
insect bite or sting, venomous (T63.4)

S30 Superficial injury of abdomen, lower back, pelvis and external genitals

EXCLUDES 2 *superficial injury of hip (S70.-)*

The appropriate 7th character is to be added to each code from category S30.
A initial encounter
D subsequent encounter
S sequela

S30.0 Contusion of lower back and pelvis
Contusion of buttock
S30.1 Contusion of abdominal wall
Contusion of flank
Contusion of groin
S30.2 Contusion of external genital organs
S30.20 Contusion of unspecified external genital organ
S30.201 Contusion of unspecified external genital organ, male ♂
S30.202 Contusion of unspecified external genital organ, female ♀
S30.21 Contusion of penis ♂

√x7th S30.22 Contusion of scrotum and testes ♂
√x7th S30.23 Contusion of vagina and vulva ♀
√x7th S30.3 Contusion of anus
√5th S30.8 Other superficial injuries of abdomen, lower back, pelvis and external genitals
√6th S30.81 Abrasion of abdomen, lower back, pelvis and external genitals
√7th S30.810 Abrasion of lower back and pelvis
√7th S30.811 Abrasion of abdominal wall
√7th S30.812 Abrasion of penis ♂
√7th S30.813 Abrasion of scrotum and testes ♂
√7th S30.814 Abrasion of vagina and vulva ♀
√7th S30.815 Abrasion of unspecified external genital organs, male ♂
√7th S30.816 Abrasion of unspecified external genital organs, female ♀
√7th S30.817 Abrasion of anus
√6th S30.82 Blister (nonthermal) of abdomen, lower back, pelvis and external genitals
√7th S30.820 Blister (nonthermal) of lower back and pelvis
√7th S30.821 Blister (nonthermal) of abdominal wall
√7th S30.822 Blister (nonthermal) of penis ♂
√7th S30.823 Blister (nonthermal) of scrotum and testes ♂
√7th S30.824 Blister (nonthermal) of vagina and vulva ♀
√7th S30.825 Blister (nonthermal) of unspecified external genital organs, male ♂
√7th S30.826 Blister (nonthermal) of unspecified external genital organs, female ♀
√7th S30.827 Blister (nonthermal) of anus
√6th S30.84 External constriction of abdomen, lower back, pelvis and external genitals
√7th S30.840 External constriction of lower back and pelvis
√7th S30.841 External constriction of abdominal wall
√7th S30.842 External constriction of penis ♂
Hair tourniquet syndrome of penis
Use additional cause code to identify the constricting item (W49.0-)
√7th S30.843 External constriction of scrotum and testes ♂
√7th S30.844 External constriction of vagina and vulva ♀
√7th S30.845 External constriction of unspecified external genital organs, male ♂
√7th S30.846 External constriction of unspecified external genital organs, female ♀
√6th S30.85 Superficial foreign body of abdomen, lower back, pelvis and external genitals
Splinter in the abdomen, lower back, pelvis and external genitals
√7th S30.850 Superficial foreign body of lower back and pelvis
√7th S30.851 Superficial foreign body of abdominal wall
√7th S30.852 Superficial foreign body of penis ♂
√7th S30.853 Superficial foreign body of scrotum and testes ♂
√7th S30.854 Superficial foreign body of vagina and vulva ♀
√7th S30.855 Superficial foreign body of unspecified external genital organs, male ♂
√7th S30.856 Superficial foreign body of unspecified external genital organs, female ♀
√7th S30.857 Superficial foreign body of anus
√6th S30.86 Insect bite (nonvenomous) of abdomen, lower back, pelvis and external genitals
√7th S30.860 Insect bite (nonvenomous) of lower back and pelvis
√7th S30.861 Insect bite (nonvenomous) of abdominal wall
√7th S30.862 Insect bite (nonvenomous) of penis ♂
√7th S30.863 Insect bite (nonvenomous) of scrotum and testes ♂
√7th S30.864 Insect bite (nonvenomous) of vagina and vulva ♀
√7th S30.865 Insect bite (nonvenomous) of unspecified external genital organs, male ♂
√7th S30.866 Insect bite (nonvenomous) of unspecified external genital organs, female ♀
√7th S30.867 Insect bite (nonvenomous) of anus
√6th S30.87 Other superficial bite of abdomen, lower back, pelvis and external genitals
EXCLUDES 1 *open bite of abdomen, lower back, pelvis and external genitals (S31.05, S31.15, S31.25, S31.35, S31.45, S31.55)*
√7th S30.870 Other superficial bite of lower back and pelvis
√7th S30.871 Other superficial bite of abdominal wall
√7th S30.872 Other superficial bite of penis ♂
√7th S30.873 Other superficial bite of scrotum and testes ♂
√7th S30.874 Other superficial bite of vagina and vulva ♀
√7th S30.875 Other superficial bite of unspecified external genital organs, male ♂
√7th S30.876 Other superficial bite of unspecified external genital organs, female ♀
√7th S30.877 Other superficial bite of anus
√5th S30.9 Unspecified superficial injury of abdomen, lower back, pelvis and external genitals
√x7th S30.91 Unspecified superficial injury of lower back and pelvis
√x7th S30.92 Unspecified superficial injury of abdominal wall
√x7th S30.93 Unspecified superficial injury of penis ♂
√x7th S30.94 Unspecified superficial injury of scrotum and testes ♂
√x7th S30.95 Unspecified superficial injury of vagina and vulva ♀
√x7th S30.96 Unspecified superficial injury of unspecified external genital organs, male ♂
√x7th S30.97 Unspecified superficial injury of unspecified external genital organs, female ♀
√x7th S30.98 Unspecified superficial injury of anus

√4th **S31 Open wound of abdomen, lower back, pelvis and external genitals**
Code also any associated:
spinal cord injury (S24.0, S24.1-, S34.0-, S34.1-)
wound infection
EXCLUDES 1 *traumatic amputation of part of abdomen, lower back and pelvis (S38.2-, S38.3)*
EXCLUDES 2 *open wound of hip (S71.00-S71.02)*
open fracture of pelvis (S32.1-- S32.9 with 7th character B)

The appropriate 7th character is to be added to each code from category S31.
A initial encounter
D subsequent encounter
S sequela

√5th S31.0 Open wound of lower back and pelvis
√6th S31.00 Unspecified open wound of lower back and pelvis
√7th S31.000 Unspecified open wound of lower back and pelvis without penetration into retroperitoneum
Unspecified open wound of lower back and pelvis NOS
√7th S31.001 Unspecified open wound of lower back and pelvis with penetration into retroperitoneum MCC
√6th S31.01 Laceration without foreign body of lower back and pelvis
√7th S31.010 Laceration without foreign body of lower back and pelvis without penetration into retroperitoneum
Laceration without foreign body of lower back and pelvis NOS
√7th S31.011 Laceration without foreign body of lower back and pelvis with penetration into retroperitoneum MCC

S31.02 **Laceration with foreign body of lower back and pelvis**

S31.020 **Laceration with foreign body of lower back and pelvis without penetration into retroperitoneum**
Laceration with foreign body of lower back and pelvis NOS

S31.021 **Laceration with foreign body of lower back and pelvis with penetration into retroperitoneum** MCC

S31.03 **Puncture wound without foreign body of lower back and pelvis**

S31.030 **Puncture wound without foreign body of lower back and pelvis without penetration into retroperitoneum**
Puncture wound without foreign body of lower back and pelvis NOS

S31.031 **Puncture wound without foreign body of lower back and pelvis with penetration into retroperitoneum** MCC

S31.04 **Puncture wound with foreign body of lower back and pelvis**

S31.040 **Puncture wound with foreign body of lower back and pelvis without penetration into retroperitoneum**
Puncture wound with foreign body of lower back and pelvis NOS

S31.041 **Puncture wound with foreign body of lower back and pelvis with penetration into retroperitoneum** MCC

S31.05 **Open bite of lower back and pelvis**
Bite of lower back and pelvis NOS
EXCLUDES 1 *superficial bite of lower back and pelvis (S30.860, S30.870)*

S31.050 **Open bite of lower back and pelvis without penetration into retroperitoneum**
Open bite of lower back and pelvis NOS

S31.051 **Open bite of lower back and pelvis with penetration into retroperitoneum** MCC

S31.1 **Open wound of abdominal wall without penetration into peritoneal cavity**
Open wound of abdominal wall NOS
EXCLUDES 2 *open wound of abdominal wall with penetration into peritoneal cavity (S31.6-)*

S31.10 **Unspecified open wound of abdominal wall without penetration into peritoneal cavity**

S31.100 **Unspecified open wound of abdominal wall, right upper quadrant without penetration into peritoneal cavity**

S31.101 **Unspecified open wound of abdominal wall, left upper quadrant without penetration into peritoneal cavity**

S31.102 **Unspecified open wound of abdominal wall, epigastric region without penetration into peritoneal cavity**

S31.103 **Unspecified open wound of abdominal wall, right lower quadrant without penetration into peritoneal cavity**

S31.104 **Unspecified open wound of abdominal wall, left lower quadrant without penetration into peritoneal cavity**

S31.105 **Unspecified open wound of abdominal wall, periumbilic region without penetration into peritoneal cavity**

S31.109 **Unspecified open wound of abdominal wall, unspecified quadrant without penetration into peritoneal cavity**
Unspecified open wound of abdominal wall NOS

S31.11 **Laceration without foreign body of abdominal wall without penetration into peritoneal cavity**

S31.110 **Laceration without foreign body of abdominal wall, right upper quadrant without penetration into peritoneal cavity**

S31.111 **Laceration without foreign body of abdominal wall, left upper quadrant without penetration into peritoneal cavity**

S31.112 **Laceration without foreign body of abdominal wall, epigastric region without penetration into peritoneal cavity**

S31.113 **Laceration without foreign body of abdominal wall, right lower quadrant without penetration into peritoneal cavity**

S31.114 **Laceration without foreign body of abdominal wall, left lower quadrant without penetration into peritoneal cavity**

S31.115 **Laceration without foreign body of abdominal wall, periumbilic region without penetration into peritoneal cavity**

S31.119 **Laceration without foreign body of abdominal wall, unspecified quadrant without penetration into peritoneal cavity**

S31.12 **Laceration with foreign body of abdominal wall without penetration into peritoneal cavity**

S31.120 **Laceration of abdominal wall with foreign body, right upper quadrant without penetration into peritoneal cavity**

S31.121 **Laceration of abdominal wall with foreign body, left upper quadrant without penetration into peritoneal cavity**

S31.122 **Laceration of abdominal wall with foreign body, epigastric region without penetration into peritoneal cavity**

S31.123 **Laceration of abdominal wall with foreign body, right lower quadrant without penetration into peritoneal cavity**

S31.124 **Laceration of abdominal wall with foreign body, left lower quadrant without penetration into peritoneal cavity**

S31.125 **Laceration of abdominal wall with foreign body, periumbilic region without penetration into peritoneal cavity**

S31.129 **Laceration of abdominal wall with foreign body, unspecified quadrant without penetration into peritoneal cavity**

S31.13 **Puncture wound of abdominal wall without foreign body without penetration into peritoneal cavity**

S31.130 **Puncture wound of abdominal wall without foreign body, right upper quadrant without penetration into peritoneal cavity**

S31.131 **Puncture wound of abdominal wall without foreign body, left upper quadrant without penetration into peritoneal cavity**

S31.132 **Puncture wound of abdominal wall without foreign body, epigastric region without penetration into peritoneal cavity**

S31.133 **Puncture wound of abdominal wall without foreign body, right lower quadrant without penetration into peritoneal cavity**

S31.134 **Puncture wound of abdominal wall without foreign body, left lower quadrant without penetration into peritoneal cavity**

S31.135 **Puncture wound of abdominal wall without foreign body, periumbilic region without penetration into peritoneal cavity**

S31.139 **Puncture wound of abdominal wall without foreign body, unspecified quadrant without penetration into peritoneal cavity**

S31.14 **Puncture wound of abdominal wall with foreign body without penetration into peritoneal cavity**

S31.140 **Puncture wound of abdominal wall with foreign body, right upper quadrant without penetration into peritoneal cavity**

S31.141 **Puncture wound of abdominal wall with foreign body, left upper quadrant without penetration into peritoneal cavity**

S31.142 **Puncture wound of abdominal wall with foreign body, epigastric region without penetration into peritoneal cavity**

S31.143 **Puncture wound of abdominal wall with foreign body, right lower quadrant without penetration into peritoneal cavity**

√7th **S31.144 Puncture wound of abdominal wall with foreign body, left lower quadrant without penetration into peritoneal cavity**

√7th **S31.145 Puncture wound of abdominal wall with foreign body, periumbilic region without penetration into peritoneal cavity**

√7th **S31.149 Puncture wound of abdominal wall with foreign body, unspecified quadrant without penetration into peritoneal cavity**

√6th **S31.15 Open bite of abdominal wall without penetration into peritoneal cavity**

Bite of abdominal wall NOS

EXCLUDES 1 *superficial bite of abdominal wall (S30.871)*

√7th **S31.150 Open bite of abdominal wall, right upper quadrant without penetration into peritoneal cavity**

√7th **S31.151 Open bite of abdominal wall, left upper quadrant without penetration into peritoneal cavity**

√7th **S31.152 Open bite of abdominal wall, epigastric region without penetration into peritoneal cavity**

√7th **S31.153 Open bite of abdominal wall, right lower quadrant without penetration into peritoneal cavity**

√7th **S31.154 Open bite of abdominal wall, left lower quadrant without penetration into peritoneal cavity**

√7th **S31.155 Open bite of abdominal wall, periumbilic region without penetration into peritoneal cavity**

√7th **S31.159 Open bite of abdominal wall, unspecified quadrant without penetration into peritoneal cavity**

√5th **S31.2 Open wound of penis**

√x7th **S31.20 Unspecified open wound of penis** ♂

√x7th **S31.21 Laceration without foreign body of penis** ♂

√x7th **S31.22 Laceration with foreign body of penis** ♂

√x7th **S31.23 Puncture wound without foreign body of penis** ♂

√x7th **S31.24 Puncture wound with foreign body of penis** ♂

√x7th **S31.25 Open bite of penis** ♂

Bite of penis NOS

EXCLUDES 1 *superficial bite of penis (S30.862, S30.872)*

√5th **S31.3 Open wound of scrotum and testes**

√x7th **S31.30 Unspecified open wound of scrotum and testes** ♂

√x7th **S31.31 Laceration without foreign body of scrotum and testes** ♂

√x7th **S31.32 Laceration with foreign body of scrotum and testes** ♂

√x7th **S31.33 Puncture wound without foreign body of scrotum and testes** ♂

√x7th **S31.34 Puncture wound with foreign body of scrotum and testes** ♂

√x7th **S31.35 Open bite of scrotum and testes** ♂

Bite of scrotum and testes NOS

EXCLUDES 1 *superficial bite of scrotum and testes (S30.863, S30.873)*

√5th **S31.4 Open wound of vagina and vulva**

EXCLUDES 1 *injury to vagina and vulva during delivery (O70.-, O71.4)*

√x7th **S31.40 Unspecified open wound of vagina and vulva** ♀

√x7th **S31.41 Laceration without foreign body of vagina and vulva** ♀

√x7th **S31.42 Laceration with foreign body of vagina and vulva** ♀

√x7th **S31.43 Puncture wound without foreign body of vagina and vulva** ♀

√x7th **S31.44 Puncture wound with foreign body of vagina and vulva** ♀

√x7th **S31.45 Open bite of vagina and vulva** ♀

Bite of vagina and vulva NOS

EXCLUDES 1 *superficial bite of vagina and vulva (S30.864, S30.874)*

√5th **S31.5 Open wound of unspecified external genital organs**

EXCLUDES 1 *traumatic amputation of external genital organs (S38.21, S38.22)*

√6th **S31.50 Unspecified open wound of unspecified external genital organs**

√7th **S31.501 Unspecified open wound of unspecified external genital organs, male** ♂

√7th **S31.502 Unspecified open wound of unspecified external genital organs, female** ♀

√6th **S31.51 Laceration without foreign body of unspecified external genital organs**

√7th **S31.511 Laceration without foreign body of unspecified external genital organs, male** ♂

√7th **S31.512 Laceration without foreign body of unspecified external genital organs, female** ♀

√6th **S31.52 Laceration with foreign body of unspecified external genital organs**

√7th **S31.521 Laceration with foreign body of unspecified external genital organs, male** ♂

√7th **S31.522 Laceration with foreign body of unspecified external genital organs, female** ♀

√6th **S31.53 Puncture wound without foreign body of unspecified external genital organs**

√7th **S31.531 Puncture wound without foreign body of unspecified external genital organs, male** ♂

√7th **S31.532 Puncture wound without foreign body of unspecified external genital organs, female** ♀

√6th **S31.54 Puncture wound with foreign body of unspecified external genital organs**

√7th **S31.541 Puncture wound with foreign body of unspecified external genital organs, male** ♂

√7th **S31.542 Puncture wound with foreign body of unspecified external genital organs, female** ♀

√6th **S31.55 Open bite of unspecified external genital organs**

Bite of unspecified external genital organs NOS

EXCLUDES 1 *superficial bite of unspecified external genital organs (S30.865, S30.866, S30.875, S30.876)*

√7th **S31.551 Open bite of unspecified external genital organs, male** ♂

√7th **S31.552 Open bite of unspecified external genital organs, female** ♀

√5th **S31.6 Open wound of abdominal wall with penetration into peritoneal cavity**

√6th **S31.60 Unspecified open wound of abdominal wall with penetration into peritoneal cavity**

√7th **S31.600 Unspecified open wound of abdominal wall, right upper quadrant with penetration into peritoneal cavity** MCC

√7th **S31.601 Unspecified open wound of abdominal wall, left upper quadrant with penetration into peritoneal cavity** MCC

√7th **S31.602 Unspecified open wound of abdominal wall, epigastric region with penetration into peritoneal cavity** MCC

√7th **S31.603 Unspecified open wound of abdominal wall, right lower quadrant with penetration into peritoneal cavity** MCC

√7th **S31.604 Unspecified open wound of abdominal wall, left lower quadrant with penetration into peritoneal cavity** MCC

√7th **S31.605 Unspecified open wound of abdominal wall, periumbilic region with penetration into peritoneal cavity** MCC

√7th **S31.609 Unspecified open wound of abdominal wall, unspecified quadrant with penetration into peritoneal cavity** MCC

√6th **S31.61 Laceration without foreign body of abdominal wall with penetration into peritoneal cavity**

√7th **S31.610 Laceration without foreign body of abdominal wall, right upper quadrant with penetration into peritoneal cavity** MCC

S31.611 Laceration without foreign body of abdominal wall, left upper quadrant with penetration into peritoneal cavity MCC
S31.612 Laceration without foreign body of abdominal wall, epigastric region with penetration into peritoneal cavity MCC
S31.613 Laceration without foreign body of abdominal wall, right lower quadrant with penetration into peritoneal cavity MCC
S31.614 Laceration without foreign body of abdominal wall, left lower quadrant with penetration into peritoneal cavity MCC
S31.615 Laceration without foreign body of abdominal wall, periumbilic region with penetration into peritoneal cavity MCC
S31.619 Laceration without foreign body of abdominal wall, unspecified quadrant with penetration into peritoneal cavity MCC

S31.62 Laceration with foreign body of abdominal wall with penetration into peritoneal cavity
S31.620 Laceration with foreign body of abdominal wall, right upper quadrant with penetration into peritoneal cavity MCC
S31.621 Laceration with foreign body of abdominal wall, left upper quadrant with penetration into peritoneal cavity MCC
S31.622 Laceration with foreign body of abdominal wall, epigastric region with penetration into peritoneal cavity MCC
S31.623 Laceration with foreign body of abdominal wall, right lower quadrant with penetration into peritoneal cavity MCC
S31.624 Laceration with foreign body of abdominal wall, left lower quadrant with penetration into peritoneal cavity MCC
S31.625 Laceration with foreign body of abdominal wall, periumbilic region with penetration into peritoneal cavity MCC
S31.629 Laceration with foreign body of abdominal wall, unspecified quadrant with penetration into peritoneal cavity MCC

S31.63 Puncture wound without foreign body of abdominal wall with penetration into peritoneal cavity
S31.630 Puncture wound without foreign body of abdominal wall, right upper quadrant with penetration into peritoneal cavity MCC
S31.631 Puncture wound without foreign body of abdominal wall, left upper quadrant with penetration into peritoneal cavity MCC
S31.632 Puncture wound without foreign body of abdominal wall, epigastric region with penetration into peritoneal cavity MCC
S31.633 Puncture wound without foreign body of abdominal wall, right lower quadrant with penetration into peritoneal cavity MCC
S31.634 Puncture wound without foreign body of abdominal wall, left lower quadrant with penetration into peritoneal cavity MCC
S31.635 Puncture wound without foreign body of abdominal wall, periumbilic region with penetration into peritoneal cavity MCC
S31.639 Puncture wound without foreign body of abdominal wall, unspecified quadrant with penetration into peritoneal cavity MCC

S31.64 Puncture wound with foreign body of abdominal wall with penetration into peritoneal cavity
S31.640 Puncture wound with foreign body of abdominal wall, right upper quadrant with penetration into peritoneal cavity MCC
S31.641 Puncture wound with foreign body of abdominal wall, left upper quadrant with penetration into peritoneal cavity MCC
S31.642 Puncture wound with foreign body of abdominal wall, epigastric region with penetration into peritoneal cavity MCC
S31.643 Puncture wound with foreign body of abdominal wall, right lower quadrant with penetration into peritoneal cavity MCC
S31.644 Puncture wound with foreign body of abdominal wall, left lower quadrant with penetration into peritoneal cavity MCC
S31.645 Puncture wound with foreign body of abdominal wall, periumbilic region with penetration into peritoneal cavity MCC
S31.649 Puncture wound with foreign body of abdominal wall, unspecified quadrant with penetration into peritoneal cavity MCC

S31.65 Open bite of abdominal wall with penetration into peritoneal cavity
EXCLUDES 1 *superficial bite of abdominal wall (S30.861, S30.871)*
S31.650 Open bite of abdominal wall, right upper quadrant with penetration into peritoneal cavity MCC
S31.651 Open bite of abdominal wall, left upper quadrant with penetration into peritoneal cavity MCC
S31.652 Open bite of abdominal wall, epigastric region with penetration into peritoneal cavity MCC
S31.653 Open bite of abdominal wall, right lower quadrant with penetration into peritoneal cavity MCC
S31.654 Open bite of abdominal wall, left lower quadrant with penetration into peritoneal cavity MCC
S31.655 Open bite of abdominal wall, periumbilic region with penetration into peritoneal cavity MCC
S31.659 Open bite of abdominal wall, unspecified quadrant with penetration into peritoneal cavity MCC

S31.8 Open wound of other parts of abdomen, lower back and pelvis

S31.80 Open wound of unspecified buttock
S31.801 Laceration without foreign body of unspecified buttock
S31.802 Laceration with foreign body of unspecified buttock
S31.803 Puncture wound without foreign body of unspecified buttock
S31.804 Puncture wound with foreign body of unspecified buttock
S31.805 Open bite of unspecified buttock
Bite of buttock NOS
EXCLUDES 1 *superficial bite of buttock (S30.870)*
S31.809 Unspecified open wound of unspecified buttock

S31.81 Open wound of right buttock
S31.811 Laceration without foreign body of right buttock
S31.812 Laceration with foreign body of right buttock
S31.813 Puncture wound without foreign body of right buttock
S31.814 Puncture wound with foreign body of right buttock
S31.815 Open bite of right buttock
Bite of right buttock NOS
EXCLUDES 1 *superficial bite of buttock (S30.870)*
S31.819 Unspecified open wound of right buttock

S31.82 Open wound of left buttock
S31.821 Laceration without foreign body of left buttock
S31.822 Laceration with foreign body of left buttock
S31.823 Puncture wound without foreign body of left buttock
S31.824 Puncture wound with foreign body of left buttock

✓7th **S31.825 Open bite of left buttock**
Bite of left buttock NOS
EXCLUDES 1 *superficial bite of buttock (S30.870)*

✓7th **S31.829 Unspecified open wound of left buttock**

✓6th **S31.83 Open wound of anus**

✓7th **S31.831 Laceration without foreign body of anus**

✓7th **S31.832 Laceration with foreign body of anus**

✓7th **S31.833 Puncture wound without foreign body of anus**

✓7th **S31.834 Puncture wound with foreign body of anus**

✓7th **S31.835 Open bite of anus**
Bite of anus NOS
EXCLUDES 1 *superficial bite of anus (S30.877)*

✓7th **S31.839 Unspecified open wound of anus**

✓4th **S32 Fracture of lumbar spine and pelvis**

NOTE A fracture not indicated as displaced or nondisplaced should be coded to displaced.
A fracture not indicated as opened or closed should be coded to closed.

INCLUDES fracture of lumbosacral neural arch
fracture of lumbosacral spinous process
fracture of lumbosacral transverse process
fracture of lumbosacral vertebra
fracture of lumbosacral vertebral arch

Code first any associated spinal cord and spinal nerve injury (S34.-)

EXCLUDES 1 *transection of abdomen (S38.3)*

EXCLUDES 2 *fracture of hip NOS (S72.0-)*

AHA: 2018,2Q,12; 2015,3Q,37-39; 2012,4Q,93

The appropriate 7th character is to be added to each code from category S32.
- A initial encounter for closed fracture
- B initial encounter for open fracture
- D subsequent encounter for fracture with routine healing
- G subsequent encounter for fracture with delayed healing
- K subsequent encounter for fracture with nonunion
- S sequela

✓5th **S32.0 Fracture of lumbar vertebra**
Fracture of lumbar spine NOS

✓6th **S32.00 Fracture of unspecified lumbar vertebra**

2,3,6 ✓7th **S32.000 Wedge compression fracture of unspecified lumbar vertebra** MCC CC H5 HCC

2,3,6 ✓7th **S32.001 Stable burst fracture of unspecified lumbar vertebra** MCC CC H5 HCC

2,3,6 ✓7th **S32.002 Unstable burst fracture of unspecified lumbar vertebra** MCC CC H5 HCC

2,3,6 ✓7th **S32.008 Other fracture of unspecified lumbar vertebra** MCC CC H5 HCC

2,3,6 ✓7th **S32.009 Unspecified fracture of unspecified lumbar vertebra** MCC CC H5 HCC

✓6th **S32.01 Fracture of first lumbar vertebra**

2,3,6 ✓7th **S32.010 Wedge compression fracture of first lumbar vertebra** MCC CC H5 HCC

2,3,6 ✓7th **S32.011 Stable burst fracture of first lumbar vertebra** MCC CC H5 HCC

2,3,6 ✓7th **S32.012 Unstable burst fracture of first lumbar vertebra** MCC CC H5 HCC

2,3,6 ✓7th **S32.018 Other fracture of first lumbar vertebra** MCC CC H5 HCC

2,3,6 ✓7th **S32.019 Unspecified fracture of first lumbar vertebra** MCC CC H5 HCC

✓6th **S32.02 Fracture of second lumbar vertebra**

2,3,6 ✓7th **S32.020 Wedge compression fracture of second lumbar vertebra** MCC CC H5 HCC

2,3,6 ✓7th **S32.021 Stable burst fracture of second lumbar vertebra** MCC CC H5 HCC

2,3,6 ✓7th **S32.022 Unstable burst fracture of second lumbar vertebra** MCC CC H5 HCC

2,3,6 ✓7th **S32.028 Other fracture of second lumbar vertebra** MCC CC H5 HCC

2,3,6 ✓7th **S32.029 Unspecified fracture of second lumbar vertebra** MCC CC H5 HCC

✓6th **S32.03 Fracture of third lumbar vertebra**

2,3,6 ✓7th **S32.030 Wedge compression fracture of third lumbar vertebra** MCC CC H5 HCC

2,3,6 ✓7th **S32.031 Stable burst fracture of third lumbar vertebra** MCC CC H5 HCC

2,3,6 ✓7th **S32.032 Unstable burst fracture of third lumbar vertebra** MCC CC H5 HCC

2,3,6 ✓7th **S32.038 Other fracture of third lumbar vertebra** MCC CC H5 HCC

2,3,6 ✓7th **S32.039 Unspecified fracture of third lumbar vertebra** MCC CC H5 HCC

✓6th **S32.04 Fracture of fourth lumbar vertebra**

2,3,6 ✓7th **S32.040 Wedge compression fracture of fourth lumbar vertebra** MCC CC H5 HCC

2,3,6 ✓7th **S32.041 Stable burst fracture of fourth lumbar vertebra** MCC CC H5 HCC

2,3,6 ✓7th **S32.042 Unstable burst fracture of fourth lumbar vertebra** MCC CC H5 HCC

2,3,6 ✓7th **S32.048 Other fracture of fourth lumbar vertebra** MCC CC H5 HCC

2,3,6 ✓7th **S32.049 Unspecified fracture of fourth lumbar vertebra** MCC CC H5 HCC

✓6th **S32.05 Fracture of fifth lumbar vertebra**

2,3,6 ✓7th **S32.050 Wedge compression fracture of fifth lumbar vertebra** MCC CC H5 HCC

2,3,6 ✓7th **S32.051 Stable burst fracture of fifth lumbar vertebra** MCC CC H5 HCC

2,3,6 ✓7th **S32.052 Unstable burst fracture of fifth lumbar vertebra** MCC CC H5 HCC

2,3,6 ✓7th **S32.058 Other fracture of fifth lumbar vertebra** MCC CC H5 HCC

2,3,6 ✓7th **S32.059 Unspecified fracture of fifth lumbar vertebra** MCC CC H5 HCC

✓5th **S32.1 Fracture of sacrum**

NOTE For vertical fractures, code to most medial fracture extension
Use two codes if both a vertical and transverse fracture are present

Code also any associated fracture of pelvic ring (S32.8-)

2,3,6 ✓x7th **S32.10 Unspecified fracture of sacrum** MCC CC H5 HCC

✓6th **S32.11 Zone I fracture of sacrum**
Vertical sacral ala fracture of sacrum

Vertical Sacral Fracture Zones

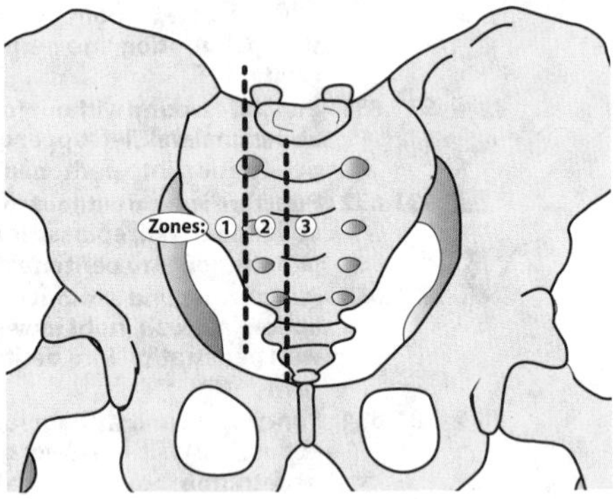

2,3,6 ✓7th **S32.110 Nondisplaced Zone I fracture of sacrum** MCC CC H5 HCC

2,3,6 ✓7th **S32.111 Minimally displaced Zone I fracture of sacrum** MCC CC H5 HCC

2,3,6 ✓7th **S32.112 Severely displaced Zone I fracture of sacrum** MCC CC H5 HCC

2,3,6 ✓7th **S32.119 Unspecified Zone I fracture of sacrum** MCC CC H5 HCC

✓6th **S32.12 Zone II fracture of sacrum**
Vertical foraminal region fracture of sacrum

2,3,6 ✓7th **S32.120 Nondisplaced Zone II fracture of sacrum** MCC CC H5 HCC

2,3,6 ✓7th **S32.121 Minimally displaced Zone II fracture of sacrum** MCC CC H5 HCC

2,3,6 ✓7th **S32.122 Severely displaced Zone II fracture of sacrum** MCC CC H5 HCC

2,3,6 ✓7th **S32.129 Unspecified Zone II fracture of sacrum** MCC CC H5 HCC

✓6th **S32.13 Zone III fracture of sacrum**

Vertical fracture into spinal canal region of sacrum

2,3,6 ✓7th **S32.130 Nondisplaced Zone III fracture of sacrum** MCC CC H5 HCC

2,3,6 ✓7th **S32.131 Minimally displaced Zone III fracture of sacrum** MCC CC H5 HCC

2,3,6 ✓7th **S32.132 Severely displaced Zone III fracture of sacrum** MCC CC H5 HCC

2,3,6 ✓7th **S32.139 Unspecified Zone III fracture of sacrum** MCC CC H5 HCC

Transverse Sacral Fracture Types

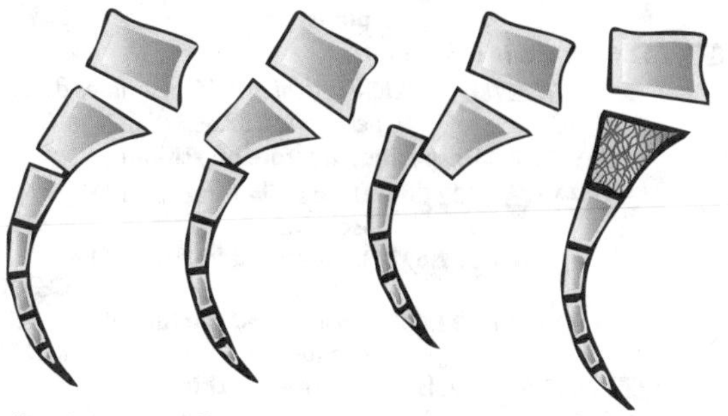

2,3,6 ✓x7th **S32.14 Type 1 fracture of sacrum** MCC CC H5 HCC

Transverse flexion fracture of sacrum without displacement

2,3,6 ✓x7th **S32.15 Type 2 fracture of sacrum** MCC CC H5 HCC

Transverse flexion fracture of sacrum with posterior displacement

2,3,6 ✓x7th **S32.16 Type 3 fracture of sacrum** MCC CC H5 HCC

Transverse extension fracture of sacrum with anterior displacement

2,3,6 ✓x7th **S32.17 Type 4 fracture of sacrum** MCC CC H5 HCC

Transverse segmental comminution of upper sacrum

2,3,6 ✓x7th **S32.19 Other fracture of sacrum** MCC CC H5 HCC

2,3,6 ✓x7th **S32.2 Fracture of coccyx** MCC CC H5 HCC

✓5th **S32.3 Fracture of ilium**

EXCLUDES 1 *fracture of ilium with associated disruption of pelvic ring (S32.8-)*

✓6th **S32.30 Unspecified fracture of ilium**

2,3,6 ✓7th **S32.301 Unspecified fracture of right ilium** MCC CC H5 HCC

2,3,6 ✓7th **S32.302 Unspecified fracture of left ilium** MCC CC H5 HCC

2,3,6 ✓7th **S32.309 Unspecified fracture of unspecified ilium** MCC CC H5 HCC

✓6th **S32.31 Avulsion fracture of ilium**

2,3,6 ✓7th **S32.311 Displaced avulsion fracture of right ilium** MCC CC H5 HCC

2,3,6 ✓7th **S32.312 Displaced avulsion fracture of left ilium** MCC CC H5 HCC

2,3,6 ✓7th **S32.313 Displaced avulsion fracture of unspecified ilium** MCC CC H5 HCC

2,3,6 ✓7th **S32.314 Nondisplaced avulsion fracture of right ilium** MCC CC H5 HCC

2,3,6 ✓7th **S32.315 Nondisplaced avulsion fracture of left ilium** MCC CC H5 HCC

2,3,6 ✓7th **S32.316 Nondisplaced avulsion fracture of unspecified ilium** MCC CC H5 HCC

✓6th **S32.39 Other fracture of ilium**

2,3,6 ✓7th **S32.391 Other fracture of right ilium** MCC CC H5 HCC

2,3,6 ✓7th **S32.392 Other fracture of left ilium** MCC CC H5 HCC

2,3,6 ✓7th **S32.399 Other fracture of unspecified ilium** MCC CC H5 HCC

✓5th **S32.4 Fracture of acetabulum**

Code also any associated fracture of pelvic ring (S32.8-)

AHA: 2016,3Q,16

✓6th **S32.40 Unspecified fracture of acetabulum**

4,6 ✓7th **S32.401 Unspecified fracture of right acetabulum** MCC CC H5 HCC

4,6 ✓7th **S32.402 Unspecified fracture of left acetabulum** MCC CC H5 HCC

4,6 ✓7th **S32.409 Unspecified fracture of unspecified acetabulum** MCC CC H5 HCC

✓6th **S32.41 Fracture of anterior wall of acetabulum**

4,6 ✓7th **S32.411 Displaced fracture of anterior wall of right acetabulum** MCC CC H5 HCC

4,6 ✓7th **S32.412 Displaced fracture of anterior wall of left acetabulum** MCC CC H5 HCC

4,6 ✓7th **S32.413 Displaced fracture of anterior wall of unspecified acetabulum** MCC CC H5 HCC

4,6 ✓7th **S32.414 Nondisplaced fracture of anterior wall of right acetabulum** MCC CC H5 HCC

4,6 ✓7th **S32.415 Nondisplaced fracture of anterior wall of left acetabulum** MCC CC H5 HCC

4,6 ✓7th **S32.416 Nondisplaced fracture of anterior wall of unspecified acetabulum** MCC CC H5 HCC

✓6th **S32.42 Fracture of posterior wall of acetabulum**

4,6 ✓7th **S32.421 Displaced fracture of posterior wall of right acetabulum** MCC CC H5 HCC

4,6 ✓7th **S32.422 Displaced fracture of posterior wall of left acetabulum** MCC CC H5 HCC

4,6 ✓7th **S32.423 Displaced fracture of posterior wall of unspecified acetabulum** MCC CC H5 HCC

4,6 ✓7th **S32.424 Nondisplaced fracture of posterior wall of right acetabulum** MCC CC H5 HCC

4,6 ✓7th **S32.425 Nondisplaced fracture of posterior wall of left acetabulum** MCC CC H5 HCC

4,6 ✓7th **S32.426 Nondisplaced fracture of posterior wall of unspecified acetabulum** MCC CC H5 HCC

✓6th **S32.43 Fracture of anterior column [iliopubic] of acetabulum**

4,6 ✓7th **S32.431 Displaced fracture of anterior column [iliopubic] of right acetabulum** MCC CC H5 HCC

4,6 ✓7th **S32.432 Displaced fracture of anterior column [iliopubic] of left acetabulum** MCC CC H5 HCC

4,6 ✓7th **S32.433 Displaced fracture of anterior column [iliopubic] of unspecified acetabulum** MCC CC H5 HCC

4,6 ✓7th **S32.434 Nondisplaced fracture of anterior column [iliopubic] of right acetabulum** MCC CC H5 HCC

4,6 ✓7th **S32.435 Nondisplaced fracture of anterior column [iliopubic] of left acetabulum** MCC CC H5 HCC

4,6 ✓7th **S32.436 Nondisplaced fracture of anterior column [iliopubic] of unspecified acetabulum** MCC CC H5 HCC

✓6th **S32.44 Fracture of posterior column [ilioischial] of acetabulum**

4,6 ✓7th **S32.441 Displaced fracture of posterior column [ilioischial] of right acetabulum** MCC CC H5 HCC

4,6 ✓7th **S32.442 Displaced fracture of posterior column [ilioischial] of left acetabulum** MCC CC H5 HCC

4,6 ✓7th **S32.443 Displaced fracture of posterior column [ilioischial] of unspecified acetabulum** MCC CC H5 HCC

4,6 ✓7th **S32.444 Nondisplaced fracture of posterior column [ilioischial] of right acetabulum** MCC CC H5 HCC

4,6 ✓7th **S32.445 Nondisplaced fracture of posterior column [ilioischial] of left acetabulum** MCC CC H5 HCC

4,6 ✓7th **S32.446 Nondisplaced fracture of posterior column [ilioischial] of unspecified acetabulum** MCC CC H5 HCC

√6th **S32.45 Transverse fracture of acetabulum**

4,6 √7th **S32.451 Displaced transverse fracture of right acetabulum** MCC CC H5 HCC

4,6 √7th **S32.452 Displaced transverse fracture of left acetabulum** MCC CC H5 HCC

4,6 √7th **S32.453 Displaced transverse fracture of unspecified acetabulum** MCC CC H5 HCC

4,6 √7th **S32.454 Nondisplaced transverse fracture of right acetabulum** MCC CC H5 HCC

4,6 √7th **S32.455 Nondisplaced transverse fracture of left acetabulum** MCC CC H5 HCC

4,6 √7th **S32.456 Nondisplaced transverse fracture of unspecified acetabulum** MCC CC H5 HCC

√6th **S32.46 Associated transverse-posterior fracture of acetabulum**

4,6 √7th **S32.461 Displaced associated transverse-posterior fracture of right acetabulum** MCC CC H5 HCC

4,6 √7th **S32.462 Displaced associated transverse-posterior fracture of left acetabulum** MCC CC H5 HCC

4,6 √7th **S32.463 Displaced associated transverse-posterior fracture of unspecified acetabulum** MCC CC H5 HCC

4,6 √7th **S32.464 Nondisplaced associated transverse-posterior fracture of right acetabulum** MCC CC H5 HCC

4,6 √7th **S32.465 Nondisplaced associated transverse-posterior fracture of left acetabulum** MCC CC H5 HCC

4,6 √7th **S32.466 Nondisplaced associated transverse-posterior fracture of unspecified acetabulum** MCC CC H5 HCC

√6th **S32.47 Fracture of medial wall of acetabulum**

4,6 √7th **S32.471 Displaced fracture of medial wall of right acetabulum** MCC CC H5 HCC

4,6 √7th **S32.472 Displaced fracture of medial wall of left acetabulum** MCC CC H5 HCC

4,6 √7th **S32.473 Displaced fracture of medial wall of unspecified acetabulum** MCC CC H5 HCC

4,6 √7th **S32.474 Nondisplaced fracture of medial wall of right acetabulum** MCC CC H5 HCC

4,6 √7th **S32.475 Nondisplaced fracture of medial wall of left acetabulum** MCC CC H5 HCC

4,6 √7th **S32.476 Nondisplaced fracture of medial wall of unspecified acetabulum** MCC CC H5 HCC

√6th **S32.48 Dome fracture of acetabulum**

4,6 √7th **S32.481 Displaced dome fracture of right acetabulum** MCC CC H5 HCC

4,6 √7th **S32.482 Displaced dome fracture of left acetabulum** MCC CC H5 HCC

4,6 √7th **S32.483 Displaced dome fracture of unspecified acetabulum** MCC CC H5 HCC

4,6 √7th **S32.484 Nondisplaced dome fracture of right acetabulum** MCC CC H5 HCC

4,6 √7th **S32.485 Nondisplaced dome fracture of left acetabulum** MCC CC H5 HCC

4,6 √7th **S32.486 Nondisplaced dome fracture of unspecified acetabulum** MCC CC H5 HCC

√6th **S32.49 Other specified fracture of acetabulum**

4,6 √7th **S32.491 Other specified fracture of right acetabulum** MCC CC H5 HCC

4,6 √7th **S32.492 Other specified fracture of left acetabulum** MCC CC H5 HCC

4,6 √7th **S32.499 Other specified fracture of unspecified acetabulum** MCC CC H5 HCC

√5th **S32.5 Fracture of pubis**

EXCLUDES 1 *fracture of pubis with associated disruption of pelvic ring (S32.8-)*

√6th **S32.50 Unspecified fracture of pubis**

2,3,6 √7th **S32.501 Unspecified fracture of right pubis** MCC CC H5 HCC

2,3,6 √7th **S32.502 Unspecified fracture of left pubis** MCC CC H5 HCC

2,3,6 √7th **S32.509 Unspecified fracture of unspecified pubis** MCC CC H5 HCC

√6th **S32.51 Fracture of superior rim of pubis**

2,3,6 √7th **S32.511 Fracture of superior rim of right pubis** MCC CC H5 HCC

2,3,6 √7th **S32.512 Fracture of superior rim of left pubis** MCC CC H5 HCC

2,3,6 √7th **S32.519 Fracture of superior rim of unspecified pubis** MCC CC H5 HCC

√6th **S32.59 Other specified fracture of pubis**

2,3,6 √7th **S32.591 Other specified fracture of right pubis** MCC CC H5 HCC

2,3,6 √7th **S32.592 Other specified fracture of left pubis** MCC CC H5 HCC

2,3,6 √7th **S32.599 Other specified fracture of unspecified pubis** MCC CC H5 HCC

√5th **S32.6 Fracture of ischium**

EXCLUDES 1 *fracture of ischium with associated disruption of pelvic ring (S32.8-)*

√6th **S32.60 Unspecified fracture of ischium**

2,3,6 √7th **S32.601 Unspecified fracture of right ischium** MCC CC H5 HCC

2,3,6 √7th **S32.602 Unspecified fracture of left ischium** MCC CC H5 HCC

2,3,6 √7th **S32.609 Unspecified fracture of unspecified ischium** MCC CC H5 HCC

√6th **S32.61 Avulsion fracture of ischium**

2,3,6 √7th **S32.611 Displaced avulsion fracture of right ischium** MCC CC H5 HCC

2,3,6 √7th **S32.612 Displaced avulsion fracture of left ischium** MCC CC H5 HCC

2,3,6 √7th **S32.613 Displaced avulsion fracture of unspecified ischium** MCC CC H5 HCC

2,3,6 √7th **S32.614 Nondisplaced avulsion fracture of right ischium** MCC CC H5 HCC

2,3,6 √7th **S32.615 Nondisplaced avulsion fracture of left ischium** MCC CC H5 HCC

2,3,6 √7th **S32.616 Nondisplaced avulsion fracture of unspecified ischium** MCC CC H5 HCC

√6th **S32.69 Other specified fracture of ischium**

2,3,6 √7th **S32.691 Other specified fracture of right ischium** MCC CC H5 HCC

2,3,6 √7th **S32.692 Other specified fracture of left ischium** MCC CC H5 HCC

2,3,6 √7th **S32.699 Other specified fracture of unspecified ischium** MCC CC H5 HCC

√5th **S32.8 Fracture of other parts of pelvis**

Code also any associated:
fracture of acetabulum (S32.4-)
sacral fracture (S32.1-)

Fractures Disrupting Pelvic Circle

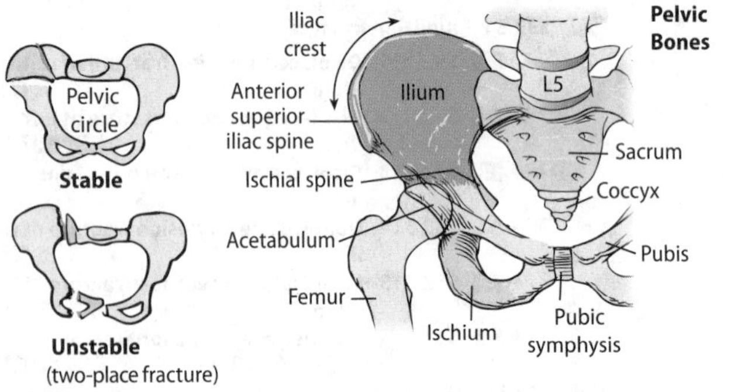

√6th **S32.81 Multiple fractures of pelvis with disruption of pelvic ring**

Multiple pelvic fractures with disruption of pelvic circle

2,3,6 √7th **S32.810 Multiple fractures of pelvis with stable disruption of pelvic ring** MCC CC H5 HCC

2,3,6 √7th **S32.811 Multiple fractures of pelvis with unstable disruption of pelvic ring** MCC CC H5 HCC

2,3,6 √x7th **S32.82 Multiple fractures of pelvis without disruption of pelvic ring** MCC CC H5 HCC

Multiple pelvic fractures without disruption of pelvic circle

2,3,6 √x7th **S32.89 Fracture of other parts of pelvis** MCC CC H5 HCC

2,3,6 √x7th **S32.9 Fracture of unspecified parts of lumbosacral spine and pelvis** MCC CC H5 HCC

Fracture of lumbosacral spine NOS

Fracture of pelvis NOS

AHA: 2012,4Q,93

√4th **S33 Dislocation and sprain of joints and ligaments of lumbar spine and pelvis**

INCLUDES avulsion of joint or ligament of lumbar spine and pelvis
laceration of cartilage, joint or ligament of lumbar spine and pelvis
sprain of cartilage, joint or ligament of lumbar spine and pelvis
traumatic hemarthrosis of joint or ligament of lumbar spine and pelvis
traumatic rupture of joint or ligament of lumbar spine and pelvis
traumatic subluxation of joint or ligament of lumbar spine and pelvis
traumatic tear of joint or ligament of lumbar spine and pelvis

Code also any associated open wound

EXCLUDES 1 *nontraumatic rupture or displacement of lumbar intervertebral disc NOS (M51.-)*
obstetric damage to pelvic joints and ligaments (O71.6)

EXCLUDES 2 *dislocation and sprain of joints and ligaments of hip (S73.-)*
strain of muscle of lower back and pelvis (S39.Ø1-)

The appropriate 7th character is to be added to each code from category S33.
A initial encounter
D subsequent encounter
S sequela

√x7th **S33.Ø Traumatic rupture of lumbar intervertebral disc**

EXCLUDES 1 *rupture or displacement (nontraumatic) of lumbar intervertebral disc NOS (M51.- with fifth character 6)*

√5th **S33.1 Subluxation and dislocation of lumbar vertebra**

Code also any associated:
open wound of abdomen, lower back and pelvis (S31)
spinal cord injury (S24.Ø, S24.1-, S34.Ø-, S34.1-)

EXCLUDES 2 *fracture of lumbar vertebrae (S32.Ø-)*

√6th **S33.1Ø Subluxation and dislocation of unspecified lumbar vertebra**

√7th **S33.1ØØ Subluxation of unspecified lumbar vertebra**

√7th **S33.1Ø1 Dislocation of unspecified lumbar vertebra**

√6th **S33.11 Subluxation and dislocation of L1/L2 lumbar vertebra**

√7th **S33.11Ø Subluxation of L1/L2 lumbar vertebra**

√7th **S33.111 Dislocation of L1/L2 lumbar vertebra**

√6th **S33.12 Subluxation and dislocation of L2/L3 lumbar vertebra**

√7th **S33.12Ø Subluxation of L2/L3 lumbar vertebra**

√7th **S33.121 Dislocation of L2/L3 lumbar vertebra**

√6th **S33.13 Subluxation and dislocation of L3/L4 lumbar vertebra**

√7th **S33.13Ø Subluxation of L3/L4 lumbar vertebra**

√7th **S33.131 Dislocation of L3/L4 lumbar vertebra**

√6th **S33.14 Subluxation and dislocation of L4/L5 lumbar vertebra**

√7th **S33.14Ø Subluxation of L4/L5 lumbar vertebra**

√7th **S33.141 Dislocation of L4/L5 lumbar vertebra**

√x7th **S33.2 Dislocation of sacroiliac and sacrococcygeal joint**

√5th **S33.3 Dislocation of other and unspecified parts of lumbar spine and pelvis**

√x7th **S33.3Ø Dislocation of unspecified parts of lumbar spine and pelvis**

√x7th **S33.39 Dislocation of other parts of lumbar spine and pelvis**

√x7th **S33.4 Traumatic rupture of symphysis pubis**

√x7th **S33.5 Sprain of ligaments of lumbar spine**

√x7th **S33.6 Sprain of sacroiliac joint**

√x7th **S33.8 Sprain of other parts of lumbar spine and pelvis**

√x7th **S33.9 Sprain of unspecified parts of lumbar spine and pelvis**

√4th **S34 Injury of lumbar and sacral spinal cord and nerves at abdomen, lower back and pelvis level**

NOTE Code to highest level of lumbar cord injury.
Injuries to the spinal cord (S34.Ø and S34.1) refer to the cord level and not bone level injury, and can affect nerve roots at and below the level given.

Code also any associated:
fracture of vertebra (S22.Ø-, S32.Ø-)
open wound of abdomen, lower back and pelvis (S31.-)
transient paralysis (R29.5)

The appropriate 7th character is to be added to each code from category S34.
A initial encounter
D subsequent encounter
S sequela

√5th **S34.Ø Concussion and edema of lumbar and sacral spinal cord**

√x7th **S34.Ø1 Concussion and edema of lumbar spinal cord** MCC HCC

√x7th **S34.Ø2 Concussion and edema of sacral spinal cord** MCC HCC

Concussion and edema of conus medullaris

√5th **S34.1 Other and unspecified injury of lumbar and sacral spinal cord**

√6th **S34.1Ø Unspecified injury to lumbar spinal cord**

√7th **S34.1Ø1 Unspecified injury to L1 level of lumbar spinal cord** MCC H5 HCC

Unspecified injury to lumbar spinal cord level 1

√7th **S34.1Ø2 Unspecified injury to L2 level of lumbar spinal cord** MCC H5 HCC

Unspecified injury to lumbar spinal cord level 2

√7th **S34.1Ø3 Unspecified injury to L3 level of lumbar spinal cord** MCC H5 HCC

Unspecified injury to lumbar spinal cord level 3

√7th **S34.1Ø4 Unspecified injury to L4 level of lumbar spinal cord** MCC H5 HCC

Unspecified injury to lumbar spinal cord level 4

√7th **S34.1Ø5 Unspecified injury to L5 level of lumbar spinal cord** MCC H5 HCC

Unspecified injury to lumbar spinal cord level 5

√7th **S34.1Ø9 Unspecified injury to unspecified level of lumbar spinal cord** MCC H5 HCC

√6th **S34.11 Complete lesion of lumbar spinal cord**

√7th **S34.111 Complete lesion of L1 level of lumbar spinal cord** MCC H5 HCC

Complete lesion of lumbar spinal cord level 1

√7th **S34.112 Complete lesion of L2 level of lumbar spinal cord** MCC H5 HCC

Complete lesion of lumbar spinal cord level 2

√7th **S34.113 Complete lesion of L3 level of lumbar spinal cord** MCC H5 HCC

Complete lesion of lumbar spinal cord level 3

√7th **S34.114 Complete lesion of L4 level of lumbar spinal cord** MCC H5 HCC

Complete lesion of lumbar spinal cord level 4

√7th **S34.115 Complete lesion of L5 level of lumbar spinal cord** MCC H5 HCC

Complete lesion of lumbar spinal cord level 5

√7th **S34.119 Complete lesion of unspecified level of lumbar spinal cord** MCC H5 HCC

√6th S34.12 **Incomplete lesion of lumbar spinal cord**

√7th S34.121 **Incomplete lesion of L1 level of lumbar spinal cord** MCC H5 HCC
Incomplete lesion of lumbar spinal cord level 1

√7th S34.122 **Incomplete lesion of L2 level of lumbar spinal cord** MCC H5 HCC
Incomplete lesion of lumbar spinal cord level 2

√7th S34.123 **Incomplete lesion of L3 level of lumbar spinal cord** MCC H5 HCC
Incomplete lesion of lumbar spinal cord level 3

√7th S34.124 **Incomplete lesion of L4 level of lumbar spinal cord** MCC H5 HCC
Incomplete lesion of lumbar spinal cord level 4

√7th S34.125 **Incomplete lesion of L5 level of lumbar spinal cord** MCC H5 HCC
Incomplete lesion of lumbar spinal cord level 5

√7th S34.129 **Incomplete lesion of unspecified level of lumbar spinal cord** MCC H5 HCC

√6th S34.13 **Other and unspecified injury to sacral spinal cord**
Other injury to conus medullaris

√7th S34.131 **Complete lesion of sacral spinal cord** MCC H5 HCC
Complete lesion of conus medullaris

√7th S34.132 **Incomplete lesion of sacral spinal cord** MCC H5 HCC
Incomplete lesion of conus medullaris

√7th S34.139 **Unspecified injury to sacral spinal cord** MCC H5 HCC
Unspecified injury of conus medullaris

√5th S34.2 **Injury of nerve root of lumbar and sacral spine**

√x7th S34.21 **Injury of nerve root of lumbar spine**

√x7th S34.22 **Injury of nerve root of sacral spine**

6 √x7th S34.3 **Injury of cauda equina** MCC H5 HCC

√x7th S34.4 **Injury of lumbosacral plexus**

√x7th S34.5 **Injury of lumbar, sacral and pelvic sympathetic nerves**
Injury of celiac ganglion or plexus
Injury of hypogastric plexus
Injury of mesenteric plexus (inferior) (superior)
Injury of splanchnic nerve

√x7th S34.6 **Injury of peripheral nerve(s) at abdomen, lower back and pelvis level**

√x7th S34.8 **Injury of other nerves at abdomen, lower back and pelvis level**

√x7th S34.9 **Injury of unspecified nerves at abdomen, lower back and pelvis level**

√4th **S35 Injury of blood vessels at abdomen, lower back and pelvis level**
Code also any associated open wound (S31.-)

The appropriate 7th character is to be added to each code from category S35.
A initial encounter
D subsequent encounter
S sequela

√5th S35.Ø **Injury of abdominal aorta**
EXCLUDES 1 *injury of aorta NOS (S25.Ø)*

√x7th S35.ØØ **Unspecified injury of abdominal aorta** MCC

√x7th S35.Ø1 **Minor laceration of abdominal aorta** MCC
Incomplete transection of abdominal aorta
Laceration of abdominal aorta NOS
Superficial laceration of abdominal aorta

√x7th S35.Ø2 **Major laceration of abdominal aorta** MCC
Complete transection of abdominal aorta
Traumatic rupture of abdominal aorta

√x7th S35.Ø9 **Other injury of abdominal aorta** MCC

√5th S35.1 **Injury of inferior vena cava**
Injury of hepatic vein
EXCLUDES 1 *injury of vena cava NOS (S25.2)*

√x7th S35.1Ø **Unspecified injury of inferior vena cava** MCC

√x7th S35.11 **Minor laceration of inferior vena cava** MCC
Incomplete transection of inferior vena cava
Laceration of inferior vena cava NOS
Superficial laceration of inferior vena cava

√x7th S35.12 **Major laceration of inferior vena cava** MCC
Complete transection of inferior vena cava
Traumatic rupture of inferior vena cava

√x7th S35.19 **Other injury of inferior vena cava** MCC

√5th S35.2 **Injury of celiac or mesenteric artery and branches**

√6th S35.21 **Injury of celiac artery**

√7th S35.211 **Minor laceration of celiac artery** MCC
Incomplete transection of celiac artery
Laceration of celiac artery NOS
Superficial laceration of celiac artery

√7th S35.212 **Major laceration of celiac artery** MCC
Complete transection of celiac artery
Traumatic rupture of celiac artery

√7th S35.218 **Other injury of celiac artery** MCC

√7th S35.219 **Unspecified injury of celiac artery** MCC

√6th S35.22 **Injury of superior mesenteric artery**

√7th S35.221 **Minor laceration of superior mesenteric artery** MCC
Incomplete transection of superior mesenteric artery
Laceration of superior mesenteric artery NOS
Superficial laceration of superior mesenteric artery

√7th S35.222 **Major laceration of superior mesenteric artery** MCC
Complete transection of superior mesenteric artery
Traumatic rupture of superior mesenteric artery

√7th S35.228 **Other injury of superior mesenteric artery** MCC

√7th S35.229 **Unspecified injury of superior mesenteric artery** MCC

√6th S35.23 **Injury of inferior mesenteric artery**

√7th S35.231 **Minor laceration of inferior mesenteric artery** MCC
Incomplete transection of inferior mesenteric artery
Laceration of inferior mesenteric artery NOS
Superficial laceration of inferior mesenteric artery

√7th S35.232 **Major laceration of inferior mesenteric artery** MCC
Complete transection of inferior mesenteric artery
Traumatic rupture of inferior mesenteric artery

√7th S35.238 **Other injury of inferior mesenteric artery** MCC

√7th S35.239 **Unspecified injury of inferior mesenteric artery** MCC

√6th S35.29 **Injury of branches of celiac and mesenteric artery**
Injury of gastric artery
Injury of gastroduodenal artery
Injury of hepatic artery
Injury of splenic artery

√7th S35.291 **Minor laceration of branches of celiac and mesenteric artery** MCC
Incomplete transection of branches of celiac and mesenteric artery
Laceration of branches of celiac and mesenteric artery NOS
Superficial laceration of branches of celiac and mesenteric artery

√7th S35.292 **Major laceration of branches of celiac and mesenteric artery** MCC
Complete transection of branches of celiac and mesenteric artery
Traumatic rupture of branches of celiac and mesenteric artery

S35.298 Other injury of branches of celiac and mesenteric artery MCC
S35.299 Unspecified injury of branches of celiac and mesenteric artery MCC

S35.3 Injury of portal or splenic vein and branches
S35.31 Injury of portal vein
S35.311 Laceration of portal vein MCC
S35.318 Other specified injury of portal vein MCC
S35.319 Unspecified injury of portal vein MCC
S35.32 Injury of splenic vein
S35.321 Laceration of splenic vein MCC
S35.328 Other specified injury of splenic vein MCC
S35.329 Unspecified injury of splenic vein MCC
S35.33 Injury of superior mesenteric vein
S35.331 Laceration of superior mesenteric vein MCC
S35.338 Other specified injury of superior mesenteric vein MCC
S35.339 Unspecified injury of superior mesenteric vein MCC
S35.34 Injury of inferior mesenteric vein
S35.341 Laceration of inferior mesenteric vein MCC
S35.348 Other specified injury of inferior mesenteric vein MCC
S35.349 Unspecified injury of inferior mesenteric vein MCC

S35.4 Injury of renal blood vessels
S35.40 Unspecified injury of renal blood vessel
S35.401 Unspecified injury of right renal artery MCC
S35.402 Unspecified injury of left renal artery MCC
S35.403 Unspecified injury of unspecified renal artery MCC
S35.404 Unspecified injury of right renal vein MCC
S35.405 Unspecified injury of left renal vein MCC
S35.406 Unspecified injury of unspecified renal vein MCC
S35.41 Laceration of renal blood vessel
S35.411 Laceration of right renal artery MCC
S35.412 Laceration of left renal artery MCC
S35.413 Laceration of unspecified renal artery MCC
S35.414 Laceration of right renal vein MCC
S35.415 Laceration of left renal vein MCC
S35.416 Laceration of unspecified renal vein MCC
S35.49 Other specified injury of renal blood vessel
S35.491 Other specified injury of right renal artery MCC
S35.492 Other specified injury of left renal artery MCC
S35.493 Other specified injury of unspecified renal artery MCC
S35.494 Other specified injury of right renal vein MCC
S35.495 Other specified injury of left renal vein MCC
S35.496 Other specified injury of unspecified renal vein MCC

S35.5 Injury of iliac blood vessels
S35.50 Injury of unspecified iliac blood vessel(s) MCC
S35.51 Injury of iliac artery or vein
Injury of hypogastric artery or vein
S35.511 Injury of right iliac artery MCC
S35.512 Injury of left iliac artery MCC
S35.513 Injury of unspecified iliac artery MCC
S35.514 Injury of right iliac vein MCC
S35.515 Injury of left iliac vein MCC
S35.516 Injury of unspecified iliac vein MCC
S35.53 Injury of uterine artery or vein
S35.531 Injury of right uterine artery CC ♀
S35.532 Injury of left uterine artery CC ♀
S35.533 Injury of unspecified uterine artery CC ♀
S35.534 Injury of right uterine vein CC ♀
S35.535 Injury of left uterine vein CC ♀
S35.536 Injury of unspecified uterine vein CC ♀
S35.59 Injury of other iliac blood vessels MCC

S35.8 Injury of other blood vessels at abdomen, lower back and pelvis level
Injury of ovarian artery or vein
S35.8X Injury of other blood vessels at abdomen, lower back and pelvis level
S35.8X1 Laceration of other blood vessels at abdomen, lower back and pelvis level CC
S35.8X8 Other specified injury of other blood vessels at abdomen, lower back and pelvis level CC
S35.8X9 Unspecified injury of other blood vessels at abdomen, lower back and pelvis level CC

S35.9 Injury of unspecified blood vessel at abdomen, lower back and pelvis level
S35.90 Unspecified injury of unspecified blood vessel at abdomen, lower back and pelvis level CC
S35.91 Laceration of unspecified blood vessel at abdomen, lower back and pelvis level CC
S35.99 Other specified injury of unspecified blood vessel at abdomen, lower back and pelvis level CC

S36 Injury of intra-abdominal organs
Code also any associated open wound (S31.-)

The appropriate 7th character is to be added to each code from category S36.
A initial encounter
D subsequent encounter
S sequela

S36.0 Injury of spleen
AHA: 2015,2Q,36; 2015,1Q,10
S36.00 Unspecified injury of spleen CC
S36.02 Contusion of spleen
TIP: When both traumatic splenic laceration and contusion are documented in the same encounter, code only the laceration, as contusions are not coded when they occur with a more severe injury in the same body site.
S36.020 Minor contusion of spleen CC
Contusion of spleen less than 2 cm
S36.021 Major contusion of spleen CC
Contusion of spleen greater than 2 cm
S36.029 Unspecified contusion of spleen CC
S36.03 Laceration of spleen
TIP: When both traumatic splenic laceration and contusion are documented in the same encounter, code only the laceration, as contusions are not coded when they occur with a more severe injury in the same body site.
S36.030 Superficial (capsular) laceration of spleen CC
Laceration of spleen less than 1 cm
Minor laceration of spleen
S36.031 Moderate laceration of spleen MCC
Laceration of spleen 1 to 3 cm
S36.032 Major laceration of spleen MCC
Avulsion of spleen
Laceration of spleen greater than 3 cm
Massive laceration of spleen
Multiple moderate lacerations of spleen
Stellate laceration of spleen
S36.039 Unspecified laceration of spleen CC
S36.09 Other injury of spleen CC

Chapter 19. Injury, Poisoning and Certain Other Consequences of External Causes
S35.298–S36.09

√5th S36.1 Injury of liver and gallbladder and bile duct
√6th S36.11 Injury of liver
√7th S36.112 Contusion of liver CC
√7th S36.113 Laceration of liver, unspecified degree CC
√7th S36.114 Minor laceration of liver CC
Laceration involving capsule only, or, without significant involvement of hepatic parenchyma [i.e., less than 1 cm deep]
√7th S36.115 Moderate laceration of liver MCC
Laceration involving parenchyma but without major disruption of parenchyma [i.e., less than 10 cm long and less than 3 cm deep]
√7th S36.116 Major laceration of liver MCC
Laceration with significant disruption of hepatic parenchyma [i.e., greater than 10 cm long and 3 cm deep]
Multiple moderate lacerations, with or without hematoma
Stellate laceration of liver
√7th S36.118 Other injury of liver CC
√7th S36.119 Unspecified injury of liver CC
√6th S36.12 Injury of gallbladder
√7th S36.122 Contusion of gallbladder CC
√7th S36.123 Laceration of gallbladder CC
√7th S36.128 Other injury of gallbladder CC
√7th S36.129 Unspecified injury of gallbladder CC
√x7th S36.13 Injury of bile duct CC
√5th S36.2 Injury of pancreas
√6th S36.20 Unspecified injury of pancreas
√7th S36.200 Unspecified injury of head of pancreas CC
√7th S36.201 Unspecified injury of body of pancreas CC
√7th S36.202 Unspecified injury of tail of pancreas CC
√7th S36.209 Unspecified injury of unspecified part of pancreas CC
√6th S36.22 Contusion of pancreas
√7th S36.220 Contusion of head of pancreas CC
√7th S36.221 Contusion of body of pancreas CC
√7th S36.222 Contusion of tail of pancreas CC
√7th S36.229 Contusion of unspecified part of pancreas CC
√6th S36.23 Laceration of pancreas, unspecified degree
√7th S36.230 Laceration of head of pancreas, unspecified degree CC
√7th S36.231 Laceration of body of pancreas, unspecified degree CC
√7th S36.232 Laceration of tail of pancreas, unspecified degree CC
√7th S36.239 Laceration of unspecified part of pancreas, unspecified degree CC
√6th S36.24 Minor laceration of pancreas
√7th S36.240 Minor laceration of head of pancreas CC
√7th S36.241 Minor laceration of body of pancreas CC
√7th S36.242 Minor laceration of tail of pancreas CC
√7th S36.249 Minor laceration of unspecified part of pancreas CC
√6th S36.25 Moderate laceration of pancreas
√7th S36.250 Moderate laceration of head of pancreas CC
√7th S36.251 Moderate laceration of body of pancreas CC
√7th S36.252 Moderate laceration of tail of pancreas CC
√7th S36.259 Moderate laceration of unspecified part of pancreas CC
√6th S36.26 Major laceration of pancreas
√7th S36.260 Major laceration of head of pancreas CC
√7th S36.261 Major laceration of body of pancreas CC
√7th S36.262 Major laceration of tail of pancreas CC
√7th S36.269 Major laceration of unspecified part of pancreas CC
√6th S36.29 Other injury of pancreas
√7th S36.290 Other injury of head of pancreas CC
√7th S36.291 Other injury of body of pancreas CC
√7th S36.292 Other injury of tail of pancreas CC
√7th S36.299 Other injury of unspecified part of pancreas CC
√5th S36.3 Injury of stomach
√x7th S36.30 Unspecified injury of stomach CC
√x7th S36.32 Contusion of stomach CC
√x7th S36.33 Laceration of stomach CC
√x7th S36.39 Other injury of stomach CC
√5th S36.4 Injury of small intestine
√6th S36.40 Unspecified injury of small intestine
√7th S36.400 Unspecified injury of duodenum CC
√7th S36.408 Unspecified injury of other part of small intestine CC
√7th S36.409 Unspecified injury of unspecified part of small intestine CC
√6th S36.41 Primary blast injury of small intestine
Blast injury of small intestine NOS
√7th S36.410 Primary blast injury of duodenum CC
√7th S36.418 Primary blast injury of other part of small intestine CC
√7th S36.419 Primary blast injury of unspecified part of small intestine CC
√6th S36.42 Contusion of small intestine
√7th S36.420 Contusion of duodenum CC
√7th S36.428 Contusion of other part of small intestine CC
√7th S36.429 Contusion of unspecified part of small intestine CC
√6th S36.43 Laceration of small intestine
√7th S36.430 Laceration of duodenum CC
√7th S36.438 Laceration of other part of small intestine CC
√7th S36.439 Laceration of unspecified part of small intestine CC
√6th S36.49 Other injury of small intestine
√7th S36.490 Other injury of duodenum CC
√7th S36.498 Other injury of other part of small intestine CC
√7th S36.499 Other injury of unspecified part of small intestine CC
√5th S36.5 Injury of colon
EXCLUDES 2 *injury of rectum (S36.6-)*
√6th S36.50 Unspecified injury of colon
√7th S36.500 Unspecified injury of ascending [right] colon CC
√7th S36.501 Unspecified injury of transverse colon CC
√7th S36.502 Unspecified injury of descending [left] colon CC
√7th S36.503 Unspecified injury of sigmoid colon CC
√7th S36.508 Unspecified injury of other part of colon CC
√7th S36.509 Unspecified injury of unspecified part of colon CC
√6th S36.51 Primary blast injury of colon
Blast injury of colon NOS
√7th S36.510 Primary blast injury of ascending [right] colon CC
√7th S36.511 Primary blast injury of transverse colon CC
√7th S36.512 Primary blast injury of descending [left] colon CC
√7th S36.513 Primary blast injury of sigmoid colon CC
√7th S36.518 Primary blast injury of other part of colon CC

S36.519 Primary blast injury of unspecified part of colon CC

S36.52 Contusion of colon

S36.52Ø Contusion of ascending [right] colon CC

S36.521 Contusion of transverse colon CC

S36.522 Contusion of descending [left] colon CC

S36.523 Contusion of sigmoid colon CC

S36.528 Contusion of other part of colon CC

S36.529 Contusion of unspecified part of colon CC

S36.53 Laceration of colon

S36.53Ø Laceration of ascending [right] colon CC

S36.531 Laceration of transverse colon CC

S36.532 Laceration of descending [left] colon CC

S36.533 Laceration of sigmoid colon CC

S36.538 Laceration of other part of colon CC

S36.539 Laceration of unspecified part of colon CC

S36.59 Other injury of colon

Secondary blast injury of colon

S36.59Ø Other injury of ascending [right] colon CC

S36.591 Other injury of transverse colon CC

S36.592 Other injury of descending [left] colon CC

S36.593 Other injury of sigmoid colon CC

S36.598 Other injury of other part of colon CC

S36.599 Other injury of unspecified part of colon CC

S36.6 Injury of rectum

S36.6Ø Unspecified injury of rectum CC

S36.61 Primary blast injury of rectum CC

Blast injury of rectum NOS

S36.62 Contusion of rectum CC

S36.63 Laceration of rectum CC

S36.69 Other injury of rectum CC

Secondary blast injury of rectum

S36.8 Injury of other intra-abdominal organs

S36.81 Injury of peritoneum CC

S36.89 Injury of other intra-abdominal organs

Injury of retroperitoneum

S36.892 Contusion of other intra-abdominal organs CC

S36.893 Laceration of other intra-abdominal organs CC

S36.898 Other injury of other intra-abdominal organs CC

S36.899 Unspecified injury of other intra-abdominal organs CC

S36.9 Injury of unspecified intra-abdominal organ

S36.9Ø Unspecified injury of unspecified intra-abdominal organ CC

S36.92 Contusion of unspecified intra-abdominal organ CC

S36.93 Laceration of unspecified intra-abdominal organ CC

S36.99 Other injury of unspecified intra-abdominal organ CC

S37 Injury of urinary and pelvic organs

Code also any associated open wound (S31.-)

EXCLUDES 1 *obstetric trauma to pelvic organs (O71.-)*

EXCLUDES 2 *injury of peritoneum (S36.81)*
injury of retroperitoneum (S36.89-)

The appropriate 7th character is to be added to each code from category S37.
A initial encounter
D subsequent encounter
S sequela

S37.Ø Injury of kidney

EXCLUDES 2 *acute kidney injury (nontraumatic) (N17.9)*

S37.ØØ Unspecified injury of kidney

S37.ØØ1 Unspecified injury of right kidney CC

S37.ØØ2 Unspecified injury of left kidney CC

S37.ØØ9 Unspecified injury of unspecified kidney CC

S37.Ø1 Minor contusion of kidney

Contusion of kidney less than 2 cm
Contusion of kidney NOS

S37.Ø11 Minor contusion of right kidney CC

S37.Ø12 Minor contusion of left kidney CC

S37.Ø19 Minor contusion of unspecified kidney CC

S37.Ø2 Major contusion of kidney

Contusion of kidney greater than 2 cm

S37.Ø21 Major contusion of right kidney CC

S37.Ø22 Major contusion of left kidney CC

S37.Ø29 Major contusion of unspecified kidney CC

S37.Ø3 Laceration of kidney, unspecified degree

S37.Ø31 Laceration of right kidney, unspecified degree CC

S37.Ø32 Laceration of left kidney, unspecified degree CC

S37.Ø39 Laceration of unspecified kidney, unspecified degree CC

S37.Ø4 Minor laceration of kidney

Laceration of kidney less than 1 cm

S37.Ø41 Minor laceration of right kidney CC

S37.Ø42 Minor laceration of left kidney CC

S37.Ø49 Minor laceration of unspecified kidney CC

S37.Ø5 Moderate laceration of kidney

Laceration of kidney 1 to 3 cm

S37.Ø51 Moderate laceration of right kidney CC

S37.Ø52 Moderate laceration of left kidney CC

S37.Ø59 Moderate laceration of unspecified kidney CC

S37.Ø6 Major laceration of kidney

Avulsion of kidney
Laceration of kidney greater than 3 cm
Massive laceration of kidney
Multiple moderate lacerations of kidney
Stellate laceration of kidney

S37.Ø61 Major laceration of right kidney MCC

S37.Ø62 Major laceration of left kidney MCC

S37.Ø69 Major laceration of unspecified kidney MCC

S37.Ø9 Other injury of kidney

S37.Ø91 Other injury of right kidney MCC

S37.Ø92 Other injury of left kidney MCC

S37.Ø99 Other injury of unspecified kidney MCC

S37.1 Injury of ureter

S37.1Ø Unspecified injury of ureter CC

S37.12 Contusion of ureter CC

S37.13 Laceration of ureter CC

S37.19 Other injury of ureter CC

S37.2 Injury of bladder

S37.2Ø Unspecified injury of bladder CC

√x7th S37.22 Contusion of bladder CC
√x7th S37.23 Laceration of bladder CC
√x7th S37.29 Other injury of bladder CC
√5th S37.3 Injury of urethra
√x7th S37.30 Unspecified injury of urethra CC
√x7th S37.32 Contusion of urethra CC
√x7th S37.33 Laceration of urethra CC
√x7th S37.39 Other injury of urethra CC
√5th S37.4 Injury of ovary
√6th S37.40 Unspecified injury of ovary
√7th S37.401 Unspecified injury of ovary, unilateral ♀
√7th S37.402 Unspecified injury of ovary, bilateral ♀
√7th S37.409 Unspecified injury of ovary, unspecified ♀
√6th S37.42 Contusion of ovary
√7th S37.421 Contusion of ovary, unilateral ♀
√7th S37.422 Contusion of ovary, bilateral ♀
√7th S37.429 Contusion of ovary, unspecified ♀
√6th S37.43 Laceration of ovary
√7th S37.431 Laceration of ovary, unilateral ♀
√7th S37.432 Laceration of ovary, bilateral ♀
√7th S37.439 Laceration of ovary, unspecified ♀
√6th S37.49 Other injury of ovary
√7th S37.491 Other injury of ovary, unilateral ♀
√7th S37.492 Other injury of ovary, bilateral ♀
√7th S37.499 Other injury of ovary, unspecified ♀
√5th S37.5 Injury of fallopian tube
√6th S37.50 Unspecified injury of fallopian tube
√7th S37.501 Unspecified injury of fallopian tube, unilateral ♀
√7th S37.502 Unspecified injury of fallopian tube, bilateral ♀
√7th S37.509 Unspecified injury of fallopian tube, unspecified ♀
√6th S37.51 Primary blast injury of fallopian tube
Blast injury of fallopian tube NOS
√7th S37.511 Primary blast injury of fallopian tube, unilateral ♀
√7th S37.512 Primary blast injury of fallopian tube, bilateral ♀
√7th S37.519 Primary blast injury of fallopian tube, unspecified ♀
√6th S37.52 Contusion of fallopian tube
√7th S37.521 Contusion of fallopian tube, unilateral ♀
√7th S37.522 Contusion of fallopian tube, bilateral ♀
√7th S37.529 Contusion of fallopian tube, unspecified ♀
√6th S37.53 Laceration of fallopian tube
√7th S37.531 Laceration of fallopian tube, unilateral ♀
√7th S37.532 Laceration of fallopian tube, bilateral ♀
√7th S37.539 Laceration of fallopian tube, unspecified ♀
√6th S37.59 Other injury of fallopian tube
Secondary blast injury of fallopian tube
√7th S37.591 Other injury of fallopian tube, unilateral ♀
√7th S37.592 Other injury of fallopian tube, bilateral ♀
√7th S37.599 Other injury of fallopian tube, unspecified ♀
√5th S37.6 Injury of uterus
EXCLUDES 1 *injury to gravid uterus (O9A.2-)*
injury to uterus during delivery (O71.-)
√x7th S37.60 Unspecified injury of uterus CC ♀
√x7th S37.62 Contusion of uterus CC ♀
√x7th S37.63 Laceration of uterus CC ♀
√x7th S37.69 Other injury of uterus CC ♀
√5th S37.8 Injury of other urinary and pelvic organs
√6th S37.81 Injury of adrenal gland
√7th S37.812 Contusion of adrenal gland CC
√7th S37.813 Laceration of adrenal gland CC
√7th S37.818 Other injury of adrenal gland CC
√7th S37.819 Unspecified injury of adrenal gland CC
√6th S37.82 Injury of prostate
√7th S37.822 Contusion of prostate ♂
√7th S37.823 Laceration of prostate ♂
√7th S37.828 Other injury of prostate ♂
√7th S37.829 Unspecified injury of prostate ♂
√6th S37.89 Injury of other urinary and pelvic organ
√7th S37.892 Contusion of other urinary and pelvic organ CC
√7th S37.893 Laceration of other urinary and pelvic organ CC
√7th S37.898 Other injury of other urinary and pelvic organ CC
√7th S37.899 Unspecified injury of other urinary and pelvic organ CC
√5th S37.9 Injury of unspecified urinary and pelvic organ
√x7th S37.90 Unspecified injury of unspecified urinary and pelvic organ CC
√x7th S37.92 Contusion of unspecified urinary and pelvic organ CC
√x7th S37.93 Laceration of unspecified urinary and pelvic organ CC
√x7th S37.99 Other injury of unspecified urinary and pelvic organ CC

√4th **S38 Crushing injury and traumatic amputation of abdomen, lower back, pelvis and external genitals**
NOTE An amputation not identified as partial or complete should be coded to complete

The appropriate 7th character is to be added to each code from category S38.
A initial encounter
D subsequent encounter
S sequela

√5th S38.0 Crushing injury of external genital organs
Use additional code for any associated injuries
√6th S38.00 Crushing injury of unspecified external genital organs
√7th S38.001 Crushing injury of unspecified external genital organs, male ♂
√7th S38.002 Crushing injury of unspecified external genital organs, female ♀
√x7th S38.01 Crushing injury of penis ♂
√x7th S38.02 Crushing injury of scrotum and testis ♂
√x7th S38.03 Crushing injury of vulva ♀
√x7th S38.1 Crushing injury of abdomen, lower back, and pelvis
Use additional code for all associated injuries, such as:
fracture of thoracic or lumbar spine and pelvis (S22.0-, S32.-)
injury to intra-abdominal organs (S36.-)
injury to urinary and pelvic organs (S37.-)
open wound of abdominal wall (S31.-)
spinal cord injury (S34.0, S34.1-)
EXCLUDES 2 *crushing injury of external genital organs (S38.0-)*
√5th S38.2 Traumatic amputation of external genital organs
√6th S38.21 Traumatic amputation of female external genital organs
Traumatic amputation of clitoris
Traumatic amputation of labium (majus) (minus)
Traumatic amputation of vulva
√7th S38.211 Complete traumatic amputation of female external genital organs ♀
√7th S38.212 Partial traumatic amputation of female external genital organs ♀
√6th S38.22 Traumatic amputation of penis
√7th S38.221 Complete traumatic amputation of penis ♂
√7th S38.222 Partial traumatic amputation of penis ♂

S38.23 Traumatic amputation of scrotum and testis
S38.231 Complete traumatic amputation of scrotum and testis ♂
S38.232 Partial traumatic amputation of scrotum and testis ♂
S38.3 Transection (partial) of abdomen

S39 Other and unspecified injuries of abdomen, lower back, pelvis and external genitals
Code also any associated open wound (S31.-)
EXCLUDES 2 *sprain of joints and ligaments of lumbar spine and pelvis (S33.-)*

The appropriate 7th character is to be added to each code from category S39.
A initial encounter
D subsequent encounter
S sequela

S39.0 Injury of muscle, fascia and tendon of abdomen, lower back and pelvis
S39.00 Unspecified injury of muscle, fascia and tendon of abdomen, lower back and pelvis
S39.001 Unspecified injury of muscle, fascia and tendon of abdomen
S39.002 Unspecified injury of muscle, fascia and tendon of lower back
S39.003 Unspecified injury of muscle, fascia and tendon of pelvis
S39.01 Strain of muscle, fascia and tendon of abdomen, lower back and pelvis
S39.011 Strain of muscle, fascia and tendon of abdomen
S39.012 Strain of muscle, fascia and tendon of lower back
S39.013 Strain of muscle, fascia and tendon of pelvis
S39.02 Laceration of muscle, fascia and tendon of abdomen, lower back and pelvis
S39.021 Laceration of muscle, fascia and tendon of abdomen
S39.022 Laceration of muscle, fascia and tendon of lower back
S39.023 Laceration of muscle, fascia and tendon of pelvis
S39.09 Other injury of muscle, fascia and tendon of abdomen, lower back and pelvis
S39.091 Other injury of muscle, fascia and tendon of abdomen
S39.092 Other injury of muscle, fascia and tendon of lower back
S39.093 Other injury of muscle, fascia and tendon of pelvis
S39.8 Other specified injuries of abdomen, lower back, pelvis and external genitals
S39.81 Other specified injuries of abdomen
S39.82 Other specified injuries of lower back
S39.83 Other specified injuries of pelvis
S39.84 Other specified injuries of external genitals
S39.840 Fracture of corpus cavernosum penis ♂
S39.848 Other specified injuries of external genitals
TIP: Assign for traumatic rupture of testis.
S39.9 Unspecified injury of abdomen, lower back, pelvis and external genitals
S39.91 Unspecified injury of abdomen
S39.92 Unspecified injury of lower back
S39.93 Unspecified injury of pelvis
S39.94 Unspecified injury of external genitals

Injuries to the shoulder and upper arm (S40-S49)

INCLUDES injuries of axilla
injuries of scapular region
EXCLUDES 2 *burns and corrosions (T20-T32)*
frostbite (T33-T34)
injuries of elbow (S50-S59)
insect bite or sting, venomous (T63.4)

S40 Superficial injury of shoulder and upper arm

The appropriate 7th character is to be added to each code from category S40.
A initial encounter
D subsequent encounter
S sequela

S40.0 Contusion of shoulder and upper arm
S40.01 Contusion of shoulder
S40.011 Contusion of right shoulder
S40.012 Contusion of left shoulder
S40.019 Contusion of unspecified shoulder
S40.02 Contusion of upper arm
S40.021 Contusion of right upper arm
S40.022 Contusion of left upper arm
S40.029 Contusion of unspecified upper arm
S40.2 Other superficial injuries of shoulder
S40.21 Abrasion of shoulder
S40.211 Abrasion of right shoulder
S40.212 Abrasion of left shoulder
S40.219 Abrasion of unspecified shoulder
S40.22 Blister (nonthermal) of shoulder
S40.221 Blister (nonthermal) of right shoulder
S40.222 Blister (nonthermal) of left shoulder
S40.229 Blister (nonthermal) of unspecified shoulder
S40.24 External constriction of shoulder
S40.241 External constriction of right shoulder
S40.242 External constriction of left shoulder
S40.249 External constriction of unspecified shoulder
S40.25 Superficial foreign body of shoulder
Splinter in the shoulder
S40.251 Superficial foreign body of right shoulder
S40.252 Superficial foreign body of left shoulder
S40.259 Superficial foreign body of unspecified shoulder
S40.26 Insect bite (nonvenomous) of shoulder
S40.261 Insect bite (nonvenomous) of right shoulder
S40.262 Insect bite (nonvenomous) of left shoulder
S40.269 Insect bite (nonvenomous) of unspecified shoulder
S40.27 Other superficial bite of shoulder
EXCLUDES 1 *open bite of shoulder (S41.05)*
S40.271 Other superficial bite of right shoulder
S40.272 Other superficial bite of left shoulder
S40.279 Other superficial bite of unspecified shoulder
S40.8 Other superficial injuries of upper arm
S40.81 Abrasion of upper arm
S40.811 Abrasion of right upper arm
S40.812 Abrasion of left upper arm
S40.819 Abrasion of unspecified upper arm
S40.82 Blister (nonthermal) of upper arm
S40.821 Blister (nonthermal) of right upper arm
S40.822 Blister (nonthermal) of left upper arm
S40.829 Blister (nonthermal) of unspecified upper arm
S40.84 External constriction of upper arm
S40.841 External constriction of right upper arm
S40.842 External constriction of left upper arm

7th **S40.849** **External constriction of unspecified upper arm**

6th **S40.85** **Superficial foreign body of upper arm**

Splinter in the upper arm

7th **S40.851** **Superficial foreign body of right upper arm**

7th **S40.852** **Superficial foreign body of left upper arm**

7th **S40.859** **Superficial foreign body of unspecified upper arm**

6th **S40.86** **Insect bite (nonvenomous) of upper arm**

7th **S40.861** **Insect bite (nonvenomous) of right upper arm**

7th **S40.862** **Insect bite (nonvenomous) of left upper arm**

7th **S40.869** **Insect bite (nonvenomous) of unspecified upper arm**

6th **S40.87** **Other superficial bite of upper arm**

EXCLUDES 1 *open bite of upper arm (S41.14)*

EXCLUDES 2 *other superficial bite of shoulder (S40.27-)*

7th **S40.871** **Other superficial bite of right upper arm**

7th **S40.872** **Other superficial bite of left upper arm**

7th **S40.879** **Other superficial bite of unspecified upper arm**

5th **S40.9** **Unspecified superficial injury of shoulder and upper arm**

6th **S40.91** **Unspecified superficial injury of shoulder**

7th **S40.911** **Unspecified superficial injury of right shoulder**

7th **S40.912** **Unspecified superficial injury of left shoulder**

7th **S40.919** **Unspecified superficial injury of unspecified shoulder**

6th **S40.92** **Unspecified superficial injury of upper arm**

7th **S40.921** **Unspecified superficial injury of right upper arm**

7th **S40.922** **Unspecified superficial injury of left upper arm**

7th **S40.929** **Unspecified superficial injury of unspecified upper arm**

4th **S41** **Open wound of shoulder and upper arm**

Code also any associated wound infection

EXCLUDES 1 *traumatic amputation of shoulder and upper arm (S48.-)*

EXCLUDES 2 *open fracture of shoulder and upper arm (S42.- with 7th character B or C)*

The appropriate 7th character is to be added to each code from category S41.
A initial encounter
D subsequent encounter
S sequela

5th **S41.0** **Open wound of shoulder**

6th **S41.00** **Unspecified open wound of shoulder**

7th **S41.001** **Unspecified open wound of right shoulder**

7th **S41.002** **Unspecified open wound of left shoulder**

7th **S41.009** **Unspecified open wound of unspecified shoulder**

6th **S41.01** **Laceration without foreign body of shoulder**

7th **S41.011** **Laceration without foreign body of right shoulder**

7th **S41.012** **Laceration without foreign body of left shoulder**

7th **S41.019** **Laceration without foreign body of unspecified shoulder**

6th **S41.02** **Laceration with foreign body of shoulder**

7th **S41.021** **Laceration with foreign body of right shoulder**

7th **S41.022** **Laceration with foreign body of left shoulder**

7th **S41.029** **Laceration with foreign body of unspecified shoulder**

6th **S41.03** **Puncture wound without foreign body of shoulder**

7th **S41.031** **Puncture wound without foreign body of right shoulder**

7th **S41.032** **Puncture wound without foreign body of left shoulder**

7th **S41.039** **Puncture wound without foreign body of unspecified shoulder**

6th **S41.04** **Puncture wound with foreign body of shoulder**

7th **S41.041** **Puncture wound with foreign body of right shoulder**

7th **S41.042** **Puncture wound with foreign body of left shoulder**

7th **S41.049** **Puncture wound with foreign body of unspecified shoulder**

6th **S41.05** **Open bite of shoulder**

Bite of shoulder NOS

EXCLUDES 1 *superficial bite of shoulder (S40.27)*

7th **S41.051** **Open bite of right shoulder**

7th **S41.052** **Open bite of left shoulder**

7th **S41.059** **Open bite of unspecified shoulder**

5th **S41.1** **Open wound of upper arm**

6th **S41.10** **Unspecified open wound of upper arm**

AHA: 2016,3Q,24

7th **S41.101** **Unspecified open wound of right upper arm**

7th **S41.102** **Unspecified open wound of left upper arm**

7th **S41.109** **Unspecified open wound of unspecified upper arm**

6th **S41.11** **Laceration without foreign body of upper arm**

7th **S41.111** **Laceration without foreign body of right upper arm**

7th **S41.112** **Laceration without foreign body of left upper arm**

7th **S41.119** **Laceration without foreign body of unspecified upper arm**

6th **S41.12** **Laceration with foreign body of upper arm**

7th **S41.121** **Laceration with foreign body of right upper arm**

7th **S41.122** **Laceration with foreign body of left upper arm**

7th **S41.129** **Laceration with foreign body of unspecified upper arm**

6th **S41.13** **Puncture wound without foreign body of upper arm**

AHA: 2016,3Q,24

7th **S41.131** **Puncture wound without foreign body of right upper arm**

7th **S41.132** **Puncture wound without foreign body of left upper arm**

7th **S41.139** **Puncture wound without foreign body of unspecified upper arm**

6th **S41.14** **Puncture wound with foreign body of upper arm**

AHA: 2016,3Q,24

7th **S41.141** **Puncture wound with foreign body of right upper arm**

7th **S41.142** **Puncture wound with foreign body of left upper arm**

7th **S41.149** **Puncture wound with foreign body of unspecified upper arm**

6th **S41.15** **Open bite of upper arm**

Bite of upper arm NOS

EXCLUDES 1 *superficial bite of upper arm (S40.87)*

7th **S41.151** **Open bite of right upper arm**

7th **S41.152** **Open bite of left upper arm**

7th **S41.159** **Open bite of unspecified upper arm**

S42 Fracture of shoulder and upper arm

NOTE A fracture not indicated as displaced or nondisplaced should be coded to displaced

A fracture not indicated as open or closed should be coded to closed

EXCLUDES 1 *traumatic amputation of shoulder and upper arm (S48.-)*

AHA: 2018,2Q,12; 2015,3Q,37-39

DEF: Diaphysis: Central shaft of a long bone.

DEF: Epiphysis: Proximal and distal rounded ends of a long bone, communicates with the joint.

DEF: Metaphysis: Section of a long bone located between the epiphysis and diaphysis at the proximal and distal ends.

DEF: Physis (growth plate): Narrow zone of cartilaginous tissue between the epiphysis and metaphysis at each end of a long bone. In childhood, proliferation of cells in this zone lengthens the bone. As the bone matures, this area thins, ossification eventually fusing into solid bone and growth stops. ***Synonyms:*** *Epiphyseal plate.*

The appropriate 7th character is to be added to all codes from category S42 [unless otherwise indicated].

- A initial encounter for closed fracture
- B initial encounter for open fracture
- D subsequent encounter for fracture with routine healing
- G subsequent encounter for fracture with delayed healing
- K subsequent encounter for fracture with nonunion
- P subsequent encounter for fracture with malunion
- S sequela

S42.0 Fracture of clavicle

S42.00 Fracture of unspecified part of clavicle

- 3 **S42.001** Fracture of unspecified part of right clavicle CC H5
- 3 **S42.002** Fracture of unspecified part of left clavicle CC H5
- 3 **S42.009** Fracture of unspecified part of unspecified clavicle CC H5
  AHA: 2012,4Q,93

S42.01 Fracture of sternal end of clavicle

- 3 **S42.011** Anterior displaced fracture of sternal end of right clavicle CC H5
- 3 **S42.012** Anterior displaced fracture of sternal end of left clavicle CC H5
- 3 **S42.013** Anterior displaced fracture of sternal end of unspecified clavicle CC H5
  Displaced fracture of sternal end of clavicle NOS
- 3 **S42.014** Posterior displaced fracture of sternal end of right clavicle CC H5
- 3 **S42.015** Posterior displaced fracture of sternal end of left clavicle CC H5
- 3 **S42.016** Posterior displaced fracture of sternal end of unspecified clavicle CC H5
- 3 **S42.017** Nondisplaced fracture of sternal end of right clavicle CC H5
- 3 **S42.018** Nondisplaced fracture of sternal end of left clavicle CC H5
- 3 **S42.019** Nondisplaced fracture of sternal end of unspecified clavicle CC H5

S42.02 Fracture of shaft of clavicle

- 3 **S42.021** Displaced fracture of shaft of right clavicle CC H5
- 3 **S42.022** Displaced fracture of shaft of left clavicle CC H5
- 3 **S42.023** Displaced fracture of shaft of unspecified clavicle CC H5
- 3 **S42.024** Nondisplaced fracture of shaft of right clavicle CC H5
- 3 **S42.025** Nondisplaced fracture of shaft of left clavicle CC H5
- 3 **S42.026** Nondisplaced fracture of shaft of unspecified clavicle CC H5

S42.03 Fracture of lateral end of clavicle

Fracture of acromial end of clavicle

- 3 **S42.031** Displaced fracture of lateral end of right clavicle CC H5
- 3 **S42.032** Displaced fracture of lateral end of left clavicle CC H5
- 3 **S42.033** Displaced fracture of lateral end of unspecified clavicle CC H5
- 3 **S42.034** Nondisplaced fracture of lateral end of right clavicle CC H5
- 3 **S42.035** Nondisplaced fracture of lateral end of left clavicle CC H5
- 3 **S42.036** Nondisplaced fracture of lateral end of unspecified clavicle CC H5

S42.1 Fracture of scapula

S42.10 Fracture of unspecified part of scapula

- 3 **S42.101** Fracture of unspecified part of scapula, right shoulder CC H5
- 3 **S42.102** Fracture of unspecified part of scapula, left shoulder CC H5
- 3 **S42.109** Fracture of unspecified part of scapula, unspecified shoulder CC H5

S42.11 Fracture of body of scapula

- 3 **S42.111** Displaced fracture of body of scapula, right shoulder CC H5
- 3 **S42.112** Displaced fracture of body of scapula, left shoulder CC H5
- 3 **S42.113** Displaced fracture of body of scapula, unspecified shoulder CC H5
- 3 **S42.114** Nondisplaced fracture of body of scapula, right shoulder CC H5
- 3 **S42.115** Nondisplaced fracture of body of scapula, left shoulder CC H5
- 3 **S42.116** Nondisplaced fracture of body of scapula, unspecified shoulder CC H5

S42.12 Fracture of acromial process

- 3 **S42.121** Displaced fracture of acromial process, right shoulder CC H5
- 3 **S42.122** Displaced fracture of acromial process, left shoulder CC H5
- 3 **S42.123** Displaced fracture of acromial process, unspecified shoulder CC H5
- 3 **S42.124** Nondisplaced fracture of acromial process, right shoulder CC H5
- 3 **S42.125** Nondisplaced fracture of acromial process, left shoulder CC H5
- 3 **S42.126** Nondisplaced fracture of acromial process, unspecified shoulder CC H5

S42.13 Fracture of coracoid process

- 3 **S42.131** Displaced fracture of coracoid process, right shoulder CC H5
- 3 **S42.132** Displaced fracture of coracoid process, left shoulder CC H5
- 3 **S42.133** Displaced fracture of coracoid process, unspecified shoulder CC H5
- 3 **S42.134** Nondisplaced fracture of coracoid process, right shoulder CC H5
- 3 **S42.135** Nondisplaced fracture of coracoid process, left shoulder CC H5
- 3 **S42.136** Nondisplaced fracture of coracoid process, unspecified shoulder CC H5

S42.14 Fracture of glenoid cavity of scapula

- 3 **S42.141** Displaced fracture of glenoid cavity of scapula, right shoulder CC H5
- 3 **S42.142** Displaced fracture of glenoid cavity of scapula, left shoulder CC H5
- 3 **S42.143** Displaced fracture of glenoid cavity of scapula, unspecified shoulder CC H5
- 3 **S42.144** Nondisplaced fracture of glenoid cavity of scapula, right shoulder CC H5
- 3 **S42.145** Nondisplaced fracture of glenoid cavity of scapula, left shoulder CC H5
- 3 **S42.146** Nondisplaced fracture of glenoid cavity of scapula, unspecified shoulder CC H5

S42.15 Fracture of neck of scapula

- 3 **S42.151** Displaced fracture of neck of scapula, right shoulder CC H5
- 3 **S42.152** Displaced fracture of neck of scapula, left shoulder CC H5
- 3 **S42.153** Displaced fracture of neck of scapula, unspecified shoulder CC H5
- 3 **S42.154** Nondisplaced fracture of neck of scapula, right shoulder CC H5
- 3 **S42.155** Nondisplaced fracture of neck of scapula, left shoulder CC H5

3 ✓7th **S42.156 Nondisplaced fracture of neck of scapula, unspecified shoulder** CC H5

✓6th **S42.19 Fracture of other part of scapula**

3 ✓7th **S42.191 Fracture of other part of scapula, right shoulder** CC H5

3 ✓7th **S42.192 Fracture of other part of scapula, left shoulder** CC H5

3 ✓7th **S42.199 Fracture of other part of scapula, unspecified shoulder** CC H5

✓5th **S42.2 Fracture of upper end of humerus**

Fracture of proximal end of humerus

EXCLUDES 2 *fracture of shaft of humerus (S42.3-)*
physeal fracture of upper end of humerus (S49.Ø-)

✓6th **S42.2Ø Unspecified fracture of upper end of humerus**

2,3 ✓7th **S42.2Ø1 Unspecified fracture of upper end of right humerus** MCC CC H5

2,3 ✓7th **S42.2Ø2 Unspecified fracture of upper end of left humerus** MCC CC H5

2,3 ✓7th **S42.2Ø9 Unspecified fracture of upper end of unspecified humerus** MCC CC H5

✓6th **S42.21 Unspecified fracture of surgical neck of humerus**

Fracture of neck of humerus NOS

2,3 ✓7th **S42.211 Unspecified displaced fracture of surgical neck of right humerus** MCC CC H5

2,3 ✓7th **S42.212 Unspecified displaced fracture of surgical neck of left humerus** MCC CC H5

2,3 ✓7th **S42.213 Unspecified displaced fracture of surgical neck of unspecified humerus** MCC CC H5

2,3 ✓7th **S42.214 Unspecified nondisplaced fracture of surgical neck of right humerus** MCC CC H5

2,3 ✓7th **S42.215 Unspecified nondisplaced fracture of surgical neck of left humerus** MCC CC H5

2,3 ✓7th **S42.216 Unspecified nondisplaced fracture of surgical neck of unspecified humerus** MCC CC H5

✓6th **S42.22 2-part fracture of surgical neck of humerus**

2,3 ✓7th **S42.221 2-part displaced fracture of surgical neck of right humerus** MCC CC H5

2,3 ✓7th **S42.222 2-part displaced fracture of surgical neck of left humerus** MCC CC H5

2,3 ✓7th **S42.223 2-part displaced fracture of surgical neck of unspecified humerus** MCC CC H5

2,3 ✓7th **S42.224 2-part nondisplaced fracture of surgical neck of right humerus** MCC CC H5

2,3 ✓7th **S42.225 2-part nondisplaced fracture of surgical neck of left humerus** MCC CC H5

2,3 ✓7th **S42.226 2-part nondisplaced fracture of surgical neck of unspecified humerus** MCC CC H5

✓6th **S42.23 3-part fracture of surgical neck of humerus**

2,3 ✓7th **S42.231 3-part fracture of surgical neck of right humerus** MCC CC H5

2,3 ✓7th **S42.232 3-part fracture of surgical neck of left humerus** MCC CC H5

2,3 ✓7th **S42.239 3-part fracture of surgical neck of unspecified humerus** MCC CC H5

✓6th **S42.24 4-part fracture of surgical neck of humerus**

2,3 ✓7th **S42.241 4-part fracture of surgical neck of right humerus** MCC CC H5

2,3 ✓7th **S42.242 4-part fracture of surgical neck of left humerus** MCC CC H5

2,3 ✓7th **S42.249 4-part fracture of surgical neck of unspecified humerus** MCC CC H5

✓6th **S42.25 Fracture of greater tuberosity of humerus**

2,3 ✓7th **S42.251 Displaced fracture of greater tuberosity of right humerus** MCC CC H5

2,3 ✓7th **S42.252 Displaced fracture of greater tuberosity of left humerus** MCC CC H5

2,3 ✓7th **S42.253 Displaced fracture of greater tuberosity of unspecified humerus** MCC CC H5

2,3 ✓7th **S42.254 Nondisplaced fracture of greater tuberosity of right humerus** MCC CC H5

2,3 ✓7th **S42.255 Nondisplaced fracture of greater tuberosity of left humerus** MCC CC H5

2,3 ✓7th **S42.256 Nondisplaced fracture of greater tuberosity of unspecified humerus** MCC CC H5

✓6th **S42.26 Fracture of lesser tuberosity of humerus**

2,3 ✓7th **S42.261 Displaced fracture of lesser tuberosity of right humerus** MCC CC H5

2,3 ✓7th **S42.262 Displaced fracture of lesser tuberosity of left humerus** MCC CC H5

2,3 ✓7th **S42.263 Displaced fracture of lesser tuberosity of unspecified humerus** MCC CC H5

2,3 ✓7th **S42.264 Nondisplaced fracture of lesser tuberosity of right humerus** MCC CC H5

2,3 ✓7th **S42.265 Nondisplaced fracture of lesser tuberosity of left humerus** MCC CC H5

2,3 ✓7th **S42.266 Nondisplaced fracture of lesser tuberosity of unspecified humerus** MCC CC H5

✓6th **S42.27 Torus fracture of upper end of humerus**

The appropriate 7th character is to be added to all codes in subcategory S42.27
- A initial encounter for closed fracture
- D subsequent encounter for fracture with routine healing
- G subsequent encounter for fracture with delayed healing
- K subsequent encounter for fracture with nonunion
- P subsequent encounter for fracture with malunion
- S sequela

3 ✓7th **S42.271 Torus fracture of upper end of right humerus** CC H5

3 ✓7th **S42.272 Torus fracture of upper end of left humerus** CC H5

3 ✓7th **S42.279 Torus fracture of upper end of unspecified humerus** CC H5

✓6th **S42.29 Other fracture of upper end of humerus**

Fracture of anatomical neck of humerus
Fracture of articular head of humerus
AHA: 2019,1Q,18

2,3 ✓7th **S42.291 Other displaced fracture of upper end of right humerus** MCC CC H5

2,3 ✓7th **S42.292 Other displaced fracture of upper end of left humerus** MCC CC H5

2,3 ✓7th **S42.293 Other displaced fracture of upper end of unspecified humerus** MCC CC H5

2,3 ✓7th **S42.294 Other nondisplaced fracture of upper end of right humerus** MCC CC H5

2,3 ✓7th **S42.295 Other nondisplaced fracture of upper end of left humerus** MCC CC H5

2,3 ✓7th **S42.296 Other nondisplaced fracture of upper end of unspecified humerus** MCC CC H5

✓5th **S42.3 Fracture of shaft of humerus**

Fracture of humerus NOS
Fracture of upper arm NOS

EXCLUDES 2 *physeal fractures of upper end of humerus (S49.Ø-)*
physeal fractures of lower end of humerus (S49.1-)

✓6th **S42.3Ø Unspecified fracture of shaft of humerus**

2,3 ✓7th **S42.3Ø1 Unspecified fracture of shaft of humerus, right arm** MCC CC H5

2,3 ✓7th **S42.3Ø2 Unspecified fracture of shaft of humerus, left arm** MCC CC H5

2,3 ✓7th **S42.3Ø9 Unspecified fracture of shaft of humerus, unspecified arm** MCC CC H5

6th S42.31 Greenstick fracture of shaft of humerus

The appropriate 7th character is to be added to all codes in subcategory S42.31
- A initial encounter for closed fracture
- D subsequent encounter for fracture with routine healing
- G subsequent encounter for fracture with delayed healing
- K subsequent encounter for fracture with nonunion
- P subsequent encounter for fracture with malunion
- S sequela

3 7th S42.311 Greenstick fracture of shaft of humerus, right arm CC H5
3 7th S42.312 Greenstick fracture of shaft of humerus, left arm CC H5
3 7th S42.319 Greenstick fracture of shaft of humerus, unspecified arm CC H5

6th S42.32 Transverse fracture of shaft of humerus
2,3 7th S42.321 Displaced transverse fracture of shaft of humerus, right arm MCC CC H5
2,3 7th S42.322 Displaced transverse fracture of shaft of humerus, left arm MCC CC H5
2,3 7th S42.323 Displaced transverse fracture of shaft of humerus, unspecified arm MCC CC H5
2,3 7th S42.324 Nondisplaced transverse fracture of shaft of humerus, right arm MCC CC H5
2,3 7th S42.325 Nondisplaced transverse fracture of shaft of humerus, left arm MCC CC H5
2,3 7th S42.326 Nondisplaced transverse fracture of shaft of humerus, unspecified arm MCC CC H5

6th S42.33 Oblique fracture of shaft of humerus
2,3 7th S42.331 Displaced oblique fracture of shaft of humerus, right arm MCC CC H5
2,3 7th S42.332 Displaced oblique fracture of shaft of humerus, left arm MCC CC H5
2,3 7th S42.333 Displaced oblique fracture of shaft of humerus, unspecified arm MCC CC H5
2,3 7th S42.334 Nondisplaced oblique fracture of shaft of humerus, right arm MCC CC H5
2,3 7th S42.335 Nondisplaced oblique fracture of shaft of humerus, left arm MCC CC H5
2,3 7th S42.336 Nondisplaced oblique fracture of shaft of humerus, unspecified arm MCC CC H5

6th S42.34 Spiral fracture of shaft of humerus
2,3 7th S42.341 Displaced spiral fracture of shaft of humerus, right arm MCC CC H5
2,3 7th S42.342 Displaced spiral fracture of shaft of humerus, left arm MCC CC H5
2,3 7th S42.343 Displaced spiral fracture of shaft of humerus, unspecified arm MCC CC H5
2,3 7th S42.344 Nondisplaced spiral fracture of shaft of humerus, right arm MCC CC H5
2,3 7th S42.345 Nondisplaced spiral fracture of shaft of humerus, left arm MCC CC H5
2,3 7th S42.346 Nondisplaced spiral fracture of shaft of humerus, unspecified arm MCC CC H5

6th S42.35 Comminuted fracture of shaft of humerus
2,3 7th S42.351 Displaced comminuted fracture of shaft of humerus, right arm MCC CC H5
2,3 7th S42.352 Displaced comminuted fracture of shaft of humerus, left arm MCC CC H5
2,3 7th S42.353 Displaced comminuted fracture of shaft of humerus, unspecified arm MCC CC H5
2,3 7th S42.354 Nondisplaced comminuted fracture of shaft of humerus, right arm MCC CC H5
2,3 7th S42.355 Nondisplaced comminuted fracture of shaft of humerus, left arm MCC CC H5
2,3 7th S42.356 Nondisplaced comminuted fracture of shaft of humerus, unspecified arm MCC CC H5

6th S42.36 Segmental fracture of shaft of humerus
2,3 7th S42.361 Displaced segmental fracture of shaft of humerus, right arm MCC CC H5
2,3 7th S42.362 Displaced segmental fracture of shaft of humerus, left arm MCC CC H5
2,3 7th S42.363 Displaced segmental fracture of shaft of humerus, unspecified arm MCC CC H5
2,3 7th S42.364 Nondisplaced segmental fracture of shaft of humerus, right arm MCC CC H5
2,3 7th S42.365 Nondisplaced segmental fracture of shaft of humerus, left arm MCC CC H5
2,3 7th S42.366 Nondisplaced segmental fracture of shaft of humerus, unspecified arm MCC CC H5

6th S42.39 Other fracture of shaft of humerus
2,3 7th S42.391 Other fracture of shaft of right humerus MCC CC H5
2,3 7th S42.392 Other fracture of shaft of left humerus MCC CC H5
2,3 7th S42.399 Other fracture of shaft of unspecified humerus MCC CC H5

5th S42.4 Fracture of lower end of humerus

Fracture of distal end of humerus

EXCLUDES 2 *fracture of shaft of humerus (S42.3-)*
physeal fracture of lower end of humerus (S49.1-)

6th S42.40 Unspecified fracture of lower end of humerus

Fracture of elbow NOS

2,3 7th S42.401 Unspecified fracture of lower end of right humerus MCC CC H5
2,3 7th S42.402 Unspecified fracture of lower end of left humerus MCC CC H5
2,3 7th S42.409 Unspecified fracture of lower end of unspecified humerus MCC CC H5

6th S42.41 Simple supracondylar fracture without intercondylar fracture of humerus
2,3 7th S42.411 Displaced simple supracondylar fracture without intercondylar fracture of right humerus MCC CC H5
2,3 7th S42.412 Displaced simple supracondylar fracture without intercondylar fracture of left humerus MCC CC H5
2,3 7th S42.413 Displaced simple supracondylar fracture without intercondylar fracture of unspecified humerus MCC CC H5
2,3 7th S42.414 Nondisplaced simple supracondylar fracture without intercondylar fracture of right humerus MCC CC H5
2,3 7th S42.415 Nondisplaced simple supracondylar fracture without intercondylar fracture of left humerus MCC CC H5
2,3 7th S42.416 Nondisplaced simple supracondylar fracture without intercondylar fracture of unspecified humerus MCC CC H5

6th S42.42 Comminuted supracondylar fracture without intercondylar fracture of humerus
2,3 7th S42.421 Displaced comminuted supracondylar fracture without intercondylar fracture of right humerus MCC CC H5
2,3 7th S42.422 Displaced comminuted supracondylar fracture without intercondylar fracture of left humerus MCC CC H5
2,3 7th S42.423 Displaced comminuted supracondylar fracture without intercondylar fracture of unspecified humerus MCC CC H5
2,3 7th S42.424 Nondisplaced comminuted supracondylar fracture without intercondylar fracture of right humerus MCC CC H5
2,3 7th S42.425 Nondisplaced comminuted supracondylar fracture without intercondylar fracture of left humerus MCC CC H5
2,3 7th S42.426 Nondisplaced comminuted supracondylar fracture without intercondylar fracture of unspecified humerus MCC CC H5

6th S42.43 Fracture (avulsion) of lateral epicondyle of humerus
2,3 7th S42.431 Displaced fracture (avulsion) of lateral epicondyle of right humerus MCC CC H5
2,3 7th S42.432 Displaced fracture (avulsion) of lateral epicondyle of left humerus MCC CC H5
2,3 7th S42.433 Displaced fracture (avulsion) of lateral epicondyle of unspecified humerus MCC CC H5

2,3 √7th **S42.434** Nondisplaced **fracture (avulsion) of lateral epicondyle of** right **humerus** MCC CC H5

2,3 √7th **S42.435** Nondisplaced **fracture (avulsion) of lateral epicondyle of** left **humerus** MCC CC H5

2,3 √7th **S42.436** Nondisplaced **fracture (avulsion) of lateral epicondyle of unspecified humerus** MCC CC H5

√6th **S42.44 Fracture (avulsion) of** medial epicondyle **of humerus**

2,3 √7th **S42.441** Displaced **fracture (avulsion) of medial epicondyle of** right **humerus** MCC CC H5

2,3 √7th **S42.442** Displaced **fracture (avulsion) of medial epicondyle of** left **humerus** MCC CC H5

2,3 √7th **S42.443** Displaced **fracture (avulsion) of medial epicondyle of unspecified humerus** MCC CC H5

2,3 √7th **S42.444** Nondisplaced **fracture (avulsion) of medial epicondyle of** right **humerus** MCC CC H5

2,3 √7th **S42.445** Nondisplaced **fracture (avulsion) of medial epicondyle of** left **humerus** MCC CC H5

2,3 √7th **S42.446** Nondisplaced **fracture (avulsion) of medial epicondyle of unspecified humerus** MCC CC H5

2,3 √7th **S42.447** Incarcerated **fracture (avulsion) of medial epicondyle of** right **humerus** MCC CC H5

2,3 √7th **S42.448** Incarcerated **fracture (avulsion) of medial epicondyle of** left **humerus** MCC CC H5

2,3 √7th **S42.449** Incarcerated **fracture (avulsion) of medial epicondyle of unspecified humerus** MCC CC H5

√6th **S42.45 Fracture of** lateral condyle **of humerus**

Fracture of capitellum of humerus

2,3 √7th **S42.451** Displaced **fracture of lateral condyle of** right **humerus** MCC CC H5

2,3 √7th **S42.452** Displaced **fracture of lateral condyle of** left **humerus** MCC CC H5

2,3 √7th **S42.453** Displaced **fracture of lateral condyle of unspecified humerus** MCC CC H5

2,3 √7th **S42.454** Nondisplaced **fracture of lateral condyle of** right **humerus** MCC CC H5

2,3 √7th **S42.455** Nondisplaced **fracture of lateral condyle of** left **humerus** MCC CC H5

2,3 √7th **S42.456** Nondisplaced **fracture of lateral condyle of unspecified humerus** MCC CC H5

√6th **S42.46 Fracture of** medial condyle **of humerus**

Trochlea fracture of humerus

2,3 √7th **S42.461** Displaced **fracture of medial condyle of** right **humerus** MCC CC H5

2,3 √7th **S42.462** Displaced **fracture of medial condyle of** left **humerus** MCC CC H5

2,3 √7th **S42.463** Displaced **fracture of medial condyle of unspecified humerus** MCC CC H5

2,3 √7th **S42.464** Nondisplaced **fracture of medial condyle of** right **humerus** MCC CC H5

2,3 √7th **S42.465** Nondisplaced **fracture of medial condyle of** left **humerus** MCC CC H5

2,3 √7th **S42.466** Nondisplaced **fracture of medial condyle of unspecified humerus** MCC CC H5

√6th **S42.47** Transcondylar **fracture of humerus**

2,3 √7th **S42.471** Displaced **transcondylar fracture of** right **humerus** MCC CC H5

2,3 √7th **S42.472** Displaced **transcondylar fracture of** left **humerus** MCC CC H5

2,3 √7th **S42.473** Displaced **transcondylar fracture of unspecified humerus** MCC CC H5

2,3 √7th **S42.474** Nondisplaced **transcondylar fracture of** right **humerus** MCC CC H5

2,3 √7th **S42.475** Nondisplaced **transcondylar fracture of** left **humerus** MCC CC H5

2,3 √7th **S42.476** Nondisplaced **transcondylar fracture of unspecified humerus** MCC CC H5

√6th **S42.48** Torus **fracture of lower end of humerus**

The appropriate 7th character is to be added to all codes in subcategory S42.48.
A initial encounter for closed fracture
D subsequent encounter for fracture with routine healing
G subsequent encounter for fracture with delayed healing
K subsequent encounter for fracture with nonunion
P subsequent encounter for fracture with malunion
S sequela

3 √7th **S42.481 Torus fracture of lower end of** right **humerus** CC H5

3 √7th **S42.482 Torus fracture of lower end of** left **humerus** CC H5

3 √7th **S42.489 Torus fracture of lower end of unspecified humerus** CC H5

√6th **S42.49 Other fracture of lower end of humerus**

2,3 √7th **S42.491 Other** displaced **fracture of lower end of** right **humerus** MCC CC H5

2,3 √7th **S42.492 Other** displaced **fracture of lower end of** left **humerus** MCC CC H5

2,3 √7th **S42.493 Other** displaced **fracture of lower end of unspecified humerus** MCC CC H5

2,3 √7th **S42.494 Other** nondisplaced **fracture of lower end of** right **humerus** MCC CC H5

2,3 √7th **S42.495 Other** nondisplaced **fracture of lower end of** left **humerus** MCC CC H5

2,3 √7th **S42.496 Other** nondisplaced **fracture of lower end of unspecified humerus** MCC CC H5

√5th **S42.9 Fracture of shoulder girdle, part unspecified**

Fracture of shoulder NOS

2,3 √x7th **S42.90 Fracture of unspecified shoulder girdle, part unspecified** MCC CC H5

2,3 √x7th **S42.91 Fracture of** right **shoulder girdle, part unspecified** MCC CC H5

2,3 √x7th **S42.92 Fracture of** left **shoulder girdle, part unspecified** MCC CC H5

√4th **S43 Dislocation and sprain of joints and ligaments of shoulder girdle**

INCLUDES avulsion of joint or ligament of shoulder girdle
laceration of cartilage, joint or ligament of shoulder girdle
sprain of cartilage, joint or ligament of shoulder girdle
traumatic hemarthrosis of joint or ligament of shoulder girdle
traumatic rupture of joint or ligament of shoulder girdle
traumatic subluxation of joint or ligament of shoulder girdle
traumatic tear of joint or ligament of shoulder girdle

Code also any associated open wound

EXCLUDES 2 *strain of muscle, fascia and tendon of shoulder and upper arm (S46.-)*

The appropriate 7th character is to be added to each code from category S43.
A initial encounter
D subsequent encounter
S sequela

√5th **S43.0 Subluxation and dislocation of** shoulder joint

Dislocation of glenohumeral joint
Subluxation of glenohumeral joint

√6th **S43.00 Unspecified subluxation and dislocation of shoulder joint**

Dislocation of humerus NOS
Subluxation of humerus NOS

√7th **S43.001 Unspecified** subluxation **of** right **shoulder joint**

√7th **S43.002 Unspecified** subluxation **of** left **shoulder joint**

√7th **S43.003 Unspecified** subluxation **of unspecified shoulder joint**

√7th **S43.004 Unspecified** dislocation **of** right **shoulder joint**

√7th **S43.005 Unspecified** dislocation **of** left **shoulder joint**

√7th **S43.006 Unspecified** dislocation **of unspecified shoulder joint**

S43.01 Anterior subluxation and dislocation of humerus
S43.011 Anterior subluxation of right humerus
S43.012 Anterior subluxation of left humerus
S43.013 Anterior subluxation of unspecified humerus
S43.014 Anterior dislocation of right humerus
S43.015 Anterior dislocation of left humerus
S43.016 Anterior dislocation of unspecified humerus
S43.02 Posterior subluxation and dislocation of humerus
S43.021 Posterior subluxation of right humerus
S43.022 Posterior subluxation of left humerus
S43.023 Posterior subluxation of unspecified humerus
S43.024 Posterior dislocation of right humerus
S43.025 Posterior dislocation of left humerus
S43.026 Posterior dislocation of unspecified humerus
S43.03 Inferior subluxation and dislocation of humerus
S43.031 Inferior subluxation of right humerus
S43.032 Inferior subluxation of left humerus
S43.033 Inferior subluxation of unspecified humerus
S43.034 Inferior dislocation of right humerus
S43.035 Inferior dislocation of left humerus
S43.036 Inferior dislocation of unspecified humerus
S43.08 Other subluxation and dislocation of shoulder joint
S43.081 Other subluxation of right shoulder joint
S43.082 Other subluxation of left shoulder joint
S43.083 Other subluxation of unspecified shoulder joint
S43.084 Other dislocation of right shoulder joint
S43.085 Other dislocation of left shoulder joint
S43.086 Other dislocation of unspecified shoulder joint
S43.1 Subluxation and dislocation of acromioclavicular joint
S43.10 Unspecified dislocation of acromioclavicular joint
S43.101 Unspecified dislocation of right acromioclavicular joint
S43.102 Unspecified dislocation of left acromioclavicular joint
S43.109 Unspecified dislocation of unspecified acromioclavicular joint
S43.11 Subluxation of acromioclavicular joint
S43.111 Subluxation of right acromioclavicular joint
S43.112 Subluxation of left acromioclavicular joint
S43.119 Subluxation of unspecified acromioclavicular joint
S43.12 Dislocation of acromioclavicular joint, 100%-200% displacement
S43.121 Dislocation of right acromioclavicular joint, 100%-200% displacement
S43.122 Dislocation of left acromioclavicular joint, 100%-200% displacement
S43.129 Dislocation of unspecified acromioclavicular joint, 100%-200% displacement
S43.13 Dislocation of acromioclavicular joint, greater than 200% displacement
S43.131 Dislocation of right acromioclavicular joint, greater than 200% displacement
S43.132 Dislocation of left acromioclavicular joint, greater than 200% displacement
S43.139 Dislocation of unspecified acromioclavicular joint, greater than 200% displacement
S43.14 Inferior dislocation of acromioclavicular joint
S43.141 Inferior dislocation of right acromioclavicular joint
S43.142 Inferior dislocation of left acromioclavicular joint
S43.149 Inferior dislocation of unspecified acromioclavicular joint
S43.15 Posterior dislocation of acromioclavicular joint
S43.151 Posterior dislocation of right acromioclavicular joint
S43.152 Posterior dislocation of left acromioclavicular joint
S43.159 Posterior dislocation of unspecified acromioclavicular joint
S43.2 Subluxation and dislocation of sternoclavicular joint
S43.20 Unspecified subluxation and dislocation of sternoclavicular joint
S43.201 Unspecified subluxation of right sternoclavicular joint CC H5
S43.202 Unspecified subluxation of left sternoclavicular joint CC H5
S43.203 Unspecified subluxation of unspecified sternoclavicular joint CC H5
S43.204 Unspecified dislocation of right sternoclavicular joint CC H5
S43.205 Unspecified dislocation of left sternoclavicular joint CC H5
S43.206 Unspecified dislocation of unspecified sternoclavicular joint CC H5
S43.21 Anterior subluxation and dislocation of sternoclavicular joint
S43.211 Anterior subluxation of right sternoclavicular joint CC H5
S43.212 Anterior subluxation of left sternoclavicular joint CC H5
S43.213 Anterior subluxation of unspecified sternoclavicular joint CC H5
S43.214 Anterior dislocation of right sternoclavicular joint CC H5
S43.215 Anterior dislocation of left sternoclavicular joint CC H5
S43.216 Anterior dislocation of unspecified sternoclavicular joint CC H5
S43.22 Posterior subluxation and dislocation of sternoclavicular joint
S43.221 Posterior subluxation of right sternoclavicular joint CC H5
S43.222 Posterior subluxation of left sternoclavicular joint CC H5
S43.223 Posterior subluxation of unspecified sternoclavicular joint CC H5
S43.224 Posterior dislocation of right sternoclavicular joint CC H5
S43.225 Posterior dislocation of left sternoclavicular joint CC H5
S43.226 Posterior dislocation of unspecified sternoclavicular joint CC H5
S43.3 Subluxation and dislocation of other and unspecified parts of shoulder girdle
S43.30 Subluxation and dislocation of unspecified parts of shoulder girdle
Dislocation of shoulder girdle NOS
Subluxation of shoulder girdle NOS
S43.301 Subluxation of unspecified parts of right shoulder girdle
S43.302 Subluxation of unspecified parts of left shoulder girdle
S43.303 Subluxation of unspecified parts of unspecified shoulder girdle
S43.304 Dislocation of unspecified parts of right shoulder girdle
S43.305 Dislocation of unspecified parts of left shoulder girdle
S43.306 Dislocation of unspecified parts of unspecified shoulder girdle
S43.31 Subluxation and dislocation of scapula
S43.311 Subluxation of right scapula
S43.312 Subluxation of left scapula
S43.313 Subluxation of unspecified scapula
S43.314 Dislocation of right scapula
S43.315 Dislocation of left scapula
S43.316 Dislocation of unspecified scapula
S43.39 Subluxation and dislocation of other parts of shoulder girdle
S43.391 Subluxation of other parts of right shoulder girdle

7th S43.392 Subluxation of other parts of left shoulder girdle
7th S43.393 Subluxation of other parts of unspecified shoulder girdle
7th S43.394 Dislocation of other parts of right shoulder girdle
7th S43.395 Dislocation of other parts of left shoulder girdle
7th S43.396 Dislocation of other parts of unspecified shoulder girdle

5th **S43.4 Sprain of shoulder joint**
6th **S43.40 Unspecified sprain of shoulder joint**
7th S43.401 Unspecified sprain of right shoulder joint
7th S43.402 Unspecified sprain of left shoulder joint
7th S43.409 Unspecified sprain of unspecified shoulder joint
6th **S43.41 Sprain of coracohumeral (ligament)**
7th S43.411 Sprain of right coracohumeral (ligament)
7th S43.412 Sprain of left coracohumeral (ligament)
7th S43.419 Sprain of unspecified coracohumeral (ligament)
6th **S43.42 Sprain of rotator cuff capsule**
EXCLUDES 1 *rotator cuff syndrome (complete) (incomplete), not specified as traumatic (M75.1-)*
EXCLUDES 2 *injury of tendon of rotator cuff (S46.Ø-)*
7th S43.421 Sprain of right rotator cuff capsule
7th S43.422 Sprain of left rotator cuff capsule
7th S43.429 Sprain of unspecified rotator cuff capsule
6th **S43.43 Superior glenoid labrum lesion**
SLAP lesion
AHA: 2019,2Q,26
DEF: Detachment injury of the superior aspect of the glenoid labrum, which is the ring of fibrocartilage attached to the rim of the glenoid cavity of the scapula.
7th S43.431 Superior glenoid labrum lesion of right shoulder
7th S43.432 Superior glenoid labrum lesion of left shoulder
7th S43.439 Superior glenoid labrum lesion of unspecified shoulder
6th **S43.49 Other sprain of shoulder joint**
7th S43.491 Other sprain of right shoulder joint
7th S43.492 Other sprain of left shoulder joint
7th S43.499 Other sprain of unspecified shoulder joint

5th **S43.5 Sprain of acromioclavicular joint**
Sprain of acromioclavicular ligament
x7th S43.50 Sprain of unspecified acromioclavicular joint
x7th S43.51 Sprain of right acromioclavicular joint
x7th S43.52 Sprain of left acromioclavicular joint

5th **S43.6 Sprain of sternoclavicular joint**
x7th S43.60 Sprain of unspecified sternoclavicular joint
x7th S43.61 Sprain of right sternoclavicular joint
x7th S43.62 Sprain of left sternoclavicular joint

5th **S43.8 Sprain of other specified parts of shoulder girdle**
x7th S43.80 Sprain of other specified parts of unspecified shoulder girdle
x7th S43.81 Sprain of other specified parts of right shoulder girdle
x7th S43.82 Sprain of other specified parts of left shoulder girdle

5th **S43.9 Sprain of unspecified parts of shoulder girdle**
x7th S43.90 Sprain of unspecified parts of unspecified shoulder girdle
Sprain of shoulder girdle NOS
x7th S43.91 Sprain of unspecified parts of right shoulder girdle
x7th S43.92 Sprain of unspecified parts of left shoulder girdle

4th **S44 Injury of nerves at shoulder and upper arm level**
Code also any associated open wound (S41.-)
EXCLUDES 2 *injury of brachial plexus (S14.3-)*

The appropriate 7th character is to be added to each code from category S44.
A initial encounter
D subsequent encounter
S sequela

5th **S44.Ø Injury of ulnar nerve at upper arm level**
EXCLUDES 1 *ulnar nerve NOS (S54.Ø)*
x7th S44.ØØ Injury of ulnar nerve at upper arm level, unspecified arm
x7th S44.Ø1 Injury of ulnar nerve at upper arm level, right arm
x7th S44.Ø2 Injury of ulnar nerve at upper arm level, left arm

5th **S44.1 Injury of median nerve at upper arm level**
EXCLUDES 1 *median nerve NOS (S54.1)*
x7th S44.1Ø Injury of median nerve at upper arm level, unspecified arm
x7th S44.11 Injury of median nerve at upper arm level, right arm
x7th S44.12 Injury of median nerve at upper arm level, left arm

5th **S44.2 Injury of radial nerve at upper arm level**
EXCLUDES 1 *radial nerve NOS (S54.2)*
x7th S44.2Ø Injury of radial nerve at upper arm level, unspecified arm
x7th S44.21 Injury of radial nerve at upper arm level, right arm
x7th S44.22 Injury of radial nerve at upper arm level, left arm

5th **S44.3 Injury of axillary nerve**
x7th S44.3Ø Injury of axillary nerve, unspecified arm
x7th S44.31 Injury of axillary nerve, right arm
x7th S44.32 Injury of axillary nerve, left arm

5th **S44.4 Injury of musculocutaneous nerve**
x7th S44.4Ø Injury of musculocutaneous nerve, unspecified arm
x7th S44.41 Injury of musculocutaneous nerve, right arm
x7th S44.42 Injury of musculocutaneous nerve, left arm

5th **S44.5 Injury of cutaneous sensory nerve at shoulder and upper arm level**
x7th S44.5Ø Injury of cutaneous sensory nerve at shoulder and upper arm level, unspecified arm
x7th S44.51 Injury of cutaneous sensory nerve at shoulder and upper arm level, right arm
x7th S44.52 Injury of cutaneous sensory nerve at shoulder and upper arm level, left arm

5th **S44.8 Injury of other nerves at shoulder and upper arm level**
6th **S44.8X Injury of other nerves at shoulder and upper arm level**
7th S44.8X1 Injury of other nerves at shoulder and upper arm level, right arm
7th S44.8X2 Injury of other nerves at shoulder and upper arm level, left arm
7th S44.8X9 Injury of other nerves at shoulder and upper arm level, unspecified arm

5th **S44.9 Injury of unspecified nerve at shoulder and upper arm level**
x7th S44.9Ø Injury of unspecified nerve at shoulder and upper arm level, unspecified arm
x7th S44.91 Injury of unspecified nerve at shoulder and upper arm level, right arm
x7th S44.92 Injury of unspecified nerve at shoulder and upper arm level, left arm

4th **S45 Injury of blood vessels at shoulder and upper arm level**
Code also any associated open wound (S41.-)
EXCLUDES 2 *injury of subclavian artery (S25.1)*
injury of subclavian vein (S25.3)

The appropriate 7th character is to be added to each code from category S45.
A initial encounter
D subsequent encounter
S sequela

5th **S45.Ø Injury of axillary artery**
6th **S45.ØØ Unspecified injury of axillary artery**
7th S45.ØØ1 Unspecified injury of axillary artery, right side MCC

Chapter 19. Injury, Poisoning and Certain Other Consequences of External Causes
S43.392–S45.ØØ1

- S45.002 Unspecified injury of axillary artery, left side MCC
- S45.009 Unspecified injury of axillary artery, unspecified side MCC

S45.01 Laceration of axillary artery
- S45.011 Laceration of axillary artery, right side MCC
- S45.012 Laceration of axillary artery, left side MCC
- S45.019 Laceration of axillary artery, unspecified side MCC

S45.09 Other specified injury of axillary artery
- S45.091 Other specified injury of axillary artery, right side MCC
- S45.092 Other specified injury of axillary artery, left side MCC
- S45.099 Other specified injury of axillary artery, unspecified side MCC

S45.1 Injury of brachial artery

S45.10 Unspecified injury of brachial artery
- S45.101 Unspecified injury of brachial artery, right side CC
- S45.102 Unspecified injury of brachial artery, left side CC
- S45.109 Unspecified injury of brachial artery, unspecified side CC

S45.11 Laceration of brachial artery
- S45.111 Laceration of brachial artery, right side CC
- S45.112 Laceration of brachial artery, left side CC
- S45.119 Laceration of brachial artery, unspecified side CC

S45.19 Other specified injury of brachial artery
- S45.191 Other specified injury of brachial artery, right side CC
- S45.192 Other specified injury of brachial artery, left side CC
- S45.199 Other specified injury of brachial artery, unspecified side CC

S45.2 Injury of axillary or brachial vein

S45.20 Unspecified injury of axillary or brachial vein
- S45.201 Unspecified injury of axillary or brachial vein, right side CC
- S45.202 Unspecified injury of axillary or brachial vein, left side CC
- S45.209 Unspecified injury of axillary or brachial vein, unspecified side CC

S45.21 Laceration of axillary or brachial vein
- S45.211 Laceration of axillary or brachial vein, right side CC
- S45.212 Laceration of axillary or brachial vein, left side CC
- S45.219 Laceration of axillary or brachial vein, unspecified side CC

S45.29 Other specified injury of axillary or brachial vein
- S45.291 Other specified injury of axillary or brachial vein, right side CC
- S45.292 Other specified injury of axillary or brachial vein, left side CC
- S45.299 Other specified injury of axillary or brachial vein, unspecified side CC

S45.3 Injury of superficial vein at shoulder and upper arm level

S45.30 Unspecified injury of superficial vein at shoulder and upper arm level
- S45.301 Unspecified injury of superficial vein at shoulder and upper arm level, right arm CC
- S45.302 Unspecified injury of superficial vein at shoulder and upper arm level, left arm CC
- S45.309 Unspecified injury of superficial vein at shoulder and upper arm level, unspecified arm CC

S45.31 Laceration of superficial vein at shoulder and upper arm level
- S45.311 Laceration of superficial vein at shoulder and upper arm level, right arm CC
- S45.312 Laceration of superficial vein at shoulder and upper arm level, left arm CC
- S45.319 Laceration of superficial vein at shoulder and upper arm level, unspecified arm CC

S45.39 Other specified injury of superficial vein at shoulder and upper arm level
- S45.391 Other specified injury of superficial vein at shoulder and upper arm level, right arm CC
- S45.392 Other specified injury of superficial vein at shoulder and upper arm level, left arm CC
- S45.399 Other specified injury of superficial vein at shoulder and upper arm level, unspecified arm CC

S45.8 Injury of other specified blood vessels at shoulder and upper arm level

S45.80 Unspecified injury of other specified blood vessels at shoulder and upper arm level
- S45.801 Unspecified injury of other specified blood vessels at shoulder and upper arm level, right arm CC
- S45.802 Unspecified injury of other specified blood vessels at shoulder and upper arm level, left arm CC
- S45.809 Unspecified injury of other specified blood vessels at shoulder and upper arm level, unspecified arm CC

S45.81 Laceration of other specified blood vessels at shoulder and upper arm level
- S45.811 Laceration of other specified blood vessels at shoulder and upper arm level, right arm CC
- S45.812 Laceration of other specified blood vessels at shoulder and upper arm level, left arm CC
- S45.819 Laceration of other specified blood vessels at shoulder and upper arm level, unspecified arm CC

S45.89 Other specified injury of other specified blood vessels at shoulder and upper arm level
- S45.891 Other specified injury of other specified blood vessels at shoulder and upper arm level, right arm CC
- S45.892 Other specified injury of other specified blood vessels at shoulder and upper arm level, left arm CC
- S45.899 Other specified injury of other specified blood vessels at shoulder and upper arm level, unspecified arm CC

S45.9 Injury of unspecified blood vessel at shoulder and upper arm level

S45.90 Unspecified injury of unspecified blood vessel at shoulder and upper arm level
- S45.901 Unspecified injury of unspecified blood vessel at shoulder and upper arm level, right arm CC
- S45.902 Unspecified injury of unspecified blood vessel at shoulder and upper arm level, left arm CC
- S45.909 Unspecified injury of unspecified blood vessel at shoulder and upper arm level, unspecified arm CC

S45.91 Laceration of unspecified blood vessel at shoulder and upper arm level
- S45.911 Laceration of unspecified blood vessel at shoulder and upper arm level, right arm CC
- S45.912 Laceration of unspecified blood vessel at shoulder and upper arm level, left arm CC
- S45.919 Laceration of unspecified blood vessel at shoulder and upper arm level, unspecified arm CC

S45.99 Other specified injury of unspecified blood vessel at shoulder and upper arm level
- S45.991 Other specified injury of unspecified blood vessel at shoulder and upper arm level, right arm CC
- S45.992 Other specified injury of unspecified blood vessel at shoulder and upper arm level, left arm CC

7th **S45.999** **Other specified injury of unspecified blood vessel at shoulder and upper arm level, unspecified arm** CC

4th **S46 Injury of muscle, fascia and tendon at shoulder and upper arm level**

Code also any associated open wound (S41.-)

EXCLUDES 2 *injury of muscle, fascia and tendon at elbow (S56.-)*
sprain of joints and ligaments of shoulder girdle (S43.9)

TIP: Refer to the Muscle/Tendon table at the beginning of this chapter.

The appropriate 7th character is to be added to each code from category S46.
A initial encounter
D subsequent encounter
S sequela

5th **S46.0** **Injury of muscle(s) and tendon(s) of the rotator cuff of shoulder**

6th **S46.00** **Unspecified injury of muscle(s) and tendon(s) of the rotator cuff of shoulder**

7th **S46.001** **Unspecified injury of muscle(s) and tendon(s) of the rotator cuff of right shoulder**

7th **S46.002** **Unspecified injury of muscle(s) and tendon(s) of the rotator cuff of left shoulder**

7th **S46.009** **Unspecified injury of muscle(s) and tendon(s) of the rotator cuff of unspecified shoulder**

6th **S46.01** **Strain of muscle(s) and tendon(s) of the rotator cuff of shoulder**

7th **S46.011** **Strain of muscle(s) and tendon(s) of the rotator cuff of right shoulder**

7th **S46.012** **Strain of muscle(s) and tendon(s) of the rotator cuff of left shoulder**

7th **S46.019** **Strain of muscle(s) and tendon(s) of the rotator cuff of unspecified shoulder**

6th **S46.02** **Laceration of muscle(s) and tendon(s) of the rotator cuff of shoulder**

7th **S46.021** **Laceration of muscle(s) and tendon(s) of the rotator cuff of right shoulder** CC

7th **S46.022** **Laceration of muscle(s) and tendon(s) of the rotator cuff of left shoulder** CC

7th **S46.029** **Laceration of muscle(s) and tendon(s) of the rotator cuff of unspecified shoulder** CC

6th **S46.09** **Other injury of muscle(s) and tendon(s) of the rotator cuff of shoulder**

7th **S46.091** **Other injury of muscle(s) and tendon(s) of the rotator cuff of right shoulder**

7th **S46.092** **Other injury of muscle(s) and tendon(s) of the rotator cuff of left shoulder**

7th **S46.099** **Other injury of muscle(s) and tendon(s) of the rotator cuff of unspecified shoulder**

5th **S46.1** **Injury of muscle, fascia and tendon of long head of biceps**

6th **S46.10** **Unspecified injury of muscle, fascia and tendon of long head of biceps**

7th **S46.101** **Unspecified injury of muscle, fascia and tendon of long head of biceps, right arm**

7th **S46.102** **Unspecified injury of muscle, fascia and tendon of long head of biceps, left arm**

7th **S46.109** **Unspecified injury of muscle, fascia and tendon of long head of biceps, unspecified arm**

6th **S46.11** **Strain of muscle, fascia and tendon of long head of biceps**

AHA: 2020,1Q,38; 2019,2Q,27

7th **S46.111** **Strain of muscle, fascia and tendon of long head of biceps, right arm**

7th **S46.112** **Strain of muscle, fascia and tendon of long head of biceps, left arm**

7th **S46.119** **Strain of muscle, fascia and tendon of long head of biceps, unspecified arm**

6th **S46.12** **Laceration of muscle, fascia and tendon of long head of biceps**

7th **S46.121** **Laceration of muscle, fascia and tendon of long head of biceps, right arm** CC

7th **S46.122** **Laceration of muscle, fascia and tendon of long head of biceps, left arm** CC

7th **S46.129** **Laceration of muscle, fascia and tendon of long head of biceps, unspecified arm** CC

6th **S46.19** **Other injury of muscle, fascia and tendon of long head of biceps**

7th **S46.191** **Other injury of muscle, fascia and tendon of long head of biceps, right arm**

7th **S46.192** **Other injury of muscle, fascia and tendon of long head of biceps, left arm**

7th **S46.199** **Other injury of muscle, fascia and tendon of long head of biceps, unspecified arm**

5th **S46.2** **Injury of muscle, fascia and tendon of other parts of biceps**

6th **S46.20** **Unspecified injury of muscle, fascia and tendon of other parts of biceps**

7th **S46.201** **Unspecified injury of muscle, fascia and tendon of other parts of biceps, right arm**

7th **S46.202** **Unspecified injury of muscle, fascia and tendon of other parts of biceps, left arm**

7th **S46.209** **Unspecified injury of muscle, fascia and tendon of other parts of biceps, unspecified arm**

6th **S46.21** **Strain of muscle, fascia and tendon of other parts of biceps**

7th **S46.211** **Strain of muscle, fascia and tendon of other parts of biceps, right arm**

7th **S46.212** **Strain of muscle, fascia and tendon of other parts of biceps, left arm**

7th **S46.219** **Strain of muscle, fascia and tendon of other parts of biceps, unspecified arm**

6th **S46.22** **Laceration of muscle, fascia and tendon of other parts of biceps**

7th **S46.221** **Laceration of muscle, fascia and tendon of other parts of biceps, right arm** CC

7th **S46.222** **Laceration of muscle, fascia and tendon of other parts of biceps, left arm** CC

7th **S46.229** **Laceration of muscle, fascia and tendon of other parts of biceps, unspecified arm** CC

6th **S46.29** **Other injury of muscle, fascia and tendon of other parts of biceps**

7th **S46.291** **Other injury of muscle, fascia and tendon of other parts of biceps, right arm**

7th **S46.292** **Other injury of muscle, fascia and tendon of other parts of biceps, left arm**

7th **S46.299** **Other injury of muscle, fascia and tendon of other parts of biceps, unspecified arm**

5th **S46.3** **Injury of muscle, fascia and tendon of triceps**

6th **S46.30** **Unspecified injury of muscle, fascia and tendon of triceps**

7th **S46.301** **Unspecified injury of muscle, fascia and tendon of triceps, right arm**

7th **S46.302** **Unspecified injury of muscle, fascia and tendon of triceps, left arm**

7th **S46.309** **Unspecified injury of muscle, fascia and tendon of triceps, unspecified arm**

6th **S46.31** **Strain of muscle, fascia and tendon of triceps**

7th **S46.311** **Strain of muscle, fascia and tendon of triceps, right arm**

7th **S46.312** **Strain of muscle, fascia and tendon of triceps, left arm**

7th **S46.319** **Strain of muscle, fascia and tendon of triceps, unspecified arm**

6th **S46.32** **Laceration of muscle, fascia and tendon of triceps**

7th **S46.321** **Laceration of muscle, fascia and tendon of triceps, right arm** CC

7th **S46.322** **Laceration of muscle, fascia and tendon of triceps, left arm** CC

7th **S46.329** **Laceration of muscle, fascia and tendon of triceps, unspecified arm** CC

6th **S46.39** **Other injury of muscle, fascia and tendon of triceps**

7th **S46.391** **Other injury of muscle, fascia and tendon of triceps, right arm**

7th **S46.392** **Other injury of muscle, fascia and tendon of triceps, left arm**

7th **S46.399** **Other injury of muscle, fascia and tendon of triceps, unspecified arm**

5th **S46.8** **Injury of other muscles, fascia and tendons at shoulder and upper arm level**

6th **S46.80** **Unspecified injury of other muscles, fascia and tendons at shoulder and upper arm level**

7th **S46.801** **Unspecified injury of other muscles, fascia and tendons at shoulder and upper arm level, right arm**

S46.802 Unspecified injury of other muscles, fascia and tendons at shoulder and upper arm level, left arm

S46.809 Unspecified injury of other muscles, fascia and tendons at shoulder and upper arm level, unspecified arm

S46.81 Strain of other muscles, fascia and tendons at shoulder and upper arm level

S46.811 Strain of other muscles, fascia and tendons at shoulder and upper arm level, right arm

S46.812 Strain of other muscles, fascia and tendons at shoulder and upper arm level, left arm

S46.819 Strain of other muscles, fascia and tendons at shoulder and upper arm level, unspecified arm

S46.82 Laceration of other muscles, fascia and tendons at shoulder and upper arm level

S46.821 Laceration of other muscles, fascia and tendons at shoulder and upper arm level, right arm CC

S46.822 Laceration of other muscles, fascia and tendons at shoulder and upper arm level, left arm CC

S46.829 Laceration of other muscles, fascia and tendons at shoulder and upper arm level, unspecified arm CC

S46.89 Other injury of other muscles, fascia and tendons at shoulder and upper arm level

S46.891 Other injury of other muscles, fascia and tendons at shoulder and upper arm level, right arm

S46.892 Other injury of other muscles, fascia and tendons at shoulder and upper arm level, left arm

S46.899 Other injury of other muscles, fascia and tendons at shoulder and upper arm level, unspecified arm

S46.9 Injury of unspecified muscle, fascia and tendon at shoulder and upper arm level

S46.90 Unspecified injury of unspecified muscle, fascia and tendon at shoulder and upper arm level

S46.901 Unspecified injury of unspecified muscle, fascia and tendon at shoulder and upper arm level, right arm

S46.902 Unspecified injury of unspecified muscle, fascia and tendon at shoulder and upper arm level, left arm

S46.909 Unspecified injury of unspecified muscle, fascia and tendon at shoulder and upper arm level, unspecified arm

S46.91 Strain of unspecified muscle, fascia and tendon at shoulder and upper arm level

S46.911 Strain of unspecified muscle, fascia and tendon at shoulder and upper arm level, right arm

S46.912 Strain of unspecified muscle, fascia and tendon at shoulder and upper arm level, left arm

S46.919 Strain of unspecified muscle, fascia and tendon at shoulder and upper arm level, unspecified arm

S46.92 Laceration of unspecified muscle, fascia and tendon at shoulder and upper arm level

S46.921 Laceration of unspecified muscle, fascia and tendon at shoulder and upper arm level, right arm CC

S46.922 Laceration of unspecified muscle, fascia and tendon at shoulder and upper arm level, left arm CC

S46.929 Laceration of unspecified muscle, fascia and tendon at shoulder and upper arm level, unspecified arm CC

S46.99 Other injury of unspecified muscle, fascia and tendon at shoulder and upper arm level

S46.991 Other injury of unspecified muscle, fascia and tendon at shoulder and upper arm level, right arm

S46.992 Other injury of unspecified muscle, fascia and tendon at shoulder and upper arm level, left arm

S46.999 Other injury of unspecified muscle, fascia and tendon at shoulder and upper arm level, unspecified arm

S47 Crushing injury of shoulder and upper arm

Use additional code for all associated injuries

EXCLUDES 2 *crushing injury of elbow (S57.0-)*

The appropriate 7th character is to be added to each code from category S47.
A initial encounter
D subsequent encounter
S sequela

S47.1 Crushing injury of right shoulder and upper arm

S47.2 Crushing injury of left shoulder and upper arm

S47.9 Crushing injury of shoulder and upper arm, unspecified arm

S48 Traumatic amputation of shoulder and upper arm

An amputation not identified as partial or complete should be coded to complete

EXCLUDES 1 *traumatic amputation at elbow level (S58.0)*

The appropriate 7th character is to be added to each code from category S48.
A initial encounter
D subsequent encounter
S sequela

S48.0 Traumatic amputation at shoulder joint

S48.01 Complete traumatic amputation at shoulder joint

S48.011 Complete traumatic amputation at right shoulder joint CC HCC

S48.012 Complete traumatic amputation at left shoulder joint CC HCC

S48.019 Complete traumatic amputation at unspecified shoulder joint CC HCC

S48.02 Partial traumatic amputation at shoulder joint

S48.021 Partial traumatic amputation at right shoulder joint CC HCC

S48.022 Partial traumatic amputation at left shoulder joint CC HCC

S48.029 Partial traumatic amputation at unspecified shoulder joint CC HCC

S48.1 Traumatic amputation at level between shoulder and elbow

S48.11 Complete traumatic amputation at level between shoulder and elbow

S48.111 Complete traumatic amputation at level between right shoulder and elbow CC HCC

S48.112 Complete traumatic amputation at level between left shoulder and elbow CC HCC

S48.119 Complete traumatic amputation at level between unspecified shoulder and elbow CC HCC

S48.12 Partial traumatic amputation at level between shoulder and elbow

S48.121 Partial traumatic amputation at level between right shoulder and elbow CC HCC

S48.122 Partial traumatic amputation at level between left shoulder and elbow CC HCC

S48.129 Partial traumatic amputation at level between unspecified shoulder and elbow CC HCC

S48.9 Traumatic amputation of shoulder and upper arm, level unspecified

S48.91 Complete traumatic amputation of shoulder and upper arm, level unspecified

S48.911 Complete traumatic amputation of right shoulder and upper arm, level unspecified CC HCC

S48.912 Complete traumatic amputation of left shoulder and upper arm, level unspecified CC HCC

S48.919 Complete traumatic amputation of unspecified shoulder and upper arm, level unspecified CC HCC

√6th S48.92 Partial traumatic amputation of shoulder and upper arm, level unspecified
7 √7th S48.921 Partial traumatic amputation of right shoulder and upper arm, level unspecified CC HCC
7 √7th S48.922 Partial traumatic amputation of left shoulder and upper arm, level unspecified CC HCC
7 √7th S48.929 Partial traumatic amputation of unspecified shoulder and upper arm, level unspecified CC HCC

√4th **S49 Other and unspecified injuries of shoulder and upper arm**

AHA: 2018,2Q,12; 2018,1Q,3

The appropriate 7th character is to be added to each code from subcategories S49.0 and S49.1.
A initial encounter for closed fracture
D subsequent encounter for fracture with routine healing
G subsequent encounter for fracture with delayed healing
K subsequent encounter for fracture with nonunion
P subsequent encounter for fracture with malunion
S sequela

√5th S49.0 Physeal fracture of upper end of humerus
AHA: 2019,4Q,56
√6th S49.00 Unspecified physeal fracture of upper end of humerus
3 √7th S49.001 Unspecified physeal fracture of upper end of humerus, right arm CC H5
3 √7th S49.002 Unspecified physeal fracture of upper end of humerus, left arm CC H5
3 √7th S49.009 Unspecified physeal fracture of upper end of humerus, unspecified arm CC H5
√6th S49.01 Salter-Harris Type I physeal fracture of upper end of humerus
3 √7th S49.011 Salter-Harris Type I physeal fracture of upper end of humerus, right arm CC H5
3 √7th S49.012 Salter-Harris Type I physeal fracture of upper end of humerus, left arm CC H5
3 √7th S49.019 Salter-Harris Type I physeal fracture of upper end of humerus, unspecified arm CC H5
√6th S49.02 Salter-Harris Type II physeal fracture of upper end of humerus
3 √7th S49.021 Salter-Harris Type II physeal fracture of upper end of humerus, right arm CC H5
3 √7th S49.022 Salter-Harris Type II physeal fracture of upper end of humerus, left arm CC H5
3 √7th S49.029 Salter-Harris Type II physeal fracture of upper end of humerus, unspecified arm CC H5
√6th S49.03 Salter-Harris Type III physeal fracture of upper end of humerus
3 √7th S49.031 Salter-Harris Type III physeal fracture of upper end of humerus, right arm CC H5
3 √7th S49.032 Salter-Harris Type III physeal fracture of upper end of humerus, left arm CC H5
3 √7th S49.039 Salter-Harris Type III physeal fracture of upper end of humerus, unspecified arm CC H5
√6th S49.04 Salter-Harris Type IV physeal fracture of upper end of humerus
3 √7th S49.041 Salter-Harris Type IV physeal fracture of upper end of humerus, right arm CC H5
3 √7th S49.042 Salter-Harris Type IV physeal fracture of upper end of humerus, left arm CC H5
3 √7th S49.049 Salter-Harris Type IV physeal fracture of upper end of humerus, unspecified arm CC H5
√6th S49.09 Other physeal fracture of upper end of humerus
3 √7th S49.091 Other physeal fracture of upper end of humerus, right arm CC H5
3 √7th S49.092 Other physeal fracture of upper end of humerus, left arm CC H5
3 √7th S49.099 Other physeal fracture of upper end of humerus, unspecified arm CC H5

√5th S49.1 Physeal fracture of lower end of humerus
AHA: 2019,4Q,56
√6th S49.10 Unspecified physeal fracture of lower end of humerus
3 √7th S49.101 Unspecified physeal fracture of lower end of humerus, right arm CC H5
3 √7th S49.102 Unspecified physeal fracture of lower end of humerus, left arm CC H5
3 √7th S49.109 Unspecified physeal fracture of lower end of humerus, unspecified arm CC H5
√6th S49.11 Salter-Harris Type I physeal fracture of lower end of humerus
3 √7th S49.111 Salter-Harris Type I physeal fracture of lower end of humerus, right arm CC H5
3 √7th S49.112 Salter-Harris Type I physeal fracture of lower end of humerus, left arm CC H5
3 √7th S49.119 Salter-Harris Type I physeal fracture of lower end of humerus, unspecified arm CC H5
√6th S49.12 Salter-Harris Type II physeal fracture of lower end of humerus
3 √7th S49.121 Salter-Harris Type II physeal fracture of lower end of humerus, right arm CC H5
3 √7th S49.122 Salter-Harris Type II physeal fracture of lower end of humerus, left arm CC H5
3 √7th S49.129 Salter-Harris Type II physeal fracture of lower end of humerus, unspecified arm CC H5
√6th S49.13 Salter-Harris Type III physeal fracture of lower end of humerus
3 √7th S49.131 Salter-Harris Type III physeal fracture of lower end of humerus, right arm CC H5
3 √7th S49.132 Salter-Harris Type III physeal fracture of lower end of humerus, left arm CC H5
3 √7th S49.139 Salter-Harris Type III physeal fracture of lower end of humerus, unspecified arm CC H5
√6th S49.14 Salter-Harris Type IV physeal fracture of lower end of humerus
3 √7th S49.141 Salter-Harris Type IV physeal fracture of lower end of humerus, right arm CC H5
3 √7th S49.142 Salter-Harris Type IV physeal fracture of lower end of humerus, left arm CC H5
3 √7th S49.149 Salter-Harris Type IV physeal fracture of lower end of humerus, unspecified arm CC H5
√6th S49.19 Other physeal fracture of lower end of humerus
3 √7th S49.191 Other physeal fracture of lower end of humerus, right arm CC H5
3 √7th S49.192 Other physeal fracture of lower end of humerus, left arm CC H5
3 √7th S49.199 Other physeal fracture of lower end of humerus, unspecified arm CC H5

√5th S49.8 Other specified injuries of shoulder and upper arm

The appropriate 7th character is to be added to each code in subcategory S49.8.
A initial encounter
D subsequent encounter
S sequela

√x7th S49.80 Other specified injuries of shoulder and upper arm, unspecified arm
√x7th S49.81 Other specified injuries of right shoulder and upper arm
√x7th S49.82 Other specified injuries of left shoulder and upper arm

√5th S49.9 Unspecified injury of shoulder and upper arm

The appropriate 7th character is to be added to each code in subcategory S49.9.
A initial encounter
D subsequent encounter
S sequela

√x7th S49.90 Unspecified injury of shoulder and upper arm, unspecified arm
√x7th S49.91 Unspecified injury of right shoulder and upper arm
√x7th S49.92 Unspecified injury of left shoulder and upper arm

Injuries to the elbow and forearm (S50-S59)

EXCLUDES 2 *burns and corrosions (T20-T32)*
frostbite (T33-T34)
injuries of wrist and hand (S60-S69)
insect bite or sting, venomous (T63.4)

S50 Superficial injury of elbow and forearm

EXCLUDES 2 *superficial injury of wrist and hand (S60.-)*

The appropriate 7th character is to be added to each code from category S50.
A initial encounter
D subsequent encounter
S sequela

S50.0 Contusion of elbow
- **S50.00 Contusion of unspecified elbow**
- **S50.01 Contusion of right elbow**
- **S50.02 Contusion of left elbow**

S50.1 Contusion of forearm
- **S50.10 Contusion of unspecified forearm**
- **S50.11 Contusion of right forearm**
- **S50.12 Contusion of left forearm**

S50.3 Other superficial injuries of elbow
- **S50.31 Abrasion of elbow**
  - **S50.311 Abrasion of right elbow**
  - **S50.312 Abrasion of left elbow**
  - **S50.319 Abrasion of unspecified elbow**
- **S50.32 Blister (nonthermal) of elbow**
  - **S50.321 Blister (nonthermal) of right elbow**
  - **S50.322 Blister (nonthermal) of left elbow**
  - **S50.329 Blister (nonthermal) of unspecified elbow**
- **S50.34 External constriction of elbow**
  - **S50.341 External constriction of right elbow**
  - **S50.342 External constriction of left elbow**
  - **S50.349 External constriction of unspecified elbow**
- **S50.35 Superficial foreign body of elbow**
  Splinter in the elbow
  - **S50.351 Superficial foreign body of right elbow**
  - **S50.352 Superficial foreign body of left elbow**
  - **S50.359 Superficial foreign body of unspecified elbow**
- **S50.36 Insect bite (nonvenomous) of elbow**
  - **S50.361 Insect bite (nonvenomous) of right elbow**
  - **S50.362 Insect bite (nonvenomous) of left elbow**
  - **S50.369 Insect bite (nonvenomous) of unspecified elbow**
- **S50.37 Other superficial bite of elbow**
  EXCLUDES 1 *open bite of elbow (S51.05)*
  - **S50.371 Other superficial bite of right elbow**
  - **S50.372 Other superficial bite of left elbow**
  - **S50.379 Other superficial bite of unspecified elbow**

S50.8 Other superficial injuries of forearm
- **S50.81 Abrasion of forearm**
  - **S50.811 Abrasion of right forearm**
  - **S50.812 Abrasion of left forearm**
  - **S50.819 Abrasion of unspecified forearm**
- **S50.82 Blister (nonthermal) of forearm**
  - **S50.821 Blister (nonthermal) of right forearm**
  - **S50.822 Blister (nonthermal) of left forearm**
  - **S50.829 Blister (nonthermal) of unspecified forearm**
- **S50.84 External constriction of forearm**
  - **S50.841 External constriction of right forearm**
  - **S50.842 External constriction of left forearm**
  - **S50.849 External constriction of unspecified forearm**
- **S50.85 Superficial foreign body of forearm**
  Splinter in the forearm
  - **S50.851 Superficial foreign body of right forearm**
  - **S50.852 Superficial foreign body of left forearm**
  - **S50.859 Superficial foreign body of unspecified forearm**
- **S50.86 Insect bite (nonvenomous) of forearm**
  - **S50.861 Insect bite (nonvenomous) of right forearm**
  - **S50.862 Insect bite (nonvenomous) of left forearm**
  - **S50.869 Insect bite (nonvenomous) of unspecified forearm**
- **S50.87 Other superficial bite of forearm**
  EXCLUDES 1 *open bite of forearm (S51.85)*
  - **S50.871 Other superficial bite of right forearm**
  - **S50.872 Other superficial bite of left forearm**
  - **S50.879 Other superficial bite of unspecified forearm**

S50.9 Unspecified superficial injury of elbow and forearm
- **S50.90 Unspecified superficial injury of elbow**
  - **S50.901 Unspecified superficial injury of right elbow**
  - **S50.902 Unspecified superficial injury of left elbow**
  - **S50.909 Unspecified superficial injury of unspecified elbow**
- **S50.91 Unspecified superficial injury of forearm**
  - **S50.911 Unspecified superficial injury of right forearm**
  - **S50.912 Unspecified superficial injury of left forearm**
  - **S50.919 Unspecified superficial injury of unspecified forearm**

S51 Open wound of elbow and forearm

Code also any associated wound infection

EXCLUDES 1 *open fracture of elbow and forearm (S52.- with open fracture 7th character)*
traumatic amputation of elbow and forearm (S58.-)

EXCLUDES 2 *open wound of wrist and hand (S61.-)*

The appropriate 7th character is to be added to each code from category S51.
A initial encounter
D subsequent encounter
S sequela

S51.0 Open wound of elbow
- **S51.00 Unspecified open wound of elbow**
  - **S51.001 Unspecified open wound of right elbow**
    AHA: 2012,4Q,108
  - **S51.002 Unspecified open wound of left elbow**
  - **S51.009 Unspecified open wound of unspecified elbow**
    Open wound of elbow NOS
- **S51.01 Laceration without foreign body of elbow**
  - **S51.011 Laceration without foreign body of right elbow**
  - **S51.012 Laceration without foreign body of left elbow**
  - **S51.019 Laceration without foreign body of unspecified elbow**
- **S51.02 Laceration with foreign body of elbow**
  - **S51.021 Laceration with foreign body of right elbow**
  - **S51.022 Laceration with foreign body of left elbow**
  - **S51.029 Laceration with foreign body of unspecified elbow**
- **S51.03 Puncture wound without foreign body of elbow**
  - **S51.031 Puncture wound without foreign body of right elbow**
  - **S51.032 Puncture wound without foreign body of left elbow**
  - **S51.039 Puncture wound without foreign body of unspecified elbow**
- **S51.04 Puncture wound with foreign body of elbow**
  - **S51.041 Puncture wound with foreign body of right elbow**

✓7th **S51.042 Puncture wound with foreign body of left elbow**

✓7th **S51.049 Puncture wound with foreign body of unspecified elbow**

✓6th **S51.05 Open bite of elbow**

Bite of elbow NOS

EXCLUDES 1 *superficial bite of elbow (S50.36, S50.37)*

✓7th **S51.051 Open bite, right elbow**

✓7th **S51.052 Open bite, left elbow**

✓7th **S51.059 Open bite, unspecified elbow**

✓5th **S51.8 Open wound of forearm**

EXCLUDES 2 *open wound of elbow (S51.0-)*

✓6th **S51.80 Unspecified open wound of forearm**

AHA: 2016,3Q,24

✓7th **S51.801 Unspecified open wound of right forearm**

✓7th **S51.802 Unspecified open wound of left forearm**

✓7th **S51.809 Unspecified open wound of unspecified forearm**

Open wound of forearm NOS

✓6th **S51.81 Laceration without foreign body of forearm**

✓7th **S51.811 Laceration without foreign body of right forearm**

✓7th **S51.812 Laceration without foreign body of left forearm**

✓7th **S51.819 Laceration without foreign body of unspecified forearm**

✓6th **S51.82 Laceration with foreign body of forearm**

✓7th **S51.821 Laceration with foreign body of right forearm**

✓7th **S51.822 Laceration with foreign body of left forearm**

✓7th **S51.829 Laceration with foreign body of unspecified forearm**

✓6th **S51.83 Puncture wound without foreign body of forearm**

AHA: 2016,3Q,24

✓7th **S51.831 Puncture wound without foreign body of right forearm**

✓7th **S51.832 Puncture wound without foreign body of left forearm**

✓7th **S51.839 Puncture wound without foreign body of unspecified forearm**

✓6th **S51.84 Puncture wound with foreign body of forearm**

AHA: 2016,3Q,24

✓7th **S51.841 Puncture wound with foreign body of right forearm**

✓7th **S51.842 Puncture wound with foreign body of left forearm**

✓7th **S51.849 Puncture wound with foreign body of unspecified forearm**

✓6th **S51.85 Open bite of forearm**

Bite of forearm NOS

EXCLUDES 1 *superficial bite of forearm (S50.86, S50.87)*

✓7th **S51.851 Open bite of right forearm**

✓7th **S51.852 Open bite of left forearm**

✓7th **S51.859 Open bite of unspecified forearm**

✓4th **S52 Fracture of forearm**

NOTE A fracture not indicated as displaced or nondisplaced should be coded to displaced.

A fracture not indicated as open or closed should be coded to closed.

The open fracture designations are based on the Gustilo open fracture classification.

EXCLUDES 1 *traumatic amputation of forearm (S58.-)*

EXCLUDES 2 *fracture at wrist and hand level (S62.-)*

AHA: 2018,2Q,12; 2016,1Q,33; 2015,3Q,37-39

DEF: Diaphysis: Central shaft of a long bone.

DEF: Epiphysis: Proximal and distal rounded ends of a long bone, communicates with the joint.

DEF: Metaphysis: Section of a long bone located between the epiphysis and diaphysis at the proximal and distal ends.

DEF: Physis (growth plate): Narrow zone of cartilaginous tissue between the epiphysis and metaphysis at each end of a long bone. In childhood, proliferation of cells in this zone lengthens the bone. As the bone matures, this area thins, ossification eventually fusing into solid bone and growth stops. ***Synonyms:*** *Epiphyseal plate.*

The appropriate 7th character is to be added to all codes from category S52 [unless otherwise indicated].

A initial encounter for closed fracture
B initial encounter for open fracture type I or II
initial encounter for open fracture NOS
C initial encounter for open fracture type IIIA, IIIB, or IIIC
D subsequent encounter for closed fracture with routine healing
E subsequent encounter for open fracture type I or II with routine healing
F subsequent encounter for open fracture type IIIA, IIIB, or IIIC with routine healing
G subsequent encounter for closed fracture with delayed healing
H subsequent encounter for open fracture type I or II with delayed healing
J subsequent encounter for open fracture type IIIA, IIIB, or IIIC with delayed healing
K subsequent encounter for closed fracture with nonunion
M subsequent encounter for open fracture type I or II with nonunion
N subsequent encounter for open fracture type IIIA, IIIB, or IIIC with nonunion
P subsequent encounter for closed fracture with malunion
Q subsequent encounter for open fracture type I or II with malunion
R subsequent encounter for open fracture type IIIA, IIIB, or IIIC with malunion
S sequela

✓5th **S52.0 Fracture of upper end of ulna**

Fracture of proximal end of ulna

EXCLUDES 2 *fracture of elbow NOS (S42.40-)*
fractures of shaft of ulna (S52.2-)

✓6th **S52.00 Unspecified fracture of upper end of ulna**

2,4 ✓7th **S52.001 Unspecified fracture of upper end of right ulna** MCC CC H5

2,4 ✓7th **S52.002 Unspecified fracture of upper end of left ulna** MCC CC H5

2,4 ✓7th **S52.009 Unspecified fracture of upper end of unspecified ulna** MCC CC H5

✓6th **S52.01 Torus fracture of upper end of ulna**

The appropriate 7th character is to be added to all codes in subcategory S52.01

A initial encounter for closed fracture
D subsequent encounter for fracture with routine healing
G subsequent encounter for fracture with delayed healing
K subsequent encounter for fracture with nonunion
P subsequent encounter for fracture with malunion
S sequela

3 ✓7th **S52.011 Torus fracture of upper end of right ulna** CC H5

3 ✓7th **S52.012 Torus fracture of upper end of left ulna** CC H5

3 ✓7th **S52.019 Torus fracture of upper end of unspecified ulna** CC H5

S52.02 Fracture of olecranon process without intraarticular extension of ulna
- 2,4 S52.021 Displaced fracture of olecranon process without intraarticular extension of right ulna MCC CC H5
- 2,4 S52.022 Displaced fracture of olecranon process without intraarticular extension of left ulna MCC CC H5
- 2,4 S52.023 Displaced fracture of olecranon process without intraarticular extension of unspecified ulna MCC CC H5
- 2,4 S52.024 Nondisplaced fracture of olecranon process without intraarticular extension of right ulna MCC CC H5
- 2,4 S52.025 Nondisplaced fracture of olecranon process without intraarticular extension of left ulna MCC CC H5
- 2,4 S52.026 Nondisplaced fracture of olecranon process without intraarticular extension of unspecified ulna MCC CC H5

S52.03 Fracture of olecranon process with intraarticular extension of ulna
- 2,4 S52.031 Displaced fracture of olecranon process with intraarticular extension of right ulna MCC CC H5
- 2,4 S52.032 Displaced fracture of olecranon process with intraarticular extension of left ulna MCC CC H5
- 2,4 S52.033 Displaced fracture of olecranon process with intraarticular extension of unspecified ulna MCC CC H5
- 2,4 S52.034 Nondisplaced fracture of olecranon process with intraarticular extension of right ulna MCC CC H5
- 2,4 S52.035 Nondisplaced fracture of olecranon process with intraarticular extension of left ulna MCC CC H5
- 2,4 S52.036 Nondisplaced fracture of olecranon process with intraarticular extension of unspecified ulna MCC CC H5

S52.04 Fracture of coronoid process of ulna
- 2,4 S52.041 Displaced fracture of coronoid process of right ulna MCC CC H5
- 2,4 S52.042 Displaced fracture of coronoid process of left ulna MCC CC H5
- 2,4 S52.043 Displaced fracture of coronoid process of unspecified ulna MCC CC H5
- 2,4 S52.044 Nondisplaced fracture of coronoid process of right ulna MCC CC H5
- 2,4 S52.045 Nondisplaced fracture of coronoid process of left ulna MCC CC H5
- 2,4 S52.046 Nondisplaced fracture of coronoid process of unspecified ulna MCC CC H5

S52.09 Other fracture of upper end of ulna
- 2,4 S52.091 Other fracture of upper end of right ulna MCC CC H5
- 2,4 S52.092 Other fracture of upper end of left ulna MCC CC H5
- 2,4 S52.099 Other fracture of upper end of unspecified ulna MCC CC H5

S52.1 Fracture of upper end of radius

Fracture of proximal end of radius

EXCLUDES 2 *physeal fractures of upper end of radius (S59.2-)*
fracture of shaft of radius (S52.3-)

S52.10 Unspecified fracture of upper end of radius
- 2,4 S52.101 Unspecified fracture of upper end of right radius MCC CC H5
- 2,4 S52.102 Unspecified fracture of upper end of left radius MCC CC H5
- 2,4 S52.109 Unspecified fracture of upper end of unspecified radius MCC CC H5

S52.11 Torus fracture of upper end of radius

The appropriate 7th character is to be added to all codes in subcategory S52.11
- A initial encounter for closed fracture
- D subsequent encounter for fracture with routine healing
- G subsequent encounter for fracture with delayed healing
- K subsequent encounter for fracture with nonunion
- P subsequent encounter for fracture with malunion
- S sequela

- 3 S52.111 Torus fracture of upper end of right radius CC H5
- 3 S52.112 Torus fracture of upper end of left radius CC H5
- 3 S52.119 Torus fracture of upper end of unspecified radius CC H5

S52.12 Fracture of head of radius
- 2,4 S52.121 Displaced fracture of head of right radius MCC CC H5
- 2,4 S52.122 Displaced fracture of head of left radius MCC CC H5
- 2,4 S52.123 Displaced fracture of head of unspecified radius MCC CC H5
- 2,4 S52.124 Nondisplaced fracture of head of right radius MCC CC H5
- 2,4 S52.125 Nondisplaced fracture of head of left radius MCC CC H5
- 2,4 S52.126 Nondisplaced fracture of head of unspecified radius MCC CC H5

S52.13 Fracture of neck of radius
- 2,4 S52.131 Displaced fracture of neck of right radius MCC CC H5
- 2,4 S52.132 Displaced fracture of neck of left radius MCC CC H5
- 2,4 S52.133 Displaced fracture of neck of unspecified radius MCC CC H5
- 2,4 S52.134 Nondisplaced fracture of neck of right radius MCC CC H5
- 2,4 S52.135 Nondisplaced fracture of neck of left radius MCC CC H5
- 2,4 S52.136 Nondisplaced fracture of neck of unspecified radius MCC CC H5

S52.18 Other fracture of upper end of radius
- 2,4 S52.181 Other fracture of upper end of right radius MCC CC H5
- 2,4 S52.182 Other fracture of upper end of left radius MCC CC H5
- 2,4 S52.189 Other fracture of upper end of unspecified radius MCC CC H5

S52.2 Fracture of shaft of ulna

S52.20 Unspecified fracture of shaft of ulna

Fracture of ulna NOS
- 2,3 S52.201 Unspecified fracture of shaft of right ulna MCC CC H5
- 2,3 S52.202 Unspecified fracture of shaft of left ulna MCC CC H5
- 2,3 S52.209 Unspecified fracture of shaft of unspecified ulna MCC CC H5

S52.21 Greenstick fracture of shaft of ulna

The appropriate 7th character is to be added to all codes in subcategory S52.21
- A initial encounter for closed fracture
- D subsequent encounter for fracture with routine healing
- G subsequent encounter for fracture with delayed healing
- K subsequent encounter for fracture with nonunion
- P subsequent encounter for fracture with malunion
- S sequela

- 3 S52.211 Greenstick fracture of shaft of right ulna CC H5

3 ✓7th S52.212 Greenstick fracture of shaft of left ulna CC H5

3 ✓7th S52.219 Greenstick fracture of shaft of unspecified ulna CC H5

✓6th S52.22 Transverse fracture of shaft of ulna

2,3 ✓7th S52.221 Displaced transverse fracture of shaft of right ulna MCC CC H5

2,3 ✓7th S52.222 Displaced transverse fracture of shaft of left ulna MCC CC H5

2,3 ✓7th S52.223 Displaced transverse fracture of shaft of unspecified ulna MCC CC H5

2,3 ✓7th S52.224 Nondisplaced transverse fracture of shaft of right ulna MCC CC H5

2,3 ✓7th S52.225 Nondisplaced transverse fracture of shaft of left ulna MCC CC H5

2,3 ✓7th S52.226 Nondisplaced transverse fracture of shaft of unspecified ulna MCC CC H5

✓6th S52.23 Oblique fracture of shaft of ulna

2,3 ✓7th S52.231 Displaced oblique fracture of shaft of right ulna MCC CC H5

2,3 ✓7th S52.232 Displaced oblique fracture of shaft of left ulna MCC CC H5

2,3 ✓7th S52.233 Displaced oblique fracture of shaft of unspecified ulna MCC CC H5

2,3 ✓7th S52.234 Nondisplaced oblique fracture of shaft of right ulna MCC CC H5

2,3 ✓7th S52.235 Nondisplaced oblique fracture of shaft of left ulna MCC CC H5

2,3 ✓7th S52.236 Nondisplaced oblique fracture of shaft of unspecified ulna MCC CC H5

✓6th S52.24 Spiral fracture of shaft of ulna

2,3 ✓7th S52.241 Displaced spiral fracture of shaft of ulna, right arm MCC CC H5

2,3 ✓7th S52.242 Displaced spiral fracture of shaft of ulna, left arm MCC CC H5

2,3 ✓7th S52.243 Displaced spiral fracture of shaft of ulna, unspecified arm MCC CC H5

2,3 ✓7th S52.244 Nondisplaced spiral fracture of shaft of ulna, right arm MCC CC H5

2,3 ✓7th S52.245 Nondisplaced spiral fracture of shaft of ulna, left arm MCC CC H5

2,3 ✓7th S52.246 Nondisplaced spiral fracture of shaft of ulna, unspecified arm MCC CC H5

✓6th S52.25 Comminuted fracture of shaft of ulna

2,3 ✓7th S52.251 Displaced comminuted fracture of shaft of ulna, right arm MCC CC H5

2,3 ✓7th S52.252 Displaced comminuted fracture of shaft of ulna, left arm MCC CC H5

2,3 ✓7th S52.253 Displaced comminuted fracture of shaft of ulna, unspecified arm MCC CC H5

2,3 ✓7th S52.254 Nondisplaced comminuted fracture of shaft of ulna, right arm MCC CC H5

2,3 ✓7th S52.255 Nondisplaced comminuted fracture of shaft of ulna, left arm MCC CC H5

2,3 ✓7th S52.256 Nondisplaced comminuted fracture of shaft of ulna, unspecified arm MCC CC H5

✓6th S52.26 Segmental fracture of shaft of ulna

2,3 ✓7th S52.261 Displaced segmental fracture of shaft of ulna, right arm MCC CC H5

2,3 ✓7th S52.262 Displaced segmental fracture of shaft of ulna, left arm MCC CC H5

2,3 ✓7th S52.263 Displaced segmental fracture of shaft of ulna, unspecified arm MCC CC H5

2,3 ✓7th S52.264 Nondisplaced segmental fracture of shaft of ulna, right arm MCC CC H5

2,3 ✓7th S52.265 Nondisplaced segmental fracture of shaft of ulna, left arm MCC CC H5

2,3 ✓7th S52.266 Nondisplaced segmental fracture of shaft of ulna, unspecified arm MCC CC H5

✓6th S52.27 Monteggia's fracture of ulna

Fracture of upper shaft of ulna with dislocation of radial head

2,4 ✓7th S52.271 Monteggia's fracture of right ulna MCC CC H5

2,4 ✓7th S52.272 Monteggia's fracture of left ulna MCC CC H5

2,4 ✓7th S52.279 Monteggia's fracture of unspecified ulna MCC CC H5

✓6th S52.28 Bent bone of ulna

2,3 ✓7th S52.281 Bent bone of right ulna MCC CC H5

2,3 ✓7th S52.282 Bent bone of left ulna MCC CC H5

2,3 ✓7th S52.283 Bent bone of unspecified ulna MCC CC H5

✓6th S52.29 Other fracture of shaft of ulna

2,3 ✓7th S52.291 Other fracture of shaft of right ulna MCC CC H5

2,3 ✓7th S52.292 Other fracture of shaft of left ulna MCC CC H5

2,3 ✓7th S52.299 Other fracture of shaft of unspecified ulna MCC CC H5

✓5th S52.3 Fracture of shaft of radius

✓6th S52.30 Unspecified fracture of shaft of radius

2,3 ✓7th S52.301 Unspecified fracture of shaft of right radius MCC CC H5

2,3 ✓7th S52.302 Unspecified fracture of shaft of left radius MCC CC H5

2,3 ✓7th S52.309 Unspecified fracture of shaft of unspecified radius MCC CC H5

✓6th S52.31 Greenstick fracture of shaft of radius

The appropriate 7th character is to be added to all codes in subcategory S52.31.

A initial encounter for closed fracture
D subsequent encounter for fracture with routine healing
G subsequent encounter for fracture with delayed healing
K subsequent encounter for fracture with nonunion
P subsequent encounter for fracture with malunion
S sequela

3 ✓7th S52.311 Greenstick fracture of shaft of radius, right arm CC H5

3 ✓7th S52.312 Greenstick fracture of shaft of radius, left arm CC H5

3 ✓7th S52.319 Greenstick fracture of shaft of radius, unspecified arm CC H5

✓6th S52.32 Transverse fracture of shaft of radius

2,3 ✓7th S52.321 Displaced transverse fracture of shaft of right radius MCC CC H5

2,3 ✓7th S52.322 Displaced transverse fracture of shaft of left radius MCC CC H5

2,3 ✓7th S52.323 Displaced transverse fracture of shaft of unspecified radius MCC CC H5

2,3 ✓7th S52.324 Nondisplaced transverse fracture of shaft of right radius MCC CC H5

2,3 ✓7th S52.325 Nondisplaced transverse fracture of shaft of left radius MCC CC H5

2,3 ✓7th S52.326 Nondisplaced transverse fracture of shaft of unspecified radius MCC CC H5

✓6th S52.33 Oblique fracture of shaft of radius

2,3 ✓7th S52.331 Displaced oblique fracture of shaft of right radius MCC CC H5

2,3 ✓7th S52.332 Displaced oblique fracture of shaft of left radius MCC CC H5

2,3 ✓7th S52.333 Displaced oblique fracture of shaft of unspecified radius MCC CC H5

2,3 ✓7th S52.334 Nondisplaced oblique fracture of shaft of right radius MCC CC H5

2,3 ✓7th S52.335 Nondisplaced oblique fracture of shaft of left radius MCC CC H5

2,3 ✓7th S52.336 Nondisplaced oblique fracture of shaft of unspecified radius MCC CC H5

✓6th S52.34 Spiral fracture of shaft of radius

2,3 ✓7th S52.341 Displaced spiral fracture of shaft of radius, right arm MCC CC H5

2,3 ✓7th S52.342 Displaced spiral fracture of shaft of radius, left arm MCC CC H5

2,3 ✓7th S52.343 Displaced spiral fracture of shaft of radius, unspecified arm MCC CC H5

2,3 ✓7th S52.344 Nondisplaced spiral fracture of shaft of radius, right arm MCC CC H5

2,3 ✓7th S52.345 Nondisplaced spiral fracture of shaft of radius, left arm MCC CC H5

2,3 ✓7th **S52.346 Nondisplaced spiral fracture of shaft of radius, unspecified arm** MCC CC H5

✓6th **S52.35 Comminuted fracture of shaft of radius**

2,3 ✓7th **S52.351 Displaced comminuted fracture of shaft of radius, right arm** MCC CC H5

2,3 ✓7th **S52.352 Displaced comminuted fracture of shaft of radius, left arm** MCC CC H5

2,3 ✓7th **S52.353 Displaced comminuted fracture of shaft of radius, unspecified arm** MCC CC H5

2,3 ✓7th **S52.354 Nondisplaced comminuted fracture of shaft of radius, right arm** MCC CC H5

2,3 ✓7th **S52.355 Nondisplaced comminuted fracture of shaft of radius, left arm** MCC CC H5

2,3 ✓7th **S52.356 Nondisplaced comminuted fracture of shaft of radius, unspecified arm** MCC CC H5

✓6th **S52.36 Segmental fracture of shaft of radius**

2,3 ✓7th **S52.361 Displaced segmental fracture of shaft of radius, right arm** MCC CC H5

2,3 ✓7th **S52.362 Displaced segmental fracture of shaft of radius, left arm** MCC CC H5

2,3 ✓7th **S52.363 Displaced segmental fracture of shaft of radius, unspecified arm** MCC CC H5

2,3 ✓7th **S52.364 Nondisplaced segmental fracture of shaft of radius, right arm** MCC CC H5

2,3 ✓7th **S52.365 Nondisplaced segmental fracture of shaft of radius, left arm** MCC CC H5

2,3 ✓7th **S52.366 Nondisplaced segmental fracture of shaft of radius, unspecified arm** MCC CC H5

✓6th **S52.37 Galeazzi's fracture**

Fracture of lower shaft of radius with radioulnar joint dislocation

2,3 ✓7th **S52.371 Galeazzi's fracture of right radius** MCC CC H5

2,3 ✓7th **S52.372 Galeazzi's fracture of left radius** MCC CC H5

2,3 ✓7th **S52.379 Galeazzi's fracture of unspecified radius** MCC CC H5

✓6th **S52.38 Bent bone of radius**

2,3 ✓7th **S52.381 Bent bone of right radius** MCC CC H5

2,3 ✓7th **S52.382 Bent bone of left radius** MCC CC H5

2,3 ✓7th **S52.389 Bent bone of unspecified radius** MCC CC H5

✓6th **S52.39 Other fracture of shaft of radius**

2,3 ✓7th **S52.391 Other fracture of shaft of radius, right arm** MCC CC H5

2,3 ✓7th **S52.392 Other fracture of shaft of radius, left arm** MCC CC H5

2,3 ✓7th **S52.399 Other fracture of shaft of radius, unspecified arm** MCC CC H5

✓5th **S52.5 Fracture of lower end of radius**

Fracture of distal end of radius

EXCLUDES 2 *physeal fractures of lower end of radius (S59.2-)*

DEF: Fracture of the distal end of the radius above the wrist, most commonly caused by a fall onto an outstretched hand.

✓6th **S52.50 Unspecified fracture of the lower end of radius**

2,3 ✓7th **S52.501 Unspecified fracture of the lower end of right radius** MCC CC H5

2,3 ✓7th **S52.502 Unspecified fracture of the lower end of left radius** MCC CC H5

2,3 ✓7th **S52.509 Unspecified fracture of the lower end of unspecified radius** MCC CC H5

✓6th **S52.51 Fracture of radial styloid process**

2,3 ✓7th **S52.511 Displaced fracture of right radial styloid process** MCC CC H5

2,3 ✓7th **S52.512 Displaced fracture of left radial styloid process** MCC CC H5

2,3 ✓7th **S52.513 Displaced fracture of unspecified radial styloid process** MCC CC H5

2,3 ✓7th **S52.514 Nondisplaced fracture of right radial styloid process** MCC CC H5

2,3 ✓7th **S52.515 Nondisplaced fracture of left radial styloid process** MCC CC H5

2,3 ✓7th **S52.516 Nondisplaced fracture of unspecified radial styloid process** MCC CC H5

✓6th **S52.52 Torus fracture of lower end of radius**

The appropriate 7th character is to be added to all codes in subcategory S52.52.
- A initial encounter for closed fracture
- D subsequent encounter for fracture with routine healing
- G subsequent encounter for fracture with delayed healing
- K subsequent encounter for fracture with nonunion
- P subsequent encounter for fracture with malunion
- S sequela

3 ✓7th **S52.521 Torus fracture of lower end of right radius** CC H5

3 ✓7th **S52.522 Torus fracture of lower end of left radius** CC H5

3 ✓7th **S52.529 Torus fracture of lower end of unspecified radius** CC H5

✓6th **S52.53 Colles' fracture**

AHA: 2016,2Q,4

DEF: Fracture of the radius at the wrist in which the distal fragment is pushed posteriorly. The dorsal angulation of the fragment results in the wrist cocking up.

2,3 ✓7th **S52.531 Colles' fracture of right radius** MCC CC H5

2,3 ✓7th **S52.532 Colles' fracture of left radius** MCC CC H5

2,3 ✓7th **S52.539 Colles' fracture of unspecified radius** MCC CC H5

✓6th **S52.54 Smith's fracture**

2,3 ✓7th **S52.541 Smith's fracture of right radius** MCC CC H5

2,3 ✓7th **S52.542 Smith's fracture of left radius** MCC CC H5

2,3 ✓7th **S52.549 Smith's fracture of unspecified radius** MCC CC H5

✓6th **S52.55 Other extraarticular fracture of lower end of radius**

2,3 ✓7th **S52.551 Other extraarticular fracture of lower end of right radius** MCC CC H5

2,3 ✓7th **S52.552 Other extraarticular fracture of lower end of left radius** MCC CC H5

2,3 ✓7th **S52.559 Other extraarticular fracture of lower end of unspecified radius** MCC CC H5

✓6th **S52.56 Barton's fracture**

2,3 ✓7th **S52.561 Barton's fracture of right radius** MCC CC H5

2,3 ✓7th **S52.562 Barton's fracture of left radius** MCC CC H5

2,3 ✓7th **S52.569 Barton's fracture of unspecified radius** MCC CC H5

✓6th **S52.57 Other intraarticular fracture of lower end of radius**

2,3 ✓7th **S52.571 Other intraarticular fracture of lower end of right radius** MCC CC H5

2,3 ✓7th **S52.572 Other intraarticular fracture of lower end of left radius** MCC CC H5

2,3 ✓7th **S52.579 Other intraarticular fracture of lower end of unspecified radius** MCC CC H5

✓6th **S52.59 Other fractures of lower end of radius**

AHA: 2019,3Q,9

2,3 ✓7th **S52.591 Other fractures of lower end of right radius** MCC CC H5

2,3 ✓7th **S52.592 Other fractures of lower end of left radius** MCC CC H5

2,3 ✓7th **S52.599 Other fractures of lower end of unspecified radius** MCC CC H5

✓5th **S52.6 Fracture of lower end of ulna**

✓6th **S52.60 Unspecified fracture of lower end of ulna**

2,3 ✓7th **S52.601 Unspecified fracture of lower end of right ulna** MCC CC H5

2,3 ✓7th **S52.602 Unspecified fracture of lower end of left ulna** MCC CC H5

2,3 ✓7th **S52.609 Unspecified fracture of lower end of unspecified ulna** MCC CC H5

√6th S52.61 Fracture of ulna styloid process
2,3 √7th S52.611 Displaced fracture of right ulna styloid process MCC CC H5
2,3 √7th S52.612 Displaced fracture of left ulna styloid process MCC CC H5
2,3 √7th S52.613 Displaced fracture of unspecified ulna styloid process MCC CC H5
2,3 √7th S52.614 Nondisplaced fracture of right ulna styloid process MCC CC H5
2,3 √7th S52.615 Nondisplaced fracture of left ulna styloid process MCC CC H5
2,3 √7th S52.616 Nondisplaced fracture of unspecified ulna styloid process MCC CC H5

√6th S52.62 Torus fracture of lower end of ulna

The appropriate 7th character is to be added to all codes in subcategory S52.62.
A initial encounter for closed fracture
D subsequent encounter for fracture with routine healing
G subsequent encounter for fracture with delayed healing
K subsequent encounter for fracture with nonunion
P subsequent encounter for fracture with malunion
S sequela

3 √7th S52.621 Torus fracture of lower end of right ulna CC H5
3 √7th S52.622 Torus fracture of lower end of left ulna CC H5
3 √7th S52.629 Torus fracture of lower end of unspecified ulna CC H5

√6th S52.69 Other fracture of lower end of ulna
AHA: 2019,3Q,9
2,3 √7th S52.691 Other fracture of lower end of right ulna MCC CC H5
2,3 √7th S52.692 Other fracture of lower end of left ulna MCC CC H5
2,3 √7th S52.699 Other fracture of lower end of unspecified ulna MCC CC H5

√5th S52.9 Unspecified fracture of forearm
2,3 √x 7th S52.90 Unspecified fracture of unspecified forearm MCC CC H5
2,3 √x 7th S52.91 Unspecified fracture of right forearm MCC CC H5
2,3 √x 7th S52.92 Unspecified fracture of left forearm MCC CC H5

√4th S53 Dislocation and sprain of joints and ligaments of elbow

INCLUDES avulsion of joint or ligament of elbow
laceration of cartilage, joint or ligament of elbow
sprain of cartilage, joint or ligament of elbow
traumatic hemarthrosis of joint or ligament of elbow
traumatic rupture of joint or ligament of elbow
traumatic subluxation of joint or ligament of elbow
traumatic tear of joint or ligament of elbow

Code also any associated open wound

EXCLUDES 2 *strain of muscle, fascia and tendon at forearm level (S56.-)*

The appropriate 7th character is to be added to each code from category S53.
A initial encounter
D subsequent encounter
S sequela

√5th S53.Ø Subluxation and dislocation of radial head
Dislocation of radiohumeral joint
Subluxation of radiohumeral joint
EXCLUDES 1 *Monteggia's fracture-dislocation (S52.27-)*

√6th S53.ØØ Unspecified subluxation and dislocation of radial head
√7th S53.ØØ1 Unspecified subluxation of right radial head
√7th S53.ØØ2 Unspecified subluxation of left radial head
√7th S53.ØØ3 Unspecified subluxation of unspecified radial head
√7th S53.ØØ4 Unspecified dislocation of right radial head
√7th S53.ØØ5 Unspecified dislocation of left radial head
√7th S53.ØØ6 Unspecified dislocation of unspecified radial head

√6th S53.Ø1 Anterior subluxation and dislocation of radial head
Anteriomedial subluxation and dislocation of radial head
√7th S53.Ø11 Anterior subluxation of right radial head
√7th S53.Ø12 Anterior subluxation of left radial head
√7th S53.Ø13 Anterior subluxation of unspecified radial head
√7th S53.Ø14 Anterior dislocation of right radial head
√7th S53.Ø15 Anterior dislocation of left radial head
√7th S53.Ø16 Anterior dislocation of unspecified radial head

√6th S53.Ø2 Posterior subluxation and dislocation of radial head
Posteriolateral subluxation and dislocation of radial head
√7th S53.Ø21 Posterior subluxation of right radial head
√7th S53.Ø22 Posterior subluxation of left radial head
√7th S53.Ø23 Posterior subluxation of unspecified radial head
√7th S53.Ø24 Posterior dislocation of right radial head
√7th S53.Ø25 Posterior dislocation of left radial head
√7th S53.Ø26 Posterior dislocation of unspecified radial head

√6th S53.Ø3 Nursemaid's elbow
√7th S53.Ø31 Nursemaid's elbow, right elbow
√7th S53.Ø32 Nursemaid's elbow, left elbow
√7th S53.Ø33 Nursemaid's elbow, unspecified elbow

√6th S53.Ø9 Other subluxation and dislocation of radial head
√7th S53.Ø91 Other subluxation of right radial head
√7th S53.Ø92 Other subluxation of left radial head
√7th S53.Ø93 Other subluxation of unspecified radial head
√7th S53.Ø94 Other dislocation of right radial head
√7th S53.Ø95 Other dislocation of left radial head
√7th S53.Ø96 Other dislocation of unspecified radial head

√5th S53.1 Subluxation and dislocation of ulnohumeral joint
Subluxation and dislocation of elbow NOS
EXCLUDES 1 *dislocation of radial head alone (S53.Ø-)*

√6th S53.1Ø Unspecified subluxation and dislocation of ulnohumeral joint
√7th S53.1Ø1 Unspecified subluxation of right ulnohumeral joint
√7th S53.1Ø2 Unspecified subluxation of left ulnohumeral joint
√7th S53.1Ø3 Unspecified subluxation of unspecified ulnohumeral joint
√7th S53.1Ø4 Unspecified dislocation of right ulnohumeral joint
√7th S53.1Ø5 Unspecified dislocation of left ulnohumeral joint
√7th S53.1Ø6 Unspecified dislocation of unspecified ulnohumeral joint

√6th S53.11 Anterior subluxation and dislocation of ulnohumeral joint
√7th S53.111 Anterior subluxation of right ulnohumeral joint
√7th S53.112 Anterior subluxation of left ulnohumeral joint
√7th S53.113 Anterior subluxation of unspecified ulnohumeral joint
√7th S53.114 Anterior dislocation of right ulnohumeral joint
AHA: 2012,4Q,108
√7th S53.115 Anterior dislocation of left ulnohumeral joint
√7th S53.116 Anterior dislocation of unspecified ulnohumeral joint

√6th S53.12 Posterior subluxation and dislocation of ulnohumeral joint
√7th S53.121 Posterior subluxation of right ulnohumeral joint
√7th S53.122 Posterior subluxation of left ulnohumeral joint
√7th S53.123 Posterior subluxation of unspecified ulnohumeral joint

S53.124 Posterior dislocation of right ulnohumeral joint
S53.125 Posterior dislocation of left ulnohumeral joint
S53.126 Posterior dislocation of unspecified ulnohumeral joint

S53.13 Medial subluxation and dislocation of ulnohumeral joint
S53.131 Medial subluxation of right ulnohumeral joint
S53.132 Medial subluxation of left ulnohumeral joint
S53.133 Medial subluxation of unspecified ulnohumeral joint
S53.134 Medial dislocation of right ulnohumeral joint
S53.135 Medial dislocation of left ulnohumeral joint
S53.136 Medial dislocation of unspecified ulnohumeral joint

S53.14 Lateral subluxation and dislocation of ulnohumeral joint
S53.141 Lateral subluxation of right ulnohumeral joint
S53.142 Lateral subluxation of left ulnohumeral joint
S53.143 Lateral subluxation of unspecified ulnohumeral joint
S53.144 Lateral dislocation of right ulnohumeral joint
S53.145 Lateral dislocation of left ulnohumeral joint
S53.146 Lateral dislocation of unspecified ulnohumeral joint

S53.19 Other subluxation and dislocation of ulnohumeral joint
S53.191 Other subluxation of right ulnohumeral joint
S53.192 Other subluxation of left ulnohumeral joint
S53.193 Other subluxation of unspecified ulnohumeral joint
S53.194 Other dislocation of right ulnohumeral joint
S53.195 Other dislocation of left ulnohumeral joint
S53.196 Other dislocation of unspecified ulnohumeral joint

S53.2 Traumatic rupture of radial collateral ligament

EXCLUDES 1 *sprain of radial collateral ligament NOS (S53.43-)*

S53.20 Traumatic rupture of unspecified radial collateral ligament
S53.21 Traumatic rupture of right radial collateral ligament
S53.22 Traumatic rupture of left radial collateral ligament

S53.3 Traumatic rupture of ulnar collateral ligament

EXCLUDES 1 *sprain of ulnar collateral ligament (S53.44-)*

S53.30 Traumatic rupture of unspecified ulnar collateral ligament
S53.31 Traumatic rupture of right ulnar collateral ligament
S53.32 Traumatic rupture of left ulnar collateral ligament

S53.4 Sprain of elbow

EXCLUDES 2 *traumatic rupture of radial collateral ligament (S53.2-)*
traumatic rupture of ulnar collateral ligament (S53.3-)

S53.40 Unspecified sprain of elbow
S53.401 Unspecified sprain of right elbow
S53.402 Unspecified sprain of left elbow
S53.409 Unspecified sprain of unspecified elbow
Sprain of elbow NOS

S53.41 Radiohumeral (joint) sprain
S53.411 Radiohumeral (joint) sprain of right elbow
S53.412 Radiohumeral (joint) sprain of left elbow
S53.419 Radiohumeral (joint) sprain of unspecified elbow

S53.42 Ulnohumeral (joint) sprain
S53.421 Ulnohumeral (joint) sprain of right elbow
S53.422 Ulnohumeral (joint) sprain of left elbow
S53.429 Ulnohumeral (joint) sprain of unspecified elbow

S53.43 Radial collateral ligament sprain
S53.431 Radial collateral ligament sprain of right elbow
S53.432 Radial collateral ligament sprain of left elbow
S53.439 Radial collateral ligament sprain of unspecified elbow

S53.44 Ulnar collateral ligament sprain
S53.441 Ulnar collateral ligament sprain of right elbow
S53.442 Ulnar collateral ligament sprain of left elbow
S53.449 Ulnar collateral ligament sprain of unspecified elbow

S53.49 Other sprain of elbow
S53.491 Other sprain of right elbow
S53.492 Other sprain of left elbow
S53.499 Other sprain of unspecified elbow

S54 Injury of nerves at forearm level

Code also any associated open wound (S51.-)

EXCLUDES 2 *injury of nerves at wrist and hand level (S64.-)*

The appropriate 7th character is to be added to each code from category S54.
A initial encounter
D subsequent encounter
S sequela

S54.0 Injury of ulnar nerve at forearm level
Injury of ulnar nerve NOS
S54.00 Injury of ulnar nerve at forearm level, unspecified arm
S54.01 Injury of ulnar nerve at forearm level, right arm
S54.02 Injury of ulnar nerve at forearm level, left arm

S54.1 Injury of median nerve at forearm level
Injury of median nerve NOS
S54.10 Injury of median nerve at forearm level, unspecified arm
S54.11 Injury of median nerve at forearm level, right arm
S54.12 Injury of median nerve at forearm level, left arm

S54.2 Injury of radial nerve at forearm level
Injury of radial nerve NOS
S54.20 Injury of radial nerve at forearm level, unspecified arm
S54.21 Injury of radial nerve at forearm level, right arm
S54.22 Injury of radial nerve at forearm level, left arm

S54.3 Injury of cutaneous sensory nerve at forearm level
S54.30 Injury of cutaneous sensory nerve at forearm level, unspecified arm
S54.31 Injury of cutaneous sensory nerve at forearm level, right arm
S54.32 Injury of cutaneous sensory nerve at forearm level, left arm

S54.8 Injury of other nerves at forearm level
S54.8X Injury of other nerves at forearm level
S54.8X1 Injury of other nerves at forearm level, right arm
S54.8X2 Injury of other nerves at forearm level, left arm
S54.8X9 Injury of other nerves at forearm level, unspecified arm

S54.9 Injury of unspecified nerve at forearm level
S54.90 Injury of unspecified nerve at forearm level, unspecified arm
S54.91 Injury of unspecified nerve at forearm level, right arm
S54.92 Injury of unspecified nerve at forearm level, left arm

✓4th S55 Injury of blood vessels at forearm level

Code also any associated open wound (S51.-)

EXCLUDES 2 *injury of blood vessels at wrist and hand level (S65.-)*
injury of brachial vessels (S45.1-S45.2)

The appropriate 7th character is to be added to each code from category S55.
A initial encounter
D subsequent encounter
S sequela

✓5th S55.0 Injury of ulnar artery at forearm level
- **✓6th S55.00 Unspecified injury of ulnar artery at forearm level**
  - **✓7th S55.001 Unspecified injury of ulnar artery at forearm level, right arm** CC
  - **✓7th S55.002 Unspecified injury of ulnar artery at forearm level, left arm** CC
  - **✓7th S55.009 Unspecified injury of ulnar artery at forearm level, unspecified arm** CC
- **✓6th S55.01 Laceration of ulnar artery at forearm level**
  - **✓7th S55.011 Laceration of ulnar artery at forearm level, right arm** CC
  - **✓7th S55.012 Laceration of ulnar artery at forearm level, left arm** CC
  - **✓7th S55.019 Laceration of ulnar artery at forearm level, unspecified arm** CC
- **✓6th S55.09 Other specified injury of ulnar artery at forearm level**
  - **✓7th S55.091 Other specified injury of ulnar artery at forearm level, right arm** CC
  - **✓7th S55.092 Other specified injury of ulnar artery at forearm level, left arm** CC
  - **✓7th S55.099 Other specified injury of ulnar artery at forearm level, unspecified arm** CC

✓5th S55.1 Injury of radial artery at forearm level
- **✓6th S55.10 Unspecified injury of radial artery at forearm level**
  - **✓7th S55.101 Unspecified injury of radial artery at forearm level, right arm** CC
  - **✓7th S55.102 Unspecified injury of radial artery at forearm level, left arm** CC
  - **✓7th S55.109 Unspecified injury of radial artery at forearm level, unspecified arm** CC
- **✓6th S55.11 Laceration of radial artery at forearm level**
  - **✓7th S55.111 Laceration of radial artery at forearm level, right arm** CC
  - **✓7th S55.112 Laceration of radial artery at forearm level, left arm** CC
  - **✓7th S55.119 Laceration of radial artery at forearm level, unspecified arm** CC
- **✓6th S55.19 Other specified injury of radial artery at forearm level**
  - **✓7th S55.191 Other specified injury of radial artery at forearm level, right arm** CC
  - **✓7th S55.192 Other specified injury of radial artery at forearm level, left arm** CC
  - **✓7th S55.199 Other specified injury of radial artery at forearm level, unspecified arm** CC

✓5th S55.2 Injury of vein at forearm level
- **✓6th S55.20 Unspecified injury of vein at forearm level**
  - **✓7th S55.201 Unspecified injury of vein at forearm level, right arm** CC
  - **✓7th S55.202 Unspecified injury of vein at forearm level, left arm** CC
  - **✓7th S55.209 Unspecified injury of vein at forearm level, unspecified arm** CC
- **✓6th S55.21 Laceration of vein at forearm level**
  - **✓7th S55.211 Laceration of vein at forearm level, right arm** CC
  - **✓7th S55.212 Laceration of vein at forearm level, left arm** CC
  - **✓7th S55.219 Laceration of vein at forearm level, unspecified arm** CC
- **✓6th S55.29 Other specified injury of vein at forearm level**
  - **✓7th S55.291 Other specified injury of vein at forearm level, right arm** CC
  - **✓7th S55.292 Other specified injury of vein at forearm level, left arm** CC
  - **✓7th S55.299 Other specified injury of vein at forearm level, unspecified arm** CC

✓5th S55.8 Injury of other blood vessels at forearm level
- **✓6th S55.80 Unspecified injury of other blood vessels at forearm level**
  - **✓7th S55.801 Unspecified injury of other blood vessels at forearm level, right arm** CC
  - **✓7th S55.802 Unspecified injury of other blood vessels at forearm level, left arm** CC
  - **✓7th S55.809 Unspecified injury of other blood vessels at forearm level, unspecified arm** CC
- **✓6th S55.81 Laceration of other blood vessels at forearm level**
  - **✓7th S55.811 Laceration of other blood vessels at forearm level, right arm** CC
  - **✓7th S55.812 Laceration of other blood vessels at forearm level, left arm** CC
  - **✓7th S55.819 Laceration of other blood vessels at forearm level, unspecified arm** CC
- **✓6th S55.89 Other specified injury of other blood vessels at forearm level**
  - **✓7th S55.891 Other specified injury of other blood vessels at forearm level, right arm** CC
  - **✓7th S55.892 Other specified injury of other blood vessels at forearm level, left arm** CC
  - **✓7th S55.899 Other specified injury of other blood vessels at forearm level, unspecified arm** CC

✓5th S55.9 Injury of unspecified blood vessel at forearm level
- **✓6th S55.90 Unspecified injury of unspecified blood vessel at forearm level**
  - **✓7th S55.901 Unspecified injury of unspecified blood vessel at forearm level, right arm** CC
  - **✓7th S55.902 Unspecified injury of unspecified blood vessel at forearm level, left arm** CC
  - **✓7th S55.909 Unspecified injury of unspecified blood vessel at forearm level, unspecified arm** CC
- **✓6th S55.91 Laceration of unspecified blood vessel at forearm level**
  - **✓7th S55.911 Laceration of unspecified blood vessel at forearm level, right arm** CC
  - **✓7th S55.912 Laceration of unspecified blood vessel at forearm level, left arm** CC
  - **✓7th S55.919 Laceration of unspecified blood vessel at forearm level, unspecified arm** CC
- **✓6th S55.99 Other specified injury of unspecified blood vessel at forearm level**
  - **✓7th S55.991 Other specified injury of unspecified blood vessel at forearm level, right arm** CC
  - **✓7th S55.992 Other specified injury of unspecified blood vessel at forearm level, left arm** CC
  - **✓7th S55.999 Other specified injury of unspecified blood vessel at forearm level, unspecified arm** CC

✓4th S56 Injury of muscle, fascia and tendon at forearm level

Code also any associated open wound (S51.-)

EXCLUDES 2 *injury of muscle, fascia and tendon at or below wrist (S66.-)*
sprain of joints and ligaments of elbow (S53.4-)

TIP: Refer to the Muscle/Tendon table at the beginning of this chapter

The appropriate 7th character is to be added to each code from category S56.
A initial encounter
D subsequent encounter
S sequela

✓5th S56.0 Injury of flexor muscle, fascia and tendon of thumb at forearm level
- **✓6th S56.00 Unspecified injury of flexor muscle, fascia and tendon of thumb at forearm level**
  - **✓7th S56.001 Unspecified injury of flexor muscle, fascia and tendon of right thumb at forearm level**
  - **✓7th S56.002 Unspecified injury of flexor muscle, fascia and tendon of left thumb at forearm level**
  - **✓7th S56.009 Unspecified injury of flexor muscle, fascia and tendon of unspecified thumb at forearm level**
- **✓6th S56.01 Strain of flexor muscle, fascia and tendon of thumb at forearm level**
  - **✓7th S56.011 Strain of flexor muscle, fascia and tendon of right thumb at forearm level**

S56.012 Strain of flexor muscle, fascia and tendon of left thumb at forearm level
S56.019 Strain of flexor muscle, fascia and tendon of unspecified thumb at forearm level
S56.02 Laceration of flexor muscle, fascia and tendon of thumb at forearm level
S56.021 Laceration of flexor muscle, fascia and tendon of right thumb at forearm level CC
S56.022 Laceration of flexor muscle, fascia and tendon of left thumb at forearm level CC
S56.029 Laceration of flexor muscle, fascia and tendon of unspecified thumb at forearm level CC
S56.09 Other injury of flexor muscle, fascia and tendon of thumb at forearm level
S56.091 Other injury of flexor muscle, fascia and tendon of right thumb at forearm level
S56.092 Other injury of flexor muscle, fascia and tendon of left thumb at forearm level
S56.099 Other injury of flexor muscle, fascia and tendon of unspecified thumb at forearm level
S56.1 Injury of flexor muscle, fascia and tendon of other and unspecified finger at forearm level
S56.10 Unspecified injury of flexor muscle, fascia and tendon of other and unspecified finger at forearm level
S56.101 Unspecified injury of flexor muscle, fascia and tendon of right index finger at forearm level
S56.102 Unspecified injury of flexor muscle, fascia and tendon of left index finger at forearm level
S56.103 Unspecified injury of flexor muscle, fascia and tendon of right middle finger at forearm level
S56.104 Unspecified injury of flexor muscle, fascia and tendon of left middle finger at forearm level
S56.105 Unspecified injury of flexor muscle, fascia and tendon of right ring finger at forearm level
S56.106 Unspecified injury of flexor muscle, fascia and tendon of left ring finger at forearm level
S56.107 Unspecified injury of flexor muscle, fascia and tendon of right little finger at forearm level
S56.108 Unspecified injury of flexor muscle, fascia and tendon of left little finger at forearm level
S56.109 Unspecified injury of flexor muscle, fascia and tendon of unspecified finger at forearm level
S56.11 Strain of flexor muscle, fascia and tendon of other and unspecified finger at forearm level
S56.111 Strain of flexor muscle, fascia and tendon of right index finger at forearm level
S56.112 Strain of flexor muscle, fascia and tendon of left index finger at forearm level
S56.113 Strain of flexor muscle, fascia and tendon of right middle finger at forearm level
S56.114 Strain of flexor muscle, fascia and tendon of left middle finger at forearm level
S56.115 Strain of flexor muscle, fascia and tendon of right ring finger at forearm level
S56.116 Strain of flexor muscle, fascia and tendon of left ring finger at forearm level
S56.117 Strain of flexor muscle, fascia and tendon of right little finger at forearm level
S56.118 Strain of flexor muscle, fascia and tendon of left little finger at forearm level
S56.119 Strain of flexor muscle, fascia and tendon of finger of unspecified finger at forearm level
S56.12 Laceration of flexor muscle, fascia and tendon of other and unspecified finger at forearm level
S56.121 Laceration of flexor muscle, fascia and tendon of right index finger at forearm level CC
S56.122 Laceration of flexor muscle, fascia and tendon of left index finger at forearm level CC
S56.123 Laceration of flexor muscle, fascia and tendon of right middle finger at forearm level CC
S56.124 Laceration of flexor muscle, fascia and tendon of left middle finger at forearm level CC
S56.125 Laceration of flexor muscle, fascia and tendon of right ring finger at forearm level CC
S56.126 Laceration of flexor muscle, fascia and tendon of left ring finger at forearm level CC
S56.127 Laceration of flexor muscle, fascia and tendon of right little finger at forearm level CC
S56.128 Laceration of flexor muscle, fascia and tendon of left little finger at forearm level CC
S56.129 Laceration of flexor muscle, fascia and tendon of unspecified finger at forearm level CC
S56.19 Other injury of flexor muscle, fascia and tendon of other and unspecified finger at forearm level
S56.191 Other injury of flexor muscle, fascia and tendon of right index finger at forearm level
S56.192 Other injury of flexor muscle, fascia and tendon of left index finger at forearm level
S56.193 Other injury of flexor muscle, fascia and tendon of right middle finger at forearm level
S56.194 Other injury of flexor muscle, fascia and tendon of left middle finger at forearm level
S56.195 Other injury of flexor muscle, fascia and tendon of right ring finger at forearm level
S56.196 Other injury of flexor muscle, fascia and tendon of left ring finger at forearm level
S56.197 Other injury of flexor muscle, fascia and tendon of right little finger at forearm level
S56.198 Other injury of flexor muscle, fascia and tendon of left little finger at forearm level
S56.199 Other injury of flexor muscle, fascia and tendon of unspecified finger at forearm level
S56.2 Injury of other flexor muscle, fascia and tendon at forearm level
S56.20 Unspecified injury of other flexor muscle, fascia and tendon at forearm level
S56.201 Unspecified injury of other flexor muscle, fascia and tendon at forearm level, right arm
S56.202 Unspecified injury of other flexor muscle, fascia and tendon at forearm level, left arm
S56.209 Unspecified injury of other flexor muscle, fascia and tendon at forearm level, unspecified arm
S56.21 Strain of other flexor muscle, fascia and tendon at forearm level
S56.211 Strain of other flexor muscle, fascia and tendon at forearm level, right arm
S56.212 Strain of other flexor muscle, fascia and tendon at forearm level, left arm
S56.219 Strain of other flexor muscle, fascia and tendon at forearm level, unspecified arm
S56.22 Laceration of other flexor muscle, fascia and tendon at forearm level
S56.221 Laceration of other flexor muscle, fascia and tendon at forearm level, right arm CC
S56.222 Laceration of other flexor muscle, fascia and tendon at forearm level, left arm CC
S56.229 Laceration of other flexor muscle, fascia and tendon at forearm level, unspecified arm CC

- ✓6th **S56.29 Other injury of other flexor muscle, fascia and tendon at forearm level**
  - ✓7th **S56.291 Other injury of other flexor muscle, fascia and tendon at forearm level, right arm**
  - ✓7th **S56.292 Other injury of other flexor muscle, fascia and tendon at forearm level, left arm**
  - ✓7th **S56.299 Other injury of other flexor muscle, fascia and tendon at forearm level, unspecified arm**
- ✓5th **S56.3 Injury of extensor or abductor muscles, fascia and tendons of thumb at forearm level**
  - ✓6th **S56.30 Unspecified injury of extensor or abductor muscles, fascia and tendons of thumb at forearm level**
    - ✓7th **S56.301 Unspecified injury of extensor or abductor muscles, fascia and tendons of right thumb at forearm level**
    - ✓7th **S56.302 Unspecified injury of extensor or abductor muscles, fascia and tendons of left thumb at forearm level**
    - ✓7th **S56.309 Unspecified injury of extensor or abductor muscles, fascia and tendons of unspecified thumb at forearm level**
  - ✓6th **S56.31 Strain of extensor or abductor muscles, fascia and tendons of thumb at forearm level**
    - ✓7th **S56.311 Strain of extensor or abductor muscles, fascia and tendons of right thumb at forearm level**
    - ✓7th **S56.312 Strain of extensor or abductor muscles, fascia and tendons of left thumb at forearm level**
    - ✓7th **S56.319 Strain of extensor or abductor muscles, fascia and tendons of unspecified thumb at forearm level**
  - ✓6th **S56.32 Laceration of extensor or abductor muscles, fascia and tendons of thumb at forearm level**
    - ✓7th **S56.321 Laceration of extensor or abductor muscles, fascia and tendons of right thumb at forearm level** CC
    - ✓7th **S56.322 Laceration of extensor or abductor muscles, fascia and tendons of left thumb at forearm level** CC
    - ✓7th **S56.329 Laceration of extensor or abductor muscles, fascia and tendons of unspecified thumb at forearm level** CC
  - ✓6th **S56.39 Other injury of extensor or abductor muscles, fascia and tendons of thumb at forearm level**
    - ✓7th **S56.391 Other injury of extensor or abductor muscles, fascia and tendons of right thumb at forearm level**
    - ✓7th **S56.392 Other injury of extensor or abductor muscles, fascia and tendons of left thumb at forearm level**
    - ✓7th **S56.399 Other injury of extensor or abductor muscles, fascia and tendons of unspecified thumb at forearm level**
- ✓5th **S56.4 Injury of extensor muscle, fascia and tendon of other and unspecified finger at forearm level**
  - ✓6th **S56.40 Unspecified injury of extensor muscle, fascia and tendon of other and unspecified finger at forearm level**
    - ✓7th **S56.401 Unspecified injury of extensor muscle, fascia and tendon of right index finger at forearm level**
    - ✓7th **S56.402 Unspecified injury of extensor muscle, fascia and tendon of left index finger at forearm level**
    - ✓7th **S56.403 Unspecified injury of extensor muscle, fascia and tendon of right middle finger at forearm level**
    - ✓7th **S56.404 Unspecified injury of extensor muscle, fascia and tendon of left middle finger at forearm level**
    - ✓7th **S56.405 Unspecified injury of extensor muscle, fascia and tendon of right ring finger at forearm level**
    - ✓7th **S56.406 Unspecified injury of extensor muscle, fascia and tendon of left ring finger at forearm level**
    - ✓7th **S56.407 Unspecified injury of extensor muscle, fascia and tendon of right little finger at forearm level**
    - ✓7th **S56.408 Unspecified injury of extensor muscle, fascia and tendon of left little finger at forearm level**
    - ✓7th **S56.409 Unspecified injury of extensor muscle, fascia and tendon of unspecified finger at forearm level**
  - ✓6th **S56.41 Strain of extensor muscle, fascia and tendon of other and unspecified finger at forearm level**
    - ✓7th **S56.411 Strain of extensor muscle, fascia and tendon of right index finger at forearm level**
    - ✓7th **S56.412 Strain of extensor muscle, fascia and tendon of left index finger at forearm level**
    - ✓7th **S56.413 Strain of extensor muscle, fascia and tendon of right middle finger at forearm level**
    - ✓7th **S56.414 Strain of extensor muscle, fascia and tendon of left middle finger at forearm level**
    - ✓7th **S56.415 Strain of extensor muscle, fascia and tendon of right ring finger at forearm level**
    - ✓7th **S56.416 Strain of extensor muscle, fascia and tendon of left ring finger at forearm level**
    - ✓7th **S56.417 Strain of extensor muscle, fascia and tendon of right little finger at forearm level**
    - ✓7th **S56.418 Strain of extensor muscle, fascia and tendon of left little finger at forearm level**
    - ✓7th **S56.419 Strain of extensor muscle, fascia and tendon of finger, unspecified finger at forearm level**
  - ✓6th **S56.42 Laceration of extensor muscle, fascia and tendon of other and unspecified finger at forearm level**
    - ✓7th **S56.421 Laceration of extensor muscle, fascia and tendon of right index finger at forearm level** CC
    - ✓7th **S56.422 Laceration of extensor muscle, fascia and tendon of left index finger at forearm level** CC
    - ✓7th **S56.423 Laceration of extensor muscle, fascia and tendon of right middle finger at forearm level** CC
    - ✓7th **S56.424 Laceration of extensor muscle, fascia and tendon of left middle finger at forearm level** CC
    - ✓7th **S56.425 Laceration of extensor muscle, fascia and tendon of right ring finger at forearm level** CC
    - ✓7th **S56.426 Laceration of extensor muscle, fascia and tendon of left ring finger at forearm level** CC
    - ✓7th **S56.427 Laceration of extensor muscle, fascia and tendon of right little finger at forearm level** CC
    - ✓7th **S56.428 Laceration of extensor muscle, fascia and tendon of left little finger at forearm level** CC
    - ✓7th **S56.429 Laceration of extensor muscle, fascia and tendon of unspecified finger at forearm level** CC
  - ✓6th **S56.49 Other injury of extensor muscle, fascia and tendon of other and unspecified finger at forearm level**
    - ✓7th **S56.491 Other injury of extensor muscle, fascia and tendon of right index finger at forearm level**
    - ✓7th **S56.492 Other injury of extensor muscle, fascia and tendon of left index finger at forearm level**
    - ✓7th **S56.493 Other injury of extensor muscle, fascia and tendon of right middle finger at forearm level**
    - ✓7th **S56.494 Other injury of extensor muscle, fascia and tendon of left middle finger at forearm level**
    - ✓7th **S56.495 Other injury of extensor muscle, fascia and tendon of right ring finger at forearm level**
    - ✓7th **S56.496 Other injury of extensor muscle, fascia and tendon of left ring finger at forearm level**
    - ✓7th **S56.497 Other injury of extensor muscle, fascia and tendon of right little finger at forearm level**

S56.498 Other injury of extensor muscle, fascia and tendon of left little finger at forearm level
S56.499 Other injury of extensor muscle, fascia and tendon of unspecified finger at forearm level

S56.5 Injury of other extensor muscle, fascia and tendon at forearm level
S56.50 Unspecified injury of other extensor muscle, fascia and tendon at forearm level
S56.501 Unspecified injury of other extensor muscle, fascia and tendon at forearm level, right arm
S56.502 Unspecified injury of other extensor muscle, fascia and tendon at forearm level, left arm
S56.509 Unspecified injury of other extensor muscle, fascia and tendon at forearm level, unspecified arm
S56.51 Strain of other extensor muscle, fascia and tendon at forearm level
S56.511 Strain of other extensor muscle, fascia and tendon at forearm level, right arm
S56.512 Strain of other extensor muscle, fascia and tendon at forearm level, left arm
S56.519 Strain of other extensor muscle, fascia and tendon at forearm level, unspecified arm
S56.52 Laceration of other extensor muscle, fascia and tendon at forearm level
S56.521 Laceration of other extensor muscle, fascia and tendon at forearm level, right arm CC
S56.522 Laceration of other extensor muscle, fascia and tendon at forearm level, left arm CC
S56.529 Laceration of other extensor muscle, fascia and tendon at forearm level, unspecified arm CC
S56.59 Other injury of other extensor muscle, fascia and tendon at forearm level
S56.591 Other injury of other extensor muscle, fascia and tendon at forearm level, right arm
S56.592 Other injury of other extensor muscle, fascia and tendon at forearm level, left arm
S56.599 Other injury of other extensor muscle, fascia and tendon at forearm level, unspecified arm

S56.8 Injury of other muscles, fascia and tendons at forearm level
S56.80 Unspecified injury of other muscles, fascia and tendons at forearm level
S56.801 Unspecified injury of other muscles, fascia and tendons at forearm level, right arm
S56.802 Unspecified injury of other muscles, fascia and tendons at forearm level, left arm
S56.809 Unspecified injury of other muscles, fascia and tendons at forearm level, unspecified arm
S56.81 Strain of other muscles, fascia and tendons at forearm level
S56.811 Strain of other muscles, fascia and tendons at forearm level, right arm
S56.812 Strain of other muscles, fascia and tendons at forearm level, left arm
S56.819 Strain of other muscles, fascia and tendons at forearm level, unspecified arm
S56.82 Laceration of other muscles, fascia and tendons at forearm level
S56.821 Laceration of other muscles, fascia and tendons at forearm level, right arm CC
S56.822 Laceration of other muscles, fascia and tendons at forearm level, left arm CC
S56.829 Laceration of other muscles, fascia and tendons at forearm level, unspecified arm CC
S56.89 Other injury of other muscles, fascia and tendons at forearm level
S56.891 Other injury of other muscles, fascia and tendons at forearm level, right arm
S56.892 Other injury of other muscles, fascia and tendons at forearm level, left arm
S56.899 Other injury of other muscles, fascia and tendons at forearm level, unspecified arm

S56.9 Injury of unspecified muscles, fascia and tendons at forearm level
S56.90 Unspecified injury of unspecified muscles, fascia and tendons at forearm level
S56.901 Unspecified injury of unspecified muscles, fascia and tendons at forearm level, right arm
S56.902 Unspecified injury of unspecified muscles, fascia and tendons at forearm level, left arm
S56.909 Unspecified injury of unspecified muscles, fascia and tendons at forearm level, unspecified arm
S56.91 Strain of unspecified muscles, fascia and tendons at forearm level
S56.911 Strain of unspecified muscles, fascia and tendons at forearm level, right arm
S56.912 Strain of unspecified muscles, fascia and tendons at forearm level, left arm
S56.919 Strain of unspecified muscles, fascia and tendons at forearm level, unspecified arm
S56.92 Laceration of unspecified muscles, fascia and tendons at forearm level
S56.921 Laceration of unspecified muscles, fascia and tendons at forearm level, right arm CC
S56.922 Laceration of unspecified muscles, fascia and tendons at forearm level, left arm CC
S56.929 Laceration of unspecified muscles, fascia and tendons at forearm level, unspecified arm CC
S56.99 Other injury of unspecified muscles, fascia and tendons at forearm level
S56.991 Other injury of unspecified muscles, fascia and tendons at forearm level, right arm
S56.992 Other injury of unspecified muscles, fascia and tendons at forearm level, left arm
S56.999 Other injury of unspecified muscles, fascia and tendons at forearm level, unspecified arm

S57 Crushing injury of elbow and forearm

Use additional code(s) for all associated injuries

EXCLUDES 2 *crushing injury of wrist and hand (S67.-)*

The appropriate 7th character is to be added to each code from category S57.
A initial encounter
D subsequent encounter
S sequela

S57.0 Crushing injury of elbow
S57.00 Crushing injury of unspecified elbow
S57.01 Crushing injury of right elbow
S57.02 Crushing injury of left elbow

S57.8 Crushing injury of forearm
S57.80 Crushing injury of unspecified forearm
S57.81 Crushing injury of right forearm
S57.82 Crushing injury of left forearm

S58 Traumatic amputation of elbow and forearm

An amputation not identified as partial or complete should be coded to complete

EXCLUDES 1 *traumatic amputation of wrist and hand (S68.-)*

The appropriate 7th character is to be added to each code from category S58.
A initial encounter
D subsequent encounter
S sequela

S58.0 Traumatic amputation at elbow level
S58.01 Complete traumatic amputation at elbow level
7 S58.011 Complete traumatic amputation at elbow level, right arm CC HCC
7 S58.012 Complete traumatic amputation at elbow level, left arm CC HCC

7 ✓7th **S58.Ø19** **Complete traumatic amputation at elbow level, unspecified arm** CC HCC

✓6th **S58.Ø2** **Partial traumatic amputation at elbow level**

7 ✓7th **S58.Ø21** **Partial traumatic amputation at elbow level, right arm** CC HCC

7 ✓7th **S58.Ø22** **Partial traumatic amputation at elbow level, left arm** CC HCC

7 ✓7th **S58.Ø29** **Partial traumatic amputation at elbow level, unspecified arm** CC HCC

✓5th **S58.1** **Traumatic amputation at level between elbow and wrist**

✓6th **S58.11** **Complete traumatic amputation at level between elbow and wrist**

7 ✓7th **S58.111** **Complete traumatic amputation at level between elbow and wrist, right arm** CC HCC

7 ✓7th **S58.112** **Complete traumatic amputation at level between elbow and wrist, left arm** CC HCC

7 ✓7th **S58.119** **Complete traumatic amputation at level between elbow and wrist, unspecified arm** CC HCC

✓6th **S58.12** **Partial traumatic amputation at level between elbow and wrist**

7 ✓7th **S58.121** **Partial traumatic amputation at level between elbow and wrist, right arm** CC HCC

7 ✓7th **S58.122** **Partial traumatic amputation at level between elbow and wrist, left arm** CC HCC

7 ✓7th **S58.129** **Partial traumatic amputation at level between elbow and wrist, unspecified arm** CC HCC

✓5th **S58.9** **Traumatic amputation of forearm, level unspecified**

EXCLUDES 1 *traumatic amputation of wrist (S68.-)*

✓6th **S58.91** **Complete traumatic amputation of forearm, level unspecified**

7 ✓7th **S58.911** **Complete traumatic amputation of right forearm, level unspecified** CC HCC

7 ✓7th **S58.912** **Complete traumatic amputation of left forearm, level unspecified** CC HCC

7 ✓7th **S58.919** **Complete traumatic amputation of unspecified forearm, level unspecified** CC HCC

✓6th **S58.92** **Partial traumatic amputation of forearm, level unspecified**

7 ✓7th **S58.921** **Partial traumatic amputation of right forearm, level unspecified** CC HCC

7 ✓7th **S58.922** **Partial traumatic amputation of left forearm, level unspecified** CC HCC

7 ✓7th **S58.929** **Partial traumatic amputation of unspecified forearm, level unspecified** CC HCC

✓4th **S59** **Other and unspecified injuries of elbow and forearm**

EXCLUDES 2 *other and unspecified injuries of wrist and hand (S69.-)*

AHA: 2018,2Q,12; 2018,1Q,3; 2015,3Q,37-39

The appropriate 7th character is to be added to each code from subcategories S59.Ø, S59.1, and S59.2.

- A initial encounter for closed fracture
- D subsequent encounter for fracture with routine healing
- G subsequent encounter for fracture with delayed healing
- K subsequent encounter for fracture with nonunion
- P subsequent encounter for fracture with malunion
- S sequela

✓5th **S59.Ø** **Physeal fracture of lower end of ulna**

AHA: 2019,4Q,56

✓6th **S59.ØØ** **Unspecified physeal fracture of lower end of ulna**

3 ✓7th **S59.ØØ1** **Unspecified physeal fracture of lower end of ulna, right arm** CC H5

3 ✓7th **S59.ØØ2** **Unspecified physeal fracture of lower end of ulna, left arm** CC H5

3 ✓7th **S59.ØØ9** **Unspecified physeal fracture of lower end of ulna, unspecified arm** CC H5

✓6th **S59.Ø1** **Salter-Harris Type I physeal fracture of lower end of ulna**

3 ✓7th **S59.Ø11** **Salter-Harris Type I physeal fracture of lower end of ulna, right arm** CC H5

3 ✓7th **S59.Ø12** **Salter-Harris Type I physeal fracture of lower end of ulna, left arm** CC H5

3 ✓7th **S59.Ø19** **Salter-Harris Type I physeal fracture of lower end of ulna, unspecified arm** CC H5

✓6th **S59.Ø2** **Salter-Harris Type II physeal fracture of lower end of ulna**

3 ✓7th **S59.Ø21** **Salter-Harris Type II physeal fracture of lower end of ulna, right arm** CC H5

3 ✓7th **S59.Ø22** **Salter-Harris Type II physeal fracture of lower end of ulna, left arm** CC H5

3 ✓7th **S59.Ø29** **Salter-Harris Type II physeal fracture of lower end of ulna, unspecified arm** CC H5

✓6th **S59.Ø3** **Salter-Harris Type III physeal fracture of lower end of ulna**

3 ✓7th **S59.Ø31** **Salter-Harris Type III physeal fracture of lower end of ulna, right arm** CC H5

3 ✓7th **S59.Ø32** **Salter-Harris Type III physeal fracture of lower end of ulna, left arm** CC H5

3 ✓7th **S59.Ø39** **Salter-Harris Type III physeal fracture of lower end of ulna, unspecified arm** CC H5

✓6th **S59.Ø4** **Salter-Harris Type IV physeal fracture of lower end of ulna**

3 ✓7th **S59.Ø41** **Salter-Harris Type IV physeal fracture of lower end of ulna, right arm** CC H5

3 ✓7th **S59.Ø42** **Salter-Harris Type IV physeal fracture of lower end of ulna, left arm** CC H5

3 ✓7th **S59.Ø49** **Salter-Harris Type IV physeal fracture of lower end of ulna, unspecified arm** CC H5

✓6th **S59.Ø9** **Other physeal fracture of lower end of ulna**

3 ✓7th **S59.Ø91** **Other physeal fracture of lower end of ulna, right arm** CC H5

3 ✓7th **S59.Ø92** **Other physeal fracture of lower end of ulna, left arm** CC H5

3 ✓7th **S59.Ø99** **Other physeal fracture of lower end of ulna, unspecified arm** CC H5

✓5th **S59.1** **Physeal fracture of upper end of radius**

AHA: 2019,4Q,56

✓6th **S59.1Ø** **Unspecified physeal fracture of upper end of radius**

4 ✓7th **S59.1Ø1** **Unspecified physeal fracture of upper end of radius, right arm** CC

4 ✓7th **S59.1Ø2** **Unspecified physeal fracture of upper end of radius, left arm** CC

4 ✓7th **S59.1Ø9** **Unspecified physeal fracture of upper end of radius, unspecified arm** CC

✓6th **S59.11** **Salter-Harris Type I physeal fracture of upper end of radius**

4 ✓7th **S59.111** **Salter-Harris Type I physeal fracture of upper end of radius, right arm** CC

4 ✓7th **S59.112** **Salter-Harris Type I physeal fracture of upper end of radius, left arm** CC

4 ✓7th **S59.119** **Salter-Harris Type I physeal fracture of upper end of radius, unspecified arm** CC

✓6th **S59.12** **Salter-Harris Type II physeal fracture of upper end of radius**

4 ✓7th **S59.121** **Salter-Harris Type II physeal fracture of upper end of radius, right arm** CC

4 ✓7th **S59.122** **Salter-Harris Type II physeal fracture of upper end of radius, left arm** CC

4 ✓7th **S59.129** **Salter-Harris Type II physeal fracture of upper end of radius, unspecified arm** CC

✓6th **S59.13** **Salter-Harris Type III physeal fracture of upper end of radius**

4 ✓7th **S59.131** **Salter-Harris Type III physeal fracture of upper end of radius, right arm** CC

4 ✓7th **S59.132** **Salter-Harris Type III physeal fracture of upper end of radius, left arm** CC

4 ✓7th **S59.139** **Salter-Harris Type III physeal fracture of upper end of radius, unspecified arm** CC

✓6th **S59.14** **Salter-Harris Type IV physeal fracture of upper end of radius**

4 ✓7th **S59.141** **Salter-Harris Type IV physeal fracture of upper end of radius, right arm** CC

4 ✓7th **S59.142** **Salter-Harris Type IV physeal fracture of upper end of radius, left arm** CC

4 ✓7th S59.149 Salter-Harris Type IV physeal fracture of upper end of radius, unspecified arm CC

✓6th S59.19 Other physeal fracture of upper end of radius

4 ✓7th S59.191 Other physeal fracture of upper end of radius, right arm CC

4 ✓7th S59.192 Other physeal fracture of upper end of radius, left arm CC

4 ✓7th S59.199 Other physeal fracture of upper end of radius, unspecified arm CC

✓5th S59.2 Physeal fracture of lower end of radius

AHA: 2019,4Q,56

✓6th S59.20 Unspecified physeal fracture of lower end of radius

3 ✓7th S59.201 Unspecified physeal fracture of lower end of radius, right arm CC H5

3 ✓7th S59.202 Unspecified physeal fracture of lower end of radius, left arm CC H5

3 ✓7th S59.209 Unspecified physeal fracture of lower end of radius, unspecified arm CC H5

✓6th S59.21 Salter-Harris Type I physeal fracture of lower end of radius

3 ✓7th S59.211 Salter-Harris Type I physeal fracture of lower end of radius, right arm CC H5

3 ✓7th S59.212 Salter-Harris Type I physeal fracture of lower end of radius, left arm CC H5

3 ✓7th S59.219 Salter-Harris Type I physeal fracture of lower end of radius, unspecified arm CC H5

✓6th S59.22 Salter-Harris Type II physeal fracture of lower end of radius

3 ✓7th S59.221 Salter-Harris Type II physeal fracture of lower end of radius, right arm CC H5

3 ✓7th S59.222 Salter-Harris Type II physeal fracture of lower end of radius, left arm CC H5

3 ✓7th S59.229 Salter-Harris Type II physeal fracture of lower end of radius, unspecified arm CC H5

✓6th S59.23 Salter-Harris Type III physeal fracture of lower end of radius

3 ✓7th S59.231 Salter-Harris Type III physeal fracture of lower end of radius, right arm CC H5

3 ✓7th S59.232 Salter-Harris Type III physeal fracture of lower end of radius, left arm CC H5

3 ✓7th S59.239 Salter-Harris Type III physeal fracture of lower end of radius, unspecified arm CC H5

✓6th S59.24 Salter-Harris Type IV physeal fracture of lower end of radius

3 ✓7th S59.241 Salter-Harris Type IV physeal fracture of lower end of radius, right arm CC H5

3 ✓7th S59.242 Salter-Harris Type IV physeal fracture of lower end of radius, left arm CC H5

3 ✓7th S59.249 Salter-Harris Type IV physeal fracture of lower end of radius, unspecified arm CC H5

✓6th S59.29 Other physeal fracture of lower end of radius

3 ✓7th S59.291 Other physeal fracture of lower end of radius, right arm CC H5

3 ✓7th S59.292 Other physeal fracture of lower end of radius, left arm CC H5

3 ✓7th S59.299 Other physeal fracture of lower end of radius, unspecified arm CC H5

✓5th S59.8 Other specified injuries of elbow and forearm

The appropriate 7th character is to be added to each code in subcategory S59.8.
A initial encounter
D subsequent encounter
S sequela

✓6th S59.80 Other specified injuries of elbow

✓7th S59.801 Other specified injuries of right elbow

✓7th S59.802 Other specified injuries of left elbow

✓7th S59.809 Other specified injuries of unspecified elbow

✓6th S59.81 Other specified injuries of forearm

✓7th S59.811 Other specified injuries right forearm

✓7th S59.812 Other specified injuries left forearm

✓7th S59.819 Other specified injuries unspecified forearm

✓5th S59.9 Unspecified injury of elbow and forearm

The appropriate 7th character is to be added to each code in subcategory S59.9.
A initial encounter
D subsequent encounter
S sequela

✓6th S59.90 Unspecified injury of elbow

✓7th S59.901 Unspecified injury of right elbow

✓7th S59.902 Unspecified injury of left elbow

✓7th S59.909 Unspecified injury of unspecified elbow

✓6th S59.91 Unspecified injury of forearm

✓7th S59.911 Unspecified injury of right forearm

✓7th S59.912 Unspecified injury of left forearm

✓7th S59.919 Unspecified injury of unspecified forearm

Injuries to the wrist, hand and fingers (S60-S69)

EXCLUDES 2 *burns and corrosions (T20-T32)*
frostbite (T33-T34)
insect bite or sting, venomous (T63.4)

✓4th S60 Superficial injury of wrist, hand and fingers

The appropriate 7th character is to be added to each code from category S60.
A initial encounter
D subsequent encounter
S sequela

✓5th S60.0 Contusion of finger without damage to nail

EXCLUDES 1 *contusion involving nail (matrix) (S60.1)*

✓x7th S60.00 Contusion of unspecified finger without damage to nail

Contusion of finger(s) NOS

✓6th S60.01 Contusion of thumb without damage to nail

✓7th S60.011 Contusion of right thumb without damage to nail

✓7th S60.012 Contusion of left thumb without damage to nail

✓7th S60.019 Contusion of unspecified thumb without damage to nail

✓6th S60.02 Contusion of index finger without damage to nail

✓7th S60.021 Contusion of right index finger without damage to nail

✓7th S60.022 Contusion of left index finger without damage to nail

✓7th S60.029 Contusion of unspecified index finger without damage to nail

✓6th S60.03 Contusion of middle finger without damage to nail

✓7th S60.031 Contusion of right middle finger without damage to nail

✓7th S60.032 Contusion of left middle finger without damage to nail

✓7th S60.039 Contusion of unspecified middle finger without damage to nail

✓6th S60.04 Contusion of ring finger without damage to nail

✓7th S60.041 Contusion of right ring finger without damage to nail

✓7th S60.042 Contusion of left ring finger without damage to nail

✓7th S60.049 Contusion of unspecified ring finger without damage to nail

✓6th S60.05 Contusion of little finger without damage to nail

✓7th S60.051 Contusion of right little finger without damage to nail

✓7th S60.052 Contusion of left little finger without damage to nail

✓7th S60.059 Contusion of unspecified little finger without damage to nail

✓5th S60.1 Contusion of finger with damage to nail

✓x7th S60.10 Contusion of unspecified finger with damage to nail

✓6th S60.11 Contusion of thumb with damage to nail

✓7th S60.111 Contusion of right thumb with damage to nail

✓7th S60.112 Contusion of left thumb with damage to nail

✓7th S60.119 Contusion of unspecified thumb with damage to nail

√6th **S60.12 Contusion of index finger with damage to nail**
- √7th **S60.121 Contusion of right index finger with damage to nail**
- √7th **S60.122 Contusion of left index finger with damage to nail**
- √7th **S60.129 Contusion of unspecified index finger with damage to nail**

√6th **S60.13 Contusion of middle finger with damage to nail**
- √7th **S60.131 Contusion of right middle finger with damage to nail**
- √7th **S60.132 Contusion of left middle finger with damage to nail**
- √7th **S60.139 Contusion of unspecified middle finger with damage to nail**

√6th **S60.14 Contusion of ring finger with damage to nail**
- √7th **S60.141 Contusion of right ring finger with damage to nail**
- √7th **S60.142 Contusion of left ring finger with damage to nail**
- √7th **S60.149 Contusion of unspecified ring finger with damage to nail**

√6th **S60.15 Contusion of little finger with damage to nail**
- √7th **S60.151 Contusion of right little finger with damage to nail**
- √7th **S60.152 Contusion of left little finger with damage to nail**
- √7th **S60.159 Contusion of unspecified little finger with damage to nail**

√5th **S60.2 Contusion of wrist and hand**

EXCLUDES 2 *contusion of fingers (S60.0-, S60.1-)*

√6th **S60.21 Contusion of wrist**
- √7th **S60.211 Contusion of right wrist**
- √7th **S60.212 Contusion of left wrist**
- √7th **S60.219 Contusion of unspecified wrist**

√6th **S60.22 Contusion of hand**
- √7th **S60.221 Contusion of right hand**
- √7th **S60.222 Contusion of left hand**
- √7th **S60.229 Contusion of unspecified hand**

√5th **S60.3 Other superficial injuries of thumb**

√6th **S60.31 Abrasion of thumb**
- √7th **S60.311 Abrasion of right thumb**
- √7th **S60.312 Abrasion of left thumb**
- √7th **S60.319 Abrasion of unspecified thumb**

√6th **S60.32 Blister (nonthermal) of thumb**
- √7th **S60.321 Blister (nonthermal) of right thumb**
- √7th **S60.322 Blister (nonthermal) of left thumb**
- √7th **S60.329 Blister (nonthermal) of unspecified thumb**

√6th **S60.34 External constriction of thumb**

Hair tourniquet syndrome of thumb

Use additional cause code to identify the constricting item (W49.0-)
- √7th **S60.341 External constriction of right thumb**
- √7th **S60.342 External constriction of left thumb**
- √7th **S60.349 External constriction of unspecified thumb**

√6th **S60.35 Superficial foreign body of thumb**

Splinter in the thumb
- √7th **S60.351 Superficial foreign body of right thumb**
- √7th **S60.352 Superficial foreign body of left thumb**
- √7th **S60.359 Superficial foreign body of unspecified thumb**

√6th **S60.36 Insect bite (nonvenomous) of thumb**
- √7th **S60.361 Insect bite (nonvenomous) of right thumb**
- √7th **S60.362 Insect bite (nonvenomous) of left thumb**
- √7th **S60.369 Insect bite (nonvenomous) of unspecified thumb**

√6th **S60.37 Other superficial bite of thumb**

EXCLUDES 1 *open bite of thumb (S61.05-, S61.15-)*
- √7th **S60.371 Other superficial bite of right thumb**
- √7th **S60.372 Other superficial bite of left thumb**
- √7th **S60.379 Other superficial bite of unspecified thumb**

√6th **S60.39 Other superficial injuries of thumb**
- √7th **S60.391 Other superficial injuries of right thumb**
- √7th **S60.392 Other superficial injuries of left thumb**
- √7th **S60.399 Other superficial injuries of unspecified thumb**

√5th **S60.4 Other superficial injuries of other fingers**

√6th **S60.41 Abrasion of fingers**
- √7th **S60.410 Abrasion of right index finger**
- √7th **S60.411 Abrasion of left index finger**
- √7th **S60.412 Abrasion of right middle finger**
- √7th **S60.413 Abrasion of left middle finger**
- √7th **S60.414 Abrasion of right ring finger**
- √7th **S60.415 Abrasion of left ring finger**
- √7th **S60.416 Abrasion of right little finger**
- √7th **S60.417 Abrasion of left little finger**
- √7th **S60.418 Abrasion of other finger**

  Abrasion of specified finger with unspecified laterality
- √7th **S60.419 Abrasion of unspecified finger**

√6th **S60.42 Blister (nonthermal) of fingers**
- √7th **S60.420 Blister (nonthermal) of right index finger**
- √7th **S60.421 Blister (nonthermal) of left index finger**
- √7th **S60.422 Blister (nonthermal) of right middle finger**
- √7th **S60.423 Blister (nonthermal) of left middle finger**
- √7th **S60.424 Blister (nonthermal) of right ring finger**
- √7th **S60.425 Blister (nonthermal) of left ring finger**
- √7th **S60.426 Blister (nonthermal) of right little finger**
- √7th **S60.427 Blister (nonthermal) of left little finger**
- √7th **S60.428 Blister (nonthermal) of other finger**

  Blister (nonthermal) of specified finger with unspecified laterality
- √7th **S60.429 Blister (nonthermal) of unspecified finger**

√6th **S60.44 External constriction of fingers**

Hair tourniquet syndrome of finger

Use additional cause code to identify the constricting item (W49.0-)
- √7th **S60.440 External constriction of right index finger**
- √7th **S60.441 External constriction of left index finger**
- √7th **S60.442 External constriction of right middle finger**
- √7th **S60.443 External constriction of left middle finger**
- √7th **S60.444 External constriction of right ring finger**
- √7th **S60.445 External constriction of left ring finger**
- √7th **S60.446 External constriction of right little finger**
- √7th **S60.447 External constriction of left little finger**
- √7th **S60.448 External constriction of other finger**

  External constriction of specified finger with unspecified laterality
- √7th **S60.449 External constriction of unspecified finger**

√6th **S60.45 Superficial foreign body of fingers**

Splinter in the finger(s)
- √7th **S60.450 Superficial foreign body of right index finger**
- √7th **S60.451 Superficial foreign body of left index finger**
- √7th **S60.452 Superficial foreign body of right middle finger**
- √7th **S60.453 Superficial foreign body of left middle finger**
- √7th **S60.454 Superficial foreign body of right ring finger**
- √7th **S60.455 Superficial foreign body of left ring finger**
- √7th **S60.456 Superficial foreign body of right little finger**
- √7th **S60.457 Superficial foreign body of left little finger**
- √7th **S60.458 Superficial foreign body of other finger**

  Superficial foreign body of specified finger with unspecified laterality
- √7th **S60.459 Superficial foreign body of unspecified finger**

- S60.46 Insect bite (nonvenomous) of fingers
  - S60.460 Insect bite (nonvenomous) of right index finger
  - S60.461 Insect bite (nonvenomous) of left index finger
  - S60.462 Insect bite (nonvenomous) of right middle finger
  - S60.463 Insect bite (nonvenomous) of left middle finger
  - S60.464 Insect bite (nonvenomous) of right ring finger
  - S60.465 Insect bite (nonvenomous) of left ring finger
  - S60.466 Insect bite (nonvenomous) of right little finger
  - S60.467 Insect bite (nonvenomous) of left little finger
  - S60.468 Insect bite (nonvenomous) of other finger
    Insect bite (nonvenomous) of specified finger with unspecified laterality
  - S60.469 Insect bite (nonvenomous) of unspecified finger
- S60.47 Other superficial bite of fingers
  EXCLUDES 1 *open bite of fingers (S61.25-, S61.35-)*
  - S60.470 Other superficial bite of right index finger
  - S60.471 Other superficial bite of left index finger
  - S60.472 Other superficial bite of right middle finger
  - S60.473 Other superficial bite of left middle finger
  - S60.474 Other superficial bite of right ring finger
  - S60.475 Other superficial bite of left ring finger
  - S60.476 Other superficial bite of right little finger
  - S60.477 Other superficial bite of left little finger
  - S60.478 Other superficial bite of other finger
    Other superficial bite of specified finger with unspecified laterality
  - S60.479 Other superficial bite of unspecified finger

S60.5 Other superficial injuries of hand
EXCLUDES 2 *superficial injuries of fingers (S60.3-, S60.4-)*

- S60.51 Abrasion of hand
  - S60.511 Abrasion of right hand
  - S60.512 Abrasion of left hand
  - S60.519 Abrasion of unspecified hand
- S60.52 Blister (nonthermal) of hand
  - S60.521 Blister (nonthermal) of right hand
  - S60.522 Blister (nonthermal) of left hand
  - S60.529 Blister (nonthermal) of unspecified hand
- S60.54 External constriction of hand
  - S60.541 External constriction of right hand
  - S60.542 External constriction of left hand
  - S60.549 External constriction of unspecified hand
- S60.55 Superficial foreign body of hand
  Splinter in the hand
  - S60.551 Superficial foreign body of right hand
  - S60.552 Superficial foreign body of left hand
  - S60.559 Superficial foreign body of unspecified hand
- S60.56 Insect bite (nonvenomous) of hand
  - S60.561 Insect bite (nonvenomous) of right hand
  - S60.562 Insect bite (nonvenomous) of left hand
  - S60.569 Insect bite (nonvenomous) of unspecified hand
- S60.57 Other superficial bite of hand
  EXCLUDES 1 *open bite of hand (S61.45-)*
  - S60.571 Other superficial bite of hand of right hand
  - S60.572 Other superficial bite of hand of left hand
  - S60.579 Other superficial bite of hand of unspecified hand

S60.8 Other superficial injuries of wrist

- S60.81 Abrasion of wrist
  - S60.811 Abrasion of right wrist
  - S60.812 Abrasion of left wrist
  - S60.819 Abrasion of unspecified wrist
- S60.82 Blister (nonthermal) of wrist
  - S60.821 Blister (nonthermal) of right wrist
  - S60.822 Blister (nonthermal) of left wrist
  - S60.829 Blister (nonthermal) of unspecified wrist
- S60.84 External constriction of wrist
  - S60.841 External constriction of right wrist
  - S60.842 External constriction of left wrist
  - S60.849 External constriction of unspecified wrist
- S60.85 Superficial foreign body of wrist
  Splinter in the wrist
  - S60.851 Superficial foreign body of right wrist
  - S60.852 Superficial foreign body of left wrist
  - S60.859 Superficial foreign body of unspecified wrist
- S60.86 Insect bite (nonvenomous) of wrist
  - S60.861 Insect bite (nonvenomous) of right wrist
  - S60.862 Insect bite (nonvenomous) of left wrist
  - S60.869 Insect bite (nonvenomous) of unspecified wrist
- S60.87 Other superficial bite of wrist
  EXCLUDES 1 *open bite of wrist (S61.55)*
  - S60.871 Other superficial bite of right wrist
  - S60.872 Other superficial bite of left wrist
  - S60.879 Other superficial bite of unspecified wrist

S60.9 Unspecified superficial injury of wrist, hand and fingers

- S60.91 Unspecified superficial injury of wrist
  - S60.911 Unspecified superficial injury of right wrist
  - S60.912 Unspecified superficial injury of left wrist
  - S60.919 Unspecified superficial injury of unspecified wrist
- S60.92 Unspecified superficial injury of hand
  - S60.921 Unspecified superficial injury of right hand
  - S60.922 Unspecified superficial injury of left hand
  - S60.929 Unspecified superficial injury of unspecified hand
- S60.93 Unspecified superficial injury of thumb
  - S60.931 Unspecified superficial injury of right thumb
  - S60.932 Unspecified superficial injury of left thumb
  - S60.939 Unspecified superficial injury of unspecified thumb
- S60.94 Unspecified superficial injury of other fingers
  - S60.940 Unspecified superficial injury of right index finger
  - S60.941 Unspecified superficial injury of left index finger
  - S60.942 Unspecified superficial injury of right middle finger
  - S60.943 Unspecified superficial injury of left middle finger
  - S60.944 Unspecified superficial injury of right ring finger
  - S60.945 Unspecified superficial injury of left ring finger
  - S60.946 Unspecified superficial injury of right little finger
  - S60.947 Unspecified superficial injury of left little finger
  - S60.948 Unspecified superficial injury of other finger
    Unspecified superficial injury of specified finger with unspecified laterality
  - S60.949 Unspecified superficial injury of unspecified finger

4th S61 Open wound of wrist, hand and fingers

Code also any associated wound infection

EXCLUDES 1 *open fracture of wrist, hand and finger (S62.- with 7th character B)*

traumatic amputation of wrist and hand (S68.-)

The appropriate 7th character is to be added to each code from category S61.
- A initial encounter
- D subsequent encounter
- S sequela

5th S61.Ø Open wound of thumb without damage to nail

EXCLUDES 1 *open wound of thumb with damage to nail (S61.1-)*

6th S61.ØØ Unspecified open wound of thumb without damage to nail

7th S61.ØØ1 Unspecified open wound of right thumb without damage to nail

7th S61.ØØ2 Unspecified open wound of left thumb without damage to nail

7th S61.ØØ9 Unspecified open wound of unspecified thumb without damage to nail

6th S61.Ø1 Laceration without foreign body of thumb without damage to nail

7th S61.Ø11 Laceration without foreign body of right thumb without damage to nail

7th S61.Ø12 Laceration without foreign body of left thumb without damage to nail

7th S61.Ø19 Laceration without foreign body of unspecified thumb without damage to nail

6th S61.Ø2 Laceration with foreign body of thumb without damage to nail

7th S61.Ø21 Laceration with foreign body of right thumb without damage to nail

7th S61.Ø22 Laceration with foreign body of left thumb without damage to nail

7th S61.Ø29 Laceration with foreign body of unspecified thumb without damage to nail

6th S61.Ø3 Puncture wound without foreign body of thumb without damage to nail

7th S61.Ø31 Puncture wound without foreign body of right thumb without damage to nail

7th S61.Ø32 Puncture wound without foreign body of left thumb without damage to nail

7th S61.Ø39 Puncture wound without foreign body of unspecified thumb without damage to nail

6th S61.Ø4 Puncture wound with foreign body of thumb without damage to nail

7th S61.Ø41 Puncture wound with foreign body of right thumb without damage to nail

7th S61.Ø42 Puncture wound with foreign body of left thumb without damage to nail

7th S61.Ø49 Puncture wound with foreign body of unspecified thumb without damage to nail

6th S61.Ø5 Open bite of thumb without damage to nail

Bite of thumb NOS

EXCLUDES 1 *superficial bite of thumb (S6Ø.36-, S6Ø.37-)*

7th S61.Ø51 Open bite of right thumb without damage to nail

7th S61.Ø52 Open bite of left thumb without damage to nail

7th S61.Ø59 Open bite of unspecified thumb without damage to nail

5th S61.1 Open wound of thumb with damage to nail

6th S61.1Ø Unspecified open wound of thumb with damage to nail

7th S61.1Ø1 Unspecified open wound of right thumb with damage to nail

7th S61.1Ø2 Unspecified open wound of left thumb with damage to nail

7th S61.1Ø9 Unspecified open wound of unspecified thumb with damage to nail

6th S61.11 Laceration without foreign body of thumb with damage to nail

7th S61.111 Laceration without foreign body of right thumb with damage to nail

7th S61.112 Laceration without foreign body of left thumb with damage to nail

7th S61.119 Laceration without foreign body of unspecified thumb with damage to nail

6th S61.12 Laceration with foreign body of thumb with damage to nail

7th S61.121 Laceration with foreign body of right thumb with damage to nail

7th S61.122 Laceration with foreign body of left thumb with damage to nail

7th S61.129 Laceration with foreign body of unspecified thumb with damage to nail

6th S61.13 Puncture wound without foreign body of thumb with damage to nail

7th S61.131 Puncture wound without foreign body of right thumb with damage to nail

7th S61.132 Puncture wound without foreign body of left thumb with damage to nail

7th S61.139 Puncture wound without foreign body of unspecified thumb with damage to nail

6th S61.14 Puncture wound with foreign body of thumb with damage to nail

7th S61.141 Puncture wound with foreign body of right thumb with damage to nail

7th S61.142 Puncture wound with foreign body of left thumb with damage to nail

7th S61.149 Puncture wound with foreign body of unspecified thumb with damage to nail

6th S61.15 Open bite of thumb with damage to nail

Bite of thumb with damage to nail NOS

EXCLUDES 1 *superficial bite of thumb (S6Ø.36-, S6Ø.37-)*

7th S61.151 Open bite of right thumb with damage to nail

7th S61.152 Open bite of left thumb with damage to nail

7th S61.159 Open bite of unspecified thumb with damage to nail

5th S61.2 Open wound of other finger without damage to nail

EXCLUDES 1 *open wound of finger involving nail (matrix) (S61.3-)*

EXCLUDES 2 *open wound of thumb without damage to nail (S61.Ø-)*

6th S61.2Ø Unspecified open wound of other finger without damage to nail

7th S61.2ØØ Unspecified open wound of right index finger without damage to nail

7th S61.2Ø1 Unspecified open wound of left index finger without damage to nail

7th S61.2Ø2 Unspecified open wound of right middle finger without damage to nail

7th S61.2Ø3 Unspecified open wound of left middle finger without damage to nail

7th S61.2Ø4 Unspecified open wound of right ring finger without damage to nail

7th S61.2Ø5 Unspecified open wound of left ring finger without damage to nail

7th S61.2Ø6 Unspecified open wound of right little finger without damage to nail

7th S61.2Ø7 Unspecified open wound of left little finger without damage to nail

7th S61.2Ø8 Unspecified open wound of other finger without damage to nail

Unspecified open wound of specified finger with unspecified laterality without damage to nail

7th S61.2Ø9 Unspecified open wound of unspecified finger without damage to nail

6th S61.21 Laceration without foreign body of finger without damage to nail

7th S61.21Ø Laceration without foreign body of right index finger without damage to nail

7th S61.211 Laceration without foreign body of left index finger without damage to nail

7th S61.212 Laceration without foreign body of right middle finger without damage to nail

7th S61.213 Laceration without foreign body of left middle finger without damage to nail

7th S61.214 Laceration without foreign body of right ring finger without damage to nail

7th S61.215 Laceration without foreign body of left ring finger without damage to nail

7th S61.216 Laceration without foreign body of right little finger without damage to nail

7th S61.217 Laceration without foreign body of left little finger without damage to nail

S61.218 **Laceration without foreign body of other finger without damage to nail**
Laceration without foreign body of specified finger with unspecified laterality without damage to nail

S61.219 **Laceration without foreign body of unspecified finger without damage to nail**

S61.22 **Laceration with foreign body of finger without damage to nail**

S61.220 **Laceration with foreign body of right index finger without damage to nail**

S61.221 **Laceration with foreign body of left index finger without damage to nail**

S61.222 **Laceration with foreign body of right middle finger without damage to nail**

S61.223 **Laceration with foreign body of left middle finger without damage to nail**

S61.224 **Laceration with foreign body of right ring finger without damage to nail**

S61.225 **Laceration with foreign body of left ring finger without damage to nail**

S61.226 **Laceration with foreign body of right little finger without damage to nail**

S61.227 **Laceration with foreign body of left little finger without damage to nail**

S61.228 **Laceration with foreign body of other finger without damage to nail**
Laceration with foreign body of specified finger with unspecified laterality without damage to nail

S61.229 **Laceration with foreign body of unspecified finger without damage to nail**

S61.23 **Puncture wound without foreign body of finger without damage to nail**

S61.230 **Puncture wound without foreign body of right index finger without damage to nail**

S61.231 **Puncture wound without foreign body of left index finger without damage to nail**

S61.232 **Puncture wound without foreign body of right middle finger without damage to nail**

S61.233 **Puncture wound without foreign body of left middle finger without damage to nail**

S61.234 **Puncture wound without foreign body of right ring finger without damage to nail**

S61.235 **Puncture wound without foreign body of left ring finger without damage to nail**

S61.236 **Puncture wound without foreign body of right little finger without damage to nail**

S61.237 **Puncture wound without foreign body of left little finger without damage to nail**

S61.238 **Puncture wound without foreign body of other finger without damage to nail**
Puncture wound without foreign body of specified finger with unspecified laterality without damage to nail

S61.239 **Puncture wound without foreign body of unspecified finger without damage to nail**

S61.24 **Puncture wound with foreign body of finger without damage to nail**

S61.240 **Puncture wound with foreign body of right index finger without damage to nail**

S61.241 **Puncture wound with foreign body of left index finger without damage to nail**

S61.242 **Puncture wound with foreign body of right middle finger without damage to nail**

S61.243 **Puncture wound with foreign body of left middle finger without damage to nail**

S61.244 **Puncture wound with foreign body of right ring finger without damage to nail**

S61.245 **Puncture wound with foreign body of left ring finger without damage to nail**

S61.246 **Puncture wound with foreign body of right little finger without damage to nail**

S61.247 **Puncture wound with foreign body of left little finger without damage to nail**

S61.248 **Puncture wound with foreign body of other finger without damage to nail**
Puncture wound with foreign body of specified finger with unspecified laterality without damage to nail

S61.249 **Puncture wound with foreign body of unspecified finger without damage to nail**

S61.25 **Open bite of finger without damage to nail**
Bite of finger without damage to nail NOS
EXCLUDES 1 *superficial bite of finger (S60.46-, S60.47-)*

S61.250 **Open bite of right index finger without damage to nail**

S61.251 **Open bite of left index finger without damage to nail**

S61.252 **Open bite of right middle finger without damage to nail**

S61.253 **Open bite of left middle finger without damage to nail**

S61.254 **Open bite of right ring finger without damage to nail**

S61.255 **Open bite of left ring finger without damage to nail**

S61.256 **Open bite of right little finger without damage to nail**

S61.257 **Open bite of left little finger without damage to nail**

S61.258 **Open bite of other finger without damage to nail**
Open bite of specified finger with unspecified laterality without damage to nail

S61.259 **Open bite of unspecified finger without damage to nail**

S61.3 **Open wound of other finger with damage to nail**

S61.30 **Unspecified open wound of finger with damage to nail**

S61.300 **Unspecified open wound of right index finger with damage to nail**

S61.301 **Unspecified open wound of left index finger with damage to nail**

S61.302 **Unspecified open wound of right middle finger with damage to nail**

S61.303 **Unspecified open wound of left middle finger with damage to nail**

S61.304 **Unspecified open wound of right ring finger with damage to nail**

S61.305 **Unspecified open wound of left ring finger with damage to nail**

S61.306 **Unspecified open wound of right little finger with damage to nail**

S61.307 **Unspecified open wound of left little finger with damage to nail**

S61.308 **Unspecified open wound of other finger with damage to nail**
Unspecified open wound of specified finger with unspecified laterality with damage to nail

S61.309 **Unspecified open wound of unspecified finger with damage to nail**

S61.31 **Laceration without foreign body of finger with damage to nail**

S61.310 **Laceration without foreign body of right index finger with damage to nail**

S61.311 **Laceration without foreign body of left index finger with damage to nail**

S61.312 **Laceration without foreign body of right middle finger with damage to nail**

S61.313 **Laceration without foreign body of left middle finger with damage to nail**

S61.314 **Laceration without foreign body of right ring finger with damage to nail**

S61.315 **Laceration without foreign body of left ring finger with damage to nail**

S61.316 **Laceration without foreign body of right little finger with damage to nail**

S61.317 **Laceration without foreign body of left little finger with damage to nail**

√7th **S61.318 Laceration without foreign body of other finger with damage to nail**
Laceration without foreign body of specified finger with unspecified laterality with damage to nail

√7th **S61.319 Laceration without foreign body of unspecified finger with damage to nail**

√6th **S61.32 Laceration with foreign body of finger with damage to nail**

√7th **S61.320 Laceration with foreign body of right index finger with damage to nail**

√7th **S61.321 Laceration with foreign body of left index finger with damage to nail**

√7th **S61.322 Laceration with foreign body of right middle finger with damage to nail**

√7th **S61.323 Laceration with foreign body of left middle finger with damage to nail**

√7th **S61.324 Laceration with foreign body of right ring finger with damage to nail**

√7th **S61.325 Laceration with foreign body of left ring finger with damage to nail**

√7th **S61.326 Laceration with foreign body of right little finger with damage to nail**

√7th **S61.327 Laceration with foreign body of left little finger with damage to nail**

√7th **S61.328 Laceration with foreign body of other finger with damage to nail**
Laceration with foreign body of specified finger with unspecified laterality with damage to nail

√7th **S61.329 Laceration with foreign body of unspecified finger with damage to nail**

√6th **S61.33 Puncture wound without foreign body of finger with damage to nail**

√7th **S61.330 Puncture wound without foreign body of right index finger with damage to nail**

√7th **S61.331 Puncture wound without foreign body of left index finger with damage to nail**

√7th **S61.332 Puncture wound without foreign body of right middle finger with damage to nail**

√7th **S61.333 Puncture wound without foreign body of left middle finger with damage to nail**

√7th **S61.334 Puncture wound without foreign body of right ring finger with damage to nail**

√7th **S61.335 Puncture wound without foreign body of left ring finger with damage to nail**

√7th **S61.336 Puncture wound without foreign body of right little finger with damage to nail**

√7th **S61.337 Puncture wound without foreign body of left little finger with damage to nail**

√7th **S61.338 Puncture wound without foreign body of other finger with damage to nail**
Puncture wound without foreign body of specified finger with unspecified laterality with damage to nail

√7th **S61.339 Puncture wound without foreign body of unspecified finger with damage to nail**

√6th **S61.34 Puncture wound with foreign body of finger with damage to nail**

√7th **S61.340 Puncture wound with foreign body of right index finger with damage to nail**

√7th **S61.341 Puncture wound with foreign body of left index finger with damage to nail**

√7th **S61.342 Puncture wound with foreign body of right middle finger with damage to nail**

√7th **S61.343 Puncture wound with foreign body of left middle finger with damage to nail**

√7th **S61.344 Puncture wound with foreign body of right ring finger with damage to nail**

√7th **S61.345 Puncture wound with foreign body of left ring finger with damage to nail**

√7th **S61.346 Puncture wound with foreign body of right little finger with damage to nail**

√7th **S61.347 Puncture wound with foreign body of left little finger with damage to nail**

√7th **S61.348 Puncture wound with foreign body of other finger with damage to nail**
Puncture wound with foreign body of specified finger with unspecified laterality with damage to nail

√7th **S61.349 Puncture wound with foreign body of unspecified finger with damage to nail**

√6th **S61.35 Open bite of finger with damage to nail**
Bite of finger with damage to nail NOS
EXCLUDES 1 *superficial bite of finger (S60.46-, S60.47-)*

√7th **S61.350 Open bite of right index finger with damage to nail**

√7th **S61.351 Open bite of left index finger with damage to nail**

√7th **S61.352 Open bite of right middle finger with damage to nail**

√7th **S61.353 Open bite of left middle finger with damage to nail**

√7th **S61.354 Open bite of right ring finger with damage to nail**

√7th **S61.355 Open bite of left ring finger with damage to nail**

√7th **S61.356 Open bite of right little finger with damage to nail**

√7th **S61.357 Open bite of left little finger with damage to nail**

√7th **S61.358 Open bite of other finger with damage to nail**
Open bite of specified finger with unspecified laterality with damage to nail

√7th **S61.359 Open bite of unspecified finger with damage to nail**

√5th **S61.4 Open wound of hand**

√6th **S61.40 Unspecified open wound of hand**

√7th **S61.401 Unspecified open wound of right hand**

√7th **S61.402 Unspecified open wound of left hand**

√7th **S61.409 Unspecified open wound of unspecified hand**

√6th **S61.41 Laceration without foreign body of hand**

√7th **S61.411 Laceration without foreign body of right hand**

√7th **S61.412 Laceration without foreign body of left hand**

√7th **S61.419 Laceration without foreign body of unspecified hand**

√6th **S61.42 Laceration with foreign body of hand**

√7th **S61.421 Laceration with foreign body of right hand**

√7th **S61.422 Laceration with foreign body of left hand**

√7th **S61.429 Laceration with foreign body of unspecified hand**

√6th **S61.43 Puncture wound without foreign body of hand**

√7th **S61.431 Puncture wound without foreign body of right hand**

√7th **S61.432 Puncture wound without foreign body of left hand**

√7th **S61.439 Puncture wound without foreign body of unspecified hand**

√6th **S61.44 Puncture wound with foreign body of hand**

√7th **S61.441 Puncture wound with foreign body of right hand**

√7th **S61.442 Puncture wound with foreign body of left hand**

√7th **S61.449 Puncture wound with foreign body of unspecified hand**

√6th **S61.45 Open bite of hand**
Bite of hand NOS
EXCLUDES 1 *superficial bite of hand (S60.56-, S60.57-)*

√7th **S61.451 Open bite of right hand**

√7th **S61.452 Open bite of left hand**

√7th **S61.459 Open bite of unspecified hand**

√5th **S61.5 Open wound of wrist**

√6th **S61.50 Unspecified open wound of wrist**

√7th **S61.501 Unspecified open wound of right wrist**

√7th **S61.502 Unspecified open wound of left wrist**

√7th **S61.509 Unspecified open wound of unspecified wrist**

√6th **S61.51 Laceration without foreign body of wrist**

√7th **S61.511 Laceration without foreign body of right wrist**

√7th **S61.512 Laceration without foreign body of left wrist**

S61.519 Laceration without foreign body of unspecified wrist
S61.52 Laceration with foreign body of wrist
S61.521 Laceration with foreign body of right wrist
S61.522 Laceration with foreign body of left wrist
S61.529 Laceration with foreign body of unspecified wrist
S61.53 Puncture wound without foreign body of wrist
S61.531 Puncture wound without foreign body of right wrist
S61.532 Puncture wound without foreign body of left wrist
S61.539 Puncture wound without foreign body of unspecified wrist
S61.54 Puncture wound with foreign body of wrist
S61.541 Puncture wound with foreign body of right wrist
S61.542 Puncture wound with foreign body of left wrist
S61.549 Puncture wound with foreign body of unspecified wrist
S61.55 Open bite of wrist
Bite of wrist NOS
EXCLUDES 1 *superficial bite of wrist (S6Ø.86-, S6Ø.87-)*
S61.551 Open bite of right wrist
S61.552 Open bite of left wrist
S61.559 Open bite of unspecified wrist

S62 Fracture at wrist and hand level

NOTE A fracture not indicated as displaced or nondisplaced should be coded to displaced

A fracture not indicated as open or closed should be coded to closed

EXCLUDES 1 *traumatic amputation of wrist and hand (S68.-)*
EXCLUDES 2 *fracture of distal parts of ulna and radius (S52.-)*

AHA: 2018,2Q,12; 2015,3Q,37-39

The appropriate 7th character is to be added to each code from category S62.
A initial encounter for closed fracture
B initial encounter for open fracture
D subsequent encounter for fracture with routine healing
G subsequent encounter for fracture with delayed healing
K subsequent encounter for fracture with nonunion
P subsequent encounter for fracture with malunion
S sequela

S62.Ø Fracture of navicular [scaphoid] bone of wrist
S62.ØØ Unspecified fracture of navicular [scaphoid] bone of wrist
S62.ØØ1 Unspecified fracture of navicular [scaphoid] bone of right wrist CC H5
S62.ØØ2 Unspecified fracture of navicular [scaphoid] bone of left wrist CC H5
AHA: 2012,4Q,106
S62.ØØ9 Unspecified fracture of navicular [scaphoid] bone of unspecified wrist CC H5
S62.Ø1 Fracture of distal pole of navicular [scaphoid] bone of wrist
Fracture of volar tuberosity of navicular [scaphoid] bone of wrist
S62.Ø11 Displaced fracture of distal pole of navicular [scaphoid] bone of right wrist CC H5
S62.Ø12 Displaced fracture of distal pole of navicular [scaphoid] bone of left wrist CC H5
S62.Ø13 Displaced fracture of distal pole of navicular [scaphoid] bone of unspecified wrist CC H5
S62.Ø14 Nondisplaced fracture of distal pole of navicular [scaphoid] bone of right wrist CC H5
S62.Ø15 Nondisplaced fracture of distal pole of navicular [scaphoid] bone of left wrist CC H5
S62.Ø16 Nondisplaced fracture of distal pole of navicular [scaphoid] bone of unspecified wrist CC H5
S62.Ø2 Fracture of middle third of navicular [scaphoid] bone of wrist
S62.Ø21 Displaced fracture of middle third of navicular [scaphoid] bone of right wrist CC H5
S62.Ø22 Displaced fracture of middle third of navicular [scaphoid] bone of left wrist CC H5
S62.Ø23 Displaced fracture of middle third of navicular [scaphoid] bone of unspecified wrist CC H5
S62.Ø24 Nondisplaced fracture of middle third of navicular [scaphoid] bone of right wrist CC H5
S62.Ø25 Nondisplaced fracture of middle third of navicular [scaphoid] bone of left wrist CC H5
S62.Ø26 Nondisplaced fracture of middle third of navicular [scaphoid] bone of unspecified wrist CC H5
S62.Ø3 Fracture of proximal third of navicular [scaphoid] bone of wrist
S62.Ø31 Displaced fracture of proximal third of navicular [scaphoid] bone of right wrist CC H5
S62.Ø32 Displaced fracture of proximal third of navicular [scaphoid] bone of left wrist CC H5
S62.Ø33 Displaced fracture of proximal third of navicular [scaphoid] bone of unspecified wrist CC H5
S62.Ø34 Nondisplaced fracture of proximal third of navicular [scaphoid] bone of right wrist CC H5
S62.Ø35 Nondisplaced fracture of proximal third of navicular [scaphoid] bone of left wrist CC H5
S62.Ø36 Nondisplaced fracture of proximal third of navicular [scaphoid] bone of unspecified wrist CC H5
S62.1 Fracture of other and unspecified carpal bone(s)
EXCLUDES 2 *fracture of scaphoid of wrist (S62.Ø-)*
S62.1Ø Fracture of unspecified carpal bone
Fracture of wrist NOS
S62.1Ø1 Fracture of unspecified carpal bone, right wrist CC H5
S62.1Ø2 Fracture of unspecified carpal bone, left wrist CC H5
AHA: 2012,4Q,95
S62.1Ø9 Fracture of unspecified carpal bone, unspecified wrist CC H5
S62.11 Fracture of triquetrum [cuneiform] bone of wrist
S62.111 Displaced fracture of triquetrum [cuneiform] bone, right wrist CC H5
S62.112 Displaced fracture of triquetrum [cuneiform] bone, left wrist CC H5
S62.113 Displaced fracture of triquetrum [cuneiform] bone, unspecified wrist CC H5
S62.114 Nondisplaced fracture of triquetrum [cuneiform] bone, right wrist CC H5
S62.115 Nondisplaced fracture of triquetrum [cuneiform] bone, left wrist CC H5
S62.116 Nondisplaced fracture of triquetrum [cuneiform] bone, unspecified wrist CC H5
S62.12 Fracture of lunate [semilunar]
S62.121 Displaced fracture of lunate [semilunar], right wrist CC H5
S62.122 Displaced fracture of lunate [semilunar], left wrist CC H5
S62.123 Displaced fracture of lunate [semilunar], unspecified wrist CC H5
S62.124 Nondisplaced fracture of lunate [semilunar], right wrist CC H5
S62.125 Nondisplaced fracture of lunate [semilunar], left wrist CC H5

3 ✓7th **S62.126 Nondisplaced fracture of lunate [semilunar], unspecified wrist** CC H5

✓6th **S62.13 Fracture of capitate [os magnum] bone**

3 ✓7th **S62.131 Displaced fracture of capitate [os magnum] bone, right wrist** CC H5

3 ✓7th **S62.132 Displaced fracture of capitate [os magnum] bone, left wrist** CC H5

3 ✓7th **S62.133 Displaced fracture of capitate [os magnum] bone, unspecified wrist** CC H5

3 ✓7th **S62.134 Nondisplaced fracture of capitate [os magnum] bone, right wrist** CC H5

3 ✓7th **S62.135 Nondisplaced fracture of capitate [os magnum] bone, left wrist** CC H5

3 ✓7th **S62.136 Nondisplaced fracture of capitate [os magnum] bone, unspecified wrist** CC H5

✓6th **S62.14 Fracture of body of hamate [unciform] bone**

Fracture of hamate [unciform] bone NOS

3 ✓7th **S62.141 Displaced fracture of body of hamate [unciform] bone, right wrist** CC H5

3 ✓7th **S62.142 Displaced fracture of body of hamate [unciform] bone, left wrist** CC H5

3 ✓7th **S62.143 Displaced fracture of body of hamate [unciform] bone, unspecified wrist** CC H5

3 ✓7th **S62.144 Nondisplaced fracture of body of hamate [unciform] bone, right wrist** CC H5

3 ✓7th **S62.145 Nondisplaced fracture of body of hamate [unciform] bone, left wrist** CC H5

3 ✓7th **S62.146 Nondisplaced fracture of body of hamate [unciform] bone, unspecified wrist** CC H5

✓6th **S62.15 Fracture of hook process of hamate [unciform] bone**

Fracture of unciform process of hamate [unciform] bone

3 ✓7th **S62.151 Displaced fracture of hook process of hamate [unciform] bone, right wrist** CC H5

3 ✓7th **S62.152 Displaced fracture of hook process of hamate [unciform] bone, left wrist** CC H5

3 ✓7th **S62.153 Displaced fracture of hook process of hamate [unciform] bone, unspecified wrist** CC H5

3 ✓7th **S62.154 Nondisplaced fracture of hook process of hamate [unciform] bone, right wrist** CC H5

3 ✓7th **S62.155 Nondisplaced fracture of hook process of hamate [unciform] bone, left wrist** CC H5

3 ✓7th **S62.156 Nondisplaced fracture of hook process of hamate [unciform] bone, unspecified wrist** CC H5

✓6th **S62.16 Fracture of pisiform**

3 ✓7th **S62.161 Displaced fracture of pisiform, right wrist** CC H5

3 ✓7th **S62.162 Displaced fracture of pisiform, left wrist** CC H5

3 ✓7th **S62.163 Displaced fracture of pisiform, unspecified wrist** CC H5

3 ✓7th **S62.164 Nondisplaced fracture of pisiform, right wrist** CC H5

3 ✓7th **S62.165 Nondisplaced fracture of pisiform, left wrist** CC H5

3 ✓7th **S62.166 Nondisplaced fracture of pisiform, unspecified wrist** CC H5

✓6th **S62.17 Fracture of trapezium [larger multangular]**

3 ✓7th **S62.171 Displaced fracture of trapezium [larger multangular], right wrist** CC H5

3 ✓7th **S62.172 Displaced fracture of trapezium [larger multangular], left wrist** CC H5

3 ✓7th **S62.173 Displaced fracture of trapezium [larger multangular], unspecified wrist** CC H5

3 ✓7th **S62.174 Nondisplaced fracture of trapezium [larger multangular], right wrist** CC H5

3 ✓7th **S62.175 Nondisplaced fracture of trapezium [larger multangular], left wrist** CC H5

3 ✓7th **S62.176 Nondisplaced fracture of trapezium [larger multangular], unspecified wrist** CC H5

✓6th **S62.18 Fracture of trapezoid [smaller multangular]**

3 ✓7th **S62.181 Displaced fracture of trapezoid [smaller multangular], right wrist** CC H5

3 ✓7th **S62.182 Displaced fracture of trapezoid [smaller multangular], left wrist** CC H5

3 ✓7th **S62.183 Displaced fracture of trapezoid [smaller multangular], unspecified wrist** CC H5

3 ✓7th **S62.184 Nondisplaced fracture of trapezoid [smaller multangular], right wrist** CC H5

3 ✓7th **S62.185 Nondisplaced fracture of trapezoid [smaller multangular], left wrist** CC H5

3 ✓7th **S62.186 Nondisplaced fracture of trapezoid [smaller multangular], unspecified wrist** CC H5

✓5th **S62.2 Fracture of first metacarpal bone**

✓6th **S62.20 Unspecified fracture of first metacarpal bone**

3 ✓7th **S62.201 Unspecified fracture of first metacarpal bone, right hand** CC H5

3 ✓7th **S62.202 Unspecified fracture of first metacarpal bone, left hand** CC H5

3 ✓7th **S62.209 Unspecified fracture of first metacarpal bone, unspecified hand** CC H5

✓6th **S62.21 Bennett's fracture**

DEF: Intra-articular, two-part fracture at the base of the first metacarpal bone (thumb) on the ulnar side at the carpometacarpal (CMC) joint.

3 ✓7th **S62.211 Bennett's fracture, right hand** CC H5

3 ✓7th **S62.212 Bennett's fracture, left hand** CC H5

3 ✓7th **S62.213 Bennett's fracture, unspecified hand** CC H5

✓6th **S62.22 Rolando's fracture**

DEF: Comminuted, three part intra-articular fracture at the base of the thumb metacarpal.

3 ✓7th **S62.221 Displaced Rolando's fracture, right hand** CC H5

3 ✓7th **S62.222 Displaced Rolando's fracture, left hand** CC H5

3 ✓7th **S62.223 Displaced Rolando's fracture, unspecified hand** CC H5

3 ✓7th **S62.224 Nondisplaced Rolando's fracture, right hand** CC H5

3 ✓7th **S62.225 Nondisplaced Rolando's fracture, left hand** CC H5

3 ✓7th **S62.226 Nondisplaced Rolando's fracture, unspecified hand** CC H5

✓6th **S62.23 Other fracture of base of first metacarpal bone**

3 ✓7th **S62.231 Other displaced fracture of base of first metacarpal bone, right hand** CC H5

3 ✓7th **S62.232 Other displaced fracture of base of first metacarpal bone, left hand** CC H5

3 ✓7th **S62.233 Other displaced fracture of base of first metacarpal bone, unspecified hand** CC H5

3 ✓7th **S62.234 Other nondisplaced fracture of base of first metacarpal bone, right hand** CC H5

3 ✓7th **S62.235 Other nondisplaced fracture of base of first metacarpal bone, left hand** CC H5

3 ✓7th **S62.236 Other nondisplaced fracture of base of first metacarpal bone, unspecified hand** CC H5

✓6th **S62.24 Fracture of shaft of first metacarpal bone**

3 ✓7th **S62.241 Displaced fracture of shaft of first metacarpal bone, right hand** CC H5

3 ✓7th **S62.242 Displaced fracture of shaft of first metacarpal bone, left hand** CC H5

3 ✓7th **S62.243 Displaced fracture of shaft of first metacarpal bone, unspecified hand** CC H5

3 ✓7th **S62.244 Nondisplaced fracture of shaft of first metacarpal bone, right hand** CC H5

3 ✓7th **S62.245 Nondisplaced fracture of shaft of first metacarpal bone, left hand** CC H5

3 ✓7th S62.246 Nondisplaced fracture of shaft of first metacarpal bone, unspecified hand CC H5

✓6th S62.25 Fracture of neck of first metacarpal bone

3 ✓7th S62.251 Displaced fracture of neck of first metacarpal bone, right hand CC H5

3 ✓7th S62.252 Displaced fracture of neck of first metacarpal bone, left hand CC H5

3 ✓7th S62.253 Displaced fracture of neck of first metacarpal bone, unspecified hand CC H5

3 ✓7th S62.254 Nondisplaced fracture of neck of first metacarpal bone, right hand CC H5

3 ✓7th S62.255 Nondisplaced fracture of neck of first metacarpal bone, left hand CC H5

3 ✓7th S62.256 Nondisplaced fracture of neck of first metacarpal bone, unspecified hand CC H5

✓6th S62.29 Other fracture of first metacarpal bone

3 ✓7th S62.291 Other fracture of first metacarpal bone, right hand CC H5

3 ✓7th S62.292 Other fracture of first metacarpal bone, left hand CC H5

3 ✓7th S62.299 Other fracture of first metacarpal bone, unspecified hand CC H5

✓5th S62.3 Fracture of other and unspecified metacarpal bone

EXCLUDES 2 *fracture of first metacarpal bone (S62.2-)*

✓6th S62.30 Unspecified fracture of other metacarpal bone

3 ✓7th S62.300 Unspecified fracture of second metacarpal bone, right hand CC H5

3 ✓7th S62.301 Unspecified fracture of second metacarpal bone, left hand CC H5

3 ✓7th S62.302 Unspecified fracture of third metacarpal bone, right hand CC H5

3 ✓7th S62.303 Unspecified fracture of third metacarpal bone, left hand CC H5

3 ✓7th S62.304 Unspecified fracture of fourth metacarpal bone, right hand CC H5

3 ✓7th S62.305 Unspecified fracture of fourth metacarpal bone, left hand CC H5

3 ✓7th S62.306 Unspecified fracture of fifth metacarpal bone, right hand CC H5

3 ✓7th S62.307 Unspecified fracture of fifth metacarpal bone, left hand CC H5

3 ✓7th S62.308 Unspecified fracture of other metacarpal bone CC H5

Unspecified fracture of specified metacarpal bone with unspecified laterality

3 ✓7th S62.309 Unspecified fracture of unspecified metacarpal bone CC H5

✓6th S62.31 Displaced fracture of base of other metacarpal bone

3 ✓7th S62.310 Displaced fracture of base of second metacarpal bone, right hand CC H5

3 ✓7th S62.311 Displaced fracture of base of second metacarpal bone, left hand CC H5

3 ✓7th S62.312 Displaced fracture of base of third metacarpal bone, right hand CC H5

3 ✓7th S62.313 Displaced fracture of base of third metacarpal bone, left hand CC H5

3 ✓7th S62.314 Displaced fracture of base of fourth metacarpal bone, right hand CC H5

3 ✓7th S62.315 Displaced fracture of base of fourth metacarpal bone, left hand CC H5

3 ✓7th S62.316 Displaced fracture of base of fifth metacarpal bone, right hand CC H5

3 ✓7th S62.317 Displaced fracture of base of fifth metacarpal bone, left hand CC H5

3 ✓7th S62.318 Displaced fracture of base of other metacarpal bone CC H5

Displaced fracture of base of specified metacarpal bone with unspecified laterality

3 ✓7th S62.319 Displaced fracture of base of unspecified metacarpal bone CC H5

✓6th S62.32 Displaced fracture of shaft of other metacarpal bone

3 ✓7th S62.320 Displaced fracture of shaft of second metacarpal bone, right hand CC H5

3 ✓7th S62.321 Displaced fracture of shaft of second metacarpal bone, left hand CC H5

3 ✓7th S62.322 Displaced fracture of shaft of third metacarpal bone, right hand CC H5

3 ✓7th S62.323 Displaced fracture of shaft of third metacarpal bone, left hand CC H5

3 ✓7th S62.324 Displaced fracture of shaft of fourth metacarpal bone, right hand CC H5

3 ✓7th S62.325 Displaced fracture of shaft of fourth metacarpal bone, left hand CC H5

3 ✓7th S62.326 Displaced fracture of shaft of fifth metacarpal bone, right hand CC H5

3 ✓7th S62.327 Displaced fracture of shaft of fifth metacarpal bone, left hand CC H5

3 ✓7th S62.328 Displaced fracture of shaft of other metacarpal bone CC H5

Displaced fracture of shaft of specified metacarpal bone with unspecified laterality

3 ✓7th S62.329 Displaced fracture of shaft of unspecified metacarpal bone CC H5

✓6th S62.33 Displaced fracture of neck of other metacarpal bone

3 ✓7th S62.330 Displaced fracture of neck of second metacarpal bone, right hand CC H5

3 ✓7th S62.331 Displaced fracture of neck of second metacarpal bone, left hand CC H5

3 ✓7th S62.332 Displaced fracture of neck of third metacarpal bone, right hand CC H5

3 ✓7th S62.333 Displaced fracture of neck of third metacarpal bone, left hand CC H5

3 ✓7th S62.334 Displaced fracture of neck of fourth metacarpal bone, right hand CC H5

3 ✓7th S62.335 Displaced fracture of neck of fourth metacarpal bone, left hand CC H5

3 ✓7th S62.336 Displaced fracture of neck of fifth metacarpal bone, right hand CC H5

3 ✓7th S62.337 Displaced fracture of neck of fifth metacarpal bone, left hand CC H5

3 ✓7th S62.338 Displaced fracture of neck of other metacarpal bone CC H5

Displaced fracture of neck of specified metacarpal bone with unspecified laterality

3 ✓7th S62.339 Displaced fracture of neck of unspecified metacarpal bone CC H5

✓6th S62.34 Nondisplaced fracture of base of other metacarpal bone

3 ✓7th S62.340 Nondisplaced fracture of base of second metacarpal bone, right hand CC H5

3 ✓7th S62.341 Nondisplaced fracture of base of second metacarpal bone, left hand CC H5

3 ✓7th S62.342 Nondisplaced fracture of base of third metacarpal bone, right hand CC H5

3 ✓7th S62.343 Nondisplaced fracture of base of third metacarpal bone, left hand CC H5

3 ✓7th S62.344 Nondisplaced fracture of base of fourth metacarpal bone, right hand CC H5

3 ✓7th S62.345 Nondisplaced fracture of base of fourth metacarpal bone, left hand CC H5

3 ✓7th S62.346 Nondisplaced fracture of base of fifth metacarpal bone, right hand CC H5

3 ✓7th S62.347 Nondisplaced fracture of base of fifth metacarpal bone, left hand CC H5

3 ✓7th S62.348 Nondisplaced fracture of base of other metacarpal bone CC H5

Nondisplaced fracture of base of specified metacarpal bone with unspecified laterality

3 ✓7th S62.349 Nondisplaced fracture of base of unspecified metacarpal bone CC H5

✓6th S62.35 Nondisplaced fracture of shaft of other metacarpal bone

3 ✓7th S62.350 Nondisplaced fracture of shaft of second metacarpal bone, right hand CC H5

3 ✓7th S62.351 Nondisplaced fracture of shaft of second metacarpal bone, left hand CC H5

3 ✓7th S62.352 Nondisplaced fracture of shaft of third metacarpal bone, right hand CC H5

3 ✓7th S62.353 Nondisplaced fracture of shaft of third metacarpal bone, left hand CC H5

3 ✓7th S62.354 Nondisplaced fracture of shaft of fourth metacarpal bone, right hand CC H5
3 ✓7th S62.355 Nondisplaced fracture of shaft of fourth metacarpal bone, left hand CC H5
3 ✓7th S62.356 Nondisplaced fracture of shaft of fifth metacarpal bone, right hand CC H5
3 ✓7th S62.357 Nondisplaced fracture of shaft of fifth metacarpal bone, left hand CC H5
3 ✓7th S62.358 Nondisplaced fracture of shaft of other metacarpal bone CC H5
Nondisplaced fracture of shaft of specified metacarpal bone with unspecified laterality
3 ✓7th S62.359 Nondisplaced fracture of shaft of unspecified metacarpal bone CC H5

✓6th S62.36 Nondisplaced fracture of neck of other metacarpal bone
3 ✓7th S62.360 Nondisplaced fracture of neck of second metacarpal bone, right hand CC H5
3 ✓7th S62.361 Nondisplaced fracture of neck of second metacarpal bone, left hand CC H5
3 ✓7th S62.362 Nondisplaced fracture of neck of third metacarpal bone, right hand CC H5
3 ✓7th S62.363 Nondisplaced fracture of neck of third metacarpal bone, left hand CC H5
3 ✓7th S62.364 Nondisplaced fracture of neck of fourth metacarpal bone, right hand CC H5
3 ✓7th S62.365 Nondisplaced fracture of neck of fourth metacarpal bone, left hand CC H5
3 ✓7th S62.366 Nondisplaced fracture of neck of fifth metacarpal bone, right hand CC H5
3 ✓7th S62.367 Nondisplaced fracture of neck of fifth metacarpal bone, left hand CC H5
3 ✓7th S62.368 Nondisplaced fracture of neck of other metacarpal bone CC H5
Nondisplaced fracture of neck of specified metacarpal bone with unspecified laterality
3 ✓7th S62.369 Nondisplaced fracture of neck of unspecified metacarpal bone CC H5

✓6th S62.39 Other fracture of other metacarpal bone
3 ✓7th S62.390 Other fracture of second metacarpal bone, right hand CC H5
3 ✓7th S62.391 Other fracture of second metacarpal bone, left hand CC H5
3 ✓7th S62.392 Other fracture of third metacarpal bone, right hand CC H5
3 ✓7th S62.393 Other fracture of third metacarpal bone, left hand CC H5
3 ✓7th S62.394 Other fracture of fourth metacarpal bone, right hand CC H5
3 ✓7th S62.395 Other fracture of fourth metacarpal bone, left hand CC H5
3 ✓7th S62.396 Other fracture of fifth metacarpal bone, right hand CC H5
3 ✓7th S62.397 Other fracture of fifth metacarpal bone, left hand CC H5
3 ✓7th S62.398 Other fracture of other metacarpal bone CC H5
Other fracture of specified metacarpal bone with unspecified laterality
3 ✓7th S62.399 Other fracture of unspecified metacarpal bone CC H5

✓5th S62.5 Fracture of thumb

✓6th S62.50 Fracture of unspecified phalanx of thumb
3 ✓7th S62.501 Fracture of unspecified phalanx of right thumb CC H5
3 ✓7th S62.502 Fracture of unspecified phalanx of left thumb CC H5
3 ✓7th S62.509 Fracture of unspecified phalanx of unspecified thumb CC H5

✓6th S62.51 Fracture of proximal phalanx of thumb
3 ✓7th S62.511 Displaced fracture of proximal phalanx of right thumb CC H5
3 ✓7th S62.512 Displaced fracture of proximal phalanx of left thumb CC H5
3 ✓7th S62.513 Displaced fracture of proximal phalanx of unspecified thumb CC H5
3 ✓7th S62.514 Nondisplaced fracture of proximal phalanx of right thumb CC H5
3 ✓7th S62.515 Nondisplaced fracture of proximal phalanx of left thumb CC H5
3 ✓7th S62.516 Nondisplaced fracture of proximal phalanx of unspecified thumb CC H5

✓6th S62.52 Fracture of distal phalanx of thumb
3 ✓7th S62.521 Displaced fracture of distal phalanx of right thumb CC H5
3 ✓7th S62.522 Displaced fracture of distal phalanx of left thumb CC H5
3 ✓7th S62.523 Displaced fracture of distal phalanx of unspecified thumb CC H5
3 ✓7th S62.524 Nondisplaced fracture of distal phalanx of right thumb CC H5
3 ✓7th S62.525 Nondisplaced fracture of distal phalanx of left thumb CC H5
3 ✓7th S62.526 Nondisplaced fracture of distal phalanx of unspecified thumb CC H5

✓5th S62.6 Fracture of other and unspecified finger(s)
EXCLUDES 2 *fracture of thumb (S62.5-)*

✓6th S62.60 Fracture of unspecified phalanx of finger
3 ✓7th S62.600 Fracture of unspecified phalanx of right index finger CC H5
3 ✓7th S62.601 Fracture of unspecified phalanx of left index finger CC H5
3 ✓7th S62.602 Fracture of unspecified phalanx of right middle finger CC H5
3 ✓7th S62.603 Fracture of unspecified phalanx of left middle finger CC H5
3 ✓7th S62.604 Fracture of unspecified phalanx of right ring finger CC H5
3 ✓7th S62.605 Fracture of unspecified phalanx of left ring finger CC H5
3 ✓7th S62.606 Fracture of unspecified phalanx of right little finger CC H5
3 ✓7th S62.607 Fracture of unspecified phalanx of left little finger CC H5
3 ✓7th S62.608 Fracture of unspecified phalanx of other finger CC H5
Fracture of unspecified phalanx of specified finger with unspecified laterality
3 ✓7th S62.609 Fracture of unspecified phalanx of unspecified finger CC H5

✓6th S62.61 Displaced fracture of proximal phalanx of finger
3 ✓7th S62.610 Displaced fracture of proximal phalanx of right index finger CC H5
3 ✓7th S62.611 Displaced fracture of proximal phalanx of left index finger CC H5
3 ✓7th S62.612 Displaced fracture of proximal phalanx of right middle finger CC H5
3 ✓7th S62.613 Displaced fracture of proximal phalanx of left middle finger CC H5
3 ✓7th S62.614 Displaced fracture of proximal phalanx of right ring finger CC H5
3 ✓7th S62.615 Displaced fracture of proximal phalanx of left ring finger CC H5
3 ✓7th S62.616 Displaced fracture of proximal phalanx of right little finger CC H5
3 ✓7th S62.617 Displaced fracture of proximal phalanx of left little finger CC H5
3 ✓7th S62.618 Displaced fracture of proximal phalanx of other finger CC H5
Displaced fracture of proximal phalanx of specified finger with unspecified laterality
3 ✓7th S62.619 Displaced fracture of proximal phalanx of unspecified finger CC H5

✓6th S62.62 Displaced fracture of middle phalanx of finger
3 ✓7th S62.620 Displaced fracture of middle phalanx of right index finger CC H5
3 ✓7th S62.621 Displaced fracture of middle phalanx of left index finger CC H5
3 ✓7th S62.622 Displaced fracture of middle phalanx of right middle finger CC H5
3 ✓7th S62.623 Displaced fracture of middle phalanx of left middle finger CC H5

3 √7th S62.624 **Displaced fracture of middle phalanx of right ring finger** CC H5
3 √7th S62.625 **Displaced fracture of middle phalanx of left ring finger** CC H5
3 √7th S62.626 **Displaced fracture of middle phalanx of right little finger** CC H5
3 √7th S62.627 **Displaced fracture of middle phalanx of left little finger** CC H5
3 √7th S62.628 **Displaced fracture of middle phalanx of other finger** CC H5
Displaced fracture of middle phalanx of specified finger with unspecified laterality
3 √7th S62.629 **Displaced fracture of middle phalanx of unspecified finger** CC H5

√6th S62.63 **Displaced fracture of distal phalanx of finger**
3 √7th S62.630 **Displaced fracture of distal phalanx of right index finger** CC H5
3 √7th S62.631 **Displaced fracture of distal phalanx of left index finger** CC H5
3 √7th S62.632 **Displaced fracture of distal phalanx of right middle finger** CC H5
3 √7th S62.633 **Displaced fracture of distal phalanx of left middle finger** CC H5
3 √7th S62.634 **Displaced fracture of distal phalanx of right ring finger** CC H5
3 √7th S62.635 **Displaced fracture of distal phalanx of left ring finger** CC H5
3 √7th S62.636 **Displaced fracture of distal phalanx of right little finger** CC H5
3 √7th S62.637 **Displaced fracture of distal phalanx of left little finger** CC H5
3 √7th S62.638 **Displaced fracture of distal phalanx of other finger** CC H5
Displaced fracture of distal phalanx of specified finger with unspecified laterality
3 √7th S62.639 **Displaced fracture of distal phalanx of unspecified finger** CC H5

√6th S62.64 **Nondisplaced fracture of proximal phalanx of finger**
3 √7th S62.640 **Nondisplaced fracture of proximal phalanx of right index finger** CC H5
3 √7th S62.641 **Nondisplaced fracture of proximal phalanx of left index finger** CC H5
3 √7th S62.642 **Nondisplaced fracture of proximal phalanx of right middle finger** CC H5
3 √7th S62.643 **Nondisplaced fracture of proximal phalanx of left middle finger** CC H5
3 √7th S62.644 **Nondisplaced fracture of proximal phalanx of right ring finger** CC H5
3 √7th S62.645 **Nondisplaced fracture of proximal phalanx of left ring finger** CC H5
3 √7th S62.646 **Nondisplaced fracture of proximal phalanx of right little finger** CC H5
3 √7th S62.647 **Nondisplaced fracture of proximal phalanx of left little finger** CC H5
3 √7th S62.648 **Nondisplaced fracture of proximal phalanx of other finger** CC H5
Nondisplaced fracture of proximal phalanx of specified finger with unspecified laterality
3 √7th S62.649 **Nondisplaced fracture of proximal phalanx of unspecified finger** CC H5

√6th S62.65 **Nondisplaced fracture of middle phalanx of finger**
3 √7th S62.650 **Nondisplaced fracture of middle phalanx of right index finger** CC H5
3 √7th S62.651 **Nondisplaced fracture of middle phalanx of left index finger** CC H5
3 √7th S62.652 **Nondisplaced fracture of middle phalanx of right middle finger** CC H5
3 √7th S62.653 **Nondisplaced fracture of middle phalanx of left middle finger** CC H5
3 √7th S62.654 **Nondisplaced fracture of middle phalanx of right ring finger** CC H5
3 √7th S62.655 **Nondisplaced fracture of middle phalanx of left ring finger** CC H5
3 √7th S62.656 **Nondisplaced fracture of middle phalanx of right little finger** CC H5
3 √7th S62.657 **Nondisplaced fracture of middle phalanx of left little finger** CC H5
3 √7th S62.658 **Nondisplaced fracture of middle phalanx of other finger** CC H5
Nondisplaced fracture of middle phalanx of specified finger with unspecified laterality
3 √7th S62.659 **Nondisplaced fracture of middle phalanx of unspecified finger** CC H5

√6th S62.66 **Nondisplaced fracture of distal phalanx of finger**
3 √7th S62.660 **Nondisplaced fracture of distal phalanx of right index finger** CC H5
3 √7th S62.661 **Nondisplaced fracture of distal phalanx of left index finger** CC H5
3 √7th S62.662 **Nondisplaced fracture of distal phalanx of right middle finger** CC H5
3 √7th S62.663 **Nondisplaced fracture of distal phalanx of left middle finger** CC H5
3 √7th S62.664 **Nondisplaced fracture of distal phalanx of right ring finger** CC H5
3 √7th S62.665 **Nondisplaced fracture of distal phalanx of left ring finger** CC H5
3 √7th S62.666 **Nondisplaced fracture of distal phalanx of right little finger** CC H5
3 √7th S62.667 **Nondisplaced fracture of distal phalanx of left little finger** CC H5
3 √7th S62.668 **Nondisplaced fracture of distal phalanx of other finger** CC H5
Nondisplaced fracture of distal phalanx of specified finger with unspecified laterality
3 √7th S62.669 **Nondisplaced fracture of distal phalanx of unspecified finger** CC H5

√5th S62.9 **Unspecified fracture of wrist and hand**
3 √x7th S62.90 **Unspecified fracture of unspecified wrist and hand** CC H5
3 √x7th S62.91 **Unspecified fracture of right wrist and hand** CC H5
3 √x7th S62.92 **Unspecified fracture of left wrist and hand** CC H5

√4th **S63 Dislocation and sprain of joints and ligaments at wrist and hand level**

INCLUDES avulsion of joint or ligament at wrist and hand level
laceration of cartilage, joint or ligament at wrist and hand level
sprain of cartilage, joint or ligament at wrist and hand level
traumatic hemarthrosis of joint or ligament at wrist and hand level
traumatic rupture of joint or ligament at wrist and hand level
traumatic subluxation of joint or ligament at wrist and hand level
traumatic tear of joint or ligament at wrist and hand level

Code also any associated open wound

EXCLUDES 2 *strain of muscle, fascia and tendon of wrist and hand (S66.-)*

The appropriate 7th character is to be added to each code from category S63.
A initial encounter
D subsequent encounter
S sequela

√5th S63.0 **Subluxation and dislocation of wrist and hand joints**
√6th S63.00 **Unspecified subluxation and dislocation of wrist and hand**
Dislocation of carpal bone NOS
Dislocation of distal end of radius NOS
Subluxation of carpal bone NOS
Subluxation of distal end of radius NOS
√7th S63.001 **Unspecified subluxation of right wrist and hand**
√7th S63.002 **Unspecified subluxation of left wrist and hand**
√7th S63.003 **Unspecified subluxation of unspecified wrist and hand**
√7th S63.004 **Unspecified dislocation of right wrist and hand**
√7th S63.005 **Unspecified dislocation of left wrist and hand**

✓7th **S63.006 Unspecified dislocation of unspecified wrist and hand**

✓6th **S63.01 Subluxation and dislocation of distal radioulnar joint**

✓7th **S63.011 Subluxation of distal radioulnar joint of right wrist**

✓7th **S63.012 Subluxation of distal radioulnar joint of left wrist**

✓7th **S63.013 Subluxation of distal radioulnar joint of unspecified wrist**

✓7th **S63.014 Dislocation of distal radioulnar joint of right wrist**

✓7th **S63.015 Dislocation of distal radioulnar joint of left wrist**

✓7th **S63.016 Dislocation of distal radioulnar joint of unspecified wrist**

✓6th **S63.02 Subluxation and dislocation of radiocarpal joint**

✓7th **S63.021 Subluxation of radiocarpal joint of right wrist**

✓7th **S63.022 Subluxation of radiocarpal joint of left wrist**

✓7th **S63.023 Subluxation of radiocarpal joint of unspecified wrist**

✓7th **S63.024 Dislocation of radiocarpal joint of right wrist**

✓7th **S63.025 Dislocation of radiocarpal joint of left wrist**

✓7th **S63.026 Dislocation of radiocarpal joint of unspecified wrist**

✓6th **S63.03 Subluxation and dislocation of midcarpal joint**

✓7th **S63.031 Subluxation of midcarpal joint of right wrist**

✓7th **S63.032 Subluxation of midcarpal joint of left wrist**

✓7th **S63.033 Subluxation of midcarpal joint of unspecified wrist**

✓7th **S63.034 Dislocation of midcarpal joint of right wrist**

✓7th **S63.035 Dislocation of midcarpal joint of left wrist**

✓7th **S63.036 Dislocation of midcarpal joint of unspecified wrist**

✓6th **S63.04 Subluxation and dislocation of carpometacarpal joint of thumb**

EXCLUDES 2 *interphalangeal subluxation and dislocation of thumb (S63.1-)*

✓7th **S63.041 Subluxation of carpometacarpal joint of right thumb**

✓7th **S63.042 Subluxation of carpometacarpal joint of left thumb**

✓7th **S63.043 Subluxation of carpometacarpal joint of unspecified thumb**

✓7th **S63.044 Dislocation of carpometacarpal joint of right thumb**

✓7th **S63.045 Dislocation of carpometacarpal joint of left thumb**

✓7th **S63.046 Dislocation of carpometacarpal joint of unspecified thumb**

✓6th **S63.05 Subluxation and dislocation of other carpometacarpal joint**

EXCLUDES 2 *subluxation and dislocation of carpometacarpal joint of thumb (S63.04-)*

✓7th **S63.051 Subluxation of other carpometacarpal joint of right hand**

✓7th **S63.052 Subluxation of other carpometacarpal joint of left hand**

✓7th **S63.053 Subluxation of other carpometacarpal joint of unspecified hand**

✓7th **S63.054 Dislocation of other carpometacarpal joint of right hand**

✓7th **S63.055 Dislocation of other carpometacarpal joint of left hand**

✓7th **S63.056 Dislocation of other carpometacarpal joint of unspecified hand**

✓6th **S63.06 Subluxation and dislocation of metacarpal (bone), proximal end**

✓7th **S63.061 Subluxation of metacarpal (bone), proximal end of right hand**

✓7th **S63.062 Subluxation of metacarpal (bone), proximal end of left hand**

✓7th **S63.063 Subluxation of metacarpal (bone), proximal end of unspecified hand**

✓7th **S63.064 Dislocation of metacarpal (bone), proximal end of right hand**

✓7th **S63.065 Dislocation of metacarpal (bone), proximal end of left hand**

✓7th **S63.066 Dislocation of metacarpal (bone), proximal end of unspecified hand**

✓6th **S63.07 Subluxation and dislocation of distal end of ulna**

✓7th **S63.071 Subluxation of distal end of right ulna**

✓7th **S63.072 Subluxation of distal end of left ulna**

✓7th **S63.073 Subluxation of distal end of unspecified ulna**

✓7th **S63.074 Dislocation of distal end of right ulna**

✓7th **S63.075 Dislocation of distal end of left ulna**

✓7th **S63.076 Dislocation of distal end of unspecified ulna**

✓6th **S63.09 Other subluxation and dislocation of wrist and hand**

✓7th **S63.091 Other subluxation of right wrist and hand**

✓7th **S63.092 Other subluxation of left wrist and hand**

✓7th **S63.093 Other subluxation of unspecified wrist and hand**

✓7th **S63.094 Other dislocation of right wrist and hand**

✓7th **S63.095 Other dislocation of left wrist and hand**

✓7th **S63.096 Other dislocation of unspecified wrist and hand**

✓5th **S63.1 Subluxation and dislocation of thumb**

✓6th **S63.10 Unspecified subluxation and dislocation of thumb**

✓7th **S63.101 Unspecified subluxation of right thumb**

✓7th **S63.102 Unspecified subluxation of left thumb**

✓7th **S63.103 Unspecified subluxation of unspecified thumb**

✓7th **S63.104 Unspecified dislocation of right thumb**

✓7th **S63.105 Unspecified dislocation of left thumb**

✓7th **S63.106 Unspecified dislocation of unspecified thumb**

✓6th **S63.11 Subluxation and dislocation of metacarpophalangeal joint of thumb**

✓7th **S63.111 Subluxation of metacarpophalangeal joint of right thumb**

✓7th **S63.112 Subluxation of metacarpophalangeal joint of left thumb**

✓7th **S63.113 Subluxation of metacarpophalangeal joint of unspecified thumb**

✓7th **S63.114 Dislocation of metacarpophalangeal joint of right thumb**

✓7th **S63.115 Dislocation of metacarpophalangeal joint of left thumb**

✓7th **S63.116 Dislocation of metacarpophalangeal joint of unspecified thumb**

✓6th **S63.12 Subluxation and dislocation of interphalangeal joint of thumb**

✓7th **S63.121 Subluxation of interphalangeal joint of right thumb**

✓7th **S63.122 Subluxation of interphalangeal joint of left thumb**

✓7th **S63.123 Subluxation of interphalangeal joint of unspecified thumb**

✓7th **S63.124 Dislocation of interphalangeal joint of right thumb**

✓7th **S63.125 Dislocation of interphalangeal joint of left thumb**

✓7th **S63.126 Dislocation of interphalangeal joint of unspecified thumb**

✓5th **S63.2 Subluxation and dislocation of other finger(s)**

EXCLUDES 2 *subluxation and dislocation of thumb (S63.1-)*

✓6th **S63.20 Unspecified subluxation of other finger**

✓7th **S63.200 Unspecified subluxation of right index finger**

✓7th **S63.201 Unspecified subluxation of left index finger**

✓7th **S63.202 Unspecified subluxation of right middle finger**

✓7th **S63.203 Unspecified subluxation of left middle finger**

✓7th **S63.204 Unspecified subluxation of right ring finger**

✓7th **S63.205 Unspecified subluxation of left ring finger**

✓7th **S63.206 Unspecified subluxation of right little finger**

S63.207 Unspecified subluxation of left little finger
S63.208 Unspecified subluxation of other finger
Unspecified subluxation of specified finger with unspecified laterality
S63.209 Unspecified subluxation of unspecified finger
S63.21 Subluxation of metacarpophalangeal joint of finger
S63.210 Subluxation of metacarpophalangeal joint of right index finger
S63.211 Subluxation of metacarpophalangeal joint of left index finger
S63.212 Subluxation of metacarpophalangeal joint of right middle finger
S63.213 Subluxation of metacarpophalangeal joint of left middle finger
S63.214 Subluxation of metacarpophalangeal joint of right ring finger
S63.215 Subluxation of metacarpophalangeal joint of left ring finger
S63.216 Subluxation of metacarpophalangeal joint of right little finger
S63.217 Subluxation of metacarpophalangeal joint of left little finger
S63.218 Subluxation of metacarpophalangeal joint of other finger
Subluxation of metacarpophalangeal joint of specified finger with unspecified laterality
S63.219 Subluxation of metacarpophalangeal joint of unspecified finger
S63.22 Subluxation of unspecified interphalangeal joint of finger
S63.220 Subluxation of unspecified interphalangeal joint of right index finger
S63.221 Subluxation of unspecified interphalangeal joint of left index finger
S63.222 Subluxation of unspecified interphalangeal joint of right middle finger
S63.223 Subluxation of unspecified interphalangeal joint of left middle finger
S63.224 Subluxation of unspecified interphalangeal joint of right ring finger
S63.225 Subluxation of unspecified interphalangeal joint of left ring finger
S63.226 Subluxation of unspecified interphalangeal joint of right little finger
S63.227 Subluxation of unspecified interphalangeal joint of left little finger
S63.228 Subluxation of unspecified interphalangeal joint of other finger
Subluxation of unspecified interphalangeal joint of specified finger with unspecified laterality
S63.229 Subluxation of unspecified interphalangeal joint of unspecified finger
S63.23 Subluxation of proximal interphalangeal joint of finger
S63.230 Subluxation of proximal interphalangeal joint of right index finger
S63.231 Subluxation of proximal interphalangeal joint of left index finger
S63.232 Subluxation of proximal interphalangeal joint of right middle finger
S63.233 Subluxation of proximal interphalangeal joint of left middle finger
S63.234 Subluxation of proximal interphalangeal joint of right ring finger
S63.235 Subluxation of proximal interphalangeal joint of left ring finger
S63.236 Subluxation of proximal interphalangeal joint of right little finger
S63.237 Subluxation of proximal interphalangeal joint of left little finger
S63.238 Subluxation of proximal interphalangeal joint of other finger
Subluxation of proximal interphalangeal joint of specified finger with unspecified laterality
S63.239 Subluxation of proximal interphalangeal joint of unspecified finger
S63.24 Subluxation of distal interphalangeal joint of finger
S63.240 Subluxation of distal interphalangeal joint of right index finger
S63.241 Subluxation of distal interphalangeal joint of left index finger
S63.242 Subluxation of distal interphalangeal joint of right middle finger
S63.243 Subluxation of distal interphalangeal joint of left middle finger
S63.244 Subluxation of distal interphalangeal joint of right ring finger
S63.245 Subluxation of distal interphalangeal joint of left ring finger
S63.246 Subluxation of distal interphalangeal joint of right little finger
S63.247 Subluxation of distal interphalangeal joint of left little finger
S63.248 Subluxation of distal interphalangeal joint of other finger
Subluxation of distal interphalangeal joint of specified finger with unspecified laterality
S63.249 Subluxation of distal interphalangeal joint of unspecified finger
S63.25 Unspecified dislocation of other finger
S63.250 Unspecified dislocation of right index finger
S63.251 Unspecified dislocation of left index finger
S63.252 Unspecified dislocation of right middle finger
S63.253 Unspecified dislocation of left middle finger
S63.254 Unspecified dislocation of right ring finger
S63.255 Unspecified dislocation of left ring finger
S63.256 Unspecified dislocation of right little finger
S63.257 Unspecified dislocation of left little finger
S63.258 Unspecified dislocation of other finger
Unspecified dislocation of specified finger with unspecified laterality
S63.259 Unspecified dislocation of unspecified finger
Unspecified dislocation of unspecified finger with unspecified laterality
S63.26 Dislocation of metacarpophalangeal joint of finger
S63.260 Dislocation of metacarpophalangeal joint of right index finger
S63.261 Dislocation of metacarpophalangeal joint of left index finger
S63.262 Dislocation of metacarpophalangeal joint of right middle finger
S63.263 Dislocation of metacarpophalangeal joint of left middle finger
S63.264 Dislocation of metacarpophalangeal joint of right ring finger
S63.265 Dislocation of metacarpophalangeal joint of left ring finger
S63.266 Dislocation of metacarpophalangeal joint of right little finger
S63.267 Dislocation of metacarpophalangeal joint of left little finger
S63.268 Dislocation of metacarpophalangeal joint of other finger
Dislocation of metacarpophalangeal joint of specified finger with unspecified laterality
S63.269 Dislocation of metacarpophalangeal joint of unspecified finger
S63.27 Dislocation of unspecified interphalangeal joint of finger
S63.270 Dislocation of unspecified interphalangeal joint of right index finger
S63.271 Dislocation of unspecified interphalangeal joint of left index finger
S63.272 Dislocation of unspecified interphalangeal joint of right middle finger

√7th **S63.273** **Dislocation of unspecified interphalangeal joint of left middle finger**

√7th **S63.274** **Dislocation of unspecified interphalangeal joint of right ring finger**

√7th **S63.275** **Dislocation of unspecified interphalangeal joint of left ring finger**

√7th **S63.276** **Dislocation of unspecified interphalangeal joint of right little finger**

√7th **S63.277** **Dislocation of unspecified interphalangeal joint of left little finger**

√7th **S63.278** **Dislocation of unspecified interphalangeal joint of other finger**
Dislocation of unspecified interphalangeal joint of specified finger with unspecified laterality

√7th **S63.279** **Dislocation of unspecified interphalangeal joint of unspecified finger**
Dislocation of unspecified interphalangeal joint of unspecified finger without specified laterality

√6th **S63.28** **Dislocation of proximal interphalangeal joint of finger**

√7th **S63.280** **Dislocation of proximal interphalangeal joint of right index finger**

√7th **S63.281** **Dislocation of proximal interphalangeal joint of left index finger**

√7th **S63.282** **Dislocation of proximal interphalangeal joint of right middle finger**

√7th **S63.283** **Dislocation of proximal interphalangeal joint of left middle finger**

√7th **S63.284** **Dislocation of proximal interphalangeal joint of right ring finger**

√7th **S63.285** **Dislocation of proximal interphalangeal joint of left ring finger**

√7th **S63.286** **Dislocation of proximal interphalangeal joint of right little finger**

√7th **S63.287** **Dislocation of proximal interphalangeal joint of left little finger**

√7th **S63.288** **Dislocation of proximal interphalangeal joint of other finger**
Dislocation of proximal interphalangeal joint of specified finger with unspecified laterality

√7th **S63.289** **Dislocation of proximal interphalangeal joint of unspecified finger**

√6th **S63.29** **Dislocation of distal interphalangeal joint of finger**

√7th **S63.290** **Dislocation of distal interphalangeal joint of right index finger**

√7th **S63.291** **Dislocation of distal interphalangeal joint of left index finger**

√7th **S63.292** **Dislocation of distal interphalangeal joint of right middle finger**

√7th **S63.293** **Dislocation of distal interphalangeal joint of left middle finger**

√7th **S63.294** **Dislocation of distal interphalangeal joint of right ring finger**

√7th **S63.295** **Dislocation of distal interphalangeal joint of left ring finger**

√7th **S63.296** **Dislocation of distal interphalangeal joint of right little finger**

√7th **S63.297** **Dislocation of distal interphalangeal joint of left little finger**

√7th **S63.298** **Dislocation of distal interphalangeal joint of other finger**
Dislocation of distal interphalangeal joint of specified finger with unspecified laterality

√7th **S63.299** **Dislocation of distal interphalangeal joint of unspecified finger**

√5th **S63.3** **Traumatic rupture of ligament of wrist**

√6th **S63.30** **Traumatic rupture of unspecified ligament of wrist**

√7th **S63.301** **Traumatic rupture of unspecified ligament of right wrist**

√7th **S63.302** **Traumatic rupture of unspecified ligament of left wrist**

√7th **S63.309** **Traumatic rupture of unspecified ligament of unspecified wrist**

√6th **S63.31** **Traumatic rupture of collateral ligament of wrist**

√7th **S63.311** **Traumatic rupture of collateral ligament of right wrist**

√7th **S63.312** **Traumatic rupture of collateral ligament of left wrist**

√7th **S63.319** **Traumatic rupture of collateral ligament of unspecified wrist**

√6th **S63.32** **Traumatic rupture of radiocarpal ligament**

√7th **S63.321** **Traumatic rupture of right radiocarpal ligament**

√7th **S63.322** **Traumatic rupture of left radiocarpal ligament**

√7th **S63.329** **Traumatic rupture of unspecified radiocarpal ligament**

√6th **S63.33** **Traumatic rupture of ulnocarpal (palmar) ligament**

√7th **S63.331** **Traumatic rupture of right ulnocarpal (palmar) ligament**

√7th **S63.332** **Traumatic rupture of left ulnocarpal (palmar) ligament**

√7th **S63.339** **Traumatic rupture of unspecified ulnocarpal (palmar) ligament**

√6th **S63.39** **Traumatic rupture of other ligament of wrist**

√7th **S63.391** **Traumatic rupture of other ligament of right wrist**

√7th **S63.392** **Traumatic rupture of other ligament of left wrist**

√7th **S63.399** **Traumatic rupture of other ligament of unspecified wrist**

√5th **S63.4** **Traumatic rupture of ligament of finger at metacarpophalangeal and interphalangeal joint(s)**

√6th **S63.40** **Traumatic rupture of unspecified ligament of finger at metacarpophalangeal and interphalangeal joint**

√7th **S63.400** **Traumatic rupture of unspecified ligament of right index finger at metacarpophalangeal and interphalangeal joint**

√7th **S63.401** **Traumatic rupture of unspecified ligament of left index finger at metacarpophalangeal and interphalangeal joint**

√7th **S63.402** **Traumatic rupture of unspecified ligament of right middle finger at metacarpophalangeal and interphalangeal joint**

√7th **S63.403** **Traumatic rupture of unspecified ligament of left middle finger at metacarpophalangeal and interphalangeal joint**

√7th **S63.404** **Traumatic rupture of unspecified ligament of right ring finger at metacarpophalangeal and interphalangeal joint**

√7th **S63.405** **Traumatic rupture of unspecified ligament of left ring finger at metacarpophalangeal and interphalangeal joint**

√7th **S63.406** **Traumatic rupture of unspecified ligament of right little finger at metacarpophalangeal and interphalangeal joint**

√7th **S63.407** **Traumatic rupture of unspecified ligament of left little finger at metacarpophalangeal and interphalangeal joint**

√7th **S63.408** **Traumatic rupture of unspecified ligament of other finger at metacarpophalangeal and interphalangeal joint**
Traumatic rupture of unspecified ligament of specified finger with unspecified laterality at metacarpophalangeal and interphalangeal joint

√7th **S63.409** **Traumatic rupture of unspecified ligament of unspecified finger at metacarpophalangeal and interphalangeal joint**

√6th **S63.41** **Traumatic rupture of collateral ligament of finger at metacarpophalangeal and interphalangeal joint**

√7th **S63.410** **Traumatic rupture of collateral ligament of right index finger at metacarpophalangeal and interphalangeal joint**

√7th **S63.411** **Traumatic rupture of collateral ligament of left index finger at metacarpophalangeal and interphalangeal joint**

√7th S63.412 **Traumatic rupture of collateral ligament of right middle finger at metacarpophalangeal and interphalangeal joint**

√7th S63.413 **Traumatic rupture of collateral ligament of left middle finger at metacarpophalangeal and interphalangeal joint**

√7th S63.414 **Traumatic rupture of collateral ligament of right ring finger at metacarpophalangeal and interphalangeal joint**

√7th S63.415 **Traumatic rupture of collateral ligament of left ring finger at metacarpophalangeal and interphalangeal joint**

√7th S63.416 **Traumatic rupture of collateral ligament of right little finger at metacarpophalangeal and interphalangeal joint**

√7th S63.417 **Traumatic rupture of collateral ligament of left little finger at metacarpophalangeal and interphalangeal joint**

√7th S63.418 **Traumatic rupture of collateral ligament of other finger at metacarpophalangeal and interphalangeal joint**

Traumatic rupture of collateral ligament of specified finger with unspecified laterality at metacarpophalangeal and interphalangeal joint

√7th S63.419 **Traumatic rupture of collateral ligament of unspecified finger at metacarpophalangeal and interphalangeal joint**

√6th S63.42 **Traumatic rupture of palmar ligament of finger at metacarpophalangeal and interphalangeal joint**

√7th S63.420 **Traumatic rupture of palmar ligament of right index finger at metacarpophalangeal and interphalangeal joint**

√7th S63.421 **Traumatic rupture of palmar ligament of left index finger at metacarpophalangeal and interphalangeal joint**

√7th S63.422 **Traumatic rupture of palmar ligament of right middle finger at metacarpophalangeal and interphalangeal joint**

√7th S63.423 **Traumatic rupture of palmar ligament of left middle finger at metacarpophalangeal and interphalangeal joint**

√7th S63.424 **Traumatic rupture of palmar ligament of right ring finger at metacarpophalangeal and interphalangeal joint**

√7th S63.425 **Traumatic rupture of palmar ligament of left ring finger at metacarpophalangeal and interphalangeal joint**

√7th S63.426 **Traumatic rupture of palmar ligament of right little finger at metacarpophalangeal and interphalangeal joint**

√7th S63.427 **Traumatic rupture of palmar ligament of left little finger at metacarpophalangeal and interphalangeal joint**

√7th S63.428 **Traumatic rupture of palmar ligament of other finger at metacarpophalangeal and interphalangeal joint**

Traumatic rupture of palmar ligament of specified finger with unspecified laterality at metacarpophalangeal and interphalangeal joint

√7th S63.429 **Traumatic rupture of palmar ligament of unspecified finger at metacarpophalangeal and interphalangeal joint**

√6th S63.43 **Traumatic rupture of volar plate of finger at metacarpophalangeal and interphalangeal joint**

√7th S63.430 **Traumatic rupture of volar plate of right index finger at metacarpophalangeal and interphalangeal joint**

√7th S63.431 **Traumatic rupture of volar plate of left index finger at metacarpophalangeal and interphalangeal joint**

√7th S63.432 **Traumatic rupture of volar plate of right middle finger at metacarpophalangeal and interphalangeal joint**

√7th S63.433 **Traumatic rupture of volar plate of left middle finger at metacarpophalangeal and interphalangeal joint**

√7th S63.434 **Traumatic rupture of volar plate of right ring finger at metacarpophalangeal and interphalangeal joint**

√7th S63.435 **Traumatic rupture of volar plate of left ring finger at metacarpophalangeal and interphalangeal joint**

√7th S63.436 **Traumatic rupture of volar plate of right little finger at metacarpophalangeal and interphalangeal joint**

√7th S63.437 **Traumatic rupture of volar plate of left little finger at metacarpophalangeal and interphalangeal joint**

√7th S63.438 **Traumatic rupture of volar plate of other finger at metacarpophalangeal and interphalangeal joint**

Traumatic rupture of volar plate of specified finger with unspecified laterality at metacarpophalangeal and interphalangeal joint

√7th S63.439 **Traumatic rupture of volar plate of unspecified finger at metacarpophalangeal and interphalangeal joint**

√6th S63.49 **Traumatic rupture of other ligament of finger at metacarpophalangeal and interphalangeal joint**

√7th S63.490 **Traumatic rupture of other ligament of right index finger at metacarpophalangeal and interphalangeal joint**

√7th S63.491 **Traumatic rupture of other ligament of left index finger at metacarpophalangeal and interphalangeal joint**

√7th S63.492 **Traumatic rupture of other ligament of right middle finger at metacarpophalangeal and interphalangeal joint**

√7th S63.493 **Traumatic rupture of other ligament of left middle finger at metacarpophalangeal and interphalangeal joint**

√7th S63.494 **Traumatic rupture of other ligament of right ring finger at metacarpophalangeal and interphalangeal joint**

√7th S63.495 **Traumatic rupture of other ligament of left ring finger at metacarpophalangeal and interphalangeal joint**

√7th S63.496 **Traumatic rupture of other ligament of right little finger at metacarpophalangeal and interphalangeal joint**

√7th S63.497 **Traumatic rupture of other ligament of left little finger at metacarpophalangeal and interphalangeal joint**

√7th S63.498 **Traumatic rupture of other ligament of other finger at metacarpophalangeal and interphalangeal joint**

Traumatic rupture of ligament of specified finger with unspecified laterality at metacarpophalangeal and interphalangeal joint

√7th S63.499 **Traumatic rupture of other ligament of unspecified finger at metacarpophalangeal and interphalangeal joint**

√5th S63.5 **Other and unspecified sprain of wrist**

√6th S63.50 **Unspecified sprain of wrist**

√7th S63.501 **Unspecified sprain of right wrist**

√7th S63.502 **Unspecified sprain of left wrist**

√7th S63.509 **Unspecified sprain of unspecified wrist**

√6th S63.51 **Sprain of carpal (joint)**

√7th S63.511 **Sprain of carpal joint of right wrist**

√7th S63.512 **Sprain of carpal joint of left wrist**

√7th S63.519 **Sprain of carpal joint of unspecified wrist**

√6th **S63.52 Sprain of radiocarpal joint**
EXCLUDES 1 *traumatic rupture of radiocarpal ligament (S63.32-)*
√7th **S63.521 Sprain of radiocarpal joint of right wrist**
√7th **S63.522 Sprain of radiocarpal joint of left wrist**
√7th **S63.529 Sprain of radiocarpal joint of unspecified wrist**
√6th **S63.59 Other specified sprain of wrist**
√7th **S63.591 Other specified sprain of right wrist**
√7th **S63.592 Other specified sprain of left wrist**
√7th **S63.599 Other specified sprain of unspecified wrist**
√5th **S63.6 Other and unspecified sprain of finger(s)**
EXCLUDES 1 *traumatic rupture of ligament of finger at metacarpophalangeal and interphalangeal joint(s) (S63.4-)*
√6th **S63.60 Unspecified sprain of thumb**
√7th **S63.601 Unspecified sprain of right thumb**
√7th **S63.602 Unspecified sprain of left thumb**
√7th **S63.609 Unspecified sprain of unspecified thumb**
√6th **S63.61 Unspecified sprain of other and unspecified finger(s)**
√7th **S63.610 Unspecified sprain of right index finger**
√7th **S63.611 Unspecified sprain of left index finger**
√7th **S63.612 Unspecified sprain of right middle finger**
√7th **S63.613 Unspecified sprain of left middle finger**
√7th **S63.614 Unspecified sprain of right ring finger**
√7th **S63.615 Unspecified sprain of left ring finger**
√7th **S63.616 Unspecified sprain of right little finger**
√7th **S63.617 Unspecified sprain of left little finger**
√7th **S63.618 Unspecified sprain of other finger**
Unspecified sprain of specified finger with unspecified laterality
√7th **S63.619 Unspecified sprain of unspecified finger**
√6th **S63.62 Sprain of interphalangeal joint of thumb**
√7th **S63.621 Sprain of interphalangeal joint of right thumb**
√7th **S63.622 Sprain of interphalangeal joint of left thumb**
√7th **S63.629 Sprain of interphalangeal joint of unspecified thumb**
√6th **S63.63 Sprain of interphalangeal joint of other and unspecified finger(s)**
√7th **S63.630 Sprain of interphalangeal joint of right index finger**
√7th **S63.631 Sprain of interphalangeal joint of left index finger**
√7th **S63.632 Sprain of interphalangeal joint of right middle finger**
√7th **S63.633 Sprain of interphalangeal joint of left middle finger**
√7th **S63.634 Sprain of interphalangeal joint of right ring finger**
√7th **S63.635 Sprain of interphalangeal joint of left ring finger**
√7th **S63.636 Sprain of interphalangeal joint of right little finger**
√7th **S63.637 Sprain of interphalangeal joint of left little finger**
√7th **S63.638 Sprain of interphalangeal joint of other finger**
√7th **S63.639 Sprain of interphalangeal joint of unspecified finger**
√6th **S63.64 Sprain of metacarpophalangeal joint of thumb**
√7th **S63.641 Sprain of metacarpophalangeal joint of right thumb**
√7th **S63.642 Sprain of metacarpophalangeal joint of left thumb**
√7th **S63.649 Sprain of metacarpophalangeal joint of unspecified thumb**
√6th **S63.65 Sprain of metacarpophalangeal joint of other and unspecified finger(s)**
√7th **S63.650 Sprain of metacarpophalangeal joint of right index finger**
√7th **S63.651 Sprain of metacarpophalangeal joint of left index finger**
√7th **S63.652 Sprain of metacarpophalangeal joint of right middle finger**
√7th **S63.653 Sprain of metacarpophalangeal joint of left middle finger**
√7th **S63.654 Sprain of metacarpophalangeal joint of right ring finger**
√7th **S63.655 Sprain of metacarpophalangeal joint of left ring finger**
√7th **S63.656 Sprain of metacarpophalangeal joint of right little finger**
√7th **S63.657 Sprain of metacarpophalangeal joint of left little finger**
√7th **S63.658 Sprain of metacarpophalangeal joint of other finger**
Sprain of metacarpophalangeal joint of specified finger with unspecified laterality
√7th **S63.659 Sprain of metacarpophalangeal joint of unspecified finger**
√6th **S63.68 Other sprain of thumb**
√7th **S63.681 Other sprain of right thumb**
√7th **S63.682 Other sprain of left thumb**
√7th **S63.689 Other sprain of unspecified thumb**
√6th **S63.69 Other sprain of other and unspecified finger(s)**
√7th **S63.690 Other sprain of right index finger**
√7th **S63.691 Other sprain of left index finger**
√7th **S63.692 Other sprain of right middle finger**
√7th **S63.693 Other sprain of left middle finger**
√7th **S63.694 Other sprain of right ring finger**
√7th **S63.695 Other sprain of left ring finger**
√7th **S63.696 Other sprain of right little finger**
√7th **S63.697 Other sprain of left little finger**
√7th **S63.698 Other sprain of other finger**
Other sprain of specified finger with unspecified laterality
√7th **S63.699 Other sprain of unspecified finger**
√5th **S63.8 Sprain of other part of wrist and hand**
√6th **S63.8X Sprain of other part of wrist and hand**
√7th **S63.8X1 Sprain of other part of right wrist and hand**
√7th **S63.8X2 Sprain of other part of left wrist and hand**
√7th **S63.8X9 Sprain of other part of unspecified wrist and hand**
√5th **S63.9 Sprain of unspecified part of wrist and hand**
√x7th **S63.90 Sprain of unspecified part of unspecified wrist and hand**
√x7th **S63.91 Sprain of unspecified part of right wrist and hand**
√x7th **S63.92 Sprain of unspecified part of left wrist and hand**

√4th **S64 Injury of nerves at wrist and hand level**
Code also any associated open wound (S61.-)

The appropriate 7th character is to be added to each code from category S64.
A initial encounter
D subsequent encounter
S sequela

√5th **S64.0 Injury of ulnar nerve at wrist and hand level**
√x7th **S64.00 Injury of ulnar nerve at wrist and hand level of unspecified arm**
√x7th **S64.01 Injury of ulnar nerve at wrist and hand level of right arm**
√x7th **S64.02 Injury of ulnar nerve at wrist and hand level of left arm**
√5th **S64.1 Injury of median nerve at wrist and hand level**
√x7th **S64.10 Injury of median nerve at wrist and hand level of unspecified arm**
√x7th **S64.11 Injury of median nerve at wrist and hand level of right arm**
√x7th **S64.12 Injury of median nerve at wrist and hand level of left arm**
√5th **S64.2 Injury of radial nerve at wrist and hand level**
√x7th **S64.20 Injury of radial nerve at wrist and hand level of unspecified arm**
√x7th **S64.21 Injury of radial nerve at wrist and hand level of right arm**

S64.22 Injury of radial nerve at wrist and hand level of left arm

S64.3 Injury of digital nerve of thumb

S64.30 Injury of digital nerve of unspecified thumb

S64.31 Injury of digital nerve of right thumb

S64.32 Injury of digital nerve of left thumb

S64.4 Injury of digital nerve of other and unspecified finger

S64.40 Injury of digital nerve of unspecified finger

S64.49 Injury of digital nerve of other finger

S64.490 Injury of digital nerve of right index finger

S64.491 Injury of digital nerve of left index finger

S64.492 Injury of digital nerve of right middle finger

S64.493 Injury of digital nerve of left middle finger

S64.494 Injury of digital nerve of right ring finger

S64.495 Injury of digital nerve of left ring finger

S64.496 Injury of digital nerve of right little finger

S64.497 Injury of digital nerve of left little finger

S64.498 Injury of digital nerve of other finger

Injury of digital nerve of specified finger with unspecified laterality

S64.8 Injury of other nerves at wrist and hand level

S64.8X Injury of other nerves at wrist and hand level

S64.8X1 Injury of other nerves at wrist and hand level of right arm

S64.8X2 Injury of other nerves at wrist and hand level of left arm

S64.8X9 Injury of other nerves at wrist and hand level of unspecified arm

S64.9 Injury of unspecified nerve at wrist and hand level

S64.90 Injury of unspecified nerve at wrist and hand level of unspecified arm

S64.91 Injury of unspecified nerve at wrist and hand level of right arm

S64.92 Injury of unspecified nerve at wrist and hand level of left arm

S65 Injury of blood vessels at wrist and hand level

Code also any associated open wound (S61.-)

The appropriate 7th character is to be added to each code from category S65.

A initial encounter
D subsequent encounter
S sequela

S65.0 Injury of ulnar artery at wrist and hand level

S65.00 Unspecified injury of ulnar artery at wrist and hand level

S65.001 Unspecified injury of ulnar artery at wrist and hand level of right arm CC

S65.002 Unspecified injury of ulnar artery at wrist and hand level of left arm CC

S65.009 Unspecified injury of ulnar artery at wrist and hand level of unspecified arm CC

S65.01 Laceration of ulnar artery at wrist and hand level

S65.011 Laceration of ulnar artery at wrist and hand level of right arm CC

S65.012 Laceration of ulnar artery at wrist and hand level of left arm CC

S65.019 Laceration of ulnar artery at wrist and hand level of unspecified arm CC

S65.09 Other specified injury of ulnar artery at wrist and hand level

S65.091 Other specified injury of ulnar artery at wrist and hand level of right arm CC

S65.092 Other specified injury of ulnar artery at wrist and hand level of left arm CC

S65.099 Other specified injury of ulnar artery at wrist and hand level of unspecified arm CC

S65.1 Injury of radial artery at wrist and hand level

S65.10 Unspecified injury of radial artery at wrist and hand level

S65.101 Unspecified injury of radial artery at wrist and hand level of right arm CC

S65.102 Unspecified injury of radial artery at wrist and hand level of left arm CC

S65.109 Unspecified injury of radial artery at wrist and hand level of unspecified arm CC

S65.11 Laceration of radial artery at wrist and hand level

S65.111 Laceration of radial artery at wrist and hand level of right arm CC

S65.112 Laceration of radial artery at wrist and hand level of left arm CC

S65.119 Laceration of radial artery at wrist and hand level of unspecified arm CC

S65.19 Other specified injury of radial artery at wrist and hand level

S65.191 Other specified injury of radial artery at wrist and hand level of right arm CC

S65.192 Other specified injury of radial artery at wrist and hand level of left arm CC

S65.199 Other specified injury of radial artery at wrist and hand level of unspecified arm CC

S65.2 Injury of superficial palmar arch

S65.20 Unspecified injury of superficial palmar arch

S65.201 Unspecified injury of superficial palmar arch of right hand CC

S65.202 Unspecified injury of superficial palmar arch of left hand CC

S65.209 Unspecified injury of superficial palmar arch of unspecified hand CC

S65.21 Laceration of superficial palmar arch

S65.211 Laceration of superficial palmar arch of right hand CC

S65.212 Laceration of superficial palmar arch of left hand CC

S65.219 Laceration of superficial palmar arch of unspecified hand CC

S65.29 Other specified injury of superficial palmar arch

S65.291 Other specified injury of superficial palmar arch of right hand CC

S65.292 Other specified injury of superficial palmar arch of left hand CC

S65.299 Other specified injury of superficial palmar arch of unspecified hand CC

S65.3 Injury of deep palmar arch

S65.30 Unspecified injury of deep palmar arch

S65.301 Unspecified injury of deep palmar arch of right hand CC

S65.302 Unspecified injury of deep palmar arch of left hand CC

S65.309 Unspecified injury of deep palmar arch of unspecified hand CC

S65.31 Laceration of deep palmar arch

S65.311 Laceration of deep palmar arch of right hand CC

S65.312 Laceration of deep palmar arch of left hand CC

S65.319 Laceration of deep palmar arch of unspecified hand CC

S65.39 Other specified injury of deep palmar arch

S65.391 Other specified injury of deep palmar arch of right hand CC

S65.392 Other specified injury of deep palmar arch of left hand CC

S65.399 Other specified injury of deep palmar arch of unspecified hand CC

S65.4 Injury of blood vessel of thumb

S65.40 Unspecified injury of blood vessel of thumb

S65.401 Unspecified injury of blood vessel of right thumb CC

S65.402 Unspecified injury of blood vessel of left thumb CC

S65.409 Unspecified injury of blood vessel of unspecified thumb CC

S65.41 Laceration of blood vessel of thumb

S65.411 Laceration of blood vessel of right thumb CC

S65.412 Laceration of blood vessel of left thumb CC

✓7th S65.419 Laceration of blood vessel of unspecified thumb CC

✓6th S65.49 Other specified injury of blood vessel of thumb

✓7th S65.491 Other specified injury of blood vessel of right thumb CC

✓7th S65.492 Other specified injury of blood vessel of left thumb CC

✓7th S65.499 Other specified injury of blood vessel of unspecified thumb CC

✓5th S65.5 Injury of blood vessel of other and unspecified finger

✓6th S65.50 Unspecified injury of blood vessel of other and unspecified finger

✓7th S65.500 Unspecified injury of blood vessel of right index finger CC

✓7th S65.501 Unspecified injury of blood vessel of left index finger CC

✓7th S65.502 Unspecified injury of blood vessel of right middle finger CC

✓7th S65.503 Unspecified injury of blood vessel of left middle finger CC

✓7th S65.504 Unspecified injury of blood vessel of right ring finger CC

✓7th S65.505 Unspecified injury of blood vessel of left ring finger CC

✓7th S65.506 Unspecified injury of blood vessel of right little finger CC

✓7th S65.507 Unspecified injury of blood vessel of left little finger CC

✓7th S65.508 Unspecified injury of blood vessel of other finger CC

Unspecified injury of blood vessel of specified finger with unspecified laterality

✓7th S65.509 Unspecified injury of blood vessel of unspecified finger CC

✓6th S65.51 Laceration of blood vessel of other and unspecified finger

✓7th S65.510 Laceration of blood vessel of right index finger CC

✓7th S65.511 Laceration of blood vessel of left index finger CC

✓7th S65.512 Laceration of blood vessel of right middle finger CC

✓7th S65.513 Laceration of blood vessel of left middle finger CC

✓7th S65.514 Laceration of blood vessel of right ring finger CC

✓7th S65.515 Laceration of blood vessel of left ring finger CC

✓7th S65.516 Laceration of blood vessel of right little finger CC

✓7th S65.517 Laceration of blood vessel of left little finger CC

✓7th S65.518 Laceration of blood vessel of other finger CC

Laceration of blood vessel of specified finger with unspecified laterality

✓7th S65.519 Laceration of blood vessel of unspecified finger CC

✓6th S65.59 Other specified injury of blood vessel of other and unspecified finger

✓7th S65.590 Other specified injury of blood vessel of right index finger CC

✓7th S65.591 Other specified injury of blood vessel of left index finger CC

✓7th S65.592 Other specified injury of blood vessel of right middle finger CC

✓7th S65.593 Other specified injury of blood vessel of left middle finger CC

✓7th S65.594 Other specified injury of blood vessel of right ring finger CC

✓7th S65.595 Other specified injury of blood vessel of left ring finger CC

✓7th S65.596 Other specified injury of blood vessel of right little finger CC

✓7th S65.597 Other specified injury of blood vessel of left little finger CC

✓7th S65.598 Other specified injury of blood vessel of other finger CC

Other specified injury of blood vessel of specified finger with unspecified laterality

✓7th S65.599 Other specified injury of blood vessel of unspecified finger CC

✓5th S65.8 Injury of other blood vessels at wrist and hand level

✓6th S65.80 Unspecified injury of other blood vessels at wrist and hand level

✓7th S65.801 Unspecified injury of other blood vessels at wrist and hand level of right arm CC

✓7th S65.802 Unspecified injury of other blood vessels at wrist and hand level of left arm CC

✓7th S65.809 Unspecified injury of other blood vessels at wrist and hand level of unspecified arm CC

✓6th S65.81 Laceration of other blood vessels at wrist and hand level

✓7th S65.811 Laceration of other blood vessels at wrist and hand level of right arm CC

✓7th S65.812 Laceration of other blood vessels at wrist and hand level of left arm CC

✓7th S65.819 Laceration of other blood vessels at wrist and hand level of unspecified arm CC

✓6th S65.89 Other specified injury of other blood vessels at wrist and hand level

✓7th S65.891 Other specified injury of other blood vessels at wrist and hand level of right arm CC

✓7th S65.892 Other specified injury of other blood vessels at wrist and hand level of left arm CC

✓7th S65.899 Other specified injury of other blood vessels at wrist and hand level of unspecified arm CC

✓5th S65.9 Injury of unspecified blood vessel at wrist and hand level

✓6th S65.90 Unspecified injury of unspecified blood vessel at wrist and hand level

✓7th S65.901 Unspecified injury of unspecified blood vessel at wrist and hand level of right arm CC

✓7th S65.902 Unspecified injury of unspecified blood vessel at wrist and hand level of left arm CC

✓7th S65.909 Unspecified injury of unspecified blood vessel at wrist and hand level of unspecified arm CC

✓6th S65.91 Laceration of unspecified blood vessel at wrist and hand level

✓7th S65.911 Laceration of unspecified blood vessel at wrist and hand level of right arm CC

✓7th S65.912 Laceration of unspecified blood vessel at wrist and hand level of left arm CC

✓7th S65.919 Laceration of unspecified blood vessel at wrist and hand level of unspecified arm CC

✓6th S65.99 Other specified injury of unspecified blood vessel at wrist and hand level

✓7th S65.991 Other specified injury of unspecified blood vessel at wrist and hand of right arm CC

✓7th S65.992 Other specified injury of unspecified blood vessel at wrist and hand of left arm CC

✓7th S65.999 Other specified injury of unspecified blood vessel at wrist and hand of unspecified arm CC

S66 Injury of muscle, fascia and tendon at wrist and hand level

Code also any associated open wound (S61.-)

EXCLUDES 2 *sprain of joints and ligaments of wrist and hand (S63.-)*

TIP: Refer to the Muscle/Tendon table at the beginning of this chapter.

The appropriate 7th character is to be added to each code from category S66.
A initial encounter
D subsequent encounter
S sequela

S66.0 Injury of long flexor muscle, fascia and tendon of thumb at wrist and hand level

S66.00 Unspecified injury of long flexor muscle, fascia and tendon of thumb at wrist and hand level

S66.001 Unspecified injury of long flexor muscle, fascia and tendon of right thumb at wrist and hand level

S66.002 Unspecified injury of long flexor muscle, fascia and tendon of left thumb at wrist and hand level

S66.009 Unspecified injury of long flexor muscle, fascia and tendon of unspecified thumb at wrist and hand level

S66.01 Strain of long flexor muscle, fascia and tendon of thumb at wrist and hand level

S66.011 Strain of long flexor muscle, fascia and tendon of right thumb at wrist and hand level

S66.012 Strain of long flexor muscle, fascia and tendon of left thumb at wrist and hand level

S66.019 Strain of long flexor muscle, fascia and tendon of unspecified thumb at wrist and hand level

S66.02 Laceration of long flexor muscle, fascia and tendon of thumb at wrist and hand level

S66.021 Laceration of long flexor muscle, fascia and tendon of right thumb at wrist and hand level CC

S66.022 Laceration of long flexor muscle, fascia and tendon of left thumb at wrist and hand level CC

S66.029 Laceration of long flexor muscle, fascia and tendon of unspecified thumb at wrist and hand level CC

S66.09 Other specified injury of long flexor muscle, fascia and tendon of thumb at wrist and hand level

S66.091 Other specified injury of long flexor muscle, fascia and tendon of right thumb at wrist and hand level

S66.092 Other specified injury of long flexor muscle, fascia and tendon of left thumb at wrist and hand level

S66.099 Other specified injury of long flexor muscle, fascia and tendon of unspecified thumb at wrist and hand level

S66.1 Injury of flexor muscle, fascia and tendon of other and unspecified finger at wrist and hand level

EXCLUDES 2 *injury of long flexor muscle, fascia and tendon of thumb at wrist and hand level (S66.0-)*

S66.10 Unspecified injury of flexor muscle, fascia and tendon of other and unspecified finger at wrist and hand level

S66.100 Unspecified injury of flexor muscle, fascia and tendon of right index finger at wrist and hand level

S66.101 Unspecified injury of flexor muscle, fascia and tendon of left index finger at wrist and hand level

S66.102 Unspecified injury of flexor muscle, fascia and tendon of right middle finger at wrist and hand level

S66.103 Unspecified injury of flexor muscle, fascia and tendon of left middle finger at wrist and hand level

S66.104 Unspecified injury of flexor muscle, fascia and tendon of right ring finger at wrist and hand level

S66.105 Unspecified injury of flexor muscle, fascia and tendon of left ring finger at wrist and hand level

S66.106 Unspecified injury of flexor muscle, fascia and tendon of right little finger at wrist and hand level

S66.107 Unspecified injury of flexor muscle, fascia and tendon of left little finger at wrist and hand level

S66.108 Unspecified injury of flexor muscle, fascia and tendon of other finger at wrist and hand level

Unspecified injury of flexor muscle, fascia and tendon of specified finger with unspecified laterality at wrist and hand level

S66.109 Unspecified injury of flexor muscle, fascia and tendon of unspecified finger at wrist and hand level

S66.11 Strain of flexor muscle, fascia and tendon of other and unspecified finger at wrist and hand level

S66.110 Strain of flexor muscle, fascia and tendon of right index finger at wrist and hand level

S66.111 Strain of flexor muscle, fascia and tendon of left index finger at wrist and hand level

S66.112 Strain of flexor muscle, fascia and tendon of right middle finger at wrist and hand level

S66.113 Strain of flexor muscle, fascia and tendon of left middle finger at wrist and hand level

S66.114 Strain of flexor muscle, fascia and tendon of right ring finger at wrist and hand level

S66.115 Strain of flexor muscle, fascia and tendon of left ring finger at wrist and hand level

S66.116 Strain of flexor muscle, fascia and tendon of right little finger at wrist and hand level

S66.117 Strain of flexor muscle, fascia and tendon of left little finger at wrist and hand level

S66.118 Strain of flexor muscle, fascia and tendon of other finger at wrist and hand level

Strain of flexor muscle, fascia and tendon of specified finger with unspecified laterality at wrist and hand level

S66.119 Strain of flexor muscle, fascia and tendon of unspecified finger at wrist and hand level

S66.12 Laceration of flexor muscle, fascia and tendon of other and unspecified finger at wrist and hand level

S66.120 Laceration of flexor muscle, fascia and tendon of right index finger at wrist and hand level CC

S66.121 Laceration of flexor muscle, fascia and tendon of left index finger at wrist and hand level CC

S66.122 Laceration of flexor muscle, fascia and tendon of right middle finger at wrist and hand level CC

S66.123 Laceration of flexor muscle, fascia and tendon of left middle finger at wrist and hand level CC

S66.124 Laceration of flexor muscle, fascia and tendon of right ring finger at wrist and hand level CC

S66.125 Laceration of flexor muscle, fascia and tendon of left ring finger at wrist and hand level CC

S66.126 Laceration of flexor muscle, fascia and tendon of right little finger at wrist and hand level CC

S66.127 Laceration of flexor muscle, fascia and tendon of left little finger at wrist and hand level CC

S66.128 Laceration of flexor muscle, fascia and tendon of other finger at wrist and hand level CC

Laceration of flexor muscle, fascia and tendon of specified finger with unspecified laterality at wrist and hand level

S66.129 Laceration of flexor muscle, fascia and tendon of unspecified finger at wrist and hand level CC

6th S66.19 Other injury of flexor muscle, fascia and tendon of other and unspecified finger at wrist and hand level

7th S66.190 Other injury of flexor muscle, fascia and tendon of right index finger at wrist and hand level

7th S66.191 Other injury of flexor muscle, fascia and tendon of left index finger at wrist and hand level

7th S66.192 Other injury of flexor muscle, fascia and tendon of right middle finger at wrist and hand level

7th S66.193 Other injury of flexor muscle, fascia and tendon of left middle finger at wrist and hand level

7th S66.194 Other injury of flexor muscle, fascia and tendon of right ring finger at wrist and hand level

7th S66.195 Other injury of flexor muscle, fascia and tendon of left ring finger at wrist and hand level

7th S66.196 Other injury of flexor muscle, fascia and tendon of right little finger at wrist and hand level

7th S66.197 Other injury of flexor muscle, fascia and tendon of left little finger at wrist and hand level

7th S66.198 Other injury of flexor muscle, fascia and tendon of other finger at wrist and hand level

Other injury of flexor muscle, fascia and tendon of specified finger with unspecified laterality at wrist and hand level

7th S66.199 Other injury of flexor muscle, fascia and tendon of unspecified finger at wrist and hand level

5th S66.2 Injury of extensor muscle, fascia and tendon of thumb at wrist and hand level

6th S66.20 Unspecified injury of extensor muscle, fascia and tendon of thumb at wrist and hand level

7th S66.201 Unspecified injury of extensor muscle, fascia and tendon of right thumb at wrist and hand level

7th S66.202 Unspecified injury of extensor muscle, fascia and tendon of left thumb at wrist and hand level

7th S66.209 Unspecified injury of extensor muscle, fascia and tendon of unspecified thumb at wrist and hand level

6th S66.21 Strain of extensor muscle, fascia and tendon of thumb at wrist and hand level

7th S66.211 Strain of extensor muscle, fascia and tendon of right thumb at wrist and hand level

7th S66.212 Strain of extensor muscle, fascia and tendon of left thumb at wrist and hand level

7th S66.219 Strain of extensor muscle, fascia and tendon of unspecified thumb at wrist and hand level

6th S66.22 Laceration of extensor muscle, fascia and tendon of thumb at wrist and hand level

7th S66.221 Laceration of extensor muscle, fascia and tendon of right thumb at wrist and hand level CC

7th S66.222 Laceration of extensor muscle, fascia and tendon of left thumb at wrist and hand level CC

7th S66.229 Laceration of extensor muscle, fascia and tendon of unspecified thumb at wrist and hand level CC

6th S66.29 Other specified injury of extensor muscle, fascia and tendon of thumb at wrist and hand level

7th S66.291 Other specified injury of extensor muscle, fascia and tendon of right thumb at wrist and hand level

7th S66.292 Other specified injury of extensor muscle, fascia and tendon of left thumb at wrist and hand level

7th S66.299 Other specified injury of extensor muscle, fascia and tendon of unspecified thumb at wrist and hand level

5th S66.3 Injury of extensor muscle, fascia and tendon of other and unspecified finger at wrist and hand level

EXCLUDES 2 *injury of extensor muscle, fascia and tendon of thumb at wrist and hand level (S66.2-)*

6th S66.30 Unspecified injury of extensor muscle, fascia and tendon of other and unspecified finger at wrist and hand level

7th S66.300 Unspecified injury of extensor muscle, fascia and tendon of right index finger at wrist and hand level

7th S66.301 Unspecified injury of extensor muscle, fascia and tendon of left index finger at wrist and hand level

7th S66.302 Unspecified injury of extensor muscle, fascia and tendon of right middle finger at wrist and hand level

7th S66.303 Unspecified injury of extensor muscle, fascia and tendon of left middle finger at wrist and hand level

7th S66.304 Unspecified injury of extensor muscle, fascia and tendon of right ring finger at wrist and hand level

7th S66.305 Unspecified injury of extensor muscle, fascia and tendon of left ring finger at wrist and hand level

7th S66.306 Unspecified injury of extensor muscle, fascia and tendon of right little finger at wrist and hand level

7th S66.307 Unspecified injury of extensor muscle, fascia and tendon of left little finger at wrist and hand level

7th S66.308 Unspecified injury of extensor muscle, fascia and tendon of other finger at wrist and hand level

Unspecified injury of extensor muscle, fascia and tendon of specified finger with unspecified laterality at wrist and hand level

7th S66.309 Unspecified injury of extensor muscle, fascia and tendon of unspecified finger at wrist and hand level

6th S66.31 Strain of extensor muscle, fascia and tendon of other and unspecified finger at wrist and hand level

7th S66.310 Strain of extensor muscle, fascia and tendon of right index finger at wrist and hand level

7th S66.311 Strain of extensor muscle, fascia and tendon of left index finger at wrist and hand level

7th S66.312 Strain of extensor muscle, fascia and tendon of right middle finger at wrist and hand level

7th S66.313 Strain of extensor muscle, fascia and tendon of left middle finger at wrist and hand level

7th S66.314 Strain of extensor muscle, fascia and tendon of right ring finger at wrist and hand level

7th S66.315 Strain of extensor muscle, fascia and tendon of left ring finger at wrist and hand level

7th S66.316 Strain of extensor muscle, fascia and tendon of right little finger at wrist and hand level

7th S66.317 Strain of extensor muscle, fascia and tendon of left little finger at wrist and hand level

7th S66.318 Strain of extensor muscle, fascia and tendon of other finger at wrist and hand level

Strain of extensor muscle, fascia and tendon of specified finger with unspecified laterality at wrist and hand level

7th S66.319 Strain of extensor muscle, fascia and tendon of unspecified finger at wrist and hand level

6th S66.32 Laceration of extensor muscle, fascia and tendon of other and unspecified finger at wrist and hand level

7th S66.320 Laceration of extensor muscle, fascia and tendon of right index finger at wrist and hand level CC

✓7th **S66.321 Laceration of extensor muscle, fascia and tendon of left index finger at wrist and hand level** CC

✓7th **S66.322 Laceration of extensor muscle, fascia and tendon of right middle finger at wrist and hand level** CC

✓7th **S66.323 Laceration of extensor muscle, fascia and tendon of left middle finger at wrist and hand level** CC

✓7th **S66.324 Laceration of extensor muscle, fascia and tendon of right ring finger at wrist and hand level** CC

✓7th **S66.325 Laceration of extensor muscle, fascia and tendon of left ring finger at wrist and hand level** CC

✓7th **S66.326 Laceration of extensor muscle, fascia and tendon of right little finger at wrist and hand level** CC

✓7th **S66.327 Laceration of extensor muscle, fascia and tendon of left little finger at wrist and hand level** CC

✓7th **S66.328 Laceration of extensor muscle, fascia and tendon of other finger at wrist and hand level** CC

Laceration of extensor muscle, fascia and tendon of specified finger with unspecified laterality at wrist and hand level

✓7th **S66.329 Laceration of extensor muscle, fascia and tendon of unspecified finger at wrist and hand level** CC

✓6th **S66.39 Other injury of extensor muscle, fascia and tendon of other and unspecified finger at wrist and hand level**

✓7th **S66.390 Other injury of extensor muscle, fascia and tendon of right index finger at wrist and hand level**

✓7th **S66.391 Other injury of extensor muscle, fascia and tendon of left index finger at wrist and hand level**

✓7th **S66.392 Other injury of extensor muscle, fascia and tendon of right middle finger at wrist and hand level**

✓7th **S66.393 Other injury of extensor muscle, fascia and tendon of left middle finger at wrist and hand level**

✓7th **S66.394 Other injury of extensor muscle, fascia and tendon of right ring finger at wrist and hand level**

✓7th **S66.395 Other injury of extensor muscle, fascia and tendon of left ring finger at wrist and hand level**

✓7th **S66.396 Other injury of extensor muscle, fascia and tendon of right little finger at wrist and hand level**

✓7th **S66.397 Other injury of extensor muscle, fascia and tendon of left little finger at wrist and hand level**

✓7th **S66.398 Other injury of extensor muscle, fascia and tendon of other finger at wrist and hand level**

Other injury of extensor muscle, fascia and tendon of specified finger with unspecified laterality at wrist and hand level

✓7th **S66.399 Other injury of extensor muscle, fascia and tendon of unspecified finger at wrist and hand level**

✓5th **S66.4 Injury of intrinsic muscle, fascia and tendon of thumb at wrist and hand level**

✓6th **S66.40 Unspecified injury of intrinsic muscle, fascia and tendon of thumb at wrist and hand level**

✓7th **S66.401 Unspecified injury of intrinsic muscle, fascia and tendon of right thumb at wrist and hand level**

✓7th **S66.402 Unspecified injury of intrinsic muscle, fascia and tendon of left thumb at wrist and hand level**

✓7th **S66.409 Unspecified injury of intrinsic muscle, fascia and tendon of unspecified thumb at wrist and hand level**

✓6th **S66.41 Strain of intrinsic muscle, fascia and tendon of thumb at wrist and hand level**

✓7th **S66.411 Strain of intrinsic muscle, fascia and tendon of right thumb at wrist and hand level**

✓7th **S66.412 Strain of intrinsic muscle, fascia and tendon of left thumb at wrist and hand level**

✓7th **S66.419 Strain of intrinsic muscle, fascia and tendon of unspecified thumb at wrist and hand level**

✓6th **S66.42 Laceration of intrinsic muscle, fascia and tendon of thumb at wrist and hand level**

✓7th **S66.421 Laceration of intrinsic muscle, fascia and tendon of right thumb at wrist and hand level** CC

✓7th **S66.422 Laceration of intrinsic muscle, fascia and tendon of left thumb at wrist and hand level** CC

✓7th **S66.429 Laceration of intrinsic muscle, fascia and tendon of unspecified thumb at wrist and hand level** CC

✓6th **S66.49 Other specified injury of intrinsic muscle, fascia and tendon of thumb at wrist and hand level**

✓7th **S66.491 Other specified injury of intrinsic muscle, fascia and tendon of right thumb at wrist and hand level**

✓7th **S66.492 Other specified injury of intrinsic muscle, fascia and tendon of left thumb at wrist and hand level**

✓7th **S66.499 Other specified injury of intrinsic muscle, fascia and tendon of unspecified thumb at wrist and hand level**

✓5th **S66.5 Injury of intrinsic muscle, fascia and tendon of other and unspecified finger at wrist and hand level**

EXCLUDES 2 *injury of intrinsic muscle, fascia and tendon of thumb at wrist and hand level (S66.4-)*

✓6th **S66.50 Unspecified injury of intrinsic muscle, fascia and tendon of other and unspecified finger at wrist and hand level**

✓7th **S66.500 Unspecified injury of intrinsic muscle, fascia and tendon of right index finger at wrist and hand level**

✓7th **S66.501 Unspecified injury of intrinsic muscle, fascia and tendon of left index finger at wrist and hand level**

✓7th **S66.502 Unspecified injury of intrinsic muscle, fascia and tendon of right middle finger at wrist and hand level**

✓7th **S66.503 Unspecified injury of intrinsic muscle, fascia and tendon of left middle finger at wrist and hand level**

✓7th **S66.504 Unspecified injury of intrinsic muscle, fascia and tendon of right ring finger at wrist and hand level**

✓7th **S66.505 Unspecified injury of intrinsic muscle, fascia and tendon of left ring finger at wrist and hand level**

✓7th **S66.506 Unspecified injury of intrinsic muscle, fascia and tendon of right little finger at wrist and hand level**

✓7th **S66.507 Unspecified injury of intrinsic muscle, fascia and tendon of left little finger at wrist and hand level**

✓7th **S66.508 Unspecified injury of intrinsic muscle, fascia and tendon of other finger at wrist and hand level**

Unspecified injury of intrinsic muscle, fascia and tendon of specified finger with unspecified laterality at wrist and hand level

✓7th **S66.509 Unspecified injury of intrinsic muscle, fascia and tendon of unspecified finger at wrist and hand level**

✓6th **S66.51 Strain of intrinsic muscle, fascia and tendon of other and unspecified finger at wrist and hand level**

✓7th **S66.510 Strain of intrinsic muscle, fascia and tendon of right index finger at wrist and hand level**

✓7th **S66.511 Strain of intrinsic muscle, fascia and tendon of left index finger at wrist and hand level**

7th **S66.512 Strain of intrinsic muscle, fascia and tendon of right middle finger at wrist and hand level**

7th **S66.513 Strain of intrinsic muscle, fascia and tendon of left middle finger at wrist and hand level**

7th **S66.514 Strain of intrinsic muscle, fascia and tendon of right ring finger at wrist and hand level**

7th **S66.515 Strain of intrinsic muscle, fascia and tendon of left ring finger at wrist and hand level**

7th **S66.516 Strain of intrinsic muscle, fascia and tendon of right little finger at wrist and hand level**

7th **S66.517 Strain of intrinsic muscle, fascia and tendon of left little finger at wrist and hand level**

7th **S66.518 Strain of intrinsic muscle, fascia and tendon of other finger at wrist and hand level**

Strain of intrinsic muscle, fascia and tendon of specified finger with unspecified laterality at wrist and hand level

7th **S66.519 Strain of intrinsic muscle, fascia and tendon of unspecified finger at wrist and hand level**

6th **S66.52 Laceration of intrinsic muscle, fascia and tendon of other and unspecified finger at wrist and hand level**

7th **S66.520 Laceration of intrinsic muscle, fascia and tendon of right index finger at wrist and hand level** CC

7th **S66.521 Laceration of intrinsic muscle, fascia and tendon of left index finger at wrist and hand level** CC

7th **S66.522 Laceration of intrinsic muscle, fascia and tendon of right middle finger at wrist and hand level** CC

7th **S66.523 Laceration of intrinsic muscle, fascia and tendon of left middle finger at wrist and hand level** CC

7th **S66.524 Laceration of intrinsic muscle, fascia and tendon of right ring finger at wrist and hand level** CC

7th **S66.525 Laceration of intrinsic muscle, fascia and tendon of left ring finger at wrist and hand level** CC

7th **S66.526 Laceration of intrinsic muscle, fascia and tendon of right little finger at wrist and hand level** CC

7th **S66.527 Laceration of intrinsic muscle, fascia and tendon of left little finger at wrist and hand level** CC

7th **S66.528 Laceration of intrinsic muscle, fascia and tendon of other finger at wrist and hand level** CC

Laceration of intrinsic muscle, fascia and tendon of specified finger with unspecified laterality at wrist and hand level

7th **S66.529 Laceration of intrinsic muscle, fascia and tendon of unspecified finger at wrist and hand level** CC

6th **S66.59 Other injury of intrinsic muscle, fascia and tendon of other and unspecified finger at wrist and hand level**

7th **S66.590 Other injury of intrinsic muscle, fascia and tendon of right index finger at wrist and hand level**

7th **S66.591 Other injury of intrinsic muscle, fascia and tendon of left index finger at wrist and hand level**

7th **S66.592 Other injury of intrinsic muscle, fascia and tendon of right middle finger at wrist and hand level**

7th **S66.593 Other injury of intrinsic muscle, fascia and tendon of left middle finger at wrist and hand level**

7th **S66.594 Other injury of intrinsic muscle, fascia and tendon of right ring finger at wrist and hand level**

7th **S66.595 Other injury of intrinsic muscle, fascia and tendon of left ring finger at wrist and hand level**

7th **S66.596 Other injury of intrinsic muscle, fascia and tendon of right little finger at wrist and hand level**

7th **S66.597 Other injury of intrinsic muscle, fascia and tendon of left little finger at wrist and hand level**

7th **S66.598 Other injury of intrinsic muscle, fascia and tendon of other finger at wrist and hand level**

Other injury of intrinsic muscle, fascia and tendon of specified finger with unspecified laterality at wrist and hand level

7th **S66.599 Other injury of intrinsic muscle, fascia and tendon of unspecified finger at wrist and hand level**

5th **S66.8 Injury of other specified muscles, fascia and tendons at wrist and hand level**

6th **S66.80 Unspecified injury of other specified muscles, fascia and tendons at wrist and hand level**

7th **S66.801 Unspecified injury of other specified muscles, fascia and tendons at wrist and hand level, right hand**

7th **S66.802 Unspecified injury of other specified muscles, fascia and tendons at wrist and hand level, left hand**

7th **S66.809 Unspecified injury of other specified muscles, fascia and tendons at wrist and hand level, unspecified hand**

6th **S66.81 Strain of other specified muscles, fascia and tendons at wrist and hand level**

7th **S66.811 Strain of other specified muscles, fascia and tendons at wrist and hand level, right hand**

7th **S66.812 Strain of other specified muscles, fascia and tendons at wrist and hand level, left hand**

7th **S66.819 Strain of other specified muscles, fascia and tendons at wrist and hand level, unspecified hand**

6th **S66.82 Laceration of other specified muscles, fascia and tendons at wrist and hand level**

7th **S66.821 Laceration of other specified muscles, fascia and tendons at wrist and hand level, right hand** CC

7th **S66.822 Laceration of other specified muscles, fascia and tendons at wrist and hand level, left hand** CC

7th **S66.829 Laceration of other specified muscles, fascia and tendons at wrist and hand level, unspecified hand** CC

6th **S66.89 Other injury of other specified muscles, fascia and tendons at wrist and hand level**

7th **S66.891 Other injury of other specified muscles, fascia and tendons at wrist and hand level, right hand**

7th **S66.892 Other injury of other specified muscles, fascia and tendons at wrist and hand level, left hand**

7th **S66.899 Other injury of other specified muscles, fascia and tendons at wrist and hand level, unspecified hand**

5th **S66.9 Injury of unspecified muscle, fascia and tendon at wrist and hand level**

6th **S66.90 Unspecified injury of unspecified muscle, fascia and tendon at wrist and hand level**

7th **S66.901 Unspecified injury of unspecified muscle, fascia and tendon at wrist and hand level, right hand**

7th **S66.902 Unspecified injury of unspecified muscle, fascia and tendon at wrist and hand level, left hand**

7th **S66.909 Unspecified injury of unspecified muscle, fascia and tendon at wrist and hand level, unspecified hand**

6th **S66.91 Strain of unspecified muscle, fascia and tendon at wrist and hand level**

7th **S66.911 Strain of unspecified muscle, fascia and tendon at wrist and hand level, right hand**

7th **S66.912 Strain of unspecified muscle, fascia and tendon at wrist and hand level, left hand**

S66.919 Strain of unspecified muscle, fascia and tendon at wrist and hand level, unspecified hand

S66.92 Laceration of unspecified muscle, fascia and tendon at wrist and hand level

S66.921 Laceration of unspecified muscle, fascia and tendon at wrist and hand level, right hand CC

S66.922 Laceration of unspecified muscle, fascia and tendon at wrist and hand level, left hand CC

S66.929 Laceration of unspecified muscle, fascia and tendon at wrist and hand level, unspecified hand CC

S66.99 Other injury of unspecified muscle, fascia and tendon at wrist and hand level

S66.991 Other injury of unspecified muscle, fascia and tendon at wrist and hand level, right hand

S66.992 Other injury of unspecified muscle, fascia and tendon at wrist and hand level, left hand

S66.999 Other injury of unspecified muscle, fascia and tendon at wrist and hand level, unspecified hand

S67 Crushing injury of wrist, hand and fingers

Use additional code for all associated injuries, such as:
fracture of wrist and hand (S62.-)
open wound of wrist and hand (S61.-)

The appropriate 7th character is to be added to each code from category S67.
A initial encounter
D subsequent encounter
S sequela

S67.Ø Crushing injury of thumb

S67.ØØ Crushing injury of unspecified thumb

S67.Ø1 Crushing injury of right thumb

S67.Ø2 Crushing injury of left thumb

S67.1 Crushing injury of other and unspecified finger(s)

EXCLUDES 2 *crushing injury of thumb (S67.Ø-)*

S67.1Ø Crushing injury of unspecified finger(s)

S67.19 Crushing injury of other finger(s)

S67.19Ø Crushing injury of right index finger

S67.191 Crushing injury of left index finger

S67.192 Crushing injury of right middle finger

S67.193 Crushing injury of left middle finger

S67.194 Crushing injury of right ring finger

S67.195 Crushing injury of left ring finger

S67.196 Crushing injury of right little finger

S67.197 Crushing injury of left little finger

S67.198 Crushing injury of other finger

Crushing injury of specified finger with unspecified laterality

S67.2 Crushing injury of hand

EXCLUDES 2 *crushing injury of fingers (S67.1-)*
crushing injury of thumb (S67.Ø-)

S67.2Ø Crushing injury of unspecified hand

S67.21 Crushing injury of right hand

S67.22 Crushing injury of left hand

S67.3 Crushing injury of wrist

S67.3Ø Crushing injury of unspecified wrist

S67.31 Crushing injury of right wrist

S67.32 Crushing injury of left wrist

S67.4 Crushing injury of wrist and hand

EXCLUDES 1 *crushing injury of hand alone (S67.2-)*
crushing injury of wrist alone (S67.3-)

EXCLUDES 2 *crushing injury of fingers (S67.1-)*
crushing injury of thumb (S67.Ø-)

S67.4Ø Crushing injury of unspecified wrist and hand

S67.41 Crushing injury of right wrist and hand

S67.42 Crushing injury of left wrist and hand

S67.9 Crushing injury of unspecified part(s) of wrist, hand and fingers

S67.9Ø Crushing injury of unspecified part(s) of unspecified wrist, hand and fingers

S67.91 Crushing injury of unspecified part(s) of right wrist, hand and fingers

S67.92 Crushing injury of unspecified part(s) of left wrist, hand and fingers

S68 Traumatic amputation of wrist, hand and fingers

An amputation not identified as partial or complete should be coded to complete.

The appropriate 7th character is to be added to each code from category S68.
A initial encounter
D subsequent encounter
S sequela

S68.Ø Traumatic metacarpophalangeal amputation of thumb

Traumatic amputation of thumb NOS

S68.Ø1 Complete traumatic metacarpophalangeal amputation of thumb

8 S68.Ø11 Complete traumatic metacarpophalangeal amputation of right thumb HCC

8 S68.Ø12 Complete traumatic metacarpophalangeal amputation of left thumb HCC

8 S68.Ø19 Complete traumatic metacarpophalangeal amputation of unspecified thumb HCC

S68.Ø2 Partial traumatic metacarpophalangeal amputation of thumb

8 S68.Ø21 Partial traumatic metacarpophalangeal amputation of right thumb HCC

8 S68.Ø22 Partial traumatic metacarpophalangeal amputation of left thumb HCC

8 S68.Ø29 Partial traumatic metacarpophalangeal amputation of unspecified thumb HCC

S68.1 Traumatic metacarpophalangeal amputation of other and unspecified finger

Traumatic amputation of finger NOS

EXCLUDES 2 *traumatic metacarpophalangeal amputation of thumb (S68.Ø-)*

S68.11 Complete traumatic metacarpophalangeal amputation of other and unspecified finger

8 S68.11Ø Complete traumatic metacarpophalangeal amputation of right index finger HCC

8 S68.111 Complete traumatic metacarpophalangeal amputation of left index finger HCC

8 S68.112 Complete traumatic metacarpophalangeal amputation of right middle finger HCC

8 S68.113 Complete traumatic metacarpophalangeal amputation of left middle finger HCC

8 S68.114 Complete traumatic metacarpophalangeal amputation of right ring finger HCC

8 S68.115 Complete traumatic metacarpophalangeal amputation of left ring finger HCC

8 S68.116 Complete traumatic metacarpophalangeal amputation of right little finger HCC

8 S68.117 Complete traumatic metacarpophalangeal amputation of left little finger HCC

8 S68.118 Complete traumatic metacarpophalangeal amputation of other finger HCC

Complete traumatic metacarpophalangeal amputation of specified finger with unspecified laterality

8 S68.119 Complete traumatic metacarpophalangeal amputation of unspecified finger HCC

S68.12 Partial traumatic metacarpophalangeal amputation of other and unspecified finger

8 S68.12Ø Partial traumatic metacarpophalangeal amputation of right index finger HCC

8 ✓7th **S68.121 Partial traumatic metacarpophalangeal amputation of left index finger** HCC
8 ✓7th **S68.122 Partial traumatic metacarpophalangeal amputation of right middle finger** HCC
8 ✓7th **S68.123 Partial traumatic metacarpophalangeal amputation of left middle finger** HCC
8 ✓7th **S68.124 Partial traumatic metacarpophalangeal amputation of right ring finger** HCC
8 ✓7th **S68.125 Partial traumatic metacarpophalangeal amputation of left ring finger** HCC
8 ✓7th **S68.126 Partial traumatic metacarpophalangeal amputation of right little finger** HCC
8 ✓7th **S68.127 Partial traumatic metacarpophalangeal amputation of left little finger** HCC
8 ✓7th **S68.128 Partial traumatic metacarpophalangeal amputation of other finger** HCC
Partial traumatic metacarpophalangeal amputation of specified finger with unspecified laterality
8 ✓7th **S68.129 Partial traumatic metacarpophalangeal amputation of unspecified finger** HCC

✓5th **S68.4 Traumatic amputation of hand at wrist level**
Traumatic amputation of hand NOS
Traumatic amputation of wrist

✓6th **S68.41 Complete traumatic amputation of hand at wrist level**
7 ✓7th **S68.411 Complete traumatic amputation of right hand at wrist level** CC HCC
7 ✓7th **S68.412 Complete traumatic amputation of left hand at wrist level** CC HCC
7 ✓7th **S68.419 Complete traumatic amputation of unspecified hand at wrist level** CC HCC

✓6th **S68.42 Partial traumatic amputation of hand at wrist level**
7 ✓7th **S68.421 Partial traumatic amputation of right hand at wrist level** CC HCC
7 ✓7th **S68.422 Partial traumatic amputation of left hand at wrist level** CC HCC
7 ✓7th **S68.429 Partial traumatic amputation of unspecified hand at wrist level** CC HCC

✓5th **S68.5 Traumatic transphalangeal amputation of thumb**
Traumatic interphalangeal joint amputation of thumb

✓6th **S68.51 Complete traumatic transphalangeal amputation of thumb**
8 ✓7th **S68.511 Complete traumatic transphalangeal amputation of right thumb** HCC
8 ✓7th **S68.512 Complete traumatic transphalangeal amputation of left thumb** HCC
8 ✓7th **S68.519 Complete traumatic transphalangeal amputation of unspecified thumb** HCC

✓6th **S68.52 Partial traumatic transphalangeal amputation of thumb**
8 ✓7th **S68.521 Partial traumatic transphalangeal amputation of right thumb** HCC
8 ✓7th **S68.522 Partial traumatic transphalangeal amputation of left thumb** HCC
8 ✓7th **S68.529 Partial traumatic transphalangeal amputation of unspecified thumb** HCC

✓5th **S68.6 Traumatic transphalangeal amputation of other and unspecified finger**

✓6th **S68.61 Complete traumatic transphalangeal amputation of other and unspecified finger(s)**
8 ✓7th **S68.610 Complete traumatic transphalangeal amputation of right index finger** HCC
8 ✓7th **S68.611 Complete traumatic transphalangeal amputation of left index finger** HCC
8 ✓7th **S68.612 Complete traumatic transphalangeal amputation of right middle finger** HCC
8 ✓7th **S68.613 Complete traumatic transphalangeal amputation of left middle finger** HCC
8 ✓7th **S68.614 Complete traumatic transphalangeal amputation of right ring finger** HCC
8 ✓7th **S68.615 Complete traumatic transphalangeal amputation of left ring finger** HCC
8 ✓7th **S68.616 Complete traumatic transphalangeal amputation of right little finger** HCC
8 ✓7th **S68.617 Complete traumatic transphalangeal amputation of left little finger** HCC
8 ✓7th **S68.618 Complete traumatic transphalangeal amputation of other finger** HCC
Complete traumatic transphalangeal amputation of specified finger with unspecified laterality
8 ✓7th **S68.619 Complete traumatic transphalangeal amputation of unspecified finger** HCC

✓6th **S68.62 Partial traumatic transphalangeal amputation of other and unspecified finger**
8 ✓7th **S68.620 Partial traumatic transphalangeal amputation of right index finger** HCC
8 ✓7th **S68.621 Partial traumatic transphalangeal amputation of left index finger** HCC
8 ✓7th **S68.622 Partial traumatic transphalangeal amputation of right middle finger** HCC
8 ✓7th **S68.623 Partial traumatic transphalangeal amputation of left middle finger** HCC
8 ✓7th **S68.624 Partial traumatic transphalangeal amputation of right ring finger** HCC
8 ✓7th **S68.625 Partial traumatic transphalangeal amputation of left ring finger** HCC
8 ✓7th **S68.626 Partial traumatic transphalangeal amputation of right little finger** HCC
8 ✓7th **S68.627 Partial traumatic transphalangeal amputation of left little finger** HCC
8 ✓7th **S68.628 Partial traumatic transphalangeal amputation of other finger** HCC
Partial traumatic transphalangeal amputation of specified finger with unspecified laterality
8 ✓7th **S68.629 Partial traumatic transphalangeal amputation of unspecified finger** HCC

✓5th **S68.7 Traumatic transmetacarpal amputation of hand**

✓6th **S68.71 Complete traumatic transmetacarpal amputation of hand**
7 ✓7th **S68.711 Complete traumatic transmetacarpal amputation of right hand** CC HCC
7 ✓7th **S68.712 Complete traumatic transmetacarpal amputation of left hand** CC HCC
7 ✓7th **S68.719 Complete traumatic transmetacarpal amputation of unspecified hand** CC HCC

✓6th **S68.72 Partial traumatic transmetacarpal amputation of hand**
7 ✓7th **S68.721 Partial traumatic transmetacarpal amputation of right hand** CC HCC
7 ✓7th **S68.722 Partial traumatic transmetacarpal amputation of left hand** CC HCC
7 ✓7th **S68.729 Partial traumatic transmetacarpal amputation of unspecified hand** CC HCC

✓4th **S69 Other and unspecified injuries of wrist, hand and finger(s)**

The appropriate 7th character is to be added to each code from category S69.
A initial encounter
D subsequent encounter
S sequela

✓5th **S69.8 Other specified injuries of wrist, hand and finger(s)**
✓x 7th **S69.80 Other specified injuries of unspecified wrist, hand and finger(s)**
✓x 7th **S69.81 Other specified injuries of right wrist, hand and finger(s)**
✓x 7th **S69.82 Other specified injuries of left wrist, hand and finger(s)**

✓5th **S69.9 Unspecified injury of wrist, hand and finger(s)**
✓x 7th **S69.90 Unspecified injury of unspecified wrist, hand and finger(s)**
✓x 7th **S69.91 Unspecified injury of right wrist, hand and finger(s)**
✓x 7th **S69.92 Unspecified injury of left wrist, hand and finger(s)**

Injuries to the hip and thigh (S70-S79)

EXCLUDES 2 *burns and corrosions (T20-T32)*
frostbite (T33-T34)
snake bite (T63.0-)
venomous insect bite or sting (T63.4-)

S70 Superficial injury of hip and thigh

The appropriate 7th character is to be added to each code from category S70.
A initial encounter
D subsequent encounter
S sequela

- **S70.0 Contusion of hip**
  - **S70.00 Contusion of unspecified hip**
  - **S70.01 Contusion of right hip**
  - **S70.02 Contusion of left hip**
- **S70.1 Contusion of thigh**
  - **S70.10 Contusion of unspecified thigh**
  - **S70.11 Contusion of right thigh**
  - **S70.12 Contusion of left thigh**
- **S70.2 Other superficial injuries of hip**
  - **S70.21 Abrasion of hip**
    - **S70.211 Abrasion, right hip**
    - **S70.212 Abrasion, left hip**
    - **S70.219 Abrasion, unspecified hip**
  - **S70.22 Blister (nonthermal) of hip**
    - **S70.221 Blister (nonthermal), right hip**
    - **S70.222 Blister (nonthermal), left hip**
    - **S70.229 Blister (nonthermal), unspecified hip**
  - **S70.24 External constriction of hip**
    - **S70.241 External constriction, right hip**
    - **S70.242 External constriction, left hip**
    - **S70.249 External constriction, unspecified hip**
  - **S70.25 Superficial foreign body of hip**
    Splinter in the hip
    - **S70.251 Superficial foreign body, right hip**
    - **S70.252 Superficial foreign body, left hip**
    - **S70.259 Superficial foreign body, unspecified hip**
  - **S70.26 Insect bite (nonvenomous) of hip**
    - **S70.261 Insect bite (nonvenomous), right hip**
    - **S70.262 Insect bite (nonvenomous), left hip**
    - **S70.269 Insect bite (nonvenomous), unspecified hip**
  - **S70.27 Other superficial bite of hip**
    EXCLUDES 1 *open bite of hip (S71.05-)*
    - **S70.271 Other superficial bite of hip, right hip**
    - **S70.272 Other superficial bite of hip, left hip**
    - **S70.279 Other superficial bite of hip, unspecified hip**
- **S70.3 Other superficial injuries of thigh**
  - **S70.31 Abrasion of thigh**
    - **S70.311 Abrasion, right thigh**
    - **S70.312 Abrasion, left thigh**
    - **S70.319 Abrasion, unspecified thigh**
  - **S70.32 Blister (nonthermal) of thigh**
    - **S70.321 Blister (nonthermal), right thigh**
    - **S70.322 Blister (nonthermal), left thigh**
    - **S70.329 Blister (nonthermal), unspecified thigh**
  - **S70.34 External constriction of thigh**
    - **S70.341 External constriction, right thigh**
    - **S70.342 External constriction, left thigh**
    - **S70.349 External constriction, unspecified thigh**
  - **S70.35 Superficial foreign body of thigh**
    Splinter in the thigh
    - **S70.351 Superficial foreign body, right thigh**
    - **S70.352 Superficial foreign body, left thigh**
    - **S70.359 Superficial foreign body, unspecified thigh**
  - **S70.36 Insect bite (nonvenomous) of thigh**
    - **S70.361 Insect bite (nonvenomous), right thigh**
    - **S70.362 Insect bite (nonvenomous), left thigh**
    - **S70.369 Insect bite (nonvenomous), unspecified thigh**
  - **S70.37 Other superficial bite of thigh**
    EXCLUDES 1 *open bite of thigh (S71.15)*
    - **S70.371 Other superficial bite of right thigh**
    - **S70.372 Other superficial bite of left thigh**
    - **S70.379 Other superficial bite of unspecified thigh**
- **S70.9 Unspecified superficial injury of hip and thigh**
  - **S70.91 Unspecified superficial injury of hip**
    - **S70.911 Unspecified superficial injury of right hip**
    - **S70.912 Unspecified superficial injury of left hip**
    - **S70.919 Unspecified superficial injury of unspecified hip**
  - **S70.92 Unspecified superficial injury of thigh**
    - **S70.921 Unspecified superficial injury of right thigh**
    - **S70.922 Unspecified superficial injury of left thigh**
    - **S70.929 Unspecified superficial injury of unspecified thigh**

S71 Open wound of hip and thigh

Code also any associated wound infection

EXCLUDES 1 *open fracture of hip and thigh (S72.-)*
traumatic amputation of hip and thigh (S78.-)

EXCLUDES 2 *bite of venomous animal (T63.-)*
open wound of ankle, foot and toes (S91.-)
open wound of knee and lower leg (S81.-)

The appropriate 7th character is to be added to each code from category S71.
A initial encounter
D subsequent encounter
S sequela

- **S71.0 Open wound of hip**
  - **S71.00 Unspecified open wound of hip**
    - **S71.001 Unspecified open wound, right hip**
    - **S71.002 Unspecified open wound, left hip**
    - **S71.009 Unspecified open wound, unspecified hip**
  - **S71.01 Laceration without foreign body of hip**
    - **S71.011 Laceration without foreign body, right hip**
    - **S71.012 Laceration without foreign body, left hip**
    - **S71.019 Laceration without foreign body, unspecified hip**
  - **S71.02 Laceration with foreign body of hip**
    - **S71.021 Laceration with foreign body, right hip**
    - **S71.022 Laceration with foreign body, left hip**
    - **S71.029 Laceration with foreign body, unspecified hip**
  - **S71.03 Puncture wound without foreign body of hip**
    - **S71.031 Puncture wound without foreign body, right hip**
    - **S71.032 Puncture wound without foreign body, left hip**
    - **S71.039 Puncture wound without foreign body, unspecified hip**
  - **S71.04 Puncture wound with foreign body of hip**
    - **S71.041 Puncture wound with foreign body, right hip**
    - **S71.042 Puncture wound with foreign body, left hip**
    - **S71.049 Puncture wound with foreign body, unspecified hip**
  - **S71.05 Open bite of hip**
    Bite of hip NOS
    EXCLUDES 1 *superficial bite of hip (S70.26, S70.27)*
    - **S71.051 Open bite, right hip**
    - **S71.052 Open bite, left hip**
    - **S71.059 Open bite, unspecified hip**

√5th **S71.1 Open wound of thigh**

√6th **S71.10 Unspecified open wound of thigh**
AHA: 2016,3Q,24
√7th **S71.101 Unspecified open wound, right thigh**
√7th **S71.102 Unspecified open wound, left thigh**
√7th **S71.109 Unspecified open wound, unspecified thigh**

√6th **S71.11 Laceration without foreign body of thigh**
√7th **S71.111 Laceration without foreign body, right thigh**
√7th **S71.112 Laceration without foreign body, left thigh**
√7th **S71.119 Laceration without foreign body, unspecified thigh**

√6th **S71.12 Laceration with foreign body of thigh**
√7th **S71.121 Laceration with foreign body, right thigh**
√7th **S71.122 Laceration with foreign body, left thigh**
√7th **S71.129 Laceration with foreign body, unspecified thigh**

√6th **S71.13 Puncture wound without foreign body of thigh**
AHA: 2016,3Q,24
√7th **S71.131 Puncture wound without foreign body, right thigh**
√7th **S71.132 Puncture wound without foreign body, left thigh**
√7th **S71.139 Puncture wound without foreign body, unspecified thigh**

√6th **S71.14 Puncture wound with foreign body of thigh**
AHA: 2016,3Q,24
√7th **S71.141 Puncture wound with foreign body, right thigh**
√7th **S71.142 Puncture wound with foreign body, left thigh**
√7th **S71.149 Puncture wound with foreign body, unspecified thigh**

√6th **S71.15 Open bite of thigh**
Bite of thigh NOS
EXCLUDES 1 *superficial bite of thigh (S70.37-)*
√7th **S71.151 Open bite, right thigh**
√7th **S71.152 Open bite, left thigh**
√7th **S71.159 Open bite, unspecified thigh**

√4th **S72 Fracture of femur**

NOTE A fracture not indicated as displaced or nondisplaced should be coded to displaced.
A fracture not indicated as open or closed should be coded to closed.
The open fracture designations are based on the Gustilo open fracture classification.

EXCLUDES 1 *traumatic amputation of hip and thigh (S78.-)*
EXCLUDES 2 *fracture of lower leg and ankle (S82.-)*
fracture of foot (S92.-)
periprosthetic fracture of prosthetic implant of hip (M97.0-)

AHA: 2018,2Q,12; 2016,1Q,33; 2015,3Q,37-39; 2015,1Q,17; 2013,4Q,128
DEF: Diaphysis: Central shaft of a long bone.
DEF: Epiphysis: Proximal and distal rounded ends of a long bone communicates with the joint.
DEF: Metaphysis: Section of a long bone located between the epiphysis and diaphysis at the proximal and distal ends.
DEF: Physis (growth plate): Narrow zone of cartilaginous tissue between the epiphysis and metaphysis at each end of a long bone. In childhood, proliferation of cells in this zone lengthens the bone. As the bone matures, this area thins, ossification eventually fusing into solid bone and growth stops. ***Synonyms:*** *Epiphyseal plate.*

The appropriate 7th character is to be added to all codes from category S72 [unless otherwise indicated].
A initial encounter for closed fracture
B initial encounter for open fracture type I or II
initial encounter for open fracture NOS
C initial encounter for open fracture type IIIA, IIIB, or IIIC
D subsequent encounter for closed fracture with routine healing
E subsequent encounter for open fracture type I or II with routine healing
F subsequent encounter for open fracture type IIIA, IIIB, or IIIC with routine healing
G subsequent encounter for closed fracture with delayed healing
H subsequent encounter for open fracture type I or II with delayed healing
J subsequent encounter for open fracture type IIIA, IIIB, or IIIC with delayed healing
K subsequent encounter for closed fracture with nonunion
M subsequent encounter for open fracture type I or II with nonunion
N subsequent encounter for open fracture type IIIA, IIIB, or IIIC with nonunion
P subsequent encounter for closed fracture with malunion
Q subsequent encounter for open fracture type I or II with malunion
R subsequent encounter for open fracture type IIIA, IIIB, or IIIC with malunion
S sequela

√5th **S72.0 Fracture of head and neck of femur**
EXCLUDES 2 *physeal fracture of upper end of femur (S79.0-)*
AHA: 2016,3Q,16

√6th **S72.00 Fracture of unspecified part of neck of femur**
Fracture of hip NOS
Fracture of neck of femur NOS
4,6 √7th **S72.001 Fracture of unspecified part of neck of right femur** MCC CC H5 HCC
4,6 √7th **S72.002 Fracture of unspecified part of neck of left femur** MCC CC H5 HCC
4,6 √7th **S72.009 Fracture of unspecified part of neck of unspecified femur** MCC CC H5 HCC

√6th **S72.01 Unspecified intracapsular fracture of femur**
Subcapital fracture of femur
4,6 √7th **S72.011 Unspecified intracapsular fracture of right femur** MCC CC H5 HCC
4,6 √7th **S72.012 Unspecified intracapsular fracture of left femur** MCC CC H5 HCC
4,6 √7th **S72.019 Unspecified intracapsular fracture of unspecified femur** MCC CC H5 HCC

√6th **S72.02 Fracture of epiphysis (separation) (upper) of femur**
Transepiphyseal fracture of femur
EXCLUDES 1 *capital femoral epiphyseal fracture (pediatric) of femur (S79.01-)*
Salter-Harris Type I physeal fracture of upper end of femur (S79.01-)
4,6 √7th **S72.021 Displaced fracture of epiphysis (separation) (upper) of right femur** MCC CC H5 HCC

- 4,6 7th **S72.022** Displaced fracture of epiphysis (separation) (upper) of left femur MCC CC H5 HCC
- 4,6 7th **S72.023** Displaced fracture of epiphysis (separation) (upper) of unspecified femur MCC CC H5 HCC
- 4,6 7th **S72.024** Nondisplaced fracture of epiphysis (separation) (upper) of right femur MCC CC H5 HCC
- 4,6 7th **S72.025** Nondisplaced fracture of epiphysis (separation) (upper) of left femur MCC CC H5 HCC
- 4,6 7th **S72.026** Nondisplaced fracture of epiphysis (separation) (upper) of unspecified femur MCC CC H5 HCC

6th **S72.03 Midcervical fracture of femur**

Transcervical fracture of femur NOS

- 4,6 7th **S72.031** Displaced midcervical fracture of right femur MCC CC H5 HCC
- 4,6 7th **S72.032** Displaced midcervical fracture of left femur MCC CC H5 HCC
- 4,6 7th **S72.033** Displaced midcervical fracture of unspecified femur MCC CC H5 HCC
- 4,6 7th **S72.034** Nondisplaced midcervical fracture of right femur MCC CC H5 HCC
- 4,6 7th **S72.035** Nondisplaced midcervical fracture of left femur MCC CC H5 HCC
- 4,6 7th **S72.036** Nondisplaced midcervical fracture of unspecified femur MCC CC H5 HCC

6th **S72.04 Fracture of base of neck of femur**

Cervicotrochanteric fracture of femur

- 4,6 7th **S72.041** Displaced fracture of base of neck of right femur MCC CC H5 HCC
- 4,6 7th **S72.042** Displaced fracture of base of neck of left femur MCC CC H5 HCC
- 4,6 7th **S72.043** Displaced fracture of base of neck of unspecified femur MCC CC H5 HCC
- 4,6 7th **S72.044** Nondisplaced fracture of base of neck of right femur MCC CC H5 HCC
- 4,6 7th **S72.045** Nondisplaced fracture of base of neck of left femur MCC CC H5 HCC
- 4,6 7th **S72.046** Nondisplaced fracture of base of neck of unspecified femur MCC CC H5 HCC

6th **S72.05 Unspecified fracture of head of femur**

Fracture of head of femur NOS

- 4,6 7th **S72.051** Unspecified fracture of head of right femur MCC CC H5 HCC
- 4,6 7th **S72.052** Unspecified fracture of head of left femur MCC CC H5 HCC
- 4,6 7th **S72.059** Unspecified fracture of head of unspecified femur MCC CC H5 HCC

6th **S72.06 Articular fracture of head of femur**

- 4,6 7th **S72.061** Displaced articular fracture of head of right femur MCC CC H5 HCC
- 4,6 7th **S72.062** Displaced articular fracture of head of left femur MCC CC H5 HCC
- 4,6 7th **S72.063** Displaced articular fracture of head of unspecified femur MCC CC H5 HCC
- 4,6 7th **S72.064** Nondisplaced articular fracture of head of right femur MCC CC H5 HCC
- 4,6 7th **S72.065** Nondisplaced articular fracture of head of left femur MCC CC H5 HCC
- 4,6 7th **S72.066** Nondisplaced articular fracture of head of unspecified femur MCC CC H5 HCC

6th **S72.09 Other fracture of head and neck of femur**

- 4,6 7th **S72.091** Other fracture of head and neck of right femur MCC CC H5 HCC
- 4,6 7th **S72.092** Other fracture of head and neck of left femur MCC CC H5 HCC
- 4,6 7th **S72.099** Other fracture of head and neck of unspecified femur MCC CC H5 HCC

5th **S72.1 Pertrochanteric fracture**

AHA: 2016,3Q,16

6th **S72.10 Unspecified trochanteric fracture of femur**

Fracture of trochanter NOS

- 4,6 7th **S72.101** Unspecified trochanteric fracture of right femur MCC CC H5 HCC
- 4,6 7th **S72.102** Unspecified trochanteric fracture of left femur MCC CC H5 HCC
- 4,6 7th **S72.109** Unspecified trochanteric fracture of unspecified femur MCC CC H5 HCC

6th **S72.11 Fracture of greater trochanter of femur**

- 4,6 7th **S72.111** Displaced fracture of greater trochanter of right femur MCC CC H5 HCC
- 4,6 7th **S72.112** Displaced fracture of greater trochanter of left femur MCC CC H5 HCC
- 4,6 7th **S72.113** Displaced fracture of greater trochanter of unspecified femur MCC CC H5 HCC
- 4,6 7th **S72.114** Nondisplaced fracture of greater trochanter of right femur MCC CC H5 HCC
- 4,6 7th **S72.115** Nondisplaced fracture of greater trochanter of left femur MCC CC H5 HCC
- 4,6 7th **S72.116** Nondisplaced fracture of greater trochanter of unspecified femur MCC CC H5 HCC

6th **S72.12 Fracture of lesser trochanter of femur**

- 4,6 7th **S72.121** Displaced fracture of lesser trochanter of right femur MCC CC H5 HCC
- 4,6 7th **S72.122** Displaced fracture of lesser trochanter of left femur MCC CC H5 HCC
- 4,6 7th **S72.123** Displaced fracture of lesser trochanter of unspecified femur MCC CC H5 HCC
- 4,6 7th **S72.124** Nondisplaced fracture of lesser trochanter of right femur MCC CC H5 HCC
- 4,6 7th **S72.125** Nondisplaced fracture of lesser trochanter of left femur MCC CC H5 HCC
- 4,6 7th **S72.126** Nondisplaced fracture of lesser trochanter of unspecified femur MCC CC H5 HCC

6th **S72.13 Apophyseal fracture of femur**

EXCLUDES 1 *chronic (nontraumatic) slipped upper femoral epiphysis (M93.0-)*

- 4,6 7th **S72.131** Displaced apophyseal fracture of right femur MCC CC H5 HCC
- 4,6 7th **S72.132** Displaced apophyseal fracture of left femur MCC CC H5 HCC
- 4,6 7th **S72.133** Displaced apophyseal fracture of unspecified femur MCC CC H5 HCC
- 4,6 7th **S72.134** Nondisplaced apophyseal fracture of right femur MCC CC H5 HCC
- 4,6 7th **S72.135** Nondisplaced apophyseal fracture of left femur MCC CC H5 HCC
- 4,6 7th **S72.136** Nondisplaced apophyseal fracture of unspecified femur MCC CC H5 HCC

6th **S72.14 Intertrochanteric fracture of femur**

- 4,6 7th **S72.141** Displaced intertrochanteric fracture of right femur MCC CC H5 HCC
- 4,6 7th **S72.142** Displaced intertrochanteric fracture of left femur MCC CC H5 HCC
- 4,6 7th **S72.143** Displaced intertrochanteric fracture of unspecified femur MCC CC H5 HCC
- 4,6 7th **S72.144** Nondisplaced intertrochanteric fracture of right femur MCC CC H5 HCC
- 4,6 7th **S72.145** Nondisplaced intertrochanteric fracture of left femur MCC CC H5 HCC
- 4,6 7th **S72.146** Nondisplaced intertrochanteric fracture of unspecified femur MCC CC H5 HCC

5th **S72.2 Subtrochanteric fracture of femur**

- 4,6 x7th **S72.21** Displaced subtrochanteric fracture of right femur MCC CC H5 HCC
- 4,6 x7th **S72.22** Displaced subtrochanteric fracture of left femur MCC CC H5 HCC
- 4,6 x7th **S72.23** Displaced subtrochanteric fracture of unspecified femur MCC CC H5 HCC
- 4,6 x7th **S72.24** Nondisplaced subtrochanteric fracture of right femur MCC CC H5 HCC
- 4,6 x7th **S72.25** Nondisplaced subtrochanteric fracture of left femur MCC CC H5 HCC
- 4,6 x7th **S72.26** Nondisplaced subtrochanteric fracture of unspecified femur MCC CC H5 HCC

5th **S72.3 Fracture of shaft of femur**

6th **S72.30 Unspecified fracture of shaft of femur**

- 4,6 7th **S72.301** Unspecified fracture of shaft of right femur MCC CC H5 HCC

Chapter 19. Injury, Poisoning and Certain Other Consequences of External Causes

S72.022–S72.301

4,6 7th **S72.302 Unspecified fracture of shaft of left femur** MCC CC H5 HCC
4,6 7th **S72.309 Unspecified fracture of shaft of unspecified femur** MCC CC H5 HCC
6th **S72.32 Transverse fracture of shaft of femur**
4,6 7th **S72.321 Displaced transverse fracture of shaft of right femur** MCC CC H5 HCC
4,6 7th **S72.322 Displaced transverse fracture of shaft of left femur** MCC CC H5 HCC
4,6 7th **S72.323 Displaced transverse fracture of shaft of unspecified femur** MCC CC H5 HCC
4,6 7th **S72.324 Nondisplaced transverse fracture of shaft of right femur** MCC CC H5 HCC
4,6 7th **S72.325 Nondisplaced transverse fracture of shaft of left femur** MCC CC H5 HCC
4,6 7th **S72.326 Nondisplaced transverse fracture of shaft of unspecified femur** MCC CC H5 HCC
6th **S72.33 Oblique fracture of shaft of femur**
4,6 7th **S72.331 Displaced oblique fracture of shaft of right femur** MCC CC H5 HCC
4,6 7th **S72.332 Displaced oblique fracture of shaft of left femur** MCC CC H5 HCC
4,6 7th **S72.333 Displaced oblique fracture of shaft of unspecified femur** MCC CC H5 HCC
4,6 7th **S72.334 Nondisplaced oblique fracture of shaft of right femur** MCC CC H5 HCC
4,6 7th **S72.335 Nondisplaced oblique fracture of shaft of left femur** MCC CC H5 HCC
4,6 7th **S72.336 Nondisplaced oblique fracture of shaft of unspecified femur** MCC CC H5 HCC
6th **S72.34 Spiral fracture of shaft of femur**
4,6 7th **S72.341 Displaced spiral fracture of shaft of right femur** MCC CC H5 HCC
4,6 7th **S72.342 Displaced spiral fracture of shaft of left femur** MCC CC H5 HCC
4,6 7th **S72.343 Displaced spiral fracture of shaft of unspecified femur** MCC CC H5 HCC
4,6 7th **S72.344 Nondisplaced spiral fracture of shaft of right femur** MCC CC H5 HCC
4,6 7th **S72.345 Nondisplaced spiral fracture of shaft of left femur** MCC CC H5 HCC
4,6 7th **S72.346 Nondisplaced spiral fracture of shaft of unspecified femur** MCC CC H5 HCC
6th **S72.35 Comminuted fracture of shaft of femur**
4,6 7th **S72.351 Displaced comminuted fracture of shaft of right femur** MCC CC H5 HCC
4,6 7th **S72.352 Displaced comminuted fracture of shaft of left femur** MCC CC H5 HCC
4,6 7th **S72.353 Displaced comminuted fracture of shaft of unspecified femur** MCC CC H5 HCC
4,6 7th **S72.354 Nondisplaced comminuted fracture of shaft of right femur** MCC CC H5 HCC
4,6 7th **S72.355 Nondisplaced comminuted fracture of shaft of left femur** MCC CC H5 HCC
4,6 7th **S72.356 Nondisplaced comminuted fracture of shaft of unspecified femur** MCC CC H5 HCC
6th **S72.36 Segmental fracture of shaft of femur**
4,6 7th **S72.361 Displaced segmental fracture of shaft of right femur** MCC CC H5 HCC
4,6 7th **S72.362 Displaced segmental fracture of shaft of left femur** MCC CC H5 HCC
4,6 7th **S72.363 Displaced segmental fracture of shaft of unspecified femur** MCC CC H5 HCC
4,6 7th **S72.364 Nondisplaced segmental fracture of shaft of right femur** MCC CC H5 HCC
4,6 7th **S72.365 Nondisplaced segmental fracture of shaft of left femur** MCC CC H5 HCC
4,6 7th **S72.366 Nondisplaced segmental fracture of shaft of unspecified femur** MCC CC H5 HCC
6th **S72.39 Other fracture of shaft of femur**
4,6 7th **S72.391 Other fracture of shaft of right femur** MCC CC H5 HCC
4,6 7th **S72.392 Other fracture of shaft of left femur** MCC CC H5 HCC
4,6 7th **S72.399 Other fracture of shaft of unspecified femur** MCC CC H5 HCC

5th **S72.4 Fracture of lower end of femur**
Fracture of distal end of femur
EXCLUDES 2 *fracture of shaft of femur (S72.3-)*
physeal fracture of lower end of femur (S79.1-)
AHA: 2016,4Q,42
6th **S72.40 Unspecified fracture of lower end of femur**
AHA: 2018,1Q,21; 2016,4Q,42
2,3,6 7th **S72.401 Unspecified fracture of lower end of right femur** MCC CC H5 HCC
2,3,6 7th **S72.402 Unspecified fracture of lower end of left femur** MCC CC H5 HCC
2,3,6 7th **S72.409 Unspecified fracture of lower end of unspecified femur** MCC CC H5 HCC
6th **S72.41 Unspecified condyle fracture of lower end of femur**
Condyle fracture of femur NOS
2,3,6 7th **S72.411 Displaced unspecified condyle fracture of lower end of right femur** MCC CC H5 HCC
2,3,6 7th **S72.412 Displaced unspecified condyle fracture of lower end of left femur** MCC CC H5 HCC
2,3,6 7th **S72.413 Displaced unspecified condyle fracture of lower end of unspecified femur** MCC CC H5 HCC
2,3,6 7th **S72.414 Nondisplaced unspecified condyle fracture of lower end of right femur** MCC CC H5 HCC
2,3,6 7th **S72.415 Nondisplaced unspecified condyle fracture of lower end of left femur** MCC CC H5 HCC
2,3,6 7th **S72.416 Nondisplaced unspecified condyle fracture of lower end of unspecified femur** MCC CC H5 HCC
6th **S72.42 Fracture of lateral condyle of femur**
2,3,6 7th **S72.421 Displaced fracture of lateral condyle of right femur** MCC CC H5 HCC
2,3,6 7th **S72.422 Displaced fracture of lateral condyle of left femur** MCC CC H5 HCC
2,3,6 7th **S72.423 Displaced fracture of lateral condyle of unspecified femur** MCC CC H5 HCC
2,3,6 7th **S72.424 Nondisplaced fracture of lateral condyle of right femur** MCC CC H5 HCC
2,3,6 7th **S72.425 Nondisplaced fracture of lateral condyle of left femur** MCC CC H5 HCC
2,3,6 7th **S72.426 Nondisplaced fracture of lateral condyle of unspecified femur** MCC CC H5 HCC
6th **S72.43 Fracture of medial condyle of femur**
2,3,6 7th **S72.431 Displaced fracture of medial condyle of right femur** MCC CC H5 HCC
2,3,6 7th **S72.432 Displaced fracture of medial condyle of left femur** MCC CC H5 HCC
2,3,6 7th **S72.433 Displaced fracture of medial condyle of unspecified femur** MCC CC H5 HCC
2,3,6 7th **S72.434 Nondisplaced fracture of medial condyle of right femur** MCC CC H5 HCC
2,3,6 7th **S72.435 Nondisplaced fracture of medial condyle of left femur** MCC CC H5 HCC
2,3,6 7th **S72.436 Nondisplaced fracture of medial condyle of unspecified femur** MCC CC H5 HCC
6th **S72.44 Fracture of lower epiphysis (separation) of femur**
EXCLUDES 1 *Salter-Harris Type I physeal fracture of lower end of femur (S79.11-)*
2,3,6 7th **S72.441 Displaced fracture of lower epiphysis (separation) of right femur** MCC CC H5 HCC
2,3,6 7th **S72.442 Displaced fracture of lower epiphysis (separation) of left femur** MCC CC H5 HCC
2,3,6 7th **S72.443 Displaced fracture of lower epiphysis (separation) of unspecified femur** MCC CC H5 HCC
2,3,6 7th **S72.444 Nondisplaced fracture of lower epiphysis (separation) of right femur** MCC CC H5 HCC
2,3,6 7th **S72.445 Nondisplaced fracture of lower epiphysis (separation) of left femur** MCC CC H5 HCC

2,3,6 ✓7th **S72.446 Nondisplaced fracture of lower epiphysis (separation) of unspecified femur** MCC CC H5 HCC

✓6th **S72.45 Supracondylar fracture without intracondylar extension of lower end of femur**
Supracondylar fracture of lower end of femur NOS
EXCLUDES 1 *supracondylar fracture with intracondylar extension of lower end of femur (S72.46-)*

2,3,6 ✓7th **S72.451 Displaced supracondylar fracture without intracondylar extension of lower end of right femur** MCC CC H5 HCC

2,3,6 ✓7th **S72.452 Displaced supracondylar fracture without intracondylar extension of lower end of left femur** MCC CC H5 HCC

2,3,6 ✓7th **S72.453 Displaced supracondylar fracture without intracondylar extension of lower end of unspecified femur** MCC CC H5 HCC

2,3,6 ✓7th **S72.454 Nondisplaced supracondylar fracture without intracondylar extension of lower end of right femur** MCC CC H5 HCC

2,3,6 ✓7th **S72.455 Nondisplaced supracondylar fracture without intracondylar extension of lower end of left femur** MCC CC H5 HCC

2,3,6 ✓7th **S72.456 Nondisplaced supracondylar fracture without intracondylar extension of lower end of unspecified femur** MCC CC H5 HCC

✓6th **S72.46 Supracondylar fracture with intracondylar extension of lower end of femur**
EXCLUDES 1 *supracondylar fracture without intracondylar extension of lower end of femur (S72.45-)*

2,3,6 ✓7th **S72.461 Displaced supracondylar fracture with intracondylar extension of lower end of right femur** MCC CC H5 HCC

2,3,6 ✓7th **S72.462 Displaced supracondylar fracture with intracondylar extension of lower end of left femur** MCC CC H5 HCC

2,3,6 ✓7th **S72.463 Displaced supracondylar fracture with intracondylar extension of lower end of unspecified femur** MCC CC H5 HCC

2,3,6 ✓7th **S72.464 Nondisplaced supracondylar fracture with intracondylar extension of lower end of right femur** MCC CC H5 HCC

2,3,6 ✓7th **S72.465 Nondisplaced supracondylar fracture with intracondylar extension of lower end of left femur** MCC CC H5 HCC

2,3,6 ✓7th **S72.466 Nondisplaced supracondylar fracture with intracondylar extension of lower end of unspecified femur** MCC CC H5 HCC

✓6th **S72.47 Torus fracture of lower end of femur**

The appropriate 7th character is to be added to all codes in subcategory S72.47.
A initial encounter for closed fracture
D subsequent encounter for fracture with routine healing
G subsequent encounter for fracture with delayed healing
K subsequent encounter for fracture with nonunion
P subsequent encounter for fracture with malunion
S sequela

3,6 ✓7th **S72.471 Torus fracture of lower end of right femur** CC H5 HCC

3,6 ✓7th **S72.472 Torus fracture of lower end of left femur** CC H5 HCC

3,6 ✓7th **S72.479 Torus fracture of lower end of unspecified femur** CC H5 HCC

✓6th **S72.49 Other fracture of lower end of femur**

2,3,6 ✓7th **S72.491 Other fracture of lower end of right femur** MCC CC H5 HCC

2,3,6 ✓7th **S72.492 Other fracture of lower end of left femur** MCC CC H5 HCC

2,3,6 ✓7th **S72.499 Other fracture of lower end of unspecified femur** MCC CC H5 HCC

✓5th **S72.8 Other fracture of femur**

✓6th **S72.8X Other fracture of femur**

4,6 ✓7th **S72.8X1 Other fracture of right femur** MCC CC H5 HCC

4,6 ✓7th **S72.8X2 Other fracture of left femur** MCC CC H5 HCC

4,6 ✓7th **S72.8X9 Other fracture of unspecified femur** MCC CC H5 HCC

✓5th **S72.9 Unspecified fracture of femur**
Fracture of thigh NOS
Fracture of upper leg NOS
EXCLUDES 1 *fracture of hip NOS (S72.00-, S72.01-)*

4,6 ✓x7th **S72.90 Unspecified fracture of unspecified femur** MCC CC H5 HCC
AHA: 2012,4Q,93

4,6 ✓x7th **S72.91 Unspecified fracture of right femur** MCC CC H5 HCC

4,6 ✓x7th **S72.92 Unspecified fracture of left femur** MCC CC H5 HCC

✓4th **S73 Dislocation and sprain of joint and ligaments of hip**

INCLUDES avulsion of joint or ligament of hip
laceration of cartilage, joint or ligament of hip
sprain of cartilage, joint or ligament of hip
traumatic hemarthrosis of joint or ligament of hip
traumatic rupture of joint or ligament of hip
traumatic subluxation of joint or ligament of hip
traumatic tear of joint or ligament of hip

Code also any associated open wound
EXCLUDES 2 *strain of muscle, fascia and tendon of hip and thigh (S76.-)*

The appropriate 7th character is to be added to each code from category S73.
A initial encounter
D subsequent encounter
S sequela

✓5th **S73.0 Subluxation and dislocation of hip**
EXCLUDES 2 *dislocation and subluxation of hip prosthesis (T84.020, T84.021)*

✓6th **S73.00 Unspecified subluxation and dislocation of hip**
Dislocation of hip NOS
Subluxation of hip NOS

6 ✓7th **S73.001 Unspecified subluxation of right hip** CC H5 HCC

6 ✓7th **S73.002 Unspecified subluxation of left hip** CC H5 HCC

6 ✓7th **S73.003 Unspecified subluxation of unspecified hip** CC H5 HCC

6 ✓7th **S73.004 Unspecified dislocation of right hip** CC H5 HCC

6 ✓7th **S73.005 Unspecified dislocation of left hip** CC H5 HCC

6 ✓7th **S73.006 Unspecified dislocation of unspecified hip** CC H5 HCC

✓6th **S73.01 Posterior subluxation and dislocation of hip**

6 ✓7th **S73.011 Posterior subluxation of right hip** CC H5 HCC

6 ✓7th **S73.012 Posterior subluxation of left hip** CC H5 HCC

6 ✓7th **S73.013 Posterior subluxation of unspecified hip** CC H5 HCC

6 ✓7th **S73.014 Posterior dislocation of right hip** CC H5 HCC

6 ✓7th **S73.015 Posterior dislocation of left hip** CC H5 HCC

6 ✓7th **S73.016 Posterior dislocation of unspecified hip** CC H5 HCC

✓6th **S73.02 Obturator subluxation and dislocation of hip**

6 ✓7th **S73.021 Obturator subluxation of right hip** CC H5 HCC

6 ✓7th **S73.022 Obturator subluxation of left hip** CC H5 HCC

6 ✓7th **S73.023 Obturator subluxation of unspecified hip** CC H5 HCC

6 ✓7th **S73.024 Obturator dislocation of right hip** CC H5 HCC

6 ✓7th **S73.025 Obturator dislocation of left hip** CC H5 HCC

6 ✓7th S73.026 Obturator dislocation of unspecified hip CC H5 HCC

✓6th S73.03 Other anterior subluxation and dislocation of hip

6 ✓7th S73.031 Other anterior subluxation of right hip CC H5 HCC

6 ✓7th S73.032 Other anterior subluxation of left hip CC H5 HCC

6 ✓7th S73.033 Other anterior subluxation of unspecified hip CC H5 HCC

6 ✓7th S73.034 Other anterior dislocation of right hip CC H5 HCC

6 ✓7th S73.035 Other anterior dislocation of left hip CC H5 HCC

6 ✓7th S73.036 Other anterior dislocation of unspecified hip CC H5 HCC

✓6th S73.04 Central subluxation and dislocation of hip

6 ✓7th S73.041 Central subluxation of right hip CC H5 HCC

6 ✓7th S73.042 Central subluxation of left hip CC H5 HCC

6 ✓7th S73.043 Central subluxation of unspecified hip CC H5 HCC

6 ✓7th S73.044 Central dislocation of right hip CC H5 HCC

6 ✓7th S73.045 Central dislocation of left hip CC H5 HCC

6 ✓7th S73.046 Central dislocation of unspecified hip CC H5 HCC

✓5th S73.1 Sprain of hip

AHA: 2014,4Q,25

✓6th S73.10 Unspecified sprain of hip

✓7th S73.101 Unspecified sprain of right hip

✓7th S73.102 Unspecified sprain of left hip

✓7th S73.109 Unspecified sprain of unspecified hip

✓6th S73.11 Iliofemoral ligament sprain of hip

✓7th S73.111 Iliofemoral ligament sprain of right hip

✓7th S73.112 Iliofemoral ligament sprain of left hip

✓7th S73.119 Iliofemoral ligament sprain of unspecified hip

✓6th S73.12 Ischiocapsular (ligament) sprain of hip

✓7th S73.121 Ischiocapsular ligament sprain of right hip

✓7th S73.122 Ischiocapsular ligament sprain of left hip

✓7th S73.129 Ischiocapsular ligament sprain of unspecified hip

✓6th S73.19 Other sprain of hip

✓7th S73.191 Other sprain of right hip

✓7th S73.192 Other sprain of left hip

✓7th S73.199 Other sprain of unspecified hip

✓4th S74 Injury of nerves at hip and thigh level

Code also any associated open wound (S71.-)

EXCLUDES 2 *injury of nerves at ankle and foot level (S94.-)*
injury of nerves at lower leg level (S84.-)

The appropriate 7th character is to be added to each code from category S74.
A initial encounter
D subsequent encounter
S sequela

✓5th S74.0 Injury of sciatic nerve at hip and thigh level

✓x7th S74.00 Injury of sciatic nerve at hip and thigh level, unspecified leg

✓x7th S74.01 Injury of sciatic nerve at hip and thigh level, right leg

✓x7th S74.02 Injury of sciatic nerve at hip and thigh level, left leg

✓5th S74.1 Injury of femoral nerve at hip and thigh level

✓x7th S74.10 Injury of femoral nerve at hip and thigh level, unspecified leg

✓x7th S74.11 Injury of femoral nerve at hip and thigh level, right leg

✓x7th S74.12 Injury of femoral nerve at hip and thigh level, left leg

✓5th S74.2 Injury of cutaneous sensory nerve at hip and thigh level

✓x7th S74.20 Injury of cutaneous sensory nerve at hip and thigh level, unspecified leg

✓x7th S74.21 Injury of cutaneous sensory nerve at hip and high level, right leg

✓x7th S74.22 Injury of cutaneous sensory nerve at hip and thigh level, left leg

✓5th S74.8 Injury of other nerves at hip and thigh level

✓6th S74.8X Injury of other nerves at hip and thigh level

✓7th S74.8X1 Injury of other nerves at hip and thigh level, right leg

✓7th S74.8X2 Injury of other nerves at hip and thigh level, left leg

✓7th S74.8X9 Injury of other nerves at hip and thigh level, unspecified leg

✓5th S74.9 Injury of unspecified nerve at hip and thigh level

✓x7th S74.90 Injury of unspecified nerve at hip and thigh level, unspecified leg

✓x7th S74.91 Injury of unspecified nerve at hip and thigh level, right leg

✓x7th S74.92 Injury of unspecified nerve at hip and thigh level, left leg

✓4th S75 Injury of blood vessels at hip and thigh level

Code also any associated open wound (S71.-)

EXCLUDES 2 *injury of blood vessels at lower leg level (S85.-)*
injury of popliteal artery (S85.0)

The appropriate 7th character is to be added to each code from category S75.
A initial encounter
D subsequent encounter
S sequela

✓5th S75.0 Injury of femoral artery

✓6th S75.00 Unspecified injury of femoral artery

✓7th S75.001 Unspecified injury of femoral artery, right leg MCC

✓7th S75.002 Unspecified injury of femoral artery, left leg MCC

✓7th S75.009 Unspecified injury of femoral artery, unspecified leg MCC

✓6th S75.01 Minor laceration of femoral artery

Incomplete transection of femoral artery
Laceration of femoral artery NOS
Superficial laceration of femoral artery

✓7th S75.011 Minor laceration of femoral artery, right leg MCC

✓7th S75.012 Minor laceration of femoral artery, left leg MCC

✓7th S75.019 Minor laceration of femoral artery, unspecified leg MCC

✓6th S75.02 Major laceration of femoral artery

Complete transection of femoral artery
Traumatic rupture of femoral artery

✓7th S75.021 Major laceration of femoral artery, right leg MCC

✓7th S75.022 Major laceration of femoral artery, left leg MCC

✓7th S75.029 Major laceration of femoral artery, unspecified leg MCC

✓6th S75.09 Other specified injury of femoral artery

✓7th S75.091 Other specified injury of femoral artery, right leg MCC

✓7th S75.092 Other specified injury of femoral artery, left leg MCC

✓7th S75.099 Other specified injury of femoral artery, unspecified leg MCC

✓5th S75.1 Injury of femoral vein at hip and thigh level

✓6th S75.10 Unspecified injury of femoral vein at hip and thigh level

✓7th S75.101 Unspecified injury of femoral vein at hip and thigh level, right leg MCC

✓7th S75.102 Unspecified injury of femoral vein at hip and thigh level, left leg MCC

✓7th S75.109 Unspecified injury of femoral vein at hip and thigh level, unspecified leg MCC

S75.11 **Minor laceration of femoral vein at hip and thigh level**
Incomplete transection of femoral vein at hip and thigh level
Laceration of femoral vein at hip and thigh level NOS
Superficial laceration of femoral vein at hip and thigh level
S75.111 **Minor laceration of femoral vein at hip and thigh level, right leg** MCC
S75.112 **Minor laceration of femoral vein at hip and thigh level, left leg** MCC
S75.119 **Minor laceration of femoral vein at hip and thigh level, unspecified leg** MCC
S75.12 **Major laceration of femoral vein at hip and thigh level**
Complete transection of femoral vein at hip and thigh level
Traumatic rupture of femoral vein at hip and thigh level
S75.121 **Major laceration of femoral vein at hip and thigh level, right leg** MCC
S75.122 **Major laceration of femoral vein at hip and thigh level, left leg** MCC
S75.129 **Major laceration of femoral vein at hip and thigh level, unspecified leg** MCC
S75.19 **Other specified injury of femoral vein at hip and thigh level**
S75.191 **Other specified injury of femoral vein at hip and thigh level, right leg** MCC
S75.192 **Other specified injury of femoral vein at hip and thigh level, left leg** MCC
S75.199 **Other specified injury of femoral vein at hip and thigh level, unspecified leg** MCC
S75.2 **Injury of greater saphenous vein at hip and thigh level**
EXCLUDES 1 *greater saphenous vein NOS (S85.3)*
S75.20 **Unspecified injury of greater saphenous vein at hip and thigh level**
S75.201 **Unspecified injury of greater saphenous vein at hip and thigh level, right leg** CC
S75.202 **Unspecified injury of greater saphenous vein at hip and thigh level, left leg** CC
S75.209 **Unspecified injury of greater saphenous vein at hip and thigh level, unspecified leg** CC
S75.21 **Minor laceration of greater saphenous vein at hip and thigh level**
Incomplete transection of greater saphenous vein at hip and thigh level
Laceration of greater saphenous vein at hip and thigh level NOS
Superficial laceration of greater saphenous vein at hip and thigh level
S75.211 **Minor laceration of greater saphenous vein at hip and thigh level, right leg** CC
S75.212 **Minor laceration of greater saphenous vein at hip and thigh level, left leg** CC
S75.219 **Minor laceration of greater saphenous vein at hip and thigh level, unspecified leg** CC
S75.22 **Major laceration of greater saphenous vein at hip and thigh level**
Complete transection of greater saphenous vein at hip and thigh level
Traumatic rupture of greater saphenous vein at hip and thigh level
S75.221 **Major laceration of greater saphenous vein at hip and thigh level, right leg** CC
S75.222 **Major laceration of greater saphenous vein at hip and thigh level, left leg** CC
S75.229 **Major laceration of greater saphenous vein at hip and thigh level, unspecified leg** CC
S75.29 **Other specified injury of greater saphenous vein at hip and thigh level**
S75.291 **Other specified injury of greater saphenous vein at hip and thigh level, right leg** CC
S75.292 **Other specified injury of greater saphenous vein at hip and thigh level, left leg** CC
S75.299 **Other specified injury of greater saphenous vein at hip and thigh level, unspecified leg** CC
S75.8 **Injury of other blood vessels at hip and thigh level**
S75.80 **Unspecified injury of other blood vessels at hip and thigh level**
S75.801 **Unspecified injury of other blood vessels at hip and thigh level, right leg** CC
S75.802 **Unspecified injury of other blood vessels at hip and thigh level, left leg** CC
S75.809 **Unspecified injury of other blood vessels at hip and thigh level, unspecified leg** CC
S75.81 **Laceration of other blood vessels at hip and thigh level**
S75.811 **Laceration of other blood vessels at hip and thigh level, right leg** CC
S75.812 **Laceration of other blood vessels at hip and thigh level, left leg** CC
S75.819 **Laceration of other blood vessels at hip and thigh level, unspecified leg** CC
S75.89 **Other specified injury of other blood vessels at hip and thigh level**
S75.891 **Other specified injury of other blood vessels at hip and thigh level, right leg** CC
S75.892 **Other specified injury of other blood vessels at hip and thigh level, left leg** CC
S75.899 **Other specified injury of other blood vessels at hip and thigh level, unspecified leg** CC
S75.9 **Injury of unspecified blood vessel at hip and thigh level**
S75.90 **Unspecified injury of unspecified blood vessel at hip and thigh level**
S75.901 **Unspecified injury of unspecified blood vessel at hip and thigh level, right leg** CC
S75.902 **Unspecified injury of unspecified blood vessel at hip and thigh level, left leg** CC
S75.909 **Unspecified injury of unspecified blood vessel at hip and thigh level, unspecified leg** CC
S75.91 **Laceration of unspecified blood vessel at hip and thigh level**
S75.911 **Laceration of unspecified blood vessel at hip and thigh level, right leg** CC
S75.912 **Laceration of unspecified blood vessel at hip and thigh level, left leg** CC
S75.919 **Laceration of unspecified blood vessel at hip and thigh level, unspecified leg** CC
S75.99 **Other specified injury of unspecified blood vessel at hip and thigh level**
S75.991 **Other specified injury of unspecified blood vessel at hip and thigh level, right leg** CC
S75.992 **Other specified injury of unspecified blood vessel at hip and thigh level, left leg** CC
S75.999 **Other specified injury of unspecified blood vessel at hip and thigh level, unspecified leg** CC

4th S76 Injury of muscle, fascia and tendon at hip and thigh level

Code also any associated open wound (S71.-)

EXCLUDES 2 *injury of muscle, fascia and tendon at lower leg level (S86)*
sprain of joint and ligament of hip (S73.1)

TIP: Refer to the Muscle/Tendon table at the beginning of this chapter.

The appropriate 7th character is to be added to each code from category S76.
A initial encounter
D subsequent encounter
S sequela

5th S76.0 Injury of muscle, fascia and tendon of hip
- **6th S76.00 Unspecified injury of muscle, fascia and tendon of hip**
  - **7th S76.001 Unspecified injury of muscle, fascia and tendon of right hip**
  - **7th S76.002 Unspecified injury of muscle, fascia and tendon of left hip**
  - **7th S76.009 Unspecified injury of muscle, fascia and tendon of unspecified hip**
- **6th S76.01 Strain of muscle, fascia and tendon of hip**
  - **7th S76.011 Strain of muscle, fascia and tendon of right hip**
  - **7th S76.012 Strain of muscle, fascia and tendon of left hip**
  - **7th S76.019 Strain of muscle, fascia and tendon of unspecified hip**
- **6th S76.02 Laceration of muscle, fascia and tendon of hip**
  - **7th S76.021 Laceration of muscle, fascia and tendon of right hip** CC
  - **7th S76.022 Laceration of muscle, fascia and tendon of left hip** CC
  - **7th S76.029 Laceration of muscle, fascia and tendon of unspecified hip** CC
- **6th S76.09 Other specified injury of muscle, fascia and tendon of hip**
  - **7th S76.091 Other specified injury of muscle, fascia and tendon of right hip**
  - **7th S76.092 Other specified injury of muscle, fascia and tendon of left hip**
  - **7th S76.099 Other specified injury of muscle, fascia and tendon of unspecified hip**

5th S76.1 Injury of quadriceps muscle, fascia and tendon

Injury of patellar ligament (tendon)
- **6th S76.10 Unspecified injury of quadriceps muscle, fascia and tendon**
  - **7th S76.101 Unspecified injury of right quadriceps muscle, fascia and tendon**
  - **7th S76.102 Unspecified injury of left quadriceps muscle, fascia and tendon**
  - **7th S76.109 Unspecified injury of unspecified quadriceps muscle, fascia and tendon**
- **6th S76.11 Strain of quadriceps muscle, fascia and tendon**
  - **7th S76.111 Strain of right quadriceps muscle, fascia and tendon**
  - **7th S76.112 Strain of left quadriceps muscle, fascia and tendon**
  - **7th S76.119 Strain of unspecified quadriceps muscle, fascia and tendon**
- **6th S76.12 Laceration of quadriceps muscle, fascia and tendon**
  - **7th S76.121 Laceration of right quadriceps muscle, fascia and tendon** CC
  - **7th S76.122 Laceration of left quadriceps muscle, fascia and tendon** CC
  - **7th S76.129 Laceration of unspecified quadriceps muscle, fascia and tendon** CC
- **6th S76.19 Other specified injury of quadriceps muscle, fascia and tendon**
  - **7th S76.191 Other specified injury of right quadriceps muscle, fascia and tendon**
  - **7th S76.192 Other specified injury of left quadriceps muscle, fascia and tendon**
  - **7th S76.199 Other specified injury of unspecified quadriceps muscle, fascia and tendon**

5th S76.2 Injury of adductor muscle, fascia and tendon of thigh
- **6th S76.20 Unspecified injury of adductor muscle, fascia and tendon of thigh**
  - **7th S76.201 Unspecified injury of adductor muscle, fascia and tendon of right thigh**
  - **7th S76.202 Unspecified injury of adductor muscle, fascia and tendon of left thigh**
  - **7th S76.209 Unspecified injury of adductor muscle, fascia and tendon of unspecified thigh**
- **6th S76.21 Strain of adductor muscle, fascia and tendon of thigh**
  - **7th S76.211 Strain of adductor muscle, fascia and tendon of right thigh**
  - **7th S76.212 Strain of adductor muscle, fascia and tendon of left thigh**
  - **7th S76.219 Strain of adductor muscle, fascia and tendon of unspecified thigh**
- **6th S76.22 Laceration of adductor muscle, fascia and tendon of thigh**
  - **7th S76.221 Laceration of adductor muscle, fascia and tendon of right thigh** CC
  - **7th S76.222 Laceration of adductor muscle, fascia and tendon of left thigh** CC
  - **7th S76.229 Laceration of adductor muscle, fascia and tendon of unspecified thigh** CC
- **6th S76.29 Other injury of adductor muscle, fascia and tendon of thigh**
  - **7th S76.291 Other injury of adductor muscle, fascia and tendon of right thigh**
  - **7th S76.292 Other injury of adductor muscle, fascia and tendon of left thigh**
  - **7th S76.299 Other injury of adductor muscle, fascia and tendon of unspecified thigh**

5th S76.3 Injury of muscle, fascia and tendon of the posterior muscle group at thigh level
- **6th S76.30 Unspecified injury of muscle, fascia and tendon of the posterior muscle group at thigh level**
  - **7th S76.301 Unspecified injury of muscle, fascia and tendon of the posterior muscle group at thigh level, right thigh**
  - **7th S76.302 Unspecified injury of muscle, fascia and tendon of the posterior muscle group at thigh level, left thigh**
  - **7th S76.309 Unspecified injury of muscle, fascia and tendon of the posterior muscle group at thigh level, unspecified thigh**
- **6th S76.31 Strain of muscle, fascia and tendon of the posterior muscle group at thigh level**
  - **7th S76.311 Strain of muscle, fascia and tendon of the posterior muscle group at thigh level, right thigh**
  - **7th S76.312 Strain of muscle, fascia and tendon of the posterior muscle group at thigh level, left thigh**
  - **7th S76.319 Strain of muscle, fascia and tendon of the posterior muscle group at thigh level, unspecified thigh**
- **6th S76.32 Laceration of muscle, fascia and tendon of the posterior muscle group at thigh level**
  - **7th S76.321 Laceration of muscle, fascia and tendon of the posterior muscle group at thigh level, right thigh** CC
  - **7th S76.322 Laceration of muscle, fascia and tendon of the posterior muscle group at thigh level, left thigh** CC
  - **7th S76.329 Laceration of muscle, fascia and tendon of the posterior muscle group at thigh level, unspecified thigh** CC
- **6th S76.39 Other specified injury of muscle, fascia and tendon of the posterior muscle group at thigh level**
  - **7th S76.391 Other specified injury of muscle, fascia and tendon of the posterior muscle group at thigh level, right thigh**
  - **7th S76.392 Other specified injury of muscle, fascia and tendon of the posterior muscle group at thigh level, left thigh**
  - **7th S76.399 Other specified injury of muscle, fascia and tendon of the posterior muscle group at thigh level, unspecified thigh**

5th S76.8 Injury of other specified muscles, fascia and tendons at thigh level
- **6th S76.80 Unspecified injury of other specified muscles, fascia and tendons at thigh level**
  - **7th S76.801 Unspecified injury of other specified muscles, fascia and tendons at thigh level, right thigh**
  - **7th S76.802 Unspecified injury of other specified muscles, fascia and tendons at thigh level, left thigh**

S76.809 Unspecified injury of other specified muscles, fascia and tendons at thigh level, unspecified thigh

S76.81 Strain of other specified muscles, fascia and tendons at thigh level

S76.811 Strain of other specified muscles, fascia and tendons at thigh level, right thigh

S76.812 Strain of other specified muscles, fascia and tendons at thigh level, left thigh

S76.819 Strain of other specified muscles, fascia and tendons at thigh level, unspecified thigh

S76.82 Laceration of other specified muscles, fascia and tendons at thigh level

S76.821 Laceration of other specified muscles, fascia and tendons at thigh level, right thigh CC

S76.822 Laceration of other specified muscles, fascia and tendons at thigh level, left thigh CC

S76.829 Laceration of other specified muscles, fascia and tendons at thigh level, unspecified thigh CC

S76.89 Other injury of other specified muscles, fascia and tendons at thigh level

S76.891 Other injury of other specified muscles, fascia and tendons at thigh level, right thigh

S76.892 Other injury of other specified muscles, fascia and tendons at thigh level, left thigh

S76.899 Other injury of other specified muscles, fascia and tendons at thigh level, unspecified thigh

S76.9 Injury of unspecified muscles, fascia and tendons at thigh level

S76.90 Unspecified injury of unspecified muscles, fascia and tendons at thigh level

S76.901 Unspecified injury of unspecified muscles, fascia and tendons at thigh level, right thigh

S76.902 Unspecified injury of unspecified muscles, fascia and tendons at thigh level, left thigh

S76.909 Unspecified injury of unspecified muscles, fascia and tendons at thigh level, unspecified thigh

S76.91 Strain of unspecified muscles, fascia and tendons at thigh level

S76.911 Strain of unspecified muscles, fascia and tendons at thigh level, right thigh

S76.912 Strain of unspecified muscles, fascia and tendons at thigh level, left thigh

S76.919 Strain of unspecified muscles, fascia and tendons at thigh level, unspecified thigh

S76.92 Laceration of unspecified muscles, fascia and tendons at thigh level

S76.921 Laceration of unspecified muscles, fascia and tendons at thigh level, right thigh CC

S76.922 Laceration of unspecified muscles, fascia and tendons at thigh level, left thigh CC

S76.929 Laceration of unspecified muscles, fascia and tendons at thigh level, unspecified thigh CC

S76.99 Other specified injury of unspecified muscles, fascia and tendons at thigh level

S76.991 Other specified injury of unspecified muscles, fascia and tendons at thigh level, right thigh

S76.992 Other specified injury of unspecified muscles, fascia and tendons at thigh level, left thigh

S76.999 Other specified injury of unspecified muscles, fascia and tendons at thigh level, unspecified thigh

S77 Crushing injury of hip and thigh

Use additional code(s) for all associated injuries

EXCLUDES 2 *crushing injury of ankle and foot (S97.-)*
crushing injury of lower leg (S87.-)

The appropriate 7th character is to be added to each code from category S77.
A initial encounter
D subsequent encounter
S sequela

S77.0 Crushing injury of hip

S77.00 Crushing injury of unspecified hip CC H5

S77.01 Crushing injury of right hip CC H5

S77.02 Crushing injury of left hip CC H5

S77.1 Crushing injury of thigh

S77.10 Crushing injury of unspecified thigh CC H5

S77.11 Crushing injury of right thigh CC H5

S77.12 Crushing injury of left thigh CC H5

S77.2 Crushing injury of hip with thigh

S77.20 Crushing injury of unspecified hip with thigh

S77.21 Crushing injury of right hip with thigh

S77.22 Crushing injury of left hip with thigh

S78 Traumatic amputation of hip and thigh

An amputation not identified as partial or complete should be coded to complete

EXCLUDES 1 *traumatic amputation of knee (S88.0-)*

The appropriate 7th character is to be added to each code from category S78.
A initial encounter
D subsequent encounter
S sequela

S78.0 Traumatic amputation at hip joint

S78.01 Complete traumatic amputation at hip joint

S78.011 Complete traumatic amputation at right hip joint CC HCC

S78.012 Complete traumatic amputation at left hip joint CC HCC

S78.019 Complete traumatic amputation at unspecified hip joint CC HCC

S78.02 Partial traumatic amputation at hip joint

S78.021 Partial traumatic amputation at right hip joint CC HCC

S78.022 Partial traumatic amputation at left hip joint CC HCC

S78.029 Partial traumatic amputation at unspecified hip joint CC HCC

S78.1 Traumatic amputation at level between hip and knee

EXCLUDES 1 *traumatic amputation of knee (S88.0-)*

S78.11 Complete traumatic amputation at level between hip and knee

S78.111 Complete traumatic amputation at level between right hip and knee CC HCC

S78.112 Complete traumatic amputation at level between left hip and knee CC HCC

S78.119 Complete traumatic amputation at level between unspecified hip and knee CC HCC

S78.12 Partial traumatic amputation at level between hip and knee

S78.121 Partial traumatic amputation at level between right hip and knee CC HCC

S78.122 Partial traumatic amputation at level between left hip and knee CC HCC

S78.129 Partial traumatic amputation at level between unspecified hip and knee CC HCC

S78.9 Traumatic amputation of hip and thigh, level unspecified

S78.91 Complete traumatic amputation of hip and thigh, level unspecified

S78.911 Complete traumatic amputation of right hip and thigh, level unspecified CC HCC

S78.912 Complete traumatic amputation of left hip and thigh, level unspecified CC HCC

✓7th **S78.919** **Complete traumatic amputation of unspecified hip and thigh, level unspecified** CC HCC

✓6th **S78.92** **Partial traumatic amputation of hip and thigh, level unspecified**

✓7th **S78.921** **Partial traumatic amputation of right hip and thigh, level unspecified** CC HCC

✓7th **S78.922** **Partial traumatic amputation of left hip and thigh, level unspecified** CC HCC

✓7th **S78.929** **Partial traumatic amputation of unspecified hip and thigh, level unspecified** CC HCC

✓4th **S79 Other and unspecified injuries of hip and thigh**

NOTE A fracture not indicated as open or closed should be coded to closed

AHA: 2018,2Q,12; 2018,1Q,3; 2015,3Q,37-39

The appropriate 7th character is to be added to each code from subcategories S79.Ø and S79.1.
- A initial encounter for closed fracture
- D subsequent encounter for fracture with routine healing
- G subsequent encounter for fracture with delayed healing
- K subsequent encounter for fracture with nonunion
- P subsequent encounter for fracture with malunion
- S sequela

✓5th **S79.Ø** **Physeal fracture of upper end of femur**

EXCLUDES 1 *apophyseal fracture of upper end of femur (S72.13-)*
nontraumatic slipped upper femoral epiphysis (M93.Ø-)

AHA: 2019,4Q,56

✓6th **S79.ØØ** **Unspecified physeal fracture of upper end of femur**

4,6 ✓7th **S79.ØØ1** **Unspecified physeal fracture of upper end of right femur** MCC CC H5 HCC

4,6 ✓7th **S79.ØØ2** **Unspecified physeal fracture of upper end of left femur** MCC CC H5 HCC

4,6 ✓7th **S79.ØØ9** **Unspecified physeal fracture of upper end of unspecified femur** MCC CC H5 HCC

✓6th **S79.Ø1** **Salter-Harris Type I physeal fracture of upper end of femur**

Acute on chronic slipped capital femoral epiphysis (traumatic)
Acute slipped capital femoral epiphysis (traumatic)
Capital femoral epiphyseal fracture

EXCLUDES 1 *chronic slipped upper femoral epiphysis (nontraumatic) (M93.Ø2-)*

4,6 ✓7th **S79.Ø11** **Salter-Harris Type I physeal fracture of upper end of right femur** MCC CC H5 HCC

4,6 ✓7th **S79.Ø12** **Salter-Harris Type I physeal fracture of upper end of left femur** MCC CC H5 HCC

4,6 ✓7th **S79.Ø19** **Salter-Harris Type I physeal fracture of upper end of unspecified femur** MCC CC H5 HCC

✓6th **S79.Ø9** **Other physeal fracture of upper end of femur**

4,6 ✓7th **S79.Ø91** **Other physeal fracture of upper end of right femur** MCC CC H5 HCC

4,6 ✓7th **S79.Ø92** **Other physeal fracture of upper end of left femur** MCC CC H5 HCC

4,6 ✓7th **S79.Ø99** **Other physeal fracture of upper end of unspecified femur** MCC CC H5 HCC

✓5th **S79.1** **Physeal fracture of lower end of femur**

AHA: 2019,4Q,56

✓6th **S79.1Ø** **Unspecified physeal fracture of lower end of femur**

3,6 ✓7th **S79.1Ø1** **Unspecified physeal fracture of lower end of right femur** CC H5 HCC

3,6 ✓7th **S79.1Ø2** **Unspecified physeal fracture of lower end of left femur** CC H5 HCC

3,6 ✓7th **S79.1Ø9** **Unspecified physeal fracture of lower end of unspecified femur** CC H5 HCC

✓6th **S79.11** **Salter-Harris Type I physeal fracture of lower end of femur**

3,6 ✓7th **S79.111** **Salter-Harris Type I physeal fracture of lower end of right femur** CC H5 HCC

3,6 ✓7th **S79.112** **Salter-Harris Type I physeal fracture of lower end of left femur** CC H5 HCC

3,6 ✓7th **S79.119** **Salter-Harris Type I physeal fracture of lower end of unspecified femur** CC H5 HCC

✓6th **S79.12** **Salter-Harris Type II physeal fracture of lower end of femur**

3,6 ✓7th **S79.121** **Salter-Harris Type II physeal fracture of lower end of right femur** CC H5 HCC

3,6 ✓7th **S79.122** **Salter-Harris Type II physeal fracture of lower end of left femur** CC H5 HCC

3,6 ✓7th **S79.129** **Salter-Harris Type II physeal fracture of lower end of unspecified femur** CC H5 HCC

✓6th **S79.13** **Salter-Harris Type III physeal fracture of lower end of femur**

3,6 ✓7th **S79.131** **Salter-Harris Type III physeal fracture of lower end of right femur** CC H5 HCC

3,6 ✓7th **S79.132** **Salter-Harris Type III physeal fracture of lower end of left femur** CC H5 HCC

3,6 ✓7th **S79.139** **Salter-Harris Type III physeal fracture of lower end of unspecified femur** CC H5 HCC

✓6th **S79.14** **Salter-Harris Type IV physeal fracture of lower end of femur**

3,6 ✓7th **S79.141** **Salter-Harris Type IV physeal fracture of lower end of right femur** CC H5 HCC

3,6 ✓7th **S79.142** **Salter-Harris Type IV physeal fracture of lower end of left femur** CC H5 HCC

3,6 ✓7th **S79.149** **Salter-Harris Type IV physeal fracture of lower end of unspecified femur** CC H5 HCC

✓6th **S79.19** **Other physeal fracture of lower end of femur**

3,6 ✓7th **S79.191** **Other physeal fracture of lower end of right femur** CC H5 HCC

3,6 ✓7th **S79.192** **Other physeal fracture of lower end of left femur** CC H5 HCC

3,6 ✓7th **S79.199** **Other physeal fracture of lower end of unspecified femur** CC H5 HCC

✓5th **S79.8** **Other specified injuries of hip and thigh**

The appropriate 7th character is to be added to each code in subcategory S79.8.
- A initial encounter
- D subsequent encounter
- S sequela

✓6th **S79.81** **Other specified injuries of hip**

✓7th **S79.811** **Other specified injuries of right hip**

✓7th **S79.812** **Other specified injuries of left hip**

✓7th **S79.819** **Other specified injuries of unspecified hip**

✓6th **S79.82** **Other specified injuries of thigh**

✓7th **S79.821** **Other specified injuries of right thigh**

✓7th **S79.822** **Other specified injuries of left thigh**

✓7th **S79.829** **Other specified injuries of unspecified thigh**

✓5th **S79.9** **Unspecified injury of hip and thigh**

The appropriate 7th character is to be added to each code in subcategory S79.9.
- A initial encounter
- D subsequent encounter
- S sequela

✓6th **S79.91** **Unspecified injury of hip**

✓7th **S79.911** **Unspecified injury of right hip**

✓7th **S79.912** **Unspecified injury of left hip**

✓7th **S79.919** **Unspecified injury of unspecified hip**

✓6th **S79.92** **Unspecified injury of thigh**

✓7th **S79.921** **Unspecified injury of right thigh**

✓7th **S79.922** **Unspecified injury of left thigh**

✓7th **S79.929** **Unspecified injury of unspecified thigh**

Injuries to the knee and lower leg (S80-S89)

EXCLUDES 2 *burns and corrosions (T20-T32)*
frostbite (T33-T34)
injuries of ankle and foot, except fracture of ankle and malleolus (S90-S99)
insect bite or sting, venomous (T63.4)

4th S80 Superficial injury of knee and lower leg

EXCLUDES 2 *superficial injury of ankle and foot (S90.-)*

The appropriate 7th character is to be added to each code from category S80.
A initial encounter
D subsequent encounter
S sequela

5th S80.0 Contusion of knee
- x7th **S80.00 Contusion of unspecified knee**
- x7th **S80.01 Contusion of right knee**
- x7th **S80.02 Contusion of left knee**

5th S80.1 Contusion of lower leg
- x7th **S80.10 Contusion of unspecified lower leg**
- x7th **S80.11 Contusion of right lower leg**
- x7th **S80.12 Contusion of left lower leg**

5th S80.2 Other superficial injuries of knee

6th S80.21 Abrasion of knee
- 7th **S80.211 Abrasion, right knee**
- 7th **S80.212 Abrasion, left knee**
- 7th **S80.219 Abrasion, unspecified knee**

6th S80.22 Blister (nonthermal) of knee
- 7th **S80.221 Blister (nonthermal), right knee**
- 7th **S80.222 Blister (nonthermal), left knee**
- 7th **S80.229 Blister (nonthermal), unspecified knee**

6th S80.24 External constriction of knee
- 7th **S80.241 External constriction, right knee**
- 7th **S80.242 External constriction, left knee**
- 7th **S80.249 External constriction, unspecified knee**

6th S80.25 Superficial foreign body of knee

Splinter in the knee
- 7th **S80.251 Superficial foreign body, right knee**
- 7th **S80.252 Superficial foreign body, left knee**
- 7th **S80.259 Superficial foreign body, unspecified knee**

6th S80.26 Insect bite (nonvenomous) of knee
- 7th **S80.261 Insect bite (nonvenomous), right knee**
- 7th **S80.262 Insect bite (nonvenomous), left knee**
- 7th **S80.269 Insect bite (nonvenomous), unspecified knee**

6th S80.27 Other superficial bite of knee

EXCLUDES 1 *open bite of knee (S81.05-)*
- 7th **S80.271 Other superficial bite of right knee**
- 7th **S80.272 Other superficial bite of left knee**
- 7th **S80.279 Other superficial bite of unspecified knee**

5th S80.8 Other superficial injuries of lower leg

6th S80.81 Abrasion of lower leg
- 7th **S80.811 Abrasion, right lower leg**
- 7th **S80.812 Abrasion, left lower leg**
- 7th **S80.819 Abrasion, unspecified lower leg**

6th S80.82 Blister (nonthermal) of lower leg
- 7th **S80.821 Blister (nonthermal), right lower leg**
- 7th **S80.822 Blister (nonthermal), left lower leg**
- 7th **S80.829 Blister (nonthermal), unspecified lower leg**

6th S80.84 External constriction of lower leg
- 7th **S80.841 External constriction, right lower leg**
- 7th **S80.842 External constriction, left lower leg**
- 7th **S80.849 External constriction, unspecified lower leg**

6th S80.85 Superficial foreign body of lower leg

Splinter in the lower leg
- 7th **S80.851 Superficial foreign body, right lower leg**
- 7th **S80.852 Superficial foreign body, left lower leg**
- 7th **S80.859 Superficial foreign body, unspecified lower leg**

6th S80.86 Insect bite (nonvenomous) of lower leg
- 7th **S80.861 Insect bite (nonvenomous), right lower leg**
- 7th **S80.862 Insect bite (nonvenomous), left lower leg**
- 7th **S80.869 Insect bite (nonvenomous), unspecified lower leg**

6th S80.87 Other superficial bite of lower leg

EXCLUDES 1 *open bite of lower leg (S81.85-)*
- 7th **S80.871 Other superficial bite, right lower leg**
- 7th **S80.872 Other superficial bite, left lower leg**
- 7th **S80.879 Other superficial bite, unspecified lower leg**

5th S80.9 Unspecified superficial injury of knee and lower leg

6th S80.91 Unspecified superficial injury of knee
- 7th **S80.911 Unspecified superficial injury of right knee**
- 7th **S80.912 Unspecified superficial injury of left knee**
- 7th **S80.919 Unspecified superficial injury of unspecified knee**

6th S80.92 Unspecified superficial injury of lower leg
- 7th **S80.921 Unspecified superficial injury of right lower leg**
- 7th **S80.922 Unspecified superficial injury of left lower leg**
- 7th **S80.929 Unspecified superficial injury of unspecified lower leg**

4th S81 Open wound of knee and lower leg

Code also any associated wound infection

EXCLUDES 1 *open fracture of knee and lower leg (S82.-)*
traumatic amputation of lower leg (S88.-)

EXCLUDES 2 *open wound of ankle and foot (S91.-)*

The appropriate 7th character is to be added to each code from category S81.
A initial encounter
D subsequent encounter
S sequela

5th S81.0 Open wound of knee

6th S81.00 Unspecified open wound of knee
- 7th **S81.001 Unspecified open wound, right knee**
- 7th **S81.002 Unspecified open wound, left knee**
- 7th **S81.009 Unspecified open wound, unspecified knee**

6th S81.01 Laceration without foreign body of knee
- 7th **S81.011 Laceration without foreign body, right knee**
- 7th **S81.012 Laceration without foreign body, left knee**
- 7th **S81.019 Laceration without foreign body, unspecified knee**

6th S81.02 Laceration with foreign body of knee
- 7th **S81.021 Laceration with foreign body, right knee**
- 7th **S81.022 Laceration with foreign body, left knee**
- 7th **S81.029 Laceration with foreign body, unspecified knee**

6th S81.03 Puncture wound without foreign body of knee
- 7th **S81.031 Puncture wound without foreign body, right knee**
- 7th **S81.032 Puncture wound without foreign body, left knee**
- 7th **S81.039 Puncture wound without foreign body, unspecified knee**

6th S81.04 Puncture wound with foreign body of knee
- 7th **S81.041 Puncture wound with foreign body, right knee**
- 7th **S81.042 Puncture wound with foreign body, left knee**
- 7th **S81.049 Puncture wound with foreign body, unspecified knee**

6th S81.05 Open bite of knee

Bite of knee NOS

EXCLUDES 1 *superficial bite of knee (S80.27-)*
- 7th **S81.051 Open bite, right knee**

√7th **S81.052 Open bite, left knee**

√7th **S81.059 Open bite, unspecified knee**

√5th **S81.8 Open wound of lower leg**

√6th **S81.80 Unspecified open wound of lower leg**

AHA: 2016,3Q,24

√7th **S81.801 Unspecified open wound, right lower leg**

√7th **S81.802 Unspecified open wound, left lower leg**

√7th **S81.809 Unspecified open wound, unspecified lower leg**

√6th **S81.81 Laceration without foreign body of lower leg**

√7th **S81.811 Laceration without foreign body, right lower leg**

√7th **S81.812 Laceration without foreign body, left lower leg**

√7th **S81.819 Laceration without foreign body, unspecified lower leg**

√6th **S81.82 Laceration with foreign body of lower leg**

√7th **S81.821 Laceration with foreign body, right lower leg**

√7th **S81.822 Laceration with foreign body, left lower leg**

√7th **S81.829 Laceration with foreign body, unspecified lower leg**

√6th **S81.83 Puncture wound without foreign body of lower leg**

AHA: 2016,3Q,24

√7th **S81.831 Puncture wound without foreign body, right lower leg**

√7th **S81.832 Puncture wound without foreign body, left lower leg**

√7th **S81.839 Puncture wound without foreign body, unspecified lower leg**

√6th **S81.84 Puncture wound with foreign body of lower leg**

AHA: 2016,3Q,24

√7th **S81.841 Puncture wound with foreign body, right lower leg**

√7th **S81.842 Puncture wound with foreign body, left lower leg**

√7th **S81.849 Puncture wound with foreign body, unspecified lower leg**

√6th **S81.85 Open bite of lower leg**

Bite of lower leg NOS

EXCLUDES 1 *superficial bite of lower leg (S80.86-, S80.87-)*

√7th **S81.851 Open bite, right lower leg**

√7th **S81.852 Open bite, left lower leg**

√7th **S81.859 Open bite, unspecified lower leg**

√4th **S82 Fracture of lower leg, including ankle**

NOTE A fracture not indicated as displaced or nondisplaced should be coded to displaced

A fracture not indicated as open or closed should be coded to closed

The open fracture designations are based on the Gustilo open fracture classification.

INCLUDES fracture of malleolus

EXCLUDES 1 *traumatic amputation of lower leg (S88.-)*

EXCLUDES 2 *fracture of foot, except ankle (S92.-)*

periprosthetic fracture of prosthetic implant of knee (M97.0-)

AHA: 2018,2Q,12; 2016,1Q,33; 2015,3Q,37-39

DEF: Diaphysis: Central shaft of a long bone.

DEF: Epiphysis: Proximal and distal rounded ends of a long bone, communicates with the joint.

DEF: Metaphysis: Section of a long bone located between the epiphysis and diaphysis at the proximal and distal ends.

DEF: Physis (growth plate): Narrow zone of cartilaginous tissue between the epiphysis and metaphysis at each end of a long bone. In childhood, proliferation of cells in this zone lengthens the bone. As the bone matures, this area thins, ossification eventually fusing into solid bone and growth stops. ***Synonyms:*** *Epiphyseal plate.*

The appropriate 7th character is to be added to all codes from category S82 [unless otherwise indicated].

- A initial encounter for closed fracture
- B initial encounter for open fracture type I or II
  initial encounter for open fracture NOS
- C initial encounter for open fracture type IIIA, IIIB, or IIIC
- D subsequent encounter for closed fracture with routine healing
- E subsequent encounter for open fracture type I or II with routine healing
- F subsequent encounter for open fracture type IIIA, IIIB, or IIIC with routine healing
- G subsequent encounter for closed fracture with delayed healing
- H subsequent encounter for open fracture type I or II with delayed healing
- J subsequent encounter for open fracture type IIIA, IIIB, or IIIC with delayed healing
- K subsequent encounter for closed fracture with nonunion
- M subsequent encounter for open fracture type I or II with nonunion
- N subsequent encounter for open fracture type IIIA, IIIB, or IIIC with nonunion
- P subsequent encounter for closed fracture with malunion
- Q subsequent encounter for open fracture type I or II with malunion
- R subsequent encounter for open fracture type IIIA, IIIB, or IIIC with malunion
- S sequela

√5th **S82.0 Fracture of patella**

Knee cap

√6th **S82.00 Unspecified fracture of patella**

3 √7th **S82.001 Unspecified fracture of right patella** CC H5

3 √7th **S82.002 Unspecified fracture of left patella** CC H5

3 √7th **S82.009 Unspecified fracture of unspecified patella** CC H5

√6th **S82.01 Osteochondral fracture of patella**

3 √7th **S82.011 Displaced osteochondral fracture of right patella** CC H5

3 √7th **S82.012 Displaced osteochondral fracture of left patella** CC H5

3 √7th **S82.013 Displaced osteochondral fracture of unspecified patella** CC H5

3 √7th **S82.014 Nondisplaced osteochondral fracture of right patella** CC H5

3 √7th **S82.015 Nondisplaced osteochondral fracture of left patella** CC H5

3 √7th **S82.016 Nondisplaced osteochondral fracture of unspecified patella** CC H5

√6th **S82.02 Longitudinal fracture of patella**

3 √7th **S82.021 Displaced longitudinal fracture of right patella** CC H5

3 √7th **S82.022 Displaced longitudinal fracture of left patella** CC H5

3 √7th **S82.023 Displaced longitudinal fracture of unspecified patella** CC H5

3 ✓7th S82.024 Nondisplaced longitudinal fracture of right patella CC H5
3 ✓7th S82.025 Nondisplaced longitudinal fracture of left patella CC H5
3 ✓7th S82.026 Nondisplaced longitudinal fracture of unspecified patella CC H5
✓6th S82.03 Transverse fracture of patella
3 ✓7th S82.031 Displaced transverse fracture of right patella CC H5
3 ✓7th S82.032 Displaced transverse fracture of left patella CC H5
3 ✓7th S82.033 Displaced transverse fracture of unspecified patella CC H5
3 ✓7th S82.034 Nondisplaced transverse fracture of right patella CC H5
3 ✓7th S82.035 Nondisplaced transverse fracture of left patella CC H5
3 ✓7th S82.036 Nondisplaced transverse fracture of unspecified patella CC H5
✓6th S82.04 Comminuted fracture of patella
3 ✓7th S82.041 Displaced comminuted fracture of right patella CC H5
3 ✓7th S82.042 Displaced comminuted fracture of left patella CC H5
3 ✓7th S82.043 Displaced comminuted fracture of unspecified patella CC H5
3 ✓7th S82.044 Nondisplaced comminuted fracture of right patella CC H5
3 ✓7th S82.045 Nondisplaced comminuted fracture of left patella CC H5
3 ✓7th S82.046 Nondisplaced comminuted fracture of unspecified patella CC H5
✓6th S82.09 Other fracture of patella
3 ✓7th S82.091 Other fracture of right patella CC H5
3 ✓7th S82.092 Other fracture of left patella CC H5
3 ✓7th S82.099 Other fracture of unspecified patella CC H5
✓5th S82.1 Fracture of upper end of tibia
Fracture of proximal end of tibia
EXCLUDES 2 *fracture of shaft of tibia (S82.2-)*
physeal fracture of upper end of tibia (S89.Ø-)
✓6th S82.10 Unspecified fracture of upper end of tibia
2,3 ✓7th S82.101 Unspecified fracture of upper end of right tibia MCC CC H5
2,3 ✓7th S82.102 Unspecified fracture of upper end of left tibia MCC CC H5
2,3 ✓7th S82.109 Unspecified fracture of upper end of unspecified tibia MCC CC H5
✓6th S82.11 Fracture of tibial spine
2,3 ✓7th S82.111 Displaced fracture of right tibial spine MCC CC H5
2,3 ✓7th S82.112 Displaced fracture of left tibial spine MCC CC H5
2,3 ✓7th S82.113 Displaced fracture of unspecified tibial spine MCC CC H5
2,3 ✓7th S82.114 Nondisplaced fracture of right tibial spine MCC CC H5
2,3 ✓7th S82.115 Nondisplaced fracture of left tibial spine MCC CC H5
2,3 ✓7th S82.116 Nondisplaced fracture of unspecified tibial spine MCC CC H5
✓6th S82.12 Fracture of lateral condyle of tibia
2,3 ✓7th S82.121 Displaced fracture of lateral condyle of right tibia MCC CC H5
2,3 ✓7th S82.122 Displaced fracture of lateral condyle of left tibia MCC CC H5
2,3 ✓7th S82.123 Displaced fracture of lateral condyle of unspecified tibia MCC CC H5
2,3 ✓7th S82.124 Nondisplaced fracture of lateral condyle of right tibia MCC CC H5
2,3 ✓7th S82.125 Nondisplaced fracture of lateral condyle of left tibia MCC CC H5
2,3 ✓7th S82.126 Nondisplaced fracture of lateral condyle of unspecified tibia MCC CC H5
✓6th S82.13 Fracture of medial condyle of tibia
2,3 ✓7th S82.131 Displaced fracture of medial condyle of right tibia MCC CC H5
2,3 ✓7th S82.132 Displaced fracture of medial condyle of left tibia MCC CC H5
2,3 ✓7th S82.133 Displaced fracture of medial condyle of unspecified tibia MCC CC H5
2,3 ✓7th S82.134 Nondisplaced fracture of medial condyle of right tibia MCC CC H5
2,3 ✓7th S82.135 Nondisplaced fracture of medial condyle of left tibia MCC CC H5
2,3 ✓7th S82.136 Nondisplaced fracture of medial condyle of unspecified tibia MCC CC H5
✓6th S82.14 Bicondylar fracture of tibia
Fracture of tibial plateau NOS
2,3 ✓7th S82.141 Displaced bicondylar fracture of right tibia MCC CC H5
2,3 ✓7th S82.142 Displaced bicondylar fracture of left tibia MCC CC H5
2,3 ✓7th S82.143 Displaced bicondylar fracture of unspecified tibia MCC CC H5
2,3 ✓7th S82.144 Nondisplaced bicondylar fracture of right tibia MCC CC H5
2,3 ✓7th S82.145 Nondisplaced bicondylar fracture of left tibia MCC CC H5
2,3 ✓7th S82.146 Nondisplaced bicondylar fracture of unspecified tibia MCC CC H5
✓6th S82.15 Fracture of tibial tuberosity
2,3 ✓7th S82.151 Displaced fracture of right tibial tuberosity MCC CC H5
2,3 ✓7th S82.152 Displaced fracture of left tibial tuberosity MCC CC H5
2,3 ✓7th S82.153 Displaced fracture of unspecified tibial tuberosity MCC CC H5
2,3 ✓7th S82.154 Nondisplaced fracture of right tibial tuberosity MCC CC H5
2,3 ✓7th S82.155 Nondisplaced fracture of left tibial tuberosity MCC CC H5
2,3 ✓7th S82.156 Nondisplaced fracture of unspecified tibial tuberosity MCC CC H5
✓6th S82.16 Torus fracture of upper end of tibia

The appropriate 7th character is to be added to all codes in subcategory S82.16.
A initial encounter for closed fracture
D subsequent encounter for fracture with routine healing
G subsequent encounter for fracture with delayed healing
K subsequent encounter for fracture with nonunion
P subsequent encounter for fracture with malunion
S sequela

3 ✓7th S82.161 Torus fracture of upper end of right tibia CC H5
3 ✓7th S82.162 Torus fracture of upper end of left tibia CC H5
3 ✓7th S82.169 Torus fracture of upper end of unspecified tibia CC H5
✓6th S82.19 Other fracture of upper end of tibia
2,3 ✓7th S82.191 Other fracture of upper end of right tibia MCC CC H5
2,3 ✓7th S82.192 Other fracture of upper end of left tibia MCC CC H5
2,3 ✓7th S82.199 Other fracture of upper end of unspecified tibia MCC CC H5
✓5th S82.2 Fracture of shaft of tibia
✓6th S82.20 Unspecified fracture of shaft of tibia
Fracture of tibia NOS
2,3 ✓7th S82.201 Unspecified fracture of shaft of right tibia MCC CC H5
2,3 ✓7th S82.202 Unspecified fracture of shaft of left tibia MCC CC H5
2,3 ✓7th S82.209 Unspecified fracture of shaft of unspecified tibia MCC CC H5
✓6th S82.22 Transverse fracture of shaft of tibia
2,3 ✓7th S82.221 Displaced transverse fracture of shaft of right tibia MCC CC H5
2,3 ✓7th S82.222 Displaced transverse fracture of shaft of left tibia MCC CC H5

2,3 ✓7th **S82.223** Displaced transverse fracture of shaft of unspecified tibia MCC CC H5
2,3 ✓7th **S82.224** Nondisplaced transverse fracture of shaft of right tibia MCC CC H5
2,3 ✓7th **S82.225** Nondisplaced transverse fracture of shaft of left tibia MCC CC H5
2,3 ✓7th **S82.226** Nondisplaced transverse fracture of shaft of unspecified tibia MCC CC H5

✓6th **S82.23** Oblique fracture of shaft of tibia
2,3 ✓7th **S82.231** Displaced oblique fracture of shaft of right tibia MCC CC H5
2,3 ✓7th **S82.232** Displaced oblique fracture of shaft of left tibia MCC CC H5
2,3 ✓7th **S82.233** Displaced oblique fracture of shaft of unspecified tibia MCC CC H5
2,3 ✓7th **S82.234** Nondisplaced oblique fracture of shaft of right tibia MCC CC H5
2,3 ✓7th **S82.235** Nondisplaced oblique fracture of shaft of left tibia MCC CC H5
2,3 ✓7th **S82.236** Nondisplaced oblique fracture of shaft of unspecified tibia MCC CC H5

✓6th **S82.24** Spiral fracture of shaft of tibia
Toddler fracture
2,3 ✓7th **S82.241** Displaced spiral fracture of shaft of right tibia MCC CC H5
2,3 ✓7th **S82.242** Displaced spiral fracture of shaft of left tibia MCC CC H5
2,3 ✓7th **S82.243** Displaced spiral fracture of shaft of unspecified tibia MCC CC H5
2,3 ✓7th **S82.244** Nondisplaced spiral fracture of shaft of right tibia MCC CC H5
2,3 ✓7th **S82.245** Nondisplaced spiral fracture of shaft of left tibia MCC CC H5
2,3 ✓7th **S82.246** Nondisplaced spiral fracture of shaft of unspecified tibia MCC CC H5

✓6th **S82.25** Comminuted fracture of shaft of tibia
2,3 ✓7th **S82.251** Displaced comminuted fracture of shaft of right tibia MCC CC H5
2,3 ✓7th **S82.252** Displaced comminuted fracture of shaft of left tibia MCC CC H5
2,3 ✓7th **S82.253** Displaced comminuted fracture of shaft of unspecified tibia MCC CC H5
2,3 ✓7th **S82.254** Nondisplaced comminuted fracture of shaft of right tibia MCC CC H5
2,3 ✓7th **S82.255** Nondisplaced comminuted fracture of shaft of left tibia MCC CC H5
2,3 ✓7th **S82.256** Nondisplaced comminuted fracture of shaft of unspecified tibia MCC CC H5

✓6th **S82.26** Segmental fracture of shaft of tibia
2,3 ✓7th **S82.261** Displaced segmental fracture of shaft of right tibia MCC CC H5
2,3 ✓7th **S82.262** Displaced segmental fracture of shaft of left tibia MCC CC H5
2,3 ✓7th **S82.263** Displaced segmental fracture of shaft of unspecified tibia MCC CC H5
2,3 ✓7th **S82.264** Nondisplaced segmental fracture of shaft of right tibia MCC CC H5
2,3 ✓7th **S82.265** Nondisplaced segmental fracture of shaft of left tibia MCC CC H5
2,3 ✓7th **S82.266** Nondisplaced segmental fracture of shaft of unspecified tibia MCC CC H5

✓6th **S82.29** Other fracture of shaft of tibia
2,3 ✓7th **S82.291** Other fracture of shaft of right tibia MCC CC H5
2,3 ✓7th **S82.292** Other fracture of shaft of left tibia MCC CC H5
2,3 ✓7th **S82.299** Other fracture of shaft of unspecified tibia MCC CC H5

✓5th **S82.3** Fracture of lower end of tibia
EXCLUDES 1 *bimalleolar fracture of lower leg (S82.84-)*
fracture of medial malleolus alone (S82.5-)
Maisonneuve's fracture (S82.86-)
pilon fracture of distal tibia (S82.87-)
trimalleolar fractures of lower leg (S82.85-)

✓6th **S82.30** Unspecified fracture of lower end of tibia
3 ✓7th **S82.301** Unspecified fracture of lower end of right tibia CC H5
3 ✓7th **S82.302** Unspecified fracture of lower end of left tibia CC H5
3 ✓7th **S82.309** Unspecified fracture of lower end of unspecified tibia CC H5

✓6th **S82.31** Torus fracture of lower end of tibia

The appropriate 7th character is to be added to all codes in subcategory S82.31.
A initial encounter for closed fracture
D subsequent encounter for fracture with routine healing
G subsequent encounter for fracture with delayed healing
K subsequent encounter for fracture with nonunion
P subsequent encounter for fracture with malunion
S sequela

3 ✓7th **S82.311** Torus fracture of lower end of right tibia CC H5
3 ✓7th **S82.312** Torus fracture of lower end of left tibia CC H5
3 ✓7th **S82.319** Torus fracture of lower end of unspecified tibia CC H5

✓6th **S82.39** Other fracture of lower end of tibia
AHA: 2015,1Q,25
3 ✓7th **S82.391** Other fracture of lower end of right tibia CC H5
3 ✓7th **S82.392** Other fracture of lower end of left tibia CC H5
3 ✓7th **S82.399** Other fracture of lower end of unspecified tibia CC H5

✓5th **S82.4** Fracture of shaft of fibula
EXCLUDES 2 *fracture of lateral malleolus alone (S82.6-)*

✓6th **S82.40** Unspecified fracture of shaft of fibula
2,4 ✓7th **S82.401** Unspecified fracture of shaft of right fibula MCC CC H5
2,4 ✓7th **S82.402** Unspecified fracture of shaft of left fibula MCC CC H5
2,4 ✓7th **S82.409** Unspecified fracture of shaft of unspecified fibula MCC CC H5

✓6th **S82.42** Transverse fracture of shaft of fibula
2,4 ✓7th **S82.421** Displaced transverse fracture of shaft of right fibula MCC CC H5
2,4 ✓7th **S82.422** Displaced transverse fracture of shaft of left fibula MCC CC H5
2,4 ✓7th **S82.423** Displaced transverse fracture of shaft of unspecified fibula MCC CC H5
2,4 ✓7th **S82.424** Nondisplaced transverse fracture of shaft of right fibula MCC CC H5
2,4 ✓7th **S82.425** Nondisplaced transverse fracture of shaft of left fibula MCC CC H5
2,4 ✓7th **S82.426** Nondisplaced transverse fracture of shaft of unspecified fibula MCC CC H5

✓6th **S82.43** Oblique fracture of shaft of fibula
2,4 ✓7th **S82.431** Displaced oblique fracture of shaft of right fibula MCC CC H5
2,4 ✓7th **S82.432** Displaced oblique fracture of shaft of left fibula MCC CC H5
2,4 ✓7th **S82.433** Displaced oblique fracture of shaft of unspecified fibula MCC CC H5
2,4 ✓7th **S82.434** Nondisplaced oblique fracture of shaft of right fibula MCC CC H5
2,4 ✓7th **S82.435** Nondisplaced oblique fracture of shaft of left fibula MCC CC H5
2,4 ✓7th **S82.436** Nondisplaced oblique fracture of shaft of unspecified fibula MCC CC H5

✓6th **S82.44** Spiral fracture of shaft of fibula
2,4 ✓7th **S82.441** Displaced spiral fracture of shaft of right fibula MCC CC H5
2,4 ✓7th **S82.442** Displaced spiral fracture of shaft of left fibula MCC CC H5
2,4 ✓7th **S82.443** Displaced spiral fracture of shaft of unspecified fibula MCC CC H5
2,4 ✓7th **S82.444** Nondisplaced spiral fracture of shaft of right fibula MCC CC H5
2,4 ✓7th **S82.445** Nondisplaced spiral fracture of shaft of left fibula MCC CC H5

2,4 √7th **S82.446** Nondisplaced spiral fracture of shaft of unspecified fibula MCC CC H5

√6th **S82.45** Comminuted fracture of shaft of fibula

2,4 √7th **S82.451** Displaced comminuted fracture of shaft of right fibula MCC CC H5

2,4 √7th **S82.452** Displaced comminuted fracture of shaft of left fibula MCC CC H5

2,4 √7th **S82.453** Displaced comminuted fracture of shaft of unspecified fibula MCC CC H5

2,4 √7th **S82.454** Nondisplaced comminuted fracture of shaft of right fibula MCC CC H5

2,4 √7th **S82.455** Nondisplaced comminuted fracture of shaft of left fibula MCC CC H5

2,4 √7th **S82.456** Nondisplaced comminuted fracture of shaft of unspecified fibula MCC CC H5

√6th **S82.46** Segmental fracture of shaft of fibula

2,4 √7th **S82.461** Displaced segmental fracture of shaft of right fibula MCC CC H5

2,4 √7th **S82.462** Displaced segmental fracture of shaft of left fibula MCC CC H5

2,4 √7th **S82.463** Displaced segmental fracture of shaft of unspecified fibula MCC CC H5

2,4 √7th **S82.464** Nondisplaced segmental fracture of shaft of right fibula MCC CC H5

2,4 √7th **S82.465** Nondisplaced segmental fracture of shaft of left fibula MCC CC H5

2,4 √7th **S82.466** Nondisplaced segmental fracture of shaft of unspecified fibula MCC CC H5

√6th **S82.49** Other fracture of shaft of fibula

2,4 √7th **S82.491** Other fracture of shaft of right fibula MCC CC H5

2,4 √7th **S82.492** Other fracture of shaft of left fibula MCC CC H5

2,4 √7th **S82.499** Other fracture of shaft of unspecified fibula MCC CC H5

√5th **S82.5 Fracture of medial malleolus**

EXCLUDES 1 *pilon fracture of distal tibia (S82.87-)*
Salter-Harris type III of lower end of tibia (S89.13-)
Salter-Harris type IV of lower end of tibia (S89.14-)

3 √x7th **S82.51** Displaced fracture of medial malleolus of right tibia CC H5

3 √x7th **S82.52** Displaced fracture of medial malleolus of left tibia CC H5

3 √x7th **S82.53** Displaced fracture of medial malleolus of unspecified tibia CC H5

3 √x7th **S82.54** Nondisplaced fracture of medial malleolus of right tibia CC H5

3 √x7th **S82.55** Nondisplaced fracture of medial malleolus of left tibia CC H5

3 √x7th **S82.56** Nondisplaced fracture of medial malleolus of unspecified tibia CC H5

√5th **S82.6 Fracture of lateral malleolus**

EXCLUDES 1 *pilon fracture of distal tibia (S82.87-)*

3 √x7th **S82.61** Displaced fracture of lateral malleolus of right fibula CC H5

3 √x7th **S82.62** Displaced fracture of lateral malleolus of left fibula CC H5

3 √x7th **S82.63** Displaced fracture of lateral malleolus of unspecified fibula CC H5

3 √x7th **S82.64** Nondisplaced fracture of lateral malleolus of right fibula CC H5

3 √x7th **S82.65** Nondisplaced fracture of lateral malleolus of left fibula CC H5

3 √x7th **S82.66** Nondisplaced fracture of lateral malleolus of unspecified fibula CC H5

√5th **S82.8 Other fractures of lower leg**

√6th **S82.81** Torus fracture of upper end of fibula

The appropriate 7th character is to be added to all codes in subcategory S82.81
- A initial encounter for closed fracture
- D subsequent encounter for fracture with routine healing
- G subsequent encounter for fracture with delayed healing
- K subsequent encounter for fracture with nonunion
- P subsequent encounter for fracture with malunion
- S sequela

4 √7th **S82.811** Torus fracture of upper end of right fibula CC

4 √7th **S82.812** Torus fracture of upper end of left fibula CC

4 √7th **S82.819** Torus fracture of upper end of unspecified fibula CC

√6th **S82.82** Torus fracture of lower end of fibula

The appropriate 7th character is to be added to all codes in subcategory S82.82.
- A initial encounter for closed fracture
- D subsequent encounter for fracture with routine healing
- G subsequent encounter for fracture with delayed healing
- K subsequent encounter for fracture with nonunion
- P subsequent encounter for fracture with malunion
- S sequela

4 √7th **S82.821** Torus fracture of lower end of right fibula CC

4 √7th **S82.822** Torus fracture of lower end of left fibula CC

4 √7th **S82.829** Torus fracture of lower end of unspecified fibula CC

√6th **S82.83** Other fracture of upper and lower end of fibula

AHA: 2015,1Q,25

2,4 √7th **S82.831** Other fracture of upper and lower end of right fibula MCC CC H5

2,4 √7th **S82.832** Other fracture of upper and lower end of left fibula MCC CC H5

2,4 √7th **S82.839** Other fracture of upper and lower end of unspecified fibula MCC CC H5

Chapter 19. Injury, Poisoning and Certain Other Consequences of External Causes

S82.446–S82.839

✓6th **S82.84 Bimalleolar fracture of lower leg**

Right Bimalleolar Fracture

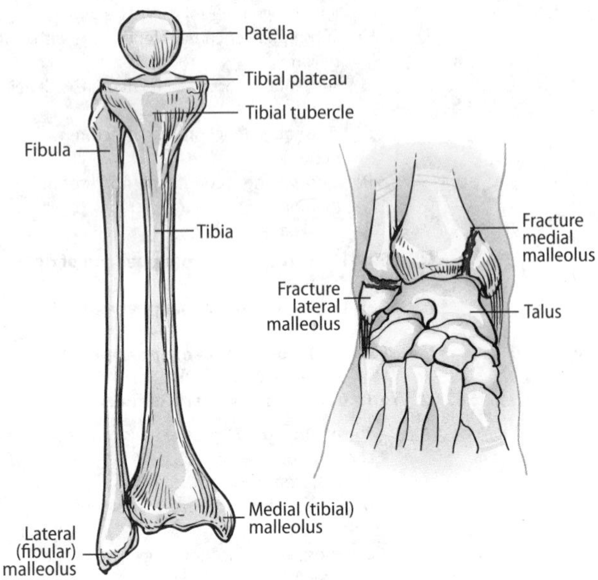

3 ✓7th **S82.841 Displaced bimalleolar fracture of right lower leg** CC H5

3 ✓7th **S82.842 Displaced bimalleolar fracture of left lower leg** CC H5

3 ✓7th **S82.843 Displaced bimalleolar fracture of unspecified lower leg** CC H5

3 ✓7th **S82.844 Nondisplaced bimalleolar fracture of right lower leg** CC H5

3 ✓7th **S82.845 Nondisplaced bimalleolar fracture of left lower leg** CC H5

3 ✓7th **S82.846 Nondisplaced bimalleolar fracture of unspecified lower leg** CC H5

✓6th **S82.85 Trimalleolar fracture of lower leg**

3 ✓7th **S82.851 Displaced trimalleolar fracture of right lower leg** CC H5

3 ✓7th **S82.852 Displaced trimalleolar fracture of left lower leg** CC H5

3 ✓7th **S82.853 Displaced trimalleolar fracture of unspecified lower leg** CC H5

3 ✓7th **S82.854 Nondisplaced trimalleolar fracture of right lower leg** CC H5

3 ✓7th **S82.855 Nondisplaced trimalleolar fracture of left lower leg** CC H5

3 ✓7th **S82.856 Nondisplaced trimalleolar fracture of unspecified lower leg** CC H5

✓6th **S82.86 Maisonneuve's fracture**

2,4 ✓7th **S82.861 Displaced Maisonneuve's fracture of right leg** MCC CC H5

2,4 ✓7th **S82.862 Displaced Maisonneuve's fracture of left leg** MCC CC H5

2,4 ✓7th **S82.863 Displaced Maisonneuve's fracture of unspecified leg** MCC CC H5

2,4 ✓7th **S82.864 Nondisplaced Maisonneuve's fracture of right leg** MCC CC H5

2,4 ✓7th **S82.865 Nondisplaced Maisonneuve's fracture of left leg** MCC CC H5

2,4 ✓7th **S82.866 Nondisplaced Maisonneuve's fracture of unspecified leg** MCC CC H5

✓6th **S82.87 Pilon fracture of tibia**

3 ✓7th **S82.871 Displaced pilon fracture of right tibia** CC H5

3 ✓7th **S82.872 Displaced pilon fracture of left tibia** CC H5

3 ✓7th **S82.873 Displaced pilon fracture of unspecified tibia** CC H5

3 ✓7th **S82.874 Nondisplaced pilon fracture of right tibia** CC H5

3 ✓7th **S82.875 Nondisplaced pilon fracture of left tibia** CC H5

3 ✓7th **S82.876 Nondisplaced pilon fracture of unspecified tibia** CC H5

✓6th **S82.89 Other fractures of lower leg**

Fracture of ankle NOS

3 ✓7th **S82.891 Other fracture of right lower leg** CC H5

3 ✓7th **S82.892 Other fracture of left lower leg** CC H5

3 ✓7th **S82.899 Other fracture of unspecified lower leg** CC H5

✓5th **S82.9 Unspecified fracture of lower leg**

3 ✓x7th **S82.9Ø Unspecified fracture of unspecified lower leg** CC H5

3 ✓x7th **S82.91 Unspecified fracture of right lower leg** CC H5

3 ✓x7th **S82.92 Unspecified fracture of left lower leg** CC H5

✓4th **S83 Dislocation and sprain of joints and ligaments of knee**

INCLUDES avulsion of joint or ligament of knee
laceration of cartilage, joint or ligament of knee
sprain of cartilage, joint or ligament of knee
traumatic hemarthrosis of joint or ligament of knee
traumatic rupture of joint or ligament of knee
traumatic subluxation of joint or ligament of knee
traumatic tear of joint or ligament of knee

Code also any associated open wound

EXCLUDES 1 ~~*derangement of patella (M22.Ø-M22.3)*~~
~~*injury of patellar ligament (tendon) (S76.1-)*~~
~~*internal derangement of knee (M23.-)*~~
~~*old dislocation of knee (M23.8X)*~~
~~*pathological dislocation of knee (M24.36)*~~
~~*recurrent dislocation of knee (M22.Ø)*~~

EXCLUDES 2 ▶*derangement of patella (M22.Ø-M22.3)*◀
▶*injury of patellar ligament (tendon) (S76.1-)*◀
▶*internal derangement of knee (M23.-)*◀
▶*old dislocation of knee (M24.36)*◀
▶*pathological dislocation of knee (M24.36)*◀
▶*recurrent dislocation of knee (M22.Ø)*◀
strain of muscle, fascia and tendon of lower leg (S86.-)

The appropriate 7th character is to be added to each code from category S83.
A initial encounter
D subsequent encounter
S sequela

✓5th **S83.Ø Subluxation and dislocation of patella**

✓6th **S83.ØØ Unspecified subluxation and dislocation of patella**

✓7th **S83.ØØ1 Unspecified subluxation of right patella**

✓7th **S83.ØØ2 Unspecified subluxation of left patella**

✓7th **S83.ØØ3 Unspecified subluxation of unspecified patella**

✓7th **S83.ØØ4 Unspecified dislocation of right patella**

✓7th **S83.ØØ5 Unspecified dislocation of left patella**

✓7th **S83.ØØ6 Unspecified dislocation of unspecified patella**

✓6th **S83.Ø1 Lateral subluxation and dislocation of patella**

✓7th **S83.Ø11 Lateral subluxation of right patella**

✓7th **S83.Ø12 Lateral subluxation of left patella**

✓7th **S83.Ø13 Lateral subluxation of unspecified patella**

✓7th **S83.Ø14 Lateral dislocation of right patella**

✓7th **S83.Ø15 Lateral dislocation of left patella**

✓7th **S83.Ø16 Lateral dislocation of unspecified patella**

✓6th **S83.Ø9 Other subluxation and dislocation of patella**

✓7th **S83.Ø91 Other subluxation of right patella**

✓7th **S83.Ø92 Other subluxation of left patella**

✓7th **S83.Ø93 Other subluxation of unspecified patella**

✓7th **S83.Ø94 Other dislocation of right patella**

✓7th **S83.Ø95 Other dislocation of left patella**

✓7th **S83.Ø96 Other dislocation of unspecified patella**

✓5th **S83.1 Subluxation and dislocation of knee**

EXCLUDES 2 *instability of knee prosthesis (T84.Ø22, T84.Ø23)*

✓6th **S83.1Ø Unspecified subluxation and dislocation of knee**

✓7th **S83.1Ø1 Unspecified subluxation of right knee**

✓7th **S83.1Ø2 Unspecified subluxation of left knee**

✓7th **S83.1Ø3 Unspecified subluxation of unspecified knee**

S83.104 Unspecified dislocation of right knee
S83.105 Unspecified dislocation of left knee
S83.106 Unspecified dislocation of unspecified knee

S83.11 Anterior subluxation and dislocation of proximal end of tibia
Posterior subluxation and dislocation of distal end of femur
S83.111 Anterior subluxation of proximal end of tibia, right knee
S83.112 Anterior subluxation of proximal end of tibia, left knee
S83.113 Anterior subluxation of proximal end of tibia, unspecified knee
S83.114 Anterior dislocation of proximal end of tibia, right knee
S83.115 Anterior dislocation of proximal end of tibia, left knee
S83.116 Anterior dislocation of proximal end of tibia, unspecified knee

S83.12 Posterior subluxation and dislocation of proximal end of tibia
Anterior dislocation of distal end of femur
S83.121 Posterior subluxation of proximal end of tibia, right knee
S83.122 Posterior subluxation of proximal end of tibia, left knee
S83.123 Posterior subluxation of proximal end of tibia, unspecified knee
S83.124 Posterior dislocation of proximal end of tibia, right knee
S83.125 Posterior dislocation of proximal end of tibia, left knee
S83.126 Posterior dislocation of proximal end of tibia, unspecified knee

S83.13 Medial subluxation and dislocation of proximal end of tibia
S83.131 Medial subluxation of proximal end of tibia, right knee
S83.132 Medial subluxation of proximal end of tibia, left knee
S83.133 Medial subluxation of proximal end of tibia, unspecified knee
S83.134 Medial dislocation of proximal end of tibia, right knee
S83.135 Medial dislocation of proximal end of tibia, left knee
S83.136 Medial dislocation of proximal end of tibia, unspecified knee

S83.14 Lateral subluxation and dislocation of proximal end of tibia
S83.141 Lateral subluxation of proximal end of tibia, right knee
S83.142 Lateral subluxation of proximal end of tibia, left knee
S83.143 Lateral subluxation of proximal end of tibia, unspecified knee
S83.144 Lateral dislocation of proximal end of tibia, right knee
S83.145 Lateral dislocation of proximal end of tibia, left knee
S83.146 Lateral dislocation of proximal end of tibia, unspecified knee

S83.19 Other subluxation and dislocation of knee
S83.191 Other subluxation of right knee
S83.192 Other subluxation of left knee
S83.193 Other subluxation of unspecified knee
S83.194 Other dislocation of right knee
S83.195 Other dislocation of left knee
S83.196 Other dislocation of unspecified knee

S83.2 Tear of meniscus, current injury
EXCLUDES 1 *old bucket-handle tear (M23.2)*
AHA: 2019,2Q,26

S83.20 Tear of unspecified meniscus, current injury
Tear of meniscus of knee NOS
S83.200 Bucket-handle tear of unspecified meniscus, current injury, right knee
S83.201 Bucket-handle tear of unspecified meniscus, current injury, left knee
S83.202 Bucket-handle tear of unspecified meniscus, current injury, unspecified knee
S83.203 Other tear of unspecified meniscus, current injury, right knee
S83.204 Other tear of unspecified meniscus, current injury, left knee
S83.205 Other tear of unspecified meniscus, current injury, unspecified knee
S83.206 Unspecified tear of unspecified meniscus, current injury, right knee
S83.207 Unspecified tear of unspecified meniscus, current injury, left knee
S83.209 Unspecified tear of unspecified meniscus, current injury, unspecified knee

S83.21 Bucket-handle tear of medial meniscus, current injury
S83.211 Bucket-handle tear of medial meniscus, current injury, right knee
S83.212 Bucket-handle tear of medial meniscus, current injury, left knee
S83.219 Bucket-handle tear of medial meniscus, current injury, unspecified knee

S83.22 Peripheral tear of medial meniscus, current injury
S83.221 Peripheral tear of medial meniscus, current injury, right knee
S83.222 Peripheral tear of medial meniscus, current injury, left knee
S83.229 Peripheral tear of medial meniscus, current injury, unspecified knee

S83.23 Complex tear of medial meniscus, current injury
S83.231 Complex tear of medial meniscus, current injury, right knee
S83.232 Complex tear of medial meniscus, current injury, left knee
S83.239 Complex tear of medial meniscus, current injury, unspecified knee

S83.24 Other tear of medial meniscus, current injury
S83.241 Other tear of medial meniscus, current injury, right knee
S83.242 Other tear of medial meniscus, current injury, left knee
S83.249 Other tear of medial meniscus, current injury, unspecified knee

S83.25 Bucket-handle tear of lateral meniscus, current injury
S83.251 Bucket-handle tear of lateral meniscus, current injury, right knee
S83.252 Bucket-handle tear of lateral meniscus, current injury, left knee
S83.259 Bucket-handle tear of lateral meniscus, current injury, unspecified knee

S83.26 Peripheral tear of lateral meniscus, current injury
S83.261 Peripheral tear of lateral meniscus, current injury, right knee
S83.262 Peripheral tear of lateral meniscus, current injury, left knee
S83.269 Peripheral tear of lateral meniscus, current injury, unspecified knee

S83.27 Complex tear of lateral meniscus, current injury
S83.271 Complex tear of lateral meniscus, current injury, right knee
S83.272 Complex tear of lateral meniscus, current injury, left knee
S83.279 Complex tear of lateral meniscus, current injury, unspecified knee

S83.28 Other tear of lateral meniscus, current injury
S83.281 Other tear of lateral meniscus, current injury, right knee
S83.282 Other tear of lateral meniscus, current injury, left knee
S83.289 Other tear of lateral meniscus, current injury, unspecified knee

S83.3 Tear of articular cartilage of knee, current
S83.30 Tear of articular cartilage of unspecified knee, current
S83.31 Tear of articular cartilage of right knee, current
S83.32 Tear of articular cartilage of left knee, current

√5th S83.4 **Sprain of collateral ligament of knee**

√6th S83.40 **Sprain of unspecified collateral ligament of knee**

√7th S83.401 **Sprain of unspecified collateral ligament of right knee**

√7th S83.402 **Sprain of unspecified collateral ligament of left knee**

√7th S83.409 **Sprain of unspecified collateral ligament of unspecified knee**

√6th S83.41 **Sprain of medial collateral ligament of knee**

Sprain of tibial collateral ligament

√7th S83.411 **Sprain of medial collateral ligament of right knee**

√7th S83.412 **Sprain of medial collateral ligament of left knee**

√7th S83.419 **Sprain of medial collateral ligament of unspecified knee**

√6th S83.42 **Sprain of lateral collateral ligament of knee**

Sprain of fibular collateral ligament

√7th S83.421 **Sprain of lateral collateral ligament of right knee**

√7th S83.422 **Sprain of lateral collateral ligament of left knee**

√7th S83.429 **Sprain of lateral collateral ligament of unspecified knee**

√5th S83.5 **Sprain of cruciate ligament of knee**

AHA: 2016,2Q,3

√6th S83.50 **Sprain of unspecified cruciate ligament of knee**

√7th S83.501 **Sprain of unspecified cruciate ligament of right knee**

√7th S83.502 **Sprain of unspecified cruciate ligament of left knee**

√7th S83.509 **Sprain of unspecified cruciate ligament of unspecified knee**

√6th S83.51 **Sprain of anterior cruciate ligament of knee**

√7th S83.511 **Sprain of anterior cruciate ligament of right knee**

√7th S83.512 **Sprain of anterior cruciate ligament of left knee**

√7th S83.519 **Sprain of anterior cruciate ligament of unspecified knee**

√6th S83.52 **Sprain of posterior cruciate ligament of knee**

√7th S83.521 **Sprain of posterior cruciate ligament of right knee**

√7th S83.522 **Sprain of posterior cruciate ligament of left knee**

√7th S83.529 **Sprain of posterior cruciate ligament of unspecified knee**

√5th S83.6 **Sprain of the superior tibiofibular joint and ligament**

√x7th S83.60 **Sprain of the superior tibiofibular joint and ligament, unspecified knee**

√x7th S83.61 **Sprain of the superior tibiofibular joint and ligament, right knee**

√x7th S83.62 **Sprain of the superior tibiofibular joint and ligament, left knee**

√5th S83.8 **Sprain of other specified parts of knee**

√6th S83.8X **Sprain of other specified parts of knee**

√7th S83.8X1 **Sprain of other specified parts of right knee**

√7th S83.8X2 **Sprain of other specified parts of left knee**

√7th S83.8X9 **Sprain of other specified parts of unspecified knee**

√5th S83.9 **Sprain of unspecified site of knee**

√x7th S83.90 **Sprain of unspecified site of unspecified knee**

√x7th S83.91 **Sprain of unspecified site of right knee**

√x7th S83.92 **Sprain of unspecified site of left knee**

√4th **S84 Injury of nerves at lower leg level**

Code also any associated open wound (S81.-)

EXCLUDES 2 *injury of nerves at ankle and foot level (S94.-)*

The appropriate 7th character is to be added to each code from category S84.
A initial encounter
D subsequent encounter
S sequela

√5th S84.0 **Injury of tibial nerve at lower leg level**

√x7th S84.00 **Injury of tibial nerve at lower leg level, unspecified leg**

√x7th S84.01 **Injury of tibial nerve at lower leg level, right leg**

√x7th S84.02 **Injury of tibial nerve at lower leg level, left leg**

√5th S84.1 **Injury of peroneal nerve at lower leg level**

√x7th S84.10 **Injury of peroneal nerve at lower leg level, unspecified leg**

√x7th S84.11 **Injury of peroneal nerve at lower leg level, right leg**

√x7th S84.12 **Injury of peroneal nerve at lower leg level, left leg**

√5th S84.2 **Injury of cutaneous sensory nerve at lower leg level**

√x7th S84.20 **Injury of cutaneous sensory nerve at lower leg level, unspecified leg**

√x7th S84.21 **Injury of cutaneous sensory nerve at lower leg level, right leg**

√x7th S84.22 **Injury of cutaneous sensory nerve at lower leg level, left leg**

√5th S84.8 **Injury of other nerves at lower leg level**

√6th S84.80 **Injury of other nerves at lower leg level**

√7th S84.801 **Injury of other nerves at lower leg level, right leg**

√7th S84.802 **Injury of other nerves at lower leg level, left leg**

√7th S84.809 **Injury of other nerves at lower leg level, unspecified leg**

√5th S84.9 **Injury of unspecified nerve at lower leg level**

√x7th S84.90 **Injury of unspecified nerve at lower leg level, unspecified leg**

√x7th S84.91 **Injury of unspecified nerve at lower leg level, right leg**

√x7th S84.92 **Injury of unspecified nerve at lower leg level, left leg**

√4th **S85 Injury of blood vessels at lower leg level**

Code also any associated open wound (S81.-)

EXCLUDES 2 *injury of blood vessels at ankle and foot level (S95.-)*

The appropriate 7th character is to be added to each code from category S85.
A initial encounter
D subsequent encounter
S sequela

√5th S85.0 **Injury of popliteal artery**

√6th S85.00 **Unspecified injury of popliteal artery**

√7th S85.001 **Unspecified injury of popliteal artery, right leg** MCC

√7th S85.002 **Unspecified injury of popliteal artery, left leg** MCC

√7th S85.009 **Unspecified injury of popliteal artery, unspecified leg** MCC

√6th S85.01 **Laceration of popliteal artery**

√7th S85.011 **Laceration of popliteal artery, right leg** MCC

√7th S85.012 **Laceration of popliteal artery, left leg** MCC

√7th S85.019 **Laceration of popliteal artery, unspecified leg** MCC

√6th S85.09 **Other specified injury of popliteal artery**

√7th S85.091 **Other specified injury of popliteal artery, right leg** MCC

√7th S85.092 **Other specified injury of popliteal artery, left leg** MCC

√7th S85.099 **Other specified injury of popliteal artery, unspecified leg** MCC

√5th S85.1 **Injury of tibial artery**

√6th S85.10 **Unspecified injury of unspecified tibial artery**

Injury of tibial artery NOS

√7th S85.101 **Unspecified injury of unspecified tibial artery, right leg** CC

√7th S85.102 **Unspecified injury of unspecified tibial artery, left leg** CC

√7th S85.109 **Unspecified injury of unspecified tibial artery, unspecified leg** CC

√6th S85.11 **Laceration of unspecified tibial artery**

√7th S85.111 **Laceration of unspecified tibial artery, right leg** CC

√7th S85.112 **Laceration of unspecified tibial artery, left leg** CC

√7th S85.119 **Laceration of unspecified tibial artery, unspecified leg** CC

S85.12 Other specified injury of unspecified tibial artery
- S85.121 Other specified injury of unspecified tibial artery, right leg CC
- S85.122 Other specified injury of unspecified tibial artery, left leg CC
- S85.129 Other specified injury of unspecified tibial artery, unspecified leg CC

S85.13 Unspecified injury of anterior tibial artery
- S85.131 Unspecified injury of anterior tibial artery, right leg CC
- S85.132 Unspecified injury of anterior tibial artery, left leg CC
- S85.139 Unspecified injury of anterior tibial artery, unspecified leg CC

S85.14 Laceration of anterior tibial artery
- S85.141 Laceration of anterior tibial artery, right leg CC
- S85.142 Laceration of anterior tibial artery, left leg CC
- S85.149 Laceration of anterior tibial artery, unspecified leg CC

S85.15 Other specified injury of anterior tibial artery
- S85.151 Other specified injury of anterior tibial artery, right leg CC
- S85.152 Other specified injury of anterior tibial artery, left leg CC
- S85.159 Other specified injury of anterior tibial artery, unspecified leg CC

S85.16 Unspecified injury of posterior tibial artery
- S85.161 Unspecified injury of posterior tibial artery, right leg CC
- S85.162 Unspecified injury of posterior tibial artery, left leg CC
- S85.169 Unspecified injury of posterior tibial artery, unspecified leg CC

S85.17 Laceration of posterior tibial artery
- S85.171 Laceration of posterior tibial artery, right leg CC
- S85.172 Laceration of posterior tibial artery, left leg CC
- S85.179 Laceration of posterior tibial artery, unspecified leg CC

S85.18 Other specified injury of posterior tibial artery
- S85.181 Other specified injury of posterior tibial artery, right leg CC
- S85.182 Other specified injury of posterior tibial artery, left leg CC
- S85.189 Other specified injury of posterior tibial artery, unspecified leg CC

S85.2 Injury of peroneal artery

S85.20 Unspecified injury of peroneal artery
- S85.201 Unspecified injury of peroneal artery, right leg CC
- S85.202 Unspecified injury of peroneal artery, left leg CC
- S85.209 Unspecified injury of peroneal artery, unspecified leg CC

S85.21 Laceration of peroneal artery
- S85.211 Laceration of peroneal artery, right leg CC
- S85.212 Laceration of peroneal artery, left leg CC
- S85.219 Laceration of peroneal artery, unspecified leg CC

S85.29 Other specified injury of peroneal artery
- S85.291 Other specified injury of peroneal artery, right leg CC
- S85.292 Other specified injury of peroneal artery, left leg CC
- S85.299 Other specified injury of peroneal artery, unspecified leg CC

S85.3 Injury of greater saphenous vein at lower leg level

Injury of greater saphenous vein NOS
Injury of saphenous vein NOS

S85.30 Unspecified injury of greater saphenous vein at lower leg level
- S85.301 Unspecified injury of greater saphenous vein at lower leg level, right leg CC
- S85.302 Unspecified injury of greater saphenous vein at lower leg level, left leg CC
- S85.309 Unspecified injury of greater saphenous vein at lower leg level, unspecified leg CC

S85.31 Laceration of greater saphenous vein at lower leg level
- S85.311 Laceration of greater saphenous vein at lower leg level, right leg CC
- S85.312 Laceration of greater saphenous vein at lower leg level, left leg CC
- S85.319 Laceration of greater saphenous vein at lower leg level, unspecified leg CC

S85.39 Other specified injury of greater saphenous vein at lower leg level
- S85.391 Other specified injury of greater saphenous vein at lower leg level, right leg CC
- S85.392 Other specified injury of greater saphenous vein at lower leg level, left leg CC
- S85.399 Other specified injury of greater saphenous vein at lower leg level, unspecified leg CC

S85.4 Injury of lesser saphenous vein at lower leg level

S85.40 Unspecified injury of lesser saphenous vein at lower leg level
- S85.401 Unspecified injury of lesser saphenous vein at lower leg level, right leg CC
- S85.402 Unspecified injury of lesser saphenous vein at lower leg level, left leg CC
- S85.409 Unspecified injury of lesser saphenous vein at lower leg level, unspecified leg CC

S85.41 Laceration of lesser saphenous vein at lower leg level
- S85.411 Laceration of lesser saphenous vein at lower leg level, right leg CC
- S85.412 Laceration of lesser saphenous vein at lower leg level, left leg CC
- S85.419 Laceration of lesser saphenous vein at lower leg level, unspecified leg CC

S85.49 Other specified injury of lesser saphenous vein at lower leg level
- S85.491 Other specified injury of lesser saphenous vein at lower leg level, right leg CC
- S85.492 Other specified injury of lesser saphenous vein at lower leg level, left leg CC
- S85.499 Other specified injury of lesser saphenous vein at lower leg level, unspecified leg CC

S85.5 Injury of popliteal vein

S85.50 Unspecified injury of popliteal vein
- S85.501 Unspecified injury of popliteal vein, right leg MCC
- S85.502 Unspecified injury of popliteal vein, left leg MCC
- S85.509 Unspecified injury of popliteal vein, unspecified leg MCC

S85.51 Laceration of popliteal vein
- S85.511 Laceration of popliteal vein, right leg MCC
- S85.512 Laceration of popliteal vein, left leg MCC
- S85.519 Laceration of popliteal vein, unspecified leg MCC

S85.59 Other specified injury of popliteal vein
- S85.591 Other specified injury of popliteal vein, right leg MCC
- S85.592 Other specified injury of popliteal vein, left leg MCC
- S85.599 Other specified injury of popliteal vein, unspecified leg MCC

S85.8 Injury of other blood vessels at lower leg level

S85.80 Unspecified injury of other blood vessels at lower leg level
- S85.801 Unspecified injury of other blood vessels at lower leg level, right leg CC
- S85.802 Unspecified injury of other blood vessels at lower leg level, left leg CC

✓7th **S85.809 Unspecified injury of other blood vessels at lower leg level, unspecified leg** CC

✓6th **S85.81 Laceration of other blood vessels at lower leg level**

✓7th **S85.811 Laceration of other blood vessels at lower leg level, right leg** CC

✓7th **S85.812 Laceration of other blood vessels at lower leg level, left leg** CC

✓7th **S85.819 Laceration of other blood vessels at lower leg level, unspecified leg** CC

✓6th **S85.89 Other specified injury of other blood vessels at lower leg level**

✓7th **S85.891 Other specified injury of other blood vessels at lower leg level, right leg** CC

✓7th **S85.892 Other specified injury of other blood vessels at lower leg level, left leg** CC

✓7th **S85.899 Other specified injury of other blood vessels at lower leg level, unspecified leg** CC

✓5th **S85.9 Injury of unspecified blood vessel at lower leg level**

✓6th **S85.90 Unspecified injury of unspecified blood vessel at lower leg level**

✓7th **S85.901 Unspecified injury of unspecified blood vessel at lower leg level, right leg** CC

✓7th **S85.902 Unspecified injury of unspecified blood vessel at lower leg level, left leg** CC

✓7th **S85.909 Unspecified injury of unspecified blood vessel at lower leg level, unspecified leg** CC

✓6th **S85.91 Laceration of unspecified blood vessel at lower leg level**

✓7th **S85.911 Laceration of unspecified blood vessel at lower leg level, right leg** CC

✓7th **S85.912 Laceration of unspecified blood vessel at lower leg level, left leg** CC

✓7th **S85.919 Laceration of unspecified blood vessel at lower leg level, unspecified leg** CC

✓6th **S85.99 Other specified injury of unspecified blood vessel at lower leg level**

✓7th **S85.991 Other specified injury of unspecified blood vessel at lower leg level, right leg** CC

✓7th **S85.992 Other specified injury of unspecified blood vessel at lower leg level, left leg** CC

✓7th **S85.999 Other specified injury of unspecified blood vessel at lower leg level, unspecified leg** CC

✓4th **S86 Injury of muscle, fascia and tendon at lower leg level**

Code also any associated open wound (S81.-)

EXCLUDES 2 *injury of muscle, fascia and tendon at ankle (S96.-)*
injury of patellar ligament (tendon) (S76.1-)
sprain of joints and ligaments of knee (S83.-)

TIP: Refer to the Muscle/Tendon table at the beginning of this chapter.

The appropriate 7th character is to be added to each code from category S86.
A initial encounter
D subsequent encounter
S sequela

✓5th **S86.0 Injury of Achilles tendon**

✓6th **S86.00 Unspecified injury of Achilles tendon**

✓7th **S86.001 Unspecified injury of right Achilles tendon**

✓7th **S86.002 Unspecified injury of left Achilles tendon**

✓7th **S86.009 Unspecified injury of unspecified Achilles tendon**

✓6th **S86.01 Strain of Achilles tendon**

✓7th **S86.011 Strain of right Achilles tendon**

✓7th **S86.012 Strain of left Achilles tendon**

✓7th **S86.019 Strain of unspecified Achilles tendon**

✓6th **S86.02 Laceration of Achilles tendon**

✓7th **S86.021 Laceration of right Achilles tendon** CC

✓7th **S86.022 Laceration of left Achilles tendon** CC

✓7th **S86.029 Laceration of unspecified Achilles tendon** CC

✓6th **S86.09 Other specified injury of Achilles tendon**

✓7th **S86.091 Other specified injury of right Achilles tendon**

✓7th **S86.092 Other specified injury of left Achilles tendon**

✓7th **S86.099 Other specified injury of unspecified Achilles tendon**

✓5th **S86.1 Injury of other muscle(s) and tendon(s) of posterior muscle group at lower leg level**

✓6th **S86.10 Unspecified injury of other muscle(s) and tendon(s) of posterior muscle group at lower leg level**

✓7th **S86.101 Unspecified injury of other muscle(s) and tendon(s) of posterior muscle group at lower leg level, right leg**

✓7th **S86.102 Unspecified injury of other muscle(s) and tendon(s) of posterior muscle group at lower leg level, left leg**

✓7th **S86.109 Unspecified injury of other muscle(s) and tendon(s) of posterior muscle group at lower leg level, unspecified leg**

✓6th **S86.11 Strain of other muscle(s) and tendon(s) of posterior muscle group at lower leg level**

✓7th **S86.111 Strain of other muscle(s) and tendon(s) of posterior muscle group at lower leg level, right leg**

✓7th **S86.112 Strain of other muscle(s) and tendon(s) of posterior muscle group at lower leg level, left leg**

✓7th **S86.119 Strain of other muscle(s) and tendon(s) of posterior muscle group at lower leg level, unspecified leg**

✓6th **S86.12 Laceration of other muscle(s) and tendon(s) of posterior muscle group at lower leg level**

✓7th **S86.121 Laceration of other muscle(s) and tendon(s) of posterior muscle group at lower leg level, right leg** CC

✓7th **S86.122 Laceration of other muscle(s) and tendon(s) of posterior muscle group at lower leg level, left leg** CC

✓7th **S86.129 Laceration of other muscle(s) and tendon(s) of posterior muscle group at lower leg level, unspecified leg** CC

✓6th **S86.19 Other injury of other muscle(s) and tendon(s) of posterior muscle group at lower leg level**

✓7th **S86.191 Other injury of other muscle(s) and tendon(s) of posterior muscle group at lower leg level, right leg**

✓7th **S86.192 Other injury of other muscle(s) and tendon(s) of posterior muscle group at lower leg level, left leg**

✓7th **S86.199 Other injury of other muscle(s) and tendon(s) of posterior muscle group at lower leg level, unspecified leg**

✓5th **S86.2 Injury of muscle(s) and tendon(s) of anterior muscle group at lower leg level**

✓6th **S86.20 Unspecified injury of muscle(s) and tendon(s) of anterior muscle group at lower leg level**

✓7th **S86.201 Unspecified injury of muscle(s) and tendon(s) of anterior muscle group at lower leg level, right leg**

✓7th **S86.202 Unspecified injury of muscle(s) and tendon(s) of anterior muscle group at lower leg level, left leg**

✓7th **S86.209 Unspecified injury of muscle(s) and tendon(s) of anterior muscle group at lower leg level, unspecified leg**

✓6th **S86.21 Strain of muscle(s) and tendon(s) of anterior muscle group at lower leg level**

✓7th **S86.211 Strain of muscle(s) and tendon(s) of anterior muscle group at lower leg level, right leg**

✓7th **S86.212 Strain of muscle(s) and tendon(s) of anterior muscle group at lower leg level, left leg**

✓7th **S86.219 Strain of muscle(s) and tendon(s) of anterior muscle group at lower leg level, unspecified leg**

✓6th **S86.22 Laceration of muscle(s) and tendon(s) of anterior muscle group at lower leg level**

✓7th **S86.221 Laceration of muscle(s) and tendon(s) of anterior muscle group at lower leg level, right leg** CC

✓7th **S86.222 Laceration of muscle(s) and tendon(s) of anterior muscle group at lower leg level, left leg** CC

7th S86.229 Laceration of muscle(s) and tendon(s) of anterior muscle group at lower leg level, unspecified leg CC

6th S86.29 Other injury of muscle(s) and tendon(s) of anterior muscle group at lower leg level

7th S86.291 Other injury of muscle(s) and tendon(s) of anterior muscle group at lower leg level, right leg

7th S86.292 Other injury of muscle(s) and tendon(s) of anterior muscle group at lower leg level, left leg

7th S86.299 Other injury of muscle(s) and tendon(s) of anterior muscle group at lower leg level, unspecified leg

5th S86.3 Injury of muscle(s) and tendon(s) of peroneal muscle group at lower leg level

6th S86.30 Unspecified injury of muscle(s) and tendon(s) of peroneal muscle group at lower leg level

7th S86.301 Unspecified injury of muscle(s) and tendon(s) of peroneal muscle group at lower leg level, right leg

7th S86.302 Unspecified injury of muscle(s) and tendon(s) of peroneal muscle group at lower leg level, left leg

7th S86.309 Unspecified injury of muscle(s) and tendon(s) of peroneal muscle group at lower leg level, unspecified leg

6th S86.31 Strain of muscle(s) and tendon(s) of peroneal muscle group at lower leg level

7th S86.311 Strain of muscle(s) and tendon(s) of peroneal muscle group at lower leg level, right leg

7th S86.312 Strain of muscle(s) and tendon(s) of peroneal muscle group at lower leg level, left leg

7th S86.319 Strain of muscle(s) and tendon(s) of peroneal muscle group at lower leg level, unspecified leg

6th S86.32 Laceration of muscle(s) and tendon(s) of peroneal muscle group at lower leg level

7th S86.321 Laceration of muscle(s) and tendon(s) of peroneal muscle group at lower leg level, right leg CC

7th S86.322 Laceration of muscle(s) and tendon(s) of peroneal muscle group at lower leg level, left leg CC

7th S86.329 Laceration of muscle(s) and tendon(s) of peroneal muscle group at lower leg level, unspecified leg CC

6th S86.39 Other injury of muscle(s) and tendon(s) of peroneal muscle group at lower leg level

7th S86.391 Other injury of muscle(s) and tendon(s) of peroneal muscle group at lower leg level, right leg

7th S86.392 Other injury of muscle(s) and tendon(s) of peroneal muscle group at lower leg level, left leg

7th S86.399 Other injury of muscle(s) and tendon(s) of peroneal muscle group at lower leg level, unspecified leg

5th S86.8 Injury of other muscles and tendons at lower leg level

6th S86.80 Unspecified injury of other muscles and tendons at lower leg level

7th S86.801 Unspecified injury of other muscle(s) and tendon(s) at lower leg level, right leg

7th S86.802 Unspecified injury of other muscle(s) and tendon(s) at lower leg level, left leg

7th S86.809 Unspecified injury of other muscle(s) and tendon(s) at lower leg level, unspecified leg

6th S86.81 Strain of other muscles and tendons at lower leg level

7th S86.811 Strain of other muscle(s) and tendon(s) at lower leg level, right leg

7th S86.812 Strain of other muscle(s) and tendon(s) at lower leg level, left leg

7th S86.819 Strain of other muscle(s) and tendon(s) at lower leg level, unspecified leg

6th S86.82 Laceration of other muscles and tendons at lower leg level

7th S86.821 Laceration of other muscle(s) and tendon(s) at lower leg level, right leg CC

7th S86.822 Laceration of other muscle(s) and tendon(s) at lower leg level, left leg CC

7th S86.829 Laceration of other muscle(s) and tendon(s) at lower leg level, unspecified leg CC

6th S86.89 Other injury of other muscles and tendons at lower leg level

7th S86.891 Other injury of other muscle(s) and tendon(s) at lower leg level, right leg

7th S86.892 Other injury of other muscle(s) and tendon(s) at lower leg level, left leg

7th S86.899 Other injury of other muscle(s) and tendon(s) at lower leg level, unspecified leg

5th S86.9 Injury of unspecified muscle and tendon at lower leg level

6th S86.90 Unspecified injury of unspecified muscle and tendon at lower leg level

7th S86.901 Unspecified injury of unspecified muscle(s) and tendon(s) at lower leg level, right leg

7th S86.902 Unspecified injury of unspecified muscle(s) and tendon(s) at lower leg level, left leg

7th S86.909 Unspecified injury of unspecified muscle(s) and tendon(s) at lower leg level, unspecified leg

6th S86.91 Strain of unspecified muscle and tendon at lower leg level

7th S86.911 Strain of unspecified muscle(s) and tendon(s) at lower leg level, right leg

7th S86.912 Strain of unspecified muscle(s) and tendon(s) at lower leg level, left leg

7th S86.919 Strain of unspecified muscle(s) and tendon(s) at lower leg level, unspecified leg

6th S86.92 Laceration of unspecified muscle and tendon at lower leg level

7th S86.921 Laceration of unspecified muscle(s) and tendon(s) at lower leg level, right leg CC

7th S86.922 Laceration of unspecified muscle(s) and tendon(s) at lower leg level, left leg CC

7th S86.929 Laceration of unspecified muscle(s) and tendon(s) at lower leg level, unspecified leg CC

6th S86.99 Other injury of unspecified muscle and tendon at lower leg level

7th S86.991 Other injury of unspecified muscle(s) and tendon(s) at lower leg level, right leg

7th S86.992 Other injury of unspecified muscle(s) and tendon(s) at lower leg level, left leg

7th S86.999 Other injury of unspecified muscle(s) and tendon(s) at lower leg level, unspecified leg

4th **S87 Crushing injury of lower leg**

Use additional code(s) for all associated injuries

EXCLUDES 2 *crushing injury of ankle and foot (S97.-)*

The appropriate 7th character is to be added to each code from category S87.
A initial encounter
D subsequent encounter
S sequela

5th S87.0 Crushing injury of knee

x7th S87.00 Crushing injury of unspecified knee

x7th S87.01 Crushing injury of right knee

x7th S87.02 Crushing injury of left knee

5th S87.8 Crushing injury of lower leg

x7th S87.80 Crushing injury of unspecified lower leg

x7th S87.81 Crushing injury of right lower leg

x7th S87.82 Crushing injury of left lower leg

4th S88 Traumatic amputation of lower leg

An amputation not identified as partial or complete should be coded to complete

EXCLUDES 1 *traumatic amputation of ankle and foot (S98.-)*

The appropriate 7th character is to be added to each code from category S88.
A initial encounter
D subsequent encounter
S sequela

5th S88.Ø Traumatic amputation at knee level

6th S88.Ø1 Complete traumatic amputation at knee level

7th S88.Ø11 Complete traumatic amputation at knee level, right lower leg CC HCC

7th S88.Ø12 Complete traumatic amputation at knee level, left lower leg CC HCC

7th S88.Ø19 Complete traumatic amputation at knee level, unspecified lower leg CC HCC

6th S88.Ø2 Partial traumatic amputation at knee level

7th S88.Ø21 Partial traumatic amputation at knee level, right lower leg CC HCC

7th S88.Ø22 Partial traumatic amputation at knee level, left lower leg CC HCC

7th S88.Ø29 Partial traumatic amputation at knee level, unspecified lower leg CC HCC

5th S88.1 Traumatic amputation at level between knee and ankle

6th S88.11 Complete traumatic amputation at level between knee and ankle

7th S88.111 Complete traumatic amputation at level between knee and ankle, right lower leg CC HCC

7th S88.112 Complete traumatic amputation at level between knee and ankle, left lower leg CC HCC

7th S88.119 Complete traumatic amputation at level between knee and ankle, unspecified lower leg CC HCC

6th S88.12 Partial traumatic amputation at level between knee and ankle

7th S88.121 Partial traumatic amputation at level between knee and ankle, right lower leg CC HCC

7th S88.122 Partial traumatic amputation at level between knee and ankle, left lower leg CC HCC

7th S88.129 Partial traumatic amputation at level between knee and ankle, unspecified lower leg CC HCC

5th S88.9 Traumatic amputation of lower leg, level unspecified

6th S88.91 Complete traumatic amputation of lower leg, level unspecified

7th S88.911 Complete traumatic amputation of right lower leg, level unspecified CC HCC

7th S88.912 Complete traumatic amputation of left lower leg, level unspecified CC HCC

7th S88.919 Complete traumatic amputation of unspecified lower leg, level unspecified CC HCC

6th S88.92 Partial traumatic amputation of lower leg, level unspecified

7th S88.921 Partial traumatic amputation of right lower leg, level unspecified CC HCC

7th S88.922 Partial traumatic amputation of left lower leg, level unspecified CC HCC

7th S88.929 Partial traumatic amputation of unspecified lower leg, level unspecified CC HCC

4th S89 Other and unspecified injuries of lower leg

NOTE A fracture not indicated as open or closed should be coded to closed.

EXCLUDES 2 *other and unspecified injuries of ankle and foot (S99.-)*

AHA: 2018,2Q,12; 2018,1Q,3; 2015,3Q,37-39

The appropriate 7th character is to be added to each code from subcategories S89.Ø, S89.1, S89.2, and S89.3.
A initial encounter for closed fracture
D subsequent encounter for fracture with routine healing
G subsequent encounter for fracture with delayed healing
K subsequent encounter for fracture with nonunion
P subsequent encounter for fracture with malunion
S sequela

5th S89.Ø Physeal fracture of upper end of tibia

AHA: 2019,4Q,56

6th S89.ØØ Unspecified physeal fracture of upper end of tibia

3 **7th S89.ØØ1 Unspecified physeal fracture of upper end of right tibia** CC H5

3 **7th S89.ØØ2 Unspecified physeal fracture of upper end of left tibia** CC H5

3 **7th S89.ØØ9 Unspecified physeal fracture of upper end of unspecified tibia** CC H5

6th S89.Ø1 Salter-Harris Type I physeal fracture of upper end of tibia

3 **7th S89.Ø11 Salter-Harris Type I physeal fracture of upper end of right tibia** CC H5

3 **7th S89.Ø12 Salter-Harris Type I physeal fracture of upper end of left tibia** CC H5

3 **7th S89.Ø19 Salter-Harris Type I physeal fracture of upper end of unspecified tibia** CC H5

6th S89.Ø2 Salter-Harris Type II physeal fracture of upper end of tibia

3 **7th S89.Ø21 Salter-Harris Type II physeal fracture of upper end of right tibia** CC H5

3 **7th S89.Ø22 Salter-Harris Type II physeal fracture of upper end of left tibia** CC H5

3 **7th S89.Ø29 Salter-Harris Type II physeal fracture of upper end of unspecified tibia** CC H5

6th S89.Ø3 Salter-Harris Type III physeal fracture of upper end of tibia

3 **7th S89.Ø31 Salter-Harris Type III physeal fracture of upper end of right tibia** CC H5

3 **7th S89.Ø32 Salter-Harris Type III physeal fracture of upper end of left tibia** CC H5

3 **7th S89.Ø39 Salter-Harris Type III physeal fracture of upper end of unspecified tibia** CC H5

6th S89.Ø4 Salter-Harris Type IV physeal fracture of upper end of tibia

3 **7th S89.Ø41 Salter-Harris Type IV physeal fracture of upper end of right tibia** CC H5

3 **7th S89.Ø42 Salter-Harris Type IV physeal fracture of upper end of left tibia** CC H5

3 **7th S89.Ø49 Salter-Harris Type IV physeal fracture of upper end of unspecified tibia** CC H5

6th S89.Ø9 Other physeal fracture of upper end of tibia

3 **7th S89.Ø91 Other physeal fracture of upper end of right tibia** CC H5

3 **7th S89.Ø92 Other physeal fracture of upper end of left tibia** CC H5

3 **7th S89.Ø99 Other physeal fracture of upper end of unspecified tibia** CC H5

5th S89.1 Physeal fracture of lower end of tibia

AHA: 2019,4Q,56

6th S89.1Ø Unspecified physeal fracture of lower end of tibia

4 **7th S89.1Ø1 Unspecified physeal fracture of lower end of right tibia** CC

4 **7th S89.1Ø2 Unspecified physeal fracture of lower end of left tibia** CC

4 **7th S89.1Ø9 Unspecified physeal fracture of lower end of unspecified tibia** CC

6th S89.11 Salter-Harris Type I physeal fracture of lower end of tibia

4 **7th S89.111 Salter-Harris Type I physeal fracture of lower end of right tibia** CC

4 **7th S89.112 Salter-Harris Type I physeal fracture of lower end of left tibia** CC

4 **7th S89.119 Salter-Harris Type I physeal fracture of lower end of unspecified tibia** CC

S89.12 Salter-Harris Type II physeal fracture of lower end of tibia
S89.121 Salter-Harris Type II physeal fracture of lower end of right tibia CC
S89.122 Salter-Harris Type II physeal fracture of lower end of left tibia CC
S89.129 Salter-Harris Type II physeal fracture of lower end of unspecified tibia CC

S89.13 Salter-Harris Type III physeal fracture of lower end of tibia
EXCLUDES 1 *fracture of medial malleolus (adult) (S82.5-)*
S89.131 Salter-Harris Type III physeal fracture of lower end of right tibia CC
S89.132 Salter-Harris Type III physeal fracture of lower end of left tibia CC
S89.139 Salter-Harris Type III physeal fracture of lower end of unspecified tibia CC

S89.14 Salter-Harris Type IV physeal fracture of lower end of tibia
EXCLUDES 1 *fracture of medial malleolus (adult) (S82.5-)*
S89.141 Salter-Harris Type IV physeal fracture of lower end of right tibia CC
S89.142 Salter-Harris Type IV physeal fracture of lower end of left tibia CC
S89.149 Salter-Harris Type IV physeal fracture of lower end of unspecified tibia CC

S89.19 Other physeal fracture of lower end of tibia
S89.191 Other physeal fracture of lower end of right tibia CC
S89.192 Other physeal fracture of lower end of left tibia CC
S89.199 Other physeal fracture of lower end of unspecified tibia CC

S89.2 Physeal fracture of upper end of fibula
AHA: 2019,4Q,56
S89.20 Unspecified physeal fracture of upper end of fibula
S89.201 Unspecified physeal fracture of upper end of right fibula CC
S89.202 Unspecified physeal fracture of upper end of left fibula CC
S89.209 Unspecified physeal fracture of upper end of unspecified fibula CC

S89.21 Salter-Harris Type I physeal fracture of upper end of fibula
S89.211 Salter-Harris Type I physeal fracture of upper end of right fibula CC
S89.212 Salter-Harris Type I physeal fracture of upper end of left fibula CC
S89.219 Salter-Harris Type I physeal fracture of upper end of unspecified fibula CC

S89.22 Salter-Harris Type II physeal fracture of upper end of fibula
S89.221 Salter-Harris Type II physeal fracture of upper end of right fibula CC
S89.222 Salter-Harris Type II physeal fracture of upper end of left fibula CC
S89.229 Salter-Harris Type II physeal fracture of upper end of unspecified fibula CC

S89.29 Other physeal fracture of upper end of fibula
S89.291 Other physeal fracture of upper end of right fibula CC
S89.292 Other physeal fracture of upper end of left fibula CC
S89.299 Other physeal fracture of upper end of unspecified fibula CC

S89.3 Physeal fracture of lower end of fibula
AHA: 2019,4Q,56
S89.30 Unspecified physeal fracture of lower end of fibula
S89.301 Unspecified physeal fracture of lower end of right fibula CC
S89.302 Unspecified physeal fracture of lower end of left fibula CC
S89.309 Unspecified physeal fracture of lower end of unspecified fibula CC

S89.31 Salter-Harris Type I physeal fracture of lower end of fibula
S89.311 Salter-Harris Type I physeal fracture of lower end of right fibula CC
S89.312 Salter-Harris Type I physeal fracture of lower end of left fibula CC
S89.319 Salter-Harris Type I physeal fracture of lower end of unspecified fibula CC

S89.32 Salter-Harris Type II physeal fracture of lower end of fibula
S89.321 Salter-Harris Type II physeal fracture of lower end of right fibula CC
S89.322 Salter-Harris Type II physeal fracture of lower end of left fibula CC
S89.329 Salter-Harris Type II physeal fracture of lower end of unspecified fibula CC

S89.39 Other physeal fracture of lower end of fibula
S89.391 Other physeal fracture of lower end of right fibula CC
S89.392 Other physeal fracture of lower end of left fibula CC
S89.399 Other physeal fracture of lower end of unspecified fibula CC

S89.8 Other specified injuries of lower leg

The appropriate 7th character is to be added to each code in subcategory S89.8.
A initial encounter
D subsequent encounter
S sequela

S89.80 Other specified injuries of unspecified lower leg
S89.81 Other specified injuries of right lower leg
S89.82 Other specified injuries of left lower leg

S89.9 Unspecified injury of lower leg

The appropriate 7th character is to be added to each code in subcategory S89.9.
A initial encounter
D subsequent encounter
S sequela

S89.90 Unspecified injury of unspecified lower leg
S89.91 Unspecified injury of right lower leg
S89.92 Unspecified injury of left lower leg

Injuries to the ankle and foot (S90-S99)

EXCLUDES 2 *burns and corrosions (T20-T32)*
fracture of ankle and malleolus (S82.-)
frostbite (T33-T34)
insect bite or sting, venomous (T63.4)

S90 Superficial injury of ankle, foot and toes

The appropriate 7th character is to be added to each code from category S90.
A initial encounter
D subsequent encounter
S sequela

S90.0 Contusion of ankle
S90.00 Contusion of unspecified ankle
S90.01 Contusion of right ankle
S90.02 Contusion of left ankle

S90.1 Contusion of toe without damage to nail
S90.11 Contusion of great toe without damage to nail
S90.111 Contusion of right great toe without damage to nail
S90.112 Contusion of left great toe without damage to nail
S90.119 Contusion of unspecified great toe without damage to nail

S90.12 Contusion of lesser toe without damage to nail
S90.121 Contusion of right lesser toe(s) without damage to nail
S90.122 Contusion of left lesser toe(s) without damage to nail
S90.129 Contusion of unspecified lesser toe(s) without damage to nail
Contusion of toe NOS

S90.2 Contusion of toe with damage to nail
S90.21 Contusion of great toe with damage to nail
S90.211 Contusion of right great toe with damage to nail

✓7th S90.212 Contusion of left great toe with damage to nail
✓7th S90.219 Contusion of unspecified great toe with damage to nail
✓6th S90.22 Contusion of lesser toe with damage to nail
✓7th S90.221 Contusion of right lesser toe(s) with damage to nail
✓7th S90.222 Contusion of left lesser toe(s) with damage to nail
✓7th S90.229 Contusion of unspecified lesser toe(s) with damage to nail
✓5th S90.3 Contusion of foot
EXCLUDES 2 *contusion of toes (S90.1-, S90.2-)*
✓x7th S90.30 Contusion of unspecified foot
Contusion of foot NOS
✓x7th S90.31 Contusion of right foot
✓x7th S90.32 Contusion of left foot
✓5th S90.4 Other superficial injuries of toe
✓6th S90.41 Abrasion of toe
✓7th S90.411 Abrasion, right great toe
✓7th S90.412 Abrasion, left great toe
✓7th S90.413 Abrasion, unspecified great toe
✓7th S90.414 Abrasion, right lesser toe(s)
✓7th S90.415 Abrasion, left lesser toe(s)
✓7th S90.416 Abrasion, unspecified lesser toe(s)
✓6th S90.42 Blister (nonthermal) of toe
✓7th S90.421 Blister (nonthermal), right great toe
✓7th S90.422 Blister (nonthermal), left great toe
✓7th S90.423 Blister (nonthermal), unspecified great toe
✓7th S90.424 Blister (nonthermal), right lesser toe(s)
✓7th S90.425 Blister (nonthermal), left lesser toe(s)
✓7th S90.426 Blister (nonthermal), unspecified lesser toe(s)
✓6th S90.44 External constriction of toe
Hair tourniquet syndrome of toe
✓7th S90.441 External constriction, right great toe
✓7th S90.442 External constriction, left great toe
✓7th S90.443 External constriction, unspecified great toe
✓7th S90.444 External constriction, right lesser toe(s)
✓7th S90.445 External constriction, left lesser toe(s)
✓7th S90.446 External constriction, unspecified lesser toe(s)
✓6th S90.45 Superficial foreign body of toe
Splinter in the toe
✓7th S90.451 Superficial foreign body, right great toe
✓7th S90.452 Superficial foreign body, left great toe
✓7th S90.453 Superficial foreign body, unspecified great toe
✓7th S90.454 Superficial foreign body, right lesser toe(s)
✓7th S90.455 Superficial foreign body, left lesser toe(s)
✓7th S90.456 Superficial foreign body, unspecified lesser toe(s)
✓6th S90.46 Insect bite (nonvenomous) of toe
✓7th S90.461 Insect bite (nonvenomous), right great toe
✓7th S90.462 Insect bite (nonvenomous), left great toe
✓7th S90.463 Insect bite (nonvenomous), unspecified great toe
✓7th S90.464 Insect bite (nonvenomous), right lesser toe(s)
✓7th S90.465 Insect bite (nonvenomous), left lesser toe(s)
✓7th S90.466 Insect bite (nonvenomous), unspecified lesser toe(s)
✓6th S90.47 Other superficial bite of toe
EXCLUDES 1 *open bite of toe (S91.15-, S91.25-)*
✓7th S90.471 Other superficial bite of right great toe
✓7th S90.472 Other superficial bite of left great toe
✓7th S90.473 Other superficial bite of unspecified great toe
✓7th S90.474 Other superficial bite of right lesser toe(s)
✓7th S90.475 Other superficial bite of left lesser toe(s)
✓7th S90.476 Other superficial bite of unspecified lesser toe(s)
✓5th S90.5 Other superficial injuries of ankle
✓6th S90.51 Abrasion of ankle
✓7th S90.511 Abrasion, right ankle
✓7th S90.512 Abrasion, left ankle
✓7th S90.519 Abrasion, unspecified ankle
✓6th S90.52 Blister (nonthermal) of ankle
✓7th S90.521 Blister (nonthermal), right ankle
✓7th S90.522 Blister (nonthermal), left ankle
✓7th S90.529 Blister (nonthermal), unspecified ankle
✓6th S90.54 External constriction of ankle
✓7th S90.541 External constriction, right ankle
✓7th S90.542 External constriction, left ankle
✓7th S90.549 External constriction, unspecified ankle
✓6th S90.55 Superficial foreign body of ankle
Splinter in the ankle
✓7th S90.551 Superficial foreign body, right ankle
✓7th S90.552 Superficial foreign body, left ankle
✓7th S90.559 Superficial foreign body, unspecified ankle
✓6th S90.56 Insect bite (nonvenomous) of ankle
✓7th S90.561 Insect bite (nonvenomous), right ankle
✓7th S90.562 Insect bite (nonvenomous), left ankle
✓7th S90.569 Insect bite (nonvenomous), unspecified ankle
✓6th S90.57 Other superficial bite of ankle
EXCLUDES 1 *open bite of ankle (S91.05-)*
✓7th S90.571 Other superficial bite of ankle, right ankle
✓7th S90.572 Other superficial bite of ankle, left ankle
✓7th S90.579 Other superficial bite of ankle, unspecified ankle
✓5th S90.8 Other superficial injuries of foot
✓6th S90.81 Abrasion of foot
✓7th S90.811 Abrasion, right foot
✓7th S90.812 Abrasion, left foot
✓7th S90.819 Abrasion, unspecified foot
✓6th S90.82 Blister (nonthermal) of foot
✓7th S90.821 Blister (nonthermal), right foot
✓7th S90.822 Blister (nonthermal), left foot
✓7th S90.829 Blister (nonthermal), unspecified foot
✓6th S90.84 External constriction of foot
✓7th S90.841 External constriction, right foot
✓7th S90.842 External constriction, left foot
✓7th S90.849 External constriction, unspecified foot
✓6th S90.85 Superficial foreign body of foot
Splinter in the foot
✓7th S90.851 Superficial foreign body, right foot
✓7th S90.852 Superficial foreign body, left foot
✓7th S90.859 Superficial foreign body, unspecified foot
✓6th S90.86 Insect bite (nonvenomous) of foot
✓7th S90.861 Insect bite (nonvenomous), right foot
✓7th S90.862 Insect bite (nonvenomous), left foot
✓7th S90.869 Insect bite (nonvenomous), unspecified foot
✓6th S90.87 Other superficial bite of foot
EXCLUDES 1 *open bite of foot (S91.35-)*
✓7th S90.871 Other superficial bite of right foot
✓7th S90.872 Other superficial bite of left foot
✓7th S90.879 Other superficial bite of unspecified foot
✓5th S90.9 Unspecified superficial injury of ankle, foot and toe
✓6th S90.91 Unspecified superficial injury of ankle
✓7th S90.911 Unspecified superficial injury of right ankle
✓7th S90.912 Unspecified superficial injury of left ankle
✓7th S90.919 Unspecified superficial injury of unspecified ankle

N Newborn: 0 P Pediatric: 0-17 M Maternity: 9-64 A Adult: 15-124 MCC Major Complication/Comorbidity CC Complication/Comorbidity SW Severe Wound Dx

S90.92 Unspecified superficial injury of foot
S90.921 Unspecified superficial injury of right foot
S90.922 Unspecified superficial injury of left foot
S90.929 Unspecified superficial injury of unspecified foot
S90.93 Unspecified superficial injury of toes
S90.931 Unspecified superficial injury of right great toe
S90.932 Unspecified superficial injury of left great toe
S90.933 Unspecified superficial injury of unspecified great toe
S90.934 Unspecified superficial injury of right lesser toe(s)
S90.935 Unspecified superficial injury of left lesser toe(s)
S90.936 Unspecified superficial injury of unspecified lesser toe(s)

S91 Open wound of ankle, foot and toes

Code also any associated wound infection

EXCLUDES 1 *open fracture of ankle, foot and toes (S92.- with 7th character B)*
traumatic amputation of ankle and foot (S98.-)

The appropriate 7th character is to be added to each code from category S91.
A initial encounter
D subsequent encounter
S sequela

S91.0 Open wound of ankle
S91.00 Unspecified open wound of ankle
S91.001 Unspecified open wound, right ankle
S91.002 Unspecified open wound, left ankle
S91.009 Unspecified open wound, unspecified ankle
S91.01 Laceration without foreign body of ankle
S91.011 Laceration without foreign body, right ankle
S91.012 Laceration without foreign body, left ankle
S91.019 Laceration without foreign body, unspecified ankle
S91.02 Laceration with foreign body of ankle
S91.021 Laceration with foreign body, right ankle
S91.022 Laceration with foreign body, left ankle
S91.029 Laceration with foreign body, unspecified ankle
S91.03 Puncture wound without foreign body of ankle
S91.031 Puncture wound without foreign body, right ankle
S91.032 Puncture wound without foreign body, left ankle
S91.039 Puncture wound without foreign body, unspecified ankle
S91.04 Puncture wound with foreign body of ankle
S91.041 Puncture wound with foreign body, right ankle
S91.042 Puncture wound with foreign body, left ankle
S91.049 Puncture wound with foreign body, unspecified ankle
S91.05 Open bite of ankle

EXCLUDES 1 *superficial bite of ankle (S90.56-, S90.57-)*

S91.051 Open bite, right ankle
S91.052 Open bite, left ankle
S91.059 Open bite, unspecified ankle
S91.1 Open wound of toe without damage to nail
S91.10 Unspecified open wound of toe without damage to nail
S91.101 Unspecified open wound of right great toe without damage to nail
S91.102 Unspecified open wound of left great toe without damage to nail
S91.103 Unspecified open wound of unspecified great toe without damage to nail
S91.104 Unspecified open wound of right lesser toe(s) without damage to nail
S91.105 Unspecified open wound of left lesser toe(s) without damage to nail
S91.106 Unspecified open wound of unspecified lesser toe(s) without damage to nail
S91.109 Unspecified open wound of unspecified toe(s) without damage to nail
S91.11 Laceration without foreign body of toe without damage to nail
S91.111 Laceration without foreign body of right great toe without damage to nail
S91.112 Laceration without foreign body of left great toe without damage to nail
S91.113 Laceration without foreign body of unspecified great toe without damage to nail
S91.114 Laceration without foreign body of right lesser toe(s) without damage to nail
S91.115 Laceration without foreign body of left lesser toe(s) without damage to nail
S91.116 Laceration without foreign body of unspecified lesser toe(s) without damage to nail
S91.119 Laceration without foreign body of unspecified toe without damage to nail
S91.12 Laceration with foreign body of toe without damage to nail
S91.121 Laceration with foreign body of right great toe without damage to nail
S91.122 Laceration with foreign body of left great toe without damage to nail
S91.123 Laceration with foreign body of unspecified great toe without damage to nail
S91.124 Laceration with foreign body of right lesser toe(s) without damage to nail
S91.125 Laceration with foreign body of left lesser toe(s) without damage to nail
S91.126 Laceration with foreign body of unspecified lesser toe(s) without damage to nail
S91.129 Laceration with foreign body of unspecified toe(s) without damage to nail
S91.13 Puncture wound without foreign body of toe without damage to nail
S91.131 Puncture wound without foreign body of right great toe without damage to nail
S91.132 Puncture wound without foreign body of left great toe without damage to nail
S91.133 Puncture wound without foreign body of unspecified great toe without damage to nail
S91.134 Puncture wound without foreign body of right lesser toe(s) without damage to nail
S91.135 Puncture wound without foreign body of left lesser toe(s) without damage to nail
S91.136 Puncture wound without foreign body of unspecified lesser toe(s) without damage to nail
S91.139 Puncture wound without foreign body of unspecified toe(s) without damage to nail
S91.14 Puncture wound with foreign body of toe without damage to nail
S91.141 Puncture wound with foreign body of right great toe without damage to nail
S91.142 Puncture wound with foreign body of left great toe without damage to nail
S91.143 Puncture wound with foreign body of unspecified great toe without damage to nail
S91.144 Puncture wound with foreign body of right lesser toe(s) without damage to nail
S91.145 Puncture wound with foreign body of left lesser toe(s) without damage to nail
S91.146 Puncture wound with foreign body of unspecified lesser toe(s) without damage to nail
S91.149 Puncture wound with foreign body of unspecified toe(s) without damage to nail
S91.15 Open bite of toe without damage to nail

Bite of toe NOS

EXCLUDES 1 *superficial bite of toe (S90.46-, S90.47-)*

S91.151 Open bite of right great toe without damage to nail

- 7th S91.152 Open bite of left great toe without damage to nail
- 7th S91.153 Open bite of unspecified great toe without damage to nail
- 7th S91.154 Open bite of right lesser toe(s) without damage to nail
- 7th S91.155 Open bite of left lesser toe(s) without damage to nail
- 7th S91.156 Open bite of unspecified lesser toe(s) without damage to nail
- 7th S91.159 Open bite of unspecified toe(s) without damage to nail

5th S91.2 Open wound of toe with damage to nail

6th S91.20 Unspecified open wound of toe with damage to nail
- 7th S91.201 Unspecified open wound of right great toe with damage to nail
- 7th S91.202 Unspecified open wound of left great toe with damage to nail
- 7th S91.203 Unspecified open wound of unspecified great toe with damage to nail
- 7th S91.204 Unspecified open wound of right lesser toe(s) with damage to nail
- 7th S91.205 Unspecified open wound of left lesser toe(s) with damage to nail
- 7th S91.206 Unspecified open wound of unspecified lesser toe(s) with damage to nail
- 7th S91.209 Unspecified open wound of unspecified toe(s) with damage to nail

6th S91.21 Laceration without foreign body of toe with damage to nail
- 7th S91.211 Laceration without foreign body of right great toe with damage to nail
- 7th S91.212 Laceration without foreign body of left great toe with damage to nail
- 7th S91.213 Laceration without foreign body of unspecified great toe with damage to nail
- 7th S91.214 Laceration without foreign body of right lesser toe(s) with damage to nail
- 7th S91.215 Laceration without foreign body of left lesser toe(s) with damage to nail
- 7th S91.216 Laceration without foreign body of unspecified lesser toe(s) with damage to nail
- 7th S91.219 Laceration without foreign body of unspecified toe(s) with damage to nail

6th S91.22 Laceration with foreign body of toe with damage to nail
- 7th S91.221 Laceration with foreign body of right great toe with damage to nail
- 7th S91.222 Laceration with foreign body of left great toe with damage to nail
- 7th S91.223 Laceration with foreign body of unspecified great toe with damage to nail
- 7th S91.224 Laceration with foreign body of right lesser toe(s) with damage to nail
- 7th S91.225 Laceration with foreign body of left lesser toe(s) with damage to nail
- 7th S91.226 Laceration with foreign body of unspecified lesser toe(s) with damage to nail
- 7th S91.229 Laceration with foreign body of unspecified toe(s) with damage to nail

6th S91.23 Puncture wound without foreign body of toe with damage to nail
- 7th S91.231 Puncture wound without foreign body of right great toe with damage to nail
- 7th S91.232 Puncture wound without foreign body of left great toe with damage to nail
- 7th S91.233 Puncture wound without foreign body of unspecified great toe with damage to nail
- 7th S91.234 Puncture wound without foreign body of right lesser toe(s) with damage to nail
- 7th S91.235 Puncture wound without foreign body of left lesser toe(s) with damage to nail
- 7th S91.236 Puncture wound without foreign body of unspecified lesser toe(s) with damage to nail
- 7th S91.239 Puncture wound without foreign body of unspecified toe(s) with damage to nail

6th S91.24 Puncture wound with foreign body of toe with damage to nail
- 7th S91.241 Puncture wound with foreign body of right great toe with damage to nail
- 7th S91.242 Puncture wound with foreign body of left great toe with damage to nail
- 7th S91.243 Puncture wound with foreign body of unspecified great toe with damage to nail
- 7th S91.244 Puncture wound with foreign body of right lesser toe(s) with damage to nail
- 7th S91.245 Puncture wound with foreign body of left lesser toe(s) with damage to nail
- 7th S91.246 Puncture wound with foreign body of unspecified lesser toe(s) with damage to nail
- 7th S91.249 Puncture wound with foreign body of unspecified toe(s) with damage to nail

6th S91.25 Open bite of toe with damage to nail

Bite of toe with damage to nail NOS

EXCLUDES 1 *superficial bite of toe (S90.46-, S90.47-)*

- 7th S91.251 Open bite of right great toe with damage to nail
- 7th S91.252 Open bite of left great toe with damage to nail
- 7th S91.253 Open bite of unspecified great toe with damage to nail
- 7th S91.254 Open bite of right lesser toe(s) with damage to nail
- 7th S91.255 Open bite of left lesser toe(s) with damage to nail
- 7th S91.256 Open bite of unspecified lesser toe(s) with damage to nail
- 7th S91.259 Open bite of unspecified toe(s) with damage to nail

5th S91.3 Open wound of foot

6th S91.30 Unspecified open wound of foot
- 7th S91.301 Unspecified open wound, right foot
- 7th S91.302 Unspecified open wound, left foot
- 7th S91.309 Unspecified open wound, unspecified foot

6th S91.31 Laceration without foreign body of foot
- 7th S91.311 Laceration without foreign body, right foot
- 7th S91.312 Laceration without foreign body, left foot
- 7th S91.319 Laceration without foreign body, unspecified foot

6th S91.32 Laceration with foreign body of foot
- 7th S91.321 Laceration with foreign body, right foot
- 7th S91.322 Laceration with foreign body, left foot
- 7th S91.329 Laceration with foreign body, unspecified foot

6th S91.33 Puncture wound without foreign body of foot
- 7th S91.331 Puncture wound without foreign body, right foot
- 7th S91.332 Puncture wound without foreign body, left foot
- 7th S91.339 Puncture wound without foreign body, unspecified foot

6th S91.34 Puncture wound with foreign body of foot
- 7th S91.341 Puncture wound with foreign body, right foot
- 7th S91.342 Puncture wound with foreign body, left foot
- 7th S91.349 Puncture wound with foreign body, unspecified foot

6th S91.35 Open bite of foot

EXCLUDES 1 *superficial bite of foot (S90.86-, S90.87-)*

- 7th S91.351 Open bite, right foot
- 7th S91.352 Open bite, left foot
- 7th S91.359 Open bite, unspecified foot

S92 Fracture of foot and toe, except ankle

NOTE A fracture not indicated as displaced or nondisplaced should be coded to displaced

A fracture not indicated as open or closed should be coded to closed.

EXCLUDES 1 *traumatic amputation of ankle and foot (S98.-)*

EXCLUDES 2 *fracture of ankle (S82.-)*

fracture of malleolus (S82.-)

AHA: 2018,2Q,12; 2015,3Q,37-39

The appropriate 7th character is to be added to each code from category S92.

- A initial encounter for closed fracture
- B initial encounter for open fracture
- D subsequent encounter for fracture with routine healing
- G subsequent encounter for fracture with delayed healing
- K subsequent encounter for fracture with nonunion
- P subsequent encounter for fracture with malunion
- S sequela

S92.Ø Fracture of calcaneus

Heel bone

Os calcis

EXCLUDES 2 *physeal fracture of calcaneus (S99.Ø-)*

S92.ØØ Unspecified fracture of calcaneus
- 3 S92.ØØ1 Unspecified fracture of right calcaneus CC H5
- 3 S92.ØØ2 Unspecified fracture of left calcaneus CC H5
- 3 S92.ØØ9 Unspecified fracture of unspecified calcaneus CC H5

S92.Ø1 Fracture of body of calcaneus
- 3 S92.Ø11 Displaced fracture of body of right calcaneus CC H5
- 3 S92.Ø12 Displaced fracture of body of left calcaneus CC H5
- 3 S92.Ø13 Displaced fracture of body of unspecified calcaneus CC H5
- 3 S92.Ø14 Nondisplaced fracture of body of right calcaneus CC H5
- 3 S92.Ø15 Nondisplaced fracture of body of left calcaneus CC H5
- 3 S92.Ø16 Nondisplaced fracture of body of unspecified calcaneus CC H5

S92.Ø2 Fracture of anterior process of calcaneus
- 3 S92.Ø21 Displaced fracture of anterior process of right calcaneus CC H5
- 3 S92.Ø22 Displaced fracture of anterior process of left calcaneus CC H5
- 3 S92.Ø23 Displaced fracture of anterior process of unspecified calcaneus CC H5
- 3 S92.Ø24 Nondisplaced fracture of anterior process of right calcaneus CC H5
- 3 S92.Ø25 Nondisplaced fracture of anterior process of left calcaneus CC H5
- 3 S92.Ø26 Nondisplaced fracture of anterior process of unspecified calcaneus CC H5

S92.Ø3 Avulsion fracture of tuberosity of calcaneus
- 3 S92.Ø31 Displaced avulsion fracture of tuberosity of right calcaneus CC H5
- 3 S92.Ø32 Displaced avulsion fracture of tuberosity of left calcaneus CC H5
- 3 S92.Ø33 Displaced avulsion fracture of tuberosity of unspecified calcaneus CC H5
- 3 S92.Ø34 Nondisplaced avulsion fracture of tuberosity of right calcaneus CC H5
- 3 S92.Ø35 Nondisplaced avulsion fracture of tuberosity of left calcaneus CC H5
- 3 S92.Ø36 Nondisplaced avulsion fracture of tuberosity of unspecified calcaneus CC H5

S92.Ø4 Other fracture of tuberosity of calcaneus
- 3 S92.Ø41 Displaced other fracture of tuberosity of right calcaneus CC H5
- 3 S92.Ø42 Displaced other fracture of tuberosity of left calcaneus CC H5
- 3 S92.Ø43 Displaced other fracture of tuberosity of unspecified calcaneus CC H5
- 3 S92.Ø44 Nondisplaced other fracture of tuberosity of right calcaneus CC H5
- 3 S92.Ø45 Nondisplaced other fracture of tuberosity of left calcaneus CC H5
- 3 S92.Ø46 Nondisplaced other fracture of tuberosity of unspecified calcaneus CC H5

S92.Ø5 Other extraarticular fracture of calcaneus
- 3 S92.Ø51 Displaced other extraarticular fracture of right calcaneus CC H5
- 3 S92.Ø52 Displaced other extraarticular fracture of left calcaneus CC H5
- 3 S92.Ø53 Displaced other extraarticular fracture of unspecified calcaneus CC H5
- 3 S92.Ø54 Nondisplaced other extraarticular fracture of right calcaneus CC H5
- 3 S92.Ø55 Nondisplaced other extraarticular fracture of left calcaneus CC H5
- 3 S92.Ø56 Nondisplaced other extraarticular fracture of unspecified calcaneus CC H5

S92.Ø6 Intraarticular fracture of calcaneus
- 3 S92.Ø61 Displaced intraarticular fracture of right calcaneus CC H5
- 3 S92.Ø62 Displaced intraarticular fracture of left calcaneus CC H5
- 3 S92.Ø63 Displaced intraarticular fracture of unspecified calcaneus CC H5
- 3 S92.Ø64 Nondisplaced intraarticular fracture of right calcaneus CC H5
- 3 S92.Ø65 Nondisplaced intraarticular fracture of left calcaneus CC H5
- 3 S92.Ø66 Nondisplaced intraarticular fracture of unspecified calcaneus CC H5

S92.1 Fracture of talus

Astragalus

S92.1Ø Unspecified fracture of talus
- 3 S92.1Ø1 Unspecified fracture of right talus CC H5
- 3 S92.1Ø2 Unspecified fracture of left talus CC H5
- 3 S92.1Ø9 Unspecified fracture of unspecified talus CC H5

S92.11 Fracture of neck of talus
- 3 S92.111 Displaced fracture of neck of right talus CC H5
- 3 S92.112 Displaced fracture of neck of left talus CC H5
- 3 S92.113 Displaced fracture of neck of unspecified talus CC H5
- 3 S92.114 Nondisplaced fracture of neck of right talus CC H5
- 3 S92.115 Nondisplaced fracture of neck of left talus CC H5
- 3 S92.116 Nondisplaced fracture of neck of unspecified talus CC H5

S92.12 Fracture of body of talus
- 3 S92.121 Displaced fracture of body of right talus CC H5
- 3 S92.122 Displaced fracture of body of left talus CC H5
- 3 S92.123 Displaced fracture of body of unspecified talus CC H5
- 3 S92.124 Nondisplaced fracture of body of right talus CC H5
- 3 S92.125 Nondisplaced fracture of body of left talus CC H5
- 3 S92.126 Nondisplaced fracture of body of unspecified talus CC H5

S92.13 Fracture of posterior process of talus
- 3 S92.131 Displaced fracture of posterior process of right talus CC H5
- 3 S92.132 Displaced fracture of posterior process of left talus CC H5
- 3 S92.133 Displaced fracture of posterior process of unspecified talus CC H5
- 3 S92.134 Nondisplaced fracture of posterior process of right talus CC H5

3 ✓7th S92.135 Nondisplaced fracture of posterior process of left talus CC H5
3 ✓7th S92.136 Nondisplaced fracture of posterior process of unspecified talus CC H5
✓6th S92.14 Dome fracture of talus
EXCLUDES 1 *osteochondritis dissecans (M93.2)*
3 ✓7th S92.141 Displaced dome fracture of right talus CC H5
3 ✓7th S92.142 Displaced dome fracture of left talus CC H5
3 ✓7th S92.143 Displaced dome fracture of unspecified talus CC H5
3 ✓7th S92.144 Nondisplaced dome fracture of right talus CC H5
3 ✓7th S92.145 Nondisplaced dome fracture of left talus CC H5
3 ✓7th S92.146 Nondisplaced dome fracture of unspecified talus CC H5
✓6th S92.15 Avulsion fracture (chip fracture) of talus
3 ✓7th S92.151 Displaced avulsion fracture (chip fracture) of right talus CC H5
3 ✓7th S92.152 Displaced avulsion fracture (chip fracture) of left talus CC H5
3 ✓7th S92.153 Displaced avulsion fracture (chip fracture) of unspecified talus CC H5
3 ✓7th S92.154 Nondisplaced avulsion fracture (chip fracture) of right talus CC H5
3 ✓7th S92.155 Nondisplaced avulsion fracture (chip fracture) of left talus CC H5
3 ✓7th S92.156 Nondisplaced avulsion fracture (chip fracture) of unspecified talus CC H5
✓6th S92.19 Other fracture of talus
3 ✓7th S92.191 Other fracture of right talus CC H5
3 ✓7th S92.192 Other fracture of left talus CC H5
3 ✓7th S92.199 Other fracture of unspecified talus CC H5
✓5th S92.2 Fracture of other and unspecified tarsal bone(s)
✓6th S92.20 Fracture of unspecified tarsal bone(s)
3 ✓7th S92.201 Fracture of unspecified tarsal bone(s) of right foot CC H5
3 ✓7th S92.202 Fracture of unspecified tarsal bone(s) of left foot CC H5
3 ✓7th S92.209 Fracture of unspecified tarsal bone(s) of unspecified foot CC H5
✓6th S92.21 Fracture of cuboid bone
3 ✓7th S92.211 Displaced fracture of cuboid bone of right foot CC H5
3 ✓7th S92.212 Displaced fracture of cuboid bone of left foot CC H5
3 ✓7th S92.213 Displaced fracture of cuboid bone of unspecified foot CC H5
3 ✓7th S92.214 Nondisplaced fracture of cuboid bone of right foot CC H5
3 ✓7th S92.215 Nondisplaced fracture of cuboid bone of left foot CC H5
3 ✓7th S92.216 Nondisplaced fracture of cuboid bone of unspecified foot CC H5
✓6th S92.22 Fracture of lateral cuneiform
3 ✓7th S92.221 Displaced fracture of lateral cuneiform of right foot CC H5
3 ✓7th S92.222 Displaced fracture of lateral cuneiform of left foot CC H5
3 ✓7th S92.223 Displaced fracture of lateral cuneiform of unspecified foot CC H5
3 ✓7th S92.224 Nondisplaced fracture of lateral cuneiform of right foot CC H5
3 ✓7th S92.225 Nondisplaced fracture of lateral cuneiform of left foot CC H5
3 ✓7th S92.226 Nondisplaced fracture of lateral cuneiform of unspecified foot CC H5
✓6th S92.23 Fracture of intermediate cuneiform
3 ✓7th S92.231 Displaced fracture of intermediate cuneiform of right foot CC H5
3 ✓7th S92.232 Displaced fracture of intermediate cuneiform of left foot CC H5
3 ✓7th S92.233 Displaced fracture of intermediate cuneiform of unspecified foot CC H5
3 ✓7th S92.234 Nondisplaced fracture of intermediate cuneiform of right foot CC H5
3 ✓7th S92.235 Nondisplaced fracture of intermediate cuneiform of left foot CC H5
3 ✓7th S92.236 Nondisplaced fracture of intermediate cuneiform of unspecified foot CC H5
✓6th S92.24 Fracture of medial cuneiform
3 ✓7th S92.241 Displaced fracture of medial cuneiform of right foot CC H5
3 ✓7th S92.242 Displaced fracture of medial cuneiform of left foot CC H5
3 ✓7th S92.243 Displaced fracture of medial cuneiform of unspecified foot CC H5
3 ✓7th S92.244 Nondisplaced fracture of medial cuneiform of right foot CC H5
3 ✓7th S92.245 Nondisplaced fracture of medial cuneiform of left foot CC H5
3 ✓7th S92.246 Nondisplaced fracture of medial cuneiform of unspecified foot CC H5
✓6th S92.25 Fracture of navicular [scaphoid] of foot
3 ✓7th S92.251 Displaced fracture of navicular [scaphoid] of right foot CC H5
3 ✓7th S92.252 Displaced fracture of navicular [scaphoid] of left foot CC H5
3 ✓7th S92.253 Displaced fracture of navicular [scaphoid] of unspecified foot CC H5
3 ✓7th S92.254 Nondisplaced fracture of navicular [scaphoid] of right foot CC H5
3 ✓7th S92.255 Nondisplaced fracture of navicular [scaphoid] of left foot CC H5
3 ✓7th S92.256 Nondisplaced fracture of navicular [scaphoid] of unspecified foot CC H5
✓5th S92.3 Fracture of metatarsal bone(s)
EXCLUDES 2 *physeal fracture of metatarsal (S99.1-)*
AHA: 2018,1Q,3
✓6th S92.30 Fracture of unspecified metatarsal bone(s)
3 ✓7th S92.301 Fracture of unspecified metatarsal bone(s), right foot CC H5
3 ✓7th S92.302 Fracture of unspecified metatarsal bone(s), left foot CC H5
3 ✓7th S92.309 Fracture of unspecified metatarsal bone(s), unspecified foot CC H5
✓6th S92.31 Fracture of first metatarsal bone
3 ✓7th S92.311 Displaced fracture of first metatarsal bone, right foot CC H5
3 ✓7th S92.312 Displaced fracture of first metatarsal bone, left foot CC H5
3 ✓7th S92.313 Displaced fracture of first metatarsal bone, unspecified foot CC H5
3 ✓7th S92.314 Nondisplaced fracture of first metatarsal bone, right foot CC H5
3 ✓7th S92.315 Nondisplaced fracture of first metatarsal bone, left foot CC H5
3 ✓7th S92.316 Nondisplaced fracture of first metatarsal bone, unspecified foot CC H5
✓6th S92.32 Fracture of second metatarsal bone
3 ✓7th S92.321 Displaced fracture of second metatarsal bone, right foot CC H5
3 ✓7th S92.322 Displaced fracture of second metatarsal bone, left foot CC H5
3 ✓7th S92.323 Displaced fracture of second metatarsal bone, unspecified foot CC H5
3 ✓7th S92.324 Nondisplaced fracture of second metatarsal bone, right foot CC H5
3 ✓7th S92.325 Nondisplaced fracture of second metatarsal bone, left foot CC H5
3 ✓7th S92.326 Nondisplaced fracture of second metatarsal bone, unspecified foot CC H5
✓6th S92.33 Fracture of third metatarsal bone
3 ✓7th S92.331 Displaced fracture of third metatarsal bone, right foot CC H5
3 ✓7th S92.332 Displaced fracture of third metatarsal bone, left foot CC H5
3 ✓7th S92.333 Displaced fracture of third metatarsal bone, unspecified foot CC H5
3 ✓7th S92.334 Nondisplaced fracture of third metatarsal bone, right foot CC H5

3 7th S92.335 Nondisplaced fracture of third metatarsal bone, left foot CC H5
3 7th S92.336 Nondisplaced fracture of third metatarsal bone, unspecified foot CC H5
6th S92.34 Fracture of fourth metatarsal bone
3 7th S92.341 Displaced fracture of fourth metatarsal bone, right foot CC H5
3 7th S92.342 Displaced fracture of fourth metatarsal bone, left foot CC H5
3 7th S92.343 Displaced fracture of fourth metatarsal bone, unspecified foot CC H5
3 7th S92.344 Nondisplaced fracture of fourth metatarsal bone, right foot CC H5
3 7th S92.345 Nondisplaced fracture of fourth metatarsal bone, left foot CC H5
3 7th S92.346 Nondisplaced fracture of fourth metatarsal bone, unspecified foot CC H5
6th S92.35 Fracture of fifth metatarsal bone
3 7th S92.351 Displaced fracture of fifth metatarsal bone, right foot CC H5
3 7th S92.352 Displaced fracture of fifth metatarsal bone, left foot CC H5
3 7th S92.353 Displaced fracture of fifth metatarsal bone, unspecified foot CC H5
3 7th S92.354 Nondisplaced fracture of fifth metatarsal bone, right foot CC H5
3 7th S92.355 Nondisplaced fracture of fifth metatarsal bone, left foot CC H5
3 7th S92.356 Nondisplaced fracture of fifth metatarsal bone, unspecified foot CC H5
5th S92.4 Fracture of great toe
EXCLUDES 2 *physeal fracture of phalanx of toe (S99.2-)*
6th S92.40 Unspecified fracture of great toe
4 7th S92.401 Displaced unspecified fracture of right great toe CC
4 7th S92.402 Displaced unspecified fracture of left great toe CC
4 7th S92.403 Displaced unspecified fracture of unspecified great toe CC
4 7th S92.404 Nondisplaced unspecified fracture of right great toe CC
4 7th S92.405 Nondisplaced unspecified fracture of left great toe CC
4 7th S92.406 Nondisplaced unspecified fracture of unspecified great toe CC
6th S92.41 Fracture of proximal phalanx of great toe
4 7th S92.411 Displaced fracture of proximal phalanx of right great toe CC
4 7th S92.412 Displaced fracture of proximal phalanx of left great toe CC
4 7th S92.413 Displaced fracture of proximal phalanx of unspecified great toe CC
4 7th S92.414 Nondisplaced fracture of proximal phalanx of right great toe CC
4 7th S92.415 Nondisplaced fracture of proximal phalanx of left great toe CC
4 7th S92.416 Nondisplaced fracture of proximal phalanx of unspecified great toe CC
6th S92.42 Fracture of distal phalanx of great toe
4 7th S92.421 Displaced fracture of distal phalanx of right great toe CC
4 7th S92.422 Displaced fracture of distal phalanx of left great toe CC
4 7th S92.423 Displaced fracture of distal phalanx of unspecified great toe CC
4 7th S92.424 Nondisplaced fracture of distal phalanx of right great toe CC
4 7th S92.425 Nondisplaced fracture of distal phalanx of left great toe CC
4 7th S92.426 Nondisplaced fracture of distal phalanx of unspecified great toe CC
6th S92.49 Other fracture of great toe
4 7th S92.491 Other fracture of right great toe CC
4 7th S92.492 Other fracture of left great toe CC
4 7th S92.499 Other fracture of unspecified great toe CC

5th S92.5 Fracture of lesser toe(s)
EXCLUDES 2 *physeal fracture of phalanx of toe (S99.2-)*
6th S92.50 Unspecified fracture of lesser toe(s)
4 7th S92.501 Displaced unspecified fracture of right lesser toe(s) CC
4 7th S92.502 Displaced unspecified fracture of left lesser toe(s) CC
4 7th S92.503 Displaced unspecified fracture of unspecified lesser toe(s) CC
4 7th S92.504 Nondisplaced unspecified fracture of right lesser toe(s) CC
4 7th S92.505 Nondisplaced unspecified fracture of left lesser toe(s) CC
4 7th S92.506 Nondisplaced unspecified fracture of unspecified lesser toe(s) CC
6th S92.51 Fracture of proximal phalanx of lesser toe(s)
4 7th S92.511 Displaced fracture of proximal phalanx of right lesser toe(s) CC
4 7th S92.512 Displaced fracture of proximal phalanx of left lesser toe(s) CC
4 7th S92.513 Displaced fracture of proximal phalanx of unspecified lesser toe(s) CC
4 7th S92.514 Nondisplaced fracture of proximal phalanx of right lesser toe(s) CC
4 7th S92.515 Nondisplaced fracture of proximal phalanx of left lesser toe(s)) CC
4 7th S92.516 Nondisplaced fracture of proximal phalanx of unspecified lesser toe(s) CC
6th S92.52 Fracture of middle phalanx of lesser toe(s)
4 7th S92.521 Displaced fracture of middle phalanx of right lesser toe(s) CC
4 7th S92.522 Displaced fracture of middle phalanx of left lesser toe(s) CC
4 7th S92.523 Displaced fracture of middle phalanx of unspecified lesser toe(s) CC
4 7th S92.524 Nondisplaced fracture of middle phalanx of right lesser toe(s) CC
4 7th S92.525 Nondisplaced fracture of middle phalanx of left lesser toe(s) CC
4 7th S92.526 Nondisplaced fracture of middle phalanx of unspecified lesser toe(s) CC
6th S92.53 Fracture of distal phalanx of lesser toe(s)
4 7th S92.531 Displaced fracture of distal phalanx of right lesser toe(s) CC
4 7th S92.532 Displaced fracture of distal phalanx of left lesser toe(s) CC
4 7th S92.533 Displaced fracture of distal phalanx of unspecified lesser toe(s) CC
4 7th S92.534 Nondisplaced fracture of distal phalanx of right lesser toe(s) CC
4 7th S92.535 Nondisplaced fracture of distal phalanx of left lesser toe(s) CC
4 7th S92.536 Nondisplaced fracture of distal phalanx of unspecified lesser toe(s) CC
6th S92.59 Other fracture of lesser toe(s)
4 7th S92.591 Other fracture of right lesser toe(s) CC
4 7th S92.592 Other fracture of left lesser toe(s) CC
4 7th S92.599 Other fracture of unspecified lesser toe(s) CC
5th S92.8 Other fracture of foot, except ankle
6th S92.81 Other fracture of foot
Sesamoid fracture of foot
AHA: 2016,4Q,68
3 7th S92.811 Other fracture of right foot CC H5
3 7th S92.812 Other fracture of left foot CC H5
3 7th S92.819 Other fracture of unspecified foot CC H5
5th S92.9 Unspecified fracture of foot and toe
6th S92.90 Unspecified fracture of foot
3 7th S92.901 Unspecified fracture of right foot CC H5
3 7th S92.902 Unspecified fracture of left foot CC H5
3 7th S92.909 Unspecified fracture of unspecified foot CC H5
6th S92.91 Unspecified fracture of toe
4 7th S92.911 Unspecified fracture of right toe(s) CC

4 ✓7th **S92.912 Unspecified fracture of left toe(s)** CC

4 ✓7th **S92.919 Unspecified fracture of unspecified toe(s)** CC

✓4th **S93 Dislocation and sprain of joints and ligaments at ankle, foot and toe level**

INCLUDES avulsion of joint or ligament of ankle, foot and toe
laceration of cartilage, joint or ligament of ankle, foot and toe
sprain of cartilage, joint or ligament of ankle, foot and toe
traumatic hemarthrosis of joint or ligament of ankle, foot and toe
traumatic rupture of joint or ligament of ankle, foot and toe
traumatic subluxation of joint or ligament of ankle, foot and toe
traumatic tear of joint or ligament of ankle, foot and toe

Code also any associated open wound

EXCLUDES 2 *strain of muscle and tendon of ankle and foot (S96.-)*

The appropriate 7th character is to be added to each code from category S93.
A initial encounter
D subsequent encounter
S sequela

✓5th **S93.0 Subluxation and dislocation of ankle joint**
Subluxation and dislocation of astragalus
Subluxation and dislocation of fibula, lower end
Subluxation and dislocation of talus
Subluxation and dislocation of tibia, lower end

✓x7th **S93.01 Subluxation of right ankle joint**
✓x7th **S93.02 Subluxation of left ankle joint**
✓x7th **S93.03 Subluxation of unspecified ankle joint**
✓x7th **S93.04 Dislocation of right ankle joint**
✓x7th **S93.05 Dislocation of left ankle joint**
✓x7th **S93.06 Dislocation of unspecified ankle joint**

✓5th **S93.1 Subluxation and dislocation of toe**

✓6th **S93.10 Unspecified subluxation and dislocation of toe**
Dislocation of toe NOS
Subluxation of toe NOS

✓7th **S93.101 Unspecified subluxation of right toe(s)**
✓7th **S93.102 Unspecified subluxation of left toe(s)**
✓7th **S93.103 Unspecified subluxation of unspecified toe(s)**
✓7th **S93.104 Unspecified dislocation of right toe(s)**
✓7th **S93.105 Unspecified dislocation of left toe(s)**
✓7th **S93.106 Unspecified dislocation of unspecified toe(s)**

✓6th **S93.11 Dislocation of interphalangeal joint**

✓7th **S93.111 Dislocation of interphalangeal joint of right great toe**
✓7th **S93.112 Dislocation of interphalangeal joint of left great toe**
✓7th **S93.113 Dislocation of interphalangeal joint of unspecified great toe**
✓7th **S93.114 Dislocation of interphalangeal joint of right lesser toe(s)**
✓7th **S93.115 Dislocation of interphalangeal joint of left lesser toe(s)**
✓7th **S93.116 Dislocation of interphalangeal joint of unspecified lesser toe(s)**
✓7th **S93.119 Dislocation of interphalangeal joint of unspecified toe(s)**

✓6th **S93.12 Dislocation of metatarsophalangeal joint**

✓7th **S93.121 Dislocation of metatarsophalangeal joint of right great toe**
✓7th **S93.122 Dislocation of metatarsophalangeal joint of left great toe**
✓7th **S93.123 Dislocation of metatarsophalangeal joint of unspecified great toe**
✓7th **S93.124 Dislocation of metatarsophalangeal joint of right lesser toe(s)**
✓7th **S93.125 Dislocation of metatarsophalangeal joint of left lesser toe(s)**
✓7th **S93.126 Dislocation of metatarsophalangeal joint of unspecified lesser toe(s)**
✓7th **S93.129 Dislocation of metatarsophalangeal joint of unspecified toe(s)**

✓6th **S93.13 Subluxation of interphalangeal joint**

✓7th **S93.131 Subluxation of interphalangeal joint of right great toe**
✓7th **S93.132 Subluxation of interphalangeal joint of left great toe**
✓7th **S93.133 Subluxation of interphalangeal joint of unspecified great toe**
✓7th **S93.134 Subluxation of interphalangeal joint of right lesser toe(s)**
✓7th **S93.135 Subluxation of interphalangeal joint of left lesser toe(s)**
✓7th **S93.136 Subluxation of interphalangeal joint of unspecified lesser toe(s)**
✓7th **S93.139 Subluxation of interphalangeal joint of unspecified toe(s)**

✓6th **S93.14 Subluxation of metatarsophalangeal joint**

✓7th **S93.141 Subluxation of metatarsophalangeal joint of right great toe**
✓7th **S93.142 Subluxation of metatarsophalangeal joint of left great toe**
✓7th **S93.143 Subluxation of metatarsophalangeal joint of unspecified great toe**
✓7th **S93.144 Subluxation of metatarsophalangeal joint of right lesser toe(s)**
✓7th **S93.145 Subluxation of metatarsophalangeal joint of left lesser toe(s)**
✓7th **S93.146 Subluxation of metatarsophalangeal joint of unspecified lesser toe(s)**
✓7th **S93.149 Subluxation of metatarsophalangeal joint of unspecified toe(s)**

✓5th **S93.3 Subluxation and dislocation of foot**

EXCLUDES 2 *dislocation of toe (S93.1-)*

✓6th **S93.30 Unspecified subluxation and dislocation of foot**
Dislocation of foot NOS
Subluxation of foot NOS

✓7th **S93.301 Unspecified subluxation of right foot**
✓7th **S93.302 Unspecified subluxation of left foot**
✓7th **S93.303 Unspecified subluxation of unspecified foot**
✓7th **S93.304 Unspecified dislocation of right foot**
✓7th **S93.305 Unspecified dislocation of left foot**
✓7th **S93.306 Unspecified dislocation of unspecified foot**

✓6th **S93.31 Subluxation and dislocation of tarsal joint**

✓7th **S93.311 Subluxation of tarsal joint of right foot**
✓7th **S93.312 Subluxation of tarsal joint of left foot**
✓7th **S93.313 Subluxation of tarsal joint of unspecified foot**
✓7th **S93.314 Dislocation of tarsal joint of right foot**
✓7th **S93.315 Dislocation of tarsal joint of left foot**
✓7th **S93.316 Dislocation of tarsal joint of unspecified foot**

✓6th **S93.32 Subluxation and dislocation of tarsometatarsal joint**

✓7th **S93.321 Subluxation of tarsometatarsal joint of right foot**
✓7th **S93.322 Subluxation of tarsometatarsal joint of left foot**
✓7th **S93.323 Subluxation of tarsometatarsal joint of unspecified foot**
✓7th **S93.324 Dislocation of tarsometatarsal joint of right foot**
✓7th **S93.325 Dislocation of tarsometatarsal joint of left foot**
✓7th **S93.326 Dislocation of tarsometatarsal joint of unspecified foot**

✓6th **S93.33 Other subluxation and dislocation of foot**

✓7th **S93.331 Other subluxation of right foot**
✓7th **S93.332 Other subluxation of left foot**
✓7th **S93.333 Other subluxation of unspecified foot**
✓7th **S93.334 Other dislocation of right foot**
✓7th **S93.335 Other dislocation of left foot**
✓7th **S93.336 Other dislocation of unspecified foot**

S93.4 Sprain of ankle
EXCLUDES 2 *injury of Achilles tendon (S86.0-)*
S93.40 Sprain of unspecified ligament of ankle
Sprain of ankle NOS
Sprained ankle NOS
S93.401 Sprain of unspecified ligament of right ankle
S93.402 Sprain of unspecified ligament of left ankle
S93.409 Sprain of unspecified ligament of unspecified ankle
S93.41 Sprain of calcaneofibular ligament
S93.411 Sprain of calcaneofibular ligament of right ankle
S93.412 Sprain of calcaneofibular ligament of left ankle
S93.419 Sprain of calcaneofibular ligament of unspecified ankle
S93.42 Sprain of deltoid ligament
S93.421 Sprain of deltoid ligament of right ankle
S93.422 Sprain of deltoid ligament of left ankle
S93.429 Sprain of deltoid ligament of unspecified ankle
S93.43 Sprain of tibiofibular ligament
S93.431 Sprain of tibiofibular ligament of right ankle
S93.432 Sprain of tibiofibular ligament of left ankle
S93.439 Sprain of tibiofibular ligament of unspecified ankle
S93.49 Sprain of other ligament of ankle
Sprain of internal collateral ligament
Sprain of talofibular ligament
S93.491 Sprain of other ligament of right ankle
S93.492 Sprain of other ligament of left ankle
S93.499 Sprain of other ligament of unspecified ankle
S93.5 Sprain of toe
S93.50 Unspecified sprain of toe
S93.501 Unspecified sprain of right great toe
S93.502 Unspecified sprain of left great toe
S93.503 Unspecified sprain of unspecified great toe
S93.504 Unspecified sprain of right lesser toe(s)
S93.505 Unspecified sprain of left lesser toe(s)
S93.506 Unspecified sprain of unspecified lesser toe(s)
S93.509 Unspecified sprain of unspecified toe(s)
S93.51 Sprain of interphalangeal joint of toe
S93.511 Sprain of interphalangeal joint of right great toe
S93.512 Sprain of interphalangeal joint of left great toe
S93.513 Sprain of interphalangeal joint of unspecified great toe
S93.514 Sprain of interphalangeal joint of right lesser toe(s)
S93.515 Sprain of interphalangeal joint of left lesser toe(s)
S93.516 Sprain of interphalangeal joint of unspecified lesser toe(s)
S93.519 Sprain of interphalangeal joint of unspecified toe(s)
S93.52 Sprain of metatarsophalangeal joint of toe
S93.521 Sprain of metatarsophalangeal joint of right great toe
S93.522 Sprain of metatarsophalangeal joint of left great toe
S93.523 Sprain of metatarsophalangeal joint of unspecified great toe
S93.524 Sprain of metatarsophalangeal joint of right lesser toe(s)
S93.525 Sprain of metatarsophalangeal joint of left lesser toe(s)
S93.526 Sprain of metatarsophalangeal joint of unspecified lesser toe(s)
S93.529 Sprain of metatarsophalangeal joint of unspecified toe(s)
S93.6 Sprain of foot
EXCLUDES 2 *sprain of metatarsophalangeal joint of toe (S93.52-)*
sprain of toe (S93.5-)
S93.60 Unspecified sprain of foot
S93.601 Unspecified sprain of right foot
S93.602 Unspecified sprain of left foot
S93.609 Unspecified sprain of unspecified foot
S93.61 Sprain of tarsal ligament of foot
S93.611 Sprain of tarsal ligament of right foot
S93.612 Sprain of tarsal ligament of left foot
S93.619 Sprain of tarsal ligament of unspecified foot
S93.62 Sprain of tarsometatarsal ligament of foot
S93.621 Sprain of tarsometatarsal ligament of right foot
S93.622 Sprain of tarsometatarsal ligament of left foot
S93.629 Sprain of tarsometatarsal ligament of unspecified foot
S93.69 Other sprain of foot
S93.691 Other sprain of right foot
S93.692 Other sprain of left foot
S93.699 Other sprain of unspecified foot

S94 Injury of nerves at ankle and foot level
Code also any associated open wound (S91.-)
The appropriate 7th character is to be added to each code from category S94.
A initial encounter
D subsequent encounter
S sequela
S94.0 Injury of lateral plantar nerve
S94.00 Injury of lateral plantar nerve, unspecified leg
S94.01 Injury of lateral plantar nerve, right leg
S94.02 Injury of lateral plantar nerve, left leg
S94.1 Injury of medial plantar nerve
S94.10 Injury of medial plantar nerve, unspecified leg
S94.11 Injury of medial plantar nerve, right leg
S94.12 Injury of medial plantar nerve, left leg
S94.2 Injury of deep peroneal nerve at ankle and foot level
Injury of terminal, lateral branch of deep peroneal nerve
S94.20 Injury of deep peroneal nerve at ankle and foot level, unspecified leg
S94.21 Injury of deep peroneal nerve at ankle and foot level, right leg
S94.22 Injury of deep peroneal nerve at ankle and foot level, left leg
S94.3 Injury of cutaneous sensory nerve at ankle and foot level
S94.30 Injury of cutaneous sensory nerve at ankle and foot level, unspecified leg
S94.31 Injury of cutaneous sensory nerve at ankle and foot level, right leg
S94.32 Injury of cutaneous sensory nerve at ankle and foot level, left leg
S94.8 Injury of other nerves at ankle and foot level
S94.8X Injury of other nerves at ankle and foot level
S94.8X1 Injury of other nerves at ankle and foot level, right leg
S94.8X2 Injury of other nerves at ankle and foot level, left leg
S94.8X9 Injury of other nerves at ankle and foot level, unspecified leg
S94.9 Injury of unspecified nerve at ankle and foot level
S94.90 Injury of unspecified nerve at ankle and foot level, unspecified leg
S94.91 Injury of unspecified nerve at ankle and foot level, right leg
S94.92 Injury of unspecified nerve at ankle and foot level, left leg

Chapter 19. Injury, Poisoning and Certain Other Consequences of External Causes
S93.4–S94.92

S95 Injury of blood vessels at ankle and foot level

Code also any associated open wound (S91.-)

EXCLUDES 2 *injury of posterior tibial artery and vein (S85.1-, S85.8-)*

The appropriate 7th character is to be added to each code from category S95.
A initial encounter
D subsequent encounter
S sequela

S95.0 Injury of dorsal artery of foot
- **S95.00 Unspecified injury of dorsal artery of foot**
  - **S95.001 Unspecified injury of dorsal artery of right foot** CC
  - **S95.002 Unspecified injury of dorsal artery of left foot** CC
  - **S95.009 Unspecified injury of dorsal artery of unspecified foot** CC
- **S95.01 Laceration of dorsal artery of foot**
  - **S95.011 Laceration of dorsal artery of right foot** CC
  - **S95.012 Laceration of dorsal artery of left foot** CC
  - **S95.019 Laceration of dorsal artery of unspecified foot** CC
- **S95.09 Other specified injury of dorsal artery of foot**
  - **S95.091 Other specified injury of dorsal artery of right foot** CC
  - **S95.092 Other specified injury of dorsal artery of left foot** CC
  - **S95.099 Other specified injury of dorsal artery of unspecified foot** CC

S95.1 Injury of plantar artery of foot
- **S95.10 Unspecified injury of plantar artery of foot**
  - **S95.101 Unspecified injury of plantar artery of right foot** CC
  - **S95.102 Unspecified injury of plantar artery of left foot** CC
  - **S95.109 Unspecified injury of plantar artery of unspecified foot** CC
- **S95.11 Laceration of plantar artery of foot**
  - **S95.111 Laceration of plantar artery of right foot** CC
  - **S95.112 Laceration of plantar artery of left foot** CC
  - **S95.119 Laceration of plantar artery of unspecified foot** CC
- **S95.19 Other specified injury of plantar artery of foot**
  - **S95.191 Other specified injury of plantar artery of right foot** CC
  - **S95.192 Other specified injury of plantar artery of left foot** CC
  - **S95.199 Other specified injury of plantar artery of unspecified foot** CC

S95.2 Injury of dorsal vein of foot
- **S95.20 Unspecified injury of dorsal vein of foot**
  - **S95.201 Unspecified injury of dorsal vein of right foot** CC
  - **S95.202 Unspecified injury of dorsal vein of left foot** CC
  - **S95.209 Unspecified injury of dorsal vein of unspecified foot** CC
- **S95.21 Laceration of dorsal vein of foot**
  - **S95.211 Laceration of dorsal vein of right foot** CC
  - **S95.212 Laceration of dorsal vein of left foot** CC
  - **S95.219 Laceration of dorsal vein of unspecified foot** CC
- **S95.29 Other specified injury of dorsal vein of foot**
  - **S95.291 Other specified injury of dorsal vein of right foot** CC
  - **S95.292 Other specified injury of dorsal vein of left foot** CC
  - **S95.299 Other specified injury of dorsal vein of unspecified foot** CC

S95.8 Injury of other blood vessels at ankle and foot level
- **S95.80 Unspecified injury of other blood vessels at ankle and foot level**
  - **S95.801 Unspecified injury of other blood vessels at ankle and foot level, right leg** CC
  - **S95.802 Unspecified injury of other blood vessels at ankle and foot level, left leg** CC
  - **S95.809 Unspecified injury of other blood vessels at ankle and foot level, unspecified leg** CC
- **S95.81 Laceration of other blood vessels at ankle and foot level**
  - **S95.811 Laceration of other blood vessels at ankle and foot level, right leg** CC
  - **S95.812 Laceration of other blood vessels at ankle and foot level, left leg** CC
  - **S95.819 Laceration of other blood vessels at ankle and foot level, unspecified leg** CC
- **S95.89 Other specified injury of other blood vessels at ankle and foot level**
  - **S95.891 Other specified injury of other blood vessels at ankle and foot level, right leg** CC
  - **S95.892 Other specified injury of other blood vessels at ankle and foot level, left leg** CC
  - **S95.899 Other specified injury of other blood vessels at ankle and foot level, unspecified leg** CC

S95.9 Injury of unspecified blood vessel at ankle and foot level
- **S95.90 Unspecified injury of unspecified blood vessel at ankle and foot level**
  - **S95.901 Unspecified injury of unspecified blood vessel at ankle and foot level, right leg** CC
  - **S95.902 Unspecified injury of unspecified blood vessel at ankle and foot level, left leg** CC
  - **S95.909 Unspecified injury of unspecified blood vessel at ankle and foot level, unspecified leg** CC
- **S95.91 Laceration of unspecified blood vessel at ankle and foot level**
  - **S95.911 Laceration of unspecified blood vessel at ankle and foot level, right leg** CC
  - **S95.912 Laceration of unspecified blood vessel at ankle and foot level, left leg** CC
  - **S95.919 Laceration of unspecified blood vessel at ankle and foot level, unspecified leg** CC
- **S95.99 Other specified injury of unspecified blood vessel at ankle and foot level**
  - **S95.991 Other specified injury of unspecified blood vessel at ankle and foot level, right leg** CC
  - **S95.992 Other specified injury of unspecified blood vessel at ankle and foot level, left leg** CC
  - **S95.999 Other specified injury of unspecified blood vessel at ankle and foot level, unspecified leg** CC

S96 Injury of muscle and tendon at ankle and foot level

Code also any associated open wound (S91.-)

EXCLUDES 2 *injury of Achilles tendon (S86.0-)*
sprain of joints and ligaments of ankle and foot (S93.-)

TIP: Refer to the Muscle/Tendon table at the beginning of this chapter.

The appropriate 7th character is to be added to each code from category S96.
A initial encounter
D subsequent encounter
S sequela

S96.0 Injury of muscle and tendon of long flexor muscle of toe at ankle and foot level
- **S96.00 Unspecified injury of muscle and tendon of long flexor muscle of toe at ankle and foot level**
  - **S96.001 Unspecified injury of muscle and tendon of long flexor muscle of toe at ankle and foot level, right foot**
  - **S96.002 Unspecified injury of muscle and tendon of long flexor muscle of toe at ankle and foot level, left foot**

S96.009 Unspecified injury of muscle and tendon of long flexor muscle of toe at ankle and foot level, unspecified foot

S96.01 Strain of muscle and tendon of long flexor muscle of toe at ankle and foot level

S96.011 Strain of muscle and tendon of long flexor muscle of toe at ankle and foot level, right foot

S96.012 Strain of muscle and tendon of long flexor muscle of toe at ankle and foot level, left foot

S96.019 Strain of muscle and tendon of long flexor muscle of toe at ankle and foot level, unspecified foot

S96.02 Laceration of muscle and tendon of long flexor muscle of toe at ankle and foot level

S96.021 Laceration of muscle and tendon of long flexor muscle of toe at ankle and foot level, right foot CC

S96.022 Laceration of muscle and tendon of long flexor muscle of toe at ankle and foot level, left foot CC

S96.029 Laceration of muscle and tendon of long flexor muscle of toe at ankle and foot level, unspecified foot CC

S96.09 Other injury of muscle and tendon of long flexor muscle of toe at ankle and foot level

S96.091 Other injury of muscle and tendon of long flexor muscle of toe at ankle and foot level, right foot

S96.092 Other injury of muscle and tendon of long flexor muscle of toe at ankle and foot level, left foot

S96.099 Other injury of muscle and tendon of long flexor muscle of toe at ankle and foot level, unspecified foot

S96.1 Injury of muscle and tendon of long extensor muscle of toe at ankle and foot level

S96.10 Unspecified injury of muscle and tendon of long extensor muscle of toe at ankle and foot level

S96.101 Unspecified injury of muscle and tendon of long extensor muscle of toe at ankle and foot level, right foot

S96.102 Unspecified injury of muscle and tendon of long extensor muscle of toe at ankle and foot level, left foot

S96.109 Unspecified injury of muscle and tendon of long extensor muscle of toe at ankle and foot level, unspecified foot

S96.11 Strain of muscle and tendon of long extensor muscle of toe at ankle and foot level

S96.111 Strain of muscle and tendon of long extensor muscle of toe at ankle and foot level, right foot

S96.112 Strain of muscle and tendon of long extensor muscle of toe at ankle and foot level, left foot

S96.119 Strain of muscle and tendon of long extensor muscle of toe at ankle and foot level, unspecified foot

S96.12 Laceration of muscle and tendon of long extensor muscle of toe at ankle and foot level

S96.121 Laceration of muscle and tendon of long extensor muscle of toe at ankle and foot level, right foot CC

S96.122 Laceration of muscle and tendon of long extensor muscle of toe at ankle and foot level, left foot CC

S96.129 Laceration of muscle and tendon of long extensor muscle of toe at ankle and foot level, unspecified foot CC

S96.19 Other specified injury of muscle and tendon of long extensor muscle of toe at ankle and foot level

S96.191 Other specified injury of muscle and tendon of long extensor muscle of toe at ankle and foot level, right foot

S96.192 Other specified injury of muscle and tendon of long extensor muscle of toe at ankle and foot level, left foot

S96.199 Other specified injury of muscle and tendon of long extensor muscle of toe at ankle and foot level, unspecified foot

S96.2 Injury of intrinsic muscle and tendon at ankle and foot level

S96.20 Unspecified injury of intrinsic muscle and tendon at ankle and foot level

S96.201 Unspecified injury of intrinsic muscle and tendon at ankle and foot level, right foot

S96.202 Unspecified injury of intrinsic muscle and tendon at ankle and foot level, left foot

S96.209 Unspecified injury of intrinsic muscle and tendon at ankle and foot level, unspecified foot

S96.21 Strain of intrinsic muscle and tendon at ankle and foot level

S96.211 Strain of intrinsic muscle and tendon at ankle and foot level, right foot

S96.212 Strain of intrinsic muscle and tendon at ankle and foot level, left foot

S96.219 Strain of intrinsic muscle and tendon at ankle and foot level, unspecified foot

S96.22 Laceration of intrinsic muscle and tendon at ankle and foot level

S96.221 Laceration of intrinsic muscle and tendon at ankle and foot level, right foot CC

S96.222 Laceration of intrinsic muscle and tendon at ankle and foot level, left foot CC

S96.229 Laceration of intrinsic muscle and tendon at ankle and foot level, unspecified foot CC

S96.29 Other specified injury of intrinsic muscle and tendon at ankle and foot level

S96.291 Other specified injury of intrinsic muscle and tendon at ankle and foot level, right foot

S96.292 Other specified injury of intrinsic muscle and tendon at ankle and foot level, left foot

S96.299 Other specified injury of intrinsic muscle and tendon at ankle and foot level, unspecified foot

S96.8 Injury of other specified muscles and tendons at ankle and foot level

S96.80 Unspecified injury of other specified muscles and tendons at ankle and foot level

S96.801 Unspecified injury of other specified muscles and tendons at ankle and foot level, right foot

S96.802 Unspecified injury of other specified muscles and tendons at ankle and foot level, left foot

S96.809 Unspecified injury of other specified muscles and tendons at ankle and foot level, unspecified foot

S96.81 Strain of other specified muscles and tendons at ankle and foot level

S96.811 Strain of other specified muscles and tendons at ankle and foot level, right foot

S96.812 Strain of other specified muscles and tendons at ankle and foot level, left foot

S96.819 Strain of other specified muscles and tendons at ankle and foot level, unspecified foot

S96.82 Laceration of other specified muscles and tendons at ankle and foot level

S96.821 Laceration of other specified muscles and tendons at ankle and foot level, right foot CC

S96.822 Laceration of other specified muscles and tendons at ankle and foot level, left foot CC

S96.829 Laceration of other specified muscles and tendons at ankle and foot level, unspecified foot CC

S96.89 Other specified injury of other specified muscles and tendons at ankle and foot level

S96.891 Other specified injury of other specified muscles and tendons at ankle and foot level, right foot

S96.892 Other specified injury of other specified muscles and tendons at ankle and foot level, left foot

S96.899 Other specified injury of other specified muscles and tendons at ankle and foot level, unspecified foot

✓5th **S96.9 Injury of unspecified muscle and tendon at ankle and foot level**

✓6th **S96.90 Unspecified injury of unspecified muscle and tendon at ankle and foot level**

✓7th **S96.901 Unspecified injury of unspecified muscle and tendon at ankle and foot level, right foot**

✓7th **S96.902 Unspecified injury of unspecified muscle and tendon at ankle and foot level, left foot**

✓7th **S96.909 Unspecified injury of unspecified muscle and tendon at ankle and foot level, unspecified foot**

✓6th **S96.91 Strain of unspecified muscle and tendon at ankle and foot level**

✓7th **S96.911 Strain of unspecified muscle and tendon at ankle and foot level, right foot**

✓7th **S96.912 Strain of unspecified muscle and tendon at ankle and foot level, left foot**

✓7th **S96.919 Strain of unspecified muscle and tendon at ankle and foot level, unspecified foot**

✓6th **S96.92 Laceration of unspecified muscle and tendon at ankle and foot level**

✓7th **S96.921 Laceration of unspecified muscle and tendon at ankle and foot level, right foot** CC

✓7th **S96.922 Laceration of unspecified muscle and tendon at ankle and foot level, left foot** CC

✓7th **S96.929 Laceration of unspecified muscle and tendon at ankle and foot level, unspecified foot** CC

✓6th **S96.99 Other specified injury of unspecified muscle and tendon at ankle and foot level**

✓7th **S96.991 Other specified injury of unspecified muscle and tendon at ankle and foot level, right foot**

✓7th **S96.992 Other specified injury of unspecified muscle and tendon at ankle and foot level, left foot**

✓7th **S96.999 Other specified injury of unspecified muscle and tendon at ankle and foot level, unspecified foot**

✓4th **S97 Crushing injury of ankle and foot**

Use additional code(s) for all associated injuries

The appropriate 7th character is to be added to each code from category S97.
A initial encounter
D subsequent encounter
S sequela

✓5th **S97.0 Crushing injury of ankle**

✓x7th **S97.00 Crushing injury of unspecified ankle**

✓x7th **S97.01 Crushing injury of right ankle**

✓x7th **S97.02 Crushing injury of left ankle**

✓5th **S97.1 Crushing injury of toe**

✓6th **S97.10 Crushing injury of unspecified toe(s)**

✓7th **S97.101 Crushing injury of unspecified right toe(s)**

✓7th **S97.102 Crushing injury of unspecified left toe(s)**

✓7th **S97.109 Crushing injury of unspecified toe(s)**
Crushing injury of toe NOS

✓6th **S97.11 Crushing injury of great toe**

✓7th **S97.111 Crushing injury of right great toe**

✓7th **S97.112 Crushing injury of left great toe**

✓7th **S97.119 Crushing injury of unspecified great toe**

✓6th **S97.12 Crushing injury of lesser toe(s)**

✓7th **S97.121 Crushing injury of right lesser toe(s)**

✓7th **S97.122 Crushing injury of left lesser toe(s)**

✓7th **S97.129 Crushing injury of unspecified lesser toe(s)**

✓5th **S97.8 Crushing injury of foot**

✓x7th **S97.80 Crushing injury of unspecified foot**
Crushing injury of foot NOS

✓x7th **S97.81 Crushing injury of right foot**

✓x7th **S97.82 Crushing injury of left foot**

✓4th **S98 Traumatic amputation of ankle and foot**

An amputation not identified as partial or complete should be coded to complete

The appropriate 7th character is to be added to each code from category S98.
A initial encounter
D subsequent encounter
S sequela

✓5th **S98.0 Traumatic amputation of foot at ankle level**

✓6th **S98.01 Complete traumatic amputation of foot at ankle level**

✓7th **S98.011 Complete traumatic amputation of right foot at ankle level** CC HCC

✓7th **S98.012 Complete traumatic amputation of left foot at ankle level** CC HCC

✓7th **S98.019 Complete traumatic amputation of unspecified foot at ankle level** CC HCC

✓6th **S98.02 Partial traumatic amputation of foot at ankle level**

✓7th **S98.021 Partial traumatic amputation of right foot at ankle level** CC HCC

✓7th **S98.022 Partial traumatic amputation of left foot at ankle level** CC HCC

✓7th **S98.029 Partial traumatic amputation of unspecified foot at ankle level** CC HCC

✓5th **S98.1 Traumatic amputation of one toe**

✓6th **S98.11 Complete traumatic amputation of great toe**

✓7th **S98.111 Complete traumatic amputation of right great toe** HCC

✓7th **S98.112 Complete traumatic amputation of left great toe** HCC

✓7th **S98.119 Complete traumatic amputation of unspecified great toe** HCC

✓6th **S98.12 Partial traumatic amputation of great toe**

✓7th **S98.121 Partial traumatic amputation of right great toe** HCC

✓7th **S98.122 Partial traumatic amputation of left great toe** HCC

✓7th **S98.129 Partial traumatic amputation of unspecified great toe** HCC

✓6th **S98.13 Complete traumatic amputation of one lesser toe**
Traumatic amputation of toe NOS

✓7th **S98.131 Complete traumatic amputation of one right lesser toe** HCC

✓7th **S98.132 Complete traumatic amputation of one left lesser toe** HCC

✓7th **S98.139 Complete traumatic amputation of one unspecified lesser toe** HCC

✓6th **S98.14 Partial traumatic amputation of one lesser toe**

✓7th **S98.141 Partial traumatic amputation of one right lesser toe** HCC

✓7th **S98.142 Partial traumatic amputation of one left lesser toe** HCC

✓7th **S98.149 Partial traumatic amputation of one unspecified lesser toe** HCC

✓5th **S98.2 Traumatic amputation of two or more lesser toes**

✓6th **S98.21 Complete traumatic amputation of two or more lesser toes**

✓7th **S98.211 Complete traumatic amputation of two or more right lesser toes** HCC

✓7th **S98.212 Complete traumatic amputation of two or more left lesser toes** HCC

✓7th **S98.219 Complete traumatic amputation of two or more unspecified lesser toes** HCC

✓6th **S98.22 Partial traumatic amputation of two or more lesser toes**

✓7th **S98.221 Partial traumatic amputation of two or more right lesser toes** HCC

✓7th **S98.222 Partial traumatic amputation of two or more left lesser toes** HCC

✓7th **S98.229 Partial traumatic amputation of two or more unspecified lesser toes** HCC

✓5th **S98.3 Traumatic amputation of midfoot**

✓6th **S98.31 Complete traumatic amputation of midfoot**

✓7th **S98.311 Complete traumatic amputation of right midfoot** CC HCC

✓7th **S98.312 Complete traumatic amputation of left midfoot** CC HCC

✓7th **S98.319** **Complete traumatic amputation of unspecified midfoot** CC HCC

✓6th **S98.32** **Partial traumatic amputation of midfoot**

✓7th **S98.321** **Partial traumatic amputation of right midfoot** CC HCC

✓7th **S98.322** **Partial traumatic amputation of left midfoot** CC HCC

✓7th **S98.329** **Partial traumatic amputation of unspecified midfoot** CC HCC

✓5th **S98.9** **Traumatic amputation of foot, level unspecified**

✓6th **S98.91** **Complete traumatic amputation of foot, level unspecified**

✓7th **S98.911** **Complete traumatic amputation of right foot, level unspecified** CC HCC

✓7th **S98.912** **Complete traumatic amputation of left foot, level unspecified** CC HCC

✓7th **S98.919** **Complete traumatic amputation of unspecified foot, level unspecified** CC HCC

✓6th **S98.92** **Partial traumatic amputation of foot, level unspecified**

✓7th **S98.921** **Partial traumatic amputation of right foot, level unspecified** CC HCC

✓7th **S98.922** **Partial traumatic amputation of left foot, level unspecified** CC HCC

✓7th **S98.929** **Partial traumatic amputation of unspecified foot, level unspecified** CC HCC

✓4th **S99** **Other and unspecified injuries of ankle and foot**

AHA: 2018,2Q,12; 2018,1Q,3; 2016,4Q,68-69

✓5th **S99.Ø** **Physeal fracture of calcaneus**

AHA: 2019,4Q,56

The appropriate 7th character is to be added to each code from subcategory S99.Ø.
- A initial encounter for closed fracture
- B initial encounter for open fracture
- D subsequent encounter for fracture with routine healing
- G subsequent encounter for fracture with delayed healing
- K subsequent encounter for fracture with nonunion
- P subsequent encounter for fracture with malunion
- S sequela

✓6th **S99.ØØ** **Unspecified physeal fracture of calcaneus**

✓7th **S99.ØØ1** **Unspecified physeal fracture of right calcaneus**

✓7th **S99.ØØ2** **Unspecified physeal fracture of left calcaneus**

✓7th **S99.ØØ9** **Unspecified physeal fracture of unspecified calcaneus**

✓6th **S99.Ø1** **Salter-Harris Type I physeal fracture of calcaneus**

✓7th **S99.Ø11** **Salter-Harris Type I physeal fracture of right calcaneus**

✓7th **S99.Ø12** **Salter-Harris Type I physeal fracture of left calcaneus**

✓7th **S99.Ø19** **Salter-Harris Type I physeal fracture of unspecified calcaneus**

✓6th **S99.Ø2** **Salter-Harris Type II physeal fracture of calcaneus**

✓7th **S99.Ø21** **Salter-Harris Type II physeal fracture of right calcaneus**

✓7th **S99.Ø22** **Salter-Harris Type II physeal fracture of left calcaneus**

✓7th **S99.Ø29** **Salter-Harris Type II physeal fracture of unspecified calcaneus**

✓6th **S99.Ø3** **Salter-Harris Type III physeal fracture of calcaneus**

✓7th **S99.Ø31** **Salter-Harris Type III physeal fracture of right calcaneus**

✓7th **S99.Ø32** **Salter-Harris Type III physeal fracture of left calcaneus**

✓7th **S99.Ø39** **Salter-Harris Type III physeal fracture of unspecified calcaneus**

✓6th **S99.Ø4** **Salter-Harris Type IV physeal fracture of calcaneus**

✓7th **S99.Ø41** **Salter-Harris Type IV physeal fracture of right calcaneus**

✓7th **S99.Ø42** **Salter-Harris Type IV physeal fracture of left calcaneus**

✓7th **S99.Ø49** **Salter-Harris Type IV physeal fracture of unspecified calcaneus**

✓6th **S99.Ø9** **Other physeal fracture of calcaneus**

✓7th **S99.Ø91** **Other physeal fracture of right calcaneus**

✓7th **S99.Ø92** **Other physeal fracture of left calcaneus**

✓7th **S99.Ø99** **Other physeal fracture of unspecified calcaneus**

✓5th **S99.1** **Physeal fracture of metatarsal**

AHA: 2019,4Q,56

The appropriate 7th character is to be added to each code from subcategory S99.1
- A initial encounter for closed fracture
- B initial encounter for open fracture
- D subsequent encounter for fracture with routine healing
- G subsequent encounter for fracture with delayed healing
- K subsequent encounter for fracture with nonunion
- P subsequent encounter for fracture with malunion
- S sequela

✓6th **S99.1Ø** **Unspecified physeal fracture of metatarsal**

✓7th **S99.1Ø1** **Unspecified physeal fracture of right metatarsal**

✓7th **S99.1Ø2** **Unspecified physeal fracture of left metatarsal**

✓7th **S99.1Ø9** **Unspecified physeal fracture of unspecified metatarsal**

✓6th **S99.11** **Salter-Harris Type I physeal fracture of metatarsal**

✓7th **S99.111** **Salter-Harris Type I physeal fracture of right metatarsal**

✓7th **S99.112** **Salter-Harris Type I physeal fracture of left metatarsal**

✓7th **S99.119** **Salter-Harris Type I physeal fracture of unspecified metatarsal**

✓6th **S99.12** **Salter-Harris Type II physeal fracture of metatarsal**

✓7th **S99.121** **Salter-Harris Type II physeal fracture of right metatarsal**

✓7th **S99.122** **Salter-Harris Type II physeal fracture of left metatarsal**

✓7th **S99.129** **Salter-Harris Type II physeal fracture of unspecified metatarsal**

✓6th **S99.13** **Salter-Harris Type III physeal fracture of metatarsal**

✓7th **S99.131** **Salter-Harris Type III physeal fracture of right metatarsal**

✓7th **S99.132** **Salter-Harris Type III physeal fracture of left metatarsal**

✓7th **S99.139** **Salter-Harris Type III physeal fracture of unspecified metatarsal**

✓6th **S99.14** **Salter-Harris Type IV physeal fracture of metatarsal**

✓7th **S99.141** **Salter-Harris Type IV physeal fracture of right metatarsal**

✓7th **S99.142** **Salter-Harris Type IV physeal fracture of left metatarsal**

✓7th **S99.149** **Salter-Harris Type IV physeal fracture of unspecified metatarsal**

✓6th **S99.19** **Other physeal fracture of metatarsal**

✓7th **S99.191** **Other physeal fracture of right metatarsal**

✓7th **S99.192** **Other physeal fracture of left metatarsal**

✓7th **S99.199** **Other physeal fracture of unspecified metatarsal**

✓5th **S99.2** **Physeal fracture of phalanx of toe**

AHA: 2019,4Q,56

The appropriate 7th character is to be added to each code from subcategories S99.2.
- A initial encounter for closed fracture
- B initial encounter for open fracture
- D subsequent encounter for fracture with routine healing
- G subsequent encounter for fracture with delayed healing
- K subsequent encounter for fracture with nonunion
- P subsequent encounter for fracture with malunion
- S sequela

✓6th **S99.2Ø** **Unspecified physeal fracture of phalanx of toe**

✓7th **S99.2Ø1** **Unspecified physeal fracture of phalanx of right toe**

✓7th **S99.2Ø2** **Unspecified physeal fracture of phalanx of left toe**

✓7th **S99.2Ø9** **Unspecified physeal fracture of phalanx of unspecified toe**

✓6th **S99.21** **Salter-Harris Type I physeal fracture of phalanx of toe**

✓7th **S99.211** **Salter-Harris Type I physeal fracture of phalanx of right toe**

✓7th **S99.212** **Salter-Harris Type I physeal fracture of phalanx of left toe**

√7th **S99.219 Salter-Harris Type I physeal fracture of phalanx of unspecified toe**

√6th **S99.22 Salter-Harris Type II physeal fracture of phalanx of toe**

√7th **S99.221 Salter-Harris Type II physeal fracture of phalanx of right toe**

√7th **S99.222 Salter-Harris Type II physeal fracture of phalanx of left toe**

√7th **S99.229 Salter-Harris Type II physeal fracture of phalanx of unspecified toe**

√6th **S99.23 Salter-Harris Type III physeal fracture of phalanx of toe**

√7th **S99.231 Salter-Harris Type III physeal fracture of phalanx of right toe**

√7th **S99.232 Salter-Harris Type III physeal fracture of phalanx of left toe**

√7th **S99.239 Salter-Harris Type III physeal fracture of phalanx of unspecified toe**

√6th **S99.24 Salter-Harris Type IV physeal fracture of phalanx of toe**

√7th **S99.241 Salter-Harris Type IV physeal fracture of phalanx of right toe**

√7th **S99.242 Salter-Harris Type IV physeal fracture of phalanx of left toe**

√7th **S99.249 Salter-Harris Type IV physeal fracture of phalanx of unspecified toe**

√6th **S99.29 Other physeal fracture of phalanx of toe**

√7th **S99.291 Other physeal fracture of phalanx of right toe**

√7th **S99.292 Other physeal fracture of phalanx of left toe**

√7th **S99.299 Other physeal fracture of phalanx of unspecified toe**

√5th **S99.8 Other specified injuries of ankle and foot**

The appropriate 7th character is to be added to each code from subcategory S99.8.
A initial encounter
D subsequent encounter
S sequela

√6th **S99.81 Other specified injuries of ankle**

√7th **S99.811 Other specified injuries of right ankle**

√7th **S99.812 Other specified injuries of left ankle**

√7th **S99.819 Other specified injuries of unspecified ankle**

√6th **S99.82 Other specified injuries of foot**

√7th **S99.821 Other specified injuries of right foot**

√7th **S99.822 Other specified injuries of left foot**

√7th **S99.829 Other specified injuries of unspecified foot**

√5th **S99.9 Unspecified injury of ankle and foot**

The appropriate 7th character is to be added to each code from subcategory S99.9.
A initial encounter
D subsequent encounter
S sequela

√6th **S99.91 Unspecified injury of ankle**

√7th **S99.911 Unspecified injury of right ankle**

√7th **S99.912 Unspecified injury of left ankle**

√7th **S99.919 Unspecified injury of unspecified ankle**

√6th **S99.92 Unspecified injury of foot**

√7th **S99.921 Unspecified injury of right foot**

√7th **S99.922 Unspecified injury of left foot**

√7th **S99.929 Unspecified injury of unspecified foot**

INJURY, POISONING AND CERTAIN OTHER CONSEQUENCES OF EXTERNAL CAUSES (T07-T88)

Injuries involving multiple body regions (T07)

EXCLUDES 1 *burns and corrosions (T20-T32)*
frostbite (T33-T34)
insect bite or sting, venomous (T63.4)
sunburn (L55.-)

√x7th **T07 Unspecified multiple injuries**

EXCLUDES 1 *injury NOS (T14.90)*

AHA: 2017,4Q,26

The appropriate 7th character is to be added to code T07.
A initial encounter
D subsequent encounter
S sequela

Injury of unspecified body region (T14)

√4th **T14 Injury of unspecified body region**

EXCLUDES 1 *multiple unspecified injuries (T07)*

AHA: 2017,4Q,26

The appropriate 7th character is to be added to each code from category T14.
A initial encounter
D subsequent encounter
S sequela

√x7th **T14.8 Other injury of unspecified body region**

Abrasion NOS
Contusion NOS
Crush injury NOS
Fracture NOS
Skin injury NOS
Vascular injury NOS
Wound NOS

√5th **T14.9 Unspecified injury**

√x7th **T14.90 Injury, unspecified**

Injury NOS

√x7th **T14.91 Suicide attempt** HCC

Attempted suicide NOS

Effects of foreign body entering through natural orifice (T15-T19)

EXCLUDES 2 *foreign body accidentally left in operation wound (T81.5-)*
foreign body in penetrating wound — see open wound by body region
residual foreign body in soft tissue (M79.5)
splinter, without open wound — see superficial injury by body region

√4th **T15 Foreign body on external eye**

EXCLUDES 2 *foreign body in penetrating wound of orbit and eye ball (S05.4-, S05.5-)*
open wound of eyelid and periocular area (S01.1-)
retained foreign body in eyelid (H02.8-)
retained (old) foreign body in penetrating wound of orbit and eye ball (H05.5-, H44.6-, H44.7-)
superficial foreign body of eyelid and periocular area (S00.25-)

The appropriate 7th character is to be added to each code from category T15.
A initial encounter
D subsequent encounter
S sequela

√5th **T15.0 Foreign body in cornea**

√x7th **T15.00 Foreign body in cornea, unspecified eye**

√x7th **T15.01 Foreign body in cornea, right eye**

√x7th **T15.02 Foreign body in cornea, left eye**

√5th **T15.1 Foreign body in conjunctival sac**

√x7th **T15.10 Foreign body in conjunctival sac, unspecified eye**

√x7th **T15.11 Foreign body in conjunctival sac, right eye**

√x7th **T15.12 Foreign body in conjunctival sac, left eye**

√5th **T15.8 Foreign body in other and multiple parts of external eye**

Foreign body in lacrimal punctum

√x7th **T15.80 Foreign body in other and multiple parts of external eye, unspecified eye**

T15.81 Foreign body in other and multiple parts of external eye, right eye
T15.82 Foreign body in other and multiple parts of external eye, left eye
T15.9 Foreign body on external eye, part unspecified
T15.90 Foreign body on external eye, part unspecified, unspecified eye
T15.91 Foreign body on external eye, part unspecified, right eye
T15.92 Foreign body on external eye, part unspecified, left eye

T16 Foreign body in ear

INCLUDES foreign body in auditory canal

The appropriate 7th character is to be added to each code from category T16.
A initial encounter
D subsequent encounter
S sequela

T16.1 Foreign body in right ear
T16.2 Foreign body in left ear
T16.9 Foreign body in ear, unspecified ear

T17 Foreign body in respiratory tract

The appropriate 7th character is to be added to each code from category T17.
A initial encounter
D subsequent encounter
S sequela

T17.0 Foreign body in nasal sinus
T17.1 Foreign body in nostril
Foreign body in nose NOS
T17.2 Foreign body in pharynx
Foreign body in nasopharynx
Foreign body in throat NOS
T17.20 Unspecified foreign body in pharynx
T17.200 Unspecified foreign body in pharynx causing asphyxiation
T17.208 Unspecified foreign body in pharynx causing other injury
T17.21 Gastric contents in pharynx
Aspiration of gastric contents into pharynx
Vomitus in pharynx
T17.210 Gastric contents in pharynx causing asphyxiation
T17.218 Gastric contents in pharynx causing other injury
T17.22 Food in pharynx
Bones in pharynx
Seeds in pharynx
T17.220 Food in pharynx causing asphyxiation
T17.228 Food in pharynx causing other injury
T17.29 Other foreign object in pharynx
T17.290 Other foreign object in pharynx causing asphyxiation
T17.298 Other foreign object in pharynx causing other injury
T17.3 Foreign body in larynx
T17.30 Unspecified foreign body in larynx
T17.300 Unspecified foreign body in larynx causing asphyxiation
T17.308 Unspecified foreign body in larynx causing other injury
T17.31 Gastric contents in larynx
Aspiration of gastric contents into larynx
Vomitus in larynx
T17.310 Gastric contents in larynx causing asphyxiation
T17.318 Gastric contents in larynx causing other injury
T17.32 Food in larynx
Bones in larynx
Seeds in larynx
T17.320 Food in larynx causing asphyxiation
T17.328 Food in larynx causing other injury
T17.39 Other foreign object in larynx
T17.390 Other foreign object in larynx causing asphyxiation
T17.398 Other foreign object in larynx causing other injury
T17.4 Foreign body in trachea
T17.40 Unspecified foreign body in trachea
T17.400 Unspecified foreign body in trachea causing asphyxiation CC
T17.408 Unspecified foreign body in trachea causing other injury CC
T17.41 Gastric contents in trachea
Aspiration of gastric contents into trachea
Vomitus in trachea
T17.410 Gastric contents in trachea causing asphyxiation CC
T17.418 Gastric contents in trachea causing other injury CC
T17.42 Food in trachea
Bones in trachea
Seeds in trachea
T17.420 Food in trachea causing asphyxiation CC
T17.428 Food in trachea causing other injury CC
T17.49 Other foreign object in trachea
T17.490 Other foreign object in trachea causing asphyxiation CC
T17.498 Other foreign object in trachea causing other injury CC
T17.5 Foreign body in bronchus
T17.50 Unspecified foreign body in bronchus
T17.500 Unspecified foreign body in bronchus causing asphyxiation CC
T17.508 Unspecified foreign body in bronchus causing other injury CC
T17.51 Gastric contents in bronchus
Aspiration of gastric contents into bronchus
Vomitus in bronchus
T17.510 Gastric contents in bronchus causing asphyxiation CC
T17.518 Gastric contents in bronchus causing other injury CC
T17.52 Food in bronchus
Bones in bronchus
Seeds in bronchus
T17.520 Food in bronchus causing asphyxiation CC
T17.528 Food in bronchus causing other injury CC
T17.59 Other foreign object in bronchus
T17.590 Other foreign object in bronchus causing asphyxiation CC
T17.598 Other foreign object in bronchus causing other injury CC
T17.8 Foreign body in other parts of respiratory tract
Foreign body in bronchioles
Foreign body in lung
T17.80 Unspecified foreign body in other parts of respiratory tract
T17.800 Unspecified foreign body in other parts of respiratory tract causing asphyxiation CC
T17.808 Unspecified foreign body in other parts of respiratory tract causing other injury CC
T17.81 Gastric contents in other parts of respiratory tract
Aspiration of gastric contents into other parts of respiratory tract
Vomitus in other parts of respiratory tract
T17.810 Gastric contents in other parts of respiratory tract causing asphyxiation CC
T17.818 Gastric contents in other parts of respiratory tract causing other injury CC

√6th **T17.82 Food in other parts of respiratory tract**
Bones in other parts of respiratory tract
Seeds in other parts of respiratory tract
√7th **T17.820 Food in other parts of respiratory tract causing asphyxiation** CC
√7th **T17.828 Food in other parts of respiratory tract causing other injury** CC
√6th **T17.89 Other foreign object in other parts of respiratory tract**
√7th **T17.890 Other foreign object in other parts of respiratory tract causing asphyxiation** CC
√7th **T17.898 Other foreign object in other parts of respiratory tract causing other injury** CC
√5th **T17.9 Foreign body in respiratory tract, part unspecified**
√6th **T17.90 Unspecified foreign body in respiratory tract, part unspecified**
√7th **T17.900 Unspecified foreign body in respiratory tract, part unspecified causing asphyxiation**
√7th **T17.908 Unspecified foreign body in respiratory tract, part unspecified causing other injury**
√6th **T17.91 Gastric contents in respiratory tract, part unspecified**
Aspiration of gastric contents into respiratory tract, part unspecified
Vomitus in trachea respiratory tract, part unspecified
√7th **T17.910 Gastric contents in respiratory tract, part unspecified causing asphyxiation**
√7th **T17.918 Gastric contents in respiratory tract, part unspecified causing other injury**
√6th **T17.92 Food in respiratory tract, part unspecified**
Bones in respiratory tract, part unspecified
Seeds in respiratory tract, part unspecified
√7th **T17.920 Food in respiratory tract, part unspecified causing asphyxiation**
√7th **T17.928 Food in respiratory tract, part unspecified causing other injury**
√6th **T17.99 Other foreign object in respiratory tract, part unspecified**
√7th **T17.990 Other foreign object in respiratory tract, part unspecified in causing asphyxiation**
AHA: 2019,3Q,15
√7th **T17.998 Other foreign object in respiratory tract, part unspecified causing other injury**

√4th **T18 Foreign body in alimentary tract**
EXCLUDES 2 *foreign body in pharynx (T17.2-)*

The appropriate 7th character is to be added to each code from category T18.
A initial encounter
D subsequent encounter
S sequela

√x7th **T18.0 Foreign body in mouth**
√5th **T18.1 Foreign body in esophagus**
EXCLUDES 2 *foreign body in respiratory tract (T17.-)*
√6th **T18.10 Unspecified foreign body in esophagus**
√7th **T18.100 Unspecified foreign body in esophagus causing compression of trachea**
Unspecified foreign body in esophagus causing obstruction of respiration
√7th **T18.108 Unspecified foreign body in esophagus causing other injury**
√6th **T18.11 Gastric contents in esophagus**
Vomitus in esophagus
√7th **T18.110 Gastric contents in esophagus causing compression of trachea**
Gastric contents in esophagus causing obstruction of respiration
√7th **T18.118 Gastric contents in esophagus causing other injury**
√6th **T18.12 Food in esophagus**
Bones in esophagus
Seeds in esophagus
√7th **T18.120 Food in esophagus causing compression of trachea**
Food in esophagus causing obstruction of respiration
√7th **T18.128 Food in esophagus causing other injury**
√6th **T18.19 Other foreign object in esophagus**
AHA: 2015,1Q,23
√7th **T18.190 Other foreign object in esophagus causing compression of trachea**
Other foreign body in esophagus causing obstruction of respiration
TIP: Any foreign object lodged in the esophagus requires immediate treatment and is considered an injury. Assign this code when there is respiratory compromise or compression.
√7th **T18.198 Other foreign object in esophagus causing other injury**
TIP: Any foreign object lodged in the esophagus requires immediate treatment and is considered an injury. Assign this code when there is no respiratory compromise or compression.
√x7th **T18.2 Foreign body in stomach**
√x7th **T18.3 Foreign body in small intestine**
√x7th **T18.4 Foreign body in colon**
√x7th **T18.5 Foreign body in anus and rectum**
Foreign body in rectosigmoid (junction)
√x7th **T18.8 Foreign body in other parts of alimentary tract**
√x7th **T18.9 Foreign body of alimentary tract, part unspecified**
Foreign body in digestive system NOS
Swallowed foreign body NOS

√4th **T19 Foreign body in genitourinary tract**
EXCLUDES 2 *complications due to implanted mesh (T83.7-)*
mechanical complications of contraceptive device (intrauterine) (vaginal) (T83.3-)
presence of contraceptive device (intrauterine) (vaginal) (Z97.5)

The appropriate 7th character is to be added to each code from category T19.
A initial encounter
D subsequent encounter
S sequela

√x7th **T19.0 Foreign body in urethra**
√x7th **T19.1 Foreign body in bladder**
√x7th **T19.2 Foreign body in vulva and vagina** ♀
√x7th **T19.3 Foreign body in uterus** ♀
√x7th **T19.4 Foreign body in penis** ♂
√x7th **T19.8 Foreign body in other parts of genitourinary tract**
√x7th **T19.9 Foreign body in genitourinary tract, part unspecified**

BURNS AND CORROSIONS (T2Ø-T32)

INCLUDES burns (thermal) from electrical heating appliances
burns (thermal) from electricity
burns (thermal) from flame
burns (thermal) from friction
burns (thermal) from hot air and hot gases
burns (thermal) from hot objects
burns (thermal) from lightning
burns (thermal) from radiation
chemical burn [corrosion] (external) (internal)
scalds

EXCLUDES 2 *erythema [dermatitis] ab igne (L59.Ø)*
radiation-related disorders of the skin and subcutaneous tissue (L55-L59)
sunburn (L55.-)

AHA: 2016,2Q,4

Burns and corrosions of external body surface, specified by site (T2Ø-T25)

INCLUDES burns and corrosions of first degree [erythema]
burns and corrosions of second degree [blisters] [epidermal loss]
burns and corrosions of third degree [deep necrosis of underlying tissue] [full-thickness skin loss]

Use additional code from category T31 or T32 to identify extent of body surface involved

✓4th T2Ø Burn and corrosion of head, face, and neck

EXCLUDES 2 *burn and corrosion of ear drum (T28.41, T28.91)*
burn and corrosion of eye and adnexa (T26.-)
burn and corrosion of mouth and pharynx (T28.Ø)

AHA: 2015,1Q,18-19

The appropriate 7th character is to be added to each code from category T2Ø.
A initial encounter
D subsequent encounter
S sequela

✓5th T2Ø.Ø Burn of unspecified degree of head, face, and neck

Use additional external cause code to identify the source, place and intent of the burn (XØØ-X19, X75-X77, X96-X98, Y92)

✓x7th T2Ø.ØØ Burn of unspecified degree of head, face, and neck, unspecified site

✓6th T2Ø.Ø1 Burn of unspecified degree of ear [any part, except ear drum]

EXCLUDES 2 *burn of ear drum (T28.41-)*

✓7th T2Ø.Ø11 Burn of unspecified degree of right ear [any part, except ear drum]

✓7th T2Ø.Ø12 Burn of unspecified degree of left ear [any part, except ear drum]

✓7th T2Ø.Ø19 Burn of unspecified degree of unspecified ear [any part, except ear drum]

✓x7th T2Ø.Ø2 Burn of unspecified degree of lip(s)

✓x7th T2Ø.Ø3 Burn of unspecified degree of chin

✓x7th T2Ø.Ø4 Burn of unspecified degree of nose (septum)

✓x7th T2Ø.Ø5 Burn of unspecified degree of scalp [any part]

✓x7th T2Ø.Ø6 Burn of unspecified degree of forehead and cheek

✓x7th T2Ø.Ø7 Burn of unspecified degree of neck

✓x7th T2Ø.Ø9 Burn of unspecified degree of multiple sites of head, face, and neck

✓5th T2Ø.1 Burn of first degree of head, face, and neck

Use additional external cause code to identify the source, place and intent of the burn (XØØ-X19, X75-X77, X96-X98, Y92)

✓x7th T2Ø.1Ø Burn of first degree of head, face, and neck, unspecified site

✓6th T2Ø.11 Burn of first degree of ear [any part, except ear drum]

EXCLUDES 2 *burn of ear drum (T28.41-)*

✓7th T2Ø.111 Burn of first degree of right ear [any part, except ear drum]

✓7th T2Ø.112 Burn of first degree of left ear [any part, except ear drum]

✓7th T2Ø.119 Burn of first degree of unspecified ear [any part, except ear drum]

✓x7th T2Ø.12 Burn of first degree of lip(s)

✓x7th T2Ø.13 Burn of first degree of chin

✓x7th T2Ø.14 Burn of first degree of nose (septum)

✓x7th T2Ø.15 Burn of first degree of scalp [any part]

✓x7th T2Ø.16 Burn of first degree of forehead and cheek

✓x7th T2Ø.17 Burn of first degree of neck

✓x7th T2Ø.19 Burn of first degree of multiple sites of head, face, and neck

Degree of Burns

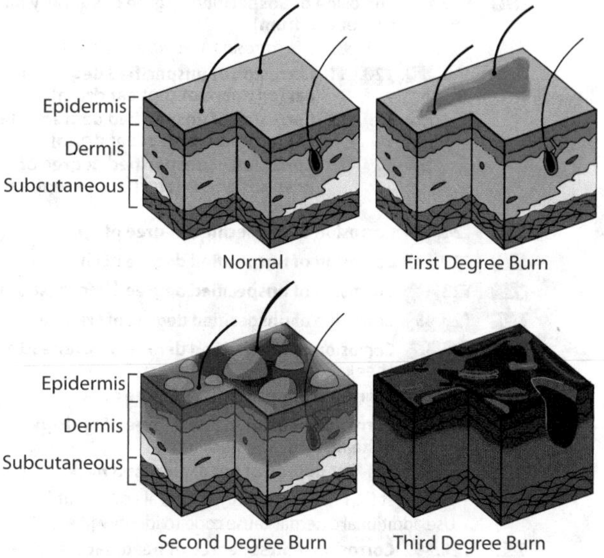

✓5th T2Ø.2 Burn of second degree of head, face, and neck

Use additional external cause code to identify the source, place and intent of the burn (XØØ-X19, X75-X77, X96-X98, Y92)

✓x7th T2Ø.2Ø Burn of second degree of head, face, and neck, unspecified site

✓6th T2Ø.21 Burn of second degree of ear [any part, except ear drum]

EXCLUDES 2 *burn of ear drum (T28.41-)*

✓7th T2Ø.211 Burn of second degree of right ear [any part, except ear drum]

✓7th T2Ø.212 Burn of second degree of left ear [any part, except ear drum]

✓7th T2Ø.219 Burn of second degree of unspecified ear [any part, except ear drum]

✓x7th T2Ø.22 Burn of second degree of lip(s)

✓x7th T2Ø.23 Burn of second degree of chin

✓x7th T2Ø.24 Burn of second degree of nose (septum)

✓x7th T2Ø.25 Burn of second degree of scalp [any part]

✓x7th T2Ø.26 Burn of second degree of forehead and cheek

✓x7th T2Ø.27 Burn of second degree of neck

✓x7th T2Ø.29 Burn of second degree of multiple sites of head, face, and neck

✓5th T2Ø.3 Burn of third degree of head, face, and neck

Use additional external cause code to identify the source, place and intent of the burn (XØØ-X19, X75-X77, X96-X98, Y92)

✓x7th T2Ø.3Ø Burn of third degree of head, face, and neck, unspecified site CC H5 SW

✓6th T2Ø.31 Burn of third degree of ear [any part, except ear drum]

EXCLUDES 2 *burn of ear drum (T28.41-)*

AHA: 2015,1Q,18

✓7th T2Ø.311 Burn of third degree of right ear [any part, except ear drum] CC H5 SW

✓7th T2Ø.312 Burn of third degree of left ear [any part, except ear drum] CC H5 SW

✓7th T2Ø.319 Burn of third degree of unspecified ear [any part, except ear drum] CC H5 SW

✓x7th T2Ø.32 Burn of third degree of lip(s) CC H5 SW

✓x7th T2Ø.33 Burn of third degree of chin CC H5 SW

✓x7th T2Ø.34 Burn of third degree of nose (septum) CC H5 SW

✓x7th T2Ø.35 Burn of third degree of scalp [any part] CC H5 SW

✓x7th T2Ø.36 Burn of third degree of forehead and cheek CC H5 SW

✓x7th T2Ø.37 Burn of third degree of neck CC H5 SW

✓x7th T2Ø.39 Burn of third degree of multiple sites of head, face, and neck CC H5 SW

√5th **T20.4 Corrosion of unspecified degree of head, face, and neck**
Code first (T51-T65) to identify chemical and intent
Use additional external cause code to identify place (Y92)

√x7th **T20.40 Corrosion of unspecified degree of head, face, and neck, unspecified site**

√6th **T20.41 Corrosion of unspecified degree of ear [any part, except ear drum]**
EXCLUDES 2 *corrosion of ear drum (T28.91-)*

√7th **T20.411 Corrosion of unspecified degree of right ear [any part, except ear drum]**

√7th **T20.412 Corrosion of unspecified degree of left ear [any part, except ear drum]**

√7th **T20.419 Corrosion of unspecified degree of unspecified ear [any part, except ear drum]**

√x7th **T20.42 Corrosion of unspecified degree of lip(s)**

√x7th **T20.43 Corrosion of unspecified degree of chin**

√x7th **T20.44 Corrosion of unspecified degree of nose (septum)**

√x7th **T20.45 Corrosion of unspecified degree of scalp [any part]**

√x7th **T20.46 Corrosion of unspecified degree of forehead and cheek**

√x7th **T20.47 Corrosion of unspecified degree of neck**

√x7th **T20.49 Corrosion of unspecified degree of multiple sites of head, face, and neck**

√5th **T20.5 Corrosion of first degree of head, face, and neck**
Code first (T51-T65) to identify chemical and intent
Use additional external cause code to identify place (Y92)

√x7th **T20.50 Corrosion of first degree of head, face, and neck, unspecified site**

√6th **T20.51 Corrosion of first degree of ear [any part, except ear drum]**
EXCLUDES 2 *corrosion of ear drum (T28.91-)*

√7th **T20.511 Corrosion of first degree of right ear [any part, except ear drum]**

√7th **T20.512 Corrosion of first degree of left ear [any part, except ear drum]**

√7th **T20.519 Corrosion of first degree of unspecified ear [any part, except ear drum]**

√x7th **T20.52 Corrosion of first degree of lip(s)**

√x7th **T20.53 Corrosion of first degree of chin**

√x7th **T20.54 Corrosion of first degree of nose (septum)**

√x7th **T20.55 Corrosion of first degree of scalp [any part]**

√x7th **T20.56 Corrosion of first degree of forehead and cheek**

√x7th **T20.57 Corrosion of first degree of neck**

√x7th **T20.59 Corrosion of first degree of multiple sites of head, face, and neck**

√5th **T20.6 Corrosion of second degree of head, face, and neck**
Code first (T51-T65) to identify chemical and intent
Use additional external cause code to identify place (Y92)

√x7th **T20.60 Corrosion of second degree of head, face, and neck, unspecified site**

√6th **T20.61 Corrosion of second degree of ear [any part, except ear drum]**
EXCLUDES 2 *corrosion of ear drum (T28.91-)*

√7th **T20.611 Corrosion of second degree of right ear [any part, except ear drum]**

√7th **T20.612 Corrosion of second degree of left ear [any part, except ear drum]**

√7th **T20.619 Corrosion of second degree of unspecified ear [any part, except ear drum]**

√x7th **T20.62 Corrosion of second degree of lip(s)**

√x7th **T20.63 Corrosion of second degree of chin**

√x7th **T20.64 Corrosion of second degree of nose (septum)**

√x7th **T20.65 Corrosion of second degree of scalp [any part]**

√x7th **T20.66 Corrosion of second degree of forehead and cheek**

√x7th **T20.67 Corrosion of second degree of neck**

√x7th **T20.69 Corrosion of second degree of multiple sites of head, face, and neck**

√5th **T20.7 Corrosion of third degree of head, face, and neck**
Code first (T51-T65) to identify chemical and intent
Use additional external cause code to identify place (Y92)

√x7th **T20.70 Corrosion of third degree of head, face, and neck, unspecified site** CC H5 SW

√6th **T20.71 Corrosion of third degree of ear [any part, except ear drum]**
EXCLUDES 2 *corrosion of ear drum (T28.91-)*

√7th **T20.711 Corrosion of third degree of right ear [any part, except ear drum]** CC H5 SW

√7th **T20.712 Corrosion of third degree of left ear [any part, except ear drum]** CC H5 SW

√7th **T20.719 Corrosion of third degree of unspecified ear [any part, except ear drum]** CC H5 SW

√x7th **T20.72 Corrosion of third degree of lip(s)** CC H5 SW

√x7th **T20.73 Corrosion of third degree of chin** CC H5 SW

√x7th **T20.74 Corrosion of third degree of nose (septum)** CC H5 SW

√x7th **T20.75 Corrosion of third degree of scalp [any part]** CC H5 SW

√x7th **T20.76 Corrosion of third degree of forehead and cheek** CC H5 SW

√x7th **T20.77 Corrosion of third degree of neck** CC H5 SW

√x7th **T20.79 Corrosion of third degree of multiple sites of head, face, and neck** CC H5 SW

√4th **T21 Burn and corrosion of trunk**
INCLUDES burns and corrosion of hip region
EXCLUDES 2 *burns and corrosion of axilla (T22.- with fifth character 4)*
burns and corrosion of scapular region (T22.- with fifth character 6)
burns and corrosion of shoulder (T22.- with fifth character 5)

The appropriate 7th character is to be added to each code from category T21.
A initial encounter
D subsequent encounter
S sequela

√5th **T21.0 Burn of unspecified degree of trunk**
Use additional external cause code to identify the source, place and intent of the burn (X00-X19, X75-X77, X96-X98, Y92)

√x7th **T21.00 Burn of unspecified degree of trunk, unspecified site**

√x7th **T21.01 Burn of unspecified degree of chest wall**
Burn of unspecified degree of breast

√x7th **T21.02 Burn of unspecified degree of abdominal wall**
Burn of unspecified degree of flank
Burn of unspecified degree of groin

√x7th **T21.03 Burn of unspecified degree of upper back**
Burn of unspecified degree of interscapular region

√x7th **T21.04 Burn of unspecified degree of lower back**

√x7th **T21.05 Burn of unspecified degree of buttock**
Burn of unspecified degree of anus

√x7th **T21.06 Burn of unspecified degree of male genital region** ♂
Burn of unspecified degree of penis
Burn of unspecified degree of scrotum
Burn of unspecified degree of testis

√x7th **T21.07 Burn of unspecified degree of female genital region** ♀
Burn of unspecified degree of labium (majus) (minus)
Burn of unspecified degree of perineum
Burn of unspecified degree of vulva
EXCLUDES 2 *burn of vagina (T28.3)*

√x7th **T21.09 Burn of unspecified degree of other site of trunk**

√5th **T21.1 Burn of first degree of trunk**
Use additional external cause code to identify the source, place and intent of the burn (X00-X19, X75-X77, X96-X98, Y92)

√x7th **T21.10 Burn of first degree of trunk, unspecified site**

√x7th **T21.11 Burn of first degree of chest wall**
Burn of first degree of breast

√x7th **T21.12 Burn of first degree of abdominal wall**
Burn of first degree of flank
Burn of first degree of groin

√x7th **T21.13 Burn of first degree of upper back**
Burn of first degree of interscapular region

√x7th **T21.14 Burn of first degree of lower back**

√x7th **T21.15 Burn of first degree of buttock**
Burn of first degree of anus

√x7th **T21.16 Burn of first degree of male genital region** ♂
Burn of first degree of penis
Burn of first degree of scrotum
Burn of first degree of testis

√x7th **T21.17 Burn of first degree of female genital region** ♀
Burn of first degree of labium (majus) (minus)
Burn of first degree of perineum
Burn of first degree of vulva
EXCLUDES 2 *burn of vagina (T28.3)*

√x7th **T21.19 Burn of first degree of other site of trunk**

√5th **T21.2 Burn of second degree of trunk**
Use additional external cause code to identify the source, place and intent of the burn (X00-X19, X75-X77, X96-X98, Y92)

√x7th **T21.20 Burn of second degree of trunk, unspecified site**

√x7th **T21.21 Burn of second degree of chest wall**
Burn of second degree of breast

√x7th **T21.22 Burn of second degree of abdominal wall**
Burn of second degree of flank
Burn of second degree of groin

√x7th **T21.23 Burn of second degree of upper back**
Burn of second degree of interscapular region

√x7th **T21.24 Burn of second degree of lower back**

√x7th **T21.25 Burn of second degree of buttock**
Burn of second degree of anus

√x7th **T21.26 Burn of second degree of male genital region** ♂
Burn of second degree of penis
Burn of second degree of scrotum
Burn of second degree of testis

√x7th **T21.27 Burn of second degree of female genital region** ♀
Burn of second degree of labium (majus) (minus)
Burn of second degree of perineum
Burn of second degree of vulva
EXCLUDES 2 *burn of vagina (T28.3)*

√x7th **T21.29 Burn of second degree of other site of trunk**

√5th **T21.3 Burn of third degree of trunk**
Use additional external cause code to identify the source, place and intent of the burn (X00-X19, X75-X77, X96-X98, Y92)

√x7th **T21.30 Burn of third degree of trunk, unspecified site** CC H5 SW

√x7th **T21.31 Burn of third degree of chest wall** CC H5 SW
Burn of third degree of breast
AHA: 2016,2Q,5

√x7th **T21.32 Burn of third degree of abdominal wall** CC H5 SW
Burn of third degree of flank
Burn of third degree of groin

√x7th **T21.33 Burn of third degree of upper back** CC H5 SW
Burn of third degree of interscapular region

√x7th **T21.34 Burn of third degree of lower back** CC H5 SW

√x7th **T21.35 Burn of third degree of buttock** CC H5 SW
Burn of third degree of anus

√x7th **T21.36 Burn of third degree of male genital region** CC H5 SW ♂
Burn of third degree of penis
Burn of third degree of scrotum
Burn of third degree of testis

√x7th **T21.37 Burn of third degree of female genital region** CC H5 SW ♀
Burn of third degree of labium (majus) (minus)
Burn of third degree of perineum
Burn of third degree of vulva
EXCLUDES 2 *burn of vagina (T28.3)*

√x7th **T21.39 Burn of third degree of other site of trunk** CC H5 SW

√5th **T21.4 Corrosion of unspecified degree of trunk**
Code first (T51-T65) to identify chemical and intent
Use additional external cause code to identify place (Y92)

√x7th **T21.40 Corrosion of unspecified degree of trunk, unspecified site**

√x7th **T21.41 Corrosion of unspecified degree of chest wall**
Corrosion of unspecified degree of breast

√x7th **T21.42 Corrosion of unspecified degree of abdominal wall**
Corrosion of unspecified degree of flank
Corrosion of unspecified degree of groin

√x7th **T21.43 Corrosion of unspecified degree of upper back**
Corrosion of unspecified degree of interscapular region

√x7th **T21.44 Corrosion of unspecified degree of lower back**

√x7th **T21.45 Corrosion of unspecified degree of buttock**
Corrosion of unspecified degree of anus

√x7th **T21.46 Corrosion of unspecified degree of male genital region** ♂
Corrosion of unspecified degree of penis
Corrosion of unspecified degree of scrotum
Corrosion of unspecified degree of testis

√x7th **T21.47 Corrosion of unspecified degree of female genital region** ♀
Corrosion of unspecified degree of labium (majus) (minus)
Corrosion of unspecified degree of perineum
Corrosion of unspecified degree of vulva
EXCLUDES 2 *corrosion of vagina (T28.8)*

√x7th **T21.49 Corrosion of unspecified degree of other site of trunk**

√5th **T21.5 Corrosion of first degree of trunk**
Code first (T51-T65) to identify chemical and intent
Use additional external cause code to identify place (Y92)

√x7th **T21.50 Corrosion of first degree of trunk, unspecified site**

√x7th **T21.51 Corrosion of first degree of chest wall**
Corrosion of first degree of breast

√x7th **T21.52 Corrosion of first degree of abdominal wall**
Corrosion of first degree of flank
Corrosion of first degree of groin

√x7th **T21.53 Corrosion of first degree of upper back**
Corrosion of first degree of interscapular region

√x7th **T21.54 Corrosion of first degree of lower back**

√x7th **T21.55 Corrosion of first degree of buttock**
Corrosion of first degree of anus

√x7th **T21.56 Corrosion of first degree of male genital region** ♂
Corrosion of first degree of penis
Corrosion of first degree of scrotum
Corrosion of first degree of testis

√x7th **T21.57 Corrosion of first degree of female genital region** ♀
Corrosion of first degree of labium (majus) (minus)
Corrosion of first degree of perineum
Corrosion of first degree of vulva
EXCLUDES 2 *corrosion of vagina (T28.8)*

√x7th **T21.59 Corrosion of first degree of other site of trunk**

√5th **T21.6 Corrosion of second degree of trunk**
Code first (T51-T65) to identify chemical and intent
Use additional external cause code to identify place (Y92)

√x7th **T21.60 Corrosion of second degree of trunk, unspecified site**

√x7th **T21.61 Corrosion of second degree of chest wall**
Corrosion of second degree of breast

√x7th **T21.62 Corrosion of second degree of abdominal wall**
Corrosion of second degree of flank
Corrosion of second degree of groin

√x7th **T21.63 Corrosion of second degree of upper back**
Corrosion of second degree of interscapular region

√x7th **T21.64 Corrosion of second degree of lower back**

√x7th **T21.65 Corrosion of second degree of buttock**
Corrosion of second degree of anus

√x7th **T21.66 Corrosion of second degree of male genital region** ♂
Corrosion of second degree of penis
Corrosion of second degree of scrotum
Corrosion of second degree of testis

T21.67 Corrosion of second degree of female genital region ♀
Corrosion of second degree of labium (majus) (minus)
Corrosion of second degree of perineum
Corrosion of second degree of vulva
EXCLUDES 2 *corrosion of vagina (T28.8)*

T21.69 Corrosion of second degree of other site of trunk

T21.7 Corrosion of third degree of trunk
Code first (T51-T65) to identify chemical and intent
Use additional external cause code to identify place (Y92)

T21.70 Corrosion of third degree of trunk, unspecified site CC HS SW

T21.71 Corrosion of third degree of chest wall CC HS SW
Corrosion of third degree of breast

T21.72 Corrosion of third degree of abdominal wall CC HS SW
Corrosion of third degree of flank
Corrosion of third degree of groin

T21.73 Corrosion of third degree of upper back CC HS SW
Corrosion of third degree of interscapular region

T21.74 Corrosion of third degree of lower back CC HS SW

T21.75 Corrosion of third degree of buttock CC HS SW
Corrosion of third degree of anus

T21.76 Corrosion of third degree of male genital region CC HS SW ♂
Corrosion of third degree of penis
Corrosion of third degree of scrotum
Corrosion of third degree of testis

T21.77 Corrosion of third degree of female genital region CC HS SW ♀
Corrosion of third degree of labium (majus) (minus)
Corrosion of third degree of perineum
Corrosion of third degree of vulva
EXCLUDES 2 *corrosion of vagina (T28.8)*

T21.79 Corrosion of third degree of other site of trunk CC HS SW

T22 Burn and corrosion of shoulder and upper limb, except wrist and hand
EXCLUDES 2 *burn and corrosion of interscapular region (T21.-)*
burn and corrosion of wrist and hand (T23.-)

The appropriate 7th character is to be added to each code from category T22.
A initial encounter
D subsequent encounter
S sequela

T22.0 Burn of unspecified degree of shoulder and upper limb, except wrist and hand
Use additional external cause code to identify the source, place and intent of the burn (X00-X19, X75-X77, X96-X98, Y92)

T22.00 Burn of unspecified degree of shoulder and upper limb, except wrist and hand, unspecified site

T22.01 Burn of unspecified degree of forearm
- **T22.011 Burn of unspecified degree of right forearm**
- **T22.012 Burn of unspecified degree of left forearm**
- **T22.019 Burn of unspecified degree of unspecified forearm**

T22.02 Burn of unspecified degree of elbow
- **T22.021 Burn of unspecified degree of right elbow**
- **T22.022 Burn of unspecified degree of left elbow**
- **T22.029 Burn of unspecified degree of unspecified elbow**

T22.03 Burn of unspecified degree of upper arm
- **T22.031 Burn of unspecified degree of right upper arm**
- **T22.032 Burn of unspecified degree of left upper arm**
- **T22.039 Burn of unspecified degree of unspecified upper arm**

T22.04 Burn of unspecified degree of axilla
- **T22.041 Burn of unspecified degree of right axilla**
- **T22.042 Burn of unspecified degree of left axilla**
- **T22.049 Burn of unspecified degree of unspecified axilla**

T22.05 Burn of unspecified degree of shoulder
- **T22.051 Burn of unspecified degree of right shoulder**
- **T22.052 Burn of unspecified degree of left shoulder**
- **T22.059 Burn of unspecified degree of unspecified shoulder**

T22.06 Burn of unspecified degree of scapular region
- **T22.061 Burn of unspecified degree of right scapular region**
- **T22.062 Burn of unspecified degree of left scapular region**
- **T22.069 Burn of unspecified degree of unspecified scapular region**

T22.09 Burn of unspecified degree of multiple sites of shoulder and upper limb, except wrist and hand
- **T22.091 Burn of unspecified degree of multiple sites of right shoulder and upper limb, except wrist and hand**
- **T22.092 Burn of unspecified degree of multiple sites of left shoulder and upper limb, except wrist and hand**
- **T22.099 Burn of unspecified degree of multiple sites of unspecified shoulder and upper limb, except wrist and hand**

T22.1 Burn of first degree of shoulder and upper limb, except wrist and hand
Use additional external cause code to identify the source, place and intent of the burn (X00-X19, X75-X77, X96-X98, Y92)

T22.10 Burn of first degree of shoulder and upper limb, except wrist and hand, unspecified site

T22.11 Burn of first degree of forearm
- **T22.111 Burn of first degree of right forearm**
- **T22.112 Burn of first degree of left forearm**
- **T22.119 Burn of first degree of unspecified forearm**

T22.12 Burn of first degree of elbow
- **T22.121 Burn of first degree of right elbow**
- **T22.122 Burn of first degree of left elbow**
- **T22.129 Burn of first degree of unspecified elbow**

T22.13 Burn of first degree of upper arm
- **T22.131 Burn of first degree of right upper arm**
- **T22.132 Burn of first degree of left upper arm**
- **T22.139 Burn of first degree of unspecified upper arm**

T22.14 Burn of first degree of axilla
- **T22.141 Burn of first degree of right axilla**
- **T22.142 Burn of first degree of left axilla**
- **T22.149 Burn of first degree of unspecified axilla**

T22.15 Burn of first degree of shoulder
- **T22.151 Burn of first degree of right shoulder**
- **T22.152 Burn of first degree of left shoulder**
- **T22.159 Burn of first degree of unspecified shoulder**

T22.16 Burn of first degree of scapular region
- **T22.161 Burn of first degree of right scapular region**
- **T22.162 Burn of first degree of left scapular region**
- **T22.169 Burn of first degree of unspecified scapular region**

T22.19 Burn of first degree of multiple sites of shoulder and upper limb, except wrist and hand
- **T22.191 Burn of first degree of multiple sites of right shoulder and upper limb, except wrist and hand**
- **T22.192 Burn of first degree of multiple sites of left shoulder and upper limb, except wrist and hand**
- **T22.199 Burn of first degree of multiple sites of unspecified shoulder and upper limb, except wrist and hand**

T22.2 Burn of second degree of shoulder and upper limb, except wrist and hand
Use additional external cause code to identify the source, place and intent of the burn (X00-X19, X75-X77, X96-X98, Y92)

T22.20 Burn of second degree of shoulder and upper limb, except wrist and hand, unspecified site

T22.21 Burn of second degree of forearm
T22.211 Burn of second degree of right forearm
T22.212 Burn of second degree of left forearm
T22.219 Burn of second degree of unspecified forearm
T22.22 Burn of second degree of elbow
T22.221 Burn of second degree of right elbow
T22.222 Burn of second degree of left elbow
T22.229 Burn of second degree of unspecified elbow
T22.23 Burn of second degree of upper arm
T22.231 Burn of second degree of right upper arm
T22.232 Burn of second degree of left upper arm
T22.239 Burn of second degree of unspecified upper arm
T22.24 Burn of second degree of axilla
T22.241 Burn of second degree of right axilla
T22.242 Burn of second degree of left axilla
T22.249 Burn of second degree of unspecified axilla
T22.25 Burn of second degree of shoulder
T22.251 Burn of second degree of right shoulder
T22.252 Burn of second degree of left shoulder
T22.259 Burn of second degree of unspecified shoulder
T22.26 Burn of second degree of scapular region
T22.261 Burn of second degree of right scapular region
T22.262 Burn of second degree of left scapular region
T22.269 Burn of second degree of unspecified scapular region
T22.29 Burn of second degree of multiple sites of shoulder and upper limb, except wrist and hand
T22.291 Burn of second degree of multiple sites of right shoulder and upper limb, except wrist and hand
T22.292 Burn of second degree of multiple sites of left shoulder and upper limb, except wrist and hand
T22.299 Burn of second degree of multiple sites of unspecified shoulder and upper limb, except wrist and hand

T22.3 Burn of third degree of shoulder and upper limb, except wrist and hand
Use additional external cause code to identify the source, place and intent of the burn (XØØ-X19, X75-X77, X96-X98, Y92)
T22.3Ø Burn of third degree of shoulder and upper limb, except wrist and hand, unspecified site CC H5 SW
T22.31 Burn of third degree of forearm
T22.311 Burn of third degree of right forearm CC H5 SW
T22.312 Burn of third degree of left forearm CC H5 SW
T22.319 Burn of third degree of unspecified forearm CC H5 SW
T22.32 Burn of third degree of elbow
T22.321 Burn of third degree of right elbow CC H5 SW
T22.322 Burn of third degree of left elbow CC H5 SW
T22.329 Burn of third degree of unspecified elbow CC H5 SW
T22.33 Burn of third degree of upper arm
T22.331 Burn of third degree of right upper arm CC H5 SW
T22.332 Burn of third degree of left upper arm CC H5 SW
T22.339 Burn of third degree of unspecified upper arm CC H5 SW
T22.34 Burn of third degree of axilla
T22.341 Burn of third degree of right axilla CC H5 SW
T22.342 Burn of third degree of left axilla CC H5 SW
T22.349 Burn of third degree of unspecified axilla CC H5 SW
T22.35 Burn of third degree of shoulder
T22.351 Burn of third degree of right shoulder CC H5 SW
T22.352 Burn of third degree of left shoulder CC H5 SW
T22.359 Burn of third degree of unspecified shoulder CC H5 SW
T22.36 Burn of third degree of scapular region
T22.361 Burn of third degree of right scapular region CC H5 SW
T22.362 Burn of third degree of left scapular region CC H5 SW
T22.369 Burn of third degree of unspecified scapular region CC H5 SW
T22.39 Burn of third degree of multiple sites of shoulder and upper limb, except wrist and hand
T22.391 Burn of third degree of multiple sites of right shoulder and upper limb, except wrist and hand CC H5 SW
T22.392 Burn of third degree of multiple sites of left shoulder and upper limb, except wrist and hand CC H5 SW
T22.399 Burn of third degree of multiple sites of unspecified shoulder and upper limb, except wrist and hand CC H5 SW

T22.4 Corrosion of unspecified degree of shoulder and upper limb, except wrist and hand
Code first (T51-T65) to identify chemical and intent
Use additional external cause code to identify place (Y92)
T22.4Ø Corrosion of unspecified degree of shoulder and upper limb, except wrist and hand, unspecified site
T22.41 Corrosion of unspecified degree of forearm
T22.411 Corrosion of unspecified degree of right forearm
T22.412 Corrosion of unspecified degree of left forearm
T22.419 Corrosion of unspecified degree of unspecified forearm
T22.42 Corrosion of unspecified degree of elbow
T22.421 Corrosion of unspecified degree of right elbow
T22.422 Corrosion of unspecified degree of left elbow
T22.429 Corrosion of unspecified degree of unspecified elbow
T22.43 Corrosion of unspecified degree of upper arm
T22.431 Corrosion of unspecified degree of right upper arm
T22.432 Corrosion of unspecified degree of left upper arm
T22.439 Corrosion of unspecified degree of unspecified upper arm
T22.44 Corrosion of unspecified degree of axilla
T22.441 Corrosion of unspecified degree of right axilla
T22.442 Corrosion of unspecified degree of left axilla
T22.449 Corrosion of unspecified degree of unspecified axilla
T22.45 Corrosion of unspecified degree of shoulder
T22.451 Corrosion of unspecified degree of right shoulder
T22.452 Corrosion of unspecified degree of left shoulder
T22.459 Corrosion of unspecified degree of unspecified shoulder
T22.46 Corrosion of unspecified degree of scapular region
T22.461 Corrosion of unspecified degree of right scapular region
T22.462 Corrosion of unspecified degree of left scapular region
T22.469 Corrosion of unspecified degree of unspecified scapular region
T22.49 Corrosion of unspecified degree of multiple sites of shoulder and upper limb, except wrist and hand
T22.491 Corrosion of unspecified degree of multiple sites of right shoulder and upper limb, except wrist and hand

√7th **T22.492 Corrosion of unspecified degree of multiple sites of left shoulder and upper limb, except wrist and hand**

√7th **T22.499 Corrosion of unspecified degree of multiple sites of unspecified shoulder and upper limb, except wrist and hand**

√5th **T22.5 Corrosion of first degree of shoulder and upper limb, except wrist and hand**

Code first (T51-T65) to identify chemical and intent

Use additional external cause code to identify place (Y92)

√x7th **T22.50 Corrosion of first degree of shoulder and upper limb, except wrist and hand unspecified site**

√6th **T22.51 Corrosion of first degree of forearm**

√7th **T22.511 Corrosion of first degree of right forearm**

√7th **T22.512 Corrosion of first degree of left forearm**

√7th **T22.519 Corrosion of first degree of unspecified forearm**

√6th **T22.52 Corrosion of first degree of elbow**

√7th **T22.521 Corrosion of first degree of right elbow**

√7th **T22.522 Corrosion of first degree of left elbow**

√7th **T22.529 Corrosion of first degree of unspecified elbow**

√6th **T22.53 Corrosion of first degree of upper arm**

√7th **T22.531 Corrosion of first degree of right upper arm**

√7th **T22.532 Corrosion of first degree of left upper arm**

√7th **T22.539 Corrosion of first degree of unspecified upper arm**

√6th **T22.54 Corrosion of first degree of axilla**

√7th **T22.541 Corrosion of first degree of right axilla**

√7th **T22.542 Corrosion of first degree of left axilla**

√7th **T22.549 Corrosion of first degree of unspecified axilla**

√6th **T22.55 Corrosion of first degree of shoulder**

√7th **T22.551 Corrosion of first degree of right shoulder**

√7th **T22.552 Corrosion of first degree of left shoulder**

√7th **T22.559 Corrosion of first degree of unspecified shoulder**

√6th **T22.56 Corrosion of first degree of scapular region**

√7th **T22.561 Corrosion of first degree of right scapular region**

√7th **T22.562 Corrosion of first degree of left scapular region**

√7th **T22.569 Corrosion of first degree of unspecified scapular region**

√6th **T22.59 Corrosion of first degree of multiple sites of shoulder and upper limb, except wrist and hand**

√7th **T22.591 Corrosion of first degree of multiple sites of right shoulder and upper limb, except wrist and hand**

√7th **T22.592 Corrosion of first degree of multiple sites of left shoulder and upper limb, except wrist and hand**

√7th **T22.599 Corrosion of first degree of multiple sites of unspecified shoulder and upper limb, except wrist and hand**

√5th **T22.6 Corrosion of second degree of shoulder and upper limb, except wrist and hand**

Code first (T51-T65) to identify chemical and intent

Use additional external cause code to identify place (Y92)

√x7th **T22.60 Corrosion of second degree of shoulder and upper limb, except wrist and hand, unspecified site**

√6th **T22.61 Corrosion of second degree of forearm**

√7th **T22.611 Corrosion of second degree of right forearm**

√7th **T22.612 Corrosion of second degree of left forearm**

√7th **T22.619 Corrosion of second degree of unspecified forearm**

√6th **T22.62 Corrosion of second degree of elbow**

√7th **T22.621 Corrosion of second degree of right elbow**

√7th **T22.622 Corrosion of second degree of left elbow**

√7th **T22.629 Corrosion of second degree of unspecified elbow**

√6th **T22.63 Corrosion of second degree of upper arm**

√7th **T22.631 Corrosion of second degree of right upper arm**

√7th **T22.632 Corrosion of second degree of left upper arm**

√7th **T22.639 Corrosion of second degree of unspecified upper arm**

√6th **T22.64 Corrosion of second degree of axilla**

√7th **T22.641 Corrosion of second degree of right axilla**

√7th **T22.642 Corrosion of second degree of left axilla**

√7th **T22.649 Corrosion of second degree of unspecified axilla**

√6th **T22.65 Corrosion of second degree of shoulder**

√7th **T22.651 Corrosion of second degree of right shoulder**

√7th **T22.652 Corrosion of second degree of left shoulder**

√7th **T22.659 Corrosion of second degree of unspecified shoulder**

√6th **T22.66 Corrosion of second degree of scapular region**

√7th **T22.661 Corrosion of second degree of right scapular region**

√7th **T22.662 Corrosion of second degree of left scapular region**

√7th **T22.669 Corrosion of second degree of unspecified scapular region**

√6th **T22.69 Corrosion of second degree of multiple sites of shoulder and upper limb, except wrist and hand**

√7th **T22.691 Corrosion of second degree of multiple sites of right shoulder and upper limb, except wrist and hand**

√7th **T22.692 Corrosion of second degree of multiple sites of left shoulder and upper limb, except wrist and hand**

√7th **T22.699 Corrosion of second degree of multiple sites of unspecified shoulder and upper limb, except wrist and hand**

√5th **T22.7 Corrosion of third degree of shoulder and upper limb, except wrist and hand**

Code first (T51-T65) to identify chemical and intent

Use additional external cause code to identify place (Y92)

√x7th **T22.70 Corrosion of third degree of shoulder and upper limb, except wrist and hand, unspecified site** CC HS SW

√6th **T22.71 Corrosion of third degree of forearm**

√7th **T22.711 Corrosion of third degree of right forearm** CC HS SW

√7th **T22.712 Corrosion of third degree of left forearm** CC HS SW

√7th **T22.719 Corrosion of third degree of unspecified forearm** CC HS SW

√6th **T22.72 Corrosion of third degree of elbow**

√7th **T22.721 Corrosion of third degree of right elbow** CC HS SW

√7th **T22.722 Corrosion of third degree of left elbow** CC HS SW

√7th **T22.729 Corrosion of third degree of unspecified elbow** CC HS SW

√6th **T22.73 Corrosion of third degree of upper arm**

√7th **T22.731 Corrosion of third degree of right upper arm** CC HS SW

√7th **T22.732 Corrosion of third degree of left upper arm** CC HS SW

√7th **T22.739 Corrosion of third degree of unspecified upper arm** CC HS SW

√6th **T22.74 Corrosion of third degree of axilla**

√7th **T22.741 Corrosion of third degree of right axilla** CC HS SW

√7th **T22.742 Corrosion of third degree of left axilla** CC HS SW

√7th **T22.749 Corrosion of third degree of unspecified axilla** CC HS SW

√6th **T22.75 Corrosion of third degree of shoulder**

√7th **T22.751 Corrosion of third degree of right shoulder** CC HS SW

√7th **T22.752 Corrosion of third degree of left shoulder** CC HS SW

√7th **T22.759 Corrosion of third degree of unspecified shoulder** CC HS SW

√6th **T22.76 Corrosion of third degree of scapular region**

√7th **T22.761 Corrosion of third degree of right scapular region** CC HS SW

T22.762 Corrosion of third degree of left scapular region CC H5 SW
T22.769 Corrosion of third degree of unspecified scapular region CC H5 SW
T22.79 Corrosion of third degree of multiple sites of shoulder and upper limb, except wrist and hand
T22.791 Corrosion of third degree of multiple sites of right shoulder and upper limb, except wrist and hand CC H5 SW
T22.792 Corrosion of third degree of multiple sites of left shoulder and upper limb, except wrist and hand CC H5 SW
T22.799 Corrosion of third degree of multiple sites of unspecified shoulder and upper limb, except wrist and hand CC H5 SW

T23 Burn and corrosion of wrist and hand

AHA: 2015,1Q,19

The appropriate 7th character is to be added to each code from category T23.
A initial encounter
D subsequent encounter
S sequela

T23.0 Burn of unspecified degree of wrist and hand
Use additional external cause code to identify the source, place and intent of the burn (X00-X19, X75-X77, X96-X98, Y92)
T23.00 Burn of unspecified degree of hand, unspecified site
T23.001 Burn of unspecified degree of right hand, unspecified site
T23.002 Burn of unspecified degree of left hand, unspecified site
T23.009 Burn of unspecified degree of unspecified hand, unspecified site
T23.01 Burn of unspecified degree of thumb (nail)
T23.011 Burn of unspecified degree of right thumb (nail)
T23.012 Burn of unspecified degree of left thumb (nail)
T23.019 Burn of unspecified degree of unspecified thumb (nail)
T23.02 Burn of unspecified degree of single finger (nail) except thumb
T23.021 Burn of unspecified degree of single right finger (nail) except thumb
T23.022 Burn of unspecified degree of single left finger (nail) except thumb
T23.029 Burn of unspecified degree of unspecified single finger (nail) except thumb
T23.03 Burn of unspecified degree of multiple fingers (nail), not including thumb
T23.031 Burn of unspecified degree of multiple right fingers (nail), not including thumb
T23.032 Burn of unspecified degree of multiple left fingers (nail), not including thumb
T23.039 Burn of unspecified degree of unspecified multiple fingers (nail), not including thumb
T23.04 Burn of unspecified degree of multiple fingers (nail), including thumb
T23.041 Burn of unspecified degree of multiple right fingers (nail), including thumb
T23.042 Burn of unspecified degree of multiple left fingers (nail), including thumb
T23.049 Burn of unspecified degree of unspecified multiple fingers (nail), including thumb
T23.05 Burn of unspecified degree of palm
T23.051 Burn of unspecified degree of right palm
T23.052 Burn of unspecified degree of left palm
T23.059 Burn of unspecified degree of unspecified palm
T23.06 Burn of unspecified degree of back of hand
T23.061 Burn of unspecified degree of back of right hand
T23.062 Burn of unspecified degree of back of left hand
T23.069 Burn of unspecified degree of back of unspecified hand
T23.07 Burn of unspecified degree of wrist
T23.071 Burn of unspecified degree of right wrist
T23.072 Burn of unspecified degree of left wrist
T23.079 Burn of unspecified degree of unspecified wrist
T23.09 Burn of unspecified degree of multiple sites of wrist and hand
T23.091 Burn of unspecified degree of multiple sites of right wrist and hand
T23.092 Burn of unspecified degree of multiple sites of left wrist and hand
T23.099 Burn of unspecified degree of multiple sites of unspecified wrist and hand

T23.1 Burn of first degree of wrist and hand
Use additional external cause code to identify the source, place and intent of the burn (X00-X19, X75-X77, X96-X98, Y92)
T23.10 Burn of first degree of hand, unspecified site
T23.101 Burn of first degree of right hand, unspecified site
T23.102 Burn of first degree of left hand, unspecified site
T23.109 Burn of first degree of unspecified hand, unspecified site
T23.11 Burn of first degree of thumb (nail)
T23.111 Burn of first degree of right thumb (nail)
T23.112 Burn of first degree of left thumb (nail)
T23.119 Burn of first degree of unspecified thumb (nail)
T23.12 Burn of first degree of single finger (nail) except thumb
T23.121 Burn of first degree of single right finger (nail) except thumb
T23.122 Burn of first degree of single left finger (nail) except thumb
T23.129 Burn of first degree of unspecified single finger (nail) except thumb
T23.13 Burn of first degree of multiple fingers (nail), not including thumb
T23.131 Burn of first degree of multiple right fingers (nail), not including thumb
T23.132 Burn of first degree of multiple left fingers (nail), not including thumb
T23.139 Burn of first degree of unspecified multiple fingers (nail), not including thumb
T23.14 Burn of first degree of multiple fingers (nail), including thumb
T23.141 Burn of first degree of multiple right fingers (nail), including thumb
T23.142 Burn of first degree of multiple left fingers (nail), including thumb
T23.149 Burn of first degree of unspecified multiple fingers (nail), including thumb
T23.15 Burn of first degree of palm
T23.151 Burn of first degree of right palm
T23.152 Burn of first degree of left palm
T23.159 Burn of first degree of unspecified palm
T23.16 Burn of first degree of back of hand
T23.161 Burn of first degree of back of right hand
T23.162 Burn of first degree of back of left hand
T23.169 Burn of first degree of back of unspecified hand
T23.17 Burn of first degree of wrist
T23.171 Burn of first degree of right wrist
T23.172 Burn of first degree of left wrist
T23.179 Burn of first degree of unspecified wrist
T23.19 Burn of first degree of multiple sites of wrist and hand
T23.191 Burn of first degree of multiple sites of right wrist and hand
T23.192 Burn of first degree of multiple sites of left wrist and hand
T23.199 Burn of first degree of multiple sites of unspecified wrist and hand

T23.2 Burn of second degree of wrist and hand
Use additional external cause code to identify the source, place and intent of the burn (X00-X19, X75-X77, X96-X98, Y92)
T23.20 Burn of second degree of hand, unspecified site
T23.201 Burn of second degree of right hand, unspecified site

- T23.202 Burn of second degree of left hand, unspecified site
- T23.209 Burn of second degree of unspecified hand, unspecified site

T23.21 Burn of second degree of thumb (nail)
- T23.211 Burn of second degree of right thumb (nail)
- T23.212 Burn of second degree of left thumb (nail)
- T23.219 Burn of second degree of unspecified thumb (nail)

T23.22 Burn of second degree of single finger (nail) except thumb
- T23.221 Burn of second degree of single right finger (nail) except thumb
- T23.222 Burn of second degree of single left finger (nail) except thumb
- T23.229 Burn of second degree of unspecified single finger (nail) except thumb

T23.23 Burn of second degree of multiple fingers (nail), not including thumb
- T23.231 Burn of second degree of multiple right fingers (nail), not including thumb
- T23.232 Burn of second degree of multiple left fingers (nail), not including thumb
- T23.239 Burn of second degree of unspecified multiple fingers (nail), not including thumb

T23.24 Burn of second degree of multiple fingers (nail), including thumb
- T23.241 Burn of second degree of multiple right fingers (nail), including thumb
- T23.242 Burn of second degree of multiple left fingers (nail), including thumb
- T23.249 Burn of second degree of unspecified multiple fingers (nail), including thumb

T23.25 Burn of second degree of palm
- T23.251 Burn of second degree of right palm
- T23.252 Burn of second degree of left palm
- T23.259 Burn of second degree of unspecified palm

T23.26 Burn of second degree of back of hand
- T23.261 Burn of second degree of back of right hand
- T23.262 Burn of second degree of back of left hand
- T23.269 Burn of second degree of back of unspecified hand

T23.27 Burn of second degree of wrist
- T23.271 Burn of second degree of right wrist
- T23.272 Burn of second degree of left wrist
- T23.279 Burn of second degree of unspecified wrist

T23.29 Burn of second degree of multiple sites of wrist and hand
- T23.291 Burn of second degree of multiple sites of right wrist and hand
- T23.292 Burn of second degree of multiple sites of left wrist and hand
- T23.299 Burn of second degree of multiple sites of unspecified wrist and hand

T23.3 Burn of third degree of wrist and hand

Use additional external cause code to identify the source, place and intent of the burn (X00-X19, X75-X77, X96-X98, Y92)

T23.30 Burn of third degree of hand, unspecified site

AHA: 2016,2Q,5

- T23.301 Burn of third degree of right hand, unspecified site CC H5 SW
- T23.302 Burn of third degree of left hand, unspecified site CC H5 SW
- T23.309 Burn of third degree of unspecified hand, unspecified site CC H5 SW

T23.31 Burn of third degree of thumb (nail)
- T23.311 Burn of third degree of right thumb (nail) CC H5 SW
- T23.312 Burn of third degree of left thumb (nail) CC H5 SW
- T23.319 Burn of third degree of unspecified thumb (nail) CC H5 SW

T23.32 Burn of third degree of single finger (nail) except thumb
- T23.321 Burn of third degree of single right finger (nail) except thumb CC H5 SW
- T23.322 Burn of third degree of single left finger (nail) except thumb CC H5 SW
- T23.329 Burn of third degree of unspecified single finger (nail) except thumb CC H5 SW

T23.33 Burn of third degree of multiple fingers (nail), not including thumb
- T23.331 Burn of third degree of multiple right fingers (nail), not including thumb CC H5 SW
- T23.332 Burn of third degree of multiple left fingers (nail), not including thumb CC H5 SW
- T23.339 Burn of third degree of unspecified multiple fingers (nail), not including thumb CC H5 SW

T23.34 Burn of third degree of multiple fingers (nail), including thumb
- T23.341 Burn of third degree of multiple right fingers (nail), including thumb CC H5 SW
- T23.342 Burn of third degree of multiple left fingers (nail), including thumb CC H5 SW
- T23.349 Burn of third degree of unspecified multiple fingers (nail), including thumb CC H5 SW

T23.35 Burn of third degree of palm
- T23.351 Burn of third degree of right palm CC H5 SW
- T23.352 Burn of third degree of left palm CC H5 SW
- T23.359 Burn of third degree of unspecified palm CC H5 SW

T23.36 Burn of third degree of back of hand
- T23.361 Burn of third degree of back of right hand CC H5 SW
- T23.362 Burn of third degree of back of left hand CC H5 SW
- T23.369 Burn of third degree of back of unspecified hand CC H5 SW

T23.37 Burn of third degree of wrist
- T23.371 Burn of third degree of right wrist CC H5 SW
- T23.372 Burn of third degree of left wrist CC H5 SW
- T23.379 Burn of third degree of unspecified wrist CC H5 SW

T23.39 Burn of third degree of multiple sites of wrist and hand
- T23.391 Burn of third degree of multiple sites of right wrist and hand CC H5 SW
- T23.392 Burn of third degree of multiple sites of left wrist and hand CC H5 SW
- T23.399 Burn of third degree of multiple sites of unspecified wrist and hand CC H5 SW

T23.4 Corrosion of unspecified degree of wrist and hand

Code first (T51-T65) to identify chemical and intent

Use additional external cause code to identify place (Y92)

T23.40 Corrosion of unspecified degree of hand, unspecified site
- T23.401 Corrosion of unspecified degree of right hand, unspecified site
- T23.402 Corrosion of unspecified degree of left hand, unspecified site
- T23.409 Corrosion of unspecified degree of unspecified hand, unspecified site

T23.41 Corrosion of unspecified degree of thumb (nail)
- T23.411 Corrosion of unspecified degree of right thumb (nail)
- T23.412 Corrosion of unspecified degree of left thumb (nail)
- T23.419 Corrosion of unspecified degree of unspecified thumb (nail)

T23.42 Corrosion of unspecified degree of single finger (nail) except thumb
- T23.421 Corrosion of unspecified degree of single right finger (nail) except thumb
- T23.422 Corrosion of unspecified degree of single left finger (nail) except thumb
- T23.429 Corrosion of unspecified degree of unspecified single finger (nail) except thumb

T23.43 Corrosion of unspecified degree of multiple fingers (nail), not including thumb
- T23.431 Corrosion of unspecified degree of multiple right fingers (nail), not including thumb
- T23.432 Corrosion of unspecified degree of multiple left fingers (nail), not including thumb
- T23.439 Corrosion of unspecified degree of unspecified multiple fingers (nail), not including thumb

T23.44 Corrosion of unspecified degree of multiple fingers (nail), including thumb
- T23.441 Corrosion of unspecified degree of multiple right fingers (nail), including thumb
- T23.442 Corrosion of unspecified degree of multiple left fingers (nail), including thumb
- T23.449 Corrosion of unspecified degree of unspecified multiple fingers (nail), including thumb

T23.45 Corrosion of unspecified degree of palm
- T23.451 Corrosion of unspecified degree of right palm
- T23.452 Corrosion of unspecified degree of left palm
- T23.459 Corrosion of unspecified degree of unspecified palm

T23.46 Corrosion of unspecified degree of back of hand
- T23.461 Corrosion of unspecified degree of back of right hand
- T23.462 Corrosion of unspecified degree of back of left hand
- T23.469 Corrosion of unspecified degree of back of unspecified hand

T23.47 Corrosion of unspecified degree of wrist
- T23.471 Corrosion of unspecified degree of right wrist
- T23.472 Corrosion of unspecified degree of left wrist
- T23.479 Corrosion of unspecified degree of unspecified wrist

T23.49 Corrosion of unspecified degree of multiple sites of wrist and hand
- T23.491 Corrosion of unspecified degree of multiple sites of right wrist and hand
- T23.492 Corrosion of unspecified degree of multiple sites of left wrist and hand
- T23.499 Corrosion of unspecified degree of multiple sites of unspecified wrist and hand

T23.5 Corrosion of first degree of wrist and hand

Code first (T51-T65) to identify chemical and intent
Use additional external cause code to identify place (Y92)

T23.50 Corrosion of first degree of hand, unspecified site
- T23.501 Corrosion of first degree of right hand, unspecified site
- T23.502 Corrosion of first degree of left hand, unspecified site
- T23.509 Corrosion of first degree of unspecified hand, unspecified site

T23.51 Corrosion of first degree of thumb (nail)
- T23.511 Corrosion of first degree of right thumb (nail)
- T23.512 Corrosion of first degree of left thumb (nail)
- T23.519 Corrosion of first degree of unspecified thumb (nail)

T23.52 Corrosion of first degree of single finger (nail) except thumb
- T23.521 Corrosion of first degree of single right finger (nail) except thumb
- T23.522 Corrosion of first degree of single left finger (nail) except thumb
- T23.529 Corrosion of first degree of unspecified single finger (nail) except thumb

T23.53 Corrosion of first degree of multiple fingers (nail), not including thumb
- T23.531 Corrosion of first degree of multiple right fingers (nail), not including thumb
- T23.532 Corrosion of first degree of multiple left fingers (nail), not including thumb
- T23.539 Corrosion of first degree of unspecified multiple fingers (nail), not including thumb

T23.54 Corrosion of first degree of multiple fingers (nail), including thumb
- T23.541 Corrosion of first degree of multiple right fingers (nail), including thumb
- T23.542 Corrosion of first degree of multiple left fingers (nail), including thumb
- T23.549 Corrosion of first degree of unspecified multiple fingers (nail), including thumb

T23.55 Corrosion of first degree of palm
- T23.551 Corrosion of first degree of right palm
- T23.552 Corrosion of first degree of left palm
- T23.559 Corrosion of first degree of unspecified palm

T23.56 Corrosion of first degree of back of hand
- T23.561 Corrosion of first degree of back of right hand
- T23.562 Corrosion of first degree of back of left hand
- T23.569 Corrosion of first degree of back of unspecified hand

T23.57 Corrosion of first degree of wrist
- T23.571 Corrosion of first degree of right wrist
- T23.572 Corrosion of first degree of left wrist
- T23.579 Corrosion of first degree of unspecified wrist

T23.59 Corrosion of first degree of multiple sites of wrist and hand
- T23.591 Corrosion of first degree of multiple sites of right wrist and hand
- T23.592 Corrosion of first degree of multiple sites of left wrist and hand
- T23.599 Corrosion of first degree of multiple sites of unspecified wrist and hand

T23.6 Corrosion of second degree of wrist and hand

Code first (T51-T65) to identify chemical and intent
Use additional external cause code to identify place (Y92)

T23.60 Corrosion of second degree of hand, unspecified site
- T23.601 Corrosion of second degree of right hand, unspecified site
- T23.602 Corrosion of second degree of left hand, unspecified site
- T23.609 Corrosion of second degree of unspecified hand, unspecified site

T23.61 Corrosion of second degree of thumb (nail)
- T23.611 Corrosion of second degree of right thumb (nail)
- T23.612 Corrosion of second degree of left thumb (nail)
- T23.619 Corrosion of second degree of unspecified thumb (nail)

T23.62 Corrosion of second degree of single finger (nail) except thumb
- T23.621 Corrosion of second degree of single right finger (nail) except thumb
- T23.622 Corrosion of second degree of single left finger (nail) except thumb
- T23.629 Corrosion of second degree of unspecified single finger (nail) except thumb

T23.63 Corrosion of second degree of multiple fingers (nail), not including thumb
- T23.631 Corrosion of second degree of multiple right fingers (nail), not including thumb
- T23.632 Corrosion of second degree of multiple left fingers (nail), not including thumb
- T23.639 Corrosion of second degree of unspecified multiple fingers (nail), not including thumb

✓6th **T23.64 Corrosion of second degree of multiple fingers (nail), including thumb**
- ✓7th **T23.641 Corrosion of second degree of multiple right fingers (nail), including thumb**
- ✓7th **T23.642 Corrosion of second degree of multiple left fingers (nail), including thumb**
- ✓7th **T23.649 Corrosion of second degree of unspecified multiple fingers (nail), including thumb**

✓6th **T23.65 Corrosion of second degree of palm**
- ✓7th **T23.651 Corrosion of second degree of right palm**
- ✓7th **T23.652 Corrosion of second degree of left palm**
- ✓7th **T23.659 Corrosion of second degree of unspecified palm**

✓6th **T23.66 Corrosion of second degree of back of hand**
- ✓7th **T23.661 Corrosion of second degree back of right hand**
- ✓7th **T23.662 Corrosion of second degree back of left hand**
- ✓7th **T23.669 Corrosion of second degree back of unspecified hand**

✓6th **T23.67 Corrosion of second degree of wrist**
- ✓7th **T23.671 Corrosion of second degree of right wrist**
- ✓7th **T23.672 Corrosion of second degree of left wrist**
- ✓7th **T23.679 Corrosion of second degree of unspecified wrist**

✓6th **T23.69 Corrosion of second degree of multiple sites of wrist and hand**
- ✓7th **T23.691 Corrosion of second degree of multiple sites of right wrist and hand**
- ✓7th **T23.692 Corrosion of second degree of multiple sites of left wrist and hand**
- ✓7th **T23.699 Corrosion of second degree of multiple sites of unspecified wrist and hand**

✓5th **T23.7 Corrosion of third degree of wrist and hand**

Code first (T51-T65) to identify chemical and intent
Use additional external cause code to identify place (Y92)

✓6th **T23.7Ø Corrosion of third degree of hand, unspecified site**
- ✓7th **T23.7Ø1 Corrosion of third degree of right hand, unspecified site** CC H5 SW
- ✓7th **T23.7Ø2 Corrosion of third degree of left hand, unspecified site** CC H5 SW
- ✓7th **T23.7Ø9 Corrosion of third degree of unspecified hand, unspecified site** CC H5 SW

✓6th **T23.71 Corrosion of third degree of thumb (nail)**
- ✓7th **T23.711 Corrosion of third degree of right thumb (nail)** CC H5 SW
- ✓7th **T23.712 Corrosion of third degree of left thumb (nail)** CC H5 SW
- ✓7th **T23.719 Corrosion of third degree of unspecified thumb (nail)** CC H5 SW

✓6th **T23.72 Corrosion of third degree of single finger (nail) except thumb**
- ✓7th **T23.721 Corrosion of third degree of single right finger (nail) except thumb** CC H5 SW
- ✓7th **T23.722 Corrosion of third degree of single left finger (nail) except thumb** CC H5 SW
- ✓7th **T23.729 Corrosion of third degree of unspecified single finger (nail) except thumb** CC H5 SW

✓6th **T23.73 Corrosion of third degree of multiple fingers (nail), not including thumb**
- ✓7th **T23.731 Corrosion of third degree of multiple right fingers (nail), not including thumb** CC H5 SW
- ✓7th **T23.732 Corrosion of third degree of multiple left fingers (nail), not including thumb** CC H5 SW
- ✓7th **T23.739 Corrosion of third degree of unspecified multiple fingers (nail), not including thumb** CC H5 SW

✓6th **T23.74 Corrosion of third degree of multiple fingers (nail), including thumb**
- ✓7th **T23.741 Corrosion of third degree of multiple right fingers (nail), including thumb** CC H5 SW
- ✓7th **T23.742 Corrosion of third degree of multiple left fingers (nail), including thumb** CC H5 SW
- ✓7th **T23.749 Corrosion of third degree of unspecified multiple fingers (nail), including thumb** CC H5 SW

✓6th **T23.75 Corrosion of third degree of palm**
- ✓7th **T23.751 Corrosion of third degree of right palm** CC H5 SW
- ✓7th **T23.752 Corrosion of third degree of left palm** CC H5 SW
- ✓7th **T23.759 Corrosion of third degree of unspecified palm** CC H5 SW

✓6th **T23.76 Corrosion of third degree of back of hand**
- ✓7th **T23.761 Corrosion of third degree of back of right hand** CC H5 SW
- ✓7th **T23.762 Corrosion of third degree of back of left hand** CC H5 SW
- ✓7th **T23.769 Corrosion of third degree back of unspecified hand** CC H5 SW

✓6th **T23.77 Corrosion of third degree of wrist**
- ✓7th **T23.771 Corrosion of third degree of right wrist** CC H5 SW
- ✓7th **T23.772 Corrosion of third degree of left wrist** CC H5 SW
- ✓7th **T23.779 Corrosion of third degree of unspecified wrist** CC H5 SW

✓6th **T23.79 Corrosion of third degree of multiple sites of wrist and hand**
- ✓7th **T23.791 Corrosion of third degree of multiple sites of right wrist and hand** CC H5 SW
- ✓7th **T23.792 Corrosion of third degree of multiple sites of left wrist and hand** CC H5 SW
- ✓7th **T23.799 Corrosion of third degree of multiple sites of unspecified wrist and hand** CC H5 SW

✓4th T24 Burn and corrosion of lower limb, except ankle and foot

EXCLUDES 2 *burn and corrosion of ankle and foot (T25.-)*
burn and corrosion of hip region (T21.-)

The appropriate 7th character is to be added to each code from category T24.
- A initial encounter
- D subsequent encounter
- S sequela

✓5th **T24.Ø Burn of unspecified degree of lower limb, except ankle and foot**

Use additional external cause code to identify the source, place and intent of the burn (XØØ-X19, X75-X77, X96-X98, Y92)

✓6th **T24.ØØ Burn of unspecified degree of unspecified site of lower limb, except ankle and foot**
- ✓7th **T24.ØØ1 Burn of unspecified degree of unspecified site of right lower limb, except ankle and foot**
- ✓7th **T24.ØØ2 Burn of unspecified degree of unspecified site of left lower limb, except ankle and foot**
- ✓7th **T24.ØØ9 Burn of unspecified degree of unspecified site of unspecified lower limb, except ankle and foot**

✓6th **T24.Ø1 Burn of unspecified degree of thigh**
- ✓7th **T24.Ø11 Burn of unspecified degree of right thigh**
- ✓7th **T24.Ø12 Burn of unspecified degree of left thigh**
- ✓7th **T24.Ø19 Burn of unspecified degree of unspecified thigh**

✓6th **T24.Ø2 Burn of unspecified degree of knee**
- ✓7th **T24.Ø21 Burn of unspecified degree of right knee**
- ✓7th **T24.Ø22 Burn of unspecified degree of left knee**
- ✓7th **T24.Ø29 Burn of unspecified degree of unspecified knee**

✓6th **T24.Ø3 Burn of unspecified degree of lower leg**
- ✓7th **T24.Ø31 Burn of unspecified degree of right lower leg**
- ✓7th **T24.Ø32 Burn of unspecified degree of left lower leg**
- ✓7th **T24.Ø39 Burn of unspecified degree of unspecified lower leg**

✓6th **T24.Ø9 Burn of unspecified degree of multiple sites of lower limb, except ankle and foot**
- ✓7th **T24.Ø91 Burn of unspecified degree of multiple sites of right lower limb, except ankle and foot**

T24.092 Burn of unspecified degree of multiple sites of left lower limb, except ankle and foot

T24.099 Burn of unspecified degree of multiple sites of unspecified lower limb, except ankle and foot

T24.1 Burn of first degree of lower limb, except ankle and foot

Use additional external cause code to identify the source, place and intent of the burn (X00-X19, X75-X77, X96-X98, Y92)

T24.10 Burn of first degree of unspecified site of lower limb, except ankle and foot

T24.101 Burn of first degree of unspecified site of right lower limb, except ankle and foot

T24.102 Burn of first degree of unspecified site of left lower limb, except ankle and foot

T24.109 Burn of first degree of unspecified site of unspecified lower limb, except ankle and foot

T24.11 Burn of first degree of thigh

T24.111 Burn of first degree of right thigh

T24.112 Burn of first degree of left thigh

T24.119 Burn of first degree of unspecified thigh

T24.12 Burn of first degree of knee

T24.121 Burn of first degree of right knee

T24.122 Burn of first degree of left knee

T24.129 Burn of first degree of unspecified knee

T24.13 Burn of first degree of lower leg

T24.131 Burn of first degree of right lower leg

T24.132 Burn of first degree of left lower leg

T24.139 Burn of first degree of unspecified lower leg

T24.19 Burn of first degree of multiple sites of lower limb, except ankle and foot

T24.191 Burn of first degree of multiple sites of right lower limb, except ankle and foot

T24.192 Burn of first degree of multiple sites of left lower limb, except ankle and foot

T24.199 Burn of first degree of multiple sites of unspecified lower limb, except ankle and foot

T24.2 Burn of second degree of lower limb, except ankle and foot

Use additional external cause code to identify the source, place and intent of the burn (X00-X19, X75-X77, X96-X98, Y92)

T24.20 Burn of second degree of unspecified site of lower limb, except ankle and foot

T24.201 Burn of second degree of unspecified site of right lower limb, except ankle and foot

T24.202 Burn of second degree of unspecified site of left lower limb, except ankle and foot

T24.209 Burn of second degree of unspecified site of unspecified lower limb, except ankle and foot

T24.21 Burn of second degree of thigh

T24.211 Burn of second degree of right thigh

T24.212 Burn of second degree of left thigh

T24.219 Burn of second degree of unspecified thigh

T24.22 Burn of second degree of knee

T24.221 Burn of second degree of right knee

T24.222 Burn of second degree of left knee

T24.229 Burn of second degree of unspecified knee

T24.23 Burn of second degree of lower leg

T24.231 Burn of second degree of right lower leg

T24.232 Burn of second degree of left lower leg

T24.239 Burn of second degree of unspecified lower leg

T24.29 Burn of second degree of multiple sites of lower limb, except ankle and foot

T24.291 Burn of second degree of multiple sites of right lower limb, except ankle and foot

T24.292 Burn of second degree of multiple sites of left lower limb, except ankle and foot

T24.299 Burn of second degree of multiple sites of unspecified lower limb, except ankle and foot

T24.3 Burn of third degree of lower limb, except ankle and foot

Use additional external cause code to identify the source, place and intent of the burn (X00-X19, X75-X77, X96-X98, Y92)

T24.30 Burn of third degree of unspecified site of lower limb, except ankle and foot

T24.301 Burn of third degree of unspecified site of right lower limb, except ankle and foot CC HS SW

T24.302 Burn of third degree of unspecified site of left lower limb, except ankle and foot CC HS SW

T24.309 Burn of third degree of unspecified site of unspecified lower limb, except ankle and foot CC HS SW

T24.31 Burn of third degree of thigh

T24.311 Burn of third degree of right thigh CC HS SW

T24.312 Burn of third degree of left thigh CC HS SW

T24.319 Burn of third degree of unspecified thigh CC HS SW

T24.32 Burn of third degree of knee

T24.321 Burn of third degree of right knee CC HS SW

T24.322 Burn of third degree of left knee CC HS SW

T24.329 Burn of third degree of unspecified knee CC HS SW

T24.33 Burn of third degree of lower leg

T24.331 Burn of third degree of right lower leg CC HS SW

T24.332 Burn of third degree of left lower leg CC HS SW

T24.339 Burn of third degree of unspecified lower leg CC HS SW

T24.39 Burn of third degree of multiple sites of lower limb, except ankle and foot

AHA: 2016,2Q,4

T24.391 Burn of third degree of multiple sites of right lower limb, except ankle and foot CC HS SW

T24.392 Burn of third degree of multiple sites of left lower limb, except ankle and foot CC HS SW

T24.399 Burn of third degree of multiple sites of unspecified lower limb, except ankle and foot CC HS SW

T24.4 Corrosion of unspecified degree of lower limb, except ankle and foot

Code first (T51-T65) to identify chemical and intent

Use additional external cause code to identify place (Y92)

T24.40 Corrosion of unspecified degree of unspecified site of lower limb, except ankle and foot

T24.401 Corrosion of unspecified degree of unspecified site of right lower limb, except ankle and foot

T24.402 Corrosion of unspecified degree of unspecified site of left lower limb, except ankle and foot

T24.409 Corrosion of unspecified degree of unspecified site of unspecified lower limb, except ankle and foot

T24.41 Corrosion of unspecified degree of thigh

T24.411 Corrosion of unspecified degree of right thigh

T24.412 Corrosion of unspecified degree of left thigh

T24.419 Corrosion of unspecified degree of unspecified thigh

T24.42 Corrosion of unspecified degree of knee

T24.421 Corrosion of unspecified degree of right knee

T24.422 Corrosion of unspecified degree of left knee

T24.429 Corrosion of unspecified degree of unspecified knee

T24.43 Corrosion of unspecified degree of lower leg

T24.431 Corrosion of unspecified degree of right lower leg

✓7th T24.432 Corrosion of unspecified degree of left lower leg
✓7th T24.439 Corrosion of unspecified degree of unspecified lower leg
✓6th T24.49 Corrosion of unspecified degree of multiple sites of lower limb, except ankle and foot
✓7th T24.491 Corrosion of unspecified degree of multiple sites of right lower limb, except ankle and foot
✓7th T24.492 Corrosion of unspecified degree of multiple sites of left lower limb, except ankle and foot
✓7th T24.499 Corrosion of unspecified degree of multiple sites of unspecified lower limb, except ankle and foot
✓5th T24.5 Corrosion of first degree of lower limb, except ankle and foot
Code first (T51-T65) to identify chemical and intent
Use additional external cause code to identify place (Y92)
✓6th T24.50 Corrosion of first degree of unspecified site of lower limb, except ankle and foot
✓7th T24.501 Corrosion of first degree of unspecified site of right lower limb, except ankle and foot
✓7th T24.502 Corrosion of first degree of unspecified site of left lower limb, except ankle and foot
✓7th T24.509 Corrosion of first degree of unspecified site of unspecified lower limb, except ankle and foot
✓6th T24.51 Corrosion of first degree of thigh
✓7th T24.511 Corrosion of first degree of right thigh
✓7th T24.512 Corrosion of first degree of left thigh
✓7th T24.519 Corrosion of first degree of unspecified thigh
✓6th T24.52 Corrosion of first degree of knee
✓7th T24.521 Corrosion of first degree of right knee
✓7th T24.522 Corrosion of first degree of left knee
✓7th T24.529 Corrosion of first degree of unspecified knee
✓6th T24.53 Corrosion of first degree of lower leg
✓7th T24.531 Corrosion of first degree of right lower leg
✓7th T24.532 Corrosion of first degree of left lower leg
✓7th T24.539 Corrosion of first degree of unspecified lower leg
✓6th T24.59 Corrosion of first degree of multiple sites of lower limb, except ankle and foot
✓7th T24.591 Corrosion of first degree of multiple sites of right lower limb, except ankle and foot
✓7th T24.592 Corrosion of first degree of multiple sites of left lower limb, except ankle and foot
✓7th T24.599 Corrosion of first degree of multiple sites of unspecified lower limb, except ankle and foot
✓5th T24.6 Corrosion of second degree of lower limb, except ankle and foot
Code first (T51-T65) to identify chemical and intent
Use additional external cause code to identify place (Y92)
✓6th T24.60 Corrosion of second degree of unspecified site of lower limb, except ankle and foot
✓7th T24.601 Corrosion of second degree of unspecified site of right lower limb, except ankle and foot
✓7th T24.602 Corrosion of second degree of unspecified site of left lower limb, except ankle and foot
✓7th T24.609 Corrosion of second degree of unspecified site of unspecified lower limb, except ankle and foot
✓6th T24.61 Corrosion of second degree of thigh
✓7th T24.611 Corrosion of second degree of right thigh
✓7th T24.612 Corrosion of second degree of left thigh
✓7th T24.619 Corrosion of second degree of unspecified thigh
✓6th T24.62 Corrosion of second degree of knee
✓7th T24.621 Corrosion of second degree of right knee
✓7th T24.622 Corrosion of second degree of left knee
✓7th T24.629 Corrosion of second degree of unspecified knee
✓6th T24.63 Corrosion of second degree of lower leg
✓7th T24.631 Corrosion of second degree of right lower leg
✓7th T24.632 Corrosion of second degree of left lower leg
✓7th T24.639 Corrosion of second degree of unspecified lower leg
✓6th T24.69 Corrosion of second degree of multiple sites of lower limb, except ankle and foot
✓7th T24.691 Corrosion of second degree of multiple sites of right lower limb, except ankle and foot
✓7th T24.692 Corrosion of second degree of multiple sites of left lower limb, except ankle and foot
✓7th T24.699 Corrosion of second degree of multiple sites of unspecified lower limb, except ankle and foot
✓5th T24.7 Corrosion of third degree of lower limb, except ankle and foot
Code first (T51-T65) to identify chemical and intent
Use additional external cause code to identify place (Y92)
✓6th T24.70 Corrosion of third degree of unspecified site of lower limb, except ankle and foot
✓7th T24.701 Corrosion of third degree of unspecified site of right lower limb, except ankle and foot CC HS SW
✓7th T24.702 Corrosion of third degree of unspecified site of left lower limb, except ankle and foot CC HS SW
✓7th T24.709 Corrosion of third degree of unspecified site of unspecified lower limb, except ankle and foot CC HS SW
✓6th T24.71 Corrosion of third degree of thigh
✓7th T24.711 Corrosion of third degree of right thigh CC HS SW
✓7th T24.712 Corrosion of third degree of left thigh CC HS SW
✓7th T24.719 Corrosion of third degree of unspecified thigh CC HS SW
✓6th T24.72 Corrosion of third degree of knee
✓7th T24.721 Corrosion of third degree of right knee CC HS SW
✓7th T24.722 Corrosion of third degree of left knee CC HS SW
✓7th T24.729 Corrosion of third degree of unspecified knee CC HS SW
✓6th T24.73 Corrosion of third degree of lower leg
✓7th T24.731 Corrosion of third degree of right lower leg CC HS SW
✓7th T24.732 Corrosion of third degree of left lower leg CC HS SW
✓7th T24.739 Corrosion of third degree of unspecified lower leg CC HS SW
✓6th T24.79 Corrosion of third degree of multiple sites of lower limb, except ankle and foot
✓7th T24.791 Corrosion of third degree of multiple sites of right lower limb, except ankle and foot CC HS SW
✓7th T24.792 Corrosion of third degree of multiple sites of left lower limb, except ankle and foot CC HS SW
✓7th T24.799 Corrosion of third degree of multiple sites of unspecified lower limb, except ankle and foot CC HS SW
✓4th T25 Burn and corrosion of ankle and foot

The appropriate 7th character is to be added to each code from category T25.
A initial encounter
D subsequent encounter
S sequela

✓5th T25.0 Burn of unspecified degree of ankle and foot
Use additional external cause code to identify the source, place and intent of the burn (X00-X19, X75-X77, X96-X98, Y92)
✓6th T25.01 Burn of unspecified degree of ankle
✓7th T25.011 Burn of unspecified degree of right ankle
✓7th T25.012 Burn of unspecified degree of left ankle
✓7th T25.019 Burn of unspecified degree of unspecified ankle

T25.02 Burn of unspecified degree of foot
EXCLUDES 2 burn of unspecified degree of toe(s) (nail) (T25.03-)
T25.021 Burn of unspecified degree of right foot
T25.022 Burn of unspecified degree of left foot
T25.029 Burn of unspecified degree of unspecified foot
T25.03 Burn of unspecified degree of toe(s) (nail)
T25.031 Burn of unspecified degree of right toe(s) (nail)
T25.032 Burn of unspecified degree of left toe(s) (nail)
T25.039 Burn of unspecified degree of unspecified toe(s) (nail)
T25.09 Burn of unspecified degree of multiple sites of ankle and foot
T25.091 Burn of unspecified degree of multiple sites of right ankle and foot
T25.092 Burn of unspecified degree of multiple sites of left ankle and foot
T25.099 Burn of unspecified degree of multiple sites of unspecified ankle and foot
T25.1 Burn of first degree of ankle and foot
Use additional external cause code to identify the source, place and intent of the burn (X00-X19, X75-X77, X96-X98, Y92)
T25.11 Burn of first degree of ankle
T25.111 Burn of first degree of right ankle
T25.112 Burn of first degree of left ankle
T25.119 Burn of first degree of unspecified ankle
T25.12 Burn of first degree of foot
EXCLUDES 2 burn of first degree of toe(s) (nail) (T25.13-)
T25.121 Burn of first degree of right foot
T25.122 Burn of first degree of left foot
T25.129 Burn of first degree of unspecified foot
T25.13 Burn of first degree of toe(s) (nail)
T25.131 Burn of first degree of right toe(s) (nail)
T25.132 Burn of first degree of left toe(s) (nail)
T25.139 Burn of first degree of unspecified toe(s) (nail)
T25.19 Burn of first degree of multiple sites of ankle and foot
T25.191 Burn of first degree of multiple sites of right ankle and foot
T25.192 Burn of first degree of multiple sites of left ankle and foot
T25.199 Burn of first degree of multiple sites of unspecified ankle and foot
T25.2 Burn of second degree of ankle and foot
Use additional external cause code to identify the source, place and intent of the burn (X00-X19, X75-X77, X96-X98, Y92)
T25.21 Burn of second degree of ankle
T25.211 Burn of second degree of right ankle
T25.212 Burn of second degree of left ankle
T25.219 Burn of second degree of unspecified ankle
T25.22 Burn of second degree of foot
EXCLUDES 2 burn of second degree of toe(s) (nail) (T25.23-)
T25.221 Burn of second degree of right foot
T25.222 Burn of second degree of left foot
T25.229 Burn of second degree of unspecified foot
T25.23 Burn of second degree of toe(s) (nail)
T25.231 Burn of second degree of right toe(s) (nail)
T25.232 Burn of second degree of left toe(s) (nail)
T25.239 Burn of second degree of unspecified toe(s) (nail)
T25.29 Burn of second degree of multiple sites of ankle and foot
T25.291 Burn of second degree of multiple sites of right ankle and foot
T25.292 Burn of second degree of multiple sites of left ankle and foot
T25.299 Burn of second degree of multiple sites of unspecified ankle and foot
T25.3 Burn of third degree of ankle and foot
Use additional external cause code to identify the source, place and intent of the burn (X00-X19, X75-X77, X96-X98, Y92)
T25.31 Burn of third degree of ankle
T25.311 Burn of third degree of right ankle CC H5 SW
T25.312 Burn of third degree of left ankle CC H5 SW
T25.319 Burn of third degree of unspecified ankle CC H5 SW
T25.32 Burn of third degree of foot
EXCLUDES 2 burn of third degree of toe(s) (nail) (T25.33-)
T25.321 Burn of third degree of right foot CC H5 SW
T25.322 Burn of third degree of left foot CC H5 SW
T25.329 Burn of third degree of unspecified foot CC H5 SW
T25.33 Burn of third degree of toe(s) (nail)
T25.331 Burn of third degree of right toe(s) (nail) CC H5 SW
T25.332 Burn of third degree of left toe(s) (nail) CC H5 SW
T25.339 Burn of third degree of unspecified toe(s) (nail) CC H5 SW
T25.39 Burn of third degree of multiple sites of ankle and foot
T25.391 Burn of third degree of multiple sites of right ankle and foot CC H5 SW
T25.392 Burn of third degree of multiple sites of left ankle and foot CC H5 SW
T25.399 Burn of third degree of multiple sites of unspecified ankle and foot CC H5 SW
T25.4 Corrosion of unspecified degree of ankle and foot
Code first (T51-T65) to identify chemical and intent
Use additional external cause code to identify place (Y92)
T25.41 Corrosion of unspecified degree of ankle
T25.411 Corrosion of unspecified degree of right ankle
T25.412 Corrosion of unspecified degree of left ankle
T25.419 Corrosion of unspecified degree of unspecified ankle
T25.42 Corrosion of unspecified degree of foot
EXCLUDES 2 corrosion of unspecified degree of toe(s) (nail) (T25.43-)
T25.421 Corrosion of unspecified degree of right foot
T25.422 Corrosion of unspecified degree of left foot
T25.429 Corrosion of unspecified degree of unspecified foot
T25.43 Corrosion of unspecified degree of toe(s) (nail)
T25.431 Corrosion of unspecified degree of right toe(s) (nail)
T25.432 Corrosion of unspecified degree of left toe(s) (nail)
T25.439 Corrosion of unspecified degree of unspecified toe(s) (nail)
T25.49 Corrosion of unspecified degree of multiple sites of ankle and foot
T25.491 Corrosion of unspecified degree of multiple sites of right ankle and foot
T25.492 Corrosion of unspecified degree of multiple sites of left ankle and foot
T25.499 Corrosion of unspecified degree of multiple sites of unspecified ankle and foot
T25.5 Corrosion of first degree of ankle and foot
Code first (T51-T65) to identify chemical and intent
Use additional external cause code to identify place (Y92)
T25.51 Corrosion of first degree of ankle
T25.511 Corrosion of first degree of right ankle
T25.512 Corrosion of first degree of left ankle
T25.519 Corrosion of first degree of unspecified ankle

√6th T25.52 **Corrosion of first degree of foot**
EXCLUDES 2 *corrosion of first degree of toe(s) (nail) (T25.53-)*
√7th T25.521 **Corrosion of first degree of right foot**
√7th T25.522 **Corrosion of first degree of left foot**
√7th T25.529 **Corrosion of first degree of unspecified foot**
√6th T25.53 **Corrosion of first degree of toe(s) (nail)**
√7th T25.531 **Corrosion of first degree of right toe(s) (nail)**
√7th T25.532 **Corrosion of first degree of left toe(s) (nail)**
√7th T25.539 **Corrosion of first degree of unspecified toe(s) (nail)**
√6th T25.59 **Corrosion of first degree of multiple sites of ankle and foot**
√7th T25.591 **Corrosion of first degree of multiple sites of right ankle and foot**
√7th T25.592 **Corrosion of first degree of multiple sites of left ankle and foot**
√7th T25.599 **Corrosion of first degree of multiple sites of unspecified ankle and foot**
√5th T25.6 **Corrosion of second degree of ankle and foot**
Code first (T51-T65) to identify chemical and intent
Use additional external cause code to identify place (Y92)
√6th T25.61 **Corrosion of second degree of ankle**
√7th T25.611 **Corrosion of second degree of right ankle**
√7th T25.612 **Corrosion of second degree of left ankle**
√7th T25.619 **Corrosion of second degree of unspecified ankle**
√6th T25.62 **Corrosion of second degree of foot**
EXCLUDES 2 *corrosion of second degree of toe(s) (nail) (T25.63-)*
√7th T25.621 **Corrosion of second degree of right foot**
√7th T25.622 **Corrosion of second degree of left foot**
√7th T25.629 **Corrosion of second degree of unspecified foot**
√6th T25.63 **Corrosion of second degree of toe(s) (nail)**
√7th T25.631 **Corrosion of second degree of right toe(s) (nail)**
√7th T25.632 **Corrosion of second degree of left toe(s) (nail)**
√7th T25.639 **Corrosion of second degree of unspecified toe(s) (nail)**
√6th T25.69 **Corrosion of second degree of multiple sites of ankle and foot**
√7th T25.691 **Corrosion of second degree of right ankle and foot**
√7th T25.692 **Corrosion of second degree of left ankle and foot**
√7th T25.699 **Corrosion of second degree of unspecified ankle and foot**
√5th T25.7 **Corrosion of third degree of ankle and foot**
Code first (T51-T65) to identify chemical and intent
Use additional external cause code to identify place (Y92)
√6th T25.71 **Corrosion of third degree of ankle**
√7th T25.711 **Corrosion of third degree of right ankle** CC H5 SW
√7th T25.712 **Corrosion of third degree of left ankle** CC H5 SW
√7th T25.719 **Corrosion of third degree of unspecified ankle** CC H5 SW
√6th T25.72 **Corrosion of third degree of foot**
EXCLUDES 2 *corrosion of third degree of toe(s) (nail) (T25.73-)*
√7th T25.721 **Corrosion of third degree of right foot** CC H5 SW
√7th T25.722 **Corrosion of third degree of left foot** CC H5 SW
√7th T25.729 **Corrosion of third degree of unspecified foot** CC H5 SW
√6th T25.73 **Corrosion of third degree of toe(s) (nail)**
√7th T25.731 **Corrosion of third degree of right toe(s) (nail)** CC H5 SW
√7th T25.732 **Corrosion of third degree of left toe(s) (nail)** CC H5 SW
√7th T25.739 **Corrosion of third degree of unspecified toe(s) (nail)** CC H5 SW
√6th T25.79 **Corrosion of third degree of multiple sites of ankle and foot**
√7th T25.791 **Corrosion of third degree of multiple sites of right ankle and foot** CC H5 SW
√7th T25.792 **Corrosion of third degree of multiple sites of left ankle and foot** CC H5 SW
√7th T25.799 **Corrosion of third degree of multiple sites of unspecified ankle and foot** CC H5 SW

Burns and corrosions confined to eye and internal organs (T26-T28)

√4th **T26 Burn and corrosion confined to eye and adnexa**

The appropriate 7th character is to be added to each code from category T26.
A initial encounter
D subsequent encounter
S sequela

√5th T26.0 **Burn of eyelid and periocular area**
Use additional external cause code to identify the source, place and intent of the burn (X00-X19, X75-X77, X96-X98, Y92)
√x7th T26.00 **Burn of unspecified eyelid and periocular area**
√x7th T26.01 **Burn of right eyelid and periocular area**
√x7th T26.02 **Burn of left eyelid and periocular area**
√5th T26.1 **Burn of cornea and conjunctival sac**
Use additional external cause code to identify the source, place and intent of the burn (X00-X19, X75-X77, X96-X98, Y92)
√x7th T26.10 **Burn of cornea and conjunctival sac, unspecified eye**
√x7th T26.11 **Burn of cornea and conjunctival sac, right eye**
√x7th T26.12 **Burn of cornea and conjunctival sac, left eye**
√5th T26.2 **Burn with resulting rupture and destruction of eyeball**
Use additional external cause code to identify the source, place and intent of the burn (X00-X19, X75-X77, X96-X98, Y92)
√x7th T26.20 **Burn with resulting rupture and destruction of unspecified eyeball** CC H5
√x7th T26.21 **Burn with resulting rupture and destruction of right eyeball** CC H5
√x7th T26.22 **Burn with resulting rupture and destruction of left eyeball** CC H5
√5th T26.3 **Burns of other specified parts of eye and adnexa**
Use additional external cause code to identify the source, place and intent of the burn (X00-X19, X75-X77, X96-X98, Y92)
√x7th T26.30 **Burns of other specified parts of unspecified eye and adnexa**
√x7th T26.31 **Burns of other specified parts of right eye and adnexa**
√x7th T26.32 **Burns of other specified parts of left eye and adnexa**
√5th T26.4 **Burn of eye and adnexa, part unspecified**
Use additional external cause code to identify the source, place and intent of the burn (X00-X19, X75-X77, X96-X98, Y92)
√x7th T26.40 **Burn of unspecified eye and adnexa, part unspecified**
√x7th T26.41 **Burn of right eye and adnexa, part unspecified**
√x7th T26.42 **Burn of left eye and adnexa, part unspecified**
√5th T26.5 **Corrosion of eyelid and periocular area**
Code first (T51-T65) to identify chemical and intent
Use additional external cause code to identify place (Y92)
√x7th T26.50 **Corrosion of unspecified eyelid and periocular area**
√x7th T26.51 **Corrosion of right eyelid and periocular area**
√x7th T26.52 **Corrosion of left eyelid and periocular area**
√5th T26.6 **Corrosion of cornea and conjunctival sac**
Code first (T51-T65) to identify chemical and intent
Use additional external cause code to identify place (Y92)
√x7th T26.60 **Corrosion of cornea and conjunctival sac, unspecified eye**
√x7th T26.61 **Corrosion of cornea and conjunctival sac, right eye**
√x7th T26.62 **Corrosion of cornea and conjunctival sac, left eye**

T26.7 Corrosion with resulting rupture and destruction of eyeball
Code first (T51-T65) to identify chemical and intent
Use additional external cause code to identify place (Y92)
T26.70 Corrosion with resulting rupture and destruction of unspecified eyeball CC H5
T26.71 Corrosion with resulting rupture and destruction of right eyeball CC H5
T26.72 Corrosion with resulting rupture and destruction of left eyeball CC H5
T26.8 Corrosions of other specified parts of eye and adnexa
Code first (T51-T65) to identify chemical and intent
Use additional external cause code to identify place (Y92)
T26.80 Corrosions of other specified parts of unspecified eye and adnexa
T26.81 Corrosions of other specified parts of right eye and adnexa
T26.82 Corrosions of other specified parts of left eye and adnexa
T26.9 Corrosion of eye and adnexa, part unspecified
Code first (T51-T65) to identify chemical and intent
Use additional external cause code to identify place (Y92)
T26.90 Corrosion of unspecified eye and adnexa, part unspecified
T26.91 Corrosion of right eye and adnexa, part unspecified
T26.92 Corrosion of left eye and adnexa, part unspecified

T27 Burn and corrosion of respiratory tract
Use additional external cause code to identify the source and intent of the burn (X00-X19, X75-X77, X96-X98)
Use additional external cause code to identify place (Y92)

The appropriate 7th character is to be added to each code from category T27.
A initial encounter
D subsequent encounter
S sequela

T27.0 Burn of larynx and trachea CC H5
T27.1 Burn involving larynx and trachea with lung CC H5
T27.2 Burn of other parts of respiratory tract CC H5
Burn of thoracic cavity
T27.3 Burn of respiratory tract, part unspecified CC H5
T27.4 Corrosion of larynx and trachea CC H5
Code first (T51-T65) to identify chemical and intent
T27.5 Corrosion involving larynx and trachea with lung CC H5
Code first (T51-T65) to identify chemical and intent
T27.6 Corrosion of other parts of respiratory tract CC H5
Code first (T51-T65) to identify chemical and intent
T27.7 Corrosion of respiratory tract, part unspecified CC H5
Code first (T51-T65) to identify chemical and intent

T28 Burn and corrosion of other internal organs
Use additional external cause code to identify the source and intent of the burn (X00-X19, X75-X77, X96-X98)
Use additional external cause code to identify place (Y92)

The appropriate 7th character is to be added to each code from category T28.
A initial encounter
D subsequent encounter
S sequela

T28.0 Burn of mouth and pharynx
T28.1 Burn of esophagus CC H5
T28.2 Burn of other parts of alimentary tract CC H5
T28.3 Burn of internal genitourinary organs
T28.4 Burns of other and unspecified internal organs
T28.40 Burn of unspecified internal organ
T28.41 Burn of ear drum
T28.411 Burn of right ear drum
T28.412 Burn of left ear drum
T28.419 Burn of unspecified ear drum
T28.49 Burn of other internal organ
T28.5 Corrosion of mouth and pharynx
Code first (T51-T65) to identify chemical and intent
T28.6 Corrosion of esophagus CC H5
Code first (T51-T65) to identify chemical and intent
T28.7 Corrosion of other parts of alimentary tract CC H5
Code first (T51-T65) to identify chemical and intent
T28.8 Corrosion of internal genitourinary organs
Code first (T51-T65) to identify chemical and intent
T28.9 Corrosions of other and unspecified internal organs
Code first (T51-T65) to identify chemical and intent
T28.90 Corrosions of unspecified internal organs
T28.91 Corrosions of ear drum
T28.911 Corrosions of right ear drum
T28.912 Corrosions of left ear drum
T28.919 Corrosions of unspecified ear drum
T28.99 Corrosions of other internal organs

Burns and corrosions of multiple and unspecified body regions (T30-T32)

T30 Burn and corrosion, body region unspecified
T30.0 Burn of unspecified body region, unspecified degree
This code is not for inpatient use. Code to specified site and degree of burns
Burn NOS
Multiple burns NOS
T30.4 Corrosion of unspecified body region, unspecified degree
This code is not for inpatient use. Code to specified site and degree of corrosion
Corrosion NOS
Multiple corrosion NOS

T31 Burns classified according to extent of body surface involved
NOTE This category is to be used as the primary code only when the site of the burn is unspecified. It should be used as a supplementary code with categories T20-T25 when the site is specified.

T31.0 Burns involving less than 10% of body surface
T31.1 Burns involving 10-19% of body surface
T31.10 Burns involving 10-19% of body surface with 0% to 9% third degree burns CC H5
Burns involving 10-19% of body surface NOS
T31.11 Burns involving 10-19% of body surface with 10-19% third degree burns CC H5 HCC
T31.2 Burns involving 20-29% of body surface
T31.20 Burns involving 20-29% of body surface with 0% to 9% third degree burns CC H5
Burns involving 20-29% of body surface NOS
T31.21 Burns involving 20-29% of body surface with 10-19% third degree burns MCC H5 HCC
T31.22 Burns involving 20-29% of body surface with 20-29% third degree burns MCC H5 HCC
T31.3 Burns involving 30-39% of body surface
T31.30 Burns involving 30-39% of body surface with 0% to 9% third degree burns CC H5
Burns involving 30-39% of body surface NOS
T31.31 Burns involving 30-39% of body surface with 10-19% third degree burns MCC H5 HCC
T31.32 Burns involving 30-39% of body surface with 20-29% third degree burns MCC H5 HCC
T31.33 Burns involving 30-39% of body surface with 30-39% third degree burns MCC H5 HCC
T31.4 Burns involving 40-49% of body surface
T31.40 Burns involving 40-49% of body surface with 0% to 9% third degree burns CC H5
Burns involving 40-49% of body surface NOS
T31.41 Burns involving 40-49% of body surface with 10-19% third degree burns MCC H5 HCC
T31.42 Burns involving 40-49% of body surface with 20-29% third degree burns MCC H5 HCC
T31.43 Burns involving 40-49% of body surface with 30-39% third degree burns MCC H5 HCC
T31.44 Burns involving 40-49% of body surface with 40-49% third degree burns MCC H5 HCC

√5th **T31.5 Burns involving 5Ø-59% of body surface**

T31.5Ø Burns involving 5Ø-59% of body surface with Ø% to 9% third degree burns CC H5
Burns involving 5Ø-59% of body surface NOS

T31.51 Burns involving 5Ø-59% of body surface with 1Ø-19% third degree burns MCC H5 HCC

T31.52 Burns involving 5Ø-59% of body surface with 2Ø-29% third degree burns MCC H5 HCC

T31.53 Burns involving 5Ø-59% of body surface with 3Ø-39% third degree burns MCC H5 HCC

T31.54 Burns involving 5Ø-59% of body surface with 4Ø-49% third degree burns MCC H5 HCC

T31.55 Burns involving 5Ø-59% of body surface with 5Ø-59% third degree burns MCC H5 HCC

√5th **T31.6 Burns involving 6Ø-69% of body surface**

T31.6Ø Burns involving 6Ø-69% of body surface with Ø% to 9% third degree burns CC H5
Burns involving 6Ø-69% of body surface NOS

T31.61 Burns involving 6Ø-69% of body surface with 1Ø-19% third degree burns MCC H5 HCC

T31.62 Burns involving 6Ø-69% of body surface with 2Ø-29% third degree burns MCC H5 HCC

T31.63 Burns involving 6Ø-69% of body surface with 3Ø-39% third degree burns MCC H5 HCC

T31.64 Burns involving 6Ø-69% of body surface with 4Ø-49% third degree burns MCC H5 HCC

T31.65 Burns involving 6Ø-69% of body surface with 5Ø-59% third degree burns MCC H5 HCC

T31.66 Burns involving 6Ø-69% of body surface with 6Ø-69% third degree burns MCC H5 HCC

√5th **T31.7 Burns involving 7Ø-79% of body surface**

T31.7Ø Burns involving 7Ø-79% of body surface with Ø% to 9% third degree burns CC H5
Burns involving 7Ø-79% of body surface NOS

T31.71 Burns involving 7Ø-79% of body surface with 1Ø-19% third degree burns MCC H5 HCC

T31.72 Burns involving 7Ø-79% of body surface with 2Ø-29% third degree burns MCC H5 HCC

T31.73 Burns involving 7Ø-79% of body surface with 3Ø-39% third degree burns MCC H5 HCC

T31.74 Burns involving 7Ø-79% of body surface with 4Ø-49% third degree burns MCC H5 HCC

T31.75 Burns involving 7Ø-79% of body surface with 5Ø-59% third degree burns MCC H5 HCC

T31.76 Burns involving 7Ø-79% of body surface with 6Ø-69% third degree burns MCC H5 HCC

T31.77 Burns involving 7Ø-79% of body surface with 7Ø-79% third degree burns MCC H5 HCC

√5th **T31.8 Burns involving 8Ø-89% of body surface**

T31.8Ø Burns involving 8Ø-89% of body surface with Ø% to 9% third degree burns CC H5
Burns involving 8Ø-89% of body surface NOS

T31.81 Burns involving 8Ø-89% of body surface with 1Ø-19% third degree burns MCC H5 HCC

T31.82 Burns involving 8Ø-89% of body surface with 2Ø-29% third degree burns MCC H5 HCC

T31.83 Burns involving 8Ø-89% of body surface with 3Ø-39% third degree burns MCC H5 HCC

T31.84 Burns involving 8Ø-89% of body surface with 4Ø-49% third degree burns MCC H5 HCC

T31.85 Burns involving 8Ø-89% of body surface with 5Ø-59% third degree burns MCC H5 HCC

T31.86 Burns involving 8Ø-89% of body surface with 6Ø-69% third degree burns MCC H5 HCC

T31.87 Burns involving 8Ø-89% of body surface with 7Ø-79% third degree burns MCC H5 HCC

T31.88 Burns involving 8Ø-89% of body surface with 8Ø-89% third degree burns MCC H5 HCC

√5th **T31.9 Burns involving 9Ø% or more of body surface**

T31.9Ø Burns involving 9Ø% or more of body surface with Ø% to 9% third degree burns CC H5
Burns involving 9Ø% or more of body surface NOS

T31.91 Burns involving 9Ø% or more of body surface with 1Ø-19% third degree burns MCC H5 HCC

T31.92 Burns involving 9Ø% or more of body surface with 2Ø-29% third degree burns MCC H5 HCC

T31.93 Burns involving 9Ø% or more of body surface with 3Ø-39% third degree burns MCC H5 HCC

T31.94 Burns involving 9Ø% or more of body surface with 4Ø-49% third degree burns MCC H5 HCC

T31.95 Burns involving 9Ø% or more of body surface with 5Ø-59% third degree burns MCC H5 HCC

T31.96 Burns involving 9Ø% or more of body surface with 6Ø-69% third degree burns MCC H5 HCC

T31.97 Burns involving 9Ø% or more of body surface with 7Ø-79% third degree burns MCC H5 HCC

T31.98 Burns involving 9Ø% or more of body surface with 8Ø-89% third degree burns MCC H5 HCC

T31.99 Burns involving 9Ø% or more of body surface with 9Ø% or more third degree burns MCC H5 HCC

Rule of Nines Estimation of Total Body Surface Burned

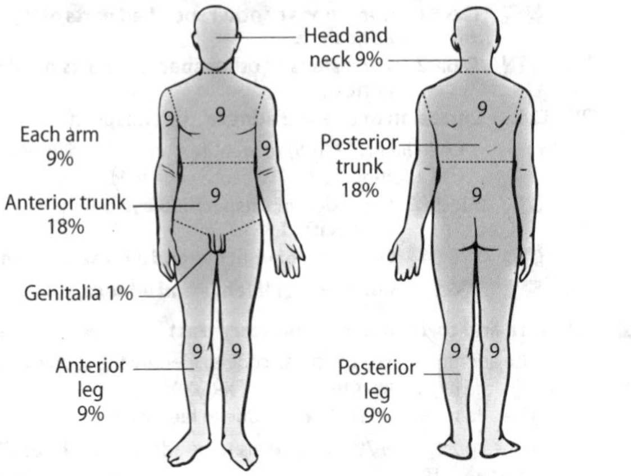

√4th **T32 Corrosions classified according to extent of body surface involved**

NOTE This category is to be used as the primary code only when the site of the corrosion is unspecified. It may be used as a supplementary code with categories T2Ø-T25 when the site is specified.

T32.Ø Corrosions involving less than 1Ø% of body surface

√5th **T32.1 Corrosions involving 1Ø-19% of body surface**

T32.1Ø Corrosions involving 1Ø-19% of body surface with Ø% to 9% third degree corrosion CC H5
Corrosions involving 1Ø-19% of body surface NOS

T32.11 Corrosions involving 1Ø-19% of body surface with 1Ø-19% third degree corrosion CC H5 HCC

√5th **T32.2 Corrosions involving 2Ø-29% of body surface**

T32.2Ø Corrosions involving 2Ø-29% of body surface with Ø% to 9% third degree corrosion CC H5

T32.21 Corrosions involving 2Ø-29% of body surface with 1Ø-19% third degree corrosion MCC H5 HCC

T32.22 Corrosions involving 2Ø-29% of body surface with 2Ø-29% third degree corrosion MCC H5 HCC

√5th **T32.3 Corrosions involving 3Ø-39% of body surface**

T32.3Ø Corrosions involving 3Ø-39% of body surface with Ø% to 9% third degree corrosion CC H5

T32.31 Corrosions involving 3Ø-39% of body surface with 1Ø-19% third degree corrosion MCC H5 HCC

T32.32 Corrosions involving 3Ø-39% of body surface with 2Ø-29% third degree corrosion MCC H5 HCC

T32.33 Corrosions involving 3Ø-39% of body surface with 3Ø-39% third degree corrosion MCC H5 HCC

√5th **T32.4 Corrosions involving 4Ø-49% of body surface**

T32.4Ø Corrosions involving 4Ø-49% of body surface with Ø% to 9% third degree corrosion CC H5

T32.41 Corrosions involving 4Ø-49% of body surface with 1Ø-19% third degree corrosion MCC H5 HCC

T32.42 Corrosions involving 4Ø-49% of body surface with 2Ø-29% third degree corrosion MCC H5 HCC

T32.43 Corrosions involving 4Ø-49% of body surface with 3Ø-39% third degree corrosion MCC H5 HCC

T32.44 Corrosions involving 4Ø-49% of body surface with 4Ø-49% third degree corrosion MCC H5 HCC

√5th **T32.5 Corrosions involving 5Ø-59% of body surface**

T32.5Ø Corrosions involving 5Ø-59% of body surface with Ø% to 9% third degree corrosion CC H5

T32.51 Corrosions involving 5Ø-59% of body surface with 1Ø-19% third degree corrosion MCC H5 HCC

T32.52 Corrosions involving 50-59% of body surface with 20-29% third degree corrosion MCC H5 HCC
T32.53 Corrosions involving 50-59% of body surface with 30-39% third degree corrosion MCC H5 HCC
T32.54 Corrosions involving 50-59% of body surface with 40-49% third degree corrosion MCC H5 HCC
T32.55 Corrosions involving 50-59% of body surface with 50-59% third degree corrosion MCC H5 HCC

T32.6 Corrosions involving 60-69% of body surface
T32.60 Corrosions involving 60-69% of body surface with 0% to 9% third degree corrosion CC H5
T32.61 Corrosions involving 60-69% of body surface with 10-19% third degree corrosion MCC H5 HCC
T32.62 Corrosions involving 60-69% of body surface with 20-29% third degree corrosion MCC H5 HCC
T32.63 Corrosions involving 60-69% of body surface with 30-39% third degree corrosion MCC H5 HCC
T32.64 Corrosions involving 60-69% of body surface with 40-49% third degree corrosion MCC H5 HCC
T32.65 Corrosions involving 60-69% of body surface with 50-59% third degree corrosion MCC H5 HCC
T32.66 Corrosions involving 60-69% of body surface with 60-69% third degree corrosion MCC H5 HCC

T32.7 Corrosions involving 70-79% of body surface
T32.70 Corrosions involving 70-79% of body surface with 0% to 9% third degree corrosion CC H5
T32.71 Corrosions involving 70-79% of body surface with 10-19% third degree corrosion MCC H5 HCC
T32.72 Corrosions involving 70-79% of body surface with 20-29% third degree corrosion MCC H5 HCC
T32.73 Corrosions involving 70-79% of body surface with 30-39% third degree corrosion MCC H5 HCC
T32.74 Corrosions involving 70-79% of body surface with 40-49% third degree corrosion MCC H5 HCC
T32.75 Corrosions involving 70-79% of body surface with 50-59% third degree corrosion MCC H5 HCC
T32.76 Corrosions involving 70-79% of body surface with 60-69% third degree corrosion MCC H5 HCC
T32.77 Corrosions involving 70-79% of body surface with 70-79% third degree corrosion MCC H5 HCC

T32.8 Corrosions involving 80-89% of body surface
T32.80 Corrosions involving 80-89% of body surface with 0% to 9% third degree corrosion CC H5
T32.81 Corrosions involving 80-89% of body surface with 10-19% third degree corrosion MCC H5 HCC
T32.82 Corrosions involving 80-89% of body surface with 20-29% third degree corrosion MCC H5 HCC
T32.83 Corrosions involving 80-89% of body surface with 30-39% third degree corrosion MCC H5 HCC
T32.84 Corrosions involving 80-89% of body surface with 40-49% third degree corrosion MCC H5 HCC
T32.85 Corrosions involving 80-89% of body surface with 50-59% third degree corrosion MCC H5 HCC
T32.86 Corrosions involving 80-89% of body surface with 60-69% third degree corrosion MCC H5 HCC
T32.87 Corrosions involving 80-89% of body surface with 70-79% third degree corrosion MCC H5 HCC
T32.88 Corrosions involving 80-89% of body surface with 80-89% third degree corrosion MCC H5 HCC

T32.9 Corrosions involving 90% or more of body surface
T32.90 Corrosions involving 90% or more of body surface with 0% to 9% third degree corrosion CC H5
T32.91 Corrosions involving 90% or more of body surface with 10-19% third degree corrosion MCC H5 HCC
T32.92 Corrosions involving 90% or more of body surface with 20-29% third degree corrosion MCC H5 HCC
T32.93 Corrosions involving 90% or more of body surface with 30-39% third degree corrosion MCC H5 HCC
T32.94 Corrosions involving 90% or more of body surface with 40-49% third degree corrosion MCC H5 HCC
T32.95 Corrosions involving 90% or more of body surface with 50-59% third degree corrosion MCC H5 HCC
T32.96 Corrosions involving 90% or more of body surface with 60-69% third degree corrosion MCC H5 HCC
T32.97 Corrosions involving 90% or more of body surface with 70-79% third degree corrosion MCC H5 HCC
T32.98 Corrosions involving 90% or more of body surface with 80-89% third degree corrosion MCC H5 HCC
T32.99 Corrosions involving 90% or more of body surface with 90% or more third degree corrosion MCC H5 HCC

Frostbite (T33-T34)

EXCLUDES 2 *hypothermia and other effects of reduced temperature (T68, T69.-)*

T33 Superficial frostbite

INCLUDES frostbite with partial thickness skin loss

The appropriate 7th character is to be added to each code from category T33.
- A initial encounter
- D subsequent encounter
- S sequela

T33.0 Superficial frostbite of head
T33.01 Superficial frostbite of ear
T33.011 Superficial frostbite of right ear CC H5
T33.012 Superficial frostbite of left ear CC H5
T33.019 Superficial frostbite of unspecified ear CC H5
T33.02 Superficial frostbite of nose CC H5
T33.09 Superficial frostbite of other part of head CC H5
T33.1 Superficial frostbite of neck CC H5
T33.2 Superficial frostbite of thorax CC H5
T33.3 Superficial frostbite of abdominal wall, lower back and pelvis CC H5
T33.4 Superficial frostbite of arm
EXCLUDES 2 *superficial frostbite of wrist and hand (T33.5-)*
T33.40 Superficial frostbite of unspecified arm CC H5
T33.41 Superficial frostbite of right arm CC H5
T33.42 Superficial frostbite of left arm CC H5
T33.5 Superficial frostbite of wrist, hand, and fingers
T33.51 Superficial frostbite of wrist
T33.511 Superficial frostbite of right wrist CC H5
T33.512 Superficial frostbite of left wrist CC H5
T33.519 Superficial frostbite of unspecified wrist CC H5
T33.52 Superficial frostbite of hand
EXCLUDES 2 *superficial frostbite of fingers (T33.53-)*
T33.521 Superficial frostbite of right hand CC H5
T33.522 Superficial frostbite of left hand CC H5
T33.529 Superficial frostbite of unspecified hand CC H5
T33.53 Superficial frostbite of finger(s)
T33.531 Superficial frostbite of right finger(s) CC H5
T33.532 Superficial frostbite of left finger(s) CC H5
T33.539 Superficial frostbite of unspecified finger(s) CC H5
T33.6 Superficial frostbite of hip and thigh
T33.60 Superficial frostbite of unspecified hip and thigh CC H5
T33.61 Superficial frostbite of right hip and thigh CC H5
T33.62 Superficial frostbite of left hip and thigh CC H5
T33.7 Superficial frostbite of knee and lower leg
EXCLUDES 2 *superficial frostbite of ankle and foot (T33.8-)*
T33.70 Superficial frostbite of unspecified knee and lower leg CC H5
T33.71 Superficial frostbite of right knee and lower leg CC H5
T33.72 Superficial frostbite of left knee and lower leg CC H5
T33.8 Superficial frostbite of ankle, foot, and toe(s)
T33.81 Superficial frostbite of ankle
T33.811 Superficial frostbite of right ankle CC H5
T33.812 Superficial frostbite of left ankle CC H5

√7th T33.819 Superficial frostbite of unspecified ankle CC H5
√6th T33.82 Superficial frostbite of foot
√7th T33.821 Superficial frostbite of right foot CC H5
√7th T33.822 Superficial frostbite of left foot CC H5
√7th T33.829 Superficial frostbite of unspecified foot CC H5
√6th T33.83 Superficial frostbite of toe(s)
√7th T33.831 Superficial frostbite of right toe(s) CC H5
√7th T33.832 Superficial frostbite of left toe(s) CC H5
√7th T33.839 Superficial frostbite of unspecified toe(s) CC H5
√5th T33.9 Superficial frostbite of other and unspecified sites
√x7th T33.90 Superficial frostbite of unspecified sites CC H5
Superficial frostbite NOS
√x7th T33.99 Superficial frostbite of other sites CC H5
Superficial frostbite of leg NOS
Superficial frostbite of trunk NOS

√4th **T34 Frostbite with tissue necrosis**

The appropriate 7th character is to be added to each code from category T34.
A initial encounter
D subsequent encounter
S sequela

√5th T34.0 Frostbite with tissue necrosis of head
√6th T34.01 Frostbite with tissue necrosis of ear
√7th T34.011 Frostbite with tissue necrosis of right ear CC H5
√7th T34.012 Frostbite with tissue necrosis of left ear CC H5
√7th T34.019 Frostbite with tissue necrosis of unspecified ear CC H5
√x7th T34.02 Frostbite with tissue necrosis of nose CC H5
√x7th T34.09 Frostbite with tissue necrosis of other part of head CC H5
√x7th T34.1 Frostbite with tissue necrosis of neck CC H5
√x7th T34.2 Frostbite with tissue necrosis of thorax CC H5
√x7th T34.3 Frostbite with tissue necrosis of abdominal wall, lower back and pelvis CC H5
√5th T34.4 Frostbite with tissue necrosis of arm
EXCLUDES 2 *frostbite with tissue necrosis of wrist and hand (T34.5-)*
√x7th T34.40 Frostbite with tissue necrosis of unspecified arm CC H5
√x7th T34.41 Frostbite with tissue necrosis of right arm CC H5
√x7th T34.42 Frostbite with tissue necrosis of left arm CC H5
√5th T34.5 Frostbite with tissue necrosis of wrist, hand, and finger(s)
√6th T34.51 Frostbite with tissue necrosis of wrist
√7th T34.511 Frostbite with tissue necrosis of right wrist CC H5
√7th T34.512 Frostbite with tissue necrosis of left wrist CC H5
√7th T34.519 Frostbite with tissue necrosis of unspecified wrist CC H5
√6th T34.52 Frostbite with tissue necrosis of hand
EXCLUDES 2 *frostbite with tissue necrosis of finger(s) (T34.53-)*
√7th T34.521 Frostbite with tissue necrosis of right hand CC H5
√7th T34.522 Frostbite with tissue necrosis of left hand CC H5
√7th T34.529 Frostbite with tissue necrosis of unspecified hand CC H5
√6th T34.53 Frostbite with tissue necrosis of finger(s)
√7th T34.531 Frostbite with tissue necrosis of right finger(s) CC H5
√7th T34.532 Frostbite with tissue necrosis of left finger(s) CC H5
√7th T34.539 Frostbite with tissue necrosis of unspecified finger(s) CC H5
√5th T34.6 Frostbite with tissue necrosis of hip and thigh
√x7th T34.60 Frostbite with tissue necrosis of unspecified hip and thigh CC H5
√x7th T34.61 Frostbite with tissue necrosis of right hip and thigh CC H5
√x7th T34.62 Frostbite with tissue necrosis of left hip and thigh CC H5
√5th T34.7 Frostbite with tissue necrosis of knee and lower leg
EXCLUDES 2 *frostbite with tissue necrosis of ankle and foot (T34.8-)*
√x7th T34.70 Frostbite with tissue necrosis of unspecified knee and lower leg CC H5
√x7th T34.71 Frostbite with tissue necrosis of right knee and lower leg CC H5
√x7th T34.72 Frostbite with tissue necrosis of left knee and lower leg CC H5
√5th T34.8 Frostbite with tissue necrosis of ankle, foot, and toe(s)
√6th T34.81 Frostbite with tissue necrosis of ankle
√7th T34.811 Frostbite with tissue necrosis of right ankle CC H5
√7th T34.812 Frostbite with tissue necrosis of left ankle CC H5
√7th T34.819 Frostbite with tissue necrosis of unspecified ankle CC H5
√6th T34.82 Frostbite with tissue necrosis of foot
√7th T34.821 Frostbite with tissue necrosis of right foot CC H5
√7th T34.822 Frostbite with tissue necrosis of left foot CC H5
√7th T34.829 Frostbite with tissue necrosis of unspecified foot CC H5
√6th T34.83 Frostbite with tissue necrosis of toe(s)
√7th T34.831 Frostbite with tissue necrosis of right toe(s) CC H5
√7th T34.832 Frostbite with tissue necrosis of left toe(s) CC H5
√7th T34.839 Frostbite with tissue necrosis of unspecified toe(s) CC H5
√5th T34.9 Frostbite with tissue necrosis of other and unspecified sites
√x7th T34.90 Frostbite with tissue necrosis of unspecified sites CC H5
Frostbite with tissue necrosis NOS
√x7th T34.99 Frostbite with tissue necrosis of other sites CC H5
Frostbite with tissue necrosis of leg NOS
Frostbite with tissue necrosis of trunk NOS

Poisoning by, adverse effects of and underdosing of drugs, medicaments and biological substances (T36-T5Ø)

INCLUDES adverse effect of correct substance properly administered
poisoning by overdose of substance
poisoning by wrong substance given or taken in error
underdosing by (inadvertently) (deliberately) taking less substance than prescribed or instructed

Code first, for adverse effects, the nature of the adverse effect, such as:
adverse effect NOS (T88.7)
aspirin gastritis (K29.-)
blood disorders (D56-D76)
contact dermatitis (L23-L25)
dermatitis due to substances taken internally (L27.-)
nephropathy (N14.Ø-N14.2)

NOTE The drug giving rise to the adverse effect should be identified by use of codes from categories T36-T5Ø with fifth or sixth character 5.

Use additional code(s) to specify:
manifestations of poisoning
underdosing or failure in dosage during medical and surgical care (Y63.6, Y63.8-Y63.9)
underdosing of medication regimen (Z91.12-, Z91.13-)

EXCLUDES 1 *toxic reaction to local anesthesia in pregnancy (O29.3-)*
EXCLUDES 2 *abuse and dependence of psychoactive substances (F1Ø-F19)*
abuse of non-dependence-producing substances (F55.-)
drug reaction and poisoning affecting newborn (PØØ-P96)
▶*immunodeficiency due to drugs (D84.821)*◀
pathological drug intoxication (inebriation) (F1Ø-F19)

AHA: 2018,4Q,71; 2016,2Q,8; 2015,3Q,22

T36 Poisoning by, adverse effect of and underdosing of systemic antibiotics

EXCLUDES 1 *antineoplastic antibiotics (T45.1-)*
locally applied antibiotic NEC (T49.Ø)
topically used antibiotic for ear, nose and throat (T49.6)
topically used antibiotic for eye (T49.5)

The appropriate 7th character is to be added to each code from category T36.
A initial encounter
D subsequent encounter
S sequela

T36.Ø Poisoning by, adverse effect of and underdosing of penicillins
T36.ØX Poisoning by, adverse effect of and underdosing of penicillins
T36.ØX1 Poisoning by penicillins, accidental (unintentional)
Poisoning by penicillins NOS
7 **T36.ØX2 Poisoning by penicillins, intentional self-harm** HCC
T36.ØX3 Poisoning by penicillins, assault
T36.ØX4 Poisoning by penicillins, undetermined
T36.ØX5 Adverse effect of penicillins
T36.ØX6 Underdosing of penicillins

T36.1 Poisoning by, adverse effect of and underdosing of cephalosporins and other beta-lactam antibiotics
T36.1X Poisoning by, adverse effect of and underdosing of cephalosporins and other beta-lactam antibiotics
T36.1X1 Poisoning by cephalosporins and other beta-lactam antibiotics, accidental (unintentional)
Poisoning by cephalosporins and other beta-lactam antibiotics NOS
7 **T36.1X2 Poisoning by cephalosporins and other beta-lactam antibiotics, intentional self-harm** HCC
T36.1X3 Poisoning by cephalosporins and other beta-lactam antibiotics, assault
T36.1X4 Poisoning by cephalosporins and other beta-lactam antibiotics, undetermined
T36.1X5 Adverse effect of cephalosporins and other beta-lactam antibiotics
T36.1X6 Underdosing of cephalosporins and other beta-lactam antibiotics

T36.2 Poisoning by, adverse effect of and underdosing of chloramphenicol group
T36.2X Poisoning by, adverse effect of and underdosing of chloramphenicol group
T36.2X1 Poisoning by chloramphenicol group, accidental (unintentional)
Poisoning by chloramphenicol group NOS
7 **T36.2X2 Poisoning by chloramphenicol group, intentional self-harm** HCC
T36.2X3 Poisoning by chloramphenicol group, assault
T36.2X4 Poisoning by chloramphenicol group, undetermined
T36.2X5 Adverse effect of chloramphenicol group
T36.2X6 Underdosing of chloramphenicol group

T36.3 Poisoning by, adverse effect of and underdosing of macrolides
T36.3X Poisoning by, adverse effect of and underdosing of macrolides
T36.3X1 Poisoning by macrolides, accidental (unintentional)
Poisoning by macrolides NOS
7 **T36.3X2 Poisoning by macrolides, intentional self-harm** HCC
T36.3X3 Poisoning by macrolides, assault
T36.3X4 Poisoning by macrolides, undetermined
T36.3X5 Adverse effect of macrolides
T36.3X6 Underdosing of macrolides

T36.4 Poisoning by, adverse effect of and underdosing of tetracyclines
T36.4X Poisoning by, adverse effect of and underdosing of tetracyclines
T36.4X1 Poisoning by tetracyclines, accidental (unintentional)
Poisoning by tetracyclines NOS
7 **T36.4X2 Poisoning by tetracyclines, intentional self-harm** HCC
T36.4X3 Poisoning by tetracyclines, assault
T36.4X4 Poisoning by tetracyclines, undetermined
T36.4X5 Adverse effect of tetracyclines
T36.4X6 Underdosing of tetracyclines

T36.5 Poisoning by, adverse effect of and underdosing of aminoglycosides
Poisoning by, adverse effect of and underdosing of streptomycin
T36.5X Poisoning by, adverse effect of and underdosing of aminoglycosides
T36.5X1 Poisoning by aminoglycosides, accidental (unintentional)
Poisoning by aminoglycosides NOS
7 **T36.5X2 Poisoning by aminoglycosides, intentional self-harm** HCC
T36.5X3 Poisoning by aminoglycosides, assault
T36.5X4 Poisoning by aminoglycosides, undetermined
T36.5X5 Adverse effect of aminoglycosides
T36.5X6 Underdosing of aminoglycosides

T36.6 Poisoning by, adverse effect of and underdosing of rifampicins
T36.6X Poisoning by, adverse effect of and underdosing of rifampicins
T36.6X1 Poisoning by rifampicins, accidental (unintentional)
Poisoning by rifampicins NOS
7 **T36.6X2 Poisoning by rifampicins, intentional self-harm** HCC
T36.6X3 Poisoning by rifampicins, assault
T36.6X4 Poisoning by rifampicins, undetermined
T36.6X5 Adverse effect of rifampicins
T36.6X6 Underdosing of rifampicins

T36.7 Poisoning by, adverse effect of and underdosing of antifungal antibiotics, systemically used
T36.7X Poisoning by, adverse effect of and underdosing of antifungal antibiotics, systemically used
T36.7X1 Poisoning by antifungal antibiotics, systemically used, accidental (unintentional)
Poisoning by antifungal antibiotics, systemically used NOS
7 **T36.7X2 Poisoning by antifungal antibiotics, systemically used, intentional self-harm** HCC
T36.7X3 Poisoning by antifungal antibiotics, systemically used, assault
T36.7X4 Poisoning by antifungal antibiotics, systemically used, undetermined

√7th **T36.7X5 Adverse effect of antifungal antibiotics, systemically used**

√7th **T36.7X6 Underdosing of antifungal antibiotics, systemically used**

√5th **T36.8 Poisoning by, adverse effect of and underdosing of other systemic antibiotics**

√6th **T36.8X Poisoning by, adverse effect of and underdosing of other systemic antibiotics**

AHA: 2017,1Q,39

√7th **T36.8X1 Poisoning by other systemic antibiotics, accidental (unintentional)**

Poisoning by other systemic antibiotics NOS

7 √7th **T36.8X2 Poisoning by other systemic antibiotics, intentional self-harm** HCC

√7th **T36.8X3 Poisoning by other systemic antibiotics, assault**

√7th **T36.8X4 Poisoning by other systemic antibiotics, undetermined**

√7th **T36.8X5 Adverse effect of other systemic antibiotics**

√7th **T36.8X6 Underdosing of other systemic antibiotics**

√5th **T36.9 Poisoning by, adverse effect of and underdosing of unspecified systemic antibiotic**

√x 7th **T36.91 Poisoning by unspecified systemic antibiotic, accidental (unintentional)**

Poisoning by systemic antibiotic NOS

7 √x 7th **T36.92 Poisoning by unspecified systemic antibiotic, intentional self-harm** HCC

√x 7th **T36.93 Poisoning by unspecified systemic antibiotic, assault**

√x 7th **T36.94 Poisoning by unspecified systemic antibiotic, undetermined**

√x 7th **T36.95 Adverse effect of unspecified systemic antibiotic**

√x 7th **T36.96 Underdosing of unspecified systemic antibiotic**

√4th **T37 Poisoning by, adverse effect of and underdosing of other systemic anti-infectives and antiparasitics**

EXCLUDES 1 *anti-infectives topically used for ear, nose and throat (T49.6-)*
anti-infectives topically used for eye (T49.5-)
locally applied anti-infectives NEC (T49.Ø-)

The appropriate 7th character is to be added to each code from category T37.
A initial encounter
D subsequent encounter
S sequela

√5th **T37.Ø Poisoning by, adverse effect of and underdosing of sulfonamides**

√6th **T37.ØX Poisoning by, adverse effect of and underdosing of sulfonamides**

√7th **T37.ØX1 Poisoning by sulfonamides, accidental (unintentional)**

Poisoning by sulfonamides NOS

7 √7th **T37.ØX2 Poisoning by sulfonamides, intentional self-harm** HCC

√7th **T37.ØX3 Poisoning by sulfonamides, assault**

√7th **T37.ØX4 Poisoning by sulfonamides, undetermined**

√7th **T37.ØX5 Adverse effect of sulfonamides**

√7th **T37.ØX6 Underdosing of sulfonamides**

√5th **T37.1 Poisoning by, adverse effect of and underdosing of antimycobacterial drugs**

EXCLUDES 1 *rifampicins (T36.6-)*
streptomycin (T36.5-)

√6th **T37.1X Poisoning by, adverse effect of and underdosing of antimycobacterial drugs**

√7th **T37.1X1 Poisoning by antimycobacterial drugs, accidental (unintentional)**

Poisoning by antimycobacterial drugs NOS

7 √7th **T37.1X2 Poisoning by antimycobacterial drugs, intentional self-harm** HCC

√7th **T37.1X3 Poisoning by antimycobacterial drugs, assault**

√7th **T37.1X4 Poisoning by antimycobacterial drugs, undetermined**

√7th **T37.1X5 Adverse effect of antimycobacterial drugs**

√7th **T37.1X6 Underdosing of antimycobacterial drugs**

√5th **T37.2 Poisoning by, adverse effect of and underdosing of antimalarials and drugs acting on other blood protozoa**

EXCLUDES 1 *hydroxyquinoline derivatives (T37.8-)*

√6th **T37.2X Poisoning by, adverse effect of and underdosing of antimalarials and drugs acting on other blood protozoa**

√7th **T37.2X1 Poisoning by antimalarials and drugs acting on other blood protozoa, accidental (unintentional)**

Poisoning by antimalarials and drugs acting on other blood protozoa NOS

7 √7th **T37.2X2 Poisoning by antimalarials and drugs acting on other blood protozoa, intentional self-harm** HCC

√7th **T37.2X3 Poisoning by antimalarials and drugs acting on other blood protozoa, assault**

√7th **T37.2X4 Poisoning by antimalarials and drugs acting on other blood protozoa, undetermined**

√7th **T37.2X5 Adverse effect of antimalarials and drugs acting on other blood protozoa**

√7th **T37.2X6 Underdosing of antimalarials and drugs acting on other blood protozoa**

√5th **T37.3 Poisoning by, adverse effect of and underdosing of other antiprotozoal drugs**

√6th **T37.3X Poisoning by, adverse effect of and underdosing of other antiprotozoal drugs**

√7th **T37.3X1 Poisoning by other antiprotozoal drugs, accidental (unintentional)**

Poisoning by other antiprotozoal drugs NOS

7 √7th **T37.3X2 Poisoning by other antiprotozoal drugs, intentional self-harm** HCC

√7th **T37.3X3 Poisoning by other antiprotozoal drugs, assault**

√7th **T37.3X4 Poisoning by other antiprotozoal drugs, undetermined**

√7th **T37.3X5 Adverse effect of other antiprotozoal drugs**

√7th **T37.3X6 Underdosing of other antiprotozoal drugs**

√5th **T37.4 Poisoning by, adverse effect of and underdosing of anthelminthics**

√6th **T37.4X Poisoning by, adverse effect of and underdosing of anthelminthics**

√7th **T37.4X1 Poisoning by anthelminthics, accidental (unintentional)**

Poisoning by anthelminthics NOS

7 √7th **T37.4X2 Poisoning by anthelminthics, intentional self-harm** HCC

√7th **T37.4X3 Poisoning by anthelminthics, assault**

√7th **T37.4X4 Poisoning by anthelminthics, undetermined**

√7th **T37.4X5 Adverse effect of anthelminthics**

√7th **T37.4X6 Underdosing of anthelminthics**

√5th **T37.5 Poisoning by, adverse effect of and underdosing of antiviral drugs**

EXCLUDES 1 *amantadine (T42.8-)*
cytarabine (T45.1-)

√6th **T37.5X Poisoning by, adverse effect of and underdosing of antiviral drugs**

√7th **T37.5X1 Poisoning by antiviral drugs, accidental (unintentional)**

Poisoning by antiviral drugs NOS

7 √7th **T37.5X2 Poisoning by antiviral drugs, intentional self-harm** HCC

√7th **T37.5X3 Poisoning by antiviral drugs, assault**

√7th **T37.5X4 Poisoning by antiviral drugs, undetermined**

√7th **T37.5X5 Adverse effect of antiviral drugs**

√7th **T37.5X6 Underdosing of antiviral drugs**

T37.8 Poisoning by, adverse effect of and underdosing of other specified systemic anti-infectives and antiparasitics
Poisoning by, adverse effect of and underdosing of hydroxyquinoline derivatives
EXCLUDES 1 *antimalarial drugs (T37.2-)*

T37.8X Poisoning by, adverse effect of and underdosing of other specified systemic anti-infectives and antiparasitics

T37.8X1 Poisoning by other specified systemic anti-infectives and antiparasitics, accidental (unintentional)
Poisoning by other specified systemic anti-infectives and antiparasitics NOS

7 **T37.8X2 Poisoning by other specified systemic anti-infectives and antiparasitics, intentional self-harm** HCC

T37.8X3 Poisoning by other specified systemic anti-infectives and antiparasitics, assault

T37.8X4 Poisoning by other specified systemic anti-infectives and antiparasitics, undetermined

T37.8X5 Adverse effect of other specified systemic anti-infectives and antiparasitics

T37.8X6 Underdosing of other specified systemic anti-infectives and antiparasitics

T37.9 Poisoning by, adverse effect of and underdosing of unspecified systemic anti-infective and antiparasitics

T37.91 Poisoning by unspecified systemic anti-infective and antiparasitics, accidental (unintentional)
Poisoning by, adverse effect of and underdosing of systemic anti-infective and antiparasitics NOS

7 **T37.92 Poisoning by unspecified systemic anti-infective and antiparasitics, intentional self-harm** HCC

T37.93 Poisoning by unspecified systemic anti-infective and antiparasitics, assault

T37.94 Poisoning by unspecified systemic anti-infective and antiparasitics, undetermined

T37.95 Adverse effect of unspecified systemic anti-infective and antiparasitic

T37.96 Underdosing of unspecified systemic anti-infectives and antiparasitics

T38 Poisoning by, adverse effect of and underdosing of hormones and their synthetic substitutes and antagonists, not elsewhere classified

EXCLUDES 1 *mineralocorticoids and their antagonists (T50.0-)*
oxytocic hormones (T48.0-)
parathyroid hormones and derivatives (T50.9-)

The appropriate 7th character is to be added to each code from category T38.
A initial encounter
D subsequent encounter
S sequela

T38.0 Poisoning by, adverse effect of and underdosing of glucocorticoids and synthetic analogues
EXCLUDES 1 *glucocorticoids, topically used (T49.-)*

T38.0X Poisoning by, adverse effect of and underdosing of glucocorticoids and synthetic analogues

T38.0X1 Poisoning by glucocorticoids and synthetic analogues, accidental (unintentional)
Poisoning by glucocorticoids and synthetic analogues NOS

7 **T38.0X2 Poisoning by glucocorticoids and synthetic analogues, intentional self-harm** HCC

T38.0X3 Poisoning by glucocorticoids and synthetic analogues, assault

T38.0X4 Poisoning by glucocorticoids and synthetic analogues, undetermined

T38.0X5 Adverse effect of glucocorticoids and synthetic analogues

T38.0X6 Underdosing of glucocorticoids and synthetic analogues

T38.1 Poisoning by, adverse effect of and underdosing of thyroid hormones and substitutes

T38.1X Poisoning by, adverse effect of and underdosing of thyroid hormones and substitutes

T38.1X1 Poisoning by thyroid hormones and substitutes, accidental (unintentional)
Poisoning by thyroid hormones and substitutes NOS

7 **T38.1X2 Poisoning by thyroid hormones and substitutes, intentional self-harm** HCC

T38.1X3 Poisoning by thyroid hormones and substitutes, assault

T38.1X4 Poisoning by thyroid hormones and substitutes, undetermined

T38.1X5 Adverse effect of thyroid hormones and substitutes

T38.1X6 Underdosing of thyroid hormones and substitutes

T38.2 Poisoning by, adverse effect of and underdosing of antithyroid drugs

T38.2X Poisoning by, adverse effect of and underdosing of antithyroid drugs

T38.2X1 Poisoning by antithyroid drugs, accidental (unintentional)
Poisoning by antithyroid drugs NOS

7 **T38.2X2 Poisoning by antithyroid drugs, intentional self-harm** HCC

T38.2X3 Poisoning by antithyroid drugs, assault

T38.2X4 Poisoning by antithyroid drugs, undetermined

T38.2X5 Adverse effect of antithyroid drugs

T38.2X6 Underdosing of antithyroid drugs

T38.3 Poisoning by, adverse effect of and underdosing of insulin and oral hypoglycemic [antidiabetic] drugs

T38.3X Poisoning by, adverse effect of and underdosing of insulin and oral hypoglycemic [antidiabetic] drugs

T38.3X1 Poisoning by insulin and oral hypoglycemic [antidiabetic] drugs, accidental (unintentional)
Poisoning by insulin and oral hypoglycemic [antidiabetic] drugs NOS

7 **T38.3X2 Poisoning by insulin and oral hypoglycemic [antidiabetic] drugs, intentional self-harm** HCC

T38.3X3 Poisoning by insulin and oral hypoglycemic [antidiabetic] drugs, assault

T38.3X4 Poisoning by insulin and oral hypoglycemic [antidiabetic] drugs, undetermined

T38.3X5 Adverse effect of insulin and oral hypoglycemic [antidiabetic] drugs

T38.3X6 Underdosing of insulin and oral hypoglycemic [antidiabetic] drugs

T38.4 Poisoning by, adverse effect of and underdosing of oral contraceptives
Poisoning by, adverse effect of and underdosing of multiple- and single-ingredient oral contraceptive preparations

T38.4X Poisoning by, adverse effect of and underdosing of oral contraceptives

T38.4X1 Poisoning by oral contraceptives, accidental (unintentional)
Poisoning by oral contraceptives NOS

7 **T38.4X2 Poisoning by oral contraceptives, intentional self-harm** HCC

T38.4X3 Poisoning by oral contraceptives, assault

T38.4X4 Poisoning by oral contraceptives, undetermined

T38.4X5 Adverse effect of oral contraceptives

T38.4X6 Underdosing of oral contraceptives

√5th **T38.5 Poisoning by, adverse effect of and underdosing of other estrogens and progestogens**
Poisoning by, adverse effect of and underdosing of estrogens and progestogens mixtures and substitutes
√6th **T38.5X Poisoning by, adverse effect of and underdosing of other estrogens and progestogens**
√7th **T38.5X1 Poisoning by other estrogens and progestogens, accidental (unintentional)**
Poisoning by other estrogens and progestogens NOS
7 √7th **T38.5X2 Poisoning by other estrogens and progestogens, intentional self-harm** HCC
√7th **T38.5X3 Poisoning by other estrogens and progestogens, assault**
√7th **T38.5X4 Poisoning by other estrogens and progestogens, undetermined**
√7th **T38.5X5 Adverse effect of other estrogens and progestogens**
√7th **T38.5X6 Underdosing of other estrogens and progestogens**
√5th **T38.6 Poisoning by, adverse effect of and underdosing of antigonadotrophins, antiestrogens, antiandrogens, not elsewhere classified**
Poisoning by, adverse effect of and underdosing of tamoxifen
√6th **T38.6X Poisoning by, adverse effect of and underdosing of antigonadotrophins, antiestrogens, antiandrogens, not elsewhere classified**
√7th **T38.6X1 Poisoning by antigonadotrophins, antiestrogens, antiandrogens, not elsewhere classified, accidental (unintentional)**
Poisoning by antigonadotrophins, antiestrogens, antiandrogens, not elsewhere classified NOS
7 √7th **T38.6X2 Poisoning by antigonadotrophins, antiestrogens, antiandrogens, not elsewhere classified, intentional self-harm** HCC
√7th **T38.6X3 Poisoning by antigonadotrophins, antiestrogens, antiandrogens, not elsewhere classified, assault**
√7th **T38.6X4 Poisoning by antigonadotrophins, antiestrogens, antiandrogens, not elsewhere classified, undetermined**
√7th **T38.6X5 Adverse effect of antigonadotrophins, antiestrogens, antiandrogens, not elsewhere classified**
√7th **T38.6X6 Underdosing of antigonadotrophins, antiestrogens, antiandrogens, not elsewhere classified**
√5th **T38.7 Poisoning by, adverse effect of and underdosing of androgens and anabolic congeners**
√6th **T38.7X Poisoning by, adverse effect of and underdosing of androgens and anabolic congeners**
√7th **T38.7X1 Poisoning by androgens and anabolic congeners, accidental (unintentional)**
Poisoning by androgens and anabolic congeners NOS
7 √7th **T38.7X2 Poisoning by androgens and anabolic congeners, intentional self-harm** HCC
√7th **T38.7X3 Poisoning by androgens and anabolic congeners, assault**
√7th **T38.7X4 Poisoning by androgens and anabolic congeners, undetermined**
√7th **T38.7X5 Adverse effect of androgens and anabolic congeners**
√7th **T38.7X6 Underdosing of androgens and anabolic congeners**
√5th **T38.8 Poisoning by, adverse effect of and underdosing of other and unspecified hormones and synthetic substitutes**
√6th **T38.80 Poisoning by, adverse effect of and underdosing of unspecified hormones and synthetic substitutes**
√7th **T38.801 Poisoning by unspecified hormones and synthetic substitutes, accidental (unintentional)**
Poisoning by unspecified hormones and synthetic substitutes NOS
7 √7th **T38.802 Poisoning by unspecified hormones and synthetic substitutes, intentional self-harm** HCC
√7th **T38.803 Poisoning by unspecified hormones and synthetic substitutes, assault**
√7th **T38.804 Poisoning by unspecified hormones and synthetic substitutes, undetermined**
√7th **T38.805 Adverse effect of unspecified hormones and synthetic substitutes**
√7th **T38.806 Underdosing of unspecified hormones and synthetic substitutes**
√6th **T38.81 Poisoning by, adverse effect of and underdosing of anterior pituitary [adenohypophyseal] hormones**
√7th **T38.811 Poisoning by anterior pituitary [adenohypophyseal] hormones, accidental (unintentional)**
Poisoning by anterior pituitary [adenohypophyseal] hormones NOS
7 √7th **T38.812 Poisoning by anterior pituitary [adenohypophyseal] hormones, intentional self-harm** HCC
√7th **T38.813 Poisoning by anterior pituitary [adenohypophyseal] hormones, assault**
√7th **T38.814 Poisoning by anterior pituitary [adenohypophyseal] hormones, undetermined**
√7th **T38.815 Adverse effect of anterior pituitary [adenohypophyseal] hormones**
√7th **T38.816 Underdosing of anterior pituitary [adenohypophyseal] hormones**
√6th **T38.89 Poisoning by, adverse effect of and underdosing of other hormones and synthetic substitutes**
√7th **T38.891 Poisoning by other hormones and synthetic substitutes, accidental (unintentional)**
Poisoning by other hormones and synthetic substitutes NOS
7 √7th **T38.892 Poisoning by other hormones and synthetic substitutes, intentional self-harm** HCC
√7th **T38.893 Poisoning by other hormones and synthetic substitutes, assault**
√7th **T38.894 Poisoning by other hormones and synthetic substitutes, undetermined**
√7th **T38.895 Adverse effect of other hormones and synthetic substitutes**
√7th **T38.896 Underdosing of other hormones and synthetic substitutes**
√5th **T38.9 Poisoning by, adverse effect of and underdosing of other and unspecified hormone antagonists**
√6th **T38.90 Poisoning by, adverse effect of and underdosing of unspecified hormone antagonists**
√7th **T38.901 Poisoning by unspecified hormone antagonists, accidental (unintentional)**
Poisoning by unspecified hormone antagonists NOS
7 √7th **T38.902 Poisoning by unspecified hormone antagonists, intentional self-harm** HCC
√7th **T38.903 Poisoning by unspecified hormone antagonists, assault**
√7th **T38.904 Poisoning by unspecified hormone antagonists, undetermined**
√7th **T38.905 Adverse effect of unspecified hormone antagonists**
√7th **T38.906 Underdosing of unspecified hormone antagonists**
√6th **T38.99 Poisoning by, adverse effect of and underdosing of other hormone antagonists**
√7th **T38.991 Poisoning by other hormone antagonists, accidental (unintentional)**
Poisoning by other hormone antagonists NOS
7 √7th **T38.992 Poisoning by other hormone antagonists, intentional self-harm** HCC
√7th **T38.993 Poisoning by other hormone antagonists, assault**
√7th **T38.994 Poisoning by other hormone antagonists, undetermined**
√7th **T38.995 Adverse effect of other hormone antagonists**
√7th **T38.996 Underdosing of other hormone antagonists**

T39 Poisoning by, adverse effect of and underdosing of nonopioid analgesics, antipyretics and antirheumatics

The appropriate 7th character is to be added to each code from category T39.
A initial encounter
D subsequent encounter
S sequela

T39.Ø Poisoning by, adverse effect of and underdosing of salicylates

T39.Ø1 Poisoning by, adverse effect of and underdosing of aspirin
Poisoning by, adverse effect of and underdosing of acetylsalicylic acid

T39.Ø11 Poisoning by aspirin, accidental (unintentional)
7 **T39.Ø12 Poisoning by aspirin, intentional self-harm** HCC
T39.Ø13 Poisoning by aspirin, assault
T39.Ø14 Poisoning by aspirin, undetermined
T39.Ø15 Adverse effect of aspirin
AHA: 2016,1Q,15
T39.Ø16 Underdosing of aspirin

T39.Ø9 Poisoning by, adverse effect of and underdosing of other salicylates

T39.Ø91 Poisoning by salicylates, accidental (unintentional)
Poisoning by salicylates NOS
7 **T39.Ø92 Poisoning by salicylates, intentional self-harm** HCC
T39.Ø93 Poisoning by salicylates, assault
T39.Ø94 Poisoning by salicylates, undetermined
T39.Ø95 Adverse effect of salicylates
T39.Ø96 Underdosing of salicylates

T39.1 Poisoning by, adverse effect of and underdosing of 4-Aminophenol derivatives

T39.1X Poisoning by, adverse effect of and underdosing of 4-Aminophenol derivatives

T39.1X1 Poisoning by 4-Aminophenol derivatives, accidental (unintentional)
Poisoning by 4-Aminophenol derivatives NOS
7 **T39.1X2 Poisoning by 4-Aminophenol derivatives, intentional self-harm** HCC
T39.1X3 Poisoning by 4-Aminophenol derivatives, assault
T39.1X4 Poisoning by 4-Aminophenol derivatives, undetermined
T39.1X5 Adverse effect of 4-Aminophenol derivatives
T39.1X6 Underdosing of 4-Aminophenol derivatives

T39.2 Poisoning by, adverse effect of and underdosing of pyrazolone derivatives

T39.2X Poisoning by, adverse effect of and underdosing of pyrazolone derivatives

T39.2X1 Poisoning by pyrazolone derivatives, accidental (unintentional)
Poisoning by pyrazolone derivatives NOS
7 **T39.2X2 Poisoning by pyrazolone derivatives, intentional self-harm** HCC
T39.2X3 Poisoning by pyrazolone derivatives, assault
T39.2X4 Poisoning by pyrazolone derivatives, undetermined
T39.2X5 Adverse effect of pyrazolone derivatives
T39.2X6 Underdosing of pyrazolone derivatives

T39.3 Poisoning by, adverse effect of and underdosing of other nonsteroidal anti-inflammatory drugs [NSAID]

T39.31 Poisoning by, adverse effect of and underdosing of propionic acid derivatives
Poisoning by, adverse effect of and underdosing of fenoprofen
Poisoning by, adverse effect of and underdosing of flurbiprofen
Poisoning by, adverse effect of and underdosing of ibuprofen
Poisoning by, adverse effect of and underdosing of ketoprofen
Poisoning by, adverse effect of and underdosing of naproxen
Poisoning by, adverse effect of and underdosing of oxaprozin

T39.311 Poisoning by propionic acid derivatives, accidental (unintentional)
7 **T39.312 Poisoning by propionic acid derivatives, intentional self-harm** HCC
T39.313 Poisoning by propionic acid derivatives, assault
T39.314 Poisoning by propionic acid derivatives, undetermined
T39.315 Adverse effect of propionic acid derivatives
T39.316 Underdosing of propionic acid derivatives

T39.39 Poisoning by, adverse effect of and underdosing of other nonsteroidal anti-inflammatory drugs [NSAID]

T39.391 Poisoning by other nonsteroidal anti-inflammatory drugs [NSAID], accidental (unintentional)
Poisoning by other nonsteroidal anti-inflammatory drugs NOS
7 **T39.392 Poisoning by other nonsteroidal anti-inflammatory drugs [NSAID], intentional self-harm** HCC
T39.393 Poisoning by other nonsteroidal anti-inflammatory drugs [NSAID], assault
T39.394 Poisoning by other nonsteroidal anti-inflammatory drugs [NSAID], undetermined
T39.395 Adverse effect of other nonsteroidal anti-inflammatory drugs [NSAID]
T39.396 Underdosing of other nonsteroidal anti-inflammatory drugs [NSAID]

T39.4 Poisoning by, adverse effect of and underdosing of antirheumatics, not elsewhere classified

EXCLUDES 1 *poisoning by, adverse effect of and underdosing of glucocorticoids (T38.Ø-)*
poisoning by, adverse effect of and underdosing of salicylates (T39.Ø-)

T39.4X Poisoning by, adverse effect of and underdosing of antirheumatics, not elsewhere classified

T39.4X1 Poisoning by antirheumatics, not elsewhere classified, accidental (unintentional)
Poisoning by antirheumatics, not elsewhere classified NOS
7 **T39.4X2 Poisoning by antirheumatics, not elsewhere classified, intentional self-harm** HCC
T39.4X3 Poisoning by antirheumatics, not elsewhere classified, assault
T39.4X4 Poisoning by antirheumatics, not elsewhere classified, undetermined
T39.4X5 Adverse effect of antirheumatics, not elsewhere classified
T39.4X6 Underdosing of antirheumatics, not elsewhere classified

✓5th **T39.8 Poisoning by, adverse effect of and underdosing of other nonopioid analgesics and antipyretics, not elsewhere classified**

✓6th **T39.8X Poisoning by, adverse effect of and underdosing of other nonopioid analgesics and antipyretics, not elsewhere classified**

✓7th **T39.8X1 Poisoning by other nonopioid analgesics and antipyretics, not elsewhere classified, accidental (unintentional)**
Poisoning by other nonopioid analgesics and antipyretics, not elsewhere classified NOS

7 ✓7th **T39.8X2 Poisoning by other nonopioid analgesics and antipyretics, not elsewhere classified, intentional self-harm** HCC

✓7th **T39.8X3 Poisoning by other nonopioid analgesics and antipyretics, not elsewhere classified, assault**

✓7th **T39.8X4 Poisoning by other nonopioid analgesics and antipyretics, not elsewhere classified, undetermined**

✓7th **T39.8X5 Adverse effect of other nonopioid analgesics and antipyretics, not elsewhere classified**

✓7th **T39.8X6 Underdosing of other nonopioid analgesics and antipyretics, not elsewhere classified**

✓5th **T39.9 Poisoning by, adverse effect of and underdosing of unspecified nonopioid analgesic, antipyretic and antirheumatic**

✓x7th **T39.91 Poisoning by unspecified nonopioid analgesic, antipyretic and antirheumatic, accidental (unintentional)**
Poisoning by nonopioid analgesic, antipyretic and antirheumatic NOS

7 ✓x7th **T39.92 Poisoning by unspecified nonopioid analgesic, antipyretic and antirheumatic, intentional self-harm** HCC

✓x7th **T39.93 Poisoning by unspecified nonopioid analgesic, antipyretic and antirheumatic, assault**

✓x7th **T39.94 Poisoning by unspecified nonopioid analgesic, antipyretic and antirheumatic, undetermined**

✓x7th **T39.95 Adverse effect of unspecified nonopioid analgesic, antipyretic and antirheumatic**

✓x7th **T39.96 Underdosing of unspecified nonopioid analgesic, antipyretic and antirheumatic**

✓4th **T4Ø Poisoning by, adverse effect of and underdosing of narcotics and psychodysleptics [hallucinogens]**

EXCLUDES 2 *drug dependence and related mental and behavioral disorders due to psychoactive substance use (F1Ø.-F19.-)*

The appropriate 7th character is to be added to each code from category T4Ø.
A initial encounter
D subsequent encounter
S sequela

✓5th **T4Ø.Ø Poisoning by, adverse effect of and underdosing of opium**

✓6th **T4Ø.ØX Poisoning by, adverse effect of and underdosing of opium**

6 ✓7th **T4Ø.ØX1 Poisoning by opium, accidental (unintentional)** HCC
Poisoning by opium NOS

7 ✓7th **T4Ø.ØX2 Poisoning by opium, intentional self-harm** HCC

✓7th **T4Ø.ØX3 Poisoning by opium, assault**

6 ✓7th **T4Ø.ØX4 Poisoning by opium, undetermined** HCC

✓7th **T4Ø.ØX5 Adverse effect of opium**

✓7th **T4Ø.ØX6 Underdosing of opium**

✓5th **T4Ø.1 Poisoning by and adverse effect of heroin**

✓6th **T4Ø.1X Poisoning by and adverse effect of heroin**

6 ✓7th **T4Ø.1X1 Poisoning by heroin, accidental (unintentional)** HCC
Poisoning by heroin NOS

7 ✓7th **T4Ø.1X2 Poisoning by heroin, intentional self-harm** HCC

✓7th **T4Ø.1X3 Poisoning by heroin, assault**

6 ✓7th **T4Ø.1X4 Poisoning by heroin, undetermined** HCC

✓5th **T4Ø.2 Poisoning by, adverse effect of and underdosing of other opioids**

✓6th **T4Ø.2X Poisoning by, adverse effect of and underdosing of other opioids**

6 ✓7th **T4Ø.2X1 Poisoning by other opioids, accidental (unintentional)** HCC
Poisoning by other opioids NOS

7 ✓7th **T4Ø.2X2 Poisoning by other opioids, intentional self-harm** HCC

✓7th **T4Ø.2X3 Poisoning by other opioids, assault**

6 ✓7th **T4Ø.2X4 Poisoning by other opioids, undetermined** HCC

✓7th **T4Ø.2X5 Adverse effect of other opioids**
AHA: 2020,2Q,24

✓7th **T4Ø.2X6 Underdosing of other opioids**

✓5th **T4Ø.3 Poisoning by, adverse effect of and underdosing of methadone**

✓6th **T4Ø.3X Poisoning by, adverse effect of and underdosing of methadone**

6 ✓7th **T4Ø.3X1 Poisoning by methadone, accidental (unintentional)** HCC
Poisoning by methadone NOS

7 ✓7th **T4Ø.3X2 Poisoning by methadone, intentional self-harm** HCC

✓7th **T4Ø.3X3 Poisoning by methadone, assault**

6 ✓7th **T4Ø.3X4 Poisoning by methadone, undetermined** HCC

✓7th **T4Ø.3X5 Adverse effect of methadone**

✓7th **T4Ø.3X6 Underdosing of methadone**

✓5th **T4Ø.4 Poisoning by, adverse effect of and underdosing of other synthetic narcotics**

~~**T4Ø.4X Poisoning by, adverse effect of and underdosing of other synthetic narcotics**~~

~~**T4Ø.4X1 Poisoning by other synthetic narcotics, accidental (unintentional)**~~

~~**T4Ø.4X2 Poisoning by other synthetic narcotics, intentional self-harm**~~

~~**T4Ø.4X3 Poisoning by other synthetic narcotics, assault**~~

~~**T4Ø.4X4 Poisoning by other synthetic narcotics, undetermined**~~

~~**T4Ø.4X5 Adverse effect of other synthetic narcotics**~~

~~**T4Ø.4X6 Underdosing of other synthetic narcotics**~~

• ✓6th **T4Ø.41 Poisoning by, adverse effect of and underdosing of fentanyl or fentanyl analogs**

• ✓7th **T4Ø.411 Poisoning by fentanyl or fentanyl analogs, accidental (unintentional)**

• ✓7th **T4Ø.412 Poisoning by fentanyl or fentanyl analogs, intentional self-harm**

• ✓7th **T4Ø.413 Poisoning by fentanyl or fentanyl analogs, assault**

• ✓7th **T4Ø.414 Poisoning by fentanyl or fentanyl analogs, undetermined**

• ✓7th **T4Ø.415 Adverse effect of fentanyl or fentanyl analogs**

• ✓7th **T4Ø.416 Underdosing of fentanyl or fentanyl analogs**

• ✓6th **T4Ø.42 Poisoning by, adverse effect of and underdosing of tramadol**

• ✓7th **T4Ø.421 Poisoning by tramadol, accidental (unintentional)**

• ✓7th **T4Ø.422 Poisoning by tramadol, intentional self-harm**

• ✓7th **T4Ø.423 Poisoning by tramadol, assault**

• ✓7th **T4Ø.424 Poisoning by tramadol, undetermined**

• ✓7th **T4Ø.425 Adverse effect of tramadol**

• ✓7th **T4Ø.426 Underdosing of tramadol**

• ✓6th **T4Ø.49 Poisoning by, adverse effect of and underdosing of other synthetic narcotics**

• ✓7th **T4Ø.491 Poisoning by other synthetic narcotics, accidental (unintentional)**

• ✓7th **T4Ø.492 Poisoning by other synthetic narcotics, intentional self-harm**

• ✓7th **T4Ø.493 Poisoning by other synthetic narcotics, assault**

• ✓7th **T4Ø.494 Poisoning by other synthetic narcotics, undetermined**

• ✓7th **T4Ø.495 Adverse effect of other synthetic narcotics**

● T40.496 Underdosing of other synthetic narcotics

T40.5 Poisoning by, adverse effect of and underdosing of cocaine

T40.5X Poisoning by, adverse effect of and underdosing of cocaine

T40.5X1 Poisoning by cocaine, accidental (unintentional) HCC
Poisoning by cocaine NOS
AHA: 2016,2Q,8

T40.5X2 Poisoning by cocaine, intentional self-harm HCC

T40.5X3 Poisoning by cocaine, assault

T40.5X4 Poisoning by cocaine, undetermined HCC

T40.5X5 Adverse effect of cocaine

T40.5X6 Underdosing of cocaine

T40.6 Poisoning by, adverse effect of and underdosing of other and unspecified narcotics

T40.60 Poisoning by, adverse effect of and underdosing of unspecified narcotics

T40.601 Poisoning by unspecified narcotics, accidental (unintentional) HCC
Poisoning by narcotics NOS

T40.602 Poisoning by unspecified narcotics, intentional self-harm HCC

T40.603 Poisoning by unspecified narcotics, assault

T40.604 Poisoning by unspecified narcotics, undetermined HCC

T40.605 Adverse effect of unspecified narcotics

T40.606 Underdosing of unspecified narcotics

T40.69 Poisoning by, adverse effect of and underdosing of other narcotics

T40.691 Poisoning by other narcotics, accidental (unintentional) HCC
Poisoning by other narcotics NOS

T40.692 Poisoning by other narcotics, intentional self-harm HCC

T40.693 Poisoning by other narcotics, assault

T40.694 Poisoning by other narcotics, undetermined HCC

T40.695 Adverse effect of other narcotics

T40.696 Underdosing of other narcotics

T40.7 Poisoning by, adverse effect of and underdosing of cannabis (derivatives)

T40.7X Poisoning by, adverse effect of and underdosing of cannabis (derivatives)

T40.7X1 Poisoning by cannabis (derivatives), accidental (unintentional)
Poisoning by cannabis NOS
AHA: 2020,1Q,8

T40.7X2 Poisoning by cannabis (derivatives), intentional self-harm HCC

T40.7X3 Poisoning by cannabis (derivatives), assault

T40.7X4 Poisoning by cannabis (derivatives), undetermined

T40.7X5 Adverse effect of cannabis (derivatives)

T40.7X6 Underdosing of cannabis (derivatives)

T40.8 Poisoning by and adverse effect of lysergide [LSD]

T40.8X Poisoning by and adverse effect of lysergide [LSD]

T40.8X1 Poisoning by lysergide [LSD], accidental (unintentional) HCC
Poisoning by lysergide [LSD] NOS

T40.8X2 Poisoning by lysergide [LSD], intentional self-harm HCC

T40.8X3 Poisoning by lysergide [LSD], assault

T40.8X4 Poisoning by lysergide [LSD], undetermined HCC

T40.9 Poisoning by, adverse effect of and underdosing of other and unspecified psychodysleptics [hallucinogens]

T40.90 Poisoning by, adverse effect of and underdosing of unspecified psychodysleptics [hallucinogens]

T40.901 Poisoning by unspecified psychodysleptics [hallucinogens], accidental (unintentional) HCC

T40.902 Poisoning by unspecified psychodysleptics [hallucinogens], intentional self-harm HCC

T40.903 Poisoning by unspecified psychodysleptics [hallucinogens], assault

T40.904 Poisoning by unspecified psychodysleptics [hallucinogens], undetermined HCC

T40.905 Adverse effect of unspecified psychodysleptics [hallucinogens]

T40.906 Underdosing of unspecified psychodysleptics [hallucinogens]

T40.99 Poisoning by, adverse effect of and underdosing of other psychodysleptics [hallucinogens]

T40.991 Poisoning by other psychodysleptics [hallucinogens], accidental (unintentional) HCC
Poisoning by other psychodysleptics [hallucinogens] NOS

T40.992 Poisoning by other psychodysleptics [hallucinogens], intentional self-harm HCC

T40.993 Poisoning by other psychodysleptics [hallucinogens], assault

T40.994 Poisoning by other psychodysleptics [hallucinogens], undetermined HCC

T40.995 Adverse effect of other psychodysleptics [hallucinogens]

T40.996 Underdosing of other psychodysleptics [hallucinogens]

T41 Poisoning by, adverse effect of and underdosing of anesthetics and therapeutic gases

EXCLUDES 1 *benzodiazepines (T42.4-)*
cocaine (T40.5-)
complications of anesthesia during labor and delivery (O74.-)
complications of anesthesia during pregnancy (O29.-)
complications of anesthesia during the puerperium (O89.-)
opioids (T40.0-T40.2-)

The appropriate 7th character is to be added to each code from category T41.
A initial encounter
D subsequent encounter
S sequela

T41.0 Poisoning by, adverse effect of and underdosing of inhaled anesthetics

EXCLUDES 1 *oxygen (T41.5-)*

T41.0X Poisoning by, adverse effect of and underdosing of inhaled anesthetics

T41.0X1 Poisoning by inhaled anesthetics, accidental (unintentional)
Poisoning by inhaled anesthetics NOS

T41.0X2 Poisoning by inhaled anesthetics, intentional self-harm HCC

T41.0X3 Poisoning by inhaled anesthetics, assault

T41.0X4 Poisoning by inhaled anesthetics, undetermined

T41.0X5 Adverse effect of inhaled anesthetics

T41.0X6 Underdosing of inhaled anesthetics

T41.1 Poisoning by, adverse effect of and underdosing of intravenous anesthetics
Poisoning by, adverse effect of and underdosing of thiobarbiturates

T41.1X Poisoning by, adverse effect of and underdosing of intravenous anesthetics

T41.1X1 Poisoning by intravenous anesthetics, accidental (unintentional)
Poisoning by intravenous anesthetics NOS

T41.1X2 Poisoning by intravenous anesthetics, intentional self-harm HCC

T41.1X3 Poisoning by intravenous anesthetics, assault

T41.1X4 Poisoning by intravenous anesthetics, undetermined

T41.1X5 Adverse effect of intravenous anesthetics

T41.1X6 Underdosing of intravenous anesthetics

T41.2 Poisoning by, adverse effect of and underdosing of other and unspecified general anesthetics

T41.20 Poisoning by, adverse effect of and underdosing of unspecified general anesthetics

T41.201 Poisoning by unspecified general anesthetics, accidental (unintentional)
Poisoning by general anesthetics NOS

7 **T41.202 Poisoning by unspecified general anesthetics, intentional self-harm** HCC

T41.203 Poisoning by unspecified general anesthetics, assault

T41.204 Poisoning by unspecified general anesthetics, undetermined

T41.205 Adverse effect of unspecified general anesthetics
AHA: 2016,4Q,73

T41.206 Underdosing of unspecified general anesthetics

T41.29 Poisoning by, adverse effect of and underdosing of other general anesthetics

T41.291 Poisoning by other general anesthetics, accidental (unintentional)
Poisoning by other general anesthetics NOS

7 **T41.292 Poisoning by other general anesthetics, intentional self-harm** HCC

T41.293 Poisoning by other general anesthetics, assault

T41.294 Poisoning by other general anesthetics, undetermined

T41.295 Adverse effect of other general anesthetics

T41.296 Underdosing of other general anesthetics

T41.3 Poisoning by, adverse effect of and underdosing of local anesthetics
Cocaine (topical)
EXCLUDES 2 *poisoning by cocaine used as a central nervous system stimulant (T40.5X1-T40.5X4)*

T41.3X Poisoning by, adverse effect of and underdosing of local anesthetics

T41.3X1 Poisoning by local anesthetics, accidental (unintentional)
Poisoning by local anesthetics NOS

7 **T41.3X2 Poisoning by local anesthetics, intentional self-harm** HCC

T41.3X3 Poisoning by local anesthetics, assault

T41.3X4 Poisoning by local anesthetics, undetermined

T41.3X5 Adverse effect of local anesthetics

T41.3X6 Underdosing of local anesthetics

T41.4 Poisoning by, adverse effect of and underdosing of unspecified anesthetic

T41.41 Poisoning by unspecified anesthetic, accidental (unintentional)
Poisoning by anesthetic NOS

7 **T41.42 Poisoning by unspecified anesthetic, intentional self-harm** HCC

T41.43 Poisoning by unspecified anesthetic, assault

T41.44 Poisoning by unspecified anesthetic, undetermined

T41.45 Adverse effect of unspecified anesthetic

T41.46 Underdosing of unspecified anesthetics

T41.5 Poisoning by, adverse effect of and underdosing of therapeutic gases

T41.5X Poisoning by, adverse effect of and underdosing of therapeutic gases

T41.5X1 Poisoning by therapeutic gases, accidental (unintentional)
Poisoning by therapeutic gases NOS

7 **T41.5X2 Poisoning by therapeutic gases, intentional self-harm** HCC

T41.5X3 Poisoning by therapeutic gases, assault

T41.5X4 Poisoning by therapeutic gases, undetermined

T41.5X5 Adverse effect of therapeutic gases

T41.5X6 Underdosing of therapeutic gases

T42 Poisoning by, adverse effect of and underdosing of antiepileptic, sedative- hypnotic and antiparkinsonism drugs
EXCLUDES 2 *drug dependence and related mental and behavioral disorders due to psychoactive substance use (F10.- – F19.-)*

The appropriate 7th character is to be added to each code from category T42.
A initial encounter
D subsequent encounter
S sequela

T42.0 Poisoning by, adverse effect of and underdosing of hydantoin derivatives

T42.0X Poisoning by, adverse effect of and underdosing of hydantoin derivatives

T42.0X1 Poisoning by hydantoin derivatives, accidental (unintentional)
Poisoning by hydantoin derivatives NOS

7 **T42.0X2 Poisoning by hydantoin derivatives, intentional self-harm** HCC

T42.0X3 Poisoning by hydantoin derivatives, assault

T42.0X4 Poisoning by hydantoin derivatives, undetermined

T42.0X5 Adverse effect of hydantoin derivatives

T42.0X6 Underdosing of hydantoin derivatives

T42.1 Poisoning by, adverse effect of and underdosing of iminostilbenes
Poisoning by, adverse effect of and underdosing of carbamazepine

T42.1X Poisoning by, adverse effect of and underdosing of iminostilbenes

T42.1X1 Poisoning by iminostilbenes, accidental (unintentional)
Poisoning by iminostilbenes NOS

7 **T42.1X2 Poisoning by iminostilbenes, intentional self-harm** HCC

T42.1X3 Poisoning by iminostilbenes, assault

T42.1X4 Poisoning by iminostilbenes, undetermined

T42.1X5 Adverse effect of iminostilbenes

T42.1X6 Underdosing of iminostilbenes

T42.2 Poisoning by, adverse effect of and underdosing of succinimides and oxazolidinediones

T42.2X Poisoning by, adverse effect of and underdosing of succinimides and oxazolidinediones

T42.2X1 Poisoning by succinimides and oxazolidinediones, accidental (unintentional)
Poisoning by succinimides and oxazolidinediones NOS

7 **T42.2X2 Poisoning by succinimides and oxazolidinediones, intentional self-harm** HCC

T42.2X3 Poisoning by succinimides and oxazolidinediones, assault

T42.2X4 Poisoning by succinimides and oxazolidinediones, undetermined

T42.2X5 Adverse effect of succinimides and oxazolidinediones

T42.2X6 Underdosing of succinimides and oxazolidinediones

T42.3 Poisoning by, adverse effect of and underdosing of barbiturates
EXCLUDES 1 *poisoning by, adverse effect of and underdosing of thiobarbiturates (T41.1-)*

T42.3X Poisoning by, adverse effect of and underdosing of barbiturates

T42.3X1 Poisoning by barbiturates, accidental (unintentional)
Poisoning by barbiturates NOS

7 **T42.3X2 Poisoning by barbiturates, intentional self-harm** HCC

T42.3X3 Poisoning by barbiturates, assault

T42.3X4 Poisoning by barbiturates, undetermined

T42.3X5 Adverse effect of barbiturates

T42.3X6 Underdosing of barbiturates

T42.4 Poisoning by, adverse effect of and underdosing of benzodiazepines

T42.4X Poisoning by, adverse effect of and underdosing of benzodiazepines

T42.4X1 Poisoning by benzodiazepines, accidental (unintentional)
Poisoning by benzodiazepines NOS

7 **T42.4X2 Poisoning by benzodiazepines, intentional self-harm** HCC

T42.4X3 Poisoning by benzodiazepines, assault

T42.4X4 Poisoning by benzodiazepines, undetermined

T42.4X5 Adverse effect of benzodiazepines

T42.4X6 Underdosing of benzodiazepines

T42.5 Poisoning by, adverse effect of and underdosing of mixed antiepileptics

T42.5X Poisoning by, adverse effect of and underdosing of antiepileptics

T42.5X1 Poisoning by mixed antiepileptics, accidental (unintentional)
Poisoning by mixed antiepileptics NOS

7 **T42.5X2 Poisoning by mixed antiepileptics, intentional self-harm** HCC

T42.5X3 Poisoning by mixed antiepileptics, assault

T42.5X4 Poisoning by mixed antiepileptics, undetermined

T42.5X5 Adverse effect of mixed antiepileptics

T42.5X6 Underdosing of mixed antiepileptics

T42.6 Poisoning by, adverse effect of and underdosing of other antiepileptic and sedative-hypnotic drugs
Poisoning by, adverse effect of and underdosing of methaqualone
Poisoning by, adverse effect of and underdosing of valproic acid
EXCLUDES 1 *poisoning by, adverse effect of and underdosing of carbamazepine (T42.1-)*

T42.6X Poisoning by, adverse effect of and underdosing of other antiepileptic and sedative-hypnotic drugs

T42.6X1 Poisoning by other antiepileptic and sedative-hypnotic drugs, accidental (unintentional)
Poisoning by other antiepileptic and sedative-hypnotic drugs NOS

7 **T42.6X2 Poisoning by other antiepileptic and sedative-hypnotic drugs, intentional self-harm** HCC

T42.6X3 Poisoning by other antiepileptic and sedative-hypnotic drugs, assault

T42.6X4 Poisoning by other antiepileptic and sedative-hypnotic drugs, undetermined

T42.6X5 Adverse effect of other antiepileptic and sedative-hypnotic drugs

T42.6X6 Underdosing of other antiepileptic and sedative-hypnotic drugs

T42.7 Poisoning by, adverse effect of and underdosing of unspecified antiepileptic and sedative-hypnotic drugs

T42.71 Poisoning by unspecified antiepileptic and sedative-hypnotic drugs, accidental (unintentional)
Poisoning by antiepileptic and sedative-hypnotic drugs NOS

7 **T42.72 Poisoning by unspecified antiepileptic and sedative-hypnotic drugs, intentional self-harm** HCC

T42.73 Poisoning by unspecified antiepileptic and sedative-hypnotic drugs, assault

T42.74 Poisoning by unspecified antiepileptic and sedative-hypnotic drugs, undetermined

T42.75 Adverse effect of unspecified antiepileptic and sedative-hypnotic drugs

T42.76 Underdosing of unspecified antiepileptic and sedative-hypnotic drugs

T42.8 Poisoning by, adverse effect of and underdosing of antiparkinsonism drugs and other central muscle-tone depressants
Poisoning by, adverse effect of and underdosing of amantadine

T42.8X Poisoning by, adverse effect of and underdosing of antiparkinsonism drugs and other central muscle-tone depressants

T42.8X1 Poisoning by antiparkinsonism drugs and other central muscle-tone depressants, accidental (unintentional)
Poisoning by antiparkinsonism drugs and other central muscle-tone depressants NOS

7 **T42.8X2 Poisoning by antiparkinsonism drugs and other central muscle-tone depressants, intentional self-harm** HCC

T42.8X3 Poisoning by antiparkinsonism drugs and other central muscle-tone depressants, assault

T42.8X4 Poisoning by antiparkinsonism drugs and other central muscle-tone depressants, undetermined

T42.8X5 Adverse effect of antiparkinsonism drugs and other central muscle-tone depressants

T42.8X6 Underdosing of antiparkinsonism drugs and other central muscle-tone depressants

T43 Poisoning by, adverse effect of and underdosing of psychotropic drugs, not elsewhere classified
EXCLUDES 1 *appetite depressants (T50.5-)*
barbiturates (T42.3-)
benzodiazepines (T42.4-)
methaqualone (T42.6-)
psychodysleptics [hallucinogens] (T40.7-T40.9-)
EXCLUDES 2 *drug dependence and related mental and behavioral disorders due to psychoactive substance use (F10.- – F19.-)*

The appropriate 7th character is to be added to each code from category T43.
A initial encounter
D subsequent encounter
S sequela

T43.0 Poisoning by, adverse effect of and underdosing of tricyclic and tetracyclic antidepressants

T43.01 Poisoning by, adverse effect of and underdosing of tricyclic antidepressants

T43.011 Poisoning by tricyclic antidepressants, accidental (unintentional)
Poisoning by tricyclic antidepressants NOS

7 **T43.012 Poisoning by tricyclic antidepressants, intentional self-harm** HCC

T43.013 Poisoning by tricyclic antidepressants, assault

T43.014 Poisoning by tricyclic antidepressants, undetermined

T43.015 Adverse effect of tricyclic antidepressants

T43.016 Underdosing of tricyclic antidepressants

T43.02 Poisoning by, adverse effect of and underdosing of tetracyclic antidepressants

T43.021 Poisoning by tetracyclic antidepressants, accidental (unintentional)
Poisoning by tetracyclic antidepressants NOS

7 **T43.022 Poisoning by tetracyclic antidepressants, intentional self-harm** HCC

T43.023 Poisoning by tetracyclic antidepressants, assault

T43.024 Poisoning by tetracyclic antidepressants, undetermined

T43.025 Adverse effect of tetracyclic antidepressants

T43.026 Underdosing of tetracyclic antidepressants

5th **T43.1 Poisoning by, adverse effect of and underdosing of monoamine-oxidase-inhibitor antidepressants**

6th **T43.1X Poisoning by, adverse effect of and underdosing of monoamine-oxidase-inhibitor antidepressants**

7th **T43.1X1 Poisoning by monoamine-oxidase-inhibitor antidepressants, accidental (unintentional)**

Poisoning by monoamine-oxidase-inhibitor antidepressants NOS

7 7th **T43.1X2 Poisoning by monoamine-oxidase-inhibitor antidepressants, intentional self-harm** HCC

7th **T43.1X3 Poisoning by monoamine-oxidase-inhibitor antidepressants, assault**

7th **T43.1X4 Poisoning by monoamine-oxidase-inhibitor antidepressants, undetermined**

7th **T43.1X5 Adverse effect of monoamine-oxidase-inhibitor antidepressants**

7th **T43.1X6 Underdosing of monoamine-oxidase-inhibitor antidepressants**

5th **T43.2 Poisoning by, adverse effect of and underdosing of other and unspecified antidepressants**

6th **T43.20 Poisoning by, adverse effect of and underdosing of unspecified antidepressants**

7th **T43.201 Poisoning by unspecified antidepressants, accidental (unintentional)**

Poisoning by antidepressants NOS

7 7th **T43.202 Poisoning by unspecified antidepressants, intentional self-harm** HCC

7th **T43.203 Poisoning by unspecified antidepressants, assault**

7th **T43.204 Poisoning by unspecified antidepressants, undetermined**

7th **T43.205 Adverse effect of unspecified antidepressants**

Antidepressant discontinuation syndrome

7th **T43.206 Underdosing of unspecified antidepressants**

6th **T43.21 Poisoning by, adverse effect of and underdosing of selective serotonin and norepinephrine reuptake inhibitors**

Poisoning by, adverse effect of and underdosing of SSNRI antidepressants

7th **T43.211 Poisoning by selective serotonin and norepinephrine reuptake inhibitors, accidental (unintentional)**

7 7th **T43.212 Poisoning by selective serotonin and norepinephrine reuptake inhibitors, intentional self-harm** HCC

7th **T43.213 Poisoning by selective serotonin and norepinephrine reuptake inhibitors, assault**

7th **T43.214 Poisoning by selective serotonin and norepinephrine reuptake inhibitors, undetermined**

7th **T43.215 Adverse effect of selective serotonin and norepinephrine reuptake inhibitors**

7th **T43.216 Underdosing of selective serotonin and norepinephrine reuptake inhibitors**

6th **T43.22 Poisoning by, adverse effect of and underdosing of selective serotonin reuptake inhibitors**

Poisoning by, adverse effect of and underdosing of SSRI antidepressants

7th **T43.221 Poisoning by selective serotonin reuptake inhibitors, accidental (unintentional)**

7 7th **T43.222 Poisoning by selective serotonin reuptake inhibitors, intentional self-harm** HCC

7th **T43.223 Poisoning by selective serotonin reuptake inhibitors, assault**

7th **T43.224 Poisoning by selective serotonin reuptake inhibitors, undetermined**

7th **T43.225 Adverse effect of selective serotonin reuptake inhibitors**

7th **T43.226 Underdosing of selective serotonin reuptake inhibitors**

6th **T43.29 Poisoning by, adverse effect of and underdosing of other antidepressants**

7th **T43.291 Poisoning by other antidepressants, accidental (unintentional)**

Poisoning by other antidepressants NOS

7 7th **T43.292 Poisoning by other antidepressants, intentional self-harm** HCC

7th **T43.293 Poisoning by other antidepressants, assault**

7th **T43.294 Poisoning by other antidepressants, undetermined**

7th **T43.295 Adverse effect of other antidepressants**

7th **T43.296 Underdosing of other antidepressants**

5th **T43.3 Poisoning by, adverse effect of and underdosing of phenothiazine antipsychotics and neuroleptics**

6th **T43.3X Poisoning by, adverse effect of and underdosing of phenothiazine antipsychotics and neuroleptics**

7th **T43.3X1 Poisoning by phenothiazine antipsychotics and neuroleptics, accidental (unintentional)**

Poisoning by phenothiazine antipsychotics and neuroleptics NOS

7 7th **T43.3X2 Poisoning by phenothiazine antipsychotics and neuroleptics, intentional self-harm** HCC

7th **T43.3X3 Poisoning by phenothiazine antipsychotics and neuroleptics, assault**

7th **T43.3X4 Poisoning by phenothiazine antipsychotics and neuroleptics, undetermined**

7th **T43.3X5 Adverse effect of phenothiazine antipsychotics and neuroleptics**

7th **T43.3X6 Underdosing of phenothiazine antipsychotics and neuroleptics**

5th **T43.4 Poisoning by, adverse effect of and underdosing of butyrophenone and thiothixene neuroleptics**

6th **T43.4X Poisoning by, adverse effect of and underdosing of butyrophenone and thiothixene neuroleptics**

7th **T43.4X1 Poisoning by butyrophenone and thiothixene neuroleptics, accidental (unintentional)**

Poisoning by butyrophenone and thiothixene neuroleptics NOS

7 7th **T43.4X2 Poisoning by butyrophenone and thiothixene neuroleptics, intentional self-harm** HCC

7th **T43.4X3 Poisoning by butyrophenone and thiothixene neuroleptics, assault**

7th **T43.4X4 Poisoning by butyrophenone and thiothixene neuroleptics, undetermined**

7th **T43.4X5 Adverse effect of butyrophenone and thiothixene neuroleptics**

7th **T43.4X6 Underdosing of butyrophenone and thiothixene neuroleptics**

5th **T43.5 Poisoning by, adverse effect of and underdosing of other and unspecified antipsychotics and neuroleptics**

EXCLUDES 1 *poisoning by, adverse effect of and underdosing of rauwolfia (T46.5-)*

6th **T43.50 Poisoning by, adverse effect of and underdosing of unspecified antipsychotics and neuroleptics**

7th **T43.501 Poisoning by unspecified antipsychotics and neuroleptics, accidental (unintentional)**

Poisoning by antipsychotics and neuroleptics NOS

7 7th **T43.502 Poisoning by unspecified antipsychotics and neuroleptics, intentional self-harm** HCC

7th **T43.503 Poisoning by unspecified antipsychotics and neuroleptics, assault**

7th **T43.504 Poisoning by unspecified antipsychotics and neuroleptics, undetermined**

7th **T43.505 Adverse effect of unspecified antipsychotics and neuroleptics**

7th **T43.506 Underdosing of unspecified antipsychotics and neuroleptics**

√6th T43.59 **Poisoning by, adverse effect of and underdosing of other antipsychotics and neuroleptics**
AHA: 2017,1Q,40

√7th T43.591 **Poisoning by other antipsychotics and neuroleptics, accidental (unintentional)**
Poisoning by other antipsychotics and neuroleptics NOS

7 √7th T43.592 **Poisoning by other antipsychotics and neuroleptics, intentional self-harm** HCC

√7th T43.593 **Poisoning by other antipsychotics and neuroleptics, assault**

√7th T43.594 **Poisoning by other antipsychotics and neuroleptics, undetermined**

√7th T43.595 **Adverse effect of other antipsychotics and neuroleptics**

√7th T43.596 **Underdosing of other antipsychotics and neuroleptics**

√5th T43.6 **Poisoning by, adverse effect of and underdosing of psychostimulants**
EXCLUDES 1 *poisoning by, adverse effect of and underdosing of cocaine (T4Ø.5-)*

√6th T43.6Ø **Poisoning by, adverse effect of and underdosing of unspecified psychostimulant**

6 √7th T43.6Ø1 **Poisoning by unspecified psychostimulants, accidental (unintentional)** HCC
Poisoning by psychostimulants NOS

7 √7th T43.6Ø2 **Poisoning by unspecified psychostimulants, intentional self-harm** HCC

√7th T43.6Ø3 **Poisoning by unspecified psychostimulants, assault**

6 √7th T43.6Ø4 **Poisoning by unspecified psychostimulants, undetermined** HCC

√7th T43.6Ø5 **Adverse effect of unspecified psychostimulants**

√7th T43.6Ø6 **Underdosing of unspecified psychostimulants**

√6th T43.61 **Poisoning by, adverse effect of and underdosing of caffeine**

6 √7th T43.611 **Poisoning by caffeine, accidental (unintentional)** HCC
Poisoning by caffeine NOS

7 √7th T43.612 **Poisoning by caffeine, intentional self-harm** HCC

√7th T43.613 **Poisoning by caffeine, assault**

6 √7th T43.614 **Poisoning by caffeine, undetermined** HCC

√7th T43.615 **Adverse effect of caffeine**

√7th T43.616 **Underdosing of caffeine**

√6th T43.62 **Poisoning by, adverse effect of and underdosing of amphetamines**
Poisoning by, adverse effect of and underdosing of methamphetamines

6 √7th T43.621 **Poisoning by amphetamines, accidental (unintentional)** HCC
Poisoning by amphetamines NOS

7 √7th T43.622 **Poisoning by amphetamines, intentional self-harm** HCC

√7th T43.623 **Poisoning by amphetamines, assault**

6 √7th T43.624 **Poisoning by amphetamines, undetermined** HCC

√7th T43.625 **Adverse effect of amphetamines**

√7th T43.626 **Underdosing of amphetamines**

√6th T43.63 **Poisoning by, adverse effect of and underdosing of methylphenidate**

6 √7th T43.631 **Poisoning by methylphenidate, accidental (unintentional)** HCC
Poisoning by methylphenidate NOS

7 √7th T43.632 **Poisoning by methylphenidate, intentional self-harm** HCC

√7th T43.633 **Poisoning by methylphenidate, assault**

6 √7th T43.634 **Poisoning by methylphenidate, undetermined** HCC

√7th T43.635 **Adverse effect of methylphenidate**

√7th T43.636 **Underdosing of methylphenidate**

√6th T43.64 **Poisoning by ecstasy**
Poisoning by MDMA
Poisoning by 3,4-methylenedioxymethamphetamine
AHA: 2018,4Q,30-31

6 √7th T43.641 **Poisoning by ecstasy, accidental (unintentional)** HCC
Poisoning by ecstasy NOS

7 √7th T43.642 **Poisoning by ecstasy, intentional self-harm** HCC

√7th T43.643 **Poisoning by ecstasy, assault**

6 √7th T43.644 **Poisoning by ecstasy, undetermined** HCC

√6th T43.69 **Poisoning by, adverse effect of and underdosing of other psychostimulants**

6 √7th T43.691 **Poisoning by other psychostimulants, accidental (unintentional)** HCC
Poisoning by other psychostimulants NOS

7 √7th T43.692 **Poisoning by other psychostimulants, intentional self-harm** HCC

√7th T43.693 **Poisoning by other psychostimulants, assault**

6 √7th T43.694 **Poisoning by other psychostimulants, undetermined** HCC

√7th T43.695 **Adverse effect of other psychostimulants**

√7th T43.696 **Underdosing of other psychostimulants**

√5th T43.8 **Poisoning by, adverse effect of and underdosing of other psychotropic drugs**

√6th T43.8X **Poisoning by, adverse effect of and underdosing of other psychotropic drugs**

√7th T43.8X1 **Poisoning by other psychotropic drugs, accidental (unintentional)**
Poisoning by other psychotropic drugs NOS

7 √7th T43.8X2 **Poisoning by other psychotropic drugs, intentional self-harm** HCC

√7th T43.8X3 **Poisoning by other psychotropic drugs, assault**

√7th T43.8X4 **Poisoning by other psychotropic drugs, undetermined**

√7th T43.8X5 **Adverse effect of other psychotropic drugs**

√7th T43.8X6 **Underdosing of other psychotropic drugs**

√5th T43.9 **Poisoning by, adverse effect of and underdosing of unspecified psychotropic drug**

√x7th T43.91 **Poisoning by unspecified psychotropic drug, accidental (unintentional)**
Poisoning by psychotropic drug NOS

7 √x7th T43.92 **Poisoning by unspecified psychotropic drug, intentional self-harm** HCC

√x7th T43.93 **Poisoning by unspecified psychotropic drug, assault**

√x7th T43.94 **Poisoning by unspecified psychotropic drug, undetermined**

√x7th T43.95 **Adverse effect of unspecified psychotropic drug**

√x7th T43.96 **Underdosing of unspecified psychotropic drug**

√4th **T44 Poisoning by, adverse effect of and underdosing of drugs primarily affecting the autonomic nervous system**

The appropriate 7th character is to be added to each code from category T44.
A initial encounter
D subsequent encounter
S sequela

√5th T44.Ø **Poisoning by, adverse effect of and underdosing of anticholinesterase agents**

√6th T44.ØX **Poisoning by, adverse effect of and underdosing of anticholinesterase agents**

√7th T44.ØX1 **Poisoning by anticholinesterase agents, accidental (unintentional)**
Poisoning by anticholinesterase agents NOS

7 √7th T44.ØX2 **Poisoning by anticholinesterase agents, intentional self-harm** HCC

√7th T44.ØX3 **Poisoning by anticholinesterase agents, assault**

√7th T44.ØX4 **Poisoning by anticholinesterase agents, undetermined**

√7th T44.ØX5 **Adverse effect of anticholinesterase agents**

√7th T44.ØX6 **Underdosing of anticholinesterase agents**

√5th **T44.1 Poisoning by, adverse effect of and underdosing of other parasympathomimetics [cholinergics]**

√6th **T44.1X Poisoning by, adverse effect of and underdosing of other parasympathomimetics [cholinergics]**

√7th **T44.1X1 Poisoning by other parasympathomimetics [cholinergics], accidental (unintentional)**
Poisoning by other parasympathomimetics [cholinergics] NOS

7 √7th **T44.1X2 Poisoning by other parasympathomimetics [cholinergics], intentional self-harm** HCC

√7th **T44.1X3 Poisoning by other parasympathomimetics [cholinergics], assault**

√7th **T44.1X4 Poisoning by other parasympathomimetics [cholinergics], undetermined**

√7th **T44.1X5 Adverse effect of other parasympathomimetics [cholinergics]**

√7th **T44.1X6 Underdosing of other parasympathomimetics [cholinergics]**

√5th **T44.2 Poisoning by, adverse effect of and underdosing of ganglionic blocking drugs**

√6th **T44.2X Poisoning by, adverse effect of and underdosing of ganglionic blocking drugs**

√7th **T44.2X1 Poisoning by ganglionic blocking drugs, accidental (unintentional)**
Poisoning by ganglionic blocking drugs NOS

7 √7th **T44.2X2 Poisoning by ganglionic blocking drugs, intentional self-harm** HCC

√7th **T44.2X3 Poisoning by ganglionic blocking drugs, assault**

√7th **T44.2X4 Poisoning by ganglionic blocking drugs, undetermined**

√7th **T44.2X5 Adverse effect of ganglionic blocking drugs**

√7th **T44.2X6 Underdosing of ganglionic blocking drugs**

√5th **T44.3 Poisoning by, adverse effect of and underdosing of other parasympatholytics [anticholinergics and antimuscarinics] and spasmolytics**
Poisoning by, adverse effect of and underdosing of papaverine

√6th **T44.3X Poisoning by, adverse effect of and underdosing of other parasympatholytics [anticholinergics and antimuscarinics] and spasmolytics**

√7th **T44.3X1 Poisoning by other parasympatholytics [anticholinergics and antimuscarinics] and spasmolytics, accidental (unintentional)**
Poisoning by other parasympatholytics [anticholinergics and antimuscarinics] and spasmolytics NOS

7 √7th **T44.3X2 Poisoning by other parasympatholytics [anticholinergics and antimuscarinics] and spasmolytics, intentional self-harm** HCC

√7th **T44.3X3 Poisoning by other parasympatholytics [anticholinergics and antimuscarinics] and spasmolytics, assault**

√7th **T44.3X4 Poisoning by other parasympatholytics [anticholinergics and antimuscarinics] and spasmolytics, undetermined**

√7th **T44.3X5 Adverse effect of other parasympatholytics [anticholinergics and antimuscarinics] and spasmolytics**

√7th **T44.3X6 Underdosing of other parasympatholytics [anticholinergics and antimuscarinics] and spasmolytics**

√5th **T44.4 Poisoning by, adverse effect of and underdosing of predominantly alpha-adrenoreceptor agonists**
Poisoning by, adverse effect of and underdosing of metaraminol

√6th **T44.4X Poisoning by, adverse effect of and underdosing of predominantly alpha-adrenoreceptor agonists**

√7th **T44.4X1 Poisoning by predominantly alpha-adrenoreceptor agonists, accidental (unintentional)**
Poisoning by predominantly alpha-adrenoreceptor agonists NOS

7 √7th **T44.4X2 Poisoning by predominantly alpha-adrenoreceptor agonists, intentional self-harm** HCC

√7th **T44.4X3 Poisoning by predominantly alpha-adrenoreceptor agonists, assault**

√7th **T44.4X4 Poisoning by predominantly alpha-adrenoreceptor agonists, undetermined**

√7th **T44.4X5 Adverse effect of predominantly alpha-adrenoreceptor agonists**

√7th **T44.4X6 Underdosing of predominantly alpha-adrenoreceptor agonists**

√5th **T44.5 Poisoning by, adverse effect of and underdosing of predominantly beta-adrenoreceptor agonists**
EXCLUDES 1 *poisoning by, adverse effect of and underdosing of beta-adrenoreceptor agonists used in asthma therapy (T48.6-)*

√6th **T44.5X Poisoning by, adverse effect of and underdosing of predominantly beta-adrenoreceptor agonists**

√7th **T44.5X1 Poisoning by predominantly beta-adrenoreceptor agonists, accidental (unintentional)**
Poisoning by predominantly beta-adrenoreceptor agonists NOS

7 √7th **T44.5X2 Poisoning by predominantly beta-adrenoreceptor agonists, intentional self-harm** HCC

√7th **T44.5X3 Poisoning by predominantly beta-adrenoreceptor agonists, assault**

√7th **T44.5X4 Poisoning by predominantly beta-adrenoreceptor agonists, undetermined**

√7th **T44.5X5 Adverse effect of predominantly beta-adrenoreceptor agonists**

√7th **T44.5X6 Underdosing of predominantly beta-adrenoreceptor agonists**

√5th **T44.6 Poisoning by, adverse effect of and underdosing of alpha-adrenoreceptor antagonists**
EXCLUDES 1 *poisoning by, adverse effect of and underdosing of ergot alkaloids (T48.Ø)*

√6th **T44.6X Poisoning by, adverse effect of and underdosing of alpha-adrenoreceptor antagonists**

√7th **T44.6X1 Poisoning by alpha-adrenoreceptor antagonists, accidental (unintentional)**
Poisoning by alpha-adrenoreceptor antagonists NOS

7 √7th **T44.6X2 Poisoning by alpha-adrenoreceptor antagonists, intentional self-harm** HCC

√7th **T44.6X3 Poisoning by alpha-adrenoreceptor antagonists, assault**

√7th **T44.6X4 Poisoning by alpha-adrenoreceptor antagonists, undetermined**

√7th **T44.6X5 Adverse effect of alpha-adrenoreceptor antagonists**

√7th **T44.6X6 Underdosing of alpha-adrenoreceptor antagonists**

√5th **T44.7 Poisoning by, adverse effect of and underdosing of beta-adrenoreceptor antagonists**

√6th **T44.7X Poisoning by, adverse effect of and underdosing of beta-adrenoreceptor antagonists**

√7th **T44.7X1 Poisoning by beta-adrenoreceptor antagonists, accidental (unintentional)**
Poisoning by beta-adrenoreceptor antagonists NOS

7 √7th **T44.7X2 Poisoning by beta-adrenoreceptor antagonists, intentional self-harm** HCC

√7th **T44.7X3 Poisoning by beta-adrenoreceptor antagonists, assault**

√7th **T44.7X4 Poisoning by beta-adrenoreceptor antagonists, undetermined**

√7th **T44.7X5 Adverse effect of beta-adrenoreceptor antagonists**

√7th **T44.7X6 Underdosing of beta-adrenoreceptor antagonists**

T44.8 Poisoning by, adverse effect of and underdosing of centrally-acting and adrenergic-neuron- blocking agents

EXCLUDES 1 *poisoning by, adverse effect of and underdosing of clonidine (T46.5)*
poisoning by, adverse effect of and underdosing of guanethidine (T46.5)

T44.8X Poisoning by, adverse effect of and underdosing of centrally-acting and adrenergic- neuron-blocking agents

T44.8X1 Poisoning by centrally-acting and adrenergic-neuron-blocking agents, accidental (unintentional)
Poisoning by centrally-acting and adrenergic-neuron-blocking agents NOS

7 **T44.8X2 Poisoning by centrally-acting and adrenergic-neuron-blocking agents, intentional self-harm** HCC

T44.8X3 Poisoning by centrally-acting and adrenergic-neuron-blocking agents, assault

T44.8X4 Poisoning by centrally-acting and adrenergic-neuron-blocking agents, undetermined

T44.8X5 Adverse effect of centrally-acting and adrenergic-neuron-blocking agents

T44.8X6 Underdosing of centrally-acting and adrenergic-neuron-blocking agents

T44.9 Poisoning by, adverse effect of and underdosing of other and unspecified drugs primarily affecting the autonomic nervous system
Poisoning by, adverse effect of and underdosing of drug stimulating both alpha and beta-adrenoreceptors

T44.90 Poisoning by, adverse effect of and underdosing of unspecified drugs primarily affecting the autonomic nervous system

T44.901 Poisoning by unspecified drugs primarily affecting the autonomic nervous system, accidental (unintentional)
Poisoning by unspecified drugs primarily affecting the autonomic nervous system NOS

7 **T44.902 Poisoning by unspecified drugs primarily affecting the autonomic nervous system, intentional self-harm** HCC

T44.903 Poisoning by unspecified drugs primarily affecting the autonomic nervous system, assault

T44.904 Poisoning by unspecified drugs primarily affecting the autonomic nervous system, undetermined

T44.905 Adverse effect of unspecified drugs primarily affecting the autonomic nervous system

T44.906 Underdosing of unspecified drugs primarily affecting the autonomic nervous system

T44.99 Poisoning by, adverse effect of and underdosing of other drugs primarily affecting the autonomic nervous system

T44.991 Poisoning by other drug primarily affecting the autonomic nervous system, accidental (unintentional)
Poisoning by other drugs primarily affecting the autonomic nervous system NOS

7 **T44.992 Poisoning by other drug primarily affecting the autonomic nervous system, intentional self-harm** HCC

T44.993 Poisoning by other drug primarily affecting the autonomic nervous system, assault

T44.994 Poisoning by other drug primarily affecting the autonomic nervous system, undetermined

T44.995 Adverse effect of other drug primarily affecting the autonomic nervous system

T44.996 Underdosing of other drug primarily affecting the autonomic nervous system

T45 Poisoning by, adverse effect of and underdosing of primarily systemic and hematological agents, not elsewhere classified

The appropriate 7th character is to be added to each code from category T45.
A initial encounter
D subsequent encounter
S sequela

T45.0 Poisoning by, adverse effect of and underdosing of antiallergic and antiemetic drugs

EXCLUDES 1 *poisoning by, adverse effect of and underdosing of phenothiazine-based neuroleptics (T43.3)*

T45.0X Poisoning by, adverse effect of and underdosing of antiallergic and antiemetic drugs

T45.0X1 Poisoning by antiallergic and antiemetic drugs, accidental (unintentional)
Poisoning by antiallergic and antiemetic drugs NOS

7 **T45.0X2 Poisoning by antiallergic and antiemetic drugs, intentional self-harm** HCC

T45.0X3 Poisoning by antiallergic and antiemetic drugs, assault

T45.0X4 Poisoning by antiallergic and antiemetic drugs, undetermined

T45.0X5 Adverse effect of antiallergic and antiemetic drugs

T45.0X6 Underdosing of antiallergic and antiemetic drugs

T45.1 Poisoning by, adverse effect of and underdosing of antineoplastic and immunosuppressive drugs

EXCLUDES 1 *poisoning by, adverse effect of and underdosing of tamoxifen (T38.6)*

AHA: 2019,1Q,17,20; 2014,4Q,22

T45.1X Poisoning by, adverse effect of and underdosing of antineoplastic and immunosuppressive drugs

T45.1X1 Poisoning by antineoplastic and immunosuppressive drugs, accidental (unintentional)
Poisoning by antineoplastic and immunosuppressive drugs NOS

7 **T45.1X2 Poisoning by antineoplastic and immunosuppressive drugs, intentional self-harm** HCC

T45.1X3 Poisoning by antineoplastic and immunosuppressive drugs, assault

T45.1X4 Poisoning by antineoplastic and immunosuppressive drugs, undetermined

T45.1X5 Adverse effect of antineoplastic and immunosuppressive drugs
AHA: 2019,2Q,24,28

T45.1X6 Underdosing of antineoplastic and immunosuppressive drugs

T45.2 Poisoning by, adverse effect of and underdosing of vitamins

EXCLUDES 2 *poisoning by, adverse effect of and underdosing of iron (T45.4)*
poisoning by, adverse effect of and underdosing of nicotinic acid (derivatives) (T46.7)
poisoning by, adverse effect of and underdosing of vitamin K (T45.7)

T45.2X Poisoning by, adverse effect of and underdosing of vitamins

T45.2X1 Poisoning by vitamins, accidental (unintentional)
Poisoning by vitamins NOS

7 **T45.2X2 Poisoning by vitamins, intentional self-harm** HCC

T45.2X3 Poisoning by vitamins, assault

T45.2X4 Poisoning by vitamins, undetermined

T45.2X5 Adverse effect of vitamins

T45.2X6 Underdosing of vitamins

EXCLUDES 1 *vitamin deficiencies (E50-E56)*

T45.3 Poisoning by, adverse effect of and underdosing of enzymes

T45.3X Poisoning by, adverse effect of and underdosing of enzymes

T45.3X1 Poisoning by enzymes, accidental (unintentional)
Poisoning by enzymes NOS

7 **T45.3X2 Poisoning by enzymes, intentional self-harm** HCC

7th T45.3X3 **Poisoning by enzymes, assault**
7th T45.3X4 **Poisoning by enzymes, undetermined**
7th T45.3X5 **Adverse effect of enzymes**
7th T45.3X6 **Underdosing of enzymes**

5th **T45.4 Poisoning by, adverse effect of and underdosing of iron and its compounds**

6th **T45.4X Poisoning by, adverse effect of and underdosing of iron and its compounds**

7th T45.4X1 **Poisoning by iron and its compounds, accidental (unintentional)**
Poisoning by iron and its compounds NOS

7 7th T45.4X2 **Poisoning by iron and its compounds, intentional self-harm** HCC
7th T45.4X3 **Poisoning by iron and its compounds, assault**
7th T45.4X4 **Poisoning by iron and its compounds, undetermined**
7th T45.4X5 **Adverse effect of iron and its compounds**
7th T45.4X6 **Underdosing of iron and its compounds**
EXCLUDES 1 *iron deficiency (E61.1)*

5th **T45.5 Poisoning by, adverse effect of and underdosing of anticoagulants and antithrombotic drugs**

6th **T45.51 Poisoning by, adverse effect of and underdosing of anticoagulants**

7th T45.511 **Poisoning by anticoagulants, accidental (unintentional)**
Poisoning by anticoagulants NOS

7 7th T45.512 **Poisoning by anticoagulants, intentional self-harm** HCC
7th T45.513 **Poisoning by anticoagulants, assault**
7th T45.514 **Poisoning by anticoagulants, undetermined**
7th T45.515 **Adverse effect of anticoagulants**
AHA: 2016,1Q,14; 2013,2Q,34
7th T45.516 **Underdosing of anticoagulants**

6th **T45.52 Poisoning by, adverse effect of and underdosing of antithrombotic drugs**
Poisoning by, adverse effect of and underdosing of antiplatelet drugs
EXCLUDES 2 *poisoning by, adverse effect of and underdosing of aspirin (T39.01-)*
poisoning by, adverse effect of and underdosing of acetylsalicylic acid (T39.01-)

7th T45.521 **Poisoning by antithrombotic drugs, accidental (unintentional)**
Poisoning by antithrombotic drug NOS

7 7th T45.522 **Poisoning by antithrombotic drugs, intentional self-harm** HCC
7th T45.523 **Poisoning by antithrombotic drugs, assault**
7th T45.524 **Poisoning by antithrombotic drugs, undetermined**
7th T45.525 **Adverse effect of antithrombotic drugs**
AHA: 2016,1Q,15
7th T45.526 **Underdosing of antithrombotic drugs**

5th **T45.6 Poisoning by, adverse effect of and underdosing of fibrinolysis-affecting drugs**

6th **T45.60 Poisoning by, adverse effect of and underdosing of unspecified fibrinolysis-affecting drugs**

7th T45.601 **Poisoning by unspecified fibrinolysis-affecting drugs, accidental (unintentional)**
Poisoning by fibrinolysis-affecting drug NOS

7 7th T45.602 **Poisoning by unspecified fibrinolysis-affecting drugs, intentional self-harm** HCC
7th T45.603 **Poisoning by unspecified fibrinolysis-affecting drugs, assault**
7th T45.604 **Poisoning by unspecified fibrinolysis-affecting drugs, undetermined**
7th T45.605 **Adverse effect of unspecified fibrinolysis-affecting drugs**
7th T45.606 **Underdosing of unspecified fibrinolysis-affecting drugs**

6th **T45.61 Poisoning by, adverse effect of and underdosing of thrombolytic drugs**

7th T45.611 **Poisoning by thrombolytic drug, accidental (unintentional)**
Poisoning by thrombolytic drug NOS

7 7th T45.612 **Poisoning by thrombolytic drug, intentional self-harm** HCC
7th T45.613 **Poisoning by thrombolytic drug, assault**
7th T45.614 **Poisoning by thrombolytic drug, undetermined**
7th T45.615 **Adverse effect of thrombolytic drugs**
AHA: 2017,2Q,9
7th T45.616 **Underdosing of thrombolytic drugs**

6th **T45.62 Poisoning by, adverse effect of and underdosing of hemostatic drugs**

7th T45.621 **Poisoning by hemostatic drug, accidental (unintentional)**
Poisoning by hemostatic drug NOS

7 7th T45.622 **Poisoning by hemostatic drug, intentional self-harm** HCC
7th T45.623 **Poisoning by hemostatic drug, assault**
7th T45.624 **Poisoning by hemostatic drug, undetermined**
7th T45.625 **Adverse effect of hemostatic drug**
7th T45.626 **Underdosing of hemostatic drugs**

6th **T45.69 Poisoning by, adverse effect of and underdosing of other fibrinolysis-affecting drugs**

7th T45.691 **Poisoning by other fibrinolysis-affecting drugs, accidental (unintentional)**
Poisoning by other fibrinolysis-affecting drug NOS

7 7th T45.692 **Poisoning by other fibrinolysis-affecting drugs, intentional self-harm** HCC
7th T45.693 **Poisoning by other fibrinolysis-affecting drugs, assault**
7th T45.694 **Poisoning by other fibrinolysis-affecting drugs, undetermined**
7th T45.695 **Adverse effect of other fibrinolysis-affecting drugs**
7th T45.696 **Underdosing of other fibrinolysis-affecting drugs**

5th **T45.7 Poisoning by, adverse effect of and underdosing of anticoagulant antagonists, vitamin K and other coagulants**

6th **T45.7X Poisoning by, adverse effect of and underdosing of anticoagulant antagonists, vitamin K and other coagulants**

7th T45.7X1 **Poisoning by anticoagulant antagonists, vitamin K and other coagulants, accidental (unintentional)**
Poisoning by anticoagulant antagonists, vitamin K and other coagulants NOS

7 7th T45.7X2 **Poisoning by anticoagulant antagonists, vitamin K and other coagulants, intentional self-harm** HCC
7th T45.7X3 **Poisoning by anticoagulant antagonists, vitamin K and other coagulants, assault**
7th T45.7X4 **Poisoning by anticoagulant antagonists, vitamin K and other coagulants, undetermined**
7th T45.7X5 **Adverse effect of anticoagulant antagonists, vitamin K and other coagulants**
7th T45.7X6 **Underdosing of anticoagulant antagonist, vitamin K and other coagulants**
EXCLUDES 1 *vitamin K deficiency (E56.1)*

Chapter 19. Injury, Poisoning and Certain Other Consequences of External Causes
T45.3X3–T45.7X6

T45.8 Poisoning by, adverse effect of and underdosing of other primarily systemic and hematological agents
Poisoning by, adverse effect of and underdosing of liver preparations and other antianemic agents
Poisoning by, adverse effect of and underdosing of natural blood and blood products
Poisoning by, adverse effect of and underdosing of plasma substitute
EXCLUDES 2 *poisoning by, adverse effect of and underdosing of immunoglobulin (T5Ø.Z1)*
poisoning by, adverse effect of and underdosing of iron (T45.4)
transfusion reactions (T8Ø.-)

T45.8X Poisoning by, adverse effect of and underdosing of other primarily systemic and hematological agents
T45.8X1 Poisoning by other primarily systemic and hematological agents, accidental (unintentional)
Poisoning by other primarily systemic and hematological agents NOS
7 **T45.8X2 Poisoning by other primarily systemic and hematological agents, intentional self-harm** HCC
T45.8X3 Poisoning by other primarily systemic and hematological agents, assault
T45.8X4 Poisoning by other primarily systemic and hematological agents, undetermined
T45.8X5 Adverse effect of other primarily systemic and hematological agents
AHA: 2016,4Q,42
T45.8X6 Underdosing of other primarily systemic and hematological agents

T45.9 Poisoning by, adverse effect of and underdosing of unspecified primarily systemic and hematological agent
T45.91 Poisoning by unspecified primarily systemic and hematological agent, accidental (unintentional)
Poisoning by primarily systemic and hematological agent NOS
7 **T45.92 Poisoning by unspecified primarily systemic and hematological agent, intentional self-harm** HCC
T45.93 Poisoning by unspecified primarily systemic and hematological agent, assault
T45.94 Poisoning by unspecified primarily systemic and hematological agent, undetermined
T45.95 Adverse effect of unspecified primarily systemic and hematological agent
T45.96 Underdosing of unspecified primarily systemic and hematological agent

T46 Poisoning by, adverse effect of and underdosing of agents primarily affecting the cardiovascular system
EXCLUDES 1 *poisoning by, adverse effect of and underdosing of metaraminol (T44.4)*

The appropriate 7th character is to be added to each code from category T46.
A initial encounter
D subsequent encounter
S sequela

T46.Ø Poisoning by, adverse effect of and underdosing of cardiac-stimulant glycosides and drugs of similar action
T46.ØX Poisoning by, adverse effect of and underdosing of cardiac-stimulant glycosides and drugs of similar action
T46.ØX1 Poisoning by cardiac-stimulant glycosides and drugs of similar action, accidental (unintentional)
Poisoning by cardiac-stimulant glycosides and drugs of similar action NOS
7 **T46.ØX2 Poisoning by cardiac-stimulant glycosides and drugs of similar action, intentional self-harm** HCC
T46.ØX3 Poisoning by cardiac-stimulant glycosides and drugs of similar action, assault
T46.ØX4 Poisoning by cardiac-stimulant glycosides and drugs of similar action, undetermined
T46.ØX5 Adverse effect of cardiac-stimulant glycosides and drugs of similar action
T46.ØX6 Underdosing of cardiac-stimulant glycosides and drugs of similar action

T46.1 Poisoning by, adverse effect of and underdosing of calcium-channel blockers
T46.1X Poisoning by, adverse effect of and underdosing of calcium-channel blockers
T46.1X1 Poisoning by calcium-channel blockers, accidental (unintentional)
Poisoning by calcium-channel blockers NOS
7 **T46.1X2 Poisoning by calcium-channel blockers, intentional self-harm** HCC
T46.1X3 Poisoning by calcium-channel blockers, assault
T46.1X4 Poisoning by calcium-channel blockers, undetermined
T46.1X5 Adverse effect of calcium-channel blockers
T46.1X6 Underdosing of calcium-channel blockers

T46.2 Poisoning by, adverse effect of and underdosing of other antidysrhythmic drugs, not elsewhere classified
EXCLUDES 1 *poisoning by, adverse effect of and underdosing of beta-adrenoreceptor antagonists (T44.7-)*
T46.2X Poisoning by, adverse effect of and underdosing of other antidysrhythmic drugs
T46.2X1 Poisoning by other antidysrhythmic drugs, accidental (unintentional)
Poisoning by other antidysrhythmic drugs NOS
7 **T46.2X2 Poisoning by other antidysrhythmic drugs, intentional self-harm** HCC
T46.2X3 Poisoning by other antidysrhythmic drugs, assault
T46.2X4 Poisoning by other antidysrhythmic drugs, undetermined
T46.2X5 Adverse effect of other antidysrhythmic drugs
T46.2X6 Underdosing of other antidysrhythmic drugs

T46.3 Poisoning by, adverse effect of and underdosing of coronary vasodilators
Poisoning by, adverse effect of and underdosing of dipyridamole
EXCLUDES 1 *poisoning by, adverse effect of and underdosing of calcium-channel blockers (T46.1)*
T46.3X Poisoning by, adverse effect of and underdosing of coronary vasodilators
T46.3X1 Poisoning by coronary vasodilators, accidental (unintentional)
Poisoning by coronary vasodilators NOS
7 **T46.3X2 Poisoning by coronary vasodilators, intentional self-harm** HCC
T46.3X3 Poisoning by coronary vasodilators, assault
T46.3X4 Poisoning by coronary vasodilators, undetermined
T46.3X5 Adverse effect of coronary vasodilators
T46.3X6 Underdosing of coronary vasodilators

T46.4 Poisoning by, adverse effect of and underdosing of angiotensin-converting-enzyme inhibitors
T46.4X Poisoning by, adverse effect of and underdosing of angiotensin-converting-enzyme inhibitors
T46.4X1 Poisoning by angiotensin-converting-enzyme inhibitors, accidental (unintentional)
Poisoning by angiotensin-converting-enzyme inhibitors NOS
7 **T46.4X2 Poisoning by angiotensin-converting-enzyme inhibitors, intentional self-harm** HCC
T46.4X3 Poisoning by angiotensin-converting-enzyme inhibitors, assault
T46.4X4 Poisoning by angiotensin-converting-enzyme inhibitors, undetermined
T46.4X5 Adverse effect of angiotensin-converting-enzyme inhibitors
T46.4X6 Underdosing of angiotensin-converting-enzyme inhibitors

√5th **T46.5 Poisoning by, adverse effect of and underdosing of other antihypertensive drugs**

EXCLUDES 2 *poisoning by, adverse effect of and underdosing of beta-adrenoreceptor antagonists (T44.7)*
poisoning by, adverse effect of and underdosing of calcium-channel blockers (T46.1)
poisoning by, adverse effect of and underdosing of diuretics (T50.0-T50.2)

√6th **T46.5X Poisoning by, adverse effect of and underdosing of other antihypertensive drugs**

√7th **T46.5X1 Poisoning by other antihypertensive drugs, accidental (unintentional)**
Poisoning by other antihypertensive drugs NOS

7 √7th **T46.5X2 Poisoning by other antihypertensive drugs, intentional self-harm** HCC

√7th **T46.5X3 Poisoning by other antihypertensive drugs, assault**

√7th **T46.5X4 Poisoning by other antihypertensive drugs, undetermined**

√7th **T46.5X5 Adverse effect of other antihypertensive drugs**

√7th **T46.5X6 Underdosing of other antihypertensive drugs**

√5th **T46.6 Poisoning by, adverse effect of and underdosing of antihyperlipidemic and antiarteriosclerotic drugs**

√6th **T46.6X Poisoning by, adverse effect of and underdosing of antihyperlipidemic and antiarteriosclerotic drugs**

√7th **T46.6X1 Poisoning by antihyperlipidemic and antiarteriosclerotic drugs, accidental (unintentional)**
Poisoning by antihyperlipidemic and antiarteriosclerotic drugs NOS

7 √7th **T46.6X2 Poisoning by antihyperlipidemic and antiarteriosclerotic drugs, intentional self-harm** HCC

√7th **T46.6X3 Poisoning by antihyperlipidemic and antiarteriosclerotic drugs, assault**

√7th **T46.6X4 Poisoning by antihyperlipidemic and antiarteriosclerotic drugs, undetermined**

√7th **T46.6X5 Adverse effect of antihyperlipidemic and antiarteriosclerotic drugs**

√7th **T46.6X6 Underdosing of antihyperlipidemic and antiarteriosclerotic drugs**

√5th **T46.7 Poisoning by, adverse effect of and underdosing of peripheral vasodilators**
Poisoning by, adverse effect of and underdosing of nicotinic acid (derivatives)

EXCLUDES 1 *poisoning by, adverse effect of and underdosing of papaverine (T44.3)*

√6th **T46.7X Poisoning by, adverse effect of and underdosing of peripheral vasodilators**

√7th **T46.7X1 Poisoning by peripheral vasodilators, accidental (unintentional)**
Poisoning by peripheral vasodilators NOS

7 √7th **T46.7X2 Poisoning by peripheral vasodilators, intentional self-harm** HCC

√7th **T46.7X3 Poisoning by peripheral vasodilators, assault**

√7th **T46.7X4 Poisoning by peripheral vasodilators, undetermined**

√7th **T46.7X5 Adverse effect of peripheral vasodilators**

√7th **T46.7X6 Underdosing of peripheral vasodilators**

√5th **T46.8 Poisoning by, adverse effect of and underdosing of antivaricose drugs, including sclerosing agents**

√6th **T46.8X Poisoning by, adverse effect of and underdosing of antivaricose drugs, including sclerosing agents**

√7th **T46.8X1 Poisoning by antivaricose drugs, including sclerosing agents, accidental (unintentional)**
Poisoning by antivaricose drugs, including sclerosing agents NOS

7 √7th **T46.8X2 Poisoning by antivaricose drugs, including sclerosing agents, intentional self-harm** HCC

√7th **T46.8X3 Poisoning by antivaricose drugs, including sclerosing agents, assault**

√7th **T46.8X4 Poisoning by antivaricose drugs, including sclerosing agents, undetermined**

√7th **T46.8X5 Adverse effect of antivaricose drugs, including sclerosing agents**

√7th **T46.8X6 Underdosing of antivaricose drugs, including sclerosing agents**

√5th **T46.9 Poisoning by, adverse effect of and underdosing of other and unspecified agents primarily affecting the cardiovascular system**

√6th **T46.90 Poisoning by, adverse effect of and underdosing of unspecified agents primarily affecting the cardiovascular system**

√7th **T46.901 Poisoning by unspecified agents primarily affecting the cardiovascular system, accidental (unintentional)**

7 √7th **T46.902 Poisoning by unspecified agents primarily affecting the cardiovascular system, intentional self-harm** HCC

√7th **T46.903 Poisoning by unspecified agents primarily affecting the cardiovascular system, assault**

√7th **T46.904 Poisoning by unspecified agents primarily affecting the cardiovascular system, undetermined**

√7th **T46.905 Adverse effect of unspecified agents primarily affecting the cardiovascular system**

√7th **T46.906 Underdosing of unspecified agents primarily affecting the cardiovascular system**

√6th **T46.99 Poisoning by, adverse effect of and underdosing of other agents primarily affecting the cardiovascular system**

√7th **T46.991 Poisoning by other agents primarily affecting the cardiovascular system, accidental (unintentional)**

7 √7th **T46.992 Poisoning by other agents primarily affecting the cardiovascular system, intentional self-harm** HCC

√7th **T46.993 Poisoning by other agents primarily affecting the cardiovascular system, assault**

√7th **T46.994 Poisoning by other agents primarily affecting the cardiovascular system, undetermined**

√7th **T46.995 Adverse effect of other agents primarily affecting the cardiovascular system**

√7th **T46.996 Underdosing of other agents primarily affecting the cardiovascular system**

√4th **T47 Poisoning by, adverse effect of and underdosing of agents primarily affecting the gastrointestinal system**

The appropriate 7th character is to be added to each code from category T47.
A initial encounter
D subsequent encounter
S sequela

√5th **T47.0 Poisoning by, adverse effect of and underdosing of histamine H2-receptor blockers**

√6th **T47.0X Poisoning by, adverse effect of and underdosing of histamine H2-receptor blockers**

√7th **T47.0X1 Poisoning by histamine H2-receptor blockers, accidental (unintentional)**
Poisoning by histamine H2-receptor blockers NOS

7 √7th **T47.0X2 Poisoning by histamine H2-receptor blockers, intentional self-harm** HCC

√7th **T47.0X3 Poisoning by histamine H2-receptor blockers, assault**

√7th **T47.0X4 Poisoning by histamine H2-receptor blockers, undetermined**

√7th **T47.0X5 Adverse effect of histamine H2-receptor blockers**

√7th **T47.0X6 Underdosing of histamine H2-receptor blockers**

√5th **T47.1 Poisoning by, adverse effect of and underdosing of other antacids and anti-gastric-secretion drugs**

√6th **T47.1X Poisoning by, adverse effect of and underdosing of other antacids and anti-gastric-secretion drugs**

√7th **T47.1X1 Poisoning by other antacids and anti-gastric-secretion drugs, accidental (unintentional)**
Poisoning by other antacids and anti-gastric-secretion drugs NOS

7 √7th **T47.1X2 Poisoning by other antacids and anti-gastric-secretion drugs, intentional self-harm** HCC

T47.1X3 Poisoning by other antacids and anti-gastric-secretion drugs, assault
T47.1X4 Poisoning by other antacids and anti-gastric-secretion drugs, undetermined
T47.1X5 Adverse effect of other antacids and anti-gastric-secretion drugs
T47.1X6 Underdosing of other antacids and anti-gastric-secretion drugs

T47.2 Poisoning by, adverse effect of and underdosing of stimulant laxatives
T47.2X Poisoning by, adverse effect of and underdosing of stimulant laxatives
T47.2X1 Poisoning by stimulant laxatives, accidental (unintentional)
Poisoning by stimulant laxatives NOS
7 T47.2X2 Poisoning by stimulant laxatives, intentional self-harm HCC
T47.2X3 Poisoning by stimulant laxatives, assault
T47.2X4 Poisoning by stimulant laxatives, undetermined
T47.2X5 Adverse effect of stimulant laxatives
T47.2X6 Underdosing of stimulant laxatives

T47.3 Poisoning by, adverse effect of and underdosing of saline and osmotic laxatives
T47.3X Poisoning by and adverse effect of saline and osmotic laxatives
T47.3X1 Poisoning by saline and osmotic laxatives, accidental (unintentional)
Poisoning by saline and osmotic laxatives NOS
7 T47.3X2 Poisoning by saline and osmotic laxatives, intentional self-harm HCC
T47.3X3 Poisoning by saline and osmotic laxatives, assault
T47.3X4 Poisoning by saline and osmotic laxatives, undetermined
T47.3X5 Adverse effect of saline and osmotic laxatives
T47.3X6 Underdosing of saline and osmotic laxatives

T47.4 Poisoning by, adverse effect of and underdosing of other laxatives
T47.4X Poisoning by, adverse effect of and underdosing of other laxatives
T47.4X1 Poisoning by other laxatives, accidental (unintentional)
Poisoning by other laxatives NOS
7 T47.4X2 Poisoning by other laxatives, intentional self-harm HCC
T47.4X3 Poisoning by other laxatives, assault
T47.4X4 Poisoning by other laxatives, undetermined
T47.4X5 Adverse effect of other laxatives
T47.4X6 Underdosing of other laxatives

T47.5 Poisoning by, adverse effect of and underdosing of digestants
T47.5X Poisoning by, adverse effect of and underdosing of digestants
T47.5X1 Poisoning by digestants, accidental (unintentional)
Poisoning by digestants NOS
7 T47.5X2 Poisoning by digestants, intentional self-harm HCC
T47.5X3 Poisoning by digestants, assault
T47.5X4 Poisoning by digestants, undetermined
T47.5X5 Adverse effect of digestants
T47.5X6 Underdosing of digestants

T47.6 Poisoning by, adverse effect of and underdosing of antidiarrheal drugs
EXCLUDES 2 *poisoning by, adverse effect of and underdosing of systemic antibiotics and other anti-infectives (T36-T37)*
T47.6X Poisoning by, adverse effect of and underdosing of antidiarrheal drugs
T47.6X1 Poisoning by antidiarrheal drugs, accidental (unintentional)
Poisoning by antidiarrheal drugs NOS
7 T47.6X2 Poisoning by antidiarrheal drugs, intentional self-harm HCC
T47.6X3 Poisoning by antidiarrheal drugs, assault
T47.6X4 Poisoning by antidiarrheal drugs, undetermined
T47.6X5 Adverse effect of antidiarrheal drugs
T47.6X6 Underdosing of antidiarrheal drugs

T47.7 Poisoning by, adverse effect of and underdosing of emetics
T47.7X Poisoning by, adverse effect of and underdosing of emetics
T47.7X1 Poisoning by emetics, accidental (unintentional)
Poisoning by emetics NOS
7 T47.7X2 Poisoning by emetics, intentional self-harm HCC
T47.7X3 Poisoning by emetics, assault
T47.7X4 Poisoning by emetics, undetermined
T47.7X5 Adverse effect of emetics
T47.7X6 Underdosing of emetics

T47.8 Poisoning by, adverse effect of and underdosing of other agents primarily affecting gastrointestinal system
T47.8X Poisoning by, adverse effect of and underdosing of other agents primarily affecting gastrointestinal system
T47.8X1 Poisoning by other agents primarily affecting gastrointestinal system, accidental (unintentional)
Poisoning by other agents primarily affecting gastrointestinal system NOS
7 T47.8X2 Poisoning by other agents primarily affecting gastrointestinal system, intentional self-harm HCC
T47.8X3 Poisoning by other agents primarily affecting gastrointestinal system, assault
T47.8X4 Poisoning by other agents primarily affecting gastrointestinal system, undetermined
T47.8X5 Adverse effect of other agents primarily affecting gastrointestinal system
T47.8X6 Underdosing of other agents primarily affecting gastrointestinal system

T47.9 Poisoning by, adverse effect of and underdosing of unspecified agents primarily affecting the gastrointestinal system
T47.91 Poisoning by unspecified agents primarily affecting the gastrointestinal system, accidental (unintentional)
Poisoning by agents primarily affecting the gastrointestinal system NOS
7 T47.92 Poisoning by unspecified agents primarily affecting the gastrointestinal system, intentional self-harm HCC
T47.93 Poisoning by unspecified agents primarily affecting the gastrointestinal system, assault
T47.94 Poisoning by unspecified agents primarily affecting the gastrointestinal system, undetermined
T47.95 Adverse effect of unspecified agents primarily affecting the gastrointestinal system
T47.96 Underdosing of unspecified agents primarily affecting the gastrointestinal system

T48 Poisoning by, adverse effect of and underdosing of agents primarily acting on smooth and skeletal muscles and the respiratory system

The appropriate 7th character is to be added to each code from category T48.
A initial encounter
D subsequent encounter
S sequela

T48.Ø Poisoning by, adverse effect of and underdosing of oxytocic drugs
EXCLUDES 1 *poisoning by, adverse effect of and underdosing of estrogens, progestogens and antagonists (T38.4-T38.6)*
T48.ØX Poisoning by, adverse effect of and underdosing of oxytocic drugs
T48.ØX1 Poisoning by oxytocic drugs, accidental (unintentional)
Poisoning by oxytocic drugs NOS
7 T48.ØX2 Poisoning by oxytocic drugs, intentional self-harm HCC
T48.ØX3 Poisoning by oxytocic drugs, assault

√7th T48.ØX4 Poisoning by oxytocic drugs, undetermined

√7th T48.ØX5 Adverse effect of oxytocic drugs

√7th T48.ØX6 Underdosing of oxytocic drugs

√5th T48.1 Poisoning by, adverse effect of and underdosing of skeletal muscle relaxants [neuromuscular blocking agents]

√6th T48.1X Poisoning by, adverse effect of and underdosing of skeletal muscle relaxants [neuromuscular blocking agents]

√7th T48.1X1 Poisoning by skeletal muscle relaxants [neuromuscular blocking agents], accidental (unintentional)
Poisoning by skeletal muscle relaxants [neuromuscular blocking agents] NOS

7 √7th T48.1X2 Poisoning by skeletal muscle relaxants [neuromuscular blocking agents], intentional self-harm HCC

√7th T48.1X3 Poisoning by skeletal muscle relaxants [neuromuscular blocking agents], assault

√7th T48.1X4 Poisoning by skeletal muscle relaxants [neuromuscular blocking agents], undetermined

√7th T48.1X5 Adverse effect of skeletal muscle relaxants [neuromuscular blocking agents]

√7th T48.1X6 Underdosing of skeletal muscle relaxants [neuromuscular blocking agents]

√5th T48.2 Poisoning by, adverse effect of and underdosing of other and unspecified drugs acting on muscles

√6th T48.2Ø Poisoning by, adverse effect of and underdosing of unspecified drugs acting on muscles

√7th T48.2Ø1 Poisoning by unspecified drugs acting on muscles, accidental (unintentional)
Poisoning by unspecified drugs acting on muscles NOS

7 √7th T48.2Ø2 Poisoning by unspecified drugs acting on muscles, intentional self-harm HCC

√7th T48.2Ø3 Poisoning by unspecified drugs acting on muscles, assault

√7th T48.2Ø4 Poisoning by unspecified drugs acting on muscles, undetermined

√7th T48.2Ø5 Adverse effect of unspecified drugs acting on muscles

√7th T48.2Ø6 Underdosing of unspecified drugs acting on muscles

√6th T48.29 Poisoning by, adverse effect of and underdosing of other drugs acting on muscles

√7th T48.291 Poisoning by other drugs acting on muscles, accidental (unintentional)
Poisoning by other drugs acting on muscles NOS

7 √7th T48.292 Poisoning by other drugs acting on muscles, intentional self-harm HCC

√7th T48.293 Poisoning by other drugs acting on muscles, assault

√7th T48.294 Poisoning by other drugs acting on muscles, undetermined

√7th T48.295 Adverse effect of other drugs acting on muscles

√7th T48.296 Underdosing of other drugs acting on muscles

√5th T48.3 Poisoning by, adverse effect of and underdosing of antitussives

√6th T48.3X Poisoning by, adverse effect of and underdosing of antitussives

√7th T48.3X1 Poisoning by antitussives, accidental (unintentional)
Poisoning by antitussives NOS

7 √7th T48.3X2 Poisoning by antitussives, intentional self-harm HCC

√7th T48.3X3 Poisoning by antitussives, assault

√7th T48.3X4 Poisoning by antitussives, undetermined

√7th T48.3X5 Adverse effect of antitussives

√7th T48.3X6 Underdosing of antitussives

√5th T48.4 Poisoning by, adverse effect of and underdosing of expectorants

√6th T48.4X Poisoning by, adverse effect of and underdosing of expectorants

√7th T48.4X1 Poisoning by expectorants, accidental (unintentional)
Poisoning by expectorants NOS

7 √7th T48.4X2 Poisoning by expectorants, intentional self-harm HCC

√7th T48.4X3 Poisoning by expectorants, assault

√7th T48.4X4 Poisoning by expectorants, undetermined

√7th T48.4X5 Adverse effect of expectorants

√7th T48.4X6 Underdosing of expectorants

√5th T48.5 Poisoning by, adverse effect of and underdosing of other anti-common-cold drugs
Poisoning by, adverse effect of and underdosing of decongestants

EXCLUDES 2 *poisoning by, adverse effect of and underdosing of antipyretics, NEC (T39.9-)*
poisoning by, adverse effect of and underdosing of non-steroidal antiinflammatory drugs (T39.3-)
poisoning by, adverse effect of and underdosing of salicylates (T39.Ø-)

√6th T48.5X Poisoning by, adverse effect of and underdosing of other anti-common-cold drugs

√7th T48.5X1 Poisoning by other anti-common-cold drugs, accidental (unintentional)
Poisoning by other anti-common-cold drugs NOS

7 √7th T48.5X2 Poisoning by other anti-common-cold drugs, intentional self-harm HCC

√7th T48.5X3 Poisoning by other anti-common-cold drugs, assault

√7th T48.5X4 Poisoning by other anti-common-cold drugs, undetermined

√7th T48.5X5 Adverse effect of other anti-common-cold drugs

√7th T48.5X6 Underdosing of other anti-common-cold drugs

√5th T48.6 Poisoning by, adverse effect of and underdosing of antiasthmatics, not elsewhere classified
Poisoning by, adverse effect of and underdosing of beta-adrenoreceptor agonists used in asthma therapy

EXCLUDES 1 *poisoning by, adverse effect of and underdosing of anterior pituitary [adenohypophyseal] hormones (T38.8)*
poisoning by, adverse effect of and underdosing of beta-adrenoreceptor agonists not used in asthma therapy (T44.5)

√6th T48.6X Poisoning by, adverse effect of and underdosing of antiasthmatics

√7th T48.6X1 Poisoning by antiasthmatics, accidental (unintentional)
Poisoning by antiasthmatics NOS

7 √7th T48.6X2 Poisoning by antiasthmatics, intentional self-harm HCC

√7th T48.6X3 Poisoning by antiasthmatics, assault

√7th T48.6X4 Poisoning by antiasthmatics, undetermined

√7th T48.6X5 Adverse effect of antiasthmatics

√7th T48.6X6 Underdosing of antiasthmatics

√5th T48.9 Poisoning by, adverse effect of and underdosing of other and unspecified agents primarily acting on the respiratory system

√6th T48.9Ø Poisoning by, adverse effect of and underdosing of unspecified agents primarily acting on the respiratory system

√7th T48.9Ø1 Poisoning by unspecified agents primarily acting on the respiratory system, accidental (unintentional)

7 √7th T48.9Ø2 Poisoning by unspecified agents primarily acting on the respiratory system, intentional self-harm HCC

√7th T48.9Ø3 Poisoning by unspecified agents primarily acting on the respiratory system, assault

√7th T48.9Ø4 Poisoning by unspecified agents primarily acting on the respiratory system, undetermined

T48.905 Adverse effect of unspecified agents primarily acting on the respiratory system
T48.906 Underdosing of unspecified agents primarily acting on the respiratory system
T48.99 Poisoning by, adverse effect of and underdosing of other agents primarily acting on the respiratory system
T48.991 Poisoning by other agents primarily acting on the respiratory system, accidental (unintentional)
7 T48.992 Poisoning by other agents primarily acting on the respiratory system, intentional self-harm HCC
T48.993 Poisoning by other agents primarily acting on the respiratory system, assault
T48.994 Poisoning by other agents primarily acting on the respiratory system, undetermined
T48.995 Adverse effect of other agents primarily acting on the respiratory system
T48.996 Underdosing of other agents primarily acting on the respiratory system

T49 Poisoning by, adverse effect of and underdosing of topical agents primarily affecting skin and mucous membrane and by ophthalmological, otorhinolaryngological and dental drugs

INCLUDES poisoning by, adverse effect of and underdosing of glucocorticoids, topically used

The appropriate 7th character is to be added to each code from category T49.
A initial encounter
D subsequent encounter
S sequela

T49.Ø Poisoning by, adverse effect of and underdosing of local antifungal, anti-infective and anti-inflammatory drugs
T49.ØX Poisoning by, adverse effect of and underdosing of local antifungal, anti-infective and anti-inflammatory drugs
T49.ØX1 Poisoning by local antifungal, anti-infective and anti-inflammatory drugs, accidental (unintentional)
Poisoning by local antifungal, anti-infective and anti-inflammatory drugs NOS
7 T49.ØX2 Poisoning by local antifungal, anti-infective and anti-inflammatory drugs, intentional self-harm HCC
T49.ØX3 Poisoning by local antifungal, anti-infective and anti-inflammatory drugs, assault
T49.ØX4 Poisoning by local antifungal, anti-infective and anti-inflammatory drugs, undetermined
T49.ØX5 Adverse effect of local antifungal, anti-infective and anti-inflammatory drugs
T49.ØX6 Underdosing of local antifungal, anti-infective and anti-inflammatory drugs

T49.1 Poisoning by, adverse effect of and underdosing of antipruritics
T49.1X Poisoning by, adverse effect of and underdosing of antipruritics
T49.1X1 Poisoning by antipruritics, accidental (unintentional)
Poisoning by antipruritics NOS
7 T49.1X2 Poisoning by antipruritics, intentional self-harm HCC
T49.1X3 Poisoning by antipruritics, assault
T49.1X4 Poisoning by antipruritics, undetermined
T49.1X5 Adverse effect of antipruritics
T49.1X6 Underdosing of antipruritics

T49.2 Poisoning by, adverse effect of and underdosing of local astringents and local detergents
T49.2X Poisoning by, adverse effect of and underdosing of local astringents and local detergents
T49.2X1 Poisoning by local astringents and local detergents, accidental (unintentional)
Poisoning by local astringents and local detergents NOS
7 T49.2X2 Poisoning by local astringents and local detergents, intentional self-harm HCC
T49.2X3 Poisoning by local astringents and local detergents, assault
T49.2X4 Poisoning by local astringents and local detergents, undetermined
T49.2X5 Adverse effect of local astringents and local detergents
T49.2X6 Underdosing of local astringents and local detergents

T49.3 Poisoning by, adverse effect of and underdosing of emollients, demulcents and protectants
T49.3X Poisoning by, adverse effect of and underdosing of emollients, demulcents and protectants
T49.3X1 Poisoning by emollients, demulcents and protectants, accidental (unintentional)
Poisoning by emollients, demulcents and protectants NOS
7 T49.3X2 Poisoning by emollients, demulcents and protectants, intentional self-harm HCC
T49.3X3 Poisoning by emollients, demulcents and protectants, assault
T49.3X4 Poisoning by emollients, demulcents and protectants, undetermined
T49.3X5 Adverse effect of emollients, demulcents and protectants
T49.3X6 Underdosing of emollients, demulcents and protectants

T49.4 Poisoning by, adverse effect of and underdosing of keratolytics, keratoplastics, and other hair treatment drugs and preparations
T49.4X Poisoning by, adverse effect of and underdosing of keratolytics, keratoplastics, and other hair treatment drugs and preparations
T49.4X1 Poisoning by keratolytics, keratoplastics, and other hair treatment drugs and preparations, accidental (unintentional)
Poisoning by keratolytics, keratoplastics, and other hair treatment drugs and preparations NOS
7 T49.4X2 Poisoning by keratolytics, keratoplastics, and other hair treatment drugs and preparations, intentional self-harm HCC
T49.4X3 Poisoning by keratolytics, keratoplastics, and other hair treatment drugs and preparations, assault
T49.4X4 Poisoning by keratolytics, keratoplastics, and other hair treatment drugs and preparations, undetermined
T49.4X5 Adverse effect of keratolytics, keratoplastics, and other hair treatment drugs and preparations
T49.4X6 Underdosing of keratolytics, keratoplastics, and other hair treatment drugs and preparations

T49.5 Poisoning by, adverse effect of and underdosing of ophthalmological drugs and preparations
T49.5X Poisoning by, adverse effect of and underdosing of ophthalmological drugs and preparations
T49.5X1 Poisoning by ophthalmological drugs and preparations, accidental (unintentional)
Poisoning by ophthalmological drugs and preparations NOS
7 T49.5X2 Poisoning by ophthalmological drugs and preparations, intentional self-harm HCC
T49.5X3 Poisoning by ophthalmological drugs and preparations, assault
T49.5X4 Poisoning by ophthalmological drugs and preparations, undetermined
T49.5X5 Adverse effect of ophthalmological drugs and preparations
T49.5X6 Underdosing of ophthalmological drugs and preparations

T49.6 Poisoning by, adverse effect of and underdosing of otorhinolaryngological drugs and preparations
T49.6X Poisoning by, adverse effect of and underdosing of otorhinolaryngological drugs and preparations
T49.6X1 Poisoning by otorhinolaryngological drugs and preparations, accidental (unintentional)
Poisoning by otorhinolaryngological drugs and preparations NOS

7 √7th T49.6X2 **Poisoning by otorhinolaryngological drugs and preparations, intentional self-harm** HCC
√7th T49.6X3 **Poisoning by otorhinolaryngological drugs and preparations, assault**
√7th T49.6X4 **Poisoning by otorhinolaryngological drugs and preparations, undetermined**
√7th T49.6X5 **Adverse effect of otorhinolaryngological drugs and preparations**
√7th T49.6X6 **Underdosing of otorhinolaryngological drugs and preparations**

√5th T49.7 **Poisoning by, adverse effect of and underdosing of dental drugs, topically applied**
√6th T49.7X **Poisoning by, adverse effect of and underdosing of dental drugs, topically applied**
√7th T49.7X1 **Poisoning by dental drugs, topically applied, accidental (unintentional)**
Poisoning by dental drugs, topically applied NOS
7 √7th T49.7X2 **Poisoning by dental drugs, topically applied, intentional self-harm** HCC
√7th T49.7X3 **Poisoning by dental drugs, topically applied, assault**
√7th T49.7X4 **Poisoning by dental drugs, topically applied, undetermined**
√7th T49.7X5 **Adverse effect of dental drugs, topically applied**
√7th T49.7X6 **Underdosing of dental drugs, topically applied**

√5th T49.8 **Poisoning by, adverse effect of and underdosing of other topical agents**
Poisoning by, adverse effect of and underdosing of spermicides
√6th T49.8X **Poisoning by, adverse effect of and underdosing of other topical agents**
√7th T49.8X1 **Poisoning by other topical agents, accidental (unintentional)**
Poisoning by other topical agents NOS
7 √7th T49.8X2 **Poisoning by other topical agents, intentional self-harm** HCC
√7th T49.8X3 **Poisoning by other topical agents, assault**
√7th T49.8X4 **Poisoning by other topical agents, undetermined**
√7th T49.8X5 **Adverse effect of other topical agents**
√7th T49.8X6 **Underdosing of other topical agents**

√5th T49.9 **Poisoning by, adverse effect of and underdosing of unspecified topical agent**
√x7th T49.91 **Poisoning by unspecified topical agent, accidental (unintentional)**
7 √x7th T49.92 **Poisoning by unspecified topical agent, intentional self-harm** HCC
√x7th T49.93 **Poisoning by unspecified topical agent, assault**
√x7th T49.94 **Poisoning by unspecified topical agent, undetermined**
√x7th T49.95 **Adverse effect of unspecified topical agent**
√x7th T49.96 **Underdosing of unspecified topical agent**

√4th T50 **Poisoning by, adverse effect of and underdosing of diuretics and other and unspecified drugs, medicaments and biological substances**

The appropriate 7th character is to be added to each code from category T50.
A initial encounter
D subsequent encounter
S sequela

√5th T50.0 **Poisoning by, adverse effect of and underdosing of mineralocorticoids and their antagonists**
√6th T50.0X **Poisoning by, adverse effect of and underdosing of mineralocorticoids and their antagonists**
√7th T50.0X1 **Poisoning by mineralocorticoids and their antagonists, accidental (unintentional)**
Poisoning by mineralocorticoids and their antagonists NOS
7 √7th T50.0X2 **Poisoning by mineralocorticoids and their antagonists, intentional self-harm** HCC
√7th T50.0X3 **Poisoning by mineralocorticoids and their antagonists, assault**
√7th T50.0X4 **Poisoning by mineralocorticoids and their antagonists, undetermined**
√7th T50.0X5 **Adverse effect of mineralocorticoids and their antagonists**
√7th T50.0X6 **Underdosing of mineralocorticoids and their antagonists**

√5th T50.1 **Poisoning by, adverse effect of and underdosing of loop [high-ceiling] diuretics**
√6th T50.1X **Poisoning by, adverse effect of and underdosing of loop [high-ceiling] diuretics**
√7th T50.1X1 **Poisoning by loop [high-ceiling] diuretics, accidental (unintentional)**
Poisoning by loop [high-ceiling] diuretics NOS
7 √7th T50.1X2 **Poisoning by loop [high-ceiling] diuretics, intentional self-harm** HCC
√7th T50.1X3 **Poisoning by loop [high-ceiling] diuretics, assault**
√7th T50.1X4 **Poisoning by loop [high-ceiling] diuretics, undetermined**
√7th T50.1X5 **Adverse effect of loop [high-ceiling] diuretics**
√7th T50.1X6 **Underdosing of loop [high-ceiling] diuretics**

√5th T50.2 **Poisoning by, adverse effect of and underdosing of carbonic-anhydrase inhibitors, benzothiadiazides and other diuretics**
Poisoning by, adverse effect of and underdosing of acetazolamide
√6th T50.2X **Poisoning by, adverse effect of and underdosing of carbonic-anhydrase inhibitors, benzothiadiazides and other diuretics**
√7th T50.2X1 **Poisoning by carbonic-anhydrase inhibitors, benzothiadiazides and other diuretics, accidental (unintentional)**
Poisoning by carbonic-anhydrase inhibitors, benzothiadiazides and other diuretics NOS
7 √7th T50.2X2 **Poisoning by carbonic-anhydrase inhibitors, benzothiadiazides and other diuretics, intentional self-harm** HCC
√7th T50.2X3 **Poisoning by carbonic-anhydrase inhibitors, benzothiadiazides and other diuretics, assault**
√7th T50.2X4 **Poisoning by carbonic-anhydrase inhibitors, benzothiadiazides and other diuretics, undetermined**
√7th T50.2X5 **Adverse effect of carbonic-anhydrase inhibitors, benzothiadiazides and other diuretics**
√7th T50.2X6 **Underdosing of carbonic-anhydrase inhibitors, benzothiadiazides and other diuretics**

√5th T50.3 **Poisoning by, adverse effect of and underdosing of electrolytic, caloric and water-balance agents**
Poisoning by, adverse effect of and underdosing of oral rehydration salts
√6th T50.3X **Poisoning by, adverse effect of and underdosing of electrolytic, caloric and water-balance agents**
√7th T50.3X1 **Poisoning by electrolytic, caloric and water-balance agents, accidental (unintentional)**
Poisoning by electrolytic, caloric and water-balance agents NOS
7 √7th T50.3X2 **Poisoning by electrolytic, caloric and water-balance agents, intentional self-harm** HCC
√7th T50.3X3 **Poisoning by electrolytic, caloric and water-balance agents, assault**
√7th T50.3X4 **Poisoning by electrolytic, caloric and water-balance agents, undetermined**
√7th T50.3X5 **Adverse effect of electrolytic, caloric and water-balance agents**
√7th T50.3X6 **Underdosing of electrolytic, caloric and water-balance agents**

√5th T50.4 **Poisoning by, adverse effect of and underdosing of drugs affecting uric acid metabolism**
√6th T50.4X **Poisoning by, adverse effect of and underdosing of drugs affecting uric acid metabolism**
√7th T50.4X1 **Poisoning by drugs affecting uric acid metabolism, accidental (unintentional)**
Poisoning by drugs affecting uric acid metabolism NOS
7 √7th T50.4X2 **Poisoning by drugs affecting uric acid metabolism, intentional self-harm** HCC
√7th T50.4X3 **Poisoning by drugs affecting uric acid metabolism, assault**

T50.4X4 **Poisoning by drugs affecting uric acid metabolism, undetermined**
T50.4X5 **Adverse effect of drugs affecting uric acid metabolism**
T50.4X6 **Underdosing of drugs affecting uric acid metabolism**

T50.5 **Poisoning by, adverse effect of and underdosing of appetite depressants**
T50.5X **Poisoning by, adverse effect of and underdosing of appetite depressants**
T50.5X1 **Poisoning by appetite depressants, accidental (unintentional)**
Poisoning by appetite depressants NOS
7 T50.5X2 **Poisoning by appetite depressants, intentional self-harm** HCC
T50.5X3 **Poisoning by appetite depressants, assault**
T50.5X4 **Poisoning by appetite depressants, undetermined**
T50.5X5 **Adverse effect of appetite depressants**
T50.5X6 **Underdosing of appetite depressants**

T50.6 **Poisoning by, adverse effect of and underdosing of antidotes and chelating agents**
Poisoning by, adverse effect of and underdosing of alcohol deterrents
T50.6X **Poisoning by, adverse effect of and underdosing of antidotes and chelating agents**
T50.6X1 **Poisoning by antidotes and chelating agents, accidental (unintentional)**
Poisoning by antidotes and chelating agents NOS
7 T50.6X2 **Poisoning by antidotes and chelating agents, intentional self-harm** HCC
T50.6X3 **Poisoning by antidotes and chelating agents, assault**
T50.6X4 **Poisoning by antidotes and chelating agents, undetermined**
T50.6X5 **Adverse effect of antidotes and chelating agents**
T50.6X6 **Underdosing of antidotes and chelating agents**

T50.7 **Poisoning by, adverse effect of and underdosing of analeptics and opioid receptor antagonists**
T50.7X **Poisoning by, adverse effect of and underdosing of analeptics and opioid receptor antagonists**
T50.7X1 **Poisoning by analeptics and opioid receptor antagonists, accidental (unintentional)**
Poisoning by analeptics and opioid receptor antagonists NOS
7 T50.7X2 **Poisoning by analeptics and opioid receptor antagonists, intentional self-harm** HCC
T50.7X3 **Poisoning by analeptics and opioid receptor antagonists, assault**
T50.7X4 **Poisoning by analeptics and opioid receptor antagonists, undetermined**
T50.7X5 **Adverse effect of analeptics and opioid receptor antagonists**
T50.7X6 **Underdosing of analeptics and opioid receptor antagonists**

T50.8 **Poisoning by, adverse effect of and underdosing of diagnostic agents**
T50.8X **Poisoning by, adverse effect of and underdosing of diagnostic agents**
T50.8X1 **Poisoning by diagnostic agents, accidental (unintentional)**
Poisoning by diagnostic agents NOS
7 T50.8X2 **Poisoning by diagnostic agents, intentional self-harm** HCC
T50.8X3 **Poisoning by diagnostic agents, assault**
T50.8X4 **Poisoning by diagnostic agents, undetermined**
T50.8X5 **Adverse effect of diagnostic agents**
T50.8X6 **Underdosing of diagnostic agents**

T50.A **Poisoning by, adverse effect of and underdosing of bacterial vaccines**
T50.A1 **Poisoning by, adverse effect of and underdosing of pertussis vaccine, including combinations with a pertussis component**
T50.A11 **Poisoning by pertussis vaccine, including combinations with a pertussis component, accidental (unintentional)**
7 T50.A12 **Poisoning by pertussis vaccine, including combinations with a pertussis component, intentional self-harm** HCC
T50.A13 **Poisoning by pertussis vaccine, including combinations with a pertussis component, assault**
T50.A14 **Poisoning by pertussis vaccine, including combinations with a pertussis component, undetermined**
T50.A15 **Adverse effect of pertussis vaccine, including combinations with a pertussis component**
T50.A16 **Underdosing of pertussis vaccine, including combinations with a pertussis component**
T50.A2 **Poisoning by, adverse effect of and underdosing of mixed bacterial vaccines without a pertussis component**
T50.A21 **Poisoning by mixed bacterial vaccines without a pertussis component, accidental (unintentional)**
7 T50.A22 **Poisoning by mixed bacterial vaccines without a pertussis component, intentional self-harm** HCC
T50.A23 **Poisoning by mixed bacterial vaccines without a pertussis component, assault**
T50.A24 **Poisoning by mixed bacterial vaccines without a pertussis component, undetermined**
T50.A25 **Adverse effect of mixed bacterial vaccines without a pertussis component**
T50.A26 **Underdosing of mixed bacterial vaccines without a pertussis component**
T50.A9 **Poisoning by, adverse effect of and underdosing of other bacterial vaccines**
T50.A91 **Poisoning by other bacterial vaccines, accidental (unintentional)**
7 T50.A92 **Poisoning by other bacterial vaccines, intentional self-harm** HCC
T50.A93 **Poisoning by other bacterial vaccines, assault**
T50.A94 **Poisoning by other bacterial vaccines, undetermined**
T50.A95 **Adverse effect of other bacterial vaccines**
T50.A96 **Underdosing of other bacterial vaccines**

T50.B **Poisoning by, adverse effect of and underdosing of viral vaccines**
T50.B1 **Poisoning by, adverse effect of and underdosing of smallpox vaccines**
T50.B11 **Poisoning by smallpox vaccines, accidental (unintentional)**
7 T50.B12 **Poisoning by smallpox vaccines, intentional self-harm** HCC
T50.B13 **Poisoning by smallpox vaccines, assault**
T50.B14 **Poisoning by smallpox vaccines, undetermined**
T50.B15 **Adverse effect of smallpox vaccines**
T50.B16 **Underdosing of smallpox vaccines**
T50.B9 **Poisoning by, adverse effect of and underdosing of other viral vaccines**
T50.B91 **Poisoning by other viral vaccines, accidental (unintentional)**
T50.90 **Poisoning by, adverse effect of and underdosing of unspecified drugs, medicaments and biological substances**
7 T50.B92 **Poisoning by other viral vaccines, intentional self-harm** HCC
T50.B93 **Poisoning by other viral vaccines, assault**
T50.B94 **Poisoning by other viral vaccines, undetermined**
T50.B95 **Adverse effect of other viral vaccines**
T50.B96 **Underdosing of other viral vaccines**

5th **T50.Z Poisoning by, adverse effect of and underdosing of other vaccines and biological substances**

6th **T50.Z1 Poisoning by, adverse effect of and underdosing of immunoglobulin**

7th **T50.Z11 Poisoning by immunoglobulin, accidental (unintentional)**

7 7th **T50.Z12 Poisoning by immunoglobulin, intentional self-harm** HCC

7th **T50.Z13 Poisoning by immunoglobulin, assault**

7th **T50.Z14 Poisoning by immunoglobulin, undetermined**

7th **T50.Z15 Adverse effect of immunoglobulin**

7th **T50.Z16 Underdosing of immunoglobulin**

6th **T50.Z9 Poisoning by, adverse effect of and underdosing of other vaccines and biological substances**

7th **T50.Z91 Poisoning by other vaccines and biological substances, accidental (unintentional)**

7 7th **T50.Z92 Poisoning by other vaccines and biological substances, intentional self-harm** HCC

7th **T50.Z93 Poisoning by other vaccines and biological substances, assault**

7th **T50.Z94 Poisoning by other vaccines and biological substances, undetermined**

7th **T50.Z95 Adverse effect of other vaccines and biological substances**
AHA: 2020,1Q,18

7th **T50.Z96 Underdosing of other vaccines and biological substances**

5th **T50.9 Poisoning by, adverse effect of and underdosing of other and unspecified drugs, medicaments and biological substances**

7th **T50.901 Poisoning by unspecified drugs, medicaments and biological substances, accidental (unintentional)**

7 7th **T50.902 Poisoning by unspecified drugs, medicaments and biological substances, intentional self-harm** HCC

7th **T50.903 Poisoning by unspecified drugs, medicaments and biological substances, assault**

7th **T50.904 Poisoning by unspecified drugs, medicaments and biological substances, undetermined**

7th **T50.905 Adverse effect of unspecified drugs, medicaments and biological substances**

7th **T50.906 Underdosing of unspecified drugs, medicaments and biological substances**

6th **T50.91 Poisoning by, adverse effect of and underdosing of multiple unspecified drugs, medicaments and biological substances**
Multiple drug ingestion NOS
Code also any specific drugs, medicaments and biological substances

7th **T50.911 Poisoning by multiple unspecified drugs, medicaments and biological substances, accidental (unintentional)**

7 7th **T50.912 Poisoning by multiple unspecified drugs, medicaments and biological substances, intentional self-harm** HCC

7th **T50.913 Poisoning by multiple unspecified drugs, medicaments and biological substances, assault**

7th **T50.914 Poisoning by multiple unspecified drugs, medicaments and biological substances, undetermined**

7th **T50.915 Adverse effect of multiple unspecified drugs, medicaments and biological substances**

7th **T50.916 Underdosing of multiple unspecified drugs, medicaments and biological substances**

6th **T50.99 Poisoning by, adverse effect of and underdosing of other drugs, medicaments and biological substances**

7th **T50.991 Poisoning by other drugs, medicaments and biological substances, accidental (unintentional)**

7 7th **T50.992 Poisoning by other drugs, medicaments and biological substances, intentional self-harm** HCC

7th **T50.993 Poisoning by other drugs, medicaments and biological substances, assault**

7th **T50.994 Poisoning by other drugs, medicaments and biological substances, undetermined**

7th **T50.995 Adverse effect of other drugs, medicaments and biological substances**

7th **T50.996 Underdosing of other drugs, medicaments and biological substances**

Toxic effects of substances chiefly nonmedicinal as to source (T51-T65)

NOTE When no intent is indicated code to accidental. Undetermined intent is only for use when there is specific documentation in the record that the intent of the toxic effect cannot be determined.

Use additional code(s) for all associated manifestations of toxic effect, such as:
personal history of foreign body fully removed (Z87.821)
respiratory conditions due to external agents (J60-J70)
to identify any retained foreign body, if applicable (Z18.-)

EXCLUDES 1 *contact with and (suspected) exposure to toxic substances (Z77.-)*

AHA: 2017,1Q,39-40

4th **T51 Toxic effect of alcohol**

The appropriate 7th character is to be added to each code from category T51.
A initial encounter
D subsequent encounter
S sequela

5th **T51.0 Toxic effect of ethanol**
Toxic effect of ethyl alcohol
EXCLUDES 2 *acute alcohol intoxication or "hangover" effects (F10.129, F10.229, F10.929)*
drunkenness (F10.129, F10.229, F10.929)
pathological alcohol intoxication (F10.129, F10.229, F10.929)

6th **T51.0X Toxic effect of ethanol**

6 7th **T51.0X1 Toxic effect of ethanol, accidental (unintentional)** HCC
Toxic effect of ethanol NOS

7 7th **T51.0X2 Toxic effect of ethanol, intentional self-harm** HCC

7th **T51.0X3 Toxic effect of ethanol, assault**

6 7th **T51.0X4 Toxic effect of ethanol, undetermined** HCC

5th **T51.1 Toxic effect of methanol**
Toxic effect of methyl alcohol

6th **T51.1X Toxic effect of methanol**

7th **T51.1X1 Toxic effect of methanol, accidental (unintentional)**
Toxic effect of methanol NOS

7 7th **T51.1X2 Toxic effect of methanol, intentional self-harm** HCC

7th **T51.1X3 Toxic effect of methanol, assault**

7th **T51.1X4 Toxic effect of methanol, undetermined**

5th **T51.2 Toxic effect of 2-Propanol**
Toxic effect of isopropyl alcohol

6th **T51.2X Toxic effect of 2-Propanol**

7th **T51.2X1 Toxic effect of 2-Propanol, accidental (unintentional)**
Toxic effect of 2-Propanol NOS

7 7th **T51.2X2 Toxic effect of 2-Propanol, intentional self-harm** HCC

7th **T51.2X3 Toxic effect of 2-Propanol, assault**

7th **T51.2X4 Toxic effect of 2-Propanol, undetermined**

5th **T51.3 Toxic effect of fusel oil**
Toxic effect of amyl alcohol
Toxic effect of butyl [1-butanol] alcohol
Toxic effect of propyl [1-propanol] alcohol

6th **T51.3X Toxic effect of fusel oil**

7th **T51.3X1 Toxic effect of fusel oil, accidental (unintentional)**
Toxic effect of fusel oil NOS

7 7th **T51.3X2 Toxic effect of fusel oil, intentional self-harm** HCC

7th **T51.3X3 Toxic effect of fusel oil, assault**

7th **T51.3X4 Toxic effect of fusel oil, undetermined**

✓5th T51.8 **Toxic effect of other alcohols**
✓6th T51.8X **Toxic effect of other alcohols**
✓7th T51.8X1 **Toxic effect of other alcohols, accidental (unintentional)**
Toxic effect of other alcohols NOS
7 ✓7th T51.8X2 **Toxic effect of other alcohols, intentional self-harm** HCC
✓7th T51.8X3 **Toxic effect of other alcohols, assault**
✓7th T51.8X4 **Toxic effect of other alcohols, undetermined**
✓5th T51.9 **Toxic effect of unspecified alcohol**
✓x7th T51.91 **Toxic effect of unspecified alcohol, accidental (unintentional)**
7 ✓x7th T51.92 **Toxic effect of unspecified alcohol, intentional self-harm** HCC
✓x7th T51.93 **Toxic effect of unspecified alcohol, assault**
✓x7th T51.94 **Toxic effect of unspecified alcohol, undetermined**

✓4th **T52 Toxic effect of organic solvents**
EXCLUDES 1 *halogen derivatives of aliphatic and aromatic hydrocarbons (T53.-)*

The appropriate 7th character is to be added to each code from category T52.
A initial encounter
D subsequent encounter
S sequela

✓5th T52.0 **Toxic effects of petroleum products**
Toxic effects of ether petroleum
Toxic effects of gasoline [petrol]
Toxic effects of kerosene [paraffin oil]
Toxic effects of naphtha petroleum
Toxic effects of paraffin wax
Toxic effects of spirit petroleum
✓6th T52.0X **Toxic effects of petroleum products**
✓7th T52.0X1 **Toxic effect of petroleum products, accidental (unintentional)**
Toxic effects of petroleum products NOS
7 ✓7th T52.0X2 **Toxic effect of petroleum products, intentional self-harm** HCC
✓7th T52.0X3 **Toxic effect of petroleum products, assault**
✓7th T52.0X4 **Toxic effect of petroleum products, undetermined**
✓5th T52.1 **Toxic effects of benzene**
EXCLUDES 1 *homologues of benzene (T52.2)*
nitroderivatives and aminoderivatives of benzene and its homologues (T65.3)
✓6th T52.1X **Toxic effects of benzene**
✓7th T52.1X1 **Toxic effect of benzene, accidental (unintentional)**
Toxic effects of benzene NOS
7 ✓7th T52.1X2 **Toxic effect of benzene, intentional self-harm** HCC
✓7th T52.1X3 **Toxic effect of benzene, assault**
✓7th T52.1X4 **Toxic effect of benzene, undetermined**
✓5th T52.2 **Toxic effects of homologues of benzene**
Toxic effects of toluene [methylbenzene]
Toxic effects of xylene [dimethylbenzene]
✓6th T52.2X **Toxic effects of homologues of benzene**
✓7th T52.2X1 **Toxic effect of homologues of benzene, accidental (unintentional)**
Toxic effects of homologues of benzene NOS
7 ✓7th T52.2X2 **Toxic effect of homologues of benzene, intentional self-harm** HCC
✓7th T52.2X3 **Toxic effect of homologues of benzene, assault**
✓7th T52.2X4 **Toxic effect of homologues of benzene, undetermined**
✓5th T52.3 **Toxic effects of glycols**
✓6th T52.3X **Toxic effects of glycols**
✓7th T52.3X1 **Toxic effect of glycols, accidental (unintentional)**
Toxic effects of glycols NOS
7 ✓7th T52.3X2 **Toxic effect of glycols, intentional self-harm** HCC
✓7th T52.3X3 **Toxic effect of glycols, assault**
✓7th T52.3X4 **Toxic effect of glycols, undetermined**
✓5th T52.4 **Toxic effects of ketones**
✓6th T52.4X **Toxic effects of ketones**
✓7th T52.4X1 **Toxic effect of ketones, accidental (unintentional)**
Toxic effects of ketones NOS
7 ✓7th T52.4X2 **Toxic effect of ketones, intentional self-harm** HCC
✓7th T52.4X3 **Toxic effect of ketones, assault**
✓7th T52.4X4 **Toxic effect of ketones, undetermined**
✓5th T52.8 **Toxic effects of other organic solvents**
✓6th T52.8X **Toxic effects of other organic solvents**
✓7th T52.8X1 **Toxic effect of other organic solvents, accidental (unintentional)**
Toxic effects of other organic solvents NOS
7 ✓7th T52.8X2 **Toxic effect of other organic solvents, intentional self-harm** HCC
✓7th T52.8X3 **Toxic effect of other organic solvents, assault**
✓7th T52.8X4 **Toxic effect of other organic solvents, undetermined**
✓5th T52.9 **Toxic effects of unspecified organic solvent**
✓x7th T52.91 **Toxic effect of unspecified organic solvent, accidental (unintentional)**
7 ✓x7th T52.92 **Toxic effect of unspecified organic solvent, intentional self-harm** HCC
✓x7th T52.93 **Toxic effect of unspecified organic solvent, assault**
✓x7th T52.94 **Toxic effect of unspecified organic solvent, undetermined**

✓4th **T53 Toxic effect of halogen derivatives of aliphatic and aromatic hydrocarbons**

The appropriate 7th character is to be added to each code from category T53.
A initial encounter
D subsequent encounter
S sequela

✓5th T53.0 **Toxic effects of carbon tetrachloride**
Toxic effects of tetrachloromethane
✓6th T53.0X **Toxic effects of carbon tetrachloride**
✓7th T53.0X1 **Toxic effect of carbon tetrachloride, accidental (unintentional)**
Toxic effects of carbon tetrachloride NOS
7 ✓7th T53.0X2 **Toxic effect of carbon tetrachloride, intentional self-harm** HCC
✓7th T53.0X3 **Toxic effect of carbon tetrachloride, assault**
✓7th T53.0X4 **Toxic effect of carbon tetrachloride, undetermined**
✓5th T53.1 **Toxic effects of chloroform**
Toxic effects of trichloromethane
✓6th T53.1X **Toxic effects of chloroform**
✓7th T53.1X1 **Toxic effect of chloroform, accidental (unintentional)**
Toxic effects of chloroform NOS
7 ✓7th T53.1X2 **Toxic effect of chloroform, intentional self-harm** HCC
✓7th T53.1X3 **Toxic effect of chloroform, assault**
✓7th T53.1X4 **Toxic effect of chloroform, undetermined**
✓5th T53.2 **Toxic effects of trichloroethylene**
Toxic effects of trichloroethene
✓6th T53.2X **Toxic effects of trichloroethylene**
✓7th T53.2X1 **Toxic effect of trichloroethylene, accidental (unintentional)**
Toxic effects of trichloroethylene NOS
7 ✓7th T53.2X2 **Toxic effect of trichloroethylene, intentional self-harm** HCC
✓7th T53.2X3 **Toxic effect of trichloroethylene, assault**
✓7th T53.2X4 **Toxic effect of trichloroethylene, undetermined**

✓5th **T53.3 Toxic effects of tetrachloroethylene**
Toxic effects of perchloroethylene
Toxic effect of tetrachloroethene

✓6th **T53.3X Toxic effects of tetrachloroethylene**

✓7th **T53.3X1 Toxic effect of tetrachloroethylene, accidental (unintentional)**
Toxic effects of tetrachloroethylene NOS

7 ✓7th **T53.3X2 Toxic effect of tetrachloroethylene, intentional self-harm** HCC

✓7th **T53.3X3 Toxic effect of tetrachloroethylene, assault**

✓7th **T53.3X4 Toxic effect of tetrachloroethylene, undetermined**

✓5th **T53.4 Toxic effects of dichloromethane**
Toxic effects of methylene chloride

✓6th **T53.4X Toxic effects of dichloromethane**

✓7th **T53.4X1 Toxic effect of dichloromethane, accidental (unintentional)**
Toxic effects of dichloromethane NOS

7 ✓7th **T53.4X2 Toxic effect of dichloromethane, intentional self-harm** HCC

✓7th **T53.4X3 Toxic effect of dichloromethane, assault**

✓7th **T53.4X4 Toxic effect of dichloromethane, undetermined**

✓5th **T53.5 Toxic effects of chlorofluorocarbons**

✓6th **T53.5X Toxic effects of chlorofluorocarbons**

✓7th **T53.5X1 Toxic effect of chlorofluorocarbons, accidental (unintentional)**
Toxic effects of chlorofluorocarbons NOS

7 ✓7th **T53.5X2 Toxic effect of chlorofluorocarbons, intentional self-harm** HCC

✓7th **T53.5X3 Toxic effect of chlorofluorocarbons, assault**

✓7th **T53.5X4 Toxic effect of chlorofluorocarbons, undetermined**

✓5th **T53.6 Toxic effects of other halogen derivatives of aliphatic hydrocarbons**

✓6th **T53.6X Toxic effects of other halogen derivatives of aliphatic hydrocarbons**

✓7th **T53.6X1 Toxic effect of other halogen derivatives of aliphatic hydrocarbons, accidental (unintentional)**
Toxic effects of other halogen derivatives of aliphatic hydrocarbons NOS

7 ✓7th **T53.6X2 Toxic effect of other halogen derivatives of aliphatic hydrocarbons, intentional self-harm** HCC

✓7th **T53.6X3 Toxic effect of other halogen derivatives of aliphatic hydrocarbons, assault**

✓7th **T53.6X4 Toxic effect of other halogen derivatives of aliphatic hydrocarbons, undetermined**

✓5th **T53.7 Toxic effects of other halogen derivatives of aromatic hydrocarbons**

✓6th **T53.7X Toxic effects of other halogen derivatives of aromatic hydrocarbons**

✓7th **T53.7X1 Toxic effect of other halogen derivatives of aromatic hydrocarbons, accidental (unintentional)**
Toxic effects of other halogen derivatives of aromatic hydrocarbons NOS

7 ✓7th **T53.7X2 Toxic effect of other halogen derivatives of aromatic hydrocarbons, intentional self-harm** HCC

✓7th **T53.7X3 Toxic effect of other halogen derivatives of aromatic hydrocarbons, assault**

✓7th **T53.7X4 Toxic effect of other halogen derivatives of aromatic hydrocarbons, undetermined**

✓5th **T53.9 Toxic effects of unspecified halogen derivatives of aliphatic and aromatic hydrocarbons**

✓x7th **T53.91 Toxic effect of unspecified halogen derivatives of aliphatic and aromatic hydrocarbons, accidental (unintentional)**

7 ✓x7th **T53.92 Toxic effect of unspecified halogen derivatives of aliphatic and aromatic hydrocarbons, intentional self-harm** HCC

✓x7th **T53.93 Toxic effect of unspecified halogen derivatives of aliphatic and aromatic hydrocarbons, assault**

✓x7th **T53.94 Toxic effect of unspecified halogen derivatives of aliphatic and aromatic hydrocarbons, undetermined**

✓4th **T54 Toxic effect of corrosive substances**

The appropriate 7th character is to be added to each code from category T54.
A initial encounter
D subsequent encounter
S sequela

✓5th **T54.Ø Toxic effects of phenol and phenol homologues**

✓6th **T54.ØX Toxic effects of phenol and phenol homologues**

✓7th **T54.ØX1 Toxic effect of phenol and phenol homologues, accidental (unintentional)**
Toxic effects of phenol and phenol homologues NOS

7 ✓7th **T54.ØX2 Toxic effect of phenol and phenol homologues, intentional self-harm** HCC

✓7th **T54.ØX3 Toxic effect of phenol and phenol homologues, assault**

✓7th **T54.ØX4 Toxic effect of phenol and phenol homologues, undetermined**

✓5th **T54.1 Toxic effects of other corrosive organic compounds**

✓6th **T54.1X Toxic effects of other corrosive organic compounds**

✓7th **T54.1X1 Toxic effect of other corrosive organic compounds, accidental (unintentional)**
Toxic effects of other corrosive organic compounds NOS

7 ✓7th **T54.1X2 Toxic effect of other corrosive organic compounds, intentional self-harm** HCC

✓7th **T54.1X3 Toxic effect of other corrosive organic compounds, assault**

✓7th **T54.1X4 Toxic effect of other corrosive organic compounds, undetermined**

✓5th **T54.2 Toxic effects of corrosive acids and acid-like substances**
Toxic effects of hydrochloric acid
Toxic effects of sulfuric acid

✓6th **T54.2X Toxic effects of corrosive acids and acid-like substances**

✓7th **T54.2X1 Toxic effect of corrosive acids and acid-like substances, accidental (unintentional)**
Toxic effects of corrosive acids and acid-like substances NOS

7 ✓7th **T54.2X2 Toxic effect of corrosive acids and acid-like substances, intentional self-harm** HCC

✓7th **T54.2X3 Toxic effect of corrosive acids and acid-like substances, assault**

✓7th **T54.2X4 Toxic effect of corrosive acids and acid-like substances, undetermined**

✓5th **T54.3 Toxic effects of corrosive alkalis and alkali-like substances**
Toxic effects of potassium hydroxide
Toxic effects of sodium hydroxide

✓6th **T54.3X Toxic effects of corrosive alkalis and alkali-like substances**

✓7th **T54.3X1 Toxic effect of corrosive alkalis and alkali-like substances, accidental (unintentional)**
Toxic effects of corrosive alkalis and alkali-like substances NOS

7 ✓7th **T54.3X2 Toxic effect of corrosive alkalis and alkali-like substances, intentional self-harm** HCC

✓7th **T54.3X3 Toxic effect of corrosive alkalis and alkali-like substances, assault**

✓7th **T54.3X4 Toxic effect of corrosive alkalis and alkali-like substances, undetermined**

✓5th **T54.9 Toxic effects of unspecified corrosive substance**

✓x7th **T54.91 Toxic effect of unspecified corrosive substance, accidental (unintentional)**

7 ✓x7th **T54.92 Toxic effect of unspecified corrosive substance, intentional self-harm** HCC

✓x7th **T54.93 Toxic effect of unspecified corrosive substance, assault**

✓x7th **T54.94 Toxic effect of unspecified corrosive substance, undetermined**

T55 Toxic effect of soaps and detergents

The appropriate 7th character is to be added to each code from category T55.
A initial encounter
D subsequent encounter
S sequela

T55.Ø Toxic effect of soaps

T55.ØX Toxic effect of soaps

T55.ØX1 Toxic effect of soaps, accidental (unintentional)
Toxic effect of soaps NOS

7 **T55.ØX2 Toxic effect of soaps, intentional self-harm** HCC

T55.ØX3 Toxic effect of soaps, assault

T55.ØX4 Toxic effect of soaps, undetermined

T55.1 Toxic effect of detergents

T55.1X Toxic effect of detergents

T55.1X1 Toxic effect of detergents, accidental (unintentional)
Toxic effect of detergents NOS

7 **T55.1X2 Toxic effect of detergents, intentional self-harm** HCC

T55.1X3 Toxic effect of detergents, assault

T55.1X4 Toxic effect of detergents, undetermined

T56 Toxic effect of metals

INCLUDES toxic effects of fumes and vapors of metals
toxic effects of metals from all sources, except medicinal substances

Use additional code to identify any retained metal foreign body, if applicable (Z18.Ø-, T18.1-)

EXCLUDES 1 *arsenic and its compounds (T57.Ø)*
manganese and its compounds (T57.2)

The appropriate 7th character is to be added to each code from category T56.
A initial encounter
D subsequent encounter
S sequela

T56.Ø Toxic effects of lead and its compounds

T56.ØX Toxic effects of lead and its compounds

T56.ØX1 Toxic effect of lead and its compounds, accidental (unintentional)
Toxic effects of lead and its compounds NOS

7 **T56.ØX2 Toxic effect of lead and its compounds, intentional self-harm** HCC

T56.ØX3 Toxic effect of lead and its compounds, assault

T56.ØX4 Toxic effect of lead and its compounds, undetermined

T56.1 Toxic effects of mercury and its compounds

T56.1X Toxic effects of mercury and its compounds

T56.1X1 Toxic effect of mercury and its compounds, accidental (unintentional)
Toxic effects of mercury and its compounds NOS

7 **T56.1X2 Toxic effect of mercury and its compounds, intentional self-harm** HCC

T56.1X3 Toxic effect of mercury and its compounds, assault

T56.1X4 Toxic effect of mercury and its compounds, undetermined

T56.2 Toxic effects of chromium and its compounds

T56.2X Toxic effects of chromium and its compounds

T56.2X1 Toxic effect of chromium and its compounds, accidental (unintentional)
Toxic effects of chromium and its compounds NOS

7 **T56.2X2 Toxic effect of chromium and its compounds, intentional self-harm** HCC

T56.2X3 Toxic effect of chromium and its compounds, assault

T56.2X4 Toxic effect of chromium and its compounds, undetermined

T56.3 Toxic effects of cadmium and its compounds

T56.3X Toxic effects of cadmium and its compounds

T56.3X1 Toxic effect of cadmium and its compounds, accidental (unintentional)
Toxic effects of cadmium and its compounds NOS

7 **T56.3X2 Toxic effect of cadmium and its compounds, intentional self-harm** HCC

T56.3X3 Toxic effect of cadmium and its compounds, assault

T56.3X4 Toxic effect of cadmium and its compounds, undetermined

T56.4 Toxic effects of copper and its compounds

T56.4X Toxic effects of copper and its compounds

T56.4X1 Toxic effect of copper and its compounds, accidental (unintentional)
Toxic effects of copper and its compounds NOS

7 **T56.4X2 Toxic effect of copper and its compounds, intentional self-harm** HCC

T56.4X3 Toxic effect of copper and its compounds, assault

T56.4X4 Toxic effect of copper and its compounds, undetermined

T56.5 Toxic effects of zinc and its compounds

T56.5X Toxic effects of zinc and its compounds

T56.5X1 Toxic effect of zinc and its compounds, accidental (unintentional)
Toxic effects of zinc and its compounds NOS

7 **T56.5X2 Toxic effect of zinc and its compounds, intentional self-harm** HCC

T56.5X3 Toxic effect of zinc and its compounds, assault

T56.5X4 Toxic effect of zinc and its compounds, undetermined

T56.6 Toxic effects of tin and its compounds

T56.6X Toxic effects of tin and its compounds

T56.6X1 Toxic effect of tin and its compounds, accidental (unintentional)
Toxic effects of tin and its compounds NOS

7 **T56.6X2 Toxic effect of tin and its compounds, intentional self-harm** HCC

T56.6X3 Toxic effect of tin and its compounds, assault

T56.6X4 Toxic effect of tin and its compounds, undetermined

T56.7 Toxic effects of beryllium and its compounds

T56.7X Toxic effects of beryllium and its compounds

T56.7X1 Toxic effect of beryllium and its compounds, accidental (unintentional)
Toxic effects of beryllium and its compounds NOS

7 **T56.7X2 Toxic effect of beryllium and its compounds, intentional self-harm** HCC

T56.7X3 Toxic effect of beryllium and its compounds, assault

T56.7X4 Toxic effect of beryllium and its compounds, undetermined

T56.8 Toxic effects of other metals

T56.81 Toxic effect of thallium

T56.811 Toxic effect of thallium, accidental (unintentional)
Toxic effect of thallium NOS

7 **T56.812 Toxic effect of thallium, intentional self-harm** HCC

T56.813 Toxic effect of thallium, assault

T56.814 Toxic effect of thallium, undetermined

T56.89 Toxic effects of other metals

T56.891 Toxic effect of other metals, accidental (unintentional)
Toxic effects of other metals NOS

7 **T56.892 Toxic effect of other metals, intentional self-harm** HCC

T56.893 Toxic effect of other metals, assault

T56.894 Toxic effect of other metals, undetermined

✓5th T56.9 Toxic effects of unspecified metal
✓x7th T56.91 Toxic effect of unspecified metal, accidental (unintentional)
7 ✓x7th T56.92 Toxic effect of unspecified metal, intentional self-harm HCC
✓x7th T56.93 Toxic effect of unspecified metal, assault
✓x7th T56.94 Toxic effect of unspecified metal, undetermined

✓4th **T57 Toxic effect of other inorganic substances**

The appropriate 7th character is to be added to each code from category T57.
A initial encounter
D subsequent encounter
S sequela

✓5th T57.0 Toxic effect of arsenic and its compounds
✓6th T57.0X Toxic effect of arsenic and its compounds
✓7th T57.0X1 Toxic effect of arsenic and its compounds, accidental (unintentional)
Toxic effect of arsenic and its compounds NOS
7 ✓7th T57.0X2 Toxic effect of arsenic and its compounds, intentional self-harm HCC
✓7th T57.0X3 Toxic effect of arsenic and its compounds, assault
✓7th T57.0X4 Toxic effect of arsenic and its compounds, undetermined

✓5th T57.1 Toxic effect of phosphorus and its compounds
EXCLUDES 1 *organophosphate insecticides (T60.0)*
✓6th T57.1X Toxic effect of phosphorus and its compounds
✓7th T57.1X1 Toxic effect of phosphorus and its compounds, accidental (unintentional)
Toxic effect of phosphorus and its compounds NOS
7 ✓7th T57.1X2 Toxic effect of phosphorus and its compounds, intentional self-harm HCC
✓7th T57.1X3 Toxic effect of phosphorus and its compounds, assault
✓7th T57.1X4 Toxic effect of phosphorus and its compounds, undetermined

✓5th T57.2 Toxic effect of manganese and its compounds
✓6th T57.2X Toxic effect of manganese and its compounds
✓7th T57.2X1 Toxic effect of manganese and its compounds, accidental (unintentional)
Toxic effect of manganese and its compounds NOS
7 ✓7th T57.2X2 Toxic effect of manganese and its compounds, intentional self-harm HCC
✓7th T57.2X3 Toxic effect of manganese and its compounds, assault
✓7th T57.2X4 Toxic effect of manganese and its compounds, undetermined

✓5th T57.3 Toxic effect of hydrogen cyanide
✓6th T57.3X Toxic effect of hydrogen cyanide
✓7th T57.3X1 Toxic effect of hydrogen cyanide, accidental (unintentional)
Toxic effect of hydrogen cyanide NOS
7 ✓7th T57.3X2 Toxic effect of hydrogen cyanide, intentional self-harm HCC
✓7th T57.3X3 Toxic effect of hydrogen cyanide, assault
✓7th T57.3X4 Toxic effect of hydrogen cyanide, undetermined

✓5th T57.8 Toxic effect of other specified inorganic substances
✓6th T57.8X Toxic effect of other specified inorganic substances
✓7th T57.8X1 Toxic effect of other specified inorganic substances, accidental (unintentional)
Toxic effect of other specified inorganic substances NOS
7 ✓7th T57.8X2 Toxic effect of other specified inorganic substances, intentional self-harm HCC
✓7th T57.8X3 Toxic effect of other specified inorganic substances, assault
✓7th T57.8X4 Toxic effect of other specified inorganic substances, undetermined

✓5th T57.9 Toxic effect of unspecified inorganic substance
✓x7th T57.91 Toxic effect of unspecified inorganic substance, accidental (unintentional)
7 ✓x7th T57.92 Toxic effect of unspecified inorganic substance, intentional self-harm HCC
✓x7th T57.93 Toxic effect of unspecified inorganic substance, assault
✓x7th T57.94 Toxic effect of unspecified inorganic substance, undetermined

✓4th **T58 Toxic effect of carbon monoxide**
INCLUDES asphyxiation from carbon monoxide
toxic effect of carbon monoxide from all sources

The appropriate 7th character is to be added to each code from category T58.
A initial encounter
D subsequent encounter
S sequela

✓5th T58.0 Toxic effect of carbon monoxide from motor vehicle exhaust
Toxic effect of exhaust gas from gas engine
Toxic effect of exhaust gas from motor pump
✓x7th T58.01 Toxic effect of carbon monoxide from motor vehicle exhaust, accidental (unintentional)
7 ✓x7th T58.02 Toxic effect of carbon monoxide from motor vehicle exhaust, intentional self-harm HCC
✓x7th T58.03 Toxic effect of carbon monoxide from motor vehicle exhaust, assault
✓x7th T58.04 Toxic effect of carbon monoxide from motor vehicle exhaust, undetermined

✓5th T58.1 Toxic effect of carbon monoxide from utility gas
Toxic effect of acetylene
Toxic effect of gas NOS used for lighting, heating, cooking
Toxic effect of water gas
✓x7th T58.11 Toxic effect of carbon monoxide from utility gas, accidental (unintentional)
7 ✓x7th T58.12 Toxic effect of carbon monoxide from utility gas, intentional self-harm HCC
✓x7th T58.13 Toxic effect of carbon monoxide from utility gas, assault
✓x7th T58.14 Toxic effect of carbon monoxide from utility gas, undetermined

✓5th T58.2 Toxic effect of carbon monoxide from incomplete combustion of other domestic fuels
Toxic effect of carbon monoxide from incomplete combustion of coal, coke, kerosene, wood
✓6th T58.2X Toxic effect of carbon monoxide from incomplete combustion of other domestic fuels
✓7th T58.2X1 Toxic effect of carbon monoxide from incomplete combustion of other domestic fuels, accidental (unintentional)
7 ✓7th T58.2X2 Toxic effect of carbon monoxide from incomplete combustion of other domestic fuels, intentional self-harm HCC
✓7th T58.2X3 Toxic effect of carbon monoxide from incomplete combustion of other domestic fuels, assault
✓7th T58.2X4 Toxic effect of carbon monoxide from incomplete combustion of other domestic fuels, undetermined

✓5th T58.8 Toxic effect of carbon monoxide from other source
Toxic effect of carbon monoxide from blast furnace gas
Toxic effect of carbon monoxide from fuels in industrial use
Toxic effect of carbon monoxide from kiln vapor
✓6th T58.8X Toxic effect of carbon monoxide from other source
✓7th T58.8X1 Toxic effect of carbon monoxide from other source, accidental (unintentional)
7 ✓7th T58.8X2 Toxic effect of carbon monoxide from other source, intentional self-harm HCC
✓7th T58.8X3 Toxic effect of carbon monoxide from other source, assault
✓7th T58.8X4 Toxic effect of carbon monoxide from other source, undetermined

✓5th T58.9 Toxic effect of carbon monoxide from unspecified source
✓x7th T58.91 Toxic effect of carbon monoxide from unspecified source, accidental (unintentional)
7 ✓x7th T58.92 Toxic effect of carbon monoxide from unspecified source, intentional self-harm HCC
✓x7th T58.93 Toxic effect of carbon monoxide from unspecified source, assault
✓x7th T58.94 Toxic effect of carbon monoxide from unspecified source, undetermined

T59 Toxic effect of other gases, fumes and vapors

INCLUDES aerosol propellants

EXCLUDES 1 *chlorofluorocarbons (T53.5)*

The appropriate 7th character is to be added to each code from category T59.
A initial encounter
D subsequent encounter
S sequela

T59.0 Toxic effect of nitrogen oxides

T59.0X Toxic effect of nitrogen oxides

T59.0X1 Toxic effect of nitrogen oxides, accidental (unintentional)
Toxic effect of nitrogen oxides NOS

7 **T59.0X2 Toxic effect of nitrogen oxides, intentional self-harm** HCC

T59.0X3 Toxic effect of nitrogen oxides, assault

T59.0X4 Toxic effect of nitrogen oxides, undetermined

T59.1 Toxic effect of sulfur dioxide

T59.1X Toxic effect of sulfur dioxide

T59.1X1 Toxic effect of sulfur dioxide, accidental (unintentional)
Toxic effect of sulfur dioxide NOS

7 **T59.1X2 Toxic effect of sulfur dioxide, intentional self-harm** HCC

T59.1X3 Toxic effect of sulfur dioxide, assault

T59.1X4 Toxic effect of sulfur dioxide, undetermined

T59.2 Toxic effect of formaldehyde

T59.2X Toxic effect of formaldehyde

T59.2X1 Toxic effect of formaldehyde, accidental (unintentional)
Toxic effect of formaldehyde NOS

7 **T59.2X2 Toxic effect of formaldehyde, intentional self-harm** HCC

T59.2X3 Toxic effect of formaldehyde, assault

T59.2X4 Toxic effect of formaldehyde, undetermined

T59.3 Toxic effect of lacrimogenic gas
Toxic effect of tear gas

T59.3X Toxic effect of lacrimogenic gas

T59.3X1 Toxic effect of lacrimogenic gas, accidental (unintentional)
Toxic effect of lacrimogenic gas NOS

7 **T59.3X2 Toxic effect of lacrimogenic gas, intentional self-harm** HCC

T59.3X3 Toxic effect of lacrimogenic gas, assault

T59.3X4 Toxic effect of lacrimogenic gas, undetermined

T59.4 Toxic effect of chlorine gas

T59.4X Toxic effect of chlorine gas

T59.4X1 Toxic effect of chlorine gas, accidental (unintentional)
Toxic effect of chlorine gas NOS

7 **T59.4X2 Toxic effect of chlorine gas, intentional self-harm** HCC

T59.4X3 Toxic effect of chlorine gas, assault

T59.4X4 Toxic effect of chlorine gas, undetermined

T59.5 Toxic effect of fluorine gas and hydrogen fluoride

T59.5X Toxic effect of fluorine gas and hydrogen fluoride

T59.5X1 Toxic effect of fluorine gas and hydrogen fluoride, accidental (unintentional)
Toxic effect of fluorine gas and hydrogen fluoride NOS

7 **T59.5X2 Toxic effect of fluorine gas and hydrogen fluoride, intentional self-harm** HCC

T59.5X3 Toxic effect of fluorine gas and hydrogen fluoride, assault

T59.5X4 Toxic effect of fluorine gas and hydrogen fluoride, undetermined

T59.6 Toxic effect of hydrogen sulfide

T59.6X Toxic effect of hydrogen sulfide

T59.6X1 Toxic effect of hydrogen sulfide, accidental (unintentional)
Toxic effect of hydrogen sulfide NOS

7 **T59.6X2 Toxic effect of hydrogen sulfide, intentional self-harm** HCC

T59.6X3 Toxic effect of hydrogen sulfide, assault

T59.6X4 Toxic effect of hydrogen sulfide, undetermined

T59.7 Toxic effect of carbon dioxide

T59.7X Toxic effect of carbon dioxide

T59.7X1 Toxic effect of carbon dioxide, accidental (unintentional)
Toxic effect of carbon dioxide NOS

7 **T59.7X2 Toxic effect of carbon dioxide, intentional self-harm** HCC

T59.7X3 Toxic effect of carbon dioxide, assault

T59.7X4 Toxic effect of carbon dioxide, undetermined

T59.8 Toxic effect of other specified gases, fumes and vapors

T59.81 Toxic effect of smoke
Smoke inhalation

EXCLUDES 2 *toxic effect of cigarette (tobacco) smoke (T65.22-)*

T59.811 Toxic effect of smoke, accidental (unintentional)
Toxic effect of smoke NOS
AHA: 2013,4Q,121

7 **T59.812 Toxic effect of smoke, intentional self-harm** HCC

T59.813 Toxic effect of smoke, assault

T59.814 Toxic effect of smoke, undetermined

T59.89 Toxic effect of other specified gases, fumes and vapors

T59.891 Toxic effect of other specified gases, fumes and vapors, accidental (unintentional)

7 **T59.892 Toxic effect of other specified gases, fumes and vapors, intentional self-harm** HCC

T59.893 Toxic effect of other specified gases, fumes and vapors, assault

T59.894 Toxic effect of other specified gases, fumes and vapors, undetermined

T59.9 Toxic effect of unspecified gases, fumes and vapors

T59.91 Toxic effect of unspecified gases, fumes and vapors, accidental (unintentional)

7 **T59.92 Toxic effect of unspecified gases, fumes and vapors, intentional self-harm** HCC

T59.93 Toxic effect of unspecified gases, fumes and vapors, assault

T59.94 Toxic effect of unspecified gases, fumes and vapors, undetermined

T60 Toxic effect of pesticides

INCLUDES toxic effect of wood preservatives

The appropriate 7th character is to be added to each code from category T60.
A initial encounter
D subsequent encounter
S sequela

T60.0 Toxic effect of organophosphate and carbamate insecticides

T60.0X Toxic effect of organophosphate and carbamate insecticides

T60.0X1 Toxic effect of organophosphate and carbamate insecticides, accidental (unintentional)
Toxic effect of organophosphate and carbamate insecticides NOS

7 **T60.0X2 Toxic effect of organophosphate and carbamate insecticides, intentional self-harm** HCC

T60.0X3 Toxic effect of organophosphate and carbamate insecticides, assault

T60.0X4 Toxic effect of organophosphate and carbamate insecticides, undetermined

√5th **T60.1 Toxic effect of halogenated insecticides**

EXCLUDES 1 *chlorinated hydrocarbon (T53.-)*

√6th **T60.1X Toxic effect of halogenated insecticides**

√7th **T60.1X1 Toxic effect of halogenated insecticides, accidental (unintentional)**
Toxic effect of halogenated insecticides NOS

7 √7th **T60.1X2 Toxic effect of halogenated insecticides, intentional self-harm** HCC

√7th **T60.1X3 Toxic effect of halogenated insecticides, assault**

√7th **T60.1X4 Toxic effect of halogenated insecticides, undetermined**

√5th **T60.2 Toxic effect of other insecticides**

√6th **T60.2X Toxic effect of other insecticides**

√7th **T60.2X1 Toxic effect of other insecticides, accidental (unintentional)**
Toxic effect of other insecticides NOS

7 √7th **T60.2X2 Toxic effect of other insecticides, intentional self-harm** HCC

√7th **T60.2X3 Toxic effect of other insecticides, assault**

√7th **T60.2X4 Toxic effect of other insecticides, undetermined**

√5th **T60.3 Toxic effect of herbicides and fungicides**

√6th **T60.3X Toxic effect of herbicides and fungicides**

√7th **T60.3X1 Toxic effect of herbicides and fungicides, accidental (unintentional)**
Toxic effect of herbicides and fungicides NOS

7 √7th **T60.3X2 Toxic effect of herbicides and fungicides, intentional self-harm** HCC

√7th **T60.3X3 Toxic effect of herbicides and fungicides, assault**

√7th **T60.3X4 Toxic effect of herbicides and fungicides, undetermined**

√5th **T60.4 Toxic effect of rodenticides**

EXCLUDES 1 *strychnine and its salts (T65.1)*
thallium (T56.81-)

√6th **T60.4X Toxic effect of rodenticides**

√7th **T60.4X1 Toxic effect of rodenticides, accidental (unintentional)**
Toxic effect of rodenticides NOS

7 √7th **T60.4X2 Toxic effect of rodenticides, intentional self-harm** HCC

√7th **T60.4X3 Toxic effect of rodenticides, assault**

√7th **T60.4X4 Toxic effect of rodenticides, undetermined**

√5th **T60.8 Toxic effect of other pesticides**

√6th **T60.8X Toxic effect of other pesticides**

√7th **T60.8X1 Toxic effect of other pesticides, accidental (unintentional)**
Toxic effect of other pesticides NOS

7 √7th **T60.8X2 Toxic effect of other pesticides, intentional self-harm** HCC

√7th **T60.8X3 Toxic effect of other pesticides, assault**

√7th **T60.8X4 Toxic effect of other pesticides, undetermined**

√5th **T60.9 Toxic effect of unspecified pesticide**

√x7th **T60.91 Toxic effect of unspecified pesticide, accidental (unintentional)**

7 √x7th **T60.92 Toxic effect of unspecified pesticide, intentional self-harm** HCC

√x7th **T60.93 Toxic effect of unspecified pesticide, assault**

√x7th **T60.94 Toxic effect of unspecified pesticide, undetermined**

√4th **T61 Toxic effect of noxious substances eaten as seafood**

EXCLUDES 1 *allergic reaction to food, such as:*
anaphylactic reaction or shock due to adverse food reaction (T78.0-)
bacterial foodborne intoxications (A05.-)
dermatitis (L23.6, L25.4, L27.2)
food protein-induced enterocolitis syndrome (K52.21)
food protein-induced enteropathy (K52.22)
gastroenteritis (noninfective) (K52.29)
toxic effect of aflatoxin and other mycotoxins (T64)
toxic effect of cyanides (T65.0-)
toxic effect of harmful algae bloom (T65.82-)
toxic effect of hydrogen cyanide (T57.3-)
toxic effect of mercury (T56.1-)
toxic effect of red tide (T65.82-)

The appropriate 7th character is to be added to each code from category T61.
A initial encounter
D subsequent encounter
S sequela

√5th **T61.0 Ciguatera fish poisoning**

√x7th **T61.01 Ciguatera fish poisoning, accidental (unintentional)**

7 √x7th **T61.02 Ciguatera fish poisoning, intentional self-harm** HCC

√x7th **T61.03 Ciguatera fish poisoning, assault**

√x7th **T61.04 Ciguatera fish poisoning, undetermined**

√5th **T61.1 Scombroid fish poisoning**
Histamine-like syndrome

√x7th **T61.11 Scombroid fish poisoning, accidental (unintentional)**

7 √x7th **T61.12 Scombroid fish poisoning, intentional self-harm** HCC

√x7th **T61.13 Scombroid fish poisoning, assault**

√x7th **T61.14 Scombroid fish poisoning, undetermined**

√5th **T61.7 Other fish and shellfish poisoning**

√6th **T61.77 Other fish poisoning**

√7th **T61.771 Other fish poisoning, accidental (unintentional)**

7 √7th **T61.772 Other fish poisoning, intentional self-harm** HCC

√7th **T61.773 Other fish poisoning, assault**

√7th **T61.774 Other fish poisoning, undetermined**

√6th **T61.78 Other shellfish poisoning**

√7th **T61.781 Other shellfish poisoning, accidental (unintentional)**

7 √7th **T61.782 Other shellfish poisoning, intentional self-harm** HCC

√7th **T61.783 Other shellfish poisoning, assault**

√7th **T61.784 Other shellfish poisoning, undetermined**

√5th **T61.8 Toxic effect of other seafood**

√6th **T61.8X Toxic effect of other seafood**

√7th **T61.8X1 Toxic effect of other seafood, accidental (unintentional)**

7 √7th **T61.8X2 Toxic effect of other seafood, intentional self-harm** HCC

√7th **T61.8X3 Toxic effect of other seafood, assault**

√7th **T61.8X4 Toxic effect of other seafood, undetermined**

√5th **T61.9 Toxic effect of unspecified seafood**

√x7th **T61.91 Toxic effect of unspecified seafood, accidental (unintentional)**

7 √x7th **T61.92 Toxic effect of unspecified seafood, intentional self-harm** HCC

√x7th **T61.93 Toxic effect of unspecified seafood, assault**

√x7th **T61.94 Toxic effect of unspecified seafood, undetermined**

T62 Toxic effect of other noxious substances eaten as food

EXCLUDES 1 *allergic reaction to food, such as:*
anaphylactic shock (reaction) due to adverse food reaction (T78.Ø-)
bacterial food borne intoxications (AØ5.-)
dermatitis (L23.6, L25.4, L27.2)
food protein-induced enterocolitis syndrome (K52.21)
food protein-induced enteropathy (K52.22)
gastroenteritis (noninfective) (K52.29)
toxic effect of aflatoxin and other mycotoxins (T64)
toxic effect of cyanides (T65.Ø-)
toxic effect of hydrogen cyanide (T57.3-)
toxic effect of mercury (T56.1-)

The appropriate 7th character is to be added to each code from category T62.
A initial encounter
D subsequent encounter
S sequela

T62.Ø Toxic effect of ingested mushrooms
T62.ØX Toxic effect of ingested mushrooms
T62.ØX1 Toxic effect of ingested mushrooms, accidental (unintentional)
Toxic effect of ingested mushrooms NOS
7 **T62.ØX2 Toxic effect of ingested mushrooms, intentional self-harm** HCC
T62.ØX3 Toxic effect of ingested mushrooms, assault
T62.ØX4 Toxic effect of ingested mushrooms, undetermined

T62.1 Toxic effect of ingested berries
T62.1X Toxic effect of ingested berries
T62.1X1 Toxic effect of ingested berries, accidental (unintentional)
Toxic effect of ingested berries NOS
7 **T62.1X2 Toxic effect of ingested berries, intentional self-harm** HCC
T62.1X3 Toxic effect of ingested berries, assault
T62.1X4 Toxic effect of ingested berries, undetermined

T62.2 Toxic effect of other ingested (parts of) plant(s)
T62.2X Toxic effect of other ingested (parts of) plant(s)
T62.2X1 Toxic effect of other ingested (parts of) plant(s), accidental (unintentional)
Toxic effect of other ingested (parts of) plant(s) NOS
7 **T62.2X2 Toxic effect of other ingested (parts of) plant(s), intentional self-harm** HCC
T62.2X3 Toxic effect of other ingested (parts of) plant(s), assault
T62.2X4 Toxic effect of other ingested (parts of) plant(s), undetermined

T62.8 Toxic effect of other specified noxious substances eaten as food
T62.8X Toxic effect of other specified noxious substances eaten as food
T62.8X1 Toxic effect of other specified noxious substances eaten as food, accidental (unintentional)
Toxic effect of other specified noxious substances eaten as food NOS
7 **T62.8X2 Toxic effect of other specified noxious substances eaten as food, intentional self-harm** HCC
T62.8X3 Toxic effect of other specified noxious substances eaten as food, assault
T62.8X4 Toxic effect of other specified noxious substances eaten as food, undetermined

T62.9 Toxic effect of unspecified noxious substance eaten as food
T62.91 Toxic effect of unspecified noxious substance eaten as food, accidental (unintentional)
Toxic effect of unspecified noxious substance eaten as food NOS
7 **T62.92 Toxic effect of unspecified noxious substance eaten as food, intentional self-harm** HCC
T62.93 Toxic effect of unspecified noxious substance eaten as food, assault
T62.94 Toxic effect of unspecified noxious substance eaten as food, undetermined

T63 Toxic effect of contact with venomous animals and plants

INCLUDES bite or touch of venomous animal
pricked or stuck by thorn or leaf

EXCLUDES 2 *ingestion of toxic animal or plant (T61.-, T62.-)*

The appropriate 7th character is to be added to each code from category T63.
A initial encounter
D subsequent encounter
S sequela

T63.Ø Toxic effect of snake venom
T63.ØØ Toxic effect of unspecified snake venom
T63.ØØ1 Toxic effect of unspecified snake venom, accidental (unintentional)
Toxic effect of unspecified snake venom NOS
7 **T63.ØØ2 Toxic effect of unspecified snake venom, intentional self-harm** HCC
T63.ØØ3 Toxic effect of unspecified snake venom, assault
T63.ØØ4 Toxic effect of unspecified snake venom, undetermined

T63.Ø1 Toxic effect of rattlesnake venom
T63.Ø11 Toxic effect of rattlesnake venom, accidental (unintentional)
Toxic effect of rattlesnake venom NOS
7 **T63.Ø12 Toxic effect of rattlesnake venom, intentional self-harm** HCC
T63.Ø13 Toxic effect of rattlesnake venom, assault
T63.Ø14 Toxic effect of rattlesnake venom, undetermined

T63.Ø2 Toxic effect of coral snake venom
T63.Ø21 Toxic effect of coral snake venom, accidental (unintentional)
Toxic effect of coral snake venom NOS
7 **T63.Ø22 Toxic effect of coral snake venom, intentional self-harm** HCC
T63.Ø23 Toxic effect of coral snake venom, assault
T63.Ø24 Toxic effect of coral snake venom, undetermined

T63.Ø3 Toxic effect of taipan venom
T63.Ø31 Toxic effect of taipan venom, accidental (unintentional)
Toxic effect of taipan venom NOS
7 **T63.Ø32 Toxic effect of taipan venom, intentional self-harm** HCC
T63.Ø33 Toxic effect of taipan venom, assault
T63.Ø34 Toxic effect of taipan venom, undetermined

T63.Ø4 Toxic effect of cobra venom
T63.Ø41 Toxic effect of cobra venom, accidental (unintentional)
Toxic effect of cobra venom NOS
7 **T63.Ø42 Toxic effect of cobra venom, intentional self-harm** HCC
T63.Ø43 Toxic effect of cobra venom, assault
T63.Ø44 Toxic effect of cobra venom, undetermined

T63.Ø6 Toxic effect of venom of other North and South American snake
T63.Ø61 Toxic effect of venom of other North and South American snake, accidental (unintentional)
Toxic effect of venom of other North and South American snake NOS
7 **T63.Ø62 Toxic effect of venom of other North and South American snake, intentional self-harm** HCC
T63.Ø63 Toxic effect of venom of other North and South American snake, assault
T63.Ø64 Toxic effect of venom of other North and South American snake, undetermined

T63.Ø7 Toxic effect of venom of other Australian snake
T63.Ø71 Toxic effect of venom of other Australian snake, accidental (unintentional)
Toxic effect of venom of other Australian snake NOS
7 **T63.Ø72 Toxic effect of venom of other Australian snake, intentional self-harm** HCC

✓7th T63.073 **Toxic effect of venom of other Australian snake, assault**
✓7th T63.074 **Toxic effect of venom of other Australian snake, undetermined**
✓6th T63.08 **Toxic effect of venom of other African and Asian snake**
✓7th T63.081 **Toxic effect of venom of other African and Asian snake, accidental (unintentional)**
Toxic effect of venom of other African and Asian snake NOS
7 ✓7th T63.082 **Toxic effect of venom of other African and Asian snake, intentional self-harm** HCC
✓7th T63.083 **Toxic effect of venom of other African and Asian snake, assault**
✓7th T63.084 **Toxic effect of venom of other African and Asian snake, undetermined**
✓6th T63.09 **Toxic effect of venom of other snake**
✓7th T63.091 **Toxic effect of venom of other snake, accidental (unintentional)**
Toxic effect of venom of other snake NOS
7 ✓7th T63.092 **Toxic effect of venom of other snake, intentional self-harm** HCC
✓7th T63.093 **Toxic effect of venom of other snake, assault**
✓7th T63.094 **Toxic effect of venom of other snake, undetermined**
✓5th T63.1 **Toxic effect of venom of other reptiles**
✓6th T63.11 **Toxic effect of venom of gila monster**
✓7th T63.111 **Toxic effect of venom of gila monster, accidental (unintentional)**
Toxic effect of venom of gila monster NOS
7 ✓7th T63.112 **Toxic effect of venom of gila monster, intentional self-harm** HCC
✓7th T63.113 **Toxic effect of venom of gila monster, assault**
✓7th T63.114 **Toxic effect of venom of gila monster, undetermined**
✓6th T63.12 **Toxic effect of venom of other venomous lizard**
✓7th T63.121 **Toxic effect of venom of other venomous lizard, accidental (unintentional)**
Toxic effect of venom of other venomous lizard NOS
7 ✓7th T63.122 **Toxic effect of venom of other venomous lizard, intentional self-harm** HCC
✓7th T63.123 **Toxic effect of venom of other venomous lizard, assault**
✓7th T63.124 **Toxic effect of venom of other venomous lizard, undetermined**
✓6th T63.19 **Toxic effect of venom of other reptiles**
✓7th T63.191 **Toxic effect of venom of other reptiles, accidental (unintentional)**
Toxic effect of venom of other reptiles NOS
7 ✓7th T63.192 **Toxic effect of venom of other reptiles, intentional self-harm** HCC
✓7th T63.193 **Toxic effect of venom of other reptiles, assault**
✓7th T63.194 **Toxic effect of venom of other reptiles, undetermined**
✓5th T63.2 **Toxic effect of venom of scorpion**
✓6th T63.2X **Toxic effect of venom of scorpion**
✓7th T63.2X1 **Toxic effect of venom of scorpion, accidental (unintentional)**
Toxic effect of venom of scorpion NOS
7 ✓7th T63.2X2 **Toxic effect of venom of scorpion, intentional self-harm** HCC
✓7th T63.2X3 **Toxic effect of venom of scorpion, assault**
✓7th T63.2X4 **Toxic effect of venom of scorpion, undetermined**
✓5th T63.3 **Toxic effect of venom of spider**
✓6th T63.30 **Toxic effect of unspecified spider venom**
✓7th T63.301 **Toxic effect of unspecified spider venom, accidental (unintentional)**
7 ✓7th T63.302 **Toxic effect of unspecified spider venom, intentional self-harm** HCC
✓7th T63.303 **Toxic effect of unspecified spider venom, assault**
✓7th T63.304 **Toxic effect of unspecified spider venom, undetermined**
✓6th T63.31 **Toxic effect of venom of black widow spider**
✓7th T63.311 **Toxic effect of venom of black widow spider, accidental (unintentional)**
7 ✓7th T63.312 **Toxic effect of venom of black widow spider, intentional self-harm** HCC
✓7th T63.313 **Toxic effect of venom of black widow spider, assault**
✓7th T63.314 **Toxic effect of venom of black widow spider, undetermined**
✓6th T63.32 **Toxic effect of venom of tarantula**
✓7th T63.321 **Toxic effect of venom of tarantula, accidental (unintentional)**
7 ✓7th T63.322 **Toxic effect of venom of tarantula, intentional self-harm** HCC
✓7th T63.323 **Toxic effect of venom of tarantula, assault**
✓7th T63.324 **Toxic effect of venom of tarantula, undetermined**
✓6th T63.33 **Toxic effect of venom of brown recluse spider**
✓7th T63.331 **Toxic effect of venom of brown recluse spider, accidental (unintentional)**
7 ✓7th T63.332 **Toxic effect of venom of brown recluse spider, intentional self-harm** HCC
✓7th T63.333 **Toxic effect of venom of brown recluse spider, assault**
✓7th T63.334 **Toxic effect of venom of brown recluse spider, undetermined**
✓6th T63.39 **Toxic effect of venom of other spider**
✓7th T63.391 **Toxic effect of venom of other spider, accidental (unintentional)**
7 ✓7th T63.392 **Toxic effect of venom of other spider, intentional self-harm** HCC
✓7th T63.393 **Toxic effect of venom of other spider, assault**
✓7th T63.394 **Toxic effect of venom of other spider, undetermined**
✓5th T63.4 **Toxic effect of venom of other arthropods**
✓6th T63.41 **Toxic effect of venom of centipedes and venomous millipedes**
✓7th T63.411 **Toxic effect of venom of centipedes and venomous millipedes, accidental (unintentional)**
7 ✓7th T63.412 **Toxic effect of venom of centipedes and venomous millipedes, intentional self-harm** HCC
✓7th T63.413 **Toxic effect of venom of centipedes and venomous millipedes, assault**
✓7th T63.414 **Toxic effect of venom of centipedes and venomous millipedes, undetermined**
✓6th T63.42 **Toxic effect of venom of ants**
✓7th T63.421 **Toxic effect of venom of ants, accidental (unintentional)**
7 ✓7th T63.422 **Toxic effect of venom of ants, intentional self-harm** HCC
✓7th T63.423 **Toxic effect of venom of ants, assault**
✓7th T63.424 **Toxic effect of venom of ants, undetermined**
✓6th T63.43 **Toxic effect of venom of caterpillars**
✓7th T63.431 **Toxic effect of venom of caterpillars, accidental (unintentional)**
7 ✓7th T63.432 **Toxic effect of venom of caterpillars, intentional self-harm** HCC
✓7th T63.433 **Toxic effect of venom of caterpillars, assault**
✓7th T63.434 **Toxic effect of venom of caterpillars, undetermined**
✓6th T63.44 **Toxic effect of venom of bees**
✓7th T63.441 **Toxic effect of venom of bees, accidental (unintentional)**
7 ✓7th T63.442 **Toxic effect of venom of bees, intentional self-harm** HCC
✓7th T63.443 **Toxic effect of venom of bees, assault**
✓7th T63.444 **Toxic effect of venom of bees, undetermined**
✓6th T63.45 **Toxic effect of venom of hornets**
✓7th T63.451 **Toxic effect of venom of hornets, accidental (unintentional)**
7 ✓7th T63.452 **Toxic effect of venom of hornets, intentional self-harm** HCC
✓7th T63.453 **Toxic effect of venom of hornets, assault**

T63.454 Toxic effect of venom of hornets, undetermined

T63.46 Toxic effect of venom of wasps

Toxic effect of yellow jacket

T63.461 Toxic effect of venom of wasps, accidental (unintentional)

7 T63.462 Toxic effect of venom of wasps, intentional self-harm HCC

T63.463 Toxic effect of venom of wasps, assault

T63.464 Toxic effect of venom of wasps, undetermined

T63.48 Toxic effect of venom of other arthropod

T63.481 Toxic effect of venom of other arthropod, accidental (unintentional)

7 T63.482 Toxic effect of venom of other arthropod, intentional self-harm HCC

T63.483 Toxic effect of venom of other arthropod, assault

T63.484 Toxic effect of venom of other arthropod, undetermined

T63.5 Toxic effect of contact with venomous fish

EXCLUDES 2 *poisoning by ingestion of fish (T61.-)*

T63.51 Toxic effect of contact with stingray

T63.511 Toxic effect of contact with stingray, accidental (unintentional)

7 T63.512 Toxic effect of contact with stingray, intentional self-harm HCC

T63.513 Toxic effect of contact with stingray, assault

T63.514 Toxic effect of contact with stingray, undetermined

T63.59 Toxic effect of contact with other venomous fish

T63.591 Toxic effect of contact with other venomous fish, accidental (unintentional)

7 T63.592 Toxic effect of contact with other venomous fish, intentional self-harm HCC

T63.593 Toxic effect of contact with other venomous fish, assault

T63.594 Toxic effect of contact with other venomous fish, undetermined

T63.6 Toxic effect of contact with other venomous marine animals

EXCLUDES 1 *sea-snake venom (T63.Ø9)*

EXCLUDES 2 *poisoning by ingestion of shellfish (T61.78-)*

T63.61 Toxic effect of contact with Portugese Man-o-war

Toxic effect of contact with bluebottle

T63.611 Toxic effect of contact with Portugese Man-o-war, accidental (unintentional)

7 T63.612 Toxic effect of contact with Portugese Man-o-war, intentional self-harm HCC

T63.613 Toxic effect of contact with Portugese Man-o-war, assault

T63.614 Toxic effect of contact with Portugese Man-o-war, undetermined

T63.62 Toxic effect of contact with other jellyfish

T63.621 Toxic effect of contact with other jellyfish, accidental (unintentional)

7 T63.622 Toxic effect of contact with other jellyfish, intentional self-harm HCC

T63.623 Toxic effect of contact with other jellyfish, assault

T63.624 Toxic effect of contact with other jellyfish, undetermined

T63.63 Toxic effect of contact with sea anemone

T63.631 Toxic effect of contact with sea anemone, accidental (unintentional)

7 T63.632 Toxic effect of contact with sea anemone, intentional self-harm HCC

T63.633 Toxic effect of contact with sea anemone, assault

T63.634 Toxic effect of contact with sea anemone, undetermined

T63.69 Toxic effect of contact with other venomous marine animals

T63.691 Toxic effect of contact with other venomous marine animals, accidental (unintentional)

7 T63.692 Toxic effect of contact with other venomous marine animals, intentional self-harm HCC

T63.693 Toxic effect of contact with other venomous marine animals, assault

T63.694 Toxic effect of contact with other venomous marine animals, undetermined

T63.7 Toxic effect of contact with venomous plant

T63.71 Toxic effect of contact with venomous marine plant

T63.711 Toxic effect of contact with venomous marine plant, accidental (unintentional)

7 T63.712 Toxic effect of contact with venomous marine plant, intentional self-harm HCC

T63.713 Toxic effect of contact with venomous marine plant, assault

T63.714 Toxic effect of contact with venomous marine plant, undetermined

T63.79 Toxic effect of contact with other venomous plant

T63.791 Toxic effect of contact with other venomous plant, accidental (unintentional)

7 T63.792 Toxic effect of contact with other venomous plant, intentional self-harm HCC

T63.793 Toxic effect of contact with other venomous plant, assault

T63.794 Toxic effect of contact with other venomous plant, undetermined

T63.8 Toxic effect of contact with other venomous animals

T63.81 Toxic effect of contact with venomous frog

EXCLUDES 1 *contact with nonvenomous frog (W62.Ø)*

T63.811 Toxic effect of contact with venomous frog, accidental (unintentional)

7 T63.812 Toxic effect of contact with venomous frog, intentional self-harm HCC

T63.813 Toxic effect of contact with venomous frog, assault

T63.814 Toxic effect of contact with venomous frog, undetermined

T63.82 Toxic effect of contact with venomous toad

EXCLUDES 1 *contact with nonvenomous toad (W62.1)*

T63.821 Toxic effect of contact with venomous toad, accidental (unintentional)

7 T63.822 Toxic effect of contact with venomous toad, intentional self-harm HCC

T63.823 Toxic effect of contact with venomous toad, assault

T63.824 Toxic effect of contact with venomous toad, undetermined

T63.83 Toxic effect of contact with other venomous amphibian

EXCLUDES 1 *contact with nonvenomous amphibian (W62.9)*

T63.831 Toxic effect of contact with other venomous amphibian, accidental (unintentional)

7 T63.832 Toxic effect of contact with other venomous amphibian, intentional self-harm HCC

T63.833 Toxic effect of contact with other venomous amphibian, assault

T63.834 Toxic effect of contact with other venomous amphibian, undetermined

T63.89 Toxic effect of contact with other venomous animals

T63.891 Toxic effect of contact with other venomous animals, accidental (unintentional)

7 T63.892 Toxic effect of contact with other venomous animals, intentional self-harm HCC

T63.893 Toxic effect of contact with other venomous animals, assault

T63.894 Toxic effect of contact with other venomous animals, undetermined

T63.9 Toxic effect of contact with unspecified venomous animal

T63.91 Toxic effect of contact with unspecified venomous animal, accidental (unintentional)

7 T63.92 Toxic effect of contact with unspecified venomous animal, intentional self-harm HCC

T63.93 Toxic effect of contact with unspecified venomous animal, assault

T63.94 Toxic effect of contact with unspecified venomous animal, undetermined

T64 Toxic effect of aflatoxin and other mycotoxin food contaminants

The appropriate 7th character is to be added to each code from category T64.
A initial encounter
D subsequent encounter
S sequela

T64.Ø Toxic effect of aflatoxin
T64.Ø1 Toxic effect of aflatoxin, accidental (unintentional)
7 **T64.Ø2 Toxic effect of aflatoxin, intentional self-harm** HCC
T64.Ø3 Toxic effect of aflatoxin, assault
T64.Ø4 Toxic effect of aflatoxin, undetermined

T64.8 Toxic effect of other mycotoxin food contaminants
T64.81 Toxic effect of other mycotoxin food contaminants, accidental (unintentional)
7 **T64.82 Toxic effect of other mycotoxin food contaminants, intentional self-harm** HCC
T64.83 Toxic effect of other mycotoxin food contaminants, assault
T64.84 Toxic effect of other mycotoxin food contaminants, undetermined

T65 Toxic effect of other and unspecified substances

The appropriate 7th character is to be added to each code from category T65.
A initial encounter
D subsequent encounter
S sequela

T65.Ø Toxic effect of cyanides
EXCLUDES 1 *hydrogen cyanide (T57.3-)*
T65.ØX Toxic effect of cyanides
T65.ØX1 Toxic effect of cyanides, accidental (unintentional)
Toxic effect of cyanides NOS
7 **T65.ØX2 Toxic effect of cyanides, intentional self-harm** HCC
T65.ØX3 Toxic effect of cyanides, assault
T65.ØX4 Toxic effect of cyanides, undetermined

T65.1 Toxic effect of strychnine and its salts
T65.1X Toxic effect of strychnine and its salts
T65.1X1 Toxic effect of strychnine and its salts, accidental (unintentional)
Toxic effect of strychnine and its salts NOS
7 **T65.1X2 Toxic effect of strychnine and its salts, intentional self-harm** HCC
T65.1X3 Toxic effect of strychnine and its salts, assault
T65.1X4 Toxic effect of strychnine and its salts, undetermined

T65.2 Toxic effect of tobacco and nicotine
EXCLUDES 2 *nicotine dependence (F17.-)*
T65.21 Toxic effect of chewing tobacco
T65.211 Toxic effect of chewing tobacco, accidental (unintentional)
Toxic effect of chewing tobacco NOS
7 **T65.212 Toxic effect of chewing tobacco, intentional self-harm** HCC
T65.213 Toxic effect of chewing tobacco, assault
T65.214 Toxic effect of chewing tobacco, undetermined
T65.22 Toxic effect of tobacco cigarettes
Toxic effect of tobacco smoke
Use additional code for exposure to second hand tobacco smoke (Z57.31, Z77.22)
T65.221 Toxic effect of tobacco cigarettes, accidental (unintentional)
Toxic effect of tobacco cigarettes NOS
7 **T65.222 Toxic effect of tobacco cigarettes, intentional self-harm** HCC
T65.223 Toxic effect of tobacco cigarettes, assault
T65.224 Toxic effect of tobacco cigarettes, undetermined
T65.29 Toxic effect of other tobacco and nicotine
T65.291 Toxic effect of other tobacco and nicotine, accidental (unintentional)
Toxic effect of other tobacco and nicotine NOS
7 **T65.292 Toxic effect of other tobacco and nicotine, intentional self-harm** HCC
T65.293 Toxic effect of other tobacco and nicotine, assault
T65.294 Toxic effect of other tobacco and nicotine, undetermined

T65.3 Toxic effect of nitroderivatives and aminoderivatives of benzene and its homologues
Toxic effect of anilin [benzenamine]
Toxic effect of nitrobenzene
Toxic effect of trinitrotoluene
T65.3X Toxic effect of nitroderivatives and aminoderivatives of benzene and its homologues
T65.3X1 Toxic effect of nitroderivatives and aminoderivatives of benzene and its homologues, accidental (unintentional)
Toxic effect of nitroderivatives and aminoderivatives of benzene and its homologues NOS
7 **T65.3X2 Toxic effect of nitroderivatives and aminoderivatives of benzene and its homologues, intentional self-harm** HCC
T65.3X3 Toxic effect of nitroderivatives and aminoderivatives of benzene and its homologues, assault
T65.3X4 Toxic effect of nitroderivatives and aminoderivatives of benzene and its homologues, undetermined

T65.4 Toxic effect of carbon disulfide
T65.4X Toxic effect of carbon disulfide
T65.4X1 Toxic effect of carbon disulfide, accidental (unintentional)
Toxic effect of carbon disulfide NOS
7 **T65.4X2 Toxic effect of carbon disulfide, intentional self-harm** HCC
T65.4X3 Toxic effect of carbon disulfide, assault
T65.4X4 Toxic effect of carbon disulfide, undetermined

T65.5 Toxic effect of nitroglycerin and other nitric acids and esters
Toxic effect of 1,2,3-Propanetriol trinitrate
T65.5X Toxic effect of nitroglycerin and other nitric acids and esters
T65.5X1 Toxic effect of nitroglycerin and other nitric acids and esters, accidental (unintentional)
Toxic effect of nitroglycerin and other nitric acids and esters NOS
7 **T65.5X2 Toxic effect of nitroglycerin and other nitric acids and esters, intentional self-harm** HCC
T65.5X3 Toxic effect of nitroglycerin and other nitric acids and esters, assault
T65.5X4 Toxic effect of nitroglycerin and other nitric acids and esters, undetermined

T65.6 Toxic effect of paints and dyes, not elsewhere classified
T65.6X Toxic effect of paints and dyes, not elsewhere classified
T65.6X1 Toxic effect of paints and dyes, not elsewhere classified, accidental (unintentional)
Toxic effect of paints and dyes NOS
7 **T65.6X2 Toxic effect of paints and dyes, not elsewhere classified, intentional self-harm** HCC
T65.6X3 Toxic effect of paints and dyes, not elsewhere classified, assault
T65.6X4 Toxic effect of paints and dyes, not elsewhere classified, undetermined

T65.8 Toxic effect of other specified substances
T65.81 Toxic effect of latex
T65.811 Toxic effect of latex, accidental (unintentional)
Toxic effect of latex NOS

7 ✓7th **T65.812 Toxic effect of latex, intentional self-harm** HCC

✓7th **T65.813 Toxic effect of latex, assault**

✓7th **T65.814 Toxic effect of latex, undetermined**

✓6th **T65.82 Toxic effect of harmful algae and algae toxins**

Toxic effect of (harmful) algae bloom NOS
Toxic effect of blue-green algae bloom
Toxic effect of brown tide
Toxic effect of cyanobacteria bloom
Toxic effect of Florida red tide
Toxic effect of pfiesteria piscicida
Toxic effect of red tide

✓7th **T65.821 Toxic effect of harmful algae and algae toxins, accidental (unintentional)**

Toxic effect of harmful algae and algae toxins NOS

7 ✓7th **T65.822 Toxic effect of harmful algae and algae toxins, intentional self-harm** HCC

✓7th **T65.823 Toxic effect of harmful algae and algae toxins, assault**

✓7th **T65.824 Toxic effect of harmful algae and algae toxins, undetermined**

✓6th **T65.83 Toxic effect of fiberglass**

✓7th **T65.831 Toxic effect of fiberglass, accidental (unintentional)**

Toxic effect of fiberglass NOS

7 ✓7th **T65.832 Toxic effect of fiberglass, intentional self-harm** HCC

✓7th **T65.833 Toxic effect of fiberglass, assault**

✓7th **T65.834 Toxic effect of fiberglass, undetermined**

✓6th **T65.89 Toxic effect of other specified substances**

✓7th **T65.891 Toxic effect of other specified substances, accidental (unintentional)**

Toxic effect of other specified substances NOS

AHA: 2018,1Q,5

7 ✓7th **T65.892 Toxic effect of other specified substances, intentional self-harm** HCC

✓7th **T65.893 Toxic effect of other specified substances, assault**

✓7th **T65.894 Toxic effect of other specified substances, undetermined**

✓5th **T65.9 Toxic effect of unspecified substance**

✓x7th **T65.91 Toxic effect of unspecified substance, accidental (unintentional)**

Poisoning NOS

7 ✓x7th **T65.92 Toxic effect of unspecified substance, intentional self-harm** HCC

✓x7th **T65.93 Toxic effect of unspecified substance, assault**

✓x7th **T65.94 Toxic effect of unspecified substance, undetermined**

Other and unspecified effects of external causes (T66-T78)

✓x7th **T66 Radiation sickness, unspecified**

EXCLUDES 1 *specified adverse effects of radiation, such as:*
burns (T20-T31)
leukemia (C91-C95)
radiation gastroenteritis and colitis (K52.0)
radiation pneumonitis (J70.0)
radiation related disorders of the skin and subcutaneous tissue (L55-L59)
radiation sunburn (L55.-)

The appropriate 7th character is to be added to code T66.
A initial encounter
D subsequent encounter
S sequela

✓4th **T67 Effects of heat and light**

EXCLUDES 1 *erythema [dermatitis] ab igne (L59.0)*
malignant hyperpyrexia due to anesthesia (T88.3)
radiation-related disorders of the skin and subcutaneous tissue (L55-L59)

EXCLUDES 2 *burns (T20-T31)*
sunburn (L55.-)
sweat disorder due to heat (L74-L75)

The appropriate 7th character is to be added to each code from category T67.
A initial encounter
D subsequent encounter
S sequela

✓5th **T67.0 Heatstroke and sunstroke**

Use additional code(s) to identify any associated complications of heatstroke, such as:
coma and stupor (R40.-)
rhabdomyolysis (M62.82)
systemic inflammatory response syndrome (R65.1-)

AHA: 2019,4Q,17-18

DEF: Headache, vertigo, cramps, and elevated body temperature due to prolonged exposure to high environmental temperatures that requires emergency intervention.

✓x7th **T67.01 Heatstroke and sunstroke** CC H5

Heat apoplexy
Heat pyrexia
Siriasis
Thermoplegia

✓x7th **T67.02 Exertional heatstroke** CC H5

✓x7th **T67.09 Other heatstroke and sunstroke** CC H5

✓x7th **T67.1 Heat syncope**

Heat collapse

✓x7th **T67.2 Heat cramp**

✓x7th **T67.3 Heat exhaustion, anhydrotic**

Heat prostration due to water depletion

EXCLUDES 1 *heat exhaustion due to salt depletion (T67.4)*

✓x7th **T67.4 Heat exhaustion due to salt depletion**

Heat prostration due to salt (and water) depletion

✓x7th **T67.5 Heat exhaustion, unspecified**

Heat prostration NOS

✓x7th **T67.6 Heat fatigue, transient**

✓x7th **T67.7 Heat edema**

✓x7th **T67.8 Other effects of heat and light**

✓x7th **T67.9 Effect of heat and light, unspecified**

✓x7th **T68 Hypothermia**

Accidental hypothermia
Hypothermia NOS
Use additional code to identify source of exposure:
exposure to excessive cold of man-made origin (W93)
exposure to excessive cold of natural origin (X31)

EXCLUDES 1 *hypothermia following anesthesia (T88.51)*
hypothermia not associated with low environmental temperature (R68.0)
hypothermia of newborn (P80.-)

EXCLUDES 2 *frostbite (T33-T34)*

The appropriate 7th character is to be added to code T68.
A initial encounter
D subsequent encounter
S sequela

✓4th **T69 Other effects of reduced temperature**

Use additional code to identify source of exposure:
exposure to excessive cold of man-made origin (W93)
exposure to excessive cold of natural origin (X31)

EXCLUDES 2 *frostbite (T33-T34)*

The appropriate 7th character is to be added to each code from category T69.
A initial encounter
D subsequent encounter
S sequela

✓5th **T69.0 Immersion hand and foot**

✓6th **T69.01 Immersion hand**

✓7th **T69.011 Immersion hand, right hand**

√7th T69.012 Immersion hand, left hand

√7th T69.019 Immersion hand, unspecified hand

√6th T69.02 Immersion foot

Trench foot

√7th T69.021 Immersion foot, right foot CC H5

√7th T69.022 Immersion foot, left foot CC H5

√7th T69.029 Immersion foot, unspecified foot CC H5

√x7th T69.1 Chilblains

DEF: Red, swollen, itchy skin primarily affecting the fingers and toes, nose and ears, and legs. Chilblains follows damp-cold exposure, and can also be associated with pruritus and a burning feeling.

√x7th T69.8 Other specified effects of reduced temperature

√x7th T69.9 Effect of reduced temperature, unspecified

√4th **T70 Effects of air pressure and water pressure**

The appropriate 7th character is to be added to each code from category T70.
A initial encounter
D subsequent encounter
S sequela

√x7th T70.0 Otitic barotrauma

Aero-otitis media
Effects of change in ambient atmospheric pressure or water pressure on ears

√x7th T70.1 Sinus barotrauma

Aerosinusitis
Effects of change in ambient atmospheric pressure on sinuses

√5th T70.2 Other and unspecified effects of high altitude

EXCLUDES 2 *polycythemia due to high altitude (D75.1)*

√x7th T70.20 Unspecified effects of high altitude

√x7th T70.29 Other effects of high altitude

Alpine sickness
Anoxia due to high altitude
Barotrauma NOS
Hypobaropathy
Mountain sickness

√x7th T70.3 Caisson disease [decompression sickness] CC H5

Compressed-air disease
Diver's palsy or paralysis
DEF: Rapid reduction in air pressure while breathing compressed air. Symptoms include skin lesions, joint pains, and respiratory and neurological problems.

√x7th T70.4 Effects of high-pressure fluids

Hydraulic jet injection (industrial)
Pneumatic jet injection (industrial)
Traumatic jet injection (industrial)

√x7th T70.8 Other effects of air pressure and water pressure

√x7th T70.9 Effect of air pressure and water pressure, unspecified

√4th **T71 Asphyxiation**

Mechanical suffocation
Traumatic suffocation

EXCLUDES 1 *acute respiratory distress (syndrome) (J80)*
anoxia due to high altitude (T70.2)
asphyxia NOS (R09.01)
asphyxia from carbon monoxide (T58.-)
asphyxia from inhalation of food or foreign body (T17.-)
asphyxia from other gases, fumes and vapors (T59.-)
respiratory distress (syndrome) in newborn (P22.-)

The appropriate 7th character is to be added to each code from category T71.
A initial encounter
D subsequent encounter
S sequela

√5th T71.1 Asphyxiation due to mechanical threat to breathing

Suffocation due to mechanical threat to breathing

√6th T71.11 Asphyxiation due to smothering under pillow

√7th T71.111 Asphyxiation due to smothering under pillow, accidental CC H5

Asphyxiation due to smothering under pillow NOS

7 √7th T71.112 Asphyxiation due to smothering under pillow, intentional self-harm CC H5 HCC

√7th T71.113 Asphyxiation due to smothering under pillow, assault CC H5

√7th T71.114 Asphyxiation due to smothering under pillow, undetermined CC H5

√6th T71.12 Asphyxiation due to plastic bag

√7th T71.121 Asphyxiation due to plastic bag, accidental CC H5

Asphyxiation due to plastic bag NOS

7 √7th T71.122 Asphyxiation due to plastic bag, intentional self-harm CC H5 HCC

√7th T71.123 Asphyxiation due to plastic bag, assault CC H5

√7th T71.124 Asphyxiation due to plastic bag, undetermined CC H5

√6th T71.13 Asphyxiation due to being trapped in bed linens

√7th T71.131 Asphyxiation due to being trapped in bed linens, accidental CC H5

Asphyxiation due to being trapped in bed linens NOS

7 √7th T71.132 Asphyxiation due to being trapped in bed linens, intentional self-harm CC H5 HCC

√7th T71.133 Asphyxiation due to being trapped in bed linens, assault CC H5

√7th T71.134 Asphyxiation due to being trapped in bed linens, undetermined CC H5

√6th T71.14 Asphyxiation due to smothering under another person's body (in bed)

√7th T71.141 Asphyxiation due to smothering under another person's body (in bed), accidental CC H5

Asphyxiation due to smothering under another person's body (in bed) NOS

√7th T71.143 Asphyxiation due to smothering under another person's body (in bed), assault CC H5

√7th T71.144 Asphyxiation due to smothering under another person's body (in bed), undetermined CC H5

√6th T71.15 Asphyxiation due to smothering in furniture

√7th T71.151 Asphyxiation due to smothering in furniture, accidental CC H5

Asphyxiation due to smothering in furniture NOS

7 √7th T71.152 Asphyxiation due to smothering in furniture, intentional self-harm CC H5 HCC

√7th T71.153 Asphyxiation due to smothering in furniture, assault CC H5

√7th T71.154 Asphyxiation due to smothering in furniture, undetermined CC H5

√6th T71.16 Asphyxiation due to hanging

Hanging by window shade cord
Use additional code for any associated injuries, such as:
crushing injury of neck (S17.-)
fracture of cervical vertebrae (S12.0-S12.2-)
open wound of neck (S11.-)

√7th T71.161 Asphyxiation due to hanging, accidental CC H5

Asphyxiation due to hanging NOS
Hanging NOS

7 √7th T71.162 Asphyxiation due to hanging, intentional self-harm CC H5 HCC

√7th T71.163 Asphyxiation due to hanging, assault CC H5

√7th T71.164 Asphyxiation due to hanging, undetermined CC H5

√6th T71.19 Asphyxiation due to mechanical threat to breathing due to other causes

√7th T71.191 Asphyxiation due to mechanical threat to breathing due to other causes, accidental CC H5

Asphyxiation due to other causes NOS

7 √7th T71.192 Asphyxiation due to mechanical threat to breathing due to other causes, intentional self-harm CC H5 HCC

T71.193 Asphyxiation due to mechanical threat to breathing due to other causes, assault CC H5

T71.194 Asphyxiation due to mechanical threat to breathing due to other causes, undetermined CC H5

T71.2 Asphyxiation due to systemic oxygen deficiency due to low oxygen content in ambient air

Suffocation due to systemic oxygen deficiency due to low oxygen content in ambient air

T71.20 Asphyxiation due to systemic oxygen deficiency due to low oxygen content in ambient air due to unspecified cause CC H5

T71.21 Asphyxiation due to cave-in or falling earth CC H5

Use additional code for any associated cataclysm (X34-X38)

T71.22 Asphyxiation due to being trapped in a car trunk

T71.221 Asphyxiation due to being trapped in a car trunk, accidental CC

7 **T71.222 Asphyxiation due to being trapped in a car trunk, intentional self-harm** CC HCC

T71.223 Asphyxiation due to being trapped in a car trunk, assault CC

T71.224 Asphyxiation due to being trapped in a car trunk, undetermined CC

T71.23 Asphyxiation due to being trapped in a (discarded) refrigerator

T71.231 Asphyxiation due to being trapped in a (discarded) refrigerator, accidental CC

7 **T71.232 Asphyxiation due to being trapped in a (discarded) refrigerator, intentional self-harm** CC HCC

T71.233 Asphyxiation due to being trapped in a (discarded) refrigerator, assault CC

T71.234 Asphyxiation due to being trapped in a (discarded) refrigerator, undetermined CC

T71.29 Asphyxiation due to being trapped in other low oxygen environment CC H5

T71.9 Asphyxiation due to unspecified cause CC H5

Suffocation (by strangulation) due to unspecified cause
Suffocation NOS
Systemic oxygen deficiency due to low oxygen content in ambient air due to unspecified cause
Systemic oxygen deficiency due to mechanical threat to breathing due to unspecified cause
Traumatic asphyxia NOS

T73 Effects of other deprivation

The appropriate 7th character is to be added to each code from category T73.
A initial encounter
D subsequent encounter
S sequela

T73.0 Starvation

Deprivation of food

T73.1 Deprivation of water

T73.2 Exhaustion due to exposure

T73.3 Exhaustion due to excessive exertion

Exhaustion due to overexertion

T73.8 Other effects of deprivation

T73.9 Effect of deprivation, unspecified

T74 Adult and child abuse, neglect and other maltreatment, confirmed

Use additional code, if applicable, to identify any associated current injury
Use additional external cause code to identify perpetrator, if known (Y07.-)

EXCLUDES 1 *abuse and maltreatment in pregnancy (O9A.3-, O9A.4-, O9A.5-)*
adult and child maltreatment, suspected (T76.-)

The appropriate 7th character is to be added to each code from category T74.
A initial encounter
D subsequent encounter
S sequela

T74.0 Neglect or abandonment, confirmed

T74.01 Adult neglect or abandonment, confirmed CC A

T74.02 Child neglect or abandonment, confirmed CC P

T74.1 Physical abuse, confirmed

EXCLUDES 2 *sexual abuse (T74.2-)*

T74.11 Adult physical abuse, confirmed CC A

T74.12 Child physical abuse, confirmed CC P

EXCLUDES 2 *shaken infant syndrome (T74.4)*

T74.2 Sexual abuse, confirmed

Rape, confirmed
Sexual assault, confirmed

T74.21 Adult sexual abuse, confirmed CC A

T74.22 Child sexual abuse, confirmed CC P

T74.3 Psychological abuse, confirmed

Bullying and intimidation, confirmed
Intimidation through social media, confirmed

T74.31 Adult psychological abuse, confirmed A

T74.32 Child psychological abuse, confirmed CC P

T74.4 Shaken infant syndrome CC P

T74.5 Forced sexual exploitation, confirmed

AHA: 2018,4Q,32-33,65

T74.51 Adult forced sexual exploitation, confirmed CC A

T74.52 Child sexual exploitation, confirmed CC P

T74.6 Forced labor exploitation, confirmed

AHA: 2018,4Q,32-33,65

T74.61 Adult forced labor exploitation, confirmed CC A

T74.62 Child forced labor exploitation, confirmed CC P

T74.9 Unspecified maltreatment, confirmed

T74.91 Unspecified adult maltreatment, confirmed CC A

T74.92 Unspecified child maltreatment, confirmed CC P

T75 Other and unspecified effects of other external causes

EXCLUDES 1 *adverse effects NEC (T78.-)*
EXCLUDES 2 *burns (electric) (T20-T31)*

The appropriate 7th character is to be added to each code from category T75.
A initial encounter
D subsequent encounter
S sequela

T75.0 Effects of lightning

Struck by lightning

T75.00 Unspecified effects of lightning

Struck by lightning NOS

T75.01 Shock due to being struck by lightning

T75.09 Other effects of lightning

Use additional code for other effects of lightning

T75.1 Unspecified effects of drowning and nonfatal submersion CC H5

Immersion

EXCLUDES 1 *specified effects of drowning — code to effects*

T75.2 Effects of vibration

T75.20 Unspecified effects of vibration

T75.21 Pneumatic hammer syndrome

T75.22 Traumatic vasospastic syndrome

√x7th **T75.23 Vertigo from infrasound**
EXCLUDES 1 *vertigo NOS (R42)*

√x7th **T75.29 Other effects of vibration**

√x7th **T75.3 Motion sickness**
Airsickness
Seasickness
Travel sickness
Use additional external cause code to identify vehicle or type of motion (Y92.81-, Y93.5-)

√x7th **T75.4 Electrocution**
Shock from electric current
Shock from electroshock gun (taser)

√5th **T75.8 Other specified effects of external causes**

√x7th **T75.81 Effects of abnormal gravitation [G] forces**

√x7th **T75.82 Effects of weightlessness**

√x7th **T75.89 Other specified effects of external causes**

√4th **T76 Adult and child abuse, neglect and other maltreatment, suspected**
Use additional code, if applicable, to identify any associated current injury
EXCLUDES 1 *adult and child maltreatment, confirmed (T74.-)*
suspected abuse and maltreatment in pregnancy (O9A.3-, O9A.4-, O9A.5-)
suspected adult physical abuse, ruled out (Z04.71)
suspected adult sexual abuse, ruled out (Z04.41)
suspected child physical abuse, ruled out (Z04.72)
suspected child sexual abuse, ruled out (Z04.42)

AHA: 2018,4Q,72

The appropriate 7th character is to be added to each code from category T76.
A initial encounter
D subsequent encounter
S sequela

√5th **T76.0 Neglect or abandonment, suspected**

√x7th **T76.01 Adult neglect or abandonment, suspected** CC A

√x7th **T76.02 Child neglect or abandonment, suspected** CC P

√5th **T76.1 Physical abuse, suspected**

√x7th **T76.11 Adult physical abuse, suspected** CC A

√x7th **T76.12 Child physical abuse, suspected** CC P
AHA: 2019,2Q,12

√5th **T76.2 Sexual abuse, suspected**
Rape, suspected
EXCLUDES 1 *alleged abuse, ruled out (Z04.7)*

√x7th **T76.21 Adult sexual abuse, suspected** CC A

√x7th **T76.22 Child sexual abuse, suspected** CC P

√5th **T76.3 Psychological abuse, suspected**
Bullying and intimidation, suspected
Intimidation through social media, suspected

√x7th **T76.31 Adult psychological abuse, suspected** A

√x7th **T76.32 Child psychological abuse, suspected** CC P

√5th **T76.5 Forced sexual exploitation, suspected**
AHA: 2018,4Q,32-33,65

√x7th **T76.51 Adult forced sexual exploitation, suspected** CC A

√x7th **T76.52 Child sexual exploitation, suspected** CC P

√5th **T76.6 Forced labor exploitation, suspected**
AHA: 2018,4Q,32-33,65

√x7th **T76.61 Adult forced labor exploitation, suspected** CC A

√x7th **T76.62 Child forced labor exploitation, suspected** CC P

√5th **T76.9 Unspecified maltreatment, suspected**

√x7th **T76.91 Unspecified adult maltreatment, suspected** CC A

√x7th **T76.92 Unspecified child maltreatment, suspected** CC P

√4th **T78 Adverse effects, not elsewhere classified**
EXCLUDES 2 *complications of surgical and medical care NEC (T80-T88)*

The appropriate 7th character is to be added to each code from category T78.
A initial encounter
D subsequent encounter
S sequela

√5th **T78.0 Anaphylactic reaction due to food**
Anaphylactic reaction due to adverse food reaction
Anaphylactic shock or reaction due to nonpoisonous foods
Anaphylactoid reaction due to food

√x7th **T78.00 Anaphylactic reaction due to unspecified food** CC

√x7th **T78.01 Anaphylactic reaction due to peanuts** CC

√x7th **T78.02 Anaphylactic reaction due to shellfish (crustaceans)** CC

√x7th **T78.03 Anaphylactic reaction due to other fish** CC

√x7th **T78.04 Anaphylactic reaction due to fruits and vegetables** CC

√x7th **T78.05 Anaphylactic reaction due to tree nuts and seeds** CC
EXCLUDES 2 *anaphylactic reaction due to peanuts (T78.01)*

√x7th **T78.06 Anaphylactic reaction due to food additives** CC

√x7th **T78.07 Anaphylactic reaction due to milk and dairy products** CC

√x7th **T78.08 Anaphylactic reaction due to eggs** CC

√x7th **T78.09 Anaphylactic reaction due to other food products** CC

√x7th **T78.1 Other adverse food reactions, not elsewhere classified**
Use additional code to identify the type of reaction, if applicable
EXCLUDES 1 *anaphylactic reaction or shock due to adverse food reaction (T78.0-)*
anaphylactic reaction due to food (T78.0-)
bacterial food borne intoxications (A05.-)
EXCLUDES 2 *allergic and dietetic gastroenteritis and colitis (K52.29)*
allergic rhinitis due to food (J30.5)
dermatitis due to food in contact with skin (L23.6, L24.6, L25.4)
dermatitis due to ingested food (L27.2)
food protein-induced enterocolitis syndrome (K52.21)
food protein-induced enteropathy (K52.22)

√x7th **T78.2 Anaphylactic shock, unspecified** CC
Allergic shock
Anaphylactic reaction
Anaphylaxis
EXCLUDES 1 *anaphylactic reaction or shock due to adverse effect of correct medicinal substance properly administered (T88.6)*
anaphylactic reaction or shock due to adverse food reaction (T78.0-)
anaphylactic reaction or shock due to serum (T80.5-)

√x7th **T78.3 Angioneurotic edema**
Allergic angioedema
Giant urticaria
Quincke's edema
EXCLUDES 1 *serum urticaria (T80.6-)*
urticaria (L50.-)

√5th **T78.4 Other and unspecified allergy**
EXCLUDES 1 *specified types of allergic reaction such as:*
allergic diarrhea (K52.29)
allergic gastroenteritis and colitis (K52.29)
dermatitis (L23-L25, L27.-)
food protein-induced enterocolitis syndrome (K52.21)
food protein-induced enteropathy (K52.22)
hay fever (J30.1)

√x7th **T78.40 Allergy, unspecified**
Allergic reaction NOS
Hypersensitivity NOS

√x7th **T78.41 Arthus phenomenon**
Arthus reaction

√x7th **T78.49 Other allergy**

√x7th **T78.8 Other adverse effects, not elsewhere classified**

Certain early complications of trauma (T79)

√4th **T79 Certain early complications of trauma, not elsewhere classified**

EXCLUDES 2 *acute respiratory distress syndrome (J8Ø)*
complications occurring during or following medical procedures (T8Ø-T88)
complications of surgical and medical care NEC (T8Ø-T88)
newborn respiratory distress syndrome (P22.Ø)

The appropriate 7th character is to be added to each code from category T79.
A initial encounter
D subsequent encounter
S sequela

6 √x7th **T79.Ø Air embolism (traumatic)** MCC HCC
EXCLUDES 1 *air embolism complicating abortion or ectopic or molar pregnancy (OØØ-OØ7, OØ8.2)*
air embolism complicating pregnancy, childbirth and the puerperium (O88.Ø)
air embolism following infusion, transfusion, and therapeutic injection (T8Ø.Ø)
air embolism following procedure NEC (T81.7-)
DEF: Arterial or venous obstruction due to the introduction of air bubbles into the blood vessels following surgery or trauma.

6 √x7th **T79.1 Fat embolism (traumatic)** MCC HCC
EXCLUDES 1 *fat embolism complicating:*
abortion or ectopic or molar pregnancy (OØØ-OØ7, OØ8.2)
pregnancy, childbirth and the puerperium (O88.8)
DEF: Arterial blockage due to the entrance of fat into the circulatory system after a fracture of the large bones or administration of corticosteroids.

6 √x7th **T79.2 Traumatic secondary and recurrent hemorrhage and seroma** CC HCC

6 √x7th **T79.4 Traumatic shock** MCC HCC
Shock (immediate) (delayed) following injury
EXCLUDES 1 *anaphylactic shock due to adverse food reaction (T78.Ø-)*
anaphylactic shock due to correct medicinal substance properly administered (T88.6)
anaphylactic shock due to serum (T8Ø.5-)
anaphylactic shock NOS (T78.2)
anesthetic shock (T88.2)
electric shock (T75.4)
nontraumatic shock NEC (R57.-)
obstetric shock (O75.1)
postprocedural shock (T81.1-)
septic shock (R65.21)
shock complicating abortion or ectopic or molar pregnancy (OØØ-OØ7, OØ8.3)
shock due to lightning (T75.Ø1)
shock NOS (R57.9)

6 √x7th **T79.5 Traumatic anuria** MCC HCC
Crush syndrome
Renal failure following crushing

6 √x7th **T79.6 Traumatic ischemia of muscle** HCC
Traumatic rhabdomyolysis
Volkmann's ischemic contracture
EXCLUDES 2 *anterior tibial syndrome (M76.8)*
compartment syndrome (traumatic) (T79.A-)
nontraumatic ischemia of muscle (M62.2-)
AHA: 2019,2Q,12

6 √x7th **T79.7 Traumatic subcutaneous emphysema** CC HCC
EXCLUDES 1 ~~*emphysema NOS (J43)*~~
~~*emphysema (subcutaneous) resulting from a procedure (T81.82)*~~
EXCLUDES 2 ►*emphysema NOS (J43)*◄
►*emphysema (subcutaneous) resulting from a procedure (T81.82)*◄

√5th **T79.A Traumatic compartment syndrome**
EXCLUDES 1 *fibromyalgia (M79.7)*
nontraumatic compartment syndrome (M79.A-)
EXCLUDES 2 *traumatic ischemic infarction of muscle (T79.6)*
DEF: Compression of nerves and blood vessels within an enclosed muscle space due to previous trauma, which leads to impaired blood flow and muscle and nerve damage.

6 √x7th **T79.AØ Compartment syndrome, unspecified** CC HCC
Compartment syndrome NOS

√6th **T79.A1 Traumatic compartment syndrome of upper extremity**
Traumatic compartment syndrome of shoulder, arm, forearm, wrist, hand, and fingers

6 √7th **T79.A11 Traumatic compartment syndrome of right upper extremity** CC HCC
6 √7th **T79.A12 Traumatic compartment syndrome of left upper extremity** CC HCC
6 √7th **T79.A19 Traumatic compartment syndrome of unspecified upper extremity** CC HCC

√6th **T79.A2 Traumatic compartment syndrome of lower extremity**
Traumatic compartment syndrome of hip, buttock, thigh, leg, foot, and toes

6 √7th **T79.A21 Traumatic compartment syndrome of right lower extremity** CC HCC
6 √7th **T79.A22 Traumatic compartment syndrome of left lower extremity** CC HCC
6 √7th **T79.A29 Traumatic compartment syndrome of unspecified lower extremity** CC HCC

6 √x7th **T79.A3 Traumatic compartment syndrome of abdomen** CC HCC

6 √x7th **T79.A9 Traumatic compartment syndrome of other sites** CC HCC

6 √x7th **T79.8 Other early complications of trauma** HCC

6 √x7th **T79.9 Unspecified early complication of trauma** HCC

Chapter 19. Injury, Poisoning and Certain Other Consequences of External Causes

T78.8–T79.9

Complications of surgical and medical care, not elsewhere classified (T80-T88)

Use additional code for adverse effect, if applicable, to identify drug (T36-T50 with fifth or sixth character 5)
Use additional code(s) to identify the specified condition resulting from the complication
Use additional code to identify devices involved and details of circumstances (Y62-Y82)

EXCLUDES 2 *any encounters with medical care for postprocedural conditions in which no complications are present, such as:*
artificial opening status (Z93.-)
closure of external stoma (Z43.-)
fitting and adjustment of external prosthetic device (Z44.-)
burns and corrosions from local applications and irradiation (T20-T32)
complications of surgical procedures during pregnancy, childbirth and the puerperium (O00-O9A)
mechanical complication of respirator [ventilator] (J95.850)
poisoning and toxic effects of drugs and chemicals (T36-T65 with fifth or sixth character 1-4 or 6)
postprocedural fever (R50.82)
specified complications classified elsewhere, such as:
cerebrospinal fluid leak from spinal puncture (G97.0)
colostomy malfunction (K94.0-)
disorders of fluid and electrolyte imbalance (E86-E87)
functional disturbances following cardiac surgery (I97.0-I97.1)
intraoperative and postprocedural complications of specified body systems (D78.-, E36.-, E89.-, G97.3-, G97.4, H59.3-, H59.-, H95.2-, H95.3, I97.4-, I97.5, J95.6-, J95.7, K91.6-, L76.-, M96.-, N99.-)
ostomy complications (J95.0-, K94.-, N99.5-)
postgastric surgery syndromes (K91.1)
postlaminectomy syndrome NEC (M96.1)
postmastectomy lymphedema syndrome (I97.2)
postsurgical blind-loop syndrome (K91.2)
ventilator associated pneumonia (J95.851)

AHA: 2015,1Q,15

√4th **T80 Complications following infusion, transfusion and therapeutic injection**

INCLUDES complications following perfusion

EXCLUDES 2 *bone marrow transplant rejection (T86.01)*
febrile nonhemolytic transfusion reaction (R50.84)
fluid overload due to transfusion (E87.71)
posttransfusion purpura (D69.51)
transfusion associated circulatory overload (TACO) (E87.71)
transfusion (red blood cell) associated hemochromatosis (E83.111)
transfusion related acute lung injury (TRALI) (J95.84)

The appropriate 7th character is to be added to each code from category T80.
A initial encounter
D subsequent encounter
S sequela

√x7th **T80.0 Air embolism following infusion, transfusion and therapeutic injection** MCC H2

√x7th **T80.1 Vascular complications following infusion, transfusion and therapeutic injection** CC

Use additional code to identify the vascular complication

EXCLUDES 2 *extravasation of vesicant agent (T80.81-)*
infiltration of vesicant agent (T80.81-)
postprocedural vascular complications (T81.7-)
vascular complications specified as due to prosthetic devices, implants and grafts (T82.8-, T83.8-, T84.8-, T85.8-)

√5th **T80.2 Infections following infusion, transfusion and therapeutic injection**

Use additional code to identify the specific infection, such as: sepsis (A41.9)
Use additional code (R65.2-) to identify severe sepsis, if applicable

EXCLUDES 2 *infections specified as due to prosthetic devices, implants and grafts (T82.6-T82.7, T83.5-T83.6, T84.5-T84.7, T85.7)*
postprocedural infections (T81.4-)

AHA: 2018,4Q,62

√6th **T80.21 Infection due to central venous catheter**

Infection due to pulmonary artery catheter (Swan-Ganz catheter)

AHA: 2019,1Q,13-14

TIP: Only centrally placed catheters are captured with this subcategory. Infections resulting from catheters that are not central lines, including those used for hemodialysis, should be coded to T82.7-.

√7th **T80.211 Bloodstream infection due to central venous catheter** CC H7

Catheter-related bloodstream infection (CRBSI) NOS
Central line-associated bloodstream infection (CLABSI)
Bloodstream infection due to Hickman catheter
Bloodstream infection due to peripherally inserted central catheter (PICC)
Bloodstream infection due to portacath (port-a-cath)
Bloodstream infection due to pulmonary artery catheter
Bloodstream infection due to triple lumen catheter
Bloodstream infection due to umbilical venous catheter

AHA: 2019,1Q,13,14; 2018,4Q,89

√7th **T80.212 Local infection due to central venous catheter** CC H7

Exit or insertion site infection
Local infection due to Hickman catheter
Local infection due to peripherally inserted central catheter (PICC)
Local infection due to portacath (port-a-cath)
Local infection due to pulmonary artery catheter
Local infection due to triple lumen catheter
Local infection due to umbilical venous catheter
Port or reservoir infection
Tunnel infection

√7th **T80.218 Other infection due to central venous catheter** CC H7

Other central line-associated infection
Other infection due to Hickman catheter
Other infection due to peripherally inserted central catheter (PICC)
Other infection due to portacath (port-a-cath)
Other infection due to pulmonary artery catheter
Other infection due to triple lumen catheter
Other infection due to umbilical venous catheter

T80.219 **Unspecified infection due to central venous catheter** CC H7
- Central line-associated infection NOS
- Unspecified infection due to Hickman catheter
- Unspecified infection due to peripherally inserted central catheter (PICC)
- Unspecified infection due to portacath (port-a-cath)
- Unspecified infection due to pulmonary artery catheter
- Unspecified infection due to triple lumen catheter
- Unspecified infection due to umbilical venous catheter

T80.22 **Acute infection following transfusion, infusion, or injection of blood and blood products** CC

T80.29 **Infection following other infusion, transfusion and therapeutic injection** CC

T80.3 **ABO incompatibility reaction due to transfusion of blood or blood products**

EXCLUDES 1 *minor blood group antigens reactions (Duffy) (E) (K) (Kell) (Kidd) (Lewis) (M) (N) (P) (S) (T80.A-)*

T80.30 **ABO incompatibility reaction due to transfusion of blood or blood products, unspecified** CC H3
- ABO incompatibility blood transfusion NOS
- Reaction to ABO incompatibility from transfusion NOS

T80.31 **ABO incompatibility with hemolytic transfusion reaction**

T80.310 **ABO incompatibility with acute hemolytic transfusion reaction** CC H3
- ABO incompatibility with hemolytic transfusion reaction less than 24 hours after transfusion
- Acute hemolytic transfusion reaction (AHTR) due to ABO incompatibility

T80.311 **ABO incompatibility with delayed hemolytic transfusion reaction** CC H3
- ABO incompatibility with hemolytic transfusion reaction 24 hours or more after transfusion
- Delayed hemolytic transfusion reaction (DHTR) due to ABO incompatibility

T80.319 **ABO incompatibility with hemolytic transfusion reaction, unspecified** CC H3
- ABO incompatibility with hemolytic transfusion reaction at unspecified time after transfusion
- Hemolytic transfusion reaction (HTR) due to ABO incompatibility NOS

T80.39 **Other ABO incompatibility reaction due to transfusion of blood or blood products** CC H3
- Delayed serologic transfusion reaction (DSTR) from ABO incompatibility
- Other ABO incompatible blood transfusion
- Other reaction to ABO incompatible blood transfusion

T80.4 **Rh incompatibility reaction due to transfusion of blood or blood products**

Reaction due to incompatibility of Rh antigens (C) (c) (D) (E) (e)

T80.40 **Rh incompatibility reaction due to transfusion of blood or blood products, unspecified** CC
- Reaction due to Rh factor in transfusion NOS
- Rh incompatible blood transfusion NOS

T80.41 **Rh incompatibility with hemolytic transfusion reaction**

T80.410 **Rh incompatibility with acute hemolytic transfusion reaction** CC
- Acute hemolytic transfusion reaction (AHTR) due to Rh incompatibility
- Rh incompatibility with hemolytic transfusion reaction less than 24 hours after transfusion

T80.411 **Rh incompatibility with delayed hemolytic transfusion reaction** CC
- Delayed hemolytic transfusion reaction (DHTR) due to Rh incompatibility
- Rh incompatibility with hemolytic transfusion reaction 24 hours or more after transfusion

T80.419 **Rh incompatibility with hemolytic transfusion reaction, unspecified** CC
- Rh incompatibility with hemolytic transfusion reaction at unspecified time after transfusion
- Hemolytic transfusion reaction (HTR) due to Rh incompatibility NOS

T80.49 **Other Rh incompatibility reaction due to transfusion of blood or blood products** CC
- Delayed serologic transfusion reaction (DSTR) from Rh incompatibility
- Other reaction to Rh incompatible blood transfusion

T80.A **Non-ABO incompatibility reaction due to transfusion of blood or blood products**

Reaction due to incompatibility of minor antigens (Duffy) (Kell) (Kidd) (Lewis) (M) (N) (P) (S)

T80.A0 **Non-ABO incompatibility reaction due to transfusion of blood or blood products, unspecified** CC
- Non-ABO antigen incompatibility reaction from transfusion NOS

T80.A1 **Non-ABO incompatibility with hemolytic transfusion reaction**

T80.A10 **Non-ABO incompatibility with acute hemolytic transfusion reaction** CC
- Acute hemolytic transfusion reaction (AHTR) due to non-ABO incompatibility
- Non-ABO incompatibility with hemolytic transfusion reaction less than 24 hours after transfusion

T80.A11 **Non-ABO incompatibility with delayed hemolytic transfusion reaction** CC
- Delayed hemolytic transfusion reaction (DHTR) due to non-ABO incompatibility
- Non-ABO incompatibility with hemolytic transfusion reaction 24 or more hours after transfusion

T80.A19 **Non-ABO incompatibility with hemolytic transfusion reaction, unspecified** CC
- Hemolytic transfusion reaction (HTR) due to non-ABO incompatibility NOS
- Non-ABO incompatibility with hemolytic transfusion reaction at unspecified time after transfusion

T80.A9 **Other non-ABO incompatibility reaction due to transfusion of blood or blood products** CC
- Delayed serologic transfusion reaction (DSTR) from non-ABO incompatibility
- Other reaction to non-ABO incompatible blood transfusion

T80.5 **Anaphylactic reaction due to serum**
- Allergic shock due to serum
- Anaphylactic shock due to serum
- Anaphylactoid reaction due to serum
- Anaphylaxis due to serum

EXCLUDES 1 *ABO incompatibility reaction due to transfusion of blood or blood products (T80.3-)*
allergic reaction or shock NOS (T78.2)
anaphylactic reaction or shock NOS (T78.2)
anaphylactic reaction or shock due to adverse effect of correct medicinal substance properly administered (T88.6)
other serum reaction (T80.6-)

DEF: Life-threatening hypersensitivity to a foreign serum causing respiratory distress, vascular collapse, and shock.

T80.51 **Anaphylactic reaction due to administration of blood and blood products** CC

T80.52 **Anaphylactic reaction due to vaccination** CC

T80.59 **Anaphylactic reaction due to other serum** CC

T80.6 Other serum reactions

Intoxication by serum
Protein sickness
Serum rash
Serum sickness
Serum urticaria

EXCLUDES 2 *serum hepatitis (B16-B19)*

DEF: Serum sickness: Hypersensitivity to a foreign serum that causes fever, hives, swelling, and lymphadenopathy.

T80.61 Other serum reaction due to administration of blood and blood products CC

T80.62 Other serum reaction due to vaccination CC

T80.69 Other serum reaction due to other serum CC

Code also, if applicable, arthropathy in hypersensitivity reactions classified elsewhere (M36.4)

T80.8 Other complications following infusion, transfusion and therapeutic injection

T80.81 Extravasation of vesicant agent

Infiltration of vesicant agent

T80.810 Extravasation of vesicant antineoplastic chemotherapy CC

Infiltration of vesicant antineoplastic chemotherapy

T80.818 Extravasation of other vesicant agent CC

Infiltration of other vesicant agent

T80.89 Other complications following infusion, transfusion and therapeutic injection

Delayed serologic transfusion reaction (DSTR), unspecified incompatibility

Use additional code to identify graft-versus-host reaction, if applicable, (D89.81-)

T80.9 Unspecified complication following infusion, transfusion and therapeutic injection

T80.90 Unspecified complication following infusion and therapeutic injection

T80.91 Hemolytic transfusion reaction, unspecified incompatibility

EXCLUDES 1 *ABO incompatibility with hemolytic transfusion reaction (T80.31-)*
non-ABO incompatibility with hemolytic transfusion reaction (T80.A1-)
Rh incompatibility with hemolytic transfusion reaction (T80.41-)

T80.910 Acute hemolytic transfusion reaction, unspecified incompatibility CC

T80.911 Delayed hemolytic transfusion reaction, unspecified incompatibility CC

T80.919 Hemolytic transfusion reaction, unspecified incompatibility, unspecified as acute or delayed CC

Hemolytic transfusion reaction NOS

T80.92 Unspecified transfusion reaction

Transfusion reaction NOS

T81 Complications of procedures, not elsewhere classified

Use additional code for adverse effect, if applicable, to identify drug (T36-T50 with fifth or sixth character 5)

EXCLUDES 2 *complications following immunization (T88.0-T88.1)*
complications following infusion, transfusion and therapeutic injection (T80.-)
complications of transplanted organs and tissue (T86.-)
specified complications classified elsewhere, such as:
complication of prosthetic devices, implants and grafts (T82-T85)
dermatitis due to drugs and medicaments (L23.3, L24.4, L25.1, L27.0-L27.1)
endosseous dental implant failure (M27.6-)
floppy iris syndrome (IFIS) (intraoperative) (H21.81)
intraoperative and postprocedural complications of specific body system (D78.-, E36.-, E89.-, G97.3-, G97.4, H59.3-, H59.-, H95.2-, H95.3, I97.4-, I97.5, J95, K91.-, L76.-, M96.-, N99.-)
ostomy complications (J95.0-, K94.-, N99.5-)
plateau iris syndrome (post-iridectomy) (postprocedural) H21.82
poisoning and toxic effects of drugs and chemicals (T36-T65 with fifth or sixth character 1-4 or 6)

AHA: 2019,2Q,21

The appropriate 7th character is to be added to each code from category T81.
A initial encounter
D subsequent encounter
S sequela

T81.1 Postprocedural shock

Shock during or resulting from a procedure, not elsewhere classified

EXCLUDES 1 *anaphylactic shock due to correct substance properly administered (T88.6)*
anaphylactic shock due to serum (T80.5-)
anaphylactic shock NOS (T78.2)
anesthetic shock (T88.2)
electric shock (T75.4)
obstetric shock (O75.1)
septic shock (R65.21)
shock following abortion or ectopic or molar pregnancy (O00-O07, O08.3)
traumatic shock (T79.4)

T81.10 Postprocedural shock unspecified CC

Collapse NOS during or resulting from a procedure, not elsewhere classified
Postprocedural failure of peripheral circulation
Postprocedural shock NOS

6 **T81.11 Postprocedural cardiogenic shock** MCC HCC

6 **T81.12 Postprocedural septic shock** MCC HCC

Postprocedural endotoxic shock resulting from a procedure, not elsewhere classified
Postprocedural gram-negative shock resulting from a procedure, not elsewhere classified
Code first underlying infection
Use additional code, to identify any associated acute organ dysfunction, if applicable

AHA: 2018,4Q,63

T81.19 Other postprocedural shock MCC

Postprocedural hypovolemic shock

T81.3 Disruption of wound, not elsewhere classified

Disruption of any suture materials or other closure methods

EXCLUDES 1 *breakdown (mechanical) of permanent sutures (T85.612)*
displacement of permanent sutures (T85.622)
disruption of cesarean delivery wound (O90.0)
disruption of perineal obstetric wound (O90.1)
mechanical complication of permanent sutures NEC (T85.692)

AHA: 2014,1Q,23

T81.30 Disruption of wound, unspecified CC SW

Disruption of wound NOS

T81.31 **Disruption of external operation (surgical) wound, not elsewhere classified** CC SW
Dehiscence of operation wound NOS
Disruption of operation wound NOS
Disruption or dehiscence of closure of cornea
Disruption or dehiscence of closure of mucosa
Disruption or dehiscence of closure of skin and subcutaneous tissue
Full-thickness skin disruption or dehiscence
Superficial disruption or dehiscence of operation wound
EXCLUDES 1 *dehiscence of amputation stump (T87.81)*

T81.32 **Disruption of internal operation (surgical) wound, not elsewhere classified** CC SW
Deep disruption or dehiscence of operation wound NOS
Disruption or dehiscence of closure of internal organ or other internal tissue
Disruption or dehiscence of closure of muscle or muscle flap
Disruption or dehiscence of closure of ribs or rib cage
Disruption or dehiscence of closure of skull or craniotomy
Disruption or dehiscence of closure of sternum or sternotomy
Disruption or dehiscence of closure of tendon or ligament
Disruption or dehiscence of closure of superficial or muscular fascia
AHA: 2020,2Q,22; 2017,3Q,4

T81.33 **Disruption of traumatic injury wound repair** CC
Disruption or dehiscence of closure of traumatic laceration (external) (internal)

T81.4 Infection following a procedure
Wound abscess following a procedure
Use additional code to identify infection
Use additional code (R65.2-) to identify severe sepsis, if applicable
EXCLUDES 2 *bleb associated endophthalmitis (H59.4-)*
infection due to infusion, transfusion and therapeutic injection (T80.2-)
infection due to prosthetic devices, implants and grafts (T82.6-T82.7, T83.5-T83.6, T84.5-T84.7, T85.7)
obstetric surgical wound infection (O86.0-)
postprocedural fever NOS (R50.82)
postprocedural retroperitoneal abscess (K68.11)
AHA: 2018,4Q,33-34,62; 2014,1Q,23

T81.40 **Infection following a procedure, unspecified** CC H11 H12 H13

T81.41 **Infection following a procedure, superficial incisional surgical site** CC H11 H12 H13
Subcutaneous abscess following a procedure
Stitch abscess following a procedure

T81.42 **Infection following a procedure, deep incisional surgical site** CC H11 H12 H13
Intra-muscular abscess following a procedure

T81.43 **Infection following a procedure, organ and space surgical site** CC H11 H12 H13
Intra-abdominal abscess following a procedure
Subphrenic abscess following a procedure

6 T81.44 **Sepsis following a procedure** CC H11 H12 H13 HCC
Use additional code to identify the sepsis

T81.49 **Infection following a procedure, other surgical site** CC H11 H12 H13

T81.5 Complications of foreign body accidentally left in body following procedure
AHA: 2014,4Q,24

T81.50 **Unspecified complication of foreign body accidentally left in body following procedure**

T81.500 **Unspecified complication of foreign body accidentally left in body following surgical operation** CC H1

T81.501 **Unspecified complication of foreign body accidentally left in body following infusion or transfusion** CC H1

T81.502 **Unspecified complication of foreign body accidentally left in body following kidney dialysis** CC H1 HCC

T81.503 **Unspecified complication of foreign body accidentally left in body following injection or immunization** CC H1

T81.504 **Unspecified complication of foreign body accidentally left in body following endoscopic examination** CC H1

T81.505 **Unspecified complication of foreign body accidentally left in body following heart catheterization** CC H1

T81.506 **Unspecified complication of foreign body accidentally left in body following aspiration, puncture or other catheterization** CC H1

T81.507 **Unspecified complication of foreign body accidentally left in body following removal of catheter or packing** CC H1

T81.508 **Unspecified complication of foreign body accidentally left in body following other procedure** CC H1

T81.509 **Unspecified complication of foreign body accidentally left in body following unspecified procedure** CC H1

T81.51 **Adhesions due to foreign body accidentally left in body following procedure**

T81.510 **Adhesions due to foreign body accidentally left in body following surgical operation** CC H1

T81.511 **Adhesions due to foreign body accidentally left in body following infusion or transfusion** CC H1

T81.512 **Adhesions due to foreign body accidentally left in body following kidney dialysis** CC H1 HCC

T81.513 **Adhesions due to foreign body accidentally left in body following injection or immunization** CC H1

T81.514 **Adhesions due to foreign body accidentally left in body following endoscopic examination** CC H1

T81.515 **Adhesions due to foreign body accidentally left in body following heart catheterization** CC H1

T81.516 **Adhesions due to foreign body accidentally left in body following aspiration, puncture or other catheterization** CC H1

T81.517 **Adhesions due to foreign body accidentally left in body following removal of catheter or packing** CC H1

T81.518 **Adhesions due to foreign body accidentally left in body following other procedure** CC H1

T81.519 **Adhesions due to foreign body accidentally left in body following unspecified procedure** CC H1

T81.52 **Obstruction due to foreign body accidentally left in body following procedure**

T81.520 **Obstruction due to foreign body accidentally left in body following surgical operation** CC H1

T81.521 **Obstruction due to foreign body accidentally left in body following infusion or transfusion** CC H1

T81.522 **Obstruction due to foreign body accidentally left in body following kidney dialysis** CC H1 HCC

T81.523 **Obstruction due to foreign body accidentally left in body following injection or immunization** CC H1

T81.524 **Obstruction due to foreign body accidentally left in body following endoscopic examination** CC H1

T81.525 **Obstruction due to foreign body accidentally left in body following heart catheterization** CC H1

T81.526 **Obstruction due to foreign body accidentally left in body following aspiration, puncture or other catheterization** CC H1

T81.527 Obstruction due to foreign body accidentally left in body following removal of catheter or packing CC H1

T81.528 Obstruction due to foreign body accidentally left in body following other procedure CC H1

T81.529 Obstruction due to foreign body accidentally left in body following unspecified procedure CC H1

T81.53 Perforation due to foreign body accidentally left in body following procedure

T81.530 Perforation due to foreign body accidentally left in body following surgical operation CC H1

T81.531 Perforation due to foreign body accidentally left in body following infusion or transfusion CC H1

T81.532 Perforation due to foreign body accidentally left in body following kidney dialysis CC H1 HCC

T81.533 Perforation due to foreign body accidentally left in body following injection or immunization CC H1

T81.534 Perforation due to foreign body accidentally left in body following endoscopic examination CC H1

T81.535 Perforation due to foreign body accidentally left in body following heart catheterization CC H1

T81.536 Perforation due to foreign body accidentally left in body following aspiration, puncture or other catheterization CC H1

T81.537 Perforation due to foreign body accidentally left in body following removal of catheter or packing CC H1

T81.538 Perforation due to foreign body accidentally left in body following other procedure CC H1

T81.539 Perforation due to foreign body accidentally left in body following unspecified procedure CC H1

T81.59 Other complications of foreign body accidentally left in body following procedure

EXCLUDES 2 *obstruction or perforation due to prosthetic devices and implants intentionally left in body (T82.Ø-T82.5, T83.Ø-T83.4, T83.7, T84.Ø-T84.4, T85.Ø-T85.6)*

T81.590 Other complications of foreign body accidentally left in body following surgical operation CC H1

T81.591 Other complications of foreign body accidentally left in body following infusion or transfusion CC H1

T81.592 Other complications of foreign body accidentally left in body following kidney dialysis CC H1 HCC

T81.593 Other complications of foreign body accidentally left in body following injection or immunization CC H1

T81.594 Other complications of foreign body accidentally left in body following endoscopic examination CC H1

T81.595 Other complications of foreign body accidentally left in body following heart catheterization CC H1

T81.596 Other complications of foreign body accidentally left in body following aspiration, puncture or other catheterization CC H1

T81.597 Other complications of foreign body accidentally left in body following removal of catheter or packing CC H1

T81.598 Other complications of foreign body accidentally left in body following other procedure CC H1

T81.599 Other complications of foreign body accidentally left in body following unspecified procedure CC H1

T81.6 Acute reaction to foreign substance accidentally left during a procedure

EXCLUDES 2 *complications of foreign body accidentally left in body cavity or operation wound following procedure (T81.5-)*

T81.6Ø Unspecified acute reaction to foreign substance accidentally left during a procedure CC H1

T81.61 Aseptic peritonitis due to foreign substance accidentally left during a procedure CC H1

Chemical peritonitis

T81.69 Other acute reaction to foreign substance accidentally left during a procedure CC H1

T81.7 Vascular complications following a procedure, not elsewhere classified

Air embolism following procedure NEC

Phlebitis or thrombophlebitis resulting from a procedure

EXCLUDES 1 *embolism complicating abortion or ectopic or molar pregnancy (OØØ-OØ7, OØ8.2)*

embolism complicating pregnancy, childbirth and the puerperium (O88.-)

traumatic embolism (T79.Ø)

EXCLUDES 2 *embolism due to prosthetic devices, implants and grafts (T82.8-, T83.81, T84.8-, T85.81-)*

embolism following infusion, transfusion and therapeutic injection (T80.Ø)

AHA: 2019,2Q,22

T81.71 Complication of artery following a procedure, not elsewhere classified

T81.71Ø Complication of mesenteric artery following a procedure, not elsewhere classified CC

T81.711 Complication of renal artery following a procedure, not elsewhere classified CC

T81.718 Complication of other artery following a procedure, not elsewhere classified CC

AHA: 2019,2Q,21-22

T81.719 Complication of unspecified artery following a procedure, not elsewhere classified CC

T81.72 Complication of vein following a procedure, not elsewhere classified CC

T81.8 Other complications of procedures, not elsewhere classified

EXCLUDES 2 *hypothermia following anesthesia (T88.51)*

malignant hyperpyrexia due to anesthesia (T88.3)

T81.81 Complication of inhalation therapy

T81.82 Emphysema (subcutaneous) resulting from a procedure

T81.83 Persistent postprocedural fistula CC SW

AHA: 2017,3Q,3-4

T81.89 Other complications of procedures, not elsewhere classified SW

Use additional code to specify complication, such as: postprocedural delirium (FØ5)

AHA: 2014,1Q,23

T81.9 Unspecified complication of procedure

T82 Complications of cardiac and vascular prosthetic devices, implants and grafts

EXCLUDES 2 *failure and rejection of transplanted organs and tissue (T86.-)*

The appropriate 7th character is to be added to each code from category T82.

A initial encounter
D subsequent encounter
S sequela

T82.Ø Mechanical complication of heart valve prosthesis

Mechanical complication of artificial heart valve

EXCLUDES 1 *mechanical complication of biological heart valve graft (T82.22-)*

T82.Ø1 Breakdown (mechanical) of heart valve prosthesis CC

T82.Ø2 Displacement of heart valve prosthesis CC

Malposition of heart valve prosthesis

T82.Ø3 Leakage of heart valve prosthesis CC

√x7th T82.09 **Other mechanical complication of heart valve prosthesis** CC
Obstruction (mechanical) of heart valve prosthesis
Perforation of heart valve prosthesis
Protrusion of heart valve prosthesis

√5th **T82.1 Mechanical complication of cardiac electronic device**

√6th **T82.11 Breakdown (mechanical) of cardiac electronic device**
√7th T82.110 **Breakdown (mechanical) of cardiac electrode** CC
√7th T82.111 **Breakdown (mechanical) of cardiac pulse generator (battery)** CC
√7th T82.118 **Breakdown (mechanical) of other cardiac electronic device** CC
√7th T82.119 **Breakdown (mechanical) of unspecified cardiac electronic device** CC

√6th **T82.12 Displacement of cardiac electronic device**
Malposition of cardiac electronic device
√7th T82.120 **Displacement of cardiac electrode** CC
√7th T82.121 **Displacement of cardiac pulse generator (battery)** CC
√7th T82.128 **Displacement of other cardiac electronic device** CC
√7th T82.129 **Displacement of unspecified cardiac electronic device** CC

√6th **T82.19 Other mechanical complication of cardiac electronic device**
Leakage of cardiac electronic device
Obstruction of cardiac electronic device
Perforation of cardiac electronic device
Protrusion of cardiac electronic device
√7th T82.190 **Other mechanical complication of cardiac electrode** CC
√7th T82.191 **Other mechanical complication of cardiac pulse generator (battery)** CC
√7th T82.198 **Other mechanical complication of other cardiac electronic device** CC
√7th T82.199 **Other mechanical complication of unspecified cardiac device** CC

√5th **T82.2 Mechanical complication of coronary artery bypass graft and biological heart valve graft**
EXCLUDES 1 *mechanical complication of artificial heart valve prosthesis (T82.0-)*

√6th **T82.21 Mechanical complication of coronary artery bypass graft**
√7th T82.211 **Breakdown (mechanical) of coronary artery bypass graft** CC
√7th T82.212 **Displacement of coronary artery bypass graft** CC
Malposition of coronary artery bypass graft
√7th T82.213 **Leakage of coronary artery bypass graft** CC
√7th T82.218 **Other mechanical complication of coronary artery bypass graft** CC
Obstruction, mechanical of coronary artery bypass graft
Perforation of coronary artery bypass graft
Protrusion of coronary artery bypass graft

√6th **T82.22 Mechanical complication of biological heart valve graft**
√7th T82.221 **Breakdown (mechanical) of biological heart valve graft** CC
√7th T82.222 **Displacement of biological heart valve graft** CC
Malposition of biological heart valve graft
√7th T82.223 **Leakage of biological heart valve graft** CC
√7th T82.228 **Other mechanical complication of biological heart valve graft** CC
Obstruction of biological heart valve graft
Perforation of biological heart valve graft
Protrusion of biological heart valve graft

√5th **T82.3 Mechanical complication of other vascular grafts**

√6th **T82.31 Breakdown (mechanical) of other vascular grafts**
6 √7th T82.310 **Breakdown (mechanical) of aortic (bifurcation) graft (replacement)** CC HCC
6 √7th T82.311 **Breakdown (mechanical) of carotid arterial graft (bypass)** CC HCC
6 √7th T82.312 **Breakdown (mechanical) of femoral arterial graft (bypass)** CC HCC
6 √7th T82.318 **Breakdown (mechanical) of other vascular grafts** CC HCC
6 √7th T82.319 **Breakdown (mechanical) of unspecified vascular grafts** CC HCC

√6th **T82.32 Displacement of other vascular grafts**
Malposition of other vascular grafts
6 √7th T82.320 **Displacement of aortic (bifurcation) graft (replacement)** CC HCC
6 √7th T82.321 **Displacement of carotid arterial graft (bypass)** CC HCC
6 √7th T82.322 **Displacement of femoral arterial graft (bypass)** CC HCC
6 √7th T82.328 **Displacement of other vascular grafts** CC HCC
6 √7th T82.329 **Displacement of unspecified vascular grafts** CC HCC

√6th **T82.33 Leakage of other vascular grafts**
6 √7th T82.330 **Leakage of aortic (bifurcation) graft (replacement)** CC HCC
6 √7th T82.331 **Leakage of carotid arterial graft (bypass)** CC HCC
6 √7th T82.332 **Leakage of femoral arterial graft (bypass)** CC HCC
6 √7th T82.338 **Leakage of other vascular grafts** CC HCC
6 √7th T82.339 **Leakage of unspecified vascular graft** CC HCC

√6th **T82.39 Other mechanical complication of other vascular grafts**
Obstruction (mechanical) of other vascular grafts
Perforation of other vascular grafts
Protrusion of other vascular grafts
6 √7th T82.390 **Other mechanical complication of aortic (bifurcation) graft (replacement)** CC HCC
6 √7th T82.391 **Other mechanical complication of carotid arterial graft (bypass)** CC HCC
6 √7th T82.392 **Other mechanical complication of femoral arterial graft (bypass)** CC HCC
6 √7th T82.398 **Other mechanical complication of other vascular grafts** CC HCC
6 √7th T82.399 **Other mechanical complication of unspecified vascular grafts** CC HCC

√5th **T82.4 Mechanical complication of vascular dialysis catheter**
Mechanical complication of hemodialysis catheter
EXCLUDES 1 *mechanical complication of intraperitoneal dialysis catheter (T85.62)*

√x7th **T82.41 Breakdown (mechanical) of vascular dialysis catheter** CC HCC
√x7th **T82.42 Displacement of vascular dialysis catheter** CC HCC
Malposition of vascular dialysis catheter
√x7th **T82.43 Leakage of vascular dialysis catheter** CC HCC
√x7th **T82.49 Other complication of vascular dialysis catheter** CC HCC
Obstruction (mechanical) of vascular dialysis catheter
Perforation of vascular dialysis catheter
Protrusion of vascular dialysis catheter

√5th **T82.5 Mechanical complication of other cardiac and vascular devices and implants**
EXCLUDES 2 *mechanical complication of epidural and subdural infusion catheter (T85.61)*

√6th **T82.51 Breakdown (mechanical) of other cardiac and vascular devices and implants**
6 √7th T82.510 **Breakdown (mechanical) of surgically created arteriovenous fistula** CC HCC
6 √7th T82.511 **Breakdown (mechanical) of surgically created arteriovenous shunt** CC HCC
√7th T82.512 **Breakdown (mechanical) of artificial heart** CC
6 √7th T82.513 **Breakdown (mechanical) of balloon (counterpulsation) device** CC HCC
6 √7th T82.514 **Breakdown (mechanical) of infusion catheter** CC HCC
6 √7th T82.515 **Breakdown (mechanical) of umbrella device** CC HCC

6 ✓7th **T82.518 Breakdown (mechanical) of other cardiac and vascular devices and implants** CC HCC

✓7th **T82.519 Breakdown (mechanical) of unspecified cardiac and vascular devices and implants** CC

✓6th **T82.52 Displacement of other cardiac and vascular devices and implants**

Malposition of other cardiac and vascular devices and implants

6 ✓7th **T82.52Ø Displacement of surgically created arteriovenous fistula** CC HCC

6 ✓7th **T82.521 Displacement of surgically created arteriovenous shunt** CC HCC

✓7th **T82.522 Displacement of artificial heart** CC

6 ✓7th **T82.523 Displacement of balloon (counterpulsation) device** CC HCC

6 ✓7th **T82.524 Displacement of infusion catheter** CC HCC

AHA: 2020,2Q,21; 2019,3Q,15

6 ✓7th **T82.525 Displacement of umbrella device** CC HCC

6 ✓7th **T82.528 Displacement of other cardiac and vascular devices and implants** CC HCC

✓7th **T82.529 Displacement of unspecified cardiac and vascular devices and implants** CC

✓6th **T82.53 Leakage of other cardiac and vascular devices and implants**

6 ✓7th **T82.53Ø Leakage of surgically created arteriovenous fistula** CC HCC

6 ✓7th **T82.531 Leakage of surgically created arteriovenous shunt** CC HCC

✓7th **T82.532 Leakage of artificial heart** CC

6 ✓7th **T82.533 Leakage of balloon (counterpulsation) device** CC HCC

6 ✓7th **T82.534 Leakage of infusion catheter** CC HCC

6 ✓7th **T82.535 Leakage of umbrella device** CC HCC

6 ✓7th **T82.538 Leakage of other cardiac and vascular devices and implants** CC HCC

✓7th **T82.539 Leakage of unspecified cardiac and vascular devices and implants** CC

✓6th **T82.59 Other mechanical complication of other cardiac and vascular devices and implants**

Obstruction (mechanical) of other cardiac and vascular devices and implants

Perforation of other cardiac and vascular devices and implants

Protrusion of other cardiac and vascular devices and implants

6 ✓7th **T82.59Ø Other mechanical complication of surgically created arteriovenous fistula** CC HCC

6 ✓7th **T82.591 Other mechanical complication of surgically created arteriovenous shunt** CC HCC

✓7th **T82.592 Other mechanical complication of artificial heart** CC

6 ✓7th **T82.593 Other mechanical complication of balloon (counterpulsation) device** CC HCC

6 ✓7th **T82.594 Other mechanical complication of infusion catheter** CC HCC

6 ✓7th **T82.595 Other mechanical complication of umbrella device** CC HCC

6 ✓7th **T82.598 Other mechanical complication of other cardiac and vascular devices and implants** CC HCC

✓7th **T82.599 Other mechanical complication of unspecified cardiac and vascular devices and implants** CC

6 ✓x7th **T82.6 Infection and inflammatory reaction due to cardiac valve prosthesis** CC H13 HCC

Use additional code to identify infection

6 ✓x7th **T82.7 Infection and inflammatory reaction due to other cardiac and vascular devices, implants and grafts** CC H13 HCC

Use additional code to identify infection

AHA: 2019,1Q,13-14

TIP: Assign this code for infections and/or cellulitis resulting from catheters that are not centrally placed (e.g., midline catheters).

✓5th **T82.8 Other specified complications of cardiac and vascular prosthetic devices, implants and grafts**

AHA: 2016,4Q,70

✓6th **T82.81 Embolism due to cardiac and vascular prosthetic devices, implants and grafts**

✓7th **T82.817 Embolism due to cardiac prosthetic devices, implants and grafts** CC

6 ✓7th **T82.818 Embolism due to vascular prosthetic devices, implants and grafts** CC HCC

✓6th **T82.82 Fibrosis due to cardiac and vascular prosthetic devices, implants and grafts**

✓7th **T82.827 Fibrosis due to cardiac prosthetic devices, implants and grafts** CC

6 ✓7th **T82.828 Fibrosis due vascular prosthetic devices, implants and grafts** CC HCC

✓6th **T82.83 Hemorrhage due to cardiac and vascular prosthetic devices, implants and grafts**

✓7th **T82.837 Hemorrhage due to cardiac prosthetic devices, implants and grafts** CC

6 ✓7th **T82.838 Hemorrhage due to vascular prosthetic devices, implants and grafts** CC HCC

✓6th **T82.84 Pain due to cardiac and vascular prosthetic devices, implants and grafts**

✓7th **T82.847 Pain due to cardiac prosthetic devices, implants and grafts** CC

6 ✓7th **T82.848 Pain due to vascular prosthetic devices, implants and grafts** CC HCC

✓6th **T82.85 Stenosis due to cardiac and vascular prosthetic devices, implants and grafts**

✓7th **T82.855 Stenosis of coronary artery stent** CC

In-stent stenosis (restenosis) of coronary artery stent

Restenosis of coronary artery stent

6 ✓7th **T82.856 Stenosis of peripheral vascular stent** CC HCC

In-stent stenosis (restenosis) of peripheral vascular stent

Restenosis of peripheral vascular stent

✓7th **T82.857 Stenosis of other cardiac prosthetic devices, implants and grafts** CC

6 ✓7th **T82.858 Stenosis of other vascular prosthetic devices, implants and grafts** CC HCC

✓6th **T82.86 Thrombosis of cardiac and vascular prosthetic devices, implants and grafts**

✓7th **T82.867 Thrombosis due to cardiac prosthetic devices, implants and grafts** CC

6 ✓7th **T82.868 Thrombosis due to vascular prosthetic devices, implants and grafts** CC HCC

✓6th **T82.89 Other specified complication of cardiac and vascular prosthetic devices, implants and grafts**

✓7th **T82.897 Other specified complication of cardiac prosthetic devices, implants and grafts** CC

AHA: 2019,2Q,33

6 ✓7th **T82.898 Other specified complication of vascular prosthetic devices, implants and grafts** CC HCC

✓x7th **T82.9 Unspecified complication of cardiac and vascular prosthetic device, implant and graft** CC

✓4th **T83 Complications of genitourinary prosthetic devices, implants and grafts**

EXCLUDES 2 *failure and rejection of transplanted organs and tissue (T86.-)*

AHA: 2016,4Q,70-71

The appropriate 7th character is to be added to each code from category T83.
A initial encounter
D subsequent encounter
S sequela

✓5th **T83.Ø Mechanical complication of urinary catheter**

EXCLUDES 2 *complications of stoma of urinary tract (N99.5-)*

✓6th **T83.Ø1 Breakdown (mechanical) of urinary catheter**

6 ✓7th **T83.Ø1Ø Breakdown (mechanical) of cystostomy catheter** CC HCC

6 ✓7th **T83.Ø11 Breakdown (mechanical) of indwelling urethral catheter** HCC

6 ✓7th **T83.Ø12 Breakdown (mechanical) of nephrostomy catheter** HCC

6 ✓7th **T83.Ø18 Breakdown (mechanical) of other urinary catheter** HCC
Breakdown (mechanical) of Hopkins catheter
Breakdown (mechanical) of ileostomy catheter
Breakdown (mechanical) urostomy catheter

✓6th **T83.Ø2 Displacement of urinary catheter**
Malposition of urinary catheter

6 ✓7th **T83.Ø20 Displacement of cystostomy catheter** CC HCC

6 ✓7th **T83.Ø21 Displacement of indwelling urethral catheter** HCC

6 ✓7th **T83.Ø22 Displacement of nephrostomy catheter** HCC

6 ✓7th **T83.Ø28 Displacement of other urinary catheter** HCC
Displacement of Hopkins catheter
Displacement of ileostomy catheter
Displacement of urostomy catheter

✓6th **T83.Ø3 Leakage of urinary catheter**

6 ✓7th **T83.Ø30 Leakage of cystostomy catheter** CC HCC

6 ✓7th **T83.Ø31 Leakage of indwelling urethral catheter** HCC

6 ✓7th **T83.Ø32 Leakage of nephrostomy catheter** HCC

6 ✓7th **T83.Ø38 Leakage of other urinary catheter** HCC
Leakage of Hopkins catheter
Leakage of ileostomy catheter
Leakage of urostomy catheter

✓6th **T83.Ø9 Other mechanical complication of urinary catheter**
Obstruction (mechanical) of urinary catheter
Perforation of urinary catheter
Protrusion of urinary catheter

6 ✓7th **T83.Ø9Ø Other mechanical complication of cystostomy catheter** CC HCC

6 ✓7th **T83.Ø91 Other mechanical complication of indwelling urethral catheter** HCC

6 ✓7th **T83.Ø92 Other mechanical complication of nephrostomy catheter** HCC

6 ✓7th **T83.Ø98 Other mechanical complication of other urinary catheter** HCC
Other mechanical complication of Hopkins catheter
Other mechanical complication of ileostomy catheter
Other mechanical complication of urostomy catheter

✓5th **T83.1 Mechanical complication of other urinary devices and implants**

✓6th **T83.11 Breakdown (mechanical) of other urinary devices and implants**

6 ✓7th **T83.11Ø Breakdown (mechanical) of urinary electronic stimulator device** CC HCC
EXCLUDES 2 *breakdown (mechanical) of electrode (lead) for sacral nerve neurostimulator (T85.111)*
breakdown (mechanical) of implanted electronic sacral neurostimulator, pulse generator or receiver (T85.113)

6 ✓7th **T83.111 Breakdown (mechanical) of implanted urinary sphincter** CC HCC

6 ✓7th **T83.112 Breakdown (mechanical) of indwelling ureteral stent** CC HCC

6 ✓7th **T83.113 Breakdown (mechanical) of other urinary stents** CC HCC
Breakdown (mechanical) of ileal conduit stent
Breakdown (mechanical) of nephroureteral stent

6 ✓7th **T83.118 Breakdown (mechanical) of other urinary devices and implants** CC HCC

✓6th **T83.12 Displacement of other urinary devices and implants**
Malposition of other urinary devices and implants

6 ✓7th **T83.12Ø Displacement of urinary electronic stimulator device** CC HCC
EXCLUDES 2 *displacement of electrode (lead) for sacral nerve neurostimulator (T85.121)*
displacement of implanted electronic sacral neurostimulator, pulse generator or receiver (T85.123)

6 ✓7th **T83.121 Displacement of implanted urinary sphincter** CC HCC

6 ✓7th **T83.122 Displacement of indwelling ureteral stent** CC HCC

6 ✓7th **T83.123 Displacement of other urinary stents** CC HCC
Displacement of ileal conduit stent
Displacement of nephroureteral stent

6 ✓7th **T83.128 Displacement of other urinary devices and implants** CC HCC

✓6th **T83.19 Other mechanical complication of other urinary devices and implants**
Leakage of other urinary devices and implants
Obstruction (mechanical) of other urinary devices and implants
Perforation of other urinary devices and implants
Protrusion of other urinary devices and implants

6 ✓7th **T83.19Ø Other mechanical complication of urinary electronic stimulator device** CC HCC
EXCLUDES 2 *other mechanical complication of electrode (lead) for sacral nerve neurostimulator (T85.191)*
other mechanical complication of implanted electronic sacral neurostimulator, pulse generator or receiver (T85.193)

6 ✓7th **T83.191 Other mechanical complication of implanted urinary sphincter** CC HCC

6 ✓7th **T83.192 Other mechanical complication of indwelling ureteral stent** CC HCC

6 ✓7th **T83.193 Other mechanical complication of other urinary stent** CC HCC
Other mechanical complication of ileal conduit stent
Other mechanical complication of nephroureteral stent

6 ✓7th **T83.198 Other mechanical complication of other urinary devices and implants** CC HCC

✓5th **T83.2 Mechanical complication of graft of urinary organ**

6 ✓x7th **T83.21 Breakdown (mechanical) of graft of urinary organ** CC HCC

6 ✓x7th **T83.22 Displacement of graft of urinary organ** CC HCC
Malposition of graft of urinary organ

6 ✓x7th **T83.23 Leakage of graft of urinary organ** CC HCC

6 ✓x7th **T83.24 Erosion of graft of urinary organ** CC HCC

6 ✓x7th **T83.25 Exposure of graft of urinary organ** CC HCC

6 ✓x7th **T83.29 Other mechanical complication of graft of urinary organ** CC HCC
Obstruction (mechanical) of graft of urinary organ
Perforation of graft of urinary organ
Protrusion of graft of urinary organ

✓5th **T83.3 Mechanical complication of intrauterine contraceptive device**

✓x7th **T83.31 Breakdown (mechanical) of intrauterine contraceptive device** ♀

✓x7th **T83.32 Displacement of intrauterine contraceptive device** ♀
Malposition of intrauterine contraceptive device
Missing string of intrauterine contraceptive device
AHA: 2018,1Q,5

✓x7th **T83.39 Other mechanical complication of intrauterine contraceptive device** ♀
Leakage of intrauterine contraceptive device
Obstruction (mechanical) of intrauterine contraceptive device
Perforation of intrauterine contraceptive device
Protrusion of intrauterine contraceptive device

✓5th **T83.4 Mechanical complication of other prosthetic devices, implants and grafts of genital tract**

✓6th **T83.41 Breakdown (mechanical) of other prosthetic devices, implants and grafts of genital tract**

6 ✓7th **T83.410 Breakdown (mechanical) of implanted penile prosthesis** CC HCC ♂
Breakdown (mechanical) of penile prosthesis cylinder
Breakdown (mechanical) of penile prosthesis pump
Breakdown (mechanical) of penile prosthesis reservoir

6 ✓7th **T83.411 Breakdown (mechanical) of implanted testicular prosthesis** CC HCC

6 ✓7th **T83.418 Breakdown (mechanical) of other prosthetic devices, implants and grafts of genital tract** CC HCC

✓6th **T83.42 Displacement of other prosthetic devices, implants and grafts of genital tract**
Malposition of other prosthetic devices, implants and grafts of genital tract

6 ✓7th **T83.420 Displacement of implanted penile prosthesis** CC HCC ♂
Displacement of penile prosthesis cylinder
Displacement of penile prosthesis pump
Displacement of penile prosthesis reservoir

6 ✓7th **T83.421 Displacement of implanted testicular prosthesis** CC HCC

6 ✓7th **T83.428 Displacement of other prosthetic devices, implants and grafts of genital tract** CC HCC
AHA: 2018,1Q,5

✓6th **T83.49 Other mechanical complication of other prosthetic devices, implants and grafts of genital tract**
Leakage of other prosthetic devices, implants and grafts of genital tract
Obstruction, mechanical of other prosthetic devices, implants and grafts of genital tract
Perforation of other prosthetic devices, implants and grafts of genital tract
Protrusion of other prosthetic devices, implants and grafts of genital tract

6 ✓7th **T83.490 Other mechanical complication of implanted penile prosthesis** CC HCC ♂
Other mechanical complication of penile prosthesis cylinder
Other mechanical complication of penile prosthesis pump
Other mechanical complication of penile prosthesis reservoir

6 ✓7th **T83.491 Other mechanical complication of implanted testicular prosthesis** CC HCC

6 ✓7th **T83.498 Other mechanical complication of other prosthetic devices, implants and grafts of genital tract** CC HCC

✓5th **T83.5 Infection and inflammatory reaction due to prosthetic device, implant and graft in urinary system**
Use additional code to identify infection

✓6th **T83.51 Infection and inflammatory reaction due to urinary catheter**
EXCLUDES 2 *complications of stoma of urinary tract (N99.5-)*
AHA: 2019,3Q,17

6 ✓7th **T83.510 Infection and inflammatory reaction due to cystostomy catheter** CC HCC

6 ✓7th **T83.511 Infection and inflammatory reaction due to indwelling urethral catheter** CC H6 HCC

6 ✓7th **T83.512 Infection and inflammatory reaction due to nephrostomy catheter** CC HCC

6 ✓7th **T83.518 Infection and inflammatory reaction due to other urinary catheter** CC H6 HCC
Infection and inflammatory reaction due to Hopkins catheter
Infection and inflammatory reaction due to ileostomy catheter
Infection and inflammatory reaction due to urostomy catheter

✓6th **T83.59 Infection and inflammatory reaction due to prosthetic device, implant and graft in urinary system**

6 ✓7th **T83.590 Infection and inflammatory reaction due to implanted urinary neurostimulation device** CC HCC
EXCLUDES 2 *infection and inflammatory reaction due to electrode lead of sacral nerve neurostimulator (T85.732)*
infection and inflammatory reaction due to pulse generator or receiver of sacral nerve neurostimulator (T85.734)

6 ✓7th **T83.591 Infection and inflammatory reaction due to implanted urinary sphincter** CC HCC

6 ✓7th **T83.592 Infection and inflammatory reaction due to indwelling ureteral stent** CC HCC

6 ✓7th **T83.593 Infection and inflammatory reaction due to other urinary stents** CC HCC
Infection and inflammatory reaction due to ileal conduit stents
Infection and inflammatory reaction due to nephroureteral stent

6 ✓7th **T83.598 Infection and inflammatory reaction due to other prosthetic device, implant and graft in urinary system** CC HCC

✓5th **T83.6 Infection and inflammatory reaction due to prosthetic device, implant and graft in genital tract**
Use additional code to identify infection

6 ✓x7th **T83.61 Infection and inflammatory reaction due to implanted penile prosthesis** CC HCC
Infection and inflammatory reaction due to penile prosthesis cylinder
Infection and inflammatory reaction due to penile prosthesis pump
Infection and inflammatory reaction due to penile prosthesis reservoir

6 ✓x7th **T83.62 Infection and inflammatory reaction due to implanted testicular prosthesis** CC HCC

6 ✓x7th **T83.69 Infection and inflammatory reaction due to other prosthetic device, implant and graft in genital tract** CC HCC

✓5th **T83.7 Complications due to implanted mesh and other prosthetic materials**

✓6th **T83.71 Erosion of implanted mesh and other prosthetic materials**

6 ✓7th **T83.711 Erosion of implanted vaginal mesh to surrounding organ or tissue** HCC ♀
Erosion of implanted vaginal mesh into pelvic floor muscles

6 ✓7th **T83.712 Erosion of implanted urethral mesh to surrounding organ or tissue** CC HCC
Erosion of implanted female urethral sling
Erosion of implanted male urethral sling
Erosion of implanted urethral mesh into pelvic floor muscles

6 ✓7th **T83.713 Erosion of implanted urethral bulking agent to surrounding organ or tissue** CC HCC

6 ✓7th **T83.714 Erosion of implanted ureteral bulking agent to surrounding organ or tissue** CC HCC

6 ✓7th **T83.718 Erosion of other implanted mesh to organ or tissue** CC HCC

6 ✓7th **T83.719 Erosion of other prosthetic materials to surrounding organ or tissue** CC HCC

✓6th T83.72 Exposure of implanted mesh and other prosthetic materials into surrounding organ or tissue
Extrusion of implanted mesh
6 ✓7th T83.721 Exposure of implanted vaginal mesh into vagina HCC ♀
Exposure of implanted vaginal mesh through vaginal wall
6 ✓7th T83.722 Exposure of implanted urethral mesh into urethra CC HCC
Exposure of implanted female urethral sling
Exposure of implanted male urethral sling
Exposure of implanted urethral mesh through urethral wall
6 ✓7th T83.723 Exposure of implanted urethral bulking agent into urethra CC HCC
6 ✓7th T83.724 Exposure of implanted ureteral bulking agent into ureter CC HCC
6 ✓7th T83.728 Exposure of other implanted mesh into organ or tissue CC HCC
6 ✓7th T83.729 Exposure of other prosthetic materials into organ or tissue CC HCC
6 ✓x7th T83.79 Other specified complications due to other genitourinary prosthetic materials CC HCC
✓5th T83.8 Other specified complications of genitourinary prosthetic devices, implants and grafts
6 ✓x7th T83.81 Embolism due to genitourinary prosthetic devices, implants and grafts CC HCC
6 ✓x7th T83.82 Fibrosis due to genitourinary prosthetic devices, implants and grafts CC HCC
6 ✓x7th T83.83 Hemorrhage due to genitourinary prosthetic devices, implants and grafts CC HCC
6 ✓x7th T83.84 Pain due to genitourinary prosthetic devices, implants and grafts CC HCC
6 ✓x7th T83.85 Stenosis due to genitourinary prosthetic devices, implants and grafts CC HCC
6 ✓x7th T83.86 Thrombosis due to genitourinary prosthetic devices, implants and grafts CC HCC
6 ✓x7th T83.89 Other specified complication of genitourinary prosthetic devices, implants and grafts CC HCC
6 ✓x7th T83.9 Unspecified complication of genitourinary prosthetic device, implant and graft CC HCC

✓4th **T84 Complications of internal orthopedic prosthetic devices, implants and grafts**
EXCLUDES 2 *failure and rejection of transplanted organs and tissues (T86.-)*
fracture of bone following insertion of orthopedic implant, joint prosthesis or bone plate (M96.6)

The appropriate 7th character is to be added to each code from category T84.
A initial encounter
D subsequent encounter
S sequela

✓5th T84.0 Mechanical complication of internal joint prosthesis
✓6th T84.01 Broken internal joint prosthesis
Breakage (fracture) of prosthetic joint
Broken prosthetic joint implant
EXCLUDES 1 *periprosthetic joint implant fracture ▶(M97.-)◀*
AHA: 2016,4Q,42
6 ✓7th T84.010 Broken internal right hip prosthesis CC HCC
6 ✓7th T84.011 Broken internal left hip prosthesis CC HCC
6 ✓7th T84.012 Broken internal right knee prosthesis CC HCC
6 ✓7th T84.013 Broken internal left knee prosthesis CC HCC
6 ✓7th T84.018 Broken internal joint prosthesis, other site CC HCC
Use additional code to identify the joint (Z96.6-)
6 ✓7th T84.019 Broken internal joint prosthesis, unspecified site CC HCC
✓6th T84.02 Dislocation of internal joint prosthesis
Instability of internal joint prosthesis
Subluxation of internal joint prosthesis
AHA: 2019,2Q,27
6 ✓7th T84.020 Dislocation of internal right hip prosthesis CC HCC
6 ✓7th T84.021 Dislocation of internal left hip prosthesis CC HCC
6 ✓7th T84.022 Instability of internal right knee prosthesis CC HCC
6 ✓7th T84.023 Instability of internal left knee prosthesis CC HCC
6 ✓7th T84.028 Dislocation of other internal joint prosthesis CC HCC
Use additional code to identify the joint (Z96.6-)
6 ✓7th T84.029 Dislocation of unspecified internal joint prosthesis CC HCC
✓6th T84.03 Mechanical loosening of internal prosthetic joint
Aseptic loosening of prosthetic joint
6 ✓7th T84.030 Mechanical loosening of internal right hip prosthetic joint CC HCC
6 ✓7th T84.031 Mechanical loosening of internal left hip prosthetic joint CC HCC
6 ✓7th T84.032 Mechanical loosening of internal right knee prosthetic joint CC HCC
6 ✓7th T84.033 Mechanical loosening of internal left knee prosthetic joint CC HCC
6 ✓7th T84.038 Mechanical loosening of other internal prosthetic joint CC HCC
Use additional code to identify the joint (Z96.6-)
6 ✓7th T84.039 Mechanical loosening of unspecified internal prosthetic joint CC HCC
✓6th T84.05 Periprosthetic osteolysis of internal prosthetic joint
Use additional code to identify major osseous defect, if applicable (M89.7-)
6 ✓7th T84.050 Periprosthetic osteolysis of internal prosthetic right hip joint CC HCC
6 ✓7th T84.051 Periprosthetic osteolysis of internal prosthetic left hip joint CC HCC
6 ✓7th T84.052 Periprosthetic osteolysis of internal prosthetic right knee joint CC HCC
6 ✓7th T84.053 Periprosthetic osteolysis of internal prosthetic left knee joint CC HCC
6 ✓7th T84.058 Periprosthetic osteolysis of other internal prosthetic joint CC HCC
Use additional code to identify the joint (Z96.6-)
6 ✓7th T84.059 Periprosthetic osteolysis of unspecified internal prosthetic joint CC HCC
✓6th T84.06 Wear of articular bearing surface of internal prosthetic joint
6 ✓7th T84.060 Wear of articular bearing surface of internal prosthetic right hip joint CC HCC
6 ✓7th T84.061 Wear of articular bearing surface of internal prosthetic left hip joint CC HCC
6 ✓7th T84.062 Wear of articular bearing surface of internal prosthetic right knee joint CC HCC
6 ✓7th T84.063 Wear of articular bearing surface of internal prosthetic left knee joint CC HCC
6 ✓7th T84.068 Wear of articular bearing surface of other internal prosthetic joint CC HCC
Use additional code to identify the joint (Z96.6-)
6 ✓7th T84.069 Wear of articular bearing surface of unspecified internal prosthetic joint CC HCC
✓6th T84.09 Other mechanical complication of internal joint prosthesis
Prosthetic joint implant failure NOS
AHA: 2019,1Q,20
6 ✓7th T84.090 Other mechanical complication of internal right hip prosthesis CC HCC
6 ✓7th T84.091 Other mechanical complication of internal left hip prosthesis CC HCC

Chapter 19. Injury, Poisoning and Certain Other Consequences of External Causes
T83.72–T84.091

6 ✓7th **T84.092 Other mechanical complication of internal right knee prosthesis** CC HCC

6 ✓7th **T84.093 Other mechanical complication of internal left knee prosthesis** CC HCC

6 ✓7th **T84.098 Other mechanical complication of other internal joint prosthesis** CC HCC
Use additional code to identify the joint (Z96.6-)

6 ✓7th **T84.099 Other mechanical complication of unspecified internal joint prosthesis** CC HCC

✓5th **T84.1 Mechanical complication of internal fixation device of bones of limb**
EXCLUDES 2 *mechanical complication of internal fixation device of bones of feet (T84.2-)*
mechanical complication of internal fixation device of bones of fingers (T84.2-)
mechanical complication of internal fixation device of bones of hands (T84.2-)
mechanical complication of internal fixation device of bones of toes (T84.2-)

✓6th **T84.11 Breakdown (mechanical) of internal fixation device of bones of limb**

6 ✓7th **T84.110 Breakdown (mechanical) of internal fixation device of right humerus** CC HCC

6 ✓7th **T84.111 Breakdown (mechanical) of internal fixation device of left humerus** CC HCC

6 ✓7th **T84.112 Breakdown (mechanical) of internal fixation device of bone of right forearm** CC HCC

6 ✓7th **T84.113 Breakdown (mechanical) of internal fixation device of bone of left forearm** CC HCC

6 ✓7th **T84.114 Breakdown (mechanical) of internal fixation device of right femur** CC HCC

6 ✓7th **T84.115 Breakdown (mechanical) of internal fixation device of left femur** CC HCC

6 ✓7th **T84.116 Breakdown (mechanical) of internal fixation device of bone of right lower leg** CC HCC

6 ✓7th **T84.117 Breakdown (mechanical) of internal fixation device of bone of left lower leg** CC HCC

6 ✓7th **T84.119 Breakdown (mechanical) of internal fixation device of unspecified bone of limb** CC HCC

✓6th **T84.12 Displacement of internal fixation device of bones of limb**
Malposition of internal fixation device of bones of limb

6 ✓7th **T84.120 Displacement of internal fixation device of right humerus** CC HCC

6 ✓7th **T84.121 Displacement of internal fixation device of left humerus** CC HCC

6 ✓7th **T84.122 Displacement of internal fixation device of bone of right forearm** CC HCC

6 ✓7th **T84.123 Displacement of internal fixation device of bone of left forearm** CC HCC

6 ✓7th **T84.124 Displacement of internal fixation device of right femur** CC HCC

6 ✓7th **T84.125 Displacement of internal fixation device of left femur** CC HCC

6 ✓7th **T84.126 Displacement of internal fixation device of bone of right lower leg** CC HCC

6 ✓7th **T84.127 Displacement of internal fixation device of bone of left lower leg** CC HCC

6 ✓7th **T84.129 Displacement of internal fixation device of unspecified bone of limb** CC HCC

✓6th **T84.19 Other mechanical complication of internal fixation device of bones of limb**
Obstruction (mechanical) of internal fixation device of bones of limb
Perforation of internal fixation device of bones of limb
Protrusion of internal fixation device of bones of limb

6 ✓7th **T84.190 Other mechanical complication of internal fixation device of right humerus** CC HCC

6 ✓7th **T84.191 Other mechanical complication of internal fixation device of left humerus** CC HCC

6 ✓7th **T84.192 Other mechanical complication of internal fixation device of bone of right forearm** CC HCC

6 ✓7th **T84.193 Other mechanical complication of internal fixation device of bone of left forearm** CC HCC

6 ✓7th **T84.194 Other mechanical complication of internal fixation device of right femur** CC HCC

6 ✓7th **T84.195 Other mechanical complication of internal fixation device of left femur** CC HCC

6 ✓7th **T84.196 Other mechanical complication of internal fixation device of bone of right lower leg** CC HCC

6 ✓7th **T84.197 Other mechanical complication of internal fixation device of bone of left lower leg** CC HCC

6 ✓7th **T84.199 Other mechanical complication of internal fixation device of unspecified bone of limb** CC HCC

✓5th **T84.2 Mechanical complication of internal fixation device of other bones**

✓6th **T84.21 Breakdown (mechanical) of internal fixation device of other bones**

6 ✓7th **T84.210 Breakdown (mechanical) of internal fixation device of bones of hand and fingers** CC HCC

6 ✓7th **T84.213 Breakdown (mechanical) of internal fixation device of bones of foot and toes** CC HCC

6 ✓7th **T84.216 Breakdown (mechanical) of internal fixation device of vertebrae** CC HCC

6 ✓7th **T84.218 Breakdown (mechanical) of internal fixation device of other bones** CC HCC

✓6th **T84.22 Displacement of internal fixation device of other bones**
Malposition of internal fixation device of other bones

6 ✓7th **T84.220 Displacement of internal fixation device of bones of hand and fingers** CC HCC

6 ✓7th **T84.223 Displacement of internal fixation device of bones of foot and toes** CC HCC

6 ✓7th **T84.226 Displacement of internal fixation device of vertebrae** CC HCC

6 ✓7th **T84.228 Displacement of internal fixation device of other bones** CC HCC

✓6th **T84.29 Other mechanical complication of internal fixation device of other bones**
Obstruction (mechanical) of internal fixation device of other bones
Perforation of internal fixation device of other bones
Protrusion of internal fixation device of other bones

6 ✓7th **T84.290 Other mechanical complication of internal fixation device of bones of hand and fingers** CC HCC

6 ✓7th **T84.293 Other mechanical complication of internal fixation device of bones of foot and toes** CC HCC

6 ✓7th **T84.296 Other mechanical complication of internal fixation device of vertebrae** CC HCC

6 ✓7th **T84.298 Other mechanical complication of internal fixation device of other bones** CC HCC

✓5th **T84.3 Mechanical complication of other bone devices, implants and grafts**
EXCLUDES 2 *other complications of bone graft (T86.83-)*

✓6th **T84.31 Breakdown (mechanical) of other bone devices, implants and grafts**

6 ✓7th **T84.310 Breakdown (mechanical) of electronic bone stimulator** CC HCC

6 ✓7th **T84.318 Breakdown (mechanical) of other bone devices, implants and grafts** CC HCC

✓6th **T84.32 Displacement of other bone devices, implants and grafts**
Malposition of other bone devices, implants and grafts

6 ✓7th **T84.320 Displacement of electronic bone stimulator** CC HCC

6 ✓7th T84.328 **Displacement of other bone devices, implants and grafts** CC HCC
AHA: 2014,4Q,28

✓6th T84.39 **Other mechanical complication of other bone devices, implants and grafts**
Obstruction (mechanical) of other bone devices, implants and grafts
Perforation of other bone devices, implants and grafts
Protrusion of other bone devices, implants and grafts

6 ✓7th T84.39Ø **Other mechanical complication of electronic bone stimulator** CC HCC

6 ✓7th T84.398 **Other mechanical complication of other bone devices, implants and grafts** CC HCC

✓5th T84.4 **Mechanical complication of other internal orthopedic devices, implants and grafts**

✓6th T84.41 **Breakdown (mechanical) of other internal orthopedic devices, implants and grafts**

6 ✓7th T84.41Ø **Breakdown (mechanical) of muscle and tendon graft** CC HCC

6 ✓7th T84.418 **Breakdown (mechanical) of other internal orthopedic devices, implants and grafts** CC HCC

✓6th T84.42 **Displacement of other internal orthopedic devices, implants and grafts**
Malposition of other internal orthopedic devices, implants and grafts

6 ✓7th T84.42Ø **Displacement of muscle and tendon graft** CC HCC

6 ✓7th T84.428 **Displacement of other internal orthopedic devices, implants and grafts** CC HCC

✓6th T84.49 **Other mechanical complication of other internal orthopedic devices, implants and grafts**
Mechanical complication of other internal orthopedic devices, implants and grafts NOS
Obstruction (mechanical) of other internal orthopedic devices, implants and grafts
Perforation of other internal orthopedic devices, implants and grafts
Protrusion of other internal orthopedic devices, implants and grafts

6 ✓7th T84.49Ø **Other mechanical complication of muscle and tendon graft** CC HCC

6 ✓7th T84.498 **Other mechanical complication of other internal orthopedic devices, implants and grafts** CC HCC

✓5th T84.5 **Infection and inflammatory reaction due to internal joint prosthesis**
Use additional code to identify infection
AHA: 2019,3Q,16; 2015,1Q,16

6 ✓x7th T84.5Ø **Infection and inflammatory reaction due to unspecified internal joint prosthesis** CC HCC

6 ✓x7th T84.51 **Infection and inflammatory reaction due to internal right hip prosthesis** CC HCC

6 ✓x7th T84.52 **Infection and inflammatory reaction due to internal left hip prosthesis** CC HCC

6 ✓x7th T84.53 **Infection and inflammatory reaction due to internal right knee prosthesis** CC HCC

6 ✓x7th T84.54 **Infection and inflammatory reaction due to internal left knee prosthesis** CC HCC

6 ✓x7th T84.59 **Infection and inflammatory reaction due to other internal joint prosthesis** CC HCC

✓5th T84.6 **Infection and inflammatory reaction due to internal fixation device**
Use additional code to identify infection

6 ✓x7th T84.6Ø **Infection and inflammatory reaction due to internal fixation device of unspecified site** CC H12 HCC

✓6th T84.61 **Infection and inflammatory reaction due to internal fixation device of arm**

6 ✓7th T84.61Ø **Infection and inflammatory reaction due to internal fixation device of right humerus** CC H12 HCC

6 ✓7th T84.611 **Infection and inflammatory reaction due to internal fixation device of left humerus** CC H12 HCC

6 ✓7th T84.612 **Infection and inflammatory reaction due to internal fixation device of right radius** CC H12 HCC

6 ✓7th T84.613 **Infection and inflammatory reaction due to internal fixation device of left radius** CC H12 HCC

6 ✓7th T84.614 **Infection and inflammatory reaction due to internal fixation device of right ulna** CC H12 HCC

6 ✓7th T84.615 **Infection and inflammatory reaction due to internal fixation device of left ulna** CC H12 HCC

6 ✓7th T84.619 **Infection and inflammatory reaction due to internal fixation device of unspecified bone of arm** CC H12 HCC

✓6th T84.62 **Infection and inflammatory reaction due to internal fixation device of leg**

6 ✓7th T84.62Ø **Infection and inflammatory reaction due to internal fixation device of right femur** CC HCC

6 ✓7th T84.621 **Infection and inflammatory reaction due to internal fixation device of left femur** CC HCC

6 ✓7th T84.622 **Infection and inflammatory reaction due to internal fixation device of right tibia** CC HCC

6 ✓7th T84.623 **Infection and inflammatory reaction due to internal fixation device of left tibia** CC HCC

6 ✓7th T84.624 **Infection and inflammatory reaction due to internal fixation device of right fibula** CC HCC

6 ✓7th T84.625 **Infection and inflammatory reaction due to internal fixation device of left fibula** CC HCC

6 ✓7th T84.629 **Infection and inflammatory reaction due to internal fixation device of unspecified bone of leg** CC HCC

6 ✓x7th T84.63 **Infection and inflammatory reaction due to internal fixation device of spine** CC H12 HCC

6 ✓x7th T84.69 **Infection and inflammatory reaction due to internal fixation device of other site** CC H12 HCC

6 ✓x7th T84.7 **Infection and inflammatory reaction due to other internal orthopedic prosthetic devices, implants and grafts** CC H12 HCC
Use additional code to identify infection

✓5th T84.8 **Other specified complications of internal orthopedic prosthetic devices, implants and grafts**

6 ✓x7th T84.81 **Embolism due to internal orthopedic prosthetic devices, implants and grafts** CC HCC

6 ✓x7th T84.82 **Fibrosis due to internal orthopedic prosthetic devices, implants and grafts** CC HCC

6 ✓x7th T84.83 **Hemorrhage due to internal orthopedic prosthetic devices, implants and grafts** CC HCC

6 ✓x7th T84.84 **Pain due to internal orthopedic prosthetic devices, implants and grafts** CC HCC

6 ✓x7th T84.85 **Stenosis due to internal orthopedic prosthetic devices, implants and grafts** CC HCC

6 ✓x7th T84.86 **Thrombosis due to internal orthopedic prosthetic devices, implants and grafts** CC HCC

6 ✓x7th T84.89 **Other specified complication of internal orthopedic prosthetic devices, implants and grafts** CC HCC

6 ✓x7th T84.9 **Unspecified complication of internal orthopedic prosthetic device, implant and graft** CC HCC

✓4th T85 **Complications of other internal prosthetic devices, implants and grafts**
EXCLUDES 2 *failure and rejection of transplanted organs and tissue (T86.-)*
AHA: 2016,4Q,71-72

The appropriate 7th character is to be added to each code from category T85.
A initial encounter
D subsequent encounter
S sequela

✓5th T85.Ø **Mechanical complication of ventricular intracranial (communicating) shunt**

6 ✓x7th T85.Ø1 **Breakdown (mechanical) of ventricular intracranial (communicating) shunt** CC HCC

6 ✓x7th T85.Ø2 **Displacement of ventricular intracranial (communicating) shunt** CC HCC
Malposition of ventricular intracranial (communicating) shunt

6 ✓x7th T85.Ø3 **Leakage of ventricular intracranial (communicating) shunt** CC HCC

6 √x7th **T85.09 Other mechanical complication of ventricular intracranial (communicating) shunt** CC HCC
Obstruction (mechanical) of ventricular intracranial (communicating) shunt
Perforation of ventricular intracranial (communicating) shunt
Protrusion of ventricular intracranial (communicating) shunt

√5th **T85.1 Mechanical complication of implanted electronic stimulator of nervous system**

√6th **T85.11 Breakdown (mechanical) of implanted electronic stimulator of nervous system**

6 √7th **T85.110 Breakdown (mechanical) of implanted electronic neurostimulator of brain electrode (lead)** CC HCC

6 √7th **T85.111 Breakdown (mechanical) of implanted electronic neurostimulator of peripheral nerve electrode (lead)** CC HCC
Breakdown of electrode (lead) for cranial nerve neurostimulators
Breakdown of electrode (lead) for gastric neurostimulator
Breakdown of electrode (lead) for sacral nerve neurostimulator
Breakdown of electrode (lead) for vagal nerve neurostimulators

6 √7th **T85.112 Breakdown (mechanical) of implanted electronic neurostimulator of spinal cord electrode (lead)** CC HCC

6 √7th **T85.113 Breakdown (mechanical) of implanted electronic neurostimulator, generator** CC HCC
Breakdown (mechanical) of implanted electronic neurostimulator generator, brain, peripheral, gastric, spinal
Breakdown (mechanical) of implanted electronic sacral neurostimulator, pulse generator or receiver

6 √7th **T85.118 Breakdown (mechanical) of other implanted electronic stimulator of nervous system** CC HCC

√6th **T85.12 Displacement of implanted electronic stimulator of nervous system**
Malposition of implanted electronic stimulator of nervous system

6 √7th **T85.120 Displacement of implanted electronic neurostimulator of brain electrode (lead)** CC HCC

6 √7th **T85.121 Displacement of implanted electronic neurostimulator of peripheral nerve electrode (lead)** CC HCC
Displacement of electrode (lead) for cranial nerve neurostimulators
Displacement of electrode (lead) for gastric neurostimulator
Displacement of electrode (lead) for sacral nerve neurostimulator
Displacement of electrode (lead) for vagal nerve neurostimulators

6 √7th **T85.122 Displacement of implanted electronic neurostimulator of spinal cord electrode (lead)** CC HCC

6 √7th **T85.123 Displacement of implanted electronic neurostimulator, generator** CC HCC
Displacement of implanted electronic neurostimulator generator, brain, peripheral, gastric, spinal
Displacement of implanted electronic sacral neurostimulator, pulse generator or receiver

6 √7th **T85.128 Displacement of other implanted electronic stimulator of nervous system** CC HCC

√6th **T85.19 Other mechanical complication of implanted electronic stimulator of nervous system**
Leakage of implanted electronic stimulator of nervous system
Obstruction (mechanical) of implanted electronic stimulator of nervous system
Perforation of implanted electronic stimulator of nervous system
Protrusion of implanted electronic stimulator of nervous system

6 √7th **T85.190 Other mechanical complication of implanted electronic neurostimulator of brain electrode (lead)** CC HCC

6 √7th **T85.191 Other mechanical complication of implanted electronic neurostimulator of peripheral nerve electrode (lead)** CC HCC
Other mechanical complication of electrode (lead) for cranial nerve neurostimulators
Other mechanical complication of electrode (lead) for gastric neurostimulator
Other mechanical complication of electrode (lead) for sacral nerve neurostimulator
Other mechanical complication of electrode (lead) for vagal nerve neurostimulators

6 √7th **T85.192 Other mechanical complication of implanted electronic neurostimulator of spinal cord electrode (lead)** CC HCC

6 √7th **T85.193 Other mechanical complication of implanted electronic neurostimulator, generator** CC HCC
Other mechanical complication of implanted electronic neurostimulator generator, brain, peripheral, gastric, spinal
Other mechanical complication of implanted electronic sacral neurostimulator, pulse generator or receiver

6 √7th **T85.199 Other mechanical complication of other implanted electronic stimulator of nervous system** CC HCC

√5th **T85.2 Mechanical complication of intraocular lens**

√x7th **T85.21 Breakdown (mechanical) of intraocular lens** CC

√x7th **T85.22 Displacement of intraocular lens** CC
Malposition of intraocular lens

√x7th **T85.29 Other mechanical complication of intraocular lens** CC
Obstruction (mechanical) of intraocular lens
Perforation of intraocular lens
Protrusion of intraocular lens

√5th **T85.3 Mechanical complication of other ocular prosthetic devices, implants and grafts**
EXCLUDES 2 *other complications of corneal graft (T86.84-)*

√6th **T85.31 Breakdown (mechanical) of other ocular prosthetic devices, implants and grafts**

√7th **T85.310 Breakdown (mechanical) of prosthetic orbit of right eye** CC

√7th **T85.311 Breakdown (mechanical) of prosthetic orbit of left eye** CC

√7th **T85.318 Breakdown (mechanical) of other ocular prosthetic devices, implants and grafts**

√6th **T85.32 Displacement of other ocular prosthetic devices, implants and grafts**
Malposition of other ocular prosthetic devices, implants and grafts

√7th **T85.320 Displacement of prosthetic orbit of right eye** CC

√7th **T85.321 Displacement of prosthetic orbit of left eye** CC

√7th **T85.328 Displacement of other ocular prosthetic devices, implants and grafts**

✓6th **T85.39 Other mechanical complication of other ocular prosthetic devices, implants and grafts**
Obstruction (mechanical) of other ocular prosthetic devices, implants and grafts
Perforation of other ocular prosthetic devices, implants and grafts
Protrusion of other ocular prosthetic devices, implants and grafts

✓7th **T85.390 Other mechanical complication of prosthetic orbit of right eye** CC

✓7th **T85.391 Other mechanical complication of prosthetic orbit of left eye** CC

✓7th **T85.398 Other mechanical complication of other ocular prosthetic devices, implants and grafts**

✓5th **T85.4 Mechanical complication of breast prosthesis and implant**

✓x7th **T85.41 Breakdown (mechanical) of breast prosthesis and implant** CC

✓x7th **T85.42 Displacement of breast prosthesis and implant** CC
Malposition of breast prosthesis and implant

✓x7th **T85.43 Leakage of breast prosthesis and implant** CC

✓x7th **T85.44 Capsular contracture of breast implant** CC

✓x7th **T85.49 Other mechanical complication of breast prosthesis and implant** CC
Obstruction (mechanical) of breast prosthesis and implant
Perforation of breast prosthesis and implant
Protrusion of breast prosthesis and implant

✓5th **T85.5 Mechanical complication of gastrointestinal prosthetic devices, implants and grafts**

✓6th **T85.51 Breakdown (mechanical) of gastrointestinal prosthetic devices, implants and grafts**

✓7th **T85.510 Breakdown (mechanical) of bile duct prosthesis** CC

✓7th **T85.511 Breakdown (mechanical) of esophageal anti-reflux device** CC

✓7th **T85.518 Breakdown (mechanical) of other gastrointestinal prosthetic devices, implants and grafts** CC

✓6th **T85.52 Displacement of gastrointestinal prosthetic devices, implants and grafts**
Malposition of gastrointestinal prosthetic devices, implants and grafts

✓7th **T85.520 Displacement of bile duct prosthesis** CC

✓7th **T85.521 Displacement of esophageal anti-reflux device** CC

✓7th **T85.528 Displacement of other gastrointestinal prosthetic devices, implants and grafts** CC

✓6th **T85.59 Other mechanical complication of gastrointestinal prosthetic devices, implants and**
Obstruction, mechanical of gastrointestinal prosthetic devices, implants and grafts
Perforation of gastrointestinal prosthetic devices, implants and grafts
Protrusion of gastrointestinal prosthetic devices, implants and grafts

✓7th **T85.590 Other mechanical complication of bile duct prosthesis** CC

✓7th **T85.591 Other mechanical complication of esophageal anti-reflux device** CC

✓7th **T85.598 Other mechanical complication of other gastrointestinal prosthetic devices, implants and grafts** CC

✓5th **T85.6 Mechanical complication of other specified internal and external prosthetic devices, implants and grafts**

✓6th **T85.61 Breakdown (mechanical) of other specified internal prosthetic devices, implants and grafts**

✓7th **T85.610 Breakdown (mechanical) of cranial or spinal infusion catheter** CC
Breakdown (mechanical) of epidural infusion catheter
Breakdown (mechanical) of intrathecal infusion catheter
Breakdown (mechanical) of subarachnoid infusion catheter
Breakdown (mechanical) of subdural infusion catheter

✓7th **T85.611 Breakdown (mechanical) of intraperitoneal dialysis catheter** CC HCC
EXCLUDES 1 *mechanical complication of vascular dialysis catheter (T82.4-)*

✓7th **T85.612 Breakdown (mechanical) of permanent sutures** CC
EXCLUDES 1 *mechanical complication of permanent (wire) suture used in bone repair (T84.1-T84.2)*

✓7th **T85.613 Breakdown (mechanical) of artificial skin graft and decellularized allodermis** CC
Failure of artificial skin graft and decellularized allodermis
Non-adherence of artificial skin graft and decellularized allodermis
Poor incorporation of artificial skin graft and decellularized allodermis
Shearing of artificial skin graft and decellularized allodermis

✓7th **T85.614 Breakdown (mechanical) of insulin pump** CC

6 ✓7th **T85.615 Breakdown (mechanical) of other nervous system device, implant or graft** CC HCC
Breakdown (mechanical) of intrathecal infusion pump

✓7th **T85.618 Breakdown (mechanical) of other specified internal prosthetic devices, implants and grafts** CC

✓6th **T85.62 Displacement of other specified internal prosthetic devices, implants and grafts**
Malposition of other specified internal prosthetic devices, implants and grafts

✓7th **T85.620 Displacement of cranial or spinal infusion catheter** CC
Displacement of epidural infusion catheter
Displacement of intrathecal infusion catheter
Displacement of subarachnoid infusion catheter
Displacement of subdural infusion catheter

✓7th **T85.621 Displacement of intraperitoneal dialysis catheter** CC HCC
EXCLUDES 1 *mechanical complication of vascular dialysis catheter (T82.4-)*

✓7th **T85.622 Displacement of permanent sutures** CC
EXCLUDES 1 *mechanical complication of permanent (wire) suture used in bone repair (T84.1-T84.2)*

✓7th **T85.623 Displacement of artificial skin graft and decellularized allodermis** CC
Dislodgement of artificial skin graft and decellularized allodermis

✓7th **T85.624 Displacement of insulin pump** CC

6 ✓7th **T85.625 Displacement of other nervous system device, implant or graft** CC HCC
Displacement of intrathecal infusion pump

✓7th **T85.628 Displacement of other specified internal prosthetic devices, implants and grafts** CC

√6th **T85.63 Leakage of other specified internal prosthetic devices, implants and grafts**

√7th **T85.630 Leakage of cranial or spinal infusion catheter** CC
Leakage of epidural infusion catheter
Leakage of intrathecal infusion catheter infusion catheter
Leakage of subdural infusion catheter
Leakage of subarachnoid infusion catheter

√7th **T85.631 Leakage of intraperitoneal dialysis catheter** CC HCC
EXCLUDES 1 *mechanical complication of vascular dialysis catheter (T82.4)*

√7th **T85.633 Leakage of insulin pump** CC

6 √7th **T85.635 Leakage of other nervous system device, implant or graft** CC HCC
Leakage of intrathecal infusion pump

√7th **T85.638 Leakage of other specified internal prosthetic devices, implants and grafts** CC

√6th **T85.69 Other mechanical complication of other specified internal prosthetic devices, implants and grafts**
Obstruction, mechanical of other specified internal prosthetic devices, implants and grafts
Perforation of other specified internal prosthetic devices, implants and grafts
Protrusion of other specified internal prosthetic devices, implants and grafts

√7th **T85.690 Other mechanical complication of cranial or spinal infusion catheter** CC
Other mechanical complication of epidural infusion catheter
Other mechanical complication of intrathecal infusion catheter
Other mechanical complication of subarachnoid infusion catheter
Other mechanical complication of subdural infusion catheter

√7th **T85.691 Other mechanical complication of intraperitoneal dialysis catheter** CC HCC
EXCLUDES 1 *mechanical complication of vascular dialysis catheter (T82.4)*

√7th **T85.692 Other mechanical complication of permanent sutures** CC
EXCLUDES 1 *mechanical complication of permanent (wire) suture used in bone repair (T84.1-T84.2)*

√7th **T85.693 Other mechanical complication of artificial skin graft and decellularized allodermis** CC

√7th **T85.694 Other mechanical complication of insulin pump** CC

6 √7th **T85.695 Other mechanical complication of other nervous system device, implant or graft** CC HCC
Other mechanical complication of intrathecal infusion pump

√7th **T85.698 Other mechanical complication of other specified internal prosthetic devices, implants and grafts** CC
Mechanical complication of nonabsorbable surgical material NOS

√5th **T85.7 Infection and inflammatory reaction due to other internal prosthetic devices, implants and grafts**
Use additional code to identify infection

√x7th **T85.71 Infection and inflammatory reaction due to peritoneal dialysis catheter** CC HCC

6 √x7th **T85.72 Infection and inflammatory reaction due to insulin pump** CC HCC

√6th **T85.73 Infection and inflammatory reaction due to nervous system devices, implants and graft**

6 √7th **T85.730 Infection and inflammatory reaction due to ventricular intracranial (communicating) shunt** CC HCC

6 √7th **T85.731 Infection and inflammatory reaction due to implanted electronic neurostimulator of brain, electrode (lead)** CC HCC

6 √7th **T85.732 Infection and inflammatory reaction due to implanted electronic neurostimulator of peripheral nerve, electrode (lead)** CC HCC
Infection and inflammatory reaction due to electrode (lead) for cranial nerve neurostimulators
Infection and inflammatory reaction due to electrode (lead) for gastric neurostimulator
Infection and inflammatory reaction due to electrode (lead) for sacral nerve neurostimulator
Infection and inflammatory reaction due to electrode (lead) for vagal nerve neurostimulators

6 √7th **T85.733 Infection and inflammatory reaction due to implanted electronic neurostimulator of spinal cord, electrode (lead)** CC HCC

6 √7th **T85.734 Infection and inflammatory reaction due to implanted electronic neurostimulator, generator** CC HCC
Generator pocket infection

6 √7th **T85.735 Infection and inflammatory reaction due to cranial or spinal infusion catheter** CC HCC
Infection and inflammatory reaction due to epidural catheter
Infection and inflammatory reaction due to intrathecal infusion catheter
Infection and inflammatory reaction due to subarachnoid catheter
Infection and inflammatory reaction due to subdural catheter

6 √7th **T85.738 Infection and inflammatory reaction due to other nervous system device, implant or graft** CC HCC
Infection and inflammatory reaction due to intrathecal infusion pump

6 √x7th **T85.79 Infection and inflammatory reaction due to other internal prosthetic devices, implants and grafts** CC HCC

√5th **T85.8 Other specified complications of internal prosthetic devices, implants and grafts, not elsewhere classified**

√6th **T85.81 Embolism due to internal prosthetic devices, implants and grafts, not elsewhere classified**

5,6 √7th **T85.810 Embolism due to nervous system prosthetic devices, implants and grafts** CC HCC

√7th **T85.818 Embolism due to other internal prosthetic devices, implants and grafts**

√6th **T85.82 Fibrosis due to internal prosthetic devices, implants and grafts, not elsewhere classified**

5,6 √7th **T85.820 Fibrosis due to nervous system prosthetic devices, implants and grafts** CC HCC

√7th **T85.828 Fibrosis due to other internal prosthetic devices, implants and grafts**

√6th **T85.83 Hemorrhage due to internal prosthetic devices, implants and grafts, not elsewhere classified**

5,6 √7th **T85.830 Hemorrhage due to nervous system prosthetic devices, implants and grafts** CC HCC

√7th **T85.838 Hemorrhage due to other internal prosthetic devices, implants and grafts**

√6th **T85.84 Pain due to internal prosthetic devices, implants and grafts, not elsewhere classified**

5,6 √7th **T85.840 Pain due to nervous system prosthetic devices, implants and grafts** CC HCC

√7th **T85.848 Pain due to other internal prosthetic devices, implants and grafts**

√6th **T85.85 Stenosis due to internal prosthetic devices, implants and grafts, not elsewhere classified**

5,6 √7th **T85.850 Stenosis due to nervous system prosthetic devices, implants and grafts** CC HCC

√7th **T85.858 Stenosis due to other internal prosthetic devices, implants and grafts**

✓6th **T85.86 Thrombosis due to internal prosthetic devices, implants and grafts, not elsewhere classified**

5,6 ✓7th **T85.860 Thrombosis due to nervous system prosthetic devices, implants and grafts** CC HCC

✓7th **T85.868 Thrombosis due to other internal prosthetic devices, implants and grafts**

✓6th **T85.89 Other specified complication of internal prosthetic devices, implants and grafts, not elsewhere classified**

Erosion or breakdown of subcutaneous device pocket

5,6 ✓7th **T85.890 Other specified complication of nervous system prosthetic devices, implants and grafts** CC HCC

✓7th **T85.898 Other specified complication of other internal prosthetic devices, implants and grafts**

✓x7th **T85.9 Unspecified complication of internal prosthetic device, implant and graft**

Complication of internal prosthetic device, implant and graft NOS

✓4th **T86 Complications of transplanted organs and tissue**

Use additional code to identify other transplant complications, such as:
- graft-versus-host disease (D89.81-)
- malignancy associated with organ transplant (C80.2)
- post-transplant lymphoproliferative disorders (PTLD) (D47.Z1)

AHA: 2020,1Q,18

✓5th **T86.0 Complications of bone marrow transplant**

T86.00 Unspecified complication of bone marrow transplant CC HCC

T86.01 Bone marrow transplant rejection CC HCC

T86.02 Bone marrow transplant failure CC HCC

T86.03 Bone marrow transplant infection CC HCC

T86.09 Other complications of bone marrow transplant CC HCC

✓5th **T86.1 Complications of kidney transplant**

T86.10 Unspecified complication of kidney transplant CC

T86.11 Kidney transplant rejection CC

T86.12 Kidney transplant failure CC

AHA: 2013,1Q,24

T86.13 Kidney transplant infection CC

Use additional code to specify infection

T86.19 Other complication of kidney transplant CC

AHA: 2019,2Q,7

✓5th **T86.2 Complications of heart transplant**

EXCLUDES 1 *complication of:*
artificial heart device (T82.5)
heart-lung transplant (T86.3)

T86.20 Unspecified complication of heart transplant CC HCC

T86.21 Heart transplant rejection CC HCC

T86.22 Heart transplant failure CC HCC

T86.23 Heart transplant infection CC HCC

Use additional code to specify infection

✓6th **T86.29 Other complications of heart transplant**

T86.290 Cardiac allograft vasculopathy CC HCC

EXCLUDES 1 *atherosclerosis of coronary arteries (I25.75-, I25.76-, I25.81-)*

T86.298 Other complications of heart transplant CC HCC

✓5th **T86.3 Complications of heart-lung transplant**

T86.30 Unspecified complication of heart-lung transplant CC HCC

T86.31 Heart-lung transplant rejection CC HCC

T86.32 Heart-lung transplant failure CC HCC

T86.33 Heart-lung transplant infection CC HCC

Use additional code to specify infection

T86.39 Other complications of heart-lung transplant CC HCC

✓5th **T86.4 Complications of liver transplant**

T86.40 Unspecified complication of liver transplant CC HCC

T86.41 Liver transplant rejection CC HCC

T86.42 Liver transplant failure CC HCC

T86.43 Liver transplant infection CC HCC

Use additional code to identify infection, such as:
cytomegalovirus (CMV) infection (B25.-)

T86.49 Other complications of liver transplant CC HCC

T86.5 Complications of stem cell transplant CC HCC

Complications from stem cells from peripheral blood
Complications from stem cells from umbilical cord

✓5th **T86.8 Complications of other transplanted organs and tissues**

✓6th **T86.81 Complications of lung transplant**

EXCLUDES 1 *complication of heart-lung transplant (T86.3-)*

T86.810 Lung transplant rejection CC HCC

T86.811 Lung transplant failure CC HCC

T86.812 Lung transplant infection CC HCC

Use additional code to specify infection

T86.818 Other complications of lung transplant CC HCC

AHA: 2019,2Q,6

T86.819 Unspecified complication of lung transplant CC HCC

✓6th **T86.82 Complications of skin graft (allograft) (autograft)**

EXCLUDES 2 *complication of artificial skin graft (T85.693)*

T86.820 Skin graft (allograft) rejection CC

T86.821 Skin graft (allograft) (autograft) failure CC

T86.822 Skin graft (allograft) (autograft) infection CC

Use additional code to specify infection

T86.828 Other complications of skin graft (allograft) (autograft) CC

T86.829 Unspecified complication of skin graft (allograft) (autograft) CC

✓6th **T86.83 Complications of bone graft**

EXCLUDES 2 *mechanical complications of bone graft (T84.3-)*

T86.830 Bone graft rejection CC

T86.831 Bone graft failure CC

T86.832 Bone graft infection CC

Use additional code to specify infection

T86.838 Other complications of bone graft CC

T86.839 Unspecified complication of bone graft CC

✓6th **T86.84 Complications of corneal transplant**

EXCLUDES 2 *mechanical complications of corneal graft (T85.3-)*

▲ ✓7th **T86.840 Corneal transplant rejection**

● **T86.8401 Corneal transplant rejection, right eye** CC

● **T86.8402 Corneal transplant rejection, left eye** CC

● **T86.8403 Corneal transplant rejection, bilateral** CC

● **T86.8409 Corneal transplant rejection, unspecified eye** CC

▲ ✓7th **T86.841 Corneal transplant failure**

● **T86.8411 Corneal transplant failure, right eye** CC

● **T86.8412 Corneal transplant failure, left eye** CC

● **T86.8413 Corneal transplant failure, bilateral** CC

● **T86.8419 Corneal transplant failure, unspecified eye** CC

▲ ✓7th **T86.842 Corneal transplant infection**

Use additional code to specify infection

● **T86.8421 Corneal transplant infection, right eye** CC

● **T86.8422 Corneal transplant infection, left eye** CC

● **T86.8423 Corneal transplant infection, bilateral** CC

● **T86.8429 Corneal transplant infection, unspecified eye** CC

▲ ✓7th **T86.848 Other complications of corneal transplant**

● **T86.8481 Other complications of corneal transplant, right eye** CC

● T86.8482 Other complications of corneal transplant, left eye CC
● T86.8483 Other complications of corneal transplant, bilateral CC
● T86.8489 Other complications of corneal transplant, unspecified eye CC
▲ √7th T86.849 Unspecified complication of corneal transplant
● T86.8491 Unspecified complication of corneal transplant, right eye CC
● T86.8492 Unspecified complication of corneal transplant, left eye CC
● T86.8493 Unspecified complication of corneal transplant, bilateral CC
● T86.8499 Unspecified complication of corneal transplant, unspecified eye CC

√6th T86.85 Complication of intestine transplant
T86.850 Intestine transplant rejection CC HCC
T86.851 Intestine transplant failure CC HCC
T86.852 Intestine transplant infection CC HCC
Use additional code to specify infection
T86.858 Other complications of intestine transplant CC HCC
T86.859 Unspecified complication of intestine transplant CC HCC

√6th T86.89 Complications of other transplanted tissue
Transplant failure or rejection of pancreas
AHA: 2020,1Q,18
T86.890 Other transplanted tissue rejection CC
T86.891 Other transplanted tissue failure CC
T86.892 Other transplanted tissue infection CC
Use additional code to specify infection
T86.898 Other complications of other transplanted tissue CC
T86.899 Unspecified complication of other transplanted tissue CC

√5th T86.9 Complication of unspecified transplanted organ and tissue
T86.90 Unspecified complication of unspecified transplanted organ and tissue CC
T86.91 Unspecified transplanted organ and tissue rejection CC
T86.92 Unspecified transplanted organ and tissue failure CC
T86.93 Unspecified transplanted organ and tissue infection CC
Use additional code to specify infection
T86.99 Other complications of unspecified transplanted organ and tissue CC

√4th **T87 Complications peculiar to reattachment and amputation**

√5th T87.0 Complications of reattached (part of) upper extremity
√6th T87.0X Complications of reattached (part of) upper extremity
T87.0X1 Complications of reattached (part of) right upper extremity CC HCC
T87.0X2 Complications of reattached (part of) left upper extremity CC HCC
T87.0X9 Complications of reattached (part of) unspecified upper extremity CC HCC

√5th T87.1 Complications of reattached (part of) lower extremity
√6th T87.1X Complications of reattached (part of) lower extremity
T87.1X1 Complications of reattached (part of) right lower extremity CC HCC
T87.1X2 Complications of reattached (part of) left lower extremity CC HCC
T87.1X9 Complications of reattached (part of) unspecified lower extremity CC HCC

T87.2 Complications of other reattached body part CC HCC

√5th T87.3 Neuroma of amputation stump
DEF: Non-neoplastic tumor generated at the proximal end of severed, partially transected, or injured nerve following amputation.
T87.30 Neuroma of amputation stump, unspecified extremity HCC
T87.31 Neuroma of amputation stump, right upper extremity HCC
T87.32 Neuroma of amputation stump, left upper extremity HCC
T87.33 Neuroma of amputation stump, right lower extremity HCC
T87.34 Neuroma of amputation stump, left lower extremity HCC

√5th T87.4 Infection of amputation stump
T87.40 Infection of amputation stump, unspecified extremity CC HCC
T87.41 Infection of amputation stump, right upper extremity CC HCC
T87.42 Infection of amputation stump, left upper extremity CC HCC
T87.43 Infection of amputation stump, right lower extremity CC HCC
T87.44 Infection of amputation stump, left lower extremity CC HCC

√5th T87.5 Necrosis of amputation stump
T87.50 Necrosis of amputation stump, unspecified extremity HCC
T87.51 Necrosis of amputation stump, right upper extremity HCC
T87.52 Necrosis of amputation stump, left upper extremity HCC
T87.53 Necrosis of amputation stump, right lower extremity HCC
T87.54 Necrosis of amputation stump, left lower extremity HCC

√5th T87.8 Other complications of amputation stump
T87.81 Dehiscence of amputation stump HCC
T87.89 Other complications of amputation stump HCC
Amputation stump contracture
Amputation stump contracture of next proximal joint
Amputation stump flexion
Amputation stump edema
Amputation stump hematoma
EXCLUDES 2 *phantom limb syndrome (G54.6-G54.7)*

T87.9 Unspecified complications of amputation stump HCC

√4th **T88 Other complications of surgical and medical care, not elsewhere classified**
EXCLUDES 2 *complication following infusion, transfusion and therapeutic injection (T80.-)*
complication following procedure NEC (T81.-)
complications of anesthesia in labor and delivery (O74.-)
complications of anesthesia in pregnancy (O29.-)
complications of anesthesia in puerperium (O89.-)
complications of devices, implants and grafts (T82-T85)
complications of obstetric surgery and procedure (O75.4)
dermatitis due to drugs and medicaments (L23.3, L24.4, L25.1, L27.0-L27.1)
poisoning and toxic effects of drugs and chemicals (T36-T65 with fifth or sixth character 1-4 or 6)
specified complications classified elsewhere

The appropriate 7th character is to be added to each code from category T88.
A initial encounter
D subsequent encounter
S sequela

√x 7th T88.0 Infection following immunization CC
Sepsis following immunization
AHA: 2018,4Q,62-63

√x 7th T88.1 Other complications following immunization, not elsewhere classified CC
Generalized vaccinia
Rash following immunization
EXCLUDES 1 *vaccinia not from vaccine (B08.011)*
EXCLUDES 2 *anaphylactic shock due to serum (T80.5-)*
other serum reactions (T80.6-)
postimmunization arthropathy (M02.2)
postimmunization encephalitis (G04.02)
postimmunization fever (R50.83)

√x 7th **T88.2 Shock due to anesthesia** CC

Use additional code for adverse effect, if applicable, to identify drug (T41.- with fifth or sixth character 5)

EXCLUDES 1 *complications of anesthesia (in):*
labor and delivery (O74.-)
postprocedural shock NOS (T81.1-)
pregnancy (O29.-)
puerperium (O89.-)

√x 7th **T88.3 Malignant hyperthermia due to anesthesia** CC

Use additional code for adverse effect, if applicable, to identify drug (T41.- with fifth or sixth character 5)

√x 7th **T88.4 Failed or difficult intubation**

√5th **T88.5 Other complications of anesthesia**

Use additional code for adverse effect, if applicable, to identify drug (T41.- with fifth or sixth character 5)

√x 7th **T88.51 Hypothermia following anesthesia**

√x 7th **T88.52 Failed moderate sedation during procedure**

Failed conscious sedation during procedure

EXCLUDES 2 *personal history of failed moderate sedation (Z92.83)*

√x 7th **T88.53 Unintended awareness under general anesthesia during procedure**

EXCLUDES 2 *personal history of unintended awareness under general anesthesia (Z92.84)*

AHA: 2016,4Q,72-73

√x 7th **T88.59 Other complications of anesthesia**

√x 7th **T88.6 Anaphylactic reaction due to adverse effect of correct drug or medicament properly administered** CC

Anaphylactic shock due to adverse effect of correct drug or medicament properly administered

Anaphylactoid reaction NOS

Use additional code for adverse effect, if applicable, to identify drug (T36-T5Ø with fifth or sixth character 5)

EXCLUDES 1 *anaphylactic reaction due to serum (T8Ø.5-)*
anaphylactic shock or reaction due to adverse food reaction (T78.Ø-)

AHA: 2020,1Q,18

√x 7th **T88.7 Unspecified adverse effect of drug or medicament**

Drug hypersensitivity NOS

Drug reaction NOS

Use additional code for adverse effect, if applicable, to identify drug (T36-T5Ø with fifth or sixth character 5)

EXCLUDES 1 *specified adverse effects of drugs and medicaments (AØØ-R94 and T8Ø-T88.6, T88.8)*

√x 7th **T88.8 Other specified complications of surgical and medical care, not elsewhere classified**

Use additional code to identify the complication

√x 7th **T88.9 Complication of surgical and medical care, unspecified**

Chapter 20. External Causes of Morbidity (VØØ–Y99)

Chapter-specific Guidelines with Coding Examples

The chapter-specific guidelines from the ICD-10-CM Official Guidelines for Coding and Reporting have been provided below. Along with these guidelines are coding examples, contained in the shaded boxes, that have been developed to help illustrate the coding and/or sequencing guidance found in these guidelines.

The external causes of morbidity codes should never be sequenced as the first-listed or principal diagnosis.

External cause codes are intended to provide data for injury research and evaluation of injury prevention strategies. These codes capture how the injury or health condition happened (cause), the intent (unintentional or accidental; or intentional, such as suicide or assault), the place where the event occurred the activity of the patient at the time of the event, and the person's status (e.g., civilian, military).

There is no national requirement for mandatory ICD-10-CM external cause code reporting. Unless a provider is subject to a state-based external cause code reporting mandate or these codes are required by a particular payer, reporting of ICD-10-CM codes in Chapter 20, External Causes of Morbidity, is not required. In the absence of a mandatory reporting requirement, providers are encouraged to voluntarily report external cause codes, as they provide valuable data for injury research and evaluation of injury prevention strategies.

a. General external cause coding guidelines

1) Used with any code in the range of AØØ.Ø–T88.9, ZØØ–Z99

An external cause code may be used with any code in the range of AØØ.Ø-T88.9, ZØØ-Z99, classification that represents a health condition due to an external cause. Though they are most applicable to injuries, they are also valid for use with such things as infections or diseases due to an external source, and other health conditions, such as a heart attack that occurs during strenuous physical activity.

> Actinic reticuloid due to tanning bed use
>
> **L57.1** **Actinic reticuloid**
>
> **W89.1XXA** **Exposure to tanning bed, initial encounter**
>
> *Explanation:* An external cause code may be used with any code in the range of AØØ.Ø–T88.9, ZØØ–Z99, classifications that describe health conditions due to an external cause. Code W89.1 Exposure to tanning bed requires a seventh character of A to report this initial encounter, with a placeholder X for the fifth and sixth characters.

2) External cause code used for length of treatment

Assign the external cause code, with the appropriate 7th character (initial encounter, subsequent encounter or sequela) for each encounter for which the injury or condition is being treated.

Most categories in chapter 20 have a 7th character requirement for each applicable code. Most categories in this chapter have three 7th character values: A, initial encounter, D, subsequent encounter and S, sequela. While the patient may be seen by a new or different provider over the course of treatment for an injury or condition, assignment of the 7th character for external cause should match the 7th character of the code assigned for the associated injury or condition for the encounter.

3) Use the full range of external cause codes

Use the full range of external cause codes to completely describe the cause, the intent, the place of occurrence, and if applicable, the activity of the patient at the time of the event, and the patient's status, for all injuries, and other health conditions due to an external cause.

4) Assign as many external cause codes as necessary

Assign as many external cause codes as necessary to fully explain each cause. If only one external code can be recorded, assign the code most related to the principal diagnosis.

5) The selection of the appropriate external cause code

The selection of the appropriate external cause code is guided by the Alphabetic Index of External Causes and by Inclusion and Exclusion notes in the Tabular List.

6) External cause code can never be a principal diagnosis

An external cause code can never be a principal (first-listed) diagnosis.

7) Combination external cause codes

Certain of the external cause codes are combination codes that identify sequential events that result in an injury, such as a fall which results in striking against an object. The injury may be due to either event or both. The combination external cause code used should correspond to the sequence of events regardless of which caused the most serious injury.

> Toddler tripped and fell while walking and struck his head on an end table, sustaining a scalp contusion
>
> **SØØ.Ø3XA** **Contusion of scalp, initial encounter**
>
> **WØ1.19ØA** **Fall on same level from slipping, tripping and stumbling with subsequent striking against furniture, initial encounter**
>
> *Explanation:* Combination external cause codes identify sequential events that result in an injury, such as a fall resulting in striking against an object. The injury may be due to either or both events.

8) No external cause code needed in certain circumstances

No external cause code from Chapter 20 is needed if the external cause and intent are included in a code from another chapter (e.g. T36.ØX1-Poisoning by penicillins, accidental (unintentional)).

b. Place of occurrence guideline

Codes from category Y92, Place of occurrence of the external cause, are secondary codes for use after other external cause codes to identify the location of the patient at the time of injury or other condition.

Generally, a place of occurrence code is assigned only once, at the initial encounter for treatment. However, in the rare instance that a new injury occurs during hospitalization, an additional place of occurrence code may be assigned. No 7th characters are used for Y92.

Do not use place of occurrence code Y92.9 if the place is not stated or is not applicable.

> A farmer was working in his barn and sustained a foot contusion when the horse stepped on his left foot
>
> **S9Ø.32XA** **Contusion of left foot, initial encounter**
>
> **W55.19XA** **Other contact with horse, initial encounter**
>
> **Y92.71** **Barn as the place of occurrence of the external cause**
>
> *Explanation:* A place-of-occurrence code from category Y92 is assigned at the initial encounter to identify the location of the patient at the time the injury occurred.

c. Activity code

Assign a code from category Y93, Activity code, to describe the activity of the patient at the time the injury or other health condition occurred.

An activity code is used only once, at the initial encounter for treatment. Only one code from Y93 should be recorded on a medical record.

The activity codes are not applicable to poisonings, adverse effects, misadventures or sequela.

Do not assign Y93.9, Unspecified activity, if the activity is not stated.

A code from category Y93 is appropriate for use with external cause and intent codes if identifying the activity provides additional information about the event.

> Ranch hand who was grooming a horse sustained a foot contusion when the horse stepped on his left foot
>
> **S9Ø.32XA** **Contusion of left foot, initial encounter**
>
> **W55.19XA** **Other contact with horse, initial encounter**
>
> **Y93.K3** **Activity, grooming and shearing an animal**
>
> *Explanation:* One activity code from category Y93 is assigned at the initial encounter only to describe the activity of the patient at the time the injury occurred.

d. Place of occurrence, activity, and status codes used with other external cause code

When applicable, place of occurrence, activity, and external cause status codes are sequenced after the main external cause code(s). Regardless of the number of external cause codes assigned, generally there should be only one place of occurrence code, one activity code, and one external cause status code assigned to an encounter. However, in the rare instance that a new injury occurs during hospitalization, an additional place of occurrence code may be assigned.

e. If the reporting format limits the number of external cause codes

If the reporting format limits the number of external cause codes that can be used in reporting clinical data, report the code for the cause/intent most related to the principal diagnosis. If the format permits capture of additional external cause codes, the cause/intent, including medical misadventures, of the additional events should be reported rather than the codes for place, activity, or external status.

f. Multiple external cause coding guidelines

More than one external cause code is required to fully describe the external cause of an illness or injury. The assignment of external cause codes should be sequenced in the following priority:

If two or more events cause separate injuries, an external cause code should be assigned for each cause. The first-listed external cause code will be selected in the following order:

External codes for child and adult abuse take priority over all other external cause codes.

See Section I.C.19., Child and Adult abuse guidelines.

External cause codes for terrorism events take priority over all other external cause codes except child and adult abuse.

External cause codes for cataclysmic events take priority over all other external cause codes except child and adult abuse and terrorism.

External cause codes for transport accidents take priority over all other external cause codes except cataclysmic events, child and adult abuse and terrorism.

Activity and external cause status codes are assigned following all causal (intent) external cause codes.

The first-listed external cause code should correspond to the cause of the most serious diagnosis due to an assault, accident, or self-harm, following the order of hierarchy listed above..

30-year-old man accidentally discharged his hunting rifle, sustaining an open gunshot wound to the right thigh, which caused him to fall down the stairs, resulting in closed displaced comminuted fracture of his left radial shaft

S71.131A	**Puncture wound without foreign body, right thigh, initial encounter**
W33.02XA	**Accidental discharge of hunting rifle, initial encounter**
S52.352A	**Displaced comminuted fracture of shaft of radius, left arm, initial encounter for closed fracture**
W10.9XXA	**Fall (on) (from) unspecified stairs and steps, initial encounter**

Explanation: If two or more events cause separate injuries, an external cause code should be assigned for each cause.

g. Child and adult abuse guideline

Adult and child abuse, neglect and maltreatment are classified as assault. Any of the assault codes may be used to indicate the external cause of any injury resulting from the confirmed abuse.

For confirmed cases of abuse, neglect and maltreatment, when the perpetrator is known, a code from Y07, Perpetrator of maltreatment and neglect, should accompany any other assault codes.

See Section I.C.19. Adult and child abuse, neglect and other maltreatment

h. Unknown or undetermined intent guideline

If the intent (accident, self-harm, assault) of the cause of an injury or other condition is unknown or unspecified, code the intent as accidental intent. All transport accident categories assume accidental intent.

1) Use of undetermined intent

External cause codes for events of undetermined intent are only for use if the documentation in the record specifies that the intent cannot be determined.

i. Sequelae (late effects) of external cause guidelines

1) Sequelae external cause codes

Sequela are reported using the external cause code with the 7th character "S" for sequela. These codes should be used with any report of a late effect or sequela resulting from a previous injury.

See Section I.B.10 Sequela (Late Effects)

2) Sequela external cause code with a related current injury

A sequela external cause code should never be used with a related current nature of injury code.

3) Use of sequela external cause codes for subsequent visits

Use a late effect external cause code for subsequent visits when a late effect of the initial injury is being treated. Do not use a late effect external cause code for subsequent visits for follow-up care (e.g., to assess healing, to receive rehabilitative therapy) of the injury when no late effect of the injury has been documented.

j. Terrorism guidelines

1) Cause of injury identified by the Federal Government (FBI) as terrorism

When the cause of an injury is identified by the Federal Government (FBI) as terrorism, the first-listed external cause code should be a code from category Y38, Terrorism. The definition of terrorism employed by the FBI is found at the inclusion note at the beginning of category Y38. Use additional code for place of occurrence (Y92.-). More than one Y38 code may be assigned if the injury is the result of more than one mechanism of terrorism.

2) Cause of an injury is suspected to be the result of terrorism

When the cause of an injury is suspected to be the result of terrorism a code from category Y38 should not be assigned. Suspected cases should be classified as assault.

3) Code Y38.9, Terrorism, secondary effects

Assign code Y38.9, Terrorism, secondary effects, for conditions occurring subsequent to the terrorist event. This code should not be assigned for conditions that are due to the initial terrorist act.

It is acceptable to assign code Y38.9 with another code from Y38 if there is an injury due to the initial terrorist event and an injury that is a subsequent result of the terrorist event.

k. External cause status

A code from category Y99, External cause status, should be assigned whenever any other external cause code is assigned for an encounter, including an Activity code, except for the events noted below. Assign a code from category Y99, External cause status, to indicate the work status of the person at the time the event occurred. The status code indicates whether the event occurred during military activity, whether a non-military person was at work, whether an individual including a student or volunteer was involved in a non-work activity at the time of the causal event.

A code from Y99, External cause status, should be assigned, when applicable, with other external cause codes, such as transport accidents and falls. The external cause status codes are not applicable to poisonings, adverse effects, misadventures or late effects.

Do not assign a code from category Y99 if no other external cause codes (cause, activity) are applicable for the encounter.

An external cause status code is used only once, at the initial encounter for treatment. Only one code from Y99 should be recorded on a medical record.

Do not assign code Y99.9, Unspecified external cause status, if the status is not stated.

Chapter 2Ø. External Causes of Morbidity (VØØ-Y99)

NOTE This chapter permits the classification of environmental events and circumstances as the cause of injury, and other adverse effects. Where a code from this section is applicable, it is intended that it shall be used secondary to a code from another chapter of the Classification indicating the nature of the condition. Most often, the condition will be classifiable to Chapter 19, Injury, poisoning and certain other consequences of external causes (SØØ-T88). Other conditions that may be stated to be due to external causes are classified in Chapters I to XVIII. For these conditions, codes from Chapter 2Ø should be used to provide additional information as to the cause of the condition.

AHA: 2018,4Q,58-60

This chapter contains the following blocks:

VØØ-X58 Accidents
VØØ-V99 Transport accidents
VØØ-VØ9 Pedestrian injured in transport accident
V1Ø-V19 Pedal cycle rider injured in transport accident
V2Ø-V29 Motorcycle rider injured in transport accident
V3Ø-V39 Occupant of three-wheeled motor vehicle injured in transport accident
V4Ø-V49 Car occupant injured in transport accident
V5Ø-V59 Occupant of pick-up truck or van injured in transport accident
V6Ø-V69 Occupant of heavy transport vehicle injured in transport accident
V7Ø-V79 Bus occupant injured in transport accident
V8Ø-V89 Other land transport accidents
V9Ø-V94 Water transport accidents
V95-V97 Air and space transport accidents
V98-V99 Other and unspecified transport accidents
WØØ-X58 Other external causes of accidental injury
WØØ-W19 Slipping, tripping, stumbling and falls
W2Ø-W49 Exposure to inanimate mechanical forces
W5Ø-W64 Exposure to animate mechanical forces
W65-W74 Accidental non-transport drowning and submersion
W85-W99 Exposure to electric current, radiation and extreme ambient air temperature and pressure
XØØ-XØ8 Exposure to smoke, fire and flames
X1Ø-X19 Contact with heat and hot substances
X3Ø-X39 Exposure to forces of nature
X5Ø Overexertion and strenuous or repetitive movements
X52-X58 Accidental exposure to other specified factors
X71-X83 Intentional self-harm
X92-YØ9 Assault
Y21-Y33 Event of undetermined intent
Y35-Y38 Legal intervention, operations of war, military operations, and terrorism
Y62-Y84 Complications of medical and surgical care
Y62-Y69 Misadventures to patients during surgical and medical care
Y7Ø-Y82 Medical devices associated with adverse incidents in diagnostic and therapeutic use
Y83-Y84 Surgical and other medical procedures as the cause of abnormal reaction of the patient, or of later complication, without mention of misadventure at the time of the procedure
Y9Ø-Y99 Supplementary factors related to causes of morbidity classified elsewhere

ACCIDENTS (VØØ-X58)

AHA: 2018,2Q,7-8

Transport accidents (VØØ-V99)

NOTE This section is structured in 12 groups. Those relating to land transport accidents (VØØ-V89) reflect the victim's mode of transport and are subdivided to identify the victim's 'counterpart' or the type of event. The vehicle of which the injured person is an occupant is identified in the first two characters since it is seen as the most important factor to identify for prevention purposes. A transport accident is one in which the vehicle involved must be moving or running or in use for transport purposes at the time of the accident.

Use additional code to identify:
airbag injury (W22.1)
type of street or road (Y92.4-)
use of cellular telephone and other electronic equipment at the time of the transport accident (Y93.C-)

EXCLUDES 1 *agricultural vehicles in stationary use or maintenance (W31.-)*
assault by crashing of motor vehicle (YØ3.-)
automobile or motor cycle in stationary use or maintenance — code to type of accident
crashing of motor vehicle, undetermined intent (Y32)
intentional self-harm by crashing of motor vehicle (X82)

EXCLUDES 2 *transport accidents due to cataclysm (X34-X38)*

NOTE Definitions related to transport accidents:

(a) A transport accident (VØØ-V99) is any accident involving a device designed primarily for, or used at the time primarily for, conveying persons or good from one place to another.

(b) A public highway [trafficway] or street is the entire width between property lines (or other boundary lines) of land open to the public as a matter of right or custom for purposes of moving persons or property from one place to another. A roadway is that part of the public highway designed, improved and customarily used for vehicular traffic.

(c) A traffic accident is any vehicle accident occurring on the public highway [i.e. originating on, terminating on, or involving a vehicle partially on the highway]. A vehicle accident is assumed to have occurred on the public highway unless another place is specified, except in the case of accidents involving only off-road motor vehicles, which are classified as nontraffic accidents unless the contrary is stated.

(d) A nontraffic accident is any vehicle accident that occurs entirely in any place other than a public highway.

(e) A pedestrian is any person involved in an accident who was not at the time of the accident riding in or on a motor vehicle, railway train, streetcar or animal-drawn or other vehicle, or on a pedal cycle or animal. This includes, a person changing a tire, working on a parked car, or a person on foot. It also includes the user of a pedestrian conveyance such as a baby stroller, ice-skates, skis, sled, roller skates, a skateboard, nonmotorized or motorized wheelchair, motorized mobility scooter, or nonmotorized scooter.

(f) A driver is an occupant of a transport vehicle who is operating or intending to operate it.

(g) A passenger is any occupant of a transport vehicle other than the driver, except a person traveling on the outside of the vehicle.

(h) A person on the outside of a vehicle is any person being transported by a vehicle but not occupying the space normally reserved for the driver or passengers, or the space intended for the transport of property. This includes a person travelling on the bodywork, bumper, fender, roof, running board or step of a vehicle, as well as, hanging on the outside of the vehicle.

(i) A pedal cycle is any land transport vehicle operated solely by nonmotorized pedals including a bicycle or tricycle.

(j) A pedal cyclist is any person riding a pedal cycle or in a sidecar or trailer attached to a pedal cycle.

(k) A motorcycle is a two-wheeled motor vehicle with one or two riding saddles and sometimes with a third wheel for the support of a sidecar. The sidecar is considered part of the motorcycle. This includes a moped, motor scooter, or motorized bicycle.

(l) A motorcycle rider is any person riding a motorcycle or in a sidecar or trailer attached to the motorcycle.

(m) A three-wheeled motor vehicle is a motorized tricycle designed primarily for on-road use. This includes a motor-driven tricycle, a motorized rickshaw, or a three-wheeled motor car.

(n) A car [automobile] is a four-wheeled motor vehicle designed primarily for carrying up to 7 persons. A trailer being towed by the car is considered part of the car. It does not include a van or minivan — see definition (o).

(o) A pick-up truck or van is a four or six-wheeled motor vehicle designed for carrying passengers as well as property or cargo weighing less than the local limit for classification as a heavy goods vehicle, and not requiring a special driver's license. This includes a minivan and a sport-utility vehicle (SUV).

(p) A heavy transport vehicle is a motor vehicle designed primarily for carrying property, meeting local criteria for classification as a heavy goods vehicle in terms of weight and requiring a special driver's license.

(q) A bus (coach) is a motor vehicle designed or adapted primarily for carrying more than 1Ø passengers, and requiring a special driver's license.

(r) A railway train or railway vehicle is any device, with or without freight or passenger cars couple to it, designed for traffic on a railway track. This includes subterranean (subways) or elevated trains.

(s) A streetcar, is a device designed and used primarily for transporting passengers within a municipality, running on rails, usually subject to normal traffic control signals, and operated principally on a right-of-way that forms part of the roadway. This includes a tram or trolley that runs on rails. A trailer being towed by a streetcar is considered part of the streetcar.

(t) A special vehicle mainly used on industrial premises is a motor vehicle designed primarily for use within the buildings and premises of industrial or commercial establishments. This includes battery-powered airport passenger vehicles or baggage/mail trucks, forklifts, coal-cars in a coal mine, logging cars and trucks used in mines or quarries.

(u) A special vehicle mainly used in agriculture is a motor vehicle designed specifically for use in farming and agriculture

Chapter 20. External Causes of Morbidity

(horticulture), to work the land, tend and harvest crops and transport materials on the farm. This includes harvesters, farm machinery and tractor and trailers.

(v) A special construction vehicle is a motor vehicle designed specifically for use on construction and demolition sites. This includes bulldozers, diggers, earth levellers, dump trucks. backhoes, front-end loaders, pavers, and mechanical shovels.

(w) A special all-terrain vehicle is a motor vehicle of special design to enable it to negotiate over rough or soft terrain, snow or sand. Examples of special design are high construction, special wheels and tires, tracks, and support on a cushion of air. This includes snow mobiles, All-terrain vehicles (ATV), and dune buggies. It does not include passenger vehicle designated as Sport Utility Vehicles. (SUV)

(x) A watercraft is any device designed for transporting passengers or goods on water. This includes motor or sailboats, ships, and hovercraft.

(y) An aircraft is any device for transporting passengers or goods in the air. This includes hot-air balloons, gliders, helicopters and airplanes.

(z) A military vehicle is any motorized vehicle operating on a public roadway owned by the military and being operated by a member of the military.

Pedestrian injured in transport accident (V00-V09)

INCLUDES person changing tire on transport vehicle
person examining engine of vehicle broken down in (on side of) road

EXCLUDES 1 *fall due to non-transport collision with other person (W03)*
pedestrian on foot falling (slipping) on ice and snow (W00.-)
struck or bumped by another person (W51)

The appropriate 7th character is to be added to each code from categories V00-V09.
A initial encounter
D subsequent encounter
S sequela

✓4th V00 Pedestrian conveyance accident

Use additional place of occurrence and activity external cause codes, if known (Y92.-, Y93.-)

EXCLUDES 1 *collision with another person without fall (W51)*
fall due to person on foot colliding with another person on foot (W03)
fall from non-moving wheelchair, nonmotorized scooter and motorized mobility scooter without collision (W05.-)
pedestrian (conveyance) collision with other land transport vehicle (V01-V09)
pedestrian on foot falling (slipping) on ice and snow (W00.-)

✓5th V00.0 Pedestrian on foot injured in collision with pedestrian conveyance

✓x7th V00.01 Pedestrian on foot injured in collision with roller-skater

✓x7th V00.02 Pedestrian on foot injured in collision with skateboarder

● **✓6th V00.03 Pedestrian on foot injured in collision with standing micro-mobility pedestrian conveyance**

● **✓7th V00.031 Pedestrian on foot injured in collision with rider of standing electric scooter**

● **✓7th V00.038 Pedestrian on foot injured in collision with rider of other standing micro-mobility pedestrian conveyance**
Pedestrian on foot injured in collision with rider of hoverboard
Pedestrian on foot injured in collision with rider of segway

✓x7th V00.09 Pedestrian on foot injured in collision with other pedestrian conveyance

✓5th V00.1 Rolling-type pedestrian conveyance accident

EXCLUDES 1 *accident with baby stroller (V00.82-)*
accident with motorized mobility scooter (V00.83-)
accident with wheelchair (powered) (V00.81-)

✓6th V00.11 In-line roller-skate accident

✓7th V00.111 Fall from in-line roller-skates

✓7th V00.112 In-line roller-skater colliding with stationary object

✓7th V00.118 Other in-line roller-skate accident

EXCLUDES 1 *roller-skater collision with other land transport vehicle (V01-V09 with 5th character 1)*

✓6th V00.12 Non-in-line roller-skate accident

✓7th V00.121 Fall from non-in-line roller-skates

✓7th V00.122 Non-in-line roller-skater colliding with stationary object

✓7th V00.128 Other non-in-line roller-skating accident

EXCLUDES 1 *roller-skater collision with other land transport vehicle (V01-V09 with 5th character 1)*

✓6th V00.13 Skateboard accident

✓7th V00.131 Fall from skateboard

✓7th V00.132 Skateboarder colliding with stationary object

✓7th V00.138 Other skateboard accident

EXCLUDES 1 *skateboarder collision with other land transport vehicle (V01-V09 with 5th character 2)*

✓6th V00.14 Scooter (nonmotorized) accident

EXCLUDES 1 *motor scooter accident (V20-V29)*

✓7th V00.141 Fall from scooter (nonmotorized)

✓7th V00.142 Scooter (nonmotorized) colliding with stationary object

✓7th V00.148 Other scooter (nonmotorized) accident

EXCLUDES 1 *scooter (nonmotorized) collision with other land transport vehicle (V01-V09 with fifth character 9)*

✓6th V00.15 Heelies accident
Rolling shoe
Wheeled shoe
Wheelies accident

✓7th V00.151 Fall from heelies

✓7th V00.152 Heelies colliding with stationary object

✓7th V00.158 Other heelies accident

✓6th V00.18 Accident on other rolling-type pedestrian conveyance

✓7th V00.181 Fall from other rolling-type pedestrian conveyance

✓7th V00.182 Pedestrian on other rolling-type pedestrian conveyance colliding with stationary object

✓7th V00.188 Other accident on other rolling-type pedestrian conveyance

✓5th V00.2 Gliding-type pedestrian conveyance accident

✓6th V00.21 Ice-skates accident

✓7th V00.211 Fall from ice-skates

✓7th V00.212 Ice-skater colliding with stationary object

✓7th V00.218 Other ice-skates accident

EXCLUDES 1 *ice-skater collision with other land transport vehicle (V01-V09 with 5th character 9)*

✓6th V00.22 Sled accident

✓7th V00.221 Fall from sled

✓7th V00.222 Sledder colliding with stationary object

✓7th V00.228 Other sled accident

EXCLUDES 1 *sled collision with other land transport vehicle (V01-V09 with 5th character 9)*

✓6th V00.28 Other gliding-type pedestrian conveyance accident

✓7th V00.281 Fall from other gliding-type pedestrian conveyance

✓7th V00.282 Pedestrian on other gliding-type pedestrian conveyance colliding with stationary object

7th V00.288 **Other accident on other gliding-type pedestrian conveyance**
EXCLUDES 1 *gliding-type pedestrian conveyance collision with other land transport vehicle (V01-V09 with 5th character 9)*

5th V00.3 **Flat-bottomed pedestrian conveyance accident**
6th V00.31 **Snowboard accident**
7th V00.311 **Fall from snowboard**
7th V00.312 **Snowboarder colliding with stationary object**
7th V00.318 **Other snowboard accident**
EXCLUDES 1 *snowboarder collision with other land transport vehicle (V01-V09 with 5th character 9)*
6th V00.32 **Snow-ski accident**
7th V00.321 **Fall from snow-skis**
7th V00.322 **Snow-skier colliding with stationary object**
7th V00.328 **Other snow-ski accident**
EXCLUDES 1 *snow-skier collision with other land transport vehicle (V01-V09 with 5th character 9)*
6th V00.38 **Other flat-bottomed pedestrian conveyance accident**
7th V00.381 **Fall from other flat-bottomed pedestrian conveyance**
7th V00.382 **Pedestrian on other flat-bottomed pedestrian conveyance colliding with stationary object**
7th V00.388 **Other accident on other flat-bottomed pedestrian conveyance**

5th V00.8 **Accident on other pedestrian conveyance**
6th V00.81 **Accident with wheelchair (powered)**
7th V00.811 **Fall from moving wheelchair (powered)**
EXCLUDES 1 *fall from non-moving wheelchair (W05.0)*
7th V00.812 **Wheelchair (powered) colliding with stationary object**
7th V00.818 **Other accident with wheelchair (powered)**
6th V00.82 **Accident with baby stroller**
7th V00.821 **Fall from baby stroller**
7th V00.822 **Baby stroller colliding with stationary object**
7th V00.828 **Other accident with baby stroller**
6th V00.83 **Accident with motorized mobility scooter**
7th V00.831 **Fall from motorized mobility scooter**
EXCLUDES 1 *fall from non-moving motorized mobility scooter (W05.2)*
7th V00.832 **Motorized mobility scooter colliding with stationary object**
7th V00.838 **Other accident with motorized mobility scooter**
● 6th V00.84 **Accident with standing micro-mobility pedestrian conveyance**
● 7th V00.841 **Fall from standing electric scooter**
● 7th V00.842 **Pedestrian on standing electric scooter colliding with stationary object**
● 7th V00.848 **Other accident with standing micro-mobility pedestrian conveyance**
Accident with hoverboard
Accident with segway
6th V00.89 **Accident on other pedestrian conveyance**
7th V00.891 **Fall from other pedestrian conveyance**
7th V00.892 **Pedestrian on other pedestrian conveyance colliding with stationary object**
7th V00.898 **Other accident on other pedestrian conveyance**
EXCLUDES 1 *other pedestrian (conveyance) collision with other land transport vehicle (V01-V09 with 5th character 9)*

4th V01 **Pedestrian injured in collision with pedal cycle**
5th V01.0 **Pedestrian injured in collision with pedal cycle in nontraffic accident**
x7th V01.00 **Pedestrian on foot injured in collision with pedal cycle in nontraffic accident**
Pedestrian NOS injured in collision with pedal cycle in nontraffic accident
x7th V01.01 **Pedestrian on roller-skates injured in collision with pedal cycle in nontraffic accident**
x7th V01.02 **Pedestrian on skateboard injured in collision with pedal cycle in nontraffic accident**
● 6th V01.03 **Pedestrian on standing micro-mobility pedestrian conveyance injured in collision with pedal cycle in nontraffic accident**
● 7th V01.031 **Pedestrian on standing electric scooter injured in collision with pedal cycle in nontraffic accident**
● 7th V01.038 **Pedestrian on other standing micro-mobility pedestrian conveyance injured in collision with pedal cycle in nontraffic accident**
Pedestrian on hoverboard injured in collision with pedal cycle in nontraffic accident
Pedestrian on segway injured in collision with pedal cycle in nontraffic accident
x7th V01.09 **Pedestrian with other conveyance injured in collision with pedal cycle in nontraffic accident**
Pedestrian with baby stroller injured in collision with pedal cycle in nontraffic accident
Pedestrian on ice-skates injured in collision with pedal cycle in nontraffic accident
Pedestrian on nonmotorized scooter injured in collision with pedal cycle in nontraffic accident
Pedestrian on sled injured in collision with pedal cycle in nontraffic accident
Pedestrian on snowboard injured in collision with pedal cycle in nontraffic accident
Pedestrian on snow-skis injured in collision with pedal cycle in nontraffic accident
Pedestrian in wheelchair (powered) injured in collision with pedal cycle in nontraffic accident
Pedestrian in motorized mobility scooter injured in collision with pedal cycle in nontraffic accident
5th V01.1 **Pedestrian injured in collision with pedal cycle in traffic accident**
x7th V01.10 **Pedestrian on foot injured in collision with pedal cycle in traffic accident**
Pedestrian NOS injured in collision with pedal cycle in traffic accident
x7th V01.11 **Pedestrian on roller-skates injured in collision with pedal cycle in traffic accident**
x7th V01.12 **Pedestrian on skateboard injured in collision with pedal cycle in traffic accident**
● 6th V01.13 **Pedestrian on standing micro-mobility pedestrian conveyance injured in collision with pedal cycle in traffic accident**
● 7th V01.131 **Pedestrian on standing electric scooter injured in collision with pedal cycle in traffic accident**
● 7th V01.138 **Pedestrian on other standing micro-mobility pedestrian conveyance injured in collision with pedal cycle in traffic accident**
Pedestrian on hoverboard injured in collision with pedal cycle in traffic accident
Pedestrian on segway injured in collision with pedal cycle in traffic accident

√x7th **VØ1.19 Pedestrian with other conveyance injured in collision with pedal cycle in traffic accident**
Pedestrian with baby stroller injured in collision with pedal cycle in traffic accident
Pedestrian on ice-skates injured in collision with pedal cycle in traffic accident
Pedestrian on nonmotorized scooter injured in collision with pedal cycle in traffic accident
Pedestrian on sled injured in collision with pedal cycle in traffic accident
Pedestrian on snowboard injured in collision with pedal cycle in traffic accident
Pedestrian on snow-skis injured in collision with pedal cycle in traffic accident
Pedestrian in wheelchair (powered) injured in collision with pedal cycle in traffic accident
Pedestrian in motorized mobility scooter injured in collision with pedal cycle in traffic accident

√5th **VØ1.9 Pedestrian injured in collision with pedal cycle, unspecified whether traffic or nontraffic accident**

√x7th **VØ1.9Ø Pedestrian on foot injured in collision with pedal cycle, unspecified whether traffic or nontraffic accident**
Pedestrian NOS injured in collision with pedal cycle, unspecified whether traffic or nontraffic accident

√x7th **VØ1.91 Pedestrian on roller-skates injured in collision with pedal cycle, unspecified whether traffic or nontraffic accident**

√x7th **VØ1.92 Pedestrian on skateboard injured in collision with pedal cycle, unspecified whether traffic or nontraffic accident**

● √6th **VØ1.93 Pedestrian on standing micro-mobility pedestrian conveyance injured in collision with pedal cycle, unspecified whether traffic or nontraffic accident**

● √7th **VØ1.931 Pedestrian on standing electric scooter injured in collision with pedal cycle, unspecified whether traffic or nontraffic accident**

● √7th **VØ1.938 Pedestrian on other standing micro-mobility pedestrian conveyance injured in collision with pedal cycle, unspecified whether traffic or nontraffic accident**
Pedestrian on hoverboard injured in collision with pedal cycle, unspecified whether traffic or nontraffic accident
Pedestrian on segway injured in collision with pedal cycle, unspecified whether traffic or nontraffic accident

√x7th **VØ1.99 Pedestrian with other conveyance injured in collision with pedal cycle, unspecified whether traffic or nontraffic accident**
Pedestrian with baby stroller injured in collision with pedal cycle, unspecified whether traffic or nontraffic accident
Pedestrian on ice-skates injured in collision with pedal cycle unspecified, whether traffic or nontraffic accident
Pedestrian on nonmotorized scooter injured in collision with pedal cycle, unspecified whether traffic or nontraffic accident
Pedestrian on sled injured in collision with pedal cycle unspecified, whether traffic or nontraffic accident
Pedestrian on snowboard injured in collision with pedal cycle, unspecified whether traffic or nontraffic accident
Pedestrian on snow-skis injured in collision with pedal cycle, unspecified whether traffic or nontraffic accident
Pedestrian in wheelchair (powered) injured in collision with pedal cycle, unspecified whether traffic or nontraffic accident
Pedestrian in motorized mobility scooter injured in collision with pedal cycle, unspecified whether traffic or nontraffic accident

√4th **VØ2 Pedestrian injured in collision with two- or three-wheeled motor vehicle**

√5th **VØ2.Ø Pedestrian injured in collision with two- or three-wheeled motor vehicle in nontraffic accident**

√x7th **VØ2.ØØ Pedestrian on foot injured in collision with two- or three-wheeled motor vehicle in nontraffic accident**
Pedestrian NOS injured in collision with two- or three-wheeled motor vehicle in nontraffic accident

√x7th **VØ2.Ø1 Pedestrian on roller-skates injured in collision with two- or three-wheeled motor vehicle in nontraffic accident**

√x7th **VØ2.Ø2 Pedestrian on skateboard injured in collision with two- or three-wheeled motor vehicle in nontraffic accident**

● √6th **VØ2.Ø3 Pedestrian on standing micro-mobility pedestrian conveyance injured in collision with two- or three-wheeled motor vehicle in nontraffic accident**

● √7th **VØ2.Ø31 Pedestrian on standing electric scooter injured in collision with two- or three-wheeled motor vehicle in nontraffic accident**

● √7th **VØ2.Ø38 Pedestrian on other standing micro-mobility pedestrian conveyance injured in collision with two- or three-wheeled motor vehicle in nontraffic accident**
Pedestrian on hoverboard injured in collision with two-or three wheeled motor vehicle in nontraffic accident
Pedestrian on segway injured in collision with two- or three-wheeled motor vehicle in nontraffic accident

√x7th **VØ2.Ø9 Pedestrian with other conveyance injured in collision with two- or three-wheeled motor vehicle in nontraffic accident**
Pedestrian with baby stroller injured in collision with two- or three-wheeled motor vehicle in nontraffic accident
Pedestrian on ice-skates injured in collision with two- or three-wheeled motor vehicle in nontraffic accident
Pedestrian on nonmotorized scooter injured in collision with two- or three-wheeled motor vehicle in nontraffic accident
Pedestrian on sled injured in collision with two- or three-wheeled motor vehicle in nontraffic accident
Pedestrian on snowboard injured in collision with two- or three-wheeled motor vehicle in nontraffic accident
Pedestrian on snow-skis injured in collision with two- or three-wheeled motor vehicle in nontraffic accident
Pedestrian in wheelchair (powered) injured in collision with two- or three-wheeled motor vehicle in nontraffic accident
Pedestrian in motorized mobility scooter injured in collision with two- or three-wheeled motor vehicle in nontraffic accident

√5th **VØ2.1 Pedestrian injured in collision with two- or three-wheeled motor vehicle in traffic accident**

√x7th **VØ2.1Ø Pedestrian on foot injured in collision with two- or three-wheeled motor vehicle in traffic accident**
Pedestrian NOS injured in collision with two- or three-wheeled motor vehicle in traffic accident

√x7th **VØ2.11 Pedestrian on roller-skates injured in collision with two- or three-wheeled motor vehicle in traffic accident**

√x7th **VØ2.12 Pedestrian on skateboard injured in collision with two- or three-wheeled motor vehicle in traffic accident**

● √6th **VØ2.13 Pedestrian on standing micro-mobility pedestrian conveyance injured in collision with two- or three-wheeled motor vehicle in traffic accident**

● √7th **VØ2.131 Pedestrian on standing electric scooter injured in collision with two- or three-wheeled motor vehicle in traffic accident**

● ✓7th **V02.138 Pedestrian on other standing micro-mobility pedestrian conveyance injured in collision with two- or three-wheeled motor vehicle in traffic accident**
Pedestrian on hoverboard injured in collision with two-or three wheeled motor vehicle in traffic accident
Pedestrian on segway injured in collision with two- or three-wheeled motor vehicle in traffic accident

✓x7th **V02.19 Pedestrian with other conveyance injured in collision with two- or three-wheeled motor vehicle in traffic accident**
Pedestrian with baby stroller injured in collision with two- or three-wheeled motor vehicle in traffic accident
Pedestrian on ice-skates injured in collision with two- or three-wheeled motor vehicle in traffic accident
Pedestrian on nonmotorized scooter injured in collision with two- or three-wheeled motor vehicle in traffic accident
Pedestrian on sled injured in collision with two- or three-wheeled motor vehicle in traffic accident
Pedestrian on snowboard injured in collision with two- or three-wheeled motor vehicle in traffic accident
Pedestrian on snow-skis injured in collision with two- or three-wheeled motor vehicle in traffic accident
Pedestrian in wheelchair (powered) injured in collision with two- or three-wheeled motor vehicle in traffic accident
Pedestrian in motorized mobility scooter injued in collision with two- or three-wheeled motor vehicle in traffic accident

✓5th **V02.9 Pedestrian injured in collision with two- or three-wheeled motor vehicle, unspecified whether traffic or nontraffic accident**

✓x7th **V02.90 Pedestrian on foot injured in collision with two- or three-wheeled motor vehicle, unspecified whether traffic or nontraffic accident**
Pedestrian NOS injured in collision with two- or three-wheeled motor vehicle, unspecified whether traffic or nontraffic accident

✓x7th **V02.91 Pedestrian on roller-skates injured in collision with two- or three-wheeled motor vehicle, unspecified whether traffic or nontraffic accident**

✓x7th **V02.92 Pedestrian on skateboard injured in collision with two- or three-wheeled motor vehicle, unspecified whether traffic or nontraffic accident**

● ✓6th **V02.93 Pedestrian on standing micro-mobility pedestrian conveyance injured in collision with two- or three-wheeled motor vehicle, unspecified whether traffic or nontraffic accident**

● ✓7th **V02.931 Pedestrian on standing electric scooter injured in collision with two- or three wheeled motor vehicle, unspecified whether traffic or nontraffic accident**

● ✓7th **V02.938 Pedestrian on other standing micro-mobility pedestrian conveyance injured in collision with two- or three wheeled motor vehicle, unspecified whether traffic or nontraffic accident**
Pedestrian on hoverboard injured in collision with two-three-wheeled motor vehicle, unspecified whether traffic or nontraffic accident
Pedestrian on segway injured in collision with two- or three wheeled motor vehicle, unspecified whether traffic or nontraffic accident

✓x7th **V02.99 Pedestrian with other conveyance injured in collision with two- or three-wheeled motor vehicle, unspecified whether traffic or nontraffic accident**
Pedestrian with baby stroller injured in collision with two- or three-wheeled motor vehicle, unspecified whether traffic or nontraffic accident
Pedestrian on ice-skates injured in collision with two- or three-wheeled motor vehicle, unspecified whether traffic or nontraffic accident
Pedestrian on nonmotorized scooter injured in collision with two- or three-wheeled motor vehicle, unspecified whether traffic or nontraffic accident
Pedestrian on sled injured in collision with two- or three-wheeled motor vehicle, unspecified whether traffic or nontraffic accident
Pedestrian on snowboard injured in collision with two- or three-wheeled motor vehicle, unspecified whether traffic or nontraffic accident
Pedestrian on snow-skis injured in collision with two- or three-wheeled motor vehicle, unspecified whether traffic or nontraffic accident
Pedestrian in wheelchair (powered) injured in collision with two- or three-wheeled motor vehicle, unspecified whether traffic or nontraffic accident
Pedestrian in motorized mobility scooter injured in collision with two- or three wheeled motor vehicle, unspecified whether traffic or nontraffic accident

✓4th **V03 Pedestrian injured in collision with car, pick-up truck or van**

✓5th **V03.0 Pedestrian injured in collision with car, pick-up truck or van in nontraffic accident**

✓x7th **V03.00 Pedestrian on foot injured in collision with car, pick-up truck or van in nontraffic accident**
Pedestrian NOS injured in collision with car, pick-up truck or van in nontraffic accident

✓x7th **V03.01 Pedestrian on roller-skates injured in collision with car, pick-up truck or van in nontraffic accident**

✓x7th **V03.02 Pedestrian on skateboard injured in collision with car, pick-up truck or van in nontraffic accident**

● ✓6th **V03.03 Pedestrian on standing micro-mobility pedestrian conveyance injured in collision with car, pick-up or van in nontraffic accident**

● ✓7th **V03.031 Pedestrian on standing electric scooter injured in collision with car, pick-up or van in nontraffic accident**

● ✓7th **V03.038 Pedestrian on other standing micro-mobility pedestrian conveyance injured in collision with car, pick-up or van in nontraffic accident**
Pedestrian on hoverboard injured in collision with car, pick-up or van in nontraffic accident
Pedestrian on segway injured in collision with car, pick-up or van in nontraffic accident

✓x7th **V03.09 Pedestrian with other conveyance injured in collision with car, pick-up truck or van in nontraffic accident**
Pedestrian with baby stroller injured in collision with car, pick-up truck or van in nontraffic accident
Pedestrian on ice-skates injured in collision with car, pick-up truck or van in nontraffic accident
Pedestrian on nonmotorized scooter injured in collision with car, pick-up truck or van in nontraffic accident
Pedestrian on sled injured in collision with car, pick-up truck or van in nontraffic accident
Pedestrian on snowboard injured in collision with car, pick-up truck or van in nontraffic accident
Pedestrian on snow-skis injured in collision with car, pick-up truck or van in nontraffic accident
Pedestrian in wheelchair (powered) injured in collision with car, pick-up truck or van in nontraffic accident
Pedestrian in motorized mobility scooter injured in collision with car, pick-up truck or van in nontraffic accident

√5th **V03.1 Pedestrian injured in collision with car, pick-up truck or van in traffic accident**

√x 7th **V03.10 Pedestrian on foot injured in collision with car, pick-up truck or van in traffic accident**
Pedestrian NOS injured in collision with car, pick-up truck or van in traffic accident

√x 7th **V03.11 Pedestrian on roller-skates injured in collision with car, pick-up truck or van in traffic accident**

√x 7th **V03.12 Pedestrian on skateboard injured in collision with car, pick-up truck or van in traffic accident**

● √6th **V03.13 Pedestrian on standing micro-mobility pedestrian conveyance injured in collision with car, pick-up or van in traffic accident**

● √7th **V03.131 Pedestrian on standing electric scooter injured in collision with car, pick-up or van in traffic accident**

● √7th **V03.138 Pedestrian on other standing micro-mobility pedestrian conveyance injured in collision with car, pick-up or van in traffic accident**
Pedestrian on hoverboard injured in collision with car, pick-up or van in traffic accident
Pedestrian on segway injured in collision with car, pick-up or van in traffic accident

√x 7th **V03.19 Pedestrian with other conveyance injured in collision with car, pick-up truck or van in traffic accident**
Pedestrian with baby stroller injured in collision with car, pick-up truck or van in traffic accident
Pedestrian on ice-skates injured in collision with car, pick-up truck or van in traffic accident
Pedestrian on nonmotorized scooter injured in collision with car, pick-up truck or van in nontraffic accident
Pedestrian on sled injured in collision with car, pick-up truck or van in traffic accident
Pedestrian on snowboard injured in collision with car, pick-up truck or van in traffic accident
Pedestrian on snow-skis injured in collision with car, pick-up truck or van in traffic accident
Pedestrian in wheelchair (powered) injured in collision with car, pick-up truck or van in traffic accident
Pedestrian in motorized mobility scooter injured in collision with car, pick-up truck or van in nontraffic accident

√5th **V03.9 Pedestrian injured in collision with car, pick-up truck or van, unspecified whether traffic or nontraffic accident**

√x 7th **V03.90 Pedestrian on foot injured in collision with car, pick-up truck or van, unspecified whether traffic or nontraffic accident**
Pedestrian NOS injured in collision with car, pick-up truck or van, unspecified whether traffic or nontraffic accident

√x 7th **V03.91 Pedestrian on roller-skates injured in collision with car, pick-up truck or van, unspecified whether traffic or nontraffic accident**

√x 7th **V03.92 Pedestrian on skateboard injured in collision with car, pick-up truck or van, unspecified whether traffic or nontraffic accident**

● √6th **V03.93 Pedestrian on standing micro-mobility pedestrian conveyance injured in collision with car, pick-up or van, unspecified whether traffic or nontraffic accident**

● √7th **V03.931 Pedestrian on standing electric scooter injured in collision with car, pick-up or van, unspecified whether traffic or nontraffic accident**

● √7th **V03.938 Pedestrian on other standing micro-mobility pedestrian conveyance injured in collision with car, pick-up or van, unspecified whether traffic or nontraffic accident**
Pedestrian on hoverboard injured in collision with car, pick-up or van, unspecified whether traffic or nontraffic accident
Pedestrian on segway injured in collision with car, pick-up or van, unspecified whether traffic or nontraffic accident

√x 7th **V03.99 Pedestrian with other conveyance injured in collision with car, pick-up truck or van, unspecified whether traffic or nontraffic accident**
Pedestrian with baby stroller injured in collision with car, pick-up truck or van, unspecified whether traffic or nontraffic accident
Pedestrian on ice-skates injured in collision with car, pick-up truck or van, unspecified whether traffic or nontraffic accident
Pedestrian on nonmotorized scooter injured in collision with car, pick-up truck or van, unspecified whether traffic or nontraffic accident
Pedestrian on sled injured in collision with car, pick-up truck or van in nontraffic accident
Pedestrian on snowboard injured in collision with car, pick-up truck or van, unspecified whether traffic or nontraffic accident
Pedestrian on snow-skis injured in collision with car, pick-up truck or van, unspecified whether traffic or nontraffic accident
Pedestrian in wheelchair (powered) injured in collision with car, pick-up truck or van, unspecified whether traffic or nontraffic accident
Pedestrian in motorized mobility scooter injured in collision with car, pick-up truck or van, unspecified whether traffic or nontraffic accident

√4th **V04 Pedestrian injured in collision with heavy transport vehicle or bus**

EXCLUDES 1 *pedestrian injured in collision with military vehicle (V09.01, V09.21)*

√5th **V04.0 Pedestrian injured in collision with heavy transport vehicle or bus in nontraffic accident**

√x 7th **V04.00 Pedestrian on foot injured in collision with heavy transport vehicle or bus in nontraffic accident**
Pedestrian NOS injured in collision with heavy transport vehicle or bus in nontraffic accident

√x 7th **V04.01 Pedestrian on roller-skates injured in collision with heavy transport vehicle or bus in nontraffic accident**

√x 7th **V04.02 Pedestrian on skateboard injured in collision with heavy transport vehicle or bus in nontraffic accident**

● √6th **V04.03 Pedestrian on standing micro-mobility pedestrian conveyance injured in collision with heavy transport vehicle or bus in nontraffic accident**

● √7th **V04.031 Pedestrian on standing electric scooter injured in collision with heavy transport vehicle or bus in nontraffic accident**

● √7th **V04.038 Pedestrian on other standing micro-mobility pedestrian conveyance injured in collision with heavy transport vehicle or bus in nontraffic accident**
Pedestrian on hoverboard injured in collision with heavy transport vehicle or bus in nontraffic accident
Pedestrian on segway injured in collision with heavy transport vehicle or bus in nontraffic accident

√x7th **V04.09 Pedestrian with other conveyance injured in collision with heavy transport vehicle or bus in nontraffic accident**
Pedestrian with baby stroller injured in collision with heavy transport vehicle or bus in nontraffic accident
Pedestrian on ice-skates injured in collision with heavy transport vehicle or bus in nontraffic accident
Pedestrian on nonmotorized scooter injured in collision with heavy transport vehicle or bus in nontraffic accident
Pedestrian on sled injured in collision with heavy transport vehicle or bus in nontraffic accident
Pedestrian on snowboard injured in collision with heavy transport vehicle or bus in nontraffic accident
Pedestrian on snow-skis injured in collision with heavy transport vehicle or bus in nontraffic accident
Pedestrian in wheelchair (powered) injured in collision with heavy transport vehicle or bus in nontraffic accident
Pedestrian in motorized mobility scooter injured in collision with heavy transport vehicle or bus in nontraffic accident

√5th **V04.1 Pedestrian injured in collision with heavy transport vehicle or bus in traffic accident**

√x7th **V04.10 Pedestrian on foot injured in collision with heavy transport vehicle or bus in traffic accident**
Pedestrian NOS injured in collision with heavy transport vehicle or bus in traffic accident

√x7th **V04.11 Pedestrian on roller-skates injured in collision with heavy transport vehicle or bus in traffic accident**

√x7th **V04.12 Pedestrian on skateboard injured in collision with heavy transport vehicle or bus in traffic accident**

● √6th **V04.13 Pedestrian on standing micro-mobility pedestrian conveyance injured in collision with heavy transport vehicle or bus in traffic accident**

● √7th **V04.131 Pedestrian on standing electric scooter injured in collision with heavy transport vehicle or bus in traffic accident**

● √7th **V04.138 Pedestrian on other standing micro-mobility pedestrian conveyance injured in collision with heavy transport vehicle or bus in traffic accident**
Pedestrian on hoverboard injured in collision with heavy transport vehicle or bus in traffic accident
Pedestrian on segway injured in collision with heavy transport vehicle or bus in traffic accident

√x7th **V04.19 Pedestrian with other conveyance injured in collision with heavy transport vehicle or bus in traffic accident**
Pedestrian with baby stroller injured in collision with heavy transport vehicle or bus in traffic accident
Pedestrian on ice-skates injured in collision with heavy transport vehicle or bus in traffic accident
Pedestrian on nonmotorized scooter injured in collision with heavy transport vehicle or bus in traffic accident
Pedestrian on sled injured in collision with heavy transport vehicle or bus in traffic accident
Pedestrian on snowboard injured in collision with heavy transport vehicle or bus in traffic accident
Pedestrian on snow-skis injured in collision with heavy transport vehicle or bus in traffic accident
Pedestrian in wheelchair (powered) injured in collision with heavy transport vehicle or bus in traffic accident
Pedestrian in motorized mobility scooter injured in collision with heavy transport vehicle or bus in traffic accident

√5th **V04.9 Pedestrian injured in collision with heavy transport vehicle or bus, unspecified whether traffic or nontraffic accident**

√x7th **V04.90 Pedestrian on foot injured in collision with heavy transport vehicle or bus, unspecified whether traffic or nontraffic accident**
Pedestrian NOS injured in collision with heavy transport vehicle or bus, unspecified whether traffic or nontraffic accident

√x7th **V04.91 Pedestrian on roller-skates injured in collision with heavy transport vehicle or bus, unspecified whether traffic or nontraffic accident**

√x7th **V04.92 Pedestrian on skateboard injured in collision with heavy transport vehicle or bus, unspecified whether traffic or nontraffic accident**

● √6th **V04.93 Pedestrian on standing micro-mobility pedestrian conveyance injured in collision with heavy transport vehicle or bus, unspecified whether traffic or nontraffic accident**

● √7th **V04.931 Pedestrian on standing electric scooter injured in collision with heavy transport vehicle or bus, unspecified whether traffic or nontraffic accident**

● √7th **V04.938 Pedestrian on other standing micro-mobility pedestrian conveyance injured in collision with heavy transport vehicle or bus, unspecified whether traffic or nontraffic accident**
Pedestrian on hoverboard injured in collision with heavy transport vehicle or bus, unspecified whether traffic or nontraffic accident
Pedestrian on segway injured in collision with heavy transport vehicle or bus, unspecified whether traffic or nontraffic accident

√x7th **V04.99 Pedestrian with other conveyance injured in collision with heavy transport vehicle or bus, unspecified whether traffic or nontraffic accident**
Pedestrian with baby stroller injured in collision with heavy transport vehicle or bus, unspecified whether traffic or nontraffic accident
Pedestrian on ice-skates injured in collision with heavy transport vehicle or bus, unspecified whether traffic or nontraffic accident
Pedestrian on nonmotorized scooter injured in collision with heavy transport vehicle or bus, unspecified whether traffic or nontraffic accident
Pedestrian on sled injured in collision with heavy transport vehicle or bus, unspecified whether traffic or nontraffic accident
Pedestrian on snowboard injured in collision with heavy transport vehicle or bus, unspecified whether traffic or nontraffic accident
Pedestrian on snow-skis injured in collision with heavy transport vehicle or bus, unspecified whether traffic or nontraffic accident
Pedestrian in wheelchair (powered) injured in collision with heavy transport vehicle or bus, unspecified whether traffic or nontraffic accident
Pedestrian in motorized mobility scooter injured in collision with heavy transport vehicle or bus, unspecified whether traffic or nontraffic accident

√4th **V05 Pedestrian injured in collision with railway train or railway vehicle**

√5th **V05.0 Pedestrian injured in collision with railway train or railway vehicle in nontraffic accident**

√x7th **V05.00 Pedestrian on foot injured in collision with railway train or railway vehicle in nontraffic accident**
Pedestrian NOS injured in collision with railway train or railway vehicle in nontraffic accident

√x7th **V05.01 Pedestrian on roller-skates injured in collision with railway train or railway vehicle in nontraffic accident**

√x7th **V05.02 Pedestrian on skateboard injured in collision with railway train or railway vehicle in nontraffic accident**

● √6th **V05.03 Pedestrian on standing micro-mobility pedestrian conveyance injured in collision with railway train or railway vehicle in nontraffic accident**

● √7th **V05.031 Pedestrian on standing electric scooter injured in collision with railway train or railway vehicle in nontraffic accident**

● V05.038 **Pedestrian on other standing micro-mobility pedestrian conveyance injured in collision with railway train or railway vehicle in nontraffic accident**
Pedestrian on hoverboard injured in collision with railway train or railway vehicle in nontraffic accident
Pedestrian on segway injured in collision with railway train or railway vehicle in nontraffic accident

V05.09 **Pedestrian with other conveyance injured in collision with railway train or railway vehicle in nontraffic accident**
Pedestrian with baby stroller injured in collision with railway train or railway vehicle in nontraffic accident
Pedestrian on ice-skates injured in collision with railway train or railway vehicle in nontraffic accident
Pedestrian on nonmotorized scooter injured in collision with railway train or railway vehicle in nontraffic accident
Pedestrian on sled injured in collision with railway train or railway vehicle in nontraffic accident
Pedestrian on snowboard injured in collision with railway train or railway vehicle in nontraffic accident
Pedestrian on snow-skis injured in collision with railway train or railway vehicle in nontraffic accident
Pedestrian in wheelchair (powered) injured in collision with railway train or railway vehicle in nontraffic accident
Pedestrian in motorized mobility scooter injured in collision with railway train or railway vehicle in nontraffic accident

V05.1 **Pedestrian injured in collision with railway train or railway vehicle in traffic accident**

V05.10 **Pedestrian on foot injured in collision with railway train or railway vehicle in traffic accident**
Pedestrian NOS injured in collision with railway train or railway vehicle in traffic accident

V05.11 **Pedestrian on roller-skates injured in collision with railway train or railway vehicle in traffic accident**

V05.12 **Pedestrian on skateboard injured in collision with railway train or railway vehicle in traffic accident**

● V05.13 **Pedestrian on standing micro-mobility pedestrian conveyance injured in collision with railway train or railway vehicle in traffic accident**

● V05.131 **Pedestrian on standing electric scooter injured in collision with railway train or railway vehicle in traffic accident**

● V05.138 **Pedestrian on other standing micro-mobility pedestrian conveyance injured in collision with railway train or railway vehicle in traffic accident**
Pedestrian on hoverboard injured in collision with railway train or railway vehicle in traffic accident
Pedestrian on segway injured in collision with railway train or railway vehicle in traffic accident

V05.19 **Pedestrian with other conveyance injured in collision with railway train or railway vehicle in traffic accident**
Pedestrian with baby stroller injured in collision with railway train or railway vehicle in traffic accident
Pedestrian on ice-skates injured in collision with railway train or railway vehicle in traffic accident
Pedestrian on nonmotorized scooter injured in collision with railway train or railway vehicle in traffic accident
Pedestrian on sled injured in collision with railway train or railway vehicle in traffic accident
Pedestrian on snowboard injured in collision with railway train or railway vehicle in traffic accident
Pedestrian on snow-skis injured in collision with railway train or railway vehicle in traffic accident
Pedestrian in wheelchair (powered) injured in collision with railway train or railway vehicle in traffic accident
Pedestrian in motorized mobility scooter injured in collision with railway train or railway vehicle in traffic accident

V05.9 **Pedestrian injured in collision with railway train or railway vehicle, unspecified whether traffic or nontraffic accident**

V05.90 **Pedestrian on foot injured in collision with railway train or railway vehicle, unspecified whether traffic or nontraffic accident**
Pedestrian NOS injured in collision with railway train or railway vehicle, unspecified whether traffic or nontraffic accident

V05.91 **Pedestrian on roller-skates injured in collision with railway train or railway vehicle, unspecified whether traffic or nontraffic accident**

V05.92 **Pedestrian on skateboard injured in collision with railway train or railway vehicle, unspecified whether traffic or nontraffic accident**

● V05.93 **Pedestrian on standing micro-mobility pedestrian conveyance injured in collision with railway train or railway vehicle, unspecified whether traffic or nontraffic accident**

● V05.931 **Pedestrian on standing electric scooter injured in collision with railway train or railway vehicle, unspecified whether traffic or nontraffic accident**

● V05.938 **Pedestrian on other standing micro-mobility pedestrian conveyance injured in collision with railway train or railway vehicle, unspecified whether traffic or nontraffic accident**
Pedestrian on hoverboard injured in collision with railway train or railway vehicle, unspecified whether traffic or nontraffic accident
Pedestrian on segway injured in collision with railway train or railway vehicle, unspecified whether traffic or nontraffic accident

√x7th **V05.99 Pedestrian with other conveyance injured in collision with railway train or railway vehicle, unspecified whether traffic or nontraffic accident**
Pedestrian with baby stroller injured in collision with railway train or railway vehicle, unspecified whether traffic or nontraffic
Pedestrian on ice-skates injured in collision with railway train or railway vehicle, unspecified whether traffic or nontraffic
Pedestrian on nonmotorized scooter injured in collision with railway train or railway vehicle, unspecified whether traffic or nontraffic
Pedestrian on sled injured in collision with railway train or railway vehicle, unspecified whether traffic or nontraffic
Pedestrian on snowboard injured in collision with railway train or railway vehicle, unspecified whether traffic or nontraffic
Pedestrian on snow-skis injured in collision with railway train or railway vehicle, unspecified whether traffic or nontraffic
Pedestrian in wheelchair (powered) injured in collision with railway train or railway vehicle, unspecified whether traffic or nontraffic
Pedestrian in motorized mobility scooter injured in collision with railway train or railway vehicle, unspecified whether traffic or nontraffic

√4th **V06 Pedestrian injured in collision with other nonmotor vehicle**
INCLUDES collision with animal-drawn vehicle, animal being ridden, nonpowered streetcar
EXCLUDES 1 *pedestrian injured in collision with pedestrian conveyance (V00.0-)*

√5th **V06.0 Pedestrian injured in collision with other nonmotor vehicle in nontraffic accident**

√x7th **V06.00 Pedestrian on foot injured in collision with other nonmotor vehicle in nontraffic accident**
Pedestrian NOS injured in collision with other nonmotor vehicle in nontraffic accident

√x7th **V06.01 Pedestrian on roller-skates injured in collision with other nonmotor vehicle in nontraffic accident**

√x7th **V06.02 Pedestrian on skateboard injured in collision with other nonmotor vehicle in nontraffic accident**

● √6th **V06.03 Pedestrian on standing micro-mobility pedestrian conveyance injured in collision with other nonmotor vehicle in nontraffic accident**

● √7th **V06.031 Pedestrian on standing electric scooter injured in collision with other nonmotor vehicle in nontraffic accident**

● √7th **V06.038 Pedestrian on other standing micro-mobility pedestrian conveyance injured in collision with other nonmotor vehicle in nontraffic accident**
Pedestrian on hoverboard injured in collision with other nonmotor vehicle in nontraffic accident
Pedestrian on segway injured in collision with other nonmotor vehicle in nontraffic accident

√x7th **V06.09 Pedestrian with other conveyance injured in collision with other nonmotor vehicle in nontraffic accident**
Pedestrian with baby stroller injured in collision with other nonmotor vehicle in nontraffic accident
Pedestrian on ice-skates injured in collision with other nonmotor vehicle in nontraffic accident
Pedestrian on nonmotorized scooter injured in collision with other nonmotor vehicle in nontraffic accident
Pedestrian on sled injured in collision with other nonmotor vehicle in nontraffic accident
Pedestrian on snowboard injured in collision with other nonmotor vehicle in nontraffic accident
Pedestrian on snow-skis injured in collision with other nonmotor vehicle in nontraffic accident
Pedestrian in wheelchair (powered) injured in collision with other nonmotor vehicle in nontraffic accident
Pedestrian in motorized mobility scooter injured in collision with other nonmotor vehicle in nontraffic accident

√5th **V06.1 Pedestrian injured in collision with other nonmotor vehicle in traffic accident**

√x7th **V06.10 Pedestrian on foot injured in collision with other nonmotor vehicle in traffic accident**
Pedestrian NOS injured in collision with other nonmotor vehicle in traffic accident

√x7th **V06.11 Pedestrian on roller-skates injured in collision with other nonmotor vehicle in traffic accident**

√x7th **V06.12 Pedestrian on skateboard injured in collision with other nonmotor vehicle in traffic accident**

● √6th **V06.13 Pedestrian on standing micro-mobility pedestrian conveyance injured in collision with other nonmotor vehicle in traffic accident**

● √7th **V06.131 Pedestrian on standing electric scooter injured in collision with other nonmotor vehicle in traffic accident**

● √7th **V06.138 Pedestrian on other standing micro-mobility pedestrian conveyance injured in collision with other nonmotor vehicle in traffic accident**
Pedestrian on hoverboard injured in collision with other nonmotor vehicle in traffic accident
Pedestrian on segway injured in collision with other nonmotor vehicle in traffic accident

√x7th **V06.19 Pedestrian with other conveyance injured in collision with other nonmotor vehicle in traffic accident**
Pedestrian with baby stroller injured in collision with other nonmotor vehicle in nontraffic accident
Pedestrian on ice-skates injured in collision with other nonmotor vehicle in traffic accident
Pedestrian on nonmotorized scooter injured in collision with other nonmotor vehicle in traffic accident
Pedestrian on sled injured in collision with other nonmotor vehicle in traffic accident
Pedestrian on snowboard injured in collision with other nonmotor vehicle in traffic accident
Pedestrian on snow-skis injured in collision with other nonmotor vehicle in traffic accident
Pedestrian in wheelchair (powered) injured in collision with other nonmotor vehicle in traffic accident
Pedestrian in motorized mobility scooter injured in collision with other nonmotor vehicle in traffic accident

√5th **V06.9 Pedestrian injured in collision with other nonmotor vehicle, unspecified whether traffic or nontraffic accident**

√x7th **V06.90 Pedestrian on foot injured in collision with other nonmotor vehicle, unspecified whether traffic or nontraffic accident**
Pedestrian NOS injured in collision with other nonmotor vehicle, unspecified whether traffic or nontraffic accident

√x7th **V06.91 Pedestrian on roller-skates injured in collision with other nonmotor vehicle, unspecified whether traffic or nontraffic accident**

√x7th **V06.92 Pedestrian on skateboard injured in collision with other nonmotor vehicle, unspecified whether traffic or nontraffic accident**

● √6th **V06.93 Pedestrian on standing micro-mobility pedestrian conveyance injured in collision with other nonmotor vehicle, unspecified whether traffic or nontraffic accident**

● √7th **V06.931 Pedestrian on standing electric scooter injured in collision with other nonmotor vehicle, unspecified whether traffic or nontraffic accident**

● √7th **V06.938 Pedestrian on other standing micro-mobility pedestrian conveyance injured in collision with other nonmotor vehicle, unspecified whether traffic or nontraffic accident**

Pedestrian on hoverboard injured in collision with other nonmotor, unspecified whether traffic or nontraffic accident

Pedestrian on segway injured in collision with other nonmotor vehicle, unspecified whether traffic or nontraffic accident

√x7th **V06.99 Pedestrian with other conveyance injured in collision with other nonmotor vehicle, unspecified whether traffic or nontraffic accident**

Pedestrian with baby stroller injured in collision with other nonmotor vehicle, unspecified whether traffic or nontraffic accident

Pedestrian on ice-skates injured in collision with other nonmotor vehicle, unspecified whether traffic or nontraffic accident

Pedestrian on nonmotorized scooter injured in collision with other nonmotor vehicle, unspecified whether traffic or nontraffic accident

Pedestrian on sled injured in collision with other nonmotor vehicle, unspecified whether traffic or nontraffic accident

Pedestrian on snowboard injured in collision with other nonmotor vehicle, unspecified whether traffic or nontraffic accident

Pedestrian on snow-skis injured in collision with other nonmotor vehicle, unspecified whether traffic or nontraffic accident

Pedestrian in wheelchair (powered) injured in collision with other nonmotor vehicle, unspecified whether traffic or nontraffic accident

Pedestrian in motorized mobility scooter injured in collision with other nonmotorized vehicle, unspecified whether traffic or nontraffic accident

√4th **V09 Pedestrian injured in other and unspecified transport accidents**

√5th **V09.0 Pedestrian injured in nontraffic accident involving other and unspecified motor vehicles**

√x7th **V09.00 Pedestrian injured in nontraffic accident involving unspecified motor vehicles**

√x7th **V09.01 Pedestrian injured in nontraffic accident involving military vehicle**

√x7th **V09.09 Pedestrian injured in nontraffic accident involving other motor vehicles**

Pedestrian injured in nontraffic accident by special vehicle

√x7th **V09.1 Pedestrian injured in unspecified nontraffic accident**

√5th **V09.2 Pedestrian injured in traffic accident involving other and unspecified motor vehicles**

√x7th **V09.20 Pedestrian injured in traffic accident involving unspecified motor vehicles**

√x7th **V09.21 Pedestrian injured in traffic accident involving military vehicle**

√x7th **V09.29 Pedestrian injured in traffic accident involving other motor vehicles**

√x7th **V09.3 Pedestrian injured in unspecified traffic accident**

√x7th **V09.9 Pedestrian injured in unspecified transport accident**

Pedal cycle rider injured in transport accident (V10-V19)

INCLUDES any non-motorized vehicle, excluding an animal-drawn vehicle, or a sidecar or trailer attached to the pedal cycle

EXCLUDES 2 *rupture of pedal cycle tire (W37.0)*

The appropriate 7th character is to be added to each code from categories V10-V19.
A initial encounter
D subsequent encounter
S sequela

√4th **V10 Pedal cycle rider injured in collision with pedestrian or animal**

EXCLUDES 1 *pedal cycle rider collision with animal-drawn vehicle or animal being ridden (V16.-)*

√x7th **V10.0 Pedal cycle driver injured in collision with pedestrian or animal in nontraffic accident**

√x7th **V10.1 Pedal cycle passenger injured in collision with pedestrian or animal in nontraffic accident**

√x7th **V10.2 Unspecified pedal cyclist injured in collision with pedestrian or animal in nontraffic accident**

√x7th **V10.3 Person boarding or alighting a pedal cycle injured in collision with pedestrian or animal**

√x7th **V10.4 Pedal cycle driver injured in collision with pedestrian or animal in traffic accident**

√x7th **V10.5 Pedal cycle passenger injured in collision with pedestrian or animal in traffic accident**

√x7th **V10.9 Unspecified pedal cyclist injured in collision with pedestrian or animal in traffic accident**

√4th **V11 Pedal cycle rider injured in collision with other pedal cycle**

√x7th **V11.0 Pedal cycle driver injured in collision with other pedal cycle in nontraffic accident**

√x7th **V11.1 Pedal cycle passenger injured in collision with other pedal cycle in nontraffic accident**

√x7th **V11.2 Unspecified pedal cyclist injured in collision with other pedal cycle in nontraffic accident**

√x7th **V11.3 Person boarding or alighting a pedal cycle injured in collision with other pedal cycle**

√x7th **V11.4 Pedal cycle driver injured in collision with other pedal cycle in traffic accident**

√x7th **V11.5 Pedal cycle passenger injured in collision with other pedal cycle in traffic accident**

√x7th **V11.9 Unspecified pedal cyclist injured in collision with other pedal cycle in traffic accident**

√4th **V12 Pedal cycle rider injured in collision with two- or three-wheeled motor vehicle**

√x7th **V12.0 Pedal cycle driver injured in collision with two- or three-wheeled motor vehicle in nontraffic accident**

√x7th **V12.1 Pedal cycle passenger injured in collision with two- or three-wheeled motor vehicle in nontraffic accident**

√x7th **V12.2 Unspecified pedal cyclist injured in collision with two- or three-wheeled motor vehicle in nontraffic accident**

√x7th **V12.3 Person boarding or alighting a pedal cycle injured in collision with two- or three-wheeled motor vehicle**

√x7th **V12.4 Pedal cycle driver injured in collision with two- or three-wheeled motor vehicle in traffic accident**

√x7th **V12.5 Pedal cycle passenger injured in collision with two- or three-wheeled motor vehicle in traffic accident**

√x7th **V12.9 Unspecified pedal cyclist injured in collision with two- or three-wheeled motor vehicle in traffic accident**

√4th **V13 Pedal cycle rider injured in collision with car, pick-up truck or van**

√x7th **V13.0 Pedal cycle driver injured in collision with car, pick-up truck or van in nontraffic accident**

√x7th **V13.1 Pedal cycle passenger injured in collision with car, pick-up truck or van in nontraffic accident**

√x7th **V13.2 Unspecified pedal cyclist injured in collision with car, pick-up truck or van in nontraffic accident**

√x7th **V13.3 Person boarding or alighting a pedal cycle injured in collision with car, pick-up truck or van**

√x7th **V13.4 Pedal cycle driver injured in collision with car, pick-up truck or van in traffic accident**

√x7th **V13.5 Pedal cycle passenger injured in collision with car, pick-up truck or van in traffic accident**

√x7th **V13.9 Unspecified pedal cyclist injured in collision with car, pick-up truck or van in traffic accident**

√4th **V14 Pedal cycle rider injured in collision with heavy transport vehicle or bus**

EXCLUDES 1 *pedal cycle rider injured in collision with military vehicle (V19.81)*

√x7th **V14.0 Pedal cycle driver injured in collision with heavy transport vehicle or bus in nontraffic accident**

V14.1 Pedal cycle passenger injured in collision with heavy transport vehicle or bus in nontraffic accident

V14.2 Unspecified pedal cyclist injured in collision with heavy transport vehicle or bus in nontraffic accident

V14.3 Person boarding or alighting a pedal cycle injured in collision with heavy transport vehicle or bus

V14.4 Pedal cycle driver injured in collision with heavy transport vehicle or bus in traffic accident

V14.5 Pedal cycle passenger injured in collision with heavy transport vehicle or bus in traffic accident

V14.9 Unspecified pedal cyclist injured in collision with heavy transport vehicle or bus in traffic accident

V15 Pedal cycle rider injured in collision with railway train or railway vehicle

V15.Ø Pedal cycle driver injured in collision with railway train or railway vehicle in nontraffic accident

V15.1 Pedal cycle passenger injured in collision with railway train or railway vehicle in nontraffic accident

V15.2 Unspecified pedal cyclist injured in collision with railway train or railway vehicle in nontraffic accident

V15.3 Person boarding or alighting a pedal cycle injured in collision with railway train or railway vehicle

V15.4 Pedal cycle driver injured in collision with railway train or railway vehicle in traffic accident

V15.5 Pedal cycle passenger injured in collision with railway train or railway vehicle in traffic accident

V15.9 Unspecified pedal cyclist injured in collision with railway train or railway vehicle in traffic accident

V16 Pedal cycle rider injured in collision with other nonmotor vehicle

INCLUDES collision with animal-drawn vehicle, animal being ridden, streetcar

V16.Ø Pedal cycle driver injured in collision with other nonmotor vehicle in nontraffic accident

V16.1 Pedal cycle passenger injured in collision with other nonmotor vehicle in nontraffic accident

V16.2 Unspecified pedal cyclist injured in collision with other nonmotor vehicle in nontraffic accident

V16.3 Person boarding or alighting a pedal cycle injured in collision with other nonmotor vehicle in nontraffic accident

V16.4 Pedal cycle driver injured in collision with other nonmotor vehicle in traffic accident

V16.5 Pedal cycle passenger injured in collision with other nonmotor vehicle in traffic accident

V16.9 Unspecified pedal cyclist injured in collision with other nonmotor vehicle in traffic accident

V17 Pedal cycle rider injured in collision with fixed or stationary object

V17.Ø Pedal cycle driver injured in collision with fixed or stationary object in nontraffic accident

V17.1 Pedal cycle passenger injured in collision with fixed or stationary object in nontraffic accident

V17.2 Unspecified pedal cyclist injured in collision with fixed or stationary object in nontraffic accident

V17.3 Person boarding or alighting a pedal cycle injured in collision with fixed or stationary object

V17.4 Pedal cycle driver injured in collision with fixed or stationary object in traffic accident

V17.5 Pedal cycle passenger injured in collision with fixed or stationary object in traffic accident

V17.9 Unspecified pedal cyclist injured in collision with fixed or stationary object in traffic accident

V18 Pedal cycle rider injured in noncollision transport accident

INCLUDES fall or thrown from pedal cycle (without antecedent collision)
overturning pedal cycle NOS
overturning pedal cycle without collision

V18.Ø Pedal cycle driver injured in noncollision transport accident in nontraffic accident

V18.1 Pedal cycle passenger injured in noncollision transport accident in nontraffic accident

V18.2 Unspecified pedal cyclist injured in noncollision transport accident in nontraffic accident

V18.3 Person boarding or alighting a pedal cycle injured in noncollision transport accident

V18.4 Pedal cycle driver injured in noncollision transport accident in traffic accident

V18.5 Pedal cycle passenger injured in noncollision transport accident in traffic accident

V18.9 Unspecified pedal cyclist injured in noncollision transport accident in traffic accident

V19 Pedal cycle rider injured in other and unspecified transport accidents

V19.Ø Pedal cycle driver injured in collision with other and unspecified motor vehicles in nontraffic accident

V19.ØØ Pedal cycle driver injured in collision with unspecified motor vehicles in nontraffic accident

V19.Ø9 Pedal cycle driver injured in collision with other motor vehicles in nontraffic accident

V19.1 Pedal cycle passenger injured in collision with other and unspecified motor vehicles in nontraffic accident

V19.1Ø Pedal cycle passenger injured in collision with unspecified motor vehicles in nontraffic accident

V19.19 Pedal cycle passenger injured in collision with other motor vehicles in nontraffic accident

V19.2 Unspecified pedal cyclist injured in collision with other and unspecified motor vehicles in nontraffic accident

V19.2Ø Unspecified pedal cyclist injured in collision with unspecified motor vehicles in nontraffic accident
Pedal cycle collision NOS, nontraffic

V19.29 Unspecified pedal cyclist injured in collision with other motor vehicles in nontraffic accident

V19.3 Pedal cyclist (driver) (passenger) injured in unspecified nontraffic accident
Pedal cycle accident NOS, nontraffic
Pedal cyclist injured in nontraffic accident NOS

V19.4 Pedal cycle driver injured in collision with other and unspecified motor vehicles in traffic accident

V19.4Ø Pedal cycle driver injured in collision with unspecified motor vehicles in traffic accident

V19.49 Pedal cycle driver injured in collision with other motor vehicles in traffic accident

V19.5 Pedal cycle passenger injured in collision with other and unspecified motor vehicles in traffic accident

V19.5Ø Pedal cycle passenger injured in collision with unspecified motor vehicles in traffic accident

V19.59 Pedal cycle passenger injured in collision with other motor vehicles in traffic accident

V19.6 Unspecified pedal cyclist injured in collision with other and unspecified motor vehicles in traffic accident

V19.6Ø Unspecified pedal cyclist injured in collision with unspecified motor vehicles in traffic accident
Pedal cycle collision NOS (traffic)

V19.69 Unspecified pedal cyclist injured in collision with other motor vehicles in traffic accident

V19.8 Pedal cyclist (driver) (passenger) injured in other specified transport accidents

V19.81 Pedal cyclist (driver) (passenger) injured in transport accident with military vehicle

V19.88 Pedal cyclist (driver) (passenger) injured in other specified transport accidents

V19.9 Pedal cyclist (driver) (passenger) injured in unspecified traffic accident
Pedal cycle accident NOS

Motorcycle rider injured in transport accident (V2Ø-V29)

INCLUDES moped
motorcycle with sidecar
motorized bicycle
motor scooter

EXCLUDES 1 *three-wheeled motor vehicle (V3Ø-V39)*

The appropriate 7th character is to be added to each code from categories V2Ø-V29.
A initial encounter
D subsequent encounter
S sequela

V2Ø Motorcycle rider injured in collision with pedestrian or animal

EXCLUDES 1 *motorcycle rider collision with animal-drawn vehicle or animal being ridden (V26.-)*

V2Ø.Ø Motorcycle driver injured in collision with pedestrian or animal in nontraffic accident

V2Ø.1 Motorcycle passenger injured in collision with pedestrian or animal in nontraffic accident

V2Ø.2 Unspecified motorcycle rider injured in collision with pedestrian or animal in nontraffic accident

V2Ø.3 Person boarding or alighting a motorcycle injured in collision with pedestrian or animal

V2Ø.4 Motorcycle driver injured in collision with pedestrian or animal in traffic accident

V2Ø.5 Motorcycle passenger injured in collision with pedestrian or animal in traffic accident

√x 7th **V20.9** Unspecified motorcycle rider injured in collision with pedestrian or animal in traffic accident

√4th **V21 Motorcycle rider injured in collision with pedal cycle**

√x 7th **V21.0** Motorcycle driver injured in collision with pedal cycle in nontraffic accident

√x 7th **V21.1** Motorcycle passenger injured in collision with pedal cycle in nontraffic accident

√x 7th **V21.2** Unspecified motorcycle rider injured in collision with pedal cycle in nontraffic accident

√x 7th **V21.3** Person boarding or alighting a motorcycle injured in collision with pedal cycle

√x 7th **V21.4** Motorcycle driver injured in collision with pedal cycle in traffic accident

√x 7th **V21.5** Motorcycle passenger injured in collision with pedal cycle in traffic accident

√x 7th **V21.9** Unspecified motorcycle rider injured in collision with pedal cycle in traffic accident

√4th **V22 Motorcycle rider injured in collision with two- or three-wheeled motor vehicle**

√x 7th **V22.0** Motorcycle driver injured in collision with two- or three-wheeled motor vehicle in nontraffic accident

√x 7th **V22.1** Motorcycle passenger injured in collision with two- or three-wheeled motor vehicle in nontraffic accident

√x 7th **V22.2** Unspecified motorcycle rider injured in collision with two- or three-wheeled motor vehicle in nontraffic accident

√x 7th **V22.3** Person boarding or alighting a motorcycle injured in collision with two- or three-wheeled motor vehicle

√x 7th **V22.4** Motorcycle driver injured in collision with two- or three-wheeled motor vehicle in traffic accident

√x 7th **V22.5** Motorcycle passenger injured in collision with two- or three-wheeled motor vehicle in traffic accident

√x 7th **V22.9** Unspecified motorcycle rider injured in collision with two- or three-wheeled motor vehicle in traffic accident

√4th **V23 Motorcycle rider injured in collision with car, pick-up truck or van**

√x 7th **V23.0** Motorcycle driver injured in collision with car, pick-up truck or van in nontraffic accident

√x 7th **V23.1** Motorcycle passenger injured in collision with car, pick-up truck or van in nontraffic accident

√x 7th **V23.2** Unspecified motorcycle rider injured in collision with car, pick-up truck or van in nontraffic accident

√x 7th **V23.3** Person boarding or alighting a motorcycle injured in collision with car, pick-up truck or van

√x 7th **V23.4** Motorcycle driver injured in collision with car, pick-up truck or van in traffic accident

√x 7th **V23.5** Motorcycle passenger injured in collision with car, pick-up truck or van in traffic accident

√x 7th **V23.9** Unspecified motorcycle rider injured in collision with car, pick-up truck or van in traffic accident

√4th **V24 Motorcycle rider injured in collision with heavy transport vehicle or bus**

EXCLUDES 1 *motorcycle rider injured in collision with military vehicle (V29.81)*

√x 7th **V24.0** Motorcycle driver injured in collision with heavy transport vehicle or bus in nontraffic accident

√x 7th **V24.1** Motorcycle passenger injured in collision with heavy transport vehicle or bus in nontraffic accident

√x 7th **V24.2** Unspecified motorcycle rider injured in collision with heavy transport vehicle or bus in nontraffic accident

√x 7th **V24.3** Person boarding or alighting a motorcycle injured in collision with heavy transport vehicle or bus

√x 7th **V24.4** Motorcycle driver injured in collision with heavy transport vehicle or bus in traffic accident

√x 7th **V24.5** Motorcycle passenger injured in collision with heavy transport vehicle or bus in traffic accident

√x 7th **V24.9** Unspecified motorcycle rider injured in collision with heavy transport vehicle or bus in traffic accident

√4th **V25 Motorcycle rider injured in collision with railway train or railway vehicle**

√x 7th **V25.0** Motorcycle driver injured in collision with railway train or railway vehicle in nontraffic accident

√x 7th **V25.1** Motorcycle passenger injured in collision with railway train or railway vehicle in nontraffic accident

√x 7th **V25.2** Unspecified motorcycle rider injured in collision with railway train or railway vehicle in nontraffic accident

√x 7th **V25.3** Person boarding or alighting a motorcycle injured in collision with railway train or railway vehicle

√x 7th **V25.4** Motorcycle driver injured in collision with railway train or railway vehicle in traffic accident

√x 7th **V25.5** Motorcycle passenger injured in collision with railway train or railway vehicle in traffic accident

√x 7th **V25.9** Unspecified motorcycle rider injured in collision with railway train or railway vehicle in traffic accident

√4th **V26 Motorcycle rider injured in collision with other nonmotor vehicle**

INCLUDES collision with animal-drawn vehicle, animal being ridden, streetcar

√x 7th **V26.0** Motorcycle driver injured in collision with other nonmotor vehicle in nontraffic accident

√x 7th **V26.1** Motorcycle passenger injured in collision with other nonmotor vehicle in nontraffic accident

√x 7th **V26.2** Unspecified motorcycle rider injured in collision with other nonmotor vehicle in nontraffic accident

√x 7th **V26.3** Person boarding or alighting a motorcycle injured in collision with other nonmotor vehicle

√x 7th **V26.4** Motorcycle driver injured in collision with other nonmotor vehicle in traffic accident

√x 7th **V26.5** Motorcycle passenger injured in collision with other nonmotor vehicle in traffic accident

√x 7th **V26.9** Unspecified motorcycle rider injured in collision with other nonmotor vehicle in traffic accident

√4th **V27 Motorcycle rider injured in collision with fixed or stationary object**

√x 7th **V27.0** Motorcycle driver injured in collision with fixed or stationary object in nontraffic accident

√x 7th **V27.1** Motorcycle passenger injured in collision with fixed or stationary object in nontraffic accident

√x 7th **V27.2** Unspecified motorcycle rider injured in collision with fixed or stationary object in nontraffic accident

√x 7th **V27.3** Person boarding or alighting a motorcycle injured in collision with fixed or stationary object

√x 7th **V27.4** Motorcycle driver injured in collision with fixed or stationary object in traffic accident

√x 7th **V27.5** Motorcycle passenger injured in collision with fixed or stationary object in traffic accident

√x 7th **V27.9** Unspecified motorcycle rider injured in collision with fixed or stationary object in traffic accident

√4th **V28 Motorcycle rider injured in noncollision transport accident**

INCLUDES fall or thrown from motorcycle (without antecedent collision)
overturning motorcycle NOS
overturning motorcycle without collision

√x 7th **V28.0** Motorcycle driver injured in noncollision transport accident in nontraffic accident

√x 7th **V28.1** Motorcycle passenger injured in noncollision transport accident in nontraffic accident

√x 7th **V28.2** Unspecified motorcycle rider injured in noncollision transport accident in nontraffic accident

√x 7th **V28.3** Person boarding or alighting a motorcycle injured in noncollision transport accident

√x 7th **V28.4** Motorcycle driver injured in noncollision transport accident in traffic accident

√x 7th **V28.5** Motorcycle passenger injured in noncollision transport accident in traffic accident

√x 7th **V28.9** Unspecified motorcycle rider injured in noncollision transport accident in traffic accident

√4th **V29 Motorcycle rider injured in other and unspecified transport accidents**

√5th **V29.0** Motorcycle driver injured in collision with other and unspecified motor vehicles in nontraffic accident

√x 7th **V29.00** Motorcycle driver injured in collision with unspecified motor vehicles in nontraffic accident

√x 7th **V29.09** Motorcycle driver injured in collision with other motor vehicles in nontraffic accident

√5th **V29.1** Motorcycle passenger injured in collision with other and unspecified motor vehicles in nontraffic accident

√x 7th **V29.10** Motorcycle passenger injured in collision with unspecified motor vehicles in nontraffic accident

√x 7th **V29.19** Motorcycle passenger injured in collision with other motor vehicles in nontraffic accident

√5th **V29.2** Unspecified motorcycle rider injured in collision with other and unspecified motor vehicles in nontraffic accident

√x 7th **V29.20** Unspecified motorcycle rider injured in collision with unspecified motor vehicles in nontraffic accident
Motorcycle collision NOS, nontraffic

√x 7th **V29.29** Unspecified motorcycle rider injured in collision with other motor vehicles in nontraffic accident

V29.3 **Motorcycle rider (driver) (passenger) injured in unspecified nontraffic accident**
Motorcycle accident NOS, nontraffic
Motorcycle rider injured in nontraffic accident NOS

V29.4 **Motorcycle driver injured in collision with other and unspecified motor vehicles in traffic accident**

V29.40 **Motorcycle driver injured in collision with unspecified motor vehicles in traffic accident**

V29.49 **Motorcycle driver injured in collision with other motor vehicles in traffic accident**

V29.5 **Motorcycle passenger injured in collision with other and unspecified motor vehicles in traffic accident**

V29.50 **Motorcycle passenger injured in collision with unspecified motor vehicles in traffic accident**

V29.59 **Motorcycle passenger injured in collision with other motor vehicles in traffic accident**

V29.6 **Unspecified motorcycle rider injured in collision with other and unspecified motor vehicles in traffic accident**

V29.60 **Unspecified motorcycle rider injured in collision with unspecified motor vehicles in traffic accident**
Motorcycle collision NOS (traffic)

V29.69 **Unspecified motorcycle rider injured in collision with other motor vehicles in traffic accident**

V29.8 **Motorcycle rider (driver) (passenger) injured in other specified transport accidents**

V29.81 **Motorcycle rider (driver) (passenger) injured in transport accident with military vehicle**

V29.88 **Motorcycle rider (driver) (passenger) injured in other specified transport accidents**

V29.9 **Motorcycle rider (driver) (passenger) injured in unspecified traffic accident**
Motorcycle accident NOS

Occupant of three-wheeled motor vehicle injured in transport accident (V30-V39)

INCLUDES motorized tricycle
motorized rickshaw
three-wheeled motor car

EXCLUDES 1 *all-terrain vehicles (V86.-)*
motorcycle with sidecar (V20-V29)
vehicle designed primarily for off-road use (V86.-)

The appropriate 7th character is to be added to each code from categories V30-V39.
A initial encounter
D subsequent encounter
S sequela

V30 **Occupant of three-wheeled motor vehicle injured in collision with pedestrian or animal**
EXCLUDES 1 *three-wheeled motor vehicle collision with animal-drawn vehicle or animal being ridden (V36.-)*

V30.0 **Driver of three-wheeled motor vehicle injured in collision with pedestrian or animal in nontraffic accident**

V30.1 **Passenger in three-wheeled motor vehicle injured in collision with pedestrian or animal in nontraffic accident**

V30.2 **Person on outside of three-wheeled motor vehicle injured in collision with pedestrian or animal in nontraffic accident**

V30.3 **Unspecified occupant of three-wheeled motor vehicle injured in collision with pedestrian or animal in nontraffic accident**

V30.4 **Person boarding or alighting a three-wheeled motor vehicle injured in collision with pedestrian or animal**

V30.5 **Driver of three-wheeled motor vehicle injured in collision with pedestrian or animal in traffic accident**

V30.6 **Passenger in three-wheeled motor vehicle injured in collision with pedestrian or animal in traffic accident**

V30.7 **Person on outside of three-wheeled motor vehicle injured in collision with pedestrian or animal in traffic accident**

V30.9 **Unspecified occupant of three-wheeled motor vehicle injured in collision with pedestrian or animal in traffic accident**

V31 **Occupant of three-wheeled motor vehicle injured in collision with pedal cycle**

V31.0 **Driver of three-wheeled motor vehicle injured in collision with pedal cycle in nontraffic accident**

V31.1 **Passenger in three-wheeled motor vehicle injured in collision with pedal cycle in nontraffic accident**

V31.2 **Person on outside of three-wheeled motor vehicle injured in collision with pedal cycle in nontraffic accident**

V31.3 **Unspecified occupant of three-wheeled motor vehicle injured in collision with pedal cycle in nontraffic accident**

V31.4 **Person boarding or alighting a three-wheeled motor vehicle injured in collision with pedal cycle**

V31.5 **Driver of three-wheeled motor vehicle injured in collision with pedal cycle in traffic accident**

V31.6 **Passenger in three-wheeled motor vehicle injured in collision with pedal cycle in traffic accident**

V31.7 **Person on outside of three-wheeled motor vehicle injured in collision with pedal cycle in traffic accident**

V31.9 **Unspecified occupant of three-wheeled motor vehicle injured in collision with pedal cycle in traffic accident**

V32 **Occupant of three-wheeled motor vehicle injured in collision with two- or three-wheeled motor vehicle**

V32.0 **Driver of three-wheeled motor vehicle injured in collision with two- or three-wheeled motor vehicle in nontraffic accident**

V32.1 **Passenger in three-wheeled motor vehicle injured in collision with two- or three-wheeled motor vehicle in nontraffic accident**

V32.2 **Person on outside of three-wheeled motor vehicle injured in collision with two- or three-wheeled motor vehicle in nontraffic accident**

V32.3 **Unspecified occupant of three-wheeled motor vehicle injured in collision with two- or three-wheeled motor vehicle in nontraffic accident**

V32.4 **Person boarding or alighting a three-wheeled motor vehicle injured in collision with two- or three-wheeled motor vehicle**

V32.5 **Driver of three-wheeled motor vehicle injured in collision with two- or three-wheeled motor vehicle in traffic accident**

V32.6 **Passenger in three-wheeled motor vehicle injured in collision with two- or three-wheeled motor vehicle in traffic accident**

V32.7 **Person on outside of three-wheeled motor vehicle injured in collision with two- or three-wheeled motor vehicle in traffic accident**

V32.9 **Unspecified occupant of three-wheeled motor vehicle injured in collision with two- or three-wheeled motor vehicle in traffic accident**

V33 **Occupant of three-wheeled motor vehicle injured in collision with car, pick-up truck or van**

V33.0 **Driver of three-wheeled motor vehicle injured in collision with car, pick-up truck or van in nontraffic accident**

V33.1 **Passenger in three-wheeled motor vehicle injured in collision with car, pick-up truck or van in nontraffic accident**

V33.2 **Person on outside of three-wheeled motor vehicle injured in collision with car, pick-up truck or van in nontraffic accident**

V33.3 **Unspecified occupant of three-wheeled motor vehicle injured in collision with car, pick-up truck or van in nontraffic accident**

V33.4 **Person boarding or alighting a three-wheeled motor vehicle injured in collision with car, pick-up truck or van**

V33.5 **Driver of three-wheeled motor vehicle injured in collision with car, pick-up truck or van in traffic accident**

V33.6 **Passenger in three-wheeled motor vehicle injured in collision with car, pick-up truck or van in traffic accident**

V33.7 **Person on outside of three-wheeled motor vehicle injured in collision with car, pick-up truck or van in traffic accident**

V33.9 **Unspecified occupant of three-wheeled motor vehicle injured in collision with car, pick-up truck or van in traffic accident**

V34 **Occupant of three-wheeled motor vehicle injured in collision with heavy transport vehicle or bus**
EXCLUDES 1 *occupant of three-wheeled motor vehicle injured in collision with military vehicle (V39.81)*

V34.0 **Driver of three-wheeled motor vehicle injured in collision with heavy transport vehicle or bus in nontraffic accident**

V34.1 **Passenger in three-wheeled motor vehicle injured in collision with heavy transport vehicle or bus in nontraffic accident**

V34.2 **Person on outside of three-wheeled motor vehicle injured in collision with heavy transport vehicle or bus in nontraffic accident**

V34.3 **Unspecified occupant of three-wheeled motor vehicle injured in collision with heavy transport vehicle or bus in nontraffic accident**

V34.4 **Person boarding or alighting a three-wheeled motor vehicle injured in collision with heavy transport vehicle or bus**

V34.5 **Driver of three-wheeled motor vehicle injured in collision with heavy transport vehicle or bus in traffic accident**

V34.6 **Passenger in three-wheeled motor vehicle injured in collision with heavy transport vehicle or bus in traffic accident**

V34.7 **Person on outside of three-wheeled motor vehicle injured in collision with heavy transport vehicle or bus in traffic accident**

V34.9 **Unspecified occupant of three-wheeled motor vehicle injured in collision with heavy transport vehicle or bus in traffic accident**

4th V35 Occupant of three-wheeled motor vehicle injured in collision with railway train or railway vehicle

√x 7th **V35.0 Driver of three-wheeled motor vehicle injured in collision with railway train or railway vehicle in nontraffic accident**

√x 7th **V35.1 Passenger in three-wheeled motor vehicle injured in collision with railway train or railway vehicle in nontraffic accident**

√x 7th **V35.2 Person on outside of three-wheeled motor vehicle injured in collision with railway train or railway vehicle in nontraffic accident**

√x 7th **V35.3 Unspecified occupant of three-wheeled motor vehicle injured in collision with railway train or railway vehicle in nontraffic accident**

√x 7th **V35.4 Person boarding or alighting a three-wheeled motor vehicle injured in collision with railway train or railway vehicle**

√x 7th **V35.5 Driver of three-wheeled motor vehicle injured in collision with railway train or railway vehicle in traffic accident**

√x 7th **V35.6 Passenger in three-wheeled motor vehicle injured in collision with railway train or railway vehicle in traffic accident**

√x 7th **V35.7 Person on outside of three-wheeled motor vehicle injured in collision with railway train or railway vehicle in traffic accident**

√x 7th **V35.9 Unspecified occupant of three-wheeled motor vehicle injured in collision with railway train or railway vehicle in traffic accident**

4th V36 Occupant of three-wheeled motor vehicle injured in collision with other nonmotor vehicle

INCLUDES collision with animal-drawn vehicle, animal being ridden, streetcar

√x 7th **V36.0 Driver of three-wheeled motor vehicle injured in collision with other nonmotor vehicle in nontraffic accident**

√x 7th **V36.1 Passenger in three-wheeled motor vehicle injured in collision with other nonmotor vehicle in nontraffic accident**

√x 7th **V36.2 Person on outside of three-wheeled motor vehicle injured in collision with other nonmotor vehicle in nontraffic accident**

√x 7th **V36.3 Unspecified occupant of three-wheeled motor vehicle injured in collision with other nonmotor vehicle in nontraffic accident**

√x 7th **V36.4 Person boarding or alighting a three-wheeled motor vehicle injured in collision with other nonmotor vehicle**

√x 7th **V36.5 Driver of three-wheeled motor vehicle injured in collision with other nonmotor vehicle in traffic accident**

√x 7th **V36.6 Passenger in three-wheeled motor vehicle injured in collision with other nonmotor vehicle in traffic accident**

√x 7th **V36.7 Person on outside of three-wheeled motor vehicle injured in collision with other nonmotor vehicle in traffic accident**

√x 7th **V36.9 Unspecified occupant of three-wheeled motor vehicle injured in collision with other nonmotor vehicle in traffic accident**

4th V37 Occupant of three-wheeled motor vehicle injured in collision with fixed or stationary object

√x 7th **V37.0 Driver of three-wheeled motor vehicle injured in collision with fixed or stationary object in nontraffic accident**

√x 7th **V37.1 Passenger in three-wheeled motor vehicle injured in collision with fixed or stationary object in nontraffic accident**

√x 7th **V37.2 Person on outside of three-wheeled motor vehicle injured in collision with fixed or stationary object in nontraffic accident**

√x 7th **V37.3 Unspecified occupant of three-wheeled motor vehicle injured in collision with fixed or stationary object in nontraffic accident**

√x 7th **V37.4 Person boarding or alighting a three-wheeled motor vehicle injured in collision with fixed or stationary object**

√x 7th **V37.5 Driver of three-wheeled motor vehicle injured in collision with fixed or stationary object in traffic accident**

√x 7th **V37.6 Passenger in three-wheeled motor vehicle injured in collision with fixed or stationary object in traffic accident**

√x 7th **V37.7 Person on outside of three-wheeled motor vehicle injured in collision with fixed or stationary object in traffic accident**

√x 7th **V37.9 Unspecified occupant of three-wheeled motor vehicle injured in collision with fixed or stationary object in traffic accident**

4th V38 Occupant of three-wheeled motor vehicle injured in noncollision transport accident

INCLUDES fall or thrown from three-wheeled motor vehicle
overturning of three-wheeled motor vehicle NOS
overturning of three-wheeled motor vehicle without collision

√x 7th **V38.0 Driver of three-wheeled motor vehicle injured in noncollision transport accident in nontraffic accident**

√x 7th **V38.1 Passenger in three-wheeled motor vehicle injured in noncollision transport accident in nontraffic accident**

√x 7th **V38.2 Person on outside of three-wheeled motor vehicle injured in noncollision transport accident in nontraffic accident**

√x 7th **V38.3 Unspecified occupant of three-wheeled motor vehicle injured in noncollision transport accident in nontraffic accident**

√x 7th **V38.4 Person boarding or alighting a three-wheeled motor vehicle injured in noncollision transport accident**

√x 7th **V38.5 Driver of three-wheeled motor vehicle injured in noncollision transport accident in traffic accident**

√x 7th **V38.6 Passenger in three-wheeled motor vehicle injured in noncollision transport accident in traffic accident**

√x 7th **V38.7 Person on outside of three-wheeled motor vehicle injured in noncollision transport accident in traffic accident**

√x 7th **V38.9 Unspecified occupant of three-wheeled motor vehicle injured in noncollision transport accident in traffic accident**

4th V39 Occupant of three-wheeled motor vehicle injured in other and unspecified transport accidents

5th **V39.0 Driver of three-wheeled motor vehicle injured in collision with other and unspecified motor vehicles in nontraffic accident**

√x 7th **V39.00 Driver of three-wheeled motor vehicle injured in collision with unspecified motor vehicles in nontraffic accident**

√x 7th **V39.09 Driver of three-wheeled motor vehicle injured in collision with other motor vehicles in nontraffic accident**

5th **V39.1 Passenger in three-wheeled motor vehicle injured in collision with other and unspecified motor vehicles in nontraffic accident**

√x 7th **V39.10 Passenger in three-wheeled motor vehicle injured in collision with unspecified motor vehicles in nontraffic accident**

√x 7th **V39.19 Passenger in three-wheeled motor vehicle injured in collision with other motor vehicles in nontraffic accident**

5th **V39.2 Unspecified occupant of three-wheeled motor vehicle injured in collision with other and unspecified motor vehicles in nontraffic accident**

√x 7th **V39.20 Unspecified occupant of three-wheeled motor vehicle injured in collision with unspecified motor vehicles in nontraffic accident**

Collision NOS involving three-wheeled motor vehicle, nontraffic

√x 7th **V39.29 Unspecified occupant of three-wheeled motor vehicle injured in collision with other motor vehicles in nontraffic accident**

√x 7th **V39.3 Occupant (driver) (passenger) of three-wheeled motor vehicle injured in unspecified nontraffic accident**

Accident NOS involving three-wheeled motor vehicle, nontraffic
Occupant of three-wheeled motor vehicle injured in nontraffic accident NOS

5th **V39.4 Driver of three-wheeled motor vehicle injured in collision with other and unspecified motor vehicles in traffic accident**

√x 7th **V39.40 Driver of three-wheeled motor vehicle injured in collision with unspecified motor vehicles in traffic accident**

√x 7th **V39.49 Driver of three-wheeled motor vehicle injured in collision with other motor vehicles in traffic accident**

5th **V39.5 Passenger in three-wheeled motor vehicle injured in collision with other and unspecified motor vehicles in traffic accident**

√x 7th **V39.50 Passenger in three-wheeled motor vehicle injured in collision with unspecified motor vehicles in traffic accident**

√x 7th **V39.59 Passenger in three-wheeled motor vehicle injured in collision with other motor vehicles in traffic accident**

5th **V39.6 Unspecified occupant of three-wheeled motor vehicle injured in collision with other and unspecified motor vehicles in traffic accident**

√x 7th **V39.60 Unspecified occupant of three-wheeled motor vehicle injured in collision with unspecified motor vehicles in traffic accident**

Collision NOS involving three-wheeled motor vehicle (traffic)

√x 7th **V39.69 Unspecified occupant of three-wheeled motor vehicle injured in collision with other motor vehicles in traffic accident**

5th **V39.8 Occupant (driver) (passenger) of three-wheeled motor vehicle injured in other specified transport accidents**

√x 7th **V39.81 Occupant (driver) (passenger) of three-wheeled motor vehicle injured in transport accident with military vehicle**

√x 7th **V39.89 Occupant (driver) (passenger) of three-wheeled motor vehicle injured in other specified transport accidents**

V39.9 Occupant (driver) (passenger) of three-wheeled motor vehicle injured in unspecified traffic accident
Accident NOS involving three-wheeled motor vehicle

Car occupant injured in transport accident (V40-V49)

INCLUDES a four-wheeled motor vehicle designed primarily for carrying passengers
automobile (pulling a trailer or camper)

EXCLUDES 1 *bus (V50-V59)*
minibus (V50-V59)
minivan (V50-V59)
motorcoach (V70-V79)
pick-up truck (V50-V59)
sport utility vehicle (SUV) (V50-V59)

The appropriate 7th character is to be added to each code from categories V40-V49.
A initial encounter
D subsequent encounter
S sequela

V40 Car occupant injured in collision with pedestrian or animal
EXCLUDES 1 *car collision with animal-drawn vehicle or animal being ridden (V46.-)*

V40.0 Car driver injured in collision with pedestrian or animal in nontraffic accident
V40.1 Car passenger injured in collision with pedestrian or animal in nontraffic accident
V40.2 Person on outside of car injured in collision with pedestrian or animal in nontraffic accident
V40.3 Unspecified car occupant injured in collision with pedestrian or animal in nontraffic accident
V40.4 Person boarding or alighting a car injured in collision with pedestrian or animal
V40.5 Car driver injured in collision with pedestrian or animal in traffic accident
V40.6 Car passenger injured in collision with pedestrian or animal in traffic accident
V40.7 Person on outside of car injured in collision with pedestrian or animal in traffic accident
V40.9 Unspecified car occupant injured in collision with pedestrian or animal in traffic accident

V41 Car occupant injured in collision with pedal cycle

V41.0 Car driver injured in collision with pedal cycle in nontraffic accident
V41.1 Car passenger injured in collision with pedal cycle in nontraffic accident
V41.2 Person on outside of car injured in collision with pedal cycle in nontraffic accident
V41.3 Unspecified car occupant injured in collision with pedal cycle in nontraffic accident
V41.4 Person boarding or alighting a car injured in collision with pedal cycle
V41.5 Car driver injured in collision with pedal cycle in traffic accident
V41.6 Car passenger injured in collision with pedal cycle in traffic accident
V41.7 Person on outside of car injured in collision with pedal cycle in traffic accident
V41.9 Unspecified car occupant injured in collision with pedal cycle in traffic accident

V42 Car occupant injured in collision with two- or three-wheeled motor vehicle

V42.0 Car driver injured in collision with two- or three-wheeled motor vehicle in nontraffic accident
V42.1 Car passenger injured in collision with two- or three-wheeled motor vehicle in nontraffic accident
V42.2 Person on outside of car injured in collision with two- or three-wheeled motor vehicle in nontraffic accident
V42.3 Unspecified car occupant injured in collision with two- or three-wheeled motor vehicle in nontraffic accident
V42.4 Person boarding or alighting a car injured in collision with two- or three-wheeled motor vehicle
V42.5 Car driver injured in collision with two- or three-wheeled motor vehicle in traffic accident
V42.6 Car passenger injured in collision with two- or three-wheeled motor vehicle in traffic accident
V42.7 Person on outside of car injured in collision with two- or three-wheeled motor vehicle in traffic accident
V42.9 Unspecified car occupant injured in collision with two- or three-wheeled motor vehicle in traffic accident

V43 Car occupant injured in collision with car, pick-up truck or van

V43.0 Car driver injured in collision with car, pick-up truck or van in nontraffic accident
V43.01 Car driver injured in collision with sport utility vehicle in nontraffic accident
V43.02 Car driver injured in collision with other type car in nontraffic accident
V43.03 Car driver injured in collision with pick-up truck in nontraffic accident
V43.04 Car driver injured in collision with van in nontraffic accident

V43.1 Car passenger injured in collision with car, pick-up truck or van in nontraffic accident
V43.11 Car passenger injured in collision with sport utility vehicle in nontraffic accident
V43.12 Car passenger injured in collision with other type car in nontraffic accident
V43.13 Car passenger injured in collision with pick-up truck in nontraffic accident
V43.14 Car passenger injured in collision with van in nontraffic accident

V43.2 Person on outside of car injured in collision with car, pick-up truck or van in nontraffic accident
V43.21 Person on outside of car injured in collision with sport utility vehicle in nontraffic accident
V43.22 Person on outside of car injured in collision with other type car in nontraffic accident
V43.23 Person on outside of car injured in collision with pick-up truck in nontraffic accident
V43.24 Person on outside of car injured in collision with van in nontraffic accident

V43.3 Unspecified car occupant injured in collision with car, pick-up truck or van in nontraffic accident
V43.31 Unspecified car occupant injured in collision with sport utility vehicle in nontraffic accident
V43.32 Unspecified car occupant injured in collision with other type car in nontraffic accident
V43.33 Unspecified car occupant injured in collision with pick-up truck in nontraffic accident
V43.34 Unspecified car occupant injured in collision with van in nontraffic accident

V43.4 Person boarding or alighting a car injured in collision with car, pick-up truck or van
V43.41 Person boarding or alighting a car injured in collision with sport utility vehicle
V43.42 Person boarding or alighting a car injured in collision with other type car
V43.43 Person boarding or alighting a car injured in collision with pick-up truck
V43.44 Person boarding or alighting a car injured in collision with van

V43.5 Car driver injured in collision with car, pick-up truck or van in traffic accident
V43.51 Car driver injured in collision with sport utility vehicle in traffic accident
V43.52 Car driver injured in collision with other type car in traffic accident
V43.53 Car driver injured in collision with pick-up truck in traffic accident
V43.54 Car driver injured in collision with van in traffic accident

V43.6 Car passenger injured in collision with car, pick-up truck or van in traffic accident
V43.61 Car passenger injured in collision with sport utility vehicle in traffic accident
V43.62 Car passenger injured in collision with other type car in traffic accident
V43.63 Car passenger injured in collision with pick-up truck in traffic accident
V43.64 Car passenger injured in collision with van in traffic accident

V43.7 Person on outside of car injured in collision with car, pick-up truck or van in traffic accident
V43.71 Person on outside of car injured in collision with sport utility vehicle in traffic accident
V43.72 Person on outside of car injured in collision with other type car in traffic accident
V43.73 Person on outside of car injured in collision with pick-up truck in traffic accident
V43.74 Person on outside of car injured in collision with van in traffic accident

√5th V43.9 **Unspecified car occupant injured in collision with car, pick-up truck or van in traffic accident**

√x7th V43.91 **Unspecified car occupant injured in collision with sport utility vehicle in traffic accident**

√x7th V43.92 **Unspecified car occupant injured in collision with other type car in traffic accident**

√x7th V43.93 **Unspecified car occupant injured in collision with pick-up truck in traffic accident**

√x7th V43.94 **Unspecified car occupant injured in collision with van in traffic accident**

√4th **V44 Car occupant injured in collision with heavy transport vehicle or bus**

EXCLUDES 1 *car occupant injured in collision with military vehicle (V49.81)*

√x7th V44.Ø **Car driver injured in collision with heavy transport vehicle or bus in nontraffic accident**

√x7th V44.1 **Car passenger injured in collision with heavy transport vehicle or bus in nontraffic accident**

√x7th V44.2 **Person on outside of car injured in collision with heavy transport vehicle or bus in nontraffic accident**

√x7th V44.3 **Unspecified car occupant injured in collision with heavy transport vehicle or bus in nontraffic accident**

√x7th V44.4 **Person boarding or alighting a car injured in collision with heavy transport vehicle or bus**

√x7th V44.5 **Car driver injured in collision with heavy transport vehicle or bus in traffic accident**

√x7th V44.6 **Car passenger injured in collision with heavy transport vehicle or bus in traffic accident**

√x7th V44.7 **Person on outside of car injured in collision with heavy transport vehicle or bus in traffic accident**

√x7th V44.9 **Unspecified car occupant injured in collision with heavy transport vehicle or bus in traffic accident**

√4th **V45 Car occupant injured in collision with railway train or railway vehicle**

√x7th V45.Ø **Car driver injured in collision with railway train or railway vehicle in nontraffic accident**

√x7th V45.1 **Car passenger injured in collision with railway train or railway vehicle in nontraffic accident**

√x7th V45.2 **Person on outside of car injured in collision with railway train or railway vehicle in nontraffic accident**

√x7th V45.3 **Unspecified car occupant injured in collision with railway train or railway vehicle in nontraffic accident**

√x7th V45.4 **Person boarding or alighting a car injured in collision with railway train or railway vehicle**

√x7th V45.5 **Car driver injured in collision with railway train or railway vehicle in traffic accident**

√x7th V45.6 **Car passenger injured in collision with railway train or railway vehicle in traffic accident**

√x7th V45.7 **Person on outside of car injured in collision with railway train or railway vehicle in traffic accident**

√x7th V45.9 **Unspecified car occupant injured in collision with railway train or railway vehicle in traffic accident**

√4th **V46 Car occupant injured in collision with other nonmotor vehicle**

INCLUDES collision with animal-drawn vehicle, animal being ridden, streetcar

√x7th V46.Ø **Car driver injured in collision with other nonmotor vehicle in nontraffic accident**

√x7th V46.1 **Car passenger injured in collision with other nonmotor vehicle in nontraffic accident**

√x7th V46.2 **Person on outside of car injured in collision with other nonmotor vehicle in nontraffic accident**

√x7th V46.3 **Unspecified car occupant injured in collision with other nonmotor vehicle in nontraffic accident**

√x7th V46.4 **Person boarding or alighting a car injured in collision with other nonmotor vehicle**

√x7th V46.5 **Car driver injured in collision with other nonmotor vehicle in traffic accident**

√x7th V46.6 **Car passenger injured in collision with other nonmotor vehicle in traffic accident**

√x7th V46.7 **Person on outside of car injured in collision with other nonmotor vehicle in traffic accident**

√x7th V46.9 **Unspecified car occupant injured in collision with other nonmotor vehicle in traffic accident**

√4th **V47 Car occupant injured in collision with fixed or stationary object**

AHA: 2016,4Q,73

√x7th V47.Ø **Car driver injured in collision with fixed or stationary object in nontraffic accident**

√x7th V47.1 **Car passenger injured in collision with fixed or stationary object in nontraffic accident**

√x7th V47.2 **Person on outside of car injured in collision with fixed or stationary object in nontraffic accident**

√x7th V47.3 **Unspecified car occupant injured in collision with fixed or stationary object in nontraffic accident**

√x7th V47.4 **Person boarding or alighting a car injured in collision with fixed or stationary object**

√x7th V47.5 **Car driver injured in collision with fixed or stationary object in traffic accident**

√x7th V47.6 **Car passenger injured in collision with fixed or stationary object in traffic accident**

√x7th V47.7 **Person on outside of car injured in collision with fixed or stationary object in traffic accident**

√x7th V47.9 **Unspecified car occupant injured in collision with fixed or stationary object in traffic accident**

√4th **V48 Car occupant injured in noncollision transport accident**

INCLUDES overturning car NOS
overturning car without collision

√x7th V48.Ø **Car driver injured in noncollision transport accident in nontraffic accident**

√x7th V48.1 **Car passenger injured in noncollision transport accident in nontraffic accident**

√x7th V48.2 **Person on outside of car injured in noncollision transport accident in nontraffic accident**

√x7th V48.3 **Unspecified car occupant injured in noncollision transport accident in nontraffic accident**

√x7th V48.4 **Person boarding or alighting a car injured in noncollision transport accident**

√x7th V48.5 **Car driver injured in noncollision transport accident in traffic accident**

√x7th V48.6 **Car passenger injured in noncollision transport accident in traffic accident**

√x7th V48.7 **Person on outside of car injured in noncollision transport accident in traffic accident**

√x7th V48.9 **Unspecified car occupant injured in noncollision transport accident in traffic accident**

√4th **V49 Car occupant injured in other and unspecified transport accidents**

√5th V49.Ø **Driver injured in collision with other and unspecified motor vehicles in nontraffic accident**

√x7th V49.ØØ **Driver injured in collision with unspecified motor vehicles in nontraffic accident**

√x7th V49.Ø9 **Driver injured in collision with other motor vehicles in nontraffic accident**

√5th V49.1 **Passenger injured in collision with other and unspecified motor vehicles in nontraffic accident**

√x7th V49.1Ø **Passenger injured in collision with unspecified motor vehicles in nontraffic accident**

√x7th V49.19 **Passenger injured in collision with other motor vehicles in nontraffic accident**

√5th V49.2 **Unspecified car occupant injured in collision with other and unspecified motor vehicles in nontraffic accident**

√x7th V49.2Ø **Unspecified car occupant injured in collision with unspecified motor vehicles in nontraffic accident**
Car collision NOS, nontraffic

√x7th V49.29 **Unspecified car occupant injured in collision with other motor vehicles in nontraffic accident**

√x7th V49.3 **Car occupant (driver) (passenger) injured in unspecified nontraffic accident**
Car accident NOS, nontraffic
Car occupant injured in nontraffic accident NOS

√5th V49.4 **Driver injured in collision with other and unspecified motor vehicles in traffic accident**

√x7th V49.4Ø **Driver injured in collision with unspecified motor vehicles in traffic accident**

√x7th V49.49 **Driver injured in collision with other motor vehicles in traffic accident**

√5th V49.5 **Passenger injured in collision with other and unspecified motor vehicles in traffic accident**

√x7th V49.5Ø **Passenger injured in collision with unspecified motor vehicles in traffic accident**

√x7th V49.59 **Passenger injured in collision with other motor vehicles in traffic accident**

√5th V49.6 **Unspecified car occupant injured in collision with other and unspecified motor vehicles in traffic accident**

√x7th V49.6Ø **Unspecified car occupant injured in collision with unspecified motor vehicles in traffic accident**
Car collision NOS (traffic)

√x7th V49.69 **Unspecified car occupant injured in collision with other motor vehicles in traffic accident**

√5th V49.8 **Car occupant (driver) (passenger) injured in other specified transport accidents**

√x7th V49.81 **Car occupant (driver) (passenger) injured in transport accident with military vehicle**

√x7th V49.88 **Car occupant (driver) (passenger) injured in other specified transport accidents**

√x7th V49.9 **Car occupant (driver) (passenger) injured in unspecified traffic accident**
Car accident NOS

Occupant of pick-up truck or van injured in transport accident (V50-V59)

INCLUDES a four or six wheel motor vehicle designed primarily for carrying passengers and property but weighing less than the local limit for classification as a heavy goods vehicle
minibus
minivan
sport utility vehicle (SUV)
truck
van

EXCLUDES 1 *heavy transport vehicle (V60-V69)*

The appropriate 7th character is to be added to each code from categories V50-V59.
A initial encounter
D subsequent encounter
S sequela

√4th **V50 Occupant of pick-up truck or van injured in collision with pedestrian or animal**
EXCLUDES 1 *pick-up truck or van collision with animal-drawn vehicle or animal being ridden (V56.-)*

√x7th V50.0 **Driver of pick-up truck or van injured in collision with pedestrian or animal in nontraffic accident**
√x7th V50.1 **Passenger in pick-up truck or van injured in collision with pedestrian or animal in nontraffic accident**
√x7th V50.2 **Person on outside of pick-up truck or van injured in collision with pedestrian or animal in nontraffic accident**
√x7th V50.3 **Unspecified occupant of pick-up truck or van injured in collision with pedestrian or animal in nontraffic accident**
√x7th V50.4 **Person boarding or alighting a pick-up truck or van injured in collision with pedestrian or animal**
√x7th V50.5 **Driver of pick-up truck or van injured in collision with pedestrian or animal in traffic accident**
√x7th V50.6 **Passenger in pick-up truck or van injured in collision with pedestrian or animal in traffic accident**
√x7th V50.7 **Person on outside of pick-up truck or van injured in collision with pedestrian or animal in traffic accident**
√x7th V50.9 **Unspecified occupant of pick-up truck or van injured in collision with pedestrian or animal in traffic accident**

√4th **V51 Occupant of pick-up truck or van injured in collision with pedal cycle**

√x7th V51.0 **Driver of pick-up truck or van injured in collision with pedal cycle in nontraffic accident**
√x7th V51.1 **Passenger in pick-up truck or van injured in collision with pedal cycle in nontraffic accident**
√x7th V51.2 **Person on outside of pick-up truck or van injured in collision with pedal cycle in nontraffic accident**
√x7th V51.3 **Unspecified occupant of pick-up truck or van injured in collision with pedal cycle in nontraffic accident**
√x7th V51.4 **Person boarding or alighting a pick-up truck or van injured in collision with pedal cycle**
√x7th V51.5 **Driver of pick-up truck or van injured in collision with pedal cycle in traffic accident**
√x7th V51.6 **Passenger in pick-up truck or van injured in collision with pedal cycle in traffic accident**
√x7th V51.7 **Person on outside of pick-up truck or van injured in collision with pedal cycle in traffic accident**
√x7th V51.9 **Unspecified occupant of pick-up truck or van injured in collision with pedal cycle in traffic accident**

√4th **V52 Occupant of pick-up truck or van injured in collision with two- or three-wheeled motor vehicle**

√x7th V52.0 **Driver of pick-up truck or van injured in collision with two- or three-wheeled motor vehicle in nontraffic accident**
√x7th V52.1 **Passenger in pick-up truck or van injured in collision with two- or three-wheeled motor vehicle in nontraffic accident**
√x7th V52.2 **Person on outside of pick-up truck or van injured in collision with two- or three-wheeled motor vehicle in nontraffic accident**
√x7th V52.3 **Unspecified occupant of pick-up truck or van injured in collision with two- or three-wheeled motor vehicle in nontraffic accident**
√x7th V52.4 **Person boarding or alighting a pick-up truck or van injured in collision with two- or three-wheeled motor vehicle**
√x7th V52.5 **Driver of pick-up truck or van injured in collision with two- or three-wheeled motor vehicle in traffic accident**
√x7th V52.6 **Passenger in pick-up truck or van injured in collision with two- or three-wheeled motor vehicle in traffic accident**
√x7th V52.7 **Person on outside of pick-up truck or van injured in collision with two- or three-wheeled motor vehicle in traffic accident**
√x7th V52.9 **Unspecified occupant of pick-up truck or van injured in collision with two- or three-wheeled motor vehicle in traffic accident**

√4th **V53 Occupant of pick-up truck or van injured in collision with car, pick-up truck or van**

√x7th V53.0 **Driver of pick-up truck or van injured in collision with car, pick-up truck or van in nontraffic accident**
√x7th V53.1 **Passenger in pick-up truck or van injured in collision with car, pick-up truck or van in nontraffic accident**
√x7th V53.2 **Person on outside of pick-up truck or van injured in collision with car, pick-up truck or van in nontraffic accident**
√x7th V53.3 **Unspecified occupant of pick-up truck or van injured in collision with car, pick-up truck or van in nontraffic accident**
√x7th V53.4 **Person boarding or alighting a pick-up truck or van injured in collision with car, pick-up truck or van**
√x7th V53.5 **Driver of pick-up truck or van injured in collision with car, pick-up truck or van in traffic accident**
√x7th V53.6 **Passenger in pick-up truck or van injured in collision with car, pick-up truck or van in traffic accident**
√x7th V53.7 **Person on outside of pick-up truck or van injured in collision with car, pick-up truck or van in traffic accident**
√x7th V53.9 **Unspecified occupant of pick-up truck or van injured in collision with car, pick-up truck or van in traffic accident**

√4th **V54 Occupant of pick-up truck or van injured in collision with heavy transport vehicle or bus**
EXCLUDES 1 *occupant of pick-up truck or van injured in collision with military vehicle (V59.81)*

√x7th V54.0 **Driver of pick-up truck or van injured in collision with heavy transport vehicle or bus in nontraffic accident**
√x7th V54.1 **Passenger in pick-up truck or van injured in collision with heavy transport vehicle or bus in nontraffic accident**
√x7th V54.2 **Person on outside of pick-up truck or van injured in collision with heavy transport vehicle or bus in nontraffic accident**
√x7th V54.3 **Unspecified occupant of pick-up truck or van injured in collision with heavy transport vehicle or bus in nontraffic accident**
√x7th V54.4 **Person boarding or alighting a pick-up truck or van injured in collision with heavy transport vehicle or bus**
√x7th V54.5 **Driver of pick-up truck or van injured in collision with heavy transport vehicle or bus in traffic accident**
√x7th V54.6 **Passenger in pick-up truck or van injured in collision with heavy transport vehicle or bus in traffic accident**
√x7th V54.7 **Person on outside of pick-up truck or van injured in collision with heavy transport vehicle or bus in traffic accident**
√x7th V54.9 **Unspecified occupant of pick-up truck or van injured in collision with heavy transport vehicle or bus in traffic accident**

√4th **V55 Occupant of pick-up truck or van injured in collision with railway train or railway vehicle**

√x7th V55.0 **Driver of pick-up truck or van injured in collision with railway train or railway vehicle in nontraffic accident**
√x7th V55.1 **Passenger in pick-up truck or van injured in collision with railway train or railway vehicle in nontraffic accident**
√x7th V55.2 **Person on outside of pick-up truck or van injured in collision with railway train or railway vehicle in nontraffic accident**
√x7th V55.3 **Unspecified occupant of pick-up truck or van injured in collision with railway train or railway vehicle in nontraffic accident**
√x7th V55.4 **Person boarding or alighting a pick-up truck or van injured in collision with railway train or railway vehicle**
√x7th V55.5 **Driver of pick-up truck or van injured in collision with railway train or railway vehicle in traffic accident**
√x7th V55.6 **Passenger in pick-up truck or van injured in collision with railway train or railway vehicle in traffic accident**
√x7th V55.7 **Person on outside of pick-up truck or van injured in collision with railway train or railway vehicle in traffic accident**
√x7th V55.9 **Unspecified occupant of pick-up truck or van injured in collision with railway train or railway vehicle in traffic accident**

√4th **V56 Occupant of pick-up truck or van injured in collision with other nonmotor vehicle**
INCLUDES collision with animal-drawn vehicle, animal being ridden, streetcar

√x7th V56.0 **Driver of pick-up truck or van injured in collision with other nonmotor vehicle in nontraffic accident**
√x7th V56.1 **Passenger in pick-up truck or van injured in collision with other nonmotor vehicle in nontraffic accident**

√x7th V56.2 Person on outside of pick-up truck or van injured in collision with other nonmotor vehicle in nontraffic accident

√x7th V56.3 Unspecified occupant of pick-up truck or van injured in collision with other nonmotor vehicle in nontraffic accident

√x7th V56.4 Person boarding or alighting a pick-up truck or van injured in collision with other nonmotor vehicle

√x7th V56.5 Driver of pick-up truck or van injured in collision with other nonmotor vehicle in traffic accident

√x7th V56.6 Passenger in pick-up truck or van injured in collision with other nonmotor vehicle in traffic accident

√x7th V56.7 Person on outside of pick-up truck or van injured in collision with other nonmotor vehicle in traffic accident

√x7th V56.9 Unspecified occupant of pick-up truck or van injured in collision with other nonmotor vehicle in traffic accident

√4th V57 Occupant of pick-up truck or van injured in collision with fixed or stationary object

√x7th V57.Ø Driver of pick-up truck or van injured in collision with fixed or stationary object in nontraffic accident

√x7th V57.1 Passenger in pick-up truck or van injured in collision with fixed or stationary object in nontraffic accident

√x7th V57.2 Person on outside of pick-up truck or van injured in collision with fixed or stationary object in nontraffic accident

√x7th V57.3 Unspecified occupant of pick-up truck or van injured in collision with fixed or stationary object in nontraffic accident

√x7th V57.4 Person boarding or alighting a pick-up truck or van injured in collision with fixed or stationary object

√x7th V57.5 Driver of pick-up truck or van injured in collision with fixed or stationary object in traffic accident

√x7th V57.6 Passenger in pick-up truck or van injured in collision with fixed or stationary object in traffic accident

√x7th V57.7 Person on outside of pick-up truck or van injured in collision with fixed or stationary object in traffic accident

√x7th V57.9 Unspecified occupant of pick-up truck or van injured in collision with fixed or stationary object in traffic accident

√4th V58 Occupant of pick-up truck or van injured in noncollision transport accident

INCLUDES overturning pick-up truck or van NOS
overturning pick-up truck or van without collision

√x7th V58.Ø Driver of pick-up truck or van injured in noncollision transport accident in nontraffic accident

√x7th V58.1 Passenger in pick-up truck or van injured in noncollision transport accident in nontraffic accident

√x7th V58.2 Person on outside of pick-up truck or van injured in noncollision transport accident in nontraffic accident

√x7th V58.3 Unspecified occupant of pick-up truck or van injured in noncollision transport accident in nontraffic accident

√x7th V58.4 Person boarding or alighting a pick-up truck or van injured in noncollision transport accident

√x7th V58.5 Driver of pick-up truck or van injured in noncollision transport accident in traffic accident

√x7th V58.6 Passenger in pick-up truck or van injured in noncollision transport accident in traffic accident

√x7th V58.7 Person on outside of pick-up truck or van injured in noncollision transport accident in traffic accident

√x7th V58.9 Unspecified occupant of pick-up truck or van injured in noncollision transport accident in traffic accident

√4th V59 Occupant of pick-up truck or van injured in other and unspecified transport accidents

√5th V59.Ø Driver of pick-up truck or van injured in collision with other and unspecified motor vehicles in nontraffic accident

√x7th V59.ØØ Driver of pick-up truck or van injured in collision with unspecified motor vehicles in nontraffic accident

√x7th V59.Ø9 Driver of pick-up truck or van injured in collision with other motor vehicles in nontraffic accident

√5th V59.1 Passenger in pick-up truck or van injured in collision with other and unspecified motor vehicles in nontraffic accident

√x7th V59.1Ø Passenger in pick-up truck or van injured in collision with unspecified motor vehicles in nontraffic accident

√x7th V59.19 Passenger in pick-up truck or van injured in collision with other motor vehicles in nontraffic accident

√5th V59.2 Unspecified occupant of pick-up truck or van injured in collision with other and unspecified motor vehicles in nontraffic accident

√x7th V59.2Ø Unspecified occupant of pick-up truck or van injured in collision with unspecified motor vehicles in nontraffic accident
Collision NOS involving pick-up truck or van, nontraffic

√x7th V59.29 Unspecified occupant of pick-up truck or van injured in collision with other motor vehicles in nontraffic accident

√x7th V59.3 Occupant (driver) (passenger) of pick-up truck or van injured in unspecified nontraffic accident
Accident NOS involving pick-up truck or van, nontraffic
Occupant of pick-up truck or van injured in nontraffic accident NOS

√5th V59.4 Driver of pick-up truck or van injured in collision with other and unspecified motor vehicles in traffic accident

√x7th V59.4Ø Driver of pick-up truck or van injured in collision with unspecified motor vehicles in traffic accident

√x7th V59.49 Driver of pick-up truck or van injured in collision with other motor vehicles in traffic accident

√5th V59.5 Passenger in pick-up truck or van injured in collision with other and unspecified motor vehicles in traffic accident

√x7th V59.5Ø Passenger in pick-up truck or van injured in collision with unspecified motor vehicles in traffic accident

√x7th V59.59 Passenger in pick-up truck or van injured in collision with other motor vehicles in traffic accident

√5th V59.6 Unspecified occupant of pick-up truck or van injured in collision with other and unspecified motor vehicles in traffic accident

√x7th V59.6Ø Unspecified occupant of pick-up truck or van injured in collision with unspecified motor vehicles in traffic accident
Collision NOS involving pick-up truck or van (traffic)

√x7th V59.69 Unspecified occupant of pick-up truck or van injured in collision with other motor vehicles in traffic accident

√5th V59.8 Occupant (driver) (passenger) of pick-up truck or van injured in other specified transport accidents

√x7th V59.81 Occupant (driver) (passenger) of pick-up truck or van injured in transport accident with military vehicle

√x7th V59.88 Occupant (driver) (passenger) of pick-up truck or van injured in other specified transport accidents

√x7th V59.9 Occupant (driver) (passenger) of pick-up truck or van injured in unspecified traffic accident
Accident NOS involving pick-up truck or van

Occupant of heavy transport vehicle injured in transport accident (V6Ø-V69)

INCLUDES 18 wheeler
armored car
panel truck

EXCLUDES 1 *bus*
motorcoach

The appropriate 7th character is to be added to each code from categories V6Ø-V69.
A initial encounter
D subsequent encounter
S sequela

√4th V6Ø Occupant of heavy transport vehicle injured in collision with pedestrian or animal

EXCLUDES 1 *heavy transport vehicle collision with animal-drawn vehicle or animal being ridden (V66.-)*

√x7th V6Ø.Ø Driver of heavy transport vehicle injured in collision with pedestrian or animal in nontraffic accident

√x7th V6Ø.1 Passenger in heavy transport vehicle injured in collision with pedestrian or animal in nontraffic accident

√x7th V6Ø.2 Person on outside of heavy transport vehicle injured in collision with pedestrian or animal in nontraffic accident

√x7th V6Ø.3 Unspecified occupant of heavy transport vehicle injured in collision with pedestrian or animal in nontraffic accident

√x7th V6Ø.4 Person boarding or alighting a heavy transport vehicle injured in collision with pedestrian or animal

√x7th V6Ø.5 Driver of heavy transport vehicle injured in collision with pedestrian or animal in traffic accident

√x7th V6Ø.6 Passenger in heavy transport vehicle injured in collision with pedestrian or animal in traffic accident

√x7th V6Ø.7 Person on outside of heavy transport vehicle injured in collision with pedestrian or animal in traffic accident

√x7th V6Ø.9 Unspecified occupant of heavy transport vehicle injured in collision with pedestrian or animal in traffic accident

√4th V61 Occupant of heavy transport vehicle injured in collision with pedal cycle

√x7th V61.Ø Driver of heavy transport vehicle injured in collision with pedal cycle in nontraffic accident

√x7th V61.1 Passenger in heavy transport vehicle injured in collision with pedal cycle in nontraffic accident

V61.2 Person on outside of heavy transport vehicle injured in collision with pedal cycle in nontraffic accident
V61.3 Unspecified occupant of heavy transport vehicle injured in collision with pedal cycle in nontraffic accident
V61.4 Person boarding or alighting a heavy transport vehicle injured in collision with pedal cycle while boarding or alighting
V61.5 Driver of heavy transport vehicle injured in collision with pedal cycle in traffic accident
V61.6 Passenger in heavy transport vehicle injured in collision with pedal cycle in traffic accident
V61.7 Person on outside of heavy transport vehicle injured in collision with pedal cycle in traffic accident
V61.9 Unspecified occupant of heavy transport vehicle injured in collision with pedal cycle in traffic accident

V62 Occupant of heavy transport vehicle injured in collision with two- or three-wheeled motor vehicle
V62.Ø Driver of heavy transport vehicle injured in collision with two- or three-wheeled motor vehicle in nontraffic accident
V62.1 Passenger in heavy transport vehicle injured in collision with two- or three-wheeled motor vehicle in nontraffic accident
V62.2 Person on outside of heavy transport vehicle injured in collision with two- or three-wheeled motor vehicle in nontraffic accident
V62.3 Unspecified occupant of heavy transport vehicle injured in collision with two- or three-wheeled motor vehicle in nontraffic accident
V62.4 Person boarding or alighting a heavy transport vehicle injured in collision with two- or three-wheeled motor vehicle
V62.5 Driver of heavy transport vehicle injured in collision with two- or three-wheeled motor vehicle in traffic accident
V62.6 Passenger in heavy transport vehicle injured in collision with two- or three-wheeled motor vehicle in traffic accident
V62.7 Person on outside of heavy transport vehicle injured in collision with two- or three-wheeled motor vehicle in traffic accident
V62.9 Unspecified occupant of heavy transport vehicle injured in collision with two- or three-wheeled motor vehicle in traffic accident

V63 Occupant of heavy transport vehicle injured in collision with car, pick-up truck or van
V63.Ø Driver of heavy transport vehicle injured in collision with car, pick-up truck or van in nontraffic accident
V63.1 Passenger in heavy transport vehicle injured in collision with car, pick-up truck or van in nontraffic accident
V63.2 Person on outside of heavy transport vehicle injured in collision with car, pick-up truck or van in nontraffic accident
V63.3 Unspecified occupant of heavy transport vehicle injured in collision with car, pick-up truck or van in nontraffic accident
V63.4 Person boarding or alighting a heavy transport vehicle injured in collision with car, pick-up truck or van
V63.5 Driver of heavy transport vehicle injured in collision with car, pick-up truck or van in traffic accident
V63.6 Passenger in heavy transport vehicle injured in collision with car, pick-up truck or van in traffic accident
V63.7 Person on outside of heavy transport vehicle injured in collision with car, pick-up truck or van in traffic accident
V63.9 Unspecified occupant of heavy transport vehicle injured in collision with car, pick-up truck or van in traffic accident

V64 Occupant of heavy transport vehicle injured in collision with heavy transport vehicle or bus
EXCLUDES 1 *occupant of heavy transport vehicle injured in collision with military vehicle (V69.81)*
V64.Ø Driver of heavy transport vehicle injured in collision with heavy transport vehicle or bus in nontraffic accident
V64.1 Passenger in heavy transport vehicle injured in collision with heavy transport vehicle or bus in nontraffic accident
V64.2 Person on outside of heavy transport vehicle injured in collision with heavy transport vehicle or bus in nontraffic accident
V64.3 Unspecified occupant of heavy transport vehicle injured in collision with heavy transport vehicle or bus in nontraffic accident
V64.4 Person boarding or alighting a heavy transport vehicle injured in collision with heavy transport vehicle or bus while boarding or alighting
V64.5 Driver of heavy transport vehicle injured in collision with heavy transport vehicle or bus in traffic accident
V64.6 Passenger in heavy transport vehicle injured in collision with heavy transport vehicle or bus in traffic accident
V64.7 Person on outside of heavy transport vehicle injured in collision with heavy transport vehicle or bus in traffic accident
V64.9 Unspecified occupant of heavy transport vehicle injured in collision with heavy transport vehicle or bus in traffic accident

V65 Occupant of heavy transport vehicle injured in collision with railway train or railway vehicle
V65.Ø Driver of heavy transport vehicle injured in collision with railway train or railway vehicle in nontraffic accident
V65.1 Passenger in heavy transport vehicle injured in collision with railway train or railway vehicle in nontraffic accident
V65.2 Person on outside of heavy transport vehicle injured in collision with railway train or railway vehicle in nontraffic accident
V65.3 Unspecified occupant of heavy transport vehicle injured in collision with railway train or railway vehicle in nontraffic accident
V65.4 Person boarding or alighting a heavy transport vehicle injured in collision with railway train or railway vehicle
V65.5 Driver of heavy transport vehicle injured in collision with railway train or railway vehicle in traffic accident
V65.6 Passenger in heavy transport vehicle injured in collision with railway train or railway vehicle in traffic accident
V65.7 Person on outside of heavy transport vehicle injured in collision with railway train or railway vehicle in traffic accident
V65.9 Unspecified occupant of heavy transport vehicle injured in collision with railway train or railway vehicle in traffic accident

V66 Occupant of heavy transport vehicle injured in collision with other nonmotor vehicle
INCLUDES collision with animal-drawn vehicle, animal being ridden, streetcar
V66.Ø Driver of heavy transport vehicle injured in collision with other nonmotor vehicle in nontraffic accident
V66.1 Passenger in heavy transport vehicle injured in collision with other nonmotor vehicle in nontraffic accident
V66.2 Person on outside of heavy transport vehicle injured in collision with other nonmotor vehicle in nontraffic accident
V66.3 Unspecified occupant of heavy transport vehicle injured in collision with other nonmotor vehicle in nontraffic accident
V66.4 Person boarding or alighting a heavy transport vehicle injured in collision with other nonmotor vehicle
V66.5 Driver of heavy transport vehicle injured in collision with other nonmotor vehicle in traffic accident
V66.6 Passenger in heavy transport vehicle injured in collision with other nonmotor vehicle in traffic accident
V66.7 Person on outside of heavy transport vehicle injured in collision with other nonmotor vehicle in traffic accident
V66.9 Unspecified occupant of heavy transport vehicle injured in collision with other nonmotor vehicle in traffic accident

V67 Occupant of heavy transport vehicle injured in collision with fixed or stationary object
V67.Ø Driver of heavy transport vehicle injured in collision with fixed or stationary object in nontraffic accident
V67.1 Passenger in heavy transport vehicle injured in collision with fixed or stationary object in nontraffic accident
V67.2 Person on outside of heavy transport vehicle injured in collision with fixed or stationary object in nontraffic accident
V67.3 Unspecified occupant of heavy transport vehicle injured in collision with fixed or stationary object in nontraffic accident
V67.4 Person boarding or alighting a heavy transport vehicle injured in collision with fixed or stationary object
V67.5 Driver of heavy transport vehicle injured in collision with fixed or stationary object in traffic accident
V67.6 Passenger in heavy transport vehicle injured in collision with fixed or stationary object in traffic accident
V67.7 Person on outside of heavy transport vehicle injured in collision with fixed or stationary object in traffic accident
V67.9 Unspecified occupant of heavy transport vehicle injured in collision with fixed or stationary object in traffic accident

V68 Occupant of heavy transport vehicle injured in noncollision transport accident
INCLUDES overturning heavy transport vehicle NOS
overturning heavy transport vehicle without collision
V68.Ø Driver of heavy transport vehicle injured in noncollision transport accident in nontraffic accident
V68.1 Passenger in heavy transport vehicle injured in noncollision transport accident in nontraffic accident

√x7th **V68.2 Person on outside of heavy transport vehicle injured in noncollision transport accident in nontraffic accident**

√x7th **V68.3 Unspecified occupant of heavy transport vehicle injured in noncollision transport accident in nontraffic accident**

√x7th **V68.4 Person boarding or alighting a heavy transport vehicle injured in noncollision transport accident**

√x7th **V68.5 Driver of heavy transport vehicle injured in noncollision transport accident in traffic accident**

√x7th **V68.6 Passenger in heavy transport vehicle injured in noncollision transport accident in traffic accident**

√x7th **V68.7 Person on outside of heavy transport vehicle injured in noncollision transport accident in traffic accident**

√x7th **V68.9 Unspecified occupant of heavy transport vehicle injured in noncollision transport accident in traffic accident**

√4th **V69 Occupant of heavy transport vehicle injured in other and unspecified transport accidents**

√5th **V69.0 Driver of heavy transport vehicle injured in collision with other and unspecified motor vehicles in nontraffic accident**

√x7th **V69.00 Driver of heavy transport vehicle injured in collision with unspecified motor vehicles in nontraffic accident**

√x7th **V69.09 Driver of heavy transport vehicle injured in collision with other motor vehicles in nontraffic accident**

√5th **V69.1 Passenger in heavy transport vehicle injured in collision with other and unspecified motor vehicles in nontraffic accident**

√x7th **V69.10 Passenger in heavy transport vehicle injured in collision with unspecified motor vehicles in nontraffic accident**

√x7th **V69.19 Passenger in heavy transport vehicle injured in collision with other motor vehicles in nontraffic accident**

√5th **V69.2 Unspecified occupant of heavy transport vehicle injured in collision with other and unspecified motor vehicles in nontraffic accident**

√x7th **V69.20 Unspecified occupant of heavy transport vehicle injured in collision with unspecified motor vehicles in nontraffic accident**

Collision NOS involving heavy transport vehicle, nontraffic

√x7th **V69.29 Unspecified occupant of heavy transport vehicle injured in collision with other motor vehicles in nontraffic accident**

√x7th **V69.3 Occupant (driver) (passenger) of heavy transport vehicle injured in unspecified nontraffic accident**

Accident NOS involving heavy transport vehicle, nontraffic
Occupant of heavy transport vehicle injured in nontraffic accident NOS

√5th **V69.4 Driver of heavy transport vehicle injured in collision with other and unspecified motor vehicles in traffic accident**

√x7th **V69.40 Driver of heavy transport vehicle injured in collision with unspecified motor vehicles in traffic accident**

√x7th **V69.49 Driver of heavy transport vehicle injured in collision with other motor vehicles in traffic accident**

√5th **V69.5 Passenger in heavy transport vehicle injured in collision with other and unspecified motor vehicles in traffic accident**

√x7th **V69.50 Passenger in heavy transport vehicle injured in collision with unspecified motor vehicles in traffic accident**

√x7th **V69.59 Passenger in heavy transport vehicle injured in collision with other motor vehicles in traffic accident**

√5th **V69.6 Unspecified occupant of heavy transport vehicle injured in collision with other and unspecified motor vehicles in traffic accident**

√x7th **V69.60 Unspecified occupant of heavy transport vehicle injured in collision with unspecified motor vehicles in traffic accident**

Collision NOS involving heavy transport vehicle (traffic)

√x7th **V69.69 Unspecified occupant of heavy transport vehicle injured in collision with other motor vehicles in traffic accident**

√5th **V69.8 Occupant (driver) (passenger) of heavy transport vehicle injured in other specified transport accidents**

√x7th **V69.81 Occupant (driver) (passenger) of heavy transport vehicle injured in transport accidents with military vehicle**

√x7th **V69.88 Occupant (driver) (passenger) of heavy transport vehicle injured in other specified transport accidents**

√x7th **V69.9 Occupant (driver) (passenger) of heavy transport vehicle injured in unspecified traffic accident**

Accident NOS involving heavy transport vehicle

Bus occupant injured in transport accident (V70-V79)

INCLUDES motorcoach

EXCLUDES 1 *minibus (V50-V59)*

The appropriate 7th character is to be added to each code from categories V70-V79.
A initial encounter
D subsequent encounter
S sequela

√4th **V70 Bus occupant injured in collision with pedestrian or animal**

EXCLUDES 1 *bus collision with animal-drawn vehicle or animal being ridden (V76.-)*

√x7th **V70.0 Driver of bus injured in collision with pedestrian or animal in nontraffic accident**

√x7th **V70.1 Passenger on bus injured in collision with pedestrian or animal in nontraffic accident**

√x7th **V70.2 Person on outside of bus injured in collision with pedestrian or animal in nontraffic accident**

√x7th **V70.3 Unspecified occupant of bus injured in collision with pedestrian or animal in nontraffic accident**

√x7th **V70.4 Person boarding or alighting from bus injured in collision with pedestrian or animal**

√x7th **V70.5 Driver of bus injured in collision with pedestrian or animal in traffic accident**

√x7th **V70.6 Passenger on bus injured in collision with pedestrian or animal in traffic accident**

√x7th **V70.7 Person on outside of bus injured in collision with pedestrian or animal in traffic accident**

√x7th **V70.9 Unspecified occupant of bus injured in collision with pedestrian or animal in traffic accident**

√4th **V71 Bus occupant injured in collision with pedal cycle**

√x7th **V71.0 Driver of bus injured in collision with pedal cycle in nontraffic accident**

√x7th **V71.1 Passenger on bus injured in collision with pedal cycle in nontraffic accident**

√x7th **V71.2 Person on outside of bus injured in collision with pedal cycle in nontraffic accident**

√x7th **V71.3 Unspecified occupant of bus injured in collision with pedal cycle in nontraffic accident**

√x7th **V71.4 Person boarding or alighting from bus injured in collision with pedal cycle**

√x7th **V71.5 Driver of bus injured in collision with pedal cycle in traffic accident**

√x7th **V71.6 Passenger on bus injured in collision with pedal cycle in traffic accident**

√x7th **V71.7 Person on outside of bus injured in collision with pedal cycle in traffic accident**

√x7th **V71.9 Unspecified occupant of bus injured in collision with pedal cycle in traffic accident**

√4th **V72 Bus occupant injured in collision with two- or three-wheeled motor vehicle**

√x7th **V72.0 Driver of bus injured in collision with two- or three-wheeled motor vehicle in nontraffic accident**

√x7th **V72.1 Passenger on bus injured in collision with two- or three-wheeled motor vehicle in nontraffic accident**

√x7th **V72.2 Person on outside of bus injured in collision with two- or three-wheeled motor vehicle in nontraffic accident**

√x7th **V72.3 Unspecified occupant of bus injured in collision with two- or three-wheeled motor vehicle in nontraffic accident**

√x7th **V72.4 Person boarding or alighting from bus injured in collision with two- or three-wheeled motor vehicle**

√x7th **V72.5 Driver of bus injured in collision with two- or three-wheeled motor vehicle in traffic accident**

√x7th **V72.6 Passenger on bus injured in collision with two- or three-wheeled motor vehicle in traffic accident**

√x7th **V72.7 Person on outside of bus injured in collision with two- or three-wheeled motor vehicle in traffic accident**

√x7th **V72.9 Unspecified occupant of bus injured in collision with two- or three-wheeled motor vehicle in traffic accident**

√4th **V73 Bus occupant injured in collision with car, pick-up truck or van**

√x7th **V73.0 Driver of bus injured in collision with car, pick-up truck or van in nontraffic accident**

√x7th **V73.1 Passenger on bus injured in collision with car, pick-up truck or van in nontraffic accident**

√x7th **V73.2 Person on outside of bus injured in collision with car, pick-up truck or van in nontraffic accident**

- V73.3 Unspecified occupant of bus injured in collision with car, pick-up truck or van in nontraffic accident
- V73.4 Person boarding or alighting from bus injured in collision with car, pick-up truck or van
- V73.5 Driver of bus injured in collision with car, pick-up truck or van in traffic accident
- V73.6 Passenger on bus injured in collision with car, pick-up truck or van in traffic accident
- V73.7 Person on outside of bus injured in collision with car, pick-up truck or van in traffic accident
- V73.9 Unspecified occupant of bus injured in collision with car, pick-up truck or van in traffic accident

V74 Bus occupant injured in collision with heavy transport vehicle or bus

EXCLUDES 1 *bus occupant injured in collision with military vehicle (V79.81)*

- V74.0 Driver of bus injured in collision with heavy transport vehicle or bus in nontraffic accident
- V74.1 Passenger on bus injured in collision with heavy transport vehicle or bus in nontraffic accident
- V74.2 Person on outside of bus injured in collision with heavy transport vehicle or bus in nontraffic accident
- V74.3 Unspecified occupant of bus injured in collision with heavy transport vehicle or bus in nontraffic accident
- V74.4 Person boarding or alighting from bus injured in collision with heavy transport vehicle or bus
- V74.5 Driver of bus injured in collision with heavy transport vehicle or bus in traffic accident
- V74.6 Passenger on bus injured in collision with heavy transport vehicle or bus in traffic accident
- V74.7 Person on outside of bus injured in collision with heavy transport vehicle or bus in traffic accident
- V74.9 Unspecified occupant of bus injured in collision with heavy transport vehicle or bus in traffic accident

V75 Bus occupant injured in collision with railway train or railway vehicle

- V75.0 Driver of bus injured in collision with railway train or railway vehicle in nontraffic accident
- V75.1 Passenger on bus injured in collision with railway train or railway vehicle in nontraffic accident
- V75.2 Person on outside of bus injured in collision with railway train or railway vehicle in nontraffic accident
- V75.3 Unspecified occupant of bus injured in collision with railway train or railway vehicle in nontraffic accident
- V75.4 Person boarding or alighting from bus injured in collision with railway train or railway vehicle
- V75.5 Driver of bus injured in collision with railway train or railway vehicle in traffic accident
- V75.6 Passenger on bus injured in collision with railway train or railway vehicle in traffic accident
- V75.7 Person on outside of bus injured in collision with railway train or railway vehicle in traffic accident
- V75.9 Unspecified occupant of bus injured in collision with railway train or railway vehicle in traffic accident

V76 Bus occupant injured in collision with other nonmotor vehicle

INCLUDES collision with animal-drawn vehicle, animal being ridden, streetcar

- V76.0 Driver of bus injured in collision with other nonmotor vehicle in nontraffic accident
- V76.1 Passenger on bus injured in collision with other nonmotor vehicle in nontraffic accident
- V76.2 Person on outside of bus injured in collision with other nonmotor vehicle in nontraffic accident
- V76.3 Unspecified occupant of bus injured in collision with other nonmotor vehicle in nontraffic accident
- V76.4 Person boarding or alighting from bus injured in collision with other nonmotor vehicle
- V76.5 Driver of bus injured in collision with other nonmotor vehicle in traffic accident
- V76.6 Passenger on bus injured in collision with other nonmotor vehicle in traffic accident
- V76.7 Person on outside of bus injured in collision with other nonmotor vehicle in traffic accident
- V76.9 Unspecified occupant of bus injured in collision with other nonmotor vehicle in traffic accident

V77 Bus occupant injured in collision with fixed or stationary object

- V77.0 Driver of bus injured in collision with fixed or stationary object in nontraffic accident
- V77.1 Passenger on bus injured in collision with fixed or stationary object in nontraffic accident
- V77.2 Person on outside of bus injured in collision with fixed or stationary object in nontraffic accident
- V77.3 Unspecified occupant of bus injured in collision with fixed or stationary object in nontraffic accident
- V77.4 Person boarding or alighting from bus injured in collision with fixed or stationary object
- V77.5 Driver of bus injured in collision with fixed or stationary object in traffic accident
- V77.6 Passenger on bus injured in collision with fixed or stationary object in traffic accident
- V77.7 Person on outside of bus injured in collision with fixed or stationary object in traffic accident
- V77.9 Unspecified occupant of bus injured in collision with fixed or stationary object in traffic accident

V78 Bus occupant injured in noncollision transport accident

INCLUDES overturning bus NOS
overturning bus without collision

- V78.0 Driver of bus injured in noncollision transport accident in nontraffic accident
- V78.1 Passenger on bus injured in noncollision transport accident in nontraffic accident
- V78.2 Person on outside of bus injured in noncollision transport accident in nontraffic accident
- V78.3 Unspecified occupant of bus injured in noncollision transport accident in nontraffic accident
- V78.4 Person boarding or alighting from bus injured in noncollision transport accident
- V78.5 Driver of bus injured in noncollision transport accident in traffic accident
- V78.6 Passenger on bus injured in noncollision transport accident in traffic accident
- V78.7 Person on outside of bus injured in noncollision transport accident in traffic accident
- V78.9 Unspecified occupant of bus injured in noncollision transport accident in traffic accident

V79 Bus occupant injured in other and unspecified transport accidents

- V79.0 Driver of bus injured in collision with other and unspecified motor vehicles in nontraffic accident
  - V79.00 Driver of bus injured in collision with unspecified motor vehicles in nontraffic accident
  - V79.09 Driver of bus injured in collision with other motor vehicles in nontraffic accident
- V79.1 Passenger on bus injured in collision with other and unspecified motor vehicles in nontraffic accident
  - V79.10 Passenger on bus injured in collision with unspecified motor vehicles in nontraffic accident
  - V79.19 Passenger on bus injured in collision with other motor vehicles in nontraffic accident
- V79.2 Unspecified bus occupant injured in collision with other and unspecified motor vehicles in nontraffic accident
  - V79.20 Unspecified bus occupant injured in collision with unspecified motor vehicles in nontraffic accident
    Bus collision NOS, nontraffic
  - V79.29 Unspecified bus occupant injured in collision with other motor vehicles in nontraffic accident
- V79.3 Bus occupant (driver) (passenger) injured in unspecified nontraffic accident
  Bus accident NOS, nontraffic
  Bus occupant injured in nontraffic accident NOS
- V79.4 Driver of bus injured in collision with other and unspecified motor vehicles in traffic accident
  - V79.40 Driver of bus injured in collision with unspecified motor vehicles in traffic accident
  - V79.49 Driver of bus injured in collision with other motor vehicles in traffic accident
- V79.5 Passenger on bus injured in collision with other and unspecified motor vehicles in traffic accident
  - V79.50 Passenger on bus injured in collision with unspecified motor vehicles in traffic accident
  - V79.59 Passenger on bus injured in collision with other motor vehicles in traffic accident
- V79.6 Unspecified bus occupant injured in collision with other and unspecified motor vehicles in traffic accident
  - V79.60 Unspecified bus occupant injured in collision with unspecified motor vehicles in traffic accident
    Bus collision NOS (traffic)
  - V79.69 Unspecified bus occupant injured in collision with other motor vehicles in traffic accident

✓5th **V79.8 Bus occupant (driver) (passenger) injured in other specified transport accidents**

✓x7th **V79.81 Bus occupant (driver) (passenger) injured in transport accidents with military vehicle**

✓x7th **V79.88 Bus occupant (driver) (passenger) injured in other specified transport accidents**

✓x7th **V79.9 Bus occupant (driver) (passenger) injured in unspecified traffic accident**
Bus accident NOS

Other land transport accidents (V80-V89)

The appropriate 7th character is to be added to each code from categories V80-V89.
A initial encounter
D subsequent encounter
S sequela

✓4th **V80 Animal-rider or occupant of animal-drawn vehicle injured in transport accident**

✓5th **V80.0 Animal-rider or occupant of animal drawn vehicle injured by fall from or being thrown from animal or animal-drawn vehicle in noncollision accident**

✓6th **V80.01 Animal-rider injured by fall from or being thrown from animal in noncollision accident**

✓7th **V80.010 Animal-rider injured by fall from or being thrown from horse in noncollision accident**

✓7th **V80.018 Animal-rider injured by fall from or being thrown from other animal in noncollision accident**

✓x7th **V80.02 Occupant of animal-drawn vehicle injured by fall from or being thrown from animal-drawn vehicle in noncollision accident**
Overturning animal-drawn vehicle NOS
Overturning animal-drawn vehicle without collision

✓5th **V80.1 Animal-rider or occupant of animal-drawn vehicle injured in collision with pedestrian or animal**
EXCLUDES 1 *animal-rider or animal-drawn vehicle collision with animal-drawn vehicle or animal being ridden (V80.7)*

✓x7th **V80.11 Animal-rider injured in collision with pedestrian or animal**

✓x7th **V80.12 Occupant of animal-drawn vehicle injured in collision with pedestrian or animal**

✓5th **V80.2 Animal-rider or occupant of animal-drawn vehicle injured in collision with pedal cycle**

✓x7th **V80.21 Animal-rider injured in collision with pedal cycle**

✓x7th **V80.22 Occupant of animal-drawn vehicle injured in collision with pedal cycle**

✓5th **V80.3 Animal-rider or occupant of animal-drawn vehicle injured in collision with two- or three-wheeled motor vehicle**

✓x7th **V80.31 Animal-rider injured in collision with two- or three-wheeled motor vehicle**

✓x7th **V80.32 Occupant of animal-drawn vehicle injured in collision with two- or three-wheeled motor vehicle**

✓5th **V80.4 Animal-rider or occupant of animal-drawn vehicle injured in collision with car, pick-up truck, van, heavy transport vehicle or bus**
EXCLUDES 1 *animal-rider injured in collision with military vehicle (V80.910)*
occupant of animal-drawn vehicle injured in collision with military vehicle (V80.920)

✓x7th **V80.41 Animal-rider injured in collision with car, pick-up truck, van, heavy transport vehicle or bus**

✓x7th **V80.42 Occupant of animal-drawn vehicle injured in collision with car, pick-up truck, van, heavy transport vehicle or bus**

✓5th **V80.5 Animal-rider or occupant of animal-drawn vehicle injured in collision with other specified motor vehicle**

✓x7th **V80.51 Animal-rider injured in collision with other specified motor vehicle**

✓x7th **V80.52 Occupant of animal-drawn vehicle injured in collision with other specified motor vehicle**

✓5th **V80.6 Animal-rider or occupant of animal-drawn vehicle injured in collision with railway train or railway vehicle**

✓x7th **V80.61 Animal-rider injured in collision with railway train or railway vehicle**

✓x7th **V80.62 Occupant of animal-drawn vehicle injured in collision with railway train or railway vehicle**

✓5th **V80.7 Animal-rider or occupant of animal-drawn vehicle injured in collision with other nonmotor vehicles**

✓6th **V80.71 Animal-rider or occupant of animal-drawn vehicle injured in collision with animal being ridden**

✓7th **V80.710 Animal-rider injured in collision with other animal being ridden**

✓7th **V80.711 Occupant of animal-drawn vehicle injured in collision with animal being ridden**

✓6th **V80.72 Animal-rider or occupant of animal-drawn vehicle injured in collision with other animal-drawn vehicle**

✓7th **V80.720 Animal-rider injured in collision with animal-drawn vehicle**

✓7th **V80.721 Occupant of animal-drawn vehicle injured in collision with other animal-drawn vehicle**

✓6th **V80.73 Animal-rider or occupant of animal-drawn vehicle injured in collision with streetcar**

✓7th **V80.730 Animal-rider injured in collision with streetcar**

✓7th **V80.731 Occupant of animal-drawn vehicle injured in collision with streetcar**

✓6th **V80.79 Animal-rider or occupant of animal-drawn vehicle injured in collision with other nonmotor vehicles**

✓7th **V80.790 Animal-rider injured in collision with other nonmotor vehicles**

✓7th **V80.791 Occupant of animal-drawn vehicle injured in collision with other nonmotor vehicles**

✓5th **V80.8 Animal-rider or occupant of animal-drawn vehicle injured in collision with fixed or stationary object**

✓x7th **V80.81 Animal-rider injured in collision with fixed or stationary object**

✓x7th **V80.82 Occupant of animal-drawn vehicle injured in collision with fixed or stationary object**

✓5th **V80.9 Animal-rider or occupant of animal-drawn vehicle injured in other and unspecified transport accidents**

✓6th **V80.91 Animal-rider injured in other and unspecified transport accidents**

✓7th **V80.910 Animal-rider injured in transport accident with military vehicle**

✓7th **V80.918 Animal-rider injured in other transport accident**

✓7th **V80.919 Animal-rider injured in unspecified transport accident**
Animal rider accident NOS

✓6th **V80.92 Occupant of animal-drawn vehicle injured in other and unspecified transport accidents**

✓7th **V80.920 Occupant of animal-drawn vehicle injured in transport accident with military vehicle**

✓7th **V80.928 Occupant of animal-drawn vehicle injured in other transport accident**

✓7th **V80.929 Occupant of animal-drawn vehicle injured in unspecified transport accident**
Animal-drawn vehicle accident NOS

✓4th **V81 Occupant of railway train or railway vehicle injured in transport accident**
INCLUDES derailment of railway train or railway vehicle
person on outside of train
EXCLUDES 1 *streetcar (V82.-)*

✓x7th **V81.0 Occupant of railway train or railway vehicle injured in collision with motor vehicle in nontraffic accident**
EXCLUDES 1 *occupant of railway train or railway vehicle injured due to collision with military vehicle (V81.83)*

✓x7th **V81.1 Occupant of railway train or railway vehicle injured in collision with motor vehicle in traffic accident**
EXCLUDES 1 *occupant of railway train or railway vehicle injured due to collision with military vehicle (V81.83)*

✓x7th **V81.2 Occupant of railway train or railway vehicle injured in collision with or hit by rolling stock**

✓x7th **V81.3 Occupant of railway train or railway vehicle injured in collision with other object**
Railway collision NOS

✓x7th **V81.4 Person injured while boarding or alighting from railway train or railway vehicle**

✓x7th **V81.5 Occupant of railway train or railway vehicle injured by fall in railway train or railway vehicle**

✓x7th **V81.6 Occupant of railway train or railway vehicle injured by fall from railway train or railway vehicle**

✓x7th **V81.7 Occupant of railway train or railway vehicle injured in derailment without antecedent collision**

V81.8 **Occupant of railway train or railway vehicle injured in other specified railway accidents**

V81.81 **Occupant of railway train or railway vehicle injured due to explosion or fire on train**

V81.82 **Occupant of railway train or railway vehicle injured due to object falling onto train**

Occupant of railway train or railway vehicle injured due to falling earth onto train

Occupant of railway train or railway vehicle injured due to falling rocks onto train

Occupant of railway train or railway vehicle injured due to falling snow onto train

Occupant of railway train or railway vehicle injured due to falling trees onto train

V81.83 **Occupant of railway train or railway vehicle injured due to collision with military vehicle**

V81.89 **Occupant of railway train or railway vehicle injured due to other specified railway accident**

V81.9 **Occupant of railway train or railway vehicle injured in unspecified railway accident**

Railway accident NOS

V82 Occupant of powered streetcar injured in transport accident

INCLUDES interurban electric car
person on outside of streetcar
tram (car)
trolley (car)

EXCLUDES 1 *bus (V70-V79)*
motorcoach (V70-V79)
nonpowered streetcar (V76.-)
train (V81.-)

V82.0 **Occupant of streetcar injured in collision with motor vehicle in nontraffic accident**

V82.1 **Occupant of streetcar injured in collision with motor vehicle in traffic accident**

V82.2 **Occupant of streetcar injured in collision with or hit by rolling stock**

V82.3 **Occupant of streetcar injured in collision with other object**

EXCLUDES 1 *collision with animal-drawn vehicle or animal being ridden (V82.8)*

V82.4 **Person injured while boarding or alighting from streetcar**

V82.5 **Occupant of streetcar injured by fall in streetcar**

EXCLUDES 1 *fall in streetcar:*
while boarding or alighting (V82.4)
with antecedent collision (V82.0-V82.3)

V82.6 **Occupant of streetcar injured by fall from streetcar**

EXCLUDES 1 *fall from streetcar:*
while boarding or alighting (V82.4)
with antecedent collision (V82.0-V82.3)

V82.7 **Occupant of streetcar injured in derailment without antecedent collision**

EXCLUDES 1 *occupant of streetcar injured in derailment with antecedent collision (V82.0-V82.3)*

V82.8 **Occupant of streetcar injured in other specified transport accidents**

Streetcar collision with military vehicle
Streetcar collision with train or nonmotor vehicles

V82.9 **Occupant of streetcar injured in unspecified traffic accident**

Streetcar accident NOS

V83 Occupant of special vehicle mainly used on industrial premises injured in transport accident

INCLUDES battery-powered airport passenger vehicle
battery-powered truck (baggage) (mail)
coal-car in mine
forklift (truck)
logging car
self-propelled industrial truck
station baggage truck (powered)
tram, truck, or tub (powered) in mine or quarry

EXCLUDES 1 *special construction vehicles (V85.-)*
special industrial vehicle in stationary use or maintenance (W31.-)

V83.0 **Driver of special industrial vehicle injured in traffic accident**

V83.1 **Passenger of special industrial vehicle injured in traffic accident**

V83.2 **Person on outside of special industrial vehicle injured in traffic accident**

V83.3 **Unspecified occupant of special industrial vehicle injured in traffic accident**

V83.4 **Person injured while boarding or alighting from special industrial vehicle**

V83.5 **Driver of special industrial vehicle injured in nontraffic accident**

V83.6 **Passenger of special industrial vehicle injured in nontraffic accident**

V83.7 **Person on outside of special industrial vehicle injured in nontraffic accident**

V83.9 **Unspecified occupant of special industrial vehicle injured in nontraffic accident**

Special-industrial-vehicle accident NOS

V84 Occupant of special vehicle mainly used in agriculture injured in transport accident

INCLUDES self-propelled farm machinery
tractor (and trailer)

EXCLUDES 1 *animal-powered farm machinery accident (W30.8-)*
contact with combine harvester (W30.0)
special agricultural vehicle in stationary use or maintenance (W30.-)

V84.0 **Driver of special agricultural vehicle injured in traffic accident**

V84.1 **Passenger of special agricultural vehicle injured in traffic accident**

V84.2 **Person on outside of special agricultural vehicle injured in traffic accident**

V84.3 **Unspecified occupant of special agricultural vehicle injured in traffic accident**

V84.4 **Person injured while boarding or alighting from special agricultural vehicle**

V84.5 **Driver of special agricultural vehicle injured in nontraffic accident**

V84.6 **Passenger of special agricultural vehicle injured in nontraffic accident**

V84.7 **Person on outside of special agricultural vehicle injured in nontraffic accident**

V84.9 **Unspecified occupant of special agricultural vehicle injured in nontraffic accident**

Special-agricultural vehicle accident NOS

V85 Occupant of special construction vehicle injured in transport accident

INCLUDES bulldozer
digger
dump truck
earth-leveller
mechanical shovel
road-roller

EXCLUDES 1 *special industrial vehicle (V83.-)*
special construction vehicle in stationary use or maintenance (W31.-)

V85.0 **Driver of special construction vehicle injured in traffic accident**

V85.1 **Passenger of special construction vehicle injured in traffic accident**

V85.2 **Person on outside of special construction vehicle injured in traffic accident**

V85.3 **Unspecified occupant of special construction vehicle injured in traffic accident**

V85.4 **Person injured while boarding or alighting from special construction vehicle**

V85.5 **Driver of special construction vehicle injured in nontraffic accident**

V85.6 **Passenger of special construction vehicle injured in nontraffic accident**

V85.7 **Person on outside of special construction vehicle injured in nontraffic accident**

V85.9 **Unspecified occupant of special construction vehicle injured in nontraffic accident**

Special-construction-vehicle accident NOS

✓4th **V86 Occupant of special all-terrain or other off-road motor vehicle, injured in transport accident**

EXCLUDES 1 *special all-terrain vehicle in stationary use or maintenance (W31.-)*
sport-utility vehicle (V5Ø-V59)
three-wheeled motor vehicle designed for on-road use (V3Ø-V39)

AHA: 2017,4Q,26

✓5th **V86.Ø Driver of special all-terrain or other off-road motor vehicle injured in traffic accident**

✓x7th **V86.Ø1 Driver of ambulance or fire engine injured in traffic accident**

✓x7th **V86.Ø2 Driver of snowmobile injured in traffic accident**

✓x7th **V86.Ø3 Driver of dune buggy injured in traffic accident**

✓x7th **V86.Ø4 Driver of military vehicle injured in traffic accident**

✓x7th **V86.Ø5 Driver of 3- or 4- wheeled all-terrain vehicle (ATV) injured in traffic accident**

✓x7th **V86.Ø6 Driver of dirt bike or motor/cross bike injured in traffic accident**

✓x7th **V86.Ø9 Driver of other special all-terrain or other off-road motor vehicle injured in traffic accident**
Driver of go cart injured in traffic accident
Driver of golf cart injured in traffic accident

✓5th **V86.1 Passenger of special all-terrain or other off-road motor vehicle injured in traffic accident**

✓x7th **V86.11 Passenger of ambulance or fire engine injured in traffic accident**

✓x7th **V86.12 Passenger of snowmobile injured in traffic accident**

✓x7th **V86.13 Passenger of dune buggy injured in traffic accident**

✓x7th **V86.14 Passenger of military vehicle injured in traffic accident**

✓x7th **V86.15 Passenger of 3- or 4- wheeled all-terrain vehicle (ATV) injured in traffic accident**

✓x7th **V86.16 Passenger of dirt bike or motor/cross bike injured in traffic accident**

✓x7th **V86.19 Passenger of other special all-terrain or other off-road motor vehicle injured in traffic accident**
Passenger of go cart injured in traffic accident
Passenger of golf cart injured in traffic accident

✓5th **V86.2 Person on outside of special all-terrain or other off-road motor vehicle injured in traffic accident**

✓x7th **V86.21 Person on outside of ambulance or fire engine injured in traffic accident**

✓x7th **V86.22 Person on outside of snowmobile injured in traffic accident**

✓x7th **V86.23 Person on outside of dune buggy injured in traffic accident**

✓x7th **V86.24 Person on outside of military vehicle injured in traffic accident**

✓x7th **V86.25 Person on outside of 3- or 4- wheeled all-terrain vehicle (ATV) injured in traffic accident**

✓x7th **V86.26 Person on outside of dirt bike or motor/cross bike injured in traffic accident**

✓x7th **V86.29 Person on outside of other special all-terrain or other off-road motor vehicle injured in traffic accident**
Person on outside of go cart in traffic accident
Person on outside of golf cart injured in traffic accident

✓5th **V86.3 Unspecified occupant of special all-terrain or other off-road motor vehicle injured in traffic accident**

✓x7th **V86.31 Unspecified occupant of ambulance or fire engine injured in traffic accident**

✓x7th **V86.32 Unspecified occupant of snowmobile injured in traffic accident**

✓x7th **V86.33 Unspecified occupant of dune buggy injured in traffic accident**

✓x7th **V86.34 Unspecified occupant of military vehicle injured in traffic accident**

✓x7th **V86.35 Unspecified occupant of 3- or 4- wheeled all-terrain vehicle (ATV) injured in traffic accident**

✓x7th **V86.36 Unspecified occupant of dirt bike or motor/cross bike injured in traffic accident**

✓x7th **V86.39 Unspecified occupant of other special all-terrain or other off-road motor vehicle injured in traffic accident**
Unspecified occupant of go cart injured in traffic accident
Unspecified occupant of golf cart injured in traffic accident

✓5th **V86.4 Person injured while boarding or alighting from special all-terrain or other off-road motor vehicle**

✓x7th **V86.41 Person injured while boarding or alighting from ambulance or fire engine**

✓x7th **V86.42 Person injured while boarding or alighting from snowmobile**

✓x7th **V86.43 Person injured while boarding or alighting from dune buggy**

✓x7th **V86.44 Person injured while boarding or alighting from military vehicle**

✓x7th **V86.45 Person injured while boarding or alighting from a 3- or 4- wheeled all-terrain vehicle (ATV)**

✓x7th **V86.46 Person injured while boarding or alighting from a dirt bike or motor/cross bike**

✓x7th **V86.49 Person injured while boarding or alighting from other special all-terrain or other off-road motor vehicle**
Person injured while boarding or alighting from go cart
Person injured while boarding or alighting from golf cart

✓5th **V86.5 Driver of special all-terrain or other off-road motor vehicle injured in nontraffic accident**

✓x7th **V86.51 Driver of ambulance or fire engine injured in nontraffic accident**

✓x7th **V86.52 Driver of snowmobile injured in nontraffic accident**

✓x7th **V86.53 Driver of dune buggy injured in nontraffic accident**

✓x7th **V86.54 Driver of military vehicle injured in nontraffic accident**

✓x7th **V86.55 Driver of 3- or 4- wheeled all-terrain vehicle (ATV) injured in nontraffic accident**

✓x7th **V86.56 Driver of dirt bike or motor/cross bike injured in nontraffic accident**

✓x7th **V86.59 Driver of other special all-terrain or other off-road motor vehicle injured in nontraffic accident**
Driver of go cart injured in nontraffic accident
Driver of golf cart injured in nontraffic accident

✓5th **V86.6 Passenger of special all-terrain or other off-road motor vehicle injured in nontraffic accident**

✓x7th **V86.61 Passenger of ambulance or fire engine injured in nontraffic accident**

✓x7th **V86.62 Passenger of snowmobile injured in nontraffic accident**

✓x7th **V86.63 Passenger of dune buggy injured in nontraffic accident**

✓x7th **V86.64 Passenger of military vehicle injured in nontraffic accident**

✓x7th **V86.65 Passenger of 3- or 4- wheeled all-terrain vehicle (ATV) injured in nontraffic accident**

✓x7th **V86.66 Passenger of dirt bike or motor/cross bike injured in nontraffic accident**

✓x7th **V86.69 Passenger of other special all-terrain or other off-road motor vehicle injured in nontraffic accident**
Passenger of go cart injured in nontraffic accident
Passenger of golf cart injured in nontraffic accident

✓5th **V86.7 Person on outside of special all-terrain or other off-road motor vehicle injured in nontraffic accident**

✓x7th **V86.71 Person on outside of ambulance or fire engine injured in nontraffic accident**

✓x7th **V86.72 Person on outside of snowmobile injured in nontraffic accident**

✓x7th **V86.73 Person on outside of dune buggy injured in nontraffic accident**

✓x7th **V86.74 Person on outside of military vehicle injured in nontraffic accident**

✓x7th **V86.75 Person on outside of 3- or 4- wheeled all-terrain vehicle (ATV) injured in nontraffic accident**

✓x7th **V86.76 Person on outside of dirt bike or motor/cross bike injured in nontraffic accident**

V86.79 Person on outside of other special all-terrain or other off-road motor vehicles injured in nontraffic accident
Person on outside of go cart injured in nontraffic accident
Person on outside of golf cart injured in nontraffic accident

V86.9 Unspecified occupant of special all-terrain or other off-road motor vehicle injured in nontraffic accident
V86.91 Unspecified occupant of ambulance or fire engine injured in nontraffic accident
V86.92 Unspecified occupant of snowmobile injured in nontraffic accident
V86.93 Unspecified occupant of dune buggy injured in nontraffic accident
V86.94 Unspecified occupant of military vehicle injured in nontraffic accident
V86.95 Unspecified occupant of 3- or 4- wheeled all-terrain vehicle (ATV) injured in nontraffic accident
V86.96 Unspecified occupant of dirt bike or motor/cross bike injured in nontraffic accident
V86.99 Unspecified occupant of other special all-terrain or other off-road motor vehicle injured in nontraffic accident
Off-road motor-vehicle accident NOS
Other motor-vehicle accident NOS
Unspecified occupant of go cart injured in nontraffic accident
Unspecified occupant of golf cart injured in nontraffic accident

V87 Traffic accident of specified type but victim's mode of transport unknown
EXCLUDES 1 *collision involving:*
pedal cycle (V10-V19)
pedestrian (V01-V09)

V87.0 Person injured in collision between car and two- or three-wheeled powered vehicle (traffic)
V87.1 Person injured in collision between other motor vehicle and two- or three-wheeled motor vehicle (traffic)
V87.2 Person injured in collision between car and pick-up truck or van (traffic)
V87.3 Person injured in collision between car and bus (traffic)
V87.4 Person injured in collision between car and heavy transport vehicle (traffic)
V87.5 Person injured in collision between heavy transport vehicle and bus (traffic)
V87.6 Person injured in collision between railway train or railway vehicle and car (traffic)
V87.7 Person injured in collision between other specified motor vehicles (traffic)
V87.8 Person injured in other specified noncollision transport accidents involving motor vehicle (traffic)
V87.9 Person injured in other specified (collision)(noncollision) transport accidents involving nonmotor vehicle (traffic)

V88 Nontraffic accident of specified type but victim's mode of transport unknown
EXCLUDES 1 *collision involving:*
pedal cycle (V10-V19)
pedestrian (V01-V09)

V88.0 Person injured in collision between car and two- or three-wheeled motor vehicle, nontraffic
V88.1 Person injured in collision between other motor vehicle and two- or three-wheeled motor vehicle, nontraffic
V88.2 Person injured in collision between car and pick-up truck or van, nontraffic
V88.3 Person injured in collision between car and bus, nontraffic
V88.4 Person injured in collision between car and heavy transport vehicle, nontraffic
V88.5 Person injured in collision between heavy transport vehicle and bus, nontraffic
V88.6 Person injured in collision between railway train or railway vehicle and car, nontraffic
V88.7 Person injured in collision between other specified motor vehicle, nontraffic
V88.8 Person injured in other specified noncollision transport accidents involving motor vehicle, nontraffic
V88.9 Person injured in other specified (collision)(noncollision) transport accidents involving nonmotor vehicle, nontraffic

V89 Motor- or nonmotor-vehicle accident, type of vehicle unspecified
V89.0 Person injured in unspecified motor-vehicle accident, nontraffic
Motor-vehicle accident NOS, nontraffic
V89.1 Person injured in unspecified nonmotor-vehicle accident, nontraffic
Nonmotor-vehicle accident NOS (nontraffic)
V89.2 Person injured in unspecified motor-vehicle accident, traffic
Motor-vehicle accident [MVA] NOS
Road (traffic) accident [RTA] NOS
V89.3 Person injured in unspecified nonmotor-vehicle accident, traffic
Nonmotor-vehicle traffic accident NOS
V89.9 Person injured in unspecified vehicle accident
Collision NOS

Water transport accidents (V90-V94)

The appropriate 7th character is to be added to each code from categories V90-V94.
A initial encounter
D subsequent encounter
S sequela

V90 Drowning and submersion due to accident to watercraft
EXCLUDES 1 *civilian water transport accident involving military watercraft (V94.81-)*
fall into water not from watercraft (W16.-)
military watercraft accident in military or war operations (Y36.0-, Y37.0-)
water-transport-related drowning or submersion without accident to watercraft (V92.-)

V90.0 Drowning and submersion due to watercraft overturning
V90.00 Drowning and submersion due to merchant ship overturning
V90.01 Drowning and submersion due to passenger ship overturning
Drowning and submersion due to Ferry-boat overturning
Drowning and submersion due to Liner overturning
V90.02 Drowning and submersion due to fishing boat overturning
V90.03 Drowning and submersion due to other powered watercraft overturning
Drowning and submersion due to Hovercraft (on open water) overturning
Drowning and submersion due to Jet ski overturning
V90.04 Drowning and submersion due to sailboat overturning
V90.05 Drowning and submersion due to canoe or kayak overturning
V90.06 Drowning and submersion due to (nonpowered) inflatable craft overturning
V90.08 Drowning and submersion due to other unpowered watercraft overturning
Drowning and submersion due to windsurfer overturning
V90.09 Drowning and submersion due to unspecified watercraft overturning
Drowning and submersion due to boat NOS overturning
Drowning and submersion due to ship NOS overturning
Drowning and submersion due to watercraft NOS overturning

V90.1 Drowning and submersion due to watercraft sinking
V90.10 Drowning and submersion due to merchant ship sinking
V90.11 Drowning and submersion due to passenger ship sinking
Drowning and submersion due to Ferry-boat sinking
Drowning and submersion due to Liner sinking
V90.12 Drowning and submersion due to fishing boat sinking
V90.13 Drowning and submersion due to other powered watercraft sinking
Drowning and submersion due to Hovercraft (on open water) sinking
Drowning and submersion due to Jet ski sinking
V90.14 Drowning and submersion due to sailboat sinking

√x7th **V90.15 Drowning and submersion due to canoe or kayak sinking**

√x7th **V90.16 Drowning and submersion due to (nonpowered) inflatable craft sinking**

√x7th **V90.18 Drowning and submersion due to other unpowered watercraft sinking**

√x7th **V90.19 Drowning and submersion due to unspecified watercraft sinking**
Drowning and submersion due to boat NOS sinking
Drowning and submersion due to ship NOS sinking
Drowning and submersion due to watercraft NOS sinking

√5th **V90.2 Drowning and submersion due to falling or jumping from burning watercraft**

√x7th **V90.20 Drowning and submersion due to falling or jumping from burning merchant ship**

√x7th **V90.21 Drowning and submersion due to falling or jumping from burning passenger ship**
Drowning and submersion due to falling or jumping from burning Ferry-boat
Drowning and submersion due to falling or jumping from burning Liner

√x7th **V90.22 Drowning and submersion due to falling or jumping from burning fishing boat**

√x7th **V90.23 Drowning and submersion due to falling or jumping from other burning powered watercraft**
Drowning and submersion due to falling and jumping from burning Hovercraft (on open water)
Drowning and submersion due to falling and jumping from burning Jet ski

√x7th **V90.24 Drowning and submersion due to falling or jumping from burning sailboat**

√x7th **V90.25 Drowning and submersion due to falling or jumping from burning canoe or kayak**

√x7th **V90.26 Drowning and submersion due to falling or jumping from burning (nonpowered) inflatable craft**

√x7th **V90.27 Drowning and submersion due to falling or jumping from burning water-skis**

√x7th **V90.28 Drowning and submersion due to falling or jumping from other burning unpowered watercraft**
Drowning and submersion due to falling and jumping from burning surf-board
Drowning and submersion due to falling and jumping from burning windsurfer

√x7th **V90.29 Drowning and submersion due to falling or jumping from unspecified burning watercraft**
Drowning and submersion due to falling or jumping from burning boat NOS
Drowning and submersion due to falling or jumping from burning ship NOS
Drowning and submersion due to falling or jumping from burning watercraft NOS

√5th **V90.3 Drowning and submersion due to falling or jumping from crushed watercraft**

√x7th **V90.30 Drowning and submersion due to falling or jumping from crushed merchant ship**

√x7th **V90.31 Drowning and submersion due to falling or jumping from crushed passenger ship**
Drowning and submersion due to falling and jumping from crushed Ferry boat
Drowning and submersion due to falling and jumping from crushed Liner

√x7th **V90.32 Drowning and submersion due to falling or jumping from crushed fishing boat**

√x7th **V90.33 Drowning and submersion due to falling or jumping from other crushed powered watercraft**
Drowning and submersion due to falling and jumping from crushed Hovercraft
Drowning and submersion due to falling and jumping from crushed Jet ski

√x7th **V90.34 Drowning and submersion due to falling or jumping from crushed sailboat**

√x7th **V90.35 Drowning and submersion due to falling or jumping from crushed canoe or kayak**

√x7th **V90.36 Drowning and submersion due to falling or jumping from crushed (nonpowered) inflatable craft**

√x7th **V90.37 Drowning and submersion due to falling or jumping from crushed water-skis**

√x7th **V90.38 Drowning and submersion due to falling or jumping from other crushed unpowered watercraft**
Drowning and submersion due to falling and jumping from crushed surf-board
Drowning and submersion due to falling and jumping from crushed windsurfer

√x7th **V90.39 Drowning and submersion due to falling or jumping from crushed unspecified watercraft**
Drowning and submersion due to falling and jumping from crushed boat NOS
Drowning and submersion due to falling and jumping from crushed ship NOS
Drowning and submersion due to falling and jumping from crushed watercraft NOS

√5th **V90.8 Drowning and submersion due to other accident to watercraft**

√x7th **V90.80 Drowning and submersion due to other accident to merchant ship**

√x7th **V90.81 Drowning and submersion due to other accident to passenger ship**
Drowning and submersion due to other accident to Ferry-boat
Drowning and submersion due to other accident to Liner

√x7th **V90.82 Drowning and submersion due to other accident to fishing boat**

√x7th **V90.83 Drowning and submersion due to other accident to other powered watercraft**
Drowning and submersion due to other accident to Hovercraft (on open water)
Drowning and submersion due to other accident to Jet ski

√x7th **V90.84 Drowning and submersion due to other accident to sailboat**

√x7th **V90.85 Drowning and submersion due to other accident to canoe or kayak**

√x7th **V90.86 Drowning and submersion due to other accident to (nonpowered) inflatable craft**

√x7th **V90.87 Drowning and submersion due to other accident to water-skis**

√x7th **V90.88 Drowning and submersion due to other accident to other unpowered watercraft**
Drowning and submersion due to other accident to surf-board
Drowning and submersion due to other accident to windsurfer

√x7th **V90.89 Drowning and submersion due to other accident to unspecified watercraft**
Drowning and submersion due to other accident to boat NOS
Drowning and submersion due to other accident to ship NOS
Drowning and submersion due to other accident to watercraft NOS

√4th **V91 Other injury due to accident to watercraft**

INCLUDES any injury except drowning and submersion as a result of an accident to watercraft

EXCLUDES 1 *civilian water transport accident involving military watercraft (V94.81-)*
military watercraft accident in military or war operations (Y36, Y37.-)

EXCLUDES 2 *drowning and submersion due to accident to watercraft (V90.-)*

√5th **V91.0 Burn due to watercraft on fire**

EXCLUDES 1 *burn from localized fire or explosion on board ship without accident to watercraft (V93.-)*

√x7th **V91.00 Burn due to merchant ship on fire**

√x7th **V91.01 Burn due to passenger ship on fire**
Burn due to Ferry-boat on fire
Burn due to Liner on fire

√x7th **V91.02 Burn due to fishing boat on fire**

√x7th **V91.03 Burn due to other powered watercraft on fire**
Burn due to Hovercraft (on open water) on fire
Burn due to Jet ski on fire

√x7th **V91.04 Burn due to sailboat on fire**

√x7th **V91.05 Burn due to canoe or kayak on fire**

√x7th **V91.06 Burn due to (nonpowered) inflatable craft on fire**

V91.07 **Burn due to water-skis on fire**

V91.08 **Burn due to other unpowered watercraft on fire**

V91.09 **Burn due to unspecified watercraft on fire**
Burn due to boat NOS on fire
Burn due to ship NOS on fire
Burn due to watercraft NOS on fire

V91.1 **Crushed between watercraft and other watercraft or other object due to collision**
Crushed by lifeboat after abandoning ship in a collision
NOTE Select the specified type of watercraft that the victim was on at the time of the collision

V91.10 **Crushed between merchant ship and other watercraft or other object due to collision**

V91.11 **Crushed between passenger ship and other watercraft or other object due to collision**
Crushed between Ferry-boat and other watercraft or other object due to collision
Crushed between Liner and other watercraft or other object due to collision

V91.12 **Crushed between fishing boat and other watercraft or other object due to collision**

V91.13 **Crushed between other powered watercraft and other watercraft or other object due to collision**
Crushed between Hovercraft (on open water) and other watercraft or other object due to collision
Crushed between Jet ski and other watercraft or other object due to collision

V91.14 **Crushed between sailboat and other watercraft or other object due to collision**

V91.15 **Crushed between canoe or kayak and other watercraft or other object due to collision**

V91.16 **Crushed between (nonpowered) inflatable craft and other watercraft or other object due to collision**

V91.18 **Crushed between other unpowered watercraft and other watercraft or other object due to collision**
Crushed between surfboard and other watercraft or other object due to collision
Crushed between windsurfer and other watercraft or other object due to collision

V91.19 **Crushed between unspecified watercraft and other watercraft or other object due to collision**
Crushed between boat NOS and other watercraft or other object due to collision
Crushed between ship NOS and other watercraft or other object due to collision
Crushed between watercraft NOS and other watercraft or other object due to collision

V91.2 **Fall due to collision between watercraft and other watercraft or other object**
Fall while remaining on watercraft after collision
NOTE Select the specified type of watercraft that the victim was on at the time of the collision
EXCLUDES 1 *crushed between watercraft and other watercraft and other object due to collision (V91.1-)*
drowning and submersion due to falling from crushed watercraft (V90.3-)

V91.20 **Fall due to collision between merchant ship and other watercraft or other object**

V91.21 **Fall due to collision between passenger ship and other watercraft or other object**
Fall due to collision between Ferry-boat and other watercraft or other object
Fall due to collision between Liner and other watercraft or other object

V91.22 **Fall due to collision between fishing boat and other watercraft or other object**

V91.23 **Fall due to collision between other powered watercraft and other watercraft or other object**
Fall due to collision between Hovercraft (on open water) and other watercraft or other object
Fall due to collision between Jet ski and other watercraft or other object

V91.24 **Fall due to collision between sailboat and other watercraft or other object**

V91.25 **Fall due to collision between canoe or kayak and other watercraft or other object**

V91.26 **Fall due to collision between (nonpowered) inflatable craft and other watercraft or other object**

V91.29 **Fall due to collision between unspecified watercraft and other watercraft or other object**
Fall due to collision between boat NOS and other watercraft or other object
Fall due to collision between ship NOS and other watercraft or other object
Fall due to collision between watercraft NOS and other watercraft or other object

V91.3 **Hit or struck by falling object due to accident to watercraft**
Hit or struck by falling object (part of damaged watercraft or other object) after falling or jumping from damaged watercraft
EXCLUDES 2 *drowning or submersion due to fall or jumping from damaged watercraft (V90.2-, V90.3-)*

V91.30 **Hit or struck by falling object due to accident to merchant ship**

V91.31 **Hit or struck by falling object due to accident to passenger ship**
Hit or struck by falling object due to accident to Ferry-boat
Hit or struck by falling object due to accident to Liner

V91.32 **Hit or struck by falling object due to accident to fishing boat**

V91.33 **Hit or struck by falling object due to accident to other powered watercraft**
Hit or struck by falling object due to accident to Hovercraft (on open water)
Hit or struck by falling object due to accident to Jet ski

V91.34 **Hit or struck by falling object due to accident to sailboat**

V91.35 **Hit or struck by falling object due to accident to canoe or kayak**

V91.36 **Hit or struck by falling object due to accident to (nonpowered) inflatable craft**

V91.37 **Hit or struck by falling object due to accident to water-skis**
Hit by water-skis after jumping off of waterskis

V91.38 **Hit or struck by falling object due to accident to other unpowered watercraft**
Hit or struck by surf-board after falling off damaged surf-board
Hit or struck by object after falling off damaged windsurfer

V91.39 **Hit or struck by falling object due to accident to unspecified watercraft**
Hit or struck by falling object due to accident to boat NOS
Hit or struck by falling object due to accident to ship NOS
Hit or struck by falling object due to accident to watercraft NOS

V91.8 **Other injury due to other accident to watercraft**

V91.80 **Other injury due to other accident to merchant ship**

V91.81 **Other injury due to other accident to passenger ship**
Other injury due to other accident to Ferry-boat
Other injury due to other accident to Liner

V91.82 **Other injury due to other accident to fishing boat**

V91.83 **Other injury due to other accident to other powered watercraft**
Other injury due to other accident to Hovercraft (on open water)
Other injury due to other accident to Jet ski

V91.84 **Other injury due to other accident to sailboat**

V91.85 **Other injury due to other accident to canoe or kayak**

V91.86 **Other injury due to other accident to (nonpowered) inflatable craft**

V91.87 **Other injury due to other accident to water-skis**

V91.88 **Other injury due to other accident to other unpowered watercraft**
Other injury due to other accident to surf-board
Other injury due to other accident to windsurfer

√x7th **V91.89 Other injury due to other accident to unspecified watercraft**
Other injury due to other accident to boat NOS
Other injury due to other accident to ship NOS
Other injury due to other accident to watercraft NOS

√4th **V92 Drowning and submersion due to accident on board watercraft, without accident to watercraft**

EXCLUDES 1 *civilian water transport accident involving military watercraft (V94.81-)*
drowning or submersion due to accident to watercraft (V90-V91)
drowning or submersion of diver who voluntarily jumps from boat not involved in an accident (W16.711, W16.721)
fall into water without watercraft (W16.-)
military watercraft accident in military or war operations (Y36, Y37)

√5th **V92.0 Drowning and submersion due to fall off watercraft**
Drowning and submersion due to fall from gangplank of watercraft
Drowning and submersion due to fall overboard watercraft
EXCLUDES 2 *hitting head on object or bottom of body of water due to fall from watercraft (V94.0-)*

√x7th **V92.00 Drowning and submersion due to fall off merchant ship**

√x7th **V92.01 Drowning and submersion due to fall off passenger ship**
Drowning and submersion due to fall off Ferry-boat
Drowning and submersion due to fall off Liner

√x7th **V92.02 Drowning and submersion due to fall off fishing boat**

√x7th **V92.03 Drowning and submersion due to fall off other powered watercraft**
Drowning and submersion due to fall off Hovercraft (on open water)
Drowning and submersion due to fall off Jet ski

√x7th **V92.04 Drowning and submersion due to fall off sailboat**

√x7th **V92.05 Drowning and submersion due to fall off canoe or kayak**

√x7th **V92.06 Drowning and submersion due to fall off (nonpowered) inflatable craft**

√x7th **V92.07 Drowning and submersion due to fall off water-skis**
EXCLUDES 1 *drowning and submersion due to falling off burning water-skis (V90.27)*
drowning and submersion due to falling off crushed water-skis (V90.37)
hit by boat while water-skiing NOS (V94.X)

√x7th **V92.08 Drowning and submersion due to fall off other unpowered watercraft**
Drowning and submersion due to fall off surf-board
Drowning and submersion due to fall off windsurfer
EXCLUDES 1 *drowning and submersion due to fall off burning unpowered watercraft (V90.28)*
drowning and submersion due to fall off crushed unpowered watercraft (V90.38)
drowning and submersion due to fall off damaged unpowered watercraft (V90.88)
drowning and submersion due to rider of nonpowered watercraft being hit by other watercraft (V94.-)
other injury due to rider of nonpowered watercraft being hit by other watercraft (V94.-)

√x7th **V92.09 Drowning and submersion due to fall off unspecified watercraft**
Drowning and submersion due to fall off boat NOS
Drowning and submersion due to fall off ship
Drowning and submersion due to fall off watercraft NOS

√5th **V92.1 Drowning and submersion due to being thrown overboard by motion of watercraft**
EXCLUDES 1 *drowning and submersion due to fall off surf-board (V92.08)*
drowning and submersion due to fall off water-skis (V92.07)
drowning and submersion due to fall off windsurfer (V92.08)

√x7th **V92.10 Drowning and submersion due to being thrown overboard by motion of merchant ship**

√x7th **V92.11 Drowning and submersion due to being thrown overboard by motion of passenger ship**
Drowning and submersion due to being thrown overboard by motion of Ferry-boat
Drowning and submersion due to being thrown overboard by motion of Liner

√x7th **V92.12 Drowning and submersion due to being thrown overboard by motion of fishing boat**

√x7th **V92.13 Drowning and submersion due to being thrown overboard by motion of other powered watercraft**
Drowning and submersion due to being thrown overboard by motion of Hovercraft

√x7th **V92.14 Drowning and submersion due to being thrown overboard by motion of sailboat**

√x7th **V92.15 Drowning and submersion due to being thrown overboard by motion of canoe or kayak**

√x7th **V92.16 Drowning and submersion due to being thrown overboard by motion of (nonpowered) inflatable craft**

√x7th **V92.19 Drowning and submersion due to being thrown overboard by motion of unspecified watercraft**
Drowning and submersion due to being thrown overboard by motion of boat NOS
Drowning and submersion due to being thrown overboard by motion of ship NOS
Drowning and submersion due to being thrown overboard by motion of watercraft NOS

√5th **V92.2 Drowning and submersion due to being washed overboard from watercraft**
Code first any associated cataclysm (X37.0-)

√x7th **V92.20 Drowning and submersion due to being washed overboard from merchant ship**

√x7th **V92.21 Drowning and submersion due to being washed overboard from passenger ship**
Drowning and submersion due to being washed overboard from Ferry-boat
Drowning and submersion due to being washed overboard from Liner

√x7th **V92.22 Drowning and submersion due to being washed overboard from fishing boat**

√x7th **V92.23 Drowning and submersion due to being washed overboard from other powered watercraft**
Drowning and submersion due to being washed overboard from Hovercraft (on open water)
Drowning and submersion due to being washed overboard from Jet ski

√x7th **V92.24 Drowning and submersion due to being washed overboard from sailboat**

√x7th **V92.25 Drowning and submersion due to being washed overboard from canoe or kayak**

√x7th **V92.26 Drowning and submersion due to being washed overboard from (nonpowered) inflatable craft**

√x7th **V92.27 Drowning and submersion due to being washed overboard from water-skis**
EXCLUDES 1 *drowning and submersion due to fall off water-skis (V92.07)*

√x7th **V92.28 Drowning and submersion due to being washed overboard from other unpowered watercraft**
Drowning and submersion due to being washed overboard from surf-board
Drowning and submersion due to being washed overboard from windsurfer

√x 7th **V92.29 Drowning and submersion due to being washed overboard from unspecified watercraft**
Drowning and submersion due to being washed overboard from boat NOS
Drowning and submersion due to being washed overboard from ship NOS
Drowning and submersion due to being washed overboard from watercraft NOS

√4th **V93 Other injury due to accident on board watercraft, without accident to watercraft**
EXCLUDES 1 *civilian water transport accident involving military watercraft (V94.81-)*
other injury due to accident to watercraft (V91.-)
military watercraft accident in military or war operations (Y36, Y37.-)
EXCLUDES 2 *drowning and submersion due to accident on board watercraft, without accident to watercraft (V92.-)*

√5th **V93.0 Burn due to localized fire on board watercraft**
EXCLUDES 1 *burn due to watercraft on fire (V91.0-)*

√x 7th **V93.00 Burn due to localized fire on board merchant vessel**

√x 7th **V93.01 Burn due to localized fire on board passenger vessel**
Burn due to localized fire on board Ferry-boat
Burn due to localized fire on board Liner

√x 7th **V93.02 Burn due to localized fire on board fishing boat**

√x 7th **V93.03 Burn due to localized fire on board other powered watercraft**
Burn due to localized fire on board Hovercraft
Burn due to localized fire on board Jet ski

√x 7th **V93.04 Burn due to localized fire on board sailboat**

√x 7th **V93.09 Burn due to localized fire on board unspecified watercraft**
Burn due to localized fire on board boat NOS
Burn due to localized fire on board ship NOS
Burn due to localized fire on board watercraft NOS

√5th **V93.1 Other burn on board watercraft**
Burn due to source other than fire on board watercraft
EXCLUDES 1 *burn due to watercraft on fire (V91.0-)*

√x 7th **V93.10 Other burn on board merchant vessel**

√x 7th **V93.11 Other burn on board passenger vessel**
Other burn on board Ferry-boat
Other burn on board Liner

√x 7th **V93.12 Other burn on board fishing boat**

√x 7th **V93.13 Other burn on board other powered watercraft**
Other burn on board Hovercraft
Other burn on board Jet ski

√x 7th **V93.14 Other burn on board sailboat**

√x 7th **V93.19 Other burn on board unspecified watercraft**
Other burn on board boat NOS
Other burn on board ship NOS
Other burn on board watercraft NOS

√5th **V93.2 Heat exposure on board watercraft**
EXCLUDES 1 *exposure to man-made heat not aboard watercraft (W92)*
exposure to natural heat while on board watercraft (X30)
exposure to sunlight while on board watercraft (X32)
EXCLUDES 2 *burn due to fire on board watercraft (V93.0-)*

√x 7th **V93.20 Heat exposure on board merchant ship**

√x 7th **V93.21 Heat exposure on board passenger ship**
Heat exposure on board Ferry-boat
Heat exposure on board Liner

√x 7th **V93.22 Heat exposure on board fishing boat**

√x 7th **V93.23 Heat exposure on board other powered watercraft**
Heat exposure on board hovercraft

√x 7th **V93.24 Heat exposure on board sailboat**

√x 7th **V93.29 Heat exposure on board unspecified watercraft**
Heat exposure on board boat NOS
Heat exposure on board ship NOS
Heat exposure on board watercraft NOS

√5th **V93.3 Fall on board watercraft**
EXCLUDES 1 *fall due to collision of watercraft (V91.2-)*

√x 7th **V93.30 Fall on board merchant ship**

√x 7th **V93.31 Fall on board passenger ship**
Fall on board Ferry-boat
Fall on board Liner

√x 7th **V93.32 Fall on board fishing boat**

√x 7th **V93.33 Fall on board other powered watercraft**
Fall on board Hovercraft (on open water)
Fall on board Jet ski

√x 7th **V93.34 Fall on board sailboat**

√x 7th **V93.35 Fall on board canoe or kayak**

√x 7th **V93.36 Fall on board (nonpowered) inflatable craft**

√x 7th **V93.38 Fall on board other unpowered watercraft**

√x 7th **V93.39 Fall on board unspecified watercraft**
Fall on board boat NOS
Fall on board ship NOS
Fall on board watercraft NOS

√5th **V93.4 Struck by falling object on board watercraft**
Hit by falling object on board watercraft
EXCLUDES 1 *struck by falling object due to accident to watercraft (V91.3)*

√x 7th **V93.40 Struck by falling object on merchant ship**

√x 7th **V93.41 Struck by falling object on passenger ship**
Struck by falling object on Ferry-boat
Struck by falling object on Liner

√x 7th **V93.42 Struck by falling object on fishing boat**

√x 7th **V93.43 Struck by falling object on other powered watercraft**
Struck by falling object on Hovercraft

√x 7th **V93.44 Struck by falling object on sailboat**

√x 7th **V93.48 Struck by falling object on other unpowered watercraft**

√x 7th **V93.49 Struck by falling object on unspecified watercraft**

√5th **V93.5 Explosion on board watercraft**
Boiler explosion on steamship
EXCLUDES 2 *fire on board watercraft (V93.0-)*

√x 7th **V93.50 Explosion on board merchant ship**

√x 7th **V93.51 Explosion on board passenger ship**
Explosion on board Ferry-boat
Explosion on board Liner

√x 7th **V93.52 Explosion on board fishing boat**

√x 7th **V93.53 Explosion on board other powered watercraft**
Explosion on board Hovercraft
Explosion on board Jet ski

√x 7th **V93.54 Explosion on board sailboat**

√x 7th **V93.59 Explosion on board unspecified watercraft**
Explosion on board boat NOS
Explosion on board ship NOS
Explosion on board watercraft NOS

√5th **V93.6 Machinery accident on board watercraft**
EXCLUDES 1 *machinery explosion on board watercraft (V93.4-)*
machinery fire on board watercraft (V93.0-)

√x 7th **V93.60 Machinery accident on board merchant ship**

√x 7th **V93.61 Machinery accident on board passenger ship**
Machinery accident on board Ferry-boat
Machinery accident on board Liner

√x 7th **V93.62 Machinery accident on board fishing boat**

√x 7th **V93.63 Machinery accident on board other powered watercraft**
Machinery accident on board Hovercraft

√x 7th **V93.64 Machinery accident on board sailboat**

√x 7th **V93.69 Machinery accident on board unspecified watercraft**
Machinery accident on board boat NOS
Machinery accident on board ship NOS
Machinery accident on board watercraft NOS

√5th **V93.8 Other injury due to other accident on board watercraft**
Accidental poisoning by gases or fumes on watercraft

√x 7th **V93.80 Other injury due to other accident on board merchant ship**

√x7th **V93.81 Other injury due to other accident on board passenger ship**
Other injury due to other accident on board Ferry-boat
Other injury due to other accident on board Liner

√x7th **V93.82 Other injury due to other accident on board fishing boat**

√x7th **V93.83 Other injury due to other accident on board other powered watercraft**
Other injury due to other accident on board Hovercraft
Other injury due to other accident on board Jet ski

√x7th **V93.84 Other injury due to other accident on board sailboat**

√x7th **V93.85 Other injury due to other accident on board canoe or kayak**

√x7th **V93.86 Other injury due to other accident on board (nonpowered) inflatable craft**

√x7th **V93.87 Other injury due to other accident on board water-skis**
Hit or struck by object while waterskiing

√x7th **V93.88 Other injury due to other accident on board other unpowered watercraft**
Hit or struck by object while surfing
Hit or struck by object while on board windsurfer

√x7th **V93.89 Other injury due to other accident on board unspecified watercraft**
Other injury due to other accident on board boat NOS
Other injury due to other accident on board ship NOS
Other injury due to other accident on board watercraft NOS

√4th **V94 Other and unspecified water transport accidents**
EXCLUDES 1 *military watercraft accidents in military or war operations (Y36, Y37)*

√x7th **V94.Ø Hitting object or bottom of body of water due to fall from watercraft**
EXCLUDES 2 *drowning and submersion due to fall from watercraft (V92.Ø-)*

√5th **V94.1 Bather struck by watercraft**
Swimmer hit by watercraft

√x7th **V94.11 Bather struck by powered watercraft**

√x7th **V94.12 Bather struck by nonpowered watercraft**

√5th **V94.2 Rider of nonpowered watercraft struck by other watercraft**

√x7th **V94.21 Rider of nonpowered watercraft struck by other nonpowered watercraft**
Canoer hit by other nonpowered watercraft
Surfer hit by other nonpowered watercraft
Windsurfer hit by other nonpowered watercraft

√x7th **V94.22 Rider of nonpowered watercraft struck by powered watercraft**
Canoer hit by motorboat
Surfer hit by motorboat
Windsurfer hit by motorboat

√5th **V94.3 Injury to rider of (inflatable) watercraft being pulled behind other watercraft**

√x7th **V94.31 Injury to rider of (inflatable) recreational watercraft being pulled behind other watercraft**
Injury to rider of inner-tube pulled behind motor boat

√x7th **V94.32 Injury to rider of non-recreational watercraft being pulled behind other watercraft**
Injury to occupant of dingy being pulled behind boat or ship
Injury to occupant of life-raft being pulled behind boat or ship

√x7th **V94.4 Injury to barefoot water-skier**
Injury to person being pulled behind boat or ship

√5th **V94.8 Other water transport accident**

√6th **V94.81 Water transport accident involving military watercraft**

√7th **V94.81Ø Civilian watercraft involved in water transport accident with military watercraft**
Passenger on civilian watercraft injured due to accident with military watercraft

√7th **V94.811 Civilian in water injured by military watercraft**

√7th **V94.818 Other water transport accident involving military watercraft**

√x7th **V94.89 Other water transport accident**

√x7th **V94.9 Unspecified water transport accident**
Water transport accident NOS

Air and space transport accidents (V95-V97)

EXCLUDES 1 *military aircraft accidents in military or war operations (Y36, Y37)*

The appropriate 7th character is to be added to each code from categories V95-V97.
A initial encounter
D subsequent encounter
S sequela

√4th **V95 Accident to powered aircraft causing injury to occupant**

√5th **V95.Ø Helicopter accident injuring occupant**

√x7th **V95.ØØ Unspecified helicopter accident injuring occupant**

√x7th **V95.Ø1 Helicopter crash injuring occupant**

√x7th **V95.Ø2 Forced landing of helicopter injuring occupant**

√x7th **V95.Ø3 Helicopter collision injuring occupant**
Helicopter collision with any object, fixed, movable or moving

√x7th **V95.Ø4 Helicopter fire injuring occupant**

√x7th **V95.Ø5 Helicopter explosion injuring occupant**

√x7th **V95.Ø9 Other helicopter accident injuring occupant**

√5th **V95.1 Ultralight, microlight or powered-glider accident injuring occupant**

√x7th **V95.1Ø Unspecified ultralight, microlight or powered-glider accident injuring occupant**

√x7th **V95.11 Ultralight, microlight or powered-glider crash injuring occupant**

√x7th **V95.12 Forced landing of ultralight, microlight or powered-glider injuring occupant**

√x7th **V95.13 Ultralight, microlight or powered-glider collision injuring occupant**
Ultralight, microlight or powered-glider collision with any object, fixed, movable or moving

√x7th **V95.14 Ultralight, microlight or powered-glider fire injuring occupant**

√x7th **V95.15 Ultralight, microlight or powered-glider explosion injuring occupant**

√x7th **V95.19 Other ultralight, microlight or powered-glider accident injuring occupant**

√5th **V95.2 Other private fixed-wing aircraft accident injuring occupant**

√x7th **V95.2Ø Unspecified accident to other private fixed-wing aircraft, injuring occupant**

√x7th **V95.21 Other private fixed-wing aircraft crash injuring occupant**

√x7th **V95.22 Forced landing of other private fixed-wing aircraft injuring occupant**

√x7th **V95.23 Other private fixed-wing aircraft collision injuring occupant**
Other private fixed-wing aircraft collision with any object, fixed, movable or moving

√x7th **V95.24 Other private fixed-wing aircraft fire injuring occupant**

√x7th **V95.25 Other private fixed-wing aircraft explosion injuring occupant**

√x7th **V95.29 Other accident to other private fixed-wing aircraft injuring occupant**

√5th **V95.3 Commercial fixed-wing aircraft accident injuring occupant**

√x7th **V95.3Ø Unspecified accident to commercial fixed-wing aircraft injuring occupant**

√x7th **V95.31 Commercial fixed-wing aircraft crash injuring occupant**

√x7th **V95.32 Forced landing of commercial fixed-wing aircraft injuring occupant**

√x7th **V95.33 Commercial fixed-wing aircraft collision injuring occupant**
Commercial fixed-wing aircraft collision with any object, fixed, movable or moving

√x7th **V95.34 Commercial fixed-wing aircraft fire injuring occupant**

√x7th **V95.35 Commercial fixed-wing aircraft explosion injuring occupant**

√x7th **V95.39 Other accident to commercial fixed-wing aircraft injuring occupant**

√5th **V95.4 Spacecraft accident injuring occupant**

√x7th **V95.4Ø Unspecified spacecraft accident injuring occupant**

√x7th **V95.41 Spacecraft crash injuring occupant**

V95.42 **Forced landing of spacecraft injuring occupant**

V95.43 **Spacecraft collision injuring occupant**

Spacecraft collision with any object, fixed, moveable or moving

V95.44 **Spacecraft fire injuring occupant**

V95.45 **Spacecraft explosion injuring occupant**

V95.49 **Other spacecraft accident injuring occupant**

V95.8 **Other powered aircraft accidents injuring occupant**

V95.9 **Unspecified aircraft accident injuring occupant**

Aircraft accident NOS

Air transport accident NOS

V96 Accident to nonpowered aircraft causing injury to occupant

V96.0 **Balloon accident injuring occupant**

V96.00 **Unspecified balloon accident injuring occupant**

V96.01 **Balloon crash injuring occupant**

V96.02 **Forced landing of balloon injuring occupant**

V96.03 **Balloon collision injuring occupant**

Balloon collision with any object, fixed, moveable or moving

V96.04 **Balloon fire injuring occupant**

V96.05 **Balloon explosion injuring occupant**

V96.09 **Other balloon accident injuring occupant**

V96.1 **Hang-glider accident injuring occupant**

V96.10 **Unspecified hang-glider accident injuring occupant**

V96.11 **Hang-glider crash injuring occupant**

V96.12 **Forced landing of hang-glider injuring occupant**

V96.13 **Hang-glider collision injuring occupant**

Hang-glider collision with any object, fixed, moveable or moving

V96.14 **Hang-glider fire injuring occupant**

V96.15 **Hang-glider explosion injuring occupant**

V96.19 **Other hang-glider accident injuring occupant**

V96.2 **Glider (nonpowered) accident injuring occupant**

V96.20 **Unspecified glider (nonpowered) accident injuring occupant**

V96.21 **Glider (nonpowered) crash injuring occupant**

V96.22 **Forced landing of glider (nonpowered) injuring occupant**

V96.23 **Glider (nonpowered) collision injuring occupant**

Glider (nonpowered) collision with any object, fixed, moveable or moving

V96.24 **Glider (nonpowered) fire injuring occupant**

V96.25 **Glider (nonpowered) explosion injuring occupant**

V96.29 **Other glider (nonpowered) accident injuring occupant**

V96.8 **Other nonpowered-aircraft accidents injuring occupant**

Kite carrying a person accident injuring occupant

V96.9 **Unspecified nonpowered-aircraft accident injuring occupant**

Nonpowered-aircraft accident NOS

V97 Other specified air transport accidents

V97.0 **Occupant of aircraft injured in other specified air transport accidents**

Fall in, on or from aircraft in air transport accident

EXCLUDES 1 *accident while boarding or alighting aircraft (V97.1)*

V97.1 **Person injured while boarding or alighting from aircraft**

V97.2 **Parachutist accident**

V97.21 **Parachutist entangled in object**

Parachutist landing in tree

V97.22 **Parachutist injured on landing**

V97.29 **Other parachutist accident**

V97.3 **Person on ground injured in air transport accident**

V97.31 **Hit by object falling from aircraft**

Hit by crashing aircraft

Injured by aircraft hitting house

Injured by aircraft hitting car

V97.32 **Injured by rotating propeller**

V97.33 **Sucked into jet engine**

V97.39 **Other injury to person on ground due to air transport accident**

V97.8 **Other air transport accidents, not elsewhere classified**

EXCLUDES 1 *aircraft accident NOS (V95.9)*

exposure to changes in air pressure during ascent or descent (W94.-)

V97.81 **Air transport accident involving military aircraft**

V97.810 **Civilian aircraft involved in air transport accident with military aircraft**

Passenger in civilian aircraft injured due to accident with military aircraft

V97.811 **Civilian injured by military aircraft**

V97.818 **Other air transport accident involving military aircraft**

V97.89 **Other air transport accidents, not elsewhere classified**

Injury from machinery on aircraft

Other and unspecified transport accidents (V98-V99)

EXCLUDES 1 *vehicle accident, type of vehicle unspecified (V89.-)*

The appropriate 7th character is to be added to each code from categories V98-V99.

A initial encounter

D subsequent encounter

S sequela

V98 Other specified transport accidents

V98.0 **Accident to, on or involving cable-car, not on rails**

Caught or dragged by cable-car, not on rails

Fall or jump from cable-car, not on rails

Object thrown from or in cable-car, not on rails

V98.1 **Accident to, on or involving land-yacht**

V98.2 **Accident to, on or involving ice yacht**

V98.3 **Accident to, on or involving ski lift**

Accident to, on or involving ski chair-lift

Accident to, on or involving ski-lift with gondola

V98.8 **Other specified transport accidents**

V99 Unspecified transport accident

OTHER EXTERNAL CAUSES OF ACCIDENTAL INJURY (W00-X58)

Slipping, tripping, stumbling and falls (W00-W19)

EXCLUDES 1 *assault involving a fall (Y01-Y02)*

fall from animal (V80.-)

fall (in) (from) machinery (in operation) (W28-W31)

fall (in) (from) transport vehicle (V01-V99)

intentional self-harm involving a fall (X80-X81)

EXCLUDES 2 *at risk for fall (history of fall) Z91.81*

fall (in) (from) burning building (X00.-)

fall into fire (X00-X04, X08)

The appropriate 7th character is to be added to each code from categories W00-W19.

A initial encounter

D subsequent encounter

S sequela

W00 Fall due to ice and snow

INCLUDES pedestrian on foot falling (slipping) on ice and snow

EXCLUDES 1 *fall on (from) ice and snow involving pedestrian conveyance (V00.-)*

fall from stairs and steps not due to ice and snow (W10.-)

AHA: 2016,2Q,4

W00.0 **Fall on same level due to ice and snow**

W00.1 **Fall from stairs and steps due to ice and snow**

W00.2 **Other fall from one level to another due to ice and snow**

W00.9 **Unspecified fall due to ice and snow**

W01 Fall on same level from slipping, tripping and stumbling
INCLUDES fall on moving sidewalk
EXCLUDES 1 *fall due to bumping (striking) against object (W18.0-)*
fall in shower or bathtub (W18.2-)
fall on same level NOS (W18.30)
fall on same level from slipping, tripping and stumbling due to ice or snow (W00.0)
fall off or from toilet (W18.1-)
slipping, tripping and stumbling NOS (W18.40)
slipping, tripping and stumbling without falling (W18.4-)

W01.0 Fall on same level from slipping, tripping and stumbling without subsequent striking against object
Falling over animal

W01.1 Fall on same level from slipping, tripping and stumbling with subsequent striking against object

W01.10 Fall on same level from slipping, tripping and stumbling with subsequent striking against unspecified object

W01.11 Fall on same level from slipping, tripping and stumbling with subsequent striking against sharp object

W01.110 Fall on same level from slipping, tripping and stumbling with subsequent striking against sharp glass

W01.111 Fall on same level from slipping, tripping and stumbling with subsequent striking against power tool or machine

W01.118 Fall on same level from slipping, tripping and stumbling with subsequent striking against other sharp object

W01.119 Fall on same level from slipping, tripping and stumbling with subsequent striking against unspecified sharp object

W01.19 Fall on same level from slipping, tripping and stumbling with subsequent striking against other object

W01.190 Fall on same level from slipping, tripping and stumbling with subsequent striking against furniture

W01.198 Fall on same level from slipping, tripping and stumbling with subsequent striking against other object

W03 Other fall on same level due to collision with another person
Fall due to non-transport collision with other person
EXCLUDES 1 *collision with another person without fall (W51)*
crushed or pushed by a crowd or human stampede (W52)
fall involving pedestrian conveyance (V00-V09)
fall due to ice or snow (W00)
fall on same level NOS (W18.30)
AHA: 2012,4Q,108

W04 Fall while being carried or supported by other persons
Accidentally dropped while being carried

W05 Fall from non-moving wheelchair, nonmotorized scooter and motorized mobility scooter
EXCLUDES 1 *fall from moving wheelchair (powered) (V00.811)*
fall from moving motorized mobility scooter (V00.831)
fall from nonmotorized scooter (V00.141)

W05.0 Fall from non-moving wheelchair
AHA: 2019,2Q,27

W05.1 Fall from non-moving nonmotorized scooter

W05.2 Fall from non-moving motorized mobility scooter

W06 Fall from bed

W07 Fall from chair

W08 Fall from other furniture

W09 Fall on and from playground equipment
EXCLUDES 1 *fall involving recreational machinery (W31)*

W09.0 Fall on or from playground slide

W09.1 Fall from playground swing

W09.2 Fall on or from jungle gym

W09.8 Fall on or from other playground equipment

W10 Fall on and from stairs and steps
EXCLUDES 1 *Fall from stairs and steps due to ice and snow (W00.1)*

W10.0 Fall (on)(from) escalator

W10.1 Fall (on)(from) sidewalk curb

W10.2 Fall (on)(from) incline
Fall (on) (from) ramp

W10.8 Fall (on) (from) other stairs and steps

W10.9 Fall (on) (from) unspecified stairs and steps

W11 Fall on and from ladder

W12 Fall on and from scaffolding

W13 Fall from, out of or through building or structure

W13.0 Fall from, out of or through balcony
Fall from, out of or through railing

W13.1 Fall from, out of or through bridge

W13.2 Fall from, out of or through roof

W13.3 Fall through floor

W13.4 Fall from, out of or through window
EXCLUDES 2 *fall with subsequent striking against sharp glass (W01.110)*

W13.8 Fall from, out of or through other building or structure
Fall from, out of or through viaduct
Fall from, out of or through wall
Fall from, out of or through flag-pole

W13.9 Fall from, out of or through building, not otherwise specified
EXCLUDES 1 *collapse of a building or structure (W20.-)*
fall or jump from burning building or structure (X00.-)

W14 Fall from tree

W15 Fall from cliff

W16 Fall, jump or diving into water
EXCLUDES 1 *accidental non-watercraft drowning and submersion not involving fall (W65-W74)*
effects of air pressure from diving (W94.-)
fall into water from watercraft (V90-V94)
hitting an object or against bottom when falling from watercraft (V94.0)
EXCLUDES 2 *striking or hitting diving board (W21.4)*

W16.0 Fall into swimming pool
Fall into swimming pool NOS
EXCLUDES 1 *fall into empty swimming pool (W17.3)*

W16.01 Fall into swimming pool striking water surface

W16.011 Fall into swimming pool striking water surface causing drowning and submersion
EXCLUDES 1 *drowning and submersion while in swimming pool without fall (W67)*

W16.012 Fall into swimming pool striking water surface causing other injury

W16.02 Fall into swimming pool striking bottom

W16.021 Fall into swimming pool striking bottom causing drowning and submersion
EXCLUDES 1 *drowning and submersion while in swimming pool without fall (W67)*

W16.022 Fall into swimming pool striking bottom causing other injury

W16.03 Fall into swimming pool striking wall

W16.031 Fall into swimming pool striking wall causing drowning and submersion
EXCLUDES 1 *drowning and submersion while in swimming pool without fall (W67)*

W16.032 Fall into swimming pool striking wall causing other injury

W16.1 Fall into natural body of water
Fall into lake
Fall into open sea
Fall into river
Fall into stream
W16.11 Fall into natural body of water striking water surface
W16.111 Fall into natural body of water striking water surface causing drowning and submersion
EXCLUDES 1 *drowning and submersion while in natural body of water without fall (W69)*
W16.112 Fall into natural body of water striking water surface causing other injury
W16.12 Fall into natural body of water striking bottom
W16.121 Fall into natural body of water striking bottom causing drowning and submersion
EXCLUDES 1 *drowning and submersion while in natural body of water without fall (W69)*
W16.122 Fall into natural body of water striking bottom causing other injury
W16.13 Fall into natural body of water striking side
W16.131 Fall into natural body of water striking side causing drowning and submersion
EXCLUDES 1 *drowning and submersion while in natural body of water without fall (W69)*
W16.132 Fall into natural body of water striking side causing other injury
W16.2 Fall in (into) filled bathtub or bucket of water
W16.21 Fall in (into) filled bathtub
EXCLUDES 1 *fall into empty bathtub (W18.2)*
W16.211 Fall in (into) filled bathtub causing drowning and submersion
EXCLUDES 1 *drowning and submersion while in filled bathtub without fall (W65)*
W16.212 Fall in (into) filled bathtub causing other injury
W16.22 Fall in (into) bucket of water
W16.221 Fall in (into) bucket of water causing drowning and submersion
W16.222 Fall in (into) bucket of water causing other injury
W16.3 Fall into other water
Fall into fountain
Fall into reservoir
W16.31 Fall into other water striking water surface
W16.311 Fall into other water striking water surface causing drowning and submersion
EXCLUDES 1 *drowning and submersion while in other water without fall (W73)*
W16.312 Fall into other water striking water surface causing other injury
W16.32 Fall into other water striking bottom
W16.321 Fall into other water striking bottom causing drowning and submersion
EXCLUDES 1 *drowning and submersion while in other water without fall (W73)*
W16.322 Fall into other water striking bottom causing other injury
W16.33 Fall into other water striking wall
W16.331 Fall into other water striking wall causing drowning and submersion
EXCLUDES 1 *drowning and submersion while in other water without fall (W73)*
W16.332 Fall into other water striking wall causing other injury
W16.4 Fall into unspecified water
W16.41 Fall into unspecified water causing drowning and submersion
W16.42 Fall into unspecified water causing other injury
W16.5 Jumping or diving into swimming pool
W16.51 Jumping or diving into swimming pool striking water surface
W16.511 Jumping or diving into swimming pool striking water surface causing drowning and submersion
EXCLUDES 1 *drowning and submersion while in swimming pool without jumping or diving (W67)*
W16.512 Jumping or diving into swimming pool striking water surface causing other injury
W16.52 Jumping or diving into swimming pool striking bottom
W16.521 Jumping or diving into swimming pool striking bottom causing drowning and submersion
EXCLUDES 1 *drowning and submersion while in swimming pool without jumping or diving (W67)*
W16.522 Jumping or diving into swimming pool striking bottom causing other injury
W16.53 Jumping or diving into swimming pool striking wall
W16.531 Jumping or diving into swimming pool striking wall causing drowning and submersion
EXCLUDES 1 *drowning and submersion while in swimming pool without jumping or diving (W67)*
W16.532 Jumping or diving into swimming pool striking wall causing other injury
W16.6 Jumping or diving into natural body of water
Jumping or diving into lake
Jumping or diving into open sea
Jumping or diving into river
Jumping or diving into stream
W16.61 Jumping or diving into natural body of water striking water surface
W16.611 Jumping or diving into natural body of water striking water surface causing drowning and submersion
EXCLUDES 1 *drowning and submersion while in natural body of water without jumping or diving (W69)*
W16.612 Jumping or diving into natural body of water striking water surface causing other injury
W16.62 Jumping or diving into natural body of water striking bottom
W16.621 Jumping or diving into natural body of water striking bottom causing drowning and submersion
EXCLUDES 1 *drowning and submersion while in natural body of water without jumping or diving (W69)*
W16.622 Jumping or diving into natural body of water striking bottom causing other injury
W16.7 Jumping or diving from boat
EXCLUDES 1 *fall from boat into water — see watercraft accident (V9Ø-V94)*
W16.71 Jumping or diving from boat striking water surface
W16.711 Jumping or diving from boat striking water surface causing drowning and submersion
W16.712 Jumping or diving from boat striking water surface causing other injury
W16.72 Jumping or diving from boat striking bottom
W16.721 Jumping or diving from boat striking bottom causing drowning and submersion
W16.722 Jumping or diving from boat striking bottom causing other injury

√5th **W16.8 Jumping or diving into other water**
Jumping or diving into fountain
Jumping or diving into reservoir

√6th **W16.81 Jumping or diving into other water striking water surface**

√7th **W16.811 Jumping or diving into other water striking water surface causing drowning and submersion**
EXCLUDES 1 *drowning and submersion while in other water without jumping or diving (W73)*

√7th **W16.812 Jumping or diving into other water striking water surface causing other injury**

√6th **W16.82 Jumping or diving into other water striking bottom**

√7th **W16.821 Jumping or diving into other water striking bottom causing drowning and submersion**
EXCLUDES 1 *drowning and submersion while in other water without jumping or diving (W73)*

√7th **W16.822 Jumping or diving into other water striking bottom causing other injury**

√6th **W16.83 Jumping or diving into other water striking wall**

√7th **W16.831 Jumping or diving into other water striking wall causing drowning and submersion**
EXCLUDES 1 *drowning and submersion while in other water without jumping or diving (W73)*

√7th **W16.832 Jumping or diving into other water striking wall causing other injury**

√5th **W16.9 Jumping or diving into unspecified water**

√x7th **W16.91 Jumping or diving into unspecified water causing drowning and submersion**

√x7th **W16.92 Jumping or diving into unspecified water causing other injury**

√4th **W17 Other fall from one level to another**

√x7th **W17.Ø Fall into well**

√x7th **W17.1 Fall into storm drain or manhole**

√x7th **W17.2 Fall into hole**
Fall into pit

√x7th **W17.3 Fall into empty swimming pool**
EXCLUDES 1 *fall into filled swimming pool (W16.Ø-)*

√x7th **W17.4 Fall from dock**

√5th **W17.8 Other fall from one level to another**

√x7th **W17.81 Fall down embankment (hill)**

√x7th **W17.82 Fall from (out of) grocery cart**
Fall due to grocery cart tipping over

√x7th **W17.89 Other fall from one level to another**
Fall from cherry picker
Fall from lifting device
Fall from mobile elevated work platform [MEWP]
Fall from sky lift
AHA: 2015,2Q,6

√4th **W18 Other slipping, tripping and stumbling and falls**

√5th **W18.Ø Fall due to bumping against object**
Striking against object with subsequent fall
EXCLUDES 1 *fall on same level due to slipping, tripping, or stumbling with subsequent striking against object (WØ1.1-)*

√x7th **W18.ØØ Striking against unspecified object with subsequent fall**

√x7th **W18.Ø1 Striking against sports equipment with subsequent fall**

√x7th **W18.Ø2 Striking against glass with subsequent fall**

√x7th **W18.Ø9 Striking against other object with subsequent fall**

√5th **W18.1 Fall from or off toilet**

√x7th **W18.11 Fall from or off toilet without subsequent striking against object**
Fall from (off) toilet NOS

√x7th **W18.12 Fall from or off toilet with subsequent striking against object**

√x7th **W18.2 Fall in (into) shower or empty bathtub**
EXCLUDES 1 *fall in full bathtub causing drowning or submersion (W16.21-)*

√5th **W18.3 Other and unspecified fall on same level**

√x7th **W18.3Ø Fall on same level, unspecified**

√x7th **W18.31 Fall on same level due to stepping on an object**
Fall on same level due to stepping on an animal
EXCLUDES 1 *slipping, tripping and stumbling without fall due to stepping on animal (W18.41)*

√x7th **W18.39 Other fall on same level**

√5th **W18.4 Slipping, tripping and stumbling without falling**
EXCLUDES 1 *collision with another person without fall (W51)*

√x7th **W18.4Ø Slipping, tripping and stumbling without falling, unspecified**

√x7th **W18.41 Slipping, tripping and stumbling without falling due to stepping on object**
Slipping, tripping and stumbling without falling due to stepping on animal
EXCLUDES 1 *slipping, tripping and stumbling with fall due to stepping on animal (W18.31)*

√x7th **W18.42 Slipping, tripping and stumbling without falling due to stepping into hole or opening**

√x7th **W18.43 Slipping, tripping and stumbling without falling due to stepping from one level to another**

√x7th **W18.49 Other slipping, tripping and stumbling without falling**

√x7th **W19 Unspecified fall**
Accidental fall NOS
AHA: 2012,4Q,95

Exposure to inanimate mechanical forces (W2Ø-W49)

EXCLUDES 1 *assault (X92-YØ9)*
contact or collision with animals or persons (W5Ø-W64)
exposure to inanimate mechanical forces involving military or war operations (Y36.-, Y37.-)
intentional self-harm (X71-X83)

The appropriate 7th character is to be added to each code from categories W2Ø-W49.
A initial encounter
D subsequent encounter
S sequela

√4th **W2Ø Struck by thrown, projected or falling object**
Code first any associated:
cataclysm (X34-X39)
lightning strike (T75.ØØ)
EXCLUDES 1 *falling object in machinery accident (W24, W28-W31)*
falling object in transport accident (VØ1-V99)
object set in motion by explosion (W35-W4Ø)
object set in motion by firearm (W32-W34)
struck by thrown sports equipment (W21.-)

√x7th **W2Ø.Ø Struck by falling object in cave-in**
EXCLUDES 2 *asphyxiation due to cave-in (T71.21)*

√x7th **W2Ø.1 Struck by object due to collapse of building**
EXCLUDES 1 *struck by object due to collapse of burning building (XØØ.2, XØ2.2)*

√x7th **W2Ø.8 Other cause of strike by thrown, projected or falling object**
EXCLUDES 1 *struck by thrown sports equipment (W21.-)*

√4th **W21 Striking against or struck by sports equipment**
EXCLUDES 1 *assault with sports equipment (YØ8.Ø-)*
striking against or struck by sports equipment with subsequent fall (W18.Ø1)

√5th **W21.Ø Struck by hit or thrown ball**

√x7th **W21.ØØ Struck by hit or thrown ball, unspecified type**

√x7th **W21.Ø1 Struck by football**

√x7th **W21.Ø2 Struck by soccer ball**

√x7th **W21.Ø3 Struck by baseball**

√x7th **W21.Ø4 Struck by golf ball**

√x7th **W21.Ø5 Struck by basketball**

√x7th **W21.Ø6 Struck by volleyball**

√x7th **W21.Ø7 Struck by softball**

W21.Ø9 **Struck by other hit or thrown ball**

W21.1 **Struck by bat, racquet or club**

W21.11 **Struck by baseball bat**

W21.12 **Struck by tennis racquet**

W21.13 **Struck by golf club**

W21.19 **Struck by other bat, racquet or club**

W21.2 **Struck by hockey stick or puck**

W21.21 **Struck by hockey stick**

W21.21Ø **Struck by ice hockey stick**

W21.211 **Struck by field hockey stick**

W21.22 **Struck by hockey puck**

W21.22Ø **Struck by ice hockey puck**

W21.221 **Struck by field hockey puck**

W21.3 **Struck by sports foot wear**

W21.31 **Struck by shoe cleats**

Stepped on by shoe cleats

W21.32 **Struck by skate blades**

Skated over by skate blades

W21.39 **Struck by other sports foot wear**

W21.4 **Striking against diving board**

Use additional code for subsequent falling into water, if applicable (W16.-)

W21.8 **Striking against or struck by other sports equipment**

W21.81 **Striking against or struck by football helmet**

W21.89 **Striking against or struck by other sports equipment**

W21.9 **Striking against or struck by unspecified sports equipment**

W22 **Striking against or struck by other objects**

EXCLUDES 1 *striking against or struck by object with subsequent fall (W18.Ø9)*

W22.Ø **Striking against stationary object**

EXCLUDES 1 *striking against stationary sports equipment (W21.8)*

W22.Ø1 **Walked into wall**

W22.Ø2 **Walked into lamppost**

W22.Ø3 **Walked into furniture**

W22.Ø4 **Striking against wall of swimming pool**

W22.Ø41 **Striking against wall of swimming pool causing drowning and submersion**

EXCLUDES 1 *drowning and submersion while swimming without striking against wall (W67)*

W22.Ø42 **Striking against wall of swimming pool causing other injury**

W22.Ø9 **Striking against other stationary object**

W22.1 **Striking against or struck by automobile airbag**

W22.1Ø **Striking against or struck by unspecified automobile airbag**

W22.11 **Striking against or struck by driver side automobile airbag**

W22.12 **Striking against or struck by front passenger side automobile airbag**

W22.19 **Striking against or struck by other automobile airbag**

W22.8 **Striking against or struck by other objects**

Striking against or struck by object NOS

EXCLUDES 1 *struck by thrown, projected or falling object (W2Ø.-)*

W23 **Caught, crushed, jammed or pinched in or between objects**

EXCLUDES 1 *injury caused by cutting or piercing instruments (W25-W27)*
injury caused by firearms malfunction (W32.1, W33.1-, W34.1-)
injury caused by lifting and transmission devices (W24.-)
injury caused by machinery (W28-W31)
injury caused by nonpowered hand tools (W27.-)
injury caused by transport vehicle being used as a means of transportation (VØ1-V99)
injury caused by struck by thrown, projected or falling object (W2Ø.-)

W23.Ø **Caught, crushed, jammed, or pinched between moving objects**

W23.1 **Caught, crushed, jammed, or pinched between stationary objects**

W24 **Contact with lifting and transmission devices, not elsewhere classified**

EXCLUDES 1 *transport accidents (VØ1-V99)*

W24.Ø **Contact with lifting devices, not elsewhere classified**

Contact with chain hoist
Contact with drive belt
Contact with pulley (block)

W24.1 **Contact with transmission devices, not elsewhere classified**

Contact with transmission belt or cable

W25 **Contact with sharp glass**

Code first any associated:
injury due to flying glass from explosion or firearm discharge (W32-W4Ø)
transport accident (VØØ-V99)

EXCLUDES 1 *fall on same level due to slipping, tripping and stumbling with subsequent striking against sharp glass (WØ1.11Ø)*
striking against sharp glass with subsequent fall (W18.Ø2)

EXCLUDES 2 *glass embedded in skin (W45)*

W26 **Contact with other sharp objects**

EXCLUDES 2 *sharp object(s) embedded in skin (W45)*

AHA: 2016,4Q,73

W26.Ø **Contact with knife**

EXCLUDES 1 *contact with electric knife (W29.1)*

W26.1 **Contact with sword or dagger**

W26.2 **Contact with edge of stiff paper**

Paper cut

W26.8 **Contact with other sharp object(s), not elsewhere classified**

Contact with tin can lid

W26.9 **Contact with unspecified sharp object(s)**

W27 **Contact with nonpowered hand tool**

W27.Ø **Contact with workbench tool**

Contact with auger
Contact with axe
Contact with chisel
Contact with handsaw
Contact with screwdriver

W27.1 **Contact with garden tool**

Contact with hoe
Contact with nonpowered lawn mower
Contact with pitchfork
Contact with rake

W27.2 **Contact with scissors**

W27.3 **Contact with needle (sewing)**

EXCLUDES 1 *contact with hypodermic needle (W46.-)*

W27.4 **Contact with kitchen utensil**

Contact with fork
Contact with ice-pick
Contact with can-opener NOS

W27.5 **Contact with paper-cutter**

W27.8 **Contact with other nonpowered hand tool**

Contact with nonpowered sewing machine
Contact with shovel

W28 **Contact with powered lawn mower**

Powered lawn mower (commercial) (residential)

EXCLUDES 1 *contact with nonpowered lawn mower (W27.1)*

EXCLUDES 2 *exposure to electric current (W86.-)*

W29 **Contact with other powered hand tools and household machinery**

EXCLUDES 1 *contact with commercial machinery (W31.82)*
contact with hot household appliance (X15)
contact with nonpowered hand tool (W27.-)
exposure to electric current (W86)

W29.Ø **Contact with powered kitchen appliance**

Contact with blender
Contact with can-opener
Contact with garbage disposal
Contact with mixer

W29.1 **Contact with electric knife**

√x7th **W29.2 Contact with other powered household machinery**
Contact with electric fan
Contact with powered dryer (clothes) (powered) (spin)
Contact with washing-machine
Contact with sewing machine

√x7th **W29.3 Contact with powered garden and outdoor hand tools and machinery**
Contact with chainsaw
Contact with edger
Contact with garden cultivator (tiller)
Contact with hedge trimmer
Contact with other powered garden tool
EXCLUDES 1 *contact with powered lawn mower (W28)*

√x7th **W29.4 Contact with nail gun**

√x7th **W29.8 Contact with other powered hand tools and household machinery**
Contact with do-it-yourself tool NOS

√4th **W3Ø Contact with agricultural machinery**
INCLUDES animal-powered farm machine
EXCLUDES 1 *agricultural transport vehicle accident (VØ1-V99)*
explosion of grain store (W4Ø.8)
exposure to electric current (W86.-)

√x7th **W3Ø.Ø Contact with combine harvester**
Contact with reaper
Contact with thresher

√x7th **W3Ø.1 Contact with power take-off devices (PTO)**

√x7th **W3Ø.2 Contact with hay derrick**

√x7th **W3Ø.3 Contact with grain storage elevator**
EXCLUDES 1 *explosion of grain store (W4Ø.8)*

√5th **W3Ø.8 Contact with other specified agricultural machinery**

√x7th **W3Ø.81 Contact with agricultural transport vehicle in stationary use**
Contact with agricultural transport vehicle under repair, not on public roadway
EXCLUDES 1 *agricultural transport vehicle accident (VØ1-V99)*

√x7th **W3Ø.89 Contact with other specified agricultural machinery**

√x7th **W3Ø.9 Contact with unspecified agricultural machinery**
Contact with farm machinery NOS

√4th **W31 Contact with other and unspecified machinery**
EXCLUDES 1 *contact with agricultural machinery (W3Ø.-)*
contact with machinery in transport under own power or being towed by a vehicle (VØ1-V99)
exposure to electric current (W86)

√x7th **W31.Ø Contact with mining and earth-drilling machinery**
Contact with bore or drill (land) (seabed)
Contact with shaft hoist
Contact with shaft lift
Contact with undercutter

√x7th **W31.1 Contact with metalworking machines**
Contact with abrasive wheel
Contact with forging machine
Contact with lathe
Contact with mechanical shears
Contact with metal drilling machine
Contact with milling machine
Contact with power press
Contact with rolling-mill
Contact with metal sawing machine

√x7th **W31.2 Contact with powered woodworking and forming machines**
Contact with band saw
Contact with bench saw
Contact with circular saw
Contact with molding machine
Contact with overhead plane
Contact with powered saw
Contact with radial saw
Contact with sander
EXCLUDES 1 *nonpowered woodworking tools (W27.Ø)*

√x7th **W31.3 Contact with prime movers**
Contact with gas turbine
Contact with internal combustion engine
Contact with steam engine
Contact with water driven turbine

√5th **W31.8 Contact with other specified machinery**

√x7th **W31.81 Contact with recreational machinery**
Contact with roller coaster

√x7th **W31.82 Contact with other commercial machinery**
Contact with commercial electric fan
Contact with commercial kitchen appliances
Contact with commercial powered dryer (clothes) (powered) (spin)
Contact with commercial washing-machine
Contact with commercial sewing machine
EXCLUDES 1 *contact with household machinery (W29.-)*
contact with powered lawn mower (W28)

√x7th **W31.83 Contact with special construction vehicle in stationary use**
Contact with special construction vehicle under repair, not on public roadway
EXCLUDES 1 *special construction vehicle accident (VØ1-V99)*

√x7th **W31.89 Contact with other specified machinery**

√x7th **W31.9 Contact with unspecified machinery**
Contact with machinery NOS

√4th **W32 Accidental handgun discharge and malfunction**
INCLUDES accidental discharge and malfunction of gun for single hand use
accidental discharge and malfunction of pistol
accidental discharge and malfunction of revolver
handgun discharge and malfunction NOS
EXCLUDES 1 *accidental airgun discharge and malfunction (W34.Ø1Ø, W34.11Ø)*
accidental BB gun discharge and malfunction (W34.Ø1Ø, W34.11Ø)
accidental pellet gun discharge and malfunction (W34.Ø1Ø, W34.11Ø)
accidental shotgun discharge and malfunction (W33.Ø1, W33.11)
assault by handgun discharge (X93)
handgun discharge involving legal intervention (Y35.Ø-)
handgun discharge involving military or war operations (Y36.4-)
intentional self-harm by handgun discharge (X72)
Very pistol discharge and malfunction (W34.Ø9, W34.19)

√x7th **W32.Ø Accidental handgun discharge**

√x7th **W32.1 Accidental handgun malfunction**
Injury due to explosion of handgun (parts)
Injury due to malfunction of mechanism or component of handgun
Injury due to recoil of handgun
Powder burn from handgun

√4th **W33 Accidental rifle, shotgun and larger firearm discharge and malfunction**
INCLUDES rifle, shotgun and larger firearm discharge and malfunction NOS
EXCLUDES 1 *accidental airgun discharge and malfunction (W34.Ø1Ø, W34.11Ø)*
accidental BB gun discharge and malfunction (W34.Ø1Ø, W34.11Ø)
accidental handgun discharge and malfunction (W32.-)
accidental pellet gun discharge and malfunction (W34.Ø1Ø, W34.11Ø)
assault by rifle, shotgun and larger firearm discharge (X94)
firearm discharge involving legal intervention (Y35.Ø-)
firearm discharge involving military or war operations (Y36.4-)
intentional self-harm by rifle, shotgun and larger firearm discharge (X73)

√5th **W33.Ø Accidental rifle, shotgun and larger firearm discharge**

√x7th **W33.ØØ Accidental discharge of unspecified larger firearm**
Discharge of unspecified larger firearm NOS

W33.01 **Accidental discharge of shotgun**
Discharge of shotgun NOS
W33.02 **Accidental discharge of hunting rifle**
Discharge of hunting rifle NOS
W33.03 **Accidental discharge of machine gun**
Discharge of machine gun NOS
W33.09 **Accidental discharge of other larger firearm**
Discharge of other larger firearm NOS
W33.1 **Accidental rifle, shotgun and larger firearm malfunction**
Injury due to explosion of rifle, shotgun and larger firearm (parts)
Injury due to malfunction of mechanism or component of rifle, shotgun and larger firearm
Injury due to piercing, cutting, crushing or pinching due to (by) slide trigger mechanism, scope or other gun part
Injury due to recoil of rifle, shotgun and larger firearm
Powder burn from rifle, shotgun and larger firearm
W33.10 **Accidental malfunction of unspecified larger firearm**
Malfunction of unspecified larger firearm NOS
W33.11 **Accidental malfunction of shotgun**
Malfunction of shotgun NOS
W33.12 **Accidental malfunction of hunting rifle**
Malfunction of hunting rifle NOS
W33.13 **Accidental malfunction of machine gun**
Malfunction of machine gun NOS
W33.19 **Accidental malfunction of other larger firearm**
Malfunction of other larger firearm NOS
W34 **Accidental discharge and malfunction from other and unspecified firearms and guns**
W34.0 **Accidental discharge from other and unspecified firearms and guns**
W34.00 **Accidental discharge from unspecified firearms or gun**
Discharge from firearm NOS
Gunshot wound NOS
Shot NOS
W34.01 **Accidental discharge of gas, air or spring-operated guns**
W34.010 **Accidental discharge of airgun**
Accidental discharge of BB gun
Accidental discharge of pellet gun
W34.011 **Accidental discharge of paintball gun**
Accidental injury due to paintball discharge
W34.018 **Accidental discharge of other gas, air or spring-operated gun**
W34.09 **Accidental discharge from other specified firearms**
Accidental discharge from Very pistol [flare]
W34.1 **Accidental malfunction from other and unspecified firearms and guns**
W34.10 **Accidental malfunction from unspecified firearms or gun**
Firearm malfunction NOS
W34.11 **Accidental malfunction of gas, air or spring-operated guns**
W34.110 **Accidental malfunction of airgun**
Accidental malfunction of BB gun
Accidental malfunction of pellet gun
W34.111 **Accidental malfunction of paintball gun**
Accidental injury due to paintball gun malfunction
W34.118 **Accidental malfunction of other gas, air or spring-operated gun**
W34.19 **Accidental malfunction from other specified firearms**
Accidental malfunction from Very pistol [flare]
W35 **Explosion and rupture of boiler**
EXCLUDES 1 *explosion and rupture of boiler on watercraft (V93.4)*
W36 **Explosion and rupture of gas cylinder**
W36.1 **Explosion and rupture of aerosol can**
W36.2 **Explosion and rupture of air tank**
W36.3 **Explosion and rupture of pressurized-gas tank**
W36.8 **Explosion and rupture of other gas cylinder**
W36.9 **Explosion and rupture of unspecified gas cylinder**
W37 **Explosion and rupture of pressurized tire, pipe or hose**
W37.0 **Explosion of bicycle tire**
W37.8 **Explosion and rupture of other pressurized tire, pipe or hose**
W38 **Explosion and rupture of other specified pressurized devices**
W39 **Discharge of firework**
W40 **Explosion of other materials**
EXCLUDES 1 *assault by explosive material (X96)*
explosion involving legal intervention (Y35.1-)
explosion involving military or war operations (Y36.0-, Y36.2-)
intentional self-harm by explosive material (X75)
W40.0 **Explosion of blasting material**
Explosion of blasting cap
Explosion of detonator
Explosion of dynamite
Explosion of explosive (any) used in blasting operations
W40.1 **Explosion of explosive gases**
Explosion of acetylene
Explosion of butane
Explosion of coal gas
Explosion in mine NOS
Explosion of explosive gas
Explosion of fire damp
Explosion of gasoline fumes
Explosion of methane
Explosion of propane
W40.8 **Explosion of other specified explosive materials**
Explosion in dump NOS
Explosion in factory NOS
Explosion in grain store
Explosion in munitions
EXCLUDES 1 *explosion involving legal intervention (Y35.1-)*
explosion involving military or war operations (Y36.0-, Y36.2-)
W40.9 **Explosion of unspecified explosive materials**
Explosion NOS
W42 **Exposure to noise**
W42.0 **Exposure to supersonic waves**
W42.9 **Exposure to other noise**
Exposure to sound waves NOS
W45 **Foreign body or object entering through skin**
INCLUDES foreign body or object embedded in skin
nail embedded in skin
EXCLUDES 2 *contact with hand tools (nonpowered) (powered) (W27-W29)*
contact with other sharp objects (W26.-)
contact with sharp glass (W25.-)
struck by objects (W20-W22)
W45.0 **Nail entering through skin**
W45.8 **Other foreign body or object entering through skin**
Splinter in skin NOS
W46 **Contact with hypodermic needle**
W46.0 **Contact with hypodermic needle**
Hypodermic needle stick NOS
W46.1 **Contact with contaminated hypodermic needle**
W49 **Exposure to other inanimate mechanical forces**
INCLUDES exposure to abnormal gravitational [G] forces
exposure to inanimate mechanical forces NEC
EXCLUDES 1 *exposure to inanimate mechanical forces involving military or war operations (Y36.-, Y37.-)*
W49.0 **Item causing external constriction**
W49.01 **Hair causing external constriction**
W49.02 **String or thread causing external constriction**
W49.03 **Rubber band causing external constriction**
W49.04 **Ring or other jewelry causing external constriction**
W49.09 **Other specified item causing external constriction**
W49.9 **Exposure to other inanimate mechanical forces**

Exposure to animate mechanical forces (W50-W64)

EXCLUDES 1 *toxic effect of contact with venomous animals and plants (T63.-)*

The appropriate 7th character is to be added to each code from categories W50-W64.
A initial encounter
D subsequent encounter
S sequela

W50 Accidental hit, strike, kick, twist, bite or scratch by another person
INCLUDES hit, strike, kick, twist, bite, or scratch by another person NOS
EXCLUDES 1 *assault by bodily force (Y04)*
struck by objects (W20-W22)

W50.0 Accidental hit or strike by another person
Hit or strike by another person NOS

W50.1 Accidental kick by another person
Kick by another person NOS

W50.2 Accidental twist by another person
Twist by another person NOS

W50.3 Accidental bite by another person
Human bite
Bite by another person NOS

W50.4 Accidental scratch by another person
Scratch by another person NOS

W51 Accidental striking against or bumped into by another person
EXCLUDES 1 *assault by striking against or bumping into by another person (Y04.2)*
fall due to collision with another person (W03)

W52 Crushed, pushed or stepped on by crowd or human stampede
Crushed, pushed or stepped on by crowd or human stampede with or without fall

W53 Contact with rodent
INCLUDES contact with saliva, feces or urine of rodent

W53.0 Contact with mouse
W53.01 Bitten by mouse
W53.09 Other contact with mouse

W53.1 Contact with rat
W53.11 Bitten by rat
W53.19 Other contact with rat

W53.2 Contact with squirrel
W53.21 Bitten by squirrel
W53.29 Other contact with squirrel

W53.8 Contact with other rodent
W53.81 Bitten by other rodent
W53.89 Other contact with other rodent

W54 Contact with dog
INCLUDES contact with saliva, feces or urine of dog

W54.0 Bitten by dog

W54.1 Struck by dog
Knocked over by dog

W54.8 Other contact with dog

W55 Contact with other mammals
INCLUDES contact with saliva, feces or urine of mammal
EXCLUDES 1 *animal being ridden — see transport accidents*
bitten or struck by dog (W54)
bitten or struck by rodent (W53.-)
contact with marine mammals (W56.-)

W55.0 Contact with cat
W55.01 Bitten by cat
W55.03 Scratched by cat
W55.09 Other contact with cat

W55.1 Contact with horse
W55.11 Bitten by horse
W55.12 Struck by horse
W55.19 Other contact with horse

W55.2 Contact with cow
Contact with bull
W55.21 Bitten by cow
W55.22 Struck by cow
Gored by bull
W55.29 Other contact with cow

W55.3 Contact with other hoof stock
Contact with goats
Contact with sheep
W55.31 Bitten by other hoof stock
W55.32 Struck by other hoof stock
Gored by goat
Gored by ram
W55.39 Other contact with other hoof stock

W55.4 Contact with pig
W55.41 Bitten by pig
W55.42 Struck by pig
W55.49 Other contact with pig

W55.5 Contact with raccoon
W55.51 Bitten by raccoon
W55.52 Struck by raccoon
W55.59 Other contact with raccoon

W55.8 Contact with other mammals
W55.81 Bitten by other mammals
W55.82 Struck by other mammals
W55.89 Other contact with other mammals

W56 Contact with nonvenomous marine animal
EXCLUDES 1 *contact with venomous marine animal (T63.-)*

W56.0 Contact with dolphin
W56.01 Bitten by dolphin
W56.02 Struck by dolphin
W56.09 Other contact with dolphin

W56.1 Contact with sea lion
W56.11 Bitten by sea lion
W56.12 Struck by sea lion
W56.19 Other contact with sea lion

W56.2 Contact with orca
Contact with killer whale
W56.21 Bitten by orca
W56.22 Struck by orca
W56.29 Other contact with orca

W56.3 Contact with other marine mammals
W56.31 Bitten by other marine mammals
W56.32 Struck by other marine mammals
W56.39 Other contact with other marine mammals

W56.4 Contact with shark
W56.41 Bitten by shark
W56.42 Struck by shark
W56.49 Other contact with shark

W56.5 Contact with other fish
W56.51 Bitten by other fish
W56.52 Struck by other fish
W56.59 Other contact with other fish

W56.8 Contact with other nonvenomous marine animals
W56.81 Bitten by other nonvenomous marine animals
W56.82 Struck by other nonvenomous marine animals
W56.89 Other contact with other nonvenomous marine animals

W57 Bitten or stung by nonvenomous insect and other nonvenomous arthropods
EXCLUDES 1 *contact with venomous insects and arthropods (T63.2-, T63.3-, T63.4-)*

W58 Contact with crocodile or alligator

W58.0 Contact with alligator
W58.01 Bitten by alligator
W58.02 Struck by alligator
W58.03 Crushed by alligator
W58.09 Other contact with alligator

W58.1 Contact with crocodile
- W58.11 Bitten by crocodile
- W58.12 Struck by crocodile
- W58.13 Crushed by crocodile
- W58.19 Other contact with crocodile

W59 Contact with other nonvenomous reptiles

EXCLUDES 1 *contact with venomous reptile (T63.Ø-, T63.1-)*

W59.Ø Contact with nonvenomous lizards
- W59.Ø1 Bitten by nonvenomous lizards
- W59.Ø2 Struck by nonvenomous lizards
- W59.Ø9 Other contact with nonvenomous lizards
  - Exposure to nonvenomous lizards

W59.1 Contact with nonvenomous snakes
- W59.11 Bitten by nonvenomous snake
- W59.12 Struck by nonvenomous snake
- W59.13 Crushed by nonvenomous snake
- W59.19 Other contact with nonvenomous snake

W59.2 Contact with turtles

EXCLUDES 1 *contact with tortoises (W59.8-)*

- W59.21 Bitten by turtle
- W59.22 Struck by turtle
- W59.29 Other contact with turtle
  - Exposure to turtles

W59.8 Contact with other nonvenomous reptiles
- W59.81 Bitten by other nonvenomous reptiles
- W59.82 Struck by other nonvenomous reptiles
- W59.83 Crushed by other nonvenomous reptiles
- W59.89 Other contact with other nonvenomous reptiles

W6Ø Contact with nonvenomous plant thorns and spines and sharp leaves

EXCLUDES 1 *contact with venomous plants (T63.7-)*

W61 Contact with birds (domestic) (wild)

INCLUDES contact with excreta of birds

W61.Ø Contact with parrot
- W61.Ø1 Bitten by parrot
- W61.Ø2 Struck by parrot
- W61.Ø9 Other contact with parrot
  - Exposure to parrots

W61.1 Contact with macaw
- W61.11 Bitten by macaw
- W61.12 Struck by macaw
- W61.19 Other contact with macaw
  - Exposure to macaws

W61.2 Contact with other psittacines
- W61.21 Bitten by other psittacines
- W61.22 Struck by other psittacines
- W61.29 Other contact with other psittacines
  - Exposure to other psittacines

W61.3 Contact with chicken
- W61.32 Struck by chicken
- W61.33 Pecked by chicken
- W61.39 Other contact with chicken
  - Exposure to chickens

W61.4 Contact with turkey
- W61.42 Struck by turkey
- W61.43 Pecked by turkey
- W61.49 Other contact with turkey

W61.5 Contact with goose
- W61.51 Bitten by goose
- W61.52 Struck by goose
- W61.59 Other contact with goose

W61.6 Contact with duck
- W61.61 Bitten by duck
- W61.62 Struck by duck
- W61.69 Other contact with duck

W61.9 Contact with other birds
- W61.91 Bitten by other birds
- W61.92 Struck by other birds
- W61.99 Other contact with other birds
  - Contact with bird NOS

W62 Contact with nonvenomous amphibians

EXCLUDES 1 *contact with venomous amphibians (T63.81-R63.83)*

- W62.Ø Contact with nonvenomous frogs
- W62.1 Contact with nonvenomous toads
- W62.9 Contact with other nonvenomous amphibians

W64 Exposure to other animate mechanical forces

INCLUDES exposure to nonvenomous animal NOS

EXCLUDES 1 *contact with venomous animal (T63.-)*

Accidental non-transport drowning and submersion (W65-W74)

EXCLUDES 1 *accidental drowning and submersion due to fall into water (W16.-)*
accidental drowning and submersion due to water transport accident (V9Ø.-, V92.-)

EXCLUDES 2 *accidental drowning and submersion due to cataclysm (X34-X39)*

The appropriate 7th character is to be added to each code from categories W65-W74.
A initial encounter
D subsequent encounter
S sequela

W65 Accidental drowning and submersion while in bath-tub

EXCLUDES 1 *accidental drowning and submersion due to fall in (into) bathtub (W16.211)*

W67 Accidental drowning and submersion while in swimming-pool

EXCLUDES 1 *accidental drowning and submersion due to fall into swimming pool (W16.Ø11, W16.Ø21, W16.Ø31)*
accidental drowning and submersion due to striking into wall of swimming pool (W22.Ø41)

W69 Accidental drowning and submersion while in natural water

Accidental drowning and submersion while in lake
Accidental drowning and submersion while in open sea
Accidental drowning and submersion while in river
Accidental drowning and submersion while in stream

EXCLUDES 1 *accidental drowning and submersion due to fall into natural body of water (W16.111, W16.121, W16.131)*

W73 Other specified cause of accidental non-transport drowning and submersion

Accidental drowning and submersion while in quenching tank
Accidental drowning and submersion while in reservoir

EXCLUDES 1 *accidental drowning and submersion due to fall into other water (W16.311, W16.321, W16.331)*

W74 Unspecified cause of accidental drowning and submersion

Drowning NOS

Exposure to electric current, radiation and extreme ambient air temperature and pressure (W85-W99)

EXCLUDES 1 *exposure to:*
failure in dosage of radiation or temperature during surgical and medical care (Y63.2-Y63.5)
lightning (T75.Ø-)
natural cold (X31)
natural heat (X3Ø)
natural radiation NOS (X39)
radiological procedure and radiotherapy (Y84.2)
sunlight (X32)

AHA: 2018,2Q,7-8

The appropriate 7th character is to be added to each code from categories W85-W99.
A initial encounter
D subsequent encounter
S sequela

W85 Exposure to electric transmission lines

Broken power line

W86 Exposure to other specified electric current

- W86.Ø Exposure to domestic wiring and appliances

√x7th **W86.1 Exposure to industrial wiring, appliances and electrical machinery**
Exposure to conductors
Exposure to control apparatus
Exposure to electrical equipment and machinery
Exposure to transformers

√x7th **W86.8 Exposure to other electric current**
Exposure to wiring and appliances in or on farm (not farmhouse)
Exposure to wiring and appliances outdoors
Exposure to wiring and appliances in or on public building
Exposure to wiring and appliances in or on residential institutions
Exposure to wiring and appliances in or on schools

√4th **W88 Exposure to ionizing radiation**
EXCLUDES 1 *exposure to sunlight (X32)*

√x7th **W88.Ø Exposure to X-rays**

√x7th **W88.1 Exposure to radioactive isotopes**

√x7th **W88.8 Exposure to other ionizing radiation**

√4th **W89 Exposure to man-made visible and ultraviolet light**
INCLUDES exposure to welding light (arc)
EXCLUDES 1 ~~*exposure to sunlight (X32)*~~
EXCLUDES 2 ►*exposure to sunlight (X32)*◄

√x7th **W89.Ø Exposure to welding light (arc)**

√x7th **W89.1 Exposure to tanning bed**

√x7th **W89.8 Exposure to other man-made visible and ultraviolet light**

√x7th **W89.9 Exposure to unspecified man-made visible and ultraviolet light**

√4th **W9Ø Exposure to other nonionizing radiation**
EXCLUDES 1 ~~*exposure to sunlight (X32)*~~
EXCLUDES 2 ►*exposure to sunlight (X32)*◄
AHA: 2019,1Q,21

√x7th **W9Ø.Ø Exposure to radiofrequency**

√x7th **W9Ø.1 Exposure to infrared radiation**

√x7th **W9Ø.2 Exposure to laser radiation**

√x7th **W9Ø.8 Exposure to other nonionizing radiation**

√x7th **W92 Exposure to excessive heat of man-made origin**

√4th **W93 Exposure to excessive cold of man-made origin**

√5th **W93.Ø Contact with or inhalation of dry ice**

√x7th **W93.Ø1 Contact with dry ice**

√x7th **W93.Ø2 Inhalation of dry ice**

√5th **W93.1 Contact with or inhalation of liquid air**

√x7th **W93.11 Contact with liquid air**
Contact with liquid hydrogen
Contact with liquid nitrogen

√x7th **W93.12 Inhalation of liquid air**
Inhalation of liquid hydrogen
Inhalation of liquid nitrogen

√x7th **W93.2 Prolonged exposure in deep freeze unit or refrigerator**

√x7th **W93.8 Exposure to other excessive cold of man-made origin**

√4th **W94 Exposure to high and low air pressure and changes in air pressure**

√x7th **W94.Ø Exposure to prolonged high air pressure**

√5th **W94.1 Exposure to prolonged low air pressure**

√x7th **W94.11 Exposure to residence or prolonged visit at high altitude**

√x7th **W94.12 Exposure to other prolonged low air pressure**

√5th **W94.2 Exposure to rapid changes in air pressure during ascent**

√x7th **W94.21 Exposure to reduction in atmospheric pressure while surfacing from deep-water diving**

√x7th **W94.22 Exposure to reduction in atmospheric pressure while surfacing from underground**

√x7th **W94.23 Exposure to sudden change in air pressure in aircraft during ascent**

√x7th **W94.29 Exposure to other rapid changes in air pressure during ascent**

√5th **W94.3 Exposure to rapid changes in air pressure during descent**

√x7th **W94.31 Exposure to sudden change in air pressure in aircraft during descent**

√x7th **W94.32 Exposure to high air pressure from rapid descent in water**

√x7th **W94.39 Exposure to other rapid changes in air pressure during descent**

√x7th **W99 Exposure to other man-made environmental factors**

Exposure to smoke, fire and flames (XØØ-XØ8)

EXCLUDES 1 *arson (X97)*
EXCLUDES 2 *explosions (W35-W4Ø)*
lightning (T75.Ø-)
transport accident (VØ1-V99)
AHA: 2018,2Q,7-8

The appropriate 7th character is to be added to each code from categories XØØ-XØ8.
A initial encounter
D subsequent encounter
S sequela

√4th **XØØ Exposure to uncontrolled fire in building or structure**
INCLUDES conflagration in building or structure
Code first any associated cataclysm
EXCLUDES 2 *exposure to ignition or melting of nightwear (XØ5)*
exposure to ignition or melting of other clothing and apparel (XØ6.-)
exposure to other specified smoke, fire and flames (XØ8.-)
AHA: 2016,2Q,5

√x7th **XØØ.Ø Exposure to flames in uncontrolled fire in building or structure**

√x7th **XØØ.1 Exposure to smoke in uncontrolled fire in building or structure**

√x7th **XØØ.2 Injury due to collapse of burning building or structure in uncontrolled fire**
EXCLUDES 1 *injury due to collapse of building not on fire (W2Ø.1)*

√x7th **XØØ.3 Fall from burning building or structure in uncontrolled fire**

√x7th **XØØ.4 Hit by object from burning building or structure in uncontrolled fire**
AHA: 2016,2Q,4

√x7th **XØØ.5 Jump from burning building or structure in uncontrolled fire**

√x7th **XØØ.8 Other exposure to uncontrolled fire in building or structure**

√4th **XØ1 Exposure to uncontrolled fire, not in building or structure**
INCLUDES exposure to forest fire

√x7th **XØ1.Ø Exposure to flames in uncontrolled fire, not in building or structure**

√x7th **XØ1.1 Exposure to smoke in uncontrolled fire, not in building or structure**

√x7th **XØ1.3 Fall due to uncontrolled fire, not in building or structure**

√x7th **XØ1.4 Hit by object due to uncontrolled fire, not in building or structure**

√x7th **XØ1.8 Other exposure to uncontrolled fire, not in building or structure**

√4th **XØ2 Exposure to controlled fire in building or structure**
INCLUDES exposure to fire in fireplace
exposure to fire in stove

√x7th **XØ2.Ø Exposure to flames in controlled fire in building or structure**

√x7th **XØ2.1 Exposure to smoke in controlled fire in building or structure**

√x7th **XØ2.2 Injury due to collapse of burning building or structure in controlled fire**
EXCLUDES 1 *injury due to collapse of building not on fire (W2Ø.1)*

√x7th **XØ2.3 Fall from burning building or structure in controlled fire**

√x7th **XØ2.4 Hit by object from burning building or structure in controlled fire**

√x7th **XØ2.5 Jump from burning building or structure in controlled fire**

√x7th **XØ2.8 Other exposure to controlled fire in building or structure**

√4th **XØ3 Exposure to controlled fire, not in building or structure**
INCLUDES exposure to bon fire
exposure to camp-fire
exposure to trash fire

√x7th **XØ3.Ø Exposure to flames in controlled fire, not in building or structure**

√x7th **XØ3.1 Exposure to smoke in controlled fire, not in building or structure**

√x7th **XØ3.3 Fall due to controlled fire, not in building or structure**

√x7th **XØ3.4 Hit by object due to controlled fire, not in building or structure**

√x7th **XØ3.8 Other exposure to controlled fire, not in building or structure**

X04 Exposure to ignition of highly flammable material
Exposure to ignition of gasoline
Exposure to ignition of kerosene
Exposure to ignition of petrol
EXCLUDES 2 *exposure to ignition or melting of nightwear (X05)*
exposure to ignition or melting of other clothing and apparel (X06)
AHA: 2016,2Q,4

X05 Exposure to ignition or melting of nightwear
EXCLUDES 2 *exposure to uncontrolled fire in building or structure (X00.-)*
exposure to uncontrolled fire, not in building or structure (X01.-)
exposure to controlled fire in building or structure (X02.-)
exposure to controlled fire, not in building or structure (X03.-)
exposure to ignition of highly flammable materials (X04.-)

X06 Exposure to ignition or melting of other clothing and apparel
EXCLUDES 2 *exposure to uncontrolled fire in building or structure (X00.-)*
exposure to uncontrolled fire, not in building or structure (X01.-)
exposure to controlled fire in building or structure (X02.-)
exposure to controlled fire, not in building or structure (X03.-)
exposure to ignition of highly flammable materials (X04.-)
X06.0 Exposure to ignition of plastic jewelry
X06.1 Exposure to melting of plastic jewelry
X06.2 Exposure to ignition of other clothing and apparel
X06.3 Exposure to melting of other clothing and apparel

X08 Exposure to other specified smoke, fire and flames
X08.0 Exposure to bed fire
Exposure to mattress fire
X08.00 Exposure to bed fire due to unspecified burning material
X08.01 Exposure to bed fire due to burning cigarette
X08.09 Exposure to bed fire due to other burning material
X08.1 Exposure to sofa fire
X08.10 Exposure to sofa fire due to unspecified burning material
X08.11 Exposure to sofa fire due to burning cigarette
X08.19 Exposure to sofa fire due to other burning material
X08.2 Exposure to other furniture fire
X08.20 Exposure to other furniture fire due to unspecified burning material
X08.21 Exposure to other furniture fire due to burning cigarette
X08.29 Exposure to other furniture fire due to other burning material
X08.8 Exposure to other specified smoke, fire and flames

Contact with heat and hot substances (X10-X19)

EXCLUDES 1 *exposure to excessive natural heat (X30)*
exposure to fire and flames (X00-X08)
AHA: 2018,2Q,7-8

The appropriate 7th character is to be added to each code from categories X10-X19.
A initial encounter
D subsequent encounter
S sequela

X10 Contact with hot drinks, food, fats and cooking oils
X10.0 Contact with hot drinks
X10.1 Contact with hot food
X10.2 Contact with fats and cooking oils

X11 Contact with hot tap-water
INCLUDES contact with boiling tap-water
contact with boiling water NOS
EXCLUDES 1 *contact with water heated on stove (X12)*
X11.0 Contact with hot water in bath or tub
EXCLUDES 1 *contact with running hot water in bath or tub (X11.1)*
X11.1 Contact with running hot water
Contact with hot water running out of hose
Contact with hot water running out of tap
X11.8 Contact with other hot tap-water
Contact with hot water in bucket
Contact with hot tap-water NOS

X12 Contact with other hot fluids
Contact with water heated on stove
EXCLUDES 1 *hot (liquid) metals (X18)*

X13 Contact with steam and other hot vapors
X13.0 Inhalation of steam and other hot vapors
X13.1 Other contact with steam and other hot vapors

X14 Contact with hot air and other hot gases
X14.0 Inhalation of hot air and gases
X14.1 Other contact with hot air and other hot gases

X15 Contact with hot household appliances
EXCLUDES 1 *contact with heating appliances (X16)*
contact with powered household appliances (W29.-)
exposure to controlled fire in building or structure due to household appliance (X02.8)
exposure to household appliances electrical current (W86.0)
X15.0 Contact with hot stove (kitchen)
X15.1 Contact with hot toaster
X15.2 Contact with hotplate
X15.3 Contact with hot saucepan or skillet
X15.8 Contact with other hot household appliances
Contact with cooker
Contact with kettle
Contact with light bulbs

X16 Contact with hot heating appliances, radiators and pipes
EXCLUDES 1 *contact with powered appliances (W29.-)*
exposure to controlled fire in building or structure due to appliance (X02.8)
exposure to industrial appliances electrical current (W86.1)

X17 Contact with hot engines, machinery and tools
EXCLUDES 1 *contact with hot heating appliances, radiators and pipes (X16)*
contact with hot household appliances (X15)

X18 Contact with other hot metals
Contact with liquid metal

X19 Contact with other heat and hot substances
EXCLUDES 1 *objects that are not normally hot, e.g., an object made hot by a house fire (X00-X08)*

Exposure to forces of nature (X30-X39)

AHA: 2018,2Q,7-8

The appropriate 7th character is to be added to each code from categories X30-X39.
A initial encounter
D subsequent encounter
S sequela

X30 Exposure to excessive natural heat
Exposure to excessive heat as the cause of sunstroke
Exposure to heat NOS
EXCLUDES 1 *excessive heat of man-made origin (W92)*
exposure to man-made radiation (W89)
exposure to sunlight (X32)
exposure to tanning bed (W89)

X31 Exposure to excessive natural cold
Excessive cold as the cause of chilblains NOS
Excessive cold as the cause of immersion foot or hand
Exposure to cold NOS
Exposure to weather conditions
EXCLUDES 1 *cold of man-made origin (W93.-)*
contact with or inhalation of dry ice (W93.-)
contact with or inhalation of liquefied gas (W93.-)

X32 Exposure to sunlight
EXCLUDES 1 *man-made radiation (tanning bed) (W89)*
EXCLUDES 2 *radiation-related disorders of the skin and subcutaneous tissue (L55-L59)*

X34 Earthquake
EXCLUDES 2 *tidal wave (tsunami) due to earthquake (X37.41)*

X35 Volcanic eruption
EXCLUDES 2 *tidal wave (tsunami) due to volcanic eruption (X37.41)*

X36 Avalanche, landslide and other earth movements
INCLUDES victim of mudslide of cataclysmic nature
EXCLUDES 1 *earthquake (X34)*
EXCLUDES 2 *transport accident involving collision with avalanche or landslide not in motion (V01-V99)*

X36.0 Collapse of dam or man-made structure causing earth movement

X36.1 Avalanche, landslide, or mudslide

X37 Cataclysmic storm

X37.0 Hurricane
Storm surge
Typhoon

X37.1 Tornado
Cyclone
Twister

X37.2 Blizzard (snow)(ice)

X37.3 Dust storm

X37.4 Tidalwave

X37.41 Tidal wave due to earthquake or volcanic eruption
Tidal wave NOS
Tsunami

X37.42 Tidal wave due to storm

X37.43 Tidal wave due to landslide

X37.8 Other cataclysmic storms
Cloudburst
Torrential rain
EXCLUDES 2 *flood (X38)*

X37.9 Unspecified cataclysmic storm
Storm NOS
EXCLUDES 1 *collapse of dam or man-made structure causing earth movement (X36.0)*

X38 Flood
Flood arising from remote storm
Flood of cataclysmic nature arising from melting snow
Flood resulting directly from storm
EXCLUDES 1 *collapse of dam or man-made structure causing earth movement (X36.0)*
tidal wave NOS (X37.41)
tidal wave caused by storm (X37.42)

X39 Exposure to other forces of nature

X39.0 Exposure to natural radiation
EXCLUDES 1 *contact with and (suspected) exposure to radon and other naturally occurring radiation (Z77.123)*
exposure to man-made radiation (W88-W90)
exposure to sunlight (X32)

X39.01 Exposure to radon

X39.08 Exposure to other natural radiation

X39.8 Other exposure to forces of nature

Overexertion and strenuous or repetitive movements (X50)

X50 Overexertion and strenuous or repetitive movements
AHA: 2018,2Q,7-8; 2016,4Q,73-74

The appropriate 7th character is to be added to each code from category X50.
A initial encounter
D subsequent encounter
S sequela

X50.0 Overexertion from strenuous movement or load
Lifting heavy objects
Lifting weights

X50.1 Overexertion from prolonged static or awkward postures
Prolonged bending
Prolonged kneeling
Prolonged reaching
Prolonged sitting
Prolonged standing
Prolonged twisting
Static bending
Static kneeling
Static reaching
Static sitting
Static standing
Static twisting

X50.3 Overexertion from repetitive movements
Use of hand as hammer
EXCLUDES 2 *overuse from prolonged static or awkward postures (X50.1)*

X50.9 Other and unspecified overexertion or strenuous movements or postures
Contact pressure
Contact stress

Accidental exposure to other specified factors (X52-X58)

AHA: 2018,2Q,7-8

The appropriate 7th character is to be added to each code from categories X52-X58.
A initial encounter
D subsequent encounter
S sequela

X52 Prolonged stay in weightless environment
Weightlessness in spacecraft (simulator)

X58 Exposure to other specified factors
Accident NOS
Exposure NOS

Intentional self-harm (X71-X83)

Purposely self-inflicted injury
Suicide (attempted)

The appropriate 7th character is to be added to each code from categories X71-X83.
A initial encounter
D subsequent encounter
S sequela

X71 Intentional self-harm by drowning and submersion

X71.0 Intentional self-harm by drowning and submersion while in bathtub HCC

X71.1 Intentional self-harm by drowning and submersion while in swimming pool HCC

X71.2 Intentional self-harm by drowning and submersion after jump into swimming pool HCC

X71.3 Intentional self-harm by drowning and submersion in natural water HCC

X71.8 Other intentional self-harm by drowning and submersion HCC

X71.9 Intentional self-harm by drowning and submersion, unspecified HCC

X72 Intentional self-harm by handgun discharge HCC
Intentional self-harm by gun for single hand use
Intentional self-harm by pistol
Intentional self-harm by revolver
EXCLUDES 1 *Very pistol (X74.8)*

X73 Intentional self-harm by rifle, shotgun and larger firearm discharge
EXCLUDES 1 *airgun (X74.01)*

X73.0 Intentional self-harm by shotgun discharge HCC

X73.1 Intentional self-harm by hunting rifle discharge HCC

X73.2 Intentional self-harm by machine gun discharge HCC

X73.8 Intentional self-harm by other larger firearm discharge HCC

X73.9 Intentional self-harm by unspecified larger firearm discharge HCC

X74 Intentional self-harm by other and unspecified firearm and gun discharge

X74.0 Intentional self-harm by gas, air or spring-operated guns

X74.01 Intentional self-harm by airgun HCC

Intentional self-harm by BB gun discharge
Intentional self-harm by pellet gun discharge

X74.02 Intentional self-harm by paintball gun HCC

X74.09 Intentional self-harm by other gas, air or spring-operated gun HCC

X74.8 Intentional self-harm by other firearm discharge HCC

Intentional self-harm by Very pistol [flare] discharge

X74.9 Intentional self-harm by unspecified firearm discharge HCC

X75 Intentional self-harm by explosive material HCC

X76 Intentional self-harm by smoke, fire and flames HCC

X77 Intentional self-harm by steam, hot vapors and hot objects

X77.0 Intentional self-harm by steam or hot vapors HCC

X77.1 Intentional self-harm by hot tap water HCC

X77.2 Intentional self-harm by other hot fluids HCC

X77.3 Intentional self-harm by hot household appliances HCC

X77.8 Intentional self-harm by other hot objects HCC

X77.9 Intentional self-harm by unspecified hot objects HCC

X78 Intentional self-harm by sharp object

X78.0 Intentional self-harm by sharp glass HCC

X78.1 Intentional self-harm by knife HCC

X78.2 Intentional self-harm by sword or dagger HCC

X78.8 Intentional self-harm by other sharp object HCC

X78.9 Intentional self-harm by unspecified sharp object HCC

X79 Intentional self-harm by blunt object HCC

X80 Intentional self-harm by jumping from a high place HCC

Intentional fall from one level to another

X81 Intentional self-harm by jumping or lying in front of moving object

X81.0 Intentional self-harm by jumping or lying in front of motor vehicle HCC

X81.1 Intentional self-harm by jumping or lying in front of (subway) train HCC

X81.8 Intentional self-harm by jumping or lying in front of other moving object HCC

X82 Intentional self-harm by crashing of motor vehicle

X82.0 Intentional collision of motor vehicle with other motor vehicle HCC

X82.1 Intentional collision of motor vehicle with train HCC

X82.2 Intentional collision of motor vehicle with tree HCC

X82.8 Other intentional self-harm by crashing of motor vehicle HCC

X83 Intentional self-harm by other specified means

EXCLUDES 1 *intentional self-harm by poisoning or contact with toxic substance — see Table of Drugs and Chemicals*

X83.0 Intentional self-harm by crashing of aircraft HCC

X83.1 Intentional self-harm by electrocution HCC

X83.2 Intentional self-harm by exposure to extremes of cold HCC

X83.8 Intentional self-harm by other specified means HCC

Assault (X92-Y09)

INCLUDES homicide
injuries inflicted by another person with intent to injure or kill, by any means

EXCLUDES 1 *injuries due to legal intervention (Y35.-)*
injuries due to operations of war (Y36.-)
injuries due to terrorism (Y38.-)

The appropriate 7th character is to be added to each code from categories X92-Y04 and Y08.
A initial encounter
D subsequent encounter
S sequela

X92 Assault by drowning and submersion

X92.0 Assault by drowning and submersion while in bathtub

X92.1 Assault by drowning and submersion while in swimming pool

X92.2 Assault by drowning and submersion after push into swimming pool

X92.3 Assault by drowning and submersion in natural water

X92.8 Other assault by drowning and submersion

X92.9 Assault by drowning and submersion, unspecified

X93 Assault by handgun discharge

Assault by discharge of gun for single hand use
Assault by discharge of pistol
Assault by discharge of revolver

EXCLUDES 1 *Very pistol (X95.8)*

X94 Assault by rifle, shotgun and larger firearm discharge

EXCLUDES 1 *airgun (X95.01)*

X94.0 Assault by shotgun

X94.1 Assault by hunting rifle

X94.2 Assault by machine gun

X94.8 Assault by other larger firearm discharge

X94.9 Assault by unspecified larger firearm discharge

X95 Assault by other and unspecified firearm and gun discharge

X95.0 Assault by gas, air or spring-operated guns

X95.01 Assault by airgun discharge

Assault by BB gun discharge
Assault by pellet gun discharge

X95.02 Assault by paintball gun discharge

X95.09 Assault by other gas, air or spring-operated gun

X95.8 Assault by other firearm discharge

Assault by Very pistol [flare] discharge

X95.9 Assault by unspecified firearm discharge

X96 Assault by explosive material

EXCLUDES 1 *incendiary device (X97)*
terrorism involving explosive material (Y38.2-)

X96.0 Assault by antipersonnel bomb

EXCLUDES 1 *antipersonnel bomb use in military or war (Y36.2-)*

X96.1 Assault by gasoline bomb

X96.2 Assault by letter bomb

X96.3 Assault by fertilizer bomb

X96.4 Assault by pipe bomb

X96.8 Assault by other specified explosive

X96.9 Assault by unspecified explosive

X97 Assault by smoke, fire and flames

Assault by arson
Assault by cigarettes
Assault by incendiary device

X98 Assault by steam, hot vapors and hot objects

X98.0 Assault by steam or hot vapors

X98.1 Assault by hot tap water

X98.2 Assault by hot fluids

X98.3 Assault by hot household appliances

X98.8 Assault by other hot objects

X98.9 Assault by unspecified hot objects

X99 Assault by sharp object

EXCLUDES 1 *assault by strike by sports equipment (Y08.0-)*

X99.0 Assault by sharp glass

X99.1 Assault by knife

X99.2 Assault by sword or dagger

X99.8 Assault by other sharp object

X99.9 Assault by unspecified sharp object

Assault by stabbing NOS

Y00 Assault by blunt object

EXCLUDES 1 *assault by strike by sports equipment (Y08.0-)*

Y01 Assault by pushing from high place

Y02 Assault by pushing or placing victim in front of moving object

Y02.0 Assault by pushing or placing victim in front of motor vehicle

Y02.1 Assault by pushing or placing victim in front of (subway) train

√x7th **Y02.8 Assault by pushing or placing victim in front of other moving object**

√4th **Y03 Assault by crashing of motor vehicle**

√x7th **Y03.0 Assault by being hit or run over by motor vehicle**

√x7th **Y03.8 Other assault by crashing of motor vehicle**

√4th **Y04 Assault by bodily force**

EXCLUDES 1 *assault by:*
submersion (X92.-)
use of weapon (X93-X95, X99, Y00)

√x7th **Y04.0 Assault by unarmed brawl or fight**

√x7th **Y04.1 Assault by human bite**

√x7th **Y04.2 Assault by strike against or bumped into by another person**

√x7th **Y04.8 Assault by other bodily force**

Assault by bodily force NOS

√4th **Y07 Perpetrator of assault, maltreatment and neglect**

NOTE Codes from this category are for use only in cases of confirmed abuse (T74.-)

Selection of the correct perpetrator code is based on the relationship between the perpetrator and the victim

INCLUDES perpetrator of abandonment
perpetrator of emotional neglect
perpetrator of mental cruelty
perpetrator of physical abuse
perpetrator of physical neglect
perpetrator of sexual abuse
perpetrator of torture

√5th **Y07.0 Spouse or partner, perpetrator of maltreatment and neglect**

Spouse or partner, perpetrator of maltreatment and neglect against spouse or partner

Y07.01 Husband, perpetrator of maltreatment and neglect

Y07.02 Wife, perpetrator of maltreatment and neglect

Y07.03 Male partner, perpetrator of maltreatment and neglect

Y07.04 Female partner, perpetrator of maltreatment and neglect

√5th **Y07.1 Parent (adoptive) (biological), perpetrator of maltreatment and neglect**

Y07.11 Biological father, perpetrator of maltreatment and neglect

Y07.12 Biological mother, perpetrator of maltreatment and neglect

Y07.13 Adoptive father, perpetrator of maltreatment and neglect

Y07.14 Adoptive mother, perpetrator of maltreatment and neglect

√5th **Y07.4 Other family member, perpetrator of maltreatment and neglect**

√6th **Y07.41 Sibling, perpetrator of maltreatment and neglect**

EXCLUDES 1 *stepsibling, perpetrator of maltreatment and neglect (Y07.435, Y07.436)*

Y07.410 Brother, perpetrator of maltreatment and neglect

Y07.411 Sister, perpetrator of maltreatment and neglect

√6th **Y07.42 Foster parent, perpetrator of maltreatment and neglect**

Y07.420 Foster father, perpetrator of maltreatment and neglect

Y07.421 Foster mother, perpetrator of maltreatment and neglect

√6th **Y07.43 Stepparent or stepsibling, perpetrator of maltreatment and neglect**

Y07.430 Stepfather, perpetrator of maltreatment and neglect

Y07.432 Male friend of parent (co-residing in household), perpetrator of maltreatment and neglect

Y07.433 Stepmother, perpetrator of maltreatment and neglect

Y07.434 Female friend of parent (co-residing in household), perpetrator of maltreatment and neglect

Y07.435 Stepbrother, perpetrator or maltreatment and neglect

Y07.436 Stepsister, perpetrator of maltreatment and neglect

√6th **Y07.49 Other family member, perpetrator of maltreatment and neglect**

Y07.490 Male cousin, perpetrator of maltreatment and neglect

Y07.491 Female cousin, perpetrator of maltreatment and neglect

Y07.499 Other family member, perpetrator of maltreatment and neglect

√5th **Y07.5 Non-family member, perpetrator of maltreatment and neglect**

Y07.50 Unspecified non-family member, perpetrator of maltreatment and neglect

√6th **Y07.51 Daycare provider, perpetrator of maltreatment and neglect**

Y07.510 At-home childcare provider, perpetrator of maltreatment and neglect

Y07.511 Daycare center childcare provider, perpetrator of maltreatment and neglect

Y07.512 At-home adultcare provider, perpetrator of maltreatment and neglect

Y07.513 Adultcare center provider, perpetrator of maltreatment and neglect

Y07.519 Unspecified daycare provider, perpetrator of maltreatment and neglect

√6th **Y07.52 Healthcare provider, perpetrator of maltreatment and neglect**

Y07.521 Mental health provider, perpetrator of maltreatment and neglect

Y07.528 Other therapist or healthcare provider, perpetrator of maltreatment and neglect

Nurse perpetrator of maltreatment and neglect
Occupational therapist perpetrator of maltreatment and neglect
Physical therapist perpetrator of maltreatment and neglect
Speech therapist perpetrator of maltreatment and neglect

Y07.529 Unspecified healthcare provider, perpetrator of maltreatment and neglect

Y07.53 Teacher or instructor, perpetrator of maltreatment and neglect

Coach, perpetrator of maltreatment and neglect

Y07.59 Other non-family member, perpetrator of maltreatment and neglect

Y07.6 Multiple perpetrators of maltreatment and neglect

AHA: 2018,4Q,32

Y07.9 Unspecified perpetrator of maltreatment and neglect

√4th **Y08 Assault by other specified means**

√5th **Y08.0 Assault by strike by sport equipment**

√x7th **Y08.01 Assault by strike by hockey stick**

√x7th **Y08.02 Assault by strike by baseball bat**

√x7th **Y08.09 Assault by strike by other specified type of sport equipment**

√5th **Y08.8 Assault by other specified means**

√x7th **Y08.81 Assault by crashing of aircraft**

√x7th **Y08.89 Assault by other specified means**

Y09 Assault by unspecified means

Assassination (attempted) NOS
Homicide (attempted) NOS
Manslaughter (attempted) NOS
Murder (attempted) NOS

Event of undetermined intent (Y21-Y33)

Undetermined intent is only for use when there is specific documentation in the record that the intent of the injury cannot be determined. If no such documentation is present, code to accidental (unintentional).

The appropriate 7th character is to be added to each code from categories Y21-Y33.
A initial encounter
D subsequent encounter
S sequela

√4th **Y21 Drowning and submersion, undetermined intent**

√x7th **Y21.0 Drowning and submersion while in bathtub, undetermined intent**

√x7th **Y21.1 Drowning and submersion after fall into bathtub, undetermined intent**

√x7th Y21.2 **Drowning and submersion while in swimming pool, undetermined intent**

√x7th Y21.3 **Drowning and submersion after fall into swimming pool, undetermined intent**

√x7th Y21.4 **Drowning and submersion in natural water, undetermined intent**

√x7th Y21.8 **Other drowning and submersion, undetermined intent**

√x7th Y21.9 **Unspecified drowning and submersion, undetermined intent**

√x7th **Y22 Handgun discharge, undetermined intent**

Discharge of gun for single hand use, undetermined intent
Discharge of pistol, undetermined intent
Discharge of revolver, undetermined intent

EXCLUDES 2 *Very pistol (Y24.8)*

√4th **Y23 Rifle, shotgun and larger firearm discharge, undetermined intent**

EXCLUDES 2 *airgun (Y24.Ø)*

√x7th Y23.Ø **Shotgun discharge, undetermined intent**

√x7th Y23.1 **Hunting rifle discharge, undetermined intent**

√x7th Y23.2 **Military firearm discharge, undetermined intent**

√x7th Y23.3 **Machine gun discharge, undetermined intent**

√x7th Y23.8 **Other larger firearm discharge, undetermined intent**

√x7th Y23.9 **Unspecified larger firearm discharge, undetermined intent**

√4th **Y24 Other and unspecified firearm discharge, undetermined intent**

√x7th Y24.Ø **Airgun discharge, undetermined intent**

BB gun discharge, undetermined intent
Pellet gun discharge, undetermined intent

√x7th Y24.8 **Other firearm discharge, undetermined intent**

Paintball gun discharge, undetermined intent
Very pistol [flare] discharge, undetermined intent

√x7th Y24.9 **Unspecified firearm discharge, undetermined intent**

√x7th **Y25 Contact with explosive material, undetermined intent**

√x7th **Y26 Exposure to smoke, fire and flames, undetermined intent**

√4th **Y27 Contact with steam, hot vapors and hot objects, undetermined intent**

√x7th Y27.Ø **Contact with steam and hot vapors, undetermined intent**

√x7th Y27.1 **Contact with hot tap water, undetermined intent**

√x7th Y27.2 **Contact with hot fluids, undetermined intent**

√x7th Y27.3 **Contact with hot household appliance, undetermined intent**

√x7th Y27.8 **Contact with other hot objects, undetermined intent**

√x7th Y27.9 **Contact with unspecified hot objects, undetermined intent**

√4th **Y28 Contact with sharp object, undetermined intent**

√x7th Y28.Ø **Contact with sharp glass, undetermined intent**

√x7th Y28.1 **Contact with knife, undetermined intent**

√x7th Y28.2 **Contact with sword or dagger, undetermined intent**

√x7th Y28.8 **Contact with other sharp object, undetermined intent**

√x7th Y28.9 **Contact with unspecified sharp object, undetermined intent**

√x7th **Y29 Contact with blunt object, undetermined intent**

√x7th **Y3Ø Falling, jumping or pushed from a high place, undetermined intent**

Victim falling from one level to another, undetermined intent

√x7th **Y31 Falling, lying or running before or into moving object, undetermined intent**

√x7th **Y32 Crashing of motor vehicle, undetermined intent**

√x7th **Y33 Other specified events, undetermined intent**

Legal intervention, operations of war, military operations, and terrorism (Y35-Y38)

The appropriate 7th character is to be added to each code from categories Y35-Y38.
A initial encounter
D subsequent encounter
S sequela

√4th **Y35 Legal intervention**

INCLUDES any injury sustained as a result of an encounter with any law enforcement official, serving in any capacity at the time of the encounter, whether on-duty or off-duty. Includes injury to law enforcement official, suspect and bystander

AHA: 2019,4Q,18-19

√5th Y35.Ø **Legal intervention involving firearm discharge**

√6th Y35.ØØ **Legal intervention involving unspecified firearm discharge**

Legal intervention involving gunshot wound
Legal intervention involving shot NOS

√7th Y35.ØØ1 **Legal intervention involving unspecified firearm discharge, law enforcement official injured**

√7th Y35.ØØ2 **Legal intervention involving unspecified firearm discharge, bystander injured**

√7th Y35.ØØ3 **Legal intervention involving unspecified firearm discharge, suspect injured**

√7th Y35.ØØ9 **Legal intervention involving unspecified firearm discharge, unspecified person injured**

√6th Y35.Ø1 **Legal intervention involving injury by machine gun**

√7th Y35.Ø11 **Legal intervention involving injury by machine gun, law enforcement official injured**

√7th Y35.Ø12 **Legal intervention involving injury by machine gun, bystander injured**

√7th Y35.Ø13 **Legal intervention involving injury by machine gun, suspect injured**

√7th Y35.Ø19 **Legal intervention involving injury by machine gun, unspecified person injured**

√6th Y35.Ø2 **Legal intervention involving injury by handgun**

√7th Y35.Ø21 **Legal intervention involving injury by handgun, law enforcement official injured**

√7th Y35.Ø22 **Legal intervention involving injury by handgun, bystander injured**

√7th Y35.Ø23 **Legal intervention involving injury by handgun, suspect injured**

√7th Y35.Ø29 **Legal intervention involving injury by handgun, unspecified person injured**

√6th Y35.Ø3 **Legal intervention involving injury by rifle pellet**

√7th Y35.Ø31 **Legal intervention involving injury by rifle pellet, law enforcement official injured**

√7th Y35.Ø32 **Legal intervention involving injury by rifle pellet, bystander injured**

√7th Y35.Ø33 **Legal intervention involving injury by rifle pellet, suspect injured**

√7th Y35.Ø39 **Legal intervention involving injury by rifle pellet, unspecified person injured**

√6th Y35.Ø4 **Legal intervention involving injury by rubber bullet**

√7th Y35.Ø41 **Legal intervention involving injury by rubber bullet, law enforcement official injured**

√7th Y35.Ø42 **Legal intervention involving injury by rubber bullet, bystander injured**

√7th Y35.Ø43 **Legal intervention involving injury by rubber bullet, suspect injured**

√7th Y35.Ø49 **Legal intervention involving injury by rubber bullet, unspecified person injured**

√6th Y35.Ø9 **Legal intervention involving other firearm discharge**

√7th Y35.Ø91 **Legal intervention involving other firearm discharge, law enforcement official injured**

√7th Y35.Ø92 **Legal intervention involving other firearm discharge, bystander injured**

√7th Y35.Ø93 **Legal intervention involving other firearm discharge, suspect injured**

√7th **Y35.Ø99 Legal intervention involving other firearm discharge, unspecified person injured**

√5th **Y35.1 Legal intervention involving explosives**

√6th **Y35.1Ø Legal intervention involving unspecified explosives**

√7th **Y35.1Ø1 Legal intervention involving unspecified explosives, law enforcement official injured**

√7th **Y35.1Ø2 Legal intervention involving unspecified explosives, bystander injured**

√7th **Y35.1Ø3 Legal intervention involving unspecified explosives, suspect injured**

√7th **Y35.1Ø9 Legal intervention involving unspecified explosives, unspecified person injured**

√6th **Y35.11 Legal intervention involving injury by dynamite**

√7th **Y35.111 Legal intervention involving injury by dynamite, law enforcement official injured**

√7th **Y35.112 Legal intervention involving injury by dynamite, bystander injured**

√7th **Y35.113 Legal intervention involving injury by dynamite, suspect injured**

√7th **Y35.119 Legal intervention involving injury by dynamite, unspecified person injured**

√6th **Y35.12 Legal intervention involving injury by explosive shell**

√7th **Y35.121 Legal intervention involving injury by explosive shell, law enforcement official injured**

√7th **Y35.122 Legal intervention involving injury by explosive shell, bystander injured**

√7th **Y35.123 Legal intervention involving injury by explosive shell, suspect injured**

√7th **Y35.129 Legal intervention involving injury by explosive shell, unspecified person injured**

√6th **Y35.19 Legal intervention involving other explosives**

Legal intervention involving injury by grenade
Legal intervention involving injury by mortar bomb

√7th **Y35.191 Legal intervention involving other explosives, law enforcement official injured**

√7th **Y35.192 Legal intervention involving other explosives, bystander injured**

√7th **Y35.193 Legal intervention involving other explosives, suspect injured**

√7th **Y35.199 Legal intervention involving other explosives, unspecified person injured**

√5th **Y35.2 Legal intervention involving gas**

Legal intervention involving asphyxiation by gas
Legal intervention involving poisoning by gas

√6th **Y35.2Ø Legal intervention involving unspecified gas**

√7th **Y35.2Ø1 Legal intervention involving unspecified gas, law enforcement official injured**

√7th **Y35.2Ø2 Legal intervention involving unspecified gas, bystander injured**

√7th **Y35.2Ø3 Legal intervention involving unspecified gas, suspect injured**

√7th **Y35.2Ø9 Legal intervention involving unspecified gas, unspecified person injured**

√6th **Y35.21 Legal intervention involving injury by tear gas**

√7th **Y35.211 Legal intervention involving injury by tear gas, law enforcement official injured**

√7th **Y35.212 Legal intervention involving injury by tear gas, bystander injured**

√7th **Y35.213 Legal intervention involving injury by tear gas, suspect injured**

√7th **Y35.219 Legal intervention involving injury by tear gas, unspecified person injured**

√6th **Y35.29 Legal intervention involving other gas**

√7th **Y35.291 Legal intervention involving other gas, law enforcement official injured**

√7th **Y35.292 Legal intervention involving other gas, bystander injured**

√7th **Y35.293 Legal intervention involving other gas, suspect injured**

√7th **Y35.299 Legal intervention involving other gas, unspecified person injured**

√5th **Y35.3 Legal intervention involving blunt objects**

Legal intervention involving being hit or struck by blunt object

√6th **Y35.3Ø Legal intervention involving unspecified blunt objects**

√7th **Y35.3Ø1 Legal intervention involving unspecified blunt objects, law enforcement official injured**

√7th **Y35.3Ø2 Legal intervention involving unspecified blunt objects, bystander injured**

√7th **Y35.3Ø3 Legal intervention involving unspecified blunt objects, suspect injured**

√7th **Y35.3Ø9 Legal intervention involving unspecified blunt objects, unspecified person injured**

√6th **Y35.31 Legal intervention involving baton**

√7th **Y35.311 Legal intervention involving baton, law enforcement official injured**

√7th **Y35.312 Legal intervention involving baton, bystander injured**

√7th **Y35.313 Legal intervention involving baton, suspect injured**

√7th **Y35.319 Legal intervention involving baton, unspecified person injured**

√6th **Y35.39 Legal intervention involving other blunt objects**

√7th **Y35.391 Legal intervention involving other blunt objects, law enforcement official injured**

√7th **Y35.392 Legal intervention involving other blunt objects, bystander injured**

√7th **Y35.393 Legal intervention involving other blunt objects, suspect injured**

√7th **Y35.399 Legal intervention involving other blunt objects, unspecified person injured**

√5th **Y35.4 Legal intervention involving sharp objects**

Legal intervention involving being cut by sharp objects
Legal intervention involving being stabbed by sharp objects

√6th **Y35.4Ø Legal intervention involving unspecified sharp objects**

√7th **Y35.4Ø1 Legal intervention involving unspecified sharp objects, law enforcement official injured**

√7th **Y35.4Ø2 Legal intervention involving unspecified sharp objects, bystander injured**

√7th **Y35.4Ø3 Legal intervention involving unspecified sharp objects, suspect injured**

√7th **Y35.4Ø9 Legal intervention involving unspecified sharp objects, unspecified person injured**

√6th **Y35.41 Legal intervention involving bayonet**

√7th **Y35.411 Legal intervention involving bayonet, law enforcement official injured**

√7th **Y35.412 Legal intervention involving bayonet, bystander injured**

√7th **Y35.413 Legal intervention involving bayonet, suspect injured**

√7th **Y35.419 Legal intervention involving bayonet, unspecified person injured**

√6th **Y35.49 Legal intervention involving other sharp objects**

√7th **Y35.491 Legal intervention involving other sharp objects, law enforcement official injured**

√7th **Y35.492 Legal intervention involving other sharp objects, bystander injured**

√7th **Y35.493 Legal intervention involving other sharp objects, suspect injured**

√7th **Y35.499 Legal intervention involving other sharp objects, unspecified person injured**

√5th **Y35.8 Legal intervention involving other specified means**

AHA: 2019,4Q,19

√6th **Y35.81 Legal intervention involving manhandling**

√7th **Y35.811 Legal intervention involving manhandling, law enforcement official injured**

√7th **Y35.812 Legal intervention involving manhandling, bystander injured**

√7th **Y35.813 Legal intervention involving manhandling, suspect injured**

√7th **Y35.819 Legal intervention involving manhandling, unspecified person injured**

✓6th **Y35.83 Legal intervention involving a conducted energy device**
Electroshock device (taser)
Stun gun

✓7th **Y35.831 Legal intervention involving a conducted energy device, law enforcement official injured**

✓7th **Y35.832 Legal intervention involving a conducted energy device, bystander injured**

✓7th **Y35.833 Legal intervention involving a conducted energy device, suspect injured**

✓7th **Y35.839 Legal intervention involving a conducted energy device, unspecified person injured**

✓6th **Y35.89 Legal intervention involving other specified means**

✓7th **Y35.891 Legal intervention involving other specified means, law enforcement official injured**

✓7th **Y35.892 Legal intervention involving other specified means, bystander injured**

✓7th **Y35.893 Legal intervention involving other specified means, suspect injured**
AHA: 2018,1Q,5

✓5th **Y35.9 Legal intervention, means unspecified**

✓x 7th **Y35.91 Legal intervention, means unspecified, law enforcement official injured**

✓x 7th **Y35.92 Legal intervention, means unspecified, bystander injured**

✓x 7th **Y35.93 Legal intervention, means unspecified, suspect injured**

✓x 7th **Y35.99 Legal intervention, means unspecified, unspecified person injured**

✓4th **Y36 Operations of war**

INCLUDES injuries to military personnel and civilians caused by war, civil insurrection, and peacekeeping missions

EXCLUDES 1 *injury to military personnel occurring during peacetime military operations (Y37.-)*
military vehicles involved in transport accidents with non-military vehicle during peacetime (V09.01, V09.21, V19.81, V29.81, V39.81, V49.81, V59.81, V69.81, V79.81)

AHA: 2014,3Q,4

✓5th **Y36.0 War operations involving explosion of marine weapons**

✓6th **Y36.00 War operations involving explosion of unspecified marine weapon**
War operations involving underwater blast NOS

✓7th **Y36.000 War operations involving explosion of unspecified marine weapon, military personnel**

✓7th **Y36.001 War operations involving explosion of unspecified marine weapon, civilian**

✓6th **Y36.01 War operations involving explosion of depth-charge**

✓7th **Y36.010 War operations involving explosion of depth-charge, military personnel**

✓7th **Y36.011 War operations involving explosion of depth-charge, civilian**

✓6th **Y36.02 War operations involving explosion of marine mine**
War operations involving explosion of marine mine, at sea or in harbor

✓7th **Y36.020 War operations involving explosion of marine mine, military personnel**

✓7th **Y36.021 War operations involving explosion of marine mine, civilian**

✓6th **Y36.03 War operations involving explosion of sea-based artillery shell**

✓7th **Y36.030 War operations involving explosion of sea-based artillery shell, military personnel**

✓7th **Y36.031 War operations involving explosion of sea-based artillery shell, civilian**

✓6th **Y36.04 War operations involving explosion of torpedo**

✓7th **Y36.040 War operations involving explosion of torpedo, military personnel**

✓7th **Y36.041 War operations involving explosion of torpedo, civilian**

✓6th **Y36.05 War operations involving accidental detonation of onboard marine weapons**

✓7th **Y36.050 War operations involving accidental detonation of onboard marine weapons, military personnel**

✓7th **Y36.051 War operations involving accidental detonation of onboard marine weapons, civilian**

✓6th **Y36.09 War operations involving explosion of other marine weapons**

✓7th **Y36.090 War operations involving explosion of other marine weapons, military personnel**

✓7th **Y36.091 War operations involving explosion of other marine weapons, civilian**

✓5th **Y36.1 War operations involving destruction of aircraft**

✓6th **Y36.10 War operations involving unspecified destruction of aircraft**

✓7th **Y36.100 War operations involving unspecified destruction of aircraft, military personnel**

✓7th **Y36.101 War operations involving unspecified destruction of aircraft, civilian**

✓6th **Y36.11 War operations involving destruction of aircraft due to enemy fire or explosives**
War operations involving destruction of aircraft due to air to air missile
War operations involving destruction of aircraft due to explosive placed on aircraft
War operations involving destruction of aircraft due to rocket propelled grenade [RPG]
War operations involving destruction of aircraft due to small arms fire
War operations involving destruction of aircraft due to surface to air missile

✓7th **Y36.110 War operations involving destruction of aircraft due to enemy fire or explosives, military personnel**

✓7th **Y36.111 War operations involving destruction of aircraft due to enemy fire or explosives, civilian**

✓6th **Y36.12 War operations involving destruction of aircraft due to collision with other aircraft**

✓7th **Y36.120 War operations involving destruction of aircraft due to collision with other aircraft, military personnel**

✓7th **Y36.121 War operations involving destruction of aircraft due to collision with other aircraft, civilian**

✓6th **Y36.13 War operations involving destruction of aircraft due to onboard fire**

✓7th **Y36.130 War operations involving destruction of aircraft due to onboard fire, military personnel**

✓7th **Y36.131 War operations involving destruction of aircraft due to onboard fire, civilian**

✓6th **Y36.14 War operations involving destruction of aircraft due to accidental detonation of onboard munitions and explosives**

✓7th **Y36.140 War operations involving destruction of aircraft due to accidental detonation of onboard munitions and explosives, military personnel**

✓7th **Y36.141 War operations involving destruction of aircraft due to accidental detonation of onboard munitions and explosives, civilian**

✓6th **Y36.19 War operations involving other destruction of aircraft**

✓7th **Y36.190 War operations involving other destruction of aircraft, military personnel**

✓7th **Y36.191 War operations involving other destruction of aircraft, civilian**

5th Y36.2 War operations involving other explosions and fragments

EXCLUDES 1 *war operations involving explosion of aircraft (Y36.1-)*
war operations involving explosion of marine weapons (Y36.Ø-)
war operations involving explosion of nuclear weapons (Y36.5-)
war operations involving explosion occurring after cessation of hostilities (Y36.8-)

6th Y36.2Ø War operations involving unspecified explosion and fragments

War operations involving air blast NOS
War operations involving blast NOS
War operations involving blast fragments NOS
War operations involving blast wave NOS
War operations involving blast wind NOS
War operations involving explosion NOS
War operations involving explosion of bomb NOS

7th Y36.2ØØ War operations involving unspecified explosion and fragments, military personnel

7th Y36.2Ø1 War operations involving unspecified explosion and fragments, civilian

6th Y36.21 War operations involving explosion of aerial bomb

7th Y36.21Ø War operations involving explosion of aerial bomb, military personnel

7th Y36.211 War operations involving explosion of aerial bomb, civilian

6th Y36.22 War operations involving explosion of guided missile

7th Y36.22Ø War operations involving explosion of guided missile, military personnel

7th Y36.221 War operations involving explosion of guided missile, civilian

6th Y36.23 War operations involving explosion of improvised explosive device [IED]

War operations involving explosion of person-borne improvised explosive device [IED]
War operations involving explosion of vehicle-borne improvised explosive device [IED]
War operations involving explosion of roadside improvised explosive device [IED]

7th Y36.23Ø War operations involving explosion of improvised explosive device [IED], military personnel

7th Y36.231 War operations involving explosion of improvised explosive device [IED], civilian

6th Y36.24 War operations involving explosion due to accidental detonation and discharge of own munitions or munitions launch device

7th Y36.24Ø War operations involving explosion due to accidental detonation and discharge of own munitions or munitions launch device, military personnel

7th Y36.241 War operations involving explosion due to accidental detonation and discharge of own munitions or munitions launch device, civilian

6th Y36.25 War operations involving fragments from munitions

7th Y36.25Ø War operations involving fragments from munitions, military personnel

7th Y36.251 War operations involving fragments from munitions, civilian

6th Y36.26 War operations involving fragments of improvised explosive device [IED]

War operations involving fragments of person-borne improvised explosive device [IED]
War operations involving fragments of vehicle-borne improvised explosive device [IED]
War operations involving fragments of roadside improvised explosive device [IED]

7th Y36.26Ø War operations involving fragments of improvised explosive device [IED], military personnel

7th Y36.261 War operations involving fragments of improvised explosive device [IED], civilian

6th Y36.27 War operations involving fragments from weapons

7th Y36.27Ø War operations involving fragments from weapons, military personnel

7th Y36.271 War operations involving fragments from weapons, civilian

6th Y36.29 War operations involving other explosions and fragments

War operations involving explosion of grenade
War operations involving explosions of land mine
War operations involving shrapnel NOS

7th Y36.29Ø War operations involving other explosions and fragments, military personnel

7th Y36.291 War operations involving other explosions and fragments, civilian

5th Y36.3 War operations involving fires, conflagrations and hot substances

War operations involving smoke, fumes, and heat from fires, conflagrations and hot substances

EXCLUDES 1 *war operations involving fires and conflagrations aboard military aircraft (Y36.1-)*
war operations involving fires and conflagrations aboard military watercraft (Y36.Ø-)
war operations involving fires and conflagrations caused indirectly by conventional weapons (Y36.2-)
war operations involving fires and thermal effects of nuclear weapons (Y36.53-)

6th Y36.3Ø War operations involving unspecified fire, conflagration and hot substance

7th Y36.3ØØ War operations involving unspecified fire, conflagration and hot substance, military personnel

7th Y36.3Ø1 War operations involving unspecified fire, conflagration and hot substance, civilian

6th Y36.31 War operations involving gasoline bomb

War operations involving incendiary bomb
War operations involving petrol bomb

7th Y36.31Ø War operations involving gasoline bomb, military personnel

7th Y36.311 War operations involving gasoline bomb, civilian

6th Y36.32 War operations involving incendiary bullet

7th Y36.32Ø War operations involving incendiary bullet, military personnel

7th Y36.321 War operations involving incendiary bullet, civilian

6th Y36.33 War operations involving flamethrower

7th Y36.33Ø War operations involving flamethrower, military personnel

7th Y36.331 War operations involving flamethrower, civilian

6th Y36.39 War operations involving other fires, conflagrations and hot substances

7th Y36.39Ø War operations involving other fires, conflagrations and hot substances, military personnel

7th Y36.391 War operations involving other fires, conflagrations and hot substances, civilian

5th Y36.4 War operations involving firearm discharge and other forms of conventional warfare

6th Y36.41 War operations involving rubber bullets

7th Y36.41Ø War operations involving rubber bullets, military personnel

7th Y36.411 War operations involving rubber bullets, civilian

6th Y36.42 War operations involving firearms pellets

7th Y36.42Ø War operations involving firearms pellets, military personnel

7th Y36.421 War operations involving firearms pellets, civilian

6th Y36.43 War operations involving other firearms discharge

War operations involving bullets NOS

EXCLUDES 1 *war operations involving munitions fragments (Y36.25-)*
war operations involving incendiary bullets (Y36.32-)

7th Y36.43Ø War operations involving other firearms discharge, military personnel

7th Y36.431 War operations involving other firearms discharge, civilian

Y36.44 **War operations involving unarmed hand to hand combat**
EXCLUDES 1 *war operations involving combat using blunt or piercing object (Y36.45-)*
war operations involving intentional restriction of air and airway (Y36.46-)
war operations involving unintentional restriction of air and airway (Y36.47-)
Y36.440 **War operations involving unarmed hand to hand combat, military personnel**
Y36.441 **War operations involving unarmed hand to hand combat, civilian**
Y36.45 **War operations involving combat using blunt or piercing object**
Y36.450 **War operations involving combat using blunt or piercing object, military personnel**
Y36.451 **War operations involving combat using blunt or piercing object, civilian**
Y36.46 **War operations involving intentional restriction of air and airway**
Y36.460 **War operations involving intentional restriction of air and airway, military personnel**
Y36.461 **War operations involving intentional restriction of air and airway, civilian**
Y36.47 **War operations involving unintentional restriction of air and airway**
Y36.470 **War operations involving unintentional restriction of air and airway, military personnel**
Y36.471 **War operations involving unintentional restriction of air and airway, civilian**
Y36.49 **War operations involving other forms of conventional warfare**
Y36.490 **War operations involving other forms of conventional warfare, military personnel**
Y36.491 **War operations involving other forms of conventional warfare, civilian**
Y36.5 **War operations involving nuclear weapons**
War operations involving dirty bomb NOS
Y36.50 **War operations involving unspecified effect of nuclear weapon**
Y36.500 **War operations involving unspecified effect of nuclear weapon, military personnel**
Y36.501 **War operations involving unspecified effect of nuclear weapon, civilian**
Y36.51 **War operations involving direct blast effect of nuclear weapon**
War operations involving blast pressure of nuclear weapon
Y36.510 **War operations involving direct blast effect of nuclear weapon, military personnel**
Y36.511 **War operations involving direct blast effect of nuclear weapon, civilian**
Y36.52 **War operations involving indirect blast effect of nuclear weapon**
War operations involving being thrown by blast of nuclear weapon
War operations involving being struck or crushed by blast debris of nuclear weapon
Y36.520 **War operations involving indirect blast effect of nuclear weapon, military personnel**
Y36.521 **War operations involving indirect blast effect of nuclear weapon, civilian**
Y36.53 **War operations involving thermal radiation effect of nuclear weapon**
War operations involving direct heat from nuclear weapon
War operation involving fireball effects from nuclear weapon
Y36.530 **War operations involving thermal radiation effect of nuclear weapon, military personnel**
Y36.531 **War operations involving thermal radiation effect of nuclear weapon, civilian**
Y36.54 **War operation involving nuclear radiation effects of nuclear weapon**
War operation involving acute radiation exposure from nuclear weapon
War operation involving exposure to immediate ionizing radiation from nuclear weapon
War operation involving fallout exposure from nuclear weapon
War operation involving secondary effects of nuclear weapons
Y36.540 **War operation involving nuclear radiation effects of nuclear weapon, military personnel**
Y36.541 **War operation involving nuclear radiation effects of nuclear weapon, civilian**
Y36.59 **War operation involving other effects of nuclear weapons**
Y36.590 **War operation involving other effects of nuclear weapons, military personnel**
Y36.591 **War operation involving other effects of nuclear weapons, civilian**
Y36.6 **War operations involving biological weapons**
Y36.6X **War operations involving biological weapons**
Y36.6X0 **War operations involving biological weapons, military personnel**
Y36.6X1 **War operations involving biological weapons, civilian**
Y36.7 **War operations involving chemical weapons and other forms of unconventional warfare**
EXCLUDES 1 *war operations involving incendiary devices (Y36.3-, Y36.5-)*
Y36.7X **War operations involving chemical weapons and other forms of unconventional warfare**
Y36.7X0 **War operations involving chemical weapons and other forms of unconventional warfare, military personnel**
Y36.7X1 **War operations involving chemical weapons and other forms of unconventional warfare, civilian**
Y36.8 **War operations occurring after cessation of hostilities**
War operations classifiable to categories Y36.0-Y36.8 but occurring after cessation of hostilities
Y36.81 **Explosion of mine placed during war operations but exploding after cessation of hostilities**
Y36.810 **Explosion of mine placed during war operations but exploding after cessation of hostilities, military personnel**
Y36.811 **Explosion of mine placed during war operations but exploding after cessation of hostilities, civilian**
Y36.82 **Explosion of bomb placed during war operations but exploding after cessation of hostilities**
Y36.820 **Explosion of bomb placed during war operations but exploding after cessation of hostilities, military personnel**
Y36.821 **Explosion of bomb placed during war operations but exploding after cessation of hostilities, civilian**
Y36.88 **Other war operations occurring after cessation of hostilities**
Y36.880 **Other war operations occurring after cessation of hostilities, military personnel**
Y36.881 **Other war operations occurring after cessation of hostilities, civilian**
Y36.89 **Unspecified war operations occurring after cessation of hostilities**
Y36.890 **Unspecified war operations occurring after cessation of hostilities, military personnel**
Y36.891 **Unspecified war operations occurring after cessation of hostilities, civilian**
Y36.9 **Other and unspecified war operations**
Y36.90 **War operations, unspecified**
Y36.91 **War operations involving unspecified weapon of mass destruction [WMD]**
Y36.92 **War operations involving friendly fire**

Y37 Military operations

INCLUDES injuries to military personnel and civilians occurring during peacetime on military property and during routine military exercises and operations

EXCLUDES 1 *military aircraft involved in aircraft accident with civilian aircraft (V97.81-)*
military vehicles involved in transport accident with civilian vehicle (VØ9.Ø1, VØ9.21, V19.81, V29.81, V39.81, V49.81, V59.81, V69.81, V79.81)
military watercraft involved in water transport accident with civilian watercraft (V94.81-)
war operations (Y36.-)

Y37.Ø Military operations involving explosion of marine weapons

Y37.ØØ Military operations involving explosion of unspecified marine weapon
Military operations involving underwater blast NOS

Y37.ØØØ Military operations involving explosion of unspecified marine weapon, military personnel

Y37.ØØ1 Military operations involving explosion of unspecified marine weapon, civilian

Y37.Ø1 Military operations involving explosion of depth-charge

Y37.Ø1Ø Military operations involving explosion of depth-charge, military personnel

Y37.Ø11 Military operations involving explosion of depth-charge, civilian

Y37.Ø2 Military operations involving explosion of marine mine
Military operations involving explosion of marine mine, at sea or in harbor

Y37.Ø2Ø Military operations involving explosion of marine mine, military personnel

Y37.Ø21 Military operations involving explosion of marine mine, civilian

Y37.Ø3 Military operations involving explosion of sea-based artillery shell

Y37.Ø3Ø Military operations involving explosion of sea-based artillery shell, military personnel

Y37.Ø31 Military operations involving explosion of sea-based artillery shell, civilian

Y37.Ø4 Military operations involving explosion of torpedo

Y37.Ø4Ø Military operations involving explosion of torpedo, military personnel

Y37.Ø41 Military operations involving explosion of torpedo, civilian

Y37.Ø5 Military operations involving accidental detonation of onboard marine weapons

Y37.Ø5Ø Military operations involving accidental detonation of onboard marine weapons, military personnel

Y37.Ø51 Military operations involving accidental detonation of onboard marine weapons, civilian

Y37.Ø9 Military operations involving explosion of other marine weapons

Y37.Ø9Ø Military operations involving explosion of other marine weapons, military personnel

Y37.Ø91 Military operations involving explosion of other marine weapons, civilian

Y37.1 Military operations involving destruction of aircraft

Y37.1Ø Military operations involving unspecified destruction of aircraft

Y37.1ØØ Military operations involving unspecified destruction of aircraft, military personnel

Y37.1Ø1 Military operations involving unspecified destruction of aircraft, civilian

Y37.11 Military operations involving destruction of aircraft due to enemy fire or explosives
Military operations involving destruction of aircraft due to air to air missile
Military operations involving destruction of aircraft due to explosive placed on aircraft
Military operations involving destruction of aircraft due to rocket propelled grenade [RPG]
Military operations involving destruction of aircraft due to small arms fire
Military operations involving destruction of aircraft due to surface to air missile

Y37.11Ø Military operations involving destruction of aircraft due to enemy fire or explosives, military personnel

Y37.111 Military operations involving destruction of aircraft due to enemy fire or explosives, civilian

Y37.12 Military operations involving destruction of aircraft due to collision with other aircraft

Y37.12Ø Military operations involving destruction of aircraft due to collision with other aircraft, military personnel

Y37.121 Military operations involving destruction of aircraft due to collision with other aircraft, civilian

Y37.13 Military operations involving destruction of aircraft due to onboard fire

Y37.13Ø Military operations involving destruction of aircraft due to onboard fire, military personnel

Y37.131 Military operations involving destruction of aircraft due to onboard fire, civilian

Y37.14 Military operations involving destruction of aircraft due to accidental detonation of onboard munitions and explosives

Y37.14Ø Military operations involving destruction of aircraft due to accidental detonation of onboard munitions and explosives, military personnel

Y37.141 Military operations involving destruction of aircraft due to accidental detonation of onboard munitions and explosives, civilian

Y37.19 Military operations involving other destruction of aircraft

Y37.19Ø Military operations involving other destruction of aircraft, military personnel

Y37.191 Military operations involving other destruction of aircraft, civilian

Y37.2 Military operations involving other explosions and fragments

EXCLUDES 1 *military operations involving explosion of aircraft (Y37.1-)*
military operations involving explosion of marine weapons (Y37.Ø-)
military operations involving explosion of nuclear weapons (Y37.5-)

Y37.2Ø Military operations involving unspecified explosion and fragments
Military operations involving air blast NOS
Military operations involving blast NOS
Military operations involving blast fragments NOS
Military operations involving blast wave NOS
Military operations involving blast wind NOS
Military operations involving explosion NOS
Military operations involving explosion of bomb NOS

Y37.2ØØ Military operations involving unspecified explosion and fragments, military personnel

Y37.2Ø1 Military operations involving unspecified explosion and fragments, civilian

Y37.21 Military operations involving explosion of aerial bomb

Y37.21Ø Military operations involving explosion of aerial bomb, military personnel

Y37.211 Military operations involving explosion of aerial bomb, civilian

Y37.22 Military operations involving explosion of guided missile

Y37.22Ø Military operations involving explosion of guided missile, military personnel

√7th **Y37.221 Military operations involving explosion of guided missile, civilian**

√6th **Y37.23 Military operations involving explosion of improvised explosive device [IED]**
Military operations involving explosion of person-borne improvised explosive device [IED]
Military operations involving explosion of vehicle-borne improvised explosive device [IED]
Military operations involving explosion of roadside improvised explosive device [IED]

√7th **Y37.230 Military operations involving explosion of improvised explosive device [IED], military personnel**

√7th **Y37.231 Military operations involving explosion of improvised explosive device [IED], civilian**

√6th **Y37.24 Military operations involving explosion due to accidental detonation and discharge of own munitions or munitions launch device**

√7th **Y37.240 Military operations involving explosion due to accidental detonation and discharge of own munitions or munitions launch device, military personnel**

√7th **Y37.241 Military operations involving explosion due to accidental detonation and discharge of own munitions or munitions launch device, civilian**

√6th **Y37.25 Military operations involving fragments from munitions**

√7th **Y37.250 Military operations involving fragments from munitions, military personnel**

√7th **Y37.251 Military operations involving fragments from munitions, civilian**

√6th **Y37.26 Military operations involving fragments of improvised explosive device [IED]**
Military operations involving fragments of person-borne improvised explosive device [IED]
Military operations involving fragments of vehicle-borne improvised explosive device [IED]
Military operations involving fragments of roadside improvised explosive device [IED]

√7th **Y37.260 Military operations involving fragments of improvised explosive device [IED], military personnel**

√7th **Y37.261 Military operations involving fragments of improvised explosive device [IED], civilian**

√6th **Y37.27 Military operations involving fragments from weapons**

√7th **Y37.270 Military operations involving fragments from weapons, military personnel**

√7th **Y37.271 Military operations involving fragments from weapons, civilian**

√6th **Y37.29 Military operations involving other explosions and fragments**
Military operations involving explosion of grenade
Military operations involving explosions of land mine
Military operations involving shrapnel NOS

√7th **Y37.290 Military operations involving other explosions and fragments, military personnel**

√7th **Y37.291 Military operations involving other explosions and fragments, civilian**

√5th **Y37.3 Military operations involving fires, conflagrations and hot substances**
Military operations involving smoke, fumes, and heat from fires, conflagrations and hot substances

EXCLUDES 1 *military operations involving fires and conflagrations aboard military aircraft (Y37.1-)*
military operations involving fires and conflagrations aboard military watercraft (Y37.Ø-)
military operations involving fires and conflagrations caused indirectly by conventional weapons (Y37.2-)
military operations involving fires and thermal effects of nuclear weapons (Y36.53-)

√6th **Y37.3Ø Military operations involving unspecified fire, conflagration and hot substance**

√7th **Y37.3ØØ Military operations involving unspecified fire, conflagration and hot substance, military personnel**

√7th **Y37.3Ø1 Military operations involving unspecified fire, conflagration and hot substance, civilian**

√6th **Y37.31 Military operations involving gasoline bomb**
Military operations involving incendiary bomb
Military operations involving petrol bomb

√7th **Y37.31Ø Military operations involving gasoline bomb, military personnel**

√7th **Y37.311 Military operations involving gasoline bomb, civilian**

√6th **Y37.32 Military operations involving incendiary bullet**

√7th **Y37.32Ø Military operations involving incendiary bullet, military personnel**

√7th **Y37.321 Military operations involving incendiary bullet, civilian**

√6th **Y37.33 Military operations involving flamethrower**

√7th **Y37.33Ø Military operations involving flamethrower, military personnel**

√7th **Y37.331 Military operations involving flamethrower, civilian**

√6th **Y37.39 Military operations involving other fires, conflagrations and hot substances**

√7th **Y37.39Ø Military operations involving other fires, conflagrations and hot substances, military personnel**

√7th **Y37.391 Military operations involving other fires, conflagrations and hot substances, civilian**

√5th **Y37.4 Military operations involving firearm discharge and other forms of conventional warfare**

√6th **Y37.41 Military operations involving rubber bullets**

√7th **Y37.41Ø Military operations involving rubber bullets, military personnel**

√7th **Y37.411 Military operations involving rubber bullets, civilian**

√6th **Y37.42 Military operations involving firearms pellets**

√7th **Y37.42Ø Military operations involving firearms pellets, military personnel**

√7th **Y37.421 Military operations involving firearms pellets, civilian**

√6th **Y37.43 Military operations involving other firearms discharge**
Military operations involving bullets NOS

EXCLUDES 1 *military operations involving munitions fragments (Y37.25-)*
military operations involving incendiary bullets (Y37.32-)

√7th **Y37.43Ø Military operations involving other firearms discharge, military personnel**

√7th **Y37.431 Military operations involving other firearms discharge, civilian**

√6th **Y37.44 Military operations involving unarmed hand to hand combat**

EXCLUDES 1 *military operations involving combat using blunt or piercing object (Y37.45-)*
military operations involving intentional restriction of air and airway (Y37.46-)
military operations involving unintentional restriction of air and airway (Y37.47-)

√7th **Y37.44Ø Military operations involving unarmed hand to hand combat, military personnel**

√7th **Y37.441 Military operations involving unarmed hand to hand combat, civilian**

√6th **Y37.45 Military operations involving combat using blunt or piercing object**

√7th **Y37.45Ø Military operations involving combat using blunt or piercing object, military personnel**

√7th **Y37.451 Military operations involving combat using blunt or piercing object, civilian**

√6th **Y37.46 Military operations involving intentional restriction of air and airway**

√7th **Y37.46Ø Military operations involving intentional restriction of air and airway, military personnel**

√7th **Y37.461 Military operations involving intentional restriction of air and airway, civilian**

√6th **Y37.47 Military operations involving unintentional restriction of air and airway**

√7th **Y37.470 Military operations involving unintentional restriction of air and airway, military personnel**

√7th **Y37.471 Military operations involving unintentional restriction of air and airway, civilian**

√6th **Y37.49 Military operations involving other forms of conventional warfare**

√7th **Y37.490 Military operations involving other forms of conventional warfare, military personnel**

√7th **Y37.491 Military operations involving other forms of conventional warfare, civilian**

√5th **Y37.5 Military operations involving nuclear weapons**

Military operation involving dirty bomb NOS

√6th **Y37.50 Military operations involving unspecified effect of nuclear weapon**

√7th **Y37.500 Military operations involving unspecified effect of nuclear weapon, military personnel**

√7th **Y37.501 Military operations involving unspecified effect of nuclear weapon, civilian**

√6th **Y37.51 Military operations involving direct blast effect of nuclear weapon**

Military operations involving blast pressure of nuclear weapon

√7th **Y37.510 Military operations involving direct blast effect of nuclear weapon, military personnel**

√7th **Y37.511 Military operations involving direct blast effect of nuclear weapon, civilian**

√6th **Y37.52 Military operations involving indirect blast effect of nuclear weapon**

Military operations involving being thrown by blast of nuclear weapon

Military operations involving being struck or crushed by blast debris of nuclear weapon

√7th **Y37.520 Military operations involving indirect blast effect of nuclear weapon, military personnel**

√7th **Y37.521 Military operations involving indirect blast effect of nuclear weapon, civilian**

√6th **Y37.53 Military operations involving thermal radiation effect of nuclear weapon**

Military operations involving direct heat from nuclear weapon

Military operation involving fireball effects from nuclear weapon

√7th **Y37.530 Military operations involving thermal radiation effect of nuclear weapon, military personnel**

√7th **Y37.531 Military operations involving thermal radiation effect of nuclear weapon, civilian**

√6th **Y37.54 Military operation involving nuclear radiation effects of nuclear weapon**

Military operation involving acute radiation exposure from nuclear weapon

Military operation involving exposure to immediate ionizing radiation from nuclear weapon

Military operation involving fallout exposure from nuclear weapon

Military operation involving secondary effects of nuclear weapons

√7th **Y37.540 Military operation involving nuclear radiation effects of nuclear weapon, military personnel**

√7th **Y37.541 Military operation involving nuclear radiation effects of nuclear weapon, civilian**

√6th **Y37.59 Military operation involving other effects of nuclear weapons**

√7th **Y37.590 Military operation involving other effects of nuclear weapons, military personnel**

√7th **Y37.591 Military operation involving other effects of nuclear weapons, civilian**

√5th **Y37.6 Military operations involving biological weapons**

√6th **Y37.6X Military operations involving biological weapons**

√7th **Y37.6X0 Military operations involving biological weapons, military personnel**

√7th **Y37.6X1 Military operations involving biological weapons, civilian**

√5th **Y37.7 Military operations involving chemical weapons and other forms of unconventional warfare**

EXCLUDES 1 *military operations involving incendiary devices (Y36.3-, Y36.5-)*

√6th **Y37.7X Military operations involving chemical weapons and other forms of unconventional warfare**

√7th **Y37.7X0 Military operations involving chemical weapons and other forms of unconventional warfare, military personnel**

√7th **Y37.7X1 Military operations involving chemical weapons and other forms of unconventional warfare, civilian**

√5th **Y37.9 Other and unspecified military operations**

√x7th **Y37.90 Military operations, unspecified**

√x7th **Y37.91 Military operations involving unspecified weapon of mass destruction [WMD]**

√x7th **Y37.92 Military operations involving friendly fire**

√4th **Y38 Terrorism**

NOTE These codes are for use to identify injuries resulting from the unlawful use of force or violence against persons or property to intimidate or coerce a Government, the civilian population, or any segment thereof, in furtherance of political or social objective

Use additional code for place of occurrence (Y92.-)

√5th **Y38.0 Terrorism involving explosion of marine weapons**

Terrorism involving depth-charge

Terrorism involving marine mine

Terrorism involving mine NOS, at sea or in harbor

Terrorism involving sea-based artillery shell

Terrorism involving torpedo

Terrorism involving underwater blast

√6th **Y38.0X Terrorism involving explosion of marine weapons**

√7th **Y38.0X1 Terrorism involving explosion of marine weapons, public safety official injured**

√7th **Y38.0X2 Terrorism involving explosion of marine weapons, civilian injured**

√7th **Y38.0X3 Terrorism involving explosion of marine weapons, terrorist injured**

√5th **Y38.1 Terrorism involving destruction of aircraft**

Terrorism involving aircraft burned

Terrorism involving aircraft exploded

Terrorism involving aircraft being shot down

Terrorism involving aircraft used as a weapon

√6th **Y38.1X Terrorism involving destruction of aircraft**

√7th **Y38.1X1 Terrorism involving destruction of aircraft, public safety official injured**

√7th **Y38.1X2 Terrorism involving destruction of aircraft, civilian injured**

√7th **Y38.1X3 Terrorism involving destruction of aircraft, terrorist injured**

√5th **Y38.2 Terrorism involving other explosions and fragments**

Terrorism involving antipersonnel (fragments) bomb

Terrorism involving blast NOS

Terrorism involving explosion NOS

Terrorism involving explosion of breech block

Terrorism involving explosion of cannon block

Terrorism involving explosion (fragments) of artillery shell

Terrorism involving explosion (fragments) of bomb

Terrorism involving explosion (fragments) of grenade

Terrorism involving explosion (fragments) of guided missile

Terrorism involving explosion (fragments) of land mine

Terrorism involving explosion of mortar bomb

Terrorism involving explosion of munitions

Terrorism involving explosion (fragments) of rocket

Terrorism involving explosion (fragments) of shell

Terrorism involving shrapnel

Terrorism involving mine NOS, on land

EXCLUDES 1 *terrorism involving explosion of nuclear weapon (Y38.5)*

terrorism involving suicide bomber (Y38.81)

√6th **Y38.2X Terrorism involving other explosions and fragments**

√7th **Y38.2X1 Terrorism involving other explosions and fragments, public safety official injured**

✓7th **Y38.2X2 Terrorism involving other explosions and fragments, civilian injured**

✓7th **Y38.2X3 Terrorism involving other explosions and fragments, terrorist injured**

✓5th **Y38.3 Terrorism involving fires, conflagration and hot substances**

Terrorism involving conflagration NOS
Terrorism involving fire NOS
Terrorism involving petrol bomb

EXCLUDES 1 *terrorism involving fire or heat of nuclear weapon (Y38.5)*

✓6th **Y38.3X Terrorism involving fires, conflagration and hot substances**

✓7th **Y38.3X1 Terrorism involving fires, conflagration and hot substances, public safety official injured**

✓7th **Y38.3X2 Terrorism involving fires, conflagration and hot substances, civilian injured**

✓7th **Y38.3X3 Terrorism involving fires, conflagration and hot substances, terrorist injured**

✓5th **Y38.4 Terrorism involving firearms**

Terrorism involving carbine bullet
Terrorism involving machine gun bullet
Terrorism involving pellets (shotgun)
Terrorism involving pistol bullet
Terrorism involving rifle bullet
Terrorism involving rubber (rifle) bullet

✓6th **Y38.4X Terrorism involving firearms**

✓7th **Y38.4X1 Terrorism involving firearms, public safety official injured**

✓7th **Y38.4X2 Terrorism involving firearms, civilian injured**

✓7th **Y38.4X3 Terrorism involving firearms, terrorist injured**

✓5th **Y38.5 Terrorism involving nuclear weapons**

Terrorism involving blast effects of nuclear weapon
Terrorism involving exposure to ionizing radiation from nuclear weapon
Terrorism involving fireball effect of nuclear weapon
Terrorism involving heat from nuclear weapon

✓6th **Y38.5X Terrorism involving nuclear weapons**

✓7th **Y38.5X1 Terrorism involving nuclear weapons, public safety official injured**

✓7th **Y38.5X2 Terrorism involving nuclear weapons, civilian injured**

✓7th **Y38.5X3 Terrorism involving nuclear weapons, terrorist injured**

✓5th **Y38.6 Terrorism involving biological weapons**

Terrorism involving anthrax
Terrorism involving cholera
Terrorism involving smallpox

✓6th **Y38.6X Terrorism involving biological weapons**

✓7th **Y38.6X1 Terrorism involving biological weapons, public safety official injured**

✓7th **Y38.6X2 Terrorism involving biological weapons, civilian injured**

✓7th **Y38.6X3 Terrorism involving biological weapons, terrorist injured**

✓5th **Y38.7 Terrorism involving chemical weapons**

Terrorism involving gases, fumes, chemicals
Terrorism involving hydrogen cyanide
Terrorism involving phosgene
Terrorism involving sarin

✓6th **Y38.7X Terrorism involving chemical weapons**

✓7th **Y38.7X1 Terrorism involving chemical weapons, public safety official injured**

✓7th **Y38.7X2 Terrorism involving chemical weapons, civilian injured**

✓7th **Y38.7X3 Terrorism involving chemical weapons, terrorist injured**

✓5th **Y38.8 Terrorism involving other and unspecified means**

✓x7th **Y38.80 Terrorism involving unspecified means**

Terrorism NOS

✓6th **Y38.81 Terrorism involving suicide bomber**

✓7th **Y38.811 Terrorism involving suicide bomber, public safety official injured**

✓7th **Y38.812 Terrorism involving suicide bomber, civilian injured**

✓6th **Y38.89 Terrorism involving other means**

Terrorism involving drowning and submersion
Terrorism involving lasers
Terrorism involving piercing or stabbing instruments

✓7th **Y38.891 Terrorism involving other means, public safety official injured**

✓7th **Y38.892 Terrorism involving other means, civilian injured**

✓7th **Y38.893 Terrorism involving other means, terrorist injured**

✓5th **Y38.9 Terrorism, secondary effects**

NOTE This code is for use to identify conditions occurring subsequent to a terrorist attack not those that are due to the initial terrorist attack

✓6th **Y38.9X Terrorism, secondary effects**

✓7th **Y38.9X1 Terrorism, secondary effects, public safety official injured**

✓7th **Y38.9X2 Terrorism, secondary effects, civilian injured**

COMPLICATIONS OF MEDICAL AND SURGICAL CARE (Y62-Y84)

INCLUDES complications of medical devices
surgical and medical procedures as the cause of abnormal reaction of the patient, or of later complication, without mention of misadventure at the time of the procedure

Misadventures to patients during surgical and medical care (Y62-Y69)

EXCLUDES 1 *surgical and medical procedures as the cause of abnormal reaction of the patient, without mention of misadventure at the time of the procedure (Y83-Y84)*

EXCLUDES 2 *breakdown or malfunctioning of medical device (during procedure) (after implantation) (ongoing use) (Y70-Y82)*

✓4th **Y62 Failure of sterile precautions during surgical and medical care**

Y62.0 Failure of sterile precautions during surgical operation

Y62.1 Failure of sterile precautions during infusion or transfusion

Y62.2 Failure of sterile precautions during kidney dialysis and other perfusion HCC

Y62.3 Failure of sterile precautions during injection or immunization

Y62.4 Failure of sterile precautions during endoscopic examination

Y62.5 Failure of sterile precautions during heart catheterization

Y62.6 Failure of sterile precautions during aspiration, puncture and other catheterization

Y62.8 Failure of sterile precautions during other surgical and medical care

Y62.9 Failure of sterile precautions during unspecified surgical and medical care

✓4th **Y63 Failure in dosage during surgical and medical care**

EXCLUDES 2 *accidental overdose of drug or wrong drug given in error (T36-T50)*

Y63.0 Excessive amount of blood or other fluid given during transfusion or infusion

Y63.1 Incorrect dilution of fluid used during infusion

Y63.2 Overdose of radiation given during therapy

Y63.3 Inadvertent exposure of patient to radiation during medical care

Y63.4 Failure in dosage in electroshock or insulin-shock therapy

Y63.5 Inappropriate temperature in local application and packing

Y63.6 Underdosing and nonadministration of necessary drug, medicament or biological substance

AHA: 2018,4Q,72

Y63.8 Failure in dosage during other surgical and medical care

AHA: 2018,4Q,72

Y63.9 Failure in dosage during unspecified surgical and medical care

AHA: 2018,4Q,72

✓4th **Y64 Contaminated medical or biological substances**

Y64.0 Contaminated medical or biological substance, transfused or infused

Y64.1 Contaminated medical or biological substance, injected or used for immunization

Y64.8 Contaminated medical or biological substance administered by other means

Y64.9 Contaminated medical or biological substance administered by unspecified means
Administered contaminated medical or biological substance NOS

√4th **Y65 Other misadventures during surgical and medical care**
Y65.0 Mismatched blood in transfusion
Y65.1 Wrong fluid used in infusion
Y65.2 Failure in suture or ligature during surgical operation
Y65.3 Endotracheal tube wrongly placed during anesthetic procedure
Y65.4 Failure to introduce or to remove other tube or instrument
√5th **Y65.5 Performance of wrong procedure (operation)**
Y65.51 Performance of wrong procedure (operation) on correct patient
Wrong device implanted into correct surgical site
EXCLUDES 1 *performance of correct procedure (operation) on wrong side or body part (Y65.53)*
Y65.52 Performance of procedure (operation) on patient not scheduled for surgery
Performance of procedure (operation) intended for another patient
Performance of procedure (operation) on wrong patient
Y65.53 Performance of correct procedure (operation) on wrong side or body part
Performance of correct procedure (operation) on wrong side
Performance of correct procedure (operation) on wrong site
Y65.8 Other specified misadventures during surgical and medical care
AHA: 2019,2Q,23-24

Y66 Nonadministration of surgical and medical care
Premature cessation of surgical and medical care
EXCLUDES 1 *DNR status (Z66)*
palliative care (Z51.5)

Y69 Unspecified misadventure during surgical and medical care

Medical devices associated with adverse incidents in diagnostic and therapeutic use (Y70-Y82)

INCLUDES breakdown or malfunction of medical devices (during use) (after implantation) (ongoing use)
EXCLUDES 2 *later complications following use of medical devices without breakdown or malfunctioning of device (Y83-Y84)*
misadventure to patients during surgical and medical care, classifiable to (Y62-Y69)
surgical and other medical procedures as the cause of abnormal reaction of the patient, or of later complication, without mention of misadventure at the time of the procedure (Y83-Y84)

√4th **Y70 Anesthesiology devices associated with adverse incidents**
Y70.0 Diagnostic and monitoring anesthesiology devices associated with adverse incidents
Y70.1 Therapeutic (nonsurgical) and rehabilitative anesthesiology devices associated with adverse incidents
Y70.2 Prosthetic and other implants, materials and accessory anesthesiology devices associated with adverse incidents
Y70.3 Surgical instruments, materials and anesthesiology devices (including sutures) associated with adverse incidents
Y70.8 Miscellaneous anesthesiology devices associated with adverse incidents, not elsewhere classified

√4th **Y71 Cardiovascular devices associated with adverse incidents**
Y71.0 Diagnostic and monitoring cardiovascular devices associated with adverse incidents
Y71.1 Therapeutic (nonsurgical) and rehabilitative cardiovascular devices associated with adverse incidents
Y71.2 Prosthetic and other implants, materials and accessory cardiovascular devices associated with adverse incidents
Y71.3 Surgical instruments, materials and cardiovascular devices (including sutures) associated with adverse incidents
Y71.8 Miscellaneous cardiovascular devices associated with adverse incidents, not elsewhere classified

√4th **Y72 Otorhinolaryngological devices associated with adverse incidents**
Y72.0 Diagnostic and monitoring otorhinolaryngological devices associated with adverse incidents
Y72.1 Therapeutic (nonsurgical) and rehabilitative otorhinolaryngological devices associated with adverse incidents
Y72.2 Prosthetic and other implants, materials and accessory otorhinolaryngological devices associated with adverse incidents
Y72.3 Surgical instruments, materials and otorhinolaryngological devices (including sutures) associated with adverse incidents
Y72.8 Miscellaneous otorhinolaryngological devices associated with adverse incidents, not elsewhere classified

√4th **Y73 Gastroenterology and urology devices associated with adverse incidents**
Y73.0 Diagnostic and monitoring gastroenterology and urology devices associated with adverse incidents
Y73.1 Therapeutic (nonsurgical) and rehabilitative gastroenterology and urology devices associated with adverse incidents
Y73.2 Prosthetic and other implants, materials and accessory gastroenterology and urology devices associated with adverse incidents
Y73.3 Surgical instruments, materials and gastroenterology and urology devices (including sutures) associated with adverse incidents
Y73.8 Miscellaneous gastroenterology and urology devices associated with adverse incidents, not elsewhere classified

√4th **Y74 General hospital and personal-use devices associated with adverse incidents**
Y74.0 Diagnostic and monitoring general hospital and personal-use devices associated with adverse incidents
Y74.1 Therapeutic (nonsurgical) and rehabilitative general hospital and personal-use devices associated with adverse incidents
Y74.2 Prosthetic and other implants, materials and accessory general hospital and personal-use devices associated with adverse incidents
Y74.3 Surgical instruments, materials and general hospital and personal-use devices (including sutures) associated with adverse incidents
Y74.8 Miscellaneous general hospital and personal-use devices associated with adverse incidents, not elsewhere classified

√4th **Y75 Neurological devices associated with adverse incidents**
Y75.0 Diagnostic and monitoring neurological devices associated with adverse incidents
Y75.1 Therapeutic (nonsurgical) and rehabilitative neurological devices associated with adverse incidents
Y75.2 Prosthetic and other implants, materials and neurological devices associated with adverse incidents
Y75.3 Surgical instruments, materials and neurological devices (including sutures) associated with adverse incidents
Y75.8 Miscellaneous neurological devices associated with adverse incidents, not elsewhere classified

√4th **Y76 Obstetric and gynecological devices associated with adverse incidents**
Y76.0 Diagnostic and monitoring obstetric and gynecological devices associated with adverse incidents ♀
Y76.1 Therapeutic (nonsurgical) and rehabilitative obstetric and gynecological devices associated with adverse incidents ♀
Y76.2 Prosthetic and other implants, materials and accessory obstetric and gynecological devices associated with adverse incidents ♀
Y76.3 Surgical instruments, materials and obstetric and gynecological devices (including sutures) associated with adverse incidents ♀
Y76.8 Miscellaneous obstetric and gynecological devices associated with adverse incidents, not elsewhere classified ♀

√4th **Y77 Ophthalmic devices associated with adverse incidents**
Y77.0 Diagnostic and monitoring ophthalmic devices associated with adverse incidents
▲ √5th **Y77.1 Therapeutic (nonsurgical) and rehabilitative ophthalmic devices associated with adverse incidents**
● **Y77.11 Contact lens associated with adverse incidents**
Rigid gas permeable contact lens associated with adverse incidents
Soft (hydrophilic) contact lens associated with adverse incidents
● **Y77.19 Other therapeutic (nonsurgical) and rehabilitative ophthalmic devices associated with adverse incidents**
Y77.2 Prosthetic and other implants, materials and accessory ophthalmic devices associated with adverse incidents
Y77.3 Surgical instruments, materials and ophthalmic devices (including sutures) associated with adverse incidents
Y77.8 Miscellaneous ophthalmic devices associated with adverse incidents, not elsewhere classified

Y78 Radiological devices associated with adverse incidents
- Y78.0 Diagnostic and monitoring radiological devices associated with adverse incidents
- Y78.1 Therapeutic (nonsurgical) and rehabilitative radiological devices associated with adverse incidents
- Y78.2 Prosthetic and other implants, materials and accessory radiological devices associated with adverse incidents
- Y78.3 Surgical instruments, materials and radiological devices (including sutures) associated with adverse incidents
- Y78.8 Miscellaneous radiological devices associated with adverse incidents, not elsewhere classified

Y79 Orthopedic devices associated with adverse incidents
- Y79.0 Diagnostic and monitoring orthopedic devices associated with adverse incidents
- Y79.1 Therapeutic (nonsurgical) and rehabilitative orthopedic devices associated with adverse incidents
- Y79.2 Prosthetic and other implants, materials and accessory orthopedic devices associated with adverse incidents
- Y79.3 Surgical instruments, materials and orthopedic devices (including sutures) associated with adverse incidents
- Y79.8 Miscellaneous orthopedic devices associated with adverse incidents, not elsewhere classified

Y80 Physical medicine devices associated with adverse incidents
- Y80.0 Diagnostic and monitoring physical medicine devices associated with adverse incidents
- Y80.1 Therapeutic (nonsurgical) and rehabilitative physical medicine devices associated with adverse incidents
- Y80.2 Prosthetic and other implants, materials and accessory physical medicine devices associated with adverse incidents
- Y80.3 Surgical instruments, materials and physical medicine devices (including sutures) associated with adverse incidents
- Y80.8 Miscellaneous physical medicine devices associated with adverse incidents, not elsewhere classified

Y81 General- and plastic-surgery devices associated with adverse incidents
- Y81.0 Diagnostic and monitoring general- and plastic-surgery devices associated with adverse incidents
- Y81.1 Therapeutic (nonsurgical) and rehabilitative general- and plastic-surgery devices associated with adverse incidents
- Y81.2 Prosthetic and other implants, materials and accessory general- and plastic-surgery devices associated with adverse incidents
- Y81.3 Surgical instruments, materials and general- and plastic-surgery devices (including sutures) associated with adverse incidents
- Y81.8 Miscellaneous general- and plastic-surgery devices associated with adverse incidents, not elsewhere classified

Y82 Other and unspecified medical devices associated with adverse incidents
- Y82.8 Other medical devices associated with adverse incidents
- Y82.9 Unspecified medical devices associated with adverse incidents

Surgical and other medical procedures as the cause of abnormal reaction of the patient, or of later complication, without mention of misadventure at the time of the procedure (Y83-Y84)

EXCLUDES 1 *misadventures to patients during surgical and medical care, classifiable to (Y62-Y69)*

EXCLUDES 2 *breakdown or malfunctioning of medical device (during procedure) (after implantation) (ongoing use) (Y70-Y82)*

Y83 Surgical operation and other surgical procedures as the cause of abnormal reaction of the patient, or of later complication, without mention of misadventure at the time of the procedure
- Y83.0 Surgical operation with transplant of whole organ as the cause of abnormal reaction of the patient, or of later complication, without mention of misadventure at the time of the procedure
- Y83.1 Surgical operation with implant of artificial internal device as the cause of abnormal reaction of the patient, or of later complication, without mention of misadventure at the time of the procedure
- Y83.2 Surgical operation with anastomosis, bypass or graft as the cause of abnormal reaction of the patient, or of later complication, without mention of misadventure at the time of the procedure
- Y83.3 Surgical operation with formation of external stoma as the cause of abnormal reaction of the patient, or of later complication, without mention of misadventure at the time of the procedure
- Y83.4 Other reconstructive surgery as the cause of abnormal reaction of the patient, or of later complication, without mention of misadventure at the time of the procedure
- Y83.5 Amputation of limb(s) as the cause of abnormal reaction of the patient, or of later complication, without mention of misadventure at the time of the procedure
- Y83.6 Removal of other organ (partial) (total) as the cause of abnormal reaction of the patient, or of later complication, without mention of misadventure at the time of the procedure
- Y83.8 Other surgical procedures as the cause of abnormal reaction of the patient, or of later complication, without mention of misadventure at the time of the procedure
- Y83.9 Surgical procedure, unspecified as the cause of abnormal reaction of the patient, or of later complication, without mention of misadventure at the time of the procedure

Y84 Other medical procedures as the cause of abnormal reaction of the patient, or of later complication, without mention of misadventure at the time of the procedure
- Y84.0 Cardiac catheterization as the cause of abnormal reaction of the patient, or of later complication, without mention of misadventure at the time of the procedure
- Y84.1 Kidney dialysis as the cause of abnormal reaction of the patient, or of later complication, without mention of misadventure at the time of the procedure
- Y84.2 Radiological procedure and radiotherapy as the cause of abnormal reaction of the patient, or of later complication, without mention of misadventure at the time of the procedure
  AHA: 2019,1Q,21; 2017,1Q,33
- Y84.3 Shock therapy as the cause of abnormal reaction of the patient, or of later complication, without mention of misadventure at the time of the procedure
- Y84.4 Aspiration of fluid as the cause of abnormal reaction of the patient, or of later complication, without mention of misadventure at the time of the procedure
- Y84.5 Insertion of gastric or duodenal sound as the cause of abnormal reaction of the patient, or of later complication, without mention of misadventure at the time of the procedure
- Y84.6 Urinary catheterization as the cause of abnormal reaction of the patient, or of later complication, without mention of misadventure at the time of the procedure
- Y84.7 Blood-sampling as the cause of abnormal reaction of the patient, or of later complication, without mention of misadventure at the time of the procedure
- Y84.8 Other medical procedures as the cause of abnormal reaction of the patient, or of later complication, without mention of misadventure at the time of the procedure
  AHA: 2014,4Q,24
- Y84.9 Medical procedure, unspecified as the cause of abnormal reaction of the patient, or of later complication, without mention of misadventure at the time of the procedure

Supplementary factors related to causes of morbidity classified elsewhere (Y90-Y99)

NOTE These categories may be used to provide supplementary information concerning causes of morbidity. They are not to be used for single-condition coding.

Y90 Evidence of alcohol involvement determined by blood alcohol level

Code first any associated alcohol related disorders (F10)
- Y90.0 Blood alcohol level of less than 20 mg/100 ml
- Y90.1 Blood alcohol level of 20-39 mg/100 ml
- Y90.2 Blood alcohol level of 40-59 mg/100 ml
- Y90.3 Blood alcohol level of 60-79 mg/100 ml
- Y90.4 Blood alcohol level of 80-99 mg/100 ml
- Y90.5 Blood alcohol level of 100-119 mg/100 ml
- Y90.6 Blood alcohol level of 120-199 mg/100 ml
- Y90.7 Blood alcohol level of 200-239 mg/100 ml
- Y90.8 Blood alcohol level of 240 mg/100 ml or more
- Y90.9 Presence of alcohol in blood, level not specified

Y92 Place of occurrence of the external cause

The following category is for use, when relevant, to identify the place of occurrence of the external cause. Use in conjunction with an activity code.

Place of occurrence should be recorded only at the initial encounter for treatment

Y92.0 Non-institutional (private) residence as the place of occurrence of the external cause

EXCLUDES 1 *abandoned or derelict house (Y92.89)*
home under construction but not yet occupied (Y92.6-)
institutional place of residence (Y92.1-)

Y92.00 Unspecified non-institutional (private) residence as the place of occurrence of the external cause

Y92.000 Kitchen of unspecified non-institutional (private) residence as the place of occurrence of the external cause

Y92.001 Dining room of unspecified non-institutional (private) residence as the place of occurrence of the external cause

▲ **Y92.002 Bathroom of unspecified non-institutional (private) residence as the place of occurrence of the external cause**

Y92.003 Bedroom of unspecified non-institutional (private) residence as the place of occurrence of the external cause

Y92.007 Garden or yard of unspecified non-institutional (private) residence as the place of occurrence of the external cause

Y92.008 Other place in unspecified non-institutional (private) residence as the place of occurrence of the external cause

Y92.009 Unspecified place in unspecified non-institutional (private) residence as the place of occurrence of the external cause

Home (NOS) as the place of occurrence of the external cause

Y92.01 Single-family non-institutional (private) house as the place of occurrence of the external cause

Farmhouse as the place of occurrence of the external cause

EXCLUDES 1 *barn (Y92.71)*
chicken coop or hen house (Y92.72)
farm field (Y92.73)
orchard (Y92.74)
single family mobile home or trailer (Y92.02-)
slaughter house (Y92.86)

Y92.010 Kitchen of single-family (private) house as the place of occurrence of the external cause

Y92.011 Dining room of single-family (private) house as the place of occurrence of the external cause

Y92.012 Bathroom of single-family (private) house as the place of occurrence of the external cause

Y92.013 Bedroom of single-family (private) house as the place of occurrence of the external cause

Y92.014 Private driveway to single-family (private) house as the place of occurrence of the external cause

Y92.015 Private garage of single-family (private) house as the place of occurrence of the external cause

Y92.016 Swimming-pool in single-family (private) house or garden as the place of occurrence of the external cause

Y92.017 Garden or yard in single-family (private) house as the place of occurrence of the external cause

Y92.018 Other place in single-family (private) house as the place of occurrence of the external cause

Y92.019 Unspecified place in single-family (private) house as the place of occurrence of the external cause

Y92.02 Mobile home as the place of occurrence of the external cause

Y92.020 Kitchen in mobile home as the place of occurrence of the external cause

Y92.021 Dining room in mobile home as the place of occurrence of the external cause

Y92.022 Bathroom in mobile home as the place of occurrence of the external cause

Y92.023 Bedroom in mobile home as the place of occurrence of the external cause

Y92.024 Driveway of mobile home as the place of occurrence of the external cause

Y92.025 Garage of mobile home as the place of occurrence of the external cause

Y92.026 Swimming-pool of mobile home as the place of occurrence of the external cause

Y92.027 Garden or yard of mobile home as the place of occurrence of the external cause

Y92.028 Other place in mobile home as the place of occurrence of the external cause

Y92.029 Unspecified place in mobile home as the place of occurrence of the external cause

Y92.03 Apartment as the place of occurrence of the external cause

Condominium as the place of occurrence of the external cause

Co-op apartment as the place of occurrence of the external cause

Y92.030 Kitchen in apartment as the place of occurrence of the external cause

Y92.031 Bathroom in apartment as the place of occurrence of the external cause

Y92.032 Bedroom in apartment as the place of occurrence of the external cause

Y92.038 Other place in apartment as the place of occurrence of the external cause

Y92.039 Unspecified place in apartment as the place of occurrence of the external cause

Y92.04 Boarding-house as the place of occurrence of the external cause

Y92.040 Kitchen in boarding-house as the place of occurrence of the external cause

Y92.041 Bathroom in boarding-house as the place of occurrence of the external cause

Y92.042 Bedroom in boarding-house as the place of occurrence of the external cause

Y92.043 Driveway of boarding-house as the place of occurrence of the external cause

Y92.044 Garage of boarding-house as the place of occurrence of the external cause

Y92.045 Swimming-pool of boarding-house as the place of occurrence of the external cause

Y92.046 Garden or yard of boarding-house as the place of occurrence of the external cause

Y92.048 Other place in boarding-house as the place of occurrence of the external cause

Y92.049 Unspecified place in boarding-house as the place of occurrence of the external cause

Y92.09 Other non-institutional residence as the place of occurrence of the external cause

AHA: 2017,2Q,10

Y92.090 Kitchen in other non-institutional residence as the place of occurrence of the external cause

Y92.091 Bathroom in other non-institutional residence as the place of occurrence of the external cause

Y92.092 Bedroom in other non-institutional residence as the place of occurrence of the external cause

Y92.093 Driveway of other non-institutional residence as the place of occurrence of the external cause

Y92.094 Garage of other non-institutional residence as the place of occurrence of the external cause

Y92.095 Swimming-pool of other non-institutional residence as the place of occurrence of the external cause

Y92.096 Garden or yard of other non-institutional residence as the place of occurrence of the external cause

Y92.098 Other place in other non-institutional residence as the place of occurrence of the external cause

Y92.099 Unspecified place in other non-institutional residence as the place of occurrence of the external cause

✓5th Y92.1 Institutional (nonprivate) residence as the place of occurrence of the external cause

Y92.10 Unspecified residential institution as the place of occurrence of the external cause

✓6th Y92.11 Children's home and orphanage as the place of occurrence of the external cause

Y92.110 Kitchen in children's home and orphanage as the place of occurrence of the external cause

Y92.111 Bathroom in children's home and orphanage as the place of occurrence of the external cause

Y92.112 Bedroom in children's home and orphanage as the place of occurrence of the external cause

Y92.113 Driveway of children's home and orphanage as the place of occurrence of the external cause

Y92.114 Garage of children's home and orphanage as the place of occurrence of the external cause

Y92.115 Swimming-pool of children's home and orphanage as the place of occurrence of the external cause

Y92.116 Garden or yard of children's home and orphanage as the place of occurrence of the external cause

Y92.118 Other place in children's home and orphanage as the place of occurrence of the external cause

Y92.119 Unspecified place in children's home and orphanage as the place of occurrence of the external cause

✓6th Y92.12 Nursing home as the place of occurrence of the external cause

Home for the sick as the place of occurrence of the external cause

Hospice as the place of occurrence of the external cause

AHA: 2017,2Q,10

Y92.120 Kitchen in nursing home as the place of occurrence of the external cause

Y92.121 Bathroom in nursing home as the place of occurrence of the external cause

Y92.122 Bedroom in nursing home as the place of occurrence of the external cause

Y92.123 Driveway of nursing home as the place of occurrence of the external cause

Y92.124 Garage of nursing home as the place of occurrence of the external cause

Y92.125 Swimming-pool of nursing home as the place of occurrence of the external cause

Y92.126 Garden or yard of nursing home as the place of occurrence of the external cause

Y92.128 Other place in nursing home as the place of occurrence of the external cause

Y92.129 Unspecified place in nursing home as the place of occurrence of the external cause

✓6th Y92.13 Military base as the place of occurrence of the external cause

EXCLUDES 1 *military training grounds (Y92.84)*

Y92.130 Kitchen on military base as the place of occurrence of the external cause

Y92.131 Mess hall on military base as the place of occurrence of the external cause

Y92.133 Barracks on military base as the place of occurrence of the external cause

Y92.135 Garage on military base as the place of occurrence of the external cause

Y92.136 Swimming-pool on military base as the place of occurrence of the external cause

Y92.137 Garden or yard on military base as the place of occurrence of the external cause

Y92.138 Other place on military base as the place of occurrence of the external cause

Y92.139 Unspecified place military base as the place of occurrence of the external cause

✓6th Y92.14 Prison as the place of occurrence of the external cause

Y92.140 Kitchen in prison as the place of occurrence of the external cause

Y92.141 Dining room in prison as the place of occurrence of the external cause

Y92.142 Bathroom in prison as the place of occurrence of the external cause

Y92.143 Cell of prison as the place of occurrence of the external cause

Y92.146 Swimming-pool of prison as the place of occurrence of the external cause

Y92.147 Courtyard of prison as the place of occurrence of the external cause

Y92.148 Other place in prison as the place of occurrence of the external cause

Y92.149 Unspecified place in prison as the place of occurrence of the external cause

✓6th Y92.15 Reform school as the place of occurrence of the external cause

Y92.150 Kitchen in reform school as the place of occurrence of the external cause

Y92.151 Dining room in reform school as the place of occurrence of the external cause

Y92.152 Bathroom in reform school as the place of occurrence of the external cause

Y92.153 Bedroom in reform school as the place of occurrence of the external cause

Y92.154 Driveway of reform school as the place of occurrence of the external cause

Y92.155 Garage of reform school as the place of occurrence of the external cause

Y92.156 Swimming-pool of reform school as the place of occurrence of the external cause

Y92.157 Garden or yard of reform school as the place of occurrence of the external cause

Y92.158 Other place in reform school as the place of occurrence of the external cause

Y92.159 Unspecified place in reform school as the place of occurrence of the external cause

✓6th Y92.16 School dormitory as the place of occurrence of the external cause

EXCLUDES 1 *reform school as the place of occurrence of the external cause (Y92.15-)*
school buildings and grounds as the place of occurrence of the external cause (Y92.2-)
school sports and athletic areas as the place of occurrence of the external cause (Y92.3-)

Y92.160 Kitchen in school dormitory as the place of occurrence of the external cause

Y92.161 Dining room in school dormitory as the place of occurrence of the external cause

Y92.162 Bathroom in school dormitory as the place of occurrence of the external cause

Y92.163 Bedroom in school dormitory as the place of occurrence of the external cause

Y92.168 Other place in school dormitory as the place of occurrence of the external cause

Y92.169 Unspecified place in school dormitory as the place of occurrence of the external cause

✓6th Y92.19 Other specified residential institution as the place of occurrence of the external cause

AHA: 2017,2Q,10

Y92.190 Kitchen in other specified residential institution as the place of occurrence of the external cause

Y92.191 Dining room in other specified residential institution as the place of occurrence of the external cause

Y92.192 Bathroom in other specified residential institution as the place of occurrence of the external cause

Y92.193 Bedroom in other specified residential institution as the place of occurrence of the external cause

Y92.194 Driveway of other specified residential institution as the place of occurrence of the external cause

Y92.195 **Garage of other specified residential institution as the place of occurrence of the external cause**

Y92.196 **Pool of other specified residential institution as the place of occurrence of the external cause**

Y92.197 **Garden or yard of other specified residential institution as the place of occurrence of the external cause**

Y92.198 **Other place in other specified residential institution as the place of occurrence of the external cause**

Y92.199 **Unspecified place in other specified residential institution as the place of occurrence of the external cause**

✓5th **Y92.2** **School, other institution and public administrative area as the place of occurrence of the external cause**

Building and adjacent grounds used by the general public or by a particular group of the public

EXCLUDES 1 *building under construction as the place of occurrence of the external cause (Y92.6)*
residential institution as the place of occurrence of the external cause (Y92.1)
school dormitory as the place of occurrence of the external cause (Y92.16-)
sports and athletics area of schools as the place of occurrence of the external cause (Y92.3-)

✓6th **Y92.21** **School (private) (public) (state) as the place of occurrence of the external cause**

Y92.210 **Daycare center as the place of occurrence of the external cause**

Y92.211 **Elementary school as the place of occurrence of the external cause**

Kindergarten as the place of occurrence of the external cause

Y92.212 **Middle school as the place of occurrence of the external cause**

Y92.213 **High school as the place of occurrence of the external cause**

AHA: 2012,4Q,108

Y92.214 **College as the place of occurrence of the external cause**

University as the place of occurrence of the external cause

Y92.215 **Trade school as the place of occurrence of the external cause**

Y92.218 **Other school as the place of occurrence of the external cause**

Y92.219 **Unspecified school as the place of occurrence of the external cause**

Y92.22 **Religious institution as the place of occurrence of the external cause**

Church as the place of occurrence of the external cause

Mosque as the place of occurrence of the external cause

Synagogue as the place of occurrence of the external cause

✓6th **Y92.23** **Hospital as the place of occurrence of the external cause**

EXCLUDES 1 *ambulatory (outpatient) health services establishments (Y92.53-)*
home for the sick as the place of occurrence of the external cause (Y92.12-)
hospice as the place of occurrence of the external cause (Y92.12-)
nursing home as the place of occurrence of the external cause (Y92.12-)

Y92.230 **Patient room in hospital as the place of occurrence of the external cause**

Y92.231 **Patient bathroom in hospital as the place of occurrence of the external cause**

Y92.232 **Corridor of hospital as the place of occurrence of the external cause**

Y92.233 **Cafeteria of hospital as the place of occurrence of the external cause**

Y92.234 **Operating room of hospital as the place of occurrence of the external cause**

Y92.238 **Other place in hospital as the place of occurrence of the external cause**

Y92.239 **Unspecified place in hospital as the place of occurrence of the external cause**

✓6th **Y92.24** **Public administrative building as the place of occurrence of the external cause**

Y92.240 **Courthouse as the place of occurrence of the external cause**

Y92.241 **Library as the place of occurrence of the external cause**

Y92.242 **Post office as the place of occurrence of the external cause**

Y92.243 **City hall as the place of occurrence of the external cause**

Y92.248 **Other public administrative building as the place of occurrence of the external cause**

✓6th **Y92.25** **Cultural building as the place of occurrence of the external cause**

Y92.250 **Art Gallery as the place of occurrence of the external cause**

Y92.251 **Museum as the place of occurrence of the external cause**

Y92.252 **Music hall as the place of occurrence of the external cause**

Y92.253 **Opera house as the place of occurrence of the external cause**

Y92.254 **Theater (live) as the place of occurrence of the external cause**

Y92.258 **Other cultural public building as the place of occurrence of the external cause**

Y92.26 **Movie house or cinema as the place of occurrence of the external cause**

Y92.29 **Other specified public building as the place of occurrence of the external cause**

Assembly hall as the place of occurrence of the external cause

Clubhouse as the place of occurrence of the external cause

✓5th **Y92.3** **Sports and athletics area as the place of occurrence of the external cause**

✓6th **Y92.31** **Athletic court as the place of occurrence of the external cause**

EXCLUDES 1 *tennis court in private home or garden (Y92.09)*

Y92.310 **Basketball court as the place of occurrence of the external cause**

Y92.311 **Squash court as the place of occurrence of the external cause**

Y92.312 **Tennis court as the place of occurrence of the external cause**

Y92.318 **Other athletic court as the place of occurrence of the external cause**

✓6th **Y92.32** **Athletic field as the place of occurrence of the external cause**

Y92.320 **Baseball field as the place of occurrence of the external cause**

Y92.321 **Football field as the place of occurrence of the external cause**

Y92.322 **Soccer field as the place of occurrence of the external cause**

Y92.328 **Other athletic field as the place of occurrence of the external cause**

Cricket field as the place of occurrence of the external cause

Hockey field as the place of occurrence of the external cause

✓6th **Y92.33** **Skating rink as the place of occurrence of the external cause**

Y92.330 **Ice skating rink (indoor) (outdoor) as the place of occurrence of the external cause**

Y92.331 **Roller skating rink as the place of occurrence of the external cause**

Y92.34 **Swimming pool (public) as the place of occurrence of the external cause**

EXCLUDES 1 *swimming pool in private home or garden (Y92.016)*

Y92.39 Other specified sports and athletic area as the place of occurrence of the external cause
Golf-course as the place of occurrence of the external cause
Gymnasium as the place of occurrence of the external cause
Riding-school as the place of occurrence of the external cause
Stadium as the place of occurrence of the external cause

√5th **Y92.4 Street, highway and other paved roadways as the place of occurrence of the external cause**
EXCLUDES 1 *private driveway of residence (Y92.014, Y92.024, Y92.043, Y92.093, Y92.113, Y92.123, Y92.154, Y92.194)*

√6th **Y92.41 Street and highway as the place of occurrence of the external cause**
Y92.410 Unspecified street and highway as the place of occurrence of the external cause
Road NOS as the place of occurrence of the external cause
Y92.411 Interstate highway as the place of occurrence of the external cause
Freeway as the place of occurrence of the external cause
Motorway as the place of occurrence of the external cause
Y92.412 Parkway as the place of occurrence of the external cause
Y92.413 State road as the place of occurrence of the external cause
Y92.414 Local residential or business street as the place of occurrence of the external cause
Y92.415 Exit ramp or entrance ramp of street or highway as the place of occurrence of the external cause

√6th **Y92.48 Other paved roadways as the place of occurrence of the external cause**
Y92.480 Sidewalk as the place of occurrence of the external cause
Y92.481 Parking lot as the place of occurrence of the external cause
Y92.482 Bike path as the place of occurrence of the external cause
Y92.488 Other paved roadways as the place of occurrence of the external cause

√5th **Y92.5 Trade and service area as the place of occurrence of the external cause**
EXCLUDES 1 *garage in private home (Y92.015)*
schools and other public administration buildings (Y92.2-)

√6th **Y92.51 Private commercial establishments as the place of occurrence of the external cause**
Y92.510 Bank as the place of occurrence of the external cause
Y92.511 Restaurant or café as the place of occurrence of the external cause
Y92.512 Supermarket, store or market as the place of occurrence of the external cause
Y92.513 Shop (commercial) as the place of occurrence of the external cause

√6th **Y92.52 Service areas as the place of occurrence of the external cause**
Y92.520 Airport as the place of occurrence of the external cause
Y92.521 Bus station as the place of occurrence of the external cause
Y92.522 Railway station as the place of occurrence of the external cause
Y92.523 Highway rest stop as the place of occurrence of the external cause
Y92.524 Gas station as the place of occurrence of the external cause
Petroleum station as the place of occurrence of the external cause
Service station as the place of occurrence of the external cause

√6th **Y92.53 Ambulatory health services establishments as the place of occurrence of the external cause**
Y92.530 Ambulatory surgery center as the place of occurrence of the external cause
Outpatient surgery center, including that connected with a hospital as the place of occurrence of the external cause
Same day surgery center, including that connected with a hospital as the place of occurrence of the external cause
Y92.531 Health care provider office as the place of occurrence of the external cause
Physician office as the place of occurrence of the external cause
Y92.532 Urgent care center as the place of occurrence of the external cause
Y92.538 Other ambulatory health services establishments as the place of occurrence of the external cause
AHA: 2019,1Q,21

Y92.59 Other trade areas as the place of occurrence of the external cause
Office building as the place of occurrence of the external cause
Casino as the place of occurrence of the external cause
Garage (commercial) as the place of occurrence of the external cause
Hotel as the place of occurrence of the external cause
Radio or television station as the place of occurrence of the external cause
Shopping mall as the place of occurrence of the external cause
Warehouse as the place of occurrence of the external cause

√5th **Y92.6 Industrial and construction area as the place of occurrence of the external cause**
Y92.61 Building [any] under construction as the place of occurrence of the external cause
Y92.62 Dock or shipyard as the place of occurrence of the external cause
Dockyard as the place of occurrence of the external cause
Dry dock as the place of occurrence of the external cause
Shipyard as the place of occurrence of the external cause
Y92.63 Factory as the place of occurrence of the external cause
Factory building as the place of occurrence of the external cause
Factory premises as the place of occurrence of the external cause
Industrial yard as the place of occurrence of the external cause
Y92.64 Mine or pit as the place of occurrence of the external cause
Mine as the place of occurrence of the external cause
Y92.65 Oil rig as the place of occurrence of the external cause
Pit (coal) (gravel) (sand) as the place of occurrence of the external cause
Y92.69 Other specified industrial and construction area as the place of occurrence of the external cause
Gasworks as the place of occurrence of the external cause
Power-station (coal) (nuclear) (oil) as the place of occurrence of the external cause
Tunnel under construction as the place of occurrence of the external cause
Workshop as the place of occurrence of the external cause

√5th **Y92.7 Farm as the place of occurrence of the external cause**
Ranch as the place of occurrence of the external cause
EXCLUDES 1 *farmhouse and home premises of farm (Y92.01-)*
Y92.71 Barn as the place of occurrence of the external cause

Y92.72 Chicken coop as the place of occurrence of the external cause
Hen house as the place of occurrence of the external cause
Y92.73 Farm field as the place of occurrence of the external cause
Y92.74 Orchard as the place of occurrence of the external cause
Y92.79 Other farm location as the place of occurrence of the external cause

✓5th **Y92.8 Other places as the place of occurrence of the external cause**
✓6th **Y92.81 Transport vehicle as the place of occurrence of the external cause**
EXCLUDES 1 *transport accidents (VØØ-V99)*
Y92.81Ø Car as the place of occurrence of the external cause
Y92.811 Bus as the place of occurrence of the external cause
Y92.812 Truck as the place of occurrence of the external cause
Y92.813 Airplane as the place of occurrence of the external cause
Y92.814 Boat as the place of occurrence of the external cause
Y92.815 Train as the place of occurrence of the external cause
Y92.816 Subway car as the place of occurrence of the external cause
Y92.818 Other transport vehicle as the place of occurrence of the external cause
✓6th **Y92.82 Wilderness area**
Y92.82Ø Desert as the place of occurrence of the external cause
Y92.821 Forest as the place of occurrence of the external cause
Y92.828 Other wilderness area as the place of occurrence of the external cause
Swamp as the place of occurrence of the external cause
Mountain as the place of occurrence of the external cause
Marsh as the place of occurrence of the external cause
Prairie as the place of occurrence of the external cause
✓6th **Y92.83 Recreation area as the place of occurrence of the external cause**
Y92.83Ø Public park as the place of occurrence of the external cause
Y92.831 Amusement park as the place of occurrence of the external cause
Y92.832 Beach as the place of occurrence of the external cause
Seashore as the place of occurrence of the external cause
Y92.833 Campsite as the place of occurrence of the external cause
Y92.834 Zoological garden (Zoo) as the place of occurrence of the external cause
Y92.838 Other recreation area as the place of occurrence of the external cause
Y92.84 Military training ground as the place of occurrence of the external cause
Y92.85 Railroad track as the place of occurrence of the external cause
Y92.86 Slaughter house as the place of occurrence of the external cause
Y92.89 Other specified places as the place of occurrence of the external cause
Derelict house as the place of occurrence of the external cause

Y92.9 Unspecified place or not applicable

✓4th **Y93 Activity codes**

NOTE Category Y93 is provided for use to indicate the activity of the person seeking healthcare for an injury or health condition, such as a heart attack while shoveling snow, which resulted from, or was contributed to, by the activity. These codes are appropriate for use for both acute injuries, such as those from chapter 19, and conditions that are due to the long-term, cumulative effects of an activity, such as those from chapter 13. They are also appropriate for use with external cause codes for cause and intent if identifying the activity provides additional information on the event. These codes should be used in conjunction with codes for external cause status (Y99) and place of occurrence (Y92).

This section contains the following broad activity categories:

Y93.Ø	Activities involving walking and running
Y93.1	Activities involving water and water craft
Y93.2	Activities involving ice and snow
Y93.3	Activities involving climbing, rappelling, and jumping off
Y93.4	Activities involving dancing and other rhythmic movement
Y93.5	Activities involving other sports and athletics played individually
Y93.6	Activities involving other sports and athletics played as a team or group
Y93.7	Activities involving other specified sports and athletics
Y93.A	Activities involving other cardiorespiratory exercise
Y93.B	Activities involving other muscle strengthening exercises
Y93.C	Activities involving computer technology and electronic devices
Y93.D	Activities involving arts and handcrafts
Y93.E	Activities involving personal hygiene and interior property and clothing maintenance
Y93.F	Activities involving caregiving
Y93.G	Activities involving food preparation, cooking and grilling
Y93.H	Activities involving exterior property and land maintenance, building and construction
Y93.I	Activities involving roller coasters and other types of external motion
Y93.J	Activities involving playing musical instrument
Y93.K	Activities involving animal care
Y93.8	Activities, other specified
Y93.9	Activity, unspecified

✓5th **Y93.Ø Activities involving walking and running**
EXCLUDES 1 *activity, walking an animal (Y93.K1)*
activity, walking or running on a treadmill (Y93.A1)
Y93.Ø1 Activity, walking, marching and hiking
Activity, walking, marching and hiking on level or elevated terrain
EXCLUDES 1 *activity, mountain climbing (Y93.31)*
Y93.Ø2 Activity, running

✓5th **Y93.1 Activities involving water and water craft**
EXCLUDES 1 *activities involving ice (Y93.2-)*
Y93.11 Activity, swimming
Y93.12 Activity, springboard and platform diving
Y93.13 Activity, water polo
Y93.14 Activity, water aerobics and water exercise
Y93.15 Activity, underwater diving and snorkeling
Activity, SCUBA diving
Y93.16 Activity, rowing, canoeing, kayaking, rafting and tubing
Activity, canoeing, kayaking, rafting and tubing in calm and turbulent water
Y93.17 Activity, water skiing and wake boarding
Y93.18 Activity, surfing, windsurfing and boogie boarding
Activity, water sliding
Y93.19 Activity, other involving water and watercraft
Activity involving water NOS
Activity, parasailing
Activity, water survival training and testing

Y93.2 Activities involving ice and snow
EXCLUDES 1 *activity, shoveling ice and snow (Y93.H1)*

Y93.21 Activity, ice skating
Activity, figure skating (singles) (pairs)
Activity, ice dancing
EXCLUDES 1 *activity, ice hockey (Y93.22)*

Y93.22 Activity, ice hockey

Y93.23 Activity, snow (alpine) (downhill) skiing, snowboarding, sledding, tobogganing and snow tubing
EXCLUDES 1 *activity, cross country skiing (Y93.24)*

Y93.24 Activity, cross country skiing
Activity, nordic skiing

Y93.29 Activity, other involving ice and snow
Activity involving ice and snow NOS

Y93.3 Activities involving climbing, rappelling and jumping off
EXCLUDES 1 *activity, hiking on level or elevated terrain (Y93.Ø1)*
activity, jumping rope (Y93.56)
activity, trampoline jumping (Y93.44)

Y93.31 Activity, mountain climbing, rock climbing and wall climbing

Y93.32 Activity, rappelling

Y93.33 Activity, BASE jumping
Activity, Building, Antenna, Span, Earth jumping

Y93.34 Activity, bungee jumping

Y93.35 Activity, hang gliding

Y93.39 Activity, other involving climbing, rappelling and jumping off

Y93.4 Activities involving dancing and other rhythmic movement
EXCLUDES 1 *activity, martial arts (Y93.75)*

Y93.41 Activity, dancing
AHA: 2012,4Q,108

Y93.42 Activity, yoga

Y93.43 Activity, gymnastics
Activity, rhythmic gymnastics
EXCLUDES 1 *activity, trampolining (Y93.44)*

Y93.44 Activity, trampolining

Y93.45 Activity, cheerleading

Y93.49 Activity, other involving dancing and other rhythmic movements

Y93.5 Activities involving other sports and athletics played individually
EXCLUDES 1 *activity, dancing (Y93.41)*
activity, gymnastic (Y93.43)
activity, trampolining (Y93.44)
activity, yoga (Y93.42)

Y93.51 Activity, roller skating (inline) and skateboarding

Y93.52 Activity, horseback riding

Y93.53 Activity, golf

Y93.54 Activity, bowling

Y93.55 Activity, bike riding

Y93.56 Activity, jumping rope

Y93.57 Activity, non-running track and field events
EXCLUDES 1 *activity, running (any form) (Y93.Ø2)*

Y93.59 Activity, other involving other sports and athletics played individually
EXCLUDES 1 *activities involving climbing, rappelling, and jumping (Y93.3-)*
activities involving ice and snow (Y93.2-)
activities involving walking and running (Y93.Ø-)
activities involving water and watercraft (Y93.1-)

Y93.6 Activities involving other sports and athletics played as a team or group
EXCLUDES 1 *activity, ice hockey (Y93.22)*
activity, water polo (Y93.13)

Y93.61 Activity, American tackle football
Activity, football NOS

Y93.62 Activity, American flag or touch football

Y93.63 Activity, rugby

Y93.64 Activity, baseball
Activity, softball

Y93.65 Activity, lacrosse and field hockey

Y93.66 Activity, soccer

Y93.67 Activity, basketball

Y93.68 Activity, volleyball (beach) (court)

Y93.6A Activity, physical games generally associated with school recess, summer camp and children
Activity, capture the flag
Activity, dodge ball
Activity, four square
Activity, kickball

Y93.69 Activity, other involving other sports and athletics played as a team or group
Activity, cricket

Y93.7 Activities involving other specified sports and athletics

Y93.71 Activity, boxing

Y93.72 Activity, wrestling

Y93.73 Activity, racquet and hand sports
Activity, handball
Activity, racquetball
Activity, squash
Activity, tennis

Y93.74 Activity, frisbee
Activity, ultimate frisbee

Y93.75 Activity, martial arts
Activity, combatives

Y93.79 Activity, other specified sports and athletics
EXCLUDES 1 *sports and athletics activities specified in categories Y93.Ø-Y93.6*

Y93.A Activities involving other cardiorespiratory exercise
Activities involving physical training

Y93.A1 Activity, exercise machines primarily for cardiorespiratory conditioning
Activity, elliptical and stepper machines
Activity, stationary bike
Activity, treadmill

Y93.A2 Activity, calisthenics
Activity, jumping jacks
Activity, warm up and cool down

Y93.A3 Activity, aerobic and step exercise

Y93.A4 Activity, circuit training

Y93.A5 Activity, obstacle course
Activity, challenge course
Activity, confidence course

Y93.A6 Activity, grass drills
Activity, guerilla drills

Y93.A9 Activity, other involving cardiorespiratory exercise
EXCLUDES 1 *activities involving cardiorespiratory exercise specified in categories Y93.Ø-Y93.7*

Y93.B Activities involving other muscle strengthening exercises

Y93.B1 Activity, exercise machines primarily for muscle strengthening

Y93.B2 Activity, push-ups, pull-ups, sit-ups

Y93.B3 Activity, free weights
Activity, barbells
Activity, dumbbells

Y93.B4 Activity, pilates

Y93.B9 Activity, other involving muscle strengthening exercises
EXCLUDES 1 *activities involving muscle strengthening specified in categories Y93.Ø-Y93.A*

Y93.C Activities involving computer technology and electronic devices
EXCLUDES 1 *activity, electronic musical keyboard or instruments (Y93.J-)*

Y93.C1 Activity, computer keyboarding
Activity, electronic game playing using keyboard or other stationary device

Y93.C2 Activity, hand held interactive electronic device
Activity, cellular telephone and communication device
Activity, electronic game playing using interactive device
EXCLUDES 1 *activity, electronic game playing using keyboard or other stationary device (Y93.C1)*

Y93.C9 Activity, other involving computer technology and electronic devices

Y93.D Activities involving arts and handcrafts
EXCLUDES 1 *activities involving playing musical instrument (Y93.J-)*

Y93.D1 Activity, knitting and crocheting

Y93.D2 **Activity, sewing**

Y93.D3 **Activity, furniture building and finishing**
Activity, furniture repair

Y93.D9 **Activity, other involving arts and handcrafts**

✓5th **Y93.E** **Activities involving personal hygiene and interior property and clothing maintenance**
EXCLUDES 1 *activities involving cooking and grilling (Y93.G-)*
activities involving exterior property and land maintenance, building and construction (Y93.H-)
activities involving caregiving (Y93.F-)
activity, dishwashing (Y93.G1)
activity, food preparation (Y93.G1)
activity, gardening (Y93.H2)

Y93.E1 **Activity, personal bathing and showering**

Y93.E2 **Activity, laundry**

Y93.E3 **Activity, vacuuming**

Y93.E4 **Activity, ironing**

Y93.E5 **Activity, floor mopping and cleaning**

Y93.E6 **Activity, residential relocation**
Activity, packing up and unpacking involved in moving to a new residence

Y93.E8 **Activity, other personal hygiene**

Y93.E9 **Activity, other interior property and clothing maintenance**

✓5th **Y93.F** **Activities involving caregiving**
Activity involving the provider of caregiving

Y93.F1 **Activity, caregiving, bathing**

Y93.F2 **Activity, caregiving, lifting**

Y93.F9 **Activity, other caregiving**

✓5th **Y93.G** **Activities involving food preparation, cooking and grilling**

Y93.G1 **Activity, food preparation and clean up**
Activity, dishwashing

Y93.G2 **Activity, grilling and smoking food**

Y93.G3 **Activity, cooking and baking**
Activity, use of stove, oven and microwave oven

Y93.G9 **Activity, other involving cooking and grilling**

✓5th **Y93.H** **Activities involving exterior property and land maintenance, building and construction**

Y93.H1 **Activity, digging, shoveling and raking**
Activity, dirt digging
Activity, raking leaves
Activity, snow shoveling

Y93.H2 **Activity, gardening and landscaping**
Activity, pruning, trimming shrubs, weeding

Y93.H3 **Activity, building and construction**

Y93.H9 **Activity, other involving exterior property and land maintenance, building and construction**

✓5th **Y93.I** **Activities involving roller coasters and other types of external motion**

Y93.I1 **Activity, rollercoaster riding**

Y93.I9 **Activity, other involving external motion**

✓5th **Y93.J** **Activities involving playing musical instrument**
Activity involving playing electric musical instrument

Y93.J1 **Activity, piano playing**
Activity, musical keyboard (electronic) playing

Y93.J2 **Activity, drum and other percussion instrument playing**

Y93.J3 **Activity, string instrument playing**

Y93.J4 **Activity, winds and brass instrument playing**

✓5th **Y93.K** **Activities involving animal care**
EXCLUDES 1 *activity, horseback riding (Y93.52)*

Y93.K1 **Activity, walking an animal**

Y93.K2 **Activity, milking an animal**

Y93.K3 **Activity, grooming and shearing an animal**

Y93.K9 **Activity, other involving animal care**

✓5th **Y93.8** **Activities, other specified**

Y93.81 **Activity, refereeing a sports activity**

Y93.82 **Activity, spectator at an event**

Y93.83 **Activity, rough housing and horseplay**

Y93.84 **Activity, sleeping**

Y93.85 **Activity, choking game**
Activity, blackout game
Activity, fainting game
Activity, pass out game
AHA: 2016,4Q,74-76

Y93.89 **Activity, other specified**

Y93.9 **Activity, unspecified**

Y95 **Nosocomial condition**
AHA: 2013,4Q,119

✓4th **Y99** **External cause status**
NOTE A single code from category Y99 should be used in conjunction with the external cause code(s) assigned to a record to indicate the status of the person at the time the event occurred.

Y99.Ø **Civilian activity done for income or pay**
Civilian activity done for financial or other compensation
EXCLUDES 1 *military activity (Y99.1)*
volunteer activity (Y99.2)

Y99.1 **Military activity**
EXCLUDES 1 *activity of off duty military personnel (Y99.8)*

Y99.2 **Volunteer activity**
EXCLUDES 1 *activity of child or other family member assisting in compensated work of other family member (Y99.8)*

Y99.8 **Other external cause status**
Activity NEC
Activity of child or other family member assisting in compensated work of other family member
Hobby not done for income
Leisure activity
Off-duty activity of military personnel
Recreation or sport not for income or while a student
Student activity
EXCLUDES 1 *civilian activity done for income or compensation (Y99.Ø)*
military activity (Y99.1)
AHA: 2012,4Q,108

Y99.9 **Unspecified external cause status**

Chapter 21. Factors Influencing Health Status and Contact with Health Services (Z00–Z99)

Chapter-specific Guidelines with Coding Examples

The chapter-specific guidelines from the ICD-10-CM Official Guidelines for Coding and Reporting have been provided below. Along with these guidelines are coding examples, contained in the shaded boxes, that have been developed to help illustrate the coding and/or sequencing guidance found in these guidelines.

Note: The chapter-specific guidelines provide additional information about the use of Z codes for specified encounters.

a. Use of Z Codes in any healthcare setting

Z codes are for use in any healthcare setting. Z codes may be used as either a first-listed (principal diagnosis code in the inpatient setting) or secondary code, depending on the circumstances of the encounter. Certain Z codes may only be used as first-listed or principal diagnosis.

> Patient with middle lobe lung cancer admitted for initiation of chemotherapy
>
> **Z51.11 Encounter for antineoplastic chemotherapy**
>
> **C34.2 Malignant neoplasm of middle lobe, bronchus or lung**
>
> *Explanation:* A Z code can be used as first-listed in this situation based on guidelines in this chapter as well as chapter 2, "Neoplasms."

b. Z Codes indicate a reason for an encounter

Z codes are not procedure codes. A corresponding procedure code must accompany a Z code to describe any procedure performed.

c. Categories of Z Codes

1) Contact/exposure

Category Z20 indicates contact with, and suspected exposure to, communicable diseases. These codes are for patients who are suspected to have been exposed to **a disease** by close personal contact with an infected individual or are in an area where a disease is epidemic.

Category Z77, Other contact with and (suspected) exposures hazardous to health, indicates contact with and suspected exposures hazardous to health.

Contact/exposure codes may be used as a first-listed code to explain an encounter for testing, or, more commonly, as a secondary code to identify a potential risk.

2) Inoculations and vaccinations

Code Z23 is for encounters for inoculations and vaccinations. It indicates that a patient is being seen to receive a prophylactic inoculation against a disease. Procedure codes are required to identify the actual administration of the injection and the type(s) of immunizations given. Code Z23 may be used as a secondary code if the inoculation is given as a routine part of preventive health care, such as a well-baby visit.

3) Status

Status codes indicate that a patient is either a carrier of a disease or has the sequelae or residual of a past disease or condition. This includes such things as the presence of prosthetic or mechanical devices resulting from past treatment. A status code is informative, because the status may affect the course of treatment and its outcome. A status code is distinct from a history code. The history code indicates that the patient no longer has the condition.

A status code should not be used with a diagnosis code from one of the body system chapters, if the diagnosis code includes the information provided by the status code. For example, code Z94.1, Heart transplant status, should not be used with a code from subcategory T86.2, Complications of heart transplant. The status code does not provide additional information. The complication code indicates that the patient is a heart transplant patient.

For encounters for weaning from a mechanical ventilator, assign a code from subcategory J96.1, Chronic respiratory failure, followed by code Z99.11, Dependence on respirator [ventilator] status.

The status Z codes/categories are:

Z14 Genetic carrier

Genetic carrier status indicates that a person carries a gene, associated with a particular disease, which may be passed to offspring who may develop that disease. The person does not have the disease and is not at risk of developing the disease.

Z15 Genetic susceptibility to disease

Genetic susceptibility indicates that a person has a gene that increases the risk of that person developing the disease.

Codes from category Z15 should not be used as principal or first-listed codes. If the patient has the condition to which he/she is susceptible, and that condition is the reason for the current encounter, the code for the current condition should be sequenced first. If the patient is being seen for follow-up after completed treatment for this condition, and the condition no longer exists, a follow-up code should be sequenced first, followed by the appropriate personal history and genetic susceptibility codes. If the purpose of the encounter is genetic counseling associated with procreative management, code Z31.5, Encounter for genetic counseling, should be assigned as the first-listed code, followed by a code from category Z15. Additional codes should be assigned for any applicable family or personal history.

Z16 Resistance to antimicrobial drugs

This code indicates that a patient has a condition that is resistant to antimicrobial drug treatment. Sequence the infection code first.

> Penicillin resistant streptococcus pneumoniae meningitis
>
> **G00.1 Pneumococcal meningitis**
>
> **Z16.11 Resistance to penicillins**
>
> *Explanation:* The status Z code is used to describe the presence of a drug-resistant organism that most likely altered how the meningitis was treated.

Z17 Estrogen receptor status

Z18 Retained foreign body fragments

Z19 Hormone sensitivity malignancy status

Z21 Asymptomatic HIV infection status

This code indicates that a patient has tested positive for HIV but has manifested no signs or symptoms of the disease.

Z22 Carrier of infectious disease

Carrier status indicates that a person harbors the specific organisms of a disease without manifest symptoms and is capable of transmitting the infection.

Z28.3 Underimmunization status

Z33.1 Pregnant state, incidental

This code is a secondary code only for use when the pregnancy is in no way complicating the reason for visit. Otherwise, a code from the obstetric chapter is required.

Z66 Do not resuscitate

This code may be used when it is documented by the provider that a patient is on do not resuscitate status at any time during the stay.

Z67 Blood type

Z68 Body mass index (BMI)

BMI codes should only be assigned when there is an associated, reportable diagnosis (such as obesity). Do not assign BMI codes during pregnancy.

See Section I.B.14 for BMI documentation by clinicians other than the patient's provider.

Z74.01 Bed confinement status

Z76.82 Awaiting organ transplant status

Z78 Other specified health status

Code Z78.1, Physical restraint status, may be used when it is documented by the provider that a patient has been put in restraints during the current encounter. Please note that this code should not be reported when it is documented by the provider that a patient is temporarily restrained during a procedure.

Z79 Long-term (current) drug therapy

Codes from this category indicate a patient's continuous use of a prescribed drug (including such things as aspirin therapy) for the long-term treatment of a condition or for prophylactic use. It is not for use for patients who have addictions to drugs. This subcategory is not for use of medications for detoxification or maintenance programs to prevent withdrawal symptoms (e.g., methadone maintenance for opiate dependence). Assign the appropriate code for the drug **use, abuse, or** dependence instead.

Assign a code from Z79 if the patient is receiving a medication for an extended period as a prophylactic measure (such as for the prevention of deep vein thrombosis) or as treatment of a chronic condition (such as arthritis) or a disease requiring a lengthy course of treatment (such as cancer). Do not assign a code from category Z79 for medication being administered for a brief period of time to treat an acute illness or injury (such as a course of antibiotics to treat acute bronchitis).

Z88 Allergy status to drugs, medicaments and biological substances

Except: Z88.9, Allergy status to unspecified drugs, medicaments and biological substances status

Z89 Acquired absence of limb

Z9Ø Acquired absence of organs, not elsewhere classified

Z91.Ø- Allergy status, other than to drugs and biological substances

Z92.82 Status post administration of tPA (rtPA) in a different facility within the last 24 hours prior to admission to a current facility

Assign code Z92.82, Status post administration of tPA (rtPA) in a different facility within the last 24 hours prior to admission to current facility, as a secondary diagnosis when a patient is received by transfer into a facility and documentation indicates they were administered tissue plasminogen activator (tPA) within the last 24 hours prior to admission to the current facility.

This guideline applies even if the patient is still receiving the tPA at the time they are received into the current facility.

The appropriate code for the condition for which the tPA was administered (such as cerebrovascular disease or myocardial infarction) should be assigned first.

Code Z92.82 is only applicable to the receiving facility record and not to the transferring facility record.

Z93 Artificial opening status

Z94 Transplanted organ and tissue status

Z95 Presence of cardiac and vascular implants and grafts

Z96 Presence of other functional implants

Z97 Presence of other devices

Z98 Other postprocedural states

Assign code Z98.85, Transplanted organ removal status, to indicate that a transplanted organ has been previously removed. This code should not be assigned for the encounter in which the transplanted organ is removed. The complication necessitating removal of the transplant organ should be assigned for that encounter.

See section I.C19. for information on the coding of organ transplant complications.

Z99 Dependence on enabling machines and devices, not elsewhere classified

Note: Categories Z89-Z9Ø and Z93-Z99 are for use only if there are no complications or malfunctions of the organ or tissue replaced, the amputation site or the equipment on which the patient is dependent.

4) History (of)

There are two types of history Z codes, personal and family. Personal history codes explain a patient's past medical condition that no longer exists and is not receiving any treatment, but that has the potential for recurrence, and therefore may require continued monitoring.

Family history codes are for use when a patient has a family member(s) who has had a particular disease that causes the patient to be at higher risk of also contracting the disease.

Personal history codes may be used in conjunction with follow-up codes and family history codes may be used in conjunction with screening codes to explain the need for a test or procedure. History codes are also acceptable on any medical record regardless of the reason for visit. A history of an illness, even if no longer present, is important information that may alter the type of treatment ordered.

The history Z code categories are:

Z8Ø Family history of primary malignant neoplasm

Z81 Family history of mental and behavioral disorders

Z82 Family history of certain disabilities and chronic diseases (leading to disablement)

Z83 Family history of other specific disorders

Z84 Family history of other conditions

Z85 Personal history of malignant neoplasm

Z86 Personal history of certain other diseases

Z87 Personal history of other diseases and conditions

Z91.4- Personal history of psychological trauma, not elsewhere classified

Z91.5 Personal history of self-harm

Z91.81 History of falling

Z91.82 Personal history of military deployment

Z92 Personal history of medical treatment

Except: Z92.Ø, Personal history of contraception

Except: Z92.82, Status post administration of tPA (rtPA) in a different facility within the last 24 hours prior to admission to a current facility

Patient has chronic lymphocytic leukemia for which the patient had previous chemotherapy and is now in remission

C91.11 Chronic lymphocytic leukemia of B-cell type in remission

Z92.21 Personal history of antineoplastic chemotherapy

Explanation: The personal history Z code is used to describe a secondary (supplementary) diagnosis to identify that this patient has had chemotherapy in the past.

5) Screening

Screening is the testing for disease or disease precursors in seemingly well individuals so that early detection and treatment can be provided for those who test positive for the disease (e.g., screening mammogram).

The testing of a person to rule out or confirm a suspected diagnosis because the patient has some sign or symptom is a diagnostic examination, not a screening. In these cases, the sign or symptom is used to explain the reason for the test.

A screening code may be a first-listed code if the reason for the visit is specifically the screening exam. It may also be used as an additional code if the screening is done during an office visit for other health problems. A screening code is not necessary if the screening is inherent to a routine examination, such as a pap smear done during a routine pelvic examination.

Should a condition be discovered during the screening then the code for the condition may be assigned as an additional diagnosis.

The Z code indicates that a screening exam is planned. A procedure code is required to confirm that the screening was performed.

The screening Z codes/categories:

Z11 Encounter for screening for infectious and parasitic diseases

Z12 Encounter for screening for malignant neoplasms

Z13 Encounter for screening for other diseases and disorders

Except: Z13.9, Encounter for screening, unspecified

Z36 Encounter for antenatal screening for mother

6) Observation

There are three observation Z code categories. They are for use in very limited circumstances when a person is being observed for a suspected condition that is ruled out. The observation codes are not for use if an injury or illness or any signs or symptoms related to the suspected condition are present. In such cases the diagnosis/symptom code is used with the corresponding external cause code.

The observation codes are **primarily** to be used as a principal/**first-listed** diagnosis. **An observation code may be assigned as a secondary diagnosis code when the patient is being observed for a condition that is ruled out and is unrelated to the principal/first-listed diagnosis (e.g., patient presents for treatment following injuries sustained in a motor vehicle accident and is also observed for suspected COVID-19 infection that is subsequently ruled out). Also,** when the principal diagnosis is required to be a code from category Z38, Liveborn infants according to place of birth and type of delivery, **then** a code from category ZØ5, Encounter for observation and evaluation of newborn for suspected diseases and conditions ruled out, is sequenced after the Z38 code. Additional codes may be used in addition to the observation code, but only if they are unrelated to the suspected condition being observed.

Codes from subcategory Z03.7, Encounter for suspected maternal and fetal conditions ruled out, may either be used as a first-listed or as an additional code assignment depending on the case. They are for use in very limited circumstances on a maternal record when an encounter is for a suspected maternal or fetal condition that is ruled out during that encounter (for example, a maternal or fetal condition may be suspected due to an abnormal test result). These codes should not be used when the condition is confirmed. In those cases, the confirmed condition should be coded. In addition, these codes are not for use if an illness or any signs or symptoms related to the suspected condition or problem are present. In such cases the diagnosis/symptom code is used.

Additional codes may be used in addition to the code from subcategory Z03.7, but only if they are unrelated to the suspected condition being evaluated.

Codes from subcategory Z03.7 may not be used for encounters for antenatal screening of mother. *See Section I.C.21. Screening*.

For encounters for suspected fetal condition that are inconclusive following testing and evaluation, assign the appropriate code from category O35, O36, O40 or O41.

The observation Z code categories:

Z03	Encounter for medical observation for suspected diseases and conditions ruled out
Z04	Encounter for examination and observation for other reasons Except: Z04.9, Encounter for examination and observation for unspecified reason
Z05	Encounter for observation and evaluation of newborn for suspected diseases and conditions ruled out

Upon initial examination, a heart murmur was heard in a newborn infant delivered vaginally in the hospital; however, after further observation, any serious cardiac conditions were ruled out.

Z38.00 Single liveborn infant, delivered vaginally

Z05.0 Observation and evaluation of newborn for suspected cardiac condition ruled out

Explanation: Normally an observation code is used as the principal diagnosis except when the patient is a newborn. A code from category Z38 Liveborn infants according to place of birth and type of delivery code would be sequenced first, followed by the encounter for observation and evaluation of newborn for suspected diseases and conditions ruled out.

7) Aftercare

Aftercare visit codes cover situations when the initial treatment of a disease has been performed and the patient requires continued care during the healing or recovery phase, or for the long-term consequences of the disease. The aftercare Z code should not be used if treatment is directed at a current, acute disease. The diagnosis code is to be used in these cases. Exceptions to this rule are codes Z51.0, Encounter for antineoplastic radiation therapy, and codes from subcategory Z51.1, Encounter for antineoplastic chemotherapy and immunotherapy. These codes are to be first listed, followed by the diagnosis code when a patient's encounter is solely to receive radiation therapy, chemotherapy, or immunotherapy for the treatment of a neoplasm. If the reason for the encounter is more than one type of antineoplastic therapy, code Z51.0 and a code from subcategory Z51.1 may be assigned together, in which case one of these codes would be reported as a secondary diagnosis.

The aftercare Z codes should also not be used for aftercare for injuries. For aftercare of an injury, assign the acute injury code with the appropriate 7th character (for subsequent encounter).

The aftercare codes are generally first listed to explain the specific reason for the encounter. An aftercare code may be used as an additional code when some type of aftercare is provided in addition to the reason for admission and no diagnosis code is applicable. An example of this would be the closure of a colostomy during an encounter for treatment of another condition.

Aftercare codes should be used in conjunction with other aftercare codes or diagnosis codes to provide better detail on the specifics of an aftercare encounter visit, unless otherwise directed by the classification. The sequencing of multiple aftercare codes depends on the circumstances of the encounter.

Certain aftercare Z code categories need a secondary diagnosis code to describe the resolving condition or sequelae. For others, the condition is included in the code title.

Additional Z code aftercare category terms include fitting and adjustment, and attention to artificial openings.

Status Z codes may be used with aftercare Z codes to indicate the nature of the aftercare. For example code Z95.1, Presence of aortocoronary bypass graft, may be used with code Z48.812, Encounter for surgical aftercare following surgery on the circulatory system, to indicate the surgery for which the aftercare is being performed. A status code should not be used when the aftercare code indicates the type of status, such as using Z43.0, Encounter for attention to tracheostomy, with Z93.0, Tracheostomy status.

The aftercare Z category/codes:

Z42	Encounter for plastic and reconstructive surgery following medical procedure or healed injury
Z43	Encounter for attention to artificial openings
Z44	Encounter for fitting and adjustment of external prosthetic device
Z45	Encounter for adjustment and management of implanted device
Z46	Encounter for fitting and adjustment of other devices
Z47	Orthopedic aftercare
Z48	Encounter for other postprocedural aftercare
Z49	Encounter for care involving renal dialysis
Z51	Encounter for other aftercare and medical care

8) Follow-up

The follow-up codes are used to explain continuing surveillance following completed treatment of a disease, condition, or injury. They imply that the condition has been fully treated and no longer exists. They should not be confused with aftercare codes, or injury codes with a 7th character for subsequent encounter, that explain ongoing care of a healing condition or its sequelae. Follow-up codes may be used in conjunction with history codes to provide the full picture of the healed condition and its treatment. The follow-up code is sequenced first, followed by the history code.

A follow-up code may be used to explain multiple visits. Should a condition be found to have recurred on the follow-up visit, then the diagnosis code for the condition should be assigned in place of the follow-up code.

The follow-up Z code categories:

Z08	Encounter for follow-up examination after completed treatment for malignant neoplasm
Z09	Encounter for follow-up examination after completed treatment for conditions other than malignant neoplasm
Z39	Encounter for maternal postpartum care and examination

9) Donor

Codes in category Z52, Donors of organs and tissues, are used for living individuals who are donating blood or other body tissue. These codes are only for individuals donating for others, not for self-donations. They are not used to identify cadaveric donations.

10)Counseling

Counseling Z codes are used when a patient or family member receives assistance in the aftermath of an illness or injury, or when support is required in coping with family or social problems.

The counseling Z codes/categories:

Z30.0-	Encounter for general counseling and advice on contraception
Z31.5	Encounter for procreative genetic counseling
Z31.6-	Encounter for general counseling and advice on procreation
Z32.2	Encounter for childbirth instruction
Z32.3	Encounter for childcare instruction
Z69	Encounter for mental health services for victim and perpetrator of abuse
Z70	Counseling related to sexual attitude, behavior and orientation
Z71	Persons encountering health services for other counseling and medical advice, not elsewhere classified **Note:** Code Z71.84, Encounter for health counseling related to travel, is to be used for health risk and safety counseling for future travel purposes.
Z76.81	Expectant mother prebirth pediatrician visit

11)Encounters for obstetrical and reproductive services

See Section I.C.15. Pregnancy, Childbirth, and the Puerperium, for further instruction on the use of these codes.

Z codes for pregnancy are for use in those circumstances when none of the problems or complications included in the codes from the Obstetrics chapter exist (a routine prenatal visit or postpartum care). Codes in category Z34, Encounter for supervision of normal pregnancy, are always first listed and are not to be used with any other code from the OB chapter.

Codes in category Z3A, Weeks of gestation, may be assigned to provide additional information about the pregnancy. Category Z3A codes should not be assigned for pregnancies with abortive outcomes (categories O00-O08), elective termination of pregnancy (code Z33.2), nor for postpartum conditions, as category Z3A is not applicable to these conditions. The date of the admission should be used to determine weeks of gestation for inpatient admissions that encompass more than one gestational week.

The outcome of delivery, category Z37, should be included on all maternal delivery records. It is always a secondary code. Codes in category Z37 should not be used on the newborn record.

Z codes for family planning (contraceptive) or procreative management and counseling should be included on an obstetric record either during the pregnancy or the postpartum stage, if applicable.

Z codes/categories for obstetrical and reproductive services:

Z30	Encounter for contraceptive management
Z31	Encounter for procreative management
Z32.2	Encounter for childbirth instruction
Z32.3	Encounter for childcare instruction
Z33	Pregnant state
Z34	Encounter for supervision of normal pregnancy
Z36	Encounter for antenatal screening of mother
Z3A	Weeks of gestation
Z37	Outcome of delivery
Z39	Encounter for maternal postpartum care and examination
Z76.81	Expectant mother prebirth pediatrician visit

12) Newborns and infants

See Section I.C.16. Newborn (Perinatal) Guidelines, for further instruction on the use of these codes.

Newborn Z codes/categories:

Z76.1	Encounter for health supervision and care of foundling
Z00.1-	Encounter for routine child health examination
Z38	Liveborn infants according to place of birth and type of delivery

13) Routine and administrative examinations

The Z codes allow for the description of encounters for routine examinations, such as, a general check-up, or, examinations for administrative purposes, such as, a pre-employment physical. The codes are not to be used if the examination is for diagnosis of a suspected condition or for treatment purposes. In such cases the diagnosis code is used. During a routine exam, should a diagnosis or condition be discovered, it should be coded as an additional code. Pre-existing and chronic conditions and history codes may also be included as additional codes as long as the examination is for administrative purposes and not focused on any particular condition.

Some of the codes for routine health examinations distinguish between "with" and "without" abnormal findings. Code assignment depends on the information that is known at the time the encounter is being coded. For example, if no abnormal findings were found during the examination, but the encounter is being coded before test results are back, it is acceptable to assign the code for "without abnormal findings." When assigning a code for "with abnormal findings," additional code(s) should be assigned to identify the specific abnormal finding(s).

Pre-operative examination and pre-procedural laboratory examination Z codes are for use only in those situations when a patient is being cleared for a procedure or surgery and no treatment is given.

The Z codes/categories for routine and administrative examinations:

Z00	Encounter for general examination without complaint, suspected or reported diagnosis
Z01	Encounter for other special examination without complaint, suspected or reported diagnosis
Z02	Encounter for administrative examination Except: Z02.9, Encounter for administrative examinations, unspecified
Z32.0-	Encounter for pregnancy test

14) Miscellaneous Z codes

The miscellaneous Z codes capture a number of other health care encounters that do not fall into one of the other categories. Certain of these codes identify the reason for the encounter; others are for use as additional codes that provide useful information on circumstances that may affect a patient's care and treatment.

Prophylactic organ removal

For encounters specifically for prophylactic removal of an organ (such as prophylactic removal of breasts due to a genetic susceptibility to cancer or a family history of cancer), the principal or first-listed code should be a code from category Z40, Encounter for prophylactic surgery, followed by the appropriate codes to identify the associated risk factor (such as genetic susceptibility or family history).

If the patient has a malignancy of one site and is having prophylactic removal at another site to prevent either a new primary malignancy or metastatic disease, a code for the malignancy should also be assigned in addition to a code from subcategory Z40.0, Encounter for prophylactic surgery for risk factors related to malignant neoplasms. A Z40.0 code should not be assigned if the patient is having organ removal for treatment of a malignancy, such as the removal of the testes for the treatment of prostate cancer.

Female patient with cancer in lower inner quadrant of right breast and positive BRCA 1 noted on testing is admitted for mastectomy of right breast and prophylactic removal of left breast

C50.311	**Malignant neoplasm of lower-inner quadrant of right female breast**
Z40.01	**Encounter for prophylactic removal of breast**
Z15.01	**Genetic susceptibility to malignant neoplasm of breast**

Explanation: Removal of the current neoplastic disease in the right breast was the focus of treatment for this admission and is sequenced first. The removal of the left breast was not required to treat a current disease process but as a means of prevention. The two Z codes are informational; they capture the reason behind the removal of what is currently a healthy left breast.

Miscellaneous Z codes/categories:

Z28	Immunization not carried out Except: Z28.3, Underimmunization status
Z29	Encounter for other prophylactic measures
Z40	Encounter for prophylactic surgery
Z41	Encounter for procedures for purposes other than remedying health state Except: Z41.9, Encounter for procedure for purposes other than remedying health state, unspecified
Z53	Persons encountering health services for specific procedures and treatment, not carried out
Z55	Problems related to education and literacy
Z56	Problems related to employment and unemployment
Z57	Occupational exposure to risk factors
Z58	Problems related to physical environment
Z59	Problems related to housing and economic circumstances
Z60	Problems related to social environment
Z62	Problems related to upbringing
Z63	Other problems related to primary support group, including family circumstances
Z64	Problems related to certain psychosocial circumstances
Z65	Problems related to other psychosocial circumstances
Z72	Problems related to lifestyle **Note:** These codes should be assigned only when the documentation specifies that the patient has an associated problem
Z73	Problems related to life management difficulty
Z74	Problems related to care provider dependency Except: Z74.01, Bed confinement status
Z75	Problems related to medical facilities and other health care
Z76.0	Encounter for issue of repeat prescription
Z76.3	Healthy person accompanying sick person
Z76.4	Other boarder to healthcare facility
Z76.5	Malingerer [conscious simulation]
Z91.1-	Patient's noncompliance with medical treatment and regimen
Z91.83	Wandering in diseases classified elsewhere
Z91.84-	Oral health risk factors
Z91.89	Other specified personal risk factors, not elsewhere classified

See Section I.B.14 for Z55-Z65 Persons with potential health hazards related to socioeconomic and psychosocial circumstances, documentation by clinicians other than the patient's provider

15) Nonspecific Z codes

Certain Z codes are so non-specific, or potentially redundant with other codes in the classification, that there can be little justification for their use in the inpatient setting. Their use in the outpatient setting should be limited to those instances when there is no further documentation to permit more precise coding. Otherwise, any sign or symptom or any other reason for visit that is captured in another code should be used.

Nonspecific Z codes/categories:

Z02.9	Encounter for administrative examinations, unspecified
Z04.9	Encounter for examination and observation for unspecified reason
Z13.9	Encounter for screening, unspecified
Z41.9	Encounter for procedure for purposes other than remedying health state, unspecified
Z52.9	Donor of unspecified organ or tissue
Z86.59	Personal history of other mental and behavioral disorders
Z88.9	Allergy status to unspecified drugs, medicaments and biological substances status
Z92.0	Personal history of contraception

16) Z codes that may only be principal/first-listed diagnosis

The following Z codes/categories may only be reported as the principal/first-listed diagnosis, except when there are multiple encounters on the same day and the medical records for the encounters are combined:

Z00	Encounter for general examination without complaint, suspected or reported diagnosis Except: Z00.6
Z01	Encounter for other special examination without complaint, suspected or reported diagnosis
Z02	Encounter for administrative examination
Z04	Encounter for examination and observation for other reasons
Z33.2	Encounter for elective termination of pregnancy
Z31.81	Encounter for male factor infertility in female patient
Z31.83	Encounter for assisted reproductive fertility procedure cycle
Z31.84	Encounter for fertility preservation procedure
Z34	Encounter for supervision of normal pregnancy
Z39	Encounter for maternal postpartum care and examination
Z38	Liveborn infants according to place of birth and type of delivery
Z40	Encounter for prophylactic surgery
Z42	Encounter for plastic and reconstructive surgery following medical procedure or healed injury
Z51.0	Encounter for antineoplastic radiation therapy
Z51.1-	Encounter for antineoplastic chemotherapy and immunotherapy
Z52	Donors of organs and tissues Except: Z52.9, Donor of unspecified organ or tissue
Z76.1	Encounter for health supervision and care of foundling
Z76.2	Encounter for health supervision and care of other healthy infant and child
Z99.12	Encounter for respirator [ventilator] dependence during power failure

Chapter 21. Factors Influencing Health Status and Contact With Health Services (Z00-Z99)

NOTE Z codes represent reasons for encounters. A corresponding procedure code must accompany a Z code if a procedure is performed. Categories Z00-Z99 are provided for occasions when circumstances other than a disease, injury or external cause classifiable to categories A00-Y89 are recorded as "diagnoses" or "problems." This can arise in two main ways:

(a) When a person who may or may not be sick encounters the health services for some specific purpose, such as to receive limited care or service for a current condition, to donate an organ or tissue, to receive prophylactic vaccination (immunization), or to discuss a problem which is in itself not a disease or injury.

(b) When some circumstance or problem is present which influences the person's health status but is not in itself a current illness or injury.

AHA: 2018,4Q,60-61

This chapter contains the following blocks:

Z00-Z13	Persons encountering health services for examinations
Z14-Z15	Genetic carrier and genetic susceptibility to disease
Z16	Resistance to antimicrobial drugs
Z17	Estrogen receptor status
Z18	Retained foreign body fragments
Z19	Hormone sensitivity malignancy status
Z20-Z29	Persons with potential health hazards related to communicable diseases
Z30-Z39	Persons encountering health services in circumstances related to reproduction
Z40-Z53	Encounters for other specific health care
Z55-Z65	Persons with potential health hazards related to socioeconomic and psychosocial circumstances
Z66	Do not resuscitate status
Z67	Blood type
Z68	Body mass index (BMI)
Z69-Z76	Persons encountering health services in other circumstances
Z77-Z99	Persons with potential health hazards related to family and personal history and certain conditions influencing health status

Persons encountering health services for examinations (Z00-Z13)

NOTE Nonspecific abnormal findings disclosed at the time of these examinations are classified to categories R70-R94.

EXCLUDES 1 *examinations related to pregnancy and reproduction (Z30-Z36, Z39.-)*

√4th **Z00 Encounter for general examination without complaint, suspected or reported diagnosis**

EXCLUDES 1 *encounter for examination for administrative purposes (Z02.-)*

EXCLUDES 2 *encounter for pre-procedural examinations (Z01.81-)*
special screening examinations (Z11-Z13)

AHA: 2017,4Q,95

√5th **Z00.0 Encounter for general adult medical examination**

Encounter for adult periodic examination (annual) (physical) and any associated laboratory and radiologic examinations

EXCLUDES 1 *encounter for examination of sign or symptom — code to sign or symptom*
general health check-up of infant or child (Z00.12.-)

Z00.00 Encounter for general adult medical examination without abnormal findings A

Encounter for adult health check-up NOS

AHA: 2016,1Q,36

Z00.01 Encounter for general adult medical examination with abnormal findings A

Use additional code to identify abnormal findings

AHA: 2016,1Q,35-36

√5th **Z00.1 Encounter for newborn, infant and child health examinations**

√6th **Z00.11 Newborn health examination**

Health check for child under 29 days old

Use additional code to identify any abnormal findings

EXCLUDES 1 *health check for child over 28 days old (Z00.12-)*

Z00.110 Health examination for newborn under 8 days old N

Health check for newborn under 8 days old

Z00.111 Health examination for newborn 8 to 28 days old N

Health check for newborn 8 to 28 days old

Newborn weight check

√6th **Z00.12 Encounter for routine child health examination**

Health check (routine) for child over 28 days old

Immunizations appropriate for age

Routine developmental screening of infant or child

Routine vison and hearing testing

EXCLUDES 1 *health check for child under 29 days old (Z00.11-)*
health supervision of foundling or other healthy infant or child (Z76.1-Z76.2)
newborn health examination (Z00.11-)

AHA: 2018,4Q,36

Z00.121 Encounter for routine child health examination with abnormal findings P

Use additional code to identify abnormal findings

AHA: 2016,1Q,34-35

Z00.129 Encounter for routine child health examination without abnormal findings P

Encounter for routine child health examination NOS

AHA: 2016,1Q,34

Z00.2 Encounter for examination for period of rapid growth in childhood P

Z00.3 Encounter for examination for adolescent development state P

Encounter for puberty development state

Z00.5 Encounter for examination of potential donor of organ and tissue

Z00.6 Encounter for examination for normal comparison and control in clinical research program

Examination of participant or control in clinical research program

√5th **Z00.7 Encounter for examination for period of delayed growth in childhood**

Z00.70 Encounter for examination for period of delayed growth in childhood without abnormal findings P

Z00.71 Encounter for examination for period of delayed growth in childhood with abnormal findings P

Use additional code to identify abnormal findings

Z00.8 Encounter for other general examination

Encounter for health examination in population surveys

√4th **Z01 Encounter for other special examination without complaint, suspected or reported diagnosis**

INCLUDES routine examination of specific system

NOTE Codes from category Z01 represent the reason for the encounter. A separate procedure code is required to identify any examinations or procedures performed

EXCLUDES 1 *encounter for examination for administrative purposes (Z02.-)*
encounter for examination for suspected conditions, proven not to exist (Z03.-)
encounter for laboratory and radiologic examinations as a component of general medical examinations (Z00.0-)
encounter for laboratory, radiologic and imaging examinations for sign(s) and symptom(s) — code to the sign(s) or symptom(s)

EXCLUDES 2 *screening examinations (Z11-Z13)*

√5th **Z01.0 Encounter for examination of eyes and vision**

EXCLUDES 1 *examination for driving license (Z02.4)*

Z01.00 Encounter for examination of eyes and vision without abnormal findings

Encounter for examination of eyes and vision NOS

Z01.01 Encounter for examination of eyes and vision with abnormal findings

Use additional code to identify abnormal findings

AHA: 2016,4Q,21

Z01.02 Encounter for examination of eyes and vision following failed vision screening

EXCLUDES 1 *examination for examination of eyes and vision with abnormal findings (Z01.01)*
examination for examination of eyes and vision without abnormal findings (Z01.00)

AHA: 2019,4Q,20

Z01.020 Encounter for examination of eyes and vision following failed vision screening without abnormal findings

Z01.021 Encounter for examination of eyes and vision following failed vision screening with abnormal findings
Use additional code to identify abnormal findings

Z01.1 Encounter for examination of ears and hearing

Z01.10 Encounter for examination of ears and hearing without abnormal findings
Encounter for examination of ears and hearing NOS
AHA: 2016,4Q,24

Z01.11 Encounter for examination of ears and hearing with abnormal findings
AHA: 2016,3Q,17-18

Z01.110 Encounter for hearing examination following failed hearing screening

Z01.118 Encounter for examination of ears and hearing with other abnormal findings
Use additional code to identify abnormal findings

Z01.12 Encounter for hearing conservation and treatment

Z01.2 Encounter for dental examination and cleaning

Z01.20 Encounter for dental examination and cleaning without abnormal findings
Encounter for dental examination and cleaning NOS

Z01.21 Encounter for dental examination and cleaning with abnormal findings
Use additional code to identify abnormal findings

Z01.3 Encounter for examination of blood pressure

Z01.30 Encounter for examination of blood pressure without abnormal findings
Encounter for examination of blood pressure NOS

Z01.31 Encounter for examination of blood pressure with abnormal findings
Use additional code to identify abnormal findings

Z01.4 Encounter for gynecological examination

EXCLUDES 2 *pregnancy examination or test (Z32.0-)*
routine examination for contraceptive maintenance (Z30.4-)

Z01.41 Encounter for routine gynecological examination
Encounter for general gynecological examination with or without cervical smear
Encounter for gynecological examination (general) (routine) NOS
Encounter for pelvic examination (annual) (periodic)
Use additional code:
for screening for human papillomavirus, if applicable, (Z11.51)
for screening vaginal pap smear, if applicable (Z12.72)
to identify acquired absence of uterus, if applicable (Z90.71-)

EXCLUDES 1 *gynecologic examination status-post hysterectomy for malignant condition (Z08)*
screening cervical pap smear not a part of a routine gynecological examination (Z12.4)

Z01.411 Encounter for gynecological examination (general) (routine) with abnormal findings ♀
Use additional code to identify abnormal findings

Z01.419 Encounter for gynecological examination (general) (routine) without abnormal findings ♀

Z01.42 Encounter for cervical smear to confirm findings of recent normal smear following initial abnormal smear ♀

Z01.8 Encounter for other specified special examinations

Z01.81 Encounter for preprocedural examinations
Encounter for preoperative examinations
Encounter for radiological and imaging examinations as part of preprocedural examination

Z01.810 Encounter for preprocedural cardiovascular examination

Z01.811 Encounter for preprocedural respiratory examination

Z01.812 Encounter for preprocedural laboratory examination
Blood and urine tests prior to treatment or procedure

Z01.818 Encounter for other preprocedural examination
Encounter for preprocedural examination NOS
Encounter for examinations prior to antineoplastic chemotherapy

Z01.82 Encounter for allergy testing
EXCLUDES 1 *encounter for antibody response examination (Z01.84)*

Z01.83 Encounter for blood typing
Encounter for Rh typing

Z01.84 Encounter for antibody response examination
Encounter for immunity status testing
EXCLUDES 1 *encounter for allergy testing (Z01.82)*
AHA: 2020,2Q,11

Z01.89 Encounter for other specified special examinations

Z02 Encounter for administrative examination

Z02.0 Encounter for examination for admission to educational institution
Encounter for examination for admission to preschool (education)
Encounter for examination for re-admission to school following illness or medical treatment

Z02.1 Encounter for pre-employment examination

Z02.2 Encounter for examination for admission to residential institution
EXCLUDES 1 *examination for admission to prison (Z02.89)*

Z02.3 Encounter for examination for recruitment to armed forces

Z02.4 Encounter for examination for driving license

Z02.5 Encounter for examination for participation in sport
EXCLUDES 1 *blood-alcohol and blood-drug test (Z02.83)*

Z02.6 Encounter for examination for insurance purposes

Z02.7 Encounter for issue of medical certificate
EXCLUDES 1 *encounter for general medical examination (Z00-Z01, Z02.0-Z02.6, Z02.8-Z02.9)*

Z02.71 Encounter for disability determination
Encounter for issue of medical certificate of incapacity
Encounter for issue of medical certificate of invalidity

Z02.79 Encounter for issue of other medical certificate

Z02.8 Encounter for other administrative examinations

Z02.81 Encounter for paternity testing

Z02.82 Encounter for adoption services

Z02.83 Encounter for blood-alcohol and blood-drug test
Use additional code for findings of alcohol or drugs in blood (R78.-)

Z02.89 Encounter for other administrative examinations
Encounter for examination for admission to prison
Encounter for examination for admission to summer camp
Encounter for immigration examination
Encounter for naturalization examination
Encounter for premarital examination
EXCLUDES 1 *health supervision of foundling or other healthy infant or child (Z76.1-Z76.2)*

Z02.9 Encounter for administrative examinations, unspecified

Additional Character Required | Placeholder | Unacceptable PDx | Questionable PDx | Manifestation | Unspecified Dx | H1-H14 HAC | HCC CMS-HCC Dx | HIV HIV Dx

Z03 Encounter for medical observation for suspected diseases and conditions ruled out

This category is to be used when a person without a diagnosis is suspected of having an abnormal condition, without signs or symptoms, which requires study, but after examination and observation, is ruled out. This category is also for use for administrative and legal observation status.

EXCLUDES 1 *contact with and (suspected) exposures hazardous to health (Z77.-)*
encounter for observation and evaluation of newborn for suspected diseases and conditions ruled out (Z05.-)
person with feared complaint in whom no diagnosis is made (Z71.1)
signs or symptoms under study — code to signs or symptoms

AHA: 2020,2Q,8; 2018,2Q,7-8; 2017,4Q,27

Z03.6 Encounter for observation for suspected toxic effect from ingested substance ruled out
Encounter for observation for suspected adverse effect from drug
Encounter for observation for suspected poisoning

Z03.7 Encounter for suspected maternal and fetal conditions ruled out
Encounter for suspected maternal and fetal conditions not found

EXCLUDES 1 *known or suspected fetal anomalies affecting management of mother, not ruled out (O26.-, O35.-, O36.-, O40.-, O41.-)*

Z03.71 Encounter for suspected problem with amniotic cavity and membrane ruled out M ♀
Encounter for suspected oligohydramnios ruled out
Encounter for suspected polyhydramnios ruled out

Z03.72 Encounter for suspected placental problem ruled out M ♀

Z03.73 Encounter for suspected fetal anomaly ruled out M ♀

Z03.74 Encounter for suspected problem with fetal growth ruled out M ♀

Z03.75 Encounter for suspected cervical shortening ruled out M ♀

Z03.79 Encounter for other suspected maternal and fetal conditions ruled out M ♀

Z03.8 Encounter for observation for other suspected diseases and conditions ruled out

Z03.81 Encounter for observation for suspected exposure to biological agents ruled out

Z03.810 Encounter for observation for suspected exposure to anthrax ruled out

Z03.818 Encounter for observation for suspected exposure to other biological agents ruled out
AHA: 2020,2Q,8; 2020,1Q,34-36
TIP: Assign for cases in which there is concern for possible exposure to COVID-19 that is ruled out after evaluation.

● **Z03.82 Encounter for observation for suspected foreign body ruled out**

EXCLUDES 1 *retained foreign body (Z18.-)*
retained foreign body in eyelid (H02.81)
residual foreign body in soft tissue (M79.5)

EXCLUDES 2 *confirmed foreign body ingestion or aspiration including:*
foreign body in alimentary tract (T18)
foreign body in ear (T16)
foreign body on external eye (T15)
foreign body in respiratory tract (T17)

● **Z03.821 Encounter for observation for suspected ingested foreign body ruled out**

● **Z03.822 Encounter for observation for suspected aspirated (inhaled) foreign body ruled out**

● **Z03.823 Encounter for observation for suspected inserted (injected) foreign body ruled out**
Encounter for observation for suspected inserted (injected) foreign body in eye ruled out
Encounter for observation for suspected inserted (injected) foreign body in orifice ruled out
Encounter for observation for suspected inserted (injected) foreign body in skin ruled out

Z03.89 Encounter for observation for other suspected diseases and conditions ruled out

Z04 Encounter for examination and observation for other reasons

INCLUDES encounter for examination for medicolegal reasons

This category is to be used when a person without a diagnosis is suspected of having an abnormal condition, without signs or symptoms, which requires study, but after examination and observation, is ruled-out. This category is also for use for administrative and legal observation status.

AHA: 2018,2Q,7-8

Z04.1 Encounter for examination and observation following transport accident

EXCLUDES 1 *encounter for examination and observation following work accident (Z04.2)*

AHA: 2019,2Q,11; 2018,2Q,8

Z04.2 Encounter for examination and observation following work accident

Z04.3 Encounter for examination and observation following other accident

Z04.4 Encounter for examination and observation following alleged rape
Encounter for examination and observation of victim following alleged rape
Encounter for examination and observation of victim following alleged sexual abuse

Z04.41 Encounter for examination and observation following alleged adult rape A
Suspected adult rape, ruled out
Suspected adult sexual abuse, ruled out

Z04.42 Encounter for examination and observation following alleged child rape P
Suspected child rape, ruled out
Suspected child sexual abuse, ruled out

Z04.6 Encounter for general psychiatric examination, requested by authority

Z04.7 Encounter for examination and observation following alleged physical abuse

Z04.71 Encounter for examination and observation following alleged adult physical abuse A
Suspected adult physical abuse, ruled out

EXCLUDES 1 *confirmed case of adult physical abuse (T74.-)*
encounter for examination and observation following alleged adult sexual abuse (Z04.41)
suspected case of adult physical abuse, not ruled out (T76.-)

Z04.72 Encounter for examination and observation following alleged child physical abuse P
Suspected child physical abuse, ruled out

EXCLUDES 1 *confirmed case of child physical abuse (T74.-)*
encounter for examination and observation following alleged child sexual abuse (Z04.42)
suspected case of child physical abuse, not ruled out (T76.-)

Z04.8 Encounter for examination and observation for other specified reasons
Encounter for examination and observation for request for expert evidence
AHA: 2018,4Q,32,35,72

Z04.81 Encounter for examination and observation of victim following forced sexual exploitation

Z04.82 Encounter for examination and observation of victim following forced labor exploitation

Z04.89 Encounter for examination and observation for other specified reasons

Z04.9 Encounter for examination and observation for unspecified reason
Encounter for observation NOS

Z05 Encounter for observation and evaluation of newborn for suspected diseases and conditions ruled out
This category is to be used for newborns, within the neonatal period (the first 28 days of life), who are suspected of having an abnormal condition, but without signs or symptoms, and which, after examination and observation, is ruled out.
AHA: 2017,4Q,27; 2016,4Q,77

Z05.0 Observation and evaluation of newborn for suspected cardiac condition ruled out N

Z05.1 Observation and evaluation of newborn for suspected infectious condition ruled out N
AHA: 2019,2Q,10

Z05.2 Observation and evaluation of newborn for suspected neurological condition ruled out N

Z05.3 Observation and evaluation of newborn for suspected respiratory condition ruled out N

Z05.4 Observation and evaluation of newborn for suspected genetic, metabolic or immunologic condition ruled out

Z05.41 Observation and evaluation of newborn for suspected genetic condition ruled out N
AHA: 2016,4Q,55

Z05.42 Observation and evaluation of newborn for suspected metabolic condition ruled out N

Z05.43 Observation and evaluation of newborn for suspected immunologic condition ruled out N

Z05.5 Observation and evaluation of newborn for suspected gastrointestinal condition ruled out N

Z05.6 Observation and evaluation of newborn for suspected genitourinary condition ruled out N

Z05.7 Observation and evaluation of newborn for suspected skin, subcutaneous, musculoskeletal and connective tissue condition ruled out

Z05.71 Observation and evaluation of newborn for suspected skin and subcutaneous tissue condition ruled out N

Z05.72 Observation and evaluation of newborn for suspected musculoskeletal condition ruled out N

Z05.73 Observation and evaluation of newborn for suspected connective tissue condition ruled out N

Z05.8 Observation and evaluation of newborn for other specified suspected condition ruled out N

Z05.9 Observation and evaluation of newborn for unspecified suspected condition ruled out N

Z08 Encounter for follow-up examination after completed treatment for malignant neoplasm
Medical surveillance following completed treatment
Use additional code to identify any acquired absence of organs (Z90.-)
Use additional code to identify the personal history of malignant neoplasm (Z85.-)
EXCLUDES 1 *aftercare following medical care (Z43-Z49, Z51)*

Z09 Encounter for follow-up examination after completed treatment for conditions other than malignant neoplasm
Medical surveillance following completed treatment
Use additional code to identify any applicable history of disease code (Z86.-, Z87.-)
EXCLUDES 1 *aftercare following medical care (Z43-Z49, Z51)*
surveillance of contraception (Z30.4-)
surveillance of prosthetic and other medical devices (Z44-Z46)
AHA: 2020,2Q,10; 2017,1Q,9; 2015,1Q,8

Z11 Encounter for screening for infectious and parasitic diseases
Screening is the testing for disease or disease precursors in asymptomatic individuals so that early detection and treatment can be provided for those who test positive for the disease.
EXCLUDES 1 *encounter for diagnostic examination — code to sign or symptom*

Z11.0 Encounter for screening for intestinal infectious diseases

Z11.1 Encounter for screening for respiratory tuberculosis
Encounter for screening for active tuberculosis disease

Z11.2 Encounter for screening for other bacterial diseases

Z11.3 Encounter for screening for infections with a predominantly sexual mode of transmission
EXCLUDES 2 *encounter for screening for human immunodeficiency virus [HIV] (Z11.4)*
encounter for screening for human papillomavirus (Z11.51)

Z11.4 Encounter for screening for human immunodeficiency virus [HIV]

Z11.5 Encounter for screening for other viral diseases
EXCLUDES 2 *encounter for screening for viral intestinal disease (Z11.0)*

Z11.51 Encounter for screening for human papillomavirus (HPV)

Z11.59 Encounter for screening for other viral diseases

Z11.6 Encounter for screening for other protozoal diseases and helminthiases
EXCLUDES 2 *encounter for screening for protozoal intestinal disease (Z11.0)*

Z11.7 Encounter for testing for latent tuberculosis infection
AHA: 2019,4Q,20

Z11.8 Encounter for screening for other infectious and parasitic diseases
Encounter for screening for chlamydia
Encounter for screening for rickettsial
Encounter for screening for spirochetal
Encounter for screening for mycoses

Z11.9 Encounter for screening for infectious and parasitic diseases, unspecified

Z12 Encounter for screening for malignant neoplasms
Screening is the testing for disease or disease precursors in asymptomatic individuals so that early detection and treatment can be provided for those who test positive for the disease.
Use additional code to identify any family history of malignant neoplasm (Z80.-)
EXCLUDES 1 *encounter for diagnostic examination — code to sign or symptom*

Z12.0 Encounter for screening for malignant neoplasm of stomach

Z12.1 Encounter for screening for malignant neoplasm of intestinal tract
AHA: 2017,1Q,8,9

Z12.10 Encounter for screening for malignant neoplasm of intestinal tract, unspecified

Z12.11 Encounter for screening for malignant neoplasm of colon
Encounter for screening colonoscopy NOS
AHA: 2019,1Q,32-33; 2018,1Q,6

Z12.12 Encounter for screening for malignant neoplasm of rectum
AHA: 2018,1Q,6

Z12.13 Encounter for screening for malignant neoplasm of small intestine

Z12.2 Encounter for screening for malignant neoplasm of respiratory organs

Z12.3 Encounter for screening for malignant neoplasm of breast

Z12.31 Encounter for screening mammogram for malignant neoplasm of breast
EXCLUDES 1 *inconclusive mammogram (R92.2)*
AHA: 2015,1Q,24

Z12.39 Encounter for other screening for malignant neoplasm of breast

Z12.4 Encounter for screening for malignant neoplasm of cervix ♀
Encounter for screening pap smear for malignant neoplasm of cervix
EXCLUDES 1 *when screening is part of general gynecological examination (Z01.4-)*
EXCLUDES 2 *encounter for screening for human papillomavirus (Z11.51)*

Z12.5 Encounter for screening for malignant neoplasm of prostate ♂

Z12.6 Encounter for screening for malignant neoplasm of bladder

Z12.7 Encounter for screening for malignant neoplasm of other genitourinary organs

Z12.71 Encounter for screening for malignant neoplasm of testis ♂

Z12.72 **Encounter for screening for malignant neoplasm of vagina** ♀
Vaginal pap smear status-post hysterectomy for non-malignant condition
Use additional code to identify acquired absence of uterus (Z90.71-)
EXCLUDES 1 *vaginal pap smear status-post hysterectomy for malignant conditions (Z08)*

Z12.73 **Encounter for screening for malignant neoplasm of ovary** ♀

Z12.79 **Encounter for screening for malignant neoplasm of other genitourinary organs**

✓5th Z12.8 **Encounter for screening for malignant neoplasm of other sites**

Z12.81 **Encounter for screening for malignant neoplasm of oral cavity**

Z12.82 **Encounter for screening for malignant neoplasm of nervous system**

Z12.83 **Encounter for screening for malignant neoplasm of skin**

Z12.89 **Encounter for screening for malignant neoplasm of other sites**

Z12.9 **Encounter for screening for malignant neoplasm, site unspecified**

✓4th **Z13 Encounter for screening for other diseases and disorders**
Screening is the testing for disease or disease precursors in asymptomatic individuals so that early detection and treatment can be provided for those who test positive for the disease.
EXCLUDES 1 *encounter for diagnostic examination — code to sign or symptom*

Z13.0 **Encounter for screening for diseases of the blood and blood-forming organs and certain disorders involving the immune mechanism**

Z13.1 **Encounter for screening for diabetes mellitus**

✓5th Z13.2 **Encounter for screening for nutritional, metabolic and other endocrine disorders**

Z13.21 **Encounter for screening for nutritional disorder**

✓6th Z13.22 **Encounter for screening for metabolic disorder**

Z13.220 **Encounter for screening for lipoid disorders**
Encounter for screening for cholesterol level
Encounter for screening for hypercholesterolemia
Encounter for screening for hyperlipidemia

Z13.228 **Encounter for screening for other metabolic disorders**

Z13.29 **Encounter for screening for other suspected endocrine disorder**
EXCLUDES 1 *encounter for screening for diabetes mellitus (Z13.1)*

✓5th Z13.3 **Encounter for screening examination for mental health and behavioral disorders**
AHA: 2018,4Q,35-36

Z13.30 **Encounter for screening examination for mental health and behavioral disorders, unspecified**

Z13.31 **Encounter for screening for depression**
Encounter for screening for depression, adult
Encounter for screening for depression for child or adolescent

Z13.32 **Encounter for screening for maternal depression** ♀
Encounter for screening for perinatal depression

Z13.39 **Encounter for screening examination for other mental health and behavioral disorders**
Encounter for screening for alcoholism
Encounter for screening for intellectual disabilities

✓5th Z13.4 **Encounter for screening for certain developmental disorders in childhood**
Encounter for development testing of infant or child
Encounter for screening for developmental handicaps in early childhood
EXCLUDES 2 *encounter for routine child health examination (Z00.12-)*
AHA: 2018,4Q,36

Z13.40 **Encounter for screening for unspecified developmental delays**

Z13.41 **Encounter for autism screening**

Z13.42 **Encounter for screening for global developmental delays (milestones)**
Encounter for screening for developmental handicaps in early childhood

Z13.49 **Encounter for screening for other developmental delays**

Z13.5 **Encounter for screening for eye and ear disorders**
EXCLUDES 2 *encounter for general hearing examination (Z01.1-)*
encounter for general vision examination (Z01.0-)
AHA: 2016,3Q,17

Z13.6 **Encounter for screening for cardiovascular disorders**

✓5th Z13.7 **Encounter for screening for genetic and chromosomal anomalies**
EXCLUDES 1 *genetic testing for procreative management (Z31.4-)*

Z13.71 **Encounter for nonprocreative screening for genetic disease carrier status**

Z13.79 **Encounter for other screening for genetic and chromosomal anomalies**

✓5th Z13.8 **Encounter for screening for other specified diseases and disorders**
EXCLUDES 2 *screening for malignant neoplasms (Z12.-)*

✓6th Z13.81 **Encounter for screening for digestive system disorders**

Z13.810 **Encounter for screening for upper gastrointestinal disorder**

Z13.811 **Encounter for screening for lower gastrointestinal disorder**
EXCLUDES 1 *encounter for screening for intestinal infectious disease (Z11.0)*

Z13.818 **Encounter for screening for other digestive system disorders**

✓6th Z13.82 **Encounter for screening for musculoskeletal disorder**

Z13.820 **Encounter for screening for osteoporosis**

Z13.828 **Encounter for screening for other musculoskeletal disorder**

Z13.83 **Encounter for screening for respiratory disorder NEC**
EXCLUDES 1 *encounter for screening for respiratory tuberculosis (Z11.1)*

Z13.84 **Encounter for screening for dental disorders**

✓6th Z13.85 **Encounter for screening for nervous system disorders**

Z13.850 **Encounter for screening for traumatic brain injury**

Z13.858 **Encounter for screening for other nervous system disorders**

Z13.88 **Encounter for screening for disorder due to exposure to contaminants**
EXCLUDES 1 *those exposed to contaminants without suspected disorders (Z57.-, Z77.-)*

Z13.89 **Encounter for screening for other disorder**
Encounter for screening for genitourinary disorders

Z13.9 **Encounter for screening, unspecified**

Genetic carrier and genetic susceptibility to disease (Z14-Z15)

✓4th **Z14 Genetic carrier**
DEF: Individuals carrying a gene mutation associated with a certain disease that typically do not develop the disease but are able to pass the mutated genes to offspring.

✓5th Z14.0 **Hemophilia A carrier**

Z14.01 **Asymptomatic hemophilia A carrier**

Z14.02 **Symptomatic hemophilia A carrier**

Z14.1 **Cystic fibrosis carrier**

Z14.8 **Genetic carrier of other disease**

✓4th **Z15 Genetic susceptibility to disease**
INCLUDES confirmed abnormal gene
Use additional code, if applicable, for any associated family history of the disease (Z80-Z84)
EXCLUDES 1 *chromosomal anomalies (Q90-Q99)*

✓5th Z15.0 **Genetic susceptibility to malignant neoplasm**
Code first, if applicable, any current malignant neoplasm (C00-C75, C81-C96)
Use additional code, if applicable, for any personal history of malignant neoplasm (Z85.-)

Z15.01 **Genetic susceptibility to malignant neoplasm of breast**

Z15.02 Genetic susceptibility to malignant neoplasm of ovary ♀

Z15.03 Genetic susceptibility to malignant neoplasm of prostate ♂

Z15.04 Genetic susceptibility to malignant neoplasm of endometrium ♀

Z15.09 Genetic susceptibility to other malignant neoplasm

Z15.8 Genetic susceptibility to other disease (5th)

Z15.81 Genetic susceptibility to multiple endocrine neoplasia [MEN]

EXCLUDES 1 *multiple endocrine neoplasia [MEN] syndromes (E31.2-)*

DEF: Group of conditions in which several endocrine glands grow excessively (such as in adenomatous hyperplasia) and/or develop benign or malignant tumors. Tumors and hyperplasia associated with MEN often produce excess hormones, which impede normal physiology. There is no comprehensive cure known for MEN syndrome. Treatment is directed at the hyperplasia or tumors in each individual gland. Tumors are usually surgically removed and oral medications or hormonal injections are used to correct hormone imbalances.

Z15.89 Genetic susceptibility to other disease

Resistance to antimicrobial drugs (Z16)

Z16 Resistance to antimicrobial drugs (4th)

NOTE The codes in this category are provided for use as additional codes to identify the resistance and non-responsiveness of a condition to antimicrobial drugs.

Code first the infection

EXCLUDES 1 *Methicillin resistant Staphylococcus aureus infection (A49.02)*
Methicillin resistant Staphylococcus aureus pneumonia (J15.212)
sepsis due to Methicillin resistant Staphylococcus aureus (A41.02)

Z16.1 Resistance to beta lactam antibiotics (5th)

Z16.10 Resistance to unspecified beta lactam antibiotics CC

Z16.11 Resistance to penicillins CC
Resistance to amoxicillin
Resistance to ampicillin

Z16.12 Extended spectrum beta lactamase (ESBL) resistance CC

EXCLUDES 2 *Methicillin resistant Staphylococcus aureus infection in diseases classified elsewhere (B95.62)*

Z16.19 Resistance to other specified beta lactam antibiotics CC
Resistance to cephalosporins

Z16.2 Resistance to other antibiotics (5th)

Z16.20 Resistance to unspecified antibiotic CC
Resistance to antibiotics NOS

Z16.21 Resistance to vancomycin CC

Z16.22 Resistance to vancomycin related antibiotics CC

Z16.23 Resistance to quinolones and fluoroquinolones CC

Z16.24 Resistance to multiple antibiotics CC

Z16.29 Resistance to other single specified antibiotic CC
Resistance to aminoglycosides
Resistance to macrolides
Resistance to sulfonamides
Resistance to tetracyclines

Z16.3 Resistance to other antimicrobial drugs (5th)

EXCLUDES 1 *resistance to antibiotics (Z16.1-, Z16.2-)*

Z16.30 Resistance to unspecified antimicrobial drugs CC
Drug resistance NOS

Z16.31 Resistance to antiparasitic drug(s) CC
Resistance to quinine and related compounds

Z16.32 Resistance to antifungal drug(s) CC

Z16.33 Resistance to antiviral drug(s) CC

Z16.34 Resistance to antimycobacterial drug(s) (6th)
Resistance to tuberculostatics

Z16.341 Resistance to single antimycobacterial drug CC
Resistance to antimycobacterial drug NOS

Z16.342 Resistance to multiple antimycobacterial drugs CC

Z16.35 Resistance to multiple antimicrobial drugs CC

EXCLUDES 1 *resistance to multiple antibiotics only (Z16.24)*

Z16.39 Resistance to other specified antimicrobial drug CC

Estrogen receptor status (Z17)

Z17 Estrogen receptor status (4th)

Code first malignant neoplasm of breast (C50.-)

DEF: Receptor status of breast cancer cells for the hormone estrogen that is used to help determine treatment and evaluate prognosis. ER+ breast cancer responds to hormone therapies while ER- breast cancer does not.

Z17.0 Estrogen receptor positive status [ER+]

Z17.1 Estrogen receptor negative status [ER-]

Retained foreign body fragments (Z18)

Z18 Retained foreign body fragments (4th)

INCLUDES embedded fragment (status)
embedded splinter (status)
retained foreign body status

EXCLUDES 1 *artificial joint prosthesis status (Z96.6-)*
foreign body accidentally left during a procedure (T81.5-)
foreign body entering through orifice (T15-T19)
in situ cardiac device (Z95.-)
organ or tissue replaced by means other than transplant (Z96.-, Z97.-)
organ or tissue replaced by transplant (Z94.-)
personal history of retained foreign body fully removed Z87.821
superficial foreign body (non-embedded splinter) — code to superficial foreign body, by site

DEF: Embedded or retained fragment, splinter, or foreign body, natural or synthetic that can cause infection.

Z18.0 Retained radioactive fragments (5th)

Z18.01 Retained depleted uranium fragments

Z18.09 Other retained radioactive fragments
Other retained depleted isotope fragments
Retained nontherapeutic radioactive fragments

Z18.1 Retained metal fragments (5th)

EXCLUDES 1 *retained radioactive metal fragments (Z18.01-Z18.09)*

Z18.10 Retained metal fragments, unspecified
Retained metal fragment NOS

Z18.11 Retained magnetic metal fragments

Z18.12 Retained nonmagnetic metal fragments

Z18.2 Retained plastic fragments
Acrylics fragments
Diethylhexyl phthalates fragments
Isocyanate fragments

Z18.3 Retained organic fragments (5th)

Z18.31 Retained animal quills or spines

Z18.32 Retained tooth

Z18.33 Retained wood fragments

Z18.39 Other retained organic fragments

Z18.8 Other specified retained foreign body (5th)

Z18.81 Retained glass fragments

Z18.83 Retained stone or crystalline fragments
Retained concrete or cement fragments

Z18.89 Other specified retained foreign body fragments

Z18.9 Retained foreign body fragments, unspecified material

Hormone sensitivity malignancy status (Z19)

Z19 Hormone sensitivity malignancy status (4th)

Code first malignant neoplasm — see Table of Neoplasms, by site, malignant

AHA: 2016,4Q,76

Z19.1 Hormone sensitive malignancy status

Z19.2 **Hormone resistant malignancy status**
Castrate resistant prostate malignancy status

Persons with potential health hazards related to communicable diseases (Z20-Z29)

✓4th **Z20 Contact with and (suspected) exposure to communicable diseases**
EXCLUDES 1 *carrier of infectious disease (Z22.-)*
diagnosed current infectious or parasitic disease — see Alphabetic Index
EXCLUDES 2 *personal history of infectious and parasitic diseases (Z86.1-)*

✓5th **Z20.0 Contact with and (suspected) exposure to intestinal infectious diseases**
Z20.01 Contact with and (suspected) exposure to intestinal infectious diseases due to Escherichia coli (E. coli)
Z20.09 Contact with and (suspected) exposure to other intestinal infectious diseases
Z20.1 Contact with and (suspected) exposure to tuberculosis
Z20.2 Contact with and (suspected) exposure to infections with a predominantly sexual mode of transmission
Z20.3 Contact with and (suspected) exposure to rabies
Z20.4 Contact with and (suspected) exposure to rubella
Z20.5 Contact with and (suspected) exposure to viral hepatitis
Z20.6 Contact with and (suspected) exposure to human immunodeficiency virus [HIV]
EXCLUDES 1 *asymptomatic human immunodeficiency virus [HIV] HIV infection status (Z21)*
Z20.7 Contact with and (suspected) exposure to pediculosis, acariasis and other infestations
✓5th **Z20.8 Contact with and (suspected) exposure to other communicable diseases**
✓6th **Z20.81 Contact with and (suspected) exposure to other bacterial communicable diseases**
Z20.810 Contact with and (suspected) exposure to anthrax
Z20.811 Contact with and (suspected) exposure to meningococcus
Z20.818 Contact with and (suspected) exposure to other bacterial communicable diseases
AHA: 2019,2Q,10
✓6th **Z20.82 Contact with and (suspected) exposure to other viral communicable diseases**
Z20.820 Contact with and (suspected) exposure to varicella
Z20.821 Contact with and (suspected) exposure to Zika virus
AHA: 2018,4Q,35,64
Z20.828 Contact with and (suspected) exposure to other viral communicable diseases
AHA: 2020,2Q,4,8; 2020,1Q,34-36
TIP: Assign for cases in which there is actual exposure to someone who is confirmed or suspected (not ruled out) to have COVID-19 and the exposed individual either tests negative or the test results are unknown. If the exposed individual tests positive for the COVID-19 virus, assign U07.1.
Z20.89 Contact with and (suspected) exposure to other communicable diseases
Z20.9 Contact with and (suspected) exposure to unspecified communicable disease

Z21 Asymptomatic human immunodeficiency virus [HIV] infection status HCC
HIV positive NOS
Code first human immunodeficiency virus [HIV] disease complicating pregnancy, childbirth and the puerperium, if applicable (O98.7-)
EXCLUDES 1 *acquired immunodeficiency syndrome (B20)*
contact with human immunodeficiency virus [HIV] (Z20.6)
exposure to human immunodeficiency virus [HIV] (Z20.6)
human immunodeficiency virus [HIV] disease (B20)
inconclusive laboratory evidence of human immunodeficiency virus [HIV] (R75)
AHA: 2019,1Q,8-11
DEF: Phase of human immunodeficiency virus (HIV) infection with no clinical symptoms. This phase may last for 10 years or more.

✓4th **Z22 Carrier of infectious disease**
INCLUDES colonization status
suspected carrier
EXCLUDES 2 *carrier of viral hepatitis (B18.-)*
Z22.0 Carrier of typhoid
Z22.1 Carrier of other intestinal infectious diseases
Z22.2 Carrier of diphtheria
✓5th **Z22.3 Carrier of other specified bacterial diseases**
Z22.31 Carrier of bacterial disease due to meningococci
✓6th **Z22.32 Carrier of bacterial disease due to staphylococci**
Z22.321 Carrier or suspected carrier of Methicillin susceptible Staphylococcus aureus
MSSA colonization
Z22.322 Carrier or suspected carrier of Methicillin resistant Staphylococcus aureus
MRSA colonization
DEF: Carriers (colonization) of methicillin resistant *Staphylococcus aureus* (MRSA) have MRSA on their skin or in their body but do not exhibit signs of infection. These individuals are able to pass MRSA on to others who may develop an infection.
✓6th **Z22.33 Carrier of bacterial disease due to streptococci**
Z22.330 Carrier of Group B streptococcus
EXCLUDES 1 *carrier of streptococcus group B (GBS) complicating pregnancy, childbirth and the puerperium (O99.82-)*
Z22.338 Carrier of other streptococcus
Z22.39 Carrier of other specified bacterial diseases
Z22.4 Carrier of infections with a predominantly sexual mode of transmission
Z22.6 Carrier of human T-lymphotropic virus type-1 [HTLV-1] infection
Z22.7 Latent tuberculosis
Latent tuberculosis infection (LTBI)
EXCLUDES 1 *nonspecific reaction to cell mediated immunity measurement of gamma interferon antigen response without active tuberculosis (R76.12)*
nonspecific reaction to tuberculin skin test without active tuberculosis (R76.11)
AHA: 2019,4Q,19
Z22.8 Carrier of other infectious diseases
Z22.9 Carrier of infectious disease, unspecified

Z23 Encounter for immunization
Code first any routine childhood examination
NOTE Procedure codes are required to identify the types of immunizations given

✓4th **Z28 Immunization not carried out and underimmunization status**
INCLUDES vaccination not carried out
✓5th **Z28.0 Immunization not carried out because of contraindication**
DEF: Contraindication: Situation where a drug, surgery, or other procedure may negatively affect or cause harm to a patient.
Z28.01 Immunization not carried out because of acute illness of patient
Z28.02 Immunization not carried out because of chronic illness or condition of patient
Z28.03 Immunization not carried out because of immune compromised state of patient
Z28.04 Immunization not carried out because of patient allergy to vaccine or component
Z28.09 Immunization not carried out because of other contraindication
Z28.1 Immunization not carried out because of patient decision for reasons of belief or group pressure
Immunization not carried out because of religious belief
✓5th **Z28.2 Immunization not carried out because of patient decision for other and unspecified reason**
Z28.20 Immunization not carried out because of patient decision for unspecified reason
Z28.21 Immunization not carried out because of patient refusal
Z28.29 Immunization not carried out because of patient decision for other reason

Z28.3 Underimmunization status
Delinquent immunization status
Lapsed immunization schedule status

√5th **Z28.8 Immunization not carried out for other reason**

Z28.81 Immunization not carried out due to patient having had the disease

Z28.82 Immunization not carried out because of caregiver refusal
Immunization not carried out because of guardian refusal
Immunization not carried out because of parent refusal
EXCLUDES 1 *immunization not carried out because of caregiver refusal because of religious belief (Z28.1)*

Z28.83 Immunization not carried out due to unavailability of vaccine
Delay in delivery of vaccine
Lack of availability of vaccine
Manufacturer delay of vaccine
AHA: 2018,4Q,36

Z28.89 Immunization not carried out for other reason

Z28.9 Immunization not carried out for unspecified reason

√4th **Z29 Encounter for other prophylactic measures**
EXCLUDES 1 *desensitization to allergens (Z51.6)*
prophylactic surgery (Z40.-)
AHA: 2016,4Q,78-79

√5th **Z29.1 Encounter for prophylactic immunotherapy**
Encounter for administration of immunoglobulin

Z29.11 Encounter for prophylactic immunotherapy for respiratory syncytial virus (RSV)

Z29.12 Encounter for prophylactic antivenin

Z29.13 Encounter for prophylactic Rho(D) immune globulin
AHA: 2019,3Q,5

Z29.14 Encounter for prophylactic rabies immune globin

Z29.3 Encounter for prophylactic fluoride administration

Z29.8 Encounter for other specified prophylactic measures

Z29.9 Encounter for prophylactic measures, unspecified

Persons encountering health services in circumstances related to reproduction (Z30-Z39)

√4th **Z30 Encounter for contraceptive management**
AHA: 2016,4Q,78
DEF: Contraceptive management to prevent pregnancy. Methods include oral medications, intrauterine devices, and surgical procedures for males and females (sterilization).

√5th **Z30.0 Encounter for general counseling and advice on contraception**

√6th **Z30.01 Encounter for initial prescription of contraceptives**
EXCLUDES 1 *encounter for surveillance of contraceptives (Z30.4-)*

Z30.011 Encounter for initial prescription of contraceptive pills ♀

Z30.012 Encounter for prescription of emergency contraception ♀
Encounter for postcoital contraception

Z30.013 Encounter for initial prescription of injectable contraceptive ♀

Z30.014 Encounter for initial prescription of intrauterine contraceptive device ♀
EXCLUDES 1 *encounter for insertion of intrauterine contraceptive device (Z30.430, Z30.432)*

Z30.015 Encounter for initial prescription of vaginal ring hormonal contraceptive ♀

Z30.016 Encounter for initial prescription of transdermal patch hormonal contraceptive device

Z30.017 Encounter for initial prescription of implantable subdermal contraceptive

Z30.018 Encounter for initial prescription of other contraceptives ♀
Encounter for initial prescription of barrier contraception
Encounter for initial prescription of diaphragm

Z30.019 Encounter for initial prescription of contraceptives, unspecified ♀

Z30.02 Counseling and instruction in natural family planning to avoid pregnancy

Z30.09 Encounter for other general counseling and advice on contraception
Encounter for family planning advice NOS

Z30.2 Encounter for sterilization

√5th **Z30.4 Encounter for surveillance of contraceptives**

Z30.40 Encounter for surveillance of contraceptives, unspecified

Z30.41 Encounter for surveillance of contraceptive pills ♀
Encounter for repeat prescription for contraceptive pill

Z30.42 Encounter for surveillance of injectable contraceptive ♀

√6th **Z30.43 Encounter for surveillance of intrauterine contraceptive device**

Z30.430 Encounter for insertion of intrauterine contraceptive device ♀

Z30.431 Encounter for routine checking of intrauterine contraceptive device ♀

Z30.432 Encounter for removal of intrauterine contraceptive device ♀

Z30.433 Encounter for removal and reinsertion of intrauterine contraceptive device ♀
Encounter for replacement of intrauterine contraceptive device

Z30.44 Encounter for surveillance of vaginal ring hormonal contraceptive device ♀

Z30.45 Encounter for surveillance of transdermal patch hormonal contraceptive device ♀

Z30.46 Encounter for surveillance of implantable subdermal contraceptive ♀
Encounter for checking, reinsertion or removal of implantable subdermal contraceptive

Z30.49 Encounter for surveillance of other contraceptives ♀
Encounter for surveillance of barrier contraception
Encounter for surveillance of diaphragm

Z30.8 Encounter for other contraceptive management
Encounter for postvasectomy sperm count
Encounter for routine examination for contraceptive maintenance
EXCLUDES 1 *sperm count following sterilization reversal (Z31.42)*
sperm count for fertility testing (Z31.41)

Z30.9 Encounter for contraceptive management, unspecified

√4th **Z31 Encounter for procreative management**
EXCLUDES 1 *complications associated with artificial fertilization (N98.-)*
female infertility (N97.-)
male infertility (N46.-)

Z31.0 Encounter for reversal of previous sterilization

√5th **Z31.4 Encounter for procreative investigation and testing**
EXCLUDES 1 *postvasectomy sperm count (Z30.8)*

Z31.41 Encounter for fertility testing
Encounter for fallopian tube patency testing
Encounter for sperm count for fertility testing

Z31.42 Aftercare following sterilization reversal
Sperm count following sterilization reversal

√6th **Z31.43 Encounter for genetic testing of female for procreative management**
Use additional code for recurrent pregnancy loss, if applicable (N96, O26.2-)
EXCLUDES 1 *nonprocreative genetic testing (Z13.7-)*

Z31.430 Encounter of female for testing for genetic disease carrier status for procreative management ♀

Z31.438 Encounter for other genetic testing of female for procreative management ♀

✓6th **Z31.44 Encounter for genetic testing of male for procreative management**
EXCLUDES 1 *nonprocreative genetic testing (Z13.7-)*
Z31.440 Encounter of male for testing for genetic disease carrier status for procreative management ♂
Z31.441 Encounter for testing of male partner of patient with recurrent pregnancy loss A ♂
Z31.448 Encounter for other genetic testing of male for procreative management A ♂
Z31.49 Encounter for other procreative investigation and testing
Z31.5 Encounter for procreative genetic counseling
AHA: 2017,4Q,27
✓5th **Z31.6 Encounter for general counseling and advice on procreation**
Z31.61 Procreative counseling and advice using natural family planning
Z31.62 Encounter for fertility preservation counseling
Encounter for fertility preservation counseling prior to cancer therapy
Encounter for fertility preservation counseling prior to surgical removal of gonads
Z31.69 Encounter for other general counseling and advice on procreation
Z31.7 Encounter for procreative management and counseling for gestational carrier ♀
EXCLUDES 1 *pregnant state, gestational carrier (Z33.3)*
AHA: 2016,4Q,78
✓5th **Z31.8 Encounter for other procreative management**
Z31.81 Encounter for male factor infertility in female patient ♀
Z31.82 Encounter for Rh incompatibility status ♀
AHA: 2015,3Q,40; 2014,4Q,17
Z31.83 Encounter for assisted reproductive fertility procedure cycle ♀
Patient undergoing in vitro fertilization cycle
Use additional code to identify the type of infertility
EXCLUDES 1 *pre-cycle diagnosis and testing — code to reason for encounter*
Z31.84 Encounter for fertility preservation procedure
Encounter for fertility preservation procedure prior to cancer therapy
Encounter for fertility preservation procedure prior to surgical removal of gonads
Z31.89 Encounter for other procreative management
Z31.9 Encounter for procreative management, unspecified

✓4th **Z32 Encounter for pregnancy test and childbirth and childcare instruction**
✓5th **Z32.0 Encounter for pregnancy test**
Z32.00 Encounter for pregnancy test, result unknown ♀
Encounter for pregnancy test NOS
Z32.01 Encounter for pregnancy test, result positive M ♀
Z32.02 Encounter for pregnancy test, result negative ♀
Z32.2 Encounter for childbirth instruction
Z32.3 Encounter for childcare instruction
Encounter for prenatal or postpartum childcare instruction

✓4th **Z33 Pregnant state**
Z33.1 Pregnant state, incidental M ♀
►Pregnancy NOS◄
Pregnant state NOS
EXCLUDES 1 *complications of pregnancy (O00-O9A)*
pregnant state, gestational carrier (Z33.3)
Z33.2 Encounter for elective termination of pregnancy M ♀
EXCLUDES 1 *early fetal death with retention of dead fetus (O02.1)*
late fetal death (O36.4)
spontaneous abortion (O03)
TIP: Do not assign a code from category Z3A with this code.
Z33.3 Pregnant state, gestational carrier M ♀
EXCLUDES 1 *encounter for procreative management and counseling for gestational carrier (Z31.7)*
AHA: 2016,4Q,78

✓4th **Z34 Encounter for supervision of normal pregnancy**
EXCLUDES 1 *any complication of pregnancy (O00-O9A)*
encounter for pregnancy test (Z32.0-)
encounter for supervision of high risk pregnancy (O09.-)
AHA: 2019,3Q,5; 2014,4Q,17
✓5th **Z34.0 Encounter for supervision of normal first pregnancy**
Z34.00 Encounter for supervision of normal first pregnancy, unspecified trimester M ♀
Z34.01 Encounter for supervision of normal first pregnancy, first trimester M ♀
Z34.02 Encounter for supervision of normal first pregnancy, second trimester M ♀
Z34.03 Encounter for supervision of normal first pregnancy, third trimester M ♀
✓5th **Z34.8 Encounter for supervision of other normal pregnancy**
Z34.80 Encounter for supervision of other normal pregnancy, unspecified trimester M ♀
Z34.81 Encounter for supervision of other normal pregnancy, first trimester M ♀
Z34.82 Encounter for supervision of other normal pregnancy, second trimester M ♀
Z34.83 Encounter for supervision of other normal pregnancy, third trimester M ♀
✓5th **Z34.9 Encounter for supervision of normal pregnancy, unspecified**
Z34.90 Encounter for supervision of normal pregnancy, unspecified, unspecified trimester M ♀
Z34.91 Encounter for supervision of normal pregnancy, unspecified, first trimester M ♀
Z34.92 Encounter for supervision of normal pregnancy, unspecified, second trimester M ♀
Z34.93 Encounter for supervision of normal pregnancy, unspecified, third trimester M ♀

✓4th **Z36 Encounter for antenatal screening of mother**
INCLUDES encounter for placental sample (taken vaginally)
screening is the testing for disease or disease precursors in asymptomatic individuals so that early detection and treatment can be provided for those who test positive for the disease.
EXCLUDES 1 *diagnostic examination — code to sign or symptom*
encounter for suspected maternal and fetal conditions ruled out (Z03.7-)
suspected fetal condition affecting management of pregnancy — code to condition in Chapter 15
EXCLUDES 2 *abnormal findings on antenatal screening of mother (O28.-)*
genetic counseling and testing (Z31.43-, Z31.5)
routine prenatal care (Z34)
AHA: 2017,4Q,28
Z36.0 Encounter for antenatal screening for chromosomal anomalies M ♀
Z36.1 Encounter for antenatal screening for raised alphafetoprotein level M ♀
Encounter for antenatal screening for elevated maternal serum alphafetoprotein level
DEF: High levels of alpha-fetoprotein (AFP) that may indicate a possibility of spina bifida and other neural tube defects, anencephaly, or omphalocele in the fetus.
Z36.2 Encounter for other antenatal screening follow-up M ♀
Non-visualized anatomy on a previous scan
Z36.3 Encounter for antenatal screening for malformations M ♀
Screening for a suspected anomaly
Z36.4 Encounter for antenatal screening for fetal growth retardation M ♀
Intrauterine growth restriction (IUGR)/small-for-dates
Z36.5 Encounter for antenatal screening for isoimmunization M ♀
✓5th **Z36.8 Encounter for other antenatal screening**
Z36.81 Encounter for antenatal screening for hydrops fetalis M ♀
DEF: Hydrops fetalis: Abnormal accumulation of fluid in two or more parts of the fetus, such as ascites, effusion of the pleural or pericardial tissues, or edema.
Z36.82 Encounter for antenatal screening for nuchal translucency M ♀
Z36.83 Encounter for fetal screening for congenital cardiac abnormalities M ♀
Z36.84 Encounter for antenatal screening for fetal lung maturity M ♀

Z36.85 **Encounter for antenatal screening for Streptococcus B** M ♀

Z36.86 **Encounter for antenatal screening for cervical length** M ♀
Screening for risk of pre-term labor

Z36.87 **Encounter for antenatal screening for uncertain dates** M ♀

Z36.88 **Encounter for antenatal screening for fetal macrosomia** M ♀
Screening for large-for-dates

Z36.89 **Encounter for other specified antenatal screening** M ♀

Z36.8A **Encounter for antenatal screening for other genetic defects** M ♀

Z36.9 **Encounter for antenatal screening, unspecified** M ♀

✓4th **Z3A Weeks of gestation**

NOTE Codes from category Z3A are for use, only on the maternal record, to indicate the weeks of gestation of the pregnancy, if known.

Code first complications of pregnancy, childbirth and the puerperium (OØ9-O9A)

AHA: 2019,2Q,11; 2016,2Q,34; 2014,3Q,17; 2014,2Q,9; 2013,2Q,33

TIP: Do not assign a code from this category with codes from categories O00-O08 or code Z33.2.

✓5th Z3A.Ø **Weeks of gestation of pregnancy, unspecified or less than 1Ø weeks**

Z3A.ØØ **Weeks of gestation of pregnancy not specified** M ♀
Z3A.Ø1 **Less than 8 weeks gestation of pregnancy** M ♀
Z3A.Ø8 **8 weeks gestation of pregnancy** M ♀
Z3A.Ø9 **9 weeks gestation of pregnancy** M ♀

✓5th Z3A.1 **Weeks of gestation of pregnancy, weeks 1Ø-19**

Z3A.1Ø **1Ø weeks gestation of pregnancy** M ♀
Z3A.11 **11 weeks gestation of pregnancy** M ♀
Z3A.12 **12 weeks gestation of pregnancy** M ♀
Z3A.13 **13 weeks gestation of pregnancy** M ♀
Z3A.14 **14 weeks gestation of pregnancy** M ♀
Z3A.15 **15 weeks gestation of pregnancy** M ♀
Z3A.16 **16 weeks gestation of pregnancy** M ♀
Z3A.17 **17 weeks gestation of pregnancy** M ♀
Z3A.18 **18 weeks gestation of pregnancy** M ♀
Z3A.19 **19 weeks gestation of pregnancy** M ♀

✓5th Z3A.2 **Weeks of gestation of pregnancy, weeks 2Ø-29**

Z3A.2Ø **2Ø weeks gestation of pregnancy** M ♀
Z3A.21 **21 weeks gestation of pregnancy** M ♀
Z3A.22 **22 weeks gestation of pregnancy** M ♀
Z3A.23 **23 weeks gestation of pregnancy** M ♀
Z3A.24 **24 weeks gestation of pregnancy** M ♀
Z3A.25 **25 weeks gestation of pregnancy** M ♀
Z3A.26 **26 weeks gestation of pregnancy** M ♀
Z3A.27 **27 weeks gestation of pregnancy** M ♀
Z3A.28 **28 weeks gestation of pregnancy** M ♀
Z3A.29 **29 weeks gestation of pregnancy** M ♀

✓5th Z3A.3 **Weeks of gestation of pregnancy, weeks 3Ø-39**

Z3A.3Ø **3Ø weeks gestation of pregnancy** M ♀
Z3A.31 **31 weeks gestation of pregnancy** M ♀
Z3A.32 **32 weeks gestation of pregnancy** M ♀
Z3A.33 **33 weeks gestation of pregnancy** M ♀
Z3A.34 **34 weeks gestation of pregnancy** M ♀
Z3A.35 **35 weeks gestation of pregnancy** M ♀
Z3A.36 **36 weeks gestation of pregnancy** M ♀
Z3A.37 **37 weeks gestation of pregnancy** M ♀
Z3A.38 **38 weeks gestation of pregnancy** M ♀
Z3A.39 **39 weeks gestation of pregnancy** M ♀

✓5th Z3A.4 **Weeks of gestation of pregnancy, weeks 4Ø or greater**

AHA: 2014,4Q,23

Z3A.4Ø **4Ø weeks gestation of pregnancy** M ♀
Z3A.41 **41 weeks gestation of pregnancy** M ♀
Z3A.42 **42 weeks gestation of pregnancy** M ♀
Z3A.49 **Greater than 42 weeks gestation of pregnancy** M ♀

✓4th **Z37 Outcome of delivery**

This category is intended for use as an additional code to identify the outcome of delivery on the mother's record. It is not for use on the newborn record.

EXCLUDES 1 *stillbirth (P95)*

Z37.Ø **Single live birth** M ♀
AHA: 2016,2Q,34; 2014,2Q,9

Z37.1 **Single stillbirth** M ♀
Z37.2 **Twins, both liveborn** M ♀
Z37.3 **Twins, one liveborn and one stillborn** M ♀
Z37.4 **Twins, both stillborn** M ♀

✓5th Z37.5 **Other multiple births, all liveborn**

Z37.5Ø **Multiple births, unspecified, all liveborn** M ♀
Z37.51 **Triplets, all liveborn** M ♀
Z37.52 **Quadruplets, all liveborn** M ♀
Z37.53 **Quintuplets, all liveborn** M ♀
Z37.54 **Sextuplets, all liveborn** M ♀
Z37.59 **Other multiple births, all liveborn** M ♀

✓5th Z37.6 **Other multiple births, some liveborn**

Z37.6Ø **Multiple births, unspecified, some liveborn** M ♀
Z37.61 **Triplets, some liveborn** M ♀
Z37.62 **Quadruplets, some liveborn** M ♀
Z37.63 **Quintuplets, some liveborn** M ♀
Z37.64 **Sextuplets, some liveborn** M ♀
Z37.69 **Other multiple births, some liveborn** M ♀

Z37.7 **Other multiple births, all stillborn** M ♀

Z37.9 **Outcome of delivery, unspecified** M ♀
Multiple birth NOS
Single birth NOS

✓4th **Z38 Liveborn infants according to place of birth and type of delivery**

This category is for use as the principal code on the initial record of a newborn baby. It is to be used for the initial birth record only. It is not to be used on the mother's record.

AHA: 2020,2Q,13; 2017,2Q,5-7; 2016,3Q,18; 2015,2Q,15

✓5th Z38.Ø **Single liveborn infant, born in hospital**
Single liveborn infant, born in birthing center or other health care facility

Z38.ØØ **Single liveborn infant, delivered vaginally** N
Z38.Ø1 **Single liveborn infant, delivered by cesarean** N

Z38.1 **Single liveborn infant, born outside hospital** N

Z38.2 **Single liveborn infant, unspecified as to place of birth** N
Single liveborn infant NOS

✓5th Z38.3 **Twin liveborn infant, born in hospital**

Z38.3Ø **Twin liveborn infant, delivered vaginally** N
Z38.31 **Twin liveborn infant, delivered by cesarean** N

Z38.4 **Twin liveborn infant, born outside hospital** N

Z38.5 **Twin liveborn infant, unspecified as to place of birth** N

✓5th Z38.6 **Other multiple liveborn infant, born in hospital**

Z38.61 **Triplet liveborn infant, delivered vaginally** N
Z38.62 **Triplet liveborn infant, delivered by cesarean** N
Z38.63 **Quadruplet liveborn infant, delivered vaginally** N
Z38.64 **Quadruplet liveborn infant, delivered by cesarean** N
Z38.65 **Quintuplet liveborn infant, delivered vaginally** N
Z38.66 **Quintuplet liveborn infant, delivered by cesarean** N
Z38.68 **Other multiple liveborn infant, delivered vaginally** N
Z38.69 **Other multiple liveborn infant, delivered by cesarean** N

Z38.7 **Other multiple liveborn infant, born outside hospital** N

Z38.8 **Other multiple liveborn infant, unspecified as to place of birth** N

✓4th **Z39 Encounter for maternal postpartum care and examination**

Z39.Ø **Encounter for care and examination of mother immediately after delivery** M ♀
Care and observation in uncomplicated cases when the delivery occurs outside a healthcare facility

EXCLUDES 1 *care for postpartum complication — see Alphabetic Index*

Z39.1 Encounter for care and examination of lactating mother M ♀
Encounter for supervision of lactation
EXCLUDES 1 *disorders of lactation (O92.-)*

Z39.2 Encounter for routine postpartum follow-up M ♀

Encounters for other specific health care (Z40-Z53)

Categories Z40-Z53 are intended for use to indicate a reason for care. They may be used for patients who have already been treated for a disease or injury, but who are receiving aftercare or prophylactic care, or care to consolidate the treatment, or to deal with a residual state

EXCLUDES 2 *follow-up examination for medical surveillance after treatment (Z08-Z09)*

✓4th **Z40 Encounter for prophylactic surgery**
EXCLUDES 1 *organ donations (Z52.-)*
therapeutic organ removal — code to condition
DEF: Agent or treatment measure intended to prevent or ward off a disease condition.

✓5th **Z40.0 Encounter for prophylactic surgery for risk factors related to malignant neoplasms**
Admission for prophylactic organ removal
Use additional code to identify risk factor
AHA: 2017,4Q,28-29

Z40.00 Encounter for prophylactic removal of unspecified organ
Z40.01 Encounter for prophylactic removal of breast
Z40.02 Encounter for prophylactic removal of ovary(s) ♀
Encounter for prophylactic removal of ovary(s) and fallopian tube(s)
Z40.03 Encounter for prophylactic removal of fallopian tube(s) ♀
Z40.09 Encounter for prophylactic removal of other organ

Z40.8 Encounter for other prophylactic surgery
Z40.9 Encounter for prophylactic surgery, unspecified

✓4th **Z41 Encounter for procedures for purposes other than remedying health state**

Z41.1 Encounter for cosmetic surgery
Encounter for cosmetic breast implant
Encounter for cosmetic procedure
EXCLUDES 1 *encounter for plastic and reconstructive surgery following medical procedure or healed injury (Z42.-)*
encounter for post-mastectomy breast implantation (Z42.1)

Z41.2 Encounter for routine and ritual male circumcision ♂
AHA: 2018,3Q,15
TIP: Do not report this code when circumcision is performed during the birth admission.

Z41.3 Encounter for ear piercing
Z41.8 Encounter for other procedures for purposes other than remedying health state
Z41.9 Encounter for procedure for purposes other than remedying health state, unspecified

✓4th **Z42 Encounter for plastic and reconstructive surgery following medical procedure or healed injury**
EXCLUDES 1 *encounter for cosmetic plastic surgery (Z41.1)*
encounter for plastic surgery for treatment of current injury — code to relevent injury

Z42.1 Encounter for breast reconstruction following mastectomy A
EXCLUDES 1 *deformity and disproportion of reconstructed breast (N65.1-)*

Z42.8 Encounter for other plastic and reconstructive surgery following medical procedure or healed injury
AHA: 2017,1Q,42

✓4th **Z43 Encounter for attention to artificial openings**
INCLUDES closure of artificial openings
passage of sounds or bougies through artificial openings
reforming artificial openings
removal of catheter from artificial openings
toilet or cleansing of artificial openings
EXCLUDES 1 *complications of external stoma (J95.0-, K94.-, N99.5-)*
EXCLUDES 2 *fitting and adjustment of prosthetic and other devices (Z44-Z46)*
AHA: 2019,2Q,33

Z43.0 Encounter for attention to tracheostomy HCC
Z43.1 Encounter for attention to gastrostomy CC HCC
EXCLUDES 2 *artificial opening status only, without need for care (Z93.-)*
Z43.2 Encounter for attention to ileostomy HCC
Z43.3 Encounter for attention to colostomy HCC
Z43.4 Encounter for attention to other artificial openings of digestive tract HCC
Z43.5 Encounter for attention to cystostomy HCC
Z43.6 Encounter for attention to other artificial openings of urinary tract HCC
Encounter for attention to nephrostomy
Encounter for attention to ureterostomy
Encounter for attention to urethrostomy
Z43.7 Encounter for attention to artificial vagina
Z43.8 Encounter for attention to other artificial openings HCC
Z43.9 Encounter for attention to unspecified artificial opening HCC

✓4th **Z44 Encounter for fitting and adjustment of external prosthetic device**
INCLUDES removal or replacement of external prosthetic device
EXCLUDES 1 *malfunction or other complications of device — see Alphabetical Index*
presence of prosthetic device (Z97.-)

✓5th **Z44.0 Encounter for fitting and adjustment of artificial arm**

✓6th **Z44.00 Encounter for fitting and adjustment of unspecified artificial arm**
Z44.001 Encounter for fitting and adjustment of unspecified right artificial arm
Z44.002 Encounter for fitting and adjustment of unspecified left artificial arm
Z44.009 Encounter for fitting and adjustment of unspecified artificial arm, unspecified arm

✓6th **Z44.01 Encounter for fitting and adjustment of complete artificial arm**
Z44.011 Encounter for fitting and adjustment of complete right artificial arm
Z44.012 Encounter for fitting and adjustment of complete left artificial arm
Z44.019 Encounter for fitting and adjustment of complete artificial arm, unspecified arm

✓6th **Z44.02 Encounter for fitting and adjustment of partial artificial arm**
Z44.021 Encounter for fitting and adjustment of partial artificial right arm
Z44.022 Encounter for fitting and adjustment of partial artificial left arm
Z44.029 Encounter for fitting and adjustment of partial artificial arm, unspecified arm

✓5th **Z44.1 Encounter for fitting and adjustment of artificial leg**

✓6th **Z44.10 Encounter for fitting and adjustment of unspecified artificial leg**
Z44.101 Encounter for fitting and adjustment of unspecified right artificial leg HCC
Z44.102 Encounter for fitting and adjustment of unspecified left artificial leg HCC
Z44.109 Encounter for fitting and adjustment of unspecified artificial leg, unspecified leg HCC

✓6th **Z44.11 Encounter for fitting and adjustment of complete artificial leg**
Z44.111 Encounter for fitting and adjustment of complete right artificial leg HCC
Z44.112 Encounter for fitting and adjustment of complete left artificial leg HCC
Z44.119 Encounter for fitting and adjustment of complete artificial leg, unspecified leg HCC

✓6th **Z44.12 Encounter for fitting and adjustment of partial artificial leg**
Z44.121 Encounter for fitting and adjustment of partial artificial right leg HCC
Z44.122 Encounter for fitting and adjustment of partial artificial left leg HCC
Z44.129 Encounter for fitting and adjustment of partial artificial leg, unspecified leg HCC

✓5th **Z44.2 Encounter for fitting and adjustment of artificial eye**
EXCLUDES 1 *mechanical complication of ocular prosthesis (T85.3)*
Z44.20 Encounter for fitting and adjustment of artificial eye, unspecified
Z44.21 Encounter for fitting and adjustment of artificial right eye
Z44.22 Encounter for fitting and adjustment of artificial left eye

✓5th **Z44.3 Encounter for fitting and adjustment of external breast prosthesis**
EXCLUDES 1 *complications of breast implant (T85.4-)*
encounter for adjustment or removal of breast implant (Z45.81-)
encounter for initial breast implant insertion for cosmetic breast augmentation (Z41.1)
encounter for breast reconstruction following mastectomy (Z42.1)
Z44.30 Encounter for fitting and adjustment of external breast prosthesis, unspecified breast
Z44.31 Encounter for fitting and adjustment of external right breast prosthesis
Z44.32 Encounter for fitting and adjustment of external left breast prosthesis

Z44.8 Encounter for fitting and adjustment of other external prosthetic devices

Z44.9 Encounter for fitting and adjustment of unspecified external prosthetic device

✓4th **Z45 Encounter for adjustment and management of implanted device**
INCLUDES removal or replacement of implanted device
EXCLUDES 1 *malfunction or other complications of device — see Alphabetical Index*
EXCLUDES 2 *encounter for fitting and adjustment of non-implanted device (Z46.-)*

✓5th **Z45.0 Encounter for adjustment and management of cardiac device**
✓6th **Z45.01 Encounter for adjustment and management of cardiac pacemaker**
Encounter for adjustment and management of cardiac resynchronization therapy pacemaker (CRT-P)
EXCLUDES 1 *encounter for adjustment and management of automatic implantable cardiac defibrillator with synchronous cardiac pacemaker (Z45.02)*
TIP: Assign an additional code for the condition the pacemaker is controlling (e.g., sick sinus syndrome). Even though the pacemaker controls the heart rate, it does not cure the sick sinus syndrome; it is still present and a reportable chronic condition.
Z45.010 Encounter for checking and testing of cardiac pacemaker pulse generator [battery]
Encounter for replacing cardiac pacemaker pulse generator [battery]
Z45.018 Encounter for adjustment and management of other part of cardiac pacemaker
EXCLUDES 1 *presence of other part of cardiac pacemaker (Z95.0)*
EXCLUDES 2 *presence of prosthetic and other devices (Z95.1-Z95.5, Z95.811-Z97)*
Z45.02 Encounter for adjustment and management of automatic implantable cardiac defibrillator
Encounter for adjustment and management of automatic implantable cardiac defibrillator with synchronous cardiac pacemaker
Encounter for adjustment and management of cardiac resynchronization therapy defibrillator (CRT-D)
Z45.09 Encounter for adjustment and management of other cardiac device

Z45.1 Encounter for adjustment and management of infusion pump

Z45.2 Encounter for adjustment and management of vascular access device
Encounter for adjustment and management of vascular catheters
EXCLUDES 1 *encounter for adjustment and management of renal dialysis catheter (Z49.01)*
AHA: 2020,2Q,21; 2018,3Q,20

✓5th **Z45.3 Encounter for adjustment and management of implanted devices of the special senses**
Z45.31 Encounter for adjustment and management of implanted visual substitution device
✓6th **Z45.32 Encounter for adjustment and management of implanted hearing device**
EXCLUDES 1 *encounter for fitting and adjustment of hearing aide (Z46.1)*
Z45.320 Encounter for adjustment and management of bone conduction device
Z45.321 Encounter for adjustment and management of cochlear device
Z45.328 Encounter for adjustment and management of other implanted hearing device

✓5th **Z45.4 Encounter for adjustment and management of implanted nervous system device**
Z45.41 Encounter for adjustment and management of cerebrospinal fluid drainage device
Encounter for adjustment and management of cerebral ventricular (communicating) shunt
Z45.42 Encounter for adjustment and management of neurostimulator
Encounter for adjustment and management of brain neurostimulator
Encounter for adjustment and management of gastric neurostimulator
Encounter for adjustment and management of peripheral nerve neurostimulator
Encounter for adjustment and management of sacral nerve neurostimulator
Encounter for adjustment and management of spinal cord neurostimulator
Encounter for adjustment and management of vagus nerve neurostimulator
Z45.49 Encounter for adjustment and management of other implanted nervous system device
AHA: 2014,3Q,19

✓5th **Z45.8 Encounter for adjustment and management of other implanted devices**
✓6th **Z45.81 Encounter for adjustment or removal of breast implant**
Encounter for elective implant exchange (different material) (different size)
Encounter removal of tissue expander with or without synchronous insertion of permanent implant
EXCLUDES 1 *complications of breast implant (T85.4-)*
encounter for initial breast implant insertion for cosmetic breast augmentation (Z41.1)
encounter for breast reconstruction following mastectomy (Z42.1)
Z45.811 Encounter for adjustment or removal of right breast implant
Z45.812 Encounter for adjustment or removal of left breast implant
Z45.819 Encounter for adjustment or removal of unspecified breast implant
Z45.82 Encounter for adjustment or removal of myringotomy device (stent) (tube)
Z45.89 Encounter for adjustment and management of other implanted devices
AHA: 2014,4Q,26-28

Z45.9 Encounter for adjustment and management of unspecified implanted device

Z46 Encounter for fitting and adjustment of other devices

INCLUDES removal or replacement of other device

EXCLUDES 1 *malfunction or other complications of device — see Alphabetical Index*

EXCLUDES 2 *encounter for fitting and management of implanted devices (Z45.-)*
issue of repeat prescription only (Z76.Ø)
presence of prosthetic and other devices (Z95-Z97)

Z46.Ø Encounter for fitting and adjustment of spectacles and contact lenses

Z46.1 Encounter for fitting and adjustment of hearing aid
EXCLUDES 1 *encounter for adjustment and management of implanted hearing device (Z45.32-)*

Z46.2 Encounter for fitting and adjustment of other devices related to nervous system and special senses
EXCLUDES 2 *encounter for adjustment and management of implanted nervous system device (Z45.4-)*
encounter for adjustment and management of implanted visual substitution device (Z45.31)

Z46.3 Encounter for fitting and adjustment of dental prosthetic device
Encounter for fitting and adjustment of dentures

Z46.4 Encounter for fitting and adjustment of orthodontic device

Z46.5 Encounter for fitting and adjustment of other gastrointestinal appliance and device
EXCLUDES 1 *encounter for attention to artificial openings of digestive tract (Z43.1-Z43.4)*

Z46.51 Encounter for fitting and adjustment of gastric lap band

Z46.59 Encounter for fitting and adjustment of other gastrointestinal appliance and device

Z46.6 Encounter for fitting and adjustment of urinary device
EXCLUDES 2 *attention to artificial openings of urinary tract (Z43.5, Z43.6)*

Z46.8 Encounter for fitting and adjustment of other specified devices

Z46.81 Encounter for fitting and adjustment of insulin pump
Encounter for insulin pump instruction and training
Encounter for insulin pump titration

Z46.82 Encounter for fitting and adjustment of non-vascular catheter

Z46.89 Encounter for fitting and adjustment of other specified devices
Encounter for fitting and adjustment of wheelchair

Z46.9 Encounter for fitting and adjustment of unspecified device

Z47 Orthopedic aftercare

EXCLUDES 1 *aftercare for healing fracture — code to fracture with 7th character D*

Z47.1 Aftercare following joint replacement surgery
Use additional code to identify the joint (Z96.6-)
AHA: 2020,1Q,23

Z47.2 Encounter for removal of internal fixation device
EXCLUDES 1 *encounter for adjustment of internal fixation device for fracture treatment — code to fracture with appropriate 7th character*
encounter for removal of external fixation device — code to fracture with 7th character D
infection or inflammatory reaction to internal fixation device (T84.6-)
mechanical complication of internal fixation device (T84.1-)

Z47.3 Aftercare following explantation of joint prosthesis
Aftercare following explantation of joint prosthesis, staged procedure
Encounter for joint prosthesis insertion following prior explantation of joint prosthesis
AHA: 2020,1Q,23; 2015,1Q,16

Z47.31 Aftercare following explantation of shoulder joint prosthesis
EXCLUDES 1 *acquired absence of shoulder joint following prior explantation of shoulder joint prosthesis (Z89.23-)*
shoulder joint prosthesis explantation status (Z89.23-)

Z47.32 Aftercare following explantation of hip joint prosthesis
EXCLUDES 1 *acquired absence of hip joint following prior explantation of hip joint prosthesis (Z89.62-)*
hip joint prosthesis explantation status (Z89.62-)

Z47.33 Aftercare following explantation of knee joint prosthesis
EXCLUDES 1 *acquired absence of knee joint following prior explantation of knee prosthesis (Z89.52-)*
knee joint prosthesis explantation status (Z89.52-)

Z47.8 Encounter for other orthopedic aftercare

Z47.81 Encounter for orthopedic aftercare following surgical amputation
Use additional code to identify the limb amputated (Z89.-)

Z47.82 Encounter for orthopedic aftercare following scoliosis surgery

Z47.89 Encounter for other orthopedic aftercare
AHA: 2015,1Q,8

Z48 Encounter for other postprocedural aftercare

EXCLUDES 1 *encounter for aftercare following injury — code to Injury, by site, with appropriate 7th character for subsequent encounter*
encounter for follow-up examination after completed treatment (Z08-Z09)

EXCLUDES 2 *encounter for attention to artificial openings (Z43.-)*
encounter for fitting and adjustment of prosthetic and other devices (Z44-Z46)

AHA: 2015,4Q,38; 2015,1Q,6-7

Z48.Ø Encounter for attention to dressings, sutures and drains
EXCLUDES 1 *encounter for planned postprocedural wound closure (Z48.1)*

Z48.ØØ Encounter for change or removal of nonsurgical wound dressing
Encounter for change or removal of wound dressing NOS

Z48.Ø1 Encounter for change or removal of surgical wound dressing
AHA: 2019,2Q,33

Z48.Ø2 Encounter for removal of sutures
Encounter for removal of staples

Z48.Ø3 Encounter for change or removal of drains
AHA: 2019,2Q,33

Z48.1 Encounter for planned postprocedural wound closure
EXCLUDES 1 *encounter for attention to dressings and sutures (Z48.Ø-)*

Z48.2 Encounter for aftercare following organ transplant

Z48.21 Encounter for aftercare following heart transplant CC HCC

Z48.22 Encounter for aftercare following kidney transplant CC

Z48.23 Encounter for aftercare following liver transplant CC HCC

Z48.24 Encounter for aftercare following lung transplant CC HCC

Z48.28 Encounter for aftercare following multiple organ transplant

Z48.28Ø Encounter for aftercare following heart-lung transplant CC HCC

Z48.288 Encounter for aftercare following multiple organ transplant

Z48.29 Encounter for aftercare following other organ transplant

Z48.29Ø Encounter for aftercare following bone marrow transplant CC HCC

Z48.298 Encounter for aftercare following other organ transplant

Z48.3 Aftercare following surgery for neoplasm
Use additional code to identify the neoplasm

✓5th **Z48.8 Encounter for other specified postprocedural aftercare**

✓6th **Z48.81 Encounter for surgical aftercare following surgery on specified body systems**

These codes identify the body system requiring aftercare. They are for use in conjunction with other aftercare codes to fully explain the aftercare encounter. The condition treated should also be coded if still present.

EXCLUDES 1 *aftercare for injury — code the injury with 7th character D*

aftercare following surgery for neoplasm (Z48.3)

EXCLUDES 2 *aftercare following organ transplant (Z48.2-)*

orthopedic aftercare (Z47.-)

AHA: 2015,4Q,38

Z48.810 Encounter for surgical aftercare following surgery on the sense organs

Z48.811 Encounter for surgical aftercare following surgery on the nervous system

EXCLUDES 2 *encounter for surgical aftercare following surgery on the sense organs (Z48.810)*

Z48.812 Encounter for surgical aftercare following surgery on the circulatory system

AHA: 2012,4Q,96

Z48.813 Encounter for surgical aftercare following surgery on the respiratory system

AHA: 2019,2Q,33

Z48.814 Encounter for surgical aftercare following surgery on the teeth or oral cavity

Z48.815 Encounter for surgical aftercare following surgery on the digestive system

Z48.816 Encounter for surgical aftercare following surgery on the genitourinary system

EXCLUDES 1 *encounter for aftercare following sterilization reversal (Z31.42)*

Z48.817 Encounter for surgical aftercare following surgery on the skin and subcutaneous tissue

Z48.89 Encounter for other specified surgical aftercare

✓4th **Z49 Encounter for care involving renal dialysis**

Code also associated end stage renal disease (N18.6)

✓5th **Z49.0 Preparatory care for renal dialysis**

Encounter for dialysis instruction and training

Z49.01 Encounter for fitting and adjustment of extracorporeal dialysis catheter HCC

Removal or replacement of renal dialysis catheter

Toilet or cleansing of renal dialysis catheter

Z49.02 Encounter for fitting and adjustment of peritoneal dialysis catheter HCC

✓5th **Z49.3 Encounter for adequacy testing for dialysis**

Z49.31 Encounter for adequacy testing for hemodialysis HCC

Z49.32 Encounter for adequacy testing for peritoneal dialysis HCC

Encounter for peritoneal equilibration test

✓4th **Z51 Encounter for other aftercare and medical care**

Code also condition requiring care

EXCLUDES 1 *follow-up examination after treatment (Z08-Z09)*

Z51.0 Encounter for antineoplastic radiation therapy

AHA: 2017,4Q,103

TIP: Do not assign when admission is for insertion/implantation of radioactive elements. Assign a code for the malignancy instead. Any complications related to the radioactive elements should be assigned as secondary diagnoses.

✓5th **Z51.1 Encounter for antineoplastic chemotherapy and immunotherapy**

EXCLUDES 2 *encounter for chemotherapy and immunotherapy for nonneoplastic condition — code to condition*

Z51.11 Encounter for antineoplastic chemotherapy

AHA: 2015,3Q,19

Z51.12 Encounter for antineoplastic immunotherapy

Z51.5 Encounter for palliative care

AHA: 2017,1Q,48

Z51.6 Encounter for desensitization to allergens

AHA: 2016,4Q,77

✓5th **Z51.8 Encounter for other specified aftercare**

EXCLUDES 1 *holiday relief care (Z75.5)*

Z51.81 Encounter for therapeutic drug level monitoring

Code also any long-term (current) drug therapy (Z79.-)

EXCLUDES 1 *encounter for blood-drug test for administrative or medicolegal reasons (Z02.83)*

DEF: Drug monitoring: Measurement of the level of a specific drug in the body or measurement of a specific function to assess effectiveness of a drug.

Z51.89 Encounter for other specified aftercare

AHA: 2012,4Q,95-97

✓4th **Z52 Donors of organs and tissues**

INCLUDES autologous and other living donors

EXCLUDES 1 *cadaveric donor - omit code*

examination of potential donor (Z00.5)

AHA: 2012,4Q,99

✓5th **Z52.0 Blood donor**

✓6th **Z52.00 Unspecified blood donor**

Z52.000 Unspecified donor, whole blood

Z52.001 Unspecified donor, stem cells

Z52.008 Unspecified donor, other blood

✓6th **Z52.01 Autologous blood donor**

Z52.010 Autologous donor, whole blood

Z52.011 Autologous donor, stem cells

Z52.018 Autologous donor, other blood

✓6th **Z52.09 Other blood donor**

Volunteer donor

Z52.090 Other blood donor, whole blood

Z52.091 Other blood donor, stem cells

Z52.098 Other blood donor, other blood

✓5th **Z52.1 Skin donor**

Z52.10 Skin donor, unspecified

Z52.11 Skin donor, autologous

Z52.19 Skin donor, other

✓5th **Z52.2 Bone donor**

Z52.20 Bone donor, unspecified

Z52.21 Bone donor, autologous

Z52.29 Bone donor, other

Z52.3 Bone marrow donor

Z52.4 Kidney donor

Z52.5 Cornea donor

Z52.6 Liver donor

✓5th **Z52.8 Donor of other specified organs or tissues**

✓6th **Z52.81 Egg (Oocyte) donor**

Z52.810 Egg (Oocyte) donor under age 35, anonymous recipient ♀

Egg donor under age 35 NOS

Z52.811 Egg (Oocyte) donor under age 35, designated recipient ♀

Z52.812 Egg (Oocyte) donor age 35 and over, anonymous recipient ♀

Egg donor age 35 and over NOS

Z52.813 Egg (Oocyte) donor age 35 and over, designated recipient ♀

Z52.819 Egg (Oocyte) donor, unspecified ♀

Z52.89 Donor of other specified organs or tissues

Z52.9 Donor of unspecified organ or tissue

Donor NOS

✓4th **Z53 Persons encountering health services for specific procedures and treatment, not carried out**

✓5th **Z53.0 Procedure and treatment not carried out because of contraindication**

Z53.01 Procedure and treatment not carried out due to patient smoking

Z53.09 Procedure and treatment not carried out because of other contraindication

Z53.1 Procedure and treatment not carried out because of patient's decision for reasons of belief and group pressure

✓5th **Z53.2 Procedure and treatment not carried out because of patient's decision for other and unspecified reasons**

Z53.20 Procedure and treatment not carried out because of patient's decision for unspecified reasons

Z53.21 **Procedure and treatment not carried out due to patient leaving prior to being seen by health care provider**

Z53.29 **Procedure and treatment not carried out because of patient's decision for other reasons**

✓5th Z53.3 **Procedure converted to open procedure**

AHA: 2016,4Q,79

Z53.31 **Laparoscopic surgical procedure converted to open procedure**

Z53.32 **Thoracoscopic surgical procedure converted to open procedure**

Z53.33 **Arthroscopic surgical procedure converted to open procedure**

Z53.39 **Other specified procedure converted to open procedure**

Z53.8 **Procedure and treatment not carried out for other reasons**

Z53.9 **Procedure and treatment not carried out, unspecified reason**

Persons with potential health hazards related to socioeconomic and psychosocial circumstances (Z55-Z65)

AHA: 2019,4Q,66; 2018,4Q,58,73; 2018,1Q,18

TIP: Codes from this code block can be assigned based on documentation from clinicians other than the diagnosing provider.

✓4th **Z55 Problems related to education and literacy**

EXCLUDES 1 *disorders of psychological development (F80-F89)*

Z55.0 **Illiteracy and low-level literacy**

Z55.1 **Schooling unavailable and unattainable**

Z55.2 **Failed school examinations**

Z55.3 **Underachievement in school**

Z55.4 **Educational maladjustment and discord with teachers and classmates**

Z55.8 **Other problems related to education and literacy**

Problems related to inadequate teaching

Z55.9 **Problems related to education and literacy, unspecified**

Academic problems NOS

✓4th **Z56 Problems related to employment and unemployment**

EXCLUDES 2 *occupational exposure to risk factors (Z57.-)*
problems related to housing and economic circumstances (Z59.-)

Z56.0 **Unemployment, unspecified**

Z56.1 **Change of job** A

Z56.2 **Threat of job loss**

Z56.3 **Stressful work schedule**

Z56.4 **Discord with boss and workmates**

Z56.5 **Uncongenial work environment**

Difficult conditions at work

Z56.6 **Other physical and mental strain related to work**

✓5th Z56.8 **Other problems related to employment**

Z56.81 **Sexual harassment on the job**

Z56.82 **Military deployment status**

Individual (civilian or military) currently deployed in theater or in support of military war, peacekeeping and humanitarian operations

Z56.89 **Other problems related to employment**

Z56.9 **Unspecified problems related to employment**

Occupational problems NOS

✓4th **Z57 Occupational exposure to risk factors**

Z57.0 **Occupational exposure to noise**

Z57.1 **Occupational exposure to radiation**

Z57.2 **Occupational exposure to dust**

✓5th Z57.3 **Occupational exposure to other air contaminants**

Z57.31 **Occupational exposure to environmental tobacco smoke**

EXCLUDES 2 *exposure to environmental tobacco smoke (Z77.22)*

Z57.39 **Occupational exposure to other air contaminants**

Z57.4 **Occupational exposure to toxic agents in agriculture**

Occupational exposure to solids, liquids, gases or vapors in agriculture

Z57.5 **Occupational exposure to toxic agents in other industries**

Occupational exposure to solids, liquids, gases or vapors in other industries

Z57.6 **Occupational exposure to extreme temperature**

Z57.7 **Occupational exposure to vibration**

Z57.8 **Occupational exposure to other risk factors**

Z57.9 **Occupational exposure to unspecified risk factor**

✓4th **Z59 Problems related to housing and economic circumstances**

EXCLUDES 2 *problems related to upbringing (Z62.-)*

Z59.0 **Homelessness**

Z59.1 **Inadequate housing**

Lack of heating
Restriction of space
Technical defects in home preventing adequate care
Unsatisfactory surroundings

EXCLUDES 1 *problems related to the natural and physical environment (Z77.1-)*

Z59.2 **Discord with neighbors, lodgers and landlord**

Z59.3 **Problems related to living in residential institution**

Boarding-school resident

EXCLUDES 1 *institutional upbringing (Z62.2)*

Z59.4 **Lack of adequate food and safe drinking water**

Inadequate drinking water supply

EXCLUDES 1 *effects of hunger (T73.0)*
inappropriate diet or eating habits (Z72.4)
malnutrition (E40-E46)

Z59.5 **Extreme poverty**

Z59.6 **Low income**

Z59.7 **Insufficient social insurance and welfare support**

Z59.8 **Other problems related to housing and economic circumstances**

Foreclosure on loan
Isolated dwelling
Problems with creditors

Z59.9 **Problem related to housing and economic circumstances, unspecified**

✓4th **Z60 Problems related to social environment**

Z60.0 **Problems of adjustment to life-cycle transitions**

Empty nest syndrome
Phase of life problem
Problem with adjustment to retirement [pension]

Z60.2 **Problems related to living alone**

Z60.3 **Acculturation difficulty**

Problem with migration
Problem with social transplantation

DEF: Problem adapting to a different culture or environment not based on any coexisting mental disorder.

Z60.4 **Social exclusion and rejection**

Exclusion and rejection on the basis of personal characteristics, such as unusual physical appearance, illness or behavior.

EXCLUDES 1 *target of adverse discrimination such as for racial or religious reasons (Z60.5)*

Z60.5 **Target of (perceived) adverse discrimination and persecution**

EXCLUDES 1 *social exclusion and rejection (Z60.4)*

Z60.8 **Other problems related to social environment**

Z60.9 **Problem related to social environment, unspecified**

✓4th **Z62 Problems related to upbringing**

INCLUDES current and past negative life events in childhood
current and past problems of a child related to upbringing

EXCLUDES 2 *maltreatment syndrome (T74.-)*
problems related to housing and economic circumstances (Z59.-)

Z62.0 **Inadequate parental supervision and control**

Z62.1 **Parental overprotection**

✓5th Z62.2 **Upbringing away from parents**

EXCLUDES 1 *problems with boarding school (Z59.3)*

Z62.21 **Child in welfare custody** P

Child in care of non-parental family member
Child in foster care

EXCLUDES 2 *problem for parent due to child in welfare custody (Z63.5)*

Z62.22 **Institutional upbringing**

Child living in orphanage or group home

Z62.29 **Other upbringing away from parents**

Z62.3 **Hostility towards and scapegoating of child** P

Z62.6 **Inappropriate (excessive) parental pressure**

Z62.8 Other specified problems related to upbringing

Z62.81 Personal history of abuse in childhood

Z62.810 Personal history of physical and sexual abuse in childhood

EXCLUDES 1 *current child physical abuse (T74.12, T76.12)*
current child sexual abuse (T74.22, T76.22)

Z62.811 Personal history of psychological abuse in childhood

EXCLUDES 1 *current child psychological abuse (T74.32, T76.32)*

Z62.812 Personal history of neglect in childhood

EXCLUDES 1 *current child neglect (T74.02, T76.02)*

Z62.813 Personal history of forced labor or sexual exploitation in childhood

AHA: 2018,4Q,32,35

Z62.819 Personal history of unspecified abuse in childhood

EXCLUDES 1 *current child abuse NOS (T74.92, T76.92)*

Z62.82 Parent-child conflict

Z62.820 Parent-biological child conflict
Parent-child problem NOS

Z62.821 Parent-adopted child conflict

Z62.822 Parent-foster child conflict

Z62.89 Other specified problems related to upbringing

Z62.890 Parent-child estrangement NEC

Z62.891 Sibling rivalry

Z62.898 Other specified problems related to upbringing

Z62.9 Problem related to upbringing, unspecified

Z63 Other problems related to primary support group, including family circumstances

EXCLUDES 2 *maltreatment syndrome (T74.-, T76)*
parent-child problems (Z62.-)
problems related to negative life events in childhood (Z62.-)
problems related to upbringing (Z62.-)

Z63.0 Problems in relationship with spouse or partner
Relationship distress with spouse or intimate partner

EXCLUDES 1 *counseling for spousal or partner abuse problems (Z69.1)*
counseling related to sexual attitude, behavior, and orientation (Z70.-)

Z63.1 Problems in relationship with in-laws

Z63.3 Absence of family member

EXCLUDES 1 *absence of family member due to disappearance and death (Z63.4)*
absence of family member due to separation and divorce (Z63.5)

Z63.31 Absence of family member due to military deployment
Individual or family affected by other family member being on military deployment

EXCLUDES 1 *family disruption due to return of family member from military deployment (Z63.71)*

Z63.32 Other absence of family member

Z63.4 Disappearance and death of family member
Assumed death of family member
Bereavement
AHA: 2014,1Q,25

Z63.5 Disruption of family by separation and divorce
Marital estrangement

Z63.6 Dependent relative needing care at home

Z63.7 Other stressful life events affecting family and household

Z63.71 Stress on family due to return of family member from military deployment
Individual or family affected by family member having returned from military deployment (current or past conflict)

Z63.72 Alcoholism and drug addiction in family

Z63.79 Other stressful life events affecting family and household
Anxiety (normal) about sick person in family
Health problems within family
Ill or disturbed family member
Isolated family

Z63.8 Other specified problems related to primary support group
Family discord NOS
Family estrangement NOS
High expressed emotional level within family
Inadequate family support NOS
Inadequate or distorted communication within family

Z63.9 Problem related to primary support group, unspecified
Relationship disorder NOS

Z64 Problems related to certain psychosocial circumstances

Z64.0 Problems related to unwanted pregnancy ♀

Z64.1 Problems related to multiparity ♀

Z64.4 Discord with counselors
Discord with probation officer
Discord with social worker

Z65 Problems related to other psychosocial circumstances

Z65.0 Conviction in civil and criminal proceedings without imprisonment

Z65.1 Imprisonment and other incarceration

Z65.2 Problems related to release from prison

Z65.3 Problems related to other legal circumstances
Arrest
Child custody or support proceedings
Litigation
Prosecution

Z65.4 Victim of crime and terrorism
Victim of torture

Z65.5 Exposure to disaster, war and other hostilities

EXCLUDES 1 *target of perceived discrimination or persecution (Z60.5)*

Z65.8 Other specified problems related to psychosocial circumstances
Religious or spiritual problem

Z65.9 Problem related to unspecified psychosocial circumstances

Do not resuscitate status (Z66)

Z66 Do not resuscitate
DNR status
DEF: Medical order written by a physician that instructs others not to perform cardiopulmonary resuscitation (CPR), intubation, or advanced life support (ACLS). It prevents unnecessary invasive treatment to prolong life should breathing stop or cardiac arrest occur.

Blood type (Z67)

Z67 Blood type
AHA: 2015,3Q,40

Blood Types

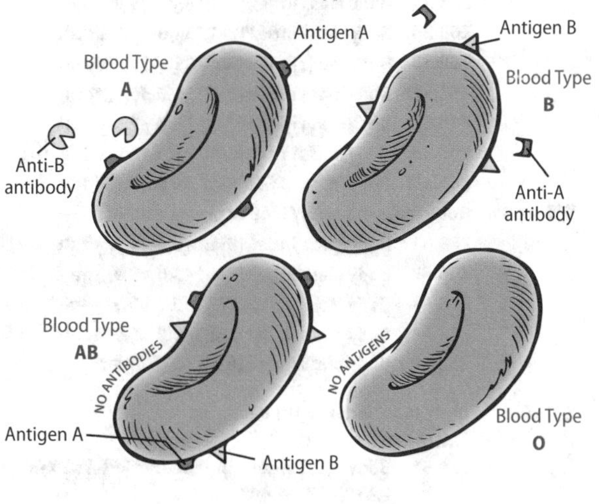

Z67.1 Type A blood

Z67.10 Type A blood, Rh positive

Z67.11 **Type A blood, Rh negative**

✓5th **Z67.2 Type B blood**

Z67.20 **Type B blood, Rh positive**

Z67.21 **Type B blood, Rh negative**

✓5th **Z67.3 Type AB blood**

Z67.30 **Type AB blood, Rh positive**

Z67.31 **Type AB blood, Rh negative**

✓5th **Z67.4 Type O blood**

Z67.40 **Type O blood, Rh positive**

Z67.41 **Type O blood, Rh negative**

✓5th **Z67.9 Unspecified blood type**

Z67.90 **Unspecified blood type, Rh positive**

Z67.91 **Unspecified blood type, Rh negative**

Body mass index [BMI] (Z68)

✓4th **Z68 Body mass index [BMI]**

Kilograms per meters squared

NOTE BMI adult codes are for use for persons 20 years of age or older

BMI pediatric codes are for use for persons 2-19 years of age.

These percentiles are based on the growth charts published by the Centers for Disease Control and Prevention (CDC)

AHA: 2019,4Q,19,57; 2018,4Q,73,77-83; 2017,1Q,39

DEF: Index used to help determine whether an individual is underweight, a healthy weight, overweight, or obese.

TIP: A BMI code may be assigned to support an associated condition based on medical record documentation from clinicians who are not the patient's provider.

TIP: Do not assign when used in association with fluctuations in body fluid during an encounter, such as fluid overload or fluid retention.

TIP: In order to assign a BMI code, the associated condition must meet the definition of a reportable diagnosis for nonoutpatient encounters, per section III of the *ICD-10-CM Official Guidelines for Coding and Reporting*.

▲ Z68.1 **Body mass index [BMI] 19.9 or less, adult** CC A

▲ ✓5th **Z68.2 Body mass index [BMI] 20-29, adult**

▲ Z68.20 **Body mass index [BMI] 20.0-20.9, adult** A

▲ Z68.21 **Body mass index [BMI] 21.0-21.9, adult** A

▲ Z68.22 **Body mass index [BMI] 22.0-22.9, adult** A

▲ Z68.23 **Body mass index [BMI] 23.0-23.9, adult** A

▲ Z68.24 **Body mass index [BMI] 24.0-24.9, adult** A

▲ Z68.25 **Body mass index [BMI] 25.0-25.9, adult** A

▲ Z68.26 **Body mass index [BMI] 26.0-26.9, adult** A

▲ Z68.27 **Body mass index [BMI] 27.0-27.9, adult** A

▲ Z68.28 **Body mass index [BMI] 28.0-28.9, adult** A

▲ Z68.29 **Body mass index [BMI] 29.0-29.9, adult** A

▲ ✓5th **Z68.3 Body mass index [BMI] 30-39, adult**

▲ Z68.30 **Body mass index [BMI] 30.0-30.9, adult** A

▲ Z68.31 **Body mass index [BMI] 31.0-31.9, adult** A

▲ Z68.32 **Body mass index [BMI] 32.0-32.9, adult** A

▲ Z68.33 **Body mass index [BMI] 33.0-33.9, adult** A

▲ Z68.34 **Body mass index [BMI] 34.0-34.9, adult** A

▲ Z68.35 **Body mass index [BMI] 35.0-35.9, adult** A

▲ Z68.36 **Body mass index [BMI] 36.0-36.9, adult** A

▲ Z68.37 **Body mass index [BMI] 37.0-37.9, adult** A

▲ Z68.38 **Body mass index [BMI] 38.0-38.9, adult** A

▲ Z68.39 **Body mass index [BMI] 39.0-39.9, adult** A

▲ ✓5th **Z68.4 Body mass index [BMI] 40 or greater, adult**

▲ Z68.41 **Body mass index [BMI] 40.0-44.9, adult** CC HCC A

▲ Z68.42 **Body mass index [BMI] 45.0-49.9, adult** CC HCC A

▲ Z68.43 **Body mass index [BMI] 50.0-59.9, adult** CC HCC A

▲ Z68.44 **Body mass index [BMI] 60.0-69.9, adult** CC HCC A

▲ Z68.45 **Body mass index [BMI] 70 or greater, adult** CC HCC A

▲ ✓5th **Z68.5 Body mass index [BMI] pediatric**

AHA: 2018,4Q,81-82

▲ Z68.51 **Body mass index [BMI] pediatric, less than 5th percentile for age**

▲ Z68.52 **Body mass index [BMI] pediatric, 5th percentile to less than 85th percentile for age**

▲ Z68.53 **Body mass index [BMI] pediatric, 85th percentile to less than 95th percentile for age**

▲ Z68.54 **Body mass index [BMI] pediatric, greater than or equal to 95th percentile for age**

Persons encountering health services in other circumstances (Z69-Z76)

✓4th **Z69 Encounter for mental health services for victim and perpetrator of abuse**

INCLUDES counseling for victims and perpetrators of abuse

✓5th **Z69.0 Encounter for mental health services for child abuse problems**

✓6th **Z69.01 Encounter for mental health services for parental child abuse**

Z69.010 **Encounter for mental health services for victim of parental child abuse** P

Encounter for mental health services for victim of child abuse by parent

Encounter for mental health services for victim of child neglect by parent

Encounter for mental health services for victim of child psychological abuse by parent

Encounter for mental health services for victim of child sexual abuse by parent

Z69.011 **Encounter for mental health services for perpetrator of parental child abuse**

Encounter for mental health services for perpetrator of parental child neglect

Encounter for mental health services for perpetrator of parental child psychological abuse

Encounter for mental health services for perpetrator of parental child sexual abuse

EXCLUDES 1 *encounter for mental health services for non-parental child abuse (Z69.02-)*

✓6th **Z69.02 Encounter for mental health services for non-parental child abuse**

Z69.020 **Encounter for mental health services for victim of non-parental child abuse** P

Encounter for mental health services for victim of non-parental child neglect

Encounter for mental health services for victim of non-parental child psychological abuse

Encounter for mental health services for victim of non-parental child sexual abuse

Z69.021 **Encounter for mental health services for perpetrator of non-parental child abuse**

Encounter for mental health services for perpetrator of non-parental child neglect

Encounter for mental health services for perpetrator of non-parental child psychological abuse

Encounter for mental health services for perpetrator of non-parental child sexual abuse

✓5th **Z69.1 Encounter for mental health services for spousal or partner abuse problems**

Z69.11 **Encounter for mental health services for victim of spousal or partner abuse**

Encounter for mental health services for victim of spouse or partner neglect

Encounter for mental health services for victim of spouse or partner psychological abuse

Encounter for mental health services for victim of spouse or partner violence, physical

Z69.12 Encounter for mental health services for perpetrator of spousal or partner abuse
Encounter for mental health services for perpetrator of spouse or partner neglect
Encounter for mental health services for perpetrator of spouse or partner psychological abuse
Encounter for mental health services for perpetrator of spouse or partner violence, physical
Encounter for mental health services for perpetrator of spouse or partner violence, sexual

Z69.8 Encounter for mental health services for victim or perpetrator of other abuse

Z69.81 Encounter for mental health services for victim of other abuse
Encounter for mental health services for victim of non-spousal adult abuse
Encounter for mental health services for victim of spouse or partner violence, sexual
Encounter for rape victim counseling

Z69.82 Encounter for mental health services for perpetrator of other abuse
Encounter for mental health services for perpetrator of non-spousal adult abuse

Z70 Counseling related to sexual attitude, behavior and orientation
INCLUDES encounter for mental health services for sexual attitude, behavior and orientation
EXCLUDES 2 *contraceptive or procreative counseling (Z30-Z31)*

Z70.0 Counseling related to sexual attitude

Z70.1 Counseling related to patient's sexual behavior and orientation
Patient concerned regarding impotence
Patient concerned regarding non-responsiveness
Patient concerned regarding promiscuity
Patient concerned regarding sexual orientation

Z70.2 Counseling related to sexual behavior and orientation of third party
Advice sought regarding sexual behavior and orientation of child
Advice sought regarding sexual behavior and orientation of partner
Advice sought regarding sexual behavior and orientation of spouse

Z70.3 Counseling related to combined concerns regarding sexual attitude, behavior and orientation

Z70.8 Other sex counseling
Encounter for sex education

Z70.9 Sex counseling, unspecified

Z71 Persons encountering health services for other counseling and medical advice, not elsewhere classified
EXCLUDES 2 *contraceptive or procreation counseling (Z30-Z31)*
sex counseling (Z70.-)

Z71.0 Person encountering health services to consult on behalf of another person
Person encountering health services to seek advice or treatment for non-attending third party
EXCLUDES 2 *anxiety (normal) about sick person in family (Z63.7)*
expectant (adoptive) parent(s) pre-birth pediatrician visit (Z76.81)

Z71.1 Person with feared health complaint in whom no diagnosis is made
Person encountering health services with feared condition which was not demonstrated
Person encountering health services in which problem was normal state
"Worried well"
EXCLUDES 1 *medical observation for suspected diseases and conditions proven not to exist (Z03.-)*

Z71.2 Person consulting for explanation of examination or test findings

Z71.3 Dietary counseling and surveillance
Use additional code for any associated underlying medical condition
Use additional code to identify body mass index (BMI), if known (Z68.-)

Z71.4 Alcohol abuse counseling and surveillance
Use additional code for alcohol abuse or dependence (F10.-)

Z71.41 Alcohol abuse counseling and surveillance of alcoholic

Z71.42 Counseling for family member of alcoholic
Counseling for significant other, partner, or friend of alcoholic

Z71.5 Drug abuse counseling and surveillance
Use additional code for drug abuse or dependence (F11-F16, F18-F19)

Z71.51 Drug abuse counseling and surveillance of drug abuser

Z71.52 Counseling for family member of drug abuser
Counseling for significant other, partner, or friend of drug abuser

Z71.6 Tobacco abuse counseling
Use additional code for nicotine dependence (F17.-)

Z71.7 Human immunodeficiency virus [HIV] counseling

Z71.8 Other specified counseling
EXCLUDES 2 *counseling for contraception (Z30.0-)*
AHA: 2017,4Q,27

Z71.81 Spiritual or religious counseling

Z71.82 Exercise counseling

Z71.83 Encounter for nonprocreative genetic counseling
EXCLUDES 1 *counseling for procreative genetics (Z31.5)*
counseling for procreative management (Z31.6)

Z71.84 Encounter for health counseling related to travel
Encounter for health risk and safety counseling for (international) travel
Code also, if applicable, encounter for immunization (Z23)
EXCLUDES 2 *encounter for administrative examination (Z02.-)*
encounter for other special examination without complaint, suspected or reported diagnosis (Z01.-)
AHA: 2019,4Q,20,57

Z71.89 Other specified counseling

Z71.9 Counseling, unspecified
Encounter for medical advice NOS

Z72 Problems related to lifestyle
EXCLUDES 2 *problems related to life-management difficulty (Z73.-)*
problems related to socioeconomic and psychosocial circumstances (Z55-Z65)

Z72.0 Tobacco use
Tobacco use NOS
EXCLUDES 1 *history of tobacco dependence (Z87.891)*
nicotine dependence (F17.2-)
tobacco dependence (F17.2-)
tobacco use during pregnancy (O99.33-)

Z72.3 Lack of physical exercise

Z72.4 Inappropriate diet and eating habits
EXCLUDES 1 *behavioral eating disorders of infancy or childhood (F98.2-F98.3)*
eating disorders (F50.-)
lack of adequate food (Z59.4)
malnutrition and other nutritional deficiencies (E40-E64)

Z72.5 High risk sexual behavior
Promiscuity
EXCLUDES 1 *paraphilias (F65)*

Z72.51 High risk heterosexual behavior

Z72.52 High risk homosexual behavior

Z72.53 High risk bisexual behavior

Z72.6 Gambling and betting
EXCLUDES 1 *compulsive or pathological gambling (F63.0)*

✓5th **Z72.8 Other problems related to lifestyle**

✓6th **Z72.81 Antisocial behavior**

EXCLUDES 1 *conduct disorders (F91.-)*

Z72.810 Child and adolescent antisocial behavior P

Antisocial behavior (child) (adolescent) without manifest psychiatric disorder

Delinquency NOS

Group delinquency

Offenses in the context of gang membership

Stealing in company with others

Truancy from school

Z72.811 Adult antisocial behavior A

Adult antisocial behavior without manifest psychiatric disorder

✓6th **Z72.82 Problems related to sleep**

Z72.820 Sleep deprivation

Lack of adequate sleep

EXCLUDES 1 *insomnia (G47.0-)*

Z72.821 Inadequate sleep hygiene

Bad sleep habits

Irregular sleep habits

Unhealthy sleep wake schedule

EXCLUDES 1 *insomnia (F51.0-, G47.0-)*

Z72.89 Other problems related to lifestyle

Self-damaging behavior

Z72.9 Problem related to lifestyle, unspecified

✓4th **Z73 Problems related to life management difficulty**

EXCLUDES 2 *problems related to socioeconomic and psychosocial circumstances (Z55-Z65)*

DEF: State of emotional, mental, and physical exhaustion causing difficulties in managing personal, school, or work circumstances. It is usually due to prolonged stress or poor interpersonal relationship skills or parenting skills.

Z73.0 Burn-out

Z73.1 Type A behavior pattern

Z73.2 Lack of relaxation and leisure

Z73.3 Stress, not elsewhere classified

Physical and mental strain NOS

EXCLUDES 1 *stress related to employment or unemployment (Z56.-)*

Z73.4 Inadequate social skills, not elsewhere classified

Z73.5 Social role conflict, not elsewhere classified

Z73.6 Limitation of activities due to disability

EXCLUDES 1 *care-provider dependency (Z74.-)*

✓5th **Z73.8 Other problems related to life management difficulty**

✓6th **Z73.81 Behavioral insomnia of childhood**

DEF: Behaviors on the part of the child or caregivers that cause negative compliance with a child's sleep schedule resulting in lack of adequate sleep.

Z73.810 Behavioral insomnia of childhood, sleep-onset association type P

Z73.811 Behavioral insomnia of childhood, limit setting type P

Z73.812 Behavioral insomnia of childhood, combined type P

Z73.819 Behavioral insomnia of childhood, unspecified type P

Z73.82 Dual sensory impairment

Z73.89 Other problems related to life management difficulty

Z73.9 Problem related to life management difficulty, unspecified

✓4th **Z74 Problems related to care provider dependency**

EXCLUDES 2 *dependence on enabling machines or devices NEC (Z99.-)*

✓5th **Z74.0 Reduced mobility**

Z74.01 Bed confinement status

Bedridden

Z74.09 Other reduced mobility

Chair ridden

Reduced mobility NOS

EXCLUDES 2 *wheelchair dependence (Z99.3)*

Z74.1 Need for assistance with personal care

Z74.2 Need for assistance at home and no other household member able to render care

Z74.3 Need for continuous supervision

Z74.8 Other problems related to care provider dependency

Z74.9 Problem related to care provider dependency, unspecified

✓4th **Z75 Problems related to medical facilities and other health care**

Z75.0 Medical services not available in home

EXCLUDES 1 *no other household member able to render care (Z74.2)*

Z75.1 Person awaiting admission to adequate facility elsewhere

Z75.2 Other waiting period for investigation and treatment

Z75.3 Unavailability and inaccessibility of health-care facilities

EXCLUDES 1 *bed unavailable (Z75.1)*

Z75.4 Unavailability and inaccessibility of other helping agencies

Z75.5 Holiday relief care

Z75.8 Other problems related to medical facilities and other health care

Z75.9 Unspecified problem related to medical facilities and other health care

✓4th **Z76 Persons encountering health services in other circumstances**

Z76.0 Encounter for issue of repeat prescription

Encounter for issue of repeat prescription for appliance

Encounter for issue of repeat prescription for medicaments

Encounter for issue of repeat prescription for spectacles

EXCLUDES 2 *issue of medical certificate (Z02.7)*

repeat prescription for contraceptive (Z30.4-)

Z76.1 Encounter for health supervision and care of foundling

Z76.2 Encounter for health supervision and care of other healthy infant and child P

Encounter for medical or nursing care or supervision of healthy infant under circumstances such as adverse socioeconomic conditions at home

Encounter for medical or nursing care or supervision of healthy infant under circumstances such as awaiting foster or adoptive placement

Encounter for medical or nursing care or supervision of healthy infant under circumstances such as maternal illness

Encounter for medical or nursing care or supervision of healthy infant under circumstances such as number of children at home preventing or interfering with normal care

Z76.3 Healthy person accompanying sick person

Z76.4 Other boarder to healthcare facility

EXCLUDES 1 *homelessness (Z59.0)*

Z76.5 Malingerer [conscious simulation]

Person feigning illness (with obvious motivation)

EXCLUDES 1 *factitious disorder (F68.1-, F68.A)*

peregrinating patient (F68.1-)

DEF: Act of intentionally exaggerating an illness or disability in order to receive personal gain or to avoid punishment or responsibility.

✓5th **Z76.8 Persons encountering health services in other specified circumstances**

Z76.81 Expectant parent(s) prebirth pediatrician visit

Pre-adoption pediatrician visit for adoptive parent(s)

Z76.82 Awaiting organ transplant status

Patient waiting for organ availability

Z76.89 Persons encountering health services in other specified circumstances

Persons encountering health services NOS

AHA: 2014,2Q,10

Persons with potential health hazards related to family and personal history and certain conditions influencing health status (Z77-Z99)

Code also any follow-up examination (Z08-Z09)

Z77 Other contact with and (suspected) exposures hazardous to health

INCLUDES contact with and (suspected) exposures to potential hazards to health

EXCLUDES 2 *contact with and (suspected) exposure to communicable diseases (Z20.-)*
exposure to (parental) (environmental) tobacco smoke in the perinatal period (P96.81)
newborn affected by noxious substances transmitted via placenta or breast milk (P04.-)
occupational exposure to risk factors (Z57.-)
retained foreign body (Z18.-)
retained foreign body fully removed (Z87.821)
toxic effects of substances chiefly nonmedicinal as to source (T51-T65)

Z77.0 Contact with and (suspected) exposure to hazardous, chiefly nonmedicinal, chemicals

Z77.01 Contact with and (suspected) exposure to hazardous metals

Z77.010 Contact with and (suspected) exposure to arsenic

Z77.011 Contact with and (suspected) exposure to lead

Z77.012 Contact with and (suspected) exposure to uranium

EXCLUDES 1 *retained depleted uranium fragments (Z18.01)*

Z77.018 Contact with and (suspected) exposure to other hazardous metals

Contact with and (suspected) exposure to chromium compounds
Contact with and (suspected) exposure to nickel dust

Z77.02 Contact with and (suspected) exposure to hazardous aromatic compounds

Z77.020 Contact with and (suspected) exposure to aromatic amines

Z77.021 Contact with and (suspected) exposure to benzene

Z77.028 Contact with and (suspected) exposure to other hazardous aromatic compounds

Aromatic dyes NOS
Polycyclic aromatic hydrocarbons

Z77.09 Contact with and (suspected) exposure to other hazardous, chiefly nonmedicinal, chemicals

Z77.090 Contact with and (suspected) exposure to asbestos

Z77.098 Contact with and (suspected) exposure to other hazardous, chiefly nonmedicinal, chemicals

Dyes NOS

Z77.1 Contact with and (suspected) exposure to environmental pollution and hazards in the physical environment

Z77.11 Contact with and (suspected) exposure to environmental pollution

Z77.110 Contact with and (suspected) exposure to air pollution

Z77.111 Contact with and (suspected) exposure to water pollution

Z77.112 Contact with and (suspected) exposure to soil pollution

Z77.118 Contact with and (suspected) exposure to other environmental pollution

Z77.12 Contact with and (suspected) exposure to hazards in the physical environment

Z77.120 Contact with and (suspected) exposure to mold (toxic)

Z77.121 Contact with and (suspected) exposure to harmful algae and algae toxins

Contact with and (suspected) exposure to (harmful) algae bloom NOS
Contact with and (suspected) exposure to blue-green algae bloom
Contact with and (suspected) exposure to brown tide
Contact with and (suspected) exposure to cyanobacteria bloom
Contact with and (suspected) exposure to Florida red tide
Contact with and (suspected) exposure to pfiesteria piscicida
Contact with and (suspected) exposure to red tide

Z77.122 Contact with and (suspected) exposure to noise

Z77.123 Contact with and (suspected) exposure to radon and other naturally occurring radiation

EXCLUDES 2 *radiation exposure as the cause of a confirmed condition (W88-W90, X39.0-)*
radiation sickness NOS (T66)

Z77.128 Contact with and (suspected) exposure to other hazards in the physical environment

Z77.2 Contact with and (suspected) exposure to other hazardous substances

Z77.21 Contact with and (suspected) exposure to potentially hazardous body fluids

Z77.22 Contact with and (suspected) exposure to environmental tobacco smoke (acute) (chronic)

Exposure to second hand tobacco smoke (acute) (chronic)
Passive smoking (acute) (chronic)

EXCLUDES 1 *nicotine dependence (F17.-)*
tobacco use (Z72.0)

EXCLUDES 2 *occupational exposure to environmental tobacco smoke (Z57.31)*

Z77.29 Contact with and (suspected) exposure to other hazardous substances

AHA: 2016,2Q,33

Z77.9 Other contact with and (suspected) exposures hazardous to health

Z78 Other specified health status

EXCLUDES 2 *asymptomatic human immunodeficiency virus [HIV] infection status (Z21)*
postprocedural status (Z93-Z99)
sex reassignment status (Z87.890)

Z78.0 Asymptomatic menopausal state A ♀

Menopausal state NOS
Postmenopausal status NOS

EXCLUDES 2 *symptomatic menopausal state (N95.1)*

Z78.1 Physical restraint status

EXCLUDES 1 *physical restraint due to a procedure — omit code*

DEF: Application of mechanical restraining devices or manual restraints to limit physical mobility of a patient.

Z78.9 Other specified health status

Z79 Long term (current) drug therapy

INCLUDES long term (current) drug use for prophylactic purposes

Code also any therapeutic drug level monitoring (Z51.81)

EXCLUDES 2 *drug abuse and dependence (F11-F19)*
drug use complicating pregnancy, childbirth, and the puerperium (O99.32-)
~~*long term (current) use of oral antidiabetic drugs (Z79.84)*~~
~~*long term (current) use of oral hypoglycemic drugs (Z79.84)*~~

Z79.0 Long term (current) use of anticoagulants and antithrombotics/antiplatelets

EXCLUDES 2 *long term (current) use of aspirin (Z79.82)*

Z79.01 Long term (current) use of anticoagulants

AHA: 2020,2Q,20

Z79.02 Long term (current) use of antithrombotics/antiplatelets

Z79.1 Long term (current) use of non-steroidal anti-inflammatories (NSAID)
EXCLUDES 2 *long term (current) use of aspirin (Z79.82)*

Z79.2 Long term (current) use of antibiotics

Z79.3 Long term (current) use of hormonal contraceptives
Long term (current) use of birth control pill or patch

Z79.4 Long term (current) use of insulin HCC
EXCLUDES 1 ▶*long term (current) use of oral antidiabetic drugs (Z79.84)*◀
▶*long term (current) use of oral hypoglycemic drugs (Z79.84)*◀
TIP: When both long-term (current) insulin and long-term (current) oral hypoglycemic use is documented, assign only a code for the long-term insulin use.

✓5th **Z79.5 Long term (current) use of steroids**

Z79.51 Long term (current) use of inhaled steroids

Z79.52 Long term (current) use of systemic steroids

✓5th **Z79.8 Other long term (current) drug therapy**

✓6th **Z79.81 Long term (current) use of agents affecting estrogen receptors and estrogen levels**
Code first, if applicable:
malignant neoplasm of breast (C5Ø.-)
malignant neoplasm of prostate (C61)
Use additional code, if applicable, to identify:
estrogen receptor positive status (Z17.Ø)
family history of breast cancer (Z8Ø.3)
genetic susceptibility to malignant neoplasm (cancer) (Z15.Ø-)
personal history of breast cancer (Z85.3)
personal history of prostate cancer (Z85.46)
postmenopausal status (Z78.Ø)
EXCLUDES 1 *hormone replacement therapy (Z79.89Ø)*

Z79.81Ø Long term (current) use of selective estrogen receptor modulators (SERMs)
Long term (current) use of raloxifene (Evista)
Long term (current) use of tamoxifen (Nolvadex)
Long term (current) use of toremifene (Fareston)

Z79.811 Long term (current) use of aromatase inhibitors
Long term (current) use of anastrozole (Arimidex)
Long term (current) use of exemestane (Aromasin)
Long term (current) use of letrozole (Femara)

Z79.818 Long term (current) use of other agents affecting estrogen receptors and estrogen levels
Long term (current) use of estrogen receptor downregulators
Long term (current) use of fulvestrant (Faslodex)
Long term (current) use of gonadotropin-releasing hormone (GnRH) agonist
Long term (current) use of goserelin acetate (Zoladex)
Long term (current) use of leuprolide acetate (leuprorelin) (Lupron)
Long term (current) use of megestrol acetate (Megace)

Z79.82 Long term (current) use of aspirin

Z79.83 Long term (current) use of bisphosphonates
AHA: 2016,4Q,42

Z79.84 Long term (current) use of oral hypoglycemic drugs
Long term (current) use of oral antidiabetic drugs
EXCLUDES 2 *long term (current) use of insulin (Z79.4)*
AHA: 2016,4Q,76
TIP: When both long-term (current) insulin and long-term (current) oral hypoglycemic use is documented, assign only code Z79.4 for the long-term insulin use.

✓6th **Z79.89 Other long term (current) drug therapy**

Z79.89Ø Hormone replacement therapy

Z79.891 Long term (current) use of opiate analgesic
Long term (current) use of methadone for pain management
EXCLUDES 1 *methodone use NOS (F11.9-)*
use of methodone for treatment of heroin addiction (F11.2-)

Z79.899 Other long term (current) drug therapy
AHA: 2020,2Q,14; 2015,4Q,34; 2015,3Q,21

✓4th **Z8Ø Family history of primary malignant neoplasm**

Z8Ø.Ø Family history of malignant neoplasm of digestive organs
Conditions classifiable to C15-C26
AHA: 2018,1Q,6

Z8Ø.1 Family history of malignant neoplasm of trachea, bronchus and lung
Conditions classifiable to C33-C34

Z8Ø.2 Family history of malignant neoplasm of other respiratory and intrathoracic organs
Conditions classifiable to C3Ø-C32, C37-C39

Z8Ø.3 Family history of malignant neoplasm of breast
Conditions classifiable to C5Ø.-

✓5th **Z8Ø.4 Family history of malignant neoplasm of genital organs**
Conditions classifiable to C51-C63

Z8Ø.41 Family history of malignant neoplasm of ovary

Z8Ø.42 Family history of malignant neoplasm of prostate

Z8Ø.43 Family history of malignant neoplasm of testis

Z8Ø.49 Family history of malignant neoplasm of other genital organs

✓5th **Z8Ø.5 Family history of malignant neoplasm of urinary tract**
Conditions classifiable to C64-C68

Z8Ø.51 Family history of malignant neoplasm of kidney

Z8Ø.52 Family history of malignant neoplasm of bladder

Z8Ø.59 Family history of malignant neoplasm of other urinary tract organ

Z8Ø.6 Family history of leukemia
Conditions classifiable to C91-C95

Z8Ø.7 Family history of other malignant neoplasms of lymphoid, hematopoietic and related tissues
Conditions classifiable to C81-C9Ø, C96.-

Z8Ø.8 Family history of malignant neoplasm of other organs or systems
Conditions classifiable to CØØ-C14, C4Ø-C49, C69-C79

Z8Ø.9 Family history of malignant neoplasm, unspecified
Conditions classifiable to C8Ø.1

✓4th **Z81 Family history of mental and behavioral disorders**

Z81.Ø Family history of intellectual disabilities
Conditions classifiable to F7Ø-F79

Z81.1 Family history of alcohol abuse and dependence
Conditions classifiable to F1Ø.-

Z81.2 Family history of tobacco abuse and dependence
Conditions classifiable to F17.-

Z81.3 Family history of other psychoactive substance abuse and dependence
Conditions classifiable to F11-F16, F18-F19

Z81.4 Family history of other substance abuse and dependence
Conditions classifiable to F55

Z81.8 Family history of other mental and behavioral disorders
Conditions classifiable elsewhere in FØ1-F99

✓4th **Z82 Family history of certain disabilities and chronic diseases (leading to disablement)**

Z82.Ø Family history of epilepsy and other diseases of the nervous system
Conditions classifiable to GØØ-G99

Z82.1 Family history of blindness and visual loss
Conditions classifiable to H54.-

Z82.2 Family history of deafness and hearing loss
Conditions classifiable to H9Ø-H91

Z82.3 Family history of stroke
Conditions classifiable to I6Ø-I64

✓5th **Z82.4 Family history of ischemic heart disease and other diseases of the circulatory system**
Conditions classifiable to IØØ-I52, I65-I99

Z82.41 Family history of sudden cardiac death

Z82.49 Family history of ischemic heart disease and other diseases of the circulatory system

Z82.5 Family history of asthma and other chronic lower respiratory diseases
Conditions classifiable to J40-J47
EXCLUDES 2 *family history of other diseases of the respiratory system (Z83.6)*

Z82.6 Family history of arthritis and other diseases of the musculoskeletal system and connective tissue
Conditions classifiable to M00-M99

Z82.61 Family history of arthritis

Z82.62 Family history of osteoporosis

Z82.69 Family history of other diseases of the musculoskeletal system and connective tissue

Z82.7 Family history of congenital malformations, deformations and chromosomal abnormalities
Conditions classifiable to Q00-Q99

Z82.71 Family history of polycystic kidney

Z82.79 Family history of other congenital malformations, deformations and chromosomal abnormalities

Z82.8 Family history of other disabilities and chronic diseases leading to disablement, not elsewhere classified

Z83 Family history of other specific disorders
EXCLUDES 2 *contact with and (suspected) exposure to communicable disease in the family (Z20.-)*

Z83.0 Family history of human immunodeficiency virus [HIV] disease
Conditions classifiable to B20

Z83.1 Family history of other infectious and parasitic diseases
Conditions classifiable to A00-B19, B25-B94, B99

Z83.2 Family history of diseases of the blood and blood-forming organs and certain disorders involving the immune mechanism
Conditions classifiable to D50-D89

Z83.3 Family history of diabetes mellitus
Conditions classifiable to E08-E13

Z83.4 Family history of other endocrine, nutritional and metabolic diseases
Conditions classifiable to E00-E07, E15-E88

Z83.41 Family history of multiple endocrine neoplasia [MEN] syndrome

Z83.42 Family history of familial hypercholesterolemia
AHA: 2016,4Q,77

Z83.43 Family history of other disorder of lipoprotein metabolism and other lipidemias
AHA: 2018,4Q,6,35

Z83.430 Family history of elevated lipoprotein(a)
Family history of elevated Lp(a)

Z83.438 Family history of other disorder of lipoprotein metabolism and other lipidemia
Family history of familial combined hyperlipidemia

Z83.49 Family history of other endocrine, nutritional and metabolic diseases

Z83.5 Family history of eye and ear disorders

Z83.51 Family history of eye disorders
Conditions classifiable to H00-H53, H55-H59
EXCLUDES 2 *family history of blindness and visual loss (Z82.1)*

Z83.511 Family history of glaucoma

Z83.518 Family history of other specified eye disorder

Z83.52 Family history of ear disorders
Conditions classifiable to H60-H83, H92-H95
EXCLUDES 2 *family history of deafness and hearing loss (Z82.2)*

Z83.6 Family history of other diseases of the respiratory system
Conditions classifiable to J00-J39, J60-J99
EXCLUDES 2 *family history of asthma and other chronic lower respiratory diseases (Z82.5)*

Z83.7 Family history of diseases of the digestive system
Conditions classifiable to K00-K93

Z83.71 Family history of colonic polyps
EXCLUDES 2 *family history of malignant neoplasm of digestive organs (Z80.0)*

Z83.79 Family history of other diseases of the digestive system

Z84 Family history of other conditions

Z84.0 Family history of diseases of the skin and subcutaneous tissue
Conditions classifiable to L00-L99

Z84.1 Family history of disorders of kidney and ureter
Conditions classifiable to N00-N29

Z84.2 Family history of other diseases of the genitourinary system
Conditions classifiable to N30-N99

Z84.3 Family history of consanguinity

Z84.8 Family history of other specified conditions

Z84.81 Family history of carrier of genetic disease

Z84.82 Family history of sudden infant death syndrome
Family history of SIDS
AHA: 2016,4Q,77

Z84.89 Family history of other specified conditions

Z85 Personal history of malignant neoplasm
Code first any follow-up examination after treatment of malignant neoplasm (Z08)
Use additional code to identify:
- alcohol use and dependence (F10.-)
- exposure to environmental tobacco smoke (Z77.22)
- history of tobacco dependence (Z87.891)
- occupational exposure to environmental tobacco smoke (Z57.31)
- tobacco dependence (F17.-)
- tobacco use (Z72.0)

EXCLUDES 2 *personal history of benign neoplasm (Z86.01-)*
personal history of carcinoma-in-situ (Z86.00-)
AHA: 2018,4Q,64

Z85.0 Personal history of malignant neoplasm of digestive organs
AHA: 2017,1Q,9

Z85.00 Personal history of malignant neoplasm of unspecified digestive organ

Z85.01 Personal history of malignant neoplasm of esophagus
Conditions classifiable to C15

Z85.02 Personal history of malignant neoplasm of stomach

Z85.020 Personal history of malignant carcinoid tumor of stomach
Conditions classifiable to C7A.092

Z85.028 Personal history of other malignant neoplasm of stomach
Conditions classifiable to C16

Z85.03 Personal history of malignant neoplasm of large intestine

Z85.030 Personal history of malignant carcinoid tumor of large intestine
Conditions classifiable to C7A.022-C7A.025, C7A.029

Z85.038 Personal history of other malignant neoplasm of large intestine
Conditions classifiable to C18

Z85.04 Personal history of malignant neoplasm of rectum, rectosigmoid junction, and anus

Z85.040 Personal history of malignant carcinoid tumor of rectum
Conditions classifiable to C7A.026

Z85.048 Personal history of other malignant neoplasm of rectum, rectosigmoid junction, and anus
Conditions classifiable to C19-C21

Z85.05 Personal history of malignant neoplasm of liver
Conditions classifiable to C22

Z85.06 Personal history of malignant neoplasm of small intestine

Z85.060 Personal history of malignant carcinoid tumor of small intestine
Conditions classifiable to C7A.01-

Z85.068 Personal history of other malignant neoplasm of small intestine
Conditions classifiable to C17

Z85.07 Personal history of malignant neoplasm of pancreas
Conditions classifiable to C25

Z85.09 Personal history of malignant neoplasm of other digestive organs

✓5th **Z85.1 Personal history of malignant neoplasm of trachea, bronchus and lung**

✓6th **Z85.11 Personal history of malignant neoplasm of bronchus and lung**

Z85.110 Personal history of malignant carcinoid tumor of bronchus and lung
Conditions classifiable to C7A.090

Z85.118 Personal history of other malignant neoplasm of bronchus and lung
Conditions classifiable to C34

Z85.12 Personal history of malignant neoplasm of trachea
Conditions classifiable to C33

✓5th **Z85.2 Personal history of malignant neoplasm of other respiratory and intrathoracic organs**

Z85.20 Personal history of malignant neoplasm of unspecified respiratory organ

Z85.21 Personal history of malignant neoplasm of larynx
Conditions classifiable to C32

Z85.22 Personal history of malignant neoplasm of nasal cavities, middle ear, and accessory sinuses
Conditions classifiable to C30-C31

✓6th **Z85.23 Personal history of malignant neoplasm of thymus**

Z85.230 Personal history of malignant carcinoid tumor of thymus
Conditions classifiable to C7A.091

Z85.238 Personal history of other malignant neoplasm of thymus
Conditions classifiable to C37

Z85.29 Personal history of malignant neoplasm of other respiratory and intrathoracic organs

Z85.3 Personal history of malignant neoplasm of breast
Conditions classifiable to C50.-

✓5th **Z85.4 Personal history of malignant neoplasm of genital organs**
Conditions classifiable to C51-C63

Z85.40 Personal history of malignant neoplasm of unspecified female genital organ ♀

Z85.41 Personal history of malignant neoplasm of cervix uteri ♀

Z85.42 Personal history of malignant neoplasm of other parts of uterus ♀

Z85.43 Personal history of malignant neoplasm of ovary ♀

Z85.44 Personal history of malignant neoplasm of other female genital organs ♀

Z85.45 Personal history of malignant neoplasm of unspecified male genital organ ♂

Z85.46 Personal history of malignant neoplasm of prostate ♂

Z85.47 Personal history of malignant neoplasm of testis ♂

Z85.48 Personal history of malignant neoplasm of epididymis ♂

Z85.49 Personal history of malignant neoplasm of other male genital organs ♂

✓5th **Z85.5 Personal history of malignant neoplasm of urinary tract**
Conditions classifiable to C64-C68

Z85.50 Personal history of malignant neoplasm of unspecified urinary tract organ

Z85.51 Personal history of malignant neoplasm of bladder

✓6th **Z85.52 Personal history of malignant neoplasm of kidney**

EXCLUDES 1 *personal history of malignant neoplasm of renal pelvis (Z85.53)*

Z85.520 Personal history of malignant carcinoid tumor of kidney
Conditions classifiable to C7A.093

Z85.528 Personal history of other malignant neoplasm of kidney
Conditions classifiable to C64

Z85.53 Personal history of malignant neoplasm of renal pelvis

Z85.54 Personal history of malignant neoplasm of ureter

Z85.59 Personal history of malignant neoplasm of other urinary tract organ

Z85.6 Personal history of leukemia
Conditions classifiable to C91-C95

EXCLUDES 1 *leukemia in remission C91.0-C95.9 with 5th character 1*

✓5th **Z85.7 Personal history of other malignant neoplasms of lymphoid, hematopoietic and related tissues**

Z85.71 Personal history of Hodgkin lymphoma
Conditions classifiable to C81

Z85.72 Personal history of non-Hodgkin lymphomas
Conditions classifiable to C82-C85

Z85.79 Personal history of other malignant neoplasms of lymphoid, hematopoietic and related tissues
Conditions classifiable to C88-C90, C96

EXCLUDES 1 *multiple myeloma in remission (C90.01)*
plasma cell leukemia in remission (C90.11)
plasmacytoma in remission (C90.21)

✓5th **Z85.8 Personal history of malignant neoplasms of other organs and systems**
Conditions classifiable to C00-C14, C40-C49, C69-C75, C7A.098, C76-C79

✓6th **Z85.81 Personal history of malignant neoplasm of lip, oral cavity, and pharynx**
▶Conditions classifiable to C00-C14◀

Z85.810 Personal history of malignant neoplasm of tongue

Z85.818 Personal history of malignant neoplasm of other sites of lip, oral cavity, and pharynx

Z85.819 Personal history of malignant neoplasm of unspecified site of lip, oral cavity, and pharynx

✓6th **Z85.82 Personal history of malignant neoplasm of skin**

Z85.820 Personal history of malignant melanoma of skin
Conditions classifiable to C43

Z85.821 Personal history of Merkel cell carcinoma
Conditions classifiable to C4A

Z85.828 Personal history of other malignant neoplasm of skin
Conditions classifiable to C44

✓6th **Z85.83 Personal history of malignant neoplasm of bone and soft tissue**
▶Conditions classifiable to C40-C41; C45-C49◀

Z85.830 Personal history of malignant neoplasm of bone

Z85.831 Personal history of malignant neoplasm of soft tissue

EXCLUDES 2 *personal history of malignant neoplasm of skin (Z85.82-)*

✓6th **Z85.84 Personal history of malignant neoplasm of eye and nervous tissue**
▶Conditions classifiable to C69-C72◀

Z85.840 Personal history of malignant neoplasm of eye

Z85.841 Personal history of malignant neoplasm of brain

Z85.848 Personal history of malignant neoplasm of other parts of nervous tissue

✓6th **Z85.85 Personal history of malignant neoplasm of endocrine glands**
▶Conditions classifiable to C73-C75◀

Z85.850 Personal history of malignant neoplasm of thyroid

Z85.858 Personal history of malignant neoplasm of other endocrine glands

Z85.89 Personal history of malignant neoplasm of other organs and systems
▶Conditions classifiable to C7A.098, C76, C77-C79◀

Z85.9 Personal history of malignant neoplasm, unspecified
Conditions classifiable to C7A.00, C80.1

✓4th **Z86 Personal history of certain other diseases**
Code first any follow-up examination after treatment (Z09)

✓5th **Z86.0 Personal history of in-situ and benign neoplasms and neoplasms of uncertain behavior**

EXCLUDES 2 *personal history of malignant neoplasms (Z85.-)*

AHA: 2017,1Q,9

✓6th **Z86.00 Personal history of in-situ neoplasm**
Conditions classifiable to D00-D09
AHA: 2019,4Q,20

Z86.000 Personal history of in-situ neoplasm of breast
Conditions classifiable to D05

Z86.ØØ1 Personal history of in-situ neoplasm of cervix uteri ♀
Conditions classifiable to DØ6
Personal history of cervical intraepithelial neoplasia III [CIN III]

Z86.ØØ2 Personal history of in-situ neoplasm of other and unspecified genital organs
Conditions classifiable to DØ7
Personal history of high-grade prostatic intraepithelial neoplasia III [HGPIN III]
Personal history of vaginal intraepithelial neoplasia III [VAIN III]
Personal history of vulvar intraepithelial neoplasia III [VIN III]

Z86.ØØ3 Personal history of in-situ neoplasm of oral cavity, esophagus and stomach
Conditions classifiable to DØØ

Z86.ØØ4 Personal history of in-situ neoplasm of other and unspecified digestive organs
Conditions classifiable to DØ1
Personal history of anal intraepithelial neoplasia (AIN III)

Z86.ØØ5 Personal history of in-situ neoplasm of middle ear and respiratory system
Conditions classifiable to DØ2

Z86.ØØ6 Personal history of melanoma in-situ
Conditions classifiable to DØ3
EXCLUDES 2 *sites other than skin — code to personal history of in-situ neoplasm of the site*

Z86.ØØ7 Personal history of in-situ neoplasm of skin
Conditions classifiable to DØ4
Personal history of carcinoma in situ of skin

Z86.ØØ8 Personal history of in-situ neoplasm of other site
Conditions classifiable to DØ9

✓6th **Z86.Ø1 Personal history of benign neoplasm**

Z86.Ø1Ø Personal history of colonic polyps
AHA: 2017,1Q,14

Z86.Ø11 Personal history of benign neoplasm of the brain

Z86.Ø12 Personal history of benign carcinoid tumor

Z86.Ø18 Personal history of other benign neoplasm
AHA: 2017,1Q,14

Z86.Ø3 Personal history of neoplasm of uncertain behavior

✓5th **Z86.1 Personal history of infectious and parasitic diseases**
Conditions classifiable to AØØ-B89, B99
EXCLUDES 1 *personal history of infectious diseases specific to a body system*
sequelae of infectious and parasitic diseases (B9Ø-B94)

Z86.11 Personal history of tuberculosis

Z86.12 Personal history of poliomyelitis

Z86.13 Personal history of malaria

Z86.14 Personal history of Methicillin resistant Staphylococcus aureus infection
Personal history of MRSA infection

Z86.15 Personal history of latent tuberculosis infection

Z86.19 Personal history of other infectious and parasitic diseases
AHA: 2020,2Q,10,12

Z86.2 Personal history of diseases of the blood and blood-forming organs and certain disorders involving the immune mechanism
Conditions classifiable to D5Ø-D89

✓5th **Z86.3 Personal history of endocrine, nutritional and metabolic diseases**
Conditions classifiable to EØØ-E88

Z86.31 Personal history of diabetic foot ulcer
EXCLUDES 2 *current diabetic foot ulcer (EØ8.621, EØ9.621, E1Ø.621, E11.621, E13.621)*

Z86.32 Personal history of gestational diabetes ♀
Personal history of conditions classifiable to O24.4-
EXCLUDES 1 *gestational diabetes mellitus in current pregnancy (O24.4-)*

Z86.39 Personal history of other endocrine, nutritional and metabolic disease
AHA: 2020,1Q,12

✓5th **Z86.5 Personal history of mental and behavioral disorders**
Conditions classifiable to F4Ø-F59

Z86.51 Personal history of combat and operational stress reaction A

Z86.59 Personal history of other mental and behavioral disorders

✓5th **Z86.6 Personal history of diseases of the nervous system and sense organs**
Conditions classifiable to GØØ-G99, HØØ-H95

Z86.61 Personal history of infections of the central nervous system
Personal history of encephalitis
Personal history of meningitis

Z86.69 Personal history of other diseases of the nervous system and sense organs
AHA: 2016,4Q,24

✓5th **Z86.7 Personal history of diseases of the circulatory system**
Conditions classifiable to IØØ-I99
EXCLUDES 2 *old myocardial infarction (I25.2)*
personal history of anaphylactic shock (Z87.892)
postmyocardial infarction syndrome (I24.1)

✓6th **Z86.71 Personal history of venous thrombosis and embolism**

Z86.711 Personal history of pulmonary embolism

Z86.718 Personal history of other venous thrombosis and embolism
AHA: 2020,2Q,20

Z86.72 Personal history of thrombophlebitis

Z86.73 Personal history of transient ischemic attack (TIA), and cerebral infarction without residual deficits
Personal history of prolonged reversible ischemic neurological deficit (PRIND)
Personal history of stroke NOS without residual deficits
EXCLUDES 1 *personal history of traumatic brain injury (Z87.82Ø)*
sequelae of cerebrovascular disease (I69.-)
AHA: 2012,4Q,92

Z86.74 Personal history of sudden cardiac arrest
Personal history of sudden cardiac death successfully resuscitated

Z86.79 Personal history of other diseases of the circulatory system
AHA: 2020,1Q,12

✓4th **Z87 Personal history of other diseases and conditions**
Code first any follow-up examination after treatment (ZØ9)

✓5th **Z87.Ø Personal history of diseases of the respiratory system**
Conditions classifiable to JØØ-J99

Z87.Ø1 Personal history of pneumonia (recurrent)

Z87.Ø9 Personal history of other diseases of the respiratory system

✓5th **Z87.1 Personal history of diseases of the digestive system**
Conditions classifiable to KØØ-K93

Z87.11 Personal history of peptic ulcer disease

Z87.19 Personal history of other diseases of the digestive system
AHA: 2017,1Q,14

Z87.2 Personal history of diseases of the skin and subcutaneous tissue
Conditions classifiable to LØØ-L99
EXCLUDES 2 *personal history of diabetic foot ulcer (Z86.31)*

√5th **Z87.3 Personal history of diseases of the musculoskeletal system and connective tissue**
Conditions classifiable to M00-M99
EXCLUDES 2 *personal history of (healed) traumatic fracture (Z87.81)*

√6th **Z87.31 Personal history of (healed) nontraumatic fracture**

Z87.310 Personal history of (healed) osteoporosis fracture
Personal history of (healed) fragility fracture
Personal history of (healed) collapsed vertebra due to osteoporosis
TIP: Assign for history of osteoporosis fractures that have resolved, even when a code from category M80 indicating current osteoporosis fracture is also reported.

Z87.311 Personal history of (healed) other pathological fracture
Personal history of (healed) collapsed vertebra NOS
EXCLUDES 2 *personal history of osteoporosis fracture (Z87.310)*

Z87.312 Personal history of (healed) stress fracture
Personal history of (healed) fatigue fracture

Z87.39 Personal history of other diseases of the musculoskeletal system and connective tissue

√5th **Z87.4 Personal history of diseases of the genitourinary system**
Conditions classifiable to N00-N99

√6th **Z87.41 Personal history of dysplasia of the female genital tract**
EXCLUDES 1 *personal history of intraepithelial neoplasia III of female genital tract (Z86.001, Z86.008)*
personal history of malignant neoplasm of female genital tract (Z85.40-Z85.44)

Z87.410 Personal history of cervical dysplasia ♀

Z87.411 Personal history of vaginal dysplasia ♀

Z87.412 Personal history of vulvar dysplasia ♀

Z87.42 Personal history of other diseases of the female genital tract ♀

√6th **Z87.43 Personal history of diseases of the male genital organs**

Z87.430 Personal history of prostatic dysplasia ♂
EXCLUDES 1 *personal history of malignant neoplasm of prostate (Z85.46)*

Z87.438 Personal history of other diseases of male genital organs ♂

√6th **Z87.44 Personal history of diseases of the urinary system**
EXCLUDES 1 *personal history of malignant neoplasm of cervix uteri (Z85.41)*

Z87.440 Personal history of urinary (tract) infections

Z87.441 Personal history of nephrotic syndrome

Z87.442 Personal history of urinary calculi
Personal history of kidney stones

Z87.448 Personal history of other diseases of urinary system

√5th **Z87.5 Personal history of complications of pregnancy, childbirth and the puerperium**
Conditions classifiable to O00-O9A
EXCLUDES 2 *recurrent pregnancy loss (N96)*

Z87.51 Personal history of pre-term labor ♀
EXCLUDES 1 *current pregnancy with history of pre-term labor (O09.21-)*

Z87.59 Personal history of other complications of pregnancy, childbirth and the puerperium ♀
Personal history of trophoblastic disease

√5th **Z87.7 Personal history of (corrected) congenital malformations**
Conditions classifiable to Q00-Q89 that have been repaired or corrected
EXCLUDES 1 *congenital malformations that have been partially corrected or repair but which still require medical treatment — code to condition*
EXCLUDES 2 *other postprocedural states (Z98.-)*
personal history of medical treatment (Z92.-)
presence of cardiac and vascular implants and grafts (Z95.-)
presence of other devices (Z97.-)
presence of other functional implants (Z96.-)
transplanted organ and tissue status (Z94.-)

√6th **Z87.71 Personal history of (corrected) congenital malformations of genitourinary system**

Z87.710 Personal history of (corrected) hypospadias ♂

Z87.718 Personal history of other specified (corrected) congenital malformations of genitourinary system

√6th **Z87.72 Personal history of (corrected) congenital malformations of nervous system and sense organs**

Z87.720 Personal history of (corrected) congenital malformations of eye

Z87.721 Personal history of (corrected) congenital malformations of ear

Z87.728 Personal history of other specified (corrected) congenital malformations of nervous system and sense organs

√6th **Z87.73 Personal history of (corrected) congenital malformations of digestive system**

Z87.730 Personal history of (corrected) cleft lip and palate

Z87.738 Personal history of other specified (corrected) congenital malformations of digestive system

Z87.74 Personal history of (corrected) congenital malformations of heart and circulatory system

Z87.75 Personal history of (corrected) congenital malformations of respiratory system

Z87.76 Personal history of (corrected) congenital malformations of integument, limbs and musculoskeletal system

√6th **Z87.79 Personal history of other (corrected) congenital malformations**

Z87.790 Personal history of (corrected) congenital malformations of face and neck

Z87.798 Personal history of other (corrected) congenital malformations

√5th **Z87.8 Personal history of other specified conditions**
EXCLUDES 2 *personal history of self harm (Z91.5)*

Z87.81 Personal history of (healed) traumatic fracture
EXCLUDES 2 *personal history of (healed) nontraumatic fracture (Z87.31-)*

√6th **Z87.82 Personal history of other (healed) physical injury and trauma**
Conditions classifiable to S00-T88, except traumatic fractures

Z87.820 Personal history of traumatic brain injury
EXCLUDES 1 *personal history of transient ischemic attack (TIA), and cerebral infarction without residual deficits (Z86.73)*

Z87.821 Personal history of retained foreign body fully removed

Z87.828 Personal history of other (healed) physical injury and trauma

√6th **Z87.89 Personal history of other specified conditions**

Z87.890 Personal history of sex reassignment

Z87.891 Personal history of nicotine dependence
EXCLUDES 1 *current nicotine dependence (F17.2-)*
AHA: 2017,2Q,27

Z87.892 **Personal history of anaphylaxis**
Code also allergy status such as:
allergy status to drugs, medicaments and biological substances (Z88.-)
allergy status, other than to drugs and biological substances (Z91.0-)

Z87.898 **Personal history of other specified conditions**
AHA: 2013,1Q,21

Z88 Allergy status to drugs, medicaments and biological substances
EXCLUDES 2 *allergy status, other than to drugs and biological substances (Z91.0-)*
AHA: 2015,3Q,23

Z88.0 **Allergy status to penicillin**
▲ Z88.1 **Allergy status to other antibiotic agents**
▲ Z88.2 **Allergy status to sulfonamides**
▲ Z88.3 **Allergy status to other anti-infective agents**
▲ Z88.4 **Allergy status to anesthetic agent**
▲ Z88.5 **Allergy status to narcotic agent**
▲ Z88.6 **Allergy status to analgesic agent**
▲ Z88.7 **Allergy status to serum and vaccine**
▲ Z88.8 **Allergy status to other drugs, medicaments and biological substances**
▲ Z88.9 **Allergy status to unspecified drugs, medicaments and biological substances**

Z89 Acquired absence of limb
INCLUDES amputation status
postprocedural loss of limb
post-traumatic loss of limb
EXCLUDES 1 *acquired deformities of limbs (M20-M21)*
congenital absence of limbs (Q71-Q73)

Z89.0 **Acquired absence of thumb and other finger(s)**
Z89.01 **Acquired absence of thumb**
Z89.011 **Acquired absence of right thumb**
Z89.012 **Acquired absence of left thumb**
Z89.019 **Acquired absence of unspecified thumb**
Z89.02 **Acquired absence of other finger(s)**
EXCLUDES 2 *acquired absence of thumb (Z89.01-)*
Z89.021 **Acquired absence of right finger(s)**
Z89.022 **Acquired absence of left finger(s)**
Z89.029 **Acquired absence of unspecified finger(s)**
Z89.1 **Acquired absence of hand and wrist**
Z89.11 **Acquired absence of hand**
Z89.111 **Acquired absence of right hand**
Z89.112 **Acquired absence of left hand**
Z89.119 **Acquired absence of unspecified hand**
Z89.12 **Acquired absence of wrist**
Disarticulation at wrist
Z89.121 **Acquired absence of right wrist**
Z89.122 **Acquired absence of left wrist**
Z89.129 **Acquired absence of unspecified wrist**
Z89.2 **Acquired absence of upper limb above wrist**
Z89.20 **Acquired absence of upper limb, unspecified level**
Z89.201 **Acquired absence of right upper limb, unspecified level**
Z89.202 **Acquired absence of left upper limb, unspecified level**
Z89.209 **Acquired absence of unspecified upper limb, unspecified level**
Acquired absence of arm NOS
Z89.21 **Acquired absence of upper limb below elbow**
Z89.211 **Acquired absence of right upper limb below elbow**
Z89.212 **Acquired absence of left upper limb below elbow**
Z89.219 **Acquired absence of unspecified upper limb below elbow**
Z89.22 **Acquired absence of upper limb above elbow**
Disarticulation at elbow
Z89.221 **Acquired absence of right upper limb above elbow**
Z89.222 **Acquired absence of left upper limb above elbow**
Z89.229 **Acquired absence of unspecified upper limb above elbow**
Z89.23 **Acquired absence of shoulder**
Acquired absence of shoulder joint following explantation of shoulder joint prosthesis, with or without presence of antibiotic-impregnated cement spacer
Z89.231 **Acquired absence of right shoulder**
Z89.232 **Acquired absence of left shoulder**
Z89.239 **Acquired absence of unspecified shoulder**
Z89.4 **Acquired absence of toe(s), foot, and ankle**
Z89.41 **Acquired absence of great toe**
Z89.411 **Acquired absence of right great toe** HCC
Z89.412 **Acquired absence of left great toe** HCC
Z89.419 **Acquired absence of unspecified great toe** HCC
Z89.42 **Acquired absence of other toe(s)**
EXCLUDES 2 *acquired absence of great toe (Z89.41-)*
Z89.421 **Acquired absence of other right toe(s)** HCC
Z89.422 **Acquired absence of other left toe(s)** HCC
Z89.429 **Acquired absence of other toe(s), unspecified side** HCC
Z89.43 **Acquired absence of foot**
Z89.431 **Acquired absence of right foot** HCC
Z89.432 **Acquired absence of left foot** HCC
Z89.439 **Acquired absence of unspecified foot** HCC
Z89.44 **Acquired absence of ankle**
Disarticulation of ankle
Z89.441 **Acquired absence of right ankle** HCC
Z89.442 **Acquired absence of left ankle** HCC
Z89.449 **Acquired absence of unspecified ankle** HCC
Z89.5 **Acquired absence of leg below knee**
Z89.51 **Acquired absence of leg below knee**
Z89.511 **Acquired absence of right leg below knee** HCC
Z89.512 **Acquired absence of left leg below knee** HCC
Z89.519 **Acquired absence of unspecified leg below knee** HCC
Z89.52 **Acquired absence of knee**
Acquired absence of knee joint following explantation of knee joint prosthesis, with or without presence of antibiotic-impregnated cement spacer
Z89.521 **Acquired absence of right knee**
Z89.522 **Acquired absence of left knee**
Z89.529 **Acquired absence of unspecified knee**
Z89.6 **Acquired absence of leg above knee**
Z89.61 **Acquired absence of leg above knee**
Acquired absence of leg NOS
Disarticulation at knee
Z89.611 **Acquired absence of right leg above knee** HCC
Z89.612 **Acquired absence of left leg above knee** HCC
Z89.619 **Acquired absence of unspecified leg above knee** HCC
Z89.62 **Acquired absence of hip**
Acquired absence of hip joint following explantation of hip joint prosthesis, with or without presence of antibiotic-impregnated cement spacer
Disarticulation at hip
Z89.621 **Acquired absence of right hip joint**
Z89.622 **Acquired absence of left hip joint**
Z89.629 **Acquired absence of unspecified hip joint**
Z89.9 **Acquired absence of limb, unspecified**

Z90 Acquired absence of organs, not elsewhere classified
INCLUDES postprocedural or post-traumatic loss of body part NEC
EXCLUDES 1 *congenital absence — see Alphabetical Index*
EXCLUDES 2 *postprocedural absence of endocrine glands (E89.-)*

Z90.0 **Acquired absence of part of head and neck**
Z90.01 **Acquired absence of eye**
Z90.02 **Acquired absence of larynx**

Z90.09 **Acquired absence of other part of head and neck**
Acquired absence of nose
EXCLUDES 2 *teeth (K08.1)*

✓5th Z90.1 Acquired absence of breast and nipple
Z90.10 **Acquired absence of unspecified breast and nipple**
Z90.11 **Acquired absence of right breast and nipple**
Z90.12 **Acquired absence of left breast and nipple**
Z90.13 **Acquired absence of bilateral breasts and nipples**

Z90.2 **Acquired absence of lung [part of]**

Z90.3 **Acquired absence of stomach [part of]**

✓5th Z90.4 **Acquired absence of other specified parts of digestive tract**
✓6th Z90.41 Acquired absence of pancreas
Code also exocrine pancreatic insufficiency (K86.81)
Use additional code to identify any associated:
diabetes mellitus, postpancreatectomy (E13.-)
insulin use (Z79.4)
Z90.410 **Acquired total absence of pancreas**
Acquired absence of pancreas NOS
Z90.411 **Acquired partial absence of pancreas**
Z90.49 **Acquired absence of other specified parts of digestive tract**

Z90.5 **Acquired absence of kidney**

Z90.6 **Acquired absence of other parts of urinary tract**
Acquired absence of bladder

✓5th Z90.7 Acquired absence of genital organ(s)
EXCLUDES 1 *personal history of sex reassignment (Z87.890)*
EXCLUDES 2 *female genital mutilation status (N90.81-)*
✓6th Z90.71 Acquired absence of cervix and uterus
Z90.710 **Acquired absence of both cervix and uterus** ♀
Acquired absence of uterus NOS
Status post total hysterectomy
Z90.711 **Acquired absence of uterus with remaining cervical stump** ♀
Status post partial hysterectomy with remaining cervical stump
Z90.712 **Acquired absence of cervix with remaining uterus** ♀
✓6th Z90.72 Acquired absence of ovaries
Z90.721 **Acquired absence of ovaries, unilateral** ♀
Z90.722 **Acquired absence of ovaries, bilateral** ♀
Z90.79 **Acquired absence of other genital organ(s)**

✓5th Z90.8 Acquired absence of other organs
Z90.81 **Acquired absence of spleen**
Z90.89 **Acquired absence of other organs**

✓4th Z91 Personal risk factors, not elsewhere classified

EXCLUDES 2 *contact with and (suspected) exposures hazardous to health (Z77.-)*
exposure to pollution and other problems related to physical environment (Z77.1-)
female genital mutilation status (N90.81-)
personal history of physical injury and trauma (Z87.81, Z87.82-)
occupational exposure to risk factors (Z57.-)

✓5th Z91.0 Allergy status, other than to drugs and biological substances
EXCLUDES 2 *allergy status to drugs, medicaments, and biological substances (Z88.-)*
✓6th Z91.01 Food allergy status
EXCLUDES 2 *food additives allergy status (Z91.02)*
Z91.010 **Allergy to peanuts**
Z91.011 **Allergy to milk products**
EXCLUDES 1 *lactose intolerance (E73.-)*
Z91.012 **Allergy to eggs**
Z91.013 **Allergy to seafood**
Allergy to shellfish
Allergy to octopus or squid ink
Z91.018 **Allergy to other foods**
Allergy to nuts other than peanuts
Z91.02 **Food additives allergy status**
✓6th Z91.03 Insect allergy status
Z91.030 **Bee allergy status**
Z91.038 **Other insect allergy status**
✓6th Z91.04 Nonmedicinal substance allergy status
Z91.040 **Latex allergy status**
Latex sensitivity status
Z91.041 **Radiographic dye allergy status**
Allergy status to contrast media used for diagnostic X-ray procedure
Z91.048 **Other nonmedicinal substance allergy status**
Z91.09 **Other allergy status, other than to drugs and biological substances**

✓5th Z91.1 Patient's noncompliance with medical treatment and regimen
Z91.11 **Patient's noncompliance with dietary regimen**
✓6th Z91.12 Patient's intentional underdosing of medication regimen
Code first underdosing of medication (T36-T50) with fifth or sixth character 6
EXCLUDES 1 *adverse effect of prescribed drug taken as directed — code to adverse effect*
poisoning (overdose) — code to poisoning
AHA: 2018,4Q,72
Z91.120 **Patient's intentional underdosing of medication regimen due to financial hardship**
Z91.128 **Patient's intentional underdosing of medication regimen for other reason**
✓6th Z91.13 Patient's unintentional underdosing of medication regimen
Code first underdosing of medication (T36-T50) with fifth or sixth character 6
EXCLUDES 1 *adverse effect of prescribed drug taken as directed — code to adverse effect*
poisoning (overdose) — code to poisoning
AHA: 2018,4Q,72
Z91.130 **Patient's unintentional underdosing of medication regimen due to age-related debility**
Z91.138 **Patient's unintentional underdosing of medication regimen for other reason**
Z91.14 **Patient's other noncompliance with medication regimen**
Patient's underdosing of medication NOS
AHA: 2018,4Q,72
Z91.15 **Patient's noncompliance with renal dialysis** HCC
Z91.19 **Patient's noncompliance with other medical treatment and regimen**
Nonadherence to medical treatment

✓5th Z91.4 Personal history of psychological trauma, not elsewhere classified
✓6th Z91.41 Personal history of adult abuse
EXCLUDES 2 *personal history of abuse in childhood (Z62.81-)*
Z91.410 **Personal history of adult physical and sexual abuse** A
EXCLUDES 1 *current adult physical abuse (T74.11, T76.11)*
current adult sexual abuse (T74.21, T76.11)
Z91.411 **Personal history of adult psychological abuse** A
Z91.412 **Personal history of adult neglect** A
EXCLUDES 1 *current adult neglect (T74.01, T76.01)*
Z91.419 **Personal history of unspecified adult abuse** A
Z91.42 **Personal history of forced labor or sexual exploitation**
AHA: 2018,4Q,32,35
Z91.49 **Other personal history of psychological trauma, not elsewhere classified**

Z91.5 **Personal history of self-harm**
Personal history of parasuicide
Personal history of self-poisoning
Personal history of suicide attempt

✓5th Z91.8 Other specified personal risk factors, not elsewhere classified
Z91.81 **History of falling**
At risk for falling

Z91.82 Personal history of military deployment A
Individual (civilian or military) with past history of military war, peacekeeping and humanitarian deployment (current or past conflict)
Returned from military deployment

Z91.83 Wandering in diseases classified elsewhere
Code first underlying disorder such as:
Alzheimer's disease (G30.-)
autism or pervasive developmental disorder (F84.-)
intellectual disabilities (F70-F79)
unspecified dementia with behavioral disturbance (F03.9-)

✓6th **Z91.84 Oral health risk factors**
AHA: 2017,4Q,29
Z91.841 Risk for dental caries, low
Z91.842 Risk for dental caries, moderate
Z91.843 Risk for dental caries, high
Z91.849 Unspecified risk for dental caries

Z91.89 Other specified personal risk factors, not elsewhere classified
AHA: 2017,1Q,45

✓4th **Z92 Personal history of medical treatment**
EXCLUDES 2 *postprocedural states (Z98.-)*

Z92.0 Personal history of contraception
EXCLUDES 1 *counseling or management of current contraceptive practices (Z30.-)*
long term (current) use of contraception (Z79.3)
presence of (intrauterine) contraceptive device (Z97.5)

✓5th **Z92.2 Personal history of drug therapy**
EXCLUDES 2 *long term (current) drug therapy (Z79.-)*
Z92.21 Personal history of antineoplastic chemotherapy
Z92.22 Personal history of monoclonal drug therapy
Z92.23 Personal history of estrogen therapy
✓6th **Z92.24 Personal history of steroid therapy**
Z92.240 Personal history of inhaled steroid therapy
Z92.241 Personal history of systemic steroid therapy
Personal history of steroid therapy NOS
Z92.25 Personal history of immunosupression therapy
EXCLUDES 2 *personal history of steroid therapy (Z92.24)*
Z92.29 Personal history of other drug therapy

Z92.3 Personal history of irradiation
Personal history of exposure to therapeutic radiation
EXCLUDES 1 *exposure to radiation in the physical environment (Z77.12)*
occupational exposure to radiation (Z57.1)

✓5th **Z92.8 Personal history of other medical treatment**
Z92.81 Personal history of extracorporeal membrane oxygenation (ECMO)
Z92.82 Status post administration of tPA (rtPA) in a different facility within the last 24 hours prior to admission to current facility
Code first condition requiring tPA administration, such as:
acute cerebral infarction (I63.-)
acute myocardial infarction (I21.-, I22.-)
AHA: 2013,4Q,124
Z92.83 Personal history of failed moderate sedation
Personal history of failed conscious sedation
EXCLUDES 2 *failed moderate sedation during procedure (T88.52)*
Z92.84 Personal history of unintended awareness under general anesthesia
EXCLUDES 2 *unintended awareness under general anesthesia during procedure (T88.53)*
AHA: 2016,4Q,72-73,77
Z92.89 Personal history of other medical treatment
AHA: 2020,1Q,18

✓4th **Z93 Artificial opening status**
EXCLUDES 1 *artificial openings requiring attention or management (Z43.-)*
complications of external stoma (J95.0-, K94.-, N99.5-)

Z93.0 Tracheostomy status HCC
AHA: 2013,4Q,129
Z93.1 Gastrostomy status HCC
Z93.2 Ileostomy status HCC
Z93.3 Colostomy status HCC
Z93.4 Other artificial openings of gastrointestinal tract status HCC
✓5th **Z93.5 Cystostomy status**
Z93.50 Unspecified cystostomy status HCC
Z93.51 Cutaneous-vesicostomy status HCC
Z93.52 Appendico-vesicostomy status HCC
Z93.59 Other cystostomy status HCC
Z93.6 Other artificial openings of urinary tract status HCC
Nephrostomy status
Ureterostomy status
Urethrostomy status
Z93.8 Other artificial opening status HCC
Z93.9 Artificial opening status, unspecified HCC

✓4th **Z94 Transplanted organ and tissue status**
INCLUDES organ or tissue replaced by heterogenous or homogenous transplant
EXCLUDES 1 *complications of transplanted organ or tissue — see Alphabetical Index*
EXCLUDES 2 *presence of vascular grafts (Z95.-)*

Z94.0 Kidney transplant status CC
Z94.1 Heart transplant status CC HCC
EXCLUDES 1 *artificial heart status (Z95.812)*
heart-valve replacement status (Z95.2-Z95.4)
Z94.2 Lung transplant status CC HCC
Z94.3 Heart and lungs transplant status CC HCC
Z94.4 Liver transplant status CC HCC
Z94.5 Skin transplant status
Autogenous skin transplant status
Z94.6 Bone transplant status
Z94.7 Corneal transplant status
✓5th **Z94.8 Other transplanted organ and tissue status**
Z94.81 Bone marrow transplant status CC HCC
Z94.82 Intestine transplant status CC HCC
Z94.83 Pancreas transplant status CC HCC
Z94.84 Stem cells transplant status CC HCC
Z94.89 Other transplanted organ and tissue status
Z94.9 Transplanted organ and tissue status, unspecified

✓4th **Z95 Presence of cardiac and vascular implants and grafts**
EXCLUDES 2 *complications of cardiac and vascular devices, implants and grafts (T82.-)*

Z95.0 Presence of cardiac pacemaker
Presence of cardiac resynchronization therapy (CRT-P) pacemaker
EXCLUDES 1 *adjustment or management of cardiac device (Z45.0-)*
adjustment or management of cardiac pacemaker (Z45.0)
presence of automatic (implantable) cardiac defibrillator with synchronous cardiac pacemaker (Z95.810)
AHA: 2019,1Q,33
TIP: Assign an additional code for the condition the pacemaker is controlling (e.g., sick sinus syndrome). Even though the pacemaker controls the heart rate, it does not cure the sick sinus syndrome; it is still present and a reportable chronic condition.
Z95.1 Presence of aortocoronary bypass graft
Presence of coronary artery bypass graft
Z95.2 Presence of prosthetic heart valve
Presence of heart valve NOS
Z95.3 Presence of xenogenic heart valve
Z95.4 Presence of other heart-valve replacement
Z95.5 Presence of coronary angioplasty implant and graft
EXCLUDES 1 *coronary angioplasty status without implant and graft (Z98.61)*

√5th **Z95.8 Presence of other cardiac and vascular implants and grafts**

√6th **Z95.81 Presence of other cardiac implants and grafts**

Z95.810 Presence of automatic (implantable) cardiac defibrillator
Presence of automatic (implantable) cardiac defibrillator with synchronous cardiac pacemaker
Presence of cardiac resynchronization therapy defibrillator (CRT-D)
Presence of cardioverter-defibrillator (ICD)

Z95.811 Presence of heart assist device CC HCC

Z95.812 Presence of fully implantable artificial heart CC HCC

Z95.818 Presence of other cardiac implants and grafts

√6th **Z95.82 Presence of other vascular implants and grafts**

Z95.820 Peripheral vascular angioplasty status with implants and grafts
EXCLUDES 1 *peripheral vascular angioplasty without implant and graft (Z98.62)*

Z95.828 Presence of other vascular implants and grafts
Presence of intravascular prosthesis NEC

Z95.9 Presence of cardiac and vascular implant and graft, unspecified

√4th **Z96 Presence of other functional implants**

EXCLUDES 2 *complications of internal prosthetic devices, implants and grafts (T82-T85)*
fitting and adjustment of prosthetic and other devices (Z44-Z46)

Z96.0 Presence of urogenital implants

Z96.1 Presence of intraocular lens
Presence of pseudophakia

√5th **Z96.2 Presence of otological and audiological implants**

Z96.20 Presence of otological and audiological implant, unspecified

Z96.21 Cochlear implant status

Z96.22 Myringotomy tube(s) status

Z96.29 Presence of other otological and audiological implants
Presence of bone-conduction hearing device
Presence of eustachian tube stent
Stapes replacement

Z96.3 Presence of artificial larynx

√5th **Z96.4 Presence of endocrine implants**

Z96.41 Presence of insulin pump (external) (internal)

Z96.49 Presence of other endocrine implants

Z96.5 Presence of tooth-root and mandibular implants

√5th **Z96.6 Presence of orthopedic joint implants**
AHA: 2019,3Q,16

Z96.60 Presence of unspecified orthopedic joint implant

√6th **Z96.61 Presence of artificial shoulder joint**

Z96.611 Presence of right artificial shoulder joint

Z96.612 Presence of left artificial shoulder joint

Z96.619 Presence of unspecified artificial shoulder joint

√6th **Z96.62 Presence of artificial elbow joint**

Z96.621 Presence of right artificial elbow joint

Z96.622 Presence of left artificial elbow joint

Z96.629 Presence of unspecified artificial elbow joint

√6th **Z96.63 Presence of artificial wrist joint**

Z96.631 Presence of right artificial wrist joint

Z96.632 Presence of left artificial wrist joint

Z96.639 Presence of unspecified artificial wrist joint

√6th **Z96.64 Presence of artificial hip joint**
Hip-joint replacement (partial) (total)

Z96.641 Presence of right artificial hip joint

Z96.642 Presence of left artificial hip joint

Z96.643 Presence of artificial hip joint, bilateral

Z96.649 Presence of unspecified artificial hip joint

√6th **Z96.65 Presence of artificial knee joint**

Z96.651 Presence of right artificial knee joint

Z96.652 Presence of left artificial knee joint

Z96.653 Presence of artificial knee joint, bilateral

Z96.659 Presence of unspecified artificial knee joint

√6th **Z96.66 Presence of artificial ankle joint**

Z96.661 Presence of right artificial ankle joint

Z96.662 Presence of left artificial ankle joint

Z96.669 Presence of unspecified artificial ankle joint

√6th **Z96.69 Presence of other orthopedic joint implants**

Z96.691 Finger-joint replacement of right hand

Z96.692 Finger-joint replacement of left hand

Z96.693 Finger-joint replacement, bilateral

Z96.698 Presence of other orthopedic joint implants

Z96.7 Presence of other bone and tendon implants
Presence of skull plate

√5th **Z96.8 Presence of other specified functional implants**

Z96.81 Presence of artificial skin

Z96.82 Presence of neurostimulator
Presence of brain neurostimulator
Presence of gastric neurostimulator
Presence of peripheral nerve neurostimulator
Presence of sacral nerve neurostimulator
Presence of spinal cord neurostimulator
Presence of vagus nerve neurostimulator
AHA: 2019,4Q,19

Z96.89 Presence of other specified functional implants

Z96.9 Presence of functional implant, unspecified

√4th **Z97 Presence of other devices**

EXCLUDES 1 *complications of internal prosthetic devices, implants and grafts (T82-T85)*
EXCLUDES 2 *fitting and adjustment of prosthetic and other devices (Z44-Z46)*
presence of cerebrospinal fluid drainage device (Z98.2)

Z97.0 Presence of artificial eye

√5th **Z97.1 Presence of artificial limb (complete) (partial)**

Z97.10 Presence of artificial limb (complete) (partial), unspecified

Z97.11 Presence of artificial right arm (complete) (partial)

Z97.12 Presence of artificial left arm (complete) (partial)

Z97.13 Presence of artificial right leg (complete) (partial)

Z97.14 Presence of artificial left leg (complete) (partial)

Z97.15 Presence of artificial arms, bilateral (complete) (partial)

Z97.16 Presence of artificial legs, bilateral (complete) (partial)

Z97.2 Presence of dental prosthetic device (complete) (partial)
Presence of dentures (complete) (partial)

Z97.3 Presence of spectacles and contact lenses

Z97.4 Presence of external hearing-aid

Z97.5 Presence of (intrauterine) contraceptive device ♀
EXCLUDES 1 *checking, reinsertion or removal of implantable subdermal contraceptive (Z30.46)*
checking, reinsertion or removal of intrauterine contraceptive device (Z30.43-)

Z97.8 Presence of other specified devices

√4th **Z98 Other postprocedural states**

EXCLUDES 2 *aftercare (Z43-Z49, Z51)*
follow-up medical care (Z08-Z09)
postprocedural complication — see Alphabetical Index

Z98.0 Intestinal bypass and anastomosis status
EXCLUDES 2 *bariatric surgery status (Z98.84)*
gastric bypass status (Z98.84)
obesity surgery status (Z98.84)

Z98.1 Arthrodesis status

Z98.2 Presence of cerebrospinal fluid drainage device
Presence of CSF shunt

Z98.3 Post therapeutic collapse of lung status
Code first underlying disease

√5th **Z98.4 Cataract extraction status**
Use additional code to identify intraocular lens implant status (Z96.1)
EXCLUDES 1 *aphakia (H27.0)*

Z98.41 Cataract extraction status, right eye

Z98.42 Cataract extraction status, left eye

Z98.49 Cataract extraction status, unspecified eye

Z98.5 Sterilization status
EXCLUDES 1 *female infertility (N97.-)*
male infertility (N46.-)

Z98.51 Tubal ligation status ♀

Z98.52 Vasectomy status A ♂

Z98.6 Angioplasty status

Z98.61 Coronary angioplasty status
EXCLUDES 1 *coronary angioplasty status with implant and graft (Z95.5)*

Z98.62 Peripheral vascular angioplasty status
EXCLUDES 1 *peripheral vascular angioplasty status with implant and graft (Z95.820)*

Z98.8 Other specified postprocedural states

Z98.81 Dental procedure status

Z98.810 Dental sealant status

Z98.811 Dental restoration status
Dental crown status
Dental fillings status

Z98.818 Other dental procedure status

Z98.82 Breast implant status
EXCLUDES 1 *breast implant removal status (Z98.86)*

Z98.83 Filtering (vitreous) bleb after glaucoma surgery status
EXCLUDES 1 *inflammation (infection) of postprocedural bleb (H59.4-)*

Z98.84 Bariatric surgery status
Gastric banding status
Gastric bypass status for obesity
Obesity surgery status
EXCLUDES 1 *bariatric surgery status complicating pregnancy, childbirth, or the puerperium (O99.84)*
EXCLUDES 2 *intestinal bypass and anastomosis status (Z98.0)*
AHA: 2020,1Q,12

Z98.85 Transplanted organ removal status
Transplanted organ previously removed due to complication, failure, rejection or infection
EXCLUDES 1 *encounter for removal of transplanted organ — code to complication of transplanted organ (T86.-)*

Z98.86 Personal history of breast implant removal

Z98.87 Personal history of in utero procedure

Z98.870 Personal history of in utero procedure during pregnancy ♀
EXCLUDES 2 *complications from in utero procedure for current pregnancy (O35.7)*
supervision of current pregnancy with history of in utero procedure during previous pregnancy (O09.82-)

Z98.871 Personal history of in utero procedure while a fetus

Z98.89 Other specified postprocedural states

Z98.890 Other specified postprocedural states
Personal history of surgery, not elsewhere classified

Z98.891 History of uterine scar from previous surgery ♀
EXCLUDES 1 *maternal care due to uterine scar from previous surgery (O34.2-)*
AHA: 2016,4Q,51-52,76

Z99 Dependence on enabling machines and devices, not elsewhere classified
EXCLUDES 1 *cardiac pacemaker status (Z95.0)*
AHA: 2020,1Q,11

Z99.0 Dependence on aspirator

Z99.1 Dependence on respirator
Dependence on ventilator

Z99.11 Dependence on respirator [ventilator] status CC HCC
AHA: 2015,1Q,21

Z99.12 Encounter for respirator [ventilator] dependence during power failure CC HCC
EXCLUDES 1 *mechanical complication of respirator [ventilator] (J95.850)*

Z99.2 Dependence on renal dialysis HCC
Hemodialysis status
Peritoneal dialysis status
Presence of arteriovenous shunt for dialysis
Renal dialysis status NOS
EXCLUDES 1 *encounter for fitting and adjustment of dialysis catheter (Z49.0-)*
EXCLUDES 2 *noncompliance with renal dialysis (Z91.15)*
AHA: 2016,1Q,12; 2013,4Q,125

Z99.3 Dependence on wheelchair
Wheelchair confinement status
Code first cause of dependence, such as:
muscular dystrophy (G71.0-)
obesity (E66.-)

Z99.8 Dependence on other enabling machines and devices

Z99.81 Dependence on supplemental oxygen
Dependence on long-term oxygen
AHA: 2013,4Q,129

Z99.89 Dependence on other enabling machines and devices
Dependence on machine or device NOS
AHA: 2020,1Q,11

Chapter 22. Codes for Special Purposes (UØØ–U85)

Chapter-specific Guidelines with Coding Examples

UØ7.Ø Vaping-related disorder (see Section I.C.1Ø.e., Vaping-related disorders)

UØ7.1 COVID-19 (see Section I.C.1.g.1., COVID-19 infection)

Chapter 22. Codes for Special Purposes (U00-U85)

This chapter contains the following blocks:

U00-U49 Provisional assignment of new diseases of uncertain etiology or emergency use

Provisional assignment of new diseases of uncertain etiology or emergency use (U00-U49)

4th **U07 Emergency use of U07**

● **U07.0 Vaping-related disorder**

Dabbing related lung damage
Dabbing related lung injury
E-cigarette, or vaping, product use associated lung injury [EVALI]
Electronic cigarette related lung damage
Electronic cigarette related lung injury
Use additional code, to identify manifestations, such as:
- abdominal pain (R10.84)
- acute respiratory distress syndrome (J80)
- diarrhea (R19.7)
- drug-induced interstitial lung disorder (J70.4)
- lipoid pneumonia (J69.1)
- weight loss (R63.4)

DEF: Respiratory illness or injury caused by harmful aerosolized substances and chemicals produced by electronic cigarettes, vapes, e-pipes, and other battery-powered vaping devices. Symptoms may include shortness of breath and fever, while some patients experience severe, sometimes fatal, lung damage. ***Synonyms:*** *e-cigarette and vaping product use-associated lung injury, EVALI.*

● **U07.1 COVID-19** HIV MCC

Use additional code to identify pneumonia or other manifestations

EXCLUDES 1 *coronavirus infection, unspecified (B34.2)*
coronavirus as the cause of diseases classified elsewhere (B97.2-)
pneumonia due to SARS-associated coronavirus (J12.81)

AHA: 2020,2Q,3-13

DEF: First diagnosed in December 2019 in China, coronavirus disease 2019 (COVID-19) is a respiratory infection caused by a newly identified (novel) virus not previously seen in humans, known as severe acute respiratory syndrome coronavirus 2 (SARS-CoV-2). Symptoms of this lower respiratory illness include fever, dry cough, and tiredness that may progress to include difficulty breathing. Older patients and those with high blood pressure, heart problems, and diabetes are more likely to develop serious symptoms of the illness. ***Synonyms:*** *2019 novel coronavirus, 2019-nCoV, coronavirus, SARS-CoV-2, Wuhan coronavirus.*

TIP: Only a confirmed diagnosis of COVID-19 can be coded to U07.1; a positive COVID-19 test result or documentation by the provider that the disease is confirmed is sufficient.

TIP: Assign for asymptomatic individuals who test positive for COVID-19. Even though asymptomatic, the individual is considered to have the COVID-19 infection due to the positive test result.

TIP: Assign appropriate codes for presenting signs/symptoms associated with COVID-19 (cough, fever, shortness of breath), instead of U07.1, if a definitive diagnosis has not been established.

Appendix A: Valid 3-Character ICD-10-CM Codes

AØ9	Infectious gastroenteritis and colitis, unspecified
A33	Tetanus neonatorum
A34	Obstetrical tetanus
A35	Other tetanus
A46	Erysipelas
A55	Chlamydial lymphogranuloma (venereum)
A57	Chancroid
A58	Granuloma inguinale
A64	Unspecified sexually transmitted disease
A65	Nonvenereal syphilis
A7Ø	Chlamydia psittaci infections
A78	Q fever
A86	Unspecified viral encephalitis
A89	Unspecified viral infection of central nervous system
A9Ø	Dengue fever [classical dengue]
A91	Dengue hemorrhagic fever
A94	Unspecified arthropod-borne viral fever
A99	Unspecified viral hemorrhagic fever
BØ3	Smallpox
BØ4	Monkeypox
BØ9	Unspecified viral infection characterized by skin and mucous membrane lesions
B2Ø	Human immunodeficiency virus [HIV] disease
B49	Unspecified mycosis
B54	Unspecified malaria
B59	Pneumocystosis
B64	Unspecified protozoal disease
B72	Dracunculiasis
B75	Trichinellosis
B79	Trichuriasis
B8Ø	Enterobiasis
B86	Scabies
B89	Unspecified parasitic disease
B91	Sequelae of poliomyelitis
B92	Sequelae of leprosy
CØ1	Malignant neoplasm of base of tongue
CØ7	Malignant neoplasm of parotid gland
C12	Malignant neoplasm of pyriform sinus
C19	Malignant neoplasm of rectosigmoid junction
C2Ø	Malignant neoplasm of rectum
C23	Malignant neoplasm of gallbladder
C33	Malignant neoplasm of trachea
C37	Malignant neoplasm of thymus
C52	Malignant neoplasm of vagina
C55	Malignant neoplasm of uterus, part unspecified
C58	Malignant neoplasm of placenta
C61	Malignant neoplasm of prostate
C73	Malignant neoplasm of thyroid gland
D34	Benign neoplasm of thyroid gland
D45	Polycythemia vera
D62	Acute posthemorrhagic anemia
D65	Disseminated intravascular coagulation [defibrination A syndrome]
D66	Hereditary factor VIII deficiency
D67	Hereditary factor IX deficiency
D71	Functional disorders of polymorphonuclear neutrophils
D77	Other disorders of blood and blood-forming organs in diseases classified elsewhere
EØ2	Subclinical iodine-deficiency hypothyroidism
E15	Nondiabetic hypoglycemic coma
E35	Disorders of endocrine glands in diseases classified elsewhere
E4Ø	Kwashiorkor
E41	Nutritional marasmus
E42	Marasmic kwashiorkor
E43	Unspecified severe protein-calorie malnutrition
E45	Retarded development following protein-calorie malnutrition
E46	Unspecified protein-calorie malnutrition
E52	Niacin deficiency [pellagra]
E54	Ascorbic acid deficiency
E58	Dietary calcium deficiency
E59	Dietary selenium deficiency
E6Ø	Dietary zinc deficiency
E65	Localized adiposity
E68	Sequelae of hyperalimentation
FØ4	Amnestic disorder due to known physiological condition
FØ5	Delirium due to known physiological condition
FØ9	Unspecified mental disorder due to known physiological condition
F21	Schizotypal disorder
F22	Delusional disorders
F23	Brief psychotic disorder
F24	Shared psychotic disorder
F28	Other psychotic disorder not due to a substance or known physiological condition
F29	Unspecified psychosis not due to a substance or known physiological condition
F39	Unspecified mood [affective] disorder
F54	Psychological and behavioral factors associated with disorders or diseases classified elsewhere
F59	Unspecified behavioral syndromes associated with physiological disturbances and physical factors
F66	Other sexual disorders
F69	Unspecified disorder of adult personality and behavior
F7Ø	Mild intellectual disabilities
F71	Moderate intellectual disabilities
F72	Severe intellectual disabilities
F73	Profound intellectual disabilities
F78	Other intellectual disabilities
F79	Unspecified intellectual disabilities
F82	Specific developmental disorder of motor function
F88	Other disorders of psychological development
F89	Unspecified disorder of psychological development
F99	Mental disorder, not otherwise specified
GØ1	Meningitis in bacterial diseases classified elsewhere
GØ2	Meningitis in other infectious and parasitic diseases classified elsewhere
GØ7	Intracranial and intraspinal abscess and granuloma in diseases classified elsewhere
GØ8	Intracranial and intraspinal phlebitis and thrombophlebitis
GØ9	Sequelae of inflammatory diseases of central nervous system
G1Ø	Huntington's disease
G14	Postpolio syndrome
G2Ø	Parkinson's disease
G26	Extrapyramidal and movement disorders in diseases classified elsewhere
G35	Multiple sclerosis
G53	Cranial nerve disorders in diseases classified elsewhere
G55	Nerve root and plexus compressions in diseases classified elsewhere
G59	Mononeuropathy in diseases classified elsewhere
G63	Polyneuropathy in diseases classified elsewhere
G64	Other disorders of peripheral nervous system
G92	Toxic encephalopathy
G94	Other disorders of brain in diseases classified elsewhere
H22	Disorders of iris and ciliary body in diseases classified elsewhere
H28	Cataract in diseases classified elsewhere
H32	Chorioretinal disorders in diseases classified elsewhere
H36	Retinal disorders in diseases classified elsewhere
H42	Glaucoma in diseases classified elsewhere
IØØ	Rheumatic fever without heart involvement
I1Ø	Essential (primary) hypertension
I32	Pericarditis in diseases classified elsewhere
I38	Endocarditis, valve unspecified

I39	Endocarditis and heart valve disorders in diseases classified elsewhere
I41	Myocarditis in diseases classified elsewhere
I43	Cardiomyopathy in diseases classified elsewhere
I52	Other heart disorders in diseases classified elsewhere
I76	Septic arterial embolism
I81	Portal vein thrombosis
I96	Gangrene, not elsewhere classified
JØØ	Acute nasopharyngitis (common cold)
J13	Pneumonia due to Streptococcus pneumoniae
J14	Pneumonia due to Hemophilus influenzae
J17	Pneumonia in diseases classified elsewhere
J22	Unspecified acute lower respiratory infection
J36	Peritonsillar abscess
J4Ø	Bronchitis, not specified as acute or chronic
J42	Unspecified chronic bronchitis
J6Ø	Coalworker's pneumoconiosis
J61	Pneumoconiosis due to asbestos and other mineral fibers
J64	Unspecified pneumoconiosis
J65	Pneumoconiosis associated with tuberculosis
J8Ø	Acute respiratory distress syndrome
J9Ø	Pleural effusion, not elsewhere classified
J99	Respiratory disorders in diseases classified elsewhere
K23	Disorders of esophagus in diseases classified elsewhere
K3Ø	Functional dyspepsia
K36	Other appendicitis
K37	Unspecified appendicitis
K67	Disorders of peritoneum in infectious diseases classified elsewhere
K77	Liver disorders in diseases classified elsewhere
K87	Disorders of gallbladder, biliary tract and pancreas in diseases classified elsewhere
LØØ	Staphylococcal scalded skin syndrome
L14	Bullous disorders in diseases classified elsewhere
L22	Diaper dermatitis
L26	Exfoliative dermatitis
L42	Pityriasis rosea
L45	Papulosquamous disorders in diseases classified elsewhere
L52	Erythema nodosum
L54	Erythema in diseases classified elsewhere
L62	Nail disorders in diseases classified elsewhere
L8Ø	Vitiligo
L83	Acanthosis nigricans
L84	Corns and callosities
L86	Keratoderma in diseases classified elsewhere
L88	Pyoderma gangrenosum
L99	Other disorders of skin and subcutaneous tissue in diseases classified elsewhere
NØ8	Glomerular disorders in diseases classified elsewhere
N1Ø	Acute tubulo-interstitial nephritis
N12	Tubulo-interstitial nephritis, not specified as acute or chronic
N16	Renal tubulo-interstitial disorders in diseases classified elsewhere
N19	Unspecified kidney failure
N22	Calculus of urinary tract in diseases classified elsewhere
N23	Unspecified renal colic
N29	Other disorders of kidney and ureter in diseases classified elsewhere
N33	Bladder disorders in diseases classified elsewhere
N37	Urethral disorders in diseases classified elsewhere
N51	Disorders of male genital organs in diseases classified elsewhere
N62	Hypertrophy of breast
N72	Inflammatory disease of cervix uteri
N74	Female pelvic inflammatory disorders in diseases classified elsewhere
N86	Erosion and ectropion of cervix uteri
N96	Recurrent pregnancy loss
O68	Labor and delivery complicated by abnormality of fetal acid-base balance
O76	Abnormality in fetal heart rate and rhythm complicating labor and delivery
O8Ø	Encounter for full-term uncomplicated delivery
O82	Encounter for cesarean delivery without indication
O85	Puerperal sepsis
O94	Sequelae of complication of pregnancy, childbirth, and the puerperium
PØ9	Abnormal findings on neonatal screening
P53	Hemorrhagic disease of newborn
P6Ø	Disseminated intravascular coagulation of newborn
P84	Other problems with newborn
P9Ø	Convulsions of newborn
P95	Stillbirth
QØ2	Microcephaly
RØ5	Cough
R12	Heartburn
R17	Unspecified jaundice
R21	Rash and other nonspecific skin eruption
R32	Unspecified urinary incontinence
R34	Anuria and oliguria
R37	Sexual dysfunction, unspecified
R42	Dizziness and giddiness
R52	Pain, unspecified
R54	Age-related physical debility
R55	Syncope and collapse
R58	Hemorrhage, not elsewhere classified
R61	Generalized hyperhidrosis
R64	Cachexia
R69	Illness, unspecified
R75	Inconclusive laboratory evidence of human immunodeficiency virus [HIV]
R81	Glycosuria
R99	Ill-defined and unknown cause of mortality
YØ9	Assault by unspecified means
Y66	Nonadministration of surgical and medical care
Y69	Unspecified misadventure during surgical and medical care
Y95	Nosocomial condition
ZØ8	Encounter for follow-up examination after completed treatment for malignant neoplasm
ZØ9	Encounter for follow-up examination after completed treatment for conditions other than malignant neoplasm
Z21	Asymptomatic human immunodeficiency virus [HIV] infection status
Z23	Encounter for immunization
Z66	Do not resuscitate

Appendix B: Pharmacology List 2021

This section enables the coder to quickly review drugs, drug actions, and indications that are often associated with overlooked or undocumented diagnoses. The coder should review the patient's medication record and know what condition the physician is treating with the prescribed medication based on documentation in the medical record. When documentation is lacking, the coder can reference this section to locate the drug, determine the drug action, confirm drug indications, and when necessary query the physician. When applicable, some of the drugs provided in this resource have also been mapped to their appropriate Z code for long-term drug use.

Drug	Z Code	Drug Action/Classification	Indications
Abilify [aripiprazole]		Antipsychotic	Depression, bipolar disorder, schizophrenia, autism symptoms
Acarbose [acarbose]	Z79.84	Oral hypoglycemic	Diabetes mellitus
Accupril [quinapril hydrochloride]		ACE inhibitor	Congestive heart failure; hypertension
Acetaminophen with codeine [acetaminophen/codeine phosphate]	Z79.891	Analgesic, narcotic	Pain, moderate to severe
Actemra [tocilizumab]		Antirheumatic	Rheumatoid arthritis
Actimmune [interferon gamma-1b]	Z79.899	Antineoplastic interferons; antiviral interferons	Chronic granulomatous disease; malignant osteopetrosis
Activella [estradiol/norethindrone acetate]	Z79.890	Estrogen therapy	Menopause symptoms; vaginal and vulvar atrophy; osteoporosis prevention
Actonel [risedronate sodium]	Z79.83	Bisphosphonate	Decrease in bone loss in multiple myeloma patients; Paget's disease; hyperparathyroidism; osteoporosis
Actoplus Met [metformin hydrochloride/pioglitazone hydrochloride]	Z79.84	Oral hypoglycemic	Diabetes mellitus
Actos [pioglitazone hydrochloride]	Z79.84	Oral hypoglycemic	Diabetes mellitus
Aczone [dapsone]		Acne agent, topical	Acne vulgaris
Adalat CC [nifedipine]		Calcium channel blocker	Vasospastic angina; chronic stable angina; hypertension
Adderall XR [amphetamine aspartate and sulfate/dextroamphetamine saccharate and sulfate]		CNS stimulant	Attention deficit hyperactivity disorder (ADHD)
Admelog [insulin lispro]	Z79.4	Insulin	Diabetes mellitus
Advair [fluticasone propionate/salmeterol xinafoate]	Z79.51	Corticosteroid – inhaled; antiasthmatic	Prophylaxis and treatment of asthma and COPD
Advil [ibuprofen]	Z79.1	Nonsteroidal anti-inflammatory drug (NSAID)	Pain or fever relief
Afrezza [human insulin recombinant]	Z79.4	Insulin – inhaled	Diabetes mellitus
Aggrastat [tirofiban hydrochloride]	Z79.02	Antiplatelet	Unstable angina; heart attacks
Aggrenox [aspirin/dipyridamole]	Z79.02	Antiplatelet	Lessening of the chance of heart attack or stroke
Aimovig [erenumab-aooe]		Antimigraine	Migraine headache
AirDuo RespiClick [fluticasone propionate/salmeterol xinafoate]	Z79.51	Corticosteroid – inhaled; antiasthmatic	Asthma
Aklief [trifarotene]		Acne agent, topical	Acne vulgaris
Aldactone [spironolactone]		Cardiovascular agent; antihypertensive agent; diuretic; electrolytic and renal agent	Severe heart failure; ascites associated with cirrhosis; hypokalemia
Aleve [naproxen sodium]	Z79.1	Nonsteroidal anti-inflammatory drug (NSAID)	Reduction of temporary aches and pains
Allegra allergy [fexofenadine hydrochloride]		Antihistamine	Seasonal allergic rhinitis
Allopurinol [allopurinol]		Antigout	Gouty arthritis, renal calculus, hyperuricemia, hyperuricemia secondary to leukemia, hyperuricemia secondary to lymphoma
Alora [estradiol]	Z79.890	Estrogen therapy	Menopause symptoms
Alphagan P [brimonidine tartrate]		Antiglaucoma agent (ophthalmic); antihypertensive, ocular	Open angle glaucoma or another condition in which pressure in the eye is too high (ocular hypertension)
Alprazolam [alprazolam]		Antianxiety; sedative/hypnotic	
Altabax [retapamulin]	Z79.2	Antibiotic, topical	Skin infections
Altace [ramipril]		ACE inhibitor	Congestive heart failure; hypertension
Altavera [ethinyl estradiol/levonorgestrel]	Z79.3	Contraceptive	Prevention of pregnancy
Alvesco [ciclesonide]	Z79.51	Corticosteroid – inhaled; antiasthmatic	Prophylaxis and treatment of asthma

Drug	Z Code	Drug Action/Classification	Indications
Alyacen [ethinyl estradiol/norethindrone]	Z79.3	Contraceptive	Prevention of pregnancy
Amaryl [glimepiride]	Z79.84	Oral hypoglycemic	Diabetes mellitus
Ambien [zolpidem tartrate]		CNS depressant; anxiolytic/sedative/hypnotic	Insomnia
Amikacin [amikacin sulfate]	Z79.2	Antibiotic	Gram-negative bacterial infections such as Pseudomonas, Escherichia coli (E. coli), Proteus, Klebsiella-Enterobacter-Serratia
Amitriptyline HCl [amitriptyline hydrochloride]		Antidepressant	Depression
Amoxicillin [amoxicillin]	Z79.2	Antibiotic	Treatment of infections with a broad spectrum of bactericidal activity against many gram-positive and gram-negative micro-organisms; otitis media, gonorrhea, skin, respiratory, gastrointestinal, and genitourinary infections
Ampicillin [ampicillin sodium]	Z79.2	Antibiotic	Bacterial infections
Ampyra [dalfampridine]		Potassium channel blocker	Improvement in walking in patients with multiple sclerosis
Amrix [cyclobenzaprine hydrochloride]		Muscle relaxant	Adjunct to rest and physical therapy for muscle spasms
Anaprox DS [naproxen sodium]	Z79.1	Nonsteroidal anti-inflammatory drug (NSAID)	Pain, inflammation or fever relief
Anastrozole [anastrozole]	Z79.811	Aromatase inhibitor	Postmenopausal breast cancer
Ancef [cefazolin sodium]	Z79.2	Antibiotic	Respiratory tract infections due to Streptococcus pneumoniae, Klebsiella species, Haemophilus influenzae (H. influenzae), Staphylococcus aureus, and group A betahemolytic streptococci; urinary tract infections due to E. coli, Proteus mirabilis, Klebsiella species and some strains of Enterobacter and enterococci; skin and skin structure infections, biliary tract infections, bone and joint infections, genital infections, septicemia, and endocarditis
Androderm [testosterone]	Z79.89Ø	Testosterone therapy – topical	Primary hypogonadism, hypogonadotropic hypogonadism
AndroGel [testosterone]	Z79.89Ø	Testosterone therapy – topical	Primary hypogonadism, hypogonadotropic hypogonadism
Angeliq [drospirenone/estradiol]	Z79.89Ø	Estrogen therapy	Menopause symptoms
Angiomax [bivalirudin]	Z79.Ø1	Anticoagulant	Prevention of blood clots
Antabuse [disulfiram]		Alcohol treatment	Alcoholism
Antineoplastic/chemotherapy	Z79.899	Antineoplastic	Cancer
Apidra [insulin glulisine recombinant]	Z79.4	Insulin	Diabetes mellitus
Aranelle [ethinyl estradiol/norethindrone]	Z79.3	Contraceptive	Prevention of pregnancy; acne
Aranesp [darbepoetin alfa]		Erythropoiesis-stimulating agent (ESA)	Treatment of lower than normal blood cells (anemia) from disorders such as CKD and neoplasms
Argatroban [argatroban]	Z79.Ø1	Anticoagulant	Prophylaxis and treatment of venous thrombosis in thrombocytopenia patients
Aricept [donepezil hydrochloride]		Acetylcholinesterase/cholinesterase inhibitors	Symptoms of mild to moderate Alzheimer's disease; can improve thinking ability in some patients
Arimidex [anastrozole]	Z79.811	Aromatase inhibitor	Postmenopausal breast cancer
Aristospan [triamcinolone hexacetonide]	Z79.52	Corticosteroid	Severe inflammation
Arixtra [fondaparinux sodium]	Z79.Ø1	Anticoagulant	Venous thrombosis and pulmonary embolism
Arnuity Ellipta [fluticasone furoate]	Z79.51	Corticosteroid – inhaled; antiasthmatic	Prophylaxis and treatment of asthma
Aromasin [exemestane]	Z79.811	Aromatase inhibitor	Postmenopausal breast cancer
Arthrotec [diclofenac sodium/misoprostol]	Z79.1	Nonsteroidal anti-inflammatory drug (NSAID)-prostaglandin combo	Treatment of patients with arthritis who may develop stomach ulcers from taking nonsteroidal anti-inflammatory drugs (NSAIDs) alone; used to help relieve some symptoms of arthritis, such as inflammation, swelling, stiffness, and joint pain
Asacol HD [mesalamine]		Anti-inflammatory	Ulcerative colitis
Ashlyna [ethinyl estradiol/levonorgestrel]	Z79.3	Contraceptive	Prevention of pregnancy
Asmanex [mometasone furoate]	Z79.51	Corticosteroid – inhaled; antiasthmatic	Prophylaxis and treatment of asthma
Astagraf XL [tacrolimus]	Z79.899	Immunosuppressant	Prophylaxis of organ transplant rejection
Atelvia [risedronate sodium]	Z79.83	Bisphosphonate	Prevention of thinning of the bones (osteoporosis)

Drug	Z Code	Drug Action/Classification	Indications
Atenolol [atenolol]		Beta blocker	Angina pectoris; hypertension; acute myocardial infarction
Ativan [lorazepam]		Antianxiety; sedative/hypnotic	Anxiety disorder associated with depressive symptoms; controls tension, agitation, irritability, and insomnia
Atripla [efavirenz/emtricitabine/tenofovir disoproxil fumarate]	Z79.899	Antiviral	HIV
Atrovent HFA [ipratropium bromide]		Antiasthmatic/bronchodilator	Chronic bronchitis, emphysema; bronchial asthma
Augmentin [amoxicillin/clavulanate potassium]	Z79.2	Antibiotic	Middle ear, lower respiratory, sinus, skin and skin structures, and urinary tract infections
Avandia [rosiglitazone maleate]	Z79.84	Oral hypoglycemic	Diabetes mellitus
Avapro [irbesartan]		Antihypertensive	Hypertension
Avelox [moxifloxacin hydrochloride]	Z79.2	Antibiotic	Bacterial infections, specifically pneumonia; skin; intra-abdominal; plague; acute sinusitis; acute chronic bronchitis
Aviane-28 [ethinyl estradiol/levonorgestrel]	Z79.3	Contraceptive	Prevention of pregnancy
Avonex [interferon beta-1a]	Z79.899	Antiviral	Treatment of relapsing multiple sclerosis
Axid AR [nizatidine]		Histamine H2-receptor antagonist	Acid/peptic disorder; gastroesophageal reflux; duodenal, gastric, and peptic ulcers
Ayvakit [avapritinib]		Multikinase inhibitor	Unresectable or metastatic gastrointestinal stromal tumor (GIST)
Azactam [aztreonam]	Z79.2	Antibiotic	Severe bacterial infections
Azithromycin [azithromycin]	Z79.2	Antibiotic	Bacterial infections
Bactrim [sulfamethoxazole/trimethoprim]	Z79.2	Antibiotic	Treatment of urinary tract infections, acute otitis media, acute exacerbation of chronic bronchitis, shigellosis, and pneumocystis carinii
Balziva-28 [ethinyl estradiol/norethindrone]	Z79.3	Contraceptive	Prevention of pregnancy
Basaglar [insulin glargine]	Z79.4	Insulin	Diabetes mellitus
Bayer [acetylsalicylic acid]	Z79.82	Aspirin	Prophylaxis and treatment of heart attacks, angina or strokes; reduction of fever, pain and inflammation
Beconase AQ [beclomethasone dipropionate monohydrate]	Z79.899	Corticosteroid – intranasal	Perennial and seasonal allergies; vasomotor rhinitis
Bekyree [desogestrel/ethinyl estradiol]	Z79.3	Contraceptive	Prevention of pregnancy
Betaseron [interferon beta-1b]	Z79.899	Antiviral	Treatment of relapsing multiple sclerosis
Betoptic [betaxolol hydrochloride]		Beta blocker; ophthalmic glaucoma agent	Lowering of intraocular pressure; also used for treatment of ocular hypertension and chronic open-angle glaucoma
Bevyxxa	Z79.Ø1	Anticoagulant	Prophylaxis of venous thromboembolism
Beyaz [drospirenone/ethinyl estradiol/levomefolate calcium]	Z79.3	Contraceptive	Prevention of pregnancy; acne
Biaxin XL [clarithromycin]	Z79.2	Antibiotic	Acid/peptic disorder or ulcer, acute exacerbation chronic bronchitis, human immunodeficiency virus, lower and upper respiratory tract infection, sinus infection, prophylaxis mycobacterium avium complex, pharyngitis, pneumonia, tonsillitis
Bijuva [estradiol/progesterone]	Z79.89Ø	Estrogen/progesterone therapy	Menopausal symptoms
Biltricide [praziquantel]		Antiparasitic	Infections from Schistosoma species and liver flukes
Binosto [alendronate sodium]	Z79.83	Bisphosphonate	Prevention of thinning of the bones (osteoporosis)
Boniva [ibandronate sodium]	Z79.83	Bisphosphonate	Prevention of thinning of the bones (osteoporosis)
Breo Ellipta [fluticasone furoate/vilanterol trifenatate]	Z79.51	Corticosteroid – inhaled; anitasthmatic	Maintenance treatment of asthma and COPD
Brevicon 28-day [ethinyl estradiol/norethindrone]	Z79.3	Contraceptive	Prevention of pregnancy; acne
Briellyn [ethinyl estradiol/norethindrone]	Z79.3	Contraceptive	Prevention of pregnancy
Brilinta [ticagrelor]	Z79.Ø2	Antiplatelet	Unstable angina; heart attacks; prevention of blood clots
Brisdelle [paroxetine]		Selective serotonin reuptake inhibitor (SSRI)	Vasomotor symptoms related to menopause
Buprenex [buprenorphine hydrochloride]	Z79.891	Analgesic, narcotic	Moderate to severe pain

Drug	Z Code	Drug Action/Classification	Indications
Buprenorphine HCl and Naloxone HCl [buprenorphine hydrochloride/naloxone hydrochloride]	Z79.891	Analgesic, narcotic	Moderate to severe pain
Buspirone HCl [buspirone hydrochloride]		Antianxiety	Generalized anxiety disorder
Butorphanol tartrate [butorphanol tartrate]	Z79.891	Analgesic, narcotic	Moderate to severe postsurgical pain
Butrans [buprenorphine]	Z79.891	Analgesic, narcotic	Chronic pain
Byetta [exenatide]	Z79.899	Antidiabetic – noninsulin injectable	Diabetes mellitus
Calan [verapamil hydrochloride]		Calcium channel blocker	Angina pectoris at rest and chronic stable, arrhythmia, atrial fibrillation, atrial flutter, paroxysmal supraventricular tachycardia, ventricular arrhythmia, Hypertension
Caldolor [ibuprofen]	Z79.1	Nonsteroidal anti-inflammatory drug (NSAID)	Pain or fever relief
Cambia [diclofenac potassium]	Z79.1	Nonsteroidal anti-inflammatory drug (NSAID)	Migraine headaches
Camila [norethindrone]	Z79.3	Contraceptive	Prevention of pregnancy; menstrual disorders
Caplyta [lumateperone]		Antipsychotic	Schizophrenia
Cardizem CD [diltiazem hydrochloride]		Calcium channel blocker	Chronic stable angina, atrial fibrillation, atrial flutter, hypertension, paroxysmal supraventricular tachycardia
Cardura [doxazosin mesylate]		Antihypertensive	Benign prostatic hyperplasia; hypertension
Catapres [clonidine hydrochloride]		Antihypertensive	Hypertension
Cefprozil [cefprozil]	Z79.2	Antibiotic	Acute exacerbation and chronic bronchitis, lower respiratory tract infection, upper respiratory tract infection, pharyngitis, tonsillitis
Ceftriaxone [ceftriaxone sodium]	Z79.2	Antibiotic	Bacterial infections
Celebrex [celecoxib]	Z79.1	Nonsteroidal anti-inflammatory drug (NSAID)	Relief of some symptoms caused by arthritis, such as inflammation, swelling, stiffness, and joint pain
Celestone Soluspan [betamethasone acetate/betamethasone sodium phosphate]	Z79.52	Corticosteroid; antiasthmatic	Asthma; severe inflammation
Celexa [citalopram hydrobromide]		Antidepressant	Depression
Cellcept [mycophenolate mofetil]	Z79.899	Immunosuppressant	Prophylaxis of organ transplant rejection
Centany [mupirocin]	Z79.2	Antibiotic	Skin infections
Cephalexin [cephalexin]	Z79.2	Antibiotic	Bacterial infections
Chantix [varenicline tartrate]		Smoking cessation aid	Nicotine addiction, smoking
Cimduo [lamivudine/tenofovir disoproxil fumarate]	Z79.899	Antiviral	HIV
Cipro [ciprofloxacin hydrochloride]	Z79.2	Antibiotic	Cystitis, infectious diarrhea, gonorrhea, bone and joint infection, gastrointestinal tract infection, lower and upper respiratory tract infection, sinus infection, urinary tract infection, nosocomial pneumonia, chronic prostatitis
Ciprofloxacin [ciprofloxacin]	Z79.2	Antibiotic	Bacterial infections
Clarithromycin [clarithromycin]	Z79.2	Antibiotic	Skin and respiratory bacterial infections
Claritin [loratadine]		Antihistamine	Seasonal allergic rhinitis; chronic idiopathic urticaria
Cleocin [clindamycin phosphate]	Z79.2	Antibiotic	Bacterial infections
Climara [estradiol]	Z79.890	Estrogen therapy	Osteoporosis prevention and to treat menopausal symptoms; vaginal and vulvar atrophy; hypoestrogenism; ovarian failure
Clindamycin [clindamycin phosphate]	Z79.2	Antibiotic	Bacterial infections
Clonazepam [clonazepam]		Anticonvulsant	Absence, akinetic and myoclonic epilepsy, Lennox-Gastaut syndrome
Clonidine HCl [clonidine hydrochloride]		Antihypertensive	Hypertension
Clopidogrel bisulfate [clopidogrel bisulfate]	Z79.02	Antiplatelet	Unstable angina; heart attacks; prevention of blood clots
Codeine [codeine sulfate]	Z79.891	Analgesic, narcotic	Mild to moderate pain
Cogentin [benztropine mesylate]		Antiparkinsonism	Parkinson's disease
Colace [docusate sodium]		Gastrointestinal agent; laxative, stool softener	Constipation

Drug	Z Code	Drug Action/Classification	Indications
Colocort [hydrocortisone]	Z79.52	Corticosteroid	Inflammation of the colon
CombiPatch [ethinyl estradiol/norethindrone acetate]	Z79.890	Estrogen therapy	Menopause symptoms; vaginal and vulvar atrophy; osteoporosis prevention
Combivent respimat [ipratropium bromide/albuterol sulfate]		Antiasthmatic/bronchodilator	Chronic bronchitis, emphysema; bronchial asthma
Compro [prochlorperazine]		Antiemetic; antipsychotic	Nausea, vomiting, and manic phase of bipolar syndrome or schizophrenia
Conjupri [levamlodipine maleate]		Antihypertensive	Hypertension
Copaxone [glatiramer acetate]		Immunostimulant	Treatment of relapsing multiple sclerosis
Coreg [carvedilol]		Beta blocker	Hypertension; chronic heart failure; left ventricular dysfunction following myocardial infarction
Coreg CR [carvedilol phosphate]		Beta blocker	Hypertension; chronic heart failure; left ventricular dysfunction following myocardial infarction
Cortef [hydrocortisone]	Z79.52	Corticosteroid	Severe inflammation
Cortenema [hydrocortisone]	Z79.52	Corticosteroid	Inflammation of the colon
Cortifoam [hydrocortisone acetate]	Z79.52	Corticosteroid	Colon and rectum inflammation
Cortisone acetate [cortisone acetate]	Z79.52	Corticosteroid	Inflammation
Cortisporin [hydrocortisone acetate/neomycin sulfate/polymyxin B sulfate]		Topical anti-infective, topical steroid	Dermatosis
Cosentyx [secukinumab]	Z79.899	Immunosuppressant	Plaque psoriasis; psoriatic arthritis; ankylosing spondylitis
Coumadin [warfarin sodium]	Z79.01	Anticoagulant	Prophylaxis and treatment of venous thrombosis, treatment of atrial fibrillation with embolization (pulmonary embolism), arrhythmias, myocardial infarction, and stroke prevention
Cozaar [losartan potassium]		Antihypertensive	Hypertension
Crestor [rosuvastatin calcium]		HMG-CoA reductase inhibitor (statin)	Hypercholesterolemia; hyperlipidemia; hyperproteinemia
Crixivan [indinavir sulfate]	Z79.899	Antiviral	HIV, asymptomatic HIV
Cryselle [ethinyl estradiol/norgestrel]	Z79.3	Contraceptive	Prevention of pregnancy
Cubicin [daptomycin]	Z79.2	Antibiotic	Bacterial skin infections; Staphylococcus aureus bloodstream infections
Cyclafem [ethinyl estradiol/norethindrone]	Z79.3	Contraceptive	Prevention of pregnancy
Cyclessa [desogestrel/ethinyl estradiol]	Z79.3	Contraceptive	Prevention of pregnancy
Cyclosporine [cyclosporine]	Z79.899	Immunosuppressant	Prophylaxis of organ transplant rejection
Cyltezo [adalimumab-abdm]	Z79.899	Antirheumatic	Rheumatoid arthritis; juvenile idiopathic arthritis; psoriatic arthritis; Crohn's disease; ulcerative colitis; plaque psoriasis
Cymbalta [duloxetine hydrochloride]		Antidepressant, serotonin and norepinephrine reuptake inhibitor (SNRI)	Major depressive disorder; general anxiety disorder; fibromyalgia; diabetic peripheral neuropathy; chronic musculoskeletal pain
Cytomel [liothyronine sodium]		Thyroid hormone	Hypothyroidism or prevention of euthyroid goiters
Daptomycin [daptomycin]	Z79.2	Antibiotic	Skin and underlying tissue bacterial infections
Dasetta [ethinyl estradiol/norethindrone]	Z79.3	Contraceptive	Prevention of pregnancy
Daypro [oxaprozin]	Z79.1	Nonsteroidal anti-inflammatory drug (NSAID)	Osteoarthritis and rheumatoid arthritis
Daysee [ethinyl estradiol/levonorgestrel]	Z79.3	Contraceptive	Prevention of pregnancy
Delestrogen [estradiol valerate]	Z79.890	Estrogen therapy	Menopause symptoms
Demerol [meperidine hydrochloride]	Z79.891	Analgesic, narcotic	Moderate to severe pain
Depakote [divalproex sodium]		Anticonvulsant	Bipolar affective disorder; complex absence, complex partial and mixed pattern epilepsy; migraine headache
Depo-Medrol [methylprednisolone acetate]	Z79.52	Corticosteroid	Arthritis; joint disorders
Depo-Provera [medroxyprogesterone acetate]	Z79.3, Z79.890	Antineoplastic; contraceptive; progestin	Amenorrhea; carcinoma, endometrium, adjunct; carcinoma, renal; Prevention of pregnancy; hemorrhage
Depo-SubQ Provera [medroxyprogesterone acetate]	Z79.3	Contraceptive	Prevention of pregnancy; menstrual disorder pain

Drug	Z Code	Drug Action/Classification	Indications
Descovy [emtricitabine/tenofovir alafenamide]	Z79.899	Antiretroviral	HIV
Desogestrel; Ethinyl [desogestrel/ethinyl estradiol]	Z79.3	Contraceptive	Prevention of pregnancy
Detrol [tolterodine tartrate]		Muscarinic receptor antagonist	Overactive bladders in patients with urinary frequency, urgency, or urge incontinence
Dexamethasone Intensol [dexamethasone]	Z79.52	Corticosteroid	Arthritis; allergic disorders; breathing disorders; lupus
Dexilant [dexlansoprazole]		Proton pump inhibitor	Healing of erosive esophagitis; relieve of heartburn; treatment of non-erosive gastroesophageal reflux disease
Diaβeta [glyburide]	Z79.84	Oral hypoglycemic	Diabetes mellitus
Diclegis [doxylamine succinate/pyridoxine hydrochloride]		Antiemetic	Nausea/vomiting in pregnancy
Dificid [fidaxomicin]	Z79.2	Antibiotic	Clostridium difficile
Diflucan [fluconazole]		Antifungal	Oropharyngeal and esophageal candidiasis and cryptococcal meningitis in AIDS patients
Digoxin [digoxin]		Cardiotonic glycoside	Heart failure, atrial flutter, atrial fibrillation, and supraventricular tachycardia
Dilantin [phenytoin sodium]		Anticonvulsant	Grand mal and psychomotor seizures
Dilaudid [hydromorphone hydrochloride]	Z79.891	Analgesic, narcotic	Moderate to severe pain
Diovan [valsartan]		Antihypertensive	Hypertension
Diskets [methadone hydrochloride]		Opioid agonist	Treatment of opioid addiction
Divigel [estradiol]	Z79.890	Estrogen therapy – topical	Menopause symptoms
Dolophine HCl [methadone hydrochloride]	Z79.891	Analgesic, narcotic; opioid agonist	Pain; treatment of opioid addiction
Doxycycline [doxycycline]	Z79.2	Antibiotic	Bacterial infections; acne
Duavee [bazedoxifene acetate/conjugated estrogens]	Z79.890	Estrogen therapy	Menopause symptoms; osteoporosis prevention
Duetact [glimepiride/pioglitazone hydrochloride]	Z79.84	Oral hypoglycemic	Diabetes mellitus
Duexis [famotidine/ibuprofen]	Z79.1	Nonsteroidal anti-inflammatory drug (NSAID)	Symptomatic treatment of osteoarthritis and rheumatoid arthritis; reduce risk of ulcers
Dulera [formoterol fumarate/mometasone furoate]	Z79.51	Corticosteroid – inhaled; antiasthmatic	Prophylaxis and treatment of asthma
Duragesic [fentanyl]	Z79.891	Analgesic, narcotic	Chronic pain
Duramorph PF [morphine sulfate]	Z79.891	Analgesic, narcotic	Moderate to severe pain
Durlaza [aspirin]	Z79.82	Aspirin	Prevention of heart attack, stroke, angina
Dynacin [minocycline hydrochloride]	Z79.2	Antibiotic	Severe acne treatment
E.E.S. [erythromycin ethylsuccinate]	Z79.2	Antibiotic	Bacterial infections
Effexor XR [venlafaxine hydrochloride]		Antidepressant, serotonin and norepinephrine reuptake inhibitors (SNRIs)	Major depressive disorder; social anxiety disorder; panic disorder
Effient [prasugrel hydrochloride]	Z79.02	Antiplatelet	Lessening of the chance of heart attack or stroke
Elestrin [estradiol]	Z79.890	Estrogen therapy	Menopause symptoms
Eligard [leuprolide acetate]	Z79.818	Agents affecting estrogen receptors and estrogen levels	Palliative treatment of prostate cancer symptoms
Elinest [norgestrel/ethinyl estradiol]	Z79.3	Contraceptive	Prevention of pregnancy
Eliquis [apixaban]	Z79.01	Anticoagulant	Venous thrombosis
Emoquette [ethinyl estradiol/desogestrel]	Z79.3	Contraceptive	Prevention of pregnancy
Emtriva [emtricitabine]	Z79.899	Antiretroviral	HIV
Enbrel [etanercept]	Z79.899	Antirheumatic	Rheumatoid arthritis; polyarticular juvenile idiopathic arthritis; psoriatic arthritis; ankylosing spondylitis, plaque psoriasis
Enpresse-28 [ethinyl estradiol/levonorgestrel]	Z79.3	Contraceptive	Prevention of pregnancy

Drug	Z Code	Drug Action/Classification	Indications
Enskyce [desogestrel/ethinyl estradiol]	Z79.3	Contraceptive	Prevention of pregnancy
Entocort EC [budesonide]	Z79.52	Corticosteroid	Crohn's disease; ulcerative colitis
Entresto [sacubitril/valsartan]		Angiotensin II receptor blocker; neprilysin inhibitor	Chronic heart failure
Entyvio [vedolizumab]	Z79.899	Immunosuppressant	Ulcerative colitis; Crohn's disease
Envarsus XR [tacrolimus]	Z79.899	Immunosuppressant	Prophylaxis of organ transplant rejection
Epinephrine [epinephrine]		Bronchodilator, cardiotonic	Most commonly, relief of distress due to bronchospasm and restoration of cardiac rhythm in cardiac arrest
Epivir, Epivir-HBV [lamivudine]	Z79.899	Antiretroviral	HIV, hepatitis B (HBV), asymptomatic HIV
Erelzi [etanercept-szzs]	Z79.899	Antirheumatic	Rheumatoid arthritis; polyarticular juvenile idiopathic arthritis; psoriatic arthritis; ankylosing spondylitis, plaque psoriasis
Errin [norethindrone]	Z79.3	Contraceptive	Prevention of pregnancy
Ertapenem [ertapenem sodium]	Z79.2	Antibiotic	Stomach, urinary tract, pelvis, skin and lung infections
ERYC [erythromycin]	Z79.2	Antibiotic	Respiratory tract infections
Erygel [erythromycin]	Z79.2	Antibiotic, topical	Bacterial skin infections
EryPed [erythromycin ethylsuccinate]	Z79.2	Antibiotic	Bacterial infections; rheumatic fever attacks
Ery-Tab [erythromycin]	Z79.2	Antibiotic	Bacterial infections
Erythrocin [erythromycin lactobionate]	Z79.2	Antibiotic	Bacterial infections
Erythromycin [erythromycin]	Z79.2	Antibiotic	Respiratory tract infections
Estarylla [ethinyl estradiol/norgestimate]	Z79.3	Contraceptive	Prevention of pregnancy
Estrace [estradiol]	Z79.890	Estrogen therapy	Vaginal cream for treatment of vaginal and vulvar atrophy
EstroGel [estradiol]	Z79.890	Estrogen therapy – topical	Menopause symptoms
Estrostep Fe [ethinyl estradiol/norethindrone acetate]	Z79.3	Contraceptive	Prevention of pregnancy
Evista [raloxifene hydrochloride]	Z79.810	Selective estrogen receptor modulator (SERM)	Prevention of thinning of the bones (osteoporosis) only in postmenopausal women
Exemestane [exemestane]	Z79.811	Aromatase inhibitor	Postmenopausal breast cancer
Factive [gemifloxacin mesylate]	Z79.2	Antibiotic	Bacterial lung infections
Falmina [ethinyl estradiol/levonorgestrel]	Z79.3	Contraceptive	Prevention of pregnancy
Fareston [toremifene citrate]	Z79.810	Selective estrogen receptor modulator (SERM)	Treatment of metastatic breast cancer in postmenopausal women
Farxiga [dapagliflozin propanediol]	Z79.84	Oral hypoglycemic	Diabetes mellitus
Faslodex [fulvestrant]	Z79.818	Agents affecting estrogen receptors and estrogen levels	Hormone-related breast cancer; metastatic breast cancer
Feldene [piroxicam]	Z79.1	Nonsteroidal anti-inflammatory drug (NSAID)	Treatment of pain and inflammation due to arthritis
Femara [letrozole]	Z79.811	Aromatase inhibitor	Postmenopausal breast cancer
Femhrt [ethinyl estradiol/norethindrone acetate]	Z79.3, Z79.890	Contraceptive; estrogen therapy	Prevention of pregnancy; menopause symptoms; osteoporosis prevention
Femring [estradiol acetate]	Z79.890	Estrogen therapy	Osteoporosis prevention and to treat menopausal symptoms; hypoestrogenism; ovarian failure
Fentanyl citrate [fentanyl citrate]	Z79.891	Analgesic, narcotic	Postprocedural or chronic pain
Fentora [fentanyl citrate]	Z79.891	Analgesic, narcotic	Breakthrough cancer pain
Fetroja [cefiderocol]	Z79.2	Antibiotic	Complicated urinary tract infections; pyelonephritis
Fiasp [insulin aspart]	Z79.4	Insulin	Diabetes mellitus
Fioricet with codeine [acetaminophen/butalbital/caffeine/codeine phosphate]	Z79.891	Analgesic, narcotic	Tension headaches
Firmagon [degarelix]	Z79.890	Hormone therapy	Prostate cancer
Flagyl [metronidazole]	Z79.2	Antibiotic	Bacterial infections
Flavoxate HCl [flavoxate hydrochloride]		Urinary tract spasmolytic	Relief of dysuria, urgency, nocturia, suprapubic pain, frequency, and incontinence associated with cystitis, prostatitis, urethritis, and urethrocystitis/urethrotrigonitis

Drug	Z Code	Drug Action/Classification	Indications
Flomax [tamsulosin hydrochloride]		Antiadrenergic	Benign prostatic hyperplasia
Flonase allergy relief [fluticasone propionate]	Z79.899	Corticosteroid – intranasal	Perennial and seasonal allergic rhinitis
Flovent HFA [fluticasone propionate]	Z79.51	Corticosteroid – inhaled; antiasthmatic	Asthma
Fortaz [ceftazidime]	Z79.2	Antibiotic	Pneumonia and lower respiratory infections
Fosamax [alendronate sodium]	Z79.83	Bisphosphonate	Osteoporosis; Paget's disease
Fosinopril sodium [fosinopril sodium]		ACE inhibitor	Hypertension
Fosrenol [lanthanum carbonate]		Phosphate binder	End-stage renal disease (ESRD)
Fragmin [dalteparin sodium]	Z79.Ø1	Anticoagulant	Prophylaxis and treatment of blood clots
Gengraf [cyclosporine]	Z79.899	Immunosuppressant	Prophylaxis of organ transplant rejection
Gentamicin sulfate [gentamicin sulfate]	Z79.2	Antibiotic	Severe bacterial infections
Gildagia [ethinyl estradiol/norethindrone]	Z79.3	Contraceptive	Prevention of pregnancy
Gildess [ethinyl estradiol/norethindrone acetate]	Z79.3	Contraceptive	Prevention of pregnancy
Glimepiride [glimepiride]	Z79.84	Oral hypoglycemic	Diabetes mellitus
Glucotrol [glipizide]	Z79.84	Oral hypoglycemic	Diabetes mellitus
Glumetza [metformin hydrochloride]	Z79.84	Oral hypoglycemic	Diabetes mellitus
Glyburide (micronized) [glyburide]	Z79.84	Oral hypoglycemic	Diabetes mellitus
Glynase [glyburide]	Z79.84	Oral hypoglycemic	Diabetes mellitus
Glyset [miglitol]	Z79.84	Oral hypoglycemic	Diabetes mellitus
Harvoni [ledipasvir/sofosbuvir]	Z79.899	Antiviral	Chronic hepatitis C
Heparin sodium [heparin sodium]	Z79.Ø1	Anticoagulant	Prophylaxis and treatment of venous thrombosis, pulmonary embolism; prevention of cerebral thrombosis, and treatment of consumptive coagulopathies
Humalog [insulin lispro recombinant]	Z79.4	Insulin	Diabetes mellitus
Humira [adalimumab]	Z79.899	Antirheumatic	Rheumatoid arthritis; juvenile idiopathic arthritis; psoriatic arthritis; Crohn's disease; ulcerative colitis; plaque psoriasis; hidradenitis suppurativa; uveitis
Humulin R [insulin recombinant]	Z79.4	Insulin	Diabetes mellitus
Hydrochlorothiazide [hydrochlorothiazide]		Diuretic; antihypertensive	Management of hypertension and in adjunctive therapy for edema associated with congestive heart failure; hepatic cirrhosis; corticosteroid, and estrogen therapy
Hydrocodone [acetaminophen/hydrocodone bitartrate]	Z79.891	Analgesic, narcotic	Moderate to severe pain
Hydrocodone bitartrate and acetaminophen [acetaminophen/ hydrocodone bitartrate]	Z79.891	Analgesic, narcotic	Pain, moderate to severe
Hydrocortisone [hydrocortisone]	Z79.52	Corticosteroid	Addison's disease; arthritis; immune disorders; allergies; breathing problems
Hydromorphone HCl [hydromorphone hydrochloride]	Z79.891	Analgesic, narcotic	Moderate to severe pain
Hyrimoz [adalimumab-adaz]	Z79.899	Antirheumatic	Rheumatoid arthritis; juvenile idiopathic arthritis; psoriatic arthritis; Crohn's disease; ulcerative colitis; plaque psoriasis
Hyzaar [hydrochlorothiazide/ losartan potassium]		Antihypertensive	Hypertension
Ibsrela [tenapanor hydrochloride]		NHE-3 inhibitor	Irritable bowel syndrome with constipation (IBS-C)
Ibuprofen [ibuprofen]	Z79.1	Nonsteroidal anti-inflammatory drug (NSAID)	Pain or fever relief
Imitrex [sumatriptan succinate]		Antimigraine	Migraine headache
Imuran [azathioprine]	Z79.899	Immunosuppressant	Rheumatoid arthritis
Inderal [propranolol hydrochloride]		Beta blocker	Angina pectoris; hypertension; cardiac arrhythmias
Indocin [indomethacin]	Z79.1	Nonsteroidal anti-inflammatory drug (NSAID)	Treatment of pain and inflammation

Drug	Z Code	Drug Action/Classification	Indications
Integrilin [eptifibatide]	Z79.Ø2	Antiplatelet	Unstable angina; heart attacks; prevention of blood clots
Intron A [interferon alfa 2-b]	Z79.899	Antineoplastic interferons; antiviral interferons	Cancer; hepatitis
Introvale [levonorgestrel/ethinyl estradiol]	Z79.3	Contraceptive	Prevention of pregnancy
Invanz [ertapeneum sodium]	Z79.2	Antibiotic	Stomach, urinary tract, pelvis, skin and lung infections
Invokamet [canagliflozin/metformin hydrochloride]	Z79.84	Oral hypoglycemic	Diabetes mellitus
Invokana [canagliflozin]	Z79.84	Oral hypoglycemic	Diabetes mellitus
Isoniazid [isoniazid]	Z79.2	Antibiotic	Tuberculosis
Isopto carpine [pilocarpine hydrochloride]		Cholinergic parasympathomimetic agent	Reduction of intraocular pressure in open-angle glaucoma or ocular hypertension; management of acute angle-closure glaucoma
Isordil [isosorbide dinitrate]		Smooth muscle relaxant	Acute anginal attacks
Isturisa [osilodrostat]		Cortisol synthesis inhibitor	Cushing's disease in adults
Isuprel [isoproterenol hydrochloride]		Adrenergic agent	Bronchodilator for asthma, chronic pulmonary emphysema, bronchitis, and other conditions accompanied by bronchospasm; can be used in cardiogenic shock cases
Jantoven [warfarin sodium]	Z79.Ø1	Anticoagulant	Prophylaxis and treatment of venous thrombosis, pulmonary embolism; prevention of cerebral thrombosis, and treatment of consumptive coagulopathies
Janumet [metformin hydrochloride/sitagliptin phosphate]	Z79.84	Oral hypoglycemic	Diabetes mellitus
Januvia [sitagliptin phosphate]	Z79.84	Oral hypoglycemic	Diabetes mellitus
Jencycla [norethindrone]	Z79.3	Contraceptive	Prevention of pregnancy
Jentadueto [linagliptin/metformin hydrochloride]]	Z79.84	Oral hypoglycemic	Diabetes mellitus
Junel [ethinyl estradiol/norethindrone acetate]	Z79.3	Contraceptive	Prevention of pregnancy
Kadian [morphine sulfate]	Z79.891	Analgesic, narcotic	Moderate to severe pain
Kariva [desogestrel/ethinyl estradiol]	Z79.3	Contraceptive	Prevention of pregnancy
Katerzia [amlodipine benzoate]		Antihypertensive	Hypertension; coronary artery disease (CAD); chronic stable angina; prinzmetal's angina; variant angina
Kazano [alogliptin benzoate/metformin hydrochloride]	Z79.84	Oral hypoglycemic	Diabetes mellitus
Keflex [cephalexin]	Z79.2	Antibiotic	Bone, middle ear, skin and skin structures, upper respiratory tract and urinary tract infections; acute prostatitis
Kelnor [ethynodiol diacetate/ethinyl estradiol]	Z79.3	Contraceptive	Prevention of pregnancy
Kenalog-10; Kenalog-40 [triamcinolone acetonide]	Z79.52	Corticosteroid	Gouty arthritis; bursitis; tenosynovitis; epicondylitis; rheumatoid arthritis; synovitis; osteoarthritis
Keytruda [pembrolizumab]	Z79.899	Antineoplastic	Cancer
Kimidess [ethinyl estradiol/desogestrel]	Z79.3	Contraceptive	Prevention of pregnancy
Klaron [sulfacetamide sodium]	Z79.2	Antibiotic, topical	Acne vulgaris
Klonopin [clonazepam]		Anticonvulsant; CNS depressant	Epilepsy; seizures; panic disorder
Klor-Con [potassium chloride]		Replaces potassium and maintains potassium level	Hypokalemia
Kombiglyze [metformin hydrochloride/saxagliptin hydrochloride]	Z79.84	Oral hypoglycemic	Diabetes mellitus
K-Tab [potassium chloride]		Replaces potassium and maintains potassium level	Hypokalemia
Kurvelo [ethinyl estradiol/levonorgestrel]	Z79.3	Contraceptive	Prevention of pregnancy; menstrual disorders
Kyleena [levonorgestrel]	Z79.3	Contraceptive	Prevention of pregnancy
Lamisil [terbinafine hydrochloride]		Antifungal	Tinea cruris (jock itch), T. pedis (athlete's foot), T. corporis (ringworm)

Drug	Z Code	Drug Action/Classification	Indications
Lanoxin [digoxin]		Cardiotonic glycoside	Congestive heart failure
Lantus [insulin glargine recombinant]	Z79.4	Insulin	Diabetes mellitus
Larin [ethinyl estradiol/norethindrone acetate]	Z79.3	Contraceptive	Prevention of pregnancy
Lasix [furosemide]		Antihypertensive; diuretic	Management of edema associated with congestive heart failure, renal disease, including nephrotic syndrome and hypertension
Lazanda [fentanyl citrate]	Z79.891	Analgesics, narcotic	Breakthrough cancer pain
Lescol XL [fluvastatin sodium]		HMG-CoA reductase inhibitor (statin)	Hypercholesterolemia; hyperlipidemia; hyperlipoproteinemia
Lessina-28 [ethinyl estradiol/levonorgestrel]	Z79.3	Contraceptive	Prevention of pregnancy
Letrozole [letrozole]	Z79.811	Aromatase inhibitor	Postmenopausal breast cancer
Levemir [insulin detemir recombinant]	Z79.4	Insulin	Diabetes mellitus
Levonest [levonorgestrel/ethinyl estradiol]	Z79.3	Contraceptive	Prevention of pregnancy; menstrual disorders; acne
Levora [levonorgestrel/ethinyl estradiol]	Z79.3	Contraceptive	Prevention of pregnancy
Levothroid [levothyroxine sodium]		Thyroid hormone	Hypothyroidism
Levoxyl [levothyroxine sodium]		Thyroid hormone	Euthyroid goiter; hypothyroidism
Lexapro [escitalopram oxalate]		Antidepressant, selective serotonin reuptake inhibitor (SSRI)	Depression; anxiety
Lialda [mesalamine]		Anti-inflammatory	Ulcerative colitis
Librium [chlordiazepoxide hydrochloride]		Antianxiety	Acute withdrawal symptoms, especially from alcohol, or for other anxiety-producing conditions
Lidocaine HCl [lidocaine hydrochloride]		Antiarrhythmic	Management of ventricular arrhythmias or during cardiac manipulation, such as cardiac surgery
Liletta [levonorgestrel]	Z79.3	Contraceptive	Intrauterine device to Prevention of pregnancy
Lincocin [lincocin hydrochloride]	Z79.2	Antibiotic	Severe bacterial infections
Lipitor [atorvastatin calcium]		HMG-CoA reductase inhibitor (statin)	Hypercholesterolemia; hyperlipidemia; hyperproteinemia
Lithium carbonate [lithium carbonate]		Antimanic	Control of manic episodes in bipolar disorders
Lo Loestrin Fe [ethinyl estradiol/norethindrone acetate]	Z79.3	Contraceptive	Prevention of pregnancy
Locoid [hydrocotisone butyrate]	Z79.52	Corticosteroid – topical	Atopic dermatitis; other dermatoses
Loestrin [ethinyl estradiol/norethindrone acetate]	Z79.3	Contraceptive	Prevention of pregnancy
Lomotil [diphenoxylate hydrochloride/atropine sulfate]		Antidiarrheal	Symptoms of chronic and functional diarrhea
Lopid [gemfibrozil]		Lipid regulating agent	Hypercholesterolemia, hyperlipidemia, hyperlipoproteinemia, hypertriglyceridemia
Lopressor [metoprolol tartrate]		Beta blocker	Angina pectoris; hypertension; acute myocardial infarction
Lorazepam [lorazepam]		Antianxiety; sedative/hypnotic	Anxiety disorder associated with depressive symptoms; controls tension, agitation, irritability, and insomnia
Loryna [drospirenone/ethinyl estradiol]	Z79.3	Contraceptive	Prevention of pregnancy
LoSeasonique [ethinyl estradiol/levonorgestrel]	Z79.3	Contraceptive	Prevention of pregnancy
Lotensin [benazepril hydrochloride]		ACE inhibitor	Hypertension
Lotrel [amlodipine besylate/benazepril hydrochloride]		Antihypertensive	Hypertension
Lotrisone [clotrimazole/ betamethasone dipropionate]		Antifungal-corticosteroid	Relief of redness, swelling, itching, and other discomfort of fungus infections
Lovastatin [lovastatin]		HMG-CoA reductase inhibitor (statin)	Hypercholesterolemia; hyperlipidemia; hyperlipoproteinemia
Lovenox [enoxaparin sodium]	Z79.Ø1	Anticoagulant	Prophylaxis and treatment of venous thrombosis and pulmonary embolism
Low-Ogestrel-28 [norgestrel/ethinyl estradiol]	Z79.3	Contraceptive	Prevention of pregnancy
Lupron Depot [leuprolide acetate]	Z79.818	Agents affecting estrogen receptors and estrogen levels	Endometriosis symptoms; uterine fibroids

Drug	Z Code	Drug Action/Classification	Indications
Macrobid [nitrofuantoin]	Z79.2	Antibiotic	Urinary tract infections
Macrodantin [nitrofurantoin]	Z79.2	Antibiotic	Urinary tract infections
Marlissa [ethinyl estradiol/levonorgestrel]	Z79.3	Contraceptive	Prevention of pregnancy
Maxipime [cefepime hydrochloride]	Z79.2	Antibiotic	Bacterial infections
Meclizine hydrochloride [meclizine hydrochloride]		Antihistamine	Nausea and vomiting, and dizziness associated with motion sickness
Medrol [methylprednisolone]	Z79.52	Corticosteroid	Endocrine, rheumatic, hematologic disorders; collagen, dermatological, ophthalmic, respiratory, neoplastic, gastrointestinal, nervous system disorders; allergic and edematous states
Mefoxin [cefoxitin sodium]	Z79.2	Antibiotic	Bacterial infections
Megace ES [megestrol acetate]	Z79.818	Agents affecting estrogen receptors and estrogen levels	Endometrial or advanced breast cancers; weight loss due to AIDS
Menest [esteriefied estrogens]	Z79.890	Estrogen therapy	Menopause symptoms; ovarian failure
Menostar [estradiol]	Z79.890	Estrogen therapy	Menopause symptoms; osteoporosis prevention
Mepron [atovaquone]	Z79.2	Antibiotic	Pneumonia due to penumocystis jiroveci
Merrem [meropenem]	Z79.2	Antibiotic	Bacterial infections of skin or stomach; bacterial meningitis
Metformin [metformin hydrochloride]	Z79.84	Oral hypoglycemic	Diabetes mellitus
Methadone HCl [methadone hydrochloride]	Z79.891	Analgesic, narcotic; opioid agonist	Pain; treatment of opioid addiction
Methadose [methadone hydrochloride]	Z79.891	Analgesic, narcotic	Acute and chronic pain
Methergine [methylergonovine maleate]		Oxytocic agent	Routine management of postpartum hemorrhage after delivery of placenta
Methylprednisolone [methylprednisolone]	Z79.52	Corticosteroid	Inflammatory disorders
Metronidazole [metronidazole]	Z79.2	Antibiotic	Bacterial infections
Miacalcin [calcitonin salmon]		Calcitonin; a peptide hormone	Hypercalcemia, osteoporosis, postmenopausal symptoms, Paget's disease
Microgestin [ethinyl estradiol/norethindrone acetate]	Z79.3	Contraceptive	Prevention of pregnancy
Minastrin [ethinyl estradiol/norethindrone acetate]	Z79.3	Contraceptive	Prevention of pregnancy
Minivelle [estradiol]	Z79.890	Estrogen therapy	Menopause symptoms; osteoporosis prevention
Minocin [minocycline hydrochloride]	Z79.2	Antibiotic	Bacterial infections; acne
Mirena [levonorgestrel]	Z79.3	Contraceptive	Intrauterine device for prevention of pregnancy; menstrual disorders
Mobic [meloxicam]	Z79.1	Nonsteroidal anti-inflammatory drug (NSAID)	Treatment of pain and inflammation due to osteoarthritis and rheumatoid arthritis
Monoclonal antibodies	Z79.899	Monoclonal antibodies	Cancer; prophylaxis of organ transplant rejection
Monodox [doxycycline]	Z79.2	Antibiotic	Bacterial infections; acne
Monoket [isosorbide mononitrate]		Antianginal; coronary vasodilator, nitrate	Angina pectoris
Mono-Linyah [norgestimate/ethinyl estradiol]	Z79.3	Contraceptive	Prevention of pregnancy; menstrual disorders; acne
Monurol [fosfomycin tromethamine]	Z79.2	Antibiotic	Bacterial bladder infections
Morphabond ER [morphine sulfate]	Z79.891	Analgesics, narcotic	Pain
Morphine sulfate [morphine sulfate]	Z79.891	Analgesic, narcotic	Moderate to severe pain
Motrin IB [ibuprofen]	Z79.1	Nonsteroidal anti-inflammatory drug (NSAID)	Pain or fever relief
MS Contin [morphine sulfate]	Z79.891	Analgesic, narcotic	Moderate to severe pain
Multaq [dronedarone hydrochloride]		Cardiac rhythm regulator	Treatment of patients with recent episodes of atrial fibrillation or atrial flutter
Mycobutin [rifabutin]	Z79.2	Antibiotic	Mycobacterium avium complex (MAC) prophylactic in HIV patients
Mytesi [crofelemer]		Antidiarrheal	Diarrhea occurring in HIV/AIDs patient's on anti-retroviral therapy
Myzilra [ethinyl estradiol/levonorgestrel]	Z79.3	Contraceptive	Prevention of pregnancy

Drug	Z Code	Drug Action/Classification	Indications
Nabumetone [nabumetone]	Z79.1	Nonsteroidal anti-inflammatory drug (NSAID)	Osteoarthritis and rheumatoid arthritis
Nalfon [fenoprofen calcium]	Z79.1	Nonsteroidal anti-inflammatory drug (NSAID)	Pain or inflammation relief
Namzaric [memantine/donepezil hydrochlroides]		Acetylcholinesterase/cholinesterase inhibitors	Dementia due to Alzheimer's
Naprelan [naproxen sodium]	Z79.1	Nonsteroidal anti-inflammatory drug (NSAID)	Pain or inflammation relief
Naprosyn [naproxen]	Z79.1	Nonsteroidal anti-inflammatory drug (NSAID)	Rheumatoid, gouty arthritis and osteoarthritis; ankylosing spondylitis; bursitis; dysmenorrhea; pain, mild to moderate; tendonitis
Natazia [estradiol valerate/dienogest]	Z79.3	Contraceptive	Prevention of pregnancy; menstrual disorders
Nebupent [pentamidine isethionate]	Z79.2	Antibiotic	Severe bacterial lung infection in high risk patients with HIV
Nefazodone HCl [nefazodone hydrochloride]		Antidepressant	Depression
Nembutal sodium [pentobarbital sodium]		Sedative/hypnotic	Adjunct medication in diagnostic procedures or for emergency use with convulsive disorders
NeoProfen [ibuprofen lysine]	Z79.1	Nonsteroidal anti-inflammatory drug (NSAID)	Pain or fever relief
Neoral [cyclosporine]	Z79.899	Immunosuppressant	Prophylaxis of organ transplant rejection
Neurontin [gabapentin]		Anticonvulsant	Epilepsy, partial
Nexium [esomeprazole magnesium]		Proton pump inhibitor	Gastroesophageal reflux disease (GERD), erosive esophagitis
Nexplanon [etonogestrel]	Z79.3	Contraceptive	Implantable device used for prevention of pregnancy
Nitrofurantoin [nitrofurantoin]	Z79.2	Antibiotic	Bacterial urinary tract infections
Nitropress [sodium nitroprusside]		Vasodilator	Potent, rapid action in reducing blood pressure in hypertensive crisis or for controlling bleeding during anesthesia by producing controlled hypotension
Nitrostat [nitroglycerin]		Muscle relaxant; antianginal; antihypertensive; coronary vasodilator	Prophylaxis and treatment of angina pectoris; heart failure associated with myocardial infarction; hypertension, perioperative; surgery, adjunct
Norco [acetaminophen/hydrocodone bitartrate]	Z79.891	Analgesic, narcotic	Moderate to severe pain
Norinyl [mestranol/norethisterone]	Z79.3	Contraceptive	Prevention of pregnancy
Norpace [disopyramide phosphate]		Antiarrhythmic	Coronary artery disease, for prevention, recurrence and control of unifocal, multifocal, and paired PVCs
Nor-QD [norethindrone]	Z79.3	Contraceptive	Prevention of pregnancy
Nortrel [ethinyl estradiol/norethindrone]	Z79.3	Contraceptive	Prevention of pregnancy
Norvasc [amlodipine besylate]		Antihypertensive	Hypertension; coronary artery disease (CAD); chronic stable angina; prinzmetal's angina; variant angina
Novolin [insulin recombinant]	Z79.4	Insulin	Diabetes mellitus
Novolog [insulin aspart recombinant]	Z79.4	Insulin	Diabetes mellitus
Nucynta [tapentadol hydrochloride]	Z79.891	Analgesic, narcotic	Moderate to severe pain
NuvaRing [etonogestrel/ethinyl estradiol]	Z79.3	Contraceptive	Vaginal ring to Prevention of pregnancy
Ogestrel [norgestrel/ethinyl estradiol]	Z79.3	Contraceptive	Prevention of pregnancy
Onglyza [saxagliptin hydrochloride]	Z79.84	Oral hypoglycemic	Diabetes mellitus
Oracea [doxycycline]	Z79.2	Antibiotic	Rosacea
Orapred ODT [prednisolone sodium phosphate]	Z79.52	Corticosteroid	Inflammatory disorders
Orbactiv [oritavancin diphosphate]	Z79.2	Antibiotic	Bacterial skin infections
Orencia [abatacept]	Z79.899	Antirheumatic	Rheumatoid arthritis; polyarticular juvenile idiopathic arthritis; psoriatic arthritis
Orilissa [elagolix]	Z79.890	Hormone therapy	Pain associated with endometriosis
Orphenadrine citrate [orphenadrine citrate]		Muscle relaxant	Acute spasms, tension, and post-trauma cases

Drug	Z Code	Drug Action/Classification	Indications
Orsythia [ethinyl estradiol/levonorgestrel]	Z79.3	Contraceptive	Prevention of pregnancy
Ortho-Novum [norethindrone/ethinyl estradiol]	Z79.3	Contraceptive	Prevention of pregnancy
Ortho-Tri-Cyclen [ethinyl estradiol/norgestimate]	Z79.3	Contraceptive	Prevention of pregnancy
Oseni [alogliptin benzoate/pioglitazone hydrochloride]	Z79.84	Oral hypoglycemic	Diabetes mellitus
Osphena [ospemifene]	Z79.81Ø, Z79.89Ø	Selective estrogen receptor modulator (SERM)	Postmenopausal dyspareunia due to vaginal atrophy; osteoporosis prevention and treatment of menopausal symptoms
Otezla [apremilast]	Z79.899	Antirheumatic	Psoriatic arthritis; plaque psoriasis
Oxazepam [oxazepam]		Antianxiety	Anxiety, tension, and alcohol withdrawal
Oxbryta [voxelotor]		Hemoglobin S polymerization inhibitor	Sickle cell disease
Oxycodone HCl [oxycodone hydrochloride]	Z79.891	Analgesic, narcotic	Moderate to severe pain
OxyContin [oxycodone hydrochloride]	Z79.891	Analgesic, narcotic	Moderate to severe pain
Ozempic [semaglutide]	Z79.899	Antidiabetic – noninsulin injectable	Diabetes mellitus
Paxil [paroxetine hydrochloride]		Antidepressant	Anxiety with panic disorder and depression; obsessive-compulsive disorder
PediaPred [prednisolone sodium phosphate]	Z79.52	Corticosteroid	Inflammatory disorders
Pegintron [peginterferon alfa-2b]	Z79.899	Antiviral	Hepatitis C
Penicillin-VK [penicillin V potassium]	Z79.2	Antibiotic	Chorea, prevention; endocarditis, prevention, secondary to tooth extraction; erysipelas; infections of the skin and skin structures, upper respiratory tract; rheumatic fever, prophylaxis; scarlet fever; Vincent's gingivitis; Vincent's pharyngitis
Pentam [pentamidine isethionate]	Z79.2	Antibiotic	Severe bacterial lung infections
Pepcid [famotidine]		Histamine H2-receptor inhibitor	Acid/peptic disorder; adenoma, secretory; gastroesophageal reflux; duodenal and gastric ulcer; Zollinger-Ellison syndrome
Percocet [oxycodone hydrochloride/acetaminophen]	Z79.891	Analgesic, narcotic	Pain, moderate to severe
Persantine [dipyridamole]	Z79.Ø2	Antiplatelet	Therapy for chronic angina pectoris, preventing clots post heart valve surgery
Pfizerpen [penicillin g potassium]	Z79.2	Antibiotic	Severe bacterial infections
Phenobarbital [phenobarbital sodium]		Anticonvulsant	Grand mal epilepsy
Philith [ethinyl estradiol/norethindrone]	Z79.3	Contraceptive	Prevention of pregnancy
Pimtrea [desogestrel/ethinyl estradiol]	Z79.3	Contraceptive	Prevention of pregnancy
Piqray [alpelisib]		Kinase inhibitor	Postmenopausal advanced or metastatic breast cancer that is HR positive, HER2 negative
Pirmella [ethinyl estradiol/norethindrone]	Z79.3	Contraceptive	Prevention of pregnancy
Pitocin [oxytocin]		Uterotonic	Induction or stimulation of labor at term
Plan B One-Step [levonorgestrel]	Z79.3	Contraceptive	Prevention of pregnancy
Plavix [clopidogrel bisulfate]	Z79.Ø2	Antiplatelet	Lessening of the chance of heart attack or stroke
Ponstel [mefenamic acid]	Z79.1	Nonsteroidal anti-inflammatory drug (NSAID)	Treatment of pain
Portia-28 [ethinyl estradiol/levonorgestrel]	Z79.3	Contraceptive	Prevention of pregnancy
Pradaxa [dabigatran etexilate mesylate]	Z79.Ø1	Anticoagulant	Prophylaxis and treatment of blood clots in patients with atrial fibrillation
Prasugrel [prasugrel hydrocloride]	Z79.Ø2	Antiplatelet	Lessening the chance of heart attack or stroke
Pravachol [pravastatin sodium]		HMG-CoA reductase inhibitor (statin)	Hypercholesterolemia; hyperlipidemia; hyperlipoproteinemia
Prednisolone [prednisolone]	Z79.52	Corticosteroid	Inflammatory disorders
Prednisone [prednisone]	Z79.52	Corticosteroid	Used for its immunosuppressant effects and for relief of inflammation; used in arthritis, polymyositis and other systemic diseases

Drug	Z Code	Drug Action/Classification	Indications
Pregnyl [chorionic gonadotropin]		Gonadotropic hormone	Prepubertal cryptorchidism; hypogonadism; corpus luteum insufficiency and infertility
Prelone [prednisolone]	Z79.52	Corticosteroid	Inflammatory disorders
Prempro [conjugated estrogens/medroxyprogesterone acetate]	Z79.890	Estrogen/progesterone therapy	Menopause; osteoporosis; atrophic vaginitis
Prevacid [lansoprazole]		Proton pump inhibitor	Acid/peptic disorder, erosive esophagitis, duodenal ulcer, Zollinger-Ellison syndrome
Previfem [ethinyl estradiol/norgestimate]	Z79.3	Contraceptive	Prevention of pregnancy
Prezcobix [darunavir/cobicistat]	Z79.899	Antiviral	HIV
Prezista [darunavir ethanolate]	Z79.899	Antiviral	HIV
Priftin [rifapentine]	Z79.2	Antibiotic	Tuberculosis
Prilosec [omeprazole magnesium]		Proton pump inhibitor	Acid/peptic disorder; endocrine adenoma; erosive esophagitis; systemic mastocytosis; gastroesophageal reflux; duodenal, peptic and gastric ulcer; Zollinger-Ellison syndrome
Primaxin [cilastatin sodium/imipenem]	Z79.2	Antibiotic	Skin, stomach, female reproductive organs or lower respiratory tract infections
Prinivil [lisinopril]		ACE inhibitor	Congestive heart failure; hypertension
Pristiq [desvenlafaxine]		Antidepressant; serotonin and norepinephrine reuptake inhibitor (SNRI)	Major depressive disorder
Procardia [nifedipine]		Calcium channel blocker	Management of vasospastic angina and chronic stable angina, hypertension
Prograf [tacrolimus]	Z79.899	Immunosuppressant	Prophylaxis of organ transplant rejection
Prolia [denosumab]	Z79.899	Monoclonal antibody	Treatment and prevention of bone resorption and prevention of bone fracture
Promethazine hydrochloride [promethazine hydrochloride]		Anesthesia, adjunct to; antiemetic; antihistamine; antitussive/expectorant; sedative/hypnotic; vertigo/motion sickness/vomiting	Anesthesia; adjunct; angioedema; conjunctivitis; dermographism; hypersensitivity, motion sickness; pain; perennial, seasonal, and allergic rhinitis; sedation, obstetrical; urticaria
Protonix [pantoprazole]		Proton pump inhibitor	Short-term treatment and maintenance therapy of erosive esophagitis associated with gastroesophageal reflux disease (GERD)
Protopic [tacrolimus]	Z79.899	Immunosuppressant	Atomic dermatitis (eczema)
Proventil-HFA [albuterol sulfate]		Antiasthmatic/bronchodilator	Asthma
Provera [medroxyprogesterone acetate]	Z79.3, Z79.890	Antineoplastic; contraceptive; progestin	Amenorrhea; carcinoma, endometrium, adjunct; carcinoma, renal; Prevention of pregnancy; hemorrhage
Prozac [fluoxetine hydrochloride]		Selective serotonin reuptake inhibitor (SSRI)	Bulimia nervosa; depression; obsessive-compulsive disorder
Pulmicort [budesonide]	Z79.51	Corticosteroid – inhaled; antiasthmatic	Prophylaxis and treatment of asthma
Qnasl [beclomethasone dipropionate]	Z79.899	Corticosteroid – intranasal	Perennial and seasonal allergies; vasomotor rhinitis
Qtern [dapagliflozin propanediol/saxagliptin hydrochloride]	Z79.84	Oral hypoglycemic	Diabetes mellitus
Quartette [levonorgestrel/ethinyl estradiol]	Z79.3	Contraceptive	Prevention of pregnancy
Quasense [ethinyl estradiol/levonorgestrel]	Z79.3	Contraceptive	Prevention of pregnancy
Quinidine gluconate [quinidine gluconate]		Antiarrhythmic	Management of cardiac arrhythmias
Qvar Redihaler [beclomethasone dipropionate]	Z79.51	Corticosteroid – inhaled; antiasthmatic	Prophylaxis and treatment of asthma
Raloxifene HCl [raloxifene hydrochloride]	Z79.810	Selective estrogen receptor modulator (SERM)	Prevention of thinning of the bones (osteoporosis) only in postmenopausal women
Rapaflo [silodosin]		Antiadrenergic	Benign prostatic hyperplasia
Rapamune [sirolimus]	Z79.899	Immunosuppressant	Prophylaxis of organ transplant rejection
Rayos [prednisone]	Z79.52	Corticosteroid; antiasthmatic	Arthritis; blood disorders; allergies; asthma
Rebetol [ribavirin]	Z79.899	Antiviral	Chronic hepatitis C
Rebif [interferon beta-1a]	Z79.899	Antiviral	Treatment of relapsing multiple sclerosis

Drug	Z Code	Drug Action/Classification	Indications
Reclast [zoledronic acid]	Z79.83	Bisphosphonate	Prevention of thinning of the bones (osteoporosis); Paget's disease; bone cancer
Relenza [zanamivir]		Antiviral	Treat and prevent influenza A and B
Renvela [sevelamer carbonate]		Phosphate binder	Chronic kidney disease (CKD) on dialysis
Repaglinide [repaglinide]	Z79.84	Oral hypoglycemic	Diabetes mellitus
Reprexain [hydrocodone bitartrate/ibuprofen]	Z79.891	Analgesic, narcotic; nonsteroidal anti-inflammatory drug (NSAID)	Pain, inflammation or fever relief
Restasis [cyclosporine ophthalmic emulsion]		Anti-inflammatory, ophthalmic	Ocular inflammation due to keratoconjunctivitis sicca
Restoril [temazepam]		Sedative/hypnotic	Insomnia
Retrovir [zidovudine]	Z79.899	Antiretroviral	Indicated in symptomatic HIV infection
Reyvow [lasmiditan]		Serotonin 1F receptor agonist	Migraine with or without aura
Rifadin [rifampin]	Z79.2	Antibiotic	Tuberculosis
Rimactane [rifampin]	Z79.2	Antibiotic	Tuberculosis
Rinvoq [upadacitinib]	Z79.899	Antirheumatic	Rheumatoid arthritis
Riomet [metformin hydrochloride]	Z79.84	Oral hypoglycemic	Diabetes mellitus
Risperdal [risperidone]		Antipsychotic/antimanic	Schizophrenia; bipolar I disorder
Ritalin [methylphenidate hydrochloride]		CNS stimulant	Depression; hyperkinetic activity in children
Roxicet [oxycodone hydrochloride/acetaminophen]	Z79.891	Analgesic, narcotic	Pain, moderate to severe
Roxicodone [oxycodone hydrochloride]	Z79.891	Analgesic, narcotic	Pain relief
Rybelsus [semaglutide]	Z79.84	Oral hypoglycemic	Diabetes mellitus
Sabril [vigabatrin]		Anticonvulsant	Refractory complex partial seizures
Safyral [drospirenone/ethinyl estradiol/levomefolate calcium]	Z79.3	Contraceptive	Prevention of pregnancy
Sandimmune [cyclosporine]	Z79.899	Immunosuppressant	Prophylaxis of organ transplant rejection
Sarafem [fluoxetine hydrochloride]		Selective serotonin reuptake inhibitor (SSRI)	Premenstrual dysphoric disorder (PMDD)
Savaysa [edoxaban tosylate]	Z79.Ø1	Anticoagulant	Prophylaxis and treatment of venous thrombosis, pulmonary embolism; prevention of blood clots due to atrial fibrillation
Seasonale [levonorgestrel/ethinyl estradiol]	Z79.3	Contraceptive	Prevention of pregnancy
Seasonique [ethinyl estradiol/levonorgestrel]	Z79.3	Contraceptive	Prevention of pregnancy
Selfemra [fluoxetine hydrochloride]		Selective serotonin reuptake inhibitor (SSRI)	Premenstrual dysphoric disorder (PMDD)
Septra [sulfamethoxazole trimethoprim]	Z79.2	Antibiotic	Urinary tract infections, acute otitis media, acute exacerbations of chronic bronchitis, and shigellosis
Serevent [salmeterol xinafoate]		Bronchodilator	Asthma
Seromycin [cycloserine]	Z79.2	Antibiotic	Tuberculosis; urinary tract infections
Seroquel XR [quetiapine fumarate]		Antipsychotic	Schizophrenia; bipolar disorder; major depressive disorder
Setlakin [ethinyl estradiol/levonorgestrel]	Z79.3	Contraceptive	Prevention of pregnancy
Silvadene [silver sulfadiazine]	Z79.2	Antibiotic, topical	Wound sepsis due to second/third degree burns
Simulect [basiliximab]	Z79.899	Immunosuppressant	Prophylaxis of organ transplant rejection
Sinemet [carbidopa/levodopa]		Antiparkinsonism	Parkinson's disease
Singulair [montelukast sodium]		Antiasthmatic	Asthma; exercise-induced bronchoconstriction; perennial and seasonal allergic rhinitis
Sirolimus [sirolimus]	Z79.899	Immunosuppressant	Prophylaxis of organ transplant rejection
Sitagliptin [sitagliptin/metformin hydrochloride]	Z79.84	Oral hypoglycemic	Diabetes mellitus
Sivextro [tedizolid phosphate]	Z79.2	Antibiotic	Skin infections including MRSA
Skyla [levonorgestrel]	Z79.3	Contraceptive	Intrauterine device to Prevention of pregnancy
Soliqua [insulin glargine/lixisenatide]	Z79.4	Insulin	Diabetes mellitus
Solodyn [minocycline hydrochloride]	Z79.2	Antibiotic	Bacterial infections

Drug	Z Code	Drug Action/Classification	Indications
Soltamox [tamoxifen citrate]	Z79.810	Selective estrogen receptor modulator (SERM)	Breast cancer
Solu-Cortef [hydrocortisone sodium succinate]	Z79.52	Corticosteroid; antiasthmatic	Asthma; severe inflammation; allergic reactions
Solu-Medrol [methylprednisolone sodium succinate]	Z79.52	Corticosteroid	Anti-inflammatory and antiallergenic for shock and ulcerative colitis
Spiriva [tiotropium bromide]		Antiasthmatic/bronchodilator	Chronic obstructive pulmonary disease (COPD); asthma
Sprintec [norgestimate/ethinyl estradiol]	Z79.3	Contraceptive	Prevention of pregnancy
Strattera [atomexetine hydrochloride]		CNS stimulant	Attention deficit hyperactivity disorder (ADHD)
Streptomycin sulfate [streptomycin sulfate]	Z79.2	Antibiotic	Severe bacterial infections
Sublimaze preservative free [fentanyl citrate]	Z79.891	Analgesic, narcotic	Pain relief
Supprelin LA [histrelin acetate]	Z79.818	Agents affecting estrogen receptors and estrogen levels	Precocious puberty
Suprax [cefixime]	Z79.2	Antibiotic	Bacterial infections
Sustiva [efavirenz]	Z79.899	Antiviral	HIV/AIDs
Syeda [drospirenone/ethinyl estradiol]	Z79.3	Contraceptive	Prevention of pregnancy
Sylatron [peginterferon alfa-2b]	Z79.899	Antineoplastic interferons; antiviral interferons	Prevention of recurrent malignant melanoma
Symbicort [budesonide/formoterol fumarate dihydrate]	Z79.51	Corticosteroid – inhaled; antiasthmatic	Prophylaxis and treatment of asthma and COPD
Symbyax [olanzapine/fluoxetine]		Antidepressant	Acute depressive episodes associated with bipolar I disorder; treatment resistant depression
Symtuza [darunavir/cobicistat/emtricitabine/tenofovir alafenamide]	Z79.899	Antiretroviral	HIV
Synarel [nafarelin acetate]	Z79.818	Agents affecting estrogen receptors and estrogen levels	Endometriosis symptoms; precocious puberty
Synercid [dalfopristin/quinupristin]	Z79.2	Antibiotic	Severe blood infections
Synjardy [empagliflozin/metformin hydrochloride]	Z79.84	Oral hypoglycemic	Diabetes mellitus
Synthroid [levothyroxine sodium]		Thyroid hormone	Hypothyroidism
Tacrolimus [tacrolimus]	Z79.899	Immunosuppressant	Prophylaxis of organ transplant rejection
Talicia [omeprazole magnesium/amoxicillin/rifabutin]	Z79.2	Combination antibiotic	Helicobacter pylori infection
Tamiflu [oseltamivir phosphate]		Antiviral	Treatment and prevention of influenza A and B
Tamoxifen citrate [tamoxifen citrate]	Z79.810	Selective estrogen receptor modulator (SERM)	Metastatic breast cancer in postmenopausal women
Tazicef [ceftazidime]	Z79.2	Antibiotic	Confirmed or suspected bacterial infections
Teflaro [ceftaroline fosamil]	Z79.2	Antibiotic	Bacterial skin infections; pneumonia
Tegretol [carbamazepine]		Anticonvulsant; analgesic	Epilepsy, especially with complex symptomatology; specific analgesic for trigeminal neuralgia
Tenormin [atenolol]		Beta blocker	Angina pectoris; hypertension; acute myocardial infarction
Terazosin HCl [terazosin hydrochloride]		Antiadrenergic	Benign prostatic hypertrophy; hypertension
Testim [testosterone]	Z79.890	Testosterone therapy – topical	Primary hypogonadism; hypogonadotropic hypogonadism
Tetracycline HCl [tetracycline hydrochloride]	Z79.2	Antibiotic	Bacterial infections
Tiazac [diltiazem hydrochloride]		Calcium channel blocker	Chronic stable angina, atrial fibrillation, atrial flutter, hypertension, paroxysmal supraventricular tachycardia
Tivorbex [indomethacin]	Z79.1	Nonsteroidal anti-inflammatory drug (NSAID)	Treatment of pain, inflammation and joint stiffness
Tobradex [tobramycin/dexamethasone]		Aminoglycoside ocular anti-infective; anti-inflammatory	Infectious conjunctivitis; dermatosis, corticosteroid-responsive with secondary infection; foreign body in eye; corneal inflammation; uveitis

Drug	Z Code	Drug Action/Classification	Indications
Tobramycin [dexamethasone/tobramycin]	Z79.2	Antibiotic	Bacterial eye infections
Topamax [topiramate]		Anticonvulsant	Epilepsy; primary generalized tonic-clonic seizures; seizures associated with Lennox-Gastaut syndrome; migraine headache
Toprol-XL [metoprolol succinate]		Beta blocker	Angina pectoris; hypertension
Toremifene citrate [toremifene citrate]	Z79.810	Selective estrogen receptor modulator (SERM)	Metastatic breast cancer in postmenopausal women
Torisel [temsirolimus]	Z79.899	Antineoplastic	Renal cell carcinoma
Toujeo Solostar [insulin glargine recombinant]	Z79.4	Insulin	Diabetes mellitus
Tradjenta [linagliptin]	Z79.84	Oral hypoglycemic	Diabetes mellitus
Trazodone HCl [trazodone hydrochloride]		Antidepressant	Depression
Trelegy Ellipta [fluticasone furoate/umeclidinium bromide/vilanterol trifenatate]	Z79.51	Corticosteroid – inhaled; anitasthmatic	COPD
Trelstar [triptorelin pamoate]	Z79.818	Agents affecting estrogen receptors and estrogen levels	Palliative treatment of prostate cancer symptoms
Tresiba [insulin degludec]	Z79.4	Insulin	Diabetes mellitus
Triamterene and hydrochlorothiazide [triamterene/ hydrochlorothiazide]		Antihypertensive; diuretic	Edema; hypertension
Tri-Estarylla [ethinyl estradiol/norgestimate]	Z79.3	Contraceptive	Prevention of pregnancy; acne
Trijardy XR [empagliflozin/linagliptin/metformin hydrochloride]	Z79.84	Oral hypoglycemic	Diabetes mellitus
Tri-Legest [ethinyl estradiol/norethindrone acetate]	Z79.3	Contraceptive	Prevention of pregnancy
Tri-Linyah [ethinyl estradiol/norgestimate]	Z79.3	Contraceptive	Prevention of pregnancy
Tri-Lo-Estarylla [ethinyl estradiol/norgestimate]	Z79.3	Contraceptive	Prevention of pregnancy
Tri-Lo-Sprintec [ethinyl estradiol/norgestimate]	Z79.3	Contraceptive	Prevention of pregnancy
Trimethoprim [trimethoprim]	Z79.2	Antibiotic	Acute exacerbation chronic bronchitis; travelers' diarrhea; infections of the middle, lower respiratory tract, and urinary tract; pneumonia, pneumocystis; shigellosis
Tri-Norinyl 28-day [ethinyl estradiol/norethindrone]	Z79.3	Contraceptive	Prevention of pregnancy
Tri-Previfem [ethinyl estradiol/norgestimate]	Z79.3	Contraceptive	Prevention of pregnancy
Triptodur [triptorelin]	Z79.818	Agents affecting estrogen receptors and estrogen levels	Precocious puberty
Tri-Sprintec [ethinyl estradiol/norgestimate]	Z79.3	Contraceptive	Prevention of pregnancy; acne
Trivora-28 [ethinyl estradiol/ levonorgestrel]	Z79.3	Contraceptive	Prevention of pregnancy
Trokendi XR [topiramate]		Anticonvulsant	Epilepsy; primary generalized tonic-clonic seizures; seizures associated with Lennox-Gastaut syndrome; migraine headache
Trulicity [dulaglutide]	Z79.899	Antidiabetic – noninsulin injectable	Diabetes mellitus
Truvada [emtricitabine/ tenofovir disoproxil fumarate]	Z79.899	Antiviral	Treatment and prevention of HIV
Turalio [pexidartinib]		Kinase inhibitor	Symptomatic tenosynovial giant cell tumor
Tygacil [tigecycline]	Z79.2	Antibiotic	Bacterial skin or digestive system infections; pneumonia
Tylenol with codeine [acetaminophen/codeine phosphate]	Z79.891	Analgesic, narcotic	Pain and cough
Ubrelvy [ubrogepant]		Antimigraine	Migraine with or without aura
Ultram [tramadol hydrochloride]	Z79.891	Analgesic, non-narcotic (opiate, narcotic-like)	Moderate to severe pain

Drug	Z Code	Drug Action/Classification	Indications
Unasyn [ampicillin sodium/sulbactam sodium]	Z79.2	Antibiotic	Bacterial infections
Vabomere [meropenem; vaborbactam]	Z79.2	Antibiotic	Complicated urinary tract infections; pyelonephritis
Vagifem [estradiol]	Z79.890	Estrogen therapy	Menopause symptoms
Valium [diazepam]		Antianxiety; muscle relaxant; anticonvulsant	Anxiety, tension, withdrawal from alcohol, muscle spasms and anticonvulsant therapy; epilepsy, generalized tonic-clonic; status epilepticus; stiff-man syndrome; tetanus
Vancocin HCl [vancomycin hydrochloride]	Z79.2	Antibiotic	Severe bacterial infections
Vancomycin HCl [vancomycin hydrochloride]	Z79.2	Antibiotic	Severe bacterial infections
Vantas [histrelin acetate]	Z79.818	Agents affecting estrogen receptors and estrogen levels	Palliative treatment of prostate cancer symptoms
Vasotec [enalaprilat maleate]		ACE inhibitor	Congestive heart failure; hypertension
Velivet [desogestrel/ethinyl estradiol]	Z79.3	Contraceptive	Prevention of pregnancy
Venlafaxine HCl [venlafaxine hydrochloride]		Antidepressant, serotonin and norepinephrine reuptake inhibitor (SNRI)	Major depressive disorder; social anxiety disorder; panic disorder
Ventolin HFA [albuterol sulfate]		Antiasthmatic/bronchodilator	Asthma
Verapamil HCL [verapamil hydrochloride]		Calcium channel blocker	Angina pectoris, chronic stable angina, atrial fibrillation, atrial flutter, paroxysmal supraventricular tachycardia, ventricular arrhythmia, hypertension
Viagra [sildenafil citrate]		Phosphodiesterase-5 (PDE5) inhibitor	Erectile dysfunction
Vibativ [telavancin hydrochloride]	Z79.2	Antibiotic	Pneumonia; severe bacterial skin infections
Vibramycin [doxycycline calcium]	Z79.2	Antibiotic	Bacterial infections
Victoza [liraglutide]	Z79.899	Antidiabetic – noninsulin injectable	Diabetes mellitus
Vienva [ethinyl estradiol/levonorgestrel]	Z79.3	Contraceptive	Prevention of pregnancy
Viorele [desogestrel/ethinyl estradiol]	Z79.3	Contraceptive	Prevention of pregnancy
Virazole [ribavirin]	Z79.899	Antiviral	Respiratory syncytial virus (RSV)
Viread [tenofovir disoproxil fumarate]	Z79.899	Antiviral	HIV; chronic hepatitis B
Vistaril [hydroxyzine pamoate]		Antianxiety; antiemetic	Treatment of nausea and vomiting, for reducing narcotic requirement in surgery and as tranquilizer for tension, anxiety, or agitation states
Vivelle [estradiol]	Z79.890	Estrogen therapy	Menopause symptoms; osteoporosis prevention
Voltaren [diclofenac sodium]	Z79.1	Nonsteroidal anti-inflammatory drug (NSAID)	Treatment of pain, inflammation and joint stiffness due to arthritis
Vumerity [diroximel fumarate]		Immunostimulant	Relapsing forms of multiple sclerosis (MS)
Vytorin [ezetimibe/simvastatin]		HMG-CoA reductase inhibitor (statin); cholesterol absorption inhibitor	Hyperlipidemia; hypercholesterolemia
Wakix [pitolisant hydrochloride]		CNS stimulant	Narcolepsy
Warfarin [warfarin sodium]	Z79.01	Anticoagulant	Prophylaxis and treatment of venous thrombosis, treatment of atrial fibrillation with embolization (pulmonary embolism), arrhythmias, myocardial infarction, and stroke prevention
Wellbutrin SR, Wellbutrin XL [bupropion hydrochloride]		Antidepressant	Depression
Wera [ethinyl estradiol/norethindrone]	Z79.3	Contraceptive	Prevention of pregnancy
Xalatan [latanoprost]		Prostaglandin F2α analogue	Glaucoma, open-angle; ocular hypertension
Xanax, Xanax XR [alprazolam]		Antianxiety; sedative/hypnotic	Anxiety disorders with panic disorder and depression
Xarelto [rivaraxaban]	Z79.01	Anticoagulant	Prophylaxis and treatment of venous thrombosis, pulmonary embolism; prevention of blood clots due to atrial fibrillation
Xeljanz [tofacitinib citrate]	Z79.899	Antirheumatic	Rheumatoid arthritis; psoriatic arthritis
Xenleta [lefamulin acetate]	Z79.2	Antibiotic	Community-acquired bacterial pneumonia
Xgeva [denosumab]	Z79.899	Monoclonal antibody	Treatment and prevention of bone resorption and prevention of bone fracture
Xifaxan [rifaximin]	Z79.2	Antibiotic	E. coli diarrhea

Drug	Z Code	Drug Action/Classification	Indications
Xigduo [dapagliflozin propanediol/metformin hydrochloride]	Z79.84	Oral hypoglycemic	Diabetes mellitus
Xpovio [selinexor]	Z79.899	Antineoplastic	Multiple myeloma in adults
Xultophy [insulin degludec/liraglutide]	Z79.4	Insulin	Diabetes mellitus
Xyrem [sodium oxybate]		CNS depressant; anxiolytic/sedative/hypnotic	Cataplexy and/or excessive daytime sleepiness in narcolepsy
Xyzal [levocetirizine dihydrochloride]		Antihistamine	Perennial allergic rhinitis; chronic idiopathic urticaria
Yasmin [drospirenone/ethinyl estradiol]	Z79.3	Contraceptive	Prevention of pregnancy
Yaz [drospirenone/ethinyl estradiol]	Z79.3	Contraceptive	Prevention of pregnancy; menstrual disorders
Zantac [ranitidine hydrochloride]		Histamine H2-receptors inhibitor	Acid/peptic disorder, erosive esophagitis, gastrointestinal hypersecretion, mastocytosis, gastroesophageal reflux, peptic ulcer, Zollinger-Ellison syndrome
Zerbaxa [ceftolozane sulfate/tazobactam sodium]	Z79.2	Antibiotic	Complicated urinary tract and intra-abdominal infections
Zestoretic [lisinopril/hydrochlorothiazide]		ACE inhibitor	Congestive heart failure; hypertension
Zestril [lisinopril]		ACE inhibitor	Congestive heart failure; hypertension
Zetia [exetimibe]		Antihyperlipidemic	Hypercholesterolemia; sitosterolemia
Ziac [bisoprolol fumarate/ hydrochlorothiazide]		Antihypertensive	Hypertension
Zinacef [cefuroxime sodium]	Z79.2	Antibiotic	Bacterial infections
Zipsor [diclofenac potassium]	Z79.1	Nonsteroidal anti-inflammatory drug (NSAID)	Pain and inflammation relief
Zithromax [azithromycin]	Z79.2	Antibiotic	Infections of the cervix, lower respiratory tract, skin and skin structures, urethra, nongonococcal; mycobacterium avium complex; pharyngitis, streptococcal pneumonia; tonsillitis
Zocor [simvastatin]		HMG-CoA reductase inhibitor (statin)	Hypercholesterolemia; hyperlipidemia; hyperlipoproteinemia; hypertriglyceridemia
Zoladex [goserelin acetate]	Z79.818	Agents affecting estrogen receptors and estrogen levels	Palliative treatment of prostate cancer and breast cancer symptoms; endometriosis
Zoloft [sertraline hydrochloride]		Antidepressant	Anxiety with panic disorder and depression; obsessive-compulsive disorder
Zometa [zoledronic acid]	Z79.83	Bisphosphonate	Multiple myeloma; Paget's disease
Zorvolex [diclofenac]	Z79.1	Nonsteroidal anti-inflammatory drug (NSAID)	Pain, inflammation or fever relief
Zosyn [piperacillin sodium/tazobactam sodium]	Z79.2	Antibiotic	Bacterial infections
Zovia [ethynodiol diacetate/ethinyl estradiol]	Z79.3	Contraceptive	Prevention of pregnancy
Zovirax [acyclovir]		Antiviral	Genital herpes and herpes zoster infections
Zubsolv [buprenorphine/naloxone]		Opioid agonist	Treatment of opioid addiction
Zyban [bupropion hydrochloride]		Smoking cessation aid	Nicotine addiction, smoking
Zyflo [zileuton]		Antiasthmatic	Asthma
Zyloprim [allopurinol]		Antigout	Gouty arthritis, renal calculus, hyperuricemia, hyperuricemia secondary to leukemia, hyperuricemia secondary to lymphoma
Zyprexa [olanzapine]		Antipsychotic/antimanic	Psychotic disorders; schizophrenia
Zyrtec allergy [cetirizine hydrochloride]		Antihistamine	Perennial and seasonal allergic rhinitis; chronic urticaria
Zyvox [linezolid]	Z79.2	Antibiotic	Severe bacterial infections

Appendix C: Z Codes for Long-Term Drug Use with Associated Drugs

This resource correlates the Z codes that are used to identify current long-term drug use with a list of drugs that are typically categorized to that class of drug. These lists are not all-inclusive, providing only the more commonly used drugs.

Z79.Ø1 Long term (current) use of anticoagulants

Angiomax
Argatroban
Arixtra
Bevyxxa
Coumadin
Eliquis
Fragmin
Heparin
Jantoven
Lovenox
Pradaxa
Savaysa
Warfarin
Xarelto

Z79.Ø2 Long term (current) use of antithrombotics/antiplatelets

Aggrastat
Aggrenox
Brilinta
Clopidogrel bisulfate
Effient
Integrilin
Persantine
Plavix
Prasugrel

Z79.1 Long term (current) use of non-steroidal anti-inflammatories (NSAID)

Advil
Aleve
Anaprox DS
Arthrotec
Caldolor
Cambia
Celebrex
Daypro
Duexis
Feldene
Ibuprofen
Indocin
Mobic
Motrin IB
Nabumetone
Nalfon
Naprelan
Naprosyn
NeoProfen
Ponstel
Tivorbex
Voltaren
Zipsor
Zorvolex

Z79.2 Long term (current) use of antibiotics

Altabax
Amikacin
Amoxicillin
Ampicillin
Ancef
Augmentin
Avelox
Azactam
Azithromycin
Bactrim
Biaxin XL
Cefprozil
Ceftriaxone
Centany
Cephalexin
Cipro
Ciprofloxacin
Clarithromycin
Cleocin
Clindamycin
Cubicin
Daptomycin
Dificid
Doxycycline
Dynacin
E.E.S.
Ertapenem
ERYC
Erygel
EryPed
Ery-Tab
Erythrocin
Erythromycin
Factive
Fetroja
Flagyl
Fortaz
Gentamicin sulfate
Invanz
Isoniazid
Keflex
Klaron
Lincocin
Macrobid
Macrodantin
Maxipime
Mefoxin
Mepron
Merrem
Metronidazole
Minocin
Monodox
Monurol
Mycobutin
Nebupent
Nitrofurantoin
Oracea
Orbactiv
Penicillin-VK
Pentam
Pfizerpen
Priftin
Primaxin
Rifadin
Rimactane
Septra
Seromycin
Silvadene
Sivextro
Solodyn
Streptomycin sulfate
Suprax
Synercid
Talicia
Tazicef
Teflaro
Tetracycline HCl
Tobramycin
Trimethoprim
Tygacil
Unasyn
Vabomere
Vancocin HCl
Vancomycin HCl
Vibativ
Vibramycin
Xenleta
Xifaxan
Zerbaxa
Zinacef
Zithromax
Zosyn
Zyvox

Z79.3 Long term (current) use of hormonal contraceptives

Altavera
Alyacen
Aranelle
Ashlyna
Aviane-28
Balziva-28
Bekyree
Beyaz
Brevicon 28-day
Briellyn
Camila
Cryselle
Cyclafem
Cyclessa
Dasetta
Daysee
Depo-Provera
Depo-SubQ Provera
Desogestrel:
  Ethinyl
Elinest
Emoquette
Enpresse-28
Enskyce
Errin
Estarylla
Estrostep Fe
Falmina
Femhrt
Gildagia
Gildess
Introvale
Jencycla
Junel
Kariva
Kelnor
Kimidess
Kurvelo
Kyleena
Larin
Lessina-28
Levonest

Levora
Liletta
Lo Loestrin Fe
Loestrin
Loryna
LoSeasonique
Low-Ogestrel-28
Marlissa
Microgestin
Minastrin
Mirena
Mono-Linyah
Myzilra
Natazia
Nexplanon
Norinyl
Nor-QD
Nortrel
NuvaRing
Ogestrel
Orsythia
Ortho-Novum
Ortho-Tri-Cyclen-28
Philith
Pimtrea
Pirmella
Plan B One-Step
Portia-28
Previfem
Provera
Quartette
Quasense
Safyral
Seasonale
Seasonique
Setlakin
Skyla
Sprintec
Syeda
Tri-Estarylla
Tri-Legest
Tri-Linyah
Tri-Lo-Estarylla
Tri-Lo-Sprintec
Tri-Norinyl 28-day
Tri-Previfem
Tri-Sprintec
Trivora-28
Velivet
Vienva
Viorele
Wera
Yasmin
Yaz
Zovia

Z79.4 Long term (current) use of insulin
Admelog
Afrezza
Apidra
Basaglar
Fiasp
Humalog
Humulin R
Lantus
Levemir
Novolin
Novolog
Soliqua
Toujeo Solostar
Tresiba
Xultophy

Z79.51 Long term (current) use of inhaled steroids
Advair
Airduo Respiclick
Alvesco
Arnuity Ellipta
Asmanex
Breo Ellipta
Dulera
Flovent
Pulmicort
Qvar Redihaler
Symbicort
Trelegy Ellipta

Z79.52 Long term (current) use of systemic steroids
Aristospan
Celestone Soluspan
Colocort
Cortef
Cortenema
Cortifoam
Cortisone acetate
Depo-Medrol
Dexamethasone Intensol
Entocort EC
Hydrocortisone
Kenalog-10
Kenalog-40
Locoid
Medrol
Methylprednisolone
Orapred ODT
PediaPred
Prednisolone
Prednisone
Prelone
Rayos
Solu-Cortef
Solu-Medrol

Z79.810 Long term (current) use of selective estrogen receptor modulators (SERMs)
Evista
Fareston
Osphena
Raloxifene HCI
Soltamox
Tamoxifen Citrate
Toremifene Citrate

Z79.811 Long term (current) use of aromatase inhibitors
Anastrozole
Arimidex
Aromasin
Exemestane
Femara
Letrozole

Z79.818 Long term (current) use of other agents affecting estrogen receptors and estrogen levels
Eligard
Faslodex
Lupron Depot
Megace ES
Supprelin LA
Synarel
Trelstar
Triptodur
Vantas
Zoladex

Z79.82 Long term (current) use of aspirin
Bayer
Durlaza

Z79.83 Long term (current) use of bisphosphonates
Actonel
Atelvia
Binosto
Boniva
Fosamax
Reclast
Zometa

Z79.84 Long term (current) use of oral hypoglycemic drugs
Acarbose
Actoplus Met
Actos
Amaryl
Avandia
DiaBeta
Duetact
Farxiga
Glimepiride
Glucotrol
Glumetza
Glyburide
Glynase
Glyset
Invokamet
Invokana
Janumet
Januvia
Jentadueto
Kazano
Kombiglyze
Metformin
Onglyza
Oseni
Qtern
Repaglinide
Riomet
Rybelsus
Sitagliptin
Synjardy
Tradjenta
Trijardy XR
Xigduo

Z79.890 Hormone replacement therapy
Activella
Alora
Androderm
AndroGel
Angeliq
Bijuva
Climara
CombiPatch
Delestrogen
Depo-Provera
Divigel

Duavee
Elestrin
Estrace
EstroGel
Femhrt
Femring
Firmagon
Menest
Menostar
Minivelle
Orlissa
Osphena
Prempro
Provera
Testim
Vagifem
Vivelle

Z79.891 Long term (current) use of opiate analgesic

Acetaminophen with codeine
Buprenex
Buprenorphine HCl and Naloxone HCl
Butorphanol tartrate
Butrans
Codeine
Demerol
Dilaudid
Dolophine HCl
Duragesic
Duramorph PF
Fentanyl Citrate
Fentora
Fioricet with codeine
Hydrocodone
Hydrocodone bitartrate and acetaminophen
Hydromorphone HCl
Kadian
Lazanda
Methadone HCl
Methadose
Morphabond ER
Morphine Sulfate
MS Contin
Norco
Nucynta
Oxycodone HCl
OxyContin
Percocet
Reprexain
Roxicet
Roxicodone
Sublimaze Preservative Free
Tylenol with codeine
Ultram

Z79.899 Other long term (current) drug therapy

Actimmune
Antineoplastic/chemotherapy
Astagraf XL
Atripla
Avonex
Beconase AQ
Betaseron
Byetta
Cellcept
Cimduo
Cosentyx
Crixivan
Cyclosporine
Cyltezo
Descovy
Emtriva
Enbrel
Entyvio
Envarsus XR
Epivir
Erelzi
Flonase
Gengraf
Harvoni
Humira
Hyrimoz
Imuran
Intron A
Keytruda
Monoclonal antibodies
Neoral
Orencia
Otezla
Ozempic
Pegintron
Prezcobix
Prezista
Prograf
Prolia
Protopic
Qnasl
Rapamune
Rebetol
Rebif
Retrovir
Rinvoq
Sandimmune
Simulect
Sirolimus
Sustiva
Sylatron
Symtuza
Tacrolimus
Torisel
Trulicity
Truvada
Victoza
Virazole
Viread
Xeljanz
Xgeva
Xpovio

Appendix D: Major Complication and Comorbidity (MCC) Code List

Note: The following is a comprehensive list of ICD-10-CM codes designated as MCCs in the tabular section of this manual. Codes listed in this resource and identified as MCCs in the tabular section reflect the most current information that was available at the time of publication. Because the fiscal 2021 IPPS final rule was not available at the time this book was printed, the ICD-10-CM codes designated as MCCs are based on the proposed, version 38, MS-DRG Grouper software and Definitions Manual files published with the fiscal 2021 IPPS proposed rule.

For the most current list of MCC designations based on the final version of the MS-DRG Grouper software and MS-DRG Definitions Manual files, Optum360 has provided an easily searchable data file that can be accessed at the following:

https://www.optum360coding.com/ProductUpdates/
Title: "2021 ICD-10-CM for Hospital IPPS Data File"
Password: Hospital21

A02.1
A02.21
A02.22
A06.4
A06.5
A06.6
A17.0
A17.1
A17.81
A17.82
A17.83
A17.89
A18.31
A19.0
A19.1
A19.2
A19.8
A19.9
A20.0
A20.1
A20.2
A20.3
A20.7
A20.8
A20.9
A22.1
A22.7
A26.7
A27.81
A32.7
A33
A35
A37.01
A37.11
A37.81
A37.91
A39.0
A39.1
A39.2
A39.3
A39.4
A39.50
A39.51
A39.52
A39.53
A39.81
A40.0
A40.1
A40.3
A40.8
A40.9
A41.01
A41.02
A41.1
A41.2
A41.3
A41.4
A41.50
A41.51
A41.52
A41.53
A41.59
A41.81
A41.89
A41.9
A42.7
A48.0
A48.1
A48.3
A50.41
A50.42
A51.41
A52.13
A52.14
A54.81
A54.86
A80.0
A80.1
A80.2
A80.30
A80.39
A83.0
A83.1
A83.2
A83.3
A83.4
A83.5
A83.6
A83.8
A83.9
A84.0
A84.1
A84.81
A84.89
A84.9
A85.2
A92.30
A92.31
A92.32
A92.39
B00.3
B00.4
B00.7
B00.82
B01.11
B01.12
B01.2
B02.1
B02.24
B05.0
B05.2
B06.01
B10.01
B10.09
B15.0
B16.0
B16.2
B17.11
B19.0
B19.11
B19.21
B25.0
B25.2
B26.1
B26.2
B37.1
B37.5
B37.6
B37.7
B38.4
B39.0
B39.1
B39.2
B44.0
B45.1
B46.0
B46.1
B46.2
B46.3
B46.4
B46.5
B46.8
B46.9
B50.9
B58.2
B58.3
B58.81
B59
B77.81
D57.00
D57.01
D57.02
D57.03
D57.09
D57.211
D57.212
D57.213
D57.218
D57.219
D57.411
D57.412
D57.413
D57.418
D57.419
D57.431
D57.432
D57.433
D57.438
D57.439
D57.451
D57.452
D57.453
D57.458
D57.459
D57.811
D57.812
D57.813
D57.818
D57.819
D59.3
D60.0
D60.1
D60.8
D60.9
D61.1
D61.2
D61.3
D61.810
D61.811
D61.89
D65
D66
D67
E03.5
E05.01
E05.11
E05.21
E05.31
E05.41
E05.81
E05.91
E08.00
E08.01
E08.10
E08.11
E08.641
E09.00
E09.01
E09.10
E09.11
E09.641
E10.10
E10.11
E10.641
E11.00
E11.01
E11.10
E11.11
E11.641
E13.00
E13.01
E13.10
E13.11
E13.641
E40
E41
E42
E43
E84.0
E84.11
E88.3
G00.0
G00.1
G00.2
G00.3
G00.8
G00.9
G01
G02
G03.0
G03.8
G03.9
G04.00
G04.01
G04.02
G04.2
G04.30
G04.31
G04.32
G04.39
G04.81
G04.89
G04.90
G04.91
G05.3
G05.4
G06.0
G06.1
G06.2
G07
G08
G21.0
G37.4
G40.301
G40.311
G40.319
G70.01
G80.0
G82.50
G82.51
G82.52
G82.53
G82.54
G83.5
G92
G93.41
G93.5
G93.6
G93.7
G93.82
G95.11
G95.19
I21.01
I21.02
I21.09
I21.11
I21.19
I21.21
I21.29
I21.3
I21.4
I21.9
I21.A1
I21.A9
I22.0
I22.1
I22.2
I22.8
I22.9
I23.4
I23.5
I25.42
I26.01
I26.02
I26.09
I26.90
I26.92
I26.93
I26.94
I26.99
I33.0
I33.9
I40.0
I40.1
I40.8
I40.9
I41
I46.2
I46.8
I46.9
I49.01
I49.02
I50.21
I50.23
I50.31
I50.33
I50.41
I50.43
I51.1
I51.2
I60.00
I60.01
I60.02
I60.10
I60.11
I60.12
I60.2
I60.30
I60.31
I60.32
I60.4
I60.50
I60.51
I60.52
I60.6
I60.7
I60.8
I60.9
I61.0
I61.1
I61.2
I61.3
I61.4
I61.5
I61.6
I61.8
I61.9
I62.00
I62.01
I62.02
I62.03
I62.1
I63.00
I63.011
I63.012
I63.013
I63.019
I63.02
I63.031
I63.032
I63.033
I63.039
I63.09
I63.10
I63.111
I63.112
I63.113
I63.119
I63.12
I63.131
I63.132
I63.133
I63.139
I63.19
I63.20
I63.211
I63.212
I63.213
I63.219
I63.22
I63.231
I63.232
I63.233
I63.239
I63.29
I63.30
I63.311
I63.312
I63.313
I63.319
I63.321
I63.322
I63.323
I63.329
I63.331
I63.332
I63.333
I63.339
I63.341
I63.342
I63.343
I63.349
I63.39
I63.40
I63.411
I63.412
I63.413
I63.419
I63.421
I63.422
I63.423
I63.429
I63.431
I63.432
I63.433
I63.439
I63.441
I63.442
I63.443
I63.449
I63.49
I63.50
I63.511
I63.512
I63.513
I63.519
I63.521
I63.522
I63.523
I63.529
I63.531
I63.532
I63.533
I63.539
I63.541
I63.542
I63.543
I63.549
I63.59
I63.6
I63.81
I63.89
I63.9
I67.0
I67.83
I71.00
I71.01
I71.02
I71.03
I71.1
I71.3
I71.5
I71.8
I74.01
I77.70
I77.71
I77.72
I77.73
I77.74
I77.75
I77.76
I77.77
I77.79
I81
I82.0
I82.220
I82.221
I85.01
I85.11
J04.11
J04.31
J05.11
J09.X1
J10.00
J10.01
J10.08
J11.00
J11.08
J12.0
J12.1
J12.2
J12.3
J12.81
J12.89
J12.9
J13
J14
J15.0
J15.1
J15.20
J15.211
J15.212
J15.29
J15.3
J15.4
J15.5
J15.6
J15.7
J15.8
J15.9
J16.0
J16.8
J17
J18.0
J18.1
J18.8
J18.9
J68.1
J69.0
J69.1
J69.8
J80
J81.0
J84.81
J84.83
J84.841
J84.842
J84.843
J84.848
J85.0
J85.1
J85.2
J85.3
J86.0
J86.9
J93.0
J95.1
J95.2
J95.3
J95.821
J95.822
J96.00
J96.01
J96.02
J96.20
J96.21
J96.22
J96.90
J96.91

J96.92
J98.51
J98.59
K20.81
K20.91
K21.01
K22.11
K22.3
K22.6
K25.0
K25.1
K25.2
K25.4
K25.5
K25.6
K26.0
K26.1
K26.2
K26.4
K26.5
K26.6
K27.0
K27.1
K27.2
K27.4
K27.5
K27.6
K28.0
K28.1
K28.2
K28.4
K28.5
K28.6
K29.01
K29.21
K29.31
K29.41
K29.51
K29.61
K29.71
K29.81
K29.91
K31.811
K31.82
K35.21
K35.32
K35.33
K40.10
K40.11
K40.40
K40.41
K41.10
K41.11
K41.40
K41.41
K42.1
K43.1
K43.4
K43.7
K44.1
K45.1
K46.1
K55.011
K55.012
K55.019
K55.021
K55.022
K55.029
K55.031
K55.032
K55.039
K55.041
K55.042
K55.049
K55.051
K55.052
K55.059
K55.061
K55.062
K55.069
K55.21
K55.30
K55.31
K55.32
K55.33
K56.2
K57.01
K57.11
K57.13
K57.21
K57.31
K57.33
K57.41
K57.51
K57.53
K57.81
K57.91
K57.93
K63.1
K63.81
K65.0
K65.1
K65.2
K65.3
K65.8
K65.9
K66.1
K67
K68.12
K68.19
K68.9
K70.41
K71.11
K72.00
K72.01
K72.11
K72.91
K75.0
K75.1
K76.2
K76.3
K76.7
K80.67
K82.2
K83.1
K83.2
K85.00
K85.01
K85.02
K85.10
K85.11
K85.12
K85.20
K85.21
K85.22
K85.30
K85.31
K85.32
K85.80
K85.81
K85.82
K85.90
K85.91
K85.92
L89.003
L89.004
L89.013
L89.014
L89.023
L89.024
L89.103
L89.104
L89.113
L89.114
L89.123
L89.124
L89.133
L89.134
L89.143
L89.144
L89.153
L89.154
L89.203
L89.204
L89.213
L89.214
L89.223
L89.224
L89.303
L89.304
L89.313
L89.314
L89.323
L89.324
L89.43
L89.44
L89.503
L89.504
L89.513
L89.514
L89.523
L89.524
L89.603
L89.604
L89.613
L89.614
L89.623
L89.624
L89.813
L89.814
L89.893
L89.894
L89.93
L89.94
M31.1
M72.6
N00.0
N00.1
N00.2
N00.3
N00.4
N00.5
N00.6
N00.7
N00.8
N00.9
N00.A
N01.0
N01.1
N01.2
N01.3
N01.4
N01.5
N01.6
N01.7
N01.8
N01.9
N01.A
N15.1
N17.0
N17.1
N17.2
N18.6
N73.3
O03.2
O03.31
O03.32
O03.81
O03.82
O04.7
O04.81
O04.82
O07.2
O07.31
O07.32
O08.2
O08.3
O08.4
O10.42
O11.1
O11.2
O11.3
O14.12
O14.13
O14.22
O14.23
O15.02
O15.03
O15.1
O15.2
O22.31
O22.32
O22.33
O24.02
O24.12
O24.32
O24.82
O34.31
O34.32
O34.33
O41.1010
O41.1011
O41.1012
O41.1013
O41.1014
O41.1015
O41.1019
O41.1020
O41.1021
O41.1022
O41.1023
O41.1024
O41.1025
O41.1029
O41.1030
O41.1031
O41.1032
O41.1033
O41.1034
O41.1035
O41.1039
O41.1210
O41.1211
O41.1212
O41.1213
O41.1214
O41.1215
O41.1219
O41.1220
O41.1221
O41.1222
O41.1223
O41.1224
O41.1225
O41.1229
O41.1230
O41.1231
O41.1232
O41.1233
O41.1234
O41.1235
O41.1239
O41.1410
O41.1411
O41.1412
O41.1413
O41.1414
O41.1415
O41.1419
O41.1420
O41.1421
O41.1422
O41.1423
O41.1424
O41.1425
O41.1429
O41.1430
O41.1431
O41.1432
O41.1433
O41.1434
O41.1435
O41.1439
O44.11
O44.12
O44.13
O44.31
O44.32
O44.33
O44.51
O44.52
O44.53
O45.001
O45.002
O45.003
O45.011
O45.012
O45.013
O45.021
O45.022
O45.023
O45.091
O45.092
O45.093
O45.8X1
O45.8X2
O45.8X3
O45.91
O45.92
O45.93
O46.001
O46.002
O46.003
O46.011
O46.012
O46.013
O46.021
O46.022
O46.023
O46.091
O46.092
O46.093
O60.02
O60.03
O60.12X0
O60.12X1
O60.12X2
O60.12X3
O60.12X4
O60.12X5
O60.12X9
O60.13X0
O60.13X1
O60.13X2
O60.13X3
O60.13X4
O60.13X5
O60.13X9
O60.14X0
O60.14X1
O60.14X2
O60.14X3
O60.14X4
O60.14X5
O60.14X9
O60.22X0
O60.22X1
O60.22X2
O60.22X3
O60.22X4
O60.22X5
O60.22X9
O60.23X0
O60.23X1
O60.23X2
O60.23X3
O60.23X4
O60.23X5
O60.23X9
O67.0
O71.02
O71.03
O71.1
O75.1
O75.3
O85
O86.04
O86.81
O86.89
O87.1
O88.011
O88.012
O88.013
O88.02
O88.03
O88.111
O88.112
O88.113
O88.12
O88.13
O88.211
O88.212
O88.213
O88.22
O88.23
O88.311
O88.312
O88.313
O88.32
O88.33
O88.811
O88.812
O88.813
O88.82
O88.83
O90.3
O90.4
O99.42
P10.0
P10.1
P10.3
P10.4
P10.8
P10.9
P11.0
P11.2
P11.9
P22.0
P23.0
P23.1
P23.2
P23.3
P23.4
P23.5
P23.6
P23.8
P23.9
P24.01
P24.11
P24.21
P24.31
P24.81
P25.0
P25.1
P25.2
P25.3
P25.8
P26.0
P26.1
P26.8
P26.9
P27.0
P27.1
P27.8
P27.9
P28.5
P28.81
P29.30
P29.38
P29.81
P35.1
P35.2
P35.3
P35.4
P35.8
P35.9
P36.0
P36.10
P36.19
P36.2
P36.30
P36.39
P36.4
P36.5
P36.8
P36.9
P37.0
P37.1
P37.2
P37.3
P37.4
P37.8
P37.9
P52.21
P52.22
P52.4
P52.5
P52.6
P52.8
P52.9
P54.1
P54.2
P54.3
P56.0
P56.90
P56.99
P57.0
P57.8
P57.9
P59.1
P59.20
P59.29
P60
P61.0
P61.5
P74.0
P77.1
P77.2
P77.3
P77.9
P78.0
P83.2
P90
P91.0
P91.1
P91.2
P91.3
P91.4
P91.5
P91.63
P91.821
P91.822
P91.823
P91.829
P92.01
Q00.0
Q00.1
Q00.2
Q04.0
Q04.1
Q04.2
Q04.3
Q20.0
Q20.1
Q20.2
Q20.3
Q20.4
Q21.3
Q22.0
Q22.4
Q22.5
Q22.6
Q22.8
Q22.9
Q23.4
Q24.2
Q24.4
Q24.6
Q25.5
Q25.6
Q25.71
Q25.72
Q25.79
Q28.2
Q28.3
Q33.2
Q33.3
Q33.6
Q39.0
Q39.1
Q39.2
Q39.3
Q39.4
Q44.2
Q44.3
Q79.0
Q79.1
Q79.2
Q79.3
Q79.4
Q79.51
Q79.59
Q89.4
Q93.81
R09.2
R40.20
R40.2110
R40.2111
R40.2112
R40.2113
R40.2114
R40.2120
R40.2121
R40.2122
R40.2123
R40.2124
R40.2210
R40.2211
R40.2212
R40.2213
R40.2214
R40.2220
R40.2221
R40.2222
R40.2223
R40.2224
R40.2310
R40.2311
R40.2312
R40.2313
R40.2314
R40.2320
R40.2321
R40.2322
R40.2323
R40.2324
R40.2340
R40.2341
R40.2342
R40.2343
R40.2344
R53.2
R57.0
R57.1
R57.8
R65.11
R65.20
R65.21
S02.0XXB
S02.101B
S02.102B
S02.109B
S02.110B
S02.111B
S02.112B
S02.113B
S02.118B
S02.119B
S02.11AB
S02.11BB
S02.11CB
S02.11DB
S02.11EB
S02.11FB
S02.11GB
S02.11HB
S02.121B
S02.122B
S02.129B
S02.19XB
S02.91XB
S06.1X0A
S06.1X1A
S06.1X2A
S06.1X3A
S06.1X4A
S06.1X5A
S06.1X6A
S06.1X7A
S06.1X8A
S06.1X9A
S06.2X6A
S06.2X7A
S06.2X8A
S06.306A
S06.307A
S06.308A
S06.310A
S06.311A
S06.312A
S06.313A
S06.314A
S06.315A
S06.316A
S06.317A
S06.318A
S06.319A
S06.320A
S06.321A
S06.322A
S06.323A
S06.324A
S06.325A

S06.326A
S06.327A
S06.328A
S06.329A
S06.33ØA
S06.331A
S06.332A
S06.333A
S06.334A
S06.335A
S06.336A
S06.337A
S06.338A
S06.339A
S06.34ØA
S06.341A
S06.342A
S06.343A
S06.344A
S06.345A
S06.346A
S06.347A
S06.348A
S06.349A
S06.35ØA
S06.351A
S06.352A
S06.353A
S06.354A
S06.355A
S06.356A
S06.357A
S06.358A
S06.359A
S06.36ØA
S06.361A
S06.362A
S06.363A
S06.364A
S06.365A
S06.366A
S06.367A
S06.368A
S06.369A
S06.37ØA
S06.376A
S06.377A
S06.378A
S06.38ØA
S06.386A
S06.387A
S06.388A
S06.4XØA
S06.4X1A
S06.4X2A
S06.4X3A
S06.4X4A
S06.4X5A
S06.4X6A
S06.4X7A
S06.4X8A
S06.4X9A
S06.5XØA
S06.5X1A
S06.5X2A
S06.5X3A
S06.5X4A
S06.5X5A
S06.5X6A
S06.5X7A
S06.5X8A
S06.5X9A
S06.6XØA
S06.6X1A
S06.6X2A
S06.6X3A
S06.6X4A
S06.6X5A
S06.6X6A
S06.6X7A
S06.6X8A
S06.6X9A
S06.816A
S06.817A
S06.818A
S06.826A
S06.827A
S06.828A
S06.896A
S06.897A
S06.898A
S06.9X6A
S06.9X7A
S06.9X8A
S11.Ø11A
S11.Ø12A
S11.Ø13A
S11.Ø14A
S11.Ø15A
S11.Ø19A
S11.Ø21A
S11.Ø22A
S11.Ø23A
S11.Ø24A
S11.Ø25A
S11.Ø29A
S11.Ø31A
S11.Ø32A
S11.Ø33A
S11.Ø34A
S11.Ø35A
S11.Ø39A
S12.ØØØB
S12.ØØ1B
S12.Ø1XB
S12.Ø2XB
S12.Ø3ØB
S12.Ø31B
S12.Ø4ØB
S12.Ø41B
S12.Ø9ØB
S12.Ø91B
S12.1ØØB
S12.1Ø1B
S12.11ØB
S12.111B
S12.112B
S12.12ØB
S12.121B
S12.13ØB
S12.131B
S12.14XB
S12.15ØB
S12.151B
S12.19ØB
S12.191B
S12.2ØØB
S12.2Ø1B
S12.23ØB
S12.231B
S12.24XB
S12.25ØB
S12.251B
S12.29ØB
S12.291B
S12.3ØØB
S12.3Ø1B
S12.33ØB
S12.331B
S12.34XB
S12.35ØB
S12.351B
S12.39ØB
S12.391B
S12.4ØØB
S12.4Ø1B
S12.43ØB
S12.431B
S12.44XB
S12.45ØB
S12.451B
S12.49ØB
S12.491B
S12.5ØØB
S12.5Ø1B
S12.53ØB
S12.531B
S12.54XB
S12.55ØB
S12.551B
S12.59ØB
S12.591B
S12.6ØØB
S12.6Ø1B
S12.63ØB
S12.631B
S12.64XB
S12.65ØB
S12.651B
S12.69ØB
S12.691B
S12.8XXA
S14.ØXXA
S14.1Ø1A
S14.1Ø2A
S14.1Ø3A
S14.1Ø4A
S14.1Ø5A
S14.1Ø6A
S14.1Ø7A
S14.1Ø8A
S14.111A
S14.112A
S14.113A
S14.114A
S14.115A
S14.116A
S14.117A
S14.118A
S14.121A
S14.122A
S14.123A
S14.124A
S14.125A
S14.126A
S14.127A
S14.128A
S14.131A
S14.132A
S14.133A
S14.134A
S14.135A
S14.136A
S14.137A
S14.138A
S14.141A
S14.142A
S14.143A
S14.144A
S14.145A
S14.146A
S14.147A
S14.148A
S14.151A
S14.152A
S14.153A
S14.154A
S14.155A
S14.156A
S14.157A
S14.158A
S21.3Ø1A
S21.3Ø2A
S21.3Ø9A
S21.311A
S21.312A
S21.319A
S21.321A
S21.322A
S21.329A
S21.331A
S21.332A
S21.339A
S21.341A
S21.342A
S21.349A
S21.351A
S21.352A
S21.359A
S21.4Ø1A
S21.4Ø2A
S21.4Ø9A
S21.411A
S21.412A
S21.419A
S21.421A
S21.422A
S21.429A
S21.431A
S21.432A
S21.439A
S21.441A
S21.442A
S21.449A
S21.451A
S21.452A
S21.459A
S22.ØØØB
S22.ØØ1B
S22.ØØ2B
S22.ØØ8B
S22.ØØ9B
S22.Ø1ØB
S22.Ø11B
S22.Ø12B
S22.Ø18B
S22.Ø19B
S22.Ø2ØB
S22.Ø21B
S22.Ø22B
S22.Ø28B
S22.Ø29B
S22.Ø3ØB
S22.Ø31B
S22.Ø32B
S22.Ø38B
S22.Ø39B
S22.Ø4ØB
S22.Ø41B
S22.Ø42B
S22.Ø48B
S22.Ø49B
S22.Ø5ØB
S22.Ø51B
S22.Ø52B
S22.Ø58B
S22.Ø59B
S22.Ø6ØB
S22.Ø61B
S22.Ø62B
S22.Ø68B
S22.Ø69B
S22.Ø7ØB
S22.Ø71B
S22.Ø72B
S22.Ø78B
S22.Ø79B
S22.Ø8ØB
S22.Ø81B
S22.Ø82B
S22.Ø88B
S22.Ø89B
S22.2ØXB
S22.21XB
S22.22XB
S22.23XB
S22.24XB
S22.31XB
S22.32XB
S22.39XB
S22.41XB
S22.42XB
S22.43XB
S22.49XB
S22.5XXA
S22.5XXB
S22.9XXB
S24.ØXXA
S24.1Ø1A
S24.1Ø2A
S24.1Ø3A
S24.1Ø4A
S24.111A
S24.112A
S24.113A
S24.114A
S24.131A
S24.132A
S24.133A
S24.134A
S24.141A
S24.142A
S24.143A
S24.144A
S24.151A
S24.152A
S24.153A
S24.154A
S25.ØØXA
S25.Ø1XA
S25.Ø2XA
S25.Ø9XA
S25.1Ø1A
S25.1Ø2A
S25.1Ø9A
S25.111A
S25.112A
S25.119A
S25.121A
S25.122A
S25.129A
S25.191A
S25.192A
S25.199A
S25.2ØXA
S25.21XA
S25.22XA
S25.29XA
S25.3Ø1A
S25.3Ø2A
S25.3Ø9A
S25.311A
S25.312A
S25.319A
S25.321A
S25.322A
S25.329A
S25.391A
S25.392A
S25.399A
S25.4Ø1A
S25.4Ø2A
S25.4Ø9A
S25.411A
S25.412A
S25.419A
S25.421A
S25.422A
S25.429A
S25.491A
S25.492A
S25.499A
S26.Ø2ØA
S26.Ø21A
S26.Ø22A
S26.12XA
S26.92XA
S27.1XXA
S27.2XXA
S27.331A
S27.332A
S27.339A
S27.4Ø1A
S27.4Ø2A
S27.4Ø9A
S27.411A
S27.412A
S27.419A
S27.421A
S27.422A
S27.429A
S27.431A
S27.432A
S27.439A
S27.491A
S27.492A
S27.499A
S27.812A
S27.813A
S27.818A
S27.819A
S31.ØØ1A
S31.Ø11A
S31.Ø21A
S31.Ø31A
S31.Ø41A
S31.Ø51A
S31.6ØØA
S31.6Ø1A
S31.6Ø2A
S31.6Ø3A
S31.6Ø4A
S31.6Ø5A
S31.6Ø9A
S31.61ØA
S31.611A
S31.612A
S31.613A
S31.614A
S31.615A
S31.619A
S31.62ØA
S31.621A
S31.622A
S31.623A
S31.624A
S31.625A
S31.629A
S31.63ØA
S31.631A
S31.632A
S31.633A
S31.634A
S31.635A
S31.639A
S31.64ØA
S31.641A
S31.642A
S31.643A
S31.644A
S31.645A
S31.649A
S31.65ØA
S31.651A
S31.652A
S31.653A
S31.654A
S31.655A
S31.659A
S32.ØØØB
S32.ØØ1B
S32.ØØ2B
S32.ØØ8B
S32.ØØ9B
S32.Ø1ØB
S32.Ø11B
S32.Ø12B
S32.Ø18B
S32.Ø19B
S32.Ø2ØB
S32.Ø21B
S32.Ø22B
S32.Ø28B
S32.Ø29B
S32.Ø3ØB
S32.Ø31B
S32.Ø32B
S32.Ø38B
S32.Ø39B
S32.Ø4ØB
S32.Ø41B
S32.Ø42B
S32.Ø48B
S32.Ø49B
S32.Ø5ØB
S32.Ø51B
S32.Ø52B
S32.Ø58B
S32.Ø59B
S32.1ØXB
S32.11ØB
S32.111B
S32.112B
S32.119B
S32.12ØB
S32.121B
S32.122B
S32.129B
S32.13ØB
S32.131B
S32.132B
S32.139B
S32.14XB
S32.15XB
S32.16XB
S32.17XB
S32.19XB
S32.2XXB
S32.3Ø1B
S32.3Ø2B
S32.3Ø9B
S32.311B
S32.312B
S32.313B
S32.314B
S32.315B
S32.316B
S32.391B
S32.392B
S32.399B
S32.4Ø1A
S32.4Ø1B
S32.4Ø2A
S32.4Ø2B
S32.4Ø9A
S32.4Ø9B
S32.411A
S32.411B
S32.412A
S32.412B
S32.413A
S32.413B
S32.414A
S32.414B
S32.415A
S32.415B
S32.416A
S32.416B
S32.421A
S32.421B
S32.422A
S32.422B
S32.423A
S32.423B
S32.424A
S32.424B
S32.425A
S32.425B
S32.426A
S32.426B
S32.431A
S32.431B
S32.432A
S32.432B
S32.433A
S32.433B
S32.434A
S32.434B
S32.435A
S32.435B
S32.436A
S32.436B
S32.441A
S32.441B
S32.442A
S32.442B
S32.443A
S32.443B
S32.444A
S32.444B
S32.445A
S32.445B
S32.446A
S32.446B
S32.451A
S32.451B
S32.452A
S32.452B
S32.453A
S32.453B
S32.454A
S32.454B
S32.455A
S32.455B
S32.456A
S32.456B
S32.461A
S32.461B
S32.462A
S32.462B
S32.463A
S32.463B
S32.464A
S32.464B
S32.465A
S32.465B
S32.466A
S32.466B
S32.471A
S32.471B
S32.472A
S32.472B
S32.473A
S32.473B
S32.474A
S32.474B
S32.475A
S32.475B
S32.476A
S32.476B
S32.481A
S32.481B
S32.482A
S32.482B
S32.483A
S32.483B
S32.484A
S32.484B
S32.485A
S32.485B
S32.486A
S32.486B
S32.491A
S32.491B
S32.492A
S32.492B
S32.499A
S32.499B
S32.5Ø1B
S32.5Ø2B
S32.5Ø9B
S32.511B
S32.512B
S32.519B
S32.591B
S32.592B
S32.599B
S32.6Ø1B
S32.6Ø2B
S32.6Ø9B
S32.611B
S32.612B
S32.613B
S32.614B
S32.615B
S32.616B
S32.691B
S32.692B
S32.699B
S32.81ØB
S32.811B
S32.82XB
S32.89XB
S32.9XXB
S34.Ø1XA
S34.Ø2XA
S34.1Ø1A
S34.1Ø2A
S34.1Ø3A
S34.1Ø4A
S34.1Ø5A
S34.1Ø9A
S34.111A
S34.112A
S34.113A
S34.114A
S34.115A
S34.119A
S34.121A
S34.122A
S34.123A
S34.124A
S34.125A
S34.129A
S34.131A
S34.132A
S34.139A
S34.3XXA
S35.ØØXA
S35.Ø1XA
S35.Ø2XA
S35.Ø9XA
S35.1ØXA

Appendix D: Major Complication and Comorbidity (MCC) Code List

S35.4Ø1A
S35.4Ø2A
S35.4Ø3A
S35.4Ø4A
S35.4Ø5A
S35.4Ø6A
S35.411A
S35.412A
S35.413A
S35.414A
S35.415A
S35.416A
S35.491A
S35.492A
S35.493A
S35.494A
S35.495A
S35.496A
S35.5ØXA
S35.511A
S35.512A
S35.513A
S35.514A
S35.515A
S35.516A
S35.59XA
S36.Ø31A
S36.Ø32A
S36.115A
S36.116A
S37.Ø61A
S37.Ø62A
S37.Ø69A
S37.Ø91A
S37.Ø92A
S37.Ø99A
S42.2Ø1B
S42.2Ø2B
S42.2Ø9B
S42.211B
S42.212B
S42.213B
S42.214B
S42.215B
S42.216B
S42.221B
S42.222B
S42.223B
S42.224B
S42.225B
S42.226B
S42.231B
S42.232B
S42.239B
S42.241B
S42.242B
S42.249B
S42.251B
S42.252B
S42.253B
S42.254B
S42.255B
S42.256B
S42.261B
S42.262B
S42.263B
S42.264B
S42.265B
S42.266B
S42.291B
S42.292B
S42.293B
S42.294B
S42.295B
S42.296B
S42.3Ø1B
S42.3Ø2B
S42.3Ø9B
S42.321B
S42.322B
S42.323B
S42.324B
S42.325B
S42.326B
S42.331B
S42.332B
S42.333B
S42.334B
S42.335B
S42.336B
S42.341B
S42.342B
S42.343B
S42.344B
S42.345B
S42.346B
S42.351B
S42.352B
S42.353B
S42.354B
S42.355B
S42.356B
S42.361B
S42.362B
S42.363B
S42.364B
S42.365B
S42.366B
S42.391B
S42.392B
S42.399B
S42.4Ø1B
S42.4Ø2B
S42.4Ø9B
S42.411B
S42.412B
S42.413B
S42.414B
S42.415B
S42.416B
S42.421B
S42.422B
S42.423B
S42.424B
S42.425B
S42.426B
S42.431B
S42.432B
S42.433B
S42.434B
S42.435B
S42.436B
S42.441B
S42.442B
S42.443B
S42.444B
S42.445B
S42.446B
S42.447B
S42.448B
S42.449B
S42.451B
S42.452B
S42.453B
S42.454B
S42.455B
S42.456B
S42.461B
S42.462B
S42.463B
S42.464B
S42.465B
S42.466B
S42.471B
S42.472B
S42.473B
S42.474B
S42.475B
S42.476B
S42.491B
S42.492B
S42.493B
S42.494B
S42.495B
S42.496B
S42.9ØXB
S42.91XB
S42.92XB
S45.ØØ1A
S45.ØØ2A
S45.ØØ9A
S45.Ø11A
S45.Ø12A
S45.Ø19A
S45.Ø91A
S45.Ø92A
S45.Ø99A
S52.ØØ1B
S52.ØØ1C
S52.ØØ2B
S52.ØØ2C
S52.ØØ9B
S52.ØØ9C
S52.Ø21B
S52.Ø21C
S52.Ø22B
S52.Ø22C
S52.Ø23B
S52.Ø23C
S52.Ø24B
S52.Ø24C
S52.Ø25B
S52.Ø25C
S52.Ø26B
S52.Ø26C
S52.Ø31B
S52.Ø31C
S52.Ø32B
S52.Ø32C
S52.Ø33B
S52.Ø33C
S52.Ø34B
S52.Ø34C
S52.Ø35B
S52.Ø35C
S52.Ø36B
S52.Ø36C
S52.Ø41B
S52.Ø41C
S52.Ø42B
S52.Ø42C
S52.Ø43B
S52.Ø43C
S52.Ø44B
S52.Ø44C
S52.Ø45B
S52.Ø45C
S52.Ø46B
S52.Ø46C
S52.Ø91B
S52.Ø91C
S52.Ø92B
S52.Ø92C
S52.Ø99B
S52.Ø99C
S52.1Ø1B
S52.1Ø1C
S52.1Ø2B
S52.1Ø2C
S52.1Ø9B
S52.1Ø9C
S52.121B
S52.121C
S52.122B
S52.122C
S52.123B
S52.123C
S52.124B
S52.124C
S52.125B
S52.125C
S52.126B
S52.126C
S52.131B
S52.131C
S52.132B
S52.132C
S52.133B
S52.133C
S52.134B
S52.134C
S52.135B
S52.135C
S52.136B
S52.136C
S52.181B
S52.181C
S52.182B
S52.182C
S52.189B
S52.189C
S52.2Ø1B
S52.2Ø1C
S52.2Ø2B
S52.2Ø2C
S52.2Ø9B
S52.2Ø9C
S52.221B
S52.221C
S52.222B
S52.222C
S52.223B
S52.223C
S52.224B
S52.224C
S52.225B
S52.225C
S52.226B
S52.226C
S52.231B
S52.231C
S52.232B
S52.232C
S52.233B
S52.233C
S52.234B
S52.234C
S52.235B
S52.235C
S52.236B
S52.236C
S52.241B
S52.241C
S52.242B
S52.242C
S52.243B
S52.243C
S52.244B
S52.244C
S52.245B
S52.245C
S52.246B
S52.246C
S52.251B
S52.251C
S52.252B
S52.252C
S52.253B
S52.253C
S52.254B
S52.254C
S52.255B
S52.255C
S52.256B
S52.256C
S52.261B
S52.261C
S52.262B
S52.262C
S52.263B
S52.263C
S52.264B
S52.264C
S52.265B
S52.265C
S52.266B
S52.266C
S52.271B
S52.271C
S52.272B
S52.272C
S52.279B
S52.279C
S52.281B
S52.281C
S52.282B
S52.282C
S52.283B
S52.283C
S52.291B
S52.291C
S52.292B
S52.292C
S52.299B
S52.299C
S52.3Ø1B
S52.3Ø1C
S52.3Ø2B
S52.3Ø2C
S52.3Ø9B
S52.3Ø9C
S52.321B
S52.321C
S52.322B
S52.322C
S52.323B
S52.323C
S52.324B
S52.324C
S52.325B
S52.325C
S52.326B
S52.326C
S52.331B
S52.331C
S52.332B
S52.332C
S52.333B
S52.333C
S52.334B
S52.334C
S52.335B
S52.335C
S52.336B
S52.336C
S52.341B
S52.341C
S52.342B
S52.342C
S52.343B
S52.343C
S52.344B
S52.344C
S52.345B
S52.345C
S52.346B
S52.346C
S52.351B
S52.351C
S52.352B
S52.352C
S52.353B
S52.353C
S52.354B
S52.354C
S52.355B
S52.355C
S52.356B
S52.356C
S52.361B
S52.361C
S52.362B
S52.362C
S52.363B
S52.363C
S52.364B
S52.364C
S52.365B
S52.365C
S52.366B
S52.366C
S52.371B
S52.371C
S52.372B
S52.372C
S52.379B
S52.379C
S52.381B
S52.381C
S52.382B
S52.382C
S52.389B
S52.389C
S52.391B
S52.391C
S52.392B
S52.392C
S52.399B
S52.399C
S52.5Ø1B
S52.5Ø1C
S52.5Ø2B
S52.5Ø2C
S52.5Ø9B
S52.5Ø9C
S52.511B
S52.511C
S52.512B
S52.512C
S52.513B
S52.513C
S52.514B
S52.514C
S52.515B
S52.515C
S52.516B
S52.516C
S52.531B
S52.531C
S52.532B
S52.532C
S52.539B
S52.539C
S52.541B
S52.541C
S52.542B
S52.542C
S52.549B
S52.549C
S52.551B
S52.551C
S52.552B
S52.552C
S52.559B
S52.559C
S52.561B
S52.561C
S52.562B
S52.562C
S52.569B
S52.569C
S52.571B
S52.571C
S52.572B
S52.572C
S52.579B
S52.579C
S52.591B
S52.591C
S52.592B
S52.592C
S52.599B
S52.599C
S52.6Ø1B
S52.6Ø1C
S52.6Ø2B
S52.6Ø2C
S52.6Ø9B
S52.6Ø9C
S52.611B
S52.611C
S52.612B
S52.612C
S52.613B
S52.613C
S52.614B
S52.614C
S52.615B
S52.615C
S52.616B
S52.616C
S52.691B
S52.691C
S52.692B
S52.692C
S52.699B
S52.699C
S52.9ØXB
S52.9ØXC
S52.91XB
S52.91XC
S52.92XB
S52.92XC
S72.ØØ1A
S72.ØØ1B
S72.ØØ1C
S72.ØØ2A
S72.ØØ2B
S72.ØØ2C
S72.ØØ9A
S72.ØØ9B
S72.ØØ9C
S72.Ø11A
S72.Ø11B
S72.Ø11C
S72.Ø12A
S72.Ø12B
S72.Ø12C
S72.Ø19A
S72.Ø19B
S72.Ø19C
S72.Ø21A
S72.Ø21B
S72.Ø21C
S72.Ø22A
S72.Ø22B
S72.Ø22C
S72.Ø23A
S72.Ø23B
S72.Ø23C
S72.Ø24A
S72.Ø24B
S72.Ø24C
S72.Ø25A
S72.Ø25B
S72.Ø25C
S72.Ø26A
S72.Ø26B
S72.Ø26C
S72.Ø31A
S72.Ø31B
S72.Ø31C
S72.Ø32A
S72.Ø32B
S72.Ø32C
S72.Ø33A
S72.Ø33B
S72.Ø33C
S72.Ø34A
S72.Ø34B
S72.Ø34C
S72.Ø35A
S72.Ø35B
S72.Ø35C
S72.Ø36A
S72.Ø36B
S72.Ø36C
S72.Ø41A
S72.Ø41B
S72.Ø41C
S72.Ø42A
S72.Ø42B
S72.Ø42C
S72.Ø43A
S72.Ø43B
S72.Ø43C
S72.Ø44A
S72.Ø44B
S72.Ø44C
S72.Ø45A
S72.Ø45B
S72.Ø45C
S72.Ø46A
S72.Ø46B
S72.Ø46C
S72.Ø51A
S72.Ø51B
S72.Ø51C
S72.Ø52A
S72.Ø52B
S72.Ø52C
S72.Ø59A
S72.Ø59B
S72.Ø59C
S72.Ø61A
S72.Ø61B
S72.Ø61C
S72.Ø62A
S72.Ø62B
S72.Ø62C
S72.Ø63A
S72.Ø63B
S72.Ø63C
S72.Ø64A
S72.Ø64B
S72.Ø64C
S72.Ø65A
S72.Ø65B
S72.Ø65C
S72.Ø66A
S72.Ø66B
S72.Ø66C
S72.Ø91A
S72.Ø91B
S72.Ø91C
S72.Ø92A
S72.Ø92B
S72.Ø92C
S72.Ø99A
S72.Ø99B
S72.Ø99C
S72.1Ø1A
S72.1Ø1B
S72.1Ø1C
S72.1Ø2A
S72.1Ø2B
S72.1Ø2C
S72.1Ø9A
S72.1Ø9B
S72.1Ø9C
S72.111A
S72.111B
S72.111C
S72.112A
S72.112B
S72.112C
S72.113A
S72.113B
S72.113C
S72.114A
S72.114B
S72.114C
S72.115A
S72.115B
S72.115C
S72.116A
S72.116B
S72.116C
S72.121A
S72.121B
S72.121C
S72.122A
S72.122B
S72.122C
S72.123A
S72.123B
S72.123C
S72.124A
S72.124B
S72.124C
S72.125A
S72.125B

S72.125C
S72.126A
S72.126B
S72.126C
S72.131A
S72.131B
S72.131C
S72.132A
S72.132B
S72.132C
S72.133A
S72.133B
S72.133C
S72.134A
S72.134B
S72.134C
S72.135A
S72.135B
S72.135C
S72.136A
S72.136B
S72.136C
S72.141A
S72.141B
S72.141C
S72.142A
S72.142B
S72.142C
S72.143A
S72.143B
S72.143C
S72.144A
S72.144B
S72.144C
S72.145A
S72.145B
S72.145C
S72.146A
S72.146B
S72.146C
S72.21XA
S72.21XB
S72.21XC
S72.22XA
S72.22XB
S72.22XC
S72.23XA
S72.23XB
S72.23XC
S72.24XA
S72.24XB
S72.24XC
S72.25XA
S72.25XB
S72.25XC
S72.26XA
S72.26XB
S72.26XC
S72.3Ø1A
S72.3Ø1B
S72.3Ø1C
S72.3Ø2A
S72.3Ø2B
S72.3Ø2C
S72.3Ø9A
S72.3Ø9B
S72.3Ø9C
S72.321A
S72.321B
S72.321C
S72.322A
S72.322B
S72.322C
S72.323A
S72.323B
S72.323C
S72.324A
S72.324B
S72.324C
S72.325A
S72.325B
S72.325C
S72.326A
S72.326B
S72.326C
S72.331A
S72.331B
S72.331C
S72.332A
S72.332B
S72.332C
S72.333A
S72.333B
S72.333C
S72.334A
S72.334B
S72.334C
S72.335A
S72.335B
S72.335C
S72.336A
S72.336B
S72.336C
S72.341A
S72.341B
S72.341C
S72.342A
S72.342B
S72.342C
S72.343A
S72.343B
S72.343C
S72.344A
S72.344B
S72.344C
S72.345A
S72.345B
S72.345C
S72.346A
S72.346B
S72.346C
S72.351A
S72.351B
S72.351C
S72.352A
S72.352B
S72.352C
S72.353A
S72.353B
S72.353C
S72.354A
S72.354B
S72.354C
S72.355A
S72.355B
S72.355C
S72.356A
S72.356B
S72.356C
S72.361A
S72.361B
S72.361C
S72.362A
S72.362B
S72.362C
S72.363A
S72.363B
S72.363C
S72.364A
S72.364B
S72.364C
S72.365A
S72.365B
S72.365C
S72.366A
S72.366B
S72.366C
S72.391A
S72.391B
S72.391C
S72.392A
S72.392B
S72.392C
S72.399A
S72.399B
S72.399C
S72.4Ø1B
S72.4Ø1C
S72.4Ø2B
S72.4Ø2C
S72.4Ø9B
S72.4Ø9C
S72.411B
S72.411C
S72.412B
S72.412C
S72.413B
S72.413C
S72.414B
S72.414C
S72.415B
S72.415C
S72.416B
S72.416C
S72.421B
S72.421C
S72.422B
S72.422C
S72.423B
S72.423C
S72.424B
S72.424C
S72.425B
S72.425C
S72.426B
S72.426C
S72.431B
S72.431C
S72.432B
S72.432C
S72.433B
S72.433C
S72.434B
S72.434C
S72.435B
S72.435C
S72.436B
S72.436C
S72.441B
S72.441C
S72.442B
S72.442C
S72.443B
S72.443C
S72.444B
S72.444C
S72.445B
S72.445C
S72.446B
S72.446C
S72.451B
S72.451C
S72.452B
S72.452C
S72.453B
S72.453C
S72.454B
S72.454C
S72.455B
S72.455C
S72.456B
S72.456C
S72.461B
S72.461C
S72.462B
S72.462C
S72.463B
S72.463C
S72.464B
S72.464C
S72.465B
S72.465C
S72.466B
S72.466C
S72.491B
S72.491C
S72.492B
S72.492C
S72.499B
S72.499C
S72.8X1A
S72.8X1B
S72.8X1C
S72.8X2A
S72.8X2B
S72.8X2C
S72.8X9A
S72.8X9B
S72.8X9C
S72.9ØXA
S72.9ØXB
S72.9ØXC
S72.91XA
S72.91XB
S72.91XC
S72.92XA
S72.92XB
S72.92XC
S75.ØØ1A
S75.ØØ2A
S75.ØØ9A
S75.Ø11A
S75.Ø12A
S75.Ø19A
S75.Ø21A
S75.Ø22A
S75.Ø29A
S75.Ø91A
S75.Ø92A
S75.Ø99A
S75.1Ø1A
S75.1Ø2A
S75.1Ø9A
S75.111A
S75.112A
S75.119A
S75.121A
S75.122A
S75.129A
S75.191A
S75.192A
S75.199A
S79.ØØ1A
S79.ØØ2A
S79.ØØ9A
S79.Ø11A
S79.Ø12A
S79.Ø19A
S79.Ø91A
S79.Ø92A
S79.Ø99A
S82.1Ø1B
S82.1Ø1C
S82.1Ø2B
S82.1Ø2C
S82.1Ø9B
S82.1Ø9C
S82.111B
S82.111C
S82.112B
S82.112C
S82.113B
S82.113C
S82.114B
S82.114C
S82.115B
S82.115C
S82.116B
S82.116C
S82.121B
S82.121C
S82.122B
S82.122C
S82.123B
S82.123C
S82.124B
S82.124C
S82.125B
S82.125C
S82.126B
S82.126C
S82.131B
S82.131C
S82.132B
S82.132C
S82.133B
S82.133C
S82.134B
S82.134C
S82.135B
S82.135C
S82.136B
S82.136C
S82.141B
S82.141C
S82.142B
S82.142C
S82.143B
S82.143C
S82.144B
S82.144C
S82.145B
S82.145C
S82.146B
S82.146C
S82.151B
S82.151C
S82.152B
S82.152C
S82.153B
S82.153C
S82.154B
S82.154C
S82.155B
S82.155C
S82.156B
S82.156C
S82.191B
S82.191C
S82.192B
S82.192C
S82.199B
S82.199C
S82.2Ø1B
S82.2Ø1C
S82.2Ø2B
S82.2Ø2C
S82.2Ø9B
S82.2Ø9C
S82.221B
S82.221C
S82.222B
S82.222C
S82.223B
S82.223C
S82.224B
S82.224C
S82.225B
S82.225C
S82.226B
S82.226C
S82.231B
S82.231C
S82.232B
S82.232C
S82.233B
S82.233C
S82.234B
S82.234C
S82.235B
S82.235C
S82.236B
S82.236C
S82.241B
S82.241C
S82.242B
S82.242C
S82.243B
S82.243C
S82.244B
S82.244C
S82.245B
S82.245C
S82.246B
S82.246C
S82.251B
S82.251C
S82.252B
S82.252C
S82.253B
S82.253C
S82.254B
S82.254C
S82.255B
S82.255C
S82.256B
S82.256C
S82.261B
S82.261C
S82.262B
S82.262C
S82.263B
S82.263C
S82.264B
S82.264C
S82.265B
S82.265C
S82.266B
S82.266C
S82.291B
S82.291C
S82.292B
S82.292C
S82.299B
S82.299C
S82.4Ø1B
S82.4Ø1C
S82.4Ø2B
S82.4Ø2C
S82.4Ø9B
S82.4Ø9C
S82.421B
S82.421C
S82.422B
S82.422C
S82.423B
S82.423C
S82.424B
S82.424C
S82.425B
S82.425C
S82.426B
S82.426C
S82.431B
S82.431C
S82.432B
S82.432C
S82.433B
S82.433C
S82.434B
S82.434C
S82.435B
S82.435C
S82.436B
S82.436C
S82.441B
S82.441C
S82.442B
S82.442C
S82.443B
S82.443C
S82.444B
S82.444C
S82.445B
S82.445C
S82.446B
S82.446C
S82.451B
S82.451C
S82.452B
S82.452C
S82.453B
S82.453C
S82.454B
S82.454C
S82.455B
S82.455C
S82.456B
S82.456C
S82.461B
S82.461C
S82.462B
S82.462C
S82.463B
S82.463C
S82.464B
S82.464C
S82.465B
S82.465C
S82.466B
S82.466C
S82.491B
S82.491C
S82.492B
S82.492C
S82.499B
S82.499C
S82.831B
S82.831C
S82.832B
S82.832C
S82.839B
S82.839C
S82.861B
S82.861C
S82.862B
S82.862C
S82.863B
S82.863C
S82.864B
S82.864C
S82.865B
S82.865C
S82.866B
S82.866C
S85.ØØ1A
S85.ØØ2A
S85.ØØ9A
S85.Ø11A
S85.Ø12A
S85.Ø19A
S85.Ø91A
S85.Ø92A
S85.Ø99A
S85.5Ø1A
S85.5Ø2A
S85.5Ø9A
S85.511A
S85.512A
S85.519A
S85.591A
S85.592A
S85.599A
T31.21
T31.22
T31.31
T31.32
T31.33
T31.41
T31.42
T31.43
T31.44
T31.51
T31.52
T31.53
T31.54
T31.55
T31.61
T31.62
T31.63
T31.64
T31.65
T31.66
T31.71
T31.72
T31.73
T31.74
T31.75
T31.76
T31.77
T31.81
T31.82
T31.83
T31.84
T31.85
T31.86
T31.87
T31.88
T31.91
T31.92
T31.93
T31.94
T31.95
T31.96
T31.97
T31.98
T31.99
T32.21
T32.22
T32.31
T32.32
T32.33
T32.41
T32.42
T32.43
T32.44
T32.51
T32.52
T32.53
T32.54
T32.55
T32.61
T32.62
T32.63
T32.64
T32.65
T32.66
T32.71
T32.72
T32.73
T32.74
T32.75
T32.76
T32.77
T32.81
T32.82
T32.83
T32.84
T32.85
T32.86
T32.87
T32.88
T32.91
T32.92
T32.93
T32.94
T32.95
T32.96
T32.97
T32.98
T32.99
T79.ØXXA
T79.1XXA
T79.4XXA
T79.5XXA
T8Ø.ØXXA
T81.11XA
T81.12XA
T81.19XA
UØ7.1

Appendix E: Complication and Comorbidity (CC) Code List

Note: The following is a comprehensive list of ICD-10-CM codes designated as CCs in the tabular section of this manual. Codes listed in this resource and identified as CCs in the tabular section reflect the most current information that was available at the time of publication. Because the fiscal 2021 IPPS final rule was not available at the time this book was printed, the ICD-10-CM codes designated as CCs are based on the proposed, version 38, MS-DRG Grouper software and Definitions Manual files published with the fiscal 2021 IPPS proposed rule.

For the most current list of CC designations based on the final version of the MS-DRG Grouper software and MS-DRG Definitions Manual files, Optum360 has provided an easily searchable data file that can be accessed at the following:

https://www.optum360coding.com/ProductUpdates/
Title: "2021 ICD-10-CM for Hospital IPPS Data File"
Password: Hospital21

AØØ.Ø
AØØ.1
AØØ.9
AØ1.ØØ
AØ1.Ø1
AØ1.Ø2
AØ1.Ø3
AØ1.Ø4
AØ1.Ø5
AØ1.Ø9
AØ1.1
AØ1.2
AØ1.3
AØ1.4
AØ2.Ø
AØ2.23
AØ2.24
AØ2.25
AØ2.29
AØ2.8
AØ2.9
AØ3.Ø
AØ4.Ø
AØ4.1
AØ4.2
AØ4.3
AØ4.4
AØ4.5
AØ4.6
AØ4.71
AØ4.72
AØ4.8
AØ4.9
AØ5.Ø
AØ5.1
AØ5.2
AØ5.3
AØ5.4
AØ5.5
AØ5.8
AØ6.Ø
AØ6.1
AØ6.2
AØ6.3
AØ6.81
AØ6.82
AØ6.89
AØ7.1
AØ7.2
AØ7.3
AØ7.4
AØ7.8
AØ7.9
AØ8.Ø
AØ8.11
AØ8.19
AØ8.2
AØ8.31
AØ8.32
AØ8.39
AØ9

A15.Ø
A15.4
A15.5
A15.6
A15.7
A15.8
A15.9
A17.9
A18.Ø1
A18.Ø2
A18.Ø3
A18.Ø9
A18.1Ø
A18.11
A18.12
A18.13
A18.14
A18.15
A18.16
A18.17
A18.18
A18.2
A18.32
A18.39
A18.4
A18.5Ø
A18.51
A18.52
A18.53
A18.54
A18.59
A18.6
A18.7
A18.81
A18.82
A18.83
A18.84
A18.85
A18.89
A21.Ø
A21.1
A21.2
A21.3
A21.7
A21.8
A21.9
A22.Ø
A22.2
A22.8
A22.9
A23.8
A23.9
A24.Ø
A24.1
A24.2
A24.3
A24.9
A25.Ø
A25.1
A25.9
A27.Ø

A27.89
A27.9
A28.Ø
A28.1
A28.2
A28.8
A28.9
A3Ø.Ø
A3Ø.1
A3Ø.2
A3Ø.3
A3Ø.4
A3Ø.5
A3Ø.8
A3Ø.9
A31.Ø
A31.1
A31.2
A31.8
A31.9
A32.Ø
A32.11
A32.12
A32.81
A32.82
A32.89
A32.9
A34
A36.Ø
A36.1
A36.2
A36.3
A36.81
A36.82
A36.83
A36.84
A36.85
A36.86
A36.89
A36.9
A37.ØØ
A37.1Ø
A37.8Ø
A37.9Ø
A38.Ø
A38.1
A38.8
A38.9
A39.82
A39.83
A39.84
A39.89
A39.9
A42.Ø
A42.1
A42.2
A42.81
A42.82
A42.89
A42.9
A43.Ø

A43.1
A43.8
A43.9
A44.Ø
A44.1
A44.8
A44.9
A48.51
A48.52
A5Ø.Ø1
A5Ø.Ø2
A5Ø.Ø3
A5Ø.Ø4
A5Ø.Ø5
A5Ø.Ø6
A5Ø.Ø7
A5Ø.Ø8
A5Ø.Ø9
A5Ø.2
A5Ø.3Ø
A5Ø.31
A5Ø.32
A5Ø.39
A5Ø.4Ø
A5Ø.43
A5Ø.44
A5Ø.45
A5Ø.49
A5Ø.51
A5Ø.52
A5Ø.53
A5Ø.54
A5Ø.55
A5Ø.56
A5Ø.57
A5Ø.59
A51.31
A51.32
A51.39
A51.42
A51.43
A51.44
A51.45
A51.46
A51.49
A52.ØØ
A52.Ø1
A52.Ø2
A52.Ø3
A52.Ø4
A52.Ø5
A52.Ø6
A52.Ø9
A52.1Ø
A52.11
A52.12
A52.15
A52.16
A52.17
A52.19
A52.2

A52.3
A52.71
A52.72
A52.73
A52.74
A52.75
A52.76
A52.77
A52.78
A52.79
A54.ØØ
A54.Ø1
A54.Ø2
A54.Ø3
A54.Ø9
A54.1
A54.21
A54.22
A54.23
A54.24
A54.29
A54.3Ø
A54.31
A54.32
A54.33
A54.39
A54.4Ø
A54.41
A54.42
A54.43
A54.49
A54.82
A54.83
A54.84
A54.85
A54.89
A54.9
A68.Ø
A68.1
A68.9
A69.1
A69.2Ø
A69.21
A69.22
A69.23
A69.29
A7Ø
A75.Ø
A75.1
A75.2
A75.3
A75.9
A77.Ø
A77.1
A77.2
A77.3
A77.4Ø
A77.41
A77.49
A77.8
A77.9

A78
A79.Ø
A79.1
A79.81
A79.89
A79.9
A81.ØØ
A81.Ø1
A81.Ø9
A81.1
A81.2
A81.81
A81.82
A81.83
A81.89
A81.9
A82.Ø
A82.1
A82.9
A85.Ø
A85.1
A85.8
A86
A87.Ø
A87.1
A87.2
A87.8
A87.9
A88.Ø
A88.8
A89
A9Ø
A91
A92.Ø
A92.1
A92.2
A92.4
A92.5
A92.8
A92.9
A93.Ø
A93.1
A93.2
A93.8
A94
A95.Ø
A95.1
A95.9
A96.Ø
A96.1
A96.8
A96.9
A98.Ø
A98.1
A98.2
A98.5
A98.8
A99
BØØ.2
BØØ.5Ø
BØØ.51

BØØ.52
BØØ.53
BØØ.59
BØØ.81
BØØ.89
BØ1.Ø
BØ1.81
BØ1.89
BØ1.9
BØ2.Ø
BØ2.21
BØ2.22
BØ2.23
BØ2.29
BØ2.3Ø
BØ2.31
BØ2.32
BØ2.33
BØ2.34
BØ2.39
BØ2.7
BØ2.8
BØ3
BØ4
BØ5.1
BØ5.4
BØ5.81
BØ5.89
BØ6.ØØ
BØ6.Ø2
BØ6.Ø9
BØ6.81
BØ6.82
BØ6.89
BØ8.3
BØ8.71
B15.9
B16.1
B16.9
B17.Ø
B17.1Ø
B17.2
B17.8
B17.9
B18.Ø
B18.1
B18.8
B18.9
B19.1Ø
B19.9
B2Ø
B25.1
B25.8
B25.9
B26.Ø
B26.3
B26.81
B26.82
B26.83
B26.84
B26.85

B26.89
B33.1
B33.2Ø
B33.21
B33.22
B33.23
B33.4
B34.3
B37.Ø
B37.41
B37.49
B37.81
B37.82
B37.83
B37.84
B37.89
B38.Ø
B38.1
B38.2
B38.3
B38.7
B38.81
B38.89
B38.9
B39.3
B4Ø.Ø
B4Ø.1
B4Ø.2
B4Ø.3
B4Ø.7
B4Ø.81
B4Ø.89
B4Ø.9
B41.Ø
B41.7
B41.8
B41.9
B44.1
B44.2
B44.7
B44.81
B44.89
B44.9
B45.Ø
B45.2
B45.3
B45.7
B45.8
B45.9
B47.Ø
B47.1
B47.9
B48.2
B48.3
B48.4
B48.8
B49
B5Ø.Ø
B5Ø.8
B51.Ø
B51.8

B51.9
B52.Ø
B52.8
B52.9
B53.Ø
B53.1
B53.8
B54
B55.Ø
B55.1
B55.2
B55.9
B56.Ø
B56.1
B56.9
B57.Ø
B57.1
B57.2
B57.3Ø
B57.31
B57.32
B57.39
B57.4Ø
B57.41
B57.42
B57.49
B57.5
B58.ØØ
B58.Ø1
B58.Ø9
B58.1
B58.82
B58.83
B58.89
B58.9
B6Ø.ØØ
B6Ø.Ø1
B6Ø.Ø2
B6Ø.Ø3
B6Ø.Ø9
B6Ø.1Ø
B6Ø.19
B6Ø.2
B65.Ø
B65.1
B65.2
B65.3
B65.8
B65.9
B66.Ø
B66.1
B66.2
B66.3
B66.4
B66.5
B66.8
B67.Ø
B67.1
B67.2
B67.31
B67.32

B67.39
B67.4
B67.5
B67.61
B67.69
B67.7
B67.8
B67.9Ø
B67.99
B68.Ø
B68.1
B68.9
B69.Ø
B69.1
B69.81
B69.89
B69.9
B7Ø.Ø
B7Ø.1
B71.Ø
B71.1
B71.8
B72
B73.ØØ
B73.Ø1
B73.Ø2
B73.Ø9
B73.1
B74.Ø
B74.1
B74.2
B74.3
B74.4
B74.8
B74.9
B75
B76.Ø
B76.1
B76.8
B76.9
B77.Ø
B77.89
B77.9
B78.Ø
B78.7
B78.9
B79
B8Ø
B81.Ø
B81.1
B81.2
B81.3
B81.4
B81.8
B82.Ø
B97.21
B97.33
B97.34
B97.35
C15.3
C15.4
C15.5
C15.8
C15.9
C16.Ø
C16.1
C16.2
C16.3
C16.4
C16.5
C16.6
C16.8
C16.9
C17.Ø
C17.1
C17.2
C17.3
C17.8
C17.9
C18.Ø
C18.1
C18.2
C18.3
C18.4
C18.5
C18.6
C18.7
C18.8
C18.9
C19
C2Ø
C21.Ø
C21.1
C21.2
C21.8
C22.Ø
C22.1
C22.2
C22.3
C22.4
C22.7
C22.8
C22.9
C23
C24.Ø
C24.1
C24.8
C24.9
C25.Ø
C25.1
C25.2
C25.3
C25.4
C25.7
C25.8
C25.9
C33
C34.ØØ
C34.Ø1
C34.Ø2
C34.1Ø
C34.11
C34.12
C34.2
C34.3Ø
C34.31
C34.32
C34.8Ø
C34.81
C34.82
C34.9Ø
C34.91
C34.92
C37
C38.Ø
C38.1
C38.2
C38.3
C38.4
C38.8
C4Ø.ØØ
C4Ø.Ø1
C4Ø.Ø2
C4Ø.1Ø
C4Ø.11
C4Ø.12
C4Ø.2Ø
C4Ø.21
C4Ø.22
C4Ø.3Ø
C4Ø.31
C4Ø.32
C4Ø.8Ø
C4Ø.81
C4Ø.82
C4Ø.9Ø
C4Ø.91
C4Ø.92
C41.Ø
C41.1
C41.2
C41.3
C41.4
C41.9
C45.Ø
C45.1
C45.2
C46.Ø
C46.1
C46.2
C46.3
C46.4
C46.5Ø
C46.51
C46.52
C46.7
C46.9
C47.Ø
C47.1Ø
C47.11
C47.12
C47.2Ø
C47.21
C47.22
C47.3
C47.4
C47.5
C47.6
C47.8
C47.9
C48.Ø
C48.1
C48.2
C48.8
C49.Ø
C49.1Ø
C49.11
C49.12
C49.2Ø
C49.21
C49.22
C49.3
C49.4
C49.5
C49.6
C49.8
C49.9
C49.AØ
C49.A1
C49.A2
C49.A3
C49.A4
C49.A5
C49.A9
C56.1
C56.2
C56.9
C64.1
C64.2
C64.9
C65.1
C65.2
C65.9
C66.1
C66.2
C66.9
C68.Ø
C68.1
C68.8
C68.9
C7Ø.Ø
C7Ø.1
C7Ø.9
C71.Ø
C71.1
C71.2
C71.3
C71.4
C71.5
C71.6
C71.7
C71.8
C71.9
C72.Ø
C72.1
C72.2Ø
C72.21
C72.22
C72.3Ø
C72.31
C72.32
C72.4Ø
C72.41
C72.42
C72.5Ø
C72.59
C72.9
C74.ØØ
C74.Ø1
C74.Ø2
C74.1Ø
C74.11
C74.12
C74.9Ø
C74.91
C74.92
C75.Ø
C75.1
C75.2
C75.3
C75.4
C75.5
C75.8
C75.9
C77.Ø
C77.1
C77.2
C77.3
C77.4
C77.5
C77.8
C77.9
C78.ØØ
C78.Ø1
C78.Ø2
C78.1
C78.2
C78.3Ø
C78.39
C78.4
C78.5
C78.6
C78.7
C78.8Ø
C78.89
C79.ØØ
C79.Ø1
C79.Ø2
C79.1Ø
C79.11
C79.19
C79.2
C79.31
C79.32
C79.4Ø
C79.49
C79.51
C79.52
C79.6Ø
C79.61
C79.62
C79.7Ø
C79.71
C79.72
C79.81
C79.82
C79.89
C79.9
C7A.ØØ
C7A.Ø1Ø
C7A.Ø11
C7A.Ø12
C7A.Ø19
C7A.Ø2Ø
C7A.Ø21
C7A.Ø22
C7A.Ø23
C7A.Ø24
C7A.Ø25
C7A.Ø26
C7A.Ø29
C7A.Ø9Ø
C7A.Ø91
C7A.Ø92
C7A.Ø93
C7A.Ø94
C7A.Ø95
C7A.Ø96
C7A.Ø98
C7A.1
C7A.8
C7B.Ø1
C7B.Ø2
C7B.Ø3
C7B.Ø4
C7B.Ø9
C7B.8
C8Ø.Ø
C8Ø.2
C81.ØØ
C81.Ø1
C81.Ø2
C81.Ø3
C81.Ø4
C81.Ø5
C81.Ø6
C81.Ø7
C81.Ø8
C81.Ø9
C81.1Ø
C81.11
C81.12
C81.13
C81.14
C81.15
C81.16
C81.17
C81.18
C81.19
C81.2Ø
C81.21
C81.22
C81.23
C81.24
C81.25
C81.26
C81.27
C81.28
C81.29
C81.3Ø
C81.31
C81.32
C81.33
C81.34
C81.35
C81.36
C81.37
C81.38
C81.39
C81.4Ø
C81.41
C81.42
C81.43
C81.44
C81.45
C81.46
C81.47
C81.48
C81.49
C81.7Ø
C81.71
C81.72
C81.73
C81.74
C81.75
C81.76
C81.77
C81.78
C81.79
C81.9Ø
C81.91
C81.92
C81.93
C81.94
C81.95
C81.96
C81.97
C81.98
C81.99
C82.ØØ
C82.Ø1
C82.Ø2
C82.Ø3
C82.Ø4
C82.Ø5
C82.Ø6
C82.Ø7
C82.Ø8
C82.Ø9
C82.1Ø
C82.11
C82.12
C82.13
C82.14
C82.15
C82.16
C82.17
C82.18
C82.19
C82.2Ø
C82.21
C82.22
C82.23
C82.24
C82.25
C82.26
C82.27
C82.28
C82.29
C82.3Ø
C82.31
C82.32
C82.33
C82.34
C82.35
C82.36
C82.37
C82.38
C82.39
C82.4Ø
C82.41
C82.42
C82.43
C82.44
C82.45
C82.46
C82.47
C82.48
C82.49
C82.5Ø
C82.51
C82.52
C82.53
C82.54
C82.55
C82.56
C82.57
C82.58
C82.59
C82.6Ø
C82.61
C82.62
C82.63
C82.64
C82.65
C82.66
C82.67
C82.68
C82.69
C82.8Ø
C82.81
C82.82
C82.83
C82.84
C82.85
C82.86
C82.87
C82.88
C82.89
C82.9Ø
C82.91
C82.92
C82.93
C82.94
C82.95
C82.96
C82.97
C82.98
C82.99
C83.ØØ
C83.Ø1
C83.Ø2
C83.Ø3
C83.Ø4
C83.Ø5
C83.Ø6
C83.Ø7
C83.Ø8
C83.Ø9
C83.1Ø
C83.11
C83.12
C83.13
C83.14
C83.15
C83.16
C83.17
C83.18
C83.19
C83.3Ø
C83.31
C83.32
C83.33
C83.34
C83.35
C83.36
C83.37
C83.38
C83.39
C83.5Ø
C83.51
C83.52
C83.53
C83.54
C83.55
C83.56
C83.57
C83.58
C83.59
C83.7Ø
C83.71
C83.72
C83.73
C83.74
C83.75
C83.76
C83.77
C83.78
C83.79
C83.8Ø
C83.81
C83.82
C83.83
C83.84
C83.85
C83.86
C83.87
C83.88
C83.89
C83.9Ø
C83.91
C83.92
C83.93
C83.94
C83.95
C83.96
C83.97
C83.98
C83.99
C84.ØØ
C84.Ø1
C84.Ø2
C84.Ø3
C84.Ø4
C84.Ø5
C84.Ø6
C84.Ø7
C84.Ø8
C84.Ø9
C84.1Ø
C84.11
C84.12
C84.13
C84.14
C84.15
C84.16
C84.17
C84.18
C84.19
C84.4Ø
C84.41
C84.42
C84.43
C84.44
C84.45
C84.46
C84.47
C84.48
C84.49
C84.6Ø
C84.61
C84.62
C84.63
C84.64
C84.65
C84.66
C84.67
C84.68
C84.69
C84.7Ø
C84.71
C84.72
C84.73
C84.74
C84.75
C84.76
C84.77
C84.78
C84.79
C84.9Ø
C84.91
C84.92
C84.93
C84.94
C84.95
C84.96
C84.97
C84.98
C84.99
C84.AØ
C84.A1
C84.A2
C84.A3
C84.A4
C84.A5
C84.A6
C84.A7
C84.A8
C84.A9
C84.ZØ
C84.Z1
C84.Z2
C84.Z3
C84.Z4
C84.Z5
C84.Z6
C84.Z7
C84.Z8
C84.Z9
C85.1Ø
C85.11
C85.12
C85.13
C85.14
C85.15
C85.16
C85.17
C85.18
C85.19
C85.2Ø
C85.21
C85.22
C85.23
C85.24
C85.25
C85.26
C85.27
C85.28
C85.29
C85.8Ø
C85.81
C85.82
C85.83
C85.84
C85.85
C85.86
C85.87
C85.88
C85.89
C85.9Ø
C85.91
C85.92
C85.93

C85.94
C85.95
C85.96
C85.97
C85.98
C85.99
C86.0
C86.1
C86.2
C86.3
C86.4
C86.5
C86.6
C88.2
C88.3
C88.4
C88.8
C88.9
C90.00
C90.01
C90.02
C90.10
C90.11
C90.12
C90.20
C90.21
C90.22
C90.30
C90.31
C90.32
C91.00
C91.01
C91.02
C91.10
C91.11
C91.12
C91.30
C91.31
C91.32
C91.40
C91.41
C91.42
C91.50
C91.51
C91.52
C91.60
C91.61
C91.62
C91.90
C91.91
C91.92
C91.A0
C91.A1
C91.A2
C91.Z0
C91.Z1
C91.Z2
C92.00
C92.01
C92.02
C92.10
C92.11
C92.12
C92.20
C92.21
C92.22
C92.30
C92.31
C92.32
C92.40
C92.41
C92.42
C92.50
C92.51
C92.52
C92.60
C92.61
C92.62
C92.90
C92.91
C92.92
C92.A0
C92.A1
C92.A2
C92.Z0
C92.Z1
C92.Z2
C93.00
C93.01
C93.02
C93.10
C93.11
C93.12
C93.30
C93.31
C93.32
C93.90
C93.91
C93.92
C93.Z0
C93.Z1
C93.Z2
C94.00
C94.01
C94.02
C94.20
C94.21
C94.22
C94.30
C94.31
C94.32
C94.40
C94.41
C94.42
C94.6
C94.80
C94.81
C94.82
C95.00
C95.01
C95.02
C95.10
C95.11
C95.12
C95.90
C95.91
C95.92
C96.0
C96.20
C96.21
C96.22
C96.29
C96.4
C96.5
C96.6
C96.9
C96.A
C96.Z
D46.22
D46.C
D47.01
D47.02
D47.09
D47.1
D47.9
D47.Z1
D47.Z2
D47.Z9
D58.8
D58.9
D59.0
D59.10
D59.11
D59.12
D59.13
D59.19
D59.2
D59.4
D59.9
D61.01
D61.09
D61.818
D61.82
D61.9
D62
D68.0
D68.1
D68.2
D68.311
D68.312
D68.318
D68.32
D68.4
D68.51
D68.52
D68.59
D68.61
D68.62
D68.69
D68.8
D68.9
D69.0
D69.3
D69.41
D69.42
D74.0
D74.8
D74.9
D75.81
D76.1
D76.2
D76.3
D78.01
D78.02
D78.11
D78.12
D78.21
D78.22
D78.31
D78.32
D78.33
D78.34
D78.81
D78.89
D80.0
D80.1
D80.2
D80.3
D80.4
D80.5
D80.6
D80.7
D80.8
D80.9
D81.0
D81.1
D81.2
D81.30
D81.31
D81.32
D81.39
D81.4
D81.5
D81.6
D81.7
D81.89
D81.9
D82.0
D82.1
D83.0
D83.1
D83.2
D83.8
D83.9
D84.81
D84.821
D84.822
D84.89
D84.9
D89.810
D89.811
D89.812
D89.813
E06.0
E08.52
E09.52
E10.52
E11.52
E13.52
E15
E22.1
E22.2
E22.8
E22.9
E23.0
E23.2
E24.0
E24.2
E24.3
E24.4
E24.8
E24.9
E27.0
E27.1
E27.2
E27.3
E27.40
E27.49
E27.5
E32.1
E34.0
E36.01
E36.02
E36.11
E36.12
E44.0
E44.1
E45
E46
E51.11
E51.12
E51.2
E51.8
E51.9
E53.0
E55.0
E64.0
E66.2
E70.0
E70.1
E70.20
E70.21
E70.29
E70.30
E70.310
E70.311
E70.318
E70.319
E70.320
E70.321
E70.328
E70.329
E70.330
E70.331
E70.338
E70.339
E70.39
E70.40
E70.41
E70.49
E70.5
E70.81
E70.89
E70.9
E71.0
E71.110
E71.111
E71.118
E71.120
E71.121
E71.128
E71.19
E71.2
E71.310
E71.311
E71.312
E71.313
E71.314
E71.318
E71.32
E71.39
E71.50
E71.510
E71.511
E71.518
E71.520
E71.521
E71.522
E71.528
E71.529
E71.53
E71.540
E71.541
E71.542
E71.548
E72.00
E72.01
E72.02
E72.03
E72.04
E72.09
E72.10
E72.11
E72.12
E72.19
E72.20
E72.21
E72.22
E72.23
E72.29
E72.3
E72.4
E72.50
E72.51
E72.52
E72.53
E72.59
E72.81
E72.89
E72.9
E74.00
E74.01
E74.02
E74.03
E74.04
E74.09
E74.20
E74.21
E74.29
E74.4
E74.810
E74.818
E74.819
E74.89
E75.00
E75.01
E75.02
E75.09
E75.10
E75.11
E75.19
E75.23
E75.25
E75.26
E75.29
E75.4
E76.01
E76.02
E76.03
E76.1
E76.210
E76.211
E76.219
E76.22
E76.29
E76.3
E76.8
E76.9
E78.71
E78.72
E79.1
E79.2
E79.8
E79.9
E80.0
E80.1
E80.20
E80.21
E80.29
E80.3
E84.19
E84.8
E84.9
E85.0
E85.1
E85.2
E85.3
E85.4
E85.81
E85.82
E85.89
E85.9
E87.0
E87.1
E87.2
E87.3
E87.4
E88.02
E88.40
E88.41
E88.42
E88.49
E89.1
E89.6
E89.810
E89.811
E89.820
E89.821
E89.822
E89.823
E89.89
F01.51
F02.81
F03.91
F05
F06.0
F06.2
F10.121
F10.130
F10.131
F10.132
F10.139
F10.14
F10.151
F10.159
F10.180
F10.181
F10.188
F10.19
F10.221
F10.230
F10.231
F10.232
F10.239
F10.24
F10.251
F10.259
F10.27
F10.280
F10.281
F10.288
F10.29
F10.921
F10.930
F10.931
F10.932
F10.939
F10.94
F10.951
F10.959
F10.980
F10.981
F10.988
F10.99
F11.121
F11.13
F11.150
F11.151
F11.20
F11.221
F11.222
F11.23
F11.250
F11.251
F11.259
F11.281
F11.282
F11.288
F11.921
F11.93
F11.950
F11.951
F12.121
F12.150
F12.151
F12.221
F12.250
F12.251
F12.921
F12.950
F12.951
F13.121
F13.130
F13.131
F13.132
F13.139
F13.150
F13.151
F13.20
F13.221
F13.230
F13.231
F13.232
F13.239
F13.250
F13.251
F13.259
F13.26
F13.27
F13.280
F13.281
F13.282
F13.288
F13.921
F13.930
F13.931
F13.932
F13.939
F13.950
F13.951
F13.97
F14.121
F14.13
F14.150
F14.151
F14.20
F14.221
F14.222
F14.229
F14.23
F14.250
F14.251
F14.259
F14.280
F14.281
F14.282
F14.288
F14.921
F14.93
F14.950
F14.951
F15.121
F15.13
F15.150
F15.151
F15.20
F15.221
F15.222
F15.23
F15.250
F15.251
F15.259
F15.280
F15.281
F15.282
F15.288
F15.921
F15.93
F15.950
F15.951
F16.121
F16.150
F16.151
F16.20
F16.221
F16.250
F16.251
F16.259
F16.280
F16.283
F16.288
F16.921
F16.950
F16.951
F17.203
F17.213
F17.223
F17.293
F18.121
F18.150
F18.151
F18.17
F18.20
F18.221
F18.250
F18.251
F18.259
F18.27
F18.280
F18.288
F18.921
F18.950
F18.951
F18.97
F19.121
F19.130
F19.131
F19.132
F19.139
F19.150
F19.151
F19.17
F19.20
F19.221
F19.222
F19.230
F19.231
F19.232
F19.239
F19.250
F19.251
F19.259
F19.26
F19.27
F19.280
F19.281
F19.282
F19.288
F19.921
F19.930
F19.931
F19.932
F19.939
F19.950
F19.951
F19.97
F20.0
F20.1
F20.2
F20.5
F20.81
F20.89
F23
F30.10
F30.11
F30.12
F30.13
F30.2
F30.9
F31.0
F31.10
F31.11
F31.12
F31.13
F31.2
F31.30
F31.31
F31.32
F31.4
F31.5
F31.60
F31.61
F31.62
F31.63
F31.64
F31.81
F31.89
F32.0
F32.1
F32.2
F32.3
F33.0
F33.1

F33.2
F33.3
F33.40
F33.8
F33.9
F34.81
F34.89
F34.9
F50.00
F50.01
F50.02
F50.2
F68.10
F68.12
F68.A
F72
F73
F84.0
F84.2
F84.3
F84.5
F84.8
F84.9
G03.1
G03.2
G04.1
G10
G11.0
G11.10
G11.11
G11.19
G11.2
G11.3
G11.4
G11.8
G11.9
G12.0
G12.1
G12.20
G12.21
G12.22
G12.23
G12.24
G12.25
G12.29
G12.8
G12.9
G21.11
G21.19
G21.2
G21.3
G21.8
G21.9
G23.0
G23.1
G23.2
G23.8
G23.9
G24.02
G24.09
G24.2
G24.8
G25.82
G25.9
G31.81
G31.82
G32.0
G32.81
G36.0
G36.1
G36.8
G36.9
G37.0
G37.1
G37.2
G37.3
G37.5
G37.8
G37.9
G40.001
G40.009
G40.011
G40.019
G40.101
G40.109
G40.111
G40.119
G40.201
G40.209
G40.211
G40.219
G40.411
G40.419
G40.501
G40.509
G40.801
G40.802
G40.803
G40.804
G40.811
G40.812
G40.813
G40.814
G40.821
G40.822
G40.823
G40.824
G40.833
G40.834
G40.89
G40.911
G40.919
G40.A11
G40.A19
G40.B01
G40.B09
G40.B11
G40.B19
G43.601
G43.609
G43.611
G43.619
G45.0
G45.1
G45.2
G45.3
G45.8
G45.9
G46.0
G46.1
G46.2
G60.1
G61.0
G61.81
G62.81
G70.80
G70.81
G71.20
G71.21
G71.220
G71.228
G71.29
G72.0
G72.1
G72.2
G72.81
G73.1
G73.3
G80.1
G80.2
G80.3
G81.00
G81.01
G81.02
G81.03
G81.04
G81.10
G81.11
G81.12
G81.13
G81.14
G81.90
G81.91
G81.92
G81.93
G81.94
G82.20
G82.21
G82.22
G83.0
G83.4
G90.3
G90.50
G90.511
G90.512
G90.513
G90.519
G90.521
G90.522
G90.523
G90.529
G90.59
G91.0
G91.1
G91.2
G91.3
G91.8
G91.9
G93.1
G93.40
G93.49
G95.0
G95.20
G95.29
G95.81
G95.89
G95.9
G96.00
G96.01
G96.02
G96.08
G96.09
G96.11
G97.0
G97.2
G97.31
G97.32
G97.41
G97.48
G97.49
G97.51
G97.52
G97.61
G97.62
G97.63
G97.64
G97.81
G97.82
G97.83
G97.84
G99.0
G99.2
H05.011
H05.012
H05.013
H05.019
H05.021
H05.022
H05.023
H05.029
H05.031
H05.032
H05.033
H05.039
H20.00
H20.011
H20.012
H20.013
H20.019
H20.021
H20.022
H20.023
H20.029
H20.031
H20.032
H20.033
H20.039
H20.9
H21.331
H21.332
H21.333
H21.339
H30.101
H30.102
H30.103
H30.109
H30.111
H30.112
H30.113
H30.119
H30.121
H30.122
H30.123
H30.129
H30.131
H30.132
H30.133
H30.139
H30.141
H30.142
H30.143
H30.149
H30.891
H30.892
H30.893
H30.899
H30.90
H30.91
H30.92
H30.93
H31.321
H31.322
H31.323
H31.329
H31.401
H31.402
H31.403
H31.409
H31.411
H31.412
H31.413
H31.419
H31.421
H31.422
H31.423
H31.429
H33.121
H33.122
H33.123
H33.129
H33.20
H33.21
H33.22
H33.23
H33.40
H33.41
H33.42
H33.43
H33.8
H34.00
H34.01
H34.02
H34.03
H34.10
H34.11
H34.12
H34.13
H34.211
H34.212
H34.213
H34.219
H34.231
H34.232
H34.233
H34.239
H34.8110
H34.8111
H34.8112
H34.8120
H34.8121
H34.8122
H34.8130
H34.8131
H34.8132
H34.8190
H34.8191
H34.8192
H34.9
H35.70
H35.721
H35.722
H35.723
H35.729
H35.731
H35.732
H35.733
H35.739
H35.82
H40.211
H40.212
H40.213
H40.219
H44.001
H44.002
H44.003
H44.009
H44.011
H44.012
H44.013
H44.019
H44.021
H44.022
H44.023
H44.029
H44.111
H44.112
H44.113
H44.119
H44.121
H44.122
H44.123
H44.129
H44.131
H44.132
H44.133
H44.139
H44.19
H46.00
H46.01
H46.02
H46.03
H46.10
H46.11
H46.12
H46.13
H46.8
H46.9
H47.10
H47.11
H47.41
H47.42
H47.43
H47.49
H47.511
H47.512
H47.519
H47.521
H47.522
H47.529
H47.531
H47.532
H47.539
H47.621
H47.622
H47.629
H47.631
H47.632
H47.639
H47.641
H47.642
H47.649
H49.811
H49.812
H49.813
H49.819
H53.121
H53.122
H53.123
H53.129
H53.131
H53.132
H53.133
H53.139
H59.011
H59.012
H59.013
H59.019
H59.031
H59.032
H59.033
H59.039
H59.091
H59.092
H59.093
H59.099
H59.111
H59.112
H59.113
H59.119
H59.121
H59.122
H59.123
H59.129
H59.211
H59.212
H59.213
H59.219
H59.221
H59.222
H59.223
H59.229
H59.311
H59.312
H59.313
H59.319
H59.321
H59.322
H59.323
H59.329
H59.331
H59.332
H59.333
H59.339
H59.341
H59.342
H59.343
H59.349
H59.351
H59.352
H59.353
H59.359
H59.361
H59.362
H59.363
H59.369
H59.811
H59.812
H59.813
H59.819
H59.88
H59.89
H60.20
H60.21
H60.22
H60.23
H70.001
H70.002
H70.003
H70.009
H70.011
H70.012
H70.013
H70.019
H70.091
H70.092
H70.093
H70.099
H95.21
H95.22
H95.31
H95.32
H95.41
H95.42
H95.51
H95.52
H95.53
H95.54
H95.811
H95.812
H95.813
H95.819
H95.88
H95.89
I01.0
I01.1
I01.2
I01.8
I01.9
I02.0
I02.9
I09.0
I09.2
I09.81
I12.0
I13.0
I13.11
I13.2
I16.1
I16.9
I20.0
I20.1
I23.0
I23.1
I23.2
I23.3
I23.6
I23.7
I23.8
I24.0
I24.1
I24.8
I24.9
I25.110
I25.3
I25.700
I25.710
I25.711
I25.718
I25.719
I25.720
I25.721
I25.728
I25.729
I25.730
I25.731
I25.738
I25.739
I25.750
I25.751
I25.758
I25.759
I25.760
I25.761
I25.768
I25.769
I25.790
I25.791
I25.798
I25.799
I25.810
I25.811
I25.812
I27.0
I27.1
I27.82
I28.0
I28.1
I30.0
I30.1
I30.8
I30.9
I31.0
I31.1
I31.2
I31.3
I31.4
I31.8
I31.9
I32
I38
I39
I42.0
I42.1
I42.2
I42.3
I42.4
I42.5
I42.6
I42.7
I42.8
I42.9
I43
I44.2
I45.2
I45.3
I45.89
I47.0
I47.1
I47.2
I48.11
I48.19
I48.20
I48.21
I48.3
I48.4
I48.92
I49.2
I50.1
I50.20
I50.22
I50.30
I50.32
I50.40
I50.42
I51.0
I51.81
I62.9
I67.3
I67.4
I67.5
I67.6
I67.7
I67.81
I67.82
I67.841
I67.848
I67.850
I67.858
I67.89
I68.2
I69.051
I69.052
I69.053
I69.054
I69.059
I69.151
I69.152
I69.153
I69.154
I69.159
I69.251
I69.252
I69.253
I69.254
I69.259
I69.351
I69.352
I69.353
I69.354
I69.359
I69.851
I69.852
I69.853
I69.854
I69.859
I69.951
I69.952
I69.953
I69.954
I69.959
I70.261
I70.262
I70.263
I70.268
I70.269
I70.331
I70.332
I70.333
I70.334
I70.338
I70.339
I70.341
I70.342
I70.343
I70.344
I70.348
I70.349
I70.361
I70.362
I70.363
I70.368
I70.369
I70.431

I70.432
I70.433
I70.434
I70.438
I70.439
I70.441
I70.442
I70.443
I70.444
I70.448
I70.449
I70.461
I70.462
I70.463
I70.468
I70.469
I70.531
I70.532
I70.533
I70.534
I70.538
I70.539
I70.541
I70.542
I70.543
I70.544
I70.548
I70.549
I70.561
I70.562
I70.563
I70.568
I70.569
I70.631
I70.632
I70.633
I70.634
I70.638
I70.639
I70.641
I70.642
I70.643
I70.644
I70.648
I70.649
I70.661
I70.662
I70.663
I70.668
I70.669
I70.731
I70.732
I70.733
I70.734
I70.738
I70.739
I70.741
I70.742
I70.743
I70.744
I70.748
I70.749
I70.761
I70.762
I70.763
I70.768
I70.769
I70.92
I73.01
I74.09
I74.10
I74.11
I74.19
I74.2
I74.3
I74.4
I74.5
I74.8
I74.9
I75.011
I75.012
I75.013
I75.019
I75.021
I75.022
I75.023
I75.029
I75.81
I75.89
I76
I77.2
I77.4
I77.5
I80.10
I80.11
I80.12
I80.13
I80.201
I80.202
I80.203
I80.209
I80.211
I80.212
I80.213
I80.219
I80.221
I80.222
I80.223
I80.229
I80.231
I80.232
I80.233
I80.239
I80.241
I80.242
I80.243
I80.249
I80.291
I80.292
I80.293
I80.299
I82.1
I82.210
I82.211
I82.290
I82.291
I82.3
I82.401
I82.402
I82.403
I82.409
I82.411
I82.412
I82.413
I82.419
I82.421
I82.422
I82.423
I82.429
I82.431
I82.432
I82.433
I82.439
I82.441
I82.442
I82.443
I82.449
I82.451
I82.452
I82.453
I82.459
I82.491
I82.492
I82.493
I82.499
I82.4Y1
I82.4Y2
I82.4Y3
I82.4Y9
I82.4Z1
I82.4Z2
I82.4Z3
I82.4Z9
I82.501
I82.502
I82.503
I82.509
I82.511
I82.512
I82.513
I82.519
I82.521
I82.522
I82.523
I82.529
I82.531
I82.532
I82.533
I82.539
I82.541
I82.542
I82.543
I82.549
I82.551
I82.552
I82.553
I82.559
I82.591
I82.592
I82.593
I82.599
I82.5Y1
I82.5Y2
I82.5Y3
I82.5Y9
I82.5Z1
I82.5Z2
I82.5Z3
I82.5Z9
I82.601
I82.602
I82.603
I82.609
I82.611
I82.612
I82.613
I82.619
I82.621
I82.622
I82.623
I82.629
I82.701
I82.702
I82.703
I82.709
I82.711
I82.712
I82.713
I82.719
I82.721
I82.722
I82.723
I82.729
I82.811
I82.812
I82.813
I82.819
I82.890
I82.891
I82.90
I82.91
I82.A11
I82.A12
I82.A13
I82.A19
I82.A21
I82.A22
I82.A23
I82.A29
I82.B11
I82.B12
I82.B13
I82.B19
I82.B21
I82.B22
I82.B23
I82.B29
I82.C11
I82.C12
I82.C13
I82.C19
I82.C21
I82.C22
I82.C23
I82.C29
I83.201
I83.202
I83.203
I83.204
I83.205
I83.208
I83.209
I83.211
I83.212
I83.213
I83.214
I83.215
I83.218
I83.219
I83.221
I83.222
I83.223
I83.224
I83.225
I83.228
I83.229
I85.00
I85.10
I87.011
I87.012
I87.013
I87.019
I87.031
I87.032
I87.033
I87.039
I87.1
I87.311
I87.312
I87.313
I87.319
I87.331
I87.332
I87.333
I87.339
I96
I97.110
I97.111
I97.120
I97.121
I97.130
I97.131
I97.190
I97.191
I97.410
I97.411
I97.418
I97.42
I97.51
I97.52
I97.610
I97.611
I97.618
I97.620
I97.621
I97.622
I97.630
I97.631
I97.638
I97.640
I97.641
I97.648
I97.710
I97.711
I97.790
I97.791
I97.810
I97.811
I97.820
I97.821
I97.88
I97.89
J05.10
J18.2
J21.0
J21.1
J21.8
J21.9
J36
J39.0
J39.1
J44.0
J44.1
J45.21
J45.22
J45.31
J45.32
J45.41
J45.42
J45.51
J45.52
J45.901
J45.902
J47.0
J47.1
J67.7
J67.8
J67.9
J68.0
J70.0
J70.1
J81.1
J82.81
J82.82
J82.83
J82.89
J84.01
J84.02
J84.03
J84.09
J84.114
J84.116
J84.117
J84.2
J84.82
J84.9
J90
J91.0
J91.8
J93.11
J93.12
J93.81
J93.82
J93.83
J93.9
J94.0
J94.2
J94.8
J95.00
J95.01
J95.02
J95.03
J95.04
J95.09
J95.4
J95.5
J95.61
J95.62
J95.71
J95.72
J95.811
J95.812
J95.830
J95.831
J95.84
J95.850
J95.851
J95.859
J95.860
J95.861
J95.862
J95.863
J95.88
J95.89
J96.10
J96.11
J96.12
J98.11
J98.19
K04.01
K04.02
K04.4
K11.3
K11.4
K12.2
K22.10
K25.3
K26.3
K27.3
K28.3
K31.0
K31.1
K31.5
K31.6
K35.20
K35.30
K35.31
K35.80
K35.890
K35.891
K40.00
K40.01
K40.30
K40.31
K41.00
K41.01
K41.30
K41.31
K42.0
K43.0
K43.3
K43.6
K44.0
K45.0
K46.0
K50.00
K50.011
K50.012
K50.013
K50.014
K50.018
K50.019
K50.10
K50.111
K50.112
K50.113
K50.114
K50.118
K50.119
K50.80
K50.811
K50.812
K50.813
K50.814
K50.818
K50.819
K50.90
K50.911
K50.912
K50.913
K50.914
K50.918
K50.919
K51.00
K51.011
K51.012
K51.013
K51.014
K51.018
K51.019
K51.20
K51.211
K51.212
K51.213
K51.214
K51.218
K51.219
K51.30
K51.311
K51.312
K51.313
K51.314
K51.318
K51.319
K51.40
K51.411
K51.412
K51.413
K51.414
K51.418
K51.419
K51.50
K51.511
K51.512
K51.513
K51.514
K51.518
K51.519
K51.80
K51.811
K51.812
K51.813
K51.814
K51.818
K51.819
K51.90
K51.911
K51.912
K51.913
K51.914
K51.918
K51.919
K52.0
K52.1
K55.1
K55.8
K55.9
K56.0
K56.1
K56.3
K56.49
K56.50
K56.51
K56.52
K56.600
K56.601
K56.609
K56.690
K56.691
K56.699
K56.7
K57.00
K57.12
K57.20
K57.32
K57.40
K57.52
K57.80
K57.92
K59.2
K59.31
K59.39
K61.0
K61.1
K61.2
K61.4
K62.5
K62.6
K63.0
K63.2
K63.3
K65.4
K68.11
K76.6
K77
K80.00
K80.01
K80.10
K80.11
K80.12
K80.13
K80.18
K80.19
K80.21
K80.30
K80.31
K80.32
K80.33
K80.34
K80.35
K80.36
K80.37
K80.40
K80.41
K80.42
K80.43
K80.44
K80.45
K80.46
K80.47
K80.51
K80.60
K80.61
K80.62
K80.63
K80.64
K80.65
K80.66
K80.71
K80.81
K81.0
K81.2
K82.0
K82.1
K82.3
K82.A2
K83.01
K83.09
K83.3
K86.0
K86.1
K86.2
K86.3
K90.1
K90.2
K90.3
K90.41
K90.49
K90.81
K90.89
K90.9
K91.2
K91.30
K91.31
K91.32
K91.61
K91.62
K91.71
K91.72
K91.81
K91.82
K91.83
K91.840
K91.841
K91.850
K91.858
K91.86
K91.870
K91.871
K91.872
K91.873
K91.89
K92.0
K92.1
K92.2
K92.81
K94.01
K94.02
K94.03
K94.09
K94.11
K94.12
K94.13
K94.19
K94.22
K94.23
K94.30
K94.31
K94.32
K94.33
K94.39
K95.01
K95.09
K95.81
K95.89
L02.01
L02.11
L02.211
L02.212
L02.213
L02.214
L02.215
L02.216
L02.219
L02.31
L02.411
L02.412
L02.413
L02.414
L02.415
L02.416
L02.419
L02.511

L02.512
L02.519
L02.611
L02.612
L02.619
L02.811
L02.818
L02.91
L03.111
L03.112
L03.113
L03.114
L03.115
L03.116
L03.119
L03.121
L03.122
L03.123
L03.124
L03.125
L03.126
L03.129
L03.211
L03.212
L03.213
L03.221
L03.222
L03.311
L03.312
L03.313
L03.314
L03.315
L03.316
L03.317
L03.319
L03.321
L03.322
L03.323
L03.324
L03.325
L03.326
L03.327
L03.329
L03.811
L03.818
L03.891
L03.898
L03.90
L03.91
L05.01
L05.02
L08.1
L10.0
L10.1
L10.2
L10.3
L10.4
L10.5
L10.81
L10.89
L10.9
L12.0
L12.30
L12.31
L12.35
L12.8
L12.9
L49.3
L49.4
L49.5
L49.6
L49.7
L49.8
L49.9
L51.1
L51.2
L51.3
L53.0
L53.1
L53.2
L53.3
L76.01
L76.02
L76.11
L76.12
L76.21
L76.22
L76.31
L76.32
L76.33
L76.34
L88
L97.101
L97.102
L97.103
L97.104
L97.105
L97.106
L97.108
L97.109
L97.111
L97.112
L97.113
L97.114
L97.115
L97.116
L97.118
L97.119
L97.121
L97.122
L97.123
L97.124
L97.125
L97.126
L97.128
L97.129
L97.201
L97.202
L97.203
L97.204
L97.205
L97.206
L97.208
L97.209
L97.211
L97.212
L97.213
L97.214
L97.215
L97.216
L97.218
L97.219
L97.221
L97.222
L97.223
L97.224
L97.225
L97.226
L97.228
L97.229
L97.301
L97.302
L97.303
L97.304
L97.305
L97.306
L97.308
L97.309
L97.311
L97.312
L97.313
L97.314
L97.315
L97.316
L97.318
L97.319
L97.321
L97.322
L97.323
L97.324
L97.325
L97.326
L97.328
L97.329
L97.401
L97.402
L97.403
L97.404
L97.405
L97.406
L97.408
L97.409
L97.411
L97.412
L97.413
L97.414
L97.415
L97.416
L97.418
L97.419
L97.421
L97.422
L97.423
L97.424
L97.425
L97.426
L97.428
L97.429
L97.505
L97.506
L97.508
L97.515
L97.516
L97.518
L97.525
L97.526
L97.528
L97.801
L97.802
L97.803
L97.804
L97.805
L97.806
L97.808
L97.809
L97.811
L97.812
L97.813
L97.814
L97.815
L97.816
L97.818
L97.819
L97.821
L97.822
L97.823
L97.824
L97.825
L97.826
L97.828
L97.829
L97.901
L97.902
L97.903
L97.904
L97.905
L97.906
L97.908
L97.909
L97.911
L97.912
L97.913
L97.914
L97.915
L97.916
L97.918
L97.919
L97.921
L97.922
L97.923
L97.924
L97.925
L97.926
L97.928
L97.929
L98.3
L98.415
L98.416
L98.418
L98.425
L98.426
L98.428
L98.495
L98.496
L98.498
M00.00
M00.011
M00.012
M00.019
M00.021
M00.022
M00.029
M00.031
M00.032
M00.039
M00.041
M00.042
M00.049
M00.051
M00.052
M00.059
M00.061
M00.062
M00.069
M00.071
M00.072
M00.079
M00.08
M00.09
M00.10
M00.111
M00.112
M00.119
M00.121
M00.122
M00.129
M00.131
M00.132
M00.139
M00.141
M00.142
M00.149
M00.151
M00.152
M00.159
M00.161
M00.162
M00.169
M00.171
M00.172
M00.179
M00.18
M00.19
M00.20
M00.211
M00.212
M00.219
M00.221
M00.222
M00.229
M00.231
M00.232
M00.239
M00.241
M00.242
M00.249
M00.251
M00.252
M00.259
M00.261
M00.262
M00.269
M00.271
M00.272
M00.279
M00.28
M00.29
M00.80
M00.811
M00.812
M00.819
M00.821
M00.822
M00.829
M00.831
M00.832
M00.839
M00.841
M00.842
M00.849
M00.851
M00.852
M00.859
M00.861
M00.862
M00.869
M00.871
M00.872
M00.879
M00.88
M00.89
M00.9
M01.X0
M01.X11
M01.X12
M01.X19
M01.X21
M01.X22
M01.X29
M01.X31
M01.X32
M01.X39
M01.X41
M01.X42
M01.X49
M01.X51
M01.X52
M01.X59
M01.X61
M01.X62
M01.X69
M01.X71
M01.X72
M01.X79
M01.X8
M01.X9
M02.10
M02.111
M02.112
M02.119
M02.121
M02.122
M02.129
M02.131
M02.132
M02.139
M02.141
M02.142
M02.149
M02.151
M02.152
M02.159
M02.161
M02.162
M02.169
M02.171
M02.172
M02.179
M02.18
M02.19
M02.30
M02.311
M02.312
M02.319
M02.321
M02.322
M02.329
M02.331
M02.332
M02.339
M02.341
M02.342
M02.349
M02.351
M02.352
M02.359
M02.361
M02.362
M02.369
M02.371
M02.372
M02.379
M02.38
M02.39
M02.80
M02.811
M02.812
M02.819
M02.821
M02.822
M02.829
M02.831
M02.832
M02.839
M02.841
M02.842
M02.849
M02.851
M02.852
M02.859
M02.861
M02.862
M02.869
M02.871
M02.872
M02.879
M02.88
M02.89
M05.40
M05.411
M05.412
M05.419
M05.421
M05.422
M05.429
M05.431
M05.432
M05.439
M05.441
M05.442
M05.449
M05.451
M05.452
M05.459
M05.461
M05.462
M05.469
M05.471
M05.472
M05.479
M05.49
M25.00
M25.011
M25.012
M25.019
M25.021
M25.022
M25.029
M25.031
M25.032
M25.039
M25.041
M25.042
M25.049
M25.051
M25.052
M25.059
M25.061
M25.062
M25.069
M25.071
M25.072
M25.073
M25.074
M25.075
M25.076
M25.08
M30.0
M30.1
M30.2
M30.3
M30.8
M31.0
M31.2
M31.30
M31.31
M31.4
M31.7
M31.8
M31.9
M32.11
M32.12
M33.00
M33.01
M33.02
M33.03
M33.09
M33.10
M33.11
M33.12
M33.13
M33.19
M33.20
M33.21
M33.22
M33.29
M33.90
M33.91
M33.92
M33.93
M33.99
M34.81
M34.82
M35.03
M35.1
M35.2
M35.5
M35.8
M36.0
M46.20
M46.21
M46.22
M46.23
M46.24
M46.25
M46.26
M46.27
M46.28
M46.30
M46.31
M46.32
M46.33
M46.34
M46.35
M46.36
M46.37
M46.38
M46.39
M47.011
M47.012
M47.013
M47.014
M47.015
M47.016
M47.019
M47.021
M47.022
M47.029
M47.10
M47.11
M47.12
M47.13
M47.14
M47.15
M47.16
M48.30
M48.31
M48.32
M48.33
M48.34
M48.35
M48.36
M48.37
M48.38
M48.50XA
M48.51XA
M48.52XA
M48.53XA
M48.54XA
M48.55XA
M48.56XA
M48.57XA
M48.58XA
M50.00
M50.01
M50.020
M50.021
M50.022
M50.023
M50.03
M51.04
M51.05
M51.06
M60.000
M60.001
M60.002
M60.003
M60.004
M60.005
M60.009
M60.011
M60.012
M60.019
M60.021
M60.022
M60.029
M60.031
M60.032
M60.039
M60.041
M60.042
M60.043
M60.044
M60.045
M60.046
M60.051
M60.052
M60.059
M60.061
M60.062
M60.069
M60.070
M60.071
M60.072
M60.073
M60.074
M60.075
M60.076
M60.077
M60.078
M60.08
M60.09
M62.82
M79.A11
M79.A12
M79.A19
M79.A21
M79.A22
M79.A29
M79.A3
M79.A9
M80.00XA
M80.00XK
M80.00XP
M80.011A
M80.011K
M80.011P
M80.012A
M80.012K
M80.012P
M80.019A
M80.019K
M80.019P
M80.021A
M80.021K
M80.021P
M80.022A
M80.022K
M80.022P
M80.029A
M80.029K
M80.029P
M80.031A
M80.031K
M80.031P
M80.032A
M80.032K
M80.032P
M80.039A
M80.039K
M80.039P
M80.041A
M80.041K
M80.041P
M80.042A
M80.042K
M80.042P
M80.049A
M80.049K
M80.049P
M80.051A
M80.051K
M80.051P

M8Ø.Ø52A
M8Ø.Ø52K
M8Ø.Ø52P
M8Ø.Ø59A
M8Ø.Ø59K
M8Ø.Ø59P
M8Ø.Ø61A
M8Ø.Ø61K
M8Ø.Ø61P
M8Ø.Ø62A
M8Ø.Ø62K
M8Ø.Ø62P
M8Ø.Ø69A
M8Ø.Ø69K
M8Ø.Ø69P
M8Ø.Ø71A
M8Ø.Ø71K
M8Ø.Ø71P
M8Ø.Ø72A
M8Ø.Ø72K
M8Ø.Ø72P
M8Ø.Ø79A
M8Ø.Ø79K
M8Ø.Ø79P
M8Ø.Ø8XA
M8Ø.Ø8XK
M8Ø.Ø8XP
M8Ø.ØAXA
M8Ø.ØAXK
M8Ø.ØAXP
M8Ø.8ØXA
M8Ø.8ØXK
M8Ø.8ØXP
M8Ø.811A
M8Ø.811K
M8Ø.811P
M8Ø.812A
M8Ø.812K
M8Ø.812P
M8Ø.819A
M8Ø.819K
M8Ø.819P
M8Ø.821A
M8Ø.821K
M8Ø.821P
M8Ø.822A
M8Ø.822K
M8Ø.822P
M8Ø.829A
M8Ø.829K
M8Ø.829P
M8Ø.831A
M8Ø.831K
M8Ø.831P
M8Ø.832A
M8Ø.832K
M8Ø.832P
M8Ø.839A
M8Ø.839K
M8Ø.839P
M8Ø.841A
M8Ø.841K
M8Ø.841P
M8Ø.842A
M8Ø.842K
M8Ø.842P
M8Ø.849A
M8Ø.849K
M8Ø.849P
M8Ø.851A
M8Ø.851K
M8Ø.851P
M8Ø.852A
M8Ø.852K
M8Ø.852P
M8Ø.859A
M8Ø.859K
M8Ø.859P
M8Ø.861A
M8Ø.861K
M8Ø.861P
M8Ø.862A
M8Ø.862K
M8Ø.862P
M8Ø.869A
M8Ø.869K
M8Ø.869P
M8Ø.871A
M8Ø.871K
M8Ø.871P
M8Ø.872A
M8Ø.872K
M8Ø.872P
M8Ø.879A
M8Ø.879K
M8Ø.879P
M8Ø.88XA
M8Ø.88XK
M8Ø.88XP
M8Ø.8AXA
M8Ø.8AXK
M8Ø.8AXP
M84.3ØXK
M84.3ØXP
M84.311K
M84.311P
M84.312K
M84.312P
M84.319K
M84.319P
M84.321K
M84.321P
M84.322K
M84.322P
M84.329K
M84.329P
M84.331K
M84.331P
M84.332K
M84.332P
M84.333K
M84.333P
M84.334K
M84.334P
M84.339K
M84.339P
M84.341K
M84.341P
M84.342K
M84.342P
M84.343K
M84.343P
M84.344K
M84.344P
M84.345K
M84.345P
M84.346K
M84.346P
M84.35ØK
M84.35ØP
M84.351K
M84.351P
M84.352K
M84.352P
M84.353K
M84.353P
M84.359K
M84.359P
M84.361K
M84.361P
M84.362K
M84.362P
M84.363K
M84.363P
M84.364K
M84.364P
M84.369K
M84.369P
M84.371K
M84.371P
M84.372K
M84.372P
M84.373K
M84.373P
M84.374K
M84.374P
M84.375K
M84.375P
M84.376K
M84.376P
M84.377K
M84.377P
M84.378K
M84.378P
M84.379K
M84.379P
M84.38XK
M84.38XP
M84.4ØXA
M84.4ØXK
M84.4ØXP
M84.411A
M84.411K
M84.411P
M84.412A
M84.412K
M84.412P
M84.419A
M84.419K
M84.419P
M84.421A
M84.421K
M84.421P
M84.422A
M84.422K
M84.422P
M84.429A
M84.429K
M84.429P
M84.431A
M84.431K
M84.431P
M84.432A
M84.432K
M84.432P
M84.433A
M84.433K
M84.433P
M84.434A
M84.434K
M84.434P
M84.439A
M84.439K
M84.439P
M84.441A
M84.441K
M84.441P
M84.442A
M84.442K
M84.442P
M84.443A
M84.443K
M84.443P
M84.444A
M84.444K
M84.444P
M84.445A
M84.445K
M84.445P
M84.446A
M84.446K
M84.446P
M84.451A
M84.451K
M84.451P
M84.452A
M84.452K
M84.452P
M84.453A
M84.453K
M84.453P
M84.454A
M84.454K
M84.454P
M84.459A
M84.459K
M84.459P
M84.461A
M84.461K
M84.461P
M84.462A
M84.462K
M84.462P
M84.463A
M84.463K
M84.463P
M84.464A
M84.464K
M84.464P
M84.469A
M84.469K
M84.469P
M84.471A
M84.471K
M84.471P
M84.472A
M84.472K
M84.472P
M84.473A
M84.473K
M84.473P
M84.474A
M84.474K
M84.474P
M84.475A
M84.475K
M84.475P
M84.476A
M84.476K
M84.476P
M84.477A
M84.477K
M84.477P
M84.478A
M84.478K
M84.478P
M84.479A
M84.479K
M84.479P
M84.48XA
M84.48XK
M84.48XP
M84.5ØXA
M84.5ØXK
M84.5ØXP
M84.511A
M84.511K
M84.511P
M84.512A
M84.512K
M84.512P
M84.519A
M84.519K
M84.519P
M84.521A
M84.521K
M84.521P
M84.522A
M84.522K
M84.522P
M84.529A
M84.529K
M84.529P
M84.531A
M84.531K
M84.531P
M84.532A
M84.532K
M84.532P
M84.533A
M84.533K
M84.533P
M84.534A
M84.534K
M84.534P
M84.539A
M84.539K
M84.539P
M84.541A
M84.541K
M84.541P
M84.542A
M84.542K
M84.542P
M84.549A
M84.549K
M84.549P
M84.55ØA
M84.55ØK
M84.55ØP
M84.551A
M84.551K
M84.551P
M84.552A
M84.552K
M84.552P
M84.553A
M84.553K
M84.553P
M84.559A
M84.559K
M84.559P
M84.561A
M84.561K
M84.561P
M84.562A
M84.562K
M84.562P
M84.563A
M84.563K
M84.563P
M84.564A
M84.564K
M84.564P
M84.569A
M84.569K
M84.569P
M84.571A
M84.571K
M84.571P
M84.572A
M84.572K
M84.572P
M84.573A
M84.573K
M84.573P
M84.574A
M84.574K
M84.574P
M84.575A
M84.575K
M84.575P
M84.576A
M84.576K
M84.576P
M84.58XA
M84.58XK
M84.58XP
M84.6ØXA
M84.6ØXK
M84.6ØXP
M84.611A
M84.611K
M84.611P
M84.612A
M84.612K
M84.612P
M84.619A
M84.619K
M84.619P
M84.621A
M84.621K
M84.621P
M84.622A
M84.622K
M84.622P
M84.629A
M84.629K
M84.629P
M84.631A
M84.631K
M84.631P
M84.632A
M84.632K
M84.632P
M84.633A
M84.633K
M84.633P
M84.634A
M84.634K
M84.634P
M84.639A
M84.639K
M84.639P
M84.641A
M84.641K
M84.641P
M84.642A
M84.642K
M84.642P
M84.649A
M84.649K
M84.649P
M84.65ØA
M84.65ØK
M84.65ØP
M84.651A
M84.651K
M84.651P
M84.652A
M84.652K
M84.652P
M84.653A
M84.653K
M84.653P
M84.659A
M84.659K
M84.659P
M84.661A
M84.661K
M84.661P
M84.662A
M84.662K
M84.662P
M84.663A
M84.663K
M84.663P
M84.664A
M84.664K
M84.664P
M84.669A
M84.669K
M84.669P
M84.671A
M84.671K
M84.671P
M84.672A
M84.672K
M84.672P
M84.673A
M84.673K
M84.673P
M84.674A
M84.674K
M84.674P
M84.675A
M84.675K
M84.675P
M84.676A
M84.676K
M84.676P
M84.68XA
M84.68XK
M84.68XP
M84.75ØA
M84.75ØK
M84.75ØP
M84.751A
M84.751K
M84.751P
M84.752A
M84.752K
M84.752P
M84.753A
M84.753K
M84.753P
M84.754A
M84.754K
M84.754P
M84.755A
M84.755K
M84.755P
M84.756A
M84.756K
M84.756P
M84.757A
M84.757K
M84.757P
M84.758A
M84.758K
M84.758P
M84.759A
M84.759K
M84.759P
M86.ØØ
M86.Ø11
M86.Ø12
M86.Ø19
M86.Ø21
M86.Ø22
M86.Ø29
M86.Ø31
M86.Ø32
M86.Ø39
M86.Ø41
M86.Ø42
M86.Ø49
M86.Ø51
M86.Ø52
M86.Ø59
M86.Ø61
M86.Ø62
M86.Ø69
M86.Ø71
M86.Ø72
M86.Ø79
M86.Ø8
M86.Ø9
M86.1Ø
M86.111
M86.112
M86.119
M86.121
M86.122
M86.129
M86.131
M86.132
M86.139
M86.141
M86.142
M86.149
M86.151
M86.152
M86.159
M86.161
M86.162
M86.169
M86.171
M86.172
M86.179
M86.18
M86.19
M86.2Ø
M86.211
M86.212
M86.219
M86.221
M86.222
M86.229
M86.231
M86.232
M86.239
M86.241
M86.242
M86.249
M86.251
M86.252
M86.259
M86.261
M86.262
M86.269
M86.271
M86.272
M86.279
M86.28
M86.29
M86.3Ø
M86.311
M86.312
M86.319
M86.321
M86.322
M86.329
M86.331
M86.332
M86.339
M86.341
M86.342
M86.349
M86.351
M86.352
M86.359
M86.361
M86.362
M86.369
M86.371
M86.372
M86.379
M86.38
M86.39
M86.4Ø
M86.411
M86.412
M86.419
M86.421
M86.422
M86.429
M86.431
M86.432
M86.439
M86.441
M86.442
M86.449
M86.451
M86.452
M86.459
M86.461
M86.462
M86.469
M86.471
M86.472
M86.479
M86.48
M86.49
M86.5Ø
M86.511
M86.512
M86.519
M86.521
M86.522
M86.529
M86.531
M86.532
M86.539
M86.541
M86.542
M86.549
M86.551
M86.552
M86.559
M86.561
M86.562
M86.569
M86.571
M86.572
M86.579
M86.58
M86.59
M86.6Ø
M86.611
M86.612
M86.619
M86.621
M86.622
M86.629
M86.631
M86.632
M86.639
M86.641
M86.642
M86.649
M86.651
M86.652
M86.659
M86.661
M86.662
M86.669
M86.671
M86.672
M86.679
M86.68
M86.69
M86.8XØ
M86.8X1
M86.8X2
M86.8X3
M86.8X4
M86.8X5
M86.8X6
M86.8X7
M86.8X8
M86.8X9
M86.9

Appendix E: Complication and Comorbidity (CC) Code List

M87.ØØ	M87.173	M87.352	M9Ø.552	NØ4.4	N76.4	OØ4.84	O23.21	O3Ø.221
M87.Ø11	M87.174	M87.353	M9Ø.559	NØ4.5	N76.81	OØ4.85	O23.22	O3Ø.222
M87.Ø12	M87.175	M87.361	M9Ø.561	NØ4.6	N82.Ø	OØ4.86	O23.23	O3Ø.223
M87.Ø19	M87.176	M87.362	M9Ø.562	NØ4.7	N82.1	OØ4.87	O23.31	O3Ø.231
M87.Ø21	M87.177	M87.363	M9Ø.569	NØ4.8	N82.2	OØ4.88	O23.32	O3Ø.232
M87.Ø22	M87.178	M87.364	M9Ø.571	NØ4.9	N82.3	OØ4.89	O23.33	O3Ø.233
M87.Ø29	M87.179	M87.365	M9Ø.572	NØ4.A	N82.4	OØ7.Ø	O23.41	O3Ø.291
M87.Ø31	M87.18Ø	M87.366	M9Ø.579	NØ5.2	N82.5	OØ7.1	O23.42	O3Ø.292
M87.Ø32	M87.188	M87.371	M9Ø.58	NØ5.3	N82.8	OØ7.3Ø	O23.43	O3Ø.293
M87.Ø33	M87.19	M87.372	M9Ø.59	NØ5.4	N82.9	OØ7.33	O23.511	O3Ø.8Ø1
M87.Ø34	M87.2Ø	M87.373	M96.Ø	NØ5.5	N83.511	OØ7.34	O23.512	O3Ø.8Ø2
M87.Ø35	M87.211	M87.374	M96.621	NØ5.A	N83.512	OØ7.35	O23.513	O3Ø.8Ø3
M87.Ø36	M87.212	M87.375	M96.622	NØ6.2	N83.519	OØ7.36	O23.521	O3Ø.811
M87.Ø37	M87.219	M87.376	M96.629	NØ6.3	N83.521	OØ7.37	O23.522	O3Ø.812
M87.Ø38	M87.221	M87.377	M96.631	NØ6.4	N83.522	OØ7.38	O23.523	O3Ø.813
M87.Ø39	M87.222	M87.378	M96.632	NØ6.5	N83.529	OØ7.39	O23.591	O3Ø.821
M87.Ø41	M87.229	M87.379	M96.639	NØ6.A	N83.53	OØ8.Ø	O23.592	O3Ø.822
M87.Ø42	M87.231	M87.38	M96.65	NØ7.2	N98.Ø	OØ8.1	O23.593	O3Ø.823
M87.Ø43	M87.232	M87.39	M96.661	NØ7.3	N98.1	OØ8.5	O23.91	O3Ø.831
M87.Ø44	M87.233	M87.8Ø	M96.662	NØ7.4	N98.2	OØ8.6	O23.92	O3Ø.832
M87.Ø45	M87.234	M87.811	M96.669	NØ7.5	N98.3	OØ8.7	O23.93	O3Ø.833
M87.Ø46	M87.235	M87.812	M96.671	NØ7.A	N98.8	OØ8.81	O24.Ø11	O3Ø.891
M87.Ø5Ø	M87.236	M87.819	M96.672	N1Ø	N98.9	OØ8.82	O24.Ø12	O3Ø.892
M87.Ø51	M87.237	M87.821	M96.679	N11.1	N99.51Ø	OØ8.83	O24.Ø13	O3Ø.893
M87.Ø52	M87.238	M87.822	M96.69	N11.8	N99.511	OØ8.89	O24.Ø19	O31.8X1Ø
M87.Ø59	M87.239	M87.829	M96.81Ø	N11.9	N99.512	OØ8.9	O24.Ø3	O31.8X11
M87.Ø61	M87.241	M87.831	M96.811	N12	N99.518	O1Ø.Ø11	O24.111	O31.8X12
M87.Ø62	M87.242	M87.832	M96.82Ø	N13.Ø	N99.61	O1Ø.Ø12	O24.112	O31.8X13
M87.Ø63	M87.243	M87.833	M96.821	N13.1	N99.62	O1Ø.Ø13	O24.113	O31.8X14
M87.Ø64	M87.244	M87.834	M96.83Ø	N13.2	N99.71	O1Ø.Ø2	O24.119	O31.8X15
M87.Ø65	M87.245	M87.835	M96.831	N13.3Ø	N99.72	O1Ø.411	O24.13	O31.8X19
M87.Ø66	M87.246	M87.836	M96.84Ø	N13.39	N99.82Ø	O1Ø.412	O24.311	O31.8X2Ø
M87.Ø71	M87.25Ø	M87.837	M96.841	N13.4	N99.821	O1Ø.413	O24.312	O31.8X21
M87.Ø72	M87.251	M87.838	M96.842	N13.6	N99.84Ø	O1Ø.43	O24.313	O31.8X22
M87.Ø73	M87.252	M87.839	M96.843	N13.8	N99.841	O1Ø.911	O24.319	O31.8X23
M87.Ø74	M87.256	M87.841	M96.89	N17.8	N99.842	O1Ø.912	O24.33	O31.8X24
M87.Ø75	M87.261	M87.842	M97.Ø1XA	N17.9	N99.843	O1Ø.913	O24.811	O31.8X25
M87.Ø76	M87.262	M87.843	M97.Ø2XA	N18.4	OØØ.ØØ	O1Ø.92	O24.812	O31.8X29
M87.Ø77	M87.263	M87.844	M97.11XA	N18.5	OØØ.Ø1	O12.11	O24.813	O31.8X3Ø
M87.Ø78	M87.264	M87.845	M97.12XA	N2Ø.1	OØØ.1Ø1	O12.12	O24.819	O31.8X31
M87.Ø79	M87.265	M87.849	M97.21XA	N2Ø.2	OØØ.1Ø2	O12.13	O24.83	O31.8X32
M87.Ø8	M87.266	M87.85Ø	M97.22XA	N25.1	OØØ.1Ø9	O12.21	O24.911	O31.8X33
M87.Ø9	M87.271	M87.851	M97.31XA	N25.81	OØØ.111	O12.22	O24.912	O31.8X34
M87.1Ø	M87.272	M87.852	M97.32XA	N28.Ø	OØØ.112	O12.23	O24.913	O31.8X35
M87.111	M87.273	M87.859	M97.41XA	N28.84	OØØ.119	O14.Ø2	O24.919	O31.8X39
M87.112	M87.274	M87.861	M97.42XA	N28.85	OØØ.2Ø1	O14.Ø3	O24.93	O33.Ø
M87.119	M87.275	M87.862	M97.8XXA	N28.86	OØØ.2Ø2	O14.92	O26.611	O36.Ø11Ø
M87.121	M87.276	M87.863	M97.9XXA	N3Ø.ØØ	OØØ.2Ø9	O14.93	O26.612	O36.Ø111
M87.122	M87.277	M87.864	M99.1Ø	N3Ø.Ø1	OØØ.211	O16.1	O26.613	O36.Ø112
M87.129	M87.278	M87.865	M99.11	N3Ø.4Ø	OØØ.212	O16.2	O26.62	O36.Ø113
M87.131	M87.279	M87.869	M99.18	N3Ø.41	OØØ.219	O16.3	O26.831	O36.Ø114
M87.132	M87.28	M87.871	NØ2.Ø	N32.1	OØØ.8Ø	O2Ø.Ø	O26.832	O36.Ø115
M87.133	M87.29	M87.872	NØ2.1	N32.2	OØØ.81	O2Ø.9	O26.833	O36.Ø119
M87.134	M87.3Ø	M87.873	NØ2.2	N34.Ø	OØØ.9Ø	O22.2Ø	O26.872	O36.Ø12Ø
M87.135	M87.311	M87.874	NØ2.3	N36.Ø	OØØ.91	O22.21	O26.873	O36.Ø121
M87.136	M87.312	M87.875	NØ2.4	N39.Ø	OØ3.Ø	O22.22	O26.879	O36.Ø122
M87.137	M87.319	M87.876	NØ2.5	N41.Ø	OØ3.3Ø	O22.23	O3Ø.1Ø1	O36.Ø123
M87.138	M87.321	M87.877	NØ2.6	N41.2	OØ3.33	O22.3Ø	O3Ø.1Ø2	O36.Ø124
M87.139	M87.322	M87.878	NØ2.7	N43.1	OØ3.34	O22.4Ø	O3Ø.1Ø3	O36.Ø125
M87.141	M87.329	M87.879	NØ2.8	N44.ØØ	OØ3.35	O22.41	O3Ø.111	O36.Ø129
M87.142	M87.331	M87.88	NØ2.9	N44.Ø1	OØ3.36	O22.42	O3Ø.112	O36.Ø13Ø
M87.143	M87.332	M87.89	NØ2.A	N44.Ø2	OØ3.37	O22.43	O3Ø.113	O36.Ø131
M87.144	M87.333	M87.9	NØ3.Ø	N44.Ø3	OØ3.38	O22.5Ø	O3Ø.121	O36.Ø132
M87.145	M87.334	M9Ø.5Ø	NØ3.1	N44.Ø4	OØ3.39	O22.51	O3Ø.122	O36.Ø133
M87.146	M87.335	M9Ø.511	NØ3.2	N45.4	OØ3.5	O22.52	O3Ø.123	O36.Ø134
M87.15Ø	M87.336	M9Ø.512	NØ3.3	N48.3Ø	OØ3.7	O22.53	O3Ø.131	O36.Ø135
M87.151	M87.337	M9Ø.519	NØ3.4	N48.31	OØ3.8Ø	O22.8X1	O3Ø.132	O36.Ø139
M87.152	M87.338	M9Ø.521	NØ3.5	N48.32	OØ3.83	O22.8X2	O3Ø.133	O36.Ø91Ø
M87.159	M87.339	M9Ø.522	NØ3.6	N48.33	OØ3.84	O22.8X3	O3Ø.191	O36.Ø911
M87.161	M87.341	M9Ø.529	NØ3.7	N48.39	OØ3.85	O22.8X9	O3Ø.192	O36.Ø912
M87.162	M87.342	M9Ø.531	NØ3.8	N7Ø.Ø1	OØ3.86	O22.9Ø	O3Ø.193	O36.Ø913
M87.163	M87.343	M9Ø.532	NØ3.9	N7Ø.Ø2	OØ3.87	O23.Ø1	O3Ø.2Ø1	O36.Ø914
M87.164	M87.344	M9Ø.539	NØ3.A	N7Ø.Ø3	OØ3.88	O23.Ø2	O3Ø.2Ø2	O36.Ø915
M87.165	M87.345	M9Ø.541	NØ4.Ø	N71.Ø	OØ3.89	O23.Ø3	O3Ø.2Ø3	O36.Ø919
M87.166	M87.346	M9Ø.542	NØ4.1	N73.Ø	OØ4.5	O23.11	O3Ø.211	O36.Ø92Ø
M87.171	M87.35Ø	M9Ø.549	NØ4.2	N73.4	OØ4.8Ø	O23.12	O3Ø.212	O36.Ø921
M87.172	M87.351	M9Ø.551	NØ4.3	N75.1	OØ4.83	O23.13	O3Ø.213	O36.Ø922

O36.0923
O36.0924
O36.0925
O36.0929
O36.0930
O36.0931
O36.0932
O36.0933
O36.0934
O36.0935
O36.0939
O36.4XX0
O36.4XX1
O36.4XX2
O36.4XX3
O36.4XX4
O36.4XX5
O36.4XX9
O41.01X0
O41.01X1
O41.01X2
O41.01X3
O41.01X4
O41.01X5
O41.01X9
O41.02X0
O41.02X1
O41.02X2
O41.02X3
O41.02X4
O41.02X5
O41.02X9
O41.03X0
O41.03X1
O41.03X2
O41.03X3
O41.03X4
O41.03X5
O41.03X9
O44.01
O44.02
O44.03
O44.21
O44.22
O44.23
O44.41
O44.42
O44.43
O47.02
O47.03
O47.1
O60.10X0
O60.10X1
O60.10X2
O60.10X3
O60.10X4
O60.10X5
O60.10X9
O60.20X0
O60.20X1
O60.20X2
O60.20X3
O60.20X4
O60.20X5
O60.20X9
O63.9
O68
O70.20
O70.21
O70.22
O70.23
O70.3
O70.4
O71.2
O71.3
O71.4
O71.5
O71.6
O71.7
O72.0
O72.1
O72.2
O75.2
O86.11
O86.12
O86.13
O86.19
O86.20
O86.21
O86.22
O86.29
O86.4
O87.0
O87.2
O87.3
O87.8
O88.319
O98.011
O98.012
O98.013
O98.02
O98.03
O98.111
O98.112
O98.113
O98.12
O98.13
O98.211
O98.212
O98.213
O98.22
O98.23
O98.311
O98.312
O98.313
O98.32
O98.33
O98.411
O98.412
O98.413
O98.42
O98.43
O98.511
O98.512
O98.513
O98.52
O98.53
O98.611
O98.612
O98.613
O98.62
O98.63
O98.711
O98.712
O98.713
O98.72
O98.73
O98.811
O98.812
O98.813
O98.82
O98.83
O98.911
O98.912
O98.913
O98.92
O98.93
O99.111
O99.112
O99.113
O99.119
O99.12
O99.13
O99.321
O99.322
O99.323
O99.324
O99.325
O99.354
O99.355
O99.411
O99.412
O99.413
O99.43
O99.830
O99.834
O99.835
P10.2
P12.2
P28.0
P28.10
P28.11
P28.19
P28.2
P28.3
P28.4
P35.0
P38.1
P38.9
P39.0
P39.2
P39.3
P39.4
P39.8
P39.9
P52.0
P52.1
P52.3
P53
P54.4
P61.2
P61.3
P61.4
P61.6
P70.2
P70.8
P71.0
P71.1
P71.2
P71.3
P71.4
P71.8
P71.9
P72.0
P72.1
P72.2
P72.8
P74.41
P74.5
P74.6
P74.8
P76.1
P83.0
P83.30
P83.39
P91.60
P91.61
P91.62
P93.0
P93.8
P94.0
P96.1
P96.2
Q01.0
Q01.1
Q01.2
Q01.8
Q01.9
Q04.4
Q04.5
Q04.6
Q04.8
Q05.0
Q05.1
Q05.2
Q05.3
Q05.4
Q07.02
Q07.03
Q20.5
Q21.0
Q21.1
Q21.2
Q22.1
Q22.2
Q22.3
Q23.0
Q23.1
Q23.2
Q23.3
Q24.0
Q24.1
Q24.3
Q24.5
Q25.0
Q25.1
Q25.21
Q25.29
Q25.3
Q25.40
Q25.41
Q25.42
Q25.43
Q25.44
Q25.45
Q25.46
Q25.47
Q25.48
Q25.49
Q25.8
Q25.9
Q26.0
Q26.1
Q26.2
Q26.3
Q26.4
Q26.8
Q26.9
Q27.30
Q27.4
Q28.0
Q28.1
Q28.8
Q28.9
Q31.1
Q31.2
Q31.3
Q31.5
Q31.8
Q31.9
Q32.0
Q32.1
Q32.2
Q32.3
Q32.4
Q33.0
Q33.4
Q39.5
Q39.6
Q39.8
Q39.9
Q41.0
Q41.1
Q41.2
Q41.8
Q41.9
Q42.0
Q42.1
Q42.2
Q42.3
Q42.8
Q42.9
Q43.1
Q43.2
Q43.3
Q43.4
Q43.5
Q43.6
Q43.7
Q43.8
Q43.9
Q44.0
Q44.1
Q44.4
Q44.5
Q44.6
Q44.7
Q45.0
Q45.1
Q45.2
Q45.3
Q60.0
Q60.1
Q60.2
Q60.3
Q60.4
Q60.5
Q60.6
Q61.00
Q61.01
Q61.02
Q61.11
Q61.19
Q61.2
Q61.3
Q61.4
Q61.5
Q61.8
Q61.9
Q62.0
Q62.10
Q62.11
Q62.12
Q62.2
Q62.31
Q62.32
Q62.39
Q64.10
Q64.11
Q64.12
Q64.19
Q64.2
Q64.31
Q64.32
Q64.33
Q64.39
Q67.5
Q67.8
Q68.1
Q74.3
Q76.3
Q76.425
Q76.426
Q76.427
Q76.428
Q76.429
Q76.6
Q76.7
Q76.8
Q76.9
Q77.2
Q78.0
Q78.2
Q79.60
Q79.61
Q79.62
Q79.63
Q79.69
Q85.1
Q85.8
Q85.9
Q87.11
Q87.19
Q87.2
Q87.3
Q87.40
Q87.410
Q87.418
Q87.42
Q87.43
Q87.5
Q87.81
Q87.82
Q87.89
Q89.01
Q89.09
Q89.3
Q89.7
Q89.8
Q91.0
Q91.1
Q91.2
Q91.3
Q91.4
Q91.5
Q91.6
Q91.7
Q93.3
Q93.4
Q93.51
Q93.59
Q93.7
Q93.82
Q93.88
Q93.89
Q93.9
R04.2
R04.81
R04.89
R04.9
R06.3
R09.01
R17
R18.0
R18.8
R29.0
R29.1
R29.5
R39.0
R40.3
R41.4
R44.0
R44.2
R44.3
R45.851
R47.01
R56.00
R56.01
R56.1
R57.9
R64
R65.10
R71.0
R78.81
R82.0
R82.1
S01.101A
S01.102A
S01.109A
S02.0XXA
S02.0XXK
S02.101A
S02.101K
S02.102A
S02.102K
S02.109A
S02.109K
S02.110A
S02.110K
S02.111A
S02.111K
S02.112A
S02.112K
S02.113A
S02.113K
S02.118A
S02.118K
S02.119A
S02.119K
S02.11AA
S02.11AK
S02.11BA
S02.11BK
S02.11CA
S02.11CK
S02.11DA
S02.11DK
S02.11EA
S02.11EK
S02.11FA
S02.11FK
S02.11GA
S02.11GK
S02.11HA
S02.11HK
S02.121A
S02.121K
S02.122A
S02.122K
S02.129A
S02.129K
S02.19XA
S02.19XK
S02.2XXB
S02.2XXK
S02.30XA
S02.30XB
S02.30XK
S02.31XA
S02.31XB
S02.31XK
S02.32XA
S02.32XB
S02.32XK
S02.400A
S02.400B
S02.400K
S02.401A
S02.401B
S02.401K
S02.402A
S02.402B
S02.402K
S02.40AA
S02.40AB
S02.40AK
S02.40BA
S02.40BB
S02.40BK
S02.40CA
S02.40CB
S02.40CK
S02.40DA
S02.40DB
S02.40DK
S02.40EA
S02.40EB
S02.40EK
S02.40FA
S02.40FB
S02.40FK
S02.411A
S02.411B
S02.411K
S02.412A
S02.412B
S02.412K
S02.413A
S02.413B
S02.413K
S02.42XA
S02.42XB
S02.42XK
S02.5XXK
S02.600A
S02.600B
S02.600K
S02.601A
S02.601B
S02.601K
S02.602A
S02.602B
S02.602K
S02.609A
S02.609B
S02.609K
S02.610A
S02.610B
S02.610K
S02.611A
S02.611B
S02.611K
S02.612A
S02.612B
S02.612K
S02.620A
S02.620B
S02.620K
S02.621A
S02.621B
S02.621K
S02.622A
S02.622B
S02.622K
S02.630A
S02.630B
S02.630K
S02.631A
S02.631B
S02.631K
S02.632A
S02.632B
S02.632K
S02.640A
S02.640B
S02.640K
S02.641A
S02.641B
S02.641K
S02.642A
S02.642B
S02.642K
S02.650A
S02.650B
S02.650K
S02.651A
S02.651B
S02.651K
S02.652A
S02.652B
S02.652K
S02.66XA
S02.66XB
S02.66XK
S02.670A
S02.670B
S02.670K
S02.671A
S02.671B
S02.671K
S02.672A
S02.672B
S02.672K
S02.69XA
S02.69XB
S02.69XK
S02.80XA
S02.80XB
S02.80XK
S02.81XA
S02.81XB
S02.81XK
S02.82XA
S02.82XB
S02.82XK
S02.831A
S02.831B
S02.831K
S02.832A
S02.832B
S02.832K
S02.839A
S02.839B
S02.839K
S02.841A
S02.841B
S02.841K
S02.842A
S02.842B
S02.842K
S02.849A
S02.849B
S02.849K
S02.85XA
S02.85XB
S02.85XK
S02.91XA
S02.91XK
S02.92XA
S02.92XB
S02.92XK
S04.011A
S04.012A
S04.019A
S04.02XA
S04.031A
S04.032A
S04.039A
S04.041A
S04.042A
S04.049A
S04.10XA
S04.11XA
S04.12XA
S04.20XA
S04.21XA
S04.22XA
S04.30XA
S04.31XA
S04.32XA
S04.40XA
S04.41XA
S04.42XA
S04.50XA
S04.51XA
S04.52XA
S04.60XA
S04.61XA
S04.62XA
S04.70XA
S04.71XA
S04.72XA
S04.811A

SØ4.812A
SØ4.819A
SØ4.891A
SØ4.892A
SØ4.899A
SØ4.9XXA
SØ5.2ØXA
SØ5.21XA
SØ5.22XA
SØ5.3ØXA
SØ5.31XA
SØ5.32XA
SØ5.4ØXA
SØ5.41XA
SØ5.42XA
SØ5.5ØXA
SØ5.51XA
SØ5.52XA
SØ5.7ØXA
SØ5.71XA
SØ5.72XA
SØ5.8X1A
SØ5.8X2A
SØ5.8X9A
SØ5.91XA
SØ5.92XA
SØ6.ØX1A
SØ6.ØX9A
SØ6.2X1A
SØ6.2X2A
SØ6.2X3A
SØ6.2X4A
SØ6.2X5A
SØ6.2X9A
SØ6.3Ø1A
SØ6.3Ø2A
SØ6.3Ø3A
SØ6.3Ø4A
SØ6.3Ø5A
SØ6.3Ø9A
SØ6.371A
SØ6.372A
SØ6.373A
SØ6.374A
SØ6.375A
SØ6.379A
SØ6.381A
SØ6.382A
SØ6.383A
SØ6.384A
SØ6.385A
SØ6.389A
SØ6.811A
SØ6.812A
SØ6.813A
SØ6.814A
SØ6.815A
SØ6.819A
SØ6.821A
SØ6.822A
SØ6.823A
SØ6.824A
SØ6.825A
SØ6.829A
SØ6.891A
SØ6.892A
SØ6.893A
SØ6.894A
SØ6.895A
SØ6.899A
SØ6.9X1A
SØ6.9X2A
SØ6.9X3A
SØ6.9X4A
SØ6.9X5A
SØ6.9X9A
SØ7.ØXXA
SØ7.1XXA
SØ7.8XXA
SØ7.9XXA
SØ9.ØXXA
SØ9.2ØXA
SØ9.21XA
SØ9.22XA
SØ9.3Ø1A
SØ9.3Ø2A
SØ9.3Ø9A
SØ9.311A
SØ9.312A
SØ9.313A
SØ9.319A
SØ9.391A
SØ9.392A
SØ9.399A
S11.1ØXA
S11.11XA
S11.12XA
S11.13XA
S11.14XA
S11.15XA
S11.2ØXA
S11.21XA
S11.22XA
S11.23XA
S11.24XA
S11.25XA
S12.ØØØA
S12.ØØØK
S12.ØØ1A
S12.ØØ1K
S12.Ø1XA
S12.Ø1XK
S12.Ø2XA
S12.Ø2XK
S12.Ø3ØA
S12.Ø3ØK
S12.Ø31A
S12.Ø31K
S12.Ø4ØA
S12.Ø4ØK
S12.Ø41A
S12.Ø41K
S12.Ø9ØA
S12.Ø9ØK
S12.Ø91A
S12.Ø91K
S12.1ØØA
S12.1ØØK
S12.1Ø1A
S12.1Ø1K
S12.11ØA
S12.11ØK
S12.111A
S12.111K
S12.112A
S12.112K
S12.12ØA
S12.12ØK
S12.121A
S12.121K
S12.13ØA
S12.13ØK
S12.131A
S12.131K
S12.14XA
S12.14XK
S12.15ØA
S12.15ØK
S12.151A
S12.151K
S12.19ØA
S12.19ØK
S12.191A
S12.191K
S12.2ØØA
S12.2ØØK
S12.2Ø1A
S12.2Ø1K
S12.23ØA
S12.23ØK
S12.231A
S12.231K
S12.24XA
S12.24XK
S12.25ØA
S12.25ØK
S12.251A
S12.251K
S12.29ØA
S12.29ØK
S12.291A
S12.291K
S12.3ØØA
S12.3ØØK
S12.3Ø1A
S12.3Ø1K
S12.33ØA
S12.33ØK
S12.331A
S12.331K
S12.34XA
S12.34XK
S12.35ØA
S12.35ØK
S12.351A
S12.351K
S12.39ØA
S12.39ØK
S12.391A
S12.391K
S12.4ØØA
S12.4ØØK
S12.4Ø1A
S12.4Ø1K
S12.43ØA
S12.43ØK
S12.431A
S12.431K
S12.44XA
S12.44XK
S12.45ØA
S12.45ØK
S12.451A
S12.451K
S12.49ØA
S12.49ØK
S12.491A
S12.491K
S12.5ØØA
S12.5ØØK
S12.5Ø1A
S12.5Ø1K
S12.53ØA
S12.53ØK
S12.531A
S12.531K
S12.54XA
S12.54XK
S12.55ØA
S12.55ØK
S12.551A
S12.551K
S12.59ØA
S12.59ØK
S12.591A
S12.591K
S12.6ØØA
S12.6ØØK
S12.6Ø1A
S12.6Ø1K
S12.63ØA
S12.63ØK
S12.631A
S12.631K
S12.64XA
S12.64XK
S12.65ØA
S12.65ØK
S12.651A
S12.651K
S12.69ØA
S12.69ØK
S12.691A
S12.691K
S12.9XXA
S13.ØXXA
S13.1ØØA
S13.1Ø1A
S13.11ØA
S13.111A
S13.12ØA
S13.121A
S13.13ØA
S13.131A
S13.14ØA
S13.141A
S13.15ØA
S13.151A
S13.16ØA
S13.161A
S13.17ØA
S13.171A
S13.18ØA
S13.181A
S13.2ØXA
S13.29XA
S15.ØØ1A
S15.ØØ2A
S15.ØØ9A
S15.Ø11A
S15.Ø12A
S15.Ø19A
S15.Ø21A
S15.Ø22A
S15.Ø29A
S15.Ø91A
S15.Ø92A
S15.Ø99A
S15.1Ø1A
S15.1Ø2A
S15.1Ø9A
S15.111A
S15.112A
S15.119A
S15.121A
S15.122A
S15.129A
S15.191A
S15.192A
S15.199A
S15.2Ø1A
S15.2Ø2A
S15.2Ø9A
S15.211A
S15.212A
S15.219A
S15.221A
S15.222A
S15.229A
S15.291A
S15.292A
S15.299A
S15.3Ø1A
S15.3Ø2A
S15.3Ø9A
S15.311A
S15.312A
S15.319A
S15.321A
S15.322A
S15.329A
S15.391A
S15.392A
S15.399A
S15.8XXA
S15.9XXA
S17.ØXXA
S17.8XXA
S17.9XXA
S21.1Ø1A
S21.1Ø2A
S21.1Ø9A
S21.111A
S21.112A
S21.119A
S21.121A
S21.122A
S21.129A
S21.131A
S21.132A
S21.139A
S21.141A
S21.142A
S21.149A
S21.151A
S21.152A
S21.159A
S21.9ØXA
S21.91XA
S21.92XA
S21.93XA
S21.94XA
S21.95XA
S22.ØØØA
S22.ØØØK
S22.ØØ1A
S22.ØØ1K
S22.ØØ2A
S22.ØØ2K
S22.ØØ8A
S22.ØØ8K
S22.ØØ9A
S22.ØØ9K
S22.Ø1ØA
S22.Ø1ØK
S22.Ø11A
S22.Ø11K
S22.Ø12A
S22.Ø12K
S22.Ø18A
S22.Ø18K
S22.Ø19A
S22.Ø19K
S22.Ø2ØA
S22.Ø2ØK
S22.Ø21A
S22.Ø21K
S22.Ø22A
S22.Ø22K
S22.Ø28A
S22.Ø28K
S22.Ø29A
S22.Ø29K
S22.Ø3ØA
S22.Ø3ØK
S22.Ø31A
S22.Ø31K
S22.Ø32A
S22.Ø32K
S22.Ø38A
S22.Ø38K
S22.Ø39A
S22.Ø39K
S22.Ø4ØA
S22.Ø4ØK
S22.Ø41A
S22.Ø41K
S22.Ø42A
S22.Ø42K
S22.Ø48A
S22.Ø48K
S22.Ø49A
S22.Ø49K
S22.Ø5ØA
S22.Ø5ØK
S22.Ø51A
S22.Ø51K
S22.Ø52A
S22.Ø52K
S22.Ø58A
S22.Ø58K
S22.Ø59A
S22.Ø59K
S22.Ø6ØA
S22.Ø6ØK
S22.Ø61A
S22.Ø61K
S22.Ø62A
S22.Ø62K
S22.Ø68A
S22.Ø68K
S22.Ø69A
S22.Ø69K
S22.Ø7ØA
S22.Ø7ØK
S22.Ø71A
S22.Ø71K
S22.Ø72A
S22.Ø72K
S22.Ø78A
S22.Ø78K
S22.Ø79A
S22.Ø79K
S22.Ø8ØA
S22.Ø8ØK
S22.Ø81A
S22.Ø81K
S22.Ø82A
S22.Ø82K
S22.Ø88A
S22.Ø88K
S22.Ø89A
S22.Ø89K
S22.2ØXA
S22.2ØXK
S22.21XA
S22.21XK
S22.22XA
S22.22XK
S22.23XA
S22.23XK
S22.24XA
S22.24XK
S22.31XA
S22.31XK
S22.32XA
S22.32XK
S22.39XA
S22.39XK
S22.41XA
S22.41XK
S22.42XA
S22.42XK
S22.43XA
S22.43XK
S22.49XA
S22.49XK
S22.5XXA
S22.5XXK
S22.9XXA
S22.9XXK
S25.5Ø1A
S25.5Ø2A
S25.5Ø9A
S25.511A
S25.512A
S25.519A
S25.591A
S25.592A
S25.599A
S25.8Ø1A
S25.8Ø2A
S25.8Ø9A
S25.811A
S25.812A
S25.819A
S25.891A
S25.892A
S25.899A
S25.9ØXA
S25.91XA
S25.99XA
S26.ØØXA
S26.Ø1XA
S26.Ø9XA
S26.1ØXA
S26.11XA
S26.19XA
S26.9ØXA
S26.91XA
S26.99XA
S27.ØXXA
S27.3Ø1A
S27.3Ø2A
S27.3Ø9A
S27.311A
S27.312A
S27.319A
S27.321A
S27.322A
S27.329A
S27.391A
S27.392A
S27.399A
S27.5ØXA
S27.51XA
S27.52XA
S27.53XA
S27.59XA
S27.6ØXA
S27.63XA
S27.69XA
S27.8Ø2A
S27.8Ø3A
S27.8Ø8A
S27.8Ø9A
S27.892A
S27.893A
S27.898A
S27.899A
S27.9XXA
S28.1XXA
S29.Ø21A
S29.Ø29A
S32.ØØØA
S32.ØØØK
S32.ØØ1A
S32.ØØ1K
S32.ØØ2A
S32.ØØ2K
S32.ØØ8A
S32.ØØ8K
S32.ØØ9A
S32.ØØ9K
S32.Ø1ØA
S32.Ø1ØK
S32.Ø11A
S32.Ø11K
S32.Ø12A
S32.Ø12K
S32.Ø18A
S32.Ø18K
S32.Ø19A
S32.Ø19K
S32.Ø2ØA
S32.Ø2ØK
S32.Ø21A
S32.Ø21K
S32.Ø22A
S32.Ø22K
S32.Ø28A
S32.Ø28K
S32.Ø29A
S32.Ø29K
S32.Ø3ØA
S32.Ø3ØK
S32.Ø31A
S32.Ø31K
S32.Ø32A
S32.Ø32K
S32.Ø38A
S32.Ø38K
S32.Ø39A
S32.Ø39K
S32.Ø4ØA
S32.Ø4ØK
S32.Ø41A
S32.Ø41K
S32.Ø42A
S32.Ø42K
S32.Ø48A
S32.Ø48K
S32.Ø49A
S32.Ø49K
S32.Ø5ØA
S32.Ø5ØK
S32.Ø51A
S32.Ø51K
S32.Ø52A
S32.Ø52K
S32.Ø58A
S32.Ø58K
S32.Ø59A
S32.Ø59K
S32.1ØXA
S32.1ØXK
S32.11ØA
S32.11ØK
S32.111A
S32.111K
S32.112A
S32.112K
S32.119A
S32.119K
S32.12ØA
S32.12ØK
S32.121A
S32.121K
S32.122A
S32.122K
S32.129A
S32.129K
S32.13ØA
S32.13ØK
S32.131A
S32.131K
S32.132A
S32.132K
S32.139A
S32.139K
S32.14XA
S32.14XK
S32.15XA
S32.15XK
S32.16XA
S32.16XK
S32.17XA
S32.17XK
S32.19XA
S32.19XK
S32.2XXA
S32.2XXK
S32.3Ø1A
S32.3Ø1K
S32.3Ø2A
S32.3Ø2K
S32.3Ø9A
S32.3Ø9K
S32.311A
S32.311K
S32.312A
S32.312K
S32.313A
S32.313K
S32.314A
S32.314K
S32.315A
S32.315K
S32.316A
S32.316K
S32.391A
S32.391K
S32.392A
S32.392K
S32.399A
S32.399K
S32.4Ø1K
S32.4Ø2K
S32.4Ø9K
S32.411K
S32.412K
S32.413K
S32.414K
S32.415K
S32.416K
S32.421K
S32.422K
S32.423K
S32.424K
S32.425K
S32.426K
S32.431K
S32.432K
S32.433K
S32.434K
S32.435K
S32.436K
S32.441K
S32.442K
S32.443K
S32.444K
S32.445K
S32.446K
S32.451K
S32.452K
S32.453K
S32.454K
S32.455K
S32.456K
S32.461K
S32.462K
S32.463K
S32.464K
S32.465K
S32.466K
S32.471K
S32.472K
S32.473K
S32.474K
S32.475K
S32.476K
S32.481K
S32.482K
S32.483K

S32.484K
S32.485K
S32.486K
S32.491K
S32.492K
S32.499K
S32.501A
S32.501K
S32.502A
S32.502K
S32.509A
S32.509K
S32.511A
S32.511K
S32.512A
S32.512K
S32.519A
S32.519K
S32.591A
S32.591K
S32.592A
S32.592K
S32.599A
S32.599K
S32.601A
S32.601K
S32.602A
S32.602K
S32.609A
S32.609K
S32.611A
S32.611K
S32.612A
S32.612K
S32.613A
S32.613K
S32.614A
S32.614K
S32.615A
S32.615K
S32.616A
S32.616K
S32.691A
S32.691K
S32.692A
S32.692K
S32.699A
S32.699K
S32.810A
S32.810K
S32.811A
S32.811K
S32.82XA
S32.82XK
S32.89XA
S32.89XK
S32.9XXA
S32.9XXK
S35.531A
S35.532A
S35.533A
S35.534A
S35.535A
S35.536A
S35.8X1A
S35.8X8A
S35.8X9A
S35.90XA
S35.91XA
S35.99XA
S36.00XA
S36.020A
S36.021A
S36.029A
S36.030A
S36.039A
S36.09XA
S36.112A
S36.113A
S36.114A
S36.118A
S36.119A
S36.122A
S36.123A
S36.128A
S36.129A
S36.13XA
S36.200A
S36.201A
S36.202A
S36.209A
S36.220A
S36.221A
S36.222A
S36.229A
S36.230A
S36.231A
S36.232A
S36.239A
S36.240A
S36.241A
S36.242A
S36.249A
S36.250A
S36.251A
S36.252A
S36.259A
S36.260A
S36.261A
S36.262A
S36.269A
S36.290A
S36.291A
S36.292A
S36.299A
S36.30XA
S36.32XA
S36.33XA
S36.39XA
S36.400A
S36.408A
S36.409A
S36.410A
S36.418A
S36.419A
S36.420A
S36.428A
S36.429A
S36.430A
S36.438A
S36.439A
S36.490A
S36.498A
S36.499A
S36.500A
S36.501A
S36.502A
S36.503A
S36.508A
S36.509A
S36.510A
S36.511A
S36.512A
S36.513A
S36.518A
S36.519A
S36.520A
S36.521A
S36.522A
S36.523A
S36.528A
S36.529A
S36.530A
S36.531A
S36.532A
S36.533A
S36.538A
S36.539A
S36.590A
S36.591A
S36.592A
S36.593A
S36.598A
S36.599A
S36.60XA
S36.61XA
S36.62XA
S36.63XA
S36.69XA
S36.81XA
S36.892A
S36.893A
S36.898A
S36.899A
S36.90XA
S36.92XA
S36.93XA
S36.99XA
S37.001A
S37.002A
S37.009A
S37.011A
S37.012A
S37.019A
S37.021A
S37.022A
S37.029A
S37.031A
S37.032A
S37.039A
S37.041A
S37.042A
S37.049A
S37.051A
S37.052A
S37.059A
S37.10XA
S37.12XA
S37.13XA
S37.19XA
S37.20XA
S37.22XA
S37.23XA
S37.29XA
S37.30XA
S37.32XA
S37.33XA
S37.39XA
S37.60XA
S37.62XA
S37.63XA
S37.69XA
S37.812A
S37.813A
S37.818A
S37.819A
S37.892A
S37.893A
S37.898A
S37.899A
S37.90XA
S37.92XA
S37.93XA
S37.99XA
S42.001B
S42.001K
S42.001P
S42.002B
S42.002K
S42.002P
S42.009B
S42.009K
S42.009P
S42.011B
S42.011K
S42.011P
S42.012B
S42.012K
S42.012P
S42.013B
S42.013K
S42.013P
S42.014B
S42.014K
S42.014P
S42.015B
S42.015K
S42.015P
S42.016B
S42.016K
S42.016P
S42.017B
S42.017K
S42.017P
S42.018B
S42.018K
S42.018P
S42.019B
S42.019K
S42.019P
S42.021B
S42.021K
S42.021P
S42.022B
S42.022K
S42.022P
S42.023B
S42.023K
S42.023P
S42.024B
S42.024K
S42.024P
S42.025B
S42.025K
S42.025P
S42.026B
S42.026K
S42.026P
S42.031B
S42.031K
S42.031P
S42.032B
S42.032K
S42.032P
S42.033B
S42.033K
S42.033P
S42.034B
S42.034K
S42.034P
S42.035B
S42.035K
S42.035P
S42.036B
S42.036K
S42.036P
S42.101B
S42.101K
S42.101P
S42.102B
S42.102K
S42.102P
S42.109B
S42.109K
S42.109P
S42.111B
S42.111K
S42.111P
S42.112B
S42.112K
S42.112P
S42.113B
S42.113K
S42.113P
S42.114B
S42.114K
S42.114P
S42.115B
S42.115K
S42.115P
S42.116B
S42.116K
S42.116P
S42.121B
S42.121K
S42.121P
S42.122B
S42.122K
S42.122P
S42.123B
S42.123K
S42.123P
S42.124B
S42.124K
S42.124P
S42.125B
S42.125K
S42.125P
S42.126B
S42.126K
S42.126P
S42.131B
S42.131K
S42.131P
S42.132B
S42.132K
S42.132P
S42.133B
S42.133K
S42.133P
S42.134B
S42.134K
S42.134P
S42.135B
S42.135K
S42.135P
S42.136B
S42.136K
S42.136P
S42.141B
S42.141K
S42.141P
S42.142B
S42.142K
S42.142P
S42.143B
S42.143K
S42.143P
S42.144B
S42.144K
S42.144P
S42.145B
S42.145K
S42.145P
S42.146B
S42.146K
S42.146P
S42.151B
S42.151K
S42.151P
S42.152B
S42.152K
S42.152P
S42.153B
S42.153K
S42.153P
S42.154B
S42.154K
S42.154P
S42.155B
S42.155K
S42.155P
S42.156B
S42.156K
S42.156P
S42.191B
S42.191K
S42.191P
S42.192B
S42.192K
S42.192P
S42.199B
S42.199K
S42.199P
S42.201A
S42.201K
S42.201P
S42.202A
S42.202K
S42.202P
S42.209A
S42.209K
S42.209P
S42.211A
S42.211K
S42.211P
S42.212A
S42.212K
S42.212P
S42.213A
S42.213K
S42.213P
S42.214A
S42.214K
S42.214P
S42.215A
S42.215K
S42.215P
S42.216A
S42.216K
S42.216P
S42.221A
S42.221K
S42.221P
S42.222A
S42.222K
S42.222P
S42.223A
S42.223K
S42.223P
S42.224A
S42.224K
S42.224P
S42.225A
S42.225K
S42.225P
S42.226A
S42.226K
S42.226P
S42.231A
S42.231K
S42.231P
S42.232A
S42.232K
S42.232P
S42.239A
S42.239K
S42.239P
S42.241A
S42.241K
S42.241P
S42.242A
S42.242K
S42.242P
S42.249A
S42.249K
S42.249P
S42.251A
S42.251K
S42.251P
S42.252A
S42.252K
S42.252P
S42.253A
S42.253K
S42.253P
S42.254A
S42.254K
S42.254P
S42.255A
S42.255K
S42.255P
S42.256A
S42.256K
S42.256P
S42.261A
S42.261K
S42.261P
S42.262A
S42.262K
S42.262P
S42.263A
S42.263K
S42.263P
S42.264A
S42.264K
S42.264P
S42.265A
S42.265K
S42.265P
S42.266A
S42.266K
S42.266P
S42.271A
S42.271K
S42.271P
S42.272A
S42.272K
S42.272P
S42.279A
S42.279K
S42.279P
S42.291A
S42.291K
S42.291P
S42.292A
S42.292K
S42.292P
S42.293A
S42.293K
S42.293P
S42.294A
S42.294K
S42.294P
S42.295A
S42.295K
S42.295P
S42.296A
S42.296K
S42.296P
S42.301A
S42.301K
S42.301P
S42.302A
S42.302K
S42.302P
S42.309A
S42.309K
S42.309P
S42.311A
S42.311K
S42.311P
S42.312A
S42.312K
S42.312P
S42.319A
S42.319K
S42.319P
S42.321A
S42.321K
S42.321P
S42.322A
S42.322K
S42.322P
S42.323A
S42.323K
S42.323P
S42.324A
S42.324K
S42.324P
S42.325A
S42.325K
S42.325P
S42.326A
S42.326K
S42.326P
S42.331A
S42.331K
S42.331P
S42.332A
S42.332K
S42.332P
S42.333A
S42.333K
S42.333P
S42.334A
S42.334K
S42.334P
S42.335A
S42.335K
S42.335P
S42.336A
S42.336K
S42.336P
S42.341A
S42.341K
S42.341P
S42.342A
S42.342K
S42.342P
S42.343A
S42.343K
S42.343P
S42.344A
S42.344K
S42.344P
S42.345A
S42.345K
S42.345P
S42.346A
S42.346K
S42.346P
S42.351A
S42.351K
S42.351P
S42.352A
S42.352K
S42.352P
S42.353A
S42.353K
S42.353P
S42.354A
S42.354K
S42.354P
S42.355A
S42.355K
S42.355P
S42.356A
S42.356K
S42.356P
S42.361A
S42.361K
S42.361P
S42.362A
S42.362K
S42.362P
S42.363A
S42.363K
S42.363P
S42.364A
S42.364K
S42.364P
S42.365A
S42.365K
S42.365P
S42.366A
S42.366K
S42.366P
S42.391A
S42.391K
S42.391P
S42.392A
S42.392K
S42.392P
S42.399A
S42.399K
S42.399P
S42.401A
S42.401K
S42.401P
S42.402A
S42.402K
S42.402P
S42.409A
S42.409K
S42.409P
S42.411A
S42.411K
S42.411P
S42.412A
S42.412K
S42.412P
S42.413A
S42.413K
S42.413P
S42.414A
S42.414K
S42.414P
S42.415A
S42.415K
S42.415P
S42.416A
S42.416K
S42.416P
S42.421A
S42.421K
S42.421P
S42.422A
S42.422K
S42.422P
S42.423A
S42.423K
S42.423P
S42.424A
S42.424K
S42.424P
S42.425A
S42.425K
S42.425P
S42.426A
S42.426K
S42.426P
S42.431A

S42.431K
S42.431P
S42.432A
S42.432K
S42.432P
S42.433A
S42.433K
S42.433P
S42.434A
S42.434K
S42.434P
S42.435A
S42.435K
S42.435P
S42.436A
S42.436K
S42.436P
S42.441A
S42.441K
S42.441P
S42.442A
S42.442K
S42.442P
S42.443A
S42.443K
S42.443P
S42.444A
S42.444K
S42.444P
S42.445A
S42.445K
S42.445P
S42.446A
S42.446K
S42.446P
S42.447A
S42.447K
S42.447P
S42.448A
S42.448K
S42.448P
S42.449A
S42.449K
S42.449P
S42.451A
S42.451K
S42.451P
S42.452A
S42.452K
S42.452P
S42.453A
S42.453K
S42.453P
S42.454A
S42.454K
S42.454P
S42.455A
S42.455K
S42.455P
S42.456A
S42.456K
S42.456P
S42.461A
S42.461K
S42.461P
S42.462A
S42.462K
S42.462P
S42.463A
S42.463K
S42.463P
S42.464A
S42.464K
S42.464P
S42.465A
S42.465K
S42.465P
S42.466A
S42.466K
S42.466P
S42.471A
S42.471K
S42.471P
S42.472A
S42.472K
S42.472P
S42.473A
S42.473K
S42.473P
S42.474A
S42.474K
S42.474P
S42.475A
S42.475K
S42.475P
S42.476A
S42.476K
S42.476P
S42.481A
S42.481K
S42.481P
S42.482A
S42.482K
S42.482P
S42.489A
S42.489K
S42.489P
S42.491A
S42.491K
S42.491P
S42.492A
S42.492K
S42.492P
S42.493A
S42.493K
S42.493P
S42.494A
S42.494K
S42.494P
S42.495A
S42.495K
S42.495P
S42.496A
S42.496K
S42.496P
S42.9ØXA
S42.9ØXK
S42.9ØXP
S42.91XA
S42.91XK
S42.91XP
S42.92XA
S42.92XK
S42.92XP
S43.2Ø1A
S43.2Ø2A
S43.2Ø3A
S43.2Ø4A
S43.2Ø5A
S43.2Ø6A
S43.211A
S43.212A
S43.213A
S43.214A
S43.215A
S43.216A
S43.221A
S43.222A
S43.223A
S43.224A
S43.225A
S43.226A
S45.1Ø1A
S45.1Ø2A
S45.1Ø9A
S45.111A
S45.112A
S45.119A
S45.191A
S45.192A
S45.199A
S45.2Ø1A
S45.2Ø2A
S45.2Ø9A
S45.211A
S45.212A
S45.219A
S45.291A
S45.292A
S45.299A
S45.3Ø1A
S45.3Ø2A
S45.3Ø9A
S45.311A
S45.312A
S45.319A
S45.391A
S45.392A
S45.399A
S45.8Ø1A
S45.8Ø2A
S45.8Ø9A
S45.811A
S45.812A
S45.819A
S45.891A
S45.892A
S45.899A
S45.9Ø1A
S45.9Ø2A
S45.9Ø9A
S45.911A
S45.912A
S45.919A
S45.991A
S45.992A
S45.999A
S46.Ø21A
S46.Ø22A
S46.Ø29A
S46.121A
S46.122A
S46.129A
S46.221A
S46.222A
S46.229A
S46.321A
S46.322A
S46.329A
S46.821A
S46.822A
S46.829A
S46.921A
S46.922A
S46.929A
S48.Ø11A
S48.Ø12A
S48.Ø19A
S48.Ø21A
S48.Ø22A
S48.Ø29A
S48.111A
S48.112A
S48.119A
S48.121A
S48.122A
S48.129A
S48.911A
S48.912A
S48.919A
S48.921A
S48.922A
S48.929A
S49.ØØ1A
S49.ØØ1K
S49.ØØ1P
S49.ØØ2A
S49.ØØ2K
S49.ØØ2P
S49.ØØ9A
S49.ØØ9K
S49.ØØ9P
S49.Ø11A
S49.Ø11K
S49.Ø11P
S49.Ø12A
S49.Ø12K
S49.Ø12P
S49.Ø19A
S49.Ø19K
S49.Ø19P
S49.Ø21A
S49.Ø21K
S49.Ø21P
S49.Ø22A
S49.Ø22K
S49.Ø22P
S49.Ø29A
S49.Ø29K
S49.Ø29P
S49.Ø31A
S49.Ø31K
S49.Ø31P
S49.Ø32A
S49.Ø32K
S49.Ø32P
S49.Ø39A
S49.Ø39K
S49.Ø39P
S49.Ø41A
S49.Ø41K
S49.Ø41P
S49.Ø42A
S49.Ø42K
S49.Ø42P
S49.Ø49A
S49.Ø49K
S49.Ø49P
S49.Ø91A
S49.Ø91K
S49.Ø91P
S49.Ø92A
S49.Ø92K
S49.Ø92P
S49.Ø99A
S49.Ø99K
S49.Ø99P
S49.1Ø1A
S49.1Ø1K
S49.1Ø1P
S49.1Ø2A
S49.1Ø2K
S49.1Ø2P
S49.1Ø9A
S49.1Ø9K
S49.1Ø9P
S49.111A
S49.111K
S49.111P
S49.112A
S49.112K
S49.112P
S49.119A
S49.119K
S49.119P
S49.121A
S49.121K
S49.121P
S49.122A
S49.122K
S49.122P
S49.129A
S49.129K
S49.129P
S49.131A
S49.131K
S49.131P
S49.132A
S49.132K
S49.132P
S49.139A
S49.139K
S49.139P
S49.141A
S49.141K
S49.141P
S49.142A
S49.142K
S49.142P
S49.149A
S49.149K
S49.149P
S49.191A
S49.191K
S49.191P
S49.192A
S49.192K
S49.192P
S49.199A
S49.199K
S49.199P
S52.ØØ1K
S52.ØØ1M
S52.ØØ1N
S52.ØØ1P
S52.ØØ1Q
S52.ØØ1R
S52.ØØ2K
S52.ØØ2M
S52.ØØ2N
S52.ØØ2P
S52.ØØ2Q
S52.ØØ2R
S52.ØØ9K
S52.ØØ9M
S52.ØØ9N
S52.ØØ9P
S52.ØØ9Q
S52.ØØ9R
S52.Ø11A
S52.Ø11K
S52.Ø11P
S52.Ø12A
S52.Ø12K
S52.Ø12P
S52.Ø19A
S52.Ø19K
S52.Ø19P
S52.Ø21K
S52.Ø21M
S52.Ø21N
S52.Ø21P
S52.Ø21Q
S52.Ø21R
S52.Ø22K
S52.Ø22M
S52.Ø22N
S52.Ø22P
S52.Ø22Q
S52.Ø22R
S52.Ø23K
S52.Ø23M
S52.Ø23N
S52.Ø23P
S52.Ø23Q
S52.Ø23R
S52.Ø24K
S52.Ø24M
S52.Ø24N
S52.Ø24P
S52.Ø24Q
S52.Ø24R
S52.Ø25K
S52.Ø25M
S52.Ø25N
S52.Ø25P
S52.Ø25Q
S52.Ø25R
S52.Ø26K
S52.Ø26M
S52.Ø26N
S52.Ø26P
S52.Ø26Q
S52.Ø26R
S52.Ø31K
S52.Ø31M
S52.Ø31N
S52.Ø31P
S52.Ø31Q
S52.Ø31R
S52.Ø32K
S52.Ø32M
S52.Ø32N
S52.Ø32P
S52.Ø32Q
S52.Ø32R
S52.Ø33K
S52.Ø33M
S52.Ø33N
S52.Ø33P
S52.Ø33Q
S52.Ø33R
S52.Ø34K
S52.Ø34M
S52.Ø34N
S52.Ø34P
S52.Ø34Q
S52.Ø34R
S52.Ø35K
S52.Ø35M
S52.Ø35N
S52.Ø35P
S52.Ø35Q
S52.Ø35R
S52.Ø36K
S52.Ø36M
S52.Ø36N
S52.Ø36P
S52.Ø36Q
S52.Ø36R
S52.Ø41K
S52.Ø41M
S52.Ø41N
S52.Ø41P
S52.Ø41Q
S52.Ø41R
S52.Ø42K
S52.Ø42M
S52.Ø42N
S52.Ø42P
S52.Ø42Q
S52.Ø42R
S52.Ø43K
S52.Ø43M
S52.Ø43N
S52.Ø43P
S52.Ø43Q
S52.Ø43R
S52.Ø44K
S52.Ø44M
S52.Ø44N
S52.Ø44P
S52.Ø44Q
S52.Ø44R
S52.Ø45K
S52.Ø45M
S52.Ø45N
S52.Ø45P
S52.Ø45Q
S52.Ø45R
S52.Ø46K
S52.Ø46M
S52.Ø46N
S52.Ø46P
S52.Ø46Q
S52.Ø46R
S52.Ø91K
S52.Ø91M
S52.Ø91N
S52.Ø91P
S52.Ø91Q
S52.Ø91R
S52.Ø92K
S52.Ø92M
S52.Ø92N
S52.Ø92P
S52.Ø92Q
S52.Ø92R
S52.Ø99K
S52.Ø99M
S52.Ø99N
S52.Ø99P
S52.Ø99Q
S52.Ø99R
S52.1Ø1K
S52.1Ø1M
S52.1Ø1N
S52.1Ø1P
S52.1Ø1Q
S52.1Ø1R
S52.1Ø2K
S52.1Ø2M
S52.1Ø2N
S52.1Ø2P
S52.1Ø2Q
S52.1Ø2R
S52.1Ø9K
S52.1Ø9M
S52.1Ø9N
S52.1Ø9P
S52.1Ø9Q
S52.1Ø9R
S52.111A
S52.111K
S52.111P
S52.112A
S52.112K
S52.112P
S52.119A
S52.119K
S52.119P
S52.121K
S52.121M
S52.121N
S52.121P
S52.121Q
S52.121R
S52.122K
S52.122M
S52.122N
S52.122P
S52.122Q
S52.122R
S52.123K
S52.123M
S52.123N
S52.123P
S52.123Q
S52.123R
S52.124K
S52.124M
S52.124N
S52.124P
S52.124Q
S52.124R
S52.125K
S52.125M
S52.125N
S52.125P
S52.125Q
S52.125R
S52.126K
S52.126M
S52.126N
S52.126P
S52.126Q
S52.126R
S52.131K
S52.131M
S52.131N
S52.131P
S52.131Q
S52.131R
S52.132K
S52.132M
S52.132N
S52.132P
S52.132Q
S52.132R
S52.133K
S52.133M
S52.133N
S52.133P
S52.133Q
S52.133R
S52.134K
S52.134M
S52.134N
S52.134P
S52.134Q
S52.134R
S52.135K
S52.135M
S52.135N
S52.135P
S52.135Q
S52.135R
S52.136K
S52.136M
S52.136N
S52.136P
S52.136Q
S52.136R
S52.181K
S52.181M
S52.181N
S52.181P
S52.181Q
S52.181R
S52.182K
S52.182M
S52.182N
S52.182P
S52.182Q
S52.182R
S52.189K
S52.189M
S52.189N
S52.189P
S52.189Q
S52.189R
S52.2Ø1A
S52.2Ø1K
S52.2Ø1M
S52.2Ø1N
S52.2Ø1P
S52.2Ø1Q
S52.2Ø1R
S52.2Ø2A
S52.2Ø2K
S52.2Ø2M
S52.2Ø2N
S52.2Ø2P
S52.2Ø2Q
S52.2Ø2R
S52.2Ø9A
S52.2Ø9K
S52.2Ø9M
S52.2Ø9N
S52.2Ø9P
S52.2Ø9Q
S52.2Ø9R
S52.211A
S52.211K
S52.211P
S52.212A
S52.212K
S52.212P
S52.219A
S52.219K
S52.219P
S52.221A
S52.221K
S52.221M
S52.221N
S52.221P
S52.221Q
S52.221R
S52.222A
S52.222K
S52.222M
S52.222N
S52.222P
S52.222Q
S52.222R
S52.223A
S52.223K
S52.223M
S52.223N
S52.223P
S52.223Q
S52.223R
S52.224A
S52.224K
S52.224M
S52.224N
S52.224P
S52.224Q
S52.224R
S52.225A
S52.225K
S52.225M
S52.225N
S52.225P
S52.225Q
S52.225R
S52.226A
S52.226K
S52.226M
S52.226N
S52.226P
S52.226Q
S52.226R
S52.231A
S52.231K
S52.231M
S52.231N
S52.231P
S52.231Q
S52.231R
S52.232A
S52.232K
S52.232M

S52.232N
S52.232P
S52.232Q
S52.232R
S52.233A
S52.233K
S52.233M
S52.233N
S52.233P
S52.233Q
S52.233R
S52.234A
S52.234K
S52.234M
S52.234N
S52.234P
S52.234Q
S52.234R
S52.235A
S52.235K
S52.235M
S52.235N
S52.235P
S52.235Q
S52.235R
S52.236A
S52.236K
S52.236M
S52.236N
S52.236P
S52.236Q
S52.236R
S52.241A
S52.241K
S52.241M
S52.241N
S52.241P
S52.241Q
S52.241R
S52.242A
S52.242K
S52.242M
S52.242N
S52.242P
S52.242Q
S52.242R
S52.243A
S52.243K
S52.243M
S52.243N
S52.243P
S52.243Q
S52.243R
S52.244A
S52.244K
S52.244M
S52.244N
S52.244P
S52.244Q
S52.244R
S52.245A
S52.245K
S52.245M
S52.245N
S52.245P
S52.245Q
S52.245R
S52.246A
S52.246K
S52.246M
S52.246N
S52.246P
S52.246Q
S52.246R
S52.251A
S52.251K
S52.251M
S52.251N
S52.251P
S52.251Q
S52.251R
S52.252A
S52.252K
S52.252M
S52.252N
S52.252P
S52.252Q
S52.252R
S52.253A
S52.253K
S52.253M
S52.253N
S52.253P
S52.253Q
S52.253R
S52.254A
S52.254K
S52.254M
S52.254N
S52.254P
S52.254Q
S52.254R
S52.255A
S52.255K
S52.255M
S52.255N
S52.255P
S52.255Q
S52.255R
S52.256A
S52.256K
S52.256M
S52.256N
S52.256P
S52.256Q
S52.256R
S52.261A
S52.261K
S52.261M
S52.261N
S52.261P
S52.261Q
S52.261R
S52.262A
S52.262K
S52.262M
S52.262N
S52.262P
S52.262Q
S52.262R
S52.263A
S52.263K
S52.263M
S52.263N
S52.263P
S52.263Q
S52.263R
S52.264A
S52.264K
S52.264M
S52.264N
S52.264P
S52.264Q
S52.264R
S52.265A
S52.265K
S52.265M
S52.265N
S52.265P
S52.265Q
S52.265R
S52.266A
S52.266K
S52.266M
S52.266N
S52.266P
S52.266Q
S52.266R
S52.271K
S52.271M
S52.271N
S52.271P
S52.271Q
S52.271R
S52.272K
S52.272M
S52.272N
S52.272P
S52.272Q
S52.272R
S52.279K
S52.279M
S52.279N
S52.279P
S52.279Q
S52.279R
S52.281A
S52.281K
S52.281M
S52.281N
S52.281P
S52.281Q
S52.281R
S52.282A
S52.282K
S52.282M
S52.282N
S52.282P
S52.282Q
S52.282R
S52.283A
S52.283K
S52.283M
S52.283N
S52.283P
S52.283Q
S52.283R
S52.291A
S52.291K
S52.291M
S52.291N
S52.291P
S52.291Q
S52.291R
S52.292A
S52.292K
S52.292M
S52.292N
S52.292P
S52.292Q
S52.292R
S52.299A
S52.299K
S52.299M
S52.299N
S52.299P
S52.299Q
S52.299R
S52.301A
S52.301K
S52.301M
S52.301N
S52.301P
S52.301Q
S52.301R
S52.302A
S52.302K
S52.302M
S52.302N
S52.302P
S52.302Q
S52.302R
S52.309A
S52.309K
S52.309M
S52.309N
S52.309P
S52.309Q
S52.309R
S52.311A
S52.311K
S52.311P
S52.312A
S52.312K
S52.312P
S52.319A
S52.319K
S52.319P
S52.321A
S52.321K
S52.321M
S52.321N
S52.321P
S52.321Q
S52.321R
S52.322A
S52.322K
S52.322M
S52.322N
S52.322P
S52.322Q
S52.322R
S52.323A
S52.323K
S52.323M
S52.323N
S52.323P
S52.323Q
S52.323R
S52.324A
S52.324K
S52.324M
S52.324N
S52.324P
S52.324Q
S52.324R
S52.325A
S52.325K
S52.325M
S52.325N
S52.325P
S52.325Q
S52.325R
S52.326A
S52.326K
S52.326M
S52.326N
S52.326P
S52.326Q
S52.326R
S52.331A
S52.331K
S52.331M
S52.331N
S52.331P
S52.331Q
S52.331R
S52.332A
S52.332K
S52.332M
S52.332N
S52.332P
S52.332Q
S52.332R
S52.333A
S52.333K
S52.333M
S52.333N
S52.333P
S52.333Q
S52.333R
S52.334A
S52.334K
S52.334M
S52.334N
S52.334P
S52.334Q
S52.334R
S52.335A
S52.335K
S52.335M
S52.335N
S52.335P
S52.335Q
S52.335R
S52.336A
S52.336K
S52.336M
S52.336N
S52.336P
S52.336Q
S52.336R
S52.341A
S52.341K
S52.341M
S52.341N
S52.341P
S52.341Q
S52.341R
S52.342A
S52.342K
S52.342M
S52.342N
S52.342P
S52.342Q
S52.342R
S52.343A
S52.343K
S52.343M
S52.343N
S52.343P
S52.343Q
S52.343R
S52.344A
S52.344K
S52.344M
S52.344N
S52.344P
S52.344Q
S52.344R
S52.345A
S52.345K
S52.345M
S52.345N
S52.345P
S52.345Q
S52.345R
S52.346A
S52.346K
S52.346M
S52.346N
S52.346P
S52.346Q
S52.346R
S52.351A
S52.351K
S52.351M
S52.351N
S52.351P
S52.351Q
S52.351R
S52.352A
S52.352K
S52.352M
S52.352N
S52.352P
S52.352Q
S52.352R
S52.353A
S52.353K
S52.353M
S52.353N
S52.353P
S52.353Q
S52.353R
S52.354A
S52.354K
S52.354M
S52.354N
S52.354P
S52.354Q
S52.354R
S52.355A
S52.355K
S52.355M
S52.355N
S52.355P
S52.355Q
S52.355R
S52.356A
S52.356K
S52.356M
S52.356N
S52.356P
S52.356Q
S52.356R
S52.361A
S52.361K
S52.361M
S52.361N
S52.361P
S52.361Q
S52.361R
S52.362A
S52.362K
S52.362M
S52.362N
S52.362P
S52.362Q
S52.362R
S52.363A
S52.363K
S52.363M
S52.363N
S52.363P
S52.363Q
S52.363R
S52.364A
S52.364K
S52.364M
S52.364N
S52.364P
S52.364Q
S52.364R
S52.365A
S52.365K
S52.365M
S52.365N
S52.365P
S52.365Q
S52.365R
S52.366A
S52.366K
S52.366M
S52.366N
S52.366P
S52.366Q
S52.366R
S52.371A
S52.371K
S52.371M
S52.371N
S52.371P
S52.371Q
S52.371R
S52.372A
S52.372K
S52.372M
S52.372N
S52.372P
S52.372Q
S52.372R
S52.379A
S52.379K
S52.379M
S52.379N
S52.379P
S52.379Q
S52.379R
S52.381A
S52.381K
S52.381M
S52.381N
S52.381P
S52.381Q
S52.381R
S52.382A
S52.382K
S52.382M
S52.382N
S52.382P
S52.382Q
S52.382R
S52.389A
S52.389K
S52.389M
S52.389N
S52.389P
S52.389Q
S52.389R
S52.391A
S52.391K
S52.391M
S52.391N
S52.391P
S52.391Q
S52.391R
S52.392A
S52.392K
S52.392M
S52.392N
S52.392P
S52.392Q
S52.392R
S52.399A
S52.399K
S52.399M
S52.399N
S52.399P
S52.399Q
S52.399R
S52.501A
S52.501K
S52.501M
S52.501N
S52.501P
S52.501Q
S52.501R
S52.502A
S52.502K
S52.502M
S52.502N
S52.502P
S52.502Q
S52.502R
S52.509A
S52.509K
S52.509M
S52.509N
S52.509P
S52.509Q
S52.509R
S52.511A
S52.511K
S52.511M
S52.511N
S52.511P
S52.511Q
S52.511R
S52.512A
S52.512K
S52.512M
S52.512N
S52.512P
S52.512Q
S52.512R
S52.513A
S52.513K
S52.513M
S52.513N
S52.513P
S52.513Q
S52.513R
S52.514A
S52.514K
S52.514M
S52.514N
S52.514P
S52.514Q
S52.514R
S52.515A
S52.515K
S52.515M
S52.515N
S52.515P
S52.515Q
S52.515R
S52.516A
S52.516K
S52.516M
S52.516N
S52.516P
S52.516Q
S52.516R
S52.521A
S52.521K
S52.521P
S52.522A
S52.522K
S52.522P
S52.529A
S52.529K
S52.529P
S52.531A
S52.531K
S52.531M
S52.531N
S52.531P
S52.531Q
S52.531R
S52.532A
S52.532K
S52.532M
S52.532N
S52.532P
S52.532Q
S52.532R
S52.539A
S52.539K
S52.539M
S52.539N
S52.539P
S52.539Q
S52.539R
S52.541A
S52.541K
S52.541M
S52.541N
S52.541P
S52.541Q
S52.541R
S52.542A
S52.542K
S52.542M
S52.542N
S52.542P
S52.542Q
S52.542R
S52.549A
S52.549K
S52.549M
S52.549N
S52.549P
S52.549Q
S52.549R
S52.551A
S52.551K
S52.551M
S52.551N
S52.551P
S52.551Q
S52.551R
S52.552A
S52.552K
S52.552M
S52.552N
S52.552P
S52.552Q
S52.552R
S52.559A
S52.559K
S52.559M
S52.559N
S52.559P
S52.559Q
S52.559R
S52.561A
S52.561K
S52.561M
S52.561N
S52.561P
S52.561Q
S52.561R
S52.562A
S52.562K
S52.562M
S52.562N
S52.562P
S52.562Q
S52.562R
S52.569A
S52.569K
S52.569M
S52.569N
S52.569P
S52.569Q
S52.569R
S52.571A
S52.571K
S52.571M
S52.571N
S52.571P
S52.571Q
S52.571R
S52.572A
S52.572K
S52.572M
S52.572N
S52.572P
S52.572Q
S52.572R
S52.579A
S52.579K

S52.579M
S52.579N
S52.579P
S52.579Q
S52.579R
S52.591A
S52.591K
S52.591M
S52.591N
S52.591P
S52.591Q
S52.591R
S52.592A
S52.592K
S52.592M
S52.592N
S52.592P
S52.592Q
S52.592R
S52.599A
S52.599K
S52.599M
S52.599N
S52.599P
S52.599Q
S52.599R
S52.601A
S52.601K
S52.601M
S52.601N
S52.601P
S52.601Q
S52.601R
S52.602A
S52.602K
S52.602M
S52.602N
S52.602P
S52.602Q
S52.602R
S52.609A
S52.609K
S52.609M
S52.609N
S52.609P
S52.609Q
S52.609R
S52.611A
S52.611K
S52.611M
S52.611N
S52.611P
S52.611Q
S52.611R
S52.612A
S52.612K
S52.612M
S52.612N
S52.612P
S52.612Q
S52.612R
S52.613A
S52.613K
S52.613M
S52.613N
S52.613P
S52.613Q
S52.613R
S52.614A
S52.614K
S52.614M
S52.614N
S52.614P
S52.614Q
S52.614R
S52.615A
S52.615K
S52.615M
S52.615N
S52.615P
S52.615Q
S52.615R
S52.616A
S52.616K
S52.616M
S52.616N
S52.616P
S52.616Q
S52.616R
S52.621A
S52.621K
S52.621P
S52.622A
S52.622K
S52.622P
S52.629A
S52.629K
S52.629P
S52.691A
S52.691K
S52.691M
S52.691N
S52.691P
S52.691Q
S52.691R
S52.692A
S52.692K
S52.692M
S52.692N
S52.692P
S52.692Q
S52.692R
S52.699A
S52.699K
S52.699M
S52.699N
S52.699P
S52.699Q
S52.699R
S52.90XA
S52.90XK
S52.90XM
S52.90XN
S52.90XP
S52.90XQ
S52.90XR
S52.91XA
S52.91XK
S52.91XM
S52.91XN
S52.91XP
S52.91XQ
S52.91XR
S52.92XA
S52.92XK
S52.92XM
S52.92XN
S52.92XP
S52.92XQ
S52.92XR
S55.001A
S55.002A
S55.009A
S55.011A
S55.012A
S55.019A
S55.091A
S55.092A
S55.099A
S55.101A
S55.102A
S55.109A
S55.111A
S55.112A
S55.119A
S55.191A
S55.192A
S55.199A
S55.201A
S55.202A
S55.209A
S55.211A
S55.212A
S55.219A
S55.291A
S55.292A
S55.299A
S55.801A
S55.802A
S55.809A
S55.811A
S55.812A
S55.819A
S55.891A
S55.892A
S55.899A
S55.901A
S55.902A
S55.909A
S55.911A
S55.912A
S55.919A
S55.991A
S55.992A
S55.999A
S56.021A
S56.022A
S56.029A
S56.121A
S56.122A
S56.123A
S56.124A
S56.125A
S56.126A
S56.127A
S56.128A
S56.129A
S56.221A
S56.222A
S56.229A
S56.321A
S56.322A
S56.329A
S56.421A
S56.422A
S56.423A
S56.424A
S56.425A
S56.426A
S56.427A
S56.428A
S56.429A
S56.521A
S56.522A
S56.529A
S56.821A
S56.822A
S56.829A
S56.921A
S56.922A
S56.929A
S58.011A
S58.012A
S58.019A
S58.021A
S58.022A
S58.029A
S58.111A
S58.112A
S58.119A
S58.121A
S58.122A
S58.129A
S58.911A
S58.912A
S58.919A
S58.921A
S58.922A
S58.929A
S59.001A
S59.001K
S59.001P
S59.002A
S59.002K
S59.002P
S59.009A
S59.009K
S59.009P
S59.011A
S59.011K
S59.011P
S59.012A
S59.012K
S59.012P
S59.019A
S59.019K
S59.019P
S59.021A
S59.021K
S59.021P
S59.022A
S59.022K
S59.022P
S59.029A
S59.029K
S59.029P
S59.031A
S59.031K
S59.031P
S59.032A
S59.032K
S59.032P
S59.039A
S59.039K
S59.039P
S59.041A
S59.041K
S59.041P
S59.042A
S59.042K
S59.042P
S59.049A
S59.049K
S59.049P
S59.091A
S59.091K
S59.091P
S59.092A
S59.092K
S59.092P
S59.099A
S59.099K
S59.099P
S59.101K
S59.101P
S59.102K
S59.102P
S59.109K
S59.109P
S59.111K
S59.111P
S59.112K
S59.112P
S59.119K
S59.119P
S59.121K
S59.121P
S59.122K
S59.122P
S59.129K
S59.129P
S59.131K
S59.131P
S59.132K
S59.132P
S59.139K
S59.139P
S59.141K
S59.141P
S59.142K
S59.142P
S59.149K
S59.149P
S59.191K
S59.191P
S59.192K
S59.192P
S59.199K
S59.199P
S59.201A
S59.201K
S59.201P
S59.202A
S59.202K
S59.202P
S59.209A
S59.209K
S59.209P
S59.211A
S59.211K
S59.211P
S59.212A
S59.212K
S59.212P
S59.219A
S59.219K
S59.219P
S59.221A
S59.221K
S59.221P
S59.222A
S59.222K
S59.222P
S59.229A
S59.229K
S59.229P
S59.231A
S59.231K
S59.231P
S59.232A
S59.232K
S59.232P
S59.239A
S59.239K
S59.239P
S59.241A
S59.241K
S59.241P
S59.242A
S59.242K
S59.242P
S59.249A
S59.249K
S59.249P
S59.291A
S59.291K
S59.291P
S59.292A
S59.292K
S59.292P
S59.299A
S59.299K
S59.299P
S62.001B
S62.001K
S62.001P
S62.002B
S62.002K
S62.002P
S62.009B
S62.009K
S62.009P
S62.011B
S62.011K
S62.011P
S62.012B
S62.012K
S62.012P
S62.013B
S62.013K
S62.013P
S62.014B
S62.014K
S62.014P
S62.015B
S62.015K
S62.015P
S62.016B
S62.016K
S62.016P
S62.021B
S62.021K
S62.021P
S62.022B
S62.022K
S62.022P
S62.023B
S62.023K
S62.023P
S62.024B
S62.024K
S62.024P
S62.025B
S62.025K
S62.025P
S62.026B
S62.026K
S62.026P
S62.031B
S62.031K
S62.031P
S62.032B
S62.032K
S62.032P
S62.033B
S62.033K
S62.033P
S62.034B
S62.034K
S62.034P
S62.035B
S62.035K
S62.035P
S62.036B
S62.036K
S62.036P
S62.101B
S62.101K
S62.101P
S62.102B
S62.102K
S62.102P
S62.109B
S62.109K
S62.109P
S62.111B
S62.111K
S62.111P
S62.112B
S62.112K
S62.112P
S62.113B
S62.113K
S62.113P
S62.114B
S62.114K
S62.114P
S62.115B
S62.115K
S62.115P
S62.116B
S62.116K
S62.116P
S62.121B
S62.121K
S62.121P
S62.122B
S62.122K
S62.122P
S62.123B
S62.123K
S62.123P
S62.124B
S62.124K
S62.124P
S62.125B
S62.125K
S62.125P
S62.126B
S62.126K
S62.126P
S62.131B
S62.131K
S62.131P
S62.132B
S62.132K
S62.132P
S62.133B
S62.133K
S62.133P
S62.134B
S62.134K
S62.134P
S62.135B
S62.135K
S62.135P
S62.136B
S62.136K
S62.136P
S62.141B
S62.141K
S62.141P
S62.142B
S62.142K
S62.142P
S62.143B
S62.143K
S62.143P
S62.144B
S62.144K
S62.144P
S62.145B
S62.145K
S62.145P
S62.146B
S62.146K
S62.146P
S62.151B
S62.151K
S62.151P
S62.152B
S62.152K
S62.152P
S62.153B
S62.153K
S62.153P
S62.154B
S62.154K
S62.154P
S62.155B
S62.155K
S62.155P
S62.156B
S62.156K
S62.156P
S62.161B
S62.161K
S62.161P
S62.162B
S62.162K
S62.162P
S62.163B
S62.163K
S62.163P
S62.164B
S62.164K
S62.164P
S62.165B
S62.165K
S62.165P
S62.166B
S62.166K
S62.166P
S62.171B
S62.171K
S62.171P
S62.172B
S62.172K
S62.172P
S62.173B
S62.173K
S62.173P
S62.174B
S62.174K
S62.174P
S62.175B
S62.175K
S62.175P
S62.176B
S62.176K
S62.176P
S62.181B
S62.181K
S62.181P
S62.182B
S62.182K
S62.182P
S62.183B
S62.183K
S62.183P
S62.184B
S62.184K
S62.184P
S62.185B
S62.185K
S62.185P
S62.186B
S62.186K
S62.186P
S62.201B
S62.201K
S62.201P
S62.202B
S62.202K
S62.202P
S62.209B
S62.209K
S62.209P
S62.211B
S62.211K
S62.211P
S62.212B
S62.212K
S62.212P
S62.213B
S62.213K
S62.213P
S62.221B
S62.221K
S62.221P
S62.222B
S62.222K
S62.222P
S62.223B
S62.223K
S62.223P
S62.224B
S62.224K
S62.224P
S62.225B
S62.225K
S62.225P
S62.226B
S62.226K
S62.226P
S62.231B
S62.231K
S62.231P
S62.232B
S62.232K
S62.232P
S62.233B
S62.233K
S62.233P
S62.234B
S62.234K
S62.234P
S62.235B
S62.235K
S62.235P
S62.236B
S62.236K
S62.236P
S62.241B
S62.241K
S62.241P
S62.242B
S62.242K
S62.242P
S62.243B
S62.243K
S62.243P
S62.244B
S62.244K
S62.244P
S62.245B
S62.245K
S62.245P
S62.246B
S62.246K
S62.246P
S62.251B
S62.251K
S62.251P
S62.252B
S62.252K
S62.252P
S62.253B
S62.253K
S62.253P
S62.254B
S62.254K
S62.254P
S62.255B
S62.255K
S62.255P
S62.256B
S62.256K
S62.256P
S62.291B
S62.291K
S62.291P
S62.292B

S62.292K
S62.292P
S62.299B
S62.299K
S62.299P
S62.300B
S62.300K
S62.300P
S62.301B
S62.301K
S62.301P
S62.302B
S62.302K
S62.302P
S62.303B
S62.303K
S62.303P
S62.304B
S62.304K
S62.304P
S62.305B
S62.305K
S62.305P
S62.306B
S62.306K
S62.306P
S62.307B
S62.307K
S62.307P
S62.308B
S62.308K
S62.308P
S62.309B
S62.309K
S62.309P
S62.310B
S62.310K
S62.310P
S62.311B
S62.311K
S62.311P
S62.312B
S62.312K
S62.312P
S62.313B
S62.313K
S62.313P
S62.314B
S62.314K
S62.314P
S62.315B
S62.315K
S62.315P
S62.316B
S62.316K
S62.316P
S62.317B
S62.317K
S62.317P
S62.318B
S62.318K
S62.318P
S62.319B
S62.319K
S62.319P
S62.320B
S62.320K
S62.320P
S62.321B
S62.321K
S62.321P
S62.322B
S62.322K
S62.322P
S62.323B
S62.323K
S62.323P
S62.324B
S62.324K
S62.324P
S62.325B
S62.325K
S62.325P
S62.326B
S62.326K
S62.326P
S62.327B
S62.327K
S62.327P
S62.328B
S62.328K
S62.328P
S62.329B
S62.329K
S62.329P
S62.330B
S62.330K
S62.330P
S62.331B
S62.331K
S62.331P
S62.332B
S62.332K
S62.332P
S62.333B
S62.333K
S62.333P
S62.334B
S62.334K
S62.334P
S62.335B
S62.335K
S62.335P
S62.336B
S62.336K
S62.336P
S62.337B
S62.337K
S62.337P
S62.338B
S62.338K
S62.338P
S62.339B
S62.339K
S62.339P
S62.340B
S62.340K
S62.340P
S62.341B
S62.341K
S62.341P
S62.342B
S62.342K
S62.342P
S62.343B
S62.343K
S62.343P
S62.344B
S62.344K
S62.344P
S62.345B
S62.345K
S62.345P
S62.346B
S62.346K
S62.346P
S62.347B
S62.347K
S62.347P
S62.348B
S62.348K
S62.348P
S62.349B
S62.349K
S62.349P
S62.350B
S62.350K
S62.350P
S62.351B
S62.351K
S62.351P
S62.352B
S62.352K
S62.352P
S62.353B
S62.353K
S62.353P
S62.354B
S62.354K
S62.354P
S62.355B
S62.355K
S62.355P
S62.356B
S62.356K
S62.356P
S62.357B
S62.357K
S62.357P
S62.358B
S62.358K
S62.358P
S62.359B
S62.359K
S62.359P
S62.360B
S62.360K
S62.360P
S62.361B
S62.361K
S62.361P
S62.362B
S62.362K
S62.362P
S62.363B
S62.363K
S62.363P
S62.364B
S62.364K
S62.364P
S62.365B
S62.365K
S62.365P
S62.366B
S62.366K
S62.366P
S62.367B
S62.367K
S62.367P
S62.368B
S62.368K
S62.368P
S62.369B
S62.369K
S62.369P
S62.390B
S62.390K
S62.390P
S62.391B
S62.391K
S62.391P
S62.392B
S62.392K
S62.392P
S62.393B
S62.393K
S62.393P
S62.394B
S62.394K
S62.394P
S62.395B
S62.395K
S62.395P
S62.396B
S62.396K
S62.396P
S62.397B
S62.397K
S62.397P
S62.398B
S62.398K
S62.398P
S62.399B
S62.399K
S62.399P
S62.501B
S62.501K
S62.501P
S62.502B
S62.502K
S62.502P
S62.509B
S62.509K
S62.509P
S62.511B
S62.511K
S62.511P
S62.512B
S62.512K
S62.512P
S62.513B
S62.513K
S62.513P
S62.514B
S62.514K
S62.514P
S62.515B
S62.515K
S62.515P
S62.516B
S62.516K
S62.516P
S62.521B
S62.521K
S62.521P
S62.522B
S62.522K
S62.522P
S62.523B
S62.523K
S62.523P
S62.524B
S62.524K
S62.524P
S62.525B
S62.525K
S62.525P
S62.526B
S62.526K
S62.526P
S62.600B
S62.600K
S62.600P
S62.601B
S62.601K
S62.601P
S62.602B
S62.602K
S62.602P
S62.603B
S62.603K
S62.603P
S62.604B
S62.604K
S62.604P
S62.605B
S62.605K
S62.605P
S62.606B
S62.606K
S62.606P
S62.607B
S62.607K
S62.607P
S62.608B
S62.608K
S62.608P
S62.609B
S62.609K
S62.609P
S62.610B
S62.610K
S62.610P
S62.611B
S62.611K
S62.611P
S62.612B
S62.612K
S62.612P
S62.613B
S62.613K
S62.613P
S62.614B
S62.614K
S62.614P
S62.615B
S62.615K
S62.615P
S62.616B
S62.616K
S62.616P
S62.617B
S62.617K
S62.617P
S62.618B
S62.618K
S62.618P
S62.619B
S62.619K
S62.619P
S62.620B
S62.620K
S62.620P
S62.621B
S62.621K
S62.621P
S62.622B
S62.622K
S62.622P
S62.623B
S62.623K
S62.623P
S62.624B
S62.624K
S62.624P
S62.625B
S62.625K
S62.625P
S62.626B
S62.626K
S62.626P
S62.627B
S62.627K
S62.627P
S62.628B
S62.628K
S62.628P
S62.629B
S62.629K
S62.629P
S62.630B
S62.630K
S62.630P
S62.631B
S62.631K
S62.631P
S62.632B
S62.632K
S62.632P
S62.633B
S62.633K
S62.633P
S62.634B
S62.634K
S62.634P
S62.635B
S62.635K
S62.635P
S62.636B
S62.636K
S62.636P
S62.637B
S62.637K
S62.637P
S62.638B
S62.638K
S62.638P
S62.639B
S62.639K
S62.639P
S62.640B
S62.640K
S62.640P
S62.641B
S62.641K
S62.641P
S62.642B
S62.642K
S62.642P
S62.643B
S62.643K
S62.643P
S62.644B
S62.644K
S62.644P
S62.645B
S62.645K
S62.645P
S62.646B
S62.646K
S62.646P
S62.647B
S62.647K
S62.647P
S62.648B
S62.648K
S62.648P
S62.649B
S62.649K
S62.649P
S62.650B
S62.650K
S62.650P
S62.651B
S62.651K
S62.651P
S62.652B
S62.652K
S62.652P
S62.653B
S62.653K
S62.653P
S62.654B
S62.654K
S62.654P
S62.655B
S62.655K
S62.655P
S62.656B
S62.656K
S62.656P
S62.657B
S62.657K
S62.657P
S62.658B
S62.658K
S62.658P
S62.659B
S62.659K
S62.659P
S62.660B
S62.660K
S62.660P
S62.661B
S62.661K
S62.661P
S62.662B
S62.662K
S62.662P
S62.663B
S62.663K
S62.663P
S62.664B
S62.664K
S62.664P
S62.665B
S62.665K
S62.665P
S62.666B
S62.666K
S62.666P
S62.667B
S62.667K
S62.667P
S62.668B
S62.668K
S62.668P
S62.669B
S62.669K
S62.669P
S62.90XB
S62.90XK
S62.90XP
S62.91XB
S62.91XK
S62.91XP
S62.92XB
S62.92XK
S62.92XP
S65.001A
S65.002A
S65.009A
S65.011A
S65.012A
S65.019A
S65.091A
S65.092A
S65.099A
S65.101A
S65.102A
S65.109A
S65.111A
S65.112A
S65.119A
S65.191A
S65.192A
S65.199A
S65.201A
S65.202A
S65.209A
S65.211A
S65.212A
S65.219A
S65.291A
S65.292A
S65.299A
S65.301A
S65.302A
S65.309A
S65.311A
S65.312A
S65.319A
S65.391A
S65.392A
S65.399A
S65.401A
S65.402A
S65.409A
S65.411A
S65.412A
S65.419A
S65.491A
S65.492A
S65.499A
S65.500A
S65.501A
S65.502A
S65.503A
S65.504A
S65.505A
S65.506A
S65.507A
S65.508A
S65.509A
S65.510A
S65.511A
S65.512A
S65.513A
S65.514A
S65.515A
S65.516A
S65.517A
S65.518A
S65.519A
S65.590A
S65.591A
S65.592A
S65.593A
S65.594A
S65.595A
S65.596A
S65.597A
S65.598A
S65.599A
S65.801A
S65.802A
S65.809A
S65.811A
S65.812A
S65.819A
S65.891A
S65.892A
S65.899A
S65.901A
S65.902A
S65.909A
S65.911A
S65.912A
S65.919A
S65.991A
S65.992A
S65.999A
S66.021A
S66.022A
S66.029A
S66.120A
S66.121A
S66.122A
S66.123A
S66.124A
S66.125A
S66.126A
S66.127A
S66.128A
S66.129A
S66.221A
S66.222A
S66.229A
S66.320A
S66.321A
S66.322A
S66.323A
S66.324A
S66.325A
S66.326A
S66.327A
S66.328A
S66.329A
S66.421A
S66.422A
S66.429A
S66.520A
S66.521A
S66.522A
S66.523A
S66.524A
S66.525A
S66.526A
S66.527A
S66.528A
S66.529A
S66.821A
S66.822A
S66.829A
S66.921A
S66.922A
S66.929A
S68.411A
S68.412A
S68.419A
S68.421A
S68.422A
S68.429A
S68.711A
S68.712A
S68.719A
S68.721A
S68.722A
S68.729A
S72.001K
S72.001M
S72.001N
S72.001P
S72.001Q
S72.001R
S72.002K
S72.002M
S72.002N
S72.002P
S72.002Q
S72.002R
S72.009K
S72.009M
S72.009N
S72.009P
S72.009Q
S72.009R
S72.011K
S72.011M
S72.011N
S72.011P
S72.011Q
S72.011R
S72.012K
S72.012M
S72.012N
S72.012P
S72.012Q
S72.012R
S72.019K
S72.019M
S72.019N
S72.019P

S72.Ø19Q
S72.Ø19R
S72.Ø21K
S72.Ø21M
S72.Ø21N
S72.Ø21P
S72.Ø21Q
S72.Ø21R
S72.Ø22K
S72.Ø22M
S72.Ø22N
S72.Ø22P
S72.Ø22Q
S72.Ø22R
S72.Ø23K
S72.Ø23M
S72.Ø23N
S72.Ø23P
S72.Ø23Q
S72.Ø23R
S72.Ø24K
S72.Ø24M
S72.Ø24N
S72.Ø24P
S72.Ø24Q
S72.Ø24R
S72.Ø25K
S72.Ø25M
S72.Ø25N
S72.Ø25P
S72.Ø25Q
S72.Ø25R
S72.Ø26K
S72.Ø26M
S72.Ø26N
S72.Ø26P
S72.Ø26Q
S72.Ø26R
S72.Ø31K
S72.Ø31M
S72.Ø31N
S72.Ø31P
S72.Ø31Q
S72.Ø31R
S72.Ø32K
S72.Ø32M
S72.Ø32N
S72.Ø32P
S72.Ø32Q
S72.Ø32R
S72.Ø33K
S72.Ø33M
S72.Ø33N
S72.Ø33P
S72.Ø33Q
S72.Ø33R
S72.Ø34K
S72.Ø34M
S72.Ø34N
S72.Ø34P
S72.Ø34Q
S72.Ø34R
S72.Ø35K
S72.Ø35M
S72.Ø35N
S72.Ø35P
S72.Ø35Q
S72.Ø35R
S72.Ø36K
S72.Ø36M
S72.Ø36N
S72.Ø36P
S72.Ø36Q
S72.Ø36R
S72.Ø41K
S72.Ø41M
S72.Ø41N
S72.Ø41P
S72.Ø41Q
S72.Ø41R
S72.Ø42K
S72.Ø42M
S72.Ø42N
S72.Ø42P
S72.Ø42Q
S72.Ø42R
S72.Ø43K
S72.Ø43M
S72.Ø43N
S72.Ø43P
S72.Ø43Q
S72.Ø43R
S72.Ø44K
S72.Ø44M
S72.Ø44N
S72.Ø44P
S72.Ø44Q
S72.Ø44R
S72.Ø45K
S72.Ø45M
S72.Ø45N
S72.Ø45P
S72.Ø45Q
S72.Ø45R
S72.Ø46K
S72.Ø46M
S72.Ø46N
S72.Ø46P
S72.Ø46Q
S72.Ø46R
S72.Ø51K
S72.Ø51M
S72.Ø51N
S72.Ø51P
S72.Ø51Q
S72.Ø51R
S72.Ø52K
S72.Ø52M
S72.Ø52N
S72.Ø52P
S72.Ø52Q
S72.Ø52R
S72.Ø59K
S72.Ø59M
S72.Ø59N
S72.Ø59P
S72.Ø59Q
S72.Ø59R
S72.Ø61K
S72.Ø61M
S72.Ø61N
S72.Ø61P
S72.Ø61Q
S72.Ø61R
S72.Ø62K
S72.Ø62M
S72.Ø62N
S72.Ø62P
S72.Ø62Q
S72.Ø62R
S72.Ø63K
S72.Ø63M
S72.Ø63N
S72.Ø63P
S72.Ø63Q
S72.Ø63R
S72.Ø64K
S72.Ø64M
S72.Ø64N
S72.Ø64P
S72.Ø64Q
S72.Ø64R
S72.Ø65K
S72.Ø65M
S72.Ø65N
S72.Ø65P
S72.Ø65Q
S72.Ø65R
S72.Ø66K
S72.Ø66M
S72.Ø66N
S72.Ø66P
S72.Ø66Q
S72.Ø66R
S72.Ø91K
S72.Ø91M
S72.Ø91N
S72.Ø91P
S72.Ø91Q
S72.Ø91R
S72.Ø92K
S72.Ø92M
S72.Ø92N
S72.Ø92P
S72.Ø92Q
S72.Ø92R
S72.Ø99K
S72.Ø99M
S72.Ø99N
S72.Ø99P
S72.Ø99Q
S72.Ø99R
S72.1Ø1K
S72.1Ø1M
S72.1Ø1N
S72.1Ø1P
S72.1Ø1Q
S72.1Ø1R
S72.1Ø2K
S72.1Ø2M
S72.1Ø2N
S72.1Ø2P
S72.1Ø2Q
S72.1Ø2R
S72.1Ø9K
S72.1Ø9M
S72.1Ø9N
S72.1Ø9P
S72.1Ø9Q
S72.1Ø9R
S72.111K
S72.111M
S72.111N
S72.111P
S72.111Q
S72.111R
S72.112K
S72.112M
S72.112N
S72.112P
S72.112Q
S72.112R
S72.113K
S72.113M
S72.113N
S72.113P
S72.113Q
S72.113R
S72.114K
S72.114M
S72.114N
S72.114P
S72.114Q
S72.114R
S72.115K
S72.115M
S72.115N
S72.115P
S72.115Q
S72.115R
S72.116K
S72.116M
S72.116N
S72.116P
S72.116Q
S72.116R
S72.121K
S72.121M
S72.121N
S72.121P
S72.121Q
S72.121R
S72.122K
S72.122M
S72.122N
S72.122P
S72.122Q
S72.122R
S72.123K
S72.123M
S72.123N
S72.123P
S72.123Q
S72.123R
S72.124K
S72.124M
S72.124N
S72.124P
S72.124Q
S72.124R
S72.125K
S72.125M
S72.125N
S72.125P
S72.125Q
S72.125R
S72.126K
S72.126M
S72.126N
S72.126P
S72.126Q
S72.126R
S72.131K
S72.131M
S72.131N
S72.131P
S72.131Q
S72.131R
S72.132K
S72.132M
S72.132N
S72.132P
S72.132Q
S72.132R
S72.133K
S72.133M
S72.133N
S72.133P
S72.133Q
S72.133R
S72.134K
S72.134M
S72.134N
S72.134P
S72.134Q
S72.134R
S72.135K
S72.135M
S72.135N
S72.135P
S72.135Q
S72.135R
S72.136K
S72.136M
S72.136N
S72.136P
S72.136Q
S72.136R
S72.141K
S72.141M
S72.141N
S72.141P
S72.141Q
S72.141R
S72.142K
S72.142M
S72.142N
S72.142P
S72.142Q
S72.142R
S72.143K
S72.143M
S72.143N
S72.143P
S72.143Q
S72.143R
S72.144K
S72.144M
S72.144N
S72.144P
S72.144Q
S72.144R
S72.145K
S72.145M
S72.145N
S72.145P
S72.145Q
S72.145R
S72.146K
S72.146M
S72.146N
S72.146P
S72.146Q
S72.146R
S72.21XK
S72.21XM
S72.21XN
S72.21XP
S72.21XQ
S72.21XR
S72.22XK
S72.22XM
S72.22XN
S72.22XP
S72.22XQ
S72.22XR
S72.23XK
S72.23XM
S72.23XN
S72.23XP
S72.23XQ
S72.23XR
S72.24XK
S72.24XM
S72.24XN
S72.24XP
S72.24XQ
S72.24XR
S72.25XK
S72.25XM
S72.25XN
S72.25XP
S72.25XQ
S72.25XR
S72.26XK
S72.26XM
S72.26XN
S72.26XP
S72.26XQ
S72.26XR
S72.3Ø1K
S72.3Ø1M
S72.3Ø1N
S72.3Ø1P
S72.3Ø1Q
S72.3Ø1R
S72.3Ø2K
S72.3Ø2M
S72.3Ø2N
S72.3Ø2P
S72.3Ø2Q
S72.3Ø2R
S72.3Ø9K
S72.3Ø9M
S72.3Ø9N
S72.3Ø9P
S72.3Ø9Q
S72.3Ø9R
S72.321K
S72.321M
S72.321N
S72.321P
S72.321Q
S72.321R
S72.322K
S72.322M
S72.322N
S72.322P
S72.322Q
S72.322R
S72.323K
S72.323M
S72.323N
S72.323P
S72.323Q
S72.323R
S72.324K
S72.324M
S72.324N
S72.324P
S72.324Q
S72.324R
S72.325K
S72.325M
S72.325N
S72.325P
S72.325Q
S72.325R
S72.326K
S72.326M
S72.326N
S72.326P
S72.326Q
S72.326R
S72.331K
S72.331M
S72.331N
S72.331P
S72.331Q
S72.331R
S72.332K
S72.332M
S72.332N
S72.332P
S72.332Q
S72.332R
S72.333K
S72.333M
S72.333N
S72.333P
S72.333Q
S72.333R
S72.334K
S72.334M
S72.334N
S72.334P
S72.334Q
S72.334R
S72.335K
S72.335M
S72.335N
S72.335P
S72.335Q
S72.335R
S72.336K
S72.336M
S72.336N
S72.336P
S72.336Q
S72.336R
S72.341K
S72.341M
S72.341N
S72.341P
S72.341Q
S72.341R
S72.342K
S72.342M
S72.342N
S72.342P
S72.342Q
S72.342R
S72.343K
S72.343M
S72.343N
S72.343P
S72.343Q
S72.343R
S72.344K
S72.344M
S72.344N
S72.344P
S72.344Q
S72.344R
S72.345K
S72.345M
S72.345N
S72.345P
S72.345Q
S72.345R
S72.346K
S72.346M
S72.346N
S72.346P
S72.346Q
S72.346R
S72.351K
S72.351M
S72.351N
S72.351P
S72.351Q
S72.351R
S72.352K
S72.352M
S72.352N
S72.352P
S72.352Q
S72.352R
S72.353K
S72.353M
S72.353N
S72.353P
S72.353Q
S72.353R
S72.354K
S72.354M
S72.354N
S72.354P
S72.354Q
S72.354R
S72.355K
S72.355M
S72.355N
S72.355P
S72.355Q
S72.355R
S72.356K
S72.356M
S72.356N
S72.356P
S72.356Q
S72.356R
S72.361K
S72.361M
S72.361N
S72.361P
S72.361Q
S72.361R
S72.362K
S72.362M
S72.362N
S72.362P
S72.362Q
S72.362R
S72.363K
S72.363M
S72.363N
S72.363P
S72.363Q
S72.363R
S72.364K
S72.364M
S72.364N
S72.364P
S72.364Q
S72.364R
S72.365K
S72.365M
S72.365N
S72.365P
S72.365Q
S72.365R
S72.366K
S72.366M
S72.366N
S72.366P
S72.366Q
S72.366R
S72.391K
S72.391M
S72.391N
S72.391P
S72.391Q
S72.391R
S72.392K
S72.392M
S72.392N
S72.392P
S72.392Q
S72.392R
S72.399K
S72.399M
S72.399N
S72.399P
S72.399Q
S72.399R
S72.4Ø1A
S72.4Ø1K
S72.4Ø1M
S72.4Ø1N
S72.4Ø1P
S72.4Ø1Q
S72.4Ø1R
S72.4Ø2A
S72.4Ø2K
S72.4Ø2M
S72.4Ø2N
S72.4Ø2P
S72.4Ø2Q
S72.4Ø2R
S72.4Ø9A
S72.4Ø9K
S72.4Ø9M
S72.4Ø9N
S72.4Ø9P
S72.4Ø9Q
S72.4Ø9R
S72.411A
S72.411K
S72.411M
S72.411N
S72.411P
S72.411Q
S72.411R
S72.412A
S72.412K
S72.412M
S72.412N
S72.412P
S72.412Q
S72.412R
S72.413A
S72.413K
S72.413M
S72.413N
S72.413P
S72.413Q
S72.413R
S72.414A
S72.414K
S72.414M
S72.414N
S72.414P
S72.414Q
S72.414R
S72.415A
S72.415K
S72.415M
S72.415N
S72.415P
S72.415Q
S72.415R
S72.416A
S72.416K
S72.416M
S72.416N
S72.416P
S72.416Q
S72.416R
S72.421A
S72.421K
S72.421M
S72.421N
S72.421P
S72.421Q
S72.421R
S72.422A
S72.422K
S72.422M
S72.422N
S72.422P
S72.422Q
S72.422R
S72.423A
S72.423K
S72.423M
S72.423N
S72.423P
S72.423Q
S72.423R
S72.424A
S72.424K
S72.424M
S72.424N
S72.424P
S72.424Q
S72.424R
S72.425A
S72.425K
S72.425M
S72.425N
S72.425P
S72.425Q

72.425R
72.426A
72.426K
72.426M
72.426N
72.426P
72.426Q
72.426R
72.431A
72.431K
72.431M
72.431N
72.431P
72.431Q
72.431R
S72.432A
S72.432K
S72.432M
S72.432N
S72.432P
S72.432Q
S72.432R
S72.433A
S72.433K
S72.433M
S72.433N
S72.433P
S72.433Q
S72.433R
S72.434A
S72.434K
S72.434M
S72.434N
S72.434P
S72.434Q
S72.434R
S72.435A
S72.435K
S72.435M
S72.435N
S72.435P
S72.435Q
S72.435R
S72.436A
S72.436K
S72.436M
S72.436N
S72.436P
S72.436Q
S72.436R
S72.441A
S72.441K
S72.441M
S72.441N
S72.441P
S72.441Q
S72.441R
S72.442A
S72.442K
S72.442M
S72.442N
S72.442P
S72.442Q
S72.442R
S72.443A
S72.443K
S72.443M
S72.443N
S72.443P
S72.443Q
S72.443R
S72.444A
S72.444K
S72.444M
S72.444N
S72.444P
S72.444Q
S72.444R
S72.445A
S72.445K
S72.445M
S72.445N
S72.445P
S72.445Q
S72.445R
S72.446A
S72.446K
S72.446M
S72.446N
S72.446P
S72.446Q
S72.446R
S72.451A
S72.451K
S72.451M
S72.451N
S72.451P
S72.451Q
S72.451R
S72.452A
S72.452K
S72.452M
S72.452N
S72.452P
S72.452Q
S72.452R
S72.453A
S72.453K
S72.453M
S72.453N
S72.453P
S72.453Q
S72.453R
S72.454A
S72.454K
S72.454M
S72.454N
S72.454P
S72.454Q
S72.454R
S72.455A
S72.455K
S72.455M
S72.455N
S72.455P
S72.455Q
S72.455R
S72.456A
S72.456K
S72.456M
S72.456N
S72.456P
S72.456Q
S72.456R
S72.461A
S72.461K
S72.461M
S72.461N
S72.461P
S72.461Q
S72.461R
S72.462A
S72.462K
S72.462M
S72.462N
S72.462P
S72.462Q
S72.462R
S72.463A
S72.463K
S72.463M
S72.463N
S72.463P
S72.463Q
S72.463R
S72.464A
S72.464K
S72.464M
S72.464N
S72.464P
S72.464Q
S72.464R
S72.465A
S72.465K
S72.465M
S72.465N
S72.465P
S72.465Q
S72.465R
S72.466A
S72.466K
S72.466M
S72.466N
S72.466P
S72.466Q
S72.466R
S72.471A
S72.471K
S72.471P
S72.472A
S72.472K
S72.472P
S72.479A
S72.479K
S72.479P
S72.491A
S72.491K
S72.491M
S72.491N
S72.491P
S72.491Q
S72.491R
S72.492A
S72.492K
S72.492M
S72.492N
S72.492P
S72.492Q
S72.492R
S72.499A
S72.499K
S72.499M
S72.499N
S72.499P
S72.499Q
S72.499R
S72.8X1K
S72.8X1M
S72.8X1N
S72.8X1P
S72.8X1Q
S72.8X1R
S72.8X2K
S72.8X2M
S72.8X2N
S72.8X2P
S72.8X2Q
S72.8X2R
S72.8X9K
S72.8X9M
S72.8X9N
S72.8X9P
S72.8X9Q
S72.8X9R
S72.9ØXK
S72.9ØXM
S72.9ØXN
S72.9ØXP
S72.9ØXQ
S72.9ØXR
S72.91XK
S72.91XM
S72.91XN
S72.91XP
S72.91XQ
S72.91XR
S72.92XK
S72.92XM
S72.92XN
S72.92XP
S72.92XQ
S72.92XR
S73.ØØ1A
S73.ØØ2A
S73.ØØ3A
S73.ØØ4A
S73.ØØ5A
S73.ØØ6A
S73.Ø11A
S73.Ø12A
S73.Ø13A
S73.Ø14A
S73.Ø15A
S73.Ø16A
S73.Ø21A
S73.Ø22A
S73.Ø23A
S73.Ø24A
S73.Ø25A
S73.Ø26A
S73.Ø31A
S73.Ø32A
S73.Ø33A
S73.Ø34A
S73.Ø35A
S73.Ø36A
S73.Ø41A
S73.Ø42A
S73.Ø43A
S73.Ø44A
S73.Ø45A
S73.Ø46A
S75.2Ø1A
S75.2Ø2A
S75.2Ø9A
S75.211A
S75.212A
S75.219A
S75.221A
S75.222A
S75.229A
S75.291A
S75.292A
S75.299A
S75.8Ø1A
S75.8Ø2A
S75.8Ø9A
S75.811A
S75.812A
S75.819A
S75.891A
S75.892A
S75.899A
S75.9Ø1A
S75.9Ø2A
S75.9Ø9A
S75.911A
S75.912A
S75.919A
S75.991A
S75.992A
S75.999A
S76.Ø21A
S76.Ø22A
S76.Ø29A
S76.121A
S76.122A
S76.129A
S76.221A
S76.222A
S76.229A
S76.321A
S76.322A
S76.329A
S76.821A
S76.822A
S76.829A
S76.921A
S76.922A
S76.929A
S77.ØØXA
S77.Ø1XA
S77.Ø2XA
S77.1ØXA
S77.11XA
S77.12XA
S78.Ø11A
S78.Ø12A
S78.Ø19A
S78.Ø21A
S78.Ø22A
S78.Ø29A
S78.111A
S78.112A
S78.119A
S78.121A
S78.122A
S78.129A
S78.911A
S78.912A
S78.919A
S78.921A
S78.922A
S78.929A
S79.ØØ1K
S79.ØØ1P
S79.ØØ2K
S79.ØØ2P
S79.ØØ9K
S79.ØØ9P
S79.Ø11K
S79.Ø11P
S79.Ø12K
S79.Ø12P
S79.Ø19K
S79.Ø19P
S79.Ø91K
S79.Ø91P
S79.Ø92K
S79.Ø92P
S79.Ø99K
S79.Ø99P
S79.1Ø1A
S79.1Ø1K
S79.1Ø1P
S79.1Ø2A
S79.1Ø2K
S79.1Ø2P
S79.1Ø9A
S79.1Ø9K
S79.1Ø9P
S79.111A
S79.111K
S79.111P
S79.112A
S79.112K
S79.112P
S79.119A
S79.119K
S79.119P
S79.121A
S79.121K
S79.121P
S79.122A
S79.122K
S79.122P
S79.129A
S79.129K
S79.129P
S79.131A
S79.131K
S79.131P
S79.132A
S79.132K
S79.132P
S79.139A
S79.139K
S79.139P
S79.141A
S79.141K
S79.141P
S79.142A
S79.142K
S79.142P
S79.149A
S79.149K
S79.149P
S79.191A
S79.191K
S79.191P
S79.192A
S79.192K
S79.192P
S79.199A
S79.199K
S79.199P
S82.ØØ1A
S82.ØØ1B
S82.ØØ1C
S82.ØØ1K
S82.ØØ1M
S82.ØØ1N
S82.ØØ1P
S82.ØØ1Q
S82.ØØ1R
S82.ØØ2A
S82.ØØ2B
S82.ØØ2C
S82.ØØ2K
S82.ØØ2M
S82.ØØ2N
S82.ØØ2P
S82.ØØ2Q
S82.ØØ2R
S82.ØØ9A
S82.ØØ9B
S82.ØØ9C
S82.ØØ9K
S82.ØØ9M
S82.ØØ9N
S82.ØØ9P
S82.ØØ9Q
S82.ØØ9R
S82.Ø11A
S82.Ø11B
S82.Ø11C
S82.Ø11K
S82.Ø11M
S82.Ø11N
S82.Ø11P
S82.Ø11Q
S82.Ø11R
S82.Ø12A
S82.Ø12B
S82.Ø12C
S82.Ø12K
S82.Ø12M
S82.Ø12N
S82.Ø12P
S82.Ø12Q
S82.Ø12R
S82.Ø13A
S82.Ø13B
S82.Ø13C
S82.Ø13K
S82.Ø13M
S82.Ø13N
S82.Ø13P
S82.Ø13Q
S82.Ø13R
S82.Ø14A
S82.Ø14B
S82.Ø14C
S82.Ø14K
S82.Ø14M
S82.Ø14N
S82.Ø14P
S82.Ø14Q
S82.Ø14R
S82.Ø15A
S82.Ø15B
S82.Ø15C
S82.Ø15K
S82.Ø15M
S82.Ø15N
S82.Ø15P
S82.Ø15Q
S82.Ø15R
S82.Ø16A
S82.Ø16B
S82.Ø16C
S82.Ø16K
S82.Ø16M
S82.Ø16N
S82.Ø16P
S82.Ø16Q
S82.Ø16R
S82.Ø21A
S82.Ø21B
S82.Ø21C
S82.Ø21K
S82.Ø21M
S82.Ø21N
S82.Ø21P
S82.Ø21Q
S82.Ø21R
S82.Ø22A
S82.Ø22B
S82.Ø22C
S82.Ø22K
S82.Ø22M
S82.Ø22N
S82.Ø22P
S82.Ø22Q
S82.Ø22R
S82.Ø23A
S82.Ø23B
S82.Ø23C
S82.Ø23K
S82.Ø23M
S82.Ø23N
S82.Ø23P
S82.Ø23Q
S82.Ø23R
S82.Ø24A
S82.Ø24B
S82.Ø24C
S82.Ø24K
S82.Ø24M
S82.Ø24N
S82.Ø24P
S82.Ø24Q
S82.Ø24R
S82.Ø25A
S82.Ø25B
S82.Ø25C
S82.Ø25K
S82.Ø25M
S82.Ø25N
S82.Ø25P
S82.Ø25Q
S82.Ø25R
S82.Ø26A
S82.Ø26B
S82.Ø26C
S82.Ø26K
S82.Ø26M
S82.Ø26N
S82.Ø26P
S82.Ø26Q
S82.Ø26R
S82.Ø31A
S82.Ø31B
S82.Ø31C
S82.Ø31K
S82.Ø31M
S82.Ø31N
S82.Ø31P
S82.Ø31Q
S82.Ø31R
S82.Ø32A
S82.Ø32B
S82.Ø32C
S82.Ø32K
S82.Ø32M
S82.Ø32N
S82.Ø32P
S82.Ø32Q
S82.Ø32R
S82.Ø33A
S82.Ø33B
S82.Ø33C
S82.Ø33K
S82.Ø33M
S82.Ø33N
S82.Ø33P
S82.Ø33Q
S82.Ø33R
S82.Ø34A
S82.Ø34B
S82.Ø34C
S82.Ø34K
S82.Ø34M
S82.Ø34N
S82.Ø34P
S82.Ø34Q
S82.Ø34R
S82.Ø35A
S82.Ø35B
S82.Ø35C
S82.Ø35K
S82.Ø35M
S82.Ø35N
S82.Ø35P
S82.Ø35Q
S82.Ø35R
S82.Ø36A
S82.Ø36B
S82.Ø36C
S82.Ø36K
S82.Ø36M
S82.Ø36N
S82.Ø36P
S82.Ø36Q
S82.Ø36R
S82.Ø41A
S82.Ø41B
S82.Ø41C
S82.Ø41K
S82.Ø41M
S82.Ø41N
S82.Ø41P
S82.Ø41Q
S82.Ø41R
S82.Ø42A
S82.Ø42B
S82.Ø42C
S82.Ø42K
S82.Ø42M
S82.Ø42N
S82.Ø42P
S82.Ø42Q
S82.Ø42R
S82.Ø43A
S82.Ø43B
S82.Ø43C
S82.Ø43K
S82.Ø43M
S82.Ø43N
S82.Ø43P
S82.Ø43Q
S82.Ø43R
S82.Ø44A
S82.Ø44B
S82.Ø44C
S82.Ø44K
S82.Ø44M
S82.Ø44N
S82.Ø44P
S82.Ø44Q
S82.Ø44R
S82.Ø45A
S82.Ø45B
S82.Ø45C
S82.Ø45K
S82.Ø45M
S82.Ø45N
S82.Ø45P
S82.Ø45Q
S82.Ø45R
S82.Ø46A
S82.Ø46B
S82.Ø46C
S82.Ø46K
S82.Ø46M
S82.Ø46N
S82.Ø46P
S82.Ø46Q
S82.Ø46R
S82.Ø91A
S82.Ø91B
S82.Ø91C
S82.Ø91K
S82.Ø91M
S82.Ø91N
S82.Ø91P
S82.Ø91Q
S82.Ø91R
S82.Ø92A
S82.Ø92B
S82.Ø92C
S82.Ø92K
S82.Ø92M
S82.Ø92N
S82.Ø92P
S82.Ø92Q
S82.Ø92R
S82.Ø99A
S82.Ø99B
S82.Ø99C
S82.Ø99K
S82.Ø99M
S82.Ø99N
S82.Ø99P
S82.Ø99Q
S82.Ø99R
S82.1Ø1A
S82.1Ø1K
S82.1Ø1M
S82.1Ø1N
S82.1Ø1P
S82.1Ø1Q
S82.1Ø1R

Appendix E: Complication and Comorbidity (CC) Code List

S82.1Ø2A
S82.1Ø2K
S82.1Ø2M
S82.1Ø2N
S82.1Ø2P
S82.1Ø2Q
S82.1Ø2R
S82.1Ø9A
S82.1Ø9K
S82.1Ø9M
S82.1Ø9N
S82.1Ø9P
S82.1Ø9Q
S82.1Ø9R
S82.111A
S82.111K
S82.111M
S82.111N
S82.111P
S82.111Q
S82.111R
S82.112A
S82.112K
S82.112M
S82.112N
S82.112P
S82.112Q
S82.112R
S82.113A
S82.113K
S82.113M
S82.113N
S82.113P
S82.113Q
S82.113R
S82.114A
S82.114K
S82.114M
S82.114N
S82.114P
S82.114Q
S82.114R
S82.115A
S82.115K
S82.115M
S82.115N
S82.115P
S82.115Q
S82.115R
S82.116A
S82.116K
S82.116M
S82.116N
S82.116P
S82.116Q
S82.116R
S82.121A
S82.121K
S82.121M
S82.121N
S82.121P
S82.121Q
S82.121R
S82.122A
S82.122K
S82.122M
S82.122N
S82.122P
S82.122Q
S82.122R
S82.123A
S82.123K
S82.123M
S82.123N
S82.123P
S82.123Q
S82.123R
S82.124A
S82.124K
S82.124M
S82.124N
S82.124P
S82.124Q
S82.124R
S82.125A
S82.125K
S82.125M
S82.125N
S82.125P
S82.125Q
S82.125R
S82.126A
S82.126K
S82.126M
S82.126N
S82.126P
S82.126Q
S82.126R
S82.131A
S82.131K
S82.131M
S82.131N
S82.131P
S82.131Q
S82.131R
S82.132A
S82.132K
S82.132M
S82.132N
S82.132P
S82.132Q
S82.132R
S82.133A
S82.133K
S82.133M
S82.133N
S82.133P
S82.133Q
S82.133R
S82.134A
S82.134K
S82.134M
S82.134N
S82.134P
S82.134Q
S82.134R
S82.135A
S82.135K
S82.135M
S82.135N
S82.135P
S82.135Q
S82.135R
S82.136A
S82.136K
S82.136M
S82.136N
S82.136P
S82.136Q
S82.136R
S82.141A
S82.141K
S82.141M
S82.141N
S82.141P
S82.141Q
S82.141R
S82.142A
S82.142K
S82.142M
S82.142N
S82.142P
S82.142Q
S82.142R
S82.143A
S82.143K
S82.143M
S82.143N
S82.143P
S82.143Q
S82.143R
S82.144A
S82.144K
S82.144M
S82.144N
S82.144P
S82.144Q
S82.144R
S82.145A
S82.145K
S82.145M
S82.145N
S82.145P
S82.145Q
S82.145R
S82.146A
S82.146K
S82.146M
S82.146N
S82.146P
S82.146Q
S82.146R
S82.151A
S82.151K
S82.151M
S82.151N
S82.151P
S82.151Q
S82.151R
S82.152A
S82.152K
S82.152M
S82.152N
S82.152P
S82.152Q
S82.152R
S82.153A
S82.153K
S82.153M
S82.153N
S82.153P
S82.153Q
S82.153R
S82.154A
S82.154K
S82.154M
S82.154N
S82.154P
S82.154Q
S82.154R
S82.155A
S82.155K
S82.155M
S82.155N
S82.155P
S82.155Q
S82.155R
S82.156A
S82.156K
S82.156M
S82.156N
S82.156P
S82.156Q
S82.156R
S82.161A
S82.161K
S82.161P
S82.162A
S82.162K
S82.162P
S82.169A
S82.169K
S82.169P
S82.191A
S82.191K
S82.191M
S82.191N
S82.191P
S82.191Q
S82.191R
S82.192A
S82.192K
S82.192M
S82.192N
S82.192P
S82.192Q
S82.192R
S82.199A
S82.199K
S82.199M
S82.199N
S82.199P
S82.199Q
S82.199R
S82.2Ø1A
S82.2Ø1K
S82.2Ø1M
S82.2Ø1N
S82.2Ø1P
S82.2Ø1Q
S82.2Ø1R
S82.2Ø2A
S82.2Ø2K
S82.2Ø2M
S82.2Ø2N
S82.2Ø2P
S82.2Ø2Q
S82.2Ø2R
S82.2Ø9A
S82.2Ø9K
S82.2Ø9M
S82.2Ø9N
S82.2Ø9P
S82.2Ø9Q
S82.2Ø9R
S82.221A
S82.221K
S82.221M
S82.221N
S82.221P
S82.221Q
S82.221R
S82.222A
S82.222K
S82.222M
S82.222N
S82.222P
S82.222Q
S82.222R
S82.223A
S82.223K
S82.223M
S82.223N
S82.223P
S82.223Q
S82.223R
S82.224A
S82.224K
S82.224M
S82.224N
S82.224P
S82.224Q
S82.224R
S82.225A
S82.225K
S82.225M
S82.225N
S82.225P
S82.225Q
S82.225R
S82.226A
S82.226K
S82.226M
S82.226N
S82.226P
S82.226Q
S82.226R
S82.231A
S82.231K
S82.231M
S82.231N
S82.231P
S82.231Q
S82.231R
S82.232A
S82.232K
S82.232M
S82.232N
S82.232P
S82.232Q
S82.232R
S82.233A
S82.233K
S82.233M
S82.233N
S82.233P
S82.233Q
S82.233R
S82.234A
S82.234K
S82.234M
S82.234N
S82.234P
S82.234Q
S82.234R
S82.235A
S82.235K
S82.235M
S82.235N
S82.235P
S82.235Q
S82.235R
S82.236A
S82.236K
S82.236M
S82.236N
S82.236P
S82.236Q
S82.236R
S82.241A
S82.241K
S82.241M
S82.241N
S82.241P
S82.241Q
S82.241R
S82.242A
S82.242K
S82.242M
S82.242N
S82.242P
S82.242Q
S82.242R
S82.243A
S82.243K
S82.243M
S82.243N
S82.243P
S82.243Q
S82.243R
S82.244A
S82.244K
S82.244M
S82.244N
S82.244P
S82.244Q
S82.244R
S82.245A
S82.245K
S82.245M
S82.245N
S82.245P
S82.245Q
S82.245R
S82.246A
S82.246K
S82.246M
S82.246N
S82.246P
S82.246Q
S82.246R
S82.251A
S82.251K
S82.251M
S82.251N
S82.251P
S82.251Q
S82.251R
S82.252A
S82.252K
S82.252M
S82.252N
S82.252P
S82.252Q
S82.252R
S82.253A
S82.253K
S82.253M
S82.253N
S82.253P
S82.253Q
S82.253R
S82.254A
S82.254K
S82.254M
S82.254N
S82.254P
S82.254Q
S82.254R
S82.255A
S82.255K
S82.255M
S82.255N
S82.255P
S82.255Q
S82.255R
S82.256A
S82.256K
S82.256M
S82.256N
S82.256P
S82.256Q
S82.256R
S82.261A
S82.261K
S82.261M
S82.261N
S82.261P
S82.261Q
S82.261R
S82.262A
S82.262K
S82.262M
S82.262N
S82.262P
S82.262Q
S82.262R
S82.263A
S82.263K
S82.263M
S82.263N
S82.263P
S82.263Q
S82.263R
S82.264A
S82.264K
S82.264M
S82.264N
S82.264P
S82.264Q
S82.264R
S82.265A
S82.265K
S82.265M
S82.265N
S82.265P
S82.265Q
S82.265R
S82.266A
S82.266K
S82.266M
S82.266N
S82.266P
S82.266Q
S82.266R
S82.291A
S82.291K
S82.291M
S82.291N
S82.291P
S82.291Q
S82.291R
S82.292A
S82.292K
S82.292M
S82.292N
S82.292P
S82.292Q
S82.292R
S82.299A
S82.299K
S82.299M
S82.299N
S82.299P
S82.299Q
S82.299R
S82.3Ø1B
S82.3Ø1C
S82.3Ø1K
S82.3Ø1M
S82.3Ø1N
S82.3Ø1P
S82.3Ø1Q
S82.3Ø1R
S82.3Ø2B
S82.3Ø2C
S82.3Ø2K
S82.3Ø2M
S82.3Ø2N
S82.3Ø2P
S82.3Ø2Q
S82.3Ø2R
S82.3Ø9B
S82.3Ø9C
S82.3Ø9K
S82.3Ø9M
S82.3Ø9N
S82.3Ø9P
S82.3Ø9Q
S82.3Ø9R
S82.311A
S82.311K
S82.311P
S82.312A
S82.312K
S82.312P
S82.319A
S82.319K
S82.319P
S82.391B
S82.391C
S82.391K
S82.391M
S82.391N
S82.391P
S82.391Q
S82.391R
S82.392B
S82.392C
S82.392K
S82.392M
S82.392N
S82.392P
S82.392Q
S82.392R
S82.399B
S82.399C
S82.399K
S82.399M
S82.399N
S82.399P
S82.399Q
S82.399R
S82.4Ø1K
S82.4Ø1M
S82.4Ø1N
S82.4Ø1P
S82.4Ø1Q
S82.4Ø1R
S82.4Ø2K
S82.4Ø2M
S82.4Ø2N
S82.4Ø2P
S82.4Ø2Q
S82.4Ø2R
S82.4Ø9K
S82.4Ø9M
S82.4Ø9N
S82.4Ø9P
S82.4Ø9Q
S82.4Ø9R
S82.421K
S82.421M
S82.421N
S82.421P
S82.421Q
S82.421R
S82.422K
S82.422M
S82.422N
S82.422P
S82.422Q
S82.422R
S82.423K
S82.423M
S82.423N
S82.423P
S82.423Q
S82.423R
S82.424K
S82.424M
S82.424N
S82.424P
S82.424Q
S82.424R
S82.425K
S82.425M
S82.425N
S82.425P
S82.425Q
S82.425R
S82.426K
S82.426M
S82.426N
S82.426P
S82.426Q
S82.426R
S82.431K
S82.431M
S82.431N
S82.431P
S82.431Q
S82.431R
S82.432K
S82.432M
S82.432N
S82.432P
S82.432Q
S82.432R
S82.433K
S82.433M
S82.433N
S82.433P
S82.433Q
S82.433R
S82.434K
S82.434M
S82.434N
S82.434P
S82.434Q
S82.434R
S82.435K
S82.435M
S82.435N
S82.435P
S82.435Q
S82.435R
S82.436K
S82.436M
S82.436N
S82.436P
S82.436Q
S82.436R
S82.441K
S82.441M
S82.441N
S82.441P
S82.441Q
S82.441R
S82.442K
S82.442M
S82.442N
S82.442P
S82.442Q
S82.442R
S82.443K
S82.443M
S82.443N
S82.443P
S82.443Q
S82.443R
S82.444K
S82.444M
S82.444N
S82.444P
S82.444Q
S82.444R
S82.445K
S82.445M
S82.445N
S82.445P
S82.445Q
S82.445R
S82.446K
S82.446M
S82.446N
S82.446P
S82.446Q
S82.446R
S82.451K
S82.451M
S82.451N
S82.451P

S82.451Q
S82.451R
S82.452K
S82.452M
S82.452N
S82.452P
S82.452Q
S82.452R
S82.453K
S82.453M
S82.453N
S82.453P
S82.453Q
S82.453R
S82.454K
S82.454M
S82.454N
S82.454P
S82.454Q
S82.454R
S82.455K
S82.455M
S82.455N
S82.455P
S82.455Q
S82.455R
S82.456K
S82.456M
S82.456N
S82.456P
S82.456Q
S82.456R
S82.461K
S82.461M
S82.461N
S82.461P
S82.461Q
S82.461R
S82.462K
S82.462M
S82.462N
S82.462P
S82.462Q
S82.462R
S82.463K
S82.463M
S82.463N
S82.463P
S82.463Q
S82.463R
S82.464K
S82.464M
S82.464N
S82.464P
S82.464Q
S82.464R
S82.465K
S82.465M
S82.465N
S82.465P
S82.465Q
S82.465R
S82.466K
S82.466M
S82.466N
S82.466P
S82.466Q
S82.466R
S82.491K
S82.491M
S82.491N
S82.491P
S82.491Q
S82.491R
S82.492K
S82.492M
S82.492N
S82.492P
S82.492Q
S82.492R
S82.499K
S82.499M
S82.499N
S82.499P
S82.499Q
S82.499R
S82.51XB
S82.51XC
S82.51XK
S82.51XM
S82.51XN
S82.51XP
S82.51XQ
S82.51XR
S82.52XB
S82.52XC
S82.52XK
S82.52XM
S82.52XN
S82.52XP
S82.52XQ
S82.52XR
S82.53XB
S82.53XC
S82.53XK
S82.53XM
S82.53XN
S82.53XP
S82.53XQ
S82.53XR
S82.54XB
S82.54XC
S82.54XK
S82.54XM
S82.54XN
S82.54XP
S82.54XQ
S82.54XR
S82.55XB
S82.55XC
S82.55XK
S82.55XM
S82.55XN
S82.55XP
S82.55XQ
S82.55XR
S82.56XB
S82.56XC
S82.56XK
S82.56XM
S82.56XN
S82.56XP
S82.56XQ
S82.56XR
S82.61XB
S82.61XC
S82.61XK
S82.61XM
S82.61XN
S82.61XP
S82.61XQ
S82.61XR
S82.62XB
S82.62XC
S82.62XK
S82.62XM
S82.62XN
S82.62XP
S82.62XQ
S82.62XR
S82.63XB
S82.63XC
S82.63XK
S82.63XM
S82.63XN
S82.63XP
S82.63XQ
S82.63XR
S82.64XB
S82.64XC
S82.64XK
S82.64XM
S82.64XN
S82.64XP
S82.64XQ
S82.64XR
S82.65XB
S82.65XC
S82.65XK
S82.65XM
S82.65XN
S82.65XP
S82.65XQ
S82.65XR
S82.66XB
S82.66XC
S82.66XK
S82.66XM
S82.66XN
S82.66XP
S82.66XQ
S82.66XR
S82.811K
S82.811P
S82.812K
S82.812P
S82.819K
S82.819P
S82.821K
S82.821P
S82.822K
S82.822P
S82.829K
S82.829P
S82.831K
S82.831M
S82.831N
S82.831P
S82.831Q
S82.831R
S82.832K
S82.832M
S82.832N
S82.832P
S82.832Q
S82.832R
S82.839K
S82.839M
S82.839N
S82.839P
S82.839Q
S82.839R
S82.841B
S82.841C
S82.841K
S82.841M
S82.841N
S82.841P
S82.841Q
S82.841R
S82.842B
S82.842C
S82.842K
S82.842M
S82.842N
S82.842P
S82.842Q
S82.842R
S82.843B
S82.843C
S82.843K
S82.843M
S82.843N
S82.843P
S82.843Q
S82.843R
S82.844B
S82.844C
S82.844K
S82.844M
S82.844N
S82.844P
S82.844Q
S82.844R
S82.845B
S82.845C
S82.845K
S82.845M
S82.845N
S82.845P
S82.845Q
S82.845R
S82.846B
S82.846C
S82.846K
S82.846M
S82.846N
S82.846P
S82.846Q
S82.846R
S82.851B
S82.851C
S82.851K
S82.851M
S82.851N
S82.851P
S82.851Q
S82.851R
S82.852B
S82.852C
S82.852K
S82.852M
S82.852N
S82.852P
S82.852Q
S82.852R
S82.853B
S82.853C
S82.853K
S82.853M
S82.853N
S82.853P
S82.853Q
S82.853R
S82.854B
S82.854C
S82.854K
S82.854M
S82.854N
S82.854P
S82.854Q
S82.854R
S82.855B
S82.855C
S82.855K
S82.855M
S82.855N
S82.855P
S82.855Q
S82.855R
S82.856B
S82.856C
S82.856K
S82.856M
S82.856N
S82.856P
S82.856Q
S82.856R
S82.861K
S82.861M
S82.861N
S82.861P
S82.861Q
S82.861R
S82.862K
S82.862M
S82.862N
S82.862P
S82.862Q
S82.862R
S82.863K
S82.863M
S82.863N
S82.863P
S82.863Q
S82.863R
S82.864K
S82.864M
S82.864N
S82.864P
S82.864Q
S82.864R
S82.865K
S82.865M
S82.865N
S82.865P
S82.865Q
S82.865R
S82.866K
S82.866M
S82.866N
S82.866P
S82.866Q
S82.866R
S82.871B
S82.871C
S82.871K
S82.871M
S82.871N
S82.871P
S82.871Q
S82.871R
S82.872B
S82.872C
S82.872K
S82.872M
S82.872N
S82.872P
S82.872Q
S82.872R
S82.873B
S82.873C
S82.873K
S82.873M
S82.873N
S82.873P
S82.873Q
S82.873R
S82.874B
S82.874C
S82.874K
S82.874M
S82.874N
S82.874P
S82.874Q
S82.874R
S82.875B
S82.875C
S82.875K
S82.875M
S82.875N
S82.875P
S82.875Q
S82.875R
S82.876B
S82.876C
S82.876K
S82.876M
S82.876N
S82.876P
S82.876Q
S82.876R
S82.891B
S82.891C
S82.891K
S82.891M
S82.891N
S82.891P
S82.891Q
S82.891R
S82.892B
S82.892C
S82.892K
S82.892M
S82.892N
S82.892P
S82.892Q
S82.892R
S82.899B
S82.899C
S82.899K
S82.899M
S82.899N
S82.899P
S82.899Q
S82.899R
S82.9ØXB
S82.9ØXC
S82.9ØXK
S82.9ØXM
S82.9ØXN
S82.9ØXP
S82.9ØXQ
S82.9ØXR
S82.91XB
S82.91XC
S82.91XK
S82.91XM
S82.91XN
S82.91XP
S82.91XQ
S82.91XR
S82.92XB
S82.92XC
S82.92XK
S82.92XM
S82.92XN
S82.92XP
S82.92XQ
S82.92XR
S85.1Ø1A
S85.1Ø2A
S85.1Ø9A
S85.111A
S85.112A
S85.119A
S85.121A
S85.122A
S85.129A
S85.131A
S85.132A
S85.139A
S85.141A
S85.142A
S85.149A
S85.151A
S85.152A
S85.159A
S85.161A
S85.162A
S85.169A
S85.171A
S85.172A
S85.179A
S85.181A
S85.182A
S85.189A
S85.2Ø1A
S85.2Ø2A
S85.2Ø9A
S85.211A
S85.212A
S85.219A
S85.291A
S85.292A
S85.299A
S85.3Ø1A
S85.3Ø2A
S85.3Ø9A
S85.311A
S85.312A
S85.319A
S85.391A
S85.392A
S85.399A
S85.4Ø1A
S85.4Ø2A
S85.4Ø9A
S85.411A
S85.412A
S85.419A
S85.491A
S85.492A
S85.499A
S85.8Ø1A
S85.8Ø2A
S85.8Ø9A
S85.811A
S85.812A
S85.819A
S85.891A
S85.892A
S85.899A
S85.9Ø1A
S85.9Ø2A
S85.9Ø9A
S85.911A
S85.912A
S85.919A
S85.991A
S85.992A
S85.999A
S86.Ø21A
S86.Ø22A
S86.Ø29A
S86.121A
S86.122A
S86.129A
S86.221A
S86.222A
S86.229A
S86.321A
S86.322A
S86.329A
S86.821A
S86.822A
S86.829A
S86.921A
S86.922A
S86.929A
S88.Ø11A
S88.Ø12A
S88.Ø19A
S88.Ø21A
S88.Ø22A
S88.Ø29A
S88.111A
S88.112A
S88.119A
S88.121A
S88.122A
S88.129A
S88.911A
S88.912A
S88.919A
S88.921A
S88.922A
S88.929A
S89.ØØ1A
S89.ØØ1K
S89.ØØ1P
S89.ØØ2A
S89.ØØ2K
S89.ØØ2P
S89.ØØ9A
S89.ØØ9K
S89.ØØ9P
S89.Ø11A
S89.Ø11K
S89.Ø11P
S89.Ø12A
S89.Ø12K
S89.Ø12P
S89.Ø19A
S89.Ø19K
S89.Ø19P
S89.Ø21A
S89.Ø21K
S89.Ø21P
S89.Ø22A
S89.Ø22K
S89.Ø22P
S89.Ø29A
S89.Ø29K
S89.Ø29P
S89.Ø31A
S89.Ø31K
S89.Ø31P
S89.Ø32A
S89.Ø32K
S89.Ø32P
S89.Ø39A
S89.Ø39K
S89.Ø39P
S89.Ø41A
S89.Ø41K
S89.Ø41P
S89.Ø42A
S89.Ø42K
S89.Ø42P
S89.Ø49A
S89.Ø49K
S89.Ø49P
S89.Ø91A
S89.Ø91K
S89.Ø91P
S89.Ø92A
S89.Ø92K
S89.Ø92P
S89.Ø99A
S89.Ø99K
S89.Ø99P
S89.1Ø1K
S89.1Ø1P
S89.1Ø2K
S89.1Ø2P
S89.1Ø9K
S89.1Ø9P
S89.111K
S89.111P
S89.112K
S89.112P
S89.119K
S89.119P
S89.121K
S89.121P
S89.122K
S89.122P
S89.129K
S89.129P
S89.131K
S89.131P
S89.132K
S89.132P
S89.139K
S89.139P
S89.141K
S89.141P
S89.142K
S89.142P
S89.149K
S89.149P
S89.191K
S89.191P
S89.192K
S89.192P
S89.199K
S89.199P
S89.2Ø1K
S89.2Ø1P
S89.2Ø2K
S89.2Ø2P
S89.2Ø9K
S89.2Ø9P
S89.211K
S89.211P
S89.212K
S89.212P
S89.219K
S89.219P
S89.221K
S89.221P
S89.222K
S89.222P
S89.229K
S89.229P
S89.291K
S89.291P
S89.292K
S89.292P
S89.299K
S89.299P
S89.3Ø1K
S89.3Ø1P
S89.3Ø2K
S89.3Ø2P
S89.3Ø9K
S89.3Ø9P
S89.311K
S89.311P
S89.312K
S89.312P
S89.319K
S89.319P
S89.321K
S89.321P
S89.322K
S89.322P
S89.329K
S89.329P
S89.391K
S89.391P
S89.392K
S89.392P
S89.399K
S89.399P
S92.ØØ1B
S92.ØØ1K
S92.ØØ1P
S92.ØØ2B
S92.ØØ2K
S92.ØØ2P
S92.ØØ9B

S92.009K
S92.009P
S92.011B
S92.011K
S92.011P
S92.012B
S92.012K
S92.012P
S92.013B
S92.013K
S92.013P
S92.014B
S92.014K
S92.014P
S92.015B
S92.015K
S92.015P
S92.016B
S92.016K
S92.016P
S92.021B
S92.021K
S92.021P
S92.022B
S92.022K
S92.022P
S92.023B
S92.023K
S92.023P
S92.024B
S92.024K
S92.024P
S92.025B
S92.025K
S92.025P
S92.026B
S92.026K
S92.026P
S92.031B
S92.031K
S92.031P
S92.032B
S92.032K
S92.032P
S92.033B
S92.033K
S92.033P
S92.034B
S92.034K
S92.034P
S92.035B
S92.035K
S92.035P
S92.036B
S92.036K
S92.036P
S92.041B
S92.041K
S92.041P
S92.042B
S92.042K
S92.042P
S92.043B
S92.043K
S92.043P
S92.044B
S92.044K
S92.044P
S92.045B
S92.045K
S92.045P
S92.046B
S92.046K
S92.046P
S92.051B
S92.051K
S92.051P
S92.052B
S92.052K
S92.052P
S92.053B
S92.053K
S92.053P
S92.054B
S92.054K
S92.054P
S92.055B
S92.055K
S92.055P
S92.056B
S92.056K
S92.056P
S92.061B
S92.061K
S92.061P
S92.062B
S92.062K
S92.062P
S92.063B
S92.063K
S92.063P
S92.064B
S92.064K
S92.064P
S92.065B
S92.065K
S92.065P
S92.066B
S92.066K
S92.066P
S92.101B
S92.101K
S92.101P
S92.102B
S92.102K
S92.102P
S92.109B
S92.109K
S92.109P
S92.111B
S92.111K
S92.111P
S92.112B
S92.112K
S92.112P
S92.113B
S92.113K
S92.113P
S92.114B
S92.114K
S92.114P
S92.115B
S92.115K
S92.115P
S92.116B
S92.116K
S92.116P
S92.121B
S92.121K
S92.121P
S92.122B
S92.122K
S92.122P
S92.123B
S92.123K
S92.123P
S92.124B
S92.124K
S92.124P
S92.125B
S92.125K
S92.125P
S92.126B
S92.126K
S92.126P
S92.131B
S92.131K
S92.131P
S92.132B
S92.132K
S92.132P
S92.133B
S92.133K
S92.133P
S92.134B
S92.134K
S92.134P
S92.135B
S92.135K
S92.135P
S92.136B
S92.136K
S92.136P
S92.141B
S92.141K
S92.141P
S92.142B
S92.142K
S92.142P
S92.143B
S92.143K
S92.143P
S92.144B
S92.144K
S92.144P
S92.145B
S92.145K
S92.145P
S92.146B
S92.146K
S92.146P
S92.151B
S92.151K
S92.151P
S92.152B
S92.152K
S92.152P
S92.153B
S92.153K
S92.153P
S92.154B
S92.154K
S92.154P
S92.155B
S92.155K
S92.155P
S92.156B
S92.156K
S92.156P
S92.191B
S92.191K
S92.191P
S92.192B
S92.192K
S92.192P
S92.199B
S92.199K
S92.199P
S92.201B
S92.201K
S92.201P
S92.202B
S92.202K
S92.202P
S92.209B
S92.209K
S92.209P
S92.211B
S92.211K
S92.211P
S92.212B
S92.212K
S92.212P
S92.213B
S92.213K
S92.213P
S92.214B
S92.214K
S92.214P
S92.215B
S92.215K
S92.215P
S92.216B
S92.216K
S92.216P
S92.221B
S92.221K
S92.221P
S92.222B
S92.222K
S92.222P
S92.223B
S92.223K
S92.223P
S92.224B
S92.224K
S92.224P
S92.225B
S92.225K
S92.225P
S92.226B
S92.226K
S92.226P
S92.231B
S92.231K
S92.231P
S92.232B
S92.232K
S92.232P
S92.233B
S92.233K
S92.233P
S92.234B
S92.234K
S92.234P
S92.235B
S92.235K
S92.235P
S92.236B
S92.236K
S92.236P
S92.241B
S92.241K
S92.241P
S92.242B
S92.242K
S92.242P
S92.243B
S92.243K
S92.243P
S92.244B
S92.244K
S92.244P
S92.245B
S92.245K
S92.245P
S92.246B
S92.246K
S92.246P
S92.251B
S92.251K
S92.251P
S92.252B
S92.252K
S92.252P
S92.253B
S92.253K
S92.253P
S92.254B
S92.254K
S92.254P
S92.255B
S92.255K
S92.255P
S92.256B
S92.256K
S92.256P
S92.301B
S92.301K
S92.301P
S92.302B
S92.302K
S92.302P
S92.309B
S92.309K
S92.309P
S92.311B
S92.311K
S92.311P
S92.312B
S92.312K
S92.312P
S92.313B
S92.313K
S92.313P
S92.314B
S92.314K
S92.314P
S92.315B
S92.315K
S92.315P
S92.316B
S92.316K
S92.316P
S92.321B
S92.321K
S92.321P
S92.322B
S92.322K
S92.322P
S92.323B
S92.323K
S92.323P
S92.324B
S92.324K
S92.324P
S92.325B
S92.325K
S92.325P
S92.326B
S92.326K
S92.326P
S92.331B
S92.331K
S92.331P
S92.332B
S92.332K
S92.332P
S92.333B
S92.333K
S92.333P
S92.334B
S92.334K
S92.334P
S92.335B
S92.335K
S92.335P
S92.336B
S92.336K
S92.336P
S92.341B
S92.341K
S92.341P
S92.342B
S92.342K
S92.342P
S92.343B
S92.343K
S92.343P
S92.344B
S92.344K
S92.344P
S92.345B
S92.345K
S92.345P
S92.346B
S92.346K
S92.346P
S92.351B
S92.351K
S92.351P
S92.352B
S92.352K
S92.352P
S92.353B
S92.353K
S92.353P
S92.354B
S92.354K
S92.354P
S92.355B
S92.355K
S92.355P
S92.356B
S92.356K
S92.356P
S92.401K
S92.401P
S92.402K
S92.402P
S92.403K
S92.403P
S92.404K
S92.404P
S92.405K
S92.405P
S92.406K
S92.406P
S92.411K
S92.411P
S92.412K
S92.412P
S92.413K
S92.413P
S92.414K
S92.414P
S92.415K
S92.415P
S92.416K
S92.416P
S92.421K
S92.421P
S92.422K
S92.422P
S92.423K
S92.423P
S92.424K
S92.424P
S92.425K
S92.425P
S92.426K
S92.426P
S92.491K
S92.491P
S92.492K
S92.492P
S92.499K
S92.499P
S92.501K
S92.501P
S92.502K
S92.502P
S92.503K
S92.503P
S92.504K
S92.504P
S92.505K
S92.505P
S92.506K
S92.506P
S92.511K
S92.511P
S92.512K
S92.512P
S92.513K
S92.513P
S92.514K
S92.514P
S92.515K
S92.515P
S92.516K
S92.516P
S92.521K
S92.521P
S92.522K
S92.522P
S92.523K
S92.523P
S92.524K
S92.524P
S92.525K
S92.525P
S92.526K
S92.526P
S92.531K
S92.531P
S92.532K
S92.532P
S92.533K
S92.533P
S92.534K
S92.534P
S92.535K
S92.535P
S92.536K
S92.536P
S92.591K
S92.591P
S92.592K
S92.592P
S92.599K
S92.599P
S92.811B
S92.811K
S92.811P
S92.812B
S92.812K
S92.812P
S92.819B
S92.819K
S92.819P
S92.901B
S92.901K
S92.901P
S92.902B
S92.902K
S92.902P
S92.909B
S92.909K
S92.909P
S92.911K
S92.911P
S92.912K
S92.912P
S92.919K
S92.919P
S95.001A
S95.002A
S95.009A
S95.011A
S95.012A
S95.019A
S95.091A
S95.092A
S95.099A
S95.101A
S95.102A
S95.109A
S95.111A
S95.112A
S95.119A
S95.191A
S95.192A
S95.199A
S95.201A
S95.202A
S95.209A
S95.211A
S95.212A
S95.219A
S95.291A
S95.292A
S95.299A
S95.801A
S95.802A
S95.809A
S95.811A
S95.812A
S95.819A
S95.891A
S95.892A
S95.899A
S95.901A
S95.902A
S95.909A
S95.911A
S95.912A
S95.919A
S95.991A
S95.992A
S95.999A
S96.021A
S96.022A
S96.029A
S96.121A
S96.122A
S96.129A
S96.221A
S96.222A
S96.229A
S96.821A
S96.822A
S96.829A
S96.921A
S96.922A
S96.929A
S98.011A
S98.012A
S98.019A
S98.021A
S98.022A
S98.029A
S98.311A
S98.312A
S98.319A
S98.321A
S98.322A
S98.329A
S98.911A
S98.912A
S98.919A
S98.921A
S98.922A
S98.929A
T17.400A
T17.408A
T17.410A
T17.418A
T17.420A
T17.428A
T17.490A
T17.498A
T17.500A
T17.508A
T17.510A
T17.518A
T17.520A
T17.528A
T17.590A
T17.598A
T17.800A
T17.808A
T17.810A
T17.818A
T17.820A
T17.828A
T17.890A
T17.898A
T20.30XA
T20.311A
T20.312A
T20.319A
T20.32XA
T20.33XA
T20.34XA
T20.35XA
T20.36XA
T20.37XA
T20.39XA
T20.70XA
T20.711A
T20.712A
T20.719A
T20.72XA
T20.73XA
T20.74XA
T20.75XA
T20.76XA
T20.77XA
T20.79XA
T21.30XA
T21.31XA
T21.32XA
T21.33XA
T21.34XA
T21.35XA
T21.36XA
T21.37XA
T21.39XA
T21.70XA
T21.71XA
T21.72XA
T21.73XA
T21.74XA
T21.75XA
T21.76XA
T21.77XA
T21.79XA
T22.30XA
T22.311A
T22.312A
T22.319A
T22.321A
T22.322A
T22.329A
T22.331A
T22.332A
T22.339A
T22.341A
T22.342A
T22.349A
T22.351A
T22.352A

T22.359A
T22.361A
T22.362A
T22.369A
T22.391A
T22.392A
T22.399A
T22.7ØXA
T22.711A
T22.712A
T22.719A
T22.721A
T22.722A
T22.729A
T22.731A
T22.732A
T22.739A
T22.741A
T22.742A
T22.749A
T22.751A
T22.752A
T22.759A
T22.761A
T22.762A
T22.769A
T22.791A
T22.792A
T22.799A
T23.3Ø1A
T23.3Ø2A
T23.3Ø9A
T23.311A
T23.312A
T23.319A
T23.321A
T23.322A
T23.329A
T23.331A
T23.332A
T23.339A
T23.341A
T23.342A
T23.349A
T23.351A
T23.352A
T23.359A
T23.361A
T23.362A
T23.369A
T23.371A
T23.372A
T23.379A
T23.391A
T23.392A
T23.399A
T23.7Ø1A
T23.7Ø2A
T23.7Ø9A
T23.711A
T23.712A
T23.719A
T23.721A
T23.722A
T23.729A
T23.731A
T23.732A
T23.739A
T23.741A
T23.742A
T23.749A
T23.751A
T23.752A
T23.759A
T23.761A
T23.762A
T23.769A
T23.771A
T23.772A
T23.779A
T23.791A
T23.792A
T23.799A
T24.3Ø1A
T24.3Ø2A
T24.3Ø9A
T24.311A
T24.312A
T24.319A
T24.321A
T24.322A
T24.329A
T24.331A
T24.332A
T24.339A
T24.391A
T24.392A
T24.399A
T24.7Ø1A
T24.7Ø2A
T24.7Ø9A
T24.711A
T24.712A
T24.719A
T24.721A
T24.722A
T24.729A
T24.731A
T24.732A
T24.739A
T24.791A
T24.792A
T24.799A
T25.311A
T25.312A
T25.319A
T25.321A
T25.322A
T25.329A
T25.331A
T25.332A
T25.339A
T25.391A
T25.392A
T25.399A
T25.711A
T25.712A
T25.719A
T25.721A
T25.722A
T25.729A
T25.731A
T25.732A
T25.739A
T25.791A
T25.792A
T25.799A
T26.2ØXA
T26.21XA
T26.22XA
T26.7ØXA
T26.71XA
T26.72XA
T27.ØXXA
T27.1XXA
T27.2XXA
T27.3XXA
T27.4XXA
T27.5XXA
T27.6XXA
T27.7XXA
T28.1XXA
T28.2XXA
T28.6XXA
T28.7XXA
T31.1Ø
T31.11
T31.2Ø
T31.3Ø
T31.4Ø
T31.5Ø
T31.6Ø
T31.7Ø
T31.8Ø
T31.9Ø
T32.1Ø
T32.11
T32.2Ø
T32.3Ø
T32.4Ø
T32.5Ø
T32.6Ø
T32.7Ø
T32.8Ø
T32.9Ø
T33.Ø11A
T33.Ø12A
T33.Ø19A
T33.Ø2XA
T33.Ø9XA
T33.1XXA
T33.2XXA
T33.3XXA
T33.4ØXA
T33.41XA
T33.42XA
T33.511A
T33.512A
T33.519A
T33.521A
T33.522A
T33.529A
T33.531A
T33.532A
T33.539A
T33.6ØXA
T33.61XA
T33.62XA
T33.7ØXA
T33.71XA
T33.72XA
T33.811A
T33.812A
T33.819A
T33.821A
T33.822A
T33.829A
T33.831A
T33.832A
T33.839A
T33.9ØXA
T33.99XA
T34.Ø11A
T34.Ø12A
T34.Ø19A
T34.Ø2XA
T34.Ø9XA
T34.1XXA
T34.2XXA
T34.3XXA
T34.4ØXA
T34.41XA
T34.42XA
T34.511A
T34.512A
T34.519A
T34.521A
T34.522A
T34.529A
T34.531A
T34.532A
T34.539A
T34.6ØXA
T34.61XA
T34.62XA
T34.7ØXA
T34.71XA
T34.72XA
T34.811A
T34.812A
T34.819A
T34.821A
T34.822A
T34.829A
T34.831A
T34.832A
T34.839A
T34.9ØXA
T34.99XA
T67.Ø1XA
T67.Ø2XA
T67.Ø9XA
T69.Ø21A
T69.Ø22A
T69.Ø29A
T7Ø.3XXA
T71.111A
T71.112A
T71.113A
T71.114A
T71.121A
T71.122A
T71.123A
T71.124A
T71.131A
T71.132A
T71.133A
T71.134A
T71.141A
T71.143A
T71.144A
T71.151A
T71.152A
T71.153A
T71.154A
T71.161A
T71.162A
T71.163A
T71.164A
T71.191A
T71.192A
T71.193A
T71.194A
T71.2ØXA
T71.21XA
T71.221A
T71.222A
T71.223A
T71.224A
T71.231A
T71.232A
T71.233A
T71.234A
T71.29XA
T71.9XXA
T74.Ø1XA
T74.Ø2XA
T74.11XA
T74.12XA
T74.21XA
T74.22XA
T74.32XA
T74.4XXA
T74.51XA
T74.52XA
T74.61XA
T74.62XA
T74.91XA
T74.92XA
T75.1XXA
T76.Ø1XA
T76.Ø2XA
T76.11XA
T76.12XA
T76.21XA
T76.22XA
T76.32XA
T76.51XA
T76.52XA
T76.61XA
T76.62XA
T76.91XA
T76.92XA
T78.ØØXA
T78.Ø1XA
T78.Ø2XA
T78.Ø3XA
T78.Ø4XA
T78.Ø5XA
T78.Ø6XA
T78.Ø7XA
T78.Ø8XA
T78.Ø9XA
T78.2XXA
T79.2XXA
T79.7XXA
T79.AØXA
T79.A11A
T79.A12A
T79.A19A
T79.A21A
T79.A22A
T79.A29A
T79.A3XA
T79.A9XA
T8Ø.1XXA
T8Ø.211A
T8Ø.212A
T8Ø.218A
T8Ø.219A
T8Ø.22XA
T8Ø.29XA
T8Ø.3ØXA
T8Ø.31ØA
T8Ø.311A
T8Ø.319A
T8Ø.39XA
T8Ø.4ØXA
T8Ø.41ØA
T8Ø.411A
T8Ø.419A
T8Ø.49XA
T8Ø.51XA
T8Ø.52XA
T8Ø.59XA
T8Ø.61XA
T8Ø.62XA
T8Ø.69XA
T8Ø.81ØA
T8Ø.818A
T8Ø.91ØA
T8Ø.911A
T8Ø.919A
T8Ø.AØXA
T8Ø.A1ØA
T8Ø.A11A
T8Ø.A19A
T8Ø.A9XA
T81.1ØXA
T81.3ØXA
T81.31XA
T81.32XA
T81.33XA
T81.4ØXA
T81.41XA
T81.42XA
T81.43XA
T81.44XA
T81.49XA
T81.5ØØA
T81.5Ø1A
T81.5Ø2A
T81.5Ø3A
T81.5Ø4A
T81.5Ø5A
T81.5Ø6A
T81.5Ø7A
T81.5Ø8A
T81.5Ø9A
T81.51ØA
T81.511A
T81.512A
T81.513A
T81.514A
T81.515A
T81.516A
T81.517A
T81.518A
T81.519A
T81.52ØA
T81.521A
T81.522A
T81.523A
T81.524A
T81.525A
T81.526A
T81.527A
T81.528A
T81.529A
T81.53ØA
T81.531A
T81.532A
T81.533A
T81.534A
T81.535A
T81.536A
T81.537A
T81.538A
T81.539A
T81.59ØA
T81.591A
T81.592A
T81.593A
T81.594A
T81.595A
T81.596A
T81.597A
T81.598A
T81.599A
T81.6ØXA
T81.61XA
T81.69XA
T81.71ØA
T81.711A
T81.718A
T81.719A
T81.72XA
T81.83XA
T82.Ø1XA
T82.Ø2XA
T82.Ø3XA
T82.Ø9XA
T82.11ØA
T82.111A
T82.118A
T82.119A
T82.12ØA
T82.121A
T82.128A
T82.129A
T82.19ØA
T82.191A
T82.198A
T82.199A
T82.211A
T82.212A
T82.213A
T82.218A
T82.221A
T82.222A
T82.223A
T82.228A
T82.31ØA
T82.311A
T82.312A
T82.318A
T82.319A
T82.32ØA
T82.321A
T82.322A
T82.328A
T82.329A
T82.33ØA
T82.331A
T82.332A
T82.338A
T82.339A
T82.39ØA
T82.391A
T82.392A
T82.398A
T82.399A
T82.41XA
T82.42XA
T82.43XA
T82.49XA
T82.51ØA
T82.511A
T82.512A
T82.513A
T82.514A
T82.515A
T82.518A
T82.519A
T82.52ØA
T82.521A
T82.522A
T82.523A
T82.524A
T82.525A
T82.528A
T82.529A
T82.53ØA
T82.531A
T82.532A
T82.533A
T82.534A
T82.535A
T82.538A
T82.539A
T82.59ØA
T82.591A
T82.592A
T82.593A
T82.594A
T82.595A
T82.598A
T82.599A
T82.6XXA
T82.7XXA
T82.817A
T82.818A
T82.827A
T82.828A
T82.837A
T82.838A
T82.847A
T82.848A
T82.855A
T82.856A
T82.857A
T82.858A
T82.867A
T82.868A
T82.897A
T82.898A
T82.9XXA
T83.Ø1ØA
T83.Ø2ØA
T83.Ø3ØA
T83.Ø9ØA
T83.11ØA
T83.111A
T83.112A
T83.113A
T83.118A
T83.12ØA
T83.121A
T83.122A
T83.123A
T83.128A
T83.19ØA
T83.191A
T83.192A
T83.193A
T83.198A
T83.21XA
T83.22XA
T83.23XA
T83.24XA
T83.25XA
T83.29XA
T83.41ØA
T83.411A
T83.418A
T83.42ØA
T83.421A
T83.428A
T83.49ØA
T83.491A
T83.498A
T83.51ØA
T83.511A
T83.512A
T83.518A
T83.59ØA
T83.591A
T83.592A
T83.593A
T83.598A
T83.61XA
T83.62XA
T83.69XA
T83.712A
T83.713A
T83.714A
T83.718A
T83.719A
T83.722A
T83.723A
T83.724A
T83.728A
T83.729A
T83.79XA
T83.81XA
T83.82XA
T83.83XA
T83.84XA
T83.85XA
T83.86XA
T83.89XA
T83.9XXA
T84.Ø1ØA
T84.Ø11A
T84.Ø12A
T84.Ø13A
T84.Ø18A
T84.Ø19A
T84.Ø2ØA
T84.Ø21A
T84.Ø22A
T84.Ø23A
T84.Ø28A
T84.Ø29A
T84.Ø3ØA
T84.Ø31A
T84.Ø32A
T84.Ø33A
T84.Ø38A
T84.Ø39A
T84.Ø5ØA
T84.Ø51A
T84.Ø52A
T84.Ø53A
T84.Ø58A
T84.Ø59A
T84.Ø6ØA
T84.Ø61A
T84.Ø62A
T84.Ø63A
T84.Ø68A
T84.Ø69A
T84.Ø9ØA
T84.Ø91A
T84.Ø92A
T84.Ø93A
T84.Ø98A
T84.Ø99A
T84.11ØA
T84.111A
T84.112A
T84.113A
T84.114A
T84.115A
T84.116A
T84.117A
T84.119A
T84.12ØA
T84.121A
T84.122A
T84.123A
T84.124A
T84.125A
T84.126A
T84.127A
T84.129A
T84.19ØA
T84.191A
T84.192A
T84.193A
T84.194A
T84.195A
T84.196A
T84.197A
T84.199A
T84.21ØA
T84.213A
T84.216A
T84.218A
T84.22ØA
T84.223A
T84.226A
T84.228A
T84.29ØA
T84.293A
T84.296A
T84.298A
T84.31ØA
T84.318A
T84.32ØA
T84.328A
T84.39ØA
T84.398A

T84.410A
T84.418A
T84.420A
T84.428A
T84.490A
T84.498A
T84.50XA
T84.51XA
T84.52XA
T84.53XA
T84.54XA
T84.59XA
T84.60XA
T84.610A
T84.611A
T84.612A
T84.613A
T84.614A
T84.615A
T84.619A
T84.620A
T84.621A
T84.622A
T84.623A
T84.624A
T84.625A
T84.629A
T84.63XA
T84.69XA
T84.7XXA
T84.81XA
T84.82XA
T84.83XA
T84.84XA
T84.85XA
T84.86XA
T84.89XA
T84.9XXA
T85.01XA
T85.02XA
T85.03XA
T85.09XA
T85.110A
T85.111A
T85.112A
T85.113A
T85.118A
T85.120A
T85.121A
T85.122A
T85.123A
T85.128A
T85.190A
T85.191A
T85.192A
T85.193A
T85.199A
T85.21XA
T85.22XA
T85.29XA
T85.310A
T85.311A
T85.320A
T85.321A
T85.390A
T85.391A
T85.41XA
T85.42XA
T85.43XA
T85.44XA
T85.49XA
T85.510A
T85.511A
T85.518A
T85.520A
T85.521A
T85.528A
T85.590A
T85.591A
T85.598A
T85.610A
T85.611A
T85.612A
T85.613A
T85.614A
T85.615A
T85.618A
T85.620A
T85.621A
T85.622A
T85.623A
T85.624A
T85.625A
T85.628A
T85.630A
T85.631A
T85.633A
T85.635A
T85.638A
T85.690A
T85.691A
T85.692A
T85.693A
T85.694A
T85.695A
T85.698A
T85.71XA
T85.72XA
T85.730A
T85.731A
T85.732A
T85.733A
T85.734A
T85.735A
T85.738A
T85.79XA
T85.810A
T85.810D
T85.820A
T85.820D
T85.830A
T85.830D
T85.840A
T85.840D
T85.850A
T85.850D
T85.860A
T85.860D
T85.890A
T85.890D
T86.00
T86.01
T86.02
T86.03
T86.09
T86.10
T86.11
T86.12
T86.13
T86.19
T86.20
T86.21
T86.22
T86.23
T86.290
T86.298
T86.30
T86.31
T86.32
T86.33
T86.39
T86.40
T86.41
T86.42
T86.43
T86.49
T86.5
T86.810
T86.811
T86.812
T86.818
T86.819
T86.820
T86.821
T86.822
T86.828
T86.829
T86.830
T86.831
T86.832
T86.838
T86.839
T86.8401
T86.8402
T86.8403
T86.8409
T86.8411
T86.8412
T86.8413
T86.8419
T86.8421
T86.8422
T86.8423
T86.8429
T86.8481
T86.8482
T86.8483
T86.8489
T86.8491
T86.8492
T86.8493
T86.8499
T86.850
T86.851
T86.852
T86.858
T86.859
T86.890
T86.891
T86.892
T86.898
T86.899
T86.90
T86.91
T86.92
T86.93
T86.99
T87.0X1
T87.0X2
T87.0X9
T87.1X1
T87.1X2
T87.1X9
T87.2
T87.40
T87.41
T87.42
T87.43
T87.44
T88.0XXA
T88.1XXA
T88.2XXA
T88.3XXA
T88.6XXA
Z16.10
Z16.11
Z16.12
Z16.19
Z16.20
Z16.21
Z16.22
Z16.23
Z16.24
Z16.29
Z16.30
Z16.31
Z16.32
Z16.33
Z16.341
Z16.342
Z16.35
Z16.39
Z43.1
Z48.21
Z48.22
Z48.23
Z48.24
Z48.280
Z48.290
Z68.1
Z68.41
Z68.42
Z68.43
Z68.44
Z68.45
Z94.0
Z94.1
Z94.2
Z94.3
Z94.4
Z94.81
Z94.82
Z94.83
Z94.84
Z95.811
Z95.812
Z99.11
Z99.12

Appendix F: Present on Admission (POA) Tutorial

Present-on-admission (POA) indicators are required on all diagnoses and external cause-of-injury codes for all inpatient acute care hospital discharges, according to the requirement outlined in the Deficit Reduction Act of 2005, section 5001(c). The only exception is for a select group of codes that have been designated as exempt from the POA regulations. Certain facilities are also exempt from this reporting requirement and include the following:

- Critical access hospitals
- Long-term care hospitals
- Cancer hospitals
- Inpatient psychiatric hospitals
- Inpatient rehabilitation facilities
- Veterans Administration/Department of Defense Hospitals
- Children's inpatient facilities

The POA indicator guidelines are not intended to replace the official *ICD-10-CM Official Guidelines for Coding and Reporting*. Nor will the POA guidelines supersede the Uniform Hospital Discharge Data Set (UHDDS) definition of principal diagnosis, defined as the condition established after study to be chiefly responsible for occasioning the admission of the patient to the hospital. The definition of "additional diagnoses" also remains the same. Coders must report all conditions that coexist at the time of admission, develop subsequently, or that affect the treatment received and/or the length of stay. This significantly affects assignment of the POA indicators. Because the POA indicator should accurately reflect the patient's conditions upon admission, review of POA guidelines as well as the *ICD-10-CM Official Guidelines for Coding and Reporting* is required.

The following is a summary of the POA guidelines:

- A POA condition is defined not only as one that is clearly present at the time of admission, but also one that was clearly present but not diagnosed until after the time of admission.
- Present on admission is defined as present at the time the order for an inpatient admission is made, whether or not the patient's episode of care originated in the emergency department, ambulatory surgery area, or other outpatient area. Conditions that develop during an outpatient encounter are considered present on admission.
- A POA indicator is assigned to the principal diagnosis, secondary diagnoses, and the external cause-of-injury codes.
- The POA guidelines are not intended to replace any of the other *ICD-10-CM Official Guidelines for Coding and Reporting.*
- The intent of the POA guidelines is not to determine whether or not a condition should be coded, but rather how to apply the POA indicator.

The following reporting options, with definitions, should be used to indicate whether a condition was POA:

Y *Yes: Present at the time of inpatient admission*

N *No: Not present at the time of inpatient admission*

U *Unknown: Documentation is insufficient to determine if condition is present at the time of inpatient admission*

W *Clinically undetermined: Provider is unable to clinically determine whether condition was or was not present at the time of inpatient admission*

Unreported/not used—(exempt from POA reporting)—Most ICD-10-CM codes require the assignment of a POA indicator. However, there are some diagnoses that are considered exempt from the POA reporting. For these exempt conditions the POA field should be left blank.

Note: *A data file of all POA exempt codes can be accessed at the following: http://www.optum360coding.com/ProductUpdates/*
Title: "2021 ICD-10-CM for Hospitals POA Exemption Data File"
Password: Hospital21

Timeframe for POA identification and documentation

There is no timeframe during the encounter in which a condition must be diagnosed to be considered present on admission. In many cases, it is not clinically possible for the provider to determine a definitive diagnosis until well into the admission, after labs, imaging, and other tests have been performed and results examined. In these cases the condition is still considered to be present on admission, indicated with Y.

Examples

- A patient was admitted for diagnostic work-up for cachexia. The final diagnosis was malignant neoplasm of lung with metastasis.

  Assign Y in the POA field for the malignant neoplasm, which was clearly present on admission, although it was not diagnosed until after the admission occurred.
- A patient with severe cough and difficulty breathing was diagnosed during his hospitalization to have lung cancer.

  Assign Y in the POA field for the lung cancer. Even though the cancer was not diagnosed until after admission, it is a chronic condition that was clearly present before the patient's admission.
- A urine culture was obtained on admission. The provider documented urinary tract infection when the culture results became available a few days later.

  Assign Y to the urinary tract infection since the diagnosis is based on test results from a specimen obtained on admission. It may not be possible for a provider to make a definitive diagnosis for a period of time after admission. There is no required timeframe as to when a provider must identify or document a condition for it to be considered present on admission.

Condition is on the "Exempt from Reporting" list

The POA field is left blank for codes excluded from POA reporting.

Examples

- A patient was admitted for inpatient surgery on a burn contracture from scar tissue from a burn five years ago.

  Assign Y for the principal condition of the scar; however, the secondary code for the specifics of the burn injury with a seventh character for sequela is left blank since it is excluded from POA reporting.
- A patient was admitted to inpatient for a PEG tube insertion because of residual dysphagia due to a recent CVA.

  No POA indicator is assigned for the dysphagia following a CVA. Codes under I69.- are defined as sequela of cerebrovascular disease and are exempt from POA reporting.
- A patient was admitted to inpatient for corrective surgery for a malunion of a closed femur fracture.

  No POA indicator is assigned for the malunion of a closed fracture because the seventh character for malunion of fractures is considered a subsequent encounter and is exempt from POA reporting.
- A patient was admitted for breast reconstruction following mastectomy.

  The POA indicator field is left blank as this Z code is exempt from POA reporting.
- A patient was admitted for changing the battery in his AICD as it is at the end of its useful life.

  The POA indicator field is left blank as this Z code is exempt from POA reporting.

POA explicitly documented

If the provider explicitly documents a condition as being present on admission or not present on admission, assign the appropriate Y or N POA indicator based on that documentation. If there is conflicting documentation by different providers, query the attending physician.

Examples

- Even though sepsis is not diagnosed in the ED, the discharge summary states that the patient presented with sepsis at the time of admission.

  The provider explicitly stated that the sepsis was present on admission and therefore the Y POA indicator should be used.
- The patient was admitted with chills and cough and two days later diagnosed with pneumonia. The discharge summary documents that the pneumonia was not present on admission.

  Although the patient showed some symptoms of pneumonia on admission, the provider may have clinical evidence (e.g., chest x-rays, cultures) that indicates that pneumonia did not develop until after admission. Since this was explicitly stated in the discharge summary, the appropriate POA indicator is N.

- A consult note states that a patient came in with renal failure while the discharge summary states that the renal failure was not present on admission.

  When in doubt and there is conflicting documentation, query the attending physician.

Conditions diagnosed prior to inpatient admission

Conditions that were diagnosed prior to admission—for example, chronic conditions such as hypertension, diabetes, and asthma—are assigned the POA indicator of Y. A tip to help establish that a condition was POA is to check the patient's medication history for drugs that are routinely prescribed for these types of chronic conditions.

Examples

- The history and physical states that the patient has a history of hypertension and seizure disorder, and it is noted that the patient is currently on Atenolol and Dilantin.

  The hypertension and seizure disorder existed prior to admission; therefore, the appropriate POA indicator is Y. Verification that the patient is on long-term use of Atenolol and Dilantin can help solidify that these conditions are currently being treated.
- A 56-year-old male was admitted as an inpatient for multi-trauma wounds. Because the patient was unconscious on admission, his medical history was unknown. A progress note two days into the stay noted that the patient was on Metformin for history of type 2 diabetes.

  The timeframe of the diagnosis is irrelevant to POA. Even though it was not discovered until two days into the encounter that the patient had a history of DM2, the DM2 was still present prior to this admission and would be identified as such with the Y POA indicator.
- A patient was admitted to an inpatient facility from the ED. The admitting provider indicated that the patient had a current history of lung cancer and chronic kidney disease.

  Both of these conditions are indicated with Y, present on admission.
- During the course of an eight-day inpatient stay with surgery, a patient was diagnosed postoperatively with hypertension and discharged on Metoprolol.

  The hypertension was not diagnosed prior to admission and would be reported with an N POA indicator.

Conditions diagnosed during the admission but clearly present before admission

The POA indicator Y is assigned for conditions that clearly presented with applicable signs and symptoms but may have not been definitively diagnosed until later on, or even at the end of the encounter. Even if the presenting diagnosis was documented on admission as suspected, possible, or rule out, or written as a differential diagnosis and later confirmed, it is still considered present on admission.

Examples

- A patient was admitted with jaundice, fatigue, and mental confusion. Differential diagnosis on admission lists possible liver failure. The definitive diagnosis of liver failure is not made until two days after admission.

  Assign Y to the liver failure since the symptoms were present on admission and the differential diagnosis listed "possible" liver failure on admission even though the final diagnosis was two days later.
- An aid worker recently returned from Afghanistan presents to the ED with hematemesis, chest pain, and fever. Patient is put into inpatient isolation with suspected TB documented on the H & P. TB is confirmed the next day.

  The POA indicator Y is assigned because, even though the TB was only "suspected" on admission, it was confirmed the next day.

Condition develops during outpatient encounter prior to inpatient admission

Assign Y for any condition that develops during an outpatient encounter such as same-day surgery, observation, or extended recovery prior to a written order for inpatient admission. This also pertains to conditions that develop in facilities such as transitional care units, skilled nursing homes, long-term care, hospice, or rehabilitation facilities with the patient transferring to inpatient hospital admission.

Examples

- A patient underwent outpatient surgery. During the recovery period, the patient developed atrial fibrillation and was subsequently admitted to the hospital as an inpatient.

  Assign Y on the POA field for the atrial fibrillation since it developed prior to a written order for inpatient admission.
- A patient was treated in observation and while in observation fell out of bed and broke a hip. The patient was subsequently admitted as an inpatient to treat the hip fracture.

  Assign Y on the POA field for the hip fracture since it developed prior to a written order for inpatient admission.
- An elderly patient underwent outpatient surgery with plans to go home after the surgery. In recovery, the patient developed shortness of breath, chest pain, and fever. A sputum sample was taken, and the surgeon decided to admit the patient to inpatient. The next day the patient was diagnosed with staphylococcal pneumonia based on sputum results and admitting chest x-ray.

  Assign Y to the staphylococcal pneumonia even though it was not diagnosed until the day following the admission. Even though the patient had undergone outpatient surgery, the sputum sample, signs, and symptoms were evident prior to the inpatient admission.

Documentation does not indicate whether condition was present on admission

If the documentation in the medical record is unclear as to the presence of a condition on admission, assign a U for unknown. This should be used sparingly and, if possible, the physician should be queried for further clarification.

Example

- A wheelchair-bound patient was admitted in respiratory failure from a long-term care facility to an inpatient hospital with severe aspiration pneumonia. A progress note three days into the admission listed a pressure ulcer stage 2 on the lower back.

  Assign U for the stage 2 pressure ulcer if unknown whether it was present on admission. Since the patient was wheelchair-bound and critically ill on admission, it is possible that the ulcer was present and not immediately addressed. The admitting physician can be queried to clarify, or a U is assigned if that is not possible.

Documentation states it cannot be determined whether the condition was or was not present on admission

A W is assigned when the documentation states that it cannot be clinically determined whether the condition was POA or not.

Examples

- An elderly patient was admitted with multi-trauma injuries from a motor vehicle accident. Two days into the admission, a urinary tract infection was diagnosed. No labs or urine cultures had been taken on admission as focus was stabilization from traumatic wounds. Documentation from the provider in a progress note stated that it was not clinically possible to determine whether the UTI was present on admission.

  Assign W for the UTI as it was specifically stated that it was not clinically possible to determine whether it was present on admission.
- A patient was admitted with high fever and pneumonia. The patient rapidly deteriorated and became septic. The discharge diagnosis listed sepsis and pneumonia. The documentation was unclear as to whether the sepsis was present on admission or developed shortly after admission.

  Query the physician as to whether the sepsis was present on admission, developed shortly after admission, or it cannot be clinically determined as to whether it was or was not present on admission.

Chronic condition with acute exacerbation during the admission

If a single code identifies only the chronic condition and not the acute exacerbation, assign Y. For instance, when there is no code for the acute exacerbation of a chronic condition as in acute exacerbation of chronic leukemia, the Y is assigned for the chronic leukemia.

For a single combination code that identifies both the chronic and acute exacerbation, see the combination code instructions.

Example

- Documentation on admission stated that the patient had chronic myelomonocytic leukemia. A progress note three days into the stay stated that the patient had, since admission, developed an acute exacerbation of his myelomonocytic leukemia.

  There is no code for an acute exacerbation of chronic myelomonocytic leukemia; therefore, assign Y since the chronic leukemia (either not specified as in remission, or in relapse) is represented by a single code and was present on admission.

Acute and chronic conditions

Assign Y to acute conditions present on admission and N to acute conditions not present at the time of admission.

Assign Y to conditions specified as chronic, even though they may not be diagnosed until after admission.

See the POA guideline "Codes that contain multiple clinical concepts" for a single code that identifies both the acute and chronic condition.

Examples

- A patient was admitted to the hospital for coronary artery bypass surgery. Postoperatively he developed a pulmonary embolism.

  Assign N in the POA field for the pulmonary embolism. This is an acute condition that was not present on admission.
- A patient admitted with sepsis due to pneumonia with acute respiratory failure, developed acute renal failure on day three.

  Assign Y for the sepsis, pneumonia, and acute respiratory failure, which were all acute conditions, present on admission. Assign N for the acute renal failure; even though it is an acute condition, it was not present until after the patient was admitted.
- A patient admitted with hypoglycemia, weakness, confusion, and slurred speech was diagnosed the next day with type 2 diabetes.

  Assign Y to the type 2 diabetes since it is a chronic condition that was present on admission, even though it was not diagnosed until the next day.

Codes that contain multiple clinical concepts

If at least one of the clinical concepts included in a code was not present on admission, assign N. If all the clinical concepts included in a code are present on admission, assign Y.

Examples

- Patient has history of gastrojejunal ulcer which started bleeding two days into the encounter.

  Assign a POA indicator of N to chronic gastrojejunal ulcer with bleeding; although the gastrojejunal ulcer is a chronic condition that was present at the time of admission, the bleeding did not occur until after the admission.
- A patient with chronic diastolic heart failure decompensated after admission.

  Assign N to the code for acute on chronic diastolic (congestive) heart failure. Although the heart failure was present on admission, the acute decompensation of the failure was not.
- A patient with viral hepatitis B progressed to hepatic coma after admission.

  Assign N for the viral hepatitis B with hepatic coma because a condition described by part of the code description did not develop until after admission.
- A patient with known systolic congestive heart failure was admitted to the hospital with decompensated systolic heart failure.

  Assign Y in the POA field for the acute on chronic systolic (congestive) heart failure as both the chronic and acute parts of the condition were present on admission.

Assign Y for infection codes that include the organism if the infection was present on admission even though the culture results are not available until after admission.

Example

- A patient was septic on admission with blood, sputum, and urine cultures taken. Two days later, *E. coli* was determined to be the causal organism.

  Assign Y even though the test results were not confirmed until after admission.

Conditions documented as possible, probable, suspected, or rule out at the time of discharge or conditions documented as impending or threatened at the time of discharge

If the final diagnosis contains language identifying a condition as possible, probable, suspected, or rule out, or as an impending or threatened diagnosis but the diagnosis is based on signs and symptoms that were present on admission, the POA indicator is Y. If those signs and symptoms were not present on admission, the appropriate POA indicator is N.

Examples

- A patient underwent inpatient surgery, after which the patient developed fever and was treated aggressively. The physician's final diagnosis documented "possible postoperative infection following surgery."

  Assign N on the POA field for the postoperative infection since final diagnoses that contain the terms "possible," "probable," "suspected," or "rule out" and that are based on symptoms or clinical findings that were not present on admission should be reported as N.
- A patient with prior cardiac intervention history was admitted with chest pain. After two days, the chest pain diminished with no underlying cause found. The discharge summary stated, "Suspected costochondritis or coronary artery spasm. Pain resolved. Follow up at regular cardiology office visit."

  Since the chest pain was present on admission, both suspected conditions of costochondritis and coronary artery spasm are represented by the POA indicator of Y.
- A patient was admitted with a known history of coronary atherosclerosis, status post myocardial infarction five years ago, and was then admitted for treatment of impending myocardial infarction. The patient was transferred to a larger facility with a cath lab. The final diagnosis was documented as "impending myocardial infarction."

  Assign Y to the impending myocardial infarction because the condition is present on admission.

Same diagnosis code for two or more conditions

When two or more separate conditions are classified to the same diagnosis code in the same encounter, assign Y if all conditions represented by the single code were present on admission and N if any of the conditions were not present on admission.

Examples

- A patient was admitted with diabetes type 2 with ketoacidosis.

  Assign Y since both the diabetes and ketoacidosis were present on admission.
- A patient involved in a car accident was admitted with hemorrhage to the abdomen secondary to the trauma; shortly after being admitted the patient also developed a seroma as a result of the trauma.

  The secondary traumatic hemorrhage was present on admission, and the traumatic seroma did not develop until after admission. Both of these conditions are classified to one code, but because both conditions were not present when the patient was admitted, a POA of N should be assigned.

Obstetrical conditions

The POA assignment for obstetrical conditions is not affected by whether the patient delivers during the encounter but rather by whether the pregnancy complication was or was not present at the time of admission. If two or more conditions are classified to a single code, all conditions represented by that single code must be present on admission to correctly assign a Y. If all conditions are not present at the time of admission, the appropriate POA indicator is N. Several obstetrics codes are listed in the POA exclusion list; for obstetrics codes that are not on the exclusion list, all applicable POA guidelines apply.

Examples

- A female patient was admitted to the hospital and underwent a normal delivery.

  Leave the "present on admission" (POA) field blank. Code O80 Normal delivery, is on the "exempt from reporting" list.
- A patient was admitted in late pregnancy due to excessive vomiting and dehydration. During admission, the patient went into premature labor.

  Assign Y for the excessive vomiting and the dehydration. Assign N for the premature labor.
- A patient was admitted in active labor. During the stay, a breast abscess was noted when the mother attempted to breastfeed. The provider was unable to clinically determine whether the abscess was present on admission.

  Assign W for the breast abscess since the provider was unable to clinically determine whether the abscess was present on admission.
- A patient was admitted in active labor. After 12 hours of labor, it was noted that the infant was in fetal distress, and a cesarean section was performed.

  Assign N for the fetal distress even if it is used for the principal diagnosis, since it did not develop until later in the admission. In obstetrics cases, the principal diagnosis may have a POA indicator of N.

Perinatal and congenital conditions

Newborns are not considered admitted until after birth; therefore all conditions that develop in utero, occur during delivery, or are present at birth are represented by the POA indicator Y. Any conditions that develop after birth and admission are represented by N.

All congenital conditions and anomalies not found in chapter 17 should have a POA indicator of Y assigned. Chapter 17 codes in categories Q00–Q99 are exempt from POA reporting. All congenital conditions, regardless of the coding chapter to which they are assigned, are considered present on admission.

Examples

- A single liveborn infant was delivered in the hospital via cesarean section. The physician documented fetal bradycardia during labor as the final diagnosis in the newborn record.

  Assign Y because the bradycardia developed prior to the newborn admission (birth).
- A newborn developed diarrhea, which was believed to be due to the hospital baby formula.

  Assign N because the diarrhea developed after admission.
- A newborn was diagnosed with cephalhematoma due to birth injury.

  Assign Y because the injury occurred during delivery.
- A newborn was diagnosed with congenital pneumonia.

  Assign Y for the congenital pneumonia. Congenital conditions from chapter 16 are always considered present on admission and require the POA indicator.
- A newborn was diagnosed with congenital hydrocephalus.

  There should be no POA indicator assigned. This condition is coded in chapter 17 and is excluded from POA reporting.
- A 10-year-old boy was admitted for complications of spina bifida with hydrocephalus.

  No POA indicator is assigned. This condition is coded in chapter 17 and is excluded from POA reporting.

External cause and injury codes

If an injury or poisoning occurred prior to or at the time of admission and the seventh character indicates an initial encounter or active treatment, the code for the injury/poisoning is reported with POA indicator Y. Injury and poisoning codes S00–T88 with the seventh character indicating subsequent or sequela are exempt from POA indicators since, in order to be a subsequent or sequela encounter, the condition must have occurred before the admission. Many of the external causes of morbidity codes from chapters V, W, and X are also exempt from POA reporting when the seventh character of S or D, representing subsequent or sequela encounters, are used.

Coders should be extremely careful in assigning the appropriate POA indicator if a patient suffers an injury while an inpatient. For example, if a patient falls from the hospital bed and fractures a hip, the codes representing that injury (along with the appropriate initial-encounter seventh character) should be assigned N for the corresponding POA indicator.

Examples

- A 12-year-old was admitted for treatment of fractured arm from falling out of a tree house.

  The injury itself and the cause of the injury are both assigned a Y POA indicator.

  Note: *The injury code and external cause code POA indicators should always match.*
- A patient admitted for pneumonia sustained a laceration of the right arm after falling and hitting his arm against a cart in the hospital room, requiring stitches.

  Assign N for the laceration for the right arm because it was not present on admission. The external cause code POA indicator should also be N.
- A patient was admitted for manipulation of a knee contracture due to a scar from a burn injury 10 years ago.

  Assign Y for the code for the scar, but leave blank the POA indicator for the burn injury with the seventh character of S for sequela. Sequela and subsequent-encounter codes in chapter 19 are exempt from POA reporting.

Appendix G: Hospital Acquired Conditions

Hospital-acquired conditions (HACs) are conditions considered reasonably preventable through the application of evidence-based guidelines. These conditions, in and of themselves, are either a complication or comorbidity (CC) or major complication or comorbidity (MCC) that as a secondary diagnosis will move the MS-DRG assignment from a lower-paying MS-DRG to a higher-paying MS-DRG. However, if these conditions are not present on admission (meaning they developed during the hospital stay), the CC or MCC designation is nullified and the case will not group to the higher-paying MS-DRG based solely upon the reporting of the HAC code.

HACs are grouped into 14 categories. ICD-10-CM codes in the tabular section of this book that are grouped to one of these HAC categories are identified by an icon specific to that category. As many of these HACs are conditional, this resource provides any additional stipulations that may be required before the code can be considered a HAC. For example, code I26.Ø2 has an H10 indicating it falls in the HAC 10 category for Deep Vein Thrombosis (DVT) or Pulmonary Embolism (PE) with Total Knee or Hip Replacement. However I26.Ø2 is not, by itself, a HAC there must also be a specific ICD-10-PCS code, such as ØSR9Ø19 Replacement of Right Hip Joint with Metal Synthetic Substitute, Cemented, Open Approach, applied in order for I26.Ø2 to act as a HAC.

Note: The resource used to compile this list is based on the proposed, version 38, MS-DRG Grouper software and Definitions Manual files published with the fiscal 2021 IPPS proposed rule. The final, version 38, MS-DRG Grouper files and MS-DRG Definitions Manual files can be found at the following: https://www.cms.gov/Medicare/Medicare-Fee-for-Service-Payment/AcuteInpatientPPS/IPPS-Regulations-and-Notices.html.

HAC 01: Foreign Object Retained After Surgery

Secondary diagnosis not POA:

T81.5ØØA
T81.5Ø1A
T81.5Ø2A
T81.5Ø3A
T81.5Ø4A
T81.5Ø5A
T81.5Ø6A
T81.5Ø7A
T81.5Ø8A
T81.5Ø9A
T81.51ØA
T81.511A
T81.512A
T81.513A
T81.514A
T81.515A
T81.516A
T81.517A
T81.518A
T81.519A
T81.52ØA
T81.521A
T81.522A
T81.523A
T81.524A
T81.525A
T81.526A
T81.527A
T81.528A
T81.529A
T81.53ØA
T81.531A
T81.532A
T81.533A
T81.534A
T81.535A
T81.536A
T81.537A
T81.538A
T81.539A
T81.59ØA
T81.591A
T81.592A
T81.593A
T81.594A
T81.595A
T81.596A
T81.597A
T81.598A
T81.599A
T81.6ØXA
T81.61XA
T81.69XA

HAC 02: Air Embolism

Secondary diagnosis not POA:

T8Ø.ØXXA

HAC 03: Blood Incompatibility

Secondary diagnosis not POA:

T8Ø.3ØXA
T8Ø.31ØA
T8Ø.311A
T8Ø.319A
T8Ø.39XA

HAC 04: Stage III and IV Pressure Ulcers

Secondary diagnosis not POA:

L89.ØØ3
L89.ØØ4
L89.Ø13
L89.Ø14
L89.Ø23
L89.Ø24
L89.1Ø3
L89.1Ø4
L89.113
L89.114
L89.123
L89.124
L89.133
L89.134
L89.143
L89.144
L89.153
L89.154
L89.2Ø3
L89.2Ø4
L89.213
L89.214
L89.223
L89.224
L89.3Ø3
L89.3Ø4
L89.313
L89.314
L89.323
L89.324
L89.43
L89.44
L89.5Ø3
L89.5Ø4
L89.513
L89.514
L89.523
L89.524
L89.6Ø3
L89.6Ø4
L89.613
L89.614
L89.623
L89.624
L89.813
L89.814
L89.893
L89.894
L89.93
L89.94

HAC 05: Falls and Trauma

Secondary diagnosis not POA:

M99.1Ø
M99.11
M99.18
SØ2.ØXXA
SØ2.ØXXB
SØ2.1Ø1A
SØ2.1Ø1B
SØ2.1Ø2A
SØ2.1Ø2B
SØ2.1Ø9A
SØ2.1Ø9B
SØ2.11ØA
SØ2.11ØB
SØ2.111A
SØ2.111B
SØ2.112A
SØ2.112B
SØ2.113A
SØ2.113B
SØ2.118A
SØ2.118B
SØ2.119A
SØ2.119B
SØ2.11AA
SØ2.11AB
SØ2.11BA
SØ2.11BB
SØ2.11CA
SØ2.11CB
SØ2.11DA
SØ2.11DB
SØ2.11EA
SØ2.11EB
SØ2.11FA
SØ2.11FB
SØ2.11GA
SØ2.11GB
SØ2.11HA
SØ2.11HB
SØ2.121A
SØ2.121B
SØ2.122A
SØ2.122B
SØ2.129A
SØ2.129B
SØ2.19XA
SØ2.19XB
SØ2.2XXB
SØ2.3ØXA
SØ2.3ØXB
SØ2.31XA
SØ2.31XB
SØ2.32XA
SØ2.32XB
SØ2.4ØØA
SØ2.4ØØB
SØ2.4Ø1A
SØ2.4Ø1B
SØ2.4Ø2A
SØ2.4Ø2B
SØ2.4ØAA
SØ2.4ØAB
SØ2.4ØBA
SØ2.4ØBB
SØ2.4ØCA
SØ2.4ØCB
SØ2.4ØDA
SØ2.4ØDB
SØ2.4ØEA
SØ2.4ØEB
SØ2.4ØFA
SØ2.4ØFB
SØ2.411A
SØ2.411B
SØ2.412A
SØ2.412B
SØ2.413A
SØ2.413B
SØ2.42XA
SØ2.42XB
SØ2.6ØØA
SØ2.6ØØB
SØ2.6Ø1A
SØ2.6Ø1B
SØ2.6Ø2A
SØ2.6Ø2B
SØ2.6Ø9A
SØ2.6Ø9B
SØ2.61ØA
SØ2.61ØB
SØ2.611A
SØ2.611B
SØ2.612A
SØ2.612B
SØ2.62ØA
SØ2.62ØB
SØ2.621A
SØ2.621B
SØ2.622A
SØ2.622B
SØ2.63ØA
SØ2.63ØB
SØ2.631A
SØ2.631B
SØ2.632A
SØ2.632B
SØ2.64ØA
SØ2.64ØB
SØ2.641A
SØ2.641B
SØ2.642A
SØ2.642B
SØ2.65ØA
SØ2.65ØB
SØ2.651A
SØ2.651B
SØ2.652A
SØ2.652B
SØ2.66XA
SØ2.66XB
SØ2.67ØA
SØ2.67ØB
SØ2.671A
SØ2.671B
SØ2.672A
SØ2.672B
SØ2.69XA
SØ2.69XB
SØ2.8ØXA
SØ2.8ØXB
SØ2.81XA
SØ2.81XB
SØ2.82XA
SØ2.82XB
SØ2.831A
SØ2.831B
SØ2.832A
SØ2.832B
SØ2.839A
SØ2.839B
SØ2.841A
SØ2.841B
SØ2.842A
SØ2.842B
SØ2.849A
SØ2.849B
SØ2.85XA
SØ2.85XB
SØ2.91XA
SØ2.91XB
SØ2.92XA
SØ2.92XB
SØ6.ØX1A
SØ6.ØX9A
SØ6.1X1A
SØ6.1X2A
SØ6.1X3A
SØ6.1X4A
SØ6.1X5A
SØ6.1X6A
SØ6.1X7A
SØ6.1X8A
SØ6.1X9A
SØ6.2X1A
SØ6.2X2A
SØ6.2X3A
SØ6.2X4A
SØ6.2X5A
SØ6.2X6A
SØ6.2X7A
SØ6.2X8A
SØ6.2X9A
SØ6.3Ø1A
SØ6.3Ø2A
SØ6.3Ø3A
SØ6.3Ø4A
SØ6.3Ø5A
SØ6.3Ø6A
SØ6.3Ø7A
SØ6.3Ø8A
SØ6.3Ø9A
SØ6.31ØA
SØ6.311A
SØ6.312A
SØ6.313A
SØ6.314A
SØ6.315A
SØ6.316A
SØ6.317A
SØ6.318A
SØ6.319A
SØ6.32ØA
SØ6.321A
SØ6.322A
SØ6.323A
SØ6.324A
SØ6.325A
SØ6.326A
SØ6.327A
SØ6.328A
SØ6.329A
SØ6.33ØA
SØ6.331A
SØ6.332A
SØ6.333A
SØ6.334A
SØ6.335A
SØ6.336A
SØ6.337A
SØ6.338A
SØ6.339A

HAC 05: Falls and Trauma (continued)

S06.340A
S06.341A
S06.342A
S06.343A
S06.344A
S06.345A
S06.346A
S06.347A
S06.348A
S06.349A
S06.350A
S06.351A
S06.352A
S06.353A
S06.354A
S06.355A
S06.356A
S06.357A
S06.358A
S06.359A
S06.360A
S06.361A
S06.362A
S06.363A
S06.364A
S06.365A
S06.366A
S06.367A
S06.368A
S06.369A
S06.370A
S06.371A
S06.372A
S06.373A
S06.374A
S06.375A
S06.376A
S06.377A
S06.378A
S06.379A
S06.380A
S06.381A
S06.382A
S06.383A
S06.384A
S06.385A
S06.386A
S06.387A
S06.388A
S06.389A
S06.4X0A
S06.4X1A
S06.4X2A
S06.4X3A
S06.4X4A
S06.4X5A
S06.4X6A
S06.4X7A
S06.4X8A
S06.4X9A
S06.5X0A
S06.5X1A
S06.5X2A
S06.5X3A
S06.5X4A
S06.5X5A
S06.5X6A
S06.5X7A
S06.5X8A
S06.5X9A
S06.6X0A
S06.6X1A
S06.6X2A
S06.6X3A
S06.6X4A
S06.6X5A
S06.6X6A
S06.6X7A
S06.6X8A
S06.6X9A
S06.811A
S06.812A
S06.813A
S06.814A
S06.815A
S06.816A
S06.817A
S06.818A
S06.819A
S06.821A
S06.822A
S06.823A
S06.824A
S06.825A
S06.826A
S06.827A
S06.828A
S06.829A
S06.891A
S06.892A
S06.893A
S06.894A
S06.895A
S06.896A
S06.897A
S06.898A
S06.899A
S06.9X1A
S06.9X2A
S06.9X3A
S06.9X4A
S06.9X5A
S06.9X6A
S06.9X7A
S06.9X8A
S06.9X9A
S07.0XXA
S07.1XXA
S07.8XXA
S07.9XXA
S12.000A
S12.000B
S12.001A
S12.001B
S12.01XA
S12.01XB
S12.02XA
S12.02XB
S12.030A
S12.030B
S12.031A
S12.031B
S12.040A
S12.040B
S12.041A
S12.041B
S12.090A
S12.090B
S12.091A
S12.091B
S12.100A
S12.100B
S12.101A
S12.101B
S12.110A
S12.110B
S12.111A
S12.111B
S12.112A
S12.112B
S12.120A
S12.120B
S12.121A
S12.121B
S12.130A
S12.130B
S12.131A
S12.131B
S12.14XA
S12.14XB
S12.150A
S12.150B
S12.151A
S12.151B
S12.190A
S12.190B
S12.191A
S12.191B
S12.200A
S12.200B
S12.201A
S12.201B
S12.230A
S12.230B
S12.231A
S12.231B
S12.24XA
S12.24XB
S12.250A
S12.250B
S12.251A
S12.251B
S12.290A
S12.290B
S12.291A
S12.291B
S12.300A
S12.300B
S12.301A
S12.301B
S12.330A
S12.330B
S12.331A
S12.331B
S12.34XA
S12.34XB
S12.350A
S12.350B
S12.351A
S12.351B
S12.390A
S12.390B
S12.391A
S12.391B
S12.400A
S12.400B
S12.401A
S12.401B
S12.430A
S12.430B
S12.431A
S12.431B
S12.44XA
S12.44XB
S12.450A
S12.450B
S12.451A
S12.451B
S12.490A
S12.490B
S12.491A
S12.491B
S12.500A
S12.500B
S12.501A
S12.501B
S12.530A
S12.530B
S12.531A
S12.531B
S12.54XA
S12.54XB
S12.550A
S12.550B
S12.551A
S12.551B
S12.590A
S12.590B
S12.591A
S12.591B
S12.600A
S12.600B
S12.601A
S12.601B
S12.630A
S12.630B
S12.631A
S12.631B
S12.64XA
S12.64XB
S12.650A
S12.650B
S12.651A
S12.651B
S12.690A
S12.690B
S12.691A
S12.691B
S12.8XXA
S12.9XXA
S13.0XXA
S13.100A
S13.101A
S13.110A
S13.111A
S13.120A
S13.121A
S13.130A
S13.131A
S13.140A
S13.141A
S13.150A
S13.151A
S13.160A
S13.161A
S13.170A
S13.171A
S13.180A
S13.181A
S13.20XA
S13.29XA
S14.101A
S14.102A
S14.103A
S14.104A
S14.105A
S14.106A
S14.107A
S14.111A
S14.112A
S14.113A
S14.114A
S14.115A
S14.116A
S14.117A
S14.121A
S14.122A
S14.123A
S14.124A
S14.125A
S14.126A
S14.127A
S14.131A
S14.132A
S14.133A
S14.134A
S14.135A
S14.136A
S14.137A
S14.151A
S14.152A
S14.153A
S14.154A
S14.155A
S14.156A
S14.157A
S17.0XXA
S17.8XXA
S17.9XXA
S22.000A
S22.000B
S22.001A
S22.001B
S22.002A
S22.002B
S22.008A
S22.008B
S22.009A
S22.009B
S22.010A
S22.010B
S22.011A
S22.011B
S22.012A
S22.012B
S22.018A
S22.018B
S22.019A
S22.019B
S22.020A
S22.020B
S22.021A
S22.021B
S22.022A
S22.022B
S22.028A
S22.028B
S22.029A
S22.029B
S22.030A
S22.030B
S22.031A
S22.031B
S22.032A
S22.032B
S22.038A
S22.038B
S22.039A
S22.039B
S22.040A
S22.040B
S22.041A
S22.041B
S22.042A
S22.042B
S22.048A
S22.048B
S22.049A
S22.049B
S22.050A
S22.050B
S22.051A
S22.051B
S22.052A
S22.052B
S22.058A
S22.058B
S22.059A
S22.059B
S22.060A
S22.060B
S22.061A
S22.061B
S22.062A
S22.062B
S22.068A
S22.068B
S22.069A
S22.069B
S22.070A
S22.070B
S22.071A
S22.071B
S22.072A
S22.072B
S22.078A
S22.078B
S22.079A
S22.079B
S22.080A
S22.080B
S22.081A
S22.081B
S22.082A
S22.082B
S22.088A
S22.088B
S22.089A
S22.089B
S22.20XA
S22.20XB
S22.21XA
S22.21XB
S22.22XA
S22.22XB
S22.23XA
S22.23XB
S22.24XA
S22.24XB
S22.31XA
S22.31XB
S22.32XA
S22.32XB
S22.39XA
S22.39XB
S22.41XA
S22.41XB
S22.42XA
S22.42XB
S22.43XA
S22.43XB
S22.49XA
S22.49XB
S22.5XXA
S22.5XXB
S22.9XXA
S22.9XXB
S24.101A
S24.102A
S24.103A
S24.104A
S24.111A
S24.112A
S24.113A
S24.114A
S24.131A
S24.132A
S24.133A
S24.134A
S24.151A
S24.152A
S24.153A
S24.154A
S32.000A
S32.000B
S32.001A
S32.001B
S32.002A
S32.002B
S32.008A

HAC 05: Falls and Trauma (continued)

S32.008B
S32.009A
S32.009B
S32.010A
S32.010B
S32.011A
S32.011B
S32.012A
S32.012B
S32.018A
S32.018B
S32.019A
S32.019B
S32.020A
S32.020B
S32.021A
S32.021B
S32.022A
S32.022B
S32.028A
S32.028B
S32.029A
S32.029B
S32.030A
S32.030B
S32.031A
S32.031B
S32.032A
S32.032B
S32.038A
S32.038B
S32.039A
S32.039B
S32.040A
S32.040B
S32.041A
S32.041B
S32.042A
S32.042B
S32.048A
S32.048B
S32.049A
S32.049B
S32.050A
S32.050B
S32.051A
S32.051B
S32.052A
S32.052B
S32.058A
S32.058B
S32.059A
S32.059B
S32.10XA
S32.10XB
S32.110A
S32.110B
S32.111A
S32.111B
S32.112A
S32.112B
S32.119A
S32.119B
S32.120A
S32.120B
S32.121A
S32.121B
S32.122A
S32.122B
S32.129A
S32.129B
S32.130A
S32.130B
S32.131A
S32.131B
S32.132A
S32.132B
S32.139A
S32.139B
S32.14XA
S32.14XB
S32.15XA
S32.15XB
S32.16XA
S32.16XB
S32.17XA
S32.17XB
S32.19XA
S32.19XB
S32.2XXA
S32.2XXB
S32.301A
S32.301B
S32.302A
S32.302B
S32.309A
S32.309B
S32.311A
S32.311B
S32.312A
S32.312B
S32.313A
S32.313B
S32.314A
S32.314B
S32.315A
S32.315B
S32.316A
S32.316B
S32.391A
S32.391B
S32.392A
S32.392B
S32.399A
S32.399B
S32.401A
S32.401B
S32.402A
S32.402B
S32.409A
S32.409B
S32.411A
S32.411B
S32.412A
S32.412B
S32.413A
S32.413B
S32.414A
S32.414B
S32.415A
S32.415B
S32.416A
S32.416B
S32.421A
S32.421B
S32.422A
S32.422B
S32.423A
S32.423B
S32.424A
S32.424B
S32.425A
S32.425B
S32.426A
S32.426B
S32.431A
S32.431B
S32.432A
S32.432B
S32.433A
S32.433B
S32.434A
S32.434B
S32.435A
S32.435B
S32.436A
S32.436B
S32.441A
S32.441B
S32.442A
S32.442B
S32.443A
S32.443B
S32.444A
S32.444B
S32.445A
S32.445B
S32.446A
S32.446B
S32.451A
S32.451B
S32.452A
S32.452B
S32.453A
S32.453B
S32.454A
S32.454B
S32.455A
S32.455B
S32.456A
S32.456B
S32.461A
S32.461B
S32.462A
S32.462B
S32.463A
S32.463B
S32.464A
S32.464B
S32.465A
S32.465B
S32.466A
S32.466B
S32.471A
S32.471B
S32.472A
S32.472B
S32.473A
S32.473B
S32.474A
S32.474B
S32.475A
S32.475B
S32.476A
S32.476B
S32.481A
S32.481B
S32.482A
S32.482B
S32.483A
S32.483B
S32.484A
S32.484B
S32.485A
S32.485B
S32.486A
S32.486B
S32.491A
S32.491B
S32.492A
S32.492B
S32.499A
S32.499B
S32.501A
S32.501B
S32.502A
S32.502B
S32.509A
S32.509B
S32.511A
S32.511B
S32.512A
S32.512B
S32.519A
S32.519B
S32.591A
S32.591B
S32.592A
S32.592B
S32.599A
S32.599B
S32.601A
S32.601B
S32.602A
S32.602B
S32.609A
S32.609B
S32.611A
S32.611B
S32.612A
S32.612B
S32.613A
S32.613B
S32.614A
S32.614B
S32.615A
S32.615B
S32.616A
S32.616B
S32.691A
S32.691B
S32.692A
S32.692B
S32.699A
S32.699B
S32.810A
S32.810B
S32.811A
S32.811B
S32.82XA
S32.82XB
S32.89XA
S32.89XB
S32.9XXA
S32.9XXB
S34.101A
S34.102A
S34.103A
S34.104A
S34.105A
S34.109A
S34.111A
S34.112A
S34.113A
S34.114A
S34.115A
S34.119A
S34.121A
S34.122A
S34.123A
S34.124A
S34.125A
S34.129A
S34.131A
S34.132A
S34.139A
S34.3XXA
S42.001B
S42.002B
S42.009B
S42.011B
S42.012B
S42.013B
S42.014B
S42.015B
S42.016B
S42.017B
S42.018B
S42.019B
S42.021B
S42.022B
S42.023B
S42.024B
S42.025B
S42.026B
S42.031B
S42.032B
S42.033B
S42.034B
S42.035B
S42.036B
S42.101B
S42.102B
S42.109B
S42.111B
S42.112B
S42.113B
S42.114B
S42.115B
S42.116B
S42.121B
S42.122B
S42.123B
S42.124B
S42.125B
S42.126B
S42.131B
S42.132B
S42.133B
S42.134B
S42.135B
S42.136B
S42.141B
S42.142B
S42.143B
S42.144B
S42.145B
S42.146B
S42.151B
S42.152B
S42.153B
S42.154B
S42.155B
S42.156B
S42.191B
S42.192B
S42.199B
S42.201A
S42.201B
S42.202A
S42.202B
S42.209A
S42.209B
S42.211A
S42.211B
S42.212A
S42.212B
S42.213A
S42.213B
S42.214A
S42.214B
S42.215A
S42.215B
S42.216A
S42.216B
S42.221A
S42.221B
S42.222A
S42.222B
S42.223A
S42.223B
S42.224A
S42.224B
S42.225A
S42.225B
S42.226A
S42.226B
S42.231A
S42.231B
S42.232A
S42.232B
S42.239A
S42.239B
S42.241A
S42.241B
S42.242A
S42.242B
S42.249A
S42.249B
S42.251A
S42.251B
S42.252A
S42.252B
S42.253A
S42.253B
S42.254A
S42.254B
S42.255A
S42.255B
S42.256A
S42.256B
S42.261A
S42.261B
S42.262A
S42.262B
S42.263A
S42.263B
S42.264A
S42.264B
S42.265A
S42.265B
S42.266A
S42.266B
S42.271A
S42.272A
S42.279A
S42.291A
S42.291B
S42.292A
S42.292B
S42.293A
S42.293B
S42.294A
S42.294B
S42.295A
S42.295B
S42.296A
S42.296B
S42.301A
S42.301B
S42.302A
S42.302B
S42.309A
S42.309B
S42.311A
S42.312A
S42.319A
S42.321A
S42.321B
S42.322A
S42.322B
S42.323A
S42.323B
S42.324A
S42.324B
S42.325A
S42.325B
S42.326A
S42.326B
S42.331A

Appendix G: Hospital Acquired Conditions

HAC 05: Falls and Trauma (continued)

S42.331B
S42.332A
S42.332B
S42.333A
S42.333B
S42.334A
S42.334B
S42.335A
S42.335B
S42.336A
S42.336B
S42.341A
S42.341B
S42.342A
S42.342B
S42.343A
S42.343B
S42.344A
S42.344B
S42.345A
S42.345B
S42.346A
S42.346B
S42.351A
S42.351B
S42.352A
S42.352B
S42.353A
S42.353B
S42.354A
S42.354B
S42.355A
S42.355B
S42.356A
S42.356B
S42.361A
S42.361B
S42.362A
S42.362B
S42.363A
S42.363B
S42.364A
S42.364B
S42.365A
S42.365B
S42.366A
S42.366B
S42.391A
S42.391B
S42.392A
S42.392B
S42.399A
S42.399B
S42.401A
S42.401B
S42.402A
S42.402B
S42.409A
S42.409B
S42.411A
S42.411B
S42.412A
S42.412B
S42.413A
S42.413B
S42.414A
S42.414B
S42.415A
S42.415B
S42.416A
S42.416B
S42.421A
S42.421B
S42.422A
S42.422B
S42.423A
S42.423B
S42.424A
S42.424B
S42.425A
S42.425B
S42.426A
S42.426B
S42.431A
S42.431B
S42.432A
S42.432B
S42.433A
S42.433B
S42.434A
S42.434B
S42.435A
S42.435B
S42.436A
S42.436B
S42.441A
S42.441B
S42.442A
S42.442B
S42.443A
S42.443B
S42.444A
S42.444B
S42.445A
S42.445B
S42.446A
S42.446B
S42.447A
S42.447B
S42.448A
S42.448B
S42.449A
S42.449B
S42.451A
S42.451B
S42.452A
S42.452B
S42.453A
S42.453B
S42.454A
S42.454B
S42.455A
S42.455B
S42.456A
S42.456B
S42.461A
S42.461B
S42.462A
S42.462B
S42.463A
S42.463B
S42.464A
S42.464B
S42.465A
S42.465B
S42.466A
S42.466B
S42.471A
S42.471B
S42.472A
S42.472B
S42.473A
S42.473B
S42.474A
S42.474B
S42.475A
S42.475B
S42.476A
S42.476B
S42.481A
S42.482A
S42.489A
S42.491A
S42.491B
S42.492A
S42.492B
S42.493A
S42.493B
S42.494A
S42.494B
S42.495A
S42.495B
S42.496A
S42.496B
S42.90XA
S42.90XB
S42.91XA
S42.91XB
S42.92XA
S42.92XB
S43.201A
S43.202A
S43.203A
S43.204A
S43.205A
S43.206A
S43.211A
S43.212A
S43.213A
S43.214A
S43.215A
S43.216A
S43.221A
S43.222A
S43.223A
S43.224A
S43.225A
S43.226A
S49.001A
S49.002A
S49.009A
S49.011A
S49.012A
S49.019A
S49.021A
S49.022A
S49.029A
S49.031A
S49.032A
S49.039A
S49.041A
S49.042A
S49.049A
S49.091A
S49.092A
S49.099A
S49.101A
S49.102A
S49.109A
S49.111A
S49.112A
S49.119A
S49.121A
S49.122A
S49.129A
S49.131A
S49.132A
S49.139A
S49.141A
S49.142A
S49.149A
S49.191A
S49.192A
S49.199A
S52.001B
S52.001C
S52.002B
S52.002C
S52.009B
S52.009C
S52.011A
S52.012A
S52.019A
S52.021B
S52.021C
S52.022B
S52.022C
S52.023B
S52.023C
S52.024B
S52.024C
S52.025B
S52.025C
S52.026B
S52.026C
S52.031B
S52.031C
S52.032B
S52.032C
S52.033B
S52.033C
S52.034B
S52.034C
S52.035B
S52.035C
S52.036B
S52.036C
S52.041B
S52.041C
S52.042B
S52.042C
S52.043B
S52.043C
S52.044B
S52.044C
S52.045B
S52.045C
S52.046B
S52.046C
S52.091B
S52.091C
S52.092B
S52.092C
S52.099B
S52.099C
S52.101B
S52.101C
S52.102B
S52.102C
S52.109B
S52.109C
S52.111A
S52.112A
S52.119A
S52.121B
S52.121C
S52.122B
S52.122C
S52.123B
S52.123C
S52.124B
S52.124C
S52.125B
S52.125C
S52.126B
S52.126C
S52.131B
S52.131C
S52.132B
S52.132C
S52.133B
S52.133C
S52.134B
S52.134C
S52.135B
S52.135C
S52.136B
S52.136C
S52.181B
S52.181C
S52.182B
S52.182C
S52.189B
S52.189C
S52.201A
S52.201B
S52.201C
S52.202A
S52.202B
S52.202C
S52.209A
S52.209B
S52.209C
S52.211A
S52.212A
S52.219A
S52.221A
S52.221B
S52.221C
S52.222A
S52.222B
S52.222C
S52.223A
S52.223B
S52.223C
S52.224A
S52.224B
S52.224C
S52.225A
S52.225B
S52.225C
S52.226A
S52.226B
S52.226C
S52.231A
S52.231B
S52.231C
S52.232A
S52.232B
S52.232C
S52.233A
S52.233B
S52.233C
S52.234A
S52.234B
S52.234C
S52.235A
S52.235B
S52.235C
S52.236A
S52.236B
S52.236C
S52.241A
S52.241B
S52.241C
S52.242A
S52.242B
S52.242C
S52.243A
S52.243B
S52.243C
S52.244A
S52.244B
S52.244C
S52.245A
S52.245B
S52.245C
S52.246A
S52.246B
S52.246C
S52.251A
S52.251B
S52.251C
S52.252A
S52.252B
S52.252C
S52.253A
S52.253B
S52.253C
S52.254A
S52.254B
S52.254C
S52.255A
S52.255B
S52.255C
S52.256A
S52.256B
S52.256C
S52.261A
S52.261B
S52.261C
S52.262A
S52.262B
S52.262C
S52.263A
S52.263B
S52.263C
S52.264A
S52.264B
S52.264C
S52.265A
S52.265B
S52.265C
S52.266A
S52.266B
S52.266C
S52.271B
S52.271C
S52.272B
S52.272C
S52.279B
S52.279C
S52.281A
S52.281B
S52.281C
S52.282A
S52.282B
S52.282C
S52.283A
S52.283B
S52.283C
S52.291A
S52.291B
S52.291C
S52.292A
S52.292B
S52.292C
S52.299A
S52.299B
S52.299C
S52.301A
S52.301B
S52.301C
S52.302A
S52.302B
S52.302C
S52.309A
S52.309B
S52.309C
S52.311A
S52.312A
S52.319A
S52.321A
S52.321B
S52.321C
S52.322A
S52.322B
S52.322C
S52.323A
S52.323B

HAC 05: Falls and Trauma (continued)

S52.323C
S52.324A
S52.324B
S52.324C
S52.325A
S52.325B
S52.325C
S52.326A
S52.326B
S52.326C
S52.331A
S52.331B
S52.331C
S52.332A
S52.332B
S52.332C
S52.333A
S52.333B
S52.333C
S52.334A
S52.334B
S52.334C
S52.335A
S52.335B
S52.335C
S52.336A
S52.336B
S52.336C
S52.341A
S52.341B
S52.341C
S52.342A
S52.342B
S52.342C
S52.343A
S52.343B
S52.343C
S52.344A
S52.344B
S52.344C
S52.345A
S52.345B
S52.345C
S52.346A
S52.346B
S52.346C
S52.351A
S52.351B
S52.351C
S52.352A
S52.352B
S52.352C
S52.353A
S52.353B
S52.353C
S52.354A
S52.354B
S52.354C
S52.355A
S52.355B
S52.355C
S52.356A
S52.356B
S52.356C
S52.361A
S52.361B
S52.361C
S52.362A
S52.362B
S52.362C
S52.363A
S52.363B
S52.363C
S52.364A
S52.364B
S52.364C
S52.365A
S52.365B
S52.365C
S52.366A
S52.366B
S52.366C
S52.371A
S52.371B
S52.371C
S52.372A
S52.372B
S52.372C
S52.379A
S52.379B
S52.379C
S52.381A
S52.381B
S52.381C
S52.382A
S52.382B
S52.382C
S52.389A
S52.389B
S52.389C
S52.391A
S52.391B
S52.391C
S52.392A
S52.392B
S52.392C
S52.399A
S52.399B
S52.399C
S52.501A
S52.501B
S52.501C
S52.502A
S52.502B
S52.502C
S52.509A
S52.509B
S52.509C
S52.511A
S52.511B
S52.511C
S52.512A
S52.512B
S52.512C
S52.513A
S52.513B
S52.513C
S52.514A
S52.514B
S52.514C
S52.515A
S52.515B
S52.515C
S52.516A
S52.516B
S52.516C
S52.521A
S52.522A
S52.529A
S52.531A
S52.531B
S52.531C
S52.532A
S52.532B
S52.532C
S52.539A
S52.539B
S52.539C
S52.541A
S52.541B
S52.541C
S52.542A
S52.542B
S52.542C
S52.549A
S52.549B
S52.549C
S52.551A
S52.551B
S52.551C
S52.552A
S52.552B
S52.552C
S52.559A
S52.559B
S52.559C
S52.561A
S52.561B
S52.561C
S52.562A
S52.562B
S52.562C
S52.569A
S52.569B
S52.569C
S52.571A
S52.571B
S52.571C
S52.572A
S52.572B
S52.572C
S52.579A
S52.579B
S52.579C
S52.591A
S52.591B
S52.591C
S52.592A
S52.592B
S52.592C
S52.599A
S52.599B
S52.599C
S52.601A
S52.601B
S52.601C
S52.602A
S52.602B
S52.602C
S52.609A
S52.609B
S52.609C
S52.611A
S52.611B
S52.611C
S52.612A
S52.612B
S52.612C
S52.613A
S52.613B
S52.613C
S52.614A
S52.614B
S52.614C
S52.615A
S52.615B
S52.615C
S52.616A
S52.616B
S52.616C
S52.621A
S52.622A
S52.629A
S52.691A
S52.691B
S52.691C
S52.692A
S52.692B
S52.692C
S52.699A
S52.699B
S52.699C
S52.90XA
S52.90XB
S52.90XC
S52.91XA
S52.91XB
S52.91XC
S52.92XA
S52.92XB
S52.92XC
S59.001A
S59.002A
S59.009A
S59.011A
S59.012A
S59.019A
S59.021A
S59.022A
S59.029A
S59.031A
S59.032A
S59.039A
S59.041A
S59.042A
S59.049A
S59.091A
S59.092A
S59.099A
S59.201A
S59.202A
S59.209A
S59.211A
S59.212A
S59.219A
S59.221A
S59.222A
S59.229A
S59.231A
S59.232A
S59.239A
S59.241A
S59.242A
S59.249A
S59.291A
S59.292A
S59.299A
S62.001B
S62.002B
S62.009B
S62.011B
S62.012B
S62.013B
S62.014B
S62.015B
S62.016B
S62.021B
S62.022B
S62.023B
S62.024B
S62.025B
S62.026B
S62.031B
S62.032B
S62.033B
S62.034B
S62.035B
S62.036B
S62.101B
S62.102B
S62.109B
S62.111B
S62.112B
S62.113B
S62.114B
S62.115B
S62.116B
S62.121B
S62.122B
S62.123B
S62.124B
S62.125B
S62.126B
S62.131B
S62.132B
S62.133B
S62.134B
S62.135B
S62.136B
S62.141B
S62.142B
S62.143B
S62.144B
S62.145B
S62.146B
S62.151B
S62.152B
S62.153B
S62.154B
S62.155B
S62.156B
S62.161B
S62.162B
S62.163B
S62.164B
S62.165B
S62.166B
S62.171B
S62.172B
S62.173B
S62.174B
S62.175B
S62.176B
S62.181B
S62.182B
S62.183B
S62.184B
S62.185B
S62.186B
S62.201B
S62.202B
S62.209B
S62.211B
S62.212B
S62.213B
S62.221B
S62.222B
S62.223B
S62.224B
S62.225B
S62.226B
S62.231B
S62.232B
S62.233B
S62.234B
S62.235B
S62.236B
S62.241B
S62.242B
S62.243B
S62.244B
S62.245B
S62.246B
S62.251B
S62.252B
S62.253B
S62.254B
S62.255B
S62.256B
S62.291B
S62.292B
S62.299B
S62.300B
S62.301B
S62.302B
S62.303B
S62.304B
S62.305B
S62.306B
S62.307B
S62.308B
S62.309B
S62.310B
S62.311B
S62.312B
S62.313B
S62.314B
S62.315B
S62.316B
S62.317B
S62.318B
S62.319B
S62.320B
S62.321B
S62.322B
S62.323B
S62.324B
S62.325B
S62.326B
S62.327B
S62.328B
S62.329B
S62.330B
S62.331B
S62.332B
S62.333B
S62.334B
S62.335B
S62.336B
S62.337B
S62.338B
S62.339B
S62.340B
S62.341B
S62.342B
S62.343B
S62.344B
S62.345B
S62.346B
S62.347B
S62.348B
S62.349B
S62.350B
S62.351B
S62.352B
S62.353B
S62.354B
S62.355B
S62.356B
S62.357B
S62.358B
S62.359B
S62.360B
S62.361B
S62.362B
S62.363B
S62.364B
S62.365B
S62.366B
S62.367B
S62.368B
S62.369B
S62.390B
S62.391B
S62.392B
S62.393B
S62.394B
S62.395B
S62.396B
S62.397B

HAC 05: Falls and Trauma (continued)

S62.398B
S62.399B
S62.5Ø1B
S62.5Ø2B
S62.5Ø9B
S62.511B
S62.512B
S62.513B
S62.514B
S62.515B
S62.516B
S62.521B
S62.522B
S62.523B
S62.524B
S62.525B
S62.526B
S62.6ØØB
S62.6Ø1B
S62.6Ø2B
S62.6Ø3B
S62.6Ø4B
S62.6Ø5B
S62.6Ø6B
S62.6Ø7B
S62.6Ø8B
S62.6Ø9B
S62.61ØB
S62.611B
S62.612B
S62.613B
S62.614B
S62.615B
S62.616B
S62.617B
S62.618B
S62.619B
S62.62ØB
S62.621B
S62.622B
S62.623B
S62.624B
S62.625B
S62.626B
S62.627B
S62.628B
S62.629B
S62.63ØB
S62.631B
S62.632B
S62.633B
S62.634B
S62.635B
S62.636B
S62.637B
S62.638B
S62.639B
S62.64ØB
S62.641B
S62.642B
S62.643B
S62.644B
S62.645B
S62.646B
S62.647B
S62.648B
S62.649B
S62.65ØB
S62.651B
S62.652B
S62.653B
S62.654B
S62.655B
S62.656B
S62.657B
S62.658B
S62.659B
S62.66ØB
S62.661B
S62.662B
S62.663B
S62.664B
S62.665B
S62.666B
S62.667B
S62.668B
S62.669B
S62.9ØXB
S62.91XB
S62.92XB
S72.ØØ1A
S72.ØØ1B
S72.ØØ1C
S72.ØØ2A
S72.ØØ2B
S72.ØØ2C
S72.ØØ9A
S72.ØØ9B
S72.ØØ9C
S72.Ø11A
S72.Ø11B
S72.Ø11C
S72.Ø12A
S72.Ø12B
S72.Ø12C
S72.Ø19A
S72.Ø19B
S72.Ø19C
S72.Ø21A
S72.Ø21B
S72.Ø21C
S72.Ø22A
S72.Ø22B
S72.Ø22C
S72.Ø23A
S72.Ø23B
S72.Ø23C
S72.Ø24A
S72.Ø24B
S72.Ø24C
S72.Ø25A
S72.Ø25B
S72.Ø25C
S72.Ø26A
S72.Ø26B
S72.Ø26C
S72.Ø31A
S72.Ø31B
S72.Ø31C
S72.Ø32A
S72.Ø32B
S72.Ø32C
S72.Ø33A
S72.Ø33B
S72.Ø33C
S72.Ø34A
S72.Ø34B
S72.Ø34C
S72.Ø35A
S72.Ø35B
S72.Ø35C
S72.Ø36A
S72.Ø36B
S72.Ø36C
S72.Ø41A
S72.Ø41B
S72.Ø41C
S72.Ø42A
S72.Ø42B
S72.Ø42C
S72.Ø43A
S72.Ø43B
S72.Ø43C
S72.Ø44A
S72.Ø44B
S72.Ø44C
S72.Ø45A
S72.Ø45B
S72.Ø45C
S72.Ø46A
S72.Ø46B
S72.Ø46C
S72.Ø51A
S72.Ø51B
S72.Ø51C
S72.Ø52A
S72.Ø52B
S72.Ø52C
S72.Ø59A
S72.Ø59B
S72.Ø59C
S72.Ø61A
S72.Ø61B
S72.Ø61C
S72.Ø62A
S72.Ø62B
S72.Ø62C
S72.Ø63A
S72.Ø63B
S72.Ø63C
S72.Ø64A
S72.Ø64B
S72.Ø64C
S72.Ø65A
S72.Ø65B
S72.Ø65C
S72.Ø66A
S72.Ø66B
S72.Ø66C
S72.Ø91A
S72.Ø91B
S72.Ø91C
S72.Ø92A
S72.Ø92B
S72.Ø92C
S72.Ø99A
S72.Ø99B
S72.Ø99C
S72.1Ø1A
S72.1Ø1B
S72.1Ø1C
S72.1Ø2A
S72.1Ø2B
S72.1Ø2C
S72.1Ø9A
S72.1Ø9B
S72.1Ø9C
S72.111A
S72.111B
S72.111C
S72.112A
S72.112B
S72.112C
S72.113A
S72.113B
S72.113C
S72.114A
S72.114B
S72.114C
S72.115A
S72.115B
S72.115C
S72.116A
S72.116B
S72.116C
S72.121A
S72.121B
S72.121C
S72.122A
S72.122B
S72.122C
S72.123A
S72.123B
S72.123C
S72.124A
S72.124B
S72.124C
S72.125A
S72.125B
S72.125C
S72.126A
S72.126B
S72.126C
S72.131A
S72.131B
S72.131C
S72.132A
S72.132B
S72.132C
S72.133A
S72.133B
S72.133C
S72.134A
S72.134B
S72.134C
S72.135A
S72.135B
S72.135C
S72.136A
S72.136B
S72.136C
S72.141A
S72.141B
S72.141C
S72.142A
S72.142B
S72.142C
S72.143A
S72.143B
S72.143C
S72.144A
S72.144B
S72.144C
S72.145A
S72.145B
S72.145C
S72.146A
S72.146B
S72.146C
S72.21XA
S72.21XB
S72.21XC
S72.22XA
S72.22XB
S72.22XC
S72.23XA
S72.23XB
S72.23XC
S72.24XA
S72.24XB
S72.24XC
S72.25XA
S72.25XB
S72.25XC
S72.26XA
S72.26XB
S72.26XC
S72.3Ø1A
S72.3Ø1B
S72.3Ø1C
S72.3Ø2A
S72.3Ø2B
S72.3Ø2C
S72.3Ø9A
S72.3Ø9B
S72.3Ø9C
S72.321A
S72.321B
S72.321C
S72.322A
S72.322B
S72.322C
S72.323A
S72.323B
S72.323C
S72.324A
S72.324B
S72.324C
S72.325A
S72.325B
S72.325C
S72.326A
S72.326B
S72.326C
S72.331A
S72.331B
S72.331C
S72.332A
S72.332B
S72.332C
S72.333A
S72.333B
S72.333C
S72.334A
S72.334B
S72.334C
S72.335A
S72.335B
S72.335C
S72.336A
S72.336B
S72.336C
S72.341A
S72.341B
S72.341C
S72.342A
S72.342B
S72.342C
S72.343A
S72.343B
S72.343C
S72.344A
S72.344B
S72.344C
S72.345A
S72.345B
S72.345C
S72.346A
S72.346B
S72.346C
S72.351A
S72.351B
S72.351C
S72.352A
S72.352B
S72.352C
S72.353A
S72.353B
S72.353C
S72.354A
S72.354B
S72.354C
S72.355A
S72.355B
S72.355C
S72.356A
S72.356B
S72.356C
S72.361A
S72.361B
S72.361C
S72.362A
S72.362B
S72.362C
S72.363A
S72.363B
S72.363C
S72.364A
S72.364B
S72.364C
S72.365A
S72.365B
S72.365C
S72.366A
S72.366B
S72.366C
S72.391A
S72.391B
S72.391C
S72.392A
S72.392B
S72.392C
S72.399A
S72.399B
S72.399C
S72.4Ø1A
S72.4Ø1B
S72.4Ø1C
S72.4Ø2A
S72.4Ø2B
S72.4Ø2C
S72.4Ø9A
S72.4Ø9B
S72.4Ø9C
S72.411A
S72.411B
S72.411C
S72.412A
S72.412B
S72.412C
S72.413A
S72.413B
S72.413C
S72.414A
S72.414B
S72.414C
S72.415A
S72.415B
S72.415C
S72.416A
S72.416B
S72.416C
S72.421A
S72.421B
S72.421C
S72.422A
S72.422B
S72.422C
S72.423A
S72.423B
S72.423C
S72.424A
S72.424B
S72.424C
S72.425A
S72.425B
S72.425C
S72.426A
S72.426B
S72.426C
S72.431A
S72.431B
S72.431C
S72.432A
S72.432B
S72.432C
S72.433A
S72.433B
S72.433C
S72.434A

HAC 05: Falls and Trauma (continued)

S72.434B
S72.434C
S72.435A
S72.435B
S72.435C
S72.436A
S72.436B
S72.436C
S72.441A
S72.441B
S72.441C
S72.442A
S72.442B
S72.442C
S72.443A
S72.443B
S72.443C
S72.444A
S72.444B
S72.444C
S72.445A
S72.445B
S72.445C
S72.446A
S72.446B
S72.446C
S72.451A
S72.451B
S72.451C
S72.452A
S72.452B
S72.452C
S72.453A
S72.453B
S72.453C
S72.454A
S72.454B
S72.454C
S72.455A
S72.455B
S72.455C
S72.456A
S72.456B
S72.456C
S72.461A
S72.461B
S72.461C
S72.462A
S72.462B
S72.462C
S72.463A
S72.463B
S72.463C
S72.464A
S72.464B
S72.464C
S72.465A
S72.465B
S72.465C
S72.466A
S72.466B
S72.466C
S72.471A
S72.472A
S72.479A
S72.491A
S72.491B
S72.491C
S72.492A
S72.492B
S72.492C
S72.499A
S72.499B
S72.499C
S72.8X1A
S72.8X1B
S72.8X1C
S72.8X2A
S72.8X2B
S72.8X2C
S72.8X9A
S72.8X9B
S72.8X9C
S72.90XA
S72.90XB
S72.90XC
S72.91XA
S72.91XB
S72.91XC
S72.92XA
S72.92XB
S72.92XC
S73.001A
S73.002A
S73.003A
S73.004A
S73.005A
S73.006A
S73.011A
S73.012A
S73.013A
S73.014A
S73.015A
S73.016A
S73.021A
S73.022A
S73.023A
S73.024A
S73.025A
S73.026A
S73.031A
S73.032A
S73.033A
S73.034A
S73.035A
S73.036A
S73.041A
S73.042A
S73.043A
S73.044A
S73.045A
S73.046A
S77.00XA
S77.01XA
S77.02XA
S77.10XA
S77.11XA
S77.12XA
S79.001A
S79.002A
S79.009A
S79.011A
S79.012A
S79.019A
S79.091A
S79.092A
S79.099A
S79.101A
S79.102A
S79.109A
S79.111A
S79.112A
S79.119A
S79.121A
S79.122A
S79.129A
S79.131A
S79.132A
S79.139A
S79.141A
S79.142A
S79.149A
S79.191A
S79.192A
S79.199A
S82.001A
S82.001B
S82.001C
S82.002A
S82.002B
S82.002C
S82.009A
S82.009B
S82.009C
S82.011A
S82.011B
S82.011C
S82.012A
S82.012B
S82.012C
S82.013A
S82.013B
S82.013C
S82.014A
S82.014B
S82.014C
S82.015A
S82.015B
S82.015C
S82.016A
S82.016B
S82.016C
S82.021A
S82.021B
S82.021C
S82.022A
S82.022B
S82.022C
S82.023A
S82.023B
S82.023C
S82.024A
S82.024B
S82.024C
S82.025A
S82.025B
S82.025C
S82.026A
S82.026B
S82.026C
S82.031A
S82.031B
S82.031C
S82.032A
S82.032B
S82.032C
S82.033A
S82.033B
S82.033C
S82.034A
S82.034B
S82.034C
S82.035A
S82.035B
S82.035C
S82.036A
S82.036B
S82.036C
S82.041A
S82.041B
S82.041C
S82.042A
S82.042B
S82.042C
S82.043A
S82.043B
S82.043C
S82.044A
S82.044B
S82.044C
S82.045A
S82.045B
S82.045C
S82.046A
S82.046B
S82.046C
S82.091A
S82.091B
S82.091C
S82.092A
S82.092B
S82.092C
S82.099A
S82.099B
S82.099C
S82.101A
S82.101B
S82.101C
S82.102A
S82.102B
S82.102C
S82.109A
S82.109B
S82.109C
S82.111A
S82.111B
S82.111C
S82.112A
S82.112B
S82.112C
S82.113A
S82.113B
S82.113C
S82.114A
S82.114B
S82.114C
S82.115A
S82.115B
S82.115C
S82.116A
S82.116B
S82.116C
S82.121A
S82.121B
S82.121C
S82.122A
S82.122B
S82.122C
S82.123A
S82.123B
S82.123C
S82.124A
S82.124B
S82.124C
S82.125A
S82.125B
S82.125C
S82.126A
S82.126B
S82.126C
S82.131A
S82.131B
S82.131C
S82.132A
S82.132B
S82.132C
S82.133A
S82.133B
S82.133C
S82.134A
S82.134B
S82.134C
S82.135A
S82.135B
S82.135C
S82.136A
S82.136B
S82.136C
S82.141A
S82.141B
S82.141C
S82.142A
S82.142B
S82.142C
S82.143A
S82.143B
S82.143C
S82.144A
S82.144B
S82.144C
S82.145A
S82.145B
S82.145C
S82.146A
S82.146B
S82.146C
S82.151A
S82.151B
S82.151C
S82.152A
S82.152B
S82.152C
S82.153A
S82.153B
S82.153C
S82.154A
S82.154B
S82.154C
S82.155A
S82.155B
S82.155C
S82.156A
S82.156B
S82.156C
S82.161A
S82.162A
S82.169A
S82.191A
S82.191B
S82.191C
S82.192A
S82.192B
S82.192C
S82.199A
S82.199B
S82.199C
S82.201A
S82.201B
S82.201C
S82.202A
S82.202B
S82.202C
S82.209A
S82.209B
S82.209C
S82.221A
S82.221B
S82.221C
S82.222A
S82.222B
S82.222C
S82.223A
S82.223B
S82.223C
S82.224A
S82.224B
S82.224C
S82.225A
S82.225B
S82.225C
S82.226A
S82.226B
S82.226C
S82.231A
S82.231B
S82.231C
S82.232A
S82.232B
S82.232C
S82.233A
S82.233B
S82.233C
S82.234A
S82.234B
S82.234C
S82.235A
S82.235B
S82.235C
S82.236A
S82.236B
S82.236C
S82.241A
S82.241B
S82.241C
S82.242A
S82.242B
S82.242C
S82.243A
S82.243B
S82.243C
S82.244A
S82.244B
S82.244C
S82.245A
S82.245B
S82.245C
S82.246A
S82.246B
S82.246C
S82.251A
S82.251B
S82.251C
S82.252A
S82.252B
S82.252C
S82.253A
S82.253B
S82.253C
S82.254A
S82.254B
S82.254C
S82.255A
S82.255B
S82.255C
S82.256A
S82.256B
S82.256C
S82.261A
S82.261B
S82.261C
S82.262A
S82.262B
S82.262C
S82.263A
S82.263B
S82.263C
S82.264A
S82.264B
S82.264C
S82.265A
S82.265B
S82.265C
S82.266A
S82.266B
S82.266C
S82.291A
S82.291B
S82.291C
S82.292A
S82.292B

Appendix G: Hospital Acquired Conditions

HAC 05: Falls and Trauma (continued)

S82.292C
S82.299A
S82.299B
S82.299C
S82.301B
S82.301C
S82.302B
S82.302C
S82.309B
S82.309C
S82.311A
S82.312A
S82.319A
S82.391B
S82.391C
S82.392B
S82.392C
S82.399B
S82.399C
S82.401B
S82.401C
S82.402B
S82.402C
S82.409B
S82.409C
S82.421B
S82.421C
S82.422B
S82.422C
S82.423B
S82.423C
S82.424B
S82.424C
S82.425B
S82.425C
S82.426B
S82.426C
S82.431B
S82.431C
S82.432B
S82.432C
S82.433B
S82.433C
S82.434B
S82.434C
S82.435B
S82.435C
S82.436B
S82.436C
S82.441B
S82.441C
S82.442B
S82.442C
S82.443B
S82.443C
S82.444B
S82.444C
S82.445B
S82.445C
S82.446B
S82.446C
S82.451B
S82.451C
S82.452B
S82.452C
S82.453B
S82.453C
S82.454B
S82.454C
S82.455B
S82.455C
S82.456B
S82.456C
S82.461B
S82.461C
S82.462B
S82.462C
S82.463B
S82.463C
S82.464B
S82.464C
S82.465B
S82.465C
S82.466B
S82.466C
S82.491B
S82.491C
S82.492B
S82.492C
S82.499B
S82.499C
S82.51XB
S82.51XC
S82.52XB
S82.52XC
S82.53XB
S82.53XC
S82.54XB
S82.54XC
S82.55XB
S82.55XC
S82.56XB
S82.56XC
S82.61XB
S82.61XC
S82.62XB
S82.62XC
S82.63XB
S82.63XC
S82.64XB
S82.64XC
S82.65XB
S82.65XC
S82.66XB
S82.66XC
S82.831B
S82.831C
S82.832B
S82.832C
S82.839B
S82.839C
S82.841B
S82.841C
S82.842B
S82.842C
S82.843B
S82.843C
S82.844B
S82.844C
S82.845B
S82.845C
S82.846B
S82.846C
S82.851B
S82.851C
S82.852B
S82.852C
S82.853B
S82.853C
S82.854B
S82.854C
S82.855B
S82.855C
S82.856B
S82.856C
S82.861B
S82.861C
S82.862B
S82.862C
S82.863B
S82.863C
S82.864B
S82.864C
S82.865B
S82.865C
S82.866B
S82.866C
S82.871B
S82.871C
S82.872B
S82.872C
S82.873B
S82.873C
S82.874B
S82.874C
S82.875B
S82.875C
S82.876B
S82.876C
S82.891B
S82.891C
S82.892B
S82.892C
S82.899B
S82.899C
S82.90XB
S82.90XC
S82.91XB
S82.91XC
S82.92XB
S82.92XC
S89.001A
S89.002A
S89.009A
S89.011A
S89.012A
S89.019A
S89.021A
S89.022A
S89.029A
S89.031A
S89.032A
S89.039A
S89.041A
S89.042A
S89.049A
S89.091A
S89.092A
S89.099A
S92.001B
S92.002B
S92.009B
S92.011B
S92.012B
S92.013B
S92.014B
S92.015B
S92.016B
S92.021B
S92.022B
S92.023B
S92.024B
S92.025B
S92.026B
S92.031B
S92.032B
S92.033B
S92.034B
S92.035B
S92.036B
S92.041B
S92.042B
S92.043B
S92.044B
S92.045B
S92.046B
S92.051B
S92.052B
S92.053B
S92.054B
S92.055B
S92.056B
S92.061B
S92.062B
S92.063B
S92.064B
S92.065B
S92.066B
S92.101B
S92.102B
S92.109B
S92.111B
S92.112B
S92.113B
S92.114B
S92.115B
S92.116B
S92.121B
S92.122B
S92.123B
S92.124B
S92.125B
S92.126B
S92.131B
S92.132B
S92.133B
S92.134B
S92.135B
S92.136B
S92.141B
S92.142B
S92.143B
S92.144B
S92.145B
S92.146B
S92.151B
S92.152B
S92.153B
S92.154B
S92.155B
S92.156B
S92.191B
S92.192B
S92.199B
S92.201B
S92.202B
S92.209B
S92.211B
S92.212B
S92.213B
S92.214B
S92.215B
S92.216B
S92.221B
S92.222B
S92.223B
S92.224B
S92.225B
S92.226B
S92.231B
S92.232B
S92.233B
S92.234B
S92.235B
S92.236B
S92.241B
S92.242B
S92.243B
S92.244B
S92.245B
S92.246B
S92.251B
S92.252B
S92.253B
S92.254B
S92.255B
S92.256B
S92.301B
S92.302B
S92.309B
S92.311B
S92.312B
S92.313B
S92.314B
S92.315B
S92.316B
S92.321B
S92.322B
S92.323B
S92.324B
S92.325B
S92.326B
S92.331B
S92.332B
S92.333B
S92.334B
S92.335B
S92.336B
S92.341B
S92.342B
S92.343B
S92.344B
S92.345B
S92.346B
S92.351B
S92.352B
S92.353B
S92.354B
S92.355B
S92.356B
S92.811B
S92.812B
S92.819B
S92.901B
S92.902B
S92.909B
T20.30XA
T20.311A
T20.312A
T20.319A
T20.32XA
T20.33XA
T20.34XA
T20.35XA
T20.36XA
T20.37XA
T20.39XA
T20.70XA
T20.711A
T20.712A
T20.719A
T20.72XA
T20.73XA
T20.74XA
T20.75XA
T20.76XA
T20.77XA
T20.79XA
T21.30XA
T21.31XA
T21.32XA
T21.33XA
T21.34XA
T21.35XA
T21.36XA
T21.37XA
T21.39XA
T21.70XA
T21.71XA
T21.72XA
T21.73XA
T21.74XA
T21.75XA
T21.76XA
T21.77XA
T21.79XA
T22.30XA
T22.311A
T22.312A
T22.319A
T22.321A
T22.322A
T22.329A
T22.331A
T22.332A
T22.339A
T22.341A
T22.342A
T22.349A
T22.351A
T22.352A
T22.359A
T22.361A
T22.362A
T22.369A
T22.391A
T22.392A
T22.399A
T22.70XA
T22.711A
T22.712A
T22.719A
T22.721A
T22.722A
T22.729A
T22.731A
T22.732A
T22.739A
T22.741A
T22.742A
T22.749A
T22.751A
T22.752A
T22.759A
T22.761A
T22.762A
T22.769A
T22.791A
T22.792A
T22.799A
T23.301A
T23.302A
T23.309A
T23.311A
T23.312A
T23.319A
T23.321A
T23.322A
T23.329A
T23.331A
T23.332A
T23.339A
T23.341A
T23.342A
T23.349A
T23.351A
T23.352A
T23.359A
T23.361A
T23.362A
T23.369A
T23.371A
T23.372A
T23.379A
T23.391A
T23.392A
T23.399A
T23.701A
T23.702A
T23.709A

HAC 05: Falls and Trauma (continued)

T23.711A
T23.712A
T23.719A
T23.721A
T23.722A
T23.729A
T23.731A
T23.732A
T23.739A
T23.741A
T23.742A
T23.749A
T23.751A
T23.752A
T23.759A
T23.761A
T23.762A
T23.769A
T23.771A
T23.772A
T23.779A
T23.791A
T23.792A
T23.799A
T24.3Ø1A
T24.3Ø2A
T24.3Ø9A
T24.311A
T24.312A
T24.319A
T24.321A
T24.322A
T24.329A
T24.331A
T24.332A
T24.339A
T24.391A
T24.392A
T24.399A
T24.7Ø1A
T24.7Ø2A
T24.7Ø9A
T24.711A
T24.712A
T24.719A
T24.721A
T24.722A
T24.729A
T24.731A
T24.732A
T24.739A
T24.791A
T24.792A
T24.799A
T25.311A
T25.312A
T25.319A
T25.321A
T25.322A
T25.329A
T25.331A
T25.332A
T25.339A
T25.391A
T25.392A
T25.399A
T25.711A
T25.712A
T25.719A
T25.721A
T25.722A
T25.729A
T25.731A
T25.732A
T25.739A
T25.791A
T25.792A
T25.799A
T26.2ØXA
T26.21XA
T26.22XA
T26.7ØXA
T26.71XA
T26.72XA
T27.ØXXA
T27.1XXA
T27.2XXA
T27.3XXA
T27.4XXA
T27.5XXA
T27.6XXA
T27.7XXA
T28.1XXA
T28.2XXA
T28.6XXA
T28.7XXA
T31.1Ø
T31.11
T31.2Ø
T31.21
T31.22
T31.3Ø
T31.31
T31.32
T31.33
T31.4Ø
T31.41
T31.42
T31.43
T31.44
T31.5Ø
T31.51
T31.52
T31.53
T31.54
T31.55
T31.6Ø
T31.61
T31.62
T31.63
T31.64
T31.65
T31.66
T31.7Ø
T31.71
T31.72
T31.73
T31.74
T31.75
T31.76
T31.77
T31.8Ø
T31.81
T31.82
T31.83
T31.84
T31.85
T31.86
T31.87
T31.88
T31.9Ø
T31.91
T31.92
T31.93
T31.94
T31.95
T31.96
T31.97
T31.98
T31.99
T32.1Ø
T32.11
T32.2Ø
T32.21
T32.22
T32.3Ø
T32.31
T32.32
T32.33
T32.4Ø
T32.41
T32.42
T32.43
T32.44
T32.5Ø
T32.51
T32.52
T32.53
T32.54
T32.55
T32.6Ø
T32.61
T32.62
T32.63
T32.64
T32.65
T32.66
T32.7Ø
T32.71
T32.72
T32.73
T32.74
T32.75
T32.76
T32.77
T32.8Ø
T32.81
T32.82
T32.83
T32.84
T32.85
T32.86
T32.87
T32.88
T32.9Ø
T32.91
T32.92
T32.93
T32.94
T32.95
T32.96
T32.97
T32.98
T32.99
T33.Ø11A
T33.Ø12A
T33.Ø19A
T33.Ø2XA
T33.Ø9XA
T33.1XXA
T33.2XXA
T33.3XXA
T33.4ØXA
T33.41XA
T33.42XA
T33.511A
T33.512A
T33.519A
T33.521A
T33.522A
T33.529A
T33.531A
T33.532A
T33.539A
T33.6ØXA
T33.61XA
T33.62XA
T33.7ØXA
T33.71XA
T33.72XA
T33.811A
T33.812A
T33.819A
T33.821A
T33.822A
T33.829A
T33.831A
T33.832A
T33.839A
T33.9ØXA
T33.99XA
T34.Ø11A
T34.Ø12A
T34.Ø19A
T34.Ø2XA
T34.Ø9XA
T34.1XXA
T34.2XXA
T34.3XXA
T34.4ØXA
T34.41XA
T34.42XA
T34.511A
T34.512A
T34.519A
T34.521A
T34.522A
T34.529A
T34.531A
T34.532A
T34.539A
T34.6ØXA
T34.61XA
T34.62XA
T34.7ØXA
T34.71XA
T34.72XA
T34.811A
T34.812A
T34.819A
T34.821A
T34.822A
T34.829A
T34.831A
T34.832A
T34.839A
T34.9ØXA
T34.99XA
T67.Ø1XA
T67.Ø2XA
T67.Ø9XA
T69.Ø21A
T69.Ø22A
T69.Ø29A
T7Ø.3XXA
T71.111A
T71.112A
T71.113A
T71.114A
T71.121A
T71.122A
T71.123A
T71.124A
T71.131A
T71.132A
T71.133A
T71.134A
T71.141A
T71.143A
T71.144A
T71.151A
T71.152A
T71.153A
T71.154A
T71.161A
T71.162A
T71.163A
T71.164A
T71.191A
T71.192A
T71.193A
T71.194A
T71.2ØXA
T71.21XA
T71.29XA
T71.9XXA
T75.1XXA

HAC 06: Catheter Associated Urinary Tract Infection (UTI)

Secondary diagnosis not POA:

T83.511A
T83.518A

With or Without

Secondary diagnosis (also not POA) of:

B37.41
B37.49
N1Ø
N11.9
N12
N13.6
N15.1
N28.84
N28.85
N28.86
N3Ø.ØØ
N3Ø.Ø1
N34.Ø
N39.Ø

HAC 07: Vascular Catheter Associated Infection

Secondary diagnosis not POA:

T8Ø.211A
T8Ø.212A
T8Ø.218A
T8Ø.219A

HAC 08: Surgical Site Infection of Mediastinitis after Coronary Bypass Graft (CABG)

Secondary diagnosis not POA:

J98.51
J98.59

AND

Any of the following procedures:

Ø210083 Bypass Coronary Artery, One Artery from Coronary Artery with Zooplastic Tissue, Open Approach
Ø210088 Bypass Coronary Artery, One Artery from Right Internal Mammary with Zooplastic Tissue, Open Approach
Ø210089 Bypass Coronary Artery, One Artery from Left Internal Mammary with Zooplastic Tissue, Open Approach
Ø21008C Bypass Coronary Artery, One Artery from Thoracic Artery with Zooplastic Tissue, Open Approach
Ø21008F Bypass Coronary Artery, One Artery from Abdominal Artery with Zooplastic Tissue, Open Approach
Ø21008W Bypass Coronary Artery, One Artery from Aorta with Zooplastic Tissue, Open Approach
Ø210093 Bypass Coronary Artery, One Artery from Coronary Artery with Autologous Venous Tissue, Open Approach
Ø210098 Bypass Coronary Artery, One Artery from Right Internal Mammary with Autologous Venous Tissue, Open Approach
Ø210099 Bypass Coronary Artery, One Artery from Left Internal Mammary with Autologous Venous Tissue, Open Approach
Ø21009C Bypass Coronary Artery, One Artery from Thoracic Artery with Autologous Venous Tissue, Open Approach
Ø21009F Bypass Coronary Artery, One Artery from Abdominal Artery with Autologous Venous Tissue, Open Approach
Ø21009W Bypass Coronary Artery, One Artery from Aorta with Autologous Venous Tissue, Open Approach
Ø2100A3 Bypass Coronary Artery, One Artery from Coronary Artery with Autologous Arterial Tissue, Open Approach
Ø2100A8 Bypass Coronary Artery, One Artery from Right Internal Mammary with Autologous Arterial Tissue, Open Approach
Ø2100A9 Bypass Coronary Artery, One Artery from Left Internal Mammary with Autologous Arterial Tissue, Open Approach
Ø2100AC Bypass Coronary Artery, One Artery from Thoracic Artery with Autologous Arterial Tissue, Open Approach
Ø2100AF Bypass Coronary Artery, One Artery from Abdominal Artery with Autologous Arterial Tissue, Open Approach
Ø2100AW Bypass Coronary Artery, One Artery from Aorta with Autologous Arterial Tissue, Open Approach
Ø2100J3 Bypass Coronary Artery, One Artery from Coronary Artery with Synthetic Substitute, Open Approach
Ø2100J8 Bypass Coronary Artery, One Artery from Right Internal Mammary with Synthetic Substitute, Open Approach
Ø2100J9 Bypass Coronary Artery, One Artery from Left Internal Mammary with Synthetic Substitute, Open Approach
Ø2100JC Bypass Coronary Artery, One Artery from Thoracic Artery with Synthetic Substitute, Open Approach
Ø2100JF Bypass Coronary Artery, One Artery from Abdominal Artery with Synthetic Substitute, Open Approach
Ø2100JW Bypass Coronary Artery, One Artery from Aorta with Synthetic Substitute, Open Approach
Ø2100K3 Bypass Coronary Artery, One Artery from Coronary Artery with Nonautologous Tissue Substitute, Open Approach
Ø2100K8 Bypass Coronary Artery, One Artery from Right Internal Mammary with Nonautologous Tissue Substitute, Open Approach
Ø2100K9 Bypass Coronary Artery, One Artery from Left Internal Mammary with Nonautologous Tissue Substitute, Open Approach
Ø2100KC Bypass Coronary Artery, One Artery from Thoracic Artery with Nonautologous Tissue Substitute, Open Approach
Ø2100KF Bypass Coronary Artery, One Artery from Abdominal Artery with Nonautologous Tissue Substitute, Open Approach
Ø2100KW Bypass Coronary Artery, One Artery from Aorta with Nonautologous Tissue Substitute, Open Approach
Ø2100Z3 Bypass Coronary Artery, One Artery from Coronary Artery, Open Approach
Ø2100Z8 Bypass Coronary Artery, One Artery from Right Internal Mammary, Open Approach
Ø2100Z9 Bypass Coronary Artery, One Artery from Left Internal Mammary, Open Approach
Ø2100ZC Bypass Coronary Artery, One Artery from Thoracic Artery, Open Approach
Ø2100ZF Bypass Coronary Artery, One Artery from Abdominal Artery, Open Approach
Ø210483 Bypass Coronary Artery, One Artery from Coronary Artery with Zooplastic Tissue, Percutaneous Endoscopic Approach
Ø210488 Bypass Coronary Artery, One Artery from Right Internal Mammary with Zooplastic Tissue, Percutaneous Endoscopic Approach
Ø210489 Bypass Coronary Artery, One Artery from Left Internal Mammary with Zooplastic Tissue, Percutaneous Endoscopic Approach
Ø21048C Bypass Coronary Artery, One Artery from Thoracic Artery with Zooplastic Tissue, Percutaneous Endoscopic Approach
Ø21048F Bypass Coronary Artery, One Artery from Abdominal Artery with Zooplastic Tissue, Percutaneous Endoscopic Approach
Ø21048W Bypass Coronary Artery, One Artery from Aorta with Zooplastic Tissue, Percutaneous Endoscopic Approach
Ø210493 Bypass Coronary Artery, One Artery from Coronary Artery with Autologous Venous Tissue, Percutaneous Endoscopic Approach
Ø210498 Bypass Coronary Artery, One Artery from Right Internal Mammary with Autologous Venous Tissue, Percutaneous Endoscopic Approach
Ø210499 Bypass Coronary Artery, One Artery from Left Internal Mammary with Autologous Venous Tissue, Percutaneous Endoscopic Approach
Ø21049C Bypass Coronary Artery, One Artery from Thoracic Artery with Autologous Venous Tissue, Percutaneous Endoscopic Approach
Ø21049F Bypass Coronary Artery, One Artery from Abdominal Artery with Autologous Venous Tissue, Percutaneous Endoscopic Approach
Ø21049W Bypass Coronary Artery, One Artery from Aorta with Autologous Venous Tissue, Percutaneous Endoscopic Approach
Ø2104A3 Bypass Coronary Artery, One Artery from Coronary Artery with Autologous Arterial Tissue, Percutaneous Endoscopic Approach
Ø2104A8 Bypass Coronary Artery, One Artery from Right Internal Mammary with Autologous Arterial Tissue, Percutaneous Endoscopic Approach
Ø2104A9 Bypass Coronary Artery, One Artery from Left Internal Mammary with Autologous Arterial Tissue, Percutaneous Endoscopic Approach
Ø2104AC Bypass Coronary Artery, One Artery from Thoracic Artery with Autologous Arterial Tissue, Percutaneous Endoscopic Approach
Ø2104AF Bypass Coronary Artery, One Artery from Abdominal Artery with Autologous Arterial Tissue, Percutaneous Endoscopic Approach
Ø2104AW Bypass Coronary Artery, One Artery from Aorta with Autologous Arterial Tissue, Percutaneous Endoscopic Approach
Ø2104J3 Bypass Coronary Artery, One Artery from Coronary Artery with Synthetic Substitute, Percutaneous Endoscopic Approach
Ø2104J8 Bypass Coronary Artery, One Artery from Right Internal Mammary with Synthetic Substitute, Percutaneous Endoscopic Approach
Ø2104J9 Bypass Coronary Artery, One Artery from Left Internal Mammary with Synthetic Substitute, Percutaneous Endoscopic Approach
Ø2104JC Bypass Coronary Artery, One Artery from Thoracic Artery with Synthetic Substitute, Percutaneous Endoscopic Approach
Ø2104JF Bypass Coronary Artery, One Artery from Abdominal Artery with Synthetic Substitute, Percutaneous Endoscopic Approach
Ø2104JW Bypass Coronary Artery, One Artery from Aorta with Synthetic Substitute, Percutaneous Endoscopic Approach
Ø2104K3 Bypass Coronary Artery, One Artery from Coronary Artery with Nonautologous Tissue Substitute, Percutaneous Endoscopic Approach
Ø2104K8 Bypass Coronary Artery, One Artery from Right Internal Mammary with Nonautologous Tissue Substitute, Percutaneous Endoscopic Approach
Ø2104K9 Bypass Coronary Artery, One Artery from Left Internal Mammary with Nonautologous Tissue Substitute, Percutaneous Endoscopic Approach
Ø2104KC Bypass Coronary Artery, One Artery from Thoracic Artery with Nonautologous Tissue Substitute, Percutaneous Endoscopic Approach
Ø2104KF Bypass Coronary Artery, One Artery from Abdominal Artery with Nonautologous Tissue Substitute, Percutaneous Endoscopic Approach
Ø2104KW Bypass Coronary Artery, One Artery from Aorta with Nonautologous Tissue Substitute, Percutaneous Endoscopic Approach
Ø2104Z3 Bypass Coronary Artery, One Artery from Coronary Artery, Percutaneous Endoscopic Approach

HAC 08: Surgical Artery Infection of Mediastinitis after Coronary Bypass Graft (CABG) (continued)

Ø2104Z8 Bypass Coronary Artery, One Artery from Right Internal Mammary, Percutaneous Endoscopic Approach
Ø2104Z9 Bypass Coronary Artery, One Artery from Left Internal Mammary, Percutaneous Endoscopic Approach
Ø2104ZC Bypass Coronary Artery, One Artery from Thoracic Artery, Percutaneous Endoscopic Approach
Ø2104ZF Bypass Coronary Artery, One Artery from Abdominal Artery, Percutaneous Endoscopic Approach
Ø211Ø83 Bypass Coronary Artery, Two Arteries from Coronary Artery with Zooplastic Tissue, Open Approach
Ø211Ø88 Bypass Coronary Artery, Two Arteries from Right Internal Mammary with Zooplastic Tissue, Open Approach
Ø211Ø89 Bypass Coronary Artery, Two Arteries from Left Internal Mammary with Zooplastic Tissue, Open Approach
Ø211Ø8C Bypass Coronary Artery, Two Arteries from Thoracic Artery with Zooplastic Tissue, Open Approach
Ø211Ø8F Bypass Coronary Artery, Two Arteries from Abdominal Artery with Zooplastic Tissue, Open Approach
Ø211Ø8W Bypass Coronary Artery, Two Arteries from Aorta with Zooplastic Tissue, Open Approach
Ø211Ø93 Bypass Coronary Artery, Two Arteries from Coronary Artery with Autologous Venous Tissue, Open Approach
Ø211Ø98 Bypass Coronary Artery, Two Arteries from Right Internal Mammary with Autologous Venous Tissue, Open Approach
Ø211Ø99 Bypass Coronary Artery, Two Arteries from Left Internal Mammary with Autologous Venous Tissue, Open Approach
Ø211Ø9C Bypass Coronary Artery, Two Arteries from Thoracic Artery with Autologous Venous Tissue, Open Approach
Ø211Ø9F Bypass Coronary Artery, Two Arteries from Abdominal Artery with Autologous Venous Tissue, Open Approach
Ø211Ø9W Bypass Coronary Artery, Two Arteries from Aorta with Autologous Venous Tissue, Open Approach
Ø211ØA3 Bypass Coronary Artery, Two Arteries from Coronary Artery with Autologous Arterial Tissue, Open Approach
Ø211ØA8 Bypass Coronary Artery, Two Arteries from Right Internal Mammary with Autologous Arterial Tissue, Open Approach
Ø211ØA9 Bypass Coronary Artery, Two Arteries from Left Internal Mammary with Autologous Arterial Tissue, Open Approach
Ø211ØAC Bypass Coronary Artery, Two Arteries from Thoracic Artery with Autologous Arterial Tissue, Open Approach
Ø211ØAF Bypass Coronary Artery, Two Arteries from Abdominal Artery with Autologous Arterial Tissue, Open Approach
Ø211ØAW Bypass Coronary Artery, Two Arteries from Aorta with Autologous Arterial Tissue, Open Approach
Ø211ØJ3 Bypass Coronary Artery, Two Arteries from Coronary Artery with Synthetic Substitute, Open Approach
Ø211ØJ8 Bypass Coronary Artery, Two Arteries from Right Internal Mammary with Synthetic Substitute, Open Approach
Ø211ØJ9 Bypass Coronary Artery, Two Arteries from Left Internal Mammary with Synthetic Substitute, Open Approach
Ø211ØJC Bypass Coronary Artery, Two Arteries from Thoracic Artery with Synthetic Substitute, Open Approach
Ø211ØJF Bypass Coronary Artery, Two Arteries from Abdominal Artery with Synthetic Substitute, Open Approach
Ø211ØJW Bypass Coronary Artery, Two Arteries from Aorta with Synthetic Substitute, Open Approach
Ø211ØK3 Bypass Coronary Artery, Two Arteries from Coronary Artery with Nonautologous Tissue Substitute, Open Approach
Ø211ØK8 Bypass Coronary Artery, Two Arteries from Right Internal Mammary with Nonautologous Tissue Substitute, Open Approach
Ø211ØK9 Bypass Coronary Artery, Two Arteries from Left Internal Mammary with Nonautologous Tissue Substitute, Open Approach
Ø211ØKC Bypass Coronary Artery, Two Arteries from Thoracic Artery with Nonautologous Tissue Substitute, Open Approach
Ø211ØKF Bypass Coronary Artery, Two Arteries from Abdominal Artery with Nonautologous Tissue Substitute, Open Approach
Ø211ØKW Bypass Coronary Artery, Two Arteries from Aorta with Nonautologous Tissue Substitute, Open Approach
Ø211ØZ3 Bypass Coronary Artery, Two Arteries from Coronary Artery, Open Approach
Ø211ØZ8 Bypass Coronary Artery, Two Arteries from Right Internal Mammary, Open Approach
Ø211ØZ9 Bypass Coronary Artery, Two Arteries from Left Internal Mammary, Open Approach
Ø211ØZC Bypass Coronary Artery, Two Arteries from Thoracic Artery, Open Approach
Ø211ØZF Bypass Coronary Artery, Two Arteries from Abdominal Artery, Open Approach
Ø211483 Bypass Coronary Artery, Two Arteries from Coronary Artery with Zooplastic Tissue, Percutaneous Endoscopic Approach
Ø211488 Bypass Coronary Artery, Two Arteries from Right Internal Mammary with Zooplastic Tissue, Percutaneous Endoscopic Approach
Ø211489 Bypass Coronary Artery, Two Arteries from Left Internal Mammary with Zooplastic Tissue, Percutaneous Endoscopic Approach
Ø21148C Bypass Coronary Artery, Two Arteries from Thoracic Artery with Zooplastic Tissue, Percutaneous Endoscopic Approach
Ø21148F Bypass Coronary Artery, Two Arteries from Abdominal Artery with Zooplastic Tissue, Percutaneous Endoscopic Approach
Ø21148W Bypass Coronary Artery, Two Arteries from Aorta with Zooplastic Tissue, Percutaneous Endoscopic Approach
Ø211493 Bypass Coronary Artery, Two Arteries from Coronary Artery with Autologous Venous Tissue, Percutaneous Endoscopic Approach
Ø211498 Bypass Coronary Artery, Two Arteries from Right Internal Mammary with Autologous Venous Tissue, Percutaneous Endoscopic Approach
Ø211499 Bypass Coronary Artery, Two Arteries from Left Internal Mammary with Autologous Venous Tissue, Percutaneous Endoscopic Approach
Ø21149C Bypass Coronary Artery, Two Arteries from Thoracic Artery with Autologous Venous Tissue, Percutaneous Endoscopic Approach
Ø21149F Bypass Coronary Artery, Two Arteries from Abdominal Artery with Autologous Venous Tissue, Percutaneous Endoscopic Approach
Ø21149W Bypass Coronary Artery, Two Arteries from Aorta with Autologous Venous Tissue, Percutaneous Endoscopic Approach
Ø2114A3 Bypass Coronary Artery, Two Arteries from Coronary Artery with Autologous Arterial Tissue, Percutaneous Endoscopic Approach
Ø2114A8 Bypass Coronary Artery, Two Arteries from Right Internal Mammary with Autologous Arterial Tissue, Percutaneous Endoscopic Approach
Ø2114A9 Bypass Coronary Artery, Two Arteries from Left Internal Mammary with Autologous Arterial Tissue, Percutaneous Endoscopic Approach
Ø2114AC Bypass Coronary Artery, Two Arteries from Thoracic Artery with Autologous Arterial Tissue, Percutaneous Endoscopic Approach
Ø2114AF Bypass Coronary Artery, Two Arteries from Abdominal Artery with Autologous Arterial Tissue, Percutaneous Endoscopic Approach
Ø2114AW Bypass Coronary Artery, Two Arteries from Aorta with Autologous Arterial Tissue, Percutaneous Endoscopic Approach
Ø2114J3 Bypass Coronary Artery, Two Arteries from Coronary Artery with Synthetic Substitute, Percutaneous Endoscopic Approach
Ø2114J8 Bypass Coronary Artery, Two Arteries from Right Internal Mammary with Synthetic Substitute, Percutaneous Endoscopic Approach
Ø2114J9 Bypass Coronary Artery, Two Arteries from Left Internal Mammary with Synthetic Substitute, Percutaneous Endoscopic Approach
Ø2114JC Bypass Coronary Artery, Two Arteries from Thoracic Artery with Synthetic Substitute, Percutaneous Endoscopic Approach
Ø2114JF Bypass Coronary Artery, Two Arteries from Abdominal Artery with Synthetic Substitute, Percutaneous Endoscopic Approach
Ø2114JW Bypass Coronary Artery, Two Arteries from Aorta with Synthetic Substitute, Percutaneous Endoscopic Approach
Ø2114K3 Bypass Coronary Artery, Two Arteries from Coronary Artery with Nonautologous Tissue Substitute, Percutaneous Endoscopic Approach
Ø2114K8 Bypass Coronary Artery, Two Arteries from Right Internal Mammary with Nonautologous Tissue Substitute, Percutaneous Endoscopic Approach

HAC 08: Surgical Site Infection of Mediastinitis after Coronary Bypass Graft (CABG) (continued)

Ø2114K9 Bypass Coronary Artery, Two Arteries from Left Internal Mammary with Nonautologous Tissue Substitute, Percutaneous Endoscopic Approach
Ø2114KC Bypass Coronary Artery, Two Arteries from Thoracic Artery with Nonautologous Tissue Substitute, Percutaneous Endoscopic Approach
Ø2114KF Bypass Coronary Artery, Two Arteries from Abdominal Artery with Nonautologous Tissue Substitute, Percutaneous Endoscopic Approach
Ø2114KW Bypass Coronary Artery, Two Arteries from Aorta with Nonautologous Tissue Substitute, Percutaneous Endoscopic Approach
Ø2114Z3 Bypass Coronary Artery, Two Arteries from Coronary Artery, Percutaneous Endoscopic Approach
Ø2114Z8 Bypass Coronary Artery, Two Arteries from Right Internal Mammary, Percutaneous Endoscopic Approach
Ø2114Z9 Bypass Coronary Artery, Two Arteries from Left Internal Mammary, Percutaneous Endoscopic Approach
Ø2114ZC Bypass Coronary Artery, Two Arteries from Thoracic Artery, Percutaneous Endoscopic Approach
Ø2114ZF Bypass Coronary Artery, Two Arteries from Abdominal Artery, Percutaneous Endoscopic Approach
Ø212Ø83 Bypass Coronary Artery, Three Arteries from Coronary Artery with Zooplastic Tissue, Open Approach
Ø212Ø88 Bypass Coronary Artery, Three Arteries from Right Internal Mammary with Zooplastic Tissue, Open Approach
Ø212Ø89 Bypass Coronary Artery, Three Arteries from Left Internal Mammary with Zooplastic Tissue, Open Approach
Ø212Ø8C Bypass Coronary Artery, Three Arteries from Thoracic Artery with Zooplastic Tissue, Open Approach
Ø212Ø8F Bypass Coronary Artery, Three Arteries from Abdominal Artery with Zooplastic Tissue, Open Approach
Ø212Ø8W Bypass Coronary Artery, Three Arteries from Aorta with Zooplastic Tissue, Open Approach
Ø212Ø93 Bypass Coronary Artery, Three Arteries from Coronary Artery with Autologous Venous Tissue, Open Approach
Ø212Ø98 Bypass Coronary Artery, Three Arteries from Right Internal Mammary with Autologous Venous Tissue, Open Approach
Ø212Ø99 Bypass Coronary Artery, Three Arteries from Left Internal Mammary with Autologous Venous Tissue, Open Approach
Ø212Ø9C Bypass Coronary Artery, Three Arteries from Thoracic Artery with Autologous Venous Tissue, Open Approach
Ø212Ø9F Bypass Coronary Artery, Three Arteries from Abdominal Artery with Autologous Venous Tissue, Open Approach
Ø212Ø9W Bypass Coronary Artery, Three Arteries from Aorta with Autologous Venous Tissue, Open Approach
Ø212ØA3 Bypass Coronary Artery, Three Arteries from Coronary Artery with Autologous Arterial Tissue, Open Approach
Ø212ØA8 Bypass Coronary Artery, Three Arteries from Right Internal Mammary with Autologous Arterial Tissue, Open Approach
Ø212ØA9 Bypass Coronary Artery, Three Arteries from Left Internal Mammary with Autologous Arterial Tissue, Open Approach
Ø212ØAC Bypass Coronary Artery, Three Arteries from Thoracic Artery with Autologous Arterial Tissue, Open Approach
Ø212ØAF Bypass Coronary Artery, Three Arteries from Abdominal Artery with Autologous Arterial Tissue, Open Approach
Ø212ØAW Bypass Coronary Artery, Three Arteries from Aorta with Autologous Arterial Tissue, Open Approach
Ø212ØJ3 Bypass Coronary Artery, Three Arteries from Coronary Artery with Synthetic Substitute, Open Approach
Ø212ØJ8 Bypass Coronary Artery, Three Arteries from Right Internal Mammary with Synthetic Substitute, Open Approach
Ø212ØJ9 Bypass Coronary Artery, Three Arteries from Left Internal Mammary with Synthetic Substitute, Open Approach
Ø212ØJC Bypass Coronary Artery, Three Arteries from Thoracic Artery with Synthetic Substitute, Open Approach
Ø212ØJF Bypass Coronary Artery, Three Arteries from Abdominal Artery with Synthetic Substitute, Open Approach
Ø212ØJW Bypass Coronary Artery, Three Arteries from Aorta with Synthetic Substitute, Open Approach
Ø212ØK3 Bypass Coronary Artery, Three Arteries from Coronary Artery with Nonautologous Tissue Substitute, Open Approach
Ø212ØK8 Bypass Coronary Artery, Three Arteries from Right Internal Mammary with Nonautologous Tissue Substitute, Open Approach
Ø212ØK9 Bypass Coronary Artery, Three Arteries from Left Internal Mammary with Nonautologous Tissue Substitute, Open Approach
Ø212ØKC Bypass Coronary Artery, Three Arteries from Thoracic Artery with Nonautologous Tissue Substitute, Open Approach
Ø212ØKF Bypass Coronary Artery, Three Arteries from Abdominal Artery with Nonautologous Tissue Substitute, Open Approach
Ø212ØKW Bypass Coronary Artery, Three Arteries from Aorta with Nonautologous Tissue Substitute, Open Approach
Ø212ØZ3 Bypass Coronary Artery, Three Arteries from Coronary Artery, Open Approach
Ø212ØZ8 Bypass Coronary Artery, Three Arteries from Right Internal Mammary, Open Approach
Ø212ØZ9 Bypass Coronary Artery, Three Arteries from Left Internal Mammary, Open Approach
Ø212ØZC Bypass Coronary Artery, Three Arteries from Thoracic Artery, Open Approach
Ø212ØZF Bypass Coronary Artery, Three Arteries from Abdominal Artery, Open Approach
Ø212483 Bypass Coronary Artery, Three Arteries from Coronary Artery with Zooplastic Tissue, Percutaneous Endoscopic Approach
Ø212488 Bypass Coronary Artery, Three Arteries from Right Internal Mammary with Zooplastic Tissue, Percutaneous Endoscopic Approach
Ø212489 Bypass Coronary Artery, Three Arteries from Left Internal Mammary with Zooplastic Tissue, Percutaneous Endoscopic Approach
Ø21248C Bypass Coronary Artery, Three Arteries from Thoracic Artery with Zooplastic Tissue, Percutaneous Endoscopic Approach
Ø21248F Bypass Coronary Artery, Three Arteries from Abdominal Artery with Zooplastic Tissue, Percutaneous Endoscopic Approach
Ø21248W Bypass Coronary Artery, Three Arteries from Aorta with Zooplastic Tissue, Percutaneous Endoscopic Approach
Ø212493 Bypass Coronary Artery, Three Arteries from Coronary Artery with Autologous Venous Tissue, Percutaneous Endoscopic Approach
Ø212498 Bypass Coronary Artery, Three Arteries from Right Internal Mammary with Autologous Venous Tissue, Percutaneous Endoscopic Approach
Ø212499 Bypass Coronary Artery, Three Arteries from Left Internal Mammary with Autologous Venous Tissue, Percutaneous Endoscopic Approach
Ø21249C Bypass Coronary Artery, Three Arteries from Thoracic Artery with Autologous Venous Tissue, Percutaneous Endoscopic Approach
Ø21249F Bypass Coronary Artery, Three Arteries from Abdominal Artery with Autologous Venous Tissue, Percutaneous Endoscopic Approach
Ø21249W Bypass Coronary Artery, Three Arteries from Aorta with Autologous Venous Tissue, Percutaneous Endoscopic Approach
Ø2124A3 Bypass Coronary Artery, Three Arteries from Coronary Artery with Autologous Arterial Tissue, Percutaneous Endoscopic Approach
Ø2124A8 Bypass Coronary Artery, Three Arteries from Right Internal Mammary with Autologous Arterial Tissue, Percutaneous Endoscopic Approach
Ø2124A9 Bypass Coronary Artery, Three Arteries from Left Internal Mammary with Autologous Arterial Tissue, Percutaneous Endoscopic Approach
Ø2124AC Bypass Coronary Artery, Three Arteries from Thoracic Artery with Autologous Arterial Tissue, Percutaneous Endoscopic Approach
Ø2124AF Bypass Coronary Artery, Three Arteries from Abdominal Artery with Autologous Arterial Tissue, Percutaneous Endoscopic Approach
Ø2124AW Bypass Coronary Artery, Three Arteries from Aorta with Autologous Arterial Tissue, Percutaneous Endoscopic Approach
Ø2124J3 Bypass Coronary Artery, Three Arteries from Coronary Artery with Synthetic Substitute, Percutaneous Endoscopic Approach
Ø2124J8 Bypass Coronary Artery, Three Arteries from Right Internal Mammary with Synthetic Substitute, Percutaneous Endoscopic Approach

HAC 08: Surgical Site Infection of Mediastinitis after Coronary Bypass Graft (CABG) (continued)

Ø2124J9 Bypass Coronary Artery, Three Arteries from Left Internal Mammary with Synthetic Substitute, Percutaneous Endoscopic Approach
Ø2124JC Bypass Coronary Artery, Three Arteries from Thoracic Artery with Synthetic Substitute, Percutaneous Endoscopic Approach
Ø2124JF Bypass Coronary Artery, Three Arteries from Abdominal Artery with Synthetic Substitute, Percutaneous Endoscopic Approach
Ø2124JW Bypass Coronary Artery, Three Arteries from Aorta with Synthetic Substitute, Percutaneous Endoscopic Approach
Ø2124K3 Bypass Coronary Artery, Three Arteries from Coronary Artery with Nonautologous Tissue Substitute, Percutaneous Endoscopic Approach
Ø2124K8 Bypass Coronary Artery, Three Arteries from Right Internal Mammary with Nonautologous Tissue Substitute, Percutaneous Endoscopic Approach
Ø2124K9 Bypass Coronary Artery, Three Arteries from Left Internal Mammary with Nonautologous Tissue Substitute, Percutaneous Endoscopic Approach
Ø2124KC Bypass Coronary Artery, Three Arteries from Thoracic Artery with Nonautologous Tissue Substitute, Percutaneous Endoscopic Approach
Ø2124KF Bypass Coronary Artery, Three Arteries from Abdominal Artery with Nonautologous Tissue Substitute, Percutaneous Endoscopic Approach
Ø2124KW Bypass Coronary Artery, Three Arteries from Aorta with Nonautologous Tissue Substitute, Percutaneous Endoscopic Approach
Ø2124Z3 Bypass Coronary Artery, Three Arteries from Coronary Artery, Percutaneous Endoscopic Approach
Ø2124Z8 Bypass Coronary Artery, Three Arteries from Right Internal Mammary, Percutaneous Endoscopic Approach
Ø2124Z9 Bypass Coronary Artery, Three Arteries from Left Internal Mammary, Percutaneous Endoscopic Approach
Ø2124ZC Bypass Coronary Artery, Three Arteries from Thoracic Artery, Percutaneous Endoscopic Approach
Ø2124ZF Bypass Coronary Artery, Three Arteries from Abdominal Artery, Percutaneous Endoscopic Approach
Ø213Ø83 Bypass Coronary Artery, Four or More Arteries from Coronary Artery with Zooplastic Tissue, Open Approach
Ø213Ø88 Bypass Coronary Artery, Four or More Arteries from Right Internal Mammary with Zooplastic Tissue, Open Approach
Ø213Ø89 Bypass Coronary Artery, Four or More Arteries from Left Internal Mammary with Zooplastic Tissue, Open Approach
Ø213Ø8C Bypass Coronary Artery, Four or More Arteries from Thoracic Artery with Zooplastic Tissue, Open Approach
Ø213Ø8F Bypass Coronary Artery, Four or More Arteries from Abdominal Artery with Zooplastic Tissue, Open Approach
Ø213Ø8W Bypass Coronary Artery, Four or More Arteries from Aorta with Zooplastic Tissue, Open Approach
Ø213Ø93 Bypass Coronary Artery, Four or More Arteries from Coronary Artery with Autologous Venous Tissue, Open Approach
Ø213Ø98 Bypass Coronary Artery, Four or More Arteries from Right Internal Mammary with Autologous Venous Tissue, Open Approach
Ø213Ø99 Bypass Coronary Artery, Four or More Arteries from Left Internal Mammary with Autologous Venous Tissue, Open Approach
Ø213Ø9C Bypass Coronary Artery, Four or More Arteries from Thoracic Artery with Autologous Venous Tissue, Open Approach
Ø213Ø9F Bypass Coronary Artery, Four or More Arteries from Abdominal Artery with Autologous Venous Tissue, Open Approach
Ø213Ø9W Bypass Coronary Artery, Four or More Arteries from Aorta with Autologous Venous Tissue, Open Approach
Ø213ØA3 Bypass Coronary Artery, Four or More Arteries from Coronary Artery with Autologous Arterial Tissue, Open Approach
Ø213ØA8 Bypass Coronary Artery, Four or More Arteries from Right Internal Mammary with Autologous Arterial Tissue, Open Approach
Ø213ØA9 Bypass Coronary Artery, Four or More Arteries from Left Internal Mammary with Autologous Arterial Tissue, Open Approach
Ø213ØAC Bypass Coronary Artery, Four or More Arteries from Thoracic Artery with Autologous Arterial Tissue, Open Approach
Ø213ØAF Bypass Coronary Artery, Four or More Arteries from Abdominal Artery with Autologous Arterial Tissue, Open Approach
Ø213ØAW Bypass Coronary Artery, Four or More Arteries from Aorta with Autologous Arterial Tissue, Open Approach
Ø213ØJ3 Bypass Coronary Artery, Four or More Arteries from Coronary Artery with Synthetic Substitute, Open Approach
Ø213ØJ8 Bypass Coronary Artery, Four or More Arteries from Right Internal Mammary with Synthetic Substitute, Open Approach
Ø213ØJ9 Bypass Coronary Artery, Four or More Arteries from Left Internal Mammary with Synthetic Substitute, Open Approach
Ø213ØJC Bypass Coronary Artery, Four or More Arteries from Thoracic Artery with Synthetic Substitute, Open Approach
Ø213ØJF Bypass Coronary Artery, Four or More Arteries from Abdominal Artery with Synthetic Substitute, Open Approach
Ø213ØJW Bypass Coronary Artery, Four or More Arteries from Aorta with Synthetic Substitute, Open Approach
Ø213ØK3 Bypass Coronary Artery, Four or More Arteries from Coronary Artery with Nonautologous Tissue Substitute, Open Approach
Ø213ØK8 Bypass Coronary Artery, Four or More Arteries from Right Internal Mammary with Nonautologous Tissue Substitute, Open Approach
Ø213ØK9 Bypass Coronary Artery, Four or More Arteries from Left Internal Mammary with Nonautologous Tissue Substitute, Open Approach
Ø213ØKC Bypass Coronary Artery, Four or More Arteries from Thoracic Artery with Nonautologous Tissue Substitute, Open Approach
Ø213ØKF Bypass Coronary Artery, Four or More Arteries from Abdominal Artery with Nonautologous Tissue Substitute, Open Approach
Ø213ØKW Bypass Coronary Artery, Four or More Arteries from Aorta with Nonautologous Tissue Substitute, Open Approach
Ø213ØZ3 Bypass Coronary Artery, Four or More Arteries from Coronary Artery, Open Approach
Ø213ØZ8 Bypass Coronary Artery, Four or More Arteries from Right Internal Mammary, Open Approach
Ø213ØZ9 Bypass Coronary Artery, Four or More Arteries from Left Internal Mammary, Open Approach
Ø213ØZC Bypass Coronary Artery, Four or More Arteries from Thoracic Artery, Open Approach
Ø213ØZF Bypass Coronary Artery, Four or More Arteries from Abdominal Artery, Open Approach
Ø213483 Bypass Coronary Artery, Four or More Arteries from Coronary Artery with Zooplastic Tissue, Percutaneous Endoscopic Approach
Ø213488 Bypass Coronary Artery, Four or More Arteries from Right Internal Mammary with Zooplastic Tissue, Percutaneous Endoscopic Approach
Ø213489 Bypass Coronary Artery, Four or More Arteries from Left Internal Mammary with Zooplastic Tissue, Percutaneous Endoscopic Approach
Ø21348C Bypass Coronary Artery, Four or More Arteries from Thoracic Artery with Zooplastic Tissue, Percutaneous Endoscopic Approach
Ø21348F Bypass Coronary Artery, Four or More Arteries from Abdominal Artery with Zooplastic Tissue, Percutaneous Endoscopic Approach
Ø21348W Bypass Coronary Artery, Four or More Arteries from Aorta with Zooplastic Tissue, Percutaneous Endoscopic Approach
Ø213493 Bypass Coronary Artery, Four or More Arteries from Coronary Artery with Autologous Venous Tissue, Percutaneous Endoscopic Approach
Ø213498 Bypass Coronary Artery, Four or More Arteries from Right Internal Mammary with Autologous Venous Tissue, Percutaneous Endoscopic Approach
Ø213499 Bypass Coronary Artery, Four or More Arteries from Left Internal Mammary with Autologous Venous Tissue, Percutaneous Endoscopic Approach
Ø21349C Bypass Coronary Artery, Four or More Arteries from Thoracic Artery with Autologous Venous Tissue, Percutaneous Endoscopic Approach
Ø21349F Bypass Coronary Artery, Four or More Arteries from Abdominal Artery with Autologous Venous Tissue, Percutaneous Endoscopic Approach
Ø21349W Bypass Coronary Artery, Four or More Arteries from Aorta with Autologous Venous Tissue, Percutaneous Endoscopic Approach

HAC 08: Surgical Site Infection of Mediastinitis after Coronary Bypass Graft (CABG) (continued)

Ø2134A3 Bypass Coronary Artery, Four or More Arteries from Coronary Artery with Autologous Arterial Tissue, Percutaneous Endoscopic Approach
Ø2134A8 Bypass Coronary Artery, Four or More Arteries from Right Internal Mammary with Autologous Arterial Tissue, Percutaneous Endoscopic Approach
Ø2134A9 Bypass Coronary Artery, Four or More Arteries from Left Internal Mammary with Autologous Arterial Tissue, Percutaneous Endoscopic Approach
Ø2134AC Bypass Coronary Artery, Four or More Arteries from Thoracic Artery with Autologous Arterial Tissue, Percutaneous Endoscopic Approach
Ø2134AF Bypass Coronary Artery, Four or More Arteries from Abdominal Artery with Autologous Arterial Tissue, Percutaneous Endoscopic Approach
Ø2134AW Bypass Coronary Artery, Four or More Arteries from Aorta with Autologous Arterial Tissue, Percutaneous Endoscopic Approach
Ø2134J3 Bypass Coronary Artery, Four or More Arteries from Coronary Artery with Synthetic Substitute, Percutaneous Endoscopic Approach
Ø2134J8 Bypass Coronary Artery, Four or More Arteries from Right Internal Mammary with Synthetic Substitute, Percutaneous Endoscopic Approach
Ø2134J9 Bypass Coronary Artery, Four or More Arteries from Left Internal Mammary with Synthetic Substitute, Percutaneous Endoscopic Approach
Ø2134JC Bypass Coronary Artery, Four or More Arteries from Thoracic Artery with Synthetic Substitute, Percutaneous Endoscopic Approach
Ø2134JF Bypass Coronary Artery, Four or More Arteries from Abdominal Artery with Synthetic Substitute, Percutaneous Endoscopic Approach
Ø2134JW Bypass Coronary Artery, Four or More Arteries from Aorta with Synthetic Substitute, Percutaneous Endoscopic Approach
Ø2134K3 Bypass Coronary Artery, Four or More Arteries from Coronary Artery with Nonautologous Tissue Substitute, Percutaneous Endoscopic Approach
Ø2134K8 Bypass Coronary Artery, Four or More Arteries from Right Internal Mammary with Nonautologous Tissue Substitute, Percutaneous Endoscopic Approach
Ø2134K9 Bypass Coronary Artery, Four or More Arteries from Left Internal Mammary with Nonautologous Tissue Substitute, Percutaneous Endoscopic Approach
Ø2134KC Bypass Coronary Artery, Four or More Arteries from Thoracic Artery with Nonautologous Tissue Substitute, Percutaneous Endoscopic Approach
Ø2134KF Bypass Coronary Artery, Four or More Arteries from Abdominal Artery with Nonautologous Tissue Substitute, Percutaneous Endoscopic Approach
Ø2134KW Bypass Coronary Artery, Four or More Arteries from Aorta with Nonautologous Tissue Substitute, Percutaneous Endoscopic Approach
Ø2134Z3 Bypass Coronary Artery, Four or More Arteries from Coronary Artery, Percutaneous Endoscopic Approach
Ø2134Z8 Bypass Coronary Artery, Four or More Arteries from Right Internal Mammary, Percutaneous Endoscopic Approach
Ø2134Z9 Bypass Coronary Artery, Four or More Arteries from Left Internal Mammary, Percutaneous Endoscopic Approach
Ø2134ZC Bypass Coronary Artery, Four or More Arteries from Thoracic Artery, Percutaneous Endoscopic Approach
Ø2134ZF Bypass Coronary Artery, Four or More Arteries from Abdominal Artery, Percutaneous Endoscopic Approach

HAC 09: Manifestations of Poor Glycemic Control

Secondary diagnosis not POA:

E08.ØØ
E08.Ø1
E08.1Ø
E09.ØØ
E09.Ø1
E09.1Ø
E1Ø.1Ø
E11.ØØ
E11.Ø1
E13.ØØ
E13.Ø1
E13.1Ø
E15

HAC 10: Deep Vein Thrombosis (DVT) or Pulmonary Embolism (PE) with Total Knee or Hip Replacement

Secondary diagnosis not POA:

I26.Ø2
I26.Ø9
I26.92
I26.93
I26.94
I26.99
I82.4Ø1
I82.4Ø2
I82.4Ø3
I82.4Ø9
I82.411
I82.412
I82.413
I82.419
I82.421
I82.422
I82.423
I82.429
I82.431
I82.432
I82.433
I82.439
I82.441
I82.442
I82.443
I82.449
I82.451
I82.452
I82.453
I82.459
I82.491
I82.492
I82.493
I82.499
I82.4Y1
I82.4Y2
I82.4Y3
I82.4Y9
I82.4Z1
I82.4Z2
I82.4Z3
I82.4Z9

AND

Any of the following procedures:

ØSR9Ø19 Replacement of Right Hip Joint with Metal Synthetic Substitute, Cemented, Open Approach
ØSR9Ø1A Replacement of Right Hip Joint with Metal Synthetic Substitute, Uncemented, Open Approach
ØSR9Ø1Z Replacement of Right Hip Joint with Metal Synthetic Substitute, Open Approach
ØSR9Ø29 Replacement of Right Hip Joint with Metal on Polyethylene Synthetic Substitute, Cemented, Open Approach
ØSR9Ø2A Replacement of Right Hip Joint with Metal on Polyethylene Synthetic Substitute, Uncemented, Open Approach
ØSR9Ø2Z Replacement of Right Hip Joint with Metal on Polyethylene Synthetic Substitute, Open Approach
ØSR9Ø39 Replacement of Right Hip Joint with Ceramic Synthetic Substitute, Cemented, Open Approach
ØSR9Ø3A Replacement of Right Hip Joint with Ceramic Synthetic Substitute, Uncemented, Open Approach
ØSR9Ø3Z Replacement of Right Hip Joint with Ceramic Synthetic Substitute, Open Approach
ØSR9Ø49 Replacement of Right Hip Joint with Ceramic on Polyethylene Synthetic Substitute, Cemented, Open Approach
ØSR9Ø4A Replacement of Right Hip Joint with Ceramic on Polyethylene Synthetic Substitute, Uncemented, Open Approach
ØSR9Ø4Z Replacement of Right Hip Joint with Ceramic on Polyethylene Synthetic Substitute, Open Approach
ØSR9Ø69 Replacement of Right Hip Joint with Oxidized Zirconium on Polyethylene Synthetic Substitute, Cemented, Open Approach
ØSR9Ø6A Replacement of Right Hip Joint with Oxidized Zirconium on Polyethylene Synthetic Substitute, Uncemented, Open Approach
ØSR9Ø6Z Replacement of Right Hip Joint with Oxidized Zirconium on Polyethylene Synthetic Substitute, Open Approach
ØSR9Ø7Z Replacement of Right Hip Joint with Autologous Tissue Substitute, Open Approach
ØSR9ØEZ Replacement of Right Hip Joint with Articulating Spacer, Open Approach
ØSR9ØJ9 Replacement of Right Hip Joint with Synthetic Substitute, Cemented, Open Approach
ØSR9ØJA Replacement of Right Hip Joint with Synthetic Substitute, Uncemented, Open Approach
ØSR9ØJZ Replacement of Right Hip Joint with Synthetic Substitute, Open Approach
ØSR9ØKZ Replacement of Right Hip Joint with Nonautologous Tissue Substitute, Open Approach
ØSRAØØ9 Replacement of Right Hip Joint, Acetabular Surface with Polyethylene Synthetic Substitute, Cemented, Open Approach
ØSRAØØA Replacement of Right Hip Joint, Acetabular Surface with Polyethylene Synthetic Substitute, Uncemented, Open Approach
ØSRAØØZ Replacement of Right Hip Joint, Acetabular Surface with Polyethylene Synthetic Substitute, Open Approach

HAC 10: Deep Vein Thrombosis (DVT) or Pulmonary Embolism (PE) with Total Knee or Hip Replacement (continued)

ØSRAØ19 Replacement of Right Hip Joint, Acetabular Surface with Metal Synthetic Substitute, Cemented, Open Approach
ØSRAØ1A Replacement of Right Hip Joint, Acetabular Surface with Metal Synthetic Substitute, Uncemented, Open Approach
ØSRAØ1Z Replacement of Right Hip Joint, Acetabular Surface with Metal Synthetic Substitute, Open Approach
ØSRAØ39 Replacement of Right Hip Joint, Acetabular Surface with Ceramic Synthetic Substitute, Cemented, Open Approach
ØSRAØ3A Replacement of Right Hip Joint, Acetabular Surface with Ceramic Synthetic Substitute, Uncemented, Open Approach
ØSRAØ3Z Replacement of Right Hip Joint, Acetabular Surface with Ceramic Synthetic Substitute, Open Approach
ØSRAØ7Z Replacement of Right Hip Joint, Acetabular Surface with Autologous Tissue Substitute, Open Approach
ØSRAØJ9 Replacement of Right Hip Joint, Acetabular Surface with Synthetic Substitute, Cemented, Open Approach
ØSRAØJA Replacement of Right Hip Joint, Acetabular Surface with Synthetic Substitute, Uncemented, Open Approach
ØSRAØJZ Replacement of Right Hip Joint, Acetabular Surface with Synthetic Substitute, Open Approach
ØSRAØKZ Replacement of Right Hip Joint, Acetabular Surface with Nonautologous Tissue Substitute, Open Approach
ØSRBØ19 Replacement of Left Hip Joint with Metal Synthetic Substitute, Cemented, Open Approach
ØSRBØ1A Replacement of Left Hip Joint with Metal Synthetic Substitute, Uncemented, Open Approach
ØSRBØ1Z Replacement of Left Hip Joint with Metal Synthetic Substitute, Open Approach
ØSRBØ29 Replacement of Left Hip Joint with Metal on Polyethylene Synthetic Substitute, Cemented, Open Approach
ØSRBØ2A Replacement of Left Hip Joint with Metal on Polyethylene Synthetic Substitute, Uncemented, Open Approach
ØSRBØ2Z Replacement of Left Hip Joint with Metal on Polyethylene Synthetic Substitute, Open Approach
ØSRBØ39 Replacement of Left Hip Joint with Ceramic Synthetic Substitute, Cemented, Open Approach
ØSRBØ3A Replacement of Left Hip Joint with Ceramic Synthetic Substitute, Uncemented, Open Approach
ØSRBØ3Z Replacement of Left Hip Joint with Ceramic Synthetic Substitute, Open Approach
ØSRBØ49 Replacement of Left Hip Joint with Ceramic on Polyethylene Synthetic Substitute, Cemented, Open Approach
ØSRBØ4A Replacement of Left Hip Joint with Ceramic on Polyethylene Synthetic Substitute, Uncemented, Open Approach
ØSRBØ4Z Replacement of Left Hip Joint with Ceramic on Polyethylene Synthetic Substitute, Open Approach
ØSRBØ69 Replacement of Left Hip Joint with Oxidized Zirconium on Polyethylene Synthetic Substitute, Cemented, Open Approach
ØSRBØ6A Replacement of Left Hip Joint with Oxidized Zirconium on Polyethylene Synthetic Substitute, Uncemented, Open Approach
ØSRBØ6Z Replacement of Left Hip Joint with Oxidized Zirconium on Polyethylene Synthetic Substitute, Open Approach
ØSRBØ7Z Replacement of Left Hip Joint with Autologous Tissue Substitute, Open Approach
ØSRBØEZ Replacement of Left Hip Joint with Articulating Spacer, Open Approach
ØSRBØJ9 Replacement of Left Hip Joint with Synthetic Substitute, Cemented, Open Approach
ØSRBØJA Replacement of Left Hip Joint with Synthetic Substitute, Uncemented, Open Approach
ØSRBØJZ Replacement of Left Hip Joint with Synthetic Substitute, Open Approach
ØSRBØKZ Replacement of Left Hip Joint with Nonautologous Tissue Substitute, Open Approach
ØSRCØ69 Replacement of Right Knee Joint with Oxidized Zirconium on Polyethylene Synthetic Substitute, Cemented, Open Approach
ØSRCØ6A Replacement of Right Knee Joint with Oxidized Zirconium on Polyethylene Synthetic Substitute, Uncemented, Open Approach
ØSRCØ6Z Replacement of Right Knee Joint with Oxidized Zirconium on Polyethylene Synthetic Substitute, Open Approach
ØSRCØ7Z Replacement of Right Knee Joint with Autologous Tissue Substitute, Open Approach
ØSRCØEZ Replacement of Right Knee Joint with Articulating Spacer, Open Approach
ØSRCØJ9 Replacement of Right Knee Joint with Synthetic Substitute, Cemented, Open Approach
ØSRCØJA Replacement of Right Knee Joint with Synthetic Substitute, Uncemented, Open Approach
ØSRCØJZ Replacement of Right Knee Joint with Synthetic Substitute, Open Approach
ØSRCØKZ Replacement of Right Knee Joint with Nonautologous Tissue Substitute, Open Approach
ØSRCØL9 Replacement of Right Knee Joint with Medial Unicondylar Synthetic Substitute, Cemented, Open Approach
ØSRCØLA Replacement of Right Knee Joint with Medial Unicondylar Synthetic Substitute, Uncemented, Open Approach
ØSRCØLZ Replacement of Right Knee Joint with Medial Unicondylar Synthetic Substitute, Open Approach
ØSRCØM9 Replacement of Right Knee Joint with Lateral Unicondylar Synthetic Substitute, Cemented, Open Approach
ØSRCØMA Replacement of Right Knee Joint with Lateral Unicondylar Synthetic Substitute, Uncemented, Open Approach
ØSRCØMZ Replacement of Right Knee Joint with Lateral Unicondylar Synthetic Substitute, Open Approach
ØSRCØN9 Replacement of Right Knee Joint with Patellofemoral Synthetic Substitute, Cemented, Open Approach
ØSRCØNA Replacement of Right Knee Joint with Patellofemoral Synthetic Substitute, Uncemented, Open Approach
ØSRCØNZ Replacement of Right Knee Joint with Patellofemoral Synthetic Substitute, Open Approach
ØSRDØ69 Replacement of Left Knee Joint with Oxidized Zirconium on Polyethylene Synthetic Substitute, Cemented, Open Approach
ØSRDØ6A Replacement of Left Knee Joint with Oxidized Zirconium on Polyethylene Synthetic Substitute, Uncemented, Open Approach
ØSRDØ6Z Replacement of Left Knee Joint with Oxidized Zirconium on Polyethylene Synthetic Substitute, Open Approach
ØSRDØ7Z Replacement of Left Knee Joint with Autologous Tissue Substitute, Open Approach
ØSRDØEZ Replacement of Left Knee Joint with Articulating Spacer, Open Approach
ØSRDØJ9 Replacement of Left Knee Joint with Synthetic Substitute, Cemented, Open Approach
ØSRDØJA Replacement of Left Knee Joint with Synthetic Substitute, Uncemented, Open Approach
ØSRDØJZ Replacement of Left Knee Joint with Synthetic Substitute, Open Approach
ØSRDØKZ Replacement of Left Knee Joint with Nonautologous Tissue Substitute, Open Approach
ØSRDØL9 Replacement of Left Knee Joint with Medial Unicondylar Synthetic Substitute, Cemented, Open Approach
ØSRDØLA Replacement of Left Knee Joint with Medial Unicondylar Synthetic Substitute, Uncemented, Open Approach
ØSRDØLZ Replacement of Left Knee Joint with Medial Unicondylar Synthetic Substitute, Open Approach
ØSRDØM9 Replacement of Left Knee Joint with Lateral Unicondylar Synthetic Substitute, Cemented, Open Approach
ØSRDØMA Replacement of Left Knee Joint with Lateral Unicondylar Synthetic Substitute, Uncemented, Open Approach
ØSRDØMZ Replacement of Left Knee Joint with Lateral Unicondylar Synthetic Substitute, Open Approach
ØSRDØN9 Replacement of Left Knee Joint with Patellofemoral Synthetic Substitute, Cemented, Open Approach
ØSRDØNA Replacement of Left Knee Joint with Patellofemoral Synthetic Substitute, Uncemented, Open Approach
ØSRDØNZ Replacement of Left Knee Joint with Patellofemoral Synthetic Substitute, Open Approach
ØSREØØ9 Replacement of Left Hip Joint, Acetabular Surface with Polyethylene Synthetic Substitute, Cemented, Open Approach
ØSREØØA Replacement of Left Hip Joint, Acetabular Surface with Polyethylene Synthetic Substitute, Uncemented, Open Approach
ØSREØØZ Replacement of Left Hip Joint, Acetabular Surface with Polyethylene Synthetic Substitute, Open Approach
ØSREØ19 Replacement of Left Hip Joint, Acetabular Surface with Metal Synthetic Substitute, Cemented, Open Approach
ØSREØ1A Replacement of Left Hip Joint, Acetabular Surface with Metal Synthetic Substitute, Uncemented, Open Approach
ØSREØ1Z Replacement of Left Hip Joint, Acetabular Surface with Metal Synthetic Substitute, Open Approach
ØSREØ39 Replacement of Left Hip Joint, Acetabular Surface with Ceramic Synthetic Substitute, Cemented, Open Approach

HAC 10: Deep Vein Thrombosis (DVT) or Pulmonary Embolism (PE) with Total Knee or Hip Replacement (continued)

ØSREØ3A Replacement of Left Hip Joint, Acetabular Surface with Ceramic Synthetic Substitute, Uncemented, Open Approach
ØSREØ3Z Replacement of Left Hip Joint, Acetabular Surface with Ceramic Synthetic Substitute, Open Approach
ØSREØ7Z Replacement of Left Hip Joint, Acetabular Surface with Autologous Tissue Substitute, Open Approach
ØSREØJ9 Replacement of Left Hip Joint, Acetabular Surface with Synthetic Substitute, Cemented, Open Approach
ØSREØJA Replacement of Left Hip Joint, Acetabular Surface with Synthetic Substitute, Uncemented, Open Approach
ØSREØJZ Replacement of Left Hip Joint, Acetabular Surface with Synthetic Substitute, Open Approach
ØSREØKZ Replacement of Left Hip Joint, Acetabular Surface with Nonautologous Tissue Substitute, Open Approach
ØSRRØ19 Replacement of Right Hip Joint, Femoral Surface with Metal Synthetic Substitute, Cemented, Open Approach
ØSRRØ1A Replacement of Right Hip Joint, Femoral Surface with Metal Synthetic Substitute, Uncemented, Open Approach
ØSRRØ1Z Replacement of Right Hip Joint, Femoral Surface with Metal Synthetic Substitute, Open Approach
ØSRRØ39 Replacement of Right Hip Joint, Femoral Surface with Ceramic Synthetic Substitute, Cemented, Open Approach
ØSRRØ3A Replacement of Right Hip Joint, Femoral Surface with Ceramic Synthetic Substitute, Uncemented, Open Approach
ØSRRØ3Z Replacement of Right Hip Joint, Femoral Surface with Ceramic Synthetic Substitute, Open Approach
ØSRRØ7Z Replacement of Right Hip Joint, Femoral Surface with Autologous Tissue Substitute, Open Approach
ØSRRØJ9 Replacement of Right Hip Joint, Femoral Surface with Synthetic Substitute, Cemented, Open Approach
ØSRRØJA Replacement of Right Hip Joint, Femoral Surface with Synthetic Substitute, Uncemented, Open Approach
ØSRRØJZ Replacement of Right Hip Joint, Femoral Surface with Synthetic Substitute, Open Approach
ØSRRØKZ Replacement of Right Hip Joint, Femoral Surface with Nonautologous Tissue Substitute, Open Approach
ØSRSØ19 Replacement of Left Hip Joint, Femoral Surface with Metal Synthetic Substitute, Cemented, Open Approach
ØSRSØ1A Replacement of Left Hip Joint, Femoral Surface with Metal Synthetic Substitute, Uncemented, Open Approach
ØSRSØ1Z Replacement of Left Hip Joint, Femoral Surface with Metal Synthetic Substitute, Open Approach
ØSRSØ39 Replacement of Left Hip Joint, Femoral Surface with Ceramic Synthetic Substitute, Cemented, Open Approach
ØSRSØ3A Replacement of Left Hip Joint, Femoral Surface with Ceramic Synthetic Substitute, Uncemented, Open Approach
ØSRSØ3Z Replacement of Left Hip Joint, Femoral Surface with Ceramic Synthetic Substitute, Open Approach
ØSRSØ7Z Replacement of Left Hip Joint, Femoral Surface with Autologous Tissue Substitute, Open Approach
ØSRSØJ9 Replacement of Left Hip Joint, Femoral Surface with Synthetic Substitute, Cemented, Open Approach
ØSRSØJA Replacement of Left Hip Joint, Femoral Surface with Synthetic Substitute, Uncemented, Open Approach
ØSRSØJZ Replacement of Left Hip Joint, Femoral Surface with Synthetic Substitute, Open Approach
ØSRSØKZ Replacement of Left Hip Joint, Femoral Surface with Nonautologous Tissue Substitute, Open Approach
ØSRTØ7Z Replacement of Right Knee Joint, Femoral Surface with Autologous Tissue Substitute, Open Approach
ØSRTØJ9 Replacement of Right Knee Joint, Femoral Surface with Synthetic Substitute, Cemented, Open Approach
ØSRTØJA Replacement of Right Knee Joint, Femoral Surface with Synthetic Substitute, Uncemented, Open Approach
ØSRTØJZ Replacement of Right Knee Joint, Femoral Surface with Synthetic Substitute, Open Approach
ØSRTØKZ Replacement of Right Knee Joint, Femoral Surface with Nonautologous Tissue Substitute, Open Approach
ØSRUØ7Z Replacement of Left Knee Joint, Femoral Surface with Autologous Tissue Substitute, Open Approach
ØSRUØJ9 Replacement of Left Knee Joint, Femoral Surface with Synthetic Substitute, Cemented, Open Approach
ØSRUØJA Replacement of Left Knee Joint, Femoral Surface with Synthetic Substitute, Uncemented, Open Approach
ØSRUØJZ Replacement of Left Knee Joint, Femoral Surface with Synthetic Substitute, Open Approach
ØSRUØKZ Replacement of Left Knee Joint, Femoral Surface with Nonautologous Tissue Substitute, Open Approach
ØSRVØ7Z Replacement of Right Knee Joint, Tibial Surface with Autologous Tissue Substitute, Open Approach
ØSRVØJ9 Replacement of Right Knee Joint, Tibial Surface with Synthetic Substitute, Cemented, Open Approach
ØSRVØJA Replacement of Right Knee Joint, Tibial Surface with Synthetic Substitute, Uncemented, Open Approach
ØSRVØJZ Replacement of Right Knee Joint, Tibial Surface with Synthetic Substitute, Open Approach
ØSRVØKZ Replacement of Right Knee Joint, Tibial Surface with Nonautologous Tissue Substitute, Open Approach
ØSRWØ7Z Replacement of Left Knee Joint, Tibial Surface with Autologous Tissue Substitute, Open Approach
ØSRWØJ9 Replacement of Left Knee Joint, Tibial Surface with Synthetic Substitute, Cemented, Open Approach
ØSRWØJA Replacement of Left Knee Joint, Tibial Surface with Synthetic Substitute, Uncemented, Open Approach
ØSRWØJZ Replacement of Left Knee Joint, Tibial Surface with Synthetic Substitute, Open Approach
ØSRWØKZ Replacement of Left Knee Joint, Tibial Surface with Nonautologous Tissue Substitute, Open Approach
ØSU9ØBZ Supplement Right Hip Joint with Resurfacing Device, Open Approach
ØSUAØBZ Supplement Right Hip Joint, Acetabular Surface with Resurfacing Device, Open Approach
ØSUBØBZ Supplement Left Hip Joint with Resurfacing Device, Open Approach
ØSUEØBZ Supplement Left Hip Joint, Acetabular Surface with Resurfacing Device, Open Approach
ØSURØBZ Supplement Right Hip Joint, Femoral Surface with Resurfacing Device, Open Approach
ØSUSØBZ Supplement Left Hip Joint, Femoral Surface with Resurfacing Device, Open Approach

HAC 11: Surgical Site Infection—Bariatric Surgery

Principal diagnosis of:

E66.Ø1

AND

Secondary diagnosis not POA:

K68.11
K95.Ø1
K95.81
T81.4ØXA
T81.41XA
T81.42XA
T81.43XA
T81.44XA
T81.49XA

AND

Any of the following procedures:

ØD16Ø79 Bypass Stomach to Duodenum with Autologous Tissue Substitute, Open Approach
ØD16Ø7A Bypass Stomach to Jejunum with Autologous Tissue Substitute, Open Approach
ØD16Ø7B Bypass Stomach to Ileum with Autologous Tissue Substitute, Open Approach
ØD16Ø7L Bypass Stomach to Transverse Colon with Autologous Tissue Substitute, Open Approach
ØD16ØJ9 Bypass Stomach to Duodenum with Synthetic Substitute, Open Approach
ØD16ØJA Bypass Stomach to Jejunum with Synthetic Substitute, Open Approach
ØD16ØJB Bypass Stomach to Ileum with Synthetic Substitute, Open Approach
ØD16ØJL Bypass Stomach to Transverse Colon with Synthetic Substitute, Open Approach
ØD16ØK9 Bypass Stomach to Duodenum with Nonautologous Tissue Substitute, Open Approach
ØD16ØKA Bypass Stomach to Jejunum with Nonautologous Tissue Substitute, Open Approach
ØD16ØKB Bypass Stomach to Ileum with Nonautologous Tissue Substitute, Open Approach
ØD16ØKL Bypass Stomach to Transverse Colon with Nonautologous Tissue Substitute, Open Approach
ØD16ØZ9 Bypass Stomach to Duodenum, Open Approach
ØD16ØZA Bypass Stomach to Jejunum, Open Approach
ØD16ØZB Bypass Stomach to Ileum, Open Approach
ØD16ØZL Bypass Stomach to Transverse Colon, Open Approach
ØD16479 Bypass Stomach to Duodenum with Autologous Tissue Substitute, Percutaneous Endoscopic Approach

HAC 11: Surgical Site Infection—Bariatric Surgery (continued)

- ØD1647A Bypass Stomach to Jejunum with Autologous Tissue Substitute, Percutaneous Endoscopic Approach
- ØD1647B Bypass Stomach to Ileum with Autologous Tissue Substitute, Percutaneous Endoscopic Approach
- ØD1647L Bypass Stomach to Transverse Colon with Autologous Tissue Substitute, Percutaneous Endoscopic Approach
- ØD164J9 Bypass Stomach to Duodenum with Synthetic Substitute, Percutaneous Endoscopic Approach
- ØD164JA Bypass Stomach to Jejunum with Synthetic Substitute, Percutaneous Endoscopic Approach
- ØD164JB Bypass Stomach to Ileum with Synthetic Substitute, Percutaneous Endoscopic Approach
- ØD164JL Bypass Stomach to Transverse Colon with Synthetic Substitute, Percutaneous Endoscopic Approach
- ØD164K9 Bypass Stomach to Duodenum with Nonautologous Tissue Substitute, Percutaneous Endoscopic Approach
- ØD164KA Bypass Stomach to Jejunum with Nonautologous Tissue Substitute, Percutaneous Endoscopic Approach
- ØD164KB Bypass Stomach to Ileum with Nonautologous Tissue Substitute, Percutaneous Endoscopic Approach
- ØD164KL Bypass Stomach to Transverse Colon with Nonautologous Tissue Substitute, Percutaneous Endoscopic Approach
- ØD164Z9 Bypass Stomach to Duodenum, Percutaneous Endoscopic Approach
- ØD164ZA Bypass Stomach to Jejunum, Percutaneous Endoscopic Approach
- ØD164ZB Bypass Stomach to Ileum, Percutaneous Endoscopic Approach
- ØD164ZL Bypass Stomach to Transverse Colon, Percutaneous Endoscopic Approach
- ØD16879 Bypass Stomach to Duodenum with Autologous Tissue Substitute, Via Natural or Artificial Opening Endoscopic
- ØD1687A Bypass Stomach to Jejunum with Autologous Tissue Substitute, Via Natural or Artificial Opening Endoscopic
- ØD1687B Bypass Stomach to Ileum with Autologous Tissue Substitute, Via Natural or Artificial Opening Endoscopic
- ØD1687L Bypass Stomach to Transverse Colon with Autologous Tissue Substitute, Via Natural or Artificial Opening Endoscopic
- ØD168J9 Bypass Stomach to Duodenum with Synthetic Substitute, Via Natural or Artificial Opening Endoscopic
- ØD168JA Bypass Stomach to Jejunum with Synthetic Substitute, Via Natural or Artificial Opening Endoscopic
- ØD168JB Bypass Stomach to Ileum with Synthetic Substitute, Via Natural or Artificial Opening Endoscopic
- ØD168JL Bypass Stomach to Transverse Colon with Synthetic Substitute, Via Natural or Artificial Opening Endoscopic
- ØD168K9 Bypass Stomach to Duodenum with Nonautologous Tissue Substitute, Via Natural or Artificial Opening Endoscopic
- ØD168KA Bypass Stomach to Jejunum with Nonautologous Tissue Substitute, Via Natural or Artificial Opening Endoscopic
- ØD168KB Bypass Stomach to Ileum with Nonautologous Tissue Substitute, Via Natural or Artificial Opening Endoscopic
- ØD168KL Bypass Stomach to Transverse Colon with Nonautologous Tissue Substitute, Via Natural or Artificial Opening Endoscopic
- ØD168Z9 Bypass Stomach to Duodenum, Via Natural or Artificial Opening Endoscopic
- ØD168ZA Bypass Stomach to Jejunum, Via Natural or Artificial Opening Endoscopic
- ØD168ZB Bypass Stomach to Ileum, Via Natural or Artificial Opening Endoscopic
- ØD168ZL Bypass Stomach to Transverse Colon, Via Natural or Artificial Opening Endoscopic
- ØDV64CZ Restriction of Stomach with Extraluminal Device, Percutaneous Endoscopic Approach

HAC 12: Surgical Site Infection—Certain Orthopedic Procedures of the Spine, Shoulder, and Elbow

Secondary diagnosis not POA:

- K68.11
- T81.40XA
- T81.41XA
- T81.42XA
- T81.43XA
- T81.44XA
- T81.49XA
- T84.60XA
- T84.610A
- T84.611A
- T84.612A
- T84.613A
- T84.614A
- T84.615A
- T84.619A
- T84.63XA
- T84.69XA
- T84.7XXA

AND

Any of the following procedures:

- ØRGØØ7Ø Fusion of Occipital-cervical Joint with Autologous Tissue Substitute, Anterior Approach, Anterior Column, Open Approach
- ØRGØØ71 Fusion of Occipital-cervical Joint with Autologous Tissue Substitute, Posterior Approach, Posterior Column, Open Approach
- ØRGØØ7J Fusion of Occipital-cervical Joint with Autologous Tissue Substitute, Posterior Approach, Anterior Column, Open Approach
- ØRGØØAØ Fusion of Occipital-cervical Joint with Interbody Fusion Device, Anterior Approach, Anterior Column, Open Approach
- ØRGØØAJ Fusion of Occipital-cervical Joint with Interbody Fusion Device, Posterior Approach, Anterior Column, Open Approach
- ØRGØØJØ Fusion of Occipital-cervical Joint with Synthetic Substitute, Anterior Approach, Anterior Column, Open Approach
- ØRGØØJ1 Fusion of Occipital-cervical Joint with Synthetic Substitute, Posterior Approach, Posterior Column, Open Approach
- ØRGØØJJ Fusion of Occipital-cervical Joint with Synthetic Substitute, Posterior Approach, Anterior Column, Open Approach
- ØRGØØKØ Fusion of Occipital-cervical Joint with Nonautologous Tissue Substitute, Anterior Approach, Anterior Column, Open Approach
- ØRGØØK1 Fusion of Occipital-cervical Joint with Nonautologous Tissue Substitute, Posterior Approach, Posterior Column, Open Approach
- ØRGØØKJ Fusion of Occipital-cervical Joint with Nonautologous Tissue Substitute, Posterior Approach, Anterior Column, Open Approach
- ØRGØ37Ø Fusion of Occipital-cervical Joint with Autologous Tissue Substitute, Anterior Approach, Anterior Column, Percutaneous Approach
- ØRGØ371 Fusion of Occipital-cervical Joint with Autologous Tissue Substitute, Posterior Approach, Posterior Column, Percutaneous Approach
- ØRGØ37J Fusion of Occipital-cervical Joint with Autologous Tissue Substitute, Posterior Approach, Anterior Column, Percutaneous Approach
- ØRGØ3AØ Fusion of Occipital-cervical Joint with Interbody Fusion Device, Anterior Approach, Anterior Column, Percutaneous Approach
- ØRGØ3AJ Fusion of Occipital-cervical Joint with Interbody Fusion Device, Posterior Approach, Anterior Column, Percutaneous Approach
- ØRGØ3JØ Fusion of Occipital-cervical Joint with Synthetic Substitute, Anterior Approach, Anterior Column, Percutaneous Approach
- ØRGØ3J1 Fusion of Occipital-cervical Joint with Synthetic Substitute, Posterior Approach, Posterior Column, Percutaneous Approach
- ØRGØ3JJ Fusion of Occipital-cervical Joint with Synthetic Substitute, Posterior Approach, Anterior Column, Percutaneous Approach
- ØRGØ3KØ Fusion of Occipital-cervical Joint with Nonautologous Tissue Substitute, Anterior Approach, Anterior Column, Percutaneous Approach
- ØRGØ3K1 Fusion of Occipital-cervical Joint with Nonautologous Tissue Substitute, Posterior Approach, Posterior Column, Percutaneous Approach
- ØRGØ3KJ Fusion of Occipital-cervical Joint with Nonautologous Tissue Substitute, Posterior Approach, Anterior Column, Percutaneous Approach
- ØRGØ47Ø Fusion of Occipital-cervical Joint with Autologous Tissue Substitute, Anterior Approach, Anterior Column, Percutaneous Endoscopic Approach
- ØRGØ471 Fusion of Occipital-cervical Joint with Autologous Tissue Substitute, Posterior Approach, Posterior Column, Percutaneous Endoscopic Approach
- ØRGØ47J Fusion of Occipital-cervical Joint with Autologous Tissue Substitute, Posterior Approach, Anterior Column, Percutaneous Endoscopic Approach
- ØRGØ4AØ Fusion of Occipital-cervical Joint with Interbody Fusion Device, Anterior Approach, Anterior Column, Percutaneous Endoscopic Approach
- ØRGØ4AJ Fusion of Occipital-cervical Joint with Interbody Fusion Device, Posterior Approach, Anterior Column, Percutaneous Endoscopic Approach
- ØRGØ4JØ Fusion of Occipital-cervical Joint with Synthetic Substitute, Anterior Approach, Anterior Column, Percutaneous Endoscopic Approach
- ØRGØ4J1 Fusion of Occipital-cervical Joint with Synthetic Substitute, Posterior Approach, Posterior Column, Percutaneous Endoscopic Approach

HAC 12: Surgical Site Infection—Certain Orthopedic Procedures of the Spine, Shoulder, and Elbow (continued)

ØRGØ4JJ Fusion of Occipital-cervical Joint with Synthetic Substitute, Posterior Approach, Anterior Column, Percutaneous Endoscopic Approach
ØRGØ4KØ Fusion of Occipital-cervical Joint with Nonautologous Tissue Substitute, Anterior Approach, Anterior Column, Percutaneous Endoscopic Approach
ØRGØ4K1 Fusion of Occipital-cervical Joint with Nonautologous Tissue Substitute, Posterior Approach, Posterior Column, Percutaneous Endoscopic Approach
ØRGØ4KJ Fusion of Occipital-cervical Joint with Nonautologous Tissue Substitute, Posterior Approach, Anterior Column, Percutaneous Endoscopic Approach
ØRG1Ø7Ø Fusion of Cervical Vertebral Joint with Autologous Tissue Substitute, Anterior Approach, Anterior Column, Open Approach
ØRG1Ø71 Fusion of Cervical Vertebral Joint with Autologous Tissue Substitute, Posterior Approach, Posterior Column, Open Approach
ØRG1Ø7J Fusion of Cervical Vertebral Joint with Autologous Tissue Substitute, Posterior Approach, Anterior Column, Open Approach
ØRG1ØAØ Fusion of Cervical Vertebral Joint with Interbody Fusion Device, Anterior Approach, Anterior Column, Open Approach
ØRG1ØAJ Fusion of Cervical Vertebral Joint with Interbody Fusion Device, Posterior Approach, Anterior Column, Open Approach
ØRG1ØJØ Fusion of Cervical Vertebral Joint with Synthetic Substitute, Anterior Approach, Anterior Column, Open Approach
ØRG1ØJ1 Fusion of Cervical Vertebral Joint with Synthetic Substitute, Posterior Approach, Posterior Column, Open Approach
ØRG1ØJJ Fusion of Cervical Vertebral Joint with Synthetic Substitute, Posterior Approach, Anterior Column, Open Approach
ØRG1ØKØ Fusion of Cervical Vertebral Joint with Nonautologous Tissue Substitute, Anterior Approach, Anterior Column, Open Approach
ØRG1ØK1 Fusion of Cervical Vertebral Joint with Nonautologous Tissue Substitute, Posterior Approach, Posterior Column, Open Approach
ØRG1ØKJ Fusion of Cervical Vertebral Joint with Nonautologous Tissue Substitute, Posterior Approach, Anterior Column, Open Approach
ØRG137Ø Fusion of Cervical Vertebral Joint with Autologous Tissue Substitute, Anterior Approach, Anterior Column, Percutaneous Approach
ØRG1371 Fusion of Cervical Vertebral Joint with Autologous Tissue Substitute, Posterior Approach, Posterior Column, Percutaneous Approach
ØRG137J Fusion of Cervical Vertebral Joint with Autologous Tissue Substitute, Posterior Approach, Anterior Column, Percutaneous Approach
ØRG13AØ Fusion of Cervical Vertebral Joint with Interbody Fusion Device, Anterior Approach, Anterior Column, Percutaneous Approach
ØRG13AJ Fusion of Cervical Vertebral Joint with Interbody Fusion Device, Posterior Approach, Anterior Column, Percutaneous Approach
ØRG13JØ Fusion of Cervical Vertebral Joint with Synthetic Substitute, Anterior Approach, Anterior Column, Percutaneous Approach
ØRG13J1 Fusion of Cervical Vertebral Joint with Synthetic Substitute, Posterior Approach, Posterior Column, Percutaneous Approach
ØRG13JJ Fusion of Cervical Vertebral Joint with Synthetic Substitute, Posterior Approach, Anterior Column, Percutaneous Approach
ØRG13KØ Fusion of Cervical Vertebral Joint with Nonautologous Tissue Substitute, Anterior Approach, Anterior Column, Percutaneous Approach
ØRG13K1 Fusion of Cervical Vertebral Joint with Nonautologous Tissue Substitute, Posterior Approach, Posterior Column, Percutaneous Approach
ØRG13KJ Fusion of Cervical Vertebral Joint with Nonautologous Tissue Substitute, Posterior Approach, Anterior Column, Percutaneous Approach
ØRG147Ø Fusion of Cervical Vertebral Joint with Autologous Tissue Substitute, Anterior Approach, Anterior Column, Percutaneous Endoscopic Approach
ØRG1471 Fusion of Cervical Vertebral Joint with Autologous Tissue Substitute, Posterior Approach, Posterior Column, Percutaneous Endoscopic Approach
ØRG147J Fusion of Cervical Vertebral Joint with Autologous Tissue Substitute, Posterior Approach, Anterior Column, Percutaneous Endoscopic Approach
ØRG14AØ Fusion of Cervical Vertebral Joint with Interbody Fusion Device, Anterior Approach, Anterior Column, Percutaneous Endoscopic Approach
ØRG14AJ Fusion of Cervical Vertebral Joint with Interbody Fusion Device, Posterior Approach, Anterior Column, Percutaneous Endoscopic Approach
ØRG14JØ Fusion of Cervical Vertebral Joint with Synthetic Substitute, Anterior Approach, Anterior Column, Percutaneous Endoscopic Approach
ØRG14J1 Fusion of Cervical Vertebral Joint with Synthetic Substitute, Posterior Approach, Posterior Column, Percutaneous Endoscopic Approach
ØRG14JJ Fusion of Cervical Vertebral Joint with Synthetic Substitute, Posterior Approach, Anterior Column, Percutaneous Endoscopic Approach
ØRG14KØ Fusion of Cervical Vertebral Joint with Nonautologous Tissue Substitute, Anterior Approach, Anterior Column, Percutaneous Endoscopic Approach
ØRG14K1 Fusion of Cervical Vertebral Joint with Nonautologous Tissue Substitute, Posterior Approach, Posterior Column, Percutaneous Endoscopic Approach
ØRG14KJ Fusion of Cervical Vertebral Joint with Nonautologous Tissue Substitute, Posterior Approach, Anterior Column, Percutaneous Endoscopic Approach
ØRG2Ø7Ø Fusion of 2 or more Cervical Vertebral Joints with Autologous Tissue Substitute, Anterior Approach, Anterior Column, Open Approach
ØRG2Ø71 Fusion of 2 or more Cervical Vertebral Joints with Autologous Tissue Substitute Posterior Approach, Posterior Column, Open Approach
ØRG2Ø7J Fusion of 2 or more Cervical Vertebral Joints with Autologous Tissue Substitute Posterior Approach, Anterior Column, Open Approach
ØRG2ØAØ Fusion of 2 or more Cervical Vertebral Joints with Interbody Fusion Device, Anterior Approach, Anterior Column, Open Approach
ØRG2ØAJ Fusion of 2 or more Cervical Vertebral Joints with Interbody Fusion Device, Posterior Approach, Anterior Column, Open Approach
ØRG2ØJØ Fusion of 2 or more Cervical Vertebral Joints with Synthetic Substitute, Anterior Approach, Anterior Column, Open Approach
ØRG2ØJ1 Fusion of 2 or more Cervical Vertebral Joints with Synthetic Substitute, Posterior Approach, Posterior Column, Open Approach
ØRG2ØJJ Fusion of 2 or more Cervical Vertebral Joints with Synthetic Substitute, Posterior Approach, Anterior Column, Open Approach
ØRG2ØKØ Fusion of 2 or more Cervical Vertebral Joints with Nonautologous Tissue Substitute, Anterior Approach, Anterior Column, Open Approach
ØRG2ØK1 Fusion of 2 or more Cervical Vertebral Joints with Nonautologous Tissue Substitute, Posterior Approach, Posterior Column, Open Approach
ØRG2ØKJ Fusion of 2 or more Cervical Vertebral Joints with Nonautologous Tissue Substitute, Posterior Approach, Anterior Column, Open Approach
ØRG237Ø Fusion of 2 or more Cervical Vertebral Joints with Autologous Tissue Substitute, Anterior Approach, Anterior Column, Percutaneous Approach
ØRG2371 Fusion of 2 or more Cervical Vertebral Joints with Autologous Tissue Substitute, Posterior Approach, Posterior Column, Percutaneous Approach
ØRG237J Fusion of 2 or more Cervical Vertebral Joints with Autologous Tissue Substitute, Posterior Approach, Anterior Column, Percutaneous Approach
ØRG23AØ Fusion of 2 or more Cervical Vertebral Joints with Interbody Fusion Device, Anterior Approach, Anterior Column, Percutaneous Approach
ØRG23AJ Fusion of 2 or more Cervical Vertebral Joints with Interbody Fusion Device, Posterior Approach, Anterior Column, Percutaneous Approach
ØRG23JØ Fusion of 2 or more Cervical Vertebral Joints with Synthetic Substitute, Anterior Approach, Anterior Column, Percutaneous Approach
ØRG23J1 Fusion of 2 or more Cervical Vertebral Joints with Synthetic Substitute, Posterior Approach, Posterior Column, Percutaneous Approach
ØRG23JJ Fusion of 2 or more Cervical Vertebral Joints with Synthetic Substitute, Posterior Approach, Anterior Column, Percutaneous Approach
ØRG23KØ Fusion of 2 or more Cervical Vertebral Joints with Nonautologous Tissue Substitute, Anterior Approach, Anterior Column, Percutaneous Approach

HAC 12: Surgical Site Infection— Certain Orthopedic Procedures of the Spine, Shoulder, and Elbow (continued)

ØRG23K1 Fusion of 2 or more Cervical Vertebral Joints with Nonautologous Tissue Substitute, Posterior Approach, Posterior Column, Percutaneous Approach
ØRG23KJ Fusion of 2 or more Cervical Vertebral Joints with Nonautologous Tissue Substitute, Posterior Approach, Anterior Column, Percutaneous Approach
ØRG247Ø Fusion of 2 or more Cervical Vertebral Joints with Autologous Tissue Substitute, Anterior Approach, Anterior Column, Percutaneous Endoscopic Approach
ØRG2471 Fusion of 2 or more Cervical Vertebral Joints with Autologous Tissue Substitute, Posterior Approach, Posterior Column, Percutaneous Endoscopic Approach
ØRG247J Fusion of 2 or more Cervical Vertebral Joints with Autologous Tissue Substitute, Posterior Approach, Anterior Column, Percutaneous Endoscopic Approach
ØRG24AØ Fusion of 2 or more Cervical Vertebral Joints with Interbody Fusion Device, Anterior Approach, Anterior Column, Percutaneous Endoscopic Approach
ØRG24AJ Fusion of 2 or more Cervical Vertebral Joints with Interbody Fusion Device, Posterior Approach, Anterior Column, Percutaneous Endoscopic Approach
ØRG24JØ Fusion of 2 or more Cervical Vertebral Joints with Synthetic Substitute, Anterior Approach, Anterior Column, Percutaneous Endoscopic Approach
ØRG24J1 Fusion of 2 or more Cervical Vertebral Joints with Synthetic Substitute, Posterior Approach, Posterior Column, Percutaneous Endoscopic Approach
ØRG24JJ Fusion of 2 or more Cervical Vertebral Joints with Synthetic Substitute, Posterior Approach, Anterior Column, Percutaneous Endoscopic Approach
ØRG24KØ Fusion of 2 or more Cervical Vertebral Joints with Nonautologous Tissue Substitute, Anterior Approach, Anterior Column, Percutaneous Endoscopic Approach
ØRG24K1 Fusion of 2 or more Cervical Vertebral Joints with Nonautologous Tissue Substitute, Posterior Approach, Posterior Column, Percutaneous Endoscopic Approach
ØRG24KJ Fusion of 2 or more Cervical Vertebral Joints with Nonautologous Tissue Substitute, Posterior Approach, Anterior Column, Percutaneous Endoscopic Approach
ØRG4Ø7Ø Fusion of Cervicothoracic Vertebral Joint with Autologous Tissue Substitute, Anterior Approach, Anterior Column, Open Approach
ØRG4Ø71 Fusion of Cervicothoracic Vertebral Joint with Autologous Tissue Substitute, Posterior Approach, Posterior Column, Open Approach
ØRG4Ø7J Fusion of Cervicothoracic Vertebral Joint with Autologous Tissue Substitute, Posterior Approach, Anterior Column, Open Approach
ØRG4ØAØ Fusion of Cervicothoracic Vertebral Joint with Interbody Fusion Device, Anterior Approach, Anterior Column, Open Approach
ØRG4ØAJ Fusion of Cervicothoracic Vertebral Joint with Interbody Fusion Device, Posterior Approach, Anterior Column, Open Approach
ØRG4ØJØ Fusion of Cervicothoracic Vertebral Joint with Synthetic Substitute, Anterior Approach, Anterior Column, Open Approach
ØRG4ØJ1 Fusion of Cervicothoracic Vertebral Joint with Synthetic Substitute, Posterior Approach, Posterior Column, Open Approach
ØRG4ØJJ Fusion of Cervicothoracic Vertebral Joint with Synthetic Substitute, Posterior Approach, Anterior Column, Open Approach
ØRG4ØKØ Fusion of Cervicothoracic Vertebral Joint with Nonautologous Tissue Substitute, Anterior Approach, Anterior Column, Open Approach
ØRG4ØK1 Fusion of Cervicothoracic Vertebral Joint with Nonautologous Tissue Substitute, Posterior Approach, Posterior Column, Open Approach
ØRG4ØKJ Fusion of Cervicothoracic Vertebral Joint with Nonautologous Tissue Substitute, Posterior Approach, Anterior Column, Open Approach
ØRG437Ø Fusion of Cervicothoracic Vertebral Joint with Autologous Tissue Substitute, Anterior Approach, Anterior Column, Percutaneous Approach
ØRG4371 Fusion of Cervicothoracic Vertebral Joint with Autologous Tissue Substitute, Posterior Approach, Posterior Column, Percutaneous Approach
ØRG437J Fusion of Cervicothoracic Vertebral Joint with Autologous Tissue Substitute, Posterior Approach, Anterior Column, Percutaneous Approach
ØRG43AØ Fusion of Cervicothoracic Vertebral Joint with Interbody Fusion Device, Anterior Approach, Anterior Column, Percutaneous Approach
ØRG43AJ Fusion of Cervicothoracic Vertebral Joint with Interbody Fusion Device, Posterior Approach, Anterior Column, Percutaneous Approach
ØRG43JØ Fusion of Cervicothoracic Vertebral Joint with Synthetic Substitute, Anterior Approach, Anterior Column, Percutaneous Approach
ØRG43J1 Fusion of Cervicothoracic Vertebral Joint with Synthetic Substitute, Posterior Approach, Posterior Column, Percutaneous Approach
ØRG43JJ Fusion of Cervicothoracic Vertebral Joint with Synthetic Substitute, Posterior Approach, Anterior Column, Percutaneous Approach
ØRG43KØ Fusion of Cervicothoracic Vertebral Joint with Nonautologous Tissue Substitute, Anterior Approach, Anterior Column, Percutaneous Approach
ØRG43K1 Fusion of Cervicothoracic Vertebral Joint with Nonautologous Tissue Substitute, Posterior Approach, Posterior Column, Percutaneous Approach
ØRG43KJ Fusion of Cervicothoracic Vertebral Joint with Nonautologous Tissue Substitute, Posterior Approach, Anterior Column, Percutaneous Approach
ØRG447Ø Fusion of Cervicothoracic Vertebral Joint with Autologous Tissue Substitute, Anterior Approach, Anterior Column, Percutaneous Endoscopic Approach
ØRG4471 Fusion of Cervicothoracic Vertebral Joint with Autologous Tissue Substitute, Posterior Approach, Posterior Column, Percutaneous Endoscopic Approach
ØRG447J Fusion of Cervicothoracic Vertebral Joint with Autologous Tissue Substitute, Posterior Approach, Anterior Column, Percutaneous Endoscopic Approach
ØRG44AØ Fusion of Cervicothoracic Vertebral Joint with Interbody Fusion Device, Anterior Approach, Anterior Column, Percutaneous Endoscopic Approach
ØRG44AJ Fusion of Cervicothoracic Vertebral Joint with Interbody Fusion Device, Posterior Approach, Anterior Column, Percutaneous Endoscopic Approach
ØRG44JØ Fusion of Cervicothoracic Vertebral Joint with Synthetic Substitute, Anterior Approach, Anterior Column, Percutaneous Endoscopic Approach
ØRG44J1 Fusion of Cervicothoracic Vertebral Joint with Synthetic Substitute, Posterior Approach, Posterior Column, Percutaneous Endoscopic Approach
ØRG44JJ Fusion of Cervicothoracic Vertebral Joint with Synthetic Substitute, Posterior Approach, Anterior Column, Percutaneous Endoscopic Approach
ØRG44KØ Fusion of Cervicothoracic Vertebral Joint with Nonautologous Tissue Substitute, Anterior Approach, Anterior Column, Percutaneous Endoscopic Approach
ØRG44K1 Fusion of Cervicothoracic Vertebral Joint with Nonautologous Tissue Substitute, Posterior Approach, Posterior Column, Percutaneous Endoscopic Approach
ØRG44KJ Fusion of Cervicothoracic Vertebral Joint with Nonautologous Tissue Substitute, Posterior Approach, Anterior Column, Percutaneous Endoscopic Approach
ØRG6Ø7Ø Fusion of Thoracic Vertebral Joint with Autologous Tissue Substitute, Anterior Approach, Anterior Column, Open Approach
ØRG6Ø71 Fusion of Thoracic Vertebral Joint with Autologous Tissue Substitute, Posterior Approach, Posterior Column, Open Approach
ØRG6Ø7J Fusion of Thoracic Vertebral Joint with Autologous Tissue Substitute, Posterior Approach, Anterior Column, Open Approach
ØRG6ØAØ Fusion of Thoracic Vertebral Joint with Interbody Fusion Device, Anterior Approach, Anterior Column, Open Approach
ØRG6ØAJ Fusion of Thoracic Vertebral Joint with Interbody Fusion Device, Posterior Approach, Anterior Column, Open Approach
ØRG6ØJØ Fusion of Thoracic Vertebral Joint with Synthetic Substitute, Anterior Approach, Anterior Column, Open Approach
ØRG6ØJ1 Fusion of Thoracic Vertebral Joint with Synthetic Substitute, Posterior Approach, Posterior Column, Open Approach
ØRG6ØJJ Fusion of Thoracic Vertebral Joint with Synthetic Substitute, Posterior Approach, Anterior Column, Open Approach
ØRG6ØKØ Fusion of Thoracic Vertebral Joint with Nonautologous Tissue Substitute, Anterior Approach, Anterior Column, Open Approach
ØRG6ØK1 Fusion of Thoracic Vertebral Joint with Nonautologous Tissue Substitute, Posterior Approach, Posterior Column, Open Approach

Appendix G: Hospital Acquired Conditions

HAC 12: Surgical Site Infection—Certain Orthopedic Procedures of the Spine, Shoulder, and Elbow (continued)

ØRG6ØKJ Fusion of Thoracic Vertebral Joint with Nonautologous Tissue Substitute, Posterior Approach, Anterior Column, Open Approach
ØRG637Ø Fusion of Thoracic Vertebral Joint with Autologous Tissue Substitute, Anterior Approach, Anterior Column, Percutaneous Approach
ØRG6371 Fusion of Thoracic Vertebral Joint with Autologous Tissue Substitute, Posterior Approach, Posterior Column, Percutaneous Approach
ØRG637J Fusion of Thoracic Vertebral Joint with Autologous Tissue Substitute, Posterior Approach, Anterior Column, Percutaneous Approach
ØRG63AØ Fusion of Thoracic Vertebral Joint with Interbody Fusion Device, Anterior Approach, Anterior Column, Percutaneous Approach
ØRG63AJ Fusion of Thoracic Vertebral Joint with Interbody Fusion Device, Posterior Approach, Anterior Column, Percutaneous Approach
ØRG63JØ Fusion of Thoracic Vertebral Joint with Synthetic Substitute, Anterior Approach, Anterior Column, Percutaneous Approach
ØRG63J1 Fusion of Thoracic Vertebral Joint with Synthetic Substitute, Posterior Approach, Posterior Column, Percutaneous Approach
ØRG63JJ Fusion of Thoracic Vertebral Joint with Synthetic Substitute, Posterior Approach, Anterior Column, Percutaneous Approach
ØRG63KØ Fusion of Thoracic Vertebral Joint with Nonautologous Tissue Substitute, Anterior Approach, Anterior Column, Percutaneous Approach
ØRG63K1 Fusion of Thoracic Vertebral Joint with Nonautologous Tissue Substitute, Posterior Approach, Posterior Column, Percutaneous Approach
ØRG63KJ Fusion of Thoracic Vertebral Joint with Nonautologous Tissue Substitute, Posterior Approach, Anterior Column, Percutaneous Approach
ØRG647Ø Fusion of Thoracic Vertebral Joint with Autologous Tissue Substitute, Anterior Approach, Anterior Column, Percutaneous Endoscopic Approach
ØRG6471 Fusion of Thoracic Vertebral Joint with Autologous Tissue Substitute, Posterior Approach, Posterior Column, Percutaneous Endoscopic Approach
ØRG647J Fusion of Thoracic Vertebral Joint with Autologous Tissue Substitute, Posterior Approach, Anterior Column, Percutaneous Endoscopic Approach
ØRG64AØ Fusion of Thoracic Vertebral Joint with Interbody Fusion Device, Anterior Approach, Anterior Column, Percutaneous Endoscopic Approach
ØRG64AJ Fusion of Thoracic Vertebral Joint with Interbody Fusion Device, Posterior Approach, Anterior Column, Percutaneous Endoscopic Approach
ØRG64JØ Fusion of Thoracic Vertebral Joint with Synthetic Substitute, Anterior Approach, Anterior Column, Percutaneous Endoscopic Approach
ØRG64J1 Fusion of Thoracic Vertebral Joint with Synthetic Substitute, Posterior Approach, Posterior Column, Percutaneous Endoscopic Approach
ØRG64JJ Fusion of Thoracic Vertebral Joint with Synthetic Substitute, Posterior Approach, Anterior Column, Percutaneous Endoscopic Approach
ØRG64KØ Fusion of Thoracic Vertebral Joint with Nonautologous Tissue Substitute, Anterior Approach, Anterior Column, Percutaneous Endoscopic Approach
ØRG64K1 Fusion of Thoracic Vertebral Joint with Nonautologous Tissue Substitute, Posterior Approach, Posterior Column, Percutaneous Endoscopic Approach
ØRG64KJ Fusion of Thoracic Vertebral Joint with Nonautologous Tissue Substitute, Posterior Approach, Anterior Column, Percutaneous Endoscopic Approach
ØRG7Ø7Ø Fusion of 2 to 7 Thoracic Vertebral Joints with Autologous Tissue Substitute, Anterior Approach, Anterior Column, Open Approach
ØRG7Ø71 Fusion of 2 to 7 Thoracic Vertebral Joints with Autologous Tissue Substitute, Posterior Approach, Posterior Column, Open Approach
ØRG7Ø7J Fusion of 2 to 7 Thoracic Vertebral Joints with Autologous Tissue Substitute, Posterior Approach, Anterior Column, Open Approach
ØRG7ØAØ Fusion of 2 to 7 Thoracic Vertebral Joints with Interbody Fusion Device, Anterior Approach, Anterior Column, Open Approach
ØRG7ØAJ Fusion of 2 to 7 Thoracic Vertebral Joints with Interbody Fusion Device, Posterior Approach, Anterior Column, Open Approach
ØRG7ØJØ Fusion of 2 to 7 Thoracic Vertebral Joints with Synthetic Substitute, Anterior Approach, Anterior Column, Open Approach
ØRG7ØJ1 Fusion of 2 to 7 Thoracic Vertebral Joints with Synthetic Substitute, Posterior Approach, Posterior Column, Open Approach
ØRG7ØJJ Fusion of 2 to 7 Thoracic Vertebral Joints with Synthetic Substitute, Posterior Approach, Anterior Column, Open Approach
ØRG7ØKØ Fusion of 2 to 7 Thoracic Vertebral Joints with Nonautologous Tissue Substitute, Anterior Approach, Anterior Column, Open Approach
ØRG7ØK1 Fusion of 2 to 7 Thoracic Vertebral Joints with Nonautologous Tissue Substitute, Posterior Approach, Posterior Column, Open Approach
ØRG7ØKJ Fusion of 2 to 7 Thoracic Vertebral Joints with Nonautologous Tissue Substitute, Posterior Approach, Anterior Column, Open Approach
ØRG737Ø Fusion of 2 to 7 Thoracic Vertebral Joints with Autologous Tissue Substitute, Anterior Approach, Anterior Column, Percutaneous Approach
ØRG7371 Fusion of 2 to 7 Thoracic Vertebral Joints with Autologous Tissue Substitute, Posterior Approach, Posterior Column, Percutaneous Approach
ØRG737J Fusion of 2 to 7 Thoracic Vertebral Joints with Autologous Tissue Substitute, Posterior Approach, Anterior Column, Percutaneous Approach
ØRG73AØ Fusion of 2 to 7 Thoracic Vertebral Joints with Interbody Fusion Device, Anterior Approach, Anterior Column, Percutaneous Approach
ØRG73AJ Fusion of 2 to 7 Thoracic Vertebral Joints with Interbody Fusion Device, Posterior Approach, Anterior Column, Percutaneous Approach
ØRG73JØ Fusion of 2 to 7 Thoracic Vertebral Joints with Synthetic Substitute, Anterior Approach, Anterior Column, Percutaneous Approach
ØRG73J1 Fusion of 2 to 7 Thoracic Vertebral Joints with Synthetic Substitute, Posterior Approach, Posterior Column, Percutaneous Approach
ØRG73JJ Fusion of 2 to 7 Thoracic Vertebral Joints with Synthetic Substitute, Posterior Approach, Anterior Column, Percutaneous Approach
ØRG73KØ Fusion of 2 to 7 Thoracic Vertebral Joints with Nonautologous Tissue Substitute, Anterior Approach, Anterior Column, Percutaneous Approach
ØRG73K1 Fusion of 2 to 7 Thoracic Vertebral Joints with Nonautologous Tissue Substitute, Posterior Approach, Posterior Column, Percutaneous Approach
ØRG73KJ Fusion of 2 to 7 Thoracic Vertebral Joints with Nonautologous Tissue Substitute, Posterior Approach, Anterior Column, Percutaneous Approach
ØRG747Ø Fusion of 2 to 7 Thoracic Vertebral Joints with Autologous Tissue Substitute, Anterior Approach, Anterior Column, Percutaneous Endoscopic Approach
ØRG7471 Fusion of 2 to 7 Thoracic Vertebral Joints with Autologous Tissue Substitute, Posterior Approach, Posterior Column, Percutaneous Endoscopic Approach
ØRG747J Fusion of 2 to 7 Thoracic Vertebral Joints with Autologous Tissue Substitute, Posterior Approach, Anterior Column, Percutaneous Endoscopic Approach
ØRG74AØ Fusion of 2 to 7 Thoracic Vertebral Joints with Interbody Fusion Device, Anterior Approach, Anterior Column, Percutaneous Endoscopic Approach
ØRG74AJ Fusion of 2 to 7 Thoracic Vertebral Joints with Interbody Fusion Device, Posterior Approach, Anterior Column, Percutaneous Endoscopic Approach
ØRG74JØ Fusion of 2 to 7 Thoracic Vertebral Joints with Synthetic Substitute, Anterior Approach, Anterior Column, Percutaneous Endoscopic Approach
ØRG74J1 Fusion of 2 to 7 Thoracic Vertebral Joints with Synthetic Substitute, Posterior Approach, Posterior Column, Percutaneous Endoscopic Approach
ØRG74JJ Fusion of 2 to 7 Thoracic Vertebral Joints with Synthetic Substitute, Posterior Approach, Anterior Column, Percutaneous Endoscopic Approach
ØRG74KØ Fusion of 2 to 7 Thoracic Vertebral Joints with Nonautologous Tissue Substitute, Anterior Approach, Anterior Column, Percutaneous Endoscopic Approach
ØRG74K1 Fusion of 2 to 7 Thoracic Vertebral Joints with Nonautologous Tissue Substitute, Posterior Approach, Posterior Column, Percutaneous Endoscopic Approach
ØRG74KJ Fusion of 2 to 7 Thoracic Vertebral Joints with Nonautologous Tissue Substitute, Posterior Approach, Anterior Column, Percutaneous Endoscopic Approach

HAC 12: Surgical Site Infection—Certain Orthopedic Procedures of the Spine, Shoulder, and Elbow (continued)

ØRG8070 Fusion of 8 or More Thoracic Vertebral Joints with Autologous Tissue Substitute, Anterior Approach, Anterior Column, Open Approach
ØRG8071 Fusion of 8 or More Thoracic Vertebral Joints with Autologous Tissue Substitute, Posterior Approach, Posterior Column, Open Approach
ØRG807J Fusion of 8 or More Thoracic Vertebral Joints with Autologous Tissue Substitute, Posterior Approach, Anterior Column, Open Approach
ØRG80AØ Fusion of 8 or More Thoracic Vertebral Joints with Interbody Fusion Device, Anterior Approach, Anterior Column, Open Approach
ØRG80AJ Fusion of 8 or More Thoracic Vertebral Joints with Interbody Fusion Device, Posterior Approach, Anterior Column, Open Approach
ØRG80JØ Fusion of 8 or More Thoracic Vertebral Joints with Synthetic Substitute, Anterior Approach, Anterior Column, Open Approach
ØRG80J1 Fusion of 8 or More Thoracic Vertebral Joints with Synthetic Substitute, Posterior Approach, Posterior Column, Open Approach
ØRG80JJ Fusion of 8 or More Thoracic Vertebral Joints with Synthetic Substitute, Posterior Approach, Anterior Column, Open Approach
ØRG80KØ Fusion of 8 or More Thoracic Vertebral Joints with Nonautologous Tissue Substitute, Anterior Approach, Anterior Column, Open Approach
ØRG80K1 Fusion of 8 or More Thoracic Vertebral Joints with Nonautologous Tissue Substitute, Posterior Approach, Posterior Column, Open Approach
ØRG80KJ Fusion of 8 or More Thoracic Vertebral Joints with Nonautologous Tissue Substitute, Posterior Approach, Anterior Column, Open Approach
ØRG8370 Fusion of 8 or More Thoracic Vertebral Joints with Autologous Tissue Substitute, Anterior Approach, Anterior Column, Percutaneous Approach
ØRG8371 Fusion of 8 or More Thoracic Vertebral Joints with Autologous Tissue Substitute, Posterior Approach, Posterior Column, Percutaneous Approach
ØRG837J Fusion of 8 or More Thoracic Vertebral Joints with Autologous Tissue Substitute, Posterior Approach, Anterior Column, Percutaneous Approach
ØRG83AØ Fusion of 8 or More Thoracic Vertebral Joints with Interbody Fusion Device, Anterior Approach, Anterior Column, Percutaneous Approach
ØRG83AJ Fusion of 8 or More Thoracic Vertebral Joints with Interbody Fusion Device, Posterior Approach, Anterior Column, Percutaneous Approach
ØRG83JØ Fusion of 8 or More Thoracic Vertebral Joints with Synthetic Substitute, Anterior Approach, Anterior Column, Percutaneous Approach
ØRG83J1 Fusion of 8 or More Thoracic Vertebral Joints with Synthetic Substitute, Posterior Approach, Posterior Column, Percutaneous Approach
ØRG83JJ Fusion of 8 or More Thoracic Vertebral Joints with Synthetic Substitute, Posterior Approach, Anterior Column, Percutaneous Approach
ØRG83KØ Fusion of 8 or More Thoracic Vertebral Joints with Nonautologous Tissue Substitute, Anterior Approach, Anterior Column, Percutaneous Approach
ØRG83K1 Fusion of 8 or More Thoracic Vertebral Joints with Nonautologous Tissue Substitute, Posterior Approach, Posterior Column, Percutaneous Approach
ØRG83KJ Fusion of 8 or More Thoracic Vertebral Joints with Nonautologous Tissue Substitute, Posterior Approach, Anterior Column, Percutaneous Approach
ØRG8470 Fusion of 8 or More Thoracic Vertebral Joints with Autologous Tissue Substitute, Anterior Approach, Anterior Column, Percutaneous Endoscopic Approach
ØRG8471 Fusion of 8 or More Thoracic Vertebral Joints with Autologous Tissue Substitute, Posterior Approach, Posterior Column, Percutaneous Endoscopic Approach
ØRG847J Fusion of 8 or More Thoracic Vertebral Joints with Autologous Tissue Substitute, Posterior Approach, Anterior Column, Percutaneous Endoscopic Approach
ØRG84AØ Fusion of 8 or More Thoracic Vertebral Joints with Interbody Fusion Device, Anterior Approach, Anterior Column, Percutaneous Endoscopic Approach
ØRG84AJ Fusion of 8 or More Thoracic Vertebral Joints with Interbody Fusion Device, Posterior Approach, Anterior Column, Percutaneous Endoscopic Approach
ØRG84JØ Fusion of 8 or More Thoracic Vertebral Joints with Synthetic Substitute, Anterior Approach, Anterior Column, Percutaneous Endoscopic Approach
ØRG84J1 Fusion of 8 or More Thoracic Vertebral Joints with Synthetic Substitute, Posterior Approach, Posterior Column, Percutaneous Endoscopic Approach
ØRG84JJ Fusion of 8 or More Thoracic Vertebral Joints with Synthetic Substitute, Posterior Approach, Anterior Column, Percutaneous Endoscopic Approach
ØRG84KØ Fusion of 8 or More Thoracic Vertebral Joints with Nonautologous Tissue Substitute, Anterior Approach, Anterior Column, Percutaneous Endoscopic Approach
ØRG84K1 Fusion of 8 or More Thoracic Vertebral Joints with Nonautologous Tissue Substitute, Posterior Approach, Posterior Column, Percutaneous Endoscopic Approach
ØRG84KJ Fusion of 8 or More Thoracic Vertebral Joints with Nonautologous Tissue Substitute, Posterior Approach, Anterior Column, Percutaneous Endoscopic Approach
ØRGA070 Fusion of Thoracolumbar Vertebral Joint with Autologous Tissue Substitute, Anterior Approach, Anterior Column, Open Approach
ØRGA071 Fusion of Thoracolumbar Vertebral Joint with Autologous Tissue Substitute, Posterior Approach, Posterior Column, Open Approach
ØRGA07J Fusion of Thoracolumbar Vertebral Joint with Autologous Tissue Substitute, Posterior Approach, Anterior Column, Open Approach
ØRGAØAØ Fusion of Thoracolumbar Vertebral Joint with Interbody Fusion Device, Anterior Approach, Anterior Column, Open Approach
ØRGAØAJ Fusion of Thoracolumbar Vertebral Joint with Interbody Fusion Device, Posterior Approach, Anterior Column, Open Approach
ØRGAØJØ Fusion of Thoracolumbar Vertebral Joint with Synthetic Substitute, Anterior Approach, Anterior Column, Open Approach
ØRGAØJ1 Fusion of Thoracolumbar Vertebral Joint with Synthetic Substitute, Posterior Approach, Posterior Column, Open Approach
ØRGAØJJ Fusion of Thoracolumbar Vertebral Joint with Synthetic Substitute, Posterior Approach, Anterior Column, Open Approach
ØRGAØKØ Fusion of Thoracolumbar Vertebral Joint with Nonautologous Tissue Substitute, Anterior Approach, Anterior Column, Open Approach
ØRGAØK1 Fusion of Thoracolumbar Vertebral Joint with Nonautologous Tissue Substitute, Posterior Approach, Posterior Column, Open Approach
ØRGAØKJ Fusion of Thoracolumbar Vertebral Joint with Nonautologous Tissue Substitute, Posterior Approach, Anterior Column, Open Approach
ØRGA370 Fusion of Thoracolumbar Vertebral Joint with Autologous Tissue Substitute, Anterior Approach, Anterior Column, Percutaneous Approach
ØRGA371 Fusion of Thoracolumbar Vertebral Joint with Autologous Tissue Substitute, Posterior Approach, Posterior Column, Percutaneous Approach
ØRGA37J Fusion of Thoracolumbar Vertebral Joint with Autologous Tissue Substitute, Posterior Approach, Anterior Column, Percutaneous Approach
ØRGA3AØ Fusion of Thoracolumbar Vertebral Joint with Interbody Fusion Device, Anterior Approach, Anterior Column, Percutaneous Approach
ØRGA3AJ Fusion of Thoracolumbar Vertebral Joint with Interbody Fusion Device, Posterior Approach, Anterior Column, Percutaneous Approach
ØRGA3JØ Fusion of Thoracolumbar Vertebral Joint with Synthetic Substitute, Anterior Approach, Anterior Column, Percutaneous Approach
ØRGA3J1 Fusion of Thoracolumbar Vertebral Joint with Synthetic Substitute, Posterior Approach, Posterior Column, Percutaneous Approach
ØRGA3JJ Fusion of Thoracolumbar Vertebral Joint with Synthetic Substitute, Posterior Approach, Anterior Column, Percutaneous Approach
ØRGA3KØ Fusion of Thoracolumbar Vertebral Joint with Nonautologous Tissue Substitute, Anterior Approach, Anterior Column, Percutaneous Approach
ØRGA3K1 Fusion of Thoracolumbar Vertebral Joint with Nonautologous Tissue Substitute, Posterior Approach, Posterior Column, Percutaneous Approach
ØRGA3KJ Fusion of Thoracolumbar Vertebral Joint with Nonautologous Tissue Substitute, Posterior Approach, Anterior Column, Percutaneous Approach

HAC 12: Surgical Site Infection—Certain Orthopedic Procedures of the Spine, Shoulder, and Elbow (continued)

ØRGA470 Fusion of Thoracolumbar Vertebral Joint with Autologous Tissue Substitute, Anterior Approach, Anterior Column, Percutaneous Endoscopic Approach
ØRGA471 Fusion of Thoracolumbar Vertebral Joint with Autologous Tissue Substitute, Posterior Approach, Posterior Column, Percutaneous Endoscopic Approach
ØRGA47J Fusion of Thoracolumbar Vertebral Joint with Autologous Tissue Substitute, Posterior Approach, Anterior Column, Percutaneous Endoscopic Approach
ØRGA4AØ Fusion of Thoracolumbar Vertebral Joint with Interbody Fusion Device, Anterior Approach, Anterior Column, Percutaneous Endoscopic Approach
ØRGA4AJ Fusion of Thoracolumbar Vertebral Joint with Interbody Fusion Device, Posterior Approach, Anterior Column, Percutaneous Endoscopic Approach
ØRGA4JØ Fusion of Thoracolumbar Vertebral Joint with Synthetic Substitute, Anterior Approach, Anterior Column, Percutaneous Endoscopic Approach
ØRGA4J1 Fusion of Thoracolumbar Vertebral Joint with Synthetic Substitute, Posterior Approach, Posterior Column, Percutaneous Endoscopic Approach
ØRGA4JJ Fusion of Thoracolumbar Vertebral Joint with Synthetic Substitute, Posterior Approach, Anterior Column, Percutaneous Endoscopic Approach
ØRGA4KØ Fusion of Thoracolumbar Vertebral Joint with Nonautologous Tissue Substitute, Anterior Approach, Anterior Column, Percutaneous Endoscopic Approach
ØRGA4K1 Fusion of Thoracolumbar Vertebral Joint with Nonautologous Tissue Substitute, Posterior Approach, Posterior Column, Percutaneous Endoscopic Approach
ØRGA4KJ Fusion of Thoracolumbar Vertebral Joint with Nonautologous Tissue Substitute, Posterior Approach, Anterior Column, Percutaneous Endoscopic Approach
ØRGEØ4Z Fusion of Right Sternoclavicular Joint with Internal Fixation Device, Open Approach
ØRGEØ7Z Fusion of Right Sternoclavicular Joint with Autologous Tissue Substitute, Open Approach
ØRGEØJZ Fusion of Right Sternoclavicular Joint with Synthetic Substitute, Open Approach
ØRGEØKZ Fusion of Right Sternoclavicular Joint with Nonautologous Tissue Substitute, Open Approach
ØRGE34Z Fusion of Right Sternoclavicular Joint with Internal Fixation Device, Percutaneous Approach
ØRGE37Z Fusion of Right Sternoclavicular Joint with Autologous Tissue Substitute, Percutaneous Approach
ØRGE3JZ Fusion of Right Sternoclavicular Joint with Synthetic Substitute, Percutaneous Approach
ØRGE3KZ Fusion of Right Sternoclavicular Joint with Nonautologous Tissue Substitute, Percutaneous Approach
ØRGE44Z Fusion of Right Sternoclavicular Joint with Internal Fixation Device, Percutaneous Endoscopic Approach
ØRGE47Z Fusion of Right Sternoclavicular Joint with Autologous Tissue Substitute, Percutaneous Endoscopic Approach
ØRGE4JZ Fusion of Right Sternoclavicular Joint with Synthetic Substitute, Percutaneous Endoscopic Approach
ØRGE4KZ Fusion of Right Sternoclavicular Joint with Nonautologous Tissue Substitute, Percutaneous Endoscopic Approach
ØRGFØ4Z Fusion of Left Sternoclavicular Joint with Internal Fixation Device, Open Approach
ØRGFØ7Z Fusion of Left Sternoclavicular Joint with Autologous Tissue Substitute, Open Approach
ØRGFØJZ Fusion of Left Sternoclavicular Joint with Synthetic Substitute, Open Approach
ØRGFØKZ Fusion of Left Sternoclavicular Joint with Nonautologous Tissue Substitute, Open Approach
ØRGF34Z Fusion of Left Sternoclavicular Joint with Internal Fixation Device, Percutaneous Approach
ØRGF37Z Fusion of Left Sternoclavicular Joint with Autologous Tissue Substitute, Percutaneous Approach
ØRGF3JZ Fusion of Left Sternoclavicular Joint with Synthetic Substitute, Percutaneous Approach
ØRGF3KZ Fusion of Left Sternoclavicular Joint with Nonautologous Tissue Substitute, Percutaneous Approach
ØRGF44Z Fusion of Left Sternoclavicular Joint with Internal Fixation Device, Percutaneous Endoscopic Approach
ØRGF47Z Fusion of Left Sternoclavicular Joint with Autologous Tissue Substitute, Percutaneous Endoscopic Approach
ØRGF4JZ Fusion of Left Sternoclavicular Joint with Synthetic Substitute, Percutaneous Endoscopic Approach
ØRGF4KZ Fusion of Left Sternoclavicular Joint with Nonautologous Tissue Substitute, Percutaneous Endoscopic Approach
ØRGGØ4Z Fusion of Right Acromioclavicular Joint with Internal Fixation Device, Open Approach
ØRGGØ7Z Fusion of Right Acromioclavicular Joint with Autologous Tissue Substitute, Open Approach
ØRGGØJZ Fusion of Right Acromioclavicular Joint with Synthetic Substitute, Open Approach
ØRGGØKZ Fusion of Right Acromioclavicular Joint with Nonautologous Tissue Substitute, Open Approach
ØRGG34Z Fusion of Right Acromioclavicular Joint with Internal Fixation Device, Percutaneous Approach
ØRGG37Z Fusion of Right Acromioclavicular Joint with Autologous Tissue Substitute, Percutaneous Approach
ØRGG3JZ Fusion of Right Acromioclavicular Joint with Synthetic Substitute, Percutaneous Approach
ØRGG3KZ Fusion of Right Acromioclavicular Joint with Nonautologous Tissue Substitute, Percutaneous Approach
ØRGG44Z Fusion of Right Acromioclavicular Joint with Internal Fixation Device, Percutaneous Endoscopic Approach
ØRGG47Z Fusion of Right Acromioclavicular Joint with Autologous Tissue Substitute, Percutaneous Endoscopic Approach
ØRGG4JZ Fusion of Right Acromioclavicular Joint with Synthetic Substitute, Percutaneous Endoscopic Approach
ØRGG4KZ Fusion of Right Acromioclavicular Joint with Nonautologous Tissue Substitute, Percutaneous Endoscopic Approach
ØRGHØ4Z Fusion of Left Acromioclavicular Joint with Internal Fixation Device, Open Approach
ØRGHØ7Z Fusion of Left Acromioclavicular Joint with Autologous Tissue Substitute, Open Approach
ØRGHØJZ Fusion of Left Acromioclavicular Joint with Synthetic Substitute, Open Approach
ØRGHØKZ Fusion of Left Acromioclavicular Joint with Nonautologous Tissue Substitute, Open Approach
ØRGH34Z Fusion of Left Acromioclavicular Joint with Internal Fixation Device, Percutaneous Approach
ØRGH37Z Fusion of Left Acromioclavicular Joint with Autologous Tissue Substitute, Percutaneous Approach
ØRGH3JZ Fusion of Left Acromioclavicular Joint with Synthetic Substitute, Percutaneous Approach
ØRGH3KZ Fusion of Left Acromioclavicular Joint with Nonautologous Tissue Substitute, Percutaneous Approach
ØRGH44Z Fusion of Left Acromioclavicular Joint with Internal Fixation Device, Percutaneous Endoscopic Approach
ØRGH47Z Fusion of Left Acromioclavicular Joint with Autologous Tissue Substitute, Percutaneous Endoscopic Approach
ØRGH4JZ Fusion of Left Acromioclavicular Joint with Synthetic Substitute, Percutaneous Endoscopic Approach
ØRGH4KZ Fusion of Left Acromioclavicular Joint with Nonautologous Tissue Substitute, Percutaneous Endoscopic Approach
ØRGJØ4Z Fusion of Right Shoulder Joint with Internal Fixation Device, Open Approach
ØRGJØ7Z Fusion of Right Shoulder Joint with Autologous Tissue Substitute, Open Approach
ØRGJØJZ Fusion of Right Shoulder Joint with Synthetic Substitute, Open Approach
ØRGJØKZ Fusion of Right Shoulder Joint with Nonautologous Tissue Substitute, Open Approach
ØRGJ34Z Fusion of Right Shoulder Joint with Internal Fixation Device, Percutaneous Approach
ØRGJ37Z Fusion of Right Shoulder Joint with Autologous Tissue Substitute, Percutaneous Approach
ØRGJ3JZ Fusion of Right Shoulder Joint with Synthetic Substitute, Percutaneous Approach
ØRGJ3KZ Fusion of Right Shoulder Joint with Nonautologous Tissue Substitute, Percutaneous Approach
ØRGJ44Z Fusion of Right Shoulder Joint with Internal Fixation Device, Percutaneous Endoscopic Approach
ØRGJ47Z Fusion of Right Shoulder Joint with Autologous Tissue Substitute, Percutaneous Endoscopic Approach
ØRGJ4JZ Fusion of Right Shoulder Joint with Synthetic Substitute, Percutaneous Endoscopic Approach
ØRGJ4KZ Fusion of Right Shoulder Joint with Nonautologous Tissue Substitute, Percutaneous Endoscopic Approach
ØRGKØ4Z Fusion of Left Shoulder Joint with Internal Fixation Device, Open Approach
ØRGKØ7Z Fusion of Left Shoulder Joint with Autologous Tissue Substitute, Open Approach
ØRGKØJZ Fusion of Left Shoulder Joint with Synthetic Substitute, Open Approach

HAC 12: Surgical Site Infection—Certain Orthopedic Procedures of the Spine, Shoulder, and Elbow (continued)

ØRGKØKZ Fusion of Left Shoulder Joint with Nonautologous Tissue Substitute, Open Approach
ØRGK34Z Fusion of Left Shoulder Joint with Internal Fixation Device, Percutaneous Approach
ØRGK37Z Fusion of Left Shoulder Joint with Autologous Tissue Substitute, Percutaneous Approach
ØRGK3JZ Fusion of Left Shoulder Joint with Synthetic Substitute, Percutaneous Approach
ØRGK3KZ Fusion of Left Shoulder Joint with Nonautologous Tissue Substitute, Percutaneous Approach
ØRGK44Z Fusion of Left Shoulder Joint with Internal Fixation Device, Percutaneous Endoscopic Approach
ØRGK47Z Fusion of Left Shoulder Joint with Autologous Tissue Substitute, Percutaneous Endoscopic Approach
ØRGK4JZ Fusion of Left Shoulder Joint with Synthetic Substitute, Percutaneous Endoscopic Approach
ØRGK4KZ Fusion of Left Shoulder Joint with Nonautologous Tissue Substitute, Percutaneous Endoscopic Approach
ØRGLØ4Z Fusion of Right Elbow Joint with Internal Fixation Device, Open Approach
ØRGLØ5Z Fusion of Right Elbow Joint with External Fixation Device, Open Approach
ØRGLØ7Z Fusion of Right Elbow Joint with Autologous Tissue Substitute, Open Approach
ØRGLØJZ Fusion of Right Elbow Joint with Synthetic Substitute, Open Approach
ØRGLØKZ Fusion of Right Elbow Joint with Nonautologous Tissue Substitute, Open Approach
ØRGL34Z Fusion of Right Elbow Joint with Internal Fixation Device, Percutaneous Approach
ØRGL35Z Fusion of Right Elbow Joint with External Fixation Device, Percutaneous Approach
ØRGL37Z Fusion of Right Elbow Joint with Autologous Tissue Substitute, Percutaneous Approach
ØRGL3JZ Fusion of Right Elbow Joint with Synthetic Substitute, Percutaneous Approach
ØRGL3KZ Fusion of Right Elbow Joint with Nonautologous Tissue Substitute, Percutaneous Approach
ØRGL44Z Fusion of Right Elbow Joint with Internal Fixation Device, Percutaneous Endoscopic Approach
ØRGL45Z Fusion of Right Elbow Joint with External Fixation Device, Percutaneous Endoscopic Approach
ØRGL47Z Fusion of Right Elbow Joint with Autologous Tissue Substitute, Percutaneous Endoscopic Approach
ØRGL4JZ Fusion of Right Elbow Joint with Synthetic Substitute, Percutaneous Endoscopic Approach
ØRGL4KZ Fusion of Right Elbow Joint with Nonautologous Tissue Substitute, Percutaneous Endoscopic Approach
ØRGMØ4Z Fusion of Left Elbow Joint with Internal Fixation Device, Open Approach
ØRGMØ5Z Fusion of Left Elbow Joint with External Fixation Device, Open Approach
ØRGMØ7Z Fusion of Left Elbow Joint with Autologous Tissue Substitute, Open Approach
ØRGMØJZ Fusion of Left Elbow Joint with Synthetic Substitute, Open Approach
ØRGMØKZ Fusion of Left Elbow Joint with Nonautologous Tissue Substitute, Open Approach
ØRGM34Z Fusion of Left Elbow Joint with Internal Fixation Device, Percutaneous Approach
ØRGM35Z Fusion of Left Elbow Joint with External Fixation Device, Percutaneous Approach
ØRGM37Z Fusion of Left Elbow Joint with Autologous Tissue Substitute, Percutaneous Approach
ØRGM3JZ Fusion of Left Elbow Joint with Synthetic Substitute, Percutaneous Approach
ØRGM3KZ Fusion of Left Elbow Joint with Nonautologous Tissue Substitute, Percutaneous Approach
ØRGM44Z Fusion of Left Elbow Joint with Internal Fixation Device, Percutaneous Endoscopic Approach
ØRGM45Z Fusion of Left Elbow Joint with External Fixation Device, Percutaneous Endoscopic Approach
ØRGM47Z Fusion of Left Elbow Joint with Autologous Tissue Substitute, Percutaneous Endoscopic Approach
ØRGM4JZ Fusion of Left Elbow Joint with Synthetic Substitute, Percutaneous Endoscopic Approach
ØRGM4KZ Fusion of Left Elbow Joint with Nonautologous Tissue Substitute, Percutaneous Endoscopic Approach
ØRQEØZZ Repair Right Sternoclavicular Joint, Open Approach
ØRQE3ZZ Repair Right Sternoclavicular Joint, Percutaneous Approach
ØRQE4ZZ Repair Right Sternoclavicular Joint, Percutaneous Endoscopic Approach
ØRQEXZZ Repair Right Sternoclavicular Joint, External Approach
ØRQFØZZ Repair Left Sternoclavicular Joint, Open Approach
ØRQF3ZZ Repair Left Sternoclavicular Joint, Percutaneous Approach
ØRQF4ZZ Repair Left Sternoclavicular Joint, Percutaneous Endoscopic Approach
ØRQFXZZ Repair Left Sternoclavicular Joint, External Approach
ØRQGØZZ Repair Right Acromioclavicular Joint, Open Approach
ØRQG3ZZ Repair Right Acromioclavicular Joint, Percutaneous Approach
ØRQG4ZZ Repair Right Acromioclavicular Joint, Percutaneous Endoscopic Approach
ØRQGXZZ Repair Right Acromioclavicular Joint, External Approach
ØRQHØZZ Repair Left Acromioclavicular Joint, Open Approach
ØRQH3ZZ Repair Left Acromioclavicular Joint, Percutaneous Approach
ØRQH4ZZ Repair Left Acromioclavicular Joint, Percutaneous Endoscopic Approach
ØRQHXZZ Repair Left Acromioclavicular Joint, External Approach
ØRQJØZZ Repair Right Shoulder Joint, Open Approach
ØRQJ3ZZ Repair Right Shoulder Joint, Percutaneous Approach
ØRQJ4ZZ Repair Right Shoulder Joint, Percutaneous Endoscopic Approach
ØRQJXZZ Repair Right Shoulder Joint, External Approach
ØRQKØZZ Repair Left Shoulder Joint, Open Approach
ØRQK3ZZ Repair Left Shoulder Joint, Percutaneous Approach
ØRQK4ZZ Repair Left Shoulder Joint, Percutaneous Endoscopic Approach
ØRQKXZZ Repair Left Shoulder Joint, External Approach
ØRQLØZZ Repair Right Elbow Joint, Open Approach
ØRQL3ZZ Repair Right Elbow Joint, Percutaneous Approach
ØRQL4ZZ Repair Right Elbow Joint, Percutaneous Endoscopic Approach
ØRQLXZZ Repair Right Elbow Joint, External Approach
ØRQMØZZ Repair Left Elbow Joint, Open Approach
ØRQM3ZZ Repair Left Elbow Joint, Percutaneous Approach
ØRQM4ZZ Repair Left Elbow Joint, Percutaneous Endoscopic Approach
ØRQMXZZ Repair Left Elbow Joint, External Approach
ØRUEØ7Z Supplement Right Sternoclavicular Joint with Autologous Tissue Substitute, Open Approach
ØRUEØJZ Supplement Right Sternoclavicular Joint with Synthetic Substitute, Open Approach
ØRUEØKZ Supplement Right Sternoclavicular Joint with Nonautologous Tissue Substitute, Open Approach
ØRUE37Z Supplement Right Sternoclavicular Joint with Autologous Tissue Substitute, Percutaneous Approach
ØRUE3JZ Supplement Right Sternoclavicular Joint with Synthetic Substitute, Percutaneous Approach
ØRUE3KZ Supplement Right Sternoclavicular Joint with Nonautologous Tissue Substitute, Percutaneous Approach
ØRUE47Z Supplement Right Sternoclavicular Joint with Autologous Tissue Substitute, Percutaneous Endoscopic Approach
ØRUE4JZ Supplement Right Sternoclavicular Joint with Synthetic Substitute, Percutaneous Endoscopic Approach
ØRUE4KZ Supplement Right Sternoclavicular Joint with Nonautologous Tissue Substitute, Percutaneous Endoscopic Approach
ØRUFØ7Z Supplement Left Sternoclavicular Joint with Autologous Tissue Substitute, Open Approach
ØRUFØJZ Supplement Left Sternoclavicular Joint with Synthetic Substitute, Open Approach
ØRUFØKZ Supplement Left Sternoclavicular Joint with Nonautologous Tissue Substitute, Open Approach
ØRUF37Z Supplement Left Sternoclavicular Joint with Autologous Tissue Substitute, Percutaneous Approach
ØRUF3JZ Supplement Left Sternoclavicular Joint with Synthetic Substitute, Percutaneous Approach
ØRUF3KZ Supplement Left Sternoclavicular Joint with Nonautologous Tissue Substitute, Percutaneous Approach
ØRUF47Z Supplement Left Sternoclavicular Joint with Autologous Tissue Substitute, Percutaneous Endoscopic Approach
ØRUF4JZ Supplement Left Sternoclavicular Joint with Synthetic Substitute, Percutaneous Endoscopic Approach
ØRUF4KZ Supplement Left Sternoclavicular Joint with Nonautologous Tissue Substitute, Percutaneous Endoscopic Approach
ØRUGØ7Z Supplement Right Acromioclavicular Joint with Autologous Tissue Substitute, Open Approach

HAC 12: Surgical Site Infection—Certain Orthopedic Procedures of the Spine, Shoulder, and Elbow (continued)

ØRUGØJZ Supplement Right Acromioclavicular Joint with Synthetic Substitute, Open Approach
ØRUGØKZ Supplement Right Acromioclavicular Joint with Nonautologous Tissue Substitute, Open Approach
ØRUG37Z Supplement Right Acromioclavicular Joint with Autologous Tissue Substitute, Percutaneous Approach
ØRUG3JZ Supplement Right Acromioclavicular Joint with Synthetic Substitute, Percutaneous Approach
ØRUG3KZ Supplement Right Acromioclavicular Joint with Nonautologous Tissue Substitute, Percutaneous Approach
ØRUG47Z Supplement Right Acromioclavicular Joint with Autologous Tissue Substitute, Percutaneous Endoscopic Approach
ØRUG4JZ Supplement Right Acromioclavicular Joint with Synthetic Substitute, Percutaneous Endoscopic Approach
ØRUG4KZ Supplement Right Acromioclavicular Joint with Nonautologous Tissue Substitute, Percutaneous Endoscopic Approach
ØRUHØ7Z Supplement Left Acromioclavicular Joint with Autologous Tissue Substitute, Open Approach
ØRUHØJZ Supplement Left Acromioclavicular Joint with Synthetic Substitute, Open Approach
ØRUHØKZ Supplement Left Acromioclavicular Joint with Nonautologous Tissue Substitute, Open Approach
ØRUH37Z Supplement Left Acromioclavicular Joint with Autologous Tissue Substitute, Percutaneous Approach
ØRUH3JZ Supplement Left Acromioclavicular Joint with Synthetic Substitute, Percutaneous Approach
ØRUH3KZ Supplement Left Acromioclavicular Joint with Nonautologous Tissue Substitute, Percutaneous Approach
ØRUH47Z Supplement Left Acromioclavicular Joint with Autologous Tissue Substitute, Percutaneous Endoscopic Approach
ØRUH4JZ Supplement Left Acromioclavicular Joint with Synthetic Substitute, Percutaneous Endoscopic Approach
ØRUH4KZ Supplement Left Acromioclavicular Joint with Nonautologous Tissue Substitute, Percutaneous Endoscopic Approach
ØRUJØ7Z Supplement Right Shoulder Joint with Autologous Tissue Substitute, Open Approach
ØRUJØJZ Supplement Right Shoulder Joint with Synthetic Substitute, Open Approach
ØRUJØKZ Supplement Right Shoulder Joint with Nonautologous Tissue Substitute, Open Approach
ØRUJ37Z Supplement Right Shoulder Joint with Autologous Tissue Substitute, Percutaneous Approach
ØRUJ3JZ Supplement Right Shoulder Joint with Synthetic Substitute, Percutaneous Approach
ØRUJ3KZ Supplement Right Shoulder Joint with Nonautologous Tissue Substitute, Percutaneous Approach
ØRUJ47Z Supplement Right Shoulder Joint with Autologous Tissue Substitute, Percutaneous Endoscopic Approach
ØRUJ4JZ Supplement Right Shoulder Joint with Synthetic Substitute, Percutaneous Endoscopic Approach
ØRUJ4KZ Supplement Right Shoulder Joint with Nonautologous Tissue Substitute, Percutaneous Endoscopic Approach
ØRUKØ7Z Supplement Left Shoulder Joint with Autologous Tissue Substitute, Open Approach
ØRUKØJZ Supplement Left Shoulder Joint with Synthetic Substitute, Open Approach
ØRUKØKZ Supplement Left Shoulder Joint with Nonautologous Tissue Substitute, Open Approach
ØRUK37Z Supplement Left Shoulder Joint with Autologous Tissue Substitute, Percutaneous Approach
ØRUK3JZ Supplement Left Shoulder Joint with Synthetic Substitute, Percutaneous Approach
ØRUK3KZ Supplement Left Shoulder Joint with Nonautologous Tissue Substitute, Percutaneous Approach
ØRUK47Z Supplement Left Shoulder Joint with Autologous Tissue Substitute, Percutaneous Endoscopic Approach
ØRUK4JZ Supplement Left Shoulder Joint with Synthetic Substitute, Percutaneous Endoscopic Approach
ØRUK4KZ Supplement Left Shoulder Joint with Nonautologous Tissue Substitute, Percutaneous Endoscopic Approach
ØRULØ7Z Supplement Right Elbow Joint with Autologous Tissue Substitute, Open Approach
ØRULØJZ Supplement Right Elbow Joint with Synthetic Substitute, Open Approach
ØRULØKZ Supplement Right Elbow Joint with Nonautologous Tissue Substitute, Open Approach
ØRUL37Z Supplement Right Elbow Joint with Autologous Tissue Substitute, Percutaneous Approach
ØRUL3JZ Supplement Right Elbow Joint with Synthetic Substitute, Percutaneous Approach
ØRUL3KZ Supplement Right Elbow Joint with Nonautologous Tissue Substitute, Percutaneous Approach
ØRUL47Z Supplement Right Elbow Joint with Autologous Tissue Substitute, Percutaneous Endoscopic Approach
ØRUL4JZ Supplement Right Elbow Joint with Synthetic Substitute, Percutaneous Endoscopic Approach
ØRUL4KZ Supplement Right Elbow Joint with Nonautologous Tissue Substitute, Percutaneous Endoscopic Approach
ØRUMØ7Z Supplement Left Elbow Joint with Autologous Tissue Substitute, Open Approach
ØRUMØJZ Supplement Left Elbow Joint with Synthetic Substitute, Open Approach
ØRUMØKZ Supplement Left Elbow Joint with Nonautologous Tissue Substitute, Open Approach
ØRUM37Z Supplement Left Elbow Joint with Autologous Tissue Substitute, Percutaneous Approach
ØRUM3JZ Supplement Left Elbow Joint with Synthetic Substitute, Percutaneous Approach
ØRUM3KZ Supplement Left Elbow Joint with Nonautologous Tissue Substitute, Percutaneous Approach
ØRUM47Z Supplement Left Elbow Joint with Autologous Tissue Substitute, Percutaneous Endoscopic Approach
ØRUM4JZ Supplement Left Elbow Joint with Synthetic Substitute, Percutaneous Endoscopic Approach
ØRUM4KZ Supplement Left Elbow Joint with Nonautologous Tissue Substitute, Percutaneous Endoscopic Approach
ØSGØØ7Ø Fusion of Lumbar Vertebral Joint with Autologous Tissue Substitute, Anterior Approach, Anterior Column, Open Approach
ØSGØØ71 Fusion of Lumbar Vertebral Joint with Autologous Tissue Substitute, Posterior Approach, Posterior Column, Open Approach
ØSGØØ7J Fusion of Lumbar Vertebral Joint with Autologous Tissue Substitute, Posterior Approach, Anterior Column, Open Approach
ØSGØØAØ Fusion of Lumbar Vertebral Joint with Interbody Fusion Device, Anterior Approach, Anterior Column, Open Approach
ØSGØØAJ Fusion of Lumbar Vertebral Joint with Interbody Fusion Device, Posterior Approach, Anterior Column, Open Approach
ØSGØØJØ Fusion of Lumbar Vertebral Joint with Synthetic Substitute, Anterior Approach, Anterior Column, Open Approach
ØSGØØJ1 Fusion of Lumbar Vertebral Joint with Synthetic Substitute, Posterior Approach, Posterior Column, Open Approach
ØSGØØJJ Fusion of Lumbar Vertebral Joint with Synthetic Substitute, Posterior Approach, Anterior Column, Open Approach
ØSGØØKØ Fusion of Lumbar Vertebral Joint with Nonautologous Tissue Substitute, Anterior Approach, Anterior Column, Open Approach
ØSGØØK1 Fusion of Lumbar Vertebral Joint with Nonautologous Tissue Substitute, Posterior Approach, Posterior Column, Open Approach
ØSGØØKJ Fusion of Lumbar Vertebral Joint with Nonautologous Tissue Substitute, Posterior Approach, Anterior Column, Open Approach
ØSGØ37Ø Fusion of Lumbar Vertebral Joint with Autologous Tissue Substitute, Anterior Approach, Anterior Column, Percutaneous Approach
ØSGØ371 Fusion of Lumbar Vertebral Joint with Autologous Tissue Substitute, Posterior Approach, Posterior Column, Percutaneous Approach
ØSGØ37J Fusion of Lumbar Vertebral Joint with Autologous Tissue Substitute, Posterior Approach, Anterior Column, Percutaneous Approach
ØSGØ3AØ Fusion of Lumbar Vertebral Joint with Interbody Fusion Device, Anterior Approach, Anterior Column, Percutaneous Approach
ØSGØ3AJ Fusion of Lumbar Vertebral Joint with Interbody Fusion Device, Posterior Approach, Anterior Column, Percutaneous Approach
ØSGØ3JØ Fusion of Lumbar Vertebral Joint with Synthetic Substitute, Anterior Approach, Anterior Column, Percutaneous Approach

HAC 12: Surgical Site Infection—Certain Orthopedic Procedures of the Spine, Shoulder, and Elbow (continued)

ØSGØ3J1 Fusion of Lumbar Vertebral Joint with Synthetic Substitute, Posterior Approach, Posterior Column, Percutaneous Approach
ØSGØ3JJ Fusion of Lumbar Vertebral Joint with Synthetic Substitute, Posterior Approach, Anterior Column, Percutaneous Approach
ØSGØ3KØ Fusion of Lumbar Vertebral Joint with Nonautologous Tissue Substitute, Anterior Approach, Anterior Column, Percutaneous Approach
ØSGØ3K1 Fusion of Lumbar Vertebral Joint with Nonautologous Tissue Substitute, Posterior Approach, Posterior Column, Percutaneous Approach
ØSGØ3KJ Fusion of Lumbar Vertebral Joint with Nonautologous Tissue Substitute, Posterior Approach, Anterior Column, Percutaneous Approach
ØSGØ47Ø Fusion of Lumbar Vertebral Joint with Autologous Tissue Substitute, Anterior Approach, Anterior Column, Percutaneous Endoscopic Approach
ØSGØ471 Fusion of Lumbar Vertebral Joint with Autologous Tissue Substitute, Posterior Approach, Posterior Column, Percutaneous Endoscopic Approach
ØSGØ47J Fusion of Lumbar Vertebral Joint with Autologous Tissue Substitute, Posterior Approach, Anterior Column, Percutaneous Endoscopic Approach
ØSGØ4AØ Fusion of Lumbar Vertebral Joint with Interbody Fusion Device, Anterior Approach, Anterior Column, Percutaneous Endoscopic Approach
ØSGØ4AJ Fusion of Lumbar Vertebral Joint with Interbody Fusion Device, Posterior Approach, Anterior Column, Percutaneous Endoscopic Approach
ØSGØ4JØ Fusion of Lumbar Vertebral Joint with Synthetic Substitute, Anterior Approach, Anterior Column, Percutaneous Endoscopic Approach
ØSGØ4J1 Fusion of Lumbar Vertebral Joint with Synthetic Substitute, Posterior Approach, Posterior Column, Percutaneous Endoscopic Approach
ØSGØ4JJ Fusion of Lumbar Vertebral Joint with Synthetic Substitute, Posterior Approach, Anterior Column, Percutaneous Endoscopic Approach
ØSGØ4KØ Fusion of Lumbar Vertebral Joint with Nonautologous Tissue Substitute, Anterior Approach, Anterior Column, Percutaneous Endoscopic Approach
ØSGØ4K1 Fusion of Lumbar Vertebral Joint with Nonautologous Tissue Substitute, Posterior Approach, Posterior Column, Percutaneous Endoscopic Approach
ØSGØ4KJ Fusion of Lumbar Vertebral Joint with Nonautologous Tissue Substitute, Posterior Approach, Anterior Column, Percutaneous Endoscopic Approach
ØSG1Ø7Ø Fusion of 2 or More Lumbar Vertebral Joints with Autologous Tissue Substitute, Anterior Approach, Anterior Column, Open Approach
ØSG1Ø71 Fusion of 2 or More Lumbar Vertebral Joints with Autologous Tissue Substitute, Posterior Approach, Posterior Column, Open Approach
ØSG1Ø7J Fusion of 2 or More Lumbar Vertebral Joints with Autologous Tissue Substitute, Posterior Approach, Anterior Column, Open Approach
ØSG1ØAØ Fusion of 2 or More Lumbar Vertebral Joints with Interbody Fusion Device, Anterior Approach, Anterior Column, Open Approach
ØSG1ØAJ Fusion of 2 or More Lumbar Vertebral Joints with Interbody Fusion Device, Posterior Approach, Anterior Column, Open Approach
ØSG1ØJØ Fusion of 2 or More Lumbar Vertebral Joints with Synthetic Substitute, Anterior Approach, Anterior Column, Open Approach
ØSG1ØJ1 Fusion of 2 or More Lumbar Vertebral Joints with Synthetic Substitute, Posterior Approach, Posterior Column, Open Approach
ØSG1ØJJ Fusion of 2 or More Lumbar Vertebral Joints with Synthetic Substitute, Posterior Approach, Anterior Column, Open Approach
ØSG1ØKØ Fusion of 2 or More Lumbar Vertebral Joints with Nonautologous Tissue Substitute, Anterior Approach, Anterior Column, Open Approach
ØSG1ØK1 Fusion of 2 or More Lumbar Vertebral Joints with Nonautologous Tissue Substitute, Posterior Approach, Posterior Column, Open Approach
ØSG1ØKJ Fusion of 2 or More Lumbar Vertebral Joints with Nonautologous Tissue Substitute, Posterior Approach, Anterior Column, Open Approach
ØSG137Ø Fusion of 2 or More Lumbar Vertebral Joints with Autologous Tissue Substitute, Anterior Approach, Anterior Column, Percutaneous Approach
ØSG1371 Fusion of 2 or More Lumbar Vertebral Joints with Autologous Tissue Substitute, Posterior Approach, Posterior Column, Percutaneous Approach
ØSG137J Fusion of 2 or More Lumbar Vertebral Joints with Autologous Tissue Substitute, Posterior Approach, Anterior Column, Percutaneous Approach
ØSG13AØ Fusion of 2 or More Lumbar Vertebral Joints with Interbody Fusion Device, Anterior Approach, Anterior Column, Percutaneous Approach
ØSG13AJ Fusion of 2 or More Lumbar Vertebral Joints with Interbody Fusion Device, Posterior Approach, Anterior Column, Percutaneous Approach
ØSG13JØ Fusion of 2 or More Lumbar Vertebral Joints with Synthetic Substitute, Anterior Approach, Anterior Column, Percutaneous Approach
ØSG13J1 Fusion of 2 or More Lumbar Vertebral Joints with Synthetic Substitute, Posterior Approach, Posterior Column, Percutaneous Approach
ØSG13JJ Fusion of 2 or More Lumbar Vertebral Joints with Synthetic Substitute, Posterior Approach, Anterior Column, Percutaneous Approach
ØSG13KØ Fusion of 2 or More Lumbar Vertebral Joints with Nonautologous Tissue Substitute, Anterior Approach, Anterior Column, Percutaneous Approach
ØSG13K1 Fusion of 2 or More Lumbar Vertebral Joints with Nonautologous Tissue Substitute, Posterior Approach, Posterior Column, Percutaneous Approach
ØSG13KJ Fusion of 2 or More Lumbar Vertebral Joints with Nonautologous Tissue Substitute, Posterior Approach, Anterior Column, Percutaneous Approach
ØSG147Ø Fusion of 2 or More Lumbar Vertebral Joints with Autologous Tissue Substitute, Anterior Approach, Anterior Column, Percutaneous Endoscopic Approach
ØSG1471 Fusion of 2 or More Lumbar Vertebral Joints with Autologous Tissue Substitute, Posterior Approach, Posterior Column, Percutaneous Endoscopic Approach
ØSG147J Fusion of 2 or More Lumbar Vertebral Joints with Autologous Tissue Substitute, Posterior Approach, Anterior Column, Percutaneous Endoscopic Approach
ØSG14AØ Fusion of 2 or More Lumbar Vertebral Joints with Interbody Fusion Device, Anterior Approach, Anterior Column, Percutaneous Endoscopic Approach
ØSG14AJ Fusion of 2 or More Lumbar Vertebral Joints with Interbody Fusion Device, Posterior Approach, Anterior Column, Percutaneous Endoscopic Approach
ØSG14JØ Fusion of 2 or More Lumbar Vertebral Joints with Synthetic Substitute, Anterior Approach, Anterior Column, Percutaneous Endoscopic Approach
ØSG14J1 Fusion of 2 or More Lumbar Vertebral Joints with Synthetic Substitute, Posterior Approach, Posterior Column, Percutaneous Endoscopic Approach
ØSG14JJ Fusion of 2 or More Lumbar Vertebral Joints with Synthetic Substitute, Posterior Approach, Anterior Column, Percutaneous Endoscopic Approach
ØSG14KØ Fusion of 2 or More Lumbar Vertebral Joints with Nonautologous Tissue Substitute, Anterior Approach, Anterior Column, Percutaneous Endoscopic Approach
ØSG14K1 Fusion of 2 or More Lumbar Vertebral Joints with Nonautologous Tissue Substitute, Posterior Approach, Posterior Column, Percutaneous Endoscopic Approach
ØSG14KJ Fusion of 2 or More Lumbar Vertebral Joints with Nonautologous Tissue Substitute, Posterior Approach, Anterior Column, Percutaneous Endoscopic Approach
ØSG3Ø7Ø Fusion of Lumbosacral Joint with Autologous Tissue Substitute, Anterior Approach, Anterior Column, Open Approach
ØSG3Ø71 Fusion of Lumbosacral Joint with Autologous Tissue Substitute, Posterior Approach, Posterior Column, Open Approach
ØSG3Ø7J Fusion of Lumbosacral Joint with Autologous Tissue Substitute, Posterior Approach, Anterior Column, Open Approach
ØSG3ØAØ Fusion of Lumbosacral Joint with Interbody Fusion Device, Anterior Approach, Anterior Column, Open Approach
ØSG3ØAJ Fusion of Lumbosacral Joint with Interbody Fusion Device, Posterior Approach, Anterior Column, Open Approach
ØSG3ØJØ Fusion of Lumbosacral Joint with Synthetic Substitute, Anterior Approach, Anterior Column, Open Approach
ØSG3ØJ1 Fusion of Lumbosacral Joint with Synthetic Substitute, Posterior Approach, Posterior Column, Open Approach

HAC 12: Surgical Site Infection—Certain Orthopedic Procedures of the Spine, Shoulder, and Elbow (continued)

ØSG3ØJJ Fusion of Lumbosacral Joint with Synthetic Substitute, Posterior Approach, Anterior Column, Open Approach
ØSG3ØKØ Fusion of Lumbosacral Joint with Nonautologous Tissue Substitute, Anterior Approach, Anterior Column, Open Approach
ØSG3ØK1 Fusion of Lumbosacral Joint with Nonautologous Tissue Substitute, Posterior Approach, Posterior Column, Open Approach
ØSG3ØKJ Fusion of Lumbosacral Joint with Nonautologous Tissue Substitute, Posterior Approach, Anterior Column, Open Approach
ØSG337Ø Fusion of Lumbosacral Joint with Autologous Tissue Substitute, Anterior Approach, Anterior Column, Percutaneous Approach
ØSG3371 Fusion of Lumbosacral Joint with Autologous Tissue Substitute, Posterior Approach, Posterior Column, Percutaneous Approach
ØSG337J Fusion of Lumbosacral Joint with Autologous Tissue Substitute, Posterior Approach, Anterior Column, Percutaneous Approach
ØSG33AØ Fusion of Lumbosacral Joint with Interbody Fusion Device, Anterior Approach, Anterior Column, Percutaneous Approach
ØSG33AJ Fusion of Lumbosacral Joint with Interbody Fusion Device, Posterior Approach, Anterior Column, Percutaneous Approach
ØSG33JØ Fusion of Lumbosacral Joint with Synthetic Substitute, Anterior Approach, Anterior Column, Percutaneous Approach
ØSG33J1 Fusion of Lumbosacral Joint with Synthetic Substitute, Posterior Approach, Posterior Column, Percutaneous Approach
ØSG33JJ Fusion of Lumbosacral Joint with Synthetic Substitute, Posterior Approach, Anterior Column, Percutaneous Approach
ØSG33KØ Fusion of Lumbosacral Joint with Nonautologous Tissue Substitute, Anterior Approach, Anterior Column, Percutaneous Approach
ØSG33K1 Fusion of Lumbosacral Joint with Nonautologous Tissue Substitute, Posterior Approach, Posterior Column, Percutaneous Approach
ØSG33KJ Fusion of Lumbosacral Joint with Nonautologous Tissue Substitute, Posterior Approach, Anterior Column, Percutaneous Approach
ØSG347Ø Fusion of Lumbosacral Joint with Autologous Tissue Substitute, Anterior Approach, Anterior Column, Percutaneous Endoscopic Approach
ØSG3471 Fusion of Lumbosacral Joint with Autologous Tissue Substitute, Posterior Approach, Posterior Column, Percutaneous Endoscopic Approach
ØSG347J Fusion of Lumbosacral Joint with Autologous Tissue Substitute, Posterior Approach, Anterior Column, Percutaneous Endoscopic Approach
ØSG34AØ Fusion of Lumbosacral Joint with Interbody Fusion Device, Anterior Approach, Anterior Column, Percutaneous Endoscopic Approach
ØSG34AJ Fusion of Lumbosacral Joint with Interbody Fusion Device, Posterior Approach, Anterior Column, Percutaneous Endoscopic Approach
ØSG34JØ Fusion of Lumbosacral Joint with Synthetic Substitute, Anterior Approach, Anterior Column, Percutaneous Endoscopic Approach
ØSG34J1 Fusion of Lumbosacral Joint with Synthetic Substitute, Posterior Approach, Posterior Column, Percutaneous Endoscopic Approach
ØSG34JJ Fusion of Lumbosacral Joint with Synthetic Substitute, Posterior Approach, Anterior Column, Percutaneous Endoscopic Approach
ØSG34KØ Fusion of Lumbosacral Joint with Nonautologous Tissue Substitute, Anterior Approach, Anterior Column, Percutaneous Endoscopic Approach
ØSG34K1 Fusion of Lumbosacral Joint with Nonautologous Tissue Substitute, Posterior Approach, Posterior Column, Percutaneous Endoscopic Approach
ØSG34KJ Fusion of Lumbosacral Joint with Nonautologous Tissue Substitute, Posterior Approach, Anterior Column, Percutaneous Endoscopic Approach
ØSG7Ø4Z Fusion of Right Sacroiliac Joint with Internal Fixation Device, Open Approach
ØSG7Ø7Z Fusion of Right Sacroiliac Joint with Autologous Tissue Substitute, Open Approach
ØSG7ØJZ Fusion of Right Sacroiliac Joint with Synthetic Substitute, Open Approach
ØSG7ØKZ Fusion of Right Sacroiliac Joint with Nonautologous Tissue Substitute, Open Approach
ØSG734Z Fusion of Right Sacroiliac Joint with Internal Fixation Device, Percutaneous Approach
ØSG737Z Fusion of Right Sacroiliac Joint with Autologous Tissue Substitute, Percutaneous Approach
ØSG73JZ Fusion of Right Sacroiliac Joint with Synthetic Substitute, Percutaneous Approach
ØSG73KZ Fusion of Right Sacroiliac Joint with Nonautologous Tissue Substitute, Percutaneous Approach
ØSG744Z Fusion of Right Sacroiliac Joint with Internal Fixation Device, Percutaneous Endoscopic Approach
ØSG747Z Fusion of Right Sacroiliac Joint with Autologous Tissue Substitute, Percutaneous Endoscopic Approach
ØSG74JZ Fusion of Right Sacroiliac Joint with Synthetic Substitute, Percutaneous Endoscopic Approach
ØSG74KZ Fusion of Right Sacroiliac Joint with Nonautologous Tissue Substitute, Percutaneous Endoscopic Approach
ØSG8Ø4Z Fusion of Left Sacroiliac Joint with Internal Fixation Device, Open Approach
ØSG8Ø7Z Fusion of Left Sacroiliac Joint with Autologous Tissue Substitute, Open Approach
ØSG8ØJZ Fusion of Left Sacroiliac Joint with Synthetic Substitute, Open Approach
ØSG8ØKZ Fusion of Left Sacroiliac Joint with Nonautologous Tissue Substitute, Open Approach
ØSG834Z Fusion of Left Sacroiliac Joint with Internal Fixation Device, Percutaneous Approach
ØSG837Z Fusion of Left Sacroiliac Joint with Autologous Tissue Substitute, Percutaneous Approach
ØSG83JZ Fusion of Left Sacroiliac Joint with Synthetic Substitute, Percutaneous Approach
ØSG83KZ Fusion of Left Sacroiliac Joint with Nonautologous Tissue Substitute, Percutaneous Approach
ØSG844Z Fusion of Left Sacroiliac Joint with Internal Fixation Device, Percutaneous Endoscopic Approach
ØSG847Z Fusion of Left Sacroiliac Joint with Autologous Tissue Substitute, Percutaneous Endoscopic Approach
ØSG84JZ Fusion of Left Sacroiliac Joint with Synthetic Substitute, Percutaneous Endoscopic Approach
ØSG84KZ Fusion of Left Sacroiliac Joint with Nonautologous Tissue Substitute, Percutaneous Endoscopic Approach
XRGØØ92 Fusion of Occipital-cervical Joint using Nanotextured Surface Interbody Fusion Device, Open Approach, New Technology Group 2
XRGØØF3 Fusion of Occipital-cervical Joint using Radiolucent Porous Interbody Fusion Device, Open Approach, New Technology Group 3
XRG1Ø92 Fusion of Cervical Vertebral Joint using Nanotextured Surface Interbody Fusion Device, Open Approach, New Technology Group 2
XRG1ØF3 Fusion of Cervical Vertebral Joint using Radiolucent Porous Interbody Fusion Device, Open Approach, New Technology Group 3
XRG2Ø92 Fusion of 2 or more Cervical Vertebral Joints using Nanotextured Surface Interbody Fusion Device, Open Approach, New Technology Group 2
XRG2ØF3 Fusion of 2 or more Cervical Vertebral Joints using Radiolucent Porous Interbody Fusion Device, Open Approach, New Technology Group 3
XRG4Ø92 Fusion of Cervicothoracic Vertebral Joint using Nanotextured Surface Interbody Fusion Device, Open Approach, New Technology Group 2
XRG4ØF3 Fusion of Cervicothoracic Vertebral Joint using Radiolucent Porous Interbody Fusion Device, Open Approach, New Technology Group 3
XRG6Ø92 Fusion of Thoracic Vertebral Joint using Nanotextured Surface Interbody Fusion Device, Open Approach, New Technology Group 2
XRG6ØF3 Fusion of Thoracic Vertebral Joint using Radiolucent Porous Interbody Fusion Device, Open Approach, New Technology Group 3
XRG7Ø92 Fusion of 2 to 7 Thoracic Vertebral Joints using Nanotextured Surface Interbody Fusion Device, Open Approach, New Technology Group 2
XRG7ØF3 Fusion of 2 to 7 Thoracic Vertebral Joints using Radiolucent Porous Interbody Fusion Device, Open Approach, New Technology Group 3
XRG8Ø92 Fusion of 8 or more Thoracic Vertebral Joints using Nanotextured Surface Interbody Fusion Device, Open Approach, New Technology Group 2

HAC 12: Surgical Site Infection—Certain Orthopedic Procedures of the Spine, Shoulder, and Elbow (continued)

XRG8ØF3 Fusion of 8 or more Thoracic Vertebral Joints using Radiolucent Porous Interbody Fusion Device, Open Approach, New Technology Group 3
XRGAØ92 Fusion of Thoracolumbar Vertebral Joint using Nanotextured Surface Interbody Fusion Device, Open Approach, New Technology Group 2
XRGAØF3 Fusion of Thoracolumbar Vertebral Joint using Radiolucent Porous Interbody Fusion Device, Open Approach, New Technology Group 3
XRGBØ92 Fusion of Lumbar Vertebral Joint using Nanotextured Surface Interbody Fusion Device, Open Approach, New Technology Group 2
XRGBØF3 Fusion of Lumbar Vertebral Joint using Radiolucent Porous Interbody Fusion Device, Open Approach, New Technology Group 3
XRGCØ92 Fusion of 2 or more Lumbar Vertebral Joints using Nanotextured Surface Interbody Fusion Device, Open Approach, New Technology Group 2
XRGCØF3 Fusion of 2 or more Lumbar Vertebral Joints using Radiolucent Porous Interbody Fusion Device, Open Approach, New Technology Group 3
XRGDØ92 Fusion of Lumbosacral Joint using Nanotextured Surface Interbody Fusion Device, Open Approach, New Technology Group 2
XRGDØF3 Fusion of Lumbosacral Joint using Radiolucent Porous Interbody Fusion Device, Open Approach, New Technology Group 3

HAC 13: Surgical Site Infection (SSI) Following Cardiac Implantable Electronic Device (CIED) Procedures

Secondary diagnosis not POA:

K68.11
T81.4ØXA
T81.41XA
T81.42XA
T81.43XA
T81.44XA
T81.49XA
T82.6XXA
T82.7XXA

AND

Any of the following procedures:

Ø2H43JZ Insertion of Pacemaker Lead into Coronary Vein, Percutaneous Approach
Ø2H43KZ Insertion of Defibrillator Lead into Coronary Vein, Percutaneous Approach
Ø2H43MZ Insertion of Cardiac Lead into Coronary Vein, Percutaneous Approach
Ø2H63JZ Insertion of Pacemaker Lead into Right Atrium, Percutaneous Approach
Ø2H63MZ Insertion of Cardiac Lead into Right Atrium, Percutaneous Approach
Ø2H73JZ Insertion of Pacemaker Lead into Left Atrium, Percutaneous Approach
Ø2H73MZ Insertion of Cardiac Lead into Left Atrium, Percutaneous Approach
Ø2HK3JZ Insertion of Pacemaker Lead into Right Ventricle, Percutaneous Approach
Ø2HL3JZ Insertion of Pacemaker Lead into Left Ventricle, Percutaneous Approach
Ø2HNØJZ Insertion of Pacemaker Lead into Pericardium, Open Approach
Ø2HNØMZ Insertion of Cardiac Lead into Pericardium, Open Approach
Ø2HN3JZ Insertion of Pacemaker Lead into Pericardium, Percutaneous Approach
Ø2HN3MZ Insertion of Cardiac Lead into Pericardium, Percutaneous Approach
Ø2HN4JZ Insertion of Pacemaker Lead into Pericardium, Percutaneous Endoscopic Approach
Ø2HN4MZ Insertion of Cardiac Lead into Pericardium, Percutaneous Endoscopic Approach
Ø2PAØMZ Removal of Cardiac Lead from Heart, Open Approach
Ø2PA3MZ Removal of Cardiac Lead from Heart, Percutaneous Approach
Ø2PA4MZ Removal of Cardiac Lead from Heart, Percutaneous Endoscopic Approach
Ø2PAXMZ Removal of Cardiac Lead from Heart, External Approach
Ø2WAØMZ Revision of Cardiac Lead in Heart, Open Approach
Ø2WA3MZ Revision of Cardiac Lead in Heart, Percutaneous Approach
Ø2WA4MZ Revision of Cardiac Lead in Heart, Percutaneous Endoscopic Approach
ØJH6Ø4Z Insertion of Pacemaker, Single Chamber into Chest Subcutaneous Tissue and Fascia, Open Approach
ØJH6Ø5Z Insertion of Pacemaker, Single Chamber Rate Responsive into Chest Subcutaneous Tissue and Fascia, Open Approach
ØJH6Ø6Z Insertion of Pacemaker, Dual Chamber into Chest Subcutaneous Tissue and Fascia, Open Approach
ØJH6Ø7Z Insertion of Cardiac Resynchronization Pacemaker Pulse Generator into Chest Subcutaneous Tissue and Fascia, Open Approach
ØJH6Ø8Z Insertion of Defibrillator Generator into Chest Subcutaneous Tissue and Fascia, Open Approach
ØJH6Ø9Z Insertion of Cardiac Resynchronization Defibrillator Pulse Generator into Chest Subcutaneous Tissue and Fascia, Open Approach
ØJH6ØPZ Insertion of Cardiac Rhythm Related Device into Chest Subcutaneous Tissue and Fascia, Open Approach
ØJH634Z Insertion of Pacemaker, Single Chamber into Chest Subcutaneous Tissue and Fascia, Percutaneous Approach
ØJH635Z Insertion of Pacemaker, Single Chamber Rate Responsive into Chest Subcutaneous Tissue and Fascia, Percutaneous Approach
ØJH636Z Insertion of Pacemaker, Dual Chamber into Chest Subcutaneous Tissue and Fascia, Percutaneous Approach
ØJH637Z Insertion of Cardiac Resynchronization Pacemaker Pulse Generator into Chest Subcutaneous Tissue and Fascia, Percutaneous Approach
ØJH638Z Insertion of Defibrillator Generator into Chest Subcutaneous Tissue and Fascia, Percutaneous Approach
ØJH639Z Insertion of Cardiac Resynchronization Defibrillator Pulse Generator into Chest Subcutaneous Tissue and Fascia, Percutaneous Approach
ØJH63PZ Insertion of Cardiac Rhythm Related Device into Chest Subcutaneous Tissue and Fascia, Percutaneous Approach
ØJH8Ø4Z Insertion of Pacemaker, Single Chamber into Abdomen Subcutaneous Tissue and Fascia, Open Approach
ØJH8Ø5Z Insertion of Pacemaker, Single Chamber Rate Responsive into Abdomen Subcutaneous Tissue and Fascia, Open Approach
ØJH8Ø6Z Insertion of Pacemaker, Dual Chamber into Abdomen Subcutaneous Tissue and Fascia, Open Approach
ØJH8Ø7Z Insertion of Cardiac Resynchronization Pacemaker Pulse Generator into Abdomen Subcutaneous Tissue and Fascia, Open Approach
ØJH8Ø8Z Insertion of Defibrillator Generator into Abdomen Subcutaneous Tissue and Fascia, Open Approach
ØJH8Ø9Z Insertion of Cardiac Resynchronization Defibrillator Pulse Generator into Abdomen Subcutaneous Tissue and Fascia, Open Approach
ØJH8ØPZ Insertion of Cardiac Rhythm Related Device into Abdomen Subcutaneous Tissue and Fascia, Open Approach
ØJH834Z Insertion of Pacemaker, Single Chamber into Abdomen Subcutaneous Tissue and Fascia, Percutaneous Approach
ØJH835Z Insertion of Pacemaker, Single Chamber Rate Responsive into Abdomen Subcutaneous Tissue and Fascia, Percutaneous Approach
ØJH836Z Insertion of Pacemaker, Dual Chamber into Abdomen Subcutaneous Tissue and Fascia, Percutaneous Approach
ØJH837Z Insertion of Cardiac Resynchronization Pacemaker Pulse Generator into Abdomen Subcutaneous Tissue and Fascia, Percutaneous Approach
ØJH838Z Insertion of Defibrillator Generator into Abdomen Subcutaneous Tissue and Fascia, Percutaneous Approach
ØJH839Z Insertion of Cardiac Resynchronization Defibrillator Pulse Generator into Abdomen Subcutaneous Tissue and Fascia, Percutaneous Approach
ØJH83PZ Insertion of Cardiac Rhythm Related Device into Abdomen Subcutaneous Tissue and Fascia, Percutaneous Approach
ØJPTØFZ Removal of Subcutaneous Defibrillator Lead from Trunk Subcutaneous Tissue and Fascia, Open Approach
ØJPTØPZ Removal of Cardiac Rhythm Related Device from Trunk Subcutaneous Tissue and Fascia, Open Approach
ØJPT3FZ Removal of Subcutaneous Defibrillator Lead from Trunk Subcutaneous Tissue and Fascia, Percutaneous Approach
ØJPT3PZ Removal of Cardiac Rhythm Related Device from Trunk Subcutaneous Tissue and Fascia, Percutaneous Approach
ØJWTØFZ Revision of Subcutaneous Defibrillator Lead in Trunk Subcutaneous Tissue and Fascia, Open Approach
ØJWTØPZ Revision of Cardiac Rhythm Related Device in Trunk Subcutaneous Tissue and Fascia, Open Approach
ØJWT3FZ Revision of Subcutaneous Defibrillator Lead in Trunk Subcutaneous Tissue and Fascia, Percutaneous Approach
ØJWT3PZ Revision of Cardiac Rhythm Related Device in Trunk Subcutaneous Tissue and Fascia, Percutaneous Approach

HAC 14: Iatrogenic Pneumothorax with Venous Catheterization

Secondary diagnosis not POA:

J95.811

AND

Any of the following procedures:

Ø2H633Z Insertion of Infusion Device into Right Atrium, Percutaneous Approach
Ø2HK33Z Insertion of Infusion Device into Right Ventricle, Percutaneous Approach
Ø2HS33Z Insertion of Infusion Device into Right Pulmonary Vein, Percutaneous Approach
Ø2HS43Z Insertion of Infusion Device into Right Pulmonary Vein, Percutaneous Endoscopic Approach
Ø2HT33Z Insertion of Infusion Device into Left Pulmonary Vein, Percutaneous Approach
Ø2HT43Z Insertion of Infusion Device into Left Pulmonary Vein, Percutaneous Endoscopic Approach
Ø2HV33Z Insertion of Infusion Device into Superior Vena Cava, Percutaneous Approach
Ø2HV43Z Insertion of Infusion Device into Superior Vena Cava, Percutaneous Endoscopic Approach
Ø5HØ33Z Insertion of Infusion Device into Azygos Vein, Percutaneous Approach
Ø5HØ43Z Insertion of Infusion Device into Azygos Vein, Percutaneous Endoscopic Approach
Ø5H133Z Insertion of Infusion Device into Hemiazygos Vein, Percutaneous Approach
Ø5H143Z Insertion of Infusion Device into Hemiazygos Vein, Percutaneous Endoscopic Approach
Ø5H333Z Insertion of Infusion Device into Right Innominate Vein, Percutaneous Approach
Ø5H343Z Insertion of Infusion Device into Right Innominate Vein, Percutaneous Endoscopic Approach
Ø5H433Z Insertion of Infusion Device into Left Innominate Vein, Percutaneous Approach
Ø5H443Z Insertion of Infusion Device into Left Innominate Vein, Percutaneous Endoscopic Approach
Ø5H533Z Insertion of Infusion Device into Right Subclavian Vein, Percutaneous Approach
Ø5H543Z Insertion of Infusion Device into Right Subclavian Vein, Percutaneous Endoscopic Approach
Ø5H633Z Insertion of Infusion Device into Left Subclavian Vein, Percutaneous Approach
Ø5H643Z Insertion of Infusion Device into Left Subclavian Vein, Percutaneous Endoscopic Approach
Ø5HM33Z Insertion of Infusion Device into Right Internal Jugular Vein, Percutaneous Approach
Ø5HN33Z Insertion of Infusion Device into Left Internal Jugular Vein, Percutaneous Approach
Ø5HP33Z Insertion of Infusion Device into Right External Jugular Vein, Percutaneous Approach
Ø5HQ33Z Insertion of Infusion Device into Left External Jugular Vein, Percutaneous Approach
ØJH63XZ Insertion of Vascular Access Device into Chest Subcutaneous Tissue and Fascia, Percutaneous Approach

Appendix H: Centers for Medicare & Medicaid Services Hierarchical Condition Categories (CMS-HCC)

In the 1970s, Medicare began demonstration projects that contracted with health maintenance organizations (HMOs) to provide care for Medicare beneficiaries in exchange for prospective payments. In 1985, this project changed from demonstration status to a regular part of the Medicare program, Medicare Part C. The Balanced Budget Act (BBA) of 1997 named Medicare's Part C managed care program Medicare+Choice, and the Medicare Modernization Act (MMA) of 2003 again renamed it to Medicare Advantage (MA).

Medicare is one of the world's largest health insurance programs, and about one-third of the beneficiaries on Medicare are enrolled in a MA private health care plan. Due to the great variance in the health status of Medicare beneficiaries, risk adjustment provides a means of adequately compensating those plans with large numbers of seriously ill patients while not overburdening other plans that have healthier individuals. Medicare Advantage (MA) plans have been using the Hierarchical Condition Category (HCC) risk adjustment model since 2004.

The Risk Adjustment Model

The primary purpose of a risk adjustment model is to predict (on average) the future health care costs for specific consortiums enrolled in Medicare Advantage (MA) health plans. CMS is then able to provide capitation payments to these private health plans. Capitation payments are an incentive for health plans to enroll not only healthier individuals but those with chronic conditions or who are more seriously ill by removing some of the financial burden.

The MA risk adjustment model uses HCCs to assess the disease burden of its enrollees. HCC diagnostic groupings were created after examining claims data so that enrollees with similar disease processes, and consequently similar health care expenditures, could be pooled into a larger data set in which an average expenditure rate could be determined. The medical conditions included in HCC categories are those that were determined to most predictably affect the health status and health care costs of any individual. Several important principles to the risk adjustment model and the development of the HCC categories include but are not limited to:

1. The HCC diagnostic categories should be clinically meaningful.
   - Diagnostic categories are well-defined.
   - Clinically specific diseases or medical conditions are grouped to each category.
2. The HCC diagnostic categories should predict medical expenditures.
   - The diagnoses grouped to a specific category should have as close to the same cost burden not only in the current year but also in the future.
3. The HCC diagnostic categories should have adequate sample sizes and discretionary categories excluded to be as accurate and stable in their estimate of costs as possible.
   - A diagnostic category that groups extremely rare diseases or conditions would not be reliably effective in determining current or future costs.
   - Codes that are not credible as cost predictors or may be subject to coding variation should be excluded, when possible.
4. The HCC diagnostic categories should be both hierarchical and additive.
   - Hierarchical measurement is used within a specific disease process.
   - Disease processes that are unrelated to each other are measured additively.
5. The diagnostic classification should encourage specificity and should not reward coding proliferation.
   - More diagnosis codes and vague diagnosis codes do not equal greater disease burden.

More than 10,000 ICD-10-CM diagnosis codes map to 86 HCCs in the current risk adjustment model. Diagnoses are excluded from mapping when they do not predict future cost or are vague or variable in diagnosis, coding, or treatment, such as symptoms or osteoarthritis. Also excluded are diagnosis codes from laboratories, radiology, and home health claims.

Risk Adjustment Factors

The CMS-HCC risk adjustment model uses "risk adjustment factors" to calculate a risk score for each member. This score summarizes that particular patient's expected cost of care relative to other members'. Each member's risk score is based on demographic and health status information and is calculated as the sum of these demographic and health factors weighted by their estimated marginal contributions to total risk. The model also takes into account where the patient resides (community or institutional), Medicaid eligibility (full or partial benefits), the patient's Medicare enrollment status (new or established), age, disability status, whether the patient is frail or has end-stage renal disease (ESRD), and even prescription drug use.

No procedure codes, ICD-10-PCS or CPT, are included in the MA risk adjustment model. The model relies solely on diagnostic and demographic data. Not all ICD-10-CM diagnoses map to an HCC, and there is no specific code sequencing involved. The CMS-HCC model is additive as well as hierarchical. The additive functionality allows a patient to have more than one HCC category assigned, providing a more complete clinical picture and prediction of resource consumption. The hierarchical aspect of the model provides a means of ranking diagnoses that are similar in disease process, by severity. The hierarchy of the condition categories ensures the patient's conditions are classified to the most severe condition within the related group. Less severe conditions within a particular hierarchy are superseded by more severe diagnoses within the same group. The hierarchy and additive relationship permits this model to characterize the person's illness level within each disease process, while still allowing the effects of unrelated disease processes to be counted in the patient's overall score.

Certain combinations of coexisting diagnoses for an individual can increase medical costs. The CMS-HCC model adjusts for these higher costs by the addition of "disease interaction" factors. For each patient, multiple HCCs assigned, along with demographic and disease interaction factors, are used to calculate a single, combined risk adjustment factor (RAF). The RAF score for an individual member represents all of the HCCs that have been submitted from all sources for that member to CMS during the course of an entire calendar year.

There are separate CMS-HCC models for new enrollees and continuing enrollees. The new enrollee model uses demographic factors only, such as age, sex, and disability status, and is used when the enrollee has less than 12 months of medical history. The community model accounts for age, sex, original reason for Medicare entitlement (age or disability), Medicaid eligibility, and clinical conditions as measured by HCCs. In the second step, expected costs are adjusted for outliers based on the member's risk score and whether the patient has ESRD.

Demographic data (age, sex, eligibility) as well as health status (diagnoses codes submitted on claims to CMS) of an MA population are used to determine the reimbursement to the health plan to care for their members.

CMS considers a RAF score of 1.0 as the benchmark to indicate the score of the average healthy patient with the same demographic and diagnostic factors. These patients are expected to use average or lower-than-average resources. When the RAF score is higher than 1.0, CMS considers the patient to be sicker than the average patient with the same criteria and expects greater-than-average resource utilization.

A low RAF score may accurately indicate a healthier patient, but it may also falsely indicate a healthier patient due to incomplete or inaccurate coding, incomplete or insufficient record documentation, or patients who fail to complete an annual assessment.

A high RAF score may accurately indicate a sicker patient, or it may be falsely inflated from overcoding due to diagnoses that are reported but not documented, or from copying and pasting from previous encounters or problem lists of resolved conditions.

Documentation Requirements

Payment is made per HCC category (not per diagnosis code). No matter how many times in the year the diagnosis codes are reported, a single payment is made to the MA plan each year. Each year the list of HCCs and the RAF for each patient is "reset." This means the annual health assessment is extremely important, and adequate documentation is critical. Accurate risk adjustment payment relies on complete medical record documentation and diagnosis coding. CMS requires that all applicable diagnosis codes be reported and that all diagnoses be reported to the highest level of specificity and that these be substantiated by the medical record.

> CMS's Guiding Principle:
>
> The risk adjustment diagnosis must be based on clinical medical record documentation from a face-to-face encounter, coded according to the *ICD-10-CM Guidelines for Coding and Reporting*; assigned based on dates of service within the data collection period, submitted to the MA

organization from an appropriate risk adjustment provider type and an appropriate risk adjustment physician data source.

A "face-to-face" health service encounter between a patient and healthcare provider describes an encounter between the patient and the provider (MD, DO), including qualified nonphysician practitioners (NPP) (e.g. nurse practitioner or physician's assistant), which is face-to-face with the patient. CMS provides a current listing of acceptable physician specialty types for risk adjustment data submission within the 2012 Regional Technical Assistance Participant Guide. The only exception to the face-to-face encounter requirement is pathology services (professional component only). Currently, CMS does not provide a listing of all services that are considered face-to-face visits for risk adjustment data, but does provide guidance on what types of services are not acceptable for risk adjustment in the Participant Guide. For example, diagnostic radiology does not qualify because diagnostic radiologists typically do not document confirmed diagnoses. Other examples of services that are not acceptable include diagnostic reports that have not been interpreted, such as laboratory reports.

It is essential that the medical record documentation show evidence by provider authentication that the direct face-to-face service was personally furnished by the physician or qualified NPP. Examples of these services include office visits, hospital visits, preoperative anesthesia assessment, and surgical and invasive procedures.

Risk adjustment relies on annual health information. Each enrollee is assigned an individual risk score based on the health status information obtained from the diagnosis codes on the claims. The CMS-HCC model relies on ICD-10-CM coding specificity for accurate risk adjustment by using the most specific code available that is substantiated by the documentation in the medical record. Providers should fully document and accurately code the evaluation and management of all severe and chronic conditions to ensure a full, complete, and accurate clinical record of the patient's condition and reflect the work involved in caring for the patient, particularly those with complex and challenging health issues. All conditions affecting the treatment or management of the patient's health should be documented at least once a year, as applicable to care provided, to accurately describe the true complexity and severity of the patient's health. If the diagnosis coding on the claim is not accurate or complete, the claim may indicate that the provider did much less medical decision-making, evaluation, and management than was actually performed.

Documentation to support or validate risk adjustment conditions may be found anywhere in the note for the face-to-face encounter. It is important to ensure that the note accurately reflects all chronic conditions that affect the health and care of the patient. Each encounter must be unique and reflect only that visit as it occurred. Insufficient documentation influences the assignment of diagnosis codes and directly affects the patient's risk score.

Documentation should properly validate all reported conditions. Each page of progress notes should be properly authenticated and include the patient's name and the date.

Providers should document each clinical diagnosis to the highest degree of specificity per encounter, including all complications and/or manifestations, including clear links to causal conditions. Only confirmed conditions should be documented—no rule-out conditions or abnormal findings without clinical significance. All known conditions, including chronic conditions, that affect the care and treatment of the patient at least once per year should be noted.

Providers should specifically document the condition and clinical significance, and any pertinent changes, using terminology such as decreased, increased, worsening, improving, or unchanged, or abnormal findings.

Documentation Tips

- Document all cause-and-effect relationships.
- Report the most specific diagnosis code available that is supported by the documentation.
- Include all current diagnoses as part of the current medical decision-making, and document for every visit.
- Identify diagnoses that are current or chronic problems rather than a past medical history or previous resolved condition.
- Document history of heart attack, status codes, etc., that affect the patient's care as "history of" or "PMH" when they no longer exist or are not current conditions.
- Ensure each progress note has the date, signature, and credentials/specialty.
- Document the thought processes used to assess each condition.
- Know high revenue HCCs that are often undiagnosed or undercoded.
- Avoid "unspecified" codes.
- Ensure the codes reported are accurate.
- Ensure each encounter is billed.
- Review rejection reports, and audit reports to assess risks.

Audits

Because reimbursement is by patient, rather than based on an average of the entire population, and is based upon documentation, there is the potential for upcoding. Audits are conducted by the MA plan and CMS recovery auditors.

Initial Validation Audit (IVA)

CMS requires that the MA plan validate HCCs. This is usually performed by an independent auditor working with the plan or a contracted vendor to validate the MA plan's data submitted to CMS.

The MA plan submits the one best medical record that supports each HCC identified for the beneficiary.

Risk Adjustment Data Validation Audit

Risk adjustment data validation (RADV) audits were introduced in 2011 and updated for 2015. They are performed by CMS to validate the integrity and accuracy of risk-adjusted payments by verifying that the diagnosis codes the MA plans submit are supported by the medical record documentation for a member

MA plans can be selected by CMS for RADV audits annually and if chosen are required to submit their members' medical records to CMS. Providers are required to assist the MA plan by providing the medical record documentation included in the audit. Even though each diagnosis needs to be reported only once in a calendar year, during a RADV audit up to five dates of service may be submitted to support any one HCC.

To be validated, medical record documentation must meet certain criteria and standards. Even if the diagnosis is documented and coded correctly, any deficiency in the documentation can make the encounter and the HCC invalid. Diagnoses that cannot be validated are considered payment errors. The results of the audit are communicated to the MA plan, which then communicates these results to the provider. Under- and overpayments are subject to payment adjustment. The results of RADV audits can be extrapolated over the MA plan population to calculate potential payment errors and overpayments/recoupments. Regulations include a RADV appeal process, a document dispute process, and a procedure for obtaining physician-signature attestations.

The following items are reviewed during the validation process:

- The record is for the correct enrollee.
- The record is from the correct calendar year for the payment year being audited.
- The record is legible.
- The date of service is present on the records and is for a face-to-face visit.
- The record is from a valid provider type.
- Valid credentials and/or a valid physician specialty are documented on the record.
- The record contains a signature from an acceptable type of physician.
- There is a diagnosis on the record.
- The diagnosis supports an HCC.
- The diagnosis supports the submitted HCC.

Mitigate audit risk by coding each reportable diagnosis each time it meets reporting guidelines. Audit regularly to assess areas of risk and in need of improvement and to capture conditions documented but not coded. Check for additional qualifying HCCs. Ensure claims are submitted and that corrected claims are submitted when indicated. There are three claims submission deadlines: January, March, and September. CMS adjusts each member's risk score twice a year, with the final reconciliation in August of the year after the plan year.

If providers emphasize correct coding and documentation and perform internal audits to determine where the risks are and prepare for audits, incorrect payment is less likely.

For additional information on risk adjustment coding, see Optum360's *Risk Adjustment Coding and HCC Guide*.

Appendix I: Long-term Care Hospital Prospective Payment System Overview

Information in this appendix is based on the Centers for Medicare and Medicaid Services (CMS) FY 2021 long-term care hospital prospective payment system (LTCH PPS) proposed rule published in the *Federal Register,* volume 85, number 104, May 29, 2020 ("Hospital Inpatient Prospective Payment Systems for Acute Care Hospitals and the Long-Term Care Hospital Prospective Payment System and Proposed Policy Changes and Fiscal Year 2021 Rates").

Classification As a Long-term Care Hospital

Under the regulations at § 412.23(e)(1), to qualify to be paid under the long-term care hospital prospective payment system (LTCH PPS), a hospital must have a provider agreement with Medicare. Furthermore, § 412.23(e)(2)(i), which implements section 1886(d)(1)(B)(iv) of the Social Security Act, requires that a hospital have an average Medicare inpatient length of stay of greater than 25 days to be paid under the LTCH PPS. In accordance with section 1206(a)(3) of the Pathway for SGR Reform Act of 2013 (Pub. L. 113–67), as amended by section 15007 of Public Law 114–255, CMS amended the regulations to specify that Medicare Advantage plans' and site-neutral payment rate discharges are excluded from the calculation of the average length of stay for all LTCHs, for discharges occurring in cost reporting period beginning on or after October 1, 2015.

The following hospitals are paid under special payment provisions, as described in § 412.22(c) and, therefore, are not subject to the LTCH PPS rules:

- Veterans Administration hospitals
- Hospitals that are reimbursed under state cost control systems approved under 42 CFR part 403
- Hospitals that are reimbursed in accordance with demonstration projects authorized under section 402(a) of the Social Security Amendments of 1967 (Pub. L. 90-248) (42 U.S.C. 1395b-1), section 222(a) of the Social Security Amendments of 1972 (Pub. L. 92-603) (42 U.S.C. 1395b-1 (note)) (statewide all-payer systems, subject to the rate-of-increase test at section 1814(b) of the Act), or section 3201 of the Patient Protection and Affordable Care Act (Pub. L. 111-148 (42 U.S.C. 1315a))
- Nonparticipating hospitals furnishing emergency services to Medicare beneficiaries

Proposed Medicare Severity Long-Term Care Diagnosis-Related Group Classification and Relative Weights for FY 2021

Background

Section 123 of the BBRA required that the secretary of the Department of Health and Human Services implement a PPS for LTCHs to replace the cost-based payment system under TEFRA. Section 307(b)(1) of the BIPA modified the requirements of section 123 of the BBRA by requiring that the HHS secretary examine the feasibility and impact of basing payment under the LTCH PPS on the use of existing (or refined) hospital DRGs that have been modified to account for different resource use of LTCH patients.

When the LTCH PPS was implemented for cost reporting periods beginning on or after October 1, 2002, CMS adopted the same DRG patient classification system used at that time under the IPPS. As a component of the LTCH PPS, CMS referred to this patient classification system as the "long-term care diagnosis-related groups (LTC-DRGs)." Although the patient classification system used under both the LTCH PPS and the IPPS are the same, the relative weights are different. The established relative weight methodology and data used under the LTCH PPS result in relative weights under the LTCH PPS that reflect the differences in patient resource use of LTCH patients, consistent with section 123(a)(1) of the BBRA (Pub. L. 106-113).

As part of CMS' efforts to better recognize severity of illness among patients, in the FY 2008 IPPS final rule with comment period (72 FR 47130), the MS-DRGs and the Medicare severity LTC-DRGs (MS-LTC-DRGs) were adopted under the IPPS and the LTCH PPS, respectively, effective beginning October 1, 2007 (FY 2008). (CMS noted, in that same final rule, that it revised the regulations at § 412.503 to specify that for LTCH discharges occurring on or after October 1, 2007, when applying the provisions of 42 CFR part 412, subpart O, applicable to LTCHs for policy descriptions and payment calculations, all references to LTC-DRGs would be considered a reference to MS-LTC-DRGs.

The MS-DRG classifications are updated annually. There are currently 761 MS-DRG groupings. For FY 2021, there would be 767 MS-DRG groupings based on the proposed changes. Consistent with section 123 of the BBRA, as amended by section 307(b)(1) of the BIPA, and § 412.515 of the regulations, CMS used information derived from LTCH PPS patient records to classify LTCH discharges into distinct MS-LTC-DRGs based on clinical characteristics and estimated resource needs. Then CMS assigned an appropriate weight to the MS-LTC-DRGs to account for the difference in resource use by patients exhibiting the case complexity and multiple medical problems characteristic of LTCHs.

For FY 2021, CMS is proposing to continue to use existing methodology to determine the MS-LTC-DRG relative weights. As previously established when CMS implemented the dual-rate LTCH PPS payment structure codified under § 412.522, which began in FY 2016, CMS is proposing that the annual recalibration of the MS-LTC-DRG relative weights be determined: (1) using only data from available LTCH PPS claims that (1) would have qualified for payment under the new LTCH PPS standard federal payment rate if that rate had been in effect at the time of discharge when claims data from time periods before the dual-rate LTCH PPS payment structure applies are used to calculate the relative weights; and (2) qualify for payment under the new LTCH PPS standard federal payment rate when claims data from time periods after the dual-rate LTCH PPS payment structure applies are used to calculate the relative weights (80 FR 49624). That is, under the current methodology, MS-LTC-DRG relative weight calculations do not use data from cases paid at the site-neutral payment rate under § 412.522(c)(1) or data from cases that would have been paid at the site-neutral payment rate if the dual-rate LTCH PPS payment structure had been in effect at the time of that discharge. In addition, for FY 2021, CMS is proposing to continue to exclude the data from all-inclusive rate providers and LTCHs paid in accordance with demonstration projects, as well as any Medicare Advantage claims from the MS-LTC-DRG relative weight calculations.

Furthermore, for FY 2021, in using data from applicable LTCH cases to establish MS-LTC-DRG relative weights, CMS is proposing to continue to establish low-volume MS-LTC-DRGs (that is, MS-LTC-DRGs with less than 25 cases) using existing quintile methodology in determining the MS-LTC-DRG relative weights because LTCHs do not typically treat the full range of diagnoses as do acute care hospitals. Therefore, for purposes of determining the relative weights for the large number of low-volume MS-LTC-DRGs, CMS grouped all of the low-volume MS-LTC-DRGs into five quintiles based on average charges per discharge. Then, under the existing methodology, CMS accounted for adjustments made to LTCH PPS standard federal payments for short-stay outlier (SSO) cases (that is, cases for which the covered length of stay at the LTCH is less than or equal to five-sixths of the geometric average length of stay for the MS-LTC-DRG), and adjustments made to account for nonmonotonically increasing weights, when necessary. The methodology is premised on more severe cases under the MS-LTC-DRG system requiring greater expenditure of medical care resources and higher average charges such that, in the severity levels within a base MS-LTC-DRG, the relative weights should increase monotonically with severity from the lowest to highest severity level.

Patient Classifications into MS-LTC-DRGs

The MS-DRGs (used under the IPPS) and the MS-LTC-DRGs (used under the LTCH PPS) are based on the CMS DRG structure. As noted previously in this section, CMS refers to the DRGs under the LTCH PPS as MS-LTC-DRGs although they are structurally identical to the MS-DRGs used under the IPPS. The MS-DRGs are organized into 25 major diagnostic categories (MDCs), most of which are based on a particular organ system of the body; the remainder involve multiple organ systems (such as MDC 22 Burns). Within most MDCs, cases are then divided into surgical DRGs and medical DRGs. Surgical DRGs are assigned based on a surgical hierarchy that orders operating room (O.R.) procedures or groups of O.R. procedures by resource intensity. The GROUPER software program does not recognize all ICD-10-PCS procedure codes as procedures affecting DRG assignment. That is, procedures that are not surgical (for example, EKGs), or minor surgical procedures (for example, a biopsy of skin and subcutaneous tissue (procedure code 0JBH3ZX)) do not affect the MS-LTC-DRG assignment based on their presence on the claim.

Generally, under the LTCH PPS, a Medicare payment is made at a predetermined specific rate for each discharge that varies based on the MS-LTC-DRG to which a beneficiary's discharge is assigned. Cases are classified into MS-LTC-DRGs for payment based on the following six data elements:

- Principal diagnosis
- Additional or secondary diagnoses
- Surgical procedures

- Age
- Sex
- Discharge status of the patient

The Health Information Portability and Accountability Act (HIPAA) requires covered entities to use the applicable medical data code set requirements when conducting HIPAA transactions (45 CFR 162.1000). Currently, upon the discharge of the patient, the LTCH must assign appropriate diagnosis and procedure codes from the most current version of ICD-10-CM for diagnosis coding and ICD-10-PCS for inpatient hospital procedure coding, both of which were required to be implemented October 1, 2015 (45 CFR 162.1002(c)(2) and (3)).

To create the MS-DRGs (and by extension, the MS-LTC-DRGs), base DRGs were subdivided according to the presence of specific secondary diagnoses designated as complications or comorbidities (CCs) into one, two, or three levels of severity, depending on the impact of the CCs on resources used for those cases. Specifically, there are sets of MS-DRGs that are split into two or three subgroups based on the presence or absence of a CC or a major complication or comorbidity (MCC).

Medicare administrative contractors (MAC) enter the clinical and demographic information submitted by LTCHs into their claims processing systems and subject this information to a series of automated screening processes called the Medicare Code Editor (MCE). These screens are designed to identify cases that require further review before being assigned into a MS-LTC-DRG. During this process, certain cases are selected for further explanation (74 FR 43949).

After screening through the MCE, each claim is classified into the appropriate MS-LTC-DRG by the Medicare LTCH Grouper software on the basis of diagnosis and procedure codes and other demographic information (age, sex, and discharge status). The Grouper software used under the LTCH PPS is the same software program used under the IPPS. Following the MS-LTC-DRG assignment, the MAC determines the prospective payment amount by using the Medicare Pricer program, which accounts for hospital-specific adjustments. Under the LTCH PPS, CMS provided an opportunity for LTCHs to review the MS-LTC-DRG assignments made by the MAC and to submit additional information within a specified timeframe as provided in § 412.513(c).

The Grouper software is used both to classify past cases to measure relative hospital resource consumption to establish the MS-LTC-DRG relative weights and to classify current cases for purposes of determining payment. The records for all Medicare hospital inpatient discharges are maintained in the MedPAR file. The data in this file are used to evaluate possible MS-DRG and MS-LTC-DRG classification changes and to recalibrate the MS-DRG and MS-LTC-DRG relative weights during the annual update under both the IPPS (§ 412.60(e)) and the LTCH PPS (§ 412.517), respectively.

Proposed Changes to the MS-LTC-DRGs for FY 2021

As specified by § 412.517(a), which require that the MS-LTC-DRG classifications and relative weights be updated annually, and consistent with our historical practice of using the same patient classification system under the LTCH PPS as is used under the IPPS, in FY 2021 proposed rule, CMS is proposing to update the MS-LTC-DRG classifications effective October 1, 2020 through September 30, 2021 (FY 2021), consistent with the proposed changes to specific MS-DRG classifications.

Accordingly, the proposed MS-LTC-DRGs for FY 2021 will be the same as the MS-DRGs that are being used under the IPPS for FY 2021. In addition, because the proposed MS-LTC-DRGs for FY 2021 are the same as the proposed MS-DRGs for FY 2021, the other proposed changes that affect MS-DRG (and by extension MS-LTC-DRG) assignments under proposed GROUPER Version 38, including the proposed changes to the MCE software and the ICD-10-CM/PCS coding system, also are applicable under the LTCH PPS for FY 2021.

Development of the Proposed MS-LTC-DRG Relative Weights for FY 2021

CMS is proposing to continue to use current methodology to determine the MS-LTC-DRG relative weights for FY 2021, including the continued application of established policies related to the hospital-specific relative value methodology, the treatment of severity levels in the MS-LTC-DRGs, low-volume and no-volume MS-LTC-DRGs, adjustments for nonmonotonicity, the steps for calculating the MS-LTC-DRG relative weights with a budget neutrality factor, and only using data from applicable LTCH cases (which includes the policy of using only cases that would meet the criteria for exclusion from the site-neutral payment rate [or, for discharges occurring prior to the implementation of the dual-rate LTCH PPS payment structure, would have met the criteria for exclusion had those criteria been in effect at the time of the discharge]).

Data

For FY 2021 IPPS/LTCH PPS proposed rule, consistent with proposals regarding the calculation of the proposed MS-LTC-DRG relative weights for FY 2021, CMS obtained total charges from FY 2019 Medicare LTCH claims data from the December 2019 update of the FY 2019 MedPAR file, which are the best available data at this time, and is proposing to use version 38 of the Grouper to classify LTCH cases. Consistent with historical practice, CMS is proposing that if more recent data become available, that data would be used, with the finalized version 38 of the Grouper, in establishing the FY 2021 MS-LTC-DRG relative weights in the final rule.

To calculate the proposed FY 2021 MS-LTC-DRG relative weights under the dual-rate LTCH PPS payment structure, CMS is proposing to continue to use applicable LTCH data, which includes the policy of using only cases that meet the criteria for exclusion from the site-neutral payment rate (or would have met the criteria had they been in effect at the time of the discharge) (80 FR 49624). Specifically, CMS began by first evaluating the LTCH claims data in the December 2019 update of the FY 2019 MedPAR file to determine which LTCH cases would meet the criteria for exclusion from the site-neutral payment rate under § 412.522(b) or had the dual-rate LTCH PPS payment structure applied to those cases at the time of discharge. CMS identified the FY 2019 LTCH cases that were not assigned to MS-LTC-DRGs 876, 880, 881, 882, 883, 884, 885, 886, 887, 894, 895, 896, 897, 945, and 946, which identify LTCH cases that do not have a principal diagnosis relating to a psychiatric diagnosis or to rehabilitation and for which one of the following is true:

- The admission to the LTCH was "immediately preceded" by discharge from a subsection (d) hospital and the immediately preceding stay in that subsection (d) hospital included at least three days in an intensive care unit (ICU), as defined under the ICU criterion.
- The admission to the LTCH was "immediately preceded" by discharge from a subsection (d) hospital and the claim for the LTCH discharge includes the applicable procedure code that indicates at least 96 hours of ventilator services were provided during the LTCH stay, as defined under the ventilator criterion. Claims data from the FY 2019 MedPAR file that reported ICD-10-PCS procedure code 5A1955Z were used to identify cases involving at least 96 hours of ventilator services in accordance with the ventilator criterion. (CMS notes that, for purposes of developing the MS-LTC-DRG relative weights, it has previously addressed the treatment of cases that would have been excluded from the site-neutral payment rate under the statutory provisions that provided for temporary exception from the site-neutral payment rate under the LTCH PPS for certain spinal cord specialty hospitals or for certain severe wound care discharges from certain LTCHs provided by sections 15009 and 15010 of Pub. L. 114-255, respectively. This temporary exception from the site-neutral payment rate for certain spinal cord specialty hospitals is effective for discharges in cost reporting periods beginning during FYs 2018 and 2019, and the temporary exception from the site-neutral payment rate for certain severe wound care discharges from certain LTCHs was effective for a discharge in cost reporting period beginning during FY 2018. These statutory provisions will no longer be in effect for any discharges occurring in FY 2021 [that is, an LTCH with a cost reporting period that begins on the last day of FY 2019, on September 30, 2019, would end on September 29, 2020, the day before the start of FY 2021 on October 1, 2020]. Therefore, CMS says it no longer needs to address the treatment of these cases for purposes of developing the MS-LTC-DRG relative weights for FY 2021 and subsequent years.)

Furthermore, consistent with historical methodology, CMS excluded any claims in the resulting data set that were submitted by LTCHs that were all-inclusive rate providers and LTCHs that are paid in accordance with demonstration projects authorized under section 402(a) of Pub. L. 90-248 or section 222(a) of Pub. L. 92-603. In addition, consistent with historical practice and policies, CMS excluded any Medicare Advantage (Part C) claims in the resulting data. Such claims were identified based on the presence of a GHO Paid indicator value of "1" in the MedPAR files. The claims that remained after these three trims (that is, the applicable LTCH data) were then used to calculate the MS-LTC-DRG relative weights for FY 2021.

In summary, in general, CMS identified the claims data used in developing the proposed FY 2021 MS-LTC-DRG relative weights in this proposed rule, by trimming claims data that were paid the site-neutral payment rate or would have been paid the site-neutral payment rate had the dual-payment-rate structure been in effect. Finally, CMS proposes to trim the claims data of all-inclusive rate providers reported in the December 2019 update of the FY 2019 MedPAR file and any Medicare Advantage claims data. There were no data from any LTCHs that are paid in accordance with a demonstration project reported in the December 2019 update of the FY 2019 MedPAR file, but, had there been any, CMS would have trimmed the claims data from those LTCHs as well, in accordance with established policy. CMS is proposing to use the remaining data (that is, the applicable LTCH data) to calculate the relative weights for FY 2021.

Steps for Determining the Proposed FY 2021 MS-LTC-DRG Relative Weights

CMS is proposing to continue to use its current methodology to determine the proposed FY 2021 MS-LTC-DRG relative weights. To determine the proposed relative weights, CMS is proposing to group applicable LTCH cases to the appropriate proposed MS-LTC-DRG, while taking into account the proposed low-volume quintiles (as described previously) and cross-walked proposed no-volume MS-LTC-DRGs. After establishing the appropriate proposed MS-LTC-DRG (or proposed low-volume quintile), CMS is proposing to calculate the proposed FY 2021 relative weights in several steps.

Step 1 Remove cases with a length of stay of seven days or less and statistical outliers

Step 2 Remove statistical outliers

Step 3 Adjust charges for the effects of short-stay outliers (SSO)

Step 4 Calculate the proposed FY 2021 MS-LTC-DRG relative weights on an iterative basis.

Step 5 Determine a proposed FY 2021 relative weight for MS-LTC-DRGs with no applicable LTCH cases

Step 6 Adjust the proposed FY 2021 MS-LTC-DRG relative weights to account for nonmonotonically increasing relative weights

Step 7Calculate the proposed FY 2021 MS-LTC-DRG reclassification and recalibration budget neutrality factor

Accordingly, in determining the proposed FY 2021 MS-LTC-DRG relative weights in this proposed rule, consistent with existing methodology, the agency is proposing to apply a normalization factor of 1.25878 and a budget neutrality factor of 0.9993445. Table 11, which is available via the internet on the CMS website, lists the proposed MS-LTC-DRGs and their respective proposed relative weights, geometric mean length of stay, and five-sixths of the geometric mean length of stay (used to identify SSO cases under § 412.529(a)) for FY 2021.

Proposed Changes to the LTCH PPS Payment Rates and Other Changes to the LTCH PPS for FY 2021

Overview

The basic methodology for determining LTCH PPS standard federal payment rates is currently set forth at 42 CFR 412.515 through 412.533 and 412.535. In this section, CMS discusses the factors it is proposing to use to update the LTCH PPS standard federal payment rate for FY 2021, that is, effective for LTCH discharges occurring on or after October 1, 2020, through September 30, 2021. Under the dual-rate LTCH PPS payment structure required by statute, beginning with discharges in cost reporting periods beginning in FY 2016, only LTCH discharges that meet the criteria for exclusion from the site-neutral payment rate are paid based on the LTCH PPS standard federal payment rate specified at § 412.523.

Before the dual-payment-rate system was implemented in FY 2016, all LTCH discharges were paid similarly to those now exempt from the site-neutral payment rate. That legacy payment rate was called the standard federal rate.

In this FY 2021 IPPS/LTCH PPS proposed rule, CMS presents proposals related to the annual update to the LTCH PPS standard federal payment rate for FY 2021. It is also proposing to adjust the LTCH PPS standard federal payment rate to account for the estimated effect of the changes to the area wage level for FY 2021 on estimated aggregate LTCH PPS payments, in accordance with § 412.523(d)(4). In addition, as discussed in the FY 2019 IPPS/LTCH PPS final rule (83 FR 41532 through 41537), CMS has eliminated the 25 percent threshold policy in a budget-neutral manner. The budget neutrality requirements are codified in the regulations at § 412.523(d)(6). Under these regulations, a temporary, one-time factor is applied to the standard federal payment rate in FY 2019 and FY 2020, and a permanent, one-time factor in FY 2021. These factors as established in the correction to the FY 2019 IPPS/LTCH PPS final rule (83 FR 41536) area as follows:

- For FY 2019, a temporary, one-time factor of 0.990878
- For FY 2020, a temporary, one-time factor of 0.990737
- For FY 2021 and subsequent years, a permanent, one-time factor of 0.991249

Therefore, in determining the FY 2021 LTCH PPS standard federal payment rate, CMS is proposing to:

- Remove the temporary, one-time factor of 0.990737 for the estimated cost of elimination of the 25-percent threshold policy in FY 2020 by applying a factor of (1/0.990737)
- Apply a permanent, one-time factor of 0.991249 for the estimated cost of the elimination of the 25-percent threshold policy in FY 2021

Proposed Annual Update to the LTCH PPS Standard Federal Payment Rate for FY 2021

CMS has used an estimated market basket increase to update the LTCH PPS. As previously noted, for FY 2021 CMS is proposing to rebase and revise the 2013-based LTCH market basket to reflect a 2017 base year. The proposed 2017-based LTCH market basket is primarily based on the Medicare cost report data submitted by LTCHs and, therefore, specifically reflects the cost structures of only LTCHs. CMS is proposing to use data from cost reports beginning in FY 2017 because these data are the latest available complete data at the time of rulemaking for purposes of calculating cost weights for the market basket. CMS believes that the proposed 2017-based LTCH market basket appropriately reflects the cost structure of LTCHs. CMS is proposing to use the proposed 2017-based LTCH market basket to update the LTCH PPS standard federal payment rate for FY 2021.

Section 1886(m)(3)(A) of the Social Security Act provides that, beginning in FY 2010, any annual update to the LTCH PPS standard federal payment rate is reduced by the adjustments specified in clauses (i) and (ii) of subparagraph (A). Clause (i) of section 1886(m)(3)(A) of the act provides for a reduction, for FY 2012 and each subsequent rate year, by the productivity adjustment described in section 1886(b)(3)(B)(xi)(II) of the act (that is, "the multifactor productivity [MFP] adjustment"). Clause (ii) of section 1886(m)(3)(A) of the act provided for a reduction, for each of FYs 2010 through 2019, by the "other adjustment" described in section 1886(m)(4)(F) of the act; therefore, it is not applicable for FY 2021.

Section 1886(m)(3)(B) of the act provides that the application of paragraph (3) of section 1886(m) of the act may result in the annual update being less than zero for a rate year and may result in payment rates for a rate year being less than such payment rates for the preceding rate year.

Appendix J: Long-Term Care Hospital Quality Reporting Program

Information in this appendix is based on:

Centers for Medicare and Medicaid Services (CMS) FY 2021 long-term care hospital prospective payment system (LTCH PPS) proposed rule published in the *Federal Register,* volume 85, number 104, May 29, 2020 ("Hospital Inpatient Prospective Payment Systems for Acute Care Hospitals and the Long-Term Care Hospital Prospective Payment System and Proposed Policy Changes and Fiscal Year 2021 Rates").

LTCH Quality Reporting Program (QRP)

https://www.cms.gov/Medicare/Quality-Initiatives-Patient-Assessment-Instruments/LTCH-Quality-Reporting

Patient Protection and Affordable Care Act (ACA) of 2010, Section 3004(a)

https://www.gpo.gov/fdsys/pkg/PLAW-111publ148/pdf/PLAW-111publ148.pdf

Improving Medicare Post-Acute Care Transformation Act of 2014 (IMPACT Act), Section 1899B

https://www.gpo.gov/fdsys/pkg/PLAW-113publ185/pdf/PLAW-113publ185.pdf

https://www.cms.gov/Medicare/Quality-Initiatives-Patient-Assessment-Instruments/Post-Acute-Care-Quality-Initiatives/IMPACT-Act-of-2014/IMPACT-Act-of-2014-Data-Standardization-and-Cross-Setting-Measures

LTCH QRP Overview

The LTCH QRP creates LTCH quality reporting requirements, as mandated by section 3004(a) of the ACA. Every year, by October 1, CMS publishes the quality measures LTCHs must report.

The IMPACT act added section 1899B to the SSA and requires the reporting of standardized patient assessment data regarding quality measures and standardized patient assessment data elements (SPADE). It requires the submission of data pertaining to quality measure, resource use, and other domains. Using standardized quality measures and standardized data, the intent of the IMPACT Act, among other obligations, is to allow for the exchange of standardized and interoperable data among post-acute providers and other providers. The IMPACT Act intends for standardized post-acute care data to improve Medicare beneficiary outcomes through shared decision-making, care coordination, and enhanced discharge planning.

For FY 2014 and each subsequent year, if an LTCH fails to submit the required quality data, the LTCH will be subject to a 2 percentage point reduction in the annual payment update. CMS strongly encourages submitting quality data prior to the deadline to allow LTCH providers an opportunity to review their data submissions for completeness and accuracy and to address any submission issues.

LTCH Continuity Assessment Record and Evaluation Data Set

The LTCH Continuity Assessment Record and Evaluation (CARE) Data Set is applicable to all patients receiving inpatient services in a facility certified as a hospital and designated as an LTCH under the Medicare program. These hospitals are certified as acute-care hospitals that treat patients requiring extended hospital-level care, typically following initial treatment at a general acute-care hospital. If a hospital is classified as an LTCH, for purposes of Medicare payments (as denoted by the last four digits of its six-digit CMS Certification Number [CCN] in the range of 2000–2299), it is subject to the requirements of the LTCH QRP. It is not applicable to patients receiving services in LTCH units that are not designated as LTCHs under the Medicare program. Data collection using the LTCH CARE Data Set is applicable regardless of patient's age, diagnosis, length of stay, or payment/payer source. Data collected must be submitted in the time frame, manner, and form established by CMS for the LTCH QRP.

Effective July 1, 2018, the data collection instrument for these measures is the LTCH CARE Data Set version 4.00.

Effective October 1, 2020, the data collection instrument for these measures is the LTCH CARE Data Set version 5.00.

Note: CMS is delaying the release of LTCH CARE Data Set version 5.00 needed to support the Transfer of Health (TOH) Information Quality Measures in order to provide maximum flexibilities for providers of LTCHs to respond to the COVID-19 pubic health emergency (PHE).

The release of updated versions of the LTCH CARE Data Set will be delayed until October 1st of the year that is at least one full fiscal year after the end of the COVID-19 PHE. For example, if the COVID-19 PHE ends on September 20, 2020, LTCHs will be required to begin collecting data using the updated versions of the item sets beginning with patients discharged on October 1, 2021.

Standardized Patient Assessment Data Elements

The IMPACT Act required CMS to develop, implement, and maintain standardized patient assessment data elements (SPADE) for post-acute care (PAC) settings. The four PAC settings specified in the IMPACT Act are home health agencies (HHAs), inpatient rehabilitation facilities (IRFs), long-term care hospitals (LTCHs), and skilled nursing facilities (SNFs). The goals of implementing cross-setting SPADEs are to facilitate care coordination, interoperability, and improve Medicare beneficiary outcomes.

The IMPACT Act further required that the assessment instruments be modified to include core data elements on health assessment categories and that such data be standardized and interoperable. Implementation of a core set of standardized assessment items across PAC settings has important implications for Medicare beneficiaries, families, providers, and policymakers.

For FY 2019 and each subsequent year, LTCHs must report standardized patient assessment data, required under section 1899B(b)(1) of the Social Security Act. Section 1899B(b)(1)(B) of the act defines standardized patient assessment data as data required for at least the quality measures described in section 1899B(c)(1) of the act and that is with respect to the following categories:

1. Functional status
2. Cognitive function
3. Special services, treatments, and interventions
4. Medical conditions and comorbidities
5. Impairments
6. Other categories deemed necessary and appropriate by the secretary of the Department of Health and Human Services

In FY 2020 IPPS/LTCH PPS final rule, CMS adopted the first five categories listed above in addition to a new category. Each category and their respective data elements are outlined in the following table.

Category	Data Elements
Functional Status	Car transfer
	Walking 10 feet on uneven surfaces
	1-step (curb)
	4 steps
	12 steps
	Picking up object
Cognitive Function	Brief interview for mental status (BIMS)
	Confusion assessment method (CAM)
	Patient health questionnaire — 2 to 9 (PHQ-2 to 9)
Special Services, Treatments, and Interventions	Chemotherapy (IV, oral, other)
	Radiation
	Oxygen therapy (intermittent, continuous, high-concentration oxygen delivery system)
	Suctioning (scheduled, as needed)
	Tracheostomy care
	Noninvasive mechanical ventilator (bilevel positive airway pressure [BiPAP]; continuous positive airway pressure [CPAP])
	Invasive mechanical ventilator
	IV medications (antibiotics, anticoagulation, vasoactive medications, other)
	Transfusions
	Dialysis (hemodialysis, peritoneal dialysis)
	IV access (peripheral IV, midline, central line)
	Parenteral/IV feeding
	Feeding tube
	Mechanically altered diet
	Therapeutic diet
	High-risk drug classes: use and indication
Medical Conditions and Comorbidities	Pain interference (pain effect on sleep, pain interference with therapy activities, and pain interference with day-to-day activities)

Category	Data Elements
Impairments	Hearing Vision
Social Determinants of Health (SDOH)	Race Ethnicity Preferred language Interpreter services Health literacy Transportation Social isolation

For the first program year in which measures or standardized patient assessment data are adopted, LTCHs will be required to report data only on patients who are admitted and discharged during the last quarter (October 1 to December 31) of the calendar year that applies to the program year. For subsequent program years, LTCHs will be required to report data on patients who are admitted and discharged during the 12-month calendar year that applies to the program year.

Note: CMS is delaying the release of new or revised SPADEs in order to provide maximum flexibilities for providers of LTCHs to respond to the COVID-19 pubic health emergency (PHE).

The release of new or revised SPADEs will be delayed until October 1st of the year that is at least one full fiscal year after the end of the COVID-19 PHE. For example, if the COVID-19 PHE ends on September 20, 2020, LTCHs will be required to begin collecting data beginning with patients discharged on October 1, 2021.

Quality Measures Currently Adopted for the FY 2022 LTCH QRP

The LTCH QRP currently has 17 measures for the FY 2022 program year, which are outlined in the following table:

Quality Measures Currently Adopted for the FY 2022 LTCH QRP	
LTCH CARE Data Set	
Short Name	**Measure Name & Data Source**
Pressure Ulcer/Injury	Changes in Skin Integrity Post-Acute Care: Pressure Ulcer/Injury
Application of Falls	Application of Percent of Residents Experiencing One or More Falls with Major Injury (Long Stay) (NQF #0674)
Functional Assessment	Percent of Long-Term Care Hospital (LTCH) Patients with an Admission and Discharge Functional Assessment and a Care Plan That Addresses Function (NQF #2631)
Application of Functional Assessment	Application of Percent of Long-Term Care Hospital (LTCH) Patients with an Admission and Discharge Functional Assessment and a Care Plan That Addresses Function (NQF #2631)
Change in Mobility	Functional Outcome Measure: Change in Mobility Among Long-Term Care Hospital (LTCH) Patients Requiring Ventilator Support (NQF #2632)
DRR	Drug Regimen Review Conducted With Follow-Up for Identified Issues—Post Acute Care (PAC) Long-Term Care Hospital (LTCH) Quality Reporting Program (QRP)
Compliance with SBT	Compliance with Spontaneous Breathing Trial (SBT) by Day 2 of the LTCH Stay
Ventilator Liberation	Ventilator Liberation Rate
TOH* – Provider	Transfer of Health Information to the Provider Post-Acute Care
TOH* – Patient	Transfer of Health Information to the Patient Post-Acute Care
NHSN	
CAUTI	National Healthcare Safety Network (NHSN) Catheter-Associated Urinary Tract Infection (CAUTI) Outcome Measure (NQF #0138)
CLABSI	National Healthcare Safety Network (NHSN) Central Line-Associated Bloodstream Infection (CLABSI) Outcome Measure (NQF #0139)
CDI	National Healthcare Safety Network (NHSN) Facility-wide Inpatient Hospital-onset *Clostridium difficile* Infection (CDI) Outcome Measure (NQF #1717)
HCP Influenza Vaccine	Influenza Vaccination Coverage among Healthcare Personnel (NQF #0431)
Claims-based	
MSPB LTCH	Medicare Spending Per Beneficiary (MSPB)—Post Acute Care (PAC) Long-Term Care Hospital (LTCH) Quality Reporting Program (QRP)
DTC	Discharge to Community—Post Acute Care (PAC) Long-Term Care Hospital (LTCH) Quality Reporting Program (QRP)
PPR	Potentially Preventable 30-Day Post-Discharge Readmission Measure for Long-Term Care Hospital (LTCH) Quality Reporting Program (QRP)

* Transfer of Health Information

Form, Manner, and Timing of Data Submission Under the LTCH QRP

Under the current CMS policy, LTCHs report data on LTCH QRP assessment-based measures and standardized patient assessment data by reporting the designated data elements for each applicable patient on the LTCH CARE Data Set patient assessment instrument and then submitting the completed instruments to CMS using the Quality Improvement and Evaluation System (QIES) Assessment and Submission Processing (ASAP) system. Data on LTCH QRP measures that are also collected by the CDC for other purposes are reported by LTCHs to the CDC through the NHSN, and the CDC then transmits the relevant data to CMS. Readers are referred to the FY 2018 IPPS/LTCH PPS final rule (82 FR 38454 through 38456) for the data collection and submission timeframes that were finalized for the LTCH QRP.

In the FY 2020 IPPS/LTCH PPS final rule, CMS finalized their proposal to move the implementation date of any new version of the LTCH CARE Data Set from April to October, beginning October 1, 2020. This would give LTCHs an additional six months (April-October) to update their systems so that they can comply with the new reporting requirements.

Appendix K: Severe Wound Diagnosis Codes by Category

The following lists the ICD-10-CM codes describing severe wound diagnoses. CMS allows for a temporary exception for certain wound care discharges from the site-neutral payment rate for certain long-term care hospitals (LTCHs). This exception applies to discharges occurring during FY2018 (that is, for cost reporting period beginning on or after October 1, 2017, and on or before September 30, 2018) from LTCHs that are grandfathered hospitals-within-hospitals (HwHs) (that is, hospitals that are described under § 412.23(e)(2)(i) that meet the criteria of § 412.22(f)) when the individual discharged "has a severe wound." Based upon the FY 2018 IPPS/LTCH final rule classification, the definition of "severe wound" has been refined to include only five categories (stage 3 wound, stage 4 wound, unstageable wound, nonhealing surgical wound, and fistula) and exclusions are limited to discharges that both meet the definition of a severe wound and are additionally grouped to certain specified MS-LTC-DRGs.

Note: An updated ICD-10-CM list was not available at the time this publication was printed and therefore does not reflect any FY 2021 code changes. An updated list of severe wound codes, effective October 1, 2020, can be found at: https://www.cms.gov/Medicare/Medicare-Fee-for-Service-Payment/LongTermCareHospitalPPS/download.html.

Stage 3 Wound

L89.003	L89.123	L89.213	L89.43	L89.613	L97.112	L97.124	L97.922	
L89.013	L89.133	L89.223	L89.503	L89.623	L97.113	L97.912	L97.923	
L89.023	L89.143	L89.303	L89.513	L89.813	L97.114	L97.913	L97.924	
L89.103	L89.153	L89.313	L89.523	L89.893	L97.122	L97.914		
L89.113	L89.203	L89.323	L89.603	L89.93	L97.123	L97.921		

Stage 4 Wound

L89.004	L89.104	L89.134	L89.204	L89.304	L89.44	L89.524	L89.624	L89.94
L89.014	L89.114	L89.144	L89.214	L89.314	L89.504	L89.604	L89.814	
L89.024	L89.124	L89.154	L89.224	L89.324	L89.514	L89.614	L89.894	

Unstageable Wound

L89.000	T20.319D	T20.72XA	T21.34XS	T21.77XD	T22.341A	T22.399S	T22.742D	T23.302A
L89.010	T20.319S	T20.72XD	T21.35XA	T21.77XS	T22.341D	T22.70XA	T22.742S	T23.302D
L89.020	T20.32XA	T20.72XS	T21.35XD	T21.79XA	T22.341S	T22.70XD	T22.749A	T23.302S
L89.100	T20.32XD	T20.73XA	T21.35XS	T21.79XD	T22.342A	T22.70XS	T22.749D	T23.309A
L89.110	T20.32XS	T20.73XD	T21.36XA	T21.79XS	T22.342D	T22.711A	T22.749S	T23.309D
L89.120	T20.33XA	T20.73XS	T21.36XD	T22.30XA	T22.342S	T22.711D	T22.751A	T23.309S
L89.130	T20.33XD	T20.74XA	T21.36XS	T22.30XD	T22.349A	T22.711S	T22.751D	T23.311A
L89.140	T20.33XS	T20.74XD	T21.37XA	T22.30XS	T22.349D	T22.712A	T22.751S	T23.311D
L89.150	T20.34XA	T20.74XS	T21.37XD	T22.311A	T22.349S	T22.712D	T22.752A	T23.311S
L89.200	T20.34XD	T20.75XA	T21.37XS	T22.311D	T22.351A	T22.712S	T22.752D	T23.312A
L89.210	T20.34XS	T20.75XD	T21.39XA	T22.311S	T22.351D	T22.719A	T22.752S	T23.312D
L89.220	T20.35XA	T20.75XS	T21.39XD	T22.312A	T22.351S	T22.719D	T22.759A	T23.312S
L89.300	T20.35XD	T20.76XA	T21.39XS	T22.312D	T22.352A	T22.719S	T22.759D	T23.319A
L89.310	T20.35XS	T20.76XD	T21.70XA	T22.312S	T22.352D	T22.721A	T22.759S	T23.319D
L89.320	T20.36XA	T20.76XS	T21.70XD	T22.319A	T22.352S	T22.721D	T22.761A	T23.319S
L89.45	T20.36XD	T20.77XA	T21.70XS	T22.319D	T22.359A	T22.721S	T22.761D	T23.321A
L89.500	T20.36XS	T20.77XD	T21.71XA	T22.319S	T22.359D	T22.722A	T22.761S	T23.321D
L89.510	T20.37XA	T20.77XS	T21.71XD	T22.321A	T22.359S	T22.722D	T22.762A	T23.321S
L89.520	T20.37XD	T20.79XA	T21.71XS	T22.321D	T22.361A	T22.722S	T22.762D	T23.322A
L89.600	T20.37XS	T20.79XD	T21.72XA	T22.321S	T22.361D	T22.729A	T22.762S	T23.322D
L89.610	T20.39XA	T20.79XS	T21.72XD	T22.322A	T22.361S	T22.729D	T22.769A	T23.322S
L89.620	T20.39XD	T21.30XA	T21.72XS	T22.322D	T22.362A	T22.729S	T22.769D	T23.329A
L89.810	T20.39XS	T21.30XD	T21.73XA	T22.322S	T22.362D	T22.731A	T22.769S	T23.329D
L89.890	T20.70XA	T21.30XS	T21.73XD	T22.329A	T22.362S	T22.731D	T22.791A	T23.329S
L89.95	T20.70XD	T21.31XA	T21.73XS	T22.329D	T22.369A	T22.731S	T22.791D	T23.331A
T20.30XA	T20.70XS	T21.31XD	T21.74XA	T22.329S	T22.369D	T22.732A	T22.791S	T23.331D
T20.30XD	T20.711A	T21.31XS	T21.74XD	T22.331A	T22.369S	T22.732D	T22.792A	T23.331S
T20.30XS	T20.711D	T21.32XA	T21.74XS	T22.331D	T22.391A	T22.732S	T22.792D	T23.332A
T20.311A	T20.711S	T21.32XD	T21.75XA	T22.331S	T22.391D	T22.739A	T22.792S	T23.332D
T20.311D	T20.712A	T21.32XS	T21.75XD	T22.332A	T22.391S	T22.739D	T22.799A	T23.332S
T20.311S	T20.712D	T21.33XA	T21.75XS	T22.332D	T22.392A	T22.739S	T22.799D	T23.339A
T20.312A	T20.712S	T21.33XD	T21.76XA	T22.332S	T22.392D	T22.741A	T22.799S	T23.339D
T20.312D	T20.719A	T21.33XS	T21.76XD	T22.339A	T22.392S	T22.741D	T23.301A	T23.339S
T20.312S	T20.719D	T21.34XA	T21.76XS	T22.339D	T22.399A	T22.741S	T23.301D	T23.341A
T20.319A	T20.719S	T21.34XD	T21.77XA	T22.339S	T22.399D	T22.742A	T23.301S	T23.341D

Unstageable Wound (continued)

T23.341S	T23.379D	T23.722A	T23.759S	T24.3Ø2D	T24.391A	T24.729A	T25.321S	T25.719D
T23.342A	T23.379S	T23.722D	T23.761A	T24.3Ø2S	T24.391D	T24.729D	T25.322A	T25.719S
T23.342D	T23.391A	T23.722S	T23.761D	T24.3Ø9A	T24.391S	T24.729S	T25.322D	T25.721A
T23.342S	T23.391D	T23.729A	T23.761S	T24.3Ø9D	T24.392A	T24.731A	T25.322S	T25.721D
T23.349A	T23.391S	T23.729D	T23.762A	T24.3Ø9S	T24.392D	T24.731D	T25.329A	T25.721S
T23.349D	T23.392A	T23.729S	T23.762D	T24.311A	T24.392S	T24.731S	T25.329D	T25.722A
T23.349S	T23.392D	T23.731A	T23.762S	T24.311D	T24.399A	T24.732A	T25.329S	T25.722D
T23.351A	T23.392S	T23.731D	T23.769A	T24.311S	T24.399D	T24.732D	T25.331A	T25.722S
T23.351D	T23.399A	T23.731S	T23.769D	T24.312A	T24.7Ø1A	T24.732S	T25.331D	T25.729A
T23.351S	T23.399D	T23.732A	T23.769S	T24.312D	T24.7Ø1D	T24.739A	T25.331S	T25.729D
T23.352A	T23.399S	T23.732D	T23.771A	T24.312S	T24.7Ø1S	T24.739D	T25.332A	T25.729S
T23.352D	T23.7Ø1A	T23.732S	T23.771D	T24.319A	T24.7Ø2A	T24.739S	T25.332D	T25.731A
T23.352S	T23.7Ø1D	T23.739A	T23.771S	T24.319D	T24.7Ø2D	T24.791A	T25.332S	T25.731D
T23.359A	T23.7Ø1S	T23.739D	T23.772A	T24.319S	T24.7Ø2S	T24.791D	T25.339A	T25.731S
T23.359D	T23.7Ø2A	T23.739S	T23.772D	T24.321A	T24.7Ø9A	T24.791S	T25.339D	T25.732A
T23.359S	T23.7Ø2D	T23.741A	T23.772S	T24.321D	T24.7Ø9D	T24.792A	T25.339S	T25.732D
T23.361A	T23.7Ø2S	T23.741D	T23.779A	T24.321S	T24.7Ø9S	T24.792D	T25.391A	T25.732S
T23.361D	T23.7Ø9A	T23.741S	T23.779D	T24.322A	T24.711A	T24.792S	T25.391D	T25.739A
T23.361S	T23.7Ø9D	T23.742A	T23.779S	T24.322D	T24.711D	T24.799A	T25.391S	T25.739D
T23.362A	T23.7Ø9S	T23.742D	T23.791A	T24.322S	T24.711S	T24.799D	T25.392A	T25.739S
T23.362D	T23.711A	T23.742S	T23.791D	T24.329A	T24.712A	T24.799S	T25.392D	T25.791A
T23.362S	T23.711D	T23.749A	T23.791S	T24.329D	T24.712D	T25.311A	T25.392S	T25.791D
T23.369A	T23.711S	T23.749D	T23.792A	T24.329S	T24.712S	T25.311D	T25.399A	T25.791S
T23.369D	T23.712A	T23.749S	T23.792D	T24.331A	T24.719A	T25.311S	T25.399D	T25.792A
T23.369S	T23.712D	T23.751A	T23.792S	T24.331D	T24.719D	T25.312A	T25.399S	T25.792D
T23.371A	T23.712S	T23.751D	T23.799A	T24.331S	T24.719S	T25.312D	T25.711A	T25.792S
T23.371D	T23.719A	T23.751S	T23.799D	T24.332A	T24.721A	T25.312S	T25.711D	T25.799A
T23.371S	T23.719D	T23.752A	T23.799S	T24.332D	T24.721D	T25.319A	T25.711S	T25.799D
T23.372A	T23.719S	T23.752D	T24.3Ø1A	T24.332S	T24.721S	T25.319D	T25.712A	T25.799S
T23.372D	T23.721A	T23.752S	T24.3Ø1D	T24.339A	T24.722A	T25.319S	T25.712D	
T23.372S	T23.721D	T23.759A	T24.3Ø1S	T24.339D	T24.722D	T25.321A	T25.712S	
T23.379A	T23.721S	T23.759D	T24.3Ø2A	T24.339S	T24.722S	T25.321D	T25.719A	

Non-Healing Surgical Wound

L97.1Ø2	L97.214	L97.313	L97.412	L97.5Ø4	L97.8Ø3	L97.9Ø2	L98.424	T81.32XA
L97.1Ø3	L97.222	L97.314	L97.413	L97.512	L97.8Ø4	L97.9Ø3	L98.492	T81.32XD
L97.1Ø4	L97.223	L97.322	L97.414	L97.513	L97.812	L97.9Ø4	L98.493	T81.89XA
L97.2Ø2	L97.224	L97.323	L97.422	L97.514	L97.813	L98.412	L98.494	T81.89XD
L97.2Ø3	L97.3Ø2	L97.324	L97.423	L97.522	L97.814	L98.413	T81.3ØXA	
L97.2Ø4	L97.3Ø3	L97.4Ø2	L97.424	L97.523	L97.822	L98.414	T81.3ØXD	
L97.212	L97.3Ø4	L97.4Ø3	L97.5Ø2	L97.524	L97.823	L98.422	T81.31XA	
L97.213	L97.312	L97.4Ø4	L97.5Ø3	L97.8Ø2	L97.824	L98.423	T81.31XD	

Fistula* (which includes osteomyelitis)

HØ4.611	H83.12	K5Ø.113	K51.813	LØ5.92	M25.131	M25.159	M25.175	Q18.1
HØ4.612	H83.13	K5Ø.813	K51.913	M25.1Ø	M25.132	M25.161	M25.176	T81.83XA
HØ4.613	H83.19	K5Ø.913	K6Ø.3	M25.111	M25.139	M25.162	M25.18	T81.83XD
HØ4.619	J86.Ø	K51.Ø13	K6Ø.4	M25.112	M25.141	M25.169	N82.Ø	T81.83XS
H7Ø.811	KØ4.6	K51.213	K6Ø.5	M25.119	M25.142	M25.171	N82.2	
H7Ø.812	K11.4	K51.313	K63.2	M25.121	M25.149	M25.172	N82.3	
H7Ø.813	K31.6	K51.413	LØ5.Ø1	M25.122	M25.151	M25.173	N82.4	
H7Ø.819	K5Ø.Ø13	K51.513	LØ5.Ø2	M25.129	M25.152	M25.174	N82.5	

Chapter 3. Diseases of the Blood and Blood-forming Organs and Certain Disorders Involving the Immune Mechanism (D5Ø–D89)

Red Blood Cells

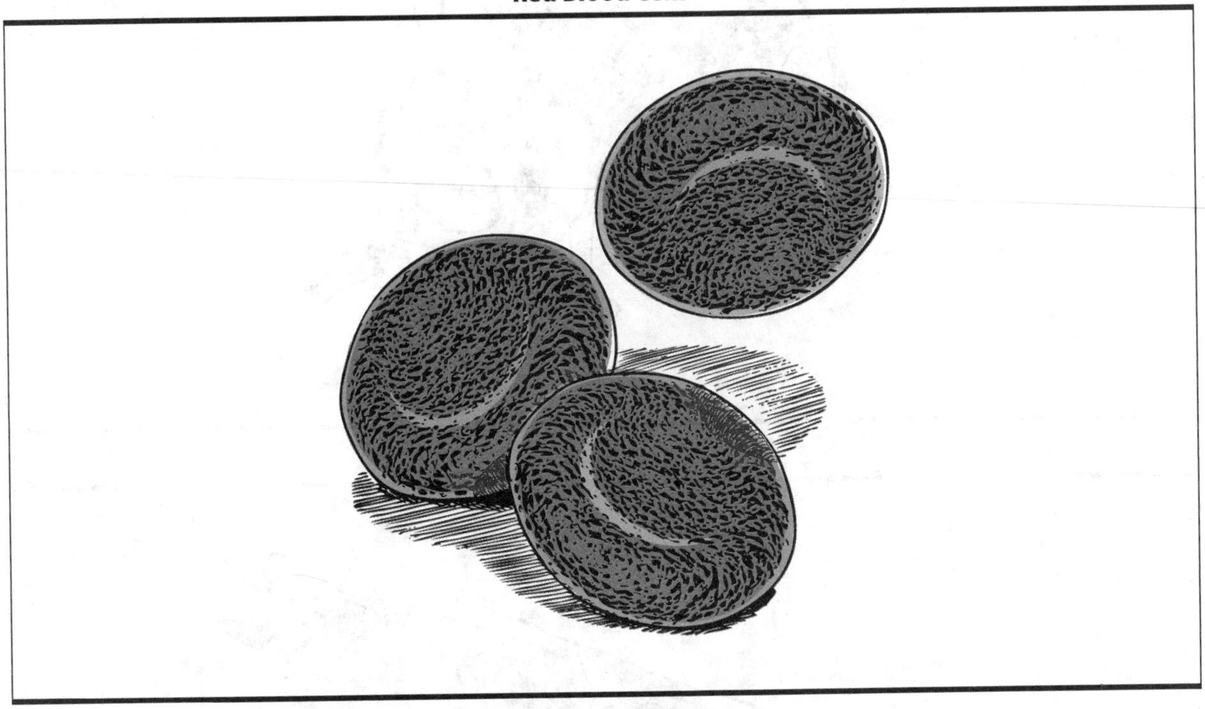

White Blood Cell

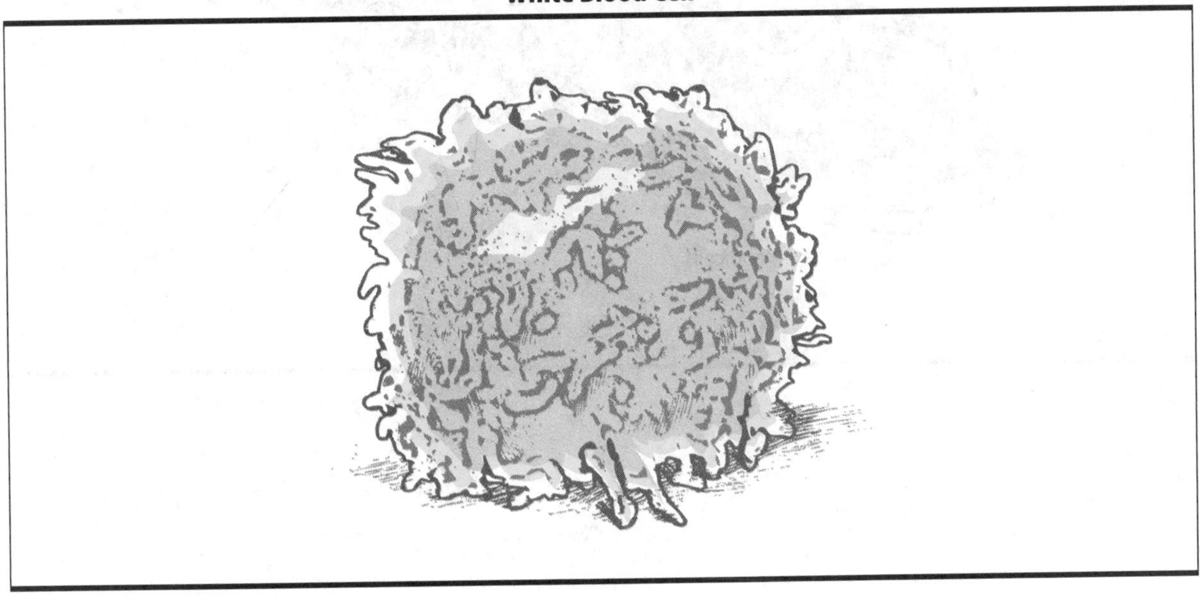

Platelet

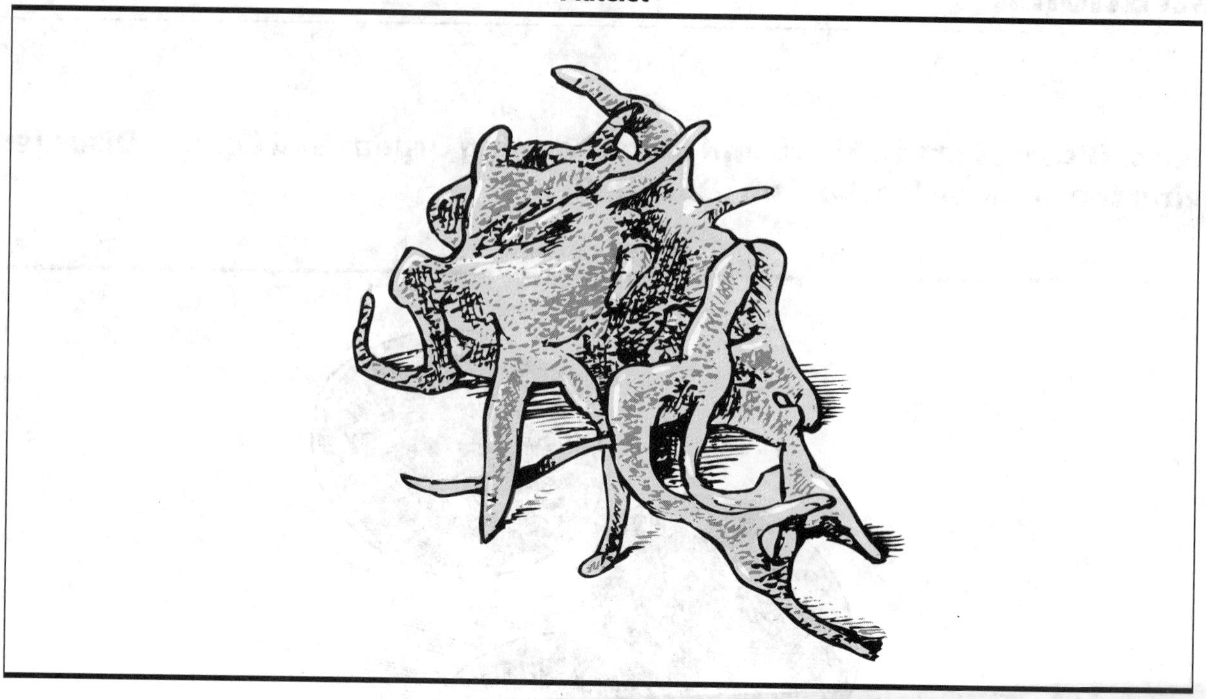

Coagulation

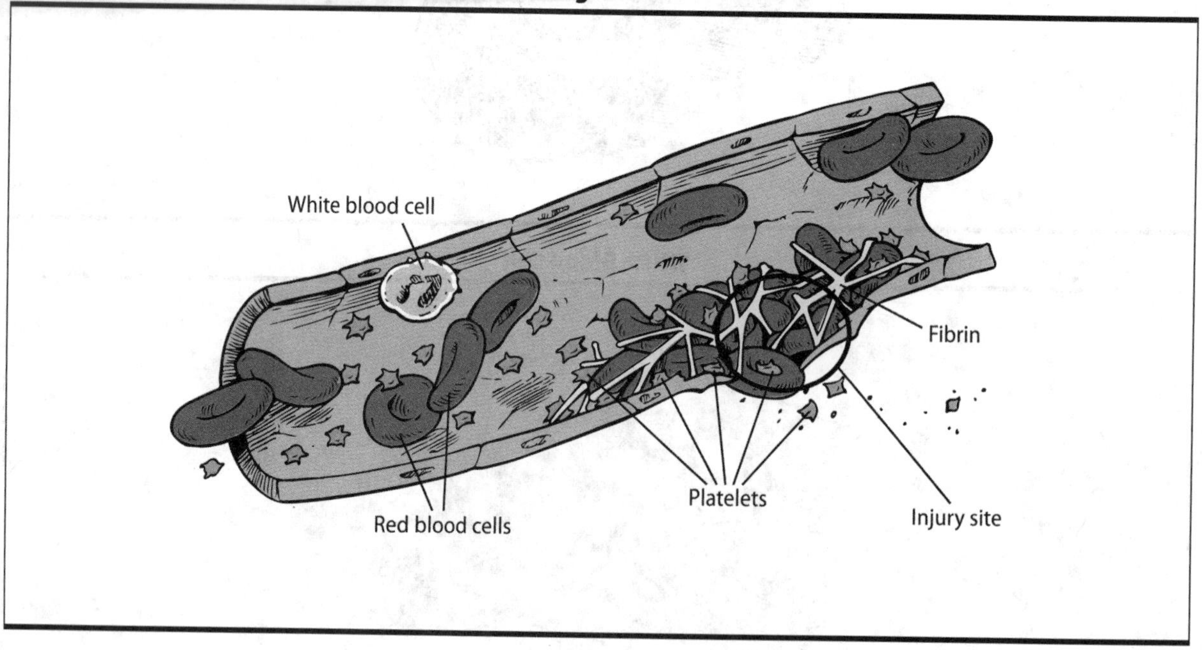

Spleen Anatomical Location and External Structures

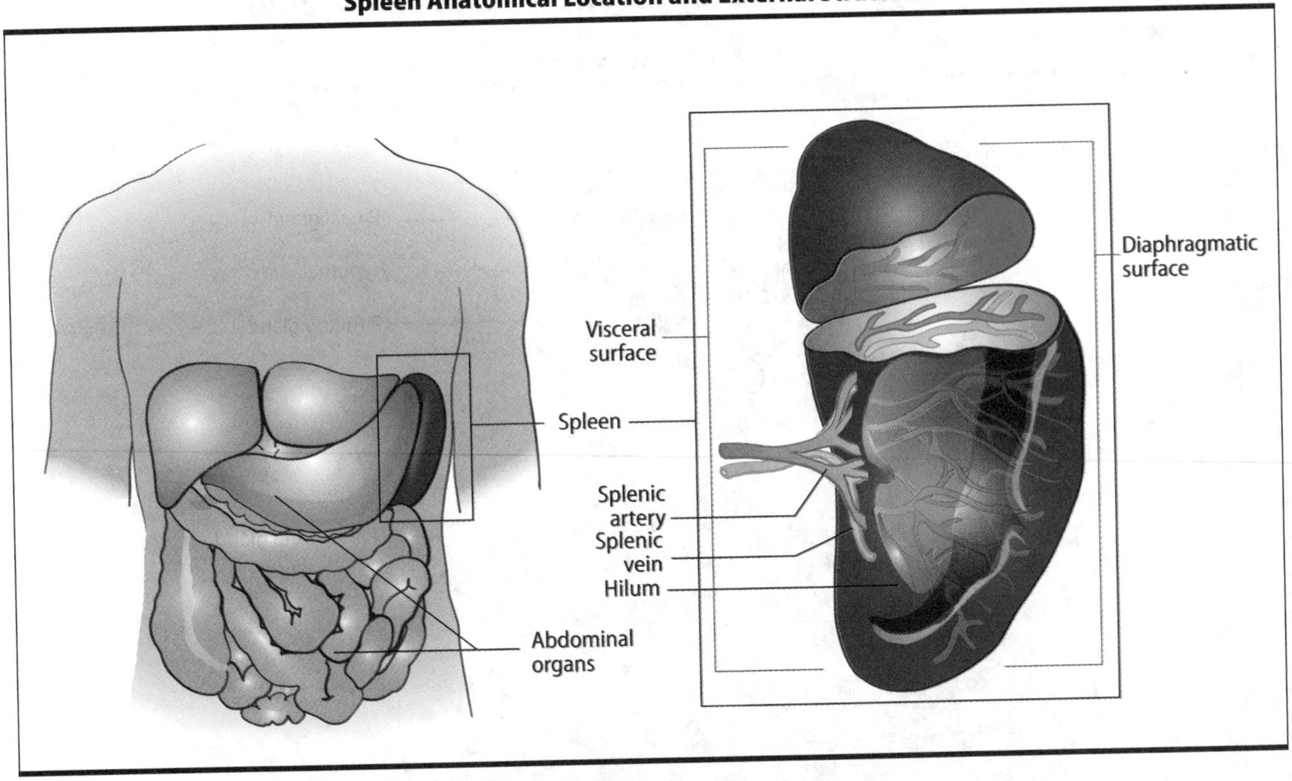

Spleen Interior Structures

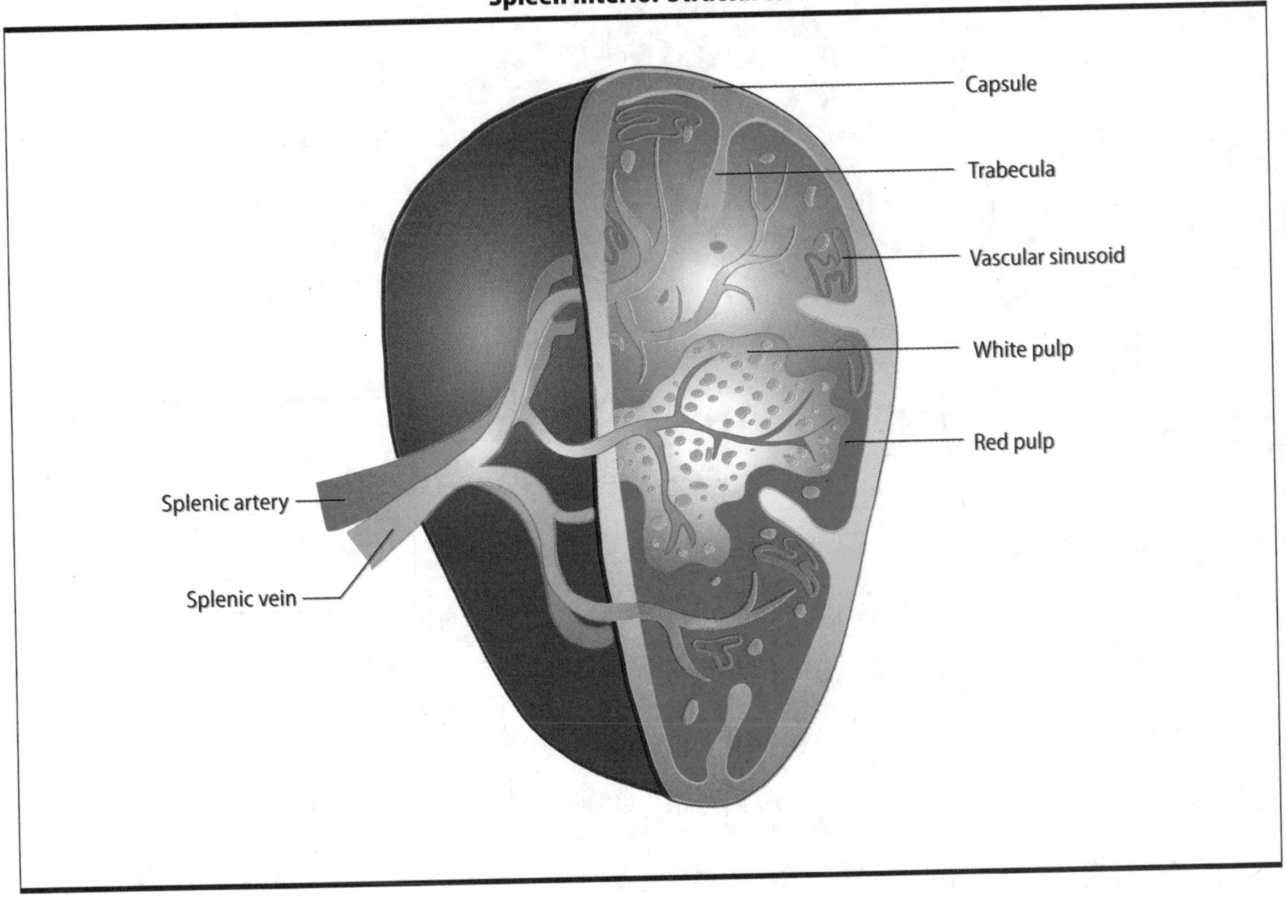

Chapter 4. Endocrine, Nutritional and Metabolic Diseases (EØØ–E89)

Endocrine System

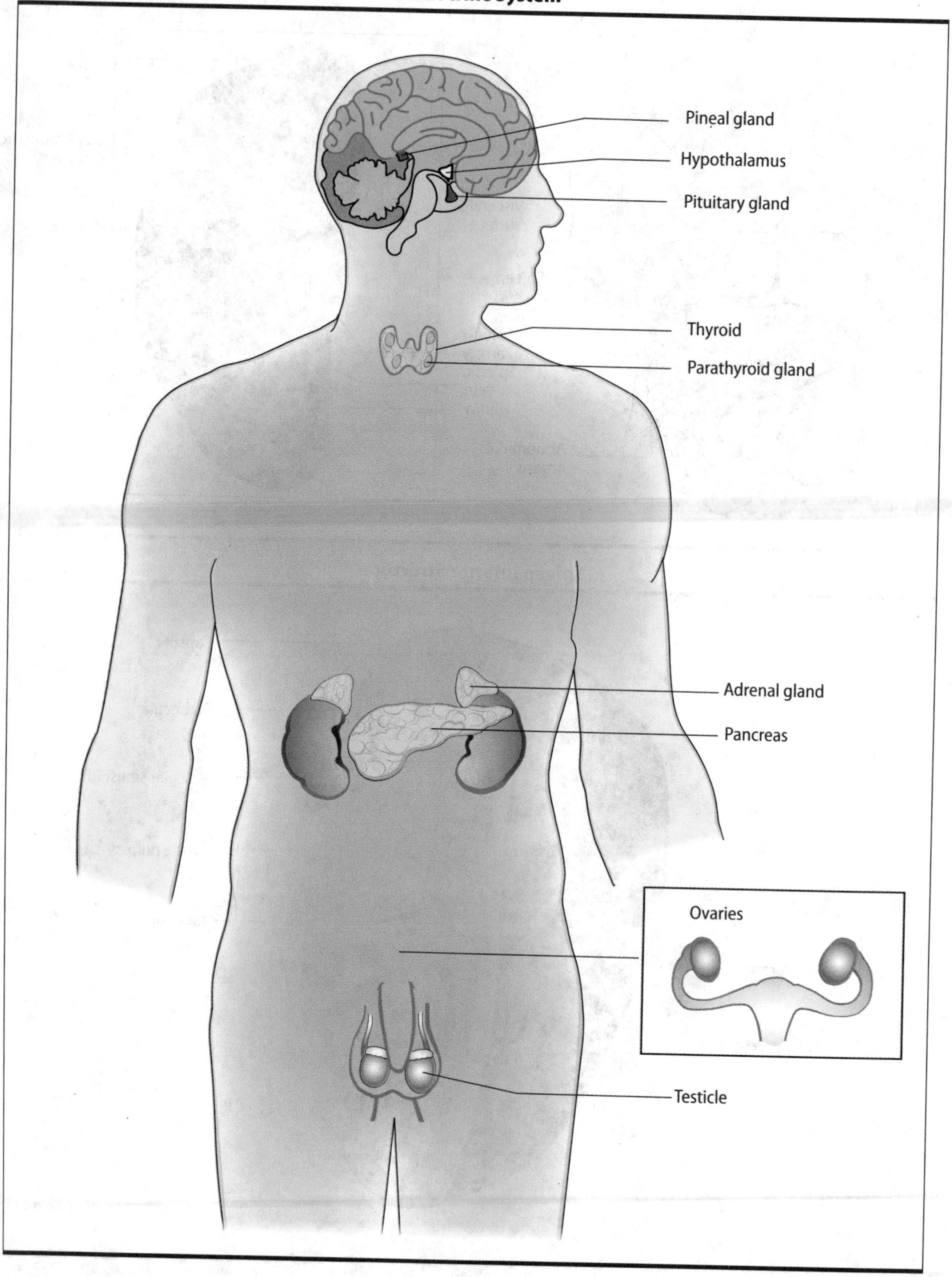

Thyroid

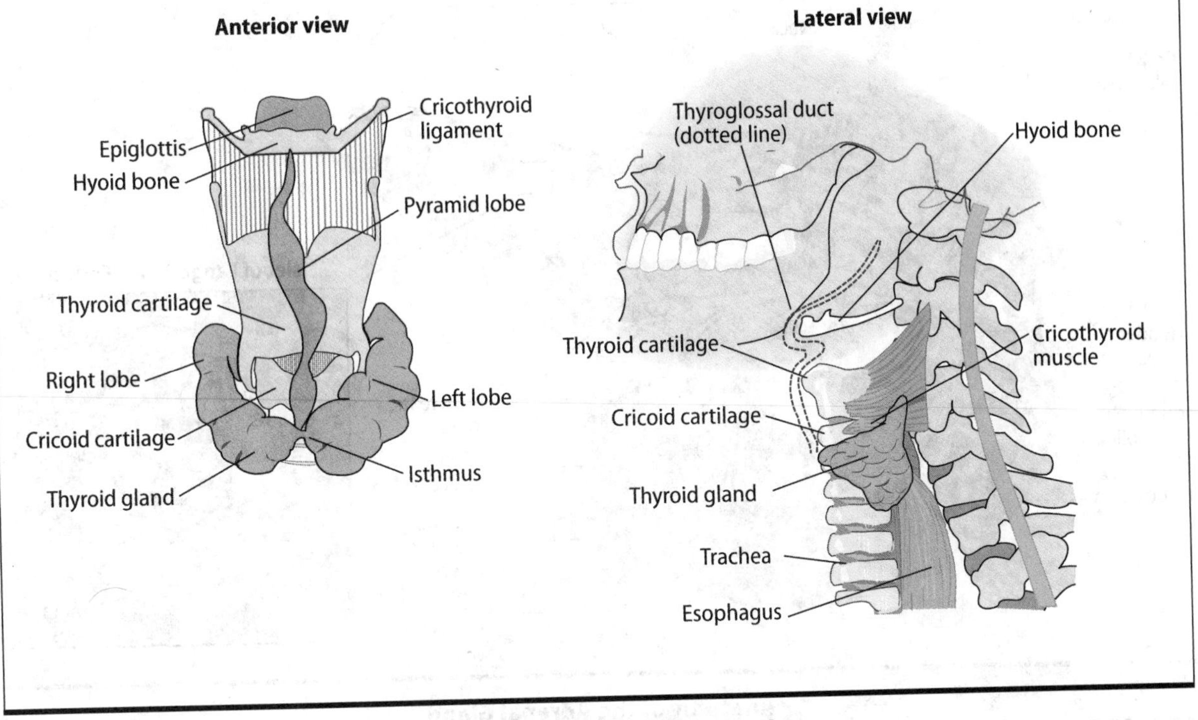

Thyroid and Parathyroid Glands

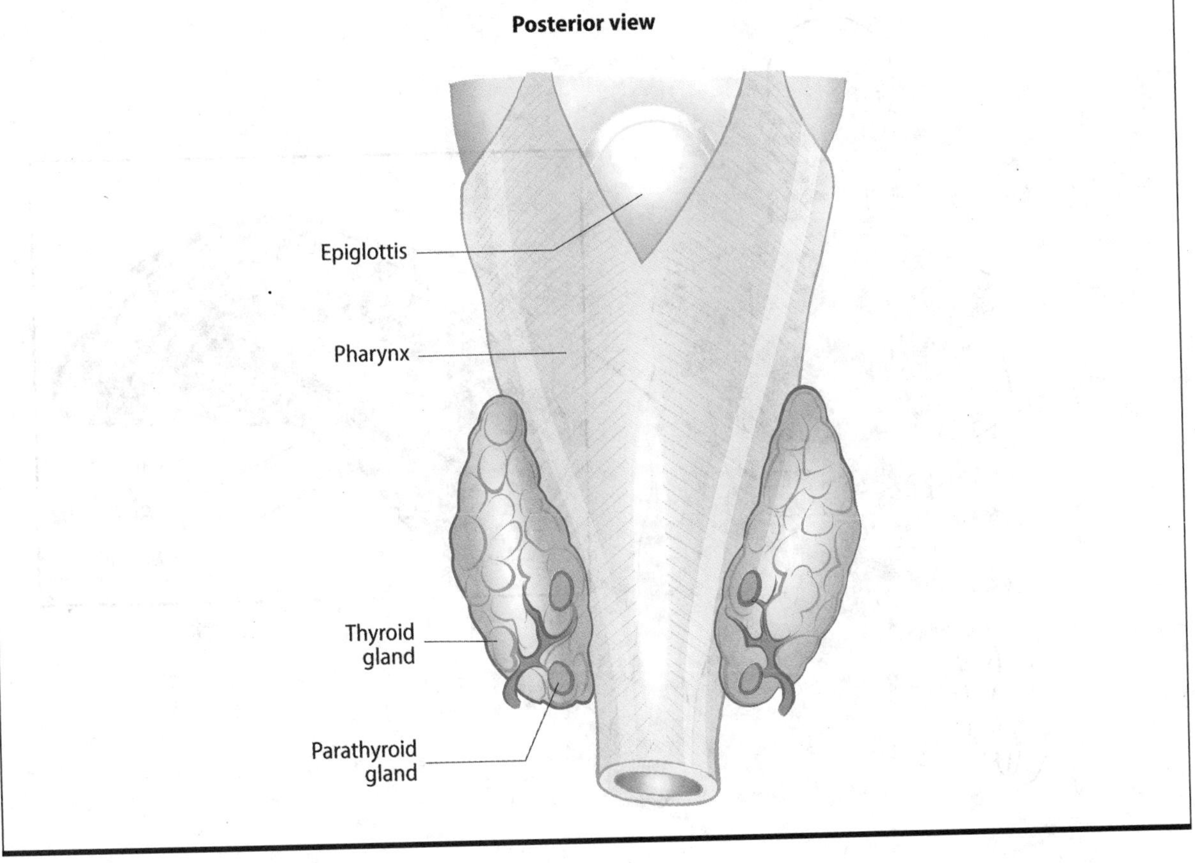

Pancreas

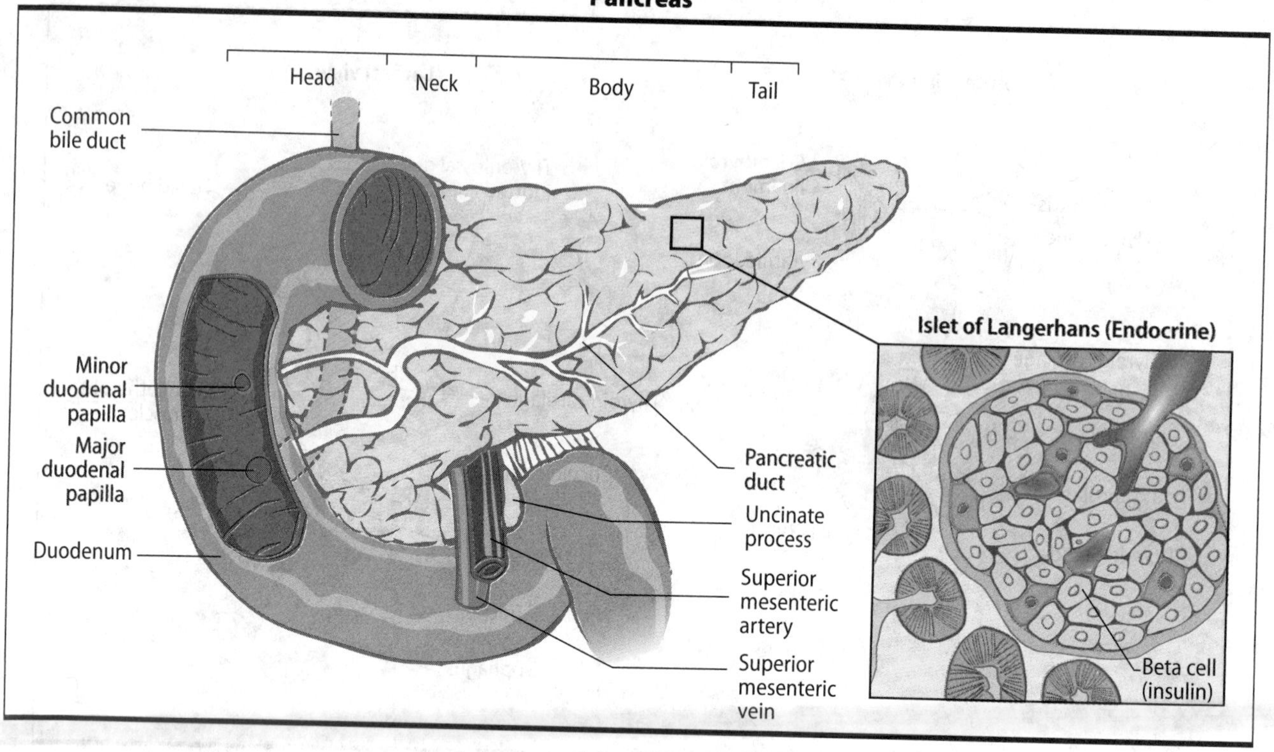

Anatomy of the Adrenal Gland

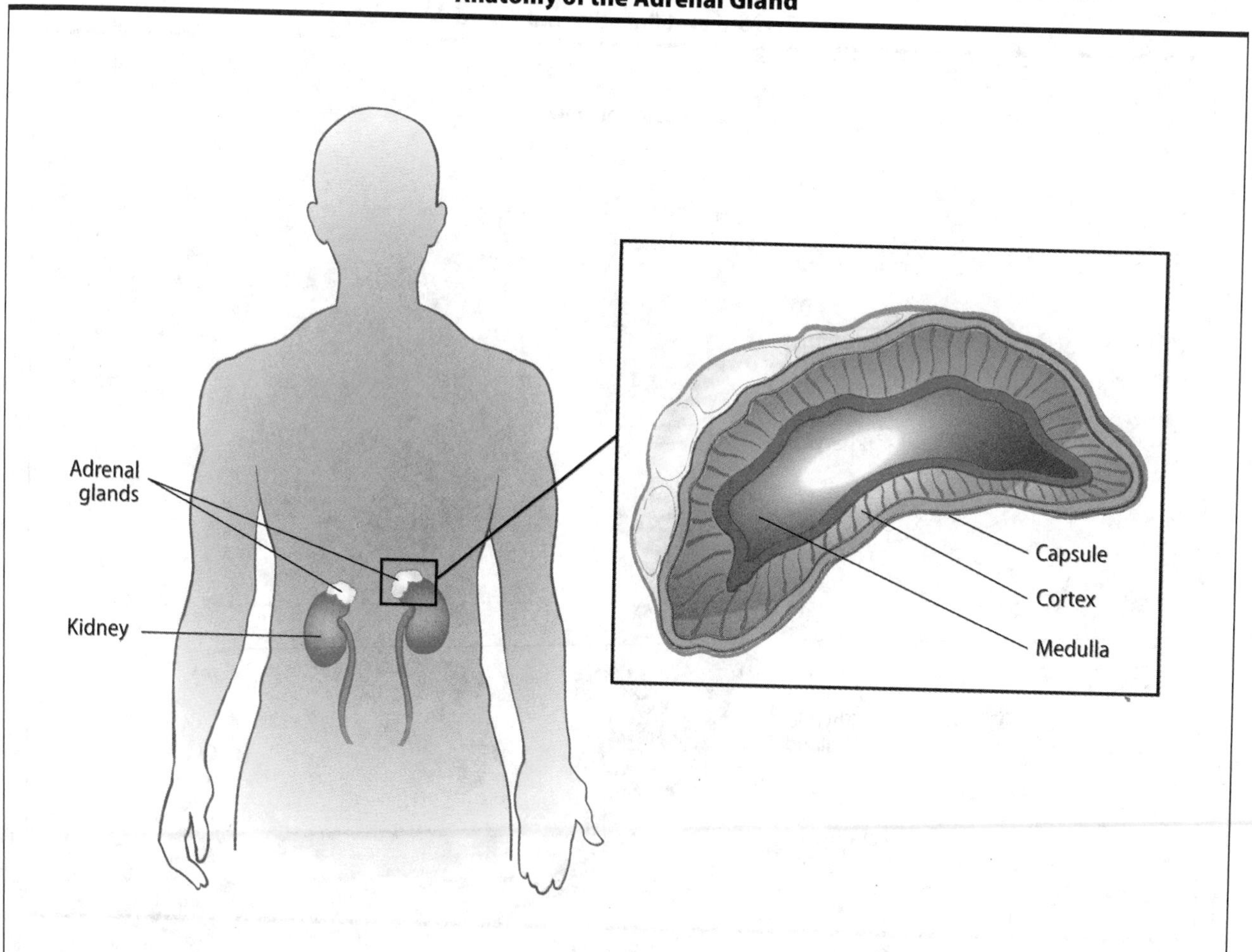

Structure of an Ovary

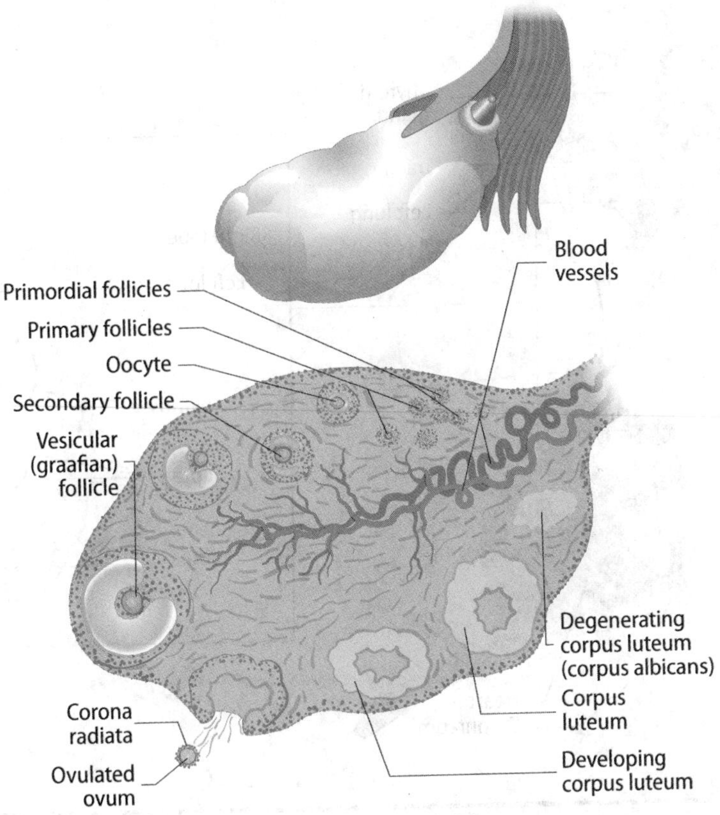

Testis and Associated Structures

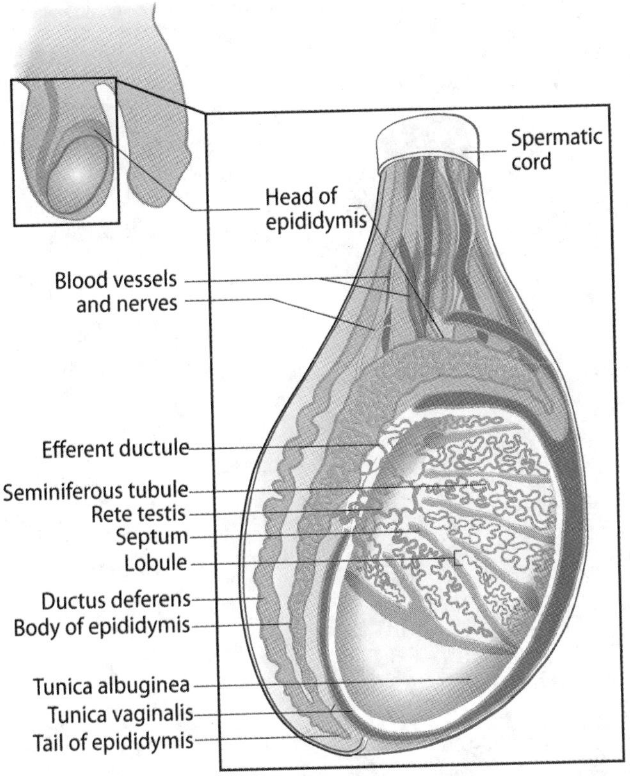

Thymus

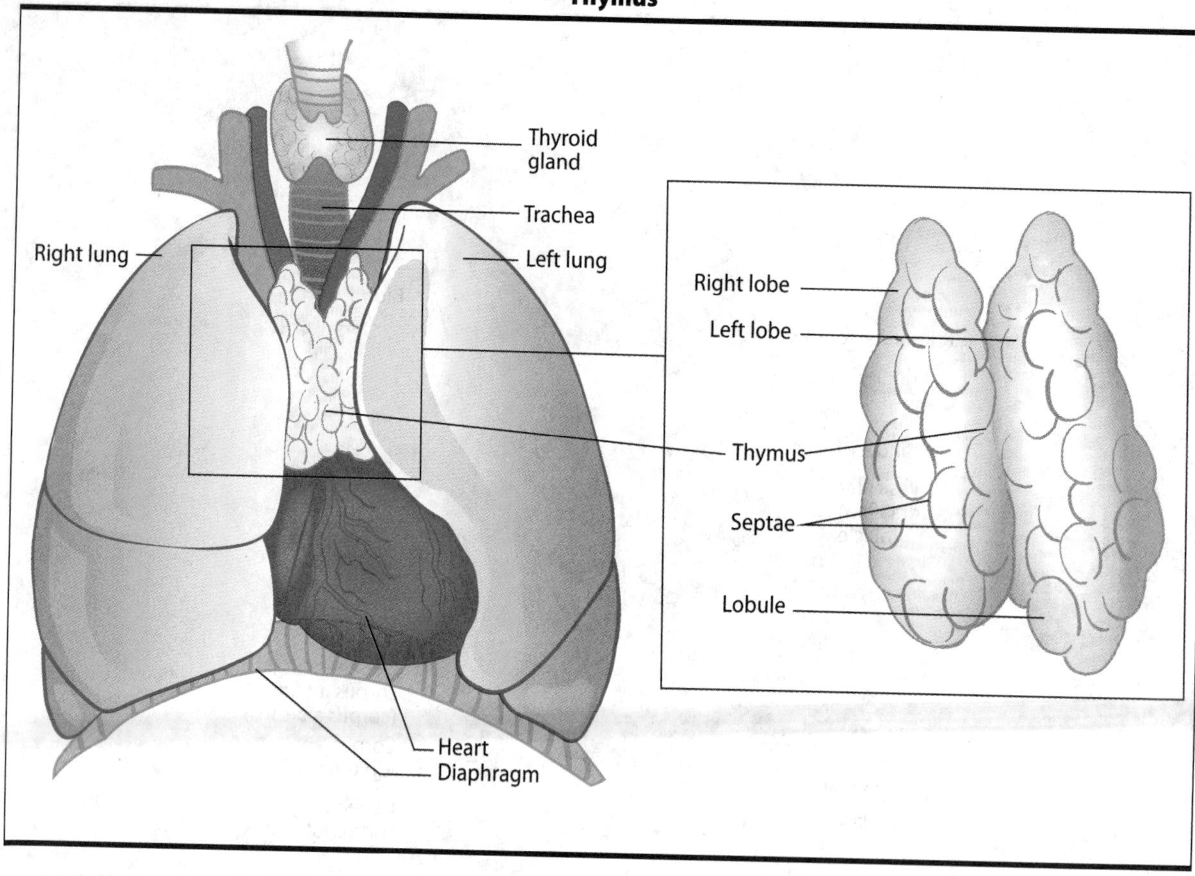
Thyroid gland
Trachea
Right lung
Left lung
Heart
Diaphragm
Right lobe
Left lobe
Thymus
Septae
Lobule

Chapter 6. Diseases of the Nervous System (GØØ–G99)

Brain

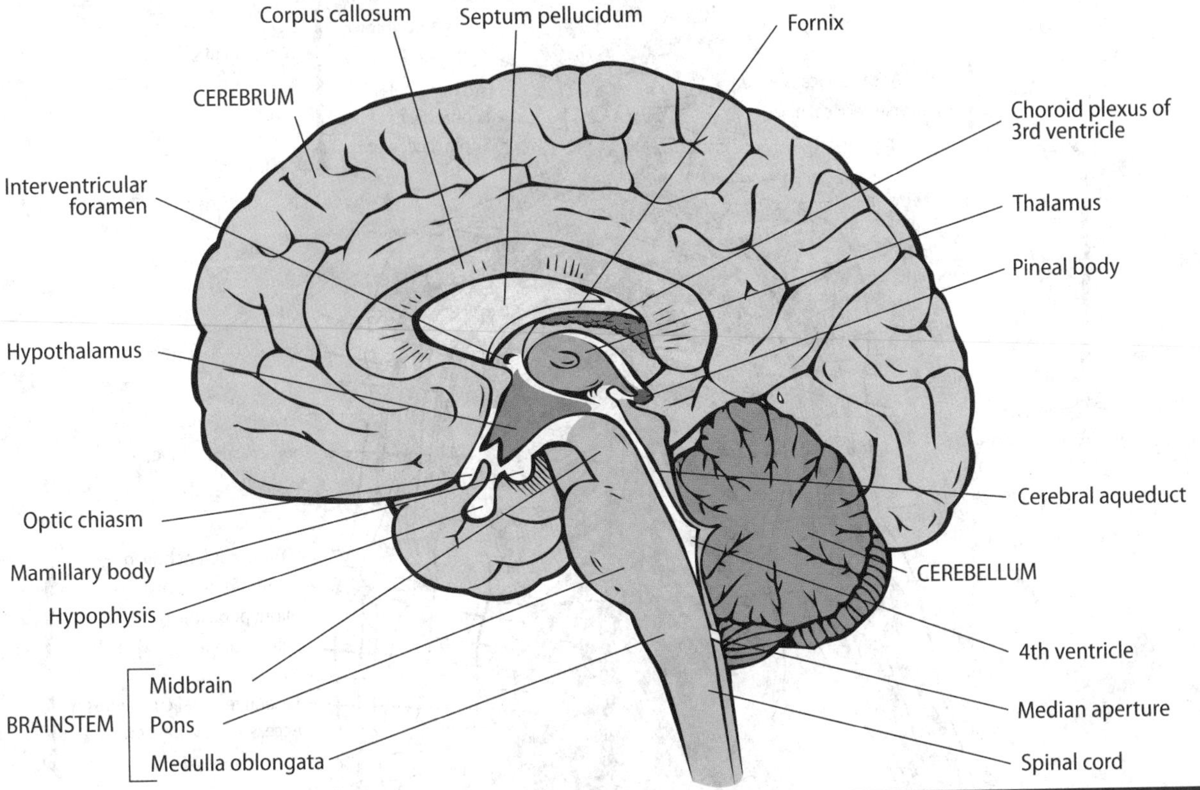

Cranial Nerves

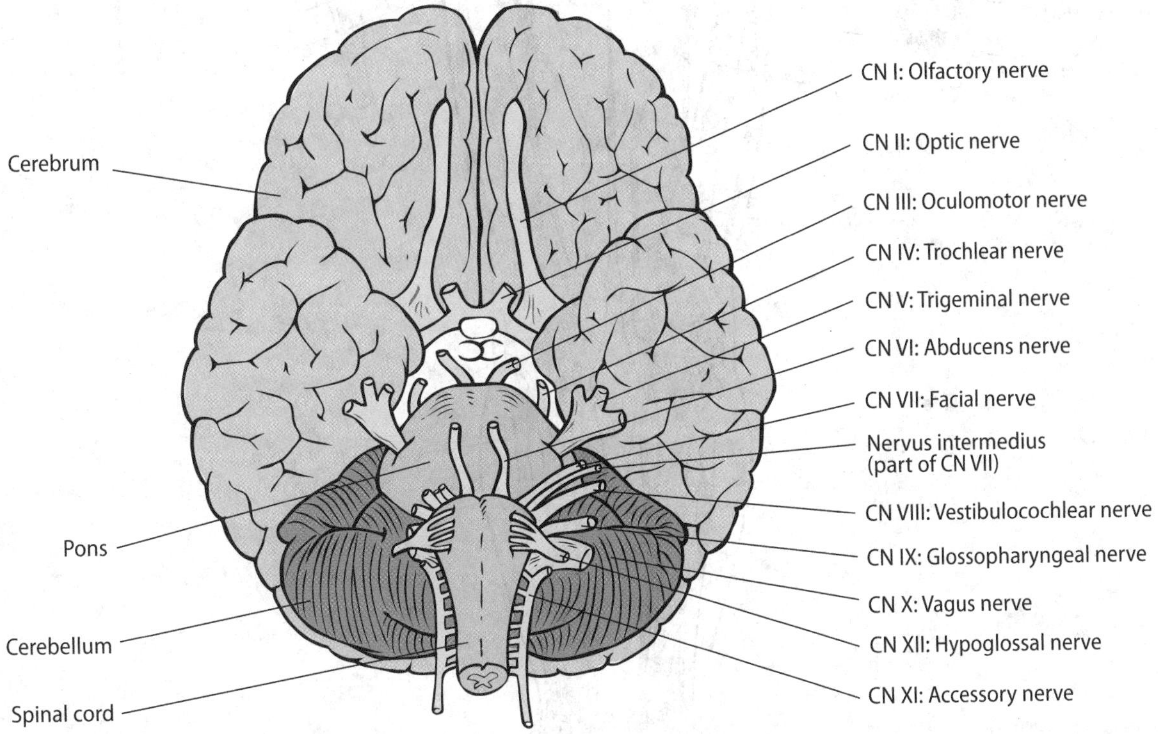

Peripheral Nervous System

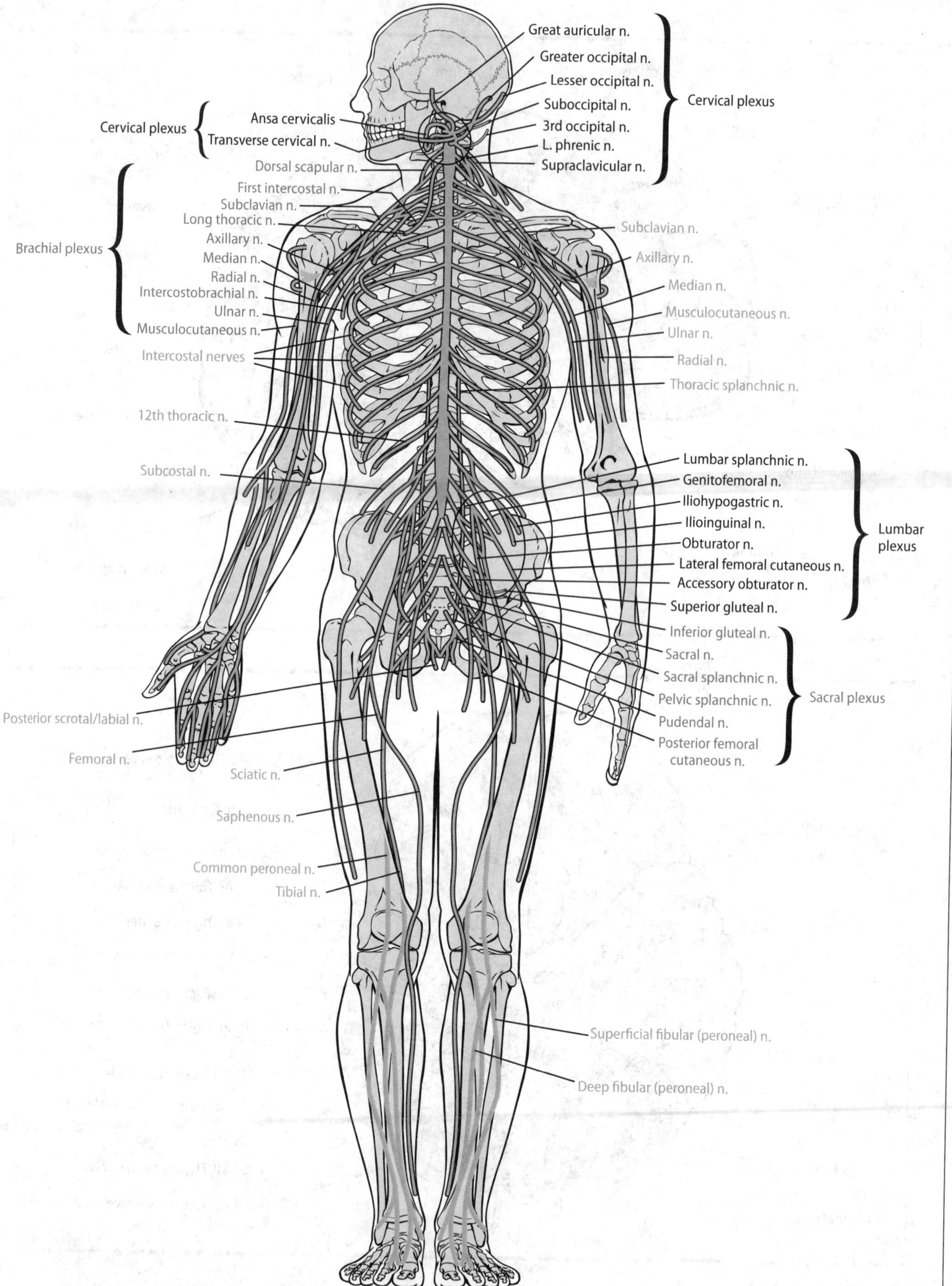

Spinal Cord and Spinal Nerves

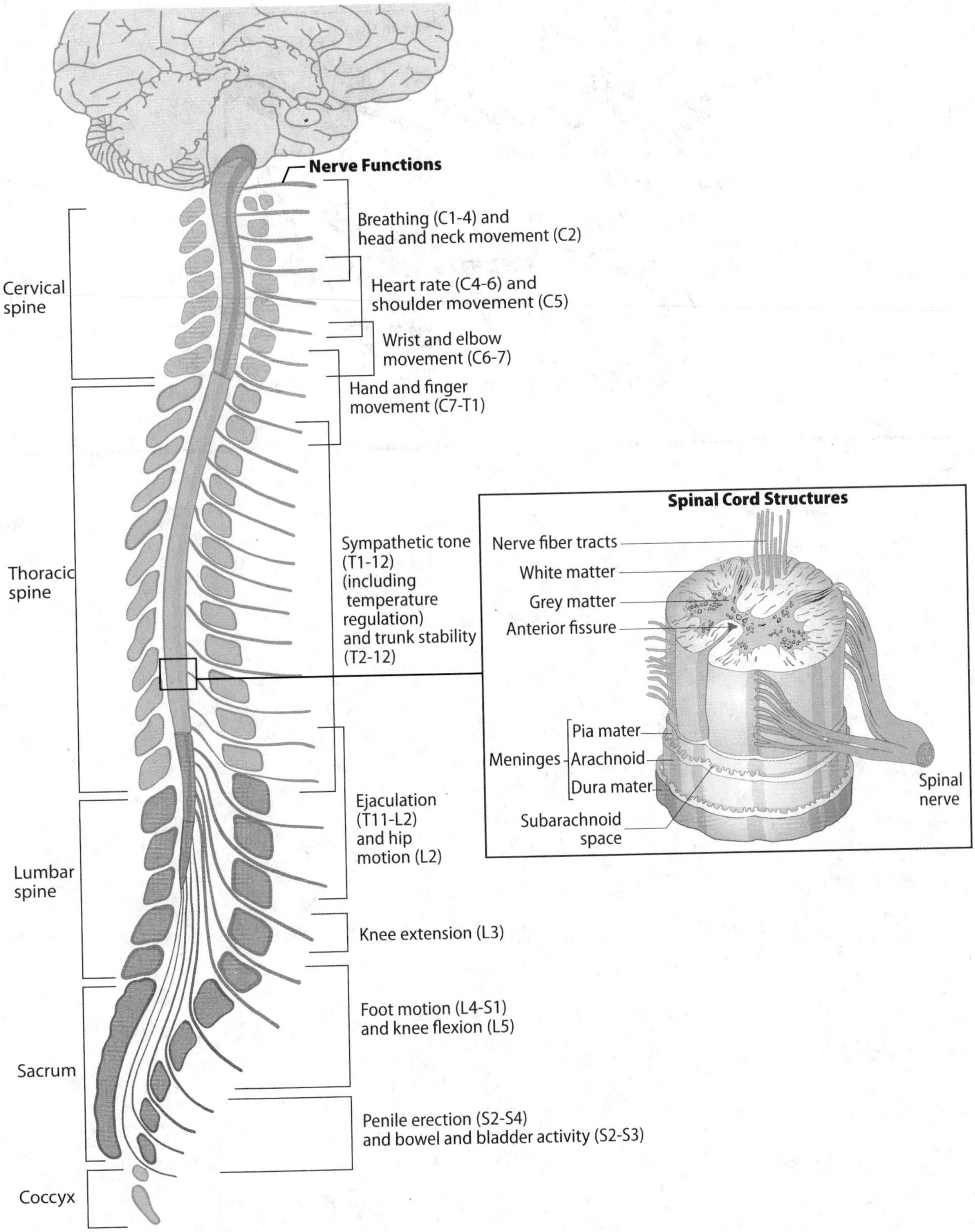

Nerve Cell

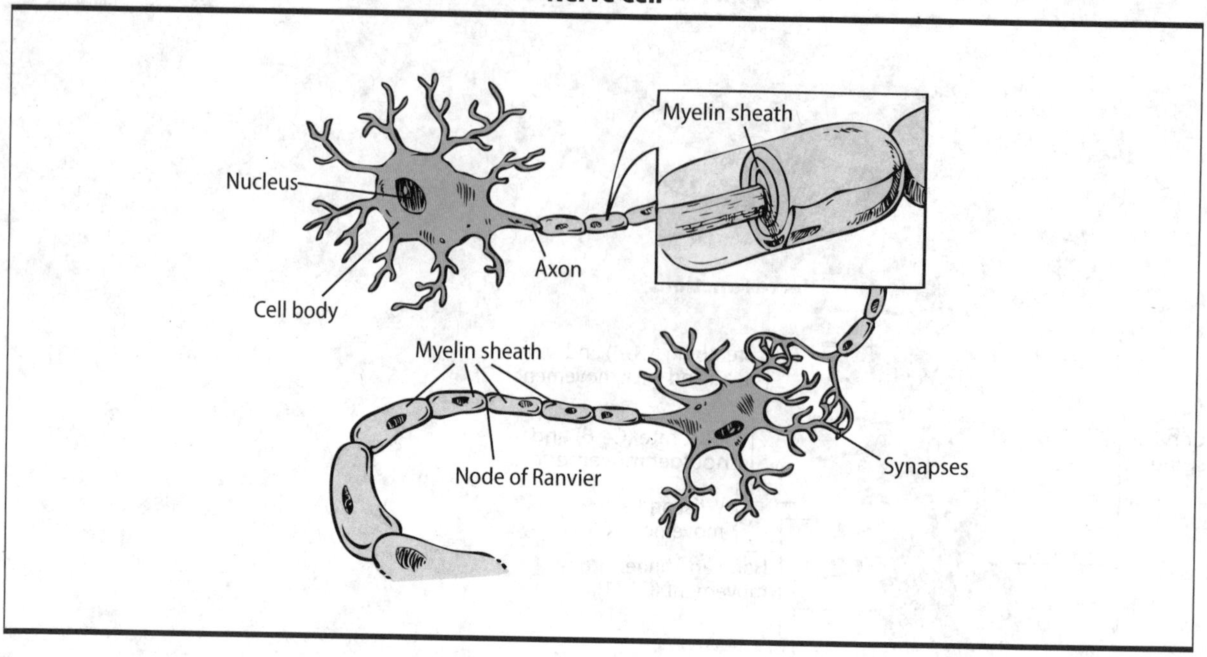
Myelin sheath
Nucleus
Axon
Cell body
Myelin sheath
Synapses
Node of Ranvier

Chapter 7. Diseases of the Eye and Adnexa (HØØ–H59)

Eye

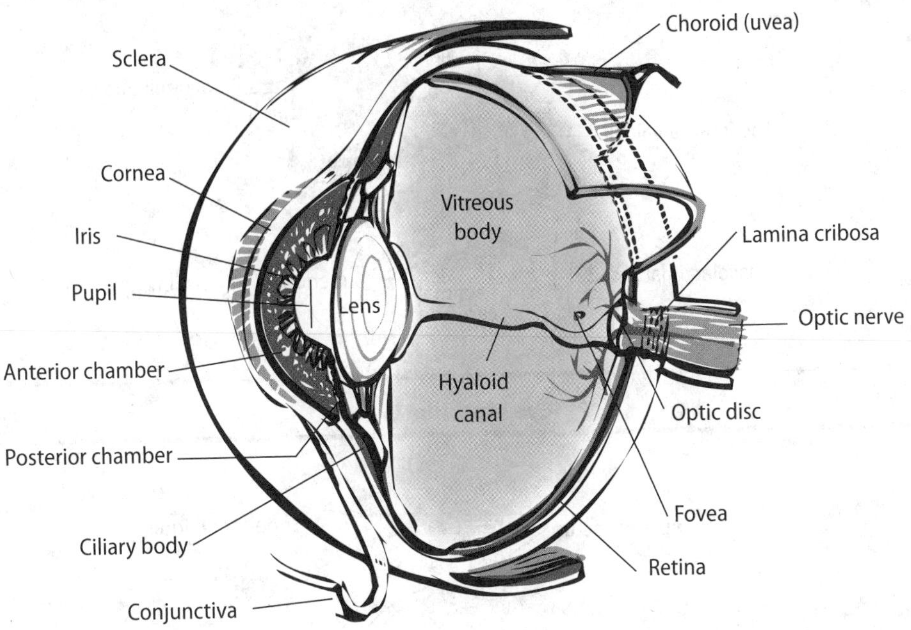

Posterior Pole of Globe/Flow of Aqueous Humor

Posterior Pole of Globe

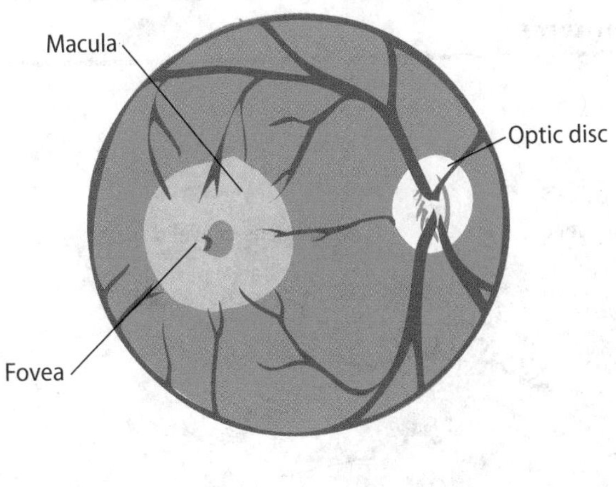

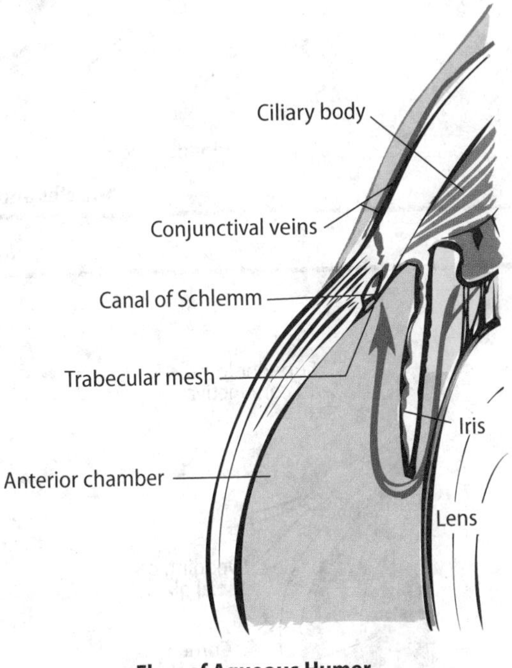

Flow of Aqueous Humor

Lacrimal System

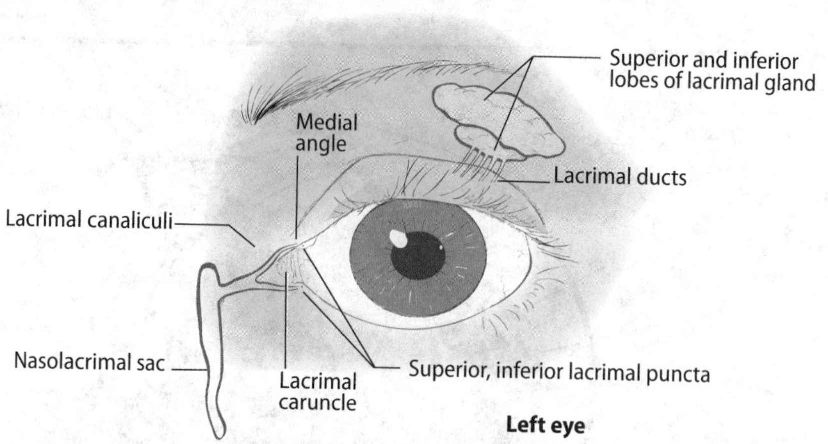

Left eye

Eye Musculature

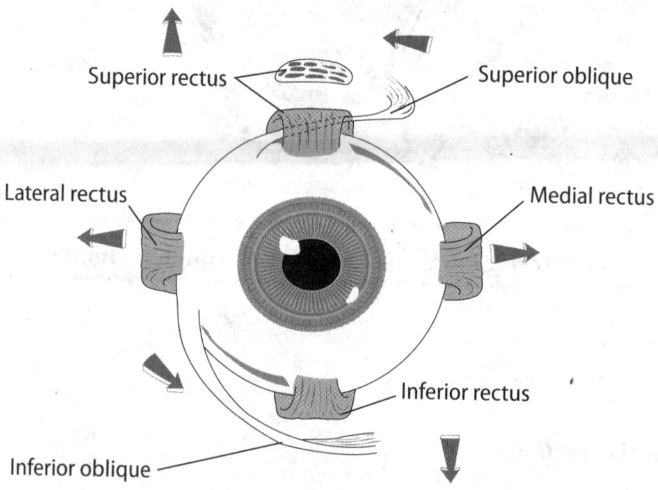

Muscles and actions (right eye)

Eyelid Structures

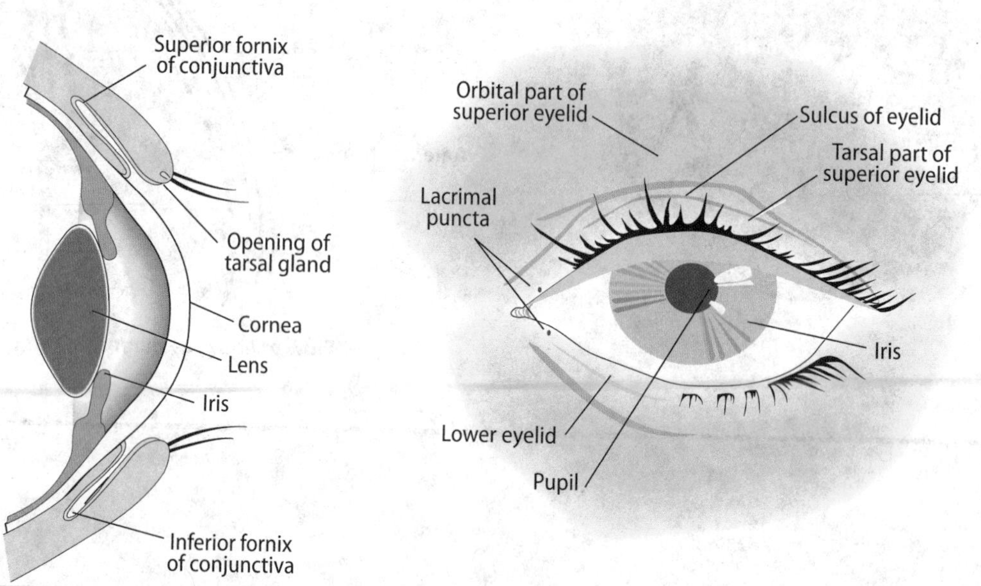

Chapter 8. Diseases of the Ear and Mastoid Process (H6Ø–H95)

Ear Anatomy

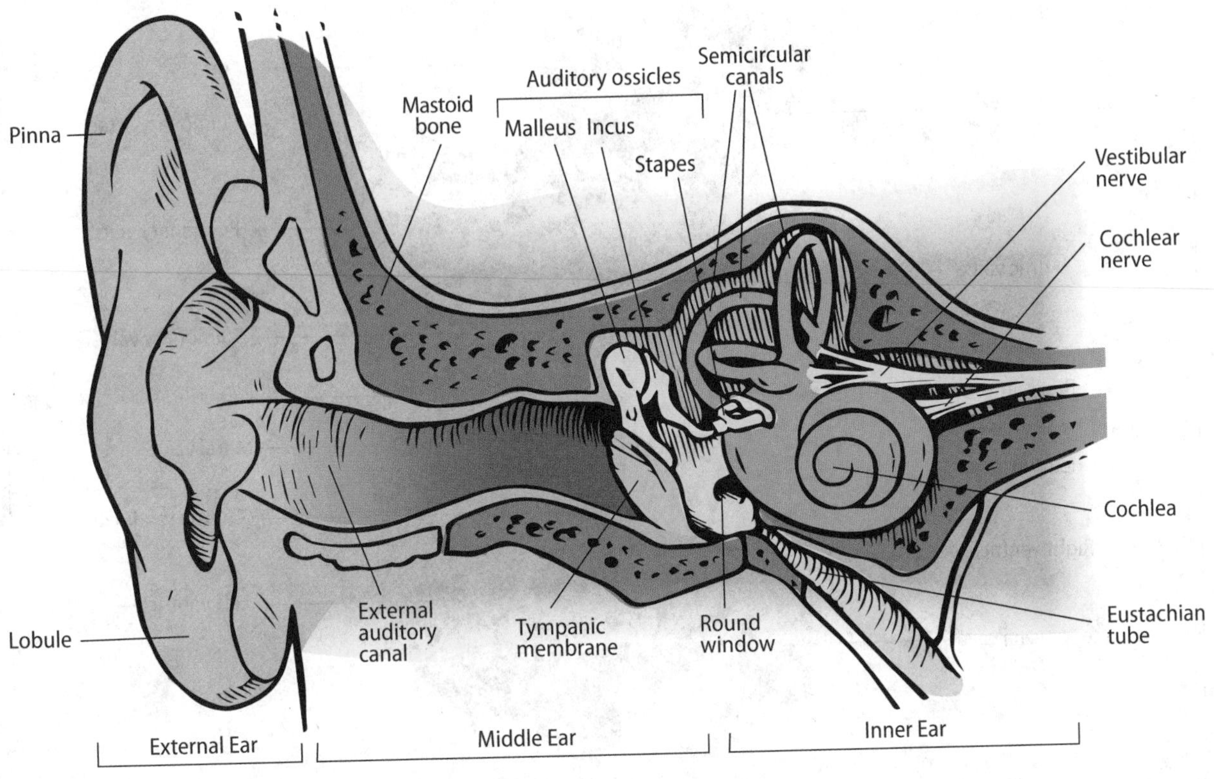

Chapter 9. Diseases of the Circulatory System (I00–I99)

Anatomy of the Heart

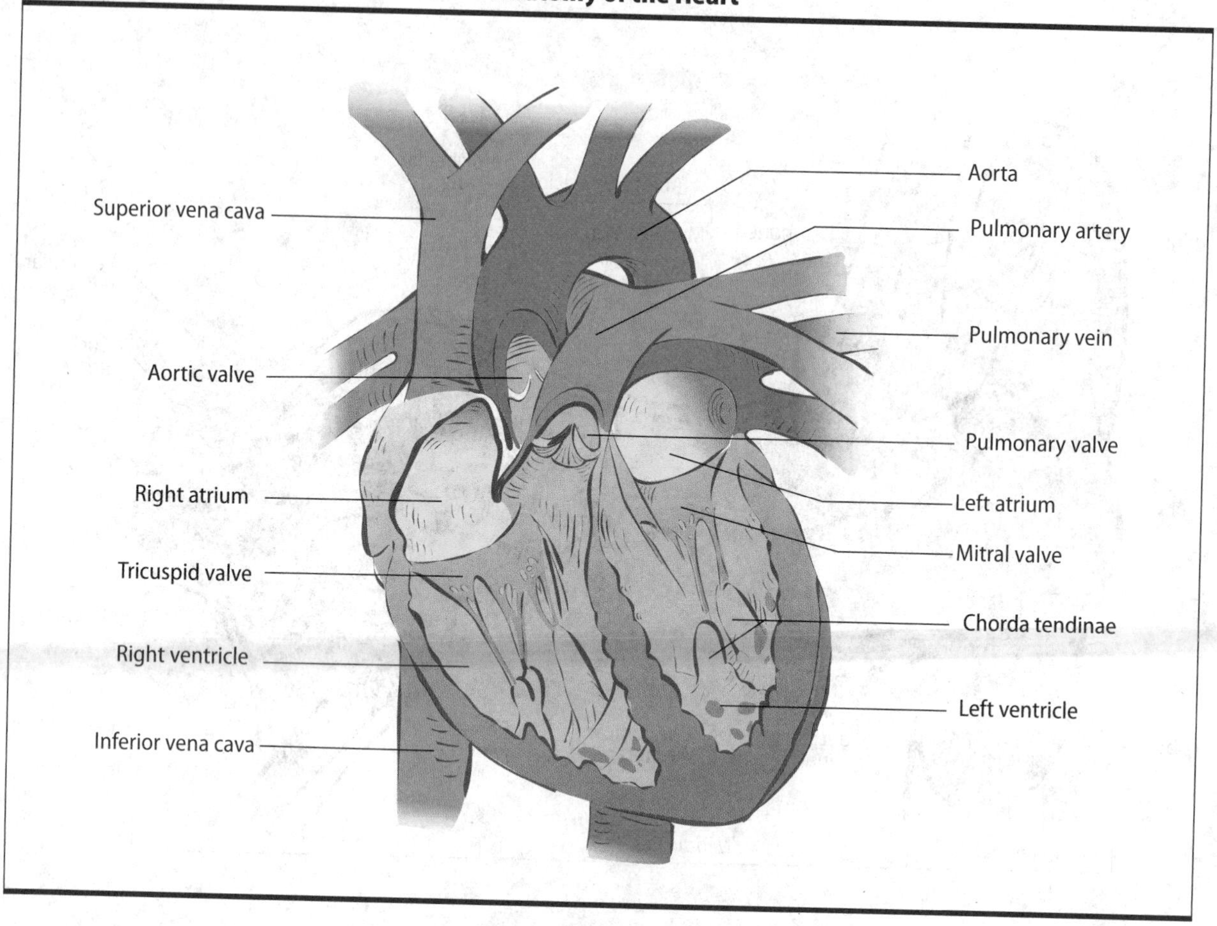

Heart Cross Section

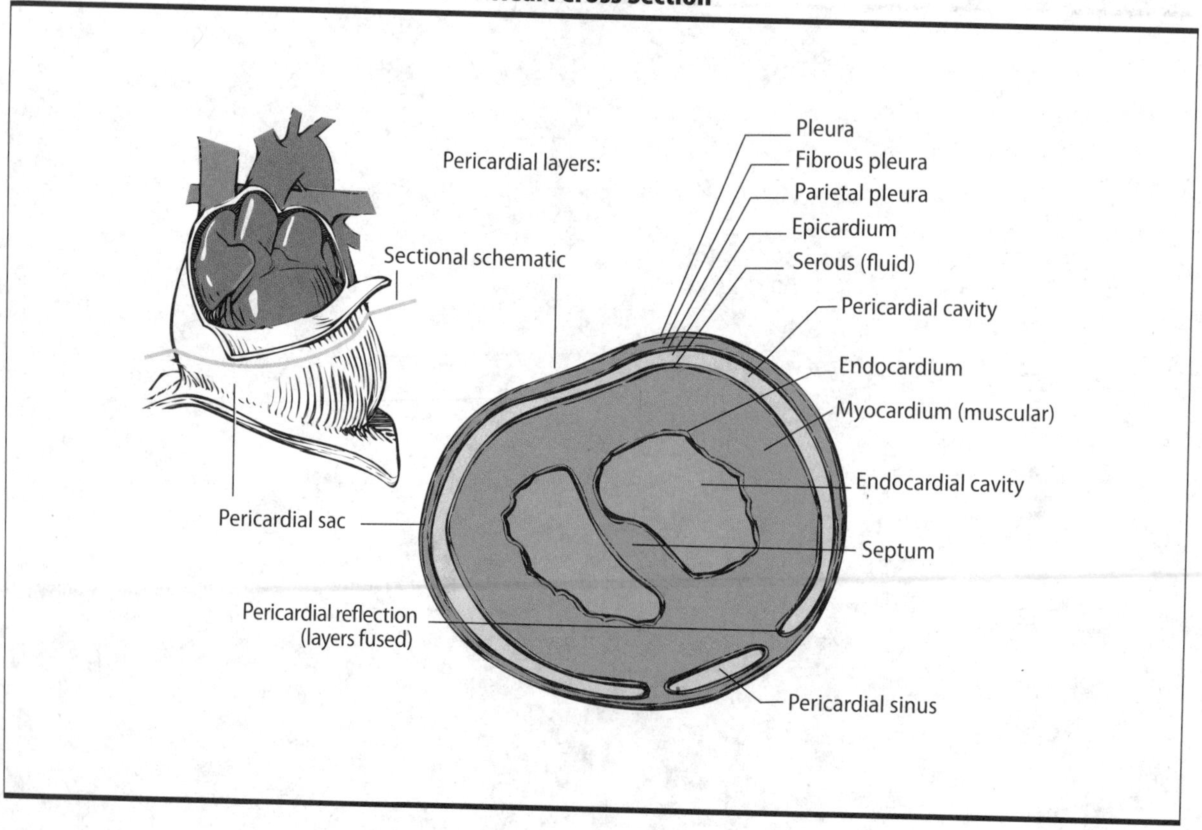

Heart Valves

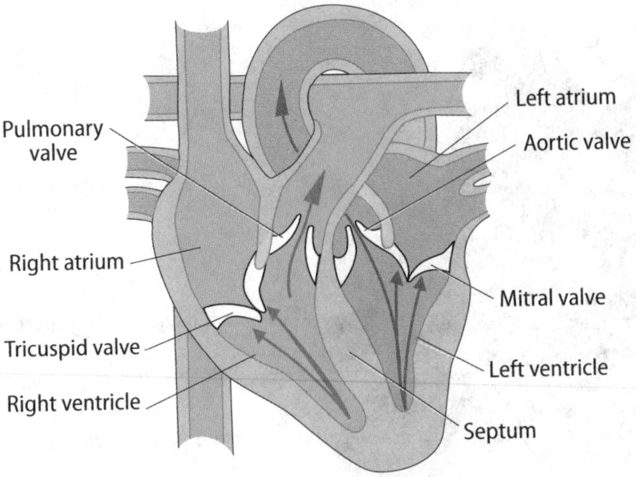

Schematic shows valves of the heart as blood is pumped out. The septum is the wall dividing the left and right ventricles. The papillary muscles and chordae tendineae (above right) function to open and close the atrioventricular valves

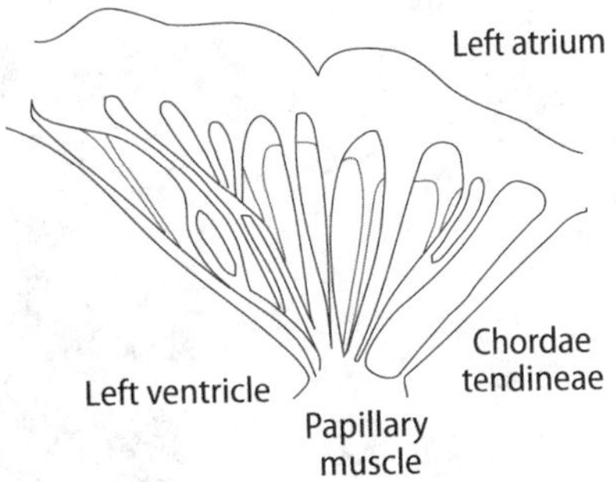

Side view of a mitral valve leaflet

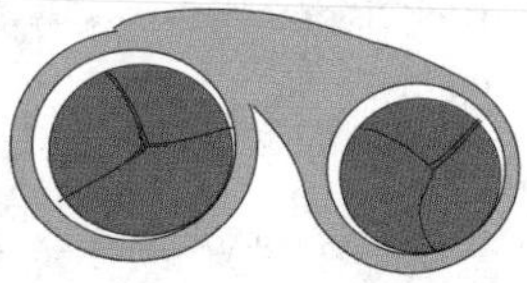

Overhead view of aortic (left) and pulmonary valves while closed

Heart Conduction System

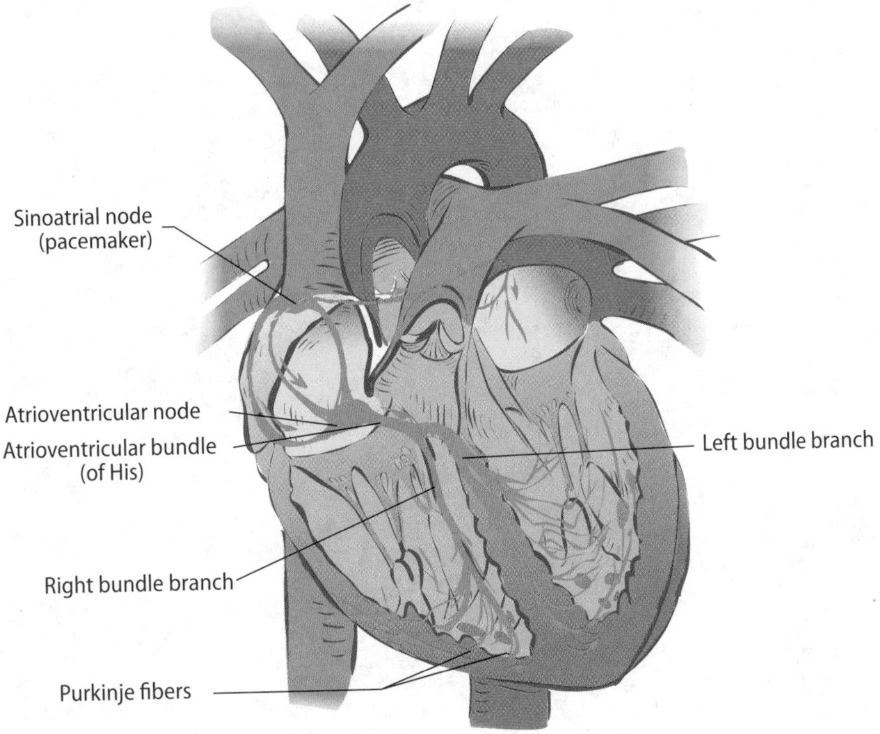

Coronary Arteries

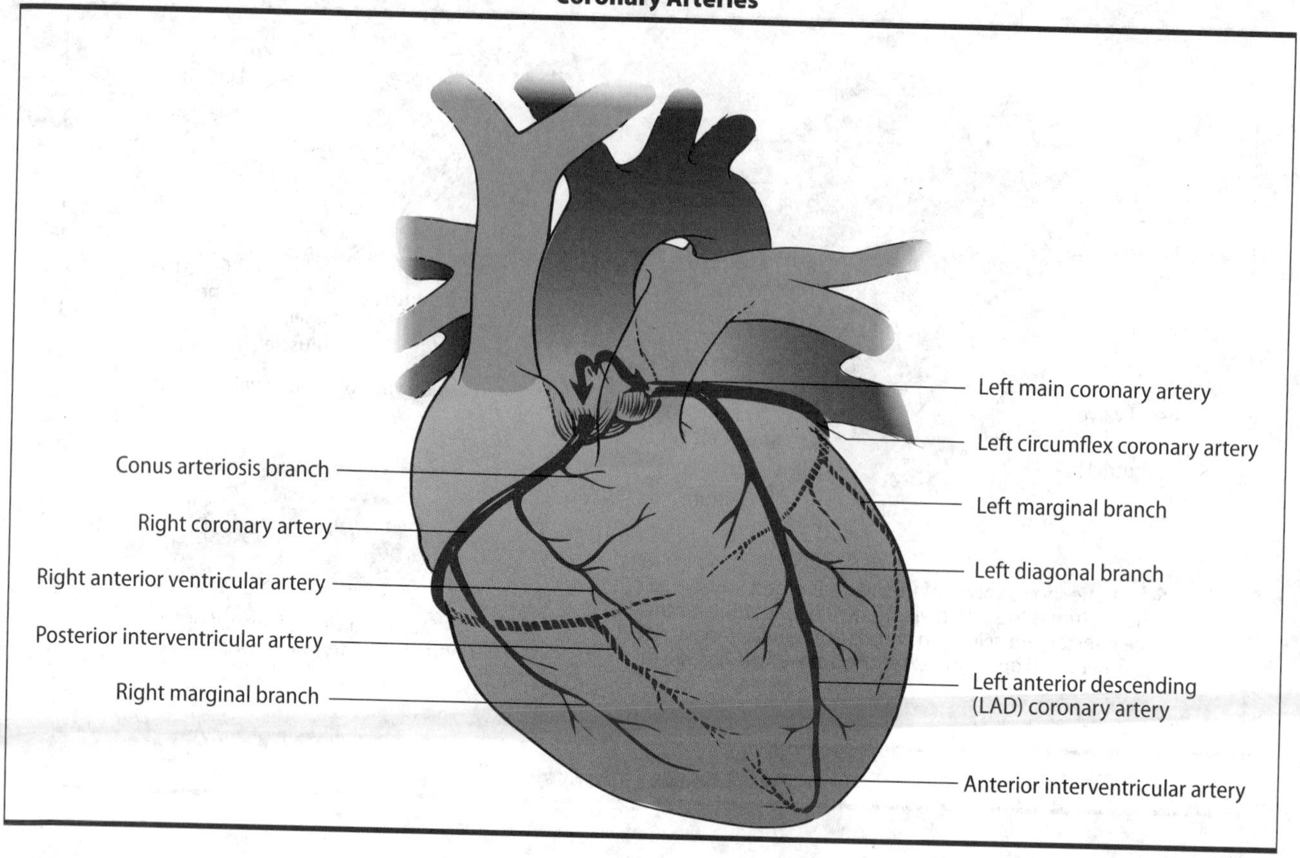

Arteries

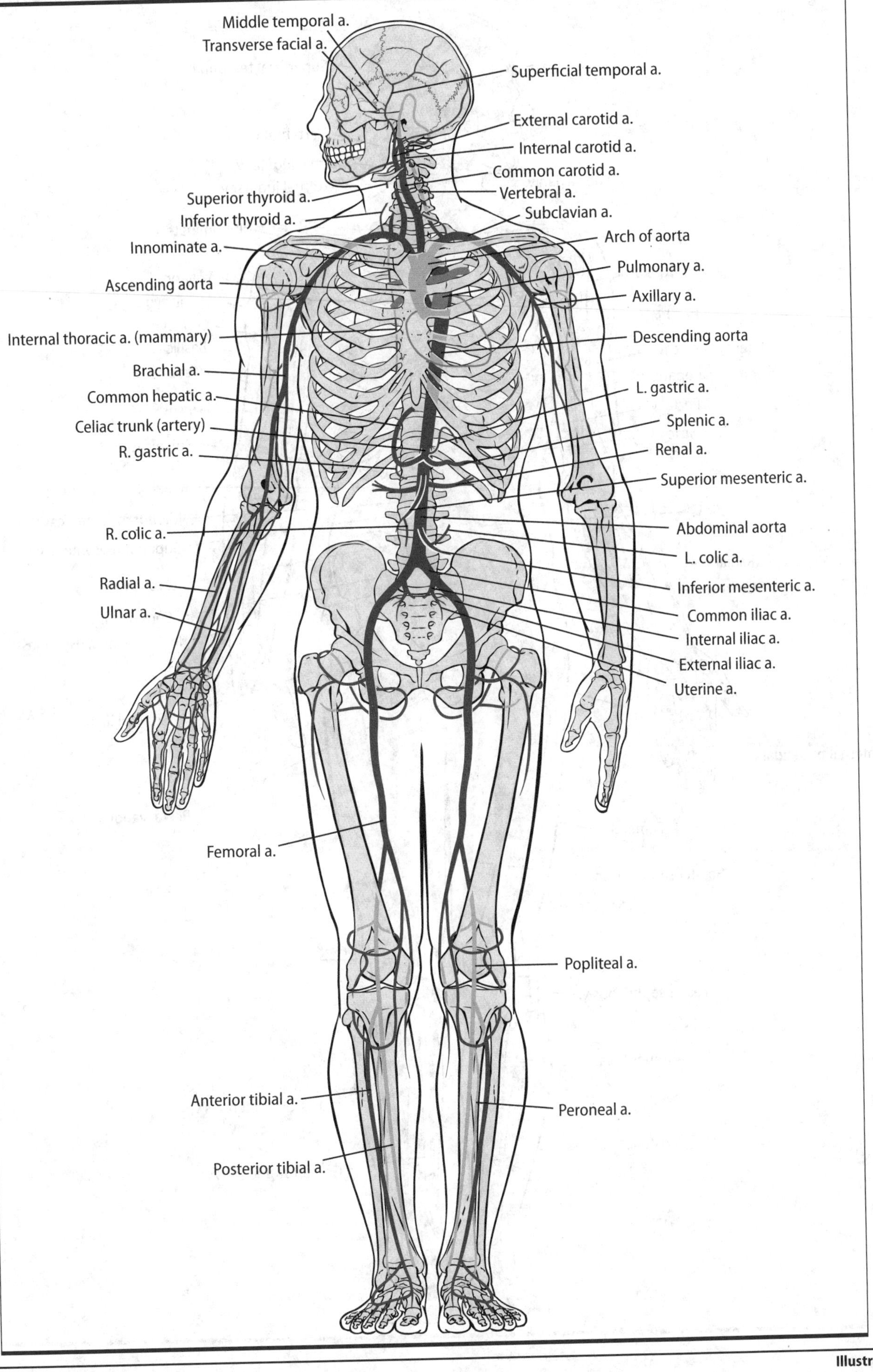
Middle temporal a.
Transverse facial a.
Superficial temporal a.
External carotid a.
Internal carotid a.
Common carotid a.
Superior thyroid a.
Vertebral a.
Inferior thyroid a.
Subclavian a.
Arch of aorta
Innominate a.
Pulmonary a.
Ascending aorta
Axillary a.
Internal thoracic a. (mammary)
Descending aorta
Brachial a.
L. gastric a.
Common hepatic a.
Splenic a.
Celiac trunk (artery)
Renal a.
R. gastric a.
Superior mesenteric a.
R. colic a.
Abdominal aorta
L. colic a.
Radial a.
Inferior mesenteric a.
Ulnar a.
Common iliac a.
Internal iliac a.
External iliac a.
Uterine a.
Femoral a.
Popliteal a.
Anterior tibial a.
Peroneal a.
Posterior tibial a.

Veins

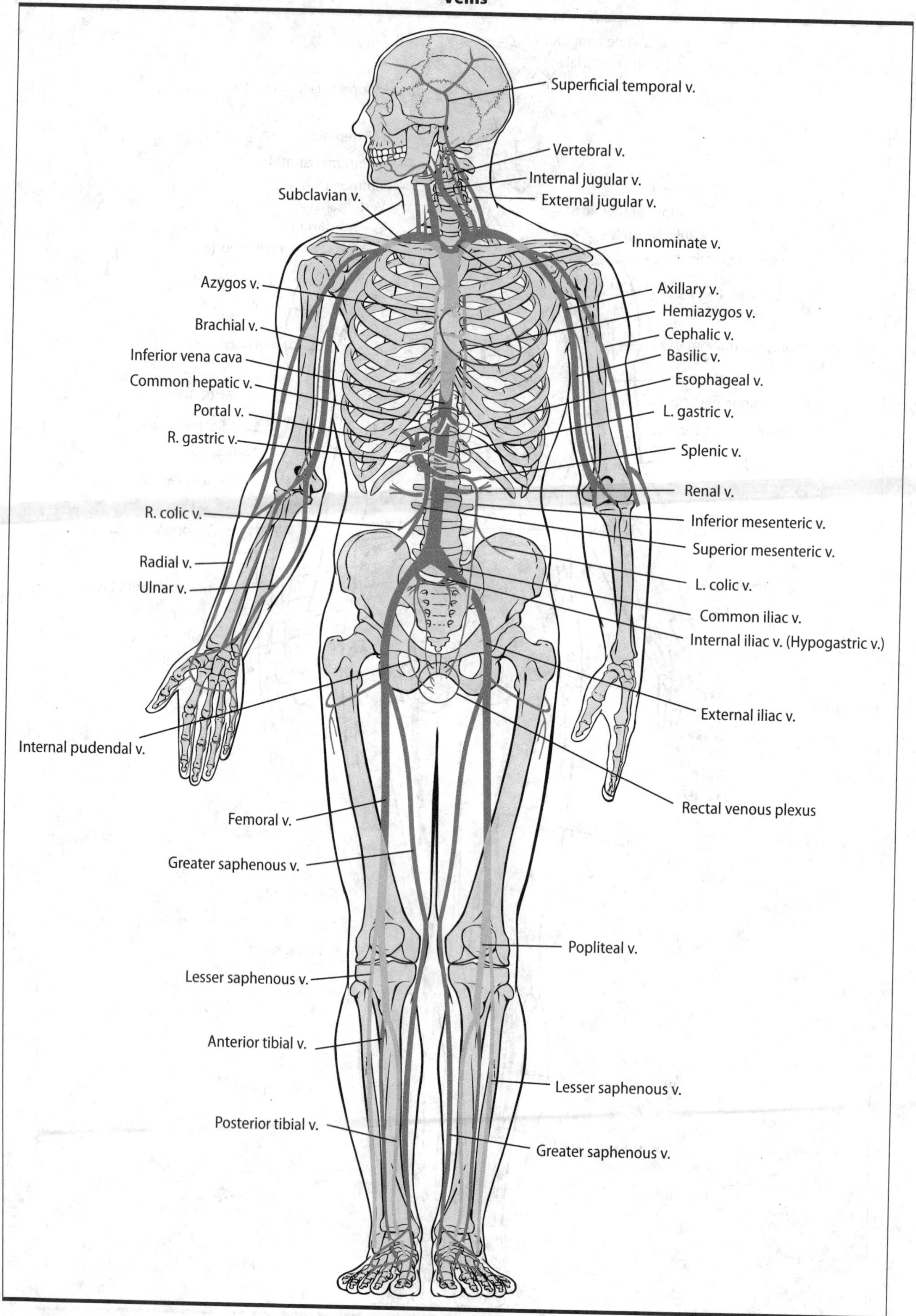
Superficial temporal v.
Vertebral v.
Internal jugular v.
External jugular v.
Subclavian v.
Innominate v.
Azygos v.
Axillary v.
Hemiazygos v.
Brachial v.
Cephalic v.
Inferior vena cava
Basilic v.
Common hepatic v.
Esophageal v.
Portal v.
L. gastric v.
R. gastric v.
Splenic v.
Renal v.
R. colic v.
Inferior mesenteric v.
Superior mesenteric v.
Radial v.
Ulnar v.
L. colic v.
Common iliac v.
Internal iliac v. (Hypogastric v.)
External iliac v.
Internal pudendal v.
Rectal venous plexus
Femoral v.
Greater saphenous v.
Popliteal v.
Lesser saphenous v.
Anterior tibial v.
Lesser saphenous v.
Posterior tibial v.
Greater saphenous v.

Internal Carotid and Vertebral Arteries and Branches

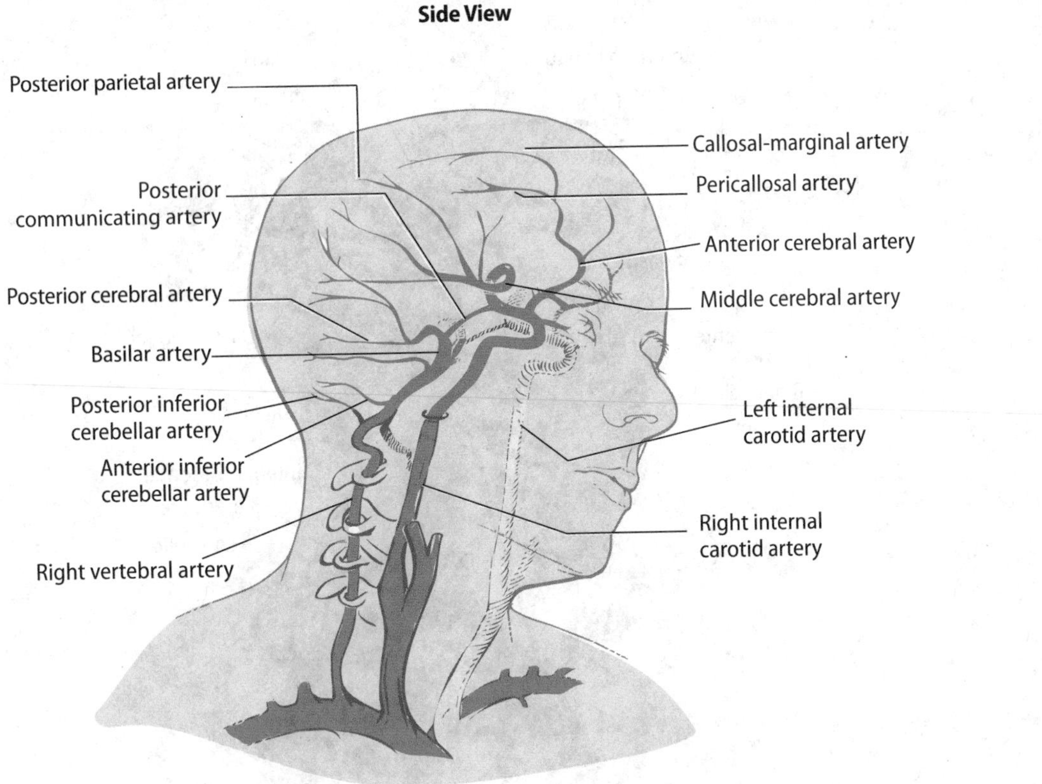

External Carotid Artery and Branches

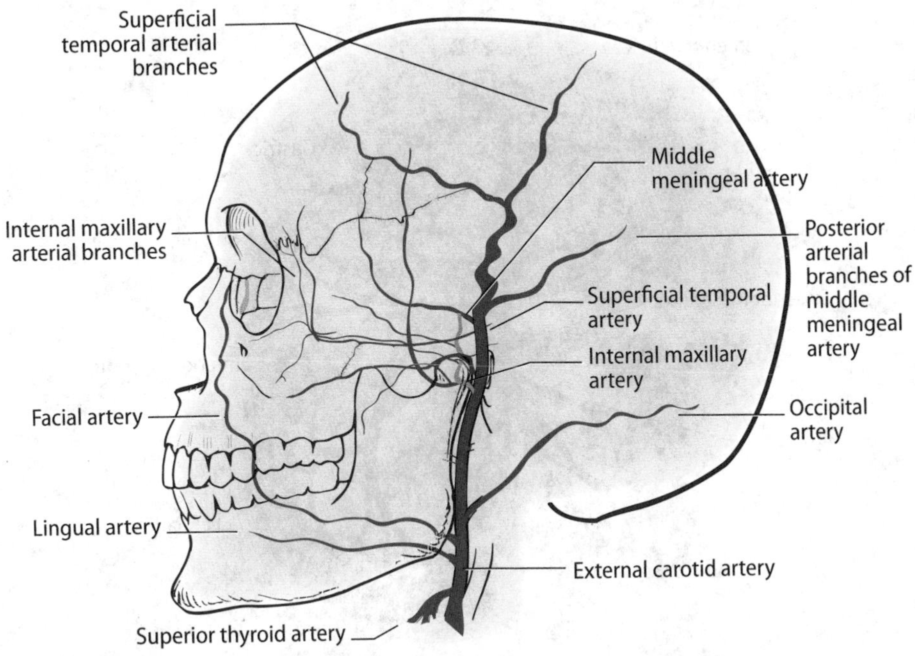

Branches of Abdominal Aorta

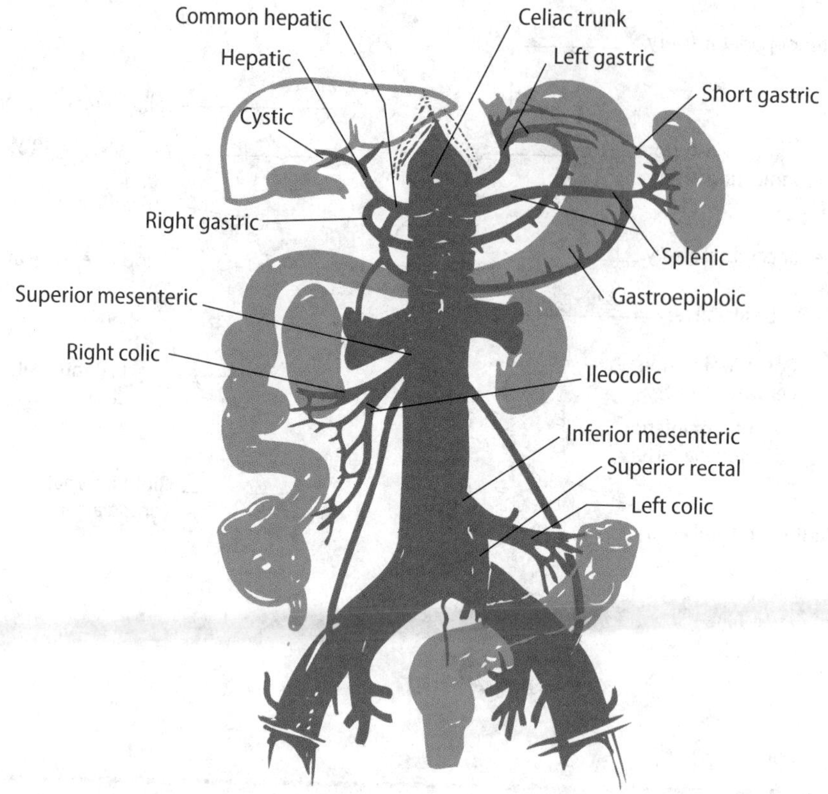

Portal Venous Circulation

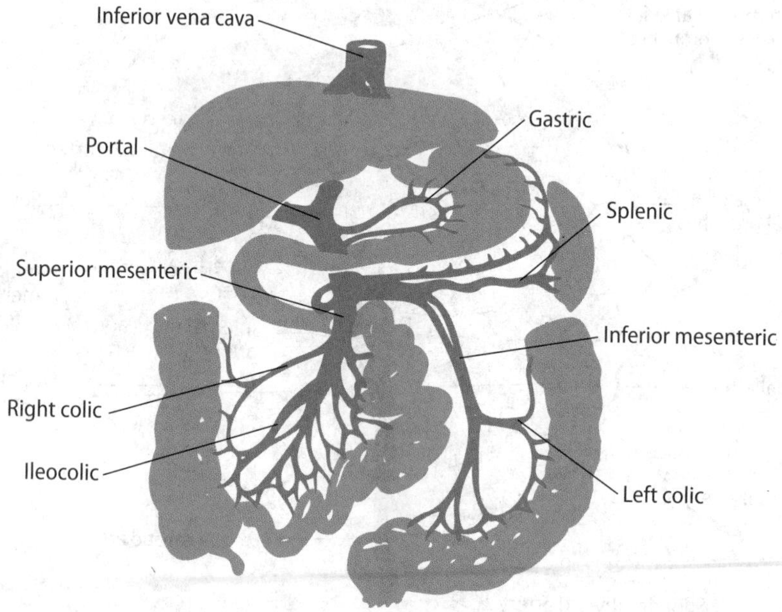

Lymphatic System

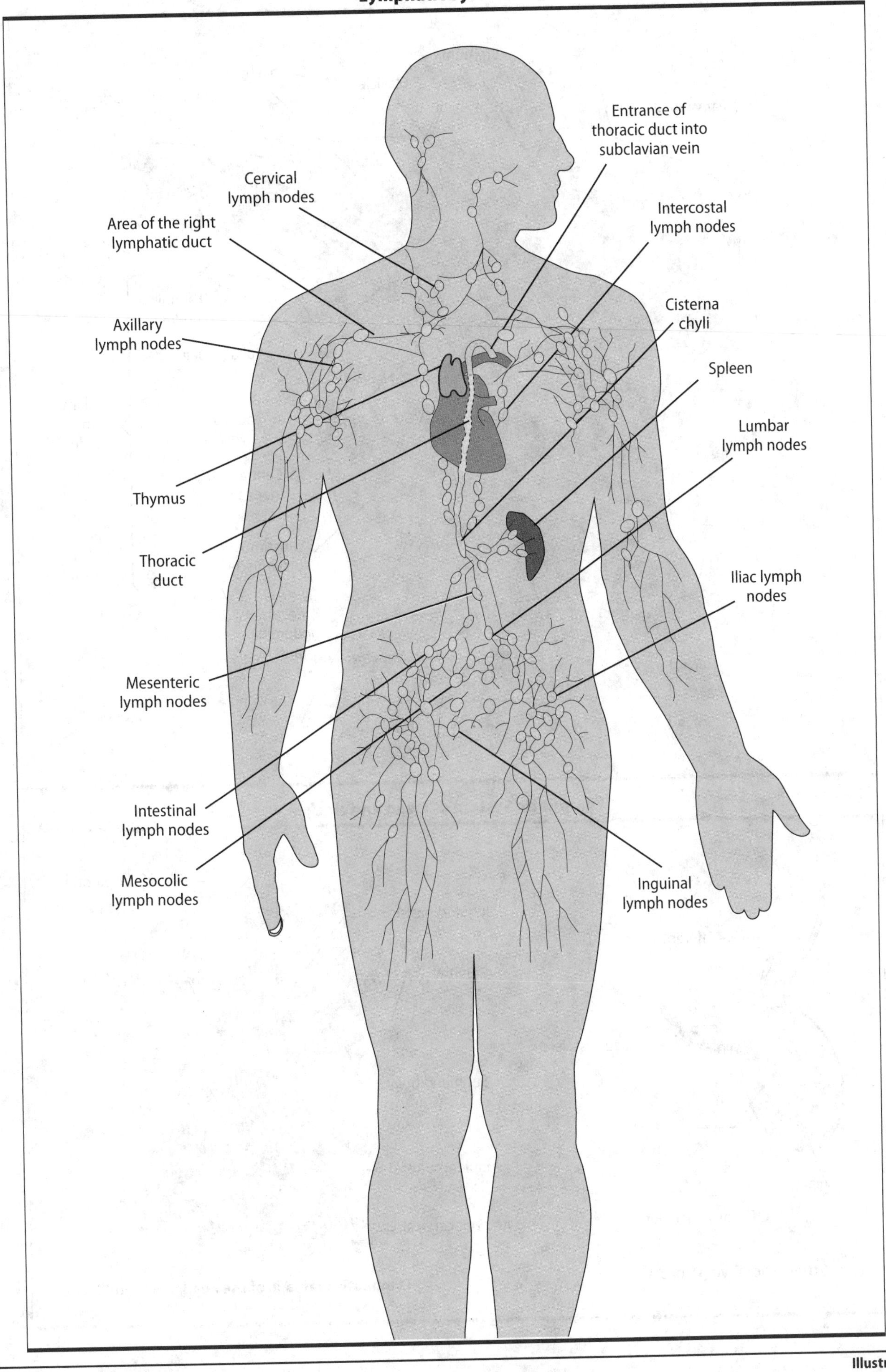

Axillary Lymph Nodes

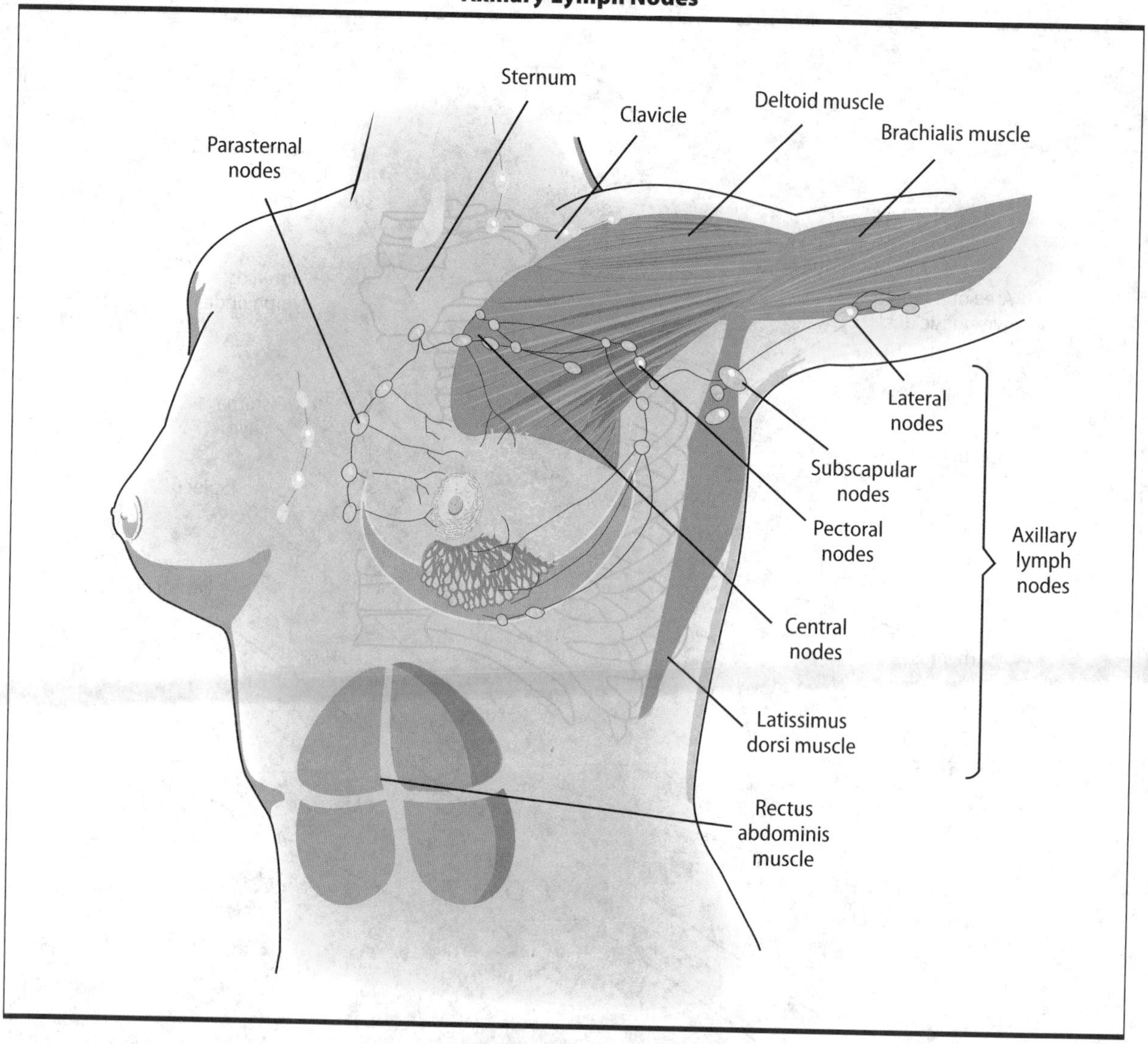

Lymphatic System of Head and Neck

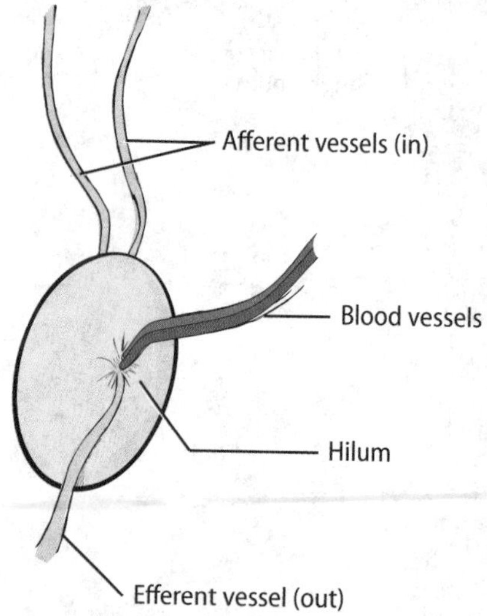

Schematic of lymph node

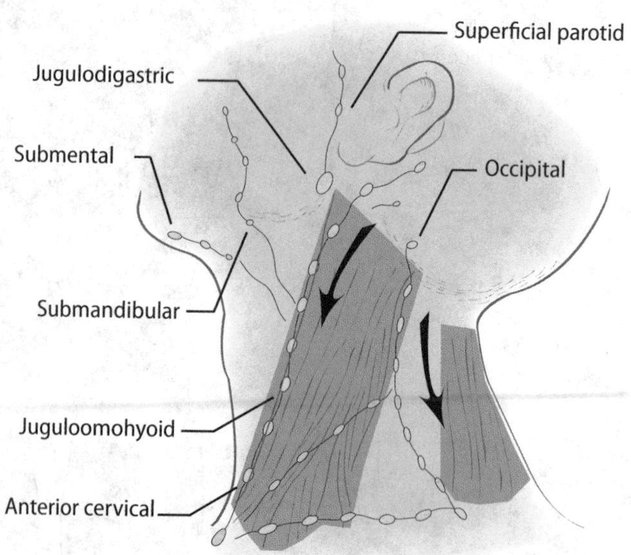

Lymphatic drainage of the head, neck, and face

Lymphatic Capillaries

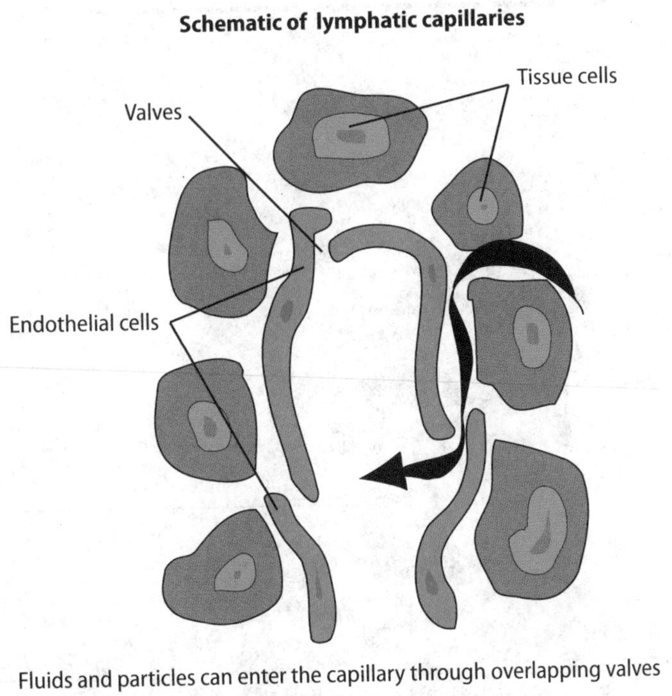

Lymphatic Drainage

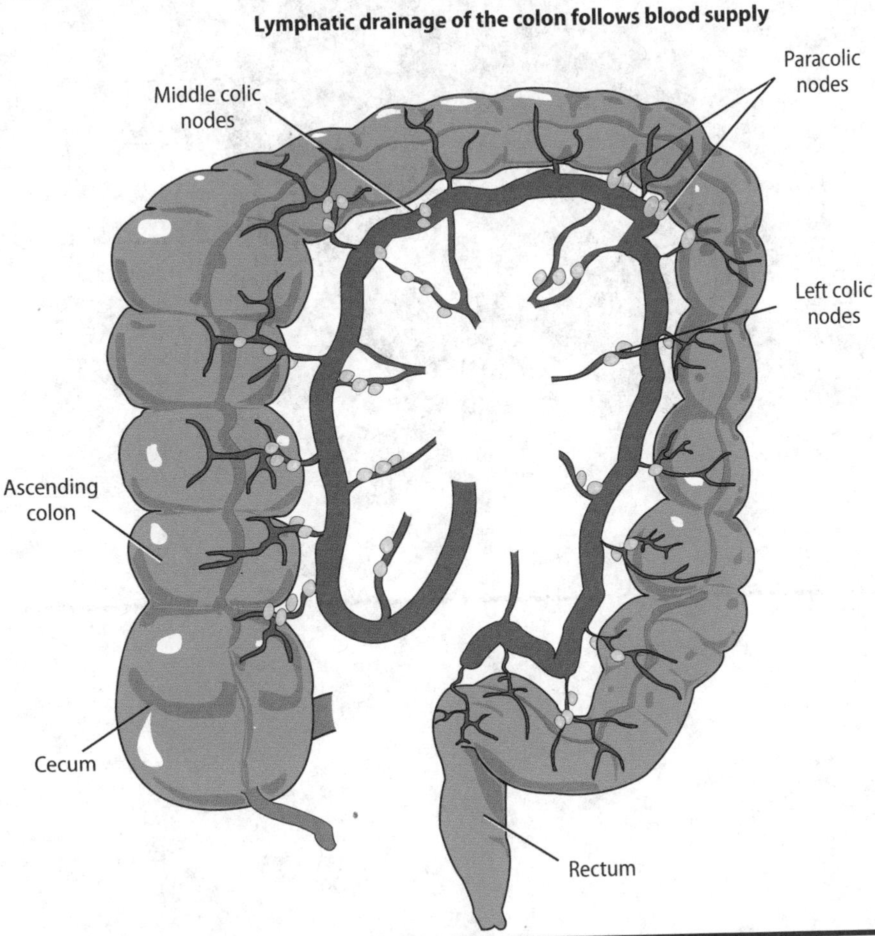

Chapter 10. Diseases of the Respiratory System (JØØ–J99)

Respiratory System

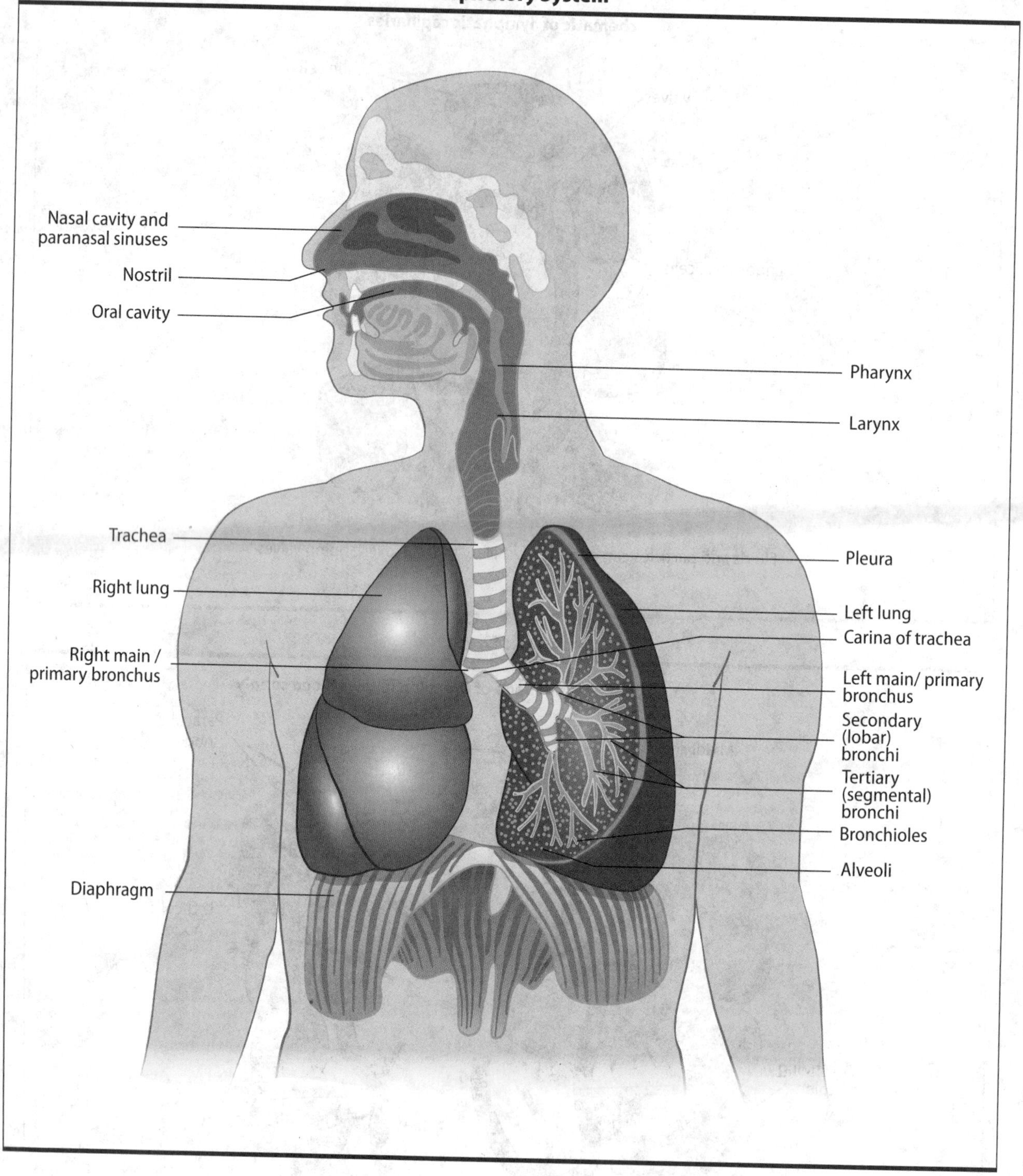

Upper Respiratory System

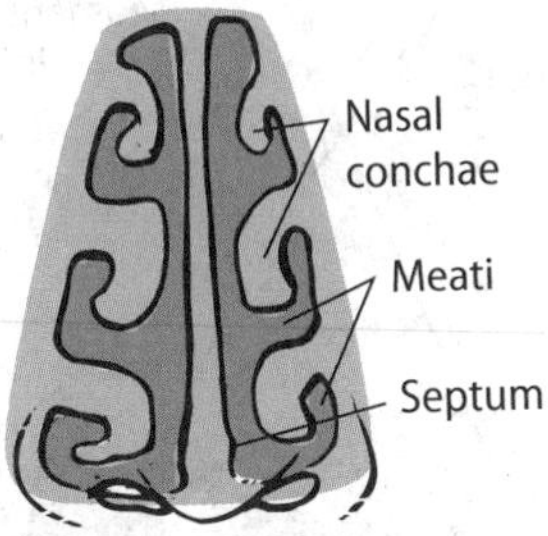

Nasal cavity from front

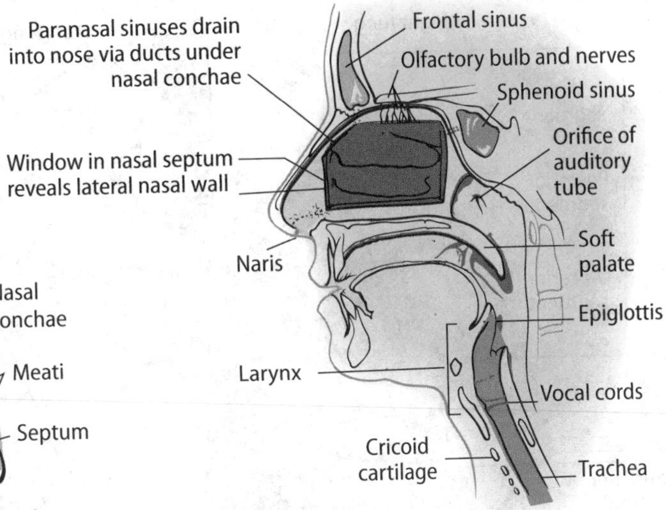

Lower Respiratory System

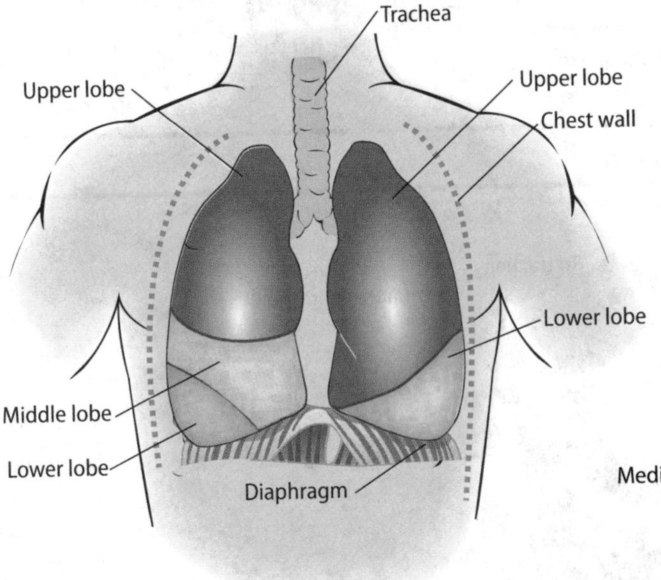

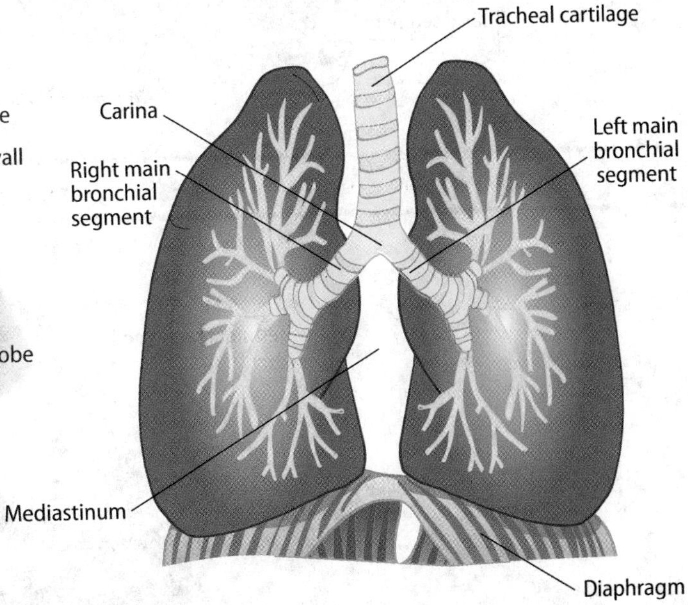

Paranasal Sinuses

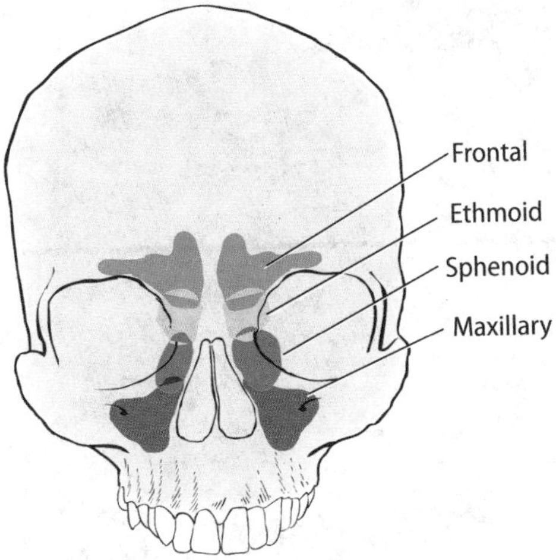

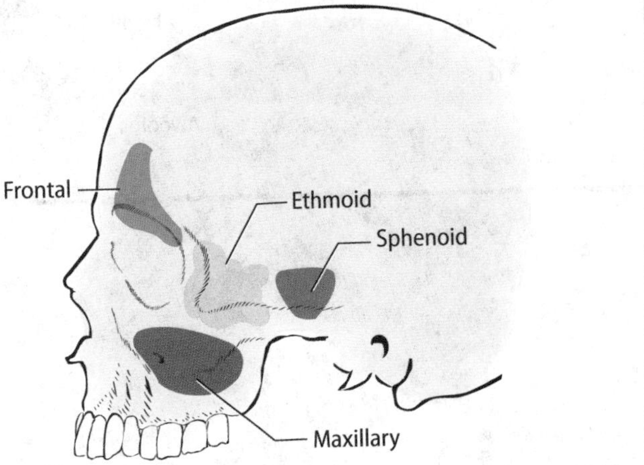

Lung Segments

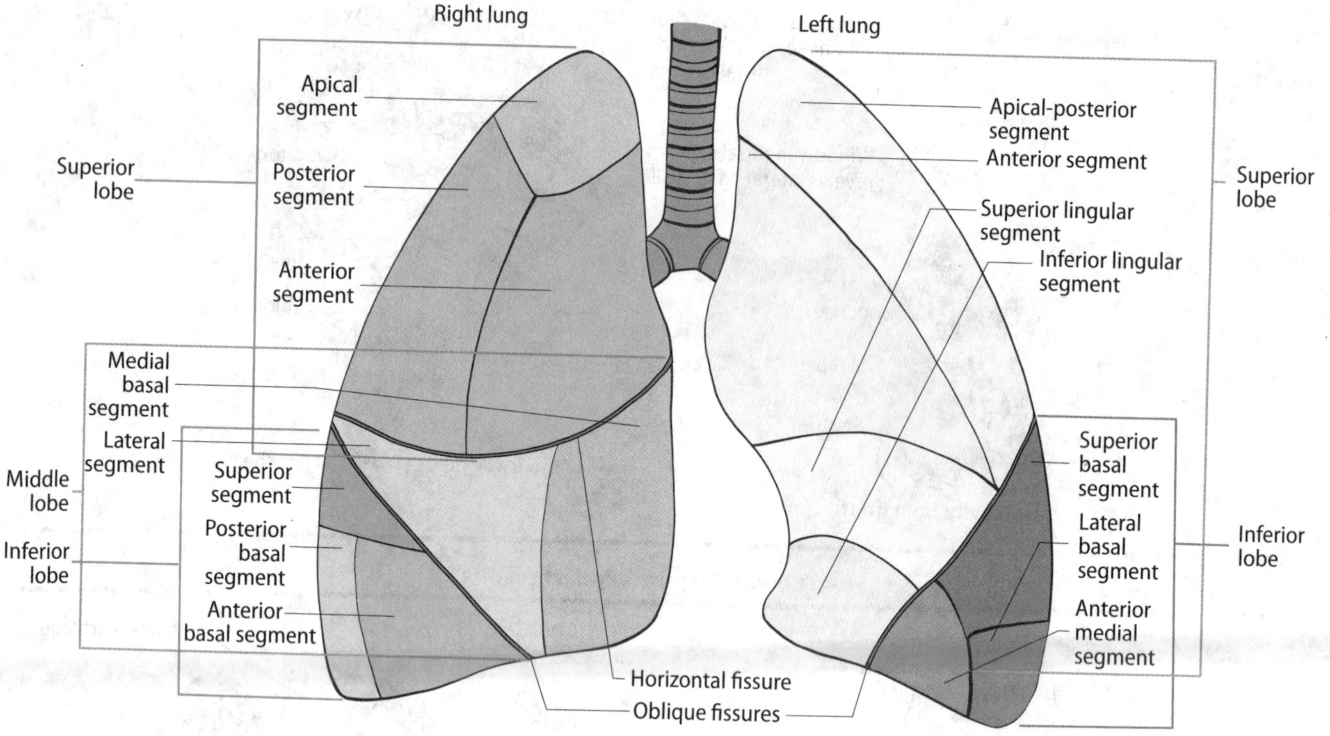

Alveoli

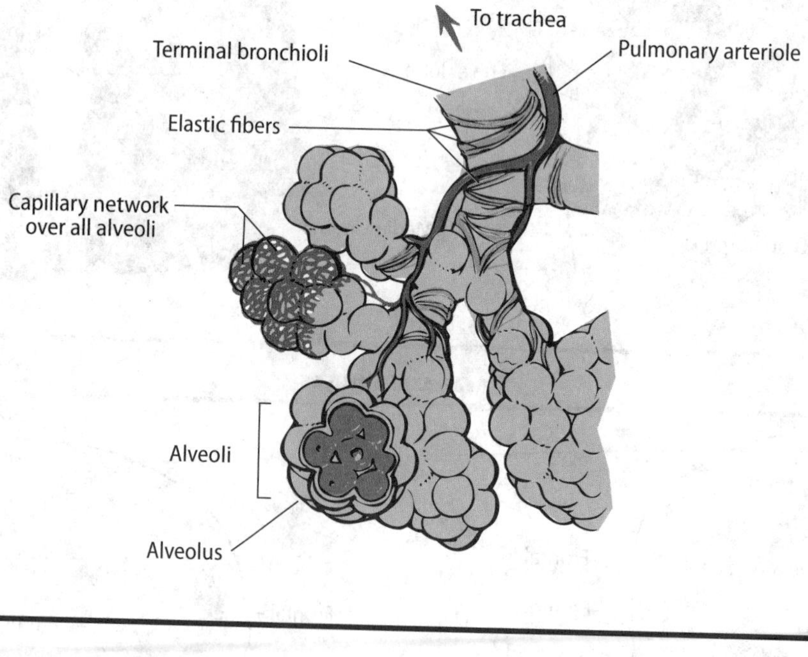

Chapter 11. Diseases of the Digestive System (KØØ–K95)

Digestive System

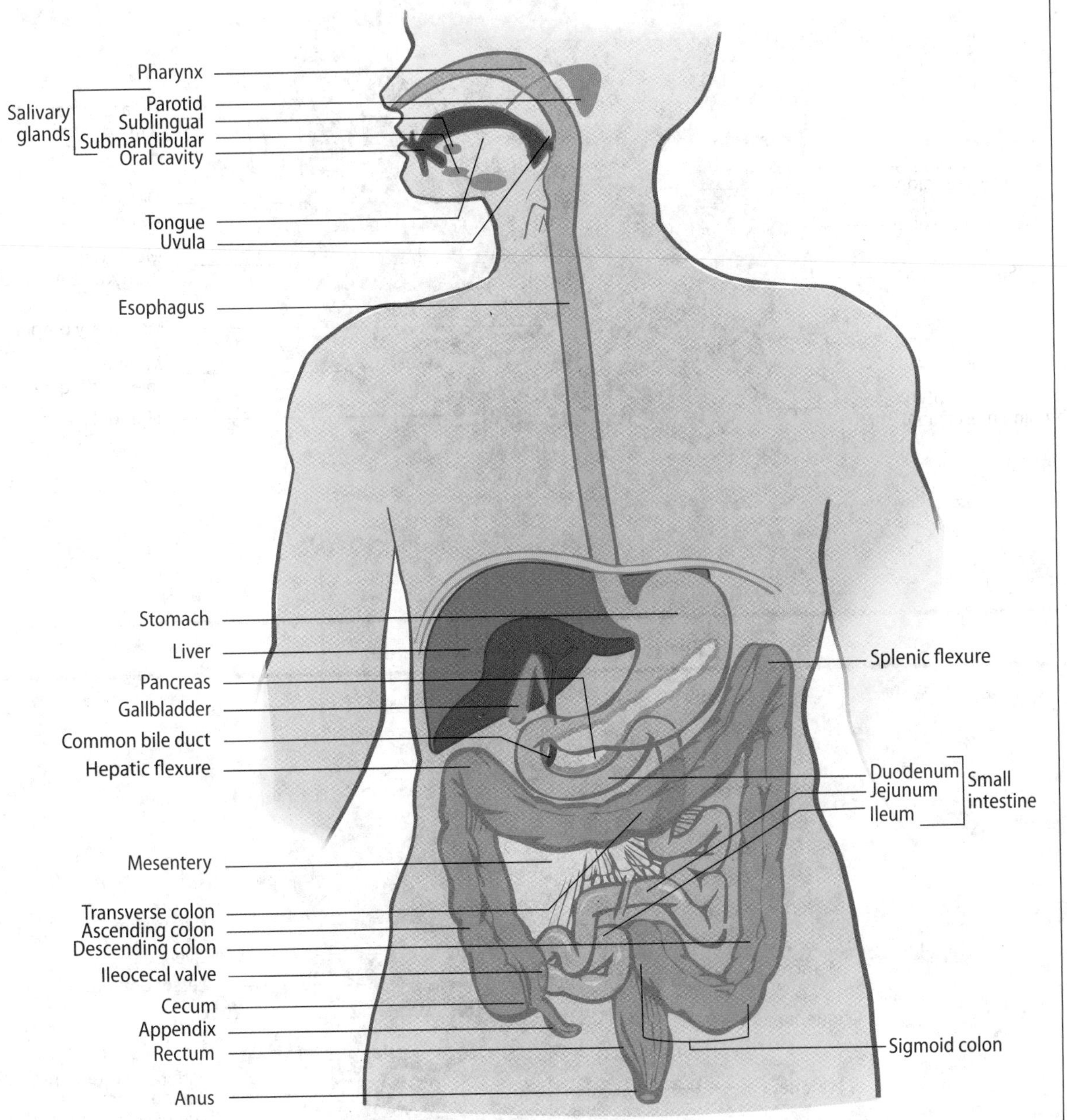

Omentum and Mesentery

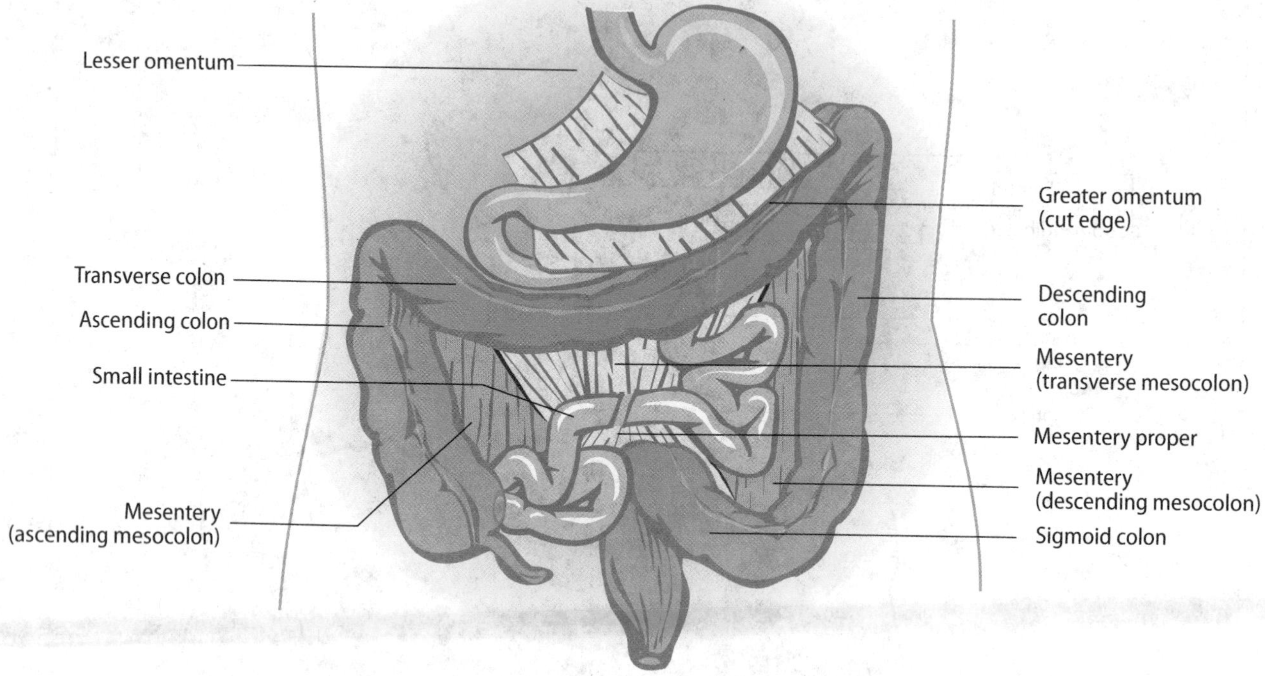

Peritoneum and Retroperitoneum

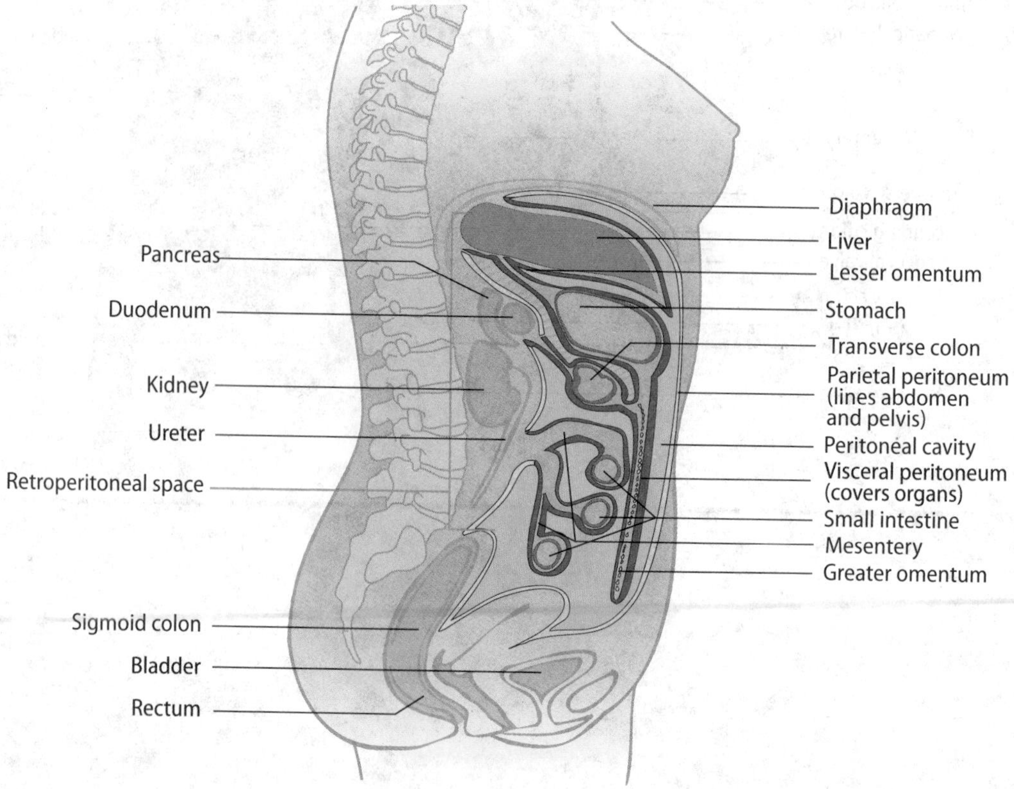

Chapter 12. Diseases of the Skin and Subcutaneous Tissue (LØØ–L99)

Nail Anatomy

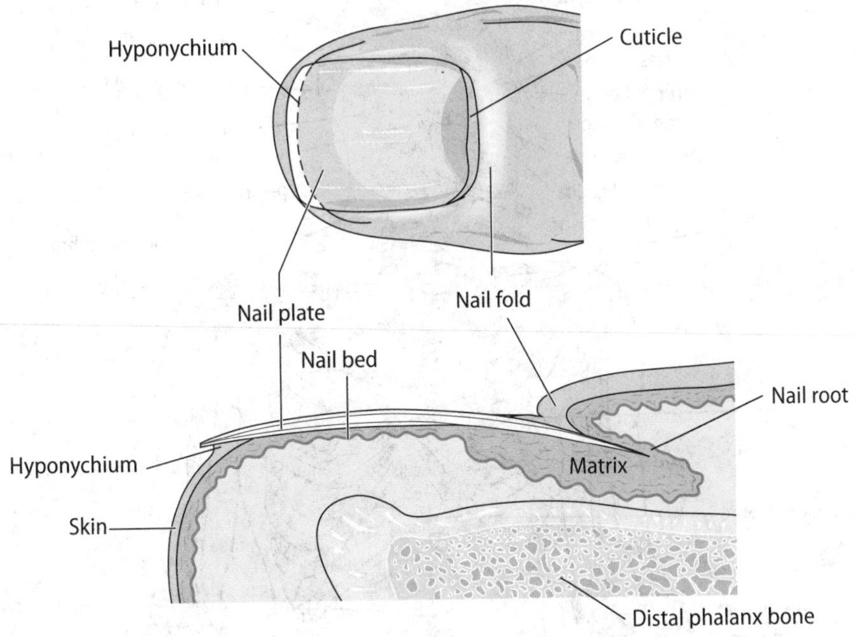

Skin and Subcutaneous Tissue

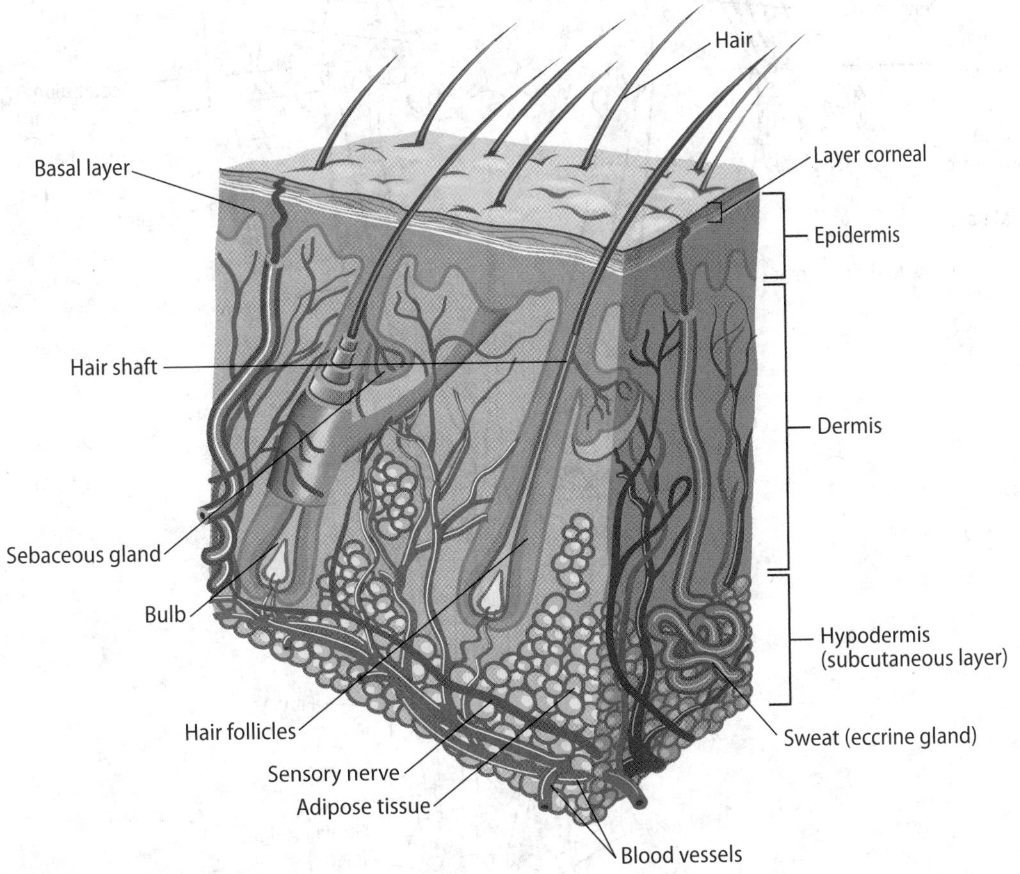

Chapter 13. Diseases of the Musculoskeletal System and Connective Tissue (MØØ–M99)

Bones and Joints

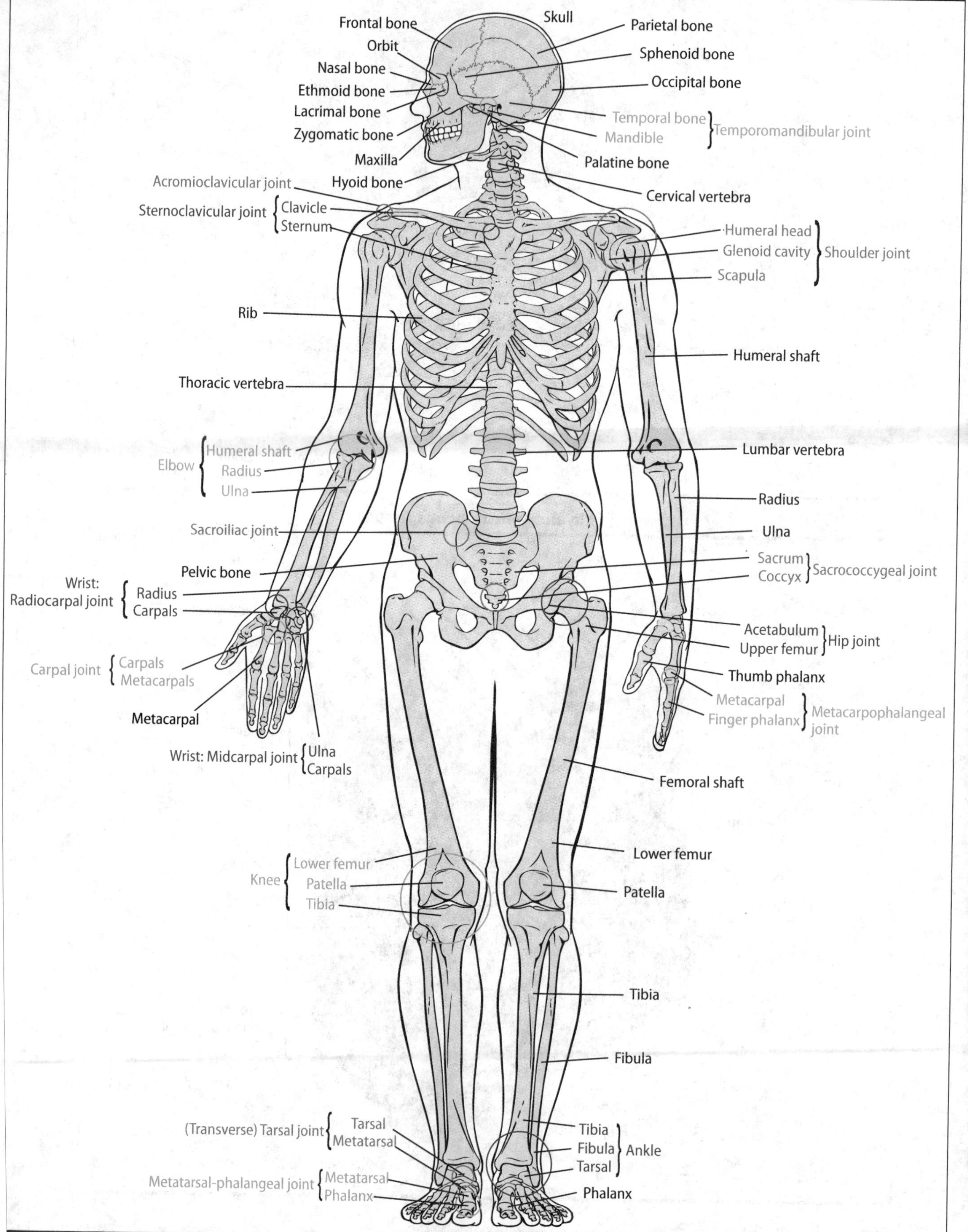

Shoulder Anterior View

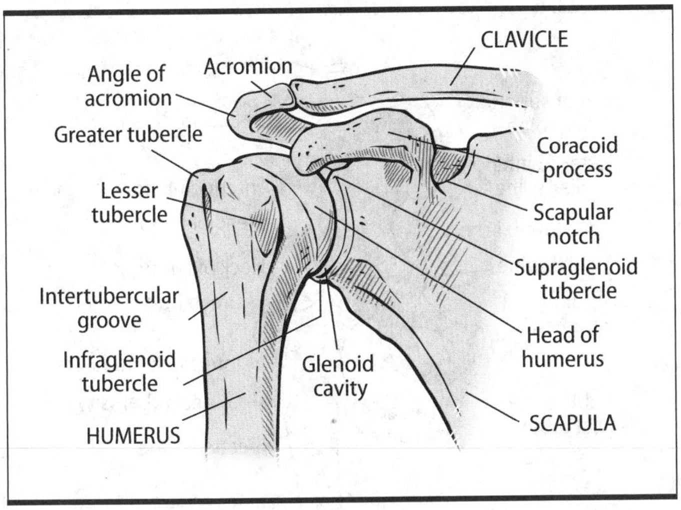

Shoulder Posterior View

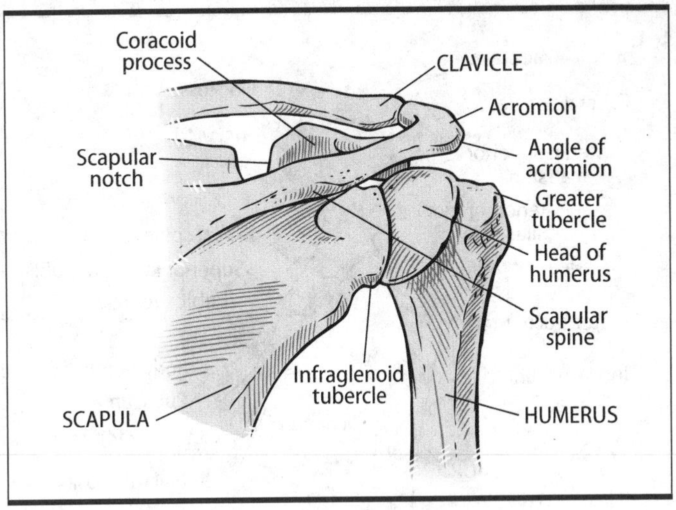

Elbow Anterior View

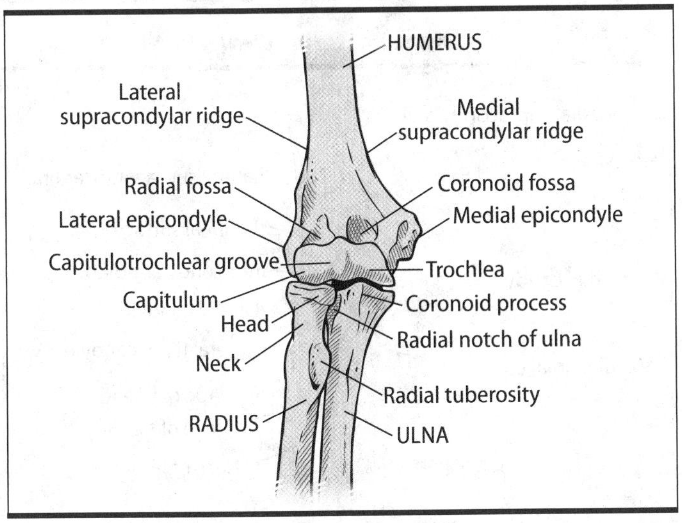

Elbow Posterior View

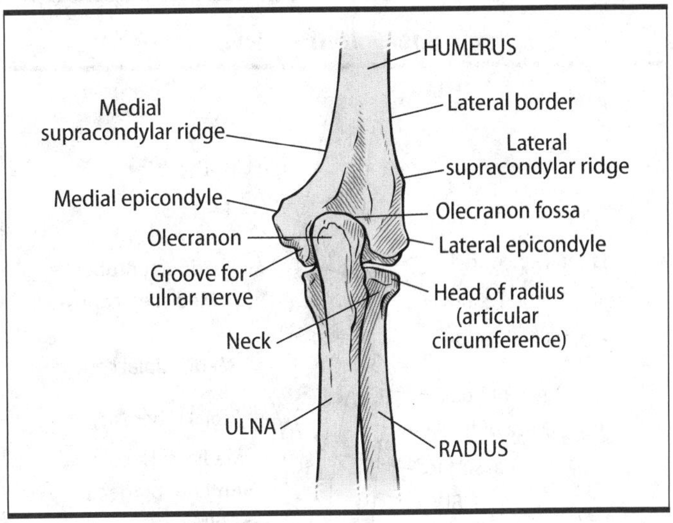

Hand

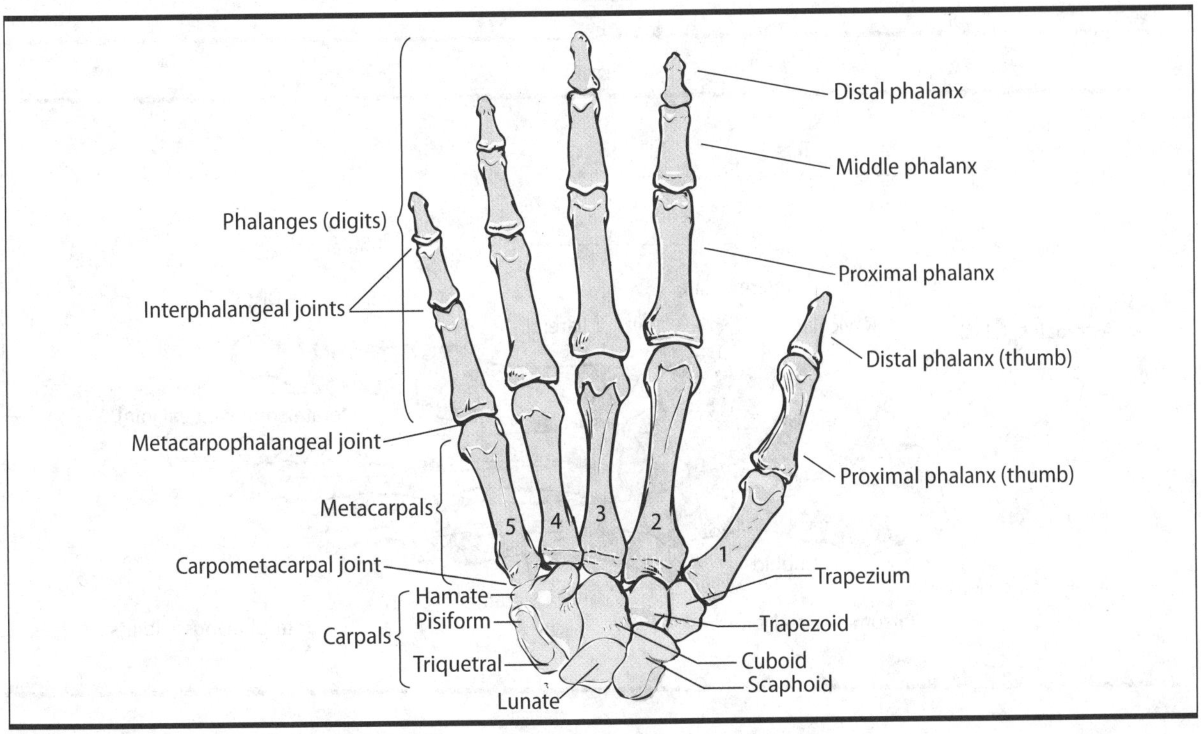

Hip Anterior View

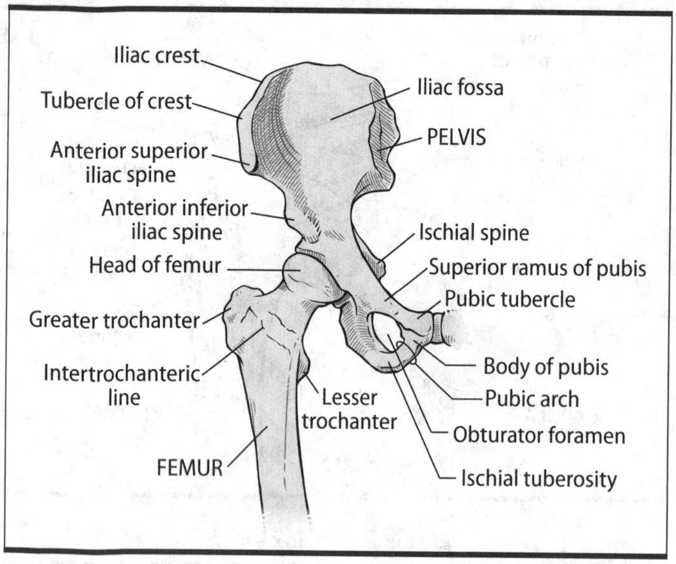

Hip Posterior View

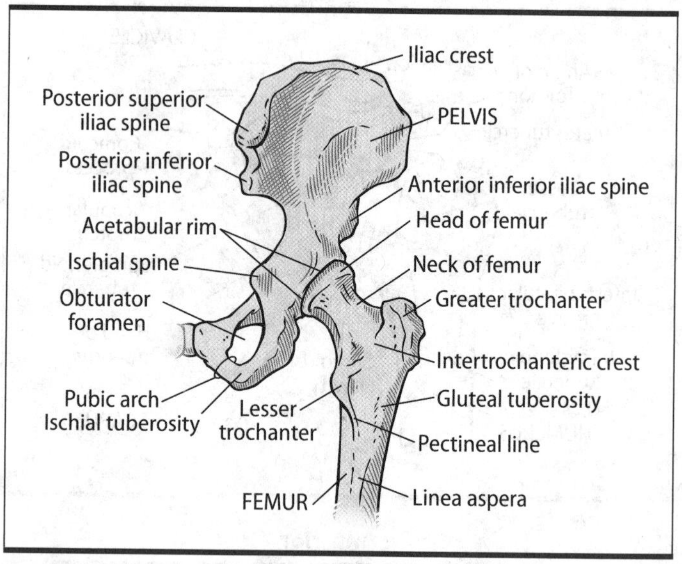

Knee Anterior View

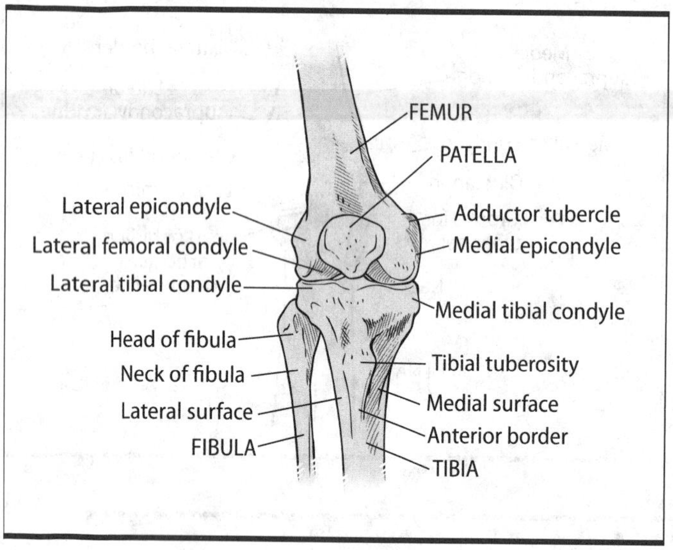

Knee Posterior View

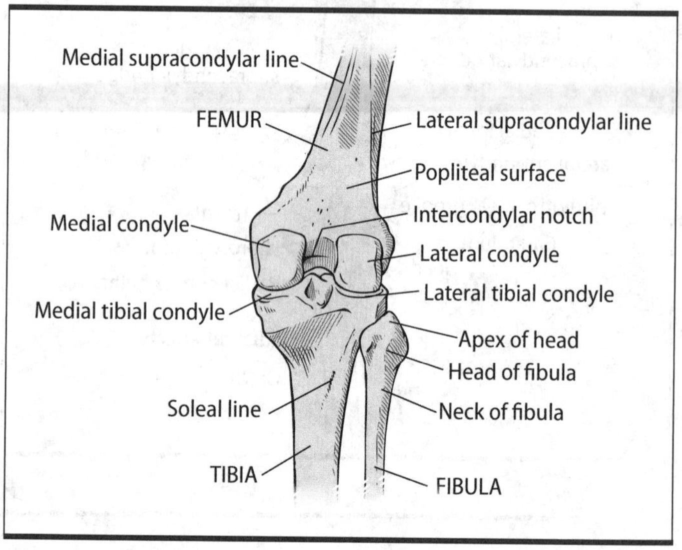

Foot

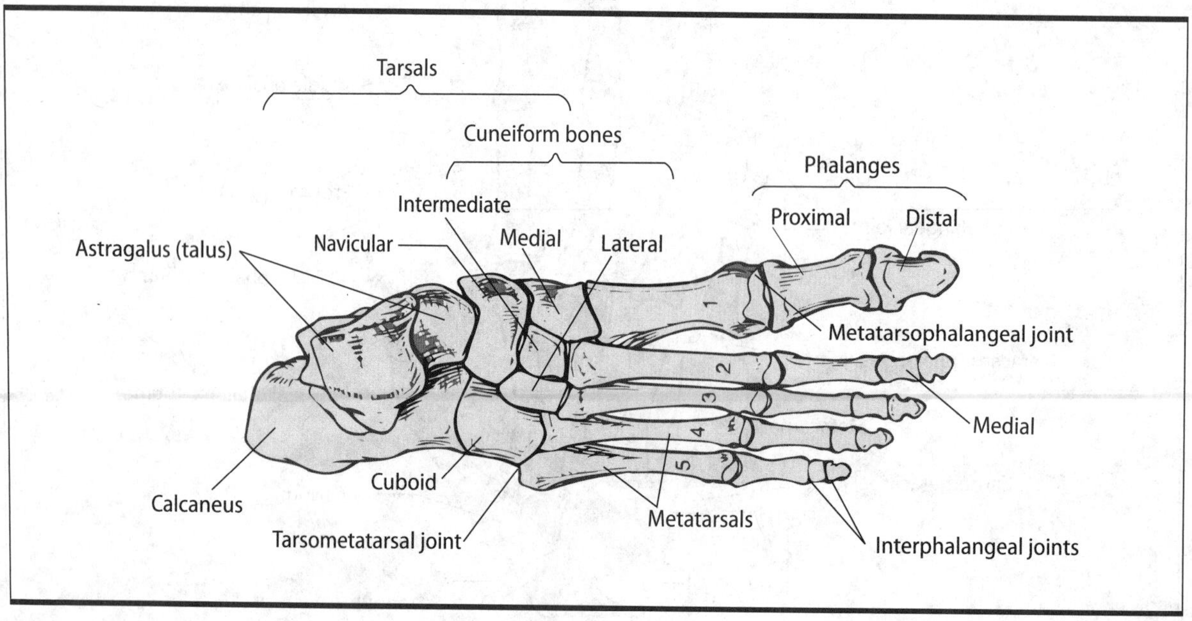

Muscles

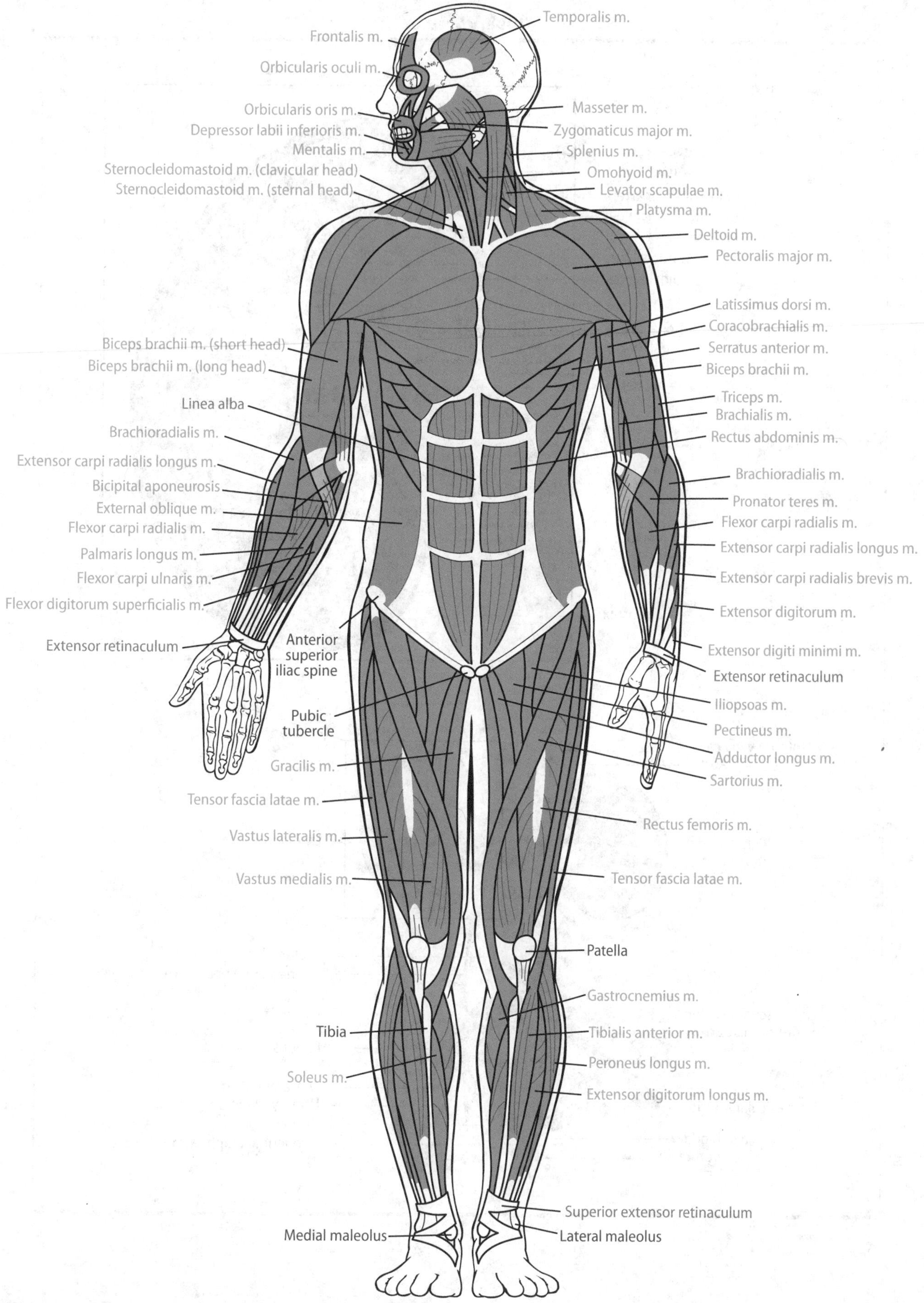

Temporalis m.
Frontalis m.
Orbicularis oculi m.
Orbicularis oris m.
Masseter m.
Depressor labii inferioris m.
Zygomaticus major m.
Mentalis m.
Splenius m.
Sternocleidomastoid m. (clavicular head)
Omohyoid m.
Sternocleidomastoid m. (sternal head)
Levator scapulae m.
Platysma m.
Deltoid m.
Pectoralis major m.
Latissimus dorsi m.
Coracobrachialis m.
Biceps brachii m. (short head)
Serratus anterior m.
Biceps brachii m. (long head)
Biceps brachii m.
Triceps m.
Linea alba
Brachialis m.
Brachioradialis m.
Rectus abdominis m.
Extensor carpi radialis longus m.
Brachioradialis m.
Bicipital aponeurosis
Pronator teres m.
External oblique m.
Flexor carpi radialis m.
Flexor carpi radialis m.
Extensor carpi radialis longus m.
Palmaris longus m.
Flexor carpi ulnaris m.
Extensor carpi radialis brevis m.
Flexor digitorum superficialis m.
Extensor digitorum m.
Extensor retinaculum
Anterior superior iliac spine
Extensor digiti minimi m.
Extensor retinaculum
Iliopsoas m.
Pubic tubercle
Pectineus m.
Adductor longus m.
Gracilis m.
Sartorius m.
Tensor fascia latae m.
Rectus femoris m.
Vastus lateralis m.
Vastus medialis m.
Tensor fascia latae m.
Patella
Gastrocnemius m.
Tibia
Tibialis anterior m.
Peroneus longus m.
Soleus m.
Extensor digitorum longus m.
Superior extensor retinaculum
Medial maleolus
Lateral maleolus

Chapter 14. Diseases of the Genitourinary System (NØØ–N99)

Urinary System

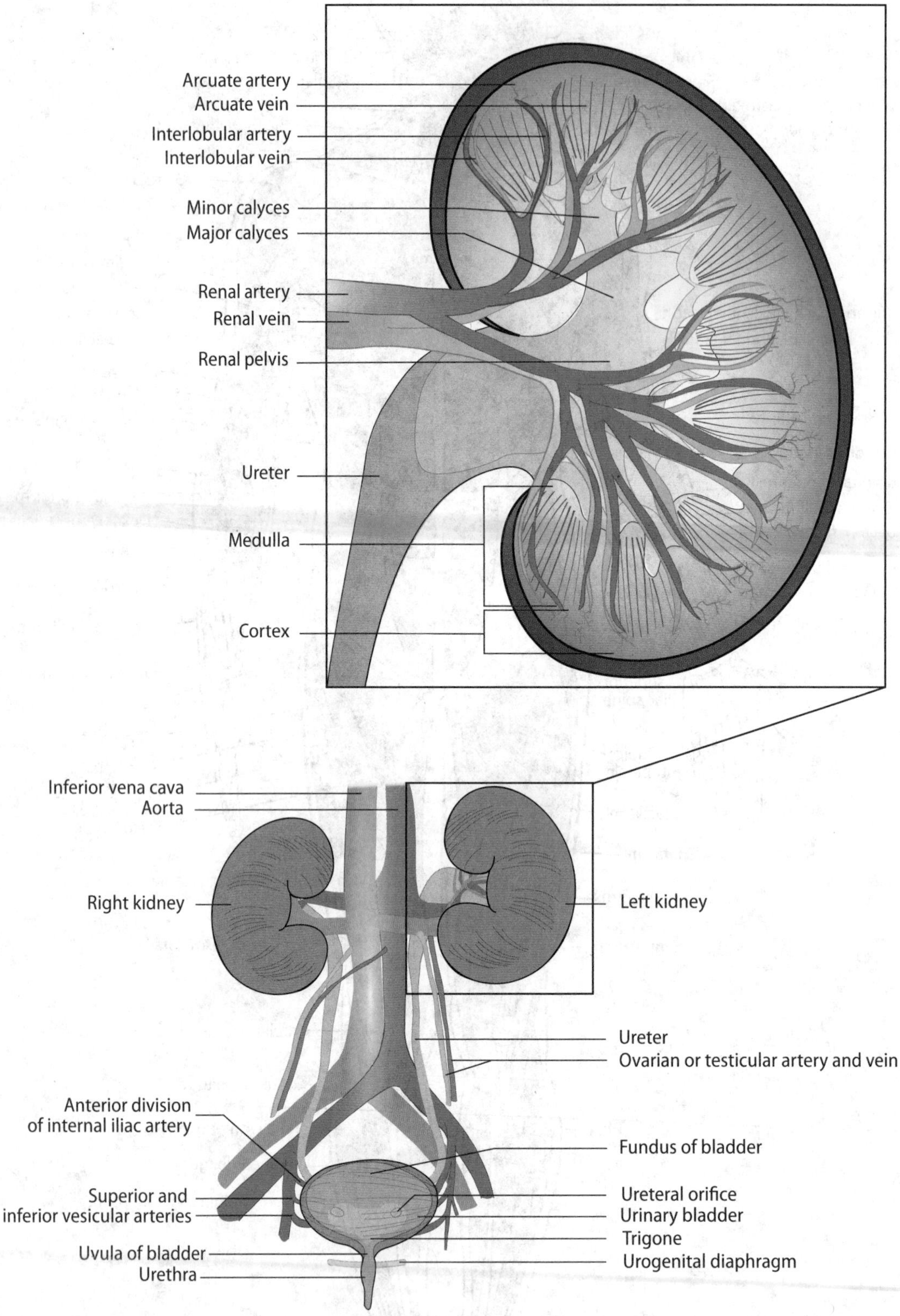

Male Genitourinary System

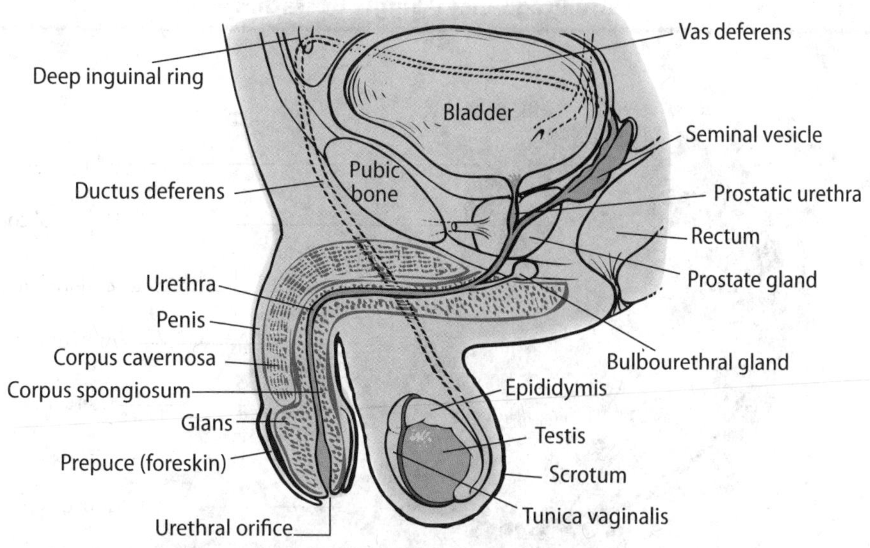

Female Internal Genitalia

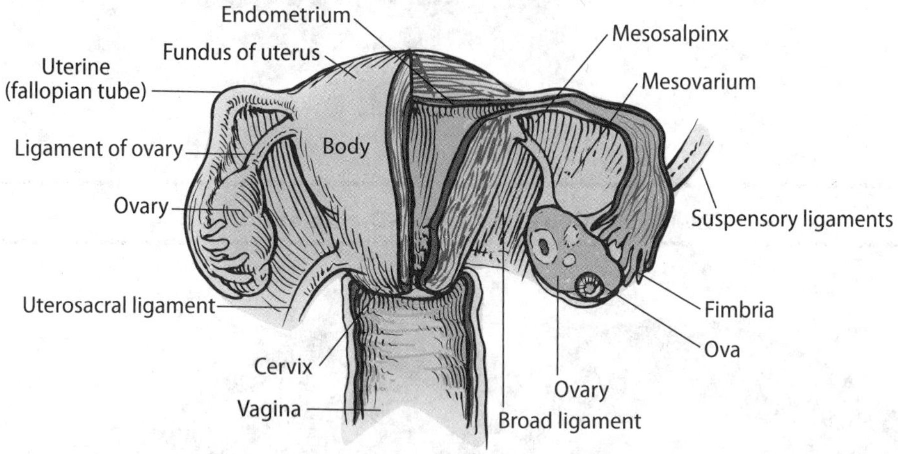

Female Genitourinary Tract Lateral View

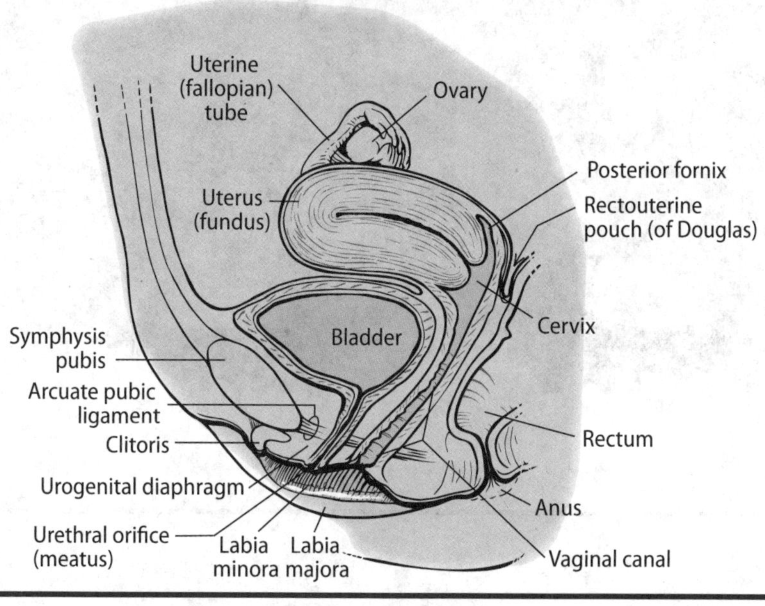

5. Pregnancy, Childbirth and the Puerperium (O00–O9A)

Term Pregnancy – Single Gestation

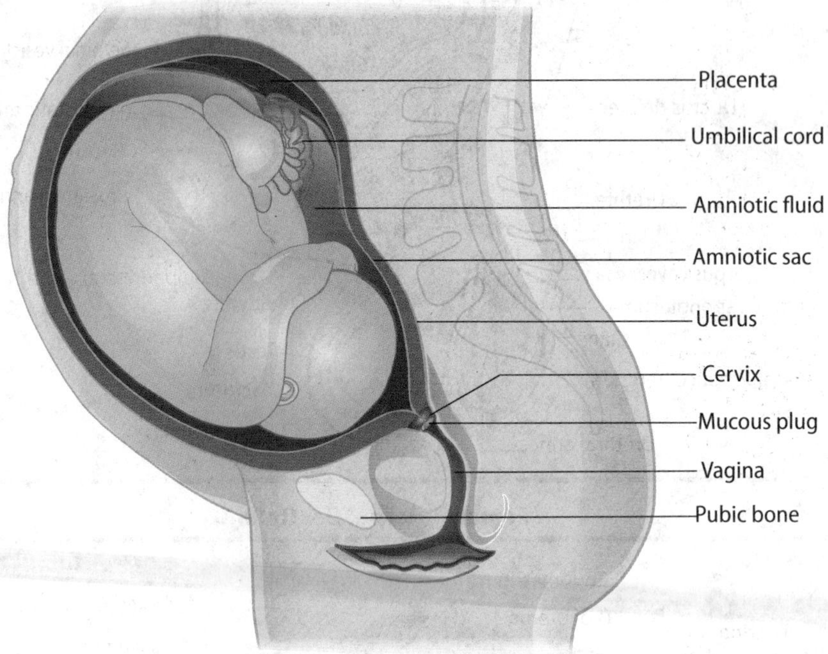

Twin Gestation–Dichorionic–Diamniotic (DI-DI)

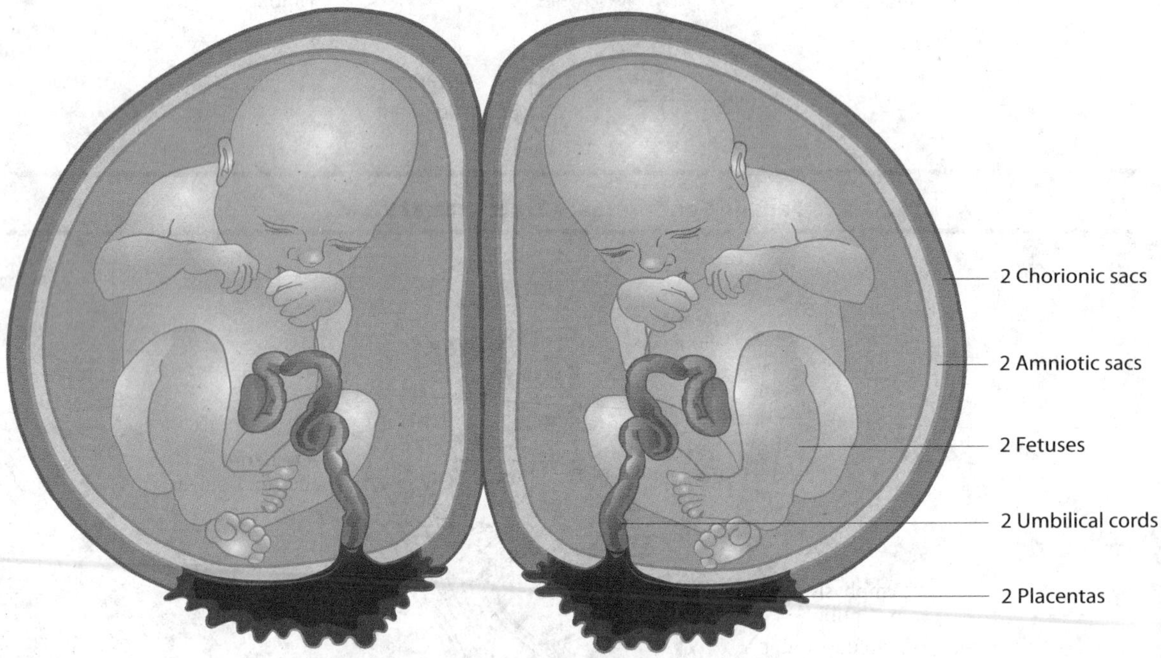